a LANGE medical book

Katzung's Basic & Clinical Pharmacology

a LANGE medical book

Katzung's Basic & Clinical Pharmacology

Sixteenth Edition

Edited by

Todd W. Vanderah, PhD

Regents Professor and Chair
Department of Pharmacology
University of Arizona College of Medicine, Tucson

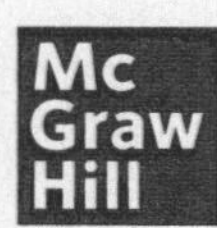

New York Chicago San Francisco Athens London Madrid Mexico City
Milan New Delhi Singapore Sydney Toronto

Katzung's Basic & Clinical Pharmacology, Sixteenth Edition

1 2 3 4 5 6 7 8 9 LWI 28 27 26 25 24 23

ISBN 978-1-260-46330-9
MHID 1-260-46330-3
ISSN 0891-2033

Notice

Medicine is an ever-changing science. As new research and clinical experience broaden our knowledge, changes in treatment and drug therapy are required. The authors and the publisher of this work have checked with sources believed to be reliable in their efforts to provide information that is complete and generally in accord with the standards accepted at the time of publication. However, in view of the possibility of human error or changes in medical sciences, neither the authors nor the publisher nor any other party who has been involved in the preparation or publication of this work warrants that the information contained herein is in every respect accurate or complete, and they disclaim all responsibility for any errors or omissions or for the results obtained from use of the information contained in this work. Readers are encouraged to confirm the information contained herein with other sources. For example and in particular, readers are advised to check the product information sheet included in the package of each drug they plan to administer to be certain that the information contained in this work is accurate and that changes have not been made in the recommended dose or in the contraindications for administration. This recommendation is of particular importance in connection with new or infrequently used drugs.

This book was set in Adobe Garamond by KnowledgeWorks Global Ltd.
The editors were Michael Weitz and Peter J. Boyle.
The production supervisor was Richard Ruzycka.
Project management provided by Tasneem Kauser, KnowledgeWorks Global Ltd.
The copy editor was Greg Feldman.
The cover designer was W2 Design.
Cover photo: Activin A protein.
Photo credit: StudioMolekuul.

This book is printed on acid-free paper.

Contents

Preface

The 16th edition of *Basic & Clinical Pharmacology* will recognize Dr. Bertram Katzung's legacy of contribution to this book by retitling the book as *Katzung's Basic & Clinical Pharmacology* and his mentorship of Dr. Todd W. Vanderah as editor for this edition. This edition continues the extensive use of full-color illustrations and expanded coverage of transporters, pharmacogenomics, and new drugs of all types emphasized in prior editions. The 16th edition also reflects the major expansion of large-molecule drugs in the pharmacopeia, with numerous new monoclonal antibodies and other biologic agents. Case studies accompany most chapters, and answers to questions posed in the case studies appear at the end of each chapter. The book is designed to provide a comprehensive, authoritative, and readable pharmacology textbook for students in the health sciences.

This edition continues the sequence used in many pharmacology courses and in integrated curricula: basic principles of drug discovery, pharmacodynamics, pharmacokinetics, and pharmacogenomics; autonomic drugs; cardiovascular-renal drugs; drugs with important actions on smooth muscle; central nervous system drugs; drugs used to treat inflammation, gout, and diseases of the blood; endocrine drugs; chemotherapeutic drugs; toxicology; and special topics. This sequence builds new information on a foundation of information already assimilated. For example, early presentation of autonomic nervous system pharmacology allows students to integrate the physiology and neuroscience they have learned elsewhere with the pharmacology they are learning and prepares them to understand the autonomic effects of other drugs. This is especially important for the cardiovascular and central nervous system drug groups. However, chapters can be used equally well in courses and curricula that present these topics in a different sequence. Within each chapter, emphasis is placed on discussion of drug groups and prototypes rather than offering repetitive detail about individual drugs. Selection of the subject matter and the order of its presentation are based on the accumulated experience of teaching this material to thousands of medical, pharmacy, dental, podiatry, nursing, and other health science students.

Health science curricula now place more emphasis on the clinical applications of therapeutic measures. Major features that make this book particularly useful in such curricula include sections that specifically address the clinical choice and use of drugs in patients and the monitoring of their effects—in other words, *clinical pharmacology* is an integral part of this text. Lists of the trade and generic names of commercial preparations available are provided at the end of each chapter for easy reference by the house officer or practitioner evaluating a patient's drug list or writing a prescription.

The 16th edition includes the novel medications that were quickly designed to prevent and overcome COVID-19 with emphasis on the importance of vaccines and antiviral drugs in pharmacology and clinical medicine.

Significant revisions in this edition include:

- Major revisions of the chapters on immunopharmacology; antiseizure, antipsychotic, antidepressant, antidiabetic, anti-inflammatory, and antiviral drugs; prostaglandins; and central nervous system neurotransmitters. Major additions on the treatment of COVID have been added in Chapter 49.
- Continued expansion of the coverage of general concepts relating to newly discovered receptors, receptor mechanisms, and drug transporters.
- Descriptions of important new drugs, especially biologicals, released through January 2022.
- Revised illustrations in full color that provide significantly more information about drug mechanisms and effects and help to clarify important concepts.

An important related educational resource is *Katzung's Pharmacology: Examination & Board Review*, 14th edition (Marieke Kruidering-Hall, Rupa L. Tuan, Todd W. Vanderah, Bertram G. Katzung, eds, McGraw Hill, 2024). This book provides a succinct review of pharmacology with almost 1000 sample examination questions and answers. It is especially helpful to students preparing for board-type examinations. A more highly condensed source of information suitable for review purposes is *USMLE Road Map: Pharmacology*, 2nd edition (Katzung BG, Trevor AJ: McGraw Hill, 2006). An extremely useful manual of toxicity due to drugs and other products is *Poisoning & Drug Overdose*, by Olson KR, ed; 8th edition, McGraw Hill, 2022.

The 16th edition marks the 42nd year of publication of *Basic & Clinical Pharmacology*. The widespread adoption of the first fifteen editions indicates that this book fills an important need. We believe that the 16th edition will satisfy this need even more successfully. Chinese, Croatian, Czech, French, Georgian, Indonesian, Italian, Japanese, Korean, Lithuanian, Portuguese, Spanish, Turkish, and Ukrainian translations of various editions are available. The publisher may be contacted for further information.

I wish to acknowledge the prior and continuing efforts of my contributing authors and the major contributions of the staff at Lange Medical Publications, Appleton & Lange, and McGraw Hill, and of our copy editor for this edition, Greg Feldman. I also wish to thank Tasneem Kauser for her contributions.

Suggestions and comments about *Katzung's Basic & Clinical Pharmacology* are always welcome. They may be sent to me in care of the publisher.

Todd W. Vanderah, PhD
Tucson, Arizona
July 2023

Authors

Michael J. Aminoff, MD, DSc, FRCP
Professor, Department of Neurology, University of California, San Francisco

Allan I. Basbaum, PhD
Professor and Chair, Department of Anatomy and W.M. Keck Foundation Center for Integrative Neuroscience, University of California, San Francisco

Camille E. Beauduy, PharmD
Assistant Clinical Professor, School of Pharmacy, University of California, San Francisco

Neal L. Benowitz, MD
Professor of Medicine and Bioengineering & Therapeutic Science, University of California, San Francisco

Nirav Bhakta, MD, PhD
Associate Professor of Clinical Medicine, University of California, San Francisco

Italo Biaggioni, MD
Professor of Pharmacology, Vanderbilt University School of Medicine, Nashville

Daniel D. Bikle, MD, PhD
Professor of Medicine, Department of Medicine, and Co-Director, Special Diagnostic and Treatment Unit, University of California, San Francisco, and Veterans Affairs Medical Center, San Francisco

Adrienne D. Briggs, MD
Clinical Director, Bone Marrow Transplant Program, Banner Good Samaritan Hospital, Phoenix

Hakan Cakmak, MD
Department of Medicine, University of California, San Francisco

Lundy Campbell, MD
Professor, Department of Anesthesiology and Perioperative Medicine, University of California San Francisco, School of Medicine, San Francisco

Theora Canonica, PharmD
University of California, San Francisco

Eugene Choo, MD
Assistant Clinical Professor, Department of Medicine, University of California San Francisco, School of Medicine, San Francisco

George P. Chrousos, MD
Professor & Chair, First Department of Pediatrics, Athens University Medical School, Athens, Greece

Edward Chu, MD
Professor of Medicine and Pharmacology & Chemical Biology; Chief, Division of Hematology-Oncology, Director, University of Pittsburgh Cancer Institute, University of Pittsburgh School of Medicine, Pittsburgh

Valerie B. Clinard, PharmD
Associate Professor, Department of Clinical Pharmacy, School of Pharmacy, University of California, San Francisco

Robin L. Corelli, PharmD
Clinical Professor, Department of Clinical Pharmacy, School of Pharmacy, University of California, San Francisco

Maria Almira Correia, PhD
Professor of Pharmacology, Pharmaceutical Chemistry and Biopharmaceutical Sciences, Department of Cellular & Molecular Pharmacology, University of California, San Francisco

Charles DeBattista, MD
Professor of Psychiatry and Behavioral Sciences, Stanford University School of Medicine, Stanford

Cathi E. Dennehy, PharmD
Professor, Department of Clinical Pharmacy, University of California, San Francisco School of Pharmacy, San Francisco

Betty J. Dong, PharmD, FASHP, FCCP, FAPHA
Professor of Clinical Pharmacy and Clinical Professor of Family and Community Medicine, Department of Clinical Pharmacy and Department of Family and Community Medicine, Schools of Pharmacy and Medicine, University of California, San Francisco

Helge Eilers, MD
Professor of Anesthesia and Perioperative Care, University of California, San Francisco

Sean P. Elliott, MD
Global MD Program, University of Arizona Health Sciences Pediatrics, Tucson Medical Center

George T. Fantry, MD
Assistant Vice President, UA/UWA Global MD Program Associate Professor of Medicine, University of Arizona College of Medicine, Tucson

Daniel E. Furst, MD
Carl M. Pearson Professor of Rheumatology, Director, Rheumatology Clinical Research Center, Department of Rheumatology, University of California, Los Angeles

Kathleen M. Giacomini, PhD
Professor of Bioengineering and Therapeutic Sciences, Schools of Pharmacy and Medicine, University of California, San Francisco

Lacrisha J. Go, DNP, FNP-C
Nurse Practitioner, Stanford University

Augustus O. Grant, MD, PhD
Professor of Medicine, Cardiovascular Division, Duke University Medical Center, Durham

John A. Gray, MD, PhD
Associate Professor, Department of Neurology, Center for Neuroscience, University of California, Davis

Vsevolod V. Gurevich, PhD
Cornelius Vanderbilt endowed Chair, Professor of Pharmacology, Vanderbilt University

Robert D. Harvey, PhD
Professor of Pharmacology and Physiology, University of Nevada School of Medicine, Reno

Jennifer E. Hibma, PharmD
Department of Bioengineering and Therapeutic Sciences, Schools of Pharmacy and Medicine, University of California, San Francisco

Nicholas H. G. Holford, MB, ChB, FRACP
Professor, Department of Pharmacology and Clinical Pharmacology, University of Auckland Medical School, Auckland

John R. Horn, PharmD, FCCP
Professor of Pharmacy, School of Pharmacy, University of Washington; Associate Director of Pharmacy Services, Department of Medicine, University of Washington Medicine, Seattle

John Hwa, MD, PhD
Professor of Medicine and Pharmacology, Yale University School of Medicine, New Haven

Mohab M. Ibrahim, MD, PhD
Professor, Department of Anesthesiology, College of Medicine-Tucson

Samie R. Jaffrey, MD, PhD
Greenberg-Starr Professor of Pharmacology, Department of Pharmacology, Cornell University Weill Medical College, New York City

John P. Kane, MD, PhD
Professor of Medicine, Department of Medicine; Professor of Biochemistry and Biophysics; Associate Director, Cardiovascular Research Institute, University of California, San Francisco

Bertram G. Katzung, MD, PhD
Professor Emeritus, Department of Cellular & Molecular Pharmacology, University of California, San Francisco

Michael J. Kosnett, MD, MPH
Associate Clinical Professor of Medicine, Division of Clinical Pharmacology and Toxicology, University of Colorado Health Sciences Center, Denver

Lisa Kroon, PharmD
Professor and Chair, Department of Clinical Pharmacy, School of Pharmacy, University of California San Francisco

Marieke Kruidering-Hall, PhD
Academy Chair in Pharmacology Education; Professor, Department of Cellular and Molecular Pharmacology, University of California, San Francisco

Douglas F. Lake, PhD
Professor, The Biodesign Institute, Arizona State University, Tempe

Harry W. Lampiris, MD
Professor of Clinical Medicine, UCSF, Interim Chief, ID Section, Medical Service, San Francisco VA Medical Center, San Francisco

Tally M. Largent-Milnes, PhD
Associate Professor, Department of Pharmacology, College of Medicine-Tucson

Rebecca M. Law, PharmD
School of Pharmacy, Memorial University of Newfoundland

Paul W. Lofholm, PharmD
Clinical Professor of Pharmacy, School of Pharmacy, University of California, San Francisco

Roger K. Long, MD
Professor of Pediatrics, Department of Pediatrics, University of California, San Francisco

Christian Lüscher, MD
Departments of Basic and Clinical Neurosciences, Medical Faculty, University Hospital of Geneva, Geneva, Switzerland

Daniel S. Maddix, PharmD[1]
Associate Clinical Professor of Pharmacy, University of California, San Francisco

[1]Deceased

Howard I. Maibach, MD
Professor of Dermatology, Department of Dermatology, University of California, San Francisco

Mary J. Malloy, MD
Clinical Professor of Pediatrics and Medicine, Departments of Pediatrics and Medicine, Cardiovascular Research Institute, University of California, San Francisco

Kathleen Martin, PhD
Professor, Yale Cardiovascular Center, Yale University, New Haven

Umesh Masharani, MBBS, MRCP (UK)
Professor of Medicine, Department of Medicine, University of California, San Francisco

Jennifer S. Mulliken, MD
Assistant Clinical Professor of Medicine, University of California, San Francisco

Ramana K. Naidu, MD
Attending Physician, Marin General Hospital, Greenbrae, California

Ahmed A. Negm, MD
Department of Medicine, University of California, Los Angeles

Saman Nematollahi, MD
Assistant Professor, Department of Medicine, University of Arizona/Banner, Tucson

Martha S. Nolte Kennedy, MD
Clinical Professor, Department of Medicine, University of California, San Francisco

David Pearce, MD
Professor of Medicine, University of California, San Francisco

Andrea I. Cesarez Ramirez
Research Associate, Division of Rheumatology, UCLA David Geffen School of Medicine, Los Angeles

Ian A. Reid, PhD
Professor Emeritus, Department of Physiology, University of California, San Francisco

Dirk B. Robertson, MD
Professor of Clinical Dermatology, Department of Dermatology, Emory University School of Medicine, Atlanta

Michael A. Rogawski, MD, PhD
Professor of Neurology, Department of Neurology, University of California, Davis

Philip J. Rosenthal, MD
Professor of Medicine, San Francisco General Hospital, University of California, San Francisco

Sharon Safrin, MD
Associate Clinical Professor, Department of Medicine, University of California, San Francisco; President, Safrin Clinical Research, Hillsborough

Ramin Sam, MD
Associate Professor, Department of Medicine, University of California, San Francisco

Mark A. Schumacher, PhD, MD
Professor, Department of Anesthesia and Perioperative Care, University of California, San Francisco

Craig Smollin, MD
Professor of Emergency Medicine, University of California, San Francisco

Daniel T. Teitelbaum, MD
Adjunct Professor of Occupational and Environmental Health, Colorado School of Public Health, Denver; and Adjunct Professor, Civil and Environmental Engineering, Colorado School of Mines, Golden

Anthony J. Trevor, PhD
Professor Emeritus, Department of Cellular & Molecular Pharmacology, University of California, San Francisco

Candy Tsourounis, PharmD
Professor of Clinical Pharmacy, Medication Outcomes Center, University of California, San Francisco School of Pharmacy, San Francisco

Todd W. Vanderah, PhD
Professor and Chair, Department of Pharmacology, University of Arizona, Tucson

Mark von Zastrow, MD, PhD
Professor, Departments of Psychiatry and Cellular & Molecular Pharmacology, University of California, San Francisco

Lisa G. Winston, MD
Clinical Professor, Department of Medicine, Division of Infectious Diseases, University of California, San Francisco; Hospital Epidemiologist, San Francisco General Hospital, San Francisco

Spencer Yost, MD
Professor, Department of Anesthesia and Perioperative Care, University of California, San Francisco; Medical Director, UCSF-Mt. Zion ICU, Chief of Anesthesia, UCSF-Mt. Zion Hospital, San Francisco

James L. Zehnder, MD
Professor of Pathology and Medicine, Pathology Department, Stanford University School of Medicine, Stanford

SECTION I BASIC PRINCIPLES

CHAPTER 1

Introduction: The Nature of Drugs & Drug Development & Regulation

Todd W. Vanderah, PhD, & Bertram G. Katzung, MD, PhD

CASE STUDY

A 78-year-old woman is brought to the hospital because of suspected aspirin overdose. She has taken aspirin for joint pain for many years without incident, but during the past year, she has exhibited signs of cognitive decline. Her caregiver finds her confused, hyperventilating, and vomiting. The caregiver finds an empty bottle of aspirin tablets and calls 9-1-1. In the emergency department, samples of venous and arterial blood are obtained while the airway, breathing, and circulation are evaluated. An intravenous (IV) drip is started, and gastrointestinal decontamination is started. After blood gas results are reported, sodium bicarbonate is administered via the IV. What is the purpose of the sodium bicarbonate?

Pharmacology can be defined as the study of substances that interact with living systems through chemical processes. These interactions usually occur by binding of the substance to regulatory molecules and activating or inhibiting normal body processes. These substances may be chemicals administered to achieve a beneficial therapeutic effect on some process within the patient or for their toxic effects on regulatory processes in parasites infecting the patient. Such deliberate therapeutic applications may be considered the proper role of **medical pharmacology,** which is often defined as the science of substances used to prevent, diagnose, and treat disease. **Toxicology** is the branch of pharmacology that deals with the undesirable effects of chemicals on living systems, from individual cells to humans to complex ecosystems (Figure 1–1). The nature of drugs—their physical properties and their interactions with biological systems—is discussed in part I of this chapter.

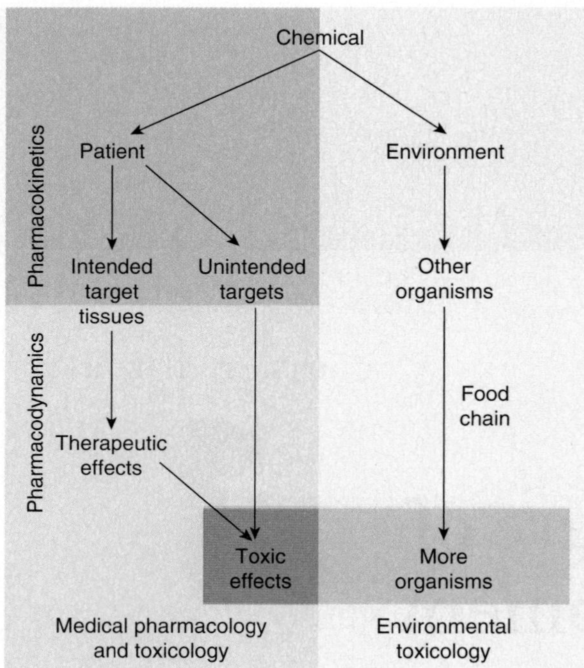

FIGURE 1–1 Major areas of study in pharmacology. The actions of chemicals can be divided into two large domains. The first (*left side*) is that of medical pharmacology and toxicology, which is aimed at understanding the actions of drugs as chemicals on individual organisms, especially humans and domestic animals. Both beneficial and toxic effects are included. Pharmacokinetics deals with the absorption, distribution, and elimination of drugs. Pharmacodynamics concerns the actions of the chemical on the organism. The second domain (*right side*) is that of environmental toxicology, which is concerned with the effects of chemicals on all organisms and their survival in groups and as species.

New drugs are added every year; they are needed for several reasons including: (1) increasing resistance by bacteria and other parasites; (2) discovery of new target processes in diseases that have not been adequately treated; and (3) recognition of new diseases. Furthermore, a dramatic increase has occurred in the number of *large molecule* drugs (especially antibodies) approved during the last two decades. The development of new drugs and their regulation by government agencies are discussed in part II.

THE HISTORY OF PHARMACOLOGY

Prehistoric people undoubtedly recognized the beneficial or toxic effects of many plant and animal materials. Early written records list remedies of many types, including a few that are still recognized as useful drugs today. Most, however, were worthless or actually harmful. Beginning about 1500 years ago, sporadic attempts were made to introduce rational methods into medicine, but none was successful owing to the dominance of systems of thought ("schools") that purported to explain all of biology and disease without the need for experimentation and observation. These schools promulgated bizarre notions such as the idea that disease was caused by excesses of bile or blood in the body, that wounds could be healed by applying a salve to the weapon that caused the wound, and so on.

Around the end of the 17th century, concepts based on observation and experimentation began to replace theorizing in physiology and clinical medicine. As the value of these methods in the study of disease became clear, physicians in Great Britain and on the Continent began to apply them systematically to the effects of traditional drugs used in their own practices. Thus, **materia medica**—the science of drug preparation and the medical uses of drugs—began to develop as the precursor to pharmacology. However, any real understanding of the mechanisms of action of drugs was prevented by the absence of methods for purifying active agents from the crude materials that were available and—even more—by the lack of methods for testing hypotheses about the nature of drug actions.

In the late 18th and early 19th centuries, François Magendie and his student Claude Bernard began to develop the methods of **experimental physiology** and **pharmacology.** Advances in chemistry and the further development of physiology in the 18th, 19th, and early 20th centuries laid the foundation needed for understanding how drugs work at the organ and cellular levels. Paradoxically, real advances in basic pharmacology during this time were accompanied by an outburst of unscientific claims by manufacturers and marketers of worthless "patent medicines." Not until the concepts of rational therapeutics, especially that of the **controlled clinical trial,** were reintroduced into medicine—only about 60 years ago—did it become possible to adequately evaluate therapeutic claims.

Around the 1940s and 1950s, a major expansion of research efforts in all areas of biology began. As new concepts and new techniques were introduced, information accumulated about drug action and the biologic substrate of that action, the **drug receptor.** During the last 60 years, many fundamentally new drug groups and new members of old groups have been introduced. The last three decades have seen an even more rapid growth of information and understanding of the molecular basis for drug action. The molecular mechanisms of action of many drugs have now been identified, and numerous receptors have been isolated, structurally characterized, and cloned. In fact, the use of receptor identification methods (described in Chapter 2) has led to the discovery of many *orphan* receptors—receptors for which no ligand has been discovered and whose function can only be guessed. Studies of the local molecular environment of receptors have shown that receptors and effectors do not function in isolation; they are strongly influenced by other receptors and by companion regulatory proteins. Most recently, it has become clear that gravitational change, radiation, and other aspects of space *outside* the Earth's environment require the development of *space medicine.* This has opened another important area for the future of pharmacology. One result of these discoveries is the confirmation that pharmacology represents an area where anatomy, biochemistry, genetics, physiology, pathology, clinical medicine, and the environment meet. Many problems that the health practitioner confronts can now be corrected or mitigated using pharmacologic tools.

Pharmacogenomics—the relation of the individual's genetic makeup to his or her response to specific drugs—is becoming an important part of therapeutics (see Chapter 5). Decoding of the genomes of many species—from bacteria to humans—has led to the recognition of unsuspected relationships between receptor families and the ways that receptor proteins have evolved. Furthermore, discovery of regulatory functions exerted by the neighbors of chromosomes and the *noncoding* regions of DNA on the expression of exons has opened a new area of possible manipulation of the genes—epigenetics—that control pharmacologic responses.

The discovery that small segments of RNA can interfere with protein synthesis with extreme selectivity has led to investigation of **small interfering RNAs (siRNAs)** and **micro-RNAs (miRNAs)** as therapeutic agents. Similarly, short nucleotide chains called **antisense oligonucleotides (ANOs),** synthesized to be complementary to natural RNA or DNA, can interfere with the readout of genes and the transcription of RNA. Recently, the development of mRNA vaccines has led to new medications by activating one's own immune system to recognize and fight off viruses. New, efficient methods of DNA editing have made possible the modification of genes that encode proteins that are critical to biological function, representing a transformative means of generating medicines. Finally, development in the production of selective monoclonal antibodies to target selective proteins has led to a dramatic increase in *large molecule* therapeutics in the last 20 years (Table 1–1).

Unfortunately, the medication-consuming public is still exposed to vast amounts of inaccurate or unscientific information regarding the pharmacologic effects of chemicals. This results in the irrational use of innumerable expensive, ineffective, and sometimes harmful remedies and the growth of a huge "alternative health care" industry. Furthermore, manipulation of the legislative process in the United States has allowed many substances promoted for health—but not promoted specifically as "drugs"—to avoid meeting the Food and Drug Administration (FDA) standards described in the second part of this chapter. Conversely, lack of understanding of basic scientific principles in biology and statistics and the absence of critical thinking about public health issues have led to rejection of medical science, including vaccines, by a segment of the public and a tendency to assume that all adverse drug effects are the result of malpractice.

General principles that the student should remember are (1) that *all* substances can under certain circumstances be toxic; (2) that the chemicals in botanicals (herbs and plant extracts, "nutraceuticals") are no different from chemicals in manufactured drugs except for the much greater proportion of impurities in botanicals; and (3) that all dietary supplements and all therapies promoted as health-enhancing should meet the same standards of efficacy and safety as conventional drugs and medical therapies. That is, there should be no artificial separation between scientific medicine and "alternative" or "complementary" medicine. Ideally, all nutritional and botanical substances should be tested by the same types of randomized controlled trials (RCTs) as synthetic compounds.

TABLE 1–1 Development of large molecule therapeutic agents as a percentage of all new drug approvals, 2000–2020.

Year	Total New Drug Approvals	New Protein Drugs (~% of new drug approvals)	New MABs (~% of new drug approvals)
2000	63	3 (5%)	1 (2%)
2008	34	5 (15%)	1 (3%)
2010	49	8 (16%)	4 (8%)
2015	69	13 (19%)	9 (13%)
2017	63	10 (16%)	9 (14%)
2020	61	? (16%)	10 (16%)

MABs, monoclonal antibodies.

GENERAL PRINCIPLES OF PHARMACOLOGY

THE NATURE OF DRUGS

In the most general sense, a drug may be defined as any substance that brings about a change in biologic function through its chemical actions. In most cases, the drug molecule interacts as an **agonist** (activator) or **antagonist** (inhibitor) with a specific target molecule that plays a regulatory role in the biologic system. This target molecule is called a **receptor.** Some of the new large molecule drugs **(biologicals)** act like receptors themselves and bind endogenous molecules. The nature of receptors is discussed more fully in Chapter 2. In a very small number of cases, drugs known as **chemical antagonists** may interact directly with other drugs, whereas a few drugs **(osmotic agents)** interact almost exclusively with water molecules. Drugs may be synthesized within the body (eg, **hormones**) or may be chemicals *not* synthesized in the patient's body (ie, **xenobiotics**). **Poisons** are drugs that have almost exclusively harmful effects. However, Paracelsus (1493–1541) famously stated that "the dose makes the poison," meaning that any substance can be harmful if taken in the wrong dosage. **Toxins** are usually defined as poisons of biologic origin, ie, synthesized by plants or animals, in contrast to inorganic poisons such as lead and arsenic.

The Physical Nature of Drugs

To interact chemically with its receptor, a drug molecule must have the appropriate size, electrical charge, shape, and atomic composition. Furthermore, a drug is often administered at a location distant from its intended site of action, eg, a pill taken orally to relieve a headache. Therefore, a useful drug must have the necessary properties to be transported from its site of administration to its site of action. Finally, a practical drug should be inactivated or excreted from the body at a reasonable rate so that its actions will be of appropriate duration.

Drugs may be solid at room temperature (eg, aspirin, atropine), liquid (eg, nicotine, ethanol), or gaseous (eg, nitrous oxide, isoflurane, xenon). These factors often determine the best route of administration. The most common routes of administration are described in Chapter 3, Table 3–3. The various classes of organic compounds—carbohydrates, proteins, lipids, and smaller molecules—are all represented in pharmacology. As noted above, many proteins and some new mRNA vaccines have been approved while some oligonucleotides have also received approval for use depending on the country's regulation agencies.

A number of inorganic elements, eg, fluoride, lithium, iron, and heavy metals, are both useful and dangerous drugs. Many organic drugs are weak acids or bases. This fact has important implications for the way they are handled by the body, because pH differences in the various compartments of the body may alter the degree of ionization of weak acids and bases (see text that follows).

Drug Size

The molecular size of drugs varies from very small (lithium ion, molecular weight [MW] 7) to very large (eg, alteplase [t-PA], a protein of MW 59,050). Many antibodies are even larger; eg, erenumab, an antibody used in the management of migraine, has a MW of more than 145,000. However, most drugs have molecular weights between 100 and 1000. The lower limit of this narrow range is probably set by the requirements for specificity of action. To have a good "fit" to only one type of receptor, a drug molecule must be sufficiently unique in shape, charge, and other properties to prevent its binding to other receptors. To achieve such selective binding, it appears that a molecule should in most cases be at least 100 MW units in size. The upper limit in molecular weight is determined primarily by the requirement that most drugs must be able to move within the body (eg, from the site of administration to the site of action and then to the site of elimination). Drugs much larger than MW 1000 do not diffuse readily between compartments of the body (discussed under Permeation, in following text). Therefore, very large drugs (usually proteins) must often be administered directly into the compartment where they have their effect. In the case of alteplase, a clot-dissolving enzyme, it is administered directly into the vascular compartment by intravenous or intra-arterial infusion.

Drug Reactivity & Drug-Receptor Bonds

Drugs interact with receptors by means of chemical forces or bonds. These are of three major types: **covalent, electrostatic,** and **hydrophobic.** Covalent bonds are very strong and in many cases not reversible under biologic conditions. Thus, the covalent bond formed between the acetyl group of acetylsalicylic acid (aspirin) and cyclooxygenase, its enzyme target in platelets, is not readily broken. The platelet aggregation–blocking effect of aspirin lasts long (days) after free acetylsalicylic acid has disappeared from the bloodstream (about 15 minutes) and is reversed only by the synthesis of new enzyme in new platelets, a process that takes several days. Other examples of highly reactive, covalent bond-forming drugs include the DNA-alkylating agents used in cancer chemotherapy to disrupt cell division in the tumor.

Electrostatic bonding is much more common than covalent bonding in drug-receptor interactions. Electrostatic bonds vary from relatively strong linkages between permanently charged ionic molecules to weaker hydrogen bonds and very weak induced dipole interactions such as van der Waals forces and similar phenomena. Electrostatic bonds are weaker than covalent bonds.

Hydrophobic bonds are usually quite weak and are probably important in the interactions of highly lipid-soluble drugs with the lipids of cell membranes and perhaps in the interaction of drugs with the internal walls of receptor "pockets."

The specific nature of a particular drug-receptor bond is of less practical importance than the fact that drugs that bind through weak bonds to their receptors are generally more selective than drugs that bind by means of very strong bonds. This is because weak bonds require a very precise fit of the drug to its receptor if an interaction is to occur. Only a few receptor types are likely to provide such a precise fit for a particular drug structure. Thus, if we wished to design a highly selective drug for a particular receptor, we would avoid highly reactive molecules that form covalent bonds and instead choose a molecule that forms weaker bonds.

A few substances that are almost completely inert in the chemical sense nevertheless have significant pharmacologic effects. For example, xenon, an "inert" gas, has anesthetic effects at elevated pressures.

Drug Shape

The shape of a drug molecule must be such as to permit binding to its target site via the bonds just described. Optimally, the drug's shape is complementary to that of the target site (usually a receptor) in the same way that a key is complementary to a lock. Furthermore, the phenomenon of **chirality (stereoisomerism)** is so common in biology that more than half of all useful drugs are chiral molecules; that is, they can exist as enantiomeric pairs. Drugs with two asymmetric centers have four diastereomers, eg, ephedrine, a sympathomimetic drug. In most cases, one of these enantiomers is much more potent than its mirror image enantiomer, reflecting a better fit to the receptor molecule. If one imagines the receptor site to be like a glove into which the drug molecule must fit to bring about its effect, it is clear why a "left-oriented" drug is more effective in binding to a left-hand receptor than its "right-oriented" enantiomer.

The more active enantiomer at one type of receptor site may not be more active at another receptor type, eg, a type that may be responsible for some other effect. For example, carvedilol, a drug that interacts with adrenoceptors, has a single chiral center and thus two enantiomers (Table 1–2). One of these enantiomers, the (*S*)(–) isomer, is a potent β-receptor blocker. The (*R*)(+) isomer is 100-fold weaker at the β receptor. However, the isomers are approximately equipotent as α-receptor blockers. Ketamine, a chiral molecule with two isomers, was introduced as an anesthetic. When administered as

TABLE 1–2 Dissociation constants (K_d) of the enantiomers and racemate of carvedilol.

Form of Carvedilol	α Receptors (K_d, nmol/L[1])	β Receptors (K_d, nmol/L)
(*R*)(+) enantiomer	14	45
(*S*)(–) enantiomer	16	0.4
(*R,S*)(±) enantiomers	11	0.9

[1]The K_d is the concentration for 50% saturation of the receptors and is inversely proportionate to the affinity of the drug for the receptors.

Data from Ruffolo RR Jr, Gellai M, Hieble JP, et al: The Pharmacology of carvedilol. Eur J Clin Pharmacol 1990;38S2:S82-88.

an anesthetic, the racemic mixture is administered intravenously. In contrast, the (*S*) enantiomer has recently been approved for use in nasal spray form as a rapid-acting antidepressant.

Finally, because enzymes are usually stereoselective, one drug enantiomer is often more susceptible than the other to drug-metabolizing enzymes. As a result, the duration of action of one enantiomer may be quite different from that of the other. Similarly, drug transporters may be stereoselective.

Unfortunately, most studies of clinical efficacy and drug elimination in humans have been carried out with racemic mixtures of drugs rather than with the separate enantiomers. At present, less than half of the chiral drugs used clinically are marketed as the active isomer—the rest are available only as racemic mixtures. As a result, a majority of patients receive drug doses of which 50% is less active or inactive. A few drugs are currently available in both the racemic and the pure, active isomer forms. However, proof that administration of the pure, active enantiomer decreases adverse effects relative to those produced by racemic formulations has not been established.

Rational Drug Design

Rational design of drugs implies the ability to predict the appropriate molecular structure of a drug on the basis of information about its biologic receptor. Until recently, no receptor was known in sufficient detail to permit such drug design. Instead, drugs were developed through random testing of chemicals or modification of drugs already known to have some effect. However, the characterization of many receptors during the past three decades has changed this picture. A few drugs now in use were developed through molecular design based on knowledge of the three-dimensional structure of the receptor site. Computer programs are now available that can iteratively optimize drug structures to fit known receptors. As more becomes known about receptor structure, rational drug design will become more common.

Receptor Nomenclature

The spectacular success of newer, more efficient ways to identify and characterize receptors (see Chapter 2) has resulted in a variety of differing, and sometimes confusing, systems for naming them. This in turn has led to a number of suggestions regarding more rational methods of naming receptors. The interested reader is referred for details to the efforts of the International Union of Pharmacology (IUPHAR) Committee on Receptor Nomenclature and Drug Classification (reported in various issues of *Pharmacological Reviews* and elsewhere) and to Alexander SP et al: The Concise guide to pharmacology 2017/18: Overview. Br J Pharmacol 2017;174:S1. The chapters in this book mainly use these sources for naming receptors.

DRUG-BODY INTERACTIONS

The interactions between a drug and the body are conveniently divided into two classes. The actions of the drug on the body are termed **pharmacodynamic** processes (see Figure 1–1); the principles of pharmacodynamics are presented in greater detail in Chapter 2. These properties determine the group in which the drug is classified, and they play the major role in deciding whether that group is appropriate therapy for a particular symptom or disease. The actions of the body on the drug are called **pharmacokinetic** processes and are described in Chapters 3 and 4. Pharmacokinetic processes govern the absorption, distribution, and elimination of drugs and are of great practical importance in the choice and administration of a particular drug for a particular patient, eg, a patient with heart failure who also has impaired renal function. The following paragraphs provide a brief introduction to pharmacodynamics and pharmacokinetics.

Pharmacodynamic Principles

Most drugs must bind to a receptor to bring about an effect. However, at the cellular level, drug binding is only the first in a sequence of possible steps:

- Drug (D) + receptor-effector (R) → drug-receptor-effector complex → effect
- D + R → drug-receptor complex → effector molecule → effect
- D + R → D-R complex → activation of coupling molecule → effector molecule → effect
- Inhibition of metabolism of endogenous activator → increased activator action on an effector molecule → increased effect

Note that the final change in function is accomplished by an **effector** mechanism. The effector may be part of the receptor molecule or may be a separate molecule. A very large number of receptors communicate with their effectors through coupling molecules, as described in Chapter 2.

A. Types of Drug-Receptor Interactions

Agonist drugs bind to and *activate* the receptor in some fashion, which directly or indirectly brings about the effect (Figure 1–2A). Receptor activation involves a change in conformation in the cases that have been studied at the molecular structure level. Some receptors incorporate effector machinery in the same molecule, so that drug binding brings about the effect directly, eg, opening of an ion channel or activation of enzyme activity. Other receptors are linked through one or more intervening coupling molecules to a separate effector molecule. The major types of drug-receptor-effector coupling systems are discussed in Chapter 2. **Pharmacologic antagonist** drugs, by binding to a receptor, compete with and prevent binding by other molecules. For example, acetylcholine receptor blockers such as atropine are antagonists because they prevent access of acetylcholine and similar agonist drugs to the acetylcholine receptor site and they stabilize the receptor in its inactive state (or some state other than the acetylcholine-activated state). These agents reduce the effects of acetylcholine and similar molecules in the body (Figure 1–2B), but their action can be overcome by increasing the dosage of agonist. Some antagonists bind very tightly to the receptor site in an irreversible or pseudoirreversible fashion and cannot be displaced by increasing the agonist concentration. Drugs that bind to the same receptor molecule but do not prevent binding of the agonist are said to act **allosterically** and may enhance (Figure 1–2C) or inhibit (Figure 1–2D) the action of

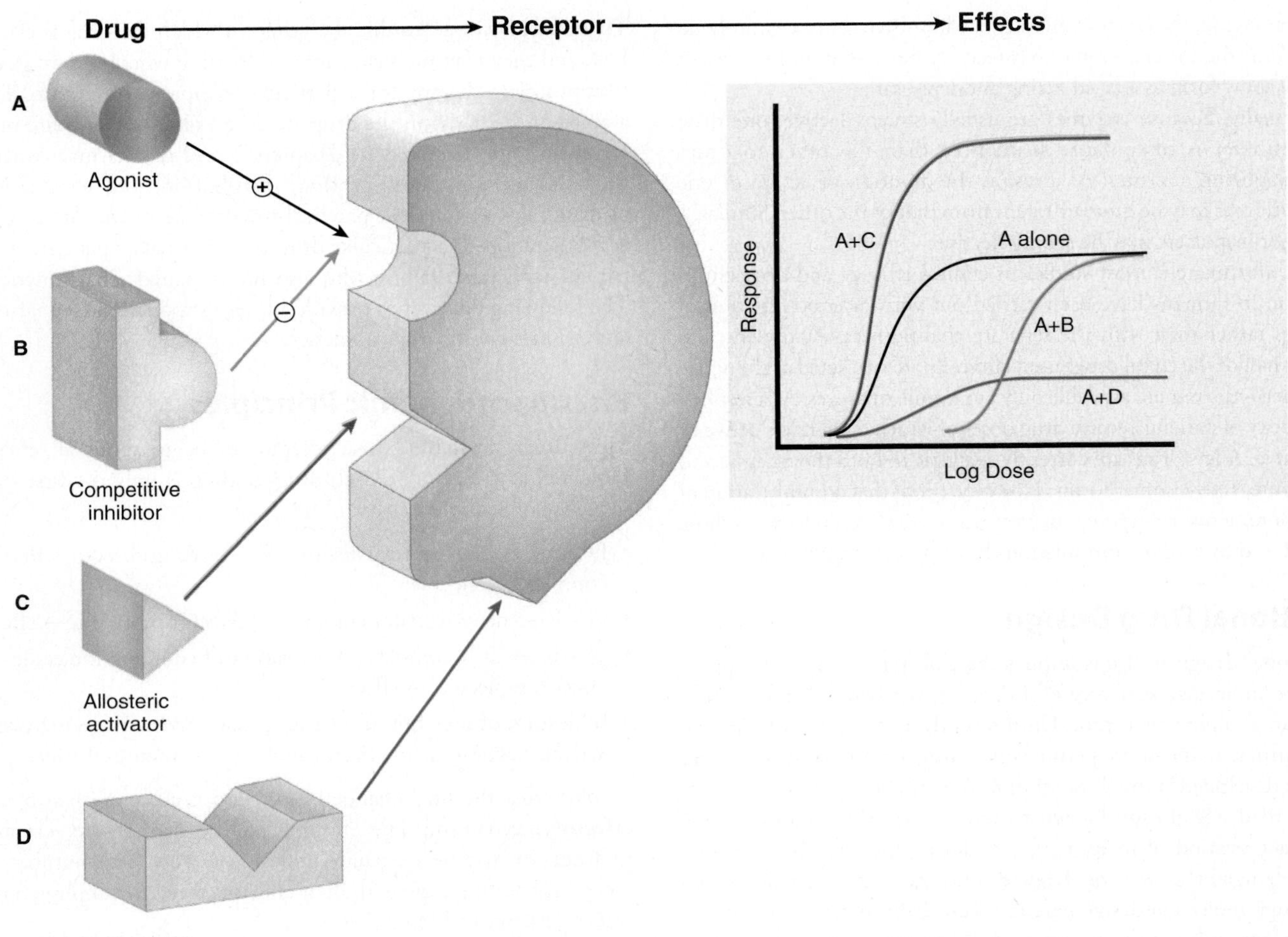

FIGURE 1–2 Drugs may interact with receptors in several ways. The effects resulting from these interactions are diagrammed in the dose-response curves at the right. Drugs that alter the agonist (**A**) response may activate the agonist binding site, compete with the agonist (competitive inhibitors, **B**), or act at separate (allosteric) sites, increasing (**C**) or decreasing (**D**) the response to the agonist. Allosteric activators (**C**) may increase the efficacy of the agonist or its binding affinity. The curve shown reflects an increase in efficacy; an increase in affinity would result in a leftward shift of the curve.

the agonist molecule. Allosteric inhibition is not usually overcome by increasing the dose of agonist.

B. Agonists That Inhibit Their Binding Molecules

Some drugs mimic agonist drugs by inhibiting the molecules responsible for terminating the action of an endogenous agonist. For example, acetylcholinesterase *inhibitors*, by slowing the destruction of endogenous acetylcholine, cause cholinomimetic effects that closely resemble the actions of cholinoceptor *agonist* molecules even though cholinesterase inhibitors do not bind or only incidentally bind to cholinoceptors (see Chapter 7). Because they amplify the effects of physiologically released endogenous agonist ligands, their effects are sometimes more selective and less toxic than those of exogenous agonists.

C. Agonists, Partial Agonists, and Inverse Agonists

Figure 1–3 describes a useful model of drug-receptor interactions. As indicated, the receptor is postulated to exist partially in the inactive, nonfunctional form (R_i) and partially in the activated form (R_a). Thermodynamic considerations indicate that even in the absence of any agonist, some of the receptor pool must exist in the R_a form some of the time and may produce the same physiologic effect as agonist-induced activity. This effect, occurring in the absence of agonist, is termed **constitutive** or **basal activity.** Agonists have a much higher affinity for the R_a configuration and stabilize it, so that a large percentage of the total pool resides in the R_a–D fraction and a large effect is produced. The recognition of constitutive activity may depend on the receptor density, the concentration of coupling molecules (if a coupled system), and the number of effectors in the system.

Many agonist drugs, when administered at concentrations sufficient to saturate the receptor pool, can activate their receptor-effector systems to the maximum extent of which the system is capable; that is, they cause a shift of almost all of the receptor pool to the R_a–D pool. Such drugs are termed **full agonists.** Other drugs, called **partial agonists,** bind to the same receptors and activate them in the same way but do not evoke as great a response, no matter how high the concentration. In the model in

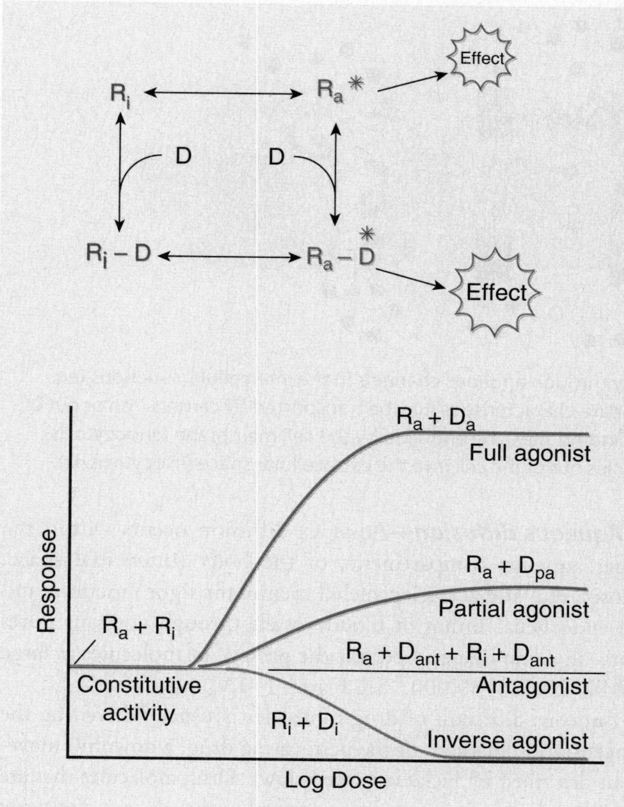

FIGURE 1–3 A model of drug-receptor interaction. The hypothetical receptor is able to assume two conformations. In the R_i conformation, it is inactive and produces no effect, even when combined with a drug molecule. In the R_a conformation, the receptor can activate downstream mechanisms that produce a small observable effect, even in the absence of drug (constitutive activity). In the absence of drugs, the two isoforms are in equilibrium, and the R_i form is favored. Conventional full agonist drugs have a much higher affinity for the R_a conformation, and mass action thus favors the formation of the R_a–D complex with a much larger observed effect. Partial agonists have an intermediate affinity for both R_i and R_a forms. Conventional antagonists, according to this hypothesis, have equal affinity for both receptor forms and maintain the same level of constitutive activity. Inverse agonists, on the other hand, have a much higher affinity for the R_i form, reduce constitutive activity, and may produce a contrasting physiologic result.

Figure 1–3, partial agonists do not stabilize the R_a configuration as fully as full agonists, so that a significant fraction of receptors exists in the R_i–D pool. Such drugs are said to have low **intrinsic efficacy.** Because they occupy the same receptor site, partial agonists can also prevent access by full agonists. Thus, pindolol, a β-adrenoceptor partial agonist, may act either as an agonist (if no full agonist is present) or as an antagonist (if a full agonist such as epinephrine is present). (See Chapter 2.) Intrinsic efficacy is independent of affinity (as usually measured) for the receptor.

In the same model, conventional antagonist action can be explained as fixing the fractions of drug-bound R_i and R_a in the same relative amounts as in the absence of any drug. In this situation, no change in activity will be observed, so the drug will appear to be without effect. However, the presence of the antagonist at the receptor site will block access of agonists to the receptor and prevent the usual agonist effect. Such blocking action can be termed **neutral antagonism.**

What will happen if a drug has a much stronger affinity for the R_i than for the R_a state and stabilizes a large fraction in the R_i–D pool? In this scenario the drug will reduce any constitutive activity, thus resulting in effects that are the opposite of the effects produced by conventional agonists at that receptor. Such drugs are termed **inverse agonists** (see Figure 1–3). One of the best documented examples of such a system is the γ-aminobutyric acid ($GABA_A$) receptor-effector (a chloride channel) in the nervous system. This receptor is activated by the endogenous transmitter GABA and causes inhibition of postsynaptic cells. Conventional exogenous agonists such as benzodiazepines also facilitate the receptor-effector system and enhance GABA-like chloride entry into cells with sedation as the therapeutic result. This sedation can be reversed by conventional neutral antagonists such as flumazenil. Inverse agonists of this receptor system cause anxiety and agitation, the inverse of sedation (see Chapter 22). Similar inverse agonists have been found for β adrenoceptors, histamine H_1 and H_2 receptors, and several other receptor systems.

D. Duration of Drug Action

Termination of drug action can result from several processes. In some cases, the effect lasts only as long as the drug occupies the receptor, and dissociation of drug from the receptor automatically terminates the effect. In many cases, however, the action may persist after the drug has dissociated because, for example, some coupling molecule is still present in activated form. In the case of drugs that bind covalently to the receptor site, the effect may persist until the drug-receptor complex is destroyed and new receptors or enzymes are synthesized, as described previously for aspirin. In addition, many receptor-effector systems incorporate desensitization mechanisms for preventing excessive activation when agonist molecules continue to be present for long periods. (See Chapter 2 for additional details.)

E. Receptors and Inert Binding Sites

To function as a receptor, an endogenous molecule must first be **selective** in choosing ligands (drug molecules) to bind; and second, it must **change its function** upon binding in such a way that the function of the biologic system (cell, tissue, etc) is altered. The selectivity characteristic is required to avoid constant activation of the receptor by promiscuous binding of many different ligands. The ability to change function is clearly necessary if the ligand is to cause a pharmacologic effect. In some cases the function of the ligand may be to inhibit the endogenous actions of the receptor (antagonist and inverse agonist). The body contains a vast array of molecules that are capable of binding drugs, however, and not all of these endogenous molecules are regulatory molecules. Binding of a drug to a nonregulatory molecule such as plasma albumin will result in no detectable change in the function of the biologic system, so this endogenous molecule can be called an **inert binding site.** Such binding is not completely without significance, however, because it affects the

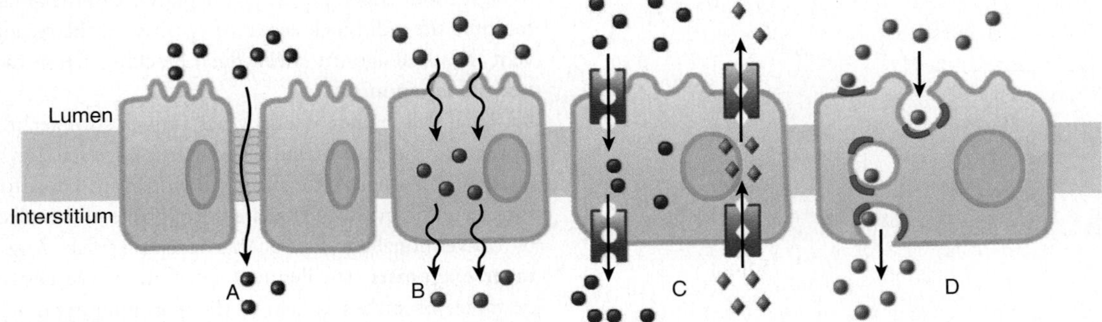

FIGURE 1–4 Mechanisms of drug permeation. Drugs may diffuse passively through aqueous channels in the intercellular junctions (eg, tight junctions, **A**), or through lipid cell membranes (**B**). Drugs with the appropriate characteristics may be transported by carriers into or out of cells (**C**). Very impermeant drugs may also bind to cell surface receptors (dark binding sites), be engulfed by the cell membrane (endocytosis), and then be released inside the cell or expelled via the membrane-limited vesicles out of the cell into the extracellular space (exocytosis, **D**).

distribution of drug within the body and determines the amount of free drug in the circulation. Both of these factors are of pharmacokinetic importance (see also Chapter 3).

Pharmacokinetic Principles

In practical therapeutics, a drug should be able to reach its intended site of action after administration by some convenient route. In many cases, the active drug molecule is sufficiently lipid-soluble and stable to be given as such. In some cases, however, an inactive precursor chemical that is readily absorbed and distributed must be administered and then converted to the active drug by biologic processes—inside the body. Such a precursor chemical is called a **prodrug.**

In only a few situations is it possible to apply a drug directly to its target tissue, eg, by topical application of an anti-inflammatory agent to inflamed skin or mucous membrane. Most often, a drug is administered into one body compartment, eg, the gut, and must move to its site of action in another compartment, eg, the brain in the case of an antiseizure medication. This requires that the drug be **absorbed** into the blood from its site of administration and **distributed** to its site of action, **permeating** through the various barriers that separate these compartments. For a drug given orally to produce an effect in the central nervous system, these barriers include the tissues that make up the wall of the intestine, the walls of the capillaries that perfuse the gut, and the blood-brain barrier, the walls of the capillaries that perfuse the brain. Finally, after bringing about its effect, a drug should be **eliminated** at a reasonable rate by metabolic inactivation, by excretion from the body, or by a combination of these processes.

A. Permeation

Drug permeation proceeds by several mechanisms. Passive diffusion in an aqueous or lipid medium is common, but active processes play a role in the movement of many drugs, especially those whose molecules are too large to diffuse readily (Figure 1–4). Drug **vehicles** can be very important in facilitating transport and permeation, eg, by encapsulating the active agent in liposomes and in regulating release, as in slow release preparations. Newer methods of facilitating transport of drugs by coupling them to **nanoparticles** are under investigation.

1. *Aqueous diffusion*—Aqueous diffusion occurs within the larger aqueous compartments of the body (interstitial space, cytosol, etc) and across epithelial membrane tight junctions and the endothelial lining of blood vessels through aqueous pores that—in some tissues—permit the passage of molecules as large as MW 20,000–30,000.* See Figure 1–4A.

Aqueous diffusion of drug molecules is usually driven by the concentration gradient of the permeating drug, a downhill movement described by Fick's law (see below). Drug molecules that are bound to large plasma proteins (eg, albumin) do not permeate most vascular aqueous pores. If the drug is charged, its flux is also influenced by electrical fields (eg, the membrane potential and—in parts of the nephron—the transtubular potential).

2. *Lipid diffusion*—Lipid diffusion is the most important limiting factor for drug permeation because of the large number of lipid barriers that separate the compartments of the body. Because these lipid barriers separate aqueous compartments, the **lipid:aqueous partition coefficient** of a drug determines how readily the molecule moves between aqueous and lipid media. In the case of weak acids and weak bases (which gain or lose electrical charge-bearing protons, depending on the pH), the ability to move from aqueous to lipid or vice versa varies with the pH of the medium, because charged molecules attract water molecules. The ratio of lipid-soluble form to water-soluble form for a weak acid or weak base is expressed by the Henderson-Hasselbalch equation (described in the following text). See Figure 1–4B.

3. *Special carriers*—Special carrier molecules exist for many substances that are important for cell function and are too large or too insoluble in lipid to diffuse passively through membranes, eg, peptides, amino acids, and glucose. These carriers bring about movement by active transport or facilitated diffusion and, unlike passive diffusion, are selective, saturable, and inhibitable. Because

*The capillaries of the brain, the testes, and some other tissues are characterized by the absence of pores that permit aqueous diffusion. They may also contain high concentrations of drug export pumps (MDR pump molecules; see text). These tissues are therefore protected or "sanctuary" sites from many circulating drugs.

many drugs are or resemble such naturally occurring peptides, amino acids, or sugars, they can use these carriers to cross membranes. See Figure 1–4C.

Many cells also contain less selective membrane carriers that are specialized for expelling foreign molecules. One large family of such transporters binds adenosine triphosphate (ATP) and is called the ABC (ATP-binding cassette) family. This family includes the **P-glycoprotein** or **multidrug resistance type 1 (MDR1) transporter** found in the brain, testes, and other tissues and in some drug-resistant neoplastic cells (Table 1–3). Similar transport molecules from the ABC family, the **multidrug resistance-associated protein (MRP)** transporters, play important roles in the excretion of some drugs or their metabolites into urine and bile and in the resistance of some tumors to chemotherapeutic drugs. Genomic variation in the expression of these transporters has a profound effect on sensitivity to these drugs (see Chapter 5). Several other transporter families have been identified that do not bind ATP but use ion gradients to drive transport. Some of these (the solute carrier [SLC] family) are particularly important in the uptake of neurotransmitters across nerve-ending membranes. The latter carriers are discussed in more detail in Chapter 6.

TABLE 1–3 Some transport molecules important in pharmacology.

Transporter	Physiologic Function	Pharmacologic Significance
NET	Norepinephrine reuptake from synapse	Target of cocaine and some tricyclic antidepressants
SERT	Serotonin reuptake from synapse	Target of selective serotonin reuptake inhibitors and some tricyclic antidepressants
VMAT	Transport of dopamine and norepinephrine into adrenergic vesicles in nerve endings	Target of reserpine and tetrabenazine
MDR1	Transport of many xenobiotics out of cells	Increased expression confers resistance to certain anticancer drugs; inhibition increases blood levels of digoxin
MRP1	Leukotriene secretion	Confers resistance to certain anticancer and antifungal drugs
OCT	Organic cationic compound uptake	Target for uptake of organic cationic compounds (acetylcholine, dopamine, norepinephrine, metformin, etc) into many tissues including the brain, liver, heart, kidney
OATP	Organic anionic and neutral compound uptake	Target for uptake of organic anionic compounds (prostaglandins, hormones, bile salts, statins, etc) into many tissues including the brain, liver, kidney, intestine

MDR1, multidrug resistance protein-1; MRP1, multidrug resistance-associated protein-1; NET, norepinephrine transporter; OATP, organic anionic transporter polypeptide; OCT, organic cationic transporter; SERT, serotonin reuptake transporter; VMAT, vesicular monoamine transporter.

4. *Endocytosis and exocytosis*—A few substances are so large or impermeant that they can enter cells only by endocytosis, the process by which the substance is bound at a cell-surface receptor, engulfed by the cell membrane, and carried into the cell by pinching off of the newly formed vesicle inside the membrane. The substance can then be released into the cytosol by breakdown of the vesicle membrane (see Figure 1–4D). This process is responsible for the transport of vitamin B_{12}, complexed with a binding protein (intrinsic factor) across the wall of the gut into the blood. Similarly, iron is transported into hemoglobin-synthesizing red blood cell precursors in association with the protein transferrin. Specific receptors for the binding proteins must be present for this process to work.

The reverse process (exocytosis) is responsible for the secretion of many substances from cells. For example, many neurotransmitter substances are stored in membrane-bound vesicles in nerve endings to protect them from metabolic destruction in the cytoplasm. Appropriate activation of the nerve ending causes fusion of the storage vesicle with the cell membrane and expulsion of its contents into the extracellular space (see Chapter 6).

B. Fick's Law of Diffusion

The passive flux of molecules down a concentration gradient is given by Fick's law:

$$\text{Flux (moles per unit time)} = (C_1 - C_2) \times \frac{\text{Area} \times \text{Permeability coefficient}}{\text{Thickness}}$$

where C_1 is the higher concentration, C_2 is the lower concentration, area is the cross-sectional area of the diffusion path, permeability coefficient is a measure of the mobility of the drug molecules in the medium of the diffusion path, and thickness is the length of the diffusion path. In the case of lipid diffusion, the lipid:aqueous partition coefficient is a major determinant of mobility of the drug because it determines how readily the drug enters the lipid membrane from the aqueous medium.

C. Ionization of Weak Acids and Weak Bases; the Henderson-Hasselbalch Equation

The electrostatic charge of an ionized molecule attracts water dipoles and results in a polar, relatively water-soluble and lipid-insoluble complex. Because lipid diffusion depends on relatively high lipid solubility, ionization of drugs may markedly reduce their ability to permeate membranes. A very large percentage of the drugs in use are weak acids or weak bases; Table 1–4 lists some examples. For drugs, a weak acid is best defined as a neutral molecule that can reversibly dissociate into an anion (a negatively charged molecule) and a proton (a hydrogen ion). For example, aspirin dissociates as follows:

$$\underset{\text{Neutral aspirin}}{C_8H_7O_2COOH} \rightleftharpoons \underset{\text{Aspirin anion}}{C_8H_7O_2COO^-} + \underset{\text{Proton}}{H^+}$$

A weak base can be defined as a neutral molecule that can form a cation (a positively charged molecule) by combining with a

TABLE 1–4 Ionization constants of some common drugs.

Drug	pK_a[1]	Drug	pK_a[1]	Drug	pK_a[1]
Weak acids		**Weak bases**		**Weak bases (cont'd)**	
Acetaminophen	9.5	Albuterol (salbutamol)	9.3	Isoproterenol	8.6
Acetazolamide	7.2	Allopurinol	9.4, 12.3[2]	Lidocaine	7.9
Ampicillin	2.5	Alprenolol	9.6	Metaraminol	8.6
Aspirin	3.5	Amiloride	8.7	Methadone	8.4
Atorvastatin	4.3	Amiodarone	6.6	Methamphetamine	10.0
Chlorothiazide	6.8, 9.4[2]	Amphetamine	9.8	Methyldopa	10.6
Chlorpropamide	5.0	Atropine	9.7	Metoprolol	9.8
Ciprofloxacin	6.1, 8.7[2]	Bupivacaine	8.1	Morphine	7.9
Cromolyn	2.0	Chlordiazepoxide	4.6	Nicotine	7.9, 3.1[2]
Ethacrynic acid	2.5	Chloroquine	10.8, 8.4	Norepinephrine	8.6
Furosemide	3.9	Chlorpheniramine	9.2	Pentazocine	7.9
Ibuprofen	4.4, 5.2[2]	Chlorpromazine	9.3	Phenylephrine	9.8
Levodopa	2.3	Clonidine	8.3	Physostigmine	7.9, 1.8[2]
Methotrexate	4.8	Cocaine	8.5	Pilocarpine	6.9, 1.4[2]
Methyldopa	2.2, 9.2[2]	Codeine	8.2	Pindolol	8.6
Penicillamine	1.8	Cyclizine	8.2	Procainamide	9.2
Pentobarbital	8.1	Desipramine	10.2	Procaine	9.0
Phenobarbital	7.4	Diazepam	3.0	Promethazine	9.1
Phenytoin	8.3	Diphenhydramine	8.8	Propranolol	9.4
Propylthiouracil	8.3	Diphenoxylate	7.1	Pseudoephedrine	9.8
Salicylic acid	3.0	Ephedrine	9.6	Pyrimethamine	7.0–7.3[3]
Sulfadiazine	6.5	Epinephrine	8.7	Quinidine	8.5, 4.4[2]
Sulfapyridine	8.4	Ergotamine	6.3	Scopolamine	8.1
Theophylline	8.8	Fluphenazine	8.0, 3.9[2]	Strychnine	8.0, 2.3[2]
Tolbutamide	5.3	Hydralazine	7.1	Terbutaline	10.1
Warfarin	5.0	Imipramine	9.5	Thioridazine	9.5

[1]The pK_a is that pH at which the concentrations of the ionized and nonionized forms are equal.

[2]More than one ionizable group.

[3]Isoelectric point.

proton. For example, pyrimethamine, an antimalarial drug, undergoes the following association-dissociation process:

$$C_{12}H_{11}ClN_3NH_3^+ \rightleftharpoons C_{12}H_{11}ClN_3NH_2 + H^+$$

Pyrimethamine cation — Neutral pyrimethamine — Proton

Note that the protonated form of a weak acid is the neutral, more lipid-soluble form, whereas the unprotonated form of a weak base is the neutral form. The law of mass action requires that these reactions move to the left in an acid environment (low pH, excess protons available) and to the right in an alkaline environment. The Henderson-Hasselbalch equation relates the ratio of protonated to unprotonated weak acid or weak base to the molecule's pK_a and the pH of the medium as follows:

$$\log \frac{\text{(Protonated)}}{\text{(Unprotonated)}} = pK_a - pH$$

This equation applies to both acidic and basic drugs. Inspection confirms that the lower the pH relative to the pK_a, the greater will be the fraction of drug in the protonated form. Because the uncharged form is the more lipid-soluble, more of a weak acid will be in the lipid-soluble form at acid pH, whereas more of a basic drug will be in the lipid-soluble form at alkaline pH.

Application of this principle is made in the manipulation of drug excretion by the kidney (see Case Study). Almost all drugs are filtered at the glomerulus. If a drug is in a lipid-soluble form during its passage down the renal tubule, a significant fraction will be reabsorbed back into the tissue by simple passive diffusion. If the goal is to accelerate excretion of the drug (eg, in a case of drug overdose), it is important to prevent its reabsorption from the tubule. This can often be accomplished by adjusting urine pH to make certain that most of the drug is in the ionized state, as shown in Figure 1–5. As a result of this partitioning effect, the drug is "trapped" in the urine. Thus, weak acids are usually excreted faster in alkaline urine; weak bases are

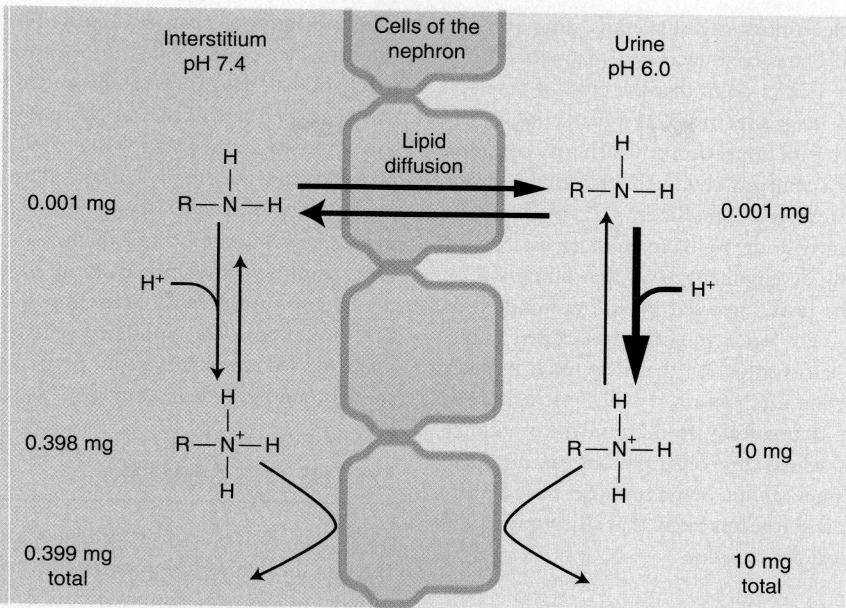

FIGURE 1–5 Trapping of a weak base (methamphetamine) in the urine when the urine is more acidic than the blood. In the hypothetical case illustrated, the diffusible uncharged form of the drug has equilibrated across the membrane, but the total concentration (charged plus uncharged) in the urine (more than 10 mg) is 25 times higher than in the blood (0.4 mg).

usually excreted faster in acidic urine. Other body fluids in which pH differences from blood pH may cause trapping or reabsorption are the contents of the stomach (normal pH 1.9–3) and small intestine (pH 7.5–8), breast milk (pH 6.4–7.6), aqueous humor (pH 6.4–7.5), and vaginal and prostatic secretions (pH 3.5–7).

As indicated by Table 1–4, a large number of drugs are weak bases. Most of these bases are amine-containing molecules. The nitrogen of a neutral amine has three atoms associated with it plus a pair of unshared electrons (see the display that follows). The three atoms may consist of one carbon or a chain of carbon atoms (designated "R") and two hydrogens (a **primary amine**), two carbons and one hydrogen (a **secondary amine**), or three carbon atoms (a **tertiary amine**). Each of these three forms may reversibly bind a proton with the unshared electrons. Some drugs have a fourth carbon-nitrogen bond; these are **quaternary amines.** However, the quaternary amine is permanently charged and has no unshared electrons with which to reversibly bind a proton. Therefore, primary, secondary, and tertiary amines may undergo reversible protonation and vary their lipid solubility with pH, but quaternary amines are always in the poorly lipid-soluble charged form.

Primary	Secondary	Tertiary	Quaternary
H	R	R	R
R:N:	R:N:	R:N:	R:N:R (+)
H	H	R	R

DRUG GROUPS

To learn each pertinent fact about each of the many hundreds of drugs mentioned in this book would be an impractical goal and, fortunately, is unnecessary. Almost all the several thousand drugs currently available can be arranged into about 70 groups. Many of the drugs within each group are very similar in pharmacodynamic actions and in their pharmacokinetic properties as well. For most groups, one or two **prototype drugs** can be identified that typify the most important characteristics of the group. This permits classification of other important drugs in the group as variants of the prototype, so that only the prototype must be learned in detail and, for the remaining drugs, only the differences from the prototype.

■ DRUG DEVELOPMENT & REGULATION

A truly new drug (one that does not simply mimic the structure and action of previously available drugs) requires the discovery of a new drug target, ie, the pathophysiologic process or substrate of a disease. Such discoveries are usually made in public sector institutions (universities and research institutes), and molecules that have beneficial effects on such targets are often discovered in the same laboratories. However, the development of new drugs usually takes place in industrial laboratories because optimization of a class of new drugs requires painstaking and expensive chemical, pharmacologic, and toxicologic research. In fact, much of the recent progress in the application of drugs to disease problems can be ascribed to the pharmaceutical industry including "big pharma," the multibillion-dollar corporations that specialize in drug development and marketing. These companies are uniquely skilled in translating basic findings into successful therapeutic breakthroughs and profit-making "blockbusters" (see https://clincalc.com/DrugStats/Top200Drugs.aspx).

Such breakthroughs come at a price, however, and the escalating cost of drugs has become a significant contributor to the increase in the cost of health care. Development of new drugs is enormously expensive, but considerable controversy surrounds drug pricing. Drug prices in the United States have increased many-fold faster than overall price inflation. Critics claim that the costs of development and marketing drugs are grossly inflated by marketing activities, advertising, and other promotional efforts, which may consume as much as 25% or more of a company's budget. Furthermore, profit margins for big pharma are relatively high. Recent drug-pricing scandals have been reported in which the rights to an older, established drug that requires no costly development have been purchased by a smaller company and the price increased by several hundred or several thousand percent. This "price gouging" has caused public outrage and attracted regulatory attention that may result in more legitimate and rational pricing mechanisms. Finally, pricing schedules for many drugs vary dramatically from country to country and even within countries, where large organizations can negotiate favorable prices and small ones cannot. Some countries have already addressed these inequities, and it seems likely that all countries will have to do so during the next few decades.

NEW DRUG DEVELOPMENT

The development of a new drug usually begins with the discovery or synthesis of a potential new drug compound or the elucidation of a new drug target. After a new drug molecule is synthesized or extracted from a natural source, subsequent steps seek an understanding of the drug's interactions with its biologic targets. Repeated application of this approach leads to synthesis of related compounds with increased efficacy, potency, and selectivity (Figure 1–6). In the United States, the safety and efficacy of drugs must be established before marketing can be legally carried out. In addition to in vitro studies, relevant biologic effects, drug metabolism, pharmacokinetic profiles, and relative safety of the drug are recommended to be characterized in vivo in animals before human drug trials can be started but not necessary if studies can be carried out in cells or alternative approaches. With regulatory approval, human testing may then go forward (usually in three phases) before the drug is considered for approval for general use. A fourth phase of data gathering and safety monitoring is becoming increasingly important and follows after approval for marketing. Once approved, the great majority of drugs become available for use by any appropriately licensed practitioner. Highly toxic drugs that are nevertheless considered valuable in lethal diseases may be approved for restricted use by practitioners who have undergone special training in their use and who maintain detailed records.

DRUG DISCOVERY

Most new drugs or drug products are discovered or developed through the following approaches: (1) screening for biologic activity of large numbers of natural products, banks of previously discovered chemical entities, or large libraries of peptides, nucleic acids, and other organic molecules; (2) chemical modification of a known active molecule, resulting in a "me-too" analog; (3) identification or elucidation of a new drug target, which suggests molecules that will hit that target; and (4) rational design of a new molecule based on an understanding of biologic mechanisms and drug receptor structure. Steps (3) and (4) are often carried out in academic research laboratories and are more likely to lead to breakthrough drugs, but the costs of steps (1) and (2) usually ensure that industry carries them out.

Once a new drug target or promising molecule has been identified, the process of moving from the basic science laboratory to the clinic begins. This **translational research** involves the preclinical and clinical

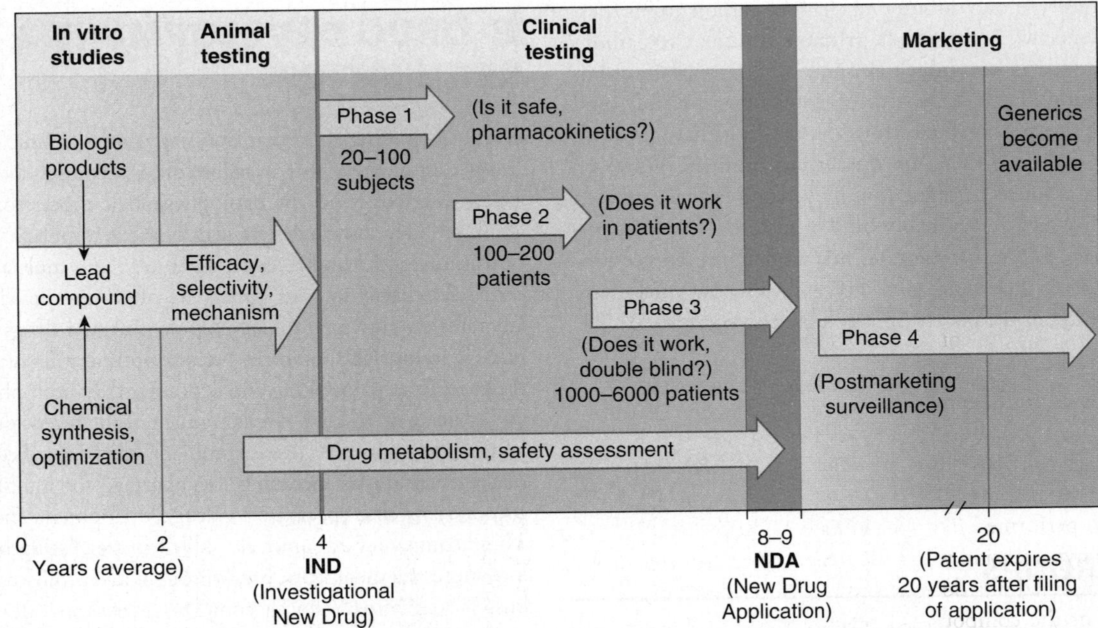

FIGURE 1–6 The development and testing process required to bring a drug to market in the USA. Some of the requirements may be different for drugs used in life-threatening diseases (see text).

steps described next. While clinical trials in humans are required only for drugs to be used in humans, all of the other steps described apply to veterinary drugs as well as drugs for human diseases.

Drug Screening

Drug screening involves a variety of assays at the molecular, cellular, organ system, and whole animal levels to define the **pharmacologic profile,** ie, the activity and selectivity of the drug. The type and number of initial screening tests depend on the pharmacologic and therapeutic goal. For example, anti-infective drugs are tested against a variety of infectious organisms, some of which are resistant to standard agents; hypoglycemic drugs are tested for their ability to lower blood sugar, etc.

The candidate molecule is also studied for a broad array of other actions to determine the mechanism of action and selectivity of the drug. This can reveal both expected and unexpected toxic effects. Occasionally, an unexpected therapeutic action is serendipitously discovered by a careful observer; for example, the era of modern diuretics was initiated by the observation that certain antimicrobial sulfonamides caused metabolic acidosis in patients. The selection of compounds for development is most efficiently conducted in animal models of human disease. Where good predictive preclinical models exist (eg, infection, hypertension, or thrombotic disease), we generally have good or excellent drugs. Good drugs or breakthrough improvements are conspicuously lacking and slow for diseases for which preclinical models are poor or not yet available, eg, autism and Alzheimer disease.

At the molecular level, the candidate compound would be screened for activity on the target, for example, receptor binding affinity to cell membranes containing the homologous animal receptors (or if possible, on the cloned human receptors). Early studies would be done to predict effects that might later cause undesired drug metabolism or toxicologic complications. For example, studies on liver cytochrome P450 enzymes would be performed to determine whether the molecule of interest is likely to be a substrate or inhibitor of these enzymes or to alter the metabolism of other drugs.

Effects on cell function determine whether the drug is an agonist, partial agonist, inverse agonist, or antagonist at relevant receptors. Isolated tissues would be used to characterize the pharmacologic activity and selectivity of the new compound in comparison with reference compounds. Comparison with other drugs would also be undertaken in a variety of in vivo studies. At each step in this process, the compound would have to meet specific performance and selectivity criteria to be carried further.

Whole animal studies are generally necessary to determine the effect of the drug on organ systems and disease models. Cardiovascular and renal function studies of new drugs are generally first performed in normal animals. Studies on disease models, if available, are then performed. For a candidate antihypertensive drug, animals with hypertension would be treated to see whether blood pressure was lowered in a dose-related manner and to characterize other effects of the compound. Evidence would be collected on duration of action and efficacy after oral and parenteral administration. If the agent possessed useful activity, it would be further studied for possible adverse effects on other organs, including the respiratory, gastrointestinal, renal, endocrine, and central nervous systems.

These studies might suggest the need for further chemical modification (compound optimization) to achieve more desirable pharmacokinetic or pharmacodynamic properties. For example, oral administration studies might show that the drug was poorly absorbed or rapidly metabolized in the liver; modification to improve bioavailability might be indicated. If the drug is to be administered long term, an assessment of tolerance development would be made. For drugs related to or having mechanisms of action similar to those known to cause physical or psychological dependence in humans, ability to cause dependence in animals would also be studied. Drug interactions would be examined.

The desired result of this screening procedure (which may have to be repeated several times with congeners of the original molecule) is a **lead compound,** ie, a leading candidate for a successful new drug. A patent application would be filed for a novel compound (a *composition of matter* patent) that is efficacious, or for a new and nonobvious therapeutic use (a *use* patent) for a previously known chemical entity.

PRECLINICAL SAFETY & TOXICITY TESTING

All chemicals are toxic in some individuals at some dose. Candidate drugs that survive the initial screening procedures must be carefully evaluated for potential risks before and during clinical testing. Depending on the proposed use of the drug, preclinical toxicity testing includes most or all of the procedures shown in Table 1–5. Although no chemical can be certified as completely "safe" (free of risk), the objective is to estimate the risk associated with exposure to the drug candidate and to consider this in the context of therapeutic needs and likely duration of drug use.

The goals of preclinical toxicity studies include identifying potential human toxicities, designing tests to further define the toxic mechanisms, and predicting the most relevant toxicities to be monitored in clinical trials. In addition to the studies shown in Table 1–5, several quantitative estimates are desirable. These include the **no-effect dose**—the maximum dose at which a specified toxic effect is not seen; the **minimum lethal dose**—the smallest dose that is observed to kill any experimental animal; and, if necessary, the **median lethal dose (LD_{50})**—the dose that kills approximately 50% of the animals in a test group. Presently, the LD_{50} is estimated from the smallest number of animals possible. These doses are used to calculate the initial dose to be tried in humans, usually taken as one hundredth to one tenth of the no-effect dose in animals.

It is important to recognize the limitations of preclinical testing. These include the following:

1. Toxicity testing is time-consuming and expensive. Two to 6 years may be required to collect and analyze data on toxicity before the drug can be considered ready for testing in humans.

TABLE 1–5 Safety tests.

Type of Test	Approach and Goals
Acute toxicity	Usually two species, two routes. Determine the no-effect dose and the maximum tolerated dose. In some cases, determine the acute dose that is lethal in approximately 50% of animals.
Subacute or subchronic toxicity	Three doses, two species. Two weeks to 3 months of testing may be required before clinical trials. The longer the duration of expected clinical use, the longer the subacute test. Determine biochemical, physiologic effects.
Chronic toxicity	Rodent and at least one nonrodent species for ≥6 months. Required when drug is intended to be used in humans for prolonged periods. Usually run concurrently with clinical trials. Determine same end points as subacute toxicity tests.
Effect on reproductive performance	Two species, usually one rodent and rabbits. Test effects on animal mating behavior, reproduction, parturition, progeny, birth defects, postnatal development.
Carcinogenic potential	Two years, two species. Required when drug is intended to be used in humans for prolonged periods. Determine gross and histologic pathology.
Mutagenic potential	Test effects on genetic stability and mutations in bacteria (Ames test) or mammalian cells in culture; dominant lethal test and clastogenicity in mice.

2. Large numbers of animals may be needed to obtain valid preclinical data. Scientists are properly concerned about this situation, and progress has been made toward reducing the numbers required while still obtaining valid data. Cell and tissue culture in vitro methods and computer modeling are increasingly being used, but their predictive value is still limited. Nevertheless, some segments of the public attempt to halt all animal testing in the unfounded belief that it has become unnecessary.
3. Extrapolations of toxicity data from animals to humans are reasonably predictive for many but not for all toxicities.
4. For statistical reasons, rare adverse effects are unlikely to be detected in preclinical testing.

EVALUATION IN HUMANS

A very small fraction of lead compounds reach clinical trials, and less than one-third of the drugs studied in humans survive clinical trials and reach the marketplace. Federal law in the USA and ethical considerations require that the study of new drugs in humans be conducted in accordance with stringent guidelines. Scientifically valid results are not guaranteed simply by conforming to government regulations, however, and the design and execution of a good clinical trial require interdisciplinary personnel including basic scientists, clinical pharmacologists, clinician specialists, statisticians, and others. The current standard for clinical trials is known as the randomized controlled trial (RCT) and is described below. The need for careful design and execution is based on three major confounding factors inherent in the study of any drug in humans.

Confounding Factors in Clinical Trials

A. The Variable Natural History of Most Diseases

Many diseases tend to wax and wane in severity; some disappear spontaneously, even, on occasion, cancer. A good experimental design takes into account the natural history of the disease by evaluating a large enough population of subjects over a sufficient period of time. Further protection against errors of interpretation caused by disease fluctuations is sometimes provided by using a **crossover design,** which consists of alternating periods of administration of test drug, placebo preparation (the control), and the previous standard treatment (positive control), if any, in each subject. These sequences are systematically varied so that different subsets of patients receive each of the possible sequences of treatment.

B. The Presence of Other Diseases and Risk Factors

Known and unknown diseases and risk factors (including lifestyles of subjects) may influence the results of a clinical study. For example, some diseases alter the pharmacokinetics of drugs (see Chapters 3 through 5). Other drugs and some foods alter the pharmacokinetics of many drugs. Concentrations of blood or tissue components being monitored as a measure of the effect of the new agent may be influenced by other diseases or other drugs. Attempts to avoid this hazard usually involve the crossover technique (when feasible) and proper selection and assignment of patients to each of the study groups. This requires obtaining accurate diagnostic tests and medical and pharmacologic histories (including use of recreational drugs, over-the-counter drugs, and "supplements") and the use of statistically valid methods of randomization in assigning subjects to particular study groups. There is growing interest in analyzing genetic variations as part of the trial that may influence whether a person responds to a particular drug. It has been shown that age, gender, and pregnancy influence the pharmacokinetics of some drugs, but these factors have not been adequately studied because of legal restrictions and reluctance to expose these populations to unknown risks.

C. Subject and Observer Bias and Other Factors

Most patients tend to respond in a positive way to any therapeutic intervention by interested, caring, and enthusiastic medical personnel. The manifestation of this phenomenon in the subject is the **placebo response** (Latin, "I shall please") and may involve objective physiologic and biochemical changes as well as changes in subjective complaints associated with the disease. The placebo response is usually quantitated by administration of an inert material with exactly the same physical appearance, odor, consistency, etc, as the active dosage form. The magnitude of the response varies considerably from patient to patient and may also be influenced by the duration of the study. In some conditions, a positive response may be noted in as many as 30–40% of subjects given placebo. Placebo adverse effects and "toxicity" also occur but usually involve subjective effects: stomach upset, insomnia, sedation, and so on.

Subject bias effects can be quantitated—and minimized relative to the response measured during active therapy—by the **single-blind** design. This involves use of a placebo as described above, administered to the same subjects in a crossover design, if possible, or to a separate control group of well-matched subjects.

Observer bias can be taken into account by disguising the identity of the medication being used—placebo or active form—from both the subjects and the personnel evaluating the subjects' responses (**double-blind** design). In this design, a third party holds the code identifying each medication packet, and the code is not broken until all the clinical data have been collected.

Drug effects seen in clinical trials are obviously affected by the patient taking the drugs at the dose and frequency prescribed. In a recent phase 2 study, one-third of the patients who said they were taking the drug were found by blood analysis to have not taken the drug. Confirmation of **compliance** with protocols (also known as **adherence**) is a necessary element to consider.

The various types of studies and the conclusions that may be drawn from them are described in the accompanying text box. (See Box: Drug Studies—The Types of Evidence.)

Drug Studies—The Types of Evidence*

As described in this chapter, drugs are studied in a variety of ways, from 30-minute test tube experiments with isolated enzymes and receptors to decades-long observations of populations of patients. The conclusions that can be drawn from such different types of studies can be summarized as follows.

Basic research is designed to answer specific, usually single, questions under tightly controlled laboratory conditions, eg, does drug *x* inhibit enzyme *y*? The basic question may then be extended, eg, if drug *x* inhibits enzyme *y*, what is the concentration-response relationship? Such experiments are usually reproducible and often lead to reliable insights into the mechanism of the drug's action.

First-in-human studies include phase 1–3 trials. Once a drug receives FDA approval for use in humans, *case reports* and *case series* consist of observations by clinicians of the effects of drug (or other) treatments in one or more patients. These results often reveal unpredictable benefits and toxicities but do not generally test a prespecified hypothesis and cannot prove cause and effect. *Analytic* epidemiologic studies consist of observations designed to test a specified hypothesis, eg, that thiazolidinedione antidiabetic drugs are associated with adverse cardiovascular events. *Cohort* epidemiologic studies utilize populations of patients that have (exposed group) and have not (control group) been exposed to the agents under study and ask whether the exposed groups show a higher or lower incidence of the effect. *Case-control* epidemiologic studies utilize populations of patients that have displayed the end point under study and ask whether they have been exposed or not exposed to the drugs in question. Such epidemiologic studies add weight to conjectures but cannot control all confounding variables and therefore cannot conclusively prove cause and effect.

Meta-analyses utilize rigorous evaluation and grouping of similar studies to increase the number of subjects studied and hence the statistical power of results obtained in multiple published studies. While the numbers may be dramatically increased by meta-analysis, the individual studies still suffer from their varying methods and end points, and a meta-analysis cannot prove cause and effect.

Large randomized controlled trials (**RCT**s) are designed to answer specific questions about the effects of medications on clinical end points or important surrogate end points, using large enough samples of patients and allocating them to control and experimental treatments using rigorous randomization methods. Randomization is the best method for distributing all foreseen confounding factors, as well as unknown confounders, equally between the experimental and control groups. When properly carried out, such studies are rarely invalidated and are considered the gold standard in evaluating drugs.

A critical factor in evaluating the data regarding a new drug is *access to all the data*. Unfortunately, many large studies are never published because the results are negative, ie, the new drug is *not* better than the standard therapy. This *missing data* phenomenon falsely exaggerates the benefits of new drugs because negative results are hidden.

*We thank Ralph Gonzales, MD, for helpful comments.

The Food & Drug Administration

The FDA is the administrative body that oversees the drug evaluation process in the USA and grants approval for marketing of new drug products. To receive FDA approval for marketing, the originating institution or company (almost always the latter) must submit evidence of safety and effectiveness. Outside the USA, the regulatory and drug approval process is generally similar to that in the USA.

As its name suggests, the FDA is also responsible for certain aspects of food safety, a role it shares with the US Department of Agriculture (USDA). Shared responsibility results in complications when questions arise regarding the use of drugs, eg, antibiotics, in food animals. A different type of problem arises when so-called food supplements are found to contain active drugs, eg, sildenafil analogs in "energy food" supplements.

The FDA's authority to regulate drugs derives from specific legislation (Table 1–6). If a drug has not been shown through adequately controlled testing to be "safe and effective" for a specific use, it cannot be marketed in interstate commerce for this use.*

*Although the FDA does not directly control drug commerce within states, a variety of state and federal laws control interstate production and marketing of drugs.

TABLE 1–6 Some major legislation pertaining to drugs in the USA.

Law	Purpose and Effect
Pure Food and Drug Act of 1906	Prohibited mislabeling and adulteration of drugs.
Opium Exclusion Act of 1909	Prohibited importation of opium.
Amendment (1912) to the Pure Food and Drug Act	Prohibited false or fraudulent advertising claims.
Harrison Narcotic Act of 1914	Established regulations for use of opium, opiates, and cocaine (marijuana added in 1937).
Food, Drug, and Cosmetic Act of 1938	Required that new drugs be safe as well as pure (but did not require proof of efficacy). Enforcement by the FDA.
Durham-Humphrey Act of 1952	Vested in the FDA the power to determine which products could be sold without prescription.
Kefauver-Harris Amendments (1962) to the Food, Drug, and Cosmetic Act	Required proof of efficacy as well as safety for new drugs and for drugs released since 1938; established guidelines for reporting of information about adverse reactions, clinical testing, and advertising of new drugs.
Comprehensive Drug Abuse Prevention and Control Act (1970)	Outlined strict controls in the manufacture, distribution, and prescribing of habit-forming drugs; established drug schedules and programs to prevent and treat drug addiction.
Orphan Drug Amendment of 1983	Provided incentives for development of drugs that treat diseases with fewer than 200,000 patients in the USA.
Drug Price Competition and Patent Restoration Act of 1984	Abbreviated new drug applications for generic drugs. Required bioequivalence data. Patent life extended by amount of time drug delayed by FDA review process. Cannot exceed 5 extra years or extend to more than 14 years post-NDA approval.
Prescription Drug User Fee Act (1992, reauthorized 2007, 2012)	Manufacturers pay user fees for certain new drug applications. "Breakthrough" products may receive special category approval after expanded phase 1 trials (2012).
Dietary Supplement Health and Education Act (1994)	Established standards with respect to dietary supplements but prohibited full FDA review of supplements and botanicals as drugs. Required the establishment of specific ingredient and nutrition information labeling that defines dietary supplements and classifies them as part of the food supply but allows unregulated advertising.
Bioterrorism Act of 2002	Enhanced controls on dangerous biologic agents and toxins. Seeks to protect safety of food, water, and drug supply.
Food and Drug Administration Amendments Act of 2007	Granted the FDA greater authority over drug marketing, labeling, and direct-to-consumer advertising; required post-approval studies, established active surveillance systems, made clinical trial operations and results more visible to the public.
Biologics Price Competition and Innovation Act of 2009	Authorized the FDA to establish a program of abbreviated pathways for approval of "biosimilar" biologics (generic versions of monoclonal antibodies, etc).
FDA Safety and Innovation Act of 2012	Renewed FDA authorization for accelerated approval of urgently needed drugs; established new accelerated process, "breakthrough therapy," in addition to "priority review," "accelerated approval," and "fast-track" procedures.
Drug Quality and Security Act of 2013	Granted the FDA more authority to regulate and monitor the manufacturing of compounded drugs.

Unfortunately, "safe" can mean different things to the patient, the physician, and society. Complete absence of risk is impossible to demonstrate, but this fact may not be understood by members of the public, who frequently assume that any medication sold with the approval of the FDA should be free of serious "side effects." This confusion is a major factor in litigation and dissatisfaction with aspects of drugs and medical care.

The history of drug regulation in the USA (see Table 1–6) reflects several health events that precipitated major shifts in public opinion. For example, the Federal Food, Drug, and Cosmetic Act of 1938 was largely a reaction to deaths associated with the use of a preparation of sulfanilamide marketed before it and its vehicle were adequately tested. Similarly, the Kefauver-Harris Amendments of 1962 were, in part, the result of a teratogenic drug disaster involving thalidomide. This agent was introduced in Europe in 1957–1958 and was marketed as a "nontoxic" hypnotic and promoted as being especially useful as a sleep aid during pregnancy. In 1961, reports were published suggesting that thalidomide was responsible for a dramatic increase in the incidence of a rare birth defect called phocomelia, a condition involving shortening or complete absence of the arms and legs. Epidemiologic studies provided strong evidence for the association of this defect with thalidomide use by women during the first trimester of pregnancy, and the drug was withdrawn from sale worldwide. An estimated 10,000 children were born with birth defects because of maternal exposure to this one agent. The tragedy led to the requirement for more extensive testing of new drugs for teratogenic effects and stimulated passage of the Kefauver-Harris Amendments of 1962, even though the drug was not then approved for use in the USA. Despite its disastrous fetal toxicity and effects in pregnancy, thalidomide is a relatively safe drug for humans other than the fetus. Even the most serious risk of toxicities may be avoided or managed if understood, and despite its toxicity, thalidomide is now approved by the FDA for limited use as a potent immunoregulatory agent and to treat certain forms of leprosy.

Clinical Trials: The IND & NDA

Once a new drug is judged ready to be studied in humans, a Notice of Claimed Investigational Exemption for a New Drug (IND) must be filed with the FDA (see Figure 1–6). The IND includes (1) information on the composition and source of the drug, (2) chemical and manufacturing information, (3) all data from animal studies, (4) proposed plans for clinical trials, (5) the names and credentials of physicians who will conduct the clinical trials, and (6) a compilation of the key preclinical data relevant to study of the drug in humans that have been made available to investigators and their institutional review boards.

It often requires 4–6 years of clinical testing to accumulate and analyze all required data. Testing in humans is begun only after sufficient acute and subacute animal toxicity studies have been completed. Chronic safety testing in animals, including carcinogenicity studies, is usually done concurrently with clinical trials. In each phase of the clinical trials, volunteers or patients must be informed of the investigational status of the drug as well as the possible risks and must be allowed to decline or to consent to participate and receive the drug. In addition to the approval of the sponsoring organization and the FDA, an interdisciplinary institutional review board (IRB) at each facility where the clinical drug trial will be conducted must review and approve the scientific and ethical plans for testing in humans.

In **phase 1,** the effects of the drug as a function of dosage are established in a small number (20–100) of healthy volunteers. If the drug is expected to have significant toxicity, as may be the case in cancer and AIDS therapy, volunteer patients with the disease participate in phase 1 rather than normal volunteers. Phase 1 trials are done to determine the probable limits of the safe clinical dosage range. These trials may be nonblind or "open"; that is, both the investigators and the subjects know what is being given. Alternatively, they may be "blinded" and placebo controlled. Many predictable toxicities are detected in this phase. Pharmacokinetic measurements of absorption, half-life, and metabolism are often done. Phase 1 studies are usually performed in research centers by specially trained clinical pharmacologists.

In **phase 2,** the drug is studied in patients with the target disease to determine its efficacy ("proof of concept" studies), and the doses to be used in any follow-on trials. A modest number of patients (100–200) are studied in detail. A single-blind design may be used, with an inert placebo medication and an established active drug (positive control) in addition to the investigational agent. Phase 2 trials are usually done in special clinical centers (eg, university hospitals). A broader range of toxicities may be detected in this phase. Phase 2 trials have the highest rate of drug failures, and only 25% of innovative drugs move on to phase 3.

In **phase 3,** the drug is evaluated in much larger numbers—usually thousands—of patients with the target disease to further establish and confirm safety and efficacy. Using information gathered in phases 1 and 2, phase 3 trials are designed to minimize errors caused by placebo effects, variable course of the disease, etc. Therefore, double-blind and crossover techniques are often used. Phase 3 trials are usually performed in settings similar to those anticipated for the ultimate use of the drug. Phase 3 studies can be difficult to design and execute and are usually expensive because of the large numbers of patients involved and the masses of data that must be collected and analyzed. The drug is formulated as intended for the market. The investigators are usually specialists in the disease being treated. Certain toxic effects, especially those caused by immunologic processes, may first become apparent in phase 3.

If phase 3 results meet expectations, application is made for permission to market the new agent. Marketing approval requires submission of a New Drug Application (NDA)—or for biologicals, a Biological License Application (BLA)—to the FDA. The application contains, often in hundreds of volumes, full reports of all preclinical and clinical data pertaining to the drug under review. The number of subjects studied in support of new drug applications has been increasing and currently averages more than 5000 patients for new drugs of novel structure (new molecular entities). The duration of the FDA review leading to approval (or denial) of the new drug application may vary from months to years. If problems arise, eg, unexpected but possibly serious toxicities, additional studies may be required and the review process may extend to several additional years.

Many phase 2 and phase 3 studies attempt to measure a new drug's "noninferiority" to the placebo or a standard treatment. Interpretation of the results may be difficult because of unexpected confounding variables, loss of subjects from some groups, or realization that results differ markedly between certain subgroups within the active treatment (new drug) group. Older statistical methods for evaluating drug trials often fail to provide definitive answers when these problems arise. Therefore, new "adaptive" statistical methods are under development that allow changes in the study design when interim data evaluation indicates the need. Preliminary results with such methods suggest that they may allow decisions regarding superiority as well as noninferiority, shortening of trial duration, discovery of new therapeutic benefits, and more reliable conclusions regarding the results (see Bhatt & Mehta, 2016).

In cases of urgent need (eg, cancer chemotherapy), the process of preclinical and clinical testing and FDA review may be accelerated. For serious diseases, the FDA may permit extensive but controlled marketing of a new drug before phase 3 studies are completed; for life-threatening diseases, it may permit controlled marketing even before phase 2 studies have been completed. "Fast track," "priority approval," and "accelerated approval" are FDA programs that are intended to speed entry of new drugs into the marketplace. In 2012, an additional special category of "breakthrough" products (eg, for cystic fibrosis) was approved for restricted marketing after expanded phase 1 trials (see Table 1–6). Roughly 50% of drugs in phase 3 trials enter early, controlled marketing. Such accelerated approval is usually granted with the requirement that careful monitoring of the effectiveness and toxicity of the drug be carried out and reported to the FDA. Unfortunately, FDA enforcement of this requirement has not always been adequate.

Once approval to market a drug has been obtained, **phase 4** begins. This constitutes monitoring the safety of the new drug under actual conditions of use in large numbers of patients. The importance of careful and complete reporting of toxicity by physicians after marketing begins can be appreciated by noting that many important drug-induced effects have an incidence of 1 in 10,000 or less and that some adverse effects may become apparent only after chronic dosing. The sample size required to disclose drug-induced events or toxicities is very large for such rare events. For example, several hundred thousand patients may have to be exposed before the first case is observed of a toxicity that occurs with an average incidence of 1 in 10,000. Therefore, low-incidence drug effects are not generally detected before phase 4 no matter how carefully phase 1, 2, and 3 studies are executed. Phase 4 has no fixed duration. As with monitoring of drugs granted accelerated approval, phase 4 monitoring has often been lax.

The time from the filing of a patent application (which usually precedes clinical trials) to approval for marketing of a new drug may be 5 years or considerably longer. Since the lifetime of a patent is 20 years in the USA, the owner of the patent (usually a pharmaceutical company) has exclusive rights for marketing the product for only a limited time after approval of the new drug application. Because the FDA review process itself can be lengthy (300–500 days for evaluation of an NDA), the time consumed by the review is sometimes added to the patent life. However, the extension (up to 5 years) cannot increase the total life of the patent to more than 14 years after approval of a new drug application. The Patient Protection and Affordable Care Act of 2010 provides for 12 years of patent protection for new drugs. After expiration of the patent, any company may produce the drug, file an abbreviated new drug application (ANDA), demonstrate required equivalence, and, with FDA approval, market the drug as a **generic** product without paying license fees to the original patent owner. Currently, more than half of prescriptions in the USA are for generic drugs. Even biotechnology-based drugs such as antibodies and other proteins are now qualifying for generic ("biosimilar") designation, and this has fueled regulatory concerns. More information on drug patents is available at the FDA website at http://www.fda.gov/Drugs/DevelopmentApprovalProcess/ucm079031.htm.

A **trademark** is a drug's proprietary trade name and is usually registered; this registered name may be legally protected as long as it is used. A generically equivalent product, unless specially licensed, cannot be sold under the trademark name and is often designated by the official generic name. Generic prescribing is described in Chapter 66.

Conflicts of Interest

Several factors in the development and marketing of drugs result in conflicts of interest. Use of pharmaceutical industry funding to support FDA approval processes raises the possibility of conflicts of interest within the FDA. Supporters of this practice point out that chronic FDA underfunding by the government allows for few alternatives. Another important source of conflicts of interest is the dependence of the FDA on outside panels of experts who are recruited from the scientific and clinical community to advise the government agency on questions regarding drug approval or withdrawal. Such experts are often recipients of grants from the companies producing the drugs in question. The need for favorable data in the new drug application leads to phase 2 and 3 trials in which the new agent is compared only to placebo, not to older, effective drugs. As a result, data regarding the efficacy and toxicity of the new drug *relative to a known effective agent* may not be available when the new drug is first marketed.

Manufacturers promoting a new agent may pay physicians to use it in preference to older drugs with which they are more familiar. Manufacturers sponsor small and often poorly designed clinical studies after marketing approval and aid in the publication of favorable results but may retard publication of unfavorable results. The need for physicians to meet continuing medical education (CME) requirements in order to maintain their licenses encourages manufacturers to sponsor conferences and courses, often in highly attractive vacation sites, and new drugs are often featured in such courses. The common practice of distributing free samples of new drugs to practicing physicians has both positive and negative effects. The samples allow physicians to try out new drugs without incurring any cost to the patient. On the other hand, new drugs are usually much more expensive than older agents, and when the free samples run out, the patient (or insurance carrier) may be forced to pay much more for treatment than if the older, cheaper, and possibly equally effective drug were used. Finally, when the patent for a drug is nearing expiration, the patent-holding manufacturer may try to extend its exclusive marketing status by paying generic manufacturers to *not* introduce a generic version ("pay to delay").

Adverse Drug Reactions

An adverse drug event (ADE) or reaction to a drug (ADR) is a harmful or unintended response. Adverse drug reactions are claimed to be the fourth leading cause of death, higher than pulmonary disease, AIDS, accidents, and automobile deaths. The FDA has further estimated that 300,000 preventable adverse events occur annually in hospitals, many as a result of confusing medical information or lack of information (eg, regarding drug incompatibilities). Adverse reactions occurring only in certain susceptible patients include intolerance, idiosyncrasy (frequently genetic in origin), and allergy (usually immunologically mediated). During IND studies and clinical trials before FDA approval, all adverse events (serious, life-threatening, disabling, reasonably drug related, or unexpected) must be reported. After FDA approval to market a drug, surveillance, evaluation, and reporting must continue for any adverse events that are related to use of the drug, including overdose, accident, failure of expected action, events occurring from drug withdrawal, and unexpected events not listed in labeling. Events that are both serious and unexpected must be reported to the FDA within 15 days. The ability to predict and avoid adverse drug reactions and optimize a drug's therapeutic index is an increasing focus of pharmacogenetic and personalized (also called "precision") medicine. It has been suggested that greater use of electronic health records will reduce some of these risks (see Chapter 66). This hope has not yet been realized.

Orphan Drugs & Treatment of Rare Diseases

Drugs for rare diseases—so-called orphan drugs—can be difficult to research, develop, and market. Proof of drug safety and efficacy in small populations must be established, but doing so is a complex process. Furthermore, because basic research in the pathophysiology and mechanisms of rare diseases receives relatively little attention or funding in both academic and industrial settings, recognized rational targets for drug action may be few. In addition, the cost of developing a drug can greatly influence priorities when the target population is relatively small. Funding for development of drugs for rare diseases or ignored diseases that do not receive priority attention from the traditional industry has received increasing support via philanthropy or similar funding from not-for-profit foundations such as the Cystic Fibrosis Foundation, the Michael J. Fox Foundation for Parkinson's Research, the Huntington's Disease Society of America, and the Gates Foundation.

The Orphan Drug Amendment of 1983 provides incentives for the development of drugs for treatment of a rare disease or condition defined as "any disease or condition which (a) affects less than 200,000 persons in the USA or (b) affects more than 200,000 persons in the USA but for which there is no reasonable expectation that the cost of developing and making available in the USA a drug for such disease or condition will be recovered from sales in the USA of such drug." Since 1983, the FDA has approved for marketing more than 300 orphan drugs to treat more than 82 rare diseases.

■ SOURCES OF INFORMATION

Students who wish to review the field of pharmacology in preparation for an examination are referred to *Pharmacology: Examination and Board Review,* by Katzung, Kruidering-Hall, Lalchandani Tuan, Vanderah, and Trevor (McGraw Hill, 2021). This book provides approximately 1000 questions and explanations in USMLE format. A short study guide is *USMLE Road Map: Pharmacology,* by Katzung and Trevor (McGraw Hill, 2006). *Road Map* contains numerous tables, figures, mnemonics, and USMLE-type clinical vignettes.

The references at the end of each chapter in this book were selected to provide reviews or classic publications of information specific to those chapters. More detailed questions relating to basic or clinical research are best answered by referring to the journals covering general pharmacology and clinical specialties. For the student and the physician, three periodicals can be recommended as especially useful sources of current information about drugs: *The New England Journal of Medicine*, which publishes much original drug-related clinical research as well as frequent reviews of topics in pharmacology; *The Medical Letter on Drugs and Therapeutics,* which publishes brief critical reviews of new and old therapies; and *Prescriber's Letter*, a monthly comparison of new and older drug therapies with much useful advice. On the Internet/World Wide Web, two sources can be particularly recommended: the Cochrane Collaboration and the FDA site (see reference list below).

Other sources of information pertinent to the United States should be mentioned as well. The "package insert" is a summary of information that the manufacturer is required to place in the prescription sales package; *Physicians' Desk Reference (PDR)* is a compendium of package inserts published annually with supplements twice a year. It is sold in bookstores and distributed to licensed physicians. The package insert consists of a brief description of the pharmacology of the product. This brochure contains much practical information, but also lists every toxic effect ever reported, no matter how rare, thus shifting responsibility for adverse drug reactions from the manufacturer to the prescriber. A black box warning, if included, is of medicolegal importance, because it indicates a potentially lethal adverse effect. *UpToDate.com* is a large subscription website containing detailed descriptions of current standards of care, including drug therapy, for a wide variety of clinical conditions. *Micromedex* and *Lexi-Comp* are extensive subscription websites. They provide downloads for personal digital assistant devices, online drug dosage and interaction information, and toxicologic information. A useful and objective quarterly handbook that presents information on drug toxicity and interactions is *Drug Interactions: Analysis and Management.* Finally, the FDA maintains an Internet website that carries news regarding recent drug approvals, withdrawals, warnings, etc. It can be accessed at http://www.fda.gov. The MedWatch drug safety program is a free e-mail notification service that provides news of FDA drug warnings and withdrawals. Subscriptions may be obtained at https://www.fda.gov/safety/medwatch-fda-safety-information-and-adverse-event-reporting-program.

REFERENCES

Alexander SPH et al: The Concise Guide to PHARMACOLOGY 2017/18: Overview. Br J Pharmacol 2017;174:S1.

Avorn J: Debate about funding comparative effectiveness research. N Engl J Med 2009;360:1927.

Avorn J: *Powerful Medicines: The Benefits and Risks and Costs of Prescription Drugs.* Alfred A. Knopf, 2004.

Bauchner H, Fontanarosa PB: Restoring confidence in the pharmaceutical industry. JAMA 2013;309:607.

Bhatt DL, Mehta C: Clinical trials series: Adaptive designs for clinical trials. N Engl J Med 2016;375:65.

Boutron I et al: Reporting and interpretation of randomized controlled trials with statistically nonsignificant results for primary outcomes. JAMA 2010; 303:2058.

Brown WA: The placebo effect. Sci Am 1998;1:91.

Cochrane Collaboration website. www.thecochranelibrary.com.

Darrow JJ, Avorn J, Kesselheim AS: FDA approval and regulation of pharmaceuticals, 1983-2018. JAMA. 2020;323:164.

Downing NS et al: Regulatory review of novel therapeutics—Comparison of three regulatory agencies. N Engl J Med 2012;366:2284.

Drug Interactions: Analysis and Management (quarterly). Wolters Kluwer Publications.

Emanuel EJ, Menikoff J: Reforming the regulations governing research with human subjects. N Engl J Med 2011;365:1145.

FDA accelerated approval website. https://www.fda.gov/patients/fast-track-breakthrough-therapy-accelerated-approval-priority-review/accelerated-approval.

FDA website. http://www.fda.gov.

Goldacre B: *Bad Pharma.* Faber & Faber, 2012.

Hennekens CMH, DeMets D: Statistical association and causation. Contributions of different types of evidence. JAMA 2011;305:1134.

Huang S-M, Temple R: Is this the drug or dose for you? Impact and consideration of ethnic factors in global drug development, regulatory review, and clinical practice. Clin Pharmacol Ther 2008;84:287.

Katzung BG et al: *Katzung & Trevor's Pharmacology: Examination & Board Review,* 13th ed. McGraw Hill, 2021.

Kesselheim AS et al: Whistle-blowers' experiences in fraud litigation against pharmaceutical companies. N Engl J Med 2010;362:1832.

Koslowski S et al: Developing the nation's biosimilar program. N Engl J Med 2011;365:385.

Landry Y, Gies J-P: Drugs and their molecular targets: An updated overview. Fund & Clin Pharmacol 2008;22:1.

The Medical Letter on Drugs and Therapeutics. The Medical Letter, Inc.

Ng R: *Drugs from Discovery to Approval*. Wiley-Blackwell, 2008.

Pharmaceutical Research and Manufacturers of America website. http://www.phrma.org.

Pharmacology: Examination & Board Review, 12th ed. McGraw Hill Education, 2019.

Prescriber's Letter. Stockton, California: prescribersletter.com.

Rockey SJ, Collins FS: Managing financial conflict of interest in biomedical research. JAMA 2010;303:2400.

Scheindlin S: Demystifying the new drug application. Mol Interventions 2004;4:188.

Sistare FD, DeGeorge JJ: Preclinical predictors of clinical safety: Opportunities for improvement. Clin Pharmacol Ther 2007;82(2):210.

Stevens AJ et al: The role of public sector research in the discovery of drugs and vaccines. N Engl J Med 2011;364:535.

Top 200 Drugs of 2019. https://clincalc.com/DrugStats/Top200Drugs.aspx

USMLE Road Map: Pharmacology. McGraw Hill Education, 2006.

World Medical Association: World Medical Association Declaration of Helsinki. Ethical principles for medical research involving human subjects. JAMA 2013;310:2191.

Zarin DA et al: Characteristics of clinical trials registered in ClinicalTrials.gov, 2007-2010. JAMA 2012;307:1838.

CASE STUDY ANSWER

Aspirin overdose commonly causes a mixed respiratory alkalosis and metabolic acidosis. Because aspirin is a weak acid, serum acidosis favors entry of the drug into tissues (increasing toxicity), and urinary acidosis favors reabsorption of excreted drug back into the blood (prolonging the effects of the overdose). Sodium bicarbonate, a weak base, is an important component of the management of aspirin overdose. It causes alkalosis, reducing entry into tissues, and increases the pH of the urine, enhancing renal clearance of the drug. See the discussion of the ionization of weak acids and weak bases in the text.

CHAPTER

2

Drug Receptors & Pharmacodynamics

Mark von Zastrow, MD, PhD

CASE STUDY

A 51-year-old man presents to the emergency department due to acute difficulty breathing. The patient is afebrile and normotensive but anxious, tachycardic, and markedly tachypneic. Auscultation of the chest reveals diffuse wheezes. The clinician provisionally makes the diagnosis of bronchial asthma and administers epinephrine by intramuscular injection, improving the patient's breathing over several minutes. A normal chest x-ray and electrocardiogram are subsequently obtained, and the medical history is remarkable only for mild hypertension that is being treated with propranolol. The clinician instructs the patient to discontinue use of propranolol and changes the patient's antihypertensive medication to verapamil. Why is the clinician correct to discontinue propranolol? Why is verapamil likely to be a more suitable choice for managing hypertension in this patient? Are there alternative pharmacotherapies that the clinician should also consider?

Therapeutic and toxic effects of drugs result from their interactions with molecules in the patient. Most drugs act by associating with specific macromolecules in ways that alter the macromolecules' biochemical or biophysical activities. This idea, more than a century old, is embodied in the term **receptor:** the component of a cell or organism that interacts with a drug and initiates the chain of events leading to the drug's observed effects.

Receptors have become the central focus of investigation of drug effects and their mechanisms of action (pharmacodynamics). The receptor concept, extended to endocrinology, immunology, and molecular biology, has proved essential for explaining many aspects of biologic regulation. Many drug receptors have been isolated and characterized in detail, thus opening the way to precise understanding of the molecular basis of drug action.

The receptor concept has important practical consequences for the development of drugs and for arriving at therapeutic decisions in clinical practice. These consequences form the basis for understanding the actions and clinical uses of drugs described in almost every chapter of this book. They may be briefly summarized as follows:

1. **Receptors largely determine the quantitative relations between dose or concentration of drug and pharmacologic effects.** The receptor's affinity for binding a drug determines the concentration of drug required to form a significant number of drug-receptor complexes, and the total number of receptors may limit the maximal effect a drug may produce.
2. **Receptors are responsible for selectivity of drug action.** The molecular size, shape, and electrical charge of a drug determine whether—and with what affinity—it will bind to a particular receptor among the vast array of chemically different binding sites available in a cell, tissue, or patient. Accordingly, changes in the chemical structure of a drug can dramatically increase or decrease a new drug's affinities for different classes of receptors, with resulting alterations in therapeutic and toxic effects.
3. **Receptors mediate the actions of pharmacologic agonists and antagonists.** Some drugs and many natural ligands, such as hormones and neurotransmitters, regulate the function of receptor macromolecules as **agonists;** this means that they activate the receptor to signal as a direct result of binding to it. Some agonists activate a single kind of receptor to produce all their biologic functions, whereas others selectively promote one receptor function more than another.

Other drugs act as pharmacologic **antagonists;** that is, they bind to receptors but do not activate generation of a signal; consequently, they interfere with the ability of an agonist to activate the receptor. Some of the most useful drugs in clinical medicine are pharmacologic antagonists. Still other drugs bind to a different site on the receptor than that bound by endogenous ligands; such drugs can produce useful and quite different clinical effects by acting as so-called **allosteric modulators** of the receptor.

MACROMOLECULAR NATURE OF DRUG RECEPTORS

Most receptors for clinically relevant drugs, and nearly all of those discussed in this chapter, are proteins. Traditionally, drug binding was used to identify or purify receptor proteins from tissue extracts; consequently, receptors were discovered after the drugs that bind to them. Advances in molecular biology and genome sequencing made it possible to identify receptors by predicted structural homology to other (previously known) receptors. This effort revealed that many known drugs bind to a larger diversity of receptors than previously anticipated and motivated efforts to develop increasingly selective drugs. It also identified **orphan receptors,** so-called because their natural ligands are presently unknown; these may prove to be useful targets for future drug development.

The best-characterized drug receptors are **regulatory proteins** that mediate the actions of endogenous chemical signals such as neurotransmitters, autacoids, and hormones. This class of receptors mediates the effects of many of the most useful therapeutic agents. The molecular structures and biochemical mechanisms of these regulatory receptors are described in a later section entitled Signaling Mechanisms & Drug Action.

Other classes of proteins have been clearly identified as drug receptors. **Enzymes** may be inhibited (or, less commonly, activated) by binding a drug. Examples include dihydrofolate reductase, the receptor for the antineoplastic drug methotrexate; 3-hydroxy-3-methylglutaryl–coenzyme A (HMG-CoA) reductase, the receptor for statins; and various protein and lipid kinases. **Transport proteins** can be useful drug targets. Examples include Na^+/K^+-ATPase, the membrane receptor for cardioactive digitalis glycosides; norepinephrine and serotonin transporter proteins that are membrane receptors for antidepressant drugs; and dopamine transporters that are membrane receptors for cocaine and a number of other psychostimulants. **Structural proteins** are also important drug targets, such as tubulin, the receptor for the anti-inflammatory agent colchicine.

This chapter deals with three aspects of drug receptor function, presented in increasing order of complexity: (1) receptors as determinants of the quantitative relation between the concentration of a drug and the pharmacologic response, (2) receptors as regulatory proteins and components of chemical signaling mechanisms that provide targets for important drugs, and (3) receptors as key determinants of the therapeutic and toxic effects of drugs in patients.

RELATION BETWEEN DRUG CONCENTRATION & RESPONSE

The relation between dose of a drug and the clinically observed response may be complex. In carefully controlled in vitro systems, however, the relation between concentration of a drug and its effect is often simple and can be described with mathematical precision. It is important to understand this idealized relation in some detail because it underlies the more complex relations between dose and effect that occur when drugs are given to patients.

Concentration-Effect Curves & Receptor Binding of Agonists

Even in intact animals or patients, responses to low doses of a drug usually increase in direct proportion to dose. As doses increase, however, the response increment diminishes; finally, doses may be reached at which no further increase in response can be achieved. This relation between drug concentration and effect is traditionally described by a hyperbolic curve (Figure 2–1A) according to the following equation:

$$E = \frac{E_{max} \times C}{C + EC_{50}}$$

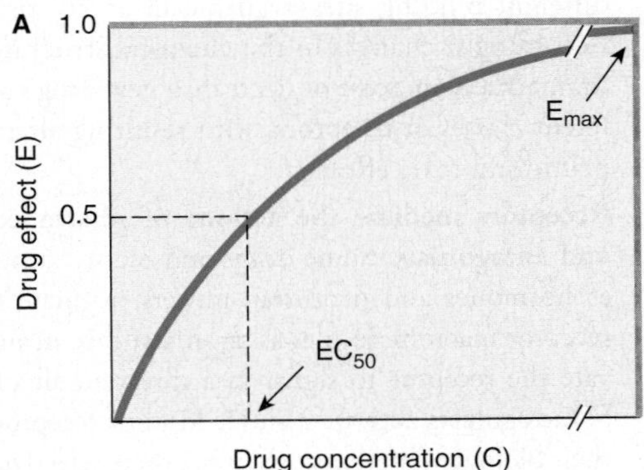

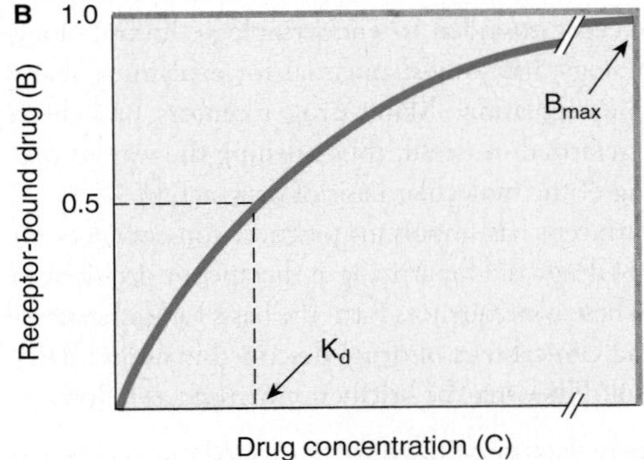

FIGURE 2–1 Relations between drug concentration and drug effect (**A**) or receptor-bound drug (**B**). The drug concentrations at which effect or receptor occupancy is half-maximal are denoted by EC_{50} and K_d, respectively.

where E is the effect observed at concentration C, E_{max} is the maximal response that can be produced by the drug, and EC_{50} is the concentration of drug that produces 50% of maximal effect.

This hyperbolic relation resembles the mass action law that describes the association between two molecules of a given affinity. This resemblance suggests that drug agonists act by binding to ("occupying") a distinct class of biologic molecules with a characteristic affinity for the drug. Radioactive receptor ligands have been used to confirm this occupancy assumption in many drug-receptor systems. In these systems, drug bound to receptors (B) relates to the concentration of free (unbound) drug (C) as depicted in Figure 2–1B and as described by an analogous equation:

$$B = \frac{B_{max} \times C}{C + K_d}$$

in which B_{max} indicates the total concentration of receptor sites (ie, sites bound to the drug at infinitely high concentrations of free drug) and K_d (the equilibrium dissociation constant) represents the concentration of free drug at which half-maximal binding is observed. This constant characterizes the receptor's affinity for binding the drug in a reciprocal fashion: If the K_d is low, binding affinity is high, and vice versa. The EC_{50} and K_d may be identical but need not be, as discussed below. Dose-response data are often presented as a plot of the drug effect (ordinate) against the *logarithm* of the dose or concentration (abscissa), transforming the hyperbolic curve of Figure 2–1 into a sigmoid curve with a linear midportion (eg, Figure 2–2). This transformation is convenient because it expands the scale of the concentration axis at low concentrations (where the effect is changing rapidly) and compresses it at high concentrations (where the effect is changing slowly), but otherwise has no biologic or pharmacologic significance.

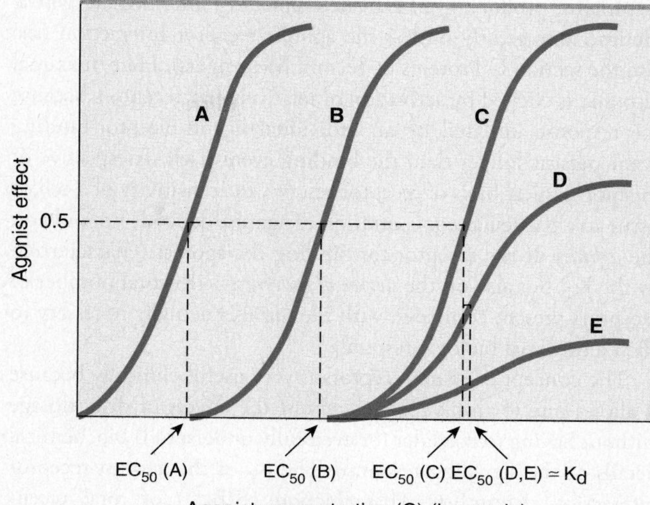

FIGURE 2–2 Logarithmic transformation of the dose axis and experimental demonstration of spare receptors, using different concentrations of an irreversible antagonist. Curve **A** shows agonist response in the absence of antagonist. After treatment with a low concentration of antagonist (curve **B**), the curve is shifted to the right. Maximal responsiveness is preserved, however, because the remaining available receptors are still in excess of the number required. In curve **C**, produced after treatment with a larger concentration of antagonist, the available receptors are no longer "spare"; instead, they are just sufficient to mediate an undiminished maximal response. Still higher concentrations of antagonist (curves **D** and **E**) reduce the number of available receptors to the point that maximal response is diminished. The apparent EC_{50} of the agonist in curves **D** and **E** may approximate the K_d that characterizes the binding affinity of the agonist for the receptor.

Receptor-Effector Coupling & Spare Receptors

When an agonist occupies a receptor, conformational changes occur in the receptor protein that represent the fundamental basis of receptor activation and the first of often many steps required to produce a pharmacologic response. The overall transduction process that links drug occupancy of receptors and pharmacologic response is called **coupling.** The relative efficiency of occupancy-response coupling is determined, in part, at the receptor itself; full agonists tend to shift the conformational equilibrium of receptors more strongly than partial agonists (described in the text that follows). Coupling is also determined by "downstream" biochemical events that transduce receptor occupancy into cellular response. For some receptors, such as ligand-gated ion channels, the relationship between drug occupancy and response can be simple because the ion current produced by a drug is often directly proportional to the number of receptors (ion channels) bound. For other receptors, such as those linked to enzymatic signal transduction cascades, the occupancy-response relationship is often more complex because the biologic response reaches a maximum before full receptor occupancy is achieved.

Many factors can contribute to nonlinear occupancy-response coupling, and often these factors are only partially understood. A useful concept for thinking about this is that of **receptor reserve** or **spare receptors.** Receptors are said to be "spare" for a given pharmacologic response if it is possible to elicit a maximal biologic response at a concentration of agonist that does not result in occupancy of all the available receptors. Experimentally, spare receptors may be demonstrated by using irreversible antagonists to prevent binding of agonist to a proportion of available receptors and showing that high concentrations of agonist can still produce an undiminished maximal response (see Figure 2–2). For example, the same maximal inotropic response of heart muscle to catecholamines can be elicited even when 90% of β adrenoceptors to which they bind are occupied by a quasi-irreversible antagonist. Accordingly, myocardial cells are said to contain a large proportion of spare β adrenoceptors.

What accounts for the phenomenon of spare receptors? In some cases, receptors may be simply *spare in number* relative to the total number of downstream signaling mediators present in the cell, so that a maximal response occurs without occupancy of all receptors. In other cases, "spareness" of receptors appears to be *temporal.* For example, β-adrenoceptor activation by an agonist promotes binding of guanosine triphosphate (GTP) to a trimeric

G protein, producing an activated signaling intermediate whose lifetime may greatly outlast the agonist-receptor interaction (see also the section G Proteins & Second Messengers). Here, maximal response is elicited by activation of relatively few receptors because the response initiated by an individual ligand-receptor-binding event persists longer than the binding event itself. Irrespective of the biochemical basis of receptor reserve, the sensitivity of a cell or tissue to a particular concentration of agonist depends not only on the *affinity* of the receptor for binding the agonist (characterized by the K_d) but also on the *degree of spareness*—the total number of receptors present compared with the number actually necessary to elicit a maximal biologic response.

The concept of spare receptors is very useful clinically because it allows one to think precisely about the effects of drug dosage without having to consider (or even fully understand) biochemical details of the signaling response. The K_d of the agonist-receptor interaction determines what fraction (B/B_{max}) of total receptors will be occupied at a given free concentration (C) of agonist regardless of the receptor concentration:

$$\frac{B}{B_{max}} = \frac{C}{C + K_d}$$

Imagine a responding cell with 100 receptors and 100 effectors. Here the number of effectors does not limit the maximal response, and the receptors are *not* spare in number. Consequently, an agonist that is present at a concentration equal to the K_d will occupy 50% of the receptors, and half of the effectors will be activated, producing a half-maximal response (ie, 50 receptors stimulate 50 effectors). Now imagine that the number of receptors increases tenfold to 1000 receptors but the total number of effectors remains constant. Most of the receptors are now spare in number. As a result, a much lower concentration of agonist suffices to occupy 50 of the 1000 receptors (5% of the receptors), and this same low concentration of agonist elicits a half-maximal response (50 of 100 effectors activated). Thus, it is possible to change the sensitivity of tissues with spare receptors by changing receptor number.

Competitive & Irreversible Antagonists

Receptor antagonists bind to receptors but do not activate them; the primary action of antagonists is to reduce the effects of agonists (other drugs or endogenous regulatory molecules) that normally activate receptors. While antagonists are traditionally thought to have no functional effect in the absence of an agonist, some antagonists exhibit "inverse agonist" activity (see Chapter 1) because they also reduce receptor activity below basal levels observed in the absence of any agonist at all. Antagonist drugs are further divided into two classes depending on whether they act *competitively* or *noncompetitively* relative to an agonist present at the same time.

In the presence of a fixed concentration of agonist, increasing concentrations of a **competitive antagonist** progressively inhibit the agonist response; high antagonist concentrations prevent the response almost completely. Conversely, sufficiently high concentrations of agonist can surmount the effect of a given concentration of the antagonist; that is, the E_{max} for the agonist remains the same for any fixed concentration of antagonist (Figure 2–3A). Because the antagonism is competitive, the presence of antagonist increases the agonist concentration required for a given degree of response, and so the agonist concentration-effect curve is shifted to the right.

The concentration (C′) of an agonist required to produce a given effect in the presence of a fixed concentration ([I]) of competitive antagonist is greater than the agonist concentration (C)

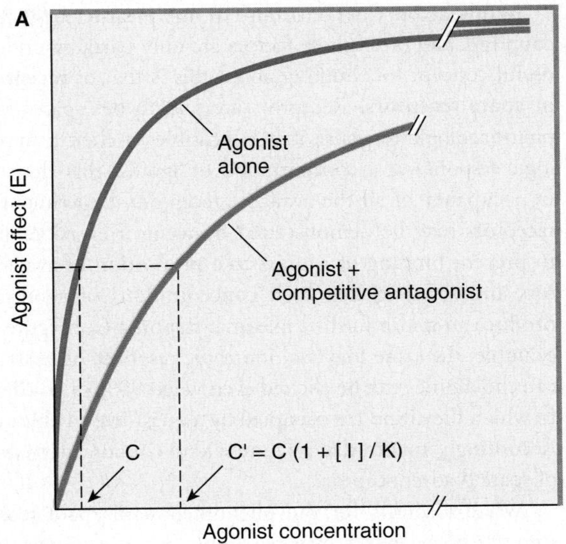

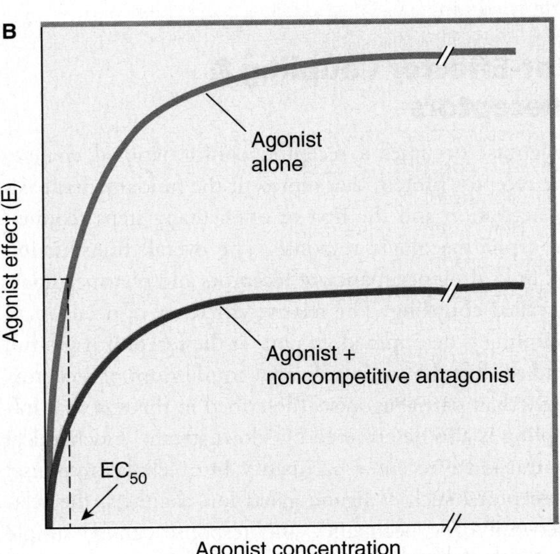

FIGURE 2–3 Changes in agonist concentration-effect curves produced by a competitive antagonist (**A**) or by an irreversible antagonist (**B**). In the presence of a competitive antagonist, higher concentrations of agonist are required to produce a given effect; thus the agonist concentration (C′) required for a given effect in the presence of concentration [I] of an antagonist is shifted to the right, as shown. High agonist concentrations can overcome inhibition by a competitive antagonist. This is not the case with an irreversible (or noncompetitive) antagonist, which reduces the maximal effect the agonist can achieve, although it may not change its EC_{50}.

required to produce the same effect in the absence of the antagonist. The ratio of these two agonist concentrations (called the dose ratio) is related to the dissociation constant (K_i) of the antagonist by the **Schild equation:**

$$\frac{C'}{C} = 1 + \frac{[I]}{K_i}$$

Pharmacologists often use this relation to determine the K_i of a competitive antagonist. Even without knowledge of the relation between agonist occupancy of the receptor and response, the K_i can be determined simply and accurately. As shown in Figure 2–3, concentration-response curves are obtained in the presence and in the absence of a fixed concentration of competitive antagonist; comparison of the agonist concentrations required to produce identical degrees of pharmacologic effect in the two situations reveals the antagonist's K_i. If C′ is twice C, for example, then $[I] = K_i$.

For the clinician, this mathematical relation has two important therapeutic implications:

1. The degree of inhibition produced by a competitive antagonist depends on the concentration of antagonist. The competitive β-adrenoceptor antagonist propranolol provides a useful example. Patients receiving a fixed dose of this drug exhibit a wide range of plasma concentrations, owing to differences among individuals in the clearance of propranolol. As a result, inhibitory effects on physiologic responses to norepinephrine and epinephrine (endogenous adrenergic receptor agonists) may vary widely, and the dose of propranolol must be adjusted accordingly.
2. Clinical response to a competitive antagonist also depends on the concentration of agonist that is competing for binding to receptors. Again, propranolol provides a useful example: When this drug is administered at moderate doses sufficient to block the effect of basal levels of the neurotransmitter norepinephrine, resting heart rate is decreased. However, the increase in the release of norepinephrine and epinephrine that occurs with exercise, postural changes, or emotional stress may suffice to overcome this competitive antagonism. Accordingly, the same dose of propranolol may have little effect under these conditions, thereby altering therapeutic response. Conversely, the same dose of propranolol that is useful for treatment of hypertension in one patient may be excessive and toxic to another, based on differences between the patients in the amount of endogenous norepinephrine and epinephrine that they produce.

The actions of a **noncompetitive antagonist** are different because, once a receptor is bound by such a drug, agonists cannot surmount the inhibitory effect irrespective of their concentration. In many cases, noncompetitive antagonists bind to the receptor in an **irreversible** or nearly irreversible fashion, sometimes by forming a covalent bond with the receptor. After occupancy of some proportion of receptors by such an antagonist, the number of remaining unoccupied receptors may be too low for the agonist (even at high concentrations) to elicit a response comparable to the previous maximal response (Figure 2–3B). If spare receptors are present, however, a lower dose of an irreversible antagonist may leave enough receptors unoccupied to allow achievement of maximum response to agonist, although a higher agonist concentration will be required (Figures 2–2B and 2–2C; see section Receptor-Effector Coupling & Spare Receptors).

Therapeutically, such irreversible antagonists present distinct advantages and disadvantages. Once the irreversible antagonist has occupied the receptor, it need not be present in unbound form to inhibit agonist responses. Consequently, the duration of action of such an irreversible antagonist is relatively independent of its own rate of elimination and more dependent on the rate of turnover of receptor molecules.

Phenoxybenzamine, an irreversible α-adrenoceptor antagonist, is used to control the hypertension caused by catecholamines released from pheochromocytoma, a tumor of the adrenal medulla. If administration of phenoxybenzamine lowers blood pressure, blockade will be maintained even when the tumor episodically releases very large amounts of catecholamine. In this case, the ability to prevent responses to varying and high concentrations of agonist is a therapeutic advantage. If overdose occurs, however, a real problem may arise. If the α-adrenoceptor blockade cannot be overcome, excess effects of the drug must be antagonized "physiologically," ie, by using a pressor agent that does not act via α adrenoceptors.

Antagonists can function noncompetitively in a different way; that is, by binding to a site on the receptor protein separate from the agonist binding site; in this way, the drug can modify receptor activity without blocking agonist binding (see Chapter 1, Figures 1–2C and 1–2D). Although these drugs act noncompetitively, their actions are often reversible. Such drugs are called *negative allosteric modulators* because they act through binding to a different (ie, "allosteric") site on the receptor relative to the classical (ie, "orthosteric") site bound by the endogenous agonist to reduce activity of the receptor. Other allosteric modulators have the opposite effect: they increase receptor activity. Benzodiazepine drugs like diazepam, for example, bind to an allosteric site on ion channels that are physiologically activated by the neurotransmitter γ-aminobutyric acid (GABA). Benzodiazepines are considered *positive allosteric modulators* of GABA receptors because they potentiate (rather than inhibit) the ability of the orthosteric agonist (GABA) to increase channel conductance. A useful feature of this allosteric mechanism is that benzodiazepines have little activating effect on their own. This contributes to making benzodiazepines relatively safe in overdose unless combined with other sedating drugs. The concept of allosteric modulators also applies to proteins that lack any known orthosteric binding site. For example, ivacaftor binds to the **cystic fibrosis transmembrane regulator (CFTR)** ion channel that is mutated in cystic fibrosis. Some mutations that cause disease by rendering this channel hypoactive can be partially rescued by ivacaftor, despite CFTR having no known physiological agonist—and thus no (presently recognized) orthosteric binding site.

Partial Agonists

Based on the maximal pharmacologic response that occurs when all receptors are occupied, agonists can be divided into two classes:

partial agonists produce a lower response, at full receptor occupancy, than do **full agonists**. Partial agonists produce concentration-effect curves that resemble those observed with full agonists in the presence of an antagonist that irreversibly blocks some of the receptor sites (compare Figures 2–2 [curve D] and 2–4B). It is important to emphasize that the failure of partial agonists to produce a maximal response is not due to decreased affinity for binding to receptors. Indeed, a partial agonist's inability to cause a maximal pharmacologic response, even when present at high concentrations that effectively saturate binding to all receptors, is indicated by the fact that partial agonists competitively inhibit the responses produced by full agonists (Figure 2–4). This mixed "agonist-antagonist" property of partial agonists can have both beneficial and deleterious effects in the clinic. For example, buprenorphine, a partial agonist of μ-opioid receptors, is a generally safer analgesic drug than morphine, a more efficacious partial agonist, and much safer than fentanyl which is a full agonist. This is because buprenorphine suppresses breathing upon binding opioid receptors (in ventilatory pacemaker neurons of the brainstem) less strongly than morphine, and much less strongly than fentanyl; breathing stops if these receptors are activated too strongly. On the other hand, buprenorphine is effectively antianalgesic when administered in combination with more efficacious opioid drugs, due to the mixed agonist-antagonist effect. In addition, buprenorphine may precipitate a severe drug withdrawal reaction in opioid-dependent individuals, due to physiologic adaptations of the nervous system that are induced after prolonged or repeated drug exposure and effectively change the "set point" for sensitivity to opioids.

Other Mechanisms of Drug Antagonism

Not all mechanisms of antagonism involve interactions of drugs or endogenous ligands at a single type of receptor, and some types of antagonism do not involve a receptor protein at all. For example, protamine, a protein that is positively charged at physiologic pH, can be used clinically as a drug to counteract the effects of heparin, a nonprotein (glycosaminoglycan) anticoagulant drug that is negatively charged. In this case, one drug acts as a **chemical antagonist** of the other simply by ionic binding that makes the other drug unavailable to interact with proteins involved in blood clotting.

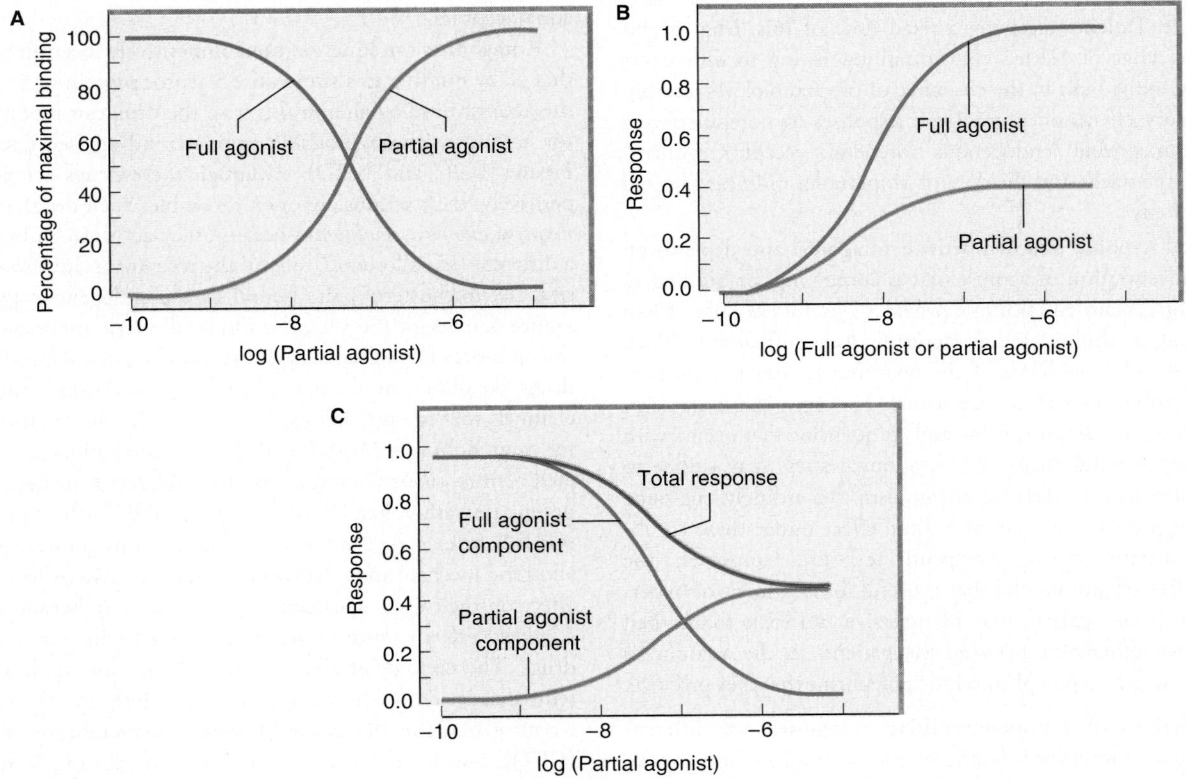

FIGURE 2–4 **A:** The percentage of receptor occupancy resulting from full agonist (present at a single concentration) binding to receptors in the presence of increasing concentrations of a partial agonist. Because the full agonist (blue line) and the partial agonist (green line) compete to bind to the same receptor sites, when occupancy by the partial agonist increases, binding of the full agonist decreases. **B:** When each of the two drugs is used alone and response is measured, occupancy of all the receptors by the partial agonist produces a lower maximal response than does similar occupancy by the full agonist. **C:** Simultaneous treatment with a single concentration of full agonist and increasing concentrations of the partial agonist produces the response patterns shown in the bottom panel. The fractional response caused by a single high concentration of the full agonist decreases as increasing concentrations of the partial agonist compete to bind to the receptor with increasing success; at the same time, the portion of the response caused by the partial agonist increases, while the total response—ie, the sum of responses to the two drugs (red line)—gradually decreases, eventually reaching the value produced by partial agonist alone (compare with B).

Another type of antagonism is **physiologic antagonism** between endogenous regulatory pathways mediated by different receptors. For example, several catabolic actions of the glucocorticoid hormones lead to increased blood glucose levels, an effect that is physiologically opposed by insulin. Although glucocorticoids and insulin act on quite distinct receptor-effector systems, the clinician must sometimes administer insulin to oppose the hyperglycemic effects of a glucocorticoid hormone, whether the latter is elevated by endogenous synthesis (eg, a tumor of the adrenal cortex) or as a result of glucocorticoid therapy.

In general, use of a drug as a physiologic antagonist produces effects that are less specific and less easy to control than are the effects of a receptor-specific antagonist. Thus, for example, to treat bradycardia caused by increased release of acetylcholine from vagus nerve endings, the clinician could use isoproterenol, a β-adrenoceptor agonist that increases heart rate by mimicking sympathetic stimulation of the heart. However, use of this physiologic antagonist would be less rational—and potentially more dangerous—than a receptor-specific antagonist such as atropine.

SIGNALING MECHANISMS & DRUG ACTION

Until now we have considered receptor interactions and drug effects in terms of equations and concentration-effect curves. We must also understand the molecular mechanisms by which drugs act. We should also consider different structural families of receptor proteins, and this allows us to ask basic questions with important clinical implications:

- Why do some drugs produce effects that persist for minutes, hours, or even days after the drug is no longer present?
- Why do responses to other drugs diminish rapidly with prolonged or repeated administration?
- How do cellular mechanisms for amplifying external chemical signals explain the phenomenon of spare receptors?
- Why do chemically similar drugs often exhibit extraordinary selectivity in their actions?
- Do these mechanisms provide targets for developing new drugs?

Most transmembrane signaling is accomplished by a small number of different molecular mechanisms. Each type of mechanism has been adapted, through the evolution of distinctive protein families, to transduce many different signals. These protein families include receptors on the cell surface and within the cell, as well as enzymes and other components that generate, amplify, coordinate, and terminate postreceptor signaling by nonprotein chemical mediators in the cell that are collectively called **second messengers**. This section first discusses mechanisms for carrying chemical information across the plasma membrane and then discusses some examples of second messenger chemicals.

Five basic mechanisms of transmembrane signaling are well understood (Figure 2–5). Each represents a different family of receptor protein and uses a different strategy to circumvent the barrier posed by the lipid bilayer of the plasma membrane. These strategies use (1) a lipid-soluble ligand that crosses the membrane and acts on an intracellular receptor; (2) a transmembrane receptor protein whose intracellular enzymatic activity is allosterically regulated by a ligand that binds to a site on the protein's extracellular domain; (3) a transmembrane receptor that binds and stimulates an intracellular protein tyrosine kinase; (4) a ligand-gated transmembrane ion channel that can be induced to open or close by the binding

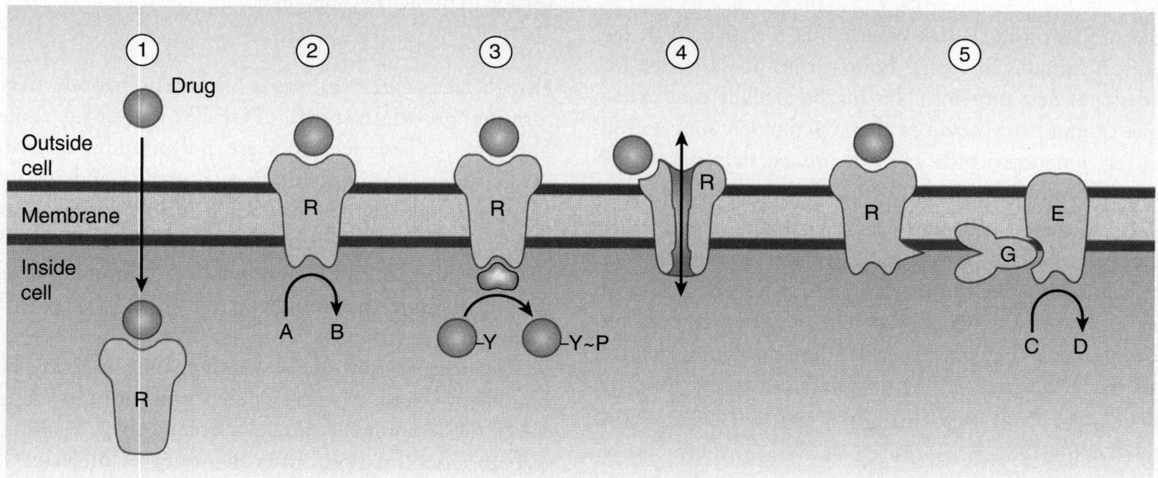

FIGURE 2–5 Known transmembrane signaling mechanisms: **1:** A lipid-soluble chemical signal crosses the plasma membrane and acts on an intracellular receptor (which may be an enzyme or a regulator of gene transcription); **2:** the signal binds to the extracellular domain of a transmembrane protein, thereby activating an enzymatic activity of its cytoplasmic domain; **3:** the signal binds to the extracellular domain of a transmembrane receptor bound to a separate protein tyrosine kinase, which it activates; **4:** the signal binds to and directly regulates the opening of an ion channel; **5:** the signal binds to a cell-surface receptor linked to an effector enzyme by a G protein. (A, C, substrates; B, D, products; R, receptor; G, G protein; E, effector [enzyme or ion channel]; Y, tyrosine; P, phosphate.)

of a ligand; and (5) a transmembrane receptor protein that stimulates a GTP-binding signal transducer protein (G protein), which in turn modulates production of an intracellular second messenger.

Although the five established mechanisms do not account for all the chemical signals conveyed across cell membranes, they do transduce many of the most important signals exploited in pharmacotherapy.

Intracellular Receptors for Lipid-Soluble Agents

Several biologic ligands are sufficiently lipid-soluble to cross the plasma membrane and act on intracellular receptors. One class of such ligands includes steroids (corticosteroids, mineralocorticoids, sex steroids, vitamin D) and thyroid hormone, whose receptors stimulate the transcription of genes by binding to specific DNA sequences (often called **response elements**) near the gene whose expression is to be regulated.

These "gene-active" receptors belong to a protein family that evolved from a common precursor. Dissection of the receptors by recombinant DNA techniques has provided insights into their molecular mechanism. For example, binding of glucocorticoid hormone to its normal receptor protein relieves an inhibitory constraint on the transcription-stimulating activity of the protein. Figure 2–6 schematically depicts the molecular mechanism of glucocorticoid action: In the absence of hormone, the receptor is bound to hsp90, a protein that prevents normal folding of several structural domains of the receptor. Binding of hormone to the ligand-binding domain triggers release of hsp90. This allows the DNA-binding and transcription-activating domains of the receptor to fold into their functionally active conformations, so that the activated receptor can initiate transcription of target genes.

The mechanism used by hormones that act by regulating gene expression has two therapeutically important consequences:

1. These hormones produce their effects after a characteristic lag period of 30 minutes to several hours—the time required for the synthesis of new proteins. This means that the gene-active hormones cannot be expected to alter a pathologic state within minutes (eg, glucocorticoids will not immediately relieve the symptoms of bronchial asthma).
2. The effects of these agents can persist for hours or days after their concentration has been reduced to zero. The persistence of effect is primarily due to the relatively slow turnover of most enzymes and proteins, which can remain active in cells for hours or days after they have been synthesized. Consequently, it means that the beneficial (or toxic) effects of a gene-active hormone usually decrease slowly when administration of the hormone is stopped.

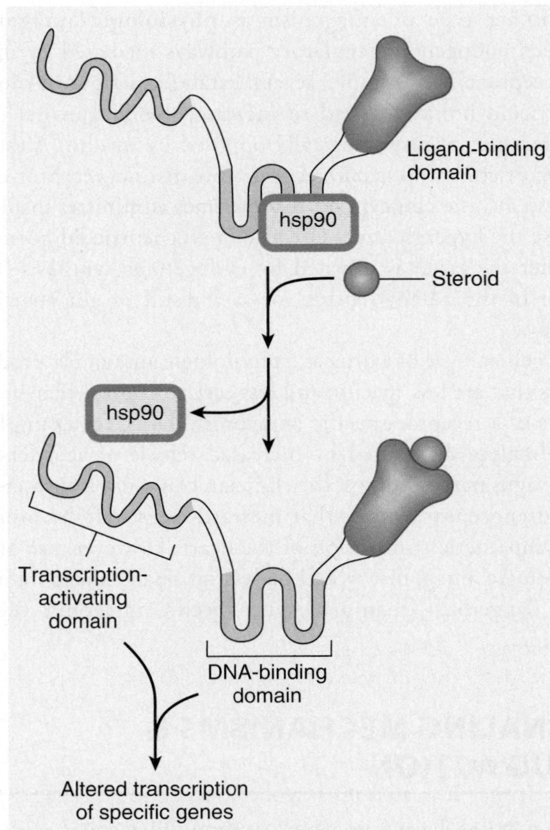

FIGURE 2–6 Mechanism of glucocorticoid action. The glucocorticoid receptor polypeptide is schematically depicted as a protein with three distinct domains. A heat-shock protein, hsp90, binds to the receptor in the absence of hormone and prevents folding into the active conformation of the receptor. Binding of a hormone ligand (steroid) causes dissociation of the hsp90 stabilizer and permits conversion to the active configuration.

Ligand-Regulated Transmembrane Enzymes Including Receptor Tyrosine Kinases

This class of receptor molecules mediates the first steps in signaling by insulin, epidermal growth factor (EGF), platelet-derived growth factor (PDGF), atrial natriuretic peptide (ANP), transforming growth factor-β (TGF-β), and many other trophic hormones. These receptors are polypeptides consisting of an extracellular hormone-binding domain and a cytoplasmic enzyme domain, which may be a protein tyrosine kinase, a serine kinase, or a guanylyl cyclase (Figure 2–7). In all these receptors, the two domains are connected by a hydrophobic segment of the polypeptide that resides in the lipid bilayer of the plasma membrane.

The receptor tyrosine kinase signaling function begins with binding of ligand, typically a polypeptide hormone or growth factor, to the receptor's extracellular domain. The resulting change in receptor conformation causes two receptor molecules to bind to one another (*dimerize*). This activates the tyrosine kinase enzyme activity present in the cytoplasmic domain of the dimer, leading to phosphorylation of the receptor as well as additional downstream signaling proteins. Activated receptors catalyze phosphorylation of tyrosine residues on different target signaling proteins, thereby allowing a single activated receptor complex to modulate a large number of biochemical processes.

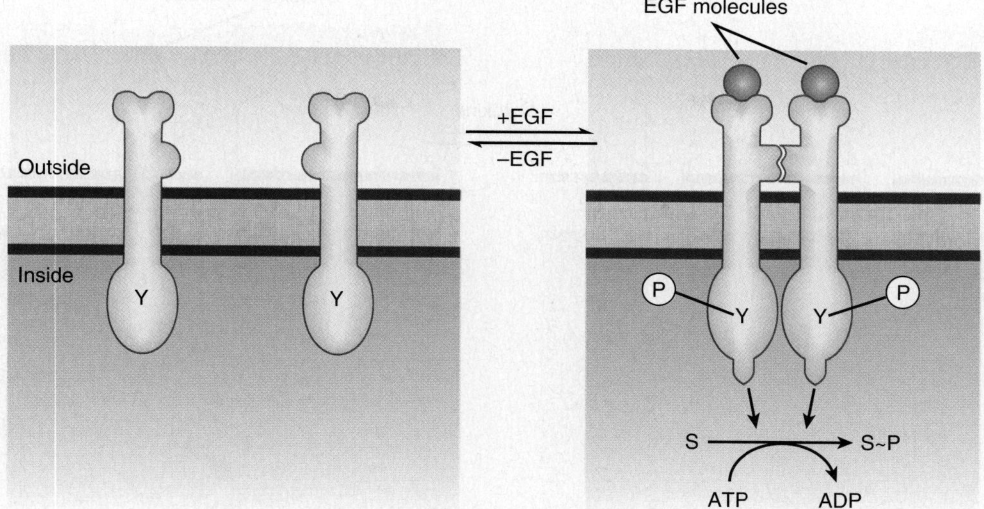

FIGURE 2–7 Mechanism of activation of the epidermal growth factor (EGF) receptor, a representative receptor tyrosine kinase. The receptor polypeptide has extracellular and cytoplasmic domains, depicted above and below the plasma membrane. Upon binding of EGF (circle), the receptor converts from its inactive monomeric state (*left*) to an active dimeric state (*right*), in which two receptor polypeptides bind noncovalently. The cytoplasmic domains become phosphorylated (P) on specific tyrosine residues (Y), and their enzymatic activities are activated, catalyzing phosphorylation of substrate proteins (S).

Insulin, for example, uses a single class of tyrosine kinase receptors to trigger increased uptake of glucose and amino acids and to regulate metabolism of glycogen and triglycerides in the cell. Activation of the receptor in specific target cells drives a complex program of cellular events ranging from altered membrane transport of ions and metabolites to changes in the expression of many genes.

Inhibitors of particular receptor tyrosine kinases are used in treating neoplastic disorders in which excessive growth factor signaling is often involved. Some of these inhibitors are monoclonal antibodies (eg, trastuzumab, cetuximab), which bind to the extracellular domain of a particular receptor and interfere with binding of growth factor. Other inhibitors are membrane-permeant small molecule chemicals (eg, gefitinib, erlotinib), which inhibit the receptor's kinase activity in the cytoplasm.

The intensity and duration of action of EGF, PDGF, and other agents that act via receptor tyrosine kinases are often limited by a process called receptor **downregulation.** This typically occurs by endocytosis of receptors from the cell surface followed by the degradation of internalized receptors (and their bound ligands). When this process occurs at a rate faster than de novo synthesis of receptors, the total number of cell-surface receptors is reduced (down-regulated), and the cell's responsiveness to ligand is correspondingly diminished. A well-understood example is the EGF receptor tyrosine kinase, whose rate of internalization from the plasma membrane is greatly accelerated after activation by EGF; internalized receptors are subsequently delivered to lysosomes and proteolyzed. This downregulation process is essential physiologically to limit the strength and duration of the endogenous growth factor signal, and genetic mutations that interfere with the downregulation process cause excessive and prolonged responses that underlie or contribute to many forms of cancer. Endocytosis of other receptor tyrosine kinases, most notably receptors for nerve growth factor, can serve a very different function. Internalized nerve growth factor receptors are not rapidly degraded but remain active in endocytic vesicles that move from the distal axon, where receptors are initially activated by nerve growth factor (released from the innervated tissue), into the neuron's cell body. In the cell body, the growth factor signal is transduced to transcription factors regulating the expression of genes controlling cell survival. This process, effectively opposite to downregulation, transports a critical survival signal from its site of initiation to the site of a critical downstream signaling effect, and can do so over a remarkably long distance—up to a meter in some neurons.

Other regulators of growth and differentiation, including TGF-β, act on another class of transmembrane receptor enzymes that phosphorylate serine and threonine residues. Atrial natriuretic peptide (ANP), an important regulator of blood volume and vascular tone, acts on a transmembrane receptor whose intracellular domain, a guanylyl cyclase, generates cGMP (see below).

Cytokine Receptors

Cytokine receptors respond to a heterogeneous group of peptide ligands, which include growth hormone, erythropoietin, several kinds of interferon, and other regulators of growth and differentiation. These receptors use a mechanism (Figure 2–8) closely resembling that of receptor tyrosine kinases, except that in this case, the protein tyrosine kinase activity is not intrinsic to the receptor molecule. Instead, a separate protein tyrosine kinase, from the Janus-kinase (JAK) family, binds noncovalently to the receptor. As in the case of the EGF receptor, cytokine receptors dimerize after they bind the activating ligand, allowing the bound JAKs to become activated and to phosphorylate tyrosine residues on the receptor.

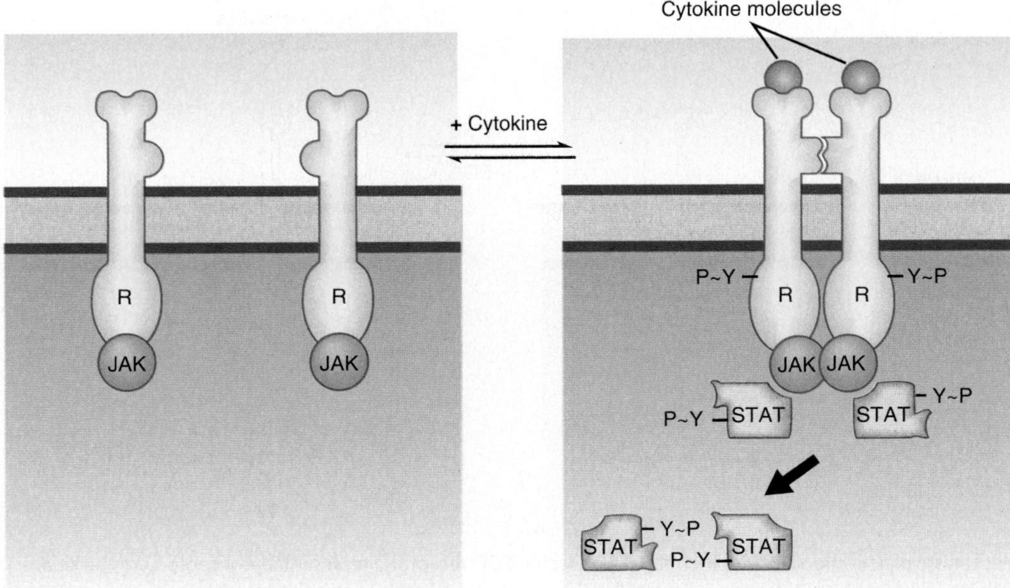

FIGURE 2–8 Cytokine receptors, like receptor tyrosine kinases, have extracellular and intracellular domains and form dimers. However, after activation by an appropriate ligand, separate mobile protein tyrosine kinase molecules (JAK) are activated, resulting in phosphorylation of signal transducers and activation of transcription (STAT) molecules. STAT dimers then travel to the nucleus, where they regulate transcription.

Phosphorylated tyrosine residues on the receptor's cytoplasmic surface then set in motion a complex signaling dance by binding another set of proteins, called STATs (signal transducers and activators of transcription). The bound STATs are themselves phosphorylated by the JAKs, two STAT molecules dimerize (attaching to one another's tyrosine phosphates), and finally the STAT/STAT dimer dissociates from the receptor and travels to the nucleus, where it regulates transcription of specific genes.

Ion Channels

Many of the most useful drugs in clinical medicine act on ion channels. For ligand-gated ion channels, drugs often mimic or block the actions of natural agonists. Natural ligands of such receptors include acetylcholine, serotonin, GABA, and glutamate; all are synaptic transmitters.

Each of their receptors transmits its signal across the plasma membrane by increasing transmembrane conductance of the relevant ion and thereby altering the electrical potential across the membrane. For example, acetylcholine causes the opening of the ion channel in the nicotinic acetylcholine receptor (nAChR), which allows Na^+ to flow down its concentration gradient into cells, producing a localized excitatory postsynaptic potential—a depolarization.

The nAChR is one of the best characterized of all cell-surface receptors for hormones or neurotransmitters (Figure 2–9). One form of this receptor is a pentamer made up of four different polypeptide subunits (eg, two α chains plus one β, one γ, and one δ chain). These polypeptides, each of which crosses the lipid bilayer four times, form a cylindrical structure that is approximately 10 nm in diameter but is impermeable to ions. When acetylcholine binds to sites on the α subunits, a conformational change occurs that results in the transient opening of a central aqueous channel, approximately 0.5 nm in diameter, through which sodium ions penetrate from the extracellular fluid to cause electrical depolarization of the cell. The structural basis for activating other

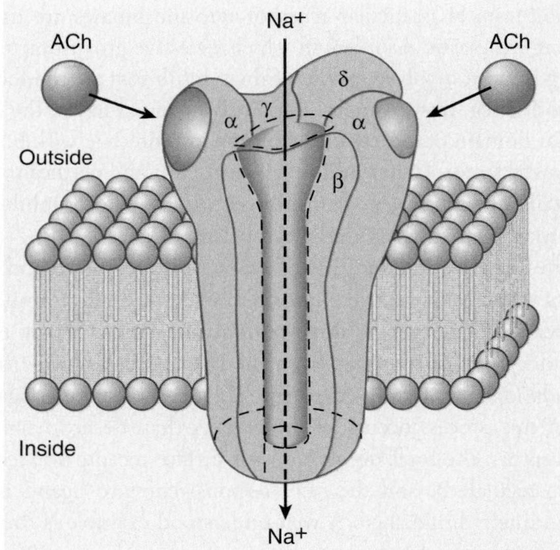

FIGURE 2–9 The nicotinic acetylcholine (ACh) receptor, a ligand-gated ion channel. The receptor molecule is depicted as embedded in a rectangular piece of plasma membrane, with extracellular fluid above and cytoplasm below. Composed of five subunits (two α, one β, one γ, and one δ), the receptor opens a central transmembrane ion channel when ACh binds to sites on the extracellular domain of its α subunits.

ligand-gated ion channels has been determined recently, and similar general principles apply, but there are differences in key details that may open new opportunities for drug design and action. For example, receptors that mediate excitatory neurotransmission at central nervous system synapses bind glutamate, a major excitatory neurotransmitter, through a large appendage domain that protrudes from the receptor and has been called a "flytrap" because it physically closes around the glutamate molecule; the glutamate-loaded flytrap domain then moves as a unit to control pore opening. Drugs can regulate the activity of such glutamate receptors by binding to the flytrap domain, to surfaces on the membrane-embedded portion around the pore, or within the pore itself.

The time elapsed between the binding of the agonist to a ligand-gated channel and the cellular response can often be measured in milliseconds. The rapidity of this signaling mechanism is crucially important for moment-to-moment transfer of information across synapses. Ligand-gated ion channels can be regulated by multiple mechanisms, including phosphorylation and endocytosis. In some cases, such as the nicotinic synapse controlling the diaphragmatic muscles mediating ventilation, these mechanisms maintain a uniform response (ie, they are homeostatic). In other cases, such as at many synapses in the central nervous system, these mechanisms can produce long-term changes in the magnitude of the response and contribute to synaptic plasticity involved in learning and memory.

Voltage-gated ion channels do not bind neurotransmitters directly but are controlled by membrane potential; such channels are also important drug targets. Drugs that regulate voltage-gated channels typically bind to a site of the receptor different from the charged amino acids that constitute the "voltage sensor" domain of the protein used for channel opening by membrane potential. For example, verapamil binds to a region in the pore of voltage-gated calcium channels that are present in the heart and in vascular smooth muscle, inhibiting the ion conductance separately from the voltage sensor, producing antiarrhythmic effects, and reducing blood pressure without mimicking or antagonizing any known endogenous transmitter. Local anesthetics such as procaine work by inhibiting voltage-sensitive sodium channels expressed in sensory neurons, probably by binding to multiple sites on the channel. Other channels, such as the CFTR, are not strongly sensitive to either a known natural ligand or voltage but are still important drug targets. Lumacaftor binds CFTR and promotes its delivery to the plasma membrane after biosynthesis. Ivacaftor binds to a different site and enhances channel conductance. Both drugs act as allosteric modulators of the CFTR and are used in the treatment of cystic fibrosis, but each has a different effect.

G Proteins & Second Messengers

Many extracellular ligands act by increasing the intracellular concentrations of second messengers such as **cyclic adenosine-3′, 5′-monophosphate (cAMP), calcium ion,** or the **phosphoinositides** (described below). In most cases, they use a transmembrane signaling system with three separate components. First, the extracellular ligand is selectively detected by a cell-surface receptor. The receptor in turn triggers the activation of a GTP-binding protein

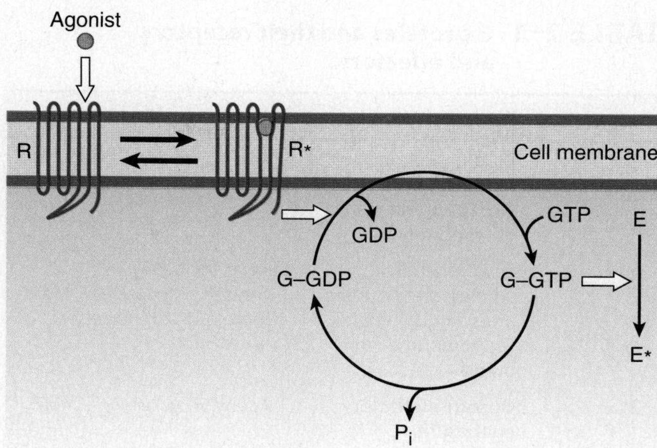

FIGURE 2–10 The guanine nucleotide-dependent activation-inactivation cycle of G proteins. The agonist activates the receptor (R→R*), which promotes release of GDP from the G protein (G), allowing entry of GTP into the nucleotide binding site. In its GTP-bound state (G–GTP), the G protein regulates activity of an effector enzyme or ion channel (E→E*). The signal is terminated by hydrolysis of GTP, followed by return of the system to the basal unstimulated state. Open arrows denote regulatory effects. (P_i, inorganic phosphate.)

(G protein) located on the cytoplasmic face of the plasma membrane. The activated G protein then changes the activity of an effector element, usually an enzyme or ion channel. This element then changes the concentration of the intracellular second messenger. For cAMP, the effector enzyme is adenylyl cyclase, a membrane protein that converts intracellular adenosine triphosphate (ATP) to cAMP. The corresponding G protein, G_s, stimulates adenylyl cyclase after being activated by hormones and neurotransmitters that act via specific G_s-coupled receptors. There are many examples of such receptors, including β adrenoceptors, glucagon receptors, thyrotropin receptors, and certain subtypes of dopamine and serotonin receptors.

G_s and other G proteins rapidly activate their downstream effectors when bound by GTP, but they also have the ability to hydrolyze GTP (Figure 2–10); this hydrolysis reaction inactivates the G protein, and the rate of GTP hydrolysis is a major determinant of both the duration and amount of downstream responses. For example, a neurotransmitter such as norepinephrine may encounter its membrane receptor for only a few tens of milliseconds. When the encounter generates a GTP-bound G_s molecule, however, the duration of activation of adenylyl cyclase depends on the longevity of GTP binding to G_s rather than on the duration of norepinephrine's binding to the receptor. Indeed, GTP-bound G_s may remain active for tens of seconds before it is inactivated by hydrolysis of the bound GTP to GDP, prolonging and enormously amplifying the original signal. The family of G proteins contains several functionally diverse subfamilies (Table 2–1), each of which mediates effects of a particular set of receptors to a distinctive group of effectors. Note that an endogenous ligand (eg, norepinephrine, acetylcholine, serotonin, many others not listed in Table 2–1) may bind and stimulate receptors that couple to different subsets of G proteins. The apparent promiscuity of such a ligand allows it to

TABLE 2–1 G proteins and their receptors and effectors.

G Protein	Receptors for	Effector/Signaling Pathway
G_s	β-Adrenergic amines, histamine, serotonin, glucagon, and many other hormones	↑ Adenylyl cyclase →↑ cAMP
G_{i1}, G_{i2}, G_{i3}	α_2-Adrenergic amines, acetylcholine (muscarinic), opioids, serotonin, and many others	Several, including: ↓ Adenylyl cyclase →↓ cAMP Open cardiac K^+ channels →↓ heart rate
G_{olf}	Odorants (olfactory epithelium)	↑ Adenylyl cyclase →↑ cAMP
G_o	Neurotransmitters in brain (not yet specifically identified)	Not yet clear
G_q	Acetylcholine (muscarinic), bombesin, serotonin (5-HT_2), and many others	↑ Phospholipase C →↑ IP_3, diacylglycerol, cytoplasmic Ca^{2+}
G_{t1}, G_{t2}	Photons (rhodopsin and color opsins in retinal rod and cone cells)	↑ cGMP phosphodiesterase →↓ cGMP (phototransduction)

cAMP, cyclic adenosine monophosphate; cGMP, cyclic guanosine monophosphate; IP_3, inositol-1,4,5-trisphosphate.

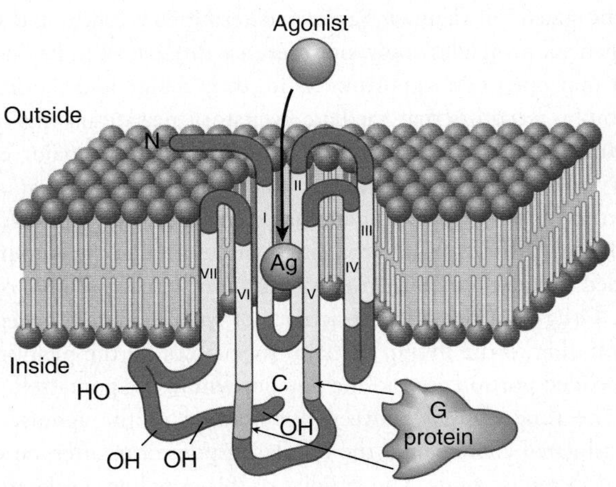

FIGURE 2–11 Transmembrane topology of a typical "serpentine" GPCR. The receptor's amino (N) terminal is extracellular (above the plane of the membrane), and its carboxyl (C) terminal intracellular, with the polypeptide chain "snaking" across the membrane seven times. The hydrophobic transmembrane segments (light color) are designated by Roman numerals (I–VII). Agonist (Ag) approaches the receptor from the extracellular fluid and binds to a site surrounded by the transmembrane regions of the receptor protein. G protein interacts with cytoplasmic regions of the receptor, especially around the third cytoplasmic loop connecting transmembrane regions V and VI. Lateral movement of these helices during activation exposes an otherwise buried cytoplasmic surface of the receptor that promotes guanine nucleotide exchange on the G protein and thereby activates the G protein, as discussed in the text. The receptor's cytoplasmic terminal tail contains numerous serine and threonine residues whose hydroxyl (-OH) groups can be phosphorylated. This phosphorylation is associated with diminished receptor–G protein coupling and can promote receptor endocytosis.

elicit different G protein–dependent responses in different cells. For instance, the body responds to danger by using catecholamines (norepinephrine and epinephrine) both to increase heart rate and to induce constriction of blood vessels in the skin, by acting on G_s-coupled β adrenoceptors and G_q-coupled α_1 adrenoceptors, respectively. Ligand promiscuity also offers opportunities in drug development (see Receptor Classes & Drug Development in the following text).

Receptors that signal via G proteins are often called "G protein–coupled receptors" **(GPCRs).** GPCRs make up the largest receptor family and are also called "seven-transmembrane" (7TM) or "serpentine" receptors because the receptor polypeptide chain "snakes" across the plasma membrane seven times (Figure 2–11). Receptors for adrenergic amines, serotonin, acetylcholine (muscarinic but not nicotinic), many peptide hormones, odorants, and light receptors (in retinal rod and cone cells) all belong to the GPCR family. A few GPCRs (eg, $GABA_B$ and metabotropic glutamate receptors) require stable assembly into *homodimers* (complexes of two identical receptor polypeptides) or *heterodimers* (complexes of different isoforms) for functional activity. However, in contrast to tyrosine kinase and cytokine receptors, oligomerization is not universally required for GPCR activation, and many GPCRs are thought to function as monomers.

GPCRs can bind agonists in a variety of ways, but they all appear to transduce signals across the plasma membrane in a similar way. Agonist binding (eg, a catecholamine or acetylcholine) stabilizes a conformational state of the receptor in which the cytoplasmic ends of the transmembrane helices spread apart by about 1 nm, opening a cavity in the receptor's cytoplasmic surface that binds a critical regulatory surface of the G protein. This reduces nucleotide affinity for the G protein, allowing GDP to dissociate and GTP to replace it (this occurs because GTP is normally present in the cytoplasm at much higher concentration than GDP). The GTP-bound form of G protein then dissociates from the receptor and can engage downstream mediators. Thus GPCR–G protein coupling involves coordinated conformational change in both proteins, allowing agonist binding to the receptor to effectively "drive" a nucleotide exchange reaction that "switches" the G protein from its inactive (GDP-bound) to active (GTP-bound) form. Figure 2–11 shows the main components schematically. Many high-resolution structures of GPCRs, and several of active-conformation GPCRs in complex with G protein, are available from the Protein Data Bank (www.rcsb.org). Such information provides deep insight into the actions and basis for specificity of existing GPCR-directed drugs, and it is beginning to be used to discover new drug leads through computational chemistry approaches.

Receptor Regulation

G protein–mediated responses to drugs and hormonal agonists often attenuate with time (Figure 2–12A). After reaching an initial high level, the response (eg, cellular cAMP accumulation, Na^+ influx, contractility, etc) diminishes over seconds or minutes, even

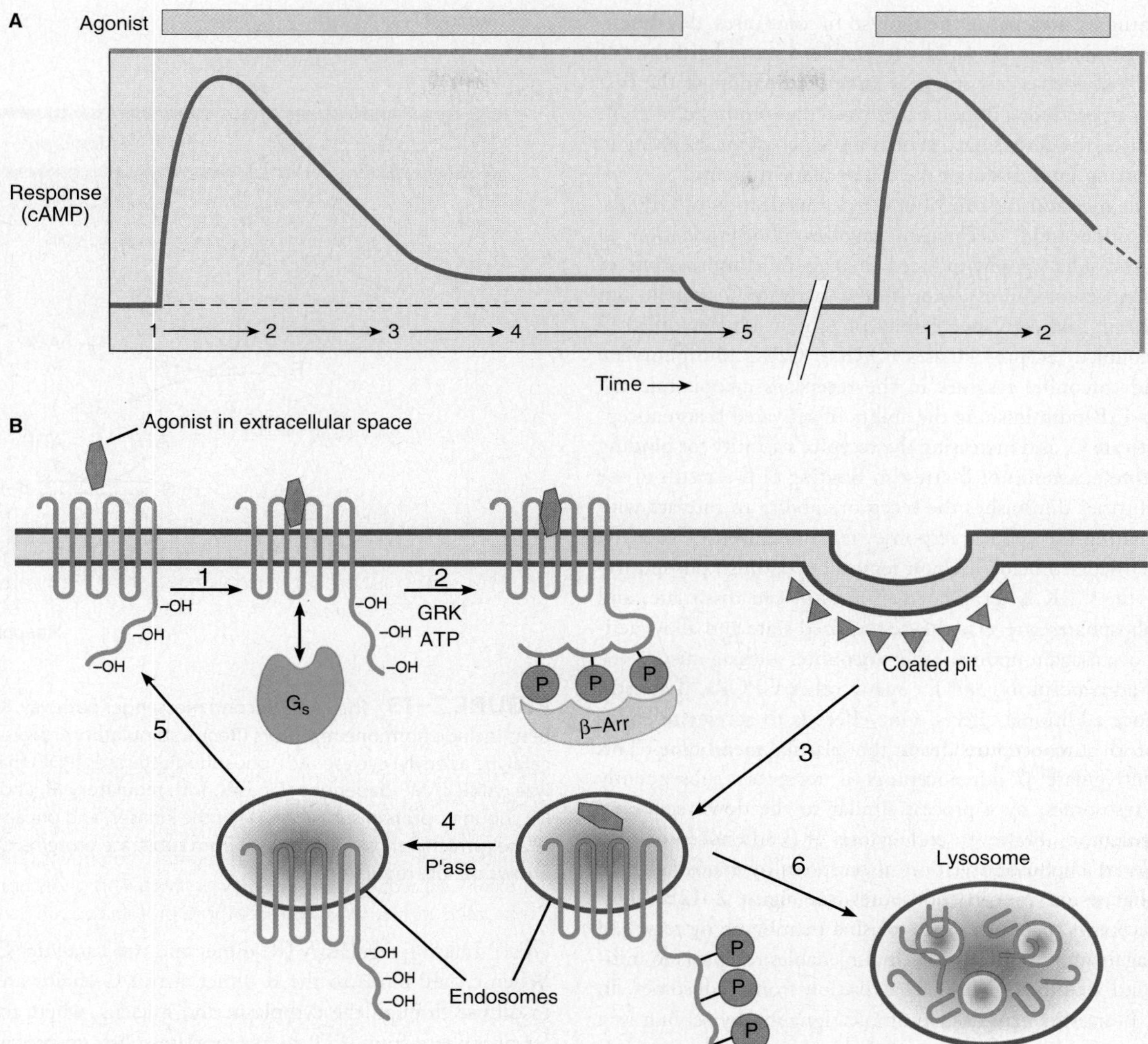

FIGURE 2–12 Rapid desensitization, resensitization, and downregulation of β adrenoceptors. **A:** Response to a β-adrenoceptor agonist (ordinate) versus time (abscissa). (Numbers refer to the phases of receptor function in B.) Exposure of cells to agonist (indicated by the light-colored bar) produces a cyclic AMP (cAMP) response. A reduced cAMP response is observed in the continued presence of agonist; this "desensitization" typically occurs within a few minutes. If agonist is removed after a short time (typically several to tens of minutes, indicated by broken line on abscissa), cells recover full responsiveness to a subsequent addition of agonist (second light-colored bar). This "resensitization" fails to occur, or occurs incompletely, if cells are exposed to agonist repeatedly or over a more prolonged time period. **B:** Agonist binding to receptors initiates signaling by promoting receptor interaction with G proteins (G_s) located in the cytoplasm (step 1 in the diagram). Agonist-activated receptors are phosphorylated by a G protein–coupled receptor kinase (GRK), preventing receptor interaction with G_s and promoting binding of a different protein, β-arrestin (β-Arr), to the receptor (step 2). The receptor-arrestin complex binds to coated pits, promoting receptor internalization (step 3). Dissociation of agonist from internalized receptors reduces β-Arr binding affinity, allowing dephosphorylation of receptors by a phosphatase (P'ase, step 4). Depending on the receptor, and on the agonist concentration achieved in the endosome, a second phase of G protein activation can occur internally before receptors recycle to the plasma membrane (step 5). Recycling of receptors serves to "resensitize" cellular responsiveness by restoring functional receptors at the cell surface, where they can initiate signaling again in response to agonist. The efficiency and rate of this recycling process depends on the GPCR, the physiological state of the cell, and on pharmacological variables including agonist concentration and duration of exposure. In general, repeated or prolonged agonist exposure favors the delivery of internalized receptors to lysosomes rather than their recycling to the cell surface (step 6), causing receptors to down-regulate and reducing, rather than recovering, cellular signaling responsiveness to agonist.

in the continued presence of the agonist. In some cases, this **desensitization** phenomenon is rapidly reversible; a second exposure to agonist, if provided a few minutes after termination of the first exposure, can produce a response similar to that produced initially. In other cases, the desensitized state is more persistent, resulting in a longer-lasting suppression of the cell or tissue response.

Multiple mechanisms contribute to desensitization of GPCRs. One well-understood mechanism involves phosphorylation of the receptor. The agonist-induced change in conformation of the β-adrenoceptor causes it not only to activate G protein, but also to recruit and activate a family of protein kinases called G protein–coupled receptor kinases (GRKs). GRKs phosphorylate serine and threonine residues in the receptor's cytoplasmic tail (Figure 2–12B), diminishing the ability of activated β adrenoceptors to activate G_s and increasing the receptor's affinity for binding a third protein, arrestin or β-arrestin. Binding of β-arrestin to the receptor further diminishes the receptor's ability to interact with G_s, attenuating the cellular response (ie, stimulation of adenylyl cyclase as discussed below). Upon removal of agonist, phosphorylation by the GRK is terminated, β-arrestin can dissociate, and cellular phosphatases reverse the desensitized state and allow activation to occur again upon another encounter with agonist.

For β adrenoceptors, and for many other GPCRs, β-arrestin can produce additional effects. One effect is to accelerate endocytosis of β adrenoceptors from the plasma membrane. This can down-regulate β adrenoceptors if receptors subsequently travel to lysosomes, by a process similar to the downregulation of EGF receptors. However, endocytosis of β adrenoceptors can also accelerate dephosphorylation of receptors by exposing them to phosphatase enzymes in endosomes (see Figure 2–12B). This enables receptors to return to the plasma membrane by recycling to signal again and, in some cases, it also enables receptors to initiate a second round of G protein activation from endosomes. In addition, β-arrestin may itself promote signaling by serving as a molecular scaffold that binds to other signaling proteins. Accordingly, β-arrestin can confer on GPCRs a great deal of flexibility in overall signaling and regulation. This may provide an opportunity to achieve additional selectivity in drug action through GPCRs, a concept called **functional selectivity** or **agonist bias**, whose clinical utility is presently under investigation.

Well-Established Second Messengers

A. Cyclic Adenosine Monophosphate (cAMP)

Acting as an intracellular second messenger, cAMP mediates such hormonal responses as the mobilization of stored energy (the breakdown of carbohydrates in liver or triglycerides in fat cells stimulated by β-adrenomimetic catecholamines), conservation of water by the kidney (mediated by vasopressin), Ca^{2+} homeostasis (regulated by parathyroid hormone), and increased rate and contractile force of heart muscle (β-adrenomimetic catecholamines). It also regulates the production of adrenal and sex steroids (in response to corticotropin or follicle-stimulating hormone), relaxation of smooth muscle, and many other endocrine and neural processes.

cAMP exerts most of its effects by stimulating cAMP-dependent protein kinases (Figure 2–13). These kinases are composed of a

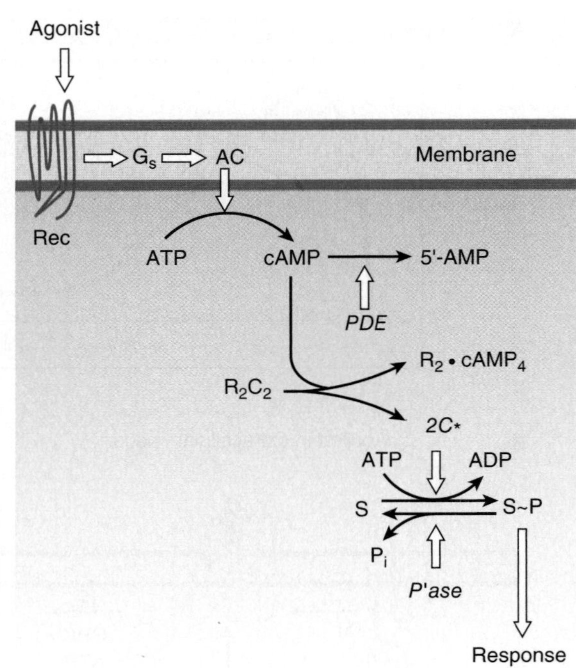

FIGURE 2–13 The cAMP second messenger pathway. Key proteins include hormone receptors (Rec), a stimulatory G protein (G_s), catalytic adenylyl cyclase (AC), phosphodiesterases (PDE) that hydrolyze cAMP, cAMP-dependent kinases, with regulatory (R) and catalytic (C) subunits, protein substrates (S) of the kinases, and phosphatases (P'ase), which remove phosphates from substrate proteins. Open arrows denote regulatory effects.

cAMP-binding regulatory (R) dimer and two catalytic (C) chains. When cAMP binds to the R dimer, active C chains are released to diffuse through the cytoplasm and nucleus, where they transfer phosphate from ATP to appropriate substrate proteins, often enzymes. The specificity of the regulatory effects of cAMP resides in the distinct protein substrates of the kinases that are expressed in different cells. For example, the liver is rich in phosphorylase kinase and glycogen synthase, enzymes whose reciprocal regulation by cAMP-dependent phosphorylation governs carbohydrate storage and release.

When the hormonal stimulus stops, the intracellular actions of cAMP are terminated by an elaborate series of enzymes. cAMP-stimulated phosphorylation of enzyme substrates is rapidly reversed by a diverse group of specific and nonspecific phosphatases. cAMP itself is degraded to 5′-AMP by several cyclic nucleotide phosphodiesterases (PDEs; see Figure 2–13). Milrinone, a selective inhibitor of type 3 phosphodiesterases that are expressed in cardiac muscle cells, has been used as an adjunctive agent in treating acute heart failure. Competitive inhibition of cAMP degradation is one way that caffeine, theophylline, and other methylxanthines produce their effects (see Chapter 20).

B. Phosphoinositides and Calcium

Another well-studied second messenger system involves hormonal stimulation of phosphoinositide hydrolysis (Figure 2–14).

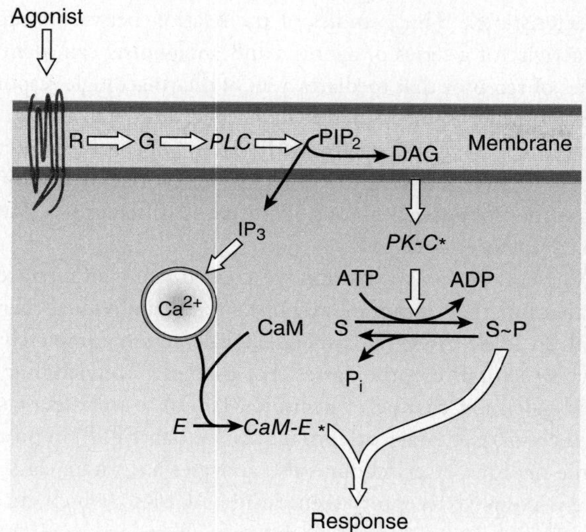

FIGURE 2–14 The Ca^{2+}-phosphoinositide signaling pathway. Key proteins include hormone receptors (R), a G protein (G), a phosphoinositide-specific phospholipase C (PLC), protein kinase C substrates of the kinase (S), calmodulin (CaM), and calmodulin-binding enzymes (E), including kinases, phosphodiesterases, etc. (PIP_2, phosphatidylinositol-4,5-bisphosphate; DAG, diacylglycerol; IP_3, inositol trisphosphate. Asterisk denotes activated state. Open arrows denote regulatory effects.)

Some of the hormones, neurotransmitters, and growth factors that trigger this pathway bind to receptors linked to G proteins, whereas others bind to receptor tyrosine kinases. In all cases, the crucial step is stimulation of a membrane enzyme, phospholipase C (PLC), which splits a minor phospholipid component of the plasma membrane, phosphatidylinositol-4,5-bisphosphate (PIP_2), into two second messengers, **diacylglycerol (DAG)** and **inositol-1,4,5-trisphosphate (IP_3 or $InsP_3$)**. Diacylglycerol is confined to the membrane, where it activates a phospholipid- and calcium-sensitive protein kinase called protein kinase C. IP_3 is water-soluble and diffuses through the cytoplasm to trigger release of Ca^{2+} by binding to ligand-gated calcium channels in the limiting membranes of internal storage vesicles. Elevated cytoplasmic Ca^{2+} concentration resulting from IP_3-promoted opening of these channels promotes the binding of Ca^{2+} to the calcium-binding protein calmodulin, which regulates activities of other enzymes, including calcium-dependent protein kinases.

With its multiple second messengers and protein kinases, the phosphoinositide signaling pathway is much more complex than the cAMP pathway. For example, different cell types may contain one or more specialized calcium- and calmodulin-dependent kinases with limited substrate specificity (eg, myosin light-chain kinase) in addition to a general calcium- and calmodulin-dependent kinase that can phosphorylate a wide variety of protein substrates. Furthermore, at least nine structurally distinct types of protein kinase C have been identified.

As in the cAMP system, multiple mechanisms damp or terminate signaling by this pathway. IP_3 is inactivated by dephosphorylation; diacylglycerol is either phosphorylated to yield phosphatidic acid, which is then converted back into phospholipids, or it is deacylated to yield arachidonic acid; Ca^{2+} is actively removed from the cytoplasm by Ca^{2+} pumps.

These and other nonreceptor elements of the calcium-phosphoinositide signaling pathway are of considerable importance in pharmacotherapy. For example, lithium ion, used in treatment of bipolar (manic-depressive) disorder, affects the cellular metabolism of phosphoinositides (see Chapter 29).

C. Cyclic Guanosine Monophosphate (cGMP)

Unlike cAMP, the ubiquitous and versatile carrier of diverse messages, cGMP has established signaling roles in only a few cell types. In the retina, cGMP mediates vision and is destroyed by hydrolysis in response to light, mediated by a phosphodiesterase stimulated by a G protein coupled to the light-activated GPCR rhodopsin. In intestinal mucosa and vascular smooth muscle, the cGMP-based signal transduction mechanism closely parallels the cAMP-mediated signaling mechanism. Ligands detected by cell-surface receptors stimulate membrane-bound guanylyl cyclase to produce cGMP, and cGMP acts by stimulating a cGMP-dependent protein kinase. The actions of cGMP in these cells are terminated by enzymatic degradation of the cyclic nucleotide and by dephosphorylation of kinase substrates.

Increased cGMP concentration causes relaxation of vascular smooth muscle by a kinase-mediated mechanism that results in dephosphorylation of myosin light chains (see Figure 12–2). In these smooth muscle cells, cGMP synthesis can be elevated by two transmembrane signaling mechanisms utilizing two different guanylyl cyclases. Atrial natriuretic peptide, a blood-borne peptide hormone, stimulates a transmembrane receptor by binding to its extracellular domain, thereby activating the guanylyl cyclase activity that resides in the receptor's intracellular domain. The other mechanism mediates responses to nitric oxide (NO; see Chapter 19), which is generated in vascular endothelial cells in response to natural vasodilator agents such as acetylcholine and histamine. After entering the target cell, nitric oxide binds to and activates a cytoplasmic guanylyl cyclase (see Figure 19–2). A number of useful vasodilating drugs, such as nitroglycerin and sodium nitroprusside used in treating cardiac ischemia and acute hypertension, act by generating or mimicking nitric oxide. Other drugs produce vasodilation by inhibiting specific phosphodiesterases, thereby interfering with the metabolic breakdown of cGMP. One such drug is sildenafil, used in treating erectile dysfunction and pulmonary hypertension (see Chapter 12).

Interplay Among Signaling Mechanisms

The calcium-phosphoinositide and cAMP signaling pathways oppose one another in some cells and are complementary in others. For example, vasopressor agents that contract smooth muscle act by IP_3-mediated mobilization of Ca^{2+}, whereas agents that relax smooth muscle often act by elevation of cAMP. In contrast, cAMP and phosphoinositide second messengers act together to stimulate glucose release from the liver.

Isolation of Signaling Mechanisms

The opposite of signal interplay is seen in some situations—an effective isolation of signaling according to location in the cell. For example, calcium signaling in the heart is highly localized because calcium released into the cytoplasm is rapidly sequestered by nearby calcium-binding proteins and is locally pumped from the cytoplasm into the sarcoplasmic reticulum. Even the second messenger cAMP can have surprisingly local effects, with signals mediated by the same messenger effectively isolated according to location. Here, it appears that signal isolation occurs by local hydrolysis of the second messenger by phosphodiesterase enzymes and by physical scaffolding of signaling pathway components into organized complexes that allow cAMP to transduce its local effects before hydrolysis. One mechanism by which phosphodiesterase inhibitor drugs produce toxic effects may be through "scrambling" local cAMP signals within the cell.

Phosphorylation: A Common Theme

Almost all second messenger signaling involves reversible phosphorylation, which performs two principal functions in signaling: amplification and flexible regulation. In **amplification,** rather like GTP bound to a G protein, the attachment of a phosphoryl group to a serine, threonine, or tyrosine residue powerfully amplifies the initial regulatory signal by recording a molecular memory that the pathway has been activated; dephosphorylation erases the memory, taking a longer time to do so than is required for dissociation of an allosteric ligand. In **flexible regulation,** differing substrate specificities of the multiple protein kinases regulated by second messengers provide branch points in signaling pathways that may be independently regulated. In this way, cAMP, Ca^{2+}, or other second messengers can use the presence or absence of particular kinases or kinase substrates to produce quite different effects in different cell types. Inhibitors of protein kinases have great potential as therapeutic agents, particularly in neoplastic diseases. Trastuzumab, an antibody that antagonizes growth factor signaling by the HER2 tyrosine kinase receptor (discussed earlier), is used for treating breast cancer. Imatinib, a small molecule inhibitor of the cytoplasmic tyrosine kinase Abl, is used for treating chronic myelogenous leukemia caused by a chromosomal translocation event that produces an inappropriate Bcr/Abl fusion protein with unregulated kinase activity.

RECEPTOR CLASSES & DRUG DEVELOPMENT

The existence of a specific drug receptor is usually inferred from studying the **structure-activity relationship** of a group of structurally similar congeners of the drug that mimic or antagonize its effects. Thus, if a series of related agonists exhibits identical relative potencies in producing two distinct effects, it is likely that the two effects are mediated by similar or identical receptor molecules. In addition, if identical receptors mediate both effects, a competitive antagonist will inhibit both responses with the same K_i; a second competitive antagonist will inhibit both responses with its own characteristic K_i. Thus, studies of the relation between structure and activity of a series of agonists and antagonists can identify a species of receptor that mediates a set of pharmacologic responses.

Exactly the same experimental procedure can show that observed effects of a drug are mediated by *different* receptors. In this case, effects mediated by different receptors may exhibit different orders of potency among agonists and different K_i values for each competitive antagonist.

Wherever we look, evolution has created many different receptors that function to mediate responses to any individual chemical signal. In some cases, the same chemical acts on completely different structural receptor classes. For example, acetylcholine uses ligand-gated ion channels (nicotinic AChRs) to initiate a fast (in milliseconds) excitatory postsynaptic potential (EPSP) in postganglionic neurons. Acetylcholine also activates a separate class of G protein–coupled receptors (muscarinic AChRs), which mediate slower (seconds to minutes) modulatory effects on the same neurons. In addition, each structural class usually includes multiple subtypes of receptor, often with significantly different signaling or regulatory properties. For example, many biogenic amines (eg, norepinephrine, acetylcholine, histamine, and serotonin) activate more than one receptor, each of which may activate a different G protein, as previously described (see also Table 2–1). The existence of many receptor classes and subtypes for the same endogenous ligand has created important opportunities for drug development. For example, propranolol, a selective antagonist of β adrenoceptors, can reduce an accelerated heart rate without preventing the sympathetic nervous system from causing vasoconstriction, an effect mediated by α_1 adrenoceptors.

The principle of drug selectivity may even apply to structurally identical receptors expressed in different cells, eg, receptors for steroids (see Figure 2–6). Different cell types express different accessory proteins, which interact with steroid receptors and change the functional effects of drug-receptor interaction. For example, tamoxifen is a drug that binds to steroid receptors naturally activated by estrogen. Tamoxifen acts as an *antagonist* on estrogen receptors expressed in mammary tissue but as an *agonist* on estrogen receptors in bone. Consequently, tamoxifen may be useful not only in the treatment of breast cancer but also in the prevention of osteoporosis by increasing bone density (see Chapters 40 and 42). Tamoxifen may create complications in postmenopausal women, however, by exerting an agonist action in the uterus, stimulating endometrial cell proliferation.

New drug development is not confined to agents that act on receptors for extracellular chemical signals. Increasingly, pharmaceutical chemists are determining whether elements of signaling pathways distal to the receptors may also serve as targets of selective and useful drugs. We have already discussed drugs that act on phosphodiesterase and some intracellular kinases. Several new kinase inhibitors and modulators are presently in therapeutic trials, and there has been recent progress in developing inhibitors of GTP-binding transducer proteins that function downstream of tyrosine kinase growth factor receptors. This includes selective inhibitors for an activated form of K-Ras (G12C mutation) that is produced (due to somatic mutation) in many tumors and that causes a pathologic stimulation of growth factor signaling pathways in the absence of upstream receptor activation. These drugs are now used in the therapy of lung cancer.

RELATION BETWEEN DRUG DOSE & CLINICAL RESPONSE

In this chapter, we have dealt with receptors as molecules and shown how receptors can quantitatively account for the relation between dose or concentration of a drug and pharmacologic responses, at least in an idealized system. When faced with a patient who needs treatment, the prescriber must make a choice among a variety of possible drugs and devise a dosage regimen that is likely to produce maximal benefit and minimal toxicity. To make rational therapeutic decisions, the prescriber must understand how drug-receptor interactions underlie the relations between dose and response in patients, the nature and causes of variation in pharmacologic responsiveness, and the clinical implications of selectivity of drug action.

Dose & Response in Patients

A. Graded Dose-Response Relations

To choose among drugs and to determine appropriate doses of a drug, the prescriber must know the relative **pharmacologic potency** and **maximal efficacy** of the drugs in relation to the desired therapeutic effect. These two important terms, often confusing to students and clinicians, can be explained by referring to Figure 2–15, which depicts graded dose-response curves that relate the dose of four different drugs to the magnitude of a particular therapeutic effect.

1. *Potency*—Drugs A and B are said to be more potent than drugs C and D because of the relative positions of their dose-response curves along the **dose axis** in Figure 2–15. Potency refers to the concentration (EC_{50}) or dose (ED_{50}) of a drug required to produce 50% of that drug's maximal effect. Thus, the pharmacologic potency of drug A in Figure 2–15 is less than that of drug B, a partial agonist because the EC_{50} of A is greater than the EC_{50} of B. Potency of a drug depends in part on the affinity (K_d) of receptors for binding the drug and in part on the efficiency with which drug-receptor interaction is coupled to response. Note that some doses of drug A can produce larger effects than any dose of drug B, despite the fact that we describe drug B as pharmacologically more potent. The reason for this is that drug A has a larger maximal efficacy (as described below).

For therapeutic purposes, the potency of a drug should be stated in dosage units, usually in terms of a particular therapeutic end point (eg, 50 mg for mild sedation, 1 mcg/kg/min for an increase in heart rate of 25 bpm). Relative potency, the ratio of equi-effective doses (0.2, 10, etc), may be used in comparing one drug with another.

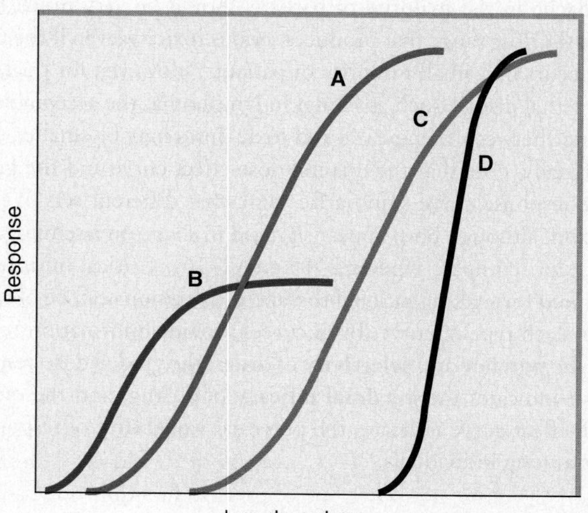

FIGURE 2–15 Graded dose-response curves for four drugs, illustrating different pharmacologic potencies and different maximal efficacies. (See text.)

2. *Maximal efficacy*—This parameter reflects the limit of the dose-response relation on the **response axis.** Drugs A, C, and D in Figure 2–15 have equal maximal efficacy, and all have greater maximal efficacy than drug B. The maximal efficacy (sometimes referred to simply as efficacy) of a drug is obviously crucial for making clinical decisions when a large response is needed. It may be determined by the drug's mode of interactions with receptors (as with partial agonists)* or by characteristics of the receptor-effector system involved.

Thus, diuretics that act on one portion of the nephron may produce much greater excretion of fluid and electrolytes than diuretics that act elsewhere. In addition, the *practical* efficacy of a drug for achieving a therapeutic end point (eg, increased cardiac contractility) may be limited by the drug's propensity to cause a toxic effect (eg, fatal cardiac arrhythmia) even if the drug could otherwise produce a greater therapeutic effect.

B. Shape of Dose-Response Curves

Although the responses depicted in curves A, B, and C of Figure 2–15 approximate the shape of a simple Michaelis–Menten relation (transformed to a logarithmic plot), some clinical responses do not. Extremely steep dose-response curves (eg, curve D) may have important clinical consequences if the upper portion of the curve represents an undesirable extent of response (eg, coma caused by a sedative-hypnotic). Steep dose-response curves in patients can result from cooperative interactions of several different actions of a drug (eg, effects on brain, heart, and peripheral vessels, all contributing to lowering of blood pressure).

*Note that "maximal efficacy," used in a therapeutic context, does not have exactly the same meaning that the term denotes in the more specialized context of drug-receptor interactions described earlier in this chapter. In an idealized in vitro system, efficacy denotes the relative maximal efficacy of agonists and partial agonists that act via the same receptor. In therapeutics, efficacy denotes the extent or degree of an effect that can be achieved in the intact patient. Thus, therapeutic efficacy may be affected by the characteristics of a particular drug-receptor interaction, but it also depends on a host of other factors as noted in the text.

C. Quantal Dose-Effect Curves

Graded dose-response curves of the sort described above have certain limitations in their application to clinical decision making. For example, such curves may be impossible to construct if the pharmacologic response is an either-or (quantal) event, such as prevention of convulsions, arrhythmia, or death. Furthermore, the clinical relevance of a quantitative dose-response relation in a single patient, no matter how precisely defined, may be limited in application to other patients, owing to the great potential variability among patients in severity of disease and responsiveness to drugs.

Some of these difficulties may be avoided by determining the dose of drug required to produce a specified magnitude of effect in a large number of individual patients or experimental animals and plotting the cumulative frequency distribution of responders versus the log dose (Figure 2–16). The specified quantal effect may be chosen on the basis of clinical relevance (eg, relief of headache) or for preservation of safety of experimental subjects (eg, using low doses of a cardiac stimulant and specifying an increase in heart rate of 20 bpm as the quantal effect), or it may be an inherently quantal event (eg, death of an experimental animal). For most drugs, the doses required to produce a specified quantal effect in individuals are lognormally distributed; that is, a frequency distribution of such responses plotted against the log of the dose produces a gaussian normal curve of variation (colored areas; see Figure 2–16). When these responses are summated, the resulting cumulative frequency distribution constitutes a quantal dose-effect curve (or dose-percent curve) of the proportion or percentage of individuals who exhibit the effect plotted as a function of log dose.

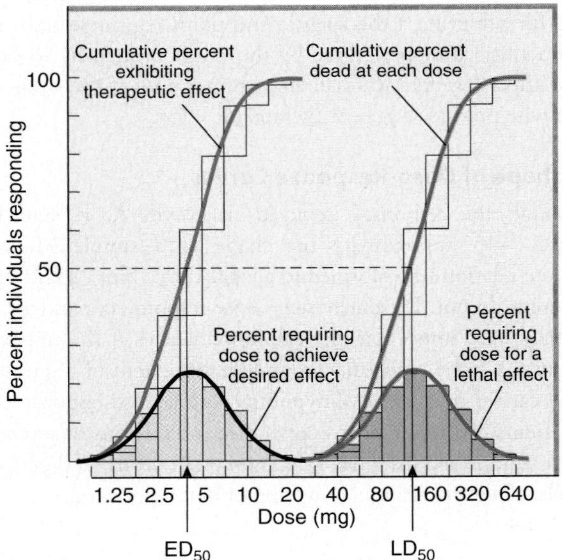

FIGURE 2–16 Quantal dose-effect plots. Shaded boxes (and the accompanying bell-shaped curves) indicate the frequency distribution of doses of drug required to produce a specified effect; that is, the percentage of animals that required a particular dose to exhibit the effect. The open boxes (and the corresponding colored curves) indicate the cumulative frequency distribution of responses, which are lognormally distributed.

The quantal dose-effect curve is often characterized by stating the **median effective dose (ED_{50})**, which is the dose at which 50% of individuals exhibit the specified quantal effect. (Note that the abbreviation ED_{50} has a different meaning in this context from its meaning in relation to graded dose-effect curves, described in previous text.) Similarly, the dose required to produce a particular toxic effect in 50% of animals is called the **median toxic dose (TD_{50}).** If the toxic effect is death of the animal, a **median lethal dose (LD_{50})** may be experimentally defined. Such values provide a convenient way of comparing the potencies of drugs in experimental and clinical settings: Thus, if the ED_{50}s of two drugs for producing a specified quantal effect are 5 and 500 mg, respectively, then the first drug can be said to be 100 times more potent than the second for that particular effect. Similarly, one can obtain a valuable index of the selectivity of a drug's action by comparing its ED_{50}s for two different quantal effects in a population (eg, cough suppression versus sedation for opioid drugs).

Quantal dose-effect curves may also be used to generate information regarding the margin of safety to be expected from a particular drug used to produce a specified effect. One measure, which relates the dose of a drug required to produce a desired effect to that which produces an undesired effect, is the **therapeutic index.** In animal studies, the therapeutic index is usually defined as the ratio of the TD_{50} to the ED_{50} for some therapeutically relevant effect. The precision possible in animal experiments may make it useful to use such a therapeutic index to estimate the potential benefit of a drug in humans. Of course, the therapeutic index of a drug in humans is almost never known with real precision; instead, drug trials and accumulated clinical experience often reveal a range of usually effective doses and a different (but sometimes overlapping) range of possibly toxic doses. The range between the minimum toxic dose and the minimum therapeutic dose is called the **therapeutic window** and is of greater practical value in choosing the dose for a patient. The clinically acceptable risk of toxicity depends critically on the severity of the disease being treated. For example, the dose range that provides relief from an ordinary headache in the majority of patients should be very much lower than the dose range that produces serious toxicity, even if the toxicity occurs in a small minority of patients. However, for treatment of a lethal disease such as Hodgkin lymphoma, the acceptable difference between therapeutic and toxic doses may be smaller.

Finally, note that the quantal dose-effect curve and the graded dose-response curve summarize somewhat different sets of information, although both appear sigmoid in shape on a semilogarithmic plot (compare Figures 2–15 and 2–16). Critical information required for making rational therapeutic decisions can be obtained from each type of curve. Both curves provide information regarding the **potency** and **selectivity** of drugs; the graded dose-response curve indicates the **maximal efficacy** of a drug, and the quantal dose-effect curve indicates the potential **variability** of responsiveness among individuals.

Variation in Drug Responsiveness

Individuals may vary considerably in their response to a drug; indeed, a single individual may respond differently to the same drug at different times during the course of treatment. Occasionally, individuals exhibit an unusual or **idiosyncratic** drug response, one that is infrequently observed in most patients. The idiosyncratic responses are usually caused by genetic differences in metabolism of the drug or by immunologic mechanisms, including allergic reactions.

Quantitative variations in drug response are, in general, more common and more clinically important. An individual patient is **hyporeactive** or **hyperreactive** to a drug in that the intensity of effect of a given dose of drug is diminished or increased compared with the effect seen in most individuals. (*Note:* The term **hypersensitivity** usually refers to allergic or other immunologic responses to drugs.) With some drugs, the intensity of response to a given dose may change during the course of therapy; in these cases, responsiveness usually decreases as a consequence of continued drug administration, producing a state of relative **tolerance** to the drug's effects. When responsiveness diminishes rapidly after administration of a drug, the response is said to be subject to **tachyphylaxis.**

Even before administering the first dose of a drug, the prescriber should consider factors that may help in predicting the direction and extent of possible variations in responsiveness. These include the propensity of a particular drug to produce tolerance or tachyphylaxis as well as the effects of age, sex, body size, disease state, genetic factors, and simultaneous administration of other drugs.

Four general mechanisms may contribute to variation in drug responsiveness among patients or within an individual patient at different times.

A. Alteration in Concentration of Drug That Reaches the Receptor

As described in Chapter 3, patients may differ in the rate of absorption of a drug, in distributing it through body compartments, or in clearing the drug from the blood. By altering the concentration of drug that reaches relevant receptors, such pharmacokinetic differences may alter the clinical response. Some differences can be predicted on the basis of age, weight, sex, disease state, and liver and kidney function, and by testing specifically for genetic differences that may result from inheritance of a functionally distinctive complement of drug-metabolizing enzymes (see Chapters 4 and 5). Another important mechanism influencing drug availability is active transport of drug from the cytoplasm, mediated by a family of membrane transporters encoded by the so-called multidrug resistance (*MDR*) genes. For example, up-regulation of *MDR* gene-encoded transporter expression is a major mechanism by which tumor cells develop resistance to anticancer drugs.

B. Variation in Concentration of an Endogenous Receptor Ligand

This mechanism contributes greatly to variability in responses to pharmacologic antagonists. Thus, propranolol, a β-adrenoceptor antagonist, markedly slows the heart rate of a patient whose endogenous catecholamines are elevated (as in pheochromocytoma) but does not affect the resting heart rate of a well-trained marathon runner. A partial agonist may exhibit even more dramatically different responses: Saralasin, a weak partial agonist at angiotensin II receptors, lowers blood pressure in patients with hypertension caused by increased angiotensin II production and raises blood pressure in patients who produce normal amounts of angiotensin.

C. Alterations in Number or Function of Receptors

Experimental studies have documented changes in drug response caused by increases or decreases in the number of receptor sites or by alterations in the efficiency of coupling of receptors to distal effector mechanisms. In some cases, the change in receptor number is caused by other hormones; for example, thyroid hormones increase both the number of β adrenoceptors in rat heart muscle and cardiac sensitivity to catecholamines. Similar changes probably contribute to the tachycardia of thyrotoxicosis in patients and may account for the usefulness of propranolol, a β-adrenoceptor antagonist, in ameliorating symptoms of this disease.

In other cases, the agonist ligand itself induces a decrease in the number (eg, downregulation) or coupling efficiency (eg, desensitization) of its receptors. These mechanisms (discussed previously under Signaling Mechanisms & Drug Action) may contribute to two clinically important phenomena: first, tachyphylaxis or tolerance to the effects of some drugs (eg, biogenic amines and their congeners), and second, the "overshoot" phenomena that follow withdrawal of certain drugs. These phenomena can occur with either agonists or antagonists. An antagonist may increase the number of receptors in a critical cell or tissue by preventing downregulation caused by an endogenous agonist. When the antagonist is withdrawn, the elevated number of receptors can produce an exaggerated response to physiologic concentrations of agonist. Potentially disastrous withdrawal symptoms can result for the opposite reason when administration of an agonist drug is discontinued. In this situation, the number of receptors, which has been decreased by drug-induced downregulation, is too low for endogenous agonist to produce effective stimulation. For example, the withdrawal of clonidine (a drug whose α_2-adrenoceptor agonist activity reduces blood pressure) can produce hypertensive crisis, probably because the drug down-regulates α_2 adrenoceptors (see Chapter 11).

The study of genetic factors determining drug response is called **pharmacogenetics,** and the use of gene sequencing or expression profile data to tailor therapies specific to an individual patient is called **personalized** or **precision medicine.** For example, somatic mutations affecting the tyrosine kinase domain of the epidermal growth factor receptor in lung cancers can confer enhanced sensitivity to kinase inhibitors such as gefitinib. This effect enhances the antineoplastic effect of the drug, and because the somatic mutation is specific to the tumor and not present in the host, the therapeutic index of these drugs can be significantly enhanced in patients whose tumors harbor such mutations. Genetic analysis can also predict drug resistance during treatment or identify new targets for therapy based on rapid mutation of the tumor in the patient.

D. Changes in Components of Response Distal to the Receptor

Although a drug initiates its actions by binding to receptors, the response observed in a patient depends on the functional integrity of biochemical processes in the responding cell and physiologic regulation by interacting organ systems. Clinically, changes in these postreceptor processes represent the largest and most important class of mechanisms that cause variation in responsiveness to drug therapy.

Before initiating therapy with a drug, the prescriber should be aware of patient characteristics that may limit the clinical response. These characteristics include the age and general health of the patient and—most importantly—the severity and pathophysiologic mechanism of the disease. The most important potential cause of failure to achieve a satisfactory response is that the diagnosis is wrong or physiologically incomplete. Drug therapy is most successful when it is accurately directed at the pathophysiologic mechanism responsible for the disease.

When the diagnosis is correct and the drug is appropriate, an unsatisfactory therapeutic response can often be traced to compensatory mechanisms in the patient that respond to and oppose the beneficial effects of the drug. Compensatory increases in sympathetic nervous tone and fluid retention by the kidney, for example, can contribute to tolerance to antihypertensive effects of a vasodilator drug. In such cases, additional drugs may be required to achieve a useful therapeutic result.

Clinical Selectivity: Beneficial Versus Toxic Effects of Drugs

Although we classify drugs according to their principal actions, it is clear that *no drug causes only a single, specific effect.* Why is this so? It is exceedingly unlikely that any kind of drug molecule will bind to only a single type of receptor molecule, if only because the number of potential receptors in every patient is astronomically large. Even if the chemical structure of a drug allowed it to bind to only one kind of receptor, the biochemical processes controlled by such receptors would take place in many cell types and would be coupled to many other biochemical functions; as a result, the patient and the prescriber would probably perceive more than one drug effect. Accordingly, drugs are only *selective*—rather than specific—in their actions, because they bind to one or a few types of receptor more tightly than to others and because these receptors control discrete processes that result in distinct effects.

It is only because of their selectivity that drugs are useful in clinical medicine. Selectivity can be measured by comparing binding affinities of a drug to different receptors or by comparing ED_{50}s for different effects of a drug in vivo. In drug development and in clinical medicine, selectivity is usually considered by separating effects into two categories: **beneficial** or **therapeutic effects** versus **toxic** or **adverse effects.** Pharmaceutical advertisements and prescribers occasionally use the term **side effect,** implying that the effect in question is insignificant or occurs via a pathway that is to one side of the principal action of the drug; such implications are frequently erroneous.

A. Beneficial and Toxic Effects Mediated by the Same Receptor-Effector Mechanism

Much of the serious drug toxicity in clinical practice represents a direct pharmacologic extension of the therapeutic actions of the drug. In some of these cases (eg, bleeding caused by anticoagulant therapy; hypoglycemic coma due to insulin), toxicity may be avoided by judicious management of the dose of drug administered, guided by careful monitoring of effect (measurements of blood coagulation or serum glucose) and aided by ancillary measures (avoiding tissue trauma that may lead to hemorrhage; regulation of carbohydrate intake). In still other cases, the toxicity may be avoided by not administering the drug at all, if the therapeutic indication is weak or if other therapy is available.

In certain situations, a drug is clearly necessary and beneficial but produces unacceptable toxicity when given in doses that produce optimal benefit. In such situations, it may be necessary to add another drug to the treatment regimen. In treating hypertension, for example, administration of a second drug often allows the prescriber to reduce the dose and toxicity of the first drug (see Chapter 11).

B. Beneficial and Toxic Effects Mediated by Identical Receptors but in Different Tissues or by Different Effector Pathways

Many drugs produce both their desired effects and adverse effects by acting on a single receptor type in different tissues. Examples discussed in this book include digitalis glycosides, which act by inhibiting Na^+/K^+-ATPase in cell membranes; methotrexate, which inhibits the enzyme dihydrofolate reductase; and glucocorticoid hormones.

Three therapeutic strategies are used to avoid or mitigate this sort of toxicity. First, the drug should always be administered at the lowest dose that produces acceptable benefit. Second, adjunctive drugs that act through different receptor mechanisms and produce different toxicities may allow lowering the dose of the first drug, thus limiting its toxicity (eg, use of other immunosuppressive agents added to glucocorticoids in treating inflammatory disorders). Third, selectivity of the drug's actions may be increased by manipulating the concentrations of drug available to receptors in different parts of the body, for example, by aerosol administration of a glucocorticoid to the bronchi in asthma.

C. Beneficial and Toxic Effects Mediated by Different Types of Receptors

Therapeutic advantages resulting from new chemical entities with improved receptor selectivity were mentioned earlier in this chapter and are described in detail in later chapters. Many receptors, such as those for catecholamines, histamine, acetylcholine, and corticosteroids, and their associated therapeutic uses were discovered by analyzing effects of the physiologic chemical signals. This approach continues to be fruitful. For example, microRNAs (miRNAs), small RNAs that regulate protein expression by binding to protein-coding (messenger) RNAs, were linked recently to Duchenne muscular dystrophy. Current preclinical investigations include the potential utility of RNA-based therapy for this and other diseases.

Other drugs were discovered by exploiting therapeutic or toxic effects of chemically similar agents observed in a clinical context. Examples include quinidine, the sulfonylureas, thiazide diuretics, tricyclic antidepressants, opioid drugs, and phenothiazine antipsychotics. Often such agents turn out to interact with receptors for endogenous substances (eg, opioids and phenothiazines for endogenous opioid and dopamine receptors, respectively). This approach is evolving toward understanding the structural details of how chemically similar agents differ in binding to receptors. For example, x-ray crystallography of β_1 and β_2 adrenoceptors shows that their orthosteric binding sites are identical; drugs discriminate between subtypes based on differences in traversing a divergent "vestibule" to access the orthosteric site. Many GPCRs have such passages, revealing a new basis for improving the selectivity of GPCR-targeted drugs.

Thus, the propensity of drugs to bind to different classes of receptor sites is not only a potentially vexing problem in treating patients, but it also presents a continuing challenge to pharmacology and an opportunity for developing new and more useful drugs.

REFERENCES

Brodlie M et al: Targeted therapies to improve CFTR function in cystic fibrosis. Genome Med 2015;7:101.

Catterall WA, Lenaeus MJ, Gamal El-Din TM: Structure and pharmacology of voltage-gated sodium and calcium channels. Ann Rev Pharmacol Toxicol 2020;60:133.

Chen Q, Tesmer JJG: G protein-coupled receptor interactions with arrestins and GPCR kinases: the unresolved issue of signal bias. J Biol Chem 2022;298:102279.

Dang CV et al: Drugging the 'undruggable' cancer targets. Nat Rev Cancer 2017;17:502.

Gouaux E, MacKinnon R: Principles of selective ion transport in channels and pumps. Science 2005;310:1461.

Hilger D et al: Structure and dynamics of GPCR signaling complexes. Nat Struct Mol Biol 2018;25:4.

Irwin JJ, Shoichet BK: Docking screens for novel ligands conferring new biology. J Med Chem 2016;59:4103.

Kenakin T: Biased receptor signaling in drug discovery. Pharmacol Rev 2019;71:267.

Kovacs E et al: A structural perspective on the regulation of the epidermal growth factor receptor. Annu Rev Biochem 2015;84:739.

Sprang SR: Activation of G proteins by GTP and the mechanism of Gα-catalyzed GTP hydrolysis. Biopolymers 2016;105:449.

Terrar DA: Calcium signaling in the heart. Adv Exp Med Biol 2020;1131:395.

Von Zastrow M, Sorkin A: Mechanisms for regulating and organizing receptor signaling by endocytosis. Annu Rev Biochem 2021;90:709.

CASE STUDY ANSWER

Propranolol, a β-adrenoceptor antagonist, is a useful antihypertensive agent because it reduces cardiac output and probably vascular resistance as well. However, it also prevents β-adrenoceptor–induced bronchodilation and therefore may precipitate bronchoconstriction in susceptible individuals. Calcium channel blockers such as verapamil also reduce blood pressure but, because they act on a different target, rarely cause bronchoconstriction or prevent bronchodilation. An alternative approach in this patient would be to use a more highly selective adrenoceptor antagonist drug (such as metoprolol) that binds preferentially to the β_1 subtype, which is a major β adrenoceptor in the heart, and has a lower affinity (ie, higher K_d) for binding the β_2 subtype that mediates bronchodilation. Selection of the most appropriate drug or drug group for one condition requires awareness of the other conditions a patient may have and the receptor selectivity of the drug groups available.

CHAPTER

3 Pharmacokinetics & Pharmacodynamics: Rational Dosing & the Time Course of Drug Action

Nicholas H. G. Holford, MB, ChB, FRACP

CASE STUDY

An 85-year-old, 60-kg woman with a serum creatinine of 1.8 mg/dL has atrial fibrillation. A decision has been made to use digoxin to control the rapid heart rate. The target concentration of digoxin for the treatment of atrial fibrillation is 1 mg/mL. Tablets of digoxin are available that contain 62.5 micrograms (mcg) and 250 mcg. What maintenance dose would you recommend?

The goal of therapeutics is to achieve a desired beneficial effect with minimal adverse effects. When a medicine has been selected for a patient, the clinician must determine the dose that most closely achieves this goal. A rational approach to this objective combines the principles of pharmacokinetics with pharmacodynamics to understand the dose-effect relationship (Figure 3–1). Pharmacodynamics governs the concentration-effect part of the relationship, whereas pharmacokinetics deals with the dose-concentration part (Holford & Sheiner, 1981). The pharmacodynamic concepts of maximum response and sensitivity determine the magnitude of the effect at a particular concentration (see E_{max} and C_{50}, Chapter 2; C_{50} is also known as EC_{50}). The pharmacokinetic processes of input, distribution, and elimination determine how rapidly and for how long the target organ will be exposed to the drug.

Figure 3–1 illustrates a fundamental hypothesis of pharmacology, namely, that a relationship exists between a beneficial or toxic effect of a drug and the concentration of the drug. This hypothesis has been documented for many drugs, as indicated by the target concentration column in Table 3–1. The target concentration is the concentration that reflects a balance between the beneficial and adverse effects. The apparent lack of such a relationship for some drugs does not weaken the basic hypothesis but points to the need to consider the time course of concentration at the actual site of pharmacologic effect (see below).

Knowing the relationship between dose, drug concentration, and effects allows the clinician to take into account the various pathologic and physiologic features of a particular patient that make him or her different from the average individual in responding to a drug. The importance of pharmacokinetics and pharmacodynamics in patient care thus rests upon the improvement in therapeutic benefit and reduction in toxicity that can be achieved by application of these principles.

PHARMACOKINETICS

The "standard" dose of a drug is based on trials in healthy subjects and patients with average ability to absorb, distribute, and eliminate the drug (see section Clinical Trials: The IND & NDA in Chapter 1).

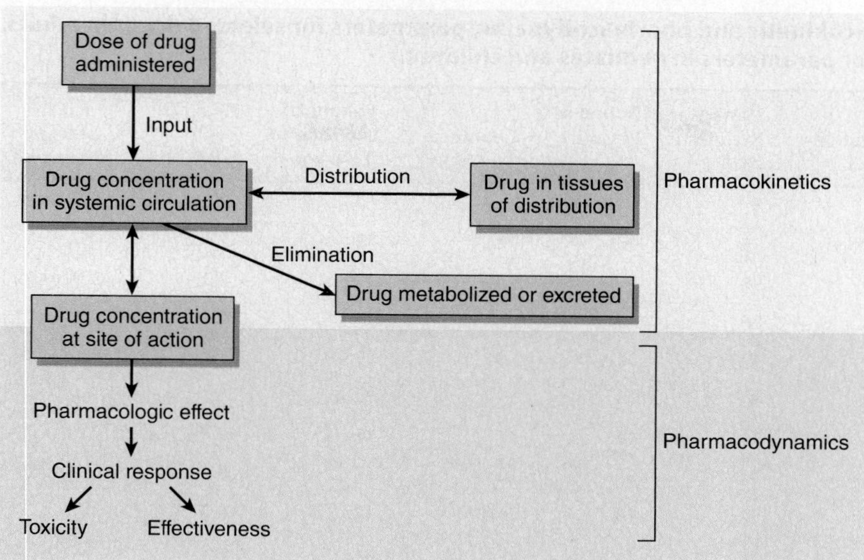

FIGURE 3–1 The relationship between dose and effect can be separated into pharmacokinetic (dose-concentration) and pharmacodynamic (concentration-effect) components. Concentration provides the link between pharmacokinetics and pharmacodynamics and is the focus of the target concentration approach to rational dosing. The three primary processes of pharmacokinetics are input, distribution, and elimination.

This dose will not be suitable for every patient. Several physiologic processes (eg, body size, maturation of organ function in neonates and infants) and pathologic processes (eg, heart failure, renal failure) may be used for dosage adjustment in individual patients. Individual differences in these physiological and pathological processes are associated with specific pharmacokinetic and pharmacodynamic properties (usually referred to as parameters) of the drug. The two basic pharmacokinetic parameters are **volume of distribution,** the measure of the apparent space in the body available to contain the drug, and **clearance,** the measure of the ability of the body to eliminate the drug. These parameters are illustrated schematically in Figure 3–2, where the volume of the beakers into which the drugs diffuse represents the volume of distribution, and the size of the outflow "drain" in Figures 3–2B and 3–2D represents the clearance.

Volume of Distribution

Volume of distribution (V) relates the amount of drug in the body to the concentration of drug (C) in blood or plasma:

$$V = \frac{\text{Amount of drug in body}}{C} \tag{1}$$

The volume of distribution may be defined with respect to blood, plasma, or water (unbound drug), depending on the concentration used in equation (1) ($C = C_b$, C_p, or C_u).

That the V calculated from equation (1) is an *apparent* volume may be appreciated by comparing the volumes of distribution of drugs such as digoxin or chloroquine (see Table 3–1) with some of the physical volumes of the body (Table 3–2). Volume of distribution often exceeds any physical volume in the body because it is the volume *apparently* necessary to contain the amount of drug *homogeneously* at the concentration found in the blood, plasma, or water. Drugs with very high volumes of distribution have much higher concentrations in extravascular tissue than in the vascular compartment, ie, they are *not* homogeneously distributed. Drugs that are completely retained within the vascular compartment, on the other hand, would have a minimum possible volume of distribution equal to the plasma component in which they are distributed, eg, 0.04 L/kg body weight or 2.8 L/70 kg (see Table 3–2) for a drug that is restricted to the plasma compartment.

Clearance

Drug clearance concepts are similar to clearance concepts of renal physiology. Clearance of a drug is the factor that predicts the rate of elimination in relation to the drug concentration (C):

$$CL = \frac{\text{Rate of elimination}}{C} \tag{2}$$

Clearance, like volume of distribution, may be defined with respect to blood (CL_b), plasma (CL_p), or unbound in water (CL_u), depending on where and how the concentration is measured.

It is important to note the additive character of clearance. Elimination of drug from the body may involve processes occurring in the kidney, the lung, the liver, and other organs. Dividing the rate of elimination at each organ by the concentration of drug yields

TABLE 3–1 Pharmacokinetic and pharmacodynamic parameters for selected drugs in adults. (See Holford et al, 2013, for parameters in neonates and children.)

Drug	Oral Availability (F) (%)	Urinary Excretion (%)[1]	Bound in Plasma (%)	Clearance (L/h/70 kg)[2]	Volume of Distribution (L/70 kg)	Half-Life (h)	Target Concentration	Toxic Concentration
Acetaminophen	88	3	0	21	67	2	15 mg/L	>300 mg/L
Acyclovir	23	75	15	19.8	48	2.4	…	…
Amikacin	…	98	4	5.46	19	2.3	10 mg/L[3]…	…
Amoxicillin	93	86	18	10.8	15	1.7	…	…
Amphotericin	…	4	90	1.92	53	18	…	…
Ampicillin	62	82	18	16.2	20	1.3	…	…
Aspirin	68	1	49	39	11	0.25	…	…
Atenolol	56	94	5	10.2	67	6.1	1 mg/L	…
Atropine	50	57	18	24.6	120	4.3	…	…
Captopril	65	38	30	50.4	57	2.2	50 ng/mL	…
Carbamazepine	70	1	74	5.34	98	15	6 mg/L	>9 mg/L
Cephalexin	90	91	14	18	18	0.9	…	…
Cephalothin	…	52	71	28.2	18	0.57	…	…
Chloramphenicol	80	25	53	10.2	66	2.7	…	…
Chlordiazepoxide	100	1	97	2.28	21	10	1 mg/L	…
Chloroquine	89	61	61	45	13,000	214	20 ng/mL	250 ng/mL
Chlorpropamide	90	20	96	0.126	6.8	33	…	…
Cimetidine	62	62	19	32.4	70	1.9	0.8 mg/L	…
Ciprofloxacin	60	65	40	25.2	130	4.1	…	…
Clonidine	95	62	20	12.6	150	12	1 ng/mL	…
Cyclosporine	30	1	98	23.9	244	15	200 ng/mL	>400 ng/mL
Diazepam	100	1	99	1.62	77	43	300 ng/mL	…
Digoxin	70	67	25	9	500	39	1 ng/mL	>2 ng/mL
Diltiazem	44	4	78	50.4	220	3.7	…	…
Disopyramide	83	55	2	5.04	41	6	3 mg/mL	>8 mg/mL
Enalapril	95	90	55	9	40	3	>0.5 ng/mL	…
Erythromycin	35	12	84	38.4	55	1.6	…	…
Ethambutol	77	79	5	36	110	3.1	…	>10 mg/L
Fluoxetine	60	3	94	40.2	2500	53	…	…
Furosemide	61	66	99	8.4	7.7	1.5	…	>25 mg/L
Gentamicin	…	76	10	4.7	20	3	3 mg/L[3]	…
Hydralazine	40	10	87	234	105	1	100 ng/mL	…
Imipramine	40	2	90	63	1600	18	200 ng/mL	>1 mg/L
Indomethacin	98	15	90	8.4	18	2.4	1 mg/L	>5 mg/L
Labetalol	18	5	50	105	660	4.9	0.1 mg/L	…
Lidocaine	35	2	70	38.4	77	1.8	3 mg/L	>6 mg/L
Lithium	100	95	0	1.5	55	22	0.7 mEq/L	>2 mEq/L
Meperidine	52	12	58	72	310	3.2	0.5 mg/L	…

(continued)

TABLE 3–1 Pharmacokinetic and pharmacodynamic parameters for selected drugs in adults. (See Holford et al, 2013, for parameters in neonates and children.) (Continued)

Drug	Oral Availability (F) (%)	Urinary Excretion (%)[1]	Bound in Plasma (%)	Clearance (L/h/70 kg)[2]	Volume of Distribution (L/70 kg)	Half-Life (h)	Target Concentration	Toxic Concentration
Methotrexate	70	48	34	9	39	7.2	750 μM-h[4,5]	>950 μM-h
Metoprolol	38	10	11	63	290	3.2	25 ng/mL	…
Metronidazole	99	10	10	5.4	52	8.5	4 mg/L	…
Midazolam	44	56	95	27.6	77	1.9	…	…
Morphine	24	8	35	60	230	1.9	15 ng/mL	…
Nifedipine	50	0	96	29.4	55	1.8	50 ng/mL	…
Nortriptyline	51	2	92	30	1300	31	100 ng/mL	>500 ng/mL
Phenobarbital	100	24	51	0.258	38	98	15 mg/L	>30 mg/L
Phenytoin	90	2	89	Conc dependent[5]	45	Conc dependent[6]	10 mg/L	>20 mg/L
Prazosin	68	1	95	12.6	42	2.9	…	…
Procainamide	83	67	16	36	130	3	5 mg/L	>14 mg/L
Propranolol	26	1	87	50.4	270	3.9	20 ng/mL	…
Pyridostigmine	14	85	…	36	77	1.9	75 ng/mL	…
Quinidine	80	18	87	19.8	190	6.2	3 mg/L	>8 mg/L
Ranitidine	52	69	15	43.8	91	2.1	100 ng/mL	…
Rifampin	?	7	89	14.4	68	3.5	…	…
Salicylic acid	100	15	85	0.84	12	13	200 mg/L	>200 mg/L
Sulfamethoxazole	100	14	62	1.32	15	10	…	…
Tacrolimus	20	…	98[7]	3[8]	133[8]	28	10 mcg/L	…
Terbutaline	14	56	20	14.4	125	14	2 ng/mL	…
Tetracycline	77	58	65	7.2	105	11	…	…
Theophylline	96	18	56	2.8	35	8.1	10 mg/L	>20 mg/L
Tobramycin	…	90	10	4.62	18	2.2	…	…
Tocainide	89	38	10	10.8	210	14	10 mg/L	…
Tolbutamide	93	0	96	1.02	7	5.9	100 mg/L	…
Trimethoprim	100	69	44	9	130	11	…	…
Tubocurarine	…	63	50	8.1	27	2	0.6 mg/L	…
Valproic acid	100	2	93	0.462	9.1	14	75 mg/L	>150 mg/L
Vancomycin	…	79	30	5.88	27	5.6	20 mg/L[3]	…
Verapamil	22	3	90	63	350	4	…	…
Warfarin	93	3	99	0.192	9.8	37	…	…
Zidovudine	63	18	25	61.8	98	1.1	…	…

[1]Assuming creatinine clearance 100 mL/min/70 kg.

[2]Convert to mL/min by multiplying the number given by 16.6.

[3]Average steady-state concentration.

[4]Target area under the concentration-time curve after a single dose.

[5]Can be estimated from measured C using $CL = V_{max}/(K_m + C)$; $V_{max} = 415$ mg/d, $K_m = 5$ mg/L. See text.

[6]Varies because of concentration-dependent clearance.

[7]Bound in whole blood (%).

[8]Based on whole blood standardized to hematocrit 45%.

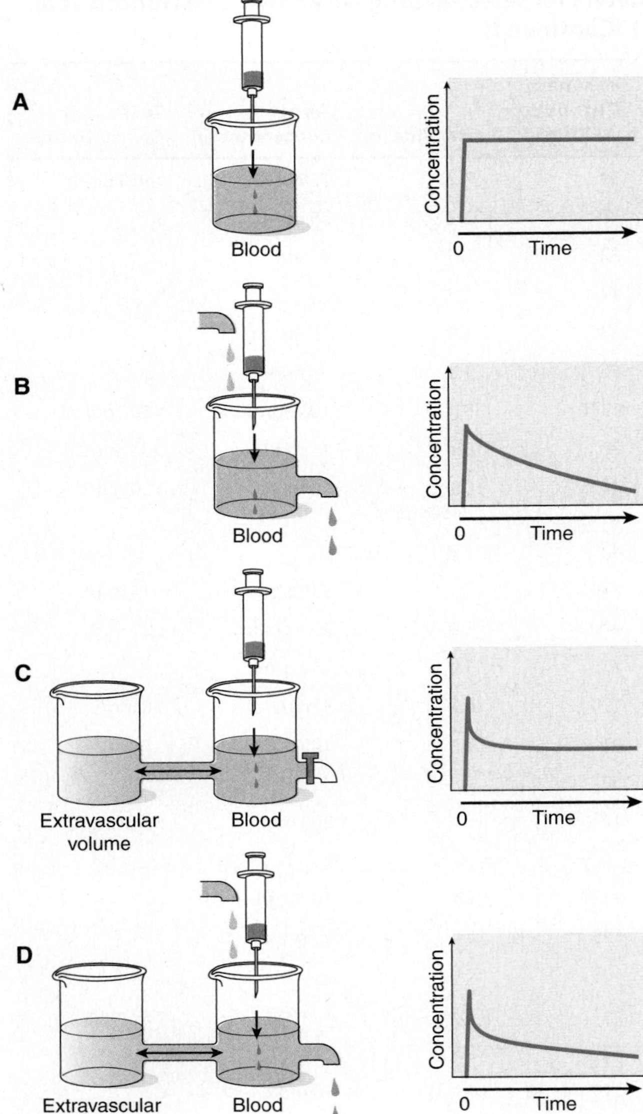

FIGURE 3–2 Models of drug distribution and elimination. The effect of adding drug to the blood by rapid intravenous injection is represented by injecting a known amount of the agent into a beaker. The time course of the amount of drug in the beaker is shown in the graphs at the right. In the first example (**A**), there is no movement of drug out of the beaker, so the graph shows only a steep rise to a maximum followed by a plateau. In the second example (**B**), a route of elimination is present, and the graph shows a slow decay after a sharp rise to a maximum. Because the amount of agent in the beaker falls, the "pressure" driving the elimination process also falls, and the slope of the curve decreases. This is an exponential decay curve. In the third model (**C**), drug placed in the first compartment ("blood") equilibrates rapidly with the second compartment ("extravascular volume") and the amount of drug in "blood" declines exponentially to a new steady state. The fourth model (**D**) illustrates a more realistic combination of elimination mechanism and extravascular equilibration. The resulting graph shows an early distribution phase followed by the slower elimination phase. Note that the volume of fluid remains constant because of a fluid input at the same rate as elimination in (**B**) and (**D**).

TABLE 3–2 Physical volumes (in L/kg body weight) of some body compartments into which drugs may be distributed.

Compartment and Volume	Examples of Drugs
Water	
Total body water (0.6 L/kg[1])	Small water-soluble molecules: eg, ethanol
Extracellular water (0.2 L/kg)	Larger water-soluble molecules: eg, gentamicin
Plasma (0.04 L/kg)	Large protein molecules: eg, antibodies
Fat (0.2–0.35 L/kg)	Highly lipid-soluble molecules: eg, diazepam
Bone (0.07 L/kg)	Certain ions: eg, lead, fluoride

[1]An average figure. Total body water in a young lean person might be 0.7 L/kg; in an obese person, 0.5 L/kg.

the respective clearance at that organ. Added together, these separate clearances equal total systemic clearance:

$$CL_{kidney} = \frac{\text{Rate of elimination}_{kidney}}{C} \tag{3a}$$

$$CL_{liver} = \frac{\text{Rate of elimination}_{liver}}{C} \tag{3b}$$

$$CL_{other} = \frac{\text{Rate of elimination}_{other}}{C} \tag{3c}$$

$$CL_{systemic} = CL_{kidney} + CL_{liver} + CL_{other} \tag{3d}$$

"Other" tissues of elimination could include the lungs and additional sites of metabolism, eg, blood or muscle.

The two major sites of drug elimination are the kidneys and the liver. Measurement of unchanged drug in the urine may be used to determine renal clearance. Within the liver, drug elimination occurs via biotransformation of parent drug to one or more metabolites, or excretion of unchanged drug into the bile, or both. Elimination of drug by the liver is difficult to measure directly, unlike renal elimination, so hepatic clearance is often assumed to be the difference between total systemic clearance and renal clearance. The pathways of biotransformation are discussed in Chapter 4. For most drugs, clearance is constant over the concentration range encountered in clinical settings, ie, elimination is not saturable, and the rate of drug elimination is directly proportional to concentration (rearranging equation [2]):

$$\text{Rate of elimination} = CL \times C \tag{4}$$

When elimination is directly proportional to C, this is called first-order elimination. When clearance is first-order, it can be estimated by calculating the **area under the curve (AUC)** of the time-concentration profile after a dose. Clearance is calculated from the dose divided by the AUC. Note that this is a convenient form of calculation—not the definition of clearance.

A. Capacity-Limited Elimination

For drugs that exhibit capacity-limited elimination (eg, phenytoin, ethanol), clearance does not remain constant but will vary depending on the concentration of drug that is achieved (see Table 3–1). Capacity-limited elimination is also known as mixed-order, saturable, nonlinear, and Michaelis-Menten elimination. It is associated with dose- or concentration-dependent clearance.

Most drug elimination pathways by metabolism will become saturated if the dose and therefore the concentration are high enough. When blood flow to an organ does not limit elimination (see below), the relation between elimination rate and concentration (C) is expressed mathematically in equation (5):

$$\text{Rate of elimination} = \frac{V_{max} \times C}{K_m + C} \qquad (5)$$

The maximum elimination capacity is V_{max}, and K_m is the drug concentration at which the rate of elimination is 50% of V_{max}. At concentrations that are high relative to the K_m, the elimination rate is almost independent of concentration—a state of "pseudo-zero order" elimination. If dosing rate exceeds elimination capacity, steady state cannot be achieved. The concentration will keep on rising as long as dosing continues. This pattern of capacity-limited elimination is important for three drugs in common use: ethanol, phenytoin, and aspirin. Clearance has no real meaning for drugs with capacity-limited elimination because it varies with concentration, and AUC should not be used to calculate clearance of such drugs.

B. Flow-Dependent Elimination

In contrast to capacity-limited drug elimination, some drugs are cleared very readily by the organ of elimination, so that at any clinically realistic concentration of the drug, most of the drug in the blood perfusing the organ is eliminated on the first pass of the drug through the organ. The elimination of these drugs will thus depend primarily on the rate of drug delivery to the organ of elimination. Such drugs (see Table 4–7) can be called "high-extraction" drugs since they are almost completely extracted from the blood by the organ. Blood flow to the organ is the main determinant of drug delivery, but plasma protein binding and blood cell partitioning may also be important for extensively bound drugs that are highly extracted.

C. Large Molecules

There are two aspects to the pharmacokinetics of proteins, often referred to as large molecules, when used as therapeutic agents. The first is that they all have much the same pharmacokinetics with a half-life of a couple of weeks. The second is that for some, but not all, the effect of the molecule is produced by binding to the target site. Elimination of the molecule is to some extent determined by the elimination of the target (eg, T cells). This is called target-mediated drug disposition. When target-mediated disposition occurs, the clearance of the molecule is increased and the half-life gets shorter. The time course of the effect of the molecule often follows the resulting changes in the time course of drug concentration.

Half-Life

Half-life ($t_{1/2}$) is the time required to change the amount of drug in the body by one-half during elimination (or during a constant infusion). In the simplest case—and the most useful in designing drug dosage regimens—the body may be considered as a single compartment (as illustrated in Figure 3–2B) of a size equal to the volume of distribution (V). The time course of drug in the body will depend on both the volume of distribution and the clearance:

$$t_{1/2} = \frac{0.7 \times V}{CL} \qquad (6)$$

Because drug elimination can be described by an exponential process, the time taken for a twofold decrease can be shown to be proportional to the natural logarithm of 2. The constant 0.7 in equation (6) is an approximation to the natural logarithm of 2.

The elimination half-life is useful because it indicates the time required to attain 50% of steady state—or to decay 50% from steady-state conditions—after a change in the rate of drug input. Figure 3–3 shows the time course of drug accumulation during a constant-rate drug infusion and the time course of drug elimination after stopping an infusion that has reached steady state.

Disease states can affect both of the physiologically related primary pharmacokinetic parameters: volume of distribution and clearance. A change in elimination half-life will not necessarily reflect a change in drug elimination. For example, patients with chronic renal failure have both decreased renal clearance of digoxin and a decreased volume of distribution; the increase in digoxin elimination half-life is not as great as might be expected based on the change in renal function. The decrease in volume of distribution is due to the decreased renal and skeletal muscle mass and consequent decreased tissue binding of digoxin to Na^+/K^+-ATPase.

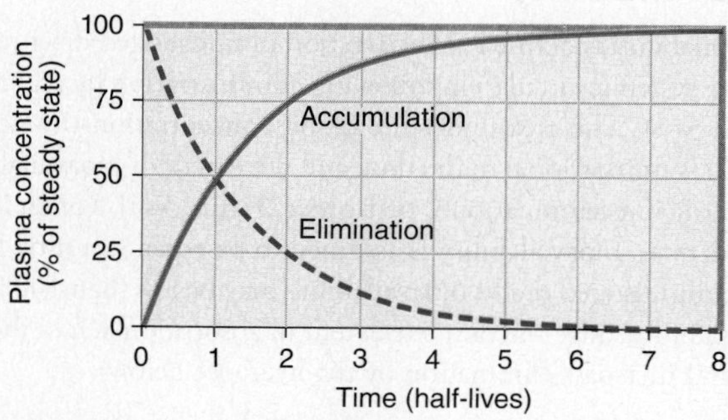

FIGURE 3–3 The time course of drug accumulation and elimination. **Solid line:** Plasma concentrations reflecting drug accumulation during a constant-rate infusion of a drug. Fifty percent of the steady-state concentration is reached after one half-life, 75% after two half-lives, and over 90% after four half-lives. **Dashed line:** Plasma concentrations reflecting drug elimination after a constant-rate infusion of a drug had reached steady state. Fifty percent of the drug is lost after one half-life, 75% after two half-lives, etc. The "rule of thumb" that four half-lives must elapse after starting a drug-dosing regimen before full effects will be seen is based on the approach of the accumulation curve to over 90% of the final steady-state concentration.

Many drugs will exhibit multicompartment pharmacokinetics (as illustrated in Figures 3–2C and 3–2D). Under these conditions, the "half-life" describing drug accumulation, as given in Table 3–1, will be greater than that calculated from equation (6).

Drug Accumulation

Whenever drug doses are repeated, the drug will accumulate in the body until dosing stops. This is because it takes an infinite time (in theory) to eliminate all of a given dose. In practical terms, this means that if the dosing interval is shorter than four half-lives, accumulation will be detectable.

Accumulation is inversely proportional to the fraction of the dose lost in each dosing interval. The fraction lost is 1 minus the fraction remaining just before the next dose. The fraction remaining can be predicted from the dosing interval and the half-life. A convenient index of accumulation is the **accumulation factor:**

$$\text{Accumulation factor} = \frac{1}{\text{Fraction lost in one dosing interval}}$$

$$\text{Accumulation factor} = \frac{1}{1 - \text{Fraction remaining}} \tag{7}$$

$$\text{Accumulation factor} = \frac{1}{1 - e^{-0.7 \times \text{Dosing interval/Half-life}}}$$

For a drug given once every half-life, the accumulation factor is 1/0.5, or 2. The accumulation factor predicts the ratio of the steady-state concentration to that seen at the same time following the first dose. Thus, the peak concentrations after intermittent doses at steady state will be equal to the peak concentration after the first dose multiplied by the accumulation factor.

Bioavailability

Bioavailability is defined as the fraction of unchanged drug reaching the systemic circulation following administration by any route (Table 3–3). The area under the blood concentration-time curve (AUC) is proportional to the dose and the extent of bioavailability for a drug if its elimination is first-order (Figure 3–4). For an intravenous dose, bioavailability is assumed to be equal to unity. For a drug administered orally, bioavailability may be less than 100% for two main reasons—incomplete extent of absorption across the gut wall and first-pass elimination by the liver (see below).

A. Extent of Absorption

After oral administration, a drug may be incompletely absorbed, eg, only 70% of a dose of digoxin reaches the systemic circulation. This is mainly due to lack of absorption from the gut. Other drugs are either too hydrophilic (eg, atenolol) or too lipophilic (eg, acyclovir) to be absorbed easily, and their low bioavailability is also due to incomplete absorption. If too hydrophilic, the drug cannot cross the lipid cell membrane; if too lipophilic, the drug is not soluble enough to cross the water layer adjacent to the cell. Drugs may not be absorbed because of a reverse transporter associated with P-glycoprotein. This process actively pumps drug out of gut wall cells back into the gut lumen. Inhibition of P-glycoprotein and gut wall metabolism, eg, by grapefruit juice, may be associated with substantially increased drug absorption.

TABLE 3–3 Routes of administration, bioavailability, and general characteristics.

Route	Bioavailability (%)	Characteristics
Intravenous (IV)	100 (by definition)	Most rapid onset
Intramuscular (IM)	75 to ≤100	Large volumes often feasible; may be painful
Subcutaneous (SC)	75 to ≤100	Smaller volumes than IM; may be painful
Oral (PO)	5 to <100	Most convenient; first-pass effect may be important
Rectal (PR)	30 to <100	Less first-pass effect than oral
Inhalation	5 to <100	Often very rapid onset
Transdermal	80 to ≤100	Usually very slow absorption; used for lack of first-pass effect; prolonged duration of action

B. First-Pass Elimination

Following absorption across the gut wall, the portal blood delivers the drug to the liver prior to entry into the systemic circulation. A drug can be metabolized in the gut wall (eg, by the CYP3A4

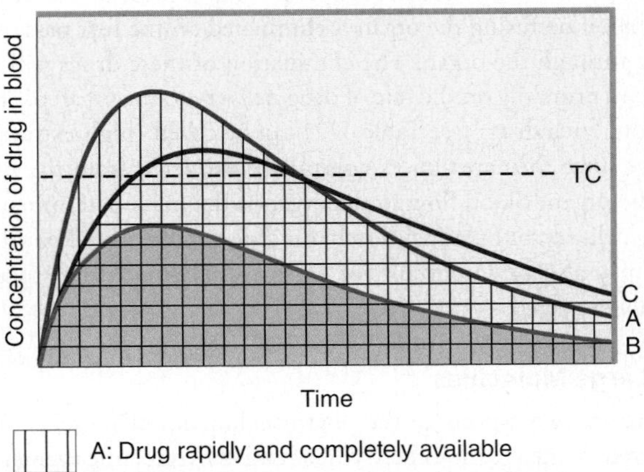

FIGURE 3–4 Blood concentration-time curves illustrating how changes in the rate of absorption and extent of bioavailability can influence both the duration of action and the effectiveness of the same total dose of a drug administered in three different formulations. The dashed line indicates the target concentration (TC) of the drug in the blood.

enzyme system) or even in the portal blood, but most commonly it is the liver that is responsible for metabolism before the drug reaches the systemic circulation. In addition, the liver can excrete the drug into the bile. Any of these sites can contribute to this reduction in bioavailability, and the overall process is known as first-pass elimination. The effect of first-pass hepatic elimination on bioavailability is expressed as the extraction ratio (ER):

$$ER = \frac{CL_{liver}}{Q} \tag{8a}$$

where CL_{liver} is the hepatic blood clearance and Q is hepatic blood flow, normally about 90 L/h in a person weighing 70 kg.

The systemic bioavailability of the drug (F) can be predicted from the extent of absorption (f) and the extraction ratio (ER):

$$F = f \times (1 - ER) \tag{8b}$$

A drug such as morphine is almost completely absorbed (f = 1), so that loss in the gut is negligible. However, the hepatic extraction ratio for morphine is morphine blood clearance (60 L/h/70 kg) divided by hepatic blood flow (90 L/h/70 kg) or 0.67. Its oral bioavailability (1 – ER) is therefore expected to be about 33%, which is close to the observed value (see Table 3–1).

Rate of Absorption

The distinction between rate and extent of absorption is shown in Figure 3–4. The rate of absorption is determined by the site of administration and the drug formulation. Both the rate of absorption and the extent of input can influence the clinical effectiveness of a drug. For the three different dosage forms depicted in Figure 3–4, differences in the intensity of clinical effect are expected. Dosage form B would require twice the dose to attain blood concentrations equivalent to those of dosage form A. Differences in rate of absorption may become important for drugs given as a single dose, such as a hypnotic used to induce sleep. In this case, drug from dosage form A would reach its target concentration earlier than drug from dosage form C; concentrations from A would also reach a higher value and remain above the target concentration for a longer period. In a multiple dosing regimen, dosage forms A and C would yield the same average blood concentrations, although dosage form A would show somewhat greater maximum and lower minimum concentrations.

The mechanism of drug absorption is said to be zero-order when the rate is independent of the amount of drug remaining in the gut, eg, when it is determined by the rate of gastric emptying or by a controlled-release drug formulation. In contrast, when the dose is dissolved in gastrointestinal fluids, the rate of absorption is usually proportional to the gastrointestinal fluid concentration and thus is first-order. The first-order rate of absorption can be described by the absorption half-life. After four absorption half-lives almost all of the dose will have been absorbed.

Extraction Ratio & the First-Pass Effect

Systemic clearance is not affected by bioavailability. However, clearance can markedly affect the extent of availability because it determines the extraction ratio (equation [8a]). Of course, therapeutic blood concentrations may still be reached by the oral route of administration if large enough doses are given. However, in this case, the concentrations of the drug *metabolites* may be increased compared with those that would occur following intravenous administration. Lidocaine and verapamil are both used to treat cardiac arrhythmias and have bioavailability less than 40%, but lidocaine is never given orally because its metabolites are believed to contribute to central nervous system toxicity. Other drugs that are highly extracted by the liver include morphine (see above), isoniazid, propranolol, and several tricyclic antidepressants (see Table 3–1).

Drugs with high extraction ratios will show marked variations in bioavailability between subjects because of differences in hepatic function and blood flow. These differences can explain some of the variation in drug concentrations that occurs among individuals given similar doses. For drugs that are highly extracted by the liver, bypassing hepatic sites of elimination (eg, in hepatic cirrhosis with portosystemic shunting) will result in substantial increases in drug availability, whereas for drugs that are poorly extracted by the liver (for which the difference between entering and exiting drug concentration is small), shunting of blood past the liver will cause little change in availability. Drugs in Table 3–1 that are poorly extracted by the liver include warfarin, diazepam, phenytoin, theophylline, tolbutamide, and chlorpropamide.

Alternative Routes of Administration & the First-Pass Effect

There are several reasons for different routes of administration used in clinical medicine (see Table 3–3)—for convenience (eg, oral), to maximize concentration at the site of action and minimize it elsewhere (eg, topical), to prolong the duration of drug absorption (eg, transdermal), or to avoid the first-pass effect (sublingual or rectal).

The hepatic first-pass effect can be avoided to a great extent by use of sublingual tablets and transdermal preparations and to a lesser extent by use of rectal suppositories. Sublingual absorption provides direct access to systemic—not portal—veins. The transdermal route offers the same advantage. Drugs absorbed from suppositories in the lower rectum enter vessels that drain into the inferior vena cava, thus bypassing the liver. However, suppositories tend to move upward in the rectum into a region where veins that lead to the liver predominate. Thus, only about 50% of a rectal dose can be assumed to bypass the liver.

Although drugs administered by inhalation bypass the hepatic first-pass effect, the lung may also serve as a site of first-pass loss by excretion and possibly metabolism for drugs administered by nongastrointestinal ("parenteral") routes.

THE TIME COURSE OF DRUG EFFECT

The principles of pharmacokinetics (discussed in this chapter) and those of pharmacodynamics (discussed in Chapter 2 and Holford & Sheiner, 1981) provide a framework for understanding the time course of drug effect.

Immediate Effects

In the simplest case, drug effects are immediately related to plasma concentrations, but this does not necessarily mean that effects simply parallel the time course of concentrations. Because the relationship between drug concentration and effect is not linear (recall the E_{max} model described in Chapter 2), the effect will not be linearly proportional to the concentration.

Consider the effect of an angiotensin-converting enzyme (ACE) inhibitor, such as enalapril, on ACE. The elimination half-life that explains the time course of ACE inhibition is about 4 hours. Enalapril is usually given once a day, so more than four of these half-lives will elapse from the time of peak concentration to the end of the dosing interval. The concentration of enalapril explaining the effect and the corresponding extent of ACE inhibition with an initial peak concentration of 100 ng/mL are shown in Figure 3–5. The extent of inhibition of ACE is calculated using the E_{max} model, where E_{max}, the maximum extent of inhibition, is 100% and the C_{50}, the concentration of enalapril associated with 50% of maximum effect, is 5 ng/mL.

Note that plasma concentrations of enalapril change by a factor of eight over the first 12 hours (three half-lives), but ACE inhibition has only decreased by about 30%. Because the concentrations over this time are so high in relation to the C_{50}, the effect on ACE is almost constant. After 24 hours (six half-lives), the concentration is about 2% of the initial peak which is just under half of the C_{50}, so ACE is still about 25% inhibited. This explains why a drug with a short half-life can be given once a day and still maintain its effect throughout the day. The key factor is a high initial concentration in relation to the C_{50}. Once-a-day dosing is common for drugs with minimal adverse effects related to peak concentrations

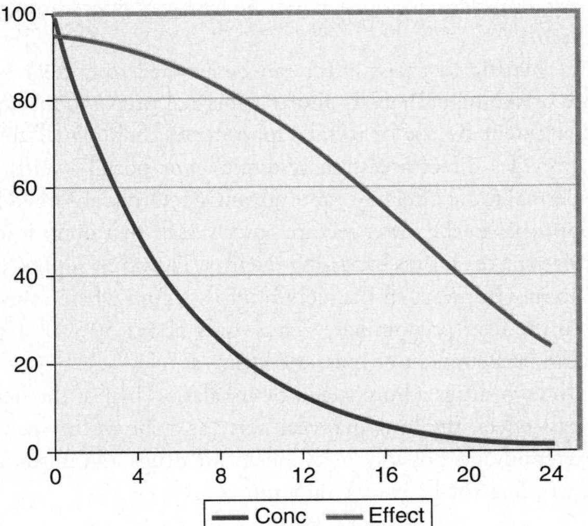

FIGURE 3–5 Time course (hours) of angiotensin-converting enzyme (ACE) inhibitor concentrations and effects. The blue line shows the plasma enalapril concentrations in nanograms per milliliter after a single oral dose. The red line indicates the percentage inhibition of its target, ACE. Note the different shapes of the concentration-time course (exponentially decreasing) and the effect-time course (linearly decreasing in its central portion).

that act on enzymes (eg, ACE inhibitors) or compete at receptors (eg, propranolol).

When concentrations are in the range between four times and one fourth of the C_{50}, the time course of effect is essentially a linear function of time. It takes four half-lives for concentrations to drop from an effect of 80% to 20% of E_{max}—15% of the effect is lost every half-life over this concentration range. At concentrations below one-fourth the C_{50}, the effect becomes almost directly proportional to concentration, and the time course of drug effect will follow the exponential decline of concentration. It is only when the concentration is low in relation to the C_{50} that the concept of a "half-life of drug effect" has any meaning.

Delayed Effects

Changes in drug effects are often delayed in relation to changes in plasma concentration. This delay may reflect the time required for the drug to distribute from plasma to the site of action. This will be the case for almost all drugs. The delay due to distribution is a pharmacokinetic phenomenon that can account for delays of a few minutes. This distributional process can account for the short delay of effects after rapid intravenous injection of central nervous system (CNS)–active agents such as thiopental.

Some drugs bind tightly to receptors, and it is the half-life of dissociation that determines the delay in effect, eg, for digoxin. Note that it is the dissociation process that controls the time to receptor equilibrium. This is exactly the same principle as the elimination process controlling the time to accumulate to steady state with a constant rate infusion (see Figure 3–3).

A common reason for more delayed drug effects—especially those that take many hours or even days to occur—is the slow turnover of a physiologic substance that is involved in the expression of the drug effect. For example, warfarin works as an anticoagulant by inhibiting vitamin K epoxide reductase (VKOR) in the liver. This action of warfarin occurs rapidly, and inhibition of the enzyme is closely related to plasma concentrations of warfarin. The clinical effect of warfarin, eg, on the international normalized ratio (INR), reflects a decrease in the concentration of the prothrombin complex of clotting factors. Inhibition of VKOR decreases the synthesis of these clotting factors, but the complex has a long elimination half-life (about 14 hours), and it is this half-life that determines how long it takes for the concentration of clotting factors to reach a new steady state and for a drug effect to reflect the average warfarin plasma concentration.

Schedule-Dependent Effects

The renal toxicity of aminoglycoside antibiotics (eg, gentamicin) is greater when administered as a constant infusion than with intermittent dosing. Even though both dosing schemes may produce the same average steady-state concentration, the intermittent dosing scheme produces much higher peak concentrations, which saturate an uptake mechanism into the renal cortex; thus, total aminoglycoside accumulation is less. The difference in toxicity is a predictable consequence of the different patterns of concentration and the saturable uptake mechanism. This is an example of schedule dependence of drug effect. It is associated with reversible drug action and a nonlinear relationship between systemic concentration and eventual response.

Cumulative Effects

Some drug effects are more obviously related to a cumulative action than to a rapidly reversible one. The effect of many drugs used to treat cancer also reflects a cumulative action—eg, the extent of binding of a drug to DNA is proportional to drug concentration and is usually irreversible. The effect on tumor growth is therefore a consequence of cumulative exposure to the drug. Measures of cumulative exposure, such as AUC, provide a means to individualize treatment.

THE TARGET CONCENTRATION APPROACH TO DESIGNING A RATIONAL DOSAGE REGIMEN

A rational dosage regimen is based on the assumption that there is a **target concentration** that will produce the desired therapeutic effect. By considering the pharmacokinetic factors that determine the dose-concentration relationship, it is possible to individualize the dose regimen to achieve the target concentration. The target concentrations shown in Table 3–1 are a guide to the concentrations measured when patients are being effectively treated. In some cases, the target concentration will also depend on the specific therapeutic objective—eg, the control of atrial fibrillation by digoxin may require a target concentration of 2 ng/mL, while heart failure is usually adequately managed with a target concentration of 1 ng/mL.

Maintenance Dose

In most clinical situations, drugs are administered in such a way as to maintain a steady state of drug in the body, ie, the amount given with each dose replaces the drug eliminated since the preceding dose. Thus, calculation of the appropriate maintenance dose is a primary goal. Clearance is the most important pharmacokinetic parameter to be considered in defining a rational steady-state drug dosage regimen. At steady state, the dosing rate ("rate in") must equal the rate of elimination ("rate out"). Substitution of the target concentration (TC) for concentration (C) in equation (4) predicts the maintenance dosing rate:

$$\begin{aligned}\text{Dosing rate}_{ss} &= \text{Rate of elimination}_{ss} \\ &= \text{CL} \times \text{TC}\end{aligned} \tag{9}$$

Thus, if the desired target concentration is known, the clearance in that patient will determine the dosing rate. If the drug is given by a route that has a bioavailability less than 100%, then the dosing rate predicted by equation (9) must be modified. For oral dosing:

$$\text{Dosing rate}_{oral} = \frac{\text{Dosing rate}}{F_{oral}} \tag{10}$$

If intermittent doses are given, the maintenance dose is calculated from:

$$\text{Maintenance dose} = \text{Dosing rate} \times \text{Dosing interval} \tag{11}$$

(See Box: Example: Maintenance Dose Calculations.)

Note that the steady-state concentration achieved by continuous infusion or the average concentration following intermittent dosing depends only on clearance. The volume of distribution and the half-life need not be known in order to determine the average plasma concentration expected from a given dosing rate or to predict the dosing rate for a desired target concentration. Figure 3–6 shows that at different dosing intervals, the concentration-time curves will have different maximum and minimum values even though the average concentration will always be 10 mg/L.

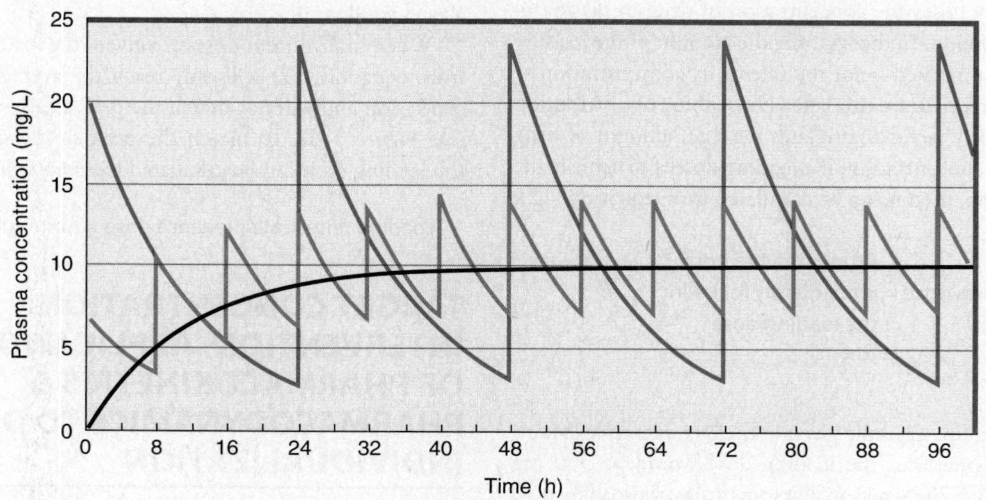

FIGURE 3–6 Relationship between frequency of dosing and maximum and minimum plasma concentrations when a steady-state theophylline plasma concentration of 10 mg/L is desired. The smoothly rising black line shows the plasma concentration achieved with an intravenous infusion of 28 mg/h. The dose for 8-hour administration (orange line) is 224 mg and for 24-hour administration (blue line) 672 mg. In each of the three cases, the mean steady-state plasma concentration is 10 mg/L.

Example: Maintenance Dose Calculations

A target plasma theophylline concentration of 10 mg/L is desired to relieve acute bronchial asthma in a patient. If the patient is a nonsmoker and otherwise normal except for asthma, we may use the mean clearance given in Table 3–1, ie, 2.8 L/h/70 kg. Since the drug will be given as an intravenous infusion, F = 1.

$$\begin{aligned}\text{Dosing rate} &= \text{CL} \times \text{TC}\\ &= 2.8\ \text{L/h/70 kg} \times 10\ \text{mg/L}\\ &= 28\ \text{mg/h/70 kg}\end{aligned}$$

Therefore, in this patient, the infusion rate would be 28 mg/h/70 kg.

If the asthma attack is relieved, the clinician might want to maintain this plasma concentration using oral theophylline, which might be given every 12 hours using an extended-release formulation to approximate a continuous intravenous infusion. According to Table 3–1, F_{oral} is 0.96. When the dosing interval is 12 hours, the size of each maintenance dose would be:

$$\begin{aligned}\text{Maintenance dose} &= \text{Dosing Rate/F} \times \text{Dosing interval}\\ &= 28\ \text{mg/h/0.96} \times 12\ \text{h}\\ &= 350\ \text{mg}\end{aligned}$$

A tablet or capsule size close to the ideal dose of 350 mg would then be prescribed at 12-hour intervals. If an 8-hour dosing interval was used, the ideal dose would be 233 mg; and if the drug was given once a day, the dose would be 700 mg. In practice, F could be omitted from the calculation since it is so close to 1.

Estimates of dosing rate and average steady-state concentrations, which may be calculated using clearance, are independent of any specific pharmacokinetic model. In contrast, the determination of maximum and minimum steady-state concentrations requires further assumptions about the pharmacokinetic model. The accumulation factor (equation [7]) assumes that the drug distribution is a one-compartment model (see Figure 3–2B), and the peak concentration prediction assumes that the absorption rate is much faster than the elimination rate. For the calculation of estimated maximum and minimum concentrations in a clinical situation, these assumptions are usually reasonable.

Loading Dose

When the time to reach steady state is appreciable, as it is for drugs with long half-lives, it may be desirable to administer a loading dose that promptly raises the concentration of drug in plasma to the target concentration. In theory, only the amount of the loading dose needs to be computed—not the rate of its administration—and, to a first approximation, this is so. The volume of distribution is the proportionality factor that relates the total amount of drug in the body to the concentration; if a loading dose is to achieve the target concentration, then it can be calculated from equation (12):

$$\begin{aligned}\text{Loading dose} &= \begin{array}{l}\text{Amount in the body}\\ \text{immediately following}\\ \text{the loading dose}\end{array}\\ &= \text{V} \times \text{TC}\end{aligned} \qquad (12)$$

For the theophylline example given in the box, Example: Maintenance Dose Calculations, the loading dose would be 350 mg (35 L × 10 mg/L) for a 70-kg person. For most drugs, the loading dose can be given as a single dose by the chosen route of administration.

Up to this point, we have ignored the fact that some drugs follow more complex multicompartment pharmacokinetics, eg, the distribution process illustrated by the two-compartment model in Figure 3–2. This is reasonable in the great majority of cases. However, in some cases the distribution phase may not be ignored, particularly in connection with the calculation of loading doses. If the rate of input is rapid relative to distribution (this is always true for rapid intravenous administration), the concentration of drug in plasma that results from an appropriate loading dose—calculated using the apparent volume of distribution—will initially be considerably higher than desired. Severe toxicity may occur, albeit transiently. This may be particularly important, eg, in the administration of an anticonvulsant drug such as phenytoin, where an almost immediate toxic response may occur. Thus, while the estimation of the *amount* of a loading dose may be quite correct, the *rate of administration* can sometimes be crucial in preventing excessive drug concentrations, and slow administration of an intravenous drug (eg, over an hour rather than seconds) is almost always prudent practice.

When intermittent doses are given, the loading dose calculated from equation (12) will only reach the average steady-state concentration and will not match the peak steady-state concentration (see Figure 3–6). To match the peak steady-state concentration, the loading dose can be calculated from equation (13):

$$\text{Loading dose} = \text{Maintenance dose} \times \text{Accumulation factor} \qquad (13)$$

TARGET CONCENTRATION INTERVENTION: APPLICATION OF PHARMACOKINETICS & PHARMACODYNAMICS TO DOSE INDIVIDUALIZATION

The basic principles outlined above can be applied to the interpretation of clinical drug concentration measurements on the basis of three major pharmacokinetic variables: rate and extent of input, clearance, and volume of distribution (and the derived variable, half-life). In addition, it may be necessary to consider two pharmacodynamic variables: maximum effect attainable in the target tissue (E_{max}) and the sensitivity (C_{50}) of the tissue to the drug. Diseases may modify all of these parameters, and the ability to predict the effect of disease states on these parameters is important in properly adjusting dosage in such cases. (See Box: The Target Concentration Strategy.)

The Target Concentration Strategy

Recognition of the essential role of concentration in linking pharmacokinetics and pharmacodynamics leads naturally to the target concentration strategy. Pharmacodynamic principles can be used to predict the concentration required to achieve a particular degree of therapeutic effect. This target concentration can then be achieved by using pharmacokinetic principles to arrive at a suitable dosing regimen (Holford, 1999). The target concentration strategy is a process for optimizing the dose in an individual on the basis of a measured surrogate response such as drug concentration:

1. Choose the target concentration, TC.
2. Predict volume of distribution (V) and clearance (CL) based on standard population values (eg, Table 3–1) with adjustments for factors such as weight and renal function.
3. Give a loading dose or maintenance dose calculated from TC, V, and CL.
4. Measure the patient's response (including, usually, drug concentration).
5. Revise V and/or CL based on the measured response.
6. Repeat steps 3–5, adjusting the predicted dose to achieve TC.

Pharmacokinetic Variables

A. Input

The amount of drug that enters the body depends on the patient's adherence to the prescribed regimen and on the rate and extent of transfer from the site of administration to the blood.

Overdosage and underdosage relative to the prescribed dosage—both aspects of failure of adherence—can frequently be detected by concentration measurements when gross deviations from expected values are obtained. If adherence is found to be adequate, absorption abnormalities in the small bowel may be the cause of abnormally low concentrations. Variations in the extent of bioavailability are rarely caused by irregularities in the manufacture of the particular drug formulation. More commonly, variations in bioavailability are due to metabolism during absorption.

B. Clearance

Abnormal clearance may be anticipated when there is major impairment of the function of the kidney, liver, or heart. Creatinine clearance is a useful quantitative indicator of renal function. Conversely, drug clearance may be a useful indicator of the functional consequences of heart, kidney, or liver failure, often with greater precision than clinical findings or other laboratory tests. For example, when renal function is changing rapidly, estimation of the clearance of aminoglycoside antibiotics may be a more accurate indicator of glomerular filtration than serum creatinine.

Hepatic disease has been shown to reduce the clearance and prolong the half-life of many drugs. However, for many other drugs known to be eliminated by hepatic processes, no changes in clearance or half-life have been noted with similar hepatic disease. This reflects the fact that hepatic disease does not always affect the hepatic intrinsic clearance. At present, there is no reliable marker of hepatic drug-metabolizing function that can be used to predict changes in liver clearance in a manner analogous to the use of creatinine clearance as a marker of renal drug clearance.

C. Volume of Distribution

The apparent volume of distribution reflects a balance between binding to tissues, which decreases plasma concentration and makes the apparent volume larger, and binding to plasma proteins, which increases plasma concentration and makes the apparent volume smaller. Changes in either tissue or plasma binding can change the apparent volume of distribution determined from plasma concentration measurements. Older people have a relative decrease in skeletal muscle mass and tend to have a smaller apparent volume of distribution of digoxin (which binds to muscle proteins). The volume of distribution may be overestimated in obese patients if based on body weight and the drug does not enter fatty tissues well, as is the case with digoxin. In contrast, theophylline has a volume of distribution similar to that of total body water. Adipose tissue has almost as much water in it as other tissues, so that the apparent total volume of distribution of theophylline is proportional to body weight even in obese patients.

Abnormal accumulation of fluid—edema, ascites, pleural effusion—can markedly increase the volume of distribution of drugs such as gentamicin that are hydrophilic and have small volumes of distribution.

D. Elimination Half-Life

The differences between clearance and elimination half-life are important in defining the underlying mechanisms for the effect of a disease state on drug disposition. For example, the elimination half-life of diazepam increases with patient age. However, in the same patients it is found that clearance of diazepam does not change with age. The increasing elimination half-life for diazepam actually results from changes in the volume of distribution with age; the metabolic processes responsible for eliminating diazepam do not change with age.

Pharmacodynamic Variables

A. Maximum Effect

All pharmacologic responses must have a maximum effect (E_{max}). No matter how high the drug concentration goes, a point will be reached beyond which no further increment in response is achieved.

If increasing the dose in a particular patient does not lead to a further clinical response, it is possible that the maximum effect has been approached. Recognition of a maximum effect is helpful in avoiding ineffectual increases of dose with the attendant risk of toxicity.

B. Sensitivity

The sensitivity of the target organ to drug concentration is reflected by the concentration required to produce 50% of maximum effect, the C_{50}. Diminished sensitivity to the drug can be detected by measuring drug concentrations that are usually associated with therapeutic response in a patient who has not responded. This may be a result of abnormal physiology—eg, hyperkalemia diminishes responsiveness to digoxin—or drug antagonism—eg, calcium channel blockers impair the inotropic response to digoxin.

Increased sensitivity to a drug is usually signaled by exaggerated responses to small or moderate doses. The pharmacodynamic nature of this sensitivity can be confirmed by measuring drug concentrations that are low in relation to the observed effect.

INTERPRETATION OF DRUG CONCENTRATION MEASUREMENTS

Clearance

Clearance is the single most important factor determining drug concentrations. The interpretation of measurements of drug concentrations depends on a clear understanding of three factors that may influence concentrations reflecting clearance: the dose, the organ blood flow, and the intrinsic function of the liver or kidneys. Each of these factors should be considered when interpreting clearance estimated from a drug concentration measurement.

It must also be recognized that changes in protein binding may lead the unwary to believe there is a change in clearance when in fact drug elimination is not altered (see Box: Plasma Protein Binding: Is It Important?). Factors affecting protein binding include the following:

1. **Albumin concentration:** Drugs such as phenytoin, salicylates, and disopyramide are extensively bound to plasma albumin. Albumin concentrations are low in many disease states, resulting in lower total drug concentrations.
2. **Alpha$_1$-acid glycoprotein concentration:** α_1-Acid glycoprotein is an important binding protein with binding sites for drugs such as quinidine, lidocaine, and propranolol. It is increased in acute inflammatory disorders and causes major changes in total plasma concentration of these drugs even though drug elimination is unchanged.
3. **Capacity-limited protein binding:** The binding of drugs to plasma proteins is capacity-limited. Therapeutic concentrations of salicylates and prednisolone show concentration-dependent protein binding. Because unbound drug concentration is determined by dosing rate and unbound clearance—which is not altered by protein binding, in the case of these low-extraction-ratio drugs—increases in dosing rate will cause corresponding changes in the pharmacodynamically important unbound concentration. In contrast, total drug concentration will increase less rapidly than the dosing rate would suggest as protein binding approaches saturation at higher concentrations.
4. **Binding to red blood cells:** Drugs such as cyclosporine and tacrolimus bind extensively inside red blood cells. Typically, whole blood concentrations are measured, and they are about 50 times higher than plasma concentration. A decrease in red blood cell concentration (reflected in the hematocrit) will cause whole blood concentration to fall without a change in pharmacologically active concentrations. Standardization of concentrations to a standard hematocrit helps to interpret the concentration-effect relationship.

Dosing History

An accurate dosing history is essential if one is to obtain maximum value from a drug concentration measurement. In fact, if the dosing history is unknown or incomplete, a drug concentration measurement loses all predictive value.

Timing of Samples for Concentration Measurement

Information about the rate and extent of drug absorption in a particular patient is rarely of great clinical importance. Absorption usually occurs during the first 2 hours after a drug dose and varies according to food intake, posture, and activity. Therefore, it is important to avoid drawing blood until absorption is complete (about 2 hours after an oral dose). Attempts to measure peak concentrations early after oral dosing are usually unsuccessful and compromise the validity of the measurement, because one cannot be certain that absorption is complete.

Plasma Protein Binding: Is It Important?

Plasma protein binding is often mentioned as a factor playing a role in pharmacokinetics, pharmacodynamics, and drug interactions. However, there are no clinically relevant examples of changes in drug disposition or effects that can be clearly ascribed to changes in plasma protein binding (Benet & Hoener, 2002). The idea that if a drug is displaced from plasma proteins it would increase the unbound drug concentration and increase the drug effect and, perhaps, produce toxicity seems a simple and obvious mechanism. Unfortunately, this simple theory, which is appropriate for a test tube, does not work in the body, which is an open system capable of eliminating unbound drug.

A seemingly dramatic change in the unbound fraction from 1% to 10% releases less than 5% of the total amount of drug in the body into the unbound pool because less than one third of the drug in the body is bound to plasma proteins even in the most extreme cases, eg, warfarin. Drug displaced from plasma protein will of course distribute throughout the volume of distribution, so that a 5% increase in the amount of unbound drug in the body produces at most a 5% increase in pharmacologically active unbound drug at the site of action.

If the amount of unbound drug in plasma increases due to displacement from plasma proteins, the rate of elimination will increase, and after four half-lives the unbound concentration will return to its previous steady-state value (if unbound clearance is unchanged). When drug interactions associated with protein binding displacement and clinically important effects have been studied, it has been found that the displacing drug is also an inhibitor of clearance, and it is the change in *clearance* of the *unbound* drug that is the relevant mechanism explaining the interaction.

The clinical importance of plasma protein binding is only to help interpretation of measured drug concentrations. When plasma proteins are lower than normal, total drug concentrations will be lower but unbound concentrations will not be affected.

Some drugs, such as digoxin and lithium, take several hours to distribute to tissues. Digoxin samples should be taken at least 6 hours after the last dose and lithium just before the next dose (usually 24 hours after the last dose). Aminoglycosides distribute quite rapidly, but it is still prudent to wait 1 hour after giving the dose before taking a sample.

Clearance is readily estimated from the dosing rate and mean steady-state concentration. Blood samples should be appropriately timed to estimate steady-state concentration. Provided steady state has been approached (at least three half-lives of constant dosing), a sample obtained near the midpoint of the dosing interval will usually be close to the mean steady-state concentration and is a better choice than a trough concentration just before the next dose.

Initial Predictions of Volume of Distribution & Clearance

A. Volume of Distribution

Volume of distribution is commonly calculated for a particular patient using body weight (70-kg body weight is assumed for the values in Table 3–1). If a patient is obese, drugs that do not readily penetrate fat (eg, gentamicin, digoxin, tacrolimus, gemcitabine) should have their volumes calculated from fat-free mass (FFM) as shown below. Total body weight (WT) is in kilograms and height (HTM) is in meters:

$$\text{For women: FFM (kg)} = \frac{37.99 \times \text{HTM}^2 \times \text{WT}}{35.98 \times \text{HTM}^2 + \text{WT}} \qquad (14a)$$

$$\text{For men: FFM (kg)} = \frac{42.92 \times \text{HTM}^2 \times \text{WT}}{30.93 \times \text{HTM}^2 + \text{WT}} \qquad (14b)$$

Patients with edema, ascites, or pleural effusions offer a larger volume of distribution to the aminoglycoside antibiotics (eg, gentamicin) than is predicted by body weight. In such patients, the weight should be corrected as follows: Subtract an estimate of the weight of the excess fluid accumulation from the measured weight. Use the resultant "normal" body weight to calculate the normal volume of distribution. Finally, this normal volume should be increased by 1 L for each estimated kilogram of excess fluid. This correction is important because of the relatively small volumes of distribution of these water-soluble drugs.

B. Clearance

Drugs cleared by the renal route often require adjustment of clearance in proportion to renal function. This can be conveniently estimated from the creatinine clearance, calculated from a single serum creatinine measurement and the predicted creatinine production rate.

The predicted creatinine production rate in women is 85% of the calculated value because they have a smaller muscle mass per kilogram, and it is muscle mass that determines creatinine production. Muscle mass as a fraction of body weight decreases with age, which is why age appears in the Cockcroft-Gault equation for estimating creatinine clearance.* The decrease of renal function with age is caused not by the decrease in creatinine production but by the progressive loss of nephrons. The loss of nephrons will reduce creatinine clearance and increase serum creatinine. This increase in serum creatinine will be reflected in estimated creatinine clearance.

*The Cockcroft-Gault equation is given in Chapter 60.

Because of the difficulty of obtaining complete urine collections, creatinine clearance calculated from serum creatinine is usually more reliable than estimates based on urine collections. The fat-free mass (equation [14]) may be considered rather than total body weight for obese patients, and correction should be made for muscle wasting in severely ill patients.

Revising Individual Estimates of Volume of Distribution & Clearance

The commonsense approach to the interpretation of drug concentrations compares predictions of pharmacokinetic parameters and expected concentrations to measured values. If measured concentrations differ by more than 20% from expected values, revised estimates of V or CL for that patient should be calculated using equation (1) or equation (2). If the change calculated is more than a 100% increase or 50% decrease in either V or CL, the assumptions made about the timing of the sample and the dosing history should be critically examined.

For example, if a patient is taking 0.25 mg of digoxin a day, a clinician may expect the digoxin concentration to be about 1 ng/mL. This is based on typical values for bioavailability of 70% and total clearance of about 7 L/h (CL_{renal} 4 L/h, $CL_{nonrenal}$ 3 L/h). If the patient has heart failure, the nonrenal (hepatic) clearance might be halved because of hepatic congestion and hypoxia, so the expected clearance would become 5.5 L/h. The concentration is then expected to be about 1.3 ng/mL. Suppose that the concentration actually measured is 2 ng/mL. Common sense would suggest halving the daily dose to achieve a target concentration of 1 ng/mL. This approach implies a revised clearance of 3.5 L/h. The smaller clearance compared with the expected value of 5.5 L/h may reflect additional renal functional impairment due to heart failure.

This technique will often be misleading if steady state has not been reached. At least a week of regular dosing (four half-lives) must elapse before the implicit method will be reliable. Dosing tools using pharmacokinetic models developed from representative patient populations should be considered for more reliable prediction of individual doses based on measured patient response (eg, www.nextdose.org).

REFERENCES

Benet LZ, Hoener B: Changes in plasma protein binding have little clinical relevance. Clin Pharmacol Ther 2002;71:115.

Holford NHG: Clinical Pharmacology, 2020. http://holford.fmhs.auckland.ac.nz/teaching/pharmacometrics/advanced.php.

Holford NHG: Target concentration intervention: Beyond Y2K. Br J Clin Pharmacol 1999;48:9.

Holford N, Heo YA, Anderson B: A pharmacokinetic standard for babies and adults. J Pharm Sci 2013;102:2941.

Holford NHG, Sheiner LB: Understanding the dose-effect relationship. Clin Pharmacokinet 1981;6:429.

CASE STUDY ANSWER

Sixty-seven percent of total standard digoxin clearance is renal, so the standard renal clearance is 0.67×9 L/h = 6 L/h/70 kg with creatinine clearance of 100 mL/min and nonrenal clearance is $(1 - 0.67) \times 9$ L/h = 3 L/h/70 kg (see Table 3–1 for standard pharmacokinetic parameters). Her predicted creatinine clearance is 22 mL/min (Cockcroft and Gault), so for digoxin, her renal clearance is $6 \times 22/100 \times 60/70 = 1.1$ L/h, nonrenal clearance $2.7 \times 60/70 = 2.6$ L/h, and total clearance 3.7 L/h. The parenteral maintenance dose rate is 1 mcg/L × 3.7 L/h = 3.7 mcg/h. Once-a-day oral dosing with bioavailability of 0.7 would require a daily maintenance dose of $3.7/0.7 \times 24 = 127$ mcg/day. A practical dose would be two 62.5-mcg tablets per day.

CHAPTER 4

Drug Biotransformation

Maria Almira Correia, PhD

CASE STUDY

A 40-year-old woman presents to the emergency department of her local hospital somewhat disoriented, complaining of midsternal chest pain, abdominal pain, shaking, and vomiting for 2 days. She admits to having taken a "handful" of Lorcet (hydrocodone/acetaminophen, an opioid/nonopioid analgesic combination), Soma (carisoprodol, a centrally acting muscle relaxant), and Cymbalta (duloxetine HCl, an antidepressant/antifibromyalgia agent) 2 days earlier. On physical examination, the sclera of her eyes shows yellow discoloration. Laboratory analyses of blood drawn within an hour of her admission reveal abnormal liver function as indicated by the increased indices: alkaline phosphatase 302 (41–133),* alanine aminotransferase (ALT) 351 (7–56),* aspartate aminotransferase (AST) 1045 (0–35),* bilirubin 3.33 mg/dL (0.1–1.2),* and prothrombin time of 19.8 seconds (11–15).* In addition, plasma bicarbonate is reduced, and she has ~45% reduced glomerular filtration rate from the normal value at her age, elevated serum creatinine, and blood urea nitrogen, markedly reduced blood glucose of 35 mg/dL, and a plasma acetaminophen concentration of 75 mcg/mL (10–20).* Her serum titer is significantly positive for hepatitis C virus (HCV). Given these data, how would you proceed with the management of this case?

*Normal values are in parentheses.

Humans are exposed daily to a wide variety of foreign compounds called **xenobiotics**—substances absorbed across the lungs or skin or, more commonly, ingested either unintentionally as compounds present in food and drink or deliberately as drugs for therapeutic or "recreational" purposes. Exposure to environmental xenobiotics may be inadvertent and accidental or—when they are present as components of air, water, and food—inescapable. Some xenobiotics are innocuous, but many can provoke biologic responses. Such biologic responses often depend on conversion of the absorbed substance into an active metabolite. The discussion that follows is applicable to xenobiotics in general (including drugs) and to some extent to endogenous compounds.

WHY IS DRUG BIOTRANSFORMATION NECESSARY?

The mammalian drug biotransformation systems are thought to have first evolved from the need to detoxify and eliminate plant and bacterial bioproducts and toxins, which later extended to drugs and other environmental xenobiotics. Renal excretion plays a pivotal role in terminating the biologic activity of some drugs, particularly those that have small molecular volumes or possess polar characteristics, such as functional groups that are fully ionized at physiologic pH. However, many drugs do not possess such physicochemical properties. Pharmacologically active organic molecules tend to be lipophilic and remain un-ionized or only partially ionized at physiologic pH; these are readily reabsorbed from the glomerular filtrate in the nephron. Certain lipophilic compounds are often strongly bound to plasma proteins and may not be readily filtered at the glomerulus. Consequently, most drugs would have a prolonged duration of action if termination of their action depended solely on renal excretion.

An alternative process that can lead to the termination or alteration of biologic activity is metabolism. In general, lipophilic xenobiotics are transformed to more polar and hence more readily excreted products. The role that metabolism plays in the inactivation of lipid-soluble drugs can be quite dramatic. For example, lipophilic barbiturates such as thiopental and pentobarbital would have extremely long half-lives if it were not for their metabolic conversion to more water-soluble compounds.

Metabolic products are often less pharmacodynamically active than the parent drug and may even be inactive. However, some biotransformation products have *enhanced* activity or toxic properties. It is noteworthy that the synthesis of endogenous substrates such as steroid hormones, cholesterol, active vitamin D congeners, and bile acids involves many pathways catalyzed by enzymes associated with the metabolism of xenobiotics. Finally, drug-metabolizing enzymes have been exploited in the design of pharmacologically inactive prodrugs that are converted to active molecules in the body.

THE ROLE OF BIOTRANSFORMATION IN DRUG DISPOSITION

Most metabolic biotransformations occur at some point between absorption of the drug into the circulation and its renal elimination. A few transformations occur in the intestinal lumen or intestinal wall. In general, all of these reactions can be assigned to one of two major categories called **phase I** and **phase II reactions** (Figure 4–1).

Phase I reactions usually convert the parent drug to a more polar metabolite by introducing or unmasking a functional group ($-OH$, $-NH_2$, $-SH$). Often these metabolites are inactive, although in some instances, activity is only modified or even enhanced.

If phase I metabolites are sufficiently polar, they may be readily excreted. However, many phase I products are not eliminated rapidly and undergo a subsequent reaction in which an endogenous substrate such as glucuronic acid, sulfuric acid, acetic acid, or an amino acid combines with the newly incorporated functional group to form a highly polar conjugate. Such conjugation or synthetic reactions are the hallmarks of phase II metabolism. A great variety of drugs undergo these sequential biotransformation reactions, although in some instances, the parent drug may already possess a functional group that may form a conjugate directly. For example, the hydrazide moiety of isoniazid is known to form an *N*-acetyl conjugate in a phase II reaction. This conjugate is then a substrate for a phase I type reaction, namely, hydrolysis to isonicotinic acid (Figure 4–2). Thus, phase II reactions may actually precede phase I reactions.

WHERE DO DRUG BIOTRANSFORMATIONS OCCUR?

Although every tissue has some ability to metabolize drugs, the liver is the principal organ of drug metabolism. Other tissues that display considerable activity include the gastrointestinal tract, the lungs, the skin, the kidneys, and the brain. After oral administration, many drugs (eg, isoproterenol, meperidine, pentazocine, morphine) are absorbed intact from the small intestine and transported first via the portal system to the liver, where they undergo extensive metabolism. This process is called the **first-pass effect** (see Chapter 3). Some orally administered drugs (eg, clonazepam, chlorpromazine, cyclosporine) are more extensively metabolized in the intestine than in the liver, while others (eg, midazolam) undergo significant (~50%) intestinal metabolism. Thus, intestinal metabolism can contribute to the overall first-pass effect, and individuals with compromised liver function may rely increasingly on such intestinal metabolism for drug elimination. Compromise of intestinal metabolism of certain drugs (eg, felodipine, cyclosporine A) can also result in significant elevation of their plasma levels and clinically relevant drug-drug interactions (**DDIs**, see below). First-pass effects may limit the bioavailability of orally administered drugs (eg, lidocaine) so greatly that alternative routes of administration must be used to achieve therapeutically effective blood levels. Furthermore, the lower gut harbors intestinal microorganisms that are capable of many biotransformation reactions. In addition, drugs may be metabolized by gastric acid (eg, penicillin), by digestive enzymes (eg, polypeptides such as insulin), or by

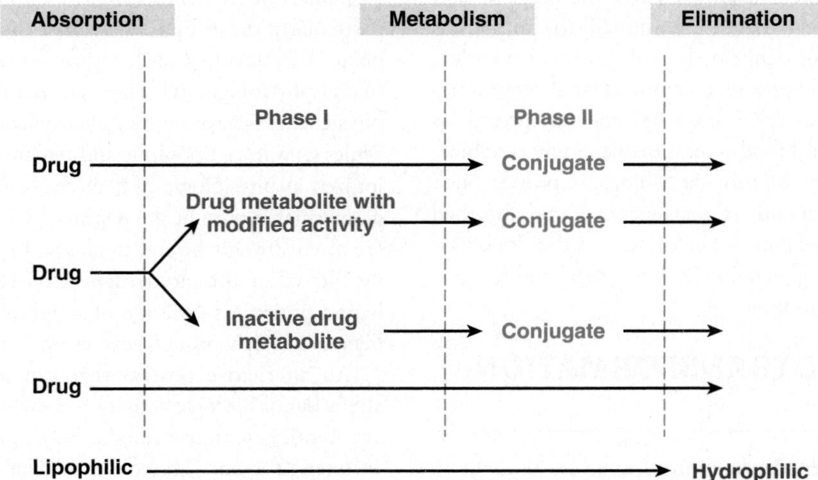

FIGURE 4–1 Phase I and phase II reactions and direct elimination, in drug biodisposition. Phase II reactions may also precede phase I reactions.

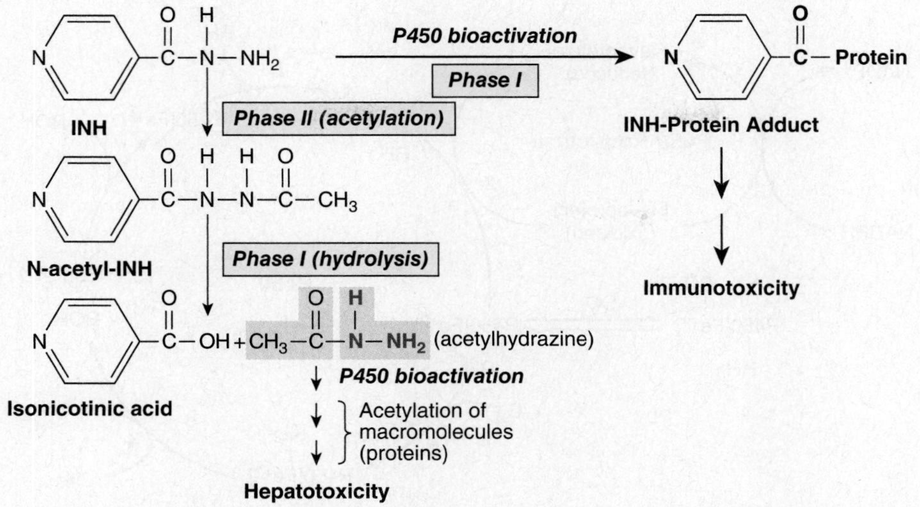

FIGURE 4–2 Phase II activation of isoniazid (INH) to a hepatotoxic metabolite. Note that INH can also undergo P450-mediated bioactivation to an isonicotinic acyl radical that can subsequently attack hepatic proteins including the P450s that metabolize it. In certain individuals, this results in idiosyncratic immunotoxicity as the INH-adducted proteins are proteolytically degraded into isonicotinic acylated peptides that act as autoantigens engendering pathogenic immunoreactive autoantibodies. Such INH-P450 autoantibodies can interact with the small fraction of the intracellular P450s that is integrated in the cell membrane but exposed extracellularly, triggering liver cell injury.

enzymes in the wall of the intestine (eg, sympathomimetic catecholamines).

Although drug biotransformation in vivo can occur by spontaneous, noncatalyzed chemical reactions, most transformations are catalyzed by specific cellular enzymes. At the subcellular level, these enzymes may be located in the endoplasmic reticulum, mitochondria, cytoplasm, lysosomes, or even the nuclear envelope or plasma membrane.

MICROSOMAL MIXED FUNCTION OXIDASE SYSTEM & PHASE I REACTIONS

Many drug-metabolizing enzymes are located in the lipophilic endoplasmic reticulum membranes of the liver and other tissues. When these lamellar membranes are isolated by homogenization and fractionation of the cell, they re-form into vesicles called **microsomes.** Microsomes retain most of the morphologic and functional characteristics of the intact membranes, including the rough and smooth surface features of the rough (ribosome-studded) and smooth (no ribosomes) endoplasmic reticulum. Whereas the rough microsomes tend to be dedicated to protein synthesis, the smooth microsomes are relatively rich in enzymes responsible for oxidative drug metabolism. In particular, they contain the important class of enzymes known as the **mixed function oxidases** (MFOs), or **monooxygenases.** The activity of these enzymes requires both a reducing agent (nicotinamide adenine dinucleotide phosphate [**NADPH**]) and molecular oxygen; in a typical reaction, one molecule of oxygen is consumed (reduced) per substrate molecule, with one oxygen atom appearing in the product and the other in the form of water.

In this oxidation-reduction process, two microsomal enzymes play a key role. The first of these is a flavoprotein, **NADPH-cytochrome P450 oxidoreductase** (**CPR**, or POR). One mole of this enzyme contains 1 mol each of flavin mononucleotide (FMN) and flavin adenine dinucleotide (FAD). The second microsomal enzyme is a hemoprotein called **cytochrome P450,** which serves as the terminal oxidase. In fact, the microsomal membrane harbors multiple forms of this hemoprotein, and this multiplicity is increased by repeated administration of or exposure to exogenous chemicals (see text that follows). The name cytochrome P450 (abbreviated as **P450** or **CYP**) is derived from the spectral properties of this hemoprotein. In its reduced (ferrous) form, it binds carbon monoxide to give a complex that absorbs light maximally at 450 nm. The relative abundance of P450s, compared with that of the reductase in the liver, contributes to making P450 heme reduction a rate-limiting step in hepatic drug oxidations.

Microsomal drug oxidations require P450, P450 reductase, NADPH, and molecular oxygen. A simplified scheme of the oxidative cycle is presented in Figure 4–3. Briefly, oxidized (Fe^{+3}) P450 combines with a drug substrate to form a binary complex (*step 1*). NADPH donates an electron to the flavoprotein P450 reductase, which in turn reduces the oxidized P450-drug complex (*step 2*). A second electron is introduced from NADPH via the same P450 reductase (or even microsomal cytochrome b_5), which serves to reduce molecular oxygen and to form an "activated oxygen"–P450–substrate complex (*step 3*). This complex in turn transfers activated oxygen to the drug substrate to form the oxidized product (*step 4*).

The potent oxidizing properties of this activated oxygen permit oxidation of a large number of substrates. Substrate specificity is very low for this enzyme complex. High lipid solubility is the only common structural feature of the wide variety of structurally

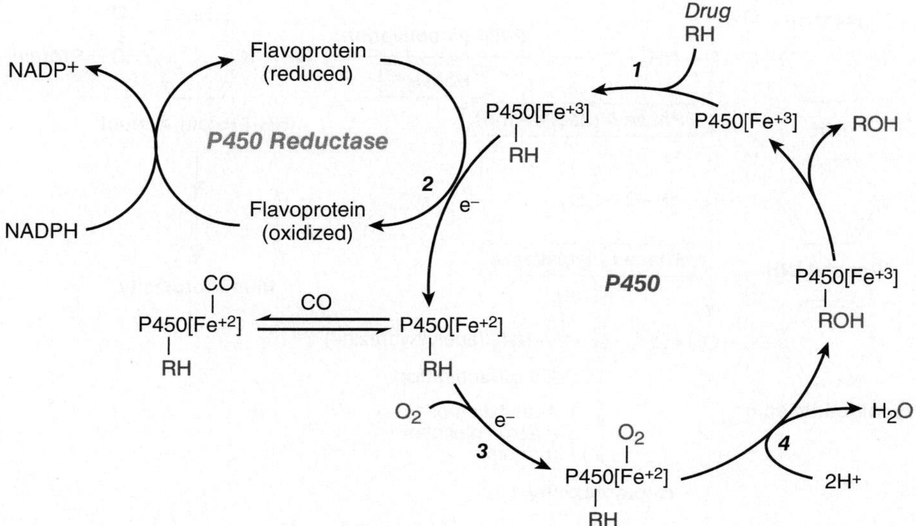

FIGURE 4–3 Cytochrome P450 cycle in drug oxidations. e⁻, electron; RH, parent drug; ROH, oxidized metabolite.

unrelated drugs and chemicals that serve as substrates in this system (Table 4–1). However, compared with many other enzymes including phase II enzymes, P450s are remarkably sluggish catalysts, and their drug biotransformation reactions are slow.

HUMAN LIVER P450 ENZYMES

Gene arrays combined with immunoblotting analyses of microsomal preparations, as well as the use of relatively selective functional markers and selective P450 inhibitors, have identified numerous P450 isoforms (CYPs: 1A2, 2A6, 2B6, 2C8, 2C9, 2C18, 2C19, 2D6, 2E1, 3A4, 3A5, 4A11, and 7) in the human liver. Of these, **CYP1A2, CYP2A6, CYP2B6, CYP2C9, CYP2D6, CYP2E1,** and **CYP3A4** appear to be the most important forms, accounting for approximately 15%, 4%, 1%, 20%, 5%, 10%, and 30%, respectively, of the total human liver P450 content. Together, they are responsible for catalyzing the bulk of the hepatic drug and xenobiotic metabolism (Table 4–2, Figure 4–4).

It is noteworthy that CYP3A4 alone is responsible for the metabolism of over 50% of the prescription drugs metabolized by the liver. The involvement of individual P450s in the metabolism of a given drug may be screened in vitro by means of selective functional markers, selective chemical P450 inhibitors, and P450 antibodies. In vivo, such screening may be accomplished by means of relatively selective noninvasive markers, which include breath tests or urinary analyses of specific metabolites after administration of a P450-selective substrate probe.

Enzyme Induction

Some of the chemically dissimilar P450 substrate drugs, on repeated administration, *induce* P450 expression by enhancing the rate of its synthesis or reducing its rate of degradation (see Table 4–2). Induction results in accelerated substrate metabolism and usually in a decrease in the pharmacologic action of the inducer and also of co-administered drugs. However, in the case of drugs metabolically transformed to reactive metabolites, enzyme induction may exacerbate metabolite-mediated toxicity.

Various substrates induce P450 isoforms having different molecular masses and exhibiting different substrate specificities and immunochemical and spectral characteristics.

Environmental chemicals and pollutants are also capable of inducing P450 enzymes. Exposure to benzo[*a*]pyrene and other polycyclic aromatic hydrocarbons, which are present in tobacco smoke, charcoal-broiled meat, and other organic pyrolysis products, is known to induce CYP1A enzymes and to alter the rates of drug metabolism. Other environmental chemicals known to induce specific P450s include the polychlorinated biphenyls (PCBs), which were once used widely in industry as insulating materials and plasticizers, and 2,3,7,8-tetrachlorodibenzo-*p*-dioxin (dioxin, TCDD), a trace byproduct of the chemical synthesis of the defoliant 2,4,5-T (see Chapter 56).

Increased P450 synthesis requires enhanced transcription and translation along with increased synthesis of heme, its prosthetic cofactor. A cytoplasmic receptor (termed AhR) for polycyclic aromatic hydrocarbons (eg, benzo[*a*]pyrene, dioxin) has been identified. The translocation of the inducer-receptor complex into the nucleus, followed by ligand-induced dimerization with Arnt, a closely related nuclear protein, leads to subsequent activation of regulatory elements of *CYP1A* genes, resulting in their induction. This is also the mechanism of CYP1A induction by cruciferous vegetables, and the proton pump inhibitor, omeprazole. A pregnane X receptor (PXR), a member of the steroid-retinoid-thyroid hormone receptor family, has recently been shown to mediate CYP3A induction by various chemicals (dexamethasone, rifampin, mifepristone, phenobarbital, atorvastatin, and hyperforin, a constituent of St. John's wort) in the liver and intestinal mucosa. A similar receptor, the constitutive androstane receptor (CAR), has been identified for the relatively large and structurally diverse phenobarbital class of inducers of CYP2B6, CYP2C9,

TABLE 4–1 Phase I reactions.

Reaction Class	Structural Change	Drug Substrate
Oxidations		
Cytochrome P450-dependent oxidations:		
Aromatic hydroxylations	(benzene ring with R → via arene epoxide intermediate → p-hydroxylated ring with R and OH)	Acetanilide, propranolol, phenobarbital, phenytoin, phenylbutazone, amphetamine, warfarin, 17α-ethinyl estradiol, naphthalene, benzpyrene
Aliphatic hydroxylations	$RCH_2CH_3 \longrightarrow RCH_2CH_2OH$ $RCH_2CH_3 \longrightarrow RCH(OH)CH_3$	Amobarbital, pentobarbital, secobarbital, chlorpropamide, ibuprofen, meprobamate, glutethimide, phenylbutazone, digitoxin
Epoxidation	$RCH{=}CHR \longrightarrow R{-}CH{-}CH{-}R$ (epoxide, O bridging the two C–H carbons)	Aldrin
Oxidative dealkylation		
N-Dealkylation	$RNHCH_3 \longrightarrow RNH_2 + CH_2O$	Morphine, ethylmorphine, benzphetamine, aminopyrine, caffeine, theophylline
O-Dealkylation	$ROCH_3 \longrightarrow ROH + CH_2O$	Codeine, *p*-nitroanisole
S-Dealkylation	$RSCH_3 \longrightarrow RSH + CH_2O$	6-Methylthiopurine, methitural
***N*-Oxidation**		
Primary amines	$RNH_2 \longrightarrow RNHOH$	Aniline, chlorphentermine
Secondary amines	$(R_1)(R_2)NH \longrightarrow (R_1)(R_2)N{-}OH$	2-Acetylaminofluorene, acetaminophen
Tertiary amines	$(R_1)(R_2)(R_3)N \longrightarrow (R_1)(R_2)(R_3)N{\rightarrow}O$	Necotine, methaqualone
***S*-Oxidation**	$(R_1)(R_2)S \longrightarrow (R_1)(R_2)S{=}O$	Thioridazine, cimetidine, chlorpromazine
Deamination	$RCH(NH_2)CH_3 \longrightarrow R{-}C(OH)(NH_2){-}CH_3 \longrightarrow R{-}C({=}O)CH_3 + NH_3$	Amphetamine, diazepam
Desulfuration	$(R_1)(R_2)C{=}S \longrightarrow (R_1)(R_2)C{=}O$	Thiopental

(*continued*)

TABLE 4–1 Phase I reactions. (Continued)

Reaction Class	Structural Change	Drug Substrate
***Cytochrome P450-dependent oxidations:* (continued)**		
	$(R_1)(R_2)P{=}S \longrightarrow (R_1)(R_2)P{=}O$	Parathion
Dechlorination	$CCl_4 \longrightarrow [CCl_3^{\cdot}] \longrightarrow CHCl_3$	Carbon tetrachloride
Cytochrome P450-independent oxidations:		
Flavin monooxygenase (Ziegler's enzyme)	$R_3N \longrightarrow R_3N^+ \rightarrow O^- \xrightarrow{H^+} R_3N^+OH$	Chlorpromazine, amitriptyline, benzphetamine
	$RCH_2N(H){-}CH_2R \longrightarrow RCH_2{-}N(OH){-}CH_2R \longrightarrow RCH{=}N(O^-){-}CH_2R$	Desipramine, nortriptyline
	$(-N)(-N)C{=}{-}SH \longrightarrow (-N)(-N)C{=}{-}SOH \longrightarrow (-N)(-N)C{=}{-}SO_2H$	Methimazole, propylthiouracil
Amine oxidases	$RCH_2NH_2 \longrightarrow RCHO + NH_3$	Phenylethylamine, epinephrine
Dehydrogenations	$RCH_2OH \longrightarrow RCHO$	Ethanol
Reductions		
Azo reductions	$RN{=}NR_1 \longrightarrow RNH{-}NHR_1 \longrightarrow RNH_2 + R1NH_2$	Prontosil, tartrazine
Nitro reductions	$RNO_2 \longrightarrow RNO \longrightarrow RNHOH \longrightarrow RNH_2$	Nitrobenzene, chloramphenicol, clonazepam, dantrolene
Carbonyl reductions	$RC({=}O)R' \longrightarrow RCH(OH)R'$	Metyrapone, methadone, naloxone
Hydrolyses		
Esters	$R_1COOR_2 \longrightarrow R_1COOH + R_2OH$	Procaine, succinylcholine, aspirin, clofibrate, methylphenidate
Amides	$RCONHR_1 \longrightarrow RCOOH + R_1NHH$[1]	Procainamide, lidocaine, indomethacin

[1]Hydrolytic reactions are generally classified as Phase I reactions, because although intracellular H_2O is utilized, it is split into its constituent H^+ and OH^- that are each singly incorporated into one or the other of the ensuing products. However, when the intact "endogenous" H_2O molecule is incorporated into a single product, ie, "water-adducted" arene-dihydrodiol generated from arene-epoxide, they are considered as Phase II reactions (Table 4–3).

and CYP3A4. Peroxisome proliferator receptor α (PPAR-α) is yet another nuclear receptor highly expressed in liver and kidneys, which uses lipid-lowering drugs (eg, fenofibrate and gemfibrozil) as ligands. Consistent with its major role in the regulation of fatty acid metabolism, PPAR-α mediates the induction of CYP4A enzymes, responsible for the metabolism of fatty acids such as arachidonic acid and its physiologically relevant derivatives. It is noteworthy that on binding of its particular ligand, PXR, CAR, and PPAR-α each form heterodimers with another nuclear receptor, the retinoid X-receptor (RXR). This heterodimer in turn binds to response elements within the promoter regions of specific *P450* genes to induce gene expression.

P450 enzymes may also be induced by **substrate stabilization,** eg, decreased degradation, as is the case with troleandomycin- or clotrimazole-mediated induction of CYP3A enzymes, the ethanol-mediated induction of CYP2E1, and the isosafrole-mediated induction of CYP1A2.

Enzyme Inhibition

Certain drug substrates inhibit cytochrome P450 enzyme activity (see Table 4–2). Imidazole-containing drugs such as cimetidine and ketoconazole bind tightly to the P450 heme iron and effectively reduce the metabolism of endogenous substrates (eg, testosterone) or other co-administered drugs through competitive inhibition.

TABLE 4–2 Human liver P450s (CYPs), and some of the drugs metabolized (substrates), inducers, and selective inhibitors. Note: Some P450 substrates can be potent competitive inhibitors and/or mechanism-based inactivators.

CYP	Substrates	Inducers	Inhibitors
1A2	Acetaminophen, alosetron, antipyrine, caffeine, clomipramine, clozapine, duloxetine, flutamide, frovatriptan, melatonin, mexiletine, mirtazapine, olanzapine, phenacetin, ramelteon, rasagiline, ropinirole, tacrine, tamoxifen, theophylline, tizanidine, triamterene, warfarin, zolmitriptan	Charcoal-broiled foods, cruciferous vegetables, grilled meat, lansoprazole, omeprazole, primidone, rifampin, smoking	Artemisinin, atazanavir, cimetidine, ciprofloxacin, enoxacin, ethinyl estradiol, fluvoxamine, furafylline, galangin, mexiletene, tacrine, thiabendazole, zileuton
2A6	Coumarin, dexmedetomidine, tobacco nitrosamines, nicotine (to cotinine and 2′-hydroxynicotine)	Efavirenz, rifampin, phenobarbital	Clotrimazole, isoniazid, ketoconazole, letrozole, menthofuran, methimazole, methoxsalen, miconazole, tranylcypromine
2B6	Artemisinin, bupropion, clopidogrel, cyclophosphamide, efavirenz, ifosfamide, irinotecan, ketamine, *S*-mephobarbital, *S*-mephenytoin (*N*-demethylation to nirvanol), methadone, nevirapine, promethazine, propofol, selegiline, sertraline, ticlopidine	Carbamazepine, cyclophosphamide, fosphenytoin, nevirapine, phenobarbital, primidone, rifampin	Amiodarone, amlodipine, clopidogrel, clotrimazole, desipramine, disulfiram, doxorubicin, ethinyl estradiol, fluoxetine, fluvoxamine, isoflurane, ketoconazole, mestranol, methimazole, nefazodone, nelfinavir, orphenadrine, paroxetine, phencyclidine, sertraline, thiotepa, ticlopidine
2C8	Amiodarone, cabazitaxel, carbamazepine, chloroquine, diclofenac, ibuprofen, paclitaxel, all-*trans*-retinoic acid, repaglinide, rosiglitazone, treprostinil	Rifampin, barbiturates	Deferasirox, gemfibrozil, lapatinib, montelukast, pioglitazone, quercetin, rosiglitazone, trimethoprim
2C9	Alosetron, bosentan, celecoxib, chlorpropamide, diclofenac, dronabinol, flurbiprofen, fluvastatin, glimepiride, glipizide, glyburide, hexobarbital, ibuprofen, indomethacin, irbesartan, losartan, meloxicam, montelukast, naproxen, nateglinide, phenobarbital, phenytoin, piroxicam, rosiglitazone, rosuvastatin, sulfamethoxazole, sulfaphenazole, ticrynafen, tolbutamide, torsemide, trimethadione, valsartan, *S*-warfarin	Aminoglutethimide, barbiturates, bosentan, carbamazepine, phenytoin, primidone, rifabutin, rifampin, rifapentine, St. John's wort	Amiodarone, clopidogrel, delavirdine, disulfiram, doxifluridine, efavirenz, fluconazole, fluvoxamine, fluorouracil, imatinib, leflunomide, metronidazole, miconazole, phenytoin, sulfamethoxazole, sulfaphenazole, sulfinpyrazone, tienilic acid, valproic acid, voriconazole
2C18	Tolbutamide, phenytoin	Phenobarbital	
2C19	Aripiprazole, carisoprodol, citalopram, clomipramine, clopidogrel, clozapine, desipramine, diazepam, diphenhydramine, doxepin, escitalopram, fluoxetine, imipramine, lansoprazole, S-mephenytoin, methadone, moclobemide, naproxen, nelfinavir, nirvanol, olanzapine, omeprazole, pantoprazole, phenobarbital, phenytoin, proguanil, propranolol, rabeprazole, sertraline, thalidomide, voriconazole, *R*-warfarin	Aminoglutethimide, artemisinin, barbiturates, carbamazepine, phenytoin, primidone, rifampin, rifapentine, St. John's wort	*N*3-Benzylnirvanol, *N*3-benzylphenobarbital, chloramphenicol, cimetidine, clopidogrel, delavirdine, efavirenz, esomeprazole, felbamate, fluconazole, fluoxetine, fluvoxamine, isoniazid, moclobemide, modafinil, nootkatone, omeprazole, ticlopidine, voriconazole
2D6	Amitriptyline, atomoxetine, bufuralol, bupranolol, carvedilol, chlorpheniramine, chlorpromazine, clomipramine, clozapine, codeine, debrisoquine, desipramine, dextromethorphan, dihydrocodeine, encainide, flecainide, fluoxetine, fluvoxamine, guanoxan, haloperidol, hydrocodone, imipramine, maprotiline, 4-methoxyamphetamine, metoclopramide, metoprolol, mexiletine, nebivolol, nortriptyline, oxycodone, palonosetron, paroxetine, perhexiline, perphenazine, phenformin, propafenone, propoxyphene, propranolol, risperidone, selegiline (deprenyl), sparteine, tamoxifen, thioridazine, timolol, tolterodine, tricyclic antidepressants, tramadol, trazodone, venlafaxine	Unknown	Bupropion, cinacalcet, chloroquine, diphenhydramine, fluoxetine, haloperidol, imatinib, paroxetine, propafenone, propoxyphene, quinidine, terbinafine, thioridazine
2E1	Acetaminophen, chlorzoxazone, dacarbazine, enflurane, ethanol (a minor pathway), halothane, isoflurane, isoniazid, sevoflurane, theophylline, trimethadione	Ethanol, isoniazid	Amitriptyline, chlorpromazine, cimetidine, clomethiazole, clotrimazole, clozapine, disulfiram, diethylthiocarbamate, diallyl sulfide, econazole, methimazole, methoxsalen, 4-methylpyrazole, miconazole, modafinil, ritonavir, selegiline, sildenafil, sulconazole, ticlopidine, tioconazole

(*continued*)

TABLE 4–2 Human liver P450s (CYPs), and some of the drugs metabolized (substrates), inducers, and selective inhibitors. Note: Some P450 substrates can be potent competitive inhibitors and/or mechanism-based inactivators. (Continued)

CYP	Substrates	Inducers	Inhibitors
3A4[1]	Acetaminophen, alfentanil, alfuzosin, almotriptan, alprazolam, amiodarone, amlodipine, aprepitant, astemizole, atazanavir, atorvastatin, bepridil, bexarotene, bosentan, bromocriptine, budesonide, buspirone, carbamazepine, cisapride, clarithromycin, clonazepam, clopidogrel, cocaine, colchicine, conivaptan, cortisol, cyclosporine, dapsone, darunavir, dasatinib, delavirdine, dexamethasone, diazepam, dihydroergotamine, dihydropyridines, diltiazem, disopyramide, doxorubicin, droperidol, dutasteride, ebastine, efavirenz, eletriptan, eplerenone, ergotamine, erlotinib, erythromycin, estazolam, eszopiclone, ethinyl estradiol, ethosuximide, etoposide, everolimus, exemestane, felodipine, fentanyl, finasteride, flurazepam, fluticasone, fosamprenavir, galantamine, gefitinib, gestodene, granisetron, halofantrine, ifosfamide, imatinib, indinavir, irinotecan, isradipine, itraconazole, ixabepilone, lapatinib, lidocaine, loperamide, lopinavir, loratadine, lovastatin, macrolides, maraviroc, mefloquine, methadone, methylprednisolone, miconazole, midazolam, mifepristone, modafinil, nefazodone, nevirapine, nicardipine, nifedipine, nimodipine, nisoldipine, paclitaxel, paricalcitol, pimozide, pioglitazone, praziquantel, prednisolone, prednisone, progesterone, quetiapine, quinacrine, quinidine, quinine, ranolazine, rapamycin, repaglinide, rifabutin, ritonavir, saquinavir, sibutramine, sildenafil, simvastatin, sirolimus, solifenacin, spironolactone, sufentanil, sulfamethoxazole, sunitinib, tacrolimus, tadalafil, tamoxifen, tamsulosin, teniposide, terfenadine, testosterone, tetrahydrocannabinol, tiagabine, tinidazole, tipranavir, tolvaptan, topiramate, triazolam, troleandomycin, vardenafil, verapamil, vinblastine, vincristine, ziprasidone, zolpidem, zonisamide, zopiclone	Aminoglutethimide, avasimibe, barbiturates, carbamazepine, efavirenz, glucocorticoids, nevirapine, pioglitazone, phenytoin, primidone, rifampin, rifapentine, St. John's wort	Amprenavir, azamulin, boceprevir, clarithromycin, conivaptan, diltiazem, erythromycin, fluconazole, grapefruit juice (furanocoumarins), indinavir, itraconazole, ketoconazole, lopinavir, mibefradil, nefazodone, nelfinavir, posaconazole, ritonavir, saquinavir, telaprevir, telithromycin, troleandomycin, verapamil, voriconazole

[1]CYP3A5 has similar substrate and inhibitor profiles but, except for a few drugs, is generally less active than CYP3A4.

Macrolide antibiotics such as troleandomycin, erythromycin, and erythromycin derivatives are metabolized, apparently by CYP3A, to metabolites that complex the cytochrome P450 heme iron and render it catalytically inactive. Another compound that acts through this mechanism is the inhibitor proadifen (SKF-525-A, used in research), which binds tightly to the heme iron and quasi-irreversibly inactivates the enzyme, thereby inhibiting the metabolism of potential substrates.

Some substrates irreversibly inhibit P450s via covalent interaction of a metabolically generated reactive intermediate that may react with the P450 apoprotein or heme moiety or even cause the heme to fragment and irreversibly modify the apoprotein. The antibiotic chloramphenicol is metabolized by CYP2B1 to a species that modifies the P450 protein and thus also inactivates the enzyme. A growing list of such **suicide inhibitors**—inactivators that attack the heme or the protein moiety—includes certain steroids (ethinyl estradiol, norethindrone, and spironolactone); fluroxene; allobarbital; the analgesic sedatives allylisopropylacetylurea, diethylpentenamide, and ethchlorvynol; carbon disulfide; grapefruit furanocoumarins; selegiline; phencyclidine; ticlopidine and clopidogrel; ritonavir; and propylthiouracil. On the other hand, the barbiturate secobarbital is found to inactivate CYP2B1 by modification of *both* its heme and protein moieties. Other metabolically activated drugs whose P450 inactivation mechanism is not fully elucidated are mifepristone, troglitazone, raloxifene, and tamoxifen.

PHASE II REACTIONS

Parent drugs or their phase I metabolites that contain suitable chemical groups often undergo coupling or conjugation reactions with an endogenous substance to yield **drug conjugates** (Table 4–3). In general, conjugates are polar molecules that are readily excreted and often inactive. Conjugate formation involves high-energy intermediates and specific transfer enzymes. Such enzymes **(transferases)** may be located in microsomes or in the cytoplasm. Of these, uridine 5′-diphosphate (UDP)-glucuronosyl transferases **(UGTs)** are the most dominant enzymes (see Figure 4–4). These microsomal enzymes catalyze the coupling of an activated endogenous substance (such as the UDP derivative of glucuronic acid) with a drug (or endogenous compound such as bilirubin, the end product of heme metabolism). Nineteen *UGT* genes (*UGT1A1* and *UGT2*) encode UGT proteins involved in the metabolism of drugs and xenobiotics. Similarly, 11 human sulfotransferases **(SULTs)** catalyze the sulfation of substrates using 3′-phosphoadenosine 5′-phosphosulfate **(PAPS)**

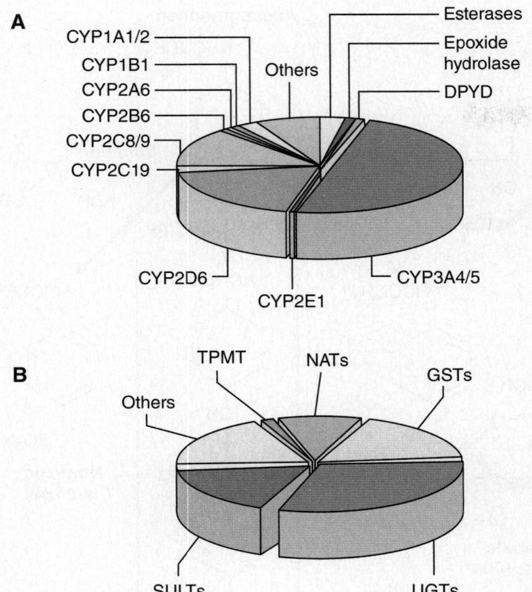

FIGURE 4–4 Relative contributions of various cytochrome P450 isoforms (**A**) and different phase II pathways (**B**) to metabolism of drugs in clinical use. Many drugs are metabolized by two or more of these pathways. Note that two pathways, CYP3A4/5 and UGT, are involved in the metabolism of more than 75% of drugs in use. DPYD, dihydropyrimidine dehydrogenase; GST, glutathione-*S*-transferase; NAT, *N*-acetyltransferase; SULT, sulfotransferase; TPMT, thiopurine methyltransferase; UGT, UDP-glucuronosyltransferase. (Reproduced with permission from Brunton LL, Chabner BA, Knollman BC: *Goodman & Gilman's The Pharmacological Basis of Therapeutics*, 12th ed. New York, NY: McGraw Hill; 2011.)

as the endogenous sulfate donor. Cytosolic and microsomal glutathione **(GSH)** transferases **(GSTs)** are also engaged in the metabolism of drugs and xenobiotics, and in that of leukotrienes and prostaglandins, respectively. Chemicals containing an aromatic amine or a hydrazine moiety (eg, isoniazid) are substrates of cytosolic *N*-acetyltransferases **(NATs),** encoded by *NAT1* and *NAT2* genes, which utilize **acetyl-CoA** as the endogenous cofactor.

S-Adenosyl-L-methionine (**SAMe**; AdoMet)-mediated *O*-, *N*-, and *S*-methylation of drugs and xenobiotics by methyltransferases **(MTs)** also occurs. Finally, endobiotic, drug, and xenobiotic epoxides generated via P450-catalyzed oxidations can also be hydrolyzed by microsomal or cytosolic epoxide hydrolases **(EHs).** Conjugation of an activated drug such as the *S*-CoA derivative of benzoic acid, with an endogenous substrate, such as glycine, also occurs. Because the endogenous substrates originate in the diet, nutrition plays a critical role in the regulation of drug conjugations.

Phase II reactions are relatively faster than P450-catalyzed reactions, thus effectively accelerating drug biotransformation.

Drug conjugations were once believed to represent terminal inactivation events and as such have been viewed as "true detoxification" reactions. However, this concept must be modified, because it is now known that certain conjugation reactions (acyl glucuronidation of nonsteroidal anti-inflammatory drugs, *O*-sulfation of *N*-hydroxyacetylaminofluorene, and *N*-acetylation of isoniazid) may lead to the formation of reactive species responsible for the toxicity of the drugs. Furthermore, sulfation is known to activate the orally active prodrug minoxidil into a very efficacious vasodilator, and morphine-6-glucuronide is more potent than morphine itself.

TABLE 4–3 Phase II reactions.

Type of Conjugation	Endogenous Reactant	Transferase (Location)	Types of Substrates	Examples
Glucuronidation	UDP glucuronic acid (UDPGA)	UDP glucuronosyl-transferase (microsomes)	Phenols, alcohols, carboxylic acids, hydroxylamines, sulfonamides	Nitrophenol, morphine, acetaminophen, diazepam, *N*-hydroxydapsone, sulfathiazole, meprobamate, digitoxin, digoxin
Acetylation	Acetyl-CoA	*N*-Acetyltransferase (cytoplasm)	Amines	Sulfonamides, isoniazid, clonazepam, dapsone, mescaline
Glutathione conjugation	Glutathione (GSH)	GSH-*S*-transferase (cytoplasm, microsomes)	Epoxides, arene oxides, nitro groups, hydroxylamines	Acetaminophen, ethacrynic acid, bromobenzene
Glycine conjugation	Glycine	Acyl-CoA glycinetransferase (mitochondria)	Acyl-CoA derivatives of carboxylic acids	Salicylic acid, benzoic acid, nicotinic acid, cinnamic acid, cholic acid, deoxycholic acid
Sulfation	Phosphoadenosyl phosphosulfate (PAPS)	Sulfotransferase (cytoplasm)	Phenols, alcohols, aromatic amines	Estrone, aniline, phenol, 3-hydroxycoumarin, acetaminophen, methyldopa
Methylation	*S*-Adenosylmethionine (SAM)	Transmethylases (cytoplasm)	Catecholamines, phenols, amines	Dopamine, epinephrine, pyridine, histamine, thiouracil
Water conjugation	Water	Epoxide hydrolase (microsomes)	Arene oxides, *cis*-disubstituted and monosubstituted oxiranes	Benzopyrene 7,8-epoxide, styrene 1,2-oxide, carbamazepine epoxide
		(cytoplasm)	Alkene oxides, fatty acid epoxides	Leukotriene A_4

METABOLISM OF DRUGS TO TOXIC PRODUCTS

Metabolism of drugs and other foreign chemicals may not always be an innocuous biochemical event leading to detoxification and elimination of the compound. Indeed, as previously noted, several compounds have been shown to be metabolically transformed to reactive intermediates that are toxic to various organs. Such toxic reactions may not be apparent at low levels of exposure to parent compounds when alternative detoxification mechanisms are not yet overwhelmed or compromised and when the availability of endogenous detoxifying cosubstrates (GSH, glucuronic acid, sulfate) is not limited. However, when these resources are exhausted, the toxic pathway may prevail, resulting in overt organ toxicity or carcinogenesis. The number of specific examples of such drug-induced toxicity is expanding rapidly. An example is acetaminophen (APAP; paracetamol)-induced hepatotoxicity (Figure 4–5). Acetaminophen, an analgesic antipyretic drug, is quite safe in therapeutic doses (1.2 g/d for an adult). It normally undergoes glucuronidation and sulfation to the corresponding conjugates, which together make up 95% of the total excreted metabolites. The alternative P450-dependent GSH conjugation pathway accounts for the remaining 5%. When acetaminophen intake far exceeds therapeutic doses, the glucuronidation and sulfation pathways are saturated, and the P450-dependent pathway becomes increasingly important. Little or no hepatotoxicity results as long as hepatic GSH is available for conjugation. However, with time, hepatic GSH is depleted faster than it can be regenerated, and a reactive, toxic metabolite accumulates. In the absence of intracellular nucleophiles such as GSH, this reactive metabolite (*N*-acetylbenzoiminoquinone) not only reacts with nucleophilic groups of cellular proteins resulting in direct hepatocellular damage, but also participates in redox cycling, thereby generating reactive O_2 species **(ROS)** and consequent oxidative stress that greatly enhance acetaminophen-induced hepatotoxicity.

The chemical and toxicologic characterization of the electrophilic nature of the reactive acetaminophen metabolite has led to the development of effective antidotes—cysteamine and *N*-acetylcysteine (NAC; Acetadote; Mucomyst). Administration of *N*-acetylcysteine (the safer of the two) within 8–16 hours after acetaminophen overdosage has been shown to protect victims from fulminant hepatotoxicity and death (see Chapter 58). Administration of GSH is not effective because it does not cross cell membranes readily.

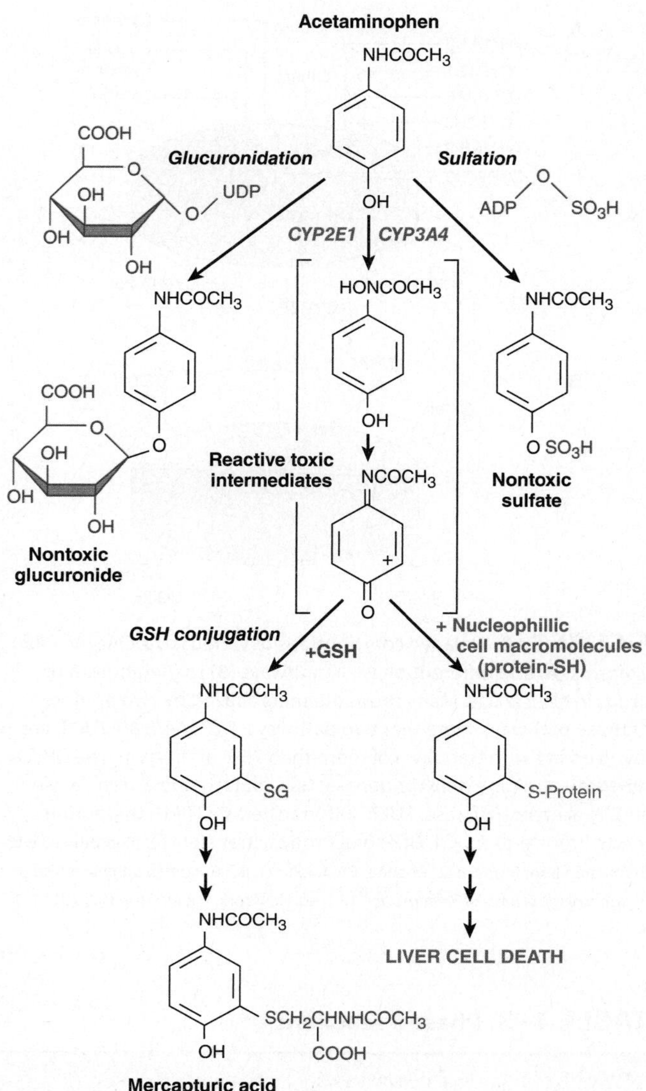

FIGURE 4–5 Metabolism of acetaminophen (top center) to hepatotoxic metabolites. GSH, glutathione; SG, glutathione moiety.

CLINICAL RELEVANCE OF DRUG METABOLISM

The dose and frequency of administration required to achieve effective therapeutic blood and tissue levels vary in different patients because of individual differences in drug distribution and rates of drug metabolism and elimination. These differences are determined by genetic factors as well as nongenetic variables, such as commensal gut microbiota, age, sex, liver size, liver function, circadian rhythm, body temperature, and nutritional and environmental factors such as concomitant exposure to inducers or inhibitors of drug metabolism. The discussion that follows summarizes the most important of these variables.

Individual Differences

Individual differences in metabolic rate depend on the nature of the drug itself. Thus, within the same population, steady-state plasma levels may reflect a 30-fold variation in the metabolism of one drug and only a twofold variation in the metabolism of another.

Genetic Factors

Genetic factors that influence enzyme levels account for some of these differences, giving rise to "genetic polymorphisms" in drug metabolism (see also Chapter 5). The first examples of drugs found to be subject to genetic polymorphisms were the muscle relaxant succinylcholine, the antituberculosis drug isoniazid, and the anticoagulant warfarin. A true genetic polymorphism is defined as the occurrence of a variant allele of a gene at a population frequency of ≥1%, resulting in altered expression or functional activity of the gene product, or both. Well-defined and clinically relevant genetic polymorphisms in both phase I and phase II drug-metabolizing enzymes exist that result in altered efficacy of drug therapy or adverse drug reactions **(ADRs).** The latter frequently necessitate dose adjustment (Table 4–4), a consideration particularly crucial for drugs with low therapeutic indices.

A. Phase I Enzyme Polymorphisms

Genetically determined defects in the phase I oxidative metabolism of several drugs have been reported (see Table 4–4; see also Chapter 5). These defects are often transmitted as autosomal recessive traits and may be expressed at any one of the multiple metabolic transformations that a chemical might undergo. Human liver P450s 3A4, 2C9, 2D6, 2C19, 1A2, and 2B6 are responsible for about 75% of all clinically relevant phase I drug metabolism (see Figure 4–4), and thus for about 60% of all physiologic drug biotransformation and elimination. Thus, genetic polymorphisms of these enzymes, by significantly influencing phase I drug metabolism, can alter their pharmacokinetics and the magnitude or the duration of drug response and associated events.

Three P450 genetic polymorphisms have been particularly well characterized, affording some insight into possible underlying molecular mechanisms, and are clinically noteworthy, as they require therapeutic dosage adjustment. The first is the **debrisoquin-sparteine oxidation** type of polymorphism, which apparently occurs in 3–10% of Caucasians and is inherited as an autosomal recessive trait. In affected individuals, the **CYP2D6**-dependent oxidations of debrisoquin and other drugs (see Table 4–2; Figure 4–6) are impaired. These defects in oxidative drug metabolism are probably co-inherited. The precise molecular basis for the defect appears to be faulty expression of the P450 protein due to either defective mRNA splicing or protein folding, resulting in little or no isoform-catalyzed drug metabolism and thereby conferring a **poor metabolizer (PM)** phenotype. This PM phenotype correlates with a higher risk of relapse in patients with breast cancer treated with tamoxifen, an anticancer drug that relies on its CYP2D6-dependent metabolic activation to endoxifen for its efficacy. More recently, however, another polymorphic genotype has been reported that results in **ultrarapid metabolism** of relevant drugs due to the presence of CYP2D6 allelic variants with up to 13 gene copies in tandem. This ultrarapid metabolizer **(UM)** genotype is most common in Ethiopians and Saudi Arabians, populations that display it in up to one third of individuals. As a result, these subjects require twofold to threefold higher daily doses of nortriptyline (an antidepressant and a CYP2D6 substrate) to achieve therapeutic plasma levels. The poor responsiveness to antidepressant therapy of the UM phenotype also clinically correlates with a higher incidence of suicides relative to that of deaths due to natural causes in this patient population. Conversely, in these UM populations, the prodrug codeine (another CYP2D6 substrate) is metabolized much faster to morphine, often resulting in undesirable adverse effects of morphine, such as abdominal pain. Indeed, intake of high doses of codeine by a mother of the ultrarapid metabolizer type was held responsible for the morphine-induced death of her breast-fed infant.

The second well-studied genetic drug polymorphism involves the stereoselective **aromatic (4)-hydroxylation** of the anticonvulsant mephenytoin, catalyzed by **CYP2C19.** This polymorphism, which is also inherited as an autosomal recessive trait, occurs in 3–5% of Caucasians and 18–23% of Japanese populations. It is genetically independent of the debrisoquin-sparteine polymorphism. In normal **extensive metabolizers** (EMs) (*S*)-mephenytoin is extensively hydroxylated by CYP2C19 at the 4-position of the phenyl ring before its glucuronidation and rapid excretion in the urine, whereas (*R*)-mephenytoin is slowly *N*-demethylated to nirvanol, an active metabolite. PMs, however, appear to totally lack the stereospecific (*S*)-mephenytoin hydroxylase activity, so both (*S*)- and (*R*)-mephenytoin enantiomers are *N*-demethylated to nirvanol, which accumulates in much higher concentrations. Thus, PMs of mephenytoin show signs of profound sedation and ataxia after doses of the drug that are well tolerated by normal metabolizers. Two defective CYP2C19 variant alleles (*CYP2C19*2* and *CYP2C19*3*), the latter predominant in Asians, are largely responsible for the PM genotype. The molecular bases include splicing defects resulting in a truncated, nonfunctional protein. CYP2C19 is responsible for the metabolism of various clinically relevant drugs (see Table 4–4). Thus, it is clinically important to recognize that the safety of each of these drugs may be severely reduced in persons with the PM phenotype. On the other hand, the PM phenotype can notably increase the therapeutic efficacy of omeprazole, a proton-pump inhibitor, in gastric ulcer and gastroesophageal reflux diseases (see Chapter 5 for additional discussion of the CYP2C19 polymorphism).

Another CYP2C19 variant allele (*CYP2C19*17*) exists that is associated with increased transcription and thus higher CYP2C19 expression and even higher functional activity than that of the wild type CYP2C19-carrying EMs. Individuals carrying this *CYP2C19*17* allele exhibit higher metabolic activation of prodrugs such as the breast cancer drug tamoxifen, the antimalarial chlorproguanil, and the antiplatelet drug clopidogrel. The former event is associated with a lower risk of breast cancer relapse, and the latter event with an increased risk of bleeding. Carriers of the *CYP2C19*17* allele are also known to enhance the metabolism and thus the elimination of drugs such as the antidepressants escitalopram and imipramine, as well as the antifungal voriconazole. This consequently impairs the therapeutic efficacy of these drugs, thus requiring clinical dosage adjustments.

The third relatively well-characterized genetic polymorphism is that of **CYP2C9.** Two well-characterized variants of this enzyme exist, each with amino acid mutations that result in altered metabolism. The *CYP2C9*2* allele encodes an Arg144Cys mutation, exhibiting impaired functional interactions with CPR. The other allelic variant, *CYP2C9*3*, encodes an enzyme with an Ile359Leu mutation that has lowered affinity for many substrates. For example, individuals displaying the *CYP2C9*3* phenotype have greatly reduced tolerance for the anticoagulant warfarin. The warfarin clearance in *CYP2C9*3*-homozygous individuals is about 10% of normal values, and these people have a much lower tolerance for the drug than those who are homozygous for the normal wild type

TABLE 4–4 Some examples of genetic polymorphisms in phase I and phase II drug metabolism.

Enzyme Involved	Defect	Genotype	Drug and Therapeutic Use	Clinical Consequences[1]
CYP1A2	*N*-Demethylation	**EM**	Caffeine (CNS stimulant)	Reduced CNS stimulation due to increased gene inducibility and thus increased metabolism/clearance in cigarette smokers and frequent ingesters of omeprazole.
	N-Demethylation	**PM**	Caffeine (CNS stimulant)	Enhanced CNS stimulation.
CYP2A6	Oxidation	**PM**	Nicotine (cholinoceptorstimulant)	Nicotine toxicity. Lesser craving for frequent cigarette smoking.
	Oxidation	**EM**	Nicotine (cholinoceptorstimulant)	Increased nicotine metabolism. Greater craving for frequent cigarette smoking.
	Oxidation	**PM**	Coumarin (anticoagulant)	Increased risk of bleeding.
	Oxidation	**EM**	Coumarin (anticoagulant)	Increased clearance. Greater risk of thrombosis.
CYP2B6	Oxidation, *N*-Dechloroethylation	**PM**	Cyclophosphamide, ifosfamide (anti-cancer)	Reduced clearance. Increased risk of ADRs.
	Oxidation	**PM**	Efavirenz, nevirapine (anti-HIV)	Reduced clearance. Increased risk of ADRs.
CYP2C8	Hydroxylation	**PM**	Repaglinide, rosiglitazone, pioglitazone (antidiabetic)	Reduced clearance. Increased risk of ADRs.
	Hydroxylation	**PM**	Paclitaxel (anti-cancer)	Reduced clearance. Increased risk of ADRs (myelosuppression).
	N-Deethylation/ *N*-Dealkylation	**PM**	Amodiaquine, chloroquine (antimalarial)	Reduced clearance. Increased risk of ADRs.
	N-Deethylation	**PM**	Amiodarone (antiarrhythmic)	Reduced clearance. Increased risk of ADRs.
CYP2C9	Hydroxylation	**PM**	Celecoxib, diclofenac, flurbiprofen, *S*-ibuprofen (NSAIDs)	Reduced clearance. Increased risk of ADRs.
	Hydroxylation	**PM**	*S*-Warfarin, *S*-acenocoumarol (anticoagulants)	Enhanced bleeding risk. Clinically highly relevant. Dose adjustment required.
	Hydroxylation	**PM**	Tolbutamide (antidiabetic)	Cardiotoxicity.
	Hydroxylation	**PM**	Phenytoin (antiepileptic)	Nystagmus, diplopia, and ataxia.
CYP2C19	*N*-Demethylation	**PM**	Amitriptyline, clomipramine (antidepressants)	Reduced clearance. Increased risk of ADRs. Dose adjustment required.
	Oxidation	**PM**	Moclobemide (MAOI)	
	N-Demethylation	**PM**	Citalopram (SSRI)	Increased risk of gastrointestinal side effects. Increased risk of QT-prolongation and Torsades de Pointes arrhythmias.
	O-Demethylation	**PM**	Omeprazole (PPI)	Increased therapeutic efficacy.
	Hydroxylation	**PM**	Mephenytoin (antiepileptic)	Overdose toxicity.
	N-Demethylation	**EM**	Escitalopram (antidepressants)	Increased gene transcription resulting in increased activity and thus reduced therapeutic efficacy.
	O-Demethylation	**EM**	Omeprazole (PPI)	Reduced therapeutic efficacy.
	Hydroxylation	**EM**	Tamoxifen (anti-cancer)	Increased metabolic activation, increased therapeutic efficacy; reduced risk of relapse. Dose adjustment required.
	Oxidative cyclization	**EM**	Chlorproguanil (antimalarial)	Increased metabolic activation, increased therapeutic efficacy. Dose adjustment required.
	Oxidation	**EM**	Clopidogrel (antiplatelet)	Increased metabolic activation, increased therapeutic efficacy. Dose adjustment required.
CYP2D6	Oxidation	**PM**	Bufuralol (β-adrenoceptor blocker)	Exacerbation of β blockade, nausea.
	O-Demethylation	**PM**	Codeine (analgesic)	Reduced metabolic activation to morphine and thus reduced analgesia.

(continued)

TABLE 4–4 Some examples of genetic polymorphisms in phase I and phase II drug metabolism. (Continued)

Enzyme Involved	Defect	Genotype	Drug and Therapeutic Use	Clinical Consequences[1]
	Oxidation	PM	Debrisoquin (antihypertensive)	Orthostatic hypotension.
	N-Demethylation	PM	Nortriptyline (antidepressant)	Reduced clearance. Increased risk of ADRs.
	Oxidation	PM	Sparteine	Oxytocic symptoms.
	O-Demethylation	PM	Dextromethorphan (antitussive)	Reduced clearance. Increased risk of ADRs.
	O-Demethylation	PM	Tramadol (analgesic)	Increased risk of seizures.
	Hydroxylation	PM	Tamoxifen (anti-cancer)	Reduced metabolic activation to the therapeutically active endoxifen and thus reduced therapeutic efficacy.
	O-Demethylation	UM	Codeine (analgesic)	Increased metabolic activation to morphine and thus increased risk of respiratory depression.
	N-Demethylation	UM	Nortriptyline (antidepressant)	Reduced therapeutic efficacy due to increased clearance.
	O-Demethylation	UM	Tramadol (analgesic)	Reduced therapeutic efficacy due to increased clearance.
CYP3A4		PM?	All drugs metabolized by this enzyme would be potentially affected	Reduced clearance. Dose adjustment may be required to avoid drugdrug interactions.
CYP3A5		PM?	Saquinavir, and other CYP3A substrates	Usually less catalytically active than CYP3A4. A higher frequency of a functional CYP3A5*1 allele is seen in Africans than in Caucasians; the latter most often carry the defective CYP3A5*3 allele. This may significantly affect therapeutics of CYP3A substrates in CYP3A5*1 or CYP3A5*3 homozygous individuals.
ALDH	Aldehyde dehydrogenation	PM	Ethanol (recreational drug)	Facial flushing, hypotension, tachycardia, nausea, vomiting.
BCHE	Ester hydrolysis	PM	Succinylcholine (muscle relaxant)	Prolonged apnea.
			Mivacurium (neuromuscular blocker)	Prolonged muscle paralysis.
			Cocaine (CNS stimulant)	Increased blood pressure, tachycardia, ventricular arrhythmias.
GST	GSH-conjugation	PM	Acetaminophen (analgesic), Busulfan (anticancer)	Impaired GSH conjugation due to gene deletion.
NAT2	*N*-Acetylation	PM	Hydralazine (antihypertensive)	Lupus erythematosus-like syndrome.
	N-Acetylation	PM	Isoniazid (antitubercular)	Peripheral neuropathy.
TPMT	*S*-Methylation	PM	6-Thiopurines (anti-cancer)	Myelotoxicity.
UGT1A1	Glucuronidation	PM	Bilirubin (heme metabolite)	Hyperbilirubinemia.
			Irinotecan (anti-cancer)	Reduced clearance. Dose adjustment may be required to avoid toxicity (GI dysfunction, immunosuppression).

[1]Observed or predictable.

ADR, adverse drug reaction; EM, extensive metabolizer; PM, poor metabolizer; UM, ultrarapid metabolizer.

allele. These individuals also have a much higher risk of adverse effects with warfarin (eg, bleeding) and with other CYP2C9 substrates such as phenytoin, losartan, tolbutamide, and some nonsteroidal anti-inflammatory drugs (see Table 4–4). Note, however, that despite the predominant role of CYP2C9 in warfarin clearance (particularly that of its pharmacologically more potent *S*-isomer), warfarin maintenance doses are largely dictated by polymorphisms in the *VKORC1* gene responsible for the expression of vitamin K epoxide reductase, the specific cellular target of warfarin, rather than by *CYP2C9*2/*3* polymorphisms alone (see Chapter 5).

Allelic variants of CYP3A4 have also been reported, but their contribution to the well-known interindividual variability in drug metabolism apparently is limited. On the other hand, the expression of **CYP3A5,** another human liver isoform, is markedly

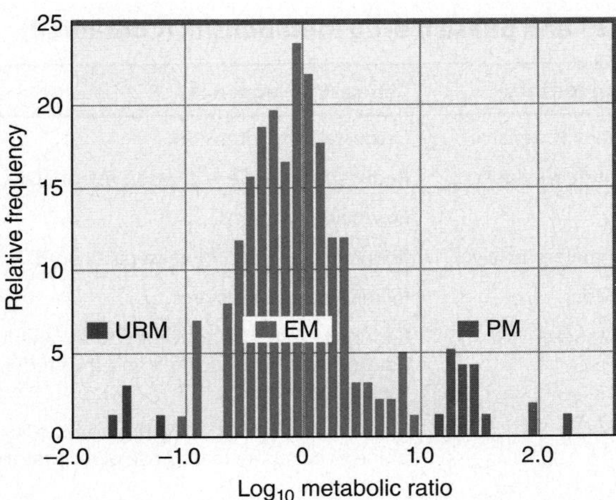

FIGURE 4–6 Genetic polymorphism in debrisoquin 4-hydroxylation by CYP2D6 in a Caucasian population. The semilog frequency distribution histogram of the metabolic ratio (MR; defined as percent of dose excreted as unchanged debrisoquin divided by the percent of dose excreted as 4-hydroxydebrisoquin metabolite) in the 8-hour urine collected after oral ingestion of 12.8 mg debrisoquin sulfate (equivalent to 10 mg free debrisoquin base). Individuals with MR values >12.6 were phenotyped as poor metabolizers (PM, *red bars*), and those with MR values <12.6 but >0.2 were designated as extensive metabolizers (EM, *blue bars*). Those with MR values <0.2 were designated as ultrarapid metabolizers (URM, *green bars*) based on the MR values (0.01–0.1) of individuals with documented multiple copies of CYP2D6 allelic variants resulting from inherited amplification of this gene. (Adapted with permission from Woolhouse NM, Andoh B, Mahgoub A, et al: Debrisoquin hydroxylation polymorphism among Ghanaians and Caucasians. Clin Pharmacol Ther 1979 Nov;26(5):584-591.)

polymorphic, ranging from 0% to 50% of the total hepatic CYP3A content. Robust CYP3A5 expression requires at the least, one normally spliced CYP3A5*1 allele. This CYP3A5 protein polymorphism is now known to result from a single nucleotide polymorphism **(SNP)** within intron 3 or 6, resulting in alternative splicing, as well as protein truncation and loss, thus enabling normally spliced CYP3A5 transcripts in just 5% of Caucasians, 29% of Japanese, 27% of Chinese, and 30% of Koreans, but 73% of African Americans. Thus, it can significantly contribute to interindividual differences in the metabolism of preferential CYP3A5 substrates such as midazolam. Two other CYP3A5 allelic variants that result in a PM phenotype also are known.

Polymorphisms in the *CYP2A6* gene have also been recently characterized, and their prevalence is apparently racially linked. CYP2A6 is responsible for nicotine oxidation, and tobacco smokers with low CYP2A6 activity consume less and have a lower incidence of lung cancer. CYP2A6 1B allelic variants associated with faster rates of nicotine metabolism have been recently discovered. It remains to be determined whether patients with these faster variants will fall into the converse paradigm of increased smoking behavior and lung cancer incidence.

Additional genetic polymorphisms in drug metabolism are being discovered. Of these, the gene for **CYP2B6** has become noteworthy as one of the most polymorphic P450 genes, with a 20- to 250-fold variation in interindividual CYP2B6 expression. Despite its low (1–5%) contribution to the total liver P450 content, these CYP2B6 polymorphisms may have a significant impact on the CYP2B6-dependent metabolism of several clinically relevant drugs such as cyclophosphamide, *S*-methadone, efavirenz, nevirapine, bupropion, selegiline, and propofol. Of clinical relevance, women (particularly Hispanic American women) express considerably higher hepatic levels of CYP2B6 protein than men.

Studies of theophylline metabolism in monozygotic and dizygotic twins that included pedigree analysis of various families have revealed that a distinct polymorphism may exist for this drug and may be inherited as a recessive genetic trait. Genetic drug metabolism polymorphisms also appear to occur for aminopyrine and carbocysteine oxidations. Regularly updated information on human P450 polymorphisms is available at https://www.pharmvar.org/.

Although genetic polymorphisms in drug oxidations often involve specific P450 enzymes, such genetic variations can also occur in other enzymes. Recently, genetic polymorphisms in CPR/POR, the essential P450 electron donor, have been reported. In particular, an allelic variant (at a 28% frequency) encoding a CPR A503V mutation (eg, *POR*10*) has been reported to result in impaired CYP17-dependent sex steroid synthesis and impaired CYP3A4- and CYP2D6-dependent drug metabolism in vitro. However, an associated impairment in drug metabolism was not always found clinically. By contrast, several other CPR/POR allelic variants (eg, *POR*5*, *POR*16*) have now been established with an associated decreased drug metabolism as their plausible clinical phenotype. Descriptions of a polymorphism in the oxidation of trimethylamine, believed to be metabolized largely by the **flavin monooxygenase (Ziegler's enzyme),** result in the "fish-odor syndrome" in slow metabolizers, thus suggesting that genetic variants of other non-P450-dependent oxidative enzymes may also contribute to such polymorphisms.

Genetic polymorphisms also exist in other Phase I enzymes, ie, esterases. Thus, succinylcholine is metabolized only half as rapidly in persons with genetically determined deficiency in pseudocholinesterase (now generally referred to as butyrylcholinesterase [**BCHE**]) as in persons with normally functioning enzyme. Different mutations, inherited as autosomal recessive traits, account for the enzyme deficiency. Deficient individuals treated with succinylcholine as a muscle relaxant may become susceptible to prolonged respiratory paralysis (succinylcholine apnea); see Chapter 27.

B. Phase II Enzyme Polymorphisms

Pharmacogenetic differences are seen in the acetylation of isoniazid. The defect in slow acetylators (of isoniazid and similar amines) appears to be caused by the synthesis of less of the NAT2 enzyme rather than of an abnormal form of it. Inherited as an autosomal recessive trait, the **slow acetylator phenotype** occurs in about 50% of blacks and whites in the USA, more frequently in Europeans living in high northern latitudes, and much less commonly in Asians and Inuit (Eskimos). The slow acetylator phenotype is also associated with a higher incidence of isoniazid-induced peripheral neuritis, drug-induced autoimmune disorders, and bicyclic aromatic amine-induced bladder cancer.

A clinically important polymorphism of the *TPMT* (thiopurine *S*-methyltransferase) gene is encountered in Europeans (frequency, 1:300), resulting in a rapidly degraded mutant enzyme and consequently deficient *S*-methylation of aromatic and heterocyclic sulfhydryl compounds including the anti-cancer thiopurine drugs 6-mercaptopurine, thioguanine, and azathioprine, required for their detoxification. Patients inheriting this polymorphism as an autosomal recessive trait are at high risk of thiopurine drug-induced fatal hematopoietic toxicity.

Genetic polymorphisms in the expression of other phase II enzymes (UGTs and GSTs) also occur. Thus, UGT polymorphisms (*UGT1A1*28*) are associated with hyperbilirubinemic diseases (Gilbert syndrome) as well as toxic effects due to impaired drug conjugation and/or elimination (eg, the anticancer drug irinotecan). Similarly, genetic polymorphisms (*GSTM1*) in GST (mu1 isoform) expression can lead to significant adverse effects and toxicities of drugs dependent on its GSH conjugation for elimination.

C. Role of Pharmacogenomic Testing in Clinically Safe & Effective Drug Therapy

Despite our improved understanding of the molecular basis of pharmacogenetic defects in drug-metabolizing enzymes, their impact on drug therapy and ADRs, and the availability of validated pharmacogenetic biomarkers to identify patients at risk, this clinically relevant information has not been effectively translated to patient care. Thus, the much-heralded potential for personalized medicine, except in a few instances of drugs with a relatively low therapeutic index (eg, warfarin), has remained largely unrealized. This is so even though 98% of US physicians are apparently aware that such genetic information may significantly influence therapy. This is partly due to the lack of adequate training in translating this knowledge to medical practice, and partly due to the logistics of genetic testing and the issue of cost-effectiveness. Severe ADRs are known to contribute to 100,000 annual US deaths, about 7% of all hospital admissions, and an increased average length of hospital stay. Genotype information could greatly enhance safe and efficacious clinical therapy through dose adjustment or alternative drug therapy, thereby curbing much of the rising ADR incidence and its associated costs. (See Chapter 5 for further discussion.)

Commensal Gut Microbiota

It is increasingly recognized that the human gut microbiome can also significantly influence drug responses. It thus serves as another relevant source of therapeutic misadventures and adverse drug-drug interactions. More than 1000 species of intestinal microorganisms have been identified, including obligate anaerobic bacteria and various yeasts that coexist in a dynamic, often symbiotic, ecological equilibrium. Their biotransformation repertoire is nonoxidative, albeit highly versatile, extending from predominantly reductive and hydrolytic reactions to decarboxylation, dehydroxylation, dealkylation, dehalogenation, and deamination. Notably, such bacterially mediated reduction of the cardiac drug digoxin significantly contributes to its metabolism and elimination. Cotreatment with antibiotics such as erythromycin or tetracycline increases digoxin serum levels twofold, increasing the risk of cardiotoxicity. Similarly, drugs that are primarily glucuronidated in the liver are excreted into the gut via the bile, whereupon they are subjected to de-glucuronidation by gut microbial β-glucuronidases (hydrolases). The pharmacologically active parent aglycone is subsequently reabsorbed into the portal circulation with consequent extension of its pharmacologic action and hepatic phase II reconjugation and subsequent enterohepatic recycling. Thus, if the parent drug is dosage limited or has a low therapeutic index, this may mean increased toxicity. For example, under normal dosage, the analgesic acetaminophen is largely metabolized via glucuronidation and sulfation, as discussed earlier, and eliminated into the hepatic sinusoidal plasma. However, upon overdosage, the increased production of these metabolites is quite likely to saturate their normal excretory transport process. Their consequently enhanced biliary excretion would subject a greater fraction of the acetaminophen-glucuronide to de-glucuronidation by intestinal microbial β-glucuronidases, which may further contribute to the toxic acetaminophen burden. This possibility is even more relevant for glucuronides of parent drugs of noted gastrointestinal toxicity. Accordingly, selective inhibition of microbial β-glucuronidases has been documented to alleviate the gastrointestinal toxicity of anticancer drugs such as irinotecan, as well as the enteropathies induced by nonsteroidal anti-inflammatory drugs (NSAIDs) such as indomethacin, ketoprofen or diclofenac, that incur substantial enterohepatic circulation. This possibility has fueled the pharmaceutical design and development of even more selective inhibitors targeted against microbial β-glucuronidases.

Diet & Environmental Factors

Diet and environmental factors contribute to individual variations in drug metabolism. Charcoal-broiled foods and cruciferous vegetables are known to induce CYP1A enzymes, whereas grapefruit juice is known to inhibit the CYP3A metabolism of co-administered drug substrates (see Table 4–2; also see below). Cigarette smokers metabolize some drugs more rapidly than nonsmokers because of enzyme induction (see previous section). Industrial workers exposed to some pesticides metabolize certain drugs more rapidly than unexposed individuals. Such differences make it difficult to determine effective and safe doses of drugs that have narrow therapeutic indices.

Age & Sex

Increased susceptibility to the pharmacologic or toxic activity of drugs has been reported in very young and very old patients compared with young adults (see Chapters 59 and 60). Although this may reflect differences in absorption, distribution, and excretion, differences in drug metabolism also play a role. Slower metabolism could be due to reduced activity of metabolic enzymes or reduced availability of essential endogenous cofactors.

Sex-dependent variations in drug metabolism have been well documented in rats but not in other rodents. Young adult male rats metabolize drugs much faster than mature female rats or prepubertal male rats. These differences in drug metabolism have been clearly associated with androgenic hormones. Clinical reports suggest that similar sex-dependent differences in drug metabolism also exist in humans for ethanol, propranolol, some benzodiazepines, estrogens, and salicylates.

TABLE 4–5 Partial list of drugs that enhance drug metabolism in humans.

Inducer	Drugs Whose Metabolism Is Enhanced
Benzo[*a*]pyrene	Theophylline
Carbamazepine	Carbamazepine, clonazepam, itraconazole
Chlorcyclizine	Steroid hormones
Ethchlorvynol	Warfarin
Glutethimide	Antipyrine, glutethimide, warfarin
Griseofulvin	Warfarin
Phenobarbital and other barbiturates[1]	Barbiturates, chloramphenicol, chlorpromazine, cortisol, coumarin anticoagulants, desmethyl imipramine, digitoxin, doxorubicin, estradiol, itraconazole, phenylbutazone, phenytoin, quinine, testosterone
Phenylbutazone	Aminopyrine, cortisol, digitoxin
Phenytoin	Cortisol, dexamethasone, digitoxin, itraconazole, theophylline
Rifampin	Coumarin anticoagulants, digitoxin, glucocorticoids, itraconazole, methadone, metoprolol, oral contraceptives, prednisone, propranolol, quinidine, saquinavir
Ritonavir[2]	Midazolam
St. John's wort[3]	Alprazolam, cyclosporine, digoxin, indinavir, oral contraceptives, ritonavir, simvastatin, tacrolimus, warfarin

[1]Secobarbital is an exception. See Table 4–6 and text.

[2]With chronic (repeated) administration; acutely, ritonavir is a potent CYP3A4 inhibitor/inactivator.

[3]For a more comprehensive list of drugs whose metabolism is enhanced by St. John's wort, see Rahimi and Abdollahi, 2012; Russo et al, 2014; and Tsai et al, 2012.

Drug-Drug Interactions (DDIs) During Metabolism

Many substrates, by virtue of their relatively high lipophilicity, are not only retained at the active site of the enzyme but remain nonspecifically bound to the lipid endoplasmic reticulum membrane. In this state, they may induce microsomal enzymes, particularly after repeated use. Acutely, depending on the residual drug levels at the active site, they also may competitively inhibit metabolism of a simultaneously administered drug.

Enzyme-inducing drugs include various sedative-hypnotics, antipsychotics, anticonvulsants, the antitubercular drug rifampin, and insecticides (Table 4–5). Patients who routinely ingest barbiturates, other sedative-hypnotics, or certain antipsychotic drugs may require considerably higher doses of warfarin to maintain a therapeutic effect. On the other hand, discontinuance of the sedative inducer may result in reduced metabolism of the anticoagulant and bleeding—a toxic effect of the ensuing enhanced plasma levels of the anticoagulant. Similar interactions have been observed in individuals receiving various combinations of drug regimens such as rifampin, antipsychotics, or sedatives with contraceptive agents, sedatives with anticonvulsant drugs, and even alcohol with hypoglycemic drugs (tolbutamide). One inducer of note is St. John's wort, a popular over-the-counter herbal medicine ingested as treatment for mild to severe depression. Because of its marked induction of hepatic CYP3A4 and, to a lesser extent, CYP2C9 and CYP2C19, St. John's wort has been linked to a large number of DDIs. Most of such DDIs stem from P450 induction by St. John's wort and entail accelerated P450-dependent metabolism of the co-ingested drug (eg, alprazolam, contraceptive estrogens, warfarin, lovastatin, delavirdine, ritonavir). In contrast, St. John's wort-mediated CYP2C19 induction may enhance the activation of the antiplatelet prodrug clopidogrel by accelerating its conversion to the active metabolite. Finally, some St. John's wort-elicited DDIs may entail decreased P450-dependent metabolism due to competitive inhibition and consequently increased plasma levels and clinical effect (eg, meperidine, hydrocodone, morphine, oxycodone). Other DDIs entail synergistic increases in serotonin levels (due to monoamine oxidase inhibition) and correspondingly increased serotonergic tone and adverse effects (eg, paroxetine, sertraline, fluoxetine, fenfluramine).

It must also be noted that an inducer may enhance not only the metabolism of other drugs but also its own metabolism. Thus, continued use of some drugs may result in a pharmacokinetic type of **tolerance**—progressively reduced therapeutic effectiveness due to enhancement of their own metabolism.

Conversely, simultaneous administration of two or more drugs may result in impaired elimination of the more slowly metabolized drug and prolongation or potentiation of its pharmacologic effects (Table 4–6). Both competitive substrate inhibition and irreversible substrate-mediated enzyme inactivation may augment plasma drug levels and lead to toxic effects from drugs with narrow therapeutic indices. Indeed, such acute interactions of terfenadine (a second-generation antihistamine) with a CYP3A4 substrate-inhibitor (ketoconazole, erythromycin, or grapefruit juice) resulted in fatal cardiac arrhythmias (torsades de pointes) requiring its withdrawal from the market. Similar DDIs with CYP3A4 substrate-inhibitors (such as the antibiotics erythromycin and clarithromycin, the antidepressant nefazodone, the antifungals itraconazole and ketoconazole, and the HIV protease inhibitors indinavir and ritonavir) and consequent cardiotoxicity led to withdrawal or restricted use of the 5-HT_4 agonist cisapride. Similarly, allopurinol both prolongs the duration and enhances the chemotherapeutic and toxic actions of mercaptopurine by competitive inhibition of xanthine oxidase. Consequently, to avoid bone marrow toxicity, the dose of mercaptopurine must be reduced in patients receiving allopurinol. Cimetidine, a drug used in the treatment of peptic ulcer, has been shown to potentiate the pharmacologic actions of anticoagulants and sedatives. The metabolism of the sedative chlordiazepoxide has been shown to be inhibited by 63% after a single dose of cimetidine; such effects are reversed within 48 hours after withdrawal of cimetidine.

Impaired metabolism may also result if a simultaneously administered drug irreversibly inactivates a common metabolizing enzyme. These inhibitors, in the course of their metabolism by cytochrome P450, inactivate the enzyme and result in impairment of their own metabolism and that of other cosubstrates. This is the case of the furanocoumarins in grapefruit juice, eg, 6′,7′-dihydroxybergamottin and bergamottin, which inactivate CYP3A4 in the intestinal mucosa and consequently enhance its

TABLE 4–6 Partial list of drugs that inhibit drug metabolism in humans.

Inhibitor[1]	Drug Whose Metabolism Is Inhibited
Allopurinol, chloramphenicol, isoniazid	Antipyrine, dicumarol, probenecid, tolbutamide
Chlorpromazine	Propranolol
Cimetidine	Chlordiazepoxide, diazepam, warfarin, others
Dicumarol	Phenytoin
Diethylpentenamide	Diethylpentenamide
Disulfiram	Antipyrine, ethanol, phenytoin, warfarin
Ethanol	Chlordiazepoxide (?), diazepam (?), methanol
Grapefruit juice[2]	Alprazolam, atorvastatin, cisapride, cyclosporine, midazolam, triazolam
Itraconazole	Alfentanil, alprazolam, astemizole, atorvastatin, buspirone, cisapride, cyclosporine, delavirdine, diazepam, digoxin, felodipine, indinavir, loratadine, lovastatin, midazolam, nisoldipine, phenytoin, quinidine, ritonavir, saquinavir, sildenafil, simvastatin, sirolimus, tacrolimus, triazolam, verapamil, warfarin
Ketoconazole	Astemizole, cyclosporine, terfenadine
Nortriptyline	Antipyrine
Oral contraceptives	Antipyrine
Phenylbutazone	Phenytoin, tolbutamide
Ritonavir	Amiodarone, cisapride, itraconazole, midazolam, triazolam
Saquinavir	Cisapride, ergot derivatives, midazolam, triazolam
Secobarbital	Secobarbital
Spironolactone	Digoxin
Troleandomycin	Theophylline, methylprednisolone

[1]While some inhibitors are selective for a given P450 enzyme, others are more general and can inhibit several P450s concurrently.

[2]Active components in grapefruit juice include furanocoumarins such as 6′,7′-dihydroxybergamottin (which inactivates both intestinal and liver CYP3A4) as well as other unknown components that inhibit P-glycoprotein-mediated intestinal drug efflux and consequently further enhance the bioavailability of certain drugs such as cyclosporine. For a more comprehensive list of drugs whose metabolism is inhibited by grapefruit juice furanocoumarins, see Bailey et al, 2013.

proteolytic degradation. This impairment of intestinal first-pass CYP3A4-dependent metabolism significantly enhances the bioavailability of drugs such as ergotamine, felodipine, nifedipine, terfenadine, verapamil, ethinylestradiol, lovastatin, saquinavir, and cyclosporine A and is associated with clinically relevant DDIs and food-drug interactions. The list of drugs subject to DDIs involving grapefruit juice is extensive and includes many drugs with a very narrow therapeutic index and a high potential for lethal adverse reactions. However, it must be borne in mind that not all commercially available grapefruit juices are equally potent, as the CYP3A4 inactivation potency is totally dependent on the amount of furanocoumarins extracted into the juice from the zest (highest), pith, and pulp of the grapefruit. Furthermore, recovery from these interactions is dependent on CYP3A4 resynthesis and thus may be slow.

Interactions Between Drugs & Endogenous Compounds

Some drugs require conjugation with endogenous substrates such as GSH, glucuronic acid, or sulfate for their inactivation. Consequently, different drugs may compete for the same endogenous substrates, and the faster-reacting drug may effectively deplete endogenous substrate levels and impair the metabolism of the slower-reacting drug. If the latter has a steep dose-response curve or a narrow margin of safety, potentiation of its therapeutic and toxic effects may result.

Diseases Affecting Drug Metabolism

Acute or chronic diseases that affect liver architecture or function markedly affect hepatic metabolism of some drugs. Such conditions include alcoholic hepatitis, active or inactive alcoholic cirrhosis, hemochromatosis, chronic active hepatitis, biliary cirrhosis, and acute viral or drug-induced hepatitis. Depending on their severity, these conditions may significantly impair hepatic drug-metabolizing enzymes, particularly microsomal oxidases, and thereby markedly affect drug elimination. For example, the half-lives of chlordiazepoxide and diazepam in patients with liver cirrhosis or acute viral hepatitis are greatly increased, with a corresponding increase in their effects. Consequently, these drugs may cause coma in patients with liver disease when given in ordinary doses.

Some drugs are metabolized so readily that even marked reduction in liver function does not significantly prolong their action. However, cardiac disease, by limiting blood flow to the liver, may impair disposition of those drugs whose metabolism is flow-limited (Table 4–7). These drugs are so readily metabolized by the liver that hepatic clearance is essentially equal to liver blood flow. The impaired enzyme activity or defective formation of enzymes associated with heavy metal poisoning or porphyria also results in reduced hepatic drug metabolism. Pulmonary disease may also affect drug metabolism, as indicated by the impaired hydrolysis of procainamide and procaine in patients with chronic respiratory insufficiency and the increased half-life of antipyrine (a P450 functional probe) in patients with lung cancer.

TABLE 4–7 Rapidly metabolized drugs whose hepatic clearance is blood flow-limited.

Alprenolol	Lidocaine
Amitriptyline	Meperidine
Clomethiazole	Morphine
Desipramine	Pentazocine
Imipramine	Propoxyphene
Isoniazid	Propranolol
Labetalol	Verapamil

Although the effects of endocrine dysfunction on drug metabolism have been well explored in experimental animal models, corresponding data for humans with endocrine disorders are scanty. Thyroid dysfunction has been associated with altered metabolism of some drugs and of some endogenous compounds as well. Hypothyroidism increases the half-life of antipyrine, digoxin, methimazole, and some β blockers, whereas hyperthyroidism has the opposite effect. A few clinical studies in diabetic patients indicate no apparent impairment of drug metabolism, although impairment has been noted in diabetic rats. Malfunctions of the pituitary, adrenal cortex, and gonads markedly reduce hepatic drug metabolism in rats. On the basis of these findings, it may be supposed that such disorders could significantly affect drug metabolism in humans. However, until sufficient evidence is obtained from clinical studies in patients, such extrapolations must be considered tentative.

Finally, the release of inflammatory mediators, cytokines, and nitric oxide associated with bacterial or viral infections, cancer, or inflammation are known to impair drug metabolism by inactivating P450s and enhancing their degradation.

Metabolism of Therapeutic Biologics

In recent decades, in addition to small chemical molecules (SMs, MW <1000 Da), large biological molecules have enriched the therapeutic armamentarium targeted to various diseases such as cancer, rheumatoid arthritis, autoimmune conditions, infections, and genetic and orphan diseases (see Chapters 36 and 55 for various pertinent examples). These include monoclonal antibodies (mAbs), cytokines (Interferons [IFN], TNFα), recombinant proteins, fusion proteins, growth factors, hormones (insulin, recombinant growth hormone), enzymes, vaccines, antibody fragments (Fabs that endow specificity and diversity), antibody-drug conjugates (ADCs), etc. The metabolism and clearance of these therapeutic agents, designed to exhibit high selectivity/affinity for their cellular targets, but possessing complex pharmacokinetic properties quite distinct from those of small molecules (SM), involve none of the drug-metabolizing/elimination pathways so far discussed for small drugs. Because of their proteinaceous nature in full (eg, mAbs) or in part (eg, PEGylated [polyethylene glycol polymer adducted] antibodies, ADCs), these biologics, much like native endogenous proteins, incur intracellular protein degradation to their constitutive amino acids, usually by lysosomes, or cellular proteases of circulating phagocytes (macrophages and monocytes), target-antigen bearing cells, or various tissue cells. However, irrespective of the cell type involved in the metabolic breakdown of the biologics, the constitutive amino acid residues are recycled into their common intracellular pool and re-utilized for de novo protein synthesis.

Biologic protein degradation requires their intracellular absorption for delivery to the target, but due to their relatively greater hydrophilicity and much larger size (~150 kDa for immunoglobulins G [IgGs]), their cellular permeability is poor and poses a major challenge. They cannot be delivered orally as they would be denatured in the acidic stomach lumen or degraded by the gastrointestinal proteases. They are therefore usually delivered parenterally via IV, IM or SC routes. Their distribution is generally limited to plasma and extracellular fluids such as the interstitial fluid and lymph. While the IV route for biologics is optimally suited for the treatment of blood cell disorders, its major impediment is the poor diffusion of such large hydrophilic molecules through the capillary endothelial cell walls to sites of cellular targets and/or protein degradation. For these reasons, large biologics (>19 kDa) are often administered via the IM or SC routes to enable them to access the tissue interstitial spaces, from where they can access the more permeable lymphatic capillaries and be delivered, albeit very slowly (120 mL/kg/h), via lymphatic convective transport into the general circulation. Thus, it is not surprising that depending on the size of the biologics in question, this relatively slow absorption means that they typically require 2–8 days to reach maximal plasma concentrations. The distribution of biologics from the systemic circulation into peripheral tissues is also very slow, involving convective transport across capillary pores as well as transcytosis from the extracellular/interstitial spaces. Such transcytosis involves receptor-mediated endocytosis, phagocytosis, and fluid-phase pinocytosis (ability of cells to take up proteins and other macromolecules from the surrounding fluid spaces through endocytosis).

Biologic protein degradation (catabolism) can occur pre-systemically upon IM and SC injection by extracellular proteases in the interstitial spaces or during their blood or lymph circulation. From the vascular or interstitial spaces, the biologics are predominantly taken up into endothelial cells or tissues by fluid-phase pinocytosis. Biologics with high affinity antigen-binding fragments (Fabs) for their pharmacological targets, eg, mAbs directed to membrane-bound antigens, can also undergo target-mediated absorption (endosomal internalization) and subsequent lysosomal catabolism within the target cell.

Partly due to the well-characterized catabolic fate of circulating endogenous IgGs, the protein degradation process is best understood for therapeutic biologics such as mAbs and IgGs, ADCs, Fabs, and antibody fusion proteins, most of which include the Fc (stem) domain of the IgGs (IgG-Fc; Chapter 55). Upon parenteral administration, IgG-Fc interacts with the Fc receptors such as the Fcγ-receptor (FcγR) or neonatal Fc-receptor (FcRn) ubiquitously expressed on the extracellular surface of various immune and nonimmune cell types, endothelial, and epithelial cells. Upon this IgG-Fc/FcRn interaction, the cell surface is endocytosed, the integral FcRn receptors sequestered within the early endosome are saturated with the available IgG-Fc molecules, and the pH drops below physiological pH (6.0–6.5), which enhances the affinity of this IgG-Fc/FcRn binding. The excess, unbound IgG-Fc fraction is degraded by the lysosome, while the bound IgG-Fc molecules are protected from lysosomal degradation. The endosome with the firmly bound IgG-Fc/FcRn complexes is then recycled to the cell surface. Upon re-exposure to the physiological pH of the extracellular fluid, the IgG-Fc/FcRn complexes dissociate, enabling the therapeutic salvage of the intact undegraded therapeutic IgGs. This FcRn-mediated recycling of endogenous and therapeutic IgGs is thought to be responsible for their extended half-life of approximately 21 days. This FcRn recycling and consequent salvage have led to the structural incorporation of this Fc-feature in the design of therapeutic Fc-fusion proteins (eg, Interferon α- or β-Fc, or factor IX-Fc fusion proteins). Fc-domains of biologics (eg, mAbs, endogenous Abs, and fusion proteins) can also interact with the similarly ubiquitously expressed cell surface FcγR, whereupon they are endosomally internalized and degraded by the lysosomes. This target-mediated degradation pathway generally favors soluble mAb-antigen complexes.

Biliary and renal excretion of biologics is also negligible due to the same issues that hinder their absorption. In contrast to their important role in SM-elimination, the kidneys play a largely metabolic rather than excretory role in the clearance of smaller (<60 kDa) biologics that can adequately incur glomerular filtration, and subsequent intraluminal catabolism, tubular reabsorption followed by intracellular lysosomal degradation, or even peritubular endocytosis with subsequent lysosomal proteolysis. To circumvent this glomerular clearance and prolong their therapeutic duration, small sized biologics are often PEGylated to increase their molecular size.

Often, for maximal therapeutic benefit, biologics are co-administered with SM drugs and although in principle inconceivable given their differential metabolism, bona fide drug-interactions (DIs) with SMs occur. Thus, certain biologics that have the potential as "foreign proteins" to trigger the release of pro-inflammatory cytokines (IL-1β, IL-6, IFN-γ, and TNFα) from circulating peripheral polymorphonuclear cells could influence the transport and metabolism of co-administered SM drugs. Such pro-inflammatory cytokines are known to influence various physiological processes by up- or down-regulating the expression of drug-transporters, transcription factors, nuclear factors (CAR, PXR, and FXR), receptors, and various drug-metabolizing P450 enzymes, thereby influencing the metabolism of co-ingested SMs and triggering DIs. Alternatively, DIs can also occur when the therapeutic proteins are aimed at targets involved in disease states that alter cytokine levels or even when these biologics are targeted to the cytokines themselves that in turn affect the P450-dependent metabolism and transport of a given SM drug. Thus, tocilizumab (rheumatoid arthritis [RA] therapy) can influence the pharmacokinetics of co-administered simvastatin by reversing the RA-associated enhanced cytokine levels. Basiliximab (B-cell lymphoma therapy) and muromonab-CD3 (immunosuppressant) increase the plasma levels of cyclosporine, through IL-2-mediated down-regulation of CYP3A4, the dominant cyclosporine-metabolizing P450. Conversely, an SM drug such as methotrexate is known to reduce the clearance of adalimumab (Humira; RA therapy), and in fact is employed clinically to extend the duration of adalimumab by as much as 19% after a single dose and by 44% after multiple doses. Similarly, mycophenolate can prolong the response of basiliximab by reducing its clearance by 50%. Many other examples of DIs exist.

REFERENCES

Bailey DG, Dresser G, Arnold JMA: Grapefruit and medication interactions: Forbidden fruit or avoidable consequences? Can Med Assoc J 2013;185:309.

Benowitz NL: Pharmacology of nicotine: Addiction, smoking-induced disease, and therapeutics. Annu Rev Pharmacol Toxicol 2009;49:57.

Clayton TA et al: Pharmacometabonomic identification of a significant host-microbiome metabolic interaction affecting human drug metabolism. Proc Natl Acad Sci USA 2009;106:14728.

Correia MA: Human and rat liver cytochromes P450: Functional markers, diagnostic inhibitor probes and parameters frequently used in P450 studies. In: Ortiz de Montellano P (editor): *Cytochrome P450: Structure, Mechanism and Biochemistry*, 3rd ed. Kluwer Academic/Plenum Press, 2005.

Correia MA, Hollenberg PF: Inhibition of cytochrome P450 enzymes. In: Ortiz de Montellano P (editor): *Cytochrome P450: Structure, Mechanism and Biochemistry*, 4th ed. Springer International, 2015.

Correia MA, Ortiz de Montellano P: Inhibition of cytochrome P450 enzymes. In: Ortiz de Montellano P (editor): *Cytochrome P450: Structure, Mechanism and Biochemistry*, 3rd ed. Kluwer Academic/Plenum Press, 2005.

Daly AK: Pharmacogenetics and human genetic polymorphisms. Biochem J 2010;429:435.

Dirks NL, Meibohm B. Population pharmacokinetics of therapeutic monoclonal antibodies. Clin Pharmacokinet 2010;49:633.

Dostalek M et al: Pharmacokinetics, pharmacodynamics and physiologically-based pharmacokinetic modelling of monoclonal antibodies. Clin Pharmacokinet 2013;52:83.

Guengerich FP: Human cytochrome P450 enzymes. In: Ortiz de Montellano P (editor): *Cytochrome P450: Structure, Mechanism and Biochemistry*, 4th ed. Springer International, 2015.

Guengerich FP: Role of cytochrome P450 enzymes in drug-drug interactions. Adv Pharmacol 1997;43:7.

Hustert E et al: The genetic determinants of the CYP3A5 polymorphism. Pharmacogenetics 2001;11:773.

Ingelman-Sundberg M: Pharmacogenetics: An opportunity for a safer and more efficient pharmacotherapy. J Intern Med 2001;250:186.

Ingelman-Sundberg M et al: Influence of cytochrome P450 polymorphisms on drug therapies: Pharmacogenetic, pharmacoepigenetic and clinical aspects. Pharmacol Ther 2007;116:496.

Ingelman-Sundberg M, Sim SC: Pharmacogenetic biomarkers as tools for improved drug therapy; emphasis on the cytochrome P450 system. Biochem Biophys Res Commun 2010;396:90.

Kang MJ et al: The effect of gut microbiota on drug metabolism. Expert Opin Drug Metab Toxicol 2013;9:1295.

Kroemer HK, Klotz U: Glucuronidation of drugs: A reevaluation of the pharmacological significance of the conjugates and modulating factors. Clin Pharmacokinet 1992;23:292.

Kuehl P et al: Sequence diversity in CYP3A promoters and characterization of the genetic basis of polymorphic CYP3A5 expression. Nat Genet 2001;27:383.

Lindenbaum J et al: Inactivation of digoxin by the gut flora: Reversal by antibiotic therapy. N Engl J Med 1981;305:789.

Lown KS et al: Grapefruit juice increases felodipine oral availability in humans by decreasing intestinal CYP3A protein expression. J Clin Invest 1997;99:2545.

Metushi I, Uetrecht J, Phillips E: Mechanism of isoniazid-induced hepatotoxicity: Then and now. Br J Clin Pharmacol 2016;81:1030.

Meyer UA: Pharmacogenetics—Five decades of therapeutic lessons from genetic diversity. Nat Rev Genet 2004;5:669.

Morgan ET et al: Regulation of drug-metabolizing enzymes and transporters in infection, inflammation, and cancer. Drug Metab Dispos 2008;36:205.

Nelson DR et al: The P450 superfamily: Update on new sequences, gene mapping, accession numbers, and nomenclature. Pharmacogenetics 1996;6:1.

Nelson DR et al: Updated human P450 sequences. http://drnelson.uthsc.edu/cytochromeP450.html.

Pirmohamed M: Drug-grapefruit juice interactions: Two mechanisms are clear but individual responses vary. Br Med J 2013;346:f1.

Posadzki P, Watson L, Ernst E: Herb-drug interactions: An overview of systematic reviews. Br J Clin Pharmacol 2013;75:603.

Rahimi R, Abdollahi M: An update on the ability of St. John's wort to affect the metabolism of other drugs. Expert Opin Drug Metab Toxicol 2012;8:691.

Rieder MJ et al: Effect of VKORC1 haplotypes on transcriptional regulation and warfarin dose. N Engl J Med 2005;352:2285.

Russo E et al: Hypericum perforatum: Pharmacokinetic, mechanism of action, tolerability, and clinical drug-drug interactions. Phytother Res 2014;28:643.

Saitta KS et al: Bacterial beta-glucuronidase inhibition protects mice against enteropathy induced by indomethacin, ketoprofen or diclofenac: Mode of action and pharmacokinetics. Xenobiotica 2014;44:28.

Shi S: Biologics: An update and challenge of their pharmacokinetics. Curr Drug Metab 2014;15:271.

Sueyoshi T, Negishi M: Phenobarbital response elements of cytochrome P450 genes and nuclear receptors. Annu Rev Pharmacol Toxicol 2001;41:123.

Ternant D et al: Clinical pharmacokinetics and pharmacodynamics of monoclonal antibodies approved to treat rheumatoid arthritis. Clin Pharmacokinet 2015;54:1107.

Thummel KE, Wilkinson GR: In vitro and in vivo drug interactions involving human CYP3A. Annu Rev Pharmacol Toxicol 1998;38:389.

Tsai HH et al: Evaluation of documented drug interactions and contraindications associated with herbs and dietary supplements: A systematic literature review. Int J Clin Pract 2012;66:1056.

Wallace BD et al: Structure and inhibition of microbiome beta-glucuronidases essential to the alleviation of cancer drug toxicity. Chem Biol 2015;22:1238.

Wang L, McLeod HL, Weinshilboum RM: Genomics and drug response. N Engl J Med 2011;364:1144.

Wang W, Wang EQ, Balthasar JP: Monoclonal antibody pharmacokinetics and pharmacodynamics. Clin Pharmacol Ther 2008;84:548.

Williams SN et al: Induction of cytochrome P450 enzymes. In: Ortiz de Montellano P (editor): *Cytochrome P450. Structure, Mechanism, and Biochemistry*. Kluwer Academic/Plenum Press, 2005; and references therein.

Willson TM, Kliewer SA: PXR, CAR and drug metabolism. Nat Rev Drug Discov 2002;1:259.

Wilson ID, Nicholson JK: The role of gut microbiota in drug response. Curr Pharm Des 2009;15:1519.

Xu C et al: CYP2A6 genetic variation and potential consequences. Adv Drug Delivery Rev 2002;54:1245.

Xu X, Vugmeyster Y: Challenges and opportunities in absorption, distribution, metabolism, and excretion studies of therapeutic biologics. AAPS J. 2012;14:781.

CASE STUDY ANSWER

Acetaminophen (APAP) is a relatively safe drug, provided it is taken at the recommended therapeutic doses. As discussed in the text, at normally ingested dosages, 95% of APAP is converted by phase II enzymes into much less toxic and more water-soluble APAP-glucuronide and APAP-sulfate, both of which are eliminated in the urine (see Figure 4–5). Five percent of parent APAP is converted by phase I P450 enzymes into a reactive toxic product that is conjugated by GSH, excreted in the urine, and thus detoxified. However, APAP's safety may be greatly compromised in mixed drug overdoses, eg, when ingested with other drugs such as hydrocodone, duloxetine, and carisoprodol, which compete with APAP for phase II-dependent elimination or for cellular cofactors (GSH, UDPGA, PAPS) involved in these processes. Accordingly, more APAP is diverted into its hepatotoxic reactive metabolite pathway, resulting in liver cell damage. Moreover, HCV infection could indeed have further compromised liver function including drug metabolism. APAP's half-life is 2 hours, and therapeutic and toxic blood levels are 15 mcg/mL and >300 mcg/mL, respectively (Chapter 3). Given that at 48 hours after ingestion (ie, 24 half-lives later), the patient's APAP blood level is 75 mcg/mL, it is obvious that her initial APAP levels were dangerously above the toxic range, and thus upon ED admission, her liver function tests are consistent with ongoing liver failure. She should be given N-acetylcysteine, the APAP-specific antidote (Acetadote, Mucomyst; see Chapter 58) and continuous intravenous glucose infusion to provide the precursor (glucose) for generating the UDPGA cofactor required for APAP glucuronidation, as well as the fluid to induce urine output and accelerate APAP-metabolite elimination.

CHAPTER

5

Pharmacogenomics

Jennifer E. Hibma, PharmD,
& Kathleen M. Giacomini, PhD

CASE STUDY

A 35-year-old man with newly diagnosed human immunodeficiency virus (HIV) infection was prescribed an antiretroviral regimen that included the protease inhibitor atazanavir 300 mg to be taken by mouth once daily, along with ritonavir, a pharmacokinetic enhancer, and two nucleoside analog antiretroviral agents. Liver function and renal function were normal. After 1 year of treatment, the patient experienced visible yellow discoloration of the skin and eyes. Blood samples were drawn, and grade 4 hyperbilirubinemia was documented. When atazanavir was discontinued and the antiretroviral regimen was modified to include lopinavir, the plasma levels of bilirubin returned to the normal range, and skin and eye color were cleared. Could a *UGT1A1*28* polymorphism have led to the adverse effects?

Pharmacogenomics, the study of genetic factors that underlie variation in drug response, is a modern term for **pharmacogenetics.** Pharmacogenomics implies a recognition that more than one genetic variant may contribute to variation in drug response. Historically, the field began with observations of severe adverse drug reactions in certain individuals, who were found to harbor genetic variants in drug-metabolizing enzymes. As a scientific field, pharmacogenomics has advanced rapidly since the sequencing of the human genome. In the last decade, powerful genome-wide association (GWA) studies, in which hundreds of thousands of genetic variants across the genome are tested for association with drug response, led to the discovery of many other important polymorphisms that underlie variation in both therapeutic and adverse drug responses. In addition to polymorphisms in genes that encode drug-metabolizing enzymes, it is now known that polymorphisms in genes that encode transporters, human leukocyte antigen (HLA) loci, cytokines, and various other proteins also are predictive of variation in therapeutic and adverse drug responses. In addition to the new discoveries that have been made, the past decade has ushered in **precision medicine,** also known as **stratified** or **personalized medicine,** in which genetic information is used to guide drug and dosing selection for subgroups of patients or individual patients in medical practice. The Clinical Pharmacogenetics Implementation Consortium (CPIC) published a series of guidelines for using genetic information in selecting medications and in dosing (https://www.pharmgkb.org/). These highly informative guidelines are being used by practitioners in prescribing drugs to more effectively treat patients. In this chapter, we begin with a case study and then describe genetic variants that are determinants of drug response. Where appropriate, CPIC recommendations are included to provide information on how to use genetic variant data appropriately in therapeutic medicine. Other expert recommendations such as those from the Dutch Pharmacogenetics Working Group (DPWG) also are available (see https://www.knmp.nl/dossiers/farmacogenetica).

The description in this chapter of DNA sequence variations in germline DNA involves a number of terms that describe the nature of the variations and their locations within the genome. A glossary of commonly used terms is presented in the Glossary Table. Some of the more common and important variations are described in the text that follows.

GLOSSARY

Term	Definition
Allele	One of two or more alternative forms of a gene that arise by mutation and are found at the same genetic locus. Example: *CYP2D6*3* is an important variant allele for a drug-metabolizing enzyme, CYP2D6.
Allele frequency	The fraction or percentage that a specific allele is observed in proportion to the total of all possible alleles in a population.
Coding single nucleotide polymorphisms (cSNPs)	A single base-pair substitution that occurs in the coding region.
Copy number variations (CNVs)	A segment of DNA in which a variable number of that segment has been found.
Haplotype	A series of alleles found in a linked locus on a chromosome.
Hardy-Weinberg equilibrium	The principle that allele frequencies will remain constant from generation to generation in the absence of evolutionary influences.
Insertion/deletion (indel)	Insertion or deletion of base pairs, which may occur in coding and noncoding regions.
Linkage disequilibrium	The nonrandom association of alleles at two or more loci that descend from a single ancestral chromosome.
Noncoding region polymorphism	Polymorphisms that occur in the 3′ and 5′ untranslated regions, intronic regions, or intergenic regions.
Nonsynonymous SNPs (nsSNPs)	A single base-pair substitution in the coding region that results in an amino acid change.
Polymorphism or variant	Any genetic variation in the DNA sequence; the terms can be used interchangeably.
PM, IM, EM, or UM	Poor, intermediate, extensive, or ultrarapid metabolizer phenotype.
SNPs	Single nucleotide polymorphisms: base-pair substitutions that occur in the genome.
Synonymous SNPs	Base-pair substitutions in the coding region that do not result in an amino acid change.

GENETIC VARIATIONS IN ENZYMES

PHASE I ENZYMES

As described in Chapter 4, biotransformation reactions mediated by P450 phase I enzymes typically modify functional groups (–OH, –SH, $-NH_2$, $-OCH_3$) of endogenous and xenobiotic compounds, resulting in an alteration of the biological activity of the compound. Phase I enzymes are involved in the biotransformation of more than 75% of prescription drugs; therefore, polymorphisms in these enzymes may significantly affect blood levels, which in turn may alter response to many drugs. Polymorphisms in drug-metabolizing enzymes dominated the field of pharmacogenomics for many years, and for some years, metabolic phenotypes such as extensive metabolizer (EM), reflecting an individual's metabolic rate of a particular drug that is a known substrate of a specific enzyme, were used to describe genetic effects on drug metabolism. After genotypic information became available, a new nomenclature was used to characterize an individual's metabolic rate. In particular, diplotypes, consisting of one maternal and one paternal allele, using star (*) allele nomenclature, have been used. Each star (*) allele is defined by specific sequence variation(s) within the gene locus, eg, single nucleotide polymorphisms (SNPs), and may be assigned a functional activity score when the functional characterization is known, eg, 0 for nonfunctional, 0.5 for reduced function, and 1.0 for fully functional. Some genes, such as *CYP2D6*, are subject to whole gene deletions, eg, *CYP2D6*5*, and whole gene duplications or multiplications, eg, **1 × N*, **2 × N*, where N is the number of copies. If more than one copy of the gene is detected, the activity score is then multiplied by the number of copies observed. Enzyme activity is generally a co-dominant or additive trait. For example, if an individual carries one normal function allele and one nonfunctional allele, he will have an intermediate metabolic activity or be considered an intermediate metabolizer (IM). The sum of allelic activity scores typically ranges between 0 and ≥3.0 and is most often used to define phenotypes as follows: 0 = PM (poor metabolizer), 0 > × > 1.25 = IM, 1.25 > × > 2.25 = EM, and >2.25 = UM (ultrarapid metabolizer). For more information regarding nomenclature, see https://www.pharmvar.org/genes.

CYP2D6

As described in Chapter 4, cytochrome P450 2D6 (CYP2D6) is involved in the metabolism of up to one-quarter of all drugs used clinically, including predominantly basic compounds such as β blockers, antidepressants, antipsychotics, and opioid analgesics. Similar to other polymorphic enzymes, four clinically defined metabolic phenotypes, ie, PMs, IMs, EMs, and UMs, are used to predict therapeutic and adverse responses following the administration of CYP2D6 substrates.

The gene encoding CYP2D6 is highly polymorphic, with more than 100 alleles defined (https://www.pharmvar.org/gene/CYP2D6); however, greater than 95% of phenotypes can be accounted for with just nine alleles, ie, *CYP2D6* alleles **3*, **4*, **5*, and **6* are nonfunctional; alleles **10*, **17*, and **41* have reduced function; and alleles **1* and **2* are fully functional. As with many polymorphisms, allele frequencies vary across populations (Table 5–1). Some genetic variants are shared among populations at similar allele frequencies, whereas others vary considerably.

TABLE 5–1 Major alleles and frequencies in African, Asian, and European populations.

Gene	Allele(s)[1]	dbSNP[2] Number	Amino Acid	Function	Activity	Fraction in African Populations	Fraction in Asian Populations	Fraction in European Populations
CYP2D6								
	**1*	Reference	—	Normal	1.0	0.39	0.34	0.54
	**1 × N*	Gene duplication or multiplication	Increased expression	Increased	1.0 × N	0.015	0.0028	0.0080
	**2*	rs16947, rs1135840	R296C, S486T	Normal	1.0	0.20	0.13	0.27
	**2 × N*	Duplication or multiplication	Increased expression	Increased	1.0 × N	0.016	0.0038	0.013
	**3*	rs35742686	Frameshift	None	0.0	0.00030	0.00	0.013
	**4*	rs1065852, rs3892097	P34S, Splicing defect	None	0.0	0.034	0.0042	0.19
	**5*	—	No enzyme	None	0.0	0.061	0.056	0.027
	**6*	rs5030655	Frameshift	None	0.0	0.031	0.0002	0.0095
	**10*	rs1065852, rs1135840	P34S, S486T	Decreased	0.25	0.068	0.42	0.032
	**17*	rs28371706, rs16947, rs1135840	T107I, R296C, S486T	Decreased	0.5	0.20	0.0001	0.0032
	**41*	rs16947, rs1135840, rs28371725	R296C, S486T, Splicing defect	Decreased	0.5	0.11	0.020	0.086
CYP2C19								
	**1*	Reference	—	Normal	—	0.68	0.60	0.63
	**2*	rs4244285	Splicing defect	None	—	0.15	0.29	0.15
	**3*	rs4986893	W212X	None	—	0.0052	0.089	0.0042
	**17*	rs12248560	Increased expression	Increased	—	0.16	0.027	0.21
CYP2C9								
	**1*	Reference	—	Normal	—			
	**2*	rs1799853	R144C	Decreased	—	0.03	0.00	0.13
	**3*	rs1057910	I359L	Decreased	—	0.02	0.04	0.07
CYP2B6								
	*1			Normal		0.36	0.58	0.53
	*4	rs2279343	K262R	Increased		0.0093	0.090	0.040
	*6	rs2279343, rs3745274	K262R , Q172H	Decreased		0.34	0.20	0.20
	*9	rs3745274	Q172H	Decreased		0.084	0.060	0.015
	*18	rs28399499	I328T	None		0.052	0.00	0.00
DPYD								
	**1*	Reference	—	Normal	1.0			
	**2A*	rs3918290	Splicing defect	None	0.0	0.0006	0.0037	0.0080
	**13*	rs55886062	I560S	None	0.0	0.00	0.00	0.0006
	—	rs67376798	D949V	Decreased	0.5	0.0006	0.0005	0.00370
	HapB3	rs56038477	E412E	Decreased	0.5	0.0018	0.0094	0.0204
UGT1A1								
	**1*	Reference	TA_6	Normal	—	0.50	0.85	0.68
	**28*	rs8175347	TA_7	Decreased	—	0.39	0.15	0.32
	**36*	rs8175347	TA_5	Increased	—	0.066	0.00	0.00
	**37*	rs8175347	TA_8	Decreased	—	0.036	0.00	0.0010

(*continued*)

TABLE 5–1 Major alleles and frequencies in African, Asian, and European populations. (Continued)

Gene	Allele(s)[1]	dbSNP[2] Number	Amino Acid	Function	Activity	Fraction in African Populations	Fraction in Asian Populations	Fraction in European Populations
TPMT								
	**1*	Reference	—	Normal	—	0.94	0.98	0.96
	**2*	rs1800462	A80P	None	—	0.00079	0.00	0.0019
	**3A*	rs1800460, rs1142345	A154T, Y240C	None	—	0.0020	0.00012	0.036
	**3B*	rs1800460	A154T	None	—	0.00	0.00	0.00046
	**3C*	rs1142345	Y240C	None	—	0.050	0.016	0.0042
G6PD								
	B	Reference	—	Normal	IV	—	—	—
	A	rs1050829	N126D	Normal	III–IV	0.31–0.35	0.00	0.00–0.060
	A- (rs1050829, rs1050828) *A-* (rs1050829, rs137852328) *A-* (rs1050829, rs76723693)		(N126D, V68M) (N126D, R227L) (N126D, L323P)	Decreased (5–10%)	III	0.117	n/a	0.00
	Mediterranean (rs5030868)		S188P	Decreased (<1%)	II	0.00–0.052	0.00	0.00–0.074
	Canton (rs72554665), Kaiping		R459L/R463H	Decreased	II	0.00	0.017	0.00
	Mahidol (rs137852314)		G163S	Decreased (5–32%)	III			
	Chinese-5 (rs137852342), Gaohe (rs72554664)		L342F H32R	Decreased	III			
SLCO1B1								
	**1a*	Reference	—	Normal	—	0.17	0.27	0.50
	**1b*	rs2306283	N130D	Normal	—	0.78	0.60	0.22
	**5*	rs4149056	V174A	Decreased	—	0.00	0.00	0.01
	**15, *17*	rs4149056, others	V174A others	Decreased	—	0.03	0.13	0.14
ABCG2								
		rs2231142	Q141K	Decreased	—	0.01	0.29	0.09
SLC22A1								
	—	rs12208357	R61C	Decreased	—	0.004	0.00	0.063
	—	rs202220802	Mdel	Decreased	—	0.045	0.005	0.184
	—	rs34130495	G401S	Decreased	—	0.003	0.001	0.02
	—	rs34059508	G465R	Decreased	—	0.00	0.00	0.02
HLA-B								
	**57:01*	—	—	positive	—	0.010	0.016	0.068
IFNL3								
	TT/CT	Reference	—	Unfavorable	—	—	—	—
	CC	rs12979860	—	Favorable	—	0.39	0.87	0.63
VKORC1								
	−1639G	Reference	—	Normal	—			
	−1639A	rs9923231	Reduced expression	Decreased	—	0.11	0.91	0.39

[1]For the official nomenclature for alleles of drug-metabolizing enzymes, see the Pharmacogene Variation Consortium (https://www.pharmvar.org/genes).

[2]The Single Nucleotide Polymorphism Database (dbSNP) is an online public repository of genomic variation established by the National Center for Biotechnology Information (NCBI).

For example, a common nonfunctional allele, *CYP2D6*4*, is observed at a frequency of approximately 20% in Europeans and is nearly absent (<1%) in Asians (see Table 5–1). Based on Hardy-Weinberg principles (see Glossary), the percentage of Europeans who are homozygous for the *CYP2D6*4* allele, ie, who carry the **4* allele on both maternal and paternal chromosomes, would be 4%, whereas that of those who are heterozygotes would be 32%. This parallels the lower number of PMs (defined as having two nonfunctional alleles, eg, PMs are homozygous for **3*, **4*, **5*, **6*, or any combination of nonfunctional alleles such as **4/*5*), observed in Asian populations (~1%) compared with European populations (~5–10%) (see Table 5–1). In contrast, the **5* gene deletion is found at similar frequencies (~3–5%) across European, African, and Asian populations, suggesting that this mutation likely took place prior to the separation of these three populations more than 100,000 years ago. *CYP2D6*17*, which consists of three SNPs in a single haplotype, constitutes a common reduced-function haplotype in populations of African ancestry. Clinically, since some genotyping platforms are specific to a single ethnicity, it is important to ensure that alleles applicable to the patient population being treated are tested. Of note, rare or previously undiscovered variants are typically not included in commercial tests, and thus novel or rare polymorphisms, which may exhibit altered function, will be missed.

Example: Codeine is a phenanthrene derivative prodrug opioid analgesic indicated for the management of mild to moderately severe pain (Chapter 31). Codeine, like its active metabolite morphine, binds to μ-opioid receptors in the central nervous system (CNS). Morphine is 200 times more potent as an agonist than codeine, and conversion of codeine into morphine is essential for codeine's analgesic activity. The enzyme responsible for the *O*-demethylation conversion of codeine into morphine is CYP2D6. Patients with normal CYP2D6 activity (ie, EMs) convert sufficient codeine to morphine (~5–10% of an administered dose) to produce the desired analgesic effect. PMs and IMs are more likely to experience insufficient pain relief, while UMs are at an increased risk for side effects, eg, drowsiness and respiratory depression, due to higher systemic concentrations of morphine. Interestingly, gastrointestinal adverse effects, eg, constipation, are decreased in PMs, whereas the central side effects, eg, sedation and dizziness, do not differ between PMs and EMs. The antitussive properties associated with codeine are not affected by CYP2D6 activity. According to CPIC guidelines, standard starting doses are recommended in EMs and IMs with close monitoring, especially in IMs, and CPIC recommends use of an alternative agent in PMs and UMs (Table 5–2).

CYP2C19

Cytochrome P450 CYP2C19 (CYP2C19) is known to preferentially metabolize acidic drugs including proton-pump inhibitors, antidepressants, antiepileptics, and antiplatelet drugs (Chapter 4). Four clinical phenotypes related to CYP2C19 activity (PM, IM, EM, and UM) are closely associated with genetic biomarkers that may assist in guiding individualized therapeutic dosing strategies. The gene that encodes CYP2C19 is highly polymorphic, with more than 35 alleles defined (https://www.pharmvar.org/genes/CYP2C19), yet just four alleles can account for the majority of phenotypic variability—ie, *CYP2C19* alleles **2* and **3* are nonfunctional, *CYP2C19* allele **1* is fully functional, and *CYP2C19*17* has increased function. Phenotypes range from PMs who have two deficient alleles, eg, **2/*3*, **2/*2*, or **3/*3*, to UMs who have increased hepatic expression levels of the CYP2C19 protein due to **1/*17* or **17/*17* alleles (see Table 5–2). Of note, the **17* increased function allele is unable to fully compensate for nonfunctional alleles, and therefore the presence of a **17* allele in combination with a nonfunctional allele would be considered an IM phenotype (see Table 5–2). The PM phenotype is more common in Asians (~16%) than in Europeans and Africans (~2–5%), which can be expected based on the inheritance patterns of variant alleles across populations—eg, the most common nonfunctional allele, *CYP2C19*2*, is observed approximately twice as frequently in Asians (~30%) compared with Africans and Europeans (~15%), while the apparent gain-of-function **17* allele is observed rarely in Asians (<3%) but more frequently in Europeans and Africans (16–21%) (see Table 5–1).

Example: Clopidogrel is a thienopyridine antiplatelet prodrug indicated for the prevention of atherothrombotic events. Active metabolites selectively and irreversibly inhibit adenosine diphosphate–induced platelet aggregation (Chapter 34). Clopidogrel is metabolized in the body via one of two main mechanisms; approximately 85% of an administered dose is rapidly hydrolyzed by hepatic esterases to its inactive carboxylic acid derivative, while the remaining ~15% is converted via two sequential CYP-mediated oxidation reactions (predominantly CYP2C19) to the active thiol metabolite responsible for antiplatelet activity.

Genetic polymorphisms in the *CYP2C19* gene that decrease active metabolite formation and consequently reduce the drug's antiplatelet activity are associated with variability in response to clopidogrel. Carriers of the nonfunctional *CYP2C19*2* alleles taking clopidogrel are at increased risk for serious adverse cardiovascular events, particularly in acute coronary syndrome managed with percutaneous coronary intervention (PCI); the hazard ratios (HRs) are 1.76 for *2/*2 genotype and 1.55 for *2 heterozygotes compared with noncarriers. The risk associated with stent thrombosis is even greater (HR 3.97 for *2/*2 genotype and 2.67 for *2 heterozygotes compared with *1 homozygotes). However, for other indications, eg, atrial fibrillation and stroke, the effects of the *CYP2C19*2* allele are less dramatic. Thus, current clinical recommendations from CPIC are specific for acute coronary syndrome with PCI: standard starting doses are recommended in EMs and UMs, and CPIC recommends use of an alternative antiplatelet agent, eg, prasugrel or ticagrelor, in PMs and IMs (see Table 5–2). The US Food and Drug Administration (FDA)-approved label for clopidogrel recommends alternative antiplatelet drugs for patients who are poor metabolizers of clopidogrel.

CYP2C9

Found in the same cluster on chromosome 10q24 as *CYP2C19*, CYP2C9 is another highly polymorphic drug-metabolizing enzyme. *CYP2C9* is discussed later in this chapter in the context of polygenic effects along with *VKORC1*.

TABLE 5–2 Gene-based dosing recommendations for selected drugs.

Gene	Drug	Diplotype[1]	Likely Phenotype (Activity Score)	Dosing Recommendation	Source of Recommendation
CYP2D6					
	Codeine	**1/*1 × N, *1/*2 × N*	UM (>2.0)	• Alternative analgesic, eg, morphine or nonopioid; increased formation of morphine following codeine administration leads to higher risk of toxicity.	CPIC[2], DPWG[3]
		**1/*1, *1/*2, *2/*2, *1/*41, *2/*5*	EM (1.0–2.0)	• Standard starting dose.	
		**4/*10, *5/*41*	IM (0.5)	• Standard starting dose; monitor closely for lack of analgesic response due to reduced morphine formation. Consider alternate analgesic, eg, morphine or nonopioid.	
		**3/*4, *4/*4, *4/*5, *5/*5, *4/*6*	PM (0.0)	• Alternative analgesic, eg, morphine or nonopioid analgesic; greatly reduced morphine formation following codeine administration, leading to insufficient pain relief. Avoid higher doses, as central side effects do not differ in PMs.	
CYP2C19					
	Clopidogrel	**1/*17, *17/*17* (UM), and **1/*1* (EM)	UM, EM	• Standard dose.	CPIC, DPWG
		**1/*2, *1/*3, *2/*17*	IM	• Alternative antiplatelet agent, eg, prasugrel or ticagrelor.	
		**2/*2, *2/*3, *3/*3*	PM	• Alternative antiplatelet agent, eg, prasugrel or ticagrelor.	
CYP2B6					
	Efavirenz	**4/*4, *22/*22, *4/*22*	UM	• Initiate efavirenz with standard dose (600 mg/day)	CPIC, DPWG
		**1/*4, *1/*22*	RM	• Initiate efavirenz with standard dose (600 mg/day)	
		**1/*1*	EM	• Initiate efavirenz with standard dose (600 mg/day)	
		**1/*6, *1/*18, *4/*6, *4/*18, *6/*22, *18/*22*	IM	• Consider initiating efavirenz with decreased dose (400 mg/day)	
		**6/*6, *18/*18, *6/*18*	PM	• Consider initiating efavirenz with decreased dose (400 or 200 mg/day)	
DPYD					
	Fluoropyrimidines	**1/*1*	Normal	• Standard dose.	CPIC
		**1/*2A, *1/*13, *1/*rs67376798A	Reduced activity	• Reduce initial dose 50% and titrate based on toxicity or on pharmacokinetic test results (if available).	
		**2A/*2A, *2A/*13, *13/*13,* rs67376798A/rs67376798A	Complete deficiency	• Different non-fluoropyrimidine anticancer agent.	
UGT1A1					
	Irinotecan	**1/*1, *1/*28*	Normal	• Standard starting dose.	
		**28/*28*	Reduced	• Reduce starting dose by at least one dose level. Or,	Drug label
				• Start with 70% of the standard dose.	DPWG
				If the patient tolerates this initial dose, the dose can be increased, guided by the neutrophil count.	
	Atazanavir	**1/*1, *1/*36, *36/*36,* rs887829 C/C	Normal	No reason to avoid prescribing atazanavir. Inform patient of risks. Based on this genotype, there is a less than 1 in 20 chance of stopping atazanavir for jaundice.	CPIC

(continued)

TABLE 5–2 Gene-based dosing recommendations for selected drugs. (Continued)

Gene	Drug	Diplotype[1]	Likely Phenotype (Activity Score)	Dosing Recommendation	Source of Recommendation
		**1/*28, *1/*37, *36/*28, *36/*37,* rs887829 C/T, **1/*6*	Intermediate	No reason to avoid prescribing atazanavir. Inform patient of risks. Based on this genotype, there is a less than 1 in 20 chance of stopping atazanavir for jaundice.	
		28/*28, *28/*37, *37/*37,* rs887829 T/T (80/*80*), **6/*6*	Reduced	Consider alternative agent. Based on this genotype, there is a high (20–60%) likelihood of developing jaundice that will result in discontinuation of atazanavir.	
TPMT					
	Thiopurines	**1/*1*	Normal, high activity	• Standard starting dose.	CPIC, DPWG
		**1/*2, *1/*3A, *1/*3B, *1/*3C, *1/*4*	Intermediate activity	• Start at 30–70% of target dose and titrate every 2–4 weeks with close clinical monitoring of tolerability, eg, white blood cell counts and liver function tests.	
		*3A/*3A, *2/*3A, *3C/*3A, *3C/*4, *3C/*2, *3A/*4*	Low activity	• Malignant disease: Drastic reduction of thiopurine doses, eg, tenfold given thrice weekly instead of daily. • Nonmalignant conditions: Alternative nonthiopurine immunosuppressive agent.	
G6PDX-linked trait	Genotype-to-phenotype predictions limited to males and homozygous females.				
	Rasburicase	*B, A*	Normal	• Standard dose.	Drug label/CPIC
		A-, Mediterranean, Canton	Deficient	• Alternative agent, eg, allopurinol: Rasburicase is contraindicated in patients with G6PD deficiency.	
		Variable	Unknown risk of hemolytic anemia	• Enzyme activity must be measured to determine G6PD status. An alternative is allopurinol.	
SLCO1B1					
	Simvastatin 40 mg	**1a/*1a, *1a/*1b, *1b/*1b*	Normal activity	• Standard dose.	CPIC
		**1a/*5, *1a/*15, *1a/*17, *1b/*5, *1b/*15, *1b/*17*	Intermediate activity	• Prescribe a lower dose or consider an alternative statin, eg, pravastatin or rosuvastatin; consider routine CK monitoring.	
		**5/*5, *5/*15, *5/*17, *15/*15, *15/*17, *17/*17*	Low activity	• Prescribe a lower dose or consider an alternative statin, eg, pravastatin or rosuvastatin; consider routine CK monitoring.	
HLA					
	Abacavir	**Other/*Other*	Negative	• Standard dose.	CPIC, DPWG
		**Other/*57:01, *57:01/*57:01*	Positive	• Alternative agent: abacavir is contraindicated in HLA-B*57:01-positive patients.	
IFNL3					
	PEG-IFN-α/RBV	rs12979860/rs12979860	Favorable	• PEG-IFN-α/RBV: Consider cure rates before initiating regimen; ~70% chance for SVR[4] after 48 weeks of therapy. • PEG-IFN-α/RBV + protease inhibitor combinations: Regimen recommended; ~90% chance for SVR after 24–48 weeks of therapy, with 80–90% chance for shortened duration of therapy.	CPIC

(*continued*)

TABLE 5–2 Gene-based dosing recommendations for selected drugs. (Continued)

Gene	Drug	Diplotype[1]	Likely Phenotype (Activity Score)	Dosing Recommendation	Source of Recommendation
		Reference/reference or reference/rs12979860	Unfavorable	• PEG-IFN-α/RBV: Consider cure rates before initiating regimen; ~30% chance for SVR after 48 weeks of therapy. • PEG-IFN-α/RBV + protease inhibitor combinations: Consider cure rates before initiating regimen; ~60% chance for SVR after 24–48 weeks of therapy, with 50% chance for shortened duration of therapy.	
CYP2C9, VKORC1					
	Warfarin	**1/*1, *1/*2, *2/*2, *2/*3, *1/*3, *3/*3,* 1639GG, 1639GA, 1639AA	Various	• Apply validated dosing algorithm, eg, www.warfarindosing.org (or IWPC[5]) for international normalized ratio target 2–3) or FDA-approved dosing table per manufacturer's labeling.	CPIC

[1]Diplotypes are shown as the two members of a chromosome pair, eg, **1/*1* indicates both chromosomes contain the **1* allele for that gene, whereas **1/*17* denotes a heterozygote with one **1* allele and one **17* allele.

[2]CPIC: Clinical Pharmacogenetics Implementation Consortium: Full drug-specific recommendations are available online at http://www.pharmgkb.org/page/cpic, https://cpicpgx.org/genes-drugs/.

[3]DPWG: Dutch Pharmacogenetics Working Group: Full drug-specific recommendations are available online at https://www.knmp.nl/patientenzorg/medicatiebewaking/farmacogenetica/pharmacogenetics-1/pharmacogenetics.

[4]SVR: sustained viral response.

[5]IWPG: International Warfarin Pharmacogenetics Consortium.

CYP2B6

CYP2B6 is highly polymorphic, with 38 known variant alleles and multiple suballeles identified (www.pharmvar.org/gene/CYP2B6). Allele frequencies vary substantially across ancestrally diverse groups (see Table 5–1). Alleles are categorized into functional groups as follows: normal function (eg, *CYP2B6*1*), decreased function (eg, *CYP2B6*6* and **9*), no function (eg, *CYP2B6*18*), and increased function (eg, *CYP2B6*4*), and phenotypes are defined based on the individual diplotype, as shown in Table 5–1. Interestingly, allele **6*, which is the most frequent (from 15% in East Asian ancestry to 62% in Oceania ancestry) and most studied allele, has demonstrated substrate-specific phenotype-diplotype associations.

Example: Efavirenz is a nonnucleoside HIV type-1 reverse transcriptase inhibitor. Efavirenz is a potent suppressor of HIV-1 replication that is indicated for treatment in HIV-positive, treatment-naïve individuals, in combination with tenofovir disoproxil fumarate and emtricitabine. Efavirenz was part of the first "one pill, once a day" treatment, and efavirenz-based regimens were "recommended" by the US Department of Health and Human Services until the year 2015. In 2015, efavirenz was designated to the "alternative" therapy category due to the more favorable tolerability profile and less drug-drug interaction potential for integrase-inhibitor-based regimens. Efavirenz remains extensively prescribed worldwide, especially in resource-limited settings, pregnant patients, patients desiring pregnancy, and patients co-infected with tuberculosis.

Efavirenz has a relatively narrow therapeutic index (suggested plasma concentration range of 1–4 mcg/mL) and large interindividual pharmacokinetic variability, due in part to variants in CYP2B6. CYP2B6 is responsible for generating efavirenz major inactive metabolite, 8-hydroxy-efavirenz. Minor metabolic pathways include other CYP-mediated hydroxylation (CYP2A6, CYP3A4, and CYP1A2) and UGT glucuronidation (UGT2B7), which may play a larger role in CYP2B6 poor metabolizers. Chronic dosing of efavirenz leads to increased expression of CYP2B6, which enhances its own metabolism in most patients, ie, **1/*1* or **1/*6* genotypes. However, patients with **6/*6* genotype are largely unaffected by CYP2B6 autoinduction.

Substantial evidence connects CYP2B6 genotype, plasma efavirenz concentration, and efavirenz adverse effects. Toxic effects of efavirenz are mainly related to the CNS—eg, sleep disorders, impaired concentration, psychosis, suicidal ideation, and depression—and typically resolve after the first few days of treatment. However, adverse effects may persist in some patients, resulting in impaired quality of life and treatment discontinuation. CPIC recommendations are provided in Table 5–2.

Dihydropyrimidine Dehydrogenase (DPD)

Dihydropyrimidine dehydrogenase (DPD, encoded by the *DPYD* gene) is the first and rate-limiting step in pyrimidine catabolism, as well as a major elimination route for fluoropyrimidine chemotherapy agents (Chapter 54). Considerable intergroup and intragroup variation exists in DPD enzyme activity. While many of the alleles identified in the *DPYD* gene either are too rare to sufficiently characterize or have shown conflicting associations with DPD activity, four alleles have been recognized clinically, ie, *DPYD *2A*, **13*, rs67376798, and HapB3. Of these variants, the **2A* and **13* allele are nonfunctional (activity score = 0) while rs67376798 and HapB3 have reduced function (activity score = 0.5). All four alleles are rare, with frequencies less than 1% in most European, African, and Asian populations, with the most common alleles being HapB3, which ranges up to 2% in Asian and European populations, and *2A, which ranges up to 3.5% in a Swedish population (see Table 5–1).

Example: Three fluoropyrimidine drugs are used clinically, namely 5-fluorouracil (5-FU), capecitabine, and tegafur (approved only in Europe). 5-FU is the pharmacologically active compound of each drug, and all are approved to treat solid tumors including colorectal and breast cancer (Chapter 54). 5-FU must be administered intravenously, while both capecitabine and tegafur are oral prodrugs that are rapidly converted to 5-FU in the body. Only 1–3% of an administered dose of the prodrug is converted to the active cytotoxic metabolites, ie, 5-fluorouridine 5′-monophosphate (5-FUMP) and 5-fluoro-2′-deoxyuridine-5′-monophosphate (5-FdUMP), which effectively target rapidly dividing cancer cells and inhibit DNA synthesis. The majority of an administered dose (~80%) is subjected to pyrimidine catabolism via DPD and is excreted in the urine. Complete or partial deficiency of DPD can lead to dramatically reduced clearances of 5-FU, increased levels of toxic metabolites 5-FUMP and 5-FdUMP, and consequently an increased risk for severe dose-dependent fluoropyrimidine toxicities, eg, myelosuppression, mucositis, neurotoxicity, hand-and-foot syndrome, and diarrhea. In a recent genotype-driven dosing study, more than 1100 patients were treated with fluoropyrimidine-based chemotherapy, including 85 (8%) heterozygous variant allele carriers of *DPYD* who received an initial dose reduction of 25% (c.2846A>T and c.1236G>A) or 50% (DPYD*2A and c.1679T>G) compared with DPYD wild-type patients. The relative risk for severe fluoropyrimidine-related toxicity was reduced with genotype-guided dosing, eg, 1.31 (95% CI 0.63–2.73) compared with 2.87 (2.14–3.86) in the historic cohort for DPYD*2A carriers. CPIC recommendations for therapeutic regimens are shown in Table 5–2.

PHASE II ENZYMES

As described in Chapter 4, phase II enzyme biotransformation reactions typically conjugate endogenous molecules, eg, sulfuric acid, glucuronic acid, and acetic acid, onto a wide variety of substrates in order to enhance their elimination from the body. Consequently, polymorphic phase II enzymes may diminish drug elimination and increase risks for toxicities. In this section, we describe key examples of polymorphic phase II enzymes and the pharmacologic consequence for selected prescription drugs.

Uridine 5′-Diphosphoglucuronosyl Transferase 1 (UGT1A1)

The uridine 5′-diphospho- (UDP) glucuronosyltransferase 1A1 (UGT1A1) enzyme, encoded by the *UGT1A1* gene, conjugates glucuronic acid onto small lipophilic molecules, eg, bilirubin, and a wide variety of therapeutic drug substrates so that they may be more readily excreted into bile (Chapter 4). The *UGT1A1* gene locus has more than 30 defined alleles, some of which lead to reduced or completely abolished UGT1A1 function. Most reduced function polymorphisms within the *UGT1A1* gene locus are quite rare; however, the **28* allele is common across three major ethnic groups (see Table 5–1). Approximately 10% of European populations are homozygous carriers of the **28* allele, ie, *UGT1A1 *28/*28* genotype, and are recognized clinically to have Gilbert syndrome. The **28* allele is characterized by an extra TA repeated in the proximal promoter region and is associated with reduced expression of the UGT1A1 enzyme. Clinically, Gilbert syndrome is generally benign; however, affected individuals may have 60–70% increased levels of circulating unconjugated bilirubin due to a ~30% reduction in UGT1A1 activity. Individuals with the *UGT1A1*28/*28* genotype are thus at an increased risk for adverse drug reactions with UGT1A1 drug substrates due to reduced biliary elimination.

Example: Irinotecan is a topoisomerase I inhibitor prodrug and is indicated as first-line chemotherapy in combination with 5-FU and leucovorin for treatment of metastatic carcinoma of the colon or rectum (Chapter 54). Irinotecan is hydrolyzed by hepatic carboxylesterase enzymes to its cytotoxic metabolite, SN-38, which inhibits topoisomerase I and eventually leads to termination of DNA replication and cell death. The active SN-38 metabolite is responsible for the majority of therapeutic action as well as the dose-limiting bone marrow and gastrointestinal toxicities. Inactivation of SN-38 occurs via the polymorphic UGT1A1 enzyme, and carriers of the *UGT1A1*6* and *UGT1A1*28* polymorphisms are consequently at increased risk for severe life-threatening toxicities, eg, neutropenia and diarrhea, due to decreased clearance of the SN-38 metabolite.

Thiopurine *S*-Methyltransferase (TPMT)

Thiopurine *S*-methyltransferase (TPMT) covalently attaches a methyl group onto aromatic and heterocyclic sulfhydryl compounds and is responsible for the pharmacologic deactivation of thiopurine drugs (Chapter 4). Genetic polymorphisms in the gene encoding TPMT may lead to three clinical TPMT activity phenotypes, ie, high, intermediate, and low activity, which are associated with differing rates of inactivation of thiopurine drugs and altered risks for toxicities. While the majority (86–97%) of the population inherits two functional *TPMT* alleles and has high TPMT activity, around 10% of Europeans and Africans inherit only one functional allele and are considered to have intermediate activity. Furthermore, about 0.3% of Europeans inherit two defective alleles and have very low to no TPMT activity (see Table 5–1). More than 90% of the phenotypic TPMT variability across populations can be accounted for with just three point mutations that are defined by four nonfunctional alleles, ie, *TPMT*2*, **3A*, **3B*, and **3C* (see Table 5–2). Most commercial genotyping platforms test for these four common genetic biomarkers and are therefore able to identify individuals with reduced TPMT activity.

Example: Three thiopurine drugs are used clinically, ie, azathioprine, 6-mercaptopurine (6-MP), and 6-thioguanine (6-TG). All share similar metabolic pathways and pharmacology. Azathioprine (a prodrug of 6-MP) and 6-MP are used for treating immunologic disorders, while 6-MP and 6-TG are important anticancer agents (Chapter 54). 6-MP and 6-TG may be activated by the salvage pathway enzyme hypoxanthine-guanine phosphoribosyltransferase (HGPRTase) to form 6-thioguanine nucleotides (TGNs), which are responsible for the majority of therapeutic efficacy as well as bone marrow toxicity. Alternatively, 6-MP and 6-TG may be inactivated by enzymes such as polymorphic TPMT and xanthine oxidase, leaving less available substrate to be activated by HGPRTase. The *TPMT* gene is a major determinant of thiopurine metabolism and exposure to cytotoxic 6-TGN metabolites and thiopurine-related toxicities. See Table 5–2 for recommended dosing strategies. Recent GWA studies have also implicated variants in the enzyme NUDT15, which catalyzes the hydrolysis of nucleotide diphosphates, as being associated with thiopurine intolerance in children from Japan, Singapore, and Guatemala.

OTHER ENZYMES

G6PD

Glucose 6-phosphate dehydrogenase (G6PD) is the first and rate-limiting step in the pentose phosphate pathway and supplies a significant amount of reduced NADPH in the body. In red blood cells (RBCs), where mitochondria are absent, G6PD is the exclusive source of NADPH and reduced glutathione, which play a critical role in the prevention of oxidative damage. Under normal conditions, G6PD in RBCs is able to detoxify unstable oxygen species while working at just 2% of its theoretical capacity. Following exposure to exogenous oxidative stressors, eg, infection, fava beans, and certain therapeutic drugs, G6PD activity in RBCs increases proportionately to meet NADPH demands and ultimately to protect hemoglobin from oxidation. Individuals with G6PD deficiency, defined as less than 60% enzyme activity, according to World Health Organization classification (Table 5–3), are at increased risk for abnormal RBC destruction, ie, hemolysis, due to reduced antioxidant capacity under oxidative pressures.

The gene that encodes the G6PD enzyme is located on the X chromosome and is highly polymorphic, with more than 180 genetic variants identified that result in enzyme deficiency. Greater than 90% of variants are single-base substitutions in the coding region that produce amino acid changes, which result in unstable proteins with reduced enzyme activity. As with most X-linked traits, males with one reference X chromosome and females with two reference X chromosomes will have equivalent "normal" G6PD activity. Similarly, hemizygous-deficient males (with a deficient copy of the *G6PD* gene on their single X chromosome) and homozygous-deficient females (with two deficient copies) express reduced activity phenotypes (see Table 5–1). However, for heterozygous females (with one deficient allele and one normal allele), genotype-to-phenotype predictions are less reliable due to the X-chromosome mosaicism, ie, where one X chromosome in each female cell is randomly inactivated, leading to G6PD activity that may range from fully functional to severely deficient. G6PD enzyme activity phenotype estimations for heterozygous females therefore may be improved with complementary G6PD activity testing.

G6PD enzyme deficiency affects more than 400 million people worldwide, and the World Health Organization has categorized G6PD activity into five classes (see Table 5–3). The majority of polymorphic *G6PD*-deficient genotypes are associated with class II for severe deficiency (<10% enzyme activity) and class III for moderate deficiency (10–60% enzyme activity). Most individuals with reduced function alleles of *G6PD* have ancestries in geographic areas of the world corresponding to areas with high malaria prevalence. Polymorphic alleles gained in frequency over time as they offered some benefit against death from malaria. The estimated frequency of G6PD deficiency is approximately 8% in malaria-endemic countries, with the milder *G6PD-A*(–) allele prevalent in Africa, and the more severe *G6PD*-Mediterranean allele widespread across western Asia (Saudi Arabia and Turkey to India). There is a much more heterogeneous distribution of variant alleles in East Asia and Asia Pacific, which complicates G6PD risk predictions; however, the most frequently identified forms in Asia include the more severe class II alleles, eg, Mediterranean, Kaiping, and Canton, as well as some class III alleles, eg, Mahidol, Chinese-5, and Gaohe (see Table 5–1).

Example: Rasburicase, a recombinant urate-oxidase enzyme, is indicated for the initial management of high uric acid levels in cancer patients receiving chemotherapy. Rasburicase alleviates the uric acid burden that often accompanies tumor-lysing treatments by converting uric acid into allantoin, a more soluble and easily excreted molecule. During the enzymatic conversion of uric acid to allantoin, hydrogen peroxide, a highly reactive oxidant, is formed. Hydrogen peroxide must be reduced by glutathione to prevent free radical formation and oxidative damage. Individuals with G6PD deficiency receiving rasburicase therapy are at greatly increased risk for severe hemolytic anemia and methemoglobinemia. The manufacturer recommends that patients at high risk (individuals of African or Mediterranean ancestry) be screened prior to the initiation of therapy and that rasburicase not be used in patients with G6PD deficiency (see Table 5–2).

TABLE 5–3 Classification of G6PD deficiency (WHO Working Group, 1989).

World Health Organization Class	Level of Deficiency	Enzyme Activity	Clinical phenotype
I	Severe	<10%	Chronic (non-spherocytic) hemolytic anemia
II	Severe	<10%	Risk of acute hemolytic anemia; intermittent hemolysis
III	Moderate	10–60%	Risk of acute hemolytic anemia; hemolysis with stressors
IV	None	60–150%	Normal
V	None	>150%	Enhanced activity

GENETIC VARIATIONS IN TRANSPORTERS

Plasma membrane transporters, located on epithelial cells of many tissues, eg, intestinal, renal, and hepatic membranes, mediate selective uptake and efflux of endogenous compounds and xenobiotics including many drug products. Transporters, which often work in concert with drug-metabolizing enzymes, play important roles in determining plasma and tissue concentrations of drugs and their metabolites. Genetic differences in transporter genes can dramatically alter drug disposition and response and thus may increase risk for toxicities. In this section, a key example of a polymorphic uptake transporter and its pharmacologic impact on statin toxicity are described.

ORGANIC ANION TRANSPORTER (OATP1B1)

The OATP1B1 transporter (encoded by the *SLCO1B1* gene) is located on the sinusoidal membrane (facing the blood) of hepatocytes and is responsible for the hepatic uptake of mainly weakly acidic drugs and endogenous compounds, eg, statins, methotrexate, and bilirubin. More than 40 nonsynonymous variants (nsSNPs) have been identified in this transporter, some of which result in decreased transport function. A common reduced-function polymorphism, rs4149056, has been shown to reduce transport of OATP1B1 substrates in vitro as well as to alter pharmacokinetic and clinical outcomes in vivo. The variant results in an amino acid change, Val174Ala, and is associated with reduced membrane expression, likely as a result of impaired trafficking capability. Allele **5* is relatively rare (rs4149056 alone; ~1%), but various other reduced-function alleles (**15* and **17*; haplotypes containing rs4149056) are common in most European and Asian populations (between 5% and 15%) (see Table 5–1).

Example: HMG-coenzyme A (CoA) reductase inhibitors (statins) are highly effective medications that are widely prescribed to reduce serum lipids for the prevention of cardiovascular events (Chapter 35). Seven statins in use currently are generally safe and well-tolerated, but skeletal muscle toxicity can limit their use. Known risk factors include high statin dose, interacting medications, advanced age, and metabolic comorbidities. Furthermore, the common variant, rs4149056 in *SLCO1B1*, increases systemic exposure of simvastatin (221% increase in plasma area under the curve for patients homozygous for the rs4149056 variant, eg, *SLCO1B1*5/*5*; **5/[*15 or *17]*; or [**15* or **17*]/[**15* or **17*]) and was identified to have the single strongest association with simvastatin-induced myopathy in a GWA analysis. For individuals receiving simvastatin with reduced OATP1B1 function (at least one nonfunctional allele), CPIC recommends a lower simvastatin dose or an alternative statin (see Table 5–2).

BREAST CANCER RESISTANCE PROTEIN (BCRP, *ABCG2*)

BCRP (encoded by the *ABCG2* gene), an efflux transporter in the ATP binding cassette (ABC) superfamily, is located on epithelial cells of the kidney, liver, and intestine as well as on the endothelial cells of the blood-brain barrier. Recent studies have implicated a reduced-function variant in *ABCG2*, which encodes an amino acid change from glutamine to lysine at position 141 of the protein (rs2231142), as a determinant of the pharmacokinetics, response, and toxicity of several drugs. The variant has a low frequency in individuals of African ancestry but is found at an allele frequency of about 30% in East Asians including Chinese and Japanese (see Table 5–1). Notably, the variant has been associated with changes in response to the xanthine oxidase inhibitor, allopurinol, and the statin rosuvastatin. In fact, the approved label of rosuvastatin, a substrate of BCRP, suggests that a lower dose (half) be given to East Asians, who have higher levels of the drug. Although still controversial, many studies speculate that the reason for the higher levels of rosuvastatin is the high allele frequency of rs2231142 in this population leading to increased bioavailability of the drug. In addition, the variant has been associated with toxicity to various anticancer drugs. Because of its high allele frequency, particularly in Asian populations, and the fact that the transporter is a determinant of the pharmacokinetics of many drugs, it is likely that this variant will become increasingly important in precision medicine.

ORGANIC CATION TRANSPORTER 1 (OCT1, *SLC22A1*)

Similar to OATP1B1, OCT1 is a transporter that is highly expressed in the liver and plays a role in drug disposition. Its substrates include many basic drugs from various pharmacologic classes such as morphine, tramadol, sumatriptan, and ondansetron. The transporter has many common reduced-function polymorphisms that are found at allele frequencies greater than 5%, particularly in Hispanics and European populations. For drugs that are metabolized in the liver, studies indicate that individuals who are compound heterozygotes for these reduced-function alleles (ie, carrying two reduced-function alleles) have on the order of twofold higher drug levels than either individuals who are heterozygous for a reduced-function allele or those who do not carry a reduced-function allele (see Table 5–1).

■ GENETIC VARIATIONS IN IMMUNE SYSTEM FUNCTION

Genetic predispositions to drug response and toxicities are not limited to genes related to pharmacokinetic processes, eg, drug-metabolizing enzymes and drug transporters. Additional genetic sources of variation may include genes involved in pharmacodynamic processes such as drug receptors and drug targets. For example, a polymorphism in HLA loci is associated with a predisposition to drug toxicity.

DRUG-INDUCED HYPERSENSITIVITY REACTIONS

Hypersensitivity reactions to various drugs can range from mild rashes to severe skin toxicities. The most severe hypersensitivity reactions are liver injury, toxic epidermal necrosis (TEN), and Stevens-Johnson syndrome (SJS), in which drugs or their metabolites form antigens.

Drug classes associated with hypersensitivity reactions include sulfonamides, nonsteroidal anti-inflammatory drugs (NSAIDs), antibiotics, steroids, antiepileptic agents, and methotrexate.

Hypersensitivity reactions have varying prevalence rates in different racial and ethnic populations. For example, carbamazepine-induced skin toxicities have an increased prevalence in East Asian populations. Population-based hypersensitivity reactions have been attributed to genetic polymorphisms in the HLA system, which are part of the major histocompatibility complex (MHC) gene family (see also Chapter 55). Of the several HLA forms, *HLA-B*, *HLA-DQ*, and *HLA-DR* polymorphisms have been associated with many drug-induced hypersensitivity reactions, including reactions to allopurinol, carbamazepine, abacavir, and flucloxacillin (Table 5–4).

Many *HLA-B* polymorphisms have been characterized and have varying allele frequencies depending on the racial and ethnic population. A polymorphism in *HLA-B* may result in altered antigen-binding sites in the HLA molecule, which in turn may recognize different peptides. The selective recognition of particular drug-bound peptides by some *HLA-B* polymorphism products results in population-selective drug hypersensitivity reactions.

Example 1: Abacavir, a nucleoside reverse transcriptase inhibitor used in the treatment of HIV, is associated with hypersensitivity reactions in the skin, particularly SJS, which for many years appeared to be idiosyncratic, ie, of unknown mechanism. Although the drug-bound peptide involved in abacavir hypersensitivity has not been isolated or identified, it appears to interact somewhat specifically with the product of *HLA-B*57:01*, an *HLA-B* polymorphism found more commonly in European populations (see Table 5–1). Other *HLA-B* polymorphisms are not associated with abacavir-induced hypersensitivity reactions. However, it is noteworthy that *HLA-B*57:01*, though necessary for SJS or TEN associated with abacavir, is not sufficient. That is, many individuals with the polymorphism do not get the hypersensitivity reaction. This lack of specificity is not understood and clearly warrants further study.

Abacavir hypersensitivity reactions are known to vary in frequency among ethnic groups, consistent with the population frequencies of the *HLA-B*57:01* allele. As a prodrug, abacavir is activated to carbovir triphosphate, a reactive molecule that may be involved in the immunogenicity of abacavir. Abacavir-induced hypersensitivity reactions are probably mediated by the activation of cytotoxic CD8 T cells. In fact, there is an increased abundance of CD8 T cells in the skin of patients with abacavir hypersensitivity reactions. Experiments demonstrating that CD8-positive T cells can be stimulated by lymphoblastoid cell lines expressing *HLA-B*57:01*, but not *HLA-B*57:02* or *HLA-B*58:01*, suggest that the HLA-B*57:01 protein may recognize and bind an abacavir-associated peptide, which is not recognized by the other polymorphisms. Alternatively, the *HLA-B*57:01* gene product complex may present the ligand-bound peptide on the cell surface in a structurally different configuration, which is recognized by cytotoxic T cells.

Because of the importance of abacavir in therapeutics, genetic testing of the *HLA-B*57:01* biomarker associated with abacavir hypersensitivity has been rapidly incorporated into clinical practice, much faster than typical genetic tests (see Figure 5–1). CPIC recommendations based on genotyping results are shown in Table 5–2.

Example 2: Flucloxacillin hypersensitivity reactions may lead to drug-induced liver toxicity. In particular, in 51 cases of flucloxacillin hepatotoxicity, a highly significant association was identified with a polymorphism linked to *HLA-B*57:01* (Figure 5–2). HLA polymorphisms also contribute to liver injury from other drugs (see Table 5–4). For example, reaction to the anticoagulant ximelagatran is associated with a *HLA-DRB1*07:01* allele. Several drugs used in the treatment of tuberculosis, including isoniazid, rifampin, and ethambutol, also cause liver injury, which appears to be related to HLA polymorphisms.

TABLE 5–4 Polymorphisms in HLA genes associated with Stevens-Johnson syndrome, toxic epidermal necrosis, or drug-induced liver injury.

Variant of *HLA* Gene	Drug and Adverse Effect
*HLA-B*57:01*	Abacavir-induced skin toxicity
*HLA-B*58:01*	Allopurinol-induced skin toxicity
*HLA-DRB1 *15:01, DRB5 *01:01, DQB1 *06:02* haplotype	Amoxicillin-clavulanate-induced liver injury
*HLA-B*15:02*	Carbamazepine-induced skin toxicity
*HLA-B *57:01*	Flucloxacillin-induced liver injury
*HLA-DQB1 *06, *02, HLA-DRB1 *15, *07*	Various drugs, subgroup analysis for cholestatic or other types of liver injury
*HLA-DRB1 *07, HLA-DQA1 *02*	Ximelagatran, increased ALT

ALT, alanine transaminase.

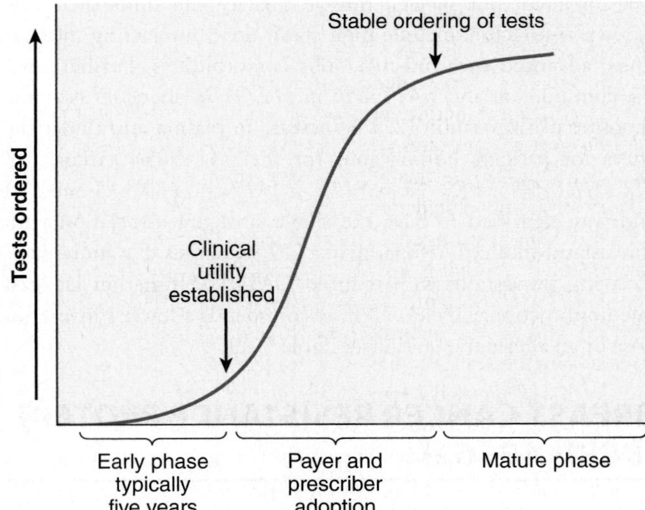

FIGURE 5–1 Increasing use of testing for genetic variants of drug metabolism over time. Adoption of testing in clinical medicine typically undergoes three phases. Testing for *HLA-B*5701* was rapidly adopted. (Reproduced with permission from Lai-Goldman M, Faruki H: Abacavir hypersensitivity: A model system for pharmacogenetic test adoption. Genet Med 2008 Dec;10(12):874-878.)

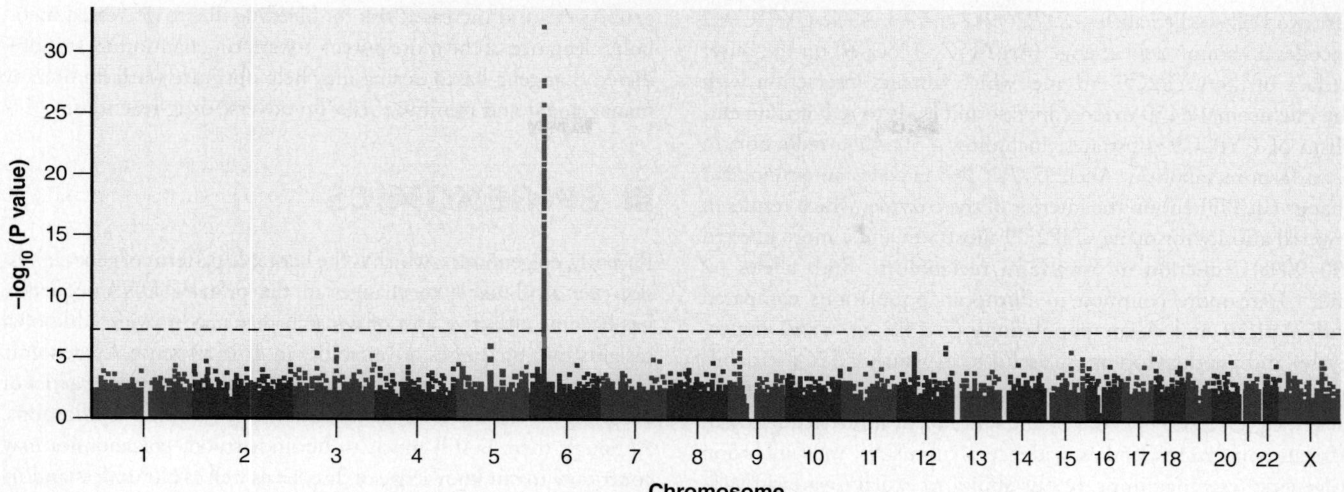

FIGURE 5–2 Results from a flucloxacillin drug-induced liver injury study. Each dot represents an SNP in a genome-wide assay. The *x* axis represents the position of the SNP on chromosomes. The *y* axis represents the magnitude of the association of each SNP with liver damage (Cochran-Armitage trend P value) in a case-control study that included 51 liver injury cases and 282 population controls. The high signal peak in chromosome 6 lies in the MHC region and indicates very strong association of injury with that SNP. The horizontal dashed line represents the commonly accepted minimum level for significance in this type of study. (Reproduced with permission from Daly AK et al: HLA-B*5701 genotype is a major determinant of drug-induced liver injury due to flucloxacillin. Nat Genet 2009 Jul;41(7):816-819.)

IFNL3 (IL-28B)

Interferon lambda-3 (IFN-λ3; also known as interleukin-28B), encoded by the *IFNL3* (or *IL28B*) gene, belongs to the family of type III IFN-λ cytokines. Type III IFNs share many therapeutic effects with type I IFNs, eg, IFN-α (Chapter 55), such as being directly induced by viruses and acting through JAK-STAT signal transduction pathways (via distinct heterodimeric receptor signaling complexes) to produce antiviral activity in cells. Type III IFNs play a role in hepatitis C virus (HCV) infection. Genetic variants near the *IFNL3* gene were found to be most significantly associated with HCV treatment response to pegylated-IFN-α (PEG-IFN-α), in combination with ribavirin (RBV). Approximately twofold greater cure rates were observed in patients with a favorable genotype. While the mechanism underlying this association has yet to be fully elucidated, the rs12979860 variant near *IFNL3* is considered the strongest baseline predictor of a cure for patients with HCV-1 receiving PEG-IFN-α/RBV. The favorable allele, the rs12979860 variant, is inherited most frequently in Asians (~90%), and least frequently in Africans (see Table 5–1). This frequency distribution is remarkably similar to rates of response to HCV PEG-IFN-α/RBV treatment among the three ethnic groups.

Pegylated interferon with ribavirin: Chronic HCV affects 160 million people worldwide and is a leading cause of cirrhosis of the liver and liver cancer. The goal for HCV antiviral therapy is to resolve the infection, defined clinically as achievement of sustained virologic response (SVR), ie, undetectable HCV RNA measured 6 months after finishing treatment. For patients receiving PEG-IFN-α/RBV regimens, which are associated with many side effects and poor response, clinical decisions of whether to initiate therapy are largely based on likelihood of SVR. Predictors of SVR include viral factors as well as patient factors. In addition, Europeans homozygous for the favorable genotype (*IFNL3 rs12979860/rs12979860*; SVR: 69%) are more likely to achieve SVR compared with the unfavorable genotype (*IFNL3 reference/reference* or *reference/rs12979860*; SVR: 33% and 27%, respectively), and similar rates are observed in African patients. Guidelines according to CPIC are shown in Table 5–2.

■ POLYGENIC EFFECTS

In the above examples, variations within single gene loci are described that are significantly associated with altered drug response or toxicity. However, it is expected that polygenic influences, ie, the combinatorial effect of multiple genes on drug response, may more accurately describe individual differences with respect to clinical outcomes. As evidence grows linking newly discovered pharmacogenetic biomarkers with therapeutic response or adverse outcomes, adequately powered clinical studies that consider the impact of newly discovered genes in the context of previously established genetic biomarkers are essential for making strong clinical recommendations. This is best exemplified by warfarin, where the effects of two genes, *CYP2C9* and *VKORC1*, on dose requirement have been clearly defined.

CYP2C9 & VKORC1

CYP2C9 is a phase I drug-metabolizing enzyme that acts primarily on acidic drugs including *S*-warfarin, phenytoin, and NSAIDs (Chapter 4). The gene that encodes CYP2C9 is highly polymorphic, with more than 50 alleles defined (https://www.pharmvar.org/gene/CYP2C9). However, much of the variability in metabolic clearance of CYP2C9 substrates may be accounted for with just two well-studied alleles, *CYP2C9*2* and **3*. Allele *CYP2C9*2* encodes an amino acid change (Arg144Cys) located on the outer surface of the CYP2C9 enzyme, which impairs interaction with the microsomal P450 oxidoreductase and leads to reduced metabolism of CYP2C9 substrates, including a 30–40% reduction in *S*-warfarin metabolism. Allele *CYP2C9*3* encodes an amino acid change (Ile359Leu) on the interior of the enzyme, which results in lowered affinity for many CYP2C9 substrates and a more marked (80–90%) reduction in *S*-warfarin metabolism. Both alleles **2* and **3* are more common in European populations compared with African and Asian populations (7–13% vs <5%, respectively) and are therefore most useful to explain *CYP2C9* variability in Europeans (see Table 5–1). Additional reduced-function alleles, eg, *CYP2C9*5*, **6*, **8*, and **11*, occur more frequently in African populations, and as evidence accumulates, their inclusion in genetic tests may improve our ability to explain warfarin variability in Africans.

Vitamin K epoxide reductase complex subunit 1 (VKORC1), encoded by the *VKORC1* gene, is the target of anticoagulant warfarin and a key enzyme in the vitamin K recycling process (Chapter 34, Figure 34–6). Activated vitamin K is an essential cofactor for activation of blood clotting factors II, VII, IX, and X, as well as endogenous anticoagulant proteins C and S. Rare genetic variants in the coding region of *VKORC1* may lead to bleeding disorders, eg, multiple coagulation factor deficiency type 2A, or warfarin resistance. A polymorphism common across all major ethnicities is located in a transcription factor–binding site, *VKORC1*-1639G>A, which results in reduced expression of VKORC1 in the liver. The most important consequences of the *VKORC1* polymorphism are increased sensitivity to warfarin (discussed below). The *VKORC1*-1639G>A polymorphism occurs most frequently in Asian populations (~90%) and least often in Africans (~10%), which explains, in part, the difference in dosing requirements among major ethnic groups (see Table 5–1).

Example: Warfarin, a vitamin K antagonist, is the oldest and most widely prescribed oral anticoagulant worldwide. Within a narrow therapeutic range, warfarin is highly effective for the prevention and treatment of thromboembolic disorders (Chapter 34). Nevertheless, interpatient differences in dosing requirements (up to 20-fold) often lead to complications from subtherapeutic anticoagulation and clotting or supratherapeutic anticoagulation and bleeding, which are among the most common causes for emergency room visits in the United States. Understanding the factors that contribute to variability in individual warfarin maintenance doses may improve therapeutic outcomes.

Warfarin dosing algorithms that include clinical and known genetic influences on warfarin dose, ie, polymorphisms in CYP2C9 and VKORC1, clearly outperform empiric-dosing approaches based on population averages, as well as dosing based on clinical factors alone (see Table 5–2). The pharmacologic action of warfarin is mediated through inactivation of VKORC1, and since the discovery of the VKORC1 gene in 2004, numerous studies have indicated that individuals with decreased VKORC1 expression, eg, carriers of the -1639G>A polymorphism, are at increased risk for excessive anticoagulation following standard warfarin dosages. Furthermore, warfarin is administered as a racemic mixture of *R*- and *S*-warfarin, and patients with reduced-function CYP2C9 genotypes are at increased risk for bleeding due to decreased metabolic clearance of the more potent *S*-warfarin enantiomer. It is predicted that gene-based dosing may help optimize warfarin therapy management and minimize risks for adverse drug reactions.

EPIGENOMICS

Recently, epigenomics, which is the heritable patterns of gene expression *not* attributable to changes in the primary DNA sequence, has become an active area of research that may provide additional insights into the causes of variability in drug response. Epigenomic mechanisms that can regulate genes involved in pharmacokinetics or drug targets include DNA methylation and histone modifications. Although there is still much to be understood, epigenomics may contribute to our knowledge of diseases as well as our understanding of individual phenotypes such as acquired drug resistance.

FUTURE DIRECTIONS

Discoveries in pharmacogenomics are increasing as new technologies for genotyping are being developed and as access to patient DNA samples along with drug response information has accelerated. Increasingly, pharmacogenomics discoveries will move beyond single SNPs to multiple SNPs that inform both adverse and therapeutic responses. It is hoped that prescriber-friendly predictive models incorporating SNPs and other biomarkers as well as information on demographics, comorbidities, epigenetic signatures, and concomitant medications will be developed to aid in drug and dose selection. CPIC guidelines and FDA-stimulated product label changes will contribute to the accelerated translation of discoveries to clinical practice.

REFERENCES

Altman RB, Whirl-Carrillo M, Klein TE: Challenges in the pharmacogenomic annotation of whole genomes. Clin Pharmacol Ther 2013;94:211.

Bertilsson DL: Geographical/interracial differences in polymorphic drug oxidation. Clin Pharmacokinet 1995;29:192.

Browning LA, Kruse JA: Hemolysis and methemoglobinemia secondary to rasburicase administration. Ann Pharmacother 2005;39:1932.

Camptosar [irinotecan product label]. New York, NY: Pfizer Inc.; 2012.

Cappellini MD, Fiorelli G: Glucose-6-phosphate dehydrogenase deficiency. Lancet 2008;371:64.

Caudle KE et al: Clinical Pharmacogenetics Implementation Consortium guidelines for dihydropyrimidine dehydrogenase genotype and fluoropyrimidine dosing. Clin Pharmacol Ther 2013;94:640.

Chasman DI et al: Genetic determinants of statin-induced low-density lipoprotein cholesterol reduction: The Justification for the Use of Statins in Prevention: An Intervention Trial Evaluating Rosuvastatin (JUPITER) trial. Circ Cardiovasc Genet 2012;5:257.

Crews KR et al: Clinical Pharmacogenetics Implementation Consortium (CPIC) guidelines for codeine therapy in the context of cytochrome P450 2D6 (CYP2D6) genotype. Clin Pharmacol Ther 2009;91:321.

Daly AK et al: HLA-B*5701 genotype is a major determinant of drug-induced liver injury due to flucloxacillin. Nat Genet 2009;41:816.

Elitek [rasburicase product label]. Bridgewater, NJ: Sanofi U.S. Inc.; 2009.

Gammal RS et al: Clinical Pharmacogenetics Implementation Consortium (CPIC) guideline for UGT1A1 and atazanavir prescribing. Clin Pharmacol Ther 2016;99:363.

Giacomini KM et al: International Transporter Consortium commentary on clinically important transporter polymorphisms. Clin Pharmacol Ther 2013;94:23.

Howes RE et al: G6PD deficiency prevalence and estimates of affected populations in malaria endemic countries: A geostatistical model-based map. PLoS Med 2012;9:e1001339.

Howes RE et al: Spatial distribution of G6PD deficiency variants across malaria-endemic regions. Malaria J 2013;12:418.

Johnson JA, Klein TE, Relling MV: Clinical implementation of pharmacogenetics: More than one gene at a time. Clin Pharmacol Ther 2013;93:384.

Johnson JA et al: Clinical Pharmacogenetics Implementation Consortium guidelines for CYP2C9 and VKORC1 genotypes and warfarin dosing. Clin Pharmacol Ther 2009;90:625.

Kim IS et al: ABCG2 Q141K polymorphism is associated with chemotherapy-induced diarrhea in patients with diffuse large B-cell lymphoma who received frontline rituximab plus cyclophosphamide/doxorubicin/vincristine/prednisone chemotherapy. Cancer Sci 2008;99:2496.

Lai-Goldman M, Faruki H: Abacavir hypersensitivity: A model system for pharmacogenetic test adoption. Genet Med 2008;10:874.

Lavanchy D: Evolving epidemiology of hepatitis C virus. Clin Microbiol Infect 2011;17:107.

Matsuura K, Watanabe T, Tanaka Y: Role of IL28B for chronic hepatitis C treatment toward personalized medicine. J Gastroenterol Hepatol 2014;29:241.

McDonagh EM et al: PharmGKB summary: Very important pharmacogene information for G6PD. Pharmacogenet Genomics 2012;22:219.

Minucci A et al: Glucose-6-phosphate dehydrogenase (G6PD) mutations database: Review of the "old" and update of the new mutations. Blood Cell Mol Dis 2012;48:154.

Moriyama T et al: NUDT15 polymorphisms alter thiopurine metabolism and hematopoietic toxicity. Nat Genet 2016;48:367.

Muir AJ et al: Clinical Pharmacogenetics Implementation Consortium (CPIC) guidelines for IFNL3 (IL28B) genotype and peginterferon alpha based regimens. Clin Pharmacol Ther 2014;95:141.

Relling MV et al: Clinical Pharmacogenetics Implementation Consortium guidelines for thiopurine methyltransferase genotype and thiopurine dosing. Clin Pharmacol Ther 2009;89:387.

Russmann S, Jetter A, Kullak-Ublick GA: Pharmacogenetics of drug-induced liver injury. Hepatology 2010;52:748.

Scott SA et al: Clinical Pharmacogenetics Implementation Consortium guidelines for CYP2C19 genotype and clopidogrel therapy: 2013 update. Clin Pharmacol Ther 2013;94:317.

Shin J: Clinical pharmacogenomics of warfarin and clopidogrel. J Pharmacy Pract 2012;25:428.

Swen JJ et al: Pharmacogenetics: From bench to byte—an update of guidelines. Clin Pharmacol Ther 2009;89:662.

Tukey RH, Strassburg CP: Human UDP-glucuronosyltransferases: Metabolism, expression, and disease. Annu Rev Pharmacol Toxicol 2000;40:581.

Tukey RH, Strassburg CP, Mackenzie PI: Pharmacogenomics of human UDP-glucuronosyltransferases and irinotecan toxicity. Mol Pharmacol 2002;62:446.

Wen CC et al: Genome-wide association study identifies ABCG2 (BCRP) as an allopurinol transporter and a determinant of drug response. Clin Pharmacol Ther 2015;97:518.

WHO Working Group: Glucose-6-phosphate dehydrogenase deficiency. Bull World Health Org 1989;67:601.

Wilke RA et al: The Clinical Pharmacogenomics Implementation Consortium: CPIC guideline for SLCO1B1 and simvastatin-induced myopathy. Clin Pharmacol Ther 2009;92:112.

Xu J-M: Severe irinotecan-induced toxicity in a patient with UGT1A1*28 and UGT1A1*6 polymorphisms. World J Gastroenterol 2013;19:3899.

Yang J et al: Influence of CYP2C9 and VKORC1 genotypes on the risk of hemorrhagic complications in warfarin-treated patients: A systematic review and meta-analysis. Int J Cardiol 2013;168:4234.

Reviews

Campbell JM et al: Irinotecan-induced toxicity pharmacogenetics: An umbrella review of systematic reviews and meta-analyses. Pharmacogenomics J 2017;17:21.

Flockhart DA, Huang SM: Clinical pharmacogenetics. In: Atkinson AJ et al (editors): *Principles of Clinical Pharmacology*, 3rd ed. Elsevier, 2012.

Huang SM, Chen L, Giacomini KM: Pharmacogenomic mechanisms of drug toxicity. In: Atkinson AJ et al (editors): *Principles of Clinical Pharmacology*, 3rd ed. Elsevier, 2012.

Meulendijks D et al: Improving safety of fluoropyrimidine chemotherapy by individualizing treatment based on dihydropyrimidine dehydrogenase activity: Ready for clinical practice? Cancer Treat Rev 2016;50:23.

Relling MV, Giacomini KM: Pharmacogenetics. In: Brunton LL, Chabner BA, Knollmann BC (editors): *Goodman & Gilman's The Pharmacological Basis of Therapeutics*, 12th ed. McGraw Hill, 2011.

Relling MV et al: Clinical Pharmacogenetics Implementation Consortium (CPIC) guidelines for rasburicase therapy in the context of G6PD deficiency genotype. Clin Pharmacol Ther 2014;96:169.

Zanger UM, Schwab M: Cytochrome P450 enzymes in drug metabolism: Regulation of gene expression, enzyme activities, and impact of genetic variation. Pharmacol Ther 2013;138:103.

CASE STUDY ANSWER

Atazanavir inhibits the polymorphic UGT1A1 enzyme, which mediates the conjugation of glucuronic acid with bilirubin. Decreased UGT1A1 activity results in the accumulation of unconjugated (indirect) bilirubin in blood and tissues. When levels are high enough, yellow discoloration of the eyes and skin, ie, jaundice, is the result. The plasma levels of indirect bilirubin concentrations are expected to increase to greater than 2.5 times the upper limit of normal (grade 3 or higher elevations) in approximately 40% of patients taking once-daily atazanavir boosted with ritonavir and at least five times the upper limit of normal (grade 4 elevation) in approximately 4.8% of patients. Carriers of the *UGT1A1* decreased-function alleles (**28/*28* or **28/*37*) have reduced enzyme activity and have an increased risk of atazanavir discontinuation. Genotyping showed that the patient was homozygous for the *UGT1A1*28* allele polymorphism. This probably led to the high levels of bilirubin and the subsequent discontinuation of atazanavir secondary to the adverse drug reaction of jaundice.

SECTION II AUTONOMIC DRUGS

CHAPTER 6

Introduction to Autonomic Pharmacology

Todd W. Vanderah, PhD, & Bertram G. Katzung, MD, PhD

CASE STUDY

A 56-year-old woman is brought to the university eye center with a complaint of "loss of vision." Because of visual impairment, she has lost her driver's license and has fallen several times in her home. Examination reveals that her eyelids close involuntarily with a frequency and duration sufficient to prevent her from seeing her surroundings for more than brief moments at a time. When she holds her eyelids open with her fingers, she can see normally. She has no other muscle dysfunction. A diagnosis of blepharospasm is made. Using a fine needle, several injections of botulinum toxin type A are made in the orbicularis oculi muscle of each eyelid. After observation in the waiting area, she is sent home. Two days later, she reports by telephone that her vision has improved dramatically. How did botulinum toxin improve her vision? How long can her vision be expected to remain normal after this single treatment?

The nervous system is anatomically divided into the central nervous system (CNS; the brain and spinal cord) and the peripheral nervous system (PNS; neuronal tissues outside the CNS). Functionally, the nervous system can be divided into two major subdivisions: **autonomic** and **somatic**. The **autonomic nervous system (ANS)** is largely independent (autonomous) in that its activities are not under direct conscious control. It is concerned primarily with control and integration of visceral functions necessary for life such as cardiac output, blood flow distribution, and digestion. Evidence is accumulating that the ANS, especially the vagus nerve, also influences immune function and some CNS functions such as seizure discharge. Remarkably, some evidence indicates that autonomic nerves can also influence cancer development and progression. The efferent (motor) portion of the **somatic** subdivision is largely concerned with consciously controlled functions such as movement, respiration, and posture. Both the autonomic and the somatic systems have important afferent (sensory) inputs that provide information regarding the internal and external environments and modify motor output through reflex arcs of varying complexity.

The nervous system has several properties in common with the endocrine system. These include high-level integration in the brain, the ability to influence processes in distant regions of the body, and extensive use of negative feedback. Both systems use chemicals for the transmission of information; the nervous system also uses electrical signaling. In the nervous system, chemical transmission occurs between nerve cells and between nerve cells and their effector cells. Chemical transmission takes place through the release of small amounts of transmitter substances from the nerve terminals into the synaptic cleft. The transmitter crosses the cleft by diffusion and activates or inhibits the postsynaptic cell by binding to a specialized receptor molecule. In a few cases, *retrograde* transmission may occur from the postsynaptic cell to the presynaptic neuron terminal and modify its subsequent activity.

By using drugs that mimic or block the actions of chemical transmitters, we can selectively modify many autonomic functions. These functions involve a variety of effector tissues, including cardiac muscle, smooth muscle, vascular endothelium, exocrine glands, and presynaptic nerve terminals. Autonomic drugs are useful in many clinical conditions. Unfortunately, a very large number of drugs used for other purposes (eg, allergies, mental illness) have unwanted effects on autonomic function.

ANATOMY OF THE AUTONOMIC NERVOUS SYSTEM

The ANS lends itself to division on anatomic grounds into two major portions: the **sympathetic (thoracolumbar)** division and the **parasympathetic** (traditionally **craniosacral,** but see Box: Sympathetic Sacral Outflow) division (Figure 6–1). Neurons in both divisions originate in nuclei within the CNS and give rise to preganglionic efferent fibers that exit from the brain stem or spinal cord and terminate in ganglia found in the periphery. The sympathetic preganglionic fibers leave the CNS through the thoracic,

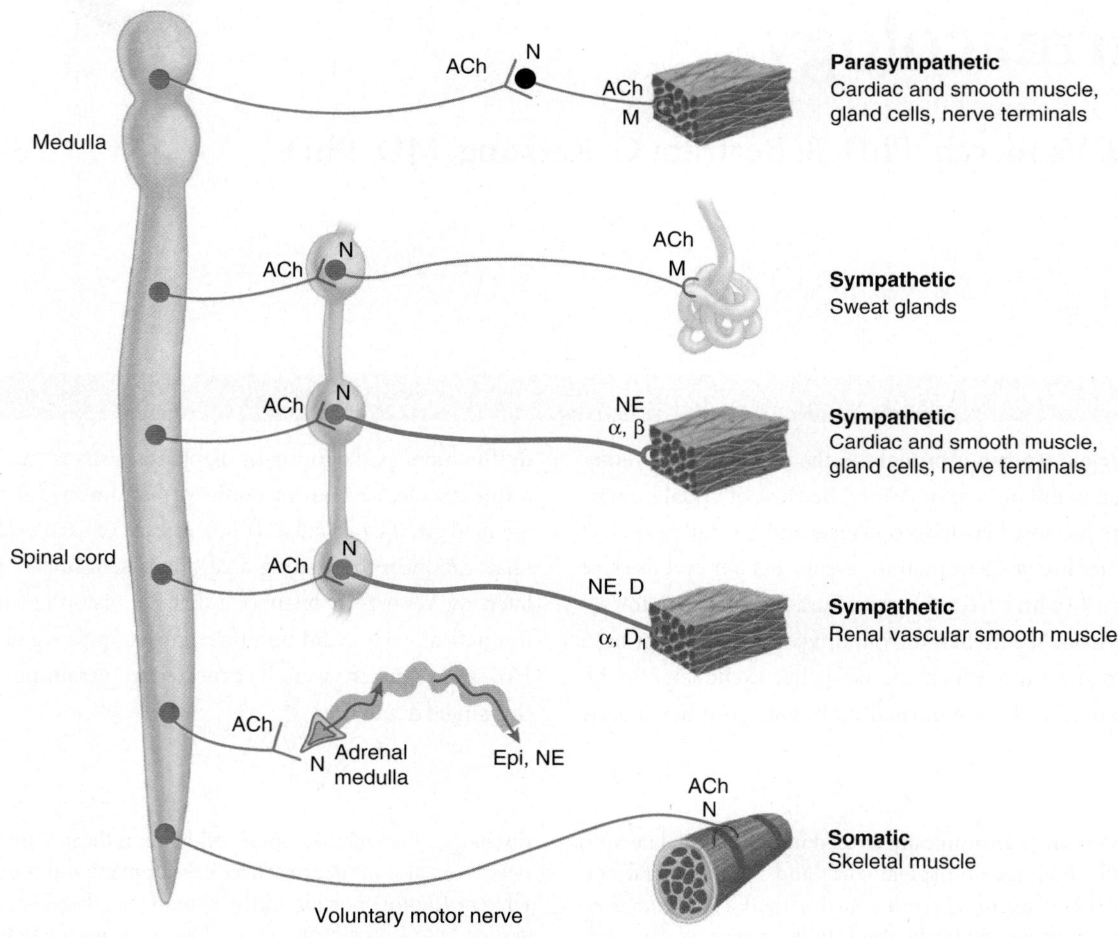

FIGURE 6–1 Schematic diagram comparing some anatomic and neurotransmitter features of autonomic and somatic motor nerves. Only the primary transmitter substances are shown. Parasympathetic ganglia are not shown because most are in or near the wall of the organ innervated. Cholinergic nerves are shown in blue, noradrenergic in red. Note that some sympathetic postganglionic fibers release acetylcholine rather than norepinephrine. Sympathetic nerves to the renal vasculature and kidney may release dopamine as well as norepinephrine during stress. The adrenal medulla, a modified sympathetic ganglion, receives sympathetic preganglionic fibers and releases epinephrine and norepinephrine into the blood. Not shown are the sacral preganglionic fibers that innervate the rectum, bladder, and genitalia. These fibers are probably sympathetic preganglionic nerves with cholinergic postganglionic fibers (see Box: Sympathetic Sacral Outflow). ACh, acetylcholine; D, dopamine; Epi, epinephrine; M, muscarinic receptors; N, nicotinic receptors; NE, norepinephrine.

lumbar, and (according to new information) sacral spinal nerves. The parasympathetic preganglionic fibers leave the CNS through the brainstem cranial nerves (cranial nerves three, seven, nine, and ten) as well as from the sacral spinal cord.

Most thoracic and lumbar sympathetic preganglionic fibers leave the intermediate gray of the spinal cord, are short, and terminate in ganglia (collection of neuron cell bodies) located in the **paravertebral** chains that lie on either side of the spinal column. The remaining sympathetic preganglionic fibers are somewhat longer and terminate in **prevertebral ganglia,** which lie in front of the vertebrae, usually on the ventral surface of the aorta. From the ganglia, postganglionic sympathetic fibers run to, and terminate on, the tissues they innervate. Some preganglionic parasympathetic fibers terminate in parasympathetic ganglia located outside the organs they innervate, including the **ciliary, pterygopalatine, submandibular,** and **otic ganglia.** However, the majority of parasympathetic preganglionic fibers terminate on ganglion cells distributed diffusely or in networks in the walls of the innervated organs. Several **pelvic ganglia** are innervated by sacral preganglionic nerves that are ontogenetically similar to sympathetic preganglionic fibers (see Box: Sympathetic Sacral Outflow). Note that the terms "sympathetic" and "parasympathetic" are anatomic designations and do not depend on the type of transmitter chemical released from the nerve endings nor on the kind of effect—excitatory or inhibitory—evoked by nerve activity.

In addition to these clearly defined peripheral motor portions of the ANS, large numbers of afferent fibers run from the periphery to integrating centers, including the enteric plexuses in the gut, the autonomic ganglia, and the CNS. Many of the sensory pathways that end in the CNS terminate in the hypothalamus and medulla and evoke reflex motor activity that is carried to the effector cells by the efferent fibers described previously. There is increasing evidence that some of these sensory fibers also have peripheral motor functions.

The **enteric nervous system (ENS)** is a large and highly organized collection of neurons located in the walls of the gastrointestinal (GI) system (Figure 6–2). With more than 150 million

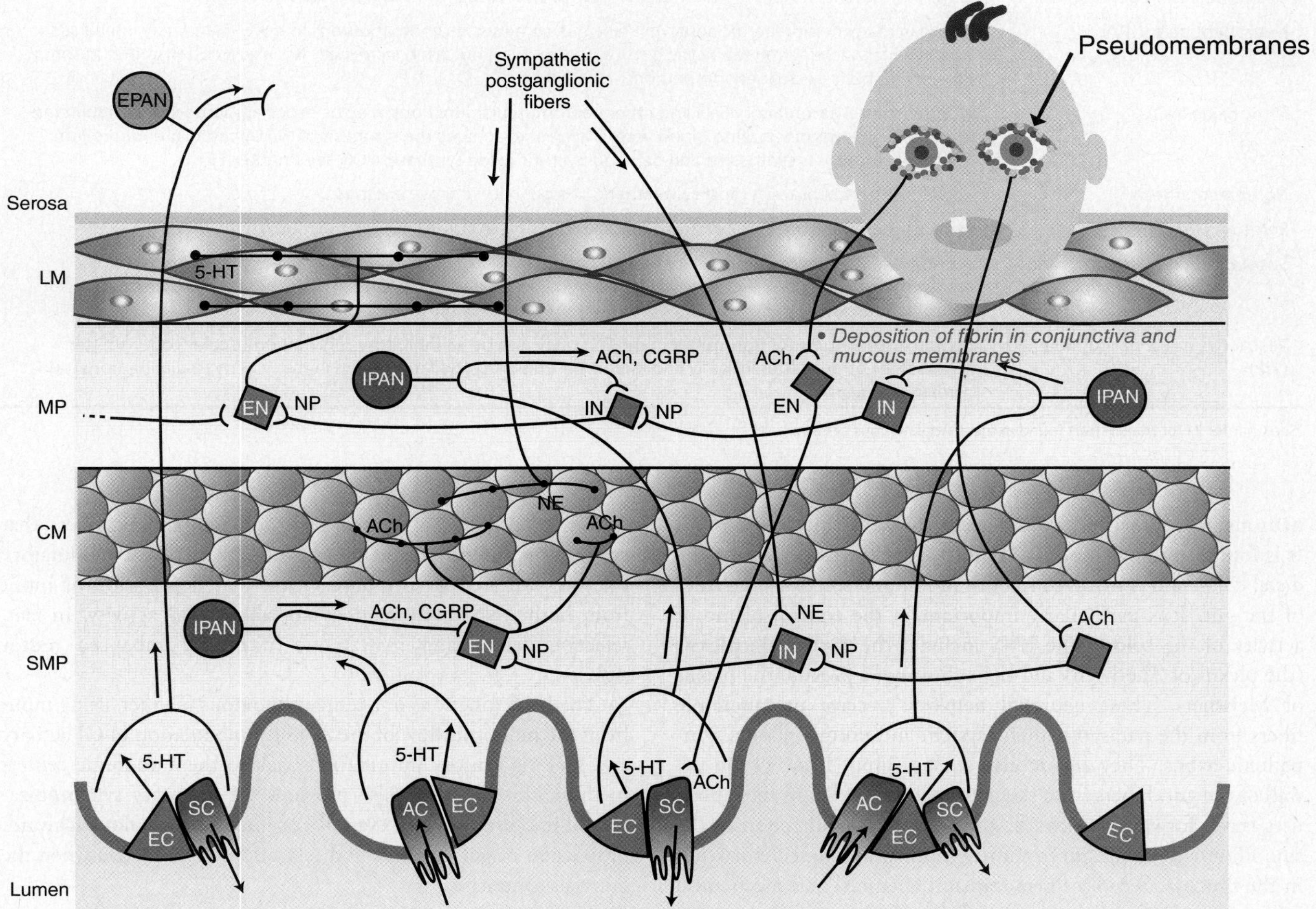

FIGURE 6–2 A highly simplified diagram of the intestinal wall and some of the circuitry of the enteric nervous system (ENS). The ENS receives input from both the sympathetic and the parasympathetic systems and sends afferent impulses to sympathetic ganglia and to the central nervous system. Many transmitter or neuromodulator substances have been identified in the ENS; see Table 6–1. ACh, acetylcholine; AC, absorptive cell; CGRP, calcitonin gene-related peptide; CM, circular muscle layer; EC, enterochromaffin cell; EN, excitatory neuron; EPAN, extrinsic primary afferent neuron; 5-HT, serotonin; IN, inhibitory neuron; IPAN, intrinsic primary afferent neuron; LM, longitudinal muscle layer; MP, myenteric plexus; NE, norepinephrine; NP, neuropeptides; SC, secretory cell; SMP, submucosal plexus. Pseudomembrane is a layer of exudate resembling a membrane, formed on the surface of the skin or of a mucous membrane, especially the conjunctiva of the eye.

TABLE 6–1 Some of the transmitter substances found in autonomic nervous system, enteric nervous system, and nonadrenergic, noncholinergic neurons.[1]

Substance	Functions
Acetylcholine (ACh)	The primary transmitter at ANS ganglia, at the somatic neuromuscular junction, and at parasympathetic postganglionic nerve endings. A primary excitatory transmitter to smooth muscle and secretory cells in the ENS. Probably also the major neuron-to-neuron ("ganglionic") transmitter in the ENS.
Adenosine triphosphate (ATP)	Acts as a transmitter or cotransmitter at many ANS-effector synapses.
Calcitonin gene-related peptide (CGRP)	Found with substance P in cardiovascular sensory nerve fibers. Present in some secretomotor ENS neurons and interneurons. A cardiac stimulant.
Cholecystokinin (CCK)	May act as a cotransmitter in some excitatory neuromuscular ENS neurons.
Dopamine	A modulatory transmitter in some ganglia and the ENS. Possibly a postganglionic sympathetic transmitter in renal blood vessels.
Enkephalin and related opioid peptides	Present in some secretomotor and interneurons in the ENS. Appear to inhibit ACh release and thereby inhibit peristalsis. May *stimulate* secretion.
Galanin	Present in secretomotor neurons; may play a role in appetite-satiety mechanisms.
GABA (γ-aminobutyric acid)	May have presynaptic effects on excitatory ENS nerve terminals. Has some relaxant effect on the gut. Probably not a major transmitter in the ENS.
Gastrin-releasing peptide (GRP)	Extremely potent excitatory transmitter to gastrin cells. Also known as mammalian bombesin.
Neuropeptide Y (NPY)	Found in many noradrenergic neurons. Present in some secretomotor neurons in the ENS and may inhibit secretion of water and electrolytes by the gut. Causes long-lasting vasoconstriction. It is also a cotransmitter in some parasympathetic postganglionic neurons.
Nitric oxide (NO)	A cotransmitter at inhibitory ENS and other neuromuscular junctions; may be especially important at sphincters. Cholinergic nerves innervating blood vessels appear to activate the synthesis of NO by vascular endothelium. NO is not stored, it is synthesized on demand by nitric oxide synthase, NOS; see Chapter 19.
Norepinephrine (NE)	The primary transmitter at most sympathetic postganglionic nerve endings.
Serotonin (5-HT)	An important transmitter or cotransmitter at excitatory neuron-to-neuron junctions in the ENS.
Substance P, related tachykinins	Substance P is an important sensory neurotransmitter in the ENS and elsewhere. Tachykinins appear to be excitatory cotransmitters with ACh at ENS neuromuscular junctions. Found with CGRP in cardiovascular sensory neurons. Substance P is a vasodilator (probably via release of nitric oxide).
Vasoactive intestinal peptide (VIP)	Excitatory secretomotor transmitter in the ENS; may also be an inhibitory ENS neuromuscular cotransmitter. A probable cotransmitter in many cholinergic neurons. A vasodilator (found in many perivascular neurons) and cardiac stimulant.

[1]See Chapter 21 for transmitters found in the central nervous system.

neurons, it is sometimes considered a third division of the ANS. It is found in the wall of the GI tract from the esophagus to the distal colon and is involved in both motor and secretory activities of the gut. It is particularly important in the control of motor activity of the colon. The ENS includes the **myenteric plexus** (the plexus of Auerbach) and the **submucous plexus** (the plexus of Meissner). These neuronal networks receive preganglionic fibers from the parasympathetic system and postganglionic sympathetic axons. They also receive sensory input from within the wall of the gut. Fibers from the neuronal cell bodies in these plexuses travel forward, backward, and in a circular direction to the smooth muscle of the gut to control motility and to secretory cells in the mucosa. Sensory fibers transmit chemical and mechanical information from the mucosa and from stretch receptors to motor neurons in the plexuses and to postganglionic neurons in the sympathetic ganglia. For example, enteroendocrine epithelial cells in the mucosal layer synapse with vagal and other sensory fibers to send information regarding gut content chemicals to the CNS. This signaling appears to utilize glutamate for rapid transmission and peptides such as cholecystokinin for slower, longer-lasting transmission. The parasympathetic and sympathetic fibers that synapse on enteric plexus neurons appear to play a modulatory role, as indicated by the observation that deprivation of input from both ANS divisions does not abolish GI activity. In fact, selective denervation may result in greatly enhanced motor activity.

The ENS functions in a semiautonomous manner, using input from the motor outflow of the ANS for modulation of GI activity and sending sensory information back to the autonomic centers in the CNS. The ENS also provides the necessary synchronization of impulses that, for example, ensures forward, not backward, propulsion of gut contents and relaxation of sphincters when the gut wall contracts.

The anatomy of autonomic synapses and junctions determines the localization of transmitter effects around nerve endings. Classic synapses such as the mammalian neuromuscular junction and most neuron-neuron synapses are relatively "tight" in that the nerve terminates in small boutons very close to the tissue innervated, so that the diffusion path from nerve terminal to postsynaptic receptors is very short. The effects are thus relatively rapid and localized.

In contrast, junctions between autonomic neuron terminals and effector cells (smooth muscle, cardiac muscle, glands) differ from classic synapses in that transmitter is often released from a chain of varicosities in the postganglionic nerve fiber in the region of the smooth muscle cells rather than from boutons, and autonomic junctional clefts are wider than somatic synaptic clefts. Effects are thus slower in onset, and discharge of a single motor fiber often activates or inhibits many effector cells.

Sympathetic Sacral Outflow

As noted in the previous editions of this book and other standard texts, it has long been believed that, like the cranial nerve cholinergic system described earlier, the cholinergic nerves that innervate the pelvic organs (rectum, bladder, and reproductive organs) are part of the parasympathetic nervous system. However, recent evidence (see Espinoza-Medina reference at the end of this chapter) suggests that the cholinergic preganglionic sacral fibers are actually derived from embryonic *sympathetic* precursor cells and that the postganglionic fibers innervated by them are therefore members of the *sympathetic cholinergic* class. This claim is based on several lines of evidence, as follows: (1) Cranial parasympathetic preganglionic neurons express the homeogene *Phox2b* and the transcription factors Tbx20, Tbx2, and Tbx3; thoracic sympathetic and sacral preganglionic neurons do not. Sacral preganglionic neurons do express transcription factor Foxp1, which is not expressed by cranial neurons. (2) Cranial parasympathetic preganglionic fibers exit the CNS via dorsolateral exit points; the sympathetic and sacral preganglionic nerves exit the spinal cord via ventral root exits. (3) At an early stage of development, cranial preganglionic neurons express the vesicular acetylcholine transporter (VAChT; VAT in Figure 6–3) but not nitric oxide synthase (NOS); sympathetic and sacral nerves at the same stage express NOS but not VAChT (even though they do express VAChT later in their development). These observations require independent confirmation but constitute strong evidence in favor of changing the traditional "craniosacral" synonym for the parasympathetic nervous system to "cranial autonomic" nervous system.

NEUROTRANSMITTER CHEMISTRY OF THE AUTONOMIC NERVOUS SYSTEM

An important traditional classification of autonomic nerves is based on the primary transmitter molecules—**acetylcholine** or **norepinephrine**—released from their terminals and varicosities. A large number of peripheral ANS fibers synthesize and release acetylcholine; they are **cholinergic** fibers; that is, they work by synthesizing and releasing acetylcholine. As shown in Figure 6–1, these include all preganglionic efferent autonomic fibers and the somatic (nonautonomic) motor fibers to skeletal muscle as well. Thus, almost all efferent fibers leaving the CNS are cholinergic. In addition, most parasympathetic postganglionic and some sympathetic postganglionic fibers are cholinergic. A significant number of parasympathetic postganglionic neurons use nitric oxide or peptides as the primary transmitter or as cotransmitters with acetylcholine.

Most postganglionic sympathetic fibers (see Figure 6–1) release norepinephrine (also known as noradrenaline); they are **noradrenergic** (often called simply "adrenergic") fibers; that is, they work by releasing norepinephrine (noradrenaline). As noted, some sympathetic fibers release acetylcholine (eg, sweat gland innervation). Dopamine is a very important transmitter in the CNS, and it may be released by some peripheral sympathetic fibers under certain circumstances. Adrenal medullary cells, which are embryologically analogous to postganglionic sympathetic neurons, receive input from preganglionic sympathetic nerves and release a mixture of epinephrine and norepinephrine into the circulation. Finally, most autonomic nerves also release several **cotransmitter** substances (described in the following text), in addition to the primary transmitters just described.

Five key features of neurotransmitter function provide potential targets for pharmacologic therapy: **synthesis, storage, release, termination of action** of the transmitter, and **receptor effects.** These processes are discussed next.

Cholinergic Transmission

The terminals and varicosities of cholinergic neurons contain large numbers of small membrane-bound vesicles concentrated near the portion of the cell membrane facing the synapse (see Figure 6–3) as well as a smaller number of large dense-cored vesicles located farther from the synaptic membrane. The large vesicles contain a high concentration of peptide cotransmitters (Table 6–1), whereas the smaller clear vesicles contain most of the acetylcholine. Vesicles may be synthesized in the neuron cell body and carried to the terminal by axonal transport. They may also be recycled several times within the terminal after each exocytotic release of transmitter. Ultrafast neuronal firing appears to be supported by rapid recycling of clathrin-coated vesicles from endosomes in the nerve terminal. Vesicles are provided with **vesicle-associated membrane proteins (VAMPs),** which serve to align them with release sites on the inner neuronal cell membrane and participate in triggering the release of transmitter. The release site on the inner surface of the nerve terminal membrane contains **synaptosomal nerve-associated proteins (SNAPs)**, which interact with VAMPs. VAMPs and SNAPs are collectively called **fusion proteins.**

Acetylcholine (ACh) is synthesized in the cytoplasm from acetyl-CoA and choline through the catalytic action of the enzyme **choline acetyltransferase (ChAT).** Acetyl-CoA is synthesized in mitochondria, which are present in large numbers in the nerve ending. Choline is transported from the extracellular fluid into the neuron terminal by a sodium-dependent membrane **choline transporter** (**CHT**; see Figure 6–3). This symporter can be blocked by a group of research drugs called **hemicholiniums.**

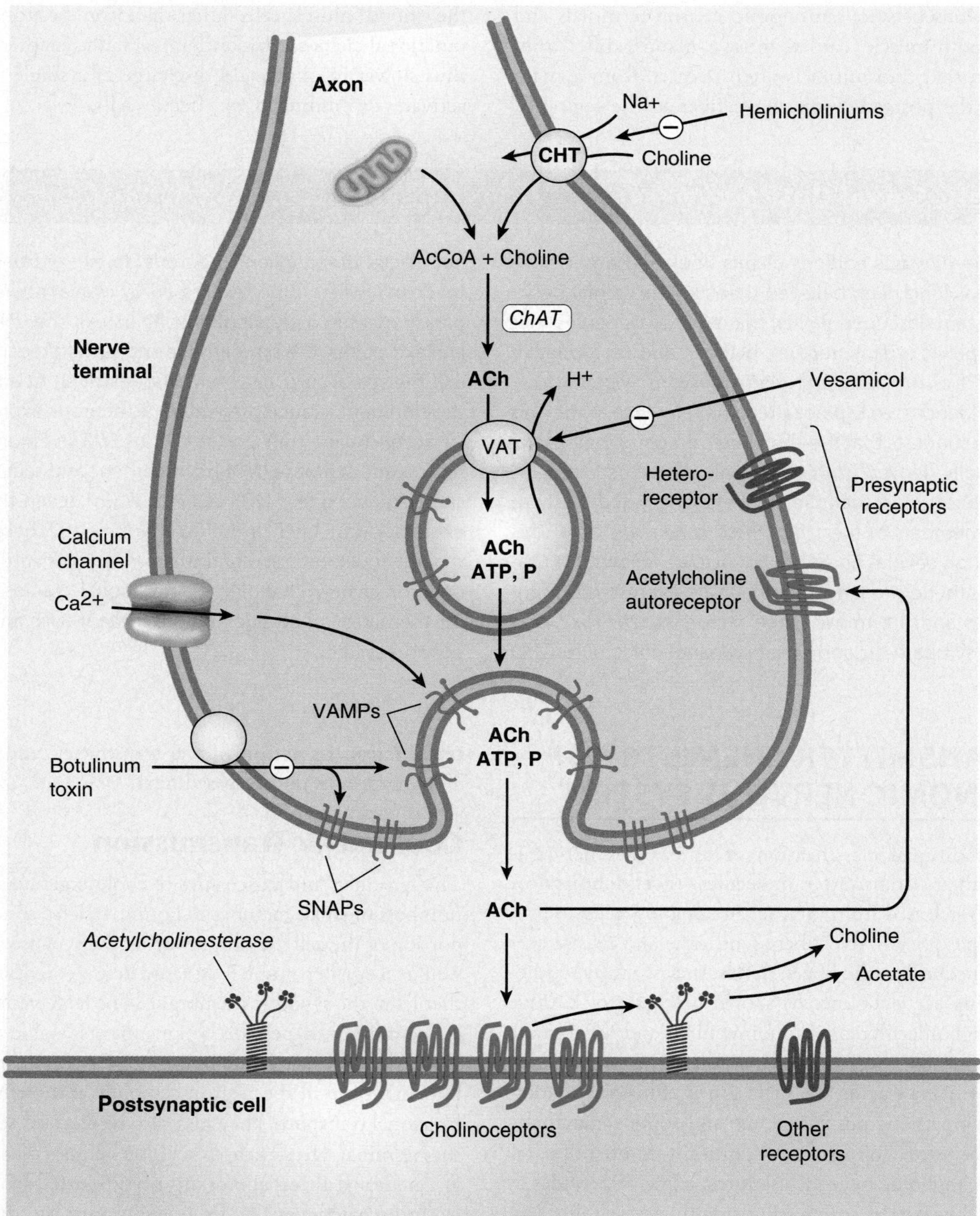

FIGURE 6–3 Schematic illustration of a generalized cholinergic junction (not to scale). Choline is transported into the presynaptic nerve terminal by a sodium-dependent choline transporter (CHT). This transporter can be inhibited by hemicholinium drugs. In the cytoplasm, acetylcholine is synthesized from choline and acetyl-CoA (AcCoA) by the enzyme choline acetyltransferase (ChAT). Acetylcholine (ACh) is then transported into the storage vesicle by a vesicle-associated transporter (VAT), which can be inhibited by vesamicol. Peptides (P), adenosine triphosphate (ATP), and proteoglycan are also stored in the vesicle. Release of transmitters occurs when voltage-sensitive calcium channels in the terminal membrane are opened, allowing an influx of calcium. The resulting increase in intracellular calcium causes fusion of vesicles with the surface membrane and exocytotic expulsion of acetylcholine and cotransmitters into the junctional cleft (see text). This step can be blocked by botulinum toxin. Acetylcholine's action is terminated by metabolism by the enzyme acetylcholinesterase. Receptors on the presynaptic nerve ending modulate transmitter release. SNAPs, synaptosomal nerve-associated proteins; VAMPs, vesicle-associated membrane proteins.

Once synthesized, acetylcholine is transported from the cytoplasm into the vesicles by a **vesicle-associated transporter (VAT)** that is driven by proton efflux (see Figure 6–3). This antiporter can be blocked by the research drug **vesamicol.** Acetylcholine synthesis is a rapid process capable of supporting a very high rate of transmitter release. Storage of acetylcholine is accomplished by the packaging of "quanta" of acetylcholine molecules (usually 1000–50,000 molecules in each vesicle). Most of the vesicular acetylcholine (a positively charged quaternary amine) is bound to negatively charged **vesicular proteoglycan (VPG).** (ACh is also synthesized in lymphocytes and may play a role in immunologic reactions to viral infection.)

Vesicles are concentrated on the inner surface of the nerve terminal facing the synapse through the interaction of so-called SNARE proteins on the vesicle (a subgroup of VAMPs called v-SNAREs, especially **synaptobrevin**) and on the inside of the terminal cell membrane (SNAPs called t-SNAREs, especially **syntaxin** and **SNAP-25**). Physiologic release of transmitter from the vesicles is dependent on extracellular calcium and occurs when an action potential reaches the terminal and triggers sufficient influx of calcium ions via N-type calcium channels. Calcium interacts with the VAMP **synaptotagmin** on the vesicle membrane and triggers fusion of the vesicle membrane with the terminal membrane and opening of a pore into the synapse. The opening of the pore and inrush of cations results in release of the acetylcholine from the proteoglycan and exocytotic expulsion into the synaptic cleft. One depolarization of a somatic motor nerve may release several hundred quanta into the synaptic cleft. One depolarization of an autonomic postganglionic nerve varicosity or terminal probably releases less and releases it over a larger area. In addition to acetylcholine, several cotransmitters are released at the same time (see Table 6–1). The acetylcholine vesicle release process is blocked by **botulinum toxin (BoNT)** through the enzymatic cleavage of two amino acids from one or more of the fusion proteins, resulting in muscle paralysis. (**Tetanus toxin [tetanospasmin, TeNT]** blocks transmitter release by a similar cleavage of fusion proteins, but it does so mainly in inhibitory neurons of the spinal cord, thus resulting in spasm, rather than paralysis, of skeletal muscle.)

After release from the presynaptic terminal, acetylcholine molecules may bind to and activate an acetylcholine receptor **(cholinoceptor).** Eventually (and usually very rapidly), all of the acetylcholine released diffuses within range of an **acetylcholinesterase (AChE)** molecule. AChE very efficiently splits acetylcholine into choline and acetate, neither of which has significant transmitter effect, and thereby terminates the action of the transmitter (see Figure 6–3). Most cholinergic synapses are richly supplied with acetylcholinesterase; the half-life of acetylcholine molecules in the synapse is therefore very short (a fraction of a second). Acetylcholinesterase is also found in other tissues, eg, red blood cells. (Other cholinesterases with a lower specificity for acetylcholine, including butyrylcholinesterase [pseudocholinesterase], are found in blood plasma, liver, glia, and many other tissues.)

Neurotransmitter Uptake Carriers

As noted in Chapters 1, 4, and 5, several large families of transport proteins have been identified. The most important of these are the ABC (ATP-binding cassette) and SLC (solute carrier) transporter families. As indicated by the name, the ABC carriers use ATP for transport. The SLC proteins are cotransporters and, in most cases, use the movement of sodium down its concentration gradient as the energy source. Under some circumstances, they also transport transmitters in the reverse direction in a sodium-independent fashion.

NET, SLC6A2, the norepinephrine transporter, is a member of the SLC family, as are similar transporters responsible for the reuptake of dopamine (**DAT,** SLC6A3) and 5-HT (serotonin, **SERT,** SLC6A4) into the neurons that release these transmitters. These transport proteins are found in peripheral tissues and in the CNS wherever neurons using these transmitters are located.

NET is important in the peripheral actions of cocaine and the amphetamines. In the CNS, NET, SERT, and DAT are important targets of several antidepressant drug classes (see Chapter 30) as well as cocaine and amphetamine use. The most important inhibitory transmitter in the CNS, γ-aminobutyric acid (GABA), is the substrate for at least three SLC transporters: GAT1, GAT2, and GAT3. GAT1 is the target of an antiseizure medication (see Chapter 24). The major excitatory CNS transmitter glutamate utilizes the excitatory amino acid transporter (EAAT) family, which are also SLC protein transporters.

Adrenergic Transmission

Adrenergic neurons (Figure 6–4) transport the precursor amino acid tyrosine into the nerve ending, convert it to dopa, and then synthesize a catecholamine transmitter (dopamine, norepinephrine, or epinephrine; Figure 6–5), and store it in membrane-bound vesicles. In most sympathetic postganglionic neurons, norepinephrine is the final product. In the adrenal medulla and certain areas of the brain, some norepinephrine is further converted to epinephrine. In dopaminergic neurons, synthesis terminates with dopamine. Several processes in these nerve terminals are potential sites of drug action. One of these, the conversion of tyrosine to dopa by tyrosine hydroxylase, is the rate-limiting step in catecholamine transmitter synthesis. It can be inhibited by the tyrosine analog **metyrosine.** A high-affinity antiporter for catecholamines located in the wall of the storage vesicle **(vesicular monoamine transporter, VMAT)** can be inhibited by the **reserpine** alkaloids. Reserpine and related drugs (tetrabenazine, deutetrabenazine) cause depletion of transmitter stores. Another transporter **(norepinephrine transporter, NET)** carries norepinephrine and similar molecules back into the cell cytoplasm from the synaptic cleft (see Figure 6–4; NET). NET is also commonly called uptake 1 or reuptake 1 and is partially responsible for the termination of synaptic activity. NET can be inhibited by **cocaine, solriamfetol,** and certain **antidepressant** drugs, resulting in an increase of transmitter activity in the synaptic cleft (see Box: Neurotransmitter Uptake Carriers).

Release of the vesicular transmitter store from noradrenergic nerve endings is similar to the calcium-dependent process previously described for cholinergic terminals. In addition to the primary transmitter (norepinephrine), adenosine triphosphate (ATP), dopamine-β-hydroxylase, and peptide cotransmitters are simultaneously released from the same vesicles. Indirectly acting and mixed-action sympathomimetics, eg, **tyramine,**

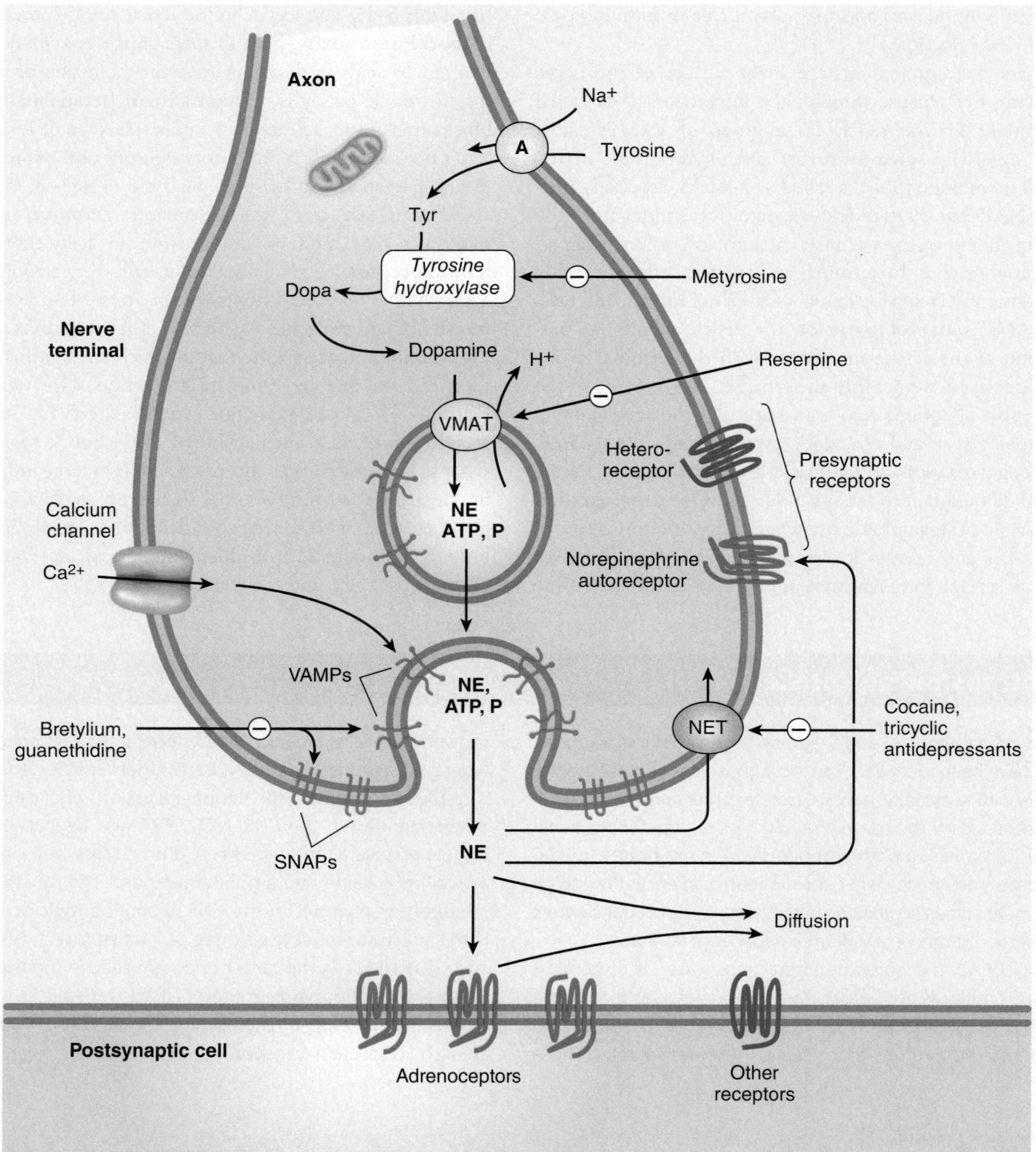

FIGURE 6–4 Schematic diagram of a generalized noradrenergic junction (not to scale). Tyrosine is transported into the noradrenergic nerve ending or varicosity by a sodium-dependent carrier (A). Tyrosine is converted to dopamine (see Figure 6–5 for details), and transported into the vesicle by the vesicular monoamine transporter (VMAT), which can be blocked by reserpine and tetrabenazine. The same carrier transports norepinephrine (NE) and several related amines into these vesicles. Dopamine is converted to NE in the vesicle by dopamine-β-hydroxylase. Physiologic release of transmitter occurs when an action potential opens voltage-sensitive calcium channels and increases intracellular calcium. Fusion of vesicles with the surface membrane results in expulsion of norepinephrine, cotransmitters, and dopamine-β-hydroxylase. Release can be blocked by drugs such as guanethidine and bretylium. After release, norepinephrine diffuses out of the cleft or is transported into the cytoplasm of the terminal by the norepinephrine transporter (NET), which can be blocked by cocaine and certain antidepressants, or into postjunctional or perijunctional cells. Regulatory receptors are present on the presynaptic terminal. SNAPs, synaptosome-associated proteins; VAMPs, vesicle-associated membrane proteins.

amphetamines, and **ephedrine,** are capable of releasing stored transmitter from noradrenergic nerve endings by a calcium-independent process. These drugs are poor agonists (some are inactive) at adrenoceptors, but they are excellent substrates for monoamine transporters. As a result, they are avidly taken up into noradrenergic nerve endings by NET. In the nerve ending, they are then transported by VMAT into the vesicles, displacing norepinephrine, which is subsequently expelled into the synaptic

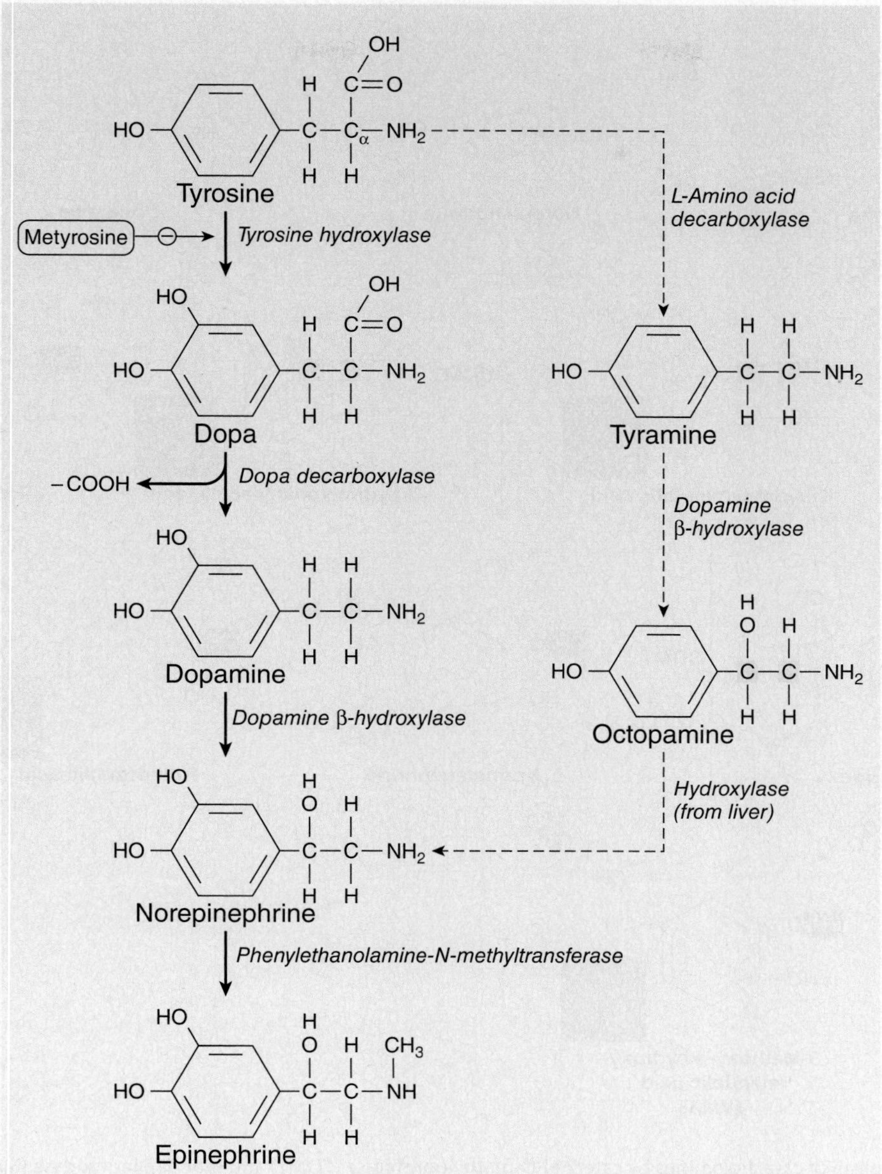

Tyrosine

Metyrosine

Tyrosine hydroxylase

L-Amino acid decarboxylase

Dopa

Tyramine

−COOH

Dopa decarboxylase

Dopamine β-hydroxylase

Dopamine

Octopamine

Dopamine β-hydroxylase

Hydroxylase (from liver)

Norepinephrine

Phenylethanolamine-N-methyltransferase

Epinephrine

FIGURE 6–5 Biosynthesis of catecholamines. The rate-limiting step, conversion of tyrosine to dopa, can be inhibited by metyrosine (α-methyltyrosine). The alternative pathway shown by the dashed arrows has not been found to be of physiologic significance in humans. However, tyramine and octopamine may accumulate in patients treated with monoamine oxidase inhibitors. (Reproduced with permission from Gardner DG, Shoback D: *Greenspan's Basic & Clinical Endocrinology*, 9th ed. New York, NY: McGraw Hill; 2011.)

space by reverse transport via NET. Amphetamines also inhibit monoamine oxidase and have other effects that result in increased norepinephrine activity in the synapse. Their action does not require vesicle exocytosis.

Norepinephrine and epinephrine can be metabolized by several enzymes, as shown in Figure 6–6. Because of the high activity of monoamine oxidase in the mitochondria of the nerve terminal, there is significant turnover of norepinephrine even in the resting terminal. Since the metabolic products are excreted in the urine, an estimate of catecholamine turnover can be obtained from measurement of total metabolites (sometimes referred to as "VMA and metanephrines") in a 24-hour urine sample. However, metabolism is not the primary mechanism for termination of action of norepinephrine physiologically released from noradrenergic nerves. Termination of noradrenergic transmission results from two processes: simple diffusion away from the receptor site (with eventual metabolism in the plasma or liver) and reuptake into the nerve terminal by NET (see Figure 6–4) or into perisynaptic glia or other cells.

Cotransmitters in Cholinergic & Adrenergic Nerves

As previously noted, the vesicles of both cholinergic and adrenergic nerves contain other substances in addition to the primary

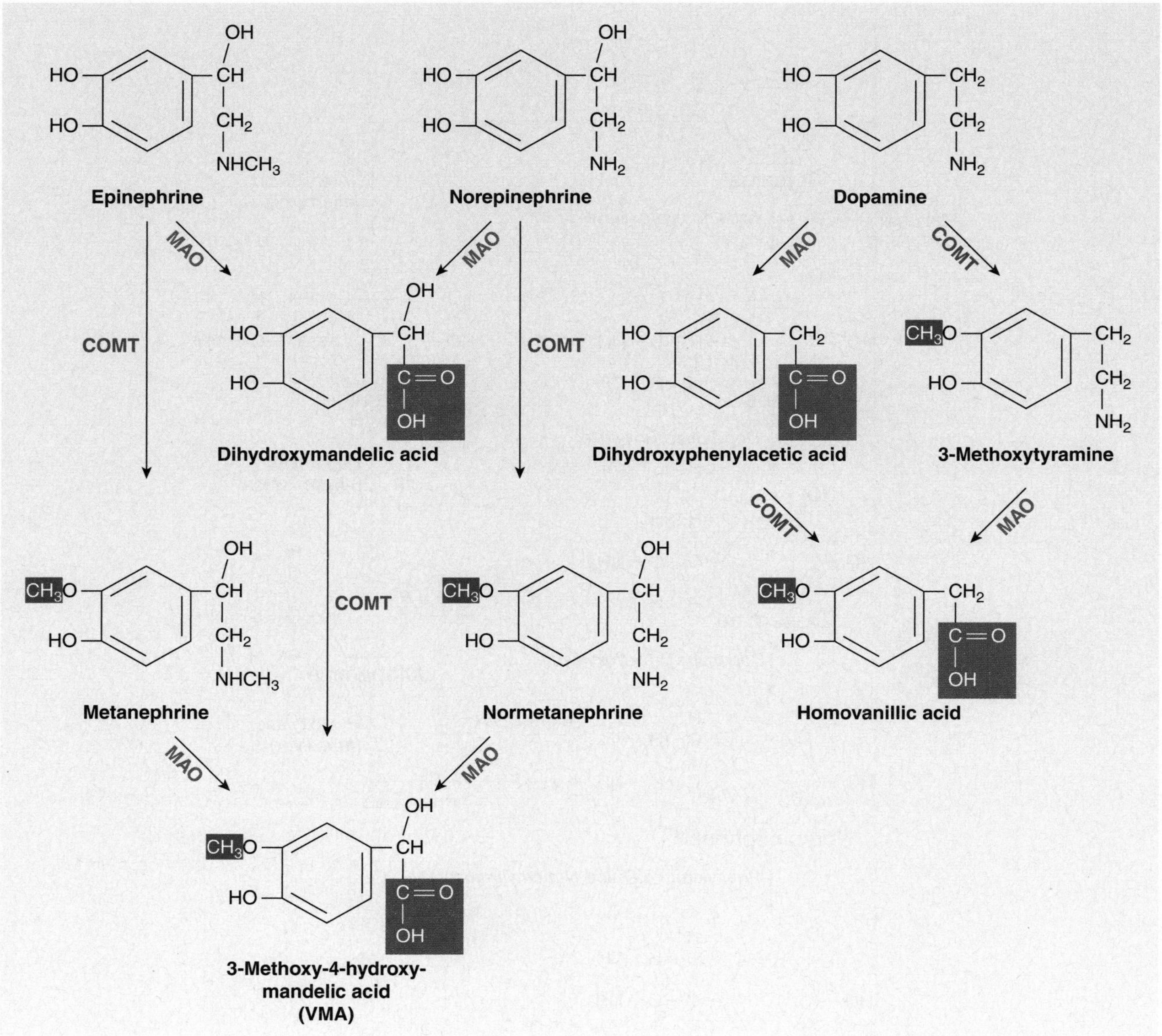

FIGURE 6–6 Metabolism of catecholamines by catechol-*O*-methyltransferase (COMT) and monoamine oxidase (MAO). (Reproduced with permission from Gardner DG, Shoback D: *Greenspan's Basic & Clinical Endocrinology*, 9th ed. New York, NY: McGraw Hill; 2011.)

transmitter, sometimes in the same vesicles and sometimes in a separate vesicle population. Some of the substances identified to date are listed in Table 6–1. Many of these substances are also *primary* transmitters in the nonadrenergic, noncholinergic nerves described in the text that follows. They appear to play several roles in the function of nerves that release acetylcholine or norepinephrine. In some cases, they provide a faster or slower action to supplement or modulate the effects of the primary transmitter. They also participate in feedback inhibition of the same and nearby nerve terminals.

Growth of neurons and transmitter expression in specific neurons is a dynamic process. For example, neurotrophic factors released from target tissues influence growth and synapse formation by neurons. In addition, the transmitters released from a specific population of neurons can change in response to environmental factors such as the light-dark cycle.

AUTONOMIC RECEPTORS

Historically, structure-activity analyses, with careful comparisons of the potency of series of autonomic agonist and antagonist analogs, led to the definition of different autonomic receptor subtypes, including muscarinic and nicotinic cholinoceptors, α, and β adrenoceptors, and dopamine receptors (Table 6–2). Subsequently, binding of isotope-labeled ligands permitted the purification and characterization of several of the receptor molecules. Molecular biology now provides techniques for the discovery and expression of genes that code for related receptors within these groups (see Chapter 2).

The primary acetylcholine receptor subtypes were named after the alkaloids originally used in their identification: muscarine and nicotine, thus **muscarinic** and **nicotinic receptors.** In the case of

TABLE 6–2 Major autonomic receptor types.

Receptor Name	Typical Locations	Result of Ligand Binding
Cholinoceptors		
Muscarinic M_1	CNS neurons, sympathetic postganglionic neurons, some presynaptic sites	Formation of IP_3 and DAG, increased intracellular calcium
Muscarinic M_2	Myocardium, smooth muscle, some presynaptic sites; CNS neurons	Opening of potassium channels, inhibition of adenylyl cyclase
Muscarinic M_3	Exocrine glands, vessels (smooth muscle and endothelium); CNS neurons	Like M_1 receptor-ligand binding
Muscarinic M_4	CNS neurons; possibly vagal nerve endings	Like M_2 receptor-ligand binding
Muscarinic M_5	Vascular endothelium, especially cerebral vessels; CNS neurons	Like M_1 receptor-ligand binding
Nicotinic N_N	Postganglionic neurons, some presynaptic cholinergic terminals; pentameric receptors typically contain α- and β-type subunits only (see Chapter 7)	Opening of Na^+, K^+ channels, depolarization
Nicotinic N_M	Skeletal muscle neuromuscular end plates; pentameric receptors typically contain two α_1- and β_1-type subunits in addition to γ and δ subunits	Opening of Na^+, K^+ channels, depolarization
Adrenoceptors		
$Alpha_1$	Postsynaptic effector cells, especially smooth muscle	Formation of IP_3 and DAG, increased intracellular calcium
$Alpha_2$	Presynaptic adrenergic nerve terminals, platelets, lipocytes, smooth muscle	Inhibition of adenylyl cyclase, decreased cAMP
$Beta_1$	Postsynaptic effector cells, especially heart, lipocytes, brain; presynaptic adrenergic and cholinergic nerve terminals, juxtaglomerular apparatus of renal tubules, ciliary body epithelium	Stimulation of adenylyl cyclase, increased cAMP
$Beta_2$	Postsynaptic effector cells, especially smooth muscle and cardiac muscle	Stimulation of adenylyl cyclase and increased cAMP. Activates cardiac G_i under some conditions.
$Beta_3$	Postsynaptic effector cells, especially lipocytes; heart	Stimulation of adenylyl cyclase and increased cAMP[1]
Dopamine receptors		
D_1 (DA_1), D_5	Brain; effector tissues, especially smooth muscle of the renal vascular bed	Stimulation of adenylyl cyclase and increased cAMP
D_2 (DA_2)	Brain; effector tissues, especially smooth muscle; presynaptic nerve terminals	Inhibition of adenylyl cyclase; increased potassium conductance
D_3	Brain	Inhibition of adenylyl cyclase
D_4	Brain, cardiovascular system	Inhibition of adenylyl cyclase

[1]Cardiac β_3-receptor function is poorly understood, but activation does *not* appear to result in stimulation of rate or force.

receptors associated with noradrenergic nerves, the use of the names of the agonists (noradrenaline, phenylephrine, isoproterenol, and others) was not practicable. Therefore, the term **adrenoceptor** is widely used to describe receptors that respond to catecholamines such as norepinephrine. By analogy, the term **cholinoceptor** denotes receptors (both muscarinic and nicotinic) that respond to acetylcholine. In North America, receptors were colloquially named after the nerves that usually innervate them; thus, **adrenergic** (or noradrenergic) **receptors** and **cholinergic receptors.** The general class of adrenoceptors can be further subdivided into **α-adrenoceptor, β-adrenoceptor,** and less thought of as an adrenoceptor, the **dopamine-receptor** types on the basis of both agonist and antagonist selectivity and on genomic grounds. Development of more selective blocking drugs has led to the naming of subclasses within these major types; for example, within the α-adrenoceptor class, α_1 and α_2 receptors differ in both agonist and antagonist selectivity. Examples of such selective drugs are given in the chapters that follow.

NONADRENERGIC, NONCHOLINERGIC (NANC) NEURONS

It has been known for many years that autonomic effector tissues (eg, gut, airways, bladder) contain nerve fibers that do not show the histochemical characteristics of either cholinergic or adrenergic fibers. Both motor and sensory NANC fibers are present in these tissues. Although peptides are the most common transmitter substances found in these nerve endings, other substances, eg, nitric oxide synthase and purines, are also present in many nerve terminals (see Table 6–1). Capsaicin, a toxin derived from chili peppers, can cause the release of transmitter (especially substance P) from such neurons and, if given in high doses, destruction of the neuron.

The enteric system in the gut wall (see Figure 6–2) is the most extensively studied system containing NANC neurons in addition to cholinergic and adrenergic fibers. In the small intestine, for example, these neurons contain one or more of the following: nitric oxide synthase (which produces nitric oxide, NO), calcitonin gene-related peptide, cholecystokinin, dynorphin, enkephalins, gastrin-releasing peptide, 5-hydroxytryptamine (5-HT, serotonin), neuropeptide Y, somatostatin, substance P, and vasoactive intestinal peptide (VIP). Some neurons contain as many as five different transmitters.

The sensory fibers in the nonadrenergic, noncholinergic systems are probably better termed "sensory-efferent" or "sensory-local effector" fibers because, when activated by a sensory input, they are capable of releasing transmitter peptides from the sensory ending itself, from local axon branches, and from collaterals that terminate in the autonomic ganglia. These peptides are potent agonists in many autonomic effector tissues.

FUNCTIONAL ORGANIZATION OF AUTONOMIC ACTIVITY

Autonomic function is integrated and regulated at many levels, from the CNS to the effector cells. Most regulation uses negative feedback, but several other mechanisms have been identified. Negative feedback is particularly important in the responses of the ANS to the administration of autonomic drugs.

Central Integration

At the highest level—midbrain and medulla—the two divisions of the ANS and the endocrine system are integrated with each other, with sensory input, and with information from higher CNS centers, including the cerebral cortex. These interactions are such that early investigators called the parasympathetic system a **trophotropic** one (ie, leading to growth) used to "rest and digest" and the sympathetic system an **ergotropic** one (ie, leading to energy expenditure), which is activated for "fight or flight." Although such terms offer little insight into the mechanisms involved, they do provide simple descriptions applicable to many of the actions of the systems (Table 6–3). For example, slowing of the heart and stimulation of digestive activity are typical energy-conserving and energy-storing actions of the parasympathetic system. In contrast, cardiac stimulation, increased blood sugar, and cutaneous vasoconstriction are responses produced by sympathetic discharge that are suited to fighting or surviving attack.

At a more subtle level of interactions in the brain stem, medulla, and spinal cord, there are important cooperative interactions between the parasympathetic and sympathetic systems. For some organs, sensory fibers associated with the parasympathetic system exert reflex control over motor outflow in the sympathetic system. Thus, the sensory carotid sinus baroreceptor fibers in the glossopharyngeal nerve have a major influence on sympathetic outflow from the vasomotor center. This example is described in greater detail in the following text. Similarly, parasympathetic sensory fibers in the wall of the urinary bladder significantly influence sympathetic inhibitory outflow to that organ. Within the ENS, sensory fibers from the wall of the gut synapse on both preganglionic and postganglionic motor neurons that control intestinal smooth muscle and secretory cells (see Figure 6–2).

A. Integration of Cardiovascular Function

Autonomic reflexes are particularly important in understanding cardiovascular responses to autonomic drugs. As indicated in Figure 6–7, the primary controlled variable in cardiovascular function is **mean arterial pressure.** In the absence of autonomic control, heart rate takes on an intrinsic value somewhat higher than normal resting rate—that is, resting heart rate in a transplanted human heart is 110–130 beats/min. This suggests that in the intact resting human, heart rate is dominated by parasympathetic tone, lowering the heart rate to the range of 70–80 beats/min. Changes in any variable contributing to mean arterial pressure (eg, a drug-induced increase in peripheral vascular resistance) evoke powerful **homeostatic** secondary responses that tend to compensate for the directly evoked change. The homeostatic response may be sufficient to reduce the change in mean arterial pressure and to reverse the drug's effects on heart rate. A slow infusion of norepinephrine provides a useful example. This agent produces direct effects on both vascular and cardiac muscle. It is a powerful vasoconstrictor and, by increasing peripheral vascular resistance, increases mean arterial pressure. In the absence of reflex control—in a patient who has had a heart transplant, for example—the drug's effect on the heart is also stimulatory; that is, it increases heart rate and contractile force. However, in a subject with intact reflexes, the negative feedback response to increased mean arterial pressure causes decreased sympathetic outflow to the heart and a powerful increase in parasympathetic (vagus nerve) discharge at the cardiac pacemaker (sinoatrial [SA] node). This response is mediated by increased firing by the baroreceptor nerves of the carotid sinus and the aortic arch. Increased baroreceptor activity causes the decreased central sympathetic outflow and increased vagal outflow. As a result, the *net* effect of ordinary pressor doses of norepinephrine in a normal subject is to produce a marked increase in peripheral vascular resistance, an increase in mean arterial pressure, and often, a *slowing* of heart rate. Bradycardia, the reflex compensatory response elicited by this agent, is the *exact opposite* of the drug's direct action; yet it is completely predictable if the integration of cardiovascular function by the ANS is understood.

B. Presynaptic Regulation

The principle of negative feedback control is also found at the presynaptic level of autonomic function. Important presynaptic feedback inhibitory control mechanisms have been shown to exist at most nerve endings. A well-documented mechanism involves the α_2 receptor located on noradrenergic nerve terminals. This receptor is activated by norepinephrine and similar molecules; activation diminishes further release of norepinephrine from these nerve endings (Table 6–4). The mechanism of this G protein–mediated effect involves inhibition of the inward calcium current that causes vesicular fusion and transmitter release. Conversely, a presynaptic β receptor appears to facilitate the release of norepinephrine from some adrenergic neurons. Presynaptic receptors that respond to the primary transmitter substance released by the nerve ending are called **autoreceptors.** Autoreceptors are usually inhibitory, but in addition to the excitatory β receptors on noradrenergic fibers, many cholinergic fibers, especially somatic motor fibers, have excitatory nicotinic autoreceptors.

TABLE 6–3 Direct effects of autonomic *nerve* activity on some organ systems. Autonomic *drug* effects are similar but not identical (see text).

	Effect of			
	Sympathetic Activity		Parasympathetic Activity	
Organ	*Action*[1]	*Receptor*[2]	*Action*	*Receptor*[2]
Eye				
Iris radial muscle	Contracts	α_1	—	—
Iris circular muscle	—	—	Contracts	M_3
Ciliary muscle	[Relaxes]	β	Contracts	M_3
Heart				
Sinoatrial node	Accelerates	β_1, β_2	Decelerates	M_2
Ectopic pacemakers	Accelerates	β_1, β_2	—	—
Contractility	Increases	β_1, β_2	Decreases (atria)	M_2
Blood vessels				
Skin, splanchnic vessels	Contracts	α	—	—
Skeletal muscle vessels	Relaxes	β_2	—	—
	[Contracts]	α	—	—
	Relaxes[3]	M_3	—	—
Endothelium of vessels in heart, brain, viscera	—	—	Synthesizes and releases EDRF[4]	M_3, M_5[5]
Bronchiolar smooth muscle	Relaxes	β_2	Contracts	M_3
Gastrointestinal tract				
Smooth muscle				
Walls	Relaxes	α_2,[6] β_2	Contracts[7]	M_3
Sphincters	Contracts	α_1	Relaxes	M_3
Secretion	[Decreases]	α_2	Increases	M_3
Genitourinary smooth muscle				
Bladder wall	Relaxes	β_2	Contracts[7]	M_3
Sphincter	Contracts	α_1	Relaxes	M_3
Uterus, pregnant	Relaxes	β_2	—	...
	Contracts	α	Contracts	M_3
Penis, seminal vesicles	Ejaculation	α	Erection	M
Skin				
Pilomotor smooth muscle	Contracts	α	—	—
Sweat glands			—	—
Eccrine	Increases	M	—	—
Apocrine (stress)	Increases	α	—	—
Metabolic functions				
Liver	Gluconeogenesis	β_2, α	—	—
Liver	Glycogenolysis	β_2, α	—	—
Fat cells	Lipolysis	β_3	—	—
Kidney	Renin release	β_1	—	—

[1]Less important actions are shown in brackets.

[2]Specific receptor type: α, alpha; β, beta; M, muscarinic.

[3]Vascular smooth muscle in skeletal muscle has sympathetic cholinergic dilator fibers.

[4]The endothelium of most blood vessels releases EDRF (endothelium-derived relaxing factor), which causes marked vasodilation, in response to muscarinic stimuli. Parasympathetic fibers innervate muscarinic receptors in vessels in the viscera and brain, and sympathetic cholinergic fibers innervate skeletal muscle blood vessels. The muscarinic receptors in the other vessels of the peripheral circulation are not innervated and respond only to circulating muscarinic agonists.

[5]Cerebral blood vessels dilate in response to M_5 receptor activation.

[6]Probably through presynaptic inhibition of parasympathetic activity.

[7]The cholinergic innervation of the rectum and the genitourinary organs may be anatomically sympathetic; see Box: Sympathetic Sacral Outflow.

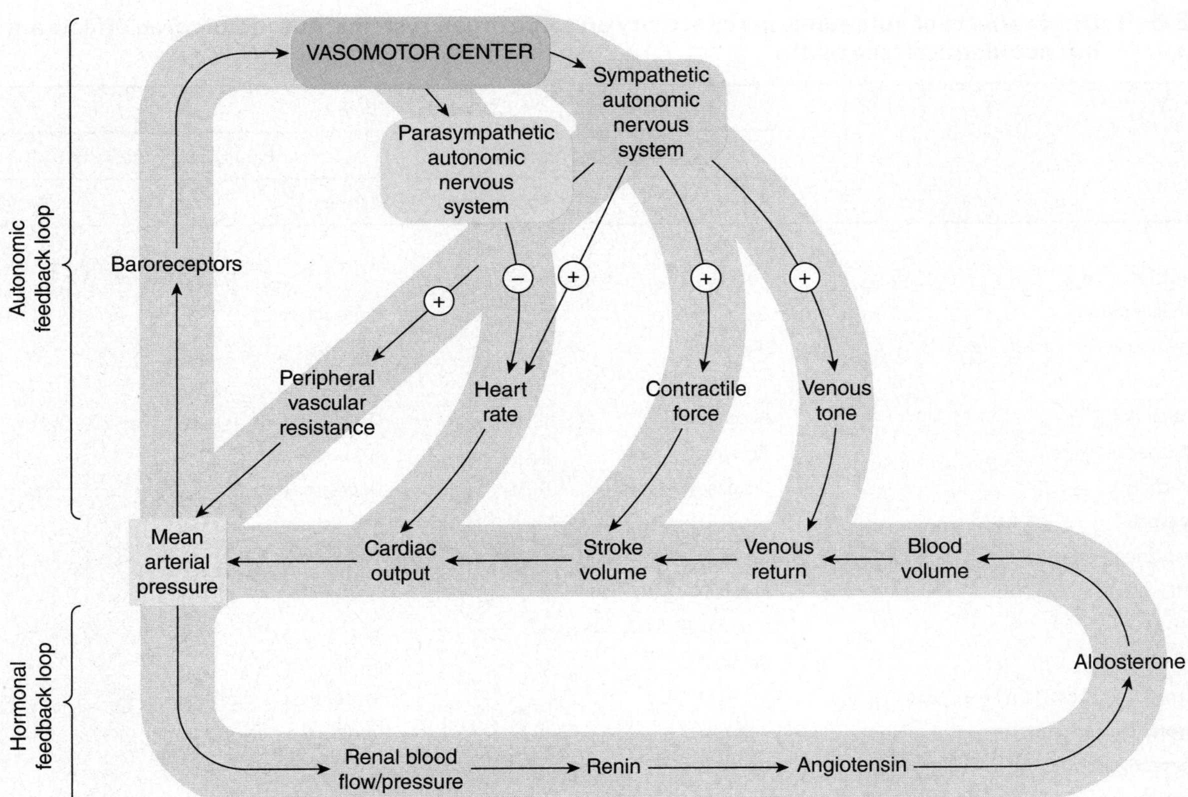

FIGURE 6–7 Autonomic and hormonal control of cardiovascular function. Note that two feedback loops are present: the autonomic nervous system loop and the hormonal loop. The sympathetic nervous system directly influences four major variables: peripheral vascular resistance, heart rate, force, and venous tone. It also directly modulates renin production (not shown). The parasympathetic nervous system directly influences heart rate. In addition to its role in stimulating aldosterone secretion, angiotensin II directly increases peripheral vascular resistance and facilitates sympathetic effects (not shown). The net feedback effect of each loop is to compensate for changes in arterial blood pressure. Thus, decreased blood pressure due to blood loss would evoke increased sympathetic outflow and renin release. Conversely, elevated pressure due to the administration of a vasoconstrictor drug would cause reduced sympathetic outflow, reduced renin release, and increased parasympathetic (vagal) outflow.

TABLE 6–4 Autoreceptor, heteroreceptor, and modulatory effects on nerve terminals in peripheral synapses.[1]

Transmitter/Modulator	Receptor Type	Neuron Terminals Where Found
Inhibitory effects		
Acetylcholine	M_2, M_4	Adrenergic, enteric nervous system
Norepinephrine	$Alpha_2$	Adrenergic
Dopamine	D_2; less evidence for D_1	Adrenergic
Serotonin (5-HT)	$5\text{-}HT_1$, $5\text{-}HT_2$, $5\text{-}HT_3$	Cholinergic preganglionic
ATP, ADP	P2Y	Adrenergic autonomic and ENS cholinergic neurons
Adenosine	A_1	Adrenergic autonomic and ENS cholinergic neurons
Histamine	H_3, possibly H_2	H_3 type identified on CNS adrenergic and serotonergic neurons
Enkephalin	Delta (also mu, kappa)	Adrenergic, ENS cholinergic
Neuropeptide Y	Y_1, Y_2 (NPY)	Adrenergic, some cholinergic
Prostaglandin E_1, E_2	EP_3	Adrenergic
Excitatory effects		
Epinephrine	$Beta_2$	Adrenergic, somatic motor cholinergic
Acetylcholine	N	Somatic motor cholinergic
Angiotensin II	AT_1	Adrenergic

[1]A provisional list. The number of transmitters and locations will undoubtedly increase with additional research.

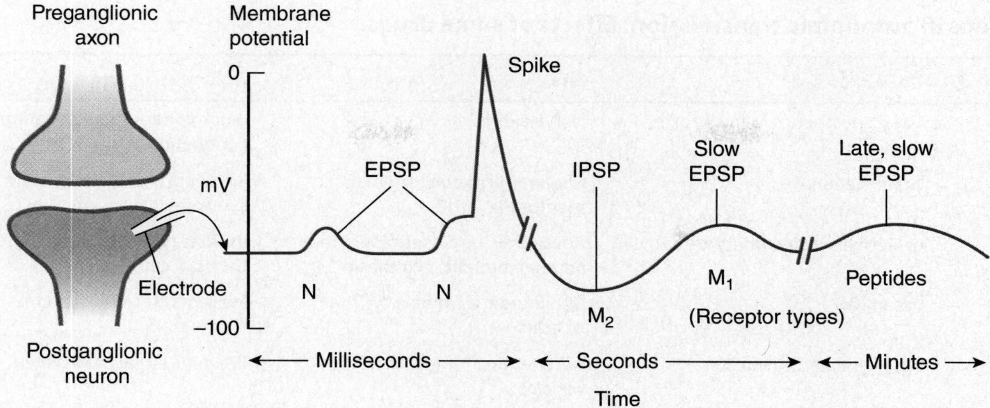

FIGURE 6–8 Excitatory and inhibitory postsynaptic potentials (EPSP and IPSP) in an autonomic ganglion cell. The postganglionic neuron shown at the left with a recording electrode might undergo the membrane potential changes shown schematically in the recording. The response begins with two EPSP responses to nicotinic (N) receptor activation, the first not reaching threshold. The second, suprathreshold, EPSP evokes an action potential, which is followed by an IPSP, probably evoked by M_2 receptor activation (with possible participation from dopamine receptor activation). The IPSP is, in turn, followed by a slower, M_1-dependent EPSP, and this is sometimes followed by a still slower peptide-induced excitatory postsynaptic potential.

Control of transmitter release is not limited to modulation by the transmitter itself. Nerve terminals also carry regulatory receptors that respond to many other substances. Such **heteroreceptors** may be activated by substances released from other nerve terminals that synapse with the nerve ending. For example, some vagal fibers in the myocardium synapse on sympathetic noradrenergic nerve terminals and inhibit norepinephrine release. Alternatively, the ligands for these receptors may diffuse to the receptors from the blood or from nearby tissues. Some of the transmitters and receptors identified to date are listed in Table 6–4. Presynaptic regulation by a variety of endogenous chemicals probably occurs at all synapses.

C. Postsynaptic Regulation

Postsynaptic regulation can be considered from two perspectives: modulation by previous activity at the primary receptor (which may up- or downregulate receptor number or desensitize receptors; see Chapter 2), and modulation by other simultaneous events.

The first mechanism has been well documented in several receptor-effector systems. Up-regulation and down-regulation are known to occur in response to decreased or increased activation, respectively, of the receptors. An extreme form of up-regulation occurs after denervation of some tissues, resulting in **denervation supersensitivity** of the tissue to activators of that receptor type. In skeletal muscle, for example, nicotinic receptors are normally restricted to the end plate regions underlying somatic motor nerve terminals. Surgical or traumatic denervation results in marked proliferation of nicotinic cholinoceptors over all parts of the fiber, including areas not previously associated with any motor nerve junctions. A pharmacologic supersensitivity related to denervation supersensitivity occurs in autonomic effector tissues after administration of drugs that deplete transmitter stores and prevent activation of the postsynaptic receptors for a sufficient period of time. For example, prolonged administration of large doses of reserpine, a norepinephrine depleter that blocks reuptake of norepinephrine into vesicles, can cause increased sensitivity of the smooth muscle and cardiac muscle effector cells served by the depleted sympathetic fibers.

The second mechanism involves modulation of the primary transmitter-receptor event by actions evoked by the same or other transmitters acting on different postsynaptic receptors. Ganglionic transmission is a good example of this phenomenon (Figure 6–8). The postganglionic cells are activated (depolarized) as a result of binding of an appropriate ligand to a neuronal nicotinic (N_N) acetylcholine receptor. The resulting fast **excitatory postsynaptic potential (EPSP)** evokes a propagated action potential if threshold is reached. This event is often followed by a small and slowly developing but longer-lasting hyperpolarizing afterpotential—a slow **inhibitory postsynaptic potential (IPSP).** This hyperpolarization involves opening of potassium channels by M_2 cholinoceptors. The IPSP is followed by a small, slow excitatory postsynaptic potential caused by closure of potassium channels linked to M_1 cholinoceptors. Finally, a late, very slow EPSP may be evoked by peptides released from other fibers. These slow potentials serve to modulate the responsiveness of the postsynaptic cell to subsequent primary excitatory presynaptic nerve activity. (See Chapter 21 for additional examples.)

PHARMACOLOGIC MODIFICATION OF AUTONOMIC FUNCTION

Because transmission involves both similar (eg, ganglionic) and different (eg, effector cell receptor) mechanisms in different segments of the ANS, some drugs produce less selective effects, whereas others are highly specific in their actions. A summary of the steps in transmission of impulses, from the CNS to the autonomic effector cells, is presented in Table 6–5. Drugs that block action potential propagation (local anesthetics and some natural

TABLE 6–5 Steps in autonomic transmission: Effects of some drugs.

Process Affected	Drug Example	Site	Action
Action potential propagation	Local anesthetics, tetrodotoxin,[1] saxitoxin[2]	Nerve axons	Block voltage-gated sodium channels; block conduction
Transmitter synthesis	Hemicholiniums	Cholinergic nerve terminals: membrane	Block uptake of choline and slow ACh synthesis
	α-Methyltyrosine (metyrosine)	Adrenergic nerve terminals and adrenal medulla: cytoplasm	Inhibits tyrosine hydroxylase and blocks synthesis of catecholamines
Transmitter storage	Vesamicol	Cholinergic terminals: VAT on vesicles	Prevents storage, depletes
	Reserpine, tetrabenazine	Adrenergic terminals: VMAT on vesicles	Prevents storage, depletes
Transmitter release	Many[3]	Nerve terminal membrane receptors	Modulate release
	ω-Conotoxin GVIA[4]	Nerve terminal calcium channels	Reduces transmitter release
	Amifampridine	Blocks nerve terminal K channels	Increases transmitter release by prolonging action potential and increasing calcium influx
	Domoic acid	Nerve terminal kainate receptors (primarily CNS; see Chapter 21)	Modulates transmitter release by altering calcium influx/release
	Botulinum toxin	Cholinergic vesicles	Prevents ACh release
	α-Latrotoxin[5]	Cholinergic and adrenergic vesicles	Causes explosive transmitter release
	Tyramine, amphetamine	Adrenergic nerve terminals	Promote transmitter release
Transmitter reuptake after release	Cocaine, tricyclic antidepressants, SNRI antidepressants[6]	Adrenergic nerve terminals, NET	Inhibit uptake; increase transmitter effect on postsynaptic receptors
Receptor activation or blockade	Norepinephrine	Receptors at adrenergic junctions	Binds and activates a receptors; causes contraction
	Phentolamine	Receptors at adrenergic junctions	Binds α receptors; prevents activation
	Isoproterenol	Receptors at adrenergic junctions	Binds β receptors; activates adenylyl cyclase
	Propranolol	Receptors at adrenergic junctions	Binds β receptors; prevents activation
	Nicotine	Receptors at nicotinic cholinergic junctions (autonomic ganglia, neuromuscular end plates)	Binds nicotinic receptors; opens ion channel in postsynaptic membrane
	Tubocurarine	Neuromuscular end plates	Prevents activation of nicotinic receptors
	Bethanechol	Receptors, parasympathetic effector cells (smooth muscle, glands)	Binds and activates muscarinic receptors
	Atropine	Receptors, parasympathetic effector cells	Binds muscarinic receptors; prevents activation
Enzymatic inactivation of transmitter	Neostigmine	Cholinergic synapses (acetylcholinesterase)	Inhibits enzyme; prolongs and intensifies transmitter action after release
	Tranylcypromine	Adrenergic nerve terminals (monoamine oxidase)	Inhibits enzyme; increases stored transmitter pool

[1]Toxin of puffer fish, California newt.

[2]Toxin of *Gonyaulax* (red tide organism).

[3]Norepinephrine, dopamine, acetylcholine, angiotensin II, various prostaglandins, etc.

[4]Toxin of marine snails of the genus *Conus*.

[5]Black widow spider venom.

[6]Serotonin, norepinephrine reuptake inhibitors.

NET, norepinephrine transporter; SNRI, serotonin-norepinephrine reuptake inhibitors; VAT, vesicle-associated transporter; VMAT, vesicular monoamine transporter.

toxins) are very nonselective in their action, since they act on a process that is common to all neurons. On the other hand, drugs that act on the biochemical processes involved in transmitter synthesis and storage are more selective, since the biochemistry of each transmitter differs, eg, norepinephrine synthesis is very different from acetylcholine synthesis. Activation or blockade of effector cell receptors offers maximum flexibility and selectivity of effect attainable with currently available drugs: adrenoceptors are easily distinguished from cholinoceptors. Furthermore, individual receptor subgroups can often be selectively activated or blocked within each major type. Some examples are given in Box: Pharmacology of the Eye. Even greater selectivity may be attainable in the future using drugs that target post-receptor processes, eg, receptors for second messengers.

Pharmacology of the Eye

The eye is an organ with multiple autonomic functions, controlled by several autonomic receptors. As shown in Figure 6–9, areas around the lens are the site of several autonomic effector tissues. These tissues include three muscles (pupillary dilator and constrictor muscles of the iris and the ciliary muscle) and the secretory epithelium of the ciliary body.

Parasympathetic nerve activity and muscarinic cholinomimetics mediate contraction of the circular pupillary constrictor muscle and of the ciliary muscle. Contraction of the pupillary constrictor muscle causes miosis, a reduction in pupil size. Miosis is usually present in patients exposed to large systemic or small topical doses of cholinomimetics, especially organophosphate cholinesterase inhibitors. Ciliary muscle contraction causes accommodation of focus for near vision. Marked contraction of the ciliary muscle, which often occurs with cholinesterase inhibitor intoxication, is called *cyclospasm*. Ciliary muscle contraction also puts tension on the trabecular meshwork, opening its pores and facilitating outflow of the aqueous humor into the canal of Schlemm. Increased outflow reduces intraocular pressure, a very useful result in patients with glaucoma. All of these effects are prevented or reversed by muscarinic blocking drugs such as atropine.

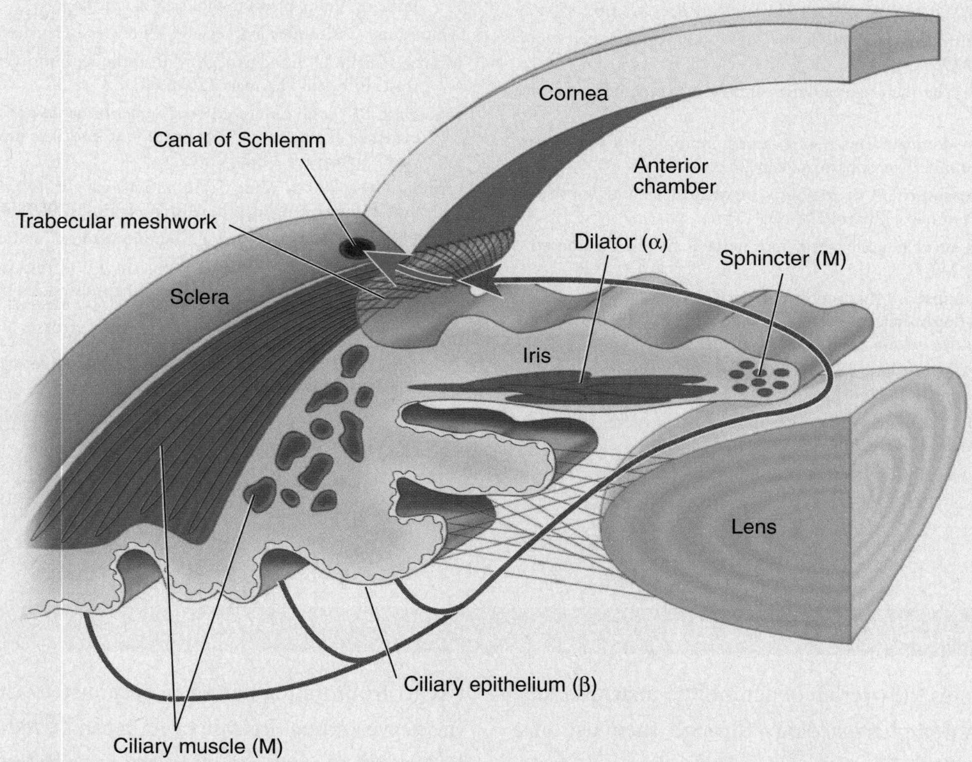

FIGURE 6–9 Structures of the anterior chamber of the eye. Tissues with significant autonomic functions and the associated ANS receptors (α, β, M) are shown in this schematic diagram. Aqueous humor is secreted by the epithelium of the ciliary body, flows into the space in front of the iris, flows through the trabecular meshwork, and exits via the canal of Schlemm (*arrow*). Blockade of the β adrenoceptors associated with the ciliary epithelium causes decreased secretion of aqueous. Blood vessels (not shown) in the sclera are also under autonomic control and influence aqueous drainage.

Alpha adrenoceptors mediate contraction of the radially oriented pupillary dilator muscle fibers in the iris and result in mydriasis (an increase in pupil size). This occurs during sympathetic discharge and when α-agonist drugs such as phenylephrine are placed in the conjunctival sac. Beta adrenoceptors on the ciliary epithelium facilitate the secretion of aqueous humor. Blocking these receptors (with β-blocking drugs) reduces the secretory activity and reduces intraocular pressure, providing another therapy for glaucoma.

The next four chapters provide many more examples of this useful diversity of autonomic control processes.

REFERENCES

Andersson K-E: Mechanisms of penile erection and basis for pharmacological treatment of erectile dysfunction. Pharmacol Rev 2011;63:811.

Barrenschee M et al: SNAP-25 is abundantly expressed in enteric neuronal networks and upregulated by the neurotrophic factor GDNF. Histochem Cell Biol 2015;143:611.

Biaggioni I: The pharmacology of autonomic failure: from hypotension to hypertension. Pharmacol Rev 2017;69:53.

Birdsall NJM: Class A GPCR heterodimers: Evidence from binding studies. Trends Pharmacol Sci 2010;31:499.

Burnstock G: Non-synaptic transmission at autonomic neuroeffector junctions. Neurochem Int 2008;52:14.

Burnstock G: Purinergic signalling in the gut. Adv Exp Med Biol 2016;891:91.

Centers for Disease Control and Prevention: Paralytic shellfish poisoning—Southeast Alaska, May-June 2011. MMWR Morb Mortal Wkly Rep 2011;60:1554.

Dulcis D et al: Neurotransmitter switching in the adult brain regulates behaviour. Science 2013;340:449.

Espinoza-Medina I et al: The sacral autonomic outflow is sympathetic. Science 2016;354:893.

Fisher J: The neurotoxin domoate causes long-lasting inhibition of the kainate receptor GluK5 subunit. Neuropharmacology 2014;85:9.

Furchgott RF: Role of endothelium in responses of vascular smooth muscle to drugs. Annu Rev Pharmacol Toxicol 1984;24:175.

Galligan JJ: Ligand-gated ion channels in the enteric nervous system. Neurogastroenterol Motil 2002;14:611.

Hills JM, Jessen KR: Transmission: γ-aminobutyric acid (GABA), 5-hydroxytryptamine (5-HT) and dopamine. In: Burnstock G, Hoyle CHV (editors): *Autonomic Neuroeffector Mechanisms*. Harwood Academic, 1992.

Holzer P et al: Neuropeptide Y, peptide YY and pancreatic polypeptide in the gut-brain axis. Neuropeptides 2012;46:261.

Johnston GR, Webster NR: Cytokines and the immunomodulatory function of the vagus nerve. Br J Anaesthesiol 2009;102:453.

Langer SZ: Presynaptic receptors regulating transmitter release. Neurochem Int 2008;52:26.

Li YC, Kavalali ET: Synaptic vesicle-recycling machinery components as potential therapeutic targets. Pharmacol Rev 2017;69:142.

Luther JA, Birren SJ: Neurotrophins and target interactions in the development and regulation of sympathetic neuron electrical and synaptic properties. Auton Neurosci 2009;151:46.

Magnon C: Autonomic nerve development contributes to prostate cancer progression. Science 2013;341:1236361.

Mikoshiba K: IP3 receptor/Ca^{2+} channel: From discovery to new signaling concepts. J Neurochem 2007;102:1426.

Pirazzini M et al: Botulinum neurotoxins: Biology, pharmacology, and toxicology. Pharmacol Rev 2017;69:200.

Raj SR, Coffin ST: Medical therapy and physical maneuvers in the treatment of the vasovagal syncope and orthostatic hypotension. Prog Cardiovasc Dis 2013;55:425.

Rizo J: Staging membrane fusion. Science 2012;337:1300.

Robertson D et al: *Primer on the Autonomic Nervous System*, 3rd ed. Academic Press, 2012.

Shibasaki M, Crandall CG: Mechanisms and controllers of eccrine sweating in humans. Front Biosci (Schol Ed) 2011;2:685.

Symposium: Gastrointestinal reviews. Curr Opin Pharmacol 2007;7:555.

Tobin G, Giglio D, Lundgren O: Muscarinic receptor subtypes in the alimentary tract. J Physiol Pharmacol 2009;60:3.

Vanderlaan RD et al: Enhanced exercise performance and survival associated with evidence of autonomic reinnervation in pediatric heart transplant recipients. Am J Transplant 2012;12:2157.

Vernino S, Hopkins S, Wang Z: Autonomic ganglia, acetylcholine antibodies, and autoimmune gangliopathy. Auton Neurosci 2009;146:3.

Verrier RL, Tan A: Heart rate, autonomic markers, and cardiac mortality. Heart Rhythm 2009;6(Suppl 11):S68.

Watanabe S et al: Clathrin regenerates synaptic vesicles from endosomes. Nature 2014;515:228.

Westfall DP, Todorov LD, Mihaylova-Todorova ST: ATP as a cotransmitter in sympathetic nerves and its inactivation by releasable enzymes. J Pharmacol Exp Ther 2002;303:439.

Whittaker VP: Some currently neglected aspects of cholinergic function. J Mol Neurosci 2010;40:7.

CASE STUDY ANSWER

This case illustrates the overlap of autonomic pharmacology with somatic motor pharmacology through their use of a common transmitter. Blepharospasm and other manifestations of involuntary muscle spasm can be disabling and, in the case of large muscles, painful. Contraction of skeletal muscle is triggered by exocytotic release of acetylcholine (ACh) from motor nerves in response to calcium influx at the nerve ending. Release of ACh can be reduced or blocked by botulinum toxin, which interferes with the fusion of nerve ending ACh vesicles with the nerve ending membrane (see text). Depending on dosage, botulinum blockade has an average duration of 1–3 months after a single administration.

CHAPTER

7

Cholinoceptor-Activating & Cholinesterase-Inhibiting Drugs

Todd W. Vanderah, PhD

CASE STUDY

In late morning, a coworker brings 43-year-old JM to the emergency department because he is agitated and unable to continue picking vegetables. His gait is unsteady, and he walks with support from his colleague. JM has difficulty speaking and swallowing, his vision is blurred, and his eyes are filled with tears. His coworker notes that JM was working in a field that had been sprayed early in the morning with a material that had the odor of sulfur. Within 3 hours after starting his work, JM complained of tightness in his chest that made breathing difficult, and he called for help before becoming disoriented.

How would you proceed to evaluate and treat JM? What should be done for his coworker?

Acetylcholine-receptor (cholinoceptor) stimulants and cholinesterase inhibitors make up a large group of drugs that mimic acetylcholine (cholinomimetics) (Figure 7–1). Cholinoceptor stimulants are classified pharmacologically by their spectrum of action, depending on the type of receptor—muscarinic or nicotinic—that is activated. Cholinomimetics are also classified by their mechanism of action because some bind directly to (and activate) cholinoceptors, whereas others act indirectly by inhibiting the hydrolysis of endogenous acetylcholine.

SPECTRUM OF ACTION OF CHOLINOMIMETIC DRUGS

Early studies of the parasympathetic nervous system showed that the alkaloid **muscarine** mimicked the effects of parasympathetic nerve discharge; that is, the effects were **parasympathomimetic.** Application of muscarine to ganglia and to autonomic effector tissues (smooth muscle, heart, exocrine glands) showed that the parasympathomimetic action of the alkaloid occurred through an action on receptors at effector cells (smooth muscle, glands), not those in ganglia. The effects of acetylcholine itself and of other cholinomimetic drugs at autonomic neuroeffector junctions are called *parasympathomimetic effects* and are mediated by **muscarinic receptors.** In contrast, low concentrations of the alkaloid **nicotine** stimulated autonomic ganglia and skeletal muscle neuromuscular junctions but not autonomic effector cells. The ganglion and skeletal muscle receptors were therefore labeled nicotinic. When acetylcholine was later identified as the physiologic transmitter at both muscarinic and **nicotinic receptors,** both receptors were recognized as acetylcholine receptor subtypes.

Cholinoceptors are members of either G protein-linked (muscarinic) or ion channel (nicotinic) families on the basis of their structure and transmembrane signaling mechanisms. Muscarinic receptors contain seven transmembrane domains whose third cytoplasmic loop is coupled to G proteins that function as transducers (see Figure 2–11). These receptors regulate the production of intracellular second messengers and modulate certain ion channels via their G proteins. Agonist selectivity is determined by the subtypes of muscarinic receptors and G proteins that are present in a given cell (Table 7–1). In native cells and in cell expression systems, muscarinic receptors form dimers or oligomers that are

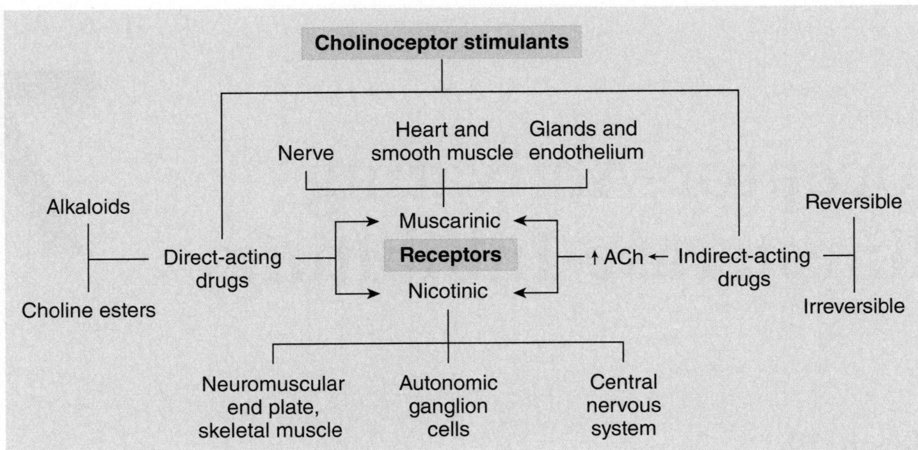

FIGURE 7–1 The major groups of cholinoceptor-activating drugs, receptors, and target tissues. ACh, acetylcholine.

thought to function in receptor movement between the endoplasmic reticulum and plasma membrane as well as in signaling. Conceivably, agonist or antagonist ligands could signal by changing the quaternary structure of the receptor, that is, the ratio of monomeric to oligomeric receptors. Muscarinic receptors are integral proteins located in plasma membranes of cells in the central nervous system, in autonomic ganglia (see Figure 6–8), in organs innervated by parasympathetic nerves, and on some tissues that are not innervated by these nerves, (eg, endothelial cells of blood vessels) (see Table 7–1), as well as on tissues innervated by postganglionic sympathetic cholinergic nerves (eg, eccrine sweat glands, blood vessels in skeletal muscles of some animals).

Nicotinic receptors are part of a transmembrane polypeptide whose five subunits form cation-selective ion channels (see Figure 2–9). The five subunits are composed of different combinations of alpha, beta, gamma, delta, or epsilon subunits. These receptors are located in plasma membranes of postganglionic cells in all autonomic ganglia, of muscles innervated by somatic motor fibers, and of some central nervous system neurons (see Figure 6–1).

Nonselective cholinoceptor stimulants in sufficient dosage can produce very diffuse and marked alterations in organ system function because acetylcholine has multiple sites of action where it initiates both excitatory and inhibitory effects. Fortunately, drugs are

TABLE 7–1 Subtypes and characteristics of cholinoceptors.

Receptor Type	Other Names	Location	Structural Features	Postreceptor Mechanism
M_1		Nerves	Seven transmembrane segments, $G_{q/11}$ protein-linked	IP_3, DAG cascade
M_2	Cardiac M_2	Heart, nerves, smooth muscle	Seven transmembrane segments, $G_{i/o}$ protein-linked	Inhibition of cAMP production, activation of K^+ channels
M_3		Glands, smooth muscle, endothelium	Seven transmembrane segments, $G_{q/11}$ protein-linked	IP_3, DAG cascade
M_4		CNS	Seven transmembrane segments, $G_{i/o}$ protein-linked	Inhibition of cAMP production
M_5		CNS	Seven transmembrane segments, $G_{q/11}$ protein-linked	IP_3, DAG cascade
N_M	Muscle type, end plate receptor	Skeletal muscle neuromuscular junction	Pentamer[1] $[(\alpha1)_2\beta1\delta\gamma]$	Na^+, K^+ depolarizing ion channel
N_N	Neuronal type, ganglion receptor	CNS, postganglionic cell body, dendrites	Pentamer[1] with α and β subunits only, eg, $(\alpha4)_2(\beta2)_3$ (CNS) or $\alpha3\alpha5(\beta2)_3$ (ganglia)	Na^+, K^+ depolarizing ion channel

[1]Pentameric structure in *Torpedo* electric organ and fetal mammalian muscle has two α1 subunits and one each of β1, δ, and γ subunits. The stoichiometry is indicated by subscripts, eg, $[(\alpha1)_2\ \beta1\ \delta\ \gamma]$. In adult muscle, the γ subunit is replaced by an ε subunit. There are 12 neuronal nicotinic receptors with nine α (α2–α10) subunits and three (β2–β4) subunits. The subunit composition varies among different mammalian tissues.

DAG, diacylglycerol; IP_3, inositol trisphosphate.

Data from Millar NS, Gotti C: Diversity of vertebrate nicotinic acetylcholine receptors. Neuropharmacology 2009 Jan;56(1):237-246.

available that have a degree of selectivity, so that desired effects can often be achieved while avoiding or minimizing adverse effects.

Selectivity of action is based on several factors. Some drugs stimulate either muscarinic receptors or nicotinic receptors. Due to the nicotinic receptors being made up of five different subunits, some agents can stimulate nicotinic receptors at neuromuscular junctions preferentially and have less effect on nicotinic receptors in ganglia that consist of different subunits. Organ selectivity can also be achieved by using appropriate routes of administration ("pharmacokinetic selectivity"). For example, muscarinic stimulants can be administered topically to the surface of the eye to modify ocular function while minimizing systemic effects.

MODE OF ACTION OF CHOLINOMIMETIC DRUGS

Direct-acting cholinomimetic agents bind to and activate muscarinic or nicotinic receptors (see Figure 7–1). Indirect-acting agents produce their primary effects by inhibiting acetylcholinesterase, which hydrolyzes acetylcholine to choline and acetic acid (see Figure 6–3). By inhibiting acetylcholinesterase, the indirect-acting drugs increase the endogenous acetylcholine concentration in synaptic clefts and neuroeffector junctions. The excess acetylcholine, in turn, stimulates cholinoceptors to evoke increased responses. These drugs act primarily where acetylcholine is physiologically released and are thus *amplifiers* of endogenous acetylcholine.

Some cholinesterase inhibitors also inhibit butyrylcholinesterase (pseudocholinesterase). However, inhibition of butyrylcholinesterase plays little role in the action of indirect-acting cholinomimetic drugs because this enzyme is not important in the physiologic termination of synaptic acetylcholine action. However, butyrylcholinesterase serves as a biological scavenger to prevent or reduce the extent of cholinesterase inhibition by organophosphate agents (see Chapter 8). Some quaternary cholinesterase inhibitors have a modest direct action as well, eg, neostigmine, which activates neuromuscular nicotinic cholinoceptors directly in addition to blocking cholinesterase. Some individuals have a mutation in the BCHE gene that is expressed as a deficient butyrylcholinesterase produced by the liver, resulting in the inability to break down certain muscle relaxants (see Chapter 27) and anesthetics (see Chapter 25). These individuals can have a severe reaction including paralysis (and apnea) due to increased concentrations of the medications.

■ BASIC PHARMACOLOGY OF THE DIRECT-ACTING CHOLINOCEPTOR STIMULANTS

The direct-acting cholinomimetic drugs can be divided on the basis of chemical structure into esters of choline (including acetylcholine) and alkaloids (such as muscarine and nicotine). Many of these drugs have effects on both receptors; acetylcholine is typical. A few of them are highly selective for the muscarinic or nicotinic receptor. However, none of the clinically useful drugs is selective for receptor subtypes within either class. Development of subtype-selective allosteric modulators could be clinically useful.

$$H_3C-\overset{O}{\overset{\|}{C}}-O-CH_2-CH_2-N^+(CH_3)_3$$

Acetylcholine

$$H_3C-\overset{O}{\overset{\|}{C}}-O-\underset{CH_3}{\underset{|}{CH}}-CH_2-N^+(CH_3)_3$$

Methacholine (acetyl-β-methylcholine)

$$H_2N-\overset{O}{\overset{\|}{C}}-O-CH_2-CH_2-N^+(CH_3)_3$$

Carbachol (carbamoylcholine)

$$H_2N-\overset{O}{\overset{\|}{C}}-O-\underset{CH_3}{\underset{|}{CH}}-CH_2-N^+(CH_3)_3$$

Bethanechol (carbamoyl-β-methylcholine)

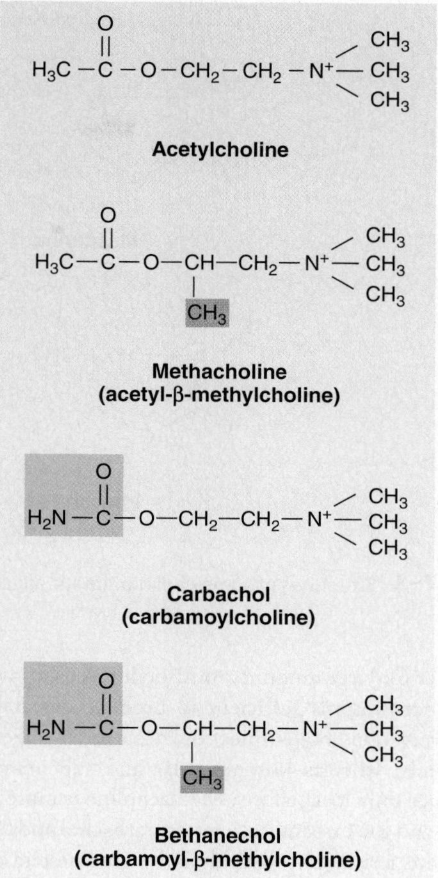

FIGURE 7–2 Molecular structures of four choline esters. Acetylcholine and methacholine are acetic acid esters of choline and β-methylcholine, respectively. Carbachol and bethanechol are carbamic acid esters of the same alcohols.

Chemistry & Pharmacokinetics

A. Structure

Four important choline esters that have been studied extensively are shown in Figure 7–2. Their permanently charged quaternary ammonium group renders them relatively insoluble in lipids. Many naturally occurring and synthetic cholinomimetic drugs that are not choline esters have been identified; a few of these are shown in Figure 7–3. The muscarinic receptor is strongly stereoselective: (*S*)-bethanechol is almost 1000 times more potent than (*R*)-bethanechol.

B. Absorption, Distribution, and Metabolism

Choline esters are poorly absorbed and poorly distributed into the central nervous system due to their hydrophilic nature. Although all are hydrolyzed in the gastrointestinal tract (and less active by the oral route), they differ markedly in their susceptibility to hydrolysis by cholinesterase. Acetylcholine is very rapidly hydrolyzed

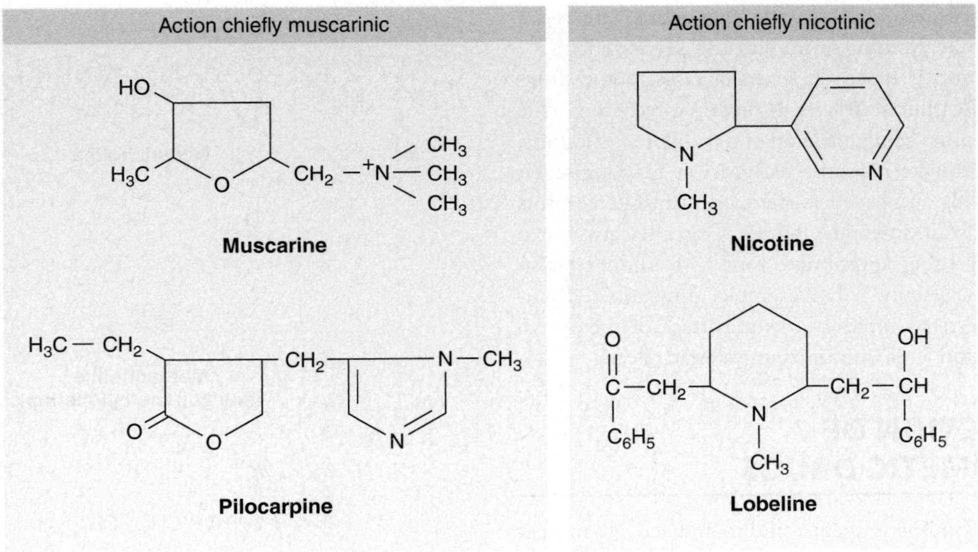

Action chiefly muscarinic

Muscarine

Pilocarpine

Action chiefly nicotinic

Nicotine

Lobeline

FIGURE 7–3 Structures of some cholinomimetic alkaloids.

(see Chapter 6); large amounts must be infused intravenously to achieve concentrations sufficient to produce detectable effects. A large intravenous bolus injection has a brief effect, typically 5–20 seconds, whereas intramuscular and subcutaneous injections produce only local effects. Methacholine is more resistant to hydrolysis, and the carbamic acid esters carbachol and bethanechol are still more resistant to hydrolysis by cholinesterase and have correspondingly longer durations of action. The β-methyl group (methacholine, bethanechol) reduces the potency of these drugs at nicotinic receptors (Table 7–2) while they maintain activity at muscarinic receptors.

The tertiary natural cholinomimetic alkaloids (pilocarpine, nicotine, lobeline) are well absorbed from most sites of administration. Nicotine, a liquid, is sufficiently lipid-soluble to be absorbed across the skin. Muscarine, a quaternary amine, is less completely absorbed from the gastrointestinal tract than the tertiary amines but is nevertheless toxic when ingested—eg, in certain mushrooms—and it even enters the brain. Lobeline is a plant derivative similar to nicotine. These amines are excreted chiefly by the kidneys. Acidification of the urine accelerates clearance of the tertiary amines (see Chapter 1).

TABLE 7–2 Properties of choline esters.

Choline Ester	Susceptibility to Cholinesterase	Muscarinic Action	Nicotinic Action
Acetylcholine chloride	++++	+++	+++
Methacholine chloride	+	++++	None
Carbachol chloride	Negligible	++	+++
Bethanechol chloride	Negligible	++	None

Pharmacodynamics

A. Mechanism of Action

Activation of the parasympathetic nervous system modifies organ function by two major mechanisms. First, acetylcholine released from parasympathetic nerves activates muscarinic receptors on effector cells to alter organ function directly. Second, acetylcholine released from parasympathetic nerves interacts with muscarinic receptors on nerve terminals to modulate the release of their neurotransmitter. By this mechanism, acetylcholine release and circulating muscarinic agonists indirectly alter organ function by modulating the effects of the parasympathetic and sympathetic nervous systems and perhaps nonadrenergic, noncholinergic (NANC) systems.

As indicated in Chapter 6, muscarinic receptor subtypes have been characterized by binding studies and cloned. Several cellular events occur when muscarinic receptors are activated, one or more of which might serve as second messengers for muscarinic activation. All muscarinic receptors appear to be of the G protein-coupled type (see Chapter 2 and Table 7–1). Muscarinic agonist binding to M_1, M_3, and M_5 receptors activates the inositol trisphosphate (IP_3), diacylglycerol (DAG) cascade. Some evidence implicates DAG in the opening of smooth muscle calcium channels; IP_3 releases calcium from endoplasmic and sarcoplasmic reticulum. Muscarinic agonists also increase cellular cGMP concentrations. Activation of muscarinic receptors also increases potassium flux across cardiac cell membranes (Figure 7–4A) and decreases it in ganglion and smooth muscle cells. This effect is mediated by the binding of an activated G protein βγ subunit directly to the channel. Finally, activation of M_2 and M_4 muscarinic receptors inhibits adenylyl cyclase activity in tissues (eg, heart, intestine). Moreover, muscarinic agonists attenuate the activation of adenylyl cyclase and decrease cAMP concentration induced by hormones such as catecholamines. These muscarinic effects on cAMP concentrations reduce the physiologic response of the organ to stimulatory hormones.

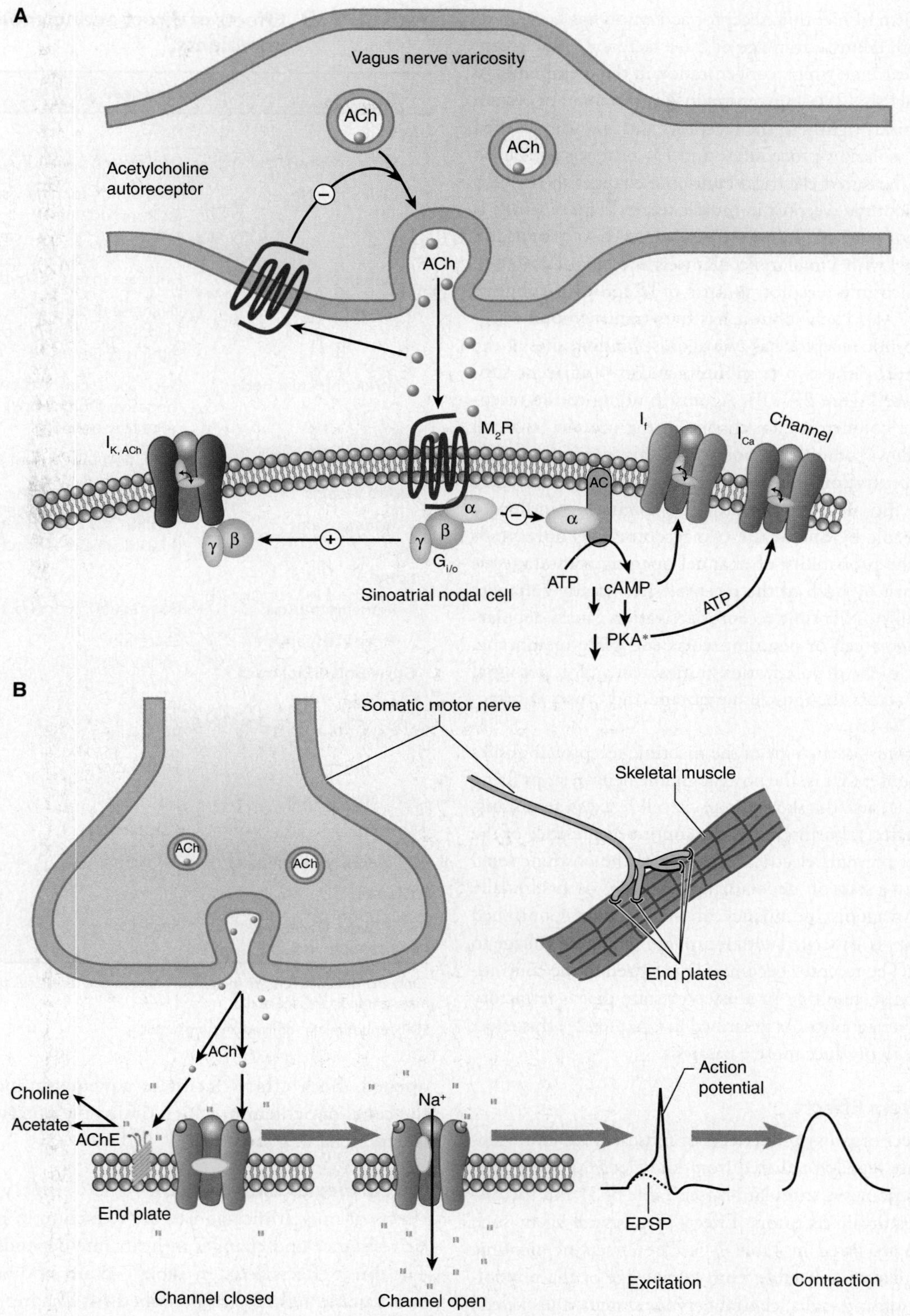

FIGURE 7–4 Muscarinic and nicotinic signaling. **A:** Muscarinic transmission to the sinoatrial node in heart. Acetylcholine (ACh) released from a varicosity of a postganglionic cholinergic axon interacts with a sinoatrial node cell muscarinic receptor (M_2R) linked via $G_{i/o}$ to K^+ channel opening, which causes hyperpolarization, and to inhibition of cAMP synthesis. Reduced cAMP shifts the voltage-dependent opening of pacemaker channels (I_f) to more negative potentials, and reduces the phosphorylation and availability of L-type Ca^{2+} channels (I_{Ca}). Released ACh also acts on an axonal muscarinic receptor (autoreceptor; see Figure 6–3) to cause inhibition of ACh release (autoinhibition). **B:** Nicotinic transmission at the skeletal neuromuscular junction. ACh released from the motor nerve terminal interacts with subunits of the pentameric nicotinic receptor to open it, allowing Na^+ influx to produce an excitatory postsynaptic potential (EPSP). The EPSP depolarizes the muscle membrane, generating an action potential, and triggering contraction. Acetylcholinesterase (AChE) in the extracellular matrix hydrolyzes ACh.

The mechanism of nicotinic receptor activation has been studied in great detail, taking advantage of three factors: (1) the receptor is present in extremely high concentration in the membranes of organs of electric fish; (2) α-bungarotoxin, a component of certain snake venoms, binds tightly to the receptors and is readily labeled as a marker for isolation procedures; and (3) receptor activation results in easily measured electrical and ionic changes in the cells involved. The nicotinic receptor in muscle tissues (Figure 7–4B) is a pentamer of four types of glycoprotein subunits (β, δ, γ, or ε, and two α monomers) with a total molecular weight of about 250,000. The neuronal nicotinic receptor consists of α and/or β subunits only (see Table 7–1). Each subunit has four transmembrane segments. The nicotinic receptor has two agonist binding sites at the interfaces formed by the two α subunits and two adjacent subunits (β, γ, ε) (see Figure 27–1B). Agonist binding to the receptor sites causes a conformational change in the protein (channel opening) that allows sodium and potassium ions to diffuse rapidly down their concentration gradients (calcium ions may also carry charge through the nicotinic receptor ion channel). Binding of an agonist molecule by one of the two receptor sites only modestly increases the probability of channel opening; simultaneous binding of agonist by both of the receptor sites greatly enhances opening probability. Nicotinic receptor activation causes depolarization of the nerve cell or neuromuscular end plate membrane. In skeletal muscle, the depolarization initiates an action potential that propagates across the muscle membrane and causes contraction (see Figure 7–4B).

Prolonged agonist occupancy of the nicotinic receptor abolishes the effector response; that is, the postganglionic neuron stops firing (ganglionic effect), and the skeletal muscle cell relaxes (neuromuscular end plate effect). Furthermore, the continued presence of the nicotinic agonist prevents electrical recovery of the postjunctional membrane. Thus, a state of "depolarizing blockade" occurs initially during persistent agonist occupancy of the receptor. Continued agonist occupancy is associated with return of membrane voltage to the resting level. The receptor becomes desensitized to the continuation of the agonist, resulting in a receptor state that is refractory to reversal by other agonists. As described in Chapter 27, this effect can be exploited to produce muscle paralysis.

TABLE 7–3 Effects of direct-acting cholinoceptor stimulants.[1]

Organ	Response
Eye	
Sphincter muscle of iris	Contraction (miosis)
Ciliary muscle	Contraction for near vision (accommodation)
Heart	
Sinoatrial node	Decrease in rate (negative chronotropy)
Atria	Decrease in contractile strength (negative inotropy). Decrease in refractory period
Atrioventricular node	Decrease in conduction velocity (negative dromotropy). Increase in refractory period
Ventricles	Small decrease in contractile strength
Blood vessels	
Arteries, veins	Dilation (via EDRF). Constriction (high-dose direct effect)
Lung	
Bronchial muscle	Contraction (bronchoconstriction)
Bronchial glands	Secretion
Gastrointestinal tract	
Motility	Increase
Sphincters	Relaxation
Secretion	Stimulation
Urinary bladder	
Detrusor	Contraction
Trigone and sphincter	Relaxation
Glands	
Sweat, salivary, lacrimal, nasopharyngeal	Secretion

[1]Only the direct effects are indicated; homeostatic responses to these direct actions may be important (see text).

EDRF, endothelium-derived relaxing factor.

B. Organ System Effects

Most of the direct organ system effects of muscarinic cholinoceptor stimulants are readily predicted from knowledge of the effects of parasympathetic nerve stimulation (see Table 6–3) and the distribution of muscarinic receptors. Effects of a typical agent such as acetylcholine are listed in Table 7–3. The effects of nicotinic agonists are similarly predictable from knowledge of the physiology of the autonomic ganglia, central nervous system, and skeletal muscle motor end plate.

1. *Eye*—Muscarinic agonists instilled into the conjunctival sac cause contraction of the smooth muscle of the iris sphincter (resulting in miosis) and of the ciliary muscle (resulting in accommodation) via M_3 receptors. As a result, the iris is pulled away from the angle of the anterior chamber, and the trabecular meshwork at the base of the ciliary muscle is opened. Both effects facilitate aqueous humor outflow into the canal of Schlemm, which drains the anterior chamber and is beneficial in glaucoma.

2. *Cardiovascular system*—The primary cardiovascular effects of muscarinic agonists are reduction in peripheral vascular resistance and changes in heart rate depending on the dose. The direct effects listed in Table 7–3 are modified by important homeostatic reflexes, as described in Chapter 6 and depicted in Figure 6–7. Intravenous infusions of minimally effective doses of acetylcholine in humans (eg, 20–50 mcg/min) cause vasodilation, resulting in a reduction in blood pressure, often accompanied by a reflex increase in heart rate. Larger doses of acetylcholine produce bradycardia and decrease atrioventricular node conduction velocity in addition to causing hypotension.

The direct cardiac actions of muscarinic stimulants include the following: (1) an increase in a potassium current ($I_{K(ACh)}$) in the cells of the sinoatrial and atrioventricular nodes, in Purkinje cells, and also in atrial and ventricular muscle cells; (2) a decrease in the slow inward calcium current (I_{Ca}) in heart cells; and (3) a reduction in the hyperpolarization-activated current (I_f) that underlies diastolic depolarization (see Figure 7–4A). All these actions are mediated by M_2 receptors and contribute to slowing the pacemaker rate. Effects (1) and (2) cause hyperpolarization, reduce action potential duration, and decrease the contractility of atrial and ventricular cells. Predictably, knockout of M_2 receptors eliminates the bradycardic effect of vagal stimulation and the negative chronotropic effect of carbachol on sinoatrial rate.

The direct slowing of sinoatrial rate and atrioventricular conduction that is produced by muscarinic agonists is often opposed by reflex sympathetic discharge, elicited by the decrease in blood pressure (see Figure 6–7). The resultant sympathetic-parasympathetic interaction is complex because muscarinic modulation of sympathetic influences occurs by inhibition of norepinephrine release and by postjunctional cellular effects. Muscarinic receptors that are present on postganglionic parasympathetic nerve terminals allow neurally released acetylcholine to inhibit its own secretion. The neuronal muscarinic receptors need not be the same subtype as found on effector cells. Therefore, the net effect on heart rate depends on local concentrations of the agonist in the heart and in the vessels and on the level of reflex responsiveness.

Parasympathetic innervation of the ventricles is much less extensive than that of the atria; activation of ventricular muscarinic receptors causes much less direct physiologic effect than that seen in atria. However, the indirect effects of muscarinic agonists on ventricular function are clearly evident during sympathetic nerve stimulation because of muscarinic modulation of sympathetic effects ("accentuated antagonism").

In the intact organism, intravascular injection of muscarinic agonists produces marked vasodilation. However, earlier studies of isolated blood vessels often showed a contractile response to these agents. It is now known that acetylcholine-induced vasodilation arises from activation of M_3 receptors and requires the presence of intact endothelium (Figure 7–5). Muscarinic agonists via M_3 release endothelium-derived relaxing factor (EDRF), identified as nitric oxide (NO), from the endothelial cells. The NO diffuses to adjacent vascular smooth muscle, where it activates guanylyl cyclase and increases cGMP, resulting in relaxation (see Figure 12–2). Isolated vessels prepared with the endothelium preserved consistently reproduce the vasodilation seen in the intact organism. The relaxing effect of acetylcholine was maximal at 3×10^{-7} M (see Figure 7–5). This effect was eliminated in the absence of endothelium, and acetylcholine, at concentrations greater than 10^{-7} M, then caused contraction. This results from a direct effect of acetylcholine on vascular smooth muscle in which activation of M_3 receptors stimulates IP_3 production and releases intracellular calcium.

Parasympathetic nerves can regulate arteriolar tone in vascular beds in thoracic and abdominal visceral organs. Acetylcholine released from postganglionic parasympathetic nerves relaxes coronary arteriolar smooth muscle via the NO/cGMP pathway in humans as described above. Damage to the endothelium, as occurs with atherosclerosis, eliminates this action, and acetylcholine is then able to contract arterial smooth muscle and produce vasoconstriction via an increase in the release of intracellular calcium. Parasympathetic nerve stimulation also causes vasodilation in cerebral blood vessels; however, the effect often appears as a result of NO released either from NANC (nitrergic) neurons or as a cotransmitter from cholinergic nerves. The relative contributions of cholinergic and NANC neurons to the vascular effects of parasympathetic nerve stimulation are not known for most viscera. Skeletal muscle receives sympathetic cholinergic vasodilator nerves, but the view that acetylcholine causes vasodilation in this vascular bed has not been verified experimentally. Nitric oxide, rather than acetylcholine, may be released from these neurons. However, this vascular bed responds to exogenous choline esters because of the presence of M_3 receptors on endothelial and smooth muscle cells.

The cardiovascular effects of all the choline esters are similar to those of acetylcholine—the main difference being in their potency and duration of action. Because of the resistance of methacholine,

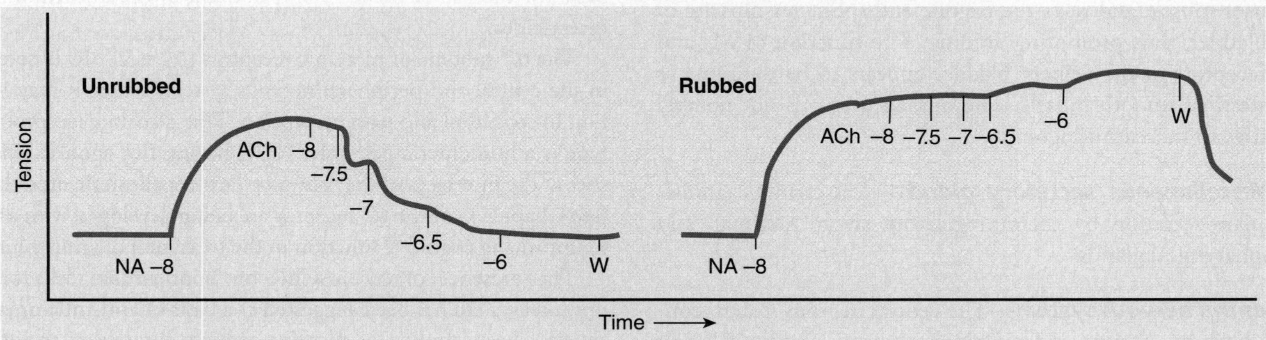

FIGURE 7–5 Activation of endothelial cell muscarinic receptors by acetylcholine (ACh) releases endothelium-derived relaxing factor (nitric oxide), which causes relaxation of vascular smooth muscle precontracted with norepinephrine, 10^{-8} M. Removal of the endothelium by rubbing eliminates the relaxant effect and reveals contraction caused by direct action of ACh on vascular smooth muscle. (NA, noradrenaline [norepinephrine]; W, wash. Numbers indicate the log molar concentration applied at the time indicated.) (Reproduced with permission from Furchgott RF, Zawadzki JV: The obligatory role of endothelial cells in the relaxation of arterial smooth muscle by acetylcholine. Nature. 1980; 288(5789):373-376.)

carbachol, and bethanechol to acetylcholinesterase, lower doses given intravenously are sufficient to produce effects similar to those of acetylcholine, and the duration of action of these synthetic choline esters is longer. The cardiovascular effects of most of the cholinomimetic natural alkaloids and the synthetic analogs also are generally similar to those of acetylcholine.

Pilocarpine is an interesting exception to the above statement due to its affinity to M_1 receptors. If given intravenously (an experimental exercise), it may produce hypertension after a brief initial hypotensive response. The longer-lasting hypertensive effect can be traced to sympathetic ganglionic discharge caused by activation of postganglionic cell membrane M_1 receptors, which close K^+ channels and elicit slow excitatory (depolarizing) postsynaptic potentials (see Figure 6–8). This effect, like the hypotensive effect, can be blocked by atropine, an antimuscarinic drug.

3. *Respiratory system*—Muscarinic stimulants contract the smooth muscle of the bronchial tree. In addition, the glands of the tracheobronchial mucosa are stimulated to secrete mucins, antimicrobial substances, and fluid. This combination of effects can occasionally cause symptoms, especially in individuals with asthma. The bronchoconstriction caused by muscarinic agonists is eliminated in knockout animals in which the M_3 receptor has been mutated.

4. *Gastrointestinal tract*—Administration of muscarinic agonists, as in parasympathetic nervous system stimulation, increases the secretory and motor activity of the gut. The salivary and gastric glands are strongly stimulated; the pancreas and small intestinal glands are stimulated less so. Peristaltic activity is increased throughout the gut, and most sphincters are relaxed. Stimulation of contraction in this organ system involves depolarization of the smooth muscle cell membrane and increased calcium influx. Muscarinic agonists do not cause contraction of the ileum in mutant mice lacking M_2 and M_3 receptors. The M_3 receptor is required for direct activation of smooth muscle contraction, whereas the M_2 receptor reduces cAMP formation and relaxation caused by sympathomimetic drugs.

5. *Genitourinary tract*—Muscarinic agonists stimulate the detrusor muscle and relax the trigone and sphincter muscles of the bladder, thus promoting voiding. The function of M_2 and M_3 receptors in the urinary bladder appears to be the same as in intestinal smooth muscle. The human uterus is not notably sensitive to muscarinic agonists.

6. *Miscellaneous secretory glands*—Muscarinic agonists stimulate secretion by thermoregulatory sweat, lacrimal, and nasopharyngeal glands.

7. *Central nervous system*—The central nervous system contains both muscarinic and nicotinic receptors, the brain being relatively richer in muscarinic sites and the spinal cord containing a preponderance of nicotinic sites. The physiologic roles of these receptors are discussed in Chapter 21.

All five muscarinic receptor subtypes have been detected in the central nervous system. The roles of M_1 through M_3 have been analyzed by means of experiments in knockout mice. The M_1 subtype is richly expressed in brain areas involved in cognition. Knockout of M_1 receptors was associated with impaired neuronal plasticity in the forebrain, and pilocarpine did not induce seizures in M_1 mutant mice. The central nervous system effects of the synthetic muscarinic agonist oxotremorine (tremor, hypothermia, and antinociception) were lacking in mice with homozygously mutated M_2 receptors. Animals lacking M_3 receptors, especially those in the hypothalamus, had reduced appetite and diminished body fat mass.

Despite the smaller ratio of nicotinic to muscarinic receptors, nicotine and lobeline (see Figure 7–3) have important effects on the brain stem and cortex. Activation of nicotinic receptors occurs at presynaptic and postsynaptic loci. Presynaptic nicotinic receptors allow acetylcholine and nicotine to regulate the release of several neurotransmitters (glutamate, serotonin, GABA, dopamine, and norepinephrine). Acetylcholine regulates norepinephrine release via $\alpha3\beta4$ nicotinic receptors in the hippocampus and inhibits acetylcholine release from neurons in the hippocampus and cortex. The $\alpha4\beta2$ oligomer is the most abundant nicotinic receptor in the brain with modulation of hippocampal and hypothalamus function and may be involved with nicotine addiction. Chronic exposure to nicotine has a dual effect at nicotinic receptors: activation (depolarization) followed by desensitization. The former effect is associated with greater release of dopamine in the mesolimbic system of humans. This effect is thought to contribute to the mild alerting action and the addictive property of nicotine absorbed from tobacco. When the $\beta2$ subunits are deleted in reconstitution experiments, acetylcholine binding is reduced, as is the release of dopamine. The later desensitization of the nicotinic receptor is accompanied by increased high-affinity agonist binding and an upregulation of nicotinic binding sites, especially those of the $\alpha4\beta2$ oligomer. Sustained desensitization may contribute to the benefits of nicotine replacement therapy in smoking cessation regimens. In high concentrations, nicotine induces tremor, emesis, and stimulation of the respiratory center. At still higher levels, nicotine causes convulsions, which may terminate in fatal coma. The lethal effects on the central nervous system and the fact that nicotine is readily absorbed form the basis for the use of nicotine and derivatives (neonicotinoids) as insecticides.

The $\alpha7$ subtype of nicotinic receptors ($\alpha7$ nAChR) is detected in the central and peripheral nervous systems where it may function in cognition and pain perception. This nicotinic receptor subtype is a homomeric pentamer $(\alpha7)_5$ having five agonist binding sites at the interfaces of the subunits. Positive allosteric modulators (see Chapter 1) of the $\alpha7$ receptor are being developed with a view to improving cognitive function in the treatment of schizophrenia.

The presence of $\alpha7$ nAChR on nonneuronal cells of the immune system has been suggested as a basis of anti-inflammatory actions. Acetylcholine or nicotine reduces the release of inflammatory cytokines via $\alpha7$ nAChR on macrophages, microglia, and astrocytes. In human volunteers, transdermal nicotine reduced markers of inflammation caused by lipopolysaccharide. The anti-inflammatory role of $\alpha7$ nAChR has gained support from such data.

8. *Peripheral nervous system*—Autonomic ganglia are important sites of nicotinic synaptic action. The α3 subtype is found in autonomic ganglia and is responsible for fast excitatory transmission. Beta2 and β4 subunits are usually present with the α3 subunit to form heteromeric subtypes in parasympathetic and sympathetic ganglia and in the adrenal medulla. Nicotinic agents cause marked activation of these nicotinic receptors and initiate action potentials in postganglionic neurons (see Figure 6–8). Nicotine itself has a somewhat greater affinity for neuronal than for skeletal muscle nicotinic receptors.

Nicotine action is the same on both parasympathetic and sympathetic ganglia. Therefore, the initial response often resembles simultaneous discharge of both the parasympathetic and sympathetic nervous systems. In the case of the cardiovascular system, the effects of nicotine are chiefly sympathomimetic. Dramatic hypertension is produced by parenteral injection of nicotine; sympathetic tachycardia may alternate with a bradycardia mediated by vagal discharge. In the gastrointestinal and urinary tracts, the effects are largely parasympathomimetic: nausea, vomiting, diarrhea, and voiding of urine are commonly observed. Prolonged exposure may result in depolarizing blockade of the ganglia.

Primary autoimmune autonomic failure provides a pathophysiologic example of the effects of **suppression** of nicotinic receptor function at autonomic ganglia. In some patients, neither diabetic neuropathy nor amyloidosis can account for the autonomic failure. In those individuals, circulating autoantibodies selective for the α3β4 nicotinic receptor subtype are present and cause orthostatic hypotension, reduced sweating, dry mouth and eyes, reduced baroreflex function, urinary retention, constipation, and erectile dysfunction. These signs of autonomic failure can be ameliorated by plasmapheresis, which also reduces the concentration of autoantibodies to the α3β4 nicotinic receptor.

Deletion of either the α3 or the β2 and β4 subunits causes widespread autonomic dysfunction and blocks the action of nicotine in experimental animals. Humans deficient in α3 subunits are afflicted with microcystis (inadequate development of the urinary bladder), microcolon, and intestinal hypoperistalsis syndrome; urinary incontinence, urinary bladder distention, and mydriasis also occur.

Neuronal nicotinic receptors are present on sensory nerve endings, especially afferent nerves in coronary arteries and the carotid and aortic bodies as well as on the glomus cells of the latter. Activation of these receptors by nicotinic stimulants and of muscarinic receptors on glomus cells by muscarinic stimulants elicits complex medullary responses, including respiratory alterations and vagal discharge.

9. *Neuromuscular junction*—The nicotinic receptors on the neuromuscular end plate apparatus are of $(\alpha1)_2\beta1\delta\varepsilon$ or $(\alpha1)_2\beta1\delta\gamma$ and function similar but not identical to the receptors in the autonomic ganglia (see Table 7–1). Both types respond to acetylcholine and nicotine. (However, as noted in Chapter 8, the receptors differ in their structural requirements for nicotinic blocking drugs.) When a nicotinic agonist is applied directly (by iontophoresis or by intra-arterial injection), an immediate depolarization of the end plate results, caused by an increase in permeability to sodium and potassium ions (see Figure 7–4B). The contractile response varies from disorganized fasciculations of independent motor units to a strong contraction of the entire muscle depending on the synchronization of depolarization of end plates throughout the muscle. Depolarizing nicotinic agents that are not rapidly hydrolyzed (like nicotine itself) cause rapid development of depolarization blockade; transmission blockade persists even when the membrane has repolarized (discussed further in Chapters 8 and 27). This latter phase of block is manifested as flaccid paralysis in the case of skeletal muscle.

■ BASIC PHARMACOLOGY OF THE INDIRECT-ACTING CHOLINOMIMETICS

The actions of acetylcholine released from autonomic and somatic motor nerves are terminated by enzymatic hydrolysis of the molecule. Hydrolysis is accomplished by the action of acetylcholinesterase, which is present in high concentrations in cholinergic synapses. The indirect-acting cholinomimetics have their primary effect at the active site of this enzyme, although some also have direct actions at nicotinic receptors. The chief differences between members of the group are chemical and pharmacokinetic—their pharmacodynamic properties are almost identical.

Chemistry & Pharmacokinetics

A. Structure

There are three chemical groups of cholinesterase inhibitors: (1) simple alcohols bearing a quaternary ammonium group, eg, edrophonium; (2) carbamic acid esters of alcohols having quaternary or tertiary ammonium groups (carbamates, eg, neostigmine); and (3) organic derivatives of phosphoric acid (organophosphates, eg, echothiophate). Examples of the first two groups are shown in Figure 7–6. Edrophonium, neostigmine, and pyridostigmine are synthetic quaternary ammonium agents used in medicine. Physostigmine (eserine) is a naturally occurring tertiary amine, and rivastigmine is synthetic and of greater lipid solubility and is also used in therapeutics (Table 7–4). Donepezil is a synthesized piperidine derivative compound used to treat dementia. Carbaryl (carbaril) is typical of a large group of carbamate insecticides designed for very high lipid solubility, so that absorption into the insect and distribution to its central nervous system are very rapid.

A few of the estimated 50,000 organophosphates are shown in Figure 7–7. Many of the organophosphates (echothiophate is an exception) are highly lipid-soluble liquids. Echothiophate, a thiocholine derivative, is of clinical value because it retains the very long duration of action of other organophosphates but is more stable in aqueous solution. Sarin is an extremely potent "nerve gas." Parathion and malathion are thiophosphate (sulfur-containing phosphate) prodrugs that are inactive as such; they are converted to the phosphate derivatives in animals and plants and are used as insecticides.

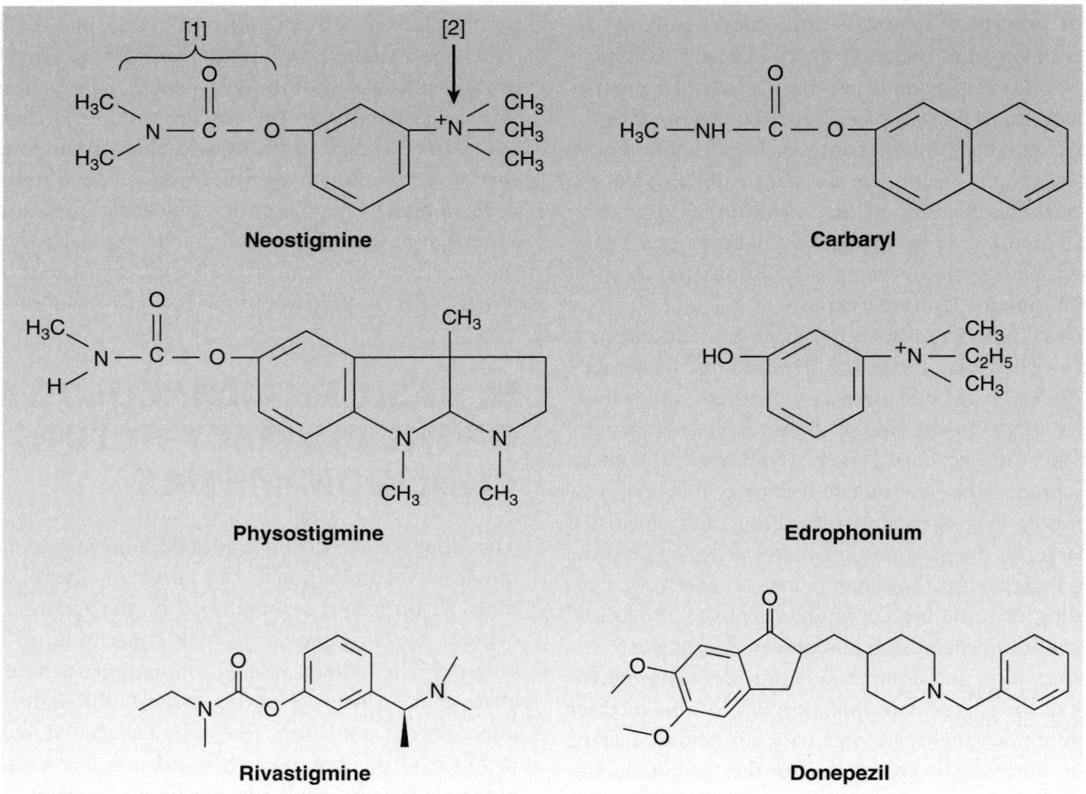

FIGURE 7–6 Cholinesterase inhibitors. Neostigmine exemplifies the typical ester composed of carbamic acid ([1]) and a phenol bearing a quaternary ammonium group ([2]). Physostigmine, a naturally occurring carbamate, is a tertiary amine. Edrophonium is not an ester but binds to the active site of the enzyme. Carbaryl is used as an insecticide.

B. Absorption, Distribution, and Metabolism

Absorption of the quaternary carbamates from the conjunctiva, skin, gut, and lungs is predictably poor, since their permanent charge renders them relatively insoluble in lipids. Thus, much larger doses are required for oral administration than for parenteral injection. Distribution into the central nervous system is negligible. Physostigmine and rivastigmine, in contrast, are well absorbed from all sites and can be used topically in the eye (see Table 7–4). They are distributed into the central nervous system and are more toxic than the more polar quaternary carbamates. The carbamates are relatively stable in aqueous solution but can be metabolized by nonspecific esterases in the body as well as by cholinesterase. However, the duration of their effect is determined chiefly by the stability of the inhibitor-enzyme complex (see later Mechanism of Action section), not by metabolism or excretion. Donepezil is well absorbed and given orally with almost 100% bioavailability and is metabolized by liver enzymes and excreted in the urine.

The organophosphate cholinesterase inhibitors (except for echothiophate) are well absorbed from the skin, lung, gut, and conjunctiva—thereby making them dangerous to humans and highly effective as insecticides. They are relatively less stable than the carbamates when dissolved in water and thus have a limited half-life in the environment (compared with another major class of insecticides, the halogenated hydrocarbons, eg, DDT). Echothiophate is highly polar and more stable than most other organophosphates. When prepared in aqueous solution for ophthalmic use, it retains activity for weeks.

The thiophosphate insecticides (parathion, malathion, and related compounds) are quite lipid-soluble and are rapidly

TABLE 7–4 Therapeutic uses and durations of action of cholinesterase inhibitors.

Group, Drug	Uses	Approximate Duration of Action
Alcohols		
Edrophonium	Myasthenia gravis, ileus, arrhythmias	5–15 minutes
Carbamates and related agents		
Neostigmine	Myasthenia gravis, ileus	0.5–4 hours
Pyridostigmine	Myasthenia gravis	4–6 hours
Physostigmine	For anticholinergic poisoning	0.5–2 hours
Rivastigmine	Mild to moderate Alzheimer dementia	8–10 hours
Donepezil	Alzheimer dementia	70–100 hours
Organophosphates		
Echothiophate	Glaucoma	100 hours

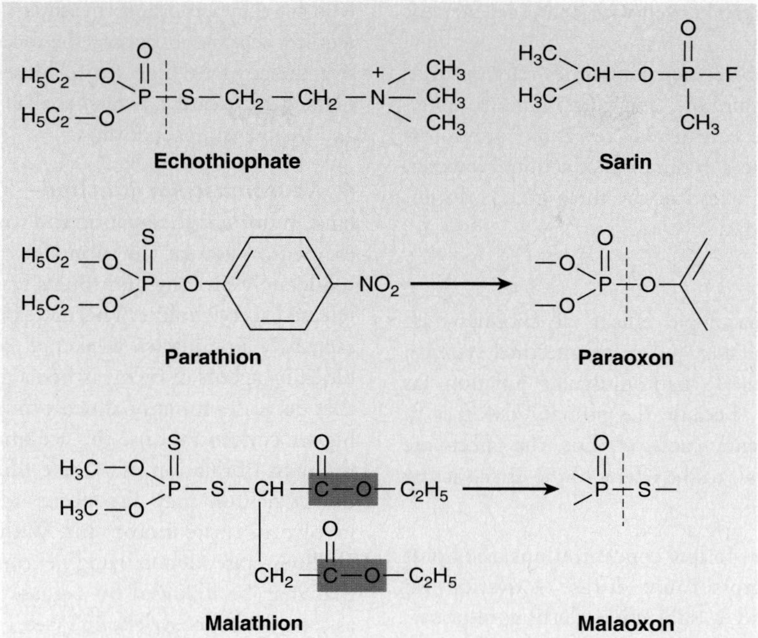

FIGURE 7–7 Structures of some organophosphate cholinesterase inhibitors. The dashed lines indicate the bond that is hydrolyzed in binding to the enzyme. The shaded ester bonds in malathion represent the points of detoxification of the molecule in mammals and birds.

absorbed by all routes. They must be activated in the body by conversion to the oxygen analogs (see Figure 7–7), a process that occurs rapidly in both insects and vertebrates. Malathion and a few other organophosphate insecticides are also rapidly metabolized by a carboxylase pathway to inactive products in birds and mammals but not in insects; these agents are therefore considered safe enough for sale to the general public. Unfortunately, fish cannot detoxify malathion, and significant numbers of fish have died from the heavy use of this agent on and near waterways. Parathion is not detoxified effectively in vertebrates; thus, it is considerably more dangerous than malathion to humans and livestock and is not available for general public use in the USA.

All the organophosphates except echothiophate are distributed to all parts of the body, including the central nervous system. Therefore, central nervous system toxicity is an important component of poisoning with these agents.

Pharmacodynamics

A. Mechanism of Action

Acetylcholinesterase is the primary target of these drugs, but butyrylcholinesterase is also inhibited. Acetylcholinesterase is an extremely active enzyme. In the initial catalytic step, acetylcholine binds to the enzyme's active site and is hydrolyzed, yielding free choline and the acetylated enzyme. In the second step, the covalent acetyl-enzyme bond is split, with the addition of water (hydration). The entire process occurs in approximately 150 microseconds.

All the cholinesterase inhibitors increase the concentration of endogenous acetylcholine at cholinoceptors by inhibiting acetylcholinesterase. However, the molecular details of their interaction with the enzyme vary according to the three chemical subgroups mentioned above.

The first group, of which edrophonium is the example, consists of quaternary alcohols. These agents reversibly bind electrostatically and by hydrogen bonds to the active site, thus preventing access of acetylcholine. The enzyme-inhibitor complex does not involve a covalent bond and is correspondingly short-lived (on the order of 2–10 minutes). The second group consists of carbamate esters, eg, neostigmine and physostigmine. These agents undergo a two-step hydrolysis sequence analogous to that described for acetylcholine. However, the covalent bond of the *carbamoylated* enzyme is considerably more resistant to the second (hydration) process, and this step is correspondingly prolonged (on the order of 30 minutes to 6 hours). The third group consists of the organophosphates. These agents also undergo initial binding and hydrolysis by the enzyme, resulting in a *phosphorylated* active site. The covalent phosphorus-enzyme bond is extremely stable and hydrolyzes in water at a very slow rate (hundreds of hours). After the initial binding-hydrolysis step, the phosphorylated enzyme complex may undergo a process called **aging.** This process apparently involves the breaking of one of the oxygen-phosphorus bonds of the inhibitor and further strengthens the phosphorus-enzyme bond. The rate of aging varies with the particular organophosphate compound. For example, aging occurs within 10 minutes with the chemical warfare agent soman, but as much as 48 hours later with the drug VX (venomous agent X). If given before aging has occurred, strong nucleophiles like pralidoxime (PAM) are able to break the phosphorus-enzyme bond and can be used as "cholinesterase regenerator" drugs for organophosphate insecticide poisoning (see Chapter 8). Once aging has occurred, the enzyme-inhibitor complex is even more stable and is more difficult to break, even with oxime regenerator compounds.

The organophosphate inhibitors are sometimes referred to as "irreversible" cholinesterase inhibitors, and edrophonium, donepezil, and the carbamates are considered "reversible" inhibitors because of the marked differences in duration of action. However, the molecular mechanisms of action of the three groups do not support this simplistic description.

B. Organ System Effects

The most prominent pharmacologic effects of cholinesterase inhibitors are on the cardiovascular and gastrointestinal systems, the eye, and the skeletal muscle neuromuscular junction (as described in the Case Study). Because the primary action is to amplify the actions of endogenous acetylcholine, the effects are similar (but not always identical) to the effects of the direct-acting cholinomimetic agonists.

1. *Central nervous system*—In low concentrations, the lipid-soluble cholinesterase inhibitors cause diffuse activation on the electroencephalogram and a subjective alerting response. In higher concentrations, they cause generalized convulsions, which may be followed by coma and respiratory arrest.

2. *Eye, respiratory tract, gastrointestinal tract, urinary tract*—The effects of the cholinesterase inhibitors on these organ systems, all of which are well innervated by the parasympathetic nervous system, are qualitatively quite similar to the effects of the direct-acting cholinomimetics (see Table 7–3).

3. *Cardiovascular system*—The cholinesterase inhibitors can increase activity in both sympathetic and parasympathetic ganglia supplying the heart and at the acetylcholine receptors on neuroeffector cells (cardiac and vascular smooth muscles) that receive cholinergic innervation.

In the heart, the effects on the parasympathetic limb predominate. Thus, cholinesterase inhibitors such as edrophonium, physostigmine, or neostigmine mimic the effects of vagal nerve activation on the heart. Negative chronotropic, dromotropic, and inotropic effects are produced, and cardiac output falls. The fall in cardiac output is attributable to bradycardia, decreased atrial contractility, and some reduction in ventricular contractility. The latter effect occurs as a result of prejunctional inhibition of norepinephrine release as well as inhibition of postjunctional cellular sympathetic effects.

Cholinesterase inhibitors have minimal effects by direct action on vascular smooth muscle because most vascular beds lack cholinergic innervation (coronary vasculature is an exception). At moderate doses, cholinesterase inhibitors cause an increase in systemic vascular resistance and blood pressure that is initiated at sympathetic ganglia in the case of quaternary nitrogen compounds and also at central sympathetic centers in the case of lipid-soluble agents. Atropine, acting in the central and peripheral nervous systems, can prevent the increase of blood pressure and the increased plasma norepinephrine.

The *net* cardiovascular effects of moderate doses of cholinesterase inhibitors therefore consist of modest bradycardia, a fall in cardiac output, and an increased vascular resistance that results in a rise in blood pressure. (Thus, in patients with Alzheimer disease who have hypertension, treatment with cholinesterase inhibitors requires that blood pressure be monitored to adjust antihypertensive therapy.) At high (toxic) doses of cholinesterase inhibitors, marked bradycardia occurs, cardiac output decreases significantly, and hypotension supervenes.

4. *Neuromuscular junction*—The cholinesterase inhibitors have important therapeutic and toxic effects at the skeletal muscle neuromuscular junction. Low (therapeutic) concentrations moderately prolong and intensify the actions of physiologically released acetylcholine. This increases the strength of contraction, especially in muscles weakened by curare-like neuromuscular blocking agents or by myasthenia gravis (an autoimmune disease that decreases functional neuromuscular nicotinic receptors). At higher concentrations, the accumulation of acetylcholine may result in fibrillation of muscle fibers. Antidromic firing of the motor neuron may also occur, resulting in fasciculations that involve an entire motor unit. With marked inhibition of acetylcholinesterase, depolarizing neuromuscular blockade occurs and that may be followed by a phase of nondepolarizing blockade as seen with succinylcholine (see Table 27–2 and Figure 27–7).

Some quaternary carbamate cholinesterase inhibitors, eg, neostigmine and pyridostigmine, have an additional *direct* nicotinic agonist effect at the neuromuscular junction. This may contribute to the effectiveness of these agents as therapy for myasthenia.

■ CLINICAL PHARMACOLOGY OF THE CHOLINOMIMETICS

The major therapeutic uses of the cholinomimetics are to treat diseases of the eye (glaucoma, accommodative esotropia), the gastrointestinal and urinary tracts (postoperative atony, neurogenic bladder), and the neuromuscular junction (myasthenia gravis, curare-induced neuromuscular paralysis), and to treat patients with Alzheimer disease. Cholinesterase inhibitors are occasionally used in the treatment of atropine overdosage and, very rarely, in the therapy of certain atrial arrhythmias.

Clinical Uses

A. The Eye

Glaucoma is a disease characterized by increased intraocular pressure. Muscarinic stimulants and cholinesterase inhibitors reduce intraocular pressure by causing contraction of the ciliary body so as to facilitate outflow of aqueous humor (see Figure 6–9). In the past, glaucoma was treated with either direct agonists (pilocarpine, methacholine, carbachol) or cholinesterase inhibitors (physostigmine, demecarium, echothiophate, isoflurophate). For chronic glaucoma, these drugs have been largely replaced by prostaglandin derivatives and topical β-adrenoceptor antagonists.

Acute angle-closure glaucoma is a medical emergency that is frequently treated initially with drugs but usually requires surgery for permanent correction. Initial therapy often consists of a combination of a direct muscarinic agonist (eg, pilocarpine) and other drugs. Once the intraocular pressure is controlled and the danger of vision loss is diminished, the patient can be prepared for corrective surgery (laser iridotomy). Open-angle glaucoma and some cases of secondary glaucoma are chronic diseases that are not amenable to traditional surgical correction, although newer laser techniques appear to be useful. Other treatments for glaucoma are described in the Box: The Treatment of Glaucoma in Chapter 10 and in Table 10–3.

Accommodative esotropia (strabismus caused by hypermetropic accommodative error) in young children is sometimes diagnosed and treated with cholinomimetic agonists. Dosage is similar to or higher than that used for glaucoma.

B. Gastrointestinal and Urinary Tracts

In clinical disorders that involve depression of smooth muscle activity without obstruction, cholinomimetic drugs with direct or indirect muscarinic effects may be helpful. These disorders include postoperative ileus (atony or paralysis of the stomach or bowel following surgical manipulation) and congenital megacolon. Urinary retention may occur postoperatively or postpartum or may be secondary to spinal cord injury or disease (neurogenic bladder). Cholinomimetics were also sometimes used to increase the tone of the lower esophageal sphincter in patients with reflux esophagitis but proton-pump inhibitors are usually indicated (see Chapter 62). Of the muscarinic agonists, bethanechol is the most widely used for these disorders. For gastrointestinal problems, it is usually administered orally in a dose of 10–25 mg three or four times daily. In patients with urinary retention, bethanechol can be given subcutaneously in a dose of 5 mg and repeated in 30 minutes if necessary. Of the cholinesterase inhibitors, neostigmine is the most widely used for these applications. For paralytic ileus or atony of the urinary bladder, neostigmine can be given subcutaneously in a dose of 0.5–1 mg. If patients are able to take the drug by mouth, neostigmine can be given orally in a dose of 15 mg. In all of these situations, the clinician must be certain that there is no mechanical obstruction to outflow before using the cholinomimetic. Otherwise, the drug may exacerbate the problem, cause urine reflux into the kidneys, and possibly cause perforation as a result of increased pressure.

Pilocarpine has long been used to increase salivary secretion. Cevimeline, a quinuclidine derivative of acetylcholine, is a newer direct-acting muscarinic agonist used for the treatment of dry mouth associated with Sjögren syndrome or caused by radiation damage of the salivary glands.

C. Neuromuscular Junction

Myasthenia gravis is an autoimmune disease affecting skeletal muscle neuromuscular junctions. In this disease, antibodies are produced against the main immunogenic region found on α1 subunits of the nicotinic receptor-channel complex. Antibodies are detected in 85% of myasthenic patients. The antibodies reduce nicotinic receptor function by (1) cross-linking receptors, a process that stimulates their internalization and degradation; (2) causing lysis of the postsynaptic membrane; and (3) binding to the nicotinic receptor and inhibiting function. Frequent findings are ptosis, diplopia, difficulty in speaking and swallowing, and extremity weakness. Severe disease may affect all the muscles, including those necessary for respiration. The disease resembles the neuromuscular paralysis produced by *d*-tubocurarine and similar nondepolarizing neuromuscular blocking drugs (see Chapter 27). Patients with myasthenia are exquisitely sensitive to the action of curariform drugs and other drugs that interfere with neuromuscular transmission, eg, aminoglycoside antibiotics.

Cholinesterase inhibitors—but not direct-acting acetylcholine receptor agonists—are extremely valuable as therapy for myasthenia. Patients with ocular myasthenia may be treated with cholinesterase inhibitors alone (see Figure 7–4B). Patients having more widespread muscle weakness are also treated with immunosuppressant drugs (steroids, cyclosporine, and azathioprine). In some patients, the thymus gland is removed; very severely affected patients may benefit from administration of immunoglobulins and from plasmapheresis.

Edrophonium is sometimes used as a diagnostic test for myasthenia. A 2-mg dose is injected intravenously after baseline muscle strength has been measured. If no reaction occurs after 45 seconds, an additional 8 mg may be injected. If the patient has myasthenia gravis, an improvement in muscle strength that lasts about 5 minutes can usually be observed.

Clinical situations in which severe myasthenia (myasthenic crisis) must be distinguished from excessive drug therapy (cholinergic crisis) usually occur in very ill myasthenic patients and must be managed in hospital with adequate emergency support systems (eg, mechanical ventilators) available. Edrophonium can be used to assess the adequacy of treatment with the longer-acting cholinesterase inhibitors usually prescribed in patients with myasthenia gravis. If excessive amounts of cholinesterase inhibitor have been used, patients may become paradoxically weak because of nicotinic depolarizing blockade of the motor end plate. These patients may also exhibit symptoms of excessive stimulation of muscarinic receptors (abdominal cramps, diarrhea, increased salivation, excessive bronchial secretions, miosis, bradycardia). Small doses of edrophonium (1–2 mg intravenously) will produce no relief or even worsen weakness if the patient is receiving excessive cholinesterase inhibitor therapy. On the other hand, if the patient improves with edrophonium, an increase in cholinesterase inhibitor dosage may be indicated.

Long-term therapy for myasthenia gravis is usually accomplished with pyridostigmine; neostigmine is an alternative. The doses are titrated to optimum levels based on changes in muscle strength. These drugs are relatively short-acting and therefore require frequent dosing (every 6 hours for pyridostigmine and every 4 hours for neostigmine; Table 7–4). Sustained-release preparations are available but should be used only at night and if needed. Longer-acting cholinesterase inhibitors such as the organophosphate agents are not used, because the dose requirement in this disease changes too rapidly to permit smooth control of symptoms with long-acting drugs.

If muscarinic effects of such therapy are prominent, they can be controlled by the administration of antimuscarinic drugs such as atropine. Frequently, tolerance to the muscarinic effects of the cholinesterase inhibitors develops, so atropine treatment is not required.

Neuromuscular blockade is frequently produced as an adjunct to surgical anesthesia, using nondepolarizing neuromuscular relaxants such as pancuronium and newer agents (see Chapter 27). After surgery, it is usually desirable to reverse this pharmacologic paralysis promptly. This can be easily accomplished with cholinesterase inhibitors; neostigmine and edrophonium are the drugs of choice. They are given intravenously or intramuscularly for prompt effect. Some snake venoms have curare-like effects, and the use of neostigmine as a nasal spray is under study to prevent respiratory arrest.

Indirect ways of increasing acetylcholine release have been utilized in conditions like Lambert-Eaton myasthenic syndrome by altering the release of acetylcholine at the neuromuscular junction (see Box: Acetylcholine Release Modulators).

D. Heart

The short-acting cholinesterase inhibitor edrophonium was used to treat supraventricular tachyarrhythmias, particularly paroxysmal supraventricular tachycardia. In this application, edrophonium has been replaced by newer drugs with different mechanisms (adenosine and the calcium channel blockers verapamil and diltiazem, see Chapter 14).

Acetylcholine Release Modulators

Amifampridine and 4-aminopyridine (fampridine and dalfampridine) are potassium channel antagonists that block the efflux of potassium in nerve terminals and can result in prolonged action potentials. In the case of Lambert-Eaton myasthenic syndrome, in which antibodies are produced that interfere with proper voltage-gated Ca^{2+} ($VGCa^{2+}$) channel function on the presynaptic nerve of the neuromuscular junction (Figure 7–8), there is a decrease in the amount of acetylcholine release at the neuromuscular junction that results in weakness. Amifampridine and 4-aminopyridine can be used to prolong the excitability by inhibiting the K^+ efflux and slowing repolarization, resulting in more $VGCa^{2+}$ activation. The end result is increased acetylcholine release and increased strength.

Amifampridine and 4-aminopyridine are both >90% bioavailable and are metabolized mainly by acetylation and excreted via the kidneys. Hence, genetic differences in acetylation rate or kidney function will alter the compounds' efficacy and side effects. Amifampridine and 4-aminopyridine, due to effects on CNS and cardiac potassium channels, may increase seizure activity and may prolong cardiac QT interval. Hence they should not be used in individuals who have a history of seizures or epilepsy or in patients with known atrial fibrillation or long QT interval. Other adverse effects include tingling (paresthesias), numbness, and insomnia.

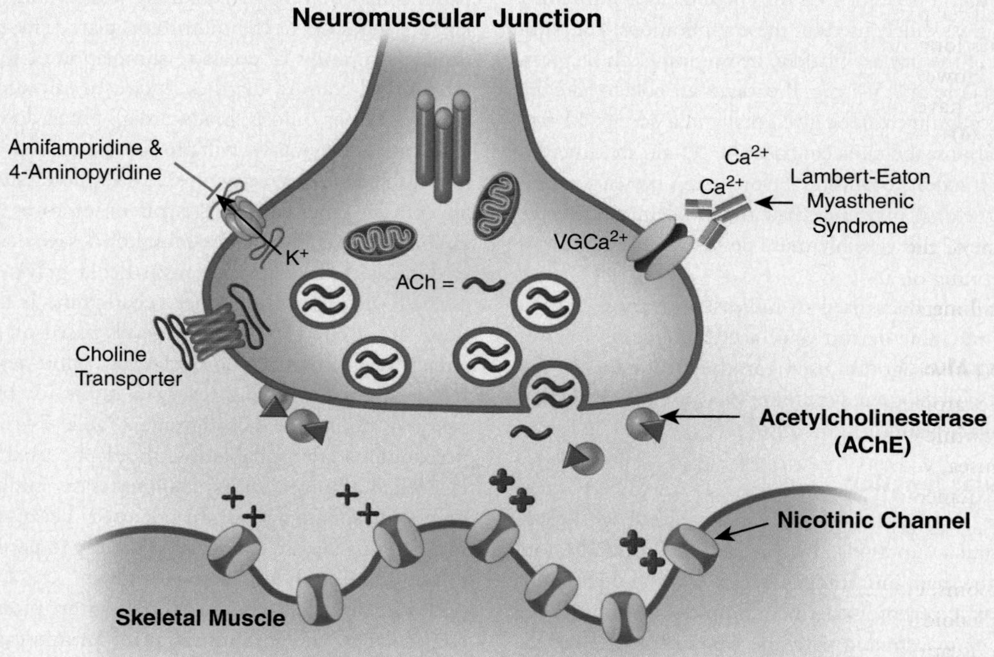

FIGURE 7–8 Schematic illustration of a neuromuscular junction demonstrating how acetylcholine release modulators act in the autoimmune disease Lambert-Eaton myasthenic syndrome (LEMS). Amifampridine and 4-aminopyridine act on the nerve terminal by blocking potassium channels and helping to maintain a positive charge in the nerve terminal that increases the release of acetylcholine (ACh). $VGCa^{2+}$, voltage-gated calcium channels.

E. Antimuscarinic Drug Intoxication

Atropine intoxication is potentially lethal in children (see Chapter 8) and may cause prolonged severe behavioral disturbances and arrhythmias in adults. The tricyclic antidepressants, when taken in overdosage (often with suicidal intent), also cause severe muscarinic blockade (see Chapter 30). The muscarinic receptor blockade produced by all these agents is competitive in nature and can be overcome by increasing the amount of endogenous acetylcholine at the neuroeffector junctions. Theoretically, a cholinesterase inhibitor could be used to reverse these effects. Physostigmine has been used for this application because it enters the central nervous system and reverses the central as well as the peripheral signs of muscarinic blockade. However, as described below, physostigmine itself can produce dangerous central nervous system effects, and such therapy is therefore used only in patients with dangerous elevation of body temperature or very rapid supraventricular tachycardia (see also Chapter 58).

F. Central Nervous System

Tacrine was the first drug with anticholinesterase and other cholinomimetic actions used for the treatment of mild to moderate Alzheimer disease. Tacrine's efficacy is slight, and hepatic toxicity is significant. Donepezil, galantamine, and rivastigmine are newer, more selective, uncharged acetylcholinesterase inhibitors that appear to have the same marginal clinical benefit as tacrine but with less toxicity in treatment of cognitive dysfunction in Alzheimer patients. Donepezil may be given once daily because of its long half-life, and it lacks the hepatotoxic effect of tacrine. However, no trials directly comparing these drugs with tacrine have been reported. These drugs are discussed in Chapter 60.

Toxicity

The toxic potential of the acetylcholine receptor stimulants varies markedly depending on their absorption, access to the central nervous system, and metabolism.

A. Direct-Acting Muscarinic Stimulants

Drugs such as pilocarpine and the choline esters cause predictable signs of muscarinic excess when given in overdosage. These effects include nausea, vomiting, diarrhea, urinary urgency, salivation, sweating, cutaneous vasodilation, and bronchial constriction. The effects are all blocked competitively by atropine and its congeners.

Certain mushrooms, especially those of the genus *Inocybe*, contain muscarinic alkaloids. Ingestion of these mushrooms causes typical signs of muscarinic excess within 15–30 minutes. These effects can be very uncomfortable but are rarely fatal. Treatment is with atropine, 1–2 mg parenterally. (*Amanita muscaria*, the first source of muscarine, contains very low concentrations of the alkaloid.)

B. Direct-Acting Nicotinic Stimulants

Nicotine itself is the only common cause of this type of poisoning. (Varenicline toxicity is discussed elsewhere in this chapter.) The acute toxicity of the alkaloid is well defined but much less important than the chronic effects associated with smoking. Nicotine was also used in insecticides but has been replaced by **neonicotinoids,** synthetic compounds that resemble nicotine only partially in structure. As nicotinic receptor agonists, neonicotinoids are more toxic for insects than for vertebrates. This advantage led to their widespread agricultural use to protect crops by coating the seeds with neonicotinoids. However, there is concern about the role of neonicotinoids in the collapse of bee colonies. In 2013 the European Commission imposed a 2-year ban on certain neonicotinoids (clothianidin, imidacloprid, thiamethoxam), and in 2018 the European Commission voted to permanently ban these three neonicotinoids for outdoor use. In 2016 the US Fish and Wildlife Service banned neonicotinoid use in wildlife refuges, and in 2019 the US Environment Protection Agency banned 12 different neonicotinoids, including the 3 listed above, due to their effect on bees and other pollinating insects. Neonicotinoids are suspected to contribute to colony collapse disorder because they suppress immunity against bee pathogens including the mite (*Varroa destructor*) that also serves as a vector for viruses and the *Nosema* species of fungi that parasitize the gut of bees. Research to ascertain the effect of neonicotinoids on pollinators such as bees and butterflies requires carefully controlled conditions. Neonicotinoid residues have a long half-life (5 months to 3 years) in the soil, and because they are systemic and enter the plant stem, leaves, and flowers, they can present a long-lasting hazard to pollinators. The Australian government's report on neonicotinoids and honey bees recounts that Australia is one of a few countries that lack *Varroa,* which therefore provides an opportunity to test neonicotinoids in the absence of compounds used to treat this mite that contributes to bee pathology.

1. *Acute toxicity*—The fatal dose of nicotine is approximately 40 mg, or 1 drop of the pure liquid. This is the amount of nicotine in two regular cigarettes. Fortunately, most of the nicotine in cigarettes is destroyed by burning or escapes via the "sidestream" smoke. Ingestion of nicotine insecticides or of tobacco by infants and children is usually followed by vomiting, limiting the amount of the alkaloid absorbed.

The toxic effects of a large dose of nicotine are simple extensions of the effects described previously. The most dangerous are (1) central stimulant actions, which cause convulsions and may progress to coma and respiratory arrest; (2) skeletal muscle end plate depolarization, which may lead to depolarization blockade and respiratory paralysis; and (3) hypertension and cardiac arrhythmias.

Treatment of acute nicotine poisoning is largely symptom-directed. Muscarinic excess resulting from parasympathetic ganglion stimulation can be controlled with atropine. Central stimulation is usually treated with parenteral anticonvulsants such as diazepam. Neuromuscular blockade is not responsive to pharmacologic treatment and may require mechanical ventilation.

Fortunately, nicotine is metabolized and excreted relatively rapidly. Patients who survive the first 4 hours usually recover completely if hypoxia and brain damage have not occurred.

2. *Chronic nicotine toxicity*—The health costs of tobacco smoking to the smoker and its socioeconomic costs to the general public are still incompletely understood. However, the 1979 *Surgeon General's Report on Health Promotion and Disease Prevention* stated that "cigarette smoking is clearly the largest single preventable cause of illness and premature death in the United States." This statement has been supported by numerous subsequent studies. Unfortunately, the fact that most of the tobacco-associated diseases are delayed in onset reduces the health incentive to stop smoking.

Clearly, the addictive power of cigarettes is directly related to their nicotine content. It is not known to what extent nicotine per se contributes to the other well-documented adverse effects of chronic tobacco use. It is highly probable that nicotine contributes to the increased risk of vascular disease and sudden coronary death associated with smoking. In addition, nicotine probably contributes to the high incidence of ulcer recurrences in smokers with peptic ulcer. These effects of smoking are not avoided by the use of electronic cigarettes ("vaping") since only the nonnicotine components ("tars") of tobacco are eliminated. The Centers for Disease Control and Prevention (CDC) report a significant increase in the use of electronic cigarettes, which deliver lower levels of carcinogens and therefore may decrease the risk of cancers due to traditional cigarette use. Thus the increase in electronic cigarette use may substantially decrease cardiovascular, lung cancer, and noncancer lung disease risks but increase the population with nicotine addiction and dependence. In 2019, a dramatic rise in acute lung injuries was reported, including several dozen deaths, due to the addition of tetrahydrocannabinol (THC) acetate ester and vitamin E acetate being added to the nicotine-containing and cannabis-containing e-cigarettes. A significant number of cases occurred in young people because **vaping** is very popular in this vulnerable population.

There are several approaches to help patients stop smoking. One approach is replacement therapy with nicotine in the form of gum, transdermal patch, nasal spray, or inhaler. All these forms have low abuse potential and are effective in patients motivated to stop smoking. Their action derives from slow absorption of nicotine that occupies $\alpha4\beta2$ receptors in the central nervous system and reduces the desire to smoke and the pleasurable feelings of smoking.

Another quite effective agent for smoking cessation is **varenicline,** a synthetic drug with partial agonist action at $\alpha4\beta2$ nicotinic receptors. Varenicline also has antagonist properties that persist because of its long half-life and high affinity for the receptor; this prevents the stimulant effect of nicotine at presynaptic $\alpha4\beta2$ receptors that causes release of dopamine. However, its use is limited by nausea and insomnia and also by exacerbation of psychiatric illnesses, including anxiety and depression. The incidence of adverse neuropsychiatric and cardiovascular events is reportedly low yet post-marketing surveillance continues. The efficacy of varenicline is superior to that of bupropion, an antidepressant (see Chapter 30) also approved for smoking cessation. Some of bupropion's efficacy in smoking cessation therapy stems from its noncompetitive antagonism (see Chapter 2) of nicotinic receptors where it displays some selectivity among neuronal subtypes.

C. Cholinesterase Inhibitors

The acute toxic effects of the cholinesterase inhibitors, like those of the direct-acting agents, are direct extensions of their pharmacologic actions. The major source of such intoxications is pesticide use in agriculture and in the home. Approximately 100 organophosphate and 20 carbamate cholinesterase inhibitors are available in pesticides and veterinary vermifuges used in the USA. Cholinesterase inhibitors used in agriculture can cause slowly or rapidly developing symptoms, as described in the Case Study, which persist for days. The cholinesterase inhibitors used as chemical warfare agents (soman, sarin, VX) induce effects rapidly because of the large concentrations present.

Acute intoxication must be recognized and treated promptly in patients with heavy exposure. The dominant initial signs are those of muscarinic excess: miosis, salivation, sweating, bronchial constriction, vomiting, and diarrhea. Central nervous system involvement (cognitive disturbances, convulsions, and coma) usually follows rapidly, accompanied by peripheral nicotinic effects, especially depolarizing neuromuscular blockade. Therapy always includes (1) maintenance of vital signs—respiration in particular may be impaired; (2) decontamination to prevent further absorption—this may require removal of all clothing and washing of the skin in cases of exposure to dusts and sprays; and (3) atropine parenterally in large doses, given as often as required to control signs of muscarinic excess. Therapy often also includes treatment with pralidoxime, as described in Chapter 8, and administration of benzodiazepines for seizures.

Preventive therapy for cholinesterase inhibitors used as chemical warfare agents has been developed to protect soldiers and civilians. Personnel are given autoinjection syringes containing a carbamate, pyridostigmine, and atropine. Protection is provided by pyridostigmine, which, by prior binding to the enzyme, impedes binding of organophosphate agents and thereby prevents prolonged inhibition of cholinesterase. The protection is limited to the peripheral nervous system because pyridostigmine does not readily enter the central nervous system. Enzyme inhibition by pyridostigmine dissipates within hours (see Table 7–4), a duration of time that allows clearance of the organophosphate agent from the body.

Chronic exposure to certain organophosphate compounds, including some organophosphate cholinesterase inhibitors, causes delayed neuropathy associated with demyelination of axons. **Triorthocresyl phosphate,** an additive in lubricating oils, is the prototype agent of this class. The effects are not caused by cholinesterase inhibition but rather by inhibition of neuropathy target esterase (NTE) whose symptoms (weakness of upper and lower extremities, unsteady gait) appear 1–2 weeks after exposure. Another nerve toxicity called intermediate syndrome occurs 1–4 days after exposure to organophosphate insecticides. This syndrome is also characterized by muscle weakness; its origin is not known but it appears to be related to cholinesterase inhibition.

SUMMARY Drugs Used for Cholinomimetic Effects

Subclass, Drug	Mechanism of Action	Effects	Clinical Applications	Pharmacokinetics, Toxicities, Interactions
DIRECT-ACTING CHOLINE ESTERS				
• Bethanechol	Muscarinic agonist • negligible effect at nicotinic receptors	Activates M_1, M_2, and M_3 receptors in all peripheral tissues • causes increased secretion, smooth muscle contraction (except vascular smooth muscle relaxes), and changes in heart rate	Postoperative and neurogenic ileus and urinary retention	Oral and parenteral, duration ~30 min • does not enter central nervous system (CNS) • *Toxicity:* Excessive parasympathomimetic effects, especially bronchospasm in asthmatics • *Interactions:* Additive with other parasympathomimetics
• *Carbachol: Nonselective muscarinic and nicotinic agonist; otherwise similar to bethanechol; used topically almost exclusively for glaucoma*				
DIRECT-ACTING MUSCARINIC ALKALOIDS OR SYNTHETICS				
• Pilocarpine	Like bethanechol, partial agonist	Like bethanechol	Glaucoma; Sjögren syndrome	Oral lozenge and topical • *Toxicity & interactions:* Like bethanechol
• *Cevimeline: Synthetic M_3-selective; similar to pilocarpine*				
DIRECT-ACTING NICOTINIC AGONISTS				
• Nicotine	Agonist at both N_N and N_M receptors	Activates autonomic postganglionic neurons (both sympathetic and parasympathetic) and skeletal muscle neuromuscular end plates • enters CNS and activates N_N receptors	Medical use in smoking cessation • nonmedical use in smoking and in insecticides	Oral gum, patch for smoking cessation • *Toxicity:* Acutely increased gastrointestinal (GI) activity, nausea, vomiting, diarrhea • increased blood pressure • high doses cause seizures • long-term GI and cardiovascular risk factor • *Interactions:* Additive with CNS stimulants
• *Varenicline: Selective partial agonist at $\alpha 4\beta 2$ nicotinic receptors; used exclusively for smoking cessation*				
SHORT-ACTING CHOLINESTERASE INHIBITOR (ALCOHOL)				
• Edrophonium	Alcohol, binds briefly to active site of acetylcholinesterase (AChE) and prevents access of acetylcholine (ACh)	Amplifies all actions of ACh • increases parasympathetic activity and somatic neuromuscular transmission	Diagnosis and acute treatment of myasthenia gravis	Parenteral • quaternary amine • does not enter CNS • *Toxicity:* Parasympathomimetic excess • *Interactions:* Additive with parasympathomimetics
INTERMEDIATE-ACTING CHOLINESTERASE INHIBITORS (CARBAMATES)				
• Neostigmine	Forms covalent bond with AChE, but hydrolyzed and released	Like edrophonium, but longer-acting	Myasthenia gravis • postoperative and neurogenic ileus and urinary retention	Oral and parenteral; quaternary amine, does not enter CNS. Duration 2–4 h • *Toxicity & interactions:* Like edrophonium
• *Pyridostigmine: Like neostigmine, but longer-acting (4–6 h); used in myasthenia*				
• *Physostigmine: Like neostigmine, but natural alkaloid tertiary amine; enters CNS*				
• *Rivastigmine: Like neostigmine, but longer acting (8–10 h) and a tertiary amine that enters CNS*				
LONG-ACTING CHOLINESTERASE INHIBITORS (ORGANOPHOSPHATES)				
• Echothiophate	Like neostigmine, but released more slowly	Like neostigmine, but longer-acting	Obsolete • was used in glaucoma	Topical only • *Toxicity:* Brow ache, uveitis, blurred vision
• *Malathion: Insecticide, relatively safe for mammals and birds because metabolized by other enzymes to inactive products; some medical use as ectoparasiticide*				
• *Parathion, others: Insecticide, dangerous for all animals; toxicity important because of agricultural use and exposure of farm workers (see text)*				
• *Sarin, others: "Nerve gas," used exclusively in warfare and terrorism*				
INDIRECT MODULATORS OF ACETYLCHOLINE RELEASE				
• Amifampridine and 4-aminopyridine	Potassium channel antagonist	Increases the excitability of the presynaptic neuron in the neuromuscular junction, resulting in increased acetylcholine release	Lambert-Eaton myasthenic syndrome; congenital myasthenic syndromes	Oral, duration ~2.5 h • acetylation, then excreted via kidneys • *Toxicity:* seizure activity • may prolong cardiac QT interval • paresthesias • numbness • insomnia

PREPARATIONS AVAILABLE

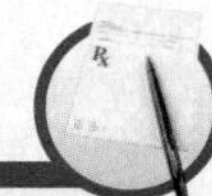

GENERIC NAME	AVAILABLE AS
DIRECT-ACTING CHOLINOMIMETICS	
Acetylcholine	Miochol-E
Bethanechol	Generic, Urecholine
Carbachol	
Ophthalmic (topical)	Isopto Carbachol, Carboptic
Ophthalmic (intraocular)	Miostat, Carbastat
Cevimeline	Generic, Evoxac
Nicotine	
Transdermal	Generic, Nicoderm CQ, Nicotrol
Inhalation	Nicotrol Inhaler, Nicotrol NS
Gum	Generic, Commit, Nicorette
Pilocarpine	
Ophthalmic (drops)1, 2, 4, 6	Generic, Isopto Carpine
Ophthalmic sustained-release inserts	Ocusert Pilo-20, Ocusert Pilo-40
Oral	Salagen
Varenicline	Chantix
CHOLINESTERASE INHIBITORS	
Donepezil	Generic, Aricept
Echothiophate	Phospholine
Edrophonium	Generic, Tensilon
Galantamine	Generic, Reminyl, Razadyne
Neostigmine	Generic, Prostigmin
Physostigmine	Generic, Eserine
Pyridostigmine	Generic, Mestinon, Regonol
Rivastigmine	Exelon
INDIRECT MODULATORS OF ACETYLCHOLINE RELEASE	
Amifampridine	Ruzurgi, Firdapse
4-aminopyridine	Fampridine, Ampyra (dalfampridine)

REFERENCES

Aaron CK: Organophosphates and carbamates. In: Shannon MW, Borron SW, Burns MJ (editors): *Haddad and Winchester's Clinical Management of Poisoning and Drug Overdose*, 4th ed. Philadelphia: Saunders, 2007:1171.

Australian Pesticides and Veterinary Medicines Authority: Overview report: Neonicotinoids and the health of honey bees in Australia. 2014. https://apvma.gov.au/node/18541.

Benowitz N: Nicotine addiction. N Engl J Med 2010;362:2295.

Brito-Zerón P et al: Primary Sjögren syndrome: An update on current pharmacotherapy options and future directions. Expert Opin Pharmacother 2013;14:279.

Cahill K et al: Pharmacological interventions for smoking cessation: An overview and network meta-analysis. Cochrane Database Syst Rev 2013:5;CD009329.

Castellão-Santana LM et al: Tetanic facilitation of neuromuscular transmission by adenosine A2A and muscarinic M1 receptors is dependent on the uptake of choline via high-affinity transporters. Pharmacology 2019;103:38.

Chen L: In pursuit of the high-resolution structure of nicotinic acetylcholine receptors. J Physiol 2010;588:557.

Corradi J, Bourzat C: Understanding the bases of function and modulation of α7 nicotinic receptors: Implications for drug discovery. Mol Pharmacol 2016;90:288.

Dineley KT et al: Nicotinic ACh receptors as therapeutic targets in CNS disorders. Trends Pharmacol Sci 2015;36:96.

Ehlert FJ: Contractile role of M2 and M3 muscarinic receptors in gastrointestinal, airway and urinary bladder smooth muscle. Life Sci 2003;74:355.

Ferré S et al: G protein-coupled receptor oligomerization revisited: Functional and pharmacological perspectives. Pharmacol Rev 2014;66:413.

Giacobini E (editor): *Cholinesterases and Cholinesterase Inhibitors*. London: Martin Dunitz, 2000.

Gilhus NE: Myasthenia gravis. N Engl J Med 2016;375:2570.

Harvey RD, Belevych AE: Muscarinic regulation of cardiac ion channels. Br J Pharmacol 2003;139:1074.

Judge S, Bever C: Potassium channel blockers in multiple sclerosis: Neuronal Kv channels and effects of symptomatic treatment. Pharmacol Ther 2006;111:224.

Kim YB et al: Effects of neuromuscular presynaptic muscarinic M1 receptor blockade on rocuronium-induced neuromuscular blockade in immobilized tibialis anterior muscles. Clin Exp Pharmacol Physiol 2018;45:1309.

Kirsch GE, Narahashi T: 3,4-diaminopyridine. A potent new potassium channel blocker. Biophys J 1978;22:507.

Lamping KG et al: Muscarinic (M) receptors in coronary circulation. Arterioscler Thromb Vasc Biol 2004;24:1253.

Lazartigues E et al: Spontaneously hypertensive rats cholinergic hyper-responsiveness: Central and peripheral pharmacological mechanisms. Br J Pharmacol 1999; 127:1657.

Picciotto MR et al: It is not "either/or": Activation and desensitization of nicotinic acetylcholine receptors both contribute to behaviors related to nicotine addiction and mood. Prog Neurobiol 2008;84:329.

Richardson CE et al: Megacystis-microcolon-intestinal hypoperistalsis syndrome and the absence of the α3 nicotinic acetylcholine receptor subunit. Gastroenterology 2001;121:350.

Sánchez-Bayo F et al: Are bee diseases linked to pesticides?—A brief review. Environ Int 2016;89-90:7.

Schroeder C et al: Plasma exchange for primary autoimmune autonomic failure. N Engl J Med 2005;353:1585.

Sharma G, Vijayaraghavan S: Nicotinic cholinergic signaling in hippocampal astrocytes involves calcium-induced calcium release from intracellular stores. Proc Natl Acad Sci USA 2001;98:4148.

Shytle RD et al: Cholinergic modulation of microglial activation by α7 nicotinic receptors. J Neurochem 2004;89:337.

Tarr TB et al: Synaptic pathophysiology and treatment of Lambert-Eaton myasthenic syndrome. Mol Neurobiol 2015;52:456.

The Surgeon General: *Smoking and Health*. US Department of Health and Human Services, 1979.

Tomizawa M, Casida JE: Neonicotinoid insecticide toxicology: Mechanisms of selective action. Annu Rev Pharmacol Toxicol 2005;45:247.

Wess J et al: Muscarinic acetylcholine receptors: Mutant mice provide new insights for drug development. Nat Rev Drug Discov 2007;6:721.

Wing VC et al: Measuring cigarette smoking-induced cortical dopamine release: A [^{11}C]FLB-457 PET study. Neuropsychopharmacology 2015;40:1417.

CASE STUDY ANSWER

The patient's presentation is characteristic of poisoning by organophosphate cholinesterase inhibitors (see Chapter 58). Ask the coworker if he can identify the agent used. Decontaminate the patient by removal of clothing and washing affected areas. Ensure an open airway and ventilate with oxygen. For muscarinic effects, administer atropine (0.5–5 mg) intravenously until signs of muscarinic excess (dyspnea, lacrimation, confusion) subside. To treat nicotinic excess, infuse 2-PAM (initially a 1–2% solution in 15–30 min) followed by infusion of 1% solution (200–500 mg/h) until muscle fasciculations cease. Respiratory support is required because 2-PAM does not enter the central nervous system and may not reactivate "aged" organophosphate-cholinesterase complex. If needed, decontaminate the coworker and isolate all contaminated clothing.

CHAPTER

8

Cholinoceptor-Blocking Drugs

Todd W. Vanderah, PhD

CASE STUDY

JH, a 63-year-old architect, complains of urinary symptoms to his family physician. He has hypertension, and during the last 8 years, he has been adequately managed with a thiazide diuretic and an angiotensin-converting enzyme inhibitor. During the same period, JH developed signs of benign prostatic hypertrophy, which eventually required prostatectomy to relieve symptoms. He now complains that he has an increased urge to urinate as well as urinary frequency, and this has disrupted the pattern of his daily life. What do you suspect is the cause of JH's problem? What information would you gather to confirm your diagnosis? What treatment steps would you initiate?

Cholinoceptor antagonists, like the agonists, are divided into muscarinic and nicotinic subgroups on the basis of their specific receptor affinities. Ganglion blockers and neuromuscular junction blockers make up the antinicotinic drugs. The ganglion-blocking drugs have little clinical use and are discussed at the end of this chapter. Neuromuscular blockers are heavily used and are discussed in Chapter 27. This chapter emphasizes drugs that block muscarinic acetylcholine receptors.

Five subtypes of muscarinic receptors have been identified, primarily on the basis of data from ligand-binding and cDNA-cloning experiments (see Chapters 6 and 7). A standard terminology (M_1 through M_5) for these subtypes is now in common use, and evidence—based mostly on selective agonists and antagonists—indicates that functional differences exist between several of these subtypes. The X-ray crystallographic structures of the M_{1-5} subtypes of muscarinic receptors have been reported. The structures of the M_{1-5} receptors are very similar in the inactive state with inverse agonist or antagonist bound to the receptor. The binding pocket for orthosteric ligands lies well within the plane of the plasma membrane, and the amino acids composing the site are conserved among muscarinic receptor subtypes. This observation underscores the difficulty in identifying subtype-selective ligands. A structure forming a "lid" separates the orthosteric binding site from an upper cavity termed the "vestibule" (Figure 8–1). The binding site for allosteric ligands is the extracellular vestibule. Among the receptor subtypes, the extracellular vestibule is comprised of different amino acids that provide distinctive sites for binding by selective allosteric modulators. The M_1 receptor subtype is located on central nervous system (CNS) neurons, autonomic postganglionic cell bodies, and many presynaptic sites. M_2 receptors are located in the myocardium, smooth muscle organs, and some neuronal sites. M_3 receptors are most common on effector cell membranes, especially glandular and smooth muscle cells. M_4 and M_5 receptors are less prominent and appear to play a greater role in the CNS than in the periphery with the M_5 receptor potentially playing a role in drug addiction.

■ BASIC PHARMACOLOGY OF THE MUSCARINIC RECEPTOR-BLOCKING DRUGS

Muscarinic antagonists are sometimes called parasympatholytic because they block the effects of parasympathetic autonomic discharge. However, the term "antimuscarinic" is preferable.

Naturally occurring compounds with antimuscarinic effects have been known and used for millennia as medicines, poisons, and cosmetics. **Atropine** is the prototype of these drugs. Many similar plant alkaloids are known, and hundreds of synthetic antimuscarinic compounds have been prepared.

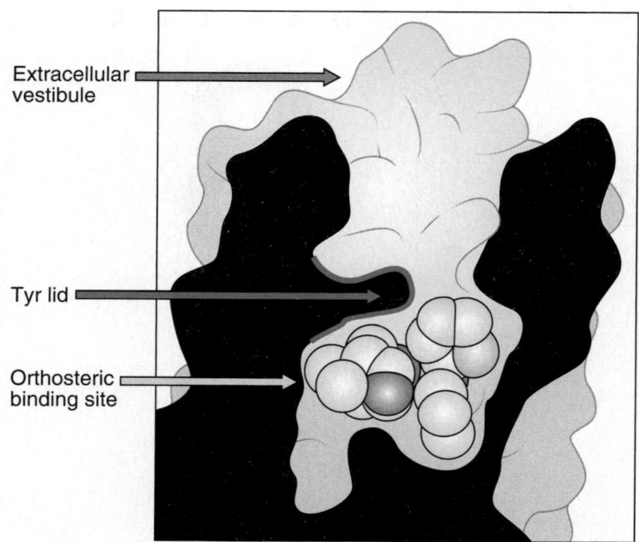

FIGURE 8–1 Upper portion of the M_3 receptor with a "lid" formed by tyrosine (Tyr) residues separating the cavity into an upper portion called the vestibule from the lower portion, with the orthosteric binding site depicted as occupied by tiotropium. The receptor is in black, tiotropium is in yellow, and the receptor surface is in green. (Reproduced with permission from Kruse AC, Hu J, Pan AC, et al. Structure and dynamics of the M3 muscarinic acetylcholine receptor. Nature. 2012;482(7386):552-556.)

Chemistry & Pharmacokinetics

A. Source and Chemistry

Atropine and its naturally occurring congeners are tertiary amine alkaloid esters of tropic acid (Figure 8–2). Atropine (hyoscyamine) is found in the plant *Atropa belladonna*, or deadly nightshade, and in *Datura stramonium*, also known as jimson-weed (Jamestown weed), sacred Datura, or thorn apple. **Scopolamine** (hyoscine) occurs in *Hyoscyamus niger*, or henbane, as the *l*(–) stereoisomer. Naturally occurring atropine is *l*(–)-hyoscyamine, but the compound readily racemizes, so the commercial material is racemic *d,l*-hyoscyamine. The *l*(–) isomers of both alkaloids are at least 100 times more potent than the *d*(+) isomers.

A variety of semisynthetic and fully synthetic molecules have antimuscarinic effects. The tertiary members of these classes (Figure 8–3) are often used for their effects on the eye or the CNS. Many antihistaminic (see Chapter 16), antipsychotic (see Chapter 29), and antidepressant (see Chapter 30) drugs have similar structures and, predictably, significant antimuscarinic effects.

Quaternary amine antimuscarinic agents (see Figure 8–3) have been developed to produce more peripheral effects and reduced CNS effects.

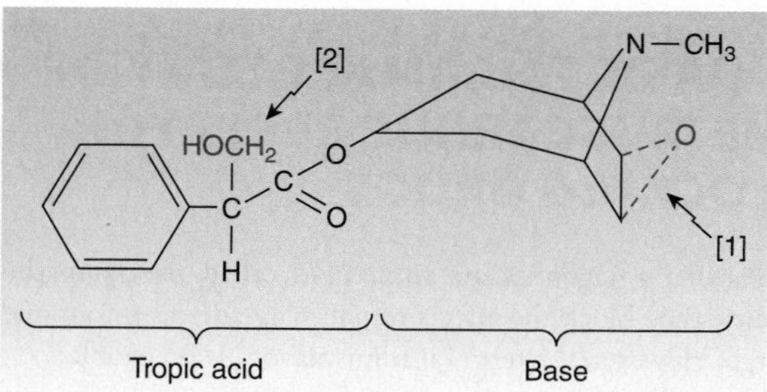

FIGURE 8–2 The structure of atropine (oxygen [red] at *[1]* is missing) or scopolamine (oxygen present). In homatropine, the hydroxymethyl at *[2]* is replaced by a hydroxyl group, and the oxygen at *[1]* is absent.

B. Absorption

Natural alkaloids and most tertiary antimuscarinic drugs are well absorbed from the gut and conjunctival membranes. When applied in a suitable vehicle, some (eg, scopolamine) are even absorbed across the skin (transdermal route). In contrast, only 10–30% of a dose of a quaternary antimuscarinic drug is absorbed after oral administration, reflecting the decreased lipid solubility of the charged molecule.

C. Distribution

Atropine and the other tertiary agents are widely distributed in the body. Significant levels are achieved in the CNS within 30 minutes to 1 hour, and this can limit the dose tolerated when the drug is taken for its peripheral effects. Scopolamine is rapidly and fully distributed into the CNS, where it has greater effects than most other antimuscarinic drugs. In contrast, the quaternary derivatives are poorly taken up by the brain and therefore are relatively free—at low doses—of CNS effects.

D. Metabolism and Excretion

After administration, the elimination of atropine from the blood occurs in two phases: the half-life ($t_{1/2}$) of the rapid phase is 2 hours and that of the slow phase is approximately 13 hours. About 50% of the dose is excreted unchanged in the urine. Most of the rest appears in the urine as hydrolysis and conjugation products. The drug's effect on parasympathetic function declines rapidly in all organs except the eye. Effects on the iris and ciliary muscle persist for ≥72 hours.

Pharmacodynamics

A. Mechanism of Action

Atropine causes reversible (surmountable) blockade (see Chapter 2) of cholinomimetic actions at muscarinic receptors; that is, blockade by a small dose of atropine can be overcome by a larger concentration of acetylcholine or equivalent muscarinic agonist. Mutation experiments suggest that aspartate in the third transmembrane segment of the heptahelical receptor forms an ionic bond with the nitrogen atom of acetylcholine; this amino acid is also required for binding of antimuscarinic drugs. When atropine binds to the muscarinic receptor, it prevents actions such as the release of inositol trisphosphate (IP_3) and the inhibition of adenylyl cyclase that are caused by muscarinic agonists (see Chapter 7). Muscarinic antagonists were traditionally viewed as neutral compounds that occupied the receptor and prevented agonist binding. Recent evidence indicates that muscarinic receptors are constitutively active, and most drugs that block the actions of acetylcholine

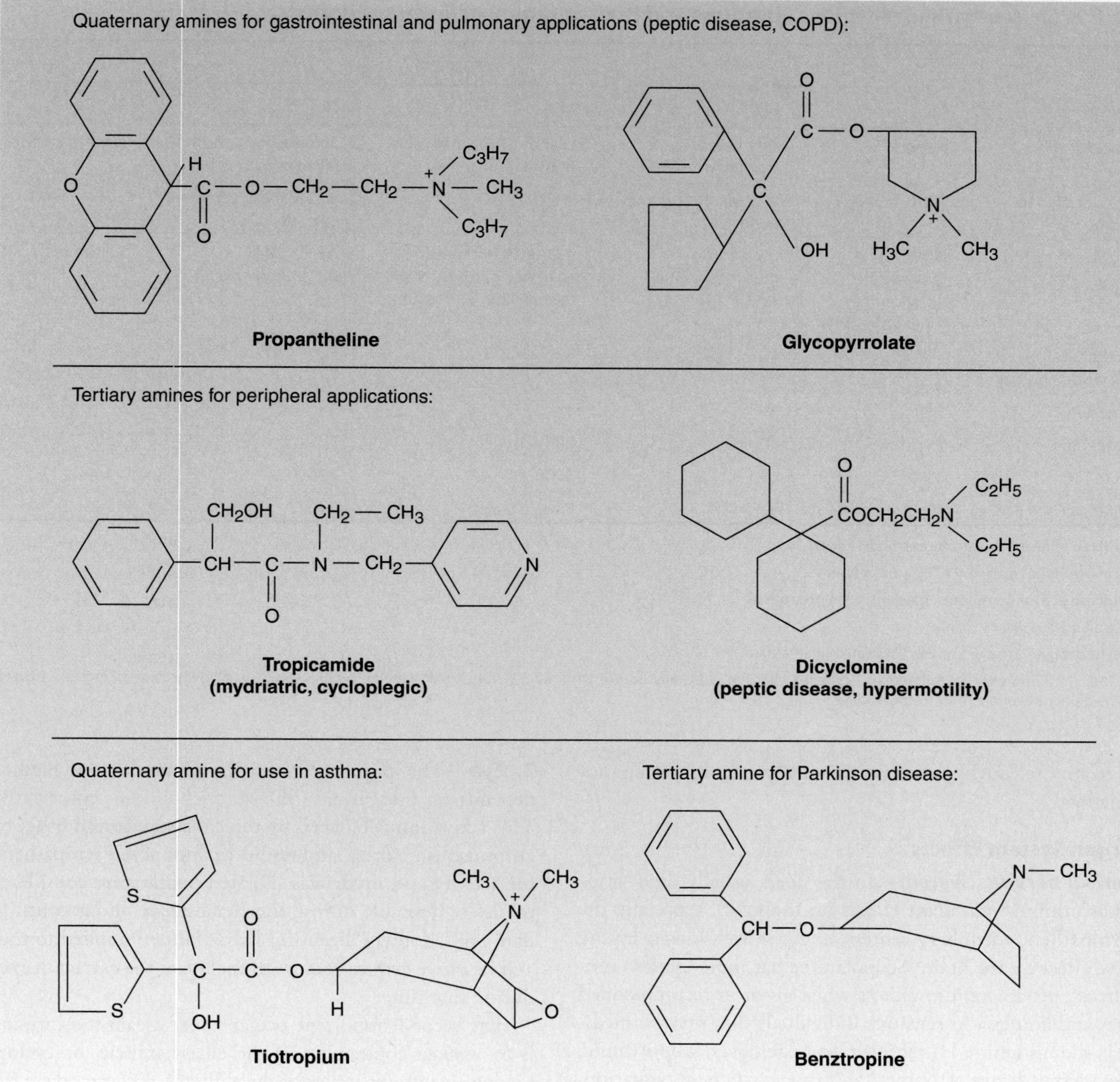

FIGURE 8–3 Structures of some semisynthetic and synthetic antimuscarinic drugs.

are inverse agonists (see Chapter 1) that shift the equilibrium to the inactive state of the receptor. Muscarinic blocking drugs that are antagonists or inverse agonists include atropine, pirenzepine, trihexyphenidyl, tiotropium, ipratropium, glycopyrrolate, dicyclomine, methscopolamine, as well as several experimental compounds, including AF-DX 116, AF-DX 384, 4-DAMP, ML381, and PCS1055 (Table 8–1).

The effectiveness of antimuscarinic drugs varies with the tissue and with the source of agonist. Tissues most sensitive to atropine are the salivary, bronchial, and sweat glands. Secretion of acid by the gastric parietal cells is the least sensitive. In most tissues, antimuscarinic agents block exogenously administered cholinoceptor agonists more effectively than endogenously released acetylcholine.

Atropine is highly selective for muscarinic receptors. Its potency at nicotinic receptors is much lower, and actions at nonmuscarinic receptors are generally undetectable clinically.

Atropine does not distinguish among the M_1–M_5 subgroups of muscarinic receptors. In contrast, other antimuscarinic drugs are moderately selective for one or another of these subgroups (see Table 8–1). Most synthetic antimuscarinic drugs are considerably less selective than atropine in interactions with nonmuscarinic receptors. For example, some quaternary amine antimuscarinic agents have significant ganglion-blocking actions (eg, propantheline), and others are potent histamine receptor blockers (eg, diphenhydramine). The antimuscarinic effects of other agents, eg, antipsychotic and antidepressant drugs, are noted as side effects and can be severe.

TABLE 8–1 Muscarinic receptor subgroups and their antagonists/inverse agonists.

	Subgroup				
Property	**M_1**	**M_2**	**M_3**	**M_4**	**M_5**
Primary locations	Nerves	Heart, nerves, smooth muscle	Glands, smooth muscle, endothelium	Spleen, duodenum, small intestine, testis	Placenta, testis
Dominant effector system	↑ IP_3, ↑ DAG	↓ cAMP, ↑ K^+ channel current	↑ IP_3, ↑ DAG	↓ cAMP, ↑ K^+ channel current	↑ IP_3, ↑ DAG
Antagonists	Pirenzepine, telenzepine, dicyclomine,[1] trihexyphenidyl[2]	Gallamine,[3] methoctramine, AF-DX 116[4]	4-DAMP,[4] darifenacin, solifenacin, oxybutynin, tolterodine, tiotropium	AF-DX 384, dicyclomine, PCS1055	Xanomeline, ML381
Approximate dissociation constant[5]					
Atropine	1	1	1	1	1
Pirenzepine	25	300	500	17	100
AF-DX 116	2000	65	4000	>1000	>1000
Darifenacin	70	55	8	22	10

[1]In clinical use as an intestinal antispasmodic agent.

[2]In clinical use in the treatment of Parkinson disease.

[3]In clinical use as a neuromuscular blocking agent (obsolete).

[4]Compound used in research only.

[5]Relative to atropine. Smaller numbers indicate higher affinity.

AF-DX 116, 11-({2-[(diethylamino)methyl]-1-piperidinyl}acetyl)-5,11-dihydro-6*H*-pyrido-[2,3-*b*](1,4)benzodiazepine-6-one; DAG, diacylglycerol; IP3, inositol trisphosphate; 4-DAMP, 4-diphenylacetoxy-*N*-methylpiperidine.

Their relative selectivity for muscarinic receptor subtypes has not been defined.

B. Organ System Effects

1. *Central nervous system*—In the doses usually used, atropine has minimal stimulant effects on the CNS, especially the parasympathetic medullary centers, and a slower, longer-lasting sedative effect on the brain. Scopolamine has more marked central effects, producing drowsiness when given in recommended dosages and amnesia in sensitive individuals that may be mediated via the histamine H_3 receptor. In toxic doses, scopolamine, and to a lesser degree atropine, can cause excitement, agitation, hallucinations, and coma.

The tremor of Parkinson disease is reduced by centrally acting antimuscarinic drugs, and atropine—in the form of belladonna extract—was one of the first drugs used in the therapy of this disease. As discussed in Chapter 28, parkinsonian tremor and rigidity seem to result from a *relative* excess of cholinergic activity because of a deficiency of dopaminergic activity in the basal ganglia-striatum system. The combination of an antimuscarinic agent with a dopamine precursor drug (levodopa) can sometimes provide more effective therapy than either drug alone. These antimuscarinic agents also reduce extrapyramidal symptoms and dystonias due to typical antipsychotic medications.

Vestibular disturbances thought to originate from the inner ear, especially motion sickness, appear to involve muscarinic (M_3 and M_4) cholinergic transmission and the production of endolymph. Scopolamine is often effective in preventing or reversing these disturbances.

2. *Eye*—The pupillary constrictor muscle (see Figure 6–9) depends on muscarinic (M_3) acetylcholine receptor activation. This activation is blocked by topical atropine and other tertiary antimuscarinic drugs and results in unopposed sympathetic dilator activity and **mydriasis**. Dilated pupils were considered cosmetically desirable during the Renaissance and account for the name belladonna ("beautiful lady," *Italian*) applied to the plant and its active extract because of the use of the extract as eye drops during that time.

The second important ocular effect of antimuscarinic drugs is to weaken contraction of the ciliary muscle, or **cycloplegia.** Cycloplegia results in loss of the ability to accommodate; the fully atropinized eye cannot focus for near vision.

Both mydriasis and cycloplegia are useful in ophthalmology. They are also potentially hazardous, since acute glaucoma may be induced in patients with a narrow anterior chamber angle.

A third ocular effect of antimuscarinic drugs is to reduce lacrimal secretion. Patients occasionally complain of dry or "sandy" eyes when receiving large doses of antimuscarinic drugs.

3. *Cardiovascular system*—The sinoatrial node is very sensitive to muscarinic receptor blockade. Moderate to high therapeutic doses of atropine cause tachycardia in the innervated and spontaneously beating heart by blockade of vagal slowing. However, lower doses often result in initial bradycardia before the effects of peripheral vagal block become manifest (Figure 8–4). This slowing may be due to block of prejunctional M_1 receptors (autoreceptors, see Figures 6–3 and 7–4A) on vagal postganglionic fibers that normally limit acetylcholine release in the sinus

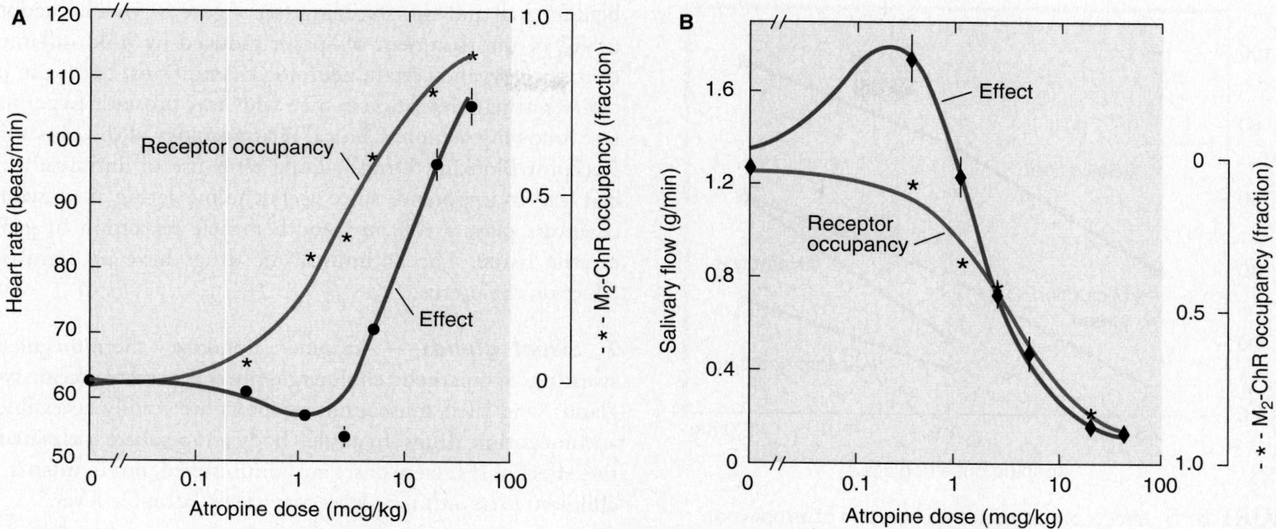

FIGURE 8–4 Effects of increasing doses of atropine on heart rate **(A)** and salivary flow **(B)** compared with muscarinic receptor occupancy in humans. The parasympathomimetic effect of low-dose atropine is attributed to blockade of prejunctional muscarinic receptors that suppress acetylcholine release. (Reproduced with permission from Wellstein A, Pitschner HF. Complex dose-response curves of atropine in man explained by different functions of M1- and M2-cholinoceptors. Naunyn Schmiedebergs Arch Pharmacol. 1988;338(1):19-27.)

node and other tissues. The same mechanisms operate in the atrioventricular node; in the presence of high vagal tone, atropine can significantly reduce the PR interval of the electrocardiogram by blocking muscarinic receptors in the atrioventricular node. Muscarinic effects on atrial muscle are similarly blocked, but these effects are of no clinical significance except in atrial flutter and fibrillation. The ventricles are less affected by antimuscarinic drugs at therapeutic levels because of a lesser degree of vagal control. In toxic concentrations, the drugs can cause intraventricular conduction block that has been attributed to a local anesthetic action.

Most blood vessels, except those in thoracic and abdominal viscera, receive no direct innervation from the parasympathetic system. However, parasympathetic nerve stimulation dilates coronary arteries, and sympathetic cholinergic nerves cause vasodilation in the skeletal muscle vascular bed (see Chapter 6). Atropine can block this vasodilation. Furthermore, almost all vessels contain endothelial muscarinic receptors that mediate vasodilation (see Chapter 7). These receptors are readily blocked by antimuscarinic drugs. At toxic doses, and in some individuals at normal doses, antimuscarinic agents cause cutaneous vasodilation, especially in the upper portion of the body. The mechanism is unknown.

The net cardiovascular effects of atropine in patients with normal hemodynamics are not dramatic: Tachycardia may occur, but there is little effect on blood pressure. However, the cardiovascular effects of administered direct-acting muscarinic agonists are easily prevented.

4. *Respiratory system*—Both smooth muscle and secretory glands of the airway receive vagal innervation and contain muscarinic receptors. Even in normal individuals, administration of atropine can cause some bronchodilation and reduce secretion. The effect is more significant in patients with airway disease, although the antimuscarinic drugs are not as useful as the β-adrenoceptor stimulants in the treatment of asthma (see Chapter 20). The effectiveness of nonselective antimuscarinic drugs in treating chronic obstructive pulmonary disease (COPD) is limited because block of autoinhibitory M_2 receptors on postganglionic parasympathetic nerves can oppose the bronchodilation caused by block of M_3 receptors on airway smooth muscle. Nevertheless, antimuscarinic agents selective for M_3 receptors are valuable in some patients with asthma and in many with COPD.

Antimuscarinic drugs are frequently used before the administration of inhalant anesthetics to reduce the accumulation of secretions in the trachea and the possibility of laryngospasm.

5. *Gastrointestinal tract*—Blockade of muscarinic receptors has dramatic effects on motility and some of the secretory functions of the gut. However, even complete muscarinic block cannot abolish activity in this organ system, since local hormones and noncholinergic neurons in the enteric nervous system (see Chapters 6 and 62) also modulate gastrointestinal function. As in other tissues, exogenously administered muscarinic stimulants are more effectively blocked than are the effects of parasympathetic (vagal) nerve activity. The removal of autoinhibition, a negative feedback mechanism by which neural acetylcholine suppresses its own release, might explain the lower efficacy of antimuscarinic drugs against the effects of endogenous acetylcholine.

Antimuscarinic drugs have marked effects on salivary secretion; dry mouth occurs frequently in patients taking antimuscarinic drugs for Parkinson disease or urinary conditions (Figure 8–5). Gastric secretion is blocked less effectively: the volume and amount of

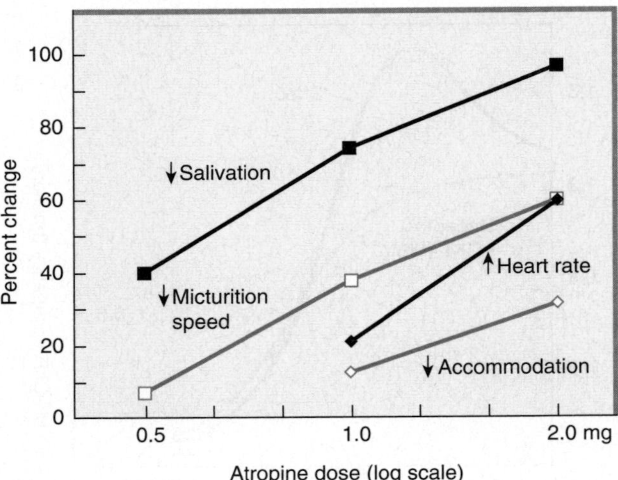

FIGURE 8–5 Effects of subcutaneous injection of atropine on salivation, speed of micturition (voiding), heart rate, and accommodation in normal adults. Note that salivation is the most sensitive of these variables, accommodation the least. (Data from Herxheimer A: A comparison of some atropine-like drugs in man with particular reference to their end-organ specificity. Br J Pharmacol Chemother 1958 Jun;13(2):184-192.)

acid, pepsin, and mucin are all reduced, but large doses of atropine may be required. Basal secretion is blocked more effectively than that stimulated by food, nicotine, or alcohol. Pirenzepine and a more potent analog, telenzepine, reduce gastric acid secretion with fewer adverse effects than atropine and other less selective agents. This was thought to result from a selective blockade of excitatory M_1 muscarinic receptors on vagal ganglion cells innervating the stomach, as suggested by their high ratio of M_1 to M_3 affinity (see Table 8–1). However, carbachol was found to stimulate gastric acid secretion in M_1 receptor knockout animals; M_3 receptors were implicated and pirenzepine opposed this effect of carbachol, an indication that pirenzepine is selective but not specific for M_1 receptors. The mechanism of vagal regulation of gastric acid secretion likely involves multiple muscarinic receptor–dependent pathways. Pirenzepine and telenzepine are investigational in the USA. Pancreatic and intestinal secretion are little affected by atropine; these processes are primarily under hormonal rather than vagal control.

Gastrointestinal smooth muscle motility is affected from the stomach to the colon. In general, antimuscarinic drugs diminish the tone and propulsive movements; the walls of the viscera are relaxed. Therefore, gastric emptying time is prolonged, and intestinal transit time is lengthened. Diarrhea due to overdosage with parasympathomimetic agents is readily stopped using antimuscarinics, and even diarrhea caused by nonautonomic agents can usually be temporarily controlled. However, intestinal "paralysis" induced by antimuscarinic drugs is temporary; local mechanisms within the enteric nervous system usually reestablish at least some peristalsis after 1–3 days of antimuscarinic drug therapy.

6. *Genitourinary tract*—The antimuscarinic action of atropine and its analogs relaxes smooth muscle of the ureters and bladder wall and slows voiding (see Figure 8–5). This action is useful in the treatment of spasm induced by mild inflammation, surgery, and certain neurologic conditions, but it can precipitate urinary retention in men who have prostatic hyperplasia (see following section, Clinical Pharmacology of the Muscarinic Receptor-Blocking Drugs). Long-term use of antimuscarinics can lead to impotence since acetylcholine acting at muscarinic receptors plays a role in smooth muscle relaxation in genital erectile tissue. The antimuscarinic drugs have no significant effect on the uterus.

7. *Sweat glands* —Atropine suppresses thermoregulatory sweating. Sympathetic cholinergic fibers innervate eccrine sweat glands, and their muscarinic receptors are readily accessible to antimuscarinic drugs. In adults, body temperature is elevated by this effect only if large doses are administered, but in infants and children, even ordinary doses may cause "atropine fever."

■ CLINICAL PHARMACOLOGY OF THE MUSCARINIC RECEPTOR-BLOCKING DRUGS

Therapeutic Applications

The antimuscarinic drugs have applications in several of the major organ systems and in the treatment of poisoning by muscarinic agonists.

A. Central Nervous System Disorders

1. *Parkinson disease*—The treatment of Parkinson disease (see Chapter 28) is often an exercise in polypharmacy, since no single agent is fully effective over the course of the disease. Most antimuscarinic drugs promoted for this application (see Table 28–1) were developed before levodopa became available. Their use is accompanied by all of the adverse effects described below, but the drugs remain useful as adjunctive therapy for reducing resting tremor in some patients.

2. *Motion sickness*—Certain vestibular disorders respond to antimuscarinic drugs (and to antihistaminic agents with antimuscarinic effects). Scopolamine is one of the oldest remedies for seasickness and is as effective as recently introduced agents. It can be given by injection or by mouth or as a transdermal patch. The patch formulation produces significant blood levels over 48–72 hours. Useful doses by any route usually cause significant sedation and dry mouth.

B. Ophthalmologic Disorders

Accurate measurement of refractive error in uncooperative patients, eg, young children, requires ciliary paralysis. Also, mydriasis greatly facilitates ophthalmoscopic examination of the retina. Therefore, antimuscarinic agents, administered topically as eye drops or ointment, are very helpful in doing a complete examination. For adults and older children, the shorter-acting drugs are preferred (Table 8–2). For younger children, the greater efficacy

TABLE 8–2 Antimuscarinic drugs used in ophthalmology.

Drug	Duration of Effect	Usual Concentration (%)
Atropine	5–6 days	0.5–1
Scopolamine	3–7 days	0.25
Homatropine	12–24 hours	2–5
Cyclopentolate	3–6 hours	0.5–2
Tropicamide	15–60 min	0.5–1

of atropine is sometimes necessary, but the possibility of antimuscarinic poisoning is correspondingly increased. Drug loss from the conjunctival sac via the nasolacrimal duct into the nasopharynx can be diminished by the use of the ointment form rather than drops. Formerly, ophthalmic antimuscarinic drugs were selected from the tertiary amine subgroup to ensure good penetration after conjunctival application. However, glycopyrrolate, a quaternary agent, is as rapid in onset and as long-lasting as atropine.

Antimuscarinic drugs should never be used for the sole purpose of mydriasis unless cycloplegia or prolonged action is required. Alpha-adrenoceptor stimulant drugs, eg, phenylephrine, produce a short-lasting mydriasis that is usually sufficient for funduscopic examination (see Chapter 9).

A second ophthalmologic use is to prevent synechia (adhesion) formation in uveitis and iritis. The longer-lasting preparations, especially homatropine, are valuable for this indication.

C. Respiratory Disorders

The use of atropine became part of routine preoperative medication when anesthetics such as ether were used, because these irritant anesthetics markedly increased airway secretions and were associated with frequent episodes of laryngospasm. Preanesthetic injection of atropine or scopolamine could prevent these hazardous effects. Scopolamine also produces significant amnesia for the events associated with surgery and obstetric delivery, an adverse effect that was considered desirable. On the other hand, urinary retention and intestinal hypomotility following surgery were often exacerbated by antimuscarinic drugs. Newer inhalational anesthetics are far less irritating to the airways.

Patients with **COPD,** a condition that occurs more frequently in older patients, particularly chronic smokers, benefit from bronchodilators, especially antimuscarinic agents. **Ipratropium, tiotropium** (see Figure 8–3), **aclidinium,** and **umeclidinium,** synthetic analogs of atropine, are used as inhalational drugs in COPD either alone or in combination with a long-acting β-adrenoceptor agonist. The aerosol route of administration has the advantage of maximal concentration at the bronchial target tissue with reduced systemic effects. This application is discussed in greater detail in Chapter 20. Tiotropium ($t_{1/2}$ 25 hours) and umeclidinium ($t_{1/2}$ 11 hours) have a longer bronchodilator action than ipratropium ($t_{1/2}$ 2 hours) and can be given once daily because they dissociate slowly from M_3 receptors. Aclidinium ($t_{1/2}$ 6 hours) is administered twice daily. Glycopyrrolate ($t_{1/2}$ 1.2 hours) is now available in inhalational form for twice-daily treatment of COPD. Tiotropium reduces the incidence of COPD exacerbations and is a useful adjunct in pulmonary rehabilitation to increase exercise tolerance. The hyperactive neural bronchoconstrictor reflex present in most individuals with **asthma** is mediated by the vagus, acting on muscarinic receptors on bronchial smooth muscle cells. Ipratropium and tiotropium are also used as inhalational drugs in asthma.

D. Cardiovascular Disorders

Marked reflex vagal discharge sometimes accompanies the pain of myocardial infarction (eg, vasovagal attack) and may depress sinoatrial or atrioventricular node function sufficiently to impair cardiac output. Parenteral atropine or a similar antimuscarinic drug is appropriate therapy in this situation. Rare individuals without other detectable cardiac disease have hyperactive carotid sinus reflexes and may experience faintness or even syncope as a result of vagal discharge in response to pressure on the neck, eg, from a tight collar. Such individuals may benefit from the judicious use of atropine or a related antimuscarinic agent.

Pathophysiology can influence muscarinic activity in other ways as well. Circulating autoantibodies against the second extracellular loop of cardiac M_2 muscarinic receptors have been detected in some patients with idiopathic dilated cardiomyopathy and those afflicted with Chagas disease caused by the protozoan *Trypanosoma cruzi*. Patients with Graves disease (hyperthyroidism) also have such autoantibodies that may facilitate the development of atrial fibrillation since these antibodies tend to act like agonists. These antibodies exert parasympathomimetic actions on the heart that are prevented by atropine. In animals immunized with a peptide from the second extracellular loop of the M_2 receptor, the antibody is an allosteric modulator of the receptor. Although their role in the pathology of heart diseases is unknown, these antibodies have provided clues to the molecular basis of receptor activation because their site of action differs from the orthosteric site where acetylcholine binds (see Chapter 2) and they favor the formation of receptor dimers.

E. Gastrointestinal Disorders

Antimuscarinic agents were used for peptic ulcer disease in the USA but are now obsolete for this indication (see Chapter 62). Antimuscarinic agents can provide some relief in the treatment of common traveler's diarrhea and other mild or self-limited conditions of hypermotility. They are often combined with an opioid antidiarrheal drug, an extremely effective therapy. In this combination, however, the very low dosage of the antimuscarinic drug functions primarily to discourage abuse of the opioid agent. The classic combination of atropine with diphenoxylate, a nonanalgesic congener of meperidine, is available under many names (eg, Lomotil) in both tablet and liquid form (see Chapter 62).

F. Urinary Disorders

Atropine and other antimuscarinic drugs have been used to provide symptomatic relief in the treatment of urinary urgency caused by minor inflammatory bladder disorders (Table 8–3). However, specific antimicrobial therapy is essential in bacterial cystitis. In the human urinary bladder, M_2 and M_3 receptors are expressed predominantly with the M_3 subtype mediating direct activation

TABLE 8–3 Antimuscarinic drugs used in gastrointestinal and genitourinary conditions.

Drug	Usual Dosage
Quaternary amines	
Anisotropine	50 mg tid
Clidinium	2.5 mg tid–qid
Mepenzolate	25–50 mg qid
Methscopolamine	2.5 mg qid
Oxyphenonium	5–10 mg qid
Propantheline	15 mg qid
Trospium	20 mg bid
Tertiary amines	
Atropine	0.4 mg tid–qid
Darifenacin	7.5 mg daily
Dicyclomine	10–20 mg qid
Oxybutynin	5 mg tid
Scopolamine	0.4 mg tid
Solifenacin	5 mg daily
Tolterodine	2 mg bid

of contraction. As in intestinal smooth muscle, the M_2 subtype appears to act indirectly by inhibiting relaxation by norepinephrine and epinephrine.

Receptors for acetylcholine on the urothelium (the epithelial lining of the urinary tract) and on afferent nerves as well as the detrusor muscle provide a broad basis for the action of antimuscarinic drugs in the treatment of overactive bladder. **Oxybutynin,** which is somewhat selective for M_3 receptors, is used to relieve bladder spasm after urologic surgery, eg, prostatectomy. It is also valuable in reducing involuntary voiding in patients with neurologic disease, eg, children with meningomyelocele. Oral oxybutynin or instillation of the drug by catheter into the bladder in such patients appears to improve bladder capacity and continence and to reduce infection and renal damage. Transdermally applied oxybutynin or its oral extended-release formulation reduces the need for multiple daily doses. **Trospium,** a nonselective antagonist, has been approved and is comparable in efficacy and adverse effects to oxybutynin. **Darifenacin** and **solifenacin** are antagonists that have greater selectivity for M_3 receptors than oxybutynin or trospium. Darifenacin and solifenacin, M_3-selective antimuscarinics, have the advantage of once-daily dosing because of their long half-lives. **Tolterodine,** an M_2- and M_3-selective antimuscarinic, and **fesoterodine,** an M_3-selective antimuscarinic that is a prodrug, are available for use in adults with urinary incontinence. They have many of the qualities of darifenacin and solifenacin and are available in extended-release tablets. **Propiverine,** a newer antimuscarinic agent with efficacy comparable to other muscarinic antagonists, has been approved for urinary incontinence in Europe but not in the USA. The convenience of the newer and longer-acting drugs has not been accompanied by improvements in overall efficacy or by reductions in adverse effects such as dry mouth. Muscarinic antagonists have an adjunct role in therapy of benign prostatic hypertrophy when bladder symptoms (increased urinary frequency) occur. Treatment with an α-adrenoceptor antagonist combined with a muscarinic antagonist resulted in a greater reduction in bladder storage problems and urinary frequency than treatment with an α-adrenoceptor antagonist alone.

An alternative treatment for urinary incontinence refractory to antimuscarinic drugs is intrabladder injection of botulinum toxin A. Botulinum toxin A is reported to reduce urinary incontinence for several months after a single treatment by interfering with the co-release of ATP with neuronal acetylcholine (see Figure 6–3). Blockade of the activation by ATP of purinergic receptors on sensory nerves in the urothelium may account for a large part of this effect. Botulinum toxin has been approved for use in patients who do not tolerate or are refractory to antimuscarinic drugs.

Imipramine, a tricyclic antidepressant drug with strong antimuscarinic actions, has long been used to reduce incontinence in institutionalized elderly patients. It is moderately effective but causes significant CNS toxicity.

Antimuscarinic agents have also been used in urolithiasis to relieve the painful ureteral smooth muscle spasm caused by passage of the stone. However, their usefulness in this condition is debatable.

G. Cholinergic Poisoning

Severe cholinergic excess is a medical emergency, especially in rural communities where cholinesterase inhibitor insecticides are commonly used and in cultures where wild mushrooms are frequently eaten. The potential use of cholinesterase inhibitors as chemical warfare "nerve gases" also requires an awareness of the methods for treating acute poisoning (see Chapter 58).

1. *Antimuscarinic therapy*—Both the nicotinic and the muscarinic effects of the cholinesterase inhibitors can be life-threatening. Unfortunately, there is no effective method for directly reversing the nicotinic effects of cholinesterase inhibition, because nicotinic agonists *and* antagonists cause blockade of transmission (see Chapter 27). To reverse the muscarinic effects, a tertiary (not quaternary) amine drug must be used (preferably atropine) to treat the CNS effects as well as the peripheral effects of the organophosphate inhibitors. Large doses of atropine may be needed to oppose the muscarinic effects of extremely potent agents like parathion and chemical warfare nerve gases: 1–2 mg of atropine sulfate may be given intravenously every 5–15 minutes until signs of effect (dry mouth, reversal of miosis) appear. The drug may have to be given many times, since the acute effects of the cholinesterase inhibitor may last 24–48 hours or longer. In this life-threatening situation, as much as 1 g of atropine per day may be required for as long as 1 month for full control of muscarinic excess.

2. *Cholinesterase regenerator compounds*—A second class of compounds, composed of substituted oximes capable of regenerating active enzyme from the organophosphorus-cholinesterase complex, also is available to treat organophosphorus

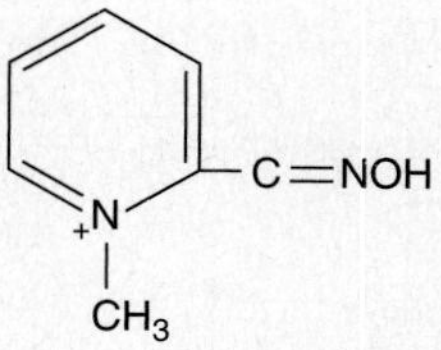

Pralidoxime 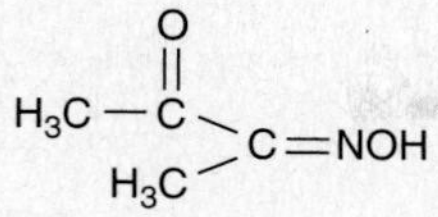 **Diacetylmonoxime**

poisoning. These oxime agents include **pralidoxime** (PAM), **diacetylmonoxime** (DAM), obidoxime, and others.

Organophosphates cause phosphorylation of the serine OH group at the active site of cholinesterase. The oxime group (=NOH) has a very high affinity for the phosphorus atom, for which it competes with serine OH. These oximes can hydrolyze the phosphorylated enzyme and regenerate active enzyme from the organophosphorus-cholinesterase complex if the complex has not "aged" (see Chapter 7). Pralidoxime is the most extensively studied—in humans—of the agents shown and the only one available for clinical use in the USA. It is most effective in regenerating the cholinesterase associated with skeletal muscle neuromuscular junctions. Pralidoxime and obidoxime are ineffective in reversing the central effects of organophosphate poisoning because each has positively charged quaternary ammonium groups that prevent entry into the CNS. Diacetylmonoxime, on the other hand, crosses the blood-brain barrier and, in experimental animals, can regenerate some of the CNS cholinesterase.

Pralidoxime is administered by intravenous infusion, 1–2 g given over 15–30 minutes. In spite of the likelihood of aging of the phosphate-enzyme complex, recent reports suggest that administration of multiple doses of pralidoxime over several days may be useful in severe poisoning. In excessive doses, pralidoxime can induce neuromuscular weakness and other adverse effects. Pralidoxime is *not* recommended for the reversal of inhibition of acetylcholinesterase by carbamate inhibitors. Further details of treatment of anticholinesterase toxicity are given in Chapter 58.

A third approach to protection against excessive acetylcholinesterase inhibition is *pretreatment* with intermediate-acting enzyme inhibitors that transiently occupy the active site to prevent binding of the much longer-acting organophosphate inhibitor. This prophylaxis can be achieved with pyridostigmine but is reserved for situations in which possibly lethal poisoning is anticipated, eg, chemical warfare (see Chapter 7). Simultaneous use of atropine is required to control muscarinic excess.

The use of biological scavengers has emerged as an adjunct to oximes in the reactivation of acetylcholinesterase inactivated by organophosphates. Human acetylcholinesterase, acting catalytically, increased the effectiveness of PAM in reactivating the enzyme. Butyrylcholinesterase can achieve the same effect, but it acts stoichiometrically, and thus large amounts of this bioscavenger are required. (Another use for butyrylcholinesterase is in the treatment of cocaine toxicity because butyrylcholinesterase displays cocaine hydrolase activity. The catalytic efficiency of human butyrylcholinesterase against cocaine has been increased by mutation of the enzyme such that it can prevent the effect of a lethal dose of cocaine in experimental animals.)

Mushroom poisoning has traditionally been divided into rapid-onset and delayed-onset types. The rapid-onset type is usually apparent within 30 minutes to 2 hours after ingestion of the mushrooms and can be caused by a variety of toxins. Some of these produce simple upset stomach; others can have disulfiram-like effects; some cause hallucinations; and a few mushrooms (eg, *Inocybe* species) can produce signs of muscarinic excess: nausea, vomiting, diarrhea, urinary urgency, sweating, salivation, and sometimes bronchoconstriction. Parenteral atropine, 1–2 mg, is effective treatment in such intoxications. Despite its name, *Amanita muscaria* contains not only muscarine (the alkaloid was named after the mushroom), but also numerous other alkaloids, including antimuscarinic agents, and ingestion of *A muscaria* often causes signs of atropine poisoning, not muscarine excess.

Delayed-onset mushroom poisoning, usually caused by *Amanita phalloides, Amanita virosa, Galerina autumnalis*, or *Galerina marginata*, manifests its first symptoms 6–12 hours after ingestion. Although the initial symptoms usually include nausea and vomiting, the major toxicity involves hepatic and renal cellular injury by amatoxins that inhibit RNA polymerase. Atropine is of no value in this form of mushroom poisoning (see Chapter 58).

H. Other Applications

Hyperhidrosis (excessive sweating) is sometimes reduced by antimuscarinic agents, eg, **propantheline bromide.** However, relief is incomplete at best, probably because apocrine rather than eccrine glands are usually involved.

Adverse Effects

Treatment with atropine or its congeners directed at one organ system almost always induces undesirable effects in other organ systems. Thus, mydriasis and cycloplegia are adverse effects when an antimuscarinic agent is used to reduce gastrointestinal secretion or motility, even though they are therapeutic effects when the drug is used in ophthalmology.

At higher concentrations, atropine causes block of all parasympathetic functions. However, atropine is a remarkably safe drug *in adults*. Atropine poisoning has occurred as a result of attempted suicide, but most cases are due to attempts to induce hallucinations. Poisoned individuals manifest dry mouth, mydriasis, tachycardia, hot and flushed skin, agitation, and delirium for as long as 1 week. Body temperature is frequently elevated. These effects are memorialized in the adage, "dry as a bone, blind as a bat, red as a beet, mad as a hatter."

Unfortunately, children, especially infants, are very sensitive to the hyperthermic effects of atropine. Although accidental administration of more than 400 mg has been followed by recovery, deaths have followed doses as small as 2 mg. Therefore, atropine should be considered a highly dangerous drug when overdose occurs in infants or children.

Overdoses of atropine or its congeners are generally treated symptomatically (see Chapter 58). Poison control experts discourage the use of physostigmine or another cholinesterase inhibitor to reverse the effects of atropine overdose because symptomatic management is more effective and less dangerous. When physostigmine is deemed necessary, *small* doses are given *slowly* intravenously (1–4 mg in adults, 0.5–1 mg in children). Symptomatic treatment may require temperature control with cooling blankets and seizure control with diazepam.

Poisoning caused by high doses of quaternary antimuscarinic drugs is associated with all of the peripheral signs of parasympathetic blockade but few or none of the CNS effects of atropine. These more polar drugs may cause significant ganglionic blockade, however, with marked orthostatic hypotension (see below). Treatment of the antimuscarinic effects, if required, can be carried out with a quaternary cholinesterase inhibitor such as neostigmine. Control of hypotension may require the administration of a sympathomimetic drug such as phenylephrine.

Recent evidence indicates that some centrally acting drugs (tricyclic antidepressants, selective serotonin reuptake inhibitors, anti-anxiety agents, antihistamines) with antimuscarinic actions impair memory and cognition in older patients.

Contraindications

Contraindications to the use of antimuscarinic drugs are relative, not absolute. Obvious muscarinic excess, especially that caused by cholinesterase inhibitors, can always be treated with atropine.

Antimuscarinic drugs are contraindicated in patients with glaucoma, especially angle-closure glaucoma. Even systemic use of moderate doses may precipitate angle closure (and acute glaucoma) in patients with shallow anterior chambers.

In elderly men, antimuscarinic drugs should always be used with caution and should be avoided in those with a history of prostatic hyperplasia.

Because the antimuscarinic drugs slow gastric emptying, they may *increase* symptoms in patients with gastric ulcer, and therefore, nonselective antimuscarinic agents should never be used to treat acid-peptic disease (see Chapter 62).

■ BASIC & CLINICAL PHARMACOLOGY OF THE GANGLION-BLOCKING DRUGS

Ganglion-blocking agents competitively block the action of acetylcholine and similar agonists at neuronal nicotinic receptors of both parasympathetic and sympathetic autonomic ganglia. Some members of the group also block the ion channel that is gated by the nicotinic cholinoceptor. The ganglion-blocking drugs are important and used in pharmacologic and physiologic research because they can block all autonomic outflow. However, their lack of selectivity confers such a broad range of undesirable effects that they have limited clinical use.

Chemistry & Pharmacokinetics

All ganglion-blocking drugs of interest are synthetic amines. **Tetraethylammonium (TEA),** the first to be recognized as having this action, has a very short duration of action. **Hexamethonium ("C6")** was developed and was introduced clinically as the first drug effective for management of hypertension. As shown in Figure 8–6, there is an obvious relationship between the structures of the agonist acetylcholine and the nicotinic antagonists tetraethylammonium and hexamethonium. Decamethonium, the "C10" analog of hexamethonium, is a depolarizing neuromuscular blocking agent.

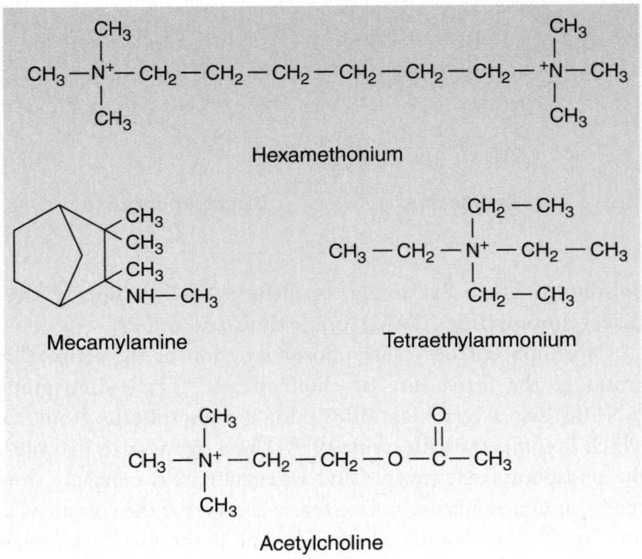

Hexamethonium: $(CH_3)_3N^+-CH_2-CH_2-CH_2-CH_2-CH_2-CH_2-{}^+N(CH_3)_3$

Mecamylamine

Tetraethylammonium: $(CH_3-CH_2)_4N^+$

Acetylcholine: $(CH_3)_3N^+-CH_2-CH_2-O-C(=O)-CH_3$

FIGURE 8–6 Some ganglion-blocking drugs. Acetylcholine is shown for reference.

Mecamylamine, a secondary amine, was developed to improve the degree and extent of absorption from the gastrointestinal tract because the quaternary amine ganglion-blocking compounds were poorly and erratically absorbed after oral administration. Trimethaphan, a short-acting, polar, ganglion-blocking drug, is no longer available for clinical use.

Pharmacodynamics

A. Mechanism of Action

Ganglionic nicotinic receptors, like those of the skeletal muscle neuromuscular junction, are subject to both depolarizing and nondepolarizing blockade (see Chapters 7 and 27). Nicotine itself, carbamoylcholine, and even acetylcholine (if amplified with a cholinesterase inhibitor) can produce depolarizing ganglion block.

Drugs now used as ganglion-blocking drugs are classified as nondepolarizing competitive antagonists. Blockade can be surmounted by increasing the concentration of an agonist, eg, acetylcholine. However, hexamethonium actually produces most of its blockade by occupying sites in or on the nicotinic ion channel, not by occupying the cholinoceptor itself.

B. Organ System Effects

1. *Central nervous system*—Mecamylamine, unlike the quaternary amine agents and trimethaphan, crosses the blood-brain barrier and readily enters the CNS. Sedation, tremor, choreiform movements, and mental aberrations have been reported as effects of mecamylamine.

2. *Eye*—The ganglion-blocking drugs cause a predictable cycloplegia with loss of accommodation because the ciliary muscle receives innervation primarily from the parasympathetic nervous system. The effect on the pupil is not so easily predicted, since the iris receives both sympathetic innervation (mediating pupillary dilation) and parasympathetic innervation (mediating pupillary constriction). Ganglionic blockade often causes moderate dilation of the pupil because parasympathetic tone usually dominates this tissue.

3. *Cardiovascular system*—Blood vessels receive chiefly vasoconstrictor fibers from the sympathetic nervous system; therefore, ganglionic blockade causes a marked decrease in arteriolar and venomotor tone. The blood pressure may fall precipitously because both peripheral vascular resistance and venous return are decreased (see Figure 6–7). Hypotension is especially marked in the upright position (orthostatic or postural hypotension), because postural reflexes that normally prevent venous pooling are blocked.

Cardiac effects include diminished contractility and, because the sinoatrial node is usually dominated by the parasympathetic nervous system, a moderate tachycardia.

4. *Gastrointestinal tract*—Secretion is reduced, although not enough to treat peptic disease effectively. Motility is profoundly inhibited, and constipation can be marked.

5. *Other systems*—Genitourinary smooth muscle is partially dependent on autonomic innervation for normal function. Therefore, ganglionic blockade causes hesitancy in urination and may precipitate urinary retention in men with prostatic hyperplasia. Sexual function is impaired in that both erection and ejaculation may be prevented by moderate doses.

Thermoregulatory sweating is reduced by the ganglion-blocking drugs. However, hyperthermia is not a problem except in very warm environments, because cutaneous vasodilation is usually sufficient to maintain a normal body temperature.

6. *Response to autonomic drugs*—Patients receiving ganglion-blocking drugs are fully responsive to autonomic drugs acting on muscarinic, α-, and β-adrenoceptors because these effector cell receptors are not blocked. In fact, responses may be exaggerated or even reversed (eg, intravenously administered norepinephrine may cause tachycardia rather than bradycardia), because homeostatic reflexes, which normally moderate autonomic responses, are absent.

Clinical Applications & Toxicity

Ganglion blocking drugs are used rarely because more selective autonomic blocking agents are available. Mecamylamine blocks central nicotinic receptors and has been advocated as a possible adjunct with the transdermal nicotine patch to reduce nicotine craving in patients attempting to quit smoking. The toxicity of the ganglion-blocking drugs is limited to the autonomic effects already described. For most patients, these effects are intolerable except for acute use.

SUMMARY Drugs with Anticholinergic Actions

Subclass, Drug	Mechanism of Action	Effects	Clinical Applications	Pharmacokinetics, Toxicities, Interactions
MOTION SICKNESS DRUGS				
• Scopolamine	Competitive antagonism at muscarinic receptors, additional $5HT_3$ antagonist mechanism in CNS	Reduces vertigo, postoperative nausea	Prevention of motion sickness and postoperative nausea and vomiting	Transdermal patch used for motion sickness • IM injection for postoperative use • *Toxicity:* Tachycardia, blurred vision, xerostomia, delirium • *Interactions:* With other antimuscarinics
GASTROINTESTINAL DISORDERS				
• Dicyclomine	Competitive antagonism at M_1 and M_4 receptors	Reduces smooth muscle and secretory activity of gut	Irritable bowel syndrome, minor diarrhea	Available in oral and parenteral forms • short $t_{½}$ but action lasts up to 6 h • *Toxicity:* Tachycardia, confusion, urinary retention, increased intraocular pressure • *Interactions:* With other antimuscarinics
• *Hyoscyamine: Longer duration of action*				
OPHTHALMOLOGY				
• Atropine	Competitive antagonism at all M receptors	Causes mydriasis and cycloplegia	Retinal examination; prevention of synechiae after surgery	Used as drops • long (5–6 days) action • *Toxicity:* Increased intraocular pressure in closed-angle glaucoma • *Interactions:* With other antimuscarinics
• *Homatropine: Shorter duration of action (12–24 h) than atropine* • *Cyclopentolate: Shorter duration of action (3–6 h)* • *Tropicamide: Shortest duration of action (15–60 min)*				

(continued)

Subclass, Drug	Mechanism of Action	Effects	Clinical Applications	Pharmacokinetics, Toxicities, Interactions
RESPIRATORY (ASTHMA, COPD)				
• Ipratropium	Competitive, nonselective antagonist at M receptors	Reduces or prevents bronchospasm	Prevention and relief of acute episodes of bronchospasm	Aerosol canister, up to qid • *Toxicity:* Xerostomia, cough • *Interactions:* With other antimuscarinics
• *Tiotropium, aclidinium, and umeclidinium: Longer duration of action; used once daily*				
URINARY				
• Oxybutynin	Slightly M_3-selective muscarinic antagonist	Reduces detrusor smooth muscle tone, spasms	Urge incontinence; postoperative spasms	Oral, IV, patch formulations • *Toxicity:* Tachycardia, constipation, increased intraocular pressure, xerostomia • Patch: Pruritus • *Interactions:* With other antimuscarinics
• *Darifenacin, solifenacin, fesoterodine, and tolterodine: Tertiary amines with somewhat greater selectivity for M_3 receptors*				
• *Trospium: Quaternary amine with less CNS effect*				
CHOLINERGIC POISONING				
• Atropine	Nonselective competitive antagonist at all muscarinic receptors in CNS and periphery	Blocks muscarinic excess at exocrine glands, heart, smooth muscle	Mandatory antidote for severe cholinesterase inhibitor poisoning	Intravenous infusion until antimuscarinic signs appear • continue as long as necessary • *Toxicity:* Insignificant as long as AChE inhibition continues
• Pralidoxime	Very high affinity for phosphorus atom but does not enter CNS	Regenerates active AChE; can relieve skeletal muscle end plate block	Usual antidote for early-stage (48 h) cholinesterase inhibitor poisoning	Intravenous every 4–6 h • *Toxicity:* Can cause muscle weakness in overdose

AChE, acetylcholinesterase; CNS, central nervous system; COPD, chronic obstructive pulmonary disease; IM, intramuscular.

PREPARATIONS AVAILABLE

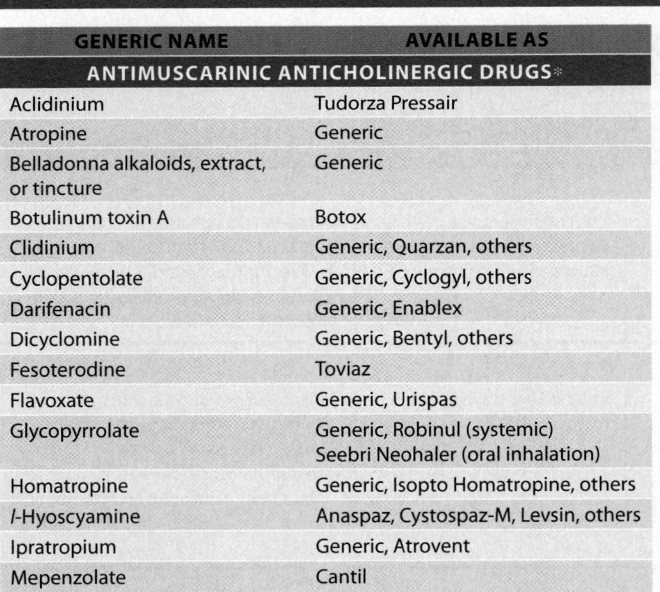

GENERIC NAME	AVAILABLE AS
ANTIMUSCARINIC ANTICHOLINERGIC DRUGS*	
Aclidinium	Tudorza Pressair
Atropine	Generic
Belladonna alkaloids, extract, or tincture	Generic
Botulinum toxin A	Botox
Clidinium	Generic, Quarzan, others
Cyclopentolate	Generic, Cyclogyl, others
Darifenacin	Generic, Enablex
Dicyclomine	Generic, Bentyl, others
Fesoterodine	Toviaz
Flavoxate	Generic, Urispas
Glycopyrrolate	Generic, Robinul (systemic) Seebri Neohaler (oral inhalation)
Homatropine	Generic, Isopto Homatropine, others
l-Hyoscyamine	Anaspaz, Cystospaz-M, Levsin, others
Ipratropium	Generic, Atrovent
Mepenzolate	Cantil

GENERIC NAME	AVAILABLE AS
Methscopolamine	Generic, Pamine
Oxybutynin	Generic, Ditropan, Gelnique, others
Propantheline	Generic, Pro-Banthine, others
Scopolamine	
Oral	Generic
Ophthalmic	Isopto Hyoscine
Transdermal	Transderm Scop
Solifenacin	Vesicare
Tiotropium	Spiriva
Tolterodine	Generic, Detrol
Tropicamide	Generic, Mydriacyl Ophthalmic, others
Trospium	Generic, Sanctura
Umeclidinium	Incruse Ellipta
GANGLION BLOCKERS	
Mecamylamine	Vecamyl
CHOLINESTERASE REGENERATOR	
Pralidoxime	Generic, Protopam

*Antimuscarinic drugs used in parkinsonism are listed in Chapter 28.

REFERENCES

Brodde OE et al: Presence, distribution and physiological function of adrenergic and muscarinic receptor subtypes in the human heart. Basic Res Cardiol 2001;96:528.

Cahill K et al: Pharmacological interventions for smoking cessation: An overview and network meta-analysis. Cochrane Database Syst Rev 2013;5:CD009329.

Carrière I et al: Drugs with anticholinergic properties, cognitive decline, and dementia in an elderly general population. Arch Intern Med 2009; 169:1317.

Casaburi R et al: Improvement in exercise tolerance with the combination of tiotropium and pulmonary rehabilitation in patients with COPD. Chest 2005;127:809.

Chapple CR et al: A comparison of the efficacy and tolerability of solifenacin succinate and extended release tolterodine at treating overactive bladder syndrome: Results of the STAR trial. Eur Urol 2005;48:464.

Cohen JS et al: Dual therapy strategies for COPD: The scientific rationale for LAMA+LABA. Int J Chron Obstruct Pulmon Dis 2016;11:785.

Ehlert FJ, Pak KJ, Griffin MT: Muscarinic agonists and antagonists: Effects on gastrointestinal function. In: Fryer AD et al (editors): *Muscarinic Receptors.* Handb Exp Pharmacol 2012;208:343.

Filson CP et al: The efficacy and safety of combined therapy with α-blockers and anticholinergics for men with benign prostatic hyperplasia: A meta-analysis. J Urol 2013;190:2013.

Fowler CJ, Griffiths D, de Groat WC: The neural control of micturition. Nat Rev Neurosci 2008;9:453.

Giovannini MG et al: Effects of histamine H3 receptor agonists and antagonists on cognitive performance and scopolamine-induced amnesia. Behav Brain Res 1999;104:147.

Kranke P et al: The efficacy and safety of transdermal scopolamine for the prevention of postoperative nausea and vomiting: A quantitative systematic review. Anesth Analg 2002;95:133.

Kruse AC et al: Muscarinic acetylcholine receptors: Novel opportunities for drug development. Nat Rev Drug Discov 2014;13:549.

Lawrence GW, Aoki KR, Dolly JO: Excitatory cholinergic and purinergic signaling in bladder are equally susceptible to botulinum neurotoxin A consistent with corelease of transmitters from efferent fibers. J Pharmacol Exp Ther 2010;334:1080.

Marquardt K: Mushrooms, amatoxin type. In: Olson K (editor): *Poisoning & Drug Overdose,* 6th ed. New York: McGraw Hill, 2012.

Moriya H et al: Affinity profiles of various muscarinic antagonists for cloned human muscarinic acetylcholine receptor (mAChR) subtypes and mAChRs in rat heart and submandibular gland. Life Sci 1999;64:2351.

Profita M et al: Smoke, choline acetyltransferase, muscarinic receptors, and fibroblast proliferation in chronic obstructive pulmonary disease. J Pharmacol Exp Ther 2009;329:753.

Rai BP et al: Anticholinergic drugs versus non-drug active therapies for non-neurogenic overactive bladder syndrome in adults. Cochrane Database Syst Rev 2012;12:CD003193.

Tauterman CS et al: Molecular basis for the long duration of action and kinetic selectivity of tiotropium for the muscarinic M3 receptor. J Med Chem 2013;56:8746.

Thai DM et al: Crystal structures of the M1 and M4 muscarinic acetylcholine receptors. Nature 2016;335:2016.

Vuckovic Z et al: Crystal structure of the M5 muscarinic acetylcholine receptor. Proc Natl Acad Sci U S A 2019;116:26001.

Wallukat G, Schimke I: Agonistic autoantibodies directed against G-protein-coupled receptors and their relationship to cardiovascular diseases. Semin Immunopathol 2014;36:351.

Young JM et al: Mecamylamine: New therapeutic uses and toxicity/risk profile. Clin Ther 2001;23:532.

Zhang L et al: A missense mutation in the CHRM2 gene is associated with familial dilated cardiomyopathy. Circ Res 2008;102:1426.

Treatment of Anticholinesterase Poisoning

Nachon F et al: Progress in the development of enzyme-based nerve agent bioscavengers. Chem Biol Interact 2013;206:536.

Thiermann H et al: Pharmacokinetics of obidoxime in patients poisoned with organophosphorus compounds. Toxicol Lett 2010;197:236.

Weinbroum AA: Pathophysiological and clinical aspects of combat anticholinesterase poisoning. Br Med Bull 2005;72:119.

CASE STUDY ANSWER

JH's symptoms are often displayed by patients following prostatectomy to relieve significant obstruction of bladder outflow. Urge incontinence can occur in patients whose prostatic hypertrophy caused instability of the detrusor muscle. JH should be advised that urinary incontinence and urinary frequency can diminish with time after prostatectomy as detrusor muscle instability subsides. JH can be helped by daily administration of a single tablet of extended-release tolterodine (4 mg/d) or oxybutynin (5–10 mg/d). A transdermal patch containing oxybutynin (3.9 mg/d) also is available.

CHAPTER

9 Adrenoceptor Agonists & Sympathomimetic Drugs

Italo Biaggioni, MD*, & Vsevolod V. Gurevich, PhD

CASE STUDY

A 68-year-old man presents with a complaint of lightheadedness on standing that is worse after meals and in hot environments. Symptoms started about 4 years ago and have slowly progressed to the point that he is disabled. He has fainted several times but always recovers consciousness almost as soon as he falls. Other symptoms include slight worsening of constipation, urinary retention out of proportion to prostate size, and decreased sweating. He is otherwise healthy with no history of hypertension, diabetes, or Parkinson disease. Because of urinary retention, he was placed on the α_{1A} antagonist tamsulosin, but the fainting spells got worse. Physical examination is unremarkable except for a blood pressure of 167/84 mm Hg supine and 106/55 mm Hg standing. There was an inadequate compensatory increase in heart rate (from 84 to 88 bpm), considering the magnitude of orthostatic hypotension. There is no evidence of peripheral neuropathy or parkinsonian features. Laboratory examinations are negative except for a low plasma norepinephrine (98 pg/mL; normal for his age 250–400 pg/mL). A diagnosis of pure autonomic failure is made, based on the clinical picture and the absence of drugs that could induce orthostatic hypotension and diseases commonly associated with autonomic neuropathy (eg, diabetes, Parkinson disease). What precautions should this patient observe in using sympathomimetic drugs? Can such drugs be used in his treatment?

The sympathetic nervous system is an important regulator of virtually all organ systems. This is particularly evident in the regulation of blood pressure. As illustrated in the case study, the sympathetic nervous system is required to maintain blood pressure stable even under relatively minor situations of stress. For example, during standing, the gravitational pooling of blood in the lower body triggers sympathetic stimulation that causes the release of norepinephrine from nerve terminals, which then activates adrenoceptors on postsynaptic sites (see Chapter 6) to restore blood pressure. Also, in response to more stressful situations (eg, hypoglycemia), sympathetic activation causes the adrenal medulla to release epinephrine, which is then transported in the blood to target tissues. In other words, epinephrine acts as a hormone, whereas norepinephrine acts as a neurotransmitter. Both have a role in the "fight or flight" response that characterizes sympathetic activation.

Drugs that mimic the actions of epinephrine or norepinephrine have traditionally been termed **sympathomimetic drugs**. The sympathomimetics can be grouped by mode of action and by the spectrum of receptors that they activate. Some of these drugs (e.g., norepinephrine and epinephrine) are *direct* agonists; they directly interact with and activate adrenoceptors. Others are *indirect* agonists because their actions are dependent on their ability to enhance the actions of endogenous catecholamines by (1) inducing the release of catecholamines by displacing them from adrenergic nerve endings (e.g., the mechanism of action of tyramine), (2) decreasing the clearance of catecholamines by inhibiting their neuronal reuptake (e.g., the mechanism of action of cocaine and certain antidepressants), or (3) preventing the enzymatic metabolism

*The author thanks David Robertson, MD, for his contributions to previous versions of this chapter.

of norepinephrine (monoamine oxidase and catechol-*O*-methyltransferase inhibitors). Some drugs have both direct and indirect actions.

Both types of sympathomimetics, direct and indirect, ultimately cause activation of adrenoceptors, leading to some or all of the characteristic effects of endogenous catecholamines. The pharmacologic effects of direct agonists depend on the route of administration, their relative affinity for adrenoceptor subtypes, and the relative expression of these receptor subtypes in target tissues. The pharmacologic effects of indirect sympathomimetics are greater under conditions of increased sympathetic activity and norepinephrine release.

MOLECULAR PHARMACOLOGY UNDERLYING THE ACTIONS OF SYMPATHOMIMETIC DRUGS

The effects of catecholamines are mediated by cell-surface receptors. Adrenoceptors are typical G protein-coupled receptors (GPCRs; see Chapter 2). The receptor protein has an extracellular N-terminus, traverses the membrane seven times (transmembrane domains) forming three extracellular and three intracellular loops, and has an intracellular C-terminus (Figure 9–1). They are coupled to G proteins that regulate various effector proteins. Each G protein is a heterotrimer consisting of α, β, and γ subunits. G proteins are classified on the basis of their distinctive α subunits. G proteins of particular importance for adrenoceptor function include G_s, the stimulatory G protein of adenylyl cyclase; G_i and G_o, the inhibitory G proteins of adenylyl cyclase; and G_q and G_{11}, the G proteins coupling α receptors to phospholipase C. The activation of G protein-coupled receptors by catecholamines promotes the dissociation of guanosine diphosphate (GDP) from the α subunit of the corresponding G protein. Guanosine triphosphate (GTP) then binds to this G protein, and the α subunit dissociates from the βγ subunit. The activated GTP-bound α subunit then regulates the activity of its effector. Effectors of adrenoceptor-activated α subunits include adenylyl cyclase, phospholipase C, and ion channels. The α subunit is inactivated by hydrolysis of the bound GTP to GDP and phosphate, and the subsequent reassociation of the α subunit with the βγ subunit. The βγ subunits have additional independent effects, acting on a variety of effectors such as ion channels and enzymes.

Adrenoceptors were originally characterized pharmacologically by their relative affinities for agonists; α receptors have the comparative potencies epinephrine ≥ norepinephrine >> isoproterenol, and β receptors have the comparative potencies isoproterenol > epinephrine ≥ norepinephrine. Molecular cloning further identified distinct subtypes of these receptors (Table 9–1).

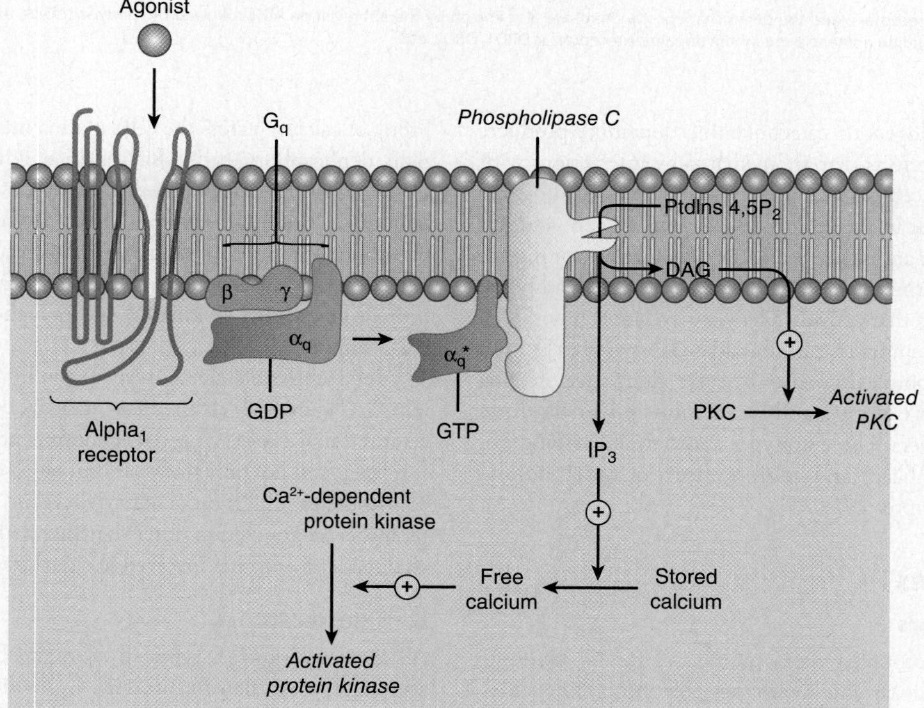

FIGURE 9–1 Activation of $α_1$ responses. Stimulation of $α_1$ receptors by catecholamines leads to the activation of a G_q-coupling protein. The activated α subunit ($α_q^*$) of this G protein activates the effector, phospholipase C, which leads to the release of IP_3 (inositol 1,4,5-trisphosphate) and DAG (diacylglycerol) from phosphatidylinositol 4,5-bisphosphate (PtdIns 4,5P_2). IP_3 stimulates the release of sequestered stores of calcium, leading to an increased concentration of cytoplasmic Ca^{2+}. Ca^{2+} may then activate Ca^{2+}-dependent protein kinases, which in turn phosphorylate their substrates. DAG activates protein kinase C (PKC). GDP, guanosine diphosphate; GTP, guanosine triphosphate. See text for additional effects of $α_1$-receptor activation.

TABLE 9–1 Adrenoceptor types and subtypes.

Receptor	Agonist	Antagonist	G Protein	Effects	Gene on Chromosome
α_1 type	Phenylephrine	Prazosin	G_q	↑ IP3, DAG common to all	
α_{1A}		Tamsulosin			C8
α_{1B}					C5
α_{1D}[1]					C20
α_2 type	Clonidine	Yohimbine	G_i	↓ cAMP common to all	
α_{2A}	Oxymetazoline				C10
α_{2B}		Prazosin			C2
α_{2C}		Prazosin			C4
β type	Isoproterenol	Propranolol	G_s	↑ cAMP common to all	
β_1	Dobutamine	Betaxolol			C10
β_2	Albuterol	Butoxamine			C5
β_3	Mirabegron				C8
Dopamine type	Dopamine				
D_1	Fenoldopam		G_s	↑ cAMP	C5
D_2	Bromocriptine		G_i	↓ cAMP	C11
D_3			G_i	↓ cAMP	C3
D_4		Clozapine	G_i	↓ cAMP	C11
D_5			G_s	↑ cAMP	C4

[1]Initially an "α_{1C}" receptor was described but was later recognized to be identical to the α_{1A} receptor. To avoid confusion, the nomenclature now omits α_{1C}.

Nomenclature: The adrenoreceptors (and the genes that encode them) are also known by the abbreviation ADR, followed by the type (ADRA, ADRB) and subtype (ADRA1A, ADRA1B, etc). The corresponding nomenclature for the dopamine receptors is DRD1, DRD2, etc.

Likewise, the endogenous catecholamine dopamine produces a variety of biologic effects that are mediated by interactions with specific dopamine receptors (see Table 9–1). These receptors are particularly important in the brain (see Chapters 21, 28, and 29) and in the splanchnic and renal vasculature. Molecular cloning has identified several distinct genes encoding five receptor subtypes: two D_1-like receptors that activate adenylate cyclase (D_1 and D_5), and three D_2-like receptors that inhibit adenylate cyclase (D_2, D_3, and D_4). Further complexity exists because alternative splicing produces D_2 receptor isoforms, and D_2 receptors might also form oligo- and heterodimers. These subtypes may have importance for understanding the efficacy and adverse effects of novel antipsychotic drugs (see Chapter 29).

Receptor Types

A. Alpha Receptors

Alpha$_1$ receptors are coupled via G proteins of the G_q family to phospholipase C. This enzyme hydrolyzes polyphosphoinositides, leading to the formation of **inositol 1,4,5-trisphosphate (IP_3)** and **diacylglycerol (DAG)** (see Table 9–1 and Figure 9–1). IP_3 promotes the release of sequestered Ca^{2+} from intracellular stores, which increases cytoplasmic free Ca^{2+} concentrations that activate various calcium-dependent protein kinases and other calmodulin-regulated proteins. Activation of these receptors may also increase influx of calcium across the cell's plasma membrane. IP_3 is sequentially dephosphorylated, which ultimately leads to the formation of free inositol. DAG cooperates with Ca^{2+} in activating protein kinase C (PKC), which modulates activity of many signaling pathways. In addition, α_1 receptors activate signal transduction pathways that stimulate tyrosine kinases such as mitogen-activated protein kinases (MAP kinases) and polyphosphoinositol-3-kinase (PI-3-kinase).

Alpha$_2$ receptors are coupled to the inhibitory regulatory protein G_i (Figure 9–2) that reduces adenylyl cyclase activity and lowers intracellular levels of cyclic adenosine monophosphate (cAMP). It is likely that not only the α subunit of G_i, but also its $\beta\gamma$ subunits, contribute to inhibition of adenylyl cyclase. It is also likely that α_2 receptors are coupled to other signaling pathways that regulate ion channels and enzymes involved in signal transduction.

B. Beta Receptors

All three receptor subtypes (β_1, β_2, and β_3) are coupled to the stimulatory regulatory protein G_s, which activates adenylyl cyclase to increase intracellular levels of cAMP (see Table 9–1 and Figure 9–2). Cyclic AMP is the second messenger that mediates most of the actions of β-receptors; in the liver cAMP mediates a cascade of events culminating in the activation of glycogen phosphorylase; in the heart, it increases the influx of calcium across the cell membrane; whereas in smooth muscle it promotes

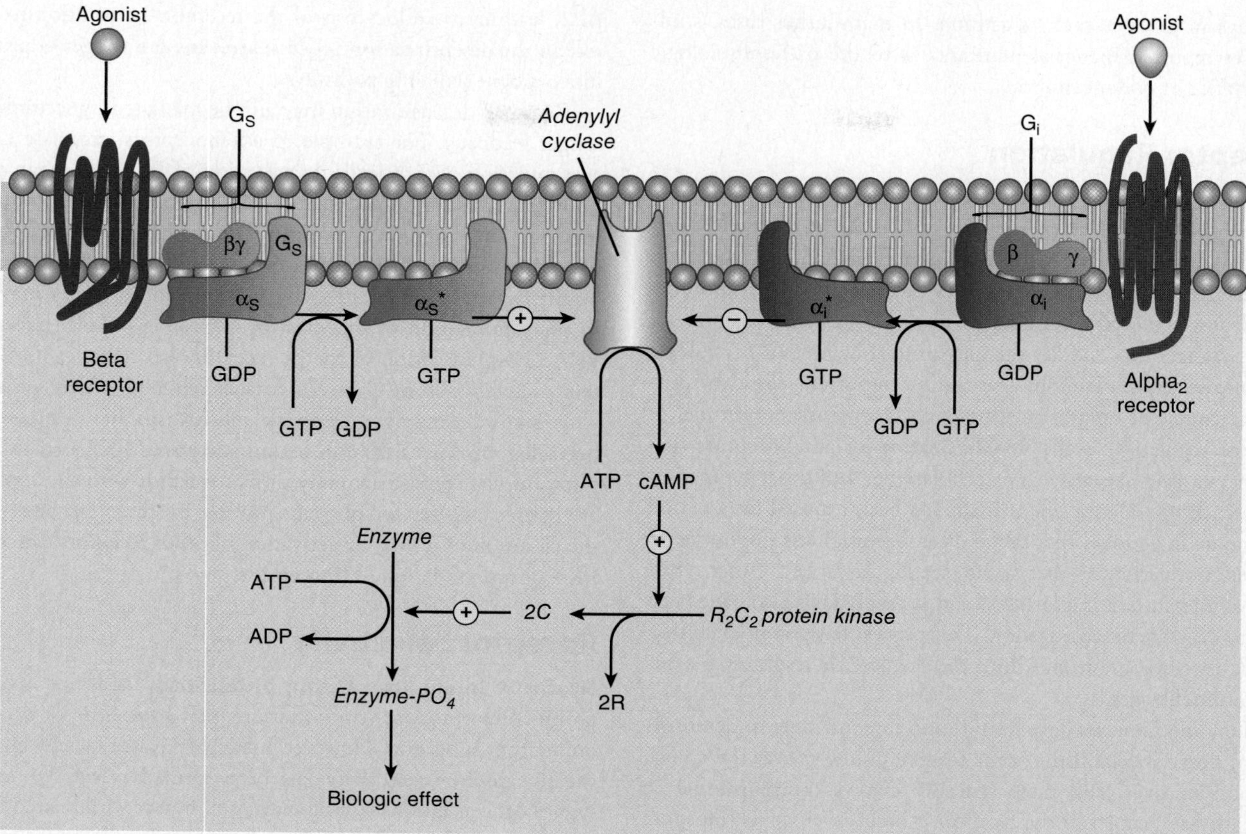

FIGURE 9–2 Activation and inhibition of adenylyl cyclase by agonists that bind to catecholamine receptors. Binding to β adrenoceptors stimulates adenylyl cyclase by activating the stimulatory G protein, G_s, which leads to the dissociation of its α subunit charged with GTP. This activated α_s subunit directly activates adenylyl cyclase, resulting in an increased rate of synthesis of cAMP. Alpha$_2$-adrenoceptor ligands inhibit adenylyl cyclase by causing dissociation of the inhibitory G protein, G_i, into its subunits—ie, an activated α_i subunit charged with GTP and a β-γ unit. The mechanism by which these subunits inhibit adenylyl cyclase is uncertain. cAMP binds to the regulatory subunit (*R*) of cAMP-dependent protein kinase, leading to the liberation of active catalytic subunits (*C*) that phosphorylate specific protein substrates and modify their activity. These catalytic units also phosphorylate the cAMP response element binding protein (CREB), which modifies gene expression. See text for other actions of β and α_2 adrenoceptors.

relaxation through phosphorylation of myosin light-chain kinase to an inactive form (see Figure 12–1). Some actions of β adrenoceptors may be mediated through different intracellular signaling pathways, via exchange proteins activated by cAMP rather than conventional protein kinase A (PKA), or via coupling to G_s but independent of cAMP, or coupling to G_q proteins and activation of MAP kinases.

The β_3 adrenoceptor is a lower-affinity receptor compared with β_1 and β_2 receptors but is more resistant to desensitization. It is found in several tissues, but its physiologic or pathologic role in humans is not clear. Beta$_3$ receptors are expressed in the detrusor muscle of the bladder and induce its relaxation, and the selective β_3 agonist **mirabegron** is used clinically for the treatment of symptoms of overactive bladder (urinary urgency and frequency).

C. Dopamine Receptors

The D_1 receptor is typically associated with the stimulation of adenylyl cyclase (see Table 9–1); for example, D_1 receptor–induced smooth muscle relaxation is presumably due to cAMP accumulation in the smooth muscle of those vascular beds in which dopamine is a vasodilator. D_2 receptors have been found to inhibit adenylyl cyclase activity, open potassium channels, and decrease calcium influx.

Adrenoceptor Polymorphisms

Since elucidation of the sequences of the genes encoding adrenoceptors, it has become clear that there are relatively common genetic **polymorphisms** (variations in the gene sequence) for many of these receptor subtypes in humans. Distinct polymorphisms may be inherited together, in combinations termed **haplotypes**. Genetic polymorphisms can result in changes in critical amino acids that may alter the function of the receptor in ways that are clinically relevant. Some polymorphisms have been shown to alter susceptibility to diseases such as heart failure, modify the propensity of a receptor to desensitize, or modulate therapeutic responses to drugs in diseases such as asthma. In many other cases, studies have reported inconsistent results as to the pathophysiologic importance of polymorphisms.

Receptor Regulation

Responses mediated by adrenoceptors are not fixed and static. The magnitude of the response depends on the number and function of adrenoceptors on the cell surface and on the regulation of these receptors by catecholamines themselves, other hormones and drugs, age, and a number of disease states (see Chapter 2). These changes may modify the magnitude of a tissue's physiologic response to catecholamines and can be important clinically during the course of treatment. One of the best-studied examples of receptor regulation is the **desensitization** of adrenoceptors that may occur after exposure to catecholamines and other sympathomimetic drugs. After a cell or tissue has been exposed for a period of time to an agonist, that tissue often becomes less responsive to further stimulation by that agent (see Figure 2–12). Other terms such as tolerance, refractoriness, and tachyphylaxis also have been used to describe desensitization. This process has potential clinical significance because it may limit the therapeutic response to sympathomimetic agents.

Many mechanisms have been found to contribute to desensitization. Some mechanisms occur relatively slowly, over the course of hours or days, and these typically involve transcriptional or translational changes in the receptor protein level, or its transport to the cell surface. Other mechanisms of desensitization occur quickly, within minutes. Rapid modulation of receptor function in desensitized cells may involve critical covalent modification of the receptor, association of these receptors with other proteins, or changes in their subcellular location.

There are two major categories of desensitization of responses mediated by G protein-coupled receptors. **Homologous** desensitization refers to loss of responsiveness exclusively of the receptors that have been exposed to repeated or sustained activation by an agonist. **Heterologous** desensitization refers to the process by which desensitization of one receptor by its agonists also results in desensitization of another receptor that has not been directly activated by the agonist in question.

A major mechanism of desensitization that occurs rapidly involves phosphorylation of receptors by members of the **G protein-coupled receptor kinase (GRK)** family, of which there are seven in most mammals, with four subtypes (GRK2, GRK3, GRK5, and GRK6) being ubiquitously expressed. Specific adrenoceptors become substrates for these kinases only when they are bound to an agonist. This mechanism is an example of homologous desensitization because it specifically affects only agonist-occupied receptors.

Phosphorylation of these receptors enhances their affinity for **arrestins,** a family of four proteins, of which the two nonvisual arrestin subtypes are widely expressed. Upon binding of arrestin, the capacity of the receptor to activate G proteins is blunted, likely as a result of steric hindrance, as suggested by the crystal structures of GPCR complexes with G proteins and arrestins (see Figure 2–12). Arrestin then interacts with clathrin and clathrin adaptor AP2, leading to endocytosis of the receptor. In addition to their role in the desensitization process, arrestins can trigger G protein-independent signaling pathways.

Receptor desensitization may also be mediated by second-messenger feedback. For example, β adrenoceptors stimulate cAMP accumulation, which leads to activation of PKA; PKA can phosphorylate residues on β receptors, resulting in inhibition of receptor function. For the β_2 receptor, PKA phosphorylation occurs on serine residues in the third cytoplasmic loop of the receptor. Similarly, activation of PKC by G_q-coupled receptors may lead to phosphorylation of this class of G protein-coupled receptors. PKA phosphorylation of the β_2 receptor also switches its G protein preference from G_s to G_i, further reducing cAMP response. This second-messenger feedback mechanism has been termed heterologous desensitization because activated PKA or PKC may phosphorylate any structurally similar receptor with the appropriate consensus sites for phosphorylation by these enzymes—e.g., the elevation of cAMP by activation of other receptors can trigger PKA phosphorylation of β receptors.

Receptor Selectivity

Selectivity means that a drug preferentially activates one subgroup of receptors at concentrations that have little or no effect on another subgroup. However, selectivity is not usually absolute (nearly absolute selectivity has been termed *specificity*), and at higher concentrations, a drug may also interact with related classes of receptors. The clinical effects of a given drug may depend not only on its selectivity to adrenoceptor types, but also on the relative expression of receptor subtypes in a given tissue. Examples of clinically useful sympathomimetic agonists that are relatively selective for α_1-, α_2-, and β-adrenoceptor subgroups are compared with some nonselective agents in Table 9–2.

TABLE 9–2 Relative receptor affinities.

	Relative Receptor Affinities
Alpha agonists	
Phenylephrine, methoxamine	$\alpha_1 > \alpha_2 >>>>> \beta$
Clonidine, methylnorepinephrine	$\alpha_2 > \alpha_1 >>>>> \beta$
Mixed alpha and beta agonists	
Norepinephrine	$\alpha_1 = \alpha_2; \beta_1 >> \beta_2$
Epinephrine	$\alpha_1 = \alpha_2; \beta_1 = \beta_2$
Beta agonists	
Dobutamine[1]	$\beta_1 > \beta_2 >>>> \alpha$
Isoproterenol	$\beta_1 = \beta_2 >>>> \alpha$
Albuterol, terbutaline, metaproterenol, ritodrine	$\beta_2 >> \beta_1 >>>> \alpha$
Dopamine agonists	
Dopamine	$D_1 = D_2 >> \beta >> \alpha$
Fenoldopam	$D_1 >> D_2$

[1]See text.

Even though each receptor subtype is coupled to a G protein that mediates most of its intracellular signaling (see Table 9–1), in many cases a receptor can be coupled to other G proteins, or signal through both G protein-dependent and G protein-independent pathways. This observation has prompted the concept of developing **biased agonists** that selectively activate one of the signaling pathways (see Box: Therapeutic Potential of Biased Agonists at Beta Receptors). There is also interest in discovering **allosteric modulators** of receptor function, i.e., ligands that bind to the receptor at a site different from the agonist binding site and modulate the response to the agonist.

Therapeutic Potential of Biased Agonists at Beta Receptors

Traditional β agonists like epinephrine activate cardiac β_1 receptors, increasing heart rate and cardiac workload through coupling with G proteins. This can be deleterious in situations such as myocardial infarction. Beta$_1$ receptors are also coupled through G protein-independent signaling pathways involving β-arrestin, which are thought to be cardioprotective. A "biased" agonist could potentially activate only the cardioprotective, β-arrestin–mediated signaling (and not the G protein–mediated signals that lead to greater cardiac workload). Such a biased agonist would be of great therapeutic potential in situations such as myocardial infarction or heart failure. In asthma, there is interest in developing biased agonists that are effective bronchial muscle relaxants but are not subject to desensitization. Biased agonists potent enough to reach these therapeutic goals have not yet been developed.

The Norepinephrine Transporter

When norepinephrine is released into the synaptic cleft, it binds to postsynaptic adrenoceptors to elicit the expected physiologic effect. However, just as the release of neurotransmitters is a tightly regulated process, the mechanisms for removal of neurotransmitter must also be highly effective. The norepinephrine transporter (**NET**) is the principal route by which this occurs. It is particularly efficient in the synapses of the heart, where up to 90% of released norepinephrine is removed by the NET. Remaining synaptic norepinephrine may escape into the extrasynaptic space and enter the bloodstream or be taken up into extraneuronal cells and metabolized by catechol-*O*-methyltransferase. In other sites such as the vasculature, where synaptic structures are less well developed, removal by NET may still be 60% or more. The NET, often situated on the presynaptic neuronal membrane, pumps the synaptic norepinephrine back into the neuron cell cytoplasm. In the cell, this norepinephrine may reenter the vesicles or undergo metabolism through monoamine oxidase to dihydroxyphenylglycol (DHPG). Elsewhere in the body similar transporters remove dopamine (dopamine transporter, DAT), serotonin (serotonin transporter, SERT), and other neurotransmitters. The NET, surprisingly, has equivalent affinity for dopamine as for norepinephrine, and it can sometimes clear dopamine in brain areas where DAT is low, like the cortex.

Blockade of the NET, e.g., by the nonselective psychostimulant cocaine or the NET-selective agents atomoxetine or reboxetine, impairs this primary site of norepinephrine removal and thus synaptic norepinephrine levels rise, leading to greater stimulation of α and β adrenoceptors. In the periphery this effect may produce a clinical picture of sympathetic activation, but it is often counterbalanced by concomitant stimulation of α_2 adrenoceptors in the brain stem that reduces sympathetic activation.

The function of the norepinephrine and dopamine transporters is complex, and drugs can interact with the NET to actually reverse the direction of transport and induce the release of intraneuronal neurotransmitter. This is illustrated in Figure 9–3. Under normal circumstances (panel A), presynaptic NET (red) inactivates and recycles norepinephrine (NE, red) released by vesicular fusion. In panel B, amphetamine (black) acts as both an NET substrate and a reuptake blocker, eliciting reverse transport and blocking normal uptake, thereby increasing NE levels in and beyond the synaptic cleft. In panel C, agents such as methylphenidate and cocaine (hexagons) block NET-mediated NE reuptake and enhance NE signaling.

■ MEDICINAL CHEMISTRY OF SYMPATHOMIMETIC DRUGS

Phenylethylamine may be considered the parent compound from which sympathomimetic drugs are derived (Figure 9–4). This compound consists of a benzene ring with an ethylamine side chain. The presence of –OH groups at the 3 and 4 positions of the benzene ring yields sympathomimetic drugs collectively known as catecholamines. Additional substitutions made on (1) the benzene ring, (2) the terminal amino group, and (3) the α or β carbons produce catechols with different affinity for α and β receptors, from almost pure α agonists (methoxamine) to almost pure β agonists (isoproterenol).

In addition to determining relative affinity to receptor subtypes, chemical structure also determines the pharmacokinetic properties and bioavailability of these molecules.

A. Substitution on the Benzene Ring

Maximal α and β activity is found with catecholamines, i.e., drugs having –OH groups at the 3 and 4 positions on the benzene ring. The absence of one or the other of these groups dramatically reduces the potency of these drugs. For example, phenylephrine (Figure 9–5) is much less potent than epinephrine; its affinity to α receptors is decreased approximately 100-fold, but because its β activity is almost negligible except at very high concentrations, it is a selective α agonist.

On the other hand, the presence of –OH groups make catecholamines subject to inactivation by catechol-*O*-methyltransferase (COMT), and because this enzyme is found in the gut and liver, catecholamines are not active orally (see Chapter 6). Absence of one or both –OH groups on the phenyl ring increases

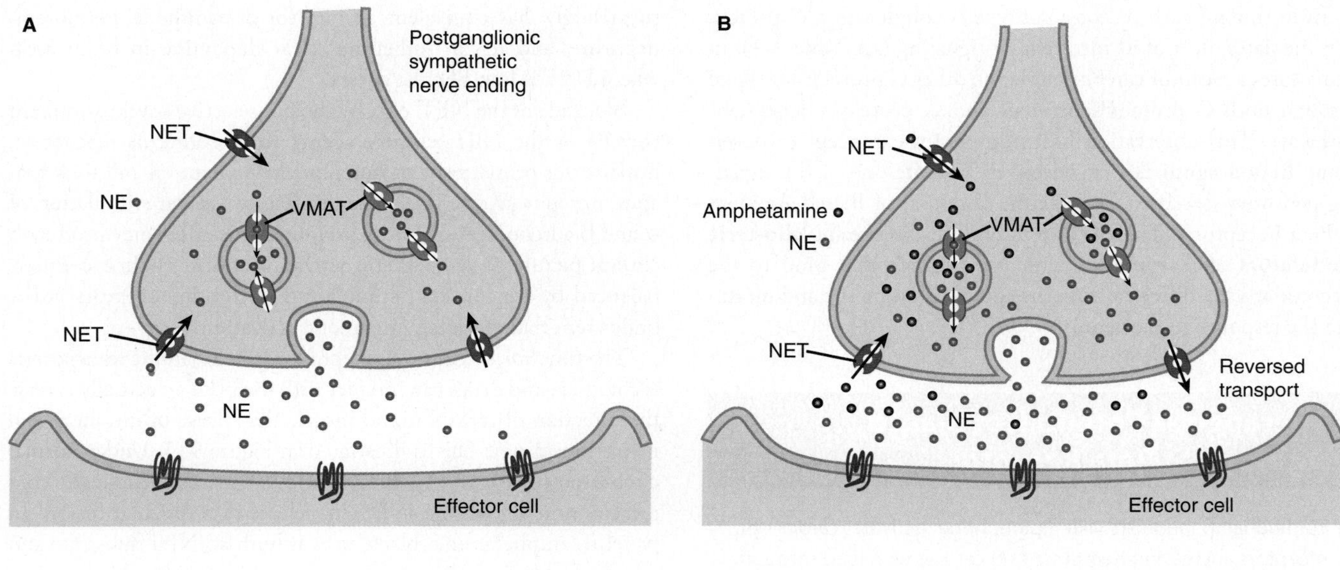

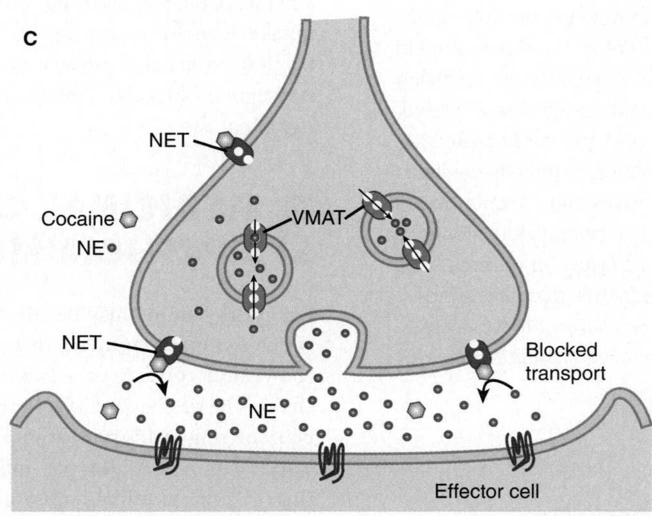

FIGURE 9–3 Pharmacologic targeting of monoamine transporters. Commonly used drugs such as antidepressants, amphetamines, and cocaine target monoamine (norepinephrine, dopamine, and serotonin) transporters with different potencies. **A** shows the mechanism of reuptake of norepinephrine (NE) back into the noradrenergic neuron via the norepinephrine transporter (NET), where a proportion is sequestered in presynaptic vesicles through the vesicular monoamine transporter (VMAT). **B** and **C** show the effects of amphetamine and cocaine on these pathways. See text for details.

the bioavailability after oral administration and prolongs the duration of action. Furthermore, absence of ring –OH groups tends to increase the distribution of the molecule to the central nervous system (CNS). For example, ephedrine and amphetamine (see Figure 9–5) are orally active, have a prolonged duration of action, and produce central nervous system effects not typically observed with the catecholamines. Methamphetamine ("crystal meth," a common drug of abuse) can be synthesized by simple dehydroxylation of ephedrine, which led to the restriction of over-the-counter distribution of its isomer pseudoephedrine.

B. Substitution on the Amino Group

Increasing the size of alkyl substituents on the amino group tends to increase β-receptor activity. For example, methyl substitution on norepinephrine (yielding epinephrine) enhances activity at β_2 receptors, and isopropyl substitution (yielding isoproterenol) increases β activity further. Conversely, the larger the substituent on the amino group, the lower is the activity at α receptors; for example, isoproterenol is very weak at α receptors. Beta$_2$-selective agonists generally require a large amino substituent group.

C. Substitution on the Alpha Carbon

Substitutions at the α carbon (e.g., ephedrine and amphetamine; see Figure 9–5) block oxidation by monoamine oxidase (MAO), thus prolonging the duration of action of these drugs. Alpha-methyl compounds are also called **phenylisopropylamines**. In addition to their resistance to oxidation by MAO, some phenylisopropylamines have an enhanced ability to displace catecholamines

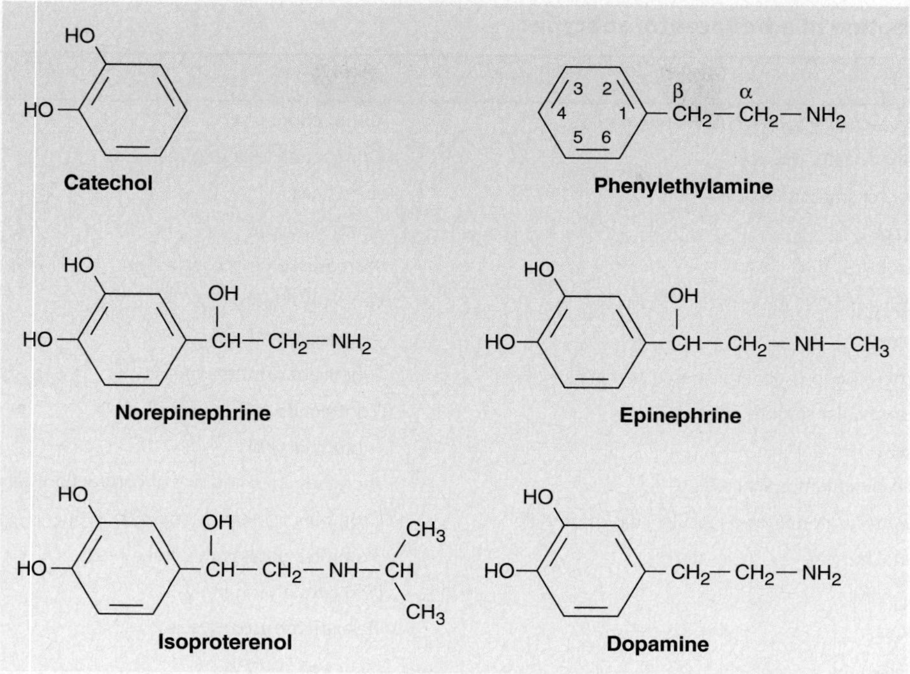

Catechol

Phenylethylamine

Norepinephrine

Epinephrine

Isoproterenol

Dopamine

FIGURE 9–4 Phenylethylamine and some important catecholamines. Catechol is shown for reference.

from storage sites in noradrenergic nerves (see Chapter 6). Therefore, a portion of their activity is dependent on the presence of normal norepinephrine stores in the body; they are indirectly acting sympathomimetics.

D. Substitution on the Beta Carbon

Direct-acting agonists typically have a β-hydroxyl group, although dopamine does not. In addition to facilitating activation of adrenoceptors, this hydroxyl group may be important for storage of sympathomimetic amines in synaptic vesicles.

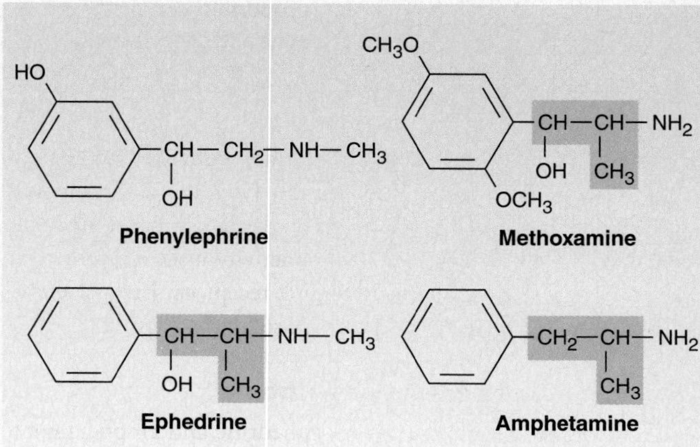

FIGURE 9–5 Some examples of noncatecholamine sympathomimetic drugs. The isopropyl group is highlighted in color. Methamphetamine is amphetamine with one of the amine hydrogens replaced by a methyl group.

ORGAN SYSTEM EFFECTS OF SYMPATHOMIMETIC DRUGS

Cardiovascular System

General outlines of the cellular actions of sympathomimetics are presented in Tables 6–3 and 9–3. Sympathomimetics have prominent cardiovascular effects because of widespread distribution of α and β adrenoceptors in the heart, blood vessels, and neural and hormonal systems involved in blood pressure regulation.

The effects of sympathomimetic drugs on blood pressure can be explained on the basis of their effects on heart rate, myocardial function, arterial vascular resistance, and venous return (see Figure 6–7 and Table 9–4). The endogenous catecholamines, norepinephrine and epinephrine, have complex cardiovascular effects because they activate both α and β receptors. It is easier to understand these actions by first describing the cardiovascular effect of sympathomimetics that are selective for a given adrenoceptor.

A. Effects of Alpha$_1$-Receptor Activation

Alpha$_1$ receptors are widely expressed in vascular beds, and their activation leads to arterial and venous vasoconstriction. Their direct effect on cardiac function is of relatively less importance. Phenylephrine and midodrine are selective α_1 agonists, and their administration increases peripheral arterial resistance (arterial vasoconstriction) and decreases venous capacitance (venous constriction). The enhanced arterial resistance usually leads to a dose-dependent rise in blood pressure (Figure 9–6). In the presence of normal cardiovascular reflexes, the rise in blood pressure elicits a baroreceptor-mediated increase in vagal tone with slowing of the heart rate, which may be quite

TABLE 9–3 Distribution of adrenoceptor subtypes.

Type	Tissue	Actions
α_1	Most vascular smooth muscle (innervated)	Contraction
	Pupillary dilator muscle	Contraction (dilates pupil)
	Pilomotor smooth muscle	Erects hair
	Prostate	Contraction
	Heart	Increases force of contraction
α_2	Postsynaptic CNS neurons	Probably multiple
	Platelets	Aggregation
	Adrenergic and cholinergic nerve terminals	Inhibits transmitter release
	Some vascular smooth muscle	Contraction
	Fat cells	Inhibits lipolysis
β_1	Heart, juxtaglomerular cells	Increases force and rate of contraction; increases renin release
β_2	Respiratory, uterine, and vascular smooth muscle	Promotes smooth muscle relaxation
	Skeletal muscle	Promotes potassium uptake
	Human liver	Activates glycogenolysis
β_3	Bladder	Relaxes detrusor muscle
	Fat cells	Activates lipolysis
D_1	Smooth muscle	Dilates renal blood vessels
D_2	Nerve endings	Modulates transmitter release

marked (Figure 9–7). However, cardiac output may not diminish in proportion to this reduction in rate, because the improved venous return increases stroke volume. Furthermore, direct α-adrenoceptor stimulation of the heart may have a modest positive inotropic action. It is important to note that any effect these agents have on blood pressure is counteracted by compensatory autonomic baroreflex mechanisms aimed at restoring homeostasis. The magnitude of the restraining effect is quite dramatic. If baroreflex function is removed

TABLE 9–4 Cardiovascular responses to sympathomimetic amines.

	Phenylephrine	Epinephrine	Isoproterenol
Vascular resistance (tone)			
Skin, mucous membranes (α)	↑↑	↑↑	0
Skeletal muscle (β_2, α)	↑	↓ or ↑	↓↓
Renal (α, D_1)	↑	↑	↓
Splanchnic (α, β)	↑↑	↓ or ↑[1]	↓
Total peripheral resistance	↑↑↑	↓ or ↑[1]	↓↓
Venous tone (α, β)	↑	↑	↓
Cardiac			
Contractility (β_1)	0 or ↑	↑↑↑	↑↑↑
Heart rate (predominantly β_1)	↓↓ (vagal reflex)	↑ or ↓	↑↑↑
Stroke volume	0, ↓, ↑	↑	↑
Cardiac output	↓	↑	↑↑
Blood pressure			
Mean	↑↑	↑	↓
Diastolic	↑↑	↓ or ↑[1]	↓↓
Systolic	↑↑	↑↑	0 or ↓
Pulse pressure	0	↑↑	↑↑

[1]Small doses decrease, large doses increase.

↑ = increase; ↓ = decrease; 0 = no change.

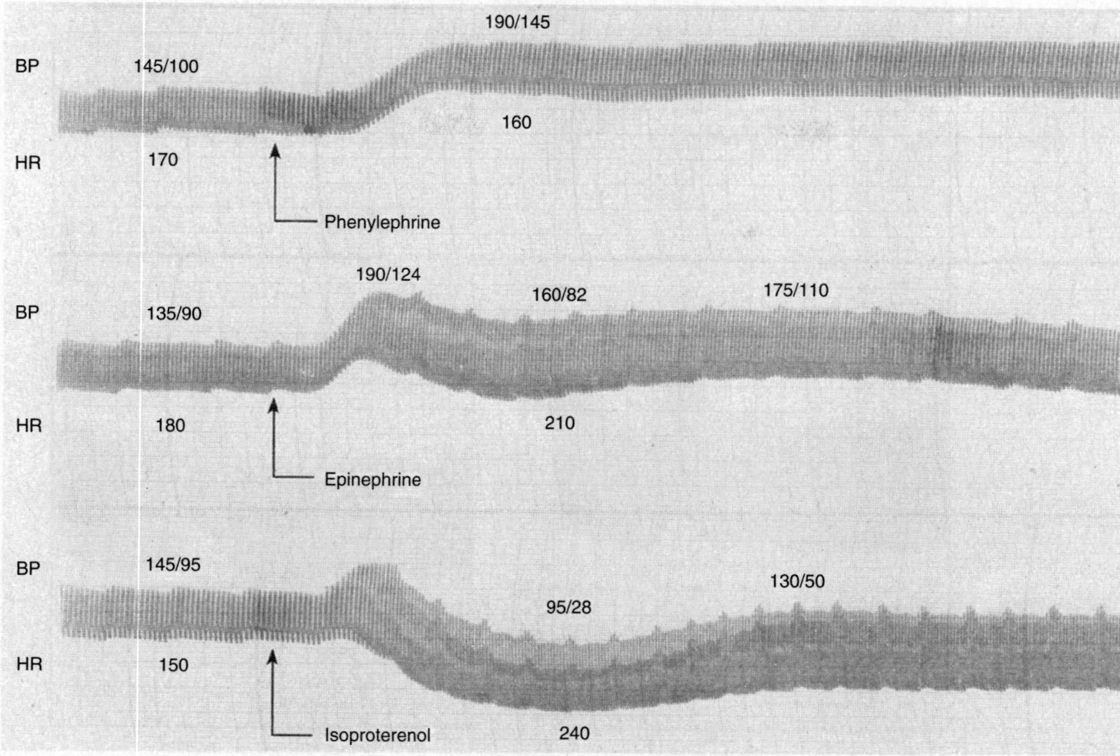

FIGURE 9–6 Effects of an α-selective (phenylephrine), β-selective (isoproterenol), and nonselective (epinephrine) sympathomimetic, given as an intravenous bolus injection to a dog. Reflexes are blunted but not eliminated in this anesthetized animal. BP, blood pressure; HR, heart rate.

by pretreatment with the ganglionic blocker trimethaphan, the pressor effect of phenylephrine is increased approximately 10-fold, and bradycardia is no longer observed (see Figure 9–7), confirming that the decrease in heart rate was reflex in nature rather than a direct effect of α_1-receptor activation.

Patients who have an impairment of autonomic function (due to pure autonomic failure as in the case study or to more common conditions such as diabetic autonomic neuropathy) exhibit this extreme hypersensitivity to most pressor and depressor stimuli, including medications. This is to a large extent due to failure of baroreflex buffering. Such patients may have exaggerated increases in heart rate or blood pressure when taking sympathomimetics. This, however, can be used as an advantage in their treatment. The α_1 agonist midodrine is commonly used to ameliorate orthostatic hypotension in these patients.

There are major differences in receptor types predominantly expressed in the various vascular beds (see Table 9–4). The skin vessels have predominantly α receptors and constrict in response to epinephrine and norepinephrine, as do the splanchnic vessels. Vessels in skeletal muscle may constrict or dilate depending on whether α or β receptors are activated. The blood vessels of the nasal mucosa express α receptors, and local vasoconstriction induced by sympathomimetics explains their decongestant action (see Therapeutic Uses of Sympathomimetic Drugs).

B. Effects of Alpha$_2$-Receptor Activation

Selective α_2 adrenoceptors agonists, such as clonidine, act in the CNS to reduce sympathetic activity ("central sympatholytics") and are used in the treatment of hypertension (see Chapter 11). Alpha$_2$ adrenoreceptors are also present in the vasculature, and their activation leads to vasoconstriction. This effect, however, is observed only when α_2 agonists are given locally, by rapid intravenous injection or in very high oral doses. When given systemically, these vascular effects are obscured by the central sympatholytic effects of α_2 receptors. In patients with pure autonomic failure, characterized by neural degeneration of postganglionic noradrenergic fibers, clonidine may increase blood pressure because the central sympatholytic effects of clonidine become irrelevant whereas the peripheral vasoconstriction remains intact.

C. Effects of Beta-Receptor Activation

The cardiovascular effects of β-adrenoceptor activation are exemplified by the response to the nonselective β agonist isoproterenol, which activates both β_1 and β_2 receptors. Stimulation of β receptors in the heart increases cardiac output by increasing contractility and by direct activation of the sinus node to increase heart rate. Beta agonists also decrease peripheral resistance by activating β_2 receptors, leading to vasodilation of certain vascular beds (see Table 9–4). The net effect is to maintain or slightly increase systolic pressure and to lower diastolic pressure, so that mean blood pressure is decreased (see Figure 9–6).

The cardiac effects of β agonists are determined largely by β_1 receptors (although β_2 and α receptors also may be involved, especially in heart failure). The prototypical β_1-selective agonist is dobutamine. Beta$_1$-receptor activation in the heart results in

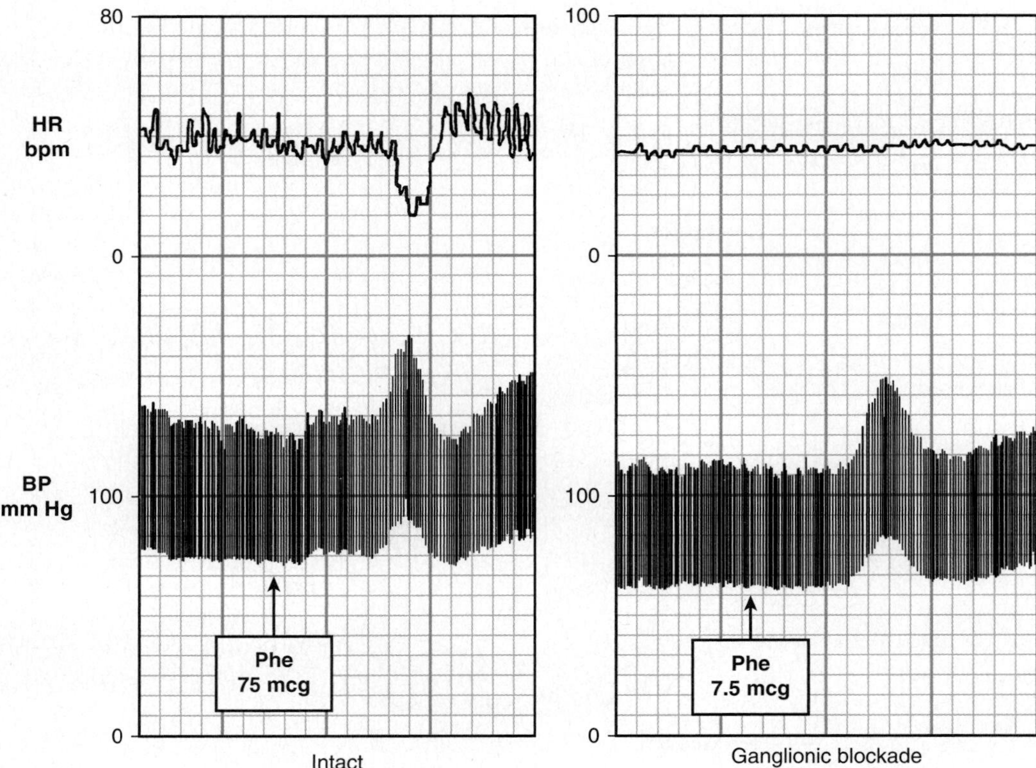

FIGURE 9–7 Effects of ganglionic blockade on the response to phenylephrine (Phe) in a human subject. **Left:** The cardiovascular effect of the selective α agonist phenylephrine when given as an intravenous bolus to a subject with intact autonomic baroreflex function. Note that the increase in blood pressure (BP) is associated with a baroreflex-mediated compensatory decrease in heart rate (HR). **Right:** The response in the same subject after autonomic reflexes were abolished by the ganglionic blocker trimethaphan. Note that resting blood pressure is decreased and heart rate is increased by trimethaphan because of sympathetic and parasympathetic withdrawal (HR scale is different). In the absence of baroreflex buffering, approximately a 10-fold lower dose of phenylephrine is required to produce a similar increase in blood pressure. Note also the lack of compensatory decrease in heart rate.

increased calcium influx in cardiac cells with both electrical and mechanical consequences. Beta$_1$ activation in the sinoatrial node increases pacemaker activity and heart rate (**positive chronotropic** effect). Beta$_1$ stimulation in the atrioventricular node increases conduction velocity (**positive dromotropic** effect) and decreases the refractory period. Beta$_1$ activation also increases intrinsic myocardial contractility (**positive inotropic** effect) and accelerates relaxation. Physiologic stimulation of the heart by catecholamines, therefore, increases heart rate and cardiac output, and it tends to increase coronary blood flow because of coronary vasodilation. Excessive stimulation of ventricular muscle and Purkinje cells can result in ventricular arrhythmias. Expression of β_3 adrenoceptors has been detected in the human heart and may be up-regulated in disease states, but the relevance of this finding is not clear.

D. Effects of Dopamine-Receptor Activation

Intravenous administration of dopamine promotes vasodilation of renal, splanchnic, coronary, cerebral, and perhaps other resistance vessels, via activation of D_1 receptors. Activation of the D_1 receptors in the renal vasculature may also induce natriuresis. The renal effects of dopamine have been used clinically to improve perfusion to the kidney in situations of oliguria (abnormally low urinary output). The activation of presynaptic D_2 receptors suppresses norepinephrine release, but it is unclear if this contributes to cardiovascular effects of dopamine.

Dopamine, however, can activate adrenoreceptors at higher concentrations. At low doses, the vasodilatory effects of dopamine receptors predominate, and peripheral resistance decreases. At moderate doses dopamine activates β_1 receptors in the heart, causing an increase in heart rate and in contractility. At higher doses dopamine activates vascular α receptors, leading to vasoconstriction, including in the renal vascular bed. Consequently, high rates of infusion of dopamine may mimic the actions of epinephrine.

Noncardiac Effects of Sympathomimetics

Adrenoceptors are distributed in virtually all organ systems. This section focuses on those actions that explain the therapeutic uses of sympathomimetics or their adverse effects. A more detailed description of the therapeutic use of sympathomimetics is given later in this chapter.

Activation of β_2 receptors in **bronchial smooth muscle** leads to bronchodilation, and β_2 agonists are important in the treatment of asthma (see Chapter 20 and Table 9–3).

In the **eye,** the radial pupillary dilator muscle of the iris contains α receptors; activation by drugs such as phenylephrine causes mydriasis (see Figure 6–9). Alpha$_2$ agonists increase the outflow of aqueous humor from the eye and can be used clinically to reduce intraocular pressure. In contrast, β agonists have little effect, but β *antagonists* decrease the production of aqueous humor and are used in the treatment of glaucoma (see Chapter 10).

In **genitourinary** organs, the bladder base, urethral sphincter, and prostate contain α_{1A} receptors that mediate contraction and therefore promote urinary continence. This effect explains why α_{1A} *antagonists* are useful in the management of symptoms of urinary flow obstruction and, conversely, why urinary retention is a potential adverse effect of administration of the α_1 agonist midodrine.

Alpha-receptor activation in the ductus deferens, seminal vesicles, and prostate plays a role in normal ejaculation and in the detumescence of erectile tissue that normally follows ejaculation. This explains why abnormal ejaculation can be seen as an adverse effect of α_{1A} antagonists.

The **salivary glands** contain adrenoceptors that regulate the secretion of amylase and water, and α_2 agonists, e.g., clonidine, produce symptoms of dry mouth. It is likely that CNS effects are responsible for this side effect, although peripheral effects may contribute.

The **apocrine sweat glands,** located on the palms of the hands and a few other areas, are nonthermoregulatory glands that respond to psychological stress and adrenoceptor stimulation with increased sweat production. (The diffusely distributed thermoregulatory eccrine sweat glands are regulated by *sympathetic cholinergic* postganglionic nerves that activate muscarinic cholinergic receptors; see Chapter 6.)

Sympathomimetic drugs have important effects on intermediary **metabolism.** Activation of β adrenoceptors in fat cells leads to increased lipolysis with enhanced release of free fatty acids and glycerol into the blood. Beta$_3$ adrenoceptors play a role in mediating this response in animals, but their role in humans is not clear. Experimentally, the β_3 agonist mirabegron stimulates brown adipose tissue in humans. The potential importance of this finding is that brown fat cells ("good fat") are thermogenic and thus have a positive metabolic function. Brown adipose tissue is present in neonates, but only remnant amounts are normally found in adult humans. Therefore, it is not clear whether β_3 agonists can be used therapeutically for the treatment of obesity. Human fat cells also contain α_2 receptors that inhibit lipolysis by decreasing intracellular cAMP. Sympathomimetic drugs enhance glycogenolysis in the liver, which leads to increased glucose release into the circulation. In the human liver, the effects of catecholamines are probably mediated mainly by β receptors, although α_1 receptors also may play a role. Activation of β_2 adrenoceptors by endogenous epinephrine or by sympathomimetic drugs promotes the uptake of potassium into cells, leading to a fall in extracellular potassium. This may result in a fall in the plasma potassium concentration during stress or protect against a rise in plasma potassium during exercise. Blockade of these receptors may accentuate the rise in plasma potassium that occurs during exercise. On the other hand, epinephrine has been used to treat hyperkalemia in certain conditions, but alternatives are more commonly used. Beta receptors and α_2 receptors that are expressed in pancreatic islets tend to increase and decrease insulin secretion, respectively, although the major regulator of insulin release is the plasma concentration of glucose.

Catecholamines are important endogenous regulators of **hormone secretion** from a number of glands. As mentioned above, insulin secretion is stimulated by β receptors and inhibited by α_2 receptors. Similarly, renin secretion is stimulated by β_1 and inhibited by α_2 receptors; indeed, β-receptor antagonist drugs may lower blood pressure in patients with hypertension at least in part by lowering plasma renin. Adrenoceptors also modulate the secretion of parathyroid hormone, calcitonin, thyroxine, and gastrin; however, the physiologic significance of these control mechanisms is probably limited. At high concentrations, epinephrine and related agents cause leukocytosis, in part by promoting demargination of sequestered white blood cells back into the general circulation.

The action of sympathomimetics on the **CNS** varies dramatically, depending on their ability to cross the blood-brain barrier. The catecholamines are almost completely excluded by this barrier, and subjective CNS effects are noted only at the highest rates of infusion. These effects have been described as ranging from "nervousness" to "an adrenaline rush" or "a feeling of impending disaster." Furthermore, peripheral effects of β-adrenoceptor agonists such as tachycardia and tremor are similar to the somatic manifestations of anxiety. In contrast, noncatecholamines with indirect actions, such as amphetamines, which readily enter the CNS from the circulation, produce qualitatively very different effects on the nervous system. These actions vary from mild alerting, with improved attention to boring tasks; through elevation of mood, insomnia, euphoria, and anorexia; to full-blown psychotic behavior. These effects are not necessarily mediated by adrenoceptor activation, and they may represent enhancement of dopamine-mediated processes or other effects of these drugs in the CNS.

SPECIFIC SYMPATHOMIMETIC DRUGS

Endogenous Catecholamines

Epinephrine (adrenaline) is released from the adrenal medulla to act as a circulating hormone. Epinephrine is an agonist at both α and β receptors. It is therefore a very potent vasoconstrictor and cardiac stimulant. The rise in systolic blood pressure that occurs after epinephrine release or administration is caused by its positive inotropic and chronotropic actions on the heart (predominantly β_1 receptors) and the vasoconstriction induced in many vascular beds (α receptors). Epinephrine also activates β_2 receptors in some vessels (e.g., skeletal muscle blood vessels), leading to vasodilation. Consequently, total peripheral resistance may actually fall, explaining the fall in diastolic pressure that is seen with epinephrine injection (see Figure 9–6 and Table 9–4). Activation of β_2 receptors in skeletal muscle contributes to increased blood flow during exercise.

Norepinephrine (levarterenol, noradrenaline) is an agonist at both α_1 and α_2 receptors. Norepinephrine also activates β_1 receptors with potency similar to epinephrine, but it has relatively little effect on β_2 receptors. Consequently, norepinephrine increases peripheral resistance and both diastolic and systolic blood pressure. Compensatory baroreflex activation tends to overcome the direct positive chronotropic effects of norepinephrine; however, the positive inotropic effects on the heart are maintained.

Dopamine is the immediate precursor in the synthesis of norepinephrine (see Figure 6–5). Its cardiovascular effects were described above. Endogenous dopamine may have more important effects in regulating sodium excretion and renal function. It is an important neurotransmitter in the CNS and is involved in the reward stimulus relevant to addiction. Its deficiency in the basal ganglia leads to Parkinson disease, which is treated with its precursor levodopa. Dopamine receptors are also targets for antipsychotic drugs.

Direct-Acting Sympathomimetics

Phenylephrine was discussed previously when describing the actions of a relatively pure α_1 agonist (see Table 9–2). Because it is not a catechol derivative (see Figure 9–5), it is not inactivated by COMT and has a longer duration of action than the catecholamines. It is an effective mydriatic and decongestant and can be used to raise the blood pressure (see Figure 9–6).

Midodrine is a prodrug that is enzymatically hydrolyzed to desglymidodrine, a selective α_1-receptor agonist. The peak concentration of desglymidodrine is achieved about 1 hour after midodrine is administered orally. The primary indication for midodrine is the treatment of orthostatic hypotension, typically due to impaired autonomic nervous system function. Midodrine increases upright blood pressure and improves orthostatic tolerance, but it may cause hypertension when the subject is supine.

Alpha$_2$-selective agonists decrease blood pressure through actions in the CNS that reduce sympathetic tone ("sympatholytics") even though direct application to a blood vessel may cause vasoconstriction. Such drugs (e.g., **clonidine, methyldopa, guanfacine, guanabenz**) are useful in the treatment of hypertension (and some other conditions) and are discussed in Chapter 11. Sedation is a recognized side effect of these drugs, but in some situations it may be beneficial. For example, **tizanidine** is used as a centrally acting muscle relaxant, and **dexmedetomidine** is used as a sedative to reduce requirements for opioids for pain control, and to induce sedation in an intensive care setting or in preparation for anesthesia. On the other hand, newer α_2 agonists (with activity also at imidazoline receptors) with fewer CNS side effects are available outside the USA for the treatment of hypertension (**moxonidine,** rilmenidine). Short-acting central sympatholytics like clonidine and tizanidine have the disadvantage that they can be associated with rebound hypertension and their effects wear off. This can be particularly relevant to tizanidine, which is marketed as a muscle relaxant and prescribed by physicians who do not realize that it can be as effective an antihypertensive as clonidine.

Oxymetazoline is a direct-acting α agonist used as a topical decongestant because of its ability to promote constriction of the vessels in the nasal mucosa and conjunctiva.

Isoproterenol (isoprenaline) is a very potent β-receptor agonist and has little effect on α receptors. Thus, the drug has positive chronotropic and inotropic actions and is a potent vasodilator. These actions lead to a marked increase in cardiac output that explains a slight increase in systolic pressure but a decrease in diastolic and mean arterial pressure (see Table 9–4 and Figure 9–6).

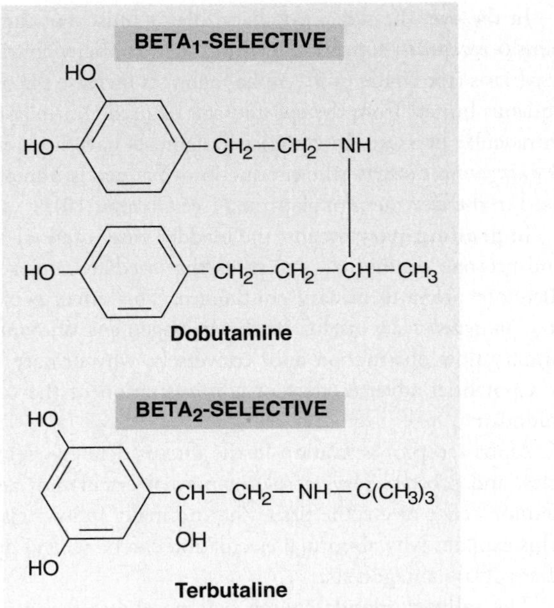

FIGURE 9–8 Examples of β_1- and β_2-selective agonists.

Beta subtype-selective agonists are very important because the separation of β_1 and β_2 effects (see Table 9–2), although incomplete, is sufficient to reduce adverse effects in several clinical applications.

Beta$_1$-selective agents (Figure 9–8) increase cardiac output without lowering diastolic blood pressure because they do not activate vasodilator β_2 receptors. **Dobutamine** was initially considered a relatively β_1-selective agonist, but its actions are more complex. Its chemical structure resembles dopamine, but its actions are mediated mostly by activation of α and β receptors. Clinical formulations of dobutamine are a racemic mixture of (–) and (+) isomers, each with contrasting activity at α_1 and α_2 receptors. The (+) isomer is a potent β_1 agonist and an α_1-receptor antagonist. The (–) isomer is a potent α_1 agonist, which is capable of causing significant vasoconstriction when given alone. The resultant cardiovascular effects of dobutamine reflect this complex pharmacology. Dobutamine has a positive inotropic action caused by the isomer with predominantly β-receptor activity. It has relatively greater inotropic than chronotropic effect compared with isoproterenol. Activation of α_1 receptors probably explains why peripheral resistance does not decrease significantly.

Beta$_2$-selective agents (see Figure 9–8) have achieved an important place in the treatment of asthma and are discussed in Chapter 20.

Mixed-Acting Sympathomimetics

Ephedrine is present in various plants and has been used in China for more than 2000 years; it was introduced into Western medicine in 1924 as the first orally active sympathomimetic drug. Ma huang, a popular herbal medication (see Chapter 64), contains ephedrine and multiple other ephedrine-like alkaloids. Because ephedrine is a noncatechol phenylisopropylamine (see Figure 9–5), it has high bioavailability and a relatively long duration of action—hours rather than minutes.

The ability of ephedrine to activate β receptors probably accounted for its earlier use in asthma. Because it gains access to the CNS, it is a mild stimulant. The US Food and Drug Administration (FDA) has banned the sale of ephedra-containing dietary supplements because of safety concerns. **Pseudoephedrine,** one of four ephedrine enantiomers, has been available over the counter as a component of many decongestant mixtures. However, the use of pseudoephedrine as a precursor in the illicit manufacture of methamphetamine has led to restrictions on the amount of drug that can be purchased.

INDIRECT-ACTING SYMPATHOMIMETICS

As noted previously, indirect-acting sympathomimetics can have one of two different mechanisms (see Figure 9–3). First, they may enter the sympathetic nerve ending and displace stored catecholamine transmitter. Such drugs have been called amphetamine-like or "displacers." Second, they may inhibit the reuptake of released transmitter by interfering with the action of the norepinephrine transporter, NET.

A. Amphetamine-Like

Amphetamine is a racemic mixture of phenylisopropylamine (see Figure 9–5) that is important chiefly because of its use and misuse as a CNS stimulant (see Chapter 32). Pharmacokinetically, it is similar to ephedrine; however, amphetamine enters the CNS even more readily, where it has marked stimulant effects on mood and alertness and a depressant effect on appetite. Its D-isomer is more potent than the L-isomer. Amphetamine's actions are mediated through the release of norepinephrine and, to some extent, dopamine.

Methamphetamine (*N*-methylamphetamine) is very similar to amphetamine, with an even higher ratio of central to peripheral actions. **Methylphenidate** is an amphetamine variant whose major pharmacologic effects and abuse potential are similar to those of amphetamine. Methylphenidate may be effective in children with attention deficit hyperactivity disorder (see Therapeutic Uses of Sympathomimetic Drugs). **Modafinil** and armodafinil are psychostimulants that differ from amphetamine in structure, neurochemical profile, and behavioral effects. Their mechanism of action is not fully known. They inhibit both norepinephrine and dopamine transporters, and increase synaptic concentrations not only of norepinephrine and dopamine, but also of serotonin and glutamate, while decreasing γ-aminobutyric acid (GABA) levels. They are used primarily to improve wakefulness in narcolepsy and some other conditions. Their use can be associated with increases in blood pressure and heart rate, although these are usually mild (see Therapeutic Uses of Sympathomimetic Drugs).

TABLE 9–5 Foods reputed to have a high content of tyramine or other sympathomimetic agents.

Food	Tyramine Content of an Average Serving
Beer	4–45 mg
Broad beans, fava beans	Negligible (but contains dopamine)
Cheese, natural or aged	Nil to 130 mg (cheddar, Gruyère, and Stilton especially high)
Chicken liver	Nil to 9 mg
Chocolate	Negligible (but contains phenylethylamine)
Sausage, fermented (eg, salami, pepperoni, summer sausage)	Nil to 74 mg
Smoked or pickled fish (eg, pickled herring)	Nil to 198 mg
Wine (red)	Nil to 3 mg
Yeast (eg, dietary brewer's yeast supplements)	2–68 mg

Note: In a patient taking an irreversible monoamine oxidase (MAO) inhibitor drug, 20–50 mg of tyramine in a meal may increase the blood pressure significantly (see also Chapter 30: Antidepressant Agents). Note that only cheese, sausage, pickled fish, and yeast supplements contain sufficient tyramine to be consistently dangerous. This does not rule out the possibility that some preparations of other foods might contain significantly greater than average amounts of tyramine. Amounts in mg as per regular food portion.

Tyramine (see Figure 6–5) is a normal byproduct of tyrosine metabolism in the body. It is an indirect sympathomimetic, inducing the release of catecholamines from noradrenergic neurons. Tyramine can be produced in high concentrations in protein-rich foods by decarboxylation of tyrosine during fermentation (Table 9–5) but is normally inactive when taken orally because it is readily metabolized by MAO in the liver (i.e., low bioavailability because of a very high first-pass effect). In patients treated with MAO inhibitors—particularly inhibitors of the MAO-A isoform—the sympathomimetic effect of tyramine may be greatly intensified, leading to marked increases in blood pressure. This occurs because of increased bioavailability of tyramine and increased neuronal stores of catecholamines. Patients taking MAO inhibitors should avoid tyramine-containing foods (aged cheese, cured meats, and pickled food). There are differences in the effects of various MAO inhibitors on tyramine bioavailability, and isoform-specific or reversible enzyme antagonists may be safer (see Chapters 28 and 30).

B. Catecholamine Reuptake Inhibitors

Many inhibitors of the amine transporters for norepinephrine, dopamine, and serotonin are used clinically. Although specificity is not absolute, some are highly selective for one of the transporters. Many antidepressants, particularly the older tricyclic antidepressants, can inhibit norepinephrine and serotonin reuptake to different degrees. Some antidepressants of this class, particularly imipramine, can induce orthostatic hypotension presumably by their clonidine-like effect or by blocking α_1 receptors, but the mechanism remains unclear.

Atomoxetine is a selective inhibitor of the norepinephrine reuptake transporter. Its actions, therefore, are mediated by potentiation of norepinephrine levels in noradrenergic synapses. It is used in the treatment of attention deficit disorders (see below). **Reboxetine** (investigational in the USA) has similar characteristics to atomoxetine but is used mainly for major depression disorder. Because reuptake inhibitors potentiate norepinephrine actions, there is concern about their cardiovascular safety. Norepinephrine reuptake is particularly important in the heart, especially during sympathetic stimulation, and this explains why atomoxetine and other norepinephrine reuptake inhibitors can cause orthostatic tachycardia. In general, however, atomoxetine produces few cardiovascular effects. This may be explained because atomoxetine has a clonidine-like effect in the CNS to decrease sympathetic outflow that may counteract the potentiating effects of norepinephrine in the periphery. In rare patients with autonomic failure due to impairment in CNS regulatory centers, the sympatholytic effects of atomoxetine are lost and blood pressure is increased by its peripheral effects.

Pharmacoepidemiologic studies have not found significant adverse cardiovascular events associated with the use of norepinephrine reuptake inhibitors and other medications used to treat attention deficit hyperactivity disorders in children and young adults. However, in patients with a history of cardiovascular disease the use of **sibutramine,** a serotonin and norepinephrine reuptake inhibitor, was associated with a small increase in cardiovascular events, including strokes. For this reason, it was taken off the market as an appetite suppressant. It is not clear if this concern applies to other serotonin and norepinephrine reuptake inhibitors widely used as antidepressants (venlafaxine, desvenlafaxine, and duloxetine; see Chapter 30), and no increase in cardiovascular risk has been reported with **duloxetine. Milnacipran,** another serotonin and norepinephrine transporter blocker, is approved for the treatment of pain in fibromyalgia (see Chapter 30).

Cocaine is a local anesthetic with a peripheral sympathomimetic action that results from inhibition of transmitter reuptake at noradrenergic synapses (see Figure 9–3). It readily enters the CNS and produces an amphetamine-like psychological effect that is shorter lasting and more intense than amphetamine. The major action of cocaine in the CNS is to inhibit dopamine reuptake into neurons in the "pleasure centers" of the brain. These properties and the fact that a rapid onset of action can be obtained when smoked, snorted, or injected have made cocaine a heavily abused drug (see Chapter 32). It is interesting that dopamine-transporter knockout mice still self-administer cocaine, suggesting that cocaine may have additional pharmacologic targets.

Dopamine Agonists

Levodopa, which is converted to dopamine in the body, and **dopamine agonists** with central actions are of considerable value in the treatment of Parkinson disease and prolactinemia. These agents are discussed in Chapters 28 and 37.

Fenoldopam is a D_1-receptor agonist that selectively leads to peripheral vasodilation in some vascular beds. The primary indication for fenoldopam is in the intravenous treatment of severe hypertension (see Chapter 11).

THERAPEUTIC USES OF SYMPATHOMIMETIC DRUGS

Cardiovascular Applications

In keeping with the critical role of the sympathetic nervous system in the control of blood pressure, a major area of application of the sympathomimetics is in cardiovascular conditions.

A. Treatment of Acute Hypotension

Acute hypotension may occur in a variety of settings such as severe hemorrhage, decreased blood volume, cardiac arrhythmias, neurologic disease, adverse reactions or overdose of medications such as antihypertensive drugs, and infections. If cerebral, renal, and cardiac perfusion is maintained, hypotension itself does not usually require vigorous direct treatment. Rather, placing the patient in the recumbent position and ensuring adequate fluid volume while the primary problem is determined and treated is usually the correct course of action. The use of sympathomimetic drugs merely to elevate a blood pressure that is not an immediate threat to the patient may increase morbidity. However, sympathomimetics may be required in cases of sustained hypotension with evidence of tissue hypoperfusion.

Shock is a complex acute cardiovascular syndrome that results in a critical reduction in perfusion of vital tissues and a wide range of systemic effects. Shock is usually associated with hypotension, an altered mental state, oliguria, and metabolic acidosis. If untreated, shock usually progresses to a refractory deteriorating state and death. The three major forms of shock are septic, cardiogenic, and hypovolemic. Volume replacement and treatment of the underlying disease are the mainstays of the treatment of shock. If vasopressors are needed, adrenergic agonists with both α and β activity are preferred. Pure β-adrenergic stimulation increases blood flow but also increases the risk of myocardial ischemia. Pure α-adrenergic stimulation increases vascular tone and blood pressure but can also decrease cardiac output and impair tissue blood flow. Norepinephrine provides an acceptable balance and is considered the vasopressor of first choice: it has predominantly α-adrenergic properties, but its modest β-adrenergic effects help to maintain cardiac output. Administration generally results in a clinically significant increase in mean arterial pressure, with little change in heart rate or cardiac output. Dopamine has no advantage over norepinephrine because it is associated with a higher incidence of arrhythmias and mortality. However, dobutamine is arguably the inotropic agent of choice when increased cardiac output is needed.

B. Chronic Orthostatic Hypotension

On standing, gravitational forces induce venous pooling, resulting in decreased venous return. Normally, a decrease in blood pressure is prevented by reflex sympathetic activation with increased heart rate, and peripheral arterial and venous vasoconstriction. Impairment of autonomic reflexes that regulate blood pressure can lead to chronic orthostatic hypotension. This is more often due to medications that can interfere with autonomic function (e.g., α blockers for the treatment of urinary retention), diabetes and other diseases causing peripheral autonomic neuropathies, and less commonly, primary degenerative disorders of the autonomic nervous system, as in the case study described at the beginning of the chapter.

Increasing peripheral resistance is one of the strategies to treat chronic orthostatic hypotension, and drugs activating α receptors can be used for this purpose. Midodrine, an orally active α_1 agonist, is frequently used for this indication. Other sympathomimetics, such as oral ephedrine or phenylephrine, can be tried. A more recent approach to treat orthostatic hypotension is **droxidopa,** a synthetic (L-threo-dihydroxyphenylserine, L-DOPS) molecule that is converted to norepinephrine by the aromatic L-amino acid decarboxylase (dopa-decarboxylase), the same enzyme that converts L-dopa to dopamine in the treatment of Parkinson disease, and is now approved for the treatment of orthostatic hypotension.

C. Cardiac Applications

Epinephrine is used during resuscitation from **cardiac arrest.** Current evidence indicates that it improves the chance of returning to spontaneous circulation, but it is less clear that it improves survival or long-term neurologic outcomes.

Dobutamine is used as a pharmacologic **cardiac stress test.** Dobutamine augments myocardial contractility and promotes coronary and systemic vasodilation. These actions lead to increased heart rate and increased myocardial work and can reveal areas of ischemia in the myocardium that are detected by echocardiogram or nuclear medicine techniques. Dobutamine can thus be used in patients unable to perform an exercise stress test.

D. Inducing Local Vasoconstriction

Reduction of local or regional blood flow is desirable for achieving hemostasis during surgery, for reducing diffusion of local anesthetics away from the site of administration, and for reducing mucous membrane congestion. In each instance, α-receptor activation is desired, and the choice of agent depends on the maximal efficacy required, the desired duration of action, and the route of administration.

Effective pharmacologic hemostasis is often necessary for facial, oral, and nasopharyngeal surgery. Epinephrine is usually applied topically in nasal packs (for epistaxis) or in a gingival string (for gingivectomy). Cocaine is still sometimes used for nasopharyngeal surgery because it combines a hemostatic effect with local anesthesia.

Combining α agonists with some local anesthetics greatly prolongs their duration of action; the total dose of local anesthetic (and the probability of systemic toxicity) can therefore be reduced. Epinephrine, 1:100,000 or 1:200,000, is the favored agent for this application. Systemic effects on the heart and peripheral vasculature may occur even with local drug administration but are usually minimal. Use of epinephrine with local anesthesia of acral vascular beds (digits, nose, and ears) has not been advised because of fear of ischemic necrosis. Recent studies suggest that it can be used (with caution) for this indication.

Alpha agonists can be used topically as mucous membrane decongestants to reduce the discomfort of allergic rhinitis or the common cold. These effects are mediated by activation of α receptors in the vasculature reducing blood flow in the nasal mucosa, thus reducing its volume. Phenylephrine and the longer-acting oxymetazoline are used in over-the-counter nasal decongestants. Unfortunately, rebound hyperemia ("rhinitis medicamentosa") may follow the use of these agents, and repeated topical use of high drug concentrations may result in ischemic changes in the mucous membranes, probably as a result of vasoconstriction of nutrient arteries. Oral administration of agents such as ephedrine and pseudoephedrine can provide a longer duration of action but at the cost of greater potential for cardiac and CNS effects.

Pulmonary Applications

One of the most important uses of sympathomimetic drugs is in the therapy of asthma and chronic obstructive pulmonary disease (COPD; discussed in more detail in Chapter 20). Beta$_2$-selective drugs (albuterol, metaproterenol, terbutaline) are used for this purpose to reduce the adverse effects that would be associated with β_1 stimulation. Short-acting preparations can be used only transiently for acute treatment of asthma symptoms. For chronic asthma treatment in adults, long-acting β_2 agonists should be used only in combination with steroids because their use in monotherapy has been associated with increased mortality. Long-acting β_2 agonists are also used in patients with COPD. **Indacaterol, olodaterol,** and **vilanterol** are newer ultralong β_2 agonists that are used with once-a-day dosing in the treatment of COPD. Nonselective drugs are now rarely used because they are likely to have more adverse effects than the selective drugs.

Anaphylaxis

Anaphylactic shock and related immediate (type I) IgE-mediated reactions affect both the respiratory and the cardiovascular systems. The syndrome of bronchospasm, mucous membrane congestion, angioedema, and severe hypotension usually responds rapidly to the parenteral administration of **epinephrine**, 0.3–0.5 mg (0.3–0.5 mL of a 1:1000 epinephrine solution). Intramuscular injection may be the preferred route of administration, since skin blood flow (and hence systemic drug absorption from subcutaneous injection) is unpredictable in hypotensive patients. In some patients with impaired cardiovascular function, intravenous injection of epinephrine may be required. The use of epinephrine for anaphylaxis precedes the era of controlled clinical trials, but extensive experimental and clinical experience supports its use as the agent of choice. Epinephrine activates α, β_1, and β_2 receptors, all of which may be important in reversing the pathophysiologic processes underlying anaphylaxis. It is recommended that patients at risk for anaphylaxis carry epinephrine in an autoinjector (EpiPen, Auvi-Q) for self-administration.

Ophthalmic Applications

Phenylephrine is an effective mydriatic agent frequently used to facilitate examination of the retina. It is also a useful decongestant for minor allergic hyperemia and itching of the conjunctival membranes. Sympathomimetics administered as ophthalmic drops are also useful in localizing the lesion in Horner syndrome. (See Box: An Application of Basic Pharmacology to a Clinical Problem.)

Glaucoma responds to a variety of sympathomimetic and sympathoplegic drugs. (See Box: The Treatment of Glaucoma, in Chapter 10.) Both α_2-selective agonists (**apraclonidine** and **brimonidine**) and β-blocking agents (timolol and others) are common topical therapies for glaucoma.

Genitourinary Applications

As noted above, β_2-selective agents (eg, **terbutaline**) relax the pregnant uterus. In the past, these agents were used to suppress premature labor. However, meta-analysis of older trials and a randomized study suggest that β-agonist therapy has no significant benefit on perinatal infant mortality and may increase maternal morbidity.

Central Nervous System Applications

The amphetamines have a mood-elevating (euphoriant) effect; this effect is the basis for the widespread abuse of this drug group (see Chapter 32). The amphetamines also have an alerting, sleep-deferring action that is manifested by improved attention to repetitive tasks and by acceleration and desynchronization of the electroencephalogram. A therapeutic application of this effect is in the treatment of narcolepsy. **Modafinil** and **armodafinil,** newer amphetamine substitutes, are approved for use in narcolepsy and are claimed to have fewer disadvantages (excessive mood changes, insomnia, and abuse potential) than amphetamine in this condition. Amphetamines have appetite-suppressing effects, but there is no evidence that long-term improvement in weight control can be achieved with amphetamines alone, especially when administered for a relatively short course. A final application of the CNS-active sympathomimetics is in the **attention deficit hyperactivity disorder (ADHD),** a behavioral syndrome consisting of short attention span, hyperkinetic physical behavior, and learning problems. Some patients with this syndrome respond well to low doses of **methylphenidate** and related agents. Extended-release formulations of methylphenidate may simplify dosing regimens and increase adherence to therapy, especially in school-age children. Slow or continuous-release preparations of the α_2 agonists clonidine and guanfacine also are effective in children with ADHD. The norepinephrine reuptake inhibitor **atomoxetine** is also used in ADHD. Clinical trials suggest that modafinil may also be useful in ADHD, but because the safety profile in children has not been defined, it has not gained approval by the FDA for this indication.

Additional Therapeutic Uses

Although the primary use of the α_2 agonist **clonidine** is in the treatment of hypertension (see Chapter 11), the drug has been found to have efficacy in the treatment of diarrhea in diabetics with autonomic neuropathy, perhaps because of its ability to enhance salt and water absorption from the intestine. In addition, clonidine has efficacy in diminishing craving for narcotics and alcohol during withdrawal and may facilitate cessation of cigarette smoking. Clonidine has also been used to diminish menopausal hot flushes. **Dexmedetomidine** is an α_2 agonist used for sedation under intensive care circumstances and during anesthesia (see Chapter 25). It blunts the sympathetic response to surgery, which may be beneficial in some situations. It lowers opioid requirements for pain control and does not depress ventilation. Clonidine is also sometimes used as a premedication before anesthesia. **Tizanidine** is an α_2 agonist closely related to clonidine that is used as a "central muscle relaxant" (see Chapter 27), but many physicians are not aware of its cardiovascular actions, which may lead to unanticipated adverse effects such as orthostatic hypotension followed by rebound hypertension.

An Application of Basic Pharmacology to a Clinical Problem

Horner syndrome is a condition—usually unilateral—that results from interruption of the sympathetic nerves to the face. This translates clinically with vasodilation, ptosis, miosis, and loss of sweating on the affected side. The syndrome can be caused by either a preganglionic or a postganglionic lesion, and knowledge of the location of the lesion (preganglionic or postganglionic) helps determine the optimal therapy.

A localized lesion in a nerve causes degeneration of the distal portion of that fiber and loss of transmitter contents from the degenerated nerve ending—without affecting neurons innervated by the fiber. Therefore, a preganglionic lesion leaves the postganglionic adrenergic neuron intact, whereas a postganglionic lesion results in degeneration of the adrenergic nerve endings and loss of stored catecholamines from them. Because indirectly acting sympathomimetics require normal stores of catecholamines, such drugs can be used to test for the presence of normal adrenergic nerve endings. The iris, because it is easily visible and responsive to topical sympathomimetics, is a convenient assay tissue in the patient.

If the lesion of Horner syndrome is postganglionic, indirectly acting sympathomimetics (e.g., cocaine, hydroxyamphetamine) will not dilate the abnormally constricted pupil because catecholamines have been lost from the nerve endings in the iris. In contrast, the pupil dilates in response to phenylephrine, which acts directly on the α receptors on the smooth muscle of the iris. A patient with a preganglionic lesion, on the other hand, shows a normal response to both drugs, since the postganglionic fibers and their catecholamine stores remain intact in this situation.

SUMMARY Sympathomimetic Drugs

Subclass, Drug	Mechanism of Action	Effects	Clinical Applications	Pharmacokinetics, Toxicities, Interactions
α_1 AGONISTS				
• Midodrine	Activates phospholipase C, resulting in increased intracellular calcium and vasoconstriction	Vascular smooth muscle contraction increasing blood pressure (BP)	Orthostatic hypotension	Oral • prodrug converted to active drug with a 1-h peak effect • *Toxicity:* Supine hypertension, piloerection (goose bumps), and urinary retention
• *Phenylephrine: Can be used IV for short-term maintenance of BP in acute hypotension and intranasally to produce local vasoconstriction as a decongestant*				
α_2 AGONISTS				
• Clonidine	Inhibits adenylyl cyclase and interacts with other intracellular pathways	Vasoconstriction is masked by central sympatholytic effect, which lowers BP	Hypertension	Oral • transdermal • peak effect 1–3 h • $t_{1/2}$ of oral drug ~12 h • produces dry mouth and sedation
• *α-Methyldopa, guanfacine, and guanabenz: Also used as central sympatholytics* • *Dexmedetomidine: Prominent sedative effects and used in anesthesia* • *Tizanidine: Used as a muscle relaxant* • *Apraclonidine and brimonidine: Used topically in glaucoma to reduce intraocular pressure*				
β_1 AGONISTS				
• Dobutamine[1]	Activates adenylyl cyclase, increasing myocardial contractility	Positive inotropic effect	Cardiogenic shock, acute heart failure	IV • requires dose titration to desired effect
A_2 AGONISTS				
• Albuterol	Activates adenylyl cyclase	Bronchial smooth muscle dilation	Asthma	Inhalation • duration 4–6 h • *Toxicity:* Tremor, tachycardia
• *See other β_2 agonists in Chapter 20*				
A_3 AGONISTS				
• Mirabegron	Activates adenylyl cyclase	Reduces bladder tone	Urinary urgency	Oral • duration 50 h • *Toxicity:* Possible hypertension
DOPAMINE AGONISTS				
D_1 AGONISTS				
• Fenoldopam	Activates adenylyl cyclase	Vascular smooth muscle relaxation	Hypertensive emergency	Requires dose titration to desired effect
D_2 AGONISTS				
• Bromocriptine	Inhibits adenylyl cyclase and interacts with other intracellular pathways	Mimics dopamine actions in the CNS	Parkinson disease, prolactinemia	Oral • *Toxicity:* Nausea, headache, orthostatic hypotension
• *See other D_2 agonists in Chapters 28 and 37*				

[1] *Dobutamine has other actions in addition to β_1-agonist effect. See text for details.*

PREPARATIONS AVAILABLE*

GENERIC NAME	AVAILABLE AS
Amphetamine, racemic mixture	Generic
1:1:1:1 mixtures of amphetamine sulfate, amphetamine aspartate, dextroamphetamine sulfate, and dextroamphetamine saccharate	Adderall
Apraclonidine	Iopidine
Armodafinil	Nuvigil
Brimonidine	Alphagan
Dexmedetomidine	Precedex
Dexmethylphenidate	Focalin
Dextroamphetamine	Generic, Dexedrine
Dobutamine	Generic, Dobutrex
Dopamine	Generic, Intropin
Droxidopa	Northera
Ephedrine	Generic
Epinephrine	Generic, Adrenalin Chloride, Primatene Mist, Bronkaid Mist, EpiPen, Auvi-Q
Fenoldopam	Corlopam
Hydroxyamphetamine	Paremyd (includes 0.25% tropicamide)
Isoproterenol	Generic, Isuprel
Metaraminol	Aramine
Methamphetamine	Desoxyn
Methylphenidate	Generic, Ritalin, Ritalin-SR
Midodrine	ProAmatine
Mirabegron	Myrbetriq
Modafinil	Provigil
Naphazoline	Generic, Privine
Norepinephrine	Generic, Levophed
Olodaterol	Striverdi Respimat
Oxymetazoline	Generic, Afrin, Neo-Synephrine 12 Hour, Visine LR
Phenylephrine	Generic, Neo-Synephrine
Pseudoephedrine	Generic, Sudafed
Tetrahydrozoline	Generic, Visine
Tizanidine	Zanaflex
Xylometazoline	Generic, Otrivin

*α_2 Agonists used in hypertension are listed in Chapter 11. β_2 Agonists used in asthma are listed in Chapter 20. Norepinephrine transporter inhibitors are listed in Chapter 30.

REFERENCES

Cooper WO et al: ADHD drugs and serious cardiovascular events in children and young adults. N Engl J Med 2011;265:1896.

Cotecchia S: The α_1-adrenergic receptors: Diversity of signaling networks and regulation. J Recept Signal Transduct Res 2010;30:410.

Guvercih VV, Guverich EV: GPCR signaling regulation: the role of GRKs and arrestins. Front Pharmacol 2019;10:125.

Gurevich VV, Gurevich EV: Biased GPCR signaling: possible mechanisms and inherent limitations. Pharmacol Ther 2020;211:107540.

Hikino K et al: A meta-analysis of the influence of ADRB2 genetic polymorphisms on albuterol (salbutamol) therapy in patients with asthma. Br J Clin Pharmacol 2021;87:1708.

Hollenberg SM: Vasoactive drugs in circulatory shock. Am J Respir Crit Care Med 2011;183:847.

Johnson JA, Liggett SB: Cardiovascular pharmacogenomics of adrenergic receptor signaling: clinical implications and future directions. Clin Pharmacol Ther 2011;89:366.

Johnson M: Molecular mechanisms of β2-adrenergic receptor function, response, and regulation. J Allergy Clin Immunol 2006;117:18.

Minzenberg MJ, Carter CS: Modafinil: A review of neurochemical actions and effects on cognition. Neuropsychopharmacology 2008;33:1477.

Sandilands AJ, O'Shaughnessy KM: The functional significance of genetic variation within the beta-adrenoceptor. Br J Clin Pharmacol 2005;60:235.

Schena G, Caplan MJ: Everything you always wanted to know about β_3-AR * (*but were afraid to ask). Cells 2019;8:357.

Seyedabadi M et al: Receptor-arrestin interactions: the GPCR perspective. Biomolecules. 2021;11:218.

Simons FE: Anaphylaxis. J Allergy Clin Immunol 2008;121:S402.

Soar J. Epinephrine for cardiac arrest: knowns, unknowns and controversies. Curr Opin Crit Care. 2020;26:590.

Vincent J-L, De Backer D: Circulatory shock. N Engl J Med 2013;369:1726.

Wisler JW et al: Biased G protein-coupled receptor signaling. Changing the paradigm of drug discovery. Circulation 2018;137:2315.

CASE STUDY ANSWER

The clinical picture is that of autonomic failure. The best indicator of this is the profound drop in orthostatic blood pressure without an adequate compensatory increase in heart rate. Pure autonomic failure is a neurodegenerative disorder selectively affecting peripheral autonomic fibers. Patients' blood pressure is critically dependent on whatever residual sympathetic tone they have, hence the symptomatic worsening of orthostatic hypotension that occurred when this patient was given the α_{1A} blocker tamsulosin. Conversely, these patients are hypersensitive to the pressor effects of α agonists and other sympathomimetics. For example, the α agonist midodrine can increase blood pressure significantly at doses that have no effect in normal subjects and can be used to treat their orthostatic hypotension. Caution should be observed in the use of sympathomimetics (including over-the-counter agents) and sympatholytic drugs.

CHAPTER

10

Adrenoceptor Antagonist Drugs

Italo Biaggioni, MD*

CASE STUDY

A 38-year-old man has been experiencing palpitations and headaches. He enjoyed good health until 1 year ago when spells of rapid heartbeat began. These became more severe and were eventually accompanied by throbbing headaches and drenching sweats. Physical examination revealed a blood pressure of 150/90 mm Hg and heart rate of 88 bpm. During the physical examination, palpation of the abdomen elicited a sudden and typical episode, with a rise in blood pressure to 210/120 mm Hg, heart rate to 122 bpm, profuse sweating, and facial pallor. This was accompanied by severe headache. What is the likely cause of his episodes? What caused the blood pressure and heart rate to rise so high during the examination? What treatments might help this patient?

Catecholamines play a role in many physiologic and pathophysiologic responses, as described in Chapter 9. Drugs that block their receptors, therefore, have important effects, some of which are of great clinical value. These effects vary dramatically according to the drug's selectivity for α and β receptors. The classification of α and β adrenoceptors subtypes and the effects of activating these receptors are discussed in Chapters 6 and 9. Blockade of peripheral dopamine receptors is of limited clinical importance at present. In contrast, modulation of central nervous system (CNS) dopamine receptors is very important, as discussed in Chapters 21, 28, and 29. This chapter deals with pharmacologic antagonist drugs whose major effect is to occupy α or β receptors and prevent their activation by catecholamines and related agonists.

Nonselective α antagonists are used in the treatment of pheochromocytoma (tumors that secrete catecholamines), and α_1-selective antagonists are used in primary hypertension and benign prostatic hyperplasia. Beta-receptor antagonist drugs are useful in a much wider variety of clinical conditions and are firmly established in the treatment of hypertension, ischemic heart disease, arrhythmias, endocrinologic and neurologic disorders, glaucoma, and other conditions.

*The author thanks David Robertson, MD, for his contributions to previous versions of this chapter.

■ BASIC PHARMACOLOGY OF THE ALPHA-RECEPTOR ANTAGONIST DRUGS

Mechanism of Action

Alpha-receptor antagonists may be reversible or irreversible in their interaction with these receptors. Reversible antagonists dissociate from receptors, and the block can be overcome with sufficiently high concentrations of agonists; irreversible drugs do not dissociate and cannot be surmounted. Phentolamine and prazosin (Figure 10–1) are examples of reversible antagonists. Phenoxybenzamine forms a reactive ethyleneimonium intermediate (see Figure 10–1) that covalently binds to α receptors, resulting in irreversible blockade. Figure 10–2 illustrates the effects of a reversible drug in comparison with those of an irreversible agent.

As discussed in Chapters 1 and 2, the duration of action of a reversible antagonist is largely dependent on the half-life of the drug in the body and the rate at which it dissociates from its receptor: The shorter the half-life, the less time it takes for the effects of the drug to dissipate. In contrast, the effects of an irreversible antagonist may persist long after the drug has been cleared from the plasma.

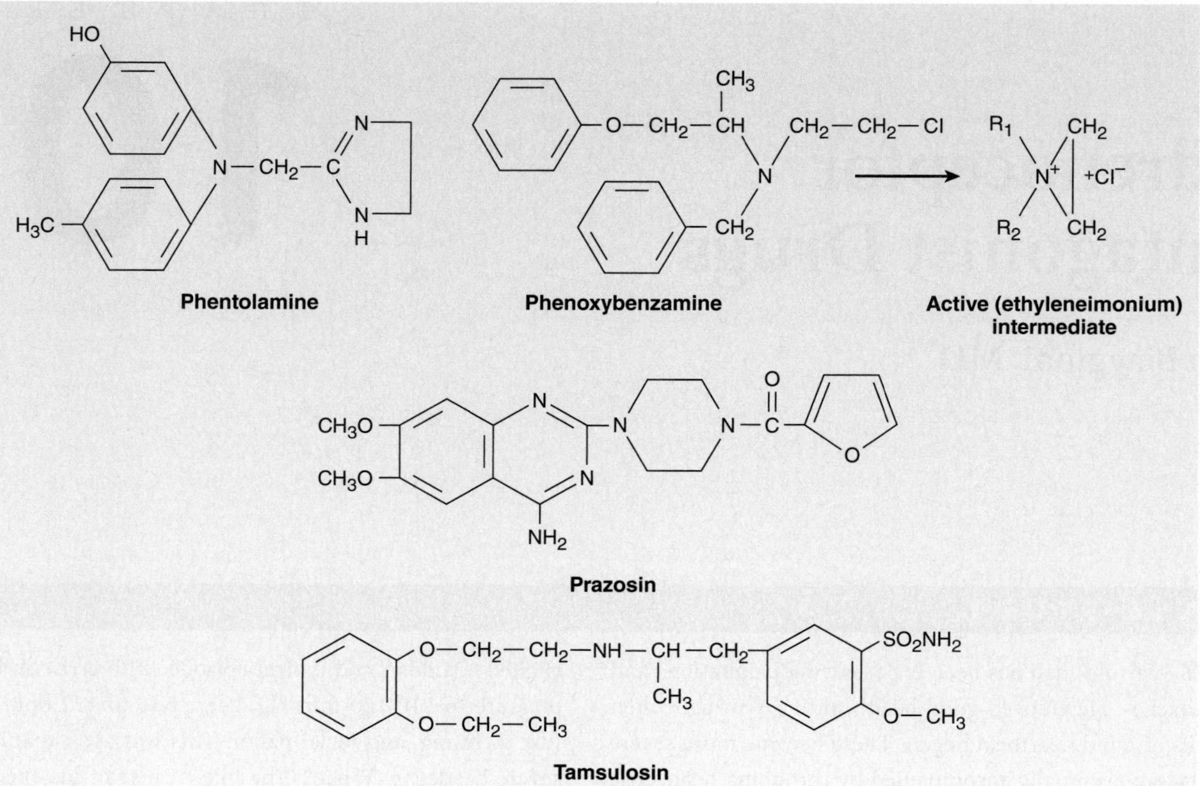

Phentolamine

Phenoxybenzamine

Active (ethyleneimonium) intermediate

Prazosin

Tamsulosin

FIGURE 10–1 Structure of several α-receptor–blocking drugs.

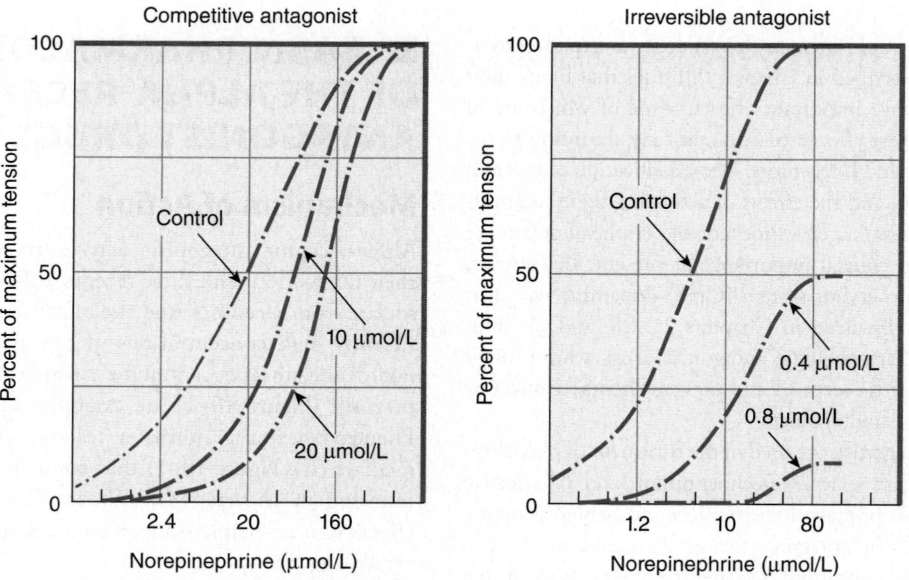

FIGURE 10–2 Dose-response curves to norepinephrine in the presence of two different α-adrenoceptor–blocking drugs. The tension produced in isolated strips of cat spleen, a tissue rich in α receptors, was measured in response to graded doses of norepinephrine. **Left:** Tolazoline, a reversible blocker, shifted the curve to the right without decreasing the maximum response when present at concentrations of 10 and 20 μmol/L. **Right:** Dibenamine, an analog of phenoxybenzamine and irreversible in its action, reduced the maximum response attainable at both concentrations tested. (Reproduced with permission from Bickerton RK: The response of isolated strips of cat spleen to sympathomimetic drugs and their antagonists. J Pharmacol Exp Ther 1963;142:99-110.)

In the case of phenoxybenzamine, the restoration of tissue responsiveness after extensive α-receptor blockade is dependent on synthesis of new receptors, which may take several days. The rate of return of α_1-adrenoceptor responsiveness may be particularly important in patients who have a sudden cardiovascular event or who become candidates for urgent surgery.

Pharmacologic Effects

A. Cardiovascular Effects

Because arteriolar and venous tone are determined to a large extent by α receptors on vascular smooth muscle, α-receptor antagonist drugs cause a lowering of peripheral vascular resistance and blood pressure (Figure 10–3). These drugs can prevent the pressor effects of usual doses of α agonists; indeed, in the case of agonists with both α and β_2 effects (eg, epinephrine), selective α-receptor antagonism may convert a pressor to a depressor response (see Figure 10–3); it illustrates how the activation of both α and β receptors in the vasculature may lead to opposite responses, and that blockade of α adrenoceptors unmasks the effects of epinephrine on β receptors. Alpha-receptor antagonists (Table 10–1) block sympathetic-mediated vasoconstriction, causing a decrease in blood pressure. The fall in blood pressure is greater in situations when blood pressure depends on increased sympathetic activity. This may occur, for example, on standing when blood pressure is maintained by sympathetic activation to compensate for gravitational pooling of blood in the lower body. Thus, α adrenoceptor antagonists can cause orthostatic hypotension by blocking sympathetically-mediated peripheral arterial vasoconstriction and splanchnic capacitance venoconstriction. Because β receptors are unopposed, this is associated with a compensatory baroreflex-mediated tachycardia.

B. Other Effects

Blockade of α receptors in noncardiac tissues elicits miosis (small pupils) and nasal stuffiness. Alpha$_1$ receptors are expressed in the base of the bladder and the prostate, and their blockade decreases resistance to the flow of urine. Alpha blockers, therefore, are used therapeutically for the treatment of urinary retention due to prostatic hyperplasia (see below).

SPECIFIC AGENTS

Phenoxybenzamine binds covalently to α receptors, causing irreversible blockade of long duration (14–48 hours or longer). It is somewhat selective for α_1 receptors but less so than prazosin (see Table 10–1). The drug also inhibits reuptake of released norepinephrine by presynaptic adrenergic nerve terminals. Phenoxybenzamine also blocks histamine (H_1), acetylcholine, and serotonin receptors (see Chapter 16), but the pharmacologic actions of phenoxybenzamine are primarily related to antagonism of α-receptor–mediated events.

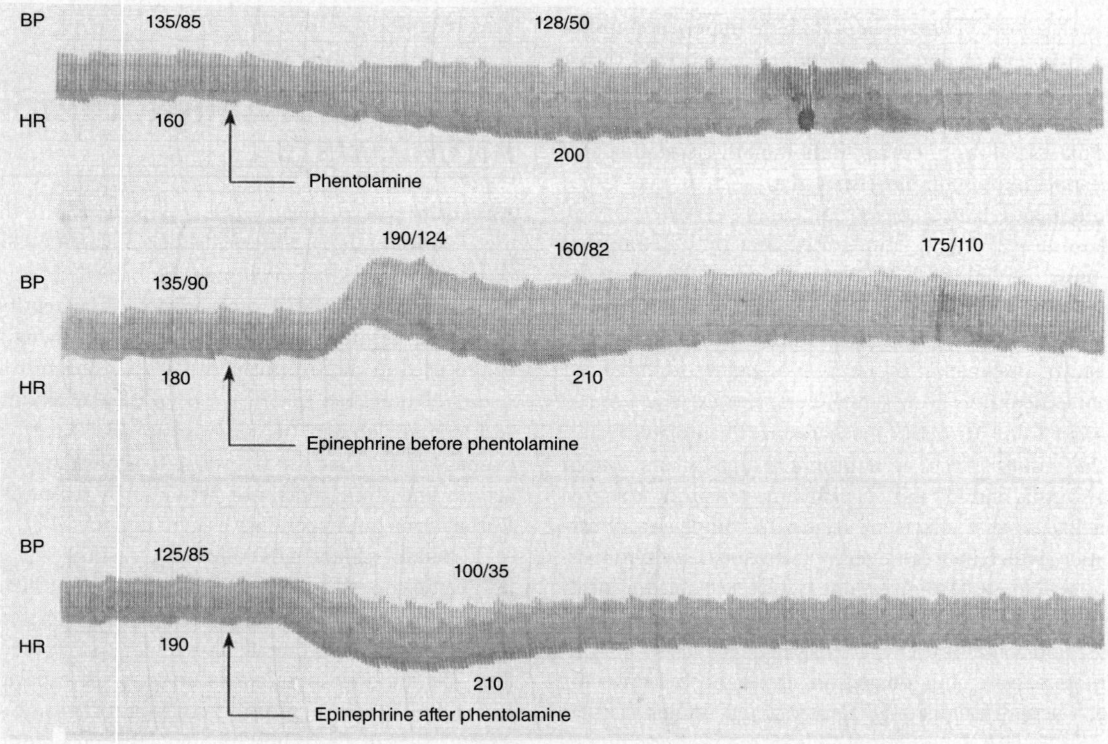

FIGURE 10–3 **Top:** Effects of phentolamine, an α-receptor–blocking drug, on blood pressure in an anesthetized dog. Epinephrine reversal is demonstrated by tracings showing the response to epinephrine before **(middle)** and after **(bottom)** phentolamine. All drugs given intravenously. BP, blood pressure; HR, heart rate.

TABLE 10–1 Relative selectivity of antagonists for adrenoceptors.

Drugs	Receptor Affinity
Alpha antagonists	
Prazosin, terazosin, doxazosin	$\alpha_1 >>>> \alpha_2$
Phenoxybenzamine	$\alpha_1 > \alpha_2$
Phentolamine	$\alpha_1 = \alpha_2$
Yohimbine, tolazoline	$\alpha_2 >> \alpha_1$
Mixed antagonists	
Labetalol, carvedilol	$\beta_1 = \beta_2 \geq \alpha_1 > \alpha_2$
Beta antagonists	
Metoprolol, acebutolol, alprenolol, atenolol, betaxolol, celiprolol, esmolol, nebivolol	$\beta_1 >>> \beta_2$
Propranolol, carteolol, nadolol, penbutolol, pindolol, timolol	$\beta_1 = \beta_2$
Butoxamine	$\beta_2 >>> \beta_1$

The most significant effect is attenuation of catecholamine-induced vasoconstriction. While phenoxybenzamine causes relatively little fall in blood pressure in normal individuals in the supine position (when sympathetic tone is low), it reduces blood pressure when sympathetic tone is high, eg, as a result of upright posture or because of reduced blood volume.

Phenoxybenzamine is absorbed after oral administration, although bioavailability is low; its other pharmacokinetic properties are not well known. Phenoxybenzamine is almost exclusively used in the treatment of pheochromocytoma (see below). Most adverse effects of phenoxybenzamine derive from its α-receptor–blocking action; the most important are orthostatic hypotension and tachycardia. Nasal stuffiness and inhibition of ejaculation also occur. Since phenoxybenzamine enters the CNS, it may cause fatigue, sedation, and nausea.

Phentolamine is a potent competitive antagonist at both α_1 and α_2 receptors (see Table 10–1). Phentolamine reduces peripheral resistance through blockade of α_1 receptors and possibly α_2 receptors on vascular smooth muscle. Its cardiac stimulation is due to antagonism of presynaptic α_2 receptors (leading to enhanced release of norepinephrine from sympathetic nerves) and sympathetic activation from baroreflex mechanisms. Phentolamine also has minor inhibitory effects at serotonin receptors and *agonist* effects at muscarinic and H_1 and H_2 histamine receptors. Phentolamine's principal adverse effects are related to compensatory cardiac stimulation, which may cause severe tachycardia, arrhythmias, and myocardial ischemia. Phentolamine is only available for intravenous administration and is now rarely used for the treatment of pheochromocytoma and other hypertensive emergencies.

Prazosin, terazosin, and **doxazosin** are highly selective for α_1 receptors. These drugs dilate both arterial and venous vascular smooth muscle, as well as smooth muscle in the prostate, due to blockade of α_1 receptors. They are used as second-line treatment for hypertension (see Chapter 11) and in men with urinary retention symptoms due to benign prostatic hyperplasia (BPH). Prazosin is extensively metabolized in humans; because of metabolic degradation by the liver, only about 50% of the drug is available after oral administration. The half-life is approximately 3 hours. Terazosin has high bioavailability but is extensively metabolized in the liver, with only a small fraction of unchanged drug excreted in the urine. The half-life of terazosin is 9–12 hours. Doxazosin has a longer half-life of about 22 hours. It has moderate bioavailability and is extensively metabolized, with very little parent drug excreted in urine or feces.

Tamsulosin is a competitive α_1 antagonist with a structure quite different from that of most other α_1-receptor blockers. It has high bioavailability and a half-life of 9–15 hours. It is metabolized extensively in the liver. Tamsulosin has higher affinity for α_{1A} and α_{1D} receptors than for the α_{1B} subtype. This results in greater potency in inhibiting contraction in *prostate* smooth muscle, which is mediated by the α_{1A} subtype versus *vascular* smooth muscle. Therefore, compared with other antagonists, tamsulosin has less effect on standing blood pressure in patients. Nevertheless, caution is appropriate in using any α antagonist in patients with diminished sympathetic nervous system function. Recent epidemiologic studies suggest an increased risk of orthostatic hypotension shortly after initiation of treatment. Patients on tamsulosin undergoing cataract surgery have a higher risk of the intraoperative floppy iris syndrome (IFIS), characterized by the billowing of a flaccid iris, propensity for iris prolapse, and progressive intraoperative pupillary constriction. These effects increase the risk of cataract surgery, and some recommend stopping tamsulosin for several weeks before cataract surgery, but the benefits of discontinuing the drug have not been proven.

OTHER ALPHA-ADRENOCEPTOR ANTAGONISTS

Alfuzosin is an α_1-selective quinazoline derivative that is approved for use in BPH. It has a bioavailability of about 60%, is extensively metabolized, and has an elimination half-life of about 5 hours. It may increase risk of QT prolongation in susceptible individuals. **Silodosin** resembles tamsulosin in blocking the α_{1A} receptor and is also used in the treatment of BPH. **Indoramin** is another α_1-selective antagonist that also has efficacy as an antihypertensive. It is not available in the USA. **Urapidil** is an α_1 antagonist (its primary effect) that also has weak α_2-agonist and 5-HT_{1A}-agonist actions and weak antagonist action at β_1 receptors. It is used in Europe as an antihypertensive agent and for BPH.

Labetalol and **carvedilol** have both α_1-selective and β-antagonistic effects; they are discussed below. Neuroleptic drugs such as **chlorpromazine** and **haloperidol** are potent dopamine receptor antagonists but are also antagonists at α receptors. Similarly, the antidepressant **trazodone** has the capacity to block α_1 receptors. This action probably contributes to some of their adverse effects, particularly orthostatic hypotension. Ergot derivatives, eg, **ergotamine** and **dihydroergotamine,** cause reversible α-receptor blockade, probably via a partial agonist action (see Chapter 16).

Yohimbine is an α_2-selective antagonist. It is sometimes used in the treatment of orthostatic hypotension because it promotes norepinephrine release through blockade of α_2 receptors in both the CNS (increasing central sympathetic activation) and the periphery (promoting norepinephrine release from noradrenergic fibers. Because it is its pharmacologic opposite, yohimbine reverses the antihypertensive effects of α_2-adrenoceptor agonists such as clonidine. It is used in veterinary medicine to reverse anesthesia produced by xylazine, an α_2 agonist. It was once widely used to treat male erectile dysfunction but has been superseded by phosphodiesterase-5 inhibitors like sildenafil (see Chapter 12), and was taken off the market in the USA solely for financial reasons. It is available as a "nutritional" supplement and through compounding pharmacies.

CLINICAL PHARMACOLOGY OF THE ALPHA-RECEPTOR–BLOCKING DRUGS

Pheochromocytoma

Pheochromocytoma is a tumor of the adrenal medulla or sympathetic ganglion cells. The tumor secretes catecholamines, especially norepinephrine and epinephrine. Patients with this tumor have many symptoms and signs of catecholamine excess, including intermittent or sustained hypertension, headaches, palpitations, and increased sweating. Release of stored catecholamines from pheochromocytomas may occur in response to physical pressure, chemical stimulation, or spontaneously. The patient in the case study at the beginning of this chapter had a left adrenal pheochromocytoma that was identified by imaging. In addition, he had elevated plasma and urinary norepinephrine, epinephrine, and their metabolites, normetanephrine and metanephrine.

The diagnosis of pheochromocytoma is confirmed on the basis of elevated plasma or urinary levels of norepinephrine, epinephrine, metanephrine, and normetanephrine (see Chapter 6). Once diagnosed biochemically, techniques to localize a pheochromocytoma include computed tomography and magnetic resonance imaging scans and scanning with radiomarkers such as ^{131}I-meta-iodobenzylguanidine (MIBG), a norepinephrine transporter substrate that is taken up by tumor cells and is therefore a useful imaging agent to identify the site of pheochromocytoma.

Alpha-receptor antagonists are most useful in the preoperative management of patients with pheochromocytoma (Figure 10–4). The major clinical use of phenoxybenzamine is in the management of pheochromocytoma. Its administration in the preoperative period helps to control hypertension and tends to reverse chronic changes resulting from excessive catecholamine secretion such as plasma volume contraction. Furthermore, it may prevent the blood pressure surges that can occur by manipulation of the tumor during surgery. Oral doses of 10 mg/d can be increased at intervals of several days until hypertension is controlled, for 1–3 weeks before surgery. A dosage of less than 100 mg/d is usually sufficient to achieve adequate α-receptor blockade, but doses up to 240 mg/d may be needed in some patients. Hypertension in patients with pheochromocytoma may also respond to reversible α_1-selective antagonists or to conventional calcium channel antagonists. Observational studies suggest that controlling hypertension without phenoxybenzamine to avoid delaying surgery is an alternative approach that can be safely implemented. Beta antagonists should not be used prior to establishing effective α-receptor blockade, since unopposed β-receptor blockade could theoretically cause blood pressure elevation from increased vasoconstriction. Beta-receptor antagonists may be required after α-receptor blockade has been instituted to reverse the cardiac effects of excessive catecholamines. Phenoxybenzamine can be very useful in the chronic treatment of inoperable or metastatic pheochromocytoma.

Pheochromocytoma is sometimes treated with **metyrosine** (α-methyltyrosine), the α-methyl analog of tyrosine. This agent is a competitive inhibitor of tyrosine hydroxylase, the rate-limiting step in the synthesis of dopamine, norepinephrine, and epinephrine (see Figure 6–5). Metyrosine is especially useful in symptomatic

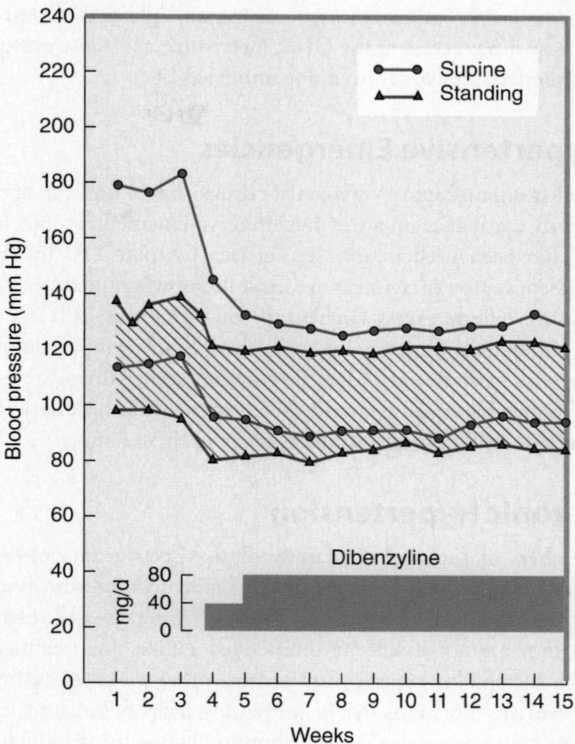

FIGURE 10–4 Effects of phenoxybenzamine (Dibenzyline) on blood pressure in a patient with pheochromocytoma. Dosage of the drug was begun in the fourth week as shown by the shaded bar. Supine systolic and diastolic pressures are indicated by the circles, and the standing pressures by triangles and the hatched area. Note that the α-blocking drug dramatically reduced blood pressure. The reduction in orthostatic hypotension, which was marked before treatment, is probably due to normalization of blood volume, a variable that is sometimes markedly reduced in patients with longstanding pheochromocytoma-induced hypertension. (From Annals of Internal Medicine, Engelman E, Sjoerdsma A: Chronic medical therapy for pheochromocytoma, 61(2):229. Copyright © 1964. All Rights Reserved. Reprinted with the permission of American College of Physicians, Inc.)

patients with inoperable or metastatic pheochromocytoma. Because it has access to the CNS, metyrosine can cause extrapyramidal effects due to reduced dopamine levels.

Hypertensive Emergencies

The α-adrenoceptor antagonist drugs have limited application in the management of hypertensive emergencies, but labetalol has been used in this setting (see Chapter 11). In theory, α-adrenoceptor antagonists are most useful when increased blood pressure reflects excess circulating concentrations of α agonists, eg, in pheochromocytoma, overdosage of sympathomimetic drugs, or clonidine withdrawal. However, other drugs are generally preferable because considerable experience is necessary to use α-adrenoceptor antagonist drugs safely in these settings.

Chronic Hypertension

Members of the prazosin family of α_1-selective antagonists are efficacious drugs in the treatment of mild to moderate systemic hypertension (see Chapter 11). They are generally well tolerated, but they are not usually recommended as first-line treatment or monotherapy for hypertension because other classes of antihypertensives are more effective in preventing heart failure and stroke. Their major adverse effect is orthostatic hypotension, which may be severe after the first few doses but is otherwise uncommon unless patients have impaired autonomic reflexes. Orthostatic changes in blood pressure should be checked routinely in any patient being treated for hypertension. Nonselective α antagonists are not used in primary hypertension.

Peripheral Vascular Disease

Alpha-receptor–blocking drugs do not seem to be effective in the treatment of peripheral vascular occlusive disease characterized by morphologic changes that limit flow in the vessels. Occasionally, individuals with Raynaud phenomenon and other conditions involving excessive reversible vasospasm in the peripheral circulation do benefit from prazosin or phenoxybenzamine, although calcium channel blockers may be preferable for most patients.

Urinary Obstruction

Benign prostatic hyperplasia is common in older men. Various surgical treatments are effective in relieving the urinary symptoms of BPH; however, drug therapy is efficacious in many patients. The mechanism of action in improving urine flow involves partial reversal of smooth muscle contraction in the enlarged prostate and in the bladder base. It has been suggested that some α_1-receptor antagonists may have additional effects on cells in the prostate that help improve symptoms.

Prazosin, doxazosin, and terazosin are all efficacious in patients with BPH. These drugs are particularly useful in patients who also have hypertension. *Subtype-selective* α_{1A}-receptor antagonists like tamsulosin may have improved efficacy and safety in treating this disease because this is the receptor subtype most important for smooth muscle contraction in the prostate. As indicated above, even though tamsulosin has less blood pressure–lowering effect, it should be used with caution in patients susceptible to orthostatic hypotension and should not be used in patients undergoing eye surgery.

Selective α_1 antagonists are also used in urolithiasis to induce ureteral dilation and facilitate the expulsion of kidney stones. It appears that this approach is less effective for smaller (5 mm or smaller) than for larger stones (>5 mm).

Applications of Alpha$_2$ Antagonists

Alpha$_2$ antagonists have relatively little clinical usefulness. Prescription drugs with this mechanism are no longer available, but extracts from the bark of the yohimbine tree are sold as dietary and health supplements, allegedly to treat erectile dysfunction, even though their efficacy is questionable.

■ BASIC PHARMACOLOGY OF THE BETA-RECEPTOR ANTAGONIST DRUGS

Beta-receptor antagonists share the common feature of antagonizing the effects of catecholamines at β adrenoceptors. Most β-blocking drugs in clinical use are pure antagonists; that is, the occupancy of a β receptor by such a drug causes no activation of the receptor. However, some are partial agonists; that is, they cause partial activation of the receptor, albeit less than that caused by the full agonists epinephrine and isoproterenol. As described in Chapter 2, partial agonists inhibit the activation of β receptors in the presence of high catecholamine concentrations but moderately activate the receptors in the absence of endogenous agonists. Finally, evidence suggests that some β blockers (eg, betaxolol, metoprolol) are *inverse agonists*—drugs that stabilize the inactive conformation of β receptors, reducing the proportion of active receptors, but the clinical significance of this property is not known.

Chemically, most β-receptor antagonist drugs (Figure 10–5) resemble isoproterenol to some degree (see Figure 9–4), even though they have opposite actions. The β-receptor–blocking drugs differ in their relative affinities for β_1 and β_2 receptors (see Table 10–1). Some have a higher affinity for β_1 than for β_2 receptors, and this selectivity may have important clinical implications. Since none of the clinically available β-receptor antagonists are absolutely specific for β_1 receptors, the selectivity is dose-related; it tends to diminish at higher drug concentrations.

Pharmacokinetic Properties of the Beta-Receptor Antagonists

A. Absorption

Most of the drugs in this class are well absorbed after oral administration; peak concentrations occur 1–3 hours after ingestion.

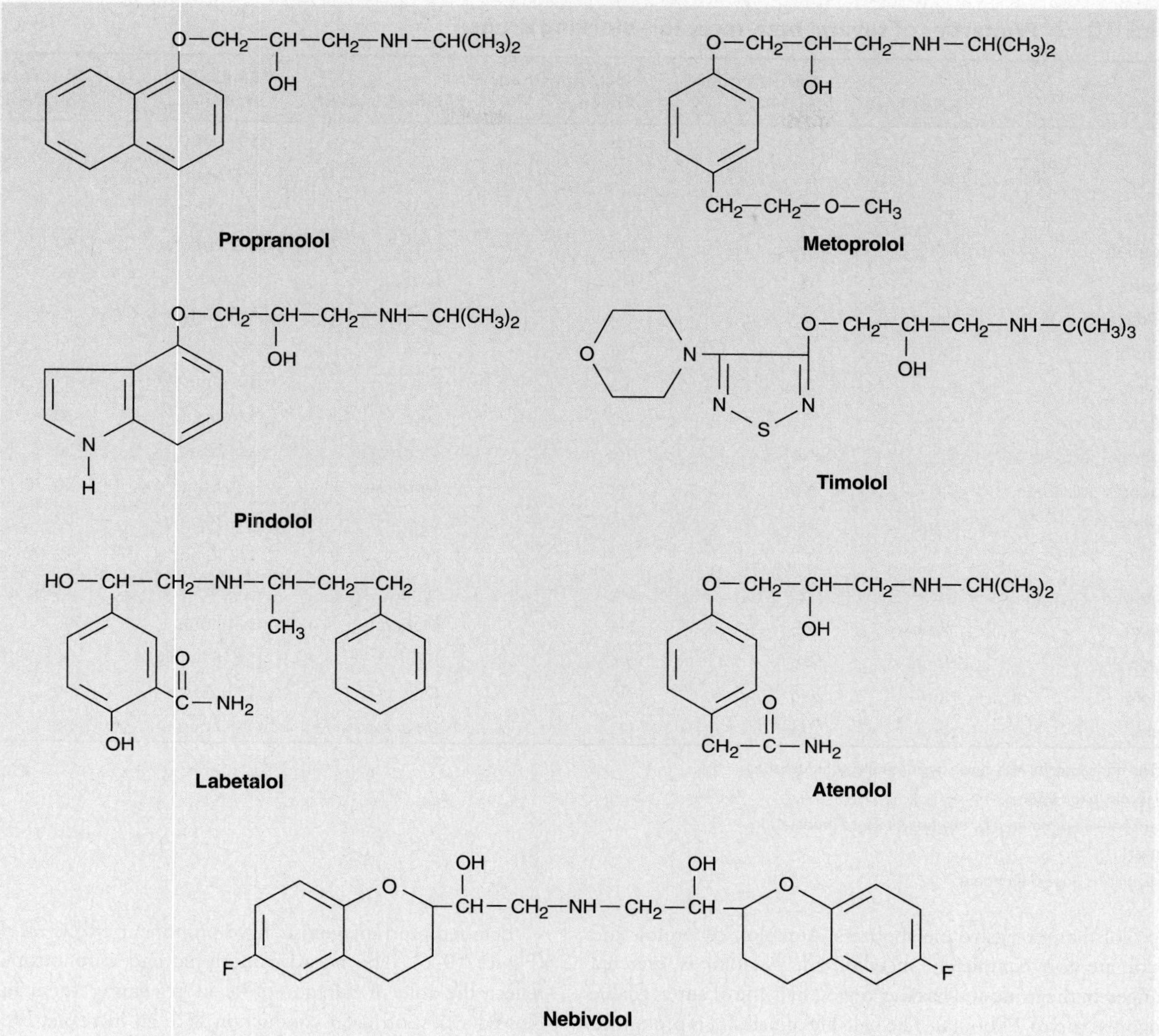

FIGURE 10–5 Structures of some β-receptor antagonists.

Sustained-release preparations of propranolol and metoprolol are available.

B. Bioavailability

Propranolol undergoes extensive hepatic (first-pass) metabolism; its bioavailability is relatively low (Table 10–2). The proportion of drug reaching the systemic circulation increases as the dose is increased, suggesting that hepatic extraction mechanisms may become saturated. A major consequence of the low bioavailability of propranolol is that oral administration of the drug leads to much lower drug concentrations than are achieved after intravenous injection of the same dose. Because the first-pass effect varies among individuals, there is great individual variability in the plasma concentrations achieved after oral propranolol. For the same reason, bioavailability is limited to varying degrees for most β antagonists with the exception of betaxolol, penbutolol, pindolol, and sotalol.

C. Distribution and Clearance

The β antagonists are rapidly distributed and have large volumes of distribution. Propranolol and penbutolol are quite lipophilic and readily cross the blood-brain barrier (see Table 10–2). Most β antagonists have half-lives in the range of 3–10 hours. A major exception is esmolol, which is rapidly hydrolyzed and has a half-life of approximately 10 minutes. Propranolol and metoprolol are extensively metabolized in the liver, with little unchanged drug appearing in the urine. The CYP2D6 genotype is a major determinant of interindividual differences in metoprolol plasma clearance (see Chapters 4 and 5). Poor metabolizers exhibit threefold to tenfold higher plasma concentrations after administration of

TABLE 10–2 Properties of several beta-receptor–blocking drugs.

Drugs	Selectivity	Partial Agonist Activity	Local Anesthetic Action	Lipid Solubility	Elimination Half-life	Approximate Bioavailability
Acebutolol	β_1	Yes	Yes	Low	3–4 hours	50
Atenolol	β_1	No	No	Low	6–9 hours	40
Betaxolol	β_1	No	Slight	Low	14–22 hours	90
Bisoprolol	β_1	No	No	Low	9–12 hours	80
Carteolol	None	Yes	No	Low	6 hours	85
Carvedilol[1]	None	No	No	Moderate	7–10 hours	25–35
Celiprolol[2]	β_1	Yes	No	Low	4–5 hours	70
Esmolol	β_1	No	No	Low	10 minutes	0
Labetalol[1]	None	Yes	Yes	Low	5 hours	30
Metoprolol Tartrate	β_1	No	Yes	Moderate	3–4 hours	50
Metoprolol Succinate	β_1	No	Yes	Moderate	~20 hours[3]	50–70
Nadolol	None	No	No	Low	14–24 hours	33
Nebivolol	β_1	?[4]	No	Low	11–30 hours	12–96
Penbutolol	None	Yes	No	High	5 hours	>90
Pindolol	None	Yes	Yes	Moderate	3–4 hours	90
Propranolol	None	No	Yes	High	3.5–6 hours	30[5]
Sotalol	None	No	No	Low	12 hours	90
Timolol	None	No	No	Moderate	4–5 hours	50

[1]Carvedilol and labetalol also cause α_1-adrenoceptor blockade.

[2]Not available in the USA.

[3]Apparent half-life prolonged by extended-release preparation.

[4]β_3 agonist.

[5]Bioavailability is dose-dependent.

metoprolol than extensive metabolizers. Atenolol, celiprolol, and pindolol are less completely metabolized. Nadolol is excreted unchanged in the urine and has the longest half-life of any available β antagonist (up to 24 hours). The half-life of nadolol is prolonged in renal failure. The elimination of drugs such as propranolol may be prolonged in the presence of liver disease, diminished hepatic blood flow, or hepatic enzyme inhibition. It is notable that the pharmacodynamic effects of these drugs are sometimes prolonged well beyond the time predicted from half-life data.

Pharmacodynamics of the Beta-Receptor Antagonist Drugs

Most of the effects of these drugs are due to occupation and blockade of β receptors. However, some actions may be due to other effects, including partial agonist activity at β receptors and local anesthetic membrane stabilizing effects, which differ among the β blockers (see Table 10–2).

A. Effects on the Cardiovascular System

Beta-blocking drugs given chronically lower blood pressure in patients with hypertension (see Chapter 11). The mechanisms involved are not fully understood but probably include suppression of renin release and effects in the CNS. These drugs do not usually cause hypotension in healthy individuals with normal blood pressure.

Beta-receptor antagonists have prominent effects on the heart (Figure 10–6). The negative inotropic and chronotropic effects reflect the role of adrenoceptors in regulating these functions. Slowed atrioventricular conduction with an increased PR interval is a related result of adrenoceptor blockade in the atrioventricular node. In the vascular system, β-receptor blockade opposes β_2-mediated vasodilation. This may acutely lead to a rise in peripheral resistance from unopposed α-receptor–mediated effects as the sympathetic nervous system discharges in response to lowered blood pressure due to the fall in cardiac output. Beta-receptor antagonists are very valuable in the treatment of angina (see Chapter 12), for chronic heart failure (see Chapter 13), and following myocardial infarction (see Chapter 14). The beneficial effects in these situations are related to blockade of the deleterious effects of catecholamines in the heart.

Overall, although the acute effects of these drugs may include a rise in peripheral resistance, chronic drug administration leads to a fall in peripheral resistance in patients with hypertension. This effect may be related to inhibition of renin release.

B. Effects on the Respiratory Tract

Blockade of the β_2 receptors in bronchial smooth muscle may lead to an increase in airway resistance, particularly in patients with asthma. Beta$_1$-receptor antagonists such as metoprolol and atenolol have an advantage over nonselective β antagonists when blockade

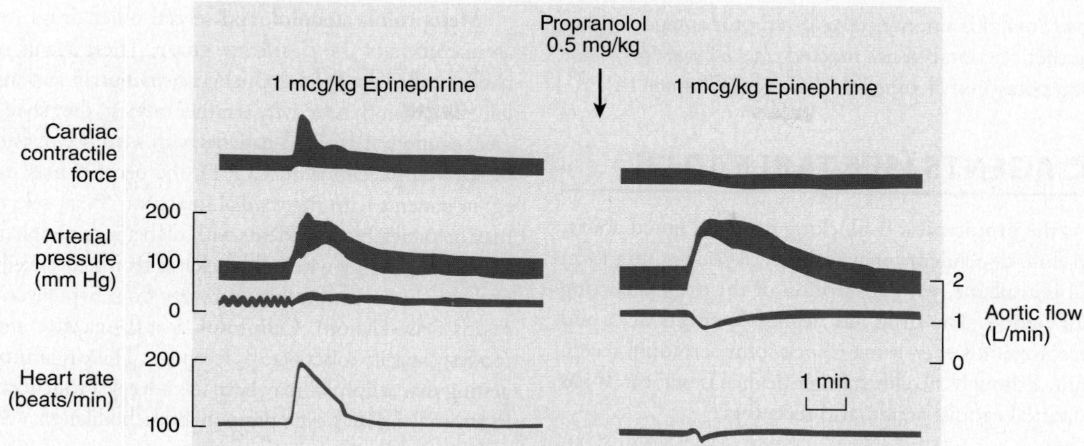

FIGURE 10–6 The effect in an anesthetized dog of the injection of epinephrine before and after propranolol. In the presence of a β-receptor–blocking agent, epinephrine no longer augments the force of contraction (measured by a strain gauge attached to the ventricular wall) nor increases cardiac rate. Blood pressure is still elevated by epinephrine because vasoconstriction is not blocked. (Reproduced with permission from Shanks RG. The pharmacology of beta sympathetic blockade. Am J Cardiol. 1966;18(3):308-316.)

of β_1 receptors in the heart is desired and β_2-receptor blockade is undesirable. However, no currently available β_1-selective antagonist is sufficiently specific to *completely* avoid interactions with β_2 adrenoceptors. Consequently, these drugs should generally be avoided in patients with asthma. However, some patients with chronic obstructive pulmonary disease (COPD) may tolerate β_1-selective blockers, and the benefits, for example in patients with concomitant ischemic heart disease, may outweigh the risks.

C. Effects on the Eye

Beta-blocking agents reduce intraocular pressure, especially in glaucoma. The likely mechanism usually is decreased aqueous humor production. (See Clinical Pharmacology and Box: The Treatment of Glaucoma.)

D. Metabolic and Endocrine Effects

Beta-receptor antagonists inhibit sympathetic nervous system stimulation of lipolysis. The effects on carbohydrate metabolism are less clear, although glycogenolysis in the human liver is at least partially inhibited after β_2-receptor blockade. Use of β-receptor antagonists can be detrimental in response to hypoglycemia, a significant clinical concern in the treatment of patients with diabetes. In part, this is because patients on β-blockers are less able to recognize the warning symptoms of hypoglycemia which includes tachycardia. Glucagon is the primary hormone used to combat hypoglycemia; it is unclear to what extent β antagonists impair recovery from hypoglycemia, but they should be used with caution in insulin-dependent diabetic patients. This may be particularly important in diabetic patients with inadequate glucagon reserve and in pancreatectomized patients since catecholamines may be the major factors in stimulating glucose release from the liver in response to hypoglycemia. Beta_1-receptor–selective drugs may be less prone to inhibit recovery from hypoglycemia.

The chronic use of β-adrenoceptor antagonists has been associated with increased plasma concentrations of very-low-density lipoproteins (VLDL) and decreased concentrations of HDL cholesterol. Both of these changes are potentially unfavorable in terms of risk of cardiovascular disease. Although low-density lipoprotein (LDL) concentrations generally do not change, there is a variable decline in the HDL cholesterol/LDL cholesterol ratio that may increase the risk of coronary artery disease. These changes tend to occur with both selective and nonselective β blockers, although they may be less likely to occur with β blockers possessing intrinsic sympathomimetic activity (partial agonists). Beta receptor antagonists also reduce resting energy expenditure, which can contribute to weight gain.

In summary, β-receptor antagonists have negative metabolic effects that can discourage its use. However, newer β–blockers such as metoprolol, carvedilol, bisoprolol, and nebivolol are less likely to have negative metabolic effects. Furthermore, the beneficial effects of these drugs, when used in patients in whom they are indicated, such as heart failure, usually overweight these concerns.

E. Effects Not Related to Beta-Blockade

Antagonists with *partial β-agonist activity* (pindolol and others noted in Table 10-2) may be desirable to prevent untoward effects such as precipitation of asthma or excessive bradycardia. However, these drugs may not be as effective as the pure antagonists in secondary prevention of myocardial infarction. Clinical trials of partial β-agonist drugs in hypertension have not confirmed increased benefit.

Local anesthetic action, also known as "membrane-stabilizing" action, is a prominent effect of several β blockers (see Table 10–2). This action is the result of typical local anesthetic blockade of sodium channels (see Chapter 26) and can be demonstrated experimentally in isolated neurons, heart muscle, and skeletal muscle membrane. However, it is unlikely that this effect is important clinically, since the concentration in plasma usually achieved by these routes is too low for the anesthetic effects to be evident.

Some β-receptor antagonists have *α–blocking effects* (carvedilol, labetalol), or promote *nitric oxide* production (nebivolol), as discussed below. Sotalol is a nonselective β-receptor antagonist that lacks local anesthetic action but has marked *class III antiarrhythmic effects*, reflecting potassium channel blockade (see Chapter 14).

SPECIFIC AGENTS (SEE TABLE 10–2)

Propranolol is the prototypical β-blocking drug. As noted above, it has low and dose-dependent bioavailability. A long-acting form of propranolol is available, with absorption of the drug occurring over a 24-hour period. The drug has negligible effects at α and muscarinic receptors; however, it may block some serotonin receptors in the brain, although the clinical significance is unclear. It has no detectable partial agonist action at β receptors.

Metoprolol, atenolol, and several other drugs (see Table 10–2) are members of the β_1*-selective* group. These agents may be safer in patients who experience bronchoconstriction in response to propranolol. Since their β_1 selectivity is rather modest, they should be used with great caution, if at all, in patients with a history of asthma. However, in selected patients with COPD, the benefits may exceed the risks, eg, in patients with myocardial infarction. Beta$_1$-selective antagonists may be preferable in patients with diabetes or peripheral vascular disease when therapy with a β blocker is required, since β_2 receptors are probably important in liver (recovery from hypoglycemia) and blood vessels (vasodilation). **Celiprolol*** is a β_1-selective antagonist with a modest capacity to activate β_2 receptors. There is limited evidence suggesting that celiprolol may have less adverse bronchoconstrictor effect in asthma and may even promote bronchodilation.

The Treatment of Glaucoma

Glaucoma is a major cause of blindness. The primary manifestation is increased intraocular pressure, which initially can be asymptomatic. Without treatment, increased intraocular pressure results in damage to the retina and optic nerve, with restriction of visual fields and, eventually, blindness. Intraocular pressure is easily measured as part of the routine ophthalmologic examination. Two major types of glaucoma are recognized: open-angle and closed-angle (also called narrow-angle). The closed-angle form is associated with a shallow anterior chamber, in which a dilated iris can occlude the outflow drainage pathway at the angle between the cornea and the ciliary body (see Figure 6–9). This form is associated with acute and painful increases of pressure, which must be controlled on an emergency basis with drugs or prevented by surgical removal of part of the iris (iridectomy). The open-angle form of glaucoma is a chronic condition, and treatment is largely pharmacologic. Because intraocular pressure is a function of the balance between fluid input and drainage out of the eye, topical medications work either by reducing aqueous humor secretion (α agonists, β blockers, carbonic anhydrase inhibitors) or by enhancing aqueous outflow (prostaglandin $F_{2\alpha}$ analogs, cholinomimetics, rho kinase inhibitors), as shown in Table 10–3. Topical prostaglandins are currently considered the drugs of choice to initiate treatment because they are effective and have a low adverse effect profile. Beta blockers are still commonly used in combination therapy and in patients who cannot afford prostaglandins.

TABLE 10–3 Topical drugs used in open-angle glaucoma.

Drugs	Mechanism	Comments
Beta Blockers		
Timolol, betaxolol, carteolol, levobunolol, metipranolol	Decreased aqueous secretion from the ciliary epithelium	Use with caution in patients with bradycardia, heart block, heart failure, asthma, or obstructive airway disease
Alpha$_2$ agonists		
Apraclonidine, brimonidine	Decreased aqueous secretion and increased outflow	May be associated with greater incidence of adverse effects
Cholinomimetics		
Pilocarpine, carbachol	Ciliary muscle contraction and opening trabecular meshwork leading to increased outflow	Higher incidence of topical adverse effects
Prostaglandins		
Latanoprost, bimatoprost, travoprost, unoprostone, tafluprost	Increased outflow	Advantage of once-daily dosing, few adverse effects
Carbonic anhydrase inhibitors*		
Dorzolamide, brinzolamide	Decreased aqueous secretion	Not as effective as other drugs
Rho kinase inhibitors		
Netarsudil	Increased outflow	Relatively new drug, less long-term experience

*Oral preparations are also available (acetazolamide and methazolamide) but can produce systemic adverse effects.

Esmolol is an ultra-short–acting *β_1-selective* adrenoceptor antagonist. The structure of esmolol contains an ester linkage; esterases in red blood cells rapidly metabolize esmolol to a metabolite that has a low affinity for β receptors. Consequently, esmolol has a short half-life (about 10 minutes) and duration of action, so that steady-state concentrations are achieved quickly during continuous infusions of esmolol and the therapeutic actions of the drug are terminated rapidly when its infusion is discontinued. Esmolol may be safer to use than longer-acting antagonists in critically ill patients who require a β-adrenoceptor antagonist. Esmolol is useful in controlling supraventricular arrhythmias, arrhythmias associated with thyrotoxicosis, perioperative hypertension, and myocardial ischemia in acutely ill patients.

Pindolol, acebutolol, penbutolol, carteolol, oxprenolol,* and **celiprolol*** are of interest because they have *partial β-agonist activity*. Although these partial agonists may be less likely to cause bradycardia and abnormalities in plasma lipids than pure antagonists, the overall clinical significance of intrinsic sympathomimetic activity remains uncertain. Pindolol also antagonizes 5-HT_{1A} serotonin receptors, and may potentiate the action of traditional antidepressant medications. Acebutolol is also a β_1-selective antagonist.

Nebivolol is the most highly selective β_1-adrenergic receptor blocker, although some of its metabolites do not have this level of specificity. Nebivolol has the additional quality of eliciting vasodilation by promoting endothelial *nitric oxide production*. Nebivolol may increase insulin sensitivity and does not adversely affect lipid profile. At equivalent beta blocking effects, nebivolol is not associated with the decrease in insulin sensitivity and increase in oxidative stress produced by metoprolol in patients with the metabolic syndrome.

Other β-blocking drugs cause vasodilation by antagonizing α-adrenoceptors. **Labetalol** is a reversible adrenoceptor antagonist available as a racemic mixture of two pairs of chiral isomers (the molecule has two centers of asymmetry). The (*S,S*)- and (*R,S*)-isomers are nearly inactive, the (*S,R*)-isomer is a potent α blocker, and the (*R,R*)-isomer is a potent β blocker. Labetalol's affinity for α receptors is less than that of phentolamine, but labetalol is α_1-selective. Its β-blocking potency is somewhat lower than that of propranolol. Hypotension induced by labetalol is accompanied by less tachycardia than occurs with phentolamine and similar α blockers.

Carvedilol, medroxalol,* and **bucindolol*** are nonselective β-receptor antagonists with some capacity to block α_1-adrenergic receptors. Carvedilol antagonizes the actions of catecholamines more potently at β receptors than at α_1 receptors. The drug has a half-life of 6–8 hours. It is extensively metabolized in the liver, and stereoselective metabolism of its two isomers is observed. Since metabolism of (*R*)-carvedilol is influenced by polymorphisms in CYP2D6 activity and by drugs that inhibit this enzyme's activity (such as quinidine and fluoxetine, see Chapter 4), drug interactions may occur. Carvedilol also appears to attenuate oxygen free radical–initiated lipid peroxidation and to inhibit vascular smooth muscle mitogenesis independently of adrenoceptor blockade. These effects may contribute to the clinical benefits of the drug in chronic heart failure (see Chapter 13).

*Not available in the USA.

Timolol is a nonselective β blocker without local anesthetic activity, a characteristic that is advantageous when given topically in the eye in the treatment of glaucoma because chronic anesthesia of the cornea, eliminating its protective reflexes, would be undesirable. **Nadolol** is noteworthy for its very long duration of action; its spectrum of action is similar to that of timolol. **Levobunolol** (nonselective) and **betaxolol** (β_1-selective) are also used for topical ophthalmic application in glaucoma; the latter drug may be less likely to induce bronchoconstriction than nonselective antagonists. **Carteolol** is a nonselective β-receptor antagonist.

Butoxamine is a selective β_2-blocking drug used in research. Beta$_2$-antagonists have not been actively developed because there is no obvious clinical application for them; none is available for clinical use.

■ CLINICAL PHARMACOLOGY OF THE BETA-RECEPTOR–BLOCKING DRUGS

Hypertension

Classic β-adrenoceptor antagonists are effective antihypertensive medications, but are not indicated as first line treatment for essential hypertension because other classes of drugs are superior in preventing stroke, particularly in patients older than 60 years. It is unclear if newer vasodilating β-adrenoceptor antagonists share the same limitation. Beta-adrenoceptor antagonists may be indicated in hypertension in special populations in whom "cardioprotection" is desirable, such as those with heart failure with reduced ejection fraction and those with coronary artery disease. Use of these agents is discussed in greater detail in Chapter 11.

Ischemic Heart Disease

Beta-adrenoceptor antagonists are first-line therapy in symptomatic management of patients with chronic stable angina (see Chapter 12). The beneficial effects are due to blockade of cardiac β receptors, resulting in decreased cardiac work, slowing and regularization of the heart rate, and reduction in oxygen demand. (Figure 10–7).

Multiple large-scale prospective studies indicate that in addition to symptomatic relief, β-adrenoceptor antagonists reduce infarct size and acute mortality when given early during acute myocardial infarct. In this setting, relative contraindications include bradycardia, hypotension, moderate or severe left ventricular failure, shock, heart block, and active airways disease. They also improve survival when given chronically to patients who have had myocardial infarction or to those with heart failure with reduced ejection fraction (Figure 10-8). The β_1-adrenoceptor antagonist **metoprolol** is commonly used for this purpose. **Atenolol** and **timolol** are also effective. Atenolol has the disadvantage that it is cleared by the kidney and its dose has to be adjusted in patients with renal failure.

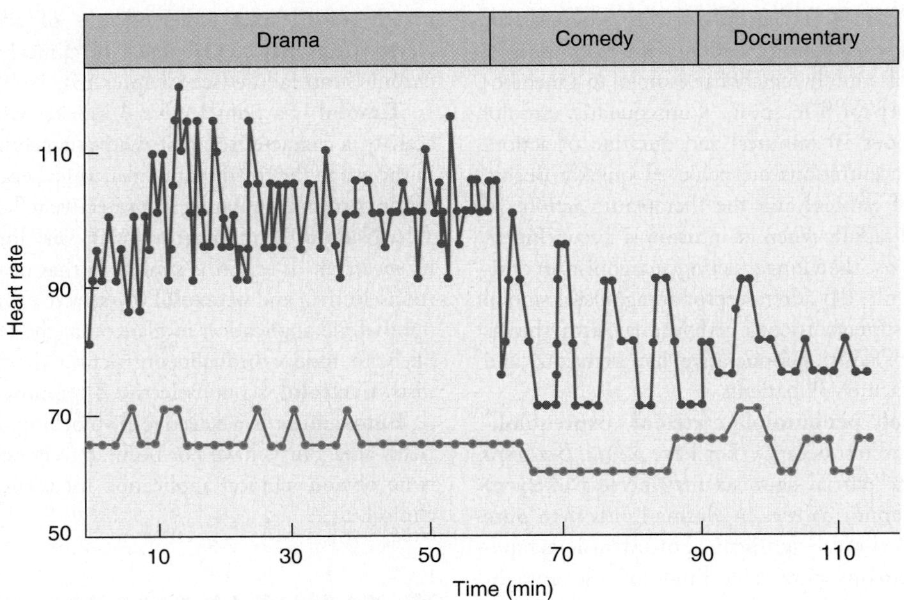

FIGURE 10–7 Heart rate in a patient with ischemic heart disease measured by telemetry while watching television. Measurements were begun 1 hour after receiving placebo (*upper line, red*) or 40 mg of oxprenolol (*lower line, blue*), a nonselective β antagonist with partial agonist activity. Not only was the heart rate decreased by the drug under the conditions of this experiment, it also varied much less in response to stimuli. (Reproduced with permission from Taylor SH. Oxprenolol in clinical practice. Am J Cardiol. 1983;52(9):34D-42D.)

Cardiac Arrhythmias

Beta antagonists are often effective in the treatment of both supraventricular and ventricular arrhythmias (see Chapter 14). It has been suggested that the improved survival following myocardial infarction in patients using β antagonists (see Figure 10–8) is due to suppression of arrhythmias. By increasing the atrioventricular nodal refractory period, β antagonists slow ventricular response rates in atrial flutter and fibrillation. These drugs can also reduce ventricular ectopic beats, particularly if the ectopic activity has been precipitated by catecholamines. Esmolol is particularly useful against acute perioperative arrhythmias because it has a short duration of action and can be given parenterally. Sotalol has antiarrhythmic effects involving ion channel blockade in addition to its β-blocking action; these are discussed in Chapter 14.

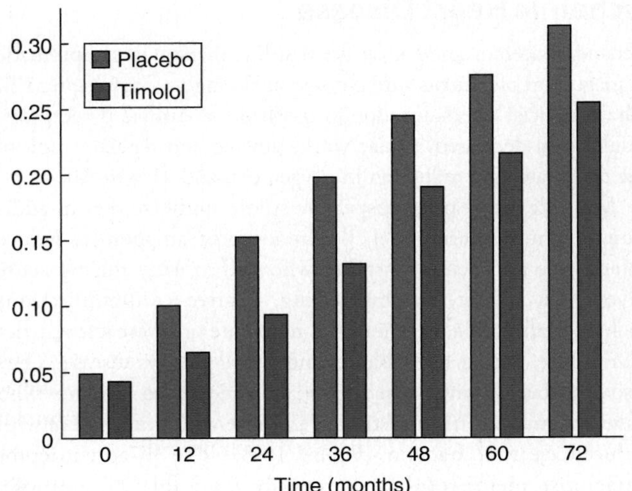

FIGURE 10–8 Effects of β-blocker therapy on life-table cumulated rates of mortality from all causes over 6 years among 1884 patients surviving myocardial infarctions. Patients were randomly assigned to treatment with placebo (*blue bar*) or timolol (*red bar*).

Heart Failure

Clinical trials have demonstrated that at least three β antagonists—metoprolol, bisoprolol, and carvedilol—are effective in reducing mortality in selected patients with chronic heart failure. In some patients, administration of these drugs may worsen acute congestive heart failure, but most patients tolerate treatment initiation with gradual dose increments. Although mechanisms are uncertain, there appear to be beneficial effects on myocardial remodeling and in decreasing the risk of sudden death (see Chapter 13).

Other Cardiovascular Disorders

Beta-receptor antagonists have been found to increase stroke volume in some patients with obstructive cardiomyopathy. This beneficial effect is thought to result from the slowing of ventricular ejection and decreased outflow resistance. Beta antagonists are indicated in the treatment of dissecting aortic aneurysms.

Glaucoma (See Box: The Treatment of Glaucoma)

Systemic administration of β-blocking drugs for other indications was found serendipitously to reduce intraocular pressure in patients with glaucoma. Subsequently, it was found that topical administration also reduces intraocular pressure. The mechanism appears to involve reduced production of aqueous humor by the ciliary body, which is physiologically activated by cAMP. Timolol and related β antagonists are suitable for local use in the eye because they lack local anesthetic properties. Beta antagonists appear to have an efficacy comparable to that of epinephrine or pilocarpine in open-angle glaucoma and are far better tolerated by most patients. While the maximal daily dose applied locally (1 mg) is small compared with the systemic doses commonly used in the treatment of hypertension or angina (10–60 mg), sufficient timolol may be absorbed from the eye to cause serious adverse effects on the heart and airways in susceptible individuals. Topical timolol may interact with orally administered verapamil and increase the risk of heart block.

Betaxolol, carteolol, levobunolol, and metipranolol are also approved for the treatment of glaucoma. Betaxolol has the potential advantage of being β_1-selective; to what extent this potential advantage might diminish systemic adverse effects remains to be determined. The drug apparently has caused worsening of pulmonary symptoms in some patients.

Hyperthyroidism

Excessive catecholamine action is an important aspect of the pathophysiology of hyperthyroidism (see Chapter 38), and β antagonists can reduce palpitations, tachycardia, tremulousness, and anxiety. They are recommended in patients diagnosed with hyperthyroidism unless a contraindication exists. Propranolol has been used extensively in patients with thyroid storm (severe hyperthyroidism); it is used cautiously in patients with this condition to control supraventricular tachycardias that often precipitate heart failure.

Neurologic Diseases

Propranolol, metoprolol, and timolol reduce the frequency and intensity of **migraine headache.** Other β-receptor antagonists with preventive efficacy include atenolol and nadolol. The mechanism is not known. Since sympathetic activity may enhance skeletal muscle tremor, it is not surprising that β antagonists have been found to reduce certain **tremors** (see Chapter 28). The somatic manifestations of anxiety may respond dramatically to low doses of propranolol, particularly when taken prophylactically. For example, benefit has been found in musicians with **performance anxiety ("stage fright").** Propranolol may contribute to the symptomatic treatment of alcohol withdrawal in some patients.

Miscellaneous

Beta-receptor antagonists have been found to diminish portal vein pressure in patients with cirrhosis. There is evidence that both propranolol and nadolol decrease the incidence of the first episode of bleeding from **esophageal varices** and decrease the mortality rate associated with bleeding in patients with cirrhosis. Nadolol in combination with isosorbide mononitrate appears to be more efficacious than sclerotherapy in preventing rebleeding in patients who have previously bled from esophageal varices. Variceal band ligation in combination with a β antagonist may be more efficacious. The potential beneficial effects of β blockers in preventing bleeding have to be balanced with the potential reduction in cardiac output and reduced blood pressure.

Infantile hemangiomas are the most common vascular tumors of infancy, and propranolol has been found to reduce their volume, color, and elevation in infants younger than 6 months and children up to 5 years of age. A retrospective analysis found improved survival of patients with **melanoma** treated with immunotherapy who happened to be taking nonselective β blockers, but not in patients taking β_1–selective antagonists or no β blockers. The significance of this finding is not yet clear. Similar putative beneficial effect have been reported in patients with breast cancer, in part because β blockers may prevent chemotherapy-induced cardiomyopathy.

CHOICE OF A BETA-ADRENOCEPTOR ANTAGONIST DRUG

In general, β_1-selective antagonists are preferred in patients with asthma, COPD, diabetes mellitus, or peripheral vascular disease. Beta blockers with intrinsic sympathetic activity may be preferred in patients with resting bradycardia. Vasodilating β blockers may be preferred in patients with heart failure or hypertension. As with other medications, patient compliance may be improved by using drugs with a longer half-life.

CLINICAL TOXICITY OF THE BETA-RECEPTOR ANTAGONIST DRUGS

The major adverse effects of β-receptor antagonist drugs relate to the predictable consequences of β blockade. Beta$_2$-receptor blockade associated with the use of nonselective agents commonly causes worsening of preexisting **asthma** and other forms of airway obstruction. β_1-selective drugs have fewer adverse effects on airways than nonselective β antagonists, and they can be used, but very cautiously, in patients with reactive airway disease.

Nonselective β blockers can induce **peripheral vasoconstriction.** Clinical symptoms can range from a sensation of cold extremities in individuals with otherwise normal circulation, to worsening of claudication in patients with peripheral vascular disease. They can also worsen Raynaud phenomenon. Beta$_1$-selective antagonists are generally better tolerated in patients with mild to moderate peripheral vascular disease, but caution is required in patients with severe peripheral vascular disease or vasospastic disorders.

Slowing of the resting heart rate and development of **sinus bradycardia** are the main pharmacological effects of β blockade, and even β blockers with intrinsic sympathetic activity are contraindicated in patients with symptomatic bradycardia and sinus node dysfunction. Beta blockers slow atrioventricular (AV) node conduction and can induce or worsen heart block, leading to potentially serious bradyarrhythmias.

Beta-receptor blockade **depresses myocardial contractility** and excitability. In patients with abnormal myocardial function, cardiac output may be dependent on sympathetic drive. If this stimulus is removed by β blockade, cardiac decompensation may ensue. Thus, caution must be exercised in starting a β-receptor antagonist in patients with compensated heart failure, but this should not deter their use; only a minority of patients with stable heart failure decompensate after cautious initiation of β blockers, and long-term use of these drugs has been shown to reduce mortality in these patients. Beta blockers may interact with the calcium antagonist verapamil; severe hypotension, bradycardia, heart failure, and cardiac conduction abnormalities have all been described. These adverse effects may even arise in susceptible patients taking a topical (ophthalmic) β blocker and oral verapamil.

Epinephrine is a critical hormone involved in the counter-regulatory response to **hypoglycemia.** β blockers can not only mask the early adrenergic warning symptoms of hypoglycemia (tachycardia, sweating and anxiety), but may delay recovery to normoglycemia. Therefore, it is not advisable to use β antagonists in insulin-dependent diabetic patients who suffer from frequent hypoglycemic episodes if alternative therapies are available. Beta$_1$-selective antagonists offer some advantage in these patients, since the rate of recovery from hypoglycemia may be faster compared with that in diabetics receiving nonselective β-adrenoceptor antagonists. There is considerable potential benefit from these drugs in diabetics after a myocardial infarction, so the balance of risk versus benefit must be evaluated in individual patients.

Fatigue, depression, and sexual dysfunction have been historically considered common adverse effects of β blockers, and these effects were thought to be less common with nonlipophilic drugs (eg, atenolol). A systematic review of the results of randomized trials, however, suggests that the risk of these effects, while present, is lower than previously thought.

The use of β blockers is associated with a small increase in **body weight** and mild negative changes in **metabolism and lipids,** with a small increase in triglycerides and a decrease in HDL. These effects are not seen with vasodilating β blockers.

Acute withdrawal of β blockers can lead to sudden onset of tachycardia and exacerbation of ischemic symptoms, and even precipitation of acute myocardial infarction. The mechanism of this effect might involve up-regulation of the number of β receptors in response to chronic exposure to an antagonist. This phenomenon can be prevented by gradual dose tapering rather than abrupt cessation when these drugs are discontinued, especially when using drugs with short half-lives.

SUMMARY Sympathetic Antagonists

Subclass, Drug	Mechanism of Action	Effects	Clinical Applications	Pharmacokinetics, Toxicities, Interactions
ALPHA-ADRENOCEPTOR ANTAGONISTS				
• Phenoxybenzamine	Irreversibly blocks α_1 and α_2 • indirect baroreflex activation	Lowers blood pressure (BP) • heart rate (HR) rises due to baroreflex activation	Pheochromocytoma • high catecholamine states	Irreversible blocker • duration > 1 day • *Toxicity:* Orthostatic hypotension • tachycardia • myocardial ischemia
• Phentolamine	Reversibly blocks α_1 and α_2	Blocks α-mediated vasoconstriction, lowers BP, increases HR (baroreflex)	Pheochromocytoma	Half-life ~45 min after IV injection
• Prazosin • Doxazosin • Terazosin	Block α_1, but not α_2	Lower BP	Hypertension • benign prostatic hyperplasia	Larger depressor effect with first dose may cause orthostatic hypotension
• Tamsulosin	Slightly selective for α_{1A}	α_{1A} blockade may relax prostatic smooth muscle more than vascular smooth muscle	Benign prostatic hyperplasia	Orthostatic hypotension may be less common with this subtype
• Yohimbine	Blocks α_2 • elicits increased central sympathetic activity • increased norepinephrine release	Raises BP and HR	Male erectile dysfunction • hypotension	May cause anxiety • excess pressor effect if norepinephrine transporter is blocked
• Labetalol (see carvedilol section below)	$\beta > \alpha_1$ block	Lowers BP with limited HR increase	Hypertension	Oral, parenteral • *Toxicity:* Less tachycardia than other α_1 agents
BETA-ADRENOCEPTOR ANTAGONISTS				
• Propranolol • Nadolol • Timolol	Block β_1 and β_2	Lower HR and BP • reduce renin	Hypertension • angina pectoris • arrhythmias • migraine • hyperthyroidism • glaucoma (topical timolol)	Oral, parenteral • *Toxicity:* Bradycardia • worsened asthma • fatigue • vivid dreams • cold hands
• Metoprolol • Atenolol • Betaxolol • Nebivolol	Block $\beta_1 > \beta_2$	Lower HR and BP • reduce renin • may be safer in asthma	Angina pectoris • hypertension • arrhythmias • glaucoma (topical betaxolol)	*Toxicity:* Bradycardia • fatigue • vivid dreams • cold hands
• Butoxamine[1]	Blocks $\beta_2 > \beta_1$	Increases peripheral resistance	No clinical indication	*Toxicity:* Asthma provocation

(continued)

Subclass, Drug	Mechanism of Action	Effects	Clinical Applications	Pharmacokinetics, Toxicities, Interactions
• Pindolol • Acebutolol • Carteolol • Bopindolol[1] • Oxprenolol[1] • Celiprolol[1] • Penbutolol	β_1, β_2, with intrinsic sympathomimetic (partial agonist) effect	Lower BP • modestly lower HR	Hypertension • arrhythmias • migraine • may avoid worsening of bradycardia	Oral • *Toxicity:* Fatigue • vivid dreams • cold hands
• Carvedilol • Medroxalol[1] • Bucindolol[1] (see labetalol above)	$\beta > \alpha_1$ block		Heart failure	Oral, long half-life • *Toxicity:* Fatigue
• Esmolol	$\beta_1 > \beta_2$	Very brief cardiac β blockade	Rapid control of BP and arrhythmias, thyrotoxicosis, and myocardial ischemia intraoperatively	Parenteral only • half-life ~10 min • *Toxicity:* Bradycardia • hypotension
TYROSINE HYDROXYLASE INHIBITOR				
• Metyrosine	Blocks tyrosine hydroxylase • reduces synthesis of dopamine, norepinephrine, and epinephrine	Lowers BP • may elicit extrapyramidal effects (due to decreased dopamine in CNS)	Pheochromocytoma	*Toxicity:* Extrapyramidal symptoms • orthostatic hypotension • crystalluria

[1]Not available in the USA.

PREPARATIONS AVAILABLE*

GENERIC NAME	AVAILABLE AS
ALPHA BLOCKERS	
Alfuzosin	Generic, Uroxatral
Doxazosin	Generic, Cardura
Phenoxybenzamine	Generic, Dibenzyline
Phentolamine	Generic
Prazosin	Generic, Minipress
Silodosin	Generic, Rapaflo
Tamsulosin	Generic, Flomax
Terazosin	Generic, Hytrin
Tolazoline	Generic, Priscoline
BETA BLOCKERS	
Acebutolol	Generic, Sectral
Atenolol	Generic, Tenormin
Betaxolol	
Oral	Generic, Kerlone
Ophthalmic	Generic, Betoptic
Bisoprolol	Generic, Zebeta
Carteolol	
Oral	Generic, Cartrol
Ophthalmic	Generic, Ocupress
Carvedilol	Generic, Coreg
Esmolol	Generic, Brevibloc
Labetalol	Generic, Normodyne, Trandate
Levobunolol	Generic, Betagan Liquifilm, others
Metipranolol	Generic, OptiPranolol
Metoprolol	Generic, Lopressor, Toprol
Nadolol	Generic, Corgard
Nebivolol	Bystolic
Penbutolol	Levatol
Pindolol	Generic, Visken
Propranolol	Generic, Inderal
Sotalol	Generic, Betapace
Timolol	
Oral	Generic, Blocadren
Ophthalmic	Generic, Timoptic
TYROSINE HYDROXYLASE INHIBITOR	
Metyrosine	Demser

*In the USA.

REFERENCES

Ambrosio G et al: β-Blockade with nebivolol for prevention of acute ischaemic events in elderly patients with heart failure. Heart 2011;97:209.

Ayers K et al: Differential effects of nebivolol and metoprolol on insulin sensitivity and plasminogen activator inhibitor in the metabolic syndrome. Hypertension 2012;59:893.

Bird ST et al: Tamsulosin treatment for benign prostatic hyperplasia and risk of severe hypotension in men aged 40-85 years in the United States: Risk window analyses using between and within patient methodology. BMJ 2013;347:f6320.

Campschroer T et al: Alpha-blockers as medical expulsive therapy for ureteral stones. Cochrane Database Syst Rev 2018;4:CD008509.

Danesh A, Gottschalk PCH: Beta-blockers for migraine prevention: a review article. Curr Treat Options Neurol. 2019;21:20.

De Nunzio C et al: Erectile dysfunction and lower urinary tract symptoms. Curr Urol Rep 2018;19:61.

Fusco et al: Alpha 1-blockers improve benign prostatic obstruction in men with lower urinary tract symptoms: A systematic review and meta-analysis of urodynamic studies. Eur Urol 2016;69:1091.

Joseph P et al: The evolution of beta-blockers in coronary artery disease and heart failure. J Am Coll Cardiol 2019;74:672.

Mancia G et al: Individualized beta-blocker treatment for high blood pressure dictated by medical comorbidities: indications beyond the 2018 European Society of Cardiology/European Society of Hypertension Guidelines. Hypertension 2022;79:1153.

Macca L et al: Update on treatment of infantile hemangiomas: what's new in the last five years? Front Pharmacol 2022;13:879602

Negri L et al: Timolol 0.1% in glaucomatous patients: efficacy, tolerance, and quality of life. J Ophthalmol 2019:4146124.

Neumann HPH et al: Pheochromocytoma and paraganglioma. N Engl J Med 2019;381:552.

Nocentini A, Supuran CT: Adrenergic agonists and antagonists as patent review (2013-2019). Exp Opin Ther Pat 2019;29:805.

Okamoto LE et al: Nebivolol, but not metoprolol lowers blood pressure in nitric oxide-sensitive human hypertension. Hypertension 2014;64:1241.

Olawi N et al: Nebivolol in the treatment of arterial hypertension. Basic Clin Pharmacol Toxicol 2019;125:189.

Phadke S, Clamon G: Beta blockade as adjunctive breast cancer therapy: A review. Crit Rev Oncol Hematol 2016;138:173.

Raj SR et al: Propranolol decreases tachycardia and improves symptoms in the postural tachycardia syndrome: Less is more. Circulation 2009;120:725.

Shah P et al: Meta-analysis comparing usefulness of beta blockers to preserve left ventricular function during anthracycline therapy. Am J Cardiol 2019;124:789.

Shanker V: Essential tremor: diagnosis and management. Br Med J 2019;366:I4485

Shibao C et al: Comparative efficacy of yohimbine against pyridostigmine for the treatment of orthostatic hypotension in autonomic failure. Hypertension 2010;56:847.

Suissa S, Ernst P: Beta-blockers in COPD: A methodological review of the observational studies. COPD 2018;15:520.

CASE STUDY ANSWER

The patient had a pheochromocytoma. This tumor secretes catecholamines, especially norepinephrine and epinephrine, resulting in increases in blood pressure (via α_1 receptors) and heart rate (via β_1 receptors). The pheochromocytoma was in the left adrenal gland and was diagnosed by elevated plasma fractionated metanephrines (catecholamine metabolites). The left adrenal tumor was identified by computer tomography and by meta-iodobenzylguanidine (MIBG) imaging, which labels tissues that have norepinephrine transporters on their cell surface (see text). In addition, he had elevated plasma and urinary norepinephrine, epinephrine, and their metabolites. The pressor episode during the physical examination was likely triggered by external pressure as the physician palpated the abdomen. His profuse sweating was typical and partly due to α_1 receptors, although the mechanism of sweating in pheochromocytoma has never been fully explained. Treatment would consist of preoperative pharmacologic control of blood pressure with α antagonists, and normalization of blood volume which is often significantly reduced, followed by surgical resection of the tumor. Control of blood pressure may be necessary during surgery as manipulation of the tumor may lead to catecholamine discharge.

SECTION III CARDIOVASCULAR-RENAL DRUGS

CHAPTER 11

Antihypertensive Agents

Neal L. Benowitz, MD

CASE STUDY

A 35-year-old man presents with a blood pressure of 140/90 mm Hg. He has been generally healthy, is sedentary, drinks several cocktails per day, and does not smoke cigarettes. He has a family history of hypertension, and his father died of a myocardial infarction at age 55. Physical examination is remarkable only for moderate obesity. Total cholesterol is 220, and high-density lipoprotein (HDL) cholesterol level is 40 mg/dL. Fasting glucose is 105 mg/dL. Chest X-ray is normal. Electrocardiogram shows left ventricular hypertrophy. How would you treat this patient?

Hypertension is the most common cardiovascular disease and the most common reason for physician office visits. Using National Health and Nutrition Examination Survey (NHANES) data from 2017 to 2018, and a definition of ≥130/90 mm Hg recommended by the 2017 ACC/AHA High Blood Pressure Clinical Practice Guideline, hypertension was found in 45% of American adults and 74% of adults age 60 years or older. The prevalence varies with age, race, education, and many other variables. Sustained arterial hypertension damages blood vessels in kidney, heart, and brain and leads to an increased incidence of renal failure, coronary disease, heart failure, stroke, and dementia. More than 50% of deaths from coronary heart disease and stroke occur in people with hypertension. Effective pharmacologic lowering of blood pressure has been shown to prevent damage to blood vessels and to substantially reduce morbidity and mortality rates. However, NHANES found that, unfortunately, only one-half of Americans with hypertension had adequate blood pressure control. Many effective drugs are available. Knowledge of their antihypertensive mechanisms and sites of action allows accurate prediction of efficacy and toxicity. The rational use of these agents, alone or in combination, can lower blood pressure with minimal risk of serious toxicity in most patients.

HYPERTENSION & REGULATION OF BLOOD PRESSURE

Diagnosis

The diagnosis of hypertension is based on repeated, reproducible measurements of elevated blood pressure (Table 11–1). Blood pressure may be elevated in the office but not at home ("white coat hypertension"), so it is best to confirm a diagnosis of hypertension with home or ambulatory blood pressure measurement. The diagnosis serves primarily as a prediction of consequences

TABLE 11–1 Blood pressure in adults.

Blood Pressure	(Systolic [mm Hg]/ Diastolic [mm Hg]
Low	70–90/40–60
Normal	90–120/60–80
Elevated	120–129/80
Hypertension	
Stage I	130–139/80–90
Stage II	>140/>90

for the patient; it seldom includes a statement about the cause of hypertension.

Epidemiologic studies indicate that the risks of damage to kidney, heart, and brain are directly related to the extent of blood pressure elevation. Even mild hypertension (blood pressure 130/80 mm Hg) increases the risk of eventual end-organ damage. Starting at 115/75 mm Hg, cardiovascular disease risk doubles with each increment of 20/10 mm Hg throughout the blood pressure range. Both systolic hypertension and diastolic hypertension are associated with end-organ damage; so-called isolated systolic hypertension is not benign. The risks—and therefore the urgency of instituting therapy—increase in proportion to the magnitude of blood pressure elevation. The risk of end-organ damage at any level of blood pressure or age is greater in African Americans and relatively less in premenopausal women than in men. Other risk factors include smoking, including exposure to secondhand smoke; diabetes; metabolic syndrome including obesity, dyslipidemia; physical inactivity; manifestations of end-organ damage at the time of diagnosis; and a family history of cardiovascular disease.

It should be noted that the diagnosis of hypertension depends on measurement of blood pressure and not on symptoms reported by the patient. In fact, hypertension is usually asymptomatic until overt end-organ damage is imminent or has already occurred.

Etiology of Hypertension

A specific cause of hypertension can be established in only 10–15% of patients. Patients in whom no specific cause of hypertension can be found are said to have *essential* or *primary hypertension.* Patients with a specific etiology are said to have *secondary hypertension.* It is important to consider specific causes in each case, however, because some of them are amenable to definitive surgical treatment: renal artery constriction, coarctation of the aorta, pheochromocytoma, Cushing disease, and primary aldosteronism.

In most cases, elevated blood pressure is associated with an overall increase in resistance to flow of blood through arterioles, whereas cardiac output is usually normal. Meticulous investigation of autonomic nervous system function, baroreceptor reflexes, the renin-angiotensin-aldosterone system, and the kidney has failed to identify a single abnormality as the cause of increased peripheral vascular resistance in essential hypertension. It appears, therefore, that elevated blood pressure is usually caused by a combination of several (multifactorial) abnormalities. Epidemiologic evidence points to genetic factors, psychological stress, environmental and dietary factors (increased salt and decreased potassium or calcium intake), alcohol consumption, and obesity as contributing to the development of hypertension. Increase in blood pressure with aging does not occur in populations with low daily sodium intake. Patients with labile hypertension appear more likely than normal controls to have blood pressure elevations after salt loading.

The heritability of essential hypertension is estimated to be about 30%. Mutations in several genes have been linked to various rare causes of hypertension, but most hypertension appears to be polygenic. Functional variations of the genes for angiotensinogen, angiotensin-converting enzyme (ACE), the angiotensin II receptor, the β_2 adrenoceptor, α adducin (a cytoskeletal protein), uromodulin (modulator of renal electrolyte transport), and others appear to contribute to some cases of essential hypertension.

Normal Regulation of Blood Pressure

According to the hydraulic equation, arterial blood pressure (BP) is directly proportionate to the product of the blood flow (cardiac output, CO) and the resistance to passage of blood through precapillary arterioles (peripheral vascular resistance, PVR):

$$BP = CO \times PVR$$

Physiologically, in both normal and hypertensive individuals, blood pressure is maintained by moment-to-moment regulation of cardiac output and peripheral vascular resistance, exerted at three anatomic sites (Figure 11–1): arterioles, postcapillary venules (capacitance vessels), and heart. A fourth anatomic control site, the kidney, contributes to maintenance of blood pressure by regulating the volume of intravascular fluid. Baroreflexes, mediated by autonomic nerves, act in combination with humoral mechanisms, including the renin-angiotensin-aldosterone system, to coordinate

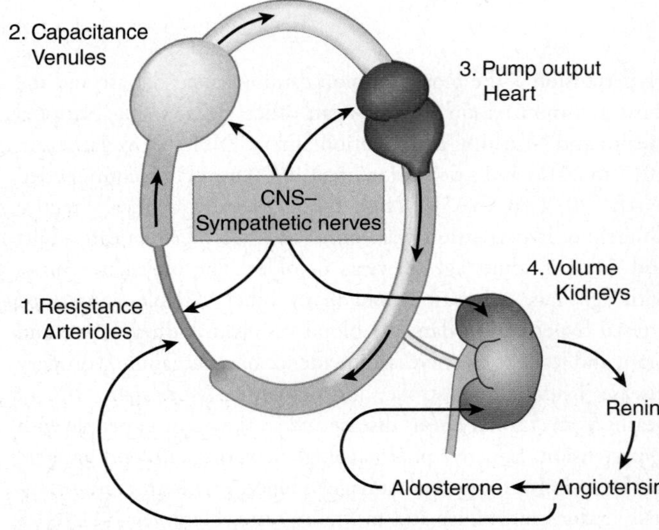

FIGURE 11–1 Anatomic sites of blood pressure control.

function at these four control sites and to maintain normal blood pressure. Finally, local release of vasoactive substances from vascular endothelium may also be involved in the regulation of vascular resistance. For example, endothelin-1 (see Chapter 17) constricts and nitric oxide (see Chapter 19) dilates blood vessels.

Blood pressure in a hypertensive patient is controlled by the same mechanisms that are operative in normotensive subjects. Regulation of blood pressure in hypertensive patients differs from healthy patients in that the baroreceptors and the renal blood volume-pressure control systems appear to be "set" at a higher level of blood pressure. All antihypertensive drugs act by interfering with these normal mechanisms, which are reviewed below.

A. Postural Baroreflex

Baroreflexes are responsible for rapid, moment-to-moment adjustments in blood pressure, such as in transition from a reclining to an upright posture (Figure 11–2). Central sympathetic neurons arising from the vasomotor area of the medulla are tonically active. Carotid baroreceptors are stimulated by the stretch of the vessel walls brought about by the internal pressure (arterial blood pressure). Baroreceptor activation inhibits central sympathetic discharge. Conversely, reduction in stretch results in a reduction in baroreceptor activity. Thus, in the case of a transition to upright posture, baroreceptors sense the reduction in arterial pressure that results from pooling of blood in the veins below the level of the heart as reduced wall stretch, and sympathetic discharge is disinhibited. The reflex increase in sympathetic outflow acts through nerve endings to increase peripheral vascular resistance (constriction of arterioles) and cardiac output (direct stimulation of the heart and constriction of capacitance vessels, which increases venous return to the heart), thereby restoring normal blood pressure. The same baroreflex acts in response to any event that lowers arterial pressure, including a primary reduction in peripheral vascular resistance (eg, caused by a vasodilating agent) or a reduction in intravascular volume (eg, due to hemorrhage or to loss of salt and water via the kidney).

B. Renal Response to Decreased Blood Pressure

By controlling blood volume, the kidney is primarily responsible for long-term blood pressure control. A reduction in renal perfusion pressure causes intrarenal redistribution of blood flow and increased reabsorption of salt and water. In addition, decreased pressure in renal arterioles as well as sympathetic neural activity (via β adrenoceptors) stimulates production of renin, which increases production of angiotensin II (see Figure 11–1 and Chapter 17). Angiotensin II causes (1) direct constriction of resistance vessels and (2) stimulation of aldosterone synthesis in the adrenal cortex, which increases renal sodium absorption and intravascular blood volume. Vasopressin released from the posterior pituitary gland also plays a role in maintenance of blood pressure through its ability to regulate water reabsorption by the kidney (see Chapters 15 and 17).

■ BASIC PHARMACOLOGY OF ANTIHYPERTENSIVE AGENTS

All antihypertensive agents act at one or more of the four anatomic control sites depicted in Figure 11–1 and produce their effects by interfering with normal mechanisms of blood pressure regulation. A useful classification of these agents categorizes them according to the principal regulatory site or mechanism on which they act (Figure 11–3). Because of their common mechanisms of action, drugs within each category tend to produce a similar spectrum of toxicities. The categories include the following:

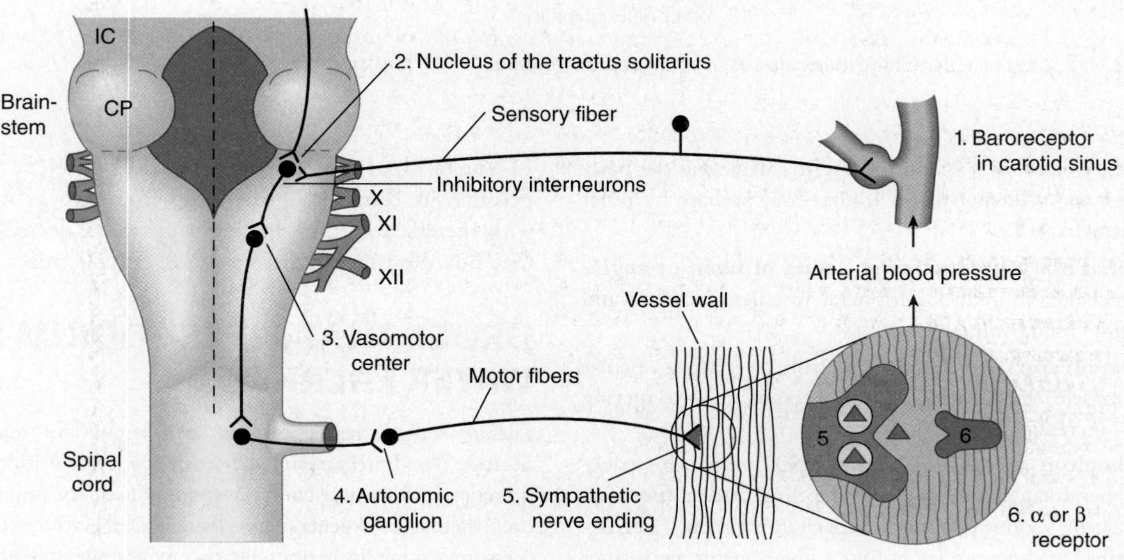

FIGURE 11–2 Baroreceptor reflex arc. CP, cerebellar peduncle; IC, inferior colliculus.

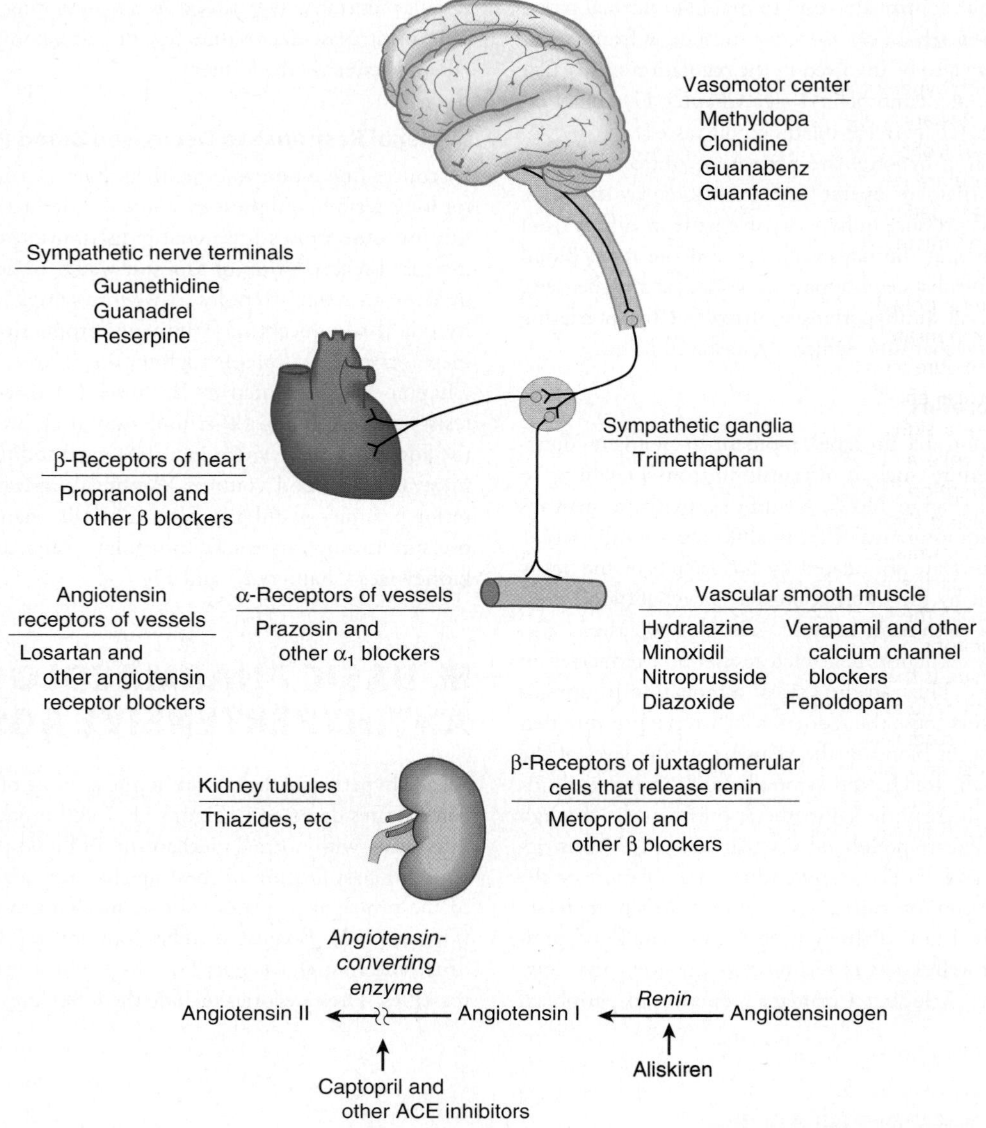

FIGURE 11–3 Sites of action of the major classes of antihypertensive drugs.

1. **Diuretics,** which lower blood pressure by depleting the body of sodium and reducing blood volume and perhaps by other mechanisms.
2. **Agents that block production or action of renin or angiotensin** and thereby reduce peripheral vascular resistance and (potentially) blood volume.
3. **Direct vasodilators,** which reduce pressure by relaxing vascular smooth muscle, thus dilating resistance vessels and—to varying degrees—increasing capacitance as well.
4. **Sympathoplegic agents,** which lower blood pressure by reducing peripheral vascular resistance, inhibiting cardiac function, and increasing venous pooling in capacitance vessels. (The latter two effects reduce cardiac output.) These agents are further subdivided according to their putative sites of action in the sympathetic reflex arc (see below).

The fact that these drug groups act by different mechanisms permits the combination of drugs from two or more groups with increased efficacy and, in some cases, decreased toxicity. (See Box: Resistant Hypertension & Polypharmacy.)

DRUGS THAT ALTER SODIUM & WATER BALANCE

Dietary sodium restriction has been known for many years to decrease blood pressure in hypertensive patients. With the advent of diuretics, sodium restriction was thought to be less important. However, there is now general agreement that dietary control of blood pressure is a relatively nontoxic therapeutic measure and may even be preventive. Even modest dietary sodium restriction lowers blood pressure (though to varying extents) in many hypertensive persons.

Resistant Hypertension & Polypharmacy

Many patients with hypertension require two or more drugs acting by different mechanisms (polypharmacy). According to some estimates, up to 40% of patients may respond inadequately even to two agents and are considered to have "resistant hypertension." Some of these patients have treatable secondary hypertension that has been missed, but most do not, and three or more drugs are required.

One rationale for polypharmacy in hypertension is that most drugs evoke compensatory regulatory mechanisms for maintaining blood pressure (see Figures 6–7 and 11–1), which may markedly limit their effect. For example, vasodilators such as hydralazine cause a significant decrease in peripheral vascular resistance, but evoke a strong compensatory tachycardia and salt and water retention (Figure 11–4) that are capable of almost completely reversing their effect. The addition of a β blocker prevents the tachycardia; addition of a diuretic (eg, hydrochlorothiazide) prevents the salt and water retention. In effect, all three drugs increase the sensitivity of the cardiovascular system to each other's actions.

A second reason is that some drugs have only modest maximum efficacy but reduction of long-term morbidity mandates their use. Many studies of angiotensin-converting enzyme (ACE) inhibitors report a maximal lowering of blood pressure of less than 10 mm Hg. In patients with more severe hypertension (pressure >160/100 mm Hg), this is inadequate to prevent all the sequelae of hypertension, but ACE inhibitors have important long-term benefits in preventing or reducing renal disease in diabetic persons and in reduction of heart failure. Finally, the toxicity of some effective drugs prevents their use at maximally effective doses.

Two approaches to treating hypertension can be considered. One may start with monotherapy, and if hypertension does not respond adequately to a regimen of one drug, a second drug from a different class with a different mechanism of action and different pattern of toxicity is added. If the response is still inadequate and compliance is known to be good, a third drug should be added. Another increasingly common approach is to use small doses of drugs two or three dugs (for example a diuretic, ACE inhibitor, or angiotensin reception blocker and/or a calcium channel blocker). If three drugs (usually including a diuretic) are inadequate, other causes of resistant hypertension such as excessive dietary sodium intake, use of nonsteroidal anti-inflammatory or stimulant drugs, or the presence of secondary hypertension should be considered. In some instances, an additional drug may be necessary, and mineralocorticoid antagonists, such as spironolactone, have been found to be particularly useful. Occasionally patients are resistant to four or more drugs, and nonpharmacologic approaches have been considered. A promising treatments that is still under investigation, particularly for patients with advanced kidney disease, is renal denervation.

Mechanisms of Action & Hemodynamic Effects of Diuretics

Diuretics lower blood pressure primarily by depleting body sodium stores. Initially, diuretics reduce blood pressure by reducing blood volume and cardiac output; peripheral vascular resistance may increase. After 6–8 weeks, cardiac output returns toward normal while peripheral vascular resistance declines. Sodium is believed to contribute to vascular resistance by increasing vessel stiffness and neural reactivity, possibly related to altered sodium-calcium exchange with a resultant increase in intracellular calcium. These effects are reversed by diuretics or dietary sodium restriction.

Diuretics are effective in lowering blood pressure by 10–15 mm Hg in most patients, and diuretics alone often provide adequate treatment for mild or moderate essential hypertension. In more severe hypertension, diuretics are used in combination with sympathoplegic and vasodilator drugs to control the tendency toward sodium retention caused by these agents. Vascular responsiveness—ie, the ability to either constrict or dilate—is diminished by sympathoplegic and vasodilator drugs, so that the vasculature behaves like an inflexible tube. As a consequence, blood pressure becomes exquisitely sensitive to blood volume. Thus, in severe hypertension, when multiple drugs are used, blood pressure may be well controlled when blood volume is 95% of normal but much too high when blood volume is 105% of normal.

Use of Diuretics

The sites of action within the kidney and the pharmacokinetics of various diuretic drugs are discussed in Chapter 15. Thiazide diuretics are appropriate for most patients with mild or moderate hypertension and normal renal and cardiac function. Chlorthalidone may be more effective than hydrochlorothiazide since it has a longer duration of action yet a recent study has shown that hydrochlorothiazide was equally effective compared to chlorthalidone with respect to cardiovascular outcomes over time in people 65 years or older. More powerful diuretics (eg, those acting on the loop of Henle) such as furosemide, bumetanide, and torsemide are necessary in severe hypertension, when multiple drugs with sodium-retaining properties are used; in renal insufficiency, when glomerular filtration rate is less than 30–40 mL/min; and in cardiac failure or cirrhosis, in which sodium retention is marked. Recent studies indicate that chlorthalidone can be effective in lowering blood pressure even in patients with advanced chronic kidney disease.

Potassium-sparing diuretics are useful both to avoid excessive potassium depletion and to enhance the natriuretic effects of other diuretics. Aldosterone receptor antagonists in particular also have a favorable effect on cardiac function in people with heart failure and as polypharmacy in patients with resistant hypertension.

Some pharmacokinetic characteristics and the initial and usual maintenance dosages of diuretics are listed in Table 11–2.

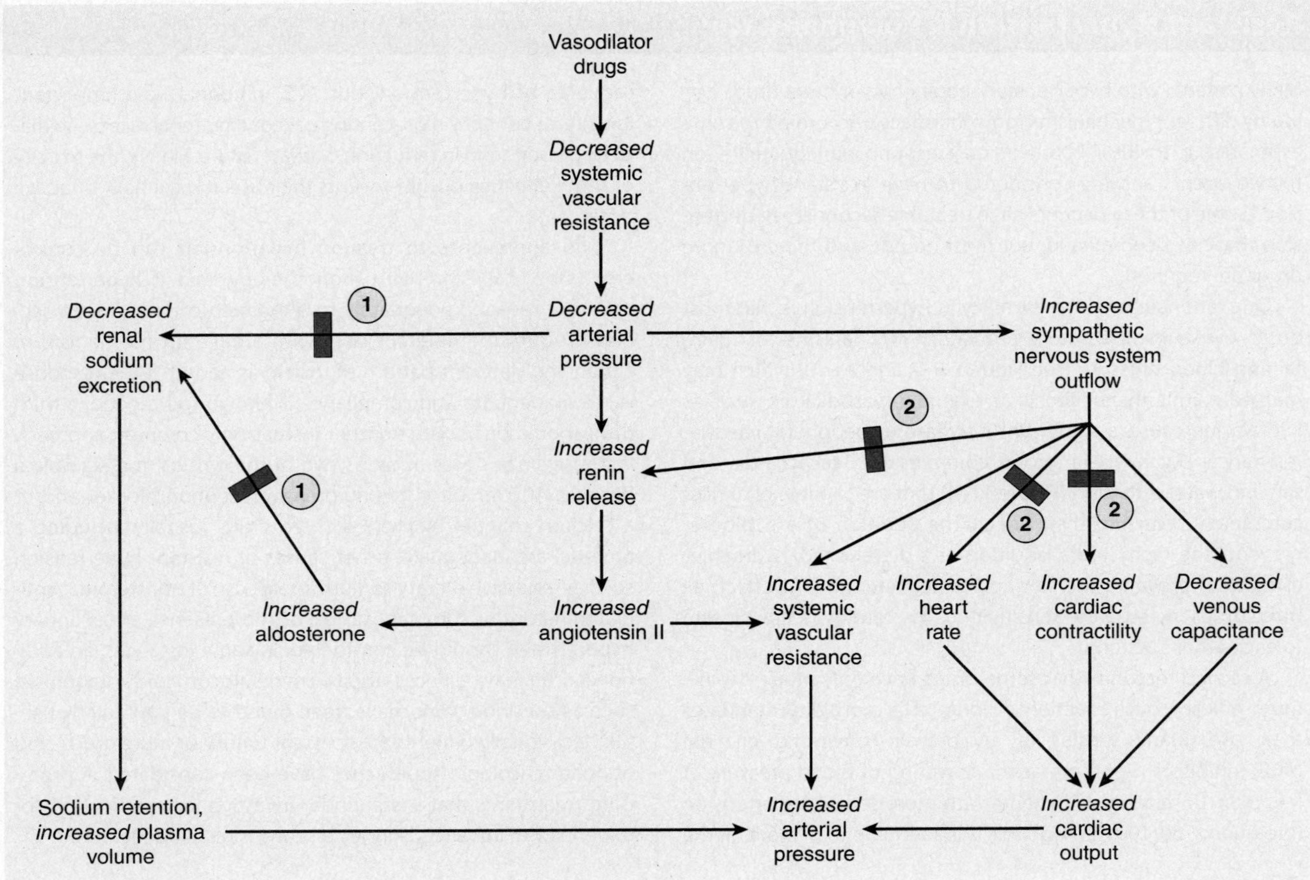

FIGURE 11–4 Compensatory responses to vasodilators; basis for combination therapy with β blockers and diuretics. ① Effect blocked by diuretics. ② Effect blocked by β blockers.

Although thiazide diuretics are more natriuretic at higher doses (up to 100–200 mg of hydrochlorothiazide), when used as a single agent, lower doses (25–50 mg) exert as much antihypertensive effect as do higher doses. In contrast to thiazides, the blood pressure response to loop diuretics continues to increase at doses many times greater than the usual therapeutic dose.

Toxicity of Diuretics

In the treatment of hypertension, the most common adverse effect of diuretics (except for potassium-sparing diuretics) is potassium depletion. Although mild degrees of hypokalemia are tolerated well by many patients, hypokalemia may be hazardous in persons taking digitalis, those who have chronic arrhythmias, or those with acute myocardial infarction or left ventricular dysfunction. Potassium loss is coupled to reabsorption of sodium, and restriction of dietary sodium intake therefore minimizes potassium loss. Diuretics may also cause magnesium depletion, impair glucose tolerance, and increase serum lipid concentrations. Diuretics increase uric acid concentrations and may precipitate gout. The use of low doses minimizes these adverse metabolic effects without impairing the antihypertensive action. Potassium-sparing diuretics may produce hyperkalemia, particularly in patients with renal insufficiency and those taking ace inhibitors or angiotensin receptor blockers; spironolactone (a steroid) is associated with gynecomastia.

INHIBITORS OF ANGIOTENSIN

Renin, angiotensin, and aldosterone play important roles in some people with essential hypertension. Approximately 20% of patients with essential hypertension have inappropriately low and 20% have inappropriately high plasma renin activity. Blood pressure of patients with high-renin hypertension responds well to drugs that interfere with the system, supporting a role for excess renin and angiotensin in this population.

Mechanism & Sites of Action

Renin release from the kidney cortex is stimulated by reduced renal arterial pressure, sympathetic neural stimulation, and reduced sodium delivery or increased sodium concentration at the distal renal tubule (see Chapter 17). Renin acts upon angiotensinogen to yield the inactive precursor decapeptide angiotensin I. Angiotensin I is then converted, primarily by endothelial ACE, to the arterial vasoconstrictor octapeptide angiotensin II (Figure 11–5), which is in turn converted in the adrenal gland to

TABLE 11–2 Pharmacokinetic characteristics and dosage of selected oral antihypertensive drugs.

Drug	Half-life (h)	Bioavailability (percent)	Suggested Initial Dose	Usual Maintenance Dose Range	Reduction of Dosage Required in Moderate Renal Insufficiency[1]
Amlodipine	35	65	2.5 mg/d	5–10 mg/d	No
Atenolol	6	60	50 mg/d	50–100 mg/d	Yes
Benazepril	0.6[2]	35	5–10 mg/d	20–40 mg/d	Yes
Captopril	2.2	65	50–75 mg/d	75–150 mg/d	Yes
Chlorthalidone	40–60	65	25 mg/d	25–50 mg/d	No
Clonidine	8–12	95	0.2 mg/d	0.2–1.2 mg/d	Yes
Diltiazem	3.5	40	120–140 mg/d	240–360 mg/d	No
Hydralazine	1.5–3	25	40 mg/d	40–200 mg/d	No
Hydrochlorothiazide	12	70	25 mg/d	25–50 mg/d	No
Lisinopril	12	25	10 mg/d	10–80 mg/d	Yes
Losartan	1–2[3]	36	50 mg/d	25–100 mg/d	No
Methyldopa	2	25	1 g/d	1–2 g/d	No
Metoprolol	3–7	40	50–100 mg/d	200–400 mg/d	No
Minoxidil	4	90	5–10 mg/d	40 mg/d	No
Nebivolol	12	Nd[4]	5 mg/d	10–40 mg/d	No
Nifedipine	2	50	30 mg/d	30–60 mg/d	No
Prazosin	3–4	70	3 mg/d	10–30 mg/d	No
Propranolol	3–5	25	80 mg/d	80–480 mg/d	No
Reserpine	24–48	50	0.25 mg/d	0.25 mg/d	No
Verapamil	4–6	22	180 mg/d	240–480 mg/d	No

[1]Creatinine clearance ≥30 mL/min. Many of these drugs do require dosage adjustment if creatinine clearance falls below 30 mL/min.

[2]The active metabolite of benazepril has a half-life of 10 hours.

[3]The active metabolite of losartan has a half-life of 3–4 hours.

[4]Nd, not determined.

angiotensin III. Angiotensin II can also be converted to angiotensin III in the brain by the enzyme aminopeptidase A. Brain angiotensin III exerts tonic control on blood pressure and is implicated in development of hypertension in animals. Angiotensin II has vasoconstrictor and sodium-retaining activity. Angiotensin II and III both stimulate aldosterone release. Angiotensin may contribute to maintaining high vascular resistance in hypertensive states associated with high plasma renin activity, such as renal arterial stenosis, some types of intrinsic renal disease, and malignant hypertension, as well as in essential hypertension after treatment with sodium restriction, diuretics, or vasodilators. However, even in low-renin hypertensive states, these drugs can lower blood pressure (see below).

A parallel system for angiotensin generation exists in several other tissues (eg, heart) and may be responsible for trophic changes such as cardiac hypertrophy. The converting enzyme involved in tissue angiotensin II synthesis is also inhibited by ACE inhibitors. Three currently marketed classes of drugs act specifically on the renin-angiotensin system: ACE inhibitors; the competitive inhibitors of angiotensin at its receptors (angiotensin receptor blockers or ARBs), including losartan and other nonpeptide antagonists; and aliskiren, an orally active renin antagonist (see Chapter 17). A fourth group of drugs, the aldosterone receptor inhibitors (eg, spironolactone, eplerenone), is discussed with the diuretics. In addition, β blockers, as noted earlier, can reduce renin secretion. The experimental drug **firibastat** inhibits brain aminopeptidase and has been shown to lower blood pressure in hypertensive overweight patients.

ANGIOTENSIN-CONVERTING ENZYME (ACE) INHIBITORS

Captopril and other drugs in this class inhibit the converting enzyme peptidyl dipeptidase that hydrolyzes angiotensin I to angiotensin II and (under the name plasma kininase) inactivates bradykinin, a potent vasodilator that works at least in part by stimulating release of nitric oxide and prostacyclin. The hypotensive activity of captopril results from both an inhibitory action on the renin-angiotensin system and a stimulating action on the kallikrein-kinin system (see Figure 11–5). The latter mechanism has been demonstrated by showing that a bradykinin receptor

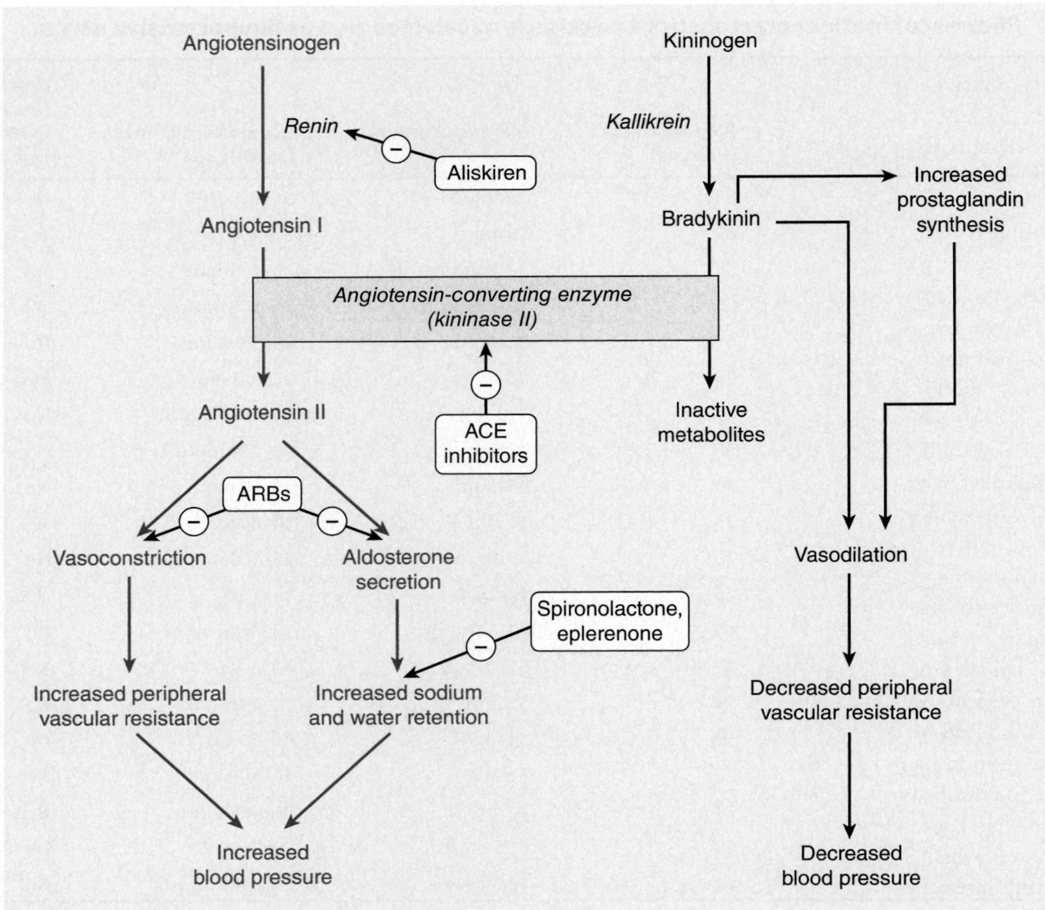

FIGURE 11–5 Sites of action of drugs that interfere with the renin-angiotensin-aldosterone system. ACE, angiotensin-converting enzyme; ARBs, angiotensin receptor blockers.

antagonist, **icatibant** (see Chapter 17), blunts the blood pressure–lowering effect of captopril.

Enalapril is an oral prodrug that is converted by hydrolysis to a converting enzyme inhibitor, enalaprilat, with effects similar to those of captopril. Enalaprilat itself is available only for intravenous use, primarily for hypertensive emergencies. Lisinopril is a lysine derivative of enalaprilat. **Benazepril, fosinopril, lisinopril, moexipril, perindopril, quinapril, ramipril,** and **trandolapril** are other long-acting members of the class. All except lisinopril are prodrugs, like enalapril, and are converted to the active agents by hydrolysis, primarily in the liver.

Angiotensin II inhibitors lower blood pressure principally by decreasing peripheral vascular resistance. Cardiac output and heart rate are not significantly changed. Unlike direct vasodilators, these agents do not result in reflex sympathetic activation and can be used safely in persons with ischemic heart disease. The absence of reflex tachycardia may be due to downward resetting of the baroreceptors or to enhanced parasympathetic activity.

Although converting enzyme inhibitors are most effective in conditions associated with high plasma renin activity, there is no good correlation among subjects between plasma renin activity and antihypertensive response. Accordingly, renin profiling is unnecessary.

ACE inhibitors have a particularly useful role in treating patients with chronic kidney disease because they diminish proteinuria and stabilize renal function (even in the absence of lowering of blood pressure). This effect is particularly valuable in diabetes, and these drugs are now recommended in diabetes even in the absence of hypertension. These benefits probably result from improved intrarenal hemodynamics, with decreased glomerular efferent arteriolar resistance and a resulting reduction of intraglomerular capillary pressure. ACE inhibitors have also proved to be extremely useful in the treatment of heart failure and as treatment after myocardial infarction, and there is evidence that ACE inhibitors reduce the incidence of diabetes in patients with high cardiovascular risk (see Chapter 13).

Pharmacokinetics & Dosage

Captopril's pharmacokinetic parameters and dosing recommendations are listed in Table 11–2. Peak concentrations of enalaprilat, the active metabolite of enalapril, occur 3–4 hours after dosing with enalapril. The half-life of enalaprilat is about 11 hours. Typical doses of enalapril are 10–20 mg once or twice daily. Lisinopril has a half-life of 12 hours. Doses of 10–80 mg once daily are effective in most patients. All of the ACE inhibitors except fosinopril and moexipril are eliminated primarily by the kidneys; doses of these drugs should be reduced in patients with renal insufficiency.

Toxicity

Severe hypotension can occur after initial doses of any ACE inhibitor in patients who are hypovolemic as a result of diuretics, salt restriction, or gastrointestinal fluid loss. Other adverse effects common to all ACE inhibitors include acute renal failure (particularly in patients with bilateral renal artery stenosis or stenosis of the renal artery of a solitary kidney), hyperkalemia, dry cough sometimes accompanied by wheezing, and angioedema. Hyperkalemia is more likely to occur in patients with renal insufficiency or diabetes. Bradykinin and substance P seem to be responsible for the cough and angioedema seen with ACE inhibition.

ACE inhibitors are contraindicated during the second and third trimesters of pregnancy because of the risk of fetal hypotension, anuria, and renal failure, sometimes associated with fetal malformations or death. Recent evidence also implicates first-trimester exposure to ACE inhibitors in increased teratogenic risk. Captopril, particularly when given in high doses to patients with renal insufficiency, may cause neutropenia or proteinuria. Minor toxic effects seen more typically include altered sense of taste, allergic skin rashes, and drug fever, which may occur in up to 10% of patients.

Important drug interactions include those with potassium supplements or potassium-sparing diuretics, which can result in hyperkalemia. Nonsteroidal anti-inflammatory drugs may impair the hypotensive effects of ACE inhibitors by blocking bradykinin-mediated vasodilation, which is at least in part prostaglandin mediated.

ANGIOTENSIN RECEPTOR-BLOCKING AGENTS

Losartan and **valsartan** were the first marketed blockers of the angiotensin II type 1 (AT_1) receptor. **Azilsartan, candesartan, eprosartan, irbesartan, olmesartan,** and **telmisartan** are also available. They have no effect on bradykinin metabolism and are therefore more selective blockers of angiotensin effects than ACE inhibitors. They also have the potential for more complete inhibition of angiotensin action compared with ACE inhibitors because there are enzymes other than ACE that are capable of generating angiotensin II. Angiotensin receptor blockers provide benefits similar to those of ACE inhibitors in patients with heart failure and chronic kidney disease. Losartan's pharmacokinetic parameters are listed in Table 11–2. The adverse effects are generally similar to those described for ACE inhibitors, including the hazard of use during pregnancy. Cough and angioedema can occur but are uncommon. In the past, angiotensin receptor-blocking drugs were most commonly used in patients who had adverse reactions such as cough or angioedema with ACE inhibitors, but now many clinicians prefer to begin with angiotensin receptor blockers to avoid such adverse reactions. Combinations of ACE inhibitors and angiotensin receptor blockers or aliskiren, which had once been considered useful for more complete inhibition of the renin-angiotensin system, are not recommended due to toxicity demonstrated in recent clinical trials. Valsartan in combination with sacubitril (a neprilysin inhibitor) is marketed for heart failure.

TABLE 11–3 Mechanisms of action of vasodilators.

Mechanism	Examples
Release of nitric oxide from drug or endothelium	Nitroprusside, hydralazine, nitrates,[1] histamine, acetylcholine
Reduction of calcium influx	Verapamil, diltiazem, nifedipine[1]
Hyperpolarization of cell membranes through opening of potassium channels	Minoxidil, diazoxide
Activation of dopamine receptors	Fenoldopam

[1]See Chapter 12.

VASODILATORS

Mechanism & Sites of Action

This class of drugs includes the oral vasodilators, hydralazine and minoxidil, which are used for long-term outpatient therapy of hypertension; the parenteral vasodilators, nitroprusside and fenoldopam, which are used to treat hypertensive emergencies; the calcium channel blockers, which are used in both circumstances; and the nitrates, which are used mainly in ischemic heart disease but sometimes also in hypertensive emergencies (Table 11–3).

Chapter 12 contains additional discussion of vasodilators. All the vasodilators that are useful in hypertension relax smooth muscle of arterioles, thereby decreasing systemic vascular resistance. Sodium nitroprusside and the nitrates also relax veins. Decreased arterial resistance and decreased mean arterial blood pressure elicit compensatory responses, mediated by baroreceptors and the sympathetic nervous system (see Figure 11–4), as well as increases in renin, angiotensin, and aldosterone. Because sympathetic reflexes are intact, vasodilator therapy does not cause orthostatic hypotension or sexual dysfunction.

Vasodilators work best in combination with other antihypertensive drugs that oppose the compensatory cardiovascular responses. (See Box: Resistant Hypertension & Polypharmacy.)

HYDRALAZINE

Hydralazine, a hydrazine derivative, dilates arterioles but not veins. It has been available for many years, although it was initially thought not to be particularly effective because tachyphylaxis to its antihypertensive effects developed rapidly. The benefits of combination therapy are now recognized, and hydralazine may be used more effectively, particularly in severe hypertension. The combination of hydralazine with nitrates is effective in heart failure and should be considered in patients with both hypertension and heart failure, especially in patients who are intolerant to angiotensin inhibiting drugs.

Pharmacokinetics & Dosage

Hydralazine is well absorbed and rapidly metabolized by the liver during the first pass, so that bioavailability is low (averaging 25%) and variable among individuals. It is metabolized in part by acetylation at a rate that appears to be bimodally distributed in the population (see Chapter 4). As a consequence, rapid acetylators have greater first-pass metabolism, lower blood levels, and less antihypertensive benefit from a given dose than do slow acetylators. The half-life of hydralazine ranges from 1.5 to 3 hours, but vascular effects persist longer than do blood concentrations, possibly due to avid binding to vascular tissue.

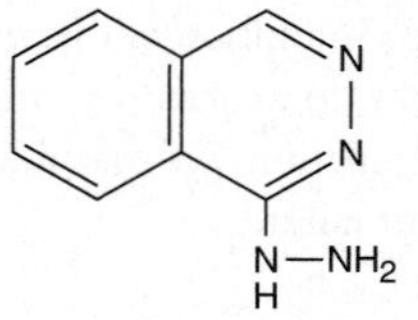

N
N
N—NH₂
H

Hydralazine

Usual dosage ranges from 40 to 200 mg/d. The higher dosage was selected as the dose at which there is a small possibility of developing the lupus erythematosus-like syndrome described in the next section. However, higher dosages result in greater vasodilation and may be used if necessary. Dosing two or three times daily provides smooth control of blood pressure.

Toxicity

The most common adverse effects of hydralazine are headache, nausea, anorexia, palpitations, sweating, and flushing. In patients with ischemic heart disease, reflex tachycardia and sympathetic stimulation may provoke angina or ischemic arrhythmias. With dosages of 400 mg/d or more, there is a 10–20% incidence—chiefly in persons who slowly acetylate the drug—of a syndrome characterized by arthralgia, myalgia, skin rashes, and fever that resembles lupus erythematosus. The syndrome is not associated with renal damage and is reversed by discontinuance of hydralazine. Peripheral neuropathy and drug fever are other serious but uncommon adverse effects.

MINOXIDIL

Minoxidil is a very efficacious orally active vasodilator. The effect results from the opening of potassium channels in smooth muscle membranes by minoxidil sulfate, the active metabolite. Increased potassium permeability stabilizes the membrane at its resting potential and makes contraction less likely. Like hydralazine, minoxidil dilates arterioles but not veins. Because of its greater potential antihypertensive effect, minoxidil should replace hydralazine when maximal doses of the latter are not effective or in patients with renal failure and severe hypertension, who do not respond well to hydralazine.

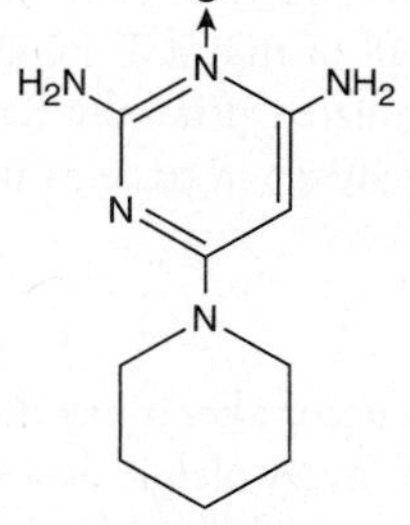

O
H_2N N NH_2
N
N

Minoxidil

Pharmacokinetics & Dosage

Pharmacokinetic parameters of minoxidil are listed in Table 11–2. Even more than with hydralazine, the use of minoxidil is associated with reflex sympathetic stimulation and sodium and fluid retention. Minoxidil must be used in combination with a β blocker and a diuretic.

Toxicity

Tachycardia, palpitations, angina, and edema are observed when doses of co-administered β blockers and diuretics are inadequate. Headache, sweating, and hypertrichosis (the latter particularly bothersome in women) are relatively common. Minoxidil illustrates how one person's toxicity may become another person's therapy. Topical minoxidil (as Rogaine) is used as a stimulant to hair growth for correction of baldness.

SODIUM NITROPRUSSIDE

Sodium nitroprusside is a powerful parenterally administered vasodilator that is used in treating hypertensive emergencies as well as severe heart failure. Nitroprusside dilates both arterial and venous vessels, resulting in reduced peripheral vascular resistance and venous return. The action occurs as a result of activation of guanylyl cyclase, either via release of nitric oxide or by direct stimulation of the enzyme. The result is increased intracellular cGMP, which relaxes vascular smooth muscle (see Figure 12–2).

In the absence of heart failure, blood pressure decreases, owing to decreased vascular resistance, whereas cardiac output does not change or decreases slightly. In patients with heart failure and low cardiac output, output often increases owing to afterload reduction.

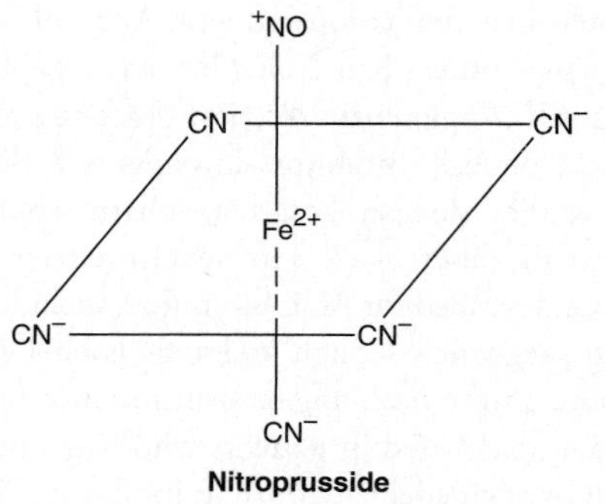

^{+}NO
CN^- CN^-
Fe^{2+}
CN^- CN^-
CN^-

Nitroprusside

Pharmacokinetics & Dosage

Nitroprusside is a complex of iron, cyanide groups, and a nitroso moiety. It is rapidly metabolized by uptake into red blood cells with release of nitric oxide and cyanide. Cyanide in turn is metabolized by the mitochondrial enzyme rhodanese, in the presence of a sulfur donor, to the less toxic thiocyanate. Thiocyanate is distributed in extracellular fluid and slowly eliminated by the kidney.

Nitroprusside rapidly lowers blood pressure, and its effects disappear within 1–10 minutes after discontinuation. The drug is given by intravenous infusion. Sodium nitroprusside in aqueous solution is sensitive to light and must therefore be made up fresh before each administration and covered with opaque foil. Infusion solutions should be changed after several hours. Dosage typically begins at 0.5 mcg/kg/min and may be increased up to 10 mcg/kg/min as necessary to control blood pressure. Higher rates of infusion, if continued for more than an hour, may result in toxicity. Because of its efficacy and rapid onset of effect, nitroprusside should be administered by infusion pump and arterial blood pressure continuously monitored via intra-arterial recording.

Toxicity

Other than excessive blood pressure lowering, the most serious toxicity is related to accumulation of cyanide; metabolic acidosis, arrhythmias, excessive hypotension, and death have resulted. In a few cases, toxicity after relatively low doses of nitroprusside suggested a defect in cyanide metabolism. Administration of sodium thiosulfate as a sulfur donor facilitates metabolism of cyanide. Hydroxocobalamin combines with cyanide to form the nontoxic cyanocobalamin. Both have been advocated for prophylaxis or treatment of cyanide poisoning during nitroprusside infusion. Thiocyanate may accumulate over the course of prolonged administration, usually several days or more, particularly in patients with renal insufficiency who do not excrete thiocyanate at a normal rate. Thiocyanate toxicity is manifested as weakness, disorientation, psychosis, muscle spasms, and convulsions, and the diagnosis is confirmed by finding serum concentrations greater than 10 mg/dL. Rarely, delayed hypothyroidism occurs, owing to thiocyanate inhibition of iodide uptake by the thyroid. Methemoglobinemia during infusion of nitroprusside has also been reported.

DIAZOXIDE

Diazoxide is an effective and relatively long-acting potassium channel opener that causes hyperpolarization in smooth muscle and pancreatic β cells. Because of its arteriolar dilating property, it was formerly used parenterally to treat hypertensive emergencies. Injection of diazoxide results in a rapid fall in systemic vascular resistance and mean arterial blood pressure. Injectable diazoxide is no longer available in the USA. Diazoxide also inhibits insulin release from the pancreas (probably by opening potassium channels in the beta cell membrane) and is used at present in the USA to treat hypoglycemia caused by hyperinsulinism secondary to insulinoma.

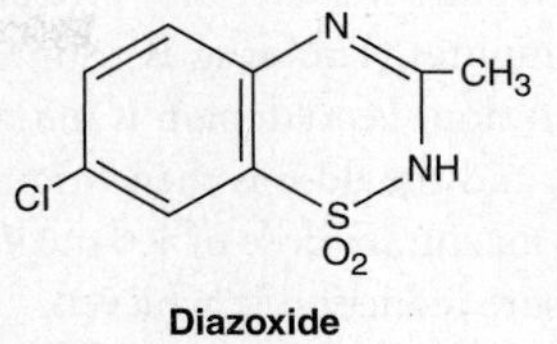

Diazoxide

Pharmacokinetics & Dosage

Oral dosage for hypoglycemia is 3–8 mg/kg/d in three divided doses, with a maximum of 15 mg/kg/d. Diazoxide is similar chemically to the thiazide diuretics but has no diuretic activity. It is bound extensively to serum albumin and to vascular tissue. Diazoxide is partially metabolized; its metabolic pathways are not well characterized. The remainder is excreted unchanged. Its half-life is approximately 24 hours, but the relationship between blood concentration and hypotensive action is not well established. The blood pressure-lowering effect after a rapid injection is established within 5 minutes and lasts for 4–12 hours.

When diazoxide was first marketed for use in hypertension, a dose of 300 mg by rapid injection was recommended. It appears, however, that excessive hypotension can be avoided by beginning with smaller doses (50–150 mg). If necessary, doses of 150 mg may be repeated every 5–15 minutes until blood pressure is lowered satisfactorily. Alternatively, diazoxide may be administered by intravenous infusion at rates of 15–30 mg/min. Because of reduced protein binding, smaller doses should be administered to persons with chronic renal failure. The hypotensive effects of diazoxide are also greater when patients are pretreated with β blockers to prevent the reflex tachycardia and associated increase in cardiac output.

Toxicity

The most significant toxicity from parenteral diazoxide has been excessive hypotension, resulting from the original recommendation to use a fixed dose of 300 mg in all patients. Such hypotension has resulted in stroke and myocardial infarction. The reflex sympathetic response can provoke angina, electrocardiographic evidence of ischemia, and cardiac failure in patients with ischemic heart disease, and diazoxide should be avoided in this situation. Occasionally, hyperglycemia complicates diazoxide use, particularly in persons with renal insufficiency.

In contrast to the structurally related thiazide diuretics, diazoxide causes renal salt and water *retention.* However, because the drug is used for short periods only, this is rarely a problem.

FENOLDOPAM

Fenoldopam is a peripheral arteriolar dilator used for hypertensive emergencies and postoperative hypertension. It acts primarily as an agonist of dopamine D_1 receptors, resulting in dilation of peripheral arteries and natriuresis. The commercial product is a racemic mixture with the (*R*)-isomer mediating the pharmacologic activity.

Fenoldopam is rapidly metabolized, primarily by conjugation. Its half-life is 10 minutes. The drug is administered by continuous intravenous infusion. Fenoldopam is initiated at a low dosage (0.1 mcg/kg/min), and the dose is then titrated upward every 15 or 20 minutes to a maximum dose of 1.6 mcg/kg/min or until the desired blood pressure reduction is achieved.

As with other direct vasodilators, the major toxicities are reflex tachycardia, headache, and flushing. Fenoldopam also increases intraocular pressure and should be avoided in patients with glaucoma.

CALCIUM CHANNEL BLOCKERS

In addition to their antianginal (see Chapter 12) and antiarrhythmic effects (see Chapter 14), calcium channel blockers also reduce peripheral resistance and blood pressure. The mechanism of action in hypertension (and, in part, in angina) is inhibition of calcium influx into arterial smooth muscle cells.

Verapamil, diltiazem, and the **dihydropyridine** family (**amlodipine, felodipine, isradipine, nicardipine, nifedipine, nisoldipine,** nimodipine, and nitrendipine [the latter two not available in the USA]) are all equally effective in lowering blood pressure. **Clevidipine** is a newer member of this group that is formulated for intravenous use only.

Hemodynamic differences among calcium channel blockers may influence the choice of a particular agent. Amlodipine and the other dihydropyridine agents are more selective as vasodilators and have less cardiac depressant effect than verapamil and diltiazem. Reflex sympathetic activation with slight tachycardia maintains or increases cardiac output in most patients given dihydropyridines. Verapamil has the greatest depressant effect on the heart and may decrease heart rate and cardiac output. Diltiazem has intermediate actions. The pharmacology and toxicity of these drugs are discussed in more detail in Chapter 12. Doses of calcium channel blockers used in treating hypertension are similar to those used in treating angina. Some epidemiologic studies reported an increased risk of myocardial infarction or mortality in patients receiving short-acting nifedipine for hypertension. It is therefore recommended that short-acting oral dihydropyridines not be used for hypertension. Sustained-release calcium blockers or calcium blockers with long half-lives provide smoother blood pressure control and are more appropriate for treatment of chronic hypertension. Intravenous nicardipine and clevidipine are available for the treatment of hypertension when oral therapy is not feasible; parenteral verapamil and diltiazem can also be used for the same indication. Nicardipine is typically infused at rates of 2–15 mg/h. Clevidipine is infused starting at 1–2 mg/h and progressing to 4–6 mg/h. It has a rapid onset of action and has been used in acute hypertension occurring during surgery. Oral short-acting nifedipine has been used in emergency management of severe hypertension.

DRUGS THAT ALTER SYMPATHETIC NERVOUS SYSTEM FUNCTION

In many patients, hypertension is initiated and sustained at least in part by sympathetic neural activation. In patients with moderate to severe hypertension, drug regimens that include an agent that inhibits function of the sympathetic nervous system may be needed for optimal blood pressure control. Drugs in this group are classified according to the site at which they impair the sympathetic reflex arc (see Figure 11–2). This neuroanatomic classification explains prominent differences in cardiovascular effects of drugs and allows the clinician to predict interactions of these drugs with one another and with other drugs.

The subclasses of sympathoplegic drugs exhibit different patterns of potential toxicity. Drugs that lower blood pressure by actions on the central nervous system tend to cause sedation and mental depression and may produce disturbances of sleep, including nightmares. Drugs that act by inhibiting transmission through autonomic ganglia (ganglion blockers) produce toxicity from inhibition of parasympathetic regulation, in addition to profound sympathetic blockade, and are no longer used. Drugs that act chiefly by reducing release of norepinephrine from sympathetic nerve endings cause effects that are similar to those of surgical sympathectomy, including inhibition of ejaculation, and hypotension that is increased by upright posture and after exercise. Drugs that block postsynaptic adrenoceptors produce a more selective spectrum of effects depending on the class of receptor to which they bind.

Finally, one should note that *all* of the agents that lower blood pressure by altering sympathetic function can elicit compensatory effects through mechanisms that are not dependent on adrenergic nerves. Thus, the antihypertensive effect of any of these agents used alone may be limited by retention of sodium by the kidney and expansion of blood volume. For this reason, sympathoplegic antihypertensive drugs are most effective when used concomitantly with a diuretic.

CENTRALLY ACTING SYMPATHOPLEGIC DRUGS

Centrally acting sympathoplegic drugs were once widely used in the treatment of hypertension. With the exception of clonidine, these drugs are rarely used today.

Mechanisms & Sites of Action

These agents reduce sympathetic outflow from vasomotor centers in the brain stem but allow these centers to retain or even increase their sensitivity to baroreceptor control. Accordingly, the antihypertensive and toxic actions of these drugs are generally less dependent on posture than are the effects of drugs that act directly on peripheral sympathetic neurons.

Methyldopa (L-α-methyl-3,4-dihydroxyphenylalanine) is an analog of L-dopa and is converted to α-methyldopamine and α-methylnorepinephrine; this pathway directly parallels the synthesis of norepinephrine from dopa illustrated in Figure 6–5. Alpha-methylnorepinephrine is stored in adrenergic nerve vesicles, where it stoichiometrically replaces norepinephrine, and is released by nerve stimulation to interact with postsynaptic adrenoceptors. However, this replacement of norepinephrine by a false transmitter in peripheral neurons is *not* responsible for methyldopa's antihypertensive effect, because the α-methylnorepinephrine released is an effective agonist at the α adrenoceptors that mediate peripheral sympathetic constriction of arterioles and venules. In fact, methyldopa's antihypertensive action appears to be due to stimulation of *central* α adrenoceptors by α-methylnorepinephrine or α-methyldopamine.

The antihypertensive action of **clonidine,** a 2-imidazoline derivative, was discovered in the course of testing the drug for use as a nasal decongestant. After intravenous injection, clonidine produces a brief rise in blood pressure followed by more prolonged hypotension. The pressor response is due to direct stimulation of α adrenoceptors in arterioles. The drug is classified as a partial agonist at α receptors because it also inhibits pressor effects of other α agonists.

The hypotensive effect of clonidine is exerted at α adrenoceptors in the medulla of the brain. In animals, the hypotensive effect of clonidine is prevented by central administration of α antagonists. Clonidine reduces sympathetic and increases parasympathetic tone, resulting in blood pressure lowering and bradycardia. The reduction in pressure is accompanied by a decrease in circulating catecholamine levels. These observations suggest that clonidine sensitizes brain stem vasomotor centers to inhibition by baroreflexes.

Thus, studies of clonidine and methyldopa suggest that normal regulation of blood pressure involves central adrenergic neurons that modulate baroreceptor reflexes. Clonidine and α-methylnorepinephrine bind more tightly to α_2 than to α_1 adrenoceptors. As noted in Chapter 6, α_2 receptors are located on presynaptic adrenergic neurons as well as some postsynaptic sites. It is possible that clonidine and α-methylnorepinephrine act in the brain to reduce norepinephrine release onto relevant receptor sites. Alternatively, these drugs may act on postsynaptic α_2 adrenoceptors to inhibit activity of appropriate neurons. Finally, clonidine also binds to a nonadrenoceptor site, the **imidazoline receptor,** which may also mediate antihypertensive effects.

Methyldopa and clonidine produce slightly different hemodynamic effects: clonidine lowers heart rate and cardiac output more than does methyldopa. This difference suggests that these two drugs do not have identical sites of action. They may act primarily on different populations of neurons in the vasomotor centers of the brain stem.

Guanabenz and **guanfacine** are centrally active antihypertensive drugs that share the central α-adrenoceptor–stimulating effects of clonidine. They do not appear to offer any advantages over clonidine and are rarely used.

METHYLDOPA

Methyldopa was widely used in the past but is now used primarily for hypertension during pregnancy. It lowers blood pressure chiefly by reducing peripheral vascular resistance, with a variable reduction in heart rate and cardiac output.

Most cardiovascular reflexes remain intact after administration of methyldopa, and blood pressure reduction is not markedly dependent on posture. Postural (orthostatic) hypotension sometimes occurs, particularly in volume-depleted patients. One potential advantage of methyldopa is that it causes reduction in renal vascular resistance.

HO, HO, OH, C=O, CH_2–C–NH_2, CH_3

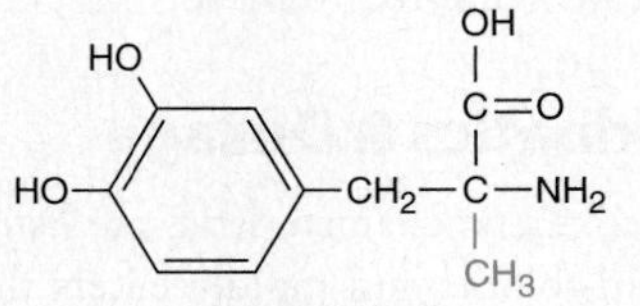

α-Methyldopa
(α-methyl group in color)

Pharmacokinetics & Dosage

Pharmacokinetic characteristics of methyldopa are listed in Table 11–2. Methyldopa enters the brain via an aromatic amino acid transporter. The usual oral dose of methyldopa produces its maximal antihypertensive effect in 4–6 hours, and the effect can persist for up to 24 hours. Because the effect depends on accumulation and storage of a metabolite (α-methylnorepinephrine) in the vesicles of nerve endings, the action persists after the parent drug has disappeared from the circulation.

Toxicity

The most common undesirable effect of methyldopa is sedation, particularly at the onset of treatment. With long-term therapy, patients may complain of persistent mental lassitude and impaired mental concentration. Nightmares, mental depression, vertigo, and extrapyramidal signs may occur but are relatively infrequent. Lactation, associated with increased prolactin secretion, can occur both in men and in women treated with methyldopa. This toxicity is probably mediated by inhibition of dopaminergic mechanisms in the hypothalamus.

Other important adverse effects of methyldopa are development of a positive Coombs test (occurring in 10–20% of patients undergoing therapy for longer than 12 months), which sometimes makes cross-matching blood for transfusion difficult and rarely is associated with hemolytic anemia, as well as hepatitis and drug fever. Discontinuation of the drug usually results in prompt reversal of these abnormalities.

CLONIDINE

Blood pressure lowering by clonidine results from reduction of cardiac output due to decreased heart rate and relaxation of capacitance vessels, as well as a reduction in peripheral vascular resistance.

Cl, NH, N, N, Cl

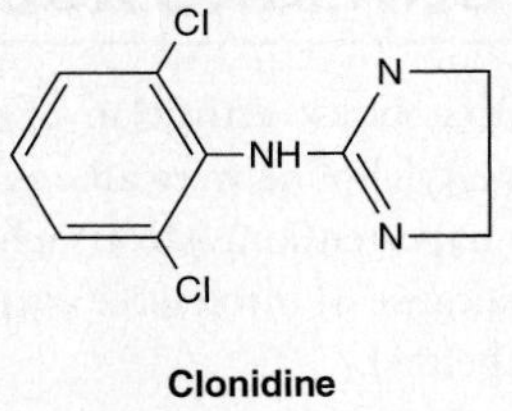

Clonidine

Reduction in arterial blood pressure by clonidine is accompanied by decreased renal vascular resistance and maintenance of renal blood flow. As with methyldopa, clonidine reduces blood pressure in the supine position and only rarely causes postural hypotension. Pressor effects of clonidine are not observed after ingestion of therapeutic doses of clonidine, but severe hypertension can complicate a massive overdose.

Pharmacokinetics & Dosage

Typical pharmacokinetic characteristics are listed in Table 11–2. Clonidine is lipid-soluble and rapidly enters the brain from the circulation. Because of its relatively short half-life and the fact that its antihypertensive effect is directly related to blood concentration, oral clonidine must be given twice a day (or as a patch, below) to maintain smooth blood pressure control. However, as is not the case with methyldopa, the dose-response curve of clonidine is such that increasing doses are more effective (but also more toxic).

A transdermal preparation of clonidine that reduces blood pressure for 7 days after a single application is also available. This preparation appears to produce less sedation than clonidine tablets but may be associated with local skin reactions.

Toxicity

Dry mouth and sedation are common. Both effects are centrally mediated and dose-dependent and coincide temporally with the drug's antihypertensive effect.

Clonidine should not be given to patients who are at risk for mental depression and should be withdrawn if depression occurs during therapy. Concomitant treatment with tricyclic antidepressants may block the antihypertensive effect of clonidine. The interaction is believed to be due to α-adrenoceptor–blocking actions of the tricyclics.

Withdrawal of clonidine after protracted use, particularly with high dosages (more than 1 mg/d), can result in life-threatening hypertensive crisis mediated by increased sympathetic nervous activity. Patients exhibit nervousness, tachycardia, headache, and sweating after omitting one or two doses of the drug. Because of the risk of severe hypertensive crisis when clonidine is suddenly withdrawn, all patients who take clonidine should be warned of this possibility. If the drug must be stopped, it should be done gradually while other antihypertensive agents are being substituted. Treatment of the hypertensive crisis consists of reinstitution of clonidine therapy or administration of α- and β-adrenoceptor–blocking agents.

GANGLION-BLOCKING AGENTS

Historically, drugs that block activation of postganglionic autonomic neurons by acetylcholine were among the first agents used in the treatment of hypertension. Most such drugs are no longer available clinically because of intolerable toxicities related to their primary action (see below).

Ganglion blockers competitively block nicotinic cholinoceptors on postganglionic neurons in both sympathetic and parasympathetic ganglia. In addition, these drugs may directly block the nicotinic acetylcholine channel, in the same fashion as neuromuscular nicotinic blockers.

The adverse effects of ganglion blockers are direct extensions of their pharmacologic effects. These effects include both sympathoplegia (excessive orthostatic hypotension and sexual dysfunction) and parasympathoplegia (constipation, urinary retention, precipitation of glaucoma, blurred vision, dry mouth, etc). These severe toxicities are the major reason for the abandonment of ganglion blockers for the therapy of hypertension.

ADRENERGIC NEURON-BLOCKING AGENTS

These drugs lower blood pressure by preventing normal physiologic release of norepinephrine from postganglionic sympathetic neurons. They have significant toxicity and are now rarely used.

Guanethidine

Guanethidine is no longer available in the USA but may be used elsewhere. In high enough doses, guanethidine can produce profound sympathoplegia. Guanethidine can thus produce all of the toxicities expected from "pharmacologic sympathectomy," including marked postural hypotension, diarrhea, and impaired ejaculation. Because of these adverse effects, guanethidine is now rarely used.

Guanethidine is too polar to enter the central nervous system. As a result, this drug has none of the central effects seen with many of the other antihypertensive agents described in this chapter.

Guanadrel is a guanethidine-like drug that is no longer used in the USA. **Bethanidine** and **debrisoquin,** antihypertensive agents not available for clinical use in the USA, are similar.

A. Mechanism and Sites of Action

Guanethidine inhibits the release of norepinephrine from sympathetic nerve endings (see Figure 6–4). This effect is probably responsible for most of the sympathoplegia that occurs in patients. Guanethidine is transported across the sympathetic nerve membrane by the same mechanism that transports norepinephrine itself (NET, uptake 1), and uptake is essential for the drug's action. Once guanethidine has entered the nerve, it is concentrated in transmitter vesicles, where it replaces norepinephrine and causes a gradual depletion of norepinephrine stores in the nerve ending.

B. Pharmacokinetics and Dosage

Because of guanethidine's long half-life (5 days), the onset of sympathoplegia is gradual (maximal effect in 1–2 weeks), and sympathoplegia persists for a comparable period after cessation of therapy. The dose should not ordinarily be increased at intervals shorter than 2 weeks.

C. Toxicity

Therapeutic use of guanethidine is often associated with symptomatic postural hypotension and hypotension following exercise, particularly when the drug is given in high doses. Guanethidine-induced sympathoplegia in men may be associated with delayed or retrograde ejaculation (into the bladder). Guanethidine commonly causes diarrhea, which results from increased gastrointestinal motility due to parasympathetic predominance in controlling the activity of intestinal smooth muscle. Interactions with other drugs may complicate guanethidine therapy.

Reserpine

Reserpine, an alkaloid extracted from the roots of an Indian plant, *Rauwolfia serpentina,* was one of the first effective drugs used on a large scale in the treatment of hypertension. Because of adverse effects, it was rarely used and is no longer available in the USA.

A. Mechanism and Sites of Action

Reserpine blocks the ability of aminergic transmitter vesicles to take up and store biogenic amines, probably by interfering with the vesicular membrane-associated transporter (VMAT, see Figure 6–4). This effect occurs throughout the body, resulting in depletion of norepinephrine, dopamine, and serotonin in both central and peripheral neurons. Chromaffin granules of the adrenal medulla are also depleted of catecholamines, although to a lesser extent than are the vesicles of neurons. Reserpine's effects on adrenergic vesicles appear irreversible; trace amounts of the drug remain bound to vesicular membranes for many days.

Depletion of peripheral amines probably accounts for much of the beneficial antihypertensive effect of reserpine, but a central component cannot be ruled out. Reserpine readily enters the brain, and depletion of cerebral amine stores causes sedation, mental depression, and parkinsonism symptoms.

At lower doses used for treatment of mild hypertension, reserpine lowers blood pressure by a combination of decreased cardiac output and decreased peripheral vascular resistance.

B. Pharmacokinetics and Dosage

See Table 11–2.

C. Toxicity

At the low doses usually administered, reserpine produces little postural hypotension. Most of the unwanted effects of reserpine result from actions on the brain or gastrointestinal tract.

High doses of reserpine characteristically produce sedation, lassitude, nightmares, and severe mental depression; occasionally, these occur even in patients receiving low doses (0.25 mg/d). Much less frequently, ordinary low doses of reserpine produce extrapyramidal effects resembling Parkinson disease, probably as a result of dopamine depletion in the corpus striatum. Patients with a history of mental depression should not receive reserpine, and the drug should be stopped if depression appears.

Reserpine rather often produces mild diarrhea and gastrointestinal cramps and increases gastric acid secretion. The drug should not be given to patients with a history of peptic ulcer.

ADRENOCEPTOR ANTAGONISTS

The detailed pharmacology of α- and β-adrenoceptor blockers is presented in Chapter 10.

BETA-ADRENOCEPTOR–BLOCKING AGENTS

Of the large number of β blockers tested, most have been shown to be effective in lowering blood pressure. The pharmacologic properties of several of these agents differ in ways that may confer therapeutic benefits in certain clinical situations.

Propranolol

Propranolol was the first β blocker shown to be effective in hypertension and ischemic heart disease. Propranolol has now been largely replaced by cardioselective β blockers such as metoprolol. All β-adrenoceptor–blocking agents are useful for lowering blood pressure in mild to moderate hypertension. In severe hypertension, β blockers are especially useful in preventing the reflex tachycardia that often results from treatment with direct vasodilators. Beta blockers have been shown to reduce mortality after a myocardial infarction and some also reduce mortality in patients with heart failure; they are particularly advantageous for treating hypertension in patients with these conditions (see Chapter 13).

A. Mechanism and Sites of Action

Propranolol's efficacy in treating hypertension as well as most of its toxic effects result from nonselective β blockade. Propranolol decreases blood pressure primarily as a result of a decrease in cardiac output. Other β blockers may decrease cardiac output or decrease peripheral vascular resistance to various degrees, depending on cardioselectivity and partial agonist activities.

Propranolol inhibits the stimulation of renin production by catecholamines (mediated by β_1 receptors). It is likely that propranolol's antihypertensive effect is due in part to depression of the renin-angiotensin-aldosterone system. Although most effective in patients with high plasma renin activity, propranolol also reduces blood pressure in hypertensive patients with normal or even low renin activity. Beta blockers might also act on peripheral presynaptic β adrenoceptors to reduce sympathetic vasoconstrictor nerve activity.

In mild to moderate hypertension, propranolol produces a significant reduction in blood pressure without prominent postural hypotension.

B. Pharmacokinetics and Dosage

See Table 11–2. Resting bradycardia and a reduction in the heart rate during exercise are indicators of propranolol's β-blocking effect, and changes in these parameters may be used as guides for regulating dosage. Propranolol can be administered twice daily, and slow-release once-daily preparations are available.

C. Toxicity

The principal toxicities of propranolol result from blockade of cardiac, vascular, or bronchial β receptors and are described in more detail in Chapter 10. The most important of these predictable extensions of the β_1-blocking action occur in patients with bradycardia or cardiac conduction disease, and those of the β_2-blocking action occur in patients with asthma, peripheral vascular insufficiency, and diabetes.

When β blockers are discontinued after prolonged regular use, some patients experience a withdrawal syndrome, manifested by nervousness, tachycardia, increased intensity of angina, and increase of blood pressure. Myocardial infarction has been reported in a few patients. Although the incidence of these complications is probably low, β blockers should not be discontinued abruptly. The withdrawal syndrome may involve up-regulation or supersensitivity of β adrenoceptors.

Metoprolol & Atenolol

Metoprolol and atenolol, which are cardioselective, are the most widely used β blockers in the treatment of hypertension. Metoprolol is approximately equipotent to propranolol in inhibiting stimulation of β_1 adrenoceptors such as those in the heart but 50- to 100-fold less potent than propranolol in blocking β_2 receptors. Relative cardioselectivity is advantageous in treating hypertensive patients who also suffer from asthma, diabetes, or peripheral vascular disease. Although cardioselectivity is not complete, metoprolol causes less bronchial constriction than propranolol at doses that produce equal inhibition of β_1-adrenoceptor responses. Metoprolol is extensively metabolized by CYP2D6 with high first-pass metabolism. The drug has a relatively short half-life of 4–6 hours, but the extended-release preparation can be dosed once daily (see Table 11–2). Sustained-release metoprolol is effective in reducing mortality from heart failure and is particularly useful in patients with hypertension and heart failure.

Atenolol is not extensively metabolized and is excreted primarily in the urine with a half-life of 6 hours; it is usually dosed once daily. Atenolol has been found to be less effective than metoprolol in preventing the complications of hypertension. A possible reason for this difference is that once-daily dosing does not maintain adequate blood levels of atenolol. The usual dosage is 50–100 mg/d. Patients with reduced renal function should receive lower doses.

Nadolol, Carteolol, Betaxolol, & Bisoprolol

Nadolol and carteolol, nonselective β-receptor antagonists, are not appreciably metabolized and are excreted to a considerable extent in the urine. Betaxolol and bisoprolol are β_1-selective blockers that are primarily metabolized in the liver but have long half-lives. Because of these relatively long half-lives, these drugs can be administered once daily. Nadolol is usually begun at a dosage of 40 mg/d, carteolol at 2.5 mg/d, betaxolol at 10 mg/d, and bisoprolol at 5 mg/d. Increases in dosage to obtain a satisfactory therapeutic effect should take place no more often than every 4 or 5 days. Patients with reduced renal function should receive correspondingly reduced doses of nadolol and carteolol.

Pindolol, Acebutolol, & Penbutolol

Pindolol, acebutolol, and penbutolol are partial agonists, ie, β blockers with some intrinsic sympathomimetic activity. They lower blood pressure but are rarely used in hypertension.

Labetalol, Carvedilol, & Nebivolol

These drugs have both β-blocking and vasodilating effects. Labetalol is formulated as a racemic mixture of four isomers (it has two centers of asymmetry). Two of these isomers—the *(S,S)*- and *(R,S)*-isomers—are relatively inactive, a third *(S,R)*- is a potent α blocker, and the last *(R,R)*- is a potent β blocker. Labetalol has a 3:1 ratio of β:α antagonism after oral dosing. Blood pressure is lowered by reduction of systemic vascular resistance (via α blockade) without significant alteration in heart rate or cardiac output. Because of its combined α- and β-blocking activity, labetalol is useful in treating the hypertension of pheochromocytoma and hypertensive emergencies. Oral daily doses of labetalol range from 200 to 2400 mg/d. Labetalol is given as repeated intravenous bolus injections of 20–80 mg to treat hypertensive emergencies.

Carvedilol, like labetalol, is administered as a racemic mixture. The *S*(−) isomer is a nonselective β-adrenoceptor blocker, but both *S*(−) and *R*(+) isomers have approximately equal α-blocking potency. The isomers are stereoselectively metabolized in the liver, which means that their elimination half-lives may differ. The average half-life is 7–10 hours. The usual starting dosage of carvedilol for ordinary hypertension is 6.25 mg twice daily. Carvedilol reduces mortality in patients with heart failure and is therefore particularly useful in patients with both heart failure and hypertension.

Nebivolol is a β_1-selective blocker with vasodilating properties that are *not* mediated by α blockade. D-Nebivolol has highly selective β_1-blocking effects, while the L-isomer causes vasodilation; the drug is marketed as a racemic mixture. The vasodilating effect may be due to an increase in endothelial release of nitric oxide via induction of endothelial nitric oxide synthase. The hemodynamic effects of nebivolol therefore differ from those of pure β blockers in that peripheral vascular resistance is acutely lowered (by nebivolol) as opposed to increased acutely (by the older agents). Nebivolol is extensively metabolized and has active metabolites. The half-life is 10–12 hours, but the drug can be given once daily. Dosing is generally started at 5 mg/d, with dose escalation as high as 40 mg/d, if necessary. The efficacy of nebivolol is similar to that of other antihypertensive agents, but several studies report fewer adverse effects.

Esmolol

Esmolol is a β_1-selective blocker that is rapidly metabolized via hydrolysis by red blood cell esterases. It has a short half-life (9–10 minutes) and is administered by intravenous infusion. Esmolol is generally administered as a loading dose (0.5–1 mg/kg), followed by a constant infusion. The infusion is typically started at 50–150 mcg/kg/min, and the dose increased every 5 minutes, up to 300 mcg/kg/min, as needed to achieve the desired therapeutic effect. Esmolol is used for management of intraoperative and postoperative hypertension, and sometimes for hypertensive emergencies, particularly when hypertension is associated with tachycardia or when there is concern about toxicity such as aggravation of severe heart failure, in which case a drug with a short duration of action that can be discontinued quickly is advantageous.

PRAZOSIN & OTHER ALPHA$_1$ BLOCKERS

Mechanism & Sites of Action

Prazosin, terazosin, and **doxazosin** produce most of their antihypertensive effects by selectively blocking α_1 receptors in arterioles and venules. These agents produce less reflex tachycardia when lowering blood pressure than do nonselective α antagonists such as phentolamine. Alpha$_1$-receptor selectivity allows norepinephrine to exert unopposed negative feedback (mediated by presynaptic α_2 receptors) on its own release (see Chapter 6); in contrast, phentolamine blocks both presynaptic and postsynaptic α receptors, with the result that reflex activation of sympathetic neurons by phentolamine's effects produces greater release of transmitter onto β receptors and correspondingly greater cardioacceleration.

Alpha blockers reduce arterial pressure by dilating both resistance and capacitance vessels. As expected, blood pressure is reduced more in the upright than in the supine position. Retention of salt and water occurs when these drugs are administered without a diuretic. The drugs are more effective when used in combination with other agents, such as a β blocker and a diuretic, than when used alone. Owing to their beneficial effects in men with prostatic hyperplasia and bladder obstruction symptoms, these drugs are used primarily in men with concurrent hypertension and benign prostatic hyperplasia.

Pharmacokinetics & Dosage

Pharmacokinetic characteristics of prazosin are listed in Table 11–2. Terazosin is also extensively metabolized but undergoes very little first-pass metabolism and has a half-life of 12 hours. Doxazosin has an intermediate bioavailability and a half-life of 22 hours.

Terazosin can often be given once daily, with doses of 5–20 mg/d. Doxazosin is usually given once daily starting at 1 mg/d and progressing to 4 mg/d or more as needed. Although long-term treatment with these α blockers causes relatively little postural hypotension, a precipitous drop in standing blood pressure develops in some patients shortly after the first dose is absorbed. For this reason, the first dose should be small and should be administered at bedtime. Although the mechanism of this first-dose phenomenon is not clear, it occurs more commonly in patients who are salt- and volume-depleted.

Aside from the first-dose phenomenon, the reported toxicities of the α_1 blockers are relatively infrequent and mild. These include dizziness, palpitations, headache, and lassitude. Some patients develop a positive test for antinuclear factor in serum while on prazosin therapy, but this has not been associated with rheumatic symptoms. The α_1 blockers do not adversely and may even beneficially affect plasma lipid profiles, but this action has not been shown to confer any benefit on clinical outcomes.

OTHER ALPHA-ADRENOCEPTOR–BLOCKING AGENTS

The nonselective agents, **phentolamine** and **phenoxybenzamine,** are useful in diagnosis and treatment of pheochromocytoma and in other clinical situations associated with exaggerated release of catecholamines (eg, phentolamine may be combined with a β blocker to treat the clonidine withdrawal syndrome, described previously). Their pharmacology is described in Chapter 10.

■ CLINICAL PHARMACOLOGY OF ANTIHYPERTENSIVE AGENTS

Hypertension presents a unique problem in therapeutics. It is usually a lifelong disease that causes few symptoms until the advanced stage. For effective treatment, medicines that may be expensive and sometimes produce adverse effects must be consumed daily. Thus, the physician must establish with certainty that hypertension is persistent and requires treatment and must exclude secondary causes of hypertension that might be treated by definitive surgical procedures. Persistence of hypertension, particularly in persons with mild elevation of blood pressure, should be established by finding an elevated blood pressure with multiple measurements on at least three different office visits. Home or ambulatory blood pressure monitoring may be the best predictor of risk and therefore of need for therapy in mild hypertension, and is recommended for initial evaluation of all patients. Isolated systolic hypertension and hypertension in the elderly also benefit from therapy.

Once the presence of hypertension is established, the question of whether to treat with medications and which drugs to use must be considered. The level of blood pressure, the age of the patient, the severity of organ damage (if any) due to high blood pressure, and the cardiovascular risk factors all must be considered. Current guidelines suggest treating people with medications for blood pressure of 140/90 mm Hg or greater if 10-year cardiovascular disease risk is less than 10%, and treatment at or above 130/80 if 10-year risk is 10% or greater. Assessment of renal function and the presence of proteinuria are useful in antihypertensive drug selection. Treatment thresholds and goals are described in Table 11–1. At this stage, the patient must be educated about the nature of hypertension and the importance of treatment so that he or she can make an informed decision regarding therapy.

Once the decision is made to treat, a therapeutic regimen must be developed. Selection of drugs is dictated by the level of blood pressure, the presence and severity of end-organ damage, and the presence of other diseases. Severe high blood pressure with life-threatening complications requires more rapid treatment with more efficacious drugs. Most patients with essential hypertension, however, have had elevated blood pressure for months or years, and therapy is best initiated in a gradual fashion.

Education about the natural history of hypertension and the importance of treatment adherence as well as potential adverse effects of drugs is essential. Obesity should be treated, and drugs that increase blood pressure (sympathomimetic decongestants, nonsteroidal anti-inflammatory drugs, estrogen-containing oral contraceptives, stimulant drug abuse, and some herbal medications) should be eliminated if possible. Follow-up visits should be frequent enough to convince the patient that the physician thinks the illness is serious. With each follow-up visit, the importance of treatment should be reinforced and questions concerning dosing or side effects of medication encouraged. Other factors that may improve compliance are simplifying dosing regimens and having the patient monitor blood pressure at home.

OUTPATIENT THERAPY OF HYPERTENSION

The initial step in treating hypertension may be nonpharmacologic. Sodium restriction may be effective treatment for some patients with mild hypertension. Weight reduction has been shown to normalize blood pressure in up to 75% of overweight patients with mild to moderate hypertension. Dietary sodium restriction should be recommended. The average American diet contains about 200 mEq of sodium per day. A reasonable dietary goal in treating hypertension is 70–100 mEq of sodium per day, which can be achieved by not salting food during or after cooking and by avoiding processed foods that contain large amounts of sodium. Eating a diet rich in fruits, vegetables, and low-fat dairy products with a reduced content of saturated and total fat, and moderation of alcohol intake (no more than two drinks per day) also lower blood pressure. Both the DASH (Dietary Approach to Stop Hypertension) and more recently the Chinese Heart-Healthy Diet have been demonstrated to reduce blood pressure in hypertensive adults. Using salt that substitutes potassium for some of the sodium reduces blood pressure and risk of future cardiovascular events. Regular exercise has been shown in some but not all studies to lower blood pressure in hypertensive patients.

For pharmacologic management of mild hypertension, blood pressure can be normalized in many patients with a single drug, although it is becoming more common to see the use of low-dose combination pharmacotherapy to improve effectiveness and reduce adverse effects. Most patients with moderate to severe hypertension require two or more antihypertensive medications (see Box: Resistant Hypertension & Polypharmacy). Thiazide diuretics, ACE inhibitors, angiotensin receptor blockers, and calcium channel blockers have all been shown to reduce complications of hypertension and may be used for initial drug therapy. There has been concern that diuretics, by adversely affecting the serum lipid profile or impairing glucose tolerance, may add to the risk of coronary disease, thereby offsetting the benefit of blood pressure reduction. However, a large clinical trial comparing different classes of antihypertensive mediations for initial therapy found that chlorthalidone (a thiazide diuretic) was as effective as other agents in reducing coronary heart disease death and nonfatal myocardial infarction, and was superior to amlodipine in preventing heart failure and superior to lisinopril in preventing stroke. Beta blockers are less effective in reducing cardiovascular events and are currently not recommended as first-line treatment for uncomplicated hypertension.

The presence of concomitant disease should influence selection of antihypertensive drugs because two diseases may benefit from a single drug. For example, drugs that inhibit the renin-angiotensin system are particularly useful in patients with diabetes or evidence of chronic kidney disease with proteinuria. Beta blockers or calcium channel blockers are useful in patients who also have angina; diuretics, ACE inhibitors, angiotensin receptor blockers, β blockers, or hydralazine combined with nitrates in patients who also have heart failure; and α_1 blockers in men who have benign prostatic hyperplasia. Race may also affect drug selection: African Americans respond better on average to diuretics and calcium channel blockers than to β blockers and ACE inhibitors. Chinese patients are more sensitive to the effects of β blockers and may require lower doses.

Drugs with different sites of action can be combined to effectively lower blood pressure while minimizing toxicity. If three drugs are required, combining a diuretic, an ACE inhibitor or angiotensin receptor blocker, and a calcium channel blocker is often effective. If a fourth drug is needed, a sympathoplegic agent such as a β blocker or clonidine should be considered. In the USA, fixed-dose drug combinations containing a β blocker, plus an ACE inhibitor or angiotensin receptor blocker, plus a thiazide; and a calcium channel blocker plus an ACE inhibitor are available. In recent studies, fixed low-dose triple combination treatment such as with telmisartan 20 mg, amlodipine 2.5 mg, and chlorthalidone 12.5 mg once daily demonstrated a high degree of efficacy in moderate hypertension with minimal side effects. Fixed three-drug combination tablets are not currently available in the USA. Fixed-dose combinations have the drawback of not allowing for titration of individual drug doses but have the advantage of allowing fewer pills to be taken, potentially enhancing compliance.

Assessment of blood pressure during office visits should include measurement of recumbent, sitting, and standing pressures. An attempt should be made to normalize blood pressure in the posture or activity level that is customary for the patient. Although there is still some debate about how much blood pressure should be lowered, the Systolic Blood Pressure Intervention Trial (SPRINT) and several meta-analyses suggest a target systolic blood pressure of 120 mm Hg for patients at high cardiovascular risk. Systolic hypertension (>150 mm Hg in the presence of normal diastolic blood pressure) is a strong cardiovascular risk factor in people older than 60 years of age and should be treated. Recent advances in outpatient treatment include home blood pressure telemonitoring with pharmacist case management, which has been shown to improve blood pressure control.

In addition to noncompliance with medication, causes of failure to respond to drug therapy include excessive sodium intake and inadequate diuretic therapy with excessive blood volume, and drugs such as tricyclic antidepressants, nonsteroidal anti-inflammatory drugs, over-the-counter sympathomimetics, abuse of stimulants (amphetamine or cocaine), or excessive doses of caffeine and oral contraceptives that can interfere with actions of some antihypertensive drugs or directly raise blood pressure.

MANAGEMENT OF HYPERTENSIVE EMERGENCIES

Despite the large number of patients with chronic hypertension, hypertensive emergencies are relatively rare. Marked or sudden elevation of blood pressure may be a serious threat to life, however, and prompt control of blood pressure is indicated. Most frequently, hypertensive emergencies occur in patients whose hypertension is severe and poorly controlled and in those who suddenly discontinue antihypertensive medications.

Clinical Presentation & Pathophysiology

Hypertensive emergencies include hypertension associated with vascular damage (termed malignant hypertension) and hypertension associated with hemodynamic complications such as heart failure, stroke, or dissecting aortic aneurysm. The underlying pathologic process in malignant hypertension is a progressive arteriopathy with inflammation and necrosis of arterioles. Vascular lesions occur in the kidney, which releases renin, which in turn stimulates production of angiotensin and aldosterone, which further increase blood pressure.

Hypertensive encephalopathy is a classic feature of malignant hypertension. Its clinical presentation consists of severe headache, mental confusion, and apprehension. Blurred vision, nausea and vomiting, and focal neurologic deficits are common. If untreated, the syndrome may progress over a period of 12–48 hours to convulsions, stupor, coma, and even death.

Treatment of Hypertensive Emergencies

The general management of hypertensive emergencies requires monitoring the patient in an intensive care unit with continuous recording of arterial blood pressure. Fluid intake and output must be monitored carefully, and body weight measured daily as an indicator of total body fluid volume during the course of therapy.

Parenteral antihypertensive medications are used to lower blood pressure rapidly (within a few hours); as soon as reasonable blood pressure control is achieved, oral antihypertensive therapy should be substituted because this allows smoother long-term management of hypertension. The goal of treatment in the first few hours or days is not complete normalization of blood pressure because chronic hypertension is associated with autoregulatory changes in cerebral blood flow. Thus, rapid normalization of blood pressure may lead to cerebral hypoperfusion and brain injury. Rather, blood pressure should be lowered by about 25%, maintaining diastolic blood pressure at no less than 100–110 mm Hg. Subsequently, blood pressure can be reduced to normal using oral medications over several weeks. The parenteral drugs used to treat hypertensive emergencies include sodium nitroprusside, nitroglycerin, labetalol, calcium channel blockers, fenoldopam, and hydralazine. Esmolol is often used to manage intraoperative and postoperative hypertension. Diuretics such as furosemide are administered to prevent the volume expansion that typically occurs during administration of powerful vasodilators.

SUMMARY Drugs Used in Hypertension

Subclass, Drug	Mechanism of Action	Effects	Clinical Applications	Pharmacokinetics, Toxicities, Interactions
DIURETICS				
• Thiazides: Hydrochlorothiazide, chlorthalidone	Block Na/Cl transporter in renal distal convoluted tubule	Reduce blood volume and poorly understood vascular effects	Hypertension, mild heart failure	See Chapter 15
• Loop diuretics: Furosemide	Block Na/K/2Cl transporter in renal loop of Henle	Like thiazides • greater efficacy	Severe hypertension, heart failure	
• Spironolactone, eplerenone	Block aldosterone receptor in renal collecting tubule	Increase Na and decrease K excretion • poorly understood reduction in heart failure mortality	Aldosteronism, heart failure, hypertension	
ANGIOTENSIN-CONVERTING ENZYME (ACE) INHIBITORS				
• Captopril, many others	Inhibit angiotensin-converting enzyme	Reduce angiotensin II levels • reduce vasoconstriction and aldosterone secretion • increase bradykinin	Hypertension • heart failure, diabetes	Oral • *Toxicity:* Cough, angioedema • hyperkalemia • renal impairment • teratogenic
ANGIOTENSIN RECEPTOR BLOCKERS (ARBs)				
• Losartan, many others	Block AT_1 angiotensin receptors	Same as ACE inhibitors but no increase in bradykinin	Hypertension • heart failure	Oral • *Toxicity:* Same as ACE inhibitors but less cough and angioedema

(continued)

Subclass, Drug	Mechanism of Action	Effects	Clinical Applications	Pharmacokinetics, Toxicities, Interactions
RENIN INHIBITOR				
• Aliskiren	Inhibits enzyme activity of renin	Reduces angiotensin I and II and aldosterone	Hypertension	Oral • *Toxicity:* Hyperkalemia, renal impairment • potential teratogen
SYMPATHOPLEGICS, CENTRALLY ACTING				
• Clonidine, methyldopa	Activate α_2 adrenoceptors	Reduce central sympathetic outflow • reduce norepinephrine release from noradrenergic nerve endings	Hypertension • clonidine also used in withdrawal from abused drugs	Oral • clonidine also as patch • *Toxicity:* sedation • methyldopa hemolytic anemia—withdrawal syndrome with sudden discontinuation of high-dose clonidine treatment
SYMPATHETIC NERVE TERMINAL BLOCKERS				
• Reserpine	Blocks vesicular amine transporter in noradrenergic nerves and depletes transmitter stores	Reduces all sympathetic effects, especially cardiovascular, and reduce blood pressure	Hypertension but rarely used	Oral • long duration (days) • *Toxicity:* Psychiatric depression, gastrointestinal disturbances
• Guanethidine, guanadrel	Interferes with amine release and replaces norepinephrine in vesicles	Same as reserpine	Same as reserpine	Severe orthostatic hypotension • sexual dysfunction • availability limited
α BLOCKERS				
• Prazosin • Terazosin • Doxazosin	Selectively block α_1 adrenoceptors	Prevent sympathetic vasoconstriction • reduce prostatic smooth muscle tone	Hypertension • benign prostatic hyperplasia	Oral • *Toxicity:* Orthostatic hypotension
β BLOCKERS				
• Metoprolol, others • Carvedilol • Nebivolol	Block β_1 receptors; carvedilol also blocks α receptors; nebivolol also releases nitric oxide	Prevent sympathetic cardiac stimulation • reduce renin secretion	Hypertension • heart failure • coronary disease	See Chapter 10
• *Propranolol: Nonselective prototype β blocker* • *Metoprolol and atenolol: Very widely used β_1-selective blockers*				
VASODILATORS				
• Verapamil • Diltiazem	Nonselective block of L-type calcium channels	Reduce cardiac rate and output • reduce vascular resistance	Hypertension, angina, arrhythmias	See Chapter 12
• Nifedipine, amlodipine, other dihydropyridines	Block vascular calcium channels > cardiac calcium channels	Reduce vascular resistance	Hypertension, angina	See Chapter 12
• Hydralazine • Minoxidil	Causes nitric oxide release Metabolite opens K channels in vascular smooth muscle	Vasodilation • reduces vascular resistance • arterioles more sensitive than veins • reflex tachycardia	Hypertension • minoxidil also used to treat hair loss	Oral • *Toxicity:* Angina, tachycardia • Hydralazine: Lupus-like syndrome • Minoxidil: Hypertrichosis
PARENTERAL AGENTS				
• Nitroprusside • Fenoldopam • Diazoxide • Labetalol	Releases nitric oxide Activates D_1 receptors Opens K channels α, β blocker	Powerful vasodilation	Hypertensive emergencies • diazoxide now used only in hypoglycemia	Parenteral • short duration • *Toxicity:* Excessive hypotension, shock

PREPARATIONS AVAILABLE

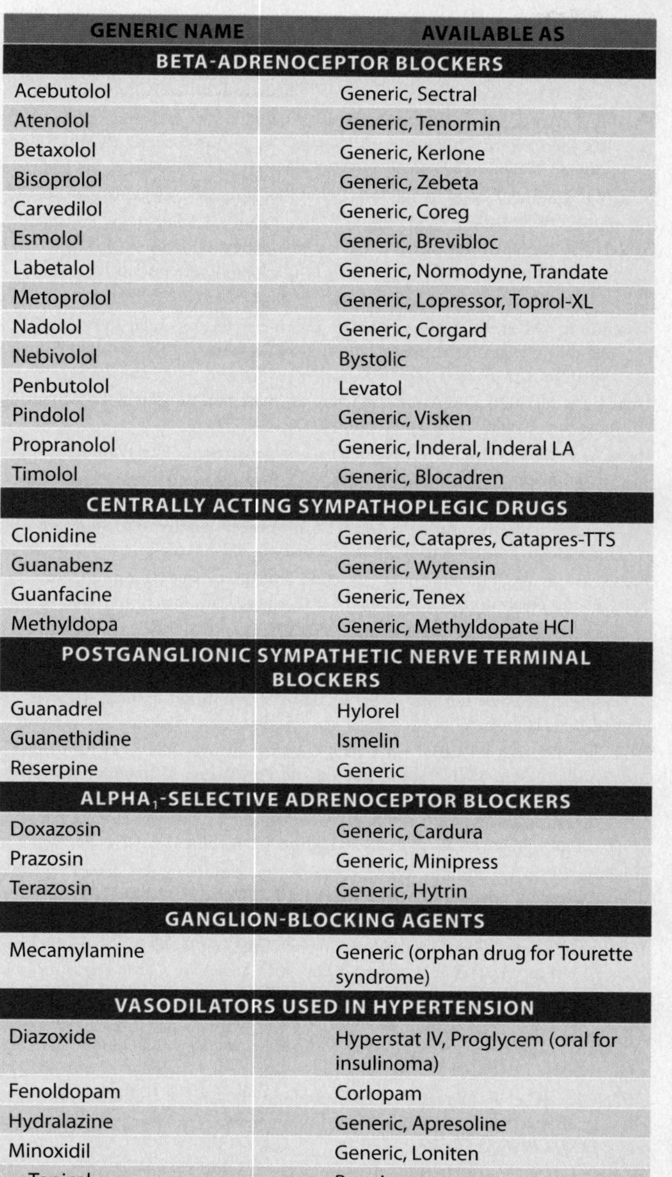

GENERIC NAME	AVAILABLE AS
BETA-ADRENOCEPTOR BLOCKERS	
Acebutolol	Generic, Sectral
Atenolol	Generic, Tenormin
Betaxolol	Generic, Kerlone
Bisoprolol	Generic, Zebeta
Carvedilol	Generic, Coreg
Esmolol	Generic, Brevibloc
Labetalol	Generic, Normodyne, Trandate
Metoprolol	Generic, Lopressor, Toprol-XL
Nadolol	Generic, Corgard
Nebivolol	Bystolic
Penbutolol	Levatol
Pindolol	Generic, Visken
Propranolol	Generic, Inderal, Inderal LA
Timolol	Generic, Blocadren
CENTRALLY ACTING SYMPATHOPLEGIC DRUGS	
Clonidine	Generic, Catapres, Catapres-TTS
Guanabenz	Generic, Wytensin
Guanfacine	Generic, Tenex
Methyldopa	Generic, Methyldopate HCl
POSTGANGLIONIC SYMPATHETIC NERVE TERMINAL BLOCKERS	
Guanadrel	Hylorel
Guanethidine	Ismelin
Reserpine	Generic
ALPHA$_1$-SELECTIVE ADRENOCEPTOR BLOCKERS	
Doxazosin	Generic, Cardura
Prazosin	Generic, Minipress
Terazosin	Generic, Hytrin
GANGLION-BLOCKING AGENTS	
Mecamylamine	Generic (orphan drug for Tourette syndrome)
VASODILATORS USED IN HYPERTENSION	
Diazoxide	Hyperstat IV, Proglycem (oral for insulinoma)
Fenoldopam	Corlopam
Hydralazine	Generic, Apresoline
Minoxidil	Generic, Loniten
Topical	Rogaine
Nitroprusside	Generic, Nitropress
CALCIUM CHANNEL BLOCKERS	
Amlodipine	Generic, Norvasc
Clevidipine	Cleviprex
Diltiazem	Generic, Cardizem, Cardizem CD, Cardizem SR, Dilacor XL
Felodipine	Generic, Plendil
Isradipine	Generic, DynaCirc, Dynacirc CR
Nicardipine	Generic, Cardene, Cardene SR, Cardene (IV)
Nifedipine	Generic, Adalat, Procardia, Adalat CC, Procardia-XL
Nisoldipine	Generic, Sular
Verapamil	Generic, Calan, Isoptin, Calan SR, Verelan
ANGIOTENSIN-CONVERTING ENZYME INHIBITORS	
Benazepril	Generic, Lotensin
Captopril	Generic, Capoten
Enalapril	Generic, Vasotec, Enalaprilat (parenteral)
Fosinopril	Generic, Monopril
Lisinopril	Generic, Prinivil, Zestril
Moexipril	Generic, Univasc
Perindopril	Generic, Aceon
Quinapril	Generic, Accupril
Ramipril	Generic, Altace
Trandolapril	Generic, Mavik
ANGIOTENSIN RECEPTOR BLOCKERS	
Azilsartan	Edarbi
Candesartan	Generic, Atacand
Eprosartan	Generic, Teveten
Irbesartan	Generic, Avapro
Losartan	Generic, Cozaar
Olmesartan	Benicar
Telmisartan	Generic, Micardis
Valsartan	Diovan
RENIN INHIBITOR	
Aliskiren	Tekturna

REFERENCES

Agarwal R et al: Chlorthalidone for hypertension in advanced chronic kidney disease. N Engl J Med 2021;385:2507.

Appel LJ et al: Intensive blood-pressure control in hypertensive chronic kidney disease. N Engl J Med 2010;363:918.

Arguedas JA et al: Blood pressure targets for hypertension in people with diabetes mellitus. Cochrane Database Syst Rev 2013;10:CD008277.

Aronow WS et al: ACCF/AHA 2011 expert consensus document on hypertension in the elderly: A report of the American College of Cardiology Foundation Task Force on Clinical Expert Consensus Documents. Circulation 2011;123:2434.

Benetos A et al: Hypertension management in older and frail older patients. Circ Res 2019;124:1045.

Bress AP et al: Potential cardiovascular disease events prevented with adoption of the 2017 American College of Cardiology/American Heart Association Blood Pressure Guideline. Circulation 2019;139:24.

Calhoun DA et al: Resistant hypertension: Diagnosis, evaluation, and treatment: A scientific statement from the American Heart Association Professional Education Committee of the Council for High Blood Pressure Research. Circulation 2008;117:e510.

Carey RM et al: Guideline-driven management of hypertension: an evidence-based update. Circ Res 2021;128:827.

Diao D et al: Pharmacotherapy for mild hypertension. Cochrane Database Syst Rev 2012;8:CD006742.

Ellison DH, Welling P: Insights into salt handling and blood pressure. N Engl J Med 2021;385:1981.

Ettehad D et al: Blood pressure lowering for prevention of cardiovascular disease and death: A systematic review and meta-analysis. Lancet 2016;387:957–67.

Ferdinand KC et al: Efficacy and safety of firibastat, a first-in-class brain aminopeptidase A inhibitor, in hypertensive overweight patients of multiple ethnic origins. Circulation 2019;140:138.

Flint AC et al: Effect of systolic and diastolic blood pressure on cardiovascular outcomes. N Engl J Med 2019 Jul 18;381(3):243–251. doi: 10.1056/NEJMoa1803180.

Garjón J et al: First-line combination therapy versus first-line monotherapy for primary hypertension. Cochrane Database Syst Rev 2020;2:CD010316.

Greene MF, Williams WW: Treating hypertension in pregnancy. N Engl J Med 2022;386:1846.

He FJ et al: Effect of longer term modest salt reduction on blood pressure: Cochrane systematic review and meta-analysis of randomised trials. BMJ 2013;346:f1325.

Hripcsak G et al: Comparison of cardiovascular and safety outcomes of chlorthalidone vs hydrochlorothiazide to treat hypertension. JAMA Intern Med 2020;180:542.

Ishani A, et al: Chlorthalidone vs. Hydrochlorothiazide for Hypertension–Cardiovascular Events. NEJM 2022;387(26)2401-2410.

James PA et al: 2014 evidence-based guideline for the management of high blood pressure in adults: Report from the panel members appointed to the Eighth Joint National Committee (JNC 8). JAMA 2014;311:507.

Kandzari DE et al: Effect of renal denervation on blood pressure in the presence of antihypertensive drugs: 6-month efficacy and safety results from the SPYRAL HTN-ON MED proof-of-concept randomised trial. Lancet 2018;391:2346.

Krause T et al: Management of hypertension: Summary of NICE guidance. BMJ 2011;343:d4891.

Lv J et al: Antihypertensive agents for preventing diabetic kidney disease. Cochrane Database Syst Rev 2012;12:CD004136.

Mancia GF et al: 2013 practice guidelines for the management of arterial hypertension of the European Society of Hypertension (ESH) and the European Society of Cardiology (ESC): ESH/ESC Task Force for the Management of Arterial Hypertension. J Hypertens 2013;31:1925.

Margolis KL et al: Effect of home blood pressure telemonitoring and pharmacist management on blood pressure control: A cluster randomized clinical trial. JAMA 2013;310:46.

Marik PE, Varon J: Hypertensive crises: Challenges and management. Chest 2007;131:1949.

Mente A et al: Associations of urinary sodium excretion with cardiovascular events in individuals with and without hypertension: A pooled analysis of data from four studies. Lancet 2016;388:465.

Muntner P et al: Trends in blood pressure control among US adults with hypertension, 1999-2000 to 2017-2018. JAMA 2020;324:1190.

Muntner P et al: Measurement of blood pressure in humans: a scientific statement from the American Heart Association. Hypertension 2019;73:e35.

Musini VM et al: Pharmacotherapy for hypertension in adults 60 years or older. Cochrane Database Syst Rev 2019;6:CD000028.

Neal B et al: Effect of salt substitution on cardiovascular events and death. N Engl J Med 2021;385:1067.

Nwankwo T et al: Hypertension among adults in the United States: National Health and Nutrition Examination Survey, 2011-2012. NCHS Data Brief 2013;133:1.

Olde Engberink RHG et al: Effects of thiazide-type and thiazide-like diuretics on cardiovascular events and mortality: Systematic review and meta-analysis. Hypertension 2015;65:1033.

Padilla Ramos A, Varon J: Current and newer agents for hypertensive emergencies. Curr Hypertens Rep 2014;16:450.

Peixoto AJ: Acute severe hypertension. N Engl J Med 2019;381:1843.

Reboussin DM et al: Systematic Review for the 2017 ACC/AHA/AAPA/ABC/ACPM/AGS/ APhA/ASH/ASPC/NMA/PCNA Guideline for the Prevention, Detection, Evaluation, and Management of High Blood Pressure in Adults: A Report of the American College of Cardiology/American Heart Association Task Force on Clinical Practice Guidelines. Circulation 2018;138:e595.

Rossignol P et al: The double challenge of resistant hypertension and chronic kidney disease. Lancet 2015;386:1588.

Roush GC, Sica DA: Diuretics for hypertension: A review and update. Am J Hypertens 2016;29:1130.

Sacks FM, Campos H: Dietary therapy in hypertension. N Engl J Med 2010; 362:2102.

Saiz LC et al: Blood pressure targets for the treatment of people with hypertension and cardiovascular disease. Cochrane Database Syst Rev 2020;9:CD010315.

Sharma P et al: Angiotensin-converting enzyme inhibitors and angiotensin receptor blockers for adults with early (stage 1 to 3) non-diabetic chronic kidney disease. Cochrane Database Syst Rev 2011;10:CD007751.

SPRINT Research Group: A randomized trial of intensive versus standard blood-pressure control. N Engl J Med 2015;373:2103.

SPRINT Research Group, Lewis CE, et al: Final report of a trial of intensive versus standard blood-pressure control. N Engl J Med 2021;384:1921.

Taler SJ: Initial treatment of hypertension. N Engl J Med 2018;378:636.

Thompson AM et al: Antihypertensive treatment and secondary prevention of cardiovascular disease events among persons without hypertension: A meta-analysis. JAMA 2011;305:913.

Unger T et al: 2020 International Society of Hypertension Global Hypertension Practice Guidelines. Hypertension 2020;75:1334.

Viera AJ et al: Does this adult patient have hypertension?: The Rational Clinical Examination Systematic Review. JAMA 2021;326:339.

Wang Y et al: Effects of cuisine-based Chinese heart-healthy diet in lowering blood pressure among adults in China: multicenter, single-blind, randomized, parallel controlled feeding trial. Circulation 2022;146:303.

Weber MA et al: Clinical practice guidelines for the management of hypertension in the community: A statement by the American Society of Hypertension and the International Society of Hypertension. J Hypertens 2014;32:3.

Webster R et al: Fixed low-dose triple combination antihypertensive medication vs usual care for blood pressure control in patients with mild to moderate hypertension in Sri Lanka: A randomized clinical trial. JAMA 2018;320:566.

Whelton PK et al: 2017 ACC/AHA/AAPA/ABC/ACPM/AGS/APhA/ASH/ASPC/NMA/ PCNA Guideline for the Prevention, Detection, Evaluation, and Management of High Blood Pressure in Adults: A Report of the American College of Cardiology/American Heart Association Task Force on Clinical Practice Guidelines. Circulation 2018;138:e484.

Whelton PK et al: Sodium, blood pressure, and cardiovascular disease: Further evidence supporting the American Heart Association sodium reduction recommendations. Circulation 2012;126:2880.

Whelton PK et al: Harmonization of the American College of Cardiology/American Heart Association and European Society of Cardiology/European Society of Hypertension Blood Pressure/Hypertension Guidelines: Comparisons, Reflections, and Recommendations. J Am Coll Cardiol 2022;80:1192.

Williams B et al: 2018 ESC/ESH Guidelines for the management of arterial hypertension. Eur Heart J 2018;39:3021.

Williamson JD et al: Intensive vs standard blood pressure control and cardiovascular disease outcomes in adults aged >/=75 years: A randomized clinical trial. JAMA 2016;315:2673.

Wiysonge CS, Opie LH: β-Blockers as initial therapy for hypertension. JAMA 2013;310:1851.

Wright JM, Musini VM, Gill R: First-line drugs for hypertension. Cochrane Database Syst Rev 2018;4:CD001841.

Xie W et al: Blood pressure-lowering drugs and secondary prevention of cardiovascular disease: Systematic review and meta-analysis. J Hypertens 2018;36:1256.

Xie X et al: Effects of intensive blood pressure lowering on cardiovascular and renal outcomes: Updated systematic review and meta-analysis. Lancet 2016;387:435.

Yang WY et al: Association of office and ambulatory blood pressure with mortality and cardiovascular outcomes. JAMA 2019;322:409.

CASE STUDY ANSWER

According to the 2017 American College of Cardiology/American Heart Association High Blood Pressure Clinical Practice Guidelines, this patient has stage 2 hypertension (see Table 11–1). The first question in management is how urgent it is to treat the hypertension. Cardiovascular risk factors in this man include family history of early coronary disease and elevated cholesterol. Evidence of end-organ impact includes left ventricular hypertrophy on electrocardiogram. The strong family history suggests that this patient has essential hypertension. However, the patient should undergo the usual screening tests including renal function, thyroid function, and serum electrolyte measurements. An echocardiogram should also be considered to determine whether the patient has left ventricular hypertrophy secondary to valvular or other structural heart disease as opposed to hypertension.

Initial management in this patient can be behavioral, including dietary changes and aerobic exercise. However, most patients like this will require medication. Thiazide diuretics in low doses are inexpensive, have relatively few side effects, and are effective in many patients with mild hypertension. Other first-line agents include angiotensin-converting enzyme inhibitors, angiotensin receptor blockers, and calcium channel blockers. Beta blockers might be considered if the patient had coronary disease or had labile hypertension. Either single agent or a combination of two agents in low doses should be prescribed and the patient reassessed in a month. If additional agents are needed, one should be a thiazide diuretic. Once blood pressure is controlled, patients should be followed periodically to reinforce the need for compliance with both lifestyle changes and medications.

CHAPTER

12 Vasodilators & the Treatment of Angina Pectoris & Coronary Syndromes

Bertram G. Katzung, MD, PhD

CASE STUDY

A 67-year-old woman presents in the emergency department of a small rural hospital with a history of chest pain and shortness of breath while watching television. While nasal oxygen is administered and an ECG is recorded, blood is drawn for high-sensitivity troponin measurement. Her husband provides the history that she has a history of exercise-induced angina pectoris and has taken nitroglycerin for relief in the past. Two doses of nitroglycerin have not relieved her pain on this occasion. She smokes and has a history of hyperlipidemia with elevated "bad cholesterol" (low-density lipoprotein [LDL]) and hypertension. Her father survived a "heart attack" at age 55, and an uncle died of some cardiac disease at age 60. On physical examination, the patient's blood pressure is 145/90 mm Hg, and her heart rate is 100 bpm. The ECG shows no ST elevation, but ST depression is present in several leads. Assuming that a dioagnosis of acute coronary syndrome (ACS) is correct, what treatment should be implemented?

Ischemic heart disease is one of the most common cardiovascular diseases in developed countries, and angina pectoris is the most common condition involving tissue ischemia in which vasodilator drugs are used. The name *angina pectoris* denotes chest pain caused by accumulation of metabolites resulting from myocardial ischemia. The organic nitrates, eg, **nitroglycerin,** are the mainstay of therapy for the immediate relief of angina. Another group of vasodilators, the **calcium channel blockers,** is also important, especially for prophylaxis, and **β blockers,** which are *not* vasodilators, are also useful in prophylaxis. Several newer drugs are available, including drugs that alter myocardial ion currents and selective cardiac rate inhibitors.

The most common cause of angina is atheromatous obstruction of the large coronary vessels (coronary artery disease, CAD). Inadequate blood flow in the presence of CAD results in **effort angina,** also known as **classic angina**. Diagnosis is usually made on the basis of the history and stress testing, sometimes supplemented by coronary angiography. Some patients have typical symptoms of angina in spite of normal epicardial coronary vessels. Previously labeled "coronary syndrome X," this condition is **coronary microvascular dysfunction.** Both types of angina are associated with diminished **coronary fractional flow reserve,** the fractional increase in coronary flow that can be achieved by maximal coronary dilation.

Transient spasm of localized portions of these vessels, usually associated with underlying atheromas, can also cause significant myocardial ischemia and pain (**vasospastic** or **variant angina**). Vasospastic angina is also called **Prinzmetal** angina. Diagnosis is usually made on the basis of history but can be confirmed by tests that provoke temporary spasm.

The primary cause of angina pectoris is an imbalance between the oxygen requirement of the heart and the oxygen supplied to it via the coronary vessels. In effort angina, the imbalance occurs when the myocardial oxygen requirement increases, especially during exercise, and coronary blood flow does not increase proportionately. The resulting ischemia with accumulation of acidic metabolites usually leads to pain. In fact, coronary flow reserve is frequently impaired in such patients because of endothelial dysfunction, which results in impaired vasodilation. As a result, ischemia may even occur at a lower level of myocardial oxygen demand. In some individuals, the ischemia is not always accompanied by pain, resulting in "silent" or "ambulatory" ischemia. In variant angina, oxygen delivery decreases as a result of reversible coronary vasospasm, which also causes ischemia and pain.

Unstable angina, an **acute coronary syndrome (ACS),** is said to be present when episodes of angina occur at rest and there is an increase in the severity, frequency, and duration of chest pain in patients with previously stable angina or an event occurs without prior history of angina. Unstable angina is caused by episodes of increased epicardial coronary artery resistance or small platelet clots occurring in the vicinity of an atherosclerotic plaque. In most cases, formation of labile partially occlusive thrombi at the site of a fissured or ulcerated plaque is the mechanism for reduction in flow. Inflammation may be a risk factor, because patients taking tumor necrosis factor inhibitors appear to have a lower risk of myocardial infarction. The course and the prognosis of unstable angina are variable, but this subset of acute coronary syndrome is associated with a high risk of myocardial infarction and death and is considered a medical emergency.

In theory, the imbalance between oxygen delivery and myocardial oxygen demand can be corrected by **decreasing oxygen demand** or by **increasing delivery** (by increasing coronary flow). In effort angina, oxygen demand can be reduced by decreasing cardiac work or, according to some studies, by shifting myocardial metabolism to substrates that require less oxygen per unit of adenosine triphosphate (ATP) produced. In variant angina, on the other hand, spasm of coronary vessels can be reversed by nitrate or calcium channel-blocking vasodilators. In unstable angina, vigorous measures are taken to achieve both—increase oxygen delivery (by medical or physical interventions) and decrease oxygen demand. Lipid-lowering drugs have become extremely important in the long-term treatment of atherosclerotic disease (see Chapter 35).

PATHOPHYSIOLOGY OF ANGINA

Determinants of Myocardial Oxygen Demand

The major determinants of myocardial oxygen requirement are listed in Table 12–1. The effects of arterial blood pressure and venous pressure are mediated through their effects on myocardial wall stress. As a consequence of its continuous activity, the heart's oxygen needs are relatively high, and it extracts approximately 75% of the available oxygen even in the absence of stress. The myocardial oxygen requirement increases when there is an increase in heart rate, contractility, arterial pressure, or ventricular volume. These hemodynamic alterations occur during physical exercise and sympathetic discharge, which often precipitate angina in patients with obstructive coronary artery disease.

Drugs that reduce cardiac size, rate, or force reduce cardiac oxygen demand. Thus, vasodilators, β blockers, and calcium blockers have predictable benefits in angina. A small, late component of sodium current helps to maintain the long plateau and prolong the calcium current of myocardial action potentials. Drugs that block this late sodium current can indirectly reduce calcium influx and consequently reduce cardiac contractile force. The heart favors fatty acids as a substrate for energy production. However, oxidation of fatty acids requires more oxygen per unit of ATP generated than oxidation of carbohydrates. Therefore, drugs that shift myocardial metabolism toward greater use of glucose (fatty acid oxidation inhibitors), at least in theory, may reduce the oxygen demand without altering hemodynamics.

TABLE 12–1 Hemodynamic determinants of myocardial oxygen consumption.

Wall stress
Intraventricular pressure
Ventricular radius (volume)
Wall thickness
Heart rate
Contractility

Determinants of Coronary Blood Flow & Myocardial Oxygen Supply

In the normal heart, increased demand for oxygen is met by augmenting coronary blood flow. Because coronary flow drops to near zero during systole, coronary blood flow is directly related to the aortic diastolic pressure and the duration of diastole. Therefore, the duration of diastole becomes a limiting factor for myocardial perfusion during tachycardia. Coronary blood flow is inversely proportional to coronary vascular resistance. Resistance is determined mainly by intrinsic factors, including metabolic products and autonomic activity, and can be modified—in normal coronary vessels—by various pharmacologic agents. Damage to the endothelium of coronary vessels has been shown to alter their ability to dilate and to increase coronary vascular resistance.

Determinants of Vascular Tone

Peripheral arteriolar and venous tone (vascular smooth muscle tension) both play a role in determining myocardial wall stress (see Table 12–1). Arteriolar tone directly controls peripheral vascular resistance and thus arterial blood pressure. In systole, intraventricular pressure must exceed aortic pressure to eject blood; arterial blood pressure thus determines the *left ventricular systolic* wall stress in an important way. Venous tone determines the capacity of the venous circulation and controls the amount of blood sequestered in the venous system versus the amount returned to the heart. Venous tone thereby determines the *right ventricular diastolic* wall stress.

The regulation of smooth muscle contraction and relaxation is shown schematically in Figure 12–1. The mechanisms of action of the major types of vasodilators are listed in Table 11–3. As shown in Figures 12–1 and 12–2, drugs may relax vascular smooth muscle in several ways:

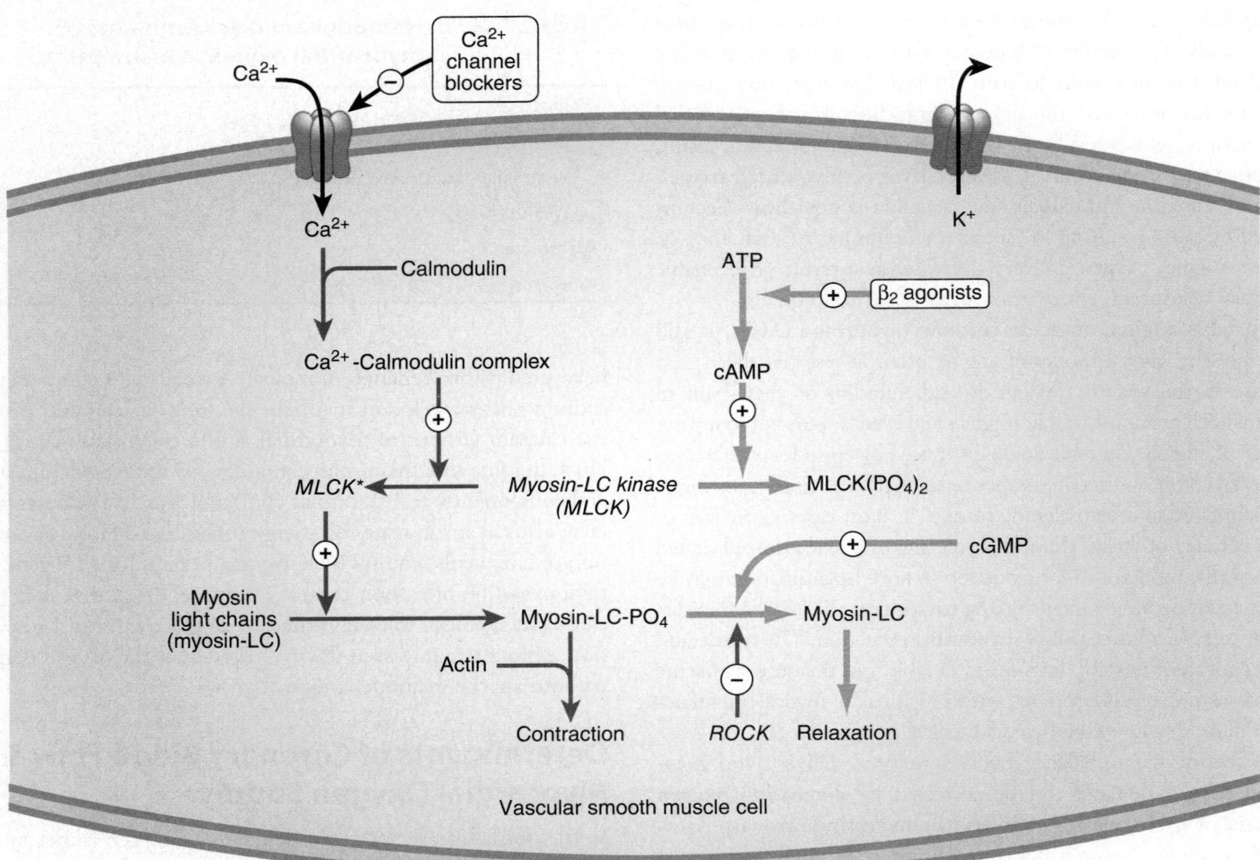

FIGURE 12–1 A simplified diagram of smooth muscle contraction and the site of action of calcium channel-blocking drugs. Contraction is triggered (red arrows) by influx of calcium (which can be blocked by calcium channel blockers) through transmembrane calcium channels. The calcium combines with calmodulin to form a complex that converts the enzyme myosin light-chain kinase to its active form (*MLCK**). The latter phosphorylates the myosin light chains, thereby initiating the interaction of myosin with actin. Other proteins, including calponin and caldesmon (not shown), inhibit the ATPase activity of myosin during the relaxation of smooth muscle. Interaction with the Ca^{2+}-calmodulin complex reduces their interaction with myosin during the contraction cycle. Beta$_2$ agonists (and other substances that increase cAMP) may cause relaxation in smooth muscle (blue arrows) by accelerating the inactivation of MLCK and by facilitating the expulsion of calcium from the cell (not shown). cGMP facilitates relaxation by the mechanism shown in Figure 12–2. ROCK, Rho kinase.

1. **Increasing cGMP:** cGMP facilitates the dephosphorylation of myosin light chains, preventing the interaction of myosin with actin. **Nitric oxide (NO)** is an effective activator of soluble guanylyl cyclase and acts mainly through increasing cGMP. Important molecular donors of nitric oxide include **nitroprusside** (used in hypertensive emergencies, see Chapter 11) and the organic **nitrates** used in angina. Atherosclerotic disease may diminish endogenous endothelial NO synthesis, thus making the vascular smooth muscle more dependent upon exogenous sources of NO.
2. **Decreasing intracellular Ca^{2+}: Calcium channel blockers** predictably cause vasodilation because they reduce intracellular Ca^{2+}, a major modulator of the activation of myosin light chain kinase (see Figure 12–1) in smooth muscle. **Beta blockers** and **calcium channel blockers** also reduce Ca^{2+} influx in cardiac muscle fibers, thereby reducing rate, contractility, and oxygen requirement under most circumstances.
3. **Stabilizing or preventing depolarization of the vascular smooth muscle cell membrane:** The membrane potential of excitable cells is stabilized near the resting potential by increasing potassium permeability. cGMP may increase permeability of Ca^{2+}-activated K+ channels. Potassium channel openers, such as minoxidil sulfate (see Chapter 11), increase the permeability of K^+ channels, probably ATP-dependent K^+ channels. Certain agents used elsewhere and under investigation in the United States (eg, **nicorandil**) may act, in part, by this mechanism.
4. **Increasing cAMP in vascular smooth muscle cells:** As shown in Figure 12–1, an increase in cAMP increases the rate of inactivation of myosin light chain kinase, the enzyme responsible for triggering the interaction of actin with myosin in these cells. This appears to be the mechanism of vasodilation caused by β_2 agonists, drugs that are *not* used in angina (because they cause too much cardiac stimulation), and by fenoldopam, a D_1 agonist used in hypertensive emergencies.

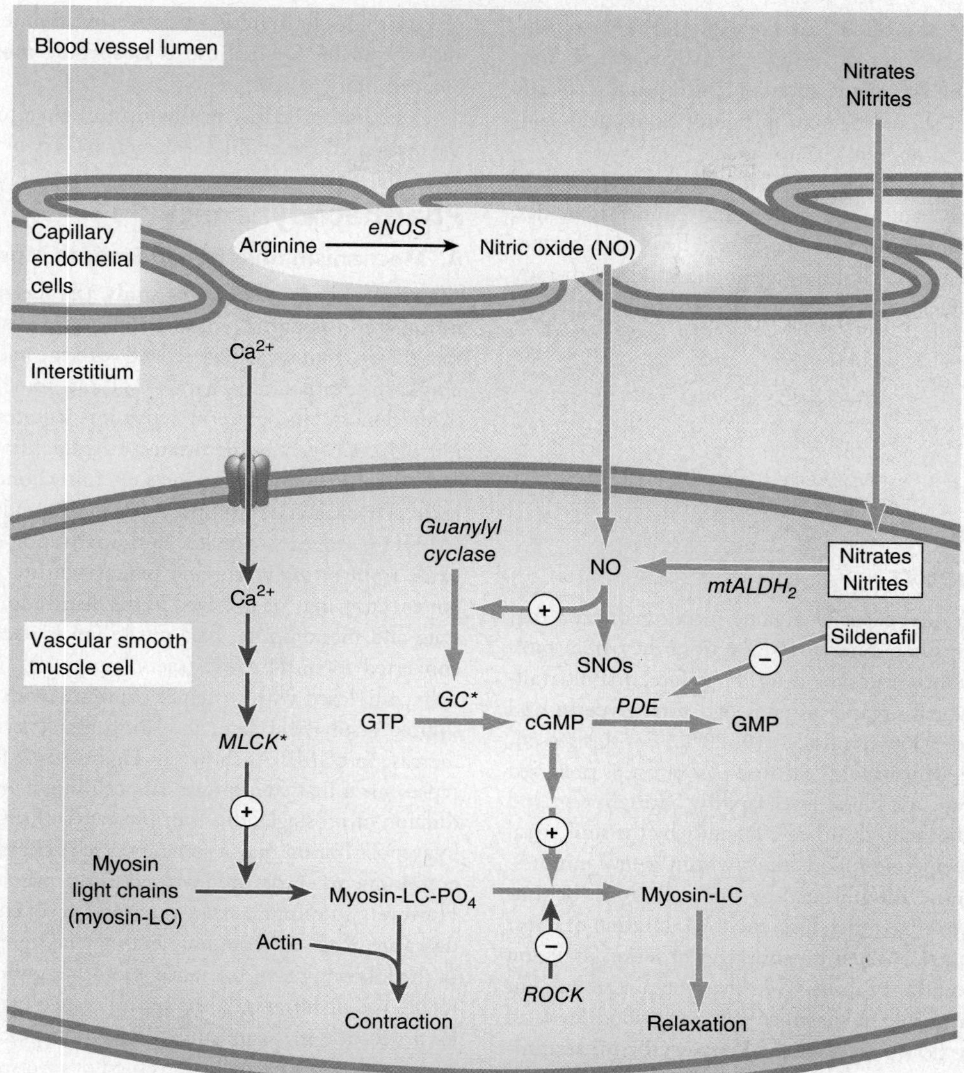

FIGURE 12–2 Mechanism of action of nitrates, nitrites, and other substances that increase the concentration of nitric oxide (NO) in vascular smooth muscle cells. Steps leading to relaxation are shown with blue arrows. MLCK∗, activated myosin light-chain kinase (see Figure 12–1). Nitrosothiols (SNOs) appear to have non-cGMP-dependent effects on potassium channels and Ca^{2+}-ATPase. eNOS, endothelial nitric oxide synthase; GC∗, activated guanylyl cyclase; mtALDH2, mitochondrial aldehyde dehydrogenase-2; PDE, phosphodiesterase; ROCK, Rho kinase.

■ BASIC PHARMACOLOGY OF DRUGS USED TO TREAT ANGINA

Drug Action in Angina

The three drug groups traditionally used in angina (organic nitrates, calcium channel blockers, and β blockers) *decrease myocardial oxygen requirement* by decreasing one or more of the major determinants of oxygen demand (heart size, heart rate, blood pressure, and contractility). In some patients, the nitrates and the calcium channel blockers may cause a redistribution of coronary flow and *increase oxygen delivery* to ischemic tissue. In variant angina, these two drug groups also increase myocardial oxygen delivery by reversing coronary artery spasm. The nitrates are used for relief of acute episodes of anginal pain and for prophylaxis. Because of their slow onset of action, calcium channel blockers and β blockers are used for prophylaxis. Newer drugs are discussed later.

NITRATES & NITRITES

Chemistry

Diets rich in inorganic nitrates are known to have a small blood pressure–lowering action but are of no value in angina. The agents useful in angina are simple organic nitric and nitrous acid esters of polyalcohols. **Nitroglycerin** is the prototype of the group and has been used in cardiovascular conditions for over 160 years. Although nitroglycerin is used in the manufacture of dynamite, the formulations used in medicine are not explosive. The conventional sublingual tablet form of nitroglycerin may lose potency when stored as a result of volatilization and adsorption to plastic surfaces. Therefore, it should be kept in tightly closed glass containers. Nitroglycerin is not sensitive to light.

All therapeutically active agents in the nitrate group appear to have identical mechanisms of action and similar toxicities, although development of tolerance may vary. Therefore, pharmacokinetic factors govern the choice of agent and mode of therapy when using the nitrates.

$$
\begin{array}{l}
H_2C-O-NO_2 \\
\quad | \\
HC-O-NO_2 \\
\quad | \\
H_2C-O-NO_2
\end{array}
$$

Nitroglycerin
(Glyceryl trinitrate)

Pharmacokinetics

The liver contains a high-capacity organic nitrate reductase that removes nitrate groups in a stepwise fashion from the parent molecule and ultimately inactivates the drug. Therefore, oral bioavailability of the traditional organic nitrates (eg, **nitroglycerin** and **isosorbide dinitrate**) is low (typically <10–20%). For this reason, the sublingual route, which avoids the first-pass effect, is preferred for achieving a therapeutic blood level rapidly. Nitroglycerin and isosorbide dinitrate both are absorbed efficiently by the sublingual route and reach therapeutic blood levels within a few minutes. However, the total dose administered by this route must be limited to avoid excessive effect; therefore, the total duration of effect is brief (15–30 minutes). When much longer duration of action is needed, oral preparations can be given that contain an amount of drug sufficient to result in sustained systemic blood levels of the parent drug plus active metabolites. **Pentaerythritol tetranitrate** (PETN) is another organic nitrate that has been promoted for oral use as a "long-acting" nitrate (>6 hours). This drug has also been reported to reduce pulmonary hypertension in experimental animals. Other routes of administration available for nitroglycerin include transdermal and buccal absorption from slow-release preparations (described below).

Amyl nitrite and related nitrites are highly volatile liquids. Amyl nitrite is available in fragile glass ampules ("poppers") packaged in a protective cloth covering. The ampule can be crushed with the fingers, resulting in rapid release of vapors inhalable through the cloth covering. The inhalation route provides very rapid absorption and, like the sublingual route, avoids the hepatic first-pass effect. Because of its unpleasant odor and extremely short duration of action, amyl nitrite is now obsolete for angina.

Once absorbed, the unchanged organic nitrate compounds have half-lives of only 2–8 minutes. The partially denitrated metabolites have much longer half-lives (up to 3 hours). Of the nitroglycerin metabolites (two dinitroglycerins and two mononitro forms), the 1,2-dinitro derivative has significant vasodilator efficacy and probably provides most of the therapeutic effect of orally administered nitroglycerin. The 5-mononitrate metabolite of isosorbide dinitrate is an active metabolite of the latter drug and is available for oral use as **isosorbide mononitrate.** It has a bioavailability of 100%.

Excretion, primarily in the form of glucuronide derivatives of the denitrated metabolites, is largely by way of the kidney.

Pharmacodynamics

A. Mechanism of Action in Smooth Muscle

After more than a century of study, the mechanism of action of nitroglycerin is partially understood. There is general agreement that the drug must be bioactivated with the release of **nitric oxide.** Unlike nitroprusside (Chapter 11) and some other direct nitric oxide donors, nitroglycerin activation requires enzymatic action. Nitroglycerin can be denitrated by glutathione *S*-transferase in smooth muscle and other cells. A mitochondrial enzyme, aldehyde dehydrogenase isoform 2 (ALDH2) and possibly isoform 3 (ALDH3), appears to be key in the activation and release of nitric oxide from nitroglycerin and pentaerythritol tetranitrate. Different enzymes may be involved in the denitration of isosorbide dinitrate and mononitrate. Free nitrite ion is released, which is then converted to nitric oxide (see Chapter 19). Nitric oxide (probably complexed with cysteine) combines with the heme group of soluble guanylyl cyclase, activating that enzyme and causing an increase in cGMP. As shown in Figure 12–2, formation of cGMP represents a first step toward smooth muscle relaxation. The production of prostaglandin E or prostacyclin (PGI_2) and membrane hyperpolarization may also be involved. There is no evidence that autonomic receptors are involved in the primary nitrate response. However, autonomic *reflex* responses, evoked when hypotensive doses are given, are common and may be significant. As described in the following text, tolerance is another important consideration in the use of nitrates. Although tolerance may be caused in part by a decrease in tissue sulfhydryl groups, eg, on cysteine, tolerance can be only partially prevented or reversed with a sulfhydryl-regenerating agent. Increased generation of free radicals during nitrate therapy may be another important mechanism of tolerance. Some evidence suggests that diminished availability of calcitonin gene-related peptide (CGRP, a potent vasodilator) is also associated with nitrate tolerance.

Nicorandil and several other antianginal agents not available in the United States appear to combine the activity of nitric oxide release with a direct potassium channel-opening action resulting in smooth muscle hyperpolarization, thus providing an additional mechanism for causing vasodilation.

B. Organ System Effects

Nitroglycerin relaxes all types of smooth muscle regardless of the cause of the preexisting muscle tone (Figure 12–3). It has practically no direct effect on cardiac or skeletal muscle.

1. Vascular smooth muscle—All segments of the vascular system from large arteries through large veins relax in response to nitroglycerin. Most evidence suggests a gradient of response, with veins responding at the lowest concentrations and arteries

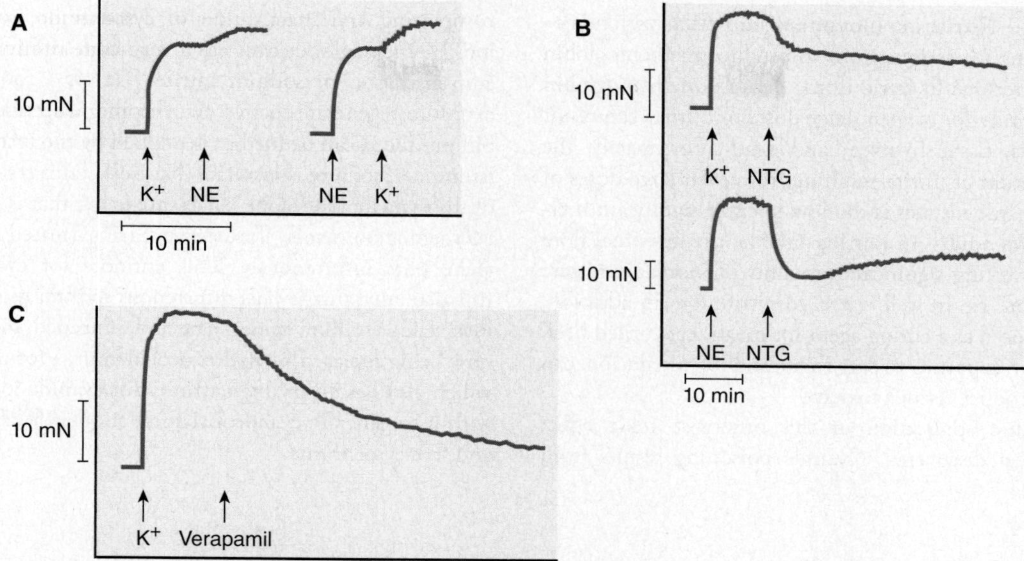

FIGURE 12–3 Effects of vasodilators on contractions of human vein segments studied in vitro. **A** shows contractions induced by two vasoconstrictor agents, norepinephrine (NE) and potassium (K^+). **B** shows the relaxation induced by nitroglycerin (NTG), 4 μmol/L. The relaxation is prompt. **C** shows the relaxation induced by verapamil, 2.2 μmol/L. The relaxation is slower but more sustained. mN, millinewtons, a measure of force. (Adapted with permission from Mikkelsen E, Andersson KE, Bengtsson B: Effects of verapamil and nitroglycerin on contractile responses to potassium and noradrenaline in isolated human peripheral veins. Acta Pharmacol Toxicol (Copenh). 1978;42(1):14-22.)

at slightly higher ones. The epicardial coronary arteries are sensitive, but concentric atheromas can prevent significant dilation. On the other hand, eccentric lesions permit an increase in flow when nitrates relax the smooth muscle on the side away from the lesion. Arterioles and precapillary sphincters are dilated least, partly because of reflex responses and partly because different vessels vary in their ability to release nitric oxide from the drug.

A primary direct result of an effective dose of nitroglycerin is marked relaxation of veins with increased venous capacitance and decreased ventricular preload. Pulmonary vascular pressures and heart size are significantly reduced. In the absence of heart failure, cardiac output is reduced. Because venous capacitance is increased, orthostatic hypotension may be marked and syncope can result. Dilation of large epicardial coronary arteries may improve oxygen delivery in the presence of eccentric atheromas or collateral vessels. Temporal artery pulsations and a throbbing headache associated with meningeal artery pulsations are common effects of nitroglycerin and amyl nitrite. In heart failure, preload is often abnormally high; the nitrates and other vasodilators, by reducing preload, may have a beneficial effect on cardiac output in this condition (see Chapter 13).

The indirect effects of nitroglycerin consist of those compensatory responses evoked by baroreceptors and hormonal mechanisms responding to decreased arterial pressure (see Figure 6–7); this often results in tachycardia and increased cardiac contractility. Retention of salt and water may also be significant, especially with intermediate- and long-acting nitrates. These compensatory responses contribute to the development of nitrate tolerance.

In normal subjects without coronary disease, nitroglycerin can induce a significant, if transient, increase in total coronary blood flow. In contrast, there is no evidence that total coronary flow is increased in patients with angina due to atherosclerotic obstructive coronary artery disease. However, some studies suggest that *redistribution* of coronary flow from normal to ischemic regions may play a role in nitroglycerin's therapeutic effect. Nitroglycerin also exerts a weak negative inotropic effect on the heart via nitric oxide.

2. Other smooth muscle organs—Relaxation of smooth muscle of the bronchi, gastrointestinal tract (including biliary system), and genitourinary tract has been demonstrated experimentally. Because of their brief duration, these actions of the nitrates are rarely of any clinical value. During recent decades, the use of amyl nitrite and isobutyl nitrite (not nitrates) by inhalation as recreational (sex-enhancing) drugs has become popular with some people. Nitrites readily release nitric oxide in erectile tissue as well as vascular smooth muscle and activate guanylyl cyclase. The resulting increase in cGMP causes dephosphorylation of myosin light chains and relaxation (see Figure 12–2), which enhances erection. This pharmacologic approach to erectile dysfunction is discussed in the Box: Drugs Used in the Treatment of Erectile Dysfunction.

3. Action on platelets—Nitric oxide released from nitroglycerin stimulates guanylyl cyclase in platelets as in smooth muscle. The increase in cGMP that results is responsible for a decrease in platelet aggregation. Unfortunately, recent prospective trials have established no survival benefit when nitroglycerin is used in acute myocardial infarction. In contrast, intravenous nitroglycerin may be of value in acute coronary syndrome, in part through its action on platelets.

***4. Other effects*—Nitrite** ion (not nitrate ion) reacts with hemoglobin (which contains ferrous iron) to produce methemoglobin (by oxidation of ferrous to ferric iron). Because methemoglobin has a very low affinity for oxygen, large doses of nitrites can result in pseudocyanosis, tissue hypoxia, and death. Fortunately, the plasma concentration of nitrite resulting from even large doses of organic and inorganic nitrates is too low to cause significant methemoglobinemia in adults. In nursing infants, the intestinal flora is capable of converting significant amounts of inorganic nitrate (sometimes present, eg, in well water) to nitrite ion. In addition, sodium nitrite is used as a curing agent for meats, eg, corned beef. Thus, inadvertent exposure to large amounts of nitrite ion can occur and may produce serious toxicity.

One therapeutic application of this otherwise toxic effect of nitrite has been discovered. Cyanide poisoning results from complexing and inactivation of cytochrome iron by the CN^- ion. Methemoglobin iron has a very high affinity for CN^-; thus, administration of sodium nitrite ($NaNO_2$) soon after cyanide exposure regenerates active cytochrome. The cyanomethemoglobin produced can be further detoxified by the intravenous administration of sodium thiosulfate ($Na_2S_2O_3$); this results in formation of thiocyanate ion (SCN^-), a less toxic ion that is readily excreted. Methemoglobinemia, if excessive, can be treated by giving methylene blue intravenously. This antidote for cyanide poisoning (inhaled amyl nitrite plus intravenous sodium nitrite, followed by intravenous sodium thiocyanate and, if needed, methylene blue) is now being replaced by hydroxocobalamin, a form of vitamin B_{12}, which also has a very high affinity for cyanide ion and combines with it to generate cyanocobalamin, another form of vitamin B_{12}, and free cytochrome.

Drugs Used in the Treatment of Erectile Dysfunction

Erectile dysfunction in men has long been the subject of research (by both amateur and professional scientists) and is heavily promoted on the internet by quacks. Among the substances used in the past and generally discredited are "Spanish Fly" (a bladder and urethral irritant), yohimbine (an α_2 antagonist; see Chapter 10), nutmeg, and mixtures containing lead, arsenic, or strychnine. Substances currently favored by practitioners of herbal medicine but of dubious value include ginseng and kava.

Scientific studies of the process have shown that erection requires *relaxation* of the nonvascular smooth muscle of the corpora cavernosa. This relaxation permits inflow of blood at nearly arterial pressure into the sinuses of the cavernosa, and it is the pressure of the blood that causes erection. (With regard to other aspects of male sexual function, ejaculation requires intact sympathetic motor function, while orgasm involves independent superficial and deep sensory nerves.) Physiologic erection occurs in response to the release of nitric oxide from nonadrenergic-noncholinergic nerves (see Chapter 6) associated with parasympathetic discharge. Thus, parasympathetic motor innervation must be intact and nitric oxide synthesis must be active. (A similar process occurs in female erectile tissues.) Certain other smooth muscle relaxants—eg, PGE_1 analogs or α-adrenoceptor antagonists—if present in high enough concentration, can independently cause sufficient cavernosal relaxation to result in erection. As noted in the text, nitric oxide activates guanylyl cyclase, which increases the concentration of cGMP, and the latter second messenger stimulates the dephosphorylation of myosin light chains (see Figure 12–2) and relaxation of the smooth muscle. Thus, any drug that increases cGMP might be of value in erectile dysfunction if normal innervation is present. **Sildenafil** (Viagra) and congeners act to increase cGMP by inhibiting its breakdown by phosphodiesterase isoform 5 (PDE-5). Three similar PDE-5 inhibitors (PDE-5I), **tadalafil, vardenafil,** and **avanafil,** are available. These drugs have been very successful in the marketplace because they can be taken orally. However, they are of little or no value in men with loss of potency due to cord injury or other damage to innervation and in men lacking libido. Furthermore, PDE-5Is potentiate the action of nitrates used for angina, and severe hypotension and a few myocardial infarctions have been reported in men taking a nitrate plus a PDE-5I. It is recommended that at least 6 hours pass between use of a nitrate and the ingestion of PDE-5 inhbitors. PDE-5Is also have effects on color vision, causing difficulty in blue-green discrimination. It is important to be aware that numerous nonprescription mail-order products that contain sildenafil analogs such as hydroxythiohomosildenafil and sulfoaildenafil have been marketed as "male enhancement" agents. These products are not approved by the Food and Drug Administration (FDA) and incur the same risk of dangerous interactions with nitrates as the approved agents.

PDE-5 inhibitors have also been studied for possible use in other conditions. Clinical studies show distinct benefit in some patients with pulmonary arterial hypertension but not in patients with advanced idiopathic pulmonary fibrosis. The drugs have possible benefit in systemic hypertension, cystic fibrosis, and benign prostatic hyperplasia. Both sildenafil and tadalafil are currently approved for pulmonary hypertension. Preclinical studies suggest that sildenafil may be useful in preventing apoptosis and cardiac remodeling after ischemia and reperfusion.

The drug most commonly used for erectile dysfunction in patients who do not respond to PDE-5Is is **alprostadil,** a PGE1 analog (see Chapter 18) that can be injected directly into the cavernosa or placed in the urethra as a minisuppository, from which it diffuses into the cavernosal tissue. Phentolamine can be used by injection into the cavernosa. These drugs will cause erection in most men who do not respond to PDE-5Is.

Toxicity & Tolerance

A. Acute Adverse Effects

The major acute toxicities of organic nitrates are direct extensions of therapeutic vasodilation: orthostatic hypotension, tachycardia, and throbbing headache. Glaucoma, once thought to be a contraindication, does not worsen, and nitrates can be used safely in the presence of increased intraocular pressure. Nitrates are contraindicated, however, if intracranial pressure is elevated. Rarely, transdermal nitroglycerin patches have ignited when external defibrillator electroshock was applied to the chest of patients in ventricular fibrillation. Such patches should be removed before use of external defibrillation to prevent superficial burns.

B. Tolerance

With continuous exposure to nitrates, isolated smooth muscle may develop complete tolerance (tachyphylaxis), and the intact human becomes progressively more tolerant when long-acting preparations (oral, transdermal) or continuous intravenous infusions are used for more than a few hours without interruption. The mechanisms by which tolerance develops are not completely understood. As previously noted, diminished release of nitric oxide resulting from reduced bioactivation may be partly responsible for tolerance to nitroglycerin. Supplementation of cysteine may partially reverse tolerance, suggesting that reduced availability of sulfhydryl donors may play a role. Systemic compensation also plays a role in tolerance in the intact human. Initially, significant sympathetic discharge occurs, and after 1 or more days of therapy with long-acting nitrates, retention of salt and water may partially reverse the favorable hemodynamic changes initially caused by nitroglycerin.

Tolerance does not occur equally with all nitric oxide donors. Nitroprusside, for example, retains activity over long periods. Other organic nitrates appear to be less susceptible than nitroglycerin to the development of tolerance. In cell-free systems, soluble guanylate cyclase is inhibited, possibly by nitrosylation of the enzyme, only after prolonged exposure to exceedingly high nitroglycerin concentrations. In contrast, treatment with antioxidants that protect ALDH2 and similar enzymes appears to prevent or reduce tolerance. This suggests that tolerance is a function of diminished bioactivation of organic nitrates and, to a lesser degree, a loss of soluble guanylate cyclase responsiveness to nitric oxide.

Continuous exposure to high levels of nitrates can occur in the chemical industry, especially where explosives are manufactured. When contamination of the workplace with volatile organic nitrate compounds is severe, workers find that upon starting their work week (Monday), they suffer headache and transient dizziness **(Monday disease).** After a day or so, these symptoms disappear owing to the development of tolerance. Over the weekend, when exposure to the chemicals is eliminated, tolerance disappears, so symptoms recur each Monday. Other hazards of industrial exposure, including dependence, have been reported. There is no evidence that physical dependence develops as a result of the *therapeutic* use of short-acting nitrates for angina, even in large doses.

C. Carcinogenicity of Nitrate and Nitrite Derivatives

Nitrosamines are small molecules with the structure R_2–N–NO formed from the combination of nitrates and nitrites with amines. Some nitrosamines are powerful carcinogens in animals, apparently through conversion to reactive derivatives. Although there is no direct proof that these agents cause cancer in humans, there is a strong epidemiologic correlation between the incidence of esophageal and gastric carcinoma and the nitrate content of food in certain cultures. Nitrosamines are also found in tobacco and in cigarette smoke. There is no evidence that the small doses of nitrates used in the treatment of angina result in significant body levels of nitrosamines.

Mechanisms of Clinical Effect

The beneficial and deleterious effects of nitrate-induced vasodilation are summarized in Table 12–2.

A. Nitrate Effects in Angina of Effort

Decreased venous return to the heart and the resulting reduction of intracardiac volume are important beneficial hemodynamic effects of nitrates. Arterial pressure also decreases. Decreased intraventricular pressure and left ventricular volume are associated with decreased wall tension (Laplace relation) and decreased myocardial oxygen requirement. In rare instances, a paradoxical *increase* in myocardial oxygen demand may occur as a result of excessive reflex tachycardia and increased contractility.

Intracoronary, intravenous, or sublingual nitrate administration consistently increases the caliber of the large epicardial coronary arteries except where blocked by concentric atheromas. Coronary arteriolar resistance tends to decrease, though to a lesser extent. However, nitrates administered by the usual systemic routes may *decrease* overall coronary blood flow (and myocardial oxygen consumption) if cardiac output is reduced due to decreased venous return.

TABLE 12–2 Beneficial and deleterious effects of nitrates in the treatment of angina.

Effect	Mechanism and Result
Potential beneficial effects	
Decreased ventricular volume Decreased arterial pressure Decreased ejection time	Decreased work and myocardial oxygen requirement
Vasodilation of epicardial coronary arteries	Relief of coronary artery spasm
Increased collateral flow	Improved perfusion of ischemic myocardium
Decreased left ventricular diastolic pressure	Improved subendocardial perfusion
Potential deleterious effects	
Reflex tachycardia	Increased myocardial oxygen requirement; decreased diastolic perfusion time and coronary perfusion
Reflex increase in contractility	Increased myocardial oxygen requirement

The reduction in oxygen demand is the major mechanism for the relief of effort angina.

B. Nitrate Effects in Variant Angina

Nitrates benefit patients with variant angina by relaxing the smooth muscle of the epicardial coronary arteries and relieving coronary artery spasm.

C. Nitrate Effects in Acute Coronary Syndromes

Nitrates are also useful in the treatment of the acute coronary syndrome of unstable angina, but the precise mechanism for their beneficial effects is not clear. Because both increased coronary vascular tone and increased myocardial oxygen demand can precipitate rest angina in these patients, nitrates may exert their beneficial effects both by dilating the epicardial coronary arteries and by simultaneously reducing myocardial oxygen demand. As previously noted, nitroglycerin also decreases platelet aggregation, and this effect may be important in acute coronary syndrome.

Clinical Use of Nitrates

Some of the forms of nitroglycerin and its congeners and their doses are listed in Table 12–3. Because of its rapid onset of action (1–3 minutes), sublingual nitroglycerin is the most frequently used agent for the immediate treatment of angina. Because its duration of action is short (not exceeding 20–30 minutes), it is not suitable for maintenance therapy. The onset of action of intravenous nitroglycerin is also rapid (minutes), but its hemodynamic effects are quickly reversed when the infusion is stopped. Clinical use of intravenous nitroglycerin is therefore restricted to the treatment of severe, recurrent rest angina. Slowly absorbed preparations of nitroglycerin include a buccal form, oral preparations, and several transdermal forms. These formulations have been shown to provide blood concentrations for long periods but, as noted above, this may lead to the development of tolerance.

The hemodynamic effects of sublingual or chewable isosorbide dinitrate and the oral organic nitrates are similar to those of nitroglycerin given by the same routes. Although transdermal administration may provide blood levels of nitroglycerin for 24 hours or more, the beneficial hemodynamic effects usually do not persist for more than 8–10 hours. The clinical efficacy of slow-release forms of nitroglycerin in maintenance therapy of angina is thus limited by the development of tolerance. Therefore, a nitrate-free period of at least 8 hours between doses of long-acting and slow-release forms should be observed to prevent tolerance.

TABLE 12–3 Nitrate and nitrite drugs used in the treatment of angina.

Drug	Dose	Duration of Action
Short-acting		
Nitroglycerin, sublingual	0.15–1.2 mg	10–30 minutes
Isosorbide dinitrate, sublingual	2.5–5 mg	10–60 minutes
Amyl nitrite, inhalant (obsolete)	0.18–0.3 mL	3–5 minutes
Long-acting		
Nitroglycerin, oral sustained-action	6.5–13 mg per 6–8 hours	6–8 hours
Nitroglycerin, 2% ointment, transdermal	1–1.5 inches per 4 hours	3–6 hours
Nitroglycerin, slow-release, buccal	1–2 mg per 4 hours	3–6 hours
Nitroglycerin, slow-release patch, transdermal	10–25 mg per 24 hours (one patch per day)	8–10 hours
Isosorbide dinitrate, sublingual	2.5–10 mg per 2 hours	1.5–2 hours
Isosorbide dinitrate, oral	10–60 mg per 4–6 hours	4–6 hours
Isosorbide dinitrate, chewable oral	5–10 mg per 2–4 hours	2–3 hours
Isosorbide mononitrate, oral	20 mg per 12 hours	6–10 hours
Pentaerythritol tetranitrate (PETN)	50 mg per 12 hours	10–12 hours

OTHER NITRO-VASODILATORS

Nicorandil is a nicotinamide nitrate ester that has vasodilating properties in normal coronary arteries but more complex effects in patients with angina. Studies in isolated myocytes indicate that the drug activates an Na^+/Ca^{2+} exchanger and reduces intracellular Ca^{2+} overload. Clinical studies suggest that it reduces both preload and afterload. It also provides some myocardial protection via preconditioning by activation of cardiac K_{ATP} channels. One large trial showed a significant reduction in relative risk of fatal and nonfatal coronary events in patients receiving the drug. Nicorandil is currently approved for use in the treatment of angina in Europe and Japan but has not been approved in the USA. **Molsidomine** is a prodrug that is converted to a nitric oxide–releasing metabolite. It is said to have efficacy comparable to that of the organic nitrates and is not subject to tolerance. Recent studies suggest that it may reduce cerebral vasospasm in stroke.

CALCIUM CHANNEL-BLOCKING DRUGS

It has been known since the late 1800s that transmembrane calcium influx is necessary for the contraction of smooth and cardiac muscle. The discovery of a calcium channel in cardiac muscle was followed by the finding of several different types of calcium channels in different tissues (Table 12–4). The discovery of these channels made possible the measurement of the transmembrane calcium current, I_{Ca}, and subsequently, the development of clinically useful blocking drugs. Although the blockers currently available for clinical use in cardiovascular conditions are exclusively L-type calcium channel blockers, selective blockers of other types of calcium channels are under investigation. Certain antiseizure drugs are thought to act, at least in part,

TABLE 12–4 Properties of several voltage-activated calcium channels.

Type	Channel Name	Where Found	Properties of the Calcium Current	Blocked By
L	$Ca_V1.1–Ca_V1.4$	Cardiac, skeletal, smooth muscle, neurons ($Ca_V1.4$ is found in retina), endocrine cells, bone	Long, large, high threshold	Verapamil, DHPs, Cd^{2+}, ω-aga-IIIA
T	$Ca_V3.1–Ca_V3.3$	Heart, neurons	Short, small, low threshold	sFTX, flunarizine, Ni^{2+} ($Ca_V3.2$ only), mibefradil[1]
N	$Ca_V2.2$	Neurons, sperm[2]	Short, high threshold	Ziconotide,[3] gabapentin,[4] ω-CTXGVIA, ω-aga-IIIA, Cd^{2+}
P/Q	$Ca_V2.1$	Neurons	Long, high threshold	ω-CTX-MVIIC, ω-aga-IVA
R	$Ca_V2.3$	Neurons, sperm[2]	Pacemaking	SNX-482, ω-aga-IIIA

[1]Antianginal drug withdrawn from market.

[2]Channel types associated with sperm flagellar activity may be of the Catsper 1–4 variety.

[3]Synthetic snail peptide analgesic (see Chapter 31).

[4]Antiseizure agent (see Chapter 24).

DHPs, dihydropyridines (eg, nifedipine); sFTX, synthetic funnel web spider toxin; ω-CTX, conotoxins extracted from several marine snails of the genus *Conus*; ω-aga-IIIA and ω-aga-IVA, toxins of the funnel web spider, *Agelenopsis aperta*; SNX-482, a toxin of the African tarantula, *Hysterocrates gigas*.

through calcium channel (especially T-type) blockade in neurons (see Chapter 24).

Chemistry & Pharmacokinetics

Verapamil, the first clinically useful member of this group, was the result of attempts to synthesize more active analogs of papaverine, a vasodilator alkaloid found in the opium poppy. Since then, dozens of agents of varying structure have been found to have the same pharmacologic action (Table 12–5). Three chemically dissimilar calcium channel blockers are shown in Figure 12–4. Nifedipine is the prototype of the dihydropyridine family of calcium channel blockers; dozens of molecules in this family have been investigated, and several are currently approved in the USA for angina, hypertension, and other indications.

The calcium channel blockers are orally active agents and are characterized by high first-pass effect, high plasma protein binding, and extensive metabolism. Verapamil and diltiazem are also used by the intravenous route.

Pharmacodynamics

A. Mechanism of Action

The *voltage-gated* L type is the dominant type of calcium channel in cardiac and smooth muscle and is known to contain several drug receptors. It consists of α1 (the larger, pore-forming subunit), α2, β, γ, and δ subunits. Four variant α1 subunits have been recognized. Nifedipine and other dihydropyridines have been demonstrated to bind to one site on the α1 subunit, whereas verapamil and diltiazem appear to bind to closely related but not identical

TABLE 12–5 Clinical pharmacology of some calcium channel–blocking drugs.

Drug	Oral Bioavailability (%)	Half-Life (hours)	Indication	Dosage
Dihydropyridines				
Amlodipine	65–90	30–50	Angina, hypertension	5–10 mg orally once daily
Felodipine	15–20	11–16	Hypertension, Raynaud phenomenon	5–10 mg orally once daily
Isradipine	15–25	8	Hypertension	2.5–10 mg orally twice daily
Nicardipine	35	2–4	Angina, hypertension	20–40 mg orally every 8 hours
Nifedipine	45–70	4	Angina, hypertension, Raynaud phenomenon	3–10 mcg/kg IV; 20–40 mg orally every 8 hours
Nisoldipine	<10	6–12	Hypertension	20–40 mg orally once daily
Nitrendipine	10–30	5–12	Investigational	20 mg orally once or twice daily
Miscellaneous				
Diltiazem	40–65	3–4	Angina, hypertension, Raynaud phenomenon	75–150 mcg/kg IV; 30–80 mg orally every 6 hours
Verapamil	20–35	6	Angina, hypertension, arrhythmias, migraine	75–150 mcg/kg IV; 80–160 mg orally every 8 hours

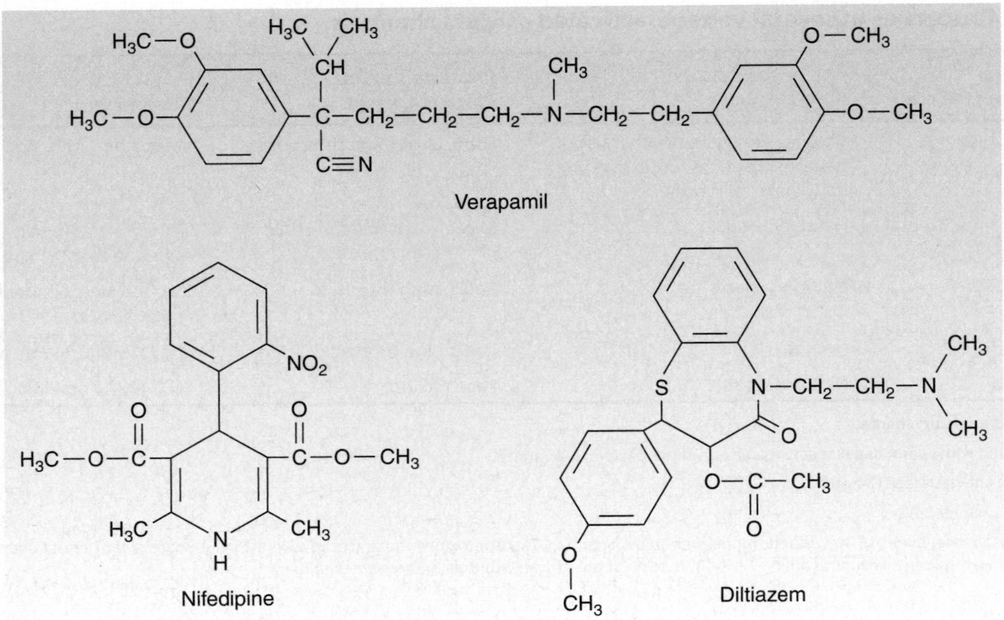

FIGURE 12–4 Chemical structures of several calcium channel-blocking drugs.

receptors in another region of the same subunit. Binding of a drug to the verapamil or diltiazem receptors allosterically affects dihydropyridine binding. These receptor regions are stereoselective, since marked differences in both stereoisomer-binding affinity and pharmacologic potency are observed for enantiomers of verapamil, diltiazem, and optically active nifedipine congeners.

Blockade of calcium channels by these drugs resembles that of sodium channel blockade by local anesthetics (see Chapters 14 and 26). The drugs act from the inner side of the membrane and bind more effectively to open channels and inactivated channels. Binding of the drug reduces the frequency of opening in response to depolarization. The result is a marked decrease in transmembrane calcium current, which in smooth muscle results in long-lasting relaxation (see Figure 12–3) and in cardiac muscle results in reduction in contractility throughout the heart and decreases in sinus node pacemaker rate and atrioventricular node conduction velocity.* Although some neuronal cells harbor L-type calcium channels, their sensitivity to these drugs is lower because the channels in these cells spend less time in the open and inactivated states.

Smooth muscle responses to calcium influx through *ligand-gated* calcium channels are also reduced by these drugs but not as markedly. The block can be partially reversed by elevating the concentration of calcium, although the levels of calcium required are not easily attainable in patients. Block can also be partially reversed by the use of drugs that increase the transmembrane flux of calcium, such as sympathomimetics.

Other types of calcium channels are less sensitive to blockade by these calcium channel blockers (see Table 12–4). Therefore, tissues in which these other channel types play a major role—neurons and most secretory glands—are much less affected by these drugs than are cardiac and smooth muscle. **Mibefradil** is a selective T-type calcium channel blocker that was introduced for antiarrhythmic use but has been withdrawn. Ion channels other than calcium channels are much less sensitive to these drugs. Potassium channels in vascular smooth muscle are inhibited by verapamil, thus limiting the vasodilation produced by this drug. Sodium channels as well as calcium channels are blocked by **bepridil,** an obsolete antiarrhythmic drug.

B. Organ System Effects

1. Smooth muscle—Most types of smooth muscle are dependent on transmembrane calcium influx for normal resting tone and contractile responses. These cells are relaxed by the calcium channel blockers (see Figure 12–3). Vascular smooth muscle appears to be the most sensitive, but similar relaxation can be shown for bronchiolar, gastrointestinal, and uterine smooth muscle. In the vascular system, arterioles appear to be more sensitive than veins; orthostatic hypotension is not a common adverse effect. Blood pressure is reduced with all calcium channel blockers (see Chapter 11). Women may be more sensitive than men to the hypotensive action of diltiazem. The reduction in peripheral vascular resistance is one mechanism by which these agents may benefit the patient with angina of effort. Reduction of coronary artery spasm has been demonstrated in patients with variant angina.

Important differences in vascular selectivity exist among the calcium channel blockers. In general, the dihydropyridines have a greater ratio of vascular smooth muscle effects relative to cardiac effects than do diltiazem and verapamil. The relatively smaller effect of verapamil on vasodilation may be the result of simultaneous blockade of vascular smooth muscle potassium channels described earlier. Furthermore, the dihydropyridines may differ in

*At very low doses and under certain circumstances, some dihydropyridines *increase* calcium influx. Some special dihydropyridines, eg, Bay K 8644, actually increase calcium influx over most of their dose range.

their potency in different vascular beds. For example, **nimodipine** is claimed to be particularly selective for cerebral blood vessels. Splice variants in the structure of the $\alpha 1$ channel subunit appear to account for these differences.

2. Cardiac muscle—Cardiac muscle is highly dependent on calcium influx during each action potential for normal function. Impulse generation in the sinoatrial node and conduction in the atrioventricular node—so-called slow-response, or calcium-dependent, action potentials—may be reduced or blocked by all of the calcium channel blockers. Excitation-contraction coupling in all cardiac cells requires calcium influx, so these drugs reduce cardiac contractility in a dose-dependent fashion. In some cases, cardiac output may also decrease. This reduction in cardiac mechanical function is another mechanism by which the calcium channel blockers can reduce the oxygen requirement in patients with angina.

Important differences between the available calcium channel blockers arise from the details of their interactions with cardiac ion channels and, as noted above, differences in their relative smooth muscle versus cardiac effects. Sodium channel block is modest with verapamil, and still less marked with diltiazem. It is negligible with nifedipine and other dihydropyridines. Verapamil and diltiazem interact kinetically with the calcium channel receptor in a different manner than the dihydropyridines; they block tachycardias in calcium-dependent cells, eg, the atrioventricular node, more selectively than do the dihydropyridines. (See Chapter 14 for additional details.) On the other hand, the dihydropyridines appear to block smooth muscle calcium channels at concentrations below those required for significant cardiac effects; they are therefore less depressant on the heart than verapamil or diltiazem.

3. Skeletal muscle—Skeletal muscle is not depressed by the calcium channel blockers because it uses intracellular pools of calcium to support excitation-contraction coupling and does not require as much transmembrane calcium influx.

4. Cerebral vasospasm and infarct following subarachnoid hemorrhage—**Nimodipine,** a member of the dihydropyridine group of calcium channel blockers, has a high affinity for cerebral blood vessels and appears to reduce morbidity after a subarachnoid hemorrhage. Nimodipine was approved for use in patients who have had a hemorrhagic stroke, but it has been withdrawn. **Nicardipine** has similar effects and is used by intravenous and intracerebral arterial infusion to prevent cerebral vasospasm associated with stroke. Verapamil, despite its lack of vasoselectivity, is also used—by the intra-arterial route—in stroke. Some evidence suggests that calcium channel blockers may also reduce cerebral damage after thromboembolic stroke.

5. Other effects—Calcium channel blockers minimally interfere with stimulus-secretion coupling in glands and nerve endings because of differences between calcium channel type and sensitivity in different tissues. Verapamil has been shown to inhibit insulin release in humans, but the dosages required are greater than those used in management of angina and other cardiovascular conditions.

A significant body of evidence suggests that the calcium channel blockers may interfere with platelet aggregation in vitro and prevent or attenuate the development of atheromatous lesions in animals. However, clinical studies have not established their role in human blood clotting and atherosclerosis.

Verapamil has been shown to block the P-glycoprotein responsible for the transport of many foreign drugs out of cancer (and other) cells (see Chapter 1); other calcium channel blockers appear to have a similar effect. This action is not stereoselective. Verapamil has been shown to partially reverse the resistance of cancer cells to many chemotherapeutic drugs in vitro. Some clinical results suggest similar effects in patients (see Chapter 54). Animal research suggests possible future roles of calcium blockers in the treatment of osteoporosis, fertility disorders and male contraception, immune modulation, and even schistosomiasis. Verapamil does not appear to block transmembrane divalent metal ion transporters such as DMT1.

Toxicity

The most important toxic effects reported for calcium channel blockers are direct extensions of their therapeutic action. Excessive inhibition of calcium influx can cause serious cardiac depression, including bradycardia, atrioventricular block, cardiac arrest, and heart failure. These effects have been rare in clinical use.

Retrospective case-control studies reported that prompt-release nifedipine increased the risk of myocardial infarction in patients with hypertension. Slow-release and long-acting dihydropyridine calcium channel blockers are usually well tolerated. However, dihydropyridines, compared with angiotensin-converting enzyme (ACE) inhibitors, have been reported to increase the risk of adverse cardiac events in patients with hypertension with or without diabetes. These results suggest that relatively short-acting calcium channel blockers such as prompt-release nifedipine have the potential to enhance the risk of adverse cardiac events and should be avoided. Patients receiving β-blocking drugs are more sensitive to the cardiodepressant effects of calcium channel blockers. Minor toxicities (troublesome but not usually requiring discontinuance of therapy) include flushing, dizziness, nausea, constipation, and peripheral edema. Constipation is particularly common with verapamil.

Mechanisms of Clinical Effects

Calcium channel blockers decrease myocardial contractile force, which reduces myocardial oxygen requirements. Calcium channel block in arterial smooth muscle decreases arterial and intraventricular pressure. Some of these drugs (eg, verapamil, diltiazem) also possess a nonspecific antiadrenergic effect, which may contribute to peripheral vasodilation. As a result of all of these effects, left ventricular wall stress declines, which reduces myocardial oxygen requirements. Decreased heart rate with the use of verapamil or diltiazem causes a further decrease in myocardial oxygen demand. Calcium channel-blocking agents also relieve and prevent focal coronary artery spasm in variant angina. Use of these agents has thus emerged as the most effective prophylactic treatment for this form of angina pectoris.

Sinoatrial and atrioventricular nodal tissues, which are mainly composed of calcium-dependent, slow-response cells, are affected markedly by verapamil, moderately by diltiazem, and much less by dihydropyridines. Thus, verapamil and diltiazem decrease atrioventricular nodal conduction and are often effective in the management of supraventricular reentry tachycardia and in decreasing ventricular rate in atrial fibrillation or flutter. Nifedipine does not affect atrioventricular conduction. Nonspecific sympathetic antagonism is most marked with diltiazem and much less with verapamil. Nifedipine does not appear to have this effect, probably because reflex tachycardia in response to hypotension occurs most frequently with nifedipine and much less so with diltiazem and verapamil. These differences in pharmacologic effects should be considered in selecting calcium channel-blocking agents for the management of angina.

Special Coronary Vasodilators

Many vasodilators can be shown to increase coronary flow in the absence of atherosclerotic disease. These include **dipyridamole** and **adenosine.** In fact, dipyridamole is an extremely effective coronary dilator, but it is not effective in angina because of coronary steal (see below). Adenosine, the naturally occurring nucleoside, acts on specific membrane-bound receptors, including at least four subtypes (A_1, A_{2A}, A_{2B}, and A_3). Adenosine, acting on A_{2A} receptors, causes a very brief but marked dilation of the coronary resistance vessels and has been used as a drug to measure maximum coronary flow **(fractional flow reserve, FFR)** in patients with coronary disease. The drug also markedly slows or blocks atrioventricular (AV) conduction in the heart and is used to convert AV nodal tachycardias to normal sinus rhythm (see Chapter 14). **Regadenoson** is a selective A_{2A} agonist and has been developed for use in stress testing in suspected coronary artery disease and for imaging the coronary circulation. It appears to have a better benefit-to-risk ratio than adenosine in these applications. Similar A_{2A} agonists (binodenoson, apadenoson) are investigational. Adenosine receptor ligands are also under investigation for anti-inflammatory and antinociceptive and other neurological applications.

Coronary steal is the term given to the action of nonselective coronary arteriolar dilators in patients with partial obstruction of a portion of the coronary vasculature. It results from the fact that in the absence of drugs, arterioles in ischemic areas of the myocardium are usually maximally dilated as a result of local control factors, whereas the resistance vessels in well-perfused regions are capable of further dilation in response to exercise. If a potent arteriolar dilator is administered, only the vessels in the well-perfused regions are capable of further dilation, so more flow is diverted ("stolen") from the ischemic region into the normal region. Dipyridamole, which acts in part by inhibiting adenosine uptake, typically produces this effect in patients with angina. In patients with unstable angina, transient coronary steal may precipitate a myocardial infarction. Adenosine and regadenoson are labeled with warnings of this effect.

Clinical Uses of Calcium Channel-Blocking Drugs

In addition to angina, calcium channel blockers have well-documented efficacy in hypertension (see Chapter 11) and supraventricular tachyarrhythmias (see Chapter 14). They also show moderate efficacy in a variety of other conditions, including hypertrophic cardiomyopathy, migraine, and Raynaud phenomenon. Nifedipine has some efficacy in preterm labor but is more toxic and not as effective as **atosiban,** an investigational oxytocin antagonist (see Chapter 37).

The pharmacokinetic properties of these drugs are set forth in Table 12–5. The choice of a particular calcium channel-blocking agent should be made with knowledge of its specific potential adverse effects as well as its pharmacologic properties. Nifedipine does not decrease atrioventricular conduction and therefore can be used more safely than verapamil or diltiazem in the presence of atrioventricular conduction abnormalities. A combination of verapamil or diltiazem with β blockers may produce atrioventricular block and depression of ventricular function. In the presence of overt heart failure, all calcium channel blockers can cause further worsening of failure as a result of their negative inotropic effect. **Amlodipine,** however, does not increase mortality in patients with heart failure due to nonischemic left ventricular systolic dysfunction and can be used safely in these patients.

In patients with relatively low blood pressure, dihydropyridines can cause further deleterious lowering of pressure. Verapamil and diltiazem appear to produce less hypotension and may be better tolerated in these circumstances. In patients with a history of atrial tachycardia, flutter, and fibrillation, verapamil and diltiazem provide a distinct advantage because of their antiarrhythmic effects. In patients receiving digitalis, verapamil should be used with caution, because it may increase digoxin blood levels through a pharmacokinetic interaction. Although increases in digoxin blood level have also been demonstrated with diltiazem and nifedipine, such interactions are less consistent than with verapamil.

In patients with unstable angina, immediate-release short-acting calcium channel blockers can increase the risk of adverse cardiac events and therefore are contraindicated (see Toxicity, above). However, in patients with non–Q-wave myocardial infarction, diltiazem can decrease the frequency of postinfarction angina and may be used.

BETA-BLOCKING DRUGS

Although they are not vasodilators (with the exception of carvedilol and nebivolol), β-blocking drugs (see Chapter 10) are extremely useful in the management of effort angina and are considered the prophylactic treatment of choice in chronic effort angina. The beneficial effects of β-blocking agents are related to their hemodynamic effects—decreased heart rate, blood pressure, and contractility—which decrease myocardial oxygen requirements at rest and during exercise. Lower heart rate is also associated with an increase in diastolic perfusion time that may increase coronary perfusion. However, reduction of heart rate and blood pressure, and consequently decreased myocardial oxygen consumption, appear to be the most important mechanisms for relief of angina and improved exercise tolerance. Beta blockers may also be valuable in treating silent or ambulatory ischemia. Because this condition causes no pain, it is usually detected by the appearance of typical electrocardiographic signs of ischemia. The total amount of "ischemic time" per day is reduced by long-term therapy with a β blocker. Beta-blocking agents decrease mortality of patients with heart failure or recent myocardial infarction and improve survival and prevent stroke in patients with hypertension. Randomized trials in patients with stable angina have shown better outcome and symptomatic improvement with β blockers compared with calcium channel blockers.

Undesirable effects of β-blocking agents in angina include an increase in end-diastolic volume and an increase in ejection time, both of which tend to increase myocardial oxygen requirement. These deleterious effects of β-blocking agents can be balanced by the concomitant use of nitrates as described below.

Contraindications to the use of β blockers are asthma and other bronchospastic conditions, severe bradycardia, atrioventricular blockade, bradycardia-tachycardia syndrome, and severe unstable left ventricular failure. Potential complications include fatigue, impaired exercise tolerance, insomnia, unpleasant dreams, worsening of claudication, and erectile dysfunction.

NEWER ANTIANGINAL DRUGS

Because of the high prevalence of angina, new drugs are actively sought for its treatment. Some of the drugs or drug groups currently under investigation are listed in Table 12–6.

TABLE 12–6 New drugs or drug groups under investigation for use in angina.

Amiloride
Capsaicin
Direct bradycardic agents, eg, ivabradine
Inhibitors of slowly inactivating sodium current, eg, ranolazine
Metabolic modulators, eg, trimetazidine
Nitric oxide donors, eg, L-arginine
Potassium channel activators, eg, nicorandil
Protein kinase G facilitators, eg, detanonoate
Rho-kinase inhibitors, eg, fasudil
Sulfonylureas, eg, glibenclamide
Thiazolidinediones
Vasopeptidase inhibitors
Xanthine oxidase inhibitors, eg, allopurinol

Ranolazine appears to act by reducing a late sodium current (INa) that facilitates calcium entry via the sodium-calcium exchanger (see Chapter 13). The reduction in intracellular calcium concentration that results from ranolazine reduces diastolic tension, cardiac contractility, and work. Ranolazine is approved for use in angina in the USA. Several studies demonstrate its effectiveness in stable angina, but its ability to reduce the incidence of death in acute coronary syndromes is unclear. Ranolazine prolongs the QT interval in patients with coronary artery disease (but shortens it in patients with long QT syndrome, LQT3). It has not been associated with torsades de pointes arrhythmia and may inhibit the metabolism of digoxin and simvastatin.

Certain metabolic modulators (eg, **trimetazidine**) are known as **pFOX inhibitors** because they partially inhibit the fatty acid oxidation pathway in myocardium. Because metabolism shifts to oxidation of fatty acids in ischemic myocardium, the oxygen requirement per unit of ATP produced increases. Partial inhibition of the enzyme required for fatty acid oxidation (long-chain 3-ketoacyl thiolase, LC-3KAT) appears to improve the metabolic status of ischemic tissue. (Ranolazine was initially assigned to this group of agents, but it lacks this action at clinically relevant concentrations.) Trimetazidine does inhibit LC-3KAT at achievable concentrations and has demonstrated efficacy in stable angina. However, it is not approved for use in the USA.

Perhexiline was found to benefit some patients with angina decades ago but was abandoned because of reports of hepatotoxicity and peripheral neuropathy. However, pharmacokinetic studies suggested that toxicity was due to variable clearance of the drug, with extremely high plasma concentrations in patients with deficient CYP2D6 activity. This drug may shift myocardial metabolism from fatty acid oxidation to more efficient glucose oxidation (like trimetazidine). Because it does not involve vasodilation, it may be useful in patients refractory to ordinary medical therapy if plasma concentration is carefully controlled. Perhexiline is currently approved in only a few countries (not the USA).

So-called *bradycardic* drugs, relatively selective I_f sodium channel blockers (eg, **ivabradine**), reduce cardiac rate by inhibiting the hyperpolarization-activated sodium channel in the sinoatrial node. No other significant hemodynamic effects have been reported. Ivabradine appears to reduce anginal attacks with an efficacy similar to that of calcium channel blockers and β blockers. The lack of effect on gastrointestinal and bronchial smooth muscle is an advantage of ivabradine, and it is approved for use in angina and heart failure outside the USA. In the USA, it is approved for heart failure and is used off-label for angina in combination with β blockers.

The Rho kinases (ROCK) comprise a family of enzymes that inhibit vascular relaxation and diverse functions of several other cell types. Excessive activity of these enzymes has been implicated in coronary spasm, pulmonary hypertension, apoptosis, and other conditions. Drugs targeting the enzyme have therefore been sought for possible clinical applications. **Fasudil** is an inhibitor of smooth muscle Rho kinase and reduces coronary vasospasm in experimental animals. In clinical trials in patients with CAD, it has improved performance in stress tests. It is investigational in angina in the USA and Europe.

Allopurinol represents another type of metabolic modifier. Allopurinol inhibits xanthine oxidase (see Chapter 36), an enzyme that contributes to oxidative stress and endothelial dysfunction in addition to reducing uric acid synthesis, its mechanism of action in gout. Studies suggest that high-dose allopurinol (eg, 600 mg/d) prolongs exercise time in patients with atherosclerotic angina. The mechanism is uncertain, but the drug appears to improve endothelium-dependent vasodilation. Allopurinol is not currently approved for use in angina.

■ CLINICAL PHARMACOLOGY OF DRUGS USED TO TREAT ANGINA

Therapy of coronary artery disease (CAD) is important because angina and other manifestations of CAD severely impact quality of life and even life itself. Several grading systems have been devised to rate the severity of disease based on the limitation of the patient's physical activity and to guide therapy (see Goldman reference). Treatment includes both medical and surgical methods. Refractory angina and acute coronary syndromes are best treated with physical revascularization, ie, percutaneous coronary intervention (PCI), with insertion of stents, or coronary artery bypass grafting (CABG). The standard of care for acute coronary syndrome (ACS) is urgent stenting. However, *prevention* of ACS and treatment of chronic angina can be accomplished in many patients with pharmacologic therapy.

Because the most common cause of angina is atherosclerotic disease of the coronaries, therapy must address the underlying causes of CAD as well as the immediate symptoms of angina. In addition to reducing the need for antianginal therapy, such primary management has been shown to reduce major cardiac events such as myocardial infarction.

First-line therapy of CAD depends on modification of risk factors such as hypertension (see Chapter 11), hyperlipidemia (see Chapter 35), obesity, smoking, and clinical depression. In addition, antiplatelet drugs (see Chapter 34) are very important.

Specific pharmacologic therapy to prevent myocardial infarction and death consists of antiplatelet agents (aspirin, ADP receptor blockers, Chapter 34) and lipid-lowering agents, especially statins (Chapter 35). Aggressive therapy with statins has been shown to reduce the incidence and severity of ischemia in patients during exercise testing and the incidence of cardiac events (including infarction and death) in clinical trials. ACE inhibitors also reduce the risk of adverse cardiac events in patients at high risk for CAD. In patients with unstable angina and non-ST-segment elevation myocardial infarction, aggressive therapy consisting of coronary stenting, antilipid drugs, heparin, and antiplatelet agents is recommended.

The treatment of established angina and other manifestations of myocardial ischemia includes the corrective measures just described as well as treatment to prevent or relieve symptoms. Treatment of symptoms is based on reduction of myocardial oxygen demand and increase of coronary blood flow to the potentially ischemic myocardium to restore the balance between myocardial oxygen supply and demand.

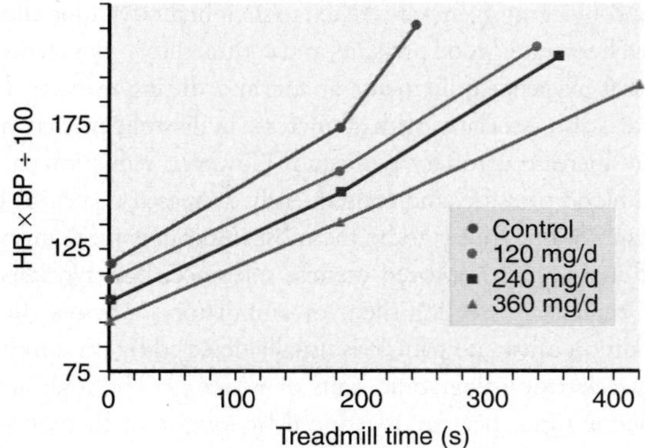

FIGURE 12–5 Effects of diltiazem on the double product (heart rate × systolic blood pressure) in a group of 20 patients with angina of effort. In a double-blind study using a standard protocol, patients were tested on a treadmill during treatment with placebo and three doses of the drug. Heart rate (HR) and systolic blood pressure (BP) were recorded at 180 seconds of exercise (midpoints of lines) and at the time of onset of anginal symptoms (rightmost points). Note that the drug treatment decreased the double product at the midpoint during exercise and prolonged the time to appearance of symptoms. (Data from Lindenberg BS, Weiner DA, McCabe CH, et al: Efficacy and safety of incremental doses of diltiazem for the treatment of stable angina pectoris. J Am Coll Cardiol 1983 Dec;2(6):1129-1133.)

Angina of Effort

Many studies have demonstrated that β blockers, nitrates, and calcium channel blockers increase time to onset of angina and ST depression during treadmill tests in patients with angina of effort (Figure 12–5). Although exercise tolerance increases, there is usually no change in the angina threshold, ie, the heart rate times blood pressure product at which symptoms occur.

For maintenance therapy of chronic stable angina, β blockers, calcium channel-blocking agents, or long-acting nitrates may be chosen; the drug of choice depends on the individual patient's response. In hypertensive patients, monotherapy with either slow-release or long-acting calcium channel blockers or β blockers may be adequate. In normotensive patients, long-acting nitrates may be suitable. The combination of a β blocker with a calcium channel blocker (eg, propranolol with nifedipine) or two different calcium channel blockers (eg, nifedipine and verapamil) has been shown to be more effective than individual drugs used alone. If a dihydropyridine is used, a longer-acting agent should be chosen (amlodipine or felodipine). If response to a single drug is inadequate, a drug from a different class should be added to maximize the beneficial reduction of cardiac work while minimizing undesirable effects (Table 12–7). Some patients may require

TABLE 12–7 Effects of nitrates alone and with β blockers or calcium channel blockers in angina pectoris.

	Nitrates Alone	Beta Blockers or Calcium Channel Blockers Alone	Combined Nitrates with Beta Blockers or Calcium Channel Blockers
Heart rate	*Reflex[1] increase*	Decrease	Decrease
Arterial pressure	Decrease	Decrease	Decrease
End-diastolic volume	Decrease	*Increase*	None or decrease
Contractility	*Reflex[1] increase*	Decrease	None
Ejection time	Decrease[1]	*Increase*	None

[1]Baroreceptor reflex.

Note: Undesirable effects are shown in italics.

therapy with all three drug groups. Addition of an ACE inhibitor may improve control of angina attacks. Ranolazine or ivabradine (off-label), combined with β blockers, may be effective in some patients refractory to traditional drugs. Most experts recommend coronary angiography and revascularization (if not contraindicated) in patients with stable chronic angina refractory to three-drug medical treatment. In the future, agents such as allopurinol or perhexiline may be useful in patients who are not candidates for revascularization.

Vasospastic Angina

Nitrates and the calcium channel blockers, but not β blockers, are effective drugs for relieving and preventing ischemic episodes in patients with variant angina. In approximately 70% of patients treated with nitrates plus calcium channel blockers, angina attacks are completely abolished; in another 20%, marked reduction of frequency of anginal episodes is observed. Prevention of coronary artery spasm (with or without fixed atherosclerotic coronary artery lesions) is the principal mechanism for this beneficial response. All presently available calcium channel blockers appear to be equally effective, and the choice of a particular drug should depend on the patient. Surgical revascularization and angioplasty are not indicated in patients with variant angina.

Unstable Angina & Acute Coronary Syndromes

In patients with unstable angina with recurrent ischemic episodes at rest, recurrent platelet-rich nonocclusive thrombus formation is the principal mechanism. Aggressive antiplatelet therapy with a combination of aspirin and clopidogrel is indicated. Evidence for the addition of intravenous heparin or subcutaneous low-molecular-weight heparin is mixed. If percutaneous coronary intervention with stenting is required (and most patients with ACS are treated with stenting), glycoprotein IIb/IIIa inhibitors such as abciximab should be added. In addition, therapy with nitroglycerin and β blockers should be considered; calcium channel blockers should be added in refractory cases for relief of myocardial ischemia. Primary lipid-lowering and ACE-inhibitor therapy should also be initiated.

TREATMENT OF PERIPHERAL ARTERY DISEASE & INTERMITTENT CLAUDICATION

Atherosclerosis can result in ischemia of peripheral muscles just as coronary artery disease causes cardiac ischemia. If blood flow is limited, pain (claudication) occurs in skeletal muscles, especially in the legs, during exercise and disappears with rest. Although claudication is not immediately life-threatening, peripheral artery disease **(PAD)** is associated with increased mortality, can severely limit exercise tolerance, and may be associated with chronic ischemic ulcers, susceptibility to infection, and the need for amputation.

Intermittent claudication results from obstruction of blood flow by atheromas in large and medium arteries. Insertion of stents in the obstructed vessels is usually indicated and can save a limb that would otherwise require amputation. Supervised exercise therapy is of benefit in reducing claudication and increasing pain-free walking distance. Medical treatment directed at reversal or control of atherosclerosis requires measurement and control of hyperlipidemia (see Chapter 35), hypertension (see Chapter 11), and obesity; cessation of smoking; and control of diabetes, if present. Physical therapy and exercise training are of proven benefit. Conventional vasodilators are of no benefit because vessels distal to the obstructive lesions are usually already dilated at rest. Antiplatelet drugs such as **aspirin** or **clopidogrel** (see Chapter 34) are often used to prevent clotting in the region of plaques and have documented benefit in reducing the risk of myocardial infarction, stroke, and vascular death even though they have little or no effect on claudication. Two drugs are used almost exclusively for PAD. **Cilostazol,** a phosphodiesterase type 3 (PDE3) inhibitor, may have selective antiplatelet and vasodilating effects. This drug has been shown to increase exercise tolerance in patients with severe claudication and is approved for use in PAD. **Naftidrofuryl,** a 5-HT_2 antagonist, is available in the UK and appears to have benefits similar to those of cilostazol. **Pentoxifylline,** a xanthine derivative, is widely promoted for use in this condition but is not recommended. It is thought to act by reducing the viscosity of blood and perhaps increasing the deformability of red blood cells, allowing blood to flow more easily through partially obstructed areas. As noted above, percutaneous angioplasty with stenting may be effective in patients with medically intractable signs and symptoms of lower limb ischemia.

SUMMARY Drugs Used In Angina Pectoris

Subclass, Drug	Mechanism of Action	Effects	Clinical Applications	Pharmacokinetics, Toxicities, Interactions
NITRATES				
• Nitroglycerin	Releases nitric oxide in smooth muscle, which activates guanylyl cyclase and increases cGMP	Smooth muscle relaxation, especially in vessels • other smooth muscle is relaxed but not as markedly • vasodilation decreases venous return and heart size • may increase coronary flow in some areas and in variant angina	Angina: Sublingual form for acute episodes • oral and transdermal forms for prophylaxis • IV form for acute coronary syndrome	High first-pass effect, so sublingual dose is much smaller than oral • high lipid solubility ensures rapid absorption • *Toxicity:* Orthostatic hypotension, tachycardia, headache • *Interactions:* Synergistic hypotension with phosphodiesterase type 5 inhibitors (sildenafil, etc)
• *Isosorbide dinitrate: Very similar to nitroglycerin, slightly longer duration of action; no transdermal form*				
• *Isosorbide mononitrate: Active metabolite of the dinitrate; used orally for prophylaxis*				
BETA BLOCKERS				
• Propranolol	Nonselective competitive antagonist at β adrenoceptors	Decreased heart rate, cardiac output, and blood pressure • decreases myocardial oxygen demand	Prophylaxis of angina • for other applications, see Chapters 10, 11, and 13	Oral and parenteral, 4–6 h duration of action • *Toxicity:* Asthma, atrioventricular block, acute heart failure, sedation • *Interactions:* Additive with all cardiac depressants
• *Atenolol, metoprolol, others: β_1-selective blockers, less risk of bronchospasm, but still significant*				
• *See* Chapters 10 *and* 11 *for other β blockers and their applications*				
CALCIUM CHANNEL BLOCKERS				
• Verapamil, diltiazem	Nonselective block of L-type calcium channels in vessels and heart	Reduced vascular resistance, cardiac rate, and cardiac force results in decreased oxygen demand	Prophylaxis of angina, hypertension, others	Oral, IV, duration 4–8 h • *Toxicity:* Atrioventricular block, acute heart failure; constipation, edema • *Interactions:* Additive with other cardiac depressants and hypotensive drugs
• Nifedipine (a dihydropyridine)	Block of vascular L-type calcium channels > cardiac channels	Like verapamil and diltiazem; less cardiac effect	Prophylaxis of angina and treatment of hypertension but *prompt release* nifedipine is *contraindicated*	Oral, duration 4–6 h • *Toxicity:* Excessive hypotension, baroreceptor reflex tachycardia • *Interactions:* Additive with other vasodilators
• *Amlodipine, felodipine, other dihydropyridines: Like nifedipine but slower onset and longer duration (up to 12 h or more)*				
MISCELLANEOUS				
• Ranolazine	Inhibits late sodium current in heart • also may modify fatty acid oxidation at much higher doses	Reduces cardiac oxygen demand • fatty acid oxidation modification could improve efficiency of cardiac oxygen utilization	Prophylaxis of angina	Oral, duration 6–8 h • *Toxicity:* QT interval prolongation (but no increase of torsades de pointes), nausea, constipation, dizziness • *Interactions:* Inhibitors of CYP3A increase ranolazine concentration and duration of action
• *Ivabradine: Inhibitor of sinoatrial pacemaker; reduction of heart rate reduces oxygen demand*				
• *Trimetazidine, allopurinol, perhexiline, fasudil: See text*				

PREPARATIONS AVAILABLE

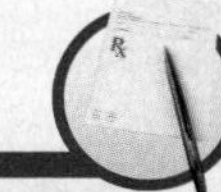

GENERIC NAME	AVAILABLE AS
NITRATES & NITRITES	
Amyl nitrite	Generic
Isosorbide dinitrate (oral, oral sustained release, sublingual)	Generic, Isordil
Isosorbide mononitrate	Ismo, others
Nitroglycerin (sublingual, buccal, oral sustained release, parenteral, transdermal patch, topical ointment)	Generic, others
CALCIUM CHANNEL BLOCKERS	
Amlodipine	Generic, Norvasc, AmVaz
Clevidipine (approved only for use in hypertensive emergencies)	Cleviprex
Diltiazem (oral, oral sustained release, parenteral)	Generic, Cardizem
Felodipine	Generic, Plendil
Isradipine (oral, oral controlled release)	DynaCirc
Nicardipine (oral, oral sustained release, parenteral)	Cardene, others
Nifedipine (oral, oral extended release)	Adalat, Procardia, others
Nisoldipine	Sular
Verapamil (oral, oral sustained release, parenteral)	Generic, Calan, Isoptin
BETA BLOCKERS	
	See Chapter 10
SODIUM CHANNEL BLOCKERS	
Ranolazine	Ranexa
DRUGS FOR ERECTILE DYSFUNCTION	
Avanafil	Stendra
Sildenafil	Viagra, Revatio
Tadalafil	Cialis, Adcirca
Vardenafil	Levitra
DRUGS FOR PERIPHERAL ARTERY DISEASE	
Cilostazol	Generic, Pletal
Pentoxifylline	Generic, Trental

REFERENCES

Bairey Merz CN et al: Ischemia and no obstructive coronary artery disease (INOCA): Developing evidence-based therapies and research agenda for the next decade. Circulation 2017;135:1075.

Bhatt DL et al: Diagnosis and treatment of acute coronary syndromes. A review. JAMA 2022;327:662.

Borer JS: Clinical effect of 'pure' heart rate slowing with a prototype If inhibitor: Placebo-controlled experience with ivabradine. Adv Cardiol 2006;43:54.

Brozovitch FV et al: Mechanisms of vascular smooth muscle contraction and the basis for pharmacologic treatment of smooth muscle disorders. Pharmacol Rev 2016;68:476.

Burashnikov A et al: Ranolazine effectively suppresses atrial fibrillation in the setting of heart failure. Circ Heart Fail 2014;7:627.

Carmichael P, Lieben J: Sudden death in explosives workers. Arch Environ Health 1963;7:50.

Catterall WA, Swanson TM: Structural basis for pharmacology of voltage-gated sodium and calcium channels. Mol Pharmacol 2015;88:141.

Chaitman BR et al: Effects of ranolazine, with atenolol, amlodipine, or diltiazem on exercise tolerance and angina frequency in patients with severe chronic angina: A randomized controlled trial. JAMA 2004;291:309.

Chang C-R, Sallustio B, Horowitz JD: Drugs that affect cardiac metabolism: Focus on perhexiline. Cardiovasc Drugs Ther 2016;30:399.

Chen Z, Zhang J, Stamler JS: Identification of the enzymatic mechanism of nitroglycerin bioactivation. Proc Natl Acad Sci 2002;99:8306.

Cooper-DeHoff RM, Chang S-W, Pepine CJ: Calcium antagonists in the treatment of coronary artery disease. Curr Opin Pharmacol 2013;13:301.

Fearon WF et al: Fractional flow reserve-guided PCI as compared with coronary bypass surgery. N Engl J Med 2022;386:128.

Fihn SD et al: Guideline for the diagnosis and management of patients with stable ischemic heart disease: Executive summary. Circulation 2012;126:3097.

Goldman L et al: Comparative reproducibility and validity of systems for assessing cardiovascular functional class: Advantages of a new specific activity scale. Circulation 1981;64:1227.

Husted SE, Ohman EM: Pharmacological and emerging therapies in the treatment of chronic angina. Lancet 2015;386:691.

Ignarro LJ et al: Mechanism of vascular smooth muscle relaxation by organic nitrates, nitrites, nitroprusside, and nitric oxide: Evidence for the involvement of S-nitrosothiols as active intermediates. J Pharmacol Exp Ther 1981;218:739.

Joshi PH, de Lemos JA: Diagnosis and management of stable angina. A review. JAMA 2021;325:1765.

Kannam JP, Aroesty JM, Gersh BJ: Overview of the management of stable angina pectoris. UpToDate, 2019. http://www.uptodate.com.

Kast R et al: Cardiovascular effects of a novel potent and highly selective asaindole-based inhibitor of Rho-kinase. Br J Pharmacol 2007;152:1070.

Lacinova L: Voltage-dependent calcium channels. Gen Physiol Biophys 2005;24(Suppl 1):1.

Li H, Föstermann U: Uncoupling of endothelial NO synthesis in atherosclerosis and vascular disease. Curr Opin Pharmacol 2013;13:161.

McGillian MM et al: Isosorbide mononitrate in heart failure with preserved ejection fraction. N Engl J Med 2015;373:2314.

McGillian MM et al: Management of patients with refractory angina: Canadian Cardiovascular Society/Canadian Pain Society joint guidelines. Can J Cardiol 2012;28(Suppl2):S20.

McLaughlin VV et al: Expert consensus document on pulmonary hypertension. J Am Coll Cardiol 2009;53:1573.

Moss AJ et al: Ranolazine shortens repolarization in patients with sustained inward sodium current due to type-3 long QT syndrome. J Cardiovasc Electrophysiol 2008;19:1289.

Münzel T et al: Physiology and pathophysiology of vascular signaling controlled by guanosine 3',5'-cyclic monophosphate-dependent protein kinase. Circulation 2003;108:2172.

Münzel T, Gori T: Nitrate therapy and nitrate tolerance in patients with coronary artery disease. Curr Opin Pharmacol 2013;13:251.

Ohman EM: Clinical practice. Chronic stable angina. N Engl J Med 2016;374:1167.

Peng J, Li Y-J: New insights into nitroglycerin effects and tolerance: Role of calcitonin gene-related peptide. Eur J Pharmacol 2008;586:9.

Rajendra NS et al: Mechanistic insights into the therapeutic use of high-dose allopurinol in angina pectoris. J Am Coll Cardiol 2011;58:820.

Sayed N et al: Nitroglycerin-induced S-nitrosylation and desensitization of soluble guanylyl cyclase contribute to nitrate tolerance. Circ Res 2008;103:606.

Simons M, Laham RJ: New therapies for angina pectoris. UpToDate 2019. http://uptodate.com.

Stevens S et al: Pentaerythritol tetranitrate in vivo treatment improves oxidative stress and vascular dysfunction by suppression of endothelin-1 signaling in monocrotaline-induced pulmonary hypertension. Oxid Med Cell Longev 2017; 2017:4353462.

Stone GW et al: A prospective natural-history study of coronary atherosclerosis. N Engl J Med 2011;364:226.

Triggle DJ: Calcium channel antagonists: Clinical uses—Past, present and future. Biochem Pharmacol 2007;74:1.

Wei J et al: Coronary microvascular dysfunction causing cardiac ischemia in women. JAMA 2019;322:2334.

CASE STUDY ANSWER

The case described is typical of acute coronary syndrome without STEMI (ST elevation myocardial infarction). Her chest pain is due to transient and possibly reversible inadequate coronary flow, probably due to rupture of an atheromatous plaque and clotting in an epicardial coronary artery. Immediate treatment to restore coronary flow is indicated. If available, percutaneous coroanary intervention (PCI) is optimal. If PCI is not available in this rural hospital, lysis of the clot should be attempted immediately with a fibrinolytic drug such as alteplase (Chapter 34). Admission to the intensive care unit is indicated, and transfer to a hospital where PCI is available also should be considered if her condition worsens.

C H A P T E R

13

Drugs Used in Heart Failure

Bertram G. Katzung, MD, PhD

CASE STUDY

A 60-year-old woman notices shortness of breath with exertion while working long hours in her bakery. She has a 20-year history of poorly controlled hypertension. The shortness of breath is accompanied by onset of swelling of the feet and ankles and increasing fatigue. On physical examination in the clinic, she is found to be mildly short of breath lying down but feels better sitting upright. Pulse is 100 bpm and regular, and blood pressure is 165/100 mm Hg. Crackles are noted at both lung bases, and her jugular venous pressure is elevated. The liver is enlarged, and there is 3+ edema of the ankles and feet. An echocardiogram shows an enlarged, poorly contracting heart with a left ventricular ejection fraction of about 30% (normal: 60%). The presumptive diagnosis is stage C, class III heart failure with reduced ejection fraction (HFrEF). What treatment is indicated?

Heart failure occurs when cardiac output is inadequate to provide the oxygen needed by the body. It is a highly lethal condition, with a 5-year mortality rate conventionally said to be about 50%. The most common cause of heart failure in the USA is coronary artery disease, with hypertension also an important factor. Two major types of failure may be distinguished. Almost 50% of younger patients have **systolic failure,** with reduced mechanical pumping action (contractility) and reduced ejection fraction **(HFrEF).** The remaining group has **diastolic failure,** with stiffening and loss of adequate relaxation playing a major role in reducing filling and cardiac output. Ejection *fraction* may be normal (preserved, **HFpEF**) in diastolic failure even though stroke *volume* is significantly reduced. The proportion of patients with diastolic failure increases with age. Because other cardiovascular conditions (especially myocardial infarction) are now being treated more effectively, more patients are surviving long enough for heart failure to develop, making heart failure one of the cardiovascular conditions that is actually increasing in prevalence in some countries. Like coronary artery disease, heart failure is disproportionately represented in underserved populations.

Heart failure is a progressive disease that is characterized by a gradual reduction in cardiac performance, punctuated in many patients by episodes of acute decompensation, often requiring hospitalization. Treatment is therefore directed at two somewhat different goals: (1) reducing symptoms and slowing progression as much as possible during relatively stable periods and (2) managing acute episodes of decompensated failure. These factors are discussed in Clinical Pharmacology of Drugs Used in Heart Failure.

Although it is believed that the primary defect in early systolic heart failure resides in the excitation-contraction coupling machinery of the myocardium, the clinical condition also involves many other processes and organs, including the baroreceptor reflex, the sympathetic nervous system, the kidneys, angiotensin II and other peptides, aldosterone, and apoptosis of cardiac cells. Recognition of these factors has resulted in a variety of drug treatment strategies (Table 13–1) that constitute the current standard of care. A rare form of amyloid cardiomyopathy, transthyretin amyloid cardiomyopathy (ATTR-CM), is associated with heart failure and can be treated with a small molecule oral drug, **tafamidis**.

Large clinical trials have shown that therapy directed at noncardiac targets is more valuable in the long-term treatment of heart failure than traditional positive inotropic agents (cardiac glycosides [digitalis]). Large trials have also shown that angiotensin-converting enzyme (ACE) inhibitors, angiotensin receptor blockers (ARBs), certain β blockers, aldosterone receptor antagonists, combined angiotensin receptor blocker plus neprilysin inhibitor (ARNI), and probably SGLT2 inhibitor therapies are the only agents in current use that actually prolong life and reduce hospitalizations in patients with chronic heart failure. These strategies are useful in both systolic and diastolic failure.

TABLE 13–1 Therapies used in heart failure.

Chronic Systolic Heart Failure	Acute Heart Failure
Diuretics	Diuretics
Aldosterone receptor antagonists	Vasodilators
Angiotensin-converting enzyme inhibitors	Beta agonists
Angiotensin receptor blockers	Bipyridines
SGLT2 inhibitors	Natriuretic peptide
Beta blockers	
Cardiac glycosides	Left ventricular assist device
Vasodilators, neprilysin inhibitor	
Resynchronization and cardioverter therapy	

Smaller studies support the use of the hydralazine-nitrate combination in African Americans and the use of ivabradine in patients with persistent tachycardia despite optimal management. Positive inotropic drugs, on the other hand, are helpful mainly in acute systolic failure. Cardiac glycosides also reduce symptoms in chronic systolic heart failure. In large clinical trials to date, other positive inotropic drugs have usually *reduced* survival in chronic failure or had no benefit, and their use is discouraged.

Control of Normal Cardiac Contractility

The vigor of contraction of heart muscle is determined by several processes that lead to the movement of actin and myosin filaments in the cardiac sarcomere (Figure 13–1). Ultimately, contraction results from the interaction of *activator* calcium (during systole) with the actin-troponin-tropomyosin system, thereby triggering the actin-myosin interaction. This activator calcium is released from the sarcoplasmic reticulum (SR). The amount released depends on the amount stored in the SR and on the amount of *trigger* calcium that enters the cell during the plateau of the action potential.

A. Sensitivity of the Contractile Proteins to Calcium and Other Contractile Protein Modifications

The determinants of calcium sensitivity, ie, the curve relating the shortening of cardiac myofibrils to the cytoplasmic calcium concentration, are incompletely understood, but several types of drugs can be shown to affect calcium sensitivity in vitro. **Levosimendan** is a drug that increases calcium sensitivity (it may also inhibit phosphodiesterase) and reduces symptoms in models of heart failure. Several reports suggest that **omecamtiv mecarbil** (CK-1827452) alters the rate of transition of myosin from a low-actin-binding state to a strongly actin-bound, force-generating state and improves ejection fraction in the failing heart. This action might increase contractility without increasing energy consumption, ie, increase efficiency.

B. Amount of Calcium Released from the Sarcoplasmic Reticulum

A small rise in free cytoplasmic calcium, brought about by calcium influx during the action potential, triggers the opening of calcium-gated, ryanodine-sensitive (RyR2) calcium channels in the membrane of the cardiac SR and the rapid release of a large amount of the ion into the cytoplasm in the vicinity of the actin-troponin-tropomyosin complex. The amount released is proportional to the amount stored in the SR and the amount of trigger calcium that enters the cell through the cell membrane. (Ryanodine is a potent negative inotropic plant alkaloid that interferes with the release of calcium through cardiac SR channels.)

C. Amount of Calcium Stored in the Sarcoplasmic Reticulum

The SR membrane contains a very efficient calcium uptake transporter known as the sarcoplasmic endoplasmic reticulum Ca^{2+}-ATPase (SERCA). This pump maintains free cytoplasmic calcium at very low levels during diastole by pumping calcium into the SR. SERCA is normally inhibited by phospholamban; phosphorylation of phospholamban by protein kinase A (activated, eg, by cAMP produced in response to β-adrenoceptor activation) removes this inhibition. (Some evidence suggests that SERCA activity is impaired in heart failure.) The amount of calcium sequestered in the SR is thus determined, in part, by the amount accessible to this transporter and the activity of the sympathetic nervous system. This in turn is dependent on the balance of calcium influx (primarily through the voltage-gated membrane L-type calcium channels) and calcium efflux, the amount removed from the cell (primarily via the sodium-calcium exchanger [NCX], a transporter in the cell membrane). The amount of Ca^{2+} released from the SR depends on the response of the RyR channels to trigger Ca^{2+}.

D. Amount of Trigger Calcium

The amount of trigger calcium that enters the cell depends on the concentration of extracellular calcium, the availability of membrane calcium channels, and the duration of their opening. As described in Chapters 6 and 9, sympathomimetics cause an increase in calcium influx through an action on these channels. Conversely, the calcium channel blockers (see Chapter 12) reduce this influx and depress contractility.

E. Activity of the Sodium-Calcium Exchanger

This antiporter (NCX) uses the inward movement of three sodium ions to move one calcium ion against its concentration gradient from the cytoplasm to the extracellular space. Extracellular concentrations of these ions are much less labile than intracellular concentrations under physiologic conditions. The sodium-calcium exchanger's ability to carry out this transport is thus strongly dependent on the intracellular concentrations of both ions, especially sodium.

F. Intracellular Sodium Concentration and Activity of Na^+/K^+-ATPase

Na^+/K^+-ATPase, by removing intracellular sodium, is the major determinant of sodium concentration in the cell. The sodium influx through voltage-gated channels, which occurs as a normal part of almost all cardiac action potentials, is another determinant, although the amount of sodium that enters with each action

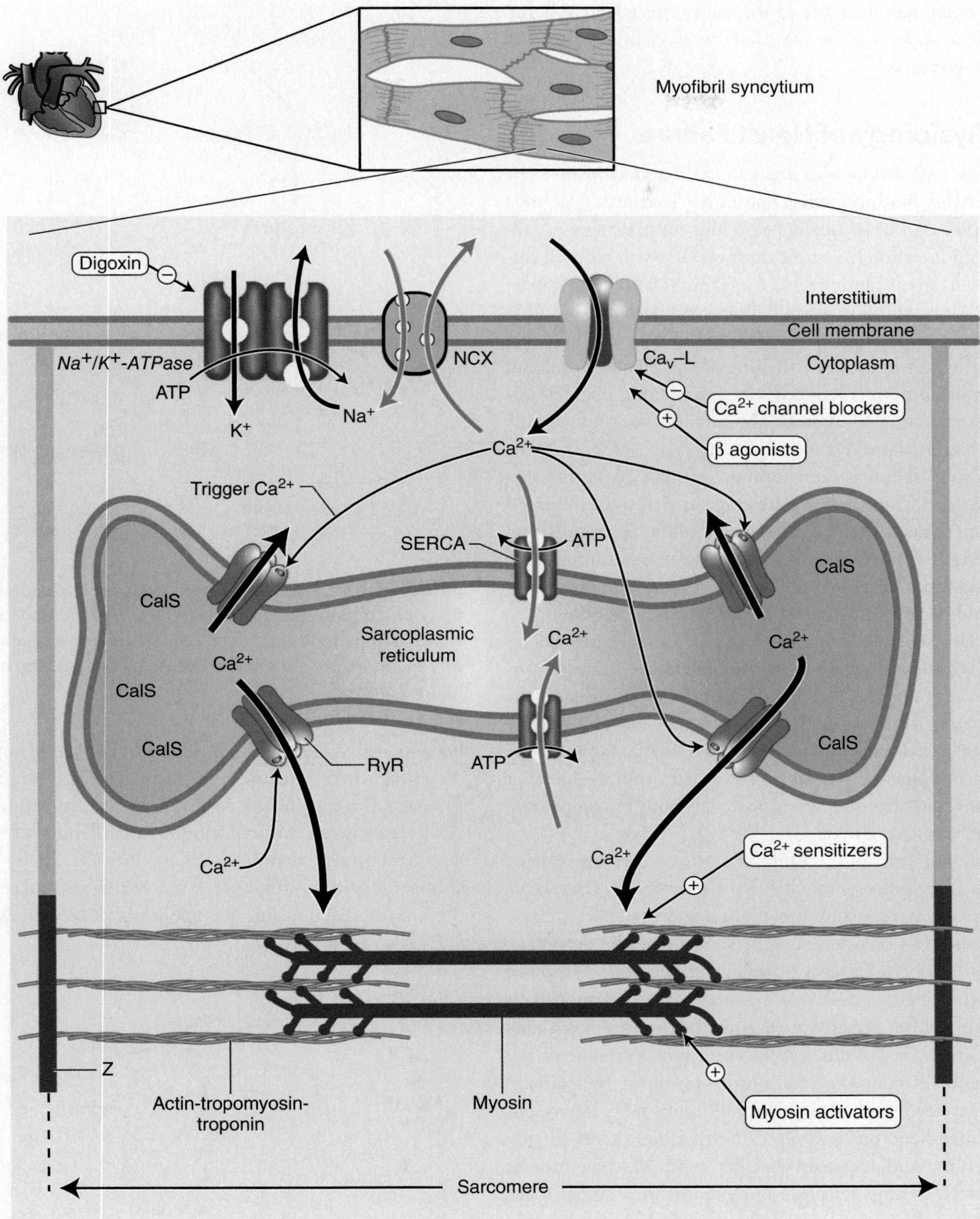

FIGURE 13–1 Schematic diagram of a cardiac muscle sarcomere, with sites of action of several drugs that alter contractility. (Mitochondria, which are critical for the generation of ATP, are omitted for simplicity.) Na^+/K^+-ATPase, the sodium pump, is the site of action of cardiac glycosides. NCX is the sodium-calcium exchanger. Ca_v-L is the voltage-gated, L-type calcium channel. SERCA (sarcoplasmic endoplasmic reticulum Ca^{2+}-ATPase) is a calcium transporter ATPase that pumps calcium into the sarcoplasmic reticulum. CalS is calcium bound to calsequestrin, a high-capacity Ca^{2+}-binding protein. RyR (ryanodine RyR2 receptor) is a calcium-activated calcium channel in the membrane of the SR that is triggered to release stored calcium. Z is the Z-line, which delimits the sarcomere. Calcium sensitizers act at the actin-troponin-tropomyosin complex where activator calcium brings about the contractile interaction of actin and myosin. *Black arrows* represent processes that initiate contraction or support basal tone. *Green arrows* represent processes that promote relaxation.

potential is much less than 1% of the total intracellular sodium. Na^+/K^+-ATPase appears to be the primary target of **digoxin** and other cardiac glycosides.

Pathophysiology of Heart Failure

Heart failure is a syndrome with many causes that may involve one or both ventricles. Normal cardiac output is ~5 L/min/70 kg body weight. Cardiac output is usually below this normal value in failure ("low-output" failure). Systolic dysfunction, with reduced cardiac output and significantly reduced ejection fraction (EF <45%; normal >60%), is typical of acute failure, especially that resulting from myocardial infarction. Diastolic dysfunction often occurs as a result of hypertrophy and stiffening of the myocardium, and although cardiac output is reduced, ejection fraction may be normal. Heart failure due to diastolic dysfunction does not usually respond optimally to positive inotropic drugs.

"High-output" failure is a rare form of heart failure. In this condition, the demands of the body are so great that even increased cardiac output is insufficient. High-output failure can result from hyperthyroidism, beriberi, anemia, or arteriovenous shunts. This form of failure responds poorly to the drugs discussed in this chapter and should be treated by correcting the underlying cause.

The primary signs and symptoms of all types of heart failure include tachycardia, decreased exercise tolerance, shortness of breath, and cardiomegaly. Peripheral and pulmonary edema (the congestion of *congestive* heart failure) are often but not always present. Decreased exercise tolerance with rapid muscular fatigue is the major direct consequence of diminished cardiac output. The other manifestations result from the attempts by the body to compensate for the intrinsic cardiac defect.

Neurohumoral (extrinsic) compensation involves two major mechanisms (previously presented in Figure 6–7)—the sympathetic nervous system and the renin-angiotensin-aldosterone hormonal response—plus several others. Some of the detrimental as well as beneficial features of these compensatory responses are illustrated in Figure 13–2. The baroreceptor reflex appears to be reset, with a lower sensitivity to arterial pressure, in patients with heart failure. As a result, baroreceptor sensory input to the vasomotor center is reduced even at normal pressures; sympathetic outflow is increased, and parasympathetic outflow is decreased. Increased sympathetic outflow causes tachycardia, increased cardiac contractility, and increased vascular tone. Vascular tone is further increased by angiotensin II and endothelin, a potent vasoconstrictor released by vascular endothelial cells. Vasoconstriction increases afterload, which further reduces ejection fraction and cardiac output. The result is a vicious cycle that is characteristic of heart failure (Figure 13–3). Neurohumoral antagonists and vasodilators attempt to reduce heart failure mortality by interrupting the cycle and slowing the downward spiral.

After a relatively short exposure to increased sympathetic drive, complex down-regulatory changes in the cardiac β_1-adrenoceptor–G protein-effector system take place that result in diminished stimulatory effects. Beta$_2$ receptors are *not* down-regulated and may develop increased coupling to the inositol 1,4,5-trisphosphate–diacylglycerol (IP_3-DAG) cascade. It has also

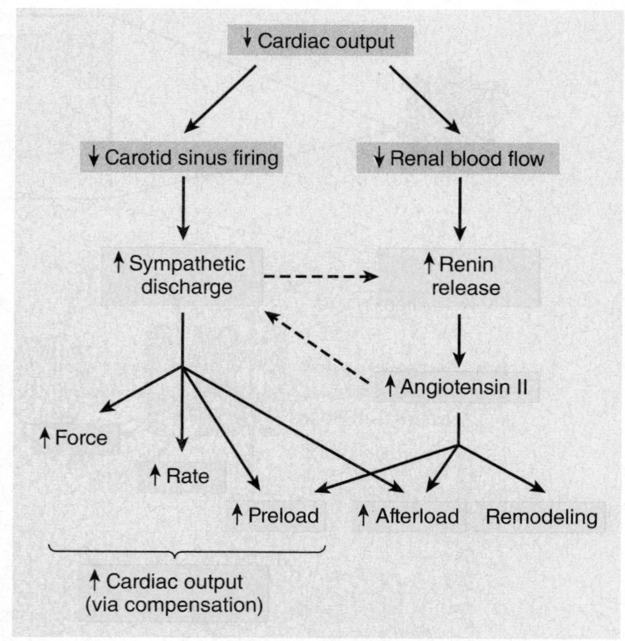

FIGURE 13–2 Some compensatory responses (orange boxes) that occur during congestive heart failure. In addition to the effects shown, sympathetic discharge facilitates renin release, and angiotensin II increases norepinephrine release by sympathetic nerve endings (*dashed arrows*).

been suggested that cardiac β_3 receptors (which do not appear to be down-regulated in failure) may mediate *negative* inotropic effects. Excessive β activation can lead to leakage of calcium from the SR via RyR channels and contributes to stiffening of the ventricles and arrhythmias. Reuptake of Ca^{2+} into the SR by SERCA may also be impaired. Prolonged β activation also increases caspases, the enzymes responsible for apoptosis. Increased angiotensin II

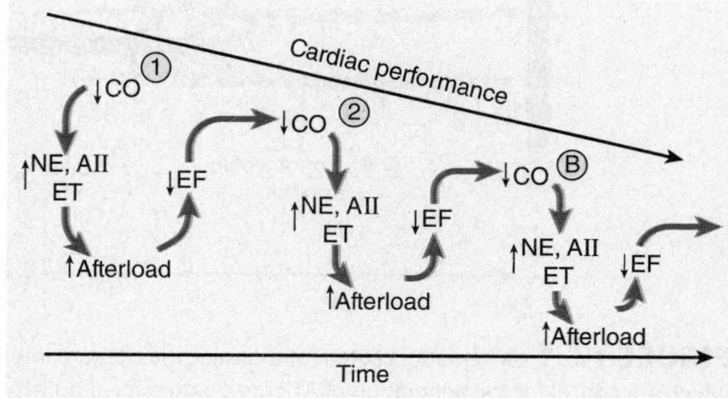

FIGURE 13–3 Vicious spiral of progression of heart failure. Decreased cardiac output (CO) activates production of neurohormones (NE, norepinephrine; AII, angiotensin II; ET, endothelin), which cause vasoconstriction and increased afterload. This further reduces ejection fraction (EF) and CO, and the cycle repeats. The downward spiral is continued until a new steady state is reached in which CO is lower and afterload is higher than is optimal for normal activity. Circled points 1, 2, and B represent points on the ventricular function curves depicted in Figure 13–4.

production leads to increased aldosterone secretion (with sodium and water retention), to increased afterload, and to remodeling of both heart and vessels. Other hormones are released, including natriuretic peptide, endothelin, and vasopressin (see Chapter 17). Of note, natriuretic peptides released from the heart and possibly other tissues include **N-terminal pro-brain natriuretic peptide (NT-proBNP),** which may be used as a surrogate marker for the presence and severity of heart failure. Within the heart, failure-induced changes have been documented in calcium handling in the SR by SERCA and phospholamban; in transcription factors that lead to hypertrophy and fibrosis; in mitochondrial function, which is critical for energy production in the overworked heart; and in ion channels, especially potassium channels, which facilitate arrhythmogenesis, a primary cause of death in heart failure. Phosphorylation of RyR channels in the SR enhances and dephosphorylation reduces Ca^{2+} release; studies in animal models indicate that the enzyme primarily responsible for RyR dephosphorylation, protein phosphatase 1 (PP1), is up-regulated in heart failure. These cellular changes provide several potential targets for future drugs.

The most obvious intrinsic compensatory mechanism is **myocardial hypertrophy.** The increase in muscle mass helps maintain cardiac performance. However, after an initial beneficial effect, hypertrophy can lead to ischemic changes, impairment of diastolic filling, and alterations in ventricular geometry. **Remodeling** is the term applied to dilation (other than that due to passive stretch) and other slow structural changes that occur in the stressed myocardium. It may include proliferation of connective tissue cells as well as abnormal myocardial cells with some biochemical characteristics of fetal myocytes. Ultimately, myocytes in the failing heart die at an accelerated rate through apoptosis, leaving the remaining myocytes subject to even greater stress.

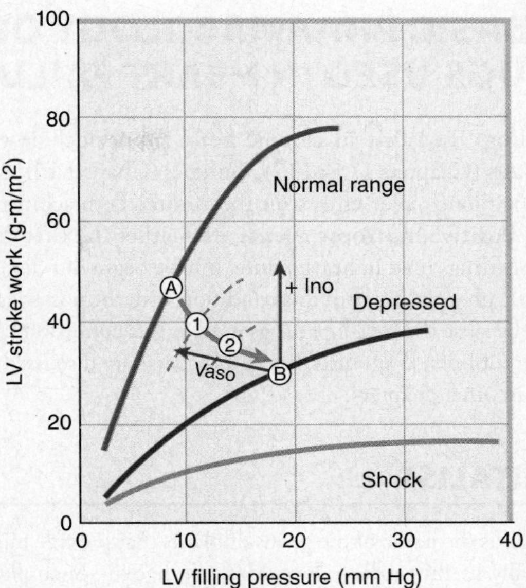

FIGURE 13–4 Relation of left ventricular (LV) performance to filling pressure in patients with acute myocardial infarction, an important cause of heart failure. The upper line indicates the range for normal, healthy individuals. At a given level of exercise, the heart operates at a stable point, eg, point A. In heart failure, function is shifted down and to the right, through points 1 and 2, finally reaching point B. A "pure" positive inotropic drug (+ Ino) would move the operating point upward by increasing cardiac stroke work. A vasodilator (Vaso) would move the point leftward by reducing filling pressure. Successful therapy usually results in both effects. (Reproduced ith permission from Sodeman WA Jr, Sodeman TM: *Pathologic Physiology*, 7th ed. Philadelphia, PA: Saunders/Elsevier; 1985.)

Pathophysiology of Cardiac Performance

Cardiac performance is a function of four primary factors:

1. **Preload:** When some measure of left ventricular performance such as stroke volume or stroke work is plotted as a function of left ventricular filling pressure or end-diastolic fiber length, the resulting graph is termed the **left ventricular function curve** (Figure 13–4). The ascending limb (<15 mm Hg filling pressure) represents the classic Frank-Starling relation described in physiology texts. Beyond approximately 15 mm Hg, there is a plateau of performance. Preloads greater than 20–25 mm Hg result in pulmonary congestion. As noted above, preload is usually increased in heart failure because of increased blood volume and venous tone. Because the function curve of the failing heart is lower, the plateau is reached at much lower values of stroke work or output. Increased fiber length or filling pressure increases oxygen demand in the myocardium, as described in Chapter 12. Reduction of high filling pressure is the goal of salt restriction and diuretic therapy in heart failure. Venodilator drugs (eg, nitroglycerin) also reduce preload by redistributing blood away from the chest into peripheral veins.
2. **Afterload:** Afterload is the resistance against which the heart must pump blood and is the result of aortic impedance and systemic vascular resistance. Systolic blood pressure is the clinically accessible measure of afterload versus stroke volume. As noted in Figure 13–2, as cardiac output falls in chronic failure, a reflex increase in systemic vascular resistance occurs, mediated in part by increased sympathetic outflow and circulating catecholamines and in part by activation of the renin-angiotensin system. Endothelin, a potent vasoconstrictor peptide, is also involved. This sets the stage for the use of drugs that reduce arteriolar tone in heart failure.
3. **Contractility:** Heart muscle obtained by biopsy from patients with chronic low-output failure demonstrates a reduction in intrinsic contractility. As contractility decreases in the heart, there is a reduction in the velocity of muscle shortening, the rate of intraventricular pressure development (dP/dt), and the stroke output achieved (see Figure 13–4). However, the heart is usually still capable of some increase in all of these measures of contractility in response to inotropic drugs.
4. **Heart rate:** The heart rate is a major determinant of cardiac output. As the intrinsic function of the heart decreases in failure and stroke volume diminishes, an increase in heart rate—through sympathetic activation of β adrenoceptors—is the first compensatory mechanism that comes into play to maintain cardiac output. However, tachycardia limits diastolic filling time and coronary flow, further stressing the heart. Thus, bradycardic drugs may benefit patients with high heart rates.

BASIC PHARMACOLOGY OF DRUGS USED IN HEART FAILURE

The drugs used first in chronic heart failure include the ACE inhibitors (Chapters 11 and 17), diuretics (Chapter 15), and other drugs without major effects on the contractile machinery of the heart. **Positive inotropic agents** are neither the first drugs nor the only drugs used in heart failure, but we begin our discussion of the basic pharmacology of this condition with the positive inotrope group because the first-line drugs used in this condition (diuretics, ACE inhibitors, β-agonists, and β-blockers) are discussed in more detail in other chapters.

DIGITALIS

Digitalis is the name of the genus of plants that provide most of the medically useful **cardiac glycosides,** eg, digoxin. Such plants have been known for thousands of years but were used erratically and with variable success until 1785, when William Withering, an English physician and botanist, published a monograph describing the clinical effects of an extract of the purple foxglove plant (*Digitalis purpurea,* a major source of these agents).

Chemistry

All of the cardiac glycosides, or cardenolides—of which **digoxin** is the prototype—combine a steroid nucleus linked to a lactone ring at the 17 position and a series of sugars at carbon 3 of the nucleus. Because they lack an easily ionizable group, their solubility is not pH-dependent. Digoxin is obtained from *Digitalis lanata,* the white foxglove, but many common plants (eg, oleander, lily of the valley, milkweed, and others) contain cardiac glycosides with similar properties and their ingestion sometimes results in poisoning.

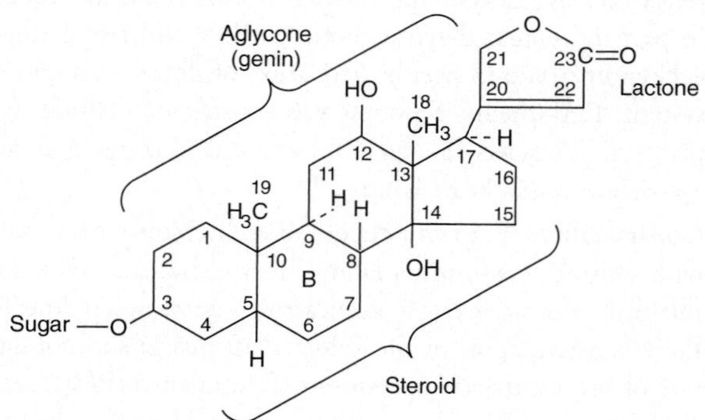

Pharmacokinetics

Digoxin, the only cardiac glycoside currently used in the USA, is 65–80% absorbed after oral administration. Absorption of other glycosides varies from zero to nearly 100%. Once present in the blood, all cardiac glycosides are widely distributed to tissues, including the central nervous system (CNS).

Digoxin is not extensively metabolized in humans; almost two thirds is excreted unchanged by the kidneys. Its renal clearance is proportional to creatinine clearance, and the half-life is 36–40 hours in patients with normal renal function. Equations and nomograms are available for adjusting digoxin dosage in patients with renal impairment, eg, https://www.ncbi.nlm.nih.gov/pmc/articles/PMC4227958/.

Pharmacodynamics

Digoxin has multiple direct and indirect cardiovascular effects, with both therapeutic and toxic consequences. In addition, it has undesirable effects on the CNS and gut.

At the molecular level, all therapeutically useful cardiac glycosides **inhibit Na^+/K^+-ATPase,** the membrane-bound transporter often called the **sodium pump** (see Figure 13–1). Although several isoforms of this ATPase occur and have varying sensitivity to cardiac glycosides, they are highly conserved in evolution, indicating the extreme importance of this activity in cell function. Inhibition of this transporter over most of the digitalis dose range has been extensively documented in all tissues studied. It is probable that this inhibitory action is largely responsible for the therapeutic effect—positive inotropy (increased contractility)—as well as a major portion of the toxicity of digitalis. Other molecular-level effects of digitalis have been studied in the heart and are discussed below. The fact that a receptor for cardiac glycosides exists on the sodium pump has prompted some investigators to propose that an endogenous digitalis-like steroid, possibly **ouabain** or **marinobufagenin,** must exist. Furthermore, additional functions of Na^+/K^+-ATPase have been postulated, involving apoptosis, cell growth and differentiation, immunity, and carbohydrate metabolism. Indirect evidence for such endogenous digitalis-like activity has been inferred from clinical studies showing some protective effect of digoxin antibodies in preeclampsia.

A. Cardiac Effects

1. Mechanical effects—Cardiac glycosides increase contraction of the cardiac sarcomere by increasing the free calcium concentration in the vicinity of the contractile proteins during systole. The increase in calcium concentration is the result of a two-step process: first, an **increase of intracellular sodium concentration** because of Na^+/K^+-ATPase inhibition; and second, a relative **reduction of calcium expulsion** from the cell by the sodium-calcium exchanger (NCX in Figure 13–1) caused by the increase in intracellular sodium. The increased cytoplasmic calcium is sequestered by SERCA in the SR for systolic release. Other mechanisms have been proposed but are not well supported.

The net result of the action of therapeutic concentrations of a cardiac glycoside in vitro is a distinctive increase in cardiac contractility (Figure 13–5, bottom trace, panels A and B). In isolated myocardial preparations, the rate of development of tension and of relaxation are both increased, with little or no change in time to peak tension. This effect occurs in both normal and failing myocardium, but in the intact patient, the responses are modified by cardiovascular reflexes and the pathophysiology of heart failure.

2. Electrical effects—The effects of digitalis on the electrical properties of the heart are a mixture of direct and autonomic actions. Direct actions include an early, brief prolongation of

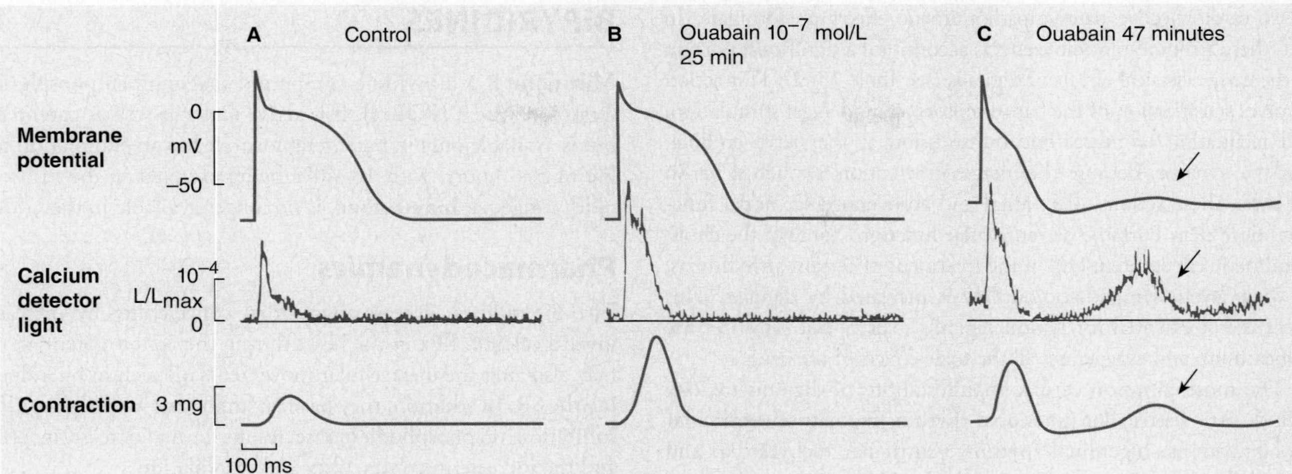

FIGURE 13–5 Effects of a cardiac glycoside, ouabain, on isolated cardiac tissue. The top tracing shows action potentials evoked during the control period (**A**), early in the "therapeutic" phase (**B**), and later, when toxicity is present (**C**). The middle tracing shows the light (L) emitted by the calcium-detecting protein aequorin (relative to the maximum possible, L_{max}) and is proportional to the free intracellular calcium concentration. The bottom tracing records the tension elicited by the action potentials. The early phase of ouabain action (**B**) shows a slight shortening of action potential and a marked increase in free intracellular calcium concentration and contractile tension. The toxic phase (**C**) is associated with depolarization of the resting potential, a marked shortening of the action potential, and the appearance of an oscillatory depolarization, calcium increment, and contraction (*arrows*). (Courtesy of P. Hess and H. Gil Wier.)

the action potential, followed by shortening (especially the plateau phase). The decrease in action potential duration is probably the result of increased potassium conductance that is caused by increased intracellular calcium (see Chapter 14). All these effects can be observed at therapeutic concentrations in the absence of overt toxicity (Table 13–2).

At higher concentrations, resting membrane potential is reduced (made less negative) as a result of inhibition of the sodium pump and reduced intracellular potassium. As toxicity progresses, oscillatory depolarizing afterpotentials appear following normally evoked action potentials (Figure 13–5, panel C). The afterpotentials (also known as **delayed after-depolarizations, DADs**) are associated with overloading of the intracellular calcium stores and oscillations in the free intracellular calcium ion concentration. When afterpotentials reach threshold, they elicit action potentials (**premature depolarizations,** ectopic "beats") that are coupled to the preceding normal action potentials. If afterpotentials in the Purkinje conducting system regularly reach threshold in this way, bigeminy will be recorded on the electrocardiogram (Figure 13–6). With further intoxication, each afterpotential-evoked action potential will itself elicit a suprathreshold afterpotential, and a self-sustaining tachycardia will be established. If allowed to progress, such a tachycardia may deteriorate into fibrillation. In the case of ventricular fibrillation, the arrhythmia will be rapidly fatal unless corrected.

Autonomic actions of cardiac glycosides on the heart involve both the parasympathetic and the sympathetic systems. At low therapeutic

TABLE 13–2 Effects of digoxin on electrical properties of cardiac tissues.

Tissue or Variable	Effects at Therapeutic Dosage	Effects at Toxic Dosage
Sinus node	↓ Rate	↓ Rate
Atrial muscle	↓ Refractory period	↓ Refractory period, arrhythmias
Atrioventricular node	↓ Conduction velocity, ↑ refractory period	↓ Refractory period, arrhythmias
Purkinje system, ventricular muscle	Slight ↓ refractory period	Extrasystoles, tachycardia, fibrillation
Electrocardiogram	↑ PR interval, ↓ QT interval	Tachycardia, fibrillation, arrest at extremely high dosage

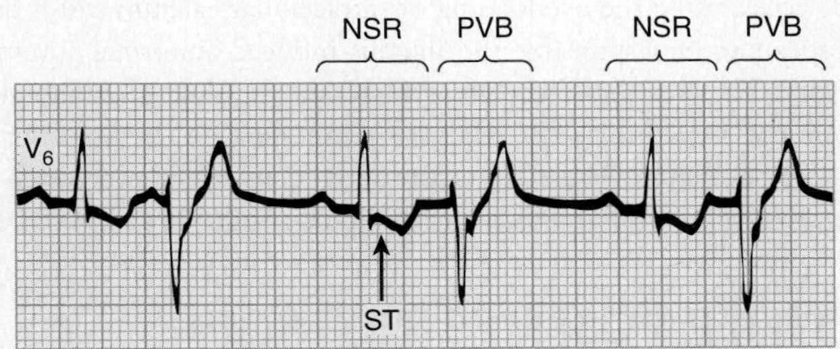

FIGURE 13–6 Electrocardiographic record showing digitalis-induced bigeminy. The complexes marked NSR are normal sinus rhythm beats; an inverted T wave and depressed ST segment are present. The complexes marked PVB are premature ventricular beats and are the electrocardiographic manifestations of depolarizations evoked by delayed oscillatory afterpotentials as shown in Figure 13–5. (Reproduced with permission from Goldman MJ: *Principles of Clinical Electrocardiography*, 12th ed. New York, NY: McGraw Hill; 1986.)

doses, cardioselective parasympathomimetic effects predominate. In fact, these atropine-blockable effects account for a significant portion of the early electrical effects of digitalis (see Table 13–2). This action involves sensitization of the baroreceptors, central vagal stimulation, and facilitation of muscarinic transmission at the nerve ending–myocyte synapse. Because cholinergic innervation is much richer in the atria, these actions affect atrial and atrioventricular nodal function more than Purkinje or ventricular function. Some of the cholinomimetic effects are useful in the treatment of certain arrhythmias. At toxic levels, sympathetic outflow is increased by digitalis. This effect is not essential for typical digitalis toxicity but sensitizes the myocardium and exaggerates all the toxic effects of the drug.

The most common cardiac manifestations of digitalis toxicity include atrioventricular junctional rhythm, premature ventricular depolarizations, bigeminal rhythm, ventricular tachycardia, and second-degree atrioventricular blockade. However, it is claimed that digitalis can cause virtually any arrhythmia.

B. Effects on Other Organs

Cardiac glycosides affect all excitable tissues, including smooth muscle and the CNS. The gastrointestinal tract is the most common site of digitalis toxicity outside the heart. The effects include anorexia, nausea, vomiting, and diarrhea. This toxicity is caused in part by direct effects on the gastrointestinal tract and in part by CNS actions.

CNS effects include vagal and chemoreceptor trigger zone stimulation. Less often, disorientation and hallucinations—especially in the elderly—and visual disturbances are noted. The latter effect may include aberrations of color perception. Gynecomastia is a rare effect reported in men taking digitalis.

C. Interactions with Potassium, Calcium, and Magnesium

Potassium and digitalis interact in two ways. First, they inhibit each other's binding to Na^+/K^+-ATPase; therefore, hyperkalemia reduces the enzyme-inhibiting actions of cardiac glycosides, whereas hypokalemia facilitates these actions. Second, increased cardiac automaticity is inhibited by hyperkalemia (see Chapter 14). Moderately increased extracellular K^+ may therefore reduce the toxic effects of digitalis.

Calcium ion facilitates the toxic actions of cardiac glycosides by accelerating the overloading of intracellular calcium stores that appears to be responsible for digitalis-induced abnormal automaticity. Hypercalcemia therefore increases the risk of a digitalis-induced arrhythmia. The effects of magnesium ion are opposite to those of calcium. These interactions mandate careful evaluation of serum electrolytes in patients with digitalis-induced arrhythmias.

OTHER POSITIVE INOTROPIC DRUGS USED IN HEART FAILURE

Major efforts are being made to find safer positive inotropic agents because cardiac glycosides have an extremely narrow therapeutic window and may not decrease mortality in chronic heart failure. Positive inotropic drugs currently available are beneficial in some patients with acute HFrEF; they are rarely beneficial, and often deleterious, in chronic failure and HFpEF.

BIPYRIDINES

Milrinone is a bipyridine compound that inhibits phosphodiesterase isozyme 3 (PDE-3). It is active orally as well as parenterally but is available only in parenteral form. It has an elimination half-life of 3–6 hours, with 10–40% being excreted in the urine. An older congener, **inamrinone,** is no longer available in the USA.

Pharmacodynamics

The bipyridines increase myocardial contractility by increasing inward calcium flux in the heart during the action potential; they may also alter the intracellular movements of calcium by influencing the SR. In addition, they have an important vasodilating effect. Inhibition of phosphodiesterase results in an increase in cAMP and the increase in contractility and vasodilation.

The toxicity of inamrinone includes nausea and vomiting; arrhythmias, thrombocytopenia, and liver enzyme changes have also been reported in a significant number of patients. As noted, this drug is not available in the USA. Milrinone appears less likely to cause bone marrow and liver toxicity, but it does cause arrhythmias. Milrinone is now used only intravenously and only for acute heart failure or severe exacerbation of chronic heart failure.

BETA-ADRENOCEPTOR AGONISTS

The general pharmacology of these agents is discussed in Chapter 9. **Dobutamine** is the selective β_1 agonist that has been most widely used in patients with acute decompensated heart failure. This parenteral drug can produce an increase in cardiac output together with a decrease in ventricular filling pressure. Some tachycardia and an increase in myocardial oxygen consumption often occurs. Therefore, the potential for producing angina or arrhythmias in patients with coronary artery disease is significant, as is the tachyphylaxis that accompanies the use of any β stimulant. Intermittent dobutamine infusion may benefit some patients with chronic heart failure.

Dopamine has also been used in acute heart failure and may be particularly helpful if there is a need to raise blood pressure.

INVESTIGATIONAL POSITIVE INOTROPIC DRUGS

Istaroxime is an investigational steroid derivative that increases contractility by inhibiting Na^+/K^+-ATPase (like cardiac glycosides) but in addition appears to facilitate sequestration of Ca^{2+} by the SR. The latter action may render the drug less arrhythmogenic than digitalis.

Levosimendan, a drug that sensitizes the troponin system to calcium, also appears to inhibit phosphodiesterase and to cause some vasodilation in addition to its inotropic effects. Some clinical trials suggest that this drug may be useful in patients with heart failure, and the drug has been approved in some countries but not in the USA.

Omecamtiv mecarbil is an investigational parenteral agent that activates cardiac myosin and prolongs systole without increasing oxygen consumption of the heart. It has been shown to reduce signs of heart failure in animal models, and clinical trials in patients with heart failure show increased systolic time and stroke volume and reduced heart rate and end-systolic and diastolic volumes. The drug is still under study.

DRUGS WITHOUT POSITIVE INOTROPIC EFFECTS USED IN HEART FAILURE

These agents—not positive inotropic drugs—are the first-line therapies for chronic heart failure. The drugs most commonly used are diuretics, ACE inhibitors, angiotensin receptor antagonists, aldosterone antagonists, and β blockers (see Table 13–1). In acute failure, diuretics and vasodilators play primary roles. The SGLT2 inhibitors are recent additions to this group.

DIURETICS

Diuretics, especially **furosemide,** are drugs of first choice in heart failure and are discussed in detail in Chapter 15. They reduce salt and water retention, reduce edema through renal effects, and reduce heart failure symptoms. They have no direct effect on cardiac contractility; their major mechanism of hemodynamic action in heart failure is to reduce venous pressure and ventricular preload. The reduction of cardiac size, which leads to improved pump efficiency, is of major importance in systolic failure. In heart failure associated with hypertension, the reduction in blood pressure also reduces afterload. Spironolactone and eplerenone, the aldosterone (mineralocorticoid) steroidal antagonist diuretics (see Chapter 15), have the additional benefit of decreasing morbidity and mortality in patients with severe heart failure who are also receiving ACE inhibitors and other standard therapy. One possible mechanism for this benefit lies in accumulating evidence that aldosterone may also cause myocardial and vascular fibrosis and baroreceptor dysfunction in addition to its renal effects. **Finerenone** is a nonsteroidal mineralocorticoid antagonist that may be less likely to induce hyperkalemia.

ANGIOTENSIN-CONVERTING ENZYME INHIBITORS, ANGIOTENSIN RECEPTOR BLOCKERS, & RELATED AGENTS

ACE inhibitors such as **captopril** were introduced in Chapter 11 and are discussed again in Chapter 17. These versatile drugs reduce peripheral resistance and thereby reduce afterload; they also reduce salt and water retention (by reducing aldosterone secretion) and in that way reduce preload. The reduction in tissue angiotensin levels also reduces sympathetic activity through diminution of angiotensin's presynaptic effects on norepinephrine release. Finally, these drugs reduce the long-term remodeling of the heart and vessels, an effect that may be responsible for the observed reduction in mortality and morbidity (see Clinical Pharmacology).

Angiotensin AT_1 receptor blockers such as **losartan** (see Chapters 11 and 17) appear to have similar beneficial effects. In combination with **sacubitril, valsartan** is now approved for HFrEF. Angiotensin receptor blockers should be considered in heart failure patients intolerant of ACE inhibitors because of incessant cough.

Aliskiren, a renin inhibitor approved for hypertension, was found to have no definitive benefit in clinical trials for heart failure.

VASODILATORS

Vasodilators are effective in acute heart failure because they provide a reduction in preload (through venodilation), or reduction in afterload (through arteriolar dilation), or both. Some evidence suggests that long-term vasodilation by **hydralazine** and **isosorbide dinitrate** can also reduce damaging remodeling of the heart. However, treatment of acute decompensation does not reliably slow progression of chronic failure in most patients.

Nesiritide, a synthetic form of the endogenous peptide brain natriuretic peptide (BNP), is approved for use in acute (not chronic) cardiac failure. This recombinant peptide increases cGMP in smooth muscle cells and reduces venous and arteriolar tone in experimental preparations. It also causes diuresis. However, large trials in patients with heart failure have failed to show a reduction in mortality or rehospitalizations. The peptide has a short half-life of about 18 minutes and is administered as a bolus intravenous dose followed by continuous infusion. Excessive hypotension is the most common adverse effect. Reports of significant renal damage and deaths have resulted in extra warnings regarding this agent, and it should be used with great caution. Similar mixed results have been obtained with **ularitide** and **serelaxin,** two other vasodilator peptides. A newer approach to modulation of the natriuretic peptide system is inhibition of the neutral endopeptidase enzyme, **neprilysin,** which is responsible for the degradation of BNP and atrial natriuretic peptide (ANP), as well as angiotensin II, bradykinin, and other peptides. **Sacubitril** is a prodrug that is metabolized to an active neprilysin inhibitor. A combination of valsartan plus sacubitril is approved for use in HFrEF. A recent large study (PIONEER-HF) confirmed that this drug combination is superior to enalapril in reducing high-sensitivity troponin-T levels and rehospitalization of patients with acute decompensated HFrEF. Unfortunately, HFpEF is not similarly improved by this combination drug.

Plasma concentrations of *endogenous* BNP rise in most patients with heart failure and are correlated with severity. Measurement of the plasma precursor NT-proBNP is a useful diagnostic or prognostic test and has been used as a surrogate marker in clinical trials.

Related peptides include ANP and urodilatin, a similar peptide produced in the kidney. **Carperitide** and **ularitide,** respectively, are investigational synthetic analogs of these endogenous peptides and are in clinical trials (see Chapter 15). **Bosentan** and **tezosentan,** orally active competitive inhibitors of endothelin (see Chapter 17), have been shown to have some benefits in experimental animal models with heart failure, but results in human trials have been disappointing. Bosentan is approved for use in pulmonary hypertension. It has significant teratogenic and hepatotoxic effects.

Several newer agents are thought to stabilize the RyR channel and may reduce Ca^{2+} leak from the SR. They are currently denoted only by code numbers (eg, TRV027, JTV519, S44121). This action, if confirmed to reduce diastolic stiffness, would be especially useful in diastolic failure with preserved ejection fraction.

BETA-ADRENOCEPTOR BLOCKERS

Most patients with chronic heart failure respond favorably to certain β blockers despite the fact that these drugs can *precipitate* acute cardiac failure (see Chapter 10). Studies with **bisoprolol, carvedilol, metoprolol,** and **nebivolol** showed a reduction in mortality in patients with stable severe heart failure, but this effect was not observed with another β blocker, bucindolol. A full understanding of the beneficial action of β blockade is lacking, but suggested mechanisms include attenuation of the adverse effects of high concentrations of endogenous catecholamines (including apoptosis), up-regulation of β receptors, decreased heart rate, and reduced remodeling through inhibition of the mitogenic activity of catecholamines.

ANTIDIABETIC DRUGS

Drugs used in type 2 diabetes have been of concern because of the association of diabetes with cardiac events. Therefore, it is of interest that two groups of these agents benefit patients with heart failure *with or without* type 2 diabetes. The gliflozins, eg, **empagliflozin** and **dapagliflozin,** are SGLT2 inhibitors that increase renal sodium excretion as well as glucose excretion (see chapter 41). They have complex effects in the heart, including inhibition of the sodium-hydrogen exchanger (NHE) and a reduction of glucose utilization for ATP production. They also slow development of chronic kidney disease. These drugs have been shown to *reduce mortality and hospitalizations for heart failure* in patients with or without type 2 diabetes. This appears to be a class effect. Empagliflozin is approved for use in both HFrEF and HFpEF; dapagliflozin is currently approved for HFrEF. **Liraglutide** and **semaglutide,** GLP-1 agonists used in diabetes (see chapter 41) and obesity (see Chapter 16), have been shown to reduce deaths from cardiovascular causes as well as the rates of myocardial infarction, nonfatal stroke, and hospitalization for heart failure. They are approved for use in HFrEF.

OTHER DRUGS

Mavacamten, an inhibitor of myosin, is approved for use in obstructive hypertrophic cardiomyopathy. This condition reduces cardiac output and is often associated with symptoms of heart failure. Mavacamten (as well as beta blockers), by slowing the contraction of the ventricles, may improve ejection and increase cardiac output. Neuroregulatory proteins appear to have cardiac as well as neural effects. The neuregulin GGF2 protein **(cimaglermin)** has been shown to benefit cardiac function in several animal models of heart failure. **Vericiguat**, a soluble guanylate cyclase stimulator, has been shown to have a small but significant benefit on death and hospitalization rates. It is approved for oral use in acute decompensated failure.

■ CLINICAL PHARMACOLOGY OF DRUGS USED IN HEART FAILURE

Detailed guidelines are issued by US and European expert groups (see References). The American College of Cardiology/American Heart Association (ACC/AHA) guidelines for management of chronic heart failure specify four stages in the development of heart failure (Table 13–3). Patients in stage A are at high risk because of other disease but have no signs or symptoms of heart failure. Stage B patients have evidence of structural heart disease but no symptoms of heart failure. Stage C patients have structural heart disease and symptoms of failure, and symptoms are responsive to ordinary therapy. Patients in stage C must often be hospitalized for acute decompensation, and after discharge, they often decompensate again, requiring rehospitalization. Stage D patients have heart failure refractory to ordinary therapy, and special interventions (eg, resynchronization therapy, transplant) are required.

Once stage C is reached, the severity of heart failure is usually described according to a scale devised by the New York Heart Association. Class I failure is associated with no limitations on ordinary activities and symptoms that occur only with greater than ordinary exercise. Class II failure is characterized by slight limitation of activities and results in fatigue and palpitations with ordinary physical activity. Class III failure results in fatigue, shortness of breath, and tachycardia with less than ordinary physical activity, but no symptoms at rest. Class IV failure is associated with symptoms even when the patient is at rest.

TABLE 13–3 Classification and treatment of chronic heart failure.

ACC/AHA Stage[1]	NYHA Class[2]	Description	Management
A	Prefailure	No symptoms but risk factors present[3]	Treat obesity, hypertension, diabetes, hyperlipidemia, etc
B	I	Symptoms with severe exercise	Diuretic, ACEI/ARB, β blocker,
C	II/III	Symptoms with marked (class II) or mild (class III) exercise	Add SGLT2I, aldosterone antagonist, digoxin; CRT, ARNI, hydralazine/nitrate[4]
D	IV	Severe symptoms at rest	Maximal medical therapy, transplant, LVAD

[1]American College of Cardiology/American Heart Association classification.

[2]New York Heart Association classification.

[3]Risk factors include hypertension, myocardial infarct, diabetes.

[4]For selected populations, eg, African Americans.

ACC, American College of Cardiology; ACEI, angiotensin-converting enzyme inhibitor; AHA, American Heart Association; ARB, angiotensin receptor blocker; ARNI, angiotensin receptor inhibitor plus neprilysin inhibitor; CRT, cardiac resynchronization therapy; LVAD, left ventricular assist device; NYHA, New York Heart Association; SGLT2I, sodium-glucose transporter-2 inhibitor.

TABLE 13–4 Differences between systolic and diastolic heart failure.

Variable or Therapy	Systolic Heart Failure	Diastolic Heart Failure
Cardiac output	Decreased	Decreased
Ejection fraction	Decreased	Normal
Diuretics	↓ Symptoms; first-line therapy if edema present	Use with caution[1]
ACEIs	↓ Mortality in chronic HF	May help to ↓ LVH
ARBs, SGLT2I	↓ Mortality in chronic HF	May be beneficial
ARNI	↓ Symptoms and NT-proBNP	↓ Symptoms and NT-proBNP
Aldosterone inhibitors	↓ Mortality in chronic HF	May be useful
Beta blockers,[2] ivabradine	Beta blocker ↓ mortality in chronic HF, ivabradine reduces hospitalizations	Useful to ↓ HR, ↓ BP
Calcium channel blockers	No or small benefit[3]	Useful to ↓ HR, ↓ BP
Digoxin	May reduce symptoms	Little or no role
Nitrates	May be useful in acute HF[4]	Use with caution[1]
PDE inhibitors	May be useful in acute HF	Very small study in chronic HF was positive
Positive inotropes	↓ Symptoms, hospitalizations	Not recommended

[1]Avoid excessive reduction of filling pressures.

[2]Limited to certain β blockers (see text).

[3]Benefit, if any, may be due to BP reduction.

[4]Useful combined with hydralazine in selected patients, especially African Americans.

ACEI, angiotensin-converting enzyme inhibitor; ARB, angiotensin receptor blocker; ARNI, angiotensin receptor inhibitor plus neprilysin inhibitor; BP, blood pressure; HF, heart failure; HR, heart rate; LVH, left ventricular hypertrophy; NT-proBNP, N-terminal pro-brain natriuretic peptide; PDE, phosphodiesterase; SGLT2I, sodium-glucose transporter 2 inhibitor.

MANAGEMENT OF CHRONIC HEART FAILURE

The major steps in the management of patients with chronic heart failure are outlined in Tables 13–3 and 13–4. Updates to the ACC/AHA guidelines suggest that treatment of patients at high risk (stages A and B) should be focused on control of hypertension, arrhythmias, hyperlipidemia, and diabetes, if present. Atrial fibrillation is increasingly common in older patients and correction of this arrhythmia can be very beneficial. Once symptoms and signs of failure are present, stage C has been entered, and active treatment of failure must be initiated.

SODIUM REMOVAL

Sodium removal—by dietary salt restriction and a diuretic—is the mainstay in management of symptomatic heart failure, especially if edema is present. The use of diuretics is discussed in greater detail in Chapter 15. In very mild failure, a **thiazide** diuretic may be tried, but a loop agent such as **furosemide** is usually required. Sodium loss causes secondary loss of potassium, which is particularly hazardous if the patient is to be given digitalis. Hypokalemia can be treated with potassium supplementation or through the addition of an ACE inhibitor or a potassium-sparing diuretic such as spironolactone. Spironolactone or eplerenone should probably be considered in all patients with moderate or severe heart failure, since both appear to reduce both morbidity and mortality. SGLT2 inhibitors also cause natriuresis, and their benefit in heart failure maybe due, in part, to this effect.

ACE INHIBITORS & ANGIOTENSIN RECEPTOR BLOCKERS

In patients with left ventricular dysfunction but no edema, an ACE inhibitor should be the first drug used. Several large studies have shown clearly that ACE inhibitors are superior both to placebo and to vasodilators and must be considered, along with diuretics, as first-line therapy for chronic heart failure. However, ACE inhibitors cannot replace digoxin in patients already receiving the glycoside because patients withdrawn from digoxin deteriorate while on ACE inhibitor therapy.

By reducing preload and afterload in asymptomatic patients, ACE inhibitors (eg, **enalapril**) slow the progress of ventricular dilation and thus slow the downward spiral of heart failure. Consequently, ACE inhibitors are beneficial in all subsets of patients—from those who are asymptomatic to those in severe chronic failure. This benefit appears to be a class effect; that is, all ACE inhibitors appear to be effective.

The angiotensin II AT_1 receptor blockers (ARBs, eg, **losartan**) produce beneficial hemodynamic effects similar to those of ACE inhibitors. However, large clinical trials suggest that when used alone, ARBs are best reserved for patients who cannot tolerate ACE inhibitors (usually because of cough). In contrast, the ARB valsartan combined with the neprilysin inhibitor sacubitril (**Entresto**) has additional benefit in HFrEF and is recommended in 2016 guidelines.

BETA BLOCKERS & ION CHANNEL BLOCKERS

Beta blocker therapy in patients with heart failure is based on the hypothesis that excessive tachycardia and adverse effects of high catecholamine levels on the heart contribute to the downward course of heart failure. The results of clinical trials clearly indicate that such therapy is beneficial if initiated cautiously at low doses, even though acutely blocking the supportive effects of catecholamines can worsen heart failure. Several months of therapy may be required before improvement is noted; this usually consists of a slight rise in ejection fraction, slower heart rate, and reduction in symptoms. As noted above, not all β blockers have proved useful, but **bisoprolol, carvedilol, metoprolol,** and **nebivolol** have been shown to reduce mortality.

In contrast, the calcium-blocking drugs appear to have no role in the treatment of patients with heart failure. Their depressant effects on the heart may worsen failure. On the other hand, slowing of heart rate with **ivabradine** (an I_f blocker, see Chapter 12) may be of benefit.

VASODILATORS

Vasodilator drugs can be divided into selective arteriolar dilators, venous dilators, and drugs with nonselective vasodilating effects. The choice of agent should be based on the patient's signs and symptoms and hemodynamic measurements. Thus, in patients with high filling pressures in whom the principal symptom is dyspnea, venous dilators such as long-acting **nitrates** will be most helpful in reducing filling pressures and the symptoms of pulmonary congestion. In patients in whom fatigue due to low left ventricular output is a primary symptom, an arteriolar dilator such as **hydralazine** may be helpful in increasing forward cardiac output. In most patients with severe chronic failure that responds poorly to other therapy, the problem usually involves both elevated filling pressures and resistance to output. In these circumstances, dilation of both arterioles and veins is required. A fixed combination of hydralazine and isosorbide dinitrate is available as isosorbide dinitrate/hydralazine **(BiDil),** and this has been recommended for use in Black persons. However, as noted above, vasodilator peptides have not been shown to reduce mortality or rehospitalizations for HFrEF.

DIGITALIS

Digoxin is indicated in patients with heart failure and atrial fibrillation. It is usually given only when diuretics and ACE inhibitors have failed to control symptoms. Only about 50% of patients with normal sinus rhythm (usually those with documented systolic dysfunction) will have relief of heart failure from digitalis. If the decision is made to use a cardiac glycoside, digoxin is the one chosen in most cases (and the only one available in the USA). When symptoms are mild, slow loading (digitalization) with 0.125–0.25 mg/d is safer and just as effective as the rapid method (0.5–0.75 mg every 8 hours for three doses, followed by 0.125–0.25 mg/d).

Determining the optimal level of digitalis effect may be difficult. Unfortunately, toxic effects may occur before therapeutic effects are detected. Measurement of plasma digoxin levels is useful in patients who appear unusually resistant or sensitive; a concentration of 1 ng/mL or less is appropriate; higher concentrations may be required in patients with atrial fibrillation.

Because it has a moderate but persistent positive inotropic effect, digitalis can, in theory, reverse all the signs and symptoms of heart failure. Although the net effect of the drug on mortality is mixed, it reduces hospitalization and deaths from progressive heart failure at the expense of an increase in sudden death. It is important to note that the mortality rate is reduced in patients with serum digoxin concentrations of less than 0.9 ng/mL but increased in those with digoxin levels greater than 1.5 ng/mL.

Other Clinical Uses of Digitalis

Digitalis is sometimes useful in the management of atrial arrhythmias because of its cardioselective parasympathomimetic effects. In atrial flutter and fibrillation, the depressant effect of the drug on atrioventricular conduction helps control an excessively high ventricular rate. Digitalis has also been used in the control of paroxysmal atrial and atrioventricular nodal tachycardia. At present, calcium channel blockers and adenosine are preferred for this application. Digoxin is explicitly *contraindicated* in patients with both Wolff-Parkinson-White syndrome and atrial fibrillation (see Chapter 14).

Toxicity

Despite its limited benefits and recognized hazards, digitalis is still often used inappropriately, and toxicity is common. Therapy for toxicity manifested as visual changes or gastrointestinal disturbances generally requires no more than reducing the dose of the drug. If cardiac arrhythmia is present, more vigorous therapy may be necessary. Serum digitalis level, potassium concentration, and the electrocardiogram should always be monitored during therapy of significant digitalis toxicity. Electrolytes should be monitored and corrected if abnormal. Digitalis-induced arrhythmias are frequently made worse by electrical cardioversion; this therapy should be reserved for ventricular fibrillation if the arrhythmia is digitalis-induced.

In severe digitalis intoxication, serum potassium will already be elevated at the time of diagnosis (because of potassium loss from the intracellular compartment of skeletal muscle and other tissues). Automaticity is usually depressed, and antiarrhythmic agents may cause cardiac arrest. Treatment should include prompt insertion of a temporary cardiac pacemaker and administration of **digitalis antibodies.** These antibodies **(digoxin immune fab)** recognize cardiac glycosides from many plants in addition to digoxin. They are extremely useful in reversing severe intoxication with most glycosides. As noted previously, they may also be useful in eclampsia and preeclampsia.

CARDIAC RESYNCHRONIZATION & CARDIAC CONTRACTILITY MODULATION THERAPY

Patients with normal sinus rhythm and a wide QRS interval, eg, greater than 120 ms, have impaired synchronization of right and left ventricular contraction. Poor synchronization of ventricular contraction results in diminished cardiac output. **Resynchronization,** with left ventricular or biventricular pacing, has been shown to reduce mortality in patients with chronic heart failure who were already receiving optimal medical therapy. Because the immediate cause of death in severe heart failure is often an arrhythmia, a combined biventricular pacemaker/cardioverter-defibrillator is usually implanted.

Application of a brief electric current through the myocardium during each QRS deflection of the electrocardiogram results in increased contractility, presumably by increasing Ca^{2+} release, in the intact heart. Preliminary clinical studies of this **cardiac contractility modulation** therapy are under way.

MANAGEMENT OF DIASTOLIC HEART FAILURE

Most authorities support the use of the drug groups described above (Table 13–4). SGLT2 inhibitors are now considered first-line therapy for HFpEF. Control of hypertension is particularly important, hyperlipidemia should be treated, and revascularization should be considered if coronary artery disease is present. ACE inhibitors and ARBs are also useful. In both reduced ejection fraction and preserved ejection fraction forms, the onset of atrial fibrillation may reduce cardiac output significantly and precipitate an episode of acute decompensation. Atrial fibrillation is common in HFpEF, and rhythm control is desirable in both forms. If the arrhythmia is resistant to correction, rate control may be helpful. Even in sinus rhythm, tachycardia limits filling time. Therefore, bradycardic drugs, eg, ivabradine, may be useful, at least in theory.

MANAGEMENT OF ACUTE HEART FAILURE

Acute heart failure occurs frequently in patients with chronic failure. Such episodes are usually associated with increased exertion, emotion, excess salt intake, nonadherence to medical therapy, or increased metabolic demand occasioned by fever, anemia, etc. A particularly common and important cause of acute failure—with or without chronic failure—is acute myocardial infarction. Measurements of arterial pressure, cardiac output, stroke work index, and pulmonary capillary wedge pressure are particularly useful in patients with acute myocardial infarction and acute heart failure. Patients with acute myocardial infarction are often treated with emergency revascularization using either coronary angioplasty and a stent, or a thrombolytic agent. Even with revascularization, acute failure may develop in such patients.

Intravenous treatment is the rule in drug therapy of acute heart failure. Among diuretics, **furosemide** is the most commonly used, usually at high dosage. A recent study suggests that addition of acetazolamide to standard high-dose furosemide has an important additive benefit. **Dopamine** or **dobutamine** are positive inotropic drugs with prompt onset and short durations of action; they are most useful in patients with failure complicated by severe hypotension. **Levosimendan** has been approved for use in acute failure in Europe, and noninferiority has been demonstrated against dobutamine. Vasodilators in use in patients with acute decompensation include **nitroprusside, nitroglycerine,** and nesiritide. Reduction in afterload often improves ejection fraction, but improved survival has not been documented. A small subset of patients in acute heart failure will have dilutional hyponatremia, presumably due to increased vasopressin activity. A V_{1a} and V_2 receptor antagonist, **conivaptan,** is approved for parenteral treatment of euvolemic hyponatremia. Some clinical trials have indicated that this drug and related V_2 antagonists **(tolvaptan)** may have a beneficial effect in some patients with acute heart failure and hyponatremia. However, vasopressin antagonists do not seem to reduce mortality. Clinical trials are under way with the myosin activator, omecamtiv mecarbil.

SUMMARY Drugs Used in Heart Failure

Subclass, Drug	Mechanism of Action	Effects	Clinical Applications	Pharmacokinetics, Toxicities, Interactions
DIURETICS				
• Furosemide	Loop diuretic: Decreases NaCl and KCl reabsorption in thick ascending limb of the loop of Henle in the nephron (see Chapter 15)	Increased excretion of salt and water • reduces cardiac preload and afterload • reduces pulmonary and peripheral edema	Acute and chronic heart failure • severe hypertension • edematous conditions	Oral and IV • duration 2–4 h • *Toxicity:* Hypovolemia, hypokalemia, orthostatic hypotension, ototoxicity, sulfonamide allergy
• SGLT2 inhibitors	Decreases sodium and glucose reabsorption in the proximal tubule; inhibits cardiac sodium-hydrogen exchanger; probable other effects (see Chapter 41)	Increased excretion of salt and water • reduces cardiac preload and afterload • reduces pulmonary and peripheral edema	Acute and chronic heart failure • Type2 diabetes	Oral • Duration 24 h • *Toxicity:* Hypovolemia, genital and urinary infection; contraindicated in type 1 diabetes
• Hydrochlorothiazide	Decreases NaCl reabsorption in the distal convoluted tubule	Same as furosemide, but much less efficacious	Mild chronic failure • mild-moderate hypertension • hypercalciuria • has not been shown to reduce mortality	Oral only • duration 10–12 h • *Toxicity:* Hyponatremia, hypokalemia, hyperglycemia, hyperuricemia, hyperlipidemia, sulfonamide allergy

- *Three other loop diuretics: Bumetanide and torsemide similar to furosemide; ethacrynic acid not a sulfonamide*
- *Many other thiazides: All basically similar to hydrochlorothiazide, differing only in pharmacokinetics*

(continued)

Subclass, Drug	Mechanism of Action	Effects	Clinical Applications	Pharmacokinetics, Toxicities, Interactions
ALDOSTERONE ANTAGONISTS				
• Spironolactone	Blocks cytoplasmic aldosterone receptors in collecting tubules of nephron • possible membrane effect	Increased salt and water excretion • reduces remodeling	Chronic heart failure • aldosteronism (cirrhosis, adrenal tumor) • hypertension • has been shown to reduce mortality	Oral • duration 24–72 h (slow onset and offset) • *Toxicity:* Hyperkalemia, antiandrogen actions
• *Eplerenone: Similar to spironolactone; more selective antimineralocorticoid effect; no significant antiandrogen action; has been shown to reduce mortality*				
ANGIOTENSIN ANTAGONISTS				
Angiotensin-converting enzyme (ACE) inhibitors: • Captopril	Inhibits ACE • reduces AngII formation by inhibiting conversion of AngI to AngII	Arteriolar and venous dilation • reduces aldosterone secretion • reduces cardiac remodeling	Chronic heart failure • hypertension • diabetic renal disease • has been shown to reduce mortality	Oral • half-life 2–4 h but given in large doses so duration 12–24 h • *Toxicity:* Cough, hyperkalemia, angioneurotic edema • *Interactions:* Additive with other angiotensin antagonists
Angiotensin receptor blockers (ARBs): • Losartan	Antagonize AngII effects at AT_1 receptors	Like ACE inhibitors	Like ACE inhibitors • used in patients intolerant to ACE inhibitors • has been shown to reduce mortality	Oral • duration 6–8 h • *Toxicity:* Hyperkalemia, angioneurotic edema • *Interactions:* Additive with other angiotensin antagonists
• *Benazepril, enalapril, many other ACE inhibitors: Like captopril* • *Candesartan, valsartan, many other ARBs: Like losartan*				
BETA BLOCKERS				
• Carvedilol	Competitively blocks β_1 receptors (see Chapter 10)	Slows heart rate • reduces blood pressure • poorly understood other effects	Chronic heart failure: To slow progression • reduce mortality in moderate and severe heart failure • many other indications in Chapter 10	Oral • duration 10–12 h • *Toxicity:* Bronchospasm, bradycardia, atrioventricular block, acute cardiac decompensation • see Chapter 10 for other toxicities and interactions
• *Metoprolol, bisoprolol, nebivolol: Select group of β blockers that have been shown to reduce heart failure mortality*				
CARDIAC GLYCOSIDE				
• Digoxin (other glycosides are used outside the USA)	Na^+/K^+-ATPase inhibition results in reduced Ca^{2+} expulsion and increased Ca^{2+} stored in sarcoplasmic reticulum	Increases cardiac contractility • cardiac parasympathomimetic effect (slowed sinus heart rate, slowed atrioventricular conduction)	Chronic symptomatic heart failure • rapid ventricular rate in atrial fibrillation • has not been shown to reduce mortality but does reduce rehospitalization	Oral, parenteral • duration 36–40 h • *Toxicity:* Nausea, vomiting, diarrhea • cardiac arrhythmias
VASODILATORS				
Venodilators: • Isosorbide dinitrate	Releases nitric oxide (NO) • activates guanylyl cyclase (see Chapter 12)	Venodilation • reduces preload and ventricular stretch	Acute and chronic heart failure • angina	Oral • duration 4–6 h • *Toxicity:* Postural hypotension, tachycardia, headache • *Interactions:* Additive with other vasodilators and synergistic with phosphodiesterase type 5 inhibitors
Arteriolar dilators: • Hydralazine	Probably increases NO synthesis in endothelium (see Chapter 11)	Reduces blood pressure and afterload • results in increased cardiac output	Hydralazine plus nitrates may reduce mortality in African Americans	Oral • duration 8–12 h • *Toxicity:* Tachycardia, fluid retention, lupus-like syndrome
Combined arteriolar and venodilator: • Nitroprusside	Releases NO spontaneously • activates guanylyl cyclase	Marked vasodilation • reduces preload and afterload	Acute cardiac decompensation • hypertensive emergencies (malignant hypertension)	IV only • duration 1–2 min • *Toxicity:* Excessive hypotension, thiocyanate and cyanide toxicity • *Interactions:* Additive with other vasodilators

(continued)

Subclass, Drug	Mechanism of Action	Effects	Clinical Applications	Pharmacokinetics, Toxicities, Interactions
BETA-ADRENOCEPTOR AGONISTS				
• Dobutamine	$Beta_1$-selective agonist • increases cAMP synthesis	Increases cardiac contractility, output	Acute decompensated heart failure	IV only • duration a few minutes • *Toxicity:* Arrhythmias • *Interactions:* Additive with other sympathomimetics
• Dopamine	Dopamine receptor agonist • higher doses activate β and α adrenoceptors	Increases renal blood flow • higher doses increase cardiac force and blood pressure	Acute decompensated heart failure • shock	IV only • duration a few minutes • *Toxicity:* Arrhythmias • *Interactions:* Additive with sympathomimetics
BIPYRIDINES				
• Milrinone	Phosphodiesterase type 3 inhibitor • decreases cAMP breakdown	Vasodilator; lower peripheral vascular resistance • also increases cardiac contractility	Acute decompensated heart failure • *increases* mortality in chronic failure	IV only • duration 3–6 h • *Toxicity:* Arrhythmias • *Interactions:* Additive with other arrhythmogenic agents
NATRIURETIC PEPTIDE				
• Nesiritide	Activates BNP receptors, increases cGMP	Vasodilation • diuresis	Acute decompensated failure • has not been shown to reduce mortality	IV only • duration 18 min • *Toxicity:* Renal damage, hypotension, may *increase* mortality
NEPRILYSIN INHIBITOR				
• Sacubitril (used only in combination with valsartan [ARNI])	Inhibits neprilysin, thus reducing breakdown of ANP and BNP; valsartan inhibits action of angiotensin on its receptors	Vasodilator	Chronic failure • combination reduces mortality and rehospitalizations in HFrEF	Oral • duration 12 h • used only in combination with ARB • *Toxicity:* Hypotension, angioedema

PREPARATIONS AVAILABLE

GENERIC NAME	AVAILABLE AS
DIURETICS	
	(See Chapter 15)
DIGITALIS	
Digoxin	Generic, Lanoxin, Lanoxicaps
DIGITALIS ANTIBODY	
Digoxin immune fab (ovine)	Digibind, DigiFab
SYMPATHOMIMETICS USED IN HEART FAILURE	
Dobutamine	Generic, DOBUTamine
Dopamine	Generic, Intropin
ANGIOTENSIN-CONVERTING ENZYME INHIBITORS	
Benazepril	Generic, Lotensin
Captopril	Generic, Capoten
Enalapril	Generic, Vasotec, Vasotec I.V.
Fosinopril	Generic, Monopril
Lisinopril	Generic, Prinivil, Zestril
Moexipril	Univasc
Perindopril	Aceon
Quinapril	Generic, Accupril
Ramipril	Generic, Altace
Trandolapril	Generic, Mavik
ANGIOTENSIN RECEPTOR BLOCKERS	
Candesartan	Atacand
Eprosartan	Generic, Teveten
Irbesartan	Generic, Avapro
Losartan	Generic, Cozaar
Olmesartan	Benicar
Telmisartan	Generic, Micardis
Valsartan	Diovan
BETA BLOCKERS	
Bisoprolol	Generic, Zebeta
Carvedilol	Generic, Coreg
Metoprolol	Generic, Lopressor, Toprol XL
Nebivolol	Bystolic
ALDOSTERONE ANTAGONISTS	
Eplerenone	Generic, Inspra
Spironolactone	Generic, Aldactone
OTHER DRUGS AND COMBINATIONS	
Bosentan	Tracleer
Dapagliflozin	Farxiga
Empagliflozin	Jardiance
Hydralazine	Generic
Hydralazine plus isosorbide dinitrate	BiDil
Isosorbide dinitrate	Generic, Isordil
Ivabradine	Corlanor
Liraglutide	Victoza
Milrinone	Generic, Primacor
Nesiritide	Natrecor
Sacubitril plus valsartan	Entresto
Semaglutide	Ozempic

REFERENCES

Ahmed A et al: Effectiveness of digoxin in reducing one-year mortality in chronic heart failure in the Digitalis Investigation Group trial. Am J Cardiol 2009;103:82.

Anker SD et al: Empagliflozin in heart failure with a preserved ejection fraction. N Engl J Med 2021;385:1451.

Borlaug BA, Colucci WS: Treatment and prognosis of heart failure with preserved ejection fraction. UpToDate 2022. http://www.UpToDate.com.

Bourge RC et al: Digoxin reduces 30-day all-cause hospital admission in older patients with chronic systolic heart failure. Am J Med 2013;126:701.

Braunwald E: Gliflozins in the management of cardiovascular disease. N Engl J Med 2022;386:2024.

Cleland JCF et al: The effect of cardiac resynchronization on morbidity and mortality in heart failure. N Engl J Med 2005;352:1539.

Cleland JCF et al: The effects of the cardiac myosin activator, omecamtiv mecarbil, on cardiac function in systolic heart failure: A double blind, placebo-controlled, crossover, dose-ranging phase 2 trial. Lancet 2011;378:676.

Colucci WS: Overview of the management of heart failure with reduced ejection fraction in adults. UpToDate 2022. http://www.UpToDate.com.

Colucci WS: Treatment of acute decompensated heart failure: Specific therapies. UpToDate, 2022. http://www.UpToDate.com.

Ellison DM, Felker GM: Diuretic treatment in heart failure. N Engl J Med 2017;377:1964.

Fitchett D et al: Heart failure outcomes with empagliflozin in patients with type 2 diabetes at high cardiovascular risk: Results of the EMPA-REG OUTCOME trial. Eur Heart J 2016;37:1526.

Hasenfuss G, Teerlink JR: Cardiac inotropes: Current agents and future directions. Eur Heart J 2011;32:1838.

Heidenreich PA et al: 2022 AHA/ACC/HFSA Guideline for the Management of Heart Failure: A Report of the American College of Cardiology/American Heart Association Joint Committee on Clinical Practice Guidelines. Circulation 2022;145:e895.

Kozhuharov N et al: Effect of a strategy of comprehensive vasodilation vs usual care on mortality and heart failure rehospitalization among patients with acute heart failure: The GALACTIC randomized clinical trial. JAMA 2019;322:2292.

Lam GK et al: Digoxin antibody fragment, antigen binding (Fab), treatment of preeclampsia in women with endogenous digitalis-like factor: A secondary analysis of the DEEP Trial. Am J Obstet Gynecol 2013;209:119.

Lingrel JB: The physiological significance of the cardiotonic steroid/ouabain-binding site of the Na, K-ATPase. Annu Rev Physiol 2010;72:395.

Lother A, Hein L: Pharmacology of heart failure: From basic science to novel therapies. Pharmacol Ther 2016;166:136.

Marso SP et al: Liraglutide and cardiovascular outcomes in type 2 diabetes. N Engl J Med 2016;375:311.

Mullens W et al: Acetazolamide in acute decompensated heart failure with volume overload. N Engl J Med 2022;387:1185

Mahtani KR et al: Reduced salt intake for heart failure: A systematic review. JAMA Intern Med 2018;178:1693.

Metra M et al: Effects of serelaxin in patients with acute heart failure. N Engl J Med 2019;381:716.

Murphy SP, Ibrahim SE, Januzzi JL: Heart failure with reduced ejection fraction: A review. JAMA 2020;324:488.

Newman RA et al: Cardiac glycosides as novel cancer therapeutic agents. Mol Interv 2008;8:36.

Packer M et al: Effect of ularitide on cardiovascular mortality in acute heart failure. N Engl J Med 2017;376:1956.

Papi L et al: Unexpected double lethal oleander poisoning. Am J Forensic Med Pathol 2012;33:93.

Parry TJ et al: Effects of neuregulin GGF2 (cimaglermin alfa) dose and treatment frequency on left ventricular function in rats following myocardial infarction. Eur J Pharmacol 2017;796:76.

Ponikowski P et al: 2016 ESC guidelines for the diagnosis and treatment of acute and chronic heart failure. Eur J Heart Fail 2016;18:2129.

Pöss J, Link M, Böhm M: Pharmacological treatment of acute heart failure: Current treatment and new targets. Clin Pharmacol Ther 2013;94:499.

Redfield MM, Borlaug BA: Heart failure with preserved ejection fraction. JAMA 2023;329:827.

Samsky MD et al: Cardiogenic shock after acute myocardial infarction. JAMA 2021;326:1840.

Singh AK, Singh R: Heart failure hospitalization with SGLT-2 inhibitors: A systematic review and meta-analysis of randomized controlled and observational studies. Expert Rev Clin Pharmacol 2019;12:299.

Solomon SD et al: Angiotensin-neprilysin inhibition in heart failure with preserved ejection fraction. N Engl J Med 2019;381:1609.

Taur Y, Frishman WH: The cardiac ryanodine receptor (RyR2) and its role in heart disease. Cardiol Rev 2005;13:142.

Teerlink JR et al: Effect of ejection fraction on clinical outcomes in patients treated with omecamtiv mecarbil in GALACTIC-HF. J Am Coll Cardiol 2021;78:97.

Turagam MK et al: Catheter ablation of atrial fibrillation in patients with heart failure: A meta-analysis of randomized controlled trials. Ann Intern Med 2019;170:41.

Velazquez EJ et al: Angiotensin-neprilysin inhibition in acute decompensated heart failure. N Engl J Med 2019;380:539.

Yancy CW et al: 2017 ACC/AHA/HFSA focused update on new pharmacological therapy for heart failure: An update of the 2013 ACCF/AHA Guideline for the Management of Heart Failure: A report of the American College of Cardiology/American Heart Association Task Force on Clinical Practice Guidelines and the Heart Failure Society of America. Circulation 2017;136:e137.

CASE STUDY ANSWER

The patient has a low ejection fraction with systolic heart failure, probably secondary to hypertension. Her heart failure must be treated first, followed by careful control of the hypertension. She was initially treated with a diuretic (furosemide, 40 mg twice daily). On this therapy, she was less short of breath on exertion and could also lie flat without dyspnea. An angiotensin-converting enzyme (ACE) inhibitor was added (enalapril, 20 mg twice daily), and over the next few weeks, she continued to feel better. Because of continued shortness of breath on exercise and mild ankle swelling, dapagliflozin 10 mg daily was added with a further modest improvement. The blood pressure stabilized at 140/90 mm Hg, and the patient will be educated regarding the relation between her hypertension and heart failure and the need for better blood pressure control. Blood lipids, which are currently in the normal range, will be monitored.

CHAPTER

14

Agents Used in Cardiac Arrhythmias

Robert D. Harvey, PhD,
& Augustus O. Grant, MD, PhD

CASE STUDY

A 69-year-old retired teacher presents with a 1-month history of palpitations, intermittent shortness of breath, and fatigue. She has a history of hypertension. An electrocardiogram (ECG) shows atrial fibrillation with a ventricular response of 122 beats/min (bpm) and signs of left ventricular hypertrophy. She is anticoagulated with rivaroxaban and started on sustained-release metoprolol, 50 mg/d. After 7 days, her rhythm reverts to normal sinus rhythm spontaneously. However, over the ensuing month, she continues to have intermittent palpitations and fatigue. Continuous ECG recording over a 48-hour period documents paroxysms of atrial fibrillation with heart rates of 88–114 bpm. An echocardiogram shows a left ventricular ejection fraction of 38% (normal ≥60%) with no localized wall motion abnormality. At this stage, would you initiate treatment with an antiarrhythmic drug to maintain normal sinus rhythm, and if so, what drug would you choose?

Cardiac arrhythmias are a common problem in clinical practice, occurring in up to 25% of patients treated with digitalis, 50% of anesthetized patients, and more than 80% of patients with acute myocardial infarction. Arrhythmias may require treatment because rhythms that are too rapid, too slow, or asynchronous can reduce cardiac output. Some arrhythmias can precipitate more serious or even lethal rhythm disturbances; for example, early premature ventricular depolarizations can precipitate ventricular fibrillation. In such patients, antiarrhythmic drugs may be lifesaving. On the other hand, the hazards of antiarrhythmic drugs—and in particular the fact that they can *precipitate* lethal arrhythmias in some patients—have led to a reevaluation of their relative risks and benefits. In general, treatment of asymptomatic or minimally symptomatic arrhythmias should be avoided for this reason.

Arrhythmias can be treated with the drugs discussed in this chapter and with nonpharmacologic therapies such as pacemakers, cardioversion, catheter ablation, and surgery. This chapter describes the pharmacology of drugs that suppress arrhythmias by a direct action on the cardiac cell membrane. Other modes of therapy are discussed briefly (see Box: The Nonpharmacologic Therapy of Cardiac Arrhythmias, later in the chapter).

ELECTROPHYSIOLOGY OF NORMAL CARDIAC RHYTHM

The electrical impulse that triggers a normal cardiac contraction originates at regular intervals in the sinoatrial (SA) node (Figure 14–1), usually at a frequency of 60–100 bpm. This impulse spreads rapidly through the atria and enters the atrioventricular (AV) node, which is normally the only conduction pathway between the atria and ventricles. Conduction through the AV node is slow, requiring about 0.15 seconds. (This delay provides time for atrial contraction to propel blood into the ventricles.) The impulse then propagates down the His-Purkinje system and invades all parts of the ventricles, beginning with the endocardial surface near the apex and ending with the epicardial surface at the base of the heart. Activation of the entire ventricular myocardium is complete in less than 0.1 seconds.

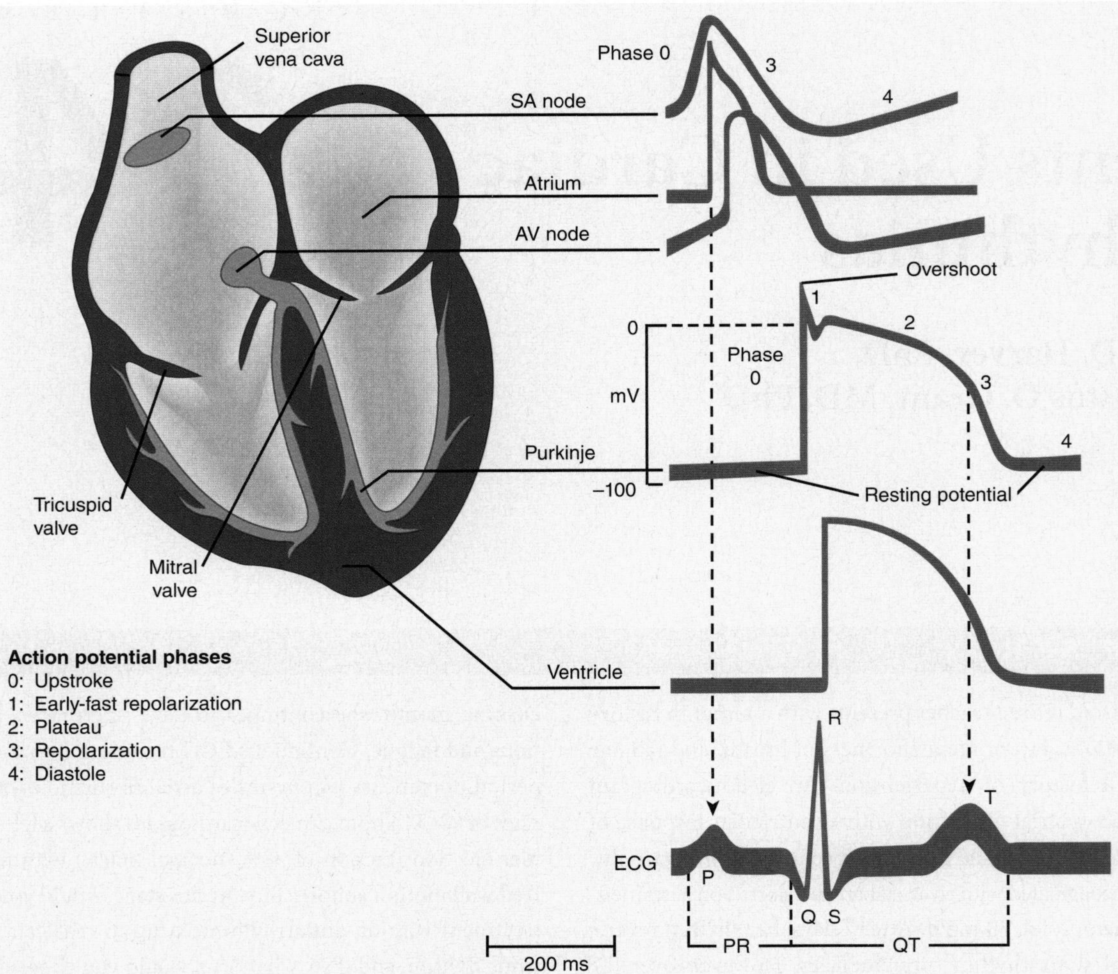

FIGURE 14–1 Schematic representation of the heart and normal cardiac electrical activity (intracellular recordings from areas indicated and electrocardiogram [ECG]). Sinoatrial (SA) node, atrioventricular (AV) node, and Purkinje cells display pacemaker activity (phase 4 depolarization). The ECG is the body surface manifestation of the depolarization and repolarization waves of the heart. The P wave is generated by atrial depolarization, the QRS by ventricular muscle depolarization, and the T wave by ventricular repolarization. Thus, the PR interval is a measure of conduction time from atrium to ventricle, and the QRS duration indicates the time required for all of the ventricular cells to be activated (ie, the intraventricular conduction time). The QT interval reflects the duration of the ventricular action potential.

As a result, ventricular contraction is synchronous and hemodynamically effective. *Arrhythmias represent electrical activity that deviates from the above description as a result of an abnormality in impulse initiation and/or impulse propagation.*

Ionic Basis of Membrane Electrical Activity

The electrical excitability of cardiac cells is a function of the unequal distribution of ions across the plasma membrane—chiefly sodium (Na^+), potassium (K^+), calcium (Ca^{2+}), and chloride (Cl^-)—and the relative permeability of the membrane to each ion. The gradients are generated by transport mechanisms that move these ions across the membrane against their concentration gradients. The most important of these transport mechanisms is the Na^+/K^+-ATPase, or sodium pump, described in Chapter 13. It is responsible for keeping the intracellular sodium concentration low and the intracellular potassium concentration high relative to their respective extracellular concentrations. Other transport mechanisms maintain the gradients for calcium and chloride.

As a result of the unequal distribution, when the membrane becomes permeable to a given ion, that ion tends to move down its concentration gradient. However, because of its charged nature, ion movement is also affected by differences in the electrical charge across the membrane, or the transmembrane potential. The potential difference that is sufficient to offset or balance the concentration gradient of an ion is referred to as the **equilibrium potential** (E_{ion}) for that ion, and for a monovalent cation at physiologic temperature, it can be calculated by a modified version of the **Nernst equation:**

$$E_{ion} = 61 \times \log\left(\frac{C_e}{C_i}\right)$$

where C_e and C_i are the extracellular and intracellular ion concentrations, respectively. Thus, the movement of an ion across the membrane of a cell is a function of the difference between the transmembrane potential and the equilibrium potential. This is also known as the "electrochemical gradient" or "driving force."

The relative permeability of the membrane to different ions determines the transmembrane potential. However, ions contributing to this potential difference are unable to freely diffuse across the lipid membrane of a cell. Their permeability relies on aqueous channels (specific pore-forming proteins). The ion channels that are thought to contribute to cardiac action potentials are illustrated in Figure 14–2. Most channels are relatively ion-specific, and the current generated by the flux of ions through them is controlled by "gates" (flexible portions of the peptide chains that make up the channel proteins). Sodium, calcium, and some potassium channels are thought to have two types of gates—one that opens or activates the channel and another that closes or inactivates the channel. For the majority of the channels responsible for the cardiac action potential, the movement of these gates is controlled by voltage changes across the cell membrane; that is, they are voltage-sensitive. However, certain channels are primarily ligand- rather than voltage-gated. Furthermore, the activity of many voltage-gated ion channels can be modulated by a variety of other factors, including permeant ion concentrations, tissue metabolic activity, and second messenger signaling pathways.

Pumps and exchangers that contribute indirectly to the membrane potential by creating ion gradients (as discussed above) can also contribute directly because of the current they generate through the unequal exchange of charged ions across the membrane. Such transporters are referred to as being "electrogenic." An important example is the sodium-calcium exchanger (NCX). Throughout most of the cardiac action potential, this exchanger couples the movement of one calcium ion out of the cell for every three sodium ions that move in, thus generating a net inward or depolarizing current. Although this current is typically small during diastole, when intracellular calcium concentrations are low, spontaneous release of calcium from intracellular storage sites can activate this exchange mechanism, generating a depolarizing current that contributes to pacemaker activity as well as arrhythmogenic events called delayed afterdepolarizations (see below).

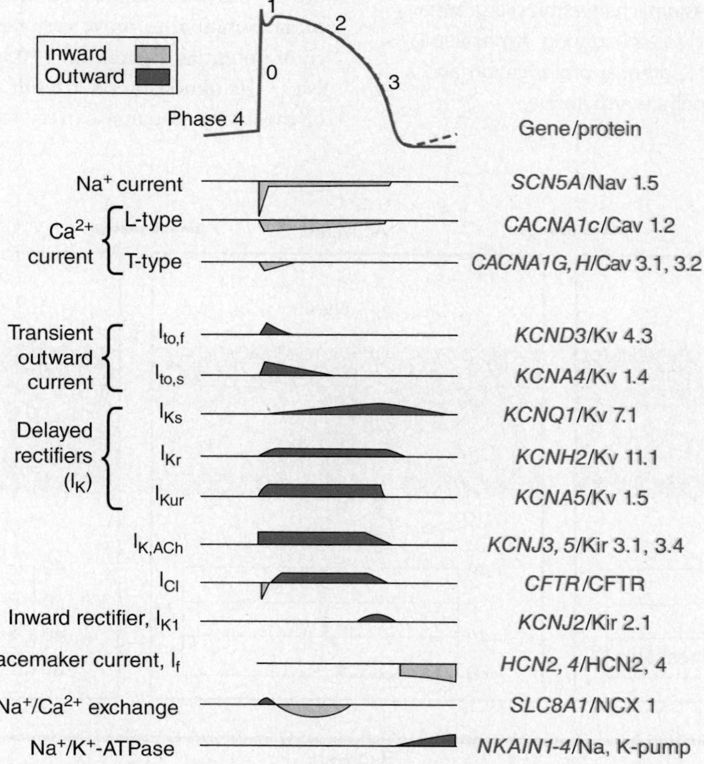

FIGURE 14–2 Schematic diagram of the ion permeability changes and transport processes that occur during an action potential. Yellow indicates inward (depolarizing) membrane currents; blue indicates outward (repolarizing) membrane currents. Multiple subtypes of potassium and calcium currents, with different sensitivities to blocking drugs, have been identified. The right side of the figure lists the genes and proteins responsible for each type of channel or transporter.

Effects of Potassium

Changes in serum potassium can have profound effects on electrical activity of the heart. An increase in serum potassium, or *hyperkalemia,* can depolarize the resting membrane potential due to changes in E_K. If the depolarization is great enough, it can inactivate some of the sodium channels, resulting in increased refractory period duration and slowed impulse propagation. Conversely, a decrease in serum potassium, or *hypokalemia,* can hyperpolarize the resting membrane potential. This can lead to an increase in pacemaker activity due to greater activation of pacemaker channels, especially in latent pacemakers (eg, Purkinje cells), which are more sensitive to changes in serum potassium than normal pacemaker cells.

In addition to effects on the potassium *electrochemical gradient*, changes in serum potassium can also produce effects that appear somewhat paradoxical, especially as they relate to action potential duration. This is because changes in serum potassium also affect the potassium *conductance* (increased potassium increases the conductance, whereas decreased potassium decreases the conductance), and this effect often predominates. As a result, *hyperkalemia* can reduce action potential duration, and *hypokalemia* can prolong action potential duration. This effect of potassium probably contributes to the observed increase in sensitivity to potassium channel-blocking antiarrhythmic agents (quinidine or sotalol) during hypokalemia, resulting in accentuated action potential prolongation and a tendency to cause torsades de pointes arrhythmia.

The Active Cell Membrane

In atrial and ventricular cells, the diastolic membrane potential (phase 4) is typically very stable. This is because it is dominated by a potassium permeability or conductance that is due to the activity of channels that generate an inward-rectifying potassium current (I_{K1}). This keeps the membrane potential near the potassium equilibrium potential, E_K (about –90 mV when K_e = 5 mmol/L and K_i = 150 mmol/L). It also explains why small changes in extracellular potassium concentration have significant effects on the resting membrane potential of these cells. For example, increasing extracellular potassium shifts the equilibrium potential in a positive direction, causing depolarization of the resting membrane potential. It is important to note, however, that potassium is unique in that changes in the extracellular concentration can also affect the permeability of potassium channels, which can produce some nonintuitive effects (see Box: Effects of Potassium).

The upstroke (phase 0) of the action potential is due to the inward sodium current (I_{Na}). From a functional point of view, the behavior of the channels responsible for this current can be described in terms of three states (Figure 14–3). It is now recognized that these states actually represent different conformations of the channel protein. Depolarization of the membrane by an impulse propagating from adjacent cells results in opening of the activation (*m*) gates of sodium channels (see Figure 14–3, middle), and sodium permeability is markedly increased. Extracellular sodium is then able to diffuse down its electrochemical gradient into the cell, causing the membrane potential to move very rapidly toward the sodium equilibrium potential, E_{Na} (about +70 mV when Na_e = 140 mmol/L and Na_i = 10 mmol/L). As a result, the maximum upstroke velocity of the action potential is very fast. This intense influx of sodium

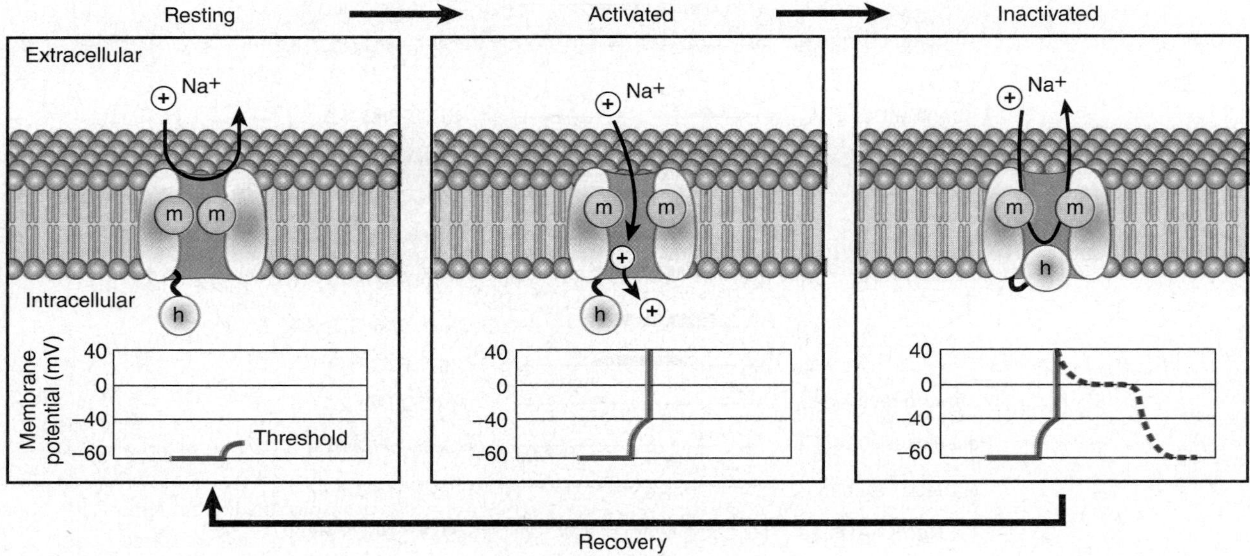

FIGURE 14–3 A schematic representation of Na^+ channels cycling through different conformational states during the cardiac action potential. Transitions between resting, activated, and inactivated states are dependent on membrane potential and time. The activation gate is shown as *m* and the inactivation gate as *h*. Potentials typical for each state are shown under each channel schematic as a function of time. The dashed line indicates that part of the action potential during which most Na^+ channels are completely or partially inactivated and unavailable for reactivation.

is very brief because opening of the *m* gates upon depolarization is promptly followed by closure of the *h* gates and inactivation of these channels (see Figure 14–3, right). This inactivation contributes to the early repolarization phase of the action potential (phase 1). In some cardiac myocytes, phase 1 is also due to a brief increase in potassium permeability due to the activity of channels generating fast and slow transient outward currents ($I_{to,f}$ and $I_{to,s}$).

A small fraction of the sodium channels activated during the upstroke may actually remain open well into the later phases of the action potential, generating a late sodium current (I_{NaL}). However, sustained depolarization during the plateau (phase 2) is due primarily to the activity of calcium channels. Because the equilibrium potential for calcium, like sodium, is very positive, these channels generate a depolarizing inward current. Cardiac calcium channels activate and inactivate in what appears to be a manner similar to sodium channels, but in the case of the most common type of calcium channel (the "L" type), the transitions occur more slowly and at more positive potentials. After activation, these channels eventually inactivate decreasing the permeability to calcium, and the permeability to potassium begins to increase, leading to final repolarization (phase 3) of the action potential. Two types of potassium channels are particularly important in phase 3 repolarization. They generate what are referred to as the rapidly activating (I_{Kr}) and slowly activating (I_{Ks}) delayed rectifier potassium currents. Repolarization, especially late in phase 3, is also aided by the inward rectifying potassium channels that are responsible for the resting membrane potential.

It is noteworthy that other delayed rectifier-type potassium currents also play important roles in repolarization of certain cardiac cell types. For example, the ultra-rapidly activating delayed rectifier potassium current (I_{Kur}) is particularly important in repolarizing the atrial action potential. The resting membrane potential and repolarization of atrial myocytes are also affected by a potassium current ($I_{K,ACh}$) generated by channels that are gated by the parasympathetic neurotransmitter acetylcholine.

Purkinje cells are similar to atrial and ventricular cells in that they generate an action potential with a fast upstroke due to the activity of sodium channels. However, unlike atrial and ventricular cells, the membrane potential during phase 4 exhibits spontaneous depolarization. This is due to the presence of pacemaker channels that generate an inward depolarizing pacemaker current. This is sometimes referred to as the "funny" current (I_f), because the channels involved have the unusual property of being activated by membrane hyperpolarization. Under some circumstances, Purkinje cells can act as pacemakers for the heart by spontaneously depolarizing and initiating an action potential that is then propagated throughout the ventricular myocardium. However, under normal conditions, the action potential in Purkinje cells is triggered by impulses that originate in the SA node and are conducted to these cells through the AV node.

Pacemaking activity in the SA node is due to spontaneous depolarization during phase 4 of the action potential as well (see Figure 14–1). This diastolic depolarization is mediated in part by the activity of pacemaker channels (I_f). It is also thought to be due to the net inward current generated by the sodium-calcium exchanger, which is activated by the spontaneous release of calcium from intracellular storage sites. Unlike the action potential in Purkinje cells, spontaneous depolarization in the SA node triggers the upstroke of an action potential that is primarily due to an increase in permeability to calcium, not sodium. Because the calcium channels involved open or activate slowly, the maximum upstroke velocity of the action potential in SA node cells is relatively slow. Repolarization occurs when the calcium channels subsequently close due to inactivation and delayed rectifier-type potassium channels open.

A similar process is involved in generating action potentials in the AV node. Although the intrinsic rate of spontaneous diastolic depolarization in the AV node is typically faster than that of Purkinje cells, it is still slower than the rate of depolarization in the SA node. Therefore, action potentials in the AV node are normally triggered by impulses that originate in the SA node and are conducted to the AV node through the atria. It is important to recognize that action potential upstroke velocity is a key determinant of impulse conduction velocity. Because the action potential upstroke in AV node cells is mediated by calcium channels, which open or activate relatively slowly, impulse conduction through the AV node is slow. This contributes to the delay between atrial and ventricular contraction.

Electrical activity in the SA node and AV node is significantly influenced by the autonomic nervous system (see Chapter 6). Sympathetic activation of β adrenoceptors speeds pacemaker activity in the SA node and impulse propagation through the AV node by enhancing pacemaker and calcium channel activity, respectively. Conversely, parasympathetic activation of muscarinic receptors slows pacemaker activity and conduction velocity by inhibiting the activity of these channels, as well as by increasing the potassium conductance by turning on acetylcholine-activated potassium channels.

The Effect of Membrane Potential on Excitability

A key factor in the pathophysiology of arrhythmias and the actions of antiarrhythmic agents is the relationship between the membrane potential and the effect it has on the ion channels responsible for excitability of the cell. During the plateau of atrial, ventricular, or Purkinje cell action potentials, most sodium channels are inactivated, rendering the cell refractory or inexcitable. Upon repolarization, recovery from inactivation takes place (in the terminology of Figure 14–3, the *h* gates reopen), making the channels available again for excitation. This is a time- and voltage-dependent process. The actual time required for enough sodium channels to recover from inactivation in order that a new propagated response can be generated is called the **refractory period.** Full recovery of excitability typically does not occur until action potential repolarization is complete. Thus, refractoriness or excitability can be affected by factors that alter either action potential duration or the resting membrane potential. This relationship can also be significantly impacted by certain classes of antiarrhythmic agents. One example is drugs that block sodium channels. They can reduce the extent and rate of recovery from inactivation (Figure 14–4). Changes in refractoriness caused by either altered recovery from inactivation or altered action potential duration can be important in the genesis or suppression of certain arrhythmias. A reduction in the number of available sodium

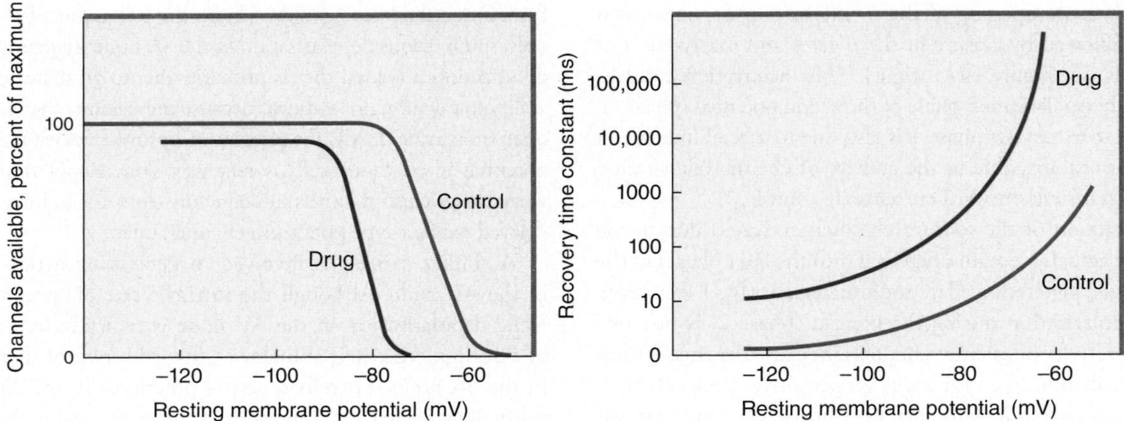

FIGURE 14–4 Dependence of sodium channel function on the membrane potential preceding the stimulus. **Left:** The fraction of sodium channels available for opening in response to a stimulus is determined by the membrane potential immediately preceding the stimulus. The decrease in the fraction available when the resting potential is depolarized in the absence of a drug (control curve) results from the voltage-dependent closure of *h* gates in the channels. The curve labeled *Drug* illustrates the effect of a typical local anesthetic antiarrhythmic drug. Most sodium channels are inactivated during the plateau of the action potential. **Right:** The time constant for recovery from inactivation after repolarization also depends on the resting potential. In the absence of drug, recovery occurs in less than 10 ms at normal resting potentials (−85 to −95 mV). Depolarized cells recover more slowly (note logarithmic scale). In the presence of a sodium channel-blocking drug, the time constant of recovery is increased, but the increase is far greater at depolarized potentials than at more negative ones.

channels can reduce excitability. In some cases, it may result in the cell being totally refractory or inexcitable. In other cases, there may be a reduction in peak sodium permeability. This can reduce the maximum upstroke velocity of the action potential, which will in turn reduce action potential conduction velocity.

In cells like those found in the SA and AV nodes, where excitability is determined by the availability of calcium channels, excitability is most sensitive to drugs that block these channels. As a result, calcium channel blockers can decrease pacemaker activity in the SA node as well as conduction velocity in the AV node.

MECHANISMS OF ARRHYTHMIAS

Many factors can precipitate or exacerbate arrhythmias: ischemia, hypoxia, acidosis or alkalosis, electrolyte abnormalities, excessive catecholamine exposure, autonomic influences, drug toxicity (eg, digitalis or antiarrhythmic drugs), overstretching of cardiac fibers, and the presence of scarred or otherwise diseased tissue. However, all arrhythmias result from (1) disturbances in impulse formation and/or (2) disturbances in impulse conduction.

Disturbances of Impulse Formation

Pacemaking activity is regulated by both sympathetic and parasympathetic activity (see above). Therefore, factors that antagonize or enhance these effects can alter normal impulse formation, producing either bradycardia or tachycardia. Genetic mutations have also been found to alter normal pacemaking activity.

Under certain circumstances, abnormal activity can be generated by latent pacemakers, cells that show slow phase 4 depolarization even under normal conditions (eg, Purkinje cells). Such cells are particularly prone to accelerated pacemaker activity, especially under conditions such as hypokalemia. Abnormalities in impulse formation can also be the result of afterdepolarizations (Figure 14–5). These can be either **early afterdepolarizations (EADs),** which occur during phase 3 of the action potential, or **delayed afterdepolarizations (DADs),** which occur during phase 4. EADs are usually triggered by factors that prolong action potential duration. When this prolongation occurs in ventricular cells, there is often a corresponding increase in the QT interval of the

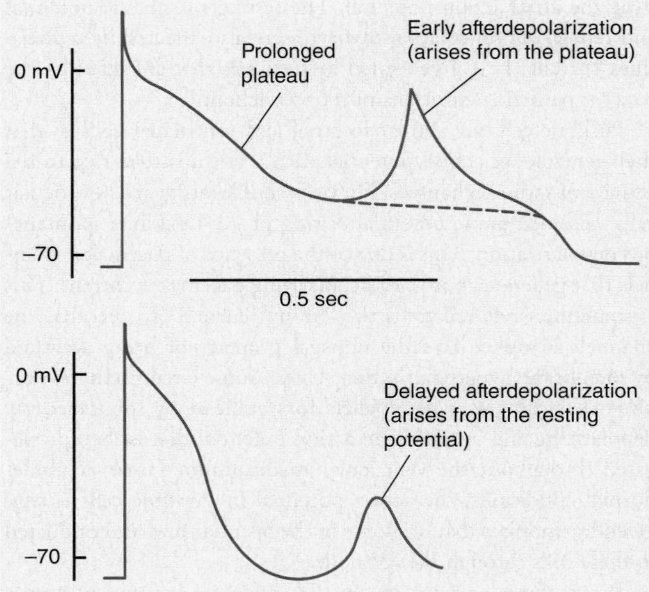

FIGURE 14–5 Two forms of abnormal activity, early (**top**) and delayed afterdepolarizations (**bottom**). In both cases, abnormal depolarizations arise during or after a normally evoked action potential. They are therefore often referred to as "triggered" automaticity; that is, they require a normal action potential for their initiation.

electrocardiogram (ECG). Such an effect can be caused by genetic mutations associated with congenital long QT (LQT) syndrome (see Box: Molecular & Genetic Basis of Cardiac Arrhythmias). A number of drugs (antiarrhythmic as well as non-antiarrhythmic agents) can produce "acquired" or drug-induced LQT syndrome, which is typically due to block of rapidly activating delayed rectifier potassium channels. Many forms of LQT syndrome are exacerbated by other factors that prolong action potential duration, including hypokalemia and *slow* heart rates. DADs, on the other hand, often occur when there is an excess accumulation of intracellular calcium (see Chapter 13), especially at *fast* heart rates. They are thought to be responsible for arrhythmias associated with digitalis toxicity, excess catecholamine stimulation, and myocardial ischemia.

Molecular & Genetic Basis of Cardiac Arrhythmias

It is now possible to define the molecular basis of several congenital and acquired cardiac arrhythmias. The best example is the polymorphic ventricular tachycardia known as torsades de pointes (Figure 14–8), which is associated with prolongation of the QT interval (especially at the onset of the tachycardia), syncope, and sudden death. This represents prolongation of the action potential of at least some ventricular cells (Figure 14–1). The effect can, in theory, be attributed to either increased inward current (gain of function) or decreased outward current (loss of function) during the plateau of the action potential. Action potential prolongation is thought to generate early afterdepolarizations (Figure 14–5) that then trigger torsades de pointes.

Molecular genetic studies have identified up to 1400 different mutations in at least 15 ion channel genes that produce congenital long QT (LQT) syndrome (Table 14–1). Loss-of-function mutations in potassium channel genes (*KCNH2, KCNE2, KCNQ1, KCNE1*, and *KCNJ2*) result in decreased outward plateau current, while gain-of-function mutations in the sodium channel gene (*SCN5A*) or calcium channel gene (*CACNA1c*) cause increases in inward plateau current. Mutations in other genes (such as *ANK2*) contribute to altered electrical activity by more complex mechanisms.

The identification of the precise molecular mechanisms underlying various forms of the LQT syndromes now raises the possibility that specific therapies may be developed for individuals with defined molecular abnormalities. Indeed, the sodium channel blocker mexiletine can correct the clinical manifestations of congenital LQT subtype 3, while β-blockers have been used to prevent arrhythmias triggered by sympathetic stimulation in patients with LQT subtype 1.

The molecular basis of several other congenital cardiac arrhythmias associated with sudden death has also been identified. At least three forms of short QT syndrome have been identified that are linked to gain-of-function mutations in different potassium channel genes (*KCNH2, KCNQ1*, and *KCNJ2*). Catecholaminergic polymorphic ventricular tachycardia, a disease that is characterized by stress- or emotion-induced syncope, can be caused by mutations in at least two different genes (*hRyR2* and *CASQ2*) of proteins expressed in the sarcoplasmic reticulum that control intracellular calcium homeostasis. Mutations in two different ion channel genes (*HCN4* and *SCN5A*) have been linked to congenital forms of sick sinus syndrome. Several forms of Brugada syndrome, which is characterized by ventricular fibrillation associated with persistent ST-segment elevation, and progressive cardiac conduction disorder (PCCD), which is characterized by impaired conduction in the His-Purkinje system and right or left bundle block leading to complete AV block, have been linked to loss-of-function mutations in the sodium channel gene (*SCN5A*). At least one form of familial atrial fibrillation is caused by a gain-of-function mutation in a potassium channel gene (*KCNQ1*).

Disturbances of Impulse Conduction

The most common form of conduction disturbance affects the AV node, causing various degrees of **heart block.** The result can be a simple slowing of impulse propagation through the AV node, which is reflected by an increase in the PR interval of the ECG. At the extreme, the result can be complete heart block, where no impulses are conducted from the atria to the ventricles. In this situation, ventricular activity must be generated by a latent pacemaker, such as a Purkinje cell, or by an artificial pacemaker. Because the AV node is typically under the tonic influence of the parasympathetic nervous system, which slows conduction, AV block can sometimes be relieved by antimuscarinic agents like atropine.

A serious form of conduction abnormality involves **reentry** (also known as "circus movement"). In this situation, one impulse reenters and excites areas of the heart more than once. The path of the reentering impulse may be confined to very small areas, such as tissue within or near the AV node or where a Purkinje fiber makes contact with the ventricular wall (Figure 14–6), or it may involve large portions of the atria or ventricles. Some forms of reentry are strictly anatomically determined. For example, in Wolff-Parkinson-White syndrome, the reentry circuit consists of atrial tissue, the AV node, ventricular tissue, and an accessory AV connection (bundle of Kent, a bypass tract). Depending on how many round trips through the pathway a reentrant impulse makes before dying out, the arrhythmia may be manifest as one or a few extra beats or as a sustained tachycardia. Circulating impulses can also give off "daughter impulses" that can spread to the rest of the heart. In cases such as atrial or ventricular fibrillation, multiple reentry circuits may meander through the heart in apparently random paths, resulting in the loss of synchronized contraction.

An example of how reentry can occur is illustrated in Figure 14–6. In this scenario, there are three key elements: (1) First is an obstacle

TABLE 14–1 Molecular and genetic basis of some cardiac arrhythmias.

Type	Chromosome Involved	Defective Gene	Ion Channel or Proteins Affected	Result
LQT-1	11	*KCNQ1*	I_{Ks}	LF
LQT-2	7	*KCNH2 (HERG)*	I_{Kr}	LF
LQT-3	3	*SCN5A*	I_{Na}	GF
LQT-4	4	*ANK2*	Ankyrin-B[1]	LF
LQT-5	21	*KCNE1*[2]	I_{Ks}	LF
LQT-6	21	*KCNE2*[3]	I_{Kr}	LF
LQT-7[4]	17	*KCNJ2*	I_{Kir}	LF
LQT-8[5]	12	*CACNA1C*	I_{Ca}	GF
SQT-1	7	*KCNH2*	I_{Kr}	GF
SQT-2	11	*KCNQ1*	I_{Ks}	GF
SQT-3	17	*KCNJ2*	I_{Kir}	GF
CPVT-1[6]	1	*RYR2*	Ryanodine receptor	GF
CPVT-2	1	*CASQ2*	Calsequestrin	LF
Sick sinus syndrome	15 or 3	*HCN4 or SCN5A*[7]	I_f or I_{Na}	LF
Brugada syndrome	3	*SCN5A*	I_{Na}	LF
PCCD	3	*SCN5A*	I_{Na}	LF
Familial atrial fibrillation	11	*KCNQ1*	I_{Ks}	GF

[1]Ankyrins are intracellular proteins that associate with a variety of transport proteins including Na^+ channels, Na^+/K^+-ATPase, Na^+, Ca^{2+} exchange, and Ca^{2+} release channels.

[2]*KCNE1* encodes an auxiliary subunit that together with the pore forming subunit encoded by *KCNQ1* creates the functional channel responsible for I_{Ks}.

[2]*KCNE2* encodes an auxiliary subunit that together with the pore forming subunit encoded by *KCNH2* creates the functional channel responsible for I_{Kr}.

[4]Also known as Andersen-Tawil syndrome; multisystem disorder, including periodic paralysis.

[5]Also known as Timothy syndrome; multisystem disorder, including autism.

[6]CPVT, catecholaminergic polymorphic ventricular tachycardia; mutations in intracellular ryanodine Ca^{2+} release channel or the Ca^{2+} buffer protein, calsequestrin, may result in enhanced sarcoplasmic reticulum Ca^{2+} leakage or enhanced Ca^{2+} release during adrenergic stimulation, causing triggered arrhythmogenesis.

[7]*HCN4* encodes a pacemaker current in sinoatrial nodal cells; mutations in sodium channel gene (*SCN5A*) cause conduction defects.

GF, gain of function; LF, loss of function; LQT, long QT syndrome; PCCD, progressive cardiac conduction disorder; SQT, short QT syndrome.

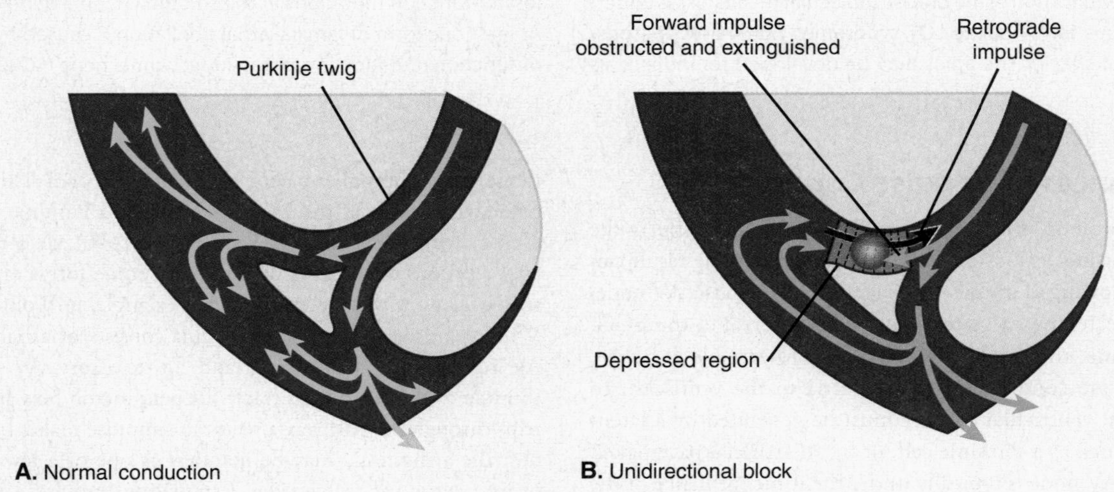

FIGURE 14–6 Schematic diagram of a reentry circuit that might occur in small bifurcating branches of the Purkinje system where they enter the ventricular wall. **A:** Normally, electrical excitation branches around the circuit, is transmitted to the ventricular branches, and becomes extinguished at the other end of the circuit due to collision of impulses. **B:** An area of unidirectional block develops in one of the branches, preventing anterograde impulse transmission at the site of block, but the retrograde impulse may be propagated through the site of block if the impulse finds excitable tissue; that is, the refractory period is shorter than the conduction time. This impulse then re-excites tissue it had previously passed through, and a reentry arrhythmia is established.

(anatomic or physiologic) to homogeneous impulse conduction, thus establishing a circuit around which the reentrant wave front can propagate. (2) The second element is unidirectional block at some point in the circuit. That is, something has occurred such that an impulse reaching the site initially encounters refractory tissue. This can occur under conditions such as ischemia, which cause an increase in extracellular potassium that partially depolarizes the resting membrane potential, slowing sodium channel recovery from inactivation and prolonging the refractory period in the affected area. (3) Finally, conduction time around the circuit must be long enough so that by the time the impulse returns to the site after traveling around the obstacle, the tissue is no longer refractory. In other words, conduction time around the circuit must exceed the effective refractory period duration in the area of unidirectional block. Representative ECGs of important arrhythmias are shown in Figures 14–7 and 14–8.

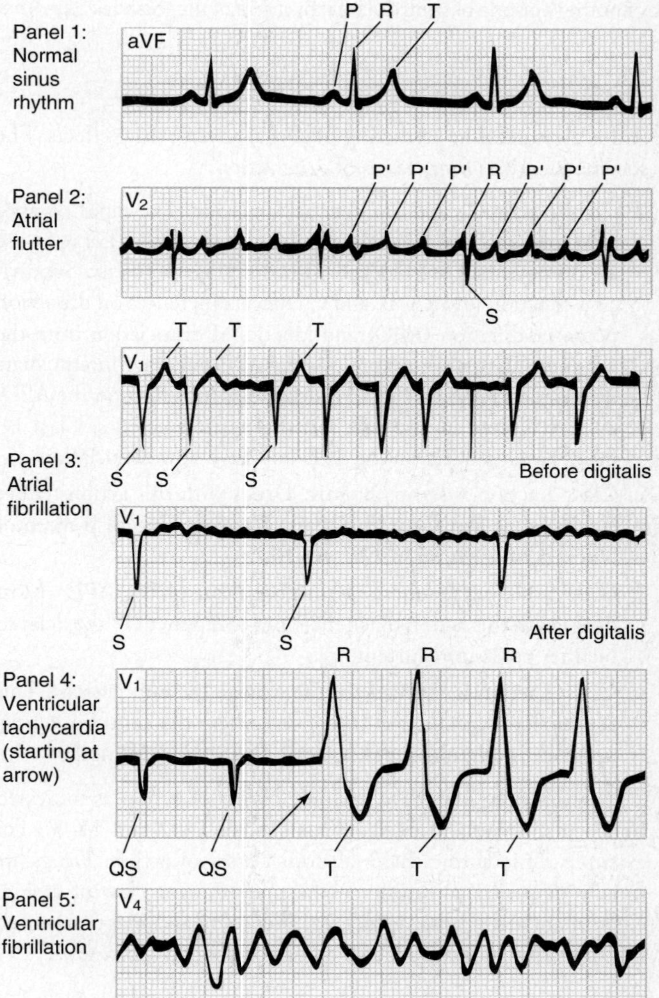

FIGURE 14–7 Electrocardiograms of normal sinus rhythm and some common arrhythmias. Major deflections (P, Q, R, S, and T) are labeled in each electrocardiographic record except in panel 5, in which electrical activity is completely disorganized and none of these deflections is recognizable. (Reproduced with permission from Goldman MJ: *Principles of Clinical Electrocardiography*. 11th ed. New York: McGraw Hill; 1982.)

Unidirectional block can be caused by prolongation of refractory period duration due to depression of sodium channel activity in atrial, ventricular, and Purkinje cells. In the AV node, it may also be a result of depressed calcium channel activity. Drugs that abolish reentry may do so by further reducing excitability by blocking sodium (see Figure 14–4) or calcium channels, thus converting an area of unidirectional block to bidirectional block. Drugs that block repolarizing potassium currents may also be effective in converting a region of unidirectional block to bidirectional block by prolonging action potential duration, and thereby increasing the refractory period duration.

BASIC PHARMACOLOGY OF THE ANTIARRHYTHMIC AGENTS

Mechanisms of Action

Arrhythmias are caused by abnormal pacemaker activity or abnormal impulse propagation. Thus, the aim of therapy of the arrhythmias is to reduce ectopic pacemaker activity and modify conduction or refractoriness in reentry circuits to disable circus movement. The major pharmacologic mechanisms currently available for accomplishing these goals are (1) sodium channel blockade, (2) blockade of sympathetic autonomic effects in the heart, (3) prolongation of the effective refractory period, and (4) calcium channel blockade.

Antiarrhythmic drugs decrease the automaticity of ectopic pacemakers more than that of the SA node. They also reduce conduction and excitability and increase the refractory period to a greater extent in depolarized tissue than in normally polarized tissue. This is accomplished chiefly by selectively blocking the sodium or calcium channels of depolarized cells (Figure 14–9). Therapeutically useful channel-blocking drugs bind readily to activated channels (ie, during phase 0) or inactivated channels (ie, during phase 2) but bind poorly or not at all to rested channels. Therefore, these drugs block electrical activity when there is a fast tachycardia (repeated cycles of activation and inactivation in a short period of time) or when there is significant loss of resting potential (many inactivated channels during rest). This type of drug action is often described as **use-dependent** or **state-dependent;** that is, channels that are being used frequently, or are in an inactivated state, are more susceptible to block. Channels in normal cells that become blocked by a drug during normal activation-inactivation cycles will rapidly lose the drug from the receptors during the resting portion of the cycle (see Figure 14–9). Channels in myocardium that is chronically depolarized (ie, has a resting potential more positive than −75 mV) recover from block very slowly if at all (see also right panel, Figure 14–4).

In cells with abnormal automaticity, most of these drugs reduce the phase 4 slope by blocking either sodium or calcium channels, thereby reducing the ratio of sodium (or calcium) permeability to potassium permeability. As a result, the membrane potential during phase 4 stabilizes closer to the potassium equilibrium potential. In addition, some agents may increase the threshold (make it more positive). Beta-adrenoceptor-blocking drugs indirectly

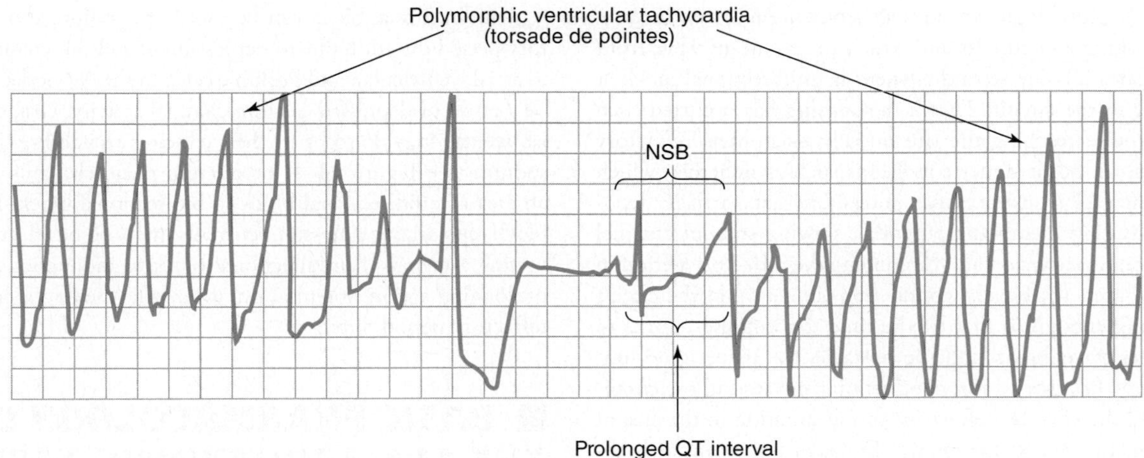

FIGURE 14–8 Electrocardiogram from a patient with long QT syndrome during two episodes of torsades de pointes. The polymorphic ventricular tachycardia is seen at the start of this tracing and spontaneously halts at the middle of the panel. A single normal sinus beat (NSB) with an extremely prolonged QT interval follows, succeeded immediately by another episode of ventricular tachycardia of the torsades type. The usual symptoms include dizziness or transient loss of consciousness.

reduce the phase 4 slope by blocking the positive chronotropic action of norepinephrine in the heart.

In reentry arrhythmias, which depend on critically depressed conduction, most antiarrhythmic agents slow conduction further by one or both of two mechanisms: (1) steady-state reduction in the number of available unblocked channels, which reduces the excitatory currents to a level below that required for propagation (see Figure 14–4, left); and (2) prolongation of recovery time of the channels still able to reach the rested and available state, which increases the effective refractory period (see Figure 14–4, right). As a result, early extrasystoles are unable to propagate at all; later impulses propagate more slowly and are subject to bidirectional conduction block.

By these mechanisms, antiarrhythmic drugs can suppress ectopic automaticity and abnormal conduction occurring in depolarized cells—rendering them electrically silent—while minimally affecting the electrical activity in normally polarized parts of the heart. However, as dosage is increased, these agents also depress conduction in normal tissue, eventually resulting in *drug-induced* arrhythmias. Furthermore, a drug concentration that is therapeutic (antiarrhythmic) under the initial circumstances of treatment may become "proarrhythmic" (arrhythmogenic) during fast heart rates (more development of block), acidosis (slower recovery from block for most drugs), hyperkalemia, or ischemia.

■ SPECIFIC ANTIARRHYTHMIC AGENTS

The Singh-Vaughan Williams classification of antiarrhythmic agents is the most widely used scheme. This classification should be viewed as a method for classifying drug actions. The scheme offers potential mechanisms of the therapeutic action of drugs and is also useful in predicting potential adverse drug effects. The scheme identifies four classes of drug action:

1. Class 1 action is sodium channel blockade. The rapid component (phase 0) and the slow component (phase 2) of fast response action potentials are blocked with differing specificity. Subdivision of action into 1A, B, and C reflects differences on the action potential duration (APD) and kinetics of dissociation from the channel. Class 1A drugs prolong the APD and have intermediate dissociation kinetics. Class 1B drugs have no effect on the APD, or may shorten it, and have fast dissociation kinetics. Class 1C drugs have no effect on the APD and have slow dissociation.
2. Class 2 action is sympatholytic. Drugs with this action reduce β-adrenergic activity in the heart. The subgroup of β-receptor blockers is discussed in Chapter 10.
3. Class 3 action manifests as prolongation of the APD. Most drugs with this action block the rapid component of the delayed rectifier potassium current, I_{Kr}.
4. Class 4 action is blockade of the cardiac calcium current. This action slows conduction in regions where the action potential upstroke is calcium dependent, eg, the SA and AV nodes.

A given drug may have multiple classes of action as indicated by its membrane and ECG effects (Tables 14–2 and 14–3). For example, amiodarone shares all four classes of action. Drugs are usually discussed according to the predominant class of action. Certain antiarrhythmic agents, eg, adenosine and magnesium, do not fit readily into this scheme and are described separately.

SODIUM CHANNEL-BLOCKING DRUGS (CLASS 1)

Drugs with local anesthetic action block sodium channels and reduce the sodium current, I_{Na}. They are the oldest group of antiarrhythmic drugs and are still widely used.

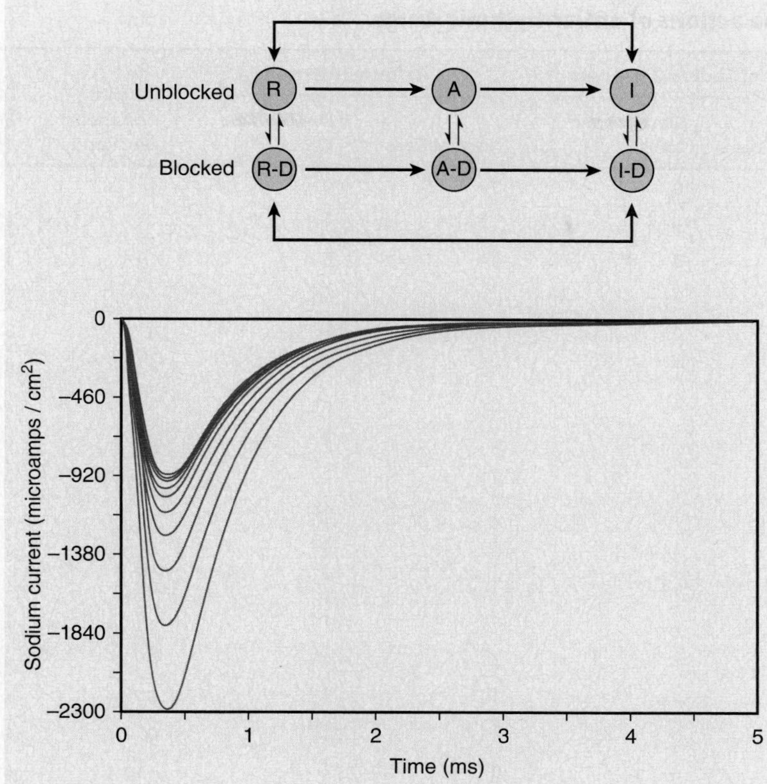

FIGURE 14–9 State- and frequency-dependent block of sodium channels by antiarrhythmic drugs. **Top:** Diagram of a mechanism for the selective depressant action of antiarrhythmic drugs on sodium channels. The upper portion of the figure shows the population of channels moving through a cycle of activity during an action potential in the absence of drugs: R (rested) → A (activated) → I (inactivated). Recovery takes place via the I → R pathway. Antiarrhythmic drugs (D) that act by blocking sodium channels can bind to their receptors in the channels, as shown by the vertical arrows, to form drug-channel complexes, indicated as R-D, A-D, and I-D. Binding of the drugs to the receptor varies with the state of the channel. Most sodium channel blockers bind to the active and inactivated channel receptor much more strongly than to the rested channel. Furthermore, recovery from the I-D state to the R-D state is much slower than from I to R. As a result, rapid activity (repeated activation and inactivation) and depolarization of the resting potential (more channels in the I state) will favor blockade of the channels and selectively suppress arrhythmic cells. **Bottom:** Progressive reduction of inward sodium current (downward deflections) in the presence of a lidocaine derivative. The largest curve is the initial sodium current elicited by a depolarizing voltage step; subsequent sodium current amplitudes are progressively reduced owing to prior accumulated block and block during each depolarization. (Reproduced with permission from Starmer CF, Grant AO, Strauss HC: Mechanisms of use-dependent block of sodium channels in excitable membranes by local anesthetics, Biophys J. 1984;46(1):15-27.)

PROCAINAMIDE (SUBGROUP 1A)

Cardiac Effects

By blocking sodium channels, procainamide slows the upstroke of the action potential, slows conduction, and prolongs the QRS duration of the ECG. The drug also prolongs the APD (a class 3 action) by nonspecific blockade of potassium channels. The drug may be somewhat less effective than quinidine (see below) in suppressing abnormal ectopic pacemaker activity but more effective in blocking sodium channels in depolarized cells.

$H_2N-C_6H_4-C(=O)-NH-CH_2-CH_2-N(C_2H_5)_2$

Procainamide

Procainamide has direct depressant actions on SA and AV nodes, and these actions are only slightly counterbalanced by drug-induced vagal block.

Extracardiac Effects

Procainamide has ganglion-blocking properties. This action reduces peripheral vascular resistance and can cause hypotension, particularly with intravenous use. However, in therapeutic concentrations, its peripheral vascular effects are less prominent than those of quinidine. Hypotension is usually associated with excessively rapid procainamide infusion or the presence of severe underlying left ventricular dysfunction.

Toxicity

Procainamide's cardiotoxic effects include excessive action potential prolongation, QT-interval prolongation, and induction of

TABLE 14–2 Membrane actions of antiarrhythmic drugs.

	Block of Sodium Channels		Refractory Period				
Drug	**Normal Cells**	**Depolarized Cells**	**Normal Cells**	**Depolarized Cells**	**Calcium Channel Blockade**	**Effect on Pacemaker Activity**	**Sympatholytic Action**
Adenosine	0	0	0	0	+	0	+
Amiodarone	+	+++	↑↑	↑↑	+	↓↓	+
Diltiazem	0	0	0	0	+++	↓↓	0
Disopyramide	+	+++	↑	↑↑	+	↓	0
Dofetilide	0	0	↑	?	0	0	0
Dronedarone	+	+	na	na	+	na	+
Esmolol	0	+	0	na	0	↓↓	+++
Flecainide	+	+++	0	↑	0	↓↓	0
Ibutilide	0	0	↑	?	0	0	0
Lidocaine	0	+++	↓	↑↑	0	↓↓	0
Mexiletine	0	+++	0	↑↑	0	↓↓	0
Procainamide	+	+++	↑	↑↑↑	0	↓	+
Propafenone	+	++	↑	↑↑	+	↓↓	+
Propranolol	0	+	↓	↑↑	0	↓↓	+++
Quinidine	+	++	↑	↑↑	0	↓↓	+
Sotalol	0	0	↑↑	↑↑↑	0	↓↓	++
Verapamil	0	+	0	↑	+++	↓↓	+
Vernakalant[1]	+	+	+	+	na	0	na

[1]Not available in the USA.

na, data not available.

torsades de pointes arrhythmia and syncope. Excessive slowing of conduction also can occur. New arrhythmias can be precipitated.

A troublesome adverse effect of long-term procainamide therapy is a syndrome resembling lupus erythematosus and usually consisting of arthralgia and arthritis. In some patients, pleuritis, pericarditis, or parenchymal pulmonary disease also occurs. Renal lupus is rarely induced by procainamide. During long-term therapy, serologic abnormalities (eg, increased antinuclear antibody titer) occur in nearly all patients, and in the absence of symptoms, these are not an indication to stop drug therapy. Approximately one third of patients receiving long-term procainamide therapy develop these reversible lupus-related symptoms.

Other adverse effects include nausea and diarrhea (in about 10% of cases), rash, fever, hepatitis (<5%), and agranulocytosis (approximately 0.2%).

Pharmacokinetics & Dosage

Procainamide can be administered safely by intravenous and intramuscular routes. The drug is now only available in intravenous form in the United States. A metabolite (*N*-acetylprocainamide, NAPA) has class 3 activity. Excessive accumulation of NAPA has been implicated in torsades de pointes during procainamide therapy, especially in patients with renal failure. Some individuals rapidly acetylate procainamide and develop high levels of NAPA. However, the lupus syndrome appears to be *less* common in these patients.

Procainamide is eliminated by hepatic metabolism to NAPA and by renal elimination in about equal proportion by each of these routes. Its half-life is only 3–4 hours, which necessitates frequent dosing or use of a slow-release formulation (the usual practice). NAPA is eliminated by the kidneys. Procainamide dosage must be reduced in patients with renal failure. The reduced volume of distribution and renal clearance associated with heart failure also require reduction in dosage. The half-life of NAPA is considerably longer than that of procainamide, and it therefore accumulates more slowly. Thus, it is important to measure plasma levels of both procainamide and NAPA, especially in patients with circulatory or renal impairment.

If a rapid procainamide effect is needed, an intravenous loading dose of up to 12 mg/kg can be given at a rate of 0.3 mg/kg/min or less rapidly. This dose is followed by a maintenance dosage of 2–5 mg/min, with careful monitoring of plasma levels. The risk of gastrointestinal (GI) or cardiac toxicity rises at plasma concentrations greater than 8 mcg/mL or NAPA concentrations greater than 20 mcg/mL.

Therapeutic Use

Procainamide is effective against most atrial and ventricular arrhythmias. Long-term use is no longer an option in the United States. Procainamide is the drug of second or third choice (after lidocaine or amiodarone) in most coronary care units for

TABLE 14–3 Clinical pharmacologic properties of antiarrhythmic drugs.

Drug	Effect on SA Nodal Rate	Effect on AV Nodal Refractory Period	PR Interval	QRS Duration	QT Interval	Usefulness in Arrhythmias: Supra-ventricular	Usefulness in Arrhythmias: Ventricular	Half-Life
Adenosine	↓↑	↑↑↑	↑↑↑	0	0	++++	?	<10 s
Amiodarone	↓↓[1]	↑↑	Variable	↑	↑↑↑↑	+++	+++	(weeks)
Diltiazem	↑↓	↑↑	↑	0	0	+++	–	4–8 h
Disopyramide	↑↓[1,2]	↑↓[2]	↑↓[2]	↑↑	↑↑	+	+++	7–8 h
Dofetilide	↓(?)	0	0	0	↑↑	++	None	7 h
Dronedarone					↑	+++	–	24 h
Esmolol	↓↓	↑↑	↑↑	0	0	+	+	10 min
Flecainide	None, ↓	↑	↑	↑↑↑	0	+[3]	++++	20 h
Ibutilide	↓(?)	0	0	0	↑↑	++	?	6 h
Lidocaine	None[1]	None	0	0	0	None[4]	+++	1–2 h
Mexiletine	None[1]	None	0	0	0	None	+++	8–20 h
Procainamide	↓[1]	↑↓[2]	↑↓[2]	↑↑	↑↑	+	+++	3–4 h
Propafenone	0, ↓	↑	↑	↑↑↑	0	+	+++	5–7 h
Propranolol	↓↓	↑↑	↑↑	0	0	+	+	5 h
Quinidine	↑↓[1,2]	↑↓[2]	↑↓[2]	↑↑	↑↑	+	+++	6 h
Sotalol	↓↓	↑↑	↑↑	0	↑↑↑	+++	+++	7–12 h
Verapamil	↓↓	↑↑	↑↑	0	0	+++	–	7 h
Vernakalant		↑	↑			+++	–	2 h

[1]May suppress diseased sinus nodes.

[2]Anticholinergic effect and direct depressant action.

[3]Especially in Wolff-Parkinson-White syndrome.

[4]May be effective in atrial arrhythmias caused by digitalis.

the treatment of sustained ventricular arrhythmias associated with acute myocardial infarction.

QUINIDINE (SUBGROUP 1A)

Cardiac Effects

Quinidine has actions similar to those of procainamide: it slows the upstroke of the action potential, slows conduction, and prolongs the QRS duration of the ECG, by blockade of sodium channels. The drug also prolongs the action potential duration by blockade of several potassium channels, including I_{TO}. Its toxic cardiac effects include excessive QT-interval prolongation and induction of torsades de pointes arrhythmia. Toxic concentrations of quinidine also produce excessive sodium channel blockade with slowed conduction throughout the heart. It also has modest antimuscarinic actions in the heart.

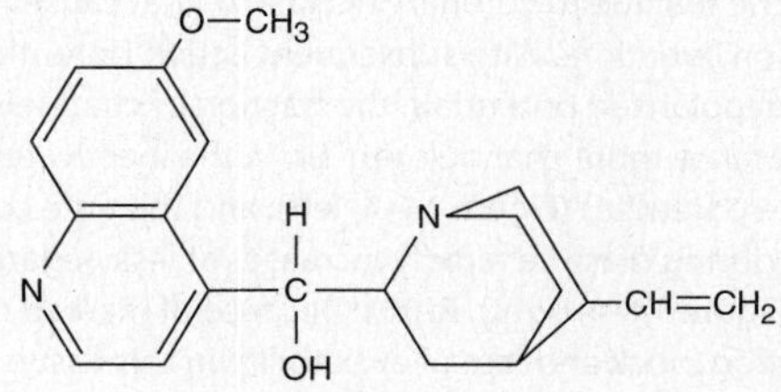

Quinidine

Extracardiac Effects

Adverse GI effects of diarrhea, nausea, and vomiting are observed in one-third to one-half of patients. A syndrome of headache, dizziness, and tinnitus **(cinchonism)** is observed at toxic drug concentrations. Idiosyncratic or immunologic reactions, including thrombocytopenia, hepatitis, angioedema, edema, and fever, are observed rarely.

Pharmacokinetics & Therapeutic Use

Quinidine is readily absorbed from the GI tract and eliminated primarily by hepatic metabolism. It is rarely used because of cardiac and extracardiac adverse effects and the availability of better-tolerated antiarrhythmic drugs. Quinidine is of benefit in treating patients with Brugada syndrome who have declined or cannot afford implantation of an implantable cardioverter defibrillator (ICD).

DISOPYRAMIDE (SUBGROUP 1A)

Cardiac Effects

The effects of disopyramide are very similar to those of procainamide and quinidine. Its cardiac antimuscarinic effects are even more marked than those of quinidine. Therefore, a drug that slows

AV conduction should be administered with disopyramide when treating atrial flutter or fibrillation.

Disopyramide

Toxicity

Toxic concentrations of disopyramide can precipitate all of the electrophysiologic disturbances described under quinidine. Because of its negative inotropic effect, disopyramide may precipitate heart failure de novo or in patients with preexisting depression of left ventricular function. Because of this effect, disopyramide is not used as a first-line antiarrhythmic agent in the USA. It should not be used in patients with heart failure.

Disopyramide's atropine-like activity accounts for most of its symptomatic adverse effects: urinary retention (most often, but not exclusively, in male patients with prostatic hyperplasia), dry mouth, blurred vision, constipation, and worsening of preexisting glaucoma. These effects may require discontinuation of the drug.

Pharmacokinetics & Dosage

In the USA, disopyramide is only available for oral use. The typical oral dosage of disopyramide is 150 mg three times a day, but up to 1 g/d has been used. In patients with renal impairment, dosage must be reduced. Because of the danger of precipitating heart failure, loading doses are not recommended.

Therapeutic Use

Disopyramide is effective in a variety of supraventricular arrhythmias. However, in the USA, it is approved only for the treatment of ventricular arrhythmias.

LIDOCAINE (SUBGROUP 1B)

Lidocaine has a low incidence of toxicity and a high degree of effectiveness in arrhythmias associated with acute myocardial infarction. For arrhythmias, it is used only by the intravenous route.

Lidocaine

Cardiac Effects

Lidocaine blocks activated and inactivated sodium channels with rapid kinetics (Figure 14–10); the inactivated state block ensures greater effects on cells with long action potentials such as Purkinje and ventricular cells, compared with atrial cells. The rapid kinetics at normal resting potentials result in recovery from block between action potentials and no effect on conduction. In depolarized cells, the increased inactivation and slower unbinding kinetics result in the selective depression of conduction. Little effect is seen on the ECG in normal sinus rhythm.

Toxicity

Lidocaine is one of the least cardiotoxic of the currently used sodium channel blockers. Proarrhythmic effects, including SA node arrest, worsening of impaired conduction, and ventricular arrhythmias, are uncommon with lidocaine use. In large doses, especially in patients with preexisting heart failure, lidocaine may cause hypotension—partly by depressing myocardial contractility.

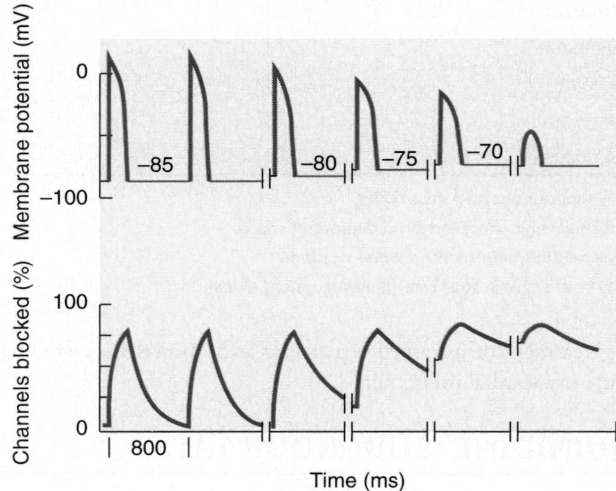

FIGURE 14–10 Computer simulation of the effect of resting membrane potential on the blocking and unblocking of sodium channels by lidocaine as the membrane depolarizes. **Upper tracing:** Action potentials in a ventricular muscle cell. **Lower tracing:** Percentage of channels blocked by the drug. An 800-ms time segment is shown. Extra passage of time is indicated by breaks in the traces. **Left side:** At the normal resting potential of –85 mV, the drug combines with open (activated) and inactivated channels during each action potential, but block is rapidly reversed during diastole because the affinity of the drug for its receptor is so low when the channel recovers to the resting state at –85 mV. **Middle:** Metabolic injury is simulated, eg, ischemia due to coronary occlusion, that causes gradual depolarization over time. With subsequent action potentials arising from more depolarized potentials, the fraction of channels blocked increases because more channels remain in the inactivated state at less negative potentials (Figure 14–4, left), and the time constant for unblocking during diastole rapidly increases at less negative resting potentials (Figure 14–4, right). **Right:** Because of marked drug binding, conduction block and loss of excitability in this tissue result; that is, the "sick" (depolarized) tissue is selectively suppressed.

Lidocaine's most common adverse effects—like those of other local anesthetics—are neurologic: paresthesia, tremor, nausea of central origin, lightheadedness, hearing disturbances, slurred speech, and convulsions. These occur most commonly in elderly or otherwise vulnerable patients or when a bolus of the drug is given too rapidly. The effects are dose-related and usually short-lived; seizures respond to intravenous diazepam. In general, if plasma levels above 9 mcg/mL are avoided, lidocaine is well tolerated.

Pharmacokinetics & Dosage

Because of its extensive first-pass hepatic metabolism, only 3% of orally administered lidocaine appears in the plasma. Thus, lidocaine must be given parenterally. Lidocaine has a half-life of 1–2 hours. In adults, a loading dose of 150–200 mg administered over about 15 minutes (as a single infusion or as a series of slow boluses) should be followed by a maintenance infusion of 2–4 mg/min to achieve a therapeutic plasma level of 2–6 mcg/mL. Determination of lidocaine plasma levels is of great value in adjusting the infusion rate. Occasional patients with myocardial infarction or other acute illness require (and tolerate) higher concentrations. This may be the result of increased plasma α_1-acid glycoprotein, an acute-phase reactant protein that binds lidocaine, making less free drug available to exert its pharmacologic effects.

In patients with heart failure, lidocaine's volume of distribution and total body clearance may both be decreased. Therefore, both loading and maintenance doses should be decreased. Since these effects counterbalance each other, the half-life may not be increased as much as predicted from clearance changes alone. In patients with liver disease, plasma clearance is markedly reduced and the volume of distribution is often increased; the elimination half-life in such cases may be increased threefold or more. In liver disease, the maintenance dose should be decreased, but usual loading doses can be given. Elimination half-life determines the time to steady state. Although steady-state concentrations may be achieved in 8–10 hours in normal patients and patients with heart failure, 24–36 hours may be required in those with liver disease. Drugs that decrease liver blood flow (eg, propranolol, cimetidine) reduce lidocaine clearance and so increase the risk of toxicity unless infusion rates are decreased. With infusions lasting more than 24 hours, clearance falls and plasma concentrations rise. Renal disease has no major effect on lidocaine disposition.

Therapeutic Use

Lidocaine is the agent of choice for termination of ventricular tachycardia and prevention of ventricular fibrillation after cardioversion in the setting of acute ischemia. However, routine *prophylactic* use of lidocaine in this setting may actually increase total mortality, possibly by increasing the incidence of asystole, and is not the standard of care. Most physicians administer IV lidocaine only to patients with arrhythmias.

MEXILETINE (SUBGROUP 1B)

Mexiletine is an orally active congener of lidocaine. Its electrophysiologic and antiarrhythmic actions are similar to those of lidocaine. (The anticonvulsant phenytoin [see Chapter 24] exerts similar electrophysiologic effects and has been used as an antiarrhythmic.) Mexiletine is used in the treatment of ventricular arrhythmias. It shortens the QT interval and may be of value in treating patients with LQT-3. The elimination half-life is 8–20 hours and permits oral administration two or three times per day. The usual daily dosage of mexiletine is 600–1200 mg/d. Dose-related adverse effects are seen frequently at therapeutic dosage. These are predominantly neurologic, including tremor, blurred vision, and lethargy. Nausea also is a common effect.

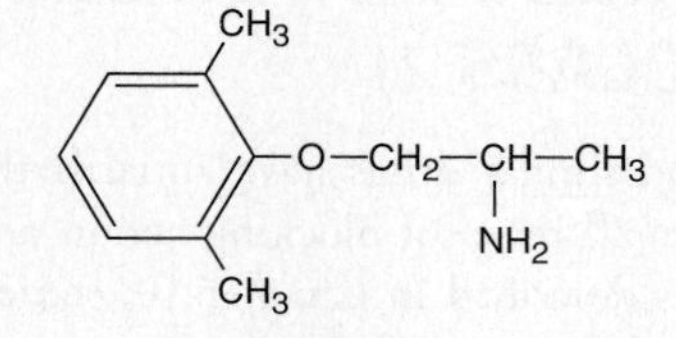

Mexiletine

Mexiletine has also shown significant efficacy in relieving chronic pain, especially pain that results from diabetic neuropathy and nerve injury. The usual dosage is 450–750 mg/d orally. This application is off label.

FLECAINIDE (SUBGROUP 1C)

Flecainide is a potent blocker of sodium and potassium channels with slow unblocking kinetics. (Note that although it does block certain potassium channels, it does not prolong the action potential or the QT interval.) It is currently used for patients with otherwise normal hearts who have supraventricular arrhythmias. It has no antimuscarinic effects.

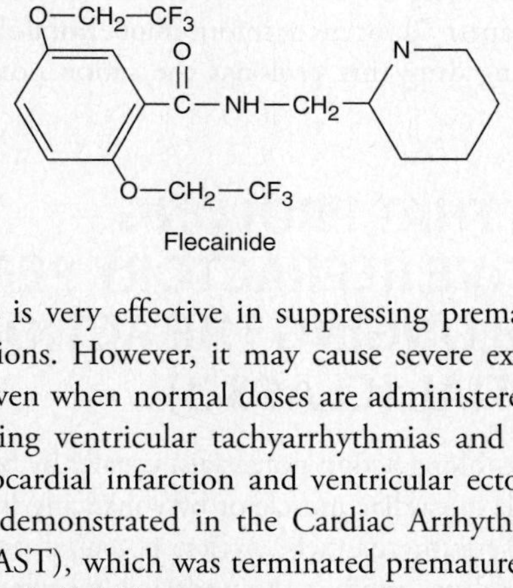

Flecainide

Flecainide is very effective in suppressing premature ventricular contractions. However, it may cause severe exacerbation of arrhythmia even when normal doses are administered to patients with preexisting ventricular tachyarrhythmias and those with a previous myocardial infarction and ventricular ectopy. This was dramatically demonstrated in the Cardiac Arrhythmia Suppression Trial (CAST), which was terminated prematurely because of a two and one-half-fold increase in mortality rate in the patients receiving flecainide and similar group 1C drugs. Flecainide is well absorbed and has a half-life of approximately 20 hours. Elimination is both by hepatic metabolism and by the kidney. The usual dosage of flecainide is 100–200 mg twice a day.

PROPAFENONE (SUBGROUP 1C)

Propafenone has some structural similarities to propranolol and possesses weak β-blocking activity. Its spectrum of action is very similar to that of quinidine, but it does not prolong the action potential. Its sodium channel-blocking kinetics are similar to those of flecainide. Propafenone is metabolized in the liver, with an average half-life of 5–7 hours. The usual daily dosage of propafenone is 450–900 mg/d in three divided doses. The drug is used primarily for supraventricular arrhythmias. The most common adverse effects are a metallic taste and constipation; arrhythmia exacerbation can also occur.

BETA-ADRENOCEPTOR-BLOCKING DRUGS (CLASS 2)

Propranolol and similar drugs have antiarrhythmic properties by virtue of their β-receptor-blocking action and direct membrane effects. As described in Chapter 10, some of these drugs have selectivity for cardiac β_1 receptors, some have intrinsic sympathomimetic activity, some have marked direct membrane effects, and some prolong the cardiac action potential. The relative contributions of the β-blocking and direct membrane effects to the antiarrhythmic effects of these drugs are not fully known. Although β-blockers are fairly well tolerated, their efficacy for suppression of ventricular ectopic depolarizations is lower than that of sodium channel blockers. However, there is good evidence that these agents can reduce the incidence of recurrent infarction and sudden death in patients recovering from acute myocardial infarction (see Chapter 10). The nonselective β-blockers such as propranolol and nadolol have proved the more effective subgroup of β-blockers for prevention and treatment of cardiac arrhythmias.

Esmolol is a short-acting β-blocker used intravenously as an antiarrhythmic drug for intraoperative and other acute arrhythmias. See Chapter 10 for more information. **Sotalol** is a nonselective β-blocking drug that prolongs the action potential (class 3 action).

DRUGS THAT PROLONG EFFECTIVE REFRACTORY PERIOD BY PROLONGING THE ACTION POTENTIAL (CLASS 3)

These drugs prolong action potentials, usually by blocking potassium channels in cardiac muscle or by enhancing inward current, eg, through sodium channels. Action potential prolongation by most of these drugs exhibits the undesirable property of "reverse use-dependence": action potential prolongation is least marked at fast rates (where it is desirable) and most marked at slow rates, where it can contribute to the risk of torsades de pointes.

Although most drugs in the class cause QT prolongation, there is considerable variability among drugs in their proarrhythmic tendency to cause torsades de pointes despite significant QT-interval prolongation. Recent studies suggest that excessive QT prolongation alone may not be the best predictor of drug-induced torsades de pointes. Other important factors in addition to QT prolongation include action potential stability and development of a triangular shape (triangulation), reverse use-dependence, and dispersion of repolarization time across the ventricles.

AMIODARONE

In the USA, amiodarone is approved for oral and intravenous use to treat serious ventricular arrhythmias. However, the drug is also highly effective in the treatment of supraventricular arrhythmias such as atrial fibrillation. Despite a broad spectrum of side effects, it is now the most commonly use drug for rhythm control in patients with atrial fibrillation. Amiodarone has unusual pharmacokinetics and important extracardiac adverse effects. **Dronedarone,** an analog that lacks iodine atoms, has US Food and Drug Administration (FDA) approval for the treatment of atrial flutter and fibrillation.

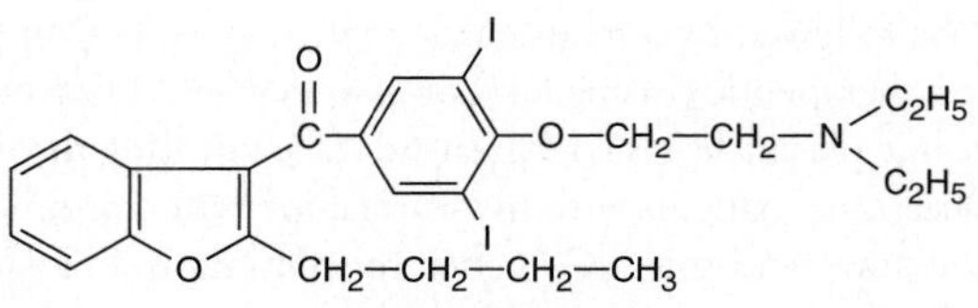

Amiodarone

Cardiac Effects

Amiodarone markedly prolongs the action potential duration (and the QT interval on the ECG) by blockade of I_{Kr}. During chronic administration, I_{Ks} is also blocked. The action potential duration is prolonged uniformly over a wide range of heart rates; that is, the drug does not have reverse use-dependent action. Despite its present classification as a class 3 agent, amiodarone also significantly blocks inactivated sodium channels. Its action potential-prolonging action reinforces this effect. Amiodarone also has weak adrenergic and calcium channel-blocking actions. Consequences of these actions include slowing of the heart rate and AV node conduction. The broad spectrum of actions may account for its relatively high efficacy and its low incidence of torsades de pointes despite significant QT-interval prolongation.

Extracardiac Effects

Amiodarone causes peripheral vasodilation. This action is prominent after intravenous administration and may be related to the action of the vehicle.

Toxicity

Amiodarone may produce symptomatic bradycardia and heart block in patients with preexisting sinus or AV node disease. The drug accumulates in many tissues, including the heart (10–50 times more so than in plasma), lung, liver, and skin, and is concentrated in tears. Dose-related pulmonary toxicity is the most important adverse effect. Even on a low dose of 200 mg/d or less, fatal pulmonary fibrosis may be observed in 1% of patients. Abnormal liver function tests and hypersensitivity hepatitis may develop during amiodarone treatment and liver function tests should be monitored regularly. The skin deposits result in a photodermatitis and a gray-blue skin discoloration in sun-exposed areas, eg, the malar regions. After a few weeks of treatment, asymptomatic corneal microdeposits are present in virtually all patients treated with amiodarone. Halos develop in the peripheral visual fields of some patients. Drug discontinuation is usually not required. Rarely, an optic neuritis may progress to blindness.

Amiodarone blocks the peripheral conversion of thyroxine (T_4) to triiodothyronine (T_3). It is also a potential source of large amounts of inorganic iodine. Amiodarone may result in hypothyroidism or hyperthyroidism. Type 1 amiodarone-induced thyrotoxicosis is the result of excessive thyroxine production and is akin to Graves disease. Type 2 amiodarone-induced thyroiditis is the result of a destructive thyroiditis. Treatment of each form of thyroiditis is different. Type 1 amiodarone-induced thyrotoxicosis is treated with thionamides; type 2 is treated with prednisolone. Thyroid function should be evaluated before initiating treatment and should be monitored periodically. Because effects have been described in virtually every organ system, amiodarone treatment should be reevaluated whenever new symptoms develop in a patient, including arrhythmia aggravation.

Pharmacokinetics

Amiodarone is variably absorbed with a bioavailability of 35–65%. It undergoes hepatic metabolism by CYP3A4, and the major metabolite, desethylamiodarone, is bioactive. The elimination half-life is complex, with a rapid component of 3–10 days (50% of the drug) and a slower component of several weeks. After discontinuation of the drug, effects are maintained for 1–3 months. Measurable tissue levels may be observed up to 1 year after discontinuation. A total loading dose of 10 g is usually achieved with 0.8–1.2 g daily doses. The maintenance dose is 200–400 mg daily. Pharmacologic effects may be achieved rapidly by intravenous loading. QT-prolonging effect is modest with this route of administration, whereas bradycardia and AV block may be significant.

Amiodarone has many important drug interactions, and all medications should be reviewed when the drug is initiated and when the dose is adjusted. Amiodarone is a substrate for liver cytochrome CYP3A4, and its levels are increased by drugs that inhibit this enzyme, eg, the histamine H_2 blocker cimetidine. Drugs that induce CYP3A4, eg, rifampin, decrease amiodarone concentration when co-administered. Amiodarone inhibits several cytochrome P450 enzymes and may result in high levels of many drugs, including statins, digoxin, and warfarin. The dose of warfarin should be reduced by one third to one half following initiation of amiodarone, and prothrombin times should be closely monitored.

Therapeutic Use

Low doses (100–200 mg/d) of amiodarone are effective in maintaining normal sinus rhythm in patients with atrial fibrillation. The drug is effective in the prevention of recurrent ventricular tachycardia. It is not associated with an increase in mortality in patients with coronary artery disease or heart failure. In many centers, the implanted cardioverter-defibrillator (ICD) has succeeded drug therapy as the primary treatment modality for ventricular tachycardia, but amiodarone may be used for ventricular tachycardia as adjuvant therapy to decrease the frequency of uncomfortable cardioverter-defibrillator discharges. The drug increases the pacing and defibrillation threshold, and these devices require retesting after a maintenance dose has been achieved. In patients with atrial fibrillation, a rapid ventricular response, and heart failure, intravenous amiodarone is useful to control the ventricular response; the calcium channel blockers may not be well tolerated in the presence of heart failure.

DRONEDARONE

Dronedarone is a structural analog of amiodarone in which the iodine atoms have been removed from the phenyl ring and a methanesulfonyl group has been added to the benzofuran ring. The design was intended to eliminate action of the parent drug on thyroxine metabolism and to modify the half-life of the drug. No thyroid dysfunction or pulmonary toxicity has been reported in short-term studies. However, liver toxicity, including two severe cases requiring liver transplantation, has been reported. Like amiodarone, dronedarone has multichannel actions, including blocking I_{Kr}, I_{Ks}, I_{Ca}, and I_{Na}. It also has β-adrenergic–blocking action. The drug has a half-life of 24 hours and can be administered twice daily at a fixed dose of 400 mg. Dronedarone absorption increases twofold to threefold when taken with food, and this information should be communicated to patients as a part of the dosing instructions. Dronedarone elimination is primarily nonrenal. It inhibits tubular secretion of creatinine, resulting in a 10–20% increase in serum creatinine; however, because the glomerular filtration rate is unchanged, no adjustments are required. Dronedarone is both a substrate and an inhibitor of CY3A4 and should not be co-administered with potent inhibitors of this enzyme, such as the azole and similar antifungal agents.

Dronedarone restores sinus rhythm in a small percentage of patients (<15%) with atrial fibrillation. It produces a 10- to 15-bpm reduction of the ventricular rate compared to placebo. In one report, dronedarone doubled the interval between episodes of atrial fibrillation recurrence in patients with paroxysmal atrial fibrillation. Initial studies suggested a reduction in mortality or hospitalization in patients with atrial fibrillation. However, a study of dronedarone's effects in permanent atrial fibrillation was terminated in 2011 because of increased risk of death, stroke, and heart failure. Use of dronedarone must be accompanied by a commitment to restore sinus rhythm. A trial of dronedarone in advanced heart failure was terminated prematurely because of an increase in mortality. The drug carries a "black box" warning against its use in acute decompensated or advanced (class IV) heart failure.

SOTALOL

Sotalol has both β-adrenergic receptor-blocking (class 2) and action potential-prolonging (class 3) actions. The drug is formulated as a racemic mixture of D- and L-sotalol. All the β-adrenergic–blocking activity resides in the L-isomer; the D- and L-isomers share action potential prolonging effects. Beta-adrenergic–blocking action is not cardioselective and is maximal at doses below those required for action potential prolongation.

OH

CH_3SO_2NH—(benzene ring)—$CHCH_2NHCH(CH_3)_2$

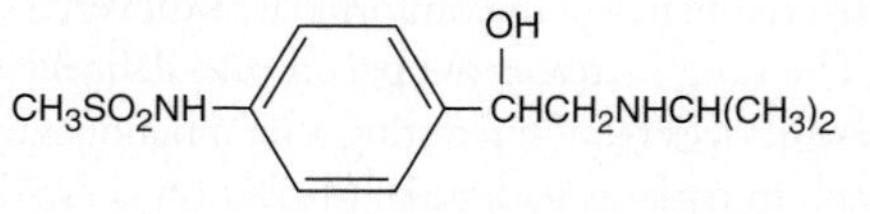

Sotalol

Sotalol is well absorbed orally with bioavailability of nearly 100%. It is not metabolized in the liver and is not bound to plasma proteins. Excretion is predominantly by the kidneys in the unchanged form with a half-life of approximately 12 hours. Because of its relatively simple pharmacokinetics, sotalol exhibits few direct drug interactions. Its most significant cardiac adverse effect is an extension of its pharmacologic action: a dose-related incidence of torsades de pointes that approaches 6% at the highest recommended daily dose. Patients with overt heart failure may experience further depression of left ventricular function during treatment with sotalol.

Sotalol is approved for the treatment of life-threatening ventricular arrhythmias and the maintenance of sinus rhythm in patients with atrial fibrillation. It is also approved for treatment of supraventricular and ventricular arrhythmias in the pediatric age group. Sotalol decreases the threshold for cardiac defibrillation.

DOFETILIDE

Dofetilide has class 3 action potential prolonging action. This action is effected by a dose-dependent blockade of the rapid component of the delayed rectifier potassium current (I_{Kr}) and the blockade of I_{Kr} increases in hypokalemia. Dofetilide produces no relevant blockade of the other potassium channels or the sodium channel. Because of the slow rate of recovery from blockade, the extent of blockade shows little dependence on stimulation frequency. However, dofetilide does show less action potential prolongation at rapid rates because of the increased importance of other potassium channels such as I_{Ks} at higher frequencies.

Dofetilide is 100% bioavailable. Verapamil increases peak plasma dofetilide concentration by increasing intestinal blood flow. Eighty percent of an oral dose is eliminated unchanged by the kidneys; the remainder is eliminated in the urine as inactive metabolites. Inhibitors of the renal cation secretion mechanism, eg, cimetidine, prolong the half-life of dofetilide. Since the QT-prolonging effects and risks of ventricular proarrhythmia are directly related to plasma concentration, dofetilide dosage must be based on the estimated creatinine clearance. Treatment with dofetilide should be initiated in hospital after baseline measurement of the rate-corrected QT interval (QT_c) and serum K^+, and Mg^{2+}. A baseline QT_c of greater than 450 ms (500 ms in the presence of an intraventricular conduction delay), bradycardia of less than 50 bpm, and hypokalemia are relative contraindications to its use. During loading, the QT_c is measured before the second and subsequent doses; an increase in the QT_c to ≥500 ms is an indication to reduce the dose or discontinue the drug.

Dofetilide is approved for the maintenance of normal sinus rhythm in patients with atrial fibrillation. It is also effective in restoring normal sinus rhythm in patients with atrial fibrillation.

IBUTILIDE

Ibutilide, like dofetilide, slows cardiac repolarization by blockade of the rapid component (I_{Kr}) of the delayed rectifier potassium current. Activation of late inward sodium current has also been suggested as an additional mechanism of action potential prolongation. After intravenous administration, ibutilide is rapidly cleared by hepatic metabolism and the elimination half-life averages 6 hours. The metabolites are excreted by the kidney.

Intravenous ibutilide is used for the acute conversion of atrial flutter and atrial fibrillation to normal sinus rhythm. The drug is more effective in atrial flutter than atrial fibrillation, with a mean time to termination of 20 minutes. The most important adverse effect is excessive QT-interval prolongation and torsades de pointes. Patients require continuous ECG monitoring for 4 hours after ibutilide infusion or until QT_c returns to baseline.

CALCIUM CHANNEL–BLOCKING DRUGS (CLASS 4)

These drugs, of which verapamil is the prototype, were first introduced as antianginal agents and are discussed in detail in Chapter 12. Verapamil and diltiazem also have antiarrhythmic effects. The dihydropyridines (eg, nifedipine) do not share antiarrhythmic efficacy and may *precipitate* arrhythmias.

VERAPAMIL

Cardiac Effects

Verapamil blocks both activated and inactivated L-type calcium channels. Thus, its effect is more marked in tissues that fire frequently, those that are less completely polarized at rest, and those in which activation depends exclusively on the calcium current, such as the SA and AV nodes. AV nodal conduction time and effective refractory period are consistently prolonged by therapeutic concentrations. Verapamil usually slows the SA node by its direct action, but its hypotensive action may occasionally result in a small reflex increase of SA rate.

Verapamil can suppress both early and delayed afterdepolarizations and may abolish slow responses arising in severely depolarized tissue.

Extracardiac Effects

Verapamil causes peripheral vasodilation, which may be beneficial in hypertension and peripheral vasospastic disorders. Its effects on smooth muscle produce a number of extracardiac effects (see Chapter 12).

Toxicity

Verapamil's cardiotoxic effects are dose-related and usually avoidable. A common error has been to administer intravenous verapamil to a patient with ventricular tachycardia misdiagnosed as supraventricular tachycardia. In this setting, hypotension and ventricular fibrillation can occur. Verapamil's negative inotropic effects may limit its clinical usefulness in diseased hearts (see Chapter 12). Verapamil can induce AV block when used in large doses or in patients with AV nodal disease. This block can be treated with atropine and β-receptor stimulants.

Adverse extracardiac effects include constipation, lassitude, nervousness, and peripheral edema.

Pharmacokinetics & Dosage

The half-life of verapamil is approximately 4–7 hours. It is extensively metabolized by the liver; after oral administration, its bioavailability is only about 20%. Therefore, verapamil must be administered with caution in patients with hepatic dysfunction or impaired hepatic perfusion.

In adult patients without heart failure or SA or AV nodal disease, parenteral verapamil can be used to terminate supraventricular tachycardia, although adenosine is the agent of first choice. Verapamil dosage is an initial bolus of 5 mg administered over 2–5 minutes, followed a few minutes later by a second 5 mg bolus if needed. Thereafter, doses of 5–10 mg can be administered every 4–6 hours, or a constant infusion of 0.4 mcg/kg/min may be used.

Effective oral dosages are higher than intravenous dosage because of first-pass metabolism and range from 120 mg to 640 mg daily, divided into three or four doses.

Therapeutic Use

Supraventricular tachycardia is the major arrhythmia indication for verapamil. Adenosine or verapamil is preferred over older treatments (propranolol, digoxin, edrophonium, vasoconstrictor agents, and cardioversion) for termination. Verapamil can also reduce the ventricular rate in atrial fibrillation and flutter ("rate control"). It only rarely converts atrial flutter and fibrillation to sinus rhythm. Verapamil is occasionally useful in ventricular arrhythmias. However, intravenous verapamil in a patient with sustained ventricular tachycardia can cause hemodynamic collapse.

DILTIAZEM

Diltiazem appears to be similar in efficacy to verapamil in the management of supraventricular arrhythmias, including rate control in atrial fibrillation. An intravenous form of diltiazem is available for the latter indication and causes hypotension or bradyarrhythmias relatively infrequently.

MISCELLANEOUS ANTIARRHYTHMIC AGENTS & OTHER DRUGS THAT ACT ON CHANNELS

Certain agents used for the treatment of arrhythmias do not fit the conventional class 1–4 organization. These include digitalis (see Chapter 13), adenosine, magnesium, and potassium. It is also becoming clear that certain non-antiarrhythmic drugs, such as drugs acting on the renin-angiotensin-aldosterone system, fish oil, and statins, can reduce recurrence of tachycardias and fibrillation in patients with coronary heart disease or congestive heart failure.

ADENOSINE

Mechanism & Clinical Use

Adenosine is a nucleoside that occurs naturally throughout the body. Its half-life in the blood is less than 10 seconds. Its cardiac mechanism of action involves activation of an inward rectifier K^+ current and inhibition of calcium current. The results of these actions are marked hyperpolarization and suppression of calcium-dependent action potentials. When given as a bolus dose, adenosine directly inhibits AV nodal conduction and increases the AV nodal refractory period but has lesser effects on the SA node. Adenosine is currently the drug of choice for prompt conversion of paroxysmal supraventricular tachycardia to sinus rhythm because of its high efficacy (90–95%) and very short duration of action. It is usually given in a bolus dose of 6 mg followed, if necessary, by a dose of 12 mg. An uncommon variant of ventricular tachycardia is adenosine-sensitive. The drug is less effective in the presence of adenosine receptor blockers such as theophylline or caffeine, and its effects are potentiated by adenosine uptake inhibitors such as dipyridamole.

The Nonpharmacologic Therapy of Cardiac Arrhythmias

It was recognized over 100 years ago that reentry in simple in vitro models (eg, rings of conducting tissues) was permanently interrupted by transecting the reentry circuit. This concept is now applied in cardiac arrhythmias with defined anatomic pathways—eg, atrioventricular reentry using accessory pathways, atrioventricular node reentry, atrial flutter, and some forms of ventricular tachycardia—by treatment with **radiofrequency catheter ablation** or extreme cold, **cryoablation.** Mapping of reentrant pathways and ablation can be carried out by means of catheters threaded into the heart from peripheral arteries and veins. Studies have also shown that paroxysmal and persistent atrial fibrillation may arise from one or more of the pulmonary veins. Both forms of atrial fibrillation can be cured by electrically isolating the pulmonary veins by radiofrequency or cryotherapy catheter ablation or during concomitant cardiac surgery. Because catheter ablation therapy can often permanently cure atrial fibrillation, and because it does not involve adverse effects of drugs, it has become a very common treatment for chronic atrial fibrillation.

Another form of nonpharmacologic therapy is the **implantable cardioverter-defibrillator (ICD),** a device that can automatically detect and treat potentially fatal arrhythmias such as ventricular fibrillation. ICDs are now widely used in patients who have been resuscitated from such arrhythmias, and several trials have shown that ICD treatment reduces mortality in patients with coronary artery disease who have an ejection fraction ≤30% and in patients with class II or III heart failure and no prior history of arrhythmias. The increasing use of nonpharmacologic antiarrhythmic therapies reflects both advances in the relevant technologies and an increasing appreciation of the dangers of long-term therapy with currently available drugs.

Toxicity

Adenosine causes flushing in about 20% of patients and shortness of breath or chest burning (perhaps related to bronchospasm) in over 10%. Induction of high-grade AV block may occur but is very short-lived. Atrial fibrillation may occur. Less common toxicities include headache, hypotension, nausea, and paresthesias.

IVABRADINE

The localized expression of the hyperpolarization-induced "funny" current I_f in the SA node and its important role in pacemaker activity provide an attractive therapeutic target for heart rate control. Ivabradine is a selective blocker of I_f. It slows pacemaker activity by decreasing diastolic depolarization of sinus node cells. It is an open channel blocker that shows use-dependent block. Unlike other heart rate-lowering agents such as β blockers, it reduces heart rate without affecting myocardial contractility, ventricular repolarization, or intracardiac conduction. At therapeutic concentrations, block of I_f is not complete. As a result, autonomic control of the sinus node pacemaker rate is retained.

Elevated heart rate is an important determinant of the ischemic threshold in patients with coronary artery disease and a prognostic indicator in patients with congestive heart failure. Antianginal and anti-ischemic effects of ivabradine have been demonstrated in patients with coronary artery disease and chronic stable angina. In controlled clinical trials, ivabradine proved as effective as β blockers in the control of angina. In patients with left ventricular dysfunction and heart rates greater than 70 bpm, ivabradine reduced mean heart rate and the composite endpoints of cardiovascular mortality and hospitalization.

Inappropriate sinus tachycardia is an uncommon disorder characterized by multiple symptoms, including palpitations, dizziness, orthostatic intolerance, and elevated heart rates. Conventional treatment includes β blockers and non-dihydropyridine calcium channel blockers. Recent case reports and one clinical trial have shown that ivabradine provides an effective alternative to slow the heart rate in patients with inappropriate sinus tachycardia. The drug is administered in doses of 5–10 mg as needed. Visual disturbances attributable to the block of the I_f channels in the retina have been described. This side effect is limited by the low permeability of ivabradine in the blood-brain barrier. Ivabradine is in use for several indications elsewhere but is currently approved only for use in heart failure in the USA.

RANOLAZINE

Ranolazine was originally developed as, and is FDA approved as, an antianginal agent. Subsequent studies have demonstrated antiarrhythmic properties that are dependent on the blockade of multiple ion channels. The drug blocks the early I_{Na} and the late component of the Na^+ current, I_{NaL}, the latter having a tenfold higher sensitivity to the drug. The block of both components of the sodium current is frequency- and voltage-dependent. Ranolazine also blocks the rapid component of the delayed rectifier K^+ current I_{Kr}. The blockade of both I_{NaL} and I_{Kr} results in opposing effects on the action potential duration (APD); the net effect depends on the relative contribution of I_{NaL} and I_{Kr} to the APD. In normal ventricular myocytes, the net effect is prolongation of the APD and the QT interval. In myocytes isolated from mice bearing long QT-associated mutations, the net effect is APD shortening. In normal atrial myocytes, the net effect is prolongation of the APD. At rapid rates, eg, during tachycardia, the atrial action potential arises from the incompletely repolarized membrane and results in voltage-dependent reduction of I_{Na}. Ranolazine has relatively little effect on I_{Ca} and the remaining K^+ currents at therapeutic concentrations.

Ranolazine had been shown to have antiarrhythmic properties in both atrial and ventricular arrhythmias. It prevents the induction of, and may terminate, atrial fibrillation. It is currently undergoing clinical trials in combination with dronedarone for the suppression of atrial fibrillation. Ranolazine has been shown to suppress ventricular tachycardia in ischemic models and in a major clinical trial of its effects in coronary artery disease. The drug has not yet received FDA approval as an antiarrhythmic drug.

VERNAKALANT

Vernakalant is a multi-ion channel blocker, placing it in several classes of antiarrhythmic action. It causes frequency- and voltage-dependent block of the early and late components of the sodium current. The muscarinic potassium current $I_{K,ACh}$, which is constitutively activated in atrial fibrillation, is blocked by vernakalant. The early-activating potassium channels I_{to} and I_{kur} are also blocked by the drug. These potassium channel currents play a more prominent role in atrial than in ventricular repolarization. As a result, vernakalant produces only mild QT-interval prolongation. It does not produce torsades de pointes. Approved in Europe but not yet approved by the FDA, vernakalant can be administered intravenously for the rapid termination of atrial fibrillation in patients with no or minimal structural heart disease. In a direct comparison trial, vernakalant proved more effective than placebo or amiodarone in terminating atrial fibrillation in a 90-minute period. This relatively rapid action decreases the required observation period for untoward side effects following drug administration. Sinus bradycardia and hypotension are the only noticeable cardiovascular adverse effects.

MAGNESIUM

Originally used for patients with digitalis-induced arrhythmias who were hypomagnesemic, magnesium infusion has been found to have antiarrhythmic effects in some patients with normal serum magnesium levels. The mechanisms of these effects are not known, but magnesium is recognized to influence Na^+/K^+-ATPase, sodium channels, certain potassium channels, and calcium channels. Magnesium therapy appears to be indicated in patients with digitalis-induced arrhythmias if hypomagnesemia is present; it is also indicated in some patients with torsades de pointes even if serum magnesium is normal. The usual dosage is 1 g (as sulfate) given intravenously over 20 minutes and repeated once if necessary. A full understanding of the action and indications for the use of magnesium as an antiarrhythmic drug awaits further investigation.

POTASSIUM

The significance of the potassium ion concentrations inside and outside the cardiac cell membrane was discussed earlier in this chapter. The effects of increasing serum K^+ can be summarized as (1) a resting potential depolarizing action and (2) a membrane potential stabilizing action, the latter caused by increased potassium permeability. Hypokalemia results in an increased risk of early and delayed afterdepolarizations, and ectopic pacemaker activity, especially in the presence of digitalis. Hyperkalemia depresses ectopic pacemakers (severe hyperkalemia is required to suppress the SA node) and slows conduction. Because both insufficient and excess potassium are potentially arrhythmogenic, potassium therapy is directed toward normalizing potassium gradients and pools in the body.

■ PRINCIPLES IN THE CLINICAL USE OF ANTIARRHYTHMIC AGENTS

The margin between efficacy and toxicity is particularly narrow for antiarrhythmic drugs. Risks and benefits must be carefully considered (see Box: Antiarrhythmic Drug-Use Principles Applied to Atrial Fibrillation).

Pretreatment Evaluation

Several important steps must be taken before initiation of any antiarrhythmic therapy:

1. **Eliminate the cause.** Precipitating factors must be recognized and eliminated if possible. These include not only abnormalities of internal homeostasis, such as hypoxia or electrolyte abnormalities (especially hypokalemia or hypomagnesemia), but also drug therapy and underlying disease states such as hyperthyroidism or cardiac disease. It is important to separate this abnormal substrate from triggering factors, such as myocardial ischemia, acute cardiac dilation, or sleep apnea, which may be treatable and reversible by different means.
2. **Make a firm diagnosis.** A firm diagnosis of arrhythmia should be established. For example, the misuse of verapamil in patients with ventricular tachycardia mistakenly diagnosed as supraventricular tachycardia can lead to catastrophic hypotension and cardiac arrest. As increasingly sophisticated methods to characterize underlying arrhythmia mechanisms become available and are validated, it may be possible to direct certain drugs toward specific arrhythmia mechanisms.
3. **Determine the baseline condition.** Underlying heart disease is a critical determinant of drug selection for a particular arrhythmia in a particular patient. A key question is whether the heart is structurally abnormal. Few antiarrhythmic drugs have documented safety in patients with congestive heart failure or ischemic heart disease. In fact, some drugs pose a documented proarrhythmic risk in certain disease states, eg, class 1C drugs in patients with ischemic heart disease. A reliable baseline should be established against which to judge the efficacy of any subsequent antiarrhythmic intervention. Several methods are now available for such baseline quantification. These include prolonged ambulatory monitoring, electrophysiologic studies that reproduce a target arrhythmia, reproduction of a target arrhythmia by treadmill exercise, or the use of transtelephonic monitoring for recording of sporadic but symptomatic arrhythmias.
4. **Question the need for therapy.** The mere identification of an abnormality of cardiac rhythm does not necessarily require that the arrhythmia be treated. An excellent justification for conservative treatment was provided by the Cardiac Arrhythmia Suppression Trial (CAST) referred to earlier.

Benefits & Risks

The benefits of antiarrhythmic therapy are difficult to establish. Two types of benefits can be envisioned: reduction of arrhythmia-related symptoms, such as palpitations, syncope, or cardiac arrest; and reduction in long-term mortality. Among drugs discussed here, only β blockers have been definitely associated with reduction of mortality in relatively asymptomatic patients, and the mechanism underlying this effect is not established (see Chapter 10).

Antiarrhythmic therapy carries with it a number of risks. In some cases, the risk of an adverse reaction is clearly related to high dosages or plasma concentrations. Examples include lidocaine-induced tremor or quinidine-induced cinchonism. In other cases, adverse reactions are unrelated to high plasma concentrations (eg, procainamide-induced agranulocytosis). For many serious adverse reactions to antiarrhythmic drugs, the *combination* of drug therapy and the underlying heart disease appears important.

Several specific syndromes of arrhythmia provocation by antiarrhythmic drugs have also been identified, each with its underlying pathophysiologic mechanism and risk factors. Drugs such as quinidine, sotalol, ibutilide, and dofetilide, which act—at least in part—by slowing repolarization and prolonging cardiac action potentials, can result in marked QT prolongation and torsades de pointes. Treatment for torsades requires recognition of the arrhythmia, withdrawal of any offending agent, correction of hypokalemia, and treatment with maneuvers to increase heart rate (pacing or isoproterenol); intravenous magnesium also appears effective, even in patients with normal magnesium levels.

Drugs that markedly slow conduction, such as flecainide, or high concentrations of quinidine can result in an increased frequency of reentry arrhythmias, notably ventricular tachycardia in patients with prior myocardial infarction in whom a potential reentry circuit may be present. Treatment here consists of recognition, withdrawal of the offending agent, and intravenous sodium to reverse unidirectional block.

Antiarrhythmic Drug-Use Principles Applied to Atrial Fibrillation

Atrial fibrillation is the most common sustained arrhythmia observed clinically. Its prevalence increases from approximately 0.5% in individuals younger than 65 years of age to 10% in individuals older than 80. Diagnosis is usually straightforward by means of an ECG. The ECG may also enable the identification of a prior myocardial infarction, left ventricular hypertrophy, and ventricular pre-excitation. Hyperthyroidism is an important treatable cause of atrial fibrillation, and a thyroid panel should be obtained at the time of diagnosis to exclude this possibility. With the clinical history and physical examination as a guide, the presence and extent of the underlying heart disease should be evaluated, preferably using noninvasive techniques such as echocardiography.

Treatment of atrial fibrillation is initiated to relieve patient symptoms and prevent the complications of thromboembolism and tachycardia-induced heart failure, the result of prolonged uncontrolled heart rates. The initial treatment objective is control of the ventricular rate. This is usually achieved by the use of a calcium channel-blocking drug alone or in combination with a β-adrenergic blocker. Digoxin may be of value in the presence of heart failure. A second objective is a restoration and maintenance of normal sinus rhythm. Several studies show that rate control (maintenance of ventricular rate in the range of 60–80 bpm) has a better benefit-to-risk outcome than rhythm control (conversion to normal sinus rhythm) in the long-term health of patients with atrial fibrillation. If rhythm control is deemed desirable, sinus rhythm is usually restored by DC cardioversion in the USA. This is also the preferred strategy in an emergency, eg, atrial fibrillation associated with hypotension or angina. For the elective restoration of sinus rhythm, a single large oral dose of propafenone or flecainide may be used, provided that safety is initially documented in a monitored setting. Intravenous ibutilide can also restore sinus rhythm promptly.

The selection of a drug to maintain normal sinus rhythm depends on the presence and type of underlying heart disease. An example of an algorithm for drug selection is given in Figure 14–11. If AF cannot be corrected or if it recurs, ablation therapy will be considered (see Box: The Nonpharmacologic Therapy of Cardiac Arrhythmias and Figure 14–11).

Antiarrhythmic drugs remain the preferred rhythm control strategy. However, a comparison of initial strategies for the maintenance of normal sinus rhythm is currently undergoing clinical trial. The essential role of oral anticoagulation in the prevention of stroke is established. Currently guidelines identify patients who are at particular risk and should undergo long-term anticoagulation.

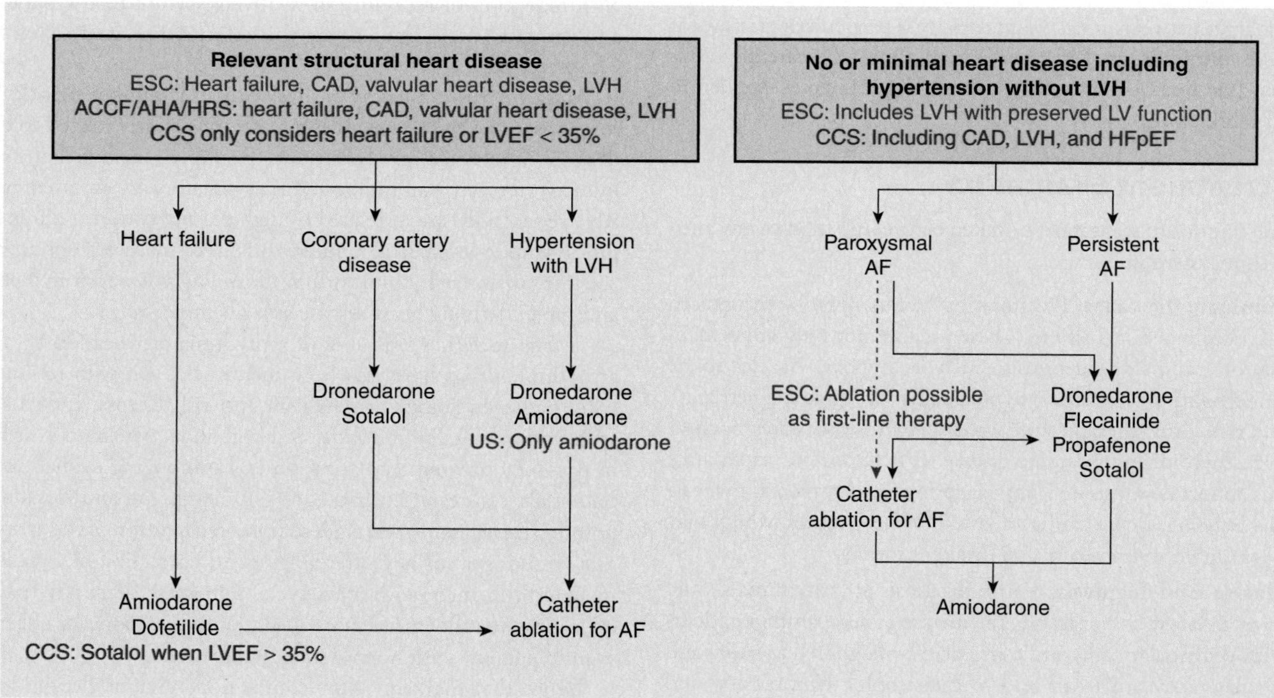

FIGURE 14–11 Selection of rhythm control therapies depends on presence and nature of any underlying heart disease. Patients may be divided into two broad categories: those with and those without underlying heart disease. Patient with heart failure, left ventricular ejection fraction (LVEF) less than 35%, coronary artery disease (CAD), valvular heart disease, and left ventricular hypertrophy (LVH) fall into the first category. The second category includes patients with mild LVH and with heart failure but a preserved ejection fraction (HFpEF). The recommendations are based on the guidelines of the American College of Cardiology Foundation (ACCF), the American Heart Association (AHA), the Heart Rhythm Society (HRS), and the Canadian Cardiology Society (CCS). AF, atrial fibrillation; ESC, European Society of Cardiology; LV, left ventricle.

Conduct of Antiarrhythmic Therapy

The urgency of the clinical situation determines the route and rate of drug initiation. When immediate drug action is required, the intravenous route is preferred. Therapeutic drug levels can be achieved by administration of multiple *slow* intravenous boluses. Drug therapy can be considered effective when the target arrhythmia is suppressed (according to the measure used to quantify it at baseline) and toxicities are absent. Conversely, drug therapy should not be considered ineffective unless toxicities occur at a time when arrhythmias are not suppressed.

Monitoring plasma drug concentrations can be a useful adjunct to managing antiarrhythmic therapy. Plasma drug concentrations are also important in establishing compliance during long-term therapy as well as in detecting drug interactions that may result in very high concentrations at low drug dosages or very low concentrations at high dosages.

Antiarrhythmic Drug Combinations

The urgency for rhythm control differs between atrial fibrillation and ventricular tachycardia or fibrillation. In atrial fibrillation, the ventricular response rate can usually be controlled with AV node–blocking drugs. Restoration of sinus rhythm may be safely deferred, or the state of atrial fibrillation may be accepted long term. In contrast, ventricular tachycardia or frequent, complex ventricular premature beats are inherently unstable and require immediate and effective therapy. The strategy of antiarrhythmic drug combinations aims to exploit the potential advantage of using two drugs with different mechanisms of action, each at a lower dose to decrease adverse effects. Sodium channel blockers are the principal class of drugs used to treat or prevent ventricular arrhythmia recurrence. Amiodarone is the most effective drug for treating ventricular arrhythmias. The multi-ion channel blocking action may be the basis of its efficacy. One strategy consists of basing the drug combination on amiodarone and adding a sodium channel blocker. An alternative strategy involves selecting another class 3 drug and a sodium channel blocker. The class 3 drug may prolong sodium channels in the inactivated state and enhance the effects of class 1 drugs. Unfortunately, there are only a few studies of antiarrhythmic drug combinations in clinical settings. One study examined the combination of amiodarone and disopyramide, flecainide, or propafenone in patients with complex ventricular ectopy. The combination of amiodarone and flecainide proved the most effective. Another study examined the combination of a low dose of sotalol with procainamide or quinidine. These drug combinations greatly prolonged refractoriness and were more effective at short coupling intervals. However, the combination of drugs was not well tolerated, with ~50% of patients discontinuing the combination. The risk of torsades de pointes would be predictably high with either combination.

The most striking difference between the atrial and ventricular action potentials is duration and the terminal phase of the action potential. As rate increases above 4/s, successive atrial action potentials are initiated at more depolarized membrane potentials. For sodium channel blockers that more readily bind inactivated channels, depolarized membrane potentials enhance channel block, making these drugs relatively more effective. This effect is enhanced by prolonging the atrial action potential duration. The drug combination of a reduced dose of dronedarone and ranolazine was examined in the HARMONY trial. This combination of ranolazine and dronedarone reduced atrial fibrillation burden in patients with paroxysmal atrial fibrillation when compared with either drug alone.

SUMMARY Antiarrhythmic Drugs

Subclass, Drug	Mechanism of Action	Effects	Clinical Applications	Pharmacokinetics, Toxicities, Interactions
CLASS 1A				
• Procainamide	I_{Na} (primary) and I_{Kr} (secondary) blockade	Slows conduction velocity and pacemaker rate • prolongs action potential duration and dissociates from I_{Na} channel with intermediate kinetics • direct depressant effects on sinoatrial (SA) and atrioventricular (AV) nodes	Pre-excited atrial arrhythmias and ventricular arrhythmias • drug of second choice for most sustained ventricular arrhythmias associated with acute myocardial infarction	Oral,* IV, IM • eliminated by hepatic metabolism to *N*-acetylprocainamide (NAPA; see text) and renal elimination • NAPA implicated in torsades de pointes in patients with renal failure • *Toxicity:* Hypotension • long-term therapy produces reversible lupus-related symptoms

*The oral formulation is no longer available in the USA.

- *Quinidine: Similar to procainamide but more toxic (cinchonism, torsades); rarely used in arrhythmias; see* Chapter 52 *for malaria*
- *Disopyramide: Similar to procainamide but significant antimuscarinic effects; may precipitate heart failure; not commonly used*

(continued)

Subclass, Drug	Mechanism of Action	Effects	Clinical Applications	Pharmacokinetics, Toxicities, Interactions
CLASS 1B				
• Lidocaine	Sodium channel (I_{Na}) blockade	Blocks activated and inactivated channels with fast kinetics • does not prolong and may shorten action potential	Ventricular tachycardias and for prevention of ventricular fibrillation after cardioversion	IV • first-pass hepatic metabolism • reduce dose in patients with heart failure or liver disease • *Toxicity:* Neurologic symptoms
• *Mexiletine: Orally active congener of lidocaine; used in ventricular arrhythmias, chronic pain syndromes*				
CLASS 1C				
• Flecainide	Sodium channel (I_{Na}) blockade	Dissociates from channel with slow kinetics • no change in action potential duration	Supraventricular arrhythmias in patients with normal heart • do not use in ischemic conditions (post-myocardial infarction)	Oral • hepatic and kidney metabolism • half-life ~20 h • *Toxicity:* Proarrhythmic
• *Propafenone: Orally active, weak β-blocking activity; supraventricular arrhythmias; hepatic metabolism*				
CLASS 2				
• Propranolol	β-Adrenoceptor blockade	Direct membrane effects (sodium channel block) and prolongation of action potential duration • slows SA node automaticity and AV nodal conduction velocity	Atrial arrhythmias and prevention of recurrent infarction and sudden death Congenital long QT syndrome	Oral, parenteral • duration 4–6 h • *Toxicity:* Asthma, AV blockade, acute heart failure • *Interactions:* With other cardiac depressants and hypotensive drugs
• *Esmolol: Short-acting, IV only; used for intraoperative and other acute arrhythmias*				
CLASS 3				
• Amiodarone	Blocks I_{Kr}, I_{Na}, $I_{Ca\text{-}L}$ channels, β adrenoceptors	Prolongs action potential duration and QT interval • slows heart rate and AV node conduction • low incidence of torsades de pointes	Serious ventricular arrhythmias and supraventricular arrhythmias	Oral, IV • variable absorption and tissue accumulation • hepatic metabolism, elimination complex and slow • *Toxicity:* Bradycardia and heart block in diseased heart, peripheral vasodilation, pulmonary and hepatic toxicity • hyper- or hypothyroidism. • *Interactions:* Many, based on CYP metabolism
• Dofetilide	I_{Kr} block	Prolongs action potential, effective refractory period	Maintenance or restoration of sinus rhythm in atrial fibrillation	Oral • renal excretion • *Toxicity:* Torsades de pointes (initiate in hospital with monitoring) • *Interactions:* Additive with other QT-prolonging drugs
• *Sotalol: β-Adrenergic and I_{Kr} blocker, direct action potential prolongation properties, use for ventricular arrhythmias, atrial fibrillation* • *Ibutilide: Potassium channel blocker, may activate inward current; IV use for conversion in atrial flutter and fibrillation* • *Dronedarone: Amiodarone derivative; multichannel actions, reduces mortality in patients with atrial fibrillation* • *Vernakalant: Investigational in the USA, multichannel actions in atria, prolongs atrial refractoriness, effective in cardioversion of atrial flutter and atrial fibrillation*				
CLASS 4				
• Verapamil	Calcium channel ($I_{Ca\text{-}L}$ type) blockade	Slows SA node automaticity and AV nodal conduction velocity • decreases cardiac contractility • reduces blood pressure	Supraventricular tachycardias, hypertension, angina	Oral, IV • hepatic metabolism • caution in patients with hepatic dysfunction • *Toxicity & Interactions:* See Chapter 12
• *Diltiazem: Similar to verapamil*				

(continued)

Subclass, Drug	Mechanism of Action	Effects	Clinical Applications	Pharmacokinetics, Toxicities, Interactions
MISCELLANEOUS				
• Adenosine	Activates inward rectifier I_K • blocks I_{Ca}	Very brief, usually complete AV blockade	Paroxysmal supraventricular tachycardias	IV only • duration 10–15 s • *Toxicity:* Flushing, chest tightness, dizziness • *Interactions:* Minimal
• Magnesium	Poorly understood • interacts with Na^+/K^+-ATPase, K^+, and Ca^{2+} channels	Normalizes or increases plasma Mg^{2+}	Torsades de pointes • digitalis-induced arrhythmias	IV • duration dependent on dosage • *Toxicity:* Muscle weakness in overdose
• Potassium	Increases K^+ permeability, K^+ currents	Slows ectopic pacemakers • slows conduction velocity in heart	Digitalis-induced arrhythmias • arrhythmias associated with hypokalemia	Oral, IV • *Toxicity:* Reentrant arrhythmias, fibrillation or arrest in overdose

PREPARATIONS AVAILABLE

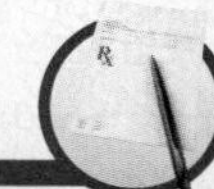

GENERIC NAME	AVAILABLE AS
SODIUM CHANNEL BLOCKERS	
Disopyramide	Generic, Norpace, Norpace CR
Flecainide	Generic, Tambocor
Lidocaine	Generic, Xylocaine
Mexiletine	Generic, Mexitil
Procainamide	Generic, Pronestyl, Procan-SR
Propafenone	Generic, Rythmol
Quinidine sulfate (83% quinidine base)	Generic
Quinidine gluconate (62% quinidine base)	Generic
Quinidine polygalacturonate (60% quinidine base)	Cardioquin
BETA BLOCKERS LABELED FOR USE AS ANTIARRHYTHMICS	
Acebutolol	Generic, Sectral
Esmolol	Generic, Brevibloc
Propranolol	Generic, Inderal
ACTION POTENTIAL–PROLONGING AGENTS	
Amiodarone	Generic, Cordarone
Dofetilide	Tikosyn
Dronedarone	Multaq
Ibutilide	Generic, Corvert
Sotalol	Generic, Betapace
CALCIUM CHANNEL BLOCKERS	
Diltiazem	Generic, Cardizem
Verapamil	Generic, Calan, Isoptin
MISCELLANEOUS	
Adenosine	Generic, Adenocard
Magnesium sulfate	Generic

REFERENCES

Anonymous: Drugs for atrial fibrillation. Med Lett 2019;61:137.

Antzelevitch C, Burashnikov A: Overview of basic mechanisms of cardiac arrhythmia. Card Electrophysiol Clin 2011;3:23.

Bezzina CR et al: Genetics of sudden cardiac death. Circ Res 2015;116:1919.

Burashnikov A, Antzelevitch C: Role of late sodium channel block in the management of atrial fibrillation. Cardiovasc Drugs Ther 2013;27:79.

Catterall WA, Lenaeus MJ, Gamal El-Din TM: Structure and pharmacology of voltage-gated sodium and calcium channels. Annu Rev Pharmacol Toxicol 2020;60:133.

Chinitz JS et al: Rate or rhythm control for atrial fibrillation: Update and controversies. Am J Med 2012;125:1049.

Cho HC, Marban E: Biological therapies for cardiac arrhythmias: Can genes and cells replace drugs and devices? Circ Res 2010;106:674.

Das MK, Zipes DP: Antiarrhythmic and nonantiarrhythmic drugs for sudden cardiac death prevention. J Cardiovasc Pharmacol 2010;55:438.

Echt DS et al, for the CAST Investigators: Mortality and morbidity in patients receiving encainide, flecainide, or placebo. The Cardiac Arrhythmia Suppression Trial. N Engl J Med 1991;324:781.

El-Sherif N, Boutjdir M: Role of pharmacotherapy in cardiac ion channelopathies. Pharmacol Ther 2015;155:132.

El-Sherif N, Turitto G: Electrolyte disorders and arrhythmogenesis. Cardiol J 2011;18:233.

Fedida D: Vernakalant (RSD1235): A novel, atrial-selective antifibrillatory agent. Expert Opin Investig Drugs 2007;16:519.

Fuster V et al: ACC/AHA/ESC Guidelines for the management of patients with atrial fibrillation. Circulation 2006;114:700.

George AL: Molecular and genetic basis of sudden cardiac death. J Clin Invest 2013;123:75.

Grant AO: Cardiac ion channels. Circ Arrhythm Electrophysiol 2009;2:185.

Hondeghem LM: Relative contributions of TRIaD and QT to proarrhythmia. J Cardiovasc Electrophysiol 2007;18:655.

Kolettis TM: Coronary artery disease and ventricular arrhythmias: Pathophysiology and treatment. Curr Opin Pharm 2013;13:210.

Lee SD et al: Electrophysiologic mechanisms of antiarrhythmic efficacy of a sotalol and class 1a drug combination: Elimination of reverse use dependence. J Am Coll Cardiol 1997;29:100.

Li A, Behr ER: Advances in the management of atrial fibrillation. Clin Med 2012;12:544.

Marrus SB, Nerbonne JM: Mechanisms linking short- and long-term electrical remodeling in the heart … Is it a stretch? Channels 2008;2:117.

Mohler PJ, Gramolini AO, Bennett V: Ankyrins. J Cell Biol 2002;115:1565.

Monfredi O, Maltsev VA, Lakatta EG: Modern concepts concerning the origin of the heartbeat. Physiology 2013;28:74.

Morady F: Catheter ablation of supraventricular arrhythmias: State of the art. J Cardiovasc Electrophysiol 2004;15:124.

Reiffel JA et al: The HARMONY TRIAL; Combined ranolazine and dronedarone in the management of atrial fibrillation: Mechanistic and therapeutic synergism. Circ Arrhythm Electrophysiol 2015;8:1048.

Roubille F, Tardif J-C: New therapeutic targets in cardiology, heart failure and arrhythmia: HCN channels. Circulation 2013;127:1986.

Starmer FC, Grant AO, Strauss HC: Mechanisms of use-dependent block of sodium channels in excitable membranes by local anesthetics. Biophys J 1984;46:15.

Veerakul G, Nademanec K: Brugada syndrome: Two decades of progress. Circ J 2012;76:2713.

Vizzardi E et al: A focus on antiarrhythmic properties of ranolazine. J Cardiovasc Pharm Ther 2012;17:353.

Wehrens XHT et al: Ryanodine receptor-targeted anti-arrhythmic therapy. NY Acad Sci 2005;1047:366.

Wolbrette D et al: Dronedarone for the treatment of atrial fibrillation and atrial flutter: Approval and efficacy. Vasc Health Risk Manag 2010;6:517.

CASE STUDY ANSWER

The patient has significant symptoms during recurrent episodes of atrial fibrillation. She has multiple risk factors for thromboembolism (age, female gender, and hypertension). Therefore, she is a candidate for lifelong anticoagulation. Warfarin was the standard drug. The factor Xa (eg, apixaban, rivaroxaban) and the direct thrombin (eg, dabigatran) inhibitors are newer classes of anticoagulants that offer more patient-acceptable alternatives but at a higher cost. The peak heart rate in this patient's atrial fibrillation is not particularly high. Maintenance of sinus rhythm appears to be important in this patient. The echocardiogram demonstrates impairment of left ventricular function. Selection of a drug that is tolerated in heart failure and has documented ability to convert or prevent atrial fibrillation, eg, dofetilide or amiodarone, would be appropriate. The patient was treated with dofetilide. A repeated echocardiogram 3 months later showed an ejection fraction of 48%. The use of catheter ablation for treatment of the initial episode of atrial fibrillation is not the standard of care but is undergoing clinical trials.

C H A P T E R

15

Diuretic Agents

Ramin Sam, MD, & David Pearce, MD

CASE STUDY

A 65-year-old man has a history of diabetes and chronic kidney disease with baseline creatinine of 2.2 mg/dL. Despite five different antihypertensive drugs, his clinic blood pressure is 176/92 mm Hg; he has mild dyspnea on exertion and 2–3+ edema on examination. He has been taking furosemide 80 mg twice a day for 1 year now. At the clinic visit, hydrochlorothiazide 25 mg daily is added for better blood pressure control and also to treat symptoms and signs of fluid overload. Two weeks later, the patient presents to the emergency department with symptoms of weakness, anorexia, and generalized malaise. His blood pressure is now 91/58 mm Hg, and he has lost 15 kg in 2 weeks. His laboratory tests are significant for a serum creatinine of 10.8 mg/dL. What has led to the acute kidney injury? What is the reason for the weight loss? What precautions could have been taken to avoid this hospitalization?

Abnormalities in fluid volume and electrolyte composition are common and important clinical disorders. Drugs that block specific transport functions of the renal tubules are valuable clinical tools in the treatment of these disorders. Although various agents that increase urine volume (diuretics) have been described since antiquity, it was not until 1937 that carbonic anhydrase inhibitors were first described and not until 1957 that a much more useful and powerful diuretic agent (chlorothiazide) became available.

Technically, a "diuretic" is an agent that increases urine volume, whereas a "natriuretic" causes an increase in renal sodium excretion and an "aquaretic" increases excretion of solute-free water. Because natriuretics almost always also increase water excretion, they are usually called diuretics. Osmotic diuretics and antidiuretic hormone antagonists (see Agents That Alter Water Excretion) are aquaretics and are not directly natriuretic; however, because they increase urine volume, diuretic is still a correct term to describe them. Most recently, an entirely new class of agents has been developed that block urea transport. These agents result in increased urine output and increased urea excretion but do not increase excretion of electrolytes. While they are technically aquaretics, they are also referred to as urearetics. These agents are not yet available for therapy but are in early investigational stages.

This chapter is divided into three sections. The first section covers major renal tubule transport mechanisms. The nephron is divided structurally and functionally into several segments (Figure 15–1, Table 15–1). Several autacoids, which exert multiple, complex effects on renal physiology (adenosine, prostaglandins, and urodilatin, a renal autacoid closely related to atrial natriuretic peptide), also are discussed. The second section describes the pharmacology of diuretic agents. Many diuretics exert their effects on specific membrane transport proteins in renal tubular epithelial cells. Other diuretics exert osmotic effects that prevent water reabsorption (mannitol), inhibit enzymes (acetazolamide), or interfere with hormone receptors in renal epithelial cells (vaptans, or vasopressin antagonists). The physiology of each nephron segment is closely linked to the basic pharmacology of the drugs acting there, which is discussed in the second section. The third section of the chapter describes the clinical applications of diuretics.

■ RENAL TUBULE TRANSPORT MECHANISMS

PROXIMAL TUBULE

Sodium bicarbonate ($NaHCO_3$), sodium chloride (NaCl), glucose, amino acids, and other organic solutes are reabsorbed via specific transport systems in the early proximal tubule (proximal convoluted tubule, **PCT**). Potassium ions (K^+) are reabsorbed via the paracellular pathway. Water is reabsorbed passively, through both a

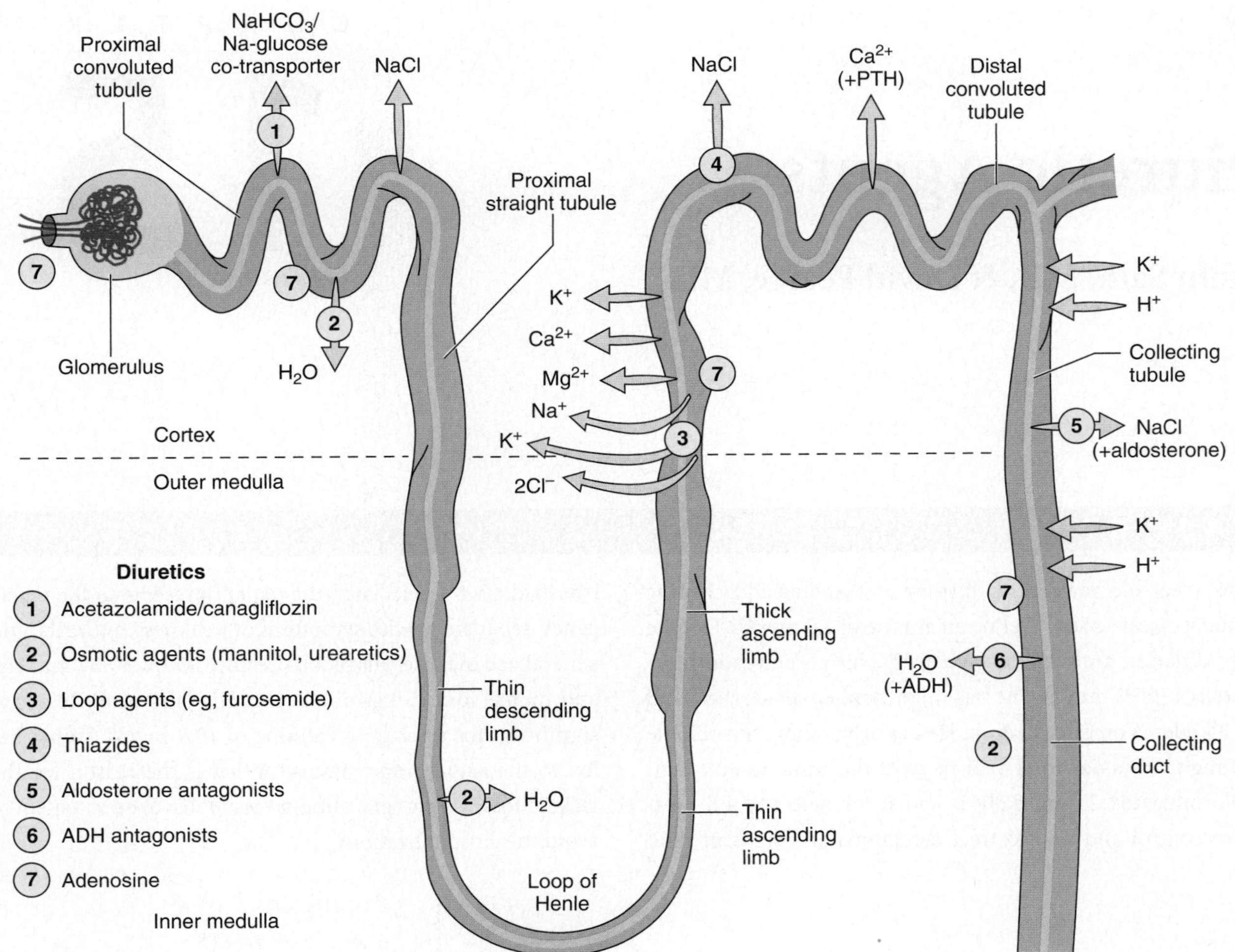

FIGURE 15–1 Tubule transport systems and sites of action of diuretics. ADH, antidiuretic hormone; PTH, parathyroid hormone.

transcellular pathway (mediated by a specific water channel, aquaporin-1 [AQP1]) and a paracellular pathway (likely mediated by claudin-2). Importantly, the water permeability of the PCT is very high, and hence, the osmolality of proximal tubular fluid is maintained at a nearly constant level, and the gradient from the tubule lumen to surrounding interstitium is very small. As tubule fluid is processed along the length of the proximal tubule, the luminal concentrations of most solutes decrease relative to the concentration of inulin, an experimental marker that is filtered but neither secreted nor absorbed by renal tubules. Approximately 66% of filtered sodium ions (Na^+), 85% of the $NaHCO_3$, 65% of the K^+, 60% of the water, and virtually all of the filtered glucose and amino acids are reabsorbed by the proximal tubule in normal humans.

Of the various solutes reabsorbed in the proximal tubule, the most relevant to diuretic action are $NaHCO_3$ and NaCl. Until recently, of the currently available diuretics, only one group (carbonic anhydrase inhibitors, which block $NaHCO_3$ reabsorption) has acted predominantly in the PCT. Sodium bicarbonate reabsorption by the PCT is initiated by the action of a **Na^+/H^+ exchanger (NHE3)** located in the luminal membrane of the proximal tubule epithelial cell (Figure 15–2). This transport system allows Na^+ to enter the cell from the tubular lumen in exchange for a proton (H^+) from inside the cell. As in all portions of the nephron, Na^+/K^+-ATPase in the basolateral membrane pumps the reabsorbed Na^+ into the interstitium in order to maintain a low intracellular Na^+ concentration. The H^+ secreted into the lumen combines with bicarbonate (HCO_3^-) to form H_2CO_3 (carbonic acid), which is rapidly dehydrated to CO_2 and H_2O by carbonic anhydrase. Carbon dioxide produced by dehydration of H_2CO_3 enters the proximal tubule cell by simple diffusion, where it is then rehydrated back to H_2CO_3, facilitated by intracellular carbonic anhydrase. After dissociation of H_2CO_3, the H^+ is available for transport by the Na^+/H^+ exchanger, and the HCO_3^- is transported out of the cell by a basolateral membrane transporter (see Figure 15–2). Bicarbonate reabsorption by the proximal tubule is thus dependent on carbonic anhydrase activity. This enzyme can be inhibited by acetazolamide and other carbonic anhydrase inhibitors.

More recently, inhibitors of the **sodium-glucose cotransporter,** isoform 2 (**SGLT2**; see Figure 15–2) have been approved to treat diabetes mellitus. The sodium-glucose cotransporter is responsible for reabsorbing much of the glucose that is filtered by the glomeruli. Although not indicated as diuretic agents, inhibition of SGLT2

TABLE 15–1 Major segments of the nephron and their functions.

Segment	Functions	Water Permeability	Primary Transporters and Drug Targets at Apical Membrane	Diuretic with Major Action
Glomerulus	Formation of glomerular filtrate	Extremely high	None	None
Proximal convoluted tubule (PCT)	Reabsorption of 65% of filtered $Na^+/K^+/CA^{2+}$, and Mg^{2+}; 85% of $NaHCO_3$, and nearly 100% of glucose and amino acids. Isosmotic reabsorption of water	Very high	Na/H[1] (NHE3), carbonic anhydrase; Na/glucose cotransporter 2 (SGLT2)	Carbonic anhydrase inhibitors, Adenosine antagonists (under investigation)
Proximal tubule, straight segments	Secretion and reabsorption of organic acids and bases, including uric acid and most diuretics	Very high	Acid (eg, uric acid) and base transporters	None
Thin descending limb of Henle's loop	Passive reabsorption of water	High	Aquaporins	None
Thick ascending limb of Henle's loop (TAL)	Active reabsorption of 15–25% of filtered $Na^+/K^+/Cl^-$; secondary reabsorption of CA^{2+} and Mg^{2+}	Very low	Na/K/2Cl (NKCC2)	Loop diuretics
Distal convoluted tubule (DCT)	Active reabsorption of 4–8% of filtered Na^+ and Cl^-; CA^{2+} reabsorption under parathyroid hormone control	Very low	Na/Cl (NCC)	Thiazides
Cortical collecting tubule (CCT)	Na^+ reabsorption (2–5%) coupled to K^+ and H^+ secretion	Variable[2]	Na channels (ENaC), K channels,[1] H^+ transporter,[1] aquaporins	K^+-sparing diuretics Adenosine antagonists (under investigation)
Medullary collecting duct	Water reabsorption under vasopressin control	Variable[2]	Aquaporins	Vasopressin antagonists

[1]Not a target of currently available drugs.

[2]Controlled by vasopressin activity.

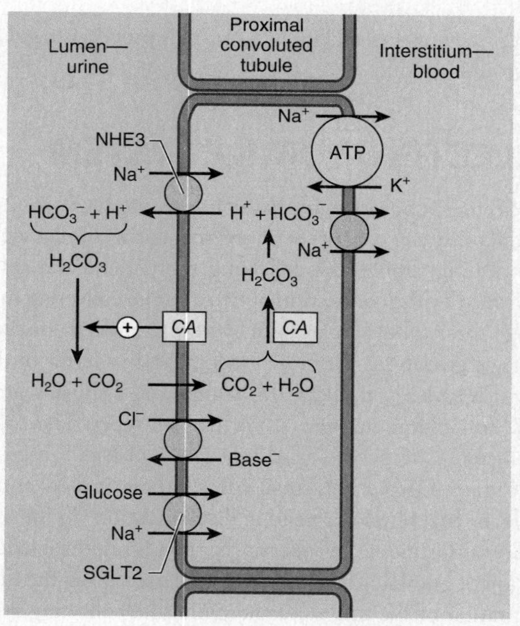

FIGURE 15–2 Apical membrane Na^+/H^+ exchange (via NHE3) and bicarbonate reabsorption in the proximal convoluted tubule cell. Na^+/K^+-ATPase is present in the basolateral membrane to maintain intracellular sodium and potassium levels within the normal range. Because of rapid equilibration, concentrations of the solutes are approximately equal in the interstitial fluid and the blood. Carbonic anhydrase (CA) is found in other locations in addition to the brush border of the luminal membrane. SGLT2, Na^+/glucose transporter.

by these drugs will be accompanied by increased sodium and glucose excretion (see below). The diuretic properties are thought to result mainly from osmotic diuresis, although these agents clearly have natriuretic properties also. It has been established recently that gliflozins do indeed reduce total body sodium content, a class effect useful in heart failure.

Organic acid secretory systems are located in the middle third of the straight part of the proximal tubule (S_2 segment). These systems secrete a variety of organic acids (uric acid, nonsteroidal anti-inflammatory drugs [NSAIDs], diuretics, antibiotics, etc) into the luminal fluid from the blood. These systems thus help deliver diuretics to the luminal side of the tubule, where most of them act. Organic base secretory systems (creatinine, choline, etc) also are present, in the early (S_1) and middle (S_2) segments of the proximal tubule.

LOOP OF HENLE

At the boundary between the inner and outer stripes of the outer medulla, the proximal tubule empties into the thin descending limb of Henle's loop. Water is extracted from the descending limb of this loop by osmotic forces found in the hypertonic medullary interstitium. As in the proximal tubule, impermeant luminal solutes such as mannitol oppose this water extraction and thus have aquaretic activity. The thin *ascending* limb is relatively water-impermeable but is permeable to some solutes.

The **thick ascending limb (TAL),** which follows the thin limb of Henle's loop, actively reabsorbs NaCl from the lumen (about

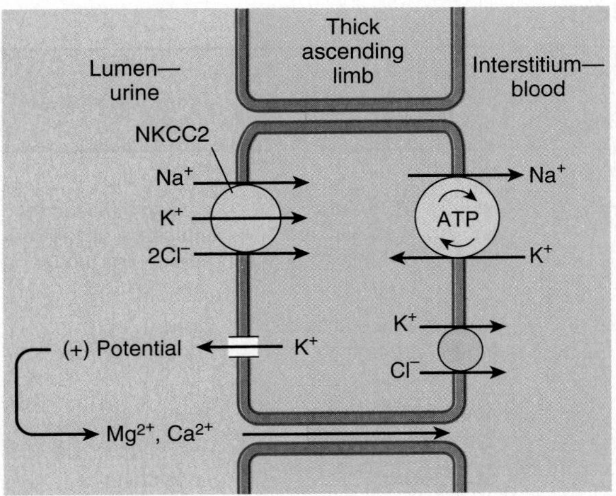

FIGURE 15–3 Ion transport pathways across the luminal and basolateral membranes of the thick ascending limb cell. The lumen positive electrical potential created by K^+ back diffusion drives divalent (and monovalent) cation reabsorption via the paracellular pathway. NKCC2 is the primary transporter in the luminal membrane.

25% of the filtered sodium), but unlike the proximal tubule and the thin descending limb of Henle's loop, it is nearly impermeable to water. Salt reabsorption in the TAL therefore dilutes the tubular fluid, and for this reason, the TAL is called a *diluting segment.* Medullary portions of the TAL contribute to medullary hypertonicity and thereby also play an important role in concentration of urine by the collecting duct.

The NaCl transport system in the luminal membrane of the TAL is the **$Na^+/K^+/2Cl^-$ cotransporter type 2** (called **NKCC2**) (Figure 15–3). This transporter is selectively blocked by diuretic agents known as loop diuretics (discussed later in the chapter). Although the $Na^+/K^+/2Cl^-$ transporter is itself electrically neutral (two cations and two anions are cotransported), the action of the transporter contributes to excess K^+ accumulation within the cell. Back diffusion of this K^+ into the tubular lumen (via the ROMK channel) causes a lumen-positive electrical potential that provides the driving force for reabsorption of cations—including magnesium and calcium—via the paracellular pathway. Thus, inhibition of salt transport in the TAL by loop diuretics, which reduces the lumen-positive potential, causes an increase in urinary excretion of divalent cations in addition to NaCl.

DISTAL CONVOLUTED TUBULE

Only about 10% of the filtered NaCl is reabsorbed in the distal convoluted tubule **(DCT).** Like the TAL of Henle's loop, this segment is relatively impermeable to water, and NaCl reabsorption further dilutes the tubular fluid. The mechanism of NaCl transport in the DCT is an electrically neutral thiazide-sensitive **Na^+/Cl^- cotransporter** (NCC; Figure 15–4).

Because K^+ does not recycle across the apical membrane of the DCT as it does in the TAL, there is no lumen-positive potential in this segment, and Ca^{2+} and Mg^{2+} are not driven out of the tubular lumen by electrical forces. Instead, Ca^{2+} is actively reabsorbed by the DCT epithelial cell via an apical Ca^{2+} channel and basolateral Na^+/Ca^{2+} exchanger (see Figure 15–4). This process is regulated by parathyroid hormone.

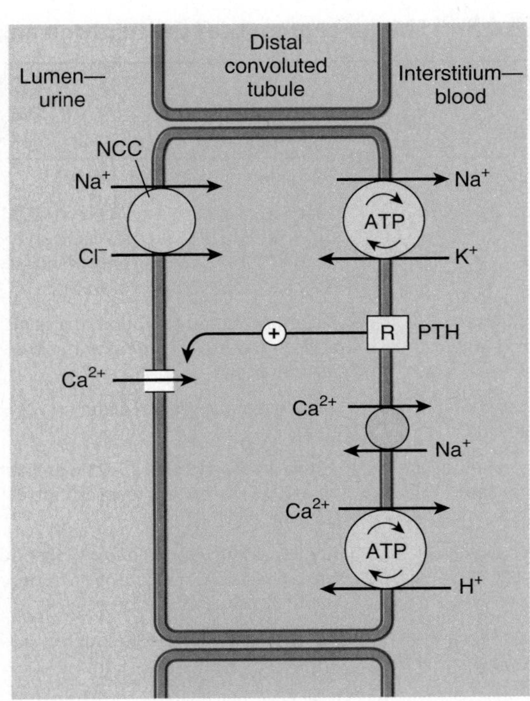

FIGURE 15–4 Ion transport pathways across the luminal and basolateral membranes of the distal convoluted tubule cell. As in all tubular cells, Na^+/K^+-ATPase is present in the basolateral membrane. NCC is the primary sodium and chloride transporter in the luminal membrane. R, parathyroid hormone (PTH) receptor.

COLLECTING TUBULE SYSTEM

The collecting tubule system that connects the DCT to the renal pelvis and the ureter consists of several sequential tubular segments: the connecting tubule, the collecting tubule, and the collecting duct (formed by the connection of two or more collecting tubules). Although these tubule segments may be anatomically distinct, the physiologic gradations are more gradual, and in terms of diuretic activity it is easier to think of this complex as a single segment of the nephron containing several distinct cell types. The collecting tubule system is responsible for only 2–5% of NaCl reabsorption by the kidney. Despite this small contribution, it plays an important role in renal physiology and in diuretic action. As the final site of NaCl reabsorption, the collecting system is responsible for tight regulation of body fluid volume and for determining the final Na^+ concentration of the urine. Furthermore, the collecting system is the site at which mineralocorticoids exert a significant influence. Lastly, this is the most important site of K^+ secretion by the kidney and the site at which virtually all diuretic-induced changes in K^+ balance occur.

The mechanism of NaCl reabsorption in the collecting tubule system is distinct from the mechanisms found in other tubule segments. The **principal cells** are the major sites of Na^+, K^+, and water transport (Figures 15–5 and 15–6), and the **intercalated**

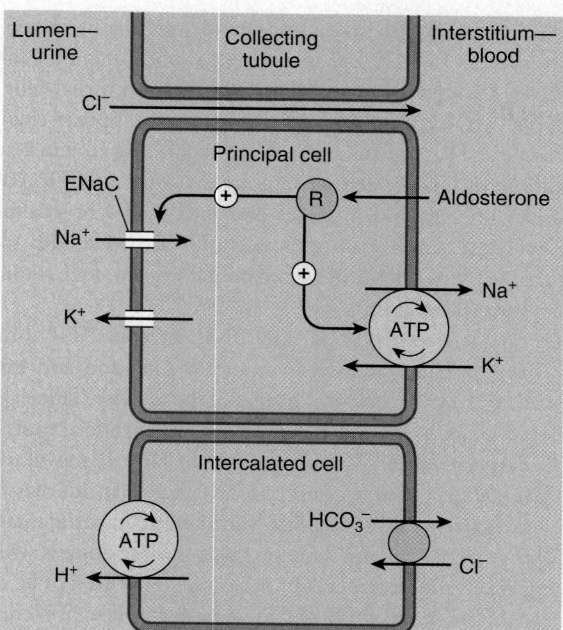

FIGURE 15–5 Ion transport pathways across the luminal and basolateral membranes of collecting tubule and collecting duct cells. Inward diffusion of Na^+ via the epithelial sodium channel (ENaC) leaves a lumen-negative potential, which drives reabsorption of Cl^- and efflux of K^+. R, aldosterone receptor.

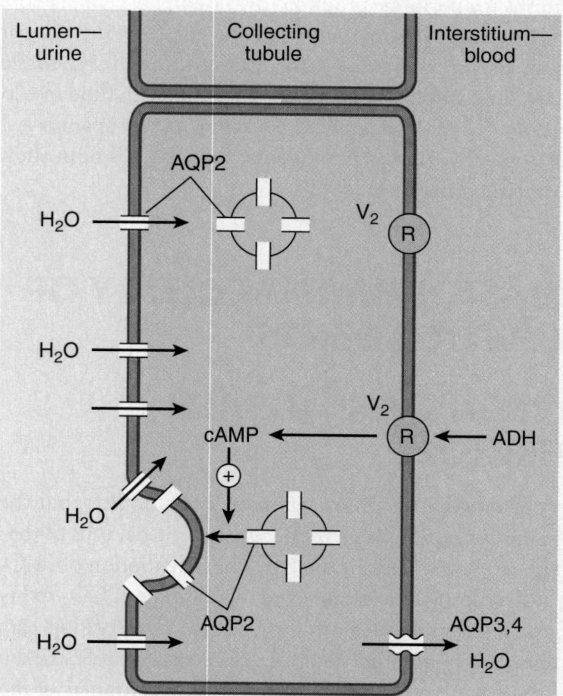

FIGURE 15–6 Water transport across the luminal and basolateral membranes of collecting duct cells. Above, low water permeability exists in the absence of antidiuretic hormone (ADH). Below, in the presence of ADH, aquaporins are inserted into the apical membrane, greatly increasing water permeability. AQP2, apical aquaporin water channels; AQP3,4, basolateral aquaporin water channels; V_2, vasopressin V_2 receptor.

cells (α, β) are the primary sites of H^+ (α cells) or bicarbonate (β cells) secretion. The α and β intercalated cells are very similar, except that the membrane locations of the H^+-ATPase and Cl^-/HCO_3^- exchanger are reversed. Principal cells do not contain apical cotransport systems for Na^+ and other ions, unlike cells in other nephron segments. Principal cell membranes exhibit separate ion channels for Na^+ and K^+. Since these channels exclude anions, transport of Na^+ or K^+ leads to a net movement of charge across the membrane. Because Na^+ entry into the principal cell predominates over K^+ secretion into the lumen, a 10- to 50-mV lumen-negative electrical potential develops. Sodium that enters the principal cell from the tubular fluid is then transported back to the blood via the basolateral Na^+/K^+-ATPase (Figure 15–5). The 10- to 50-mV lumen-negative electrical potential drives the transport of Cl^- back to the blood via the paracellular pathway and draws K^+ out of cells through the apical membrane K^+ channel. Thus, there is an important relationship between Na^+ delivery to the collecting tubule system and the resulting secretion of K^+. Upstream diuretics increase Na^+ delivery to this site and enhance K^+ secretion. If Na^+ is delivered to the collecting system with an anion that cannot be reabsorbed as readily as Cl^- (eg, HCO_3^-), the lumen-negative potential is increased, and K^+ secretion is enhanced. This mechanism, combined with enhanced aldosterone secretion due to volume depletion, is the basis for most diuretic-induced K^+ wasting. Reabsorption of Na^+ via the **epithelial Na channel (ENaC)** and its coupled secretion of K^+ are regulated by aldosterone. This steroid hormone, through its actions on gene transcription, increases the activity of both the apical membrane channels and the basolateral Na^+/K^+-ATPase. This leads to an increase in the transepithelial electrical potential and a dramatic increase in both Na^+ reabsorption and K^+ secretion.

The collecting tubule system is also the site at which the final urine concentration is determined. In addition to their role in control of Na^+ absorption and K^+ secretion (see Figure 15–5), principal cells also contain a regulated system of water channels (Figure 15–6). Antidiuretic hormone (ADH, also called arginine vasopressin, AVP) controls the permeability of these cells to water by regulating the insertion of preformed water channels **(aquaporin-2, AQP2)** into the apical membrane. Vasopressin receptors in the vasculature and central nervous system (CNS) are V_1 receptors, and those in the kidney are V_2 receptors. V_2 receptors act via a G_s protein-coupled, cAMP-mediated process. In the absence of ADH, the collecting tubule (and duct) is impermeable to water, and dilute urine is produced. ADH markedly increases water permeability, and this leads to the formation of a more concentrated urine. ADH also stimulates the insertion of urea transporter UT1 (UT-A, UTA-1) molecules into the apical membranes of collecting duct cells in the medulla.

Urea concentration in the medulla plays an important role in maintaining the high osmolarity of the medulla and subsequently in the concentration of urine. ADH secretion is regulated by serum osmolality and by volume status. A new class of drugs, the vaptans (see Agents That Alter Water Excretion), are ADH antagonists, which act at the vasopressin receptor; some vaptans are more selective than others for the V_2 receptors.

RENAL AUTACOIDS

A number of locally produced compounds exhibit physiologic effects within the kidney and are therefore referred to as *autacoids*, or *paracrine factors*. Several of these autacoids (adenosine, the prostaglandins, and urodilatin) appear to have important effects on the pharmacology of diuretics. Since these effects are complex, they will be treated independently of the individual tubule segments discussed above.

ADENOSINE

Adenosine is an unphosphorylated ribonucleoside whose actions in the kidney have been intensively studied. As in all tissues, renal adenosine concentrations rise in response to hypoxia and ATP consumption. In contrast to most other organs, in the hypoxic kidney, adenosine actually decreases blood flow and glomerular filtration rate (GFR).

There are four distinct adenosine receptors (A_1, A_{2a}, A_{2b}, and A_3), all of which have been found in the kidney. However, probably only one of these (A_1) is of importance. The adenosine A_1 receptor is found on the pre-glomerular afferent arteriole, as well as the PCT and most other tubule segments. Adenosine is known to affect ion transport in the PCT, the medullary TAL, and collecting tubules. In addition, adenosine (via A_1 receptors on the afferent arteriole) reduces blood flow to the glomerulus (and GFR) and is also the key signaling molecule in the process of tubuloglomerular feedback. Adenosine receptor antagonists have generally been found to block the enhancement of NHE3 activity and thus exhibit diuretic activity (see below). It is particularly interesting that unlike other diuretics that act upstream of the collecting tubules, adenosine antagonists do not cause wasting of K^+.

PROSTAGLANDINS

Prostaglandins contribute importantly to renal physiology and to the function of many other organs (see Chapter 18). Five prostaglandin subtypes (PGE_2, PGI_2, PGD_2, $PGF_{2\alpha}$, and thromboxane [TXA_2]) are synthesized in the kidney and have receptors in this organ. The role of some of these receptors in renal physiology is not yet completely understood. However, PGE_2 (acting on EP_1, EP_3, and possibly EP_2 receptors) has been shown to play a role in the activity of certain diuretics. Among its many actions, PGE_2 blunts Na^+ reabsorption in the TAL of Henle's loop and ADH-mediated water transport in collecting tubules. These actions of PGE_2 contribute significantly to the diuretic efficacy of loop diuretics. Blockade of prostaglandin synthesis with NSAIDs can therefore interfere with loop diuretic activity.

PEPTIDES

The natriuretic peptides (ANP, BNP, and CNP, see Chapter 17) induce natriuresis through several different mechanisms. ANP and BNP are synthesized in the heart, while CNP comes primarily from the CNS. A fourth natriuretic peptide, urodilatin, is structurally very similar to ANP but is synthesized and functions only in the kidney. Urodilatin is made in distal tubule epithelial cells and blunts Na^+ reabsorption through effects on Na^+ uptake channels and Na^+/K^+-ATPase at the downstream collecting tubule system. In addition, through effects on vascular smooth muscle, it reduces glomerular afferent and increases glomerular efferent vasomotor tone. These effects cause an increase in GFR, which adds to the natriuretic activity. Ularitide is a recombinant peptide that mimics the activity of urodilatin.

The cardiac peptides ANP and BNP increase GFR through effects on glomerular arteriolar vasomotor tone and also exhibit diuretic activity. CNP has very little diuretic activity. Three agents in this group are in clinical use or under investigation: **nesiritide** (BNP), **carperitide** (ANP, available only in Japan), and **ularitide** (urodilatin, under investigation). Intravenous ularitide has been studied extensively for use in acute heart failure. Experimentally, it can improve cardiovascular function and promote diuresis without reducing creatinine clearance, but it has not yet proved to be clinically useful. The Acute Study of Clinical Effectiveness of Nesiritide (simulating BNP) in Decompensated Heart Failure (ASCEND-HF) study did not show an improvement in outcomes with nesiritide compared with regular care in patients with heart failure.

DOPAMINE AND DOPAMINE AGONISTS

Dopamine is a hormone produced by the adrenal gland in addition to being produced in the brain and the gut. Low-dose dopamine has been shown to increase urine output through vasodilation of renal arteries. Its role in treatment of patients with fluid overload is not clearly defined and likely to be minor. Fenoldopam is a short-acting dopamine A1 receptor agonist that also has been shown to have diuretic properties.

■ BASIC PHARMACOLOGY OF DIURETIC AGENTS

CARBONIC ANHYDRASE INHIBITORS

Carbonic anhydrase is present in many nephron sites, but the predominant location of this enzyme is the epithelial cells of the PCT (see Figure 15–2), where it catalyzes the dehydration of H_2CO_3 to CO_2 at the luminal membrane and rehydration of CO_2 to H_2CO_3 in the cytoplasm as previously described. By blocking carbonic anhydrase, inhibitors blunt $NaHCO_3$ reabsorption and cause diuresis.

Carbonic anhydrase inhibitors were the forerunners of modern diuretics. They were discovered in 1937 when it was found that bacteriostatic sulfonamides caused an alkaline diuresis and hyperchloremic metabolic acidosis. With the development of newer agents, carbonic anhydrase inhibitors are now rarely used as diuretics, but they still have several specific applications that are discussed below. The prototypical carbonic anhydrase inhibitor is acetazolamide.

TABLE 15–2 Changes in urinary electrolyte patterns and body pH in response to diuretic drugs.

Group	Urinary Electrolytes			Body pH
	NaCl	$NaHCO_3$	K^+	
Carbonic anhydrase inhibitors	+	+++	+	↓
Loop agents	++++	0	+	↑
Thiazides	++	+	+	↑
Loop agents plus thiazides	+++++	+	++	↑
K^+-sparing agents	+	(+)	–	↓

+, increase; –, decrease; 0, no change; ↓, acidosis; ↑, alkalosis.

Pharmacokinetics

The carbonic anhydrase inhibitors are well absorbed after oral administration. An increase in urine pH from the HCO_3^- diuresis is apparent within 30 minutes, is maximal at 2 hours, and persists for 12 hours after a single dose. Excretion of the drug is by secretion in the proximal tubule S_2 segment. Therefore, dosing must be reduced in renal insufficiency.

Pharmacodynamics

Inhibition of carbonic anhydrase activity profoundly depresses HCO_3^- reabsorption in the PCT. At maximal safe inhibitor dosage, 85% of the HCO_3^- reabsorptive capacity of the superficial PCT is inhibited. Some HCO_3^- can still be absorbed at other nephron sites by carbonic anhydrase-independent mechanisms, so the overall effect of maximal acetazolamide dosage is only about 45% inhibition of whole kidney HCO_3^- reabsorption. Nevertheless, carbonic anhydrase inhibition causes significant HCO_3^- losses and hyperchloremic metabolic acidosis (Table 15–2). Because of reduced HCO_3^- in the glomerular filtrate and the fact that HCO_3^- depletion leads to enhanced NaCl reabsorption by the remainder of the nephron, the diuretic efficacy of acetazolamide decreases significantly with use over several days.

At present, the major clinical applications of acetazolamide involve carbonic anhydrase–dependent HCO_3^- and fluid transport at sites other than the kidney, although it is also used for diuresis if metabolic alkalosis is present, and occasionally for ventilator weaning. The ciliary body of the eye secretes HCO_3^- from the blood into the aqueous humor, and similarly, formation of cerebrospinal fluid (CSF) by the choroid plexus involves HCO_3^- secretion. Although these processes remove HCO_3^- from the blood (the direction opposite of that in the proximal tubule), they are similarly inhibited by carbonic anhydrase inhibitors.

Clinical Indications & Dosage (Table 15–3)

A. Glaucoma

The reduction of aqueous humor formation by carbonic anhydrase inhibitors decreases the intraocular pressure. This effect is valuable in the management of glaucoma in some patients, making it the most common indication for use of carbonic anhydrase inhibitors (see Table 10–3). Topically active agents, which reduce intraocular pressure without producing renal or systemic effects, are available (dorzolamide, brinzolamide).

TABLE 15–3 Carbonic anhydrase inhibitors used orally in the treatment of glaucoma.

Drug	Usual Oral Dosage
Dichlorphenamide	50 mg 1–3 times daily
Methazolamide	50–100 mg 2–3 times daily

B. Urinary Alkalinization

Uric acid and cystine are relatively insoluble and may form stones in acidic urine. Therefore, in cystinuria, a disorder of cystine reabsorption, solubility of cystine can be enhanced by increasing urinary pH to 7–7.5 with carbonic anhydrase inhibitors. In the case of uric acid, pH needs to be raised only to 6–6.5. In the absence of HCO_3^- administration, these effects of acetazolamide last only 2–3 days, so prolonged therapy requires oral HCO_3^-. As a result, these agents have proved to be of limited utility for this indication. Counterintuitively, acetazolamide has been shown to lead to acute crystal formation in some rare cases, sometimes resulting in severe acute kidney injury (eg, calcium phosphate crystals can form in alkaline urine). Acetazolamide itself may crystallize and precipitate in renal tubules and cause intratubular obstruction leading to acute kidney injury.

C. Metabolic Alkalosis

Metabolic alkalosis is generally treated by correction of abnormalities in total body K^+, intravascular volume, or mineralocorticoid levels. However, when the alkalosis is due to excessive use of diuretics in patients with severe heart failure, replacement of intravascular volume may be contraindicated. In these cases, acetazolamide can be useful in correcting the alkalosis as well as producing a small additional diuresis for correction of volume overload. Acetazolamide can also be used to rapidly correct the metabolic alkalosis that may appear following the correction of respiratory acidosis.

D. Acute Mountain Sickness

Weakness, dizziness, insomnia, headache, and nausea can occur in mountain travelers who rapidly ascend above 3000 m. The symptoms are usually mild and last for a few days. In more serious cases, rapidly progressing pulmonary or cerebral edema can be life-threatening. Acetazolamide counteracts the respiratory alkalosis that occurs with ascending to high altitudes by increasing bicarbonate excretion in the urine and thereby diminishing symptoms of mountain sickness. This mild metabolic central and CSF acidosis is also useful in the treatment of sleep apnea. It seems that doses as low as 125 mg twice daily are as effective as higher doses for treatment of acute mountain sickness; whether even smaller doses (62.5 mg twice a day) can be as effective for this indication is under investigation.

E. Other Uses

Carbonic anhydrase inhibitors have been used as adjuvants in the treatment of epilepsy and in some forms of hypokalemic periodic paralysis. They are also useful in treating patients with CSF leakage (usually caused by tumor or head trauma, but often idiopathic). By reducing the rate of CSF formation and intracranial pressure, carbonic anhydrase inhibitors can significantly slow the rate of CSF leakage. They also increase urinary phosphate excretion during severe hyperphosphatemia. Finally, acetazolamide may have a role in the treatment of Meniere disease, nephrogenic diabetes insipidus, idiopathic intracranial hypertension, central sleep apnea (likely not obstructive sleep apnea), and Kleine-Levin syndrome (episodes of hypersomnia and cognitive and behavioral abnormalities).

Toxicity

A. Hyperchloremic Metabolic Acidosis

Acidosis predictably results from chronic reduction of body HCO_3^- stores by carbonic anhydrase inhibitors (see Table 15–2) and limits the diuretic efficacy of these drugs to 2 or 3 days. Unlike the diuretic effect, acidosis persists as long as the drug is continued.

B. Renal Stones

Phosphaturia and hypercalciuria occur during the bicarbonaturic response to inhibitors of carbonic anhydrase. Renal excretion of solubilizing factors (eg, citrate) also may decline with chronic use. Calcium phosphate salts are relatively insoluble at alkaline pH, which means that the potential for renal stone formation from these salts is enhanced.

C. Renal Potassium Wasting

Potassium wasting can occur because the increased Na^+ presented to the collecting tubule (with HCO_3^-) is partially reabsorbed, increasing the lumen-negative electrical potential in that segment and enhancing K^+ secretion. This effect can be counteracted by simultaneous administration of potassium chloride or a K^+-sparing diuretic. Potassium wasting is theoretically a problem with any diuretic that increases Na^+ delivery to the collecting tubule.

In addition to potassium wasting, carbonic anhydrase inhibitors can lead to phosphorus wasting, and even symptomatic hypophosphatemia has been reported with these agents. Therefore, both serum potassium and serum phosphorus should be monitored in patients who are being treated chronically with these agents.

D. Other Toxicities

Drowsiness and paresthesias are common following large doses of acetazolamide. Carbonic anhydrase inhibitors may accumulate in patients with renal failure, leading to nervous system toxicity. Hypersensitivity reactions (fever, rashes, bone marrow suppression, and interstitial nephritis) also may occur, including DRESS syndrome.

Contraindications

Carbonic anhydrase inhibitor-induced alkalinization of the urine decreases urinary excretion of NH_4^+ (by converting it to rapidly reabsorbed NH_3) and may contribute to the development of hyperammonemia and hepatic encephalopathy in patients with cirrhosis.

SODIUM GLUCOSE COTRANSPORTER 2 (SGLT2) INHIBITORS

In the normal individual, the proximal convoluted tubule reabsorbs almost all of the glucose filtered by the glomeruli. Ninety percent of the glucose reabsorption occurs through SGLT2 (see Figure 15–2), but inhibiting this transporter using the currently available drugs will result in glucose excretion of only 30–50% of the amount filtered. Although we have known about the proximal tubule sodium/glucose cotransporter for many years, the inhibitors of this transport channel were developed only recently. Five SGLT2 inhibitors (**dapagliflozin, canagliflozin, empagliflozin, ertugliflozin,** and **ipragliflozin** [available in Japan and Russia]) are currently available. Angiotensin II has been shown to induce SGLT2 production via the AT_1 receptor. Thus, blockade of the renin-angiotensin-aldosterone axis may result in lower SGLT2 availability.

Pharmacokinetics

The SGLT2 inhibitors are rapidly absorbed by the gastrointestinal (GI) tract. The elimination half-life of dapagliflozin is 10–12 hours, and up to 70% of the given dose is excreted in the urine in the form of 3-O-glucuronide (only around 2% of the drug is excreted unchanged in the urine). Although the drug levels are higher with more severe renal failure, urinary glucose excretion would also decline as chronic kidney disease worsens. The dose of canagliflozin is recommended not to exceed 100 mg/d with an estimated GFR of 45–59. The drugs were originally not recommended in patients with more severe renal failure or advanced liver disease, although large multicenter trials including the EMPA-REG and the CREDENCE studies included patients with GFRs as low as 30 mL/min with no documented major adverse events. Whether the effectiveness of the drugs will start to wane with more advanced kidney disease is yet to be established. Drug-drug interactions are a consideration with these drugs. For example, concomitant rifampin administration reduces the total exposure to dapagliflozin by 22%.

Clinical Indications

The main approved indication for the use of these drugs has been as third-line therapy for diabetes mellitus (see Chapter 41). Cardiac and renal protection have now been clearly established with the use of these drugs and has now overtaken treatment of diabetes as their main indication. SGLT2 inhibitors will reduce the hemoglobin A1c by 0.5–1.0%, similar to other oral hypoglycemic agents. SGLT2 inhibitors have other minor effects. SGLT2 inhibitors will result in an average weight loss of 3.2 kg versus a weight gain of 1.2 kg with glipizide. It is not clearly established how much of this is due to the diuretic effect, but it is notable that SGLT2 inhibitors also induce a drop in systolic blood pressure by an average of 5.1 mm Hg, compared with an increase in systolic blood pressure of approximately 1 mm Hg after starting sitagliptin. In one study, ipragliflozin resulted in an increase in urine volume from day 1 to day 3. There was a 0.7-kg decrease in body weight by day 3 compared to day 1. Both urine sodium and urine potassium excretion increased with the use of ipragliflozin, but the serum concentrations of both electrolytes remained stable. Thus, it is likely that at least part of the weight loss is due to the diuretic effect of the drugs.

There is increasing evidence that these drugs are cardioprotective and also renoprotective in high-risk diabetic and nondiabetic patients. It has been suggested that the renoprotection stems from decreasing intraglomerular pressure similar to that produced by angiotensin-converting enzyme (ACE) inhibitors. However, the major beneficial effect may be the result of better blood pressure control. Similar to ACE inhibitors, these drugs are associated with an initial drop in GFR followed by slowed progression of chronic kidney disease. This beneficial effect is likely a class effect. In 2020, dapagliflozin was approved for use in heart failure with reduced ejection fraction, with or without diabetes. It has also been shown that dapagliflozin can increase urine output and reduce need for increasing diuretic doses in patients with acute heart failure without causing worsening of renal function. Although these results are somewhat contradictory to the well established mild increase in serum creatinine with initiation of SGLT-2 inhibitors. Another study has also shown a decreased in pulmonary artery pressure in patients with pulmonary hypertension treated with empagliflozin.

Adverse Reactions

Recently there have also been reports of acute kidney injury (AKI) with these drugs. At this time, it is unclear how much the diuretic and blood pressure–lowering effects of these drugs contribute to the reported AKI.

SGLT2 inhibitor therapy is associated with a low incidence of hypoglycemia (3.5% versus 40.8% with glipizide). There is a sixfold increased incidence of genital fungal infection in women and a slightly higher risk of urinary tract infections (8.8% versus 6.1%). All of these agents have been shown to have no or minimal effects on serum electrolyte concentrations.

LOOP DIURETICS

Loop diuretics selectively inhibit NaCl reabsorption in the TAL. Because of the large NaCl absorptive capacity of this segment and the fact that the diuretic action of these drugs is not limited by development of acidosis, as is the case with the carbonic anhydrase inhibitors, loop diuretics are the most efficacious diuretic agents currently available.

Chemistry

The two prototypical drugs of this group are **furosemide** and **ethacrynic acid** (Table 15–4). The structures of these diuretics are shown in Figure 15–7. In addition to furosemide, **bumetanide** and **torsemide** are sulfonamide-based loop diuretics.

Ethacrynic acid—not a sulfonamide derivative—is a phenoxyacetic acid derivative containing adjacent ketone and methylene groups (see Figure 15–7). The methylene group (shaded in figure) forms an adduct with the free sulfhydryl group of cysteine. The cysteine adduct appears to be the active form of the drug.

TABLE 15–4 Typical dosages of loop diuretics.

Drug	Total Daily Oral Dose[1]
Bumetanide	0.5–2 mg
Ethacrynic acid	50–200 mg
Furosemide	20–80 mg
Torsemide	5–20 mg

[1]As single dose or in two divided doses.

Organic **mercurial diuretics** also inhibit salt transport in the TAL but are no longer used because of their toxicity.

Pharmacokinetics

The loop diuretics are rapidly absorbed. Furosemide is mainly eliminated by the kidney by glomerular filtration and tubular secretion. Bumetanide elimination is 50% by the kidneys and 50% by the liver, whereas torsemide is mainly eliminated by the liver. Absorption of oral torsemide is more rapid (1 hour) than that of furosemide (2–3 hours) and is nearly as complete as with intravenous administration. Bumetanide pharmacokinetics are similar to those of torsemide, but bumetanide is a much more potent loop diuretic. The duration of effect for furosemide is usually 2–3 hours. The effect of torsemide lasts 4–6 hours. Half-life depends on renal function. Since loop agents act on the luminal side of the tubule, their diuretic activity correlates with their secretion by the proximal tubule. Reduction in the secretion of loop diuretics may result from simultaneous administration of agents such as NSAIDs or probenecid, which compete for weak acid secretion in the proximal tubule. Metabolites of ethacrynic acid and furosemide have been identified, but it is not known whether they have any diuretic activity. Torsemide has at least one active metabolite with a half-life considerably longer than that of the parent compound. Because of

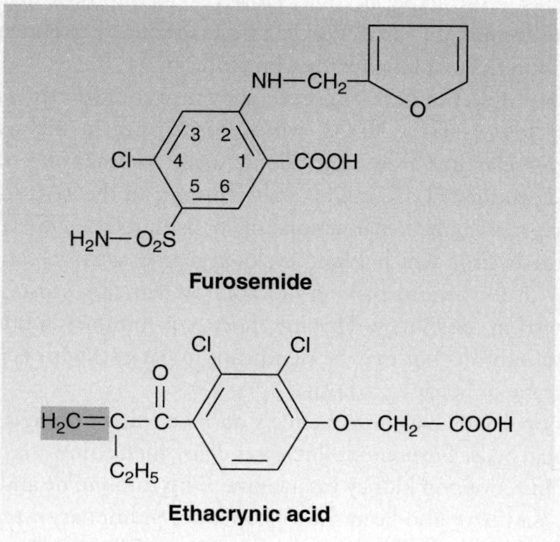

FIGURE 15–7 Two loop diuretics. The shaded methylene group on ethacrynic acid is reactive and may combine with free sulfhydryl groups.

TABLE 15–5 Relative potency of loop diuretics.

Drug	Equivalent Dose[1]
Furosemide	20 mg
Torsemide	10 mg
Bumetanide	0.5 mg
Ethacrynic acid	~50 mg

[1]Doses are approximate as bioavailability of furosemide is variable.

the variable bioavailability of furosemide and the more consistent bioavailability of torsemide and bumetanide, the equivalent dosages of these agents are unpredictable and also dependent on renal function, but estimates are presented in Table 15–5. Although study results comparing outcomes related to use of different loop diuretics have been inconsistent, there may be a benefit of using torsemide compared to furosemide and bumetanide in decreasing hospitalizations and possibly decreasing acute kidney injury episodes in heart failure patients. A mortality benefit has not been shown in any of the studies.

Pharmacodynamics

Loop diuretics inhibit NKCC2, the luminal $Na^+/K^+/2Cl^-$ transporter in the TAL of Henle's loop. By inhibiting this transporter, loop diuretics reduce the reabsorption of NaCl and also diminish the lumen-positive potential that comes from K^+ recycling (see Figure 15–3). This positive potential normally drives divalent cation reabsorption in the TAL (see Figure 15–3), and by reducing this potential, loop diuretics cause an increase in Mg^{2+} and Ca^{2+} excretion. Prolonged use can cause significant hypomagnesemia in some patients. However, the hypomagnesemia is probably not as profound as that caused by thiazide diuretics. Since vitamin D–induced intestinal absorption and parathyroid hormone–induced renal reabsorption of Ca^{2+} can be increased, loop diuretics do not generally cause hypocalcemia. However, in disorders that cause hypercalcemia, Ca^{2+} excretion can be enhanced by treatment with loop diuretics combined with saline infusion.

Loop diuretics have also been shown to induce expression of the cyclooxygenase COX-2, which participates in the synthesis of prostaglandins from arachidonic acid. At least one of these prostaglandins, PGE_2, inhibits salt transport in the TAL and thus participates in the renal actions of loop diuretics. NSAIDs (eg, indomethacin), which blunt cyclooxygenase activity, can interfere with the actions of loop diuretics by reducing prostaglandin synthesis in the kidney. This interference is minimal in otherwise normal subjects but may be significant in patients with nephrotic syndrome or hepatic cirrhosis.

Loop agents have direct effects on blood flow through several vascular beds. Furosemide increases renal blood flow via prostaglandin actions on kidney vasculature. Both furosemide and ethacrynic acid have also been shown to reduce pulmonary congestion and left ventricular filling pressures in heart failure before a measurable increase in urinary output occurs. These effects on peripheral vascular tone are also due to release of renal prostaglandins that are induced by the diuretics.

Clinical Indications & Dosage

The most important indications for the use of the loop diuretics include **acute pulmonary edema** and **other edematous conditions.** Often the treatment of the fluid overload will also serve as an effective antihypertensive agent, especially in the presence of renal insufficiency. The use of loop diuretics in these conditions is discussed below. For dosage, see Table 15-4. Other indications for loop diuretics include hypercalcemia, hyperkalemia, acute renal failure, and anion overdose.

A. Hyperkalemia

In mild hyperkalemia—or in conjunction with acute management of severe hyperkalemia by other measures (including pharmacotherapy such as dextrose plus insulin, β_2 agonists, calcium, K^+-binding substances [sodium polystyrene sulfonate, patiromer, sodium zirconium cyclosilicate], and dialysis)—loop diuretics can significantly enhance urinary K^+ excretion. If the patient is hypo- or euvolemic, loop diuretic administration should be accompanied by NaCl and water infusion, usually in the form of normal saline, both to maintain euvolemia and to enhance K^+ excretion.

B. Acute Renal Failure

Loop agents can increase the rate of urine flow and enhance K^+ excretion in acute renal failure. However, they cannot prevent or shorten the duration of renal failure. Loop agents can actually worsen cast formation in myeloma and light-chain nephropathy because increased distal Cl^- concentration enhances secretion of Tamm-Horsfall protein, which then aggregates with myeloma Bence Jones proteins.

C. Anion Overdose

Loop diuretics are useful in treating toxic ingestions of bromide, fluoride, and iodide, which are reabsorbed in the TAL. Saline solution must be administered to replace urinary losses of Na^+ and to provide Cl^-, so as to avoid extracellular fluid volume depletion.

D. Autism Spectrum Disorder

In the last 2-3 years, there have been a number of reports and studies that bumetanide may be helpful in treating autism spectrum disorder. One study found cytokine measurements can be useful to determine who will respond to therapy. Another showed improvements in communicative and cognitive abilities.

Toxicity

A. Hypokalemic Metabolic Alkalosis

By inhibiting salt reabsorption in the TAL, loop diuretics increase Na^+ delivery to the collecting duct. Increased Na^+ delivery leads to increased secretion of K^+ and H^+ by the duct, causing hypokalemic metabolic alkalosis (see Table 15–2). This toxicity is common and is a function of the magnitude of the diuresis and can be reversed by K^+ replacement and correction of hypovolemia. At least one study has found that potassium supplementation upon initiation of loop diuretics, irrespective of the serum potassium concentration, will improve survival.

B. Ototoxicity

Loop diuretics occasionally cause dose-related hearing loss that is usually reversible. It is most common in patients who have diminished renal function or who are also receiving other ototoxic agents such as aminoglycoside antibiotics. Ototoxicity is the result of inhibition of Na/Cl/K transport in the inner ear (via NKCC1), and disturbance of ion concentrations of the endolymph.

C. Hyperuricemia

Loop diuretics can cause hyperuricemia and precipitate attacks of gout. This is caused by hypovolemia-associated enhancement of uric acid reabsorption in the proximal tubule. It may be prevented by using lower doses to avoid development of hypovolemia.

D. Hypomagnesemia

Magnesium depletion is a predictable consequence of the chronic use of loop agents and occurs most often in patients with dietary magnesium deficiency. It can be reversed by administration of oral magnesium preparations, but this is often complicated by diarrhea.

E. Allergic and Other Reactions

All loop diuretics, with the exception of ethacrynic acid, are sulfonamides. Therefore, skin rash, eosinophilia, and less often, interstitial nephritis are occasional adverse effects of these drugs. Rare cases of drug reaction with eosinophilia and systemic symptoms (DRESS) syndrome also have been reported with furosemide. This toxicity usually resolves rapidly after drug withdrawal. Allergic reactions are much less common with ethacrynic acid.

Because Henle's loop is indirectly responsible for water reabsorption by the downstream collecting duct, loop diuretics can cause severe dehydration. Hyponatremia is less common than with the thiazides (see below). In fact, loop diuretics are in general protective against causing hyponatremia, but uncommonly patients who increase water intake in response to hypovolemia-induced thirst can become hyponatremic with loop agents.

Loop agents can cause hypercalciuria, which can lead to mild hypocalcemia and secondary hyperparathyroidism. On the other hand, loop agents can have the opposite effect (hypercalcemia) in volume-depleted patients who have another—previously occult—cause for hypercalcemia, such as metastatic breast or squamous cell lung carcinoma. Long-term loop diuretic therapy may worsen thiamine deficiency in patients with heart failure. Furosemide has also been reported to cause pseudoporphyria, and chronic prolonged use may increase the risk of fractures. Intravenous bumetanide administration has rarely caused superficial tenderness of the skin at the injection site, an effect not seen with other loop diuretics. In addition, continuous bumetanide infusion led to generalized musculoskeletal pain in 38% of patients who received it in one study—an effect that resolved after stopping the infusion.

Contraindications

Furosemide, bumetanide, and torsemide may exhibit allergic cross-reactivity in patients who are sensitive to other sulfonamides, but this appears to be very rare. Overzealous use of any diuretic is dangerous in hepatic cirrhosis, borderline renal failure, or heart failure.

THIAZIDES

The thiazide diuretics were discovered in 1957, as a result of efforts to synthesize more potent carbonic anhydrase inhibitors. It subsequently became clear that the thiazides inhibit NaCl rather than $NaHCO_3^-$ transport, and that their action is predominantly in the DCT rather than the PCT. Some members of this group retain significant carbonic anhydrase inhibitory activity (eg, chlorthalidone). The prototypical thiazide is **hydrochlorothiazide (HCTZ).**

Chemistry & Pharmacokinetics

Like carbonic anhydrase inhibitors and three loop diuretics, all of the thiazides have an unsubstituted sulfonamide group (Figure 15–8).

All thiazides can be administered orally, but there are differences in their metabolism. **Chlorothiazide,** the parent of the group, is not very lipid-soluble and must be given in relatively large doses. It is the only thiazide available for parenteral administration. However, one group was able to test an oil-in-water emulsion of metolazone for intravenous injection in rats with good results. HCTZ is considerably more potent and should be used in much lower doses (Table 15–6). **Chlorthalidone** is slowly absorbed and has a longer duration of action. Although indapamide is excreted primarily by the biliary system, enough of the active form is cleared by the kidney to exert its diuretic effect in the DCT. Bendroflumethiazide is likely the least prescribed thiazide diuretic. All thiazides

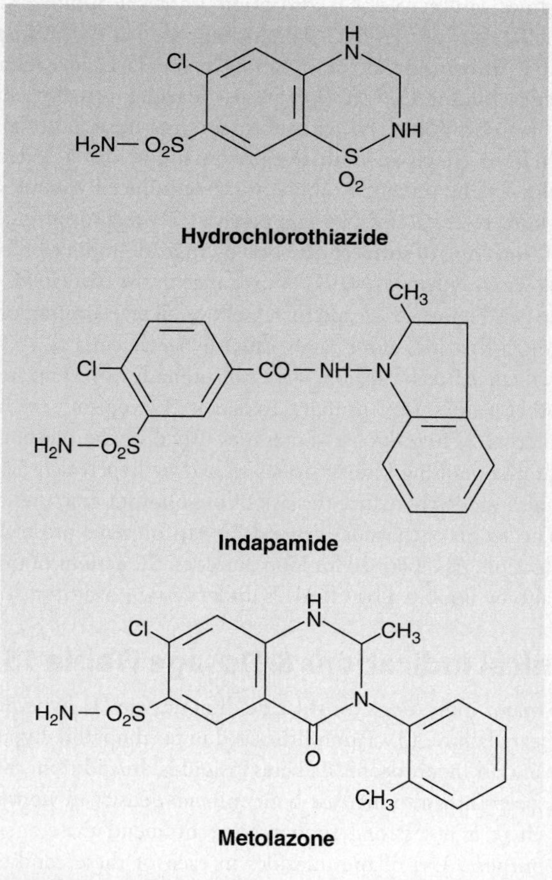

FIGURE 15–8 Hydrochlorothiazide and related agents.

TABLE 15–6 Thiazides and related diuretics.

Drug	Total Daily Oral Dose	Frequency of Daily Administration
Bendroflumethiazide	2.5–10 mg	Single dose
Chlorothiazide	0.5–2 g	Two divided doses
Chlorthalidone[1]	25–50 mg	Single dose
Hydrochlorothiazide	25–100 mg	Single dose
Hydroflumethiazide	12.5–50 mg	Two divided doses
Indapamide[1]	2.5–10 mg	Single dose
Methyclothiazide	2.5–10 mg	Single dose
Metolazone[1]	2.5–10 mg	Single dose
Polythiazide	1–4 mg	Single dose
Quinethazone[1]	25–100 mg	Single dose
Trichlormethiazide	1–4 mg	Single dose

[1]Not a thiazide but a sulfonamide qualitatively similar to the thiazides.

are secreted by the organic acid secretory system in the proximal tubule and compete with the secretion of uric acid by that system. As a result, thiazide use may blunt uric acid secretion and elevate serum uric acid level.

Pharmacodynamics

Thiazides inhibit NaCl reabsorption from the luminal side of epithelial cells in the DCT by blocking the Na^+/Cl^- transporter (NCC). In contrast to the situation in the TAL, in which loop diuretics inhibit Ca^{2+} reabsorption, thiazides actually enhance Ca^{2+} reabsorption. This enhancement has been postulated to result from effects in both the proximal and distal convoluted tubules. In the proximal tubule, thiazide-induced volume depletion leads to enhanced Na^+ and passive Ca^{2+} reabsorption. In the DCT, lowering of intracellular Na^+ by thiazide-induced blockade of Na^+ entry enhances Na^+/Ca^{2+} exchange in the basolateral membrane (see Figure 15–4) and increases overall reabsorption of Ca^{2+}. Although thiazides alone rarely cause hypercalcemia as a result of this enhanced reabsorption, they can unmask hypercalcemia due to other causes (eg, primary hyperparathyroidism, carcinoma, sarcoidosis). Thiazides are sometimes useful in the prevention of calcium-containing kidney stones caused by hypercalciuria. They may also modestly reduce the risk of osteoporotic fractures.

The action of thiazides depends in part on renal prostaglandin production. As described for loop diuretics, the actions of thiazides can also be inhibited by NSAIDs under certain conditions.

Clinical Indications & Dosage (Table 15–6)

The major indications for thiazide diuretics are (1) hypertension, (2) heart failure, (3) nephrolithiasis due to idiopathic hypercalciuria, and (4) nephrogenic diabetes insipidus. In addition, thiazides have been shown to increase bone mineral density in women, but this effect is not strong enough to recommend these agents for this purpose. Use of the thiazides in each of these conditions is described below in Clinical Pharmacology of Diuretic Agents.

Toxicity

A. Hypokalemic Metabolic Alkalosis

These toxicities are similar to those observed with loop diuretics (see previous text and Table 15–2). In one study the risk of hypokalemia was highest in women, underweight persons, and those who have been taking them for longer than 5 years.

B. Impaired Carbohydrate Tolerance

Hyperglycemia may occur in patients who are overtly diabetic or who have even mildly abnormal glucose tolerance tests. It occurs at higher doses of HCTZ (>50 mg/d) and has not been seen with doses of 12.5 mg/d or less. The effect is due to both impaired pancreatic release of insulin and diminished tissue utilization of glucose. Thiazides have a weak, dose-dependent, off-target effect to stimulate ATP-sensitive K^+ channels and cause hyperpolarization of beta cells, thereby inhibiting insulin release. This effect is exacerbated by hypokalemia, and thus thiazide-induced hyperglycemia may be partially reversed with correction of hypokalemia.

C. Hyperlipidemia

Thiazides cause a 5–15% increase in total serum cholesterol and low-density lipoproteins (LDLs). These levels may return toward baseline after prolonged use.

D. Hyponatremia

Hyponatremia is an important adverse effect of thiazide diuretics. It is caused by a combination of hypovolemia-induced elevation of ADH, reduction in the diluting capacity of the kidney, and increased thirst. It can be prevented by reducing the dose of the drug or limiting water intake. Genetic studies have shown a link between *KCNJ1* polymorphism and thiazide-induced hyponatremia. Elderly women are most prone to develop hyponatremia from thiazide use. A Swedish study found that one-quarter of patients admitted to hospital with hyponatremia had hyponatremia due to thiazide use.

E. Impaired Uric Acid Metabolism and Gout

Thiazides are the diuretics most associated with development of gout. One large study found that thiazide diuretics only increase the risk of gout in men younger than age 60 years and not in women or older men. The increased risk in this group of patients was found to be only about 1%.

F. Allergic Reactions

The thiazides are sulfonamides and share cross-reactivity with other members of this chemical group. Photosensitivity or generalized dermatitis occurs rarely. Serious allergic reactions are extremely rare but do include hemolytic anemia, thrombocytopenia, and acute necrotizing pancreatitis.

G. Skin Cancer

Thiazide diuretics are likely to increase the incidence of skin cancers. This seems to be an effect that depends on degree of exposure to the drug. It is not clear whether this is only for squamous cell and basal cell cancers or if it also includes melanomas. At least three authors have reported increased risk of melanoma, but a few have not shown this increased risk. One meta-analysis of more than 10 million people found the odds ratio of melanoma was increased by 1.10, basal cell cancer by 1.05, and squamous cell cancer by 1.35. Bendroflumethiazide may be associated with a lower risk of skin cancer.

H. Other Toxicities

Weakness, fatigability, and paresthesias similar to those of carbonic anhydrase inhibitors may occur. Impotence has been reported but is probably related to volume depletion. Cases of acute angle-closure glaucoma from hyponatremia caused by thiazide diuretics have been reported. Hypomagnesemia is more likely with thiazide diuretics than with loop diuretics and is usually seen after using the drug for more than 1 year. Rare toxicities may also include systemic lupus, acute respiratory distress syndrome, Merkel cell carcinoma, and choroidal effusion of the eyes.

Contraindications

Excessive use of any diuretic is dangerous in patients with hepatic cirrhosis, borderline renal failure, or heart failure (see text that follows).

POTASSIUM-SPARING DIURETICS

Potassium-sparing diuretics prevent K^+ secretion by antagonizing the effects of aldosterone in collecting tubules. Inhibition may occur by direct pharmacologic antagonism of mineralocorticoid receptors **(spironolactone, eplerenone)** or by inhibition of Na^+ influx through ion channels in the luminal membrane **(amiloride, triamterene)**. Finally, ularitide (recombinant urodilatin), which is currently still under investigation, blunts Na^+ uptake and Na^+/K^+-ATPase in collecting tubules and increases GFR through its vascular effects. Nesiritide, which is available for intravenous use only, increases GFR and blunts Na^+ reabsorption in both proximal and collecting tubules.

Chemistry & Pharmacokinetics

The structures of spironolactone and amiloride are shown in Figure 15–9.

Spironolactone is a synthetic steroid that acts as a competitive antagonist to aldosterone. Onset and duration of its action are determined substantially by the active metabolites canrenone and 7-α-spironolactone, which are produced in the liver and have long half-lives (12–20 and approximately 14 hours, respectively). Spironolactone binds with high affinity and potently inhibits the androgen receptor, which is an important source of side effects in males (notably, gynecomastia and decreased libido). However, it does not seem that spironolactone increases the risk of breast cancer in women and can be used to treat alopecia in women with this diagnosis. Eplerenone is a spironolactone analog with much greater selectivity for the mineralocorticoid receptor. At least one study has found eplerenone to be as effective as spironolactone for the treatment of congestive heart failure. It is several hundredfold less active on androgen and progesterone receptors than

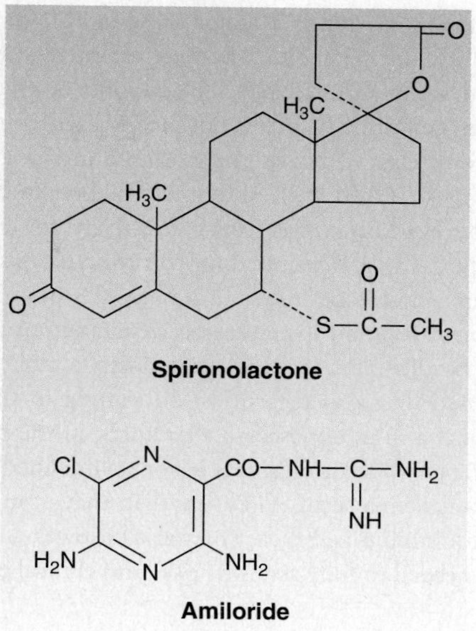

FIGURE 15–9 Potassium-sparing diuretics.

spironolactone, and therefore eplerenone has considerably fewer adverse effects (eg, gynecomastia). Canrenoate is a mineralocorticoid receptor antagonist that can be given intravenously.

Finerenone, esaxerenone, and **apararenone** are new agents in this class with apararenone still being an investigational agent. They are nonsteroidal mineralocorticoid antagonists that reduce nuclear accumulation of mineralocorticoid receptors more efficiently than spironolactone. Like eplerenone, finerenone binds less avidly to the androgen and progesterone receptors. Finerenone accumulates similarly in the heart and the kidneys, whereas eplerenone has three times higher drug concentration in the kidney than the heart and spironolactone is even more preferentially concentrated in the kidneys. Because of this effect, finerenone may prove to be useful for cardioprotection. Finerenone results in less (but still significant) hyperkalemia than spironolactone or eplerenone for poorly understood reasons but possibly from its decreased tendency to accumulate in the kidneys. It also does not have as great a blood pressure–lowering effect as spironolactone or eplerenone. A preliminary study found finerenone to be as effective as spironolactone in decreasing the ratio of urinary albumin to creatinine. The antihypertensive action of this agent may be inferior to that of the other members of the group. Esaxerenone has also been shown to reduce albuminuria in type 2 diabetics in preliminary studies. It has been available clinically in Japan since 2019. In comparison with finerenone, esaxerenone has a longer half-life and higher affinity for the mineralocorticoid receptor, and a stronger blood pressure–lowering effect. The incidence of hyperkalemia with both of these agents seems to be lower compared with steroidal mineralocorticoid receptor blockers. DSR-71167 is an investigational agent in this class that is believed to have carbonic anhydrase inhibitory activity in addition to antimineralocorticoid activity and is thus less likely to cause hyperkalemia.

Amiloride and triamterene are direct inhibitors of the Na^+ influx channel in the CCT. Triamterene is metabolized in the liver, but renal excretion is a major route of elimination for the active form and the metabolites. Because triamterene is extensively metabolized, it has a shorter half-life and must be given more frequently than amiloride (which is not metabolized).

The newest class of potassium sparing diuretics are the aldosterone synthase (CYP11b2) inhibitors. The best studied of these compounds, baxdrostat, has 100:1 selectively for CYP11b2 as compared to CYP11b1 (required for cortisol synthesis), and effectively lowers aldosterone levels. In a phase 2 study, 248 patients with treatment-resistant hypertension were randomized to receive placebo or baxdrostat at three different doses. Systolic blood pressure decreased by an average of 10-20 mmHg in the 0.5-2 mg interventional arm as opposed to 11 mmHg in the placebo arm. The diuretic effect of these agents is not well defined yet, but the risk of hyperkalemia seems to be less than that of mineralocorticoid receptor inhibitors. Efficacy may also be lower, and additional research is needed to fully assess its risks and clinical utility.

Pharmacodynamics

Potassium-sparing diuretics reduce Na^+ absorption in the collecting tubules and ducts (see Figure 15-5). Sodium absorption (and K^+ secretion) at this site is regulated by aldosterone, as described above. Aldosterone antagonists interfere with this process. Similar effects are observed with respect to H^+ handling by the intercalated cells of the collecting tubule, in part explaining the metabolic acidosis seen with aldosterone antagonists (see Table 15–2).

Spironolactone and eplerenone bind to mineralocorticoid receptors and blunt aldosterone activity. Amiloride and triamterene do not block aldosterone but instead directly interfere with Na^+ entry through the epithelial Na^+ channels (ENaC; see Figure 15–5) in the apical membrane of the collecting tubule. Since K^+ secretion is coupled with Na^+ entry in this segment, these agents are also effective K^+-sparing diuretics.

The actions of the aldosterone antagonists depend on renal prostaglandin production. The actions of K^+-sparing diuretics can be inhibited by NSAIDs under certain conditions.

Clinical Indications & Dosage (Table 15–7)

Potassium-sparing diuretics are most useful in states of mineralocorticoid excess or hyperaldosteronism (also called aldosteronism), due to either primary hypersecretion (Conn syndrome, ectopic adrenocorticotropic hormone production) or secondary hyperaldosteronism (evoked by heart failure, hepatic cirrhosis, nephrotic syndrome, or other conditions associated with diminished effective intravascular volume). Use of diuretics such as thiazides or loop agents can cause or exacerbate volume contraction and may cause secondary hyperaldosteronism. In the setting of enhanced mineralocorticoid secretion and excessive delivery of Na^+ to distal nephron sites, renal K^+ wasting occurs. Potassium-sparing diuretics of either type may be used in this setting to blunt the K^+ secretory response.

It has also been found that low doses of eplerenone (25–50 mg/d) may interfere with some of the fibrotic and inflammatory effects of aldosterone. By doing so, it can slow the progression of albuminuria in diabetic patients. It is notable that eplerenone has been found to reduce myocardial perfusion defects after myocardial infarction. In one clinical study, eplerenone reduced mortality rate by 15% (compared with placebo) in patients with mild to moderate heart failure after myocardial infarction. Spironolactone may also reduce the incidence of recurrence of atrial fibrillation in patients after radiofrequency catheter ablation, and there are data suggesting that finerenone may reduce risk of atrial fibrillation in patients with chronic kidney disease and type 2 diabetes. Likely all mineralocorticoid receptor antagonists reduce the risk of atrial fibrillation; however, it remains unclear if this is due to direct effects in cardiomyocytes or effects on serum potassium.

TABLE 15–7 Potassium-sparing diuretics and combination preparations.

Trade Name	Potassium-Sparing Agent	Hydrochlorothiazide
Aldactazide	Spironolactone 25 mg	50 mg
Aldactone	Spironolactone 25, 50, or 100 mg	—
Dyazide	Triamterene 37.5 mg	25 mg
Dyrenium	Triamterene 50 or 100 mg	—
Inspra[1]	Eplerenone 25, 50, or 100 mg	—
Maxzide	Triamterene 75 mg	50 mg
Maxzide-25 mg	Triamterene 37.5 mg	25 mg
Midamor	Amiloride 5 mg	—
Moduretic	Amiloride 5 mg	50 mg

[1]Eplerenone is currently approved for use only in hypertension.

Liddle syndrome is a rare autosomal dominant disorder caused by activating mutations in ENaC, which result in increased sodium reabsorption and potassium secretion in the collecting ducts. Amiloride has been shown to be of benefit in this condition, while spironolactone has limited efficacy as aldosterone levels are usually not elevated in this condition. Amiloride is also useful for treatment of nephrogenic diabetes insipidus, although only studied in patients with lithium-induced diabetes insipidus.

Spironolactone has also shown beneficial effects in women treated for acne and for treating female-pattern hair loss. (The effect is modest for this diagnosis.) Doses lower than 200 mg per day may still be effective. Complete response rate can be around 25%, while partial response rate is as high as 80% for treatment of acne. Spironolactone was also found to reduce the risk of prostate cancer in men being treated for heart failure with a hazard ratio of 0.55.

Toxicity

A. Hyperkalemia

Unlike most other diuretics, K^+-sparing diuretics reduce urinary excretion of K^+ (see Table 15–2) and can cause mild, moderate, or even life-threatening hyperkalemia. The risk of this complication is greatly increased by renal disease (in which maximal K^+

excretion may be reduced) or by the use of other drugs that reduce or inhibit renin (β blockers, NSAIDs, aliskiren) or angiotensin II activity (ACE inhibitors, angiotensin receptor inhibitors). Since most other diuretic agents lead to K^+ losses, hyperkalemia is more common when K^+-sparing diuretics are used as the sole diuretic agent, especially in patients with renal insufficiency. With fixed-dosage combinations of K^+-sparing and thiazide diuretics, the thiazide-induced hypokalemia and metabolic alkalosis are ameliorated. However, because of variations in the bioavailability of the components of fixed-dosage forms, the thiazide-associated adverse effects often predominate. Therefore, it is generally preferable to adjust the doses of the two drugs separately.

The Randomized Aldactone Evaluation Study (RALES) study, published in 1999, showed that patients with severe systolic heart failure can benefit from addition of spironolactone to ACE inhibitor therapy. Subsequently a large analysis demonstrated that after the publication of the RALES study, the rates of spironolactone use, hospital admission for hyperkalemia, and mortality in patients admitted for hyperkalemia all rose in the following years. Therefore, spironolactone either should not be used or should be used with extreme caution and close monitoring in patients with significant renal insufficiency.

B. Hyperchloremic Metabolic Acidosis

By inhibiting H^+ secretion in parallel with K^+ secretion, the K^+-sparing diuretics can cause acidosis similar to that seen with type IV renal tubular acidosis.

C. Gynecomastia

Synthetic steroids may cause endocrine abnormalities by actions on other steroid receptors. Gynecomastia, impotence, and benign prostatic hyperplasia (very rare) have been reported with spironolactone. Such effects have not been reported with eplerenone, presumably because it is much more selective than spironolactone for the mineralocorticoid receptor and virtually inactive on androgen or progesterone receptors.

D. Acute Renal Failure

The combination of triamterene with indomethacin has been reported to cause acute renal failure. This has not been reported with other K^+-sparing diuretics.

E. Kidney Stones

Triamterene is only slightly soluble and may precipitate in the urine, causing kidney stones.

Contraindications

Potassium-sparing agents can cause severe, even fatal, hyperkalemia in susceptible patients. Patients with chronic renal insufficiency are especially vulnerable and should rarely be treated with these diuretics. Oral K^+ administration should be discontinued if K^+-sparing diuretics are administered. Concomitant use of other agents that blunt the renin-angiotensin system (β blockers, ACE inhibitors, angiotensin receptor blockers) increases the likelihood of hyperkalemia. Patients with liver disease may have impaired metabolism of triamterene and spironolactone; therefore dosing of these agents must be carefully adjusted. Strong CYP3A4 inhibitors (eg, erythromycin, fluconazole, diltiazem, and grapefruit juice) can markedly increase blood levels of eplerenone but not spironolactone.

AGENTS THAT ALTER WATER EXCRETION (AQUARETICS)

OSMOTIC DIURETICS

The proximal tubule and descending limb of Henle's loop are freely permeable to water (see Table 15–1). Any osmotically active agent that is filtered by the glomerulus but not reabsorbed causes water to be retained in these segments and promotes a water diuresis. Such agents can be used to reduce intracranial pressure and to promote prompt removal of renal toxins. The prototypic osmotic diuretic is **mannitol.** Glucose is not used clinically as a diuretic but frequently causes osmotic diuresis (glycosuria) in patients with hyperglycemia.

Pharmacokinetics

Mannitol is poorly absorbed by the GI tract, and when administered orally, it causes osmotic diarrhea rather than diuresis. For systemic effect, mannitol must be given intravenously. Mannitol is not metabolized and is excreted by glomerular filtration within 30–60 minutes, without any important tubular reabsorption or secretion. It must be used cautiously in patients with even mild renal insufficiency (see below).

Pharmacodynamics

Osmotic diuretics have their major effect in the proximal tubule and the descending limb of Henle's loop. Through osmotic effects, they also oppose the action of ADH in the collecting tubule. The presence of a nonreabsorbable solute such as mannitol prevents the normal absorption of water by interposing a countervailing osmotic force. As a result, urine volume increases. The increase in urine flow decreases the contact time between fluid and the tubular epithelium, thus reducing Na^+ as well as water reabsorption. The resulting natriuresis is of lesser magnitude than the water diuresis, leading eventually to hypernatremia.

Clinical Indications & Dosage

A. Reduction of Intracranial and Intraocular Pressure

Osmotic diuretics alter Starling forces so that water leaves cells and reduces intracellular volume. This effect is used to reduce intracranial pressure in neurologic conditions and to reduce intraocular pressure before ophthalmologic procedures. A dose of 1–2 g/kg mannitol is administered intravenously. Intracranial pressure, which must be monitored, should fall in 60–90 minutes. At times the rapid lowering of serum osmolality at initiation of dialysis (from removal of uremic toxins) results in symptoms. Many nephrologists also use mannitol to prevent adverse reactions when first starting patients on hemodialysis. The evidence for efficacy in this setting is limited.

Toxicity

A. Extracellular Volume Expansion

Mannitol is rapidly distributed in the extracellular compartment and extracts water from cells. Prior to the diuresis, this leads to expansion of the extracellular volume and hyponatremia. This effect can complicate heart failure and may produce florid pulmonary edema. Headache, nausea, and vomiting are commonly observed in patients treated with osmotic diuretics.

B. Dehydration, Hyperkalemia, and Hypernatremia

Excessive use of mannitol without adequate water replacement can ultimately lead to severe dehydration, free water losses, and hypernatremia. As water is extracted from cells, intracellular K^+ concentration rises, leading to cellular losses and hyperkalemia. These complications can be avoided by careful attention to serum ion composition and fluid balance.

C. Hyponatremia

When used in patients with severe renal impairment, parenterally administered mannitol cannot be excreted and is retained in the blood. This causes osmotic extraction of water from cells, leading to hyponatremia without a decrease in serum osmolality.

D. Acute Renal Failure

Acute renal failure has been well described with use of mannitol. The effect is thought to be mediated by the increase in osmolality. The incidence of acute kidney injury with mannitol use has been estimated to be 6–7% of patients who receive the drug.

ANTIDIURETIC HORMONE ANTAGONISTS

A variety of medical conditions, including congestive heart failure (CHF) and the syndrome of inappropriate ADH secretion (SIADH), cause water retention as a result of excessive ADH secretion. Patients with CHF who are on diuretics frequently develop hyponatremia secondary to excessive ADH secretion.

Until recently, two nonselective agents, lithium (see Chapter 29) and demeclocycline (a tetracycline antimicrobial drug discussed in Chapter 44), were used for their well-known interference with ADH activity. The mechanism for this interference has not been completely determined for either of these agents. Demeclocycline is used more often than lithium because of the many adverse effects of lithium administration. However, demeclocycline is now being rapidly replaced by several specific ADH receptor antagonists **(vaptans),** which have yielded encouraging clinical results.

There are three known vasopressin receptors, V_{1a}, V_{1b}, and V_2. V_1 receptors are expressed in the vasculature and CNS, while V_2 receptors are expressed specifically in the kidney. **Conivaptan** (currently available only for intravenous use) exhibits activity against both V_{1a} and V_2 receptors (see below), OPC-61815 is a prodrug of tolvaptan and is being studied for intravenous use. The oral agents **tolvaptan,** lixivaptan, mozavaptan, and satavaptan are selectively active against the V_2 receptor. Mozavaptan has been approved for use in Japan since 2006, satavaptan was abandoned for further development in 2009, and lixivaptan was under investigation for the treatment of polycystic kidney disease (however, as of 2022 it has been abandoned also). Tolvaptan, which is approved by the US Food and Drug Administration (FDA), is very effective in treatment of hyponatremia and as an adjunct to standard diuretic therapy in patients with CHF.

Pharmacokinetics

The half-lives of conivaptan and demeclocycline are 5–10 hours, while that of tolvaptan is 12–24 hours.

Pharmacodynamics

Antidiuretic hormone antagonists inhibit the effects of ADH in the collecting tubule. Conivaptan and tolvaptan are direct ADH receptor antagonists, while both lithium and demeclocycline reduce ADH-induced cAMP by unknown mechanisms.

Clinical Indications & Dosage

A. Syndrome of Inappropriate ADH Secretion

Antidiuretic hormone antagonists are used to manage SIADH when water restriction has failed to correct the abnormality. This generally occurs in the outpatient setting, where water restriction cannot be enforced, but can occur in the hospital when large quantities of intravenous fluid are needed for other purposes. Demeclocycline (600–1200 mg/d) or tolvaptan (7.5–60 mg/d) can be used for SIADH. Starting with lower doses of tolvaptan may be indicated in certain situations. Appropriate plasma levels of demeclocycline (2 mcg/mL) should be maintained by monitoring, but tolvaptan levels are not routinely monitored. Unlike demeclocycline or tolvaptan, conivaptan is administered intravenously and is not suitable for chronic use in outpatients.

B. Other Causes of Elevated Antidiuretic Hormone

Antidiuretic hormone is also elevated in response to diminished effective circulating blood volume, as often occurs in heart failure. Due to the elevated ADH levels, hyponatremia may result. As in the management of SIADH, water restriction is frequently the treatment of choice. In patients with heart failure, this approach is often unsuccessful in view of increased thirst and the large number of oral medications being used. For patients with heart failure, intravenous conivaptan may be particularly useful because it has been found that the blockade of V_{1a} receptors by this drug leads to decreased peripheral vascular resistance and increased cardiac output. Tolvaptan has recently been studied as an adjunct to diuretic therapy in patients with heart failure. These studies indicate that treatment with tolvaptan will result in an increase in serum sodium concentration, an increase in urine output, a decrease in body weight, and no change in serum creatinine levels. Tolvaptan has also shown effectiveness in treating fluid overload and hyponatremia in children with nephrotic syndrome.

C. Autosomal Dominant Polycystic Kidney Disease

Cyst development in polycystic kidney disease is thought to be mediated through cAMP. Vasopressin is a major stimulus for cAMP production in the kidney. It is hypothesized that inhibition of V_2 receptors in the kidney might delay the progression of polycystic kidney disease. In a large, multicenter, prospective trial, tolvaptan was able to reduce the increase in kidney size and slow progression of kidney failure over a 3-year follow-up period. In this trial, however, the tolvaptan group experienced a 9% incidence of abnormal liver function test results compared with 2% in the placebo group. This led to discontinuation of the drug in some patients. However, the doses of tolvaptan used in this trial were significantly higher than the doses used to treat hyponatremia, and with low doses of tolvaptan used in treating hyponatremia, hepatotoxicity has not been reported.

Toxicity

A. Nephrogenic Diabetes Insipidus

If serum Na^+ is not monitored closely, any ADH antagonist can cause severe hypernatremia and nephrogenic diabetes insipidus. If lithium is being used for a psychiatric disorder, nephrogenic diabetes insipidus can be treated with a thiazide diuretic or amiloride (see the section Diabetes Insipidus). There have been at least three reports of using hydrochlorothiazide and one report of using trichlormethiazide with success to treat polyuria in patients being treated with tolvaptan for polycystic kidney disease.

B. Renal Failure

Both lithium and demeclocycline have been reported to cause acute renal failure. Long-term lithium therapy may also cause chronic interstitial nephritis.

C. Other

Dry mouth and thirst are common with many of these drugs. Tolvaptan may cause hypotension. Multiple adverse effects associated with lithium therapy have been found and are discussed in Chapter 29. Demeclocycline should be avoided in patients with liver disease (see Chapter 44) and in children younger than 12 years. Tolvaptan may also cause an elevation in liver function tests and is relatively contraindicated in patients with active hepatitis. However, tolvaptan has been used successfully to treat volume overload with less need for oral diuretics in cirrhosis.

UREARETICS

Medullary urine concentration depends in large part on urea movement in the kidney. Two families of urea transporters have been described. UT-A is present in inner medullary collecting duct cells and the thin descending limb of Henle. UT-B is present in the descending vasa recta and several extrarenal tissues. Inhibitors of both UT-A and UT-B (eg, **PU-14**) have been developed and are currently in preclinical studies. These agents are aquaretics that increase urea and water excretion but not sodium excretion. Urea transport inhibitors have been shown to blunt the increase in urine osmolality seen after desmopressin administration. These agents may prove to be useful in edematous states and even in SIADH; however, their potential clinical role as compared to that of vaptans remains to be established.

DIURETIC COMBINATIONS

LOOP AGENTS & THIAZIDES

Some patients are refractory to the usual dose of loop diuretics or become refractory after an initial response. Since these agents have a short half-life (2–6 hours), refractoriness may be due to an excessive interval between doses. Renal Na^+ retention may be greatly increased during the time period when the drug is no longer active. It is hoped that continuous loop diuretic infusions would be useful in treating patients with heart failure and diuretic resistance. One high-quality study did not show a benefit for continuous loop diuretic infusion as opposed to bolus doses in all patients with fluid overload. (The study did not restrict to patients with diuretic resistance.) However, a more recent study showed that continuous furosemide infusion in patients with moderate renal insufficiency and acute decompensated heart failure resulted in increased urine output and more weight loss than the same dose of furosemide administered in bolus doses.

After the dosing interval for loop agents is minimized or the dose is maximized, the use of two drugs acting at different nephron sites may exhibit dramatic synergy. Loop agents and thiazides in combination often produce diuresis when neither agent acting alone is even minimally effective. There are several reasons for this phenomenon.

First, salt reabsorption in either the TAL or the DCT can increase when the other is blocked. Inhibition of both can therefore produce more than an additive diuretic response. Second, thiazide diuretics often produce a mild natriuresis in the proximal tubule that is usually masked by increased reabsorption in the TAL. The combination of loop diuretics and thiazides can therefore reduce Na^+ reabsorption, to some extent, from all three segments.

Metolazone is the thiazide-like drug usually used in patients refractory to loop agents alone, but it is likely that other thiazides at equipotent doses would be just as effective. Moreover, metolazone is available only in an oral preparation, whereas chlorothiazide can be given parenterally.

The combination of loop diuretics and thiazides can mobilize large amounts of fluid, even in patients who have not responded to single agents. Therefore, close hemodynamic monitoring is essential. Routine outpatient use is not recommended but may be possible with extreme caution and close follow-up. Furthermore, K^+ wasting is extremely common and may require parenteral K^+ administration with careful monitoring of fluid and electrolyte status. The first large-scale randomized controlled trial of combination loop and thiazide diuretic therapy in patients with heart failure is currently under way in the CLOROTIC (Combination of Loop with Thiazide-type Diuretics in Patients with Decompensated Heart Failure) trial. Clinical experience suggests that in outpatients, adverse effects of thiazides as add-on therapy to loop diuretics can be mitigated by infrequent low-dose therapy. Add-on diuretic therapy with metolazone is started at 2.5 mg weekly and titrated up slowly as needed, with close monitoring of the patient's blood pressure and serum potassium concentration.

POTASSIUM-SPARING DIURETICS & PROXIMAL TUBULE DIURETICS, LOOP AGENTS, OR THIAZIDES

Hypokalemia often develops in patients taking carbonic anhydrase inhibitors, loop diuretics, or thiazides. This can usually be managed by dietary NaCl restriction or by taking dietary KCl supplements. When hypokalemia cannot be managed in this way, the addition of a K^+-sparing diuretic can significantly lower K^+ excretion. Although this approach is generally safe, it should be avoided or used with caution in patients with renal insufficiency and in those receiving angiotensin antagonists such as ACE inhibitors, in whom life-threatening hyperkalemia can develop in response to K^+-sparing diuretics. For diuresis purposes, though, it seems adding a thiazide to a loop diuretic is more effective than adding spironolactone to loop agents.

■ CLINICAL PHARMACOLOGY OF DIURETIC AGENTS

A summary of the effects of diuretics on urinary electrolyte excretion is shown in Table 15–2.

EDEMATOUS STATES

A common reason for diuretic use is for reduction of peripheral or pulmonary edema that has accumulated as a result of cardiac, renal, or vascular diseases that reduce blood flow to the kidney. This reduction is sensed as insufficient effective arterial blood volume and leads to salt and water retention, which expands blood volume and eventually causes edema formation. Judicious use of diuretics can mobilize this interstitial edema without significant reductions in plasma volume. However, excessively rapid diuretic therapy may compromise the effective arterial blood volume and reduce the perfusion of vital organs. Therefore, the use of diuretics to mobilize edema requires careful monitoring of the patient's hemodynamic status and an understanding of the pathophysiology of the underlying illness.

HEART FAILURE

When cardiac output is reduced by heart failure, the resultant changes in blood pressure and blood flow to the kidney are sensed as hypovolemia and lead to renal retention of salt and water. This physiologic response initially increases intravascular volume and venous return to the heart and may partially restore the cardiac output toward normal (see Chapter 13).

If the underlying disease causes cardiac output to deteriorate despite expansion of plasma volume, the kidney continues to retain salt and water, which then leaks from the vasculature and becomes interstitial or pulmonary edema. At this point, diuretic use becomes necessary to reduce the accumulation of edema, particularly in the lungs. Reduction of pulmonary vascular congestion with diuretics may actually improve oxygenation and thereby improve myocardial function. Reduction of preload can reduce the size of the heart, allowing it to work at a more efficient fiber length. Edema associated with heart failure is generally managed with loop diuretics. In some instances, salt and water retention may become so severe that a combination of thiazides and loop diuretics is necessary.

In treating the heart failure patient with diuretics, it must always be remembered that cardiac output in these patients is being maintained in part by high filling pressures. Therefore, excessive use of diuretics may diminish venous return and further impair cardiac output. This is especially critical in right ventricular heart failure. Systemic, rather than pulmonary, vascular congestion is the hallmark of this disorder. Diuretic-induced volume contraction predictably reduces venous return and can severely compromise cardiac output if left ventricular filling pressure is reduced below 15 mm Hg (see Chapter 13). Reduction in cardiac output, resulting from either left or right ventricular dysfunction, also eventually leads to renal dysfunction resulting from reduced perfusion pressures.

Diuretic-induced metabolic alkalosis, exacerbated by hypokalemia, is another adverse effect that may further compromise cardiac function. This complication can be treated with replacement of K^+ and restoration of intravascular volume with saline; however, severe heart failure may preclude the use of saline even in patients who have received excessive diuretic therapy. In these cases, adjunctive use of acetazolamide and/or potassium sparing diuretic helps to correct the alkalosis.

Another serious toxicity of diuretic use in the cardiac patient is hypokalemia. Hypokalemia can exacerbate underlying cardiac arrhythmias and contribute to digitalis toxicity. This can usually be avoided by having the patient reduce Na^+ intake while taking diuretics, thus decreasing Na^+ delivery to the K^+-secreting collecting tubule. Patients who do not adhere to a low-Na^+ diet must take oral KCl supplements or a K^+-sparing diuretic.

Recently, there has been interest in the use of vaptans in heart failure, not only to treat hyponatremia but also to treat volume overload. Electrolyte dysfunction is less likely with a combination of diuretics and vaptans as opposed to higher doses of the diuretics alone. There is some evidence that at least in the short term the use of vaptans in heart failure will reduce the incidence of worsening renal function, although long-term benefit is questionable.

KIDNEY DISEASE AND RENAL FAILURE

A variety of diseases interfere with the kidney's critical role in volume homeostasis. Although some renal disorders cause salt wasting, most cause retention of salt and water. When renal failure is severe (GFR < 5 mL/min), diuretic agents are of little benefit, because glomerular filtration is insufficient to generate or sustain a natriuretic response. However, a large number of patients, and even dialysis patients, with milder degrees of severe renal insufficiency (GFR of 5–15 mL/min), can be treated with diuretics with some success. There is low-quality evidence that continuation of diuretics in end-stage kidney disease patients results in reduced hospitalization, lower incidence of intradialytic hypotension, and less weight gain between dialysis sessions.

There is still interest in the question as to whether diuretic therapy can alter the severity or the outcome of acute renal failure. This is because "nonoliguric" forms of acute renal insufficiency have better outcomes than "oliguric" (<400–500 mL/24 h urine output) acute renal failure. Almost all studies done to address this question have shown that diuretic therapy helps in the short-term fluid management of some of these patients with acute renal failure, but that it has no impact on the long-term outcome.

Many glomerular diseases, such as those associated with diabetes mellitus or systemic lupus erythematosus, exhibit renal retention of salt and water. The cause of this sodium retention is not precisely known, but it probably involves disordered regulation of the renal microcirculation and tubular function through release of vasoconstrictors, prostaglandins, cytokines, and other mediators. When edema or hypertension develops in these patients, diuretic therapy can be very effective.

Certain forms of renal disease, particularly diabetic nephropathy, are frequently associated with development of hyperkalemia at a relatively early stage of renal failure. This is often due to type IV renal tubular acidosis. In these cases, a thiazide or loop diuretic will enhance K^+ excretion by increasing delivery of salt to the K^+-secreting collecting tubule.

Patients with renal diseases leading to the nephrotic syndrome often present complex problems in volume management. These patients may exhibit fluid retention in the form of ascites or edema but have reduced plasma volume due to reduced plasma oncotic pressures. This is very often the case in patients with "minimal change" nephropathy. In these patients, diuretic use may cause further reductions in plasma volume that can impair GFR and may lead to orthostatic hypotension. Most other causes of nephrotic syndrome are associated with primary retention of salt and water by the kidney, leading to expanded plasma volume and hypertension despite the low plasma oncotic pressure. In these cases, diuretic therapy may be beneficial in controlling the volume-dependent component of hypertension. Addition of a vaptan to loop diuretics may be beneficial but needs further study in patients with nephrotic syndrome.

In choosing a diuretic for the patient with kidney disease, there are a number of important limitations. Acetazolamide must usually be avoided because it causes $NaHCO_3$ excretion and can exacerbate acidosis. Potassium-sparing diuretics may cause hyperkalemia. Thiazide diuretics are thought to be ineffective when GFR falls below 30 mL/min, although the exact GFR at which they no longer prove to be beneficial is still a matter of debate and, as recently shown, may be lower than previously imagined. In addition, it has been found that thiazides can be used to significantly reduce the dose of loop diuretics needed to promote diuresis in a patient with a GFR of 5–15 mL/min. Thus, high-dose loop diuretics (up to 500 mg/d of furosemide) or a combination of metolazone (2.5–10 mg/d) with furosemide (40–80 mg/d) may be useful in treating volume overload in dialysis or predialysis patients. Finally, although excessive use of diuretics can impair renal function in all patients, the consequences are obviously more serious in patients with underlying renal disease.

HEPATIC CIRRHOSIS

Liver disease is often associated with edema and ascites in conjunction with elevated portal hydrostatic pressures and reduced plasma oncotic pressures. Mechanisms for retention of Na^+ by the kidney in this setting include diminished renal perfusion (from systemic vascular alterations), diminished plasma volume (due to ascites formation), and diminished oncotic pressure (hypoalbuminemia). In addition, there may be primary Na^+ retention due to elevated plasma aldosterone levels.

When ascites and edema become severe, diuretic therapy can be very useful. However, cirrhotic patients are often resistant to loop diuretics because of decreased secretion of the drug into the tubular fluid and because of high aldosterone levels. In contrast, cirrhotic edema is unusually responsive to spironolactone and eplerenone. The combination of loop diuretics and an aldosterone receptor antagonist may be useful in some patients. However, considerable caution is necessary in the use of aldosterone antagonists in cirrhotic patients with even mild renal insufficiency because of the potential for causing serious hyperkalemia.

It is important to note that, even more than in heart failure, overly aggressive use of diuretics in this setting can be disastrous. Vigorous diuretic therapy can cause marked depletion of intravascular volume, hypokalemia, and metabolic alkalosis. Hepatorenal syndrome and hepatic encephalopathy are the unfortunate consequences of excessive diuretic use in the cirrhotic patient. Vaptans are relatively contraindicated in patients with liver disease because a study of tolvaptan in treating patients with autosomal dominant polycystic kidney disease resulted in increased transaminases in some patients treated with high-dose tolvaptan. Low-dose tolvaptan, however, may prove to be useful in treating some patients with cirrhosis (those who do not have ongoing liver damage) who suffer from hyponatremia or fluid overload. Use of this agent was shown to reduce need for albumin infusion and the degree of ascites accumulation in a group of patients with decompensated cirrhosis. Another large study found tolvaptan to be effective in patients with decompensated cirrhosis. Thus, even though it is true that vaptans should not be used or used with extreme caution in patients with active hepatitis, in patients with burned-out liver disease and cirrhosis, they may actually be useful therapy.

IDIOPATHIC EDEMA

Idiopathic edema (fluctuating salt retention and edema) is a syndrome found most often in 20- to 30-year-old women. Despite intensive study, the pathophysiology remains obscure. Some studies suggest that surreptitious, intermittent diuretic use may actually contribute to the syndrome and should be ruled out before additional therapy is pursued. While spironolactone has been used for idiopathic edema, it should probably be managed with moderate salt restriction alone if possible. Compression stockings also have been used but appear to be of variable benefit.

NONEDEMATOUS STATES

HYPERTENSION

The diuretic and mild vasodilator actions of the thiazides are useful in treating virtually all patients with essential hypertension and may be sufficient in many (see also Chapter 11). Although hydrochlorothiazide is the most widely used diuretic for hypertension, chlorthalidone may be more effective because of its much longer half-life. Recently there have been several studies looking at whether chlorthalidone is superior to hydrochlorothiazide in treating patients with hypertension. Taken together, these studies support the conclusion that chlorthalidone is a more potent thiazide diuretic, and is more effective in controlling blood pressure, but also has more adverse effects. The largest relevant study did not show a greater reduction in cardiovascular morbidity and mortality with use of chlorthalidone as compared with hydrochlorothiazide; however the follow up period may have been too short to see an affect.

Loop diuretics are usually reserved for patients with mild renal insufficiency (GFR < 30–40 mL/min) or heart failure. Moderate restriction of dietary Na^+ intake (60–100 mEq/d) has been shown to potentiate the effects of diuretics in essential hypertension and to lessen renal K^+ wasting. A K^+-sparing diuretic can be added to reduce K^+ wasting. A recent study found chlorthalidone to still have blood pressure–lowering effects even in stage 4 chronic kidney disease.

There has been debate about whether thiazides should be used as the initial therapy in the treatment of hypertension. Their modest efficacy sometimes limits their use as monotherapy. However, a very large study of more than 30,000 participants has shown that inexpensive diuretics like thiazides result in outcomes that are similar or superior to those found with ACE inhibitor or calcium channel-blocker therapy, reinforcing the importance of thiazide therapy in hypertension.

Although diuretics are often successful as monotherapy, they also play an important role in patients who require multiple drugs to control blood pressure. Diuretics enhance the efficacy of many agents, particularly ACE inhibitors. Patients being treated with powerful vasodilators such as hydralazine or minoxidil usually require simultaneous diuretics because the vasodilators cause significant salt and water retention. There is also growing evidence showing that spironolactone may be the most effective single agent in the therapy of drug-resistant hypertension, and this effect may extend to dialysis patients.

NEPHROLITHIASIS

Approximately two thirds of kidney stones contain Ca^{2+} phosphate or Ca^{2+} oxalate. Although there are numerous medical conditions (hyperparathyroidism, hypervitaminosis D, sarcoidosis, malignancies, etc) that cause hypercalciuria, many patients with such stones exhibit a defect in proximal tubular Ca^{2+} reabsorption. This can be treated with thiazide diuretics, which enhance Ca^{2+} reabsorption in the DCT and thus reduce the urinary Ca^{2+} concentration. Fluid intake should be increased, but salt intake must be reduced, since excess dietary NaCl will overwhelm the hypocalciuric effect of thiazides. Dietary Ca^{2+} should not be restricted, as this can lead to negative total-body Ca^{2+} balance. Calcium stones may also be caused by increased intestinal absorption of Ca^{2+}, or they may be idiopathic. In these situations, thiazides are also effective but should be used as adjunctive therapy with other measures.

HYPERCALCEMIA

Hypercalcemia can be a medical emergency (see Chapter 42). Because loop diuretics reduce Ca^{2+} reabsorption significantly, they can be quite effective in promoting Ca^{2+} diuresis. However, loop diuretics alone can cause marked volume contraction. If this occurs, loop diuretics are ineffective (and potentially counterproductive) because Ca^{2+} reabsorption in the proximal tubule would be enhanced. Thus, saline must be administered simultaneously with loop diuretics if an effective Ca^{2+} diuresis is to be maintained. The usual approach is to infuse normal saline and furosemide (80–120 mg) intravenously. Once the diuresis begins, the rate of saline infusion can be matched with the urine flow rate to avoid volume depletion. Potassium chloride may be added to the saline infusion as needed.

DIABETES INSIPIDUS

Diabetes insipidus is due to either deficient production of ADH (neurogenic or central diabetes insipidus) or inadequate responsiveness to ADH (nephrogenic diabetes insipidus [NDI]). Administration of supplementary ADH or one of its analogs is effective only in central diabetes insipidus. Thiazide diuretics can reduce polyuria and polydipsia in nephrogenic diabetes insipidus, which is not responsive to ADH supplementation.

Lithium, used in the treatment of bipolar disorder, is a common cause of NDI, and thiazide diuretics have been found to be helpful in treating it. This seemingly paradoxical beneficial effect of thiazides was previously thought to be mediated through plasma volume reduction, with an associated fall in GFR, leading to enhanced proximal reabsorption of NaCl and water and decreased delivery of fluid to the downstream diluting segments. However, in the case of Li^+-induced NDI, it is now known that HCTZ causes increased osmolality in the inner medulla (papilla) and a partial correction of the Li^+-induced reduction in aquaporin-2 expression. HCTZ also leads to increased expression of Na^+ transporters in the DCT and CCT segments of the nephron. Thus, the maximum volume of dilute urine that can be produced is significantly reduced by thiazides in NDI. Dietary sodium restriction can potentiate the beneficial effects of thiazides on urine volume in this setting. Serum Li^+ levels must be carefully monitored in these patients, because diuretics may reduce renal clearance of Li^+ and raise plasma Li^+ levels into the toxic range (see Chapter 29). Lithium-induced polyuria can also be partially reversed by amiloride or even triamterene, which blocks Li^+ entry into collecting duct cells, much as it blocks Na^+ entry. As mentioned above, thiazides are also beneficial in other forms of nephrogenic diabetes insipidus. It is not yet clear whether this is via the same mechanism that has been found in Li^+-induced NDI. Acetazolamide has also shown efficacy in treating polyuria in nephrogenic diabetes insipidus with fewer adverse events.

RENAL & CARDIAC PROTECTION

Aldosterone antagonists have been shown to be cardioprotective in patients with heart disease. In addition, they may exert an additional benefit in lowering albuminuria in patients with diabetes and microalbuminuria. Their use has been limited in patients with renal dysfunction because of the increased risk of inducing hyperkalemia. In the Treatment of Preserved Cardiac Function Heart Failure with an Aldosterone Antagonist (TOPCAT) study, the risk of cardiovascular events was lower in the group treated with spironolactone but only if they had resistant hypertension. In the TOPCAT-Americas study, the subgroup of patients with congestive heart failure had a higher incidence of worsening renal function if started on spironolactone—but even among those patients there was reduced rates of cardiovascular deaths. Even in dialysis patients, low-dose mineralocorticoid receptor antagonist use was shown to reduce cardiovascular mortality.

In the Effect of Finerenone in Chronic Kidney Disease Outcomes in Type 2 Diabetes (FIDELIO-DKD) trial, finerenone decreased incidence of end-stage kidney disease and/or >40% decline in eGFR from 21.1% to 17.8%. It also decreased the incidence of CKD progression and cardiovascular outcomes. The risk of hyperkalemia with finerenone was 2.8%.

It is also shown that both amiloride and triamterene reduced proteinuria in patients with proteinuric kidney disease by 30–40% while lowering blood pressure. Hyperkalemia was again an adverse effect. As noted earlier, SGLT-2 inhibitors also have been shown to be both cardio- and renoprotective.

RISK OF HYPONATREMIA WITH DIFFERENT DIURETIC CLASSES

In one large Scandinavian study, the odds ratio of hyponatremia with loop diuretics was 0.61, with amiloride it was 1.69, and with spironolactone it was 1.96 compared with matched controls. The risk with thiazide diuretics was not studied but was assumed to be even higher. Thus, it seems that loop diuretics are likely not associated with hyponatremia and may even decrease the risk.

SUMMARY Diuretic Agents

Subclass, Drug	Mechanism of Action	Effects	Clinical Applications	Pharmacokinetics, Toxicities, Interactions
CARBONIC ANHYDRASE INHIBITORS				
• Acetazolamide, others	Inhibition of the enzyme prevents dehydration of H_2CO_3 and hydration of CO_2 in the proximal convoluted tubule	Reduce reabsorption of HCO_3^-, causing self-limited diuresis • hyperchloremic metabolic acidosis • reduce body pH, • reduce intraocular pressure	Glaucoma, mountain sickness, edema with alkalosis	Oral and topical preparations available • duration of action ~8–12 h • *Toxicity:* Metabolic acidosis, renal stones, hyperammonemia in cirrhotics
• *Brinzolamide, dorzolamide: Topical for glaucoma*				
SGLT2 INHIBITORS				
• Canagliflozin	Inhibition of sodium/glucose cotransporter (SGLT2) in the PCT results in decreased Na^+ and glucose reabsorption	Inhibition of glucose reabsorption lowers serum glucose concentration, and reduced Na^+ reabsorption causes mild diuresis	Diabetes mellitus; approved for the treatment of hyperglycemia, not as a diuretic	Available orally. Half-life 10–12 h • not recommended in severe renal or liver disease
• *Dapagliflozin, empagliflozin, etc: Similar to canagliflozin*				
LOOP DIURETICS				
• Furosemide	Inhibition of the Na/K/2Cl transporter in the ascending limb of Henle's loop	Marked increase in NaCl excretion, some K wasting, hypokalemic metabolic alkalosis, increased urine Ca and Mg	Pulmonary edema, peripheral edema, heart failure, hypertension, acute hypercalcemia, anion overdose	Oral and parenteral preparations • duration of action 2–4 h • *Toxicity:* Ototoxicity, hypovolemia, K wasting, hyperuricemia, hypomagnesemia
• *Bumetanide, torsemide: Sulfonamide loop agents like furosemide* • *Ethacrynic acid: Not a sulfonamide but has typical loop activity and some uricosuric action*				
THIAZIDES				
• Hydrochlorothiazide	Inhibition of the Na/Cl transporter in the distal convoluted tubule	Modest increase in NaCl excretion • some K wasting • hypokalemic metabolic alkalosis • decreased urine Ca	Hypertension, mild heart failure, nephrolithiasis, nephrogenic diabetes insipidus	Oral • duration 8–12 h • *Toxicity:* Hypokalemic metabolic alkalosis, hyperuricemia, hyperglycemia, hyponatremia
• *Metolazone: Popular for use with loop agents for synergistic effects* • *Chlorothiazide: Only parenteral thiazide available (IV)* • *Chlorthalidone: Long half-life (50–60 h) due to binding to red blood cells*				

(continued)

Subclass, Drug	Mechanism of Action	Effects	Clinical Applications	Pharmacokinetics, Toxicities, Interactions
POTASSIUM-SPARING DIURETICS				
• Spironolactone	Pharmacologic antagonist of aldosterone in collecting tubules • weak antagonism of androgen receptors	Reduces Na retention and K wasting in kidney • poorly understood antagonism of aldosterone in heart and vessels	Aldosteronism from any cause • hypokalemia due to other diuretics • post-myocardial infarction	Slow onset and offset of effect • duration 24–48 h • *Toxicity:* Hyperkalemia, gynecomastia (spironolactone, not eplerenone) • additive interaction with other K-retaining drugs
• Amiloride	Blocks epithelial sodium channels in collecting tubules	Reduces Na retention and K wasting • increases lithium clearance	Hypokalemia from other diuretics • reduces lithium-induced polyuria • Liddle syndrome	Orally active • duration 24 h • *Toxicity:* Hyperkalemic metabolic acidosis
• *Eplerenone, finerenone, esaxerenone: Like spironolactone, more selective for aldosterone receptor*				
• *Triamterene: Mechanism like amiloride, much less potent, more toxic*				
OSMOTIC DIURETICS				
• Mannitol	Physical osmotic effect on tissue water distribution because it is retained in the vascular compartment	Marked increase in urine flow, reduced brain volume, decreased intraocular pressure, initial hyponatremia, then hypernatremia	Renal failure due to increased solute load (rhabdomyolysis, chemotherapy), increased intracranial pressure, glaucoma	IV administration • *Toxicity:* Nausea, vomiting, headache
VASOPRESSIN (ADH) ANTAGONISTS				
• Conivaptan	Antagonist at V_{1a} and V_2 ADH receptors	Reduces water reabsorption, increases plasma Na concentration, vasodilation	Hyponatremia, congestive heart failure	IV only, usually continuous • *Toxicity:* Infusion site reactions, thirst, polyuria, hypernatremia
• Tolvaptan	Selective antagonist at V_2 ADH receptors	Reduces water reabsorption, increases plasma Na concentration	Hyponatremia, SIADH	Oral • duration 12–24 h • *Toxicity:* Polyuria (frequency), thirst, hypernatremia

PREPARATIONS AVAILABLE

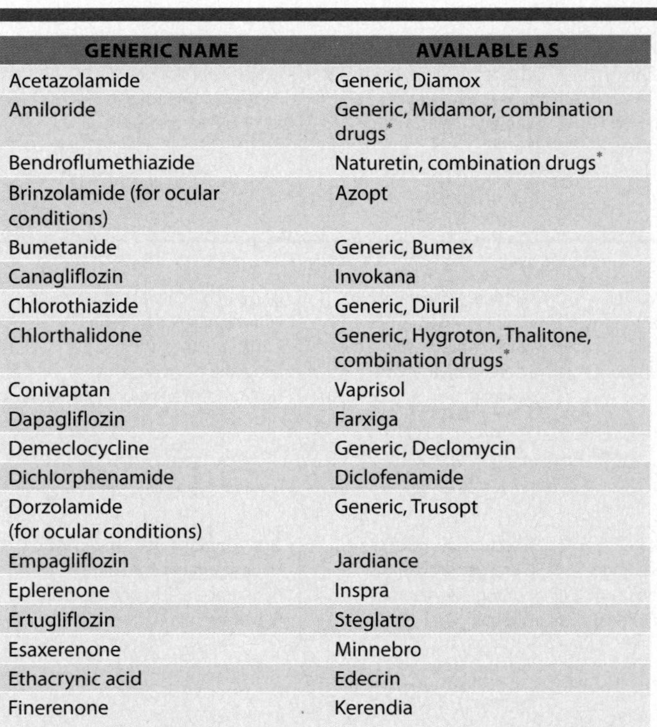

GENERIC NAME	AVAILABLE AS
Acetazolamide	Generic, Diamox
Amiloride	Generic, Midamor, combination drugs*
Bendroflumethiazide	Naturetin, combination drugs*
Brinzolamide (for ocular conditions)	Azopt
Bumetanide	Generic, Bumex
Canagliflozin	Invokana
Chlorothiazide	Generic, Diuril
Chlorthalidone	Generic, Hygroton, Thalitone, combination drugs*
Conivaptan	Vaprisol
Dapagliflozin	Farxiga
Demeclocycline	Generic, Declomycin
Dichlorphenamide	Diclofenamide
Dorzolamide (for ocular conditions)	Generic, Trusopt
Empagliflozin	Jardiance
Eplerenone	Inspra
Ertugliflozin	Steglatro
Esaxerenone	Minnebro
Ethacrynic acid	Edecrin
Finerenone	Kerendia

GENERIC NAME	AVAILABLE AS
Furosemide	Generic, Lasix, others
Hydrochlorothiazide	Generic, Esidrix, Hydro-DIURIL, combination drugs*
Hydroflumethiazide	Generic, Saluron
Indapamide	Generic, Lozol
Ipragliflozin	Suglat
Mannitol	Generic, Osmitrol
Methazolamide (for ocular conditions)	Generic, Neptazane
Methyclothiazide	Generic, Aquatensen, Enduron
Metolazone	Generic, Mykrox, Zaroxolyn (*Note:* Bioavailability of Mykrox is greater than that of Zaroxolyn)
Nesiritide	Natrecor
Polythiazide	Renese, combination drugs*
Quinethazone	Hydromox
Spironolactone	Generic, Aldactone, combination drugs*
Tolvaptan	Samsca, Jynarque
Torsemide	Generic, Demadex
Triamterene	Dyrenium
Trichlormethiazide	Generic, Diurese, Naqua, others

*Combination drugs: see Table 15–6.

REFERENCES

Abou-Mrad RM et al: Anuric acute kidney injury requiring dialysis following acetazolamide use for cataract surgery. Am J Case Rep 2021;22:e931319.

Adalsteinsson JA et al: Association between hydrochlorothiazide and the risk of in situ and invasive squamous cell skin carcinoma and basal cell carcinoma: A population-based case-controlled study. J Am Acad Dermatol 2021;84:669.

Agarwal R et al: Chlorthalidone for hypertension in advanced chronic kidney disease. N Engl J Med 2021;385:2507.

Ahlschwede KM et al. Formulation, characterization, and the diuretic effects of a new intravenous metolazone emulsion. Drug Res 2022;72:299.

Ali SB et al: Drug reaction with eosinophilia and systemic symptoms syndrome secondary to acetazolamide associated with markedly elevated procalcitonin. BMJ Case Rep 2021;14:e236966.

ALLHAT Officers and Coordinators for the ALLHAT Collaborative Research Group: Major outcomes in high-risk hypertensive patients randomized to angiotensin-converting enzyme inhibitor or calcium channel blocker vs diuretic: The Antihypertensive and Lipid-Lowering Treatment to Prevent Heart Attack Trial (ALLHAT). JAMA 2002;288:2981.

Bakris GL et al: Effect of finerenone on albuminuria in patients with diabetic nephropathy. JAMA 2015;314:884.

Bakris GL et al: Effect of finerenone on chronic kidney disease outcomes in type 2 diabetes. N Engl J Med 2020;383:2219.

Beldhuis IE et al: Spironolactone in patients with heart failure, preserved ejection fraction and worsening renal function. J Am Coll Cardiol 2021;77:1211.

Berger C et al: Patients with acute heart failure treated with the CARRESS-HF diuretic protocol in association with canrenoate potassium: Tolerance of high doses of canrenoate potassium. Arch Cardiovasc Dis 2020;113:679.

Berl T et al: Oral tolvaptan is safe and effective in chronic hyponatremia. J Am Soc Nephrol 2010;21:705.

Bokrantz T et al: Thiazide diuretics and fracture-risk among hypertensive patients. Results from the Swedish primary care cardiovascular database (SPCCD). J Hypertens 2015;33:e94.

Brater DC: Mechanism of action of diuretics. UpToDate, 2013. http://www.uptodate.com.

Brenner BM (editor): *Brenner & Rector's The Kidney*, 8th ed. Saunders, 2008.

Burns LJ et al: Spironolactone for treatment of female pattern hair loss. J Am Acad Dermatol 2020;83:276.

Cagliani JA et al: Fenoldopam increases urine output in oliguric critically ill surgical patients. Cureus 2021;13:e20445.

Carney K et al: Does hydrochlorothiazide increase the incidence of skin, lip and oral cancer in a UK population? Evid Based Dent 2022;23:38.

Cefalu WT et al: Efficacy and safety of canagliflozin versus glimepiride in patients with type 2 diabetes inadequately controlled with metformin (CANTATA-SU): 52 week results from a randomized, double-blind, phase 3 non-inferiority trial. Lancet 2014;382:941.

Charaya K et al: Impact of dapagliflozin treatment on renal function and diuretic use in acute heart failure: a pilot study. Open Heart 2022;9:e001936.

Chekka LMS et al: Race-specific comparisons of antihypertensive and metabolic effects of hydrochlorothiazide and chlorthalidone. Am J Med 2021;134:918.

Chrysant SG et al: Superior antihypertensive and cardioprotective effects of chlorthalidone compared with hydrochlorothiazide. Drugs Today 2021;57:291.

Cooper BE: Diuresis in renal failure: Treat the patient, not the urine output. Crit Care Med 2009;37:761.

Doggrell SA: Finerenone - are we there yet with a non-steroidal mineralocorticoid receptor antagonist for the treatment of diabetic chronic kidney disease? Expert Opin Pharmacother 2021;22:1253.

Drucker AM et al: Association between antihypertensive medications and risk of skin cancer in people older than 65 years: a population-based study. CMAJ 2021;193:E508.

Ellison DH: Clinical pharmacology in diuretic use. Clin J Am Soc Nephrol 2019;14:1248.

Ernst ME, Moser M: Use of diuretics in patients with hypertension. N Engl J Med 2009;361:2153.

Fernell E et al: Bumetanide for autism: open-label trial in six children. Acta Paediatr 2021;110:1548.

Filippatos G et al: Finerenone reduces new-onset atrial fibrillation in patients with chronic kidney disease and type 2 diabetes. J Am Coll Cardiol 2021;78:142.

Freeman MW et al: Phase 2 trial of baxdrostat for treatment-resistant hypertension. N Engl J Med 2023;388:395-405.

Gao D et al: Efficacy of acetazolamide for the prophylaxis of acute mountain sickness: A systematic review, meta-analysis, and trial sequential analysis of randomized clinical trials. Ann Thorac Med 2021;16:337.

Garg V et al: Long-term use of spironolactone for acne in women: a case series of 403 patients. J Am Acad Dermatol 2021;84:1348.

Ginés P, Schrier RW: Renal failure in cirrhosis. N Engl J Med 2009;361:1279.

Habel LA et al: Hydrochlorothiazide and the risk of melanoma subtypes. Pharmacoepidemiol Drug Saf 2021;30:1396.

Hao C-M, Breyer MD: Physiological regulation of prostaglandins in the kidney. Annu Rev Physiol 2008;70:357.

Hays RM: Vasopressin antagonists: Progress and promise. N Engl J Med 2006;355:146.

Herges LB et al: Pain associated with continuous intravenous infusion of bumetanide: A case series. Crit Care Nurse 2021;41:44.

Hiebert BM et al: Impact of spironolactone exposure on prostate cancer incidence amongst men with heart failure: A pharmacoepidemiological study. Br J Clin Pharmacol 2021;87:1801.

Hosui A et al: Early administration of tolvaptan can improve survival in patients with cirrhotic ascites. J Clin Med 2021;10:294.

Hripcsak G et al: Comparison of cardiovascular and safety outcomes of chlorthalidone vs hydrochlorothiazide to treat hypertension. JAMA Intern Med 2020;180:542.

Huynh HL et al: Thiazide use and skeletal microstructure: results from a multiethnic study. Bone Rep 2022;16:101589.

Inoue M et al: Triamterene in lithium-induced nephrogenic diabetes insipidus: a case report. CEN Case Rep 2021;10:64.

Ito S et al: Antihypertensive effects and safety of esaxerenone in patients with moderate kidney dysfunction. Hypertens Res 2021;44:489.

Ito S et al: Efficacy and safety of esaxerenone (CS-3150) for the treatment of type 2 diabetes with microalbuminuria. Clin J Am Soc Nephrol 2019;14:1161.

Jankovic SM et al: Clinical pharmacokinetics and pharmacodynamics of esaxerenone, a novel mineralocorticoid receptor antagonist: a review. Eur J Drug Metab Pharmacokinet 2022;47:291.

Jansson PS et al: Recurrent hydrochlorothiazide-induced acute respiratory distress syndrome treated with extracorporeal membrane oxygenation. J Emerg Med 2018;55:836.

Juurlink DN et al: Rates of hyperkalemia after publication of the randomized aldactone evaluation study. N Engl J Med 2004;351:543.

Karg MV et al: SGLT-2-inhibition with dapagliflozin reduces tissue sodium content: a randomised controlled trial. Cardiovasc Diabetol 2018;17:5.

Kieboom BCT et al: Thiazide but not loop diuretics is associated with hypomagnesaemia in the general population. Pharmacoepidemiol Drug Saf 2018;27:1166.

Kim G-H et al: Antidiuretic effect of hydrochlorothiazide in lithium-induced nephrogenic diabetes insipidus is associated with upregulation of aquaporin-2, Na-Cl co-transporter, and epithelial sodium channel. J Am Soc Nephrol 2004;15:2836.

Klein JD, Sands JM: Urea transport and clinical potential of urearetics. Curr Opin Nephrol Hypertens 2016;25:1.

Kogiso T et al: Impact of continued administration of tolvaptan on cirrhotic patients with ascites. BMC Pharmacol Toxicol 2018;19:87.

Kramers BJ et al: Case report: A thiazide diuretic to treat polyuria induced by tolvaptan. BMC Nephrol 2018;19:157.

Kramers BJ et al: Effects of hydrochlorothiazide and metformin on aquaresis and nephroprotection by a vasopressin V2 receptor antagonist in ADPKD: a randomized crossover trial. Clin J Am Soc Nephrol 2022;17:507.

Llacer P et al: Comparison of chlorthalidone and spironolactone as additional diuretic therapy in patients with acute heart failure and preserved ejection fraction. Eur Heart J Acute Cardiovasc Care 2022;11:350.

Lee C, Burnett J: Natriuretic peptides and therapeutic applications. Heart Fail Rev 2007;12:131.

Liern M et al: Antiproteinuric action of amiloride in paediatric patient with corticoresistant nephrotic syndrome. Nefrologia 2021;41:304.

Lin Z et al: Hypokalaemia associated with hydrochlorothiazide used in the treatment of hypertension in NHANES 1999-2018. J Hum Hypertens 2022. [Epub ahead of print.]

Luks AM, Swenson ER: Medication and dosage considerations in the prophylaxis and treatment of high-altitude illness. Chest 2008;133:744.

Mannheimer B et al: Association between newly initiated thiazide diuretics and hospitalization due to hyponatremia. Eur J Clin Pharmacol 2021;77:1049.

Mannheimer B et al: Non-thiazide diuretics and hospitalization due to hyponatraemia: a population-based case-control study. Clin Endocrinol 2021;95:520.

Matsue Y et al: Clinical effectiveness of tolvaptan in patients with acute heart failure and renal dysfunction: AQUAMARINE study. J Card Fail 2016;22:423.

Meena J et al: Efficacy and safety of combination therapy with tolvaptan and furosemide in children with nephrotic syndrome and refractory edema: a prospective interventional study. Indian J Pediatr 2022;89:699.

Messerli FH et al: Comparison of cardiovascular and safety outcomes of chlorthalidone vs hydrochlorothiazide to treat hypertension. JAMA Intern Med 2020;180:1133.

Nakao K et al: Long-term administration of tolvaptan ameliorates annual decline in estimated glomerular filtration rate in outpatients with chronic heart failure. Heart Vessels 2021;36:1175.

Nariai T et al: DSR-71167, a novel mineralocorticoid receptor antagonist with carbonic anhydrase inhibitory activity, separates urinary sodium excretion and serum potassium elevation in rats. Pharmacol Exp Ther 2015;354:2.

Nassif ME et al: Empagliflozin effects on pulmonary artery pressure in patients with heart failure: results from the EMBRACE-HF trial. Circulation 2021;143:1673.

Ni YN et al: The role of acetazolamide in sleep apnea at sea level: a systematic review and meta-analysis. J Clin Sleep Med 2021;17:1295.

Nijenhuis T et al: Enhanced passive Ca^{2+} reabsorption and reduced Mg^{2+} channel abundance explains thiazide-induced hypocalciuria and hypomagnesemia. J Clin Invest 2005;115:1651.

Nishino M et al: Temporal change in renoprotective effect of tolvaptan on patients with heart failure: AURORA study. J Clin Med 2022;11:977.

Nochaiwong S et al: Use of thiazide diuretics and risk of all types of skin cancers: an updated systematic review and meta-analysis. Cancers 2022;14:2566.

Olde Engberink RHG et al: Effects of thiazide-type and thiazide-like diuretics on cardiovascular events and mortality. Hypertension 2015;65:1033.

Pedersen SA et al: Hydrochlorothiazide use and risk for Merkel cell carcinoma and malignant adnexal skin tumors: A nationwide case-control study. J Am Acad Dermatol 2019;80:460.

Pei H et al: The use of a novel non-steroidal mineralocorticoid receptor antagonist finerenone for the treatment of chronic heart failure: A systematic review and meta-analysis. Medicine (Baltimore) 2018;97:e0254.

Perkovic V et al: Canagliflozin and renal outcomes in type 2 diabetes and nephropathy. N Engl J Med 2019;380:2295.

Phylactou M et al: Indapamide-induced bilateral choroidal effusion in pseudophakic patient. BMJ Case Rep 2018.

Poinas A et al: FASCE, the benefit of spironolactone for treating acne in women: study protocol for a randomized double-blind trial. Trials 2020;21:571.

Qinyang L et al: The immune-behavioural covariation associated with the treatment response to bumetanide in young children with autism spectrum disorder. Transl Psychiatry 2022;12:228.

Roberts EE et al: Use of spironolactone to treat acne in adolescent females. Pediatr Dermatol 2021;38:72.

Saimiya M et al: Efficacy of oral tolvaptan for severe edema and hyponatremia in a patient with refractory nephrotic syndrome. CEN Case Rep 2021;10:523.

Sakaida I et al: Real-world effectiveness and safety of tolvaptan in liver cirrhosis patients with hepatic edema: results from a post-marketing surveillance study (START study). J Gastroenterol 2020;55:800.

Sato N et al: Pharmacokinetics, pharmacodynamics, efficacy, and safety of OPC-61815, a prodrug of tolvaptan for intravenous administration, in patients with congestive heart failure- a phase II, multicenter, double-blind, randomized, active-controlled trial. Circ J 2022;86:699.

Schneider R et al: Risk of skin cancer in new users of thiazides and thiazide-like diuretics: a cohort study using an active comparator group. Br J Dermatol 2021;185:343.

Schnermann J, Huang Y, Mizel D: Fluid reabsorption in proximal convoluted tubules of mice with gene deletions of claudin-2 and/or aquaporin1. Am J Physiol Renal Physiol 2013;305:F1352.

Shargorodsky M et al: Treatment of hypertension with thiazides: Benefit or damage—Effect of low- and high-dose thiazide diuretics on arterial elasticity and metabolic parameters in hypertensive patients with and without glucose intolerance. J Cardiometab Syndr 2007;2:16.

Shen W et al: The effect of amiloride on proteinuria in patients with proteinuric kidney disease. Am J Nephrol 2021;52:368.

Shlipak MG, Massie BM: The clinical challenge of cardiorenal syndrome. Circulation 2004;110:1514.

Sibbel S et al: Association of continuation of loop diuretics at hemodialysis initiation with clinical outcomes. Clin J Am Soc Nephrol 2019;14:95.

Sica DA, Gehr TWB: Diuretic use in stage 5 chronic kidney disease and end-stage renal disease. Curr Opin Nephrol Hypertens 2003;12:483.

Sosenko T et al: When chest pain reveals more: A case of hydrochlorothiazide-induced systemic lupus erythematosus. Am J Case Rep 2019;20:26.

Suzuki Y et al: Tolvaptan reduces the required amount of albumin infusion in patients with decompensated cirrhosis with uncontrolled ascites: a multicenter retrospective propensity score-matched cohort study. Acta Gastroenterol Belg 2021;84:57.

Tager T et al: Comparative effectiveness of loop diuretics on mortality in the treatment of patients with chronic heart failure—A multicenter propensity score matched analysis. Int J Cardiol 2019;289:83.

Takeuchi T et al: Diuretic effects of sodium-glucose cotransporter 2 inhibitor in patients with type 2 diabetes mellitus and heart failure. Int J Cardiol 2015;201:1.

Takimura H et al: A novel validated method for predicting the risk of re-hospitalization for worsening heart failure and the effectiveness of the diuretic upgrading therapy with tolvaptan. PLoS One 2018;13.

Tovar-Palacio C et al: Ion and diuretic specificity of chimeric proteins between apical Na^+-K^+-$2Cl^-$ and Na^+-Cl^- cotransporters. Am J Physiol 2004;287:F570.

Tsujimoto T et al: Spironolactone use and improved outcomes in patients with heart failure with preserved ejection fraction with resistant hypertension. J Am Heart Assoc 2020;9:e018827.

Uchiyama k et al: The effects of trichlormethiazide in autosomal dominant polycystic kidney disease patients receiving tolvaptan: a randomized crossover controlled trial. Sci Rep 2021;11:17666.

Vaclavik J et al: Effect of spironolactone in resistant arterial hypertension: A randomized, double-blind, placebo-controlled trial (ASPIRANT-EXT). Medicine (Baltimore) 2014;93:e162.

Vasilakou D et al: Sodium-glucose cotransporter 2 inhibitors for type 2 diabetes: A systematic review and meta-analysis. Ann Intern Med 2013;159:262.

Verkman AS et al: Small-molecule inhibitors of urea transporters. Subcell Biochem 2014;73:165.

Wada T et al: Apararenone in patients with diabetic nephropathy: results of a randomized, double-blind, placebo-controlled phase 2 dose-response study and open-label extension study. Clin Exp Nephrol 2021;25:120.

Wakai A, Roberts I, Schierhout G: Mannitol for acute traumatic brain injury. Cochrane Database Syst Rev. 2007;1:CD001049.

Wan N et al: Esaxerenone, a novel nonsteroidal mineralocorticoid receptor blocker (MRB) in hypertension and chronic kidney disease. J Hum Hypertens 2021;35:148.

Wang W et al: Radiofrequency catheter ablation combined with spironolactone in the treatment of atrial fibrillation: a single center randomized controlled study. Clin Cardiol 2021;44:1120.

Wanner C et al: Empagliflozin and progression of kidney disease in type 2 diabetes. N Engl J Med 2016;375:323.

Wei C et al: Spironolactone use does not increase the risk of female breast cancer recurrence: A retrospective analysis. J Am Acad Dermatol 2020;83:1021.

Wongboonsin J et al: Acetazolamide therapy in patients with heart failure: a meta-analysis. J Clin Med 2019;8:E349.

Zheng Z et al: Continuous versus intermittent use of furosemide in patients with heart failure and moderate chronic renal dysfunction. ESC Heart Fail 2021;8:2070.

Zhu Y et al: The safety and efficacy of low-dose mineralocorticoid receptor antagonists in dialysis patients: A meta-analysis. Medicine 2021;100: e24882.

CASE STUDY ANSWER

This patient demonstrates the dramatic diuresis that can be achieved in patients on chronic loop diuretic therapy after addition of a thiazide diuretic. The drop in systolic blood pressure and the weight loss are consistent with the rapid diuresis achieved in this patient, with hypovolemia following. This effect has now led to acute kidney injury in this patient with pre-existing advanced kidney disease. This case demonstrates the need for very close monitoring of outpatients after addition of thiazide diuretics to chronic loop diuretic therapy (particularly if they have pre-existing chronic kidney disease). This is often best achieved in the inpatient setting.

SECTION IV DRUGS WITH IMPORTANT ACTIONS ON SMOOTH MUSCLE

CHAPTER 16

Histamine, Serotonin, Anti-Obesity Drugs, & the Ergot Alkaloids

Bertram G. Katzung, MD, PhD

CASE STUDY

A healthy 45-year-old physician attending a reunion in a vacation hotel developed dizziness, redness of the skin over the head and chest, and tachycardia while eating dinner in the restaurant. A short time later, another physician at the same table developed similar signs and symptoms with marked orthostatic hypotension. The menu included a green salad, sautéed fish with rice, and apple pie. What is the probable diagnosis? How would you treat these patients?

Many tissues contain substances that, when released by various stimuli, cause physiologic effects such as reddening of the skin, pain or itching, and bronchospasm. Some of these substances are also present in nervous tissue and have multiple functions. Histamine and serotonin (5-hydroxytryptamine, 5-HT) are biologically active amines that function as neurotransmitters and are also found in non-neural tissues, have complex physiologic and pathologic effects through multiple receptor subtypes, and are often released locally. Together with endogenous peptides (see Chapter 17), prostaglandins and leukotrienes (see Chapter 18), and cytokines (see Chapter 55), they constitute the **autacoid group** of drugs.

Because of their broad and largely undesirable peripheral effects, neither histamine nor serotonin has any clinical application in the treatment of disease. However, compounds that *selectively activate* certain receptor subtypes or *selectively antagonize* the actions of these amines are of considerable clinical value. This chapter therefore emphasizes the basic pharmacology of histamine and serotonin and the clinical pharmacology of the more selective agonist analogs and antagonist drugs. Obesity, a poorly understood condition, appears to involve many receptors, including some histamine and serotonin receptors. It is discussed in a special section following the discussion of serotonin and its antagonists. The ergot alkaloids, compounds with partial agonist activity at serotonin and several other receptors, are discussed at the end of the chapter.

■ HISTAMINE

Histamine was synthesized in 1907 and later isolated from mammalian tissues. Early hypotheses concerning the possible physiologic roles of tissue histamine were based on similarities between the effects of intravenously administered histamine and the symptoms of anaphylactic shock and tissue injury. Marked species variation is observed, but in humans histamine is an important mediator of immediate allergic reactions (such as urticaria) and inflammatory reactions, although it plays only a modest role in anaphylaxis. Histamine plays an important role in gastric acid secretion (see Chapter 62) and functions as a neurotransmitter and neuromodulator (see Chapters 6 and 21). Evidence indicates that histamine also plays a role in immune functions and chemotaxis of white blood cells.

BASIC PHARMACOLOGY OF HISTAMINE

Chemistry & Pharmacokinetics

Histamine occurs in plants as well as in animal tissues and is a component of some venoms and stinging secretions.

Histamine is formed by decarboxylation of the amino acid L-histidine, a reaction catalyzed in mammalian tissues by the enzyme histidine decarboxylase. Once formed, histamine is either stored or rapidly inactivated. Very little histamine is excreted unchanged. The major metabolic pathways involve conversion to *N*-methylhistamine, methylimidazoleacetic acid, and imidazoleacetic acid (IAA). Certain neoplasms (systemic mastocytosis, urticaria pigmentosa, gastric carcinoid, and occasionally myelogenous leukemia) are associated with increased numbers of mast cells or basophils and with increased excretion of histamine and its metabolites.

$CH_2—CH_2—NH_2$

HN N

Histamine

Most tissue histamine is sequestered and bound in granules (vesicles) in mast cells or basophils; the histamine content of many tissues is directly related to their mast cell content. The bound form of histamine is biologically inactive, but as noted below, many stimuli can trigger the release of mast cell histamine, allowing the free amine to exert its actions on surrounding tissues. Mast cells are especially numerous at sites of potential tissue injury—nose, mouth, and feet; internal body surfaces; and blood vessels, particularly at pressure points and bifurcations.

Non–mast cell histamine is found in several tissues, including the brain, where it functions as a neurotransmitter. Strong evidence implicates endogenous neurotransmitter histamine in many brain functions such as neuroendocrine control, cardiovascular regulation, thermal and body weight regulation, and sleep and arousal (see Chapter 21).

A second important nonneuronal site of histamine storage and release is the enterochromaffin-like (ECL) cells of the fundus of the stomach. ECL cells release histamine, one of the primary gastric acid secretagogues, to activate the acid-producing parietal cells of the mucosa (see Chapter 62).

Storage & Release of Histamine

The stores of histamine in mast cells can be released through several mechanisms.

A. Immunologic Release

Immunologic processes account for the most important pathophysiologic mechanism of mast cell and basophil histamine release. These cells, if sensitized by IgE antibodies attached to their surface membranes, degranulate explosively when exposed to the appropriate antigen (see Figure 55–5, effector phase). This type of release also requires energy and calcium. Degranulation leads to the simultaneous release of histamine, adenosine triphosphate (ATP), and other mediators that are stored together in the granules. Histamine released by this mechanism is a mediator in immediate (type I) allergic reactions, such as hay fever and acute urticaria. Substances released during IgG- or IgM-mediated immune reactions that activate the complement cascade also release histamine from mast cells and basophils.

Histamine appears to modulate its own release and that of other mediators from sensitized mast cells in some tissues by a negative feedback control mechanism mediated by H_2 receptors. In humans, mast cells in skin and basophils show this negative feedback mechanism; lung mast cells do not. Thus, histamine may act to limit the intensity of the allergic reaction in the skin and blood.

Endogenous histamine has a modulating role in a variety of inflammatory and immune responses. Upon injury to a tissue, released histamine causes local vasodilation and leakage of plasma-containing mediators of acute inflammation (complement, C-reactive protein) and antibodies. Histamine has an active chemotactic attraction for inflammatory cells (neutrophils, eosinophils, basophils, monocytes, and lymphocytes). Histamine inhibits the release of lysosome contents and several T- and B-lymphocyte functions. Most of these actions are mediated by H_2 or H_4 receptors. Release of peptides from nerves in response to inflammation is probably modulated by histamine acting on presynaptic H_3 receptors.

B. Chemical and Mechanical Release

Certain amines, including drugs such as morphine and tubocurarine, can displace histamine from its bound form within cells. This type of release does not require energy and is not associated with mast cell injury or explosive degranulation. Loss of granules from the mast cell also releases histamine, because sodium ions in the extracellular fluid rapidly displace the amine from the complex. Chemical and mechanical mast cell injury causes degranulation and histamine release. **Compound 48/80,** an experimental drug, selectively releases histamine from tissue mast cells by an exocytotic degranulation process requiring energy and calcium.

Pharmacodynamics

A. Mechanism of Action

Histamine exerts its biologic actions by combining with specific receptors located on the cell membrane. Four different histamine receptors have been characterized and are designated H_1–H_4; they are described in Table 16–1. Unlike the other amine transmitter receptors discussed in previous chapters, no subfamilies have been found within these major types, although different splice variants of several receptor types have been described.

All four histamine receptor types have been cloned and belong to the large superfamily of G protein-coupled receptors (GPCR). The structures of the H_1 and H_2 receptors differ significantly and appear to be more closely related to muscarinic and 5-HT_1 receptors, respectively, than to each other. The H_3 and H_4 receptors have about 40% homology but do not seem to be closely related to any other histamine receptor. All four histamine receptors have been shown to have constitutive activity in some systems; thus, some antihistamines previously considered to be traditional pharmacologic antagonists must now be considered to be inverse agonists (see Chapters 1 and 2). Indeed, many first- and second-generation H_1 blockers function as inverse agonists. Furthermore, a single molecule may be an agonist at one histamine receptor and an antagonist or inverse agonist at another. For example, clobenpropit, an agonist at H_4 receptors, is an antagonist or inverse agonist at H_3 receptors (see Table 16–1).

In the brain, H_1 and H_2 receptors are located on postsynaptic membranes, whereas H_3 receptors are predominantly presynaptic. Activation of H_1 receptors, which are present in endothelium, smooth muscle cells, and nerve endings, usually elicits an increase in phosphoinositol hydrolysis and an increase in inositol trisphosphate (IP_3) and intracellular calcium. Activation of H_2 receptors, present in gastric mucosa, cardiac muscle cells, and some immune cells, increases intracellular cyclic adenosine monophosphate (cAMP) via G_s. Like the β_2 adrenoceptor, under certain circumstances the H_2 receptor may couple to G_q, activating the IP_3-DAG (inositol 1,4,5-trisphosphate-diacylglycerol) cascade. Activation of H_3 receptors decreases transmitter release from histaminergic and other neurons, probably mediated by G_i with diminished cAMP, and a decrease in calcium influx through N-type calcium channels in nerve endings. H_4 receptors are found mainly on leukocytes in the bone marrow and circulating blood. H_4 receptors have very important chemotactic effects on eosinophils and mast cells. In this role, they play a part in inflammation and allergy. They may also modulate production of these cell types and they may mediate, in part, the previously recognized effects of histamine on cytokine production.

B. Tissue and Organ System Effects of Histamine

Histamine exerts powerful effects on smooth and cardiac muscle, on certain endothelial and nerve cells, on the secretory cells of the stomach, and on inflammatory cells. However, sensitivity to histamine varies greatly among species. Guinea pigs are exquisitely sensitive; humans, dogs, and cats somewhat less so; and mice and rats very much less so.

1. *Nervous system*—Histamine is a powerful stimulant of sensory nerve endings, especially those mediating pain and itching. This H_1-mediated effect is an important component of the urticarial response and reactions to insect and nettle stings. Some evidence suggests that local high concentrations can also depolarize efferent (axonal) nerve endings (see Triple Response, item 8 in this list). In the mouse, and probably in humans, respiratory neurons signaling inspiration and expiration are modulated by H_1 receptors. H_1 and H_3 receptors play important roles in appetite and satiety; antipsychotic drugs that block these receptors cause significant weight gain (see Chapter 29). These receptors may also participate in nociception. Presynaptic H_3 receptors play important roles in modulating release of several transmitters in the nervous system. H_3 agonists reduce the release of acetylcholine, amine, and peptide transmitters in various areas of the brain and in peripheral nerves. An antagonist or inverse H_3 agonist, **pitolisant** (tiprolisant, BF2649), appears to reduce drowsiness in patients with narcolepsy.

2. *Cardiovascular system*—In humans, injection or infusion of histamine causes a decrease in systolic and diastolic blood pressure and an increase in heart rate. The blood pressure changes are caused by the vasodilator action of histamine on arterioles and precapillary sphincters; the increase in heart rate

TABLE 16–1 Histamine receptor subtypes.

Receptor Subtype	Distribution	Postreceptor Mechanism	Partially Selective Agonists	Partially Selective Antagonists or Inverse Agonists
H_1	Smooth muscle, endothelium, brain	G_q, ↑ IP_3, DAG	Histaprodifen	Mepyramine,[1] triprolidine, cetirizine
H_2	Gastric mucosa, cardiac muscle, mast cells, brain	G_s, ↑ cAMP	Amthamine	Cimetidine,[1] ranitidine,[1] famotidine,[1] tiotidine
H_3	Presynaptic autoreceptors and heteroreceptors: brain, myenteric plexus, other neurons	G_i, ↓ cAMP	R-α-Methylhistamine, imetit, immepip	Thioperamide,[1] iodophenpropit, clobenpropit,[1] tiprolisant (pitolisant),[1] proxyfan
H_4	Eosinophils, neutrophils, mast cells, CD4 T cells	G_i, ↓ cAMP	Clobenpropit, imetit, clozapine	Thioperamide[1]

[1]Inverse agonist.

cAMP, cyclic adenosine monophosphate; DAG, diacylglycerol; IP_3, inositol trisphosphate.

involves both stimulatory actions of histamine on the heart and a reflex tachycardia. Flushing, a sense of warmth, and headache also may occur during histamine administration, consistent with the vasodilation. Vasodilation elicited by small doses of histamine is caused by H_1-receptor activation and is mediated mainly by release of nitric oxide from the endothelium (see Chapter 19). The decrease in blood pressure is usually accompanied by a reflex tachycardia. Higher doses of histamine activate the H_2-mediated cAMP process of vasodilation and direct cardiac stimulation. In humans, the cardiovascular effects of small doses of histamine can usually be antagonized by H_1-receptor antagonists alone.

Histamine-induced edema results from the action of the amine on H_1 receptors in the vessels of the microcirculation, especially the postcapillary vessels. The effect is associated with the separation of the endothelial cells, which permits the transudation of fluid and molecules as large as small proteins into the perivascular tissue. This effect is responsible for urticaria (hives), which signals the release of histamine in the skin. Studies of endothelial cells suggest that actin and myosin within these cells cause contraction, resulting in separation of the endothelial cells and increased permeability.

Direct cardiac effects of histamine include both increased contractility and increased pacemaker rate. These effects are mediated chiefly by H_2 receptors. In human atrial muscle, histamine can also decrease contractility; this effect is mediated by H_1 receptors. The physiologic significance of these cardiac actions is not clear. Some of the cardiovascular signs and symptoms of anaphylaxis are due to released histamine, although several other mediators are involved and are much more important than histamine in humans.

3. *Bronchiolar smooth muscle*—In both humans and guinea pigs, histamine causes bronchoconstriction mediated by H_1 receptors. In the guinea pig, this effect is the cause of death from histamine toxicity, but in humans with normal airways, bronchoconstriction following small doses of histamine is not marked. However, patients with asthma are very sensitive to histamine. The bronchoconstriction induced in these patients probably represents a hyperactive neural response, since such patients also respond excessively to many other stimuli, and the response to histamine can be blocked by autonomic blocking drugs such as ganglion blocking agents as well as by H_1-receptor antagonists (see Chapter 20). Although methacholine provocation is more commonly used, tests using small doses of inhaled histamine have been used in the diagnosis of bronchial hyperreactivity in patients with suspected asthma or cystic fibrosis. Such individuals may be 100 to 1000 times more sensitive to histamine (and methacholine) than are normal subjects. Curiously, a few species (eg, rabbit) respond to histamine with broncho*dilation*, reflecting the dominance of the H_2 receptor in their airways.

4. *Gastrointestinal tract smooth muscle*—Histamine causes contraction of intestinal smooth muscle, and histamine-induced contraction of guinea pig ileum is a standard bioassay for this amine. The human gut is not as sensitive as that of the guinea pig, but large doses of histamine may cause diarrhea, partly as a result of this effect. This action of histamine is mediated by H_1 receptors.

5. *Other smooth muscle organs*—In humans, histamine generally has insignificant effects on the smooth muscle of the eye and genitourinary tract. However, pregnant women suffering anaphylactic reactions may abort as a result of histamine-induced uterine contractions, and in some species the sensitivity of the uterus is sufficient to form the basis for a bioassay.

6. *Secretory tissue*—Histamine has long been recognized as a powerful stimulant of gastric acid secretion and, to a lesser extent, of gastric pepsin and intrinsic factor production. The effect is caused by activation of H_2 receptors on gastric parietal cells and is associated with increased adenylyl cyclase activity, cAMP concentration, and intracellular Ca^{2+} concentration. Other stimulants of gastric acid secretion such as acetylcholine and gastrin do not increase cAMP even though their maximal effects on acid output can be reduced—but not abolished—by H_2-receptor antagonists. These actions are discussed in more detail in Chapter 62. Histamine also stimulates secretion in the small and large intestine. In contrast, H_3-selective histamine agonists *inhibit* acid secretion stimulated by food or pentagastrin in several species.

Histamine has much smaller effects on the activity of other glandular tissue at ordinary concentrations. Very high concentrations can cause catecholamine release from the adrenal medulla.

7. *Metabolic effects*—Recent studies of H_3-receptor knockout mice demonstrate that absence of this receptor results in increased food intake, decreased energy expenditure, and obesity. They also show insulin resistance and increased blood levels of leptin and insulin. It is not yet known whether the H_3 receptor has a similar role in humans, but research is under way to determine whether H_3 agonists are useful in the treatment of obesity.

8. *The "triple response"*—Intradermal injection of histamine causes a characteristic red spot, edema, and flare response. The effect involves three separate cell types: smooth muscle in the microcirculation, capillary or venular endothelium, and sensory nerve endings. At the site of injection, a reddening appears owing to dilation of small vessels, followed soon by an edematous wheal at the injection site and a red irregular flare surrounding the wheal. The flare is said to be caused by an axon reflex. A sensation of itching may accompany these effects.

Similar local effects may be produced by injecting histamine liberators (compound 48/80, morphine, etc) intradermally or by applying the appropriate antigens to the skin of a sensitized person. Although most of these local effects can be prevented by adequate doses of an H_1-receptor-blocking agent, H_2 and H_3 receptors also may be involved.

9. *Other effects possibly mediated by histamine receptors*—In addition to the local stimulation of peripheral pain nerve endings via H_3 and H_1 receptors, histamine appears to play a role in nociception in the central nervous system. **Burimamide,** an early candidate for H_2-blocking action, and newer analogs with no notable effect on H_1, H_2, or H_3 receptors, have been shown to have significant analgesic action in rodents when administered into the central nervous system. The analgesia is said to be comparable to that produced by opioids, but tolerance, respiratory depression, and constipation have not been reported. Potentiation of simultaneously administered opioids may occur.

Other Histamine Agonists

Small substitutions on the imidazole ring of histamine significantly modify the selectivity of the compounds for the histamine receptor subtypes. Some of these are listed in Table 16–1.

CLINICAL PHARMACOLOGY OF HISTAMINE

Clinical Uses

In pulmonary function laboratories, histamine aerosol has rarely been used as a **provocative test** of bronchial hyperreactivity. Histamine has no other current clinical applications.

Toxicity & Contraindications

Adverse effects of histamine release, like those following administration of histamine, are dose related. Flushing, hypotension, tachycardia, headache, urticaria, bronchoconstriction, and gastrointestinal upset are noted. These effects are also observed after the ingestion of spoiled fish (scombroid fish poisoning), and histamine produced by bacterial action in the flesh of improperly stored fish is the major causative agent.

Histamine should not be given to patients with asthma (except as part of a carefully monitored test of pulmonary function) or to patients with active ulcer disease or gastrointestinal bleeding.

HISTAMINE ANTAGONISTS

The effects of histamine released in the body can be reduced in several ways. **Physiologic antagonists,** especially epinephrine, have smooth muscle actions opposite to those of histamine, but they act at different receptors. This is important clinically because injection of epinephrine can be lifesaving in systemic **anaphylaxis** and in other conditions in which massive release of histamine—and other more important mediators—occurs.

Release inhibitors reduce the degranulation of mast cells that results from immunologic triggering by antigen-IgE interaction. **Cromolyn** and **nedocromil** appear to have this effect (see Chapter 20) and have been used in the treatment of asthma. Beta$_2$-adrenoceptor agonists also appear capable of reducing histamine release.

Histamine **receptor antagonists** represent a third approach to the reduction of histamine-mediated responses. For more than 70 years, compounds have been available that competitively antagonize many of the actions of histamine on smooth muscle. However, not until the H$_2$-receptor antagonist burimamide was described in 1972 was it possible to antagonize the gastric acid–stimulating activity of histamine. The development of selective H$_2$-receptor antagonists has led to more effective therapy for peptic disease (see Chapter 62). A selective H$_3$ antagonist/inverse agonist, pitolisant (also known as tiprolisant) is approved for the treatment of narcolepsy. Selective H$_4$ antagonists are not yet available for clinical use. However, potent and partially selective experimental H$_3$-receptor antagonists or inverse agonists, thioperamide and clobenpropit, have been developed.

■ HISTAMINE RECEPTOR ANTAGONISTS

H$_1$-RECEPTOR ANTAGONISTS

Compounds that competitively block histamine or act as inverse agonists at H$_1$ receptors have been used in the treatment of allergic conditions for many years, and in the discussion that follows they are referred to as antagonists. Many H$_1$ antagonists are currently marketed in the USA. A large number are available without prescription, both alone and in combination formulations such as "cold pills" and "sleep aids" (see Chapter 64).

BASIC PHARMACOLOGY OF H$_1$-RECEPTOR ANTAGONISTS

Chemistry & Pharmacokinetics

The H$_1$ antagonists are conveniently divided into first-generation and second-generation agents. These groups are distinguished by the relatively strong sedative effects of most of the first-generation drugs. The first-generation agents are also more likely to block autonomic receptors. The second-generation H$_1$ blockers are less sedating, owing in part to reduced distribution into the central nervous system. All the H$_1$ antagonists are stable amines with the general structure illustrated in Figure 16–1. Doses of some of these drugs are given in Table 16–2.

These agents are rapidly absorbed after oral administration, with peak blood concentrations occurring in 1–2 hours. They are widely distributed throughout the body, and the first-generation H$_1$ blockers enter the central nervous system readily. Some of them are extensively metabolized, primarily by microsomal systems in the liver. Several of the second-generation agents are metabolized by the CYP3A4 system and thus are subject to important interactions when other drugs (such as ketoconazole) inhibit this subtype of P450 enzymes. Most of the drugs have an effective duration of action of 4–6 hours following a single dose, but meclizine and several second-generation agents are longer-acting, with a duration of action of 12–24 hours. The newer agents are considerably less lipid-soluble than the first-generation drugs and are substrates of the P-glycoprotein transporter in the blood-brain barrier; as a result, they enter the central nervous system with difficulty or not at all. Many H$_1$ antagonists have active metabolites. The active metabolites of hydroxyzine, terfenadine, and loratadine are available as drugs (cetirizine, fexofenadine, and desloratadine, respectively).

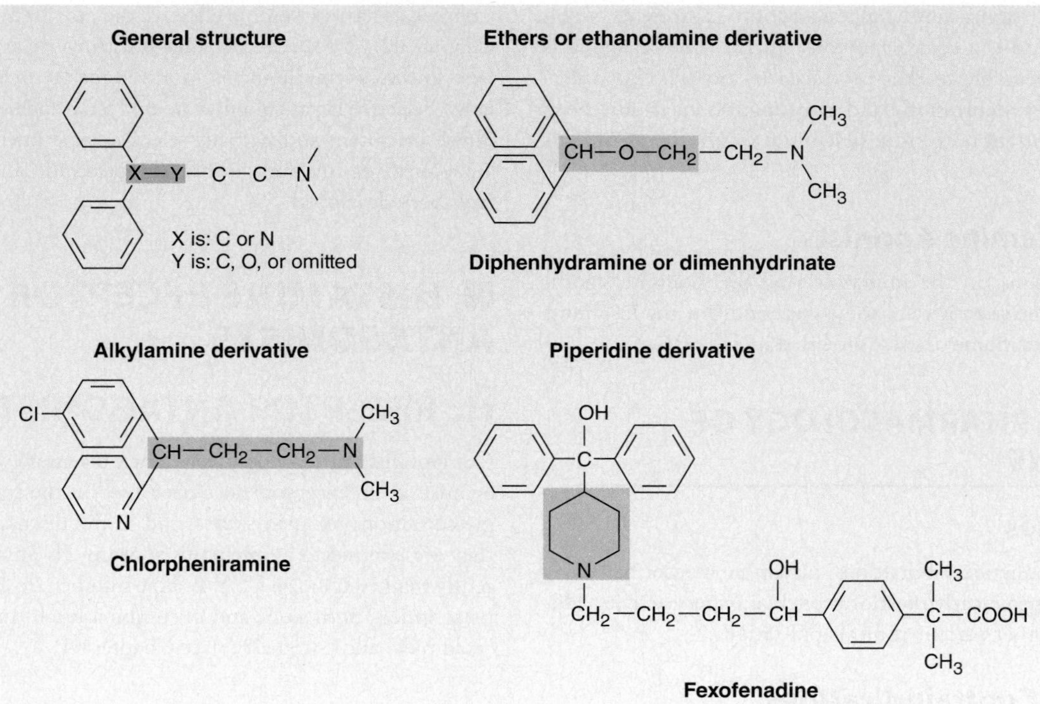

FIGURE 16–1 **General structure of H_1-antagonist drugs and examples of the major subgroups.** Subgroup names are based on the shaded moieties.

Pharmacodynamics

Both neutral H_1 antagonists and inverse H_1 agonists reduce or block the actions of histamine by reversible competitive binding to the H_1 receptor. Several have been clearly shown to be inverse agonists, and it is possible that all act by this mechanism. They have negligible potency at the H_2 receptor and little at the H_3 receptor. For example, histamine-induced contraction of bronchiolar or gastrointestinal smooth muscle can be completely blocked by these agents, but histamine-stimulated gastric acid secretion and the stimulation of the heart are unaffected.

The first-generation H_1-receptor antagonists have many actions in addition to blockade of the actions of histamine. The large number of these actions probably results from the similarity of the general structure (see Figure 16–1) to the structure of drugs that have effects at muscarinic cholinoceptor, α adrenoceptor, serotonin, and local anesthetic receptor sites. Some of these actions are of therapeutic value and some are undesirable.

1. *Sedation*—A common effect of the first-generation H_1 antagonists is sedation, but the intensity of this effect varies among chemical subgroups (see Table 16–2) and among patients as well. The effect is sufficiently prominent with some agents to make them useful as "sleep aids" (see Chapter 64) and unsuitable for daytime use. The effect resembles that of some antimuscarinic drugs and is considered very different from the disinhibited sedation produced by sedative-hypnotic drugs. Compulsive use has not been reported. At ordinary dosages, children occasionally (and adults rarely) manifest excitation rather than sedation. At very high toxic dose levels, marked stimulation, agitation, and even seizures may precede coma. The second-generation H_1 antagonists have little or no sedative or stimulant actions. These drugs (or their active metabolites) also have far fewer autonomic effects than the first-generation antihistamines.

2. *Antinausea and antiemetic actions*—Several first-generation H_1 antagonists have significant activity in preventing motion sickness (see Table 16–2). They are less effective against an episode of motion sickness already present. Certain H_1 antagonists, notably **doxylamine** (in **Bendectin**), were used widely in the past in the treatment of nausea and vomiting of pregnancy (see below). Although Bendectin was withdrawn in 1983, a similar formulation, combining doxylamine and pyridoxine **(Diclegis)**, was approved by the US Food and Drug Administration (FDA) in 2013.

3. *Antiparkinsonism effects*—Some of the H_1 antagonists, especially **diphenhydramine,** have significant acute suppressant effects on the extrapyramidal symptoms associated with certain antipsychotic drugs. This drug is given parenterally for acute dystonic reactions to antipsychotics.

4. *Antimuscarinic actions*—Many first-generation agents, especially those of the ethanolamine and ethylenediamine subgroups, have significant atropine-like effects on peripheral muscarinic receptors. This action may be responsible for some of the (uncertain) benefits reported for nonallergic rhinorrhea but may also cause urinary retention and blurred vision.

TABLE 16–2 Some H_1 antihistaminic drugs in clinical use.

Drugs	Usual Adult Dose	Anticholinergic Activity	Comments
FIRST-GENERATION ANTIHISTAMINES			
Ethanolamines			
Carbinoxamine (Clistin)	4–8 mg	+++	Slight to moderate sedation
Dimenhydrinate (salt of diphenhydramine) (Dramamine)	50 mg	+++	Marked sedation; anti-motion sickness activity
Diphenhydramine (Benadryl, etc)	25–50 mg	+++	Marked sedation; anti-motion sickness activity
Piperazine derivatives			
Hydroxyzine (Atarax, etc)	15–100 mg	nd	Marked sedation
Cyclizine (Marezine)	25–50 mg	—	Slight sedation; anti-motion sickness activity
Meclizine (Bonine, etc)	25–50 mg	—	Slight sedation; anti-motion sickness activity
Alkylamines			
Brompheniramine (Dimetane, etc)	4–8 mg	+	Slight sedation
Chlorpheniramine (Chlor-Trimeton, etc)	4–8 mg	+	Slight sedation; common component of OTC "cold" medication
Phenothiazine derivative			
Promethazine (Phenergan, etc)	10–25 mg	+++	Marked sedation; antiemetic; α-block
Miscellaneous			
Cyproheptadine (Periactin, etc)	4 mg	+	Moderate sedation; significant antiserotonin activity; mixed evidence for use as an appetite stimulant
SECOND-GENERATION ANTIHISTAMINES			
Piperidine			
Fexofenadine (Allegra, etc)	60 mg	—	
Miscellaneous			
Loratadine (Claritin, etc), desloratadine (Clarinex)	10 mg (desloratadine, 5 mg)	—	Longer action; used at 5 mg dosage
Cetirizine (Zyrtec, etc)	5–10 mg	—	

nd, no data found.

5. *Adrenoceptor-blocking actions*—Alpha-receptor–blocking effects can be demonstrated for many H_1 antagonists, especially those in the phenothiazine subgroup, eg, **promethazine.** This action may cause orthostatic hypotension in susceptible individuals. Beta-receptor blockade is not significant.

6. *Serotonin-blocking actions*—Strong blocking effects at serotonin receptors have been demonstrated for some first-generation H_1 antagonists, notably **cyproheptadine.** This drug is promoted as an antiserotonin agent and is discussed with that drug group. Nevertheless, its structure resembles that of the phenothiazine antihistamines, and it is a potent H_1-blocking agent.

7. *Local anesthesia*—Several first-generation H_1 antagonists are potent local anesthetics. They block sodium channels in excitable membranes in the same fashion as procaine and lidocaine. Diphenhydramine and promethazine are actually more potent than procaine as local anesthetics. They are occasionally used to produce local anesthesia in patients allergic to conventional local anesthetic drugs. A small number of these agents also block potassium channels; this action is discussed below (see the section Toxicity).

8. *Other actions*—Certain H_1 antagonists, eg, cetirizine, inhibit mast cell release of histamine and some other mediators of inflammation. This action is not due to H_1-receptor blockade and may reflect an H_4-receptor effect (see below). The mechanism is not fully understood but could play a role in the beneficial effects of these drugs in the treatment of allergies such as rhinitis or pruritis. A few H_1 antagonists (eg, terfenadine, acrivastine) have been shown to inhibit the P-glycoprotein transporter found in cancer cells, the epithelium of the gut, and the capillaries of the brain. The significance of this effect is not known.

CLINICAL PHARMACOLOGY OF H_1-RECEPTOR ANTAGONISTS

Clinical Uses

The first-generation H_1-receptor blockers are commonly used over-the-counter drugs. The prevalence of allergic conditions and the relative safety of the drugs contribute to this heavy use. However, the fact that they do cause sedation contributes to use of older agents (eg, doxylamine, diphenhydramine) as night-time sleep-aids as well as increasing over-the-counter use of the second-generation antihistamines to avoid the sedative action.

A. Allergic Reactions

The H_1 antihistaminic agents are often the first drugs used to prevent or treat the symptoms of allergic reactions. In **allergic rhinitis (hay fever),** the H_1 antagonists are the second-line drugs after glucocorticoids administered by nasal spray. In urticaria, in which histamine is often the primary mediator, the H_1 antagonists are the drugs of choice and are often quite effective if given before exposure. However, in bronchial asthma, which involves several mediators, the H_1 antagonists are largely ineffective.

Angioedema may be precipitated by histamine release but appears to be maintained by peptide kinins that are not affected by antihistaminic agents. For atopic dermatitis, antihistaminic drugs such as diphenhydramine are used mostly for their sedative effect, which reduces awareness of itching. H_4 antihistamines may supplant the H_1 antagonists in atopic dermatitis (see below).

The H_1 antihistamines used for treating allergic conditions such as hay fever are usually selected with the goal of minimizing sedative effects; in the USA, the drugs in widest use are the alkylamines and the second-generation nonsedating agents. However, the sedative effect and the therapeutic efficacy of different agents vary widely among individuals. In addition, the clinical effectiveness of one group may diminish with continued use, and switching to another group may restore drug effectiveness for as yet unexplained reasons.

The second-generation H_1 antagonists are used mainly for the treatment of allergic rhinitis and chronic **urticaria.** Several double-blind comparisons with older agents (eg, chlorpheniramine) indicated approximately equal therapeutic efficacy. However, sedation and interference with safe operation of machinery, which occur in about 50% of subjects taking the first-generation antihistamines, occurred in only about 7% of subjects taking the second-generation agents. The newer drugs are much more expensive, even in over-the-counter generic formulations.

B. Motion Sickness and Vestibular Disturbances

Scopolamine (see Chapter 8) and certain first-generation H_1 antagonists are the most effective agents available for the prevention of motion sickness. The antihistaminic drugs with the greatest effectiveness in this application are diphenhydramine and promethazine. Dimenhydrinate, which is promoted almost exclusively for the treatment of motion sickness, is a salt of diphenhydramine and has similar efficacy. The piperazines (cyclizine and meclizine) also have significant activity in preventing motion sickness and are less sedating than diphenhydramine in most patients. Dosage is the same as that recommended for allergic disorders (see Table 16–2). Both scopolamine and the H_1 antagonists are more effective in preventing motion sickness when combined with ephedrine or amphetamine.

It has been claimed that the antihistaminic agents effective in prophylaxis of motion sickness are also useful in Ménière syndrome, but efficacy in the latter condition is not established.

C. Nausea and Vomiting of Pregnancy

Several H_1-antagonist drugs have been studied for possible use in treating "morning sickness." The piperazine derivatives were withdrawn from such use when it was demonstrated that they have teratogenic effects in rodents. Doxylamine, an ethanolamine H_1 antagonist, was promoted for this application as a component of Bendectin, a prescription medication that also contained pyridoxine. Possible teratogenic effects of doxylamine were widely publicized in the lay press after 1978 as a result of a few case reports of fetal malformation that occurred after maternal ingestion of Bendectin. However, several large prospective studies disclosed no increase in the incidence of birth defects, thereby justifying the reintroduction of a similar product.

Toxicity

The wide spectrum of nonantihistaminic effects of the H_1 antihistamines is described above. Several of these effects (sedation, antimuscarinic action) have been used for therapeutic purposes, especially in over-the-counter remedies (see Chapter 64). Nevertheless, these two effects constitute the most common undesirable actions when these drugs are used to block peripheral histamine receptors.

Less common toxic effects of systemic use include excitation and convulsions in children, postural hypotension, and allergic responses. Drug allergy is relatively common after topical use of H_1 antagonists. The effects of severe systemic overdosage of the older agents resemble those of atropine overdosage and are treated in the same way (see Chapters 8 and 58). Overdosage of astemizole or terfenadine may induce cardiac arrhythmias; the same effect may be caused at normal dosage by interaction with enzyme inhibitors (see Drug Interactions). These drugs are no longer marketed in the USA.

Drug Interactions

Lethal ventricular arrhythmias occurred in several patients taking either of the early second-generation agents, terfenadine or astemizole, in combination with ketoconazole, itraconazole, or macrolide antibiotics such as erythromycin. These antimicrobial drugs inhibit the metabolism of many drugs by CYP3A4 and cause significant increases in blood concentrations of the antihistamines. The mechanism of this toxicity involves blockade of the HERG (I_{Kr}) potassium channels in the heart that contribute to repolarization of the action potential (see Chapter 14). The result is prolongation and a change in shape of the action potential, and these changes lead to arrhythmias. Both terfenadine and astemizole were withdrawn from the US market in recognition of these problems. Where still available, terfenadine and astemizole should be considered to be contraindicated in patients taking ketoconazole, itraconazole, or macrolides and in patients with liver disease. Grapefruit juice also inhibits CYP3A4 and has been shown to increase blood levels of terfenadine significantly.

For those H_1 antagonists that cause significant sedation, concurrent use of other drugs that cause central nervous system depression produces additive effects and is contraindicated while driving or operating machinery. Similarly, the autonomic blocking effects of older antihistamines are additive with those of antimuscarinic and α-blocking drugs.

H_2-RECEPTOR ANTAGONISTS

The development of H_2-receptor antagonists was based on the observation that H_1 antagonists had no effect on histamine-induced acid secretion in the stomach. Molecular manipulation of the histamine molecule resulted in drugs that blocked acid secretion and had no H_1 agonist or antagonist effects. Like the other histamine receptors, the H_2 receptor displays constitutive activity, and some H_2 blockers are inverse agonists.

The high prevalence of peptic ulcer disease created great interest in the therapeutic potential of the H_2-receptor antagonists when first discovered. Although these agents are not the most efficacious available, their ability to reduce gastric acid secretion with very low toxicity has made them extremely popular as over-the-counter preparations. These drugs are discussed in detail in Chapter 62.

H_3- & H_4-RECEPTOR ANTAGONISTS

Although no selective H_3 or H_4 ligands are presently available for general clinical use, there is great interest in their therapeutic potential. H_3-selective ligands may be of value in sleep disorders, narcolepsy, obesity, and cognitive and psychiatric disorders. **Tiprolisant,** an inverse H_3-receptor agonist, has been shown to reduce sleep cycles in mutant mice and in humans with narcolepsy. Increased obesity has been demonstrated in both H_1- and H_3-receptor knockout mice; however, H_3 inverse agonists decrease feeding in obese mouse models. As noted in Chapter 29, several atypical antipsychotic drugs have significant affinity for H_3 receptors (and cause weight gain).

Because of the homology between the H_3 and H_4 receptors, some H_3 ligands also have affinity for the H_4 receptor. H_4 blockers have potential in chronic inflammatory conditions such as asthma, in which eosinophils and mast cells play a prominent role. No selective H_4 ligand is approved for use in humans, but in addition to research agents listed in Table 16–1, many H_1 blockers (eg, diphenhydramine, cetirizine, loratadine) show some affinity for this receptor. Several studies have suggested that H_4-receptor antagonists may be useful in atopic dermatitis, pruritus, asthma, allergic rhinitis, and pain conditions.

■ SEROTONIN (5-HYDROXYTRYPTAMINE)

Before the identification of 5-hydroxytryptamine (5-HT), it was known that when blood is allowed to clot, a vasoconstrictor (*tonic*) substance is released from the clot into the *serum*. This substance was called serotonin. Independent studies established the existence of a smooth muscle stimulant in intestinal mucosa. This was called enteramine. The synthesis of 5-hydroxytryptamine in 1951 led to the identification of serotonin and enteramine as the same metabolite of 5-hydroxytryptophan.

Serotonin is an important neurotransmitter, a local hormone in the gut, a component of the platelet clotting process, and is thought to play a role in migraine headache and several other clinical conditions, including carcinoid syndrome. This syndrome is an unusual manifestation of carcinoid tumor, a neoplasm of enterochromaffin cells. In patients whose tumor is not surgically resectable, a serotonin antagonist may constitute a useful treatment.

BASIC PHARMACOLOGY OF SEROTONIN

Chemistry & Pharmacokinetics

Like histamine, serotonin is widely distributed in nature, being found in plant and animal tissues, venoms, and stings. It is synthesized in biologic systems from the amino acid L-tryptophan by hydroxylation of the indole ring followed by decarboxylation of the amino acid (Figure 16–2). Hydroxylation at C5 by tryptophan hydroxylase-1 is the rate-limiting step and can be blocked by *p*-chlorophenylalanine (PCPA; fenclonine) and by *p*-chloroamphetamine. These agents have been used experimentally to reduce serotonin synthesis in carcinoid syndrome but are too toxic for general clinical use. **Telotristat ethyl,** an orally active hydroxylase inhibitor, has been approved for the treatment of diarrhea due to carcinoid tumor.

After synthesis, the free amine is stored in vesicles or is rapidly inactivated, usually by oxidation by monoamine oxidase (MAO).

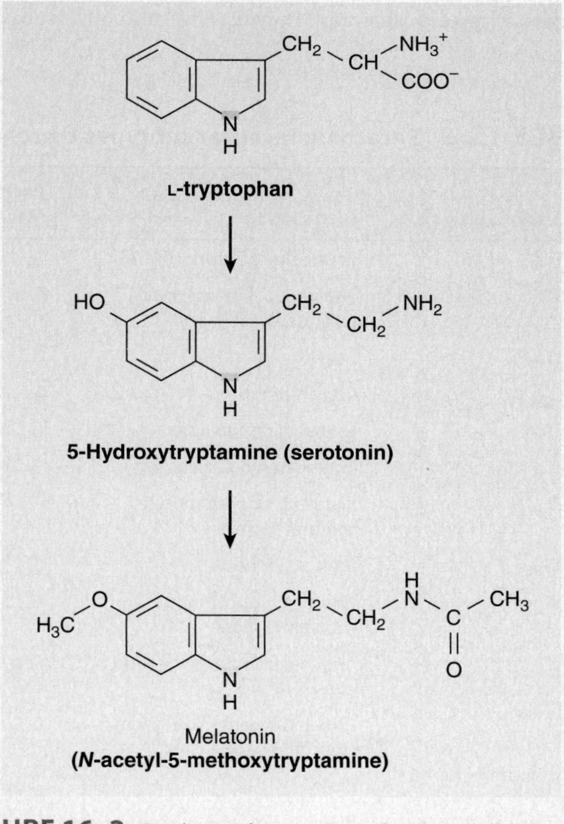

L-tryptophan

5-Hydroxytryptamine (serotonin)

Melatonin (*N*-acetyl-5-methoxytryptamine)

FIGURE 16–2 Synthesis of serotonin and melatonin from L-tryptophan.

In the pineal gland, serotonin serves as a precursor of melatonin, a melanocyte-stimulating hormone that has complex effects in several tissues. In mammals (including humans), more than 90% of the serotonin in the body is found in enterochromaffin cells in the gastrointestinal tract. In the blood, serotonin is found in platelets, which are able to concentrate the amine by means of an active serotonin transporter mechanism (SERT) similar to that in the membrane of serotonergic nerve endings. Once transported into the platelet or nerve ending, 5-HT is concentrated in vesicles by a vesicle-associated transporter (VAT) that is blocked by **reserpine.** Serotonin is also found in the raphe nuclei of the brainstem, which contain cell bodies of serotonergic neurons that synthesize, store, and release serotonin as a transmitter. Stored serotonin can be depleted by reserpine in much the same manner as this drug depletes catecholamines from vesicles in adrenergic nerves and the adrenal medulla (see Chapter 6).

Brain serotonergic neurons are involved in numerous diffuse functions such as mood, sleep, appetite, and temperature regulation, as well as the perception of pain, the regulation of blood pressure, and vomiting (see Chapter 21). Serotonin is clearly involved in psychiatric depression (see Chapter 30) and also appears to be involved in conditions such as anxiety and migraine. Serotonergic neurons are found in the enteric nervous system of the gastrointestinal tract and around blood vessels. In rodents (but not in humans), serotonin is also found in mast cells.

The function of serotonin in enterochromaffin cells is not fully understood. These cells synthesize serotonin, store the amine in a complex with adenosine triphosphate (ATP) and other substances in granules, and release serotonin in response to mechanical and neuronal stimuli. This serotonin interacts in a paracrine fashion with several different 5-HT receptors in the gut (see Chapter 62). Some of the released serotonin diffuses into blood vessels and is taken up and stored in platelets.

Serotonin is metabolized by MAO, and the intermediate product, 5-hydroxyindoleacetaldehyde, is further oxidized by aldehyde dehydrogenase to 5-hydroxyindoleacetic acid (5-HIAA). In humans consuming a normal diet, the excretion of 5-HIAA is a measure of serotonin synthesis. Therefore, the 24-hour excretion of 5-HIAA can be used as a diagnostic test for tumors that synthesize excessive quantities of serotonin, especially carcinoid tumor. A few foods (eg, bananas) contain large amounts of serotonin or its precursors and must be prohibited during such diagnostic tests.

Pharmacodynamics

A. Mechanisms of Action

Serotonin exerts many actions and, like histamine, displays many species differences, making generalizations difficult. The actions of serotonin are mediated through a remarkably large number of cell membrane receptors. The serotonin receptors that have been characterized thus far are listed in Table 16–3. Seven families of 5-HT-receptor subtypes (those given numeric subscripts 1 through 7) have been identified, six involving G protein-coupled receptors of the usual seven-transmembrane serpentine type and one a ligand-gated ion channel. The latter (5-HT_3) receptor is a member of the nicotinic family of Na^+/K^+ channel proteins.

TABLE 16–3 Serotonin receptor subtypes currently recognized. (See also Chapter 21.)

Receptor Subtype	Distribution	Postreceptor Mechanism	Partially Selective Agonists	Partially Selective Antagonists
5-HT_{1A}	Raphe nuclei, hippocampus	G_i, ↓ cAMP	8-OH-DPAT,[1] repinotan	WAY1006351
5-HT_{1B}	Substantia nigra, globus pallidus, basal ganglia	G_i, ↓ cAMP	Sumatriptan, L694247[1]	
5-HT_{1D}	Brain	G_i, ↓ cAMP	Sumatriptan, eletriptan	
5-HT_{1E}	Cortex, putamen	G_i, ↓ cAMP		
5-HT_{1F}	Cortex, hippocampus	G_i, ↓ cAMP	Lasmiditan	
5-HT_{1P}	Enteric nervous system	G_o, slow EPSP	5-Hydroxyindalpine	Renzapride
5-HT_{2A}	Platelets, smooth muscle, cerebral cortex	G_q, ↑ IP_3	α-Methyl-5-HT, DOI[1]	Ketanserin
5-HT_{2B}	Stomach fundus	G_q, ↑ IP_3	α-Methyl-5-HT, DOI[1]	RS127445[1]
5-HT_{2C}	Choroid, hippocampus, substantia nigra	G_q, ↑ IP_3	α-Methyl-5-HT, DOI,[1] lorcaserin	Mesulergine
5-HT_3	Area postrema, sensory and enteric nerves	Receptor is an Na^+/K^+ ion channel	2-Methyl-5-HT, *m*-chlorophenylbiguanide	Granisetron, ondansetron, others
5-HT_4	CNS and myenteric neurons, smooth muscle	G_s, ↑ cAMP	BIMU8,[1] renzapride, metoclopramide	GR113808[1]
5-$HT_{5A,B}$	Brain	↓ cAMP		
5-$HT_{6,7}$	Brain	G_s, ↑ cAMP		Clozapine (5-HT_7)

[1]Research agents; for chemical names see Alexander SPH, Mathie A, Peters JA: Guide to receptors and channels (GRAC). Br J Pharmacol 2011;164 (Suppl 1):S16–17, 116–117.

cAMP, cyclic adenosine monophosphate; EPSP, excitatory postsynaptic potential; IP_3, inositol trisphosphate.

Melatonin Pharmacology

Melatonin is *N*-acetyl-5-methoxytryptamine (see Figure 16–2), a simple methoxylated and *N*-acetylated product of serotonin found in the pineal gland. It is produced and released primarily at night and appears to play a role in the diurnal cycle of animals and the sleep-wake behavior of humans. Melatonin receptors have been characterized in the central nervous system and several peripheral tissues. In the brain, MT_1 and MT_2 receptors are found in membranes of neurons in the suprachiasmatic nucleus of the hypothalamus, an area associated—from lesioning experiments—with circadian rhythm. MT_1 and MT_2 are seven-transmembrane G_i protein-coupled receptors. The result of receptor binding is inhibition of adenylyl cyclase. A third receptor, MT_3, is an enzyme; binding to this molecule has a poorly defined physiologic role, possibly related to intraocular pressure. Activation of the MT_1 receptor results in sleepiness, whereas the MT_2 receptor may be related to the light-dark synchronization of the biologic clock. Melatonin has also been implicated in energy metabolism and obesity, and administration of the agent reduces body weight in certain animal models. However, its role in these processes is poorly understood, and there is no evidence that melatonin itself is of any value in obesity in humans. Other studies suggest that melatonin has antiapoptotic effects in experimental models. Recent research implicates melatonin receptors in depressive disorders. Insomnia associated with autism spectrum disorder may respond to melatonin.

Melatonin is promoted commercially as a sleep aid by the food supplement industry (see Chapter 65). Extensive literature supports its use in ameliorating jet lag. For this purpose, it is used in oral doses of 0.5–5 mg, usually administered at the destination bedtime. **Ramelteon** is a selective MT_1 and MT_2 agonist that is approved for the medical treatment of insomnia. This drug has no addiction liability (it is not a controlled substance), and it appears to be more efficacious than melatonin (but less efficacious than benzodiazepines) as a hypnotic. It is metabolized by P450 enzymes and should not be used in individuals taking CYP1A2 inhibitors. It has a half-life of 1–3 hours and an active metabolite with a half-life of up to 5 hours. Ramelteon may increase prolactin levels. **Tasimelteon** is a newer MT_1 and MT_2 agonist that is approved for non-24-hour sleep-wake disorder. **Agomelatine,** an MT_1 and MT_2 agonist and a weak $5\text{-}HT_{2B}$ and $5\text{-}HT_{2C}$ antagonist, is approved in Europe for use in major depressive disorder.

B. Tissue and Organ System Effects

1. *Nervous system*—Serotonin is present in a variety of sites in the brain. Its role as a neurotransmitter and its relation to the actions of drugs acting in the central nervous system are discussed in Chapters 21 and 30. Serotonin is also a precursor of melatonin in the pineal gland (see Figure 16–2; see Box: Melatonin Pharmacology). **Repinotan,** a $5\text{-}HT_{1A}$ agonist currently in clinical trials, appears to have some antinociceptive action at higher doses while reversing opioid-induced respiratory depression.

$5\text{-}HT_3$ receptors in the gastrointestinal tract and in the vomiting center of the medulla participate in the vomiting reflex (see Chapter 62). They are particularly important in vomiting caused by chemical triggers such as cancer chemotherapy drugs. $5\text{-}HT_{1P}$ and $5\text{-}HT_4$ receptors also play important roles in enteric nervous system function.

Like histamine, serotonin is a potent stimulant of pain and itch sensory nerve endings and is responsible for some of the symptoms caused by insect and plant stings. In addition, serotonin is a powerful activator of chemosensitive endings located in the coronary vascular bed. Activation of $5\text{-}HT_3$ receptors on these afferent vagal nerve endings is associated with the **chemoreceptor reflex** (also known as the Bezold-Jarisch reflex). The reflex response consists of marked bradycardia and hypotension, and its physiologic role is uncertain. The bradycardia is mediated by vagal outflow to the heart and can be blocked by atropine. The hypotension is a consequence of the decrease in cardiac output that results from bradycardia. A variety of other agents can activate the chemoreceptor reflex. These include nicotinic cholinoceptor agonists and some cardiac glycosides, eg, ouabain.

Although serotonergic neurons are not found below the site of injury to the adult spinal cord, constitutive activity of 5-HT receptors may play a role following such a lesion—administration of $5\text{-}HT_2$ blockers appears to reduce skeletal muscle spasm following this type of injury.

2. *Respiratory system*—Serotonin has a small direct stimulant effect on bronchiolar smooth muscle in normal humans, probably via $5\text{-}HT_{2A}$ receptors. It also appears to facilitate acetylcholine release from bronchial vagal nerve endings. In patients with carcinoid syndrome, episodes of bronchoconstriction occur in response to elevated levels of the amine or peptides released from the tumor. Serotonin may also cause hyperventilation as a result of the chemoreceptor reflex or stimulation of bronchial sensory nerve endings.

3. *Cardiovascular system*—Serotonin directly causes the contraction of vascular smooth muscle, mainly through $5\text{-}HT_2$ receptors. In humans, serotonin is a powerful vasoconstrictor except in skeletal muscle and the heart, where it dilates blood vessels.

At least part of the 5-HT-induced vasodilation requires the presence of vascular endothelial cells. When the endothelium is damaged, coronary vessels are constricted by 5-HT. As noted previously, serotonin can also elicit reflex bradycardia by activation of $5\text{-}HT_3$ receptors on chemoreceptor nerve endings. A triphasic blood pressure response is often seen following injection of serotonin in experimental animals. Initially, there is a decrease in heart rate, cardiac output, and blood pressure caused by the chemoreceptor response. After this decrease, blood pressure increases as a result of vasoconstriction. The third phase is again a decrease in blood pressure attributed to vasodilation in vessels supplying skeletal muscle. In contrast, pulmonary and renal vessels seem very sensitive to the vasoconstrictor action of serotonin.

TABLE 16–4 Characteristics of serotonin syndrome and other hyperthermic syndromes.

Syndrome	Precipitating Drugs	Clinical Presentation	Therapy[1]
Serotonin syndrome	SSRIs, second-generation antidepressants, MAOIs, linezolid, tramadol, meperidine, fentanyl, ondansetron, sumatriptan, MDMA, LSD, St. John's wort, ginseng	Hypertension, hyperreflexia, tremor, clonus, hyperthermia, hyperactive bowel sounds, diarrhea, mydriasis, agitation, coma; onset within hours	**Sedation (benzodiazepines), paralysis, intubation, and ventilation;** consider 5-HT_2 block with cyproheptadine or chlorpromazine
Neuroleptic malignant syndrome	D_2-blocking antipsychotics	Acute severe parkinsonism; hypertension, hyperthermia, normal or reduced bowel sounds; onset over 1–3 days	**Diphenhydramine** (parenteral), cooling if temperature is very high, sedation with benzodiazepines
Malignant hyperthermia	Volatile anesthetics, succinylcholine	Hyperthermia, muscle rigidity, hypertension, tachycardia; onset within minutes	**Dantrolene,** cooling

[1]Precipitating drugs should be discontinued immediately. First-line therapy is in boldface font.

LSD, lysergic acid diethylamide, MAOIs, monoamine oxidase inhibitors; MDMA, methylenedioxy-methamphetamine (ecstasy); SSRIs, selective serotonin reuptake inhibitors.

Studies in knockout mice suggest that 5-HT, acting on 5-HT_{1A}, 5-HT_2, and 5-HT_4 receptors, is needed for normal cardiac development in the fetus. On the other hand, chronic exposure of adults to 5-HT_{2B} agonists is associated with valvulopathy and adult mice lacking the 5-HT_{2B} receptor gene are protected from cardiac hypertrophy. Preliminary studies suggest that 5-HT_{2B} antagonists can prevent development of pulmonary hypertension in animal models.

Serotonin also constricts veins, and venoconstriction with increased capillary filling appears to be responsible for the flush that is observed after serotonin administration or release from a carcinoid tumor. Serotonin has small direct positive chronotropic and inotropic effects on the heart, which are probably of no clinical significance. However, prolonged elevation of the blood level of serotonin (which occurs in carcinoid syndrome) is associated with pathologic alterations in the endocardium (subendocardial fibroplasia), which may result in valvular or electrical malfunction.

Serotonin causes blood platelets to aggregate by activating 5-HT_2 receptors. This response, in contrast to aggregation induced during normal clot formation, is not accompanied by the release of serotonin stored in the platelets. The physiologic role of this effect is unclear.

4. *Gastrointestinal tract*—Serotonin is a powerful stimulant of gastrointestinal smooth muscle, increasing tone and facilitating peristalsis. This action is caused by the direct action of serotonin on 5-HT_2 smooth muscle receptors plus a stimulating action on ganglion cells located in the enteric nervous system (see Chapter 6). 5-HT_{1A} and 5-HT_7 receptors also may be involved. Activation of 5-HT_4 receptors in the enteric nervous system causes increased acetylcholine release and thereby mediates a motility-enhancing or "prokinetic" effect of selective serotonin agonists such as cisapride. These agents are useful in several gastrointestinal disorders (see Chapter 62). Overproduction of serotonin (and other substances) in carcinoid tumor is associated with severe diarrhea. Serotonin has little effect on gastrointestinal secretions, and what effects it has are generally inhibitory.

5. *Skeletal muscle and the eye*—5-HT_2 receptors are present on skeletal muscle membranes, but their physiologic role is not understood. As discussed in the box, **serotonin syndrome** is associated with skeletal muscle contractions and precipitated when MAO inhibitors are given with serotonin agonists, especially antidepressants of the selective serotonin reuptake inhibitor class (SSRIs; see Chapter 30). Although the hyperthermia of serotonin syndrome results from excessive muscle contraction, serotonin syndrome is probably caused by a central nervous system effect of these drugs (Table 16–4 and Box: Serotonin Syndrome and Similar Syndromes).

Studies in animal models of glaucoma indicate that 5-HT_{2A} agonists reduce intraocular pressure. This action can be blocked by ketanserin and similar 5-HT_2 antagonists.

Serotonin Syndrome and Similar Syndromes

Excess synaptic serotonin causes a serious, potentially fatal syndrome that is diagnosed on the basis of a history of administration of a serotonergic drug within recent weeks and physical findings. It has some characteristics in common with **neuroleptic malignant syndrome** (NMS) and **malignant hyperthermia** (MH), but its pathophysiology and management are quite different (see Table 16–4).

As suggested by the drugs that precipitate it, serotonin syndrome occurs when overdose with a single drug, or concurrent use of several drugs, results in excess serotonergic activity in the central nervous system. It is predictable and not idiosyncratic, but milder forms may easily be misdiagnosed. In experimental animal models, many of the signs of the syndrome can be reversed by administration of 5-HT_2 antagonists; however, other 5-HT receptors may be involved as well. Dantrolene is of no value, unlike the treatment of MH.

NMS is idiosyncratic rather than predictable and appears to be associated with hypersensitivity to the parkinsonism-inducing effects of D_2-blocking antipsychotics in certain individuals. MH is associated with a genetic defect in the RyR1 calcium channel of skeletal muscle sarcoplasmic reticulum that permits uncontrolled calcium release from the sarcoplasmic reticulum when precipitating drugs are given (see Chapter 27).

CLINICAL PHARMACOLOGY OF SEROTONIN

Serotonin Agonists

Serotonin has no clinical applications as a drug. However, several receptor subtype-selective agonists have proved to be of value. **Buspirone,** a 5-HT$_{1A}$ agonist, has received attention as an effective nonbenzodiazepine anxiolytic (see Chapter 22). Appetite suppression appears to be associated with agonist action at 5-HT$_{2C}$ receptors in the central nervous system, and **dexfenfluramine,** a selective 5-HT agonist, was widely used as an appetite suppressant but was withdrawn because of cardiac valvulopathy. **Lorcaserin,** a more selective 5-HT$_{2C}$ agonist, was approved by the FDA for use as a weight-loss medication but has been withdrawn (see Box: Treatment of Obesity).

Treatment of Obesity

It is said that much of the world is experiencing an "epidemic of obesity." Statistics show that in the USA and many other countries, 30–40% of the population is above optimal weight, and that the excess weight (especially abdominal fat) is often associated with the **metabolic syndrome** and increased risks of cardiovascular disease, diabetes, cancer, and dementia. Since eating behavior is an expression of endocrine, neurophysiologic, and psychological processes, prevention and treatment of obesity are challenging. Because of its prevalence, there is great scientific and financial interest in developing pharmacologic therapy for the condition.

Although obesity can be defined as excess adipose tissue, it is important to note that white fat (energy-storing), and not brown fat (energy-expending), is the tissue primarily responsible for the morbidity of obesity. Obesity is currently quantitated by means of the body mass index (BMI), calculated from BMI = weight (in kilograms)/height^2 (in meters). Using this measure, the range of normal BMI is defined as 18.5–24.9; overweight, 25–29.9; obese, 30–39.9; and morbidly obese (ie, at very high risk), ≥40. (Underweight persons, ie, those with a BMI < 18, also have an increased [but smaller] risk of health problems.) Some extremely muscular individuals may have a BMI higher than 25 and no excess fat; however, the BMI scale generally correlates with the degree of obesity and with risk of morbidity. A second metric, which may be an even better predictor of cardiovascular risk, is the ratio of waist measurement to body height; cardiovascular risk is lower if this ratio is less than 0.5. Experts consider drug therapy to be justified in patients with increased risk factors and a BMI ≥ 27 and in those without comorbidities but with a BMI ≥ 30.

Although the cause of obesity can be simply stated as energy intake (dietary calories) that exceeds energy output (resting metabolism plus exercise), the actual physiology of weight control is extremely complex, and the pathophysiology of obesity is still poorly understood. Many hormones and neuronal mechanisms regulate intake (appetite, satiety), processing (absorption, conversion to fat, glycogen, etc), and output (thermogenesis, muscle work). The fact that a large number of hormones reduce appetite might appear to offer many targets for weight-reducing drug therapy, but despite intensive research, no available pharmacologic therapy with the possible exception of the glutides has succeeded in maintaining a weight loss of over 10% for 1 year. Furthermore, the social and psychological aspects of eating are powerful influences that are independent of or only partially dependent on the physiologic control mechanisms. In contrast to drug therapy, bariatric (weight-reducing) surgery readily achieves a sustained weight loss of 10–40%. Furthermore, surgery that bypasses the stomach and upper small intestine (but not simple restrictive banding) rapidly reverses some aspects of the metabolic syndrome even before significant loss of weight. Even a 5–10% loss of weight is associated with a reduction in blood pressure and improved glycemic control. Other physical measures to reduce eating include balloons that are inflated in the stomach and retained there. Cellulose hydrogel in a capsule that dissolves in the stomach and expands as it absorbs water is the most recent addition to agents approved for use in obesity management. Gastrointestinal flora also influence metabolic efficiency, and research in mice suggests that altering the microbiome can lead to weight gain or loss.

Until approximately 15 years ago, the most popular and successful appetite suppressants were the nonselective 5-HT$_2$ agonists **fenfluramine** and **dexfenfluramine.** Combined with phentermine as **Fen-Phen** and **Dex-Phen,** they were moderately effective. However, these 5-HT$_2$ agonists were found to cause pulmonary hypertension and cardiac valve defects and were withdrawn.

Older drugs still available in the USA and some other countries include **phenylpropanolamine, benzphetamine, amphetamine, methamphetamine, phentermine, diethylpropion, mazindol,** and **phendimetrazine.** These drugs are all amphetamine mimics and are central nervous system appetite suppressants; they are generally helpful only during the first few weeks of therapy. Their toxicity is significant and includes hypertension (with a risk of cerebral hemorrhage) and addiction liability.

Semaglutide, liraglutide, orlistat, phentermine, and cellulose hydrogel are the only single-agent drugs currently approved in the USA for the treatment of obesity. In addition, combination agents (**phentermine** plus **topiramate** and **naltrexone** plus **bupropion**) are available. These drugs have been intensely studied, and some of their properties are listed in Table 16–5. Lorcaserin was withdrawn in 2020 because of evidence of carcinogenesis. Clinical trials and phase 4 reports suggest that these agents are modestly effective for the duration of therapy (up to 1 year) and are probably safer than the single-agent amphetamine mimics. **Mirabegron,** a β_3 adrenoceptor agonist approved for the treatment for overactive bladder (see Chapter 9), is of possible future interest because β_3 agonists activate brown fat to consume more energy. **Sibutramine** and **rimonabant** were marketed for several years but were withdrawn because of increasing evidence of cardiovascular and other toxicities. Much current research is aimed at peptides that mimic endogenous peptides involved in satiety and glucose homeostasis. The **glucagon-like peptide, GLP-1**, was identified early as a modulator of glucagon and insulin secretion and was found to reduce food consumption and body weight in experimental animals. Very short half-life required discovery or synthesis of modified GLP-1 analogs, and semaglutide, exenatide, lixisenatide, liraglutide, albiglutide, and dulaglutide have all been tested and appear to be the most efficacious anti-obesity drugs currently available. All are administered subcutaneously; semaglutide is also available for oral use. Further molecular modification to include glucagon, amylin, or other metabolic peptide agonism has been successfully investigated in animals. Agonist molecules that combine GLP-1 peptide structure with estrogen, dexamethasone, or thyroxin have been developed and are investigational.

Because of the moderate efficacy and the toxicity of currently available drugs, intensive research continues. Because of the redundant physiologic mechanisms for control of body weight, it seems likely that polypharmacy targeting multiple pathways will be needed to achieve success.

$5\text{-HT}_{1D/1B}$ Agonists & Other Drugs Used In Migraine Headache

After more than a century of intense study, the pathophysiology of migraine is still incompletely understood. Although the symptom pattern and duration of prodrome and headache vary markedly among patients, the severity of migraine headache justifies vigorous therapy in the great majority of cases.

The $5\text{-HT}_{1D/1B}$ agonists (**triptans, eg, sumatriptan**) are used almost exclusively for acute migraine headache. Migraine in its "classic" form is characterized by an aura or prodrome of variable duration that may involve nausea, vomiting, paresthesias, visual scotomas or even hemianopsia, and speech abnormalities; the aura is followed by a severe throbbing unilateral headache that lasts for a few hours to 1–2 days. "Common" migraine lacks the aura phase, but the headache is similar. Chronic migraine (daily or near-daily headache) is usually treated prophylactically. First-line agents for chronic migraine include propranolol, amitriptyline, topiramate, or valproic acid. Second-line agents include CGRP antagonist antibodies (second-line because of expense), botulinum toxin injection, venlafaxine, beta blockers, or calcium channel blockers.

Migraine involves the trigeminal nerve distribution to intracranial (and possibly extracranial) arteries. These nerves release peptide neurotransmitters, especially **calcitonin gene-related peptide** (CGRP; see Chapter 17), an extremely powerful vasodilator. Substance P and neurokinin A also may be involved. Extravasation of plasma and plasma proteins into the perivascular space

TABLE 16–5 Antiobesity drugs and their effects.

Drug or Drug Combination	Drug Group	Possible Mechanism of Action	Dosage	Toxicity
Cellulose-citric acid	Physical expander	Increases fullness sensation		Possible bloating, diarrhea, constipation
Orlistat	GI lipase inhibitor	Reduces lipid absorption	60–120 mg TID PO	Decreased absorption of fat-soluble vitamins, flatulence, fecal incontinence
Lorcaserin (withdrawn)	5-HT_{2c} agonist	Decreases appetite	10 mg PO BID	Headache, nausea, dry mouth, dizziness, constipation; possibly carcinogenic
Naltrexone/bupropion	Opioid antagonist + antidepressant	Unknown	32 mg/360 mg PO TID	Headache, nausea, dizziness, constipation
Phentermine	Sympathomimetic	Norepinephrine release in CNS	30–37.5 mg/d PO	Increased BP, HR; arrhythmias, insomnia, anxiety
Phentermine/topiramate	Sympathomimetic + antiseizure agent	Norepinephrine release plus unknown mechanism	3.75–15 mg/23–92 mg PO	Insomnia, dizziness, nausea, paresthesia, dysgeusia
Semaglutide	GLP-1 agonist	Decreases appetite	2.4 mg/w SC or PO/d	Nausea, vomiting
Setmelanotide	Melanocortin agonist	Corrects rare genetic deficiency	NA	Nausea, skin reactions
Tirzepatide (Phase 3 trials)	Dual insulinotropic and GLP-1 agonist	Decreases appetite	NA	Nausea

BID, twice daily; BP, blood pressure; CNS, central nervous system; GI, gastrointestinal; HR, heart rate; NA, data not available; PO, by mouth; SC, subcutaneously; TID, three times daily; w, weekly.

appears to be a common feature of animal migraine models and is found in biopsy specimens from migraine patients. This effect probably reflects the action of the neuropeptides on the vessels. The mechanical stretching caused by this perivascular edema may be the immediate cause of activation of pain nerve endings in the dura. The onset of headache is sometimes associated with a marked increase in amplitude of temporal artery pulsations, and relief of pain by administration of effective therapy is sometimes accompanied by diminution of these pulsations.

The mechanisms of action of drugs used in migraine are poorly understood, in part because they include such a wide variety of drug groups and actions. In addition to the triptans, these include anti-CGRP antibodies, oral anti-CGRP agents, nonsteroidal anti-inflammatory analgesic agents, β-adrenoceptor blockers, calcium channel blockers, tricyclic antidepressants and SSRIs, ergot alkaloids, and several antiseizure agents. Some of these drug groups are effective only for prophylaxis and not for the acute attack.

Two primary hypotheses have been proposed to explain the actions of these drugs. First, the triptans, the ergot alkaloids, and antidepressants may activate 5-$HT_{1D/1B}$ receptors on presynaptic trigeminal nerve endings to inhibit the release of vasodilating peptides, and antiseizure agents may suppress excessive firing of these nerve endings. Second, the vasoconstrictor actions of direct 5-HT agonists (triptans and ergot) may prevent vasodilation and stretching of the pain endings. It is possible that both mechanisms contribute in the case of some drugs.

Sumatriptan and its congeners are currently first-line therapy for acute severe migraine attacks in most patients (Figure 16–3). However, they should not be used in patients with coronary artery disease. Anti-inflammatory analgesics such as aspirin and ibuprofen are often helpful in controlling the pain of migraine. Rarely, parenteral opioids may be needed in refractory cases. For patients with very severe nausea and vomiting, parenteral metoclopramide may be helpful.

Sumatriptan and the other triptans are selective agonists for 5-HT_{1D} and 5-HT_{1B} receptors; the similarity of the triptan structure to that of the 5-HT nucleus can be seen in the structure below. These receptor types are found in cerebral and meningeal vessels and mediate vasoconstriction. They are also found on neurons and probably function as presynaptic inhibitory receptors.

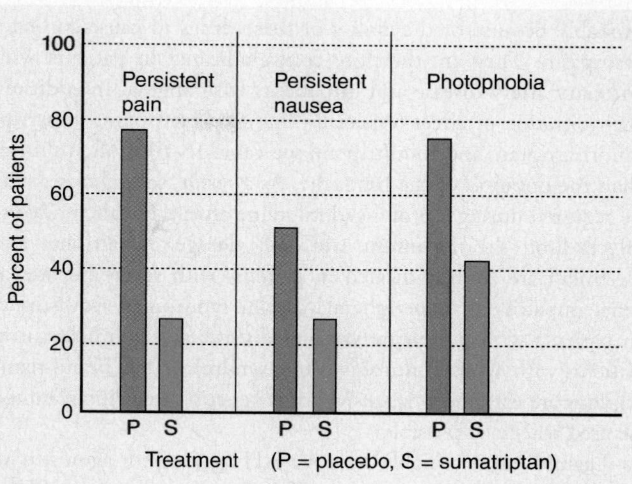

FIGURE 16–3 Effects of sumatriptan (734 patients) or placebo (370 patients) on symptoms of acute migraine headache 60 minutes after injection of 6 mg subcutaneously. All differences between placebo and sumatriptan were statistically significant. (Data from Cady RK, Wendt JK, Kirchner JR, Sargent JD, Rothrock JF, Skaggs H Jr: Treatment of acute migraine with subcutaneous sumatriptan. JAMA 1991 Jun 5;265(21):2831-2835.)

$CH_3-NH-SO_2-CH_2$ (indole ring, N) $CH_2-CH_2-N(CH_3)_2$

Sumatriptan

In population studies, all of the triptan 5-HT_1 agonists are as effective or more effective in migraine than older acute drug treatments, eg, parenteral, oral, and rectal ergot alkaloids. However, individual drugs in this class may have different efficacies in individual patients. The pharmacokinetics and potencies of the triptans differ significantly and are set forth in Table 16–6. Most adverse effects are mild and include altered sensations (tingling, warmth, etc), dizziness, muscle weakness, neck pain, and for parenteral sumatriptan, injection site reactions. Chest discomfort occurs in 1–5% of patients, and chest pain has been reported,

TABLE 16–6 Pharmacokinetics of triptans.

Drug	Routes	Time to Onset (h)	Single Dose (mg)	Maximum Dose per Day (mg)	Half-Life (h)
Almotriptan	Oral	2.6	6.25–12.5	25	3.3
Eletriptan	Oral	2	20–40	80	4
Frovatriptan	Oral	3	2.5	7.5	27
Naratriptan	Oral	2	1–2.5	5	5.5
Rizatriptan	Oral	1–2.5	5–10	30	2
Sumatriptan	Oral, nasal, subcutaneous, rectal	1.5 (0.2 for subcutaneous)	25–100 (PO), 20 nasal, 6 subcutaneous, 25 rectal	200	2
Zolmitriptan	Oral, nasal	1.5–3	2.5–5	10	2.8

probably because of the ability of these drugs to cause coronary vasospasm. They are therefore contraindicated in patients with coronary artery disease and in patients with angina. In addition, their duration of effect (especially that of almotriptan, sumatriptan, rizatriptan, and zolmitriptan; see Table 16–6) is often shorter than the duration of the headache. As a result, several doses may be required during a prolonged migraine attack, but their adverse effects limit the maximum safe daily dosage. Naratriptan and eletriptan are contraindicated in patients with severe hepatic or renal impairment or peripheral vascular syndromes; frovatriptan in patients with peripheral vascular disease; and zolmitriptan in patients with Wolff-Parkinson-White syndrome. The brand-name triptans are extremely expensive; thus generic sumatriptan should be used whenever possible.

Lasmiditan is a highly selective 5-HT_{1F} receptor agonist with significant antimigraine efficacy. This drug has very low affinity for other 5-HT receptors and all autonomic receptors tested. The agent lacks the vasoconstrictor action of the triptans, suggesting better cardiovascular safety than triptans. It reduces trigeminal nerve stimulation–induced plasma and plasma protein extravasation in dural vessels, which is thought to underlie the pain of migraine. A small molecule, lasmiditan is orally active and has a half-life of 6 h. It is metabolized by CYP2D6 and metabolites are excreted in the urine.

Other Drugs Used In Migraine

CGRP has become an important target in the *prophylaxis* and treatment of migraine and cluster headache. Several monoclonal antibodies (MABs) are currently approved for this application. **Erenumab** binds to the CGRP receptor and prevents activation by the peptide. **Fremanezumab** and **galcanezumab** bind CGRP and prevent its binding to and activation of the receptor. These drugs are given subcutaneously once per month. Because they are new, must be given subcutaneously, and very expensive, anti-CGRP antibody therapy is reserved for patients whose migraine is not adequately controlled by oral agents. **Rimegepant and ubrogepant** are newer orally active small molecule CGRP receptor antagonists. They are used only for immediate treatment of acute attacks. Adverse effects reported thus far include nausea, fatigue, and dry mouth.

Propranolol, amitriptyline, and some calcium channel blockers have been found to be effective for the prophylaxis of migraine in some patients. They are of no value in the treatment of acute migraine. The anticonvulsants **valproic acid** and **topiramate** (see Chapter 24) also have been found to have some prophylactic efficacy in migraine. **Flunarizine,** a calcium channel blocker used in Europe, has been reported in clinical trials to effectively reduce the severity of the acute attack and to prevent recurrences. **Verapamil** appears to have modest efficacy as prophylaxis against migraine.

Other Serotonin Agonists in Clinical Use

Flibanserin, a 5-HT_{1A} agonist and 5-HT_{2A} antagonist, is approved for treatment of hypoactive sexual desire disorder in women. Due to inadequate evidence of efficacy, it was refused approval in 2010 and 2013. The clinical trials that led to its approval in 2015 showed a very small but significant increase in satisfactory sexual desire and activities over several weeks of daily oral administration. Consumption of alcohol is contraindicated due to increased risk of severe hypotension. Other adverse effects include syncope, nausea, fatigue, dizziness, and somnolence. A very different drug, **bremelanotide** (a melanocortin MC3 and MC4 agonist), also is approved for hypoactive sexual desire in women (see Chapter 37).

Cisapride, a 5-HT_4 agonist, was used in the treatment of gastroesophageal reflux and motility disorders. Because of toxicity, it is now available only for compassionate use in the USA. **Tegaserod,** a 5-HT_4 partial agonist, and **prucalopride,** a high-affinity 5-HT_4 agonist, are used for irritable bowel syndrome with constipation (see Chapter 62).

Compounds such as **fluoxetine** and other SSRIs, which modulate serotonergic transmission by blocking reuptake of the transmitter, are among the most widely prescribed drugs for the management of depression and similar disorders. These drugs are discussed in Chapter 30.

SEROTONIN ANTAGONISTS

The actions of serotonin, like those of histamine, can be antagonized in several ways. Such antagonism is clearly desirable in those rare patients who have carcinoid tumor and may also be valuable in certain other conditions.

Serotonin synthesis can be inhibited by ***p*-chlorophenylalanine** and ***p*-chloroamphetamine.** However, these agents are too toxic for general use. Storage of serotonin can be inhibited by the use of **reserpine,** but the sympatholytic effects of this drug (see Chapter 11) and the high levels of circulating serotonin that result from release prevent its use in carcinoid. Therefore, receptor blockade is the major therapeutic approach to conditions of serotonin excess.

SEROTONIN RECEPTOR ANTAGONISTS

A wide variety of drugs with actions at other receptors (eg, α adrenoceptors, H_1-histamine receptors) also have serotonin receptor-blocking effects. **Phenoxybenzamine** (see Chapter 10) has a long-lasting blocking action at 5-HT_2 receptors. In addition, the ergot alkaloids discussed in the last portion of this chapter are partial agonists at serotonin receptors.

Cyproheptadine resembles the phenothiazine antihistaminic agents in chemical structure and has potent H_1-receptor-blocking as well as 5-HT_2-blocking actions. The actions of cyproheptadine are predictable from its H_1 histamine and 5-HT receptor affinities. It prevents the smooth muscle effects of both amines but has no effect on the gastric secretion stimulated by histamine. It also has significant antimuscarinic effects and causes sedation.

The major clinical applications of cyproheptadine are in the treatment of the smooth muscle manifestations of **carcinoid tumor** (see Box: Carcinoid Syndrome) and in **cold-induced urticaria.** The usual dosage in adults is 12–16 mg/d orally in three or four divided doses. It is of some value in serotonin syndrome, but because it is available only in tablet form, cyproheptadine must be crushed and administered by stomach tube in unconscious patients. The drug also appears to reduce muscle spasms following spinal cord injury, in which constitutive activity of 5-HT_{2C} receptors is associated with increases in Ca^{2+} currents leading to spasms. Anecdotal evidence suggests some efficacy as an appetite *stimulant* in cancer patients, but controlled trials have yielded mixed results.

Ketanserin blocks 5-HT_2 receptors in smooth muscle and other tissues and has little reported antagonist activity at other 5-HT or H_1 receptors. However, this drug potently blocks vascular α_1 adrenoceptors. The drug blocks 5-HT_2 receptors on platelets and antagonizes platelet aggregation promoted by serotonin. The mechanism involved in ketanserin's hypotensive action probably involves α_1 adrenoceptor blockade more than 5-HT_2 receptor blockade. Ketanserin is available in Europe for the treatment of hypertension and vasospastic conditions but has not been approved in the USA. **Ritanserin,** another 5-HT_2 antagonist, has little or no α-blocking action. It has been reported to alter bleeding time and to reduce thromboxane formation, presumably by altering platelet function.

Carcinoid Syndrome

Carcinoid syndrome is a manifestation of a type of well-differentiated neuroendocrine tumor that usually originates in the digestive tract but sometimes in the lungs, kidneys, or ovaries. It is usually metastatic at diagnosis and is poorly responsive to cytotoxic chemotherapy. Carcinoid tumor usually secretes serotonin, other amines, and peptides with smooth muscle effects, so agents that reduce secretion or block serotonin receptors are helpful in managing flushing, diarrhea, and other signs and symptoms. Chronic exposure to 5-HT is often associated with cardiac valvular and conduction defects in these patients. Somatostatin analogs (**octreotide** or **lanreotide**) are the primary antisecretory drugs used in carcinoid syndrome. **Telotristat,** an inhibitor of tyrosine hydroxylase, reduces production of serotonin and has recently been approved for use in combination with octreotide. **Everolimus** and **interferon-alpha** (see Chapter 55) also have been applied. Inhibitors of serotonin receptors such as **cyproheptadine** may be useful.

Ondansetron is the prototypical 5-HT_3 antagonist. This drug and its analogs are very important in the prevention of nausea and vomiting associated with surgery and cancer chemotherapy. They are discussed in Chapter 62.

Considering the diverse effects attributed to serotonin and the heterogeneous nature of 5-HT receptors, other selective 5-HT antagonists may prove to be clinically useful.

THE ERGOT ALKALOIDS

Ergot alkaloids are produced by *Claviceps purpurea*, a fungus that infects grasses and grains—especially rye—under damp growing or storage conditions. This versatile fungus synthesizes histamine, acetylcholine, tyramine, and other biologically active products in addition to a score or more of unique ergot alkaloids. These alkaloids affect α adrenoceptors, dopamine receptors, 5-HT receptors, and perhaps other receptor types. Similar alkaloids are produced by fungi parasitic to a number of other grass-like plants.

The accidental ingestion of ergot alkaloids in contaminated grain can be traced back more than 2000 years from descriptions of epidemics of ergot poisoning **(ergotism).** The most dramatic effects of poisoning are dementia with florid hallucinations; prolonged vasospasm, which may result in gangrene; and stimulation of uterine smooth muscle, which in pregnancy may result in abortion. In medieval times, ergot poisoning was called **St. Anthony's fire** after the saint whose help was sought in relieving the burning pain of vasospastic ischemia. Identifiable epidemics have occurred sporadically up to modern times (see Box: Ergot Poisoning: Not Just an Ancient Disease) and mandate continuous surveillance of all grains used for food. Poisoning of grazing animals is common in many areas because the fungus may grow on pasture grasses.

In addition to the effects noted above, the ergot alkaloids produce a variety of other central nervous system and peripheral effects. Detailed structure-activity analysis and appropriate semisynthetic modifications have yielded a large number of agents of experimental and clinical interest.

Ergot Poisoning: Not Just an Ancient Disease

As noted in the text, epidemics of **ergotism,** or poisoning by ergot-contaminated grain, are known to have occurred sporadically throughout history. It is easy to imagine the social chaos that might result if fiery pain, gangrene, hallucinations, convulsions, and abortions occurred simultaneously in members of a community in which all or most of the people believed in witchcraft, demonic possession, and the visitation of supernatural punishments upon humans for their misdeeds. Fortunately, such beliefs are uncommon today. However, ergotism has not disappeared. A most convincing demonstration of ergotism occurred in the small French village of Pont-Saint-Esprit in 1951. It was vividly described in the *British Medical Journal* in 1951 (Gabbai et al, 1951) and in a later book-length narrative account (Fuller, 1968). Several hundred individuals suffered symptoms of hallucinations, convulsions, and ischemia—and several died—after eating bread made from contaminated flour. Similar events have occurred even more recently when poverty, famine, or incompetence resulted in the consumption of contaminated grain. Ergot toxicity caused by excessive self-medication with pharmaceutical ergot preparations is still occasionally reported.

TABLE 16–7 Major ergoline derivatives (ergot alkaloids).

Amine alkaloids

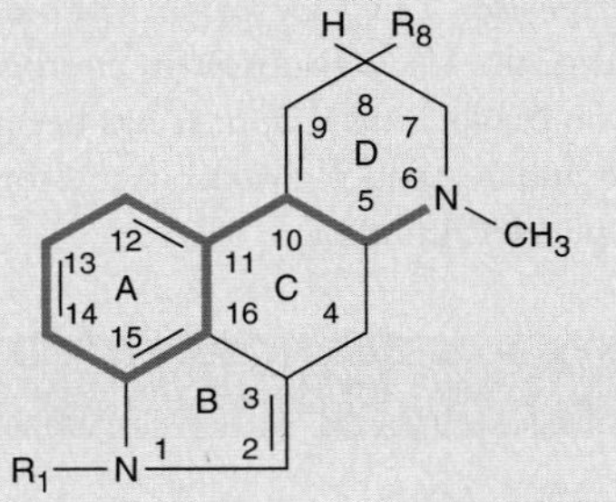

	R_1	R_8
6-Methylergoline	$-H$	$-H$
Lysergic acid	$-H$	$-COOH$
Lysergic acid diethylamide (LSD)	$-H$	$-C(=O)-N(CH_2-CH_3)_2$
Ergonovine (ergometrine)	$-H$	$-C(=O)-NHCH(CH_2OH)CH_3$

Peptide alkaloids

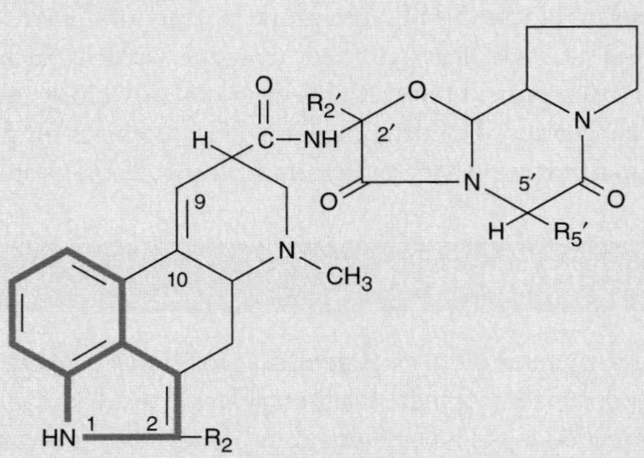

	R_2	R_2'	R_5'
Ergotamine[1]	$-H$	$-CH_3$	$-CH_2-C_6H_5$ 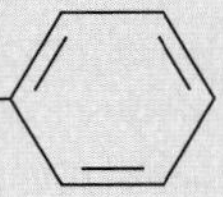
α-Ergocryptine	$-H$	$-CH(CH_3)_2$	$-CH_2-CH(CH_3)_2$
Bromocriptine	$-Br$	$-CH(CH_3)_2$	$-CH_2-CH(CH_3)_2$

[1]Dihydroergotamine lacks the double bond between carbons 9 and 10.

BASIC PHARMACOLOGY OF ERGOT ALKALOIDS

Chemistry & Pharmacokinetics

Two major families of compounds that incorporate the tetracyclic **ergoline** nucleus may be identified: the amine alkaloids and the peptide alkaloids (Table 16–7). Drugs of therapeutic and toxicologic importance are found in both groups.

The ergot alkaloids are variably absorbed from the gastrointestinal tract. The oral dose of ergotamine is about 10 times larger than the intramuscular dose, but the speed of absorption and peak blood levels after oral administration can be improved by administration with caffeine (see below). The amine alkaloids are also absorbed from the rectum and the buccal cavity and after administration by aerosol inhaler. Absorption after intramuscular injection is slow but usually reliable. Semisynthetic analogs such as bromocriptine and cabergoline are well absorbed from the gastrointestinal tract.

The ergot alkaloids are extensively metabolized in the body. The primary metabolites are hydroxylated in the A ring, and peptide alkaloids are also modified in the peptide moiety.

Pharmacodynamics

A. Mechanism of Action

The ergot alkaloids act on several types of receptors. As shown by the color outlines in Table 16–7, the nuclei of both catecholamines (phenylethylamine, left panel) and 5-HT (indolethylamine, right panel) can be discerned in the ergoline nucleus. Their effects include agonist, partial agonist, and antagonist actions at α adrenoceptors and serotonin receptors (especially 5-HT_{1A} and 5-HT_{1D}; less for 5-HT_3); and agonist or partial agonist actions at central nervous system dopamine receptors (Table 16–8). Furthermore, some members of the ergot family have a high affinity for presynaptic receptors, whereas others are more selective for postjunctional receptors. There is a powerful stimulant effect on the uterus that seems to be most closely associated with agonist or partial agonist effects at 5-HT_2 receptors. Structural variations increase the selectivity of certain members of the family for specific receptor types.

B. Organ System Effects

1. *Central nervous system*—As indicated by traditional descriptions of ergotism, certain of the naturally occurring alkaloids are powerful hallucinogens. **Lysergic acid diethylamide** (**LSD**; "acid") is a synthetic ergot compound that clearly demonstrates this action. The drug has been used in the laboratory as a potent peripheral 5-HT_2 *antagonist*, but good evidence suggests that its behavioral effects are mediated by *agonist* effects at prejunctional or postjunctional 5-HT_2 receptors in the central nervous system. In spite of extensive research, no clinical value has been discovered for LSD's dramatic central nervous system effects. Abuse of this drug has waxed and waned but is still widespread. It is discussed in Chapter 32.

Dopamine receptors in the central nervous system play important roles in extrapyramidal motor control and the regulation of

TABLE 16–8 Effects of ergot alkaloids at several receptors.[1]

Ergot Alkaloid	α Adrenoceptor	Dopamine Receptor	Serotonin Receptor (5-HT_2)	Uterine Smooth Muscle Stimulation
Bromocriptine	–	+++	–	0
Ergonovine	++	– (PA)	+++	++
Ergotamine	– – (PA)	0	+ (PA)	+++
Lysergic acid diethylamide (LSD)	0	+++	– – (++ in CNS)	+
Methysergide	+/0	+/0	– – – (PA)	+/0

[1]Agonist effects are indicated by +, antagonist by –, no effect by 0. Relative affinity for the receptor is indicated by the number of + or – signs. PA means partial agonist (both agonist and antagonist effects can be detected).

pituitary prolactin release. The actions of the peptide ergoline **bromocriptine** on the extrapyramidal system are discussed in Chapter 28. Of all the currently available ergot derivatives, bromocriptine, **cabergoline,** and **pergolide** have the highest agonist selectivity for pituitary dopamine receptors. These drugs directly suppress prolactin secretion from pituitary cells by activating regulatory dopamine receptors (see Chapter 37). They compete for binding to these sites with dopamine itself and with other dopamine agonists such as apomorphine. They bind with high affinity and dissociate slowly.

2. *Vascular smooth muscle*—The actions of ergot alkaloids on vascular smooth muscle are drug-, species-, and vessel-dependent, so few generalizations are possible. In humans, **ergotamine** and similar compounds constrict most vessels in nanomolar concentrations (Figure 16–4). The vasospasm is prolonged. This response is partially blocked by conventional α-blocking agents. However, ergotamine's effect is also associated with "epinephrine reversal" (see Chapter 10) and with *blockade* of the response to other α agonists. This dual effect reflects the drug's partial agonist action (see Table 16–8). Because ergotamine dissociates very slowly from the α receptor, it produces very long-lasting agonist and antagonist effects at this receptor. There is little or no effect at β adrenoceptors.

Although much of the vasoconstriction elicited by ergot alkaloids can be ascribed to partial agonist effects at α adrenoceptors, some may be the result of effects at 5-HT receptors. Ergotamine, ergonovine, and methysergide all have partial agonist effects at 5-HT_2 vascular receptors. The remarkably selective antimigraine action of the ergot derivatives was originally thought to be related to their actions on vascular serotonin receptors. Current hypotheses, however, emphasize their action on prejunctional neuronal 5-HT receptors.

After overdosage with ergotamine and similar agents, vasospasm is severe and prolonged (see Toxicity, below). This vasospasm is not easily reversed by α antagonists, serotonin antagonists, or combinations of both. Nitroprusside may be useful in case of severe ischemia.

Ergotamine is typical of the ergot alkaloids that have a strong vasoconstrictor action. The hydrogenation of ergot alkaloids at the 9 and 10 positions (Table 16–6) yields dihydro derivatives that have reduced serotonin partial agonist and vasoconstrictor effects and increased selective α-receptor–blocking actions.

3. *Uterine smooth muscle*—The stimulant action of ergot alkaloids on the uterus, as on vascular smooth muscle, appears to combine α agonist, serotonin agonist, and other effects.

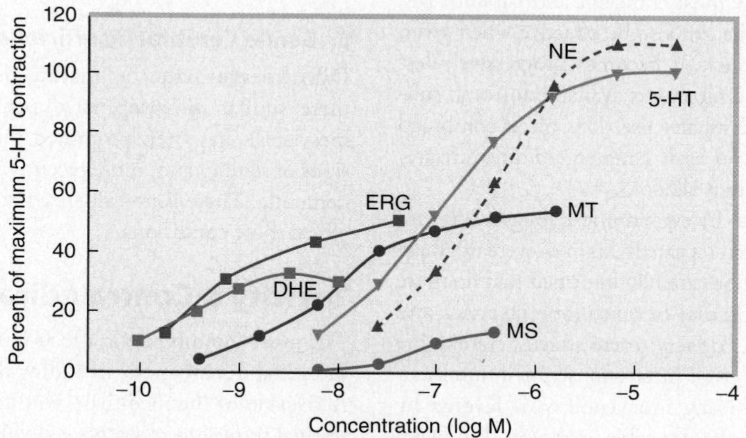

FIGURE 16–4 Effects of ergot derivatives on contraction of isolated segments of human basilar artery strips removed at surgery. All of the ergot derivatives are partial agonists; and all are more potent than the full agonists, norepinephrine and serotonin. DHE, dihydroergotamine; ERG, ergotamine; 5-HT, serotonin; MS, methysergide; MT, methylergometrine; NE, norepinephrine. (Modified with permission from Olesen J, Saxena PR: *5-Hydroxytryptamine Mechanisms in Primary Headaches*. Philadelphia, PA: Raven Press; 1992.)

Furthermore, the sensitivity of the uterus to the stimulant effects of ergot increases dramatically during pregnancy, perhaps because of increasing dominance of α_1 receptors of the uterus as pregnancy progresses. As a result, the uterus at term is more sensitive to ergot than earlier in pregnancy and far more sensitive than the nonpregnant organ.

In very small doses, ergot preparations can evoke rhythmic contraction and relaxation of the uterus. At higher concentrations, these drugs induce powerful and prolonged contracture. In patients with serious postpartum bleeding (a major cause of maternal morbidity and death), increasing doses of oxytocin are usually the first-line treatment. If necessary, this is supplemented with **tranexamic acid**, which facilitates clotting, and **carboprost**, a prostaglandin with strong smooth muscle–**stimulating action. Methylergonovine** is more selective than other ergot alkaloids in affecting the uterus and is an ergot agent of choice in controlling postpartum bleeding as an alternative to carboprost.

4. Other smooth muscle organs—In most patients, the ergot alkaloids have little or no effect on bronchiolar or urinary smooth muscle. The gastrointestinal tract, on the other hand, is quite sensitive. In some patients, nausea, vomiting, and diarrhea may be induced even by low doses. The effect is consistent with action on the central nervous system emetic center and on gastrointestinal serotonin receptors.

CLINICAL PHARMACOLOGY OF ERGOT ALKALOIDS

Clinical Uses

Despite their significant toxicities, ergot alkaloids are still used in patients with migraine headache or pituitary dysfunction. They are used only occasionally in the postpartum patient.

A. Migraine

Ergot derivatives are highly specific for migraine pain; they are not analgesic for any other condition. Although the triptan drugs discussed above are preferred by most clinicians and patients, traditional therapy with ergotamine can also be effective when given during the prodrome of an attack; it becomes progressively less effective if delayed. Ergotamine tartrate is available for oral, sublingual, rectal suppository, and inhaler use. It is often combined with caffeine (100 mg caffeine for each 1 mg ergotamine tartrate) to facilitate absorption of the ergot alkaloid.

The vasoconstriction induced by ergotamine is long-lasting and cumulative when the drug is taken repeatedly, as in a severe migraine attack. Therefore, patients must be carefully informed that no more than 6 mg of the oral preparation may be taken for each attack and no more than 10 mg per week. For very severe attacks, ergotamine tartrate, 0.25–0.5 mg, may be given intravenously or intramuscularly. Dihydroergotamine, 0.5–1 mg intravenously, is favored by some clinicians for treatment of intractable migraine. Intranasal dihydroergotamine also may be effective. Methysergide, which was used for migraine prophylaxis in the past, was withdrawn because of toxicity (see below).

B. Hyperprolactinemia

Increased serum levels of the anterior pituitary hormone prolactin are associated with secreting tumors of the gland and also with the use of centrally acting dopamine antagonists, especially the D_2-blocking antipsychotic drugs. Because of negative feedback effects, hyperprolactinemia is associated with amenorrhea and infertility in women as well as galactorrhea in both sexes. Rarely, the prolactin surge that occurs around the end-of-term pregnancy may be associated with heart failure; cabergoline has been used to treat this cardiac condition successfully.

Bromocriptine is extremely effective in reducing the high levels of prolactin that result from pituitary tumors and has even been associated with regression of the tumor in some cases. The usual dosage of bromocriptine is 2.5 mg two or three times daily. **Cabergoline** is similar but more potent. Bromocriptine has also been used in the same dosage to suppress physiologic lactation. However, serious postpartum cardiovascular toxicity has been reported in association with the latter use of bromocriptine or **pergolide,** and this application is discouraged (see Chapter 37).

C. Postpartum Hemorrhage

The uterus at term is extremely sensitive to the stimulant action of ergot, and even moderate doses produce a prolonged and powerful spasm of the muscle quite unlike natural labor. Therefore, ergot derivatives should be used only for control of postpartum uterine bleeding and should never be given before delivery. Oxytocin is the preferred agent for control of postpartum hemorrhage, but if this peptide agent is ineffective, ergonovine maleate, 0.2 mg given intramuscularly, can be tried. It is usually effective within 1–5 minutes and is less toxic than other ergot derivatives for this application. It is given at the time of delivery of the placenta or immediately afterward if bleeding is significant.

D. Diagnosis of Variant Angina

Ergonovine given intravenously has been used to produce prompt vasoconstriction during coronary angiography to diagnose variant angina if reactive segments of the coronary arteries are present. In Europe, methylergometrine has been used for this purpose.

E. Senile Cerebral Insufficiency

Dihydroergotoxine, a mixture of dihydro-α-ergocryptine and three similar dihydrogenated peptide ergot alkaloids (ergoloid mesylates), has been promoted for many years for the relief of signs of senility and, more recently, for the treatment of Alzheimer dementia. There is no evidence that this drug has significant benefit in these conditions.

Toxicity & Contraindications

The most common toxic effects of the ergot derivatives are gastrointestinal disturbances, including diarrhea, nausea, and vomiting. Activation of the medullary vomiting center and of the gastrointestinal serotonin receptors is involved. Since migraine attacks are often associated with these symptoms before therapy is begun, these adverse effects are rarely contraindications to the use of ergot.

A more dangerous toxic effect—usually associated with overdosage—of agents like ergotamine and ergonovine is prolonged vasospasm. This sign of vascular smooth muscle stimulation may result in gangrene and may require amputation. Bowel infarction also has been reported and may require resection. Vasospasm caused by ergot is refractory to most vasodilators, but infusion of large doses of nitroprusside or nitroglycerin has been successful in some cases.

Chronic therapy with **methysergide** was associated with connective tissue proliferation in the retroperitoneal space, the pleural cavity, and the endocardial tissue of the heart. These changes occurred insidiously over months and presented as hydronephrosis (from obstruction of the ureters) or a cardiac murmur (from distortion of the valves of the heart). In some cases, valve damage required surgical replacement. As a result, this drug was withdrawn from the US market. Similar fibrotic change has resulted from the chronic exposure to 5-HT in carcinoid syndrome and from the use of non-ergot 5-HT agonists promoted in the past for weight loss (fenfluramine, dexfenfluramine).

Other toxic effects of the ergot alkaloids include drowsiness and, in the case of methysergide, occasional instances of central stimulation and hallucinations. In fact, methysergide was sometimes used as a substitute for LSD by members of the so-called drug culture.

Contraindications to the use of ergot derivatives consist of the obstructive vascular diseases, especially symptomatic coronary artery disease, and collagen diseases.

There is no evidence that ordinary use of ergotamine for migraine is hazardous in pregnancy. However, most clinicians counsel restraint in the use of the ergot derivatives by pregnant patients. Use to deliberately cause abortion is contraindicated because the high doses required often cause dangerous vasoconstriction.

SUMMARY Drugs with Actions on Histamine and Serotonin Receptors; Ergot Alkaloids

Subclass, Drug	Mechanism of Action	Effects	Clinical Applications	Pharmacokinetics, Toxicities, Interactions
H_1 ANTIHISTAMINES				
First generation:				
• Diphenhydramine	Competitive antagonism/inverse agonism at H_1 receptors	Reduces or prevents histamine effects on smooth muscle, immune cells • also blocks muscarinic and α adrenoceptors • highly sedative	IgE immediate allergies; especially hay fever, urticaria • often used as a sedative, anti-emetic, and anti–motion sickness drug	Oral and parenteral • duration 4–6 h • *Toxicity:* Sedation when used in hay fever, muscarinic blockade symptoms, orthostatic hypotension • *Interactions:* Additive sedation with other sedatives, including alcohol • some inhibition of CYP2D6, may prolong action of some β blockers
Second generation:				
• Cetirizine	Competitive antagonism/inverse agonism at H_1 receptors	Reduces or prevents histamine effects on smooth muscle, immune cells	IgE immediate allergies; especially hay fever, urticaria	Oral • duration 12–24 h • *Toxicity:* Sedation and arrhythmias in overdose • *Interactions:* Minimal
• *Other first-generation H_1 blockers: Chlorpheniramine is a less sedating H_1 blocker with fewer autonomic effects. Doxylamine, a strongly sedating H_1 blocker, is available over-the-counter in many sleep-aid formulations and in Diclegis (in combination with pyridoxine) for use in nausea and vomiting of pregnancy*				
• *Other second-generation H_1 blockers: Loratadine, desloratadine, and fexofenadine are very similar to cetirizine*				
H_2 ANTIHISTAMINES				
• Cimetidine, others (see Chapter 62)				
SEROTONIN AGONISTS				
5-$HT_{1B/1D}$:				
• Sumatriptan	Partial agonist at 5-$HT_{1B/1D}$ receptors	Effects not fully understood • may reduce release of calcitonin gene-related peptide and perivascular edema in cerebral circulation	Migraine and cluster headache	Oral, nasal, parenteral • duration 2 h • *Toxicity:* Paresthesias, dizziness, coronary vasoconstriction • *Interactions:* Additive with other vasoconstrictors
• *Other triptans (almotriptan, eletriptan, frovatriptan, naratriptan, rizatriptan, zolmitriptan): Similar to sumatriptan except for pharmacokinetics (2–6 h duration of action); much more expensive than generic sumatriptan*				

(continued)

Subclass, Drug	Mechanism of Action	Effects	Clinical Applications	Pharmacokinetics, Toxicities, Interactions
5-HT1F:				
• Lasmiditan	Agonist at 5-HT_{1F} receptors	Reduces extravasation from blood vessels in the dura	Acute migraine	*Toxicity:* dizziness, vertigo, nausea, paresthesias
5-HT2C:				
• Lorcaserin (withdrawn)	Agonist at 5-HT_{2C} receptors	Appears to reduce appetite	Obesity	Oral • duration 11 h • *Toxicity:* Dizziness, headache, constipation
5-HT_4:				
• Tegaserod, prucalopride (see Chapter 62)				
SEROTONIN BLOCKERS				
5-HT_2:				
• Ketanserin (not available in USA)	Competitive blockade at 5-HT_2 receptors	Prevents vasoconstriction and bronchospasm of carcinoid syndrome	Hypertension • carcinoid syndrome associated with carcinoid tumor	Oral • duration 12–24 h • *Toxicity:* Hypotension
5-HT_3:				
• Ondansetron, others (see Chapter 62)				
ERGOT ALKALOIDS				
Vasoselective:				
• Ergotamine	Mixed partial agonist effects at 5-HT_2 and α adrenoceptors	Causes marked smooth muscle contraction but blocks α-agonist vasoconstriction	Migraine and cluster headache	Oral, parenteral • duration 12–24 h • *Toxicity:* Prolonged vasospasm causing angina, gangrene; uterine spasm
Uteroselective:				
• Ergonovine	Mixed partial agonist effects at 5-HT_2 and α adrenoceptors	Same as ergotamine • some selectivity for uterine smooth muscle	Postpartum bleeding • migraine headache	Oral, parenteral (methylergonovine) • duration 2–4 h • *Toxicity:* Same as ergotamine
CNS selective:				
• Lysergic acid diethylamide	Central nervous system 5-HT_2 and dopamine agonist • 5-HT_2 antagonist in periphery	Hallucinations • psychotomimetic	None • widely abused	Oral • duration several hours • *Toxicity:* Prolonged psychotic state, flashbacks
• *Bromocriptine, pergolide: Ergot derivatives used in Parkinson disease (see* Chapter 28) *and prolactinoma (see* Chapter 37). *Pergolide used in* equine *Cushing disease*				

PREPARATIONS AVAILABLE

GENERIC NAME	AVAILABLE AS
ANTIHISTAMINES (H_1 BLOCKERS)	
Azelastine	Generic, Astelin (nasal), Optivar (ophthalmic)
Brompheniramine	Brovex, Dimetapp, others
Buclizine	Bucladin-S Softabs
Carbinoxamine	Generic, Histex
Cetirizine	Generic, Zyrtec
Chlorpheniramine	Generic, Chlor-Trimeton
Clemastine	Generic, Tavist
Cyclizine	Generic, Marezine
Cyproheptadine	Generic, Periactin
Desloratadine	Generic, Clarinex
Dimenhydrinate[†]	Generic, Dramamine
Diphenhydramine	Generic, Benadryl
Doxylamine	Diclegis (combination with pyridoxine), Unisom Sleep Tabs
Epinastine	Generic, Elestat
Fexofenadine	Generic, Allegra
Hydroxyzine	Generic, Vistaril
Ketotifen	Generic, Zaditor
Levocabastine	Livostin
Levocetirizine	Generic, Xyzal
Loratadine	Generic, Claritin
Meclizine	Generic, Antivert, Bonine
Olopatadine	Patanol, Pataday
Phenindamine	Nolahist
Promethazine	Generic, Phenergan
Triprolidine	Generic, Zymine, Tripohist

(*continued*)

GENERIC NAME	AVAILABLE AS
H_2 BLOCKERS	
See Chapter 62.	
H_3 BLOCKERS	
Pitolisant	Wakix
5-HT AGONISTS	
Almotriptan	Axert
Eletriptan	Relpax
Flibanserin	Addyi
Frovatriptan	Frova
Lasmiditan	Reyvow
Naratriptan	Generic, Amerge
Prucalopride	Motegrity, Prudac
Rizatriptan	Generic, Maxalt, Maxalt-MLT
Sumatriptan	Generic, Imitrex
Tegaserod	Zelnorm, Zelmac
Zolmitriptan	Generic, Zomig
5-HT ANTAGONISTS	
See Chapter 62.	
TRYPTOPHAN HYDROXYLASE INHIBITOR	
Telotristat	Xermelo
MELATONIN RECEPTOR AGONISTS	
Ramelteon	Rozerem
Tasimelteon	Hetlioz

GENERIC NAME	AVAILABLE AS
ERGOT ALKALOIDS	
Dihydroergotamine	Generic, Migranal, D.H.E. 45
Ergonovine	Generic, Ergotrate
Ergotamine mixtures (include caffeine)	Generic, Cafergot
Ergotamine tartrate	Generic, Ergomar
Methylergonovine	Generic, Methergine
ANTI-CGRP AGENTS	
Erenumab	Aimovig
Galcanezumab	Emgality
Fremanezumab	Ajovy
Rimegepant	Nurtec
Ubrogepant	Ubrelvy
ANTI-OBESITY DRUGS	
Exenatide[‡]	Byetta
Cellulose–citric acid hydrogel	Plenity
Liraglutide	Saxenda, Victoza
Lorcaserin	Belviq
Naltrexone/bupropion	Contrave
Orlistat	Alli, Xenical
Phentermine	Generic, Adipex-P, Lomaira
Phentermine/topiramate	Qsymia
Semaglutide	Ozempic, Wegovy

[*]Several other antihistamines are available only in combination products with, for example, phenylephrine.

[†]Dimenhydrinate is the chlorotheophylline salt of diphenhydramine.

[‡]Off-label use.

REFERENCES

Histamine

Asero R: New-onset urticaria. UpToDate, 2022. http://www.uptodate.com.

Bond RA, Ijerman AP: Recent developments in constitutive receptor activity and inverse agonism, and their potential for GPCR drug discovery. Trend Pharmacol Sci 2006;27:92.

deShazo RD, Kemp SF: Pharmacotherapy of allergic rhinitis. UpToDate, 2018. http://www.uptodate.com.

Feng C et al: Histamine (scombroid) fish poisoning: A comprehensive review. Clin Rev Allerg Immunol 2016;50:64.

Keet C: Recognition and management of food induced anaphylaxis. Pediatr Clin North Am 2011;58:377.

Mahdy AM, Webster NR: Histamine and antihistamines. Anaest Int Care 2017;18:210.

McParlin C et al: Treatments of hyperemesis gravidarum and nausea and vomiting in pregnancy. JAMA 2016;316:1392.

Panula P et al: International Union of Basic and Clinical Pharmacology. XCVIII. Histamine receptors. Pharmacol Rev 2015;67:601.

Preuss H et al: Constitutive activity and ligand selectivity of human, guinea pig, rat, and canine histamine H2 receptors. J Pharmacol Exp Therap 2007;321:983.

Provensi G et al: The histaminergic system as a target for the prevention of obesity and metabolic syndrome. Neuropharmacology 2016;106:3.

Rapanelli M, Pittenger C: Histamine and histamine receptors in Tourette syndrome and other neuropsychiatric conditions. Neuropharmacology 2016;106:85.

Schaper-Gerhardt K et al: The role of the histamine H_4 receptor in atopic dermatitis and psoriasis. Br J Pharmacol 2020;177:490.

Theoharides TC et al: Mast cells, mastocytosis, and related disorders. N Engl J Med 2015;373:163.

Thurmond RL et al: The role of histamine H1 and H4 receptors in allergic inflammation: The search for new antihistamines. Nat Rev Drug Discov 2008;7:41.

Serotonin

Barrenetxe J et al: Physiologic and metabolic functions of melatonin. J Physiol Biochem 2004;60:61.

D'Amico JM et al: Constitutively active 5-$HT_2/\alpha 1$ receptors facilitate muscle spasms after human spinal cord injury. J Neurophysiol 2013;109:1473.

Elangbam CS: Drug-induced valvulopathy: An update. Toxicol Path 2010; 38:837.

Frank C: Recognition and treatment of serotonin syndrome. Can Fam Physician 2008;54:988.

Jaspers L et al: Efficacy and safety of flibanserin for the treatment of hypoactive sexual desire disorder in women. A systematic review and meta-analysis. JAMA Intern Med 2016;176:453.

Katus LE, Frucht SJ: Management of serotonin syndrome and neuroleptic malignant syndrome. Curr Treat Options Neurol 2016;18:39.

Kuca B et al: Lasmiditan is an effective acute treatment for migraine. Neurology 2018;91:e2222.

Loder E: Triptan therapy in migraine. N Engl J Med 2010;363:63.

Porvasnik SL et al: PRX-08066, a novel 5-hydroxytryptamine receptor 2B antagonist, reduces monocrotaline-induced pulmonary hypertension and right ventricular hypertrophy in rats. J Pharmacol Exp Therap 2010;334:364.

Thompson AJ: Recent developments in 5-HT3 receptor pharmacology. Trends Pharmacol Sci 2013;34:100.

Wang C et al: Structural basis for molecular recognition at serotonin receptors. Science 2013;340:610.

Ergot Alkaloids: Historical

Fuller JG: *The Day of St. Anthony's Fire.* Macmillan, 1968; Signet, 1969. (Historical novel)

Gabbai Dr et al: Ergot poisoning at Pont St. Esprit. Br Med J 1951;2:650.

Migraine and Postpartum Hemorrhage: Pharmacology

Belfort MA: Postpartum hemorrhage: medical and minimally invasive management. UpToDate, 2022. http://www.uptodate.com.

Dahlöf C, Van Den Brink A: Dihydroergotamine, ergotamine, methysergide and sumatriptan—Basic science in relation to migraine treatment. Headache 2012;52:707.

Dierckx RA et al: Intraarterial sodium nitroprusside infusion in the treatment of severe ergotism. Clin Neuropharmacol 1986;9:542.

Dildy GA: Postpartum hemorrhage: New management options. Clin Obstet Gynecol 2002;45:330.

Edvinsson L: CGRP and migraine: from bench to bedside. Rev Neurol (Paris). 2021;177:785.

Lipton RB et al: Efficacy and safety of eptinezumab in patients with chronic migraine: PROMISE-2. Neurollogy 2020;94:e1365.

Mantegani S et al: Ergoline derivatives: Receptor affinity and selectivity. Farmaco 1999;54:288.

Pavitt S et al: Efficacy and safety of repetitive intravenous sodium valproate in pediatric patients with refractory chronic headache disorders. Pediatr Neurol 2022;128:52.

Porter JK, Thompson FN Jr: Effects of fescue toxicosis on reproduction in livestock. J Anim Sci 1992;70:1594.

Schuster NM, Rapoport AM: Calcitonin gene-related peptide-targeted therapies for migraine and cluster headache: A review. Clin Neuropharmacol 2017;40:169.

Schwenk ES et al: Ketamine for refractory chronic migraine: An observational pilot study and metabolite analysis. J Clin Pharmacol 2021;61:1421.

VanderPluym JH et al: Acute treatments for episodic migraine in adults. A systematic review and meta-analysis. JAMA 2021;325:2357.

Obesity

Bohula EA et al: Cardiovascular safety of lorcaserin in overweight or obese patients. N Engl J Med 2018;379:1107.

Bray GA: Drug therapy of obesity. UpToDate, 2016. http://www.uptodate.com.

Cypess AM: Reassessing human adipose tissue. N Engl J Med 2022;386:768.

Heymsfield SB, Wadden TA: Mechanisms, pathophysiology, and management of obesity. N Engl J Med 2017;376:254.

Mehta MD, Istfan NW, Apovian CM: Obesity: Overview of weight management. Endocr Pract 2021;27:626.

Müller TD et al: Anti-obesity therapy: From rainbow pills to polyagonists. Pharmacol Rev 2018;70:712.

Perreault L: Obesity in adults: Drug therapy. UpToDate, 2022. http://www.uptodate.com.

Pi-Sunyer X et al: A randomized, controlled trial of 3.0 mg of liraglutide in weight management. N Engl J Med 2015;373:11.

Rubino DM et al: Effect of weekly subcutaneous semaglutide vs daily liraglutide on body weight in adults with overweight or obesity without diabetes. The STEP 8 randomized clinical trial. JAMA 2022;327:138.

Skinner AC et al: Cardiometabolic risks and severity of obesity in children and young adults. N Engl J Med 2015;373:1307.

Son JW, Kim S: Comprehensive review of current and upcoming anti-obesity drugs. Diabetes Metab J. 2020;44:802.

CASE STUDY ANSWER

These patients demonstrate typical symptoms and signs caused by histamine. Fortunately, neither patient in this episode of food poisoning had significant laryngeal edema or bronchospasm. Certain types of fish, if improperly preserved, contain large quantities of histamine, due to the conversion—by bacteria contaminating the muscle tissue—of histidine to histamine. If consumed in sufficient amount, enough histamine can be absorbed to cause the clinical picture described. This syndrome is termed *scombroid poisoning*. (The Scombridae family of fish is most commonly associated with this toxicity.) Treatment with maximal doses of histamine blockers, especially H_1 blockers, is usually sufficient to control the symptoms. Because this is not an allergic reaction, administration of epinephrine is not necessary unless hypotension or airway obstruction is severe. (See Edlow JA: *The Deadly Dinner Party: And Other Medical Detective Stories*. Yale University Press, 2009.)

CHAPTER

17

Vasoactive Peptides

Ian A. Reid, PhD

CASE STUDY

During a routine check and on two follow-up visits, a 45-year-old man was found to have high blood pressure (160–165/95–100 mm Hg). His physician initially prescribed hydrochlorothiazide, a diuretic commonly used to treat hypertension. His blood pressure was reduced by hydrochlorothiazide but remained at a hypertensive level (145/95 mm Hg), and he was referred to the university hypertension clinic. Because the patient had elevated plasma renin activity and aldosterone concentration, hydrochlorothiazide was replaced with enalapril, an angiotensin-converting enzyme inhibitor. Enalapril lowered his blood pressure to almost normotensive levels. However, after several weeks on enalapril, the patient returned complaining of a persistent cough. In addition, some signs of angioedema were detected. How does enalapril lower blood pressure? Why does it occasionally cause coughing and angioedema? What other drugs could be used to inhibit the renin-angiotensin system and decrease blood pressure, without the adverse effects of enalapril?

A wide variety of peptides play important roles in the regulation of the cardiovascular system by acting at several levels in the body. Many of the peptides act as classic hormones, being transported in the blood from their site of synthesis to act on the heart, blood vessels, and other targets. Others function as paracrine or autocrine regulators, acting close to their site of synthesis. Several of the peptides are also present in the central nervous system where they function as neurotransmitters or neuromodulators (see Chapter 21), regulating brain centers involved in cardiovascular control. Some are present in the autonomic and enteric nervous systems where they frequently function as cotransmitters, with actions on the cardiovascular, gastrointestinal, and other systems (see Chapter 6). A smaller number of neuropeptides enter the circulation and act as neurohormones.

Peptides that participate in cardiovascular control include the vasoconstrictors **angiotensin II, vasopressin, endothelins, neuropeptide Y,** and **urotensin;** and the vasodilators **bradykinin** and related **kinins, natriuretic peptides, vasoactive intestinal peptide, substance P, neurotensin, calcitonin gene-related peptide, adrenomedullin, relaxin,** and **the urocortins.** This distinction between vasoconstrictor and vasodilator is an oversimplification because, depending on their receptors and associated signaling pathways, some peptides can elicit both responses.

Although these peptides are generally considered individually, many belong to families, the members of which have similarities in structure and function and act on the same or related receptors. Examples are substance P, which belongs to the **tachykinin family;** calcitonin gene-related peptide and adrenomedullin **(calcitonin family)**; vasoactive intestinal peptide **(secretin-glucagon family)**; relaxin **(insulin superfamily)**; and urocortins **(corticotropin releasing hormone family).**

Many of these peptides were initially regarded as physiologic curiosities, but subsequent investigation showed that they play important roles not only in physiologic regulation, but also in hypertension and several cardiovascular diseases including heart failure. Moreover, many drugs that alter the biosynthesis or actions of the peptides have been developed. In previous versions of this chapter, such drugs were often referred to as "being under development" or "having promise." The present version of this chapter indicates that many are now in routine clinical use to treat cardiovascular and other diseases. Indeed, the development of drugs targeting vasoactive peptides has become a major activity of the pharmaceutical industry.

This chapter focuses on the vasoactive peptides, with emphasis on their actions on the cardiovascular system. The vasoconstrictors are considered first, followed by the vasodilators.

VASOCONSTRICTORS

■ ANGIOTENSIN

BIOSYNTHESIS OF ANGIOTENSIN

The pathway for the formation and metabolism of angiotensin II (ANG II) is summarized in Figure 17–1. The principal steps include enzymatic cleavage of angiotensin I (ANG I) from angiotensinogen by renin, conversion of ANG I to ANG II by converting enzyme, and degradation of ANG II by several peptidases.

Renin

Renin is an aspartyl protease enzyme that specifically catalyzes the hydrolytic release of the decapeptide ANG I from angiotensinogen. It is synthesized as a prepromolecule that is first processed to prorenin and then to active renin by cleavage of a 43-amino acid N-terminal prosegment. Active renin is a glycoprotein consisting of 340 amino acids.

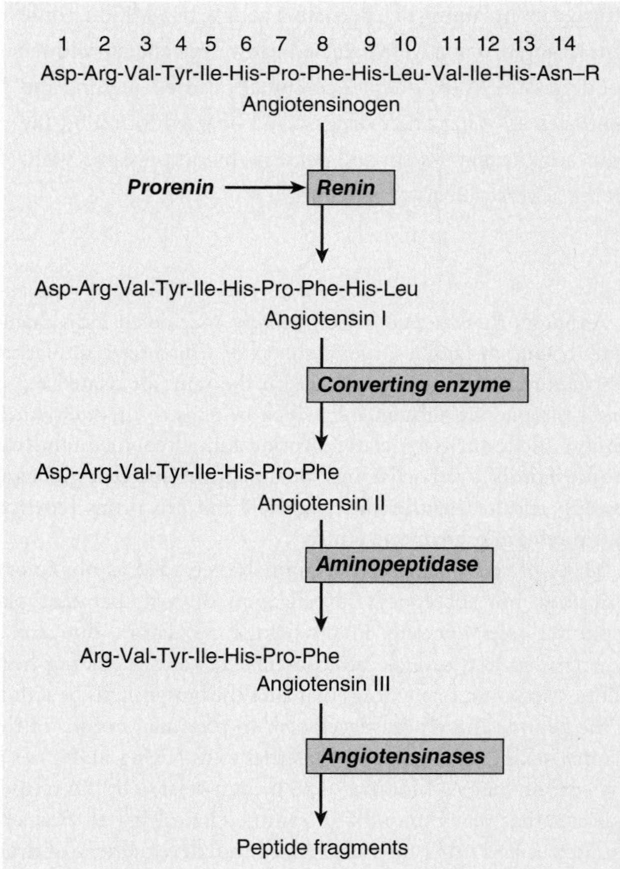

FIGURE 17–1 Chemistry of the renin-angiotensin system. The amino acid sequence of the amino terminal of human angiotensinogen is shown. R denotes the remainder of the protein molecule. See text for additional steps in the formation and metabolism of angiotensin peptides.

Active renin in the circulation originates in the kidneys and disappears entirely after nephrectomy. Within the kidney, renin is synthesized and stored in the juxtaglomerular apparatus of the nephron. Specialized granular cells called juxtaglomerular cells are the site of synthesis, storage, and release of renin. The macula densa is a specialized segment of the nephron that is closely associated with the vascular components of the juxtaglomerular apparatus. The vascular and tubular components of the juxtaglomerular apparatus, including the juxtaglomerular cells, are innervated by the sympathetic nervous system.

Prorenin is present in the circulation at levels considerably higher than those of active renin. Plasma prorenin levels decrease after nephrectomy, but significant amounts remain. The remaining prorenin is thought to originate in extrarenal tissues including the adrenal gland, ovaries, testes, placenta, and retina. Prorenin exerts a variety of actions via a unique prorenin receptor.

Control of Renin Release

The rate at which renin is released by the kidneys is the primary determinant of activity of the renin-angiotensin system. Active renin is released by exocytosis immediately upon stimulation of the juxtaglomerular apparatus. Prorenin is released constitutively, usually at a rate higher than that of active renin, thus accounting for the fact that prorenin can constitute 80–90% of the total renin in the circulation. The significance of circulating prorenin and a unique prorenin receptor is discussed at the end of this section. Active renin release is controlled by a variety of factors, including the macula densa, a renal vascular receptor, the sympathetic nervous system, and ANG II.

A. Macula Densa

Renin release is controlled in part by the macula densa, a structure that has a close anatomic association with the afferent arteriole. The initial step involves the detection of some function of NaCl concentration in, or delivery to, the distal tubule, possibly by the $Na^+/K^+/2Cl^-$ cotransporter. The macula densa then signals changes in renin release by the juxtaglomerular cells such that there is an inverse relationship between NaCl delivery or concentration and renin release. Potential candidates for signal transmission include prostaglandin E_2 (PGE_2) and nitric oxide, which stimulate renin release, and adenosine, which inhibits it. Because the sodium intake in the general population is high, macula densa-mediated renin secretion is usually at basal levels, increasing only when sodium intake decreases.

B. Renal Baroreceptor

The renal vascular baroreceptor mediates an inverse relationship between renal artery pressure and renin release. The mechanism is not completely understood, but it appears that the juxtaglomerular cells are sensitive to stretch and that increased stretch results in decreased renin release. The decrease may result from influx of calcium which, somewhat paradoxically, inhibits renin release. The paracrine factors PGE_2, nitric oxide, and adenosine have also been

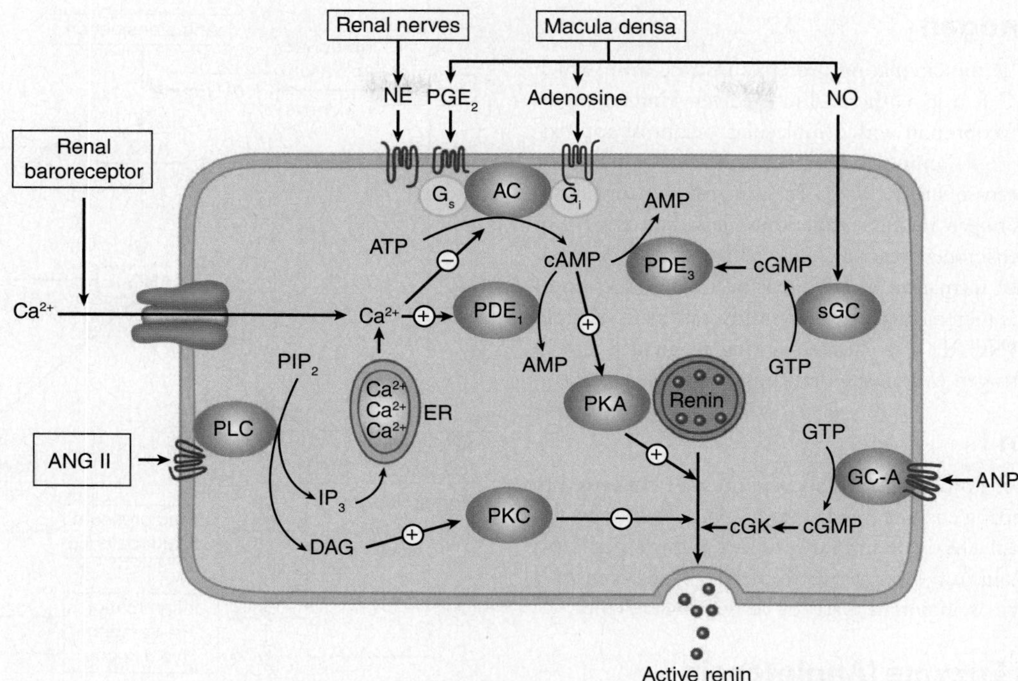

FIGURE 17–2 Major physiologic inputs to renin release and proposed integration with signaling pathways in the juxtaglomerular cell. AC, adenylyl cyclase; ANG II, angiotensin II; ANP, atrial natriuretic peptide; cGK, protein kinase G; DAG, diacylglycerol; ER, endoplasmic reticulum; GC-A, particulate guanylyl cyclase; IP_3, inositol trisphosphate; NE, norepinephrine; NO, nitric oxide; PDE, phosphodiesterase; PKA, protein kinase A; PLC, phospholipase C; sGC, soluble guanylyl cyclase. (Reproduced with permission from Castrop H, Höcherl K, Kurtz A, et al: Physiology of kidney renin. Physiol Rev 2010;90(2):607-673.)

implicated in the baroreceptor control of renin release. At normal blood pressure, renal baroreceptor-mediated renin secretion is low; it increases in hypotensive states.

C. Sympathetic Nervous System

Norepinephrine released from renal sympathetic nerves stimulates renin release indirectly by α-adrenergic activation of the renal baroreceptor and macula densa mechanisms, and directly by an action on the juxtaglomerular cells. In humans, the direct effect is mediated by β_1 adrenoceptors. Through this mechanism, reflex activation of the sympathetic nervous system by hypotension or hypovolemia leads to activation of the renin-angiotensin system.

D. Angiotensin

ANG II inhibits renin release. The inhibition results from increased blood pressure acting by way of the renal baroreceptor and macula densa mechanisms, and from a direct action of the peptide on the juxtaglomerular cells. The direct inhibition is mediated by increased intracellular Ca^{2+} concentration and forms the basis of a short-loop negative feedback mechanism controlling renin release. Interruption of this feedback with drugs that inhibit the renin-angiotensin system results in stimulation of renin release.

E. Intracellular Signaling Pathways

The release of renin by the juxtaglomerular cells is controlled by interplay among three intracellular messengers: cAMP, cyclic guanosine monophosphate (cGMP), and free cytosolic Ca^{2+} concentration (Figure 17–2). cAMP plays a major role; maneuvers that increase cAMP levels, including activation of adenylyl cyclase, inhibition of cAMP phosphodiesterases, and administration of cAMP analogs, increase renin release. In experimental studies, selective deficiency of $G_{s\alpha}$ in the juxtaglomerular cells was associated with a marked reduction in basal renin secretion and in the response to several stimuli to renin secretion.

Increases in intracellular Ca^{2+} can result from increased entry of extracellular Ca^{2+} or mobilization of Ca^{2+} from intracellular stores, while increases in cGMP levels can result from activation of soluble or particulate guanylyl cyclase. Ca^{2+} and cGMP appear to alter renin release indirectly, primarily by changing cAMP levels.

F. Pharmacologic Alteration of Renin Release

The release of renin is altered by a wide variety of pharmacologic agents. It is stimulated by vasodilators (eg, hydralazine, minoxidil, nitroprusside), β-adrenoceptor agonists, α-adrenoceptor antagonists, phosphodiesterase inhibitors (eg, theophylline, milrinone, rolipram), and most diuretics and anesthetics. This stimulation can be accounted for by the control mechanisms just described. Drugs that inhibit renin release are discussed below.

Many of the peptides reviewed in this chapter also alter renin release. Release is stimulated by adrenomedullin, bradykinin, and calcitonin gene-related peptide, and inhibited by atrial natriuretic peptide, endothelin, substance P, and vasopressin.

Angiotensinogen

Angiotensinogen is the circulating protein substrate from which renin cleaves ANG I. It is synthesized in the liver. Human angiotensinogen is a glycoprotein with a molecular weight of approximately 57,000. The 14 amino acids at the amino terminal of the molecule are shown in Figure 17–1. In humans, the concentration of angiotensinogen in the circulation is less than the K_m of the renin-angiotensinogen reaction and is therefore a determinant of the rate of formation of angiotensin. The production of angiotensinogen is increased by corticosteroids, estrogens, thyroid hormones, and ANG II. It is elevated during pregnancy and in women taking estrogen-containing oral contraceptives.

Angiotensin I

ANG I has little or no biologic activity and must be converted to ANG II by converting enzyme (see Figure 17–1). ANG I may also be acted on by plasma or tissue aminopeptidases to form [des-Asp[1]] angiotensin I; this in turn is converted to [des-Asp[1]]angiotensin II (commonly known as angiotensin III) by converting enzyme.

Converting Enzyme (Angiotensin-Converting Enzyme [ACE], Peptidyl Dipeptidase, Kininase II)

Converting enzyme is a dipeptidyl carboxypeptidase with two active sites that catalyzes the cleavage of dipeptides from the carboxyl terminal of certain peptides. Its most important substrates are ANG I, which it converts to ANG II, and bradykinin, which it inactivates (see Kinins, below). It also cleaves enkephalins and substance P, but the physiologic significance of these effects has not been established. The action of converting enzyme is prevented by a penultimate prolyl residue in the substrate, and ANG II is therefore not hydrolyzed by converting enzyme. Converting enzyme is distributed widely in the body. In most organs, converting enzyme is located on the luminal surface of vascular endothelial cells and is thus in close contact with the circulation.

A homolog of converting enzyme known as ACE2 is expressed in vascular endothelial cells of the kidneys, lungs, heart, and testes. Unlike converting enzyme, ACE2 has only one active site and functions as a carboxypeptidase rather than a dipeptidyl carboxypeptidase. It removes a single amino acid from the C-terminal of ANG I forming ANG 1-9 (Figure 17–3), which is inactive but is converted to ANG 1-7 by ACE. ACE2 also converts ANG II to ANG 1-7. ANG 1-7 has vasodilator activity, apparently mediated by the orphan heterotrimeric guanine nucleotide-binding protein–coupled receptor (Mas receptor). This vasodilation may serve to counteract the vasoconstrictor activity of ANG II. ACE2 also differs from ACE in that it does not hydrolyze bradykinin and is not inhibited by converting enzyme inhibitors (see below).

ACE2 also binds the virus SARS-CoV-2, thus, facilitating its entry into cells. Animal studies show that ACE2 is upregulated by converting enzyme inhibitors and angiotensin receptor blockers (see below), and this may have implications for the use of these drugs in Covid-19 patients. To date, neither beneficial nor adverse outcomes have been observed, although the concern has been raised that withdrawal of the drugs may be harmful in certain high-risk patients with Covid-19.

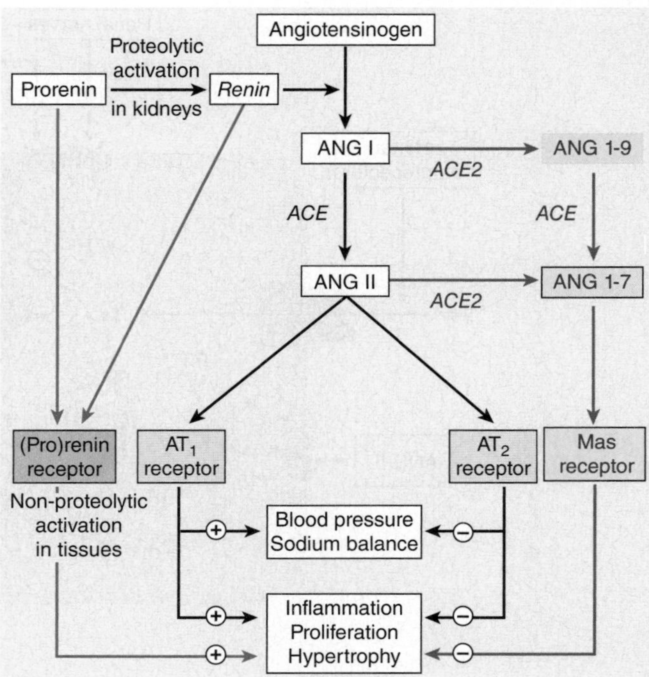

FIGURE 17–3 The renin-angiotensin system showing the established system (black) and more recently discovered pathways involving the (pro)renin receptor (red) and ANG 1-7 (blue). (Reproduced with permission from Castrop H, Höcherl K, Kurtz A, et al: Physiology of kidney renin, Physiol Rev 2010 Apr;90(2):607-673.)

Angiotensinase

ANG II, which has a plasma half-life of 15–60 seconds, is removed from the circulation by a variety of peptidases collectively referred to as angiotensinase. It is metabolized during passage through most vascular beds (a notable exception being the lung). Most metabolites of ANG II are biologically inactive, but the initial product of aminopeptidase action—[des-Asp[1]] angiotensin II or angiotensin III—retains some biologic activity. Recently another endogenous angiotensin peptide named **alamandine** was identified. It is the heptapeptide Ala[1]-ANG 1-7, and differs from ANG 1-7 only in having Ala at its N-terminal instead of Asp.

ACTIONS OF ANGIOTENSIN II

ANG II exerts important actions at vascular smooth muscle, adrenal cortex, kidney, heart, and brain via the receptors described below. Through these actions, the renin-angiotensin system plays a key role in the regulation of fluid and electrolyte balance and arterial blood pressure. Excessive activity of the renin-angiotensin system can result in hypertension and disorders of fluid and electrolyte homeostasis.

Blood Pressure

ANG II is a potent pressor agent—on a molar basis, approximately 40 times more potent than norepinephrine. The pressor response to intravenous ANG II is rapid in onset (10–15 seconds) and sustained during long-term infusions. A large component of the pressor response is due to direct contraction of vascular—especially arteriolar—smooth muscle. In addition, however, ANG II can also increase blood pressure through actions on the brain and autonomic nervous system. For example, the pressor response to ANG II is not usually accompanied by reflex bradycardia because the peptide simultaneously acts on the brain to reset the baroreceptor reflex control of heart rate to a higher pressure. This action, which is associated with reduced efferent vagal tone to the heart, effectively enhances the pressor response to ANG II.

ANG II also stimulates autonomic ganglia, increases the release of epinephrine and norepinephrine from the adrenal medulla, and facilitates sympathetic transmission by an action at adrenergic nerve terminals. The latter effect involves both increased release and reduced reuptake of norepinephrine. ANG II has a less important direct positive inotropic action on the heart. The physiologic significance of these actions remains unclear.

In patients with severe vasodilatory shock, infusion of ANG II increases arterial pressure and improves survival. It has been approved by the FDA as a vasopressor in the treatment of vasodilatory shock. It has also been used to prevent hypotension during anesthesia and following ACE inhibitor overdose, and may be beneficial in acute kidney injury and acute respiratory distress syndrome.

Adrenal Cortex & Kidney

ANG II acts directly on the zona glomerulosa of the adrenal cortex to stimulate aldosterone synthesis and release. At higher concentrations, ANG II also stimulates glucocorticoid synthesis. ANG II acts on the kidney to cause renal vasoconstriction, increase proximal tubular sodium reabsorption, and inhibit the release of renin.

Central Nervous System

In addition to its central effects on blood pressure, ANG II acts on the central nervous system to stimulate drinking (dipsogenic effect) and increase the secretion of vasopressin and adrenocorticotropic hormone (ACTH). The physiologic significance of these effects is not known.

Cell Growth

ANG II is mitogenic for vascular and cardiac muscle cells and may contribute to the development of cardiac hypertrophy. It also exerts a variety of important effects on the vascular endothelium. Indeed, overactivity of the renin-angiotensin system has been implicated as one of the most significant factors in the development of hypertensive vascular disease. Considerable evidence now indicates that inhibition of the renin-angiotensin system (see below) slows or prevents morphologic changes (remodeling) following myocardial infarction that would otherwise lead to heart failure. The stimulation of vascular and cardiac growth by ANG II is mediated by other pathways, probably receptor and nonreceptor tyrosine kinases such as the Janus tyrosine kinase Jak2, and by increased transcription of specific genes (see Chapter 2).

Inflammation

ANG II is involved in the inflammatory response associated with several diseases including atherosclerosis, arthritis, steatohepatitis, colitis, pancreatitis, and nephritis. Blockade of the renin-angiotensin system (see below) may be effective in their treatment.

ANGIOTENSIN RECEPTORS & MECHANISM OF ACTION

Angiotensin Receptors

ANG II receptors are widely distributed in the body. ANG II receptors are G protein–coupled and located on the plasma membrane of target cells, permitting rapid onset of the various actions of ANG II. Two distinct subtypes of ANG II receptors, termed **AT_1** and **AT_2**, have been identified. ANG II binds equally to both subtypes. The relative proportion of the two subtypes varies from tissue to tissue: AT_1 receptors predominate in vascular smooth muscle. Most of the known actions of ANG II are mediated by the AT_1 receptor, a G_q protein–coupled receptor. Binding of ANG II to AT_1 receptors in vascular smooth muscle results in activation of phospholipase C and generation of inositol trisphosphate and diacylglycerol (see Chapter 2). These events, which occur within seconds, result in smooth muscle contraction.

The AT_2 receptor has a structure and affinity for ANG II similar to those of the AT_1 receptor. In contrast, however, stimulation of AT_2 receptors causes vasodilation that may serve to counteract the vasoconstriction resulting from AT_1 receptor stimulation. AT_2 receptor-induced vasodilation appears to be nitric oxide-dependent and may involve the bradykinin B_2 receptor-nitric oxide-cGMP pathway. AT_2 receptors and the Mas receptor are co-localized and may form a heterodimer, which could also be important.

AT_2 receptors are present at high density in all tissues during fetal development, and may play an important role in regulating cellular differentiation and organ development by virtue of their high abundance in fetal mesenchymal tissues. AT_2 expression declines rapidly to an undetectable level in many tissues after birth, but low levels remain in the heart, adrenal gland, kidney, brain, and reproductive tissues. Up-regulation occurs in some disease states including heart failure and myocardial infarction. In animal studies, activation of AT_2 receptors has been reported to produce anti-inflammatory, antiproliferative, antihypertrophic, antifibrotic, proapoptotic, and vasodilatory effects. These effects could help to counterbalance the detrimental effects of excessive ANG II mediated via AT_1 receptors, and thereby protect against the progression of organ damage.

Prorenin Receptors

For many years, prorenin was considered to be an inactive precursor of renin, with no receptor or function of its own, despite

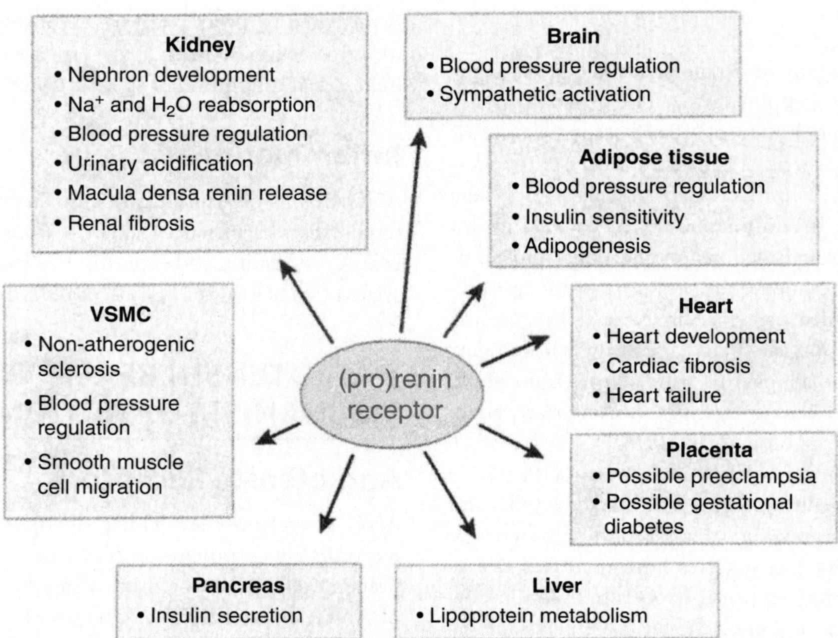

FIGURE 17–4 Potential functions of the (pro)renin receptor. (Reproduced with permission from Ramkumar N, Kohan DE: The (pro)renin receptor: An emerging player in hypertension and metabolic syndrome, Kidney Int 2019;95(5):1041-1052.)

its high levels in the circulation. However, a novel receptor has been described. This receptor binds both renin and prorenin and is therefore referred to as the (pro)renin receptor. It is a 350-amino acid protein with a single transmembrane domain that binds prorenin to a large N-terminal extracellular domain. It has been localized to several organs including the kidney, heart, vascular smooth muscle, brain, adipose tissue, liver, eye, and placenta.

When prorenin binds to the (pro)renin receptor, the prorenin undergoes a conformational change and becomes enzymatically active without cleavage of the prosegment. This is referred to as nonproteolytic to distinguish it from the proteolytic activation with prosegment removal that occurs in the kidney. Binding of prorenin to the receptor activates intracellular signaling pathways that differ depending on the cell type. For example, in mesangial and vascular smooth muscle cells, prorenin binding activates MAP kinases and expression of profibrotic molecules. Thus, elevated prorenin levels (as occur, for example, in diabetes mellitus) might have adverse effects via angiotensin-dependent and independent pathways (see Figure 17–3).

Renin inhibitors such as aliskiren (see below) do not block (pro)renin-induced signaling. However, a synthetic peptide named ***handle region peptide*** **(HRP),** which consists of the amino acid sequence corresponding to the "handle" region of the prorenin prosegment, has been synthesized and shown to competitively inhibit binding of prorenin to the (pro)renin receptor. However, it has partial agonist activity. A newer (pro)renin receptor antagonist, PRO20, is identical to the first 20 amino acids of the prorenin segment, contains all the (pro)renin receptor binding sites, and acts as a competitive antagonist.

Studies utilizing these antagonists and other approaches indicate that the (pro)renin receptor mediates a variety of effects at several sites (Figure 17–4). The receptor may be of pathologic significance in hypertension, metabolic syndrome, diabetes, and other disorders.

Note that the concentration of prorenin required to activate (pro)renin receptors is higher than that occurring under physiologic conditions.

INHIBITION OF THE RENIN-ANGIOTENSIN SYSTEM

In view of the importance of the renin-angiotensin system in heart failure, hypertension, renal, and other diseases, considerable effort has been directed to developing drugs that inhibit it. A wide variety of agents that block the formation or action of ANG II are now available. Some of these drugs block renin release, but most inhibit the enzymatic action of renin, inhibit the conversion of ANG I to ANG II **(ACE inhibitors),** or block angiotensin AT_1 receptors (angiotensin receptor blockers, **ARBs**).

Drugs That Block Renin Release

Drugs that block the sympathetic nervous system inhibit the release of renin. Examples are propranolol and other β-adrenoceptor-blocking drugs, which act by blocking the renal β receptors that mediate the sympathetic control of renin release.

Renin Inhibitors

Cleavage of angiotensinogen by renin (see Figures 17–1 and 17–3) is the rate-limiting step in the formation of ANG II and thus represents a logical target for inhibition of the renin-angiotensin system. Several nonpeptide, low-molecular-weight, orally active inhibitors are available. **Aliskiren** was the first nonpeptide renin inhibitor to be approved for the treatment of hypertension. In healthy subjects, aliskiren produces dose-dependent reductions in plasma renin activity and plasma ANG I, ANG II, and aldosterone concentrations. In patients with hypertension, some of whom have elevated plasma renin levels, aliskiren suppresses plasma renin activity and causes dose-related reductions in blood pressure similar to or larger than those produced by ACE inhibitors and ARBs (see below). The safety and tolerability of aliskiren are comparable to ARBs. It does not increase bradykinin levels and does not cause cough or angioedema. However, despite its effectiveness in decreasing blood pressure, it has not been shown to reduce mortality or cardiovascular outcomes. Aliskiren is contraindicated in pregnancy.

Inhibition of the renin-angiotensin system with ACE inhibitors or ARBs may be incomplete because the drugs disrupt the negative feedback action of ANG II on renin release and thereby increase plasma renin activity. Other antihypertensive drugs, notably hydrochlorothiazide and other diuretics, also increase plasma renin activity. Aliskiren not only decreases baseline plasma renin activity in hypertensive subjects, but also eliminates the rise produced by ACE inhibitors, ARBs, and diuretics, thereby enhancing their antihypertensive effects. For this reason, aliskiren has been used in combination with an ACE inhibitor or ARB. However, such dual blockade may not produce significant clinical benefit and may be associated with adverse effects.

Angiotensin-Converting Enzyme Inhibitors

Orally active ACE inhibitors are directed against the active site of ACE and are now extensively used. **Captopril** and **enalapril** are examples of the many ACE inhibitors that are available. These drugs differ in their structure and pharmacokinetics, but they are interchangeable in clinical use. ACE inhibitors decrease blood pressure without increasing heart rate and promote natriuresis. The absence of tachycardia results from resetting of the baroreflex to a lower pressure, the converse of the action of ANG II. This effectively enhances the antihypertensive action of ACE inhibitors (and other inhibitors of the renin-angiotensin system).

As described in Chapters 11 and 13, ACE inhibitors are effective in the treatment of hypertension, decrease morbidity and mortality in heart failure and left ventricular dysfunction after myocardial infarction, and delay the progression of diabetic nephropathy.

ACE inhibitors not only block the conversion of ANG I to ANG II but also inhibit the degradation of other substances, including bradykinin, substance P, and enkephalins. The action of ACE inhibitors to inhibit bradykinin metabolism contributes significantly to their hypotensive action (Figure 11–5); indeed, it has been proposed that increased bradykinin levels are more important than decreased ANG II levels. Bradykinin is apparently responsible for some adverse side effects, including cough and angioedema. These drugs are contraindicated in pregnancy because they cause fetal kidney damage.

Angiotensin Receptor Blockers

ANG II receptor blockers are now widely used. **Losartan, valsartan,** and several others are orally active, potent, and specific competitive antagonists at angiotensin AT_1 receptors. The efficacy of these drugs in hypertension is similar to that of ACE inhibitors, but they are associated with a lower incidence of cough. Like ACE inhibitors, ARBs slow the progression of diabetic nephropathy, and valsartan has been reported to decrease the incidence of diabetes in patients with impaired glucose tolerance. The antagonists are also effective in the treatment of heart failure and provide a useful alternative when ACE inhibitors are not well tolerated. ARBs are generally well tolerated but should not be used by patients with nondiabetic renal disease or in pregnancy. In addition, some ARBs may cause a syndrome known as sprue-like enteropathy.

Combination of ANG II receptor antagonists with a neprilysin inhibitor resulted in a new class of drugs with benefits in patients with hypertension and heart disease (see Clinical Role of Natriuretic Peptides, below).

Marfan syndrome is a connective tissue disorder associated with aortic disease and other abnormalities involving increased transforming growth factor-β (TGF-β) signaling. Since ANG II increases TGF-β levels, it was reasoned that blockade of the renin-angiotensin system might be beneficial in Marfan syndrome. Clinical studies indicate that the ARB losartan may be as effective as atenolol, the standard treatment for this syndrome. Topical administration of valsartan has been reported to enhance wound healing in diabetic mice and pigs, an action that may be mediated by AT_2 receptors (see above).

The currently available ARBs are selective for the AT_1 receptor. Since prolonged treatment with the drugs disinhibits renin release and increases circulating ANG II levels, there may be increased stimulation of AT_2 receptors. This may be significant in view of the evidence noted above that activation of the AT_2 receptor causes vasodilation and other beneficial effects. Indeed, a selective, orally active AT_2 *agonist*, **Compound 21** (C21), has been shown to produce several beneficial effects in animal models of cardiovascular disease. The drug is under clinical development and may represent the first of a new class of cardiovascular drugs.

The clinical benefits of ARBs are generally similar to those of renin inhibitors and ACE inhibitors, and it is not clear if any has significant advantages over the others.

Summary: Renin-Angiotensin System

The renin-angiotensin system is an important control system involved in the regulation of blood pressure, fluid and electrolyte balance, and other functions. Overactivity of this system has been implicated in hypertension, heart failure, and other diseases. Drugs that block the formation or actions of ANG II are used extensively in the treatment of these diseases.

More recent observations suggest that the system is even more complex than originally envisioned. Specifically, there is evidence for roles of ANG 1-7 and Ala^1-ANG 1-7, possibly acting via the Mas receptor; and for the (pro)renin receptor, acting via angiotensin-independent pathways. However, the significance of these findings remains to be defined.

VASOPRESSIN

Vasopressin **(arginine vasopressin, AVP; antidiuretic hormone, ADH)** plays an important role in the long-term control of blood pressure through its action on the kidney to increase water reabsorption. This and other aspects of the physiology of AVP are discussed in Chapters 15 and 37 and will not be reviewed here.

AVP also plays an important role in the regulation of arterial pressure by its vasoconstrictor action. Mutant mice lacking the gene for the V_{1a} receptor (see below) show significantly lower blood pressure compared with control mice. AVP increases total peripheral resistance when infused in doses less than those required to produce maximum urine concentration. Such doses do not normally increase arterial pressure because the vasopressor activity of the peptide is buffered by a reflex decrease in cardiac output. When the influence of this reflex is removed, eg, in shock, pressor sensitivity to AVP is greatly increased. Pressor sensitivity to AVP is also enhanced in patients with idiopathic orthostatic hypotension. Higher doses of AVP increase blood pressure even when baroreceptor reflexes are intact.

VASOPRESSIN RECEPTORS, AGONISTS, & ANTAGONISTS

Three subtypes of AVP receptors have been identified; all are G protein–coupled. V_{1a} receptors mediate the vasoconstrictor action of AVP; V_{1b} receptors mediate release of ACTH by pituitary corticotropes; and V_2 receptors mediate the antidiuretic action. V_{1a} effects are mediated by G_q activation of phospholipase C, formation of inositol trisphosphate, and increased intracellular calcium concentration. V_2 effects are mediated by G_s activation of adenylyl cyclase.

AVP analogs selective for vasoconstrictor or antidiuretic activity have been synthesized. The first specific V_1 vasoconstrictor agonist to be synthesized was [Phe^2, Ile^3, Orn^8]vasotocin. [Phe^2, Ile^8, Hgn^4, Orn(i-Pr)^8]vasopressin, or **selepressin,** is a newer short-acting selective V_{1a} receptor agonist. Selective V_2 antidiuretic analogs include 1-deamino[D-Arg^8]arginine vasopressin (dDAVP) and 1-deamino[Val^4, D-Arg^8]arginine vasopressin (dVDAVP).

AVP, often in combination with norepinephrine, has proved beneficial in the treatment of septic and other vasodilatory shock states, at least in part by virtue of its V1a agonist activity. Terlipressin (triglycyl lysine vasopressin), a synthetic vasopressin analog that is converted to lysine vasopressin in the body, also is effective. However, AVP and terlipressin also stimulate renal V2 receptors, and this may have undesirable effects. Therefore, interest has focused on the use of selepressin in septic shock. Two phase 2 trials are in progress, and preliminary results are positive. AVP in combination with methylprednisolone improves the return to spontaneous circulation in patients with in-hospital cardiac arrest.

Antagonists of the vasoconstrictor action of AVP also are available. The peptide antagonist d(CH2)$_5$[Tyr(Me)^2]AVP also has antioxytocic activity but does not antagonize the antidiuretic action of AVP. A related antagonist d(CH2)$_5$[Tyr(Me)^2 Dab^5]AVP lacks oxytocin antagonism but has less anti-V_1 activity. Nonpeptide, orally active V_{1a}-receptor antagonists have been developed, examples being **relcovaptan** and **SRX251.**

The V_{1a} antagonists have been particularly useful in revealing the important role that AVP plays in blood pressure regulation in situations such as dehydration and hemorrhage. They have potential as therapeutic agents for the treatment of such diverse conditions as Raynaud disease, hypertension, heart failure, brain edema, motion sickness, cancer, preterm labor, and anger management. To date, most studies have focused on heart failure; promising results have been obtained with V_2 antagonists such as **tolvaptan,** which is, however, currently approved only for use in hyponatremia. V_{1a} antagonists also have potential, and **conivaptan** (YM087), a drug with both V_{1a} and V_2 antagonist activity, has also been approved for treatment of hyponatremia (see Chapter 15).

ENDOTHELINS

The endothelium is the source of a variety of substances with vasodilator (PGI_2 and nitric oxide) and vasoconstrictor activities. The latter include the endothelin family, potent vasoconstrictor peptides that were first isolated from aortic endothelial cells.

Biosynthesis, Structure, & Clearance

Three isoforms of endothelin (ET) have been identified: the originally described ET, **ET-1,** and two similar peptides, **ET-2** and **ET-3.** Each isoform is a product of a different gene and is synthesized as a prepro form that is processed to a propeptide and then to the mature peptide. Processing to the mature peptides occurs through the action of endothelin-converting enzyme. Each ET is a 21-amino-acid peptide containing two disulfide bridges.

ETs are widely distributed in the body. ET-1 is the predominant ET secreted by the vascular endothelium. It is also produced by neurons and astrocytes in the central nervous system and in endometrial, renal mesangial, Sertoli, breast epithelial, and other cells. ET-2 is produced predominantly in the kidneys and intestine, whereas ET-3 is found in highest concentration in the brain but is also present in the gastrointestinal tract, lungs, and kidneys. ETs are present in the blood in low concentration; they appear to act in a paracrine or autocrine fashion rather than as circulating hormones.

The expression of the ET-1 gene is increased by growth factors and cytokines, including TGF-β and interleukin 1 (IL-1), vasoactive substances including ANG II and AVP, and mechanical stress. Expression is inhibited by nitric oxide, prostacyclin, and ANP.

Clearance of ETs from the circulation is rapid and involves both enzymatic degradation by neprilysin and clearance by the ET_B receptor.

Actions

Two ET receptor subtypes, termed $\mathbf{ET_A}$ and $\mathbf{ET_B}$, are widely distributed in the body. ET_A receptors have a high affinity for ET-1 and a low affinity for ET-3 and are located on smooth muscle cells, where they mediate vasoconstriction (see Figure 17–5). ET_B receptors have approximately equal affinities for ET-1 and ET-3

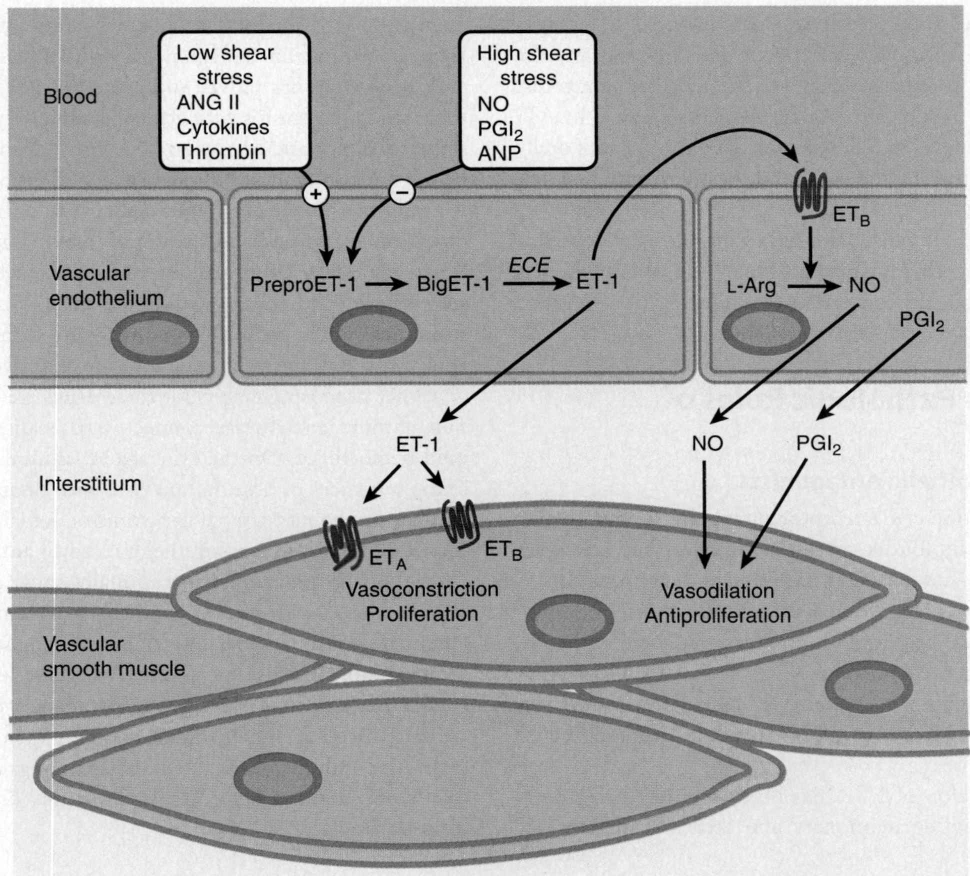

FIGURE 17–5 Generation of endothelin-1 (ET-1) in the vascular endothelium, and its direct and indirect effects on smooth muscle cells mediated by ET_A and ET_B receptors. ANG II, angiotensin II; ANP, atrial natriuretic peptide; Arg, arginine; BigET-1, proET-1; ECE, endothelial-converting enzyme; NO, nitric oxide; PreproET-1, precursor of BigET-1; PGI_2, prostaglandin I_2.

and are primarily located on vascular endothelial cells, where they mediate release of PGI_2 and nitric oxide. Some ET_B receptors are also present on smooth muscle cells and mediate vasoconstriction. The ET_B-induced release of nitric oxide and PGI_2 and resulting vasodilation serve to counterbalance the ET_A (and ET_B)-induced vasoconstriction. Both receptor subtypes belong to the G protein–coupled seven-transmembrane domain family of receptors.

ETs exert widespread actions in the body. In particular, they cause potent dose-dependent vasoconstriction in most vascular beds. Intravenous administration of ET-1 causes a rapid and transient decrease in arterial blood pressure followed by a sustained increase. The depressor response results from release of PGI_2 and nitric oxide from the vascular endothelium, whereas the pressor response is due to direct contraction of vascular smooth muscle. ETs also exert direct positive inotropic and chronotropic actions on the heart and are potent coronary vasoconstrictors. They act on the kidneys to cause vasoconstriction and decrease glomerular filtration rate and sodium and water excretion. In the respiratory system, they cause potent contraction of tracheal and bronchial smooth muscle. ETs interact with several endocrine systems, increasing the secretion of renin, aldosterone, AVP, and ANP. They exert a variety of actions on the central and peripheral nervous systems, the gastrointestinal system, the liver, the urinary tract, the reproductive system, eye, skeleton, and skin. ET-1 is a potent mitogen for vascular smooth muscle cells, cardiac myocytes, and glomerular mesangial cells.

The signal transduction mechanisms triggered by binding of ET-1 to its vascular receptors include stimulation of phospholipase C, formation of inositol trisphosphate, and release of calcium from the endoplasmic reticulum, which results in vasoconstriction. Conversely, stimulation of PGI_2 and nitric oxide synthesis results in decreased intracellular calcium concentration and vasodilation.

INHIBITORS OF ENDOTHELIN SYNTHESIS & ACTION

The ET system can be blocked with receptor antagonists and by drugs that block endothelin-converting enzyme. ET_A or ET_B receptors can be blocked selectively, or both can be blocked with nonselective ET_A-ET_B antagonists.

Bosentan is a nonselective ET receptor antagonist. It is active orally and blocks both the initial transient depressor (ET_B) and the prolonged pressor (ET_A) responses to intravenous ET. A newer dual endothelin receptor antagonist, **macitentan,** was developed by modifying the structure of bosentan. Additional ET receptor antagonists with increased selectivity include the ET_A antagonists **ambrisentan,** with ET_A selectivity, and **sitaxsentan,** the most selective ET_A antagonist. A novel ET receptor antagonist is **sparsentan**. It is made by merging elements present in AT_1 antagonists with elements in ET_A receptors, and it is the first orally active antagonist with ET_A and AT_1 receptor antagonist activities in a single compound.

The formation of ETs can be blocked by inhibiting endothelin-converting enzyme with **phosphoramidon**. Phosphoramidon is not specific for endothelin-converting enzyme, but more selective inhibitors including CGS35066 are available.

Physiologic & Pathologic Roles of Endothelin

A. Effects of Endothelin Antagonists

Systemic administration of ET receptor antagonists or endothelin-converting enzyme inhibitors causes vasodilation and decreases arterial pressure in humans and experimental animals. Intra-arterial administration of the drugs also causes slow-onset vasodilation in humans. These observations provide evidence that the ET system participates in the regulation of vascular tone under resting conditions. The activity of the system is higher in males than in females. It increases with age, an effect that can be counteracted by regular aerobic exercise.

Increased production of ET-1 has been implicated in a variety of diseases, including pulmonary and arterial hypertension, renal disease, diabetes, cancer, heart failure, and atherosclerosis. Indeed, endothelin antagonism with bosentan, ambrisentan, and macitentan has proved to be an effective and generally well-tolerated treatment for patients with pulmonary arterial hypertension, an important condition with few effective treatments (see Box: The Treatment of Pulmonary Hypertension). Hepatotoxicity is a known side effect of endothelin antagonists but is generally dose-related and reversible. Cases of idiosyncratic hepatitis resulting in acute liver failure leading to death have been reported with **sitaxsentan,** and it was withdrawn in 2010. Endothelins have structures similar to snake venom toxins (safarotoxins), and ET antagonists have been proposed for use as antivenoms.

Other promising targets for these drugs are resistant hypertension, chronic renal disease, connective tissue disease, and subarachnoid hemorrhage. On the other hand, clinical trials of the drugs in the treatment of heart failure have been disappointing. Thus, at present, pulmonary arterial hypertension remains the only clinical condition approved for endothelin receptor antagonists.

Endothelin antagonists occasionally cause systemic hypotension, increased heart rate, facial flushing or edema, and headaches. Potential gastrointestinal effects include nausea, vomiting, and constipation. Because of their teratogenic effects, endothelin antagonists are contraindicated in pregnancy. Bosentan has been associated with fatal hepatotoxicity, and patients taking this drug must have monthly liver function tests. Negative pregnancy test results are required before prescribing this drug for women of child-bearing age.

The Treatment of Pulmonary Hypertension

Idiopathic pulmonary arterial hypertension (PAH) is a progressive and potentially fatal condition; signs and symptoms include dyspnea, chest pain, syncope, cardiac arrhythmias, and right heart failure. Epithelial damage and abnormal fibroblast activity has been implicated in its genesis. Continuous nasal oxygen supplementation is required for most patients and anticoagulants are commonly used. Medical treatments directed at elevated pulmonary vascular resistance have been less successful than those used in ordinary hypertension (see Chapter 11). In addition to the endothelin antagonists mentioned in the text (**bosentan, ambrisentan,** and **macitentan** are approved for use in PAH), vasoactive agents that have been promoted for PAH include prostaglandins (epoprostenol, treprostinil, iloprost), nitric oxide, PDE-5 inhibitors (sildenafil, tadalafil), and Ca^{2+} channel blockers (nifedipine, amlodipine, diltiazem). **Riociguat,** a small-molecule activator of soluble guanylyl cyclase, increases cGMP independently of nitric oxide, reduces pulmonary vascular pressure, and increases exercise duration. Riociguat was approved in the USA in 2013. **Selexipag** is an oral nonprostanoid prodrug that is rapidly hydrolyzed to the selective prostaglandin I receptor agonist ACT-333679. It has a mechanism of action similar to prostacyclin and was approved in 2015 (see Chapter 18). It is extraordinarily expensive. **Fasudil** is an investigational selective RhoA/Rho kinase (ROCK) inhibitor that appears to reduce pulmonary artery pressure in PAH. In vitro evidence suggests that certain serum proteins may inhibit abnormal fibroblast activity. **Pirfenidone** and **nintedanib** inhibit growth factors involved in connective tissue proliferation and are approved for use in acute exacerbations of PAH. In a preliminary study, recombinant human **pentraxin 2** slowed the decline in lung function in patients with idiopathic pulmonary fibrosis. Surgical treatment for advanced disease includes creation of a right atrial to left atrial shunt and lung transplantation.

B. Dual Inhibitors of Endothelin-Converting Enzyme and Neprilysin

A newer strategy uses combined inhibition of endothelin-converting enzyme and neprilysin. **Daglutril** (SLV306) is a prodrug that is converted to the active metabolite KC-12625, a mixed inhibitor of endothelin-converting enzyme and neprilysin. Thus, it simultaneously inhibits the formation of ET and the breakdown of natriuretic peptides. Daglutril appears to be well tolerated with few or none of the side effects on liver function and edema observed with endothelin antagonists. It has been shown to have beneficial effects in heart failure and to lower blood pressure in patients with type 2 diabetes and nephropathy.

NEUROPEPTIDE Y

The neuropeptide Y family is a multiligand/multireceptor system consisting of three polypeptide agonists that bind and activate four distinct receptors with different affinity and potency. The peptides are **pancreatic polypeptide (PP), peptide YY (PYY),** and **neuropeptide Y (NPY).** Each peptide consists of 36 amino acids and has an amidated C-terminus. PP is secreted by the islets of Langerhans after food ingestion in proportion to the caloric content and appears to act mainly in the brainstem and vagus to promote appetite suppression, inhibit gastric emptying, and increase energy expenditure; it also exerts direct actions in the gut. PYY is released by entero-endocrine L cells of the distal gut in proportion to food intake and produces anorexigenic effects.

NPY is one of the most abundant neuropeptides in both the central and peripheral nervous systems. Whereas PYY and PP act as neurohormones, NPY acts as a neurotransmitter. In the sympathetic nervous system, NPY is frequently localized in noradrenergic neurons and apparently functions both as a vasoconstrictor and as a cotransmitter with norepinephrine. The remainder of this section focuses on NPY.

NPY produces a variety of central nervous system effects, including increased feeding (it is one of the most potent orexigenic molecules in the brain), hypotension, hypothermia, respiratory depression, and activation of the hypothalamic-pituitary-adrenal axis. Other effects include constriction of cerebral blood vessels, positive chronotropic and inotropic actions on the heart, and hypertension. The peptide is a potent renal vasoconstrictor, suppresses renin secretion, and can cause diuresis and natriuresis. Prejunctional neuronal actions include inhibition of transmitter release from sympathetic and parasympathetic nerves. Vascular actions include direct vasoconstriction, potentiation of the action of vasoconstrictors, and inhibition of the action of vasodilators. NPY promotes angiogenesis and cardiomyocyte remodeling.

The diverse effects of NPY (and PP and PYY) are mediated by four subtypes of NPY receptors designated Y_1, Y_2, Y_4, and Y_5. All are G_i protein–coupled receptors linked to mobilization of Ca^{2+} and inhibition of adenylyl cyclase. Y_1, Y_2, and Y_5 receptors are of most importance in the cardiovascular and other peripheral effects of the peptide. Y_4 receptors have a high affinity for pancreatic polypeptide and may be a receptor for the pancreatic peptide rather than for NPY. Y_5 receptors are found mainly in the central nervous system and may be involved in the control of food intake. They also mediate the activation of the hypothalamic-pituitary-adrenal axis by NPY.

Some selective nonpeptide NPY receptor antagonists are available for research. The first nonpeptide Y_1 receptor antagonist, BIBP3226, is also the most thoroughly studied. It has a short half-life in vivo. In animal models, it blocks the vasoconstrictor and pressor responses to NPY. Structurally related Y_1 antagonists include BIB03304 and H409/22; the latter has been tested in humans. SR120107A and SR120819A are orally active Y_1 antagonists and have a long duration of action. BIIE0246 is the first nonpeptide antagonist selective for the Y_2 receptor; it does not cross the blood-brain barrier. Useful Y_4 antagonists are not available. The Y_5 antagonists MK-0557 and S-2367 have been tested in clinical trials for obesity.

These drugs have been useful in analyzing the role of NPY in cardiovascular regulation. It now appears that the peptide is not important in the regulation of hemodynamics under normal resting conditions but may play a role in cardiovascular disorders including hypertension, atherosclerosis, myocardial ischemia and infarction, arrhythmias, and heart failure. Other studies have implicated NPY in eating disorders, obesity, alcoholism, anxiety, depression, epilepsy, pain, cancer, and bone physiology. Y_1 and particularly Y_5 receptor antagonists may have potential as antiobesity agents.

UROTENSIN

Urotensin II (UII) was originally identified in fish, but isoforms are now known to be present in the human and other mammalian species. Human UII is an 11-amino-acid peptide. An eight-amino-acid peptide, UII-related peptide (URP), which is almost identical to the C-terminal of UII, has also been identified. Major sites of UII expression in humans include the central nervous system, cardiovascular system, lungs, liver, and endocrine glands including the pituitary, pancreas, and adrenal. UII is also present in plasma, and potential sources of this circulating peptide include the heart, lungs, liver, and kidneys. The stimulus to UII release has not been identified, but increased blood pressure has been implicated in some studies.

In vitro, UII is a potent constrictor of vascular smooth muscle; its activity depends on the type of blood vessel and the species from which the vessel was obtained. Vasoconstriction occurs primarily in arterial vessels, where UII can be more potent than ET-1, making it the most potent known vasoconstrictor. However, under some conditions, UII may cause vasodilation. In vivo, UII has complex hemodynamic effects, the most prominent being regional vasoconstriction and cardiac depression. In some ways, these effects resemble those produced by ET-1. Nevertheless, the role of the peptide in the normal regulation of vascular tone and blood pressure in humans appears to be minor. In addition to its cardiovascular effects, UII exerts osmoregulatory actions, induces collagen and fibronectin accumulation, modulates the inflammatory response, and inhibits glucose-induced insulin release.

The actions of UII are mediated by a G_q protein–coupled receptor referred to as the UT receptor. UT receptors are widely distributed in the brain, spinal cord, heart, vascular smooth muscle, skeletal muscle, and pancreas. They are located at the cell surface, but specific UII-binding sites have also been observed in heart and brain cell nuclei. Some effects of the peptide including vasoconstriction are mediated by the phospholipase C, inositol trisphosphate, and diacylglycerol signal transduction pathway.

Although UII appears to play only a minor role in health, there is some evidence that it is involved in cardiovascular and other diseases. In particular, it has been reported that plasma UII levels are increased in hypertension, heart failure, atherosclerosis, diabetes mellitus, and renal failure. For this reason, the development of UII receptor antagonists was of considerable interest. **Urantide** ("urotensin antagonist peptide") is a penicillamine-substituted derivative of UII. **Palosuran** is an orally active nonpeptide antagonist of the UII receptor. It has displayed beneficial effects in animal models of renal failure but not in hypertensive patients with type 2 diabetic nephropathy. More potent UII antagonists are available. GSK1440115 has undergone phase 1 testing for the treatment of asthma but was found to be ineffective. Thus, the role of UII in disease remains to be defined.

VASODILATORS

■ KININS

BIOSYNTHESIS OF KININS

Kinins are potent vasodilator peptides formed enzymatically by the action of enzymes known as kallikreins acting on protein substrates called kininogens. The kallikrein-kinin system has several features in common with the renin-angiotensin system.

Kallikreins

Kallikreins are serine proteases present in plasma (plasma kallikrein) and in several organs (tissue kallikrein), including the kidneys, pancreas, intestine, sweat glands, and salivary glands. The two groups are secreted as zymogens and are activated by proteolytic cleavage. Plasma prekallikrein is activated by activated blood coagulation factor XII (FXIIa). The two groups differ in their gene structure, molecular weight, substrate specificity, and kinin produced. Kallikreins can convert prorenin to active renin, but the physiologic significance of this action is not known.

Kininogens

Kininogens—the substrates for kallikreins and precursors of kinins—are present in plasma, lymph, and interstitial fluid. Two kininogens are present in plasma: a low-molecular-weight form (LMW kininogen) and a high-molecular-weight form (HMW kininogen). The two forms result from differential splicing of the kininogen gene to generate proteins that differ at the C-terminus. About 15–20% of the total plasma kininogen is in the HMW form. It is thought that LMW kininogen crosses capillary walls and serves as the substrate for tissue kallikreins, whereas HMW kininogen is confined to the bloodstream and serves as the substrate for plasma kallikrein.

FORMATION & METABOLISM OF KININS

The pathway for the formation and metabolism of kinins is shown in Figure 17–6. The two major kinins in humans are **bradykinin** and **Lys-bradykinin** or **kallidin.** Bradykinin is released from HMW kininogen by plasma kallikrein, whereas kallidin is released from LMW kininogen by tissue kallikrein. Kallidin can be converted to bradykinin by an arginine aminopeptidase. The two kinins are present in plasma and urine. Bradykinin is the predominant kinin in plasma, whereas Lys-bradykinin is the major urinary form.

Kinins are metabolized rapidly (half-life < 15 seconds) by nonspecific exopeptidases or endopeptidases, commonly referred to as kininases. Two plasma kininases have been characterized. Kininase I, apparently synthesized in the liver, is a carboxypeptidase that releases the carboxyl terminal arginine residue. Kininase II is present in plasma and vascular endothelial cells throughout the body. It is identical to angiotensin-converting enzyme (ACE, peptidyl dipeptidase), discussed above. Kininase II inactivates kinins by cleaving the carboxyl terminal dipeptide phenylalanyl-arginine. Like angiotensin I, bradykinin is almost completely hydrolyzed during a single passage through the pulmonary vascular bed.

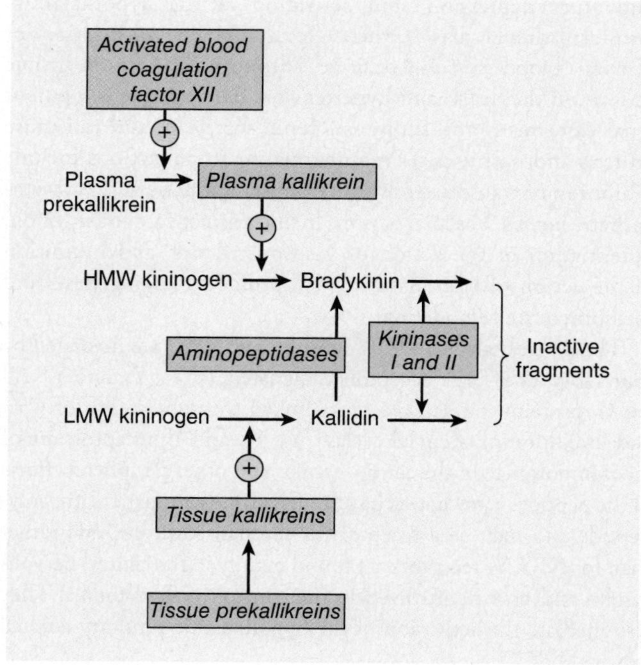

FIGURE 17–6 The kallikrein-kinin system. Kininase II is identical to converting enzyme peptidyl dipeptidase (ACE). Kallidin, lys-bradykinin.

PHYSIOLOGIC & PATHOLOGIC EFFECTS OF KININS

Effects on the Cardiovascular System

Kinins produce marked arteriolar dilation in several vascular beds, including the heart, skeletal muscle, kidney, liver, and intestine. In this respect, kinins are approximately 10 times more potent on a molar basis than histamine. The vasodilation may result from a direct inhibitory effect of kinins on arteriolar smooth muscle or may be mediated by the release of nitric oxide or vasodilator prostaglandins such as PGE_2 and PGI_2. In contrast, the predominant effect of kinins on veins is contraction; again, this may result from direct stimulation of venous smooth muscle or from the release of venoconstrictor prostaglandins such as $PGF_{2\alpha}$. Kinins also produce contraction of most visceral smooth muscle.

When injected intravenously, kinins produce a rapid but brief fall in blood pressure that is due to their arteriolar vasodilator action. Intravenous infusions of the peptide fail to produce a sustained decrease in blood pressure; prolonged hypotension can only be produced by progressively increasing the rate of infusion. The rapid reversibility of the hypotensive response to kinins is due primarily to reflex increases in heart rate, myocardial contractility, and cardiac output. In some species, bradykinin produces a biphasic change in blood pressure—an initial hypotensive response followed by an increase above the preinjection level. The increase in blood pressure may be due to a reflex activation of the sympathetic nervous system, but under some conditions, bradykinin can directly release catecholamines from the adrenal medulla and stimulate sympathetic ganglia. Bradykinin also increases blood pressure when injected into the central nervous system, but the physiologic significance of this effect is not clear, since it is unlikely that kinins cross the blood-brain barrier. (Note, however, that bradykinin can increase the permeability of the blood-brain barrier to some other substances.) Kinins have no consistent effect on sympathetic or parasympathetic nerve endings.

The arteriolar dilation produced by kinins causes an increase in pressure and flow in the capillary bed, thus favoring efflux of fluid from blood to tissues. This effect may be facilitated by increased capillary permeability resulting from contraction of endothelial cells and widening of intercellular junctions, and by increased venous pressure secondary to constriction of veins. As a result of these changes, water and solutes pass from the blood to the extracellular fluid, lymph flow increases, and edema may result.

The role that endogenous kinins play in the regulation of blood pressure is not clear. They do not appear to participate in the control of blood pressure under resting conditions but may play a role in postexercise hypotension.

Effects on Endocrine & Exocrine Glands

As noted earlier, prekallikreins and kallikreins are present in several glands, including the pancreas, kidney, intestine, salivary glands, and sweat glands, and they can be released into the secretory fluids of these glands. The function of the enzymes in these tissues is not known. Since kinins have such marked effects on smooth muscle, they may modulate the tone of salivary and pancreatic ducts, help regulate gastrointestinal motility, and act as local modulators of blood flow. Kinins also influence the transepithelial transport of water, electrolytes, glucose, and amino acids, and may regulate the transport of these substances in the gastrointestinal tract and kidney. Finally, kallikreins may play a role in the physiologic activation of certain prohormones, including proinsulin and prorenin.

Role in Inflammation & Pain

Bradykinin has long been known to produce the four classic symptoms of inflammation—redness, local heat, swelling, and pain. Kinins are rapidly generated after tissue injury and play a pivotal role in the development and maintenance of these inflammatory processes.

Kinins are potent pain-producing substances when applied to a blister base or injected intradermally. They elicit pain by stimulating nociceptive afferents in the skin and viscera.

Role in Hereditary Angioedema

Hereditary angioedema is a rare autosomal dominant disorder that results from deficiency or dysfunction of the C1 esterase inhibitor (C1-INH), a major inhibitor of proteases of the complement, coagulation, and kallikrein-kinin systems. C1-INH deficiency results in activation of kallikrein and increased formation of bradykinin, which by increasing vascular permeability and other actions causes recurrent episodes of angioedema of the airways, gastrointestinal tract, extremities, and genitalia, which can be debilitating. Hereditary angioedema can be treated with drugs that inhibit the formation or actions of bradykinin (see below).

Other Roles of Kinins

Kinins have been implicated in acute inflammatory diseases including septic shock, acute lung injury, and respiratory distress syndrome. They also appear to participate in chronic inflammatory diseases including vasculitis, inflammatory autoimmune disease, neuroinflammation, and cancer. On the other hand, kinins may play a protective role in certain cardiovascular diseases and ischemic stroke-induced brain injury. These effects are largely mediated by B_1 receptors.

KININ RECEPTORS & MECHANISMS OF ACTION

The biologic actions of kinins are mediated by specific receptors located on the membranes of the target tissues. Two types of kinin receptors, termed B_1 and B_2, have been defined based on the rank orders of agonist potencies; both are G protein–coupled receptors. (Note that B here stands for bradykinin, not for β adrenoceptor.) Bradykinin displays the highest affinity in most B_2 receptor systems, followed by Lys-bradykinin. One exception is the B_2 receptor that mediates contraction of venous smooth muscle; this appears to be more sensitive to Lys-bradykinin.

There is little expression of B_1 receptors under normal physiological conditions, but they are rapidly and highly upregulated following tissue injury, infection, or other inflammatory stimuli. They appear to be involved in the pathogenesis of some inflammatory diseases. By contrast, B_2 receptors are constitutively expressed in multiple tissues and have a widespread distribution that is consistent with the multiple effects mediated by these receptors.

B_1 and B_2 receptors belong to the G protein–coupled superfamily. Agonist binding activates phospholipase C and sets in motion multiple intracellular signaling events including mobilization of Ca^{2+}; generation of diacylglycerol, NO, and prostaglandins; and activation of MAPK. Stimulation of B_1 receptors can induce proliferative effects through ERK1/2 activation, but can also exert antiproliferative actions.

DRUGS AFFECTING THE KALLIKREIN-KININ SYSTEM

Drugs that modify the activity of the kallikrein-kinin system are available. Considerable effort has been directed toward developing kinin receptor antagonists, since such drugs have considerable therapeutic potential as anti-inflammatory and antinociceptive agents. Competitive antagonists of both B_1 and B_2 receptors are available for research use. Examples of B_1 receptor antagonists are the peptides [Leu^8-des-Arg^9]bradykinin and Lys[Leu^8-des-Arg^9] bradykinin. The first B_2 receptor antagonists to be discovered were also peptide derivatives of bradykinin. These first-generation antagonists were used extensively in animal studies of kinin receptor pharmacology. However, their half-life is short, they are not orally active, and they are almost inactive on the human B_2 receptor.

Icatibant (Firazyr) is a second-generation B_2 receptor antagonist. It is a decapeptide with an affinity for the B_2 receptor similar to that of bradykinin and acts as a competitive highly selective antagonist of these receptors. It is absorbed rapidly after subcutaneous administration. Icatibant is effective in the treatment of hereditary angioedema and can be self-administered at home. It may also be useful in other conditions including drug-induced angioedema, airway disease, thermal injury, ascites, and pancreatitis.

A third generation of B_2 receptor antagonists has been developed; examples are **FR 173657, FR 172357,** and **NPC 18884.** These antagonists are orally active nonpeptides with longer half-lives. They have been reported to inhibit bradykinin-induced bronchoconstriction in guinea pigs, carrageenan-induced inflammation in rats, and capsaicin-induced nociception in mice. These antagonists have promise for the treatment of inflammatory pain in humans.

SSR240612 is a newer, potent, selective, and orally active antagonist of B_1 receptors in humans and several animal species. It reduces obesity in diabetic rats and has analgesic and anti-inflammatory activities in mice and rats. It entered preclinical studies for the treatment of inflammatory and neurogenic pain, but its development was discontinued.

The synthesis of kinins can be inhibited with the kallikrein inhibitor **aprotinin.** Kinin synthesis can also be inhibited by two preparations of human plasma C1-INH, **cinryze** and **berinert,** and these are used for the intravenous prophylaxis or treatment of hereditary angioedema. **Ecallantide,** a more recently developed recombinant plasma kallikrein inhibitor, also is effective. It is more potent and selective than C1-INH and can be administered by subcutaneous injection. **Lanadelumab,** an antibody that inhibits plasma kallikrein, has shown promise in early clinical trials. **Donidalorsen** is a modified antisense oligonucleotide designed to inhibit the production of plasma prekallikrien (see Figure 17–6). In small phase 1 and 2 trials, donidalorsen decreased plasma prekallikrein activity and decreased the incidence of angioedema attacks.

Actions of kinins mediated by prostaglandin generation can be blocked nonspecifically with inhibitors of prostaglandin synthesis such as aspirin. Conversely, the actions of kinins can be enhanced with ACE inhibitors, which block the degradation of the peptides. Indeed, as noted above, inhibition of bradykinin metabolism by ACE inhibitors contributes significantly to their antihypertensive action.

Selective B_2 agonists are under study and have been shown to be effective in some animal models of human cardiovascular disease. These drugs have potential for the treatment of hypertension, myocardial hypertrophy, and other diseases.

■ NATRIURETIC PEPTIDES

Synthesis & Structure

The atria and other tissues of mammals contain a family of peptides with natriuretic, diuretic, vasorelaxant, and other properties. The family includes atrial natriuretic peptide (ANP), brain natriuretic peptide (BNP), and C-type natriuretic peptide (CNP). The peptides share a common 17-amino-acid disulfide ring with variable C- and N-terminals. A fourth peptide, urodilatin, has the same structure as ANP with an extension of four amino acids at the N-terminal. The renal effects of these peptides are discussed in Chapter 15.

ANP is derived from the carboxyl terminal end of a common precursor termed preproANP. ANP is synthesized primarily in cardiac atrial cells, but it is also synthesized in ventricular myocardium, by neurons in the central and peripheral nervous systems, and in the lungs. A fragment of proANP, known as mid-regional proANP (MR-proANP), is released into the circulation where it is more stable than mature ANP and is considered to be a better measure of ANP production. The most important stimulus to the release of ANP from the heart is atrial stretch via mechanosensitive ion channels. ANP release is increased by volume expansion, changing from the standing to the supine position, rapid atrial pacing, and exercise. ANP release is also increased by sympathetic stimulation via α_{1A} adrenoceptors, endothelins via the ET_A-receptor subtype (see below), glucocorticoids, ANG II, and AVP. Plasma ANP concentration increases in several pathologic states, including heart failure, atrial fibrillation, primary aldosteronism, chronic renal failure, and inappropriate ADH secretion syndrome.

Administration of ANP increases sodium excretion and urine flow. The ANP-induced natriuresis is due both to an increase in glomerular filtration rate and a decrease in proximal tubular sodium reabsorption. ANP inhibits the release of renin, aldosterone, and AVP, which would further increase sodium and water excretion. ANP also causes vasodilation, decreases arterial blood pressure, and modulates the baroreceptor reflex control of heart rate. Suppression of ANP production or blockade of its action impairs the natriuretic response to volume expansion, and increases blood pressure. In the longer term, ANP exerts antihypertrophic and antifibrotic actions. It also participates in the regulation of body metabolism, increasing lipolysis and lipid oxidation, adiponectin levels, and insulin sensitivity.

Like ANP, BNP is synthesized in the heart, but primarily in the ventricles. Also like ANP, the release of BNP appears to be volume related; indeed, the two peptides may be co-secreted. BNP exhibits natriuretic, diuretic, and hypotensive activities similar to those of ANP but circulates at a lower concentration. An N-terminal fragment of proBNP **(NT-proBNP)** is inactive but its level in plasma provides a useful index of BNP release.

Unlike ANP and BNP, CNP is expressed mainly in the vascular endothelium. It is also present in the brain, heart, chondrocytes, kidneys, and intestine. CNP levels in the circulation are low but increase in some disease states. CNP has less natriuretic and diuretic activity than ANP and BNP but is a potent vasodilator and may play a role in the regulation of peripheral resistance. It is also a potent stimulus to endochondral ossification, an action that is utilized for the treatment of children with achondroplasia (see below).

Factors that affect plasma natriuretic peptide levels include age, gender, ethnicity, and genetic variants, as well as several cardiac and noncardiac disorders.

Urodilatin is synthesized in the distal tubules of the kidneys by alternative processing of the ANP precursor. It elicits potent natriuresis and diuresis, and thereby functions as a paracrine regulator of sodium and water excretion. It also relaxes vascular smooth muscle.

In summary, the natriuretic peptide system can be regarded as a physiological regulator of blood volume, being released in response to volume expansion and in turn acting to cause natriuresis, diuresis, and vasodilation.

Pharmacodynamics & Pharmacokinetics

The biologic actions of the natriuretic peptides are mediated through association with specific high-affinity receptors located on the surface of the target cells (Figure 17–7). Three receptor subtypes termed **NPR-A** (ANP-A), **NPR-B** (ANP-B), and **NPR-C** (ANP-C) have been identified. The NPR-A and NPR-B receptors contain guanylyl cyclase at their intracellular domains. The primary ligands of the NPR-A receptor are ANP and BNP. The NPR-B receptor is similar in structure to the ANP-A receptor, but its primary ligand appears to be CNP. The NPR-C receptor may be coupled to adenylyl cyclase or phospholipase C; it binds all three natriuretic peptides and functions as a clearance receptor.

The natriuretic peptides have a short half-life in the circulation. They are metabolized in the kidneys, liver, and lungs by the ubiquitous neutral endopeptidase **neprilysin,** which is also responsible for the breakdown of other vasoactive peptides including bradykinin, adrenomedullin, endothelin, and ANG II. Urodilatin is more resistant to neprilysin than the other natriuretic peptides and therefore has a longer duration of action. Inhibition of neprilysin results in increases in circulating levels of the natriuretic peptides and, in turn, natriuresis and diuresis. The peptides are also removed from the circulation by binding to ANP-C receptors in the vascular endothelium. This receptor binds the natriuretic peptides with equal affinity. The receptor and bound peptide are

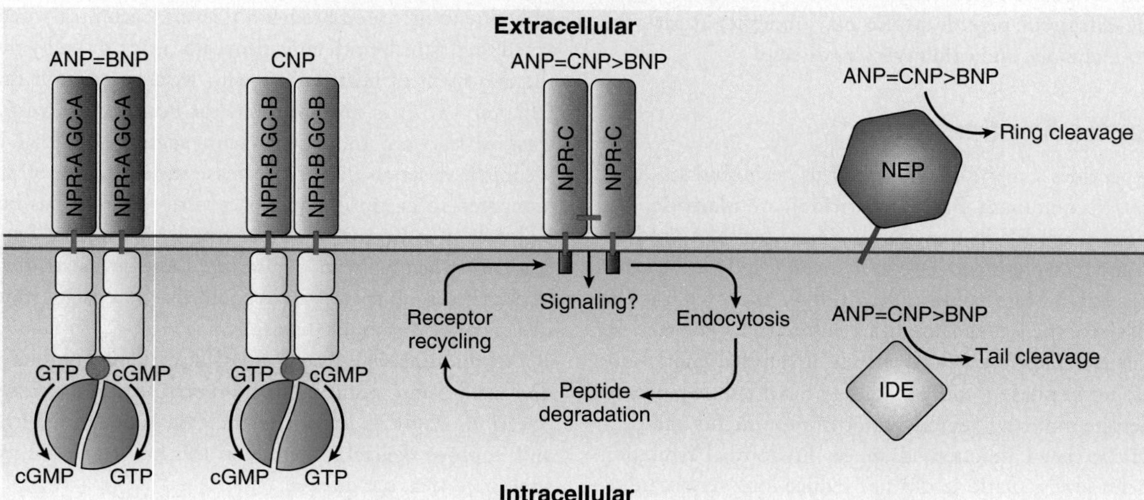

FIGURE 17–7 Natriuretic hormone receptors, intracellular signaling, and degradation processes. The expression above each receptor indicates the relative affinities of the three peptides, ANP, BNP, and CNP. GC-A, guanylate cyclase type A; GC-B, guanylate cyclase type B; IDE, insulin degrading enzyme; NEP, neprilysin. (Adapted from Volpe M, Carnovali M, Mastromarino V: The natriuretic peptides system in the pathophysiology of heart failure: From molecular basis to treatment, Clin Sci. 2016 Jan;130(2):57-77.)

internalized, the peptide is degraded enzymatically, and the receptor is returned to the cell surface.

CLINICAL ROLE OF NATRIURETIC PEPTIDES

In heart failure, release of ANP and BNP is increased in response to cardiac stretch. This represents a compensatory response that ultimately fails to prevent the sodium and water retention caused by activation of the renin-angiotensin and other neurohormonal systems. The increases in ANP and BNP are proportional to the severity of the disease, and measurement of their plasma levels (or MR-proANP or NT-proBNP) has significant diagnostic and prognostic value. Indeed, BNP and NT-proBNP are regarded by some as the gold standard for the diagnosis and stratification of heart failure, and their use is recommended by ACC/AHA guidelines.

Atrial fibrillation (AFib) is the most common cardiac arrhythmia and an important risk factor for ischemic stroke. Plasma natriuretic peptide levels are frequently increased in patients with AFib and an association between elevated ANP and the incidence of AFib and stroke has been reported. It has been recommended that natriuretic peptide, MR-proANP, or NT-proBNP levels be measured as part of the routine evaluation of patients with AFib. Successful treatment of AFib with catheter ablation is accompanied by decreased plasma ANP, and pretreatment plasma ANP may predict the effectiveness of the treatment. Increased release of natriuretic peptides during AFib may cause natriuresis and diuresis.

As noted above, ANP and BNP participate in the regulation of whole body metabolism. Furthermore, epidemiological studies suggest that these peptides are involved in some metabolic diseases. For example, natriuretic peptide deficiency may contribute to the etiology of obesity, metabolic syndrome, and type 2 diabetes. Thus the natriuretic peptide system may underlie, in part, the link between metabolic and cardiovascular disease.

Therapeutic Applications

Natriuretic peptides can be administered as recombinant ANP **(carperitide),** recombinant BNP **(nesiritide),** or **ularitide,** the synthetic form of urodilatin (see above). These peptides produce vasodilation and natriuresis and have been investigated for the treatment of congestive heart failure. Nesiritide is approved for the treatment of decompensated acute heart failure (see Chapter 13). Ularitide demonstrated beneficial effects in animal models of heart failure and in phase 1 and 2 studies in heart failure patients. However, despite inducing hemodynamic improvements and beneficial effects on renal function, dyspnea, myocardial structure, and endothelin levels, ularitide did not reduce long-term cardiovascular mortality in patients with acute heart failure.

M-ANP is a novel synthetic 40-amino acid peptide which consists of the native 28-amino acid core of ANP with a 12-amino acid extended C-terminus. M-ANP activates particulate guanylyl cyclase with equal potency to ANP and is highly resistant to degradation by neprilysin. It has potential for the treatment of acute hypertension.

The circulating levels of natriuretic peptides can also be increased by drugs that inhibit their breakdown by neprilysin. The resulting increase in ANP and BNP causes natriuresis and vasodilation, as well as a compensatory increase in renin secretion and plasma ANG II levels. Because of the increase in ANG II, these peptides are not effective as monotherapy in the treatment of heart failure. However, these observations led to the development of drugs that combine neprilysin inhibition with an ACE inhibitor in order to prevent the increase in plasma ANG II, or with an ARB to block the actions of ANG II.

Drugs that combine neprilysin inhibition with ACE inhibition, known as vasopeptidase inhibitors, include **omapatrilat, sampatrilat,** and **fasidotrilat.** Omapatrilat, which received the most attention, lowers blood pressure in animal models of hypertension as well as in hypertensive patients, and improves cardiac function in patients with heart failure. Unfortunately, omapatrilat causes a significant incidence of angioedema and cough, apparently as a result of decreased metabolism of bradykinin, and is not approved for clinical use.

The combination of an ANG II receptor antagonist with a neprilysin inhibitor **(ARNI)** increases endogenous natriuretic peptide levels while simultaneously blocking the effects of the increase in plasma ANG II. The first-in-class ARNI, **sacubitril-valsartan,** is a single molecule composed of the neprilysin inhibitor prodrug **sacubitril** and the ANG II receptor antagonist **valsartan.**

In healthy subjects, sacubitril-valsartan increased plasma ANP and cGMP levels in combination with increases in plasma renin and ANG II levels. Clinical trials in patients with heart failure demonstrated several beneficial effects of sacubitril-valsartan, and it has proved superior to ACE inhibition or angiotensin receptor blockade in reducing the risk of death and hospitalization from heart failure (Figure 17–8). Side effects include hypotension, hyperkalemia, renal impairment, and angioedema, the latter possibly due to increased bradykinin levels. Sacubitril-valsartan, marketed under the brand name **Entresto,** is approved by the FDA for the treatment of heart failure with reduced ejection fraction (see Chapter 13). It is not approved for heart failure with preserved ejection fraction. In patients with acute myocardial infarction, sacubitril-valsartan did not decrease the incidence of death when compared to ramipril alone. Sacubitril-valsartan has been shown to lower blood pressure in patients with essential hypertension, comparing favorably with valsartan. Increasing natriuretic peptide levels with sacubitril-valsartan could also be a useful strategy in the treatment of metabolic disease.

Achondroplasia is a rare genetic disease that inhibits endochondral ossification, resulting in short stature and other health complications. CNP is known to increase endochondral ossification and improve skeletal growth, and this has led to the use of CNP analogs to treat the disease.

Vosoritide is a 39-amino acid CNP analog with an extended plasma half-life due to increased resistance to neprilysin. In children with achondroplasia, once-daily subcutaneous administration of vosoritide resulted in a sustained increase in growth velocity for up to 42 months. This was accompanied by an increase in urinary

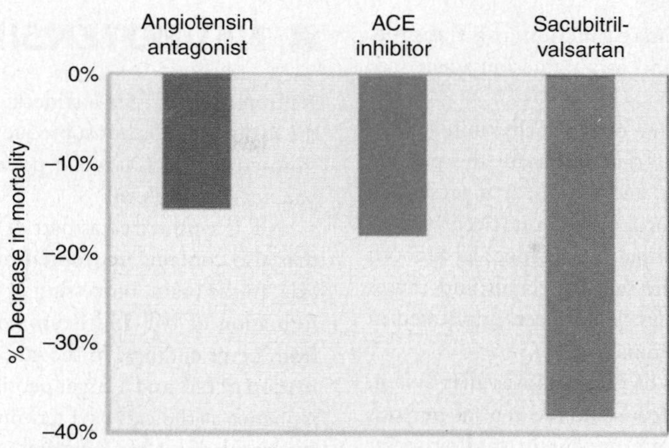

FIGURE 17–8 Comparison of the decrease in mortality produced by an angiotensin receptor antagonist, a converting enzyme inhibitor, and the combined angiotensin receptor antagonist-neprilysin inhibitor sacubitril-valsartan (Entresto) in patients with heart failure. Results for the three drugs are from separate trials. Each bar represents the drug effect versus placebo. (Adapted from Volpe M, Carnovali M, Mastromarino V: The natriuretic peptides system in the pathophysiology of heart failure: From molecular basis to treatment, Clin Sci 2016;130(2):57-77.)

cyclic GMP. Side effects included a transient reduction in blood pressure.

TransCon CNP is a 38-amino acid CNP analog conjugated to a polyethylene glycol carrier, designed to provide sustained systemic CNP levels during subcutaneous administration. In mice and monkeys, transCon CNP produced a sustained increase in plasma CNP-38 and was more effective in stimulating bone growth than either unconjugated CNP-38 or vosoritide. There was no reduction in blood pressure. This prodrug is in clinical development for the treatment of achondroplasia.

VASOACTIVE INTESTINAL PEPTIDE

Vasoactive intestinal peptide (VIP) is a 28-amino-acid peptide that belongs to the glucagon-secretin family of peptides. VIP is widely distributed in the central and peripheral nervous systems, where it functions as one of the major peptide neurotransmitters. It is present in cholinergic presynaptic neurons in the central nervous system, and in peripheral peptidergic neurons innervating diverse tissues including the heart, lungs, gastrointestinal and urogenital tracts, skin, eyes, ovaries, and thyroid gland. Many blood vessels are innervated by VIP neurons. VIP is also present in key organs of the immune system including the thymus, spleen, and lymph nodes. Although VIP is present in blood, where it undergoes rapid degradation, it does not appear to function as a hormone. VIP participates in a wide variety of biologic functions including metabolic processes, secretion of endocrine and exocrine glands, cell differentiation, smooth muscle relaxation, and modulation of the immune response.

VIP exerts significant effects on the cardiovascular system. It produces marked vasodilation in most vascular beds and in this regard is more potent on a molar basis than acetylcholine. In the heart, VIP causes coronary vasodilation and exerts positive inotropic and chronotropic effects. It may thus participate in the regulation of coronary blood flow, cardiac contraction, and heart rate.

The effects of VIP are mediated by two G protein–coupled receptors, VPAC1 and VPAC2. Both receptors are widely distributed in the central nervous system and in the heart, blood vessels, and other tissues. VIP has a high affinity for both receptor subtypes. Binding of VIP to its receptors results in activation of adenylyl cyclase and formation of cAMP, which is responsible for the vasodilation and many other effects of the peptide. Other actions may be mediated by inositol trisphosphate synthesis and calcium mobilization. VIP can also bind with low affinity to the VIP-like peptide pituitary adenylyl cyclase-activating peptide receptor, PAC1.

In view of its potent vasodilator action, VIP has potential for the treatment of systemic and pulmonary hypertension and heart failure, but this is limited by its short half-life in the circulation. However, **PB1046 (Vasomera),** a stable long-acting form of VIP that is selective for VPAC2 receptors, has been developed. Vasomera reduces blood pressure in animal models of hypertension, pulmonary arterial hypertension, and heart failure, and has been shown to be safe and well tolerated after single subcutaneous or intravenous injection in phase 1 studies in patients with essential hypertension. It has received orphan drug designation for the treatment of pulmonary arterial hypertension and cardiomyopathy associated with dystrophinopathies.

SUBSTANCE P

Substance P (SP) belongs to the **tachykinin** family of peptides, which share the common carboxyl terminal sequence Phe-Gly-Leu-Met. Other members of this family are **neurokinins A** and **B,** and three **endokinins, hemokinin-1** and **endokinins A** and **B.** SP is an undecapeptide, while neurokinins A and B are decapeptides.

SP is widely distributed in the central and peripheral nervous systems and in the cardiovascular system. It is also present in the gastrointestinal tract, where it may function as a transmitter in the enteric nervous system and as a paracrine agent (see Chapter 6).

SP is the most important member of the tachykinin family. It exerts a variety of central actions that implicate the peptide in stress, anxiety, depression, nausea, and emesis. It is present in peripheral afferent pain fibers and participates in nociception. SP causes contraction of venous, intestinal, and bronchial smooth muscle. It stimulates secretion by the salivary glands and causes diuresis and natriuresis by the kidneys. It has been implicated in immune system regulation and inflammation.

SP participates in the regulation of the cardiovascular system at both the central and peripheral levels. In the central nervous system, SP-containing nerve fibers are present in cardiovascular centers in the brain and spinal cord. In the heart, SP-containing fibers are present in both atrial and ventricular myocardium. Intravenous infusion of SP induces a dose-dependent increase in cardiac output, mostly due to increased stroke volume. In the vascular system, SP-containing nerve fibers are located around blood vessels, particularly those of the gut and skin. Vasodilation is the predominant vascular action of SP. It apparently results from an action on the vascular endothelium mediated by nitric oxide or other endothelium-derived factors. In some vascular beds, SP causes vasoconstriction.

The actions of SP and neurokinins A and B are mediated by three G_q protein–coupled tachykinin receptors designated NK_1, NK_2, and NK_3, which exhibit different affinities for the tachykinins. SP is the preferred ligand for the NK_1 receptor, which is widespread throughout the body and is the predominant tachykinin receptor in the human brain. Neurokinins A and B also possess considerable affinity for this receptor but display the highest affinity for NK_2 and NK_3. Most of the central and peripheral effects of SP including vasodilation are mediated by NK_1 receptors. In some cells SP binding leads to activation of phospholipase C; in others it activates adenylyl cyclase.

Several nonpeptide NK_1 receptor antagonists have been developed. These compounds are highly selective and orally active, and enter the brain. Recent clinical trials have shown that these antagonists may be useful in treating depression and other disorders and in preventing chemotherapy-induced emesis. The first of these to be approved for the prevention of chemotherapy-induced and postoperative nausea and vomiting is **aprepitant** (see Chapter 62). **Fosaprepitant** is a prodrug that is converted to aprepitant after intravenous administration and may be a useful parenteral alternative to oral aprepitant.

The SP-NK_1 system has also been implicated in cancer. SP and NK_1 receptors are present in a variety of tumor cells, and NK_1 receptor antagonists exert an antitumor action. Thus, drugs such as aprepitant may have potential as anticancer agents. A role for NK_1 antagonists in the treatment of cardiovascular disease has not been identified.

Novel selective nonpeptide NK_2 antagonists include **saredutant, nepadutant,** and **ibodutant.** They have undergone clinical testing for the treatment of respiratory and gastrointestinal disorders as well as anxiety, but their use is limited by their low efficacy.

NEUROTENSIN

Neurotensin (NT) is a tridecapeptide that was first isolated from the hypothalamus but subsequently found to be present in the gastrointestinal tract. It is also present in the blood, heart, lungs, liver, pancreas, and spleen.

NT is synthesized as part of a larger precursor, pro-NT/NMN, that also contains **neuromedin N,** a six-amino-acid NT-like peptide. In the brain, processing of the precursor leads primarily to the formation of NT and neuromedin N; these are released together from nerve endings. In the gut, processing leads mainly to the formation of NT and a larger peptide that contains the neuromedin N sequence at the carboxyl terminal. Both peptides are secreted into the circulation after ingestion of food. Most of the activity of NT is mediated by the six amino acids at the C-terminus, NT(8-13).

Like many other neuropeptides, NT serves a dual function as a neurotransmitter or neuromodulator in the central nervous system. When administered centrally, NT exerts potent effects including hypothermia, antinociception, and modulation of dopamine and glutamate neurotransmission. There are close associations between NT and dopamine systems, and NT may be involved in clinical disorders involving dopamine pathways such as schizophrenia, Parkinson disease, and drug abuse. Consistent with this, it has been shown that central administration of NT in rodents produces effects similar to those produced by antipsychotic drugs.

NT also participates in cardiovascular regulation. NT-containing nerve fibers make close contact with atrial and ventricular myocytes, the cardiac conduction system, and coronary vessels. NT-containing fibers are also present in the ascending aorta, aortic arch, and pulmonary veins. Intravenous administration of NT produces tachycardia, vasodilation, and hypotension. It affects coronary vascular tone, blood flow in cutaneous and adipose tissues and the gastrointestinal tract, and venous smooth muscle tone. It may also participate in cardiovascular reflexes.

There is evidence that the NT-induced decrease in blood pressure is involved in acute circulatory disorders such as shock. For example, elevated levels of NT have been found in patients with septic and cardiogenic shock and may contribute to the hypotension.

Other peripheral actions of NT include increased vascular permeability, increased secretion of several anterior pituitary hormones, hyperglycemia, inhibition of gastric acid and pepsin secretion, and inhibition of gastric motility. Actions on the immune system have also been described.

The effects of NT are mediated by three subtypes of NT receptors, designated NTR_1, NTR_2, and NTR_3, also known as NTS_1, NTS_2, and NTS_3. NTR_1 and NTR_2 belong to the G_q protein–coupled superfamily. NTR_1 has a higher affinity for NT than NTR_2 and is the major mediator of the diverse effects of NT. The NTR_3 receptor is a single-transmembrane protein that is structurally unrelated to NTR_1 or NTR_2. It belongs to a family of sorting proteins and is therefore known as NTR_3/sortilin.

The potential use of NT as an antipsychotic agent has been hampered by its rapid degradation in the circulation and inability to cross the blood-brain barrier. However, a series of analogs of NT(8-13) that exert antipsychotic-like activity in animal studies has been developed. These agonists include **NT69L,** which binds with high affinity to NTR_1 and NTR_2; and **NT79,** which preferentially binds to NTR_2. Another agonist, **PD149163,** has improved metabolic stability.

In addition to their possible role as antipsychotic drugs, these agonists may be useful in the treatment of pain, psychostimulant abuse, and Parkinson disease. Potential adverse effects include hypothermia and hypotension. Development of tolerance to some of the effects of the agonists may occur.

NT receptors can be blocked with the nonpeptide antagonists SR142948A and **meclinertant** (SR48692). SR142948A is a potent antagonist of the hypothermia and analgesia produced by centrally administered NT. It also blocks the cardiovascular effects of systemic NT.

■ CALCITONIN GENE-RELATED PEPTIDE

Calcitonin gene-related peptide (CGRP) is a member of the calcitonin family of peptides that also includes calcitonin, adrenomedullin, and amylin. In humans, CGRP exists in two isoforms termed α-CGRP and β-CGRP. α-CGRP is a 37-amino acid peptide formed by alternative splicing of the calcitonin/CGRP gene on chromosome 11. β-CGRP, which is encoded in a separate gene in the same region, differs in three amino acids. α-CGRP and β-CGRP have similar biological activity but α-CGRP is the principal form.

Like calcitonin, CGRP is present in large quantities in the C cells of the thyroid gland. It is also distributed widely in the central and peripheral nervous systems, cardiovascular and respiratory systems, and gastrointestinal tract. In the cardiovascular system, CGRP-containing neuronal fibers are more abundant around arteries than around veins and in atria than in ventricles. CGRP fibers are associated with most smooth muscles of the gastrointestinal tract. CGRP is found with substance P (see above) in some of these regions and with acetylcholine in others.

When CGRP is injected into the central nervous system, it produces a variety of effects, including hypertension and suppression of feeding. When injected into the systemic circulation, the peptide causes hypotension, tachycardia, and a positive inotropic effect. The hypotensive action of CGRP results from the potent vasodilator action of the peptide; indeed, CGRP is the most potent vasodilator yet discovered. It dilates multiple vascular beds and increases cutaneous, renal, and coronary blood flow, the coronary circulation being particularly sensitive. The vasodilation results in part from increased nitric oxide production in endothelial cells which in turn acts to relax the underlying vascular smooth muscle.

The biological effects of CGRP are mainly mediated by the CGRP receptor, a complex composed of the G protein–coupled calcitonin-like receptor (CLR) and a single transmembrane domain protein, receptor activity-modifying protein 1 (RAMP1). Some CGRP effects are mediated by the amylin-1 receptor (AMY1), a complex consisting of the calcitonin receptor (CTR) and RAMP1. Both receptors are expressed throughout the central nervous, cardiovascular, and other systems.

Despite its cardiovascular actions, CGRP does not appear to participate in the physiologic regulation of blood pressure. However, it might play a protective role in cardiovascular diseases including hypertension, where it may counteract the renin-angiotensin and sympathetic nervous systems, and in heart failure, where it could alleviate cardiac hypertrophy, inflammation, and apoptosis. Indeed, an acylated α-CGRP analog with a longer half-life than the native peptide has shown promising results in animal models of hypertension and heart failure.

There is now considerable evidence that release of CGRP from trigeminal nerves plays a central role in the pathophysiology of **migraine** (see Chapter 16). The peptide is released during migraine attacks, and successful treatment of migraine with a selective serotonin agonist normalizes cranial CGRP levels. Intravenous administration of CGRP can induce migraine-like headaches in migraineurs. Peptide and nonpeptide antagonists of the CGRP receptor have been developed. $CGRP_{8\text{-}37}$ was used extensively to investigate the actions of CGRP but displays affinity for other related receptors including those for adrenomedullin (see below). Smaller, nonpeptide CGRP receptor antagonists target the interface between CLR and RAMP1, making them more selective for the CGRP receptor. Examples are the "gepants," **olcegepant** and **telcagepant.** They are effective in the treatment of migraine, but their development was limited by concerns regarding liver toxicity.

A second generation of gepants includes **ubrogepant, rimegepant,** and **atogepant.** Ubrogepant and rimegepant are approved for acute treatment of migraine, while rimegepant and atogepant can be used for migraine prevention. **Vazegepant** is a new intranasal gepant being investigated as an acute treatment for migraine.

Monoclonal antibodies targeting CGRP or its receptor have been developed. To date, four such monoclonal antibodies have been developed and tested in humans: **erenumab,** which targets the extracellular domain of the CGRP receptor; and **eptinezumab, fremanezumab,** and **galcanezumab,** which target CGRP. These drugs are effective and have a good safety and tolerability profile but must be given subcutaneously and are very expensive.

In view of the cardioprotective effects of CGRP noted above, it will be important to monitor the cardiovascular effects of these anti-migraine drugs. No adverse effects have been reported to date.

■ ADRENOMEDULLIN

Adrenomedullin (AM) was discovered in human adrenal medullary pheochromocytoma tissue. It is a 52-amino acid peptide with a six-amino acid disulfide ring and a C-terminal amide, both of which are required for activity. Like CGRP, AM is a member of the calcitonin family of peptides. A related 47-amino acid peptide called adrenomedullin 2 or intermedin has been identified in humans and other mammals where it is expressed in several organs including the heart and kidneys.

AM is synthesized as the 185-amino acid preproAM which is cleaved, ultimately forming mature AM, proAM N-terminal 20 peptide (PAMP), and mid-regional AM **(MR-proAM).** It is expressed in virtually all tissues of the body, the highest levels occurring in the adrenal medulla, kidneys, cardiac atria, and lungs. AM is present in the hypothalamus where it may participate in the central control of blood pressure by increasing sympathetic outflow.

It is present in the circulation, the main source apparently being the vasculature. Plasma AM is metabolized by peptidases including neprilysin, resulting in a half-life of approximately 22 minutes.

Intravenous infusion of AM causes marked vasodilation which results from a direct action on resistance vessels and leads to decreased peripheral resistance and arterial pressure. The fall in blood pressure in turn elicits compensatory increases in heart rate, cardiac output, and plasma norepinephrine and renin levels. AM also acts on the kidneys to cause diuresis and natriuresis. Other actions include positive inotropy, inhibition of cardiomyocyte hypertrophy and proliferation, and reduced collagen production in cardiac fibroblasts.

The actions of AM are mediated by two receptors, AM_1 and AM_2. These receptors are formed by heterodimerization of the calcitonin receptor-like receptor (CLR) with RAMP2 and RAMP3, respectively, in a manner analogous to the formation of the CGRP receptor. The receptors are distributed widely in the body. They are present in vascular endothelial and smooth muscle cells, and AM-induced vasodilation results from actions on both. In endothelial cells, AM increases NO production, which subsequently causes dilation of the adjacent smooth muscle cells. In vascular smooth muscle cells, AM increases cAMP levels resulting in activation of protein kinase A and, in turn, vasodilation. In addition to binding to AM_1 and AM_2 receptors, AM has significant affinity for the CGRP receptor.

Circulating AM levels increase in a number of pathologic states, including sepsis, heart failure, essential and pulmonary hypertension, myocardial infarction, and renal failure. Plasma AM and MR-proAM levels increase in proportion to the severity of these diseases and show promise as prognostic markers. The roles of AM in these states remain to be defined, but it is currently thought that the peptide may serve a protective role, mitigating cardiovascular overload and injury by virtue of its vasodilator and natriuretic activity. Studies have shown that AM exerts beneficial hemodynamic, endocrine, and myocardial effects in animal models and in patients with heart failure.

Drugs are available to block or prolong the actions of AM. Its vasodilator action can be blocked by the receptor antagonist **AM(22-52).** AM can be administered intravenously as the native peptide but its effectiveness is limited by its short half-life (22 minutes). PEGylation at the N-terminus extends the half-life while leaving the C-terminus free to bind to AM receptors.

Adrecizumab is a humanized, monoclonal, non-neutralizing antibody against the N-terminus of AM. The C-terminus of antibody-bound AM remains exposed, permitting receptor binding without activation. The antibody has a half-life of 15 days. Adrecizumab partly inhibits AM signaling, but following administration of the antibody, there is a marked increase in plasma AM so that there is a net increase in AM activity in the blood. The mechanism of this increase is not clear but it has been proposed that the antibody translocates AM from the interstitium to the blood. The resulting decrease in interstitial AM would reduce its direct vasodilatory action on vascular smooth muscle, while the increase in AM in the blood (mostly antibody-bound) could help stabilize the endothelial barrier. ADZ demonstrated a promising safety profile in phase 1 studies and a phase 2 study is in progress. It is increasingly seen as a potential adjunct therapy to restore endothelial function in septic shock.

RELAXIN

Relaxin (RLX) is a member of the relaxin family of peptides (RXFPs) which, in humans, comprises three peptides RLX-1, RLX-2, and RLX-3. They are members of the insulin superfamily, being structurally related to insulin with A and B chains connected by two disulfide bonds. RLX-2 is the major form of RLX in the circulation where it has a short half-life.

RLX is an important hormone of pregnancy, being responsible for vasodilation and increased cardiac output. However, there is now a large body of evidence that its actions extend well beyond those concerned with reproduction. For example, RLX is produced not only in the reproductive system but also in the brain, heart, kidneys, lungs, and liver. Circulating RLX levels are increased in diseases including pulmonary arterial hypertension, heart failure, prostate cancer, and atrial fibrillation.

Intravenous administration of RLX causes systemic and renal vasodilation, resulting in increased cardiac output, and renal blood flow and glomerular filtration rate. It also reduces collagen synthesis and causes beneficial remodeling of the vasculature. These actions are mediated primarily by the relaxin family peptide receptor-1 (RXFP1), a G protein–coupled receptor that is expressed in brain, liver, kidneys, lungs, and cardiovascular system. Multiple signaling pathways include NO, cGMP, and cAMP (Figure 17–9).

The beneficial effects of RLX can be mimicked by **serelaxin** (RLX030) a recombinant form of the human RLX peptide. In addition to causing systemic and renal vasodilation, serelaxin

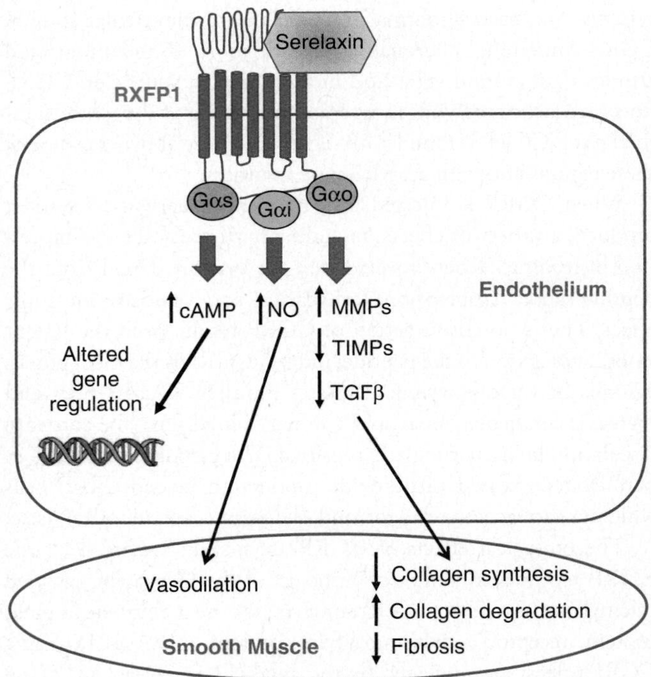

FIGURE 17–9 Mechanism of action of the relaxin analog, serelaxin. RXFP1, relaxin family peptide receptor-1; MMP, matrix metalloproteinase; TIMP, tissue inhibitor of metalloproteinase.
(Adapted from Yandrapalli S, Jolly G, Biswas M, et al. Newer hormonal pharmacotherapies for heart failure, Expert Rev Endocrinol Metab 2018 Jan;13(1):35-49.)

delivered intravenously has been reported to exert multiple beneficial effects on the cardiovascular system including suppression of arrhythmia and inflammation and reversal of fibrosis. Unfortunately, extended phase III clinical trials for the treatment of acute heart failure were generally negative.

Recently, RLX mimetics with longer half-lives and lower cost have been developed. B7-33 is a peptide consisting of residues 7-33 of the B chain of RLX. It reduces cardiac and renal fibrosis in rodent models. A newer drug, ML290 is a non-peptide agonist of the RXFP1 receptor. It exerts antifibrotic effects in a human hepatic cell line and has potential for the treatment of cardiovascular disease, at least in the short term.

Another member of the relaxin family of peptides is **insulin-like 3 peptide** (INSL3). It is expressed mainly in the gonads and acts through relaxin family peptide receptor-2 (RXFP2). This peptide and its receptor are closely related to RLX and RXFP1 but they appear to be concerned more with reproduction and bone and muscle metabolism.

■ UROCORTINS

Urocortins (UCNs) are members of the corticotropin-releasing hormone (CRH) family of peptides, which in mammals comprises CRH and three UCNs: UCN1 (40 amino acids), UCN2 (39), and UCN3 (38). UCNs are widely expressed throughout the central nervous system and in the cardiovascular, digestive, and immune systems, kidneys, adrenals, and other tissues. They are present in the circulation and urine.

In the central nervous system, UCNs are involved in anxiety, depression, and drug abuse. UCN2 participates in the control of gastric emptying via sympathetic pathways and may contribute to the control of the hypothalamic-pituitary-adrenal axis. UCN3 contributes to the control of food intake.

In the periphery, UCNs exert actions on the cardiovascular, gastrointestinal, and reproductive systems, and in the adrenal medulla. Systemic administration of UCN2 in healthy volunteers increases heart rate and cardiac output, and decreases peripheral resistance and diastolic and mean arterial pressure. Intra-arterial forearm infusion of UCN2 causes vasodilation which is at least partly mediated by NO. All three UCNs cause renal vasodilation.

UCNs modulate the actions of other vasoactive peptides including ANG II, endothelins, and natriuretic peptides. They also exert complex actions on endothelial cell function, with most evidence suggesting an endothelial-protective role.

UCNs act via two G protein–coupled receptors, CRHR1 and CRHR2. UCN1 activates both receptors but has a higher affinity for CRHR2. UCN2 and UCN3 bind specifically to CRHR2. CRHR1 is preferentially expressed in the brain and pituitary while CRHR2 is expressed in discrete brain regions and peripheral organs including all chambers of the heart, and endothelial and smooth muscle cells of arteries and veins.

Role in Heart Failure

Plasma levels of UCN2 are elevated in patients with heart failure and might serve as a biomarker for the diagnosis and prognosis of this disease. However, UCN2 does not appear to have any additional value over NT-proBNP.

Several studies have demonstrated beneficial effects of UCNs in heart failure. Intravenous administration of UCN2 in patients with congestive heart failure produced cardiovascular changes generally similar to those in healthy subjects, ie, increased cardiac output, vasodilation, and decreased blood pressure. In patients with acute decompensated heart failure, administration of UCN2 increased heart rate and cardiac output, and decreased peripheral vascular resistance and arterial pressure. Administration of UCN3 in patients with stable heart failure increased cardiac index and decreased systemic vascular resistance and diastolic pressure with no significant changes in heart rate or systolic pressure.

Role in Pulmonary Hypertension

Expression of UCN2 and CRHR2 has been reported to increase in right ventricular tissue of patients with right ventricular failure and in rats with a model of pulmonary hypertension. Chronic infusion of UCN2 attenuated pulmonary arterial hypertension and right ventricular dysfunction in the rat model.

Taken together these observations suggest that UCNs have potential for the diagnosis and treatment of heart failure and pulmonary hypertension. They may also be beneficial in other diseases including ischemic heart disease and systemic hypertension.

UCN3 is available as the investigational drug **stresscopin (RT-400).** It is in phase II development as a peptide infusion therapy for acute decompensated heart failure.

■ VASOACTIVE PEPTIDES: SUMMARY AND PERSPECTIVE

The vasoactive peptides are a diverse group of chemical messengers that participate in the control of cardiovascular function. They are not only important in physiological regulation but also cause or contribute to cardiovascular disease, and are thus important targets for drug development.

From the physiological point of view, the vasoconstrictors play an important role in defending blood pressure and volume against hypotension and hypovolemia by virtue of their actions on the cardiovascular system and kidneys. Important players here include ANG II, vasopressin, and the endothelins. From the pathological standpoint, excessive secretion of the peptides can, by the same actions, cause or exacerbate cardiovascular diseases such as hypertension, heart failure, and kidney disease. For this reason, a wide variety of drugs that block the formation of the peptides (e.g., renin and ACE inhibitors) or antagonize their receptors (e.g., ANG II receptor blockers) has been developed.

The vasodilators play a quite different role, being concerned more with defending against hypervolemia and maintaining optimal blood flow. This is largely accomplished by increasing renal sodium and water excretion, dilating blood vessels, and, in some cases, increasing cardiac output. Of significance here are the natriuretic peptides, which also play a protective role in disease states. For example, in heart failure, ANP and BNP are released in an attempt to counter the overactive renin-angiotensin and sympathetic nervous systems. Other vasodilator peptides exert a similar protective action, although their roles are less well defined.

In view of the beneficial effects of the vasodilators, considerable attention has been directed to developing drugs that mimic or enhance their actions. The use of the native peptides is generally limited by their short half-lives, but they can be helpful in short-term therapy. Another approach is to increase the circulating levels of the peptides with an inhibitor of the peptidases that metabolize the peptides, e.g., sacubitril. However, elevated levels of some of the peptides may produce undesirable effects including cough (bradykinin) and vasoconstriction (ANG II). A solution to this problem is to combine the peptidase inhibitor with a drug that blocks the unwanted effect of the peptide. An example of such a combination, sacubitril/valsartan, has proved to be of value in the treatment of heart failure.

SUMMARY Drugs that Interact with Vasoactive Peptide Systems

Subclass, Drug	Mechanism of Action	Effects	Clinical Applications
ANGIOTENSIN RECEPTOR ANTAGONISTS			
• Valsartan	Selective competitive antagonist of angiotensin AT_1 receptors	Arteriolar dilation • decreased aldosterone secretion • increased sodium and water excretion	Hypertension
• *Eprosartan, irbesartan, candesartan, olmesartan, telmisartan: Similar to valsartan*			
ANGIOTENSIN RECEPTOR AGONISTS			
• Angiotensin II	AT_1 (and AT_2) receptor agonist	Increased blood pressure	Vasodilatory shock
• Compound 21	AT_2 receptor agonist	Beneficial cardiovascular effects	Potential for treatment of cardiovascular disease
CONVERTING ENZYME INHIBITORS			
• Enalapril	Inhibits conversion of angiotensin I to angiotensin II	Arteriolar dilation • decreased aldosterone secretion • increased sodium and water excretion	Hypertension • heart failure
• *Captopril and many others: Similar to enalapril*			
RENIN INHIBITOR			
• Aliskiren	Inhibits catalytic activity of renin	Arteriolar dilation • decreased aldosterone secretion • increased sodium and water excretion	Hypertension
KININ INHIBITORS			
• Icatibant	Selective antagonist of kinin B_2 receptors	Blocks effects of kinins on pain, hyperalgesia, and inflammation	Hereditary angioedema
• *Cinryze, Berinert: Plasma C1 esterase inhibitors, decrease bradykinin formation, used in hereditary angioedema* • *Ecallantide: Plasma kallikrein inhibitor* • *Donidalorsen: Inhibits production of plasma prekallikrien*			
VASOPRESSIN AGONISTS			
• Arginine vasopressin	Agonist of vasopressin V_1 (and V_2) receptors	Vasoconstriction	Vasodilatory shock
• *Selepressin, terlipressin: More selective for V_{1a} receptor*			
VASOPRESSIN ANTAGONISTS			
• Conivaptan	Antagonist of vasopressin V_1 and V_2 receptors	Vasodilation	Potential use in hypertension and heart failure • hyponatremia
• *Relcovaptan, SRX251: Increased selectivity for V_1 receptor* • *Tolvaptan: Increased selectivity for V_2 receptor*			
NATRIURETIC PEPTIDE AGONISTS			
• Nesiritide, Carperitide, M-ANP	Agonists of natriuretic peptide receptors	Increased sodium and water excretion • vasodilation	Potential use in acute hypertension and heart failure
• Vosoritide	Agonist of C-type natriuretic peptide receptor	Increased endochondral ossification	Achondroplasia
• *Ularitide: Synthetic form of urodilatin*			

(continued)

Subclass, Drug	Mechanism of Action	Effects	Clinical Applications
COMBINED ANGIOTENSIN-CONVERTING ENZYME/NEPRILYSIN INHIBITORS (VASOPEPTIDASE INHIBITORS)			
• Omapatrilat	Decreases breakdown of natriuretic peptides and formation of angiotensin II	Vasodilation • increased sodium and water excretion	Hypertension • heart failure[1]
• *Sampatrilat, fasidotrilat: Similar to omapatrilat*			
COMBINED ANGIOTENSIN RECEPTOR ANTAGONIST/NEPRILYSIN INHIBITOR			
• Sacubitril/valsartan	Decreases breakdown of natriuretic peptides and blocks angiotensin II receptors	Vasodilation • increased sodium and water excretion	Heart failure • hypertension[1]
ENDOTHELIN ANTAGONISTS			
• Bosentan, macitentan	Nonselective antagonists of endothelin ET_A and ET_B receptors	Vasodilation	Pulmonary arterial hypertension
• Sparsentan	Combined ET_A/AT_1 antagonist	Vasodilation	
• *Sitaxsentan, ambrisentan: Selective antagonists of ET_A receptors*			
COMBINED ENDOTHELIN-CONVERTING ENZYME/NEPRILYSIN INHIBITOR			
• SLV306, daglutril	Blocks formation of endothelins and breakdown of natriuretic peptides	Vasodilation • increased sodium and water excretion	Heart failure • hypertension[1]
VASOACTIVE INTESTINAL PEPTIDE AGONIST			
• PB1046, Vasomera	Selective agonist of VPAC2 receptors	Vasodilation • multiple metabolic, endocrine, and other effects	Essential and pulmonary hypertension • cardiomyopathy[1]
SUBSTANCE P ANTAGONISTS			
• Aprepitant	Selective antagonist of tachykinin NK_1 receptors	Blocks several central nervous system effects of substance P	Prevention of chemotherapy-induced nausea and vomiting
• Saredutant, nepadutant, ibodutant	Selective antagonists of tachykinin NK_2 receptors		Potential for treatment of respiratory and gastrointestinal disorders and anxiety
• *Fosaprepitant: Prodrug that is converted to aprepitant*			
NEUROTENSIN AGONISTS			
• PD149163, NT69L, NT79	Agonists of central neurotensin receptors	Interact with central dopamine systems	Potential for treatment of schizophrenia and Parkinson disease
NEUROTENSIN ANTAGONIST			
• Meclinertant	Antagonist of central and peripheral neurotensin receptors	Blocks some central and peripheral (vasodilator) actions of neurotensin	None identified
CALCITONIN GENE-RELATED PEPTIDE AGONIST			
• Acylated alpha-CGRP	Agonist of CGRP receptors	Mimics beneficial cardiovascular effects of CGRP	Potential for treatment of hypertension and heart failure
CALCITONIN GENE-RELATED PEPTIDE ANTAGONISTS			
• Telcagepant, olcegepant	Antagonists of the calcitonin gene-related peptide (CGRP) receptor	Blocks some central and peripheral (vasodilator) actions of CGRP	Migraine[1]
• Ubrogepant, rimegepant, atogepant	Second-generation CGRP receptor antagonists	Blocks some central and peripheral (vasodilator) actions of CGRP	Migraine
• Erenumab	Monoclonal antibody against the CGRP receptor		Migraine prevention and treatment
• Eptinezumab, fremanezumab, galcanezumab	Monoclonal antibodies against CGRP		
ADRENOMEDULLIN ANTAGONIST			
• Adrecizumab	Monoclonal antibody against adrenomedullin receptors	Partly inhibits adrenomedullin signaling Increases plasma adrenomedullin levels	Septic shock[1]

(*continued*)

Subclass, Drug	Mechanism of Action	Effects	Clinical Applications
NEUROPEPTIDE Y ANTAGONISTS			
• BIBP3226	Selective antagonist of neuropeptide Y_1 receptors	Blocks vasoconstrictor response to neurotensin	Potential antiobesity agent
• *BIIE0246: Selective for Y_2 receptor*			
• *MK-0557: Selective for Y_5 receptor*			
RELAXIN AGONISTS			
• Serelaxin	Agonist of relaxin family peptide receptor-1	Vasodilation and other cardiovascular actions	Potential for treatment of heart failure and other cardiovascular diseases
• *B7-33, ML290: Longer half-lives than serelaxin*			
UROCORTIN AGONIST			
• Stresscopin, RT-400	Agonist of urocortin receptors	Vasodilation and other cardiovascular effects	Acute heart failure[1]
UROTENSIN ANTAGONISTS			
• Palosuran	Antagonist of urotensin receptors	Blocks vasoconstrictor action of urotensin	Potential for treatment of diabetic renal failure and asthma[1]
• *GSK1440115: More potent than palosuran*			

[1]Undergoing preclinical or clinical evaluation.

PREPARATIONS AVAILABLE

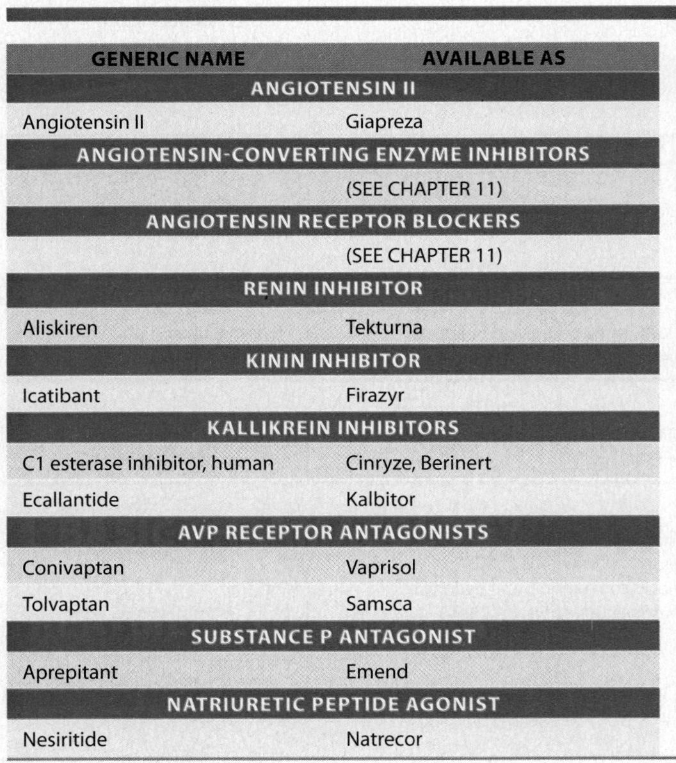

GENERIC NAME	AVAILABLE AS
ANGIOTENSIN II	
Angiotensin II	Giapreza
ANGIOTENSIN-CONVERTING ENZYME INHIBITORS	
	(SEE CHAPTER 11)
ANGIOTENSIN RECEPTOR BLOCKERS	
	(SEE CHAPTER 11)
RENIN INHIBITOR	
Aliskiren	Tekturna
KININ INHIBITOR	
Icatibant	Firazyr
KALLIKREIN INHIBITORS	
C1 esterase inhibitor, human	Cinryze, Berinert
Ecallantide	Kalbitor
AVP RECEPTOR ANTAGONISTS	
Conivaptan	Vaprisol
Tolvaptan	Samsca
SUBSTANCE P ANTAGONIST	
Aprepitant	Emend
NATRIURETIC PEPTIDE AGONIST	
Nesiritide	Natrecor

GENERIC NAME	AVAILABLE AS
COMBINED NEPRILYSIN INHIBITOR / ANGIOTENSIN RECEPTOR ANTAGONIST	
Sacubitril/valsartan	Entresto
CGRP ANTAGONISTS	
Erenumab	Aimovig
Fremanezumab	Ajovy
Galcanezumab	Emgality
Ubrogepant	Ubrelvy
DRUGS USED IN PULMONARY HYPERTENSION	
Ambrisentan	Letairis
Bosentan	Tracleer
Epoprostenol	Flolan, Veletri
Iloprost	Ventavis
Macitentan	Opsumit
Nintedanib	Ofev
Pirfenidone	Esbriet
Riociguat	Adempas
Selexipag	Uptravi
Treprostinil	Tyvaso, Remodulin

REFERENCES

Vasoconstrictors

Angiotensin

Abadir P et al: Topical reformulation of valsartan for treatment of chronic diabetic wounds. J Invest Dermatol 2018;138:434.

Bjerre HL et al: The role of aliskiren in the management of hypertension and major cardiovascular outcomes: A systematic review and meta-analysis. J Hum Hypertens 2019;33:795.

Bussard RL, Busse LW: Angiotensin II: A new therapeutic option for vasodilatory shock. Ther Clin Risk Manag 2018;14:1287.

Busse PJ, Christiansen SC: Hereditary angioedema. N Engl J Med 2020;382:1136.

Chow BS, Allen TJ: Angiotensin II type 2 receptor (AT2R) in renal and cardiovascular disease. Clin Sci (Lond) 2016;130:1307.

Cruz Rodriguez JB, Cu C, Siddiqui T. Narrative review in the current role of angiotensin receptor-neprilysin inhibitors. Ann Transl Med 2021;9:518.

Danser AH: The role of the (pro)renin receptor in hypertensive disease. Am J Hypertens 2015;28:1187.

Friis UG et al: Regulation of renin secretion by renal juxtaglomerular cells. Eur J Physiol 2013;465:25.

Karnik SS et al: International Union of Basic and Clinical Pharmacology. XCIX. Angiotensin receptors: Interpreters of pathophysiological angiotensinergic stimuli [corrected]. Pharmacol Rev 2015;67:754.

Miller AJ, Arnold AC: The renin-angiotensin system in cardiovascular autonomic control: Recent developments and clinical implications. Clin Auton Res 2019;29:231.

Packer M: Are healthcare systems now ready to adopt sacubitril/valsartan as the preferred approach to inhibiting the renin-angiotensin system in chronic heart failure? The culmination of a 20-year journey. Eur Heart J. 2019;40:3353.

Patel S, Hussain T: Dimerization of AT_2 and Mas receptors in control of blood pressure. Curr Hypertens Rep 2018;20:41.

Ramkumar N, Kohan DE: The (pro)renin receptor: An emerging player in hypertension and metabolic syndrome. Kidney Int 2019;95:1041.

Ranjbar R et al: The potential therapeutic use of renin-angiotensin system inhibitors in the treatment of inflammatory diseases. J Cell Physiol 2019;234:2277.

Vaduganathan M et al: Renin-angiotensin-aldosterone system inhibitors in patients with covid-19. N Engl J Med 2020;382:1653.

Wieruszewski PM et al: Angiotensin II Infusion for Shock: A multicenter study of postmarketing use. Chest 2021;159:596.

Xu Y et al. Effect of angiotensin-neprilysin versus renin-angiotensin system inhibition on renal outcomes: a systematic review and meta-analysis. Front Pharmacol 2021;12:604017.

Vasopressin

Asfar P et al: Selepressin in septic shock: A step toward decatecholaminization? Crit Care Med 2016;44:234.

Boucheix OB et al: Selepressin, a new V1A receptor agonist: Hemodynamic comparison to vasopressin in dogs. Shock 2013;39:533.

Jentzer JC, Hollenberg SM. Vasopressor and inotrope therapy in cardiac critical care. J Intensive Care Med 2021;36:843.

Kunkes JH et al: Vasopressin therapy in cardiac surgery. J Card Surg 2019;34:20.

Palmer BF: Vasopressin receptor antagonists. Curr Hypertens Rep 2015;17:510.

Endothelins

Correale M et al: Endothelin-receptor antagonists in the management of pulmonary arterial hypertension: Where do we stand? Vasc Health Risk Manag 2018;14:253.

Davenport AP et al: Endothelin. Pharmacol Rev 2016;68:357.

Haryono A et al. Endothelin and the cardiovascular system: the long journey and where we are going. Biology (Basel) 2022;11:759.

Maguire JJ, Davenport AP: Endothelin@25—new agonists, antagonists, inhibitors and emerging research frontiers: IUPHAR Review 12. Br J Pharmacol 2014;171:5555.

Pulido T et al: Macitentan and morbidity and mortality in pulmonary arterial hypertension. N Engl J Med 2013;369:809.

Sidharta PN, van Giersbergen PL, Dingemanse J: Safety, tolerability, pharmacokinetics, and pharmacodynamics of macitentan, an endothelin receptor antagonist, in an ascending multiple-dose study in healthy subjects. J Clin Pharmacol 2013;53:1131.

Neuropeptide Y

Saraf R et al: Neuropeptide Y is an angiogenic factor in cardiovascular regeneration. Eur J Pharmacol 2016;776:64.

Tan CMJ et al: The role of neuropeptide Y in cardiovascular health and disease. Front Physiol 2018;9:1281.

Thorsell A, Mathé AA: Neuropeptide Y in alcohol addiction and affective disorders. Front Endocrinol (Lausanne) 2017;8:178.

Zhu P et al: The role of neuropeptide Y in the pathophysiology of atherosclerotic cardiovascular disease. Int J Cardiol 2016;220:235.

Urotensin

Chatenet D et al: Update on the urotensinergic system: New trends in receptor localization, activation, and drug design. Front Endocrinol 2013;3:1.

Cheriyan J et al: The effects of urotensin II and urantide on forearm blood flow and systemic haemodynamics in humans. Br J Clin Pharmacol 2009;68:518.

Portnoy A et al: Effects of urotensin II receptor antagonist, GSK1440115, in asthma. Front Pharmacol 2013;4:54.

Sun SL, Liu LM: Urotensin II: An inflammatory cytokine. J Endocrinol. 2019;240:R107.

Svistunov AA et al: Urotensin II: Molecular mechanisms of biological activity. Curr Protein Pept Sci 2018;19:924.

Vaudry H et al: International Union of Basic and Clinical Pharmacology. XCII. Urotensin II, urotensin II-related peptide, and their receptor: From structure to function. Pharmacol Rev 2015;67:214.

Vasodilators

Kinins

Bork K: A decade of change: Recent developments in pharmacotherapy of hereditary angioedema (HAE). Clin Rev Allergy Immunol 2016;51:183.

Dutra RC: Kinin receptors: Key regulators of autoimmunity. Autoimmun Rev 2017;16:192.

Farkas H, Köhalmi KV: Icatibant for the treatment of hereditary angioedema with C1-inhibitor deficiency in adolescents and in children aged over 2 years. Expert Rev Clin Immunol 2018;14:447.

Fijen LM et al. Inhibition of prekallikrein for hereditary angioedema. N Engl J Med 2022;386:1026.

Girolami JP et al. Kinins and kinin receptors in cardiovascular and renal diseases. Pharmaceuticals (Basel) 2021;14:240.

Longhurst HJ et al: Real-world outcomes in hereditary angioedema: First experience from the Icatibant Outcome Survey in the United Kingdom. Allergy Asthma Clin Immunol 2018;14:28.

Qadri F, Bader M: Kinin B1 receptors as a therapeutic target for inflammation. Expert Opin Ther Targets 2018;22:31.

Taddei S, Bortolotto L: Unraveling the pivotal role of bradykinin in ACE inhibitor activity. Am J Cardiovasc Drugs 2016;16:309.

Natriuretic Peptides

Anker SD et al: Ularitide for the treatment of acute decompensated heart failure: From preclinical to clinical studies. Eur Heart J 2015;36:715.

Baba M, Yoshida K, Ieda M. Clinical applications of natriuretic peptides in heart failure and atrial fibrillation. Int J Mol Sci 2019;20.

Berntsson J et al: Pro-atrial natriuretic peptide and prediction of atrial fibrillation and stroke: The Malmo Preventive Project. Eur J Prev Cardiol 2017;24:788.

Breinholt VM et al: TransCon CNP, a sustained-release C-Type Natriuretic Peptide prodrug, a potentially safe and efficacious new therapeutic modality for the treatment of comorbidities associated with FGFR3-related skeletal dysplasias. J Pharmacol Exp Ther. 2019;370:459.

Cannone V et al: Atrial natriuretic peptide: A molecular target of novel therapeutic approaches to cardio-metabolic disease. Int J Mol Sci 2019;20:3265.

Castiglione V et al. Biomarkers for the diagnosis and management of heart failure. Heart Fail Rev 2022;2:625.

Hanigan S, DiDomenico RJ: Emerging therapies for acute and chronic heart failure: Hope or hype? J Pharm Pract 2016;29:46.

Hijazi Z et al: Cardiac biomarkers and left ventricular hypertrophy in relation to outcomes in patients with atrial fibrillation: experiences from the RE-LY trial. J Am Heart Assoc 2019;8:e010107.

Jhund PS, McMurray JJ: The neprilysin pathway in heart failure: A review and guide on the use of sacubitril/valsartan. Heart 2016;102:1342.

Matsuo A et al: Natriuretic peptides in human heart: Novel insight into their molecular forms, functions, and diagnostic use. Peptides 2019;111:3.

Nakanishi K et al: Pre-procedural serum atrial natriuretic peptide levels predict left atrial reverse remodeling after catheter ablation in patients with atrial fibrillation. JACC Clin Electrophysiol 2016;2:151.

Packer M et al: Effect of ularitide on cardiovascular mortality in acute heart failure. N Engl J Med 2017;376:1956.

Pfeffer MA et al. Angiotensin receptor-neprilysin inhibition in acute myocardial infarction. N Engl J Med 2021;385:1845.

Prenner SB et al: Role of angiotensin receptor-neprilysin inhibition in heart failure. Curr Atheroscler Rep 2016;18:48.

Saito Y: Roles of atrial natriuretic peptide and its therapeutic use. J Cardiol 2010;56:262.

Savarirayan R et al: C-Type natriuretic peptide analogue therapy in children with achondroplasia. N Engl J Med 2019;381:25.

Solomon, SD et al: Angiotensin receptor neprilysin inhibition in heart failure with preserved ejection fraction: Rationale and design of the PARAGON-HF trial. JACC Heart Fail 2017;5:471.

Tanase DM et al: Natriuretic peptides in heart failure with preserved left ventricular ejection fraction: From molecular evidences to clinical implications. Int J Mol Sci. 2019;20:2629.

Tsiachris D et al: Biomarkers determining prognosis of atrial fibrillation ablation. Curr Med Chem 2019;26:925.

Vilela-Martin JF: Spotlight on valsartan-sacubitril fixed-dose combination for heart failure: The evidence to date. Drug Des Devel Ther 2016;10:1627.

Volpe M et al: The natriuretic peptides system in the pathophysiology of heart failure: From molecular basis to treatment. Clin Sci (Lond) 2016;130:57.

Vasoactive Intestinal Peptide

Paulis L et al: New developments in the pharmacological treatment of hypertension: Dead-end or a glimmer at the horizon? Curr Hypertens Rep 2015;17:557.

White CM et al: Therapeutic potential of vasoactive intestinal peptide and its receptors in neurological disorders. CNS Neurol Disord Drug Targets 2010;9:661.

Substance P

Garcia-Recio S, Gascon P: Biological and pharmacological aspects of the NK1-receptor. Biomed Res Int 2015;2015:495704.

Jung HJ, Priefer R. Tachykinin NK2 antagonist for treatments of various disease states. Auton Neurosci 2021;235:102865.

Khorasani S et al. The immunomodulatory effects of tachykinins and their receptors. J Cell Biochem 2020;121:3031.

Mistrova E et al: Role of substance P in the cardiovascular system. Neuropeptides 2016;58:41.

Munoz M, Covenas R: Involvement of substance P and the NK-1 receptor in cancer progression. Peptides 2013;48C:1.

Neurotensin

Boules M et al: Diverse roles of neurotensin agonists in the central nervous system. Front Endocrinol 2013;4:36.

Hwang JI et al: Phylogenetic history, pharmacological features, and signal transduction of neurotensin receptors in vertebrates. Ann N Y Acad Sci 2009;1163:169.

Iyer MR, Kunos G. Therapeutic approaches targeting the neurotensin receptors. Expert Opin Ther Pat 2021;3:361.

Konno N: Neurotensin. In: Takei Y, Ando H, Tsutsui K (editors): *Handbook of Hormones: Comparative Endocrinology for Basic and Clinical Research*. Elsevier, 2016.

Osadchii OE: Emerging role of neurotensin in regulation of the cardiovascular system. Eur J Pharmacol 2015;762:184.

Calcitonin Gene-Related Peptide

Ailani J et al. Atogepant for the preventive treatment of migraine. N Engl J Med 2021;385:695.

Aubdool AA et al: A novel alpha-calcitonin gene-related peptide analogue protects against end-organ damage in experimental hypertension, cardiac hypertrophy, and heart failure. Circulation 2017;136:367.

Caronna E, Starling AJ. Update on preventive treatment of migraine. Neurol Clin 2021;39:1.

Hay DL, Walker CS: CGRP and its receptors. Headache 2017;57:625.

Kee Z, Kodji X, Brain SD: The role of calcitonin gene related peptide (CGRP) in neurogenic vasodilation and its cardioprotective effects. Front Physiol 2018;9:1249.

Tajti J et al: Migraine and neuropeptides. Neuropeptides 2015;2:19.

Tiseo C et al: How to integrate monoclonal antibodies targeting the calcitonin gene-related peptide or its receptor in daily clinical practice. J Headache Pain 2019;20:49.

Wrobel Goldberg S, Silberstein SD: Targeting CGRP: A new era for migraine treatment. CNS Drugs 2015;29:443.

Adrenomedullin

Deniau B et al. Adrecizumab: an investigational agent for the biomarker-guided treatment of sepsis. Expert Opin Investig Drugs 2021;30:95.

Geven C, Kox M, Pickkers P: Adrenomedullin and adrenomedullin-targeted therapy as treatment strategies relevant for sepsis. Front Immunol 2018;9:292.

Kato J, Kitamura K: Bench-to-bedside pharmacology of adrenomedullin. Eur J Pharmacol 2015;764:140.

Koyama T et al: Adrenomedullin-RAMP2 system in vascular endothelial cells. J Atheroscler Thromb 2015;22:647.

Nishikimi T, Nakagawa Y: Adrenomedullin as a biomarker of heart failure. Heart Fail Clin 2018;14:49.

Tsuruda T et al: Adrenomedullin: Continuing to explore cardioprotection. Peptides 2019;111:47.

Voors AA et al: Adrenomedullin in heart failure: Pathophysiology and therapeutic application. Eur J Heart Fail 2019;21:163.

Watkins HA et al: Receptor activity-modifying proteins 2 and 3 generate adrenomedullin receptor subtypes with distinct molecular properties. J Biol Chem 2016;291:11657.

Relaxin

Ghosh RK et al: Serelaxin in acute heart failure: Most recent update on clinical and preclinical evidence. Cardiovasc Ther 2017;35:55.

Jelinic M et al: From pregnancy to cardiovascular disease: Lessons from relaxin-deficient animals to understand relaxin actions in the vascular system. Microcirculation 2019;26:e12464.

Kanai AJ et al: Relaxin and fibrosis: Emerging targets, challenges, and future directions. Mol Cell Endocrinol 2019;487:66.

Martin B et al: Cardioprotective actions of relaxin. Mol Cell Endocrinol 2019;487:45.

Martins RC et al. Relaxin and the cardiovascular system: from basic science to clinical practice. Curr Mol Med 2020;20:167.

Ng HH et al: Relaxin and extracellular matrix remodeling: Mechanisms and signaling pathways. Mol Cell Endocrinol 2019;487:59.

Ng TM et al: Relaxin for the treatment of acute decompensated heart failure: Pharmacology, mechanisms of action, and clinical evidence. Cardiol Rev 2016;24:194.

Patil NA et al: Relaxin family peptides: Structure-activity relationship studies. Br J Pharmacol 2017;174:950.

Summers RJ: Recent progress in the understanding of relaxin family peptides and their receptors. Br J Pharmacol 2017;174:915.

Urocortins

Adao R et al: Urocortin-2 improves right ventricular function and attenuates pulmonary arterial hypertension. Cardiovasc Res 2018;114:1165.

Chatzaki E et al: Do urocortins have a role in treating cardiovascular disease? Drug Discov Today 2019;24:279.

Grieco P, Gomez-Monterrey I: Natural and synthetic peptides in the cardiovascular diseases: An update on diagnostic and therapeutic potentials. Arch Biochem Biophys 2019;662:15.

Kovacs DK et al. Assessment of clinical data on urocortins and their therapeutic potential in cardiovascular diseases: A systematic review and meta-analysis. Clin Transl Sci 2021;14:2461.

Rademaker MT, Richards AM: Urocortins: Actions in health and heart failure. Clin Chim Acta 2017;474:76.

Stenmark KR, Graham BB: Urocortin 2: Will a drug targeting both the vasculature and the right ventricle be the future of pulmonary hypertension therapy? Cardiovasc Res 2018;114:1057.

GENERAL

Lo CCW, Moosavi SM, Bubb KJ: The regulation of pulmonary vascular tone by neuropeptides and the implications for pulmonary hypertension. Front Physiol 2018;9:1167.

Oparil S, Schmieder RE: New approaches in the treatment of hypertension. Circ Res 2015;116:1074.

Perrin S et al: New pharmacotherapy options for pulmonary arterial hypertension. Expert Opin Pharmacother 2015;16:2113.

Raghu GB et al: Effect of recombinant human pentraxin 2 vs placebo on change in forced vital capacity in patients with idiopathic pulmonary fibrosis: A randomized clinical trial. JAMA 2018;319:2299.

Sommer N et al. Current and future treatments of pulmonary arterial hypertension. Br J Pharmacol 2021;178:6.

Yandrapalli S et al: Newer hormonal pharmacotherapies for heart failure. Expert Rev Endocrinol Metab 2018;13:35.

CASE STUDY ANSWER

Enalapril lowers blood pressure by blocking the conversion of angiotensin I to angiotensin II (ANG II). Since converting enzyme also inactivates bradykinin, enalapril increases bradykinin levels, and this is responsible for adverse side effects such as cough and angioedema. This problem might be avoided by using a renin inhibitor, eg, aliskiren, or an ANG II receptor antagonist, eg, valsartan, instead of an angiotensin-converting enzyme inhibitor, to block the renin-angiotensin system. A β-adrenoceptor-blocking drug might also be tried since, in addition to their cardiac action, these drugs can inhibit renin secretion.

C H A P T E R

18 The Eicosanoids: Prostaglandins, Thromboxanes, Leukotrienes, & Related Compounds

John Hwa, MD, PhD, & Kathleen Martin, PhD*

CASE STUDY

A 40-year-old woman presented to her doctor with a 6-month history of increasing shortness of breath. This was associated with poor appetite and ankle swelling. On physical examination, she had elevated jugular venous distention, a soft tricuspid regurgitation murmur, clear lungs, and mild peripheral edema. An echocardiogram revealed tricuspid regurgitation, severely elevated pulmonary pressures, and right ventricular enlargement. Cardiac catheterization confirmed the severely elevated pulmonary pressures. She was commenced on appropriate therapies. Which of the eicosanoid agonists have been demonstrated to reduce both morbidity and mortality in patients with such a diagnosis? What are the modes of action?

The eicosanoids are oxygenation (oxidation) products of polyunsaturated 20-carbon long-chain fatty acids (*eicosa*, Greek for "twenty"). They are ubiquitous in the animal kingdom and are also found in a variety of plants. They constitute a very large family of compounds that are highly potent and display an extraordinarily wide spectrum of important biologic activities. Thus, the eicosanoid ligands, their specific receptors, their synthetic enzymes and inhibitors, and their plant and fish oil precursors, are therapeutic targets for a growing list of conditions.

ARACHIDONIC ACID & OTHER POLYUNSATURATED PRECURSORS

Arachidonic acid (AA) (5,8,11,14-eicosatetraenoic acid), the most abundant of the eicosanoid precursors, is a 20-carbon (C20) polyunsaturated fatty acid containing four double bonds (C20:4(5,8,11,14)). Linoleic acid, an essential fatty acid, is converted to linolenic acid, followed by conversion to AA. The first double bond in AA occurs at 6 carbons from the methyl end, defining AA as an omega-6 fatty acid (C20:4(ω–6) or C20:4-6). AA must first be released or mobilized from the sn-2 position of membrane phospholipids by one or more lipases of the phospholipase A_2 (PLA_2) type (Figure 18–1) for eicosanoid synthesis to occur. The phospholipase A_2 superfamily consists of over 30 isoforms classified into several families, contributing to arachidonate

*The authors thank Emer M. Smyth, PhD, and Garret A. FitzGerald, MD, for their contributions to previous editions of this chapter.

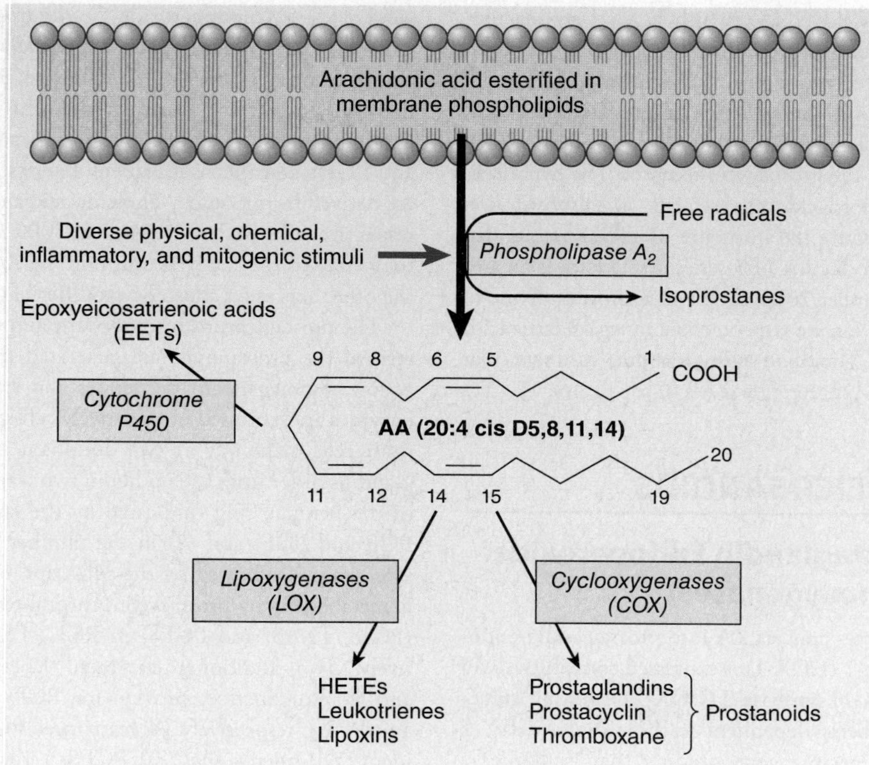

FIGURE 18–1 Pathways of arachidonic acid (AA) release and metabolism.

release from membrane lipids. The major two families are cytosolic PLA_2 ($cPLA_2$) and secretory PLA_2 ($sPLA_2$), both of which are calcium-dependent. Others include calcium-independent PLA_2 ($iPLA_2$); platelet-activating factor acetylhydrolase (PAF-AH); lysosomal PLA_2 ($LPLA_2$); PLA/acyltransferase (PLAAT); and α/β hydrolase (ABHD). Chemical and physical stimuli activate the Ca^{2+}-dependent translocation of $cPLA_2$ to the plasma membrane, where it releases arachidonate for metabolism to eicosanoids. While

ACRONYMS

AA	Arachidonic acid
COX	Cyclooxygenase
DHET	Dihydroxyeicosatrienoic acid
EET	Epoxyeicosatrienoic acid
HETE	Hydroxyeicosatetraenoic acid
HPETE	Hydroxyperoxyeicosatetraenoic acid
LTB, LTC	Leukotriene B, C, etc
LOX	Lipoxygenase
LXA, LXB	Lipoxin A, B
NSAID	Nonsteroidal anti-inflammatory drug
PGE, PGF	Prostaglandin E, F, etc
PLA, PLC	Phospholipase A, C
TXA, TXB	Thromboxane A, B

$cPLA_2$ dominates in the acute release of AA, inducible $sPLA_2$ contributes under conditions of sustained or intense stimulation of AA production. In contrast, under non-stimulated conditions, AA liberated by $iPLA_2$ is reincorporated into cell membranes, so there is negligible eicosanoid biosynthesis. AA can also be released from phospholipase C-generated diacylglycerol esters by the action of diacylglycerol and monoacylglycerol lipases.

Following mobilization, AA is oxygenated by four separate routes: enzymatically via the cyclooxygenase (COX), lipoxygenase, and P450 epoxygenase pathways; and nonenzymatically via the isoeicosanoid pathway (see Figure 18–1). Among factors determining the type of eicosanoid synthesized are (1) the substrate lipid species, (2) the cell stimulus, and (3) the cell type. The cell type-specific production of eicosanoids is largely determined by the presence of downstream "synthases" (ie, thromboxane versus prostacyclin synthase) that metabolize COX-derived endoperoxide to distinct eicosanoids. Distinct but related products can be formed from precursors other than AA. For example, an omega-6 fatty acid such as homo-γ-linoleic acid (C20:3–6), in comparison to the omega-3 fatty acid eicosapentaenoic acid (C20:5–3), yields products that differ quantitatively and qualitatively from those derived from AA. This serves as the basis for dietary manipulation of eicosanoid generation using fatty acids obtained from cold-water fish or from plants as nutritional supplements. For example, thromboxane (TXA_2), a powerful vasoconstrictor and platelet agonist, is synthesized from AA via the COX pathway. COX metabolism of eicosapentaenoic acid (an omega-3 fatty acid) yields TXA_3, which is relatively inactive. 3-Series prostaglandins, such as prostaglandin E_3 (PGE_3), can also act as partial agonists or antagonists, thereby having reduced activity in comparison to their AA-derived 2-series counterparts. Similarly, eicosapentaenoic acid can be metabolized to prostaglandin I_3, which serves as a full agonist for the prostacyclin receptor. The hypothesis that dietary eicosapentaenoic acid (omega-3 fatty acid) substitution for arachidonate could reduce the incidence of cardiovascular disease and cancer via the production of 3-series prostanoids is an area of intense study. In December 2019, the FDA approved the use of icosapent ethyl (Vascepa) (an eicosapentaenoic omega-3 fatty acid) as adjunctive therapy (e.g., add on to statin) to reduce cardiovascular risk in adults with elevated triglyceride levels (Chapter 41).

SYNTHESIS OF EICOSANOIDS

Products of Prostaglandin Endoperoxide Synthases (Cyclooxygenases)

Two unique COX isozymes convert AA into prostaglandin endoperoxides. PGH synthase-1 **(COX-1)** is expressed constitutively in most cells. In contrast, PGH synthase-2 **(COX-2)** is readily inducible, its expression levels being dependent on the stimulus. COX-2 is an immediate early-response gene product that is markedly up-regulated by shear stress, growth factors, tumor promoters, and inflammatory cytokines, consistent with the presence of multiple regulatory motifs in the promoter and 3′ untranslated regions of the COX-2 gene for several transcription factors, including NFκB, a key regulator of inflammatory gene expression. Put simply, COX-1 generates prostanoids for "housekeeping" functions, such as gastric epithelial cytoprotection, whereas COX-2 is the major source of prostanoids in inflammation and cancer. However, there are additional physiologic and pathophysiologic processes in which each enzyme is uniquely involved, and others in which they function coordinately. For example, endothelial COX-2 is the primary source of vascular prostacyclin (PGI_2), whereas renal COX-2-derived prostanoids are important for normal renal development and maintenance of function. Nonsteroidal anti-inflammatory drugs (NSAIDs; see Chapter 36) exert their therapeutic effects through inhibition of the COXs. Most older NSAIDs like indomethacin, sulindac, meclofenamate, and ibuprofen nonselectively inhibit both COX-1 and COX-2, whereas the selective COX-2 inhibitors follow the order celecoxib = diclofenac = meloxicam = etodolac < valdecoxib << rofecoxib < lumiracoxib = etoricoxib for increasing COX-2 selectivity. Aspirin acetylates and inhibits both COX-1 and COX-2 enzymes covalently and hence irreversibly. Low doses (<100 mg/d) inhibit preferentially, but not exclusively, platelet COX-1 (thus reducing thromboxane production), whereas higher doses inhibit both systemic COX-1 and COX-2. Genetic variations in human COX-2 variants have been linked with increased coronary heart disease risk, increases in some cancers, and reduced pain perception.

Both COX-1 and COX-2 function as homodimers inserted into the membrane of the endoplasmic reticulum to promote the uptake of two molecules of oxygen by cyclization of AA to yield a C_9–C_{11} endoperoxide C_{15} hydroperoxide (Figure 18–2). This product is PGG_2, which is then rapidly modified by the peroxidase moiety of the COX enzyme to add a 15-hydroxyl group that is essential for biologic activity. This product is PGH_2. Both endoperoxides are highly unstable. Analogous families—PGH_1 and PGH_3 and their subsequent 1-series and 3-series products—are derived from homo-γ-linolenic acid and eicosapentaenoic acid, respectively. In both COX-1 and COX-2 homodimers, one protomer acts as the catalytic unit binding AA for oxygenation, while the other acts as an allosteric modifier of catalytic activity.

The prostaglandins thromboxane and prostacyclin, collectively termed the prostanoids, are generated from PGH_2 through the action of downstream isomerases and synthases. These terminal enzymes are expressed in a relatively cell-specific fashion, such that most cells make one or two dominant prostanoids. The prostaglandins differ from each other in two ways: (1) in the substituents of the pentane ring (indicated by the last letter, eg, E and F in PGE and PGF) and (2) in the number of double bonds in the side chains (indicated by the subscript, eg, PGE_1, PGE_2). PGH_2 is metabolized by prostacyclin, thromboxane, and PGF synthases (PGIS, TXAS, and PGFS) to PGI_2, TXA_2, and $PGF_{2\alpha}$, respectively. Two additional enzymes, 9,11-endoperoxide reductase and 9-ketoreductase, provide for $PGF_{2\alpha}$ synthesis from PGH_2 and PGE_2, respectively. At least three PGE_2 synthases have been identified: microsomal (m) PGES-1, the more readily inducible mPGES-2, and cytosolic PGES. There are two distinct PGDS isoforms, the lipocalin-type PGDS and the hematopoietic PGDS.

Several products of the arachidonate series are in current clinical use. **Alprostadil** (PGE_1) may be used for its smooth muscle relaxing effects in the treatment of erectile dysfunction and to temporarily maintain a patent ductus arteriosus in some neonates with congenital heart disease awaiting corrective cardiac surgery. **Misoprostol,** a PGE_1 derivative, is a cytoprotective prostaglandin used in preventing peptic ulcer, for labor induction, and in combination with mifepristone (RU-486) for terminating early pregnancies. **Dinoprostone** (PGE_2) is used in obstetrics to dilate the cervix in inducing labor. **Latanoprost** and several similar compounds are topically active $PGF_{2\alpha}$ derivatives used in ophthalmology to reduce intraocular pressure in open-angle glaucoma or ocular hypertension. **Prostacyclin** (PGI_2) is synthesized mainly by the vascular endothelium and is a powerful vasodilator and inhibitor of platelet aggregation. Synthetic PGI_2 **(epoprostenol)** and PGI_2 analogs **(iloprost, treprostinil)** are used to treat pulmonary hypertension. In contrast, **thromboxane** (TXA_2) has undesirable properties (platelet aggregation, vasoconstriction). Therefore, TXA_2-receptor antagonists and synthesis inhibitors have been developed for cardiovascular indications, although these (except for aspirin) have yet to establish a place in clinical usage, because large clinical trials have failed to show superiority over low-dose aspirin for secondary stroke protection.

All the naturally occurring COX products undergo rapid metabolism to inactive products either by hydration (for PGI_2 and TXA_2) or by oxidation (of the 15-hydroxyl group to the corresponding ketone) by prostaglandin 15-hydroxy prostaglandin dehydrogenase (15-PGDH) after cellular uptake via an organic anion transporter polypeptide (OATP 2A1). Further metabolism

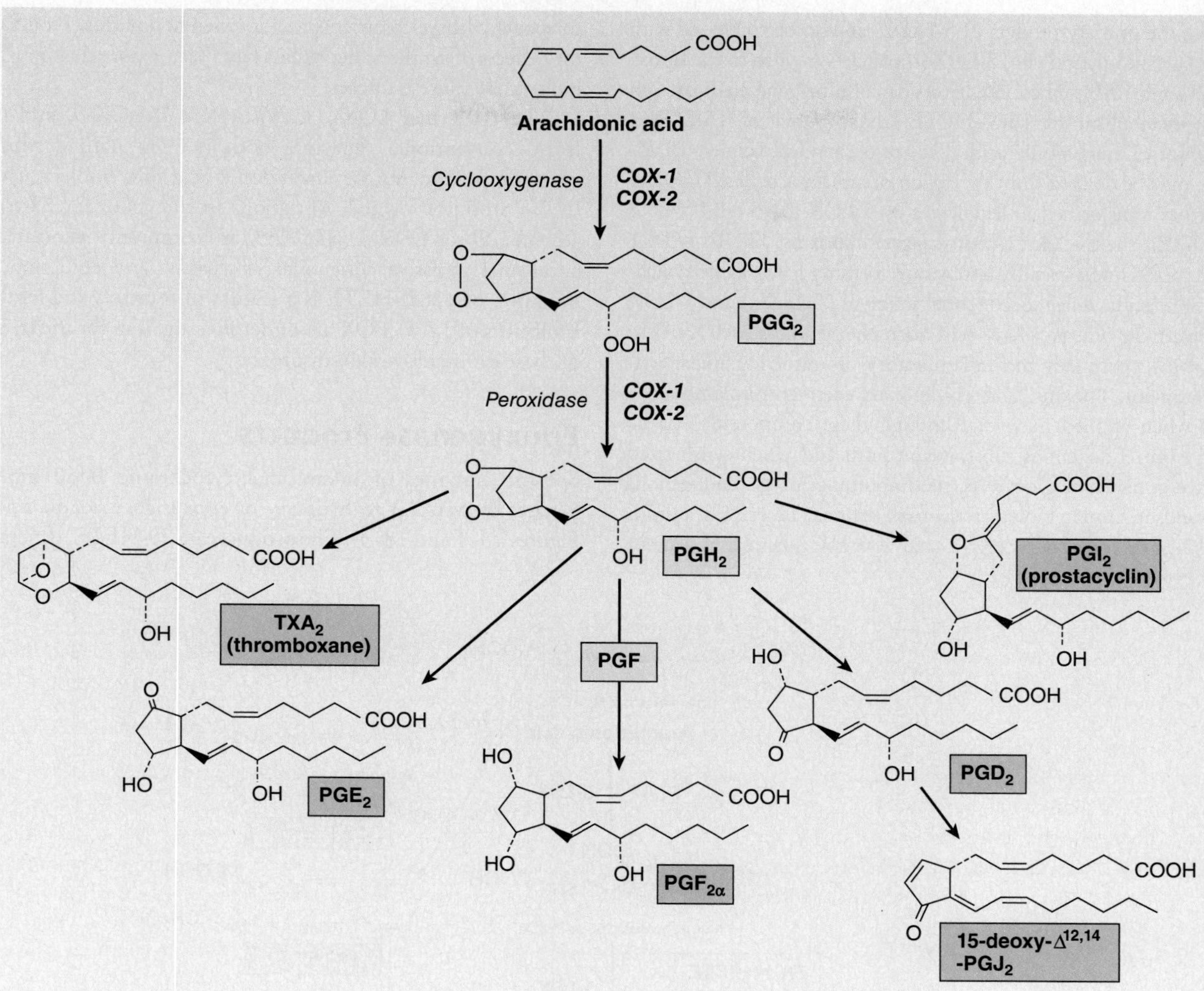

FIGURE 18–2 Prostanoid biosynthesis. Compound names are enclosed in boxes.

is by Δ^{13}-reduction, β-oxidation, and ω-oxidation. The inactive metabolites are chemically stable and can be quantified in blood and urine by immunoassay or mass spectrometry as a measure of the in vivo synthesis of their parent compounds.

Products of Lipoxygenase

The metabolism of AA by the **5-, 12-, and 15-lipoxygenases (LOX)** results in production of hydroperoxyeicosatetraenoic acids (HPETEs), which rapidly convert to hydroxy derivatives (HETEs). **5-LOX,** the most actively investigated pathway, gives rise to the leukotrienes (Figure 18–3) and is present in leukocytes (neutrophils, basophils, eosinophils, and monocyte-macrophages) and other inflammatory cells such as mast cells and dendritic cells. This pathway is of great interest because it is associated with asthma, anaphylactic shock, and cardiovascular disease. Stimulation of these cells elevates intracellular Ca^{2+} and releases arachidonate; incorporation of molecular oxygen by 5-LOX, in association with **5-LOX-activating protein (FLAP),** yields 5(*S*)-HPETE, which is then further converted by 5-LOX to the unstable epoxide leukotriene A_4 (LTA_4). This intermediate is either converted to the dihydroxy leukotriene B_4 (LTB_4), via the action of LTA_4 hydrolase, or conjugated with glutathione to yield leukotriene C_4 (LTC_4), by LTC_4 synthase. Sequential degradation of the glutathione moiety by peptidases yields LTD_4 and LTE_4. These three products, LTC_4, D_4, and E_4, are called cysteinyl leukotrienes. Although leukotrienes are predominantly generated in leukocytes, nonleukocyte cells (eg, endothelial cells) that express enzymes downstream of 5-LOX/FLAP can take up and convert leukocyte-derived LTA_4 in a process termed transcellular biosynthesis. Transcellular formation of prostaglandins has also been shown; for example, endothelial cells can use platelet PGH_2 to form PGI_2.

LTC4 and **LTD4** are potent bronchoconstrictors and are secreted in asthma and anaphylaxis. There are four current approaches to antileukotriene drug development: 5-LOX enzyme inhibitors, cysteinyl leukotriene-receptor antagonists, inhibitors of FLAP, and phospholipase A_2 inhibitors. Variants in the human 5-LOX gene (*ALOX5*) or the cysteinyl receptors (CYSLTR1 or CYSLTR2) have been linked with asthma and with altered response to antileukotriene drugs.

LTA_4, the primary product of 5-LOX, can also be converted with appropriate stimulation via 12-LOX in platelets in vitro to the **lipoxins** LXA_4 and LXB_4. These mediators can also be generated through 5-LOX metabolism of 15(*S*)-HETE, the product of 15-LOX-2 metabolism of arachidonic acid. The stereochemical isomer, 15(*R*)-HETE, may be derived from the action of aspirin-acetylated COX-2 and further transformed in leukocytes by 5-LOX to 15-epi-LXA_4 or 15-epi-LXB_4, the so-called aspirin-triggered lipoxins. The 15-LOX-1 isoform prefers linoleic acid as a substrate, forming 13(*S*)-hydroxyoctadecadienoic acid, while the sequential action of 15-LOX-1 and 5-LOX can convert the omega-3 fatty acid docosahexaenoic acid (DHA) to the resolvins, potentially anti-inflammatory, pro-resolving lipids. Synthetic resolvins, lipoxins, and epi-lipoxins exert anti-inflammatory actions when applied in vivo. Although these compounds can be formed from endogenous substrates in vitro and when synthesized may have potent biologic effects, the importance of the endogenous compounds in human biology remains ill defined. 12-HETE, a product of 12-LOX, can also undergo a catalyzed molecular rearrangement to epoxyhydroxyeicosatrienoic acids called **hepoxilins.** Proinflammatory effects of synthetic hepoxilins have been reported although their biologic relevance is unclear.

The epidermal LOXs, 12(*R*)-LOX and LOX-3, are distinct from "conventional" enzymes both in their natural substrates, which appear to not be arachidonic acid and linoleic acid, and in the products formed. Mutations in the genes for 12(*R*)-LOX *(ALOX12B)* or LOX-3 *(ALOXE3)* are commonly associated with autosomal recessive congenital ichthyosis, and epidermal accumulation of 12(*R*)-HETE is a feature of psoriasis and ichthyosis. Inhibitors of 12(*R*)-LOX are under investigation for the treatment of these proliferative skin disorders.

Epoxygenase Products

Specific isozymes of microsomal cytochrome P450 monooxygenases convert AA to hydroxy- or epoxyeicosatrienoic acids (see Figures 18–1 and 18–3). The products are 20-HETE, generated by

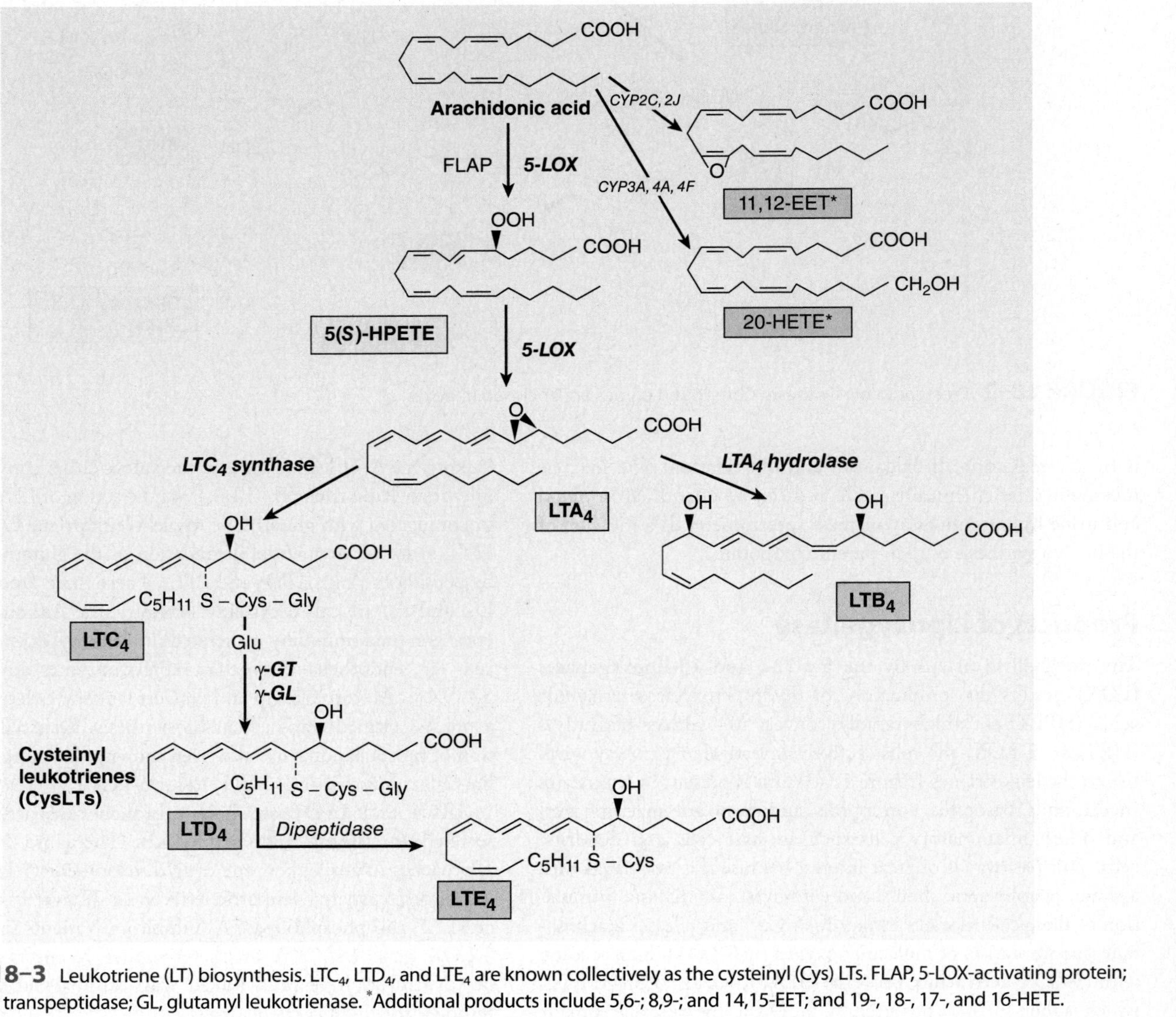

FIGURE 18–3 Leukotriene (LT) biosynthesis. LTC_4, LTD_4, and LTE_4 are known collectively as the cysteinyl (Cys) LTs. FLAP, 5-LOX-activating protein; GT, glutamyl transpeptidase; GL, glutamyl leukotrienase. *Additional products include 5,6-; 8,9-; and 14,15-EET; and 19-, 18-, 17-, and 16-HETE.

the CYP hydroxylases (CYP3A, 4A, 4F) and the 5,6-, 8,9-, 11,12-, and 14,15-epoxyeicosatrienoic acids (EETs), which arise from the CYP epoxygenase (2J, 2C). Their biosynthesis can be altered by pharmacologic, nutritional, and genetic factors that affect P450 expression. The biologic actions of the EETs are reduced by their conversion to the corresponding, and biologically less active, dihydroxyeicosatrienoic acids (DHETs) through the action of soluble epoxide hydrolase (sEH). Unlike the prostaglandins, the EETs can be esterified into phospholipids, which then act as storage sites. Intracellular fatty acid-binding proteins promote EET uptake into cells, incorporation into phospholipids, and availability to sEH. EETs are synthesized in endothelial cells and cause vasodilation in a number of vascular beds by activating the smooth muscle large conductance Ca^{2+}-activated K^+ channels. This results in smooth muscle cell hyperpolarization and vasodilation, leading to reduced blood pressure. Substantial evidence indicates that EETs may function as **endothelium-derived hyperpolarizing factors,** particularly in the coronary circulation. 15(*S*)-Hydroxy-11,12-EET, which arises from the 15-LOX pathway, is also an endothelium-derived hyperpolarizing factor and a substrate for sEH. Consequently, there is interest in inhibitors of soluble sEH as potential antithrombotic and antihypertensive drugs. Anti-inflammatory, antiapoptotic, and proangiogenic actions of the EETs have also been reported.

Isoeicosanoids

The isoeicosanoids, a family of eicosanoid isomers, are formed nonenzymatically by direct free radical-based action on AA and related lipid substrates. The **isoprostanes** thus formed are prostaglandin stereoisomers. Because prostaglandins have many asymmetric centers, they have a large number of potential stereoisomers. COX is not needed for the formation of the isoprostanes, and its inhibition with aspirin or other NSAIDs should not affect the isoprostane pathway. The primary epimerization mechanism is peroxidation of arachidonate by free radicals. Peroxidation occurs while arachidonic acid is still esterified to the membrane phospholipids. Thus, unlike prostaglandins, these stereoisomers are "stored" as part of the membrane. They are then cleaved by phospholipases, circulate, and are excreted in urine. Isoprostanes are present in relatively large amounts (tenfold greater in blood and urine than the COX-derived prostaglandins). They have potent vasoconstrictor effects when infused into renal and other vascular beds and may activate prostanoid receptors. They also may modulate other aspects of vascular function, including leukocyte and platelet adhesive interactions and angiogenesis. It has been speculated that they may contribute to the pathophysiology of inflammatory responses in a manner insensitive to COX inhibitors. A particular difficulty in assessing the likely biologic functions of isoprostanes—several of which have been shown to serve as incidental ligands at prostaglandin receptors—is that while high concentrations of individual isoprostanes may be necessary to elicit a response, multiple compounds are formed coincidentally in vivo under conditions of oxidant stress. Analogous leukotriene and EET isomers have been described.

■ BASIC PHARMACOLOGY OF EICOSANOIDS

MECHANISMS & EFFECTS OF EICOSANOIDS

Receptor Mechanisms

As a result of their short half-lives, the eicosanoids act mainly in an autocrine and a paracrine fashion, ie, close to the site of their synthesis, and not as circulating hormones. These ligands bind to receptors on the cell surface, with pharmacologic specificity determined by receptor density and type on different cells (Figure 18–4). A single gene product has been identified for each of the PGI_2 (IP), $PGF_{2\alpha}$ (FP), and TXA_2 (TP) receptors, while four distinct PGE_2 receptors (EPs 1–4) and two PGD_2 receptors (DP_1 and DP_2) have been identified. Additional isoforms of the human TP (α and β), FP (A and B), and EP_3 (eight isoforms, I through VIII) receptors can arise through differential mRNA splicing. Two receptors exist for LTB_4 (BLT_1 and BLT_2) and for LTC_4/LTD_4 ($cysLT_1$ and $cysLT_2$). The formyl peptide (fMLP)-1 receptor can be activated by lipoxin A4 and consequently has been termed the ALX receptor. Receptor heterodimerization has been reported for a number of the eicosanoid receptors, providing for additional receptor subtypes from the currently identified gene products. All of these receptors are G protein-coupled; properties of the best-studied receptors are listed in Table 18–1.

EP_2, EP_4, IP, and DP_1 receptors activate adenylyl cyclase via G_s. This leads to increased intracellular cAMP levels, which in turn activate specific protein kinases (see Chapter 2). EP_1, FP, and TP activate phosphatidylinositol metabolism, leading to the formation of inositol trisphosphate, with subsequent mobilization of Ca^{2+} stores and an increase of free intracellular Ca^{2+}. TP can also couple to multiple G proteins, including $G_{12/13}$ and G_{16}, to stimulate small G protein signaling pathways. EP_3 isoforms can couple to both increased intracellular calcium and to increased or decreased cAMP. The DP_2 receptor (also known as the chemoattractant receptor-homologous molecule expressed on TH2 cells, or CRTH2), which is unrelated to the other prostanoid receptors, is a member of the fMLP receptor superfamily. This receptor couples through a G_i-type G protein and leads to inhibition of cAMP synthesis and increases in intracellular Ca^{2+} in a variety of cell types.

LTB_4 also causes inositol trisphosphate release via the BLT_1 receptor, causing activation, degranulation, and superoxide anion generation in leukocytes. The BLT_2 receptor, a low-affinity receptor for LTB_4, is also bound with reasonable affinity by 12(*S*)- and 12(*R*)-HETE. BLT2 appears to play roles in allergic and inflammatory responses as well as progression of certain cancer cells. $CysLT_1$ and $cysLT_2$ couple to G_q, leading to increased intracellular Ca^{2+}. Studies have also placed G_i downstream of $cysLT_2$. As noted above, the EETs promote vasodilation via paracrine activation of calcium-activated potassium channels on smooth muscle cells leading to hyperpolarization and relaxation. This occurs in a manner consistent with activation of a G_s-coupled receptor. Although a specific high affinity EET receptor has yet to be

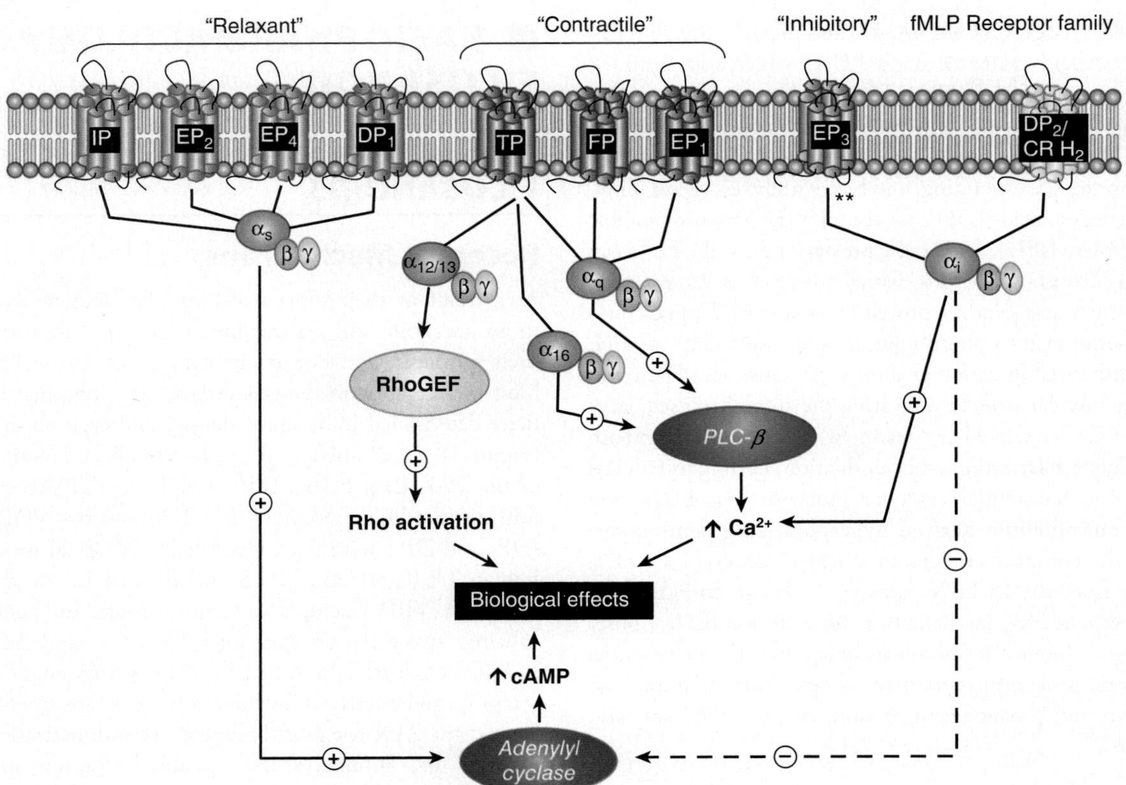

FIGURE 18–4 Prostanoid receptors and their signaling pathways. fMLP, formylated Met-Leu-Phe, a small peptide receptor; PLC-β, phospholipase C-β. All of the receptors shown are of the seven-transmembrane, G protein-coupled type. The terms "relaxant," "contractile," and "inhibitory" refer to the phylogenetic characterization of their primary effects. **, all EP_3 isoforms couple through G_i but some can also activate G_s or $G_{12/13}$ pathways. RhoGEF, rho guanine nucleotide exchange factor. See text for additional details.

identified, GPR40 (FFA1) may serve as a low affinity receptor for 11,12-EET in endothelial cells. EETs may also act in an autocrine manner directly activating endothelial transient receptor potential channels to cause endothelial hyperpolarization, which is then transferred to the smooth muscle cells by gap junctions or potassium ions. Recently, a specific G protein-coupled receptor (GPR75) for the vasoconstrictor 20-HETE has been identified and 20-HETE signaling is coupled via $G_{q/11}$. Specific receptors for isoprostanes have not been identified, and the biologic importance of their capacity to act as incidental ligands at prostaglandin receptors remains to be established.

Although prostanoids can activate peroxisome proliferator-activated receptors (PPARs) if added in sufficient concentration in vitro, it remains questionable whether these compounds ever attain concentrations sufficient to function as endogenous nuclear-receptor ligands in vivo.

Effects of Prostaglandins & Thromboxanes

The prostaglandins and thromboxanes have major effects on smooth muscle in the vasculature, airways, and gastrointestinal and reproductive tracts. Contraction of smooth muscle is mediated by the release of calcium, while relaxing effects are mediated by the generation of cAMP. Many of the eicosanoids' contractile effects on smooth muscle can be inhibited by lowering extracellular calcium or by using calcium channel-blocking drugs. Other important targets include platelets and monocytes, kidneys, the central nervous system, autonomic presynaptic nerve terminals, sensory nerve endings, endocrine organs, adipose tissue, and the eye (the effects on the eye may involve smooth muscle).

A. Smooth Muscle

1. *Vascular*—TXA_2 is a potent vasoconstrictor. It is also a smooth muscle cell mitogen and is the only eicosanoid that has convincingly been shown to have this effect. $PGF_{2\alpha}$ is also a vasoconstrictor but is not a smooth muscle mitogen. Another vasoconstrictor is the isoprostane 8-iso-$PGF_{2\alpha}$, also known as $iPF_{2\alpha}III$, which may act via the TP receptor.

Vasodilator prostaglandins, especially PGI_2 and PGE_2, promote vasodilation by increasing cAMP and decreasing smooth muscle intracellular calcium, primarily via the IP and EP_4 receptors, respectively. Vascular PGI_2 is synthesized by both smooth muscle and endothelial cells, with the COX-2 isoform in the latter cell type being the major contributor. In the microcirculation, PGE_2 is a vasodilator produced by endothelial cells. PGI_2 inhibits proliferation of smooth muscle cells, an action that may be particularly relevant in pulmonary hypertension. PGD_2 may also function as a vasodilator, in particular as a dominant mediator of flushing induced by the lipid-lowering drug niacin.

TABLE 18–1 Eicosanoid receptors.[1]

Receptor (Human)	Endogenous Ligand	Secondary Ligands	G Protein; Second Messenger	Major Phenotype(s) in Knockout Mice
DP_1	PGD_2		G_s; ↑cAMP	↓Allergic asthma
				↑Inflammatory cardiovascular disease, hypertension, thrombosis
DP_2	PGD_2	15d-PGJ_2	G_i; ↑$Ca^{2+}{}_i$, ↓cAMP	↑Allergic airway inflammation
				↓Cutaneous inflammation
EP_1	PGE_2	PGI_2	G_q; ↑$Ca^{2+}{}_i$	↓Colon carcinogenesis
EP_2	PGE_2		G_s; ↑cAMP	Impaired fertilization
				Salt-sensitive hypertension
				↓Tumorgenesis
$EP_{3\ I, II, III, IV, V, VI, e, f}$	PGE_2		G_i; ↓cAMP, ↑$Ca^{2+}{}_i$	Resistance to pyrogens
			G_s; ↑cAMP	↓Acute cutaneous inflammation
			G_q; ↑PLC, ↑$Ca^{2+}{}_i$	↑Allergic airway inflammation
			$G_{12/13}$; Rho activation	Obesity
EP_4	PGE_2		G_s; ↑cAMP	↑Myocardial infarction severity
				↑Intestinal inflammatory/immune response
				↓Colon carcinogenesis
				Patent ductus arteriosus
$FP_{A,B}$	$PGF_{2\alpha}$	isoPs	G_q; ↑PLC, ↑$Ca^{2+}{}_i$	Parturition failure
			$G_{12/13}$; Rho activation	↓Basal blood pressure; ↑Vasopressor response
				↓Atherosclerosis
IP	PGI_2	PGE_2	Gs; ↑cAMP	↑Thrombotic response
				↑Response to vascular injury
				↑Atherosclerosis
				↑Cardiac fibrosis
				Salt-sensitive hypertension
$TP_{\alpha,\beta}$	TXA_2	isoPs	G_q,$G_{12/13}$,G_{16}; ↑PLC, ↑$Ca^{2+}{}_i$, Rho activation	↑Bleeding time
				↓Response to vascular injury
				↓Atherosclerosis
				↑Survival after cardiac allograft
BLT_1	LTB_4		G_{16},G_i; ↑$Ca^{2+}{}_i$, ↓cAMP	Inflammatory responses
				↓Insulin resistance in obesity
BLT_2	LTB_4	12(*S*)-HETE	G_q-like, G_i-like, G_{12}-like, ↑$Ca^{2+}{}_i$	↓inflammatory arthritis
		12(*R*)-HETE		↑Experimental colitis
$CysLT_1$	LTD_4	LTC_4/LTE_4	G_q; ↑PLC, ↑$Ca^{2+}{}_i$	↓Innate and adaptive immune vascular permeability response
				↑Pulmonary inflammatory and fibrotic response
$CysLT_2$	LTC_4/LTD_4	LTE_4	G_q; ↑PLC, ↑$Ca^{2+}{}_i$	↓Pulmonary inflammatory and fibrotic response

[1]Splice variants for the eicosanoid receptors are indicated where appropriate.

$Ca^{2+}{}_i$, intracellular calcium; cAMP, cyclic adenosine 3′,5′-monophosphate; PLC, phospholipase C; isoPs, isoprostanes; 15d-PGJ_2, 15-deoxy-$\Delta^{12,14}$-PGJ_2.

2. *Gastrointestinal tract*—Most of the prostaglandins and thromboxanes activate gastrointestinal smooth muscle. Longitudinal muscle is contracted by PGE_2 (via EP_3) and $PGF_{2\alpha}$ (via FP), whereas circular muscle is contracted strongly by $PGF_{2\alpha}$ and weakly by PGI_2, and is relaxed by PGE_2 (via EP_4). Administration of either PGE_2 or $PGF_{2\alpha}$ thus can result in colicky cramps (see Clinical Pharmacology of Eicosanoids, below). The leukotrienes also have powerful contractile effects.

3. *Airways*—Respiratory smooth muscle is relaxed by PGE_2 and PGI_2 and contracted by PGD_2, TXA_2, and $PGF_{2\alpha}$. Studies of DP_1 and DP_2 receptor knockout mice suggest an important role of PGD_2 in asthma, although the DP_2 receptor appears more relevant to allergic airway diseases. The cysteinyl leukotrienes are also bronchoconstrictors. They act principally on smooth muscle in peripheral airways and are a thousand times more potent than histamine, both in vitro and in vivo. They also stimulate bronchial mucus secretion and cause mucosal edema. Bronchospasm occurs in about 10% of people taking NSAIDs, possibly because of a shift in arachidonate metabolism from COX metabolism to leukotriene formation.

4. *Reproductive*—The actions of prostaglandins on reproductive smooth muscle are discussed below under section D, Reproductive Organs.

B. Platelets

Platelet aggregation is markedly affected by eicosanoids. PGI_2, a major product of endothelial-derived COX-2, is a potent inhibitor of platelet aggregation. This inhibition occurs via an IP receptor-dependent elevation in G_s activity and cAMP. Dysfunctional genetic variants in the human prostacyclin receptor as well as drug inhibition of COX-2 (reducing prostacyclin signaling and production, respectively) lead to increased platelet activation and aggregation. This has recently been demonstrated to have major implications regarding adverse cardiovascular events, as described below (see Inhibition of Eicosanoid Synthesis). TXA_2 is the major product of platelet COX-1, the only COX isoform expressed in mature platelets, with COX-1-derived PGD_2 found in lesser amounts. TXA_2 is a powerful inducer of platelet aggregation. TXA_2 additionally amplifies the effects of other, more potent, platelet agonists such as thrombin. The TP-G_q signaling pathway elevates intracellular Ca^{2+} and activates protein kinase C, facilitating platelet aggregation and TXA_2 biosynthesis. Activation of G_{12}/G_{13} induces Rho/Rho-kinase–dependent regulation of myosin light chain phosphorylation leading to platelet shape change. Mutations in the human TP have been associated with mild bleeding disorders. The platelet actions of TXA_2 are restrained in vivo by PGI_2, which inhibits platelet aggregation by all recognized agonists, and PGD_2. Platelet COX-1-derived TXA_2 biosynthesis is increased during platelet activation and aggregation and is irreversibly inhibited by chronic administration of aspirin at low doses. Urinary metabolites of TXA_2 increase in clinical syndromes of platelet activation, such as diabetes mellitus, and particularly in patients with myocardial infarction and stroke. Macrophage COX-2 appears to contribute roughly 10% of the increment in TXA_2 biosynthesis observed in smokers, while the rest is derived from platelet COX-1. Low concentrations of PGE_2 enhance (via EP_3 receptors), whereas higher concentrations inhibit (via IP receptors), platelet aggregation. PGD_2 inhibits aggregation via increased cAMP generation from DP_1 activation.

C. Kidney

Both the medulla and the cortex of the kidney synthesize prostaglandins, the medulla substantially more than the cortex. COX-1 is expressed mainly in cortical and medullary collecting ducts and mesangial cells, arteriolar endothelium, and epithelial cells of Bowman's capsule. COX-2 is restricted to the renal medullary interstitial cells, the macula densa, and the cortical thick ascending limb.

The major renal eicosanoid products are PGE_2 and PGI_2, followed by $PGF_{2\alpha}$ and TXA_2. The kidney also synthesizes several hydroxyeicosatetraenoic acids, leukotrienes, cytochrome P450 products, and epoxides. Prostaglandins play important roles in maintaining blood pressure and regulating renal function, particularly in marginally functioning kidneys and volume-contracted states. Under these circumstances, renal cortical COX-2-derived PGE_2 and PGI_2 maintain renal blood flow and glomerular filtration rate through their local vasodilating effects. These prostaglandins also modulate systemic blood pressure through regulation of water and sodium excretion. Expression of medullary COX-2 and mPGES-1 is increased under conditions of high salt intake. COX-2-derived prostanoids increase medullary blood flow and inhibit tubular sodium reabsorption, while COX-1-derived products promote salt excretion in the collecting ducts. Increased water clearance probably results from an attenuation of the action of antidiuretic hormone (ADH) on adenylyl cyclase. Loss of these effects may underlie the systemic or salt-sensitive hypertension often associated with COX inhibition. A common misperception—often articulated in discussion of the cardiovascular toxicity of NSAID drugs—is that hypertension secondary to NSAID administration is somehow independent of the inhibition of prostaglandins. Loop diuretics, eg, furosemide, produce some of their effect by stimulating COX activity. In the normal kidney, this increases the synthesis of the vasodilator prostaglandins. Therefore, patient response to a loop diuretic is diminished if a COX inhibitor is administered concurrently (see Chapter 15).

There is an additional layer of complexity associated with the effects of renal prostaglandins. In contrast to the medullary enzyme, cortical COX-2 expression is increased by low salt intake, leading to increased renin release. This elevates glomerular filtration rate and contributes to enhanced sodium reabsorption and a rise in blood pressure. PGE_2 is thought to stimulate renin release through activation of EP_4 or EP_2. PGI_2 can also stimulate renin release and this may be relevant to maintenance of blood pressure in volume-contracted conditions and to the pathogenesis of renovascular hypertension. Inhibition of COX-2 may reduce blood pressure in these settings.

TXA_2 causes intrarenal vasoconstriction (and perhaps an ADH-like effect), resulting in a decline in renal function. The normal kidney synthesizes only small amounts of TXA_2. However, in renal conditions involving inflammatory cell infiltration (such as glomerulonephritis and renal transplant rejection), the inflammatory cells (monocyte-macrophages) release substantial amounts of TXA_2. Theoretically, TXA_2 synthase inhibitors or receptor antagonists should improve renal function in these patients, but no such drug is clinically available. Hypertension is associated with increased TXA_2 and decreased PGE_2 and PGI_2 synthesis in some animal models, eg, the Goldblatt kidney model. It is not known whether these changes are primary contributing factors or secondary responses. $PGF_{2\alpha}$ may elevate blood pressure by regulating renin release in the kidney.

D. Reproductive Organs

1. *Female reproductive organs*—Animal studies demonstrate a role for PGE_2 and $PGF_{2\alpha}$ in early reproductive processes such as ovulation, luteolysis, and fertilization. Uterine muscle is contracted by $PGF_{2\alpha}$, TXA_2, and low concentrations of PGE_2; PGI_2 and high concentrations of PGE_2 cause relaxation. $PGF_{2\alpha}$, together with oxytocin, is essential for the onset of parturition. PGI_2 also assists in promoting uterine smooth muscle cell maturation. The effects of prostaglandins on uterine function are discussed below (see Clinical Pharmacology of Eicosanoids).

2. *Male reproductive organs*—Prostaglandins may have a dual role in seminal fluid, with $PGF_{2\alpha}$ facilitating sperm transport through peristaltic actions in the female reproductive tract, and PGE_1/PGE_2 inducing sperm motility. Smooth muscle-relaxing prostaglandins such as PGE_1 enhance penile erection by relaxing the smooth muscle of the corpora cavernosa (see Clinical Pharmacology of Eicosanoids, below). Thus men with a low seminal fluid concentration of prostaglandins are relatively infertile. The major source of these prostaglandins is the seminal vesicle; the prostate, despite the name "prostaglandin," and the testes synthesize only small amounts. The factors that regulate the concentration of prostaglandins in human seminal plasma are not known in detail, but testosterone does promote prostaglandin production. Thromboxane and leukotrienes have not been found in seminal fluid.

E. Central and Peripheral Nervous Systems

1. *Fever*—PGE_2 increases body temperature, predominantly via EP_3, although EP_1 also plays a role. Exogenous $PGF_{2\alpha}$ and PGI_2 induce fever, whereas PGD_2 and TXA_2 do not. Endogenous pyrogens release interleukin-1, which in turn promotes the synthesis and release of PGE_2. This synthesis is blocked by aspirin, other NSAIDs, and acetaminophen, and explains how these drugs reduce fever.

2. *Sleep*—PGD_2 induces physiological sleep (as determined by electroencephalographic analysis) via activation of DP_1 receptors and secondary release of adenosine. PGE_2 may promote wakefulness.

3. *Neurotransmission*—PGE compounds inhibit the release of norepinephrine from postganglionic sympathetic nerve endings. Moreover, NSAIDs increase norepinephrine release in vivo, suggesting that the prostaglandins play a physiologic role in this process. Thus, vasoconstriction observed during treatment with COX inhibitors may be due, in part, to increased release of norepinephrine as well as to inhibition of the endothelial synthesis of the vasodilators PGE_2 and PGI_2. PGE_2 and PGI_2 sensitize the peripheral nerve endings to painful stimuli. PGE_2 acts via EP_1 and EP_4 receptors to potentiate excitatory cation channel activity and inhibit hyperpolarizing K^+ channel activity, thereby increasing membrane excitability. Prostaglandins also modulate pain centrally. Both COX-1 and COX-2 are expressed in the spinal cord and release prostaglandins in response to peripheral pain stimuli. PGE_2, and perhaps also PGD_2, PGI_2, and $PGF_{2\alpha}$, contributes to so-called central sensitization, an increase in excitability of spinal dorsal horn neurons, that augments pain intensity, widens the area of pain perception, and results in pain from normally innocuous stimuli. PGE_2 acts on the EP_2 receptor to facilitate presynaptic release of excitatory neurotransmitters and block inhibitory glycinergic neurotransmission as well as postsynaptically to enhance excitatory neurotransmitter receptor activity.

F. Inflammation and Immunity

PGE_2 and PGI_2 are the predominant prostanoids associated with inflammation. Both markedly enhance edema formation and leukocyte infiltration by promoting blood flow in the inflamed region. PGE_2 and PGI_2, through activation of EP_2 and IP, respectively, increase vascular permeability and leukocyte infiltration. PGI_2 contributes to immune suppression by interfering with dendritic cell maturation and antigen uptake for presentation to immune cells. PGE_2 suppresses the immunologic response by inhibiting differentiation of B lymphocytes into antibody-secreting plasma cells, thus depressing the humoral antibody response. It also inhibits cytotoxic T-cell function, mitogen-stimulated proliferation of T lymphocytes, and maturation and function of TH1 lymphocytes. PGE_2 can modify myeloid cell differentiation, promoting type 2 immune-suppressive macrophage and myeloid suppressor cell phenotypes. These effects likely contribute to immune escape in tumors where infiltrating myeloid-derived cells predominantly display type 2 phenotypes. TXA_2, through its action as a platelet agonist, can increase platelet-leukocyte interactions. PGE_2 and TXA_2 may play a role in T-lymphocyte development by regulating apoptosis of immature thymocytes. PGD_2, a major product of mast cells, is a potent chemoattractant for eosinophils in which it also induces degranulation and leukotriene biosynthesis. PGD_2 also induces chemotaxis and migration of TH2 lymphocytes, mainly via activation of DP_2, although a role for DP_1 has also been established. It remains unclear how these two receptors coordinate the actions of PGD_2 in inflammation and immunity. A degradation product of PGD_2, 15d-PGJ_2, at concentrations formed in vivo, may also activate eosinophils via the DP_2 (CRTH2) receptor.

G. Bone Metabolism

Prostaglandins are abundant in skeletal tissue and are produced by osteoblasts and adjacent hematopoietic cells. The major effect of prostaglandins (especially PGE_2, acting on EP_4) in vivo is to increase bone turnover, ie, stimulation of bone resorption and formation. EP_4 receptor deletion in mice results in an imbalance between bone resorption and formation, leading to a negative balance of bone mass and density in older animals. Prostaglandins may mediate the effects of mechanical forces on bones and changes in bone during inflammation. EP_4-receptor deletion and inhibition of prostaglandin biosynthesis have both been associated with impaired fracture healing in animal models. Prostaglandins may contribute to the bone loss that occurs at menopause. NSAIDs, especially those specific for inhibition of COX-2, delay bone healing in experimental models of fracture. COX inhibitors can also slow skeletal muscle healing by interfering with prostaglandin effects on myocyte proliferation, differentiation, and fibrosis in response to injury.

H. Eye

PGE, PGF, and PGD derivatives lower intraocular pressure. The mechanism of this action is unclear but probably involves increased outflow of aqueous humor from the anterior chamber via the uveoscleral pathway (see Clinical Pharmacology of Eicosanoids).

I. Cancer

There has been considerable interest in the role of prostaglandins, and in particular the COX-2 pathway, in the development of malignancies. Pharmacologic inhibition or genetic deletion of COX-2 restrains tumor formation in murine models of colon, breast, lung, and other cancers. Large human epidemiologic studies have found that the incidental use of NSAIDs is associated with significant reductions in relative risk for developing these and other cancers. The anticancer efficacy of aspirin in humans may be related to hyperactivity of the PI3 kinase/Akt pathway in tumor cells. In patients with familial polyposis coli, COX inhibitors significantly decrease polyp formation. Polymorphisms in COX-2 have been associated with increased risk of some cancers. Several studies have suggested that COX-2 expression is associated with markers of tumor progression in breast cancer. In mouse mammary tissue, COX-2 is oncogenic, whereas NSAID use is associated with a reduced risk of breast cancer in women, especially for hormone receptor-positive tumors. Despite the support for COX-2 as the predominant source of oncogenic prostaglandins, randomized clinical trials have not been performed to determine whether superior anti-oncogenic effects occur with selective inhibition of COX-2, compared with nonselective NSAIDs. Indeed, data from animal models and epidemiologic studies in humans are consistent with a role for COX-1 as well as COX-2 in the production of oncogenic prostanoids. However, ongoing clinical studies for the use of aspirin for cancer chemoprevention have been conflicting, and may arise from multiple factors including age of patient at initiation of aspirin, type of cancer, and patient comorbidities.

PGE_2, which is considered the principal oncogenic prostanoid, facilitates tumor initiation, progression, and metastasis through multiple biologic effects, increasing proliferation and angiogenesis, inhibiting apoptosis, augmenting cellular invasiveness, and modulating immunosuppression. Augmented expression of mPGES-1 is evident in tumors, and preclinical studies support the potential use of mPGES-1 inhibitors in chemoprevention or treatment. In tumors, reduced levels of OATP2A1 and 15-PGDH, which mediate cellular uptake and metabolic inactivation of PGE_2, respectively, likely contribute to sustained PGE_2 activity. The pro- and anti-oncogenic roles of other prostanoids remain under investigation, with TXA_2 emerging as another likely procarcinogenic mediator, deriving either from macrophage COX-2 or platelet COX-1. Studies in mice lacking EP_1, EP_2, or EP_4 receptors confirm reduced disease in multiple carcinogenesis models. EP_3, in contrast, plays no role or may even play a protective role in some cancers. Transactivation of epidermal growth factor receptor (EGFR) has been linked with the oncogenic activity of PGE_2. PGD_2, acting on the DP_1 receptor, may reduce angiogenesis, thereby reducing tumor progression. Despite the many potential mechanisms, until longer-term, large, randomized clinical trials (greater than 10 years to support a biological effect) are performed, definitive recommendations by the US Preventative Service Task Force will likely not be forthcoming.

Effects of Lipoxygenase & Cytochrome P450-Derived Metabolites

Lipoxygenases generate compounds that can regulate specific cellular responses that are important in inflammation and immunity. Cytochrome P450-derived metabolites affect nephron transport functions either directly or via metabolism to active compounds (see below). The biologic functions of the various forms of hydroxy- and hydroperoxyeicosaenoic acids are largely unknown, but their pharmacologic potency is impressive.

A. Blood Cells and Inflammation

LTB_4, acting at the BLT_1 receptor, is a potent chemoattractant for T lymphocytes, neutrophils, eosinophils, monocytes, and possibly mast cells. LTB_4 also contributes to activation of neutrophils and eosinophils, and to monocyte-endothelial adhesion. The cysteinyl leukotrienes are potent chemoattractants for eosinophils and T lymphocytes. Cysteinyl leukotrienes may also generate distinct sets of cytokines through activation of mast cell $cysLT_1$ and $cysLT_2$. At higher concentrations, these leukotrienes also promote eosinophil adherence, degranulation, cytokine or chemokine release, and oxygen radical formation. Cysteinyl leukotrienes also contribute to inflammation by increasing endothelial permeability, thus promoting migration of inflammatory cells to the site of inflammation. The leukotrienes have been strongly implicated in the pathogenesis of inflammation, especially in chronic diseases such as asthma and inflammatory bowel disease.

Lipoxins have diverse effects on leukocytes, including activation of monocytes and macrophages and inhibition of neutrophil, eosinophil, and lymphocyte activation. Both lipoxin A and lipoxin B inhibit natural killer cell cytotoxicity. Lipoxins, including their epimers (epi-LXA4 and LXB4), appear to act primarily to reduce and resolve inflammation.

B. Heart and Smooth Muscle

1. *Cardiovascular*—12(*S*)-HETE promotes vascular smooth muscle cell proliferation and migration at low concentrations; it may play a role in myointimal proliferation that occurs after vascular injury such as that caused by angioplasty. In vascular smooth muscle LTB_4 may cause vasoconstriction as well as smooth muscle cell migration and proliferation, possibly contributing to atherosclerosis and injury-induced neointimal proliferation. LTC_4 and LTD_4 reduce myocardial contractility and coronary blood flow, leading to depression of cardiac output. In addition to their vasodilatory action, EETs may reduce cardiac hypertrophy as well as systemic and pulmonary vascular smooth muscle proliferation and migration.

2. *Gastrointestinal*—Human colonic epithelial cells synthesize LTB_4, a chemoattractant for neutrophils. The colonic mucosa of patients with inflammatory bowel disease contains substantially increased amounts of LTB_4. It appears that activation of the BLT_2 receptor, possibly by agonists other than LTB_4, is protective in colonic epithelium and contributes to maintenance of barrier function.

3. *Airways*—The cysteinyl leukotrienes, particularly LTC_4 and LTD_4, are potent bronchoconstrictors and cause increased microvascular permeability, plasma exudation, and mucus secretion in the airways. Controversies exist over whether the pattern and specificity of the leukotriene receptors differ in animal models and humans. LTC_4-specific receptors have not been found in human lung tissue, whereas both high- and low-affinity LTD_4 receptors are present.

C. Renal System

There is substantial evidence for a role of the epoxygenase products in regulating renal function, although their exact role in the human kidney remains unclear. Both 20-HETE and the EETs are generated in renal tissue. 20-HETE, which potently blocks the smooth muscle cell Ca^{2+}-activated K^+ channel and leads to vasoconstriction of the renal arteries, has been implicated in the pathogenesis of hypertension. In contrast, studies support an antihypertensive effect of the EETs because of their vasodilating and natriuretic actions. EETs increase renal blood flow and may protect against inflammatory renal damage by limiting glomerular macrophage infiltration. Inhibitors of soluble epoxide hydrolase, which prolong the biologic activities of the EETs, are being developed as potential new antihypertensive drugs. In vitro studies, and work in animal models, support targeting sEH for blood pressure control, although the potential for pulmonary vasoconstriction and tumor promotion through antiapoptotic actions require careful investigation.

D. Miscellaneous

Leukotriene production and leukotriene receptors are present in the endometrium and myometrium. They may be involved in primary dysmenorrhea.

12-HETE stimulates the release of aldosterone from the adrenal cortex and mediates a portion of the aldosterone release stimulated by angiotensin II but not that by adrenocorticotropic hormone.

INHIBITION OF EICOSANOID SYNTHESIS

Corticosteroids block all the known pathways of eicosanoid synthesis, in part by stimulating the synthesis of several inhibitory proteins collectively called annexins or lipocortins. They inhibit phospholipase A_2 activity by interfering with phospholipid binding, thus preventing the release of arachidonic acid.

The NSAIDs (eg, **indomethacin, ibuprofen;** see Chapter 36) block both prostaglandin and thromboxane formation by reversibly inhibiting COX activity. The traditional NSAIDs are not selective for COX-1 or COX-2. The more recent, purposefully designed selective COX-2 inhibitors vary—as do the older drugs—in their degree of selectivity. Indeed, there is considerable variability between (and within) individuals in the selectivity attained by the same dose of the same NSAID. **Aspirin** is an irreversible COX inhibitor. In platelets, which lack nuclei, COX-1 (the only isoform expressed in mature platelets) cannot be restored via protein biosynthesis, resulting in extended inhibition of TXA_2 biosynthesis, and this effect is the basis of aspirin's reduction of the incidence of secondary myocardial infarction.

EP-receptor agonists and antagonists are under evaluation in the treatment of bone fracture and osteoporosis. TP-receptor antagonists investigated in the treatment of cardiovascular syndromes, however, were not superior to aspirin. Direct inhibition of PGE_2 biosynthesis through selective inhibition of the inducible mPGES-1 isoform is also under study for potential therapeutic efficacy in pain and inflammation, cardiovascular disease, and chemoprevention of cancer.

Although they remain less effective than inhaled corticosteroids, a 5-LOX inhibitor **(zileuton)** and selective antagonists of the $CysLT_1$ receptor for leukotrienes (**zafirlukast, montelukast,** and **pranlukast;** see Chapter 20) are used clinically in mild to moderate asthma. Growing evidence for a role of the leukotrienes in cardiovascular disease has expanded the potential clinical applications of leukotriene modifiers. Conflicting data have been reported in animal studies depending on the disease model used and the molecular target (5-LOX versus FLAP). Human genetic studies demonstrate a link between cardiovascular disease and polymorphisms in the leukotriene biosynthetic enzymes, and indicate an interaction between the 5-LOX and COX-2 pathways, in some populations.

NSAIDs usually do not inhibit lipoxygenase activity at concentrations attained clinically that inhibit COX activity. In fact, by preventing arachidonic acid conversion via the COX pathway, NSAIDs may cause more substrate to be metabolized through the lipoxygenase pathways, leading to an increased formation of the inflammatory and proliferative leukotrienes. Even among the COX-dependent pathways, inhibiting the synthesis of one derivative may increase the synthesis of an enzymatically related product. Therefore, drugs that inhibit both COX and lipoxygenase are being developed. One such drug, the COX-2/5-LOX inhibitor **darbufelone,** has shown promise in studies of cancer cells and in mouse tumor models. These mechanistic studies, paired with the observed up-regulation of both COX-2 and 5-LOX in multiple human tumors, including pancreatic cancer, suggest that this may be an important avenue for further investigations.

■ CLINICAL PHARMACOLOGY OF EICOSANOIDS

Several approaches have been used in the clinical application of eicosanoids. First, stable oral or parenteral long-acting analogs of the naturally occurring prostaglandins have been developed (Figure 18–5). Second, enzyme inhibitors and receptor antagonists have been developed to interfere with the synthesis or effects

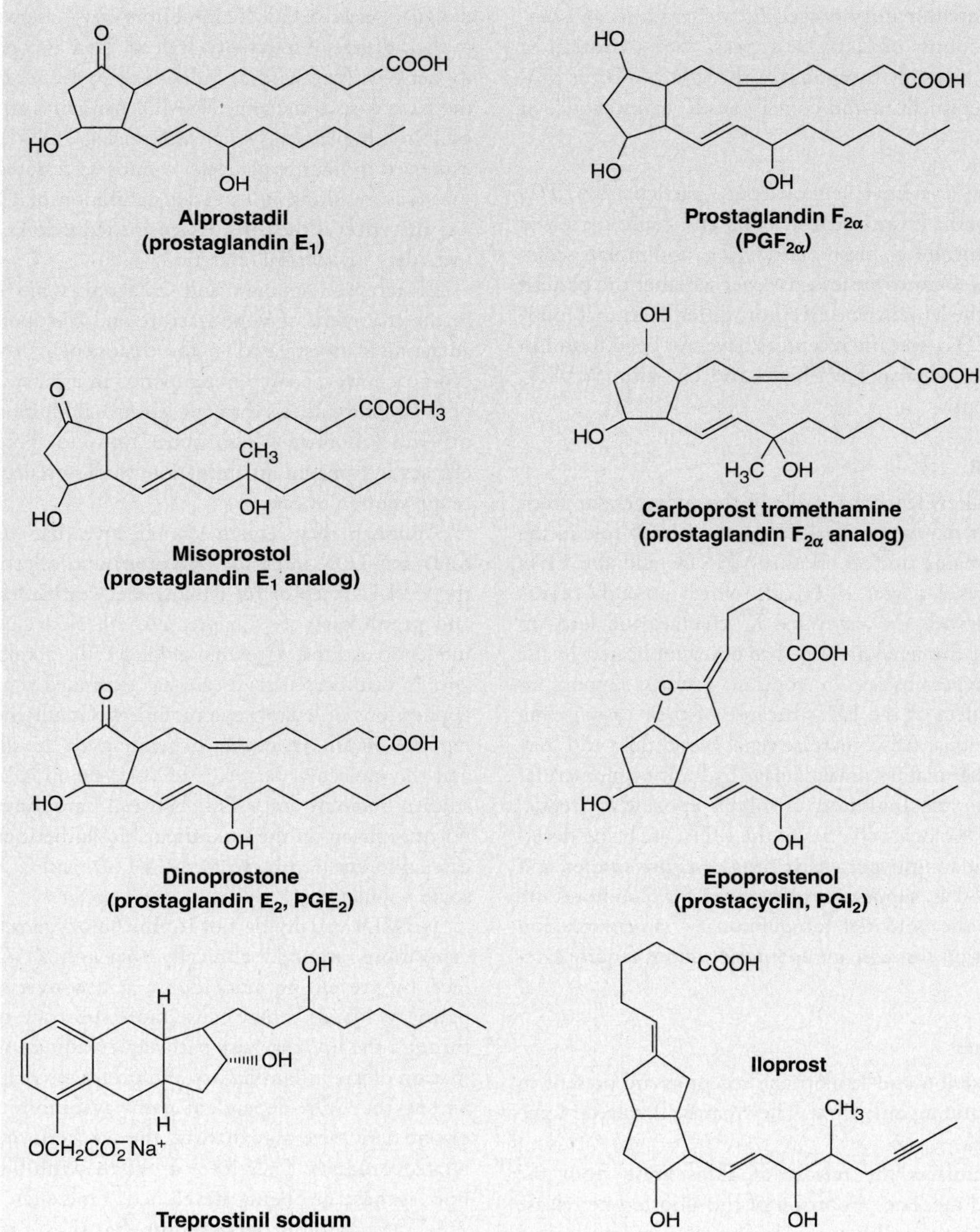

FIGURE 18–5 Chemical structures of some prostaglandins and prostaglandin analogs currently in clinical use.

of the eicosanoids. The discovery of COX-2 as a major source of inflammatory prostanoids led to the development of selective COX-2 inhibitors in an effort to preserve the gastrointestinal and renal functions directed through COX-1, thereby reducing toxicity. However, it is apparent that the marked decrease in biosynthesis of PGI_2 that follows COX-2 inhibition occurring without a concurrent inhibition of platelet COX-1-derived TXA_2 removes a protective constraint on endogenous mediators of cardiovascular dysfunction and leads to an increase in cardiovascular events in patients taking selective COX-2 inhibitors. Third, efforts at dietary manipulation—to change the polyunsaturated fatty acid precursors in the cell membrane phospholipids and so change eicosanoid synthesis—is used extensively in over-the-counter products and in diets emphasizing increased consumption of cold-water fish.

Female Reproductive System

Studies with knockout mice have confirmed a role for prostaglandins in reproduction and parturition. COX-1-derived $PGF_{2\alpha}$ appears important for luteolysis, consistent with delayed parturition in COX-1-deficient mice. A complex interplay between $PGF_{2\alpha}$

and oxytocin is critical to the onset of labor. EP_2 receptor-deficient mice demonstrate a preimplantation defect, which underlies some of the breeding difficulties seen in COX-2 knockouts. PGI_2 production leads to maturation of uterine smooth muscle cell prior to labor.

A. Abortion

PGE_2 and $PGF_{2\alpha}$ have potent oxytocic actions. The ability of the E and F prostaglandins and their analogs to terminate pregnancy at any stage by promoting uterine contractions has been adapted to common clinical use. Many studies worldwide have established that prostaglandin administration efficiently terminates pregnancy. The drugs are used for first- and second-trimester abortion and for priming or ripening the cervix before abortion. These prostaglandins appear to soften the cervix by increasing proteoglycan content and changing the biophysical properties of collagen.

Dinoprostone, a synthetic preparation of PGE_2, is administered vaginally for oxytocic use. In the USA, it is approved for inducing abortion in the second trimester of pregnancy, for missed abortion, for benign hydatidiform mole, and for ripening of the cervix for induction of labor in patients at or near term (see below). Dinoprostone stimulates the contraction of the uterus throughout pregnancy. As the pregnancy progresses, the uterus increases its contractile response, and the contractile effect of oxytocin is potentiated as well. Dinoprostone also directly affects the collagenase of the cervix, resulting in softening. Dinoprostone is metabolized in local tissues and on the first pass through the lungs (about 95%). The metabolites are mainly excreted in the urine. The plasma half-life is 2.5–5 minutes.

For abortifacient purposes, the recommended dosage is a 20-mg dinoprostone vaginal suppository repeated at 3- to 5-hour intervals depending on the response of the uterus. The mean time to abortion is 17 hours, but in more than 25% of cases, the abortion is incomplete and requires additional intervention.

Antiprogestins (eg, **mifepristone**) have been combined with an oral oxytocic synthetic analog of PGE_1 **(misoprostol)** to produce early abortion (through 70 days gestation). This regimen is available in the USA and Europe (see Chapter 40). The ease of use and the effectiveness of the combination have aroused considerable opposition in some quarters. The major toxicities are cramping pain and diarrhea. The oral and vaginal routes of administration are equally effective, but the vaginal route has been associated with an increased incidence of sepsis, so the oral route is now recommended.

An analog of $PGF_{2\alpha}$ is also used in obstetrics. This drug, **carboprost tromethamine** (15-methyl-$PGF_{2\alpha}$; the 15-methyl group prolongs the duration of action), is used to induce second-trimester abortions and to control postpartum hemorrhage that is not responding to conventional methods of management. The success rate is approximately 80%. It is administered as a single 250-mcg intramuscular injection, repeated if necessary. Vomiting and diarrhea occur commonly, probably because of gastrointestinal smooth muscle stimulation. In some patients transient bronchoconstriction can occur. Transient elevations in temperature are seen in approximately one eighth of patients.

B. Facilitation of Labor

Numerous studies have shown that PGE_2, $PGF_{2\alpha}$, and their analogs effectively initiate and stimulate labor, but $PGF_{2\alpha}$ is one tenth as potent as PGE_2. There appears to be no difference in the efficacy of PGE_2 and $PGF_{2\alpha}$ when they are administered intravenously; however, the most common usage is local application of PGE_2 analogs (dinoprostone) to promote labor through ripening of the cervix. These agents and oxytocin have similar success rates and comparable induction-to-delivery intervals. The adverse effects of the prostaglandins are moderate, with a slightly higher incidence of nausea, vomiting, and diarrhea than that produced by oxytocin. $PGF_{2\alpha}$ has more gastrointestinal toxicity than PGE_2. Neither drug has significant maternal cardiovascular toxicity in the recommended doses. In fact, PGE_2 must be infused at a rate about 20 times faster than that used for induction of labor to decrease blood pressure and increase heart rate. $PGF_{2\alpha}$ is a bronchoconstrictor and should be used with caution in women with asthma; however, neither asthma attacks nor bronchoconstriction have been observed during the induction of labor. Although both PGE_2 and $PGF_{2\alpha}$ pass the fetoplacental barrier, fetal toxicity is uncommon.

For the induction of labor or softening of the cervix, dinoprostone is used either as a gel (0.5 mg PGE_2 every 6 hours; maximum 24-hour cumulative dose of 1.5 mg) or as a controlled-release vaginal insert (10 mg PGE_2) that releases PGE_2 over 12 hours. The softening of the cervix for induction of labor substantially shortens the time to onset of labor and the delivery time. An advantage of the controlled-release formulation is a lower incidence of gastrointestinal effects (<1% versus 5.7%).

The effects of oral PGE_2 administration (0.5–1.5 mg/h) have been compared with those of intravenous oxytocin and oral demoxytocin, an oxytocin derivative, in the induction of labor. Oral PGE_2 is superior to the oral oxytocin derivative and in most studies is as efficient as intravenous oxytocin. Oral $PGF_{2\alpha}$ causes too much gastrointestinal toxicity to be useful by this route.

Theoretically, PGE_2 and $PGF_{2\alpha}$ should be superior to oxytocin for inducing labor in women with preeclampsia-eclampsia or cardiac and renal diseases because, unlike oxytocin, they have no antidiuretic effect. In addition, PGE_2 has natriuretic effects. However, the clinical benefits of these effects have not been documented. In cases of intrauterine fetal death, the prostaglandins alone or with oxytocin seem to cause delivery effectively.

C. Dysmenorrhea

Primary dysmenorrhea is attributable to increased endometrial synthesis of PGE_2 and $PGF_{2\alpha}$ during menstruation, with contractions of the uterus that lead to ischemic pain. NSAIDs successfully inhibit the formation of these prostaglandins (see Chapter 36) and so relieve dysmenorrhea in 75–85% of cases. Some of these drugs are available over the counter. Aspirin is also effective in dysmenorrhea, but because it has low potency and is quickly hydrolyzed, large doses and frequent administration are necessary. In addition, the acetylation of platelet COX, causing irreversible inhibition of platelet TXA_2 synthesis, may increase the amount of menstrual bleeding.

Male Reproductive System

Intracavernosal injection or transurethral suppository therapy with **alprostadil** (PGE_1) is a second-line treatment for erectile dysfunction. Injected doses are 2.5–25 mcg; suppositories are recommended to start at 125 mcg or 250 mcg, up to 1000 mcg. Penile pain is a frequent side effect, which may be related to the algesic effects of PGE derivatives; however, only a few patients discontinue the use because of pain. Prolonged erection and priapism are side effects that occur in less than 4% of patients and are minimized by careful titration to the minimal effective dose. When given by injection, alprostadil may be used as monotherapy or in combination with either papaverine or phentolamine.

Renal System

Increased biosynthesis of prostaglandins has been associated with one form of Bartter syndrome. This is a rare disease characterized by low-to-normal blood pressure, decreased sensitivity to angiotensin, hyperreninemia, hyperaldosteronism, and excessive loss of K^+. There also is an increased excretion of prostaglandins, especially PGE metabolites, in the urine. After long-term administration of COX inhibitors, sensitivity to angiotensin, plasma renin values, and the concentration of aldosterone in plasma return to normal. Although plasma K^+ rises, it remains low, and urinary wasting of K^+ persists. Whether an increase in prostaglandin biosynthesis is the cause of Bartter syndrome or a reflection of a more basic physiologic defect is not yet known.

Cardiovascular System

A. Pulmonary Hypertension

PGI_2 lowers peripheral, pulmonary, and coronary vascular resistance. Pulmonary hypertension is characterized by an increase in vascular resistance in the pulmonary blood vessels. PGI_2 has been used to treat pulmonary hypertension arising from primary lung disease and that arising from heart or systemic diseases. In addition, prostacyclin has been used successfully to treat portopulmonary hypertension, which arises secondary to liver disease. The first commercial preparation of PGI_2 approved for treatment of pulmonary hypertension **(epoprostenol)** improves symptoms, prolongs survival, and delays or prevents the need for lung or lung-heart transplantation. Side effects include flushing, headache, hypotension, nausea, and diarrhea. The extremely short plasma half-life (3–5 minutes) of epoprostenol necessitates continuous intravenous infusion through a central line for long-term treatment. Intravenous infusion dosage of epoprostenol is increased in a graded dose-dependent manner, based on recurrence, persistence, or worsening of symptoms. Several prostacyclin analogs with longer half-lives have been developed and used clinically. **Iloprost** (half-life about 30 minutes) is usually inhaled six to nine times per day (2.5–5 mcg/dose), although it has been delivered by intravenous administration outside the USA. **Treprostinil** (half-life about 4 hours) may be delivered by subcutaneous or intravenous infusion or by inhalation. Three oral prostacyclin receptor agonists can be used for the treatment of pulmonary hypertension: **selexipag** (a prodrug rapidly converted to active prostacyclin agonist), **treprostinil** (prostacyclin analogue), and **beraprost** (prostacyclin analogue, currently used only in Asia). Other drugs used in pulmonary hypertension are discussed in Chapter 17.

B. Peripheral Vascular Disease

A number of studies have investigated the use of PGE_1 and PGI_2 compounds in Raynaud phenomenon and peripheral arterial disease. However, these studies are mostly small and uncontrolled. Currently, these therapies do not have an established place in the treatment of peripheral vascular disease.

C. Patent Ductus Arteriosus

Patency of the fetal ductus arteriosus depends on COX-2-derived PGE_2 acting on the EP_4 receptor. At birth, reduced PGE_2 levels, a consequence of increased PGE_2 metabolism, allow ductus arteriosus closure. In certain types of congenital heart disease (eg, transposition of the great arteries, pulmonary atresia, pulmonary artery stenosis), it is important to maintain the patency of the neonate's ductus arteriosus until corrective surgery can be carried out. This can be achieved with **alprostadil** (PGE_1). Like PGE_2, PGE_1 is a vasodilator and an inhibitor of platelet aggregation, and it contracts uterine and intestinal smooth muscle. Adverse effects include apnea, bradycardia, hypotension, and hyperpyrexia. Because of rapid pulmonary clearance (the half-life is about 5–10 minutes in healthy adults and neonates), the drug must be continuously infused at an initial rate of 0.05–0.1 mcg/kg/min, which may be increased to 0.4 mcg/kg/min. Prolonged treatment has been associated with ductal fragility and rupture.

In delayed closure of the ductus arteriosus, COX inhibitors are often used to inhibit synthesis of PGE_2 and so close the ductus. Premature infants in whom respiratory distress develops due to failure of ductus closure can be treated with a high degree of success with indomethacin or ibuprofen. This treatment often precludes the need for surgical closure of the ductus.

Blood

As noted above, TXA_2 promotes platelet aggregation while PGI_2, and perhaps also PGE_2 and PGD_2, inhibits aggregation. Chronic administration of low-dose aspirin (81 mg/d) selectively and irreversibly inhibits platelet COX-1, and its dominant product TXA_2, without modifying the activity of nonplatelet COX-1 or COX-2 (see Chapter 34). TXA_2, in addition to activating platelets, amplifies the response to other platelet agonists; hence, inhibition of TXA_2 synthesis inhibits secondary aggregation of platelets induced by adenosine diphosphate, by low concentrations of thrombin and collagen, and by epinephrine. Because their effects are reversible within the typical dosing interval, nonselective NSAIDs (eg, ibuprofen) do not reproduce this effect, although naproxen, because of its variably prolonged half-life, may provide antiplatelet benefit in some individuals. Not surprisingly, given the absence of COX-2 in platelets, selective COX-2 inhibitors do not alter platelet TXA_2 biosynthesis and are not platelet inhibitors. However, COX-2-derived PGI_2 generation is substantially suppressed during selective COX-2 inhibition, removing a restraint on the cardiovascular action of TXA_2 and other platelet agonists. Selective depression of PGI_2 generation explains the increase in vascular events, particularly major coronary events, in humans treated with a coxib or nonselective NSAID. High-dose ibuprofen may confer a similar risk, whereas high-dose naproxen appears to be neutral with respect to thrombotic risk.

Large clinical studies have now clearly demonstrated secondary prevention of adverse cardiovascular events (ie, preventing a second event after an initial event) by low-dose aspirin. There is also some evidence that low-dose aspirin can confer primary cardiovascular protection (protection from an initial cardiovascular event), particularly in high cardiovascular risk populations. However, low-dose aspirin also elevates the risk of serious gastrointestinal bleeding by about twofold over placebo. The effects of aspirin on platelet function are discussed in greater detail in Chapter 34.

Respiratory System

PGE_2 is a powerful bronchodilator when given in aerosol form. Unfortunately, it also promotes coughing, and an analog that possesses only the bronchodilator properties has been difficult to generate.

$PGF_{2\alpha}$ and TXA_2 are both strong bronchoconstrictors and were once thought to be primary mediators in asthma. Polymorphisms in the genes for PGD_2 synthase, both DP receptors, and the TP receptor have been linked with asthma in humans. DP antagonists, particularly those directed against DP_2, are being investigated as potential treatments for allergic diseases including asthma. However, the cysteinyl leukotrienes—LTC_4, LTD_4, and LTE_4—probably dominate during asthmatic constriction of the airways. As described in Chapter 20, leukotriene-receptor inhibitors (eg, **zafirlukast, montelukast**) are effective in asthma. A lipoxygenase inhibitor **(zileuton)** has also been used in asthma but is not as popular as the receptor inhibitors. It remains unclear whether leukotrienes are partially responsible for acute respiratory distress syndrome.

Corticosteroids and cromolyn are also useful in asthma. Corticosteroids inhibit eicosanoid synthesis and thus limit the amounts of eicosanoid mediator available for release. Cromolyn appears to inhibit the release of eicosanoids and other mediators such as histamine and platelet-activating factor from mast cells.

Gastrointestinal System

The word "cytoprotection" was coined to signify the remarkable protective effect of the E prostaglandins against peptic ulcers in animals at doses that do not reduce acid secretion. Since then, numerous experimental and clinical investigations have shown that the PGE compounds and their analogs protect against peptic ulcers produced by either steroids or NSAIDs. **Misoprostol** is an orally active synthetic analog of PGE_1. The FDA-approved indication is for prevention of NSAID-induced peptic ulcers. This and other PGE analogs (eg, enprostil) are cytoprotective at low doses and inhibit gastric acid secretion at higher doses. Because it is also an abortifacient, misoprostol is a pregnancy category X drug. Misoprostol use is low, in part due to its adverse effects including abdominal discomfort and occasional diarrhea. Dose-dependent bone pain and hyperostosis have been described in patients with liver disease who were given long-term PGE treatment. **Lubiprostone** is a prostaglandin E_1 derivative that activates chloride channels and increases gastrointestinal secretions. It is used for irritable bowel syndrome with constipation.

Selective COX-2 inhibitors were developed in an effort to spare gastric COX-1 so that the natural cytoprotection by locally synthesized PGE_2 and PGI_2 is undisturbed (see Chapter 36). However, this benefit is seen only with highly selective inhibitors and is offset, at least at a population level, by increased cardiovascular toxicity.

Immune System

Cells of the immune system contribute substantially to eicosanoid biosynthesis during an immune reaction. T and B lymphocytes are not primary synthetic sources; however, they may supply arachidonic acid to monocyte-macrophages for eicosanoid synthesis. In addition, there is evidence for eicosanoid-mediated cell-cell interaction by platelets, erythrocytes, leukocytes, and endothelial cells.

PGE_2 and PGI_2 limit T-lymphocyte proliferation in vitro, as do corticosteroids. PGE_2 also inhibits B-lymphocyte differentiation and the antigen-presenting function of myeloid-derived cells, suppressing the immune response. T-cell clonal expansion is attenuated through inhibition of interleukin-1 and interleukin-2 and class II antigen expression by macrophages or other antigen-presenting cells. The leukotrienes, TXA_2, and platelet-activating factor stimulate T-cell clonal expansion. These compounds stimulate the formation of interleukin-1 and interleukin-2 as well as the expression of interleukin-2 receptors. The leukotrienes also promote interferon-γ release and can replace interleukin-2 as a stimulator of interferon-γ. PGD_2 induces chemotaxis and migration of TH2 lymphocytes. These in vitro effects of the eicosanoids agree with in vivo findings in animals with acute organ transplant rejection.

A. Inflammation

Aspirin has been used to treat arthritis of all types for approximately 100 years, but its mechanism of action—inhibition of COX activity—was not discovered until 1971. COX-2 appears to be the form of the enzyme most associated with cells involved in the inflammatory process, although, as outlined above, COX-1 also contributes significantly to prostaglandin biosynthesis during inflammation. Aspirin and other anti-inflammatory agents that inhibit COX are discussed in Chapter 36.

B. Rheumatoid Arthritis

In rheumatoid arthritis, immune complexes are deposited in the affected joints, causing an inflammatory response that is amplified by eicosanoids. Lymphocytes and macrophages accumulate in the synovium, whereas leukocytes localize mainly in the synovial fluid. The major eicosanoids produced by leukocytes are leukotrienes, which facilitate T-cell proliferation and act as chemoattractants. Human macrophages synthesize the COX products PGE_2 and TXA_2 and large amounts of leukotrienes.

Glaucoma

Latanoprost, a stable long-acting $PGF_{2\alpha}$ derivative, was the first prostanoid used for glaucoma. The success of latanoprost has stimulated development of similar prostanoids with ocular hypotensive effects: **bimatoprost, travoprost,** and **tafluprost** are also available. These drugs act at the FP receptor and are administered as drops into the conjunctival sac once or twice daily. Adverse effects include irreversible brown pigmentation of the iris and eyelashes, drying of the eyes, and conjunctivitis.

Hypotrichosis

Bimatoprost is FDA approved for treatment of eyelash hypotrichosis and has shown efficacy in enhancing eyelash growth after chemotherapy. The drug is applied in a 0.03% solution to the skin at the base of the upper lashes. A common but minor adverse effect is darkening of eyelid skin due to increased melanin production that is reversible with discontinuation. Recent trials have also demonstrated efficacy in eyebrow hypotrichosis, and emerging studies have suggested that this drug may have utility for treating alopecia.

DIETARY MANIPULATION OF ARACHIDONIC ACID METABOLISM

The effects of dietary manipulation on arachidonic acid metabolism have been extensively studied. Dietary intake of linoleic and α-linolenic acids, which are, respectively, omega-6 and omega-3 essential fatty acids, can modify arachidonic acid metabolism and the nature of the eicosanoids produced. Two approaches have been used. The first adds corn, safflower, and sunflower oils, which contain linoleic acid (C18:2), to the diet, allowing for generation of 1-series prostaglandins via dihomo-γ-linoleic acid. The second approach adds oils from cold-water fish that contain the omega-3 fatty acids eicosapentaenoic (C20:5) and docosahexaenoic acids (C22:6). Diets high in fish oils have been shown to impact indices of platelet and leukocyte function, blood pressure, and triglycerides with different dose-response relationships. There is an abundance of epidemiologic data relating diets high in fatty fish to a reduction in the incidence of myocardial infarction and sudden cardiac death, although there is more ambiguity with strokes. However, such epidemiologic data may be confounded by concurrent reduction in saturated fats and inclusion of other elements of a "healthy" lifestyle, raising questions about the cardiovascular benefit of dietary omega-3 fatty acids. Nevertheless, data from prospective randomized trials suggest that such dietary interventions may reduce the incidence of sudden death while experiments in vitro suggest that fish oils protect against experimentally induced arrhythmogenesis, platelet aggregation, vasomotor spasm, and dyslipidemias. The REDUCE-IT trial demonstrated that icosapent ethyl (Vascepa) reduced cardiovascular events and deaths in patients with high triglycerides in high-cardiovascular-risk patients already on statin therapy. Further intense studies on the use of omega-3 fatty acids in cardiovascular disease are ongoing.

PREPARATIONS AVAILABLE

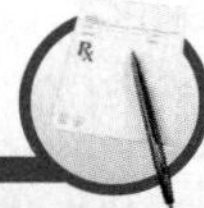

GENERIC NAME	AVAILABLE AS
NONSTEROIDAL ANTI-INFLAMMATORY DRUGS ARE LISTED IN CHAPTER 36.	
Alprostadil	
Penile injection, mini-suppository	Caverject, Edex, Muse
Parenteral	Generic, Prostin VR Pediatric
Bimatoprost	Lumigan, Latisse
Carboprost tromethamine	Hemabate
Dinoprostone [prostaglandin E_2]	Prostin E2, Prepidil, Cervidil
Epoprostenol [prostacyclin]	Generic, Flolan, Veletri
Iloprost	Ventavis
Icosapent ethyl	Vascepa
Latanoprost	Generic, Xalatan
Lubiprostone	Amizita
Misoprostol	Generic, Cytotec
Montelukast	Generic, Singulair
Selexipag	Uptravi
Tafluprost	Taflotan, Zioptan
Travoprost	Generic
Treprostinil	Remodulin, Tyvaso, Orenitram
Zafirlukast	Generic, Accolate
Zileuton	Zyflo, Zyflo CR

REFERENCES

Alexander SPH et al: The concise guide to pharmacology 2019/20: G protein-coupled receptors. Br J Pharmacol 2019;176:S21.

Bäck M et al: International Union of Basic and Clinical Pharmacology Review. Update on leukotriene, lipoxin and oxoeicosanoid receptors: IUPHAR Review 7. Br J Pharmacol 2014;171:3551.

Barnes H et al: Prostacyclin for pulmonary hypertension. Cochrane Database Syst Rev 2019;5:CD012785.

Dehmer SP et al: Aspirin use to prevent cardiovascular disease and colorectal cancer updated modeling study for the US Preventative Service Task Force. JAMA 2022;327:1598.

Dyall SC et al: Polyunsaturated fatty acids and fatty acid-derived lipid mediators: Recent advances in the understanding of their biosynthesis, structures and functions. Prog Lipid Res 2022;86:101165.

Mason RP: New insights into mechanisms of action for omega-3 fatty acids in atherothrombotic cardiovascular disease. Curr Atheroscler Rep 2019;21:2.

Mouchlis VD, Dennis EA: Phospholipase A2 catalysis and lipid mediator lipidomics. Biochim Biophys Acta Mol Cell Biol Lipids 2019;1864:766.

Norel X et al: Prostanoid receptors. IUPHAR/BPS Guide to Pharmacology. http://www.guidetopharmacology.org/GRAC/FamilyDisplayForward?familyId=58. Accessed on August 1, 2019.

Theken KN et al: The roles of lipids in SARS-CoV-2 viral replication and the host immune response. J Lipid Res 2021;62:100129.

Wang Q et al: Prostaglandin pathways: opportunities for cancer prevention and therapy. Cancer Res 2022:82:949.

CASE STUDY ANSWER

Prostacyclin analogs have been shown to be effective in the treatment of pulmonary hypertension. Multiple formulations are now available including intravenous, inhalational, and more recently, oral. These agents activate the G protein–coupled IP receptor, leading to elevated cAMP. The result is reduced proliferation of vascular smooth muscle cells and vasodilation, key strategies in the treatment of pulmonary hypertension.

CHAPTER

19 Nitric Oxide

Samie R. Jaffrey, MD, PhD

Nitric oxide (NO) is a gaseous signaling molecule that is generated by specific cells in the body and readily diffuses across cell membranes to regulate a wide range of physiologic and pathophysiologic processes including cardiovascular, inflammatory, and neuronal functions. Nitric oxide should not be confused with nitrous oxide (N_2O), an anesthetic gas, or with nitrogen dioxide (NO_2), a toxic pulmonary irritant gas.

■ DISCOVERY OF ENDOGENOUSLY GENERATED NITRIC OXIDE

The understanding that NO is an endogenously synthesized signaling molecule came from a series of discoveries that began with Italian chemist Ascanio Sobrero, who synthesized nitroglycerin in 1846 and found it to be unstable and explosive. Nevertheless, upon tasting the chemical, which was not an unusual practice at the time, he noted profound headache, which was soon understood to be caused by cerebral vasodilation. Based on this early observation, nitroglycerin was used to treat angina and hypertension within 20 years.

These and other early studies demonstrated that human cells have the capacity to detect and respond to nitroglycerin, as well as its metabolite, NO. However, the first indication that NO could be produced in the body came from studies of cultured macrophages. Treatment of these cells with inflammatory mediators such as bacterial endotoxin resulted in increased levels of nitrate and nitrite in the culture media, which are known byproducts of NO breakdown. Similarly, injection of endotoxin in animals elevated urinary nitrite and nitrate.

The second indication came from studies of vascular tissue, the well-known target of nitroglycerin. Several naturally occurring signaling molecules can be applied to blood vessels, such causing vasorelaxation. These molecules, such as acetylcholine, were found to act by stimulating the endothelial cells that cover the smooth muscle of the vessel wall since removal of these endothelial cells prevents acetylcholine-induced vasodilation (see Figure 7–5). Subsequent studies showed that endothelial cells respond to vasorelaxants by releasing a soluble **endothelial-derived relaxing factor (EDRF).** When EDRF diffuses into vascular muscle it causes vasorelaxation. These findings prompted an intense search for the identity of EDRF.

NO was suspected to be EDRF because they both have similar vasorelaxation effects. Systematic comparison of the biochemical and pharmacologic properties of EDRF and NO provided initial evidence that NO is the major bioactive component of EDRF. These findings also made it clear that exogenously applied NO and compounds that can be metabolized to NO (nitrates, nitrites, nitroprusside; see Chapters 11 and 12) elicit their effects by recruiting many of the physiologic signaling pathways that normally mediate the actions of endogenously generated NO.

■ NITRIC OXIDE SYNTHESIS, SIGNALING MECHANISMS, & INACTIVATION

Enzymatic Synthesis

NO, written as $NO^{\bullet}$ to indicate an unpaired electron in its chemical structure, or simply NO, is a highly reactive signaling molecule that is synthesized in cells by both enzymatic and non-enzymatic pathways. The enzymatic pathways for NO synthesis utilize any of three closely related NO synthase (NOS, EC 1.14.13.49) isoenzymes, each of which is encoded by a separate gene and named for the initial cell type from which it was isolated (Table 19–1). These enzymes, neuronal NOS (nNOS or NOS-1), macrophage or inducible NOS (iNOS or NOS-2), and endothelial NOS (eNOS or NOS-3), despite their names, are each expressed in a wide variety of cell types, sometimes with an overlapping distribution.

The NOS isoforms generate NO from the amino acid L-arginine in an O_2- and NADPH-dependent reaction (Figure 19–1). This enzymatic reaction involves enzyme-bound cofactors, including heme, tetrahydrobiopterin, and flavin adenine dinucleotide (FAD). The activity of nNOS and eNOS can be triggered either by phosphorylation or by neurotransmitters and signaling molecules that increase cytosolic calcium concentrations. Calcium

TABLE 19–1 Properties of the three isoforms of nitric oxide synthase (NOS).

	Isoform Names		
Property	**NOS-1**	**NOS-2**	**NOS-3**
Other names	nNOS (neuronal NOS)	iNOS (inducible NOS)	eNOS (endothelial NOS)
Tissue	Neurons, skeletal muscle	Macrophages, smooth muscle cells	Endothelial cells, neurons, platelets
Expression	Constitutive	Transcriptional induction	Constitutive and transcriptional induction/repression
Enzymatic activation	Calcium	Constitutive	Calcium and/or phosphorylation

forms complexes with calmodulin, an abundant calcium-binding protein, which in turn binds and activates eNOS and nNOS. This mechanism mediates vasorelaxation induced by experimental application of acetylcholine, which increases cytosolic calcium. However, the physiologic importance of this pathway is likely to be minimal. Instead, the major trigger for NO production by eNOS is the hemodynamic forces exerted by blood flow on endothelial cells. These shear forces activate PIEZO1, a mechanosensitive channel, leading to phosphorylation and activation of eNOS. The magnitude of NO production is further influenced by expression levels of eNOS, which are notably reduced in inflammatory disease and diabetes, leading to reduced NO and a subsequent increase in vascular tone.

In contrast, iNOS is not regulated by calcium, but instead produces NO in proportion to the expression level of iNOS. iNOS is generally not expressed at detectable levels in macrophages, neutrophils, and several other cell types, until these cells are exposed to inflammatory mediators that induce the transcription of the *iNOS* gene, resulting in accumulation of iNOS protein and synthesis of large quantities of NO.

Signaling Mechanisms

NO mediates its effects by covalent modification of proteins. The major target of NO is **soluble guanylyl cyclase (sGC),** a heme-containing enzyme that generates **cyclic guanosine monophosphate (cGMP)** from guanosine triphosphate (GTP). NO binds and activates sGC activity several hundredfold. The subsequent increase in cGMP induces smooth muscle relaxation and the vasorelaxation effect normally associated with NO. However, NO is highly reactive and can form chemical adducts with additional targets that may contribute to its biological actions (see Figure 19–1).

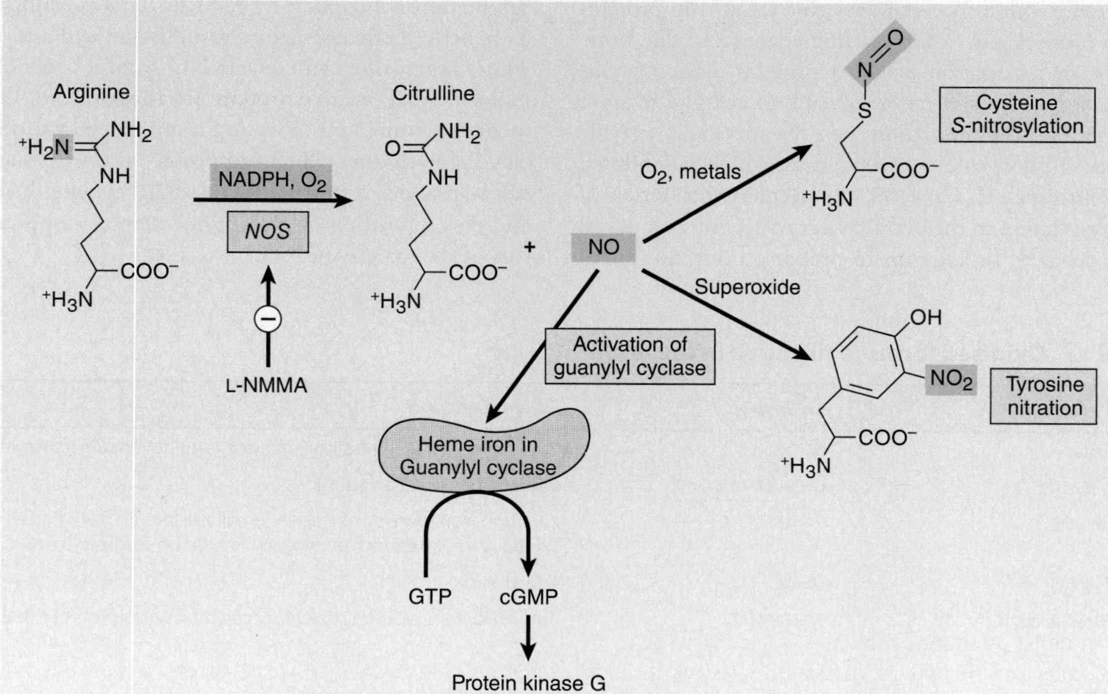

FIGURE 19–1 Synthesis and reactions of nitric oxide (NO). L-NMMA (see Table 19–3) inhibits nitric oxide synthase (NOS). NO binds to the iron in hemoproteins (eg, guanylyl cyclase), resulting in the activation of cyclic guanosine monophosphate (cGMP) synthesis and cGMP target proteins such as protein kinase G. Under conditions of oxidative stress, NO can react with superoxide to nitrate tyrosine. GTP, guanosine triphosphate.

1. *Metalloproteins*—The ability of NO to activate sGC is due to the highly efficient interaction of NO with metals, especially iron in heme, a prosthetic group in certain proteins. When NO binds the heme in sGC, the enzyme is activated, resulting in elevated intracellular cGMP levels. cGMP activates protein kinase G (PKG), which phosphorylates specific proteins. In blood vessels, NO released from endothelial cells increases cGMP and PKG activity in vascular smooth muscle cells. The elevated PKG activity results in the phosphorylation of proteins that reduce cytosolic calcium levels. Since calcium triggers contraction of smooth muscle, the NO-mediated reduction in cytosolic calcium leads to vasorelaxation. In platelets, endothelium-derived NO also activates sGC to increase cGMP. However, in these cells, elevated cGMP prevents platelet aggregation and clot formation.

NO can also inactivate metalloproteins involved in oxidative phosphorylation, such as cytochrome c oxidase. This occurs when NO is produced at high levels, eg, in activated macrophages. Inhibition of heme-containing cytochrome P450 enzymes by NO is a major pathogenic mechanism in inflammatory liver disease.

2. *Thiols*—NO can also form metal-independent interactions with proteins. The most prominent reaction of NO occurs with thiols (compounds containing the –SH group) to form nitrosothiols. In proteins, the thiol moiety is found in the amino acid cysteine. This posttranslational modification, termed *S*-nitrosylation or *S*-nitr osation, requires either metals or O_2 to catalyze the formation of the nitrosothiol adduct. *S*-nitrosylation is highly specific, with only certain cysteine residues in proteins becoming *S*-nitrosylated. *S*-nitrosylation can alter the function, stability, or localization of target proteins. Major targets of *S*-nitrosylation include H-ras, a regulator of cell proliferation that is activated by *S*-nitrosylation, and the metabolic enzyme glyceraldehyde-3-phosphate dehydrogenase, which is inhibited when it is *S*-nitrosylated. However, the overall contribution of protein *S*-nitrosylation to the overall effect of NO in various cell types is still debated. In addition to proteins, thiols are found in glutathione, a highly abundant intracellular reducing agents. Glutathione can also be *S*-nitrosylated under physiologic conditions to generate *S*-nitrosoglutathione. *S*-nitrosoglutathione may serve as an endogenous stabilized form of NO or as a carrier of NO. Vascular glutathione is decreased in diabetes mellitus and atherosclerosis, and the resulting deficiency of *S*-nitrosoglutathione may account for the increased incidence of cardiovascular complications in these conditions.

3. *Tyrosine Nitration*—NO can also undergo diverse oxidation and reduction reactions in the cell; oxidation products can be either stable or highly reactive (Table 19–2). When large amounts of both NO and superoxide are produced, they efficiently react to form peroxynitrite ($ONOO^-$), a highly reactive and short-lived oxidant. Peroxynitrite leads to nitration of tyrosine and DNA, as well as oxidation of cysteine to disulfides or to various sulfur oxides (SO_x). Peroxynitrite is more reactive and damaging to proteins than NO itself or other reactive oxygen species such as superoxide or hydrogen peroxide. Superoxide can be synthesized by several enzymes, and many of these enzymes are elevated in concert with NO synthase in inflammatory cells and neurodegenerative diseases. Numerous proteins are susceptible to peroxynitrite-catalyzed tyrosine nitration, and this irreversible modification is often associated with inhibition of protein function. Tyrosine nitration in tissue is often used as a histological marker of excessive NO and superoxide production. It is likely that tyrosine nitration contributes to the overall tissue damage seen during inflammation. The ability of superoxide to shunt NO to peroxynitrite production concomitantly reduces the availability of NO for its beneficial effects, such as vasodilation and anti-thrombosis. Thus, superoxide can convert NO from a beneficial signaling molecule to a reactive protein-nitrating species. Peroxynitrite-mediated protein modification is mitigated by intracellular levels of glutathione, which can protect against tissue damage by scavenging peroxynitrite. Factors that regulate the biosynthesis and decomposition of glutathione may be important modulators of the toxicity of NO.

TABLE 19–2 Oxidized forms of nitrogen in the body.

Name	Structure	Known Function
Nitric oxide (NO)	N=O*	Vasodilator, platelet inhibitor, immune regulator, neurotransmitter
Peroxynitrite (NO_3^-)	$O{=}N{-}O{-}O^-$	Oxidant and nitrating agent
Nitroxyl anion (NO^-)	$N^-{=}O$	Can form from nonspecific donation of an electron from metals to NO Exhibits NO-like effects, possibly by first being oxidized to NO
Nitrous oxide (N_2O)	$N^-{=}N^+{=}O$	Anesthetic
Dinitrogen trioxide (N_2O_3)	$O{=}N{-}N^+{=}O$ with O^- on N^+	Auto-oxidation product of NO that can nitrosylate protein thiols
Nitrite (NO_2^-)	$O{=}N{=}O^-$	Stable oxidation product of NO Slowly metabolized to nitrosothiols, and decomposes to NO at acidic pH
Nitrate (NO_3^-)	$O{=}N^+{-}O^-$ with O^- on N^+	Stable oxidation product of NO

Inactivation

Although NO can readily diffuse in all directions, its effects can be targeted to specific cells because NO that goes in undesired directions can be rapidly inactivated by heme, O_2, and reactive oxygen species. For example, NO that diffuses from endothelial cells into the bloodstream reacts with the oxygenated heme in hemoglobin, which facilitates the oxidation of NO to nitrate. NO is also inactivated by reaction with O_2 to form nitrogen dioxide. As noted, NO reacts with superoxide, which results in the formation of the highly reactive oxidizing species, peroxynitrite. Scavengers of superoxide anion such as superoxide dismutase may reduce peroxynitrite production, thus enhancing the potency of NO and prolonging its duration of action.

PHARMACOLOGIC MANIPULATION OF NITRIC OXIDE

Nitric Oxide Donors

NO donors, which release NO or related NO species, are used clinically to elicit smooth muscle relaxation. NO donors are prodrugs and therefore require biotransformation in order to release NO. They do not spontaneously release NO. The enzymes that convert NO donors to NO are often enriched in specific cell types, which therefore allow different NO donors to have different effects based in part on which tissues possess the metabolic pathways that convert these donors to NO.

1. *Organic nitrates*—Nitroglycerin (also called glyceryl trinitrate), which dilates veins and coronary arteries, is metabolized to NO by mitochondrial aldehyde dehydrogenase-2, an enzyme enriched in venous smooth muscle, accounting for the more prominent vasodilatory effect of this molecule in veins. Venous dilation decreases cardiac preload, which along with coronary artery dilation accounts for the antianginal effects of nitroglycerin (see also Chapter 12). Other organic nitrates, such as isosorbide dinitrate, are metabolized to an NO-releasing species through a poorly understood enzymatic pathway. Unlike NO, organic nitrates have less significant effects on aggregation of platelets, which appear to lack the enzymatic pathways necessary for rapid metabolic activation. Patients taking organic nitrates exhibit rapid tolerance during continuous administration. This nitrate tolerance may derive from the generation of reactive oxygen species that inhibit mitochondrial aldehyde dehydrogenase-2, endogenous NO synthesis, and other pathways (see Chapter 12).

2. *Organic nitrites*—Organic nitrites, such as the antianginal inhalant amyl nitrite, also require metabolic activation to elicit vasorelaxation, although the responsible enzyme has not been identified. Nitrites are arterial vasodilators and do not exhibit the rapid tolerance seen with nitrates. Amyl nitrite is abused for euphoric and sex-enhancing effects, and combining it with phosphodiesterase inhibitors, such as sildenafil, can cause lethal hypotension. In clinical medicine, amyl nitrite has been largely replaced by nitrates, such as nitroglycerin, which are more easily administered.

3. *Sodium nitroprusside*—Sodium nitroprusside, which dilates arterioles and venules, is used for rapid pressure reduction in arterial hypertension. The biotransformation of sodium nitroprusside to NO may involve interaction thiols on erythrocytes as well as reaction with oxygenated hemoglobin. This process generates five cyanide molecules and a single NO. See Chapter 11 for additional details.

4. *NO gas inhalation*—NO itself is used therapeutically in infants with hypoxic respiratory failure. Inhalation of NO results in reduced pulmonary artery resistance and pressure and improved perfusion of ventilated areas of the lung. In adults, inhaled NO is used for pulmonary hypertension, acute hypoxemia, and cardiopulmonary resuscitation, based on evidence of short-term improvements in pulmonary function. NO for inhalation is stored as a compressed gas mixture with nitrogen, which does not readily react with NO, and further diluted to the desired concentration upon administration. NO can react with O_2 to form nitrogen dioxide, a pulmonary irritant that can cause deterioration of lung function (see Chapter 56). Additionally, NO can induce the formation of methemoglobin, a form of hemoglobin containing Fe^{3+} rather than Fe^{2+}, which does not bind O_2 (see also Chapter 12). Therefore, nitrogen dioxide and methemoglobin levels are monitored during inhaled NO treatment.

Augmenting the Effects of Endogenous Nitric Oxide

In some cases, endogenous NO signaling occurs but is insufficient and the therapeutic goal is to magnify the effects of endogenous NO. Since the major effect of NO is to increase cGMP levels, strategies have been developed to slow the degradation of cGMP by phosphodiesterases or to amplify the sensitivity of sGC to NO so that more cGMP is generated.

1. *Phosphodiesterase inhibitors*—The effects of NO signaling are terminated by phosphodiesterase enzymes, which break down cGMP to GMP. Inhibiting phosphodiesterase enzymes allows cGMP to persist longer and accumulate to higher levels. Type 5 phosphodiesterase is present in vascular smooth muscle and lung as well as other tissues and is especially enriched in the corpus cavernosa of the penis. Inhibitors such as **sildenafil** allow NO-induced cGMP elevations to achieve higher cytosolic levels and result in prolongation of the duration of the cGMP elevations in these tissues (see Chapter 12). This can allow otherwise insufficient NO production to have more pronounced physiologic effects.

2. *sGC stimulators*—NO signaling can also be enhanced by increasing the synthesis of cGMP. sGC stimulators such as **riociguat** and **vericiguat** directly bind sGC, causing sGC to have increased affinity for NO and enhanced cGMP synthesis rates. sGC stimulators can therefore enhance the effects of endogenously synthesized NO. Riociguat is used for the treatment of certain forms of pulmonary hypertension. Vericiguat is approved for use in heart failure due to its ability to dilate pulmonary arteries. In this way, vericiguat reduces cardiac effort to pump blood through the lungs.

Inhibitors of Nitric Oxide Synthesis

Although numerous disease pathologies are linked to excessive NO production, NOS enzyme inhibitors have not shown efficacy in any clinical trial to date. iNOS induction is seen in sepsis and in inflammatory diseases such as arthritis. However, a clinical trial using a NOS inhibitor that targets all NOS isoforms did not show efficacy in sepsis, possibly due to inhibition of beneficial effects of eNOS. iNOS-selective inhibitors also failed to show benefit in inflammatory pain and different types of arthritis.

NITRIC OXIDE IN DISEASE

VASCULAR EFFECTS

NO is a major regulator of vascular smooth muscle tone and blood pressure. The shear force induced by blood flow along the vessel wall is a major trigger for activation of NO synthesis by inducing phosphorylation of eNOS. This homeostatic pathway leads to vasodilation and reduced blood flow rate. Numerous endothelium-dependent vasodilators, such as acetylcholine and bradykinin, act by increasing intracellular calcium levels in endothelial cells, also leading to the synthesis of NO. NO diffuses to vascular smooth muscle, leading to vasorelaxation (Figure 19–2). Mice with a knockout of the *eNOS* gene display increased vascular tone and elevated mean arterial pressure, indicating that eNOS is a fundamental regulator of blood pressure in animals.

Apart from being a vasodilator and regulating blood pressure, NO also has antithrombotic effects. Both endothelial cells and platelets contain eNOS, which acts via an NO-cGMP pathway to inhibit platelet activation, an initiator of thrombus formation. In diseases such as diabetes, endothelial cells are dysfunctional and produce reduced levels of NO, resulting in an increased propensity for abnormal platelet function and thrombosis. NO may have an additional inhibitory effect on blood coagulation by enhancing fibrinolysis via an effect on plasminogen.

NO also protects against atherogenesis through several mechanisms. A major antiatherogenic mechanism of NO involves the inhibition of proliferation and migration of vascular smooth muscle cells. In animal models, myointimal proliferation following angioplasty can be blocked by NO donors, by NOS gene transfer, and by NO inhalation. NO produced by endothelial cells also reduces the expression of adhesion molecules on the endothelial cell surface. This impairs the adherence of monocytes and leukocytes to endothelial cells, which is an early step in the development

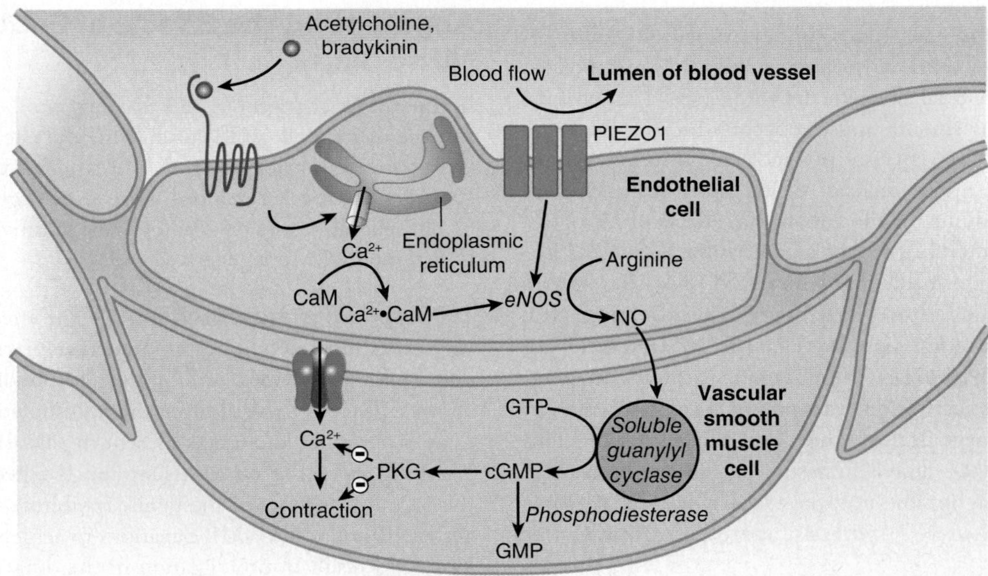

FIGURE 19–2 Regulation of vasorelaxation by endothelial-derived nitric oxide (NO). Endogenous vasodilators, eg, acetylcholine and bradykinin, cause calcium (Ca^{2+}) efflux from the endoplasmic reticulum in the luminal endothelial cells into the cytoplasm. Calcium binds to calmodulin (CaM), which activates endothelial NO synthase (eNOS), resulting in NO synthesis from L-arginine. Shear forces from blood flow activate the mechanically activated PIEZO1 channel, which promotes eNOS activation via phosphorylation. NO diffuses into smooth muscle cells, where it activates soluble guanylyl cyclase and cyclic guanosine monophosphate (cGMP) synthesis from guanosine triphosphate (GTP). cGMP binds and activates protein kinase G (PKG), resulting in an overall reduction in calcium influx, and inhibition of calcium-dependent muscle contraction. PKG can also block other pathways that lead to muscle contraction. cGMP signaling is terminated by phosphodiesterases, which convert cGMP to GMP.

of atheromatous plaques. The antiatherogenic effect of NO may also include an antioxidant effect, blocking the oxidation of low-density lipoproteins and thus preventing or reducing the formation of foam cells in the vascular wall. Plaque formation is also reduced by NO-dependent reduction of endothelial cell permeability to lipoproteins. The importance of eNOS in cardiovascular disease is supported by experiments showing increased atherosclerosis in animals treated with eNOS inhibitors. Atherosclerosis risk factors, such as smoking, hyperlipidemia, diabetes, and hypertension, are associated with decreased endothelial NO production, and thus with a loss of the diverse antiatherogenic effects of NO.

SEPTIC SHOCK

Sepsis is a systemic inflammatory response caused by infection. Endotoxin components from the bacterial wall along with endogenously generated tumor necrosis factor-α and other cytokines induce synthesis of iNOS in macrophages, neutrophils, and T cells, as well as hepatocytes, smooth muscle cells, endothelial cells, and fibroblasts. This widespread generation of NO has long been thought to contribute to the exaggerated hypotension, shock, and, in some cases, death. Although hypotension is reduced or reversed by NOS inhibitors in animal models (Table 19–3), NOS inhibitors do not lead to an overall improvement in survival in patients with gram-negative sepsis, despite some amelioration of hypotension. The absence of benefit may indicate that NO is not a key pathologic mediator in sepsis. Alternatively, the lack of benefit of NOS inhibitors may reflect the inability of the NOS inhibitors used in these trials to differentiate between NOS isoforms, and thus a loss of the beneficial effects of eNOS or other NOS isoforms.

INFECTION & INFLAMMATION

NO has both beneficial and detrimental roles in the host immune response and in inflammation. The host response to infection or injury involves the recruitment of leukocytes and the release of inflammatory mediators, such as tumor necrosis factor and interleukin-1. This leads to a marked increase in iNOS levels and activity in leukocytes, fibroblasts, and other cell types. The NO that is produced, along with peroxynitrite that forms from its interaction with superoxide, is an important microbicide. NO also appears to play an important protective role in the body via immune cell function. When challenged with foreign antigens, TH1 cells (see Chapter 55) respond by synthesizing NO, which acts to modulate signaling in these cells. The importance of NO in TH1 cell function is demonstrated by the impaired protective response to injected parasites in animal models after inhibition of iNOS. NO also stimulates the synthesis of inflammatory prostaglandins by activating cyclooxygenase isoenzyme 2 (COX-2). Through its effects on COX-2, its direct vasodilatory effects, and other mechanisms, NO generated during inflammation contributes to the erythema, vascular permeability, and subsequent edema associated with acute inflammation.

However, in both acute and chronic inflammatory conditions, prolonged or excessive NO production may exacerbate tissue injury. Indeed, psoriasis lesions, airway epithelium in asthma, and inflammatory bowel lesions in humans all demonstrate elevated levels of NO and iNOS, suggesting that persistent iNOS induction may contribute to disease pathogenesis. Moreover, these tissues also exhibit increased levels of nitrotyrosine, indicating excessive formation of peroxynitrite. In several animal models of arthritis, increasing NO production by dietary L-arginine supplementation exacerbates arthritis, whereas protection is seen with iNOS inhibitors. Thus, inhibition of the NO pathway may have a beneficial effect on a variety of acute and chronic inflammatory diseases.

TABLE 19–3 Some inhibitors of nitric oxide synthesis or action.

Inhibitor	Mechanism	Comment
N^{ω}-Monomethyl-L-arginine (L-NMMA)	Competitive inhibitor, binds arginine-binding site in NOS	Nonselective NOS inhibitor
N^{ω}-Nitro-L-arginine methyl ester (L-NAME)	Competitive inhibitor, binds arginine-binding site in NOS	Nonselective NOS inhibitor
7-Nitroindazole	Competitive inhibitor, binds both tetrahydrobiopterin and arginine-binding sites in NOS	Partially selective for NOS-1 in vivo
Methylene blue	Inhibits soluble guanylyl cyclase	
Hemoglobin	NO scavenger	

NOS, nitric oxide synthase.

THE CENTRAL NERVOUS SYSTEM

NO has an important role in the central nervous system as a neurotransmitter (see Chapter 21). Unlike classic transmitters such as glutamate or dopamine, which are stored in synaptic vesicles and released in the synaptic cleft upon vesicle fusion, NO is not stored, but rather is synthesized on demand and immediately diffuses to neighboring cells. NO synthesis is induced at postsynaptic sites in neurons, most commonly upon activation of the NMDA subtype of glutamate receptor, which results in calcium influx and activation of nNOS. In several neuronal subtypes, eNOS is also present and activated by neurotransmitter pathways that lead to calcium influx. NO synthesized postsynaptically may function as a retrograde messenger and diffuse to the presynaptic terminal to enhance the efficiency of neurotransmitter release, thereby regulating synaptic plasticity, the process of synapse strengthening that underlies learning and memory. Because aberrant NMDA receptor activation and excessive NO synthesis are linked to excitotoxic neuronal death in several neurologic diseases, including stroke, amyotrophic lateral sclerosis, and Parkinson disease, therapy with NOS inhibitors may reduce neuronal damage in these conditions. However, clinical trials have not clearly supported any benefit of NOS inhibition, which may reflect nonselectivity of the inhibitors, resulting in inhibition of the beneficial effects of eNOS.

THE PERIPHERAL NERVOUS SYSTEM

Nonadrenergic, noncholinergic (NANC) neurons are widely distributed in peripheral tissues, especially the gastrointestinal and reproductive tracts (see Chapter 6). Considerable evidence implicates NO as a mediator of certain NANC actions, and some NANC neurons appear to release NO. Penile erection is thought to be caused by the release of NO from NANC neurons; NO promotes relaxation of the smooth muscle in the corpora cavernosa—the initiating factor in penile erection—and inhibitors of NOS have been shown to prevent erection caused by pelvic nerve stimulation in the rat. An established approach in treating erectile dysfunction is to enhance the effect of NO signaling by inhibiting the breakdown of cGMP by the phosphodiesterase (PDE isoform 5) present in the smooth muscle of the corpora cavernosa with drugs such as sildenafil, tadalafil, and vardenafil (see Chapter 12).

RESPIRATORY DISORDERS

NO is administered by inhalation to newborns with hypoxic respiratory failure associated with pulmonary hypertension. The current treatment for severely defective gas exchange in the newborn is with extracorporeal membrane oxygenation (ECMO), which does not directly affect pulmonary vascular pressures. NO inhalation dilates pulmonary vessels, resulting in decreased pulmonary vascular resistance and reduced pulmonary artery pressure. Inhaled NO also improves oxygenation by reducing mismatch of ventilation and perfusion in the lung. Inhalation of NO results in dilation of pulmonary vessels in areas of the lung with better ventilation, thereby redistributing pulmonary blood flow away from poorly ventilated areas. NO inhalation does not typically exert pronounced effects on the systemic circulation. Inhaled NO has also been shown to improve cardiopulmonary function in adult patients with pulmonary artery hypertension.

An additional approach for treating pulmonary hypertension is to potentiate the actions of NO in pulmonary vascular beds. Due to the enrichment of PDE-5 in pulmonary vascular beds, PDE-5 inhibitors such as sildenafil and tadalafil induce vasodilation and marked reductions in pulmonary hypertension (see also Chapters 12 and 17). Similarly, the enrichment of sGC in pulmonary vascular smooth muscle accounts for the beneficial effects of sGC stimulators such as riociguat in pulmonary hypertension.

SUMMARY Nitric Oxide

Subclass, Drug	Mechanism of Action	Effects	Clinical Applications	Pharmacokinetics, Toxicity, Interactions
• Nitric oxide (NO)	NO activates soluble guanylyl cyclase to elevate cGMP levels in vascular smooth muscle	Vasodilator • relaxes other smooth muscle • inhalation of NO leads to increased blood flow to parts of the lung exposed to NO and decreased pulmonary vascular resistance	Hypoxic respiratory failure and pulmonary hypertension	Inhaled gas • *Toxicity:* Methemoglobinemia
• Organic nitrates, nitroglycerin, isosorbide mononitrate	Biotransformation into NO, activation of soluble guanylyl cyclase	Vasodilator • Prominent venodilation effect	Angina pectoris	Oral, sublingual • *Toxicity:* Hypotension, headache, dizziness
• Phosphodiesterase inhibitor, sildenafil	Inhibits PDE-5	Smooth muscle relaxant	Erectile dysfunction, pulmonary hypertension	Oral • *Toxicity:* Hypotension
• Soluble guanylyl cyclase activator, riociguat, vericiguat	Activates soluble guanylyl cyclase	Smooth muscle relaxant	Pulmonary hypertension, heart failure	Oral • *Toxicity:* Hypotension; GI disturbance

PREPARATIONS AVAILABLE

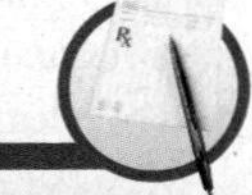

GENERIC NAME	AVAILABLE AS
Nitric oxide	INOmax

REFERENCES

Chen Z, Stamler JS: Bioactivation of nitroglycerin by the mitochondrial aldehyde dehydrogenase. Trends Cardiovasc Med 2006;16:259.

Griffiths MJ, Evans TW: Inhaled nitric oxide therapy in adults. N Engl J Med 2005;353:2683.

Guix FX et al: The physiology and pathophysiology of nitric oxide in the brain. Prog Neurobiol 2005;76:126.

Lundberg JO, Weitzberg E: Nitric oxide signaling in health and disease. Cell 2022;185:2853.

Moncada S, Higgs EA: The discovery of nitric oxide and its role in vascular biology. Br J Pharmacol 2006;147:S193.

Napoli C, Ignarro LJ: Nitric oxide-releasing drugs. Annu Rev Pharmacol Toxicol 2003;43:97.

Paige JS, Jaffrey, SR: Pharmacologic manipulation of nitric oxide signaling: Targeting NOS dimerization and protein-protein interactions. Curr Topics Med Chem 2007;7:97.

Wimalawansa SJ: Nitric oxide: New evidence for novel therapeutic indications. Expert Opin Pharmacother 2008;9:1935.

CHAPTER

20

Drugs Used in Asthma & Chronic Obstructive Pulmonary Disease

Nirav R. Bhakta, MD, PhD, & Eugene Choo, MD*

CASE STUDY

A 14-year-old girl with a history of asthma requiring daily inhaled corticosteroid therapy and allergies to house dust mites, cats, grasses, and ragweed presents to the emergency department in mid-September, reporting a recent "cold" complicated by worsening shortness of breath and audible inspiratory and expiratory wheezing. She appears frightened and refuses to lie down but is not cyanotic. Her pulse is 120 bpm, and respirations are 32/min. Her mother states that she has used her albuterol inhaler several times a day for the past 3 days and twice during the previous night. She took an additional two puffs on her way to the emergency department, but her mother states that "the inhaler didn't seem to be helping so I told her not to take any more." What emergency measures are indicated? How should her long-term management be altered?

A consistent increase in the prevalence of asthma over the past 60 years has made it an extraordinarily common disease. The reasons for this increase—most striking in people under 18 years of age and shared across all modern, "Westernized" societies—are poorly understood. The global estimate of the number of affected individuals is 300 million. In the United States alone, 17.7 million adults (7.4% of the population) and 6.3 million children (8.6% of the population) have asthma. The condition accounts for 10.5 million outpatient visits, 1.8 million emergency department visits, and 439,000 hospitalizations each year. Considering the disease's prevalence, the annual mortality in the USA is low—around 3500 deaths—but many of these deaths are considered preventable, and the number has not changed much despite improvements in treatment. Asthma prevalence and mortality disproportionately affect Black Americans, likely due to access to health care, environmental exposures (eg, pollution), racism, and biological factors.

The clinical features of asthma are recurrent episodes of shortness of breath, chest tightness, and wheezing, often associated with coughing. Its hallmark pathophysiologic features are widespread, reversible narrowing of the bronchial airways and a marked increase in bronchial responsiveness to inhaled stimuli. Its pathologic features are lymphocytic, eosinophilic inflammation of the bronchial mucosa. These changes are sometimes accompanied by "remodeling" of the bronchial wall, with thickening of the lamina reticularis beneath the epithelium and hyperplasia of the bronchial vasculature, smooth muscle, secretory glands, and goblet cells.

In mild asthma, symptoms occur only intermittently, as on exposure to allergens or airway irritants such as air pollution or tobacco smoke, on exercise, or after viral upper respiratory infection. More severe forms of asthma are associated with more frequent and severe symptoms, especially at night. Chronic airway constriction causes persistent respiratory impairment, punctuated by periodic asthma exacerbations marked by acute worsening of symptoms. These attacks are most often associated with viral respiratory infections and characterized by severe airflow obstruction from intense contraction of airway smooth muscle, inspissation of

*We thank Joshua Galanter, MD, and Homer Boushey, MD, for contributions to previous editions of this chapter.

mucus plugs in the airway lumen, and thickening of the bronchial mucosa from edema and inflammatory cell infiltration. The spectrum of asthma's severity is wide, and patients are classified based on two domains: impairment and risk. Measures of impairment are based on the frequency and severity of symptoms, the severity of airflow obstruction on pulmonary function testing, and the intensity of therapy required for maintenance of asthma control. Measures of risk are based on susceptibility to asthma exacerbations. Based on measures of impairment, patients may be classified as having "mild intermittent," "mild persistent," "moderate persistent," or "severe persistent" asthma, but will be classified in a more severe category if their history indicates they are prone to frequent or severe exacerbations ("exacerbation-prone" versus "exacerbation-resistant"). Risk factors for exacerbations include a history of one or more exacerbations in the previous year, low lung function, poor medication adherence or incorrect inhaler technique, smoking, and sputum or blood eosinophilia.

Until recently, the entire range of asthma severity was regarded as eminently treatable, because treatments for quick relief of symptoms of acute bronchoconstriction ("short-term relievers") and treatments for reduction in symptoms and prevention of attacks, especially using inhaled corticosteroids ("long-term controllers"), had been shown to be effective in many large, well-designed randomized clinical trials, pragmatic clinical trials, observational studies, and evidence-based reviews. The persistence of high medical costs for asthma, driven largely by the costs of emergency department and hospital treatment of asthma exacerbations, was thus believed to reflect underutilization of the treatments available. Reconsideration of this view was driven by recognition that the term "asthma" is applied to a variety of different disorders sharing common clinical features but fundamentally different pathophysiologic mechanisms. Attention has thus turned to the possibility that there are different asthma phenotypes, some of which are less responsive to the current mainstays of asthma controller therapy. The current view of asthma treatment may be summarized as follows: that the treatments commonly used at present are indeed effective for the most common form of the disease, as it presents in children and young adults with allergic asthma, but that there are other phenotypes of asthma for which these therapies are less effective, and that represent an unmet medical need. Accordingly, this chapter first reviews the pathophysiology of the most common form of asthma (*classic allergic asthma*) and the basic pharmacology of the agents used in its treatment. This is followed by a discussion of different forms or phenotypes of asthma and the efforts to develop effective therapies for them.

PATHOGENESIS OF ASTHMA

Classic allergic asthma is regarded as mediated by immune globulin (IgE), produced in response to exposure to foreign proteins, like those from house dust mite, cockroach, animal danders, molds, and pollens. These qualify as allergens on the basis of their induction of IgE antibody production in people exposed to them. The tendency to produce IgE is at least in part genetically determined, and asthma clusters with other allergic diseases (allergic rhinitis, atopic dermatitis, food allergy) in family groups. Once produced, IgE binds to high-affinity receptors (FCεR-1) on mast cells in the airway mucosa (Figure 20–1), so that re-exposure to the allergen triggers the release of mediators stored in the mast cells' granules and the synthesis and release of other mediators. The histamine, tryptase, leukotrienes C_4 and D_4, and prostaglandin D_2 released cause the smooth muscle contraction and vascular leakage responsible for the acute bronchoconstriction of the "early asthmatic response." This response is often followed in 3–6 hours by a second, more sustained phase of bronchoconstriction, the "late asthmatic response," associated with an influx of inflammatory cells into the bronchial mucosa and an increase in bronchial reactivity. This late response is thought to be due to cytokines characteristically produced by T2 lymphocytes, especially interleukins (IL) 4, 5, and 13. These cytokines are thought to attract and activate eosinophils, stimulate IgE production by B lymphocytes, and stimulate mucus production by bronchial epithelial cells. It is not clear whether lymphocytes or mast cells in the airway mucosa are the primary source of the mediators responsible for the late inflammatory response, but the benefits of corticosteroid therapy are attributed to their inhibition of the production of proinflammatory cytokines in the airways and of the response of airway epithelial cells to them.

A major limitation to this classic conception of asthma as an allergic disease is that it applies only to a subgroup of patients with asthma, those with evidence of allergy. Allergic asthma accounts for a great proportion of asthma that develops in childhood, but a smaller proportion of adult-onset asthma. This is implied by the use of modifying terms to describe asthma in different patients, such as "extrinsic" versus "intrinsic," "aspirin-sensitive," "adult-onset," "postviral," and "obesity-related." The allergen challenge model fails to account for all the features of the condition even in allergic asthmatics. Many pathways and mechanisms other than production of IgE and activation of mast cell degranulation are involved in asthma's pathogenesis (Figure 20–2), and most asthma attacks are not triggered by inhalation of allergens, but instead by viral respiratory infections. Asthmatic bronchospasm can also be provoked by nonallergenic stimuli such as distilled water aerosol, exercise, cold air, cigarette smoke, and sulfur dioxide. This tendency to develop bronchospasm on encountering nonallergenic stimuli—assessed by measuring the fall in maximal expiratory flow provoked by inhaling serially increasing concentrations of the aerosolized cholinergic agonist methacholine—is described as "bronchial hyperreactivity." It is considered a fundamental characteristic of asthma because it is nearly ubiquitous in patients with asthma, and its degree roughly correlates with the clinical severity of the disease.

The mechanisms underlying bronchial hyperreactivity are incompletely understood but appear to be related to inflammation of the airway mucosa. The anti-inflammatory activity of inhaled corticosteroid (ICS) treatment is credited with preventing the increase in bronchial reactivity associated with the late asthmatic response (see Figure 20–1).

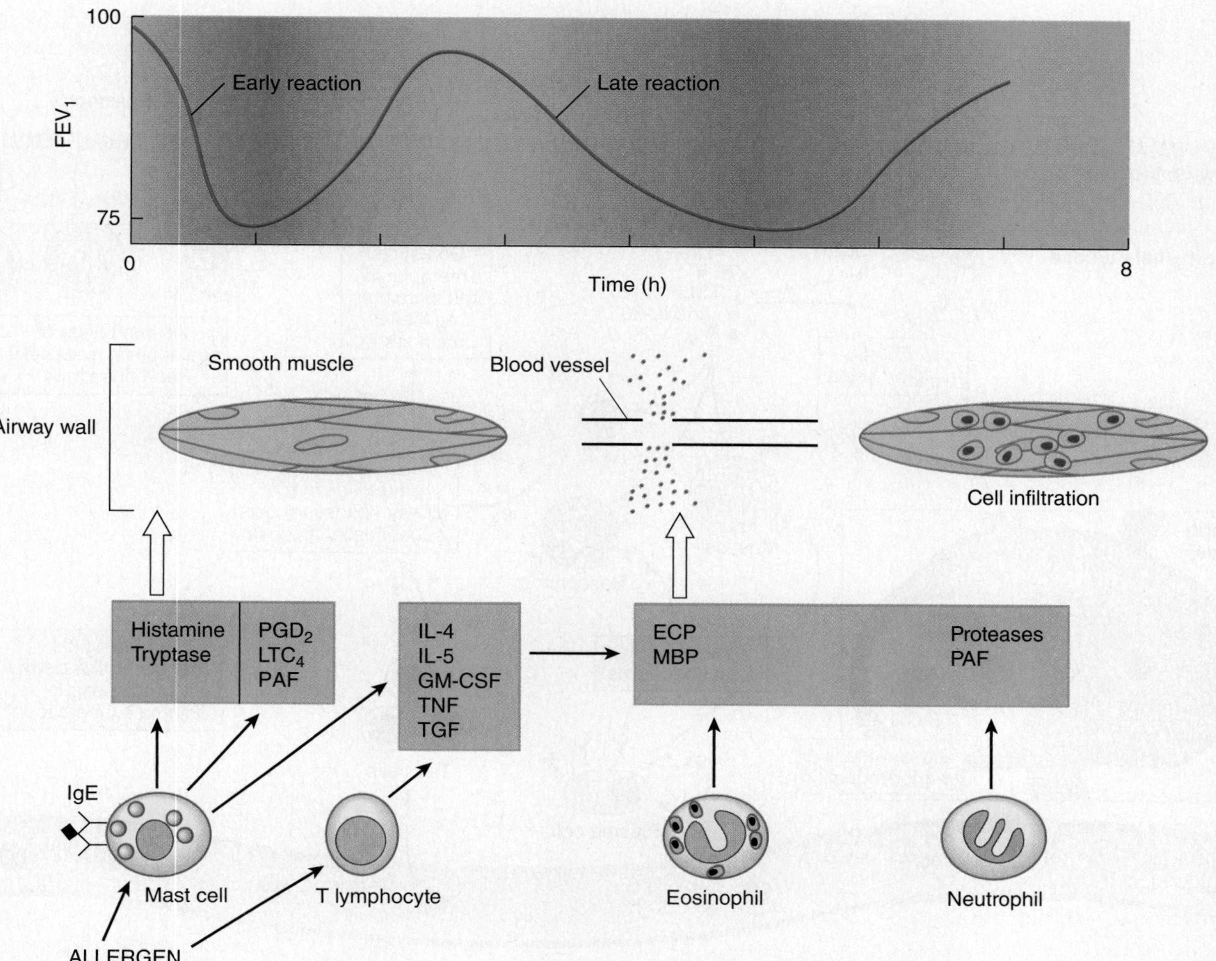

FIGURE 20–1 Conceptual model for the immunopathogenesis of asthma. Exposure to allergen causes synthesis of IgE, which binds to mast cells in the airway mucosa. On re-exposure to allergen, antigen-antibody interaction on mast cell surfaces triggers release of mediators of anaphylaxis: histamine, tryptase, prostaglandin D_2 (PGD_2), leukotriene (LT) C_4, and platelet-activating factor (PAF). These agents provoke contraction of airway smooth muscle, causing the immediate fall in forced expiratory volume in 1 second (FEV_1). Re-exposure to allergen also causes the synthesis and release of a variety of cytokines: interleukins (IL) 4 and 5, granulocyte-macrophage colony-stimulating factor (GM-CSF), tumor necrosis factor (TNF), and tissue growth factor (TGF) from T cells and mast cells. These cytokines in turn attract and activate eosinophils and neutrophils, whose products include eosinophil cationic protein (ECP), major basic protein (MBP), proteases, and platelet-activating factor. These mediators cause the edema, mucus hypersecretion, smooth muscle contraction, and increase in bronchial reactivity associated with the late asthmatic response, indicated by a second fall in FEV_1 3–6 hours after the exposure.

Whatever the mechanisms responsible for bronchial hyperreactivity, bronchoconstriction itself results not simply from the direct effect of the released mediators but also from their activation of neural pathways. This is suggested by the effectiveness of muscarinic receptor antagonists, which have no direct effect on smooth muscle contractility, in inhibiting the bronchoconstriction caused by inhalation of allergens and airway irritants.

The hypothesis suggested by this conceptual model—that asthmatic bronchospasm results from a combination of release of mediators and an exaggeration of responsiveness to their effects—predicts that drugs with different modes of action may effectively treat asthma. The bronchospasm provoked by exposure to allergens might be reversed or prevented, for example, by drugs that reduce the amount of IgE bound to mast cells (anti-IgE antibody), reduce the number and activity of eosinophils in the airway mucosa (anti-IL-5 antibody), block the receptor for IL-4 and IL-13 (anti-IL-4α receptor antibody), prevent mast cell degranulation (cromolyn or nedocromil, sympathomimetic agents, calcium channel blockers), block the action of the products released (antihistamines and leukotriene receptor antagonists), or interfere with the action of inflammatory cytokines (anti-IL-5 and anti-IL-13 monoclonal antibodies). Other drugs that might be expected to be effective in all forms of asthma are those that relax airway smooth muscle (sympathomimetic agents, phosphodiesterase inhibitors) or inhibit the effect of acetylcholine released from vagal motor nerves (muscarinic antagonists, also described as anticholinergic agents).

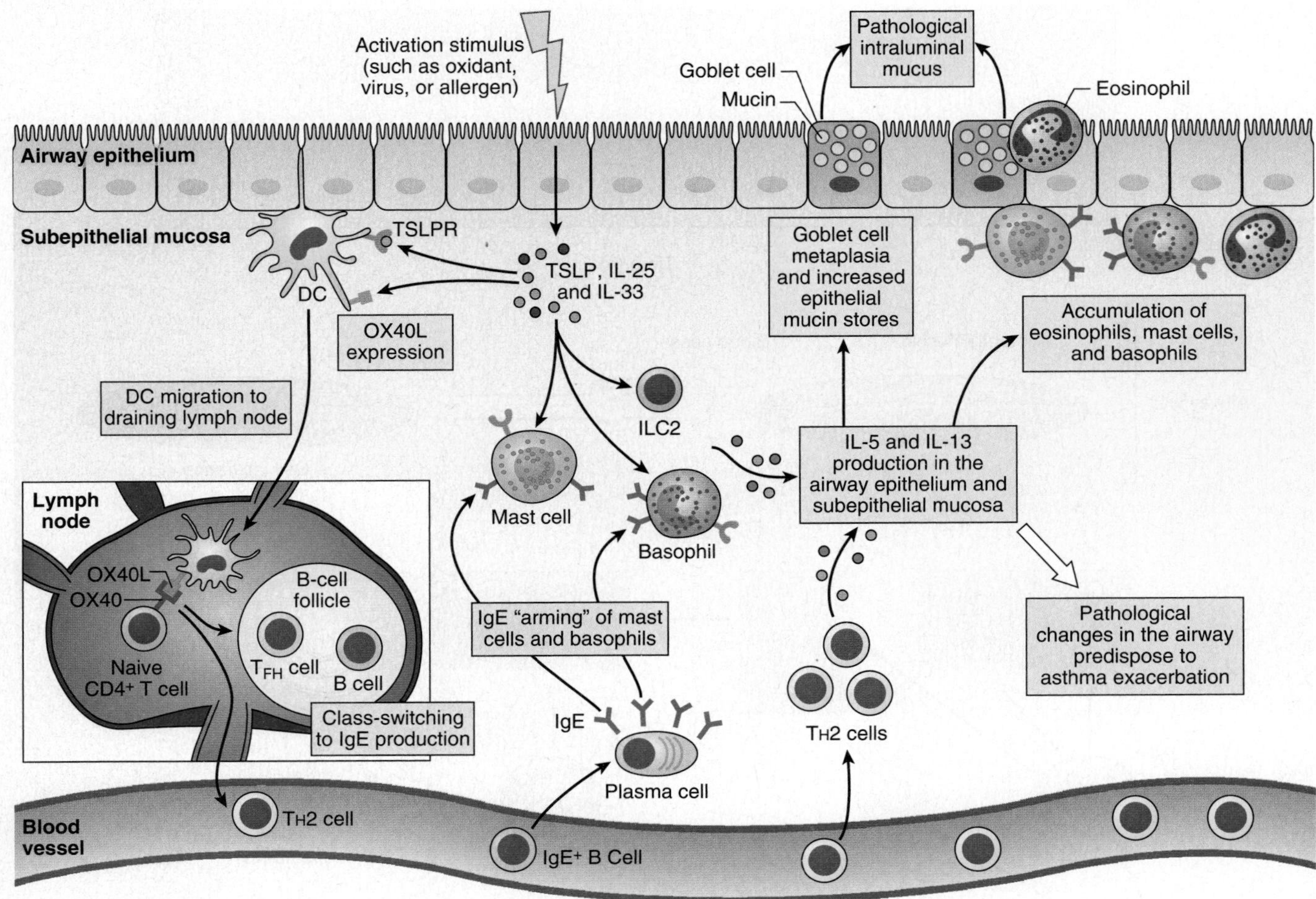

FIGURE 20–2 Inflammatory mechanism of asthma. Airway epithelial cells exposed to activation stimuli, including allergens, viruses, and irritants, release cytokines that promote dendritic cell (DC) mobilization to draining lymph nodes, where they present antigens and thereby activate naive CD4 T cells. These T cells then induce B-cell class switching and maturation into plasma cells, which produce IgE. TH2 cells also migrate into the airway subepithelial mucosa, where they release inflammatory cytokines such as IL-5 and IL-13, which induce goblet cell metaplasia and mucus production, and act as a chemokine for eosinophils, mast cells, and basophils. Unbound IgE secreted by plasma cells binds the FcεRI receptor on submucosal mast cells and basophils and, when crosslinked by an antigen, induces the release of preformed mediators such as histamine and leukotrienes, as well as the release of inflammatory cytokines. (Reproduced with permission from Fahy JV: Type 2 inflammation in asthma—present in most, absent in many. Nat Rev Immunol 2015 Jan;15(1):57-65.)

■ BASIC PHARMACOLOGY OF AGENTS USED IN THE TREATMENT OF ASTHMA

The drugs most used for asthma management are adrenoceptor agonists or sympathomimetic agents (used as "relievers" or bronchodilators) and inhaled corticosteroids (used as "controllers" or anti-inflammatory agents). Their basic pharmacology is presented elsewhere (see Chapters 9 and 39). In this chapter, we review their pharmacology relevant to asthma.

SYMPATHOMIMETIC AGENTS

Adrenoceptor agonists are mainstays in the treatment of asthma. Their binding to β-adrenergic receptors—abundant on airway smooth muscle cells—stimulates adenylyl cyclase and increases the formation of intracellular cAMP (Figure 20–3), thereby relaxing airway smooth muscle and inhibiting release of bronchoconstricting mediators from mast cells. They may also inhibit microvascular leakage and increase mucociliary transport. Adverse effects, especially of adrenoceptor agonists that activate β_1 as well as β_2 receptors, include tachycardia, skeletal muscle tremor, and decreases in serum potassium levels.

Sympathomimetic agents now widely used in the treatment of asthma include albuterol and other β_2-selective agents (Figure 20–4). The place of epinephrine and isoproterenol has markedly diminished because of their effects on the rate and force of cardiac contraction (mediated mainly by β_1 receptors).

In general, β-adrenoceptor agonists are best delivered by inhalation. This results in the greatest local effect on airway smooth muscle with the least systemic toxicity. Aerosol deposition depends on the particle size, the pattern of breathing, and the geometry of the airways. Even with particles in the optimal size range of

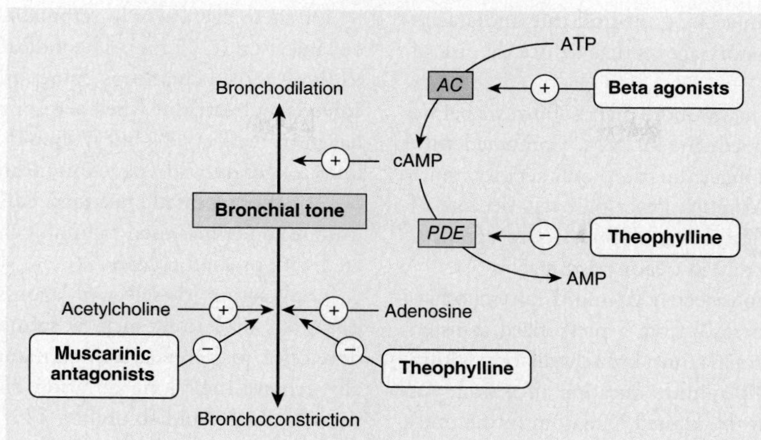

FIGURE 20–3 Bronchodilation is promoted by cAMP. Intracellular levels of cAMP can be increased by β-adrenoceptor agonists, which increase the rate of its synthesis by adenylyl cyclase (AC), or by phosphodiesterase (PDE) inhibitors such as theophylline, which slow the rate of its degradation. Bronchoconstriction can be inhibited by muscarinic antagonists and possibly by adenosine antagonists.

2–5 μm, 80–90% of the total dose of aerosol is deposited in the mouth or pharynx. Particles under 1–2 μm remain suspended and may be exhaled. Bronchial deposition of an aerosol is increased by slow inhalation of a nearly full breath and by 5 or more seconds of breath-holding at the end of inspiration.

Epinephrine is an effective, rapidly acting bronchodilator when injected subcutaneously (0.4 mL of 1 mg/mL solution) or inhaled as a microaerosol from a pressurized canister (125 mcg per puff). Maximal bronchodilation is achieved within 15 minutes after inhalation and lasts 60–90 minutes. Because epinephrine stimulates α and $β_1$ as well as $β_2$ receptors, tachycardia, arrhythmias, and worsening of angina pectoris are potentially serious adverse effects. Its current use is thus largely for treatment of the acute vasodilation and bronchospasm of anaphylaxis. Aerosol delivery of other, more β-selective agents has largely displaced its use in asthma (see below). Very recently, epinephrine was reintroduced in the USA as the only over-the-counter inhaler for asthma. Proponents of this preparation point to affordable access to a lifesaving medication. Major guidelines advise against its use and leading medical societies have opposed its sale, citing inferior effectiveness compared to

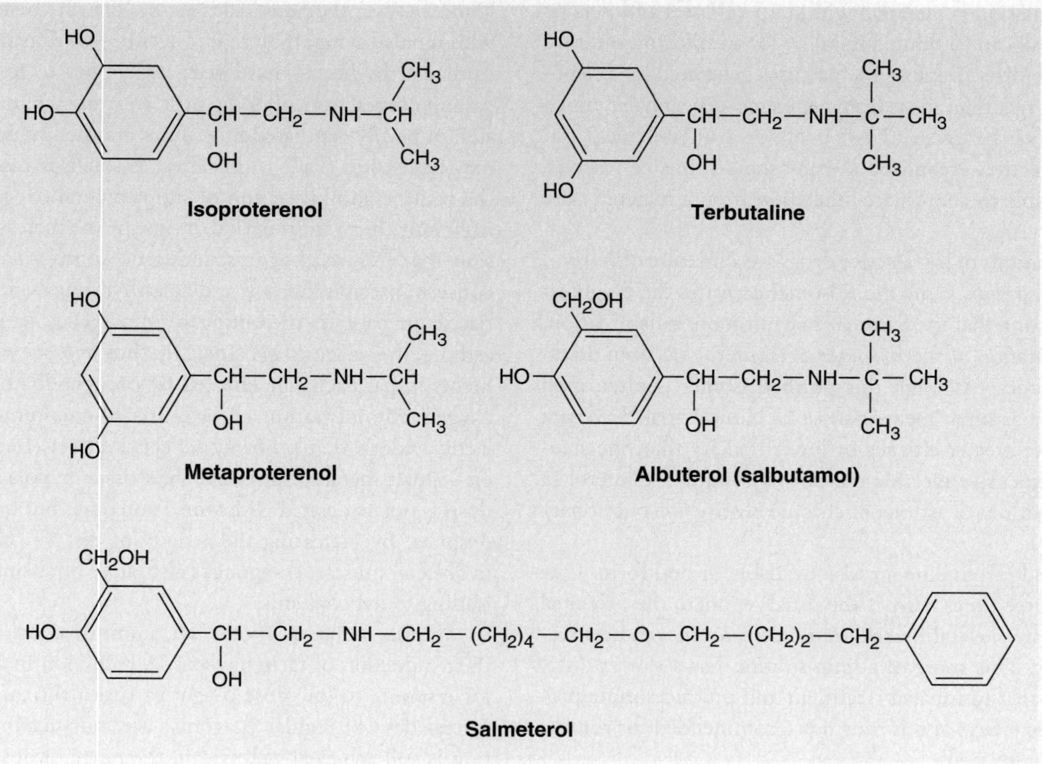

Isoproterenol

Terbutaline

Metaproterenol

Albuterol (salbutamol)

Salmeterol

FIGURE 20–4 Structures of isoproterenol and several $β_2$-selective analogs.

β-selective agents, and delays in seeking medical care and associated initiation of anti-inflammatory agents that reduce the risk of exacerbation.

Ephedrine was used in China for more than 2000 years before its introduction into Western medicine in 1924. Compared with epinephrine, ephedrine has a longer duration, oral activity, more pronounced central effects, and much lower potency. Because of the development of more efficacious and β_2-selective agonists, ephedrine is now used infrequently in treating asthma.

Isoproterenol is a potent nonselective β_1 and β_2 bronchodilator. When inhaled as a microaerosol from a pressurized canister, 80–120 mcg isoproterenol causes maximal bronchodilation within 5 minutes and has a 60- to 90-minute duration of action. An increase in asthma mortality in the United Kingdom in the mid-1960s was attributed to cardiac arrhythmias resulting from the use of high doses of inhaled isoproterenol. As a result of the availability and efficacy of β_2-selective agonists, these have displaced the use of isoproterenol for asthma.

Beta$_2$-Selective Drugs

The β_2-selective adrenoceptor agonist drugs, particularly albuterol, are now the most widely used sympathomimetics for the treatment of acute bronchoconstriction (see Figure 20–4). These agents differ structurally from epinephrine in having a larger substitution on the amino group and in the position of the hydroxyl groups on the aromatic ring. They are more effective than inhalation of epinephrine and have a longer duration of action.

Albuterol and **terbutaline** (outside the United States) are available as metered-dose inhalers. Given by inhalation, these agents cause bronchodilation equivalent to that produced by isoproterenol. Bronchodilation is maximal within 15 minutes and persists for 3–4 hours. All can be diluted in saline for administration from a hand-held nebulizer. Because the particles generated by a nebulizer are much larger than those from a metered-dose inhaler, much higher doses must be given (2.5–5.0 mg vs 100–400 mcg) but are no more effective. Nebulized therapy should thus be reserved for patients unable to coordinate inhalation from a metered-dose inhaler.

Most preparations of β_2-selective drugs are a mixture of *R* (levo) and *S* (dextro) isomers. Only the *R* isomer activates the β-agonist receptor. Reasoning that the *S* isomer may promote inflammation, a purified preparation of the *R* isomer of albuterol has been developed (levalbuterol). Although this purified isomer is often used in children with asthma, meta-analyses of clinical trials have not shown it to have greater efficacy or lower toxicity than the standard and less expensive racemic mixture of *R*- and *S*-albuterol in treating exacerbations of asthma or chronic obstructive pulmonary disease (COPD).

Albuterol and terbutaline are also available in oral form. One tablet two or three times daily is the usual regimen; the principal adverse effects are skeletal muscle tremor, nervousness, and occasional weakness. This route of administration has a slower onset of action compared to inhaled treatment and produces more pronounced adverse effects and is thus not recommended for routine use and rarely prescribed.

Of these agents, only terbutaline is available for subcutaneous injection (0.25 mg). The indications for this route are similar to those for subcutaneous epinephrine—severe asthma requiring emergency treatment when aerosolized therapy is not available or has been ineffective—but it should be remembered that terbutaline's longer duration of action means that cumulative effects may be seen after repeated injections. Large doses of parenteral terbutaline are sometimes used to inhibit the uterine contractions associated with premature labor.

Long-acting β_2-selective agonists (LABAs), with 12-hour durations of action, such as **salmeterol** and **formoterol,** were developed to facilitate asthma management. These drugs generally achieve their long duration of bronchodilating action as a result of high lipid solubility. This permits them to dissolve in the smooth muscle cell membrane in high concentrations or, possibly, attach to "mooring" molecules in the vicinity of the adrenoceptor. These drugs appear to interact with inhaled corticosteroids to improve asthma control. Because they have no anti-inflammatory action, they should not be used as monotherapy for asthma. (Of recent note, the COVID-19 antiviral combination nirmatrelvir/ritonavir [Paxlovid] may increase the serum concentration of salmeterol and should not be used with it.) Ultra-long-acting β agonists, such as **indacaterol, olodaterol, vilanterol,** and **bambuterol,** need to be taken only once a day, but because their prolonged bronchodilation masks symptoms of bronchial inflammation, they should be used only in combination with an ICS for asthma. However, they may be used as monotherapy for treatment of COPD.

Toxicities

Concerns over the potential toxicities of acute treatment of asthma with inhaled sympathomimetic agents—worsened hypoxemia and cardiac arrhythmia—have been largely put to rest. Although the vasodilating action of β_2-agonist treatment may increase perfusion of poorly ventilated lung units, transiently decreasing arterial oxygen tension (PaO_2), this effect is small, is easily overcome by the routine administration of supplemental oxygen, and is made irrelevant after a short period of time by the increase in oxygen tension that follows β-agonist-induced bronchodilation. The other concern, precipitation of cardiac arrhythmias, appears unsubstantiated. In patients presenting for emergency treatment of severe asthma, irregularities in cardiac rhythm *improve* with the improvements in gas exchange effected by bronchodilator treatment and oxygen administration. β_2-agonists also commonly produce a lactic acidosis that probably reflects a direct effect of β_2-agonists on cellular metabolism rather than tissue hypoxia. The lactic acidosis is not associated with worse outcomes but may contribute to dyspnea. By increasing the activity of the Na^+/K^+-ATPase pump in skeletal muscle, β_2-agonists also drive potassium into the cells, leading to hypokalemia.

Another concern about the administration of β-agonists is their induction of tachyphylaxis. A reduction in the bronchodilator response to low-dose β-agonist treatment can be shown after several days of regular β-agonist use, but maximal bronchodilation is still achieved well within the range of doses usually given.

Tachyphylaxis is more clearly reflected by a loss of the protection afforded by acute treatment with a β agonist against a later challenge by exercise or inhalation of allergen or an airway irritant. It remains to be demonstrated in a clinical trial, however, whether this loss of bronchoprotective efficacy is associated with adverse outcomes.

The demonstration of genetic variations in the β receptor raised the possibility that the risks of adverse effects might not be uniformly distributed among asthmatic patients. Attention first focused on a single nucleotide polymorphism (SNP) that changes the receptor's amino acid code at position 16 from glycine to arginine (Gly16Arg). Retrospective analyses of studies of regular β-agonist treatment suggested that asthma control deteriorated among patients homozygous for arginine at this locus, prompting speculation that a genetic variant may underlie the controversial reports of increased asthma mortality in studies of very large numbers of patients treated with an LABA (see below). Studies of LABA treatment have since shown, however, that differences in multiple measures of asthma control are negligible in patient groups with different genotypes at that locus. Nonetheless, it is likely that pharmacogenetic studies of asthma treatment will continue to be an active focus of research, as an approach to the development of "personalized therapy."

METHYLXANTHINE DRUGS

The three important methylxanthines are **theophylline, theobromine,** and **caffeine.** Their major source is beverages (tea, cocoa, and coffee, respectively). The use of theophylline, once a mainstay of asthma treatment, has almost ceased with demonstration of the greater efficacy of inhaled adrenoceptor agonists for acute asthma and of inhaled anti-inflammatory agents for chronic asthma. Accelerating this decline in theophylline's use are its toxicities (nausea, vomiting, tremulousness, arrhythmias) and the requirement for monitoring serum levels because of its narrow therapeutic index. This monitoring is made all the more necessary by individual differences in theophylline metabolism and frequent drug-drug interactions. Despite these disadvantages of theophylline, it is still used in some countries because of its low cost.

Chemistry

As shown below (Figure 20–5), theophylline is 1,3-dimethylxanthine; theobromine is 3,7-dimethylxanthine; and caffeine is 1,3,7-trimethylxanthine. A theophylline preparation commonly used for therapeutic purposes is **aminophylline,** a theophylline-ethylenediamine complex. The pharmacokinetics of theophylline are discussed below (see Clinical Uses). Its metabolic products, partially demethylated xanthines (not uric acid), are excreted in the urine.

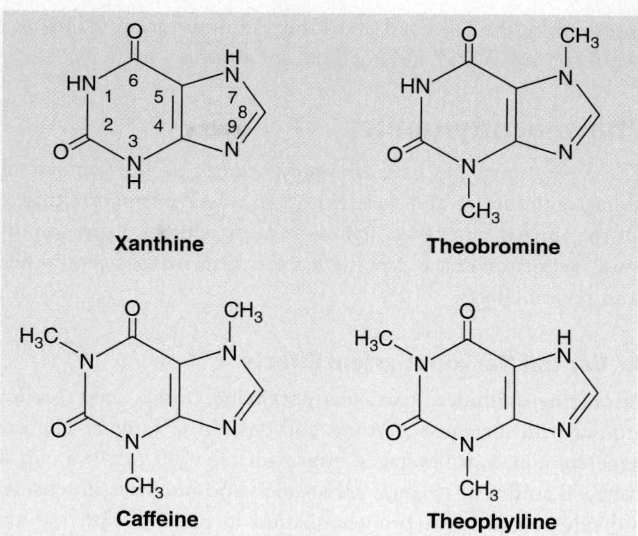

FIGURE 20–5 Structures of theophylline and other methylxanthines.

Mechanism of Action

Several mechanisms have been proposed for the actions of methylxanthines, but none has been firmly established. At high concentrations, they can be shown to inhibit several members of the phosphodiesterase (PDE) enzyme family in vitro, thereby increasing concentrations of intracellular cAMP and, in some tissues, cGMP (see Figure 20–3). Cyclic AMP regulates many cellular functions including, but not limited to, stimulation of cardiac function, relaxation of smooth muscle, and reduction in the immune and inflammatory activity of specific cells.

Another proposed mechanism for the bronchodilating action of this class of drugs is inhibition of cell surface receptors for adenosine. Adenosine has been shown to provoke contraction of isolated airway smooth muscle and release of histamine from airway mast cells. It has been shown, however, that xanthine derivatives devoid of adenosine antagonism (eg, **enprofylline**) can inhibit bronchoconstriction in asthmatic subjects.

A third proposed mechanism of action for theophylline's efficacy is enhancement of histone deacetylation. Acetylation of core histones is necessary for activation of inflammatory gene transcription. Corticosteroids act, at least in part, by recruiting histone deacetylases to the site of inflammatory gene transcription, an action enhanced by low-dose theophylline. This interaction should predict that low-dose theophylline treatment would enhance the effectiveness of corticosteroid treatment, but this approach to treating patients with asthma or COPD uncontrolled by ICS plus LABA therapy has not been widely adopted. Of the various isoforms of PDE identified, inhibition of PDE3 appears to be the most involved in relaxing airway smooth muscle and inhibition of PDE4 in inhibiting release of cytokines and chemokines, thus decreasing immune cell migration and activation. This anti-inflammatory effect is achieved at doses lower than those necessary for bronchodilation.

In an effort to reduce toxicity while maintaining therapeutic efficacy, selective inhibitors of PDE4 have been developed. Many were abandoned after clinical trials showed that they induced unacceptably frequent side effects of nausea, headache, and diarrhea. However, one, **roflumilast,** has been shown to be effective for reducing the frequency of exacerbations of COPD and is approved by the US Food and Drug Administration (FDA) as a treatment for COPD, although not for asthma.

Pharmacodynamics

The methylxanthines have effects on the central nervous system, kidney, and cardiac and skeletal muscle as well as smooth muscle. Of the three agents, theophylline is most selective in its smooth muscle effects, whereas caffeine has the most marked central nervous system effects.

A. Central Nervous System Effects

All methylxanthines, particularly caffeine, cause mild cortical arousal with increased alertness and deferral of fatigue. The caffeine contained in beverages, approximately 100 mg in a cup of coffee, is sufficient to cause nervousness and insomnia in sensitive individuals and slight bronchodilation in patients with asthma. The larger doses necessary for more effective bronchodilation cause nervousness and tremor. Very high doses, from accidental or suicidal overdose, can cause medullary stimulation, convulsions, and even death.

B. Cardiovascular Effects

Methylxanthines have positive chronotropic and inotropic effects on the heart. At low concentrations, these effects result from inhibition of presynaptic adenosine receptors in sympathetic nerves, increasing catecholamine release at nerve endings. The higher concentrations (>10 μmol/L, 2 mg/L) associated with inhibition of phosphodiesterase and increases in cAMP may result in increased influx of calcium. At much higher concentrations (>100 μmol/L), sequestration of calcium by the sarcoplasmic reticulum is impaired.

The clinical expression of these effects on cardiovascular function varies among individuals. Ordinary consumption of methylxanthine-containing beverages usually produces slight tachycardia, an increase in cardiac output, and an increase in peripheral resistance, potentially raising blood pressure slightly. In sensitive individuals, consumption of a few cups of coffee may result in arrhythmias. High doses of these agents relax vascular smooth muscle except in cerebral blood vessels, where they cause contraction.

C. Effects on Gastrointestinal Tract

The methylxanthines stimulate secretion of both gastric acid and digestive enzymes. However, even decaffeinated coffee has a potent stimulant effect on secretion, which means that the primary secretagogue in coffee is not caffeine.

D. Effects on Kidney

The methylxanthines—especially theophylline—are weak diuretics. This effect may involve both increased glomerular filtration and reduced tubular sodium reabsorption. The diuresis is not of sufficient magnitude to be therapeutically useful, although it does counteract some of the cardiovascular effects and limits the degree of hypertension produced.

E. Effects on Smooth Muscle

The bronchodilation produced by the methylxanthines is the major therapeutic action in asthma. Tolerance does not develop, but adverse effects, especially in the central nervous system, limit the dose (see below). In addition to their effect on airway smooth muscle, these agents—in sufficient concentration—inhibit antigen-induced release of histamine from lung tissue.

F. Effects on Skeletal Muscle

The respiratory actions of methylxanthines are not confined to the airways; they also improve contractility of skeletal muscle and reverse fatigue of the diaphragm in patients with COPD. This effect—rather than an effect on the respiratory center—may account for theophylline's ability to improve the ventilatory response to hypoxia and diminish dyspnea even in patients with irreversible airflow obstruction.

Clinical Uses

Of the xanthines, theophylline is the most effective bronchodilator. It relieves airflow obstruction in acute asthma and reduces the severity of symptoms in patients with chronic asthma. However, the efficacy and safety of other drugs, especially inhaled β_2-agonists and inhaled corticosteroids, and the toxicities and need for monitoring of blood concentration of theophylline have made it almost obsolete in asthma treatment.

ANTIMUSCARINIC AGENTS

Observation of the use of leaves from *Datura stramonium* for asthma treatment in India led to the discovery of atropine, a potent competitive inhibitor of acetylcholine at postganglionic muscarinic receptors, as a bronchodilator. Interest in the potential value of antimuscarinic agents increased with demonstration of the importance of the vagus nerves in bronchospastic responses of laboratory animals and with the development of **ipratropium,** a potent atropine analog that is poorly absorbed after aerosol administration and is therefore relatively free of systemic atropine-like effects.

Mechanism of Action

Muscarinic antagonists competitively inhibit the action of acetylcholine at muscarinic receptors and are therefore sometimes referred to as "anticholinergic agents" (see Chapter 8). In the airways, acetylcholine is released from efferent endings of the vagus nerve, and muscarinic antagonists block the contraction of airway smooth muscle and the increase in secretion of mucus that occurs in response to vagal activity (Figure 20–6). This selectivity of muscarinic antagonists accounts for their usefulness as investigative tools to examine the role of parasympathetic reflex pathways in bronchomotor responses but limits their usefulness in preventing bronchospasm. In the doses given, antimuscarinic agents inhibit only that portion of the response mediated by muscarinic receptors, which varies by stimulus and which further appears to vary among individual responses to the same stimulus.

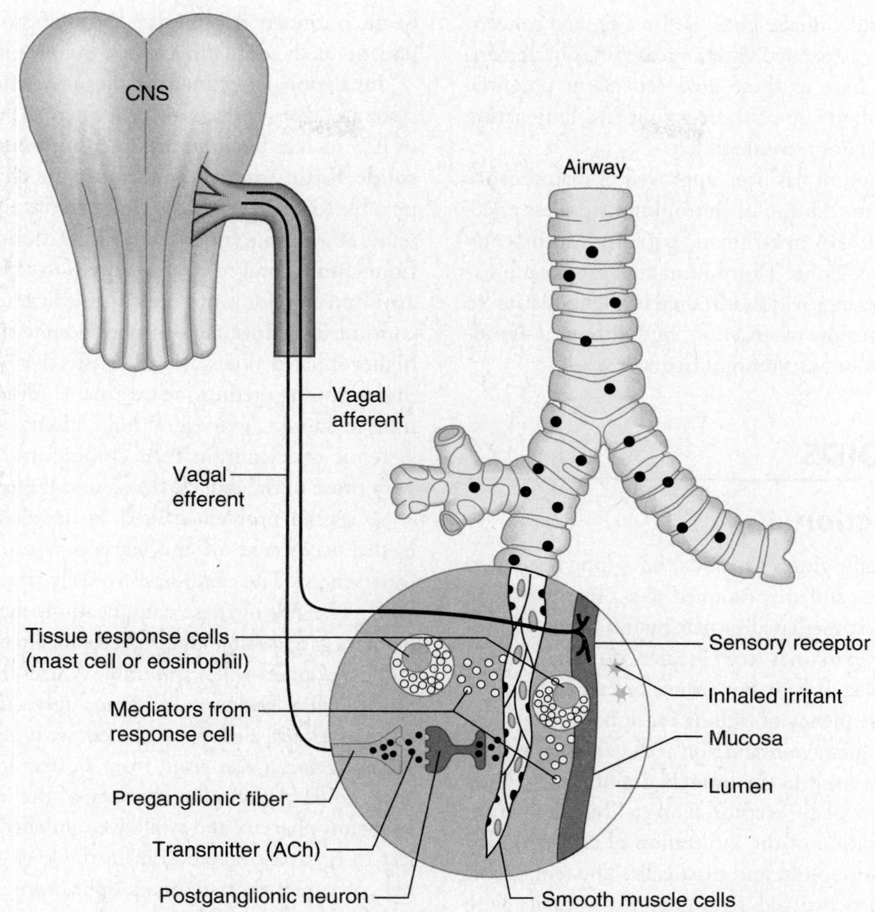

FIGURE 20–6 Mechanisms of response to inhaled irritants. The airway is represented microscopically by a cross section of the wall with branching vagal sensory endings lying adjacent to the lumen. Afferent pathways in the vagus nerves travel to the central nervous system; efferent pathways from the central nervous system travel to efferent ganglia. Postganglionic fibers release acetylcholine (ACh), which binds to muscarinic receptors on airway smooth muscle. Inhaled materials may provoke bronchoconstriction by several possible mechanisms. First, they may trigger the release of chemical mediators from mast cells. Second, they may stimulate afferent receptors to initiate reflex bronchoconstriction or to release tachykinins (eg, substance P) that directly stimulate smooth muscle contraction.

Clinical Uses

Antimuscarinic agents are effective bronchodilators. Even when administered by aerosol, the bronchodilation achievable with atropine, the prototypic muscarinic antagonist, is limited by absorption into the circulation and across the blood-brain barrier. Greater bronchodilation, with less toxicity from systemic absorption, is achieved with a selective quaternary ammonium derivative of atropine, **ipratropium bromide,** which can be inhaled in high doses because of its poor absorption into the circulation and poor entry into the central nervous system. Studies with this agent have shown that the degree of involvement of parasympathetic pathways in bronchomotor responses varies among subjects. This variation indicates that other mechanisms in addition to parasympathetic reflex pathways must be involved.

Even though the bronchodilation and inhibition of provoked bronchoconstriction afforded by antimuscarinic agents are incomplete, their use is of clinical value, especially for patients intolerant of inhaled β agonists.

Ipratropium appears to be as effective as albuterol in patients with COPD who have at least partially reversible obstruction. Longer-acting antimuscarinic agents, including **tiotropium, aclidinium, umeclidinium,** and **glycopyrrolate** are approved for maintenance therapy of COPD. These drugs bind to M_1, M_2, and M_3 receptors with equal affinity, but dissociate most rapidly from M_2 receptors, expressed on the efferent nerve ending. This means that they do not inhibit the M_2-receptor-mediated inhibition of acetylcholine release and thus benefit from a degree of receptor selectivity. They are taken by inhalation. A single dose of 18 mcg of tiotropium or 62.5 mcg of umeclidinium has a 24-hour duration of action, whereas inhalation of 400 mcg of aclidinium has a 12-hour duration of action and is thus taken twice daily. Daily inhalation of tiotropium has been shown not only to improve functional capacity of patients with COPD, but also to reduce the frequency of exacerbations of their condition. Some patients using inhaled anticholinergics experience the adverse effect of dry mouth, which can often be managed with the use of a spacer to reduce oropharyngeal deposition or by dose reduction. Rarely, there may be urinary retention in susceptible individuals. There is also a general concern that anticholinergic use is associated with increased risk of dementia with advancing age. Due to these dose-dependent potential side effects, the concomitant use of short-acting and long-acting inhaled antimuscarinics is not recommended.

Of these drugs, tiotropium has been approved as maintenance treatment for asthma. The addition of tiotropium is no less effective than addition of an LABA in asthmatic patients insufficiently controlled by ICS therapy alone. Tiotropium added to combination ICS/LABA therapy can provide additional bronchodilation in patients with persistent airflow obstruction, but without a significant change in symptoms or exacerbation frequency.

CORTICOSTEROIDS

Mechanism of Action

Corticosteroids (specifically, glucocorticoids) have long been used in the treatment of asthma and are presumed to act by their broad anti-inflammatory efficacy, mediated in part by inhibition of production of inflammatory cytokines (see Chapter 39). They do not relax airway smooth muscle directly but reduce bronchial hyperreactivity and reduce the frequency of asthma exacerbations if taken regularly. Their effect on airway obstruction is due in part to their contraction of engorged vessels in the bronchial mucosa and their potentiation of the effects of β-receptor agonists, but their most important action is inhibition of the infiltration of asthmatic airways by lymphocytes, eosinophils, and mast cells. The remarkable benefits of systemic glucocorticoid treatment for patients with severe asthma have been noted since the 1950s. So too have been its numerous and severe toxicities, especially when given repeatedly, as is necessary for a chronic disease like asthma. The development of beclomethasone in the 1970s as a topically active glucocorticoid preparation that could be taken by inhalation enabled delivery of high doses of a glucocorticoid to the target tissue—the bronchial mucosa—with little absorption into the systemic circulation. The development of ICS has transformed the treatment of all but mild, intermittent asthma, which can be treated with "as-needed" use of albuterol alone.

Clinical Uses

Clinical studies of corticosteroids consistently show them to be effective in improving all indices of asthma control: severity of symptoms, tests of airway caliber and bronchial reactivity, frequency of exacerbations, and quality of life. Because of severe adverse effects when given chronically, oral and parenteral corticosteroids are reserved for patients who require urgent treatment, ie, those who have not improved adequately with bronchodilators or who experience worsening symptoms despite high-dose maintenance therapy.

For severe asthma exacerbations, urgent treatment is often begun with an oral dose of 30–60 mg prednisone per day or an intravenous dose of 0.5–1 mg/kg methylprednisolone every 6–12 hours; the dose is decreased after airway obstruction has improved. In most patients, systemic corticosteroid therapy can be discontinued in 5–10 days, but symptoms may worsen in other patients as the dose is decreased to lower levels.

Inhalational treatment is the most effective way to avoid the systemic adverse effects of corticosteroid therapy. The introduction of ICS such as **beclomethasone, budesonide, ciclesonide, flunisolide, fluticasone, mometasone,** and **triamcinolone** has made it possible to deliver corticosteroids to the airways with minimal systemic absorption. Indeed, one of the cautions in switching patients from chronic oral to ICS therapy is to taper oral therapy slowly to avoid precipitation of adrenal insufficiency. In patients requiring continued prednisone treatment despite standard doses of an ICS, higher inhaled doses are often effective and enable tapering and discontinuing prednisone treatment. Although these high doses of inhaled steroids may cause mild adrenal suppression, the risks of systemic toxicity from their chronic use are negligible compared with those of the oral corticosteroid therapy they replace.

A special problem caused by inhaled topical corticosteroids is the occurrence of oropharyngeal candidiasis and dysphonia (hoarseness). The candidiasis is easily treated with topical clotrimazole. The risk of these complications may be reduced by having patients gargle water and expectorate after each inhaled treatment, and use a spacer when applicable. Ciclesonide, a prodrug activated by bronchial esterases, is comparably effective to other inhaled corticosteroids and is associated with less frequent candidiasis. Hoarseness can also result from a direct local effect of ICS on the vocal cords. Although a majority of the inhaled dose is deposited in the oropharynx and swallowed, inhaled corticosteroids are subject to first-pass metabolism in the liver and thus are remarkably free of other short-term complications in adults. Nonetheless, chronic use may increase the risks of osteoporosis and cataracts. In children, ICS therapy has been shown to slow the rate of growth by about 1 cm over the first year of treatment, but not the rate of growth thereafter, so that the effect on adult height is minimal.

Because of the efficacy and safety of inhaled corticosteroids, national and international guidelines for asthma management recommend their prescription for patients with persistent asthma who require more than occasional inhalations of a β agonist for relief of symptoms. This therapy is continued for 10–12 weeks and then withdrawn to determine whether more prolonged therapy is needed; inhaled corticosteroids are not curative. In most patients, the manifestations of asthma return within a few weeks after stopping therapy even if they have been taken in high doses for 2 or more years. A prospective, placebo-controlled study of the early, sustained use of inhaled corticosteroids in young children with asthma showed significantly greater improvement in asthma symptoms, pulmonary function, and frequency of asthma exacerbations over the 2 years of treatment, but no difference in overall asthma control 3 months after the end of the trial. Inhaled corticosteroids are thus properly labeled as "controllers." They are effective only so long as they are taken.

Another approach to reducing the risk of long-term, twice-daily use of ICS is to administer them only intermittently, when symptoms of asthma flare. Taking a single inhalation of an ICS with each inhalation of a short-acting β-agonist reliever (eg, an inhalation of beclomethasone for each inhalation of albuterol) or taking a 5- to 10-day course of twice-daily high-dose budesonide or beclomethasone when asthma symptoms worsen has been found to be nearly as effective as regular daily therapy in adults and children with mild to moderate asthma. Similarly, in adults and adolescents, as-needed use of a single combined inhaled corticosteroid and long-acting beta agonist (eg, budesonide-formoterol) is as effective for prevention of exacerbations and results in lower overall steroid exposure compared to twice-daily scheduled inhaled corticosteroids, but is inferior in regard to symptom control.

CROMOLYN & NEDOCROMIL

Cromolyn sodium (disodium cromoglycate) and nedocromil sodium were once widely used for asthma management, especially in children, but have now been supplanted so completely by other therapies that they are mostly of historic interest as asthma treatments. These drugs are thought to act by inhibiting mast cell degranulation and, as such, have no direct bronchodilator action, but inhibit both antigen- and exercise-induced bronchospasm in asthmatic patients. In the United States, these drugs are no longer available in inhaler formulations but solutions of cromolyn are available for nebulization; cromolyn also remains available for allergic and other mast cell disorders as a nasal spray (OTC) and oral solution, and both drugs can be prescribed as ophthalmic solutions.

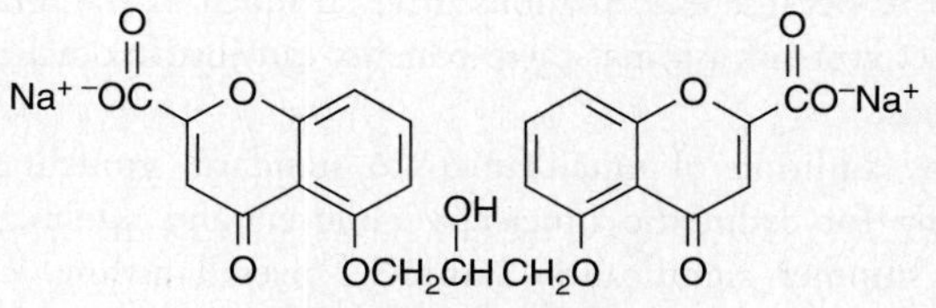

Cromolyn sodium

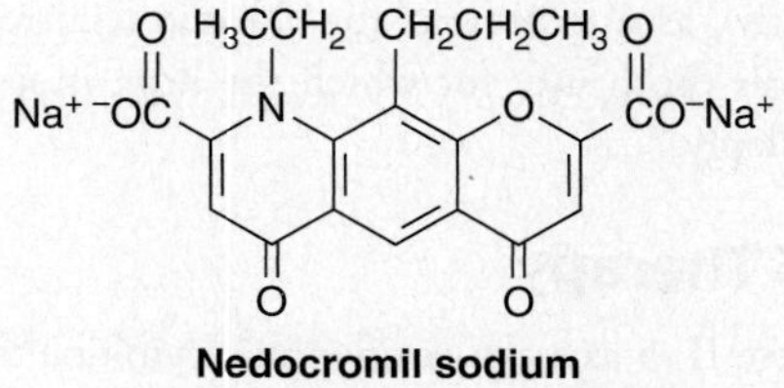

Nedocromil sodium

LEUKOTRIENE PATHWAY INHIBITORS

The involvement of leukotrienes in many inflammatory diseases (see Chapter 18) and in anaphylaxis prompted the development of drugs that block their synthesis or interaction with their receptors. Leukotrienes result from the action of 5-lipoxygenase on arachidonic acid and are synthesized by a variety of inflammatory cells in the airways, including eosinophils, mast cells, macrophages, and basophils. Leukotriene B_4 (LTB_4) is a potent neutrophil chemoattractant, and LTC_4 and LTD_4 exert many effects known to occur in asthma, including bronchoconstriction, increased bronchial reactivity, mucosal edema, and mucus hypersecretion.

Two approaches to interrupting the leukotriene pathway have been pursued: inhibition of 5-lipoxygenase, thereby preventing leukotriene synthesis; and inhibition of the binding of LTD_4 to its receptor on target tissues, thereby preventing its action. Efficacy in blocking airway responses to exercise and to antigen challenge has been shown for drugs in both categories: **zileuton,** a 5-lipoxygenase inhibitor, and **zafirlukast** and **montelukast,** LTD_4-receptor ($CysLT_1$) antagonists (Figure 20–7). All three drugs have been shown to improve asthma control and reduce the frequency of asthma exacerbations in clinical trials. They are not as effective as even low-dose ICS therapy in inducing and maintaining asthma control, but are preferred by many patients, especially the parents of asthmatic children, because of often exaggerated concerns over the toxicities of corticosteroids. They have the additional advantage of being effective when taken orally, which is an easier route of administration than aerosol inhalation in young children, and montelukast is approved for children as young as 12 months of age.

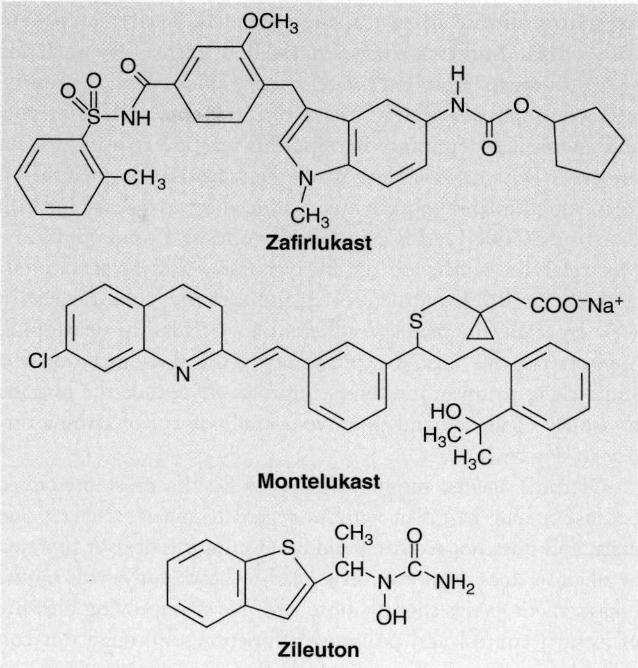

Zafirlukast

Montelukast

Zileuton

FIGURE 20–7 Structures of leukotriene receptor antagonists (montelukast, zafirlukast) and of the 5-lipoxygenase inhibitor (zileuton).

Some patients appear to have particularly favorable responses, but apart from the subclass of patients with aspirin-exacerbated respiratory disease (described below), no clinical features allow identification of "responders" before a trial of therapy. In the USA, zileuton is approved for use in an oral dosage of 1200 mg of the sustained-release form twice daily; zafirlukast, 20 mg twice daily; and montelukast, 10 mg (for adults) or 4–5 mg (for children) once daily.

Trials with leukotriene inhibitors have demonstrated an important role for leukotrienes in aspirin-exacerbated respiratory disease (AERD), a disease that combines the features of asthma, chronic rhinosinusitis with nasal polyposis, and reactions to aspirin or other nonsteroidal anti-inflammatory drugs (NSAIDs) that inhibit cyclooxygenase-1 (COX-1). Aspirin-exacerbated respiratory disease occurs in approximately 5–10% of patients with asthma. In these patients, ingestion of even a very small dose of aspirin causes profound bronchoconstriction, nasal congestion, and symptoms of systemic release of histamine, such as flushing and abdominal cramping. Because this reaction to aspirin is not associated with any evidence of allergic sensitization to aspirin or its metabolites and because it is produced by any of the NSAIDs that target COX-1, AERD is thought to result from inhibition of prostaglandin synthetase (cyclooxygenase), shifting arachidonic acid metabolism from the prostaglandin to the leukotriene pathway, especially in platelets adherent to circulating neutrophils. Support for this idea was provided by the demonstration that leukotriene pathway inhibitors impressively reduce the response to aspirin challenge and improve overall control of asthma on a day-to-day basis.

Of these agents, montelukast is by far the most prescribed, because it may be taken without regard to meals, is taken once daily, and does not require periodic monitoring of liver function, as zileuton does. However, in a head-to-head study with montelukast, zileuton was slightly more effective at improving measures of asthma control and pulmonary function. Although not considered first-line therapy, the leukotriene-modifying agents are sometimes given in lieu of inhaled corticosteroids for mild asthma when prescription of an ICS meets patient resistance. The receptor antagonists have little toxicity. Early reports of eosinophilic granulomatosis with polyangiitis (EGPA), a systemic vasculitis accompanied by worsening asthma, pulmonary infiltrates, and eosinophilia, appear to have been coincidental, with the syndrome unmasked by the reduction in prednisone dosage made possible by the addition of zafirlukast or montelukast. In 2020, the FDA required a boxed warning for montelukast about the risk of serious neuropsychiatric events, including suicidality in adults and adolescents, and nightmares and behavioral problems in children.

TARGETED (MONOCLONAL ANTIBODY) THERAPY

As the pathophysiologic mechanisms responsible for asthma have become better understood, anti-inflammatory therapy targeting specific inflammatory pathways has been developed. Specifically, monoclonal antibodies targeting IgE, IL-5, the receptor for IL-4 and IL-13, and thymic stromal lymphopoietin (TSLP) have been brought to market (Table 20–1).

TABLE 20–1 Monoclonal antibodies for use in asthma.

Antibody Name	Isotype	Target
Omalizumab	Humanized IgG1	IgE
Mepolizumab	Humanized IgG1	IL-5
Benralizumab	Humanized IgG1	IL-5 receptor
Reslizumab	Humanized IgG4	IL-5
Dupilumab	HumanIgG4	IL-4 receptor
Tezepelumab-ekko	Human IgG2	TSLP

Anti-IgE Monoclonal Antibodies

The monoclonal antibody **omalizumab** was raised in mice and then humanized, making it less likely to cause sensitization when given to human subjects (see Chapter 55). Because its specific target is the portion of IgE that binds to its receptors (Fcε-R1 and Fcε-R2 receptors) on dendritic cells, basophils, mast cells, and other inflammatory cells, omalizumab inhibits the binding of IgE but does not activate IgE already bound to its receptor and thus does not provoke mast cell degranulation.

Omalizumab's use is restricted to patients with moderate to severe asthma and evidence of perennial allergic sensitization, and the dose administered is adjusted for total IgE level and body weight. Administered by subcutaneous injection every 2–4 weeks to asthmatic patients, it lowers free plasma IgE to undetectable levels and significantly reduces the magnitude of both early and late bronchospastic responses to antigen challenge. Omalizumab's most important clinical effect is reduction in the frequency and severity of asthma exacerbations, while enabling a reduction in corticosteroid requirements. Combined analysis of several clinical trials has shown that the patients most likely to respond are those with a history of repeated exacerbations, a high requirement for corticosteroid treatment, and poor pulmonary function. Similarly, the exacerbations most often prevented are the most severe; omalizumab treatment reduced exacerbations requiring hospitalization by 88%. Because exacerbations drive so much of the direct and indirect costs of asthma, these benefits can justify omalizumab's high cost.

The addition of omalizumab to standard, guideline-based therapy for asthmatic inner-city children and adolescents in early summer significantly improved overall asthma control, reduced the need for other medications, and nearly eliminated the autumnal peak in exacerbations. Omalizumab has also been proven effective as a treatment for chronic recurrent urticaria, nasal polyposis (both uses for which the drug is approved) and for peanut allergy.

Anti-IL-5 Therapy

T2 cells secrete IL-5 as a pro-eosinophilic cytokine that results in eosinophilic airway inflammation. Although not central to the mechanisms of asthma in all patients, a substantial proportion of patients with severe asthma have airway and peripheral eosinophilia driven by up-regulation of IL-5-secreting T2 lymphocytes. Two humanized monoclonal antibodies targeting IL-5, **mepolizumab** and **reslizumab,** and another targeting the IL-5 receptor, **benralizumab,** have recently been developed for the treatment of severe eosinophilic asthma. Clinical trials with these drugs have shown them to be effective in improving pulmonary function and measures of asthma control, while preventing exacerbations in asthmatic patients with peripheral eosinophilia, leading to their approval as add-on, maintenance therapy of severe asthma in patients with an eosinophilic phenotype. Mepolizumab has also been approved for treatment of EGPA, hypereosinophilic syndrome (HES), and rhinosinusitis with nasal polyps. Mepolizumab and benralizumab are administered via subcutaneous injection, while reslizumab is given intravenously.

Like omalizumab, reslizumab carries a small (0.3%) risk of anaphylaxis, and a period of observation following infusion is recommended. Mepolizumab, although not associated with anaphylaxis, has resulted in reports of hypersensitivity. In addition, reactivation of herpes zoster has been reported in some patients who received mepolizumab.

Anti-IL-4/IL-13 Therapy

Dupilumab (an antibody directed against the IL-4α co-receptor for both IL-4 and IL-13) has also been shown to reduce exacerbation frequency and improve pulmonary function and measures of asthma control. It is a subcutaneous injection administered every other week that is approved for patients with moderate to severe asthma, whether with an eosinophilic phenotype or corticosteroid-dependent. It is also indicated for moderate to severe atopic dermatitis, prurigo nodularis, rhinosinusitis with nasal polyposis, and eosinophilic esophagitis. Of note, dupilumab may cause a peripheral eosinophilia; this is typically transient but in rare cases may persist. Due to this, some clinicians will avoid initiation if baseline eosinophils are very elevated (eg, >1500 eosinophils/μL).

Anti-TSLP Therapy

The most recent monoclonal antibody approved for severe asthma treatment is tezepelumab-ekko, which is a subcutaneous injection administered every 4 weeks. Its target, TSLP, is an epithelial cytokine; blocking it decreases several downstream inflammation-associated cytokines (IgE, Il-5, and IL-13) and biomarkers (peripheral and airway submucosal eosinophils and fractional exhalation of nitric oxide).

FUTURE DIRECTIONS OF ASTHMA THERAPY

The term "asthma" encompasses a heterogeneous collection of disorders, some of which are poorly responsive to corticosteroid treatment. The existence of different forms or subtypes of asthma has actually long been recognized, as implied by the use of modifying terms to describe asthma in particular patients. More rigorous description of asthma phenotypes, based on cluster analysis of multiple clinical, physiologic, and laboratory features, including analysis of blood and sputum inflammatory cell assessments, has identified as many as five different asthma phenotypes. The key question raised by this approach is whether the phenotypes respond differently to available asthma treatments.

The demonstration of differences in the pattern of gene expression in the airway epithelium of asthmatic and healthy subjects is persuasive evidence of the existence of different asthma phenotypes requiring different approaches to therapy. Compared with healthy controls, half of the asthmatic participants overexpressed genes for periostin, CLCA1, and serpinB2, genes known to be up-regulated in airway epithelial cells by IL-13, a signature cytokine of T2 lymphocytes. The other half of the asthmatic participants did not. These findings suggest that fundamentally different pathophysiologic mechanisms exist even among patients with mild asthma. The participants with overexpression of genes up-regulated by IL-13 are referred to as having a "T2-high molecular phenotype" of asthma. The other subjects, who did not overexpress these genes, are described as having a "non-T2" or "T2-low" molecular phenotype. The T2-high asthmatic subjects on average tended to have more sputum eosinophilia and blood eosinophilia, positive skin test results, higher levels of IgE, and greater expression of certain mucin genes. The response to ICS treatment of these two groups was quite different. Eight weeks of treatment with an ICS improved forced expiratory volume in 1 second (FEV_1) only in the T2-high subjects. The implications of these findings are far reaching because they indicate that perhaps as many as half of patients with mild to moderate asthma do not respond to ICS therapy with an improvement in lung function. These data do not address whether there is differential response to ICS in symptoms or exacerbation frequency between T2-low and high.

Current research focuses on further exploring molecular phenotypes in asthma and in finding effective treatments for each group. An NIH-sponsored prospective, double-blind multicenter trial was recently completed to compare mometasone (an ICS) and tiotropium (an antimuscarinic) in subjects with mild asthma characterized as T2-high or non-T2-high by analysis of their induced sputum samples for eosinophil number. This trial demonstrated that although subjects with T2-high asthma had a better response to mometasone than tiotropium, subjects with T2-low asthma did not respond better to one agent vs the other. Further studies are needed to determine if the benefit of either of these agents in T2-low asthma is superior to placebo. Another advance for T2-low asthma is the finding that low-dose azithromycin, given to adults with poorly controlled asthma already on a combination of inhaled corticosteroids and long-acting bronchodilators, reduced exacerbation frequency and improved quality of life equally in both eosinophilic (ie, T2-high) and non-eosinophilic (ie, T2-low) asthma. Advances in the development of novel not yet on market bronchodilators (eg, soluble guanylyl cyclase agonists and Ste20-like kinase inhibitors) also has the potential to improve the treatment of asthma across phenotypes.

The pace of advance in the scientific description of the immunopathogenesis of asthma has spurred the development of many new therapies that target different sites in the immune cascade. Beyond the monoclonal antibodies directed against cytokines (IL-4, IL-5, IL-13, and TSLP) already reviewed (see Table 20–1), these include antagonists of cell adhesion molecules, protease inhibitors, and immunomodulators aimed at shifting CD4 lymphocytes from the TH2 to the TH1 subtype or at selective inhibition of the subset of TH2 lymphocytes directed against particular antigens. Among the monoclonal antibodies in development is daclizumab, a humanized antibody that binds the CD25 subunit of the IL-2 receptor. As these new therapies are developed, it will become increasingly important to identify biomarkers of specific phenotypes of asthma that are most likely to benefit from specific therapies. This will enable truly personalized asthma therapy.

CLINICAL PHARMACOLOGY OF DRUGS USED IN THE TREATMENT OF ASTHMA

National and international guidelines for asthma emphasize the need for adjusting the intensity of asthma therapy to the underlying severity of the disease and the level of control achieved by the patient's current treatment (https://www.nhlbi.nih.gov/health-pro/guidelines/current/asthma-guidelines; ginasthma.org). An underlying principle common to these guidelines is that asthma should be considered in two time domains. In the present domain, asthma is important for the symptoms and impairments it causes—cough, nocturnal awakenings, and shortness of breath that interfere with the ability to exercise or to pursue desired activities. For mild asthma, occasional inhalation of a bronchodilator may be all that is needed to control these symptoms. For more severe asthma, treatment with a long-term controller, like an ICS, is necessary to relieve symptoms and restore function. The second domain of asthma is the risk it presents of future events, such as exacerbations or progressive loss of pulmonary function. Satisfaction with the ability to control symptoms and maintain function by frequent use of an inhaled β_2 agonist does not mean that the risk of future events is also controlled. In fact, use of two or more canisters of an inhaled β agonist per month is a marker for increased risk of asthma fatality.

The challenges of assessing severity and adjusting therapy for these two domains of asthma are different. For relief of distress in the present domain, the key information is obtained by asking specific questions about the frequency and severity of symptoms, the frequency of rescue use of an inhaled β agonist, the frequency of nocturnal awakenings, and the ability to exercise, and by measuring lung function with spirometry. The best predictor of the risk for future exacerbations is the frequency and severity of their occurrence in the past. Without such a history, estimation of risk is more difficult. In general, patients with poorly controlled symptoms have a heightened risk of exacerbations in the future, but some patients seem unaware of the severity of their airflow obstruction (sometimes described as "poor perceivers") and can be identified only by measurement of pulmonary function. Reductions in FEV_1 correlate with heightened risk of future attacks of asthma. Other possible markers of heightened risk are unstable pulmonary function (large variations in FEV_1 from visit to visit, large change with bronchodilator treatment), extreme bronchial reactivity, high numbers of eosinophils in blood or sputum, and high levels of nitric oxide in exhaled air. Assessment of these features may identify patients who need increases in therapy for protection against future exacerbations.

BRONCHODILATORS

Bronchodilators, eg, inhaled albuterol, are rapidly effective, safe, and inexpensive. Many patients with only occasional symptoms of asthma require no more than an inhaled bronchodilator taken on an as-needed basis. If symptoms require this "rescue" therapy more than twice a week, nocturnal symptoms occur more than twice a month, or the FEV_1 is less than 80% of predicted, additional treatment is needed. The treatment first recommended is a low dose of an ICS, although a leukotriene receptor antagonist may be used as an alternative.

An important caveat for patients with mild asthma is that although the risk of a severe, life-threatening attack is low, it is not zero. All patients with asthma should be instructed in a simple action plan for severe, frightening attacks: to take up to four puffs of albuterol every 20 minutes over 1 hour. If no improvement is noted after the first four puffs, additional treatments should be taken while on the way to an emergency department or other higher level of care. With the goal of improving outcomes on a population level, the non-zero risk of a life-threatening attack led one set of international guidelines (Global Initiative for Asthma) to recommend that all patients with asthma, however mild, should take doses of ICS at least on an as-needed basis; ie, every time a dose of bronchodilator is taken. Nonetheless, major guidelines diverge on this recommendation given the unclear benefit of ICS for all individuals with the mildest forms of asthma.

MUSCARINIC ANTAGONISTS

Inhaled muscarinic antagonists have so far earned a limited place in the treatment of asthma. The effects of short-acting agents (eg, ipratropium bromide) on baseline airway resistance are nearly as great as, but no greater than, those of the sympathomimetic drugs, so they are used largely as alternative therapies for patients intolerant of β-adrenoceptor agonists. The airway effects of antimuscarinic and sympathomimetic drugs given in full doses have been shown to be additive only in reducing hospitalization rates in patients with severe airflow obstruction who present for emergency care.

The long-acting antimuscarinic (LAMA) agent tiotropium, added to an ICS in asthma, is likely as effective as the addition of an LABA. The addition of tiotropium to combined ICS and LABA therapy can increase lung function and reduce exacerbations in individuals with persistent airflow obstruction, more bronchodilator responsiveness, higher symptom burden, and a history of exacerbations. As a treatment for COPD, LAMAs improve functional capacity, presumably through their action as bronchodilators, and reduce the frequency of exacerbations through currently unknown mechanisms. Studies have provided mixed data as to whether LAMAs can slow the rate of decline of lung function in COPD.

CORTICOSTEROIDS

If asthmatic symptoms occur frequently, or if significant airflow obstruction persists despite bronchodilator therapy, inhaled corticosteroids should be started. For patients with severe symptoms or severe airflow obstruction (eg, FEV_1 <50% of predicted), initial treatment with a high dose of an ICS in combination with an LABA is appropriate. Once clinical improvement is noted, usually after 3 months, the dose of treatment should be stepped down to no more than is necessary to control symptoms and maintain pulmonary function.

An issue for ICS treatment is patient adherence. Analysis of prescription renewals shows that only a minority of patients take corticosteroids regularly. This may be a function of a general "steroid phobia" fostered by emphasis in the lay press on the hazards of long-term oral corticosteroid therapy and by ignorance of the difference between glucocorticoids and anabolic steroids, taken to enhance muscle strength by now-infamous athletes. This fear of corticosteroid toxicity makes it hard to persuade patients whose symptoms have improved after starting treatment that they should continue it for protection against attacks. This context accounts for the interest in reports that instructing patients with mild but persistent asthma to take ICS therapy only when their symptoms worsen is nearly as effective in maintaining pulmonary function and preventing attacks as is taking the ICS twice each day.

Two options for asthma inadequately controlled by a standard dose of an ICS are to (1) double the dose of ICS or (2) combine it with another drug. The addition of theophylline or a leukotriene receptor antagonist modestly increases asthma control, but the most impressive benefits are afforded by addition of a *long-acting* inhaled β_2-receptor agonist (LABA, eg, salmeterol or formoterol). Many studies have shown this combination to be more effective than doubling the dose of the ICS. Combinations of an ICS and an LABA in a single inhaler are now available in fixed-dose preparations (eg, fluticasone propionate and salmeterol [Advair]; budesonide and formoterol [Symbicort]; mometasone and formoterol [Dulera]; fluticasone furoate and vilanterol [Breo]). The rapid onset of action of formoterol enables novel use of its combination with a low dose of budesonide. The combination of 80 mcg of budesonide plus 12.5 mcg of formoterol taken twice daily and additionally for relief of symptoms (ie, taken as both a "controller" and a "reliever") is as effective as inhalation twice daily of a four-times-higher dose of budesonide with albuterol alone taken for relief of symptoms. This flexible dosing strategy has been widespread in Europe for several years. Since 2020, this SMART (single maintenance and reliever therapy) paradigm has become a part of US guidelines as well, and now combined corticosteroid/formoterol inhalers are recommended for both scheduled and as needed use (whether low or medium dose).

Until recently, a shadow hung over the use of combination ICS-LABA therapy for moderate and severe asthma, generated by evidence of a statistically significant increase in the very low risk of fatal or near-fatal asthma attacks from use of an LABA even when taken in combination with an ICS. This evidence prompted the FDA to require the addition of a "black box" warning to the package insert issued with each ICS-LABA inhaler. Subsequent studies do not show an increased risk of asthma-related deaths when LABA is used in combination with an ICS, and therefore the "black box" warning has been removed from ICS-LABA preparations. Concerns remain regarding LABA monotherapy and guidelines advise against this treatment.

An interesting difference between ICS options is whether the drug is formulated as a traditional suspension or a solution. When paired with specially designed inhalers, solution formulations are capable of generating much smaller aerosol particles than is possible with suspension formulations. Two small particle ICS solution formulations are currently available: ciclesonide and beclomethasone. These solution formulations increase lung deposition of corticosteroid, decrease oropharyngeal deposition, and improve indirect measures of small airway function, presumably reflecting deeper penetration into the lung by small particles. Therefore, it is hypothesized that solution formulations can achieve asthma control with lower doses of corticosteroids and less severe side effects. This possibility, as well as additional potential benefits from increased activity on small airways, has yet to be shown to translate into better control of symptoms or reduced exacerbations.

LEUKOTRIENE ANTAGONISTS

A leukotriene pathway antagonist taken as an oral tablet is an alternative to ICS treatment in patients with symptoms occurring more than twice a week or those who are awakened from sleep by asthma more than twice a month.

The leukotriene receptor antagonist montelukast is the most widely prescribed of these treatments, especially by primary care providers. This drug, taken orally, is easy to administer and is rarely associated with troublesome adverse effects. This maintenance therapy is widely used for treating children in the USA, particularly those who have concurrent symptomatic allergic rhinitis, which is also effectively treated by montelukast.

TARGETED THERAPY

Treatment with **omalizumab,** the monoclonal humanized anti-IgE antibody, and with any of the other monoclonal anti-IL-5 antibodies is reserved for patients with moderate to severe asthma inadequately controlled by ICS/LABA treatment. Omalizumab reduces lymphocytic, eosinophilic bronchial inflammation, oral and inhaled corticosteroid dose requirements, and the frequency and severity of exacerbations. It is reserved for patients with demonstrated IgE-mediated sensitivity (by positive skin test or radioallergosorbent test [RAST] to perennial aeroallergens) and an IgE level within a range that can be reduced sufficiently by twice-weekly subcutaneous injection. Other options for treatment of severe asthma uncontrolled by ICS/LABA therapy, especially if associated with peripheral eosinophilia, are the anti-IL5 monoclonal antibodies reviewed earlier—**mepolizumab, reslizumab,** and **benralizumab. Dupilumab,** the monoclonal human anti-IL4/IL-13 receptor antibody, is targeted as adjunctive treatment for individuals with moderate to severe asthma with eosinophilia, or for patients with severe, oral corticosteroid-dependent asthma (in which case eosinophilia is not required). Finally, tezepelumab is approved for use in patients with severe asthma; no biomarkers such as eosinophilia or IgE are required.

In addition to their high cost, several factors have limited the use of targeted therapies. First, they must be given parenterally at 2- to 8-week intervals. Second, some can cause anaphylactic reactions or other hypersensitivity reactions, albeit in a small percentage (<0.5%) of patients, making some degree of monitoring important and self-administration more difficult. In addition, a small number of patients receiving mepolizumab developed herpes zoster infection, and administration of the varicella-zoster vaccine to adults age 50 or older 4 weeks prior to initiation with mepolizumab is recommended.

MANAGEMENT OF ACUTE ASTHMA

The treatment of acute attacks of asthma in patients reporting to the hospital requires close, continuous clinical assessment and repeated objective measurement of lung function. For patients with mild attacks, inhalation of a β-receptor agonist is as effective as subcutaneous injection of epinephrine. Severe attacks require treatment with oxygen, frequent or continuous administration of aerosolized albuterol, and systemic treatment with prednisone or methylprednisolone (0.5 mg/kg every 6–12 hours). Even this aggressive treatment is not invariably effective, and patients must be watched closely for signs of deterioration. General anesthesia, intubation, and mechanical ventilation of asthmatic patients cannot be undertaken lightly but may be lifesaving if respiratory failure supervenes.

PROSPECTS FOR PREVENTION

The high prevalence of asthma in the developed world and its rapid increases in the developing world call for a strategy for primary prevention. Strict antigen avoidance during infancy, once thought to be sensible, has now been shown to be ineffective. In fact, growing up from birth on a farm with domestic animals or in a household where cats or dogs are kept as pets appears to *protect* against developing asthma. The best hope seems to lie in understanding the mechanisms by which microbial exposures during infancy foster development of a balanced immune response and then mimicking the effects of natural environmental exposures through administration of harmless microbial commensals (probiotics) or nutrients that foster their growth (prebiotics) in the intestinal tract during the critical period of immune development in early infancy. Identifying the particular microbes whose growth should be fostered, or the microbial products responsible for inducing appropriate maturation of immune function, has become an active focus of epidemiologic, basic, and translational research.

TREATMENT OF CHRONIC OBSTRUCTIVE PULMONARY DISEASE (COPD)

COPD is the third most common cause of death in the United States and accounts for more than $40 billion per year in direct and indirect health care costs. COPD resembles asthma in that it is also characterized by airflow limitation, although the obstruction of COPD is not fully reversible with treatment. The airflow limitation of COPD, believed to reflect an abnormal inflammatory response of the lung to noxious particles or gases, especially to cigarette smoke, progresses if the exposure continues and may progress in some individuals, albeit more slowly, even if the exposure ceases. The belief that COPD develops in only 15–30% of habitual smokers is now challenged by radiographic demonstration of important, progressive changes in bronchial wall thickness and loss of lung tissue even in smokers with measures of pulmonary function in the normal range. Although COPD differs from asthma, many of the same drugs are used in its treatment. This section discusses the drugs that are useful in both conditions; a more comprehensive guide to their use is available in the Global Initiative for Chronic Obstructive Lung Disease (GOLD) guidelines for classification and treatment of COPD (http://goldcopd.org).

Although asthma and COPD are both characterized by airway inflammation, reduction in maximum expiratory flow, and episodic exacerbations of airflow obstruction, most often triggered by viral respiratory infection, they differ in many important respects. Compared to asthma, COPD occurs in older patients, is commonly associated with neutrophilic rather than eosinophilic inflammation, is poorly responsive even to high-dose ICS therapy, and is associated with progressive, inexorable loss of pulmonary function over time, especially with continued cigarette smoking.

Despite these differences, the approaches to treatment are similar, although the benefits expected (and achieved) are less for COPD than for asthma. For relief of acute symptoms, inhalation of a short-acting β agonist (eg, albuterol), of an anticholinergic drug (eg, ipratropium bromide), or of the two in combination is usually effective. For patients with persistent symptoms of exertional dyspnea and limitation of activities, regular use of a long-acting bronchodilator, whether an LABA or a long-acting anticholinergic, or the two together, is indicated. Despite enthusiasm for theophylline from experiments suggesting improved contractile function of the diaphragm and increased sensitivity to corticosteroids, a recent large placebo-controlled double-blind randomized trial of low-dose theophylline failed to show a benefit on exacerbation frequency. The nonmethylxanthine **roflumilast,** a selective phosphodiesterase inhibitor that improves pulmonary function and reduces exacerbation frequency, is approved as a treatment for COPD.

The place of ICS therapy is less central to treatment of COPD than asthma, in part because of its lower efficacy for this condition and in part because of reports of its use being associated with heightened risk of bacterial pneumonia. Its use is thus recommended only for patients with severe airflow obstruction or with a history of prior exacerbations, and for those with a clear history of asthma independent of smoking. Based on a similar concept to the T2-low vs T2-high molecular phenotypes of asthma, recent evidence-based international guidelines recommend using low and high blood eosinophils to assess whether a patient with COPD will have a low or reasonable likelihood of benefit from ICS use. The use of biomarkers to guide ICS therapy allows treatment decisions to be based on underlying pathology rather than based on the determination of whether there is an overlap of asthma and COPD.

COPD Exacerbations

Acute exacerbations of COPD are a major driver of the morbidity, mortality, and health care costs of COPD. Because of the greater age of the patients affected and the prevalence of comorbidities, especially cardiovascular disease, the mortality of acute COPD exacerbations is greater than that of exacerbation of asthma, but management does not differ greatly except in the routine use of antibiotics, which are given because exacerbations of COPD frequently involve bacterial infection of the lower airways. Antibiotics commonly used include β-lactams, doxycycline, and azithromycin, which are active against the prevalent COPD pathogen *Haemophilus influenzae*.

Because of their importance in driving the morbidity and mortality of COPD, much attention has been paid to approaches to prevention of COPD exacerbations. For patients with a history of two or more exacerbations per year, daily treatment with an ICS is appropriate, and a recent large study showed significant reduction in exacerbation frequency from daily treatment with azithromycin. An innovative, although initially counterintuitive, hypothesis that treatment with the selective β_1-receptor antagonist, metoprolol succinate, might reduce exacerbations in patients with moderate to severe COPD has recently been examined with negative results. Some epidemiologic surveys showed significant reductions in overall mortality and exacerbations in COPD patients taking a β-receptor antagonist. However, a large, prospective, placebo-controlled study of metoprolol treatment of COPD patients at risk for exacerbations (but without cardiovascular indications for β antagonist treatment) gave negative results.

SUMMARY Drugs Used in Asthma and COPD

Subclass, Drug	Mechanism of Action	Effects	Clinical Applications	Pharmacokinetics, Toxicities
BETA AGONISTS				
• Albuterol	Selective β_2 agonist	Prompt, efficacious bronchodilation	Asthma, chronic obstructive pulmonary disease (COPD) • drug of choice in acute asthmatic bronchospasm	Aerosol inhalation • duration several hours • also available for nebulizer and parenteral use • *Toxicity:* Tremor, tachycardia • *Overdose:* arrhythmias
• Salmeterol	Selective β_2 agonist	Slow onset, primarily preventive action; potentiates corticosteroid effects	Bronchodilation, prevention of asthma exacerbations	Aerosol inhalation • duration 12–24 h • *Toxicity:* Tremor, tachycardia • *Overdose:* arrhythmias
• *Metaproterenol, terbutaline: Similar to albuterol; terbutaline available as an oral drug*				
• *Formoterol, vilanterol: Similar to salmeterol*				
• Epinephrine	Nonselective α and β agonist	Bronchodilation plus all other sympathomimetic effects on cardiovascular and other organ systems (see Chapter 9)	Anaphylaxis, asthma, others (see Chapter 9) • rarely used for asthma (β_2-selective agents preferred)	Aerosol, nebulizer, or parenteral • see Chapter 9
• Isoproterenol	β_1 and β_2 agonist	Bronchodilation plus powerful cardiovascular effects	Asthma, but β_2-selective agents preferred	Aerosol, nebulizer, or parenteral • see Chapter 9
CORTICOSTEROIDS, INHALED				
• Fluticasone propionate	Alters gene expression	Reduces mediators of inflammation • powerful prophylaxis of exacerbations	Asthma • adjunct in COPD • rhinitis (nasal)	Aerosol • duration hours • *Toxicity:* Limited by aerosol application • candidal infection, vocal cord changes
• *Fluticasone furoate: A different molecule than fluticasone propionate and ~2x as potent, and ~2x duration of action—dosed once daily unlike other ICS*				
• *Beclomethasone, budesonide, flunisolide, others: Similar to fluticasone propionate*				
CORTICOSTEROIDS, SYSTEMIC				
• Prednisone	Like fluticasone	Like fluticasones	Asthma • adjunct in COPD	Oral • duration 12–24 h • *Toxicity:* Multiple • see Chapter 39
• *Methylprednisolone: Parenteral agent like prednisone*				

(continued)

Subclass, Drug	Mechanism of Action	Effects	Clinical Applications	Pharmacokinetics, Toxicities
STABILIZERS OF MAST AND OTHER CELLS				
• Cromolyn, nedocromil (no longer available as inhalers in the USA)	Alter function of delayed chloride channels • inhibit inflammatory cell activation	Prevention of bronchospastic response to allergen inhalation	Asthma (other routes used for ocular, nasal, and gastrointestinal allergy)	Aerosol • duration 6–8 h • *Toxicity:* Cough • not absorbed so other toxicities are minimal
METHYLXANTHINES				
• Theophylline	Uncertain: • phosphodiesterase inhibition • adenosine receptor antagonist	Bronchodilation, cardiac stimulation, increased skeletal muscle strength (diaphragm)	Asthma, COPD	Oral • duration 8–12 h but extended-release preparations often used • *Toxicity:* Multiple (see text)
• *Roflumilast: Similar to theophylline, but with better therapeutic ratio*				
LEUKOTRIENE ANTAGONISTS				
• Montelukast, zafirlukast	Block leukotriene D_4 receptors	Block airway response to exercise and antigen challenge	Prophylaxis of asthma, especially in children and in aspirin-induced asthma	Oral • duration hours • *Toxicity:* Minimal
• *Zileuton: Inhibits lipoxygenase, reduces leukotriene synthesis; slightly more effective than montelukast, but needs liver function test monitoring*				
ANTI-IGE ANTIBODY				
• Omalizumab	Humanized IgE antibody reduces circulating IgE	Reduces frequency of asthma exacerbations	Moderate to severe asthma inadequately controlled by above agents (age 6+ years), chronic spontaneous urticaria, nasal polyps	Subcutaneous • duration 2–4 weeks • *Toxicity:* Injection site reactions (anaphylaxis extremely rare)
ANTI-INTERLEUKIN-5 PATHWAY ANTIBODIES				
• Mepolizumab	Humanized anti-IL-5 antibody; reduces circulating and tissue eosinophils	Reduces frequency of asthma exacerbations; improves pulmonary function; reduced oral corticosteroid dosing	Severe asthma inadequately controlled by above agents, with associated eosinophilia (age 6+ years), EGPA, HES, rhinosinusitis with nasal polyps	Subcutaneous • duration 4 weeks • *Toxicity:* Injection site reactions (anaphylaxis extremely rare); possible increased risk of herpes zoster infection (vaccination may be advisable)
• Reslizumab	Humanized anti-IL-5 antibody; reduces circulating and tissue eosinophils	Reduces frequency of asthma exacerbations; improves pulmonary function; reduced oral corticosteroid dosing	Severe asthma inadequately controlled by above agents, with associated eosinophilia (age 18+ years)	Intravenous • duration 4 weeks • *Toxicity:* Injection site reactions, anaphylaxis rare
• Benralizumab	Humanized anti-IL-5 receptor antibody; reduces circulating and tissue eosinophils	Reduces frequency of asthma exacerbations; improves pulmonary function; reduced oral corticosteroid dosing	Severe asthma inadequately controlled by above agents (age 12+ years)	Subcutaneous • duration 4–8 weeks • *Toxicity:* Injection site reactions (anaphylaxis extremely rare)
ANTI-INTERLEUKIN 4/INTERLEUKIN 13 ANTIBODY				
• Dupilumab	Human antibody against IL-4α receptor for IL-4 and IL-13	Reduces frequency of asthma exacerbations; improves pulmonary function; reduced oral corticosteroid dosing	Moderate to severe eosinophilic or corticosteroid-dependent asthma (age 6+ years), atopic dermatitis, eosinophilic esophagitis, prurigo nodularis, rhinosinusitis with nasal polyposis	Subcutaneous • duration 2 weeks • *Toxicity:* Injection site reactions (anaphylaxis extremely rare), dermatologic and ocular effects, peripheral eosinophilia
ANTI-THYMIC STROMAL LYMPHOPOIETIN ANTIBODY				
• Tezepelumab	Human antibody against thymic stromal lymphopoietin	Reduces frequency of asthma exacerbations; improves pulmonary function; reduced oral corticosteroid dosing if blood eosinophils ≥ 150/μl	Severe asthma (age 12+ years)	Subcutaneous • duration 4 weeks • *Toxicity:* arthralgia, pharyngitis

PREPARATIONS AVAILABLE

GENERIC NAME	AVAILABLE AS
SHORT-ACTING BETA-AGONIST BRONCHODILATORS	
Albuterol	Generic, Proventil, ProAir, Ventolin
Bitolterol	Tornalate
Ephedrine	Generic
Epinephrine	Generic, Adrenaline, Primatene Mist
Levalbuterol	Xenopex
Metaproterenol	Generic, Alupent
Pirbuterol	Maxair
Terbutaline	Breathaire, Brethine
SHORT-ACTING ANTIMUSCARINIC BRONCHODILATOR	
Ipratropium	Generic, Atrovent
COMBINATION SHORT-ACTING BRONCHODILATOR	
Albuterol/ipratropium	Combivent
LONG-ACTING BETA-ADRENERGIC BRONCHODILATORS	
Formoterol	Foradil
Indacaterol	Arcapta
Olodaterol	Striverdi
Salmeterol	Serevent
Vilanterol	Only available in combination inhalers
LONG-ACTING ANTIMUSCARINIC BRONCHODILATORS	
Aclidinium	Tudorza
Tiotropium	Spiriva
Umeclidinium	Incruse
Glycopyrrolate	Lonhala Magnair
Revefenacin	Yupelri
AEROSOL CORTICOSTEROIDS	
	See also Chapter 39
Beclomethasone	QVAR, Beclovent, Vanceril
Budesonide	Pulmicort
Ciclesonide	Alvesco
Mometasone	Asmanex
Flunisolide	AeroBid, Aerospan
Fluticasone propionate	Flovent
Fluticasone furoate	Arnuity Ellipta
Triamcinolone	Azmacort
COMBINATION INHALERS	
Formoterol/budesonide	Symbicort
Formoterol/mometasone	Dulera
Salmeterol/fluticasone propionate	Advair
Vilanterol/fluticasone furoate	Breo Ellipta
Vilanterol/umeclidinium	Anoro
LEUKOTRIENE INHIBITORS	
Montelukast	Generic, Singulair
Zafirlukast	Accolate
Zileuton	Zyflo CR
PHOSPHODIESTERASE INHIBITORS, METHYLXANTHINES	
Dyphylline	Dilor, Dylix, Lufyllin
Roflumilast	Daliresp
Theophylline	Generic, Elixophyllin, Slo-Phyllin, Uniphyl, Theo-Dur, Theo-24
MONOCLONAL ANTIBODIES	
Omalizumab	Xolair (subcutaneous)
Benralizumab	Fasenra (subcutaneous every 8 weeks)
Mepolizumab	Nucala (subcutaneous)
Reslizumab	Cinqair (intravenous)
Dupilumab	Dupixent (subcutaneous)
Tezepelumab-ekko	Tezpire (subcutaneous)

REFERENCES

Pathophysiology of Airway Disease

Fahy JV: Type 2 inflammation in asthma: Present in most, absent in many. Nat Rev Immunol 2015;15:57.

Kim HY, DeKruyff RH, Umetsu DT: The many paths to asthma: Phenotype shaped by innate and adaptive immunity. Nat Immunol 2010; 7:577.

Locksley RM: Asthma and allergic inflammation. Cell 2010;140:777.

Lotvall J et al: Asthma endotypes: A new approach to classification of disease entities within the asthma syndrome. J Allergy Clin Immunol 2011; 127:355.

Martinez FD, Vercelli D: Asthma. Lancet 2013;382:1360.

Asthma Treatment

Bateman ED et al: Overall asthma control: The relationship between current control and future risk. J Allergy Clin Immunol 2010;125:600.

Bel EH: Mild asthma. N Engl J Med 2013;369:2362.

Expert Panel Working Group of the National Heart, Lung and Blood Institute: 2020 focused updates to the asthma management guidelines: a report from the National Asthma Education and Prevention Program Coordinating Committee Expert Panel Working Group. J Allergy Clin Immunol 2020; 146:1217.

Global Lung Initiative for Asthma: Global Strategy for Asthma Management and Prevention, 2022. Available from: www.ginasthma.org.

National Heart, Lung, and Blood Institute, National Asthma Education and Prevention Program: Expert Panel Report 3: Guidelines for the diagnosis and management of asthma. National Heart, Lung, and Blood Institute; Revised August 2007. NIH publication no. 07-4051. https://www.nhlbi.nih.gov/health-pro/guidelines/current/asthma-guidelines.

Beta Agonists

Busse WW et al: Combined analysis of asthma safety trials of long-acting β2-agonists. N Engl J Med 2018;378:2497.

Ducharme FM et al: Addition of long-acting beta2-agonists to inhaled steroids versus higher dose inhaled steroids in adults and children with persistent asthma. Cochrane Database Syst Rev 2010;4:CD005533.

Papi A et al: Beclomethasone-formoterol as maintenance and reliever treatment in patients with asthma: A double-blind, randomised controlled trial. Lancet Respir Med 2013;1:23.

Sadreameli SC, Brigham EP, Patel A: The surprising reintroduction of Primatene Mist in the United States. Ann Am Thorac Soc 2019;16:1234.

Stempel DA et al: Serious asthma events with fluticasone plus salmeterol versus fluticasone alone. N Engl J Med 2016;374:1822.

Stempel DA et al: Safety of adding salmeterol to fluticasone propionate in children with asthma. N Engl J Med 2016;375:840.

Methylxanthines & Roflumilast

Barnes PJ: Theophylline. Am J Respir Crit Care Med 2013;188:901.

Devereux G et al: Effect of theophylline as adjunct to inhaled corticosteroids on exacerbations in patients with COPD: A randomized clinical trial. JAMA 2018;320:1548.

Rabe KF: Roflumilast for the treatment of chronic obstructive pulmonary disease. Expert Rev Respir Med 2010;4:543.

Corticosteroids

Barnes P: How corticosteroids control inflammation: Quintiles Prize Lecture 2005. Br J Pharmacol 2006;148:245.

Bateman ED et al: As-needed budesonide-formoterol versus maintenance budesonide in mild asthma. N Engl J Med 2018;378:1877.

Beasley R et al: Combination corticosteroid/beta-agonist inhaler as reliever therapy: A solution for intermittent and mild asthma? J Allergy Clin Immunol 2014;133:39.

Boushey HA et al: Daily versus as-needed corticosteroids for mild persistent asthma. N Engl J Med 2005;352:1519.

Leach C, Colice GL, Luskin A: Particle size of inhaled corticosteroids: Does it matter? J Allergy Clin Immunol 2009;124(6 Suppl):S88.

O'Byrne PM et al: Inhaled combined budesonide-formoterol as needed in mild asthma. N Engl J Med 2018;378:1865.

Postma DS et al: Asthma-related outcomes in patients initiating extrafine ciclesonide or fine-particle inhaled corticosteroids. Allergy Asthma Immunol Res 2017;9:116.

Suissa S et al: Low-dose inhaled corticosteroids and the prevention of death from asthma. N Engl J Med 2000;343:332.

Antimuscarinic Drugs

D'Amato M et al: Anticholinergic drugs in asthma therapy. Curr Opin Pulm Med 2016;22:527.

Lazarus SC et al: Mometasone or tiotropium in mild asthma with a low sputum eosinophil level. N Engl J Med 2019;380:2009.

Lee AM, Jacoby DB, Fryer AD: Selective muscarinic receptor antagonists for airway diseases. Curr Opin Pharmacol 2001;1:223.

Peters SP et al: Tiotropium bromide step-up therapy for adults with uncontrolled asthma. N Engl J Med 2010;363:1715.

Sobieraj DM et al: Association of inhaled corticosteroids and long-acting muscarinic antagonists with asthma control in patients with uncontrolled, persistent asthma: A systematic review and meta-analysis. JAMA 2018;319:1473.

Virchow JC et al: Single inhaler extrafine triple therapy in uncontrolled asthma (TRIMARAN and TRIGGER): two double-blind, parallel-group, randomised, controlled phase 3 trials. Lancet 2019;394:1737.

Leukotriene Pathway Inhibitors

Calhoun WJ: Anti-leukotrienes for asthma. Curr Opin Pharmacol 2001;1:230.

Laidlaw TM et al: Cysteinyl leukotriene overproduction in aspirin-exacerbated respiratory disease is driven by platelet-adherent leukocytes. Blood 2012;119:3790.

Wang L et al: Cost-effectiveness analysis of fluticasone versus montelukast in children with mild-to-moderate persistent asthma in the Pediatric Asthma Controller Trial. J Allergy Clin Immunol 2011;127:161.

Anti-IgE Therapy

Busse WW et al: Randomized trial of omalizumab (anti-IgE) for asthma in inner-city children. N Engl J Med 2011;364:1005.

Walker S et al: Anti-IgE for chronic asthma in adults and children. Cochrane Database Syst Rev 2006;2:CD003559.

Targeted Monoclonal Antibody Therapy

McGregor MC et al: Role of biologics in asthma. Am J Respir Crit Care Med 2019;199:433.

Future Directions of Asthma Therapy

Chang TS et al: Childhood asthma clusters and response to therapy in clinical trials. J Allergy Clin Immunol 2014;133:363.

Haldar P et al: Cluster analysis and clinical asthma phenotypes. Am J Respir Crit Care Med 2008;178:218.

Lotvall J et al: Asthma endotypes: A new approach to classification of disease entities within the asthma syndrome. J Allergy Clin Immunol 2011;127:355.

Moore WC et al: Identification of asthma phenotypes using cluster analysis in the Severe Asthma Research Program. Am J Respir Crit Care Med 2010; 181:315.

Woodruff PG et al: T-helper type 2-driven inflammation defines major subphenotypes of asthma. Am J Respir Crit Care Med 2009;180:388.

Management of Acute Asthma

Lazarus SC: Clinical practice. Emergency treatment of asthma. N Engl J Med 2010;363:755.

Prospects for Prevention

Klauth M, Heine H: Allergy protection by cowshed bacteria: Recent findings and future prospects. Pediatr Allergy Immunol 2016;27:340.

Lynch SV et al: Effects of early-life exposure to allergens and bacteria on recurrent wheeze and atopy in urban children. J Allergy Clin Immunol 2014;134:593.

Martinez FD: New insights into the natural history of asthma: Primary prevention on the horizon. J Allergy Clin Immunol 2011;128:939.

Stein MM et al: Innate immunity and asthma risk in Amish and Hutterite farm children. N Engl J Med 2016;375:411.

Treatment of COPD

Global Initiative for Chronic Obstructive Lung Disease: Global Strategy for Diagnosis, Management, and Prevention of COPD. http://www.goldcopd.org.

Huisman EL et al: Comparative efficacy of combination bronchodilator therapies in COPD: A network meta-analysis. Int J Chron Obstruct Pulmon Dis 2015;10:1863.

Kew KM, Dias S, Cates CJ: Long-acting inhaled therapy (beta-agonists, anticholinergics and steroids) for COPD: A network meta-analysis. Cochrane Database Syst Rev 2014;1:CD010844.

Niewoehner DE: Clinical practice. Outpatient management of severe COPD. N Engl J Med 2010;362:1407.

Vogelmeier C et al: Tiotropium versus salmeterol for the prevention of exacerbations of COPD. N Engl J Med 2011;364:1093.

Dransfield MT et al: Metoprolol for the prevention of acute exacerbations of COPD. N Engl J Med 2019;381:2304.

CASE STUDY ANSWER

This patient demonstrates the destabilizing effects of a respiratory infection on asthma, and her mother's comments demonstrate the common (and dangerous) phobia about "overuse" of bronchodilator or steroid inhalers. The patient has signs of imminent respiratory failure, including her refusal to lie down, her fear, and her tachycardia, which cannot be attributed to her minimal treatment with albuterol. Critically important immediate steps are to administer high-flow oxygen and to start albuterol by nebulization. Adding ipratropium (Atrovent) to the nebulized solution is recommended. A corticosteroid (0.5–1.0 mg/kg of methylprednisolone) should be administered intravenously. It is also advisable to alert the intensive care unit, because a patient with severe bronchospasm who tires can slip into respiratory failure quickly, and intubation can be difficult.

Fortunately, most patients treated in hospital emergency departments do well. Asthma mortality is rare (fewer than 4000 deaths per year among a population of more than 20 million asthmatics in the USA), and when it occurs, it is often out of hospital. Presuming this patient recovers, she needs adjustments to her therapy before discharge. The strongest predictor of severe attacks of asthma is their occurrence in the past. Thus, this patient's therapy needs to be stepped up to a higher level, like a high-dose inhaled corticosteroid in combination with a long-acting β agonist. Both the patient and her parents need instruction on the importance of regular adherence to therapy, with reassurance that it can be "stepped down" to a lower dose of inhaled corticosteroid (although still in combination with a long-acting β agonist) once her condition stabilizes. They also need instruction on an action plan for managing severe symptoms. This can be as simple as advising that if the patient has a severe, frightening attack, she can take up to four puffs of albuterol every 15 minutes, but if the first treatment does not bring significant relief, she should take the next four puffs while on her way to an emergency department or urgent care clinic. She should also be given a prescription for prednisone, with instructions to take 40–60 mg orally for severe attacks, but not to wait for it to take effect if she remains severely short of breath even after albuterol inhalations. Asthma is a chronic disease, and good care requires close follow-up and creation of a provider-patient partnership for optimal management. If she has had several previous exacerbations, she should be considered a candidate for monoclonal anti-IgE antibody therapy with omalizumab, which effectively reduces the rate of asthma exacerbations—even those associated with viral respiratory infection—in patients with allergic asthma. Alternatively, if the patient is found to have blood eosinophilia, treatment with an anti-IL-5 monoclonal antibody (eg, mepolizumab) should be considered as well.

SECTION V DRUGS THAT ACT IN THE CENTRAL NERVOUS SYSTEM

CHAPTER 21

Introduction to the Pharmacology of CNS Drugs

John A. Gray, MD, PhD*

Drugs acting in the central nervous system (CNS) were among the first to be discovered by primitive humans and are still the most widely used group of pharmacologic agents. These include medications used to treat a wide range of neurologic and psychiatric conditions as well as drugs that relieve pain, suppress nausea, and reduce fever, among other symptoms. In addition, many CNS-acting drugs are used without prescription to increase the sense of well-being.

Due to their complexity, the mechanisms by which various drugs act in the CNS have not always been clearly understood. In recent decades, however, dramatic advances have been made in the methodology of CNS pharmacology. It is now possible to study the action of a drug on individual neurons and even single receptors within synapses. The information obtained from such studies is the basis for several major developments in studies of the CNS. First, it is clear that nearly all drugs with CNS effects act on specific receptors that modulate synaptic transmission. While a few agents such as general anesthetics and alcohol may have nonspecific actions on membranes (although these exceptions are not fully accepted), even these non–receptor-mediated actions result in demonstrable alterations in synaptic transmission.

Second, drugs are among the most valuable tools for studying CNS function, from understanding the mechanism of convulsions to the laying down of long-term memory. Both agonists that mimic natural transmitters (and in many cases are more selective than the endogenous substances) and antagonists are extremely useful in such studies. Third, unraveling the actions of drugs with known clinical efficacy has led to some of the most fruitful hypotheses regarding the mechanisms of disease. For example, information about the action of antipsychotic drugs on dopamine receptors has provided the basis for important hypotheses regarding the pathophysiology of schizophrenia. Studies of the effects of a variety of agonists and antagonists on γ-aminobutyric acid (GABA) receptors have resulted in new concepts pertaining to the pathophysiology of several diseases, including anxiety and epilepsy.

A full appreciation of the effects of a drug on the CNS requires an understanding of the multiple levels of brain organization, from genes to circuits to behavior. This chapter introduces the functional organization of the CNS and its synaptic transmitters as a basis for understanding the actions of the drugs described in the following chapters.

*The author thanks Dr. Roger A. Nicoll for his contributions to previous editions.

ORGANIZATION OF THE CNS

The CNS is composed of the brain and spinal cord and is responsible for integrating sensory information and generating motor output and other behaviors needed to successfully interact with the environment and enhance species survival. The human brain contains about 100 billion interconnected neurons surrounded by various supporting glial cells. Throughout the CNS, neurons are either clustered into groups called nuclei or are present in layered structures such as the cerebellum or hippocampus. Connections among neurons both within and among these clusters form the circuitry that regulates information flow through the CNS.

Neurons

Neurons are electrically excitable cells that process and transmit information via an electrochemical process. There are many types of neurons in the CNS, and they are classified in multiple ways: by location, by function, and by the neurotransmitter they release. A typical neuron possesses a cell body (or soma) and specialized processes called dendrites and axons (Figure 21–1). Dendrites, which form highly branched complex dendritic "trees," receive and integrate the input from other neurons and conduct this information to the cell body. The axon carries the output signal of a neuron from the cell body, sometimes over long distances. Neurons may have hundreds of dendrites but generally have only one axon, although axons may branch distally to contact multiple targets. The axon terminal makes contact with other neurons at specialized junctions called synapses where neurotransmitter chemicals are released and interact with receptors on other neurons.

Neuroglia

In addition to neurons, there are a large number of non-neuronal support cells, called glia, that perform a variety of essential functions in the CNS. Astrocytes are the most abundant cell in the brain and play homeostatic support roles, including providing metabolic nutrients to neurons and maintaining extracellular ion concentrations. Astrocyte processes are closely associated with neuronal synapses, where they are involved in the removal and recycling of neurotransmitters after release (see below). In addition, astrocytes play increasingly recognized active roles in regulating synapse formation and function. For example, astrocytes express neurotransmitter receptors and can release neuromodulators that can alter neuronal activity.

Oligodendrocytes are cells that wrap around the axons of projection neurons in the CNS forming the myelin sheath (see Figure 21–1). Similar to the Schwann cells in peripheral neurons, the myelin sheath created by the oligodendrocytes insulates the axons and increases the speed of signal propagation. Damage to oligodendrocytes occurs in multiple sclerosis, and thus they are a target of drug discovery efforts.

Microglia are specialized macrophages derived from the bone marrow that settle in the CNS and are the major immune defense system in the brain. These cells are actively involved in neuroinflammatory processes in many pathologic states including neurodegenerative diseases. In addition, roles for microglia in normal brain function are increasingly appreciated. For example, microglia engulf and eliminate synapses, a process called synaptic pruning, which is crucial for normal circuit development. Excessive microglia-mediated synapse elimination has been linked to schizophrenia and Alzheimer disease.

Blood-Brain Barrier

The blood-brain barrier (BBB) is a protective functional separation of the circulating blood from the extracellular fluid of the CNS that limits the penetration of substances, including drugs. This separation is accomplished by the presence of tight junctions between the capillary endothelial cells as well as a surrounding

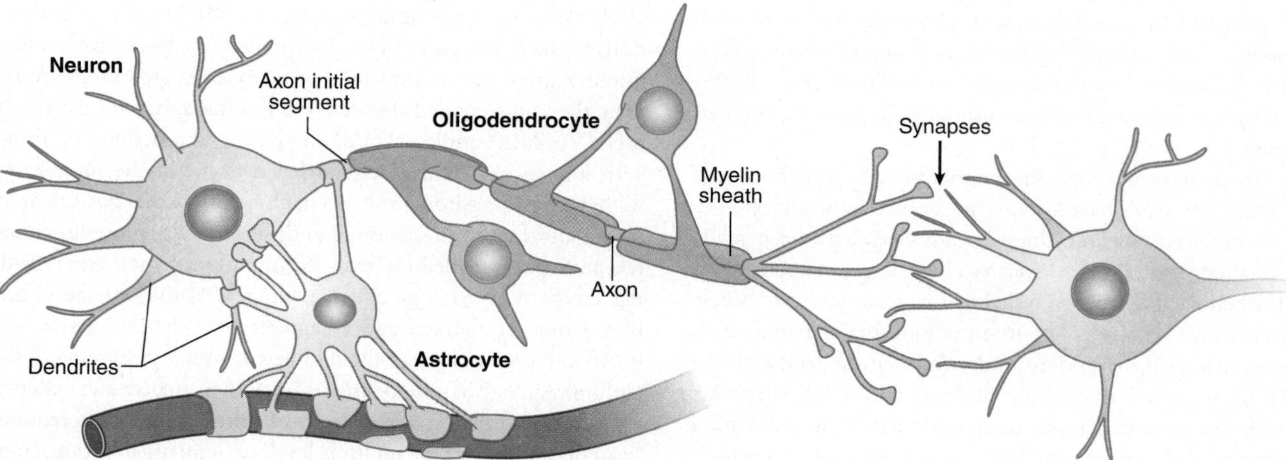

FIGURE 21–1 Neurons and glia in the CNS. A typical neuron has a cell body (or soma) that receives the synaptic responses from the dendritic tree. These synaptic responses are integrated at the axon initial segment, which has a high concentration of voltage-gated sodium channels. If an action potential is initiated, it propagates down the axon to the synaptic terminals, which contact other neurons. The axon of long-range projection neurons are insulated by a myelin sheath derived from specialized membrane processes of oligodendrocytes, analogous to the Schwann cells in the peripheral nervous system. Astrocytes perform supportive roles in the CNS, and their processes are closely associated with neuronal synapses.

layer of astrocyte end-feet. As such, to enter the CNS, drugs must either be highly hydrophobic or engage specific transport mechanisms. For example, the second-generation antihistamines cause less drowsiness because they were developed to be significantly more polar than older antihistamines, limiting their crossing of the BBB (see Chapter 16). Many nutrients, such as glucose and the essential amino acids, have specific transporters that allow them to cross the BBB. L-DOPA, a precursor of the neurotransmitter dopamine, can enter the brain using an amino acid transporter, whereas dopamine cannot cross the BBB. Thus, the orally administered drug L-DOPA, but not dopamine, can be used to boost CNS dopamine levels in the treatment of Parkinson disease. Some parts of the brain, the so-called circumventricular organs, lack a normal BBB. These include regions that sample the blood, such as the area postrema vomiting center, and regions that secrete neurohormones into the circulation.

Natural Toxins: Tools for Characterizing Ion Channels

Evolution is tireless in the development of natural toxins. A vast number of variations are possible with even a small number of amino acids in peptides, and peptides make up only one of a broad array of toxic compounds. For example, the hundreds of different species of predatory marine cone snails each kills or paralyzes its prey with a venom containing 50–200 different peptides, with very little duplication of peptides among species. Other animals with useful toxins include snakes, frogs, spiders, bees, wasps, and scorpions. Plant species with toxic (or therapeutic) substances are referred to in several other chapters of this book.

Since many toxins act on ion channels, they provide a wealth of chemical tools for studying the function of these channels. In fact, much of our current understanding of the properties of ion channels comes from studies utilizing only a small percentage of the highly potent and selective toxins that are now available. The toxins typically target voltage-sensitive ion channels, but a number of very useful toxins block ligand-gated ion channel receptors. Table 21–1 lists some of the toxins most commonly used in research, their mode of action, and their source.

ION CHANNELS & NEUROTRANSMITTER RECEPTORS

The membranes of neurons contain two types of channels defined by the mechanisms controlling their gating (opening and closing): **voltage-gated** and **ligand-gated** channels (Figure 21–2A and B). Voltage-gated channels respond to changes in the membrane potential of the cell. The voltage-gated sodium channel described in Chapter 14 for the heart is an example of this type of channel. In nerve cells, these channels are highly concentrated on the initial segment of the axon (see Figure 21–1), which initiates the all-or-nothing fast action potential, and along the length of the axon where they propagate the action potential to the nerve terminal. There are also many types of voltage-gated calcium and potassium channels on the cell body, dendrites, and initial segment, which act on a slower time scale and modulate the rate at which the neuron discharges. For example, some types of potassium channels opened by depolarization of the cell result in slowing of further depolarization and act as a brake to limit action potentials. Plant and animal toxins that target various voltage-gated ion channels have been invaluable for studying the functions of these channels (see Box: Natural Toxins: Tools for Characterizing Ion Channels; Table 21–1).

Neurotransmitters exert their effects on neurons by binding to two distinct classes of receptor. The first class is referred to as **ligand-gated channels,** or **ionotropic receptors.** These receptors consist of multiple subunits, and binding of the neurotransmitter ligand directly opens the channel, which is an integral part of the receptor complex. These channels are insensitive or only weakly sensitive to membrane potential. Activation of these channels typically results in a brief (a few milliseconds to tens of milliseconds) opening of the channel. Ligand-gated channels are responsible for fast synaptic transmission typical of hierarchical projection pathways in the CNS (see following text).

The second class of neurotransmitter receptors are referred to as **metabotropic receptors** (Figure 21–2C). These are seven-transmembrane G protein–coupled receptors (GPCRs) of the type described in Chapter 2. The binding of neurotransmitter to this type of receptor does not result in the direct gating of a channel. Rather, binding to the receptor engages a G protein, which results in the production of second messengers that mediate intracellular signaling cascades such as those described in Chapter 2.

In neurons, activation of metabotropic neurotransmitter receptors often leads to the modulation of voltage-gated channels. These interactions can occur entirely within the plane of the membrane and are referred to as **membrane-delimited** pathways (Figure 21–2D). In this case, the G protein (often the βγ subunits) interacts directly with a voltage-gated ion channel. In general, two types of voltage-gated ion channels are the targets of this type of signaling: calcium channels and potassium channels. When G proteins interact with calcium channels, they inhibit channel function. This mechanism accounts for the inhibition of neurotransmitter release that occurs when presynaptic metabotropic receptors are activated. In contrast, when these receptors are postsynaptic, they activate (cause the opening of) potassium channels, resulting in a slow postsynaptic inhibition. Metabotropic receptors can also modulate voltage-gated channels less directly by the generation of **diffusible second messengers** (Figure 21–2E). A classic example of this type of action is provided by β-adrenergic receptors, which generate cAMP via the activation of adenylyl

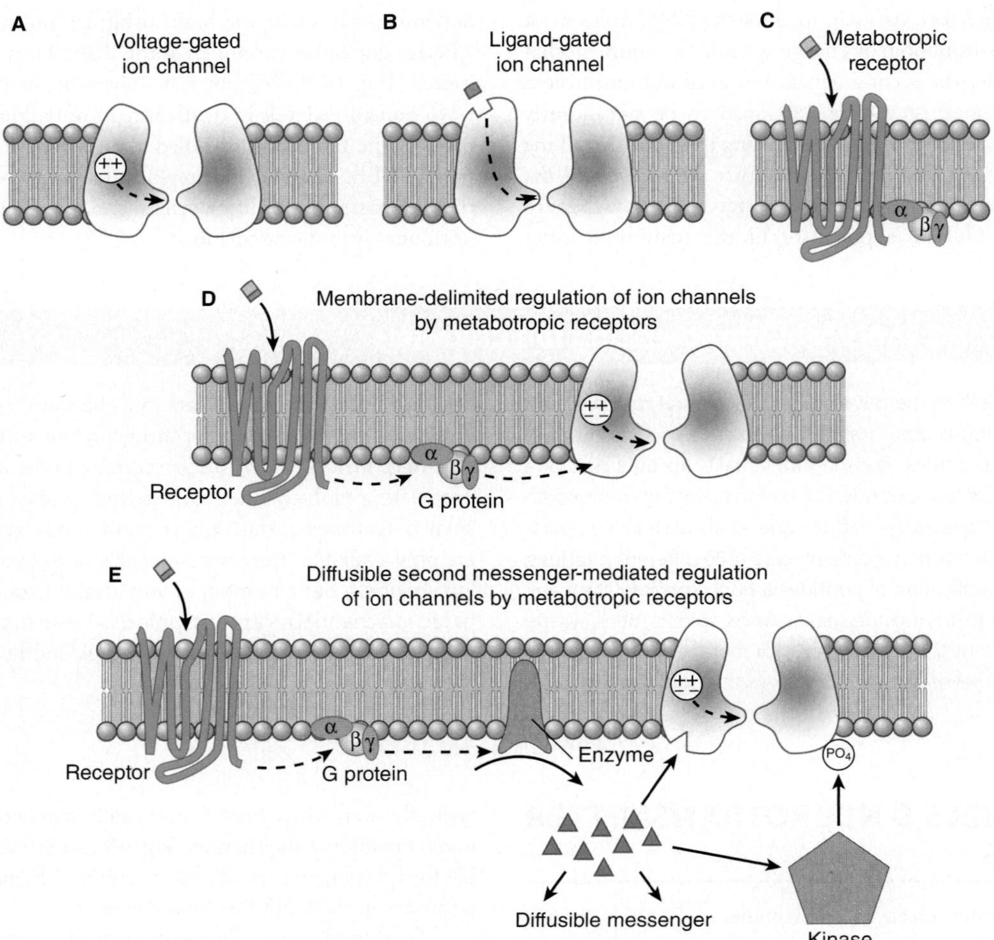

FIGURE 21–2 Types of ion channels and neurotransmitter receptors in the CNS. **A** shows a voltage-gated channel in which a voltage sensor component of the protein controls the gating (*broken arrow*) of the channel. **B** shows a ligand-gated channel in which the binding of the neurotransmitter to the ionotropic channel receptor controls the gating (*broken arrow*) of the channel. **C** shows a G protein–coupled (metabotropic) receptor, which, when bound, activates a heterotrimeric G protein. **D** and **E** show two ways metabotropic receptors can regulate ion channels. The activated G protein can interact directly to modulate an ion channel (**D**) or the G protein can activate an enzyme that generates a diffusible second messenger (**E**), eg, cAMP, which can interact with the ion channel or can activate a kinase that phosphorylates and modulates a channel.

cyclase (see Chapter 2). Whereas membrane-delimited actions occur within microdomains in the membrane, second messenger-mediated effects can occur over considerable distances. Finally, an important consequence of the involvement of G proteins in receptor signaling is that, in contrast to the brief effect of ionotropic receptors, the effects of metabotropic receptor activation can last tens of seconds to minutes. Metabotropic receptors predominate in the diffuse modulatory neuronal systems in the CNS (see below).

THE SYNAPSE & SYNAPTIC POTENTIALS

The communication between neurons in the CNS occurs through chemical synapses in the majority of cases. (A few instances of electrical coupling between neurons have been documented, and such coupling may play a role in synchronizing neuronal discharge. However, it is unlikely that these electrical synapses are an important site of drug action.) The events involved in synaptic transmission can be summarized as follows.

An action potential propagating down the axon of the presynaptic neuron enters the synaptic terminal and activates voltage-gated calcium channels in the membrane of the terminal (see Figure 6–3). The calcium channels responsible for the release of neurotransmitter are generally resistant to the calcium channel-blocking agents discussed in Chapter 12 (eg, verapamil) but are sensitive to blockade by certain marine toxins and metal ions (see Tables 21–1 and 12–4). As calcium flows into the terminal, the increased calcium concentration promotes the fusion of synaptic vesicles with the presynaptic membrane. The neurotransmitter contained in the vesicles is released into the synaptic cleft and diffuses to the receptors on the postsynaptic membrane. The neurotransmitter binds to its receptor and opens channels (either directly or indirectly as described above) causing a brief change in membrane conductance (permeability to ions) of the postsynaptic cell. The time delay from

TABLE 21–1 Some toxins used to characterize ion channels.

Channel Types	Mode of Toxin Action	Source
Voltage-gated		
Sodium channels		
Tetrodotoxin (TTX)	Blocks channel from outside	Puffer fish
Batrachotoxin (BTX)	Slows inactivation, shifts activation	Colombian frog
Potassium channels		
Apamin	Blocks "small Ca-activated" K channel	Honeybee
Charybdotoxin	Blocks "big Ca-activated" K channel	Scorpion
Calcium channels		
Omega conotoxin (ω-CTX-GVIA)	Blocks N-type channel	Pacific cone snail
Agatoxin (ω -AGAIVA)	Blocks P-type channel	Funnel web spider
Ligand-gated		
Nicotinic ACh receptor		
α-Bungarotoxin	Irreversible antagonist	Marine snake
$GABA_A$ receptor		
Picrotoxin	Blocks channel	Vine native to Southeast Asia
Glycine receptor		
Strychnine	Competitive antagonist	Tree native to Southeast Asia
AMPA receptor		
Philanthotoxin	Blocks channel	European beewolf wasp

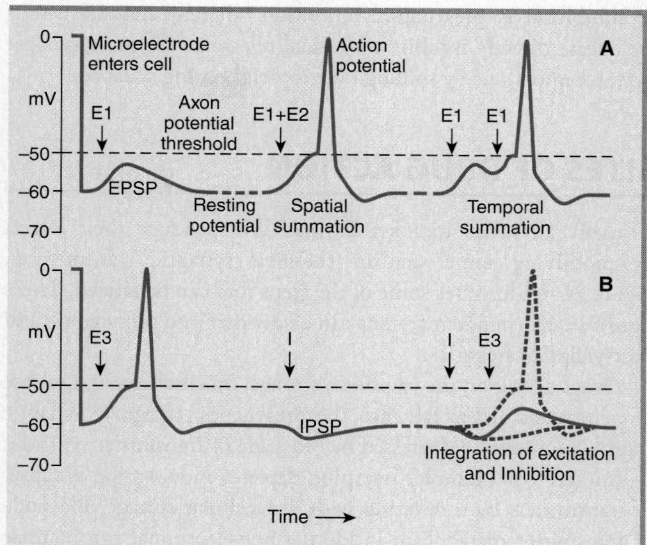

FIGURE 21–3 Postsynaptic potentials and action potential generation. **A** shows the voltage recorded upon entry of a microelectrode into a postsynaptic cell and subsequent recording of a resting membrane potential of –60 mV. Stimulation of an excitatory pathway (E1, left) generates transient depolarization called an excitatory postsynaptic potential (EPSP). Simultaneous activation of multiple excitatory synapses (E1 + E2, middle) increases the size of the depolarization, so that the threshold for action potential generation is reached. Alternatively, a train of stimuli from a single input can temporally summate to reach the threshold (E1 + E1, right). **B** demonstrates the interaction of excitatory and inhibitory synapses. On the left, a suprathreshold excitatory stimulus (E3) evokes an action potential. In the center, an inhibitory pathway (I) generates a small hyperpolarizing current called an inhibitory postsynaptic potential (IPSP). On the right, if the previously suprathreshold excitatory input (E3) is given shortly after the inhibitory input (I), the IPSP prevents the excitatory potential from reaching threshold.

the arrival of the presynaptic action potential to the onset of the postsynaptic response is approximately 0.5 ms. Most of this delay is consumed by the release process, particularly the time required for calcium channels to open.

The first systematic analysis of synaptic potentials in the CNS was in the early 1950s by Eccles and associates, who recorded intracellularly from spinal motor neurons. When a microelectrode enters a cell, there is a sudden change in the potential recorded by the electrode, which is typically about -60 mV (Figure 21–3A). This is the resting membrane potential of the neuron. Two types of pathways—excitatory and inhibitory—impinge on the motor neuron.

When an excitatory pathway is stimulated, a small depolarization or **excitatory postsynaptic potential (EPSP)** is recorded. This potential is due to the excitatory transmitter acting on an ionotropic receptor, causing an increase in cation permeability. As additional excitatory synapses are activated, there is a graded summation of the EPSPs to increase the size of the depolarization (see Figure 21–3A, spatial summation, middle). When a sufficient number of excitatory synapses are activated, the excitatory postsynaptic potential depolarizes the postsynaptic cell to threshold, and an all-or-none action potential is generated. Alternatively, if there is a repetitive firing of an excitatory input, the temporal summation of the EPSPs may also reach the action potential threshold (see Figure 21–3A, right).

When an inhibitory pathway is stimulated, the postsynaptic membrane is hyperpolarized owing to the selective opening of chloride channels, producing an **inhibitory postsynaptic potential (IPSP)** (see Figure 21–3B, middle). However, because the equilibrium potential for chloride (see Chapter 14) is only slightly more negative than the resting potential (~ -65 mV), the hyperpolarization is small and contributes only modestly to the inhibitory action. The opening of the chloride channel during the inhibitory postsynaptic potential makes the neuron "leaky" so that changes in membrane potential are more difficult to achieve. This shunting effect decreases the change in membrane potential during the excitatory postsynaptic potential. As a result, an EPSP that evoked an action potential under resting conditions fails to evoke an action potential during the IPSP (see Figure 21–3B, right). A second type of inhibition is presynaptic inhibition whereby neurotransmitter release directly inhibits additional release at the same synapse (autoreceptors), or by spilling over to neighboring synapses.

SITES OF DRUG ACTION

Virtually all drugs that act in the CNS produce their effects by modifying some step in chemical synaptic transmission. Figure 21–4 illustrates some of the steps that can be altered. These transmitter-dependent actions can be divided into presynaptic and postsynaptic categories.

Drugs acting on the synthesis, storage, metabolism, and release of neurotransmitters fall into the presynaptic category. Synaptic transmission can be depressed by blockade of transmitter synthesis or storage. For example, reserpine depletes monoamine synapses of transmitters by interfering with intracellular storage. Blockade of transmitter metabolism inside the nerve terminal can increase transmitter concentrations and has been reported to increase the amount of transmitter released per impulse. Drugs also can alter the release of transmitters. The stimulant amphetamine induces the release of catecholamines from adrenergic synapses (see Chapters 6, 9, and 32). Capsaicin causes the release of the peptide substance P from sensory neurons, and tetanus toxin blocks the release of transmitters. After a CNS transmitter has been released into the synaptic cleft, its action is terminated either by uptake or by degradation. For most neurotransmitters, there are uptake mechanisms into the presynaptic terminal and also into surrounding glia. Cocaine, for example, blocks the uptake of catecholamines at adrenergic synapses and thus potentiates the action of these amines. Acetylcholine, however, is inactivated by enzymatic degradation, not reuptake. Anticholinesterases block the degradation of acetylcholine and thereby prolong its action (see Chapter 7). No uptake mechanism has been found for any of the numerous CNS peptides, and it has yet to be demonstrated whether specific enzymatic degradation terminates the action of peptide transmitters.

In the postsynaptic region, the transmitter receptor provides the primary site of drug action. Drugs can act as neurotransmitter agonists, such as the opioids, which mimic the action of enkephalin, or they can block receptor function. Receptor antagonism is a common mechanism of action for CNS drugs. An example is strychnine's blockade of the receptor for the inhibitory transmitter glycine. This block, which underlies strychnine's convulsant action, illustrates how the blockade of inhibitory processes results in excitation. Drugs can also act directly on the ion channel of ionotropic receptors. For example, the anesthetic ketamine blocks the NMDA subtype of glutamate ionotropic receptors by binding in the ion channel pore. In the case of metabotropic receptors, drugs can act at any of the steps downstream of the receptor. Perhaps the best example is provided by the methylxanthines, which

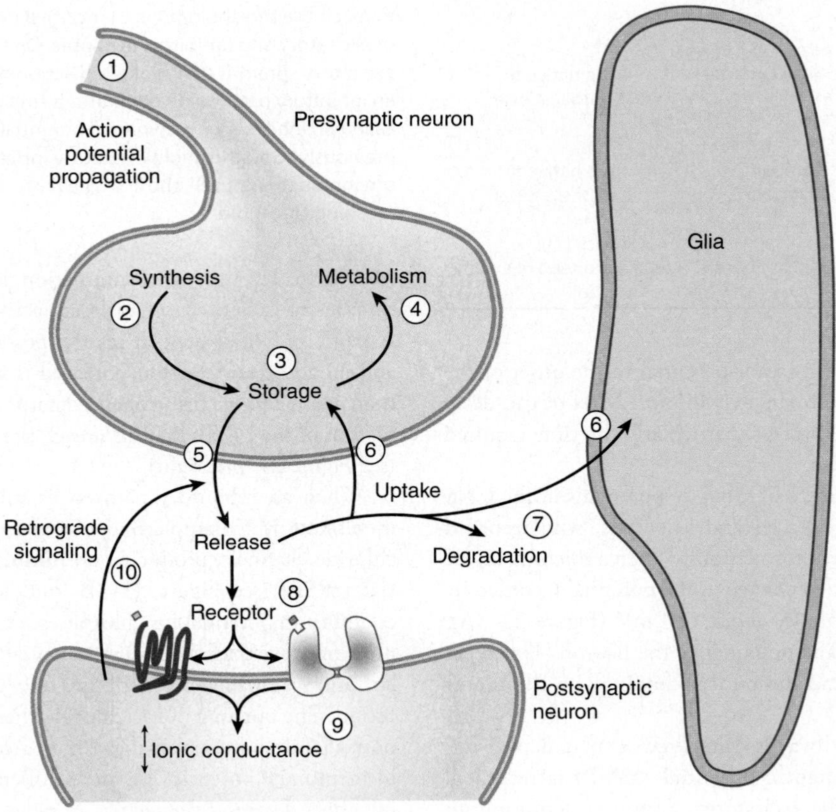

FIGURE 21–4 Sites of drug action. Schematic drawing of steps at which drugs can alter synaptic transmission. (1) Action potential in presynaptic fiber; (2) synthesis of transmitter; (3) storage; (4) metabolism; (5) release; (6) reuptake into the nerve ending or uptake into a glial cell; (7) degradation; (8) receptor for the transmitter; (9) receptor-induced increase or decrease in ionic conductance; (10) retrograde signaling.

can modify neurotransmitter responses mediated through the second-messenger cAMP. At high concentrations, the methylxanthines elevate the level of cAMP by blocking its metabolism and thereby prolonging its action.

The traditional view of the synapse is that it functions like a valve, transmitting information in one direction. However, it is now clear that the synapse can generate signals that feed back onto the presynaptic terminal to modify transmitter release. Endocannabinoids are the best documented example of such *retrograde* signaling (see below). Postsynaptic activity leads to the synthesis and release of endocannabinoids, which then bind to receptors on the presynaptic terminal. Although the gas nitric oxide (NO) has long been proposed as a retrograde messenger, its physiologic role in the CNS is still not well understood.

The selectivity of CNS drug action is based on two primary factors. First, with a few exceptions, different neurotransmitters are released by different groups of neurons. These transmitters are often segregated into neuronal systems that subserve broadly different CNS functions. This segregation provides neuroscientists with powerful pharmacologic approaches for analyzing CNS function and treating pathologic conditions. Second, there is a multiplicity of receptors for each neurotransmitter. For example, there are at least 14 different serotonin receptors encoded by different genes. These receptors often have differential cellular distributions throughout the CNS, allowing for the development of drugs that selectively target particular receptors and CNS functions.

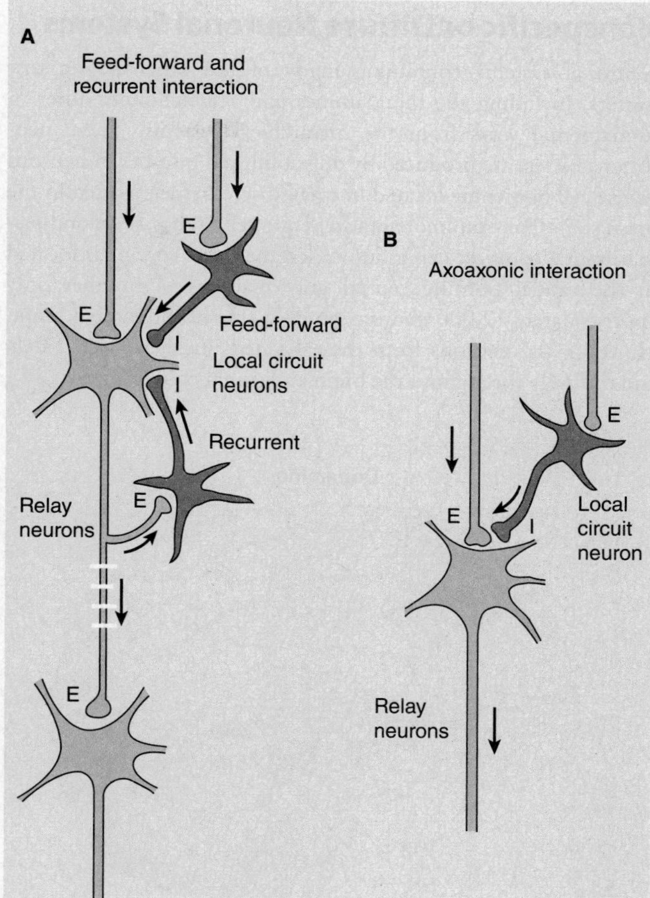

FIGURE 21–5 Hierarchical pathways in the CNS. **A** shows parts of three excitatory relay neurons (blue) and two types of local inhibitory interneuron pathways, recurrent and feed-forward. The inhibitory neurons are shown in gray. **B** shows the pathway responsible for axoaxonic presynaptic inhibition in which the axon of an inhibitory neuron (gray) synapses onto the presynaptic axon terminal of an excitatory fiber (blue) to inhibit its neurotransmitter release.

CELLULAR ORGANIZATION OF THE BRAIN

Most of the neuronal systems in the CNS can be divided into two broad categories: **hierarchical** systems and **nonspecific** or **diffuse** neuronal systems.

Hierarchical Systems

Hierarchical systems include all the pathways directly involved in sensory perception and motor control. These pathways are generally clearly delineated, being composed of large myelinated fibers that can often conduct action potentials at a rate of more than 50 m/s. The information is typically phasic and occurs in bursts of action potentials. In sensory systems, the information is processed sequentially by successive integrations at each relay nucleus on its way to the cortex. A lesion at any link incapacitates the system.

Within each nucleus and in the cortex, there are two types of cells: **relay** or **projection neurons** and **local circuit neurons** (Figure 21–5A). The projection neurons form the interconnecting pathways that transmit signals over long distances. Their cell bodies are relatively large, and their axons can project long distances but also emit small collaterals that synapse onto local interneurons. These neurons are excitatory, and their synaptic influences, which involve ionotropic receptors, are very short-lived. The excitatory transmitter released from these cells is, in most instances, **glutamate.**

Local circuit neurons are typically smaller than projection neurons, and their axons arborize in the immediate vicinity of the cell body. Most of these neurons are inhibitory, and they release either **GABA** or **glycine.** They synapse primarily on the cell body of the projection neurons but can also synapse on the dendrites of projection neurons as well as with each other. Two common types of pathways for these neurons (see Figure 21–5A) include recurrent feedback pathways and feed-forward pathways. A special class of local circuit neurons in the spinal cord forms axoaxonic synapses on the terminals of sensory axons (see Figure 21–5B). Although there are a great variety of synaptic connections in these hierarchical systems, the fact that a limited number of transmitters are used by these neurons indicates that any major pharmacologic manipulation of this system will have a profound effect on the overall excitability of the CNS. For instance, selectively blocking $GABA_A$ receptors with a drug such as picrotoxin results in generalized convulsions. Thus, although the mechanism of action of picrotoxin is specific in blocking the effects of GABA, the overall functional effect appears to be quite nonspecific, because GABA-mediated synaptic inhibition is so widely utilized in the brain.

Nonspecific or Diffuse Neuronal Systems

Neuronal systems containing many of the other neurotransmitters, including the monoamines and acetylcholine, differ in fundamental ways from the hierarchical systems. These neurotransmitters are produced by only a limited number of neurons whose cell bodies are located in small discrete nuclei, often in the brain stem. For example, noradrenergic cell bodies are found primarily in a compact cell group called the locus coeruleus located in the caudal pontine central gray matter and number only approximately 12,000 neurons on each side of the human brain. However, the neurons from these limited nuclei project widely and diffusely throughout the brain and spinal cord (Figure 21–6). Because the axons from these diffusely projecting neurons are fine and unmyelinated, they conduct very slowly, at about 0.5 m/s. The axons branch repeatedly and are extraordinarily divergent. Branches from the same neuron can innervate several functionally different parts of the CNS, synapsing onto and modulating neurons within the hierarchical systems. In the neocortex, these fibers have a tangential organization and therefore can influence large areas of cortex. In addition, most neurotransmitters utilized by diffuse neuronal systems, including norepinephrine, act predominantly on metabotropic receptors and therefore initiate long-lasting synaptic effects. Based on these observations, it is clear that the monoamine systems cannot be conveying topographically specific types of information; rather, vast areas of the CNS

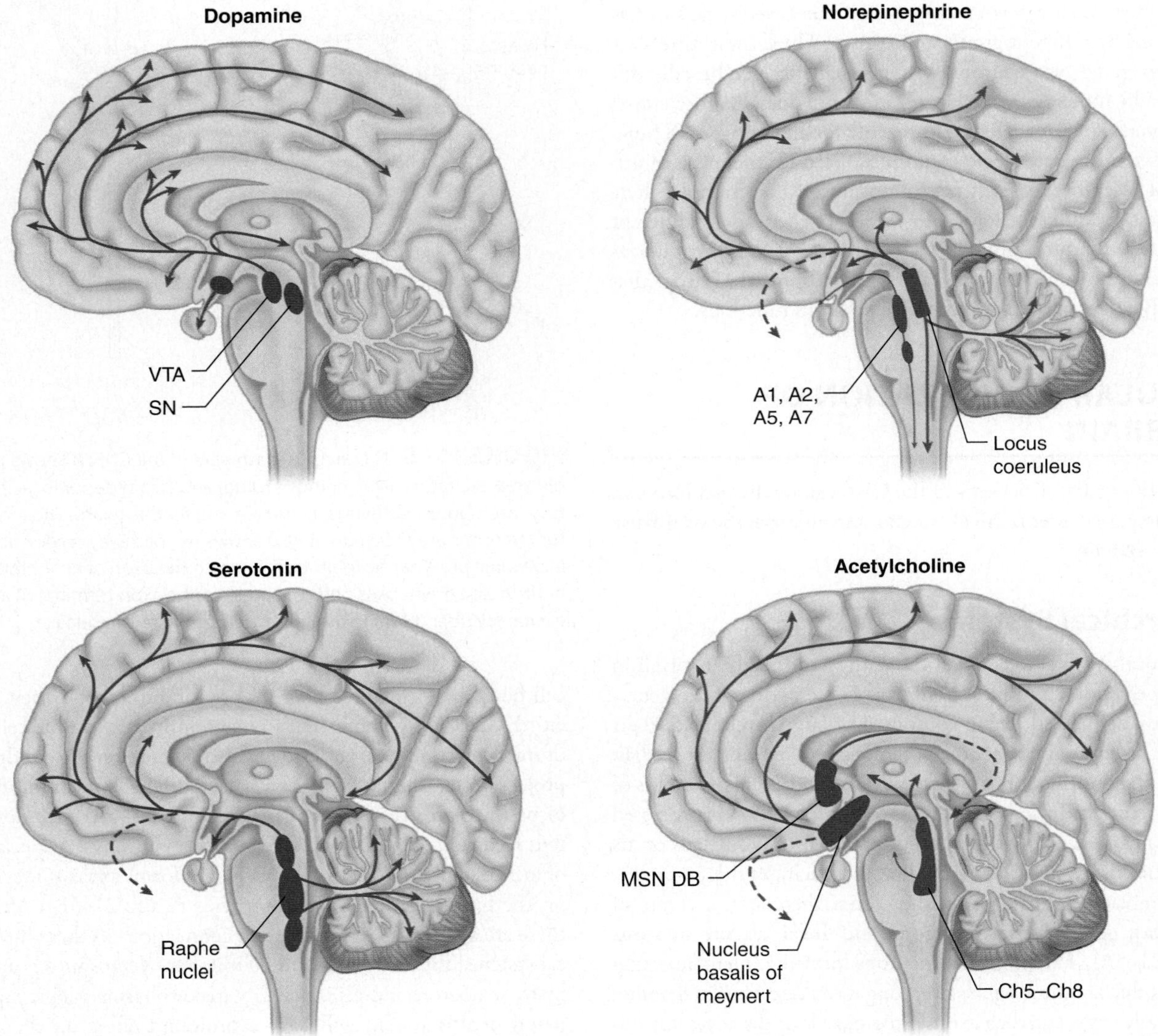

FIGURE 21–6 Diffuse neurotransmitter pathways in the CNS. For each of the neurotransmitter pathways shown, the cell bodies are located in discrete brain stem or basal forebrain nuclei and project widely throughout the CNS. These diffuse systems largely modulate the function of the hierarchical pathways. Serotonin neurons, for example, are found in the midline raphe nuclei in the forebrain and send extraordinarily divergent projections to nearly all regions of the CNS. Other diffusely projecting neurotransmitter pathways include the histamine and orexin systems (not shown). A1–A7, adrenergic brain stem nuclei; Ch5–Ch8, cholinergic brain stem nuclei; DB, diagonal band of Broca; MSN, medial septal nucleus; SN, substantia nigra; VTA, ventral tegmental area.

must be affected simultaneously and in a rather uniform way. It is not surprising, then, that these systems have been implicated in such global functions as sleeping and waking, attention, appetite, and emotional states.

CENTRAL NEUROTRANSMITTERS

Because drug selectivity is based on the fact that different pathways use different transmitters, a primary goal of neuroscience has been to identify the neurotransmitters in CNS pathways. Establishing that a chemical substance is a transmitter has been far more difficult for central synapses than for peripheral synapses. The following criteria were established for transmitter identification.

1. Localization: A suspected transmitter must reside in the presynaptic terminal of the pathway of interest.
2. Release: A suspected transmitter must be released from a neuron in response to neuronal activity and in a calcium-dependent manner.
3. Synaptic Mimicry: Application of the candidate substance should produce a response that mimics the action of the transmitter released by nerve stimulation, and application of a selective antagonist should block the response.

Using the criteria above, studies using a variety of approaches suggest that the agents listed in Table 21–2 are neurotransmitters. A brief summary of some of these compounds follows.

Amino Acid Neurotransmitters

The amino acids of primary interest to the pharmacologist fall into two categories: the acidic amino acid glutamate and the neutral amino acids glycine and GABA. These compounds are present in high concentrations in the CNS and are extremely potent modifiers of neuronal excitability.

A. Glutamate

Excitatory synaptic transmission is mediated by glutamate, which is present in very high concentrations in excitatory synaptic vesicles (~100 mM). Glutamate is released into the synaptic cleft by Ca^{2+}-dependent exocytosis. The released glutamate acts on postsynaptic glutamate receptors and is cleared by glutamate transporters present on surrounding glia (Figure 21–7). In glia, glutamate is converted to glutamine by glutamine synthetase, released from the glia, taken up by the nerve terminal, and converted back to glutamate by the enzyme glutaminase. The high concentration of glutamate in synaptic vesicles is achieved by the **vesicular glutamate transporter (VGLUT).**

Almost all neurons that have been tested are strongly excited by glutamate. This excitation is caused by the activation of both ionotropic and metabotropic receptors, which have been extensively characterized by molecular cloning. The ionotropic receptors are divided into three subtypes based on the action of selective agonists: α-amino-3-hydroxy-5-methylisoxazole-4-propionic acid **(AMPA),** kainic acid **(KA),** and *N*-methyl-D-aspartate **(NMDA).** All the ionotropic receptors are composed of four subunits. AMPA receptors, which are present on all neurons, are heterotetramers assembled from four subunits (GluA1–GluA4). The majority of AMPA receptors contain the GluA2 subunit and are permeable to Na^+ and K^+, but not to Ca^{2+}. Some AMPA receptors, typically present on inhibitory interneurons, lack the GluA2 subunit and are also permeable to Ca^{2+}.

Kainate receptors are not as uniformly distributed as AMPA receptors, being expressed at high levels in the hippocampus, cerebellum, and spinal cord. They are formed from a number of subunit combinations (GluK1–GluK5). Although GluK4 and GluK5 are unable to form channels on their own, their presence in the receptor changes the receptor's affinity and kinetics. Similar to AMPA receptors, kainate receptors are permeable to Na^+ and K^+ and in some subunit combinations can also be permeable to Ca^{2+}. **Domoic acid,** a toxin produced by algae and concentrated in shellfish, is a potent agonist at kainate and AMPA receptors. Consumption of contaminated shellfish has been implicated in illness in animals and humans.

NMDA receptors are as ubiquitous as AMPA receptors, being present on essentially all neurons in the CNS. All NMDA receptors require the presence of the subunit GluN1. The channel also contains one or two GluN2 subunits (GluN2A–GluN2D). Unlike AMPA and kainate receptors, all NMDA receptors are highly permeable to Ca^{2+} as well as to Na^+ and K^+. NMDA receptor function is controlled in a number of intriguing ways. In addition to glutamate binding, the channel also requires the binding of glycine to a separate site in order for the channel to open. However, the regulation and physiologic role of glycine binding remains unclear. Another important feature is that while AMPA and kainate receptor activation results in channel opening at resting membrane potential, NMDA receptor activation does not. This is because, at resting membrane potential, the NMDA receptor pore is blocked by extracellular Mg^{2+}. Only when the neuron is strongly depolarized, as occurs with intense activation of the synapse or by activation of neighboring synapses, is the Mg^{2+} expelled, allowing the channel to open. Thus, there are three requirements for NMDA receptor channel opening: Glutamate and glycine must bind the receptor, and the membrane must be depolarized. The rise in intracellular Ca^{2+} that accompanies NMDA receptor channel opening results in a long-lasting enhancement in synaptic strength that is referred to as **long-term potentiation (LTP).** This enhancement of synaptic strength, which is one major type of synaptic plasticity, can last for many hours or even days and is generally accepted as an important cellular mechanism underlying learning and memory.

The metabotropic glutamate receptors are G protein–coupled receptors that act indirectly on ion channels via G proteins. Metabotropic receptors (mGluR1–mGluR8) have been divided into three groups (I, II, and III). A variety of agonists and antagonists have been developed that interact selectively with the different groups. Group I receptors are typically located postsynaptically and activate phospholipase C, leading to inositol trisphosphate–mediated intracellular Ca^{2+} release. In contrast, group II and group III receptors are typically located on presynaptic nerve terminals and act as inhibitory autoreceptors. Activation of these receptors causes the inhibition of Ca^{2+} channels, resulting in inhibition of transmitter release. These receptors are activated only

TABLE 21–2 Summary of neurotransmitter pharmacology in the central nervous system.

Transmitter	Anatomy	Receptor Subtypes and Preferred Agonists	Receptor Antagonists	Mechanisms
Acetylcholine	Cell bodies at all levels; long and short connections	Muscarinic (M_1): muscarine	Pirenzepine, atropine	Excitatory: ↓ in K^+ conductance; ↑ IP_3, DAG
		Muscarinic (M_2): muscarine, bethanechol	Atropine, methoctramine	Inhibitory: ↓ K^+ conductance; ↑ cAMP
	Motoneuron-Renshaw cell synapse	Nicotinic: nicotine	Dihydro-β-erythroidine, α-bungarotoxin	Excitatory: ↑ cation conductance
Dopamine	Cell bodies at all levels; short, medium, and long connections	D_1: dihydrexidine	Phenothiazines	Inhibitory (?):↑ cAMP
		D_2: bromocriptine	Phenothiazines, butyrophenones	Inhibitory (presynaptic): ↓ Ca^{2+}; Inhibitory (postsynaptic): ↓ in K^+ conductance, ↑ cAMP
GABA	Supraspinal and spinal interneurons involved in pre- and postsynaptic inhibition	$GABA_A$: muscimol	Bicuculline, picrotoxin	Inhibitory: ↑ Cl^- conductance
		$GABA_B$: baclofen	2-OH saclofen	Inhibitory (presynaptic): ↓ Ca^{2+} conductance; Inhibitory (postsynaptic): ↑ K^+ conductance
Glutamate	Relay neurons at all levels and some interneurons	*N*-Methyl-D-aspartate (NMDA): NMDA	2-Amino-5-phosphonovalerate, dizocilpine	Excitatory: ↑ cation conductance, particularly Ca^{2+}
		AMPA: AMPA	NBQX	Excitatory: ↑ cation conductance
		Kainate: kainic acid, domoic acid	ACET	Excitatory: ↑ cation conductance
		Metabotropic: ACPD, quisqualate	MCPG	Inhibitory (presynaptic): ↓ Ca^{2+} conductance, ↓ cAMP; Excitatory: ↓ K^+ conductance, ↑ IP_3, DAG
Glycine	Spinal interneurons and some brain stem interneurons	Taurine, β-alanine	Strychnine	Inhibitory: ↑ Cl^- conductance
5-Hydroxytryptamine (serotonin)	Cell bodies in mid-brain and pons project to all levels	$5\text{-}HT_{1A}$: eptapirone	Metergoline, spiperone	Inhibitory: ↑ K^+ conductance, ↓ cAMP
		$5\text{-}HT_{2A}$: LSD	Ketanserin	Excitatory: ↓ K^+ conductance, ↑ IP_3, DAG
		$5\text{-}HT_3$: 2-methyl-5-HT	Ondansetron	Excitatory: ↑ cation conductance
		$5\text{-}HT_4$: cisapride	Piboserod	Excitatory: ↓ K^+ conductance
Norepinephrine	Cell bodies in pons and brain stem project to all levels	α_1: phenylephrine	Prazosin	Excitatory: ↓ K^+ conductance, ↑ IP_3, DAG
		α_2: clonidine	Yohimbine	Inhibitory (presynaptic): ↓ Ca^{2+} conductance; Inhibitory: ↑ K^+ conductance, ↓ cAMP
		β_1: isoproterenol, dobutamine	Atenolol, practolol	Excitatory: ↓ K^+ conductance, ↑ cAMP
		β_2: albuterol	Butoxamine	Inhibitory: may involve ↑ in electrogenic sodium pump; ↑ cAMP
Histamine	Cells in ventral posterior hypothalamus	H_1: 2(*m*-fluorophenyl)-histamine	Mepyramine	Excitatory: ↓ K^+ conductance, ↑ IP_3, DAG
		H_2: dimaprit	Ranitidine	Excitatory: ↓ K^+ conductance, ↑ cAMP
		H_3: *R*-α-methyl-histamine	Thioperamide	Inhibitory autoreceptors

(continued)

TABLE 21–2 Summary of neurotransmitter pharmacology in the central nervous system. (Continued)

Transmitter	Anatomy	Receptor Subtypes and Preferred Agonists	Receptor Antagonists	Mechanisms
Opioid peptides	Cell bodies at all levels; long and short connections	Mu: β-endorphin	Naloxone	Inhibitory (presynaptic): ↓ Ca^{2+} conductance, ↓ cAMP
		Delta: enkephalin	Naloxone	Inhibitory (postsynaptic): ↑ K^+ conductance, ↓ cAMP
		Kappa: dynorphin, salvinorin A	Naloxone	Inhibitory (postsynaptic): ↑ K^+ conductance, ↓ cAMP
Orexins	Cell bodies in hypothalamus; project widely	OX_1: orexin A	Suvorexant	Excitatory, glutamate co-release
		OX_2: orexins A and B	Suvorexant	
Tachykinins	Primary sensory neurons, cell bodies at all levels; long and short connections	NK1: substance P methylester	Aprepitant	Excitatory: ↓ K^+ conductance, ↑ IP_3, DAG
		NK2: neurokinin A	Saredutant	Excitatory: ↓ K^+ conductance, ↑ IP_3, DAG
		NK3: neurokinin B	Osanetant	Excitatory: ↓ K^+ conductance, ↑ IP_3, DAG
Endocannabinoids	Widely distributed	CB1: anandamide, 2-arachidonyglycerol	Rimonabant	Inhibitory (presynaptic): ↓ Ca^{2+} conductance, ↓ cAMP

Note: Many other central transmitters have been identified (see text).

ACET, (S)-1-(2-amino-2-carboxyethyl)-3-(2-carboxy-5-phenylthiophene-3-yl-methyl)-5-methylpyrimidine-2,4-dione; ACPD, *trans*-1-amino-cyclopentyl-1,3-dicarboxylate; AMPA, DL-α-amino-3-hydroxy-5-methylisoxazole-4-propionate; cAMP, cyclic adenosine monophosphate; DAG, diacylglycerol; IP_3, inositol trisphosphate; LSD, lysergic acid diethylamide; MCPG, α-methyl-4-carboxyphenylglycine; NBQX, 2,3-dihydroxy-6-nitro-7-sulfamoylbenzo(*f*)quinoxaline.

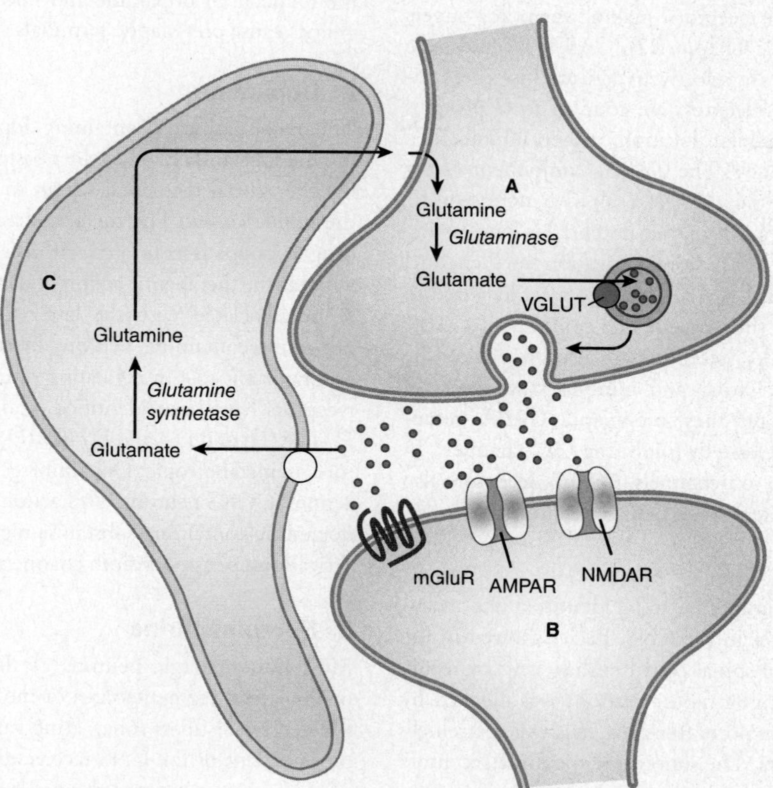

FIGURE 21–7 Schematic diagram of a glutamate synapse. Glutamine is imported into the glutamatergic neuron **(A)** and converted into glutamate by glutaminase. The glutamate is then concentrated in vesicles by the vesicular glutamate transporter (VGLUT). Upon release into the synapse, glutamate can interact with AMPA and NMDA ionotropic receptor channels (AMPAR, NMDAR) and with metabotropic receptors (mGluR) on the postsynaptic cell **(B)**. Synaptic transmission is terminated by active transport of the glutamate into a neighboring glial cell **(C)** by a glutamate transporter. It is converted into glutamine by glutamine synthetase and transported back into the glutamatergic axon terminal.

when the concentration of glutamate rises to high levels during repetitive stimulation of the synapse. Activation of these receptors also causes the inhibition of adenylyl cyclase and decreases cAMP generation.

B. GABA and Glycine

Both GABA and glycine are inhibitory neurotransmitters, which are typically released from local interneurons. Interneurons that release glycine are largely restricted to the spinal cord and brain stem, whereas interneurons releasing GABA are present throughout the CNS, including the spinal cord. Glycine receptors are pentameric structures that are selectively permeable to Cl^-. Strychnine, which is a potent spinal cord convulsant and has been used in some rat poisons, selectively blocks glycine receptors.

GABA receptors are divided into two main types: $GABA_A$ and $GABA_B$. Inhibitory postsynaptic potentials in many areas of the brain have a fast and slow component. The fast component is mediated by $GABA_A$ receptors and the slow component by $GABA_B$ receptors. The difference in kinetics stems from the differences in coupling of the receptors to ion channels. $GABA_A$ receptors are ionotropic receptors and, like glycine receptors, are pentameric structures that are selectively permeable to Cl^-. These receptors are selectively inhibited by picrotoxin and bicuculline, both of which cause generalized convulsions. A great many subunits for $GABA_A$ receptors have been cloned; this accounts for the large diversity in the pharmacology of $GABA_A$ receptors, making them key targets for clinically useful agents (see Chapter 22). $GABA_B$ receptors are metabotropic receptors that are selectively activated by the antispastic drug baclofen. These receptors are coupled to G proteins that, depending on their cellular location, either inhibit Ca^{2+} channels or activate K^+ channels. The $GABA_B$ component of the inhibitory postsynaptic potential is due to a selective increase in K^+ conductance. This inhibitory postsynaptic potential is long-lasting and slow because the coupling of receptor activation to K^+ channel opening is indirect and delayed. $GABA_B$ receptors are localized to the perisynaptic region and thus require the spillover of GABA from the synaptic cleft. $GABA_B$ receptors are also present on the axon terminals of many excitatory and inhibitory synapses. In this case, GABA spills over onto these presynaptic $GABA_B$ receptors, inhibiting transmitter release by inhibiting Ca^{2+} channels. In addition to their coupling to ion channels, $GABA_B$ receptors also inhibit adenylyl cyclase and decrease cAMP generation.

Acetylcholine

Acetylcholine was the first compound to be identified pharmacologically as a neurotransmitter in the CNS. Eccles showed in the early 1950s that excitation of spinal cord Renshaw cells by recurrent axon collaterals from spinal motor neurons was blocked by nicotinic antagonists. Furthermore, Renshaw cells were extremely sensitive to nicotinic agonists. The ionotropic nicotinic receptors in the CNS are composed of subunits entirely distinct from the nicotinic channels at the neuromuscular junction (see Chapter 27) and are widely distributed throughout the brain and spinal cord. However, most CNS responses to acetylcholine are mediated by a large family of G protein–coupled muscarinic receptors. At a few sites, acetylcholine causes slow inhibition of the neuron by activating the M_2 subtype of receptor, which opens potassium channels. A far more widespread muscarinic action in response to acetylcholine is a slow excitation that in some cases is mediated by M_1 receptors. These muscarinic effects are much slower than either nicotinic effects on Renshaw cells or the effect of amino acids. Furthermore, this M_1 muscarinic excitation is unusual in that acetylcholine produces it by *decreasing* the membrane permeability to potassium, ie, the opposite of conventional transmitter action.

Eight major CNS nuclei of acetylcholine neurons have been characterized with diffuse projections. These include neurons in the neostriatum, the medial septal nucleus, and the reticular formation that appear to play an important role in cognitive functions, especially memory. Presenile dementia of the Alzheimer type is reportedly associated with a profound loss of cholinergic neurons.

Monoamine Neurotransmitters

Monoamines include the catecholamines (dopamine and norepinephrine) and 5-hydroxytryptamine. The diamine neurotransmitter, histamine, has several similarities to these monoamines. Although these compounds are present in very small amounts in the CNS, they act widely. These pathways are the site of action of many drugs; for example, the CNS stimulants cocaine and amphetamine appear to act primarily at catecholamine synapses. Cocaine blocks the reuptake of dopamine and norepinephrine, whereas amphetamines cause presynaptic terminals to release these transmitters.

A. Dopamine

The major pathways containing dopamine are the projection linking the substantia nigra to the neostriatum and the projection linking the ventral tegmental region to limbic structures, particularly the limbic cortex. The therapeutic action of the antiparkinsonian drug levodopa is associated with the former area (see Chapter 28), whereas the therapeutic action of the antipsychotic drugs is thought to be associated with the latter (see Chapter 29). In addition, dopamine-containing neurons in the ventral hypothalamus play an important role in regulating pituitary function. Five dopamine receptors have been identified, and they fall into two categories: D_1-like (D_1 and D_5) and D_2-like (D_2, D_3, D_4). All dopamine receptors are metabotropic. Dopamine generally exerts a slow inhibitory action on CNS neurons. This action has been best characterized on dopamine-containing substantia nigra neurons, where D_2-receptor activation opens potassium channels via its G protein.

B. Norepinephrine

Most noradrenergic neurons are located in the locus coeruleus or the lateral tegmental area of the reticular formation. Although the density of fibers innervating various sites differs considerably, most regions of the CNS receive diffuse noradrenergic input. All noradrenergic receptor subtypes are metabotropic. When applied to neurons, norepinephrine can hyperpolarize them by increasing potassium conductance. This effect is mediated by α_2 receptors and has been characterized most thoroughly on locus coeruleus neurons. In many regions of the CNS, norepinephrine actually enhances excitatory inputs by both indirect and direct mechanisms.

The indirect mechanism involves disinhibition; that is, inhibitory local circuit neurons are inhibited. The direct mechanism involves blockade of potassium conductances that slow neuronal discharge. Depending on the type of neuron, this effect is mediated by either α_1 or β receptors. Facilitation of excitatory synaptic transmission is in accordance with many of the behavioral processes thought to involve noradrenergic pathways, eg, attention and arousal.

C. 5-Hydroxytryptamine

Most 5-hydroxytryptamine (5-HT, serotonin) pathways originate from neurons in the midline raphe nuclei of the pons and upper brain stem. 5-HT is contained in unmyelinated fibers that diffusely innervate most regions of the CNS, but the density of the innervation varies. 5-HT acts on more than a dozen receptor subtypes. Except for the 5-HT_3 receptor, all of these receptors are metabotropic. The ionotropic 5-HT_3 receptor exerts a rapid excitatory action at a very limited number of sites in the CNS. In most areas of the CNS, 5-HT has a strong inhibitory action. This action is mediated by 5-HT_{1A} receptors and is associated with membrane hyperpolarization caused by an increase in potassium conductance. It has been found that 5-HT_{1A} receptors and $GABA_B$ receptors activate the same population of potassium channels. Some cell types are slowly excited by 5-HT owing to its blockade of potassium channels via 5-HT_2 or 5-HT_4 receptors. Both excitatory and inhibitory actions can occur on the same neuron. 5-HT has been implicated in the regulation of virtually all brain functions, including perception, mood, anxiety, pain, sleep, appetite, temperature, neuroendocrine control, and aggression. Given the broad roles of 5-HT in CNS function and the rich molecular diversity of 5-HT receptors, it is not surprising that many therapeutic agents target the 5-HT system (see Chapters 16, 29, 30, and 32).

D. Histamine

In the CNS, histamine is exclusively made by neurons in the tuberomammillary nucleus (TMN) in the posterior hypothalamus. These neurons project widely throughout the brain and spinal cord where they modulate arousal, attention, feeding behavior, and memory (see Chapter 16). There are four histamine receptors (H_1 to H_4), all of which are metabotropic. Centrally acting antihistamines are generally used for their sedative properties, and antagonism of H_1 receptors is a common side effect of many drugs including some tricyclic antidepressants and antipsychotics.

Neuropeptides

A great many CNS peptides have been discovered that produce dramatic effects both on animal behavior and on the activity of individual neurons. In many cases, peptide hormones discovered in the periphery (see Chapter 17) also act as neurotransmitters in the CNS. As most of these peptides were initially named based on their peripheral functions, the names are often unrelated to their CNS function. The pathways for many of the peptides have been mapped with immunohistochemical techniques and include opioid peptides (eg, enkephalins, endorphins), neurotensin, substance P, somatostatin, cholecystokinin, vasoactive intestinal polypeptide, neuropeptide Y, and thyrotropin-releasing hormone.

Unlike the classic neurotransmitters above, which are packaged in small synaptic vesicles, neuropeptides are generally packaged in large, dense core vesicles. As in the peripheral autonomic nervous system, peptides often coexist with a conventional nonpeptide transmitter in the same neuron, but the release of the neuropeptides and the small-molecule neurotransmitters can be independently regulated. Released neuropeptides may act locally or may diffuse long distances and bind to distant receptors. Most neuropeptide receptors are metabotropic and, like monoamines, primarily serve modulatory roles in the nervous system. Neuropeptides have been implicated in a wide range of CNS functions including reproduction, social behaviors, appetite, arousal, pain, reward, and learning and memory. Thus, neuropeptides and their receptors are active targets of drug discovery efforts.

A good example of the approaches used to define the role of these peptides in the CNS comes from studies on substance P and its association with sensory fibers. Substance P is contained in and released from small unmyelinated primary sensory neurons in the spinal cord and brain stem and causes a slow excitatory postsynaptic potential in target neurons. These sensory fibers are known to transmit noxious stimuli, and it is therefore surprising that—although substance P receptor antagonists can modify responses to certain types of pain—they do not block the response. Glutamate, which is released with substance P from these synapses, presumably plays an important role in transmitting pain stimuli. Substance P is certainly involved in many other functions because it is found in many areas of the CNS that are unrelated to pain pathways.

Orexin

Orexins are peptide neurotransmitters produced in neurons in the lateral and posterior hypothalamus that, like the monoamine systems, project widely throughout the CNS. Orexins are also called hypocretins due to the near simultaneous discovery by two independent laboratories. Like most neuropeptides, orexin is released from large, dense core vesicles and bind to two G protein–coupled receptors. Orexin neurons also release glutamate and are thus excitatory. The orexin system, like the monoamine systems, projects widely throughout the CNS to influence physiology and behavior. In particular, orexin neurons exhibit firing patterns associated with wakefulness and project to and activate monoamine and acetylcholine neurons involved in sleep-wake cycles (see also Chapter 22). Animals lacking orexin or its receptors have narcolepsy and disrupted sleep-wake patterns. In addition to promoting wakefulness, the orexin system is involved in energy homeostasis, feeding behaviors, autonomic function, and reward.

Other Signaling Substances

A. Endocannabinoids

The primary psychoactive ingredient in cannabis, Δ^9-tetrahydrocannabinol (Δ^9-THC), affects the brain mainly by activating a specific cannabinoid receptor, CB_1. CB_1 receptors are expressed at high levels in many brain regions, and they are primarily located on presynaptic terminals (Figure 21–8). Several endogenous brain lipids, including anandamide and 2-arachidonylglycerol (2-AG), have been identified as CB_1 ligands and are

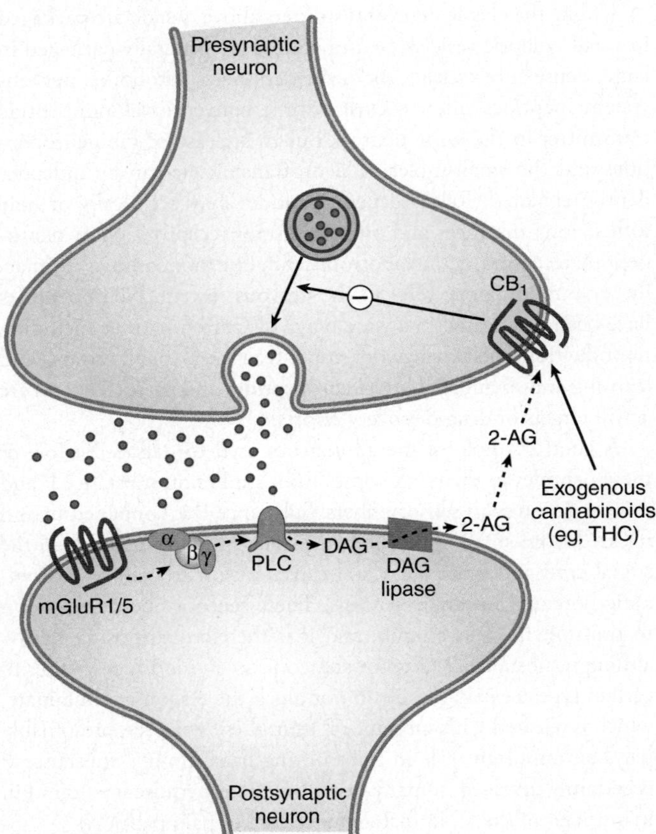

FIGURE 21–8 Endogenous cannabinoid system. Activation of postsynaptic group I metabotropic glutamate receptors (mGluR1/5) leads to the G protein-mediated membrane-delimited activation of phospholipase C (PLC) that produces the second messengers inositol trisphosphate (IP_3, not shown) and diacylglycerol (DAG). DAG can then be converted to the endogenous cannabinoid 2-arachidonoylglycerol (2-AG) by DAG lipase. 2-AG is then released by unknown mechanisms to diffuse across the synaptic cleft where it acts as a full agonist at CB_1 cannabinoid receptors on the presynaptic terminals. Activation of CB_1 receptors by either endocannabinoids or exogenous cannabinoids such as Δ^9-tetrahydrocannabinol (THC) results in the inhibition of presynaptic neurotransmitter release.

called endocannabinoids. These ligands are not stored, as are classic neurotransmitters, but instead are rapidly synthesized by neurons in response to calcium influx or activation of metabotropic receptors (eg, by acetylcholine and glutamate). In further contrast to classic neurotransmitters, endocannabinoids function as retrograde synaptic messengers: they are released from postsynaptic neurons and travel backward across synapses, activating CB_1 receptors on presynaptic neurons and suppressing transmitter release. This suppression can be transient or long lasting, depending on the pattern of activity. Cannabinoids, both endogenous and exogenous, may affect memory, cognition, and pain perception by this mechanism.

B. Nitric Oxide

The CNS contains a substantial amount of nitric oxide synthase (NOS) within certain classes of neurons. This neuronal NOS is an enzyme activated by calcium-calmodulin, and activation of NMDA receptors, which increases intracellular calcium, results in the generation of nitric oxide. Although a physiologic role for nitric oxide has been clearly established for vascular smooth muscle, its role in synaptic transmission and synaptic plasticity remains controversial. Nitric oxide diffuses freely across membranes and thus has been hypothesized to be a retrograde messenger, although this has not been demonstrated conclusively. Perhaps the strongest case for a role of nitric oxide in neuronal signaling in the CNS is for long-term depression of synaptic transmission in the cerebellum.

C. Purines

Receptors for purines, particularly adenosine, ATP, UTP, and UDP, are found throughout the body, including the CNS. High concentrations of ATP are found in and released from catecholaminergic synaptic vesicles, and ATP may be released by astrocytes to modulate neuronal function. ATP binds to two classes of receptors. The P2X family of ATP receptors includes nonselective ligand-gated cation channels, whereas the P2Y family is metabotropic. The physiologic roles for ATP release in the CNS are poorly understood, but pharmacologic studies suggest these receptors are involved in memory, wakefulness, and appetite and may play roles in multiple neuropsychiatric disorders.

Extracellular ATP also gets converted to adenosine by nucleotidases. Adenosine in the CNS acts on metabotropic A_1 and A_{2A} adenosine receptors. Presynaptic A_1 receptors inhibit calcium channels and inhibit release of both amino acid and monoamine transmitters. Postsynaptic A_{2A} receptors increase cAMP production and have a mildly excitatory effect on neurons. Increasing levels of extracellular adenosine in the CNS promote drowsiness and sleep, largely through A_{2A} receptors. Caffeine, as a nonselective antagonist at adenosine receptors, promotes wakefulness in part (see Chapter 20) through blocking the action of adenosine on A_{2A} receptors.

REFERENCES

Allen NJ: Astrocyte regulation of synaptic behavior. Annu Rev Cell Dev Biol 2014;30:439.

Berger M et al: The expanded biology of serotonin. Annu Rev Med 2009;60:355.

Castillo PE et al: Endocannabinoid signaling and synaptic function. Neuron 2012;76:70.

Catterall WA: Voltage-gated sodium channels at 60: Structure, function and pathophysiology. J Physiol 2012;590:2577.

Daneman R, Prat A: The blood-brain barrier. Cold Spring Harb Perspect Biol 2015;7:a020412.

Gotter AL et al: International Union of Basic and Clinical Pharmacology. LXXXVI. Orexin receptor function, nomenclature and pharmacology. Pharmacol Rev 2012;64:389.

Hansen KB et al: Structure, function, and pharmacology of glutamate receptor ion channels. Pharmacol Rev 2021;73:298.

Jan LY, Jan YN: Voltage-gated potassium channels and the diversity of electrical signalling. J Physiol 2012;590:2591.

Lewis RJ et al: Conus venom peptide pharmacology. Pharmacol Rev 2012;64:259.

Mody I, Pearce RA: Diversity of inhibitory neurotransmission through GABA(A) receptors. Trends Neurosci 2004;27:569.

Südhof TC, Rizo J: Synaptic vesicle exocytosis. Cold Spring Harb Perspect Biol 2011;3:a005637.

Zamponi GW et al: The physiology, pathology, and pharmacology of voltage-gated calcium channels and their future therapeutic potential. Pharmacol Rev 2015;67:821.

CHAPTER

22

Sedative-Hypnotic Drugs

Todd W. Vanderah, PhD*

CASE STUDY

At her annual physical examination, a 53-year-old middle school teacher complains that she has been having difficulty falling asleep, and after falling asleep, she awakens several times during the night. These episodes now occur almost nightly and are interfering with her ability to teach. She has tried various over-the-counter sleep remedies, but they were of little help and she experienced "hangover" effects on the day following their use. Her general health is good, she is not overweight, and she takes no prescription drugs. She drinks decaffeinated coffee but only one cup in the morning; however, she drinks as many as six cans per day of diet cola. She drinks a glass of wine with her evening meal but does not like stronger spirits. What other aspects of this patient's history would you like to know? What therapeutic measures are appropriate for this patient? What drug, or drugs, (if any) would you prescribe?

Assignment of a drug to the sedative-hypnotic class indicates that it is able to **relieve anxiety** (sedation) or to **encourage sleep** (hypnosis). This drug classification is based on clinical uses rather than on similarities in chemical structure. Anxiety states and sleep disorders are common problems, and sedative-hypnotics are widely prescribed drugs worldwide.

■ BASIC PHARMACOLOGY OF SEDATIVE-HYPNOTICS

An effective **sedative** (anxiolytic) agent should reduce anxiety and exert a calming effect. The degree of central nervous system (CNS) depression caused by a sedative should be the minimum consistent with therapeutic efficacy. A **hypnotic** drug should produce drowsiness and encourage the onset and maintenance of a state of sleep. Hypnotic effects involve more pronounced depression of the CNS than sedation, and this can be achieved with many drugs in this class simply by increasing the dose. Graded dose-dependent depression of CNS function is a characteristic of most sedative-hypnotics. However, individual drugs differ in the relationship between the dose and the degree of CNS depression. Two examples of such dose-response relationships are shown in Figure 22–1. The linear slope for drug A is typical of many of the older sedative-hypnotics, including the barbiturates and alcohols. With such drugs, an increase in dose higher than that needed for hypnosis may lead to a state of general anesthesia. At still higher doses, these sedative-hypnotics may depress respiratory and vasomotor centers in the medulla, leading to coma and death. Deviations from a linear dose-response relationship, as shown for drug B, require proportionately greater dosage increments to achieve CNS depression more profound than hypnosis. This appears to be the case for benzodiazepines and for certain newer hypnotics that have a similar mechanism of action.

CHEMICAL CLASSIFICATION

The **benzodiazepines** are widely used sedative-hypnotics. All of the structures shown in Figure 22–2 are 1,4-benzodiazepines, and most contain a carboxamide group in the seven-membered heterocyclic ring structure. A substituent in the 7 position, such as a halogen or a nitro group, is required for sedative-hypnotic activity.

*The author thanks Anthony J Trevor, PhD, the previous author of this chapter, for his contributions.

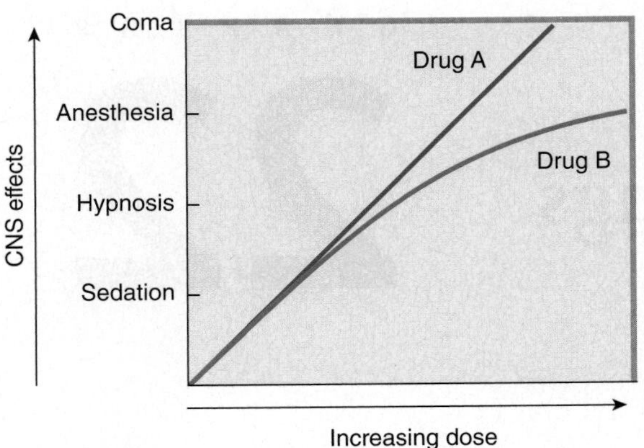

FIGURE 22–1 Dose-response curves for two hypothetical sedative-hypnotics.

The structures of triazolam and alprazolam include the addition of a triazole ring at the 1,2 position.

The chemical structures of some older and less commonly used sedative-hypnotics, including several **barbiturates,** are shown in Figure 22–3. Glutethimide and meprobamate are of distinctive chemical structure but are practically equivalent to barbiturates in their pharmacologic effects. They are rarely used. The sedative-hypnotic class also includes compounds of simpler chemical structure, including **ethanol** (see Chapter 23) and **chloral hydrate.**

Several drugs with novel chemical structures have been introduced more recently for use in sleep disorders. **Zolpidem,** an imidazopyridine; **zaleplon,** a pyrazolopyrimidine; and **eszopiclone,** a cyclopyrrolone (Figure 22–4), although structurally unrelated to benzodiazepines, share a similar mechanism of action, as

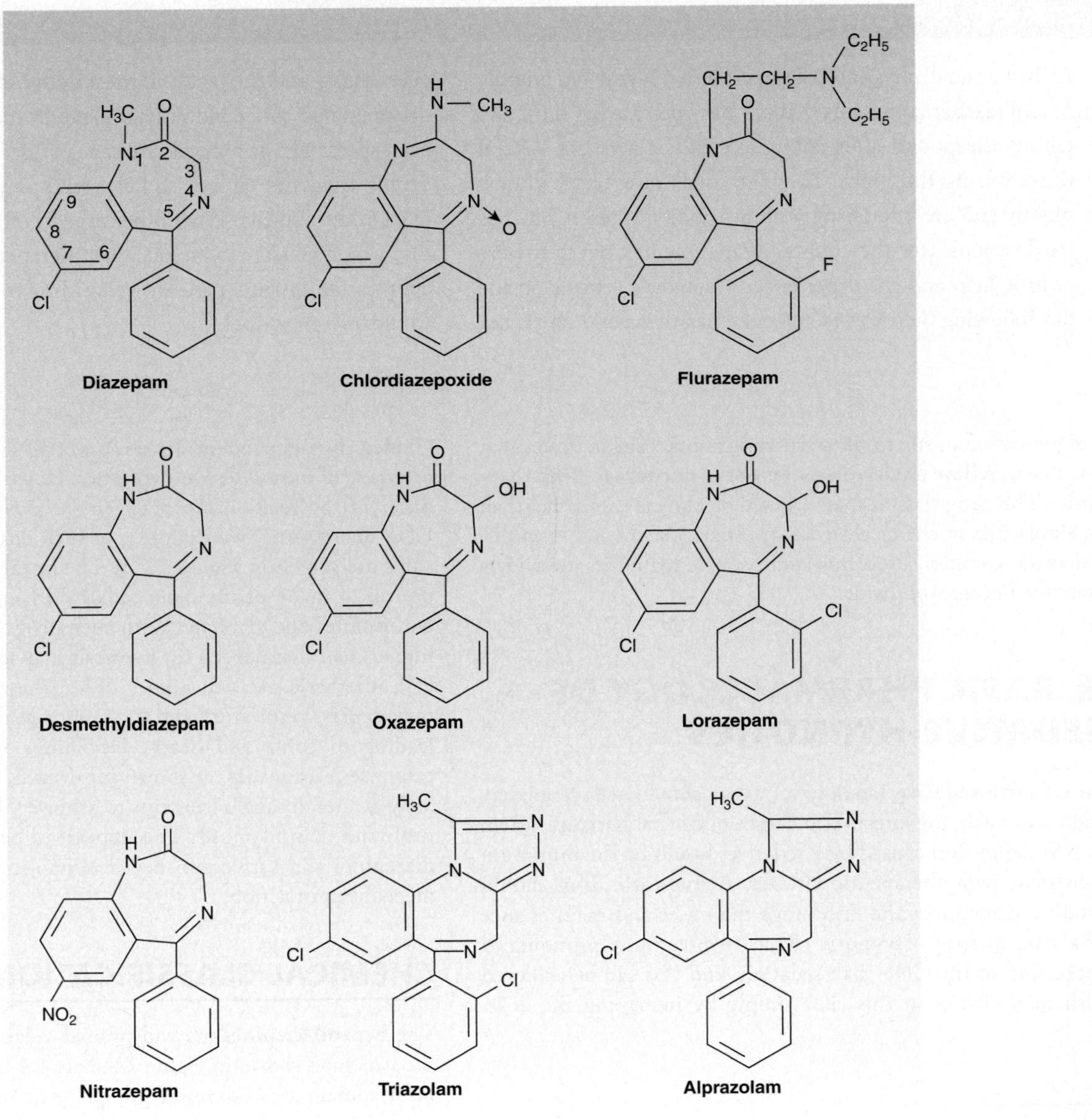

Diazepam | Chlordiazepoxide | Flurazepam

Desmethyldiazepam | Oxazepam | Lorazepam

Nitrazepam | Triazolam | Alprazolam

FIGURE 22–2 Chemical structures of some benzodiazepines.

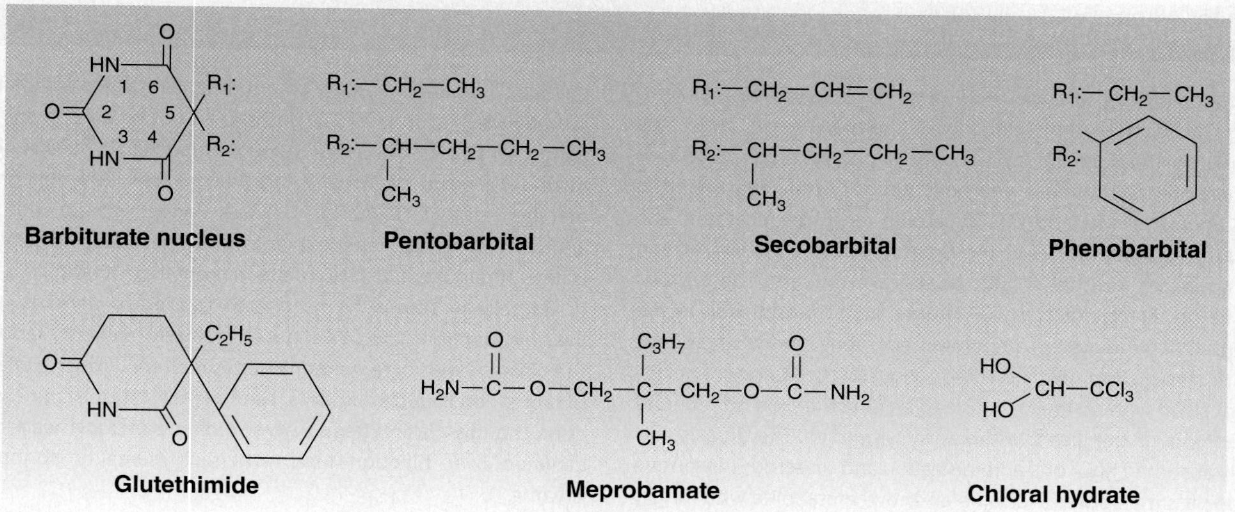

FIGURE 22–3 Chemical structures of some barbiturates and other sedative-hypnotics.

described below. Eszopiclone is the (*S*) enantiomer of zopiclone, a hypnotic drug that has been available outside the United States since 1989. **Ramelteon** and **tasimelteon,** melatonin receptor agonists, are newer hypnotic drugs (see Box: Ramelteon and Tasimelteon). **Suvorexant** and **lemborexant** are orexin antagonists that improve sleep duration. **Buspirone** is a slow-onset anxiolytic agent whose actions are quite different from those of conventional sedative-hypnotics (see Box: Buspirone).

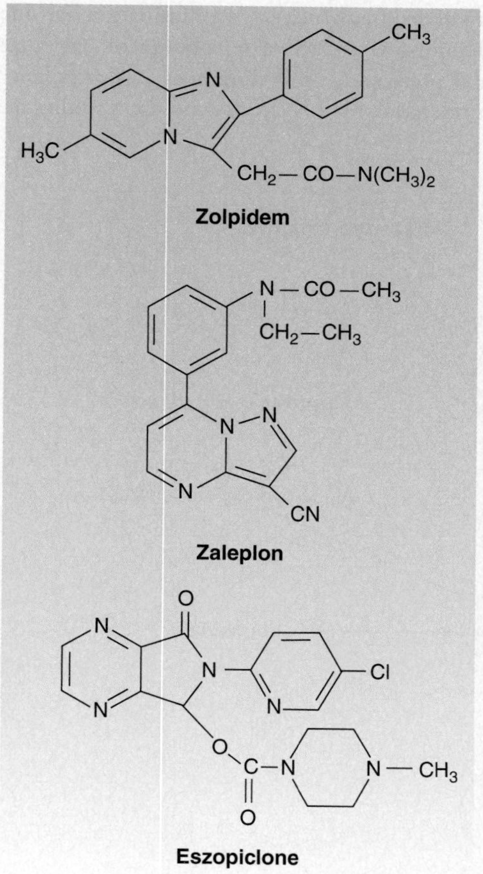

FIGURE 22–4 Chemical structures of newer hypnotics.

Other classes of drugs that exert sedative effects include antipsychotics (see Chapter 29) and many antidepressant drugs (see Chapter 30). The latter are currently used widely in management of chronic anxiety disorders. Certain antihistaminic agents including diphenhydramine, doxylamine, hydroxyzine, and promethazine (see Chapter 16) also are sedating. These agents commonly exert marked effects on the peripheral autonomic nervous system. Diphenhydramine and doxylamine are available in over-the-counter sleep aids.

Pharmacokinetics

A. Absorption and Distribution

The rates of oral absorption of sedative-hypnotics differ depending on a number of factors, including lipophilicity. For example, the absorption of triazolam is extremely rapid, and that of diazepam and the active metabolite of clorazepate is more rapid than other commonly used benzodiazepines. Clorazepate, a prodrug, is converted to its active form, desmethyldiazepam (nordiazepam), by acid hydrolysis in the stomach. Most of the barbiturates and other older sedative-hypnotics, as well as the newer hypnotics (eszopiclone, zaleplon, zolpidem, suvorexant), are absorbed rapidly into the blood following oral administration.

Lipid solubility plays a major role in determining the rate at which a particular sedative-hypnotic enters the CNS. This property is responsible for the rapid onset of the effects of triazolam, thiopental (see Chapter 25), and the newer hypnotics.

All sedative-hypnotics cross the placental barrier during pregnancy. If sedative-hypnotics are given during the predelivery period, they may contribute to the depression of neonatal vital functions. Sedative-hypnotics are also detectable in breast milk and may exert depressant effects in the nursing infant.

Ramelteon and Tasimelteon

Melatonin receptors are thought to be involved in maintaining circadian rhythms underlying the sleep-wake cycle (see Chapter 16). Ramelteon, a novel hypnotic drug prescribed specifically for patients who have difficulty in falling asleep, is an agonist at MT_1 and MT_2 melatonin receptors located in the suprachiasmatic nuclei of the brain. Tasimelteon is similar and is approved for non-24-hour sleep-wake disorder. These drugs have no direct effects on GABAergic neurotransmission in the central nervous system. In polysomnography studies of patients with chronic insomnia, ramelteon reduced the latency of persistent sleep with no effects on sleep architecture and no rebound insomnia or significant withdrawal symptoms. The drug is rapidly absorbed after oral administration and undergoes extensive first-pass metabolism, forming an active metabolite with longer half-life (2–5 hours) than the parent drug. Ramelteon is metabolized by CYP1A2 and CYP2C9 and should not be used in combination with inhibitors of CYP1A2 (eg, ciprofloxacin, fluvoxamine, tacrine, zileuton) or CYP2C9 (eg, fluconazole). Tasimelteon is metabolized by CYP1A2 and CYP3A4. Concurrent use with the antidepressant fluvoxamine increases the peak plasma concentration of ramelteon and tasimelteon more than 50-fold!

Ramelteon should be used with caution in patients with liver dysfunction. The CYP inducer rifampin markedly reduces the plasma levels of ramelteon and tasimelteon. Adverse effects of ramelteon include dizziness, somnolence, fatigue, and endocrine changes. Tasimelteon's adverse effects include headache, elevated liver function tests, and nightmares or abnormal dreams.

B. Biotransformation

Metabolic transformation to more water-soluble metabolites is necessary for clearance of sedative-hypnotics from the body. The microsomal drug-metabolizing enzyme systems of the liver are most important in this regard, so elimination half-life of these drugs depends mainly on the rate of their metabolic transformation.

1. *Benzodiazepines*—Hepatic metabolism accounts for the clearance of all benzodiazepines. The patterns and rates of metabolism depend on the individual drugs. Most benzodiazepines undergo microsomal oxidation (phase I reactions), including *N*-dealkylation and aliphatic hydroxylation catalyzed by cytochrome P450 isozymes, especially CYP3A4. The metabolites are subsequently conjugated (phase II reactions) to form glucuronides that are excreted in the urine. However, many phase I metabolites of benzodiazepines are pharmacologically active, some with long half-lives (Figure 22–5). For example, desmethyldiazepam, which has an elimination half-life of more than 40 hours, is an active metabolite of chlordiazepoxide, diazepam, prazepam, and clorazepate. Alprazolam and triazolam undergo α-hydroxylation, and the resulting metabolites

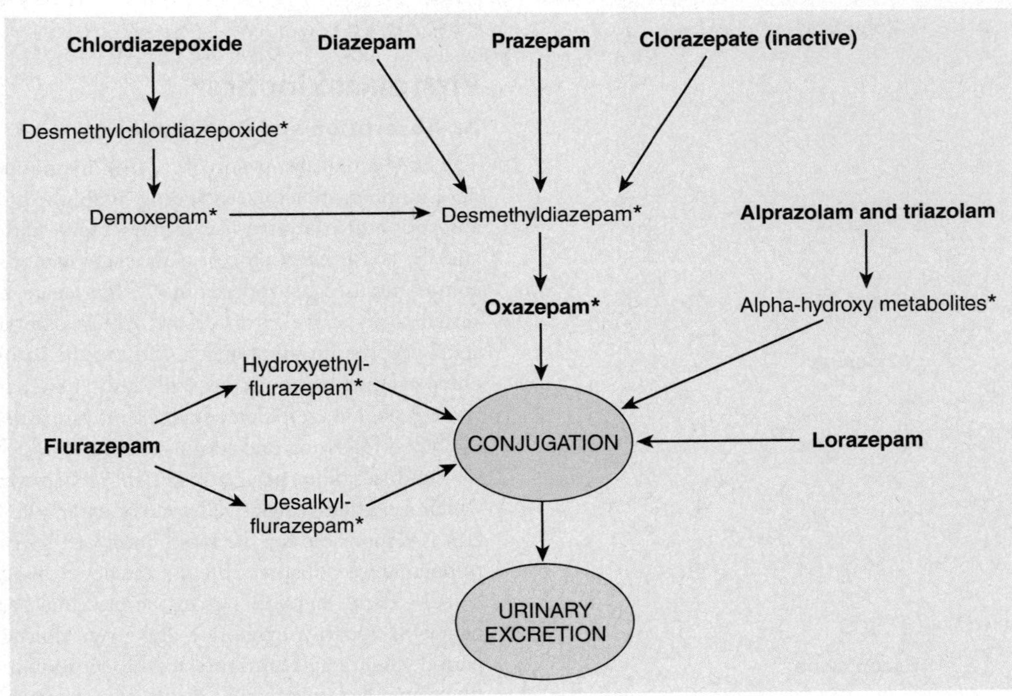

FIGURE 22–5 Biotransformation of benzodiazepines. Boldface, drugs available for clinical use in various countries; *, active metabolite.

appear to exert short-lived pharmacologic effects because they are rapidly conjugated to form inactive glucuronides. The short elimination half-life of triazolam (2–3 hours) favors its use as a hypnotic rather than as a sedative drug.

The formation of active metabolites has complicated studies on the pharmacokinetics of the benzodiazepines in humans because the elimination half-life of the parent drug may have little relation to the time course of pharmacologic effects. Benzodiazepines for which the parent drug or active metabolites have long half-lives are more likely to cause cumulative effects with multiple doses. Cumulative and residual effects such as excessive drowsiness appear to be less of a problem with such drugs as estazolam, oxazepam, and lorazepam, which have relatively short half-lives and are metabolized directly to inactive glucuronides. Some pharmacokinetic properties of selected benzodiazepines and newer hypnotics are listed in Table 22–1. The metabolism of several commonly used benzodiazepines including diazepam, midazolam, and triazolam is affected by inhibitors and inducers of hepatic P450 isozymes (see Chapter 4).

2. *Barbiturates*—With the exception of phenobarbital, only insignificant quantities of the barbiturates are excreted unchanged. The major metabolic pathways involve oxidation by hepatic enzymes to form alcohols, acids, and ketones, which appear in the urine as glucuronide conjugates. The overall rate of hepatic metabolism in humans depends on the individual drug but (with the exception of the thiobarbiturates) is usually slow. The elimination half-lives of secobarbital and pentobarbital range from 18 to 48 hours in different individuals. The elimination half-life of phenobarbital in humans is 4–5 days. Multiple dosing with these agents can lead to cumulative effects.

Buspirone

Buspirone has selective anxiolytic effects, and its pharmacologic characteristics are different from those of other drugs described in this chapter. Buspirone relieves anxiety without causing marked sedative, hypnotic, or euphoric effects. Unlike benzodiazepines, the drug has no anticonvulsant or muscle relaxant properties. Buspirone does not interact directly with GABAergic systems. It may exert its anxiolytic effects by acting as a partial agonist at brain 5-HT_{1A} receptors, but it also has affinity for brain dopamine D_2 receptors. Buspirone-treated patients show no rebound anxiety or withdrawal signs on abrupt discontinuance. The drug is not effective in blocking the acute withdrawal syndrome resulting from abrupt cessation of use of benzodiazepines or other sedative-hypnotics. Buspirone has minimal abuse liability. In marked contrast to the benzodiazepines, the anxiolytic effects of buspirone may take 3–4 weeks to become established, making the drug unsuitable for management of acute anxiety states. The drug is used in generalized anxiety states but is less effective in panic disorders.

Buspirone is rapidly absorbed orally but undergoes extensive first-pass metabolism via hydroxylation and dealkylation reactions to form several active metabolites. The major metabolite is 1-(2-pyrimidyl)-piperazine (1-PP), which has α_2-adrenoceptor-blocking actions and which enters the central nervous system to reach higher levels than the parent drug. It is not known what role (if any) 1-PP plays in the central actions of buspirone. The elimination half-life of buspirone is 2–4 hours, and liver dysfunction may slow its clearance. Rifampin, an inducer of cytochrome P450, decreases the half-life of buspirone; inhibitors of CYP3A4 (eg, erythromycin, ketoconazole, grapefruit juice, nefazodone) can markedly increase its plasma levels.

Buspirone causes less psychomotor impairment than benzodiazepines and does not affect driving skills. The drug does not potentiate effects of conventional sedative-hypnotic drugs, ethanol, or tricyclic antidepressants; and elderly patients do not appear to be more sensitive to its actions. Nonspecific chest pain, tachycardia, palpitations, dizziness, nervousness, headache, tinnitus, gastrointestinal distress, and paresthesias and a dose-dependent pupillary constriction may occur. Blood pressure may be significantly elevated in patients receiving monoamine oxidase (MAO) inhibitors. Buspirone is a US Food and Drug Administration (FDA) category B drug in terms of its use in pregnancy.

3. *Newer hypnotics*—After oral administration of the standard formulation, zolpidem reaches peak plasma levels in 1–3 hours (Table 22–1). Sublingual and oral spray formulations of zolpidem are also available. Zolpidem is rapidly metabolized to inactive metabolites via oxidation and hydroxylation by hepatic CYP3A4. The elimination half-life of the drug is greater in women and is increased significantly in the elderly. A biphasic extended-release formulation extends plasma levels by approximately 2 hours. Zaleplon is metabolized to inactive metabolites mainly by hepatic aldehyde oxidase and partly by the cytochrome P450 isoform CYP3A4 followed by glucuronidation and eliminated in the urine. Dosage should be reduced in patients with hepatic impairment and in the elderly. Cimetidine, which inhibits both aldehyde oxidase and CYP3A4, markedly increases the peak plasma level of zaleplon. Eszopiclone is metabolized by hepatic cytochromes P450 (especially CYP3A4) to form the inactive *N*-oxide derivative and weakly active desmethyleszopiclone. The elimination half-life of eszopiclone is prolonged in the elderly and in the presence of inhibitors of CYP3A4 (eg, ketoconazole). Inducers of CYP3A4 (eg, rifampin) increase the hepatic metabolism of eszopiclone. The new hypnotic orexin receptor antagonists suvorexant and lemborexant

TABLE 22–1 Pharmacokinetic properties of some benzodiazepines and newer hypnotics in humans.

Drug	Tmax (hours)[1]	$t_{1/2}$ (hours)[2]	Comments
Alprazolam	1–2	12–15	Rapid oral absorption
Chlordiazepoxide	2–4	15–40	Active metabolites; erratic bioavailability from IM injection
Clorazepate	1–2 (nordiazepam)	50–100	Prodrug; hydrolyzed to active form in stomach
Diazepam	1–2	20–80	Active metabolites; erratic bioavailability from IM injection
Estazolam	1–6	10–24	Rapid oral absorption, active metabolites
Eszopiclone	1	6	Minor active metabolites
Flurazepam	1–2	40–100	Active metabolites with long half-lives
Lorazepam	1–6	10–20	No active metabolites
Midazolam	<1	1–3	Rapid onset; short duration of cation
Oxazepam	2–4	10–20	No active metabolites
Suvorexant	2–3	8–20	No active metabolites
Temazepam	2–3	10–40	Slow oral absorption
Triazolam	1	2–3	Rapid onset; short duration of action
Zaleplon	<1	1–2	Metabolized via aldehyde oxidase
Zolpidem	1–3	1.5–3.5	No active metabolites

[1]Time to peak blood level.

[2]Includes half-lives of major metabolites.

are well absorbed orally and metabolized by CYP3A4, and their half-lives are prolonged by inhibitors of CYP3A4 including azole antifungal drugs, clarithromycin, and verapamil.

C. Excretion

The water-soluble metabolites of sedative-hypnotics, formed mostly via the phase II conjugation of phase I metabolites, are excreted mainly via the kidney. In most cases, changes in renal function do not have a marked effect on the elimination of parent drugs. Phenobarbital is excreted unchanged in the urine to a certain extent (20–30% in humans), and its elimination rate can be increased significantly by alkalinization of the urine. This is partly due to increased ionization at alkaline pH, since phenobarbital is a weak acid with a pK_a of 7.4. Suvorexant is mainly excreted in the feces, with a smaller amount eliminated in urine.

D. Factors Affecting Biodisposition

The biodisposition of sedative-hypnotics can be influenced by several factors, particularly alterations in hepatic function resulting from disease or drug-induced increases or decreases in microsomal enzyme activities (see Chapter 4).

In very old patients and in patients with severe liver disease, the elimination half-lives of these drugs are often increased significantly. In such cases, multiple normal doses of these sedative-hypnotics can result in excessive CNS effects.

The activity of hepatic microsomal drug-metabolizing enzymes may be increased in patients exposed to certain older sedative-hypnotics on a long-term basis (enzyme induction; see Chapter 4). Barbiturates (especially phenobarbital) and meprobamate are most likely to cause this effect, which may result in an increase in their hepatic metabolism as well as that of other drugs. Increased biotransformation of other pharmacologic agents as a result of enzyme induction by barbiturates is a potential mechanism underlying drug interactions (see Chapter 67). In contrast, benzodiazepines and the newer hypnotics do not change hepatic drug-metabolizing enzyme activity with continuous use.

Pharmacodynamics of Benzodiazepines, Barbiturates, & Newer Hypnotics

A. Molecular Pharmacology of the $GABA_A$ Receptor

The benzodiazepines, the barbiturates, zolpidem, zaleplon, eszopiclone, and many other drugs bind to molecular components of the $GABA_A$ receptor in neuronal membranes in the CNS. This receptor, which functions as a chloride ion channel, is activated by the inhibitory neurotransmitter GABA (see Chapter 21).

The $GABA_A$ receptor has a pentameric structure assembled from five subunits (each with four membrane-spanning domains) selected from multiple polypeptide classes (α, β, γ, δ, ε, π, ρ, etc). Multiple subunits of several of these classes have been characterized, eg, six different α, four β, and three γ. A model of the $GABA_A$ receptor–chloride ion channel macromolecular complex is shown in Figure 22–6.

A major isoform of the $GABA_A$ receptor that is found in many regions of the brain consists of two α1 subunits, two β2 subunits, and one γ2 subunit. In this isoform, the two binding sites for GABA are located between adjacent α1 and β2 subunits, and the binding pocket for benzodiazepines (the **BZ site** of the $GABA_A$ receptor) is between an α1 and the γ2 subunit. However, $GABA_A$ receptors in different areas of the CNS consist of various combinations of the essential subunits, and the benzodiazepines bind to many of these, including receptor isoforms containing α2, α3,

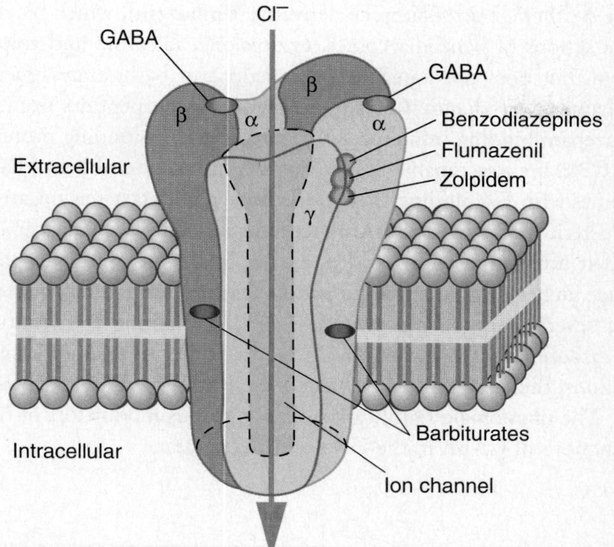

FIGURE 22–6 A model of the $GABA_A$ receptor–chloride ion channel macromolecular complex. A hetero-oligomeric glycoprotein, the complex consists of five or more membrane-spanning subunits. Multiple forms of α, β, and γ subunits are arranged in different pentameric combinations so that $GABA_A$ receptors exhibit molecular heterogeneity. GABA appears to interact at two sites between α and β subunits triggering chloride channel opening with resulting membrane hyperpolarization. Binding of benzodiazepines and the newer hypnotic drugs such as zolpidem occurs at a single site between α and γ subunits, facilitating the process of chloride ion channel opening. The benzodiazepine antagonist flumazenil also binds at this site and can reverse the hypnotic effects of zolpidem. Note that these binding sites are distinct from those of the barbiturates. (See also text and Box: The Versatility of the Chloride Channel GABA Receptor Complex.)

and α5 subunits. Barbiturates also bind to multiple isoforms of the $GABA_A$ receptor but at different sites from those with which benzodiazepines interact. In contrast to benzodiazepines, zolpidem, zaleplon, and eszopiclone bind more selectively because these drugs interact only with $GABA_A$-receptor isoforms that contain α1 subunits. The heterogeneity of $GABA_A$ receptors may constitute the molecular basis for the varied pharmacologic actions of benzodiazepines and related drugs (see Box: GABA Receptor Heterogeneity & Pharmacologic Selectivity).

In contrast to GABA itself, benzodiazepines and other sedative-hypnotics have a low affinity for $GABA_B$ receptors, which are activated by the spasmolytic drug baclofen (see Chapters 21 and 27).

B. Neuropharmacology

GABA (γ-aminobutyric acid) is a major inhibitory neurotransmitter in the CNS (see Chapter 21). Electrophysiologic studies have shown that benzodiazepines potentiate GABAergic inhibition at all levels of the neuraxis, including the spinal cord, hypothalamus, hippocampus, substantia nigra, cerebellar cortex, and cerebral cortex. Benzodiazepines appear to increase the efficiency of GABAergic synaptic inhibition. The benzodiazepines do not substitute for GABA but appear to enhance GABA's effects allosterically without directly activating $GABA_A$ receptors or opening the associated chloride channels. The enhancement in chloride ion conductance induced by the interaction of benzodiazepines with GABA takes the form of an increase in the *frequency* of channel-opening events.

Barbiturates also facilitate the actions of GABA at multiple sites in the CNS, but—in contrast to benzodiazepines—they appear to increase the *duration* of the GABA-gated chloride channel openings. Unlike benzodiazepines, at high concentrations, the barbiturates may also be GABA-mimetic, directly activating chloride channels. These effects involve a binding site or sites distinct from the benzodiazepine binding sites. Barbiturates are less selective in their actions than benzodiazepines, because they also depress the actions of the excitatory neurotransmitter glutamic acid via binding to the AMPA receptor. Barbiturates also exert nonsynaptic membrane effects in parallel with their effects on GABA and glutamate neurotransmission. This multiplicity of sites of action of barbiturates may be the basis for their ability to induce full surgical anesthesia (see Chapter 25) and for their more pronounced central depressant effects (which result in their low margin of safety) compared with benzodiazepines and the newer hypnotics.

GABA Receptor Heterogeneity & Pharmacologic Selectivity

Studies involving genetically engineered ("knockout") rodents have demonstrated that the specific pharmacologic actions elicited by benzodiazepines and other drugs that modulate GABA actions are influenced by the composition of the subunits assembled to form the $GABA_A$ receptor. Benzodiazepines interact primarily with brain $GABA_A$ receptors in which the α subunits (1, 2, 3, and 5) have a conserved histidine residue in the N-terminal domain. Strains of mice, in which a point mutation has been inserted converting histidine to arginine in the α1 subunit, show resistance to both the sedative and amnestic effects of benzodiazepines, but anxiolytic and muscle-relaxing effects are largely unchanged. These animals are also unresponsive to the hypnotic actions of zolpidem and zaleplon, drugs that bind selectively to $GABA_A$ receptors containing α1 subunits. In contrast, mice with selective histidine-arginine mutations in the α2 or α3 subunits of $GABA_A$ receptors show selective resistance to the antianxiety effects of benzodiazepines. Based on studies of this type, it has been suggested that α1 subunits in $GABA_A$ receptors mediate sedation, amnesia, and ataxic effects of benzodiazepines, whereas α2 and α3 subunits are involved in their anxiolytic and muscle-relaxing actions. Other mutation studies have led to suggestions that an α5 subtype is involved in at least some of the memory impairment caused by benzodiazepines. It should be emphasized that these studies involving genetic manipulations of the $GABA_A$ receptor utilize rodent models of the anxiolytic and amnestic actions of drugs.

C. Benzodiazepine Binding Site Ligands

The components of the $GABA_A$ receptor-chloride ion channel macromolecule that function as benzodiazepine binding sites exhibit heterogeneity (see Box: The Versatility of the Chloride Channel GABA Receptor Complex). Three types of ligand-benzodiazepine receptor interactions have been reported: (1) **Agonists** facilitate GABA actions, and this occurs at multiple BZ binding sites in the case of the benzodiazepines. As noted above, the nonbenzodiazepines zolpidem, zaleplon, and eszopiclone are selective agonists at the BZ sites that contain an α1 subunit. Endogenous agonist ligands for the BZ binding sites have been proposed, because benzodiazepine-like chemicals have been isolated from brain tissue of animals never exposed to these drugs. Nonbenzodiazepine molecules that have affinity for BZ sites on the $GABA_A$ receptor have also been detected in human brain. (2) **Antagonists** are typified by the synthetic benzodiazepine derivative **flumazenil,** which blocks the actions of benzodiazepines, eszopiclone, zaleplon, and zolpidem, but does not antagonize the actions of barbiturates, meprobamate, or ethanol. Certain endogenous neuropeptides termed diazepam binding inhibitor (DBI) and acyl-CoA-binding protein (ACBP) are also capable of blocking the interaction of benzodiazepines with BZ binding sites. (3) **Inverse agonists** act as negative allosteric modulators of GABA-receptor function (see Chapter 1). Their interaction with BZ sites on the $GABA_A$ receptor can produce anxiety and seizures, an action that has been demonstrated for several compounds, especially the β-carbolines, eg, *n*-butyl-β-carboline-3-carboxylate (β-CCB). In addition to their direct actions, these molecules can block the effects of benzodiazepines.

The physiologic significance of endogenous modulators of the functions of GABA in the CNS remains unclear.

The Versatility of the Chloride Channel GABA Receptor Complex

The $GABA_A$-chloride channel macromolecular complex is one of the most versatile drug-responsive machines in the body. In addition to the benzodiazepines, barbiturates, and the newer hypnotics (eg, zolpidem), many other drugs with central nervous system effects can modify the function of this important ionotropic receptor. These include alcohol and certain intravenous anesthetics (etomidate, propofol) in addition to thiopental. For example, etomidate and propofol (see Chapter 25) appear to act selectively at $GABA_A$ receptors that contain α2 and α3 subunits, the latter suggested to be the most important with respect to the hypnotic and muscle-relaxing actions of these anesthetic agents. The anesthetic steroid alphaxalone as well as the volatile anesthetics (eg, sevoflurane) are thought to interact with $GABA_A$ receptors. Most of these agents facilitate, allosterically modulate, or mimic the action of GABA. However, it has not been shown that all these drugs act exclusively by this mechanism while volatile anesthetics are thought to have multiple additional actions (see Chapter 25). Other drugs used in the management of seizure disorders indirectly influence the activity of the $GABA_A$-chloride channel macromolecular complex by inhibiting GABA metabolism (eg, vigabatrin) or the reuptake of the transmitter (eg, tiagabine) (see Chapter 24). Central nervous system excitatory agents that act on the chloride channel include picrotoxin and bicuculline. These convulsant drugs block the channel directly (picrotoxin) or interfere with GABA binding (bicuculline).

D. Organ-Level Effects

1. *Sedation*—Benzodiazepines, barbiturates, and most older sedative-hypnotic drugs exert calming effects with concomitant reduction of anxiety at relatively low doses. In most cases, however, the anxiolytic actions of sedative-hypnotics are accompanied by some depressant effects on psychomotor and cognitive functions. In experimental animal models, benzodiazepines and older sedative-hypnotic drugs are able to disinhibit punishment-suppressed behavior. This disinhibition has been equated with antianxiety effects of sedative-hypnotics, and it is not a characteristic of all drugs that have sedative effects, eg, the tricyclic antidepressants and antihistamines. However, the disinhibition of previously suppressed behavior may be more related to behavioral disinhibitory effects of sedative-hypnotics, including euphoria, impaired judgment, and loss of self-control, which can occur at dosages in the range of those used for management of anxiety. The benzodiazepines also exert dose-dependent anterograde amnestic effects (inability to remember events occurring during the drug's duration of action).

2. *Hypnosis*—By definition, all of the sedative-hypnotics induce sleep if high enough doses are given. The effects of sedative-hypnotics on the stages of sleep depend on several factors, including the specific drug, the dose, and the frequency of its administration. The general effects of benzodiazepines and older sedative-hypnotics on patterns of normal sleep are as follows: (1) the latency of sleep onset is decreased (time to fall asleep); (2) the duration of stage 2 NREM (non-rapid eye movement) sleep is increased; (3) the duration of REM (rapid eye movement) sleep is decreased; and (4) the duration of stage 3 NREM slow-wave sleep is decreased. The newer hypnotics all decrease the latency to persistent sleep. Zolpidem decreases REM sleep but has minimal effect on slow-wave sleep. Zaleplon decreases the latency of sleep onset with little effect on total sleep time, NREM, or REM sleep. Eszopiclone increases total sleep time, mainly via increases in stage 2 NREM sleep, and at low doses has little effect on sleep patterns. At the highest recommended dose, eszopiclone decreases REM sleep. Suvorexant decreases time to persistent sleep and increases total sleep time with a decrease in REM sleep.

More rapid onset of sleep and prolongation of stage 2 are presumably clinically useful effects. However, the significance of older sedative-hypnotic drug effects on REM and slow-wave sleep is not clear. Deliberate interruption of REM sleep causes anxiety and irritability followed by a rebound increase in REM sleep at the end of the experiment. A similar pattern of "REM rebound" can be detected following abrupt cessation of drug treatment with older sedative-hypnotics, especially when drugs with short durations of action (eg, triazolam) are used at high doses. With respect to zolpidem and the other newer hypnotics, there is little evidence of REM rebound when these drugs are discontinued after use of recommended doses. However, rebound insomnia occurs with both zolpidem and zaleplon if used at higher doses. Despite possible reductions in slow-wave sleep, there are no reports of disturbances in the secretion of pituitary or adrenal hormones when either barbiturates or benzodiazepines are used as hypnotics. The use of sedative-hypnotics for more than 1–2 weeks leads to some tolerance to their effects on sleep patterns.

3. *Anesthesia*—As shown in Figure 22–1, high doses of certain sedative-hypnotics depress the CNS to the point known as stage III of general anesthesia (see Chapter 25). However, the suitability of a particular agent as an adjunct in anesthesia depends mainly on the physicochemical properties that determine its rapidity of onset and duration of effect. Among the barbiturates, thiopental and methohexital are very lipid-soluble, penetrating brain tissue rapidly following intravenous administration, a characteristic favoring their use for the induction of anesthesia. Rapid tissue redistribution (not rapid elimination) accounts for the short duration of action of these drugs, a feature useful in recovery from anesthesia.

Benzodiazepines—including diazepam, lorazepam, and midazolam—are used intravenously in anesthesia (see Chapter 25), often in combination with other agents. Not surprisingly, benzodiazepines given in large doses as adjuncts to general anesthetics may contribute to a persistent postanesthetic respiratory depression. This is probably related to their relatively long half-lives and the formation of active metabolites. However, such depressant actions of the benzodiazepines are usually reversible with flumazenil. Zolpidem, zaleplon, and eszopiclone as well as suvorexant lack anesthetic activity.

4. *Anticonvulsant effects*—Most sedative-hypnotics are capable of inhibiting the development and spread of epileptiform electrical activity in the CNS. Some selectivity exists in that some members of the group can exert anticonvulsant effects without marked CNS depression (although psychomotor function may be impaired). Several benzodiazepines—including clonazepam, nitrazepam, lorazepam, and diazepam—are sufficiently selective to be clinically useful in the management of seizures (see Chapter 24). Of the barbiturates, phenobarbital and metharbital (converted to phenobarbital in the body) are effective in the treatment of generalized tonic-clonic seizures, though not the drugs of first choice. However, zolpidem, zaleplon, and eszopiclone lack anticonvulsant activity, presumably because of their more selective binding than that of benzodiazepines to $GABA_A$ $\alpha 1$ subunit receptor isoforms. Suvorexant, an orexin receptor antagonist, also lacks anticonvulsant activity.

5. *Muscle relaxation*—Certain drugs in the sedative-hypnotic class, particularly members of the carbamate (eg, meprobamate) and benzodiazepine groups, exert inhibitory effects on polysynaptic reflexes and internuncial transmission and at high doses may also depress transmission at the skeletal neuromuscular junction. Somewhat selective actions of this type that lead to muscle relaxation can be readily demonstrated in animals and have led to claims of usefulness for relaxing contracted voluntary muscle in muscle spasm (see Clinical Pharmacology of Sedative-Hypnotics). Some benzodiazepines are useful in the treatment of essential tremor (see Chapter 28). Muscle relaxation is not a characteristic action of zolpidem, zaleplon, eszopiclone, or suvorexant.

6. *Effects on respiration and cardiovascular function*—At hypnotic doses in healthy patients, the effects of sedative-hypnotics on respiration are comparable to changes during natural sleep. However, even at therapeutic doses, sedative-hypnotics can produce significant respiratory depression in patients with pulmonary disease. Effects on respiration are dose-related, and depression of the medullary respiratory center is the usual cause of death due to overdose of sedative-hypnotics.

At doses up to those causing hypnosis, no significant effects on the cardiovascular system are observed in healthy patients. However, in hypovolemic states, heart failure, and other diseases that impair cardiovascular function, normal doses of sedative-hypnotics may cause cardiovascular depression, probably as a result of actions on the medullary vasomotor centers. At toxic doses, myocardial contractility and vascular tone both may be depressed by central and peripheral effects, possibly via facilitation of the actions of adenosine, leading to circulatory collapse. Respiratory and cardiovascular effects are more marked when sedative-hypnotics are given intravenously. Suvorexant does not show any significant respiratory or cardiovascular effects.

Tolerance: Psychological & Physiologic Dependence

Tolerance—decreased responsiveness to a drug following repeated exposure—is a common feature of sedative-hypnotic use. It may result in the need for an increase in the dose required to maintain symptomatic improvement or to promote sleep. It is important to recognize that partial cross-tolerance occurs between the sedative-hypnotics described here and also with ethanol (see Chapter 23)—a feature of some clinical importance, as explained below. The mechanisms responsible for tolerance to sedative-hypnotics are not well understood. An increase in the rate of drug metabolism (metabolic tolerance) may be partly responsible in the case of chronic administration of barbiturates, but changes in responsiveness of the CNS (pharmacodynamic tolerance) are of greater importance for most sedative-hypnotics. In the case of benzodiazepines, the development of tolerance in animals has been associated with down-regulation of brain benzodiazepine receptors. Tolerance has been reported to occur with the extended use of zolpidem. Minimal tolerance was observed with the use of zaleplon over a 5-week period and eszopiclone over a 6-month period.

The perceived relief of anxiety, euphoria, disinhibition, and promotion of sleep have led to the compulsive misuse of virtually all sedative-hypnotics by vulnerable individuals. (See Chapter 32 for a detailed discussion.) For this reason, most sedative-hypnotic drugs are classified as Schedule III or Schedule IV drugs for prescribing purposes. The consequences of abuse of these agents can be defined in both psychological and physiologic terms. The psychological component may initially parallel simple neurotic behavior patterns difficult to differentiate from those of the inveterate coffee drinker or cigarette smoker. When the pattern of sedative-hypnotic use becomes compulsive, more serious complications develop, including physiologic dependence and tolerance.

Physiologic dependence can be described as an altered physiologic state that requires continuous drug administration to prevent an abstinence or withdrawal syndrome. In the case of sedative-hypnotics, this syndrome is characterized by states of increased anxiety, insomnia, and CNS excitability that may progress to convulsions. Most sedative-hypnotics—including benzodiazepines—are capable of causing physiologic dependence when used on a long-term basis. However, the severity of withdrawal symptoms differs among individual drugs and depends also on the magnitude of the dose used immediately before cessation of use. When higher doses of sedative-hypnotics are used, abrupt withdrawal leads to more serious withdrawal signs. Differences in the severity of withdrawal symptoms resulting from individual sedative-hypnotics relate in part to half-life, since drugs with long half-lives are eliminated slowly enough to accomplish gradual withdrawal with few physical symptoms. The use of drugs with very short half-lives for hypnotic effects may lead to signs of withdrawal even between doses. For example, triazolam, a benzodiazepine with a half-life of about 4 hours, has been reported to cause daytime anxiety when used to treat sleep disorders. The abrupt cessation of zolpidem, zaleplon, eszopiclone, or suvorexant also may result in withdrawal symptoms, though usually of less intensity than those seen with benzodiazepines. Suvorexant's relatively long half-life results in accumulation and reports of daytime sedation and fatigue.

BENZODIAZEPINE ANTAGONISTS: FLUMAZENIL

Flumazenil is one of several 1,4-benzodiazepine derivatives with a high affinity for the benzodiazepine binding site on the $GABA_A$ receptor that act as competitive antagonists. It blocks many of the actions of benzodiazepines, zolpidem, zaleplon, and eszopiclone, but does not antagonize the CNS effects of other sedative-hypnotics, ethanol, opioids, or general anesthetics. Flumazenil is approved for use in reversing the CNS depressant effects of benzodiazepine overdose and to hasten recovery following use of these drugs in anesthetic and diagnostic procedures. Although the drug reverses the sedative effects of benzodiazepines, antagonism of benzodiazepine-induced respiratory depression is less predictable. When given intravenously, flumazenil acts rapidly but has a short half-life (0.7–1.3 hours) due to rapid hepatic clearance. Because all benzodiazepines have a longer duration of action than flumazenil, sedation commonly recurs, requiring repeated administration of the antagonist.

Adverse effects of flumazenil include agitation, confusion, dizziness, and nausea. Flumazenil may cause a severe precipitated abstinence syndrome in patients who have developed physiologic benzodiazepine dependence. In patients who have ingested benzodiazepines with tricyclic antidepressants, seizures and cardiac arrhythmias may follow flumazenil administration.

■ CLINICAL PHARMACOLOGY OF SEDATIVE-HYPNOTICS

TREATMENT OF ANXIETY STATES

The psychological, behavioral, and physiologic responses that characterize anxiety can take many forms. Typically, the psychic awareness of anxiety is accompanied by enhanced vigilance, motor tension, and autonomic hyperactivity. Anxiety is often secondary to organic disease states—acute myocardial infarction, angina pectoris, cancer, etc—which themselves require specific therapy. Another class of secondary anxiety states (situational anxiety) results from circumstances that may have to be dealt with only once or a few times, including anticipation of frightening medical or dental procedures and family illness or other stressful events. Even though situational anxiety tends to be self-limiting, the short-term use of sedative-hypnotics may be appropriate for the treatment of this and certain disease-associated anxiety states. Similarly, the use of a sedative-hypnotic as premedication prior to surgery or some unpleasant medical procedure is rational and appropriate (Table 22–2).

Excessive or unreasonable anxiety about life circumstances (generalized anxiety disorder, GAD), panic disorders, and agoraphobia also are amenable to drug therapy, sometimes in conjunction with psychotherapy. The benzodiazepines continue to be widely used for the management of acute anxiety states and for rapid control of panic attacks. They are also used, though less commonly, in the long-term management of GAD and panic disorders. Anxiety symptoms may be relieved by many benzodiazepines, but it is

TABLE 22–2 Clinical uses of sedative-hypnotics.

For relief of anxiety
For insomnia
For sedation and amnesia before and during medical and surgical procedures
For treatment of epilepsy and seizure states
As a component of balanced anesthesia (intravenous administration)
For control of ethanol or other sedative-hypnotic withdrawal states
For muscle relaxation in specific neuromuscular disorders
As diagnostic aids or for treatment in psychiatry

not always easy to demonstrate the superiority of one drug over another. Alprazolam has been used in the treatment of panic disorders and agoraphobia and appears to be more selective in these conditions than other benzodiazepines. The choice of benzodiazepines for anxiety is based on several sound pharmacologic principles: (1) a rapid onset of action; (2) a relatively high therapeutic index (see drug B in Figure 22–1), plus availability of flumazenil for treatment of overdose; (3) a low risk of drug interactions based on liver enzyme induction; and (4) minimal effects on cardiovascular or autonomic functions.

Disadvantages of the benzodiazepines include the risk of dependence, depression of CNS functions, and amnestic effects. In addition, the benzodiazepines exert additive CNS depression when administered with other drugs, including ethanol. The patient should be warned of this possibility to avoid impairment of performance of any task requiring mental alertness and motor coordination. In the treatment of generalized anxiety disorders and certain phobias, newer antidepressants, including selective serotonin reuptake inhibitors (SSRIs) and serotonin-norepinephrine reuptake inhibitors (SNRIs), are now considered by many authorities to be drugs of first choice (see Chapter 30). However, these agents have a slow onset of action and thus minimal effectiveness in acute anxiety states.

Sedative-hypnotics should be used with appropriate caution to minimize adverse effects. A dose should be prescribed that does not impair mentation or motor functions during waking hours. Some patients may tolerate the drug better if most of the daily dose is given at bedtime, with smaller doses during the day. Prescriptions should be written for short periods, since there is little justification for long-term therapy (defined as use of therapeutic doses for 2 months or longer). The physician should make an effort to assess the efficacy of therapy from the patient's subjective responses. Combinations of antianxiety agents should be avoided, and people taking sedatives should be cautioned about the consumption of alcohol and the concurrent use of over-the-counter medications containing antihistaminic or anticholinergic drugs (see Chapter 64).

Orexin Receptor Antagonists: Sleep-Enabling Drugs

Orexin A and B are peptides found in specific hypothalamic neurons that are involved in the control of wakefulness and that are silent during sleep. Orexin levels increase in the day and decrease at night. Loss of orexin neurons is associated with narcolepsy, a disorder characterized by daytime sleepiness and cataplexy. Animal studies show that orexin receptor antagonists have sleep-enabling effects. This has prompted the development of a new class of hypnotic drugs, orexin antagonists, which include the drugs **lemborexant** and **suvorexant**. There are two known orexin receptors, OX_1 and OX_2. They are both G protein–coupled receptors that bind both orexin A and B, with OX_2 having 5- to 10-fold higher affinity for orexin B. Suvorexant and lemborexant act as antagonists at both OX_1 and OX_2 receptors.

TREATMENT OF SLEEP PROBLEMS

Sleep disorders are common and often result from inappropriate lifestyle, inadequate treatment of underlying medical conditions, or psychiatric illness. True primary insomnia is rare. Recent studies confirm that insufficient sleep, especially in adolescents and in the elderly, impacts many aspects of psychiatric and physical health, with 8–9 hours of sleep per 24 hours recommended for both groups. Nonpharmacologic therapies that are useful for sleep problems include proper diet and exercise, avoiding stimulants before going to sleep, ensuring a comfortable sleeping environment, and retiring at a regular time each night. In some cases, however, the patient will need and should be given a sedative-hypnotic for a limited period. The abrupt discontinuance of many drugs in the sedative-hypnotic class can lead to rebound insomnia.

Benzodiazepines can cause a dose-dependent decrease in both REM and slow-wave sleep, though to a lesser extent than the barbiturates. The newer hypnotics, zolpidem, zaleplon, eszopiclone, and suvorexant, are less likely than the benzodiazepines to change sleep patterns. However, little is known about the clinical impact of sleep pattern effects. The drug selected should be one that provides sleep of fairly rapid onset (decreased sleep latency) and sufficient duration, with minimal "hangover" effects such as drowsiness, dysphoria, and mental or motor depression the following day. Older drugs such as chloral hydrate, secobarbital, and pentobarbital may be used in special circumstances (eg, institutionalized patients), but benzodiazepines, zolpidem, zaleplon, eszopiclone, or suvorexant are preferred. Daytime sedation is more common with benzodiazepines that have slow elimination rates (eg, lorazepam) and those that are biotransformed to active metabolites (eg, flurazepam, quazepam). If benzodiazepines are used nightly, tolerance can occur, which may lead to dose increases by the patient to produce the desired effect. Anterograde amnesia occurs to some degree with all benzodiazepines used for hypnosis.

Eszopiclone, zaleplon, and zolpidem have efficacies similar to those of the hypnotic benzodiazepines in the management of sleep disorders. Favorable clinical features of zolpidem and the other newer hypnotics include rapid onset of activity and modest day-after psychomotor depression with few amnestic effects. Zolpidem, one of the most frequently prescribed hypnotic drugs in the United States, is available in a biphasic release formulation that provides sustained drug levels for sleep maintenance. Zaleplon acts rapidly, and because of its short half-life, the drug appears to have value in the management of patients who awaken early in the sleep cycle. At recommended doses, zaleplon and eszopiclone (despite a relatively long half-life) appear to cause less amnesia or day-after somnolence than zolpidem or benzodiazepines.

TABLE 22–3 Dosages of drugs used commonly for sedation and hypnosis.

Sedation		Hypnosis	
Drug	**Dosage**	**Drug**	**Dosage (at Bedtime)**
Alprazolam	0.25–0.5 mg 2–3 times daily	Chloral hydrate	500–1000 mg
Buspirone	5–10 mg 2–3 times daily	Estazolam	0.5–2 mg
		Eszopiclone	1–3 mg
Chlordiazepoxide	10–20 mg 2–3 times daily	Lemborexant	5 mg
Clorazepate	5–7.5 mg twice daily	Lorazepam	2–4 mg
		Quazepam	7.5–15 mg
Diazepam	5 mg twice daily	Secobarbital	100–200 mg
		Suvorexant	10 mg
Halazepam	20–40 mg 3–4 times daily	Tasimelteon	10 mg
Lorazepam	1–2 mg once or twice daily	Temazepam	7.5–30 mg
		Triazolam	0.125–0.5 mg
Oxazepam	15–30 mg 3–4 times daily	Zaleplon	5–20 mg
Phenobarbital	15–30 mg 2–3 times daily	Zolpidem	2.5–10 mg

Suvorexant is FDA-approved for treatment of both sleep-onset and sleep-maintenance insomnia. The most common adverse effect of suvorexant is next-day somnolence.

The drugs in this class commonly used for sedation and hypnosis are listed in Table 22–3 together with recommended doses. *Note:* The failure of insomnia to remit after 7–10 days of treatment may indicate the presence of a primary psychiatric or medical illness that should be evaluated. Long-term use of hypnotics is an irrational and dangerous medical practice.

OTHER THERAPEUTIC USES

Table 22–2 summarizes several other important clinical uses of drugs in the sedative-hypnotic class. Drugs used in the management of seizure disorders and as intravenous agents in anesthesia are discussed in Chapters 24 and 25.

For sedative and possible amnestic effects during medical or surgical procedures such as endoscopy and bronchoscopy—as well as for premedication prior to anesthesia—oral formulations of shorter-acting drugs are preferred.

Long-acting drugs such as chlordiazepoxide and diazepam and, to a lesser extent, phenobarbital are administered in progressively decreasing doses to patients during withdrawal from physiologic dependence on ethanol or other sedative-hypnotics. Parenteral lorazepam is used to suppress the symptoms of delirium tremens.

Meprobamate and the benzodiazepines have frequently been used as central muscle relaxants, though evidence for general efficacy without accompanying sedation is lacking. A possible exception is diazepam, which has useful relaxant effects in skeletal muscle spasticity of central origin (see Chapter 27).

Psychiatric uses of benzodiazepines other than treatment of anxiety states include the initial management of mania and the control of drug-induced hyperexcitability states (eg, phencyclidine intoxication). Sedative-hypnotics are also used occasionally as diagnostic aids in neurology and psychiatry.

CLINICAL TOXICOLOGY OF SEDATIVE-HYPNOTICS

Direct Toxic Actions

Many of the common adverse effects of sedative-hypnotics result from dose-related depression of the CNS. Relatively low doses may lead to drowsiness, impaired judgment, and diminished motor skills, sometimes with a significant impact on driving ability, job performance, and personal relationships. Sleep driving and other somnambulistic behavior with no memory of the event have occurred with the sedative-hypnotic drugs used in sleep disorders, prompting the FDA in 2007 to issue warnings of this potential hazard. Benzodiazepines may cause a significant dose-related anterograde amnesia; they can significantly impair ability to learn new information, particularly that involving effortful cognitive processes, while leaving the retrieval of previously learned information intact. This effect is utilized for uncomfortable clinical procedures, eg, endoscopy, because the patient is able to cooperate during the procedure but amnesic regarding it afterward. The criminal use of benzodiazepines in cases of "date rape" is based on their dose-dependent amnestic effects. Hangover effects are not uncommon following use of hypnotic drugs with long elimination half-lives. Because elderly patients are more sensitive to the effects of sedative-hypnotics, doses approximately half of those used in younger adults are safer and usually as effective. *The most common reversible cause of confusional states in the elderly is overuse of sedative-hypnotics.* At higher doses, toxicity may present as lethargy or a state of exhaustion or, alternatively, as gross symptoms equivalent to those of ethanol intoxication. The physician should be aware of variability among patients in terms of doses causing adverse effects. An increased sensitivity to sedative-hypnotics is more common in patients with cardiovascular disease, respiratory disease, or hepatic impairment and in older patients. Sedative-hypnotics can exacerbate breathing problems in patients with chronic pulmonary disease and in those with symptomatic sleep apnea.

Sedative-hypnotics are the drugs most frequently involved in deliberate overdoses, in part because of their general availability as very commonly prescribed pharmacologic agents. The benzodiazepines are considered to be safer drugs in this respect, since they have flatter dose-response curves. Epidemiologic studies on the incidence of drug-related deaths support this general assumption—eg, 0.3 deaths per million tablets of diazepam prescribed versus 11.6 deaths per million capsules of secobarbital in one study. Alprazolam is purportedly more toxic in overdose than other benzodiazepines. Many factors other than the specific sedative-hypnotic influence such data—particularly the presence of other CNS depressants, including ethanol. Most serious cases of drug overdose, intentional or accidental, involve polypharmacy; when combinations of agents are taken, the practical safety of benzodiazepines may be significantly reduced.

The lethal dose of any sedative-hypnotic varies with the patient and the circumstances (see Chapter 58). If discovery of the ingestion is made early and a conservative treatment regimen is started, the outcome is rarely fatal, even following very high doses. On the other hand, for most sedative-hypnotics—with the exception of benzodiazepines and possibly the newer hypnotic drugs that have a similar mechanism of action—a dose as low as 10 times the hypnotic dose may be fatal if the patient is not discovered or does not seek help in time. With severe toxicity, the respiratory depression from central actions of the drug may be complicated by aspiration of gastric contents in the unattended patient—an even more likely occurrence if ethanol is present. Cardiovascular depression further complicates successful resuscitation. In such patients, treatment consists of ensuring a patent airway, with mechanical ventilation if needed, and maintenance of plasma volume, renal output, and cardiac function. Use of a positive inotropic drug such as dopamine, which preserves renal blood flow, is sometimes indicated. Hemodialysis or hemoperfusion may be used to hasten elimination of some of these drugs (see Table 58–2).

Flumazenil reverses the sedative actions of benzodiazepines, and those of eszopiclone, zaleplon, and zolpidem, although experience with its use in overdose of the newer hypnotics is limited. However, its duration of action is short, its antagonism of respiratory depression is unpredictable, and there is a risk of precipitation of withdrawal symptoms in long-term users of benzodiazepines. Consequently, the use of flumazenil in benzodiazepine overdose remains controversial and *must* be accompanied by adequate monitoring and support of respiratory function. The extensive clinical use of triazolam has led to reports of serious CNS effects including behavioral disinhibition, delirium, aggression, and violence. However, behavioral disinhibition may occur with any sedative-hypnotic drug, and it does not appear to be more prevalent with triazolam than with other benzodiazepines. Disinhibitory reactions during benzodiazepine treatment are more clearly associated with the use of very high doses and the pretreatment level of patient hostility.

Adverse effects of the sedative-hypnotics that are not referable to their CNS actions occur infrequently. Hypersensitivity reactions, including skin rashes, occur only occasionally with most drugs of this class. Reports of teratogenicity leading to fetal deformation following use of certain benzodiazepines have resulted in FDA assignment of individual benzodiazepines to either category D or X in terms of pregnancy risk. Increased incidence of miscarriage, premature birth, and low birth weight has been reported for the benzodiazepines. Most barbiturates are FDA pregnancy category D. Eszopiclone, ramelteon, suvorexant, zaleplon, and zolpidem are category C, while buspirone is a category B drug in terms of use in pregnancy. Because barbiturates enhance porphyrin synthesis, they are *absolutely contraindicated* in patients with a history of acute intermittent porphyria, variegate porphyria, hereditary coproporphyria, or symptomatic porphyria.

Alterations in Drug Response

Depending on the dosage and the duration of use, tolerance occurs in varying degrees to many of the pharmacologic effects of sedative-hypnotics. However, it should not be assumed that the degree of tolerance achieved is identical for all pharmacologic effects. There is evidence that the lethal dose range is not altered significantly by the long-term use of sedative-hypnotics. Cross-tolerance between the different sedative-hypnotics, including ethanol, can lead to an unsatisfactory therapeutic response when standard doses of a drug are used in a patient with a recent history of excessive use of these agents. However, there have been very few reports of tolerance development when eszopiclone, zolpidem, or zaleplon was used for less than 4 weeks.

With the long-term use of sedative-hypnotics, especially if doses are increased, a state of physiologic dependence can occur. This may develop to a degree unparalleled by any other drug group, *including the opioids*. Withdrawal from a sedative-hypnotic can have severe and life-threatening manifestations. Withdrawal symptoms range from restlessness, anxiety, weakness, and orthostatic hypotension to hyperactive reflexes and generalized seizures. Symptoms of withdrawal are usually more severe following discontinuance of sedative-hypnotics with shorter half-lives. However, eszopiclone, zolpidem, and zaleplon appear to be exceptions to this, because withdrawal symptoms are minimal following abrupt discontinuance of these newer short-acting agents. Symptoms are less pronounced with longer-acting drugs, which may partly accomplish their own "tapered" withdrawal by virtue of their slow elimination. Cross-dependence, defined as the ability of one drug to suppress abstinence symptoms from discontinuance of another drug, is quite marked among sedative-hypnotics. This provides the rationale for therapeutic regimens in the management of withdrawal states: Longer-acting drugs such as chlordiazepoxide, diazepam, and phenobarbital can be used to alleviate withdrawal symptoms of shorter-acting drugs, including ethanol.

Drug Interactions

The most common drug interactions involving sedative-hypnotics are interactions with other CNS depressant drugs, leading to additive effects. These interactions have some therapeutic usefulness when these drugs are used as adjuvants in anesthesia practice. However, if not anticipated, such interactions can lead to serious consequences, including enhanced depression with concomitant use of many other drugs. Additive effects can be predicted with concomitant use of alcoholic beverages, opioid analgesics, anticonvulsants, antihistamines, antihypertensive agents, tricyclic antidepressants, and phenothiazines.

Interactions involving changes in the activity of hepatic drug-metabolizing enzyme systems have been discussed (see also Chapters 4 and 67).

SUMMARY Sedative-Hypnotics

Subclass, Drug	Mechanism of Action	Effects	Clinical Applications	Pharmacokinetics, Toxicities, Interactions
BENZODIAZEPINES				
• Alprazolam • Chlordiazepoxide • Clonazepam • Clorazepate • Diazepam • Estazolam • Flurazepam • Lorazepam • Midazolam • Oxazepam • Quazepam • Temazepam • Triazolam	Bind to specific $GABA_A$ receptor subunits at central nervous system (CNS) neuronal synapses facilitating GABA-mediated chloride ion channel opening frequency • enhance membrane hyperpolarization	Dose-dependent depressant effects on the CNS including sedation and relief of anxiety • amnesia • hypnosis • anesthesia • coma • and respiratory depression	Acute anxiety states • panic attacks • generalized anxiety disorder • insomnia and other sleep disorders • relaxation of skeletal muscle • anesthesia (adjunctive) • seizure disorders	Half-lives from 2 to 40 h (clorazepate longer) • oral activity • hepatic metabolism—some active metabolites • *Toxicity:* Extensions of CNS depressant effects • dependence liability • *Interactions:* Additive CNS depression with ethanol and many other drugs
BENZODIAZEPINE ANTAGONIST				
• Flumazenil	Antagonist at benzodiazepine-binding sites on the $GABA_A$ receptor	Blocks actions of benzodiazepines and zolpidem but not other sedative-hypnotic drugs	Management of benzodiazepineoverdose	IV, short half-life • *Toxicity:* Agitation, confusion • possible withdrawal symptoms in benzodiazepine dependence
BARBITURATES				
• Amobarbital • Butabarbital • Mephobarbital • Pentobarbital • Phenobarbital • Secobarbital	Bind to specific $GABA_A$ receptor subunits at CNS neuronal synapses facilitating GABA-mediated chloride ion channel opening duration • enhance membrane hyperpolarization	Dose-dependent depressant effects on the CNS including sedation and relief of anxiety • amnesia • hypnosis • anesthesia • coma and respiratory depression • steeper dose-response relationship than benzodiazepines	Anesthesia (thiopental) • insomnia (secobarbital) • seizure disorders (phenobarbital)	Half-lives from 4 to 60 h (phenobarbital longer) • oral activity • hepatic metabolism—phenobarbital 20% renal elimination • *Toxicity:* Extensions of CNS depressant effects • dependence liability > benzodiazepines • *Interactions:* Additive CNS depression with ethanol and many other drugs • induction of hepatic drug-metabolizing enzymes
NEWER HYPNOTICS				
• Eszopiclone • Zaleplon • Zolpidem	Bind selectively to a subgroup of $GABA_A$ receptors, acting like benzodiazepines to enhance membrane hyperpolarization	Rapid onset of hypnosis with few amnestic effects or day-after psychomotor depression or somnolence	Sleep disorders, especially those characterized by difficulty in falling asleep	Oral activity • short half-lives • CYP substrates • *Toxicity:* Extensions of CNS depressant effects • dependence liability • *Interactions:* Additive CNS depression with ethanol and many other drugs
MELATONIN RECEPTOR AGONISTS				
• Ramelteon	Activates MT_1 and MT_2 receptors in suprachiasmatic nuclei in the CNS	Rapid onset of sleep with minimal rebound insomnia or withdrawal symptoms	Sleep disorders, especially those characterized by difficulty in falling asleep • not a controlled substance	Oral activity • forms active metabolite via CYP1A2 • *Toxicity:* Dizziness • fatigue • endocrine changes • *Interactions:* Fluvoxamine inhibits metabolism
• *Tasimelteon: Orally active MT_1 and MT_2 agonist, recently approved for non-24-hour sleep disorder*				
OREXIN ANTAGONIST				
• Suvorexant • Lemborexant	Blocks binding of orexins to OX_1 and OX_2 receptors, neuropeptides that promote wakefulness	Promotes sleep onset and duration	Sleep disorders, especially those characterized by difficulty in falling asleep	CYP450 metabolism is inhibited by fluconazole, verapamil, and grapefruit juice • next-day somnolence and driving impairment
5-HT-RECEPTOR AGONIST				
• Buspirone	Mechanism uncertain: Partial agonist at 5-HT receptors but affinity for D_2 receptors also possible	Slow onset (1–2 weeks) of anxiolytic effects • minimal psychomotor impairment—no additive CNS depression with sedative-hypnotic drugs	Generalized anxiety states	Oral activity • forms active metabolite • short half-life • *Toxicity:* Tachycardia • paresthesias • gastrointestinal distress • *Interactions:* CYP3A4 inducers and inhibitors

PREPARATIONS AVAILABLE

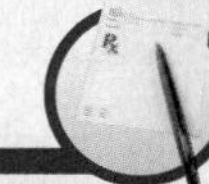

GENERIC NAME	AVAILABLE AS
BENZODIAZEPINES	
Alprazolam	Generic, Xanax
Chlordiazepoxide	Generic, Librium
Clonazepam	Generic, Tranxene
Clorazepate	Generic, Klonopin
Diazepam	Generic, Valium
Estazolam	Generic
Flurazepam	Generic
Lorazepam	Generic, Ativan
Midazolam	Generic, Versed
Oxazepam	Generic, Serax
Quazepam	Generic, Doral
Temazepam	Generic, Restoril
Triazolam	Generic, Halcion
BENZODIAZEPINE ANTAGONIST	
Flumazenil	Generic, Romazicon
BARBITURATES	
Amobarbital	Amytal
Mephobarbital	Mebaral (withdrawn)
Pentobarbital	Generic, Nembutal Sodium
Phenobarbital	Generic, Luminal Sodium
Secobarbital	Generic, Seconal
MISCELLANEOUS DRUGS	
Buspirone	Generic, BuSpar
Chloral hydrate	Generic, Aquachloral Supprettes
Eszopiclone	Generic, Lunesta
Hydroxyzine	Generic, Atarax, Vistaril
Lemborexant	Dayvigo
Meprobamate	Generic, Equanil, Miltown
Paraldehyde	Generic
Ramelteon	Rozerem
Suvorexant	Belsomra
Tasimelteon	Hetlioz
Zaleplon	Sonata
Zolpidem	Generic, Ambien, Ambien-CR, Zolpimist

REFERENCES

Ancoli-Israel S et al: Long-term use of sedative hypnotics in older patients with insomnia. Sleep Med 2005;6:107.

Anonymous: Drugs for chronic insomnia. Med Lett 2018;60:201.

Anonymous: Drugs for anxiety disorders. Med Lett 2019;61:121.

Bateson AN: The benzodiazepine site of the GABA A receptor: An old target with new potential? Sleep Med 2004;5(Suppl 1):S9.

Chouinard G: Issues in the clinical use of benzodiazepines: Potency, withdrawal, and rebound. J Clin Psychiatry 2004;65(Suppl 5):7.

Clayton T et al: An updated unified pharmacophore model of the benzodiazepine binding site on gamma-aminobutyric acid(a) receptors: Correlation with comparative models. Curr Med Chem 2007;14:2755.

Cloos JM, Ferreira V: Current use of benzodiazepines in anxiety disorders. Curr Opin Psychiatry 2009;22:90.

Craske M, Bystritsky A: Approach to treating generalized anxiety disorder in adults: Up To Date 2019; topic 101879.

Da Settimo F et al: GABA A/Bz receptor subtypes as targets for selective drugs. Curr Med Chem 2007;14:2680.

Davidson JR et al: A psychopharmacological treatment algorithm for generalized anxiety disorder. J Psychopharmacol 2010;24:3.

Dhillon S, Clarke M: Tasimelteon: first global approval. Drugs 2014;74:505.

Drover DR: Comparative pharmacokinetics and pharmacodynamics of short-acting hypnosedatives: Zaleplon, zolpidem and zopiclone. Clin Pharmacokinet 2004;43:227.

Dubey AK et al: Suvorexant: The first orexin receptor antagonist to treat insomnia. J Pharmacol Pharmacother 2015;6:118.

Erman M et al: An efficacy, safety, and dose-response study of ramelteon in patients with chronic primary insomnia. Sleep Med 2006;7:17.

Gottesmann C: GABA mechanisms and sleep. Neuroscience 2002;111:231.

Han W et al: Shisa7 is a $GABA_A$ receptor auxiliary subunit controlling benzodiazepine actions. Science 2019;366:246.

Hanson SM, Czajkowski C: Structural mechanisms underlying benzodiazepine modulation of the GABA(A) receptor. J Neurosci 2008;28:3490.

Hesse LM et al: Clinically important drug interactions with zopiclone, zolpidem and zaleplon. CNS Drugs 2003;17:513.

Jacobson LH et al: Suvorexant for the treatment of insomnia. Exp Rev Clin Pharmacol 2014;7:711.

Kato K et al: Neurochemical properties of ramelteon, a selective MT1/MT2 receptor agonist. Neuropharmacology 2005;48:301.

Kralic JE et al: GABA(A) receptor alpha-1 subunit deletion alters receptor subtype assembly, pharmacological and behavioral responses to benzodiazepines and zolpidem. Neuropharmacology 2002;43:685.

Kripke DF: Is suvorexant a better choice than alternative hypnotics? F1000Res. 2015;4:456.

Lader M, Tylee A, Donoghue J: Withdrawing benzodiazepines in primary care. CNS Drugs 2009;23:2319.

McKernan RM et al: Anxiolytic-like action of diazepam: Which GABA(A) receptor subtype is involved? Trends Pharmacol Sci 2001;22:402.

Medical Letter: Drugs for insomnia. Treat Guidel Med Lett 2012;10:57.

Morairty SR et al: The hypocretin/orexin antagonist almorexant promotes sleep without impairment of performance in rats. Front Neurosci 2014;8:3.

Rapaport MJ et al: Benzodiazepine use and driving: A meta analysis. J Clin Psychiatry 2009;70:663.

Rosenberg R et al: An assessment of the efficacy and safety of eszopiclone in the treatment of transient insomnia in healthy adults. Sleep Med 2005;6:15.

Sanger DJ: The pharmacology and mechanism of action of new generation, non-benzodiazepine hypnotic agents. CNS Drugs 2004;18(Suppl 1):9.

Shyken JM et al: Benzodiazepines in pregnancy. Clin Obstet Gynecol 2019;62:156.

Silber MH: Chronic insomnia. N Engl J Med 2005;353:803.

Walsh JK: Pharmacologic management of insomnia. J Clin Psychiatry 2004; 65(Suppl 16):41.

Winkelman JW: Insomnia disorder. N Engl J Med 2015;373:1437.

Wurtman R: Ramelteon: A novel treatment for the treatment of insomnia. Expert Rev Neurother 2006;6:957.

CASE STUDY ANSWER

As described in this chapter, nonpharmacologic factors are very important in the management of sleep problems: proper diet (and avoidance of snacks before bedtime), exercise, and a regular time and place for sleep. Avoidance of stimulants is very important, and the large intake of diet colas reported by the patient should be reduced, especially in the latter half of the day. If problems persist after these measures are implemented, one of the newer hypnotics (eszopiclone, zaleplon, or zolpidem) may be tried on a short-term basis.

CHAPTER

23

The Alcohols

Todd W. Vanderah, PhD, & Anthony J. Trevor, PhD

CASE STUDY

A 19-year-old college freshman began drinking alcohol at 8:30 PM during a hazing event at his new fraternity. Between 8:30 and approximately midnight, he and several other pledges consumed beer and a bottle of whiskey, and then he consumed most of a bottle of rum at the urging of upperclassmen. The young man complained of feeling nauseated, lay down on a couch, and began to lose consciousness. Two upperclassmen carried him to a bedroom, placed him on his stomach, and positioned a trash can nearby. Approximately 10 minutes later, the freshman was found unconscious and covered with vomit. There was a delay in treatment because the upperclassmen called the college police instead of calling 911. After the call was transferred to 911, emergency medical technicians responded quickly and discovered that the young man was not breathing and that he had choked on his vomit. He was rushed to the hospital, where he remained in a coma for 2 days before ultimately being pronounced dead. The patient's blood alcohol concentration shortly after arriving at the hospital was 510 mg/dL. What was the cause of this patient's death? If he had received medical care sooner, what treatment might have prevented his death?

Alcohol, primarily in the form of ethyl alcohol (ethanol), has occupied an important place in the history of humankind for at least 8000 years. In Western society, beer and wine were a main staple of daily life until the 19th century. These relatively dilute alcoholic beverages were preferred over water, which was known—long before the discovery of microbes—to be associated with acute and chronic illness. Partially sterilized by the fermentation process and the alcohol content, alcoholic beverages provided calories and some nutrients and served as a main source of daily liquid intake. As systems for improved sanitation and water purification were introduced in the 1800s, beer and wine became less important components of the human diet, and the consumption of alcoholic beverages, including distilled preparations with higher concentrations of alcohol, shifted toward their present-day role, in many societies, as a socially acceptable form of recreation.

Today, alcohol is widely consumed. Like other sedative-hypnotic drugs, alcohol in low to moderate amounts relieves anxiety and fosters a feeling of well-being or even euphoria. However, alcohol is also the most commonly abused drug in the world, and the cause of vast medical and societal costs. In the United States, approximately 75% of the adult population drinks alcohol regularly. The majority of this drinking population is able to enjoy the pleasurable effects of alcohol without allowing alcohol consumption to become a health risk. However, 8–10% of the general population in the United States has an **alcohol-use disorder.** Individuals who use alcohol in dangerous situations (eg, drinking and driving or combining alcohol with other medications) or continue to drink alcohol despite adverse consequences related directly to their alcohol consumption suffer from **alcohol abuse** (see also Chapter 32). Individuals with **alcohol dependence** have characteristics of alcohol abuse and additionally exhibit physical dependence on alcohol (tolerance to alcohol and signs and symptoms upon withdrawal). They also demonstrate an inability to control their drinking and devote much time to getting and using alcohol, or recovering from its effects. The alcohol-use disorders are complex, with genetic as well as environmental determinants.

The societal and medical costs of alcohol abuse are staggering. It is estimated that more than 600,000 emergency department visits and approximately 95,000 deaths (approximately 68,000 men and 27,000 women) in the USA annually are due to alcohol use. This makes alcohol use the third-leading preventable cause of death in the United States. Once in the hospital, people with chronic alcoholism generally have poorer outcomes. In addition, each year, tens of thousands of children are born with morphologic and functional defects resulting from prenatal exposure to ethanol. Despite the investment of many resources and much basic research, alcoholism remains a common chronic disease that is difficult to treat.

Ethanol and many other alcohols with potentially toxic effects are used as fuels and in industry—some in enormous quantities. In addition to ethanol, methanol and ethylene glycol toxicity occurs with sufficient frequency to warrant discussion in this chapter.

BASIC PHARMACOLOGY OF ETHANOL

Pharmacokinetics

Ethanol is a small water-soluble molecule that is absorbed rapidly from the gastrointestinal tract. After ingestion of alcohol in the fasting state, peak blood alcohol concentrations are reached within 30 minutes. The presence of food in the stomach delays absorption by slowing gastric emptying. Distribution is rapid, with tissue levels approximating the concentration in blood. The volume of distribution for ethanol approximates total body water (0.5–0.7 L/kg). After an equivalent oral dose of alcohol, women have a higher peak concentration than men, in part because women have a lower total body water content and in part because of differences in first-pass metabolism. In the central nervous system (CNS), the concentration of ethanol rises quickly, since the brain receives a large proportion of total blood flow and ethanol readily crosses biologic membranes.

More than 90% of alcohol consumed is oxidized in the liver; much of the remainder is excreted through the lungs and in the urine. The excretion of a small but consistent proportion of alcohol by the lungs can be quantified with breath alcohol tests that serve as a basis for a legal definition of "driving under the influence" (DUI) in many countries. In most states in the USA, the alcohol level for driving under the influence is set at 80 mg/dL (0.08%). At levels of ethanol usually achieved in blood, the rate of oxidation follows zero-order kinetics; that is, it is independent of time and concentration of the drug. The typical adult can metabolize 7–10 g (150–220 mmol) of alcohol per hour, the equivalent of approximately one "drink" [10 oz (300 mL) beer, 3.5 oz (105 mL) wine, or 1 oz (30 mL) distilled 80-proof spirits]. A commercial product ("Palcohol"), approved in some states in the USA in 2015, consists of a powder to be mixed to form a drink containing 10% ethanol (approximately equivalent to wine).

Two major pathways of alcohol metabolism to acetaldehyde have been identified (Figure 23–1). Acetaldehyde is then oxidized to acetate by a third metabolic process.

A. Alcohol Dehydrogenase Pathway

The primary pathway for alcohol metabolism involves alcohol dehydrogenase (ADH), a family of cytosolic enzymes that catalyze the conversion of alcohol to acetaldehyde (see Figure 23–1, left). These enzymes are located mainly in the liver, but small amounts

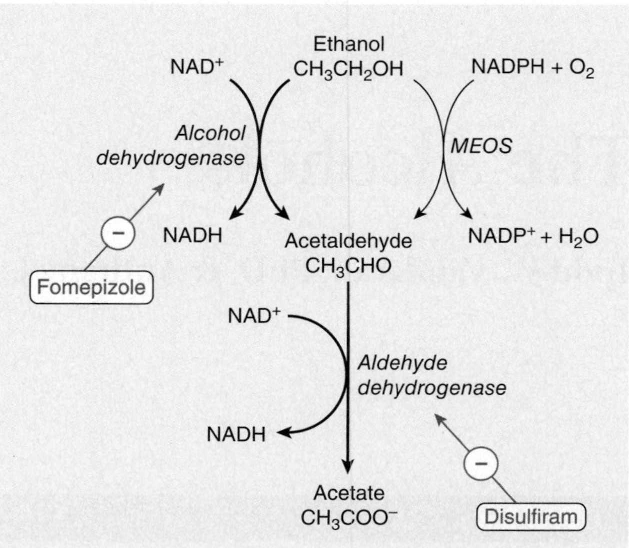

FIGURE 23–1 Metabolism of ethanol by alcohol dehydrogenase and the microsomal ethanol-oxidizing system (MEOS). Alcohol dehydrogenase and aldehyde dehydrogenase are inhibited by fomepizole and disulfiram, respectively. NAD^+, nicotinamide adenine dinucleotide; NADPH, nicotinamide adenine dinucleotide phosphate.

are found in other organs such as the brain and stomach. There is considerable genetic variation in ADH enzymes, affecting the rate of ethanol metabolism and also appearing to alter vulnerability to alcohol-abuse disorders. For example, one ADH allele (the *ADH1B*2* allele), which is associated with rapid conversion of ethanol to acetaldehyde, has been found to be protective against alcohol dependence in several ethnic populations, especially East Asians.

Some metabolism of ethanol by ADH occurs in the stomach in men, but a smaller amount occurs in women, who appear to have lower levels of the gastric enzyme. This difference in gastric metabolism of alcohol in women probably contributes to the sex-related differences in blood alcohol concentrations noted above.

During conversion of ethanol by ADH to acetaldehyde, hydrogen ion is transferred from ethanol to the cofactor nicotinamide adenine dinucleotide (NAD^+) to form NADH. As a net result, alcohol oxidation generates an excess of reducing equivalents in the liver, chiefly as NADH. The excess NADH production appears to contribute to the metabolic disorders that accompany chronic alcoholism and to both the lactic acidosis and hypoglycemia that frequently accompany acute alcohol poisoning.

B. Microsomal Ethanol-Oxidizing System (MEOS)

This enzyme system, also known as the mixed function oxidase system, uses NADPH as a cofactor in the metabolism of ethanol (see Figure 23–1, right) and consists primarily of cytochrome P450 2E1, 1A2, and 3A4 (see Chapter 4).

During chronic alcohol consumption, MEOS activity is induced. As a result, chronic alcohol consumption results in significant increases not only in ethanol metabolism but also in the clearance of other drugs eliminated by the cytochrome P450s that constitute the MEOS system, and in the generation of the toxic byproducts of cytochrome P450 reactions (toxins, free radicals, H_2O_2).

C. Acetaldehyde Metabolism

Much of the acetaldehyde formed from alcohol is oxidized in the liver in a reaction catalyzed by mitochondrial NAD-dependent aldehyde dehydrogenase (ALDH). The product of this reaction is acetate (see Figure 23–1), which can be further metabolized to CO_2 and water, or used to form acetyl-CoA.

Oxidation of acetaldehyde is inhibited by **disulfiram,** a drug that has been used to deter drinking by patients with alcohol dependence. When ethanol is consumed in the presence of disulfiram, acetaldehyde accumulates and causes an unpleasant reaction of facial flushing, nausea, vomiting, dizziness, and headache. Several other drugs (eg, metronidazole, cefotetan, trimethoprim) inhibit ALDH and have been claimed to cause a disulfiram-like reaction if combined with ethanol.

Some people, primarily of East Asian descent, have genetic deficiency in the activity of the mitochondrial form of ALDH, which is encoded by the *ALDH2* gene. When these individuals drink alcohol, they develop high blood acetaldehyde concentrations and experience a noxious reaction similar to that seen with the combination of disulfiram and ethanol. This form of reduced-activity ALDH is strongly protective against alcohol-use disorders.

Pharmacodynamics of Acute Ethanol Consumption

A. Central Nervous System

The CNS is markedly affected by acute alcohol consumption. Alcohol causes sedation, relief of anxiety and, at higher concentrations, slurred speech, ataxia, impaired judgment, and disinhibited behavior, a condition usually called intoxication or drunkenness (Table 23–1). These CNS effects are most marked as the blood level is rising, because acute tolerance to the effects of alcohol occurs after a few hours of drinking. For chronic drinkers who are tolerant to the effects of alcohol, higher concentrations are needed to elicit these CNS effects. For example, an individual with chronic alcoholism may appear sober or only slightly intoxicated with a blood alcohol concentration of 300–400 mg/dL (0.30-0.40%), whereas this level is associated with marked intoxication or even coma in a nontolerant individual. The propensity of moderate doses of alcohol to inhibit the attention and information-processing skills as well as the motor skills required for operation of motor vehicles has profound effects. Approximately 30–40% of all traffic accidents resulting in a fatality in the United States involve at least one person with blood alcohol near or above the legal level of intoxication, and drunken driving is a leading cause of death in young adults.

Like other sedative-hypnotic drugs, alcohol is a CNS depressant. At high blood concentrations, it induces coma, respiratory depression, and death.

Ethanol affects a large number of membrane proteins that participate in signaling pathways, including neurotransmitter receptors for amines, amino acids, opioids, and neuropeptides; enzymes such as Na^+/K^+-ATPase, adenylyl cyclase, phosphoinositide-specific phospholipase C; a nucleoside transporter; and ion channels. Much attention has focused on alcohol's effects on neurotransmission by glutamate and γ-aminobutyric acid (GABA), the main excitatory and inhibitory neurotransmitters in the CNS. Acute ethanol exposure enhances the action of GABA at $GABA_A$ receptors, which is consistent with the ability of GABA-mimetics to intensify many of the acute effects of alcohol and of $GABA_A$ antagonists to attenuate some of the actions of ethanol. Ethanol inhibits the ability of glutamate to open the cation channel associated with the *N*-methyl-D-aspartate (NMDA) subtype of glutamate receptors. The NMDA receptor is implicated in many aspects of cognitive function, including learning and memory. "Blackouts"—periods of memory loss that occur with high levels of alcohol—may result from inhibition of NMDA receptor activation. Experiments that use modern genetic approaches eventually will yield a more precise definition of ethanol's direct and indirect targets. In recent years, experiments with mutant strains of mice, worms, and flies have reinforced the importance of previously identified targets and helped identify new candidates, including a calcium-regulated and voltage-gated potassium channel that may be one of ethanol's direct targets (see Box: What Can Drunken Worms, Flies, and Mice Tell Us About Alcohol?).

B. Heart

Significant depression of myocardial contractility has been observed in individuals who acutely consume moderate amounts of alcohol, ie, at a blood concentration above 100 mg/dL.

C. Smooth Muscle

Ethanol is a vasodilator, probably as a result of both CNS effects (depression of the vasomotor center) and direct smooth muscle relaxation caused by its metabolite, acetaldehyde. In cases of severe overdose, hypothermia—caused by vasodilation—may be marked in cold environments. Preliminary evidence indicates that flibanserin, a drug that interacts with 5-HT receptors, augments the hypotensive effects of ethanol and may cause severe orthostatic hypotension and syncope (see Chapter 16). Ethanol also relaxes the uterus and—before the introduction of more effective and

TABLE 23–1 Blood alcohol concentration (BAC) and clinical effects in nontolerant individuals.

BAC (mg/dL)[1]	Clinical Effect
50–100	Sedation, subjective "high," slower reaction times
100–200	Impaired motor function, slurred speech, ataxia
200–300	Emesis, stupor
300–400	Coma
>400	Respiratory depression, death

[1]In many parts of the United States, a blood level above 80–100 mg/dL for adults or 5–20 mg/dL for persons under 21 is sufficient for conviction of driving while "under the influence."

safer uterine relaxants (eg, calcium channel antagonists)—was used intravenously for the suppression of premature labor.

Consequences of Chronic Alcohol Consumption

Chronic alcohol consumption profoundly affects the function of several vital organs—particularly the liver—and the nervous, gastrointestinal, cardiovascular, and immune systems. Since ethanol has low potency, it requires concentrations thousands of times higher than other misused drugs (eg, cocaine, opiates, amphetamines) to produce its intoxicating effects. As a result, ethanol is consumed in quantities that are unusually large for a pharmacologically active drug. The tissue damage caused by chronic alcohol ingestion results from a combination of the direct effects of ethanol and acetaldehyde, and the metabolic consequences of processing a heavy load of a metabolically active substance. Specific mechanisms implicated in tissue damage include increased oxidative stress coupled with depletion of glutathione, damage to mitochondria, growth factor dysregulation, and potentiation of cytokine-induced injury.

Chronic consumption of large amounts of alcohol is associated with an increased risk of death. Deaths linked to alcohol consumption are caused by liver disease, cancer, accidents, and suicide.

A. Liver and Gastrointestinal Tract

Liver disease is the most common medical complication of alcohol abuse; an estimated 15–30% of chronic heavy drinkers eventually develop severe liver disease. Alcoholic fatty liver, a reversible condition, may progress to alcoholic hepatitis and finally to cirrhosis and liver failure. In the USA, chronic alcohol abuse is the leading cause of liver cirrhosis and of the need for liver transplantation. The risk of developing liver disease is related both to the average amount of daily consumption and to the duration of alcohol abuse. Women appear to be more susceptible to alcohol hepatotoxicity than men. Concurrent infection with hepatitis B or C virus increases the risk of severe liver disease. Cirrhosis contributes to elevated portal blood pressure and esophageal and gastric venous varices. These varices may rupture and result in massive bleeding.

What Can Drunken Worms, Flies, and Mice Tell Us About Alcohol?

For a drug like ethanol, which exhibits low potency and specificity and modifies complex behaviors, the precise roles of its many direct and indirect targets are difficult to define. Increasingly, ethanol researchers are employing genetic approaches to complement standard neurobiologic experimentation. Three experimental animal systems for which powerful genetic techniques exist—mice, flies, and worms—have yielded intriguing results.

Strains of mice with abnormal sensitivity to ethanol were identified many years ago by breeding and selection programs. Using sophisticated genetic mapping and sequencing techniques, researchers have made progress in identifying the genes that confer ethanol susceptibility or resistance traits. A more targeted approach is the use of transgenic mice to test hypotheses about specific genes. For example, after earlier experiments suggested a link between brain neuropeptide Y (NPY) and ethanol, researchers used two transgenic mouse models to further investigate the link. They found that a strain of mice that lacks the gene for NPY—NPY knockout mice—consume more ethanol than control mice and are less sensitive to ethanol's sedative effects. As would be expected if increased concentrations of NPY in the brain make mice more sensitive to ethanol, a strain of mice that overexpresses NPY drinks less alcohol than the controls even though their total consumption of food and liquid is normal. Work with other transgenic knockout mice supports the central role in ethanol responses of signaling systems that have long been believed to be involved (eg, $GABA_A$, glutamate, dopamine, opioid, and serotonin receptors) and has helped build the case for newer candidates such as NPY and corticotropin-releasing hormone, cannabinoid receptors, ion channels, and protein kinase C.

It is easy to imagine mice having measurable behavioral responses to alcohol, but drunken worms and fruit flies are harder to imagine. Actually, both invertebrates respond to ethanol in ways that parallel mammalian responses. *Drosophila melanogaster* fruit flies exposed to ethanol vapor show increased locomotion at low concentrations but at higher concentrations, they become poorly coordinated, sedated, and finally immobile. These behaviors can be monitored by sophisticated laser or video tracking methods or with an ingenious "chromatography" column of air that separates relatively insensitive flies from inebriated flies, which drop to the bottom of the column. The worm *Caenorhabditis elegans* similarly exhibits increased locomotion at low ethanol concentrations and, at higher concentrations, reduced locomotion, sedation, and—something that can be turned into an effective screen for mutant worms that are resistant to ethanol—impaired egg laying. The advantage of using flies and worms as genetic models for ethanol research is their relatively simple neuroanatomy, well-established techniques for genetic manipulation, extensive libraries of well-characterized mutants, and completely or nearly completely solved genetic codes. Already, much information has accumulated about candidate proteins involved with the effects of ethanol in flies. In an elegant study on *C elegans*, researchers found evidence that a calcium-activated, voltage-gated BK potassium channel is a direct target of ethanol. This channel, which is activated by ethanol, has close homologs in flies and vertebrates, and evidence is accumulating that ethanol has similar effects in these homologs. Genetic experiments in these model systems should provide information that will help narrow and focus research into the complex and important effects of ethanol in humans.

The pathogenesis of alcoholic liver disease is a multifactorial process involving metabolic repercussions of ethanol oxidation in the liver, dysregulation of fatty acid oxidation and synthesis, and activation of the innate immune system by a combination of direct effects of ethanol and its metabolites and by bacterial endotoxins that access the liver as a result of ethanol-induced changes in the intestinal tract. Tumor necrosis factor-α appears to play a pivotal role in the progression of alcoholic liver disease and may be a fruitful therapeutic target.

Other portions of the gastrointestinal tract can also be injured. Chronic alcohol ingestion is by far the most common cause of chronic pancreatitis in the Western world. In addition to its direct toxic effect on pancreatic acinar cells, alcohol alters pancreatic epithelial permeability and promotes the formation of protein plugs and calcium carbonate-containing stones.

Individuals with chronic alcoholism are prone to gastritis and have increased susceptibility to blood and plasma protein loss during drinking, which may contribute to anemia and protein malnutrition. Alcohol also injures the small intestine, leading to diarrhea, weight loss, and multiple vitamin deficiencies.

Malnutrition from dietary deficiency and vitamin deficiencies due to malabsorption are common in alcoholism. Malabsorption of water-soluble vitamins is especially severe.

B. Nervous System

1. *Tolerance and dependence*—The consumption of alcohol in high doses over a long period results in tolerance and in physical and psychological dependence. Tolerance to the intoxicating effects of alcohol is a complex process involving poorly understood changes in the nervous system as well as the pharmacokinetic changes described earlier. As with other sedative-hypnotic drugs, there is a limit to tolerance, so that only a relatively small increase in the *lethal* dose occurs with increasing alcohol use.

Chronic alcohol drinkers, when forced to reduce or discontinue alcohol, experience a withdrawal syndrome, which indicates the existence of physical dependence. Alcohol withdrawal symptoms usually consist of hyperexcitability in mild cases and seizures, toxic psychosis, and **delirium tremens** (eg, shaking, confusion, high blood pressure, fever, hallucinations, death) in severe ones. The dose, rate, and duration of alcohol consumption determine the intensity of the withdrawal syndrome. When consumption has been very high, merely reducing the rate of consumption may lead to signs of withdrawal.

Psychological dependence on alcohol is characterized by a compulsive desire to experience the rewarding effects of alcohol and, for current drinkers, a desire to avoid the negative consequences of withdrawal. People who have recovered from alcoholism and become abstinent still experience periods of intense craving for alcohol that can be triggered by environmental cues associated in the past with drinking, such as familiar places, groups of people, or events.

The molecular basis of alcohol tolerance and dependence is not known with certainty, nor is it known whether the two phenomena reflect opposing effects on a shared molecular pathway. Tolerance may result from ethanol-induced up-regulation of a pathway in response to the continuous presence of ethanol. Dependence may result from overactivity of that same pathway after the ethanol effect dissipates and before the system has time to return to a normal ethanol-free state.

Chronic exposure of animals or cultured cells to alcohol elicits a multitude of adaptive responses involving neurotransmitters and their receptors, ion channels, and enzymes that participate in signal transduction pathways. Up-regulation of the NMDA subtype of glutamate receptors and voltage-sensitive Ca^{2+} channels may underlie the seizures that accompany the alcohol withdrawal syndrome. GABA neurotransmission is believed to play a significant role in tolerance and withdrawal because (1) sedative-hypnotic drugs that enhance GABAergic neurotransmission are able to substitute for alcohol during alcohol withdrawal, and (2) there is evidence of down-regulation of $GABA_A$-mediated responses with chronic alcohol exposure.

Like other drugs of abuse, ethanol modulates neural activity in the brain's mesolimbic dopamine reward circuit and increases dopamine release in the nucleus accumbens (see Chapter 32). Alcohol affects local concentrations of serotonin, endorphin, endocannabinoid, and dopamine—neurotransmitters involved in the brain reward system. The discovery that naltrexone, a nonselective opioid receptor antagonist, helps patients who are recovering from alcoholism abstain from drinking supports the idea that a common neurochemical reward system is shared by very different drugs associated with physical and psychological dependence. There is also convincing evidence from animal models that ethanol intake and seeking behavior are reduced by antagonists of another important regulator of the brain reward system, the cannabinoid CB_1 receptor. Two other important neuroendocrine systems that appear to play key roles in modulating ethanol-seeking activity in experimental animals are the appetite-regulating system—which uses peptides such as leptin, ghrelin, and neuropeptide Y—and the stress response system, which is controlled by corticotropin-releasing factor.

2. *Neurotoxicity*—Consumption of large amounts of alcohol over extended periods (usually years) can lead to neurologic deficits. The most common neurologic abnormality in chronic alcoholism is generalized symmetric peripheral nerve injury, which begins with distal paresthesias of the hands and feet. Degenerative changes can also result in gait disturbances and ataxia. Other neurologic disturbances associated with alcoholism include dementia and, rarely, demyelinating disease.

Wernicke-Korsakoff syndrome is a relatively uncommon but important entity characterized by paralysis of the external eye muscles, ataxia, and a confused state that can progress to hallucinations, confabulations, coma, and death. It is associated with thiamine deficiency but is rarely seen in the absence of alcoholism, although reports of Wernicke-Korsakoff have been seen in patients with gastric bypass. Because of the importance of thiamine in this pathologic condition and the absence of toxicity associated with thiamine administration, all patients suspected of having Wernicke-Korsakoff syndrome (including virtually all patients who present to the emergency department with altered consciousness, seizures, or both) should receive thiamine therapy. Often, the ocular signs, ataxia, and confusion improve promptly upon administration of thiamine. However, most patients are left with a chronic disabling memory disorder known as Korsakoff psychosis.

Alcohol may also impair visual acuity, with painless blurring that occurs over several weeks of heavy alcohol consumption. Changes are usually bilateral and symmetric and may be followed by optic nerve degeneration. Ingestion of ethanol substitutes such as methanol (see section Pharmacology of Other Alcohols) causes severe visual disturbances.

C. Cardiovascular System

1. *Cardiomyopathy and heart failure*—Alcohol has complex effects on the cardiovascular system. Heavy alcohol consumption of long duration is associated with a dilated cardiomyopathy with ventricular hypertrophy and fibrosis. In animals and humans, alcohol causes cardiac membrane disruption, depressed function of mitochondria and sarcoplasmic reticulum, intracellular accumulation of phospholipids and fatty acids, as well as upregulation of voltage-gated calcium channels. There is evidence that patients with alcohol-induced dilated cardiomyopathy do significantly worse than patients with idiopathic dilated cardiomyopathy, even though cessation of drinking is associated with a reduction in cardiac size and improved function. The poorer prognosis for patients who continue to drink appears to be due in part to interference by ethanol with the beneficial effects of β blockers and angiotensin-converting enzyme (ACE) inhibitors.

2. *Arrhythmias*—Heavy drinking—and especially "binge" drinking—are associated with both atrial and ventricular arrhythmias. Patients undergoing alcohol withdrawal syndrome can develop severe arrhythmias that may reflect abnormalities of potassium or magnesium metabolism as well as enhanced release of catecholamines. Seizures, syncope, and sudden death during alcohol withdrawal may be due to these arrhythmias.

3. *Hypertension*—A link between heavier alcohol consumption (more than three drinks per day) and hypertension has been firmly established in epidemiologic studies. Alcohol is estimated to be responsible for approximately 5% of cases of hypertension, independent of obesity, salt intake, coffee drinking, and cigarette smoking. A reduction in alcohol intake appears to be effective in lowering blood pressure in hypertensive individuals who are also heavy drinkers; the hypertension seen in this population is also responsive to standard blood pressure medications.

4. *Coronary heart disease*—Although the deleterious effects of excessive alcohol use on the cardiovascular system are well established, there is strong epidemiologic evidence that *moderate* alcohol consumption actually *prevents* coronary heart disease (CHD), ischemic stroke, and peripheral arterial disease. This type of relationship between mortality and the dose of a drug is called a "J-shaped" relationship. Results of these clinical studies are supported by ethanol's ability to raise serum levels of high-density lipoprotein (HDL) cholesterol (the form of cholesterol that appears to protect against atherosclerosis; see Chapter 35), by its ability to inhibit some of the inflammatory processes that underlie atherosclerosis while also increasing production of the endogenous anticoagulant tissue plasminogen activator (t-PA, see Chapter 34), and by the presence in some alcoholic beverages such as red wine of antioxidants (eg, resveratrol, ellagic acid) and other substances that may protect against atherosclerosis. These observational studies are intriguing, but randomized clinical trials examining the possible benefit of moderate alcohol consumption in prevention of CHD have not been carried out.

D. Blood

Alcohol indirectly affects hematopoiesis through metabolic and nutritional effects and may also directly inhibit the proliferation of all cellular elements in bone marrow. The most common hematologic disorder seen in chronic drinkers is mild anemia resulting from alcohol-related folic acid deficiency. Iron-deficiency anemia may result from gastrointestinal bleeding. Alcohol has also been implicated as a cause of several hemolytic syndromes, some of which are associated with hyperlipidemia and severe liver disease.

E. Endocrine System and Electrolyte Balance

Chronic alcohol use has important effects on the endocrine system and on fluid and electrolyte balance. Clinical reports of gynecomastia and testicular atrophy in alcoholics with or without cirrhosis suggest a derangement in steroid hormone balance.

Individuals with chronic liver disease may have disorders of fluid and electrolyte balance, including ascites, edema, and effusions. Alterations of whole body potassium induced by vomiting and diarrhea, as well as severe secondary aldosteronism, may contribute to muscle weakness and can be worsened by diuretic therapy. The metabolic derangements caused by metabolism of large amounts of ethanol can result in hypoglycemia, as a result of impaired hepatic gluconeogenesis, and in ketosis, caused by excessive lipolytic factors, especially increased cortisol and growth hormone.

F. Fetal Alcohol Syndrome

Chronic maternal alcohol abuse during pregnancy is associated with teratogenic effects, and alcohol is a leading cause of mental retardation and congenital malformation. The abnormalities that have been characterized as fetal alcohol syndrome include (1) intrauterine growth retardation, (2) microcephaly, (3) poor coordination, (4) underdevelopment of midfacial region (appearing as a flattened face), and (5) minor joint anomalies. More severe cases may include congenital heart defects and mental retardation. Although the level of alcohol intake required to cause serious neurologic deficits appears quite high, the threshold for more subtle neurologic deficits is uncertain.

The mechanisms that underlie ethanol's teratogenic effects are unknown. Ethanol rapidly crosses the placenta and reaches concentrations in the fetus that are similar to those in maternal blood. The fetal liver has little or no alcohol dehydrogenase activity, so the fetus must rely on maternal and placental enzymes for elimination of alcohol.

The neuropathologic abnormalities seen in humans and in animal models of fetal alcohol syndrome indicate that ethanol triggers apoptotic neurodegeneration and also causes aberrant neuronal and glial migration in the developing nervous system. In tissue culture systems, ethanol causes a striking reduction in neurite outgrowth.

G. Immune System

The effects of alcohol on the immune system are complex; immune function in some tissues is inhibited (eg, the lung), whereas pathologic, hyperactive immune function in other tissues is triggered (eg, liver, pancreas). In addition, acute and chronic exposure to alcohol have widely different effects on immune function. The types of immunologic changes reported for the lung include suppression of the function of alveolar macrophages, inhibition of chemotaxis of granulocytes, and reduced number and function of T cells. In the liver, there is enhanced function of key cells of the innate immune system (eg, Kupffer cells, hepatic stellate cells) and increased cytokine production. In addition to the inflammatory damage that chronic heavy alcohol use precipitates in the liver and pancreas, it predisposes to infections, especially of the lung, and worsens the morbidity and increases the mortality risk of patients with pneumonia.

H. Increased Risk of Cancer

Chronic alcohol use increases the risk for cancer of the mouth, pharynx, larynx, esophagus, and liver. Evidence also points to a small increase in the risk of breast cancer in women. A threshold level for alcohol consumption as it relates to cancer has not been determined. Alcohol itself does not appear to be a carcinogen in most test systems. However, its primary metabolite, acetaldehyde, can damage DNA, as can the reactive oxygen species produced by increased cytochrome P450 activity. Other factors implicated in the link between alcohol and cancer include changes in folate metabolism and the growth-promoting effects of chronic inflammation.

Alcohol-Drug Interactions

Interactions between ethanol and other drugs can have important clinical effects resulting from alterations in the pharmacokinetics or pharmacodynamics of the second drug.

The most common pharmacokinetic alcohol-drug interactions stem from alcohol-induced increases of drug-metabolizing enzymes, as described in Chapter 4. Thus, prolonged intake of alcohol without damage to the liver can enhance the metabolic biotransformation of other drugs. Ethanol-mediated induction of hepatic cytochrome P450 enzymes is particularly important with regard to acetaminophen. Chronic consumption of three or more drinks per day increases the risk of hepatotoxicity due to toxic or even high therapeutic levels of acetaminophen as a result of increased P450-mediated conversion of acetaminophen to reactive hepatotoxic metabolites (see Figure 4–5). Current US Food and Drug Administration (FDA) regulations require that over-the-counter products containing acetaminophen carry a warning about the relation between ethanol consumption and acetaminophen-induced hepatotoxicity.

In contrast, *acute* alcohol use can inhibit metabolism of other drugs because of decreased enzyme activity or decreased liver blood flow. Phenothiazines, tricyclic antidepressants, and sedative-hypnotic drugs are the most important drugs that interact with alcohol by this pharmacokinetic mechanism.

Pharmacodynamic interactions also are of great clinical significance. The additive CNS depression that occurs when alcohol is combined with other CNS depressants, particularly sedative-hypnotics, is most important. Alcohol also potentiates the pharmacologic effects of many nonsedative drugs, including vasodilators and oral hypoglycemic agents.

■ CLINICAL PHARMACOLOGY OF ETHANOL

Alcohol is the cause of more preventable morbidity and mortality than all other drugs combined with the exception of tobacco. Epidemiologic studies indicate that for men under 65, risk is increased by consumption of more than four drinks on any single day or more than 14 drinks per average week; for women and for men over 65, risk is increased by consumption of more than three drinks on a single day or seven drinks per week. The search for specific etiologic factors or the identification of significant predisposing variables for alcohol abuse has led to disappointing results. Personality type, severe life stresses, psychiatric disorders, and parental role models are not reliable predictors of alcohol abuse. Although environmental factors clearly play a role, evidence suggests that there is a large genetic contribution to the development of alcoholism. Not surprisingly, polymorphisms in alcohol dehydrogenase and aldehyde dehydrogenase that lead to increased aldehyde accumulation and its associated facial flushing, nausea, and hypotension appear to protect against alcoholism. Much attention in genetic mapping experiments has focused on membrane-signaling proteins known to be affected by ethanol and on protein constituents of reward pathways in the brain. Polymorphisms associated with a relative insensitivity to alcohol and presumably thereby a greater risk of alcohol abuse have been identified in genes encoding an α subunit of the $GABA_A$ receptor, an M_2 muscarinic receptor, a serotonin transporter, adenylyl cyclase, and a potassium channel. The link between a polymorphism in an opioid receptor gene and a blunted response to naltrexone raises the possibility of genotype-guided pharmacotherapy for alcohol dependence.

MANAGEMENT OF ACUTE ALCOHOL INTOXICATION

Nontolerant individuals who consume alcohol in large quantities develop typical effects of acute sedative-hypnotic drug overdose along with the cardiovascular effects previously described (vasodilation, tachycardia) and gastrointestinal irritation. Since tolerance is not absolute, even individuals with chronic alcohol dependence may become severely intoxicated if sufficient alcohol is consumed.

The most important goals in the treatment of acute alcohol intoxication are to prevent severe respiratory depression and aspiration of vomitus. Even with very high blood ethanol levels, survival is probable as long as the respiratory and cardiovascular systems can be supported. The average blood alcohol concentration in fatal cases is above 400 mg/dL; however, the lethal dose of alcohol varies because of varying degrees of tolerance.

Electrolyte imbalances often need to be corrected, and metabolic alterations may require treatment of hypoglycemia and ketoacidosis by administration of **glucose. Thiamine** is given to protect against Wernicke-Korsakoff syndrome. Patients who are dehydrated and vomiting should also receive electrolyte solutions. If vomiting is severe, large amounts of potassium may be required as long as renal function is normal.

MANAGEMENT OF ALCOHOL WITHDRAWAL SYNDROME

Abrupt alcohol discontinuation in an individual with alcohol dependence leads to a characteristic syndrome of motor agitation, anxiety, insomnia, and reduction of seizure threshold. The severity of the syndrome is usually proportionate to the degree and duration of alcohol abuse. However, this can be greatly modified by the use of other sedatives as well as by associated factors (eg, diabetes, injury). In its mildest form, the alcohol withdrawal syndrome of increased pulse and blood pressure, tremor, anxiety, and insomnia occurs 6–8 hours after alcohol consumption is stopped (Figure 23–2). These effects usually lessen in 1–2 days, although some, such as anxiety and sleep disturbances, can be seen at decreasing levels for several months. In some patients, more severe acute reactions occur, with withdrawal seizures or alcoholic hallucinations during the first 1–5 days of withdrawal. Alcohol withdrawal is one of the most common causes of seizures in adults. Several days later, individuals can develop the syndrome of **delirium tremens,** which is characterized by delirium, agitation, autonomic nervous system instability, low-grade fever, and diaphoresis.

The major objective of drug therapy in the alcohol withdrawal period is prevention of seizures, delirium, and arrhythmias. Potassium, magnesium, and phosphate balance should be restored as rapidly as is consistent with renal function. Thiamine therapy is initiated in all cases. Individuals in mild alcohol withdrawal do not need any other pharmacologic assistance.

Specific drug treatment for detoxification in more severe cases involves two basic principles: substituting a long-acting sedative-hypnotic drug for alcohol and then gradually reducing ("tapering") the dose of the long-acting drug. Because of their wide margin of safety, benzodiazepines are preferred. Long-acting benzodiazepines, including **chlordiazepoxide** and **diazepam,** have the advantage of requiring less frequent dosing. Since their pharmacologically active metabolites are eliminated slowly, the long-acting drugs provide a built-in tapering effect. A disadvantage of the long-acting drugs is that they and their active metabolites may accumulate, especially in patients with compromised liver function. Shorter-acting drugs such as **lorazepam** and **oxazepam** are rapidly converted to inactive water-soluble metabolites that will not accumulate, and for this reason the short-acting drugs are especially useful in alcoholic patients with liver disease. Benzodiazepines can be administered orally in mild or moderate cases, or parenterally for patients with more severe withdrawal reactions.

After the alcohol withdrawal syndrome has been treated acutely, sedative-hypnotic medications must be tapered slowly

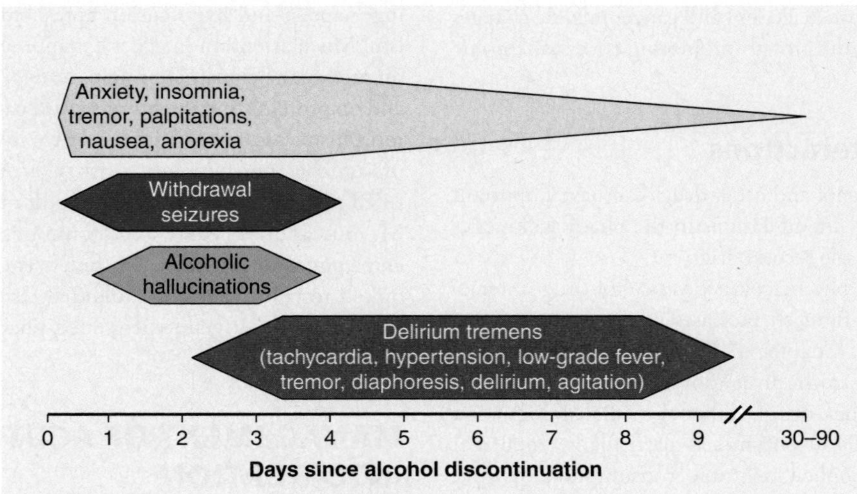

FIGURE 23–2 Time course of events during the alcohol withdrawal syndrome. The signs and symptoms that manifest earliest are anxiety, insomnia, tremor, palpitations, nausea, and anorexia as well as (in severe syndromes) hallucinations and seizures. Delirium tremens typically develops 48–72 hours after alcohol discontinuation. The earliest symptoms (anxiety, insomnia, etc) can persist, in a milder form, for several months after alcohol discontinuation.

over several weeks. Complete detoxification is not achieved with just a few days of alcohol abstinence. Several months may be required for restoration of normal nervous system function, especially sleep.

TREATMENT OF ALCOHOLISM

After detoxification, psychosocial therapy either in intensive inpatient or in outpatient rehabilitation programs serves as the primary treatment for alcohol dependence. Other psychiatric problems, most commonly depressive or anxiety disorders, often coexist with alcoholism and, if untreated, can contribute to the tendency of detoxified alcoholics to relapse. Treatment for these associated disorders with counseling and drugs can help decrease the rate of relapse for alcoholic patients.

Three drugs—naltrexone, acamprosate, and disulfiram—have FDA approval for adjunctive treatment of alcohol dependence.

Naltrexone

Naltrexone, a relatively long-acting opioid antagonist, blocks μ-opioid receptors (see Chapter 31). Alone and in combination with behavioral counseling, naltrexone has been shown in a number of short-term (12- to 16-week), placebo-controlled trials to reduce the rate of relapse to either drinking or alcohol dependence and to reduce craving for alcohol, especially in patients with high rates of naltrexone adherence. Naltrexone is approved by the FDA for treatment of alcohol dependence. Nalmefene, another opioid antagonist, appears to have similar effects in alcohol-use disorder but is not yet approved by the FDA for this indication.

Naltrexone is generally taken once a day in an oral dose of 50 mg for treatment of alcoholism. An extended-release formulation administered as an intramuscular injection once every 4 weeks also is effective. The drug can cause dose-dependent hepatotoxicity and should be used with caution in patients with elevated serum aminotransferase activity. The combination of naltrexone plus disulfiram should be avoided, since both drugs are potential hepatotoxins. Administration of naltrexone to patients who are physically dependent on opioids precipitates an acute withdrawal syndrome, so patients must be opioid-free before initiating naltrexone therapy. Naltrexone also blocks the therapeutic analgesic effects of usual doses of opioids.

Acamprosate

Acamprosate has been used in Europe for a number of years to treat alcohol dependence and is approved for this use by the FDA. Like ethanol, acamprosate has many molecular effects including actions on GABA, glutamate, serotonin, noradrenergic, and dopamine receptors. Probably its best-characterized actions are as a weak NMDA-receptor antagonist and a $GABA_A$-receptor activator. In European clinical trials, acamprosate reduced short-term and long-term (more than 6 months) relapse rates when combined with psychotherapy. However, in a large American trial that compared acamprosate with naltrexone and with combined acamprosate and naltrexone therapy (the COMBINE study), acamprosate did not show a statistically significant effect alone or in combination with naltrexone.

Acamprosate is administered as one or two enteric-coated 333-mg tablets three times daily. It is poorly absorbed, and food reduces its absorption even further. Acamprosate is widely distributed and is eliminated renally. It does not appear to participate in drug-drug interactions. The most common adverse effects are gastrointestinal (nausea, vomiting, diarrhea) and rash. It should not be used in patients with severe renal impairment.

Disulfiram

Disulfiram acts by inhibiting aldehyde dehydrogenase. Alcohol is metabolized as usual, but acetaldehyde accumulates. Thus, disulfiram causes extreme discomfort in patients who drink alcoholic beverages. Disulfiram alone has little effect, but flushing, throbbing headache, nausea, vomiting, sweating, hypotension, and confusion occur within a few minutes after an individual taking disulfiram drinks alcohol. The effects may last 30 minutes in mild cases or several hours in severe ones. Because adherence to disulfiram therapy is low and because evidence from clinical trials for its effectiveness is weak, disulfiram is no longer commonly used.

Disulfiram is rapidly and completely absorbed from the gastrointestinal tract; however, a period of 12 hours is required for its full action. Its elimination is slow, and its action may persist for several days after the last dose. The drug inhibits the metabolism of many other therapeutic agents, including phenytoin, oral anticoagulants, and isoniazid. It should not be administered with medications that contain alcohol, including nonprescription medications such as those listed in Table 64–3. Disulfiram can cause small increases in hepatic transaminases. Its safety in pregnancy has not been demonstrated.

Other Drugs

Several other drugs have shown efficacy in maintaining abstinence and reducing craving in chronic alcoholism, although none has FDA approval yet for this use. Such drugs include antiseizure agents (topiramate, gabapentin, and valproate, see Chapter 24); and baclofen, a $GABA_B$ receptor agonist used as a spasmolytic (see Chapter 27). Studies of varenicline (see Chapter 7) indicate that this nicotinic agonist drug can reduce binge drinking in mice. Clinical trials of selective serotonin reuptake inhibitors (SSRIs, see Chapter 30) and ondansetron, a 5-HT_3 antagonist (see Chapter 62) yielded negative results overall, but suggested that these agents may have benefits in certain subgroups of patients. Based on evidence from model systems, efforts are under way to explore agents that modulate cannabinoid CB_1 receptors, corticotropin-releasing factor receptors, and GABA receptor systems, as well as several other possible targets. Rimonabant, a CB_1 receptor antagonist, has been shown to suppress alcohol-related behaviors in animal models and is being tested in clinical trials of alcoholism. Cannabidiol (CBD) and spironolactone also have had recent positive studies in animal models as well as in clinical trials.

PHARMACOLOGY OF OTHER ALCOHOLS

Other alcohols related to ethanol have wide applications as industrial solvents and occasionally cause severe poisoning. Of these, **methanol** and **ethylene glycol** are two of the most common causes of intoxication. **Isopropyl alcohol** (isopropanol, rubbing alcohol) is another alcohol that is sometimes ingested when ethanol is not available. It produces coma and gastrointestinal irritation, nausea, and vomiting, but is not usually associated with retinal or renal injury.

METHANOL

Methanol (methyl alcohol, wood alcohol) is widely used in the industrial production of synthetic organic compounds and as a constituent of many commercial solvents. In the home, methanol is most frequently found in the form of "canned heat" or in windshield-washing products. Poisonings occur from accidental ingestion of methanol-containing products or when it is misguidedly ingested as an ethanol substitute.

Methanol can be absorbed through the skin or from the respiratory or gastrointestinal tract and is then distributed in body water. The primary mechanism of elimination of methanol in humans is by oxidation to formaldehyde, formic acid, and CO_2 (Figure 23–3).

Animal species show great variability in mean lethal doses of methanol. The special susceptibility of humans to methanol toxicity is due to metabolism to formate and formaldehyde, not due to methanol itself. Since the conversion of methanol to its toxic metabolites is relatively slow, there is often a delay of 6–30 hours before the appearance of severe toxicity.

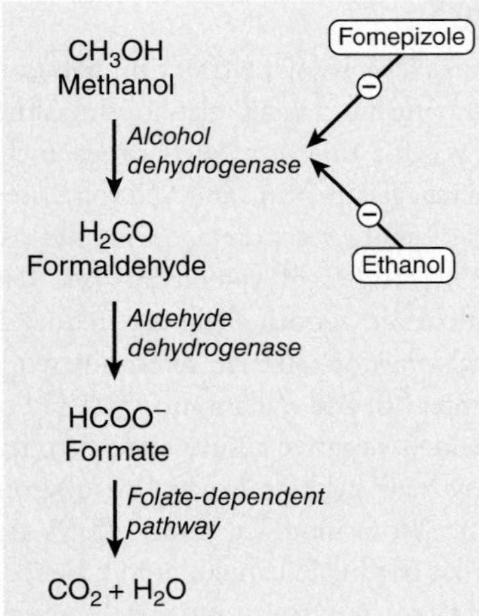

FIGURE 23–3 Methanol is converted to the toxic metabolites formaldehyde and formate by alcohol dehydrogenase and aldehyde dehydrogenase. By inhibiting alcohol dehydrogenase, fomepizole and ethanol reduce the formation of toxic metabolites.

Physical findings in early methanol poisoning are generally nonspecific, such as inebriation, gastritis, and an elevated osmolar gap (see Chapter 58). In severe cases, the odor of formaldehyde may be present on the breath or in the urine. After a delay, the most characteristic symptom in methanol poisoning—visual disturbance—occurs along with anion gap metabolic acidosis. The visual disturbance is frequently described as "like being in a snowstorm" and can progress to blindness. Changes in the retina may sometimes be detected on examination, but these are usually late. The development of bradycardia, prolonged coma, seizures, and resistant acidosis all imply a poor prognosis. The cause of death in fatal cases is sudden cessation of respiration. A serum methanol concentration higher than 20 mg/dL warrants treatment, and a concentration higher than 50 mg/dL is considered serious enough to require hemodialysis. Serum formate levels are a better indication of clinical pathology but are not widely available.

The first treatment for methanol poisoning, as in all critical poisoning situations, is support of respiration. There are three specific modalities of treatment for severe methanol poisoning: suppression of metabolism by alcohol dehydrogenase to toxic products, hemodialysis to enhance removal of methanol and its toxic products, and alkalinization to counteract metabolic acidosis.

The enzyme chiefly responsible for methanol oxidation in the liver is alcohol dehydrogenase (see Figure 23–3). **Fomepizole,** an alcohol dehydrogenase inhibitor, is approved for the treatment of methanol and ethylene glycol poisoning. It is administered intravenously in a loading dose of 15 mg/kg followed by 10 mg/kg every 12 hours for 48 hours and then 15 mg/kg every 12 hours thereafter until the serum methanol level falls below 20–30 mg/dL. The dosage increase after 48 hours is based on evidence that fomepizole rapidly induces its own metabolism by the cytochrome P450 system. Patients undergoing hemodialysis are given fomepizole more frequently (6 hours after the loading dose and every 4 hours thereafter). Fomepizole appears to be safe during the short time it is administered for treatment of methanol or ethylene glycol poisoning. The most common adverse effects are burning at the infusion site, headache, nausea, and dizziness. Intravenous ethanol is an alternative to fomepizole. It has a higher affinity than methanol for alcohol dehydrogenase; thus, saturation of the enzyme with ethanol reduces formate production. Ethanol is used intravenously as treatment for methanol and ethylene glycol poisoning. The dose-dependent characteristics of ethanol metabolism and the variability of ethanol metabolism require frequent monitoring of blood ethanol levels to ensure appropriate alcohol concentration.

In cases of severe poisoning, hemodialysis (discussed in Chapter 58) can be used to eliminate both methanol and formate from the blood. Two other measures are commonly taken. Because of profound metabolic acidosis in methanol poisoning, treatment with bicarbonate often is necessary. Since folate-dependent systems are responsible for the oxidation of formic acid to CO_2 in humans (see Figure 23–3), folinic and folic acid are often administered to patients poisoned with methanol, although this has never been fully tested in clinical studies.

ETHYLENE GLYCOL

Polyhydric alcohols such as ethylene glycol (CH_2OHCH_2OH) are used as heat exchangers, in antifreeze formulations, and as industrial solvents. Young children and animals are sometimes attracted by the sweet taste of ethylene glycol and, rarely, it is ingested intentionally as an ethanol substitute or in attempted suicide. Although ethylene glycol itself is relatively harmless and eliminated by the kidney, it is metabolized to toxic aldehydes and oxalate.

Three stages of ethylene glycol overdose occur. Within the first few hours after ingestion, there is transient excitation followed by CNS depression. After a delay of 4–12 hours, severe metabolic acidosis develops from accumulation of acid metabolites and lactate. Finally, deposition of oxalate crystals in renal tubules occurs, followed by delayed renal insufficiency. The key to the diagnosis of ethylene glycol poisoning is recognition of anion gap acidosis, osmolar gap, and oxalate crystals in the urine in a patient without visual symptoms.

As with methanol poisoning, early fomepizole is the standard treatment for ethylene glycol poisoning. Intravenous treatment with fomepizole is initiated immediately, as described above for methanol poisoning, and continued until the patient's serum ethylene glycol concentration drops below a toxic threshold (20–30 mg/dL). Intravenous ethanol is an alternative to fomepizole in ethylene glycol poisoning. Hemodialysis effectively removes ethylene glycol and its toxic metabolites and is recommended for patients with a serum ethylene glycol concentration above 50 mg/dL, significant metabolic acidosis, and significant renal impairment. Fomepizole has reduced the need for hemodialysis, especially in patients with less severe acidosis and intact renal function.

SUMMARY The Alcohols and Associated Drugs

Subclass, Drug	Mechanism of Action, Effects	Clinical Applications	Pharmacokinetics, Toxicities, Interactions
ALCOHOLS			
• Ethanol	Multiple effects on neurotransmitter receptors, ion channels, and signaling pathways	Antidote in methanol and ethylene glycol poisoning; topical antiseptic	Zero-order metabolism • duration depends on dose • *Toxicity:* Acutely, central nervous system depression and respiratory failure • chronically, damage to many systems, including liver, pancreas, gastrointestinal tract, and central and peripheral nervous systems • *Interactions:* Induces CYP2E1 • increased conversion of acetaminophen to toxic metabolite
• *Methanol: Poisonings result in toxic levels of formate, which causes characteristic visual disturbance plus coma, seizures, acidosis, and death due to respiratory failure*			
• *Ethylene glycol: Poisoning creates toxic aldehydes and oxalate, which causes kidney damage and severe acidosis*			
DRUGS USED IN ACUTE ETHANOL WITHDRAWAL			
• Benzodiazepines (eg, chlordiazepoxide, diazepam, lorazepam)	BDZ receptor agonists that facilitate GABA-mediated activation of $GABA_A$ receptors	Prevention and treatment of acute ethanol withdrawal syndrome	See Chapter 22
• Thiamine (vitamin B_1)	Essential vitamin required for synthesis of the coenzyme thiamine pyrophosphate	Administered to patients suspected of having alcoholism (those exhibiting acute alcohol intoxication or alcohol withdrawal syndrome) to prevent Wernicke-Korsakoff syndrome	Administered parenterally • *Toxicity:* None • *Interactions:* None
DRUGS USED IN CHRONIC ALCOHOLISM			
• Naltrexone	Nonselective competitive antagonist of opioid receptors	Reduced risk of relapse in individuals with alcoholism	Available as an oral or long-acting parenteral formulation • *Toxicity:* GI effects and liver toxicity; will precipitate a withdrawal reaction in individuals physically dependent on opioids and will prevent the analgesic effect of opioids
• Acamprosate	Poorly understood NMDA receptor antagonist and $GABA_A$ agonist effects	Reduced risk of relapse in individuals with alcoholism	*Toxicity:* GI effects and rash
• Disulfiram	Inhibits aldehyde dehydrogenase, resulting in aldehyde accumulation during ethanol ingestion	Deterrent to drinking in individuals with alcohol dependence; rarely used	*Toxicity:* Little effect alone but severe and potentially dangerous flushing, headache, nausea, vomiting, and hypotension when combined with ethanol

(*continued*)

Subclass, Drug	Mechanism of Action, Effects	Clinical Applications	Pharmacokinetics, Toxicities, Interactions
DRUGS USED IN ACUTE METHANOL OR ETHYLENE GLYCOL TOXICITY			
• Fomepizole	Inhibits alcohol dehydrogenase, prevents conversion of methanol and ethylene glycol to toxic metabolites	Methanol and ethylene glycol poisoning	Orphan drug • *Toxicity:* Headache, nausea, dizziness, rare allergic reactions
• *Ethanol: Higher affinity than methanol or ethylene glycol for alcohol dehydrogenase; used to reduce metabolism of methanol and ethylene glycol to toxic products*			

PREPARATIONS AVAILABLE

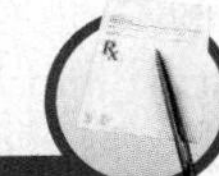

GENERIC NAME	AVAILABLE AS
DRUGS FOR THE TREATMENT OF ACUTE ALCOHOL WITHDRAWAL SYNDROME (SEE ALSO CHAPTER 22 FOR OTHER BENZODIAZEPINES)	
Chlordiazepoxide HCl	Generic, Librium
Diazepam	Generic, Valium
Lorazepam	Generic, Ativan
Oxazepam	Generic, Serax
Thiamine HCl	Generic
DRUGS FOR THE PREVENTION OF ALCOHOL ABUSE	
Acamprosate calcium	Generic, Campral
Disulfiram	Generic, Antabuse
Naltrexone HCl	Generic, Vivitrol, ReVia
DRUGS FOR THE TREATMENT OF ACUTE METHANOL OR ETHYLENE GLYCOL POISONING	
Ethanol	Generic
Fomepizole	Generic, Antizol

REFERENCES

Anton RF: Naltrexone for the management of alcohol dependence. N Engl J Med 2008;359:715.

Anton RF et al: Combined pharmacotherapies and behavioral interventions for alcohol dependence: The COMBINE study: A randomized controlled trial. JAMA 2006;295:2003.

Brent J: Fomepizole for ethylene glycol and methanol poisoning. N Engl J Med 2009;360:2216.

Brodie MS et al: Ethanol interactions with calcium-dependent potassium channels. Alcohol Clin Exp Res 2007;31:1625.

Centers for Disease Control and Prevention: Fetal alcohol spectrum disorder. https://www.cdc.gov/ncbddd/fasd/

Chan LN, Anderson GD: Pharmacokinetic and pharmacodynamics interactions with ethanol (alcohol). Clin Pharmacokinet 2014;53:1115.

Chen YC et al: Polymorphism of ethanol-metabolism genes and alcoholism: Correlation of allelic variations with the pharmacokinetic and pharmacodynamic consequences. Chem Biol Interact 2009;178:2.

Colombo G et al: The cannabinoid CB1 receptor antagonist, rimonabant, as a promising pharmacotherapy for alcohol dependence: Preclinical evidence. Mol Neurobiol 2007;36:102.

Crabbe JC et al: Alcohol-related genes: Contributions from studies with genetically engineered mice. Addict Biol 2006;11:195.

Edenberg HJ: The genetics of alcohol metabolism: Role of alcohol dehydrogenase and aldehyde dehydrogenase variants. Alcohol Res Health 2007;30:5.

Farokhnia M et al: Spironolactone as a potential new pharmacotherapy for alcohol use disorder: convergent evidence from rodent and human studies. Mol Psychiatry 2022;27:4642.

Hendricson AW et al: Aberrant synaptic activation of N-methyl-D-aspartate receptors underlies ethanol withdrawal hyperexcitability. J Pharmacol Exp Ther 2007;321:60.

Johnson BA: Pharmacotherapy for alcohol use disorder. In: Saitz R (editor): UpToDate. Waltham, MA. http://www.uptodate.com/contents/pharmacotherapy-for-alcohol-use-disorder

Johnson BA: Update on neuropharmacological treatments for alcoholism: Scientific basis and clinical findings. Biochem Pharmacol 2008;75:34.

Jonas DE et al: Pharmacotherapy for adults with alcohol use disorders in outpatient settings. A systematic review and meta-analysis. JAMA 2014;311:1889.

Karoly HC: Cannabinoids and the microbiota-gut-brain axis: emerging effects of cannabidiol and potential applications to alcohol use disorders. Alcohol Clin Exp Res 2020;44:340.

Klatsky AL: Alcohol and cardiovascular diseases. Expert Rev Cardiovasc Ther 2009;7:499.

Kraut JA, Mullins ME: Toxic alcohols. N Engl J Med 2018;378:270.

Lepik KJ et al: Adverse drug events associated with the antidotes for methanol and ethylene glycol poisoning: A comparison of ethanol and fomepizole. Ann Emerg Med 2009;53:439.

Lobo IA, Harris RA: GABA(A) receptors and alcohol. Pharmacol Biochem Behav 2008;90:90.

Mann K et al: Acamprosate: Recent findings and future research directions. Alcohol Clin Exp Res 2008;32:1105.

Mayfield RD et al: Genetic factors influencing alcohol dependence. Br J Pharmacol 2008;154:275.

Mitchell JM: Varenicline decreases alcohol consumption in heavy-drinking smokers. Psychopharmacology (Berl) 2012;223:299.

National Institutes of Health: National Institute on Alcohol Abuse and Alcoholism. http://www.niaaa.nih.gov/

O'Keefe JH et al: Alcohol and cardiovascular health: The razor-sharp double-edged sword. J Am Coll Cardiol 2007:50:1009.

Olson KR et al (editors): *Poisoning and Drug Overdose*, 8th ed. McGraw Hill, 2021.

Patkar OL et al: The effect of varenicline on binge-like ethanol consumption in mice is β4 nicotinic acetylcholine receptor-independent. Neurosci Lett 2016;633:235.

Prescriber's Letter: Alcohol and drug interactions. Chart 351106. Prescribers Lett 2019:26:64.

Qiang M et al: Chronic intermittent ethanol treatment selectively alters N-methyl-D-aspartate receptor subunit surface expression in cultured cortical neurons. Mol Pharmacol 2007;72:95.

Saitz R: Medications for alcohol use disorder and predicting severe withdrawal. JAMA 2018;320:766.

Seitz HK, Stickel F: Molecular mechanisms of alcohol-mediated carcinogenesis. Nat Rev Cancer 2007;7:599.

Srisurapanont M, Jarusuraisin N: Opioid antagonists for alcohol dependence. Cochrane Database Syst Rev 2005;1:CD001867.

Wolf FW, Heberlein U: Invertebrate models of drug abuse. J Neurobiol 2003;54:161.

CASE STUDY ANSWER

This young man exhibited classic signs and symptoms of acute alcohol poisoning, which is confirmed by the blood alcohol concentration. We do not know from the case whether the patient was tolerant to the effects of alcohol but note that his blood alcohol concentration was in the lethal range for a non-tolerant individual. Death most likely resulted from respiratory and cardiovascular collapse prior to medical treatment, complicated by a chemical pneumonitis secondary to aspiration of vomitus. The treatment of acute alcohol poisoning includes standard supportive care of airway, breathing, and circulation ("ABCs," see Chapter 58). Most importantly, the trachea would be intubated, vomitus removed, and mechanical ventilation begun. Intravenous access would be obtained and used to administer dextrose and thiamine, as well as electrolytes and vitamins. If a young, previously healthy individual receives medical care in time, supportive care will most likely be highly effective. As the patient recovers, it is important to be vigilant for signs and symptoms of the alcohol withdrawal syndrome. (For a case involving chronic alcoholism and withdrawal management, see Nejad SH et al: Case 39-2012: A man with alcoholism, recurrent seizures, and agitation. N Engl J Med 2013; 368:1163.)

CHAPTER

24 Antiseizure Medications

Michael A. Rogawski, MD, PhD

CASE STUDY

A 23-year-old woman presents for consultation regarding her antiseizure medications. Seven years ago, this otherwise healthy young woman had a tonic-clonic seizure at home. She was rushed to the emergency department, at which time she was alert but complained of headache. A consulting neurologist prescribed levetiracetam 500 mg bid. Four days later, electroencephalography (EEG) showed rare right temporal sharp waves. Magnetic resonance imaging (MRI) was normal. One year after this episode, a repeat EEG was unchanged, and levetiracetam was increased to 1000 mg bid. The patient had no adverse effects at this dose. At age 21, she had a second tonic-clonic seizure while in college. Discussion with her roommate at that time revealed that she had had two recent episodes of 1–2 minutes of altered consciousness with lip smacking (*focal impaired awareness seizure*, formerly *complex partial seizure*). A repeat EEG showed occasional right temporal spikes. What is one possible strategy for controlling her present symptoms?

Epilepsy is a chronic disorder of brain function characterized by the recurrent and unpredictable occurrence of seizures. Approximately 1% of the world's population has epilepsy, which is the fourth most common neurologic disorder after migraine, stroke, and Alzheimer disease. Seizures that occur in people with epilepsy are transitory alterations in behavior, sensation, or consciousness caused by an abnormal, synchronized electrical discharge in the brain. Many cases of epilepsy are the result of damage to the brain, as occurs in traumatic brain injury, stroke, or infections, whereas in other cases, the epilepsy is caused by a brain tumor or developmental lesion such as a cortical or vascular malformation; these epilepsies are referred to as *symptomatic*. In other cases, genetic factors are believed to be the root cause. In most cases, the inheritance is complex (oligogenic or polygenic); rarely, a single gene defect can be identified. Genetic epilepsies in which seizures are the only clinical manifestation and there is no identifiable structural or metabolic abnormality have been called *idiopathic*. The term idiopathic generalized epilepsy (IGE) was used in conjunction with generalized epilepsies with bilateral EEG discharges including childhood absence epilepsy, juvenile myoclonic epilepsy, juvenile absence epilepsy, and generalized tonic-clonic seizures alone (formerly generalized tonic-clonic seizures on awakening). These syndromes now fall under the genetic generalized epilepsy (GGE) category, but the term idiopathic generalized epilepsy may still be applied. The most severe and intractable forms of epilepsy have associated developmental and intellectual disabilities and are referred to as developmental and epileptic encephalopathies (DEEs). In some cases, the DEE is acquired. Hypoxic-ischemic encephalopathy, perinatal stroke, infections, or trauma are causes. In other circumstances the DEE is a component of a genetic syndrome, such as tuberous sclerosis complex (TSC), that has other associated structural or metabolic brain abnormalities. Other prominent DEEs include Lennox-Gastaut syndrome (multiple etiologies), Dravet syndrome (mutations in the *SCN1A* gene in ~85% of patients), CDKL5 deficiency disorder (mutations in the *CDKL5* gene), PCDH19 clustering epilepsy (mutations in the *PCDH19* gene), GLUT1 deficiency syndrome (mutations the *SLC2A* glucose transporter gene), and infantile spasms (West syndrome; multiple etiologies).

The antiseizure medications discussed in this chapter are usually used chronically to prevent the occurrence of seizures in people with epilepsy. These medications are also, on occasion, used in people who do not have epilepsy—to prevent seizures that may occur as part of an acute illness such as meningitis or in the early period following neurosurgery or traumatic brain injury. In addition, certain antiseizure medications are used to manage bouts of increased seizure frequency (referred to as *acute repetitive seizures* or *seizure clusters*) or to terminate ongoing seizures such as in status epilepticus, prolonged febrile seizures, or neonatal seizures or following exposure to seizure-inducing nerve toxins. Seizures are occasionally caused by an acute underlying toxic or metabolic disorder, such as hypocalcemia, in which case appropriate therapy should be directed toward correcting the specific abnormality.

CLASSIFICATION OF SEIZURES

Epileptic seizures are classified into two main categories: (1) *focal onset seizures* (in the past called "partial" or "partial-onset" seizures), which begin in a local cortical site, and (2) *generalized onset seizures*, which involve both brain hemispheres from the onset (Table 24–1). *Focal seizures* can transition to *bilateral tonic-clonic seizures* (formerly called "secondarily generalized"). *Focal aware seizures* (previously "simple partial seizures") have preservation of consciousness; *focal impaired awareness seizures* (formerly "complex partial seizures") have impaired consciousness. *Tonic-clonic convulsions* (previously termed "grand mal") are what most people typically think of as a seizure: the person loses consciousness, falls, stiffens (the tonic phase), and jerks (clonic phase). Tonic-clonic convulsions usually last for less than 3 minutes but are followed by confusion and tiredness of variable duration ("postictal period"). *Generalized tonic-clonic seizures* involve both hemispheres from the onset; they occur in patients with idiopathic (genetic) generalized epilepsies, in some classifications referred to as genetic generalized epilepsies, and have been referred to as primary generalized tonic-clonic seizures. *Generalized absence seizures* (formerly called "petit mal") are brief episodes of unconsciousness (4–20 seconds, usually <10 seconds) with no warning and immediate resumption of consciousness (no postictal abnormality). Generalized absence seizures (typical absence seizures) most commonly occur in children with childhood absence epilepsy, which begins between 4 and 10 years (usually 5–7 years) and mostly remits by age 12. The major seizure type in infantile spasms is the epileptic spasm, which consists of a sudden flexion, extension, or mixed extension-flexion of predominantly proximal and truncal muscles. Limited forms, such as grimacing, head nodding, or subtle eye movements, can occur. Myoclonic seizures are sudden, brief (<100 milliseconds), involuntary, single or multiple contractions of muscles or muscle groups of variable topography (axial, proximal limb, distal limb). Myoclonus is less regularly repetitive and less sustained than is clonus. Atypical absences are distinct from typical absences in that they occur in DEEs such as Lennox-Gastaut syndrome; loss of awareness begins and ends less abruptly than in typical absence seizures. Atonic seizures (drop attacks), which mainly occur in the Lennox-Gastaut syndrome, are characterized by sudden loss of muscle tone, often causing a forward fall.

TABLE 24–1 International League Against Epilepsy classification of seizure types.

Focal onset (formerly *partial onset*) seizures
Focal aware seizure (formerly *simple partial seizure*)
Focal impaired awareness seizure (formerly *complex partial seizure*)
Focal-to-bilateral tonic-clonic seizure (formerly *partial seizure secondarily generalized* or *grand mal seizure*)
Generalized onset seizures
Generalized tonic-clonic seizure (formerly *primary generalized tonic-clonic seizure* or *grand mal seizure*)
Generalized absence seizure (formerly *petit mal seizure*; occurs, for example, in absence epilepsy; atypical absence seizures occur in epileptic encephalopathies such as the Lennox-Gastaut syndrome)
Myoclonic seizure (occurs, for example, in juvenile myoclonic epilepsy and Dravet syndrome)
Atonic seizure (*drop seizure* or *astatic seizure*; occurs, for example, in the Lennox-Gastaut syndrome)
Epileptic spasms (as in infantile spasms also known as West syndrome)

Lennox-Gastaut syndrome, Dravet syndrome, and juvenile myoclonic epilepsy are epilepsy syndromes in which there are multiple different seizure types.

TREATMENT OF EPILEPSY

Antiseizure medications used in the chronic treatment of epilepsy are administered orally; the objective is to prevent the occurrence of seizures. The choice of medication depends either on the type of seizures that the patient exhibits or on the patient's syndromic classification. Appropriately chosen antiseizure medications provide adequate seizure control in about two-thirds of patients. In designing a therapeutic strategy, the use of a single medication is preferred, especially in patients who are not severely affected; such patients can benefit from the advantage of fewer adverse effects with monotherapy. For patients with hard-to-control seizures, multiple medications are usually used simultaneously. Patients who do not achieve seizure control following adequate trials with two or more appropriate medications are considered "pharmacoresistant." The basis for pharmacoresistance is not well understood. DEEs—such as Lennox-Gastaut syndrome, early infantile developmental and epileptic encephalopathy (EIDEE; Ohtahara syndrome), infantile spasms, and Dravet syndrome as well as other etiology-specific DEEs such as CDKL5 deficiency disorder—are difficult to treat with medications. Focal seizures also may be refractory to medications. In some cases, the epilepsy can be cured by surgical resection of the affected brain region. The most commonly performed epilepsy surgery is temporal lobe resection for mesial temporal lobe epilepsy; extratemporal cortical resection, when indicated, is less successful. When seizures arise from cortical injury, malformation, tumor, or a vascular lesion, lesionectomy may be curative. In addition to medications and surgery, several electrical stimulation devices are used in the treatment of epilepsy. The vagus nerve stimulator (VNS) is an implanted programmable pulse generator with a helical electrode that is wrapped around the left vagus nerve in the neck. The device, which continuously delivers open-loop stimulation according to a duty cycle, is approved for the treatment of drug-refractory focal seizures but may also be a good option for symptomatic (or cryptogenic) generalized epilepsies of the Lennox-Gastaut type, including those with intractable atonic seizures. Another device for the treatment of medically refractory focal epilepsy is the responsive neurostimulator (RNS).

The RNS is an implanted closed-loop system that detects a pattern of abnormal electrical activity in the seizure focus and then delivers electrical stimulation to prevent seizure occurrence. Deep brain stimulation (DBS) via an implanted device that applies bilateral open-loop stimulation to the anterior nuclei of the thalamus is the third brain stimulation modality approved for epilepsy therapy. DBS is indicated as adjunctive therapy to medications for reducing the frequency of seizures in epilepsy characterized by focal seizures, with or without secondary generalization (focal-to-bilateral tonic-clonic). While not currently approved, stimulation in other targets such as the centromedian nucleus of the thalamus may be more effective for generalized seizures and Lennox-Gastaut syndrome. Dietary therapies, most notably ketogenic diets that are high in fat, low in carbohydrate, and that control protein intake, may be effective in refractory epilepsy. Such dietary therapies are particularly beneficial in myoclonic epilepsies, infantile spasms, Dravet syndrome, and seizures associated with tuberous sclerosis complex, and are the recommended first-line treatment GLUT1 deficiency syndrome (De Vivo disease), associated with impaired transport of glucose into the brain. Ketogenic diets are most commonly used in children but adults may also benefit.

MECHANISMS OF ACTION

Antiseizure medications protect against seizures by interacting with one or more molecular targets in the brain. The ultimate effect of these interactions is to inhibit the local generation of seizure discharges, both by reducing the ability of neurons to fire action potentials at high rate and by reducing neuronal synchronization. In addition, antiseizure medications inhibit the spread of epileptic activity to nearby and distant sites, either by strengthening the inhibitory surround mediated by GABAergic interneurons or by reducing glutamate-mediated excitatory neurotransmission (the means through which a presynaptic neuron depolarizes and excites a postsynaptic follower neuron). The specific actions of antiseizure medications on their targets are broadly described as (1) modulation of voltage-gated sodium, calcium, or potassium channels; (2) enhancement of fast GABA-mediated synaptic inhibition; (3) modification of synaptic release processes; and (4) diminution of fast glutamate-mediated excitation. These actions can be viewed in the context of the balance between excitation mediated by glutamatergic neurons and inhibition mediated by GABAergic neurons. A propensity for seizure generation occurs when there is an imbalance favoring excitation over inhibition, which can result from either excessive excitation or diminished inhibition or both. Treatments, therefore, that either inhibit excitation or enhance inhibition have antiseizure actions to reduce seizure generation. Inhibition of excitation can be produced by effects on intrinsic excitability mechanisms in excitatory neurons (eg, sodium channel blockers) or on excitatory synaptic transmission (eg, modification of release of the excitatory neurotransmitter glutamate; AMPA receptor antagonists). Enhancement of inhibition is produced by increased activation of $GABA_A$ receptors, the mediators of inhibition in cortical areas relevant to seizures. Some drug treatments (eg, benzodiazepines, phenobarbital, ganaxolone) act as positive allosteric modulators of $GABA_A$ receptors, whereas others (eg, tiagabine, vigabatrin) lead to increased availability of neurotransmitter GABA. Voltage-gated potassium channels of the K_v7 type also serve as an inhibitory influence on epileptiform activity. Retigabine (ezogabine), an opener of K_v7 channels, exerts a unique antiseizure action by virtue of its ability to enhance the natural inhibitory influence of these channels. The specific sites at excitatory and inhibitory neurons and synapses where currently available antiseizure medications act to exert these diverse actions are illustrated in Figure 24–1. Instead of affecting mechanisms of seizure generation, a more specific approach for the treatment of epilepsy would be to target mechanisms of disease pathology, thus reducing or eliminating seizures and possibly also associated comorbidities. At present, this strategy has been successful only in tuberous sclerosis complex, an inherited neurocutaneous disorder that is characterized by hamartomatous lesions involving many organ systems, including the brain. Seizures, most commonly infantile spasms, often begin in the first year of life, but there also can be focal onset seizures and less commonly generalized onset seizures. Everolimus, a rapalog (analog of rapamycin) that reverses pathological mTOR signaling, reduces seizures in tuberous sclerosis. Table 24–2 lists the various targets at which currently available antiseizure medications are thought to act and the medications that act on those targets. For some drugs, there is no consensus as to the specific molecular target (eg, valproate, zonisamide, rufinamide) or there may be multiple targets (eg, topiramate, felbamate, cenobamate).

PHARMACOKINETICS

Chronic antiseizure medication administration prevents the occurrence of seizures, which can, on occasion, be life threatening. Therefore, adequate drug exposure must be continuously maintained. However, many antiseizure medications also have a narrow therapeutic window; dosing must therefore avoid excessive, toxic exposure. An understanding of the pharmacokinetic properties of the drugs is essential. It is also necessary for the clinician to be cognizant of special factors that affect dosing; these factors include nonlinear relationships between dose and drug exposure and the influence of hepatic or renal impairment on clearance (see Chapters 3 and 4). Further, drug-drug interactions occur with many of the agents—a special issue since the drugs are often used in combination. For some antiseizure medications, drug-drug interactions are complex (see Chapter 67). For example, addition of a new drug may affect the clearance of the current drug such that the dose of the current drug must be modified. Further, the current drug may necessitate selection of a dosing regimen for the new drug that is different from dosing in a drug-naïve subject. Many antiseizure medications are metabolized by hepatic enzymes, and some, such as carbamazepine, oxcarbazepine, eslicarbazepine acetate, phenobarbital, phenytoin, and primidone, are strong inducers of hepatic cytochrome P450 and glucuronyl transferase enzymes. A new antiseizure drug may increase the concentration of an existing drug by inhibiting its metabolism;

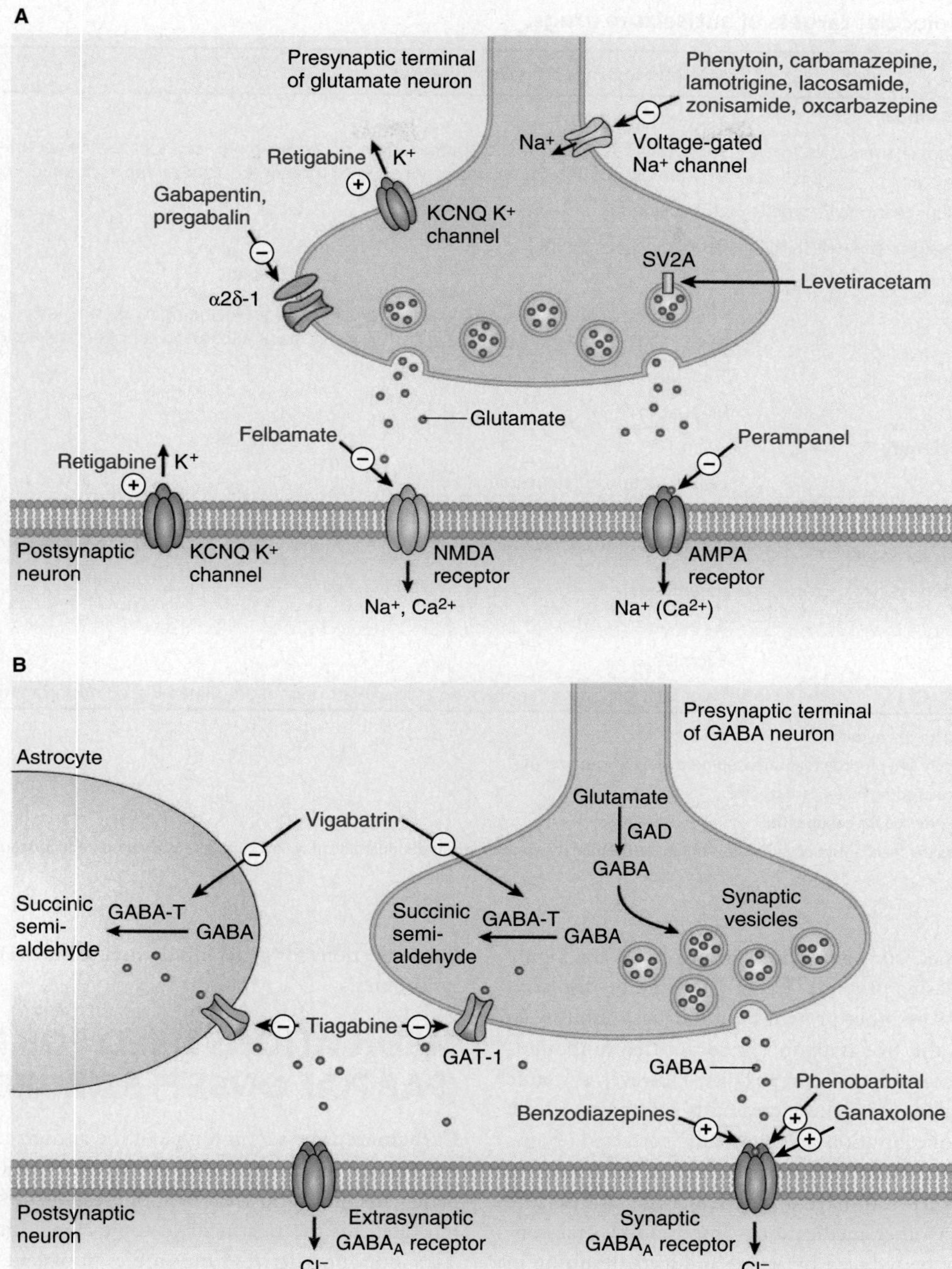

FIGURE 24–1 Molecular targets for antiseizure medications at the excitatory glutamatergic synapse (**A**) and the inhibitory GABAergic synapse (**B**). Presynaptic targets diminishing glutamate release include $Na_v1.6$ voltage-gated sodium channels (phenytoin, carbamazepine, lamotrigine, lacosamide, zonisamide, and oxcarbazepine); KCNQ (K_v7) voltage-gated potassium channels (retigabine [ezogabine]); and α2δ–1 protein (gabapentin and pregabalin), which interacts with NMDA receptors and voltage-gated calcium channels. Postsynaptic targets at excitatory synapses are AMPA receptors (perampanel) and KCNQ voltage-gated potassium channels (retigabine [ezogabine]). At inhibitory synapses and in astrocytes, vigabatrin inhibits GABA-transaminase (GABA-T) and tiagabine blocks GABA transporter 1 (GAT-1). Phenobarbital, primidone (via metabolism to phenobarbital), and benzodiazepines are positive allosteric modulators of synaptic $GABA_A$ receptors; high GABA levels resulting from blockade of GABA-T may act on extrasynaptic $GABA_A$ receptors.

alternatively, the new drug may reduce the concentration of the existing drug by inducing its metabolism. Other antiseizure medications are excreted in the kidney and are less susceptible to drug-drug interactions. Some antiseizure medications, including oxcarbazepine, carbamazepine, primidone, mephenytoin, and clobazam, have active metabolites. The extent of conversion to the active forms can be affected by the presence of other drugs. Some antiseizure medications, such as phenytoin, tiagabine, valproate,

TABLE 24–2 Molecular targets of antiseizure drugs.

Molecular Target	Antiseizure Drugs That Act on Target
Voltage-gated ion channels	
Voltage-gated sodium channels (Na_V)	Phenytoin, fosphenytoin,[1] carbamazepine, oxcarbazepine,[2] eslicarbazepine acetate,[3] lamotrigine, lacosamide; possibly (or among other actions) topiramate, zonisamide, rufinamide, cenobamate
Voltage-gated calcium channels (T-type)	Ethosuximide
Voltage-gated potassium channels (K_V7)	Retigabine (ezogabine)
GABA inhibition	
$GABA_A$ receptors	Phenobarbital, primidone, ganaxolone; benzodiazepines including diazepam, lorazepam, clonazepam, midazolam, clobazam; stiripentol; possibly topiramate, felbamate, cenobamate, Retigabine (ezogabine)
GAT-1 GABA transporter	Tiagabine
GABA transaminase	Vigabatrin
Synaptic release machinery	
SV2A	Levetiracetam, brivaracetam
$\alpha 2\delta$	Gabapentin, gabapentin enacarbil,[4] pregabalin
Ionotropic glutamate receptors	
AMPA receptor	Perampanel
Disease specific	
mTORC1 signaling	Everolimus
Mixed/unknown[5]	Valproate, felbamate, cenobamate, topiramate, zonisamide, rufinamide, adrenocorticotropin, cannabidiol

[1]Fosphenytoin is a prodrug for phenytoin.

[2]Oxcarbazepine serves largely as a prodrug for licarbazepine, mainly *S*-licarbazepine.

[3]Eslicarbazepine acetate is a prodrug for *S*-licarbazepine.

[4]Gabapentin enacarbil is a prodrug for gabapentin.

[5]There is no consensus as to the mechanism of valproate; felbamate, topiramate, zonisamide, and rufinamide may have actions on as yet unidentified targets in addition to those shown in the table.

diazepam, perampanel, stiripentol, and ganaxolone, are highly (>90%) bound to plasma proteins. These drugs can be displaced from plasma proteins by other protein-bound drugs, resulting in a temporary rise in the free fraction. Since the free (unbound) drug is active, there can be transient toxicity. However, systemic clearance increases along with the increased free fraction, so the elevation in free concentration is eventually corrected. Some antiseizure medications, notably levetiracetam, gabapentin, and pregabalin, are not known to have drug interactions. Antiseizure drugs can also affect other medications. Importantly, oral contraceptive levels may be reduced by strong inducers, resulting in failure of birth control.

Antiseizure medications must have reasonable oral bioavailability and must enter the central nervous system. These drugs are predominantly distributed into total body water. Plasma clearance is relatively slow; many antiseizure medications are therefore considered to be medium to long acting, such that they are administered twice or three times a day. Some have half-lives longer than 12 hours. A few, such as zonisamide and perampanel, can often be administered once daily. For some drugs with short half-lives, extended-release preparations are now available, which may improve compliance. In the remainder of the chapter, the most widely used antiseizure medications, as well as some that are used only in special circumstances, are reviewed. The focal (partial onset) seizure medications are described first, followed by medications for generalized onset seizures and certain epilepsy syndromes.

MEDICATIONS USED FOR FOCAL (PARTIAL ONSET) SEIZURES

Carbamazepine is a prototype of the antiseizure medications primarily used in the treatment of focal onset seizures. In addition to being effective in the treatment of focal seizures, carbamazepine is indicated for the treatment of tonic-clonic (grand mal) seizures. This indication derives from studies in patients whose focal onset seizures progressed to bilateral tonic-clonic seizures (previously called "secondarily generalized tonic-clonic seizures"). Medications like carbamazepine *exacerbate* certain seizure types in idiopathic (genetic) generalized epilepsies, including myoclonic and absence seizures, and are generally avoided in patients with such a diagnosis. There is evidence from anecdotal reports and small studies indicating that carbamazepine, phenytoin, and lacosamide may be effective and safe in the treatment of generalized tonic-clonic seizures in idiopathic generalized epilepsies. The most popular medications for the treatment of focal seizures in addition to carbamazepine are lamotrigine, lacosamide, and oxcarbazepine; levetiracetam also is frequently used. Phenobarbital is useful if cost is an issue. Vigabatrin and felbamate are third-line drugs because of risk of toxicity.

CARBAMAZEPINE

Carbamazepine is one of the most widely used antiseizure medications despite its limited range of activity as a treatment for focal (partial onset) and focal-to-bilateral tonic-clonic seizures. It was initially marketed for the treatment of trigeminal neuralgia, for which it is highly effective; it is usually the medication of first choice for this condition. In addition, carbamazepine is a mood stabilizer used to treat bipolar disorder.

Chemistry

Structurally, carbamazepine is an iminostilbene (dibenzazepine)—a tricyclic compound consisting of two benzene rings fused to an azepine group. The structure of carbamazepine is similar to that of tricyclic antidepressants such as imipramine, but unlike the tricyclic antidepressants, carbamazepine does not inhibit monoamine (serotonin and norepinephrine) transporters with high affinity; therefore, carbamazepine is not used as an antidepressant despite its ability to treat bipolar disorder.

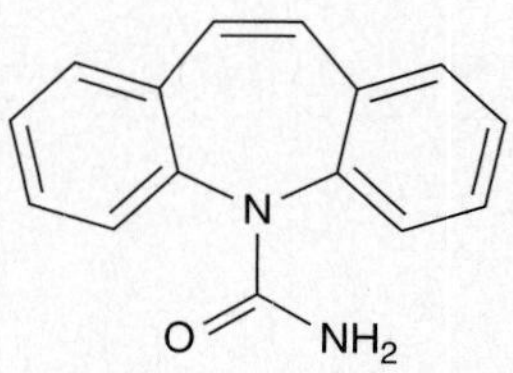

Mechanism of Action

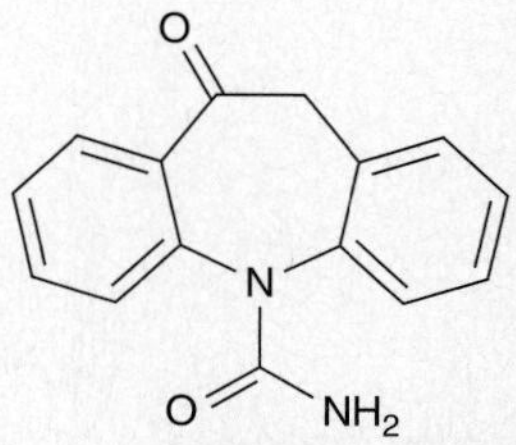

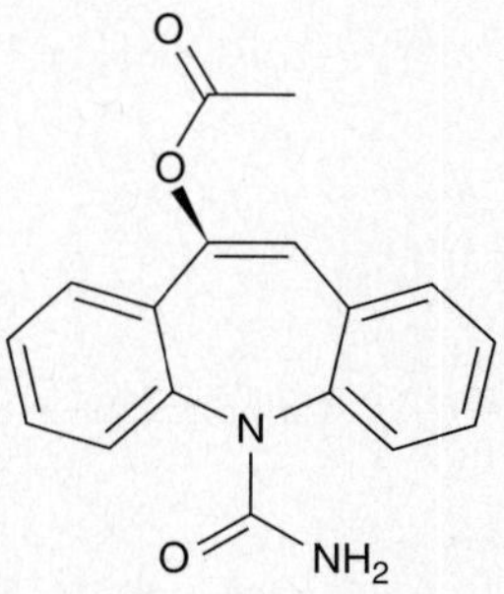

Carbamazepine is a prototypical sodium channel-blocking antiseizure medication that is thought to protect against seizures by interacting with the voltage-gated sodium channels (Na_v1) responsible for the rising phase of neuronal action potentials (see Chapters 14 and 21). In the normal state, when neurons are depolarized to action potential threshold, the sodium channel protein senses the depolarization and, within a few hundred microseconds, undergoes a conformational change (gating) that converts the channel from its closed (resting) nonconducting state to the open conducting state that permits sodium flux (Figure 24–2). Then, within less than a millisecond, the channel enters the inactivated state, terminating the flow of sodium ions. The channel must then be repolarized before it can be activated again by a subsequent depolarization. Brain sodium channels can rapidly cycle through the resting, open, and inactivated states, allowing neurons to fire high-frequency trains of action potentials.

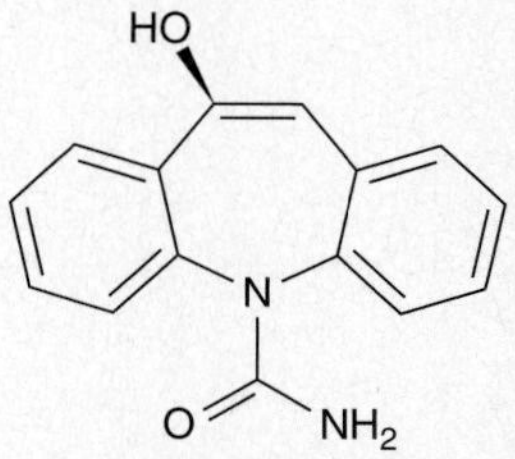

Sodium channels are multimeric protein complexes, composed of (1) a large α subunit that forms four subunit-like homologous domains (designated I–IV) and (2) one or more smaller β subunits. The ion-conducting pore is contained within the α subunit, as are the elements of the channel that undergo conformational changes in response to membrane depolarization. Carbamazepine and other sodium channel-blocking antiseizure medications such as phenytoin and lamotrigine bind preferentially to the channel when it is in the inactivated state, causing it to be stabilized in this state. During high-frequency firing, sodium channels cycle rapidly through the inactivated state, allowing the block to accumulate. This leads to a characteristic use-dependent blocking action in which high-frequency trains of action potentials are more effectively inhibited than are either individual action potentials or the firing at low frequencies (see Chapter 14, Figures 14–9 and 14–10). In addition, sodium channel-blocking antiseizure medications exhibit a voltage dependence to their blocking action because a greater fraction of sodium channels exist in the inactivated state at depolarized potentials. Thus, action potentials that are superimposed on a depolarized plateau potential (as characteristically occurs with seizures) are effectively inhibited. The use dependence and voltage dependence of the blocking action of medications like carbamazepine provide the ability to preferentially inhibit action potentials during seizure discharges and to less effectively interfere with ordinary ongoing action potential firing (Figure 24–3). Such action is thought to allow such medications to prevent the occurrence of seizures without causing unacceptable neurologic impairment. It is noteworthy that sodium channel-blocking antiseizure medications act mainly on action potential firing; the medications do not directly alter excitatory or inhibitory synaptic responses. However, the effect on action potentials translates into reduced transmitter output at synapses. Carbamazepine and other sodium channel–blocking antiseizure medications have activity in the rodent (rat or mouse) maximal electroshock (MES) but not in the pentylenetetrazol (PTZ) test; these tests are discussed later in this chapter.

Clinical Uses

Carbamazepine is effective for the treatment of focal and focal-to-bilateral tonic-clonic seizures. As noted earlier, there is anecdotal evidence that carbamazepine may be effective in the treatment of generalized tonic-clonic seizures in idiopathic (genetic) generalized epilepsies but must be used with caution as it can exacerbate absence and myoclonic seizures. Carbamazepine is also effective for the treatment of trigeminal and glossopharyngeal neuralgia, and mania in bipolar disorder.

Pharmacokinetics

Carbamazepine has nearly 100% oral bioavailability, but the rate of absorption varies widely among patients. Peak levels are usually

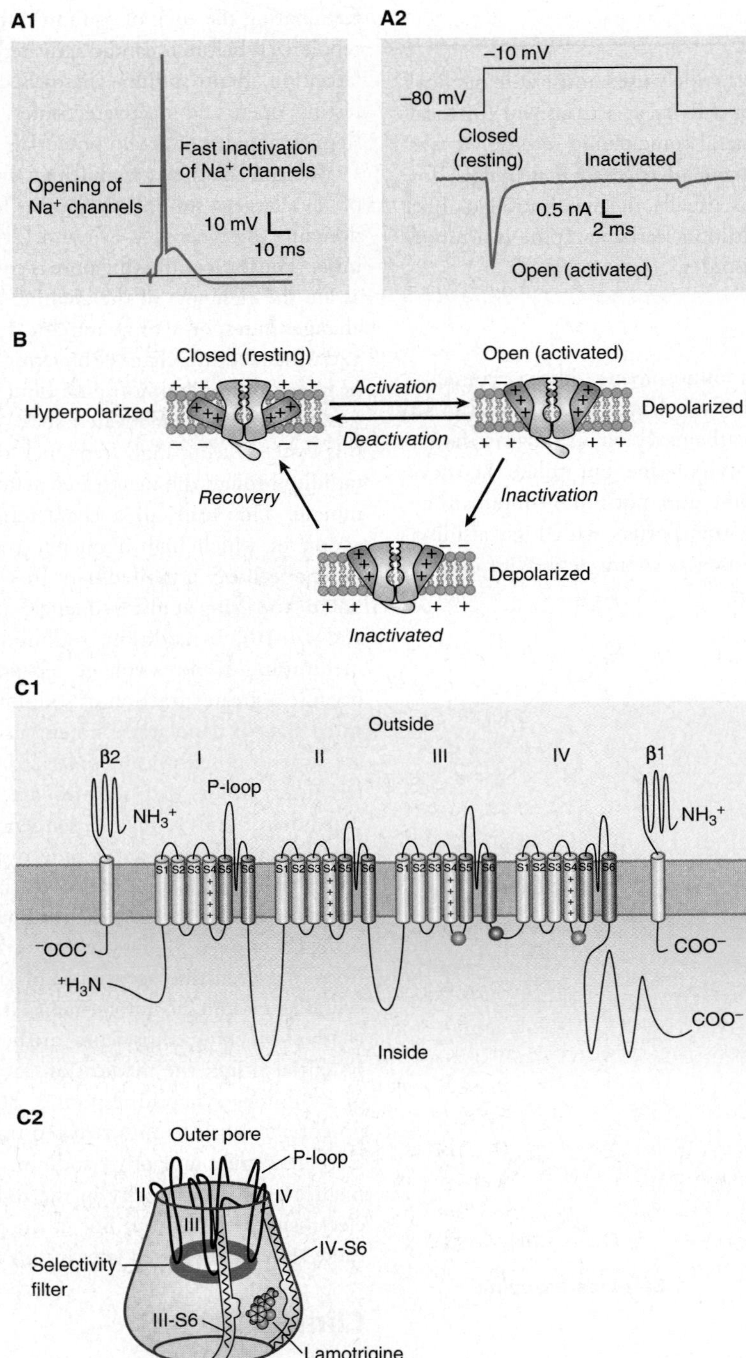

FIGURE 24–2 (**A1**) Voltage-gated sodium channels mediate the upstroke of action potentials in brain neurons. Fast inactivation of sodium channels (along with the activation of potassium channels) terminates the action potential. (**A2**) Voltage-clamp recording of sodium channel current following depolarization, illustrating the time course of sodium channel gating. (**B**) Schematic illustration of the voltage-dependent gating of sodium channels between closed, open, and inactivated states. (**C1**) Primary structures of the subunits of sodium channels. The main α subunit, consisting of four homologous repeats (I–IV), is shown flanked by the two auxiliary β subunits. Cylinders represent α-helical transmembrane segments. Blue α-helical segments (S5, S6) form the pore region. +, S4 voltage sensors; grey circles, inactivation particle in inactivation gate loop; III-S6 and IV-S6 (red) are regions where sodium channel–blocking antiseizure medications bind. (**C2**) Schematic illustration of the sodium channel pore composed of the homologous repeats arrayed around the central channel pore through which sodium flows into the neuron. The S5 and S6 transmembrane α-helical segments from each homologous repeat (I–IV) form the four walls of the pore. The outer pore mouth and ion selectivity filter are formed by re-entrant P-loops. The key α-helical S6 segments in repeat III and IV, which contain the drug binding sites, are highlighted. A lamotrigine molecule is illustrated in association with its binding site.

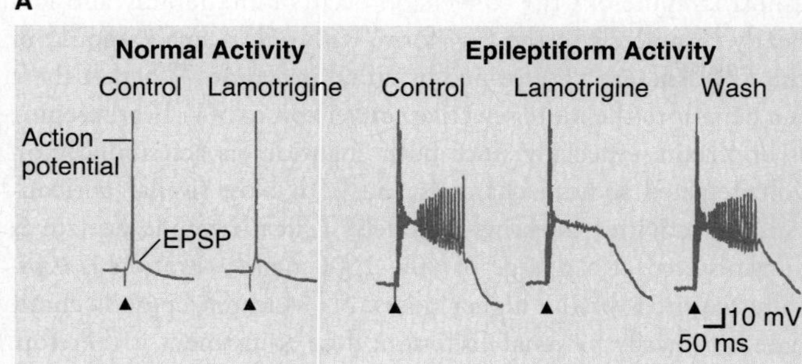

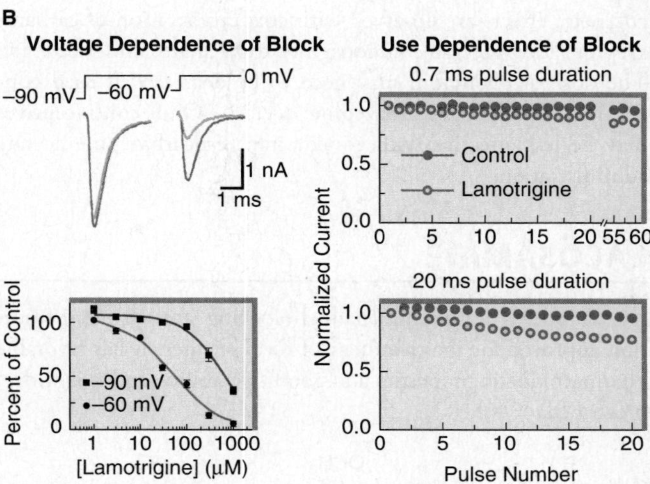

FIGURE 24–3 (**A**) Selective effect of a clinically relevant concentration of lamotrigine (50 μM) on action potentials and epileptic-like discharges in rat hippocampal neurons as assessed with intracellular recording. In normal recording conditions, lamotrigine has no effect on action potentials or on the evoked excitatory postsynaptic potentials (EPSPs) that elicit the action potential. In epileptic-like conditions (low magnesium), activation elicits initial spikes followed by repetitive epileptiform spike firing (afterdischarge). Lamotrigine inhibits the pathologic discharge but not the initial spikes. EPSPs were elicited by stimulation of the Schaffer collateral/commissural fibers (triangles). (**B**) Voltage and use dependence of block of human $Na_v1.2$ voltage-activated sodium channels. Sodium currents elicited by depolarization from a holding potential of –90 mV (where there is little inactivation) are minimally affected by 100 μM of lamotrigine, whereas there is strong block of current elicited from –60 mV (where there is more substantial inactivation). Trains of 0.7-millisecond (ms) duration pulses from –90 mV (minimal inactivation) are minimally blocked in a use-dependent fashion by 100 μM of lamotrigine, whereas 20-ms pulses (marked inactivation) show substantial use dependence. (Adapted with permission from Xie X, Hagan RM: Cellular and molecular actions of lamotrigine: Possible mechanisms of efficacy in bipolar disorder. Neuropsychobiology 1998;38(3):119-130. Copyright © 1998 Karger Publishers, Basel, Switzerland.)

achieved 6–8 hours after administration. Slowing absorption by giving the medication after meals causes a reduction in peak levels and helps the patient tolerate larger total daily doses. Extended-release formulations also may decrease the incidence of adverse effects.

Distribution is slow, and the volume of distribution is approximately 1 L/kg. Plasma protein binding is approximately 70%. Carbamazepine has a very low systemic clearance of approximately 1 L/kg/d at the start of therapy. The medication has a notable ability to induce its own metabolism, often causing serum concentrations to fall after a few weeks of treatment. Typically, the half-life of 36 hours observed in subjects after an initial single dose decreases to as little as 8–12 hours in subjects receiving continuous therapy. Considerable dosage adjustments are thus to be expected during the first weeks of therapy.

Carbamazepine is metabolized in the liver, and only about 5% of the drug is excreted unchanged. The major route of metabolism is conversion to carbamazepine-10,11-epoxide, which has been shown to have antiseizure activity. This reaction is primarily catalyzed by CYP3A4, although CYP2C8 also plays a role and CYP3A5 may be involved. The contribution of this and other metabolites to the clinical activity of carbamazepine is unknown.

Dosage Recommendations & Therapeutic Levels

Carbamazepine is available in immediate-release tablets and suspensions, and extended-release forms that are usually administered twice daily. The medication is effective in children, in whom a dosage of 15–25 mg/kg/d is appropriate. In adults, the typical daily maintenance dose is 800–1200 mg/d, and the maximum recommended dose is 1600 mg/d, but rarely patients have required doses up to 2400 mg/d. Higher dosage is achieved by giving multiple divided doses daily. In patients in whom the blood is drawn just before the morning dose (trough level), therapeutic concentrations are usually 4–8 mcg/mL. Although many patients complain of diplopia at drug levels above 7 mcg/mL, others can tolerate levels above 10 mcg/mL, especially with monotherapy. Initiation of therapy should be slow, with gradual increases in dose.

Drug Interactions

Carbamazepine stimulates the transcriptional up-regulation of CYP3A4 and CYP2B6. This autoinduction leads not only to a reduction in steady-state carbamazepine concentrations but also to an increased rate of metabolism of concomitant antiseizure medications including primidone, phenytoin, ethosuximide, valproate, clonazepam, perampanel, and ganaxolone. Some antiseizure medications such as valproate may inhibit carbamazepine clearance and increase steady-state carbamazepine blood levels. Other antiseizure medications, notably phenytoin and phenobarbital, may decrease steady-state concentrations of carbamazepine through enzyme induction. These interactions may require dosing changes. No clinically significant protein-binding interactions have been reported.

Adverse Effects

Carbamazepine may cause dose-dependent mild gastrointestinal discomfort, dizziness, blurred vision, diplopia, or ataxia; sedation occurs only at high doses, and rarely, weight gain can occur. The diplopia often occurs first and may last less than an hour during a particular time of day. Rearrangement of the divided daily dose can often remedy this complaint. A benign leukopenia occurs in many patients, but there is usually no need for intervention unless neutrophil count falls below 1000/mm^3. Rash and hyponatremia are the most common reasons for discontinuation. Stevens-Johnson syndrome is rare, but the risk is significantly higher in patients with the HLA-B*1502 allele. It is recommended that Asians, who have a 10-fold higher incidence of carbamazepine-induced Stevens-Johnson syndrome compared to other ethnic groups, be tested before starting therapy.

OXCARBAZEPINE

Oxcarbazepine is the 10-keto analog of carbamazepine. Unlike carbamazepine, it cannot form an epoxide metabolite. Although it has been hypothesized that the epoxide is associated with carbamazepine's adverse effects, little evidence is available to document the claim that oxcarbazepine is better tolerated. Orally administered oxcarbazepine is rapidly and almost completely (>95%) absorbed. It resides in the plasma for only a short time, as it is quickly converted by non-inducible arylketone reductase to the active 10-hydroxy metabolites, *S*(+)- and *R*(–)-licarbazepine (also referred to as monohydroxy derivatives or MHDs), with a half-life of only 1–2 hours. Oxcarbazepine can be considered a prodrug, as the antiseizure resides almost exclusively in these active metabolites, which are thought to protect against seizures by blocking voltage-gated sodium channels in the same way as carbamazepine. The bulk (80%) of oxcarbazepine is converted to the *S*(+) form. MHD is cleared primarily by the kidney (95%), either unchanged (two-thirds) or as the glucuronide conjugate (one-third); fecal excretion is <4% of the dose. Less than 1% of the administered dose is excreted in the urine as unchanged oxcarbazepine. In the absence of enzyme induction, the plasma half-lives of MHD are similar to that of carbamazepine (8–15 hours) while in the presence of enzyme-inducing antiseizure medications plasma half-lives are slightly shorter (7–12 hours). Oxcarbazepine does not induce its own metabolism. Drug interactions are minimal, but oxcarbazepine has the potential to reduce the effectiveness of hormonal contraceptives.

Oxcarbazepine is less potent than carbamazepine, both in animal tests and in patients; clinical doses of oxcarbazepine may need to be 50% higher than those of carbamazepine to obtain equivalent seizure control. Oxcarbazepine is administered at a starting dose of 300–600 mg/d and may be titrated to a dose of 900–2400 mg/d. Some studies report fewer hypersensitivity reactions to oxcarbazepine, and cross-reactivity with carbamazepine does not always occur. Furthermore, the drug appears to induce hepatic enzymes to a lesser extent than carbamazepine, minimizing drug interactions. Although hyponatremia may occur more commonly with oxcarbazepine than with carbamazepine, most adverse effects of oxcarbazepine are similar to those of carbamazepine.

ESLICARBAZEPINE ACETATE

Eslicarbazepine acetate, a prodrug of *S*(+)-licarbazepine, provides an alternative to oxcarbazepine, with some minor differences. Like oxcarbazepine, eslicarbazepine acetate is converted to eslicarbazepine but the conversion occurs more rapidly and it is nearly completely to the *S*(+) form, with only a small amount of the *R*(–) isomer (5%) formed by chiral inversion. Whether there is a benefit to the more selective conversion to *S*(+)-licarbazepine is uncertain, especially since both enantiomers act similarly on voltage-gated sodium channels and both have similar anticonvulsant activities in animal models. Eslicarbazepine acetate is administered at a dosage of 400–1600 mg/d; titration is typically required for the higher doses. *S*(+)-Licarbazepine is eliminated primarily by renal excretion; dose adjustment is therefore required for patients with renal impairment. Minimal pharmacokinetic effects are observed with coadministration of carbamazepine, levetiracetam, lamotrigine, topiramate, and valproate. The dose of phenytoin may need to be decreased if used concomitantly with eslicarbazepine acetate. Oral contraceptives may be less effective with concomitant eslicarbazepine acetate administration.

LACOSAMIDE

Lacosamide is a sodium channel-blocking antiseizure medication approved for the treatment of focal seizures. It has favorable pharmacokinetic properties and good tolerability, and it is widely prescribed.

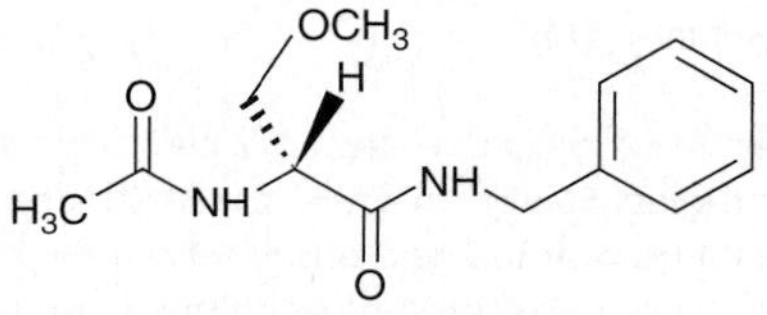

OCH_3 H O H_3C NH NH O

Lacosamide

Mechanism of Action

Early studies suggested that lacosamide enhances a poorly understood type of sodium channel inactivation called slow inactivation. Recent studies, however, contradict this view and indicate that the drug binds selectively to the fast inactivated state of sodium channels—as is the case for other sodium channel-blocking antiseizure medications, except that the binding is much slower.

Clinical Use

Lacosamide is approved for the treatment of focal onset seizures in patients age 17 years and older. In clinical trials with more than 1300 patients, lacosamide was effective at doses of 200 mg/d and had greater and roughly similar overall efficacy at 400 and 600 mg/d, respectively. Although the overall efficacy was similar at 400 and 600 mg/d, the higher dose may provide better control of focal-to-bilateral tonic-clonic (secondarily generalized) seizures; however, this dose is associated with a greater incidence of adverse effects. Adverse effects include dizziness, headache, nausea, and diplopia. Cardiac arrhythmias have been associated with lacosamide use. Lacosamide is typically administered twice daily, beginning with 50-mg doses and increasing by 100-mg increments weekly. An intravenous formulation provides short-term replacement for the oral medication. The oral solution contains aspartame, which is a source of phenylalanine and could be harmful in people with phenylketonuria.

Pharmacokinetics

Oral lacosamide is rapidly and completely absorbed in adults, with no food effect. Bioavailability is nearly 100%. The plasma concentrations are proportional to oral dosage up to 800 mg. Peak concentrations occur from 1 to 4 hours after oral dosing, with an elimination half-life of 13 hours. There are no active metabolites, and protein binding is minimal. Lacosamide does not induce or inhibit cytochrome P450 isoenzymes, so drug interactions are minimal.

PHENYTOIN

Phenytoin, first identified to have antiseizure activity in 1938, is the oldest nonsedating medication used in the treatment of epilepsy. It is prescribed for the prevention of focal seizures and generalized tonic-clonic seizures and for the acute treatment of status epilepticus. Because of its adverse effects and propensity for drug-drug interactions, phenytoin is no longer considered a first-line chronic therapy.

Chemistry

Phenytoin, sometimes referred to as diphenylhydantoin, is the 5,5-diphenyl-substituted analog of hydantoin. Hydantoin is a five-membered ring molecule similar structurally to barbiturates, which are based on a six-member ring. Phenytoin free base (pK_a = 8.06–8.33) is poorly water soluble, but phenytoin sodium does dissolve in water (17 mg/mL). Phenytoin is most commonly prescribed in an extended-release capsule containing phenytoin sodium and other excipients to provide a slow and extended rate of absorption with peak blood concentrations from 4 to 12 hours. This form differs from the prompt phenytoin sodium capsule form that provides rapid rate of absorption with peak blood concentration from 1.5 to 3 hours. In addition, the free base is available as an immediate-release suspension and chewable tablets. Phenytoin is available as an intravenous solution containing propylene glycol and alcohol adjusted to a pH of 12. Absorption after intramuscular injection is unpredictable, and some drug precipitation in the muscle occurs; this route of administration is not recommended.

With intravenous administration, there is a risk of the potentially serious "purple glove syndrome" in which a purplish-black discoloration accompanied by edema and pain occurs distal to the site of injection. **Fosphenytoin** is a water-soluble prodrug of phenytoin that may have a lower incidence of purple glove syndrome. This phosphate ester compound is rapidly converted to phenytoin in the plasma and is used for intravenous administration and treatment of status epilepticus. Fosphenytoin is well absorbed after intramuscular administration, but this route is rarely appropriate for the treatment of status epilepticus.

HN, O, NH, O
Phenytoin

HN, O, N, O, CH_2—O—P(=O)(—O^-Na^+)—O^-Na^+
Fosphenytoin

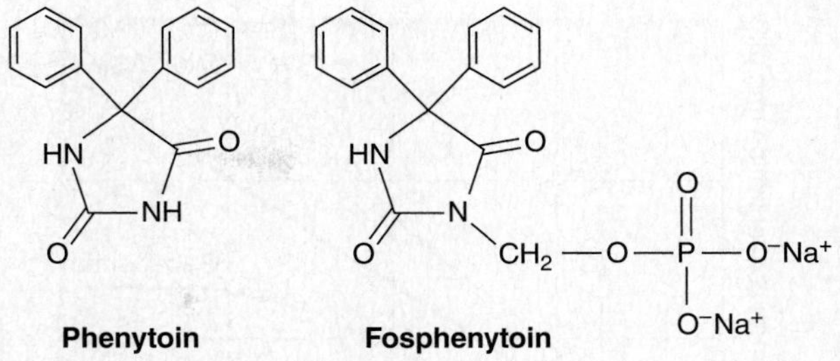

Mechanism of Action

Phenytoin is a sodium channel-blocking antiseizure medication that acts in a similar fashion to carbamazepine and other agents in the class.

Clinical Uses

Phenytoin is effective in preventing focal onset seizures and also tonic-clonic seizures, whether they are focal-to-bilateral tonic-clonic (secondarily generalized) or occurring in the setting of an idiopathic (genetic) generalized epilepsy syndrome. Phenytoin may worsen other seizure types in idiopathic generalized epilepsies, including absence epilepsy and juvenile myoclonic epilepsy, and in Dravet syndrome.

Pharmacokinetics & Drug Interactions

Absorption of phenytoin is highly dependent on the formulation. Particle size and pharmaceutical additives affect both the rate and the extent of absorption. Therefore, while absorption from the gastrointestinal tract is nearly complete in most patients, the time to peak may range from 3 to 12 hours. Phenytoin is extensively (~90%) bound to serum albumin and is prone to displacement in response to a variety of factors (eg, hyperbilirubinemia or drugs such as warfarin or valproate), which can lead to toxicity. Also, low plasma albumin (such as in liver disease or nephrotic syndrome) can result in abnormally high free concentrations and toxicity. Small changes in the bound fraction dramatically affect the amount of free (active) drug. Increased proportions of free drug are also present in the neonate and in the elderly. Some agents such as valproate, phenylbutazone, and sulfonamides can compete with phenytoin for binding to plasma proteins. Valproate also inhibits phenytoin metabolism. The combined effect can result in marked increases in free phenytoin. In all of these situations, patients may exhibit signs of toxicity when total drug levels are within the therapeutic range. Because of its high protein binding, phenytoin has a low volume of distribution (0.6–0.7 L/kg in adults).

Phenytoin is metabolized by CYP2C9 and CYP2C19 to inactive metabolites that are excreted in the urine. Only a small proportion of the dose is excreted unchanged. The elimination of phenytoin depends on the dose. At low blood levels, phenytoin metabolism follows first-order kinetics. However, as blood levels rise within the therapeutic range, the maximum capacity of the liver to metabolize the drug is approached (saturation kinetics). Even small increases in dose may be associated with large changes

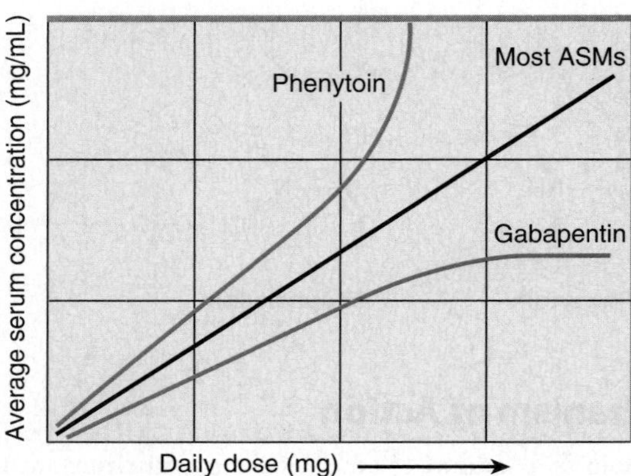

FIGURE 24–4 Relationship between dose and exposure for antiseizure medications (ASMs). Most antiseizure medications follow linear (first-order) kinetics, in which a constant fraction per unit time of the drug is eliminated (elimination is proportional to drug concentration). In the case of phenytoin, as the dose increases, there is saturation of metabolism and a shift from first-order to zero-order kinetics, in which a constant quantity per unit time is metabolized. A small increase in dose can result in a large increase in concentration. Orally administered gabapentin also exhibits zero-order kinetics, but in contrast to phenytoin where metabolism can be saturated, in the case of gabapentin, gut absorption, which is mediated by the large neutral amino acid system L transporter, is susceptible to saturation. The bioavailability of gabapentin falls at high doses as the transporter is saturated so that increases in blood levels do not keep pace with increases in dose.

in phenytoin serum concentrations (Figure 24–4). In such cases, the half-life increases markedly, steady state is not achieved in routine fashion (since the plasma level continues to rise), and patients quickly develop symptoms of toxicity.

The half-life of phenytoin in most patients varies from 12 to 36 hours, with an average of 24 hours in the low to mid therapeutic range. Much longer half-lives are observed at higher concentrations. At low blood levels, 5–7 days are needed to reach steady-state blood levels after every dosage change; at higher levels, it may be 4–6 weeks before blood levels are stable. Phenytoin—like carbamazepine, phenobarbital, and primidone—is a major enzyme-inducing antiseizure medication that stimulates the rate of metabolism of many coadministered antiseizure medications, including valproate, tiagabine, ethosuximide, lamotrigine, topiramate, oxcarbazepine and MHDs, zonisamide, felbamate, many benzodiazepines, and perampanel. Autoinduction of its own metabolism, however, is insignificant.

Therapeutic Levels & Dosing

The therapeutic plasma level of phenytoin for most patients is between 10 and 20 mcg/mL. A loading dose can be given either orally or intravenously, with either fosphenytoin sodium injection (preferred) or phenytoin sodium injection. When oral therapy is started, it is common to begin adults at a dosage of 300 mg/d, regardless of body weight. This may be acceptable in some patients, but it frequently yields steady-state blood levels below 10 mcg/mL, which is the minimum therapeutic level for most patients. If seizures continue, higher doses are usually necessary to achieve plasma levels in the upper therapeutic range. Because of the kinetic factors discussed earlier, toxic levels may occur with only small increments in dosage. The phenytoin dosage should be increased in increments of no more than 25–30 mg/d in adults, and ample time should be allowed for the new steady state to be achieved before further increasing the dosage. A common clinical error is to increase the dosage directly from 300 mg/d to 400 mg/d; toxicity frequently occurs at a variable time thereafter. In children, a dosage of 5 mg/kg/d should be followed by readjustment after steady-state plasma levels are obtained.

Two types of oral phenytoin are currently available in the USA, differing in their respective rates of dissolution. The predominant form is the sodium salt in an extended-release pill intended for once- or twice-a-day use. In addition, the free acid is available as an immediate-release suspension and chewable tablets. Although a few patients being given phenytoin on a long-term basis have been proved to have low blood levels from poor absorption or rapid metabolism, the most common cause of low levels is poor compliance. As noted, fosphenytoin sodium is available for intravenous or intramuscular use and usually replaces intravenous phenytoin sodium, a much less soluble form of the medication.

Toxicity

Early signs of phenytoin administration include nystagmus and loss of smooth extraocular pursuit movements; neither is an indication for decreasing the dose. Diplopia and ataxia are the most common dose-related adverse effects requiring dosage adjustment; sedation usually occurs only at considerably higher levels. Gingival hyperplasia and hirsutism occur to some degree in most patients; the latter can be especially unpleasant in women. Long-term use is associated in some patients with coarsening of facial features and with mild peripheral neuropathy, usually manifested by diminished deep tendon reflexes in the lower extremities. Long-term use may also result in abnormalities of vitamin D metabolism, leading to osteomalacia. Low folate levels and megaloblastic anemia have been reported, but the clinical importance of these observations is unknown.

Idiosyncratic reactions to phenytoin are relatively rare. A skin rash may indicate hypersensitivity of the patient to the medication. Fever may also occur, and in rare cases, the skin lesions may be severe and exfoliative. Lymphadenopathy may rarely occur; this must be distinguished from malignant lymphoma. Hematologic complications are exceedingly rare, although agranulocytosis has been reported in combination with fever and rash.

MEPHENYTOIN, ETHOTOIN, & PHENACEMIDE

Many analogs of phenytoin have been synthesized, but only three have been marketed in the USA, with none currently commercially available. Of the three, mephenytoin and ethotoin are hydantoins, whereas phenacemide (phenacetylurea) is a ring-opened analog of phenytoin. Like phenytoin, the analogs appear to be most effective against focal and generalized tonic-clonic seizures although no well-controlled clinical trials have documented their effectiveness. Ethotoin may avoid phenytoin-like side effects such as hirsutism and gingival hyperplasia but it can cause gastrointestinal disturbances, skin rash, and psychiatric side effects. It has a short half-life of 3 to 6 hours, so that dosing four times a day is required. Mephenytoin is metabolized to 5-ethyl-5-phenyl-hydantoin (nirvanol) via demethylation; nirvanol contributes most of the antiseizure activity of mephenytoin. The incidence of severe reactions such as dermatitis, agranulocytosis, or hepatitis is higher for mephenytoin than for phenytoin. Phenacemide has been associated with fatal aplastic anemia and hepatic failure.

GABAPENTIN & PREGABALIN

Gabapentin [1-(aminomethyl)cyclohexaneacetic acid] and pregabalin [(S)-3-(aminomethyl)-5-methylhexanoic acid], known as "gabapentinoids," are amino acid-like molecules that were originally synthesized as analogs of GABA but are now known not to act through GABA mechanisms. They are used in the treatment of focal seizures and various nonepilepsy indications, such as neuropathic pain, restless legs syndrome, and anxiety disorders.

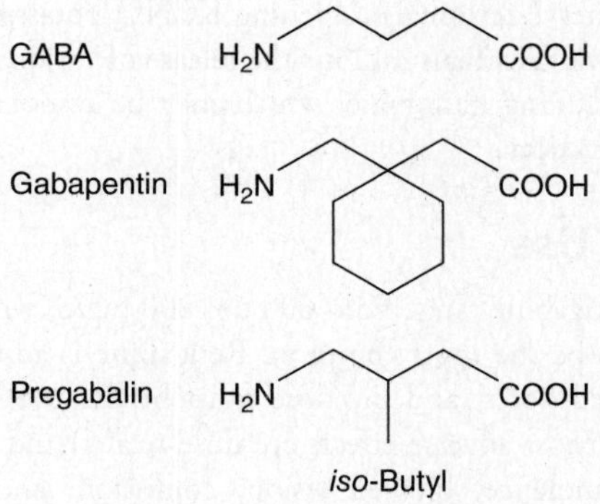

GABA H_2N COOH

Gabapentin H_2N COOH

Pregabalin H_2N COOH

iso-Butyl

Mechanism of Action

Despite their close structural resemblance to GABA, gabapentin and pregabalin do not act through effects on GABA receptors or any other mechanism related to GABA-mediated neurotransmission. Rather, gabapentinoids bind avidly to $\alpha2\delta$ proteins, specifically $\alpha2\delta$-1 and $\alpha2\delta$-2. These proteins serve as auxiliary subunits of voltage-gated calcium channels but also have other binding partners. Importantly, $\alpha2\delta$-1 forms a heteromeric complex with presynaptic *N*-methyl-D-aspartate (NMDA) receptors. The precise way in which binding of gabapentinoids to $\alpha2\delta$ proteins protects against seizures is not known but may relate to a decrease in glutamate release at excitatory synapses. Despite the binding interaction with voltage-gated calcium channels, gabapentinoids have little effect on calcium currents, suggesting that calcium channels are not the target. Rather, recent research indicates that gabapentinoids inhibit the ability of $\alpha2\delta$-1 to facilitate trafficking of presynaptic NMDA receptors to the cell surface and their incorporation into synapses, but the role of these NMDA receptors in seizures is yet to be defined.

Clinical Uses

Gabapentin and pregabalin are effective in the treatment of focal seizures; there is no evidence that they are efficacious in generalized epilepsies. Indeed, gabapentin may aggravate absence seizures and myoclonic seizures. Gabapentin is usually started at a dose of 900 mg/d (in three divided doses), but starting doses as high as 3600 mg/d can be used if a rapid response is required. Some clinicians have found that even higher dosages are needed to achieve improvement in seizure control. The recommended starting dose of pregabalin is 150 mg/d, but a lower starting dose (50–75 mg/d) may avoid adverse effects that can occur on therapy initiation; the effective maintenance dose range is 150–600 mg/d. Although comparative studies are lacking, gabapentinoids are generally considered less effective than other antiseizure medications for the treatment of focal seizures. Gabapentinoids are frequently used in the treatment of neuropathic pain conditions, including postherpetic neuralgia and painful diabetic neuropathy, and in the treatment of anxiety disorders. Pregabalin is also approved for the treatment of fibromyalgia. Gabapentin and pregabalin are generally well tolerated. The most common adverse effects are somnolence, dizziness, ataxia, headache, and tremor. These adverse effects are most troublesome at initiation of therapy and often resolve with continued dosing. Both gabapentinoids can cause weight gain and peripheral edema.

Pharmacokinetics

Gabapentin and pregabalin are not metabolized and do not induce hepatic enzymes; they are eliminated unchanged in the urine. Both medications are absorbed by the L-amino acid transport system, which is found only in the upper small intestine. The oral bioavailability of gabapentin decreases with increasing dose because of saturation of this transport system. In contrast, pregabalin exhibits linear absorption within the therapeutic dose range. This is explained, in part, by the fact that pregabalin is used at much lower doses than gabapentin so it does not saturate the transport system. Also, pregabalin may be absorbed by mechanisms other than the L-amino acid transport system. Because of dependence on the transport system, absorption of gabapentin shows patient-to-patient variability and dosing requires individualization. Pregabalin bioavailability exceeds 90% and is independent of dose so that it may produce a more predictable patient response. Gabapentinoids are not bound to plasma proteins. Drug-drug interactions are negligible. The half-life of both medications is relatively short (ranging from 5 to 8 hours for gabapentin and 4.5 to 7.0 hours for pregabalin); they are typically administered two or three times per day. Sustained-release, once-a-day preparations of gabapentin are available. The gabapentin prodrug gabapentin enacarbil also is available in an extended-release formulation. This prodrug is actively absorbed by high-capacity nutrient transporters, which are abundant throughout the intestinal tract, and then converted to gabapentin presumably within the intestine, so there is dose-proportional systemic gabapentin exposure over a wide dose range.

TIAGABINE

Tiagabine, a selective inhibitor of the GAT-1 GABA transporter, is a second-line treatment for focal seizures. It is contraindicated in generalized onset epilepsies.

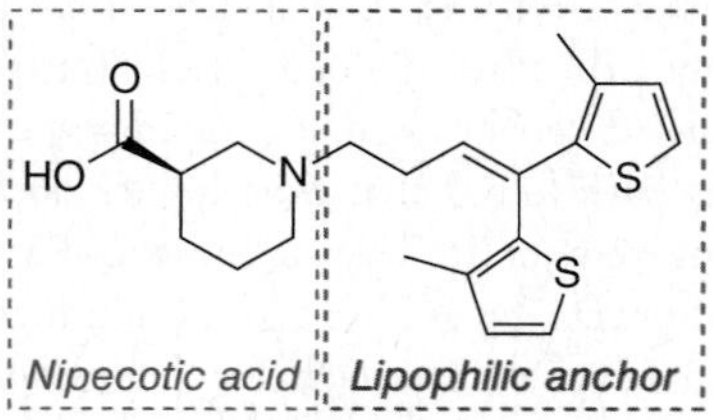

Nipecotic acid *Lipophilic anchor*

Tiagabine

Mechanism of Action

Tiagabine is a lipophilic, blood-brain barrier-permeant analog of nipecotic acid, a GABA uptake inhibitor that is not active systemically. The chemical structure of tiagabine consists of the active moiety—nipecotic acid—and a lipophilic anchor that allows the molecule to cross the blood-brain barrier. Tiagabine is highly selective for the GAT-1 GABA transporter isoform, the most abundant GABA transporter expressed in brain, and has little or no activity on the other sodium- and chloride-dependent GABA transporters, GAT-2, GAT-3, or BGT-1. The action of the GABA that is released by inhibitory neurons is normally terminated by reuptake into the neuron and surrounding glia by these transporters. Tiagabine inhibits the movement of GABA from the extracellular space—where the GABA can act on neuronal receptors—to the intracellular compartment, where it is inactive. This action of tiagabine causes prolongation of GABA-mediated inhibitory synaptic responses and potentiation of tonic inhibition; the latter is caused by the action of GABA on extrasynaptic GABA receptors. Tiagabine is considered a "rationally designed" antiseizure medication because it was developed with the understanding that potentiation of GABA action in the brain is a possible antiseizure mechanism.

Clinical Uses

Tiagabine is indicated for the adjunctive treatment of focal seizures, with or without secondary generalization (focal-to-bilateral tonic-clonic). In adults, the recommended initial dose is 4 mg/d with weekly increments of 4–8 mg/d to total doses of 16–56 mg/d. Initial dosages can be given twice a day, but a change to three times a day is recommended above 30–32 mg/d. Divided doses as often as four times daily are sometimes required. Adverse effects and apparent lack of efficacy limit the use of this medication. Minor adverse events are dose related and include nervousness, dizziness, tremor, difficulty concentrating, and depression. Excessive confusion, somnolence, or ataxia may require discontinuation. Psychosis occurs rarely. Rash is an uncommon idiosyncratic adverse effect. Tiagabine may worsen myoclonic seizures and cause nonconvulsive status epilepticus, even in patients without a history of epilepsy.

Pharmacokinetics

Tiagabine is 90–100% bioavailable, has linear kinetics, and is highly protein bound. The half-life is 5–8 hours and decreases in the presence of enzyme-inducing drugs. Food decreases the peak plasma concentration but not the area under the concentration curve (see Chapter 3). To avoid adverse effects, tiagabine should be taken with food. Hepatic impairment causes a slight decrease in clearance and may necessitate a lower dose. The drug is oxidized in the liver by CYP3A. Elimination is primarily in the feces (60–65%) and urine (25%).

RETIGABINE (EZOGABINE)

Retigabine (US Adopted Name: ezogabine), a potassium channel opener, is indicated for the treatment of focal seizures. Because retigabine causes pigment discoloration of the skin and eye, it had limited use and its sale was discontinued. It is currently not available in the USA.

Mechanism of Action

Retigabine is an allosteric opener of KCNQ2-5 ($K_v7.2$-$K_v7.5$) voltage-gated potassium channels, which are localized, in part, in axons and nerve terminals. Opening KCNQ potassium channels in presynaptic terminals inhibits the release of various neurotransmitters, including glutamate, which may be responsible for the seizure protection.

Clinical Use

Doses of retigabine range from 600 to 1200 mg/d, with 900 mg/d expected to be the most common. Retigabine is administered in three divided doses, and the dose must be titrated beginning at 300 mg/d. Most adverse effects are dose-related and include dizziness, somnolence, blurred vision, confusion, and dysarthria. Urinary symptoms, including retention, hesitation, and dysuria, believed to be due to effects of the drug on KCNQ potassium channels in detrusor smooth muscle, may occur. They are generally mild and usually do not require drug discontinuation. In 2013, reports began to appear of blue pigmentation, primarily on the skin and lips, but also on the palate, and in the eyes. The discoloration appears to be due to binding of dimers of retigabine and retigabine with its N-acetyl metabolite to melanin in the skin and uveal tract of the eye. The skin and eye discoloration has not been associated with more serious adverse effects and there is no evidence of visual impairment but the dyspigmentation may be of cosmetic significance.

Pharmacokinetics

Absorption of retigabine is not affected by food, and kinetics are linear; drug interactions are minimal. The major metabolic pathways in humans are N-glucuronidation and N-acetylation.

Retigabine neither inhibits nor induces the major CYP enzymes involved in drug metabolism.

CENOBAMATE

Cenobamate is a tetrazole alkyl monocarbamate used in the treatment of focal seizures. It has broad-spectrum antiseizure activity in animal models, but a clinical assessment of its efficacy in the treatment of generalized seizures has not yet been completed.

Cenobamate

Clinical Uses

The usual maintenance dose of cenobamate is 200 mg once daily. A dose of 400 mg once daily was studied in a clinical trial and had efficacy only modestly greater than the 200-mg dose. Seizure-free rates during the clinical trial were higher than observed in trials of other agents approved for the treatment of focal seizures. In long-term follow-up over more than 2 years, high seizure-free rates were maintained, raising the possibility that cenobamate may overcome pharmacoresistance in some cases. Cenobamate frequently causes central nervous system adverse effects including fatigue, dizziness, somnolence, diplopia, balance disorder, gait disturbance, dysarthria, nystagmus, and ataxia. The 400-mg dose tended to cause adverse effects more frequently than the 200-mg dose. During early clinical development, among the first 953 patients exposed to cenobamate, 3 confirmed cases of drug reaction with eosinophilia and systemic symptoms (DRESS) syndrome were reported, with 1 death. No cases of DRESS occurred in 1339 patients when therapy was initiated with a very low dose (12.5 mg/d) and the daily dose increased at 2-week intervals over 11 weeks to achieve a maintenance dose of 200 mg/d, with further slow increases to 400 mg/d, if required. Cenobamate may cause physical dependence and lead to a withdrawal syndrome characterized by insomnia, decreased appetite, depressed mood, tremor, and amnesia.

Pharmacokinetics

Cenobamate is well absorbed following oral administration (>88%) and reaches peak levels within 1–4 hours. It has a long terminal half-life (50–60 h), which permits once-daily dosing. Cenobamate is extensively metabolized by glucuronide conjugation and oxidation, mainly by CYP2E1, CYP2A6, and CYP2B6, and to a lesser extent by CYP2C19 and CYP3A4/5. Due to pharmacokinetic drug–drug interactions, when cenobamate is added to clobazam, phenytoin, or phenobarbital, it is advisable to proactively reduce the dose of the baseline medication.

MEDICATIONS EFFECTIVE FOR FOCAL SEIZURES & CERTAIN GENERALIZED ONSET SEIZURE TYPES

Correct diagnosis is critical to antiseizure medication selection. The medications described in the previous section are effective for the treatment of focal onset seizures, including focal-to-bilateral tonic-clonic seizures (secondarily generalized tonic-clonic seizures), but some can worsen certain seizure types in generalized epilepsy syndromes. A variety of medications were shown initially to be effective in the treatment of focal onset seizures and are primarily used to treat these types of seizures; in addition, these medications have also found uses in the treatment of certain generalized onset seizure types. These medications are described below.

LAMOTRIGINE

Lamotrigine is considered a sodium channel-blocking antiseizure medication; it is effective for the treatment of focal seizures, as are other medications in this category. In addition, clinical trials of lamotrigine have demonstrated effectiveness in the treatment of generalized tonic-clonic seizures in idiopathic (genetic) generalized epilepsies and in the treatment of generalized absence epilepsy. In the latter, lamotrigine is not as effective as ethosuximide or valproate. The medication is generally well tolerated; however, it can produce a potentially fatal rash (Stevens-Johnson syndrome). Although adverse effects are similar to those of other sodium channel-blocking antiseizure medications, lamotrigine paradoxically may cause insomnia instead of sedation. Lamotrigine causes fewer adverse cognitive effects than carbamazepine or topiramate. It can also improve depression in patients with epilepsy and reduces the risk of relapse in bipolar disorder.

Chemistry

Lamotrigine was developed when investigators thought that the antifolate effects of certain antiseizure medications such as phenytoin might contribute to their effectiveness. Several phenyltriazines were developed; although their antifolate properties were weak, some were active in seizure screening tests. The antifolate activity of lamotrigine is not believed to contribute to its therapeutic activity in epilepsy.

Lamotrigine

Mechanism of Action

The action of lamotrigine on voltage-gated sodium channels is similar to that of carbamazepine. The mechanism by which lamotrigine is effective against absence seizures is not known.

Clinical Uses

Although most controlled studies have evaluated lamotrigine as add-on therapy, the medication is effective as monotherapy for focal seizures, and lamotrigine is now widely prescribed for this indication because of its excellent tolerability. Despite being less effective than ethosuximide and valproate for absence epilepsy, lamotrigine may be prescribed because of its tolerability or in females of childbearing age because it has fewer fetal risks than valproate. Lamotrigine is also approved for primary generalized tonic-clonic seizures and generalized seizures of the Lennox-Gastaut syndrome. Adverse effects include dizziness, headache, diplopia, nausea, insomnia, somnolence, and skin rash. The rash is a typical hypersensitivity reaction. Pediatric patients are at greater risk: serious rash occurs in approximately 0.3–0.8% of children age 2–17 years, whereas in adults, the rate is 0.08–0.3%. The risk of rash may be diminished by slow dose escalation. Thus, the titration schedule to initiate lamotrigine requires more than 5 weeks. Lamotrigine, by virtue of its effects on voltage-gated sodium channels, has effects on the heart, including the potential to cause modest QRS prolongation at therapeutic doses. There is no conclusive evidence that concern is warranted when using lamotrigine in patients without a history of cardiac illness. If there is a history of conduction disorder or ventricular arrhythmia, electrocardiogram monitoring may be justified. Lamotrigine should not be used in patients with Brugada syndrome.

Pharmacokinetics

Lamotrigine is almost completely absorbed and has a volume of distribution of 1–1.4 L/kg. Protein binding is only about 55%. The drug has linear kinetics and is metaboli zed primarily by glucuronidation in the liver to the inactive 2-*N*-glucuronide, which is excreted in the urine. Lamotrigine has a half-life of approximately 24 hours in normal volunteers; this decreases to 13–15 hours in patients taking enzyme-inducing drugs. Lamotrigine is effective in the treatment of focal seizures in adults at dosages typically between 100 and 300 mg/d. The initial dose is 25 mg/d, increasing to 50 mg/d after 2 weeks; thereafter, titration can proceed by 50 mg/d every 1–2 weeks to a usual maintenance dose of 225–375 mg/d (in two divided doses). Therapeutic serum levels have not been established, but toxicity is infrequent with levels <10 mcg/mL. The combination of lamotrigine and valproate is believed to be particularly efficacious. However, valproate causes a twofold increase in the half-life of lamotrigine and can increase blood levels correspondingly, leading to a risk of skin rash if valproate is added to a stable regimen of lamotrigine. In patients receiving valproate, the initial dose of lamotrigine must be reduced to 12.5–25 mg every other day, with increases of 25–50 mg/d every 2 weeks as needed to a usual maintenance dose of 100–200 mg/d.

LEVETIRACETAM

Levetiracetam is a broad-spectrum antiseizure agent and one of the most commonly prescribed drugs for epilepsy, primarily because of its perceived favorable adverse effect profile, broad therapeutic window, favorable pharmacokinetic properties, and lack of drug-drug interactions.

Levetiracetam **Brivaracetam**

Mechanism of Action

Levetiracetam is an analog of piracetam, which is purported to be a cognition enhancer. In animal testing, levetiracetam is not active in the MES or PTZ tests, but it does have activity against seizures in the 6-Hz and kindling models. Levetiracetam binds selectively to SV2A, a ubiquitous synaptic vesicle integral membrane protein, which may function as a positive effector of synaptic vesicle exocytosis. The drug accesses the luminal side of recycling synaptic vesicles by vesicular endocytosis. Binding to SV2A in the vesicle reduces the release of the excitatory neurotransmitter glutamate during trains of high-frequency activity.

Clinical Uses

Levetiracetam is effective in the treatment of focal seizures in adults and children, primary generalized tonic-clonic seizures, and the myoclonic seizures of juvenile myoclonic epilepsy. Adult dosing can begin with 500 or 1000 mg/d. The dosage can be increased every 2–4 weeks by 1000 mg to a maximum dosage of 3000 mg/d. The drug is dosed twice daily. Adverse effects include somnolence, asthenia, ataxia, infection (colds), and dizziness. Less common but more serious are behavioral and mood changes, such as irritability, aggression, agitation, anger, anxiety, apathy, depression, and emotional lability. Oral formulations include extended-release tablets; an intravenous preparation also is available.

Pharmacokinetics

Oral absorption of levetiracetam is rapid and nearly complete, with peak plasma concentrations in 1.3 hours. Food slows the rate of absorption but does not affect the amount absorbed. Kinetics are linear. Protein binding is less than 10%. The plasma half-life is 6–8 hours but may be longer in the elderly. Two thirds of the drug is excreted unchanged in the urine and the remainder as the inactive deaminated metabolite 2-pyrrolidone-*N*-butyric acid. The metabolism of levetiracetam occurs in the blood. There is no metabolism in the liver, and drug interactions are minimal.

BRIVARACETAM

Brivaracetam, the 4-*n*-propyl analog of levetiracetam, is a high-affinity SV2A ligand recently approved for the treatment of focal (partial) onset seizures. There is no evidence that brivaracetam has superior efficacy to levetiracetam for this indication. As is the case with levetiracetam, brivaracetam use has been associated with psychiatric adverse effects including depression, insomnia, irritability, aggression, belligerence, anger, and anxiety. There is some evidence that patients experiencing such behavioral adverse effects during treatment with levetiracetam will benefit from a switch to brivaracetam. However, there is also evidence that levetiracetam may have reduced propensity for other adverse effects such as dizziness. Whether brivaracetam will prove to have the broad-spectrum activity of levetiracetam remains to be demonstrated although this seems likely given the similarity with levetiracetam. Brivaracetam is active in animal models of generalized epilepsies. It improved or abolished the photoparoxysmal response (abnormal occurrence of cortical spikes or spike and wave discharges on EEG in response to intermittent light stimulation) in patients with generalized epilepsies. In addition, the drug reduced the frequency of generalized seizures in a small number of patients with generalized epilepsy included in a clinical trial, and there have been case reports of favorable responses in additional patients with absence and myoclonic seizures. Brivaracetam exhibits linear pharmacokinetics over a wide dose range (10–600 mg, single oral dose). It is rapidly and completely absorbed after oral administration; has an elimination half-life of 7–8 hours, which allows twice-daily dosing; and has low plasma protein binding (<20%).

Coadministration of brivaracetam with carbamazepine may increase exposure to carbamazepine epoxide, the active metabolite of carbamazepine, possibly leading to adverse effects; carbamazepine dose reduction should be considered. Similarly, coadministration of brivaracetam with phenytoin may increase phenytoin levels. Coadministration of other antiseizure medications is unlikely to affect brivaracetam exposure. Brivaracetam provides no added therapeutic benefit when administered in conjunction with levetiracetam; both drugs act on SV2A.

PERAMPANEL

Perampanel is an orally active AMPA receptor antagonist approved for the treatment of focal seizures and primary generalized tonic-clonic seizures in idiopathic (genetic) generalized epilepsies.

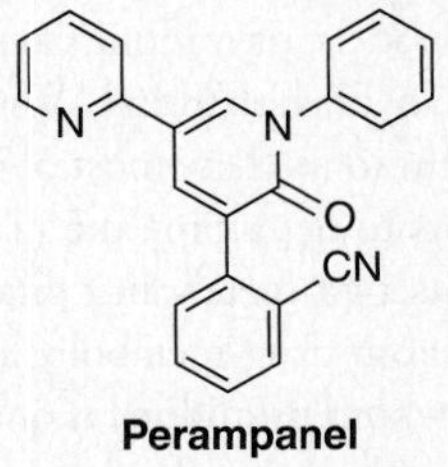

Perampanel

Mechanism of Action

Perampanel is a potent noncompetitive antagonist of the AMPA receptor, a subtype of the ionotropic glutamate receptor that is the main mediator of synaptic excitation in the central nervous system (see Figure 24–1). AMPA receptors are critical to local generation of seizure activity in epileptic foci and are also responsible for the neuron-to-neuron spread of excitation. Partial blockade of AMPA receptors by therapeutic concentrations of perampanel reduces the likelihood of seizure occurrence. In generalized convulsive seizures, whether occurring as a secondarily generalized convulsion following a focal seizure or as a primary generalized seizure, excitatory cortical neurons engage subcortical centers, including the thalamus, that relay the excitation throughout both hemispheres. This spread of excitation to distant sites is mediated by AMPA receptors at the excitatory synapses that long axons make on their distant targets. Perampanel is therefore well suited to inhibit this spread of excitation, which may account for its activity in preventing secondary (focal-to-bilateral tonic-clonic) and primary generalized convulsive seizures. Perampanel binds to an allosteric site on the extracellular side of the channel, acting as a wedge to prevent channel opening.

Clinical Use

A typical maintenance dose of perampanel for patients 12 years of age and older is 4, 6, or 8 mg/d. Higher doses may be needed in patients who are receiving CYP3A4-inducing antiseizure medications. Perampanel use is often associated with behavioral adverse reactions including aggression, hostility, irritability, and anger. The frequency of these adverse effects increases in a dose-dependent fashion, and they occur more often in younger patients and in those with learning disabilities or dementia. Alcohol use may exacerbate the level of anger. Other common adverse effects are dizziness, somnolence, and headache. Falls are more common at higher doses.

Pharmacokinetics

Perampanel has a long half-life, typically ranging from 70 to 110 hours, which permits once-daily dosing. Because of the long half-life, steady state is not achieved for 2–3 weeks; the prescriber should make dosage changes no more frequently than at 2-week (or longer) intervals. The kinetics are linear in the dose range of 2–12 mg/d. The half-life is prolonged in moderate hepatic failure. Absorption is rapid and the drug is fully bioavailable. Although food slows the rate of absorption, the extent is not affected. Perampanel is 95% bound to plasma proteins. The drug is extensively metabolized via initial oxidation by CYP3A4 and subsequent glucuronidation.

Drug Interactions

The most significant drug interactions with perampanel are with potent CYP3A4 inducer antiseizure medications such as carbamazepine, oxcarbazepine, and phenytoin. Concomitant use with such agents increases the clearance of perampanel by 50–70%, which may require the use of higher perampanel doses. Of somewhat lesser concern is the potential for strong CYP3A4 inhibitors to increase the levels of perampanel. Perampanel may decrease the effectiveness of levonorgestrel-containing hormonal contraceptives.

PHENOBARBITAL

In 1903, chemists in Germany discovered that lipophilic derivatives of barbituric acid induced sleep in dogs. Phenobarbital was introduced into the clinical market in 1912 as a sleeping aid; it was serendipitously found to be useful in the treatment of epilepsy. In comparison with anesthetic barbiturates such as pentobarbital, phenobarbital is preferred in the chronic treatment of epilepsy because it is less sedative at antiseizure doses. Intravenous pentobarbital, however, is frequently used to induce general anesthesia in the treatment of drug-refractory status epilepticus. Phenobarbital is the oldest of the currently available antiseizure medications; however, the drug is no longer a first choice in the developed world because of its sedative properties and many drug interactions. Phenobarbital has long been used as a first-line treatment for seizures in neonates, and in 2022 it was approved by the US Food and Drug Administration for the treatment of neonatal seizures in term and preterm infants.

Chemistry

Four barbituric acid derivatives were once used for epilepsy: phenobarbital, mephobarbital, metharbital, and primidone. Only phenobarbital and primidone remain in common use.

Mechanism of Action (see also Chapter 22)

Barbiturates such as phenobarbital act as positive allosteric modulators of $GABA_A$ receptors at low concentrations (see Figure 22–6); at higher concentrations, the drugs directly activate $GABA_A$ receptors. In contrast to benzodiazepines, which augment the frequency of $GABA_A$ receptor chloride channel opening, barbiturates increase the mean open duration of the channel without altering either channel conductance or opening frequency. Phenobarbital also exerts other actions on synaptic function and intrinsic neuronal excitability mechanisms; some of these could be relevant to its clinical antiseizure activity, including block of AMPA receptors or voltage-activated calcium channels.

Clinical Uses

Phenobarbital is useful in the treatment of focal seizures and generalized tonic-clonic seizures. Evidence-based comparisons of phenobarbital with phenytoin and carbamazepine have shown no difference in seizure control, but phenobarbital was more likely to be discontinued due to adverse effects. Phenobarbital may be useful in the treatment of myoclonic seizures, such as in juvenile myoclonic epilepsy, but it is not a drug of first choice. Phenobarbital may worsen absence seizures and infantile spasms. Long-term administration of phenobarbital leads to physical dependence such that seizure threshold is reduced upon withdrawal. The drug must be discontinued gradually over several weeks to avoid the occurrence of severe seizures or status epilepticus.

Pharmacokinetics, Therapeutic Levels, & Dosage

For pharmacokinetics, drug interactions, and toxicity of phenobarbital, see Chapter 22. The dose of phenobarbital is individualized based on clinical response. Dosing information from clinical trials is limited. Doses in the range of 60–200 mg, divided two or three times daily, are typically used. The minimally effective dose may be 60 mg/d, and the median effective dose range may be 100–150 mg/d. The accepted serum concentration reference range is 15–40 mcg/mL, although many patients tolerate chronic levels above 40 mcg/mL. Mean steady-state plasma phenobarbital levels with 60 and 100 mg/d dosing are 14 and 21 mcg/mL, respectively.

PRIMIDONE

Primidone (2-desoxyphenobarbital) is a derivative of phenobarbital. In the early 1950s, the drug was found to have antiseizure activity in animal models; subsequent evidence showed it to be clinically active in the treatment of epilepsy. It was widely used until the 1960s but was then largely abandoned because of its high incidence of adverse effects. It is effective for the treatment of essential tremor and is still used for this indication.

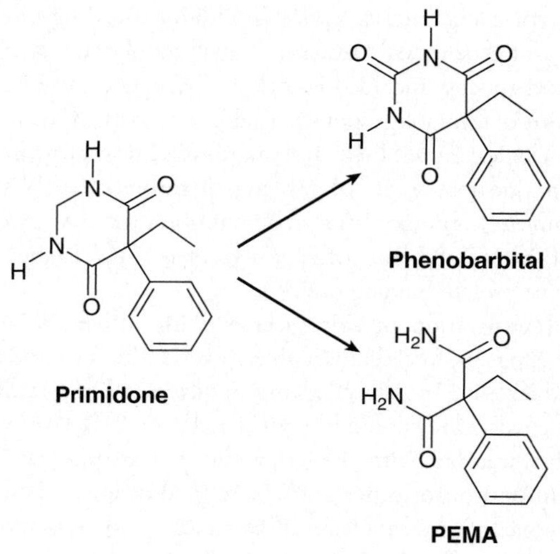

Primidone

Phenobarbital

PEMA

Mechanism of Action

Primidone is metabolized to phenobarbital and phenylethylmalonamide (PEMA). All three compounds are active antiseizure agents. Although phenobarbital is roughly equally active in the MES and PTZ animal tests, primidone has greater activity in the MES test than the PTZ test, indicating that it acts more like the sodium channel-blocking antiseizure medications than phenobarbital. Also, in animal models, primidone causes relatively less acute motor impairment than phenobarbital. With chronic treatment, phenobarbital is thought to mediate most of the antiseizure activity of primidone. Attempts to determine the relative contributions of the parent drug and its two metabolites have been conducted in newborn infants, in whom drug-metabolizing enzyme systems are very immature and in whom primidone is only slowly metabolized. In these patients, primidone is effective in controlling seizures, confirming that it has intrinsic antiseizure activity. This conclusion was reinforced by studies in older patients initiating treatment with primidone, in which seizure control was obtained before phenobarbital concentrations reached the therapeutic range.

Clinical Uses

Primidone is effective against focal seizures and generalized tonic-clonic seizures, but its overall effectiveness is less than drugs such as carbamazepine and phenytoin because of a high incidence of acute toxicity on initial administration and because of chronic sedative effects at effective doses. Use of primidone in movement disorders is discussed in Chapter 28.

Pharmacokinetics

Primidone is completely absorbed, usually reaching peak concentrations about 3 hours after oral administration. Primidone is only 30% bound to plasma proteins. The volume of distribution is 0.6 L/kg. As shown in the text figure, primidone is metabolized by oxidation to phenobarbital, which accumulates slowly, and by scission of the heterocyclic ring to form PEMA. Both primidone and phenobarbital also undergo subsequent conjugation and excretion. Primidone has a larger clearance than most other antiseizure medications (2 L/kg/d), corresponding to a half-life of 6–8 hours. PEMA clearance is approximately half that of primidone, but phenobarbital has a very low clearance (see Table 3–1). The appearance of phenobarbital corresponds to the disappearance of primidone. During chronic therapy, the phenobarbital levels derived from primidone are usually two to three times higher than the primidone levels.

Therapeutic Levels & Dosage

Primidone is most efficacious when plasma levels are in the range of 8–12 mcg/mL. Concomitant levels of its metabolite, phenobarbital, at steady state, usually vary from 15 to 30 mcg/mL. Dosages of 10–20 mg/kg/d are necessary to obtain these levels. Primidone should be started at a low daily dose, which is then gradually escalated over several days to a few weeks to avoid prominent sedation and gastrointestinal complaints. When adjusting doses of the drug, the parent drug reaches steady state rapidly (30–40 hours), but the active metabolites phenobarbital and PEMA reach steady state much more slowly, at approximately 20 days and 3–4 days, respectively.

Toxicity

The dose-related adverse effects of primidone are similar to those of its metabolite, phenobarbital, except that many patients experience severe adverse effects on initial dosing including drowsiness, dizziness, ataxia, nausea, and vomiting. Tolerance to these adverse effects develops in hours to days and can be minimized by slow titration.

FELBAMATE

Felbamate is a dicarbamate that is used in the treatment of focal seizures and in the Lennox-Gastaut syndrome. It is structurally related to the sedative-hypnotic meprobamate. Felbamate is generally well tolerated; some patients report *improved* alertness. However, because the drug can cause aplastic anemia and hepatic failure, felbamate is used only for patients with refractory seizures who respond poorly to other medications. Despite the seriousness of the adverse effects, thousands of patients worldwide use this medication.

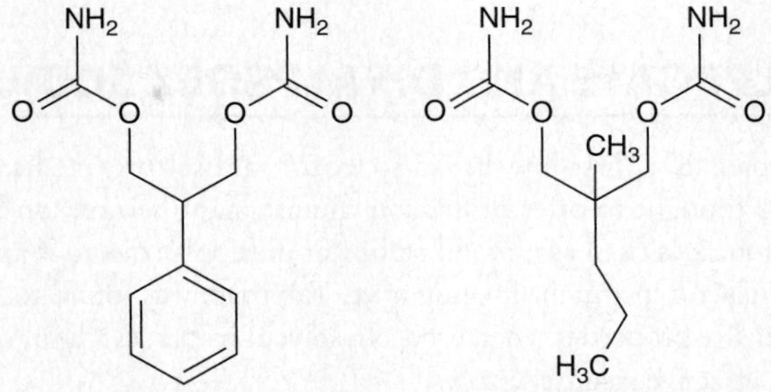

Felbamate   Meprobamate

Mechanism of Action

Felbamate appears to have multiple mechanisms of action. It produces a use-dependent block of NMDA receptors, with selectivity for those containing the GluN2B (NR2B) subunit; the drug also produces a barbiturate-like potentiation of $GABA_A$ receptor responses, but is of low efficacy.

Clinical Use

The typical starting dose of felbamate is 400 mg three times a day. The dose may be escalated slowly to a maximum dose of 3600 mg/d, although some patients have received doses as high as 6000 mg/d. Effective plasma levels range from 30 to 100 mcg/mL; optimal seizure control is believed to occur with concentrations below 60 mcg/mL. In addition to its usefulness in focal seizures, felbamate ameliorates atonic seizures as well as other seizure types in the Lennox-Gastaut syndrome.

Pharmacokinetics & Drug Interactions

Oral felbamate is well absorbed (>90%). Of the absorbed dose, 30–50% is excreted unchanged in the urine. The remainder is metabolized by CYP3A4 and CYP2E1 in the liver. The mean terminal half-life of 20 hours in monotherapy decreases to 13–14 hours in the presence of phenytoin or carbamazepine. Felbamate decreases the clearance of phenytoin (by inhibition of CYP2C19) and valproate (by inhibition of β-oxidation) and increases their blood levels; dose reductions of these drugs may be necessary when felbamate is initiated. Felbamate reduces levels of carbamazepine but increases levels of the metabolite carbamazepine epoxide, which may be associated with adverse effects including dizziness, diplopia, or headache.

MEDICATIONS EFFECTIVE FOR GENERALIZED ONSET SEIZURES

A limited number of antiseizure medications are first-line agents in the treatment of patients who exhibit multiple generalized onset seizure types. Valproate is especially effective and is considered the first-choice treatment for such patients. However, it has various troublesome side effects and is a known human teratogen; its use is avoided in women of childbearing potential. Other drugs that may have broad activity in generalized epilepsies are topiramate and zonisamide.

VALPROATE AND DIVALPROEX SODIUM

Valproate is a first-line broad-spectrum antiseizure medication that is thought to offer protection against many seizure types. In addition, it is used as a mood stabilizer in bipolar disorder and as prophylactic treatment for migraine. Valproate was found to have antiseizure properties when used as a solvent in the search for other drugs effective against seizures.

Chemistry

Valproic acid is a short-chain branched fatty acid that is liquid at room temperature; it is formulated as an oral syrup solution or in gelatin capsules. More commonly, however, the drug is used in a coordination complex—referred to as divalproex sodium—composed of equal parts of valproic acid and the salt sodium valproate. An extended-release divalproex formulation in a hydrophilic polymer matrix allows once-a-day oral administration. Valproic acid has a pK_a value of 4.56 and is therefore fully ionized at body pH; for that reason, the active form of the drug is the valproate ion, regardless of whether valproic acid or the salt of the acid is administered. Valproic acid is one of a series of fatty carboxylic acids that have antiseizure activity; this activity appears to be greatest for carbon chain lengths of five to eight atoms. The amides and esters of valproic acid also are active antiseizure agents.

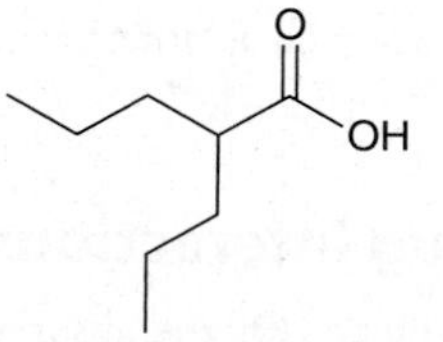

O OH O O⁻Na⁺

Valproic acid 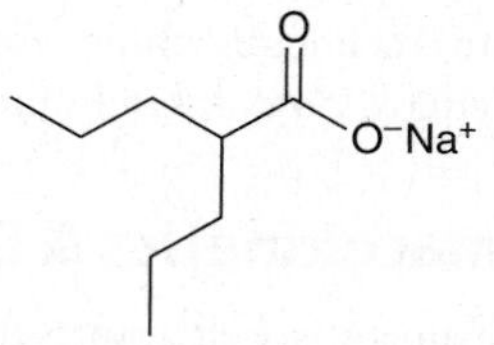 Sodium valproate

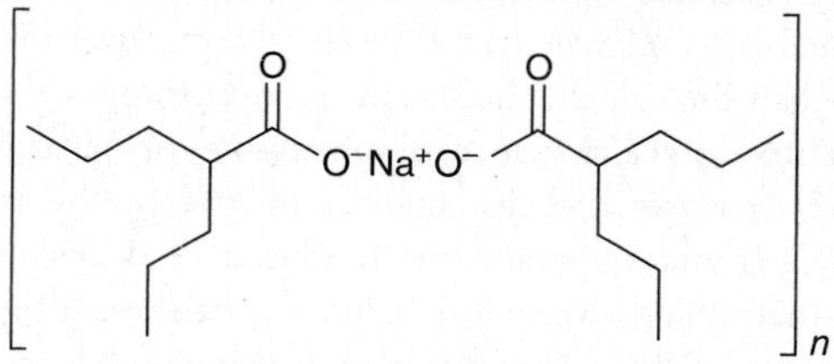

O O O⁻Na⁺O⁻ n

Divalproex sodium

Mechanism of Action

The mechanism or mechanisms whereby valproate exerts its therapeutic actions are not known. Valproate has broad-spectrum efficacy in animal models, conferring seizure protection in diverse chemoconvulsant seizure models, the MES test, and the kindling models. The time course of valproate's antiseizure activity is poorly correlated with blood or tissue levels of the parent drug, an observation that has led to speculation regarding the active species.

Clinical Uses

Valproate is one of the most versatile and effective antiseizure medications. It is widely used for myoclonic (such as in juvenile myoclonic epilepsy), atonic (as in Lennox-Gastaut syndrome), and generalized onset tonic-clonic seizures. Valproate is also effective in the treatment of generalized absence seizures and is often preferred to ethosuximide when the patient has concomitant generalized tonic-clonic seizures. Valproate is also effective in focal seizures, but it may not be as effective as carbamazepine or phenytoin. Intravenous formulations can be used to treat status epilepticus.

Pharmacokinetics

Valproate is well absorbed after an oral dose, with bioavailability greater than 80%. Peak blood levels are observed within 2 hours. Food may delay absorption, and the drug may have improved tolerability if it is administered after meals. Valproate is highly bound to plasma proteins, but protein binding becomes saturated as the concentration increases at the upper end of the therapeutic range, resulting in an increase in the plasma free fraction of valproate from 10% at plasma concentrations up to 75 mcg/mL to 30% at levels greater that 150 mcg/mL. Such increases lead to an apparent increase in the clearance of total valproate at high doses. The half-life varies from 9 to 18 hours; extended-release formulations are therefore preferred. Because valproate is highly protein bound, it is largely confined to blood plasma; the drug has a low volume of distribution of approximately 0.15 L/kg. Valproate is extensively metabolized in the liver. A major hepatic metabolite is the glucuronide conjugate, which is excreted in the urine (approximately 30–50% of the dose). Valproate also undergoes mitochondrial β-oxidation (20–40%) and hepatic microsomal cytochrome P450-mediated oxidation (approximately 10%). In excess of 25 metabolites have been identified, but apart from valproic acid glucuronide, 3-oxo-valproic acid is the most abundant.

Dosing and Therapeutic Levels

An initial daily dose of 15 mg/kg is recommended with slow titration to the therapeutic dose. Dosages of 25–30 mg/kg/d may be adequate in some patients, but others may require 60 mg/kg/d or even more. Therapeutic levels of valproate range from 50 to 100 mcg/mL, but concentrations up to 150 mcg/mL are generally tolerated and may be required.

Drug Interactions

Valproate inhibits the metabolism of several drugs, including phenobarbital and ethosuximide, leading to higher steady-state concentrations of these agents. Levels of phenobarbital may rise steeply, causing stupor or coma. Valproate displaces phenytoin from plasma proteins, causing an increase in the free fraction of phenytoin, and total phenytoin concentrations in the therapeutic range may be associated with toxicity. Although valproate does not increase levels of carbamazepine itself, levels of carbamazepine epoxide may be increased. Valproate can dramatically decrease the clearance of lamotrigine, resulting in a two- to threefold prolongation of lamotrigine's half-life.

Toxicity

The most common dose-related adverse effects of valproate are nausea, vomiting, and other gastrointestinal complaints such as abdominal pain and heartburn. The drug should be started gradually to avoid these symptoms. A fine tremor is frequently seen at higher levels. Other reversible adverse effects occurring in some patients include weight gain, increased appetite, and hair loss.

Valproate rarely causes idiosyncratic hepatic toxicity that may be severe and has been fatal. The risk is greatest for patients under 2 years of age and for those taking multiple medications. Initial aspartate aminotransferase values may not be elevated in susceptible patients, although these levels do eventually become abnormal. Most fatalities have occurred within 4 months after initiation of therapy. The other observed idiosyncratic adverse effect with valproate is thrombocytopenia, although documented cases of abnormal bleeding are lacking. Valproate can interfere with conversion of ammonia to urea. It can cause lethargy associated with increased blood ammonia concentrations. Fatal hyperammonemic encephalopathy has occurred in patients with genetic defects in urea metabolism; the drug is contraindicated in these patients.

Treatment with valproate during the first trimester of pregnancy is associated with a 1–2% risk of neural tube defects including spina bifida. In addition, an increased incidence of cardiovascular, orofacial, and digital abnormalities has been noted. Finally, cognitive impairment in offspring has been reported. These observations must be strongly considered in the choice of drugs in women of child-bearing potential.

TOPIRAMATE

Topiramate is a broad-spectrum antiseizure medication whose chemical structure is that of a sulfamate-substituted monosaccharide derived from D-fructose. It is used in the treatment of focal seizures, primary generalized seizures, and seizures in the Lennox-Gastaut syndrome. Topiramate is also commonly used for migraine headache prophylaxis.

Topiramate

Mechanism of Action

Topiramate likely acts through several cellular targets, which may account for its broad-spectrum activity in epilepsy and migraine. Possible sites of action relevant to its clinical activities are (1) voltage-gated sodium channels; (2) $GABA_A$ receptor subtypes; and (3) AMPA or kainate receptors. The drug is a weak inhibitor of carbonic anhydrase isoenzymes II and IV, but this is not thought to account for its antiseizure effects. In rare cases, the inhibition of carbonic anhydrase may cause metabolic acidosis of clinical importance.

Clinical Uses

Topiramate is effective in the treatment of focal seizures in adults and children and in primary generalized tonic-clonic seizures. The drug is approved for the Lennox-Gastaut syndrome and may be effective in juvenile myoclonic epilepsy, infantile spasms, Dravet syndrome, and even childhood absence seizures. The initial dose in newly diagnosed patients is typically 100 mg/d, but maintenance doses usually range from 200 to 400 mg/d. Most clinicians begin at a low dose (25–50 mg/d) and increase slowly to prevent adverse effects. Cognitive side effects commonly occur with topiramate and are a frequent reason for discontinuation. Affected patients experience impaired expressive language function (dysnomia and diminished verbal fluency), impaired verbal memory, and a general slowing of cognitive processing. These effects are unlike those of other antiseizure medications and often occur without sedation or mood change. The incidence of cognitive side effects increases in a dose-dependent fashion, reaching 26% at a dose of 400 mg/d; however, some patients are completely unaffected even at higher dosages. Another troublesome adverse effect that commonly occurs with topiramate is paresthesias, typically occurring during initiation of therapy or at high doses; the symptoms may resolve with continuing treatment. Other dose-related adverse effects that occur frequently in the first 4 weeks of topiramate therapy are somnolence, fatigue, dizziness, nervousness, and confusion. Acute myopia and angle-closure glaucoma may require prompt drug withdrawal. Urolithiasis occurs in 0.5–1.5% of patients on long-term therapy and is more common in men. In some patients, carbonic anhydrase inhibition is associated with reduced serum bicarbonate that is usually asymptomatic but may result in nonspecific symptoms such as fatigue, anorexia, or nausea and vomiting. The potential for chronic untreated hyperchloremic non–anion gap metabolic acidosis for bone health is unknown. Decreased sweating (oligohydrosis) and an elevation in body temperature may occur during exposure to hot weather, mostly in children. Long-term topiramate therapy is often associated with significant weight loss, primarily due to a reduction in body fat mass. In clinical trials, 85% of adults receiving topiramate lost weight, which on average amounted to 5% of mean baseline body weight. Greater weight loss occurs in those with higher pretreatment weight. Weight loss is gradual and typically peaks at 12–18 months after initiation of therapy. Beneficial changes in lipid profile, glycemic control, and blood pressure may accompany the weight loss. Data in humans suggest a link between topiramate use in the first trimester of pregnancy and oral cleft formation in newborns (relative risk 16- to 21-fold).

Pharmacokinetics

Topiramate is rapidly absorbed (about 2 hours) and is 80% bioavailable. There is minimal food effect on absorption, minimal (15%) plasma protein binding, and only moderate (20–50%) metabolism; no active metabolites are formed. The drug is primarily excreted in the urine (50–80% is unchanged). The monotherapy half-life is 20–30 hours but drops to 12–15 hours when administered with concomitant enzyme-inducing drugs. Immediate-release formulations are usually administered in two daily doses. Extended-release formulations are available that have been approved for once-daily administration. Although increased levels are seen with renal failure and hepatic impairment, there is no age or gender effect, no autoinduction, and no inhibition of metabolism, and kinetics are linear. Drug interactions do occur and can be complex, but the major effect is on topiramate levels rather than on the levels of other antiseizure medications. Birth control pills may be less effective in the presence of topiramate, and alternative modes of contraception are recommended in women taking more than 200 mg/d; however, oral contraceptives with a higher content of ethinyl estradiol (50 mcg) may be satisfactory.

ZONISAMIDE

Zonisamide is a broad-spectrum antiseizure medication that is effective for focal and generalized tonic-clonic seizures in adults and children and may also be effective in some myoclonic epilepsies and in infantile spasms. There are reports of improvement in generalized onset tonic-clonic seizures and atypical absence seizures.

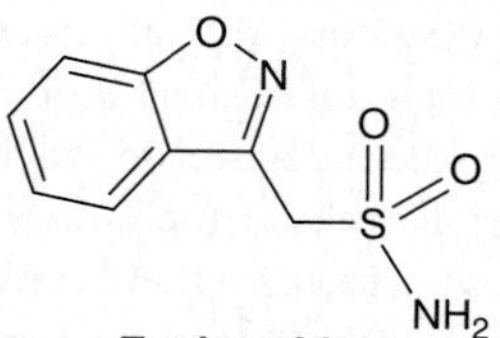

O N O O S NH$_2$

Zonisamide

There is little information on the mechanism of action of zonisamide. Although it does block voltage-gated sodium channels, other actions also may contribute to its antiseizure activity. Zonisamide has high bioavailability, modest protein binding (>50–60%), and a half-life of 1–3 days, so it can be administered once daily. The drug is extensively metabolized by acetylation to form *N*-acetyl-zonisamide, which is excreted in the urine unchanged, and by CYP3A4 to form 2-sulfamoylacetylphenol, which is excreted as the glucuronide. Maintenance doses are 200–400 mg/d in adults (maximum 600 mg/d) and 4–8 mg/kg/d in children (maximum 12 mg/kg/d). Adverse effects include drowsiness, cognitive impairment, renal stones, and potentially serious skin rashes. Zonisamide has no clinically significant effects on the pharmacokinetics of other antiseizure medications. However, antiseizure medications such as carbamazepine, phenytoin, and phenobarbital that induce CYP3A4 increase the clearance of zonisamide, shortening its half-life; concomitant use with CYP3A4-inducing agents may therefore require an increase in zonisamide dose. Zonisamide, like topiramate, contains sulfur: zonisamide is a sulfonamide, whereas topiramate contains the same sulfonamide structure but is strictly a sulfamate. They have similar pharmacologic actions, including carbonic anhydrase inhibition like acetazolamide, which also is a sulfonamide. Both zonisamide and topiramate are associated with weight loss. They also both (rarely) cause kidney stones and oligohydrosis. Whether these actions are related to the common sulfonamide structure is not known.

MEDICATIONS EFFECTIVE FOR GENERALIZED ABSENCE SEIZURES

Ethosuximide and valproate are effective and well-tolerated treatments for generalized absence seizures in childhood absence epilepsy; lamotrigine is possibly effective. Ethosuximide is considered in this section along with trimethadione, which is of historical interest.

ETHOSUXIMIDE

Ethosuximide is a first-line drug for the treatment of generalized absence seizures. It can be used as monotherapy unless generalized tonic-clonic seizures also are present, in which case valproate is preferred or ethosuximide can be combined with another drug effective against generalized tonic-clonic seizures.

Chemistry

Ethosuximide was introduced in 1958 as the third of three marketed succinimides; the other two, phensuximide and methsuximide, are rarely used. Ethosuximide and methsuximide have asymmetric carbons (asterisks in the following figure) and are used as racemates.

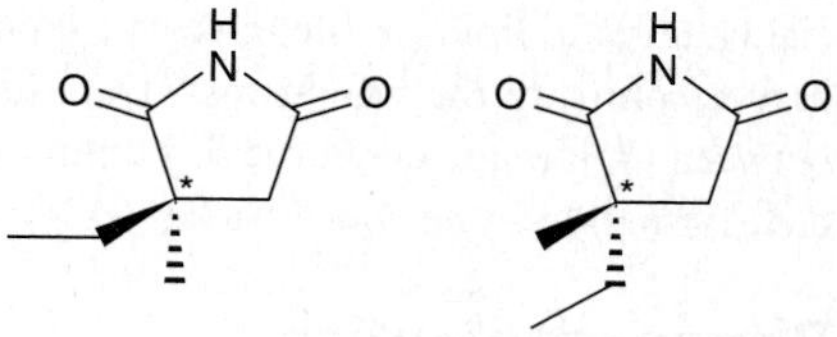

H O N O * H O N O * O N O O N O *

Ethosuximide 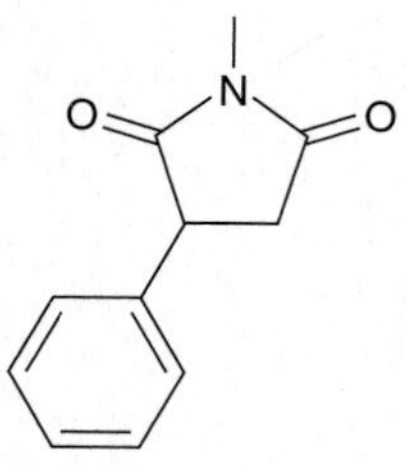 Phensuximide 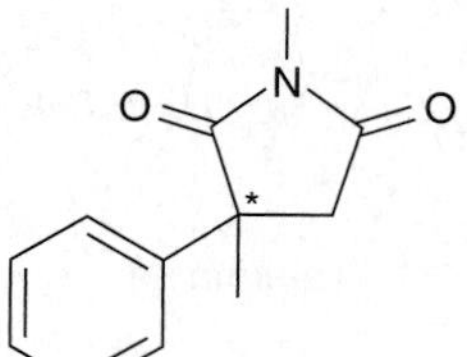 Methsuximide

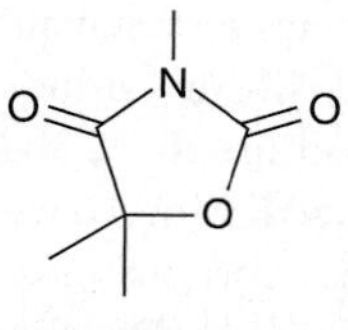

O N O O

Trimethadione

Mechanism of Action

Ethosuximide is thought to act by inhibition of low-voltage-activated T-type calcium channels in thalamocortical neurons that underlie the 3-Hz spike-wave discharges of generalized absence seizures. Other ion channels affected include voltage-gated sodium channels, calcium-activated potassium channels, and inward rectifier potassium channels; these actions may contribute to the efficacy of ethosuximide in absence epilepsy.

Clinical Uses

Studies in the mid-1970s provided evidence that monotherapy with ethosuximide is effective in the treatment of childhood generalized absence seizures. There is also evidence that it is effective in the treatment of atypical absence and epileptic negative myoclonus, a rare seizure type characterized by interruption of ongoing electromyographic activity contralateral to a lateralized spike-and-wave discharge. If ethosuximide in monotherapy does not lead to seizure control, the drug can be used in combination with valproate or other agents such as benzodiazepines.

Pharmacokinetics

Absorption is complete following administration of the oral dosage forms. Peak levels are observed 3–7 hours after oral administration of the capsules. Ethosuximide is not protein bound. During long-term administration, approximately 20% of the dose is excreted unchanged by the kidney. The remaining drug is metabolized in the liver, principally by CYP3A hydroxylation, to inactive metabolites. Ethosuximide has a very low total body clearance (0.25 L/kg/d). This corresponds to a half-life of approximately 40 hours, although values from 18 to 72 hours have been reported.

Therapeutic Levels & Dosage

In children, a common starting dose is 10–15 mg/kg/d, with titration according to clinical response to a maintenance dose of 15–40 mg/kg/d. In older children and adults, the initial dose is 250 or 500 mg/d, increasing in 250-mg increments to clinical response to a maximum of 1500 mg/d. While dosing is based on titration to maximal seizure control with acceptable tolerability, the accepted therapeutic serum concentration range is 40–100 mcg/mL (although plasma levels up to 150 mcg/mL may be necessary and tolerated in some patients). There is a linear relationship between ethosuximide dose and steady-state plasma levels. While the long half-life could allow once-daily dosing, ethosuximide is generally administered in two or even three divided doses to minimize adverse gastrointestinal effects.

Drug Interactions & Toxicity

Administration of ethosuximide with valproate results in a decrease in ethosuximide clearance and higher steady-state concentrations owing to inhibition of ethosuximide metabolism. No other important drug interactions have been reported. The most common dose-related adverse effect of ethosuximide is gastric distress, including pain, nausea, and vomiting. When an adverse effect does occur, temporary dosage reductions may allow adaptation. Other dose-related adverse effects are transient lethargy or fatigue and, much less commonly, headache, dizziness, hiccup, and euphoria. Behavioral changes are usually in the direction of improvement. Non-dose-related or idiosyncratic adverse effects of ethosuximide are extremely uncommon.

TRIMETHADIONE

Trimethadione is an oxazolidinedione antiseizure medication introduced in 1945. It is no longer marketed in the USA but is available elsewhere. Trimethadione is effective in the treatment of generalized absence seizures and was the drug of choice for this seizure type until the introduction of ethosuximide. Trimethadione has numerous dose-related and idiosyncratic side effects, including hemeralopia (day blindness). Because of the high propensity for side effects, trimethadione and the related oxazolidinediones paramethadione and dimethadione, the major metabolite of trimethadione, are now rarely used.

MEDICATIONS EFFECTIVE FOR MYOCLONIC SEIZURES SUCH AS IN THE SYNDROME OF JUVENILE MYOCLONIC EPILEPSY

Valproate is the drug of first choice for the treatment of myoclonic seizures. Other drugs effective in the treatment of this seizure type are levetiracetam, zonisamide, topiramate, and lamotrigine.

MEDICATIONS EFFECTIVE FOR ATONIC SEIZURES SUCH AS IN THE LENNOX-GASTAUT SYNDROME

Valproate in combination with lamotrigine and a benzodiazepine is the most widely used treatment for atonic seizures. Topiramate, felbamate, and lamotrigine are used in the treatment of Lennox-Gastaut syndrome; clinical trials have shown improvement in atonic seizures. Clobazam and rufinamide, discussed in this section, also are used in the treatment of seizures associated with Lennox-Gastaut syndrome and have been demonstrated in clinical trials to reduce the frequency of atonic seizures.

CLOBAZAM

Clobazam is widely used for the treatment of focal seizures in many countries, although it is not approved for that indication in the USA, where its only approved use is for treatment of seizures associated with Lennox-Gastaut syndrome in patients 2 years of age or older. Clobazam is a 1,5-benzodiazepine and structurally different from other marketed benzodiazepines, which are 1,4-benzodiazepines. Like the 1,4-benzodiazepines, however, clobazam is a positive allosteric modulator of $GABA_A$ receptors and has similar pharmacologic activities and adverse effects. In addition, while tolerance occurs to clobazam in animal models within days to weeks of chronic administration, retrospective studies assessing the extent of tolerance in the clinical setting have suggested that tolerance is not a prominent issue in clinical treatment. Side effects that occur in a dose-dependent fashion include somnolence and sedation, dysarthria, drooling, and behavioral changes, including aggression. Withdrawal symptoms may occur with abrupt discontinuation. Clobazam has a half-life of 10–30 hours and is effective at dosages of 0.5–1 mg/kg/d. Clobazam is metabolized in the liver by CYP and non-CYP transformations, with up to 14 metabolites; however, the major metabolite is N-desmethylclobazam (norclobazam), which is produced by CYP3A4. Norclobazam is then mainly metabolized by CYP2C19 except in CYP2C19-poor metabolizers with a CYP2C19 inactive allele. With long-term administration of clobazam, levels of norclobazam, which has a longer half-life than clobazam, are 8–20 times higher than those of the parent. Norclobazam has antiseizure activity, although it is weaker than clobazam. Nevertheless, because norclobazam levels are so much higher at steady state, seizure protection during chronic therapy is likely mainly due to norclobazam. Cannabidiol, via inhibition of CYP2C19, causes a threefold increase in plasma concentrations of norclobazam. When cannabidiol is added, the clobazam dose may require reduction to avoid excessive sedation. Clobazam is a moderate inhibitor of CYP2D6 and has been shown to significantly increase the levels of drugs metabolized by this isoenzyme such as phenytoin and carbamazepine. Reduced dosing may be required when these antiseizure medications are used in combination with clobazam.

RUFINAMIDE

Rufinamide is a triazole derivative identified by screening in animal seizure models. It is effective for atonic seizures in Lennox-Gastaut syndrome, but there is also some evidence of efficacy in the treatment of focal seizures. In the USA and Europe, rufinamide is only approved for treatment of seizures associated with the Lennox-Gastaut syndrome.

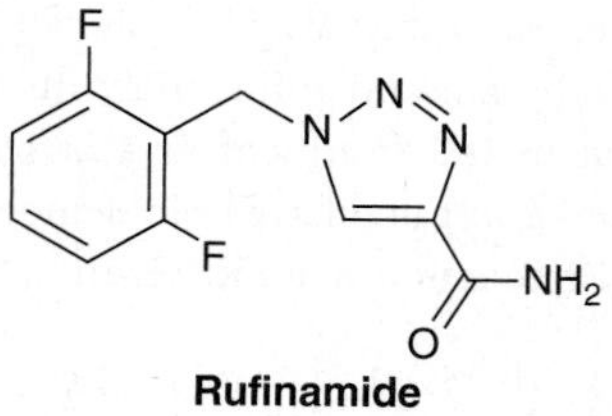

Rufinamide

Mechanism of Action

In mice and rats, rufinamide is protective in the MES test and, at higher doses, in the PTZ test. Its only known action that is relevant to seizure protection is as a blocker of voltage-gated sodium channels.

Clinical Uses

In the Lennox-Gastaut syndrome, rufinamide is effective against all seizure types but especially against atonic seizures. Some clinical data suggest it may be effective against focal seizures. Treatment in children is typically started at 10 mg/kg/d in two equally divided doses and gradually increased to 45 mg/kg/d to a maximum of 3200 mg/d. Adults can begin with 400–800 mg/d in two equally divided doses up to a maximum of 3200 mg/d as tolerated. The drug should be given with food. The most common adverse events are somnolence and vomiting.

Pharmacokinetics

Rufinamide is well absorbed, and plasma concentrations peak between 4 and 6 hours. The half-life is 6–10 hours, and minimal plasma protein binding is observed. Although cytochrome P450 enzymes are not involved, the drug is extensively metabolized to inactive products. Most of the drug is excreted in the urine; an acid metabolite accounts for about two thirds of the dose. Most drug-drug interactions are minor except that valproate may decrease the clearance of rufinamide; dosing with valproate, particularly in children, may need to be decreased, typically by 50%.

MEDICATIONS EFFECTIVE FOR DRAVET SYNDROME

Dravet syndrome (severe myoclonic epilepsy in infancy) is a rare genetic epileptic encephalopathy characterized by diverse generalized and focal seizure types, including myoclonic seizures, tonic-clonic seizures, absence seizures, atonic seizures, and one-sided hemiconvulsive and focal seizures. Mutations of the *SCN1A* gene encoding $Na_v1.1$ voltage-gated sodium channels cause 79% of diagnosed cases of Dravet syndrome. Although drugs such as clobazam, valproate, topiramate, and stiripentol (approved only in combination with clobazam in the USA and in combination with clobazam and valproate in Europe) are used, none of these is very effective. Cannabidiol is a newly available option; it and stiripentol are the only medications specifically approved for Dravet syndrome in the USA. In patients with *SCN1A* gene mutations, sodium channel-blocking antiseizure medications are contraindicated because they worsen seizures.

CANNABIDIOL

Cannabidiol, a non-psychoactive phytocannabinoid found in *Cannabis sativa,* is approved for the treatment of seizures associated with Dravet syndrome and Lennox-Gastaut syndrome. The drug has also been found to be useful in the treatment of seizures associated with tuberous sclerosis complex. In the approved medicinal product, cannabidiol is formulated in an oil-based solution for oral administration. Other cannabidiol preparations, including oil-based solutions, are available as dietary supplements but may not be legal under federal regulations in the USA.

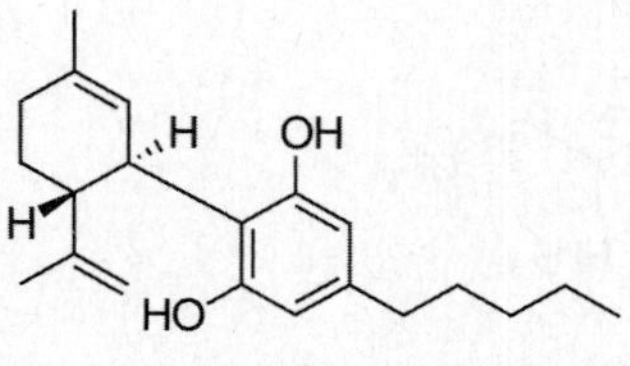

Cannabidiol **Δ^9-Tetrahydrocannabinol**

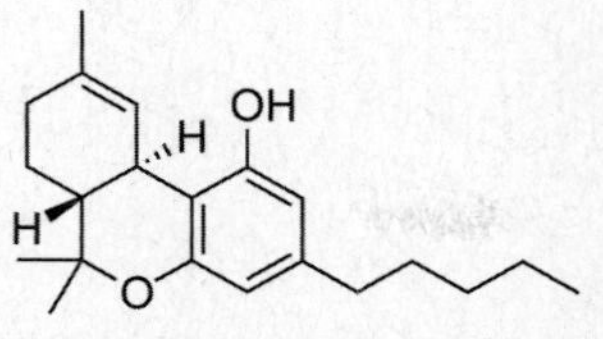

Mechanism of Action

Cannabidiol exhibits broad-spectrum antiseizure activity in animal seizure models, although the overall potency is weak. Unlike the structurally related psychoactive cannabinoid Δ^9-tetrahydrocannabinol, which acts as an agonist of CB_1 (central nervous system) and CB_2 (immune system) cannabinoid receptors, cannabidiol is not a CB_1 or CB_2 receptor agonist and it has been shown that the antiseizure activity of cannabidiol is not due to an action on brain CB_1 receptors. The basis for the antiseizure activity of cannabidiol is unknown.

Clinical Uses

In the epilepsy syndromes where it has been studied, cannabidiol is an effective option, and in some patients may be useful where other medications have failed. Reductions in convulsive seizures associated with Dravet syndrome and atonic seizures associated with Lennox-Gastaut syndrome have been observed. The main adverse events are somnolence (25%), decreased appetite (19%), diarrhea (19%), and fatigue (13%). Liver function test abnormalities occur in a dose-dependent fashion; concurrent valproate increases the risk. Cannabidiol solution is titrated to a maintenance dose of 10 mg/kg/d in two divided doses. The dose may be increased to 20 to 25 mg/kg/d if required for further seizure control.

Pharmacokinetics

The oral bioavailability of cannabidiol is very low (13–19%). The approved formulation of cannabidiol is in sesame oil (100 mg/mL), which consists largely of long-chain triglycerides. Coadministration of the highly lipophilic cannabidiol with the dietary oil results in the formation of mixed micelles as the lipid is digested. Intestinal enterocytes incorporate the micelles into chylomicrons that are transferred by intestinal lymphatics directly into the systemic circulation, bypassing first-pass metabolism in the liver. Consequently, bioavailability is increased threefold in the sesame oil formulation. Bioavailability is further increased four- to fivefold by a high-fat meal. Administration with food is recommended to reduce fluctuations in systemic exposure.

Cannabidiol is metabolized in the liver primarily by CYP2C19 and to a lesser extent by CYP3A4 isoenzymes. Cannabidiol may also be glucuronidated by several UDP-glucuronosyltransferase isoforms. 7-Carboxy-cannabidiol is the major circulating metabolite and after chronic dosing has an approximately 40-fold higher AUC than cannabidiol itself. In animal studies, 7-carboxy-cannabidiol does not exhibit antiseizure activity. Concomitant administration of cannabidiol with clobazam resulted in increased plasma concentrations of N-desmethylclobazam, likely by inhibition of CYP2C19 by cannabidiol. This can lead to excessive sedation and may require reduction in the clobazam dose.

STIRIPENTOL

Stiripentol is an aromatic allylic alcohol that has activity in the treatment of Dravet syndrome. Clinical studies indicate that it reduces the frequency of prolonged seizures in children with this condition. Stiripentol is often used in conjunction with clobazam or valproate; whether it has activity by itself has not been studied in clinical trials. The drug has various effects on GABA-mediated neurotransmission including an action as a positive allosteric modulator of $GABA_A$ receptors. Two metabolites of stiripentol have been identified: 1-(3-methoxy-4-hydroxyphenyl)-4,4-dimethyl-1-penten-3-ol, which has antiseizure activity, and 1-(3-hydroxy-4-methoxyphenyl)-4,4-dimethyl-1-penten-3-ol, which does not. Stiripentol is a potent inhibitor of CYP3A4, CYP1A2, and CYP2C19 and dramatically increases the levels of clobazam and its active metabolite norclobazam; it also inhibits valproate metabolism. These drug-drug interactions have been proposed as the basis for the clinical effectiveness of stiripentol, and elevations in concomitant drugs likely contribute to some extent to efficacy. However, stiripentol has activity in various animal seizure models, indicating that it has antiseizure activity in its own right. Dosing is complex, typically beginning with a reduction in concomitant medications. Stiripentol is then started at 10–15 mg/kg/d in 2–3 divided doses and is increased gradually to a target dose of 50 mg/kg/d over 2–4 weeks as tolerated. The most frequent adverse effects are sedation/drowsiness, reduced appetite, slowing of mental function, ataxia, diplopia, nausea, and abdominal pain. Stiripentol exhibits nonlinear pharmacokinetics, decreasing in clearance as the dose increases.

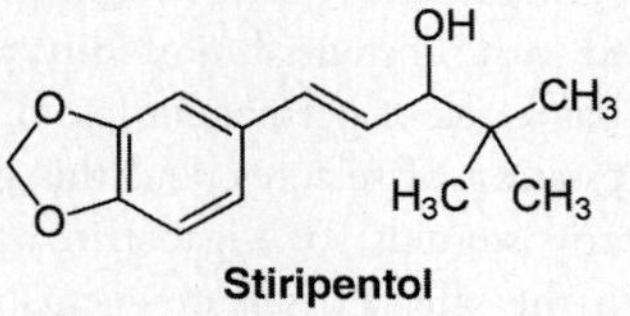

Stiripentol

FENFLURAMINE

Fenfluramine oral solution is effective for the treatment convulsive seizures in Dravet syndrome and atonic seizures in the Lennox-Gastaut syndrome. Fenfluramine, an amphetamine derivative, is an anorexigen that had been used for weight loss but was withdrawn because it induces valvular heart disease and pulmonary hypertension. Studies in patients with Dravet syndrome have shown marked reductions in convulsive seizure frequency. Common side effects are decreased appetite, diarrhea, and fatigue. Fenfluramine is a substrate of the serotonin transporter, causing inhibition of serotonin uptake and enhancing its extracellular release. Norfenfluramine, the main metabolite of fenfluramine, also causes serotonin release. The extent to which serotonin release or effects of fenfluramine on serotonin receptors or other targets contribute the antiseizure activity of the drug remains to be determined. Fenfluramine has minimal activity in rodent seizure models. Norfenfluramine activates 5-HT_{2B} receptors on heart valve and pulmonary artery interstitial cells, leading to the formation of proliferative fibromyxoid plaques that compromise tissue integrity and function. No clinically significant cardiac effects were observed in clinical trials and in long-term monitoring for up to 3 years. Stiripentol inhibits the metabolism of fenfluramine, elevating levels of the parent and reducing levels of the norfenfluramine.

Fenfluramine Norfenfluramine

MEDICATIONS EFFECTIVE FOR INFANTILE SPASMS (WEST SYNDROME)

Infantile spasms are treated with repository corticotropin injection gel by intramuscular or subcutaneous injection, or with oral corticosteroids such as prednisone, prednisolone, methylprednisolone, or dexamethasone. Corticotropin gel is a complex mixture of adrenocorticotropic hormone (ACTH) analogs (including N25-deamidated porcine $ACTH_{1-39}$) as well as other peptides derived from porcine pituitary gland. Vigabatrin also is often used and is particularly effective in cases associated with tuberous sclerosis. Other antiseizure medications that may be helpful are valproate, topiramate, zonisamide, or a benzodiazepine such as clonazepam or nitrazepam. Corticotropin gel and corticosteroids are associated with substantial morbidity, and vigabatrin, as discussed below, has a risk of permanent loss of vision. The goal of treatment is cessation of seizures, and this generally requires corticotropin, corticosteroids, or vigabatrin and is not generally achieved with the safer antiseizure agents. The mechanism of action of corticotropin and corticosteroids in the treatment of infantile spasms is unknown.

VIGABATRIN

Vigabatrin is an analog of GABA, designed as an inhibitor of GABA transaminase (GABA-T), the enzyme responsible for the metabolism of synaptically released GABA. Vigabatrin is effective in the treatment of focal seizures (but not generalized seizures) and in the treatment of infantile spasms. Because it may cause irreversible visual loss, it is usually reserved for patients with seizures refractory to other treatments.

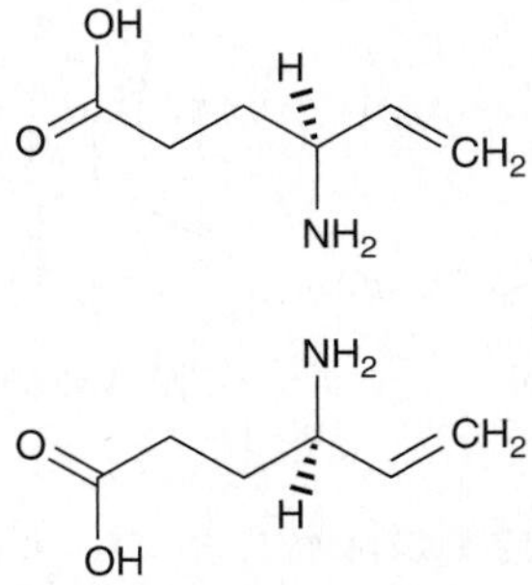

Vigabatrin enantiomers

Mechanism of Action

Vigabatrin is a specific, irreversible inhibitor of GABA-T, producing a sustained increase in the extracellular concentrations of GABA in the brain. This paradoxically leads to inhibition of synaptic $GABA_A$ receptor responses, but also prolongs the activation of extrasynaptic $GABA_A$ receptors that mediate tonic inhibition. Vigabatrin is effective in a wide range of animal seizure models. Vigabatrin is marketed as a racemate; the *S*(+) enantiomer is active and the *R*(–) enantiomer appears to be inactive.

Clinical Uses

Vigabatrin is useful in the treatment of infantile spasms, especially when associated with tuberous sclerosis. The drug is also effective against focal seizures. The half-life is approximately 6–8 hours, but the pharmacodynamic activity of the drug is more prolonged and not well correlated with the plasma half-life because recovery from the drug requires synthesis of replacement GABA-T enzyme. In infants, the dosage is 50–150 mg/kg/d. In adults, vigabatrin is started at an oral dosage of 500 mg twice daily; a total of 2–3 g/d may be required for full effectiveness. The most important adverse effect of vigabatrin is irreversible retinal dysfunction. Patients may develop permanent bilateral concentric visual field constriction that is often asymptomatic but can be disabling. Minimal evidence also suggests that vigabatrin can also damage the central retina. The onset of vision loss can occur within weeks of starting treatment or after months or years. Other adverse effects are somnolence, headache, dizziness, and weight gain. Less common but more troublesome adverse effects are agitation, confusion, and psychosis; preexisting mental illness is a relative contraindication.

EVEROLIMUS FOR FOCAL ONSET SEIZURES ASSOCIATED WITH TUBEROUS SCLEROSIS COMPLEX

The treatment of infantile spasms in tuberous sclerosis complex was discussed previously. Other seizure types that occur in tuberous sclerosis complex are treated with an antiseizure medication appropriate to the seizure type. Medication-refractory patients may benefit from alternative therapies such as the ketogenic diet, vagal nerve stimulation, or epilepsy surgery. The mTORC1 (mammalian target of rapamycin complex 1) inhibitor everolimus is now also an option to treat refractory focal onset seizures associated with the disorder.

Mechanism of Action

Tuberous sclerosis is caused by loss-of-function mutations in the *TSC1* gene encoding the protein hamartin or in the *TSC2* gene encoding tuberin. The mutations lead to constitutive mTOR activation, resulting in abnormal cerebral cortical development with multiple focal structural malformations. The aberrant mTOR signaling leads to cortical tubers and perituberal cortical tissue with dysmorphic neurons, giant cells, reactive astrocytes, and disturbed cortical layering. The development of epilepsy is believed to be related to these structural abnormalities, but the precise basis for epileptogenesis is not understood. mTOR is one member of a family of six atypical serine/threonine protein kinases, referred to as PIKKs (PIK3-related kinases). mTOR forms the catalytic subunit of the cytosolic protein complex mTORC1, which acts as a central controller of cell growth. Drugs that inhibit mTORC1, such as rapamycin (sirolimus) and the rapalog everolimus, bind to the cyclophilin protein FKBP12, a peptidyl-prolyl isomerase. The rapamycin/rapalog-FKBP12 complex then allosterically inhibits mTORC1 by binding to mTOR (when it is associated with the adaptor protein raptor and MLST8).

Clinical Use

Studies have indicated a consistent relationship between everolimus exposure and efficacy in the treatment of seizures associated with tuberous sclerosis complex. Therefore, the dosing recommendation is to target the trough (predose) everolimus whole blood concentration, initially within the range of 5–7 ng/mL and then to titrate to the range of 5–15 ng/mL in the event of an inadequate clinical response. The usual starting dose is 5 mg/m^2 orally once daily, with increments not exceeding 5 mg to achieve the desired blood concentration. The most frequent adverse reactions of everolimus are stomatitis, diarrhea, and pyrexia. Increasing the exposure did not result in an increase in reported adverse events.

Pharmacokinetics

Oral everolimus is absorbed rapidly (30% bioavailability), and reaches peak concentration after 1.3–1.8 hours. The drug is metabolized in the liver primarily by CYP3A4 and is a substrate of the P-glycoprotein (P-gp) transporter. The dosage will likely require reduction in the presence of CYP3A4 inducers such as phenobarbital, primidone, phenytoin, carbamazepine, and oxcarbazepine. The elimination half-life is 30 hours. Plasma protein binding is 74%.

GANAXOLONE

Ganaxolone is a synthetic steroid structurally related to progesterone and the endogenous progesterone metabolite allopregnanolone, and also to the related steroid anesthetic alphaxalone. Ganaxolone is available as an oral suspension for the treatment of seizures associated with CDKL5 deficiency disorder, but its mechanism of action as a $GABA_A$ receptor positive allosteric modulator is compatible with broad-spectrum antiseizure activity. Ganaxolone potentiates $GABA_A$ receptors at distinct sites on the receptor protein complex and in a functionally different way from benzodiazepines; it also acts on benzodiazepine-insensitive $GABA_A$ receptor isoforms. In support of broad clinical utility, ganaxolone confers seizure protection in a wide range of animal seizure models. In in vitro tests, ganaxolone does not interact appreciably with human steroid hormone receptors. In the treatment of CDKL5 deficiency disorder, ganaxolone reduced the occurrence of major motor seizures. There is evidence from long-term follow-up studies of undiminished efficacy for more than 1 year. Consistent with the $GABA_A$ receptor mechanism, there is a high incidence of somnolence and sedation in clinical use.

Ganaxolone has low oral bioavailability, and absorption is enhanced markedly by food; administration with food is recommended. Ganaxolone is dosed in three divided doses per day (single dose maximum 600 mg). The divided dosing schedule maintains trough levels greater than those believed to be required for seizure control. The approved dosage form exhibits nonlinear absorption such that the plasma exposure is unlikely to rise substantially with doses greater than 600 mg. Ganaxolone is highly protein bound (99%) and is metabolized in the liver by CYP3A4/5, CYP2B6, CYP2C19, and CYP2D6. An increased dose may be required when used adjunctively with CYP3A4 inducers. Mass balance studies in humans indicate that two metabolites are present in plasma at much higher concentrations than the parent: an oxy-dehydro unconjugated derivative, which is inactive at $GABA_A$ receptors, and a ganaxolone sulfate conjugate.

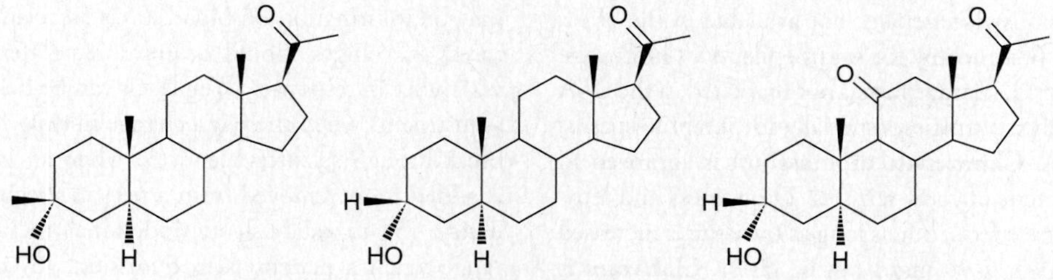

O HO H
Ganaxolone

O H HO H
Allopregnanolone

O O H HO H
Alphaxolone

OTHER MEDICATIONS USED IN MANAGEMENT OF SEIZURES AND EPILEPSY

BENZODIAZEPINES

Seven benzodiazepines play roles in the treatment of seizures and epilepsy (see also Chapter 22). All produce their functional effects by positive allosteric modulation of $GABA_A$ receptors; however, subtle structural differences among the benzodiazepines result in differences in their pharmacokinetic properties. Certain benzodiazepines are the initial acute treatment for seizures, either in status epilepticus or acute repetitive seizures (seizure clusters). However, two prominent aspects of benzodiazepines limit their usefulness in the chronic therapy of epilepsy. The first is their pronounced sedative effects; however, in children, there may be a paradoxical hyperactivity, as is the case with other sedative agents such as barbiturates. The second problem is tolerance with chronic dosing, in which seizures may respond initially but recur within a few months. As a result of these limitations, benzodiazepines are infrequently used in the chronic treatment of epilepsy.

Diazepam given intravenously is a first-line treatment for status epilepticus. It is also used in a rectal gel formulation or nasal spray for the treatment of acute repetitive seizures (seizure clusters). The drug is occasionally given orally on a long-term basis, although it is not considered very effective in this application because tolerance limits its efficacy. As discussed in more detail in Additional Topics below, **lorazepam** is more commonly used in the treatment of status epilepticus because it has a more prolonged duration of action after bolus intravenous injection. Lorazepam is also available as an oral concentrate that may be administered buccally, and in some countries a sublingual tablet is available. Lorazepam can also be administered nasally. There is evidence that intramuscular **midazolam**, which is well absorbed from muscle and rapidly acting, is preferred in the out-of-hospital treatment of status epilepticus because the delay required to achieve intravenous access may be avoided. Midazolam is available as a nasal spray for the treatment of acute repetitive seizures (seizure clusters) and in buccal (oromucosal) dosage form in some countries. **Clonazepam** is a long-acting benzodiazepine that on a milligram basis is one of the most potent antiseizure agents known. It has documented efficacy in the treatment of absence, atonic, and myoclonic seizures. As is the case for all benzodiazepines, sedation is prominent, especially on initiation of therapy; starting doses should be small. Maximal tolerated doses are usually in the range of 0.1–0.2 mg/kg/d, but many weeks of gradually increasing daily doses may be needed to achieve these dosages in some patients. Intravenous clonazepam, not available in the USA, is commonly used as a first therapy for status epilepticus in Europe and elsewhere in the world. **Nitrazepam** is not marketed in the USA but is used in many other countries, especially for infantile spasms and myoclonic seizures. **Clorazepate dipotassium** is approved in the USA for the treatment of focal seizures. Drowsiness and lethargy are common adverse effects, but as long as the drug is increased gradually, dosages as high as 90 mg/d can be given. **Clobazam** is described earlier in this chapter in the section on atonic seizures.

CARBONIC ANHYDRASE INHIBITORS

Carbonic anhydrases are enzymes that catalyze the interconversion between CO_2 and bicarbonate (see Chapter 15). Inhibitors of carbonic anhydrases, particularly the cytosolic forms CA II and CA VII, exhibit antiseizure activity. Bicarbonate efflux through $GABA_A$ receptors can exert a depolarizing (excitatory) influence that is especially relevant during intense $GABA_A$ receptor activation, as occurs during seizures, when there is diminution of the hyperpolarizing chloride gradient. Carbonic anhydrase inhibition prevents the replenishment of intracellular bicarbonate and depresses the depolarizing action of bicarbonate.

The prototypical carbonic anhydrase inhibitor is the sulfonamide **acetazolamide** (see Chapter 15), which has broad-spectrum antiseizure activity in animal models. In addition, acetazolamide is believed to have clinical antiseizure activity, at least transiently, against most types of seizures including focal and generalized tonic-clonic seizures and especially generalized absence seizures. However, acetazolamide is rarely used for chronic therapy because tolerance develops rapidly, with return of seizures usually within a few weeks. The drug is often used in the intermittent treatment of menstrual seizure exacerbations in women. The usual dosage is approximately 10 mg/kg/d to a maximum of 1000 mg/d.

Another sulfonamide carbonic anhydrase inhibitor, **sulthiame**, was introduced in Europe in the early 1960s and was used for the treatment of focal and myoclonic seizures but fell out of favor. Clinical trials and case reports have indicated that the drug is effective in benign focal epilepsy with centrotemporal spikes (BECTS) and infantile spasms; in some countries it is considered the drug of choice for BECTS. Sulthiame is available in Europe, Japan, Australia, and Israel but not in the USA.

As noted previously, topiramate and zonisamide are sulfur-containing molecules with weak carbonic anhydrase activity. There is little evidence that this activity is a major factor in their therapeutic effects.

■ ADDITIONAL TOPICS

THERAPEUTIC DRUG MONITORING

The pharmacokinetic behavior of most antiseizure medications varies markedly from patient to patient so that dosing must be individualized. Therapeutic drug concentration monitoring is often used as an aid to dosing. Established reference ranges are available for most of the older antiseizure medications (Table 24–3). Such ranges are generally not available for newer drugs, although there may be information on blood levels associated with efficacy. In all cases, the ranges should be interpreted flexibly given individual variability in response. Drug levels can be helpful (1) to guide dose adjustments when there is a change in drug formulation, (2) when breakthrough seizures occur, (3) when an interacting medication is added to or removed from a patient's regimen, (4) during pregnancy, (5) to establish an individual therapeutic concentration range when a patient is in remission, (6) to determine whether adverse effects are related to drug levels, and (7) to assess adherence.

TABLE 24–3 Blood (serum/plasma) concentration reference ranges for some antiseizure drugs.[1]

Antiseizure Drug	Reference Range[1]	
	µmol/L	mcg/mL
Acetazolamide	45–63	10–14
Brivaracetam	1–10	0.2–2
Cannabidiol[2]	1.0	0.3
Carbamazepine	15–45	4–12
Cenobamate[3]	58–88	15–23
Clobazam	Clobazam: 0.1–1 Norclobazam: 1–10	Clobazam: 0.03–0.30 Norclobazam: 0.3–3
Clonazepam	0.04–0.12	0.013–0.038
Eslicarbazepine acetate[4]	12–140	3–36
Ethosuximide	300–600	40–100
Everolimus	5.2–15.7 nmol/L	5–15 ng/mL
Felbamate	125–250	30–60
Fenfluramine[5]	<216 nmol/L	<50 ng/mL
Gabapentin	70–120	12–21
Ganaxolone[6]	241–709 nmol/L	85–250 ng/mL
Lacosamide	10–40	3–10
Lamotrigine	10–50	3–13
Levetiracetam	30–240	5–41
Oxcarbazepine[4]	12–140	3–36
Perampanel	0.1–1.1	0.05–0.4
Phenobarbital	65–172	15–40
Phenytoin	40–80	10–20
Pregabalin	10–35	2–6
Primidone	Primidone: 37–55 Phenobarbital: 65–129	Primidone: 8–12 Phenobarbital: 15–30
Retigabine (ezogabine)	No data	
Rufinamide	15–130	4–31
Stiripentol[7]	34–51	8–12
Sulthiame	7–34	2–10
Tiagabine	0.05–0.53	0.02–0.2
Topiramate	6–30	2–10
Valproate	300–600	40–100
Vigabatrin	6–279	0.8–36
Zonisamide	47–188	10–40

[1]These data are provided only as a general guideline. Many patients will respond better at different levels, and some patients may have drug-related adverse events within the listed reference ranges.

[2]No reference range available. Value given is mean plasma concentration in children and adult clinical trial responders receiving a mean dose of 27.1 mg/kg/day.

[3]No reference range available. Range bounds are mean steady-state plasma concentrations for trial subjects receiving daily doses of 200 mg and 400 mg.

[4]Monohydroxy metabolites (combination of eslicarbazepine and *R*-licarbazepine).

[5]Concentration range in clinical studies was 5.1–712.5 ng/mL (22–3081 nmol/L); most patients never had concentrations >50 ng/mL (216 nmol/L); toxicity has been associated with concentrations ≥240 ng/mL (1038 nmol/L).

[6]Range is minimum and maximum concentrations in clinical trial of seizures associated with CDKL5 deficiency disorder. Patients achieving favorable seizure control had mean levels of 120 ng/mL (340 nmol/L).

[7]Not well established; values given were associated with positive response in Dravet syndrome.

STATUS EPILEPTICUS

Status epilepticus, a serious neurological emergency, is an abnormally prolonged seizure, or repeated seizures with incomplete recovery of consciousness. Status epilepticus presents in two forms: (1) **generalized convulsive status epilepticus** characterized by prominent motor symptoms (bilateral rhythmic jerking of the limbs) and impaired consciousness, and (2) **nonconvulsive status epilepticus**, a persistent change in behavior (manifested as a change in cognition, memory, arousal, affect, motor learning, or motor behavior) with continuous epileptiform EEG activity but without major motor signs (tonic or clonic activity). Nonconvulsive status epilepticus encompasses several distinct conditions: (1) absence status epilepticus of the typical, atypical, or myoclonic forms, (2) focal status epilepticus with or without impairment of consciousness, which may have focal motor or sensory features; and (3) nonconvulsive status epilepticus in coma, which often occurs after treatment of convulsive status epilepticus.

Convulsive status epilepticus is a life-threatening emergency that requires immediate treatment. Traditionally, convulsive status epilepticus was defined as more than 30 minutes of either (1) continuous seizure activity or (2) two or more sequential seizures without full recovery of consciousness between seizures. Because persistent seizure activity is believed to cause permanent neuronal injury and because the majority of seizures terminate in 2 to 3 minutes, it is now generally accepted that treatment should be begun when the seizure duration reaches 5 minutes for generalized tonic-clonic seizures and 10 minutes for nonconvulsive seizures. It is noteworthy that convulsive status epilepticus may evolve to nonconvulsive status epilepticus. The initial treatment of convulsive and nonconvulsive status epilepticus is similar except that with the latter there is less urgency to achieve seizure control so therapy can be begun more cautiously with lower medication doses.

The initial treatment of choice is a benzodiazepine, either intravenous lorazepam or diazepam or intramuscular midazolam. Lorazepam is less lipophilic than diazepam (logP values of 2.4 and 2.8, respectively) and does not undergo redistribution from brain to peripheral tissues as rapidly as diazepam. Lorazepam has a slightly longer onset of action than diazepam, approximating 2 minutes, but a longer duration of action. Clinically effective diazepam concentrations in the brain following an intravenous bolus fall rapidly as the drug exits the central compartment into peripheral fat. Lorazepam has less extensive peripheral tissue uptake, allowing clinically effective concentrations to remain in the central compartment much longer. Although lorazepam is now used more frequently than diazepam because of the perceived pharmacokinetic advantage, recent appraisals of the clinical data have not found evidence to favor lorazepam. Intravenous clonazepam may be used as a first treatment for status epilepticus outside the USA. In the prehospital setting, rectal diazepam, intranasal midazolam, or buccal midazolam are acceptable alternative first treatments if the preferred options are not available. Because of the short effective duration of action of benzodiazepines, unless the cause of the status epilepticus has been definitively corrected, a second therapy is administered. Intravenous levetiracetam, valproate, fosphenytoin, or phenytoin are acceptable choices. They are equally effective in terminating benzodiazepine-refractory convulsive status epilepticus and have similar rates of adverse effects. Seizure cessation occurs in approximately one-half of patients receiving any of the three drugs after failure of a benzodiazepine. Intravenous phenobarbital is highly effective at terminating status epilepticus, but it has a long half-life causing persistent side effects including severe sedation, respiratory depression, and hypotension. Intravenous lacosamide also has been used as a second treatment for status epilepticus. Intravenous loading with lacosamide is usually well tolerated, but due to its effects on the heart including the potential to induce arrhythmias, electrocardiographic monitoring is prudent. If the second therapy fails to stop the seizures, an additional second therapy agent is often tried. Refractory status epilepticus occurs when seizures continue or recur at least 30 minutes after treatment with first and second therapy agents. Refractory convulsive status epilepticus is treated with anesthetic doses of pentobarbital, propofol, midazolam, or thiopental. Case reports indicate that ketamine may be effective. If status epilepticus continues or recurs 24 hours or more after the onset of anesthesia, the condition is considered super-refractory. Often, super-refractory status epilepticus is recognized when anesthetics are withdrawn and seizures recur. There are no established therapies for super-refractory status epilepticus other than to reinstitute general anesthesia.

Special considerations apply to the treatment of certain forms of nonconvulsive status epilepticus. Absence status epilepticus can often be effectively treated with a benzodiazepine followed by intravenous valproate. Long-term control is usually achieved with oral ethosuximide or valproate. Absence status epilepticus can occur when an inappropriate antiseizure medication, such as vigabatrin, tiagabine, carbamazepine, or phenytoin, is used in a patient with idiopathic (genetic) generalized epilepsy. Focal nonconvulsive status epilepticus with or without impairment of consciousness generally responds to intravenous antiseizure medications, and general anesthetics are avoided. Nonconvulsive status epilepticus in coma is often refractory to antiseizure medications and may require general anesthesia.

ACUTE REPETITIVE SEIZURES (SEIZURE CLUSTERS)

Acute repetitive seizures, also referred to as seizure clusters, are groups of seizures that occur more frequently than the patient's habitual seizure frequency. The clusters can occur rapidly over several minutes, or they may occur over a longer time period of 1 or 2 days. In acute repetitive seizures, there is complete recovery between seizures so that patients do not meet the definition of status epilepticus. However, the condition is concerning nevertheless because, in the absence of treatment, prolonged seizures or status epilepticus can occur. Acute repetitive seizures can be treated in the emergency department with intravenous benzodiazepines or other antiseizure medications. In the USA, diazepam rectal gel and midazolam and diazepam nasal sprays are approved for the out-of-hospital treatment of acute repetitive seizures. Intranasal lorazepam injection solution delivered with a nasal atomizer or instilled by drop into the nostril also has been shown to be efficacious but is not approved for this route of administration in the USA. Buccal (oromucosal) midazolam, in which the treatment solution is administered to the buccal mucosa using an oral syringe, is commonly used in Europe and elsewhere in the world. Lorazepam oral solution concentrate, available in the USA, can be administered buccally. Lorazepam solutions require refrigeration; diazepam and midazolam are stable at room temperature. Lorazepam buccal/sublingual tablets are available outside the USA. Some clinicians in the USA use oral swallowed benzodiazepine tablets on an off-label basis. Outside the USA, rectal paraldehyde is sometimes used. Administering rectal medications can be difficult, time consuming, and an embarrassing experience for the patient and caregivers; such products are generally limited to use in children because of the social stigma and the mechanical difficulties of positioning adults.

TERATOGENICITY (SEE ALSO CHAPTER 59)

Most women with epilepsy who become pregnant require continued drug therapy for seizure control. No antiseizure medication is known to be completely safe for the developing fetus. Valproate is a known human teratogen. First-trimester exposure is associated with an approximately threefold increased risk of major congenital malformations, most commonly spina bifida (absolute risk, 6–9%). Phenobarbital use during pregnancy is also associated with an elevated risk of major congenital malformation, most often cardiac defects. First-trimester in utero exposure to topiramate is associated with an approximately 10-fold increase in oral clefts risk (absolute risk, 1.4%). If possible, valproate, phenobarbital, and topiramate should be avoided in women of childbearing potential, and if the drugs cannot be eliminated, they should be used at the lowest dose possible because the risk, at least for valproate, has been shown to be dose-dependent. Other antiseizure medications may present a lower risk of major congenital malformations (or the risk is poorly understood), but the risk for most drugs, including carbamazepine, phenytoin, and levetiracetam, is not zero. In addition to congenital malformations, there is evidence that first-trimester exposure is associated with cognitive impairment. In particular, fetal exposure to valproate is associated with a dose-dependent reduction in cognitive abilities across a range of domains including IQ. Fetal exposure to lamotrigine or levetiracetam may be safer with regard to cognition than other antiseizure medications, and these two agents also have the lowest risks of major congenital malformations. Polytherapy may increase the risk of neurodevelopmental deficits, particularly when one of the drugs is valproate. In addition, there is evidence that valproate exposure may be associated with an increased risk of autism spectrum disorder.

BREASTFEEDING

Some antiepileptic drugs such as primidone, levetiracetam, gabapentin, lamotrigine, and topiramate penetrate into breast milk in relatively high concentrations. For example, in one study, plasma concentrations of lamotrigine in breastfeeding infants were 18.3% of maternal plasma concentrations. Other antiseizure medications that are highly protein bound, such as valproate, phenobarbital, phenytoin, and carbamazepine, do not penetrate into breast milk substantially. Case series have not reported adverse effects on the newborn of antiseizure medication exposure via breast milk, although there are some reports of sedation with the barbiturates and benzodiazepines. As a general rule, breastfeeding should not be discouraged given the lack of evidence of harm and the known positive benefits.

SUICIDALITY

An analysis of suicidal behavior during clinical trials of antiseizure medications was carried out by the US Food and Drug Administration in 2008. The presence of either suicidal behavior or suicidal ideation was 0.37% in patients taking active drugs and 0.24% in patients taking placebo. This led to an alert of an increased risk of suicide in people taking antiseizure medications. Following the report, several studies have addressed the issue in various ways but have not provided convincing data that, as a class, antiseizure medications induce suicide-related behaviors. In addition, an analysis of data from placebo-controlled clinical trials of more recently approved antiseizure medications (eslicarbazepine, perampanel, brivaracetam, cannabidiol, and cenobamate) where suicidality was investigated prospectively found no evidence of increased risk of suicidal ideation or suicide attempt in relation to placebo. Whether or not antiseizure medications are associated with increased suicidality, psychiatric disorders are more frequent in people with epilepsy than in the general population. The cause of death in persons with epilepsy is much more frequently suicide (11.5%) than in the population at large (1%). It is therefore crucial to routinely assess patients with epilepsy for depression and suicide risk.

WITHDRAWAL

Antiseizure medications may not need to be taken indefinitely. Children who are seizure free for periods longer than 2–4 years while on antiseizure medications will remain so when medications are withdrawn in 70% of cases. The risk of recurrence depends on the seizure syndrome. Resolution of seizures is common for generalized absence epilepsy but not for juvenile myoclonic epilepsy. Other risk factors for recurrence are an abnormal EEG, the presence of neurologic deficits, or when seizure control had been difficult to achieve. There is little information on antiseizure medication withdrawal in seizure-free adults. Withdrawal is believed to be more likely to be successful in patients with generalized epilepsies who exhibit a single seizure type, whereas longer duration of epilepsy, an abnormal neurologic examination, an abnormal EEG, and certain epilepsy syndromes, including juvenile myoclonic epilepsy, are associated with increased risk of recurrence. Medications are generally withdrawn slowly over a 1- to 3-month period or longer. Abrupt cessation may be associated with return of seizures and even a risk of status epilepticus. Some medications are more easily withdrawn than others. Physical dependence occurs with barbiturates and benzodiazepines, and there is a well-recognized risk of rebound seizures with abrupt withdrawal.

MEDICATION DEVELOPMENT FOR EPILEPSY

Most antiseizure medications have been identified by tests in rodent (rat or mouse) models. The **maximal electroshock (MES)** test, in which animals receive an electrical stimulus, with tonic hindlimb extension as the endpoint, has been the most productive model. The MES test led to the identification of many of the sodium channel–blocking antiseizure medications. Another model, the **pentylenetetrazol (PTZ)** test, in which animals receive a dose of the chemical convulsant PTZ (an antagonist of $GABA_A$ receptors) sufficient to cause clonic seizures, also has been widely used. The **6-Hz seizure test** is a distinct electrical stimulation model that responds differently to antiseizure agents than does the MES test. Immediately after the stimulation, animals (usually mice but rats can be used) exhibit a limbic-type seizure characterized by forelimb clonus followed by stereotyped, automatistic behaviors, including twitching of the vibrissae and Straub tail. In the **kindling model**, mice or rats repeatedly receive a mild electrical stimulus in the amygdala or hippocampus over the course of a number of days, causing them to develop a permanent propensity for limbic seizures when they later are stimulated. The kindling model can be used to assess the ability of a chemical compound to protect against focal seizures. Animals with a genetic susceptibility to absence-like episodes are useful in identifying drugs for the treatment of absence seizures. In addition to empirical screening of chemical compounds in such animal models, a few antiseizure medications have been identified by in vitro screening against a molecular target. Examples of targets that have been used to identify approved antiseizure medications include γ-aminobutyric acid (GABA) transaminase (vigabatrin), GAT-1 GABA transporter (tiagabine), AMPA receptors (perampanel), or the synaptic vesicle protein SV2A (brivaracetam).

ANTISEIZURE MEDICATIONS IN DEVELOPMENT

Several potential new antiseizure medications are in clinical development for the treatment of focal seizures, including XEN1101, a potent Kv7.2/Kv7.3 (KCNQ2/KCNQ3) potassium channel opener; darigabat, a subtype selective α2,α3,α5 $GABA_A$ receptor positive modulator; and NBI-921352, a potent and highly selective state-dependent Nav1.6 sodium channel inhibitor. Various small molecule and gene therapies, including antisense oligonucleotide and adeno-associated virus capsid based, are in development for diverse DEEs. Some treatments in late-stage development for acute seizures emergencies include Staccato (thermal aerosol inhaled) alprazolam to terminate acute seizures; diazepam buccal film (Libervant) for acute repetitive seizures; and ganaxolone for refractory status epilepticus.

SUMMARY Antiseizure Medications

Type, Drug	Mechanism of Action	Pharmacokinetics	Clinical Applications	Toxicities, Interactions
SODIUM CHANNEL BLOCKERS				
• Carbamazepine	Sodium channel blocker	Rapidly absorbed orally, with bioavailability 75–85% • peak levels in 4–5 h • plasma protein binding 75% • extensively metabolized in liver primarily by CYP3A4, in part to active carbamazepine-10,11-epoxide • $t_{1/2}$ of parent in adults initially 25–65 h, decreasing to 8–20 h with autoinduction	Focal and focal-to-bilateral tonic-clonic seizures; trigeminal neuralgia	*Toxicity:* Nausea, diplopia, ataxia, hyponatremia, headache • *Interactions:* Phenytoin, valproate, fluoxetine, verapamil, macrolide antibiotics, isoniazid, propoxyphene, danazol, phenobarbital, primidone, many others
• *Oxcarbazepine: Similar to carbamazepine; 100% bioavailability; active 10-hydroxycarbazepine (licarbazepine or MHD) metabolite 40% protein binding; 1–2 h $t_{1/2}$ but active metabolites with $t_{1/2}$ of 8–12 h; fewer interactions reported*				
• *Eslicarbazepine acetate: Similar pharmacokinetics to oxcarbazepine but approved by regulatory authorities for once daily dosing*				
• Lamotrigine	Sodium channel blocker	Nearly complete (~90%) absorption • peak levels in 1–3 h • protein binding 55% • extensively metabolized; no active metabolites • $t_{1/2}$ 8–35 h	Focal seizures, generalized tonic-clonic seizures, absence seizures, other generalized seizures; bipolar depression	*Toxicity:* Dizziness, headache, diplopia, rash • *Interactions:* Valproate, carbamazepine, oxcarbazepine, phenytoin, phenobarbital, primidone, succinimides, sertraline, topiramate
• Lacosamide	Sodium channel blocker, slow blocking kinetics	Complete absorption • peak levels in 1–2 h • protein binding <30% • no active metabolites • $t_{1/2}$ 12–14 h	Focal seizures	*Toxicity:* Dizziness, headache, nausea • cardiac arrhythmia • *Interactions:* Minimal
• Phenytoin, fosphenytoin	Sodium channel blocker	Absorption is formulation-dependent • highly bound to plasma proteins • no active metabolites • dose-dependent elimination, $t_{1/2}$ 12–36 h • fosphenytoin is for IV, IM routes	Focal seizures, tonic-clonic seizures	*Toxicity:* Diplopia, ataxia, gingival hyperplasia, hirsutism, neuropathy • *Interactions:* Phenobarbital, carbamazepine, isoniazid, felbamate, oxcarbazepine, topiramate, fluoxetine, fluconazole, digoxin, quinidine, cyclosporine, steroids, oral contraceptives, others
BROAD SPECTRUM				
• Valproate	Unknown	Nearly complete (>90%) absorption • peak levels formulation-dependent • highly (90%) bound to plasma proteins • extensively metabolized in liver • $t_{1/2}$ 5–16 h	Generalized tonic-clonic seizures, focal seizures, absence seizures, myoclonic seizures, other generalized seizure types; migraine prophylaxis	*Toxicity:* Nausea, tremor, weight gain, hair loss, teratogenic, hepatotoxic • *Interactions:* Phenobarbital, phenytoin, carbamazepine, lamotrigine, felbamate, rifampin, ethosuximide, primidone
• Levetiracetam	SV2A ligand	Nearly complete (~95%) absorption • peak levels in 1–2 h • not bound to plasma proteins • minimal metabolism in blood to inactive metabolite; ~66% excreted unchanged in urine • $t_{1/2}$ 6–11 h	Focal seizures, generalized tonic-clonic seizures, myoclonic seizures	*Toxicity:* Nervousness, dizziness, depression, seizures • *Interactions:* Rare
• *Brivaracetam: Similar to levetiracetam but interaction with carbamazepine*				
• Topiramate	Multiple actions	Bioavailability ~80% • peak levels in 2–4 h • minimal (15%) plasma protein binding • variable metabolism; no active metabolites; 20–70% excreted unchanged in the urine • $t_{1/2}$ 20–30 h, but decreases with concomitant drugs	Focal seizures, primary generalized seizures, Lennox-Gastaut syndrome; migraine prophylaxis	*Toxicity:* Somnolence, cognitive slowing, confusion, paresthesias • *Interactions:* Phenytoin, carbamazepine, oral contraceptives, lamotrigine, lithium
• Zonisamide	Unknown	Nearly complete (>90%) absorption • peak concentrations in 2–6 h • modest (40–60%) plasma protein binding • moderate (>50%) metabolism in liver; 30% excreted unchanged in urine • $t_{1/2}$ 50–70 h	Focal seizures, generalized tonic-clonic seizures, myoclonic seizures	*Toxicity:* Drowsiness, cognitive impairment, confusion, skin rashes • *Interactions:* Minimal

(continued)

Type, Drug	Mechanism of Action	Pharmacokinetics	Clinical Applications	Toxicities, Interactions
• Rufinamide	Sodium channel blocker and other mechanisms	Well absorbed orally (>85%) • peak concentrations in 4–6 h • low (35%) plasma protein binding • $t_{1/2}$ 6–10 h • metabolized in liver by carboxylesterase 1; no active metabolites • metabolite mostly excreted in urine (~70%)	Lennox-Gastaut syndrome, focal seizures	*Toxicity:* Somnolence, vomiting, pyrexia, diarrhea • *Interactions:* Not metabolized via P450 enzymes, but there may be interactions with other antiseizure medications
GABAPENTINOIDS				
• Gabapentin	α2δ ligand	Bioavailability 50%, decreasing with increasing doses • peak concentrations in 2–3 h • not bound to plasma proteins • not metabolized; 100% excreted unchanged in urine • $t_{1/2}$ 5–9 h	Focal seizures; neuropathic pain; postherpetic neuralgia; anxiety	*Toxicity:* Somnolence, dizziness, ataxia • *Interactions:* Minimal
• Pregabalin	α2δ ligand	Nearly complete (~90%) absorption • peak concentrations in 1–2 h • not bound to plasma proteins • not metabolized; 98% excreted unchanged in urine • $t_{1/2}$ 4.5–7 h	Focal seizures; neuropathic pain; postherpetic neuralgia; fibromyalgia; anxiety	*Toxicity:* Somnolence, dizziness, ataxia • *Interactions:* Minimal
BARBITURATES				
• Phenobarbital	Positive allosteric modulator of $GABA_A$ receptors • reduces excitatory synaptic responses	Nearly complete (>90%) absorption • peak concentrations in 0.5–4 h • modest (55%) plasma protein binding • extensively metabolized in liver; no active metabolites; 20–25% excreted unchanged in urine • $t_{1/2}$ 75–140 h	Focal seizures, generalized tonic-clonic seizures, myoclonic seizures, neonatal seizures; sedation	*Toxicity:* Sedation, cognitive impairment, ataxia, hyperactivity • *Interactions:* Valproate, carbamazepine, felbamate, phenytoin, cyclosporine, felodipine, lamotrigine, nifedipine, nimodipine, steroids, theophylline, verapamil, others
• Primidone	Sodium channel blocker-like but converted to phenobarbital	Nearly complete (>90%) absorption • minimal (10%) plasma protein binding • peak concentrations in 2–6 h • extensively metabolized in liver; 2 active metabolites (phenobarbital and phenylethylmalonamide); 65% excreted unchanged in urine • $t_{1/2}$ 10–25 h	Generalized tonic-clonic seizures, focal seizures	*Toxicity:* Sedation, cognitive impairment, ataxia, hyperactivity • *Interactions:* Similar to phenobarbital
ABSENCE SEIZURE–SPECIFIC				
• Ethosuximide	Inhibit low-threshold calcium channels (T-type)	Nearly complete (>90%) absorption • peak concentrations in 3–7 h • not bound to plasma proteins • extensively metabolized in liver; no active metabolites; 20% excreted unchanged in urine • $t_{1/2}$ 20–60 h	Absence seizures	*Toxicity:* Nausea, headache, dizziness, lethargy • *Interactions:* Valproate, phenobarbital, phenytoin, carbamazepine, rifampicin
BENZODIAZEPINES				
• Diazepam	Positive allosteric modulator of $GABA_A$ receptors	Nearly complete (>90%) oral or rectal absorption • peak concentrations in 1–1.5 h • IV for status epilepticus • highly (95–98%) bound to plasma proteins • extensively metabolized by CYP3A4 and CYP2C19 to N-desmethyldiazepam and other active metabolites • $t_{1/2}$ of N-desmethyldiazepam up to 100 h	Status epilepticus, acute repetitive seizures (seizure clusters); sedation, anxiety, muscle relaxation (muscle spasms, spasticity), acute alcohol withdrawal	*Toxicity:* Sedation • *Interactions:* Additive with sedative-hypnotics
• Clonazepam	Positive allosteric modulator of $GABA_A$ receptors	Bioavailability >80% • peak concentrations in 1–4 h • highly (86%) bound to plasma proteins • extensively metabolized in liver by CYP3A4; no active metabolites • $t_{1/2}$ 12–56 h	Absence seizures, myoclonic seizures, infantile spasms	*Toxicity:* Similar to diazepam • *Interactions:* Additive with sedative-hypnotics

(continued)

Type, Drug	Mechanism of Action	Pharmacokinetics	Clinical Applications	Toxicities, Interactions
• Clobazam	Positive allosteric modulator of $GABA_A$ receptors	Bioavailability >95% • protein binding 80–90% • extensively metabolized to N-desmethylclobazam, which is pharmacologically active • parent: $t_{1/2}$ 10–30 h • N-desmethyl metabolite: $t_{1/2}$ 36–46 h	Focal seizures, seizures associated with Lennox-Gastaut syndrome and Dravet syndrome	*Toxicity:* Somnolence, sedation, lethargy*Interactions:* Increases levels of phenytoin and carbamazepine; cannabidiol increases levels of N-desmethylclobazam
• *Lorazepam: Used for status epilepticus; rapidly conjugated to lorazepam glucuronide, which is inactive;* $t_{1/2}$ *12 h* • *Midazolam: Used for status epilepticus and acute repetitive seizures (seizure clusters); water soluble at pH <4 but becomes highly lipid soluble at physiological pH, minimizing pain on injection and contributing to rapid onset of action; converted by CYP3A isoenzymes to active metabolite 1-hydroxymidazolam;* $t_{1/2}$ *1.5–3 h*				
GABA MECHANISMS OTHER THAN BARBITURATE AND BENZODIAZEPINE				
• Tiagabine	GAT-1 GABA transporter inhibitor	Nearly complete (~90%) absorption • peak concentrations in 0.5–2 h • highly (96%) bound to plasma proteins • extensively metabolized in liver; no active metabolites; <2% excreted unchanged in urine • $t_{1/2}$ 2–9 h	Focal seizures	*Toxicity:* Nervousness, dizziness, depression, seizures • *Interactions:* Phenobarbital, phenytoin, carbamazepine, primidone
• Vigabatrin	Irreversible inhibitor of GABA transaminase	Complete absorption • peak concentrations in 1 h • not bound to plasma proteins • not metabolized; eliminated unchanged in urine • $t_{1/2}$ 5–8 h (not relevant because of irreversible action)	Focal seizures, infantile spasms	*Toxicity:* Drowsiness, dizziness, psychosis, visual field loss • *Interactions:* Minimal
• Ganaxolone	Positive allosteric modulator of $GABA_A$ receptors (non-benzodiazepine site)	Absorption increases with high fat meal • peak concentrations in 2–3 h • highly (99%) bound to plasma proteins • extensively metabolized in liver • $t_{1/2}$ 34 h	Seizures associated with cyclin-dependent kinase-like 5 (CDKL5) deficiency disorder; evidence of efficacy in other epilepsies	*Toxicity:* Symptoms of central nervous system depression, including lethargy, drowsiness, sedation, and hypersomnia • *Interactions:* CYP3A4 inducers decrease exposure
POTASSIUM CHANNEL OPENER				
• Retigabine (ezogabine)	Opens KCNQ potassium channels	Bioavailability ~60% • peak concentrations in 0.5–2 h • moderately (~80%) bound to plasma proteins • extensively metabolized in liver; 36% excreted unchanged in urine • $t_{1/2}$ 7–11 h	Focal seizures	*Toxicity:* Dizziness, somnolence, confusion, blurred vision • *Interactions:* Minimal
AMPA RECEPTOR BLOCKER				
• Perampanel	Noncompetitive block of AMPA receptors	Complete absorption • peak concentrations in 0.5–3 h • highly (95%) bound to plasma proteins • extensively metabolized in liver • $t_{1/2}$ 25–129 h	Focal and focal-to-bilateral tonic-clonic seizures, generalized tonic-clonic seizures	*Toxicity:* Dizziness, somnolence, headache; psychiatric syndromes • *Interactions:* Substantial, with increased clearance caused by CYP3A inducers
CANNABINOID				
• Cannabidiol (sesame oil formulation)	Unknown	Absorption enhanced by high-fat meal • peak concentrations in 2.5–5 h • highly (>94%) bound to plasma proteins • extensively metabolized in liver • $t_{1/2}$ 14 h (single dose study)	Seizures associated with Lennox-Gastaut syndrome, Dravet syndrome, and tuberous sclerosis complex	*Toxicity:* Diarrhea, nausea, somnolence, headache*Interactions:* Clobazam (threefold increase in N-desmethylclobazam), valproate (increased risk of liver enzyme elevation)
CARBAMATE				
• Felbamate	NMDA receptor blocker; low-efficacy positive allosteric modulator of $GABA_A$ receptors	Well absorbed (>90%) • no food effect • 22–25% bound to plasma proteins, primarily albumin • 40–50% excreted unchanged in urine • $t_{1/2}$ 20–23 h	Focal seizures; seizures associated with Lennox-Gastaut syndrome	*Toxicity:* Anorexia, nausea, vomiting, insomnia, anxiety, weight loss, dizziness, headache, somnolence, aplastic anemia, hepatic failure • *Interactions:* Increases phenytoin, valproate and phenobarbital; reduces carbamazepine but increases carbamazepine epoxide; phenytoin, carbamazepine, and phenobarbital reduce felbamate concentrations

(*continued*)

Type, Drug	Mechanism of Action	Pharmacokinetics	Clinical Applications	Toxicities, Interactions
• Cenobamate	Sodium channel blocker; low-efficacy positive allosteric modulator of $GABA_A$ receptors	Well absorbed (>88%) • no food effect • peak concentrations in 1–4 h • >60% bound to plasma proteins, primarily albumin • extensively metabolized in liver • $t_{1/2}$ 50–60 h	Focal seizures	*Toxicity:* Somnolence, dizziness, fatigue, balance disorder, gait disturbance, dysarthria, nystagmus, and ataxia; DRESS; short QT interval • *Interactions:* Increases phenytoin; may also increase phenobarbital and N-desmethylclobazam; decreases carbamazepine, lamotrigine
AROMATIC ALLYLIC ALCOHOL				
• Stiripentol	Positive allosteric modulator of $GABA_A$ receptors; increases clobazam and norclobazam levels	Used in combination with clobazam or valproate • bioavailability 30% • $t_{1/2}$ 4.5–13 h (dose-dependent) • highly (>99%) bound to plasma proteins • metabolized in liver	Dravet syndrome (USA: adjunctive use in conjunction with clobazam; European Union: adjunctive use in conjunction with clobazam and valproate)	*Toxicity:* Sedation/drowsiness, reduced appetite, slowing of mental function, ataxia, diplopia, nausea, and abdominal pain *Interactions:* Clobazam, valproate; also carbamazepine, phenobarbital, phenytoin
SUBSTITUTED AMPHETAMINE				
• Fenfluramine	Serotonin release	Bioavailability 68–74% • no food effect • peak concentration 3–5 h • $t_{1/2}$ 20 h • metabolized to norfenfluramine by CYP1A2, CYP2B6, CYP2D6	Convulsive seizures associated with Dravet syndrome; atonic seizures associated with Lennox-Gastaut syndrome	*Toxicity:* Decreased appetite, diarrhea, fatigue • *Interactions:* concomitant stiripentol increases fenfluramine exposure and reduces norfenfluramine exposure; fenfluramine does not affect valproate, stiripentol, clobazam, or norclobazam

PREPARATIONS AVAILABLE

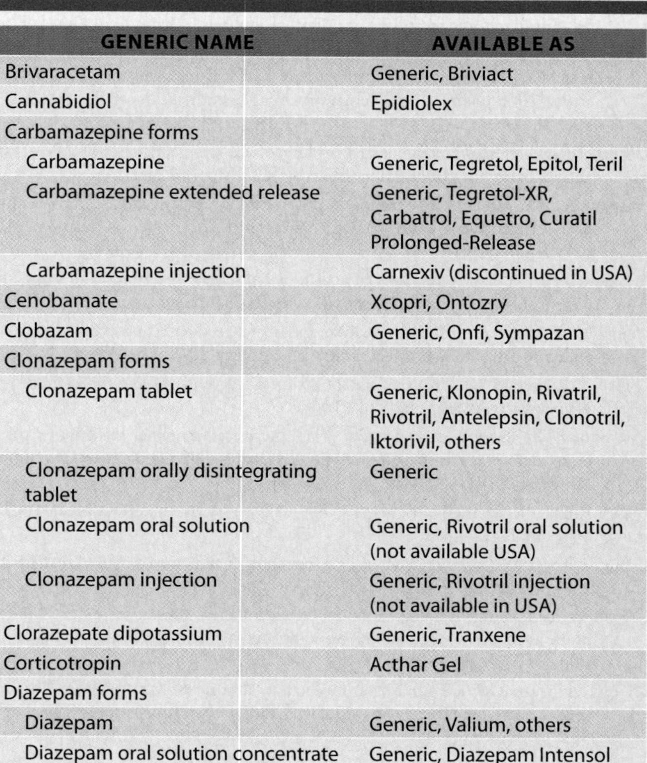

GENERIC NAME	AVAILABLE AS
Brivaracetam	Generic, Briviact
Cannabidiol	Epidiolex
Carbamazepine forms	
Carbamazepine	Generic, Tegretol, Epitol, Teril
Carbamazepine extended release	Generic, Tegretol-XR, Carbatrol, Equetro, Curatil Prolonged-Release
Carbamazepine injection	Carnexiv (discontinued in USA)
Cenobamate	Xcopri, Ontozry
Clobazam	Generic, Onfi, Sympazan
Clonazepam forms	
Clonazepam tablet	Generic, Klonopin, Rivatril, Rivotril, Antelepsin, Clonotril, Iktorivil, others
Clonazepam orally disintegrating tablet	Generic
Clonazepam oral solution	Generic, Rivotril oral solution (not available USA)
Clonazepam injection	Generic, Rivotril injection (not available in USA)
Clorazepate dipotassium	Generic, Tranxene
Corticotropin	Acthar Gel
Diazepam forms	
Diazepam	Generic, Valium, others
Diazepam oral solution concentrate	Generic, Diazepam Intensol
Diazepam injection	Generic
Diazepam rectal gel	Diastat Acudial
Diazepam intranasal	Valtoco
Eslicarbazepine acetate	Aptiom, Stedesa
Ethosuximide	Generic, Zarontin
Ethotoin	Peganone (discontinued in USA)
Everolimus	Afinitor
Felbamate	Generic, Felbatol
Fenfluramine	Fintepla
Fosphenytoin sodium injection	Generic, Cerebyx
Gabapentin	Generic, Neurontin, Gralise
Gabapentin enacarbil	Horizant
Ganaxolone	Ztalmy
Lacosamide forms	
Lacosamide	Generic, Vimpat
Lacosamide injection	Generic, Vimpat injection
Lamotrigine forms	
Lamotrigine	Generic, Lamictal
Lamotrigine extended release	Generic, Lamictal XR
Levetiracetam forms	
Levetiracetam	Generic, Keppra, Spritam
Levetiracetam extended release	Generic, Keppra XR, Elepsia XR
Levetiracetam injection	Generic, Keppra injection

(continued)

GENERIC NAME	AVAILABLE AS
Lorazepam forms	
Lorazepam	Generic, Ativan
Lorazepam oral solution concentrate	Generic, Lorazepam Intensol
Lorazepam injection	Generic, Ativan injection
Mephenytoin	Mesantoin (discontinued in USA)
Methsuximide	Celontin
Midazolam forms	
Midazolam hydrochloride injection	Generic, Versed, Seizalam
Midazolam hydrochloride syrup	Generic
Midazolam oromucosal solution (buccal)	Epistatus, Buccolam
Midazolam nasal spray	Nayzilam, Nasolam
Oxcarbazepine	Generic, Trileptal, Oxtellar XR
Pentobarbital sodium injection	Generic, Nembutal Sodium injection
Perampanel	Fycompa
Phenobarbital forms	
Phenobarbital	Generic, Luminal Sodium, others
Phenobarbital sodium injection	Generic, Sezaby
Phenytoin sodium forms	
Phenytoin sodium extended	Generic, Dilantin, Phenytek
Phenytoin sodium injectable	Generic, phenytoin sodium injection
Pregabalin forms	
Pregabalin	Generic, Lyrica
Pregabalin extended release	Generic, Lyrica CR
Primidone	Generic, Mysoline
Retigabine (ezogabine)	Potiga, Trobalt (discontinued)
Rufinamide	Generic, Banzel
Stiripentol	Diacomit
Tiagabine	Generic, Gabitril
Topiramate forms	
Topiramate	Generic, Topamax, Eprontia
Topiramate extended release	Generic, Trokendi XR, Qudexy XR
Trimethadione	Tridione (discontinued)
Valproate/valproic acid forms	
Valproic acid	Generic, Depakene
Divalproex sodium delayed release	Generic, Depakote
Divalproex sodium extended release	Generic, Depakote ER
Valproate sodium injection	Generic, Depacon
Vigabatrin	Generic, Sabril, Vigradone
Zonisamide	Generic, Zonegran, Zonisade

REFERENCES

Ettinger AB, Argoff CE: Use of antiepileptic drugs for non-epileptic conditions: Psychiatric disorders and chronic pain. Neurotherapeutics 2007;4:75.

French JA et al: Development of new treatment approaches for epilepsy: Unmet needs and opportunities. Epilepsia 2013;54(Suppl 4):3.

Glauser TA et al: Ethosuximide, valproic acid, and lamotrigine in childhood absence epilepsys. N Engl J Med 2010;362:790.

Grover EH et al: Treatment of convulsive status epilepticus. Curr Treat Options Neurol 2016;18:11.

Haut SR: Seizure clusters: Characteristics and treatment. Curr Opin Neurol 2015;28:143.

Kaminski RM et al: SV2A is a broad-spectrum anticonvulsant target: Functional correlation between protein binding and seizure protection in models of both partial and generalized epilepsy. Neuropharmacology 2008;54:715.

Kapur J et al: Randomized trial of three anticonvulsant medications for status epilepticus. N Engl J Med 2019;381:2103.

Kienitz R et al: Benzodiazepines in the management of seizures and status epilepticus: a review of routes of delivery, pharmacokinetics, efficacy, and tolerability. CNS Drugs 2022;36:951.

Klein P et al: Suicidality risk of newer antiseizure medications: a meta-analysis. JAMA Neurol 2021;78:1118.

Löscher W et al: Synaptic vesicle glycoprotein 2A ligands in the treatment of epilepsy and beyond. CNS Drugs 2016;30:1055.

Meldrum BS, Rogawski MA: Molecular targets for antiepileptic drug development. Neurotherapeutics 2007;4:18.

Patsalos PN: *Antiepileptic Drug Interactions. A Clinical Guide.* Springer International Publishing, 2016.

Patsalos PN: Drug interactions with the newer antiepileptic drugs (AEDs)—Part 1: Pharmacokinetic and pharmacodynamic interactions between AEDs. Clin Pharmacokinet 2013;52:927.

Patsalos PN et al: Therapeutic drug monitoring of antiepileptic drugs in epilepsy: A 2018 update. Ther Drug Monit 2018;40(5):526.

Porter RJ et al: AED mechanisms and principles of drug treatment. In: Stefan H, Theodore W (editors): *Handbook of Clinical Neurology, 3rd series, Epilepsies Part 2: Treatment.* Elsevier, 2012.

Reimers A et al: Reference ranges for antiepileptic drugs revisited: A practical approach to establish national guidelines. Drug Des Devel Ther 2018;12:271.

Rosenfeld WE et al: Efficacy of cenobamate by focal seizure subtypes: Post-hoc analysis of a phase 3, multicenter, open-label study. Epilepsy Res 2022;183: 106940.

Rogawski MA et al: Current understanding of the mechanism of action of the antiepileptic drug lacosamide. Epilepsy Res 2015;110:189.

Rogawski MA, Hanada T: Preclinical pharmacology of perampanel, a selective non-competitive AMPA receptor antagonist. Acta Neurol Scand 2013; 127(Suppl 197):19.

Rogawski MA et al: Mechanisms of action of antiseizure drugs and the ketogenic diet. Cold Spring Harb Perspect Med 2016;6:a022780.

Sánchez Fernández I et al: Meta-analysis and cost-effectiveness of second-line antiepileptic drugs for status epilepticus. Neurology 2019;92:e2339.

Sills GJ, Rogawski MA: Mechanisms of action of currently used antiseizure drugs. Neuropharmacology 2020;168:107966.

Steinhof BJ et al: Efficacy and safety of adjunctive perampanel for the treatment of refractory partial seizures: A pooled analysis of three phase III studies. Epilepsia 2013;54:1481.

Vélez-Ruiz NJ, Pennell PB: Issues for women with epilepsy. Neurol Clin 2016;34:411.

Wilcox KS et al: Issues related to development of new anti-seizure treatments. Epilepsia 2013;54(Suppl 4):24.

Xie X et al: Electrophysiological and pharmacological properties of the human brain type IIA Na^+ channel expressed in a stable mammalian cell line. Pflugers Arch 2001;441:425.

Xie X, Hagan RM: Cellular and molecular actions of lamotrigine: Possible mechanisms of efficacy in bipolar disorder. Neuropsychobiology 1998; 38:119.

CASE STUDY ANSWER

Lamotrigine was gradually added to the regimen to a dosage of 200 mg bid. Since then, the patient has been seizure-free for almost 2 years but now comes to the office for a medication review. Gradual discontinuation of levetiracetam is planned if the patient continues to do well for another year, although risk of recurrent seizures is always present when medications are withdrawn.

CHAPTER

25 General Anesthetics

Helge Eilers, MD, & Spencer Yost, MD

CASE STUDY

An elderly man with type 2 diabetes mellitus and ischemic pain in a lower extremity is scheduled for femoral-to-popliteal artery bypass surgery. He has a history of hypertension and coronary artery disease with symptoms of stable angina. He can walk only half a block before pain in his legs forces him to stop. He has a 50-pack-year smoking history but stopped 2 years ago. Medications include atenolol, atorvastatin, and hydrochlorothiazide.

The nurse in the preoperative holding area obtains the following vital signs: temperature 36.8°C (98.2°F), blood pressure 168/100 mm Hg, heart rate 78 bpm, oxygen saturation by pulse oximeter 96% while breathing room air; he reports pain 5/10 in the right lower leg after walking into the hospital. What anesthetic agents will you choose for his anesthetic plan? Why? Does the choice of anesthetic make a difference?

For centuries, humans relied on natural medicines and physical methods to control surgical pain. Historical texts describe the sedative effects of cannabis, henbane, mandrake, and opium poppy. Physical methods such as cold, nerve compression, carotid artery occlusion, and cerebral concussion were also employed, with variable effectiveness. Although surgery was performed under ether anesthesia as early as 1842, the first public demonstration of surgical general anesthesia in 1846 is generally accepted as the start of the modern era of anesthesia. For the first time, physicians had a reliable means to keep their patients from experiencing pain during surgical procedures.

The neurophysiologic state produced by general anesthetics is characterized by five primary effects: **unconsciousness, amnesia, analgesia, inhibition of autonomic reflexes,** and **skeletal muscle relaxation.** None of the currently available anesthetic agents used alone can achieve all five of these desired effects well. An ideal anesthetic drug should also induce rapid, smooth loss of consciousness, be rapidly reversible upon discontinuation, and possess a wide margin of safety.

The modern practice of anesthesiology relies on the use of combinations of intravenous and inhaled drugs (**balanced anesthesia** techniques) to take advantage of the favorable properties of each agent while minimizing their adverse effects. The choice of anesthetic technique is determined by the type of diagnostic, therapeutic, or surgical intervention that the patient needs. For minor superficial surgery or invasive diagnostic procedures, oral or parenteral sedatives can be combined with local anesthetics in a technique termed **monitored anesthesia care** (MAC) (see Box: Sedation & Monitored Anesthesia Care, and Chapter 26). This approach can provide profound analgesia, while retaining the patient's ability to maintain a patent airway and to respond to verbal commands. For more invasive surgical procedures, anesthesia may begin with a preoperative benzodiazepine, be induced with a rapidly acting intravenous drug (eg, propofol or thiopental), and be maintained with inhaled agents (eg, volatile agents, nitrous oxide), intravenous drugs (eg, propofol, opioid analgesics), or both.

MECHANISM OF GENERAL ANESTHETIC ACTION

General anesthetics have been in successful clinical use for more than 175 years, yet their mechanism of action remains unknown. The principal effect that is common to all anesthetic agents is suppression of the normal activity of the central nervous system (CNS). Initial research focused on identifying a single biologic site of action for these drugs. This "unitary theory" of anesthetic action has been supplanted by a more complex model of molecular targets located at multiple levels of the CNS. Ongoing research has focused on cellular, molecular, and network sites to understand the mechanism of general anesthesia.

Anesthetics affect neurons at various **cellular** locations, but the primary focus has been on the **synapse.** A presynaptic action may alter the release of neurotransmitters, whereas a postsynaptic effect may change the frequency or amplitude of impulses exiting the synapse. The cumulative effect of these actions may produce strengthened inhibition or diminished excitation within key areas of the CNS. Studies on isolated spinal cord tissue have demonstrated that excitatory transmission is impaired more strongly by anesthetics than inhibitory effects are potentiated.

The principal **molecular** targets of anesthetic action that have been studied are neuronal ion channels that mediate impulse conduction in the CNS. Chloride channels (γ-aminobutyric acid-A [$GABA_A$] and glycine receptors) and potassium channels (K_{2P}, possibly K_V, and K_{ATP} channels) remain the primary *inhibitory* ion channels considered possible sites of anesthetic action. *Excitatory* ion channel targets include those activated by acetylcholine (nicotinic and muscarinic receptors), by glutamate (amino-3-hydroxy-5-methyl-4-isoxazol-propionic acid [AMPA], kainate, and *N*-methyl-D-aspartate [NMDA] receptors), or by serotonin (5-HT_2 and 5-HT_3 receptors). Figure 25–1 depicts the relation of these inhibitory and excitatory targets of anesthetics within the context of the nerve terminal.

Recently, researchers using new investigational tools such as extended array electroencephalography and functional magnetic resonance imaging have focused on neural **networks** within the brain that are altered by general anesthetics (see Box: What Does Anesthesia Represent & How Does It Work? for more details). Nevertheless, the principal barrier to understanding the mechanism of action of anesthetic agents is the lack of a coherent, widely accepted explanation for how CNS neuronal activity gives rise to the fundamental properties of brain function such as memory, sensation, emotion, and consciousness.

INHALED ANESTHETICS

A clear distinction should be made between gaseous and volatile anesthetics, both of which are administered by inhalation. *Gaseous* anesthetics **(nitrous oxide, xenon)** have high vapor pressures and low boiling points so that they are in gas form at room temperature. *In contrast, volatile* anesthetics **(halothane, isoflurane, desflurane, sevoflurane)** have lower vapor pressures and relatively higher boiling points so that they are liquids at room temperature (20°C) and sea-level ambient pressure. The physical characteristics of volatile anesthetics determine that they need to be administered using precision vaporizers. Figure 25–2 shows the chemical structures of important, clinically used, inhaled anesthetics.

Sedation & Monitored Anesthesia Care

Many diagnostic and minor therapeutic surgical procedures can be performed without general anesthesia (GA) using sedation-based anesthetic techniques. In this setting, regional (nerve block) or local anesthesia supplemented with a benzodiazepine or propofol with or without opioid analgesics (or ketamine) will allow a patient to tolerate superficial surgical or interventional procedures. This anesthetic technique is known as **monitored anesthesia care**, abbreviated as **MAC**, and should not be confused with the minimal alveolar concentration for the comparison of potencies of inhaled anesthetics (see text and Box: What Does Anesthesia Represent & How Does It Work?). The technique typically begins with intravenous midazolam to produce anxiolysis, amnesia, and mild sedation, followed by a titrated, variable-rate propofol infusion (to provide moderate to deep levels of sedation). A potent opioid analgesic or ketamine may be added to blunt pain associated with the injection of local anesthesia and the procedure itself.

Another approach, used primarily by non-anesthesiologists, is called **conscious sedation.** This technique produces alleviation of anxiety and pain with less alteration of the level of consciousness by using smaller doses of sedative medications. In this state, the patient retains the ability to maintain a patent airway and remains responsive to verbal commands. Using intravenous anesthetic drugs such as benzodiazepines and/or opioid analgesics (eg, fentanyl) in conscious sedation protocols carries the added advantage of being rapidly reversible by specific receptor antagonist drugs (flumazenil and naloxone, respectively) if a particular patient displays unusual sensitivity to them.

MAC or conscious sedation can also help supplement regional anesthesia techniques such as peripheral nerve blocks or neuraxial anesthesia.

A specialized form of sedation is occasionally required for critically ill patients in the intensive care unit (ICU) that require invasive cardiopulmonary support such as mechanical ventilation or extracorporeal membrane oxygenation (ECMO). In this situation, sedative-hypnotic drugs and low doses of intravenous anesthetic infusions may be combined. Propofol, fentanyl, and dexmedetomidine are popular choices for this indication.

Deep sedation is similar to a light state of general anesthesia characterized by decreased consciousness from which the patient is not easily aroused. The transition from deep sedation to general anesthesia is fluid and can be difficult to define. Because deep sedation is accompanied by loss of verbal responsiveness, protective airway reflexes, and the ability to maintain a patent airway, this state may be indistinguishable from general anesthesia. A practitioner with expertise in airway management (anesthesiologist or nurse anesthetist) must be present.

Intravenous agents used in deep sedation protocols mainly include the sedative-hypnotics propofol and midazolam, sometimes in combination with potent opioid analgesics or ketamine, depending on the level of pain associated with the surgery or procedure.

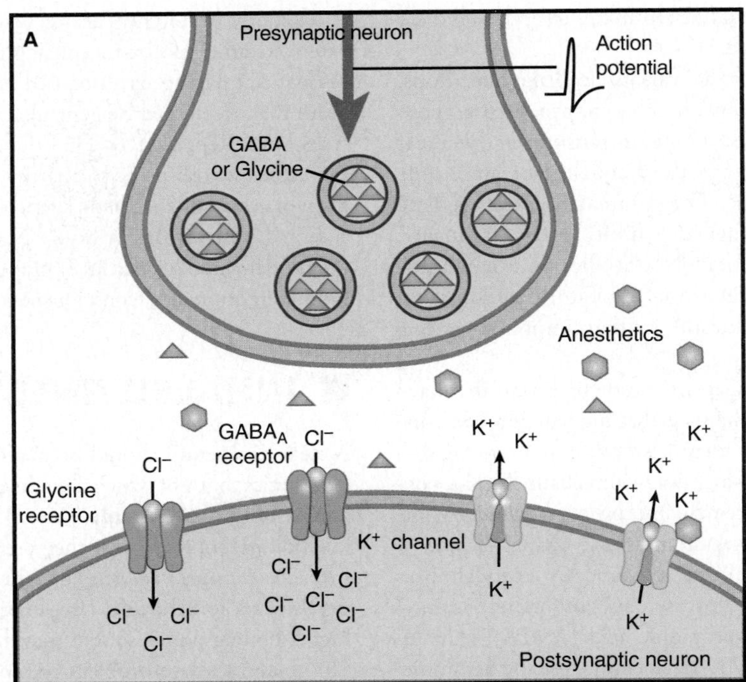

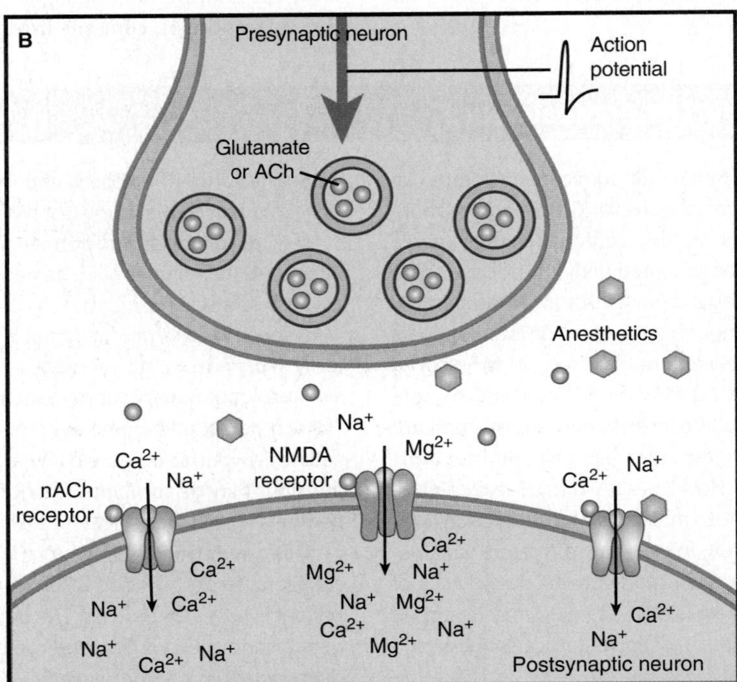

FIGURE 25–1 Putative targets of anesthetic action. Anesthetic drugs may (**A**) enhance inhibitory synaptic activity or (**B**) diminish excitatory activity. ACh, acetylcholine; GABA$_A$, γ-aminobutyric acid-A.

PHARMACOKINETICS

Inhaled anesthetics, both volatile and gaseous, are taken up through gas exchange in the alveoli of the lung for distribution to the effect compartments within the body. The kinetic goal of delivering anesthetic gases this way is to rapidly achieve an effective concentration of the agent at the lung:blood interface. When this equilibrium is reached we presume that the effect site concentration within the CNS (brain and spinal cord) has also been reached. Several factors determine how quickly the alveolar and subsequent CNS concentrations change.

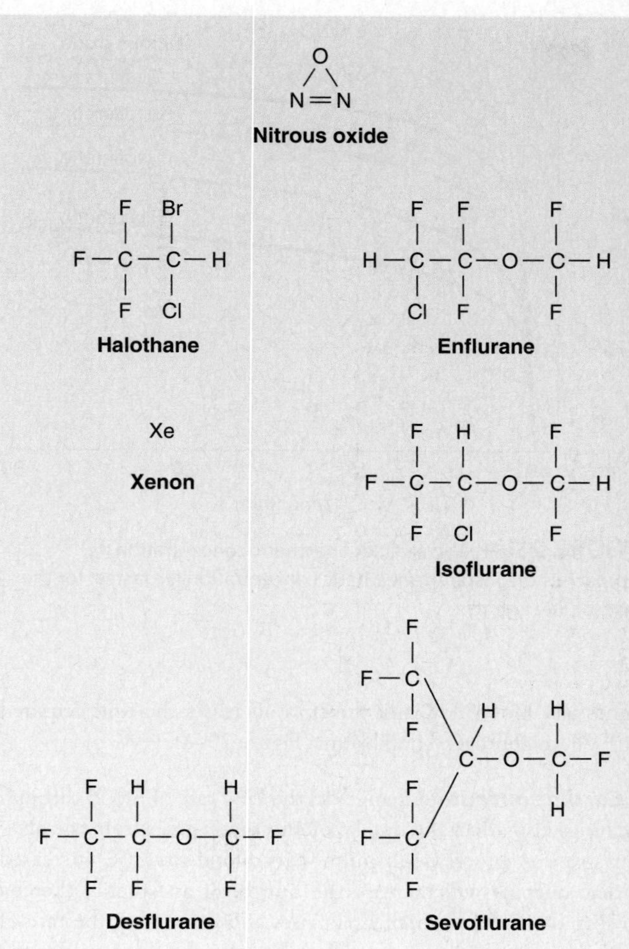

FIGURE 25–2 Chemical structures of inhaled anesthetics.

Uptake & Distribution

A. Factors Controlling Uptake

1. *Inspired concentration and ventilation*—The driving force for uptake of an inhaled anesthetic into the body is the ratio between inspired and alveolar concentration. The most important parameter that can be controlled by the anesthesiologist to change alveolar concentration quickly is the *inspired concentration* or *partial pressure*. The partial pressure is the fraction of a gas mixture that a particular component comprises. For example, a mixture of gases that may be delivered by an anesthesia machine—70% nitrous oxide, 29% oxygen, and 1% isoflurane at normal barometric pressure (760 mm Hg)—contains partial pressures of 532 mm Hg nitrous oxide, 220 mm Hg oxygen, and 7.6 mm Hg isoflurane. The partial pressure of anesthetic in the inspired gas mixture determines the maximum partial pressure that can be achieved in the alveoli as well as the rate of rise of the partial pressure in the alveoli. To accelerate induction, the anesthesiologist increases the inspired anesthetic partial pressure to create a steeper gradient between inspired and alveolar partial pressure. This fractional rise of anesthetic partial pressure during induction is expressed as a ratio of alveolar concentration (F_A) over inspired concentration (F_I); the faster F_A/F_I approaches 1 (representing inspired-to-alveolar equilibrium), the faster anesthesia onset will be during inhaled induction of anesthesia.

The other parameter under control of the anesthesiologist that directly determines the rate of rise of F_A/F_I is alveolar ventilation. By increasing the tidal volume and respiratory rate the anesthesiologist can quickly deliver a larger mass of anesthetic agent to the alveoli of the lung. The tendency for a given inhaled anesthetic to pass from the gas phase of the alveoli into pulmonary capillary blood is determined by the blood:gas partition coefficient (see the following section Solubility and Table 25–1). As increased ventilation supplies more anesthetic molecules to the alveoli, a highly soluble anesthetic (blood:gas partition coefficient >1) will traverse the alveolar capillary membrane and be taken up by the pulmonary flow, preventing a rise in its alveolar partial pressure. Thus, increased ventilation will replenish the alveolar anesthetic concentration for a highly soluble anesthetic but is not necessary for an anesthetic with low solubility. Therefore, an increase in ventilation accelerates the rise in alveolar partial pressure of an anesthetic with low blood solubility very little, but can significantly increase the partial pressure of agents with moderate to high blood solubility such as halothane. As seen in Figure 25–3, a fourfold increase in the ventilation rate almost doubles the F_A/F_I ratio

TABLE 25–1 Pharmacologic properties of inhaled anesthetics.

Anesthetic	Blood:Gas Partition Coefficient[1]	Brain:Blood Partition Coefficient[1]	Minimal Alveolar Concentration (MAC) (%)[2]	Metabolism	Comments
Nitrous oxide	0.47	1.1	>100	None	Incomplete anesthetic; rapid onset and recovery
Desflurane	0.42	1.3	6–7	<0.05%	Low volatility; poor induction agent (pungent); rapid recovery
Sevoflurane	0.69	1.7	2.0	2–5% (fluoride)	Rapid onset and recovery; unstable in soda-lime
Isoflurane	1.40	2.6	1.40	<2%	Medium rate of onset and recovery
Enflurane	1.80	1.4	1.7	8%	Medium rate of onset and recovery
Halothane	2.30	2.9	0.75	>40%	Medium rate of onset and recovery

[1]Partition coefficients (at 37°C) are from multiple literature sources.

[2]MAC is the anesthetic concentration that produces immobility in 50% of patients exposed to a noxious stimulus.

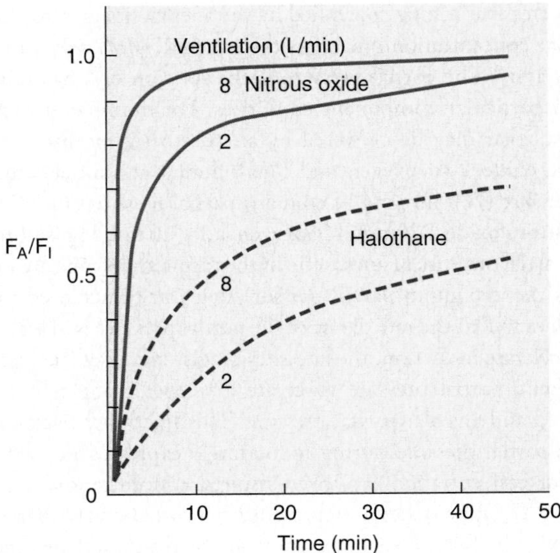

FIGURE 25–3 Effect of ventilation on F_A/F_I and induction of anesthesia. Increased ventilation (8 L/min versus 2 L/min) accelerates the rate of rise toward equilibration of both halothane and nitrous oxide but results in a larger percentage increase for halothane in the first few minutes of induction.

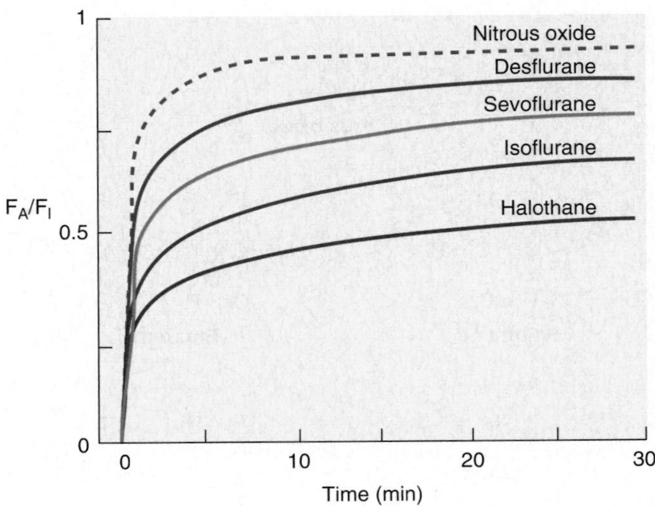

FIGURE 25–4 The alveolar anesthetic concentration (F_A) approaches the inspired anesthetic concentration (F_I) fastest for the least soluble agents.

for halothane during the first few minutes of administration but increases the F_A/F_I ratio for the low solubility gas nitrous oxide by only 15%. Thus, hyperventilation increases the speed of induction of anesthesia with inhaled anesthetics that would normally have a slow onset.

2. *Solubility*—As described above, the rate of rise of F_A/F_I is an important determinant of the speed of induction, but is opposed by the uptake of anesthetic into the blood. Uptake is determined by pharmacokinetic characteristics of each anesthetic agent as well as patient factors.

One of the most important factors influencing the transfer of an anesthetic from the lungs to the arterial blood is its solubility characteristics (see Table 25–1). As described above, the blood:gas partition coefficient is a useful index of solubility and defines the relative affinity of an anesthetic for the blood compared to the affinity for inspired gas phase. Desflurane, sevoflurane, and nitrous oxide, which are relatively insoluble in blood, display low partition coefficients. When an anesthetic with low blood solubility partitions between gas in the lung and pulmonary capillary blood, equilibrium is quickly established and the blood concentration rises rapidly (Figure 25–4, top; nitrous oxide, desflurane, sevoflurane). Conversely, for anesthetics with greater solubility (Figure 25–4, bottom; halothane, isoflurane), more molecules dissolve in the blood before partial pressure changes significantly, and arterial concentration of the gas increases less rapidly. A blood:gas partition coefficient of 0.47 for nitrous oxide means that at equilibrium, the concentration in blood is less than half the concentration in the alveolar space (gas). A larger blood:gas partition coefficient causes a greater uptake of anesthetic into the pulmonary blood flow and therefore increases the time required for F_A/F_I to approach equilibrium (Figure 25–4).

3. *Cardiac output*—Changes in the flow rate of blood through the lungs also affect the uptake of anesthetic gases from the alveolar space. An increase in pulmonary blood flow (ie, increased cardiac output) will increase the uptake of anesthetic, thereby slowing the rate by which F_A/F_I rises and decreasing the rate of induction of anesthesia. Furthermore, one should consider the effect of cardiac output in combination with the tissue distribution and uptake of anesthetic into other tissue compartments. The increased uptake of anesthetic into the blood caused by increased cardiac output will be distributed to all tissues. Since cerebral blood flow is well regulated and maintained relatively constant at clinical anesthetic concentrations, the increased anesthesia uptake caused by increased cardiac output will predominantly be distributed to tissues that are not involved in the site of action of the anesthetic. Conversely, low-cardiac-output states such as in patients with heart failure predispose to overdosage with soluble agents, as the rate of rise in alveolar concentrations will be markedly increased.

4. *Alveolar-venous partial pressure difference*—The anesthetic partial pressure difference between alveolar and mixed venous blood is dependent mainly on uptake of the anesthetic by the tissues, including non-neural tissues. Depending on the rate and extent of tissue uptake, venous blood returning to the lungs may contain significantly less anesthetic than arterial blood leaving the heart. Anesthetic uptake into tissues is influenced by factors similar to those that determine transfer of the anesthetic from the lung to the intravascular space, including tissue:blood partition coefficients (see Table 25–1), rates of blood flow to the tissues, and concentration gradients. The greater this difference in anesthetic gas concentrations, the more time it will take to achieve equilibrium with brain tissue.

During the induction phase of anesthesia (and the initial phase of the maintenance period), the tissues that exert greatest influence on the arteriovenous anesthetic concentration gradient are those that are highly perfused (eg, brain, heart, liver, kidneys, and splanchnic bed). Combined, these tissues receive over 75% of the resting cardiac output. In the case of volatile anesthetics with relatively high solubility in highly perfused tissues, venous blood concentration initially is very low, and equilibrium with the alveolar space is achieved slowly.

During maintenance of anesthesia with inhaled anesthetics, the drug continues to be transferred between various tissues at rates dependent on the solubility of the agent, the concentration gradient between the blood and the respective tissue, and the tissue blood flow. Although muscle and skin constitute 50% of the total body mass, anesthetics accumulate more slowly in these tissues than in highly perfused tissues (eg, brain) because they receive only one fifth of the resting cardiac output. Although most anesthetic agents are highly soluble in adipose (fatty) tissues, the relatively low blood perfusion to these tissues delays accumulation, and equilibrium is unlikely to occur with most anesthetics during a typical 1- to 3-hour operation.

The combined effect of ventilation, solubility in the different tissues, cardiac output, and blood flow distribution determines the rate of rise of F_A/F_I characteristic of each drug. Figure 25–5 schematically compares how uptake and distribution proceed with two widely different agents. The anesthetic state is achieved when the partial pressure of the anesthetic in the brain reaches a threshold concentration determined by its **potency** (MAC; see Table 25–1 and Box: What Does Anesthesia Represent & How Does It Work?). For relatively insoluble agents like desflurane and sevoflurane, the alveolar partial pressure can quickly equilibrate through the blood and brain compartments to reach anesthetizing concentrations.

However, for an agent like halothane, its greater solubility in blood and other tissue compartments (higher partition coefficients) results in a steeper decline in the concentration gradient from alveolus to brain, causing a slower onset of anesthesia. Therefore, administering a larger concentration of halothane and increasing alveolar ventilation are the two strategies used by anesthesiologists to speed the rate of induction with halothane.

B. Elimination

Recovery from inhalation anesthesia occurs by the same principles that are important during induction. Many of the factors that speed induction also speed recovery: high fresh gas flows, decreased solubility, high cerebral blood flow, and increased ventilation. The time to recovery from inhaled anesthetics depends on the rate of removal of the drug from the brain. One of the most important factors governing rate of recovery is again the blood:gas partition coefficient of the anesthetic agent. When the anesthesiologist discontinues the administration of the anesthetic agent to the lung, the inspired and alveolar concentrations fall rapidly. Insoluble anesthetics that prefer the gas phase over blood will then rapidly diffuse into the alveoli and be removed from the body by the process of lung ventilation. Other factors controlling rate of recovery include pulmonary blood flow (cardiac output) and tissue solubility of the anesthetic.

Two features differentiate the recovery phase from the induction phase. First, transfer of an anesthetic from the lungs to blood

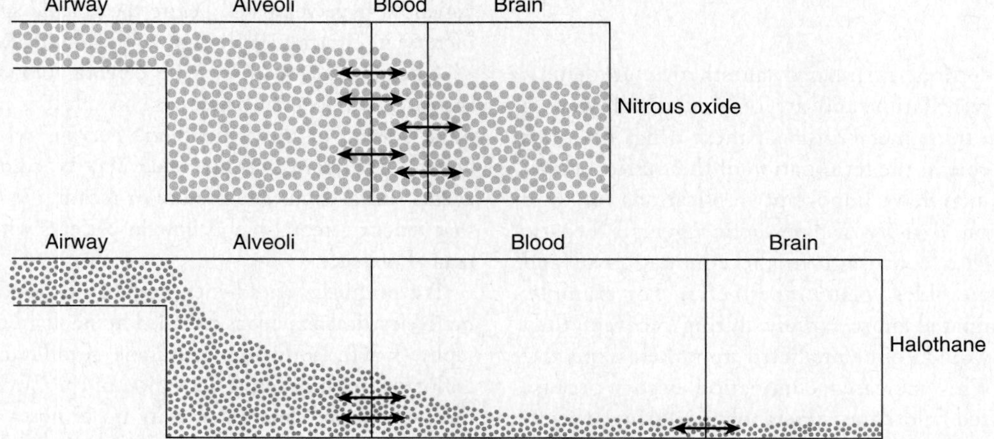

FIGURE 25–5 Why induction of anesthesia is slower with more soluble anesthetic gases. In this schematic diagram, solubility in blood is represented by the relative size of the blood compartment (the more soluble, the larger the compartment). Relative partial pressures of the agents in the compartments are indicated by the degree of filling of each compartment. For a given concentration or partial pressure of the two anesthetic gases in the inspired air, it will take much longer for the blood partial pressure of the more soluble gas (halothane) to rise to the same partial pressure as in the alveoli. Since the concentration of the anesthetic agent in the brain can rise no faster than the concentration in the blood, the onset of anesthesia will be slower with halothane than with nitrous oxide.

during induction can be enhanced by increasing its concentration in inspired air, but the reverse transfer process cannot be enhanced because the concentration in the lungs cannot be reduced below zero. Second, at the beginning of the recovery phase, the anesthetic gas tension in different tissues throughout the body may be quite variable, depending on the specific agent solubility and the duration of anesthesia. In contrast, at the start of induction of anesthesia, the initial anesthetic tension is zero in all tissues.

Inhaled anesthetics that are relatively insoluble in blood (ie, possess low blood:gas partition coefficients) and brain are eliminated faster than the more soluble anesthetics. The washout of nitrous oxide, desflurane, and sevoflurane occurs at a rapid rate, leading to a more rapid recovery from their anesthetic effects compared with halothane and isoflurane. Halothane is approximately twice as soluble in brain tissue and five times more soluble in blood than nitrous oxide and desflurane; its elimination therefore takes place more slowly, and recovery from halothane- and isoflurane-based anesthesia is predictably less rapid.

The duration of exposure to the anesthetic is a significant factor in the speed of emergence from anesthesia, especially in the case of the more soluble anesthetics. Accumulation of anesthetics in muscle, skin, and fat increases with prolonged exposure (especially in obese patients), and blood concentration may decline slowly after discontinuation as the anesthetic is slowly eliminated from these tissues. Although recovery after a short exposure to anesthesia may be rapid even with the more soluble agents, recovery is slow after prolonged administration of halothane or isoflurane.

1. *Ventilation*—Two parameters that can be manipulated by the anesthesiologist are useful in controlling the speed of induction of and recovery from inhaled anesthesia: (1) concentration of anesthetic in the inspired gas and (2) alveolar ventilation. As stated above, since the concentration of anesthetic in the inspired gas cannot be reduced below zero, hyperventilation is the only way to speed recovery.

2. *Metabolism*—Modern inhaled anesthetics are eliminated mainly by ventilation and are only metabolized to a very small extent; thus, metabolism of these drugs does not play a significant role in the termination of their effect. However, metabolism may have important implications for their toxicity (see section Toxicity of Anesthetic Agents). Hepatic metabolism may also contribute to the elimination of and recovery from some older volatile anesthetics. For example, halothane is eliminated more rapidly during recovery than enflurane, which would not be predicted from their respective tissue solubility. This increased elimination occurs because over 40% of inspired halothane is metabolized during an average anesthetic procedure, whereas less than 10% of enflurane is metabolized over the same period.

In terms of the extent of hepatic metabolism, the rank order for the inhaled anesthetics is halothane > enflurane > sevoflurane > isoflurane > desflurane > nitrous oxide (see Table 25–1). Nitrous oxide is not metabolized by human tissues. However, bacteria in the gastrointestinal tract may be able to break down the nitrous oxide molecule.

PHARMACODYNAMICS

Organ System Effects of Inhaled Anesthetics

A. CNS Effects

Anesthetic potency is currently described by the minimal alveolar concentration (MAC) required to prevent a response to a surgical incision (see Box: What Does Anesthesia Represent & How Does It Work?). This parameter was first described by investigators in the 1960s and remains the best clinical guide for administering inhaled anesthetics, especially since improved medical technology can now provide instantaneous, accurate determination of gas concentrations.

Inhaled anesthetics (and intravenous anesthetics, discussed later) decrease the metabolic activity of the brain. Decreased cerebral metabolic rate (CMR) generally causes a reduction in blood flow within the brain. However, volatile anesthetics may also produce cerebral vasodilation, which can increase cerebral blood flow. The net effect on cerebral blood flow (increase, decrease, or no change) depends on the concentration of anesthetic delivered. At 0.5 MAC, the reduction in CMR is greater than the vasodilation caused by anesthetics, so cerebral blood flow is decreased. Conversely, at 1.5 MAC, vasodilation by the anesthetic is greater than the reduction in CMR, so cerebral blood flow is increased. In between, at 1.0 MAC, the effects are balanced and cerebral blood flow is unchanged. An increase in cerebral blood flow is clinically undesirable in patients who have increased intracranial pressure because of brain tumor, intracranial hemorrhage, or head injury. Therefore, administration of high concentrations of volatile anesthetics is best avoided in patients with increased intracranial pressure. Hyperventilation can be used to attenuate this response—decreasing the Pa_{CO_2} (the partial pressure of carbon dioxide in arterial blood) through hyperventilation causes cerebral vasoconstriction. If the patient is hyperventilated before the volatile agent is started, the increase in intracranial pressure can be minimized.

Nitrous oxide can increase cerebral blood flow and cause increased intracranial pressure. This effect is most likely caused by activation of the sympathetic nervous system (as described below). Therefore, nitrous oxide may be combined with other agents (intravenous anesthetics) or techniques (hyperventilation) that reduce cerebral blood flow in patients with increased intracranial pressure.

Potent inhaled anesthetics produce a basic pattern of change to brain electrical activity as recorded by standard electroencephalography (EEG). Isoflurane, desflurane, sevoflurane, halothane, and enflurane produce initial activation of the EEG at low doses and then slowing of electrical activity up to doses of 1.0–1.5 MAC. At higher concentrations, EEG suppression increases to the point of electrical silence with isoflurane at 2.0–2.5 MAC. Isolated epileptic-like patterns may also be seen between 1.0 and 2.0 MAC, especially with sevoflurane and enflurane, but frank clinical seizure activity has been observed only with enflurane. Nitrous oxide used alone causes fast electrical oscillations emanating from the frontal cortex at doses associated with analgesia and depressed consciousness.

What Does Anesthesia Represent & How Does It Work?

Anesthetic action has three principal components: immobility, amnesia, and unconsciousness. The exact cellular, molecular, or physiologic mechanisms for producing these effects are largely unknown.

Immobility

Immobility is the easiest anesthetic end point to measure. Edmond Eger and colleagues introduced the concept of **minimal alveolar concentration (MAC)** to quantify the **potency** of an inhalational anesthetic. They defined 1.0 MAC as the alveolar partial pressure of an inhalational anesthetic at which 50% of a population of unparalyzed patients remained immobile at the time of abdominal surgery skin incision. Anesthetic immobility is mediated primarily by neural inhibition within the spinal cord but may also include inhibited nociceptive transmission to the brain. This concept is the most convenient measure by which anesthesiologists compare the potency of inhaled agents and guide the conduct of patient anesthesia.

Amnesia

The ablation of memory occurs in several locations in the CNS, including the hippocampus, amygdala, prefrontal cortex, and regions of the sensory and motor cortices. Memory researchers differentiate two types of remembrance that should be abolished under anesthesia: (1) explicit memory, ie, specific awareness or consciousness under anesthesia; and (2) implicit memory, the unconscious acquisition of information under adequate levels of anesthesia. Their studies have found that formation of both types of memory is reliably prevented at low MAC values (0.2–0.4 MAC). Prevention of explicit memory (awareness) has spurred the development of monitors such as the bispectral index, patient state index, electroencephalogram (EEG), and entropy monitor of auditory evoked potentials to help recognize inadequate depth of anesthesia.

Unconsciousness

The ability of anesthetic drugs to abolish consciousness requires action at anatomic locations responsible for the formation of human consciousness. Neuroscientists studying consciousness identify three regions in the brain involved in generating personal awareness: the cerebral cortical hemispheres, the thalamus, and the reticular activating system. Neural pathways emanating from these regions seem to synchronize as an interacting system to produce the mental state in which humans are awake, aware, and perceiving.

Our current state of understanding supports the following framework: sensory stimuli conducted through the reticular formation of the brainstem into supratentorial signaling loops, connecting the thalamus with various regions of the cortex, are the foundation of consciousness. These neural pathways involved in the development of consciousness are reversibly disrupted by anesthetic agents.

Traditionally, anesthetic effects on the brain produce four stages or levels of increasing depth of CNS depression (**Guedel's signs,** derived from observations of the effects of inhaled diethyl ether): **Stage I—analgesia:** The patient initially experiences analgesia without amnesia. Later in stage I, both analgesia and amnesia are produced. **Stage II—excitement:** During this stage, the patient appears delirious and may vocalize but is completely amnesic. Respiration is rapid, and heart rate and blood pressure increase. Duration and severity of this light stage of anesthesia are shortened by rapidly increasing the concentration of the agent. **Stage III—surgical anesthesia:** This stage begins with slowing of respiration and heart rate and extends to complete cessation of spontaneous respiration (apnea). Four planes of stage III are described based on changes in ocular movements, eye reflexes, and pupil size, indicating increasing depth of anesthesia. **Stage IV—medullary depression:** This deep stage of anesthesia represents severe depression of the CNS, including the vasomotor center in the medulla and respiratory center in the brainstem. Without circulatory and respiratory support, death would rapidly ensue in stage IV.

B. Cardiovascular Effects

Halothane, enflurane, isoflurane, desflurane, and sevoflurane all depress normal cardiac contractility (halothane and enflurane more so than isoflurane, desflurane, and sevoflurane). As a result, all volatile agents tend to decrease mean arterial pressure in direct proportion to their alveolar concentration. With halothane and enflurane, the reduced arterial pressure is caused primarily by myocardial depression (reduced cardiac output) and there is little change in systemic vascular resistance. In contrast, isoflurane, desflurane, and sevoflurane produce greater vasodilation with minimal effect on cardiac output. These differences may have important implications for patients with heart failure. Because isoflurane, desflurane, and sevoflurane better preserve cardiac output as well as reduce preload (ventricular filling) and afterload (systemic vascular resistance), these agents may be better choices for patients with impaired myocardial function.

Nitrous oxide also depresses myocardial function in a concentration-dependent manner. This depression may be significantly offset by a concomitant activation of the sympathetic nervous system resulting in preservation of cardiac output. Therefore, administration of nitrous oxide in combination with the more potent volatile anesthetics can minimize circulatory depressant effects by both anesthetic-sparing and sympathetic-activating actions.

Because all inhaled anesthetics produce a dose-dependent decrease in arterial blood pressure, activation of autonomic nervous system reflexes may trigger increased heart rate. However, halothane, enflurane, and sevoflurane have little effect on heart rate, probably because they attenuate baroreceptor input into the autonomic nervous system. Desflurane and isoflurane significantly increase heart rate because they cause less depression of the baroreceptor reflex. In addition, desflurane can trigger transient sympathetic activation—with elevated catecholamine levels—to cause marked increases in heart rate and blood pressure during administration of high desflurane concentrations or when desflurane concentrations are changed rapidly.

Inhaled anesthetics tend to reduce myocardial oxygen consumption, which reflects depression of normal cardiac contractility and decreased arterial blood pressure. In addition, inhaled anesthetics produce coronary vasodilation. The net effect of decreased oxygen demand and increased coronary flow (oxygen supply) is improved myocardial oxygenation. However, other factors, such as surgical stimulation, intravascular volume status, blood oxygen levels, and withdrawal of perioperative β blockers, may tilt the oxygen supply-demand balance toward myocardial ischemia in specific patients.

C. Respiratory Effects

All volatile anesthetics possess varying degrees of bronchodilating properties, an effect of value in patients with active wheezing and in status asthmaticus. However, airway irritation, which may provoke coughing or breath-holding, is induced by the pungency of some volatile anesthetics. The pungency of isoflurane and desflurane makes these agents less suitable for induction of anesthesia in patients with active bronchospasm. These reactions rarely occur with halothane and sevoflurane, which are considered nonpungent. Therefore, the bronchodilating action of halothane and sevoflurane makes them the agents of choice in patients with underlying airway problems. Nonpungency and rapid increases in alveolar anesthetic concentration also make sevoflurane an excellent choice for smooth and rapid inhalation inductions in pediatric and adult patients. Nitrous oxide is also nonpungent and can facilitate inhalational induction of anesthesia in a patient with bronchospasm.

The control of breathing is significantly affected by inhaled anesthetics. With the exception of nitrous oxide, all inhaled anesthetics in current use cause a dose-dependent decrease in tidal volume and an increase in respiratory rate, resulting in a rapid, shallow breathing pattern. However, the increase in respiratory rate varies among agents and does not fully compensate for the decrease in tidal volume, resulting in decreased alveolar ventilation. In addition, all volatile anesthetics are respiratory depressants, as defined by a reduced ventilatory response to increased levels of carbon dioxide in the blood. The degree of ventilatory depression varies among the volatile agents, with isoflurane and enflurane being the most depressant. By this hypoventilation mechanism, all volatile anesthetics increase the resting level of $Paco_2$ in spontaneously breathing patients.

Volatile anesthetics also raise the apneic threshold ($Paco_2$ level below which apnea occurs through lack of CO_2-driven respiratory stimulation) and decrease the ventilatory response to hypoxia. Clinically, the respiratory depressant effects of anesthetics are overcome by assisting (controlling) ventilation mechanically. The ventilatory depression produced by inhaled anesthetics may be counteracted by surgical stimulation; however, low, subanesthetic concentrations of volatile anesthetic present after surgery in the early recovery period can continue to depress the compensatory increase in ventilation normally caused by hypoxia.

Inhaled anesthetics also depress mucociliary function in the airway. During prolonged exposure to inhaled anesthetics, mucus pooling may result in atelectasis and the development of postoperative respiratory complications, including hypoxemia, mucous plugging, and respiratory infections.

D. Renal Effects

Inhaled anesthetics tend to decrease glomerular filtration rate (GFR) and urine flow. Renal blood flow may also be decreased by some agents, but filtration fraction is increased, implying that autoregulatory control of efferent arteriole tone helps compensate and limits the reduction in GFR. In general these anesthetic effects are minor compared with the stress of surgery itself and usually reversible after discontinuation of the anesthetic.

E. Hepatic Effects

Volatile anesthetics cause a concentration-dependent decrease in portal vein blood flow that parallels the decline in cardiac output produced by these agents. However, total hepatic blood flow may be relatively preserved as hepatic artery blood flow to the liver may increase or stay the same. Although transient changes in liver function tests may occur following exposure to volatile anesthetics, persistent elevation in liver enzymes is rare except following repeated exposures to halothane (see section Toxicity of Anesthetic Agents).

F. Effects on Uterine Smooth Muscle

Nitrous oxide appears to have little effect on uterine musculature. However, the halogenated anesthetics are potent uterine muscle relaxants and produce this effect in a concentration-dependent fashion. This pharmacologic effect can be helpful when profound uterine relaxation is required for intrauterine fetal manipulation or manual extraction of a retained placenta during delivery. However, it can also lead to increased uterine bleeding after delivery when uterine contraction is desired.

Toxicity of Anesthetic Agents

A. Acute Toxicity

Volatile anesthetics have a narrow therapeutic range and must be administered in a well-controlled, monitored setting by trained practitioners. When delivered in this way the risk of acute organ injury is low. The effects described below are rare or of historical interest only. However, concern over neurotoxicity of volatile anesthetics, especially in the developing brain is an active area of research.

1. *Nephrotoxicity*—Metabolism of enflurane and sevoflurane may generate compounds that are potentially nephrotoxic. Although their metabolism can liberate nephrotoxic fluoride ions, significant renal injury has been reported only for enflurane with prolonged exposure. The insolubility and rapid elimination of sevoflurane may prevent toxicity. This drug may be degraded by carbon dioxide absorbents in anesthesia machines to form a nephrotoxic vinyl ether compound termed "compound A," which, in high concentrations, has caused proximal tubular necrosis in rats. Nevertheless, there have been no reports of renal injury in humans receiving sevoflurane anesthesia. Moreover, exposure to sevoflurane does not produce any change in standard markers of renal function.

2. *Hematotoxicity*—Prolonged exposure to nitrous oxide decreases methionine synthase activity, which theoretically could cause megaloblastic anemia. Megaloblastic bone marrow changes have been observed in patients after 12-hour exposure to 50% nitrous oxide. Chronic exposure of dental personnel to nitrous oxide in inadequately ventilated dental operating suites is a potential occupational hazard.

All inhaled anesthetics can produce some carbon monoxide (CO) from their interaction with strong bases in dry carbon dioxide absorbers. CO binds to hemoglobin with high affinity, reducing oxygen delivery to tissues. Desflurane produces the most CO, and intraoperative formation of CO has been reported. CO production can be avoided simply by using fresh carbon dioxide absorbent and by preventing its complete desiccation.

3. *Malignant hyperthermia*—Malignant hyperthermia is a heritable genetic disorder of skeletal muscle that occurs in susceptible individuals exposed to volatile anesthetics while undergoing general anesthesia (see Chapter 16 and Table 16–4). The depolarizing muscle relaxant succinylcholine may also trigger malignant hyperthermia. The malignant hyperthermia syndrome consists of muscle rigidity, hyperthermia, rapid onset of tachycardia and hypercapnia, hyperkalemia, and metabolic acidosis following exposure to one or more triggering agents. Malignant hyperthermia is a rare but important cause of anesthetic morbidity and mortality. A specific biochemical abnormality—an increase in free cytosolic calcium concentration in skeletal muscle cells—may be the underlying cellular basis of malignant hyperthermia. Treatment includes administration of **dantrolene** (to reduce calcium release from the sarcoplasmic reticulum) and appropriate measures to reduce body temperature and restore electrolyte and acid-base balance (see Chapters 16 and 27). A new formulation of dantrolene with improved solubility has become available that can speed the treatment of this rare but potentially fatal reaction.

Malignant hyperthermia susceptibility is characterized by genetic heterogeneity, and several predisposing clinical myopathies have been identified. It has been associated with mutations in the gene coding for the skeletal muscle ryanodine receptor (RyR1, the calcium release channel on the sarcoplasmic reticulum), and mutant alleles of the gene encoding the α_1 subunit of the human skeletal muscle L-type voltage-dependent calcium channel. However, the genetic loci identified to date account for less than 50% of malignant hyperthermia-susceptible individuals, and genetic testing cannot definitively determine malignant hyperthermia susceptibility. Currently, the most reliable test to establish susceptibility is the in vitro caffeine-halothane contracture test using skeletal muscle biopsy samples. Genetic counseling is recommended for family members of a person who has experienced a documented malignant hyperthermia reaction in the operating room.

4. *Hepatotoxicity (halothane hepatitis)*—Hepatic dysfunction following surgery and general anesthesia is most likely caused by hypovolemic shock, infection conferred by blood transfusion, or other surgical stresses rather than by volatile anesthetic toxicity. However, a small subset of individuals previously exposed to halothane developed fulminant hepatic failure. The incidence of severe hepatotoxicity following exposure to halothane was estimated to be in the range of 1 in 20,000–35,000. The mechanisms underlying halothane hepatotoxicity remain unclear, but studies in animals implicate the formation of reactive metabolites that either cause direct hepatocellular damage (eg, free radicals) or initiate immune-mediated responses. Cases of hepatitis following exposure to other volatile anesthetics, including enflurane, isoflurane, and desflurane, have rarely been reported.

5. *Neurotoxicity*—Neuronal toxicity of volatile anesthesia in young infants whose brains are still undergoing neurogenesis is an emerging concern, first identified in animal studies. In vitro studies have also found increased levels of apoptosis in cultured neurons exposed to clinical levels of volatile anesthetics. Human data is difficult to obtain but a recently reported epidemiologic study that followed a cohort of children receiving either general anesthesia or nerve block anesthesia for hernia repair in the first 3 months of life found no difference in IQ testing at 5 years of age. The neurotoxicity of longer or multiple exposures to volatile anesthetics is unknown.

B. Chronic Toxicity

1. *Mutagenicity, teratogenicity, and reproductive effects*—Under normal conditions, inhaled anesthetics including nitrous oxide are neither mutagens nor carcinogens in patients. Nitrous oxide can be directly teratogenic in animals under conditions of extremely high exposure. Halothane, enflurane, isoflurane, desflurane, and sevoflurane may be teratogenic in rodents as a result of physiologic changes associated with the anesthesia rather than through a direct teratogenic effect.

The most consistent finding in surveys conducted to determine the reproductive success of female operating room personnel who may have low-level chronic exposure to anesthetic agents has been a questionably higher-than-expected incidence of miscarriages. However, there are several problems in interpreting these studies. The association of obstetric problems with surgery and anesthesia in pregnant patients is also an important consideration. In the United States, at least 50,000 pregnant women each year undergo anesthesia and surgery for indications unrelated to pregnancy. The risk of abortion is clearly higher following this experience. It is not obvious, however, whether the underlying disease, surgery, anesthesia, or a combination of these factors is the cause of the increased risk.

2. *Carcinogenicity*—Epidemiologic studies suggested an increase in the cancer rate in operating room personnel who were exposed to trace concentrations of anesthetic agents. However, no study has demonstrated the existence of a causal relationship between anesthetics and cancer. Many other factors might account for the questionably positive results seen after a careful review of epidemiologic data. Anesthesia machines are now equipped with gas scavenging systems to remove concentrations of anesthetics administered to patients, and operating rooms rely on high air exchange rates to remove trace concentrations of anesthetics released from anesthesia machines.

ENVIRONMENTAL IMPACT OF INHALED ANESTHETICS

The primary inhalational anesthetics in clinical use, sevoflurane, isoflurane, desflurane, and nitrous oxide, are known to act as greenhouse gases but their contribution to global temperature rise and climate change are considered small compared with other industrial processes. In current practice these gases are administered to patients, exhaled with little metabolism, and then collected by anesthesia machine scavenging systems for venting out of the building directly into the atmosphere. By their intrinsic chemical nature these compounds are hundreds to thousands of times more potent than carbon dioxide (CO_2) in their global warming potential. Moreover, each of these gases possess widely varying atmospheric lifetimes. For example, the tropospheric lifetime of sevoflurane, isoflurane, desflurane, and nitrous oxide are 1.4, 3.6, 10, and 114 years, respectively. The medical use of nitrous oxide for anesthesia has been estimated to represent 1–3% of the annual U.S. nitrous oxide emission. Because of this increased awareness, clinical guidelines for decreasing the amount of inhaled anesthetics used have been proposed. The current trend is to use the agents in ultra-low total gas flow techniques (0.5–1.0 liter per minute), to avoid adding nitrous oxide as a carrier admixture gas with room air, and to restrict the use of desflurane.

■ INTRAVENOUS ANESTHETICS

Intravenous nonopioid anesthetics play an essential role in the practice of modern anesthesia. They are used to facilitate rapid induction of anesthesia and have replaced inhalation as the preferred method of anesthesia induction in most settings except for pediatric anesthesia. Intravenous agents are also commonly used to provide sedation during monitored anesthesia care and for patients in ICU settings. With the introduction of propofol, intravenous anesthesia also became a good option for the maintenance of anesthesia. However, similar to the inhaled agents, the currently available intravenous anesthetics are not ideal anesthetic drugs in the sense of producing all and only the five desired effects (unconsciousness, amnesia, analgesia, inhibition of autonomic reflexes, and skeletal muscle relaxation). Therefore, **balanced anesthesia** employing multiple drugs (inhaled anesthetics, sedative-hypnotics, opioids, neuromuscular blocking drugs) is generally used to achieve the desired combination of effects while minimizing unwanted effects.

The intravenous anesthetics used for induction of general anesthesia are lipophilic and preferentially partition into highly perfused lipophilic tissues (brain, spinal cord), which accounts for their rapid onset of action. Regardless of the extent and speed of their metabolism, termination of the effect of a single bolus is determined by redistribution of the drug into less perfused and inactive tissues such as skeletal muscle and fat. Thus, all drugs used for induction of anesthesia have similar durations of action when administered as a single bolus dose despite significant differences in their metabolism. Figure 25–6 shows the chemical structures of common clinically used intravenous anesthetics. Table 25–2 lists pharmacokinetic properties of these and other intravenous agents.

PROPOFOL

In most countries, propofol is the drug most frequently administered for the induction of anesthesia, and it has largely replaced barbiturates in this setting. Because its pharmacokinetic profile allows for continuous infusions, propofol is a good alternative to inhaled anesthetics for maintenance of anesthesia and is also a common choice for sedation in the setting of monitored anesthesia care. When used during maintenance of anesthesia, propofol infusion can be supplemented with intravenous opioids and neuromuscular blockers as needed to completely avoid the use of inhaled anesthetics (total intravenous anesthesia, TIVA). Alternatively, a propofol infusion might be used to reduce the required concentration of inhaled anesthetics so that undesired effects can be minimized. Increasingly, propofol is also used for sedation in the ICU as well as conscious sedation and short-duration general anesthesia in locations outside the operating room (eg, interventional radiology suites, emergency department; see Box: Sedation & Monitored Anesthesia Care, earlier).

Propofol (2,6-diisopropylphenol) is an alkyl phenol with hypnotic properties that is chemically distinct from other groups of intravenous anesthetics (see Figure 25–6). Because of its poor solubility in water, it is formulated as an emulsion containing 10% soybean oil, 2.25% glycerol, and 1.2% lecithin, the major component of the egg yolk phosphatide fraction. Hence, susceptible patients may experience allergic reactions. The solution appears milky white and slightly viscous, has a pH of approximately 7, and has a propofol concentration of 1% (10 mg/mL). In some countries, a 2% formulation is available. Although retardants of bacterial growth are added to the formulations, solutions should be used as soon as possible (unused drug must be discarded 12 hours after opening the vial), and proper sterile technique is essential. The addition of metabisulfite in one of the formulations has raised concern regarding its use in patients with reactive airway disease (eg, asthma) or sulfite allergies.

The presumed mechanism of action of propofol is through potentiation of the chloride current mediated through the $GABA_A$ receptor complex.

Pharmacokinetics

Propofol is rapidly metabolized in the liver; the resulting water-soluble compounds are presumed to be inactive and are excreted through the kidneys. Plasma clearance is high and exceeds hepatic blood flow, indicating the importance of extrahepatic metabolism, which presumably occurs in the lungs and may account for

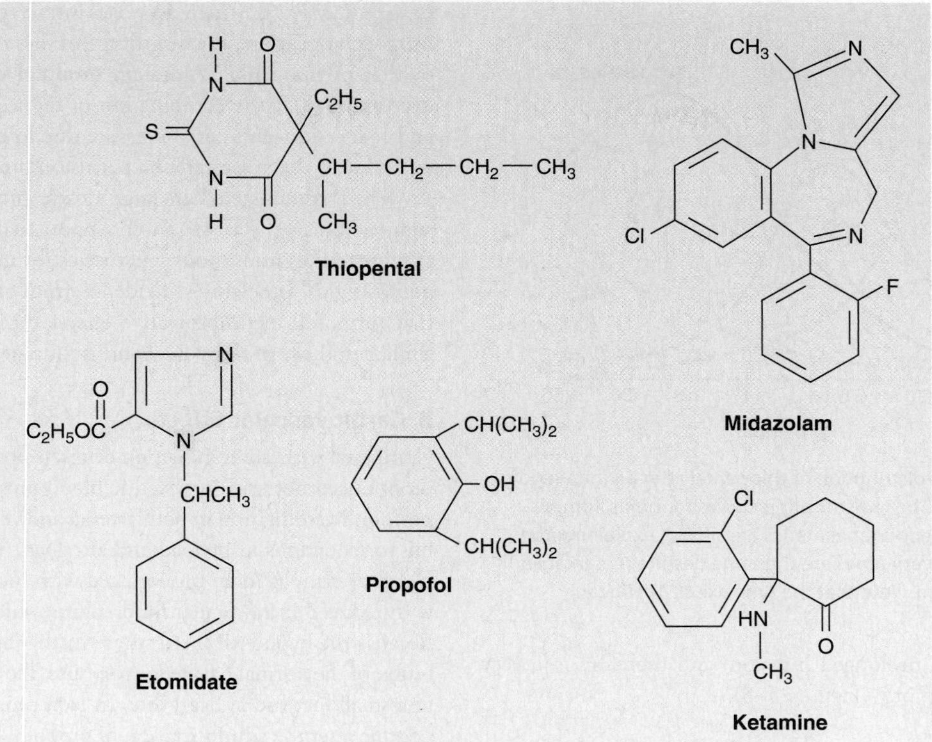

FIGURE 25–6 Chemical structures of some intravenous anesthetics.

the elimination of up to 30% of a bolus dose of the drug (see Table 25–2). The recovery from propofol is more complete, with less "hangover" than that observed with thiopental, likely due to the high plasma clearance. However, as with other intravenous drugs, transfer of propofol from the plasma (central) compartment and the associated termination of drug effect after a single bolus dose are mainly the result of redistribution from highly perfused (brain) to less-well-perfused (skeletal muscle) compartments (Figure 25–7). As with other intravenous agents, awakening after an induction dose of propofol usually occurs within 8–10 minutes. The kinetics of propofol (and other intravenous anesthetics) after a single bolus dose or continuous infusion are best described by means of a three-compartment model. Such models have been used as the basis for developing systems of target-controlled infusions.

The **context-sensitive half-time** of a drug describes the elimination half-time after discontinuation of a continuous infusion as a function of the duration of the infusion. It is an important parameter in assessing the suitability of a drug for use as maintenance anesthetic. The context-sensitive half-time of propofol

TABLE 25–2 Pharmacokinetic properties of intravenous anesthetics.

Drug	Induction Dose (mg/kg IV)	Duration of Action (min)	V_{dss} (L/kg)	$t_{½}$ Distribution (min)	Protein Binding (%)	CL (mL/kg/min)	$t_{½}$ Elimination (h)
Dexmedetomidine	NA	NA	2–3	6	94	10–30	2–3
Diazepam	0.3–0.6	15–30	0.7–1.7	…	98	0.2–0.5	20–50
Etomidate	0.2–0.3	3–8	2.5–4.5	2–4	77	18–25	2.9–5.3
Ketamine	1–2	5–10	3.1	11–16	12	12–17	2–4
Lorazepam	0.03–0.1	60–120	0.8–1.3	3–10	98	0.8–1.8	11–22
Methohexital	1–1.5	4–7	2.2	5–6	73	11	4
Midazolam	0.1–0.3	15–20	1.1–1.7	7–15	94	6.4–11	1.7–2.6
Propofol	1–2.5	3–8	2–10	2–4	97	20–30	4–23
Thiopental	3–5	5–10	2.5	2–4	83	3.4	11

Note: The duration of action reflects the duration after a typical single IV dose given for induction of anesthesia. Data are for average adult patients.

CL, clearance; NA, not applicable; V_{dss}, volume of distribution at steady state.

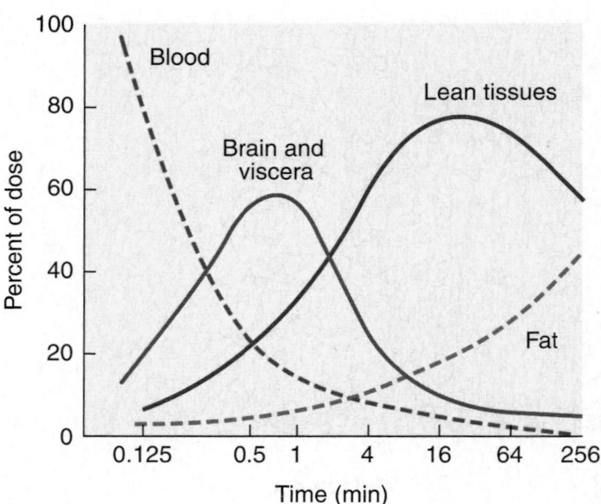

FIGURE 25–7 Redistribution of thiopental after an intravenous bolus administration. The redistribution curves for bolus administration of other intravenous anesthetics are similar, explaining the observation that recovery times are the same despite remarkable differences in metabolism. Note that the time axis is not linear.

is brief, even after a prolonged infusion, and therefore, recovery occurs relatively promptly (Figure 25–8).

Organ System Effects

A. CNS Effects

Propofol acts as hypnotic but does not have analgesic properties. Although the drug leads to a general suppression of CNS activity, excitatory effects such as twitching or spontaneous movement are occasionally observed during induction of anesthesia. These effects may resemble seizure activity; however, most studies support an anticonvulsant effect of propofol, and the drug may be safely administered to patients with seizure disorders. Propofol decreases cerebral blood flow and the cerebral metabolic rate for oxygen ($CMRO_2$), which decreases intracranial pressure (ICP) and intraocular pressure; the magnitude of these changes is comparable to that of thiopental. Although propofol can produce a desired decrease in ICP, the combination of reduced cerebral blood flow and reduced mean arterial pressure due to peripheral vasodilation can critically decrease cerebral perfusion pressure.

When administered in large doses, propofol produces burst suppression in the EEG, an end point that has been used when administering intravenous anesthetics for neuroprotection during neurosurgical procedures. Evidence from animal studies suggests that propofol's neuroprotective effects during focal ischemia are similar to those of thiopental and isoflurane.

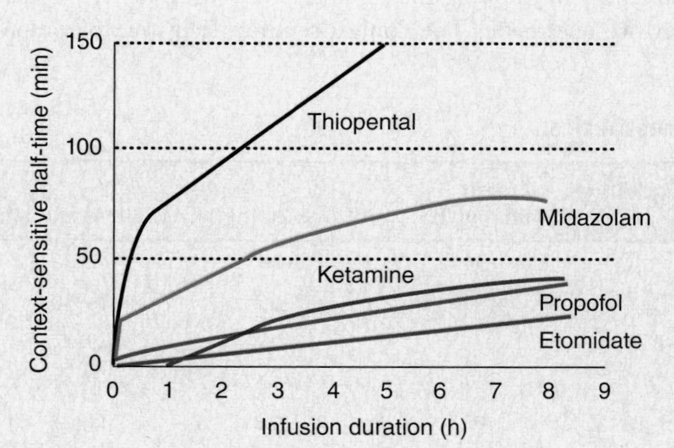

FIGURE 25–8 The context-sensitive half-time of common intravenous anesthetics. Even after a prolonged infusion, the half-time of propofol is relatively short, which makes propofol the preferred choice for intravenous maintenance of anesthesia. Ketamine and etomidate have similar characteristics, but their use is limited by other effects.

B. Cardiovascular Effects

Compared with other induction drugs, propofol produces the most pronounced decrease in systemic blood pressure; this is a result of profound vasodilation in both arterial and venous circulations leading to reductions in preload and afterload. This effect on systemic blood pressure is more pronounced with increased age, in patients with reduced intravascular fluid volume, and with rapid injection. Because the hypotensive effects are further augmented by the inhibition of the normal baroreflex response, the vasodilation only leads to a small increase in heart rate. In fact, profound bradycardia and asystole after the administration of propofol have been described in healthy adults despite prophylactic anticholinergic drugs.

C. Respiratory Effects

Propofol is a potent respiratory depressant and generally produces apnea after an induction dose. A maintenance infusion reduces minute ventilation through reductions in tidal volume and respiratory rate, with the effect on tidal volume being more pronounced. In addition, the ventilatory response to hypoxia and hypercapnia is reduced. Propofol causes a greater reduction in upper airway reflexes than thiopental does, which makes it well suited for instrumentation of the airway, such as placement of a laryngeal mask airway.

D. Other Effects

Although propofol, unlike volatile anesthetics, does not augment neuromuscular block, studies have found good intubating conditions after propofol induction without the use of neuromuscular blocking agents. Unexpected tachycardia occurring during propofol anesthesia should prompt laboratory evaluation for possible metabolic acidosis (propofol infusion syndrome). An interesting and desirable side effect of propofol is its antiemetic activity. Pain on injection is a common complaint and can be reduced by premedication with an opioid or coadministration with lidocaine. Dilution of propofol and the use of larger veins for injection can also reduce the incidence and severity of injection pain.

Clinical Uses & Dosage

The most common use of propofol is to facilitate induction of general anesthesia by bolus injection of 1–2.5 mg/kg IV. Increasing age, reduced cardiovascular reserve, or premedication with benzodiazepines or opioids reduces the required induction dose;

children require higher doses (2.5–3.5 mg/kg IV). Generally, titration of the induction dose helps to prevent severe hemodynamic changes. Propofol is often used for maintenance of anesthesia either as part of a balanced anesthesia regimen in combination with volatile anesthetics, nitrous oxide, sedative-hypnotics, and opioids or as part of a total intravenous anesthetic technique, usually in combination with opioids. Therapeutic plasma concentrations for maintenance of anesthesia normally range between 3 and 8 mcg/mL (typically requiring a continuous infusion rate between 100 and 200 mcg/kg/min) when combined with nitrous oxide or opioids. In many countries (other than the United States), propofol is frequently administered utilizing target-controlled infusion (TCI). TCI uses pharmacokinetic models based on patient characteristics (height, weight, gender, and age) to control an infusion pump based on target plasma concentrations entered by the anesthesiologist. The models incorporate context-sensitive half-time and automatically set the infusion rate to reach or maintain the target concentration entered, thereby replacing the manual administration of the boluses and infusion estimated by the anesthesiologist. Data suggest that induction using TCI provides better hemodynamic stability. TCI is often combined with the use of the bispectral index (BIS) or other monitors of processed EEG signals. Pharmacologic models also exist for other drugs such as opioid analgesics and allow TCI application for multiple drugs.

When used for sedation of mechanically ventilated patients in the ICU or for sedation during procedures, the required plasma concentration is 1–2 mcg/mL, which can be achieved with a continuous infusion at 25–75 mcg/kg/min. Because of its pronounced respiratory depressant effect and narrow therapeutic range, propofol should be administered only by individuals trained in airway management.

Subanesthetic doses of propofol can be used to treat postoperative nausea and vomiting (10–20 mg IV as bolus or 10 mcg/kg/min as an infusion).

FOSPROPOFOL

As previously noted, injection pain during administration of propofol is often perceived as severe, and the lipid emulsion has several disadvantages. Intense research has focused on finding alternative formulations or related drugs that would address some of these problems. Fospropofol is a water-soluble prodrug of propofol, is rapidly metabolized by alkaline phosphatase, and produces propofol, phosphate, and formaldehyde. The formaldehyde is metabolized by aldehyde dehydrogenase in the liver and in erythrocytes. The available fospropofol formulation is a sterile, aqueous, colorless, and clear solution that is supplied in a single-dose vial at a concentration of 35 mg/mL under the trade name Lusedra.

Pharmacokinetics & Organ System Effects

Because the active compound is propofol and fospropofol is a prodrug that requires metabolism to form propofol, the pharmacokinetics are more complex than for propofol itself. Multicompartment models with two compartments for fospropofol and three for propofol have been used to describe the kinetics.

The effect profile of fospropofol is similar to that of propofol, but onset and recovery are prolonged compared with propofol because the prodrug must first be converted into an active form. Although patients receiving fospropofol do not appear to experience the injection pain typical of propofol, a common adverse effect is the experience of paresthesia, often in the perianal region, which occurs in up to 74% of patients. The mechanism for this effect is unknown.

Clinical Uses & Dosage

Fospropofol is approved for sedation during monitored anesthesia care. Supplemental oxygen must be administered to all patients receiving the drug. As with propofol, airway compromise is a major concern. Hence, it is recommended that fospropofol be administered only by personnel trained in airway management. The recommended standard dosage is an initial bolus dose of 6.5 mg/kg IV followed by supplemental doses of 1.6 mg/kg IV as needed. For patients weighing more than 90 kg or less than 60 kg, 90 or 60 kg should be used to calculate the dose, respectively. The dose should be reduced by 25% in patients older than 65 years and in those with an American Society of Anesthesiologists status of 3 or 4.

BARBITURATES

This section focuses on the use of **thiopental** and **methohexital** for induction of general anesthesia; however, these barbiturate hypnotics have been largely replaced as induction agents by propofol. Other barbiturates and general barbiturate pharmacology are discussed in Chapter 22.

The anesthetic effect of barbiturates presumably involves a combination of enhancement of inhibitory transmission and inhibition of excitatory neurotransmission (see Figure 25–1). Although the effects on inhibitory transmission probably result from activation of the $GABA_A$ receptor complex, the effects on excitatory transmission are less well understood.

Pharmacokinetics

Thiopental and methohexital undergo hepatic metabolism, mostly by oxidation but also by *N*-dealkylation, desulfuration, and destruction of the barbituric acid ring structure. Barbiturates should not be administered to patients with acute intermittent porphyria because they increase the production of porphyrins through stimulation of aminolevulinic acid synthetase. Methohexital has a shorter elimination half-time than thiopental due to its larger plasma clearance (see Table 25–2), leading to a faster and more complete recovery after bolus injection. Although thiopental is metabolized more slowly and has a long elimination half-time, recovery after a single bolus injection is comparable to that of methohexital and propofol because it depends on redistribution to inactive tissue sites rather than on metabolism (Figure 25–7). However, if administered through repeated bolus injections or continuous infusion, recovery will be markedly prolonged because elimination will depend on metabolism under these circumstances (see also context-sensitive half-time, Figure 25–8).

Organ System Effects

A. CNS Effects

Barbiturates produce dose-dependent CNS depression ranging from sedation to general anesthesia when administered as bolus injections. They do not produce analgesia; instead, some evidence suggests they may reduce the pain threshold, causing hyperalgesia. Barbiturates are potent cerebral vasoconstrictors and produce predictable decreases in cerebral blood flow, cerebral blood volume, and ICP. As a result, they decrease $CMRO_2$ consumption in a dose-dependent manner up to a dose at which they suppress all EEG activity. The ability of barbiturates to decrease ICP and $CMRO_2$ makes these drugs useful in the management of patients with space-occupying intracranial lesions. They may provide neuroprotection from focal cerebral ischemia (stroke, surgical retraction, temporary clips during aneurysm surgery), but likely will not reduce the injury after global cerebral ischemia (eg, from cardiac arrest). Except for methohexital, barbiturates decrease electrical activity on the EEG and can be used as anticonvulsants. In contrast, methohexital activates epileptic foci and may therefore be useful to facilitate electroconvulsive therapy or during the identification of epileptic foci during surgery.

B. Cardiovascular Effects

The decrease in systemic blood pressure associated with administration of barbiturates for induction of anesthesia is primarily due to peripheral vasodilation and is usually smaller than the blood pressure decrease associated with propofol. There are also direct negative inotropic effects on the heart. However, inhibition of the baroreceptor reflex is less pronounced than with propofol; thus, compensatory increases in heart rate limit the decrease in blood pressure and make it transient. The depressant effects on systemic blood pressure are increased in patients with hypovolemia, cardiac tamponade, cardiomyopathy, coronary artery disease, or cardiac valvular disease because such patients are less able to compensate for the effects of peripheral vasodilation. Hemodynamic effects are also more pronounced with larger doses and rapid injection.

C. Respiratory Effects

Barbiturates are respiratory depressants, and a usual induction dose of thiopental or methohexital typically produces transient apnea, which will be more pronounced if other respiratory depressants are also administered. Barbiturates lead to decreased minute ventilation through reduced tidal volumes and respiratory rate and also decrease the ventilatory responses to hypercapnia and hypoxia. Resumption of spontaneous breathing after an anesthetic induction dose of a barbiturate is characterized by a slow breathing rate and decreased tidal volume. Suppression of laryngeal reflexes and cough reflexes is probably not as profound as after an equianesthetic propofol administration, which makes barbiturates an inferior choice for airway instrumentation in the absence of neuromuscular blocking drugs. Furthermore, stimulation of the upper airway or trachea (eg, by secretions, laryngeal mask airway, direct laryngoscopy, tracheal intubation) during inadequate depression of airway reflexes may result in laryngospasm or bronchospasm. This phenomenon is not unique to barbiturates but is true whenever the dose of the anesthetic drug is inadequate to suppress the airway reflexes.

D. Other Effects

Accidental intra-arterial injection of barbiturates results in excruciating pain and intense vasoconstriction, often leading to severe tissue injury involving gangrene. Approaches to treatment include blockade of the sympathetic nervous system (eg, stellate ganglion block) in the involved extremity. If extravasation occurs, some authorities recommend local injection of the area with 0.5% lidocaine (5–10 mL) in an attempt to dilute the barbiturate concentration. Life-threatening allergic reactions to barbiturates are rare, with an estimated occurrence of 1 in 30,000 patients. However, barbiturate-induced histamine release occasionally is seen.

Clinical Uses & Dosage

The principal clinical use of thiopental (3–5 mg/kg IV) or methohexital (1–1.5 mg/kg IV) is for induction of anesthesia (unconsciousness), which usually occurs in less than 30 seconds. Patients may experience a garlic or onion taste after administration. Solutions of thiopental sodium for intravenous injection have a pH range of 10–11 to maintain stability. Rapid co-injection with depolarizing and nondepolarizing muscle relaxants, which have much lower pH, may cause precipitation of insoluble thiopentone acid. Barbiturates such as methohexital (20–30 mg/kg) may be administered per rectum to facilitate induction of anesthesia in mentally challenged patients and uncooperative pediatric patients. When a barbiturate is administered with the goal of neuroprotection, an isoelectric EEG indicating maximal reduction of $CMRO_2$ has traditionally been used as the end point. More recent data demonstrating equal protection after smaller doses have challenged this practice. The use of smaller doses is less frequently associated with hypotension, thus making it easier to maintain adequate cerebral perfusion pressure, especially in the setting of increased ICP.

BENZODIAZEPINES

Benzodiazepines commonly used in the perioperative period include **midazolam, lorazepam,** and less frequently, **diazepam.** Benzodiazepines are unique among the group of intravenous anesthetics in that their action can readily be terminated by administration of their selective antagonist, flumazenil. Their most desired effects are anxiolysis and anterograde amnesia, which are extremely useful for premedication.

The chemical structure and pharmacodynamics of the benzodiazepines are discussed in detail in Chapter 22.

Pharmacokinetics in the Anesthesia Setting

The highly lipid-soluble benzodiazepines rapidly enter the CNS, which accounts for their rapid onset of action, followed by redistribution to inactive tissue sites and subsequent termination of the drug effect. Additional information regarding the pharmacokinetics of the benzodiazepines may be found in Chapter 22.

Despite its prompt passage into the brain, midazolam is considered to have a slower effect-site equilibration time than propofol and thiopental. In this regard, intravenous doses of midazolam should be sufficiently spaced to permit the peak clinical effect to be recognized before a repeat dose is considered. Midazolam has the shortest context-sensitive half-time, which makes it the only one of the three benzodiazepine drugs suitable for continuous infusion (see Figure 25–8).

Organ System Effects

A. CNS Effects

Benzodiazepines decrease $CMRO_2$ and cerebral blood flow but to a smaller extent than propofol or the barbiturates. There appears to be a ceiling effect for benzodiazepine-induced decreases in $CMRO_2$ as evidenced by midazolam's inability to produce an isoelectric EEG. Patients with decreased intracranial compliance demonstrate little or no change in ICP after the administration of midazolam. Although neuroprotective properties have not been shown for benzodiazepines, these drugs are potent anticonvulsants used in the treatment of status epilepticus, alcohol withdrawal, and local anesthetic-induced seizures. The CNS effects of benzodiazepines can be promptly terminated by administration of the selective benzodiazepine antagonist flumazenil, which improves their safety profile.

B. Cardiovascular Effects

If used for the induction of anesthesia, midazolam produces a greater decrease in systemic blood pressure than comparable doses of diazepam. These changes are most likely due to peripheral vasodilation inasmuch as cardiac output is not changed. Similar to other intravenous induction agents, midazolam's effect on systemic blood pressure is exaggerated in hypovolemic patients.

C. Respiratory Effects

Benzodiazepines alone produce minimal depression of ventilation, although transient apnea may follow rapid intravenous administration of midazolam for induction of anesthesia, especially in the presence of opioid premedication. Benzodiazepines decrease the ventilatory response to carbon dioxide, but this effect is not usually significant if they are administered alone. More severe respiratory depression can occur when benzodiazepines are administered together with opioids. Another problem affecting ventilation is airway obstruction induced by the hypnotic effects of benzodiazepines, especially in patients at risk for obstructive sleep apnea.

D. Other Effects

Pain during intravenous and intramuscular injection and subsequent thrombophlebitis are most pronounced with diazepam and reflect the poor water solubility of this benzodiazepine, which requires an organic solvent in the formulation. Despite its better solubility, eliminating the need for an organic solvent, midazolam may also produce pain on injection. Allergic reactions to benzodiazepines are rare to nonexistent.

Clinical Uses & Dosage

Benzodiazepines are most commonly used for preoperative medication, intravenous sedation, and suppression of seizure activity. Less frequently, midazolam and diazepam may also be used to induce general anesthesia. The slow onset and prolonged duration of action of lorazepam limit its usefulness as preoperative medication or for induction of anesthesia, especially when rapid and sustained awakening at the end of surgery is desirable. Although flumazenil (8–15 mcg/kg IV) may be useful for treating patients experiencing delayed awakening, its duration of action is brief (about 20 minutes) and resedation may occur.

The amnestic, anxiolytic, and sedative effects of benzodiazepines make this class of drugs the most popular choice for preoperative medication. Midazolam (1–2 mg IV) is effective for premedication, sedation during regional anesthesia, and brief therapeutic procedures. Midazolam has a more rapid onset, with greater amnesia and less postoperative sedation, than diazepam. Midazolam is also the most commonly used oral premedication for children; 0.5 mg/kg administered orally 30 minutes before induction of anesthesia provides reliable sedation and anxiolysis in children without producing delayed awakening.

The synergistic effects between benzodiazepines and other drugs, especially opioids and propofol, can be used to achieve better sedation and analgesia but may also greatly enhance their combined respiratory depression and may lead to airway obstruction or apnea. Because benzodiazepine effects are more pronounced with increasing age, dose reduction and careful titration may be necessary in elderly patients.

General anesthesia can be induced by the administration of midazolam (0.1–0.3 mg/kg IV), but the onset of unconsciousness is slower than after the administration of thiopental, propofol, or etomidate. Delayed awakening is a potential disadvantage, limiting the usefulness of benzodiazepines for induction of general anesthesia despite their advantage of less pronounced circulatory effects.

ETOMIDATE

Etomidate (see Figure 25–6) is an intravenous anesthetic with hypnotic but not analgesic effects and is often chosen for its minimal hemodynamic effects. Although its pharmacokinetics are favorable, endocrine side effects limit its use for continuous infusions. Etomidate is a carboxylated imidazole derivative that is poorly soluble in water and is therefore supplied as a 2 mg/mL solution in 35% propylene glycol. The solution has a pH of 6.9 and does not cause problems with precipitation as thiopental does. Etomidate appears to have GABA-like effects and seems to act primarily through potentiation of $GABA_A$-mediated chloride current, like most other intravenous anesthetics.

Pharmacokinetics

An induction dose of etomidate produces rapid onset of anesthesia, and recovery depends on redistribution to inactive tissue sites, comparable to thiopental and propofol. Metabolism is primarily by ester hydrolysis to inactive metabolites, which are then excreted in urine (78%) and bile (22%). Less than 3% of an administered dose of etomidate is excreted as unchanged drug in urine. Clearance of etomidate is about five times that of thiopental, as reflected by a shorter elimination half-time (see Table 25–2). The duration of action is linearly related to the dose, with each 0.1 mg/kg providing about 100 seconds of unconsciousness. Because of etomidate's minimal effects on hemodynamics and short context-sensitive half-time, larger doses, repeated boluses, or continuous infusions can safely be administered. Etomidate, like most other intravenous anesthetics, is highly protein bound (77%), primarily to albumin.

Organ System Effects

A. CNS Effects

Etomidate is a potent cerebral vasoconstrictor, as reflected by decreases in cerebral blood flow and ICP. These effects are similar to those produced by comparable doses of thiopental. Despite its reduction of $CMRO_2$, etomidate has failed to show neuroprotective properties in animal studies, and human studies are lacking. The frequency of excitatory spikes on the EEG after the administration of etomidate is greater than with thiopental. Similar to methohexital, etomidate may activate seizure foci, manifested as fast activity on the EEG, making it a useful drug in the setting of electroconvulsive therapy. In addition, spontaneous movements characterized as myoclonus occur in more than 50% of patients receiving etomidate, and this myoclonic activity may be associated with seizure-like activity on the EEG.

B. Cardiovascular Effects

A characteristic and desired feature of induction of anesthesia with etomidate is cardiovascular stability after bolus injection. In this regard, decrease in systemic blood pressure is modest or absent and principally reflects a decrease in systemic vascular resistance. Therefore, the systemic blood pressure–lowering effects of etomidate are probably exaggerated in the presence of hypovolemia, and the patient's intravascular fluid volume status should be optimized before induction of anesthesia. Etomidate produces minimal changes in heart rate and cardiac output. Its depressant effects on myocardial contractility are minimal at concentrations used for induction of anesthesia.

C. Respiratory Effects

The depressant effects of etomidate on ventilation are less pronounced than those of barbiturates, although apnea may occasionally follow rapid intravenous injection of the drug. Depression of ventilation may be exaggerated when etomidate is combined with inhaled anesthetics or opioids.

D. Endocrine Effects

Etomidate causes adrenocortical suppression by producing a dose-dependent inhibition of 11β-hydroxylase, an enzyme necessary for the conversion of cholesterol to cortisol (see Figure 39–1). This suppression lasts 4–8 hours after an induction dose of the drug. Despite concerns regarding this finding, no outcome studies have demonstrated an adverse effect when etomidate is given in a bolus dose. However, because of its endocrine effects, etomidate is not used as continuous infusion.

Clinical Uses & Dosage

Etomidate is an alternative to propofol and barbiturates for the rapid intravenous induction of anesthesia, especially in patients with compromised myocardial contractility. After a standard induction dose (0.2–0.3 mg/kg IV), the onset of unconsciousness is comparable to that achieved by thiopental and propofol. Similar to propofol, during intravenous injection of etomidate, there is a high incidence of pain, which may be followed by venous irritation. Involuntary myoclonic movements are also common but may be masked by the concomitant administration of neuromuscular blocking drugs. Awakening after a single intravenous dose of etomidate is rapid, with little evidence of any residual depressant effects. Etomidate does not produce analgesia, and postoperative nausea and vomiting may be more common than after the administration of thiopental or propofol.

KETAMINE

Ketamine (see Figure 25–6) is a partially water-soluble and highly lipid-soluble phencyclidine derivative differing from most other intravenous anesthetics in that it produces significant analgesia. The characteristic state observed after an induction dose of ketamine is known as "dissociative anesthesia," a cataleptic state wherein the patient's eyes often remain open with a slow nystagmic gaze. Of the two stereoisomers, the *S*(+) form is more potent than the *R*(–) isomer, but only the racemic mixture of ketamine is available as an injection drug in the USA. A formulation of *S*(+) ketamine (Esketamine) for intranasal administration was recently approved by the FDA for the treatment of acute depression (see Chapter 30).

Ketamine's mechanism of action is complex, but the major effect is probably produced through inhibition of the NMDA receptor complex.

Pharmacokinetics

The high lipid solubility of ketamine ensures a rapid onset of its effect. As with other intravenous induction drugs, the effect of a single bolus injection is terminated by redistribution to inactive tissue sites. Metabolism occurs primarily in the liver and involves *N*-demethylation by the cytochrome P450 system. Norketamine, the primary active metabolite, is less potent (one third to one fifth the potency of ketamine) and is subsequently hydroxylated and conjugated into water-soluble inactive metabolites that are excreted in urine. Ketamine is the only intravenous anesthetic that has low protein binding (see Table 25–2).

Organ System Effects

If ketamine is administered as the sole anesthetic, amnesia is not as complete as with the other intravenous anesthetics. Reflexes are often preserved, but it cannot be assumed that patients are able to protect the upper airway. The eyes remain open and the pupils are moderately dilated with a nystagmic gaze. Frequently, lacrimation and salivation are increased, and premedication with an anticholinergic drug may be indicated to limit this effect.

A. CNS Effects

In contrast to other intravenous anesthetics, ketamine is considered to be a cerebral vasodilator that *increases* cerebral blood flow, as well as $CMRO_2$. For these reasons, ketamine has traditionally not been recommended for use in patients with intracranial pathology, especially increased ICP. Nevertheless, these perceived undesirable effects on cerebral blood flow may be blunted by the maintenance of normocapnia. Despite the potential to produce myoclonic activity, ketamine is considered an anticonvulsant and may be recommended for treatment of status epilepticus when more conventional drugs are ineffective.

Unpleasant emergence reactions after administration are the main factor limiting ketamine's use. Such reactions may include vivid colorful dreams, hallucinations, out-of-body experiences, and increased and distorted visual, tactile, and auditory sensitivity. These reactions can be associated with fear and confusion, but a euphoric state may also be induced, which explains the potential for abuse of the drug. Children usually have a lower incidence of and less severe emergence reactions. Combination with a benzodiazepine may be indicated to limit the unpleasant emergence reactions and also increase amnesia.

B. Cardiovascular Effects

Ketamine can produce transient but significant *increases* in systemic blood pressure, heart rate, and cardiac output, presumably by centrally mediated sympathetic stimulation. These effects, which are associated with increased cardiac workload and myocardial oxygen consumption, are not always desirable and can be blunted by coadministration of benzodiazepines, opioids, or inhaled anesthetics. Although the mechanism is more controversial, ketamine is also considered to be a direct myocardial depressant. This property is usually masked by the stimulation of the sympathetic nervous system but may become apparent in critically ill patients with limited ability to increase their sympathetic nervous system activity.

C. Respiratory Effects

Ketamine is not thought to produce significant respiratory depression. When it is used as a single drug, the respiratory response to hypercapnia is preserved and blood gases remain stable. Transient hypoventilation and, in rare cases, a short period of apnea can follow rapid administration of a large intravenous dose for induction of anesthesia. The ability to protect the upper airway in the presence of ketamine cannot be assumed despite the presence of active airway reflexes. Especially in children, the risk for laryngospasm due to increased salivation must be considered; this risk can be reduced by premedication with an anticholinergic drug. Ketamine relaxes bronchial smooth muscle and may be helpful in patients with reactive airways and in the management of patients experiencing bronchoconstriction.

Clinical Uses & Dosage

Its unique properties, including profound analgesia, stimulation of the sympathetic nervous system, bronchodilation, and minimal respiratory depression, make ketamine an important alternative to the other intravenous anesthetics and a desirable adjunct in many cases despite the unpleasant psychomimetic effects. Moreover, ketamine can be administered by multiple routes (intravenous, intramuscular, oral, rectal, epidural), thus making it a useful option for premedication in mentally challenged and uncooperative pediatric patients.

Induction of anesthesia can be achieved with ketamine, 1–2 mg/kg intravenously or 4–6 mg/kg intramuscularly. Although the drug is not commonly used for maintenance of anesthesia, its short context-sensitive half-time makes ketamine a candidate for this purpose. For example, general anesthesia can be achieved with the infusion of ketamine, 15–45 mcg/kg/min, plus 50–70% nitrous oxide or by ketamine alone, 30–90 mcg/kg/min.

Small bolus doses of ketamine (0.2–0.8 mg/kg IV) may be useful during regional anesthesia when additional analgesia is needed (eg, cesarean delivery under neuraxial anesthesia with an insufficient regional block). Ketamine provides effective analgesia without compromise of the airway. An infusion of a subanalgesic dose of ketamine (3–5 mcg/kg/min) during general anesthesia and in the early postoperative period may be useful to augment opioid analgesia and reduce opioid tolerance and opioid-induced hyperalgesia. The use of ketamine has always been limited by its unpleasant psychotomimetic side effects, but its unique features make it a very valuable alternative in certain settings, mostly because of the potent analgesia with minimal respiratory depression. Most recently, it has become popular as an adjunct administered at subanalgesic doses to limit or reverse opioid tolerance, especially in patients with chronic pain.

DEXMEDETOMIDINE

Dexmedetomidine is a highly selective α_2-adrenergic agonist. Recognition of the usefulness of α_2 agonists is based on observations of decreased anesthetic requirements in patients receiving chronic clonidine therapy. The effects of dexmedetomidine can be antagonized with α_2-antagonist drugs. Dexmedetomidine is the active *S*-enantiomer of medetomidine, a highly selective α_2-adrenergic agonist imidazole derivative that is used in veterinary medicine. Dexmedetomidine is water soluble and available as a parenteral formulation.

Pharmacokinetics

Dexmedetomidine undergoes rapid hepatic metabolism involving *N*-methylation and hydroxylation, followed by conjugation. Metabolites are excreted in the urine and bile. Clearance is high, and the elimination half-time is short (see Table 25–2). However, there is a significant increase in the context-sensitive half-time from 4 minutes after a 10-minute infusion to 250 minutes after an 8-hour infusion.

Organ System Effects

A. CNS Effects

Dexmedetomidine produces its selective α_2-agonist effects through activation of CNS α_2 receptors. Hypnosis presumably results from stimulation of α_2 receptors in the locus coeruleus, and the analgesic effect originates at the level of the spinal cord. The sedative effect produced by dexmedetomidine has a different quality than that produced by other intravenous anesthetics in that it more completely resembles a physiologic sleep state through activation of endogenous sleep pathways. Dexmedetomidine is likely to be associated with a decrease in cerebral blood flow without significant changes in ICP and $CMRO_2$. It has the potential to lead to the development of tolerance and dependence.

B. Cardiovascular Effects

Dexmedetomidine infusion results in moderate decreases in heart rate and systemic vascular resistance and, consequently, a decrease in systemic blood pressure. A bolus injection may produce a transient increase in systemic blood pressure and pronounced decrease in heart rate, an effect that is probably mediated through activation of peripheral α_2 adrenoceptors. Bradycardia associated with dexmedetomidine infusion may require treatment. Heart block, severe bradycardia, and asystole have been observed and may result from unopposed vagal stimulation. The response to anticholinergic drugs is unchanged.

C. Respiratory Effects

The effects of dexmedetomidine on the respiratory system are a small to moderate decrease in tidal volume and very little change in the respiratory rate. The ventilatory response to carbon dioxide is unchanged. Although the respiratory effects are mild, upper airway obstruction as a result of sedation is possible. In addition, dexmedetomidine has a synergistic sedative effect when combined with other sedative-hypnotics.

Clinical Uses & Dosage

Dexmedetomidine is principally used for the short-term sedation of intubated and ventilated patients in an ICU setting. In the operating room, dexmedetomidine may be used as an adjunct to general anesthesia or to provide sedation, eg, during awake fiberoptic tracheal intubation or regional anesthesia. When administered during general anesthesia, dexmedetomidine (0.5–1 mcg/kg loading dose over 10–15 minutes, followed by an infusion of 0.2–0.7 mcg/kg/h) decreases the dose requirements for inhaled and injected anesthetics. Awakening and the transition to the postoperative setting may benefit from dexmedetomidine-produced sedative and analgesic effects without respiratory depression.

OPIOID ANALGESICS IN ANESTHESIA

Opioids are analgesic agents and are distinct from general anesthetics and hypnotics. Even when high doses of opioid analgesics are administered, recall cannot be prevented reliably unless hypnotic agents such as benzodiazepines are also used. Opioid analgesics are routinely used to achieve postoperative analgesia and intraoperatively as part of a balanced anesthesia regimen as described earlier (see Intravenous Anesthetics). Their pharmacology and clinical use are described in greater detail in Chapter 31.

In addition to their use as part of a balanced anesthesia regimen, opioids in large doses have been used in combination with large doses of benzodiazepines to achieve a general anesthetic state, particularly in patients with limited circulatory reserve who undergo cardiac surgery. When administered in large doses, potent opioids such as fentanyl can induce chest wall (and laryngeal) rigidity, thereby acutely impairing mechanical ventilation. Furthermore, large doses of potent opioids may speed up the development of tolerance and complicate postoperative pain management.

CURRENT CLINICAL PRACTICE

The practice of clinical anesthesia requires integrating the pharmacology and the known adverse effects of these potent drugs with the pathophysiologic state of individual patients. Every case tests the ability of the anesthesiologist to produce the depth of anesthesia required to allow invasive surgery to proceed and to achieve this safely despite frequent major medical problems.

AWARENESS DURING ANESTHESIA

As described in this chapter inhalational and intravenous agents are used alone and in combination to induce the depression of central nervous system function that allows patients to undergo painful procedures. The job of the anesthesiologist is to gauge the intensity of the noxious stimulus and deliver the appropriate amount and combination of agents to render the patient unaware of stimulus. During light and even deep sedation it is not uncommon for patients to have some memory of events.

PREPARATIONS AVAILABLE*

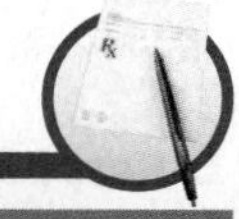

GENERIC NAME	AVAILABLE AS
Desflurane	Suprane
Dexmedetomidine	Precedex
Diazepam	Generic, Valium
Droperidol	Generic, Inapsine
Enflurane	Enflurane, Ethrane
Etomidate	Generic, Amidate
Fospropofol	Lusedra
Halothane	Generic, Fluothane
Isoflurane	Generic, Forane, Terrell
Ketamine	Generic, Ketalar
Lorazepam	Generic, Ativan
Methohexital	Generic, Brevital
Midazolam	Generic, Versed
Nitrous oxide (gas, supplied in blue cylinders)	Generic
Propofol	Generic, Diprivan
Sevoflurane	Generic, Ultane
Thiopental	Pentothal

*See Chapter 31 for names of opioid agents used in anesthesia.

REFERENCES

Allaert SE et al: First trimester anesthesia exposure and fetal outcome. A review. Acta Anaesthesiol Belg 2007;58:119.

Eger EI II: Uptake and distribution. In: Miller RD (editor): *Anesthesia*, 8th ed. Churchill Livingstone, 2015.

Fraga M et al: The effects of isoflurane and desflurane on intracranial pressure, cerebral perfusion and cerebral arteriovenous oxygen content difference in normocapnic patients with supratentorial brain tumors. Anesthesiology 2003;98:1085.

Fragen RJ: *Drug Infusions in Anesthesiology*. Lippincott Williams & Wilkins, 2005.

Hirshey Dirksen SJ et al: Future directions in malignant hyperthermia research and patient care. Anesth Analg 2011;113:1108.

Mashour GA: Top-down mechanisms of anesthetic-induced unconsciousness. Front Syst Neurosci 2014;8:1.

O'Leary JD, Orser BA: Neurodevelopment after general anaesthesia in infants. Lancet 2019;393:614.

Olkkola KT, Ahonen J: Midazolam and other benzodiazepines. Handb Exp Pharmacol 2008;182:335.

Reves JG et al: Intravenous anesthetics. In: Miller RD (editor): *Anesthesia*, 7th ed. Churchill Livingstone, 2010.

Ryan SM, Nielsen CJ: Global warming potential of inhaled anesthetics: Application to clinical use. Anesth Analg 2010;111:92.

Rudolph U et al: Sedatives, anxiolytics, and amnestics. In: Evers AS, Maze M (editors): *Anesthetic Pharmacology: Physiologic Principles and Clinical Practice*. Churchill Livingstone, 2004.

Stoelting R, Hillier S: Barbiturates. In: Stoelting RK, Hillier SC (editors): *Pharmacology and Physiology in Anesthetic Practice*. Lippincott Williams & Wilkins, 2005.

Struys MMR et al: The history of target-controlled infusion. Anesth Analg 2016;122:56.

CASE STUDY ANSWER

This patient presents with significant underlying cardiac risk and is scheduled to undergo major stressful surgery. Balanced anesthesia would begin with intravenous agents that cause minimal changes in blood pressure and heart rate such as a lowered dose of propofol or etomidate, combined with potent analgesics such as fentanyl (see Chapter 31) to block undesirable stimulation of autonomic reflexes. Maintenance of anesthesia could incorporate inhaled anesthetics that ensure unconsciousness and amnesia, additional intravenous agents to provide intraoperative and postoperative analgesia, and, if needed, neuromuscular blocking drugs (see Chapter 27) to induce muscle relaxation. The choice of inhaled agent(s) would be made based on the desire to maintain sufficient myocardial contractility, systemic blood pressure, and cardiac output for adequate perfusion of critical organs throughout the operation. If the patient's ischemic pain has been chronic and severe, a low-dose ketamine infusion may be administered for additional pain control. Rapid emergence from the combined effects of the chosen anesthetic drugs, which would facilitate the patient's return to a baseline state of heart function, breathing, and mentation, can be attained by understanding the known pharmacokinetic properties of the anesthetic agents as presented in this chapter.

CHAPTER

26 Local Anesthetics

Mohab M. Ibrahim, MD, PhD, &
Tally M. Largent-Milnes, PhD

CASE STUDY

A 67-year-old woman is scheduled for elective total knee arthroplasty. What local anesthetic agents would be most appropriate if surgical anesthesia were to be administered using a spinal or an epidural technique, and what potential complications might arise from their use? What anesthetics would be most appropriate for providing postoperative analgesia via an indwelling epidural or peripheral nerve catheter?

Simply stated, local anesthesia refers to loss of sensation in a limited region of the body. This is accomplished by disruption of afferent neural traffic via inhibition of impulse generation or propagation. Such blockade may bring with it other physiologic changes such as muscle paralysis and suppression of somatic or visceral reflexes, and these effects might be desirable or undesirable depending on the particular circumstances. Nonetheless, in most cases, it is the loss of sensation, or at least the achievement of localized analgesia, that is the primary goal.

Although local anesthetics are often used as analgesics, it is their ability to provide complete loss of all sensory modalities that is their distinguishing characteristic. The contrast with general anesthesia should be obvious, but it is perhaps worthwhile to emphasize that with local anesthesia the drug is delivered directly to the target organ, and the systemic circulation serves only to diminish or terminate its effect. Local anesthesia can also be produced by various chemical or physical means. However, in routine clinical practice, it is achieved with a rather narrow spectrum of compounds, and recovery is normally spontaneous, predictable, and without residual effects. The development of these compounds has a rich history (see Box: Historical Development of Local Anesthesia), punctuated by serendipitous observations, delayed starts, and an evolution driven more by concerns for safety than improvements in efficacy.

■ BASIC PHARMACOLOGY OF LOCAL ANESTHETICS

Chemistry

Most local anesthetic agents consist of a lipophilic group (eg, an aromatic ring) connected by an intermediate chain via an ester or amide to an ionizable group (eg, a tertiary amine) (Table 26–1). In addition to the general physical properties of the molecules, specific stereochemical configurations are associated with differences in the potency of stereoisomers (eg, levobupivacaine, ropivacaine). Because ester links are more prone to hydrolysis than amide links, esters usually have a shorter duration of action.

Local anesthetics are weak bases and are usually made available clinically as salts to increase solubility and stability. In the body, they exist either as the uncharged base or as a cation (see Chapter 1, section Ionization of Weak Acids and Weak Bases). The relative proportions of these two forms are governed by their pK_a and the pH of the body fluids according to the Henderson-Hasselbalch equation, which can be expressed as:

$$pK_a = pH - \log [base]/[conjugate\ acid]$$

If the concentration of base and conjugate acid are equal, the second portion of the right side of the equation drops out, as log 1 = 0, leaving:

$$pK_a = pH \text{ (when base concentration = conjugate acid concentration)}$$

TABLE 26–1 Structure and properties of some ester and amide local anesthetics.[1]

	Structure	Potency (Procaine = 1)	Duration of Action
Esters			
Cocaine	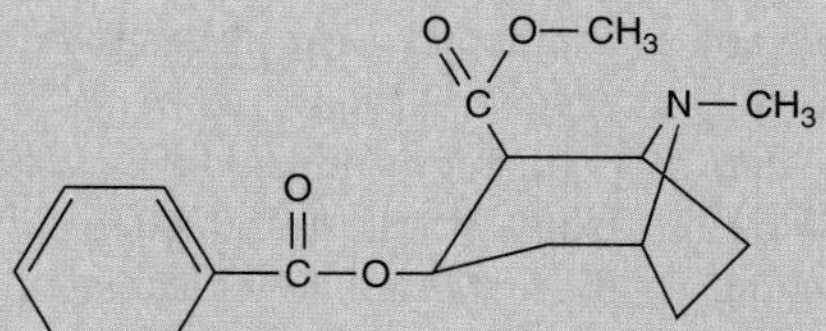	2	Medium
Procaine (Novocain)	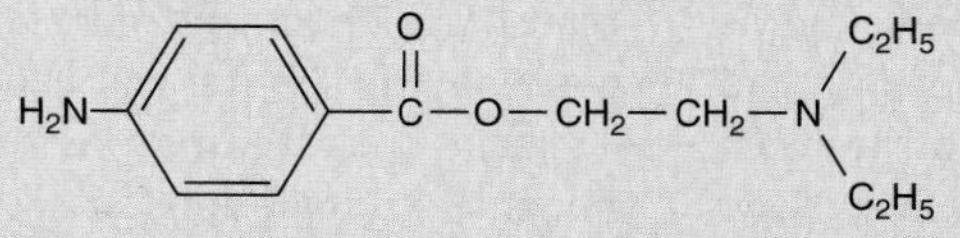	1	Short
Tetracaine (Pontocaine)	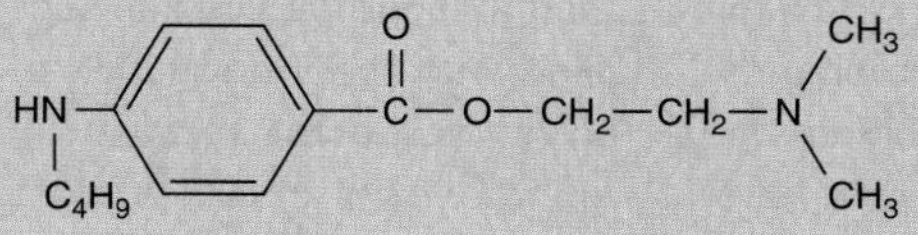	16	Long
Benzocaine	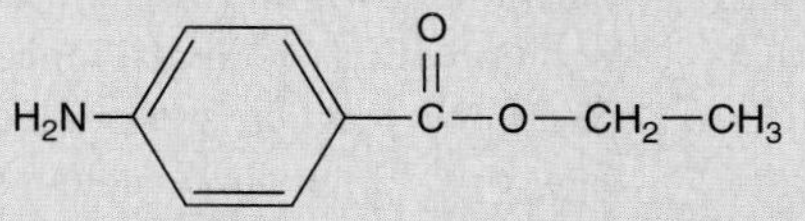	Surface use only	
Amides			
Lidocaine (Xylocaine)	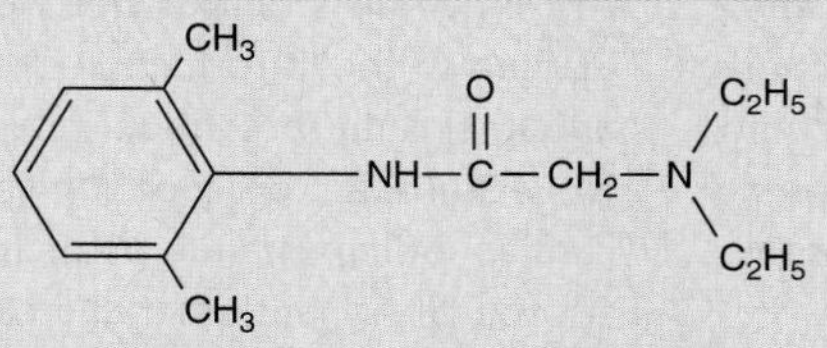	4	Medium
Mepivacaine (Carbocaine, Isocaine)	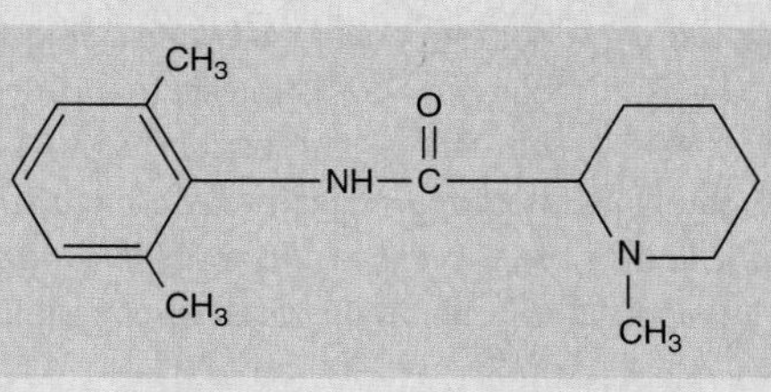	2	Medium
Bupivacaine (Marcaine), Levobupivacaine (Chirocaine)	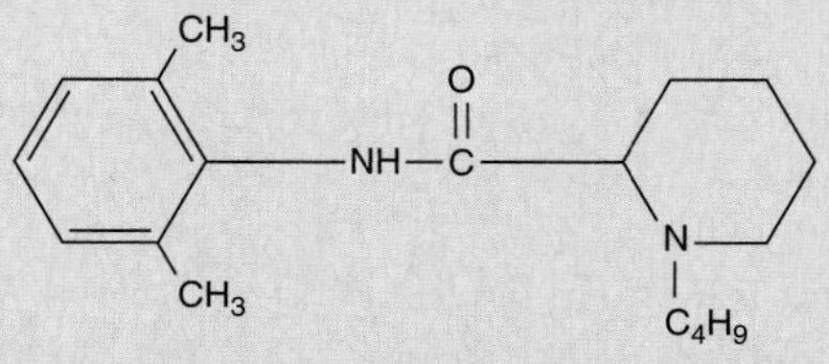	16	Long
Ropivacaine (Naropin)	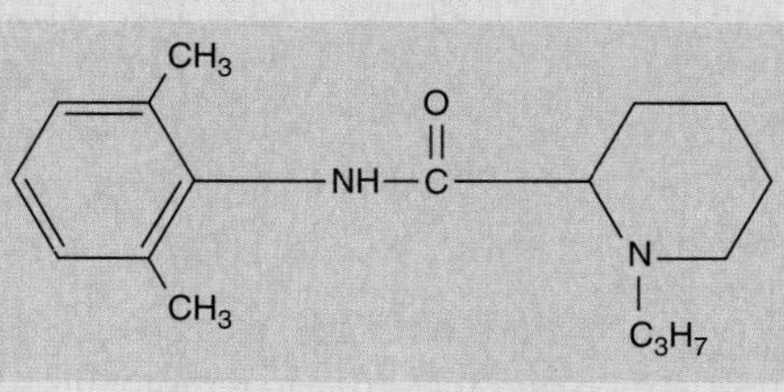	16	Long
Articaine	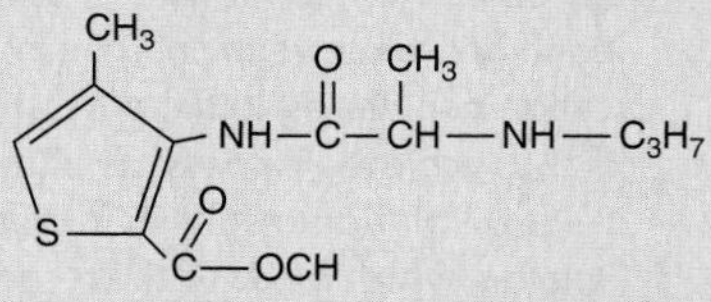	nf[2]	Medium

[1]Other chemical types are available including ethers (pramoxine), ketones (dyclonine), and phenetidine derivatives (phenacaine).

[2]Data not found.

Historical Development of Local Anesthesia

Although the numbing properties of cocaine were recognized for centuries, one might consider September 15, 1884, to mark the "birth of local anesthesia." Based on work performed by Carl Koller, cocaine's numbing effect on the cornea was demonstrated before the Ophthalmological Congress in Heidelberg, ushering in the era of surgical local anesthesia. Unfortunately, with widespread use came recognition of cocaine's significant central nervous system (CNS) and cardiac toxicity, which along with its addiction potential, tempered enthusiasm for this application. As the early investigator Mattison commented, "the risk of untoward results have robbed this peerless drug of much favor in the minds of many surgeons, and so deprived them of a most valued ally." As cocaine was known to be a benzoic acid ester, the search for alternative local anesthetics focused on this class of compounds, resulting in the identification of benzocaine shortly before the turn of the last century. However, benzocaine proved to have limited utility due to its marked hydrophobicity, and was thus relegated to topical anesthesia, a use for which it still finds limited application in current clinical practice. The first useful injectable local anesthetic, procaine, was introduced shortly thereafter by Einhorn, and its structure has served as the template for the development of the most commonly used modern local anesthetics. The three basic structural elements of these compounds can be appreciated by review of Table 26–1: an aromatic ring, conferring lipophilicity; an ionizable tertiary amine, conferring hydrophilicity; and an intermediate chain connecting these via an ester or amide linkage.

One of procaine's limitations was its short duration of action, a drawback overcome with the introduction of tetracaine in 1928. Unfortunately, tetracaine demonstrated significant toxicity when employed for high-volume peripheral blocks, ultimately reducing its common usage to spinal anesthesia. Both procaine and tetracaine shared another drawback: their ester linkage conferred instability, and particularly in the case of procaine, the free aromatic acid released during ester hydrolysis of the parent compound was believed to be the source of relatively frequent allergic reactions.

Löfgren and Lundqvist circumvented the problem of instability with the introduction of lidocaine in 1948. Lidocaine was the first in a series of amino-amide local anesthetics that would come to dominate the second half of the 20th century. Lidocaine had a longer (and more favorable) duration of action than procaine, and less systemic toxicity than tetracaine. To this day, it remains one of the most versatile and widely used anesthetics. Nonetheless, some applications required more prolonged block than that afforded by lidocaine, a pharmacologic void that was filled with the introduction of bupivacaine, a more lipophilic and more potent anesthetic. Unfortunately, bupivacaine was found to have greater propensity for significant effects on cardiac conduction and function, which at times proved lethal. Recognition of this potential for cardiac toxicity led to changes in anesthetic practice, and significant toxicity became sufficiently rare for it to remain a widely used anesthetic for nearly every regional technique in modern clinical practice. Nonetheless, this inherent cardiotoxicity would drive developmental work leading to the introduction of two additions to the anesthetic armamentarium, levobupivacaine and ropivacaine. The former is the *S*(–) enantiomer of bupivacaine, which has less affinity for cardiac sodium channels than its *R*(+) counterpart. Ropivacaine, another *S*(–) enantiomer, shares this reduced affinity for cardiac sodium channels, while being slightly less potent than bupivacaine or levobupivacaine. However, despite the reduced channel affinity, a recent advisory panel of the American Society of Regional Anesthesia concluded that in most clinical settings ropivacaine and bupivacaine probably have similar toxicity when administered on an equipotent basis.

Thus, pK_a can be seen as an effective way to consider the tendency for compounds to exist in a charged or uncharged form, ie, the lower the pK_a, the greater the percentage of uncharged weak bases at a given pH. Because the pK_a of most local anesthetics is in the range of 7.5–9.0, the charged, cationic form will constitute the larger percentage at physiologic pH. A glaring exception is benzocaine, which has a pK_a around 3.5, and thus exists solely as the nonionized base under normal physiologic conditions.

This issue of ionization is of critical importance because the cationic form is the most active at the receptor site. However, the story is a bit more complex, because the receptor site for local anesthetics is at the inner vestibule of the sodium channel, and the charged form of the anesthetic penetrates biologic membranes poorly. Thus, the uncharged form is important for cell penetration. After penetration into the cytoplasm, equilibration leads to formation and binding of the charged cation at the sodium channel, and hence the production of a clinical effect (Figure 26–1). Drug may also reach the receptor laterally through what has been

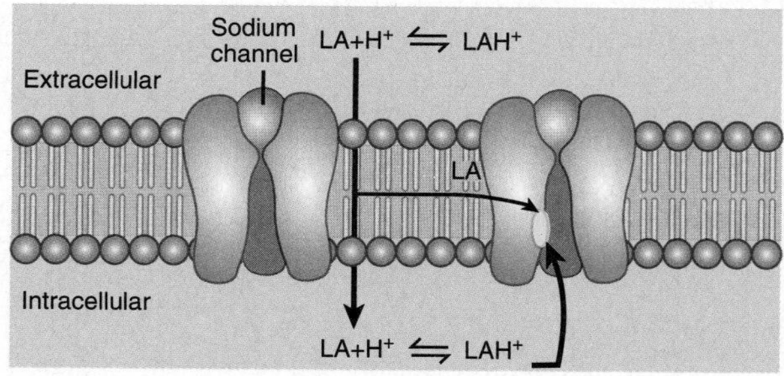

FIGURE 26–1 Schematic diagram depicting paths of local anesthetic (LA) to receptor sites. Extracellular anesthetic exists in equilibrium between charged and uncharged forms. The charged cation penetrates lipid membranes poorly; intracellular access is thus achieved by passage of the uncharged form. Intracellular re-equilibration results in formation of the more active charged species, which binds to the receptor at the inner vestibule of the sodium channel. Anesthetic may also gain access more directly by diffusing laterally within the membrane (hydrophobic pathway).

termed the hydrophobic pathway. As a clinical consequence, local anesthetics are less effective when they are injected into infected tissues because the low extracellular pH favors the charged form, with less of the neutral base available for diffusion across the membrane. Conversely, adding bicarbonate to a local anesthetic—a strategy sometimes used in clinical practice—will raise the effective concentration of the nonionized form and thus shorten the onset time of a regional block.

Pharmacokinetics

When local anesthetics are used for local, peripheral, and central neuraxial anesthesia—their most common clinical applications—systemic absorption, distribution, and elimination serve only to diminish or terminate their effect. Thus, classic pharmacokinetics plays a lesser role than with systemic therapeutics, yet remains important to the anesthetic's duration and critical to the potential development of adverse reactions, specifically cardiac and CNS toxicity.

Some pharmacokinetic properties of the commonly used amide local anesthetics are summarized in Table 26–2. The pharmacokinetics of the ester-based local anesthetics have not been extensively studied owing to their rapid breakdown in plasma (elimination half-life <1 minute).

A. Absorption

Systemic absorption of injected local anesthetic from the site of administration is determined by several factors, including dosage, site of injection, drug-tissue binding, local tissue blood flow, use of a vasoconstrictor (eg, epinephrine), and the physicochemical properties of the drug itself. Anesthetics that are more lipid soluble are generally more potent, have a longer duration of action, and take longer to achieve their clinical effect. Extensive protein binding also serves to increase the duration of action.

Application of a local anesthetic to a highly vascular area such as the tracheal mucosa or the tissue surrounding intercostal nerves results in more rapid absorption and thus higher blood levels than if the local anesthetic is injected into a poorly perfused tissue such as subcutaneous fat. When used for major conduction blocks, the peak serum levels will vary as a function of the specific site of injection, with intercostal blocks among the highest, and sciatic and femoral among the lowest (Figure 26–2). When vasoconstrictors are used with local anesthetics, the resultant reduction in blood flow serves to reduce the rate of systemic absorption and thus diminishes peak serum levels. This effect is generally most evident with the shorter-acting, less potent, and less lipid-soluble anesthetics.

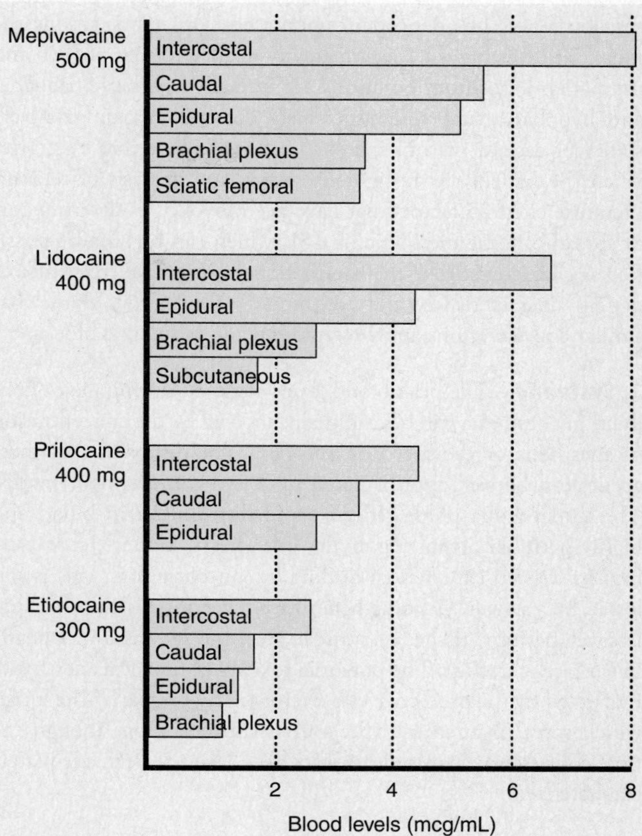

FIGURE 26–2 Comparative peak blood levels of several local anesthetic agents following administration into various anatomic sites. (This article was published in Grune & Stratton, Covino BD, Vassals HG: *Local Anesthetics: Mechanism of Action in Clinical Use*, Copyright Elsevier, 1976.)

B. Distribution

1. *Localized*—As local anesthetic is usually injected directly at the site of the target organ, distribution within this compartment plays an essential role with respect to achievement of clinical effect. For example, anesthetics delivered into the subarachnoid space will be diluted with cerebrospinal fluid (CSF) and the pattern of

TABLE 26–2 Pharmacokinetic properties of several amide local anesthetics.

Agent	$t_{1/2}$ Distribution (min)	$t_{1/2}$ Elimination (h)	V_{dss} (L)	CL (L/min)
Bupivacaine	28	3.5	72	0.47
Lidocaine	10	1.6	91	0.95
Mepivacaine	7	1.9	84	0.78
Prilocaine	5	1.5	261	2.84
Ropivacaine	23	4.2	47	0.44

CL, clearance; V_{dss}, volume of distribution at steady state per 70 kg body weight.

distribution will be dependent upon a host of factors, among the most critical being the specific gravity relative to that of CSF and the patient's position. Solutions are termed hyperbaric, isobaric, and hypobaric, and will respectively descend, remain relatively static, or ascend, within the subarachnoid space due to gravity when the patient sits upright. A review and analysis of relevant literature cited 25 factors that have been invoked as determinants of spread of local anesthetic in CSF, which can be broadly classified as characteristics of the anesthetic solution, CSF constituents, patient characteristics, and techniques of injection. Somewhat similar considerations apply to epidural and peripheral blocks.

2. *Systemic*—The peak blood levels achieved during major conduction anesthesia will be minimally affected by the concentration of anesthetic or the speed of injection. The disposition of these agents can be well approximated by a two-compartment model. The initial alpha phase reflects rapid distribution in blood and highly perfused organs (eg, brain, liver, heart, kidney), characterized by a steep exponential decline in concentration. This is followed by a slower declining beta phase reflecting distribution into less well perfused tissue (eg, muscle, gut), and may assume a nearly linear rate of decline. The potential toxicity of the local anesthetics is affected by the protective effect afforded by uptake by the lungs, which serve to attenuate the arterial concentration, though the time course and magnitude of this effect have not been adequately characterized.

C. Metabolism and Excretion

The local anesthetics are converted to more water-soluble metabolites in the liver (amide type) or in plasma (ester type), which are excreted in the urine. Since local anesthetics in the uncharged form diffuse readily through lipid membranes, little or no urinary excretion of the neutral form occurs. Acidification of urine promotes ionization of the tertiary amine base to the more water-soluble charged form, leading to more rapid elimination. Ester-type local anesthetics are hydrolyzed very rapidly in the blood by circulating butyrylcholinesterase to inactive metabolites. For example, the half-lives of procaine and chloroprocaine in plasma are less than a minute. However, excessive concentrations may accumulate in patients with reduced or absent plasma hydrolysis secondary to atypical plasma cholinesterase.

The amide local anesthetics undergo complex biotransformation in the liver, which includes hydroxylation and *N*-dealkylation by liver microsomal cytochrome P450 isozymes. There is considerable variation in the rate of liver metabolism of individual amide compounds, with prilocaine (fastest) > lidocaine > mepivacaine > ropivacaine ≈ bupivacaine and levobupivacaine (slowest). As a result, toxicity from amide-type local anesthetics is more likely to occur in patients with hepatic disease. For example, the average elimination half-life of lidocaine may be increased from 1.6 hours in normal patients ($t_{1/2}$, see Table 26–2) to more than 6 hours in patients with severe liver disease. Many other drugs used in anesthesia are metabolized by the same P450 isozymes, and concomitant administration of these competing drugs may slow the hepatic metabolism of the local anesthetics. Decreased hepatic elimination of local anesthetics would also be anticipated in patients with reduced hepatic blood flow. For example, the hepatic elimination of lidocaine in patients anesthetized with volatile anesthetics (which reduce liver blood flow) is slower than in patients anesthetized with intravenous anesthetic techniques. Delayed metabolism due to impaired hepatic blood flow may likewise occur in patients with heart failure.

Pharmacodynamics

A. Mechanism of Action

1. *Membrane potential*—The primary mechanism of action of local anesthetics is blockade of voltage-gated sodium channels (see Figure 26–1). The excitable membrane of nerve axons, like the membrane of cardiac muscle (see Chapter 14) and neuronal cell bodies (see Chapter 21), maintains a resting transmembrane potential of –90 to –60 mV. During excitation, the sodium channels open, and a fast, inward sodium current quickly depolarizes the membrane toward the sodium equilibrium potential (+40 mV). As a result of this depolarization process, the sodium channels close (inactivate) and potassium channels open. The outward flow of potassium repolarizes the membrane toward the potassium equilibrium potential (about –95 mV); repolarization returns the sodium channels to the rested state with a characteristic recovery time that determines the refractory period. The transmembrane ionic gradients are maintained by the sodium pump. These ionic fluxes are similar to, but simpler than, those in heart muscle, and local anesthetics have similar effects in both tissues.

2. *Sodium channel isoforms*—Each sodium channel consists of a single alpha subunit containing a central ion-conducting pore associated with accessory beta subunits. The pore-forming alpha subunit is actually sufficient for functional expression, but the kinetics and voltage dependence of channel gating are modified by the beta subunit. A variety of different sodium channels have been characterized by electrophysiologic recording, and subsequently isolated and cloned, while mutational analysis has allowed for identification of the essential components of the local anesthetic binding site. Nine members of a mammalian family of sodium channels have been so characterized and classified as $Na_v1.1$–$Na_v1.9$, where the chemical symbol represents the primary ion, the subscript denotes the physiologic regulator (in this case voltage), the initial number denotes the gene, and the number following the period indicates the particular isoform.

3. *Channel blockade*—Biologic toxins such as batrachotoxin, aconitine, veratridine, and some scorpion venoms bind to receptors within the channel and prevent inactivation. This results in prolonged influx of sodium through the channel and depolarization of the resting potential. The marine toxins tetrodotoxin (TTX) and saxitoxin have clinical effects that largely resemble those of local anesthetics (ie, block of conduction without a change in the resting potential). However, in contrast to the local anesthetics, the toxin binding site is located near the extracellular surface. The sensitivity of these channels to TTX varies, and subclassification based on this pharmacologic sensitivity has important physiologic and therapeutic implications. Six of the aforementioned channels are sensitive to nanomolar concentration of this biotoxin (TTX-S), while three are resistant (TTX-R). Such differences, along with their variable neuronal distribution, raise the possibility of targeting specific neuronal subpopulations. Such fine-tuned analgesic therapy has the theoretical potential of providing effective analgesia, while limiting the significant adverse effects produced by nonspecific sodium channel blockers.

When progressively increasing concentrations of a local anesthetic are applied to a nerve fiber, the threshold for excitation increases, impulse conduction slows, the rate of rise of the action potential declines, action potential amplitude decreases, and, finally, the ability to generate an action potential is completely abolished. These progressive effects result from binding of the local anesthetic to more and more sodium channels. If the sodium current is blocked over a critical length of the nerve, propagation across the blocked area is no longer possible. In myelinated nerves, the critical length appears to be two to three nodes of Ranvier. At the minimum dose required to block propagation, the resting potential is not significantly altered.

The blockade of sodium channels by most local anesthetics is both voltage- and time-dependent: Channels in the rested state, which predominate at more negative membrane potentials, have a much lower affinity for local anesthetics than activated (open state) and inactivated channels, which predominate at more positive membrane potentials (see Figure 14–10). Therefore, the effect of a given drug concentration is more marked in rapidly firing axons than in resting fibers (Figure 26–3). Between successive action potentials, a portion of the sodium channels will recover from the local anesthetic block (see Figure 14–10). The recovery from drug-induced block is 10–1000 times slower than the recovery of channels from normal inactivation (as shown for the cardiac membrane in Figure 14–4). As a result, the refractory period is lengthened and the nerve conducts fewer action potentials.

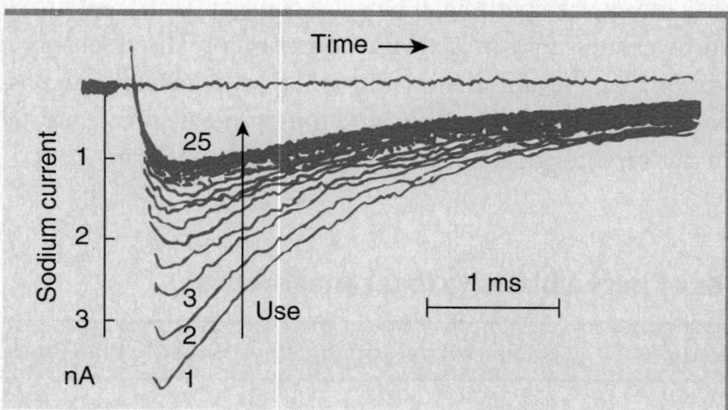

FIGURE 26–3 Effect of repetitive activity on the block of sodium current produced by a local anesthetic in a myelinated axon. A series of 25 pulses was applied, and the resulting sodium currents (downward deflections) are superimposed. Note that the current produced by the pulses rapidly decreased from the first to the 25th pulse. A long rest period after the train resulted in recovery from block, but the block could be reinstated by a subsequent train. nA, nanoamperes. (Reproduced with permission from Courtney KR: Mechanism of frequency-dependent inhibition of sodium currents in frog myelinated nerve by the lidocaine derivative GEA. J Pharmacol Exp Ther. 1975;195(2):225–236.)

Elevated extracellular calcium partially antagonizes the action of local anesthetics owing to the calcium-induced increase in the surface potential on the membrane (which favors the low-affinity rested state). Conversely, increases in extracellular potassium depolarize the membrane potential and favor the inactivated state, enhancing the effect of local anesthetics.

4. *Other effects*—Currently used local anesthetics bind to the sodium channel with low affinity and poor specificity, and there are multiple other sites for which their affinity is nearly the same as that for sodium channel binding. Thus, at clinically relevant concentrations, local anesthetics are potentially active at countless other channels (eg, potassium and calcium), enzymes (eg, adenylyl cyclase, carnitine-acylcarnitine translocase), and receptors (eg, *N*-methyl-D-aspartate [NMDA], G protein-coupled, 5-HT_3, neurokinin-1 [substance P receptor]). The role that such ancillary effects play in achievement of local anesthesia appears to be important but is poorly understood. Further, interactions with these other sites are likely the basis for numerous differences between the local anesthetics with respect to anesthetic effects (eg, differential block) and toxicities that do not parallel anesthetic potency, and thus are not adequately accounted for solely by blockade of the voltage-gated sodium channel.

The actions of circulating local anesthetics at such diverse sites exert a multitude of effects, some of which go beyond pain control, including some that are also potentially beneficial. For example, there is evidence to suggest that the blunting of the stress response and improvements in perioperative outcome that may occur with epidural anesthesia derive in part from an action of the anesthetic beyond its sodium channel block. Circulating local anesthetics also demonstrate antithrombotic effects, including having an impact on coagulation, platelet aggregation, and the microcirculation, as well as modulation of inflammation.

B. Structure-Activity Characteristics of Local Anesthetics

The smaller and more highly lipophilic local anesthetics have a faster rate of interaction with the sodium channel receptor. As previously noted, potency is also positively correlated with lipid solubility. Lidocaine, procaine, and mepivacaine are more water soluble than tetracaine, bupivacaine, and ropivacaine. The latter agents are more potent and have longer durations of local anesthetic action. These long-acting local anesthetics also bind more extensively to proteins and can be displaced from these binding sites by other protein-bound drugs. In the case of optically active agents (eg, bupivacaine), the *R*(+) isomer can usually be shown to be slightly more potent than the *S*(–) isomer (levobupivacaine).

C. Neuronal Factors Affecting Block

1. *Differential block*—Since local anesthetics are capable of blocking all nerves, their actions are not limited to the desired loss of sensation from sites of noxious (painful) stimuli. With central neuraxial techniques (spinal or epidural), motor paralysis may impair respiratory activity, and autonomic nerve blockade may promote hypotension. Further, while motor paralysis may be desirable during surgery, it may be a disadvantage in other settings. For example, motor weakness occurring as a consequence of epidural anesthesia during obstetrical labor may limit the ability of the patient to bear down (ie, "push") during delivery. Similarly, when used for postoperative analgesia, weakness may hamper ability to ambulate without assistance and pose a risk of falling, while residual autonomic blockade may interfere with bladder function, resulting in urinary retention and the need for bladder catheterization. These issues are particularly problematic in the setting of ambulatory (same-day) surgery, which represents an ever-increasing percentage of surgical caseloads.

2. *Intrinsic susceptibility of nerve fibers*—Nerve fibers differ significantly in their susceptibility to local anesthetic blockade. It has been traditionally taught, and still often cited, that local anesthetics preferentially block smaller diameter fibers first because the distance over which such fibers can passively propagate an electrical impulse is shorter. However, a variable proportion of large fibers are blocked prior to the disappearance of the small fiber component of the compound action potential. Most notably, myelinated nerves tend to be blocked before unmyelinated nerves of the same diameter. For example, preganglionic B fibers are blocked before the smaller unmyelinated C fibers involved in pain transmission (Table 26–3).

Another important factor underlying differential block derives from the state- and use-dependent mechanism of action of local anesthetics. Blockade by these drugs is more marked at higher frequencies of depolarization. Sensory (pain) fibers have a high firing rate and relatively long action potential duration. Motor fibers fire at a slower rate and have a shorter action potential duration. As type A delta and C fibers participate in high-frequency pain transmission, this characteristic may favor blockade of these fibers earlier and with lower concentrations of local anesthetics. The potential impact of such effects mandates cautious interpretation of non-physiologic experiments evaluating intrinsic susceptibility of nerves to conduction block by local anesthetics.

3. *Anatomic arrangement*—In addition to the effect of intrinsic vulnerability to local anesthetic block, the anatomic organization of the peripheral nerve bundle may impact the onset and susceptibility of its components. As one would predict based on the necessity of having proximal sensory fibers join the nerve trunk last, the core will contain sensory fibers innervating the most distal sites. Anesthetic placed outside the nerve bundle will thus reach and anesthetize the proximal fibers located at the outer portion of the bundle first, and sensory block will occur in sequence from proximal to distal.

CLINICAL PHARMACOLOGY OF LOCAL ANESTHETICS

Local anesthetics can provide highly effective analgesia in well-defined regions of the body. The most common routes of administration include a topical application (eg, nasal mucosa), wound or incision site infiltration, injection in the vicinity of peripheral nerve endings or major nerve trunks, and injection into the epidural or subarachnoid spaces surrounding the spinal cord (Figure 26–4). In addition, recent clinical practice has seen the development of truncal blocks that target fascial planes (eg, transversus abdominis or erector spinae), as well as expansion of the use of local infiltration anesthesia (LIA), particularly in the setting of total joint arthroplasty.

Clinical Block Characteristics

In clinical practice, there is generally an orderly evolution of block components beginning with sympathetic transmission and progressing to temperature, pain, light touch, and finally motor block. This is most readily appreciated during the onset of spinal anesthesia, where a spatial discrepancy can be detected in modalities, the most vulnerable components achieving greater dermatomal (cephalad) spread. Thus, loss of the sensation of cold (often assessed by a wet alcohol sponge) will be roughly two segments above the analgesic level for pinprick, which in turn will be roughly two segments rostral to loss of light touch recognition. However, because of the anatomic considerations noted earlier for peripheral nerve trunks, onset with peripheral blocks is more variable, and proximal motor weakness may precede the onset of more distal sensory loss. Additionally, the anesthetic solution is not generally deposited evenly around a nerve bundle, and longitudinal spread and radial penetration into the nerve trunk are far from uniform.

TABLE 26–3 Relative size and susceptibility of different types of nerve fibers to local anesthetics.

Fiber Type	Function	Diameter (μm)	Myelination	Conduction Velocity (m/s)	Sensitivity to Block
Type A					
Alpha	Proprioception, motor	12–20	Heavy	70–120	+
Beta	Touch, pressure	5–12	Heavy	30–70	++
Gamma	Muscle spindles	3–6	Heavy	15–30	++
Delta	Pain, temperature	2–5	Heavy	5–25	+++
Type B	Preganglionic autonomic	<3	Light	3–15	++++
Type C					
Dorsal root	Pain	0.4–1.2	None	0.5–2.3	++++
Sympathetic	Postganglionic	0.3–1.3	None	0.7–2.3	++++

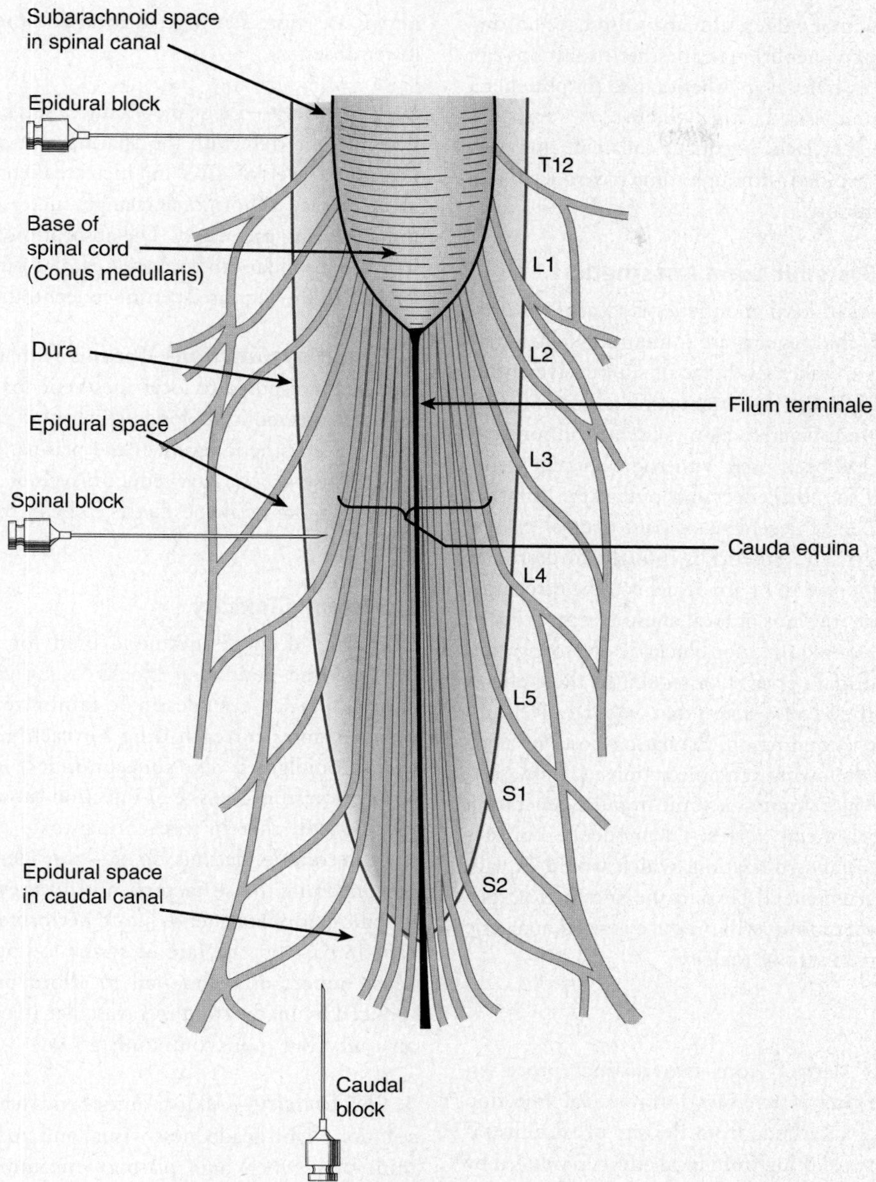

FIGURE 26–4 Schematic diagram of the typical sites of injection of local anesthetics in and around the spinal canal. When local anesthetics are injected extradurally, it is referred to as an epidural block. A caudal block is a specific type of epidural block in which a needle is inserted into the caudal canal via the sacral hiatus. Injections around peripheral nerves are known as perineural blocks (eg, paravertebral block). Finally, injection into cerebrospinal fluid in the subarachnoid (intrathecal) space is referred to as a spinal block.

With respect to differential block, it is worth noting that "successful" surgical anesthesia may require loss of tactile sensation, not just the ablation of pain, as some patients will find even the sensation of touch distressing during surgery, often fearing that the procedure may become painful. Further, while differences may exist in modalities, it is not possible with conventional techniques to produce surgical anesthesia without some loss of motor function.

A. Effect of Added Vasoconstrictors

Several benefits may be derived from addition of a vasoconstrictor to a local anesthetic. First, localized neuronal uptake is enhanced because of higher sustained local tissue concentrations that can translate clinically into a longer duration block. This may enable adequate anesthesia for more prolonged procedures, extended duration of postoperative pain control, and lower total anesthetic requirement. Second, peak blood levels will be lowered as absorption is more closely matched to metabolism and elimination, and the risk of systemic toxic effects is reduced. Moreover, when incorporated into a spinal anesthetic, epinephrine may not only contribute to the prolongation of the local anesthetic effect via its vasoconstrictor properties, but also exert a direct analgesic effect mediated by postsynaptic α_2 adrenoceptors within the spinal cord. Recognition of this potential has led to the clinical use of the α_2 agonist clonidine as a local anesthetic adjuvant for spinal anesthesia.

Conversely, the inclusion of epinephrine may also have untoward effects. The addition of epinephrine to anesthetic solutions can potentiate the neurotoxicity of local anesthetics used for peripheral nerve blocks or spinal anesthesia. Further, the use of a vasoconstrictor agent in an area that lacks adequate collateral flow (eg, digital block) is generally avoided, although some have questioned the validity of this proscription.

B. Intentional Use of Systemic Local Anesthetics

Although the principal use of local anesthetics is to achieve anesthesia in a restricted area, these agents are sometimes deliberately administered systemically to take advantage of suppressive effects on pain processing. In addition to documented reductions in anesthetic requirement and postoperative pain, systemic administration of local anesthetics has been used with some success in the treatment of chronic pain, and this effect may outlast the duration of anesthetic exposure. The achievement of pain control by systemic administration of local anesthetics is thought to derive, at least in part, from the suppression of abnormal ectopic discharge, an effect observed at concentrations of local anesthetic an order of magnitude lower than those required for blockade of propagation of action potentials in normal nerves. Consequently, these effects can be achieved without the adverse effects that would derive from the failure of normal nerve conduction. Escalating doses of anesthetic appear to exert the following systemic actions: (1) low concentrations may preferentially suppress ectopic impulse generation in chronically injured peripheral nerves; (2) moderate concentrations may suppress central sensitization, which would explain therapeutic benefit that may extend beyond the anesthetic exposure; and (3) higher concentrations will produce general analgesic effects and may culminate in serious toxicity.

Toxicity

Local anesthetic toxicity derives from two distinct processes: (1) systemic effects following inadvertent intravascular injection or absorption of the local anesthetic from the site of administration; and (2) neurotoxicity resulting from local effects produced by direct contact with neural elements.

A. Risk Factors for Local Anesthetic Toxicity

Some patients may be more predisposed to local anesthetic toxicity. Appreciating the risk factors for local anesthetic toxicity will facilitate better monitoring to decrease the incidence of adverse effects. Additionally, understanding who may be at greater risk for local anesthetics toxicity may encourage taking additional precautions to prepare resuscitation plans. The following are considered at high risk for local anesthetic toxicity.

1. *Extremes of age*—Individuals under 4 months of age or the elderly. Individuals under the age of 4 months have low hepatic clearance and low levels of alpha-1-acid glycoprotein (AAG). AAG is an acute phase protein produced by the liver and peripheral tissues with a high affinity for local anesthetics. Low levels of AAG will render more local anesthetics in the free form in the plasma. For the elderly, in addition to low hepatic clearance, nerves are more sensitive to local anesthetics, which necessitate lower doses.

2. *Pregnancy*—Pregnancy induces several physiological changes that may interfere with the pharmacokinetics of local anesthetics. Decreased levels of AAG and increased sensitivity to local anesthetics secondary to hormonal changes increase the risks of local anesthetics during pregnancy. The absorption of local anesthetics may increase secondary to increased cardiac output in pregnancy, thus leading to the increased serum concentration of local anesthetics.

3. *Organ dysfunction*—Patients with renal or hepatic disease may be predisposed to local anesthetic toxicity. Renal disease may result in metabolic acidosis, which may cause a rapid increase in the local anesthetic levels in the plasma. Patients with end-stage hepatic disease may have reduced levels of AAG and albumin, thus allowing more local anesthetics to be in the unbound form in the plasma.

B. Systemic Toxicity

The dose of local anesthetic used for epidural anesthesia or high-volume peripheral blocks is sufficient to produce major clinical toxicity, even death. To minimize risk, maximum recommended doses for each drug for each general application have been promulgated. The concept underlying this approach is that absorption from the site of injection should appropriately match metabolism, thereby preventing toxic serum levels. However, these recommendations do not consider patient characteristics or concomitant risk factors, nor do they take into account the specific peripheral nerve block performed, which has a significant impact on the rate of systemic uptake (see Figure 26–2). Most importantly, they fail to afford protection from toxicity induced by inadvertent intravascular injection (occasionally into an artery, but more commonly a vein).

1. *CNS toxicity*—All local anesthetics have the ability to produce sedation, light-headedness, visual and auditory disturbances, and restlessness when high plasma concentrations result from rapid absorption or inadvertent intravascular administration. An early symptom of local anesthetic toxicity is circumoral and tongue numbness and a metallic taste. At higher concentrations, nystagmus and muscular twitching occur, followed by tonic-clonic convulsions. Local anesthetics apparently cause depression of cortical inhibitory pathways, thereby allowing unopposed activity of excitatory neuronal pathways. This transitional stage of unbalanced excitation (ie, seizure activity) is then followed by generalized CNS depression. However, this classic pattern of evolving toxicity has been largely characterized in human volunteer studies (which are ethically constrained to low doses) and by graded administration in animal models. Deviations from such classic progression are common in clinical toxicity and will be influenced by a host of factors, including patient vulnerability, the particular local anesthetic administered, concurrent drugs, and the rate of rising of serum drug levels. For example, in a literature review of reported clinical cases of local anesthetic cardiac toxicity, prodromal signs of CNS toxicity occurred in only 18% of cases.

When large doses of a local anesthetic are required (eg, for major peripheral nerve block or local infiltration for major plastic surgery), premedication with a parenteral benzodiazepine (eg, diazepam or midazolam) may provide some prophylaxis against local anesthetic-induced CNS toxicity. However, such premedication will have little, if any, effect on cardiovascular toxicity, potentially delaying the recognition of a life-threatening overdose. If seizures do occur, it is critical to prevent hypoxemia and acidosis, which potentiate anesthetic toxicity. Rapid tracheal intubation can facilitate adequate ventilation and oxygenation, and is essential to prevent pulmonary aspiration of gastric contents in patients at risk. The effect of hyperventilation is complex, and its role in resuscitation following anesthetic overdose is somewhat controversial. While generally not recommended, it is possible that hyperventilation might offer some benefit if used to counteract significant metabolic acidosis. Seizures induced by local anesthetics should be rapidly controlled to prevent patient harm and exacerbation of acidosis. A recent practice advisory from the American Society of Regional Anesthesia considered benzodiazepines as first-line drugs. However, small doses of propofol (eg, 0.25–0.5 mg/kg) were considered acceptable alternatives, as they are often more immediately available in the setting of local anesthetic administration, while higher doses were to be avoided, particularly in the setting of hemodynamic instability. The motor activity of the seizure can be effectively terminated by the administration of a neuromuscular blocker, though this will not diminish the CNS manifestations, and efforts must include therapy directed at the underlying seizure activity.

2. *Cardiotoxicity*—The most feared complications associated with local anesthetic administration result from the profound effects these agents can have on cardiac conduction and function. In 1979, an editorial by Albright reviewed the circumstances of six deaths associated with the use of bupivacaine and etidocaine. This seminal publication suggested that these relatively new lipophilic and potent anesthetics had greater potential for cardiotoxicity and that cardiac arrest could occur concurrently or immediately following seizures and, most importantly, in the absence of hypoxia or acidosis. Although this suggestion was sharply criticized, subsequent clinical experience, unfortunately, reinforced Albright's concern—within 4 years, the US Food and Drug Administration (FDA) had received reports of 12 cases of cardiac arrest associated with the use of 0.75% bupivacaine for epidural anesthesia in obstetrics. Further support for enhanced cardiotoxicity of these anesthetics came from animal studies demonstrating that doses of bupivacaine and etidocaine as low as two-thirds of those producing convulsions could induce arrhythmias, while the margin between CNS and cardiac toxicity was less than half that for lidocaine. In response, the FDA banned the use of 0.75% bupivacaine in obstetrics. In addition, the incorporation of a test dose became ingrained as a standard of anesthetic practice, along with the practice of fractionated administration of local anesthetic.

Although the reduction in bupivacaine's anesthetic concentration and changes in anesthetic practice did much to reduce the risk of cardiotoxicity, the recognized differences in the toxicity of the stereoisomers comprising bupivacaine created an opportunity for the development of potentially safer anesthetics (see Chapter 1). Investigations demonstrated that the enantiomers of the racemic mixture bupivacaine were not equivalent with respect to cardiotoxicity, the *S*(–) enantiomer having a better therapeutic advantage, leading to the subsequent marketing of levobupivacaine. This was followed shortly thereafter by ropivacaine, a slightly less potent anesthetic than bupivacaine. It should be noted, however, that the reduction in toxicity afforded by these compounds is only modest. In fact, a recent advisory panel of the American Society of Regional Anesthesia (ASRA) concluded that in most clinical settings ropivacaine and bupivacaine likely have similar toxicity when administered on an equipotent basis. Thus, the risk of significant cardiotoxicity remains a very real concern when any of these anesthetics are administered for high-volume blocks.

3. *Reversal of bupivacaine toxicity*—Recently, a series of clinical events, serendipitous observations, systematic experimentation, and astute clinical decisions have identified a relatively simple, practical, and apparently effective therapy for resistant bupivacaine cardiotoxicity using intravenous infusion of lipid. Furthermore, this therapy appears to have applications that extend beyond bupivacaine cardiotoxicity to the cardiac or CNS toxicity induced by an overdose of any lipid-soluble drug (see Box: Lipid Resuscitation).

C. Localized Toxicity

1. *Neural injury*—From the early introduction of spinal anesthesia into clinical practice, sporadic reports of neurologic injury associated with this technique raised concern that local anesthetic agents were potentially neurotoxic. Following injuries associated with Durocaine—a spinal anesthetic formulation containing procaine—initial attention focused on the vehicle components. However, experimental studies found 10% procaine alone induced similar injuries in cats, whereas the vehicle did not. Concern for anesthetic neurotoxicity reemerged in the early 1980s with a series of reports of major neurologic injury occurring with the use of chloroprocaine for epidural anesthesia. In these cases, there was evidence that anesthetic intended for the epidural space was inadvertently administered intrathecally. As the dose required for spinal anesthesia is roughly an order of magnitude less than for epidural anesthesia, injury was apparently the result of excessive exposure of the more vulnerable subarachnoid neural elements.

With changes in vehicle formulation and in clinical practice, concern for toxicity again subsided, only to reemerge a decade later with reports of cauda equina syndrome associated with continuous spinal anesthesia (CSA). In contrast to the more common single-injection technique, CSA involves placing a catheter in the subarachnoid space to permit repetitive dosing to facilitate adequate anesthesia and maintenance of block for extended periods. In these cases, the local anesthetic was evidently administered to a relatively restricted area of the subarachnoid space; in order to extend the block to achieve adequate surgical anesthesia, multiple repetitive doses of anesthetic were then administered. By the time the block was adequate, neurotoxic concentrations had accumulated in a restricted area of the caudal region of the subarachnoid space. Most notably, the anesthetic involved in the majority of these cases was lidocaine, a drug most clinicians considered to be the least toxic of agents. This was followed by reports of neurotoxic injury occurring with lidocaine intended for epidural administration that had inadvertently been administered intrathecally, similar to the cases involving chloroprocaine a decade earlier. The occurrence of neurotoxic injury with CSA and subarachnoid administration of epidural doses of lidocaine served to establish vulnerability whenever excessive anesthetic was administered intrathecally, regardless of the specific anesthetic used. Of even more concern, subsequent reports provided evidence for injury with spinal lidocaine administered at the high end of the recommended clinical dosage, prompting recommendations for a reduction in maximum dose. These clinical reports (as well as concurrent experimental studies) served to dispel the concept that modern local anesthetics administered at clinically relevant doses and concentrations were incapable of inducing neurotoxic injury.

Lipid Resuscitation

Based on a case of apparent cardiotoxicity from a very low dose of bupivacaine in a patient with carnitine deficiency, G. L. Weinberg postulated that this metabolic derangement led to enhanced toxicity due to the accumulation of fatty acids within the cardiac myocyte. He hypothesized that administration of lipid would similarly potentiate bupivacaine cardiotoxicity, but experiments performed to test this hypothesis demonstrated exactly the opposite effect. Accordingly, he began systematic laboratory investigations, which clearly demonstrated the potential efficacy of an **intravenous lipid emulsion (ILE)** for resuscitation from bupivacaine cardiotoxicity. Clinical confirmation came 8 years later with the report of the successful resuscitation of a patient who sustained an anesthetic-induced (bupivacaine plus mepivacaine) cardiac arrest refractory to standard advanced cardiac life support procedures (ACLS). Numerous similar reports of successful resuscitations soon followed, extending this clinical experience to other anesthetics including levobupivacaine and ropivacaine local anesthetic-induced CNS toxicity, as well as toxicity induced by other classes of compounds, eg, bupropion-induced cardiovascular collapse and multiform ventricular tachycardia provoked by haloperidol. Laboratory investigations have likewise provided evidence of efficacy for treatment of diverse toxic challenges (eg, verapamil, clomipramine, and propranolol).

Our understanding of the mechanisms by which lipid is effective is incomplete, but has advanced significantly over the last two decades. Almost certainly an important effect is related to its ability to extract a lipophilic drug from aqueous plasma, thus reducing its effective concentration at tissue targets, a mechanism initially termed "lipid sink." More recently, the more dynamic term "lipid shuttle" has been favored to reflect the redistribution of drug from organs susceptible to toxicity to organs where drug might be stored, detoxified, or excreted. However, this alone does not appear adequate to account for the magnitude of clinical effect, suggesting that other mechanisms contribute to the efficacy of lipid rescue. Consistent with this, there is experimental evidence demonstrating beneficial cardiotonic and vasoconstrictive effects as well as postconditioning (through activation of prosurvival kinases).

Although numerous questions remain, the evolving evidence is sufficient to warrant administration of lipid in cases of systemic anesthetic toxicity. Its use has been promulgated by a task force of the American Society of Regional Anesthesia (https://www.asra.com/advisory-guidelines/article/3/checklist-for-treatment-of-local-anesthetic-systemic-toxicity), and administration of lipid has been incorporated into the most recent revision of ACLS guidelines for Cardiac Arrest in Special Situations. Importantly, propofol cannot be administered for this purpose, as the relatively enormous volume of this solution required for lipid therapy would deliver lethal quantities of propofol.

The mechanism of local anesthetic neurotoxicity has been extensively investigated in cell cultures, isolated axons, and in vivo models. These studies have demonstrated myriad deleterious effects including conduction failure, membrane damage, enzyme leakage, cytoskeletal disruption, accumulation of intracellular calcium, disruption of axonal transport, growth cone collapse, and apoptosis. It is not clear what role these factors or others play in clinical injury. It is clear, however, that injury does not result from the blockade of the voltage-gated sodium channel per se, and thus clinical effect and toxicity are not tightly linked.

2. *Transient neurologic symptoms (TNS)*—In addition to the very rare but devastating neural complications that can occur with neuraxial (spinal and epidural) administration of local anesthetics, a syndrome of transient pain or dysesthesia, or both, has been recently linked to use of lidocaine for spinal anesthesia. Although these symptoms are not associated with sensory loss, motor weakness, or bowel and bladder dysfunction, the pain can be quite severe, often exceeding that induced by the surgical procedure. TNS occurs even at modest doses of anesthetic and has been documented in as many as one-third of patients receiving lidocaine, with increased risk associated with certain patient positions during surgery (eg, lithotomy) and with ambulatory anesthesia. The risk with other anesthetics varies considerably. For example, the incidence is only slightly reduced with procaine or mepivacaine but appears to be negligible with bupivacaine, prilocaine, and chloroprocaine. The etiology and significance of TNS remain to be established, but differences between factors affecting TNS and experimental animal toxicity argue strongly against a common mechanism mediating these symptoms and persistent or permanent neurologic deficits. Nonetheless, the high incidence of TNS with spinal lidocaine has led to decreased use for this procedure, though lidocaine's popularity for all other applications, including epidural anesthesia, remains intact. Rather ironically, chloroprocaine, once considered a more toxic anesthetic, is now gaining popularity for short-duration spinal anesthesia as an alternative to lidocaine, a compound that had been considered the gold standard for safety for over half a century, and had been used for well over 50 million spinal anesthetic procedures.

■ COMMONLY USED LOCAL ANESTHETICS & THEIR APPLICATIONS

ARTICAINE

Approved for use in the USA as a dental anesthetic in April 2000, articaine is unique among the amino-amide anesthetics in having a thiophene, rather than a benzene ring, as well as an additional ester group that is subject to metabolism by plasma esterases (see Table 26–1). The modification of the ring serves to enhance lipophilicity, and thus improve tissue penetration, while inclusion of the ester leads to a shorter plasma half-life (approximately 20 minutes), potentially imparting a better therapeutic index with respect to systemic toxicity. These characteristics have led to widespread popularity in dental anesthesia, where it is generally considered to be more effective, and possibly safer, than lidocaine, the prior standard. Balanced against these positive attributes are concerns that the development of persistent paresthesias, while rare, may be three times more common with articaine. However, prilocaine has been associated with an even higher relative incidence (twice that of articaine). Importantly, these are the only two dental anesthetics that are formulated as 4% solutions; the others are all marketed at lower concentrations (eg, the maximum concentration of lidocaine used for dental anesthesia is 2%), and it is well established that anesthetic neurotoxicity is, to some extent, concentration-dependent. Thus, it is quite possible that enhanced risk derives from the formulation rather than from an intrinsic property of the anesthetic. In a recent survey of US and Canadian dental schools, over half of respondents indicated that 4% articaine is no longer used for mandibular nerve block.

BENZOCAINE

As previously noted, benzocaine's pronounced lipophilicity has relegated its application to topical anesthesia. However, despite over a century of use for this purpose, its popularity has recently diminished owing to increasing concerns regarding its potential to induce methemoglobinemia. Elevated levels can be due to inborn errors or can occur with exposure to an oxidizing agent, and such is the case with significant exposure to benzocaine (or nitrites, see Chapter 12). Because methemoglobin does not transport oxygen, elevated levels pose a serious risk, with severity obviously paralleling blood levels.

BUPIVACAINE

Based on concerns for cardiotoxicity, bupivacaine is often avoided for techniques that demand high volumes of concentrated anesthetics, such as epidural or peripheral nerve blocks performed for surgical anesthesia. In contrast, relatively low concentrations (≤0.25%) are frequently used to achieve prolonged peripheral anesthesia and analgesia for postoperative pain control, and the drug enjoys similar popularity where anesthetic infiltration is used to control pain from a surgical incision. It is often the agent of choice for epidural infusions used for postoperative pain control and for labor analgesia. Finally, it has a comparatively unblemished record as a spinal anesthetic, with a relatively favorable therapeutic index with respect to neurotoxicity, and little, if any, risk of TNS. However, spinal bupivacaine is not well suited for outpatient or ambulatory surgery, because its relatively long duration of action can delay recovery, resulting in a longer stay prior to discharge to home.

CHLOROPROCAINE

The introduction of chloroprocaine into clinical practice in 1951 represented a reversion to the earlier amino-ester template. Chloroprocaine gained widespread use as an epidural agent in obstetrical anesthesia where its rapid hydrolysis served to minimize risk of systemic toxicity or fetal exposure. The unfortunate reports of neurologic injury associated with apparent intrathecal misplacement of large doses intended for the epidural space led to its near abandonment. However, although chloroprocaine was never exonerated with respect to these early neurologic injuries associated with epidural anesthesia, it is now appreciated that high doses of any local anesthetic are capable of inducing neurotoxic injury.

The frequent occurrence of TNS with lidocaine administered as a spinal anesthetic created an anesthetic void that chloroprocaine appeared well suited to fill. The onset and duration of action of spinal chloroprocaine are even shorter than those of lidocaine, while presenting little, if any, risk of TNS. These favorable characteristics provoked considerable off-label use of a preservative-free (epidural) solution, and ultimately led to the approval and marketing of Clorotekal, a chloroprocaine formulation specifically indicated for spinal anesthesia. Nonetheless, documented use of chloroprocaine as a spinal anesthetic is relatively limited when compared with compounds such as lidocaine and bupivacaine, and additional experience will be required to firmly establish its safety profile. In addition to chloroprocaine's emerging use for spinal anesthesia, it still finds some current use as an epidural anesthetic, particularly in circumstances where there is an indwelling catheter and the need for quick attainment of surgical anesthesia, such as caesarian section for a laboring parturient with a compromised fetus.

COCAINE

Current clinical use of cocaine is largely restricted to topical anesthesia for ear, nose, and throat procedures, where its intense vasoconstriction can serve to reduce bleeding. Even here, use has diminished in favor of other anesthetics combined with vasoconstrictors because of concerns about systemic toxicity, as well as the inconvenience of dispensing and handling this controlled substance.

ETIDOCAINE

Introduced along with bupivacaine, etidocaine has had limited application due to its poor block characteristics. It has a tendency to produce an inverse differential block (ie, compared with other anesthetics such as bupivacaine, it produces excessive motor relative to sensory block), which is rarely a favorable attribute.

LEVOBUPIVACAINE

As previously discussed, this *S*(–) enantiomer of bupivacaine is somewhat less cardiotoxic than the racemic mixture. It is also less potent and tends to have a longer duration of action, although the magnitude of these effects is too small to have any substantial clinical significance.

LIDOCAINE

Aside from the issue of a high incidence of TNS with spinal administration, lidocaine has had an excellent record as an intermediate duration anesthetic and remains the reference standard against which most anesthetics are compared.

MEPIVACAINE

Although structurally similar to bupivacaine and ropivacaine (see Table 26–1), mepivacaine displays clinical properties that are comparable to lidocaine. However, it differs from lidocaine with respect to vasoactivity, as it has a tendency toward vasoconstriction rather than vasodilation. This characteristic likely accounts for its slightly longer duration of action, which has made it a popular choice for major peripheral blocks. Lidocaine has retained its dominance over mepivacaine for epidural anesthesia, where the routine placement of a catheter negates the importance of a longer duration. More importantly, mepivacaine is slowly metabolized by the fetus, making it a poor choice for epidural anesthesia in the parturient. When used for spinal anesthesia, mepivacaine has a slightly lower incidence of TNS than lidocaine.

PRILOCAINE

Prilocaine has the highest clearance of the amino-amide anesthetics, imparting reduced risk of systemic toxicity. Unfortunately, this is somewhat offset by its propensity to induce methemoglobinemia, which results from accumulation of one of its metabolites, ortho-toluidine, an oxidizing agent. As a spinal anesthetic, prilocaine's duration of action is slightly longer than that of lidocaine, and the limited data suggest it carries a low risk of TNS. It is gaining increasing use for spinal anesthesia in Europe, where it has been marketed specifically for this purpose. No approved formulation exists in the USA, and there is no formulation that would be appropriate to use for spinal anesthesia as an off-label indication.

ROPIVACAINE

Ropivacaine is an *S*(–) enantiomer in a homologous series that includes bupivacaine and mepivacaine, distinguished by its chirality and the propyl group off the piperidine ring (see Table 26–1). Its perceived reduced cardiotoxicity has led to widespread use for high-volume peripheral blocks. However, as previously mentioned, such reduction in toxicity is modest, and its actual advantage over bupivacaine in most clinical settings has been questioned. Nonetheless, it remains a popular choice for high-volume blocks as well as epidural infusions for control of labor or postoperative pain. Although there is some evidence to suggest that ropivacaine might produce a more favorable differential block than bupivacaine, the lack of equivalent clinical potency adds complexity to such comparisons.

EMLA

The term *eutectic* is applied to mixtures in which the combination of elements has a lower melting temperature than its component elements. Lidocaine and prilocaine can combine to form such a mixture, which is marketed as EMLA (**E**utectic **M**ixture of **L**ocal **A**nesthetics). This formulation, containing 2.5% lidocaine and 2.5% prilocaine, permits anesthetic penetration of the keratinized layer of skin, producing localized numbness. It is commonly used in pediatrics to anesthetize the skin prior to venipuncture for intravenous catheter placement.

FUTURE DEVELOPMENTS

Sustained-Release Formulations

The provision of prolonged analgesia or anesthesia, as in the case of postoperative pain management, has traditionally been accomplished by the placement of a catheter to permit continuous administration of anesthetic. More recently, efforts have focused on drug delivery systems that can slowly release anesthetic, thereby providing extended duration without the drawbacks of a catheter. Current developmental efforts have focused on diverse methods of achieving this goal, and one formulation, Exparel, which uses liposomal encapsulation for sustained release of bupivacaine, received FDA approval in 2011. Although this initial approval was limited to infiltration analgesia, it has since been expanded to include interscalene block, while other indications are likely to follow.

Less Toxic Agents; More Selective Agents

It has been clearly demonstrated that anesthetic neurotoxicity does not result from the blockade of the voltage-gated sodium channel. Thus, effect and tissue toxicity are not mediated by a common mechanism, establishing the possibility of developing compounds with considerably better therapeutic indexes. In addition, the intense binding of site 1 sodium channel biotoxins presents an alternative strategy for providing prolonged block, obviating the need for catheter placement and continuous anesthetic infusion. One such compound, **neosaxitoxin,** is currently undergoing clinical investigation.

As previously discussed, the identification and subclassification of families of neuronal sodium channels have spurred research aimed at the development of more selective sodium channel blockers. The variable neuronal distribution of these isoforms and the unique role that some play in pain signaling suggest that selective blockade of these channels may greatly improve the therapeutic index of sodium channel modulators. For example, compounds specifically targeting $Na_v1.7$ hold therapeutic promise for effective non-opiate pain control. These channels have abundant representation in dorsal root ganglia: humans with loss-of-function mutations of $Na_v1.7$ show congenital insensitivity to pain (CIP); while gain-of-function mutations are associated with severe chronic pain syndromes. A number of compounds with specificity for $Na_v1.7$ have been identified and are currently under clinical development.

SUMMARY Drugs Used for Local Anesthesia

Subclass, Drug	Mechanism of Action	Effects	Clinical Applications	Pharmacokinetics, Toxicities
AMIDES				
• Lidocaine	Blockade of sodium channels	Slows, then blocks, action potential propagation	Short-duration procedures • topical (mucosal), intravenous, infiltration, spinal, epidural, minor and major peripheral blocks	Parenteral (eg, peripheral block, but varies significantly based on specific site) • duration 1–2 h • 2–4 h with epinephrine • *Toxicity:* Central nervous system (CNS) excitation (high-volume blocks) and local neurotoxicity
• Bupivacaine	Same as lidocaine	Same as lidocaine	Longer-duration procedures (but not used topically or intravenously)	Parenteral • duration 3–6 h • *Toxicity:* CNS excitation • cardiovascular collapse (high-volume blocks)
• *Prilocaine, mepivacaine: Like lidocaine (but also risk of methemoglobinemia with prilocaine)*				
• *Articaine: Popular dental anesthetic*				
• *Ropivacaine, levobupivacaine: Like bupivacaine*				
ESTERS				
• Chloroprocaine	Like lidocaine	Like lidocaine	Very short procedures (not generally used topically or intravenously)	Parenteral • duration 30–60 min • 60–90 min with epinephrine • *Toxicity:* Like lidocaine
• Cocaine	Same as above • also has sympathomimetic effects	Same as above	Procedures requiring high surface activity and vasoconstriction	Topical or parenteral • duration 1–2 h • *Toxicity:* CNS excitation, convulsions, cardiac arrhythmias, hypertension, stroke
• *Procaine: Like chloroprocaine (but not used epidurally)*				
• *Tetracaine: Used primarily for spinal anesthesia; duration 2–3 h*				
• *Benzocaine: Used exclusively for topical anesthesia*				

PREPARATIONS AVAILABLE

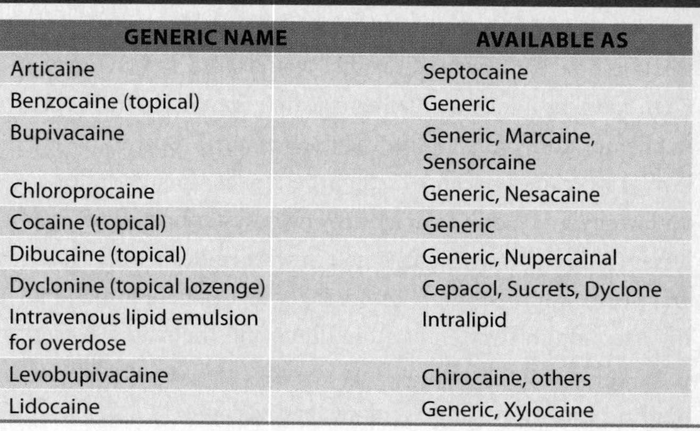

GENERIC NAME	AVAILABLE AS
Articaine	Septocaine
Benzocaine (topical)	Generic
Bupivacaine	Generic, Marcaine, Sensorcaine
Chloroprocaine	Generic, Nesacaine
Cocaine (topical)	Generic
Dibucaine (topical)	Generic, Nupercainal
Dyclonine (topical lozenge)	Cepacol, Sucrets, Dyclone
Intravenous lipid emulsion for overdose	Intralipid
Levobupivacaine	Chirocaine, others
Lidocaine	Generic, Xylocaine

GENERIC NAME	AVAILABLE AS
Lidocaine and hydrocortisone (patch)	Generic
Lidocaine and bupivacaine mixture	Duocaine
Lidocaine and prilocaine eutectic mixture (topical)	EMLA cream
Mepivacaine	Generic, Carbocaine
Pramoxine (topical)	Generic, Tronothane
Prilocaine	Citanest
Procaine	Generic, Novocain
Proparacaine (ophthalmic)	Generic, Alcaine, others
Ropivacaine	Generic, Naropin
Tetracaine	Generic, Pontocaine

REFERENCES

Albright GA: Cardiac arrest following regional anesthesia with etidocaine or bupivacaine. Anesthesiology 1979;51:285.

American Society of Regional Anesthesia and Pain Medicine: Checklist for treatment of local anesthetic systemic toxicity. 2017. https://www.asra.com/advisory-guidelines/article/3/checklist-for-treatment-of-local-anesthetic-systemic-toxicity

Anell-Olofsson M et al: Plasma concentrations of alpha-1-acid glycoprotein in preterm and term newborns: influence of mode of delivery and implications for plasma protein binding of local anaesthetics. Br J Anaesth 2018;121:427.

Auroy Y et al: Serious complications related to regional anesthesia: Results of a prospective survey in France. Anesthesiology 1997;87:479.

Balocco AL et al: Extended release bupivacaine formulations for postoperative analgesia: An update. Curr Opin Anesthesiol 2018;31:636.

Braid DP, Scott DB: The systemic absorption of local analgesic drugs. Br J Anaesth 1965;37:394.

Butterworth JF 4th, Strichartz GR: Molecular mechanisms of local anesthesia: A review. Anesthesiology 1990;72:711.

Catterall WA, Goldin AL, Waxman SG: International Union of Pharmacology. XLVII. Nomenclature and structure-function relationships of voltage-gated sodium channels. Pharmacol Rev 2005;57:397.

Cave G, Harvey M: Intravenous lipid emulsion as antidote beyond local anesthetic toxicity: A systematic review. Acad Emerg Med 2009;16:815.

de Jong RH, Ronfeld RA, DeRosa RA: Cardiovascular effects of convulsant and supraconvulsant doses of amide local anesthetics. Anesth Analg 1982;61:3.

de Lera Ruiz L, Kraus RL: Voltage-gated sodium channels: Structure, function, pharmacology, and clinical indications. J Med Chem 2015;58:7093.

Di Gregorio G et al: Clinical presentation of local anesthetic systemic toxicity: A review of published cases, 1979 to 2009. Reg Anesth Pain Med 2010;35:181.

Drasner K: Chloroprocaine spinal anesthesia: Back to the future? Anesth Analg 2005;100:549.

Drasner K: Lidocaine spinal anesthesia: A vanishing therapeutic index? Anesthesiology 1997;87:469.

Drasner K: Local anesthetic neurotoxicity: Clinical injury and strategies that may minimize risk. Reg Anesth Pain Med 2002;27:576.

Drasner K: Local anesthetic systemic toxicity: A historical perspective. Reg Anesth Pain Med 2010;35:162.

Drasner K et al: Cauda equina syndrome following intended epidural anesthesia. Anesthesiology 1992;77:582.

Drasner K et al: Persistent sacral sensory deficit induced by intrathecal local anesthetic infusion in the rat. Anesthesiology 1994;80:847.

Fettiplace MR, Weinberg G: The mechanisms underlying lipid resuscitation therapy. Reg Anesth Pain Med 2018;43:138.

Flight MH: Analgesics: Specifically attenuating pain. Nat Rev Drug Discov 2007;6:518.

Freedman JM et al: Transient neurologic symptoms after spinal anesthesia: An epidemiologic study of 1,863 patients. Anesthesiology 1998;89:633.

Gitman M, Barrington MJ: Local anesthetic systemic toxicity: A review of recent case reports and registries. Reg Anesth Pain Med. 2018;43:124.

Goldblum E, Atchabahian A: The use of 2-chloroprocaine for spinal anaesthesia. Acta Anaesthesiol Scand 2013;57:545.

Hampl KF et al: Transient neurologic symptoms after spinal anesthesia. Anesth Analg 1995;81:1148.

Hille B: Local anesthetics: Hydrophilic and hydrophobic pathways for the drug-receptor interaction. J Gen Physiol 1977;69:497.

Holmdahl MH: Xylocain (lidocaine, lignocaine), its discovery and Gordh's contribution to its clinical use. Acta Anaesthesiol Scand Suppl 1998;113:8.

Jokinen MJ et al: Pharmacokinetics of ropivacaine in patients with chronic end-stage liver disease. Anesthesiology 2007;106:43.

Kouri ME, Kopacz DJ: Spinal 2-chloroprocaine: A comparison with lidocaine in volunteers. Anesth Analg 2004;98:75.

Lahaye LA, Butterworth JF: Site-1 sodium channel blockers as local anesthetics: Will neosaxitoxin supplant the need for continuous nerve blocks? Anesthesiology 2015;123:741.

Larsson BA, Lonnqvist PA, Olsson GL: Plasma concentrations of bupivacaine in neonates after continuous epidural infusion. Anesth Analg 1997;84:501.

Mattison JB: Cocaine poisoning. Med Surg Rep 1891;115:645.

McNamara PJ, Alcorn J: Protein binding predictions in infants. AAPS PharmSci 2002;4:E4.

Meunier JF et al. Pharmacokinetics of bupivacaine after continuous epidural infusion in infants with and without biliary atresia. Anesthesiology 2001;95:87.

Neal JM et al: The Third American Society of Regional Anesthesia and Pain Medicine Practice Advisory on Local Anesthetic Systemic Toxicity: Executive Summary 2017. Reg Anesth Pain Med 2018;43:113.

Pollock JE: Transient neurologic symptoms: Etiology, risk factors, and management. Reg Anesth Pain Med 2002;27:581.

Priest BT: Future potential and status of selective sodium channel blockers for the treatment of pain. Curr Opin Drug Discov Dev 2009;12:682.

Rigler ML et al: Cauda equina syndrome after continuous spinal anesthesia. Anesth Analg 1991;72:275.

Ruetsch YA, Boni T, Borgeat A: From cocaine to ropivacaine: The history of local anesthetic drugs. Curr Top Med Chem 2001;1:175.

Sakura S et al: Local anesthetic neurotoxicity does not result from blockade of voltage-gated sodium channels. Anesth Analg 1995;81:338.

Schneider M et al: Transient neurologic toxicity after hyperbaric subarachnoid anesthesia with 5% lidocaine. Anesth Analg 1993;76:1154.

Sirianni AJ et al: Use of lipid emulsion in the resuscitation of a patient with prolonged cardiovascular collapse after overdose of bupropion and lamotrigine. Ann Emerg Med 2008;51:412.

Taniguchi M, Bollen AW, Drasner K: Sodium bisulfite: Scapegoat for chloroprocaine neurotoxicity? Anesthesiology 2004;100:85.

Tremont-Lukats IW et al: Systemic administration of local anesthetics to relieve neuropathic pain: A systematic review and meta-analysis. Anesth Analg 2005;101:1738.

Weinberg GL: Lipid emulsion infusion: Resuscitation for local anesthetic and other drug overdose. Anesthesiology 2012;117:180.

Weinberg GL et al: Pretreatment or resuscitation with a lipid infusion shifts the dose-response to bupivacaine-induced asystole in rats. Anesthesiology 1998;88:1071.

CASE STUDY ANSWER

If a spinal anesthetic technique were selected, bupivacaine would be an excellent choice. It has an adequately long duration of action and a relatively unblemished record with respect to neurotoxic injury and transient neurologic symptoms, which are the complications of most concern with spinal anesthetic technique. Although bupivacaine has greater potential for cardiotoxicity, this is not a concern when the drug is used for spinal anesthesia because of the extremely low doses required for intrathecal administration. If an epidural technique were chosen for the surgical procedure, the potential for systemic toxicity would need to be considered, making lidocaine or mepivacaine (generally with epinephrine) preferable to bupivacaine (or even ropivacaine or levobupivacaine) because of their better therapeutic indexes with respect to cardiotoxicity. However, systemic toxicity is a lesser (but not nonexistent) concern with epidural or peripheral nerve administration for postoperative pain control, as it involves administration of more dilute anesthetic at a slower rate. The most common agents used for this indication are bupivacaine, ropivacaine, and levobupivacaine.

CHAPTER

27

Skeletal Muscle Relaxants

Marieke Kruidering-Hall, PhD, &
Lundy J. Campbell, MD

CASE STUDY

An 80-kg 35-year-old woman with a BMI of 32 is undergoing right knee surgery for a meniscus tear. The surgeon and the patient both request general anesthesia for the procedure. In addition to obesity, the patient has hypertension (treated with hydrochlorothiazide) and insulin-dependent diabetes, and she takes an oral contraceptive pill. She has no known drug allergies. Her physical examination is remarkable only for obesity and a Mallampati class 3 airway (indicating extremely limited space from tongue base to roof of mouth and probable difficulty in intubating). Because of her diabetes and risk for delayed gastric emptying, you elect to use endotracheal intubation to protect her airway during the procedure.

After induction of anesthesia with propofol, you administer a dose of rocuronium to achieve skeletal muscle relaxation and to facilitate endotracheal intubation. Once fully relaxed, you attempt direct laryngoscopy but are unable to visualize her airway. You make changes to the patient's position, and use a different technique, but you are still unable to perform intubation.

You switch back to bag/mask ventilation, but it has now become more difficult to achieve adequate tidal volumes. You decide to reverse the neuromuscular blockade and wake the patient. (1) What agents could be used to reverse the neuromuscular blockade? (2) What would be the most appropriate agent to use in this scenario? (3) What problems may occur with your chosen agent?

Drugs that affect skeletal muscle function include two different therapeutic groups: those used during surgical procedures and in the intensive care unit (ICU) to produce muscle paralysis (ie, **neuromuscular blockers**), and those used to reduce spasticity in a variety of painful conditions (ie, **spasmolytics** and **antispasmodics**). Neuromuscular blocking drugs interfere with transmission at the neuromuscular end plate and lack central nervous system (CNS) activity. These compounds are used primarily as adjuncts during general anesthesia to optimize surgical conditions and to facilitate endotracheal intubation in order to ensure adequate ventilation. Drugs in the spasmolytic group have traditionally been called "centrally acting" muscle relaxants and are used primarily to treat chronic back pain and painful fibromyalgic conditions. Dantrolene, an agent that has no significant central effects and is used primarily to treat a rare anesthetic-related complication, malignant hyperthermia, is also discussed in this chapter.

NEUROMUSCULAR BLOCKING DRUGS

History

During the 16th century, European explorers found that natives in the Amazon Basin of South America were using curare, an arrow poison that produced skeletal muscle paralysis, to kill animals. The active compound, *d*-tubocurarine, and its modern synthetic analogs have had a major influence on the practice of anesthesia and surgery and have proved useful in understanding the basic mechanisms involved in neuromuscular transmission.

Normal Neuromuscular Function

The mechanism of neuromuscular transmission at the motor end plate is similar to that described for preganglionic cholinergic nerves in Chapter 6. The arrival of an action potential at the motor nerve terminal causes an influx of calcium and release of the neurotransmitter acetylcholine. Acetylcholine then diffuses across the synaptic cleft to activate nicotinic receptors located on the motor end plate, present at a density of 10,000/μm^2 in some species. As noted in Chapter 7, the adult N_M receptor is composed of five peptides: two alpha peptides, one beta, one gamma, and one delta peptide (Figure 27–1). The binding of two acetylcholine molecules to receptors on the α-β and δ-α subunits causes opening of the channel. The subsequent movement of sodium and potassium through the channel is associated with a graded depolarization of the end plate membrane (see Figure 7–4, panel B). This change in voltage is termed the motor end plate potential. The magnitude of the end plate potential is directly related to the amount of acetylcholine released. If the potential is small, the permeability and the end plate potential return to normal without an impulse being propagated from the end plate region to the rest of the muscle membrane. However, if the end plate potential is large, the adjacent muscle membrane is depolarized, and an action potential will be propagated along the entire muscle fiber. Muscle contraction is then initiated by excitation-contraction coupling. The released acetylcholine is quickly removed from the end plate region by both diffusion and enzymatic destruction by the local acetylcholinesterase enzyme.

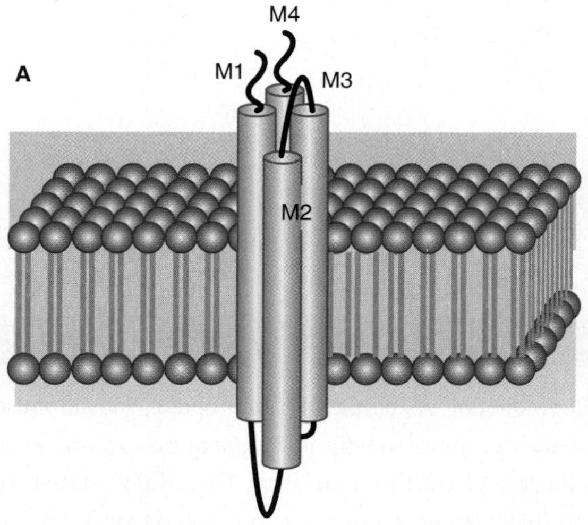

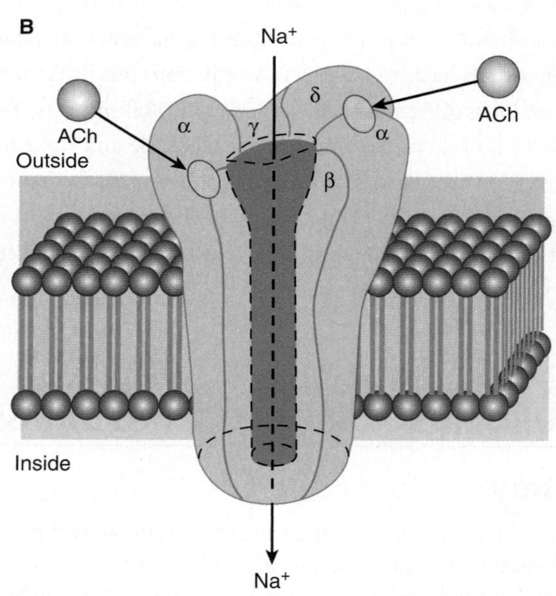

FIGURE 27–1 The adult nicotinic acetylcholine receptor (nAChR) is an intrinsic membrane protein with five distinct subunits ($\alpha_2 \beta \delta \gamma$). **(A)** Cartoon of one of five subunits of the AChR in the end plate surface of adult mammalian muscle. Each subunit contains four helical domains labeled M1–M4. The M2 domains line the channel pore. **(B)** Cartoon of the full nAChR. The N termini of two subunits cooperate to form two distinct binding pockets for acetylcholine (ACh). These pockets occur at the α-β and the δ-α subunit interfaces. Binding of one molecule of ACh enhances the receptor's affinity for the second molecule, followed by multiple intermediate steps leading to channel opening. These steps are the subject of intense investigation.

At least two additional types of acetylcholine receptors are found within the neuromuscular apparatus. One type is located on the presynaptic motor axon terminal, and activation of these receptors mobilizes additional transmitter for subsequent release by moving more acetylcholine vesicles toward the synaptic membrane. The second type of receptor is found on extrajunctional cells and is not normally involved in neuromuscular transmission. However, under certain conditions (eg, prolonged immobilization, thermal burns), these receptors may proliferate sufficiently to affect subsequent neuromuscular transmission. This proliferation of extrajunctional acetylcholine receptors may be clinically relevant when using depolarizing or nondepolarizing skeletal muscle relaxant drugs and is described later.

Skeletal muscle relaxation and paralysis can occur from interruption of function at several sites along the pathway from the CNS to myelinated somatic nerves, unmyelinated motor nerve terminals, nicotinic acetylcholine receptors, the motor end plate, the muscle membrane, and the intracellular muscular contractile apparatus itself.

Blockade of end plate function can be accomplished by two basic mechanisms. First, pharmacologic blockade of the physiologic agonist acetylcholine is characteristic of the antagonist neuromuscular blocking drugs (ie, nondepolarizing neuromuscular blocking drugs). These drugs prevent access of the transmitter to its receptor and thereby prevent depolarization. The prototype of this nondepolarizing subgroup is ***d*-tubocurarine.** The second mechanism of blockade can be produced by an excess of a depolarizing agonist, such as acetylcholine. This seemingly paradoxical effect of acetylcholine also occurs at the ganglionic nicotinic acetylcholine receptor. The prototypical depolarizing blocking drug is **succinylcholine.** A similar depolarizing block can be produced by acetylcholine itself when high local concentrations are achieved in the synaptic cleft (eg, by cholinesterase inhibitor intoxication) and by nicotine and other nicotinic agonists. However, the neuromuscular block produced by depolarizing drugs other than succinylcholine cannot be precisely controlled and is of no clinical value.

BASIC PHARMACOLOGY OF NEUROMUSCULAR BLOCKING DRUGS

Chemistry

All of the available neuromuscular blocking drugs bear a structural resemblance to acetylcholine. For example, succinylcholine is two acetylcholine molecules linked end-to-end (Figure 27–2). In contrast to the linear structure of succinylcholine and other depolarizing drugs, the nondepolarizing agents (eg, pancuronium) conceal the "double-acetylcholine" structure in one of two types of bulky, semi-rigid ring systems (see Figure 27–2).

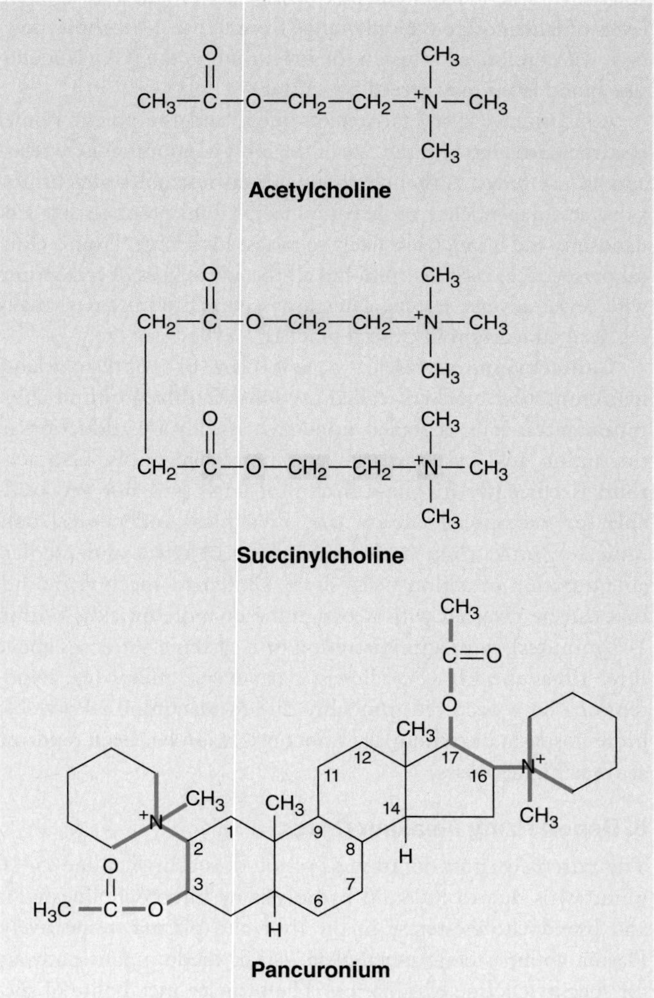

Acetylcholine

Succinylcholine

Pancuronium

FIGURE 27–2 Structural relationship of succinylcholine, a depolarizing agent, and pancuronium, a nondepolarizing agent, to acetylcholine, the neuromuscular transmitter. Succinylcholine, originally called diacetylcholine, is simply two molecules of acetylcholine linked through the acetate methyl groups. Pancuronium may be viewed as two acetylcholine-like fragments (outlined in color) oriented on a steroid nucleus.

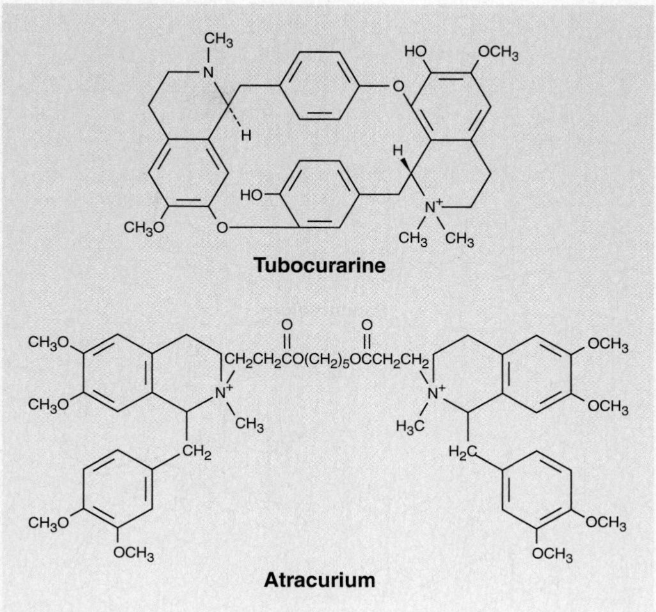

Tubocurarine

Atracurium

FIGURE 27–3 Structures of two isoquinoline neuromuscular blocking drugs. These agents are nondepolarizing muscle relaxants.

Examples of the two major families of nondepolarizing blocking drugs—the isoquinoline and steroid derivatives—are shown in Figures 27–3 and 27–4. Another feature common to all currently used neuromuscular blockers is the presence of one or two quaternary nitrogens, which makes them poorly lipid soluble and limits entry into the CNS.

Pharmacokinetics of Neuromuscular Blocking Drugs

All of the neuromuscular blocking drugs are highly polar compounds and inactive orally; they must be administered parenterally.

A. Nondepolarizing Relaxant Drugs

The rate of disappearance of a nondepolarizing neuromuscular blocking drug from the blood is characterized by a rapid initial distribution phase followed by a slower elimination phase. Neuromuscular blocking drugs are highly ionized, do not readily cross cell membranes, and are not strongly bound in peripheral tissues. Therefore, their volume of distribution (80–140 mL/kg) is only slightly larger than the blood volume.

The duration of neuromuscular blockade produced by nondepolarizing relaxants is strongly correlated with the elimination half-life. Drugs that are excreted by the kidney typically have longer half-lives, leading to longer durations of action (>35 minutes). Drugs eliminated by the liver tend to have shorter half-lives and durations of action (Table 27–1). All steroidal muscle relaxants are metabolized to their 3-hydroxy, 17-hydroxy, or 3,17-dihydroxy products in the liver. The 3-hydroxy metabolites are usually 40–80% as potent as the parent drug. Under normal circumstances, metabolites are not formed in sufficient

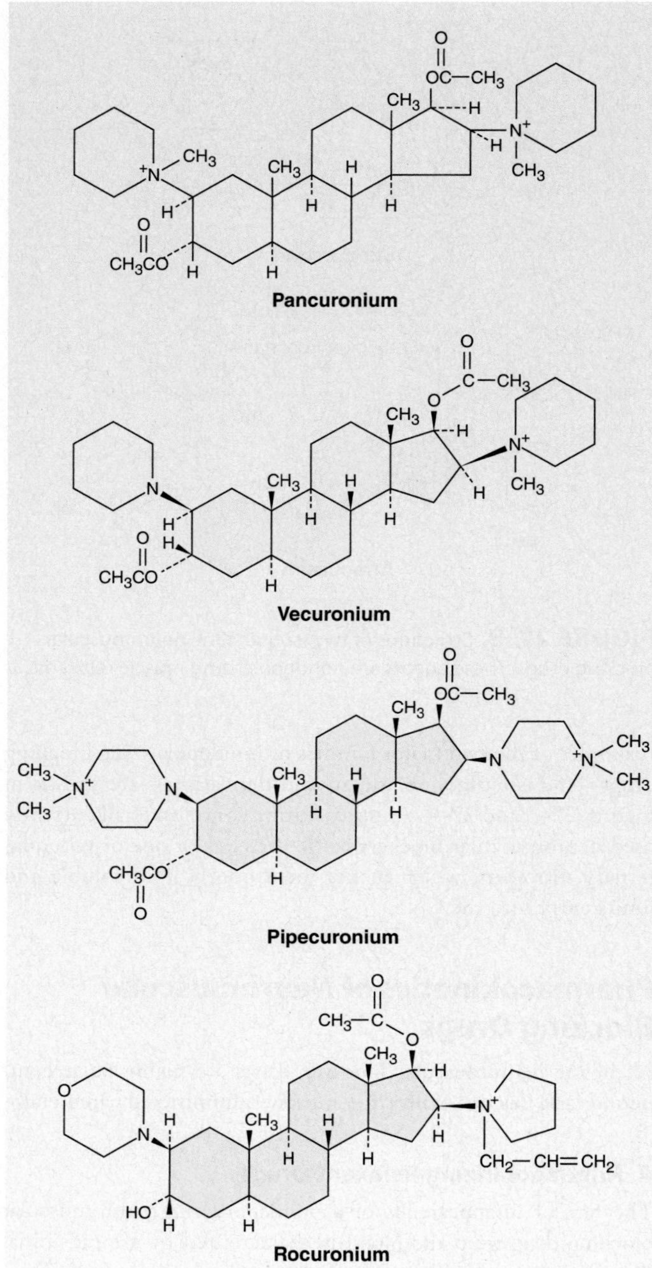

FIGURE 27–4 Structures of steroid neuromuscular blocking drugs (steroid nucleus in color). These agents are all nondepolarizing muscle relaxants.

quantities to produce a significant degree of neuromuscular blockade during or after anesthesia. However, if the parent compound is administered for several days in the ICU setting, the 3-hydroxy metabolite may accumulate and cause prolonged paralysis because it has a longer half-life than the parent compound. The remaining metabolites possess minimal neuromuscular blocking properties.

The intermediate-acting steroid muscle relaxants (eg, **vecuronium** and **rocuronium**) tend to be more dependent on biliary excretion or hepatic metabolism for their elimination. These muscle relaxants are more commonly used clinically than the long-acting steroid-based drugs (eg, **pancuronium**). The duration of action of these relaxants may be prolonged significantly in patients with impaired liver function.

Atracurium (see Figure 27–3) is an intermediate-acting isoquinoline nondepolarizing muscle relaxant that is no longer in widespread clinical use. In addition to hepatic metabolism, atracurium is inactivated by a form of spontaneous breakdown known as Hofmann elimination. The main breakdown products are laudanosine and a related quaternary acid, neither of which possesses neuromuscular blocking properties. Laudanosine is slowly metabolized by the liver and has a longer elimination half-life (ie, 150 minutes). It readily crosses the blood-brain barrier, and high blood concentrations may cause seizures and an increase in the volatile anesthetic requirement. During surgical anesthesia, blood levels of laudanosine typically range from 0.2 to 1 mcg/mL; however, with prolonged infusions of atracurium in the ICU, laudanosine blood levels may exceed 5 mcg/mL.

Atracurium has several stereoisomers, and the potent isomer **cisatracurium** has become one of the most common muscle relaxants in use today. Although cisatracurium resembles atracurium, it has less dependence on hepatic inactivation, produces less laudanosine, and is much less likely to release histamine. From a clinical perspective, cisatracurium has all the advantages of atracurium with fewer adverse effects. Therefore, cisatracurium has virtually replaced atracurium in clinical practice.

Gantacurium represents a new class of nondepolarizing neuromuscular blockers, called asymmetric mixed onium chlorofumarates. It is degraded nonenzymatically by adduction of the amino acid cysteine and ester bond hydrolysis. Gantacurium is currently in phase 3 clinical trials and not yet available for widespread clinical use. Preclinical and clinical data indicate gantacurium has a rapid onset of effect and predictable duration of action (very short, similar to succinylcholine) that can be reversed with neostigmine or more quickly (within 1–2 minutes), with administration of L-cysteine. At doses above three times the ED_{95}, cardiovascular adverse effects (eg, hypotension) have occurred, probably due to histamine release. No bronchospasm or pulmonary vasoconstriction has been reported at these higher doses.

B. Depolarizing Relaxant Drugs

The extremely short duration of action of succinylcholine (5–10 minutes) is due to its rapid hydrolysis by butyrylcholinesterase and pseudocholinesterase in the liver and plasma, respectively. Plasma cholinesterase metabolism is the predominant pathway for succinylcholine elimination. The primary metabolite of succinylcholine, succinylmonocholine, is rapidly broken down to succinic acid and choline. Because plasma cholinesterase has an enormous capacity to hydrolyze succinylcholine, only a small percentage of the original intravenous dose ever reaches the neuromuscular junction. In addition, because there is little if any plasma cholinesterase at the motor end plate, a succinylcholine-induced blockade is terminated by its diffusion away from the end plate into extracellular fluid. Therefore, the circulating levels

TABLE 27–1 Pharmacokinetic and dynamic properties of neuromuscular blocking drugs.

Drug	Elimination	Clearance (mL/kg/min)	Approximate Duration of Action (minutes)	Approximate Potency Relative to Tubocurarine
Isoquinoline derivatives				
Atracurium	Spontaneous[1]	6.6	20–35	1.5
Cisatracurium	Mostly spontaneous	5–6	25–44	1.5
Tubocurarine	Kidney (40%)	2.3–2.4	>50	1
Steroid derivatives				
Pancuronium	Kidney (80%)	1.7–1.8	>35	6
Rocuronium	Liver (75–90%) and kidney	2.9	20–35	0.8
Vecuronium	Liver (75–90%) and kidney	3–5.3	20–35	6
Depolarizing agent				
Succinylcholine	Plasma ChE[2] (100%)	>100	>8	0.4

[1]Nonenzymatic and enzymatic hydrolysis of ester bonds.

[2]Butyrylcholinesterase (pseudocholinesterase).

of plasma cholinesterase influence the duration of action of succinylcholine by determining the amount of the drug that reaches the motor end plate.

Neuromuscular blockade produced by succinylcholine can be prolonged in patients with an abnormal genetic variant of plasma cholinesterase. The ***dibucaine number*** is a measure of the ability of a patient to metabolize succinylcholine and can be used to identify at-risk patients. Under standardized test conditions, dibucaine inhibits the normal enzyme by 80% and the abnormal enzyme by only 20%. Many genetic variants of plasma cholinesterase have been identified, although the dibucaine-related variants are the most important. Given the rarity of these genetic variants, plasma cholinesterase testing is not a routine clinical procedure but may be indicated for patients with a family history of plasma cholinesterase deficiency. Another reasonable strategy is to avoid the use of succinylcholine where practical in patients with a possible family history of plasma cholinesterase deficiency.

Mechanism of Action

The interactions of drugs with the acetylcholine receptor-end plate channel have been described at the molecular level. Several modes of action of drugs on the receptor are illustrated in Figure 27–5.

A. Nondepolarizing Relaxant Drugs

All the neuromuscular blocking drugs in current use in the USA except succinylcholine are classified as nondepolarizing agents. Although it is no longer in widespread clinical use, ***d*-tubocurarine** is considered the prototype neuromuscular blocker. When small doses of nondepolarizing muscle relaxants are administered, they act predominantly at the nicotinic receptor site by competing with acetylcholine. The least potent nondepolarizing relaxants (eg, rocuronium) have the fastest onset and the shortest duration of action. In larger doses, nondepolarizing drugs can enter the pore of the ion channel (see Figure 27–5) to produce a more intense motor blockade. This action further weakens neuromuscular transmission and diminishes the ability of the acetylcholinesterase inhibitors (eg, neostigmine, edrophonium, pyridostigmine) to antagonize the effect of nondepolarizing muscle relaxants.

Nondepolarizing relaxants can also block prejunctional sodium channels. As a result of this action, muscle relaxants interfere with the mobilization of acetylcholine at the nerve ending and cause fade of evoked nerve twitch contractions (Figure 27–6 and described below). One consequence of the surmountable nature of the postsynaptic blockade produced by nondepolarizing muscle relaxants is the fact that tetanic stimulation (rapid delivery of electrical stimuli to a peripheral nerve) releases a large quantity of acetylcholine and is followed by transient posttetanic facilitation of the twitch strength (ie, relief of blockade). An important clinical consequence of this principle is the reversal of residual blockade by cholinesterase inhibitors. The characteristics of a nondepolarizing neuromuscular blockade are summarized in Table 27–2 and Figure 27–6.

B. Depolarizing Relaxant Drugs

1. *Phase I block (depolarizing)*—Succinylcholine is the only clinically useful depolarizing blocking drug. Its neuromuscular effects are like those of acetylcholine except that succinylcholine produces a longer effect at the myoneural junction. Succinylcholine reacts with the nicotinic receptor to open the channel and cause depolarization of the motor end plate, and this in turn spreads to the adjacent membranes, causing transient contractions of muscle motor units. Data from single-channel recordings indicate that depolarizing blockers can enter the channel to produce a prolonged "flickering" of the ion conductance (Figure 27–7). Because succinylcholine is not metabolized effectively at the synapse, the depolarized membranes remain depolarized and unresponsive to subsequent impulses (ie, a state of depolarizing blockade). Furthermore, because excitation-contraction coupling requires end plate repolarization ("repriming") and repetitive

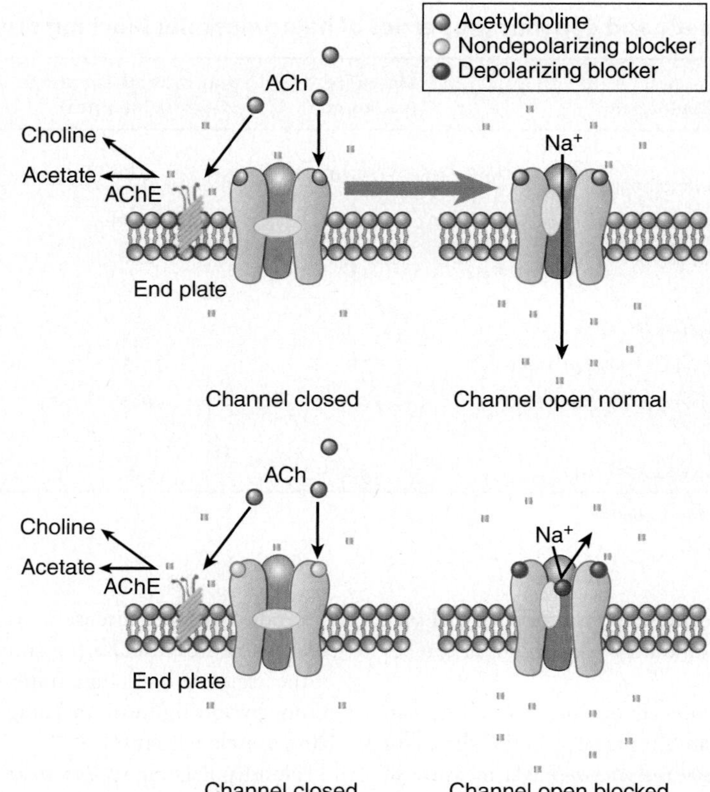

FIGURE 27–5 Schematic diagram of the interactions of drugs with the acetylcholine receptor on the end plate channel (structures are purely symbolic). **Top:** The action of the normal agonist, acetylcholine (red) in opening the channel. **Bottom, left:** A nondepolarizing blocker, eg, rocuronium (yellow), is shown as preventing the opening of the channel when it binds to the receptor. **Bottom, right:** A depolarizing blocker, eg, succinylcholine (blue), both occupying the receptor and blocking the channel. Normal closure of the channel gate is prevented, and the blocker may move rapidly in and out of the pore. Depolarizing blockers may desensitize the end plate by occupying the receptor and causing persistent depolarization. An additional effect of drugs on the end plate channel may occur through changes in the lipid environment surrounding the channel (not shown). General anesthetics and alcohols may impair neuromuscular transmission by this mechanism.

firing to maintain muscle tension, a flaccid paralysis results. In contrast to the nondepolarizing drugs, this so-called phase I (depolarizing) block is augmented, not reversed, by cholinesterase inhibitors.

The characteristics of a depolarizing neuromuscular blockade are summarized in Table 27–2 and Figure 27–6.

2. *Phase II block (desensitizing)*—With prolonged exposure to succinylcholine, the initial end plate depolarization decreases, and the membrane becomes repolarized. Despite this repolarization, the membrane cannot easily be depolarized again because it is *desensitized.* The mechanism for this desensitizing phase is unclear, but some evidence indicates that channel block may become more important than agonist action at the receptor in phase II of succinylcholine's neuromuscular blocking action. Regardless of the mechanism, the channels behave as if they are in a prolonged closed state (see Figure 27–6). Later in phase II, the characteristics of the blockade are nearly identical to those of a nondepolarizing block (ie, a nonsustained twitch response to a tetanic stimulus) (see Figure 27–6), with possible reversal by acetylcholinesterase inhibitors.

■ CLINICAL PHARMACOLOGY OF NEUROMUSCULAR BLOCKING DRUGS

Skeletal Muscle Paralysis

Before the introduction of neuromuscular blocking drugs, profound skeletal muscle relaxation for intracavitary operations could be achieved only by producing levels of volatile (inhaled) anesthesia deep enough to produce profound depressant effects on the cardiovascular and respiratory systems. The adjunctive use of neuromuscular blocking drugs makes it possible to achieve adequate muscle relaxation for all types of surgical procedures without the cardiorespiratory depressant effects produced by deep anesthesia.

Assessment of Neuromuscular Transmission

Monitoring the effect of muscle relaxants during surgery (and recovery following the administration of cholinesterase

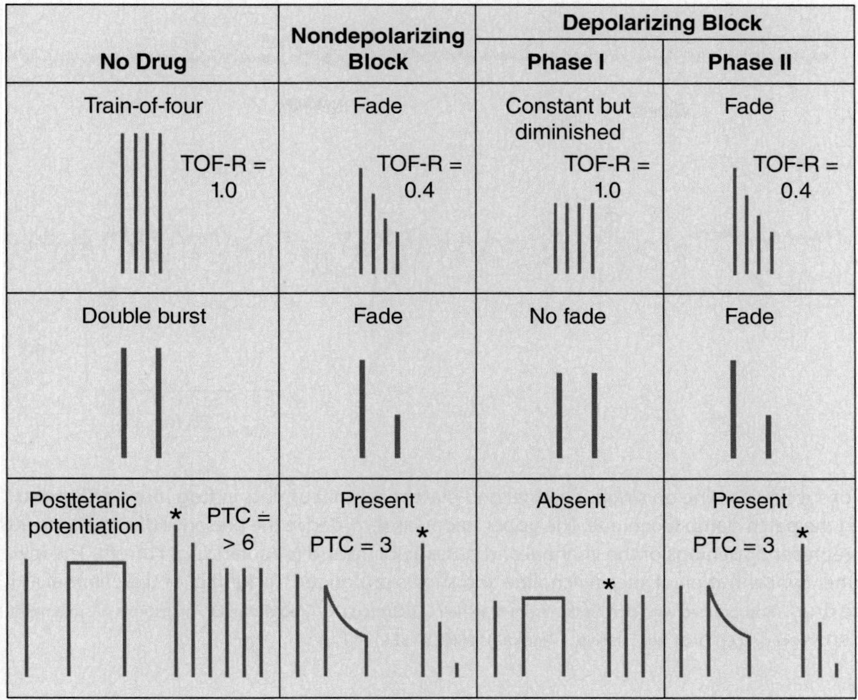

FIGURE 27–6 Muscle contraction responses to different patterns of nerve stimulation used in monitoring skeletal muscle relaxation. The alterations produced by a nondepolarizing blocker and depolarizing and desensitizing blockade by succinylcholine are shown. In the train-of-four (TOF) pattern, four stimuli are applied at 2 Hz. The TOF ratio (TOF-R) is calculated from the strength of the fourth contraction divided by that of the first. In the double-burst pattern, three stimuli are applied at 50 Hz, followed by a 700 ms rest period and then repeated. In the posttetanic potentiation pattern, several seconds of 50 Hz stimulation are applied, followed by several seconds of rest and then by single stimuli at a slow rate (eg, 0.5 Hz). The number of detectable posttetanic twitches is the posttetanic count (PTC),* first posttetanic contraction.

inhibitors) typically involves the use of a device that produces transdermal electrical stimulation of one of the peripheral nerves to the hand or facial muscles and recording of the evoked contractions (ie, twitch responses). The motor responses to different patterns of peripheral nerve stimulation can be recorded in the operating room during the procedure (see Figure 27–6). The standard approach for monitoring the clinical effects of muscle relaxants during surgery uses peripheral nerve stimulation to elicit motor responses, which are visually observed by the anesthesiologist. The three most commonly used patterns include (1) single-twitch stimulation, (2) train-of-four (TOF) stimulation, and (3) tetanic stimulation. Two other modalities are also available to monitor neuromuscular transmission: double-burst stimulation and posttetanic count.

TABLE 27–2 Comparison of a typical nondepolarizing muscle relaxant (rocuronium) and a depolarizing muscle relaxant (succinylcholine).

		Succinylcholine	
	Rocuronium	**Phase I**	**Phase II**
Administration of tubocurarine	Additive	Antagonistic	Augmented[1]
Administration of succinylcholine	Antagonistic	Additive	Augmented[1]
Effect of neostigmine	Antagonistic	Augmented[1]	Antagonistic
Initial excitatory effect on skeletal muscle	None	Fasciculations	None
Response to a tetanic stimulus	Unsustained (fade)	Sustained[2] (no fade)	Unsustained (fade)
Posttetanic facilitation	Yes	No	Yes
Rate of recovery	30–60 min[3]	4–8 min	>20 min[3]

[1]It is not known whether this interaction is additive or synergistic (super additive).

[2]The amplitude is decreased, but the response is sustained.

[3]The rate depends on the dose and on the completeness of neuromuscular blockade.

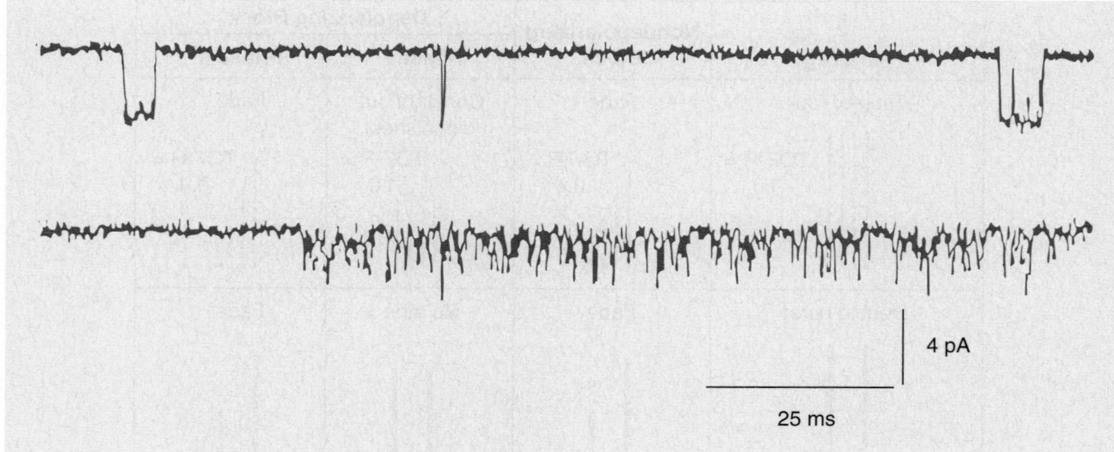

FIGURE 27–7 Action of succinylcholine on single-channel end plate receptor currents in frog muscle. Currents through a single AChR channel were recorded using the patch clamp technique. The upper trace was recorded in the presence of a low concentration of succinylcholine; the downward deflections represent openings of the channel and passage of inward (depolarizing) current. The lower trace was recorded in the presence of a much higher concentration of succinylcholine and shows prolonged "flickering" of the channel as it repetitively opens and closes or is "plugged" by the drug. (Reproduced with permission from Marshall CG, Ogden DC, Colquhoun D. The actions of suxamethonium (succinyldicholine) as an agonist and channel blocker at the nicotinic receptor of frog muscle. J Physiol. 1990;428:155–174.)

With single-twitch stimulation, a single supramaximal electrical stimulus is applied to a peripheral nerve at frequencies from 0.1 Hz to 1.0 Hz. The higher frequency is often used during induction and reversal to more accurately determine the peak (maximal) drug effect. TOF stimulation involves four successive supramaximal stimuli given at intervals of 0.5 second (2 Hz). Each stimulus in the TOF causes the muscle to contract, and the relative magnitude of the response of the fourth twitch compared with the first twitch is the TOF ratio. With a depolarizing block, all four twitches are reduced in a dose-related fashion. With a nondepolarizing block, the TOF ratio decreases ("fades") and is inversely proportional to the degree of blockade. During recovery from nondepolarizing block, the amount of fade decreases and the TOF ratio approaches 1.0. Recovery to a TOF ratio greater than 0.7 is typically necessary for resumption of spontaneous ventilation. However, complete clinical recovery from a nondepolarizing block is considered to require a TOF greater than 0.9. Fade in the TOF response after administration of succinylcholine signifies the development of a phase II block.

Tetanic stimulation consists of a very rapid (30–100 Hz) delivery of electrical stimuli for several seconds. During a nondepolarizing neuromuscular block (and a phase II block after succinylcholine), the response is not sustained, and fade of the twitch responses is observed. Fade in response to tetanic stimulation is normally considered a presynaptic event. However, the degree of fade depends primarily on the degree of neuromuscular blockade. During a partial nondepolarizing blockade, tetanic nerve stimulation is followed by an increase in the posttetanic twitch response, so-called *posttetanic facilitation* of neuromuscular transmission. During intense neuromuscular blockade, there is no response to either tetanic or posttetanic stimulation. As the intensity of the block diminishes, the response to posttetanic twitch stimulation reappears. The reappearance of the first response to twitch stimulation after tetanic stimulation reflects the duration of profound (clinical) neuromuscular blockade. To determine the posttetanic count, 5 seconds of 50 Hz tetany is applied, followed by 3 seconds of rest, followed by 1 Hz pulses for about 10 seconds (10 pulses). The counted number of muscle twitches provides an estimation of the depth of blockade. For instance, a posttetanic count of 2 suggests no twitch response (by TOF) for about 20–30 minutes, and a posttetanic count of 5 correlates to a no-twitch response (by TOF) of about 10–15 minutes (see Figure 27–6, bottom panel).

The double-burst stimulation pattern is another mode of electrical nerve stimulation developed with the goal of allowing for manual detection of residual neuromuscular blockade when it is not possible to record the responses to single-twitch, TOF, or tetanic stimulation. In this pattern, three nerve stimuli are delivered at 50 Hz followed by a 700 ms rest period and then by two or three additional stimuli at 50 Hz. It is easier to detect fade in the responses to double-burst stimulation than to TOF stimulation. The absence of fade in response to double-burst stimulation implies that clinically significant residual neuromuscular blockade does not exist.

A more quantitative approach to neuromuscular monitoring involves monitoring using a force transducer for measuring the evoked response (ie, movement) of the thumb to TOF stimulation over the ulnar nerve at the wrist. This device has the advantage of being integrated in the anesthesia machine and also provides a more accurate graphic display of the percentage of fade to TOF stimulation.

A. Nondepolarizing Relaxant Drugs

During anesthesia, administration of tubocurarine, 0.1–0.4 mg/kg IV, initially causes motor weakness, followed by the skeletal muscles becoming flaccid and inexcitable to electrical stimulation (Figure 27–8). In general, larger muscles (eg, abdominal, trunk, paraspinous, diaphragm) are more resistant to neuromuscular blockade and recover more rapidly than smaller muscles (eg, facial, foot,

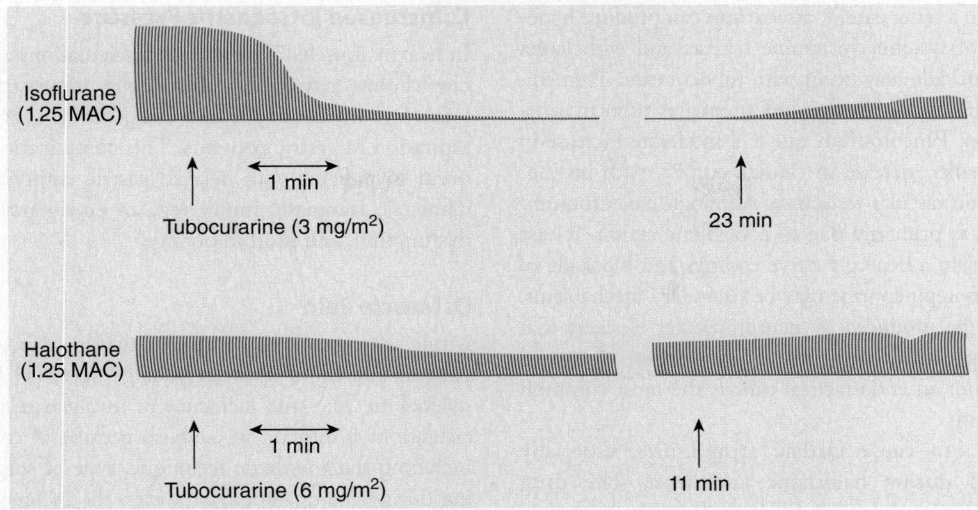

FIGURE 27–8 Neuromuscular blockade from tubocurarine during equivalent levels of isoflurane and halothane anesthesia in patients. Note that isoflurane augments the block far more than does halothane. MAC, minimal alveolar concentration.

hand). The diaphragm is usually the last muscle to be paralyzed. Assuming that ventilation is adequately maintained, no adverse effects occur with skeletal muscle paralysis. When administration of muscle relaxants is discontinued, recovery of muscles usually occurs in reverse order, with the diaphragm regaining function first. The pharmacologic effect of tubocurarine, 0.3 mg/kg IV, usually lasts 45–60 minutes. However, subtle evidence of residual muscle paralysis detected using a neuromuscular monitor may last for another hour, increasing the likelihood of adverse outcomes, eg, aspiration and decreased hypoxic drive. Potency and duration of action of the other nondepolarizing drugs are shown in Table 27–1. In addition to the duration of action, the most important property distinguishing the nondepolarizing relaxants is the time to onset of the blocking effect, which determines how rapidly the patient's trachea can be intubated. Of the currently available nondepolarizing drugs, rocuronium has the most rapid onset time (60–120 seconds).

B. Depolarizing Relaxant Drugs

Following the administration of succinylcholine, 0.75–1.5 mg/kg IV, transient muscle fasciculations occur over the chest and abdomen within 30 seconds, although general anesthesia and the prior administration of a small dose of a nondepolarizing muscle relaxant tend to attenuate them. As paralysis develops rapidly (<90 seconds), the arm, neck, and leg muscles are initially relaxed followed by the respiratory muscles. As a result of succinylcholine's rapid hydrolysis by cholinesterase in the plasma (and liver), the neuromuscular block typically lasts less than 10 minutes (see Table 27–1).

Cardiovascular Effects

Vecuronium, cisatracurium, and rocuronium have minimal, if any, cardiovascular effects. The other nondepolarizing muscle relaxants (ie, pancuronium and atracurium) produce cardiovascular effects that are mediated by autonomic or histamine receptors (Table 27–3).

TABLE 27–3 Effects of neuromuscular blocking drugs on other tissues.

Drug	Effect on Autonomic Ganglia	Effect on Cardiac Muscarinic Receptors	Tendency to Cause Histamine Release
Isoquinoline derivatives			
Atracurium	None	None	Slight
Cisatracurium	None	None	None
Tubocurarine	Weak block	None	Moderate
Steroid derivatives			
Pancuronium	None	Moderate block	None
Rocuronium[1]	None	Slight	None
Vecuronium	None	None	None
Other agents			
Gallamine	None	Strong block	None
Succinylcholine	Stimulation	Stimulation	Slight

[1]Allergic reactions have been reported.

Tubocurarine and, to a lesser extent, atracurium can produce hypotension as a result of systemic histamine release, and with larger doses, ganglionic blockade may occur with tubocurarine. Premedication with an antihistaminic compound attenuates tubocurarine-induced hypotension. Pancuronium causes a moderate increase in heart rate and a smaller increase in cardiac output, with little or no change in systemic vascular resistance. Although pancuronium-induced tachycardia is primarily due to a vagolytic action, release of norepinephrine from adrenergic nerve endings and blockade of neuronal uptake of norepinephrine may be secondary mechanisms. Bronchospasm may be produced by neuromuscular blockers that release histamine (eg, atracurium), but after induction of general anesthesia, insertion of an endotracheal tube is the most common cause of bronchospasm.

Succinylcholine can cause cardiac arrhythmias, especially when administered during halothane anesthesia. The drug stimulates autonomic cholinoceptors, including the nicotinic receptors at both sympathetic and parasympathetic ganglia and muscarinic receptors in the heart (eg, sinus node). The negative inotropic and chronotropic responses to succinylcholine can be attenuated by administration of an anticholinergic drug (eg, glycopyrrolate, atropine). With large doses of succinylcholine, positive inotropic and chronotropic effects may be observed. On the other hand, bradycardia has been repeatedly observed when a second dose of succinylcholine is given less than 5 minutes after the initial dose. This transient bradycardia can be prevented by thiopental, atropine, and ganglionic-blocking drugs, and by pretreating with a small dose of a nondepolarizing muscle relaxant (eg, rocuronium). Direct myocardial effects, increased muscarinic stimulation, and ganglionic stimulation contribute to this bradycardic response.

Other Adverse Effects of Depolarizing Blockade

A. Hyperkalemia

Patients with burns, nerve damage or neuromuscular disease, closed head injury, and other trauma may develop proliferation of extrajunctional acetylcholine receptors. During administration of succinylcholine, potassium is released from muscles, likely due to fasciculations. If the proliferation of extrajunctional receptors is great enough, sufficient potassium may be released to result in cardiac arrest. The exact time course of receptor proliferation is unknown; therefore, it is best to avoid the use of succinylcholine in these cases.

B. Increased Intraocular Pressure

Administration of succinylcholine may be associated with the rapid onset of an increase in intraocular pressure (<60 seconds), peaking at 2–4 minutes, and declining after 5 minutes. The mechanism may involve tonic contraction of myofibrils or transient dilation of ocular choroidal blood vessels. Despite the increase in intraocular pressure, the use of succinylcholine for ophthalmologic operations is not contraindicated unless the anterior chamber is open ("open globe") due to trauma.

C. Increased Intragastric Pressure

In heavily muscled patients, the fasciculations associated with succinylcholine may cause an increase in intragastric pressure ranging from 5 to 40 cm H_2O, increasing the risk for regurgitation and aspiration of gastric contents. This complication is more likely to occur in patients with delayed gastric emptying (eg, those with diabetes), traumatic injury (eg, an emergency case), esophageal dysfunction, and morbid obesity.

D. Muscle Pain

Myalgias are a common postoperative complaint of heavily muscled patients and those who receive large doses (>1.5 mg/kg) of succinylcholine. The true incidence of myalgias related to muscle fasciculations is difficult to establish because of confounding factors, including the anesthetic technique, type of surgery, and positioning during the operation. However, the incidence of myalgias has been reported to vary from less than 1% to 20%. It occurs more frequently in ambulatory than in bedridden patients. The pain is thought to be secondary to the unsynchronized contractions of adjacent muscle fibers just before the onset of paralysis. However, there is controversy over whether the incidence of muscle pain following succinylcholine is actually higher than with nondepolarizing muscle relaxants when other potentially confounding factors are taken into consideration.

Interactions with Other Drugs

A. Anesthetics

Inhaled (volatile) anesthetics potentiate the neuromuscular blockade produced by nondepolarizing muscle relaxants in a dose-dependent fashion. Of the general anesthetics that have been studied, inhaled anesthetics augment the effects of muscle relaxants in the following order: isoflurane (most), sevoflurane, desflurane, halothane, and nitrous oxide (least) (see Figure 27–8). The most important factors involved in this interaction are the following: (1) nervous system depression at sites proximal to the neuromuscular junction (ie, CNS); (2) increased muscle blood flow (ie, due to peripheral vasodilation produced by volatile anesthetics), which allows a larger fraction of the injected muscle relaxant to reach the neuromuscular junction; and (3) decreased sensitivity of the postjunctional membrane to depolarization.

A rare interaction of succinylcholine with volatile anesthetics results in **malignant hyperthermia,** a condition caused by abnormal release of calcium from stores in skeletal muscle. This condition is treated with dantrolene and is discussed below under Spasmolytic & Antispasmodic Drugs and in Chapter 16.

B. Antibiotics

Numerous reports have described enhancement of neuromuscular blockade by antibiotics (eg, aminoglycosides). Many of the antibiotics have been shown to cause a depression of evoked release of acetylcholine similar to that caused by administering magnesium. The mechanism of this prejunctional effect appears to be blockade of specific P-type calcium channels in the motor nerve terminal.

C. Local Anesthetics and Antiarrhythmic Drugs

In small doses, local anesthetics can depress posttetanic potentiation via a prejunctional neural effect. In large doses, local anesthetics can block neuromuscular transmission. With these higher doses, local anesthetics block acetylcholine-induced muscle contractions as a result of blockade of the nicotinic receptor ion channels. Experimentally, similar effects can be demonstrated with sodium channel-blocking antiarrhythmic drugs such as quinidine. However, at the doses used for cardiac arrhythmias, this interaction is of little or no clinical significance. Higher doses of bupivacaine have been associated with cardiac arrhythmias independent of the muscle relaxant used.

D. Other Neuromuscular Blocking Drugs

The end plate-depolarizing effect of succinylcholine can be antagonized by administering a small dose of a nondepolarizing blocker. To prevent the fasciculations associated with succinylcholine administration, a small nonparalyzing dose of a nondepolarizing drug can be given before succinylcholine (eg, *d*-tubocurarine, 2 mg IV, or pancuronium, 0.5 mg IV). Although this dose usually reduces fasciculations and postoperative myalgias, it can increase the amount of succinylcholine required for relaxation by 50–90% and can produce a feeling of weakness in awake patients. Therefore, "pre-curarization" before succinylcholine is no longer widely practiced.

Effects of Diseases & Aging on the Neuromuscular Response

Several diseases can diminish or augment the neuromuscular blockade produced by nondepolarizing muscle relaxants. Myasthenia gravis enhances the neuromuscular blockade produced by these drugs. Advanced age is associated with a prolonged duration of action from nondepolarizing relaxants as a result of decreased clearance of the drugs by the liver and kidneys. As a result, the dosage of neuromuscular blocking drugs should be reduced in older patients (>70 years).

Conversely, patients with severe burns and those with upper motor neuron disease are resistant to nondepolarizing muscle relaxants. This desensitization is probably caused by proliferation of extrajunctional receptors, which results in an increased dose requirement for the nondepolarizing relaxant to block a sufficient number of receptors.

Reversal of Nondepolarizing Neuromuscular Blockade

The cholinesterase inhibitors effectively antagonize the neuromuscular blockade caused by nondepolarizing drugs. Their general pharmacology is discussed in Chapter 7. **Neostigmine** and **pyridostigmine** antagonize nondepolarizing neuromuscular blockade by increasing the availability of acetylcholine at the motor end plate, mainly by inhibition of acetylcholinesterase. To a lesser extent, these cholinesterase inhibitors also increase the release of this transmitter from the motor nerve terminal. In contrast, **edrophonium** antagonizes neuromuscular blockade purely by inhibiting acetylcholinesterase activity. Edrophonium has a more rapid onset of action but may be less effective than neostigmine in reversing the effects of nondepolarizing blockers in the presence of profound neuromuscular blockade. These differences are important in determining recovery from *residual block*, the neuromuscular blockade remaining after completion of surgery and movement of the patient to the recovery room. Unsuspected residual block may result in hypoventilation, leading to hypoxia and even apnea, especially if patients have received central depressant medications in the early recovery period.

Sugammadex is a reversal agent approved for rapid reversal of the steroid neuromuscular blocking agents rocuronium and vecuronium. Although it has been in clinical use in Europe since 2008, its approval in the USA was delayed because of concerns that it causes a low incidence of anaphylaxis and hypersensitivity reactions. Sugammadex is a modified g-cyclodextrin (a large ring structure with 16 polar hydroxyl groups facing inward and 8 polar carboxyl groups facing outward) that binds tightly to rocuronium in a 1:1 ratio. By binding to plasma rocuronium, sugammadex decreases the free plasma concentration and establishes a concentration gradient for rocuronium to diffuse away from the neuromuscular junction back into the circulation, where it is quickly bound by free sugammadex.

Currently, three dose ranges are recommended for sugammadex: 2 mg/kg to reverse shallow neuromuscular blockade (spontaneous recovery has reached the second twitch in TOF stimulation), 4 mg/kg to reverse deeper blockade (1–2 posttetanic count and no response to TOF stimulation), and 16 mg/kg for immediate reversal following administration of a single dose of 1.2 mg/kg of rocuronium. In patients with normal renal function (defined as a creatinine clearance [CrCl] > 80 mL/min), the sugammadex-rocuronium complex is typically excreted unchanged in the urine within 24 hours. In patients with renal insufficiency, complete urinary elimination may take much longer. The plasma half-life of sugammadex in patients with renal impairment increases significantly as CrCl is reduced. In mild to moderate renal insufficiency (CrCl between 30 and 80 mL/min), the half-life varies between 4 and 6 hours. This increases dramatically in patients with severe renal impairment (CrCl > 30 mL/min), in whom the half-life is extended to 19 hours. The ability to dialyze sugammadex is variable, although some studies have demonstrated the ability to dialyze it using a high-flux method. Therefore, sugammadex is not recommended for use in patients with severe renal impairment unless absolutely necessary.

Sugammadex is associated with a few significant adverse reactions. Most importantly, sugammadex may cause anaphylaxis, which occurred in 0.3% of patients who received the 16 mg/kg dose in the US Food and Drug Administration (FDA) studies. Hypersensitivity reactions, such as nausea, pruritus, and urticaria, are more common than anaphylaxis, and also occur more frequently with higher doses of sugammadex. Other significant adverse reactions include marked bradycardia that may progress to cardiac arrest within minutes of administration and coagulopathy, with an approximately 25% elevation of activated partial thromboplastin time and prothrombin time/international normalized ratio values that may last up to 1 hour.

Because sugammadex binds the steroidal neuromuscular blocking agents rocuronium and vecuronium, it is not surprising that it can also block other steroidal drugs. The two most important of these drugs are progesterone-based contraceptives and the selective estrogen receptor modulator toremifene. When sugammadex is administered to a woman who is taking hormonal contraceptives that contain progesterone, the progesterone may be bound by sugammadex, and the efficacy of the contraceptive is decreased as if the woman missed one or two doses. The manufacturer recommends that an alternative nonhormonal contraceptive be used for 7 days following sugammadex administration. Sugammadex also very tightly binds toremifene, which may be used to treat metastatic breast cancer (see Chapter 40). Not only will the efficacy of toremifene be reduced, but displacement of rocuronium from sugammadex may result, and prolonged neuromuscular blockade could occur.

Uses of Neuromuscular Blocking Drugs

A. Surgical Relaxation

One of the most important applications of the neuromuscular blockers is in facilitating intracavitary surgery, especially in intra-abdominal and intrathoracic procedures.

B. Endotracheal Intubation

By relaxing the pharyngeal and laryngeal muscles, neuromuscular blocking drugs facilitate laryngoscopy and placement of an endotracheal tube. Endotracheal tube placement ensures an adequate airway and minimizes the risk of pulmonary aspiration during general anesthesia.

C. Control of Ventilation

In critically ill patients who have ventilatory failure from various causes (eg, severe bronchospasm, pneumonia, chronic obstructive airway disease), it may be necessary to control ventilation to provide adequate gas exchange and to prevent atelectasis. In the ICU, neuromuscular blocking drugs are frequently administered to reduce chest wall resistance (ie, improve thoracic compliance), decrease oxygen utilization, and improve ventilator synchrony.

D. Treatment of Convulsions

Neuromuscular blocking drugs (ie, succinylcholine) are occasionally used to attenuate the peripheral (motor) manifestations of convulsions associated with status epilepticus, local anesthetic toxicity, or electroconvulsive therapy. Although this approach is effective in eliminating the muscular manifestations of the seizures, it has no effect on the central processes because neuromuscular blocking drugs do not cross the blood-brain barrier.

SPASMOLYTIC & ANTISPASMODIC DRUGS

Skeletal muscle relaxants include neuromuscular blockers, spasmolytics, and antispasmodics. Spasmolytics and antispasmodics are used to treat two conditions: spasms from peripheral musculoskeletal conditions (antispasmodics) and spasticity from upper motor neuron lesions (spasmolytics).

Spasticity presents as intermittent or sustained involuntary contraction of skeletal muscle, causing stiffness that interferes with mobility and speech. It is characterized by an increase in tonic stretch reflexes and flexor muscle spasms (ie, increased basal muscle tone) together with muscle weakness. It is often associated with spinal injury, cerebral palsy, multiple sclerosis, and stroke. The mechanisms underlying clinical spasticity appear to involve not only the stretch reflex arc itself but also higher centers in the CNS, with damage to descending pathways in the spinal cord resulting in hyperexcitability of the alpha motor neurons in the cord. The important components involved in these processes are shown in Figure 27–9. Pharmacologic therapy may ameliorate some of the symptoms of spasticity by modifying the stretch reflex arc or by interfering directly with skeletal muscle (ie, excitation-contraction coupling).

Drugs that modify the reflex arc may modulate excitatory or inhibitory synapses (see Chapter 21). Thus, to reduce the hyperactive stretch reflex, it is desirable to reduce the activity of the Ia fibers that excite the primary motor neuron or to enhance the activity of the inhibitory internuncial neurons. These structures are shown in greater detail in Figure 27–10.

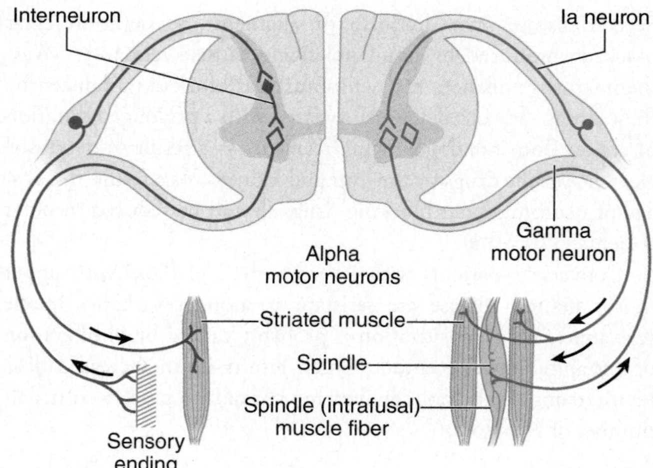

FIGURE 27–9 Schematic illustration of the structures involved in the stretch reflex (right half) showing innervation of extrafusal (striated muscle) fibers by alpha motor neurons and of intrafusal fibers (within muscle spindle) by gamma motor neurons. The left half of the diagram shows an inhibitory reflex arc, which includes an intercalated inhibitory interneuron. (Reproduced with permission from Waxman SG: *Clinical Neuroanatomy*, 26th ed. New York, NY: McGraw Hill; 2009.)

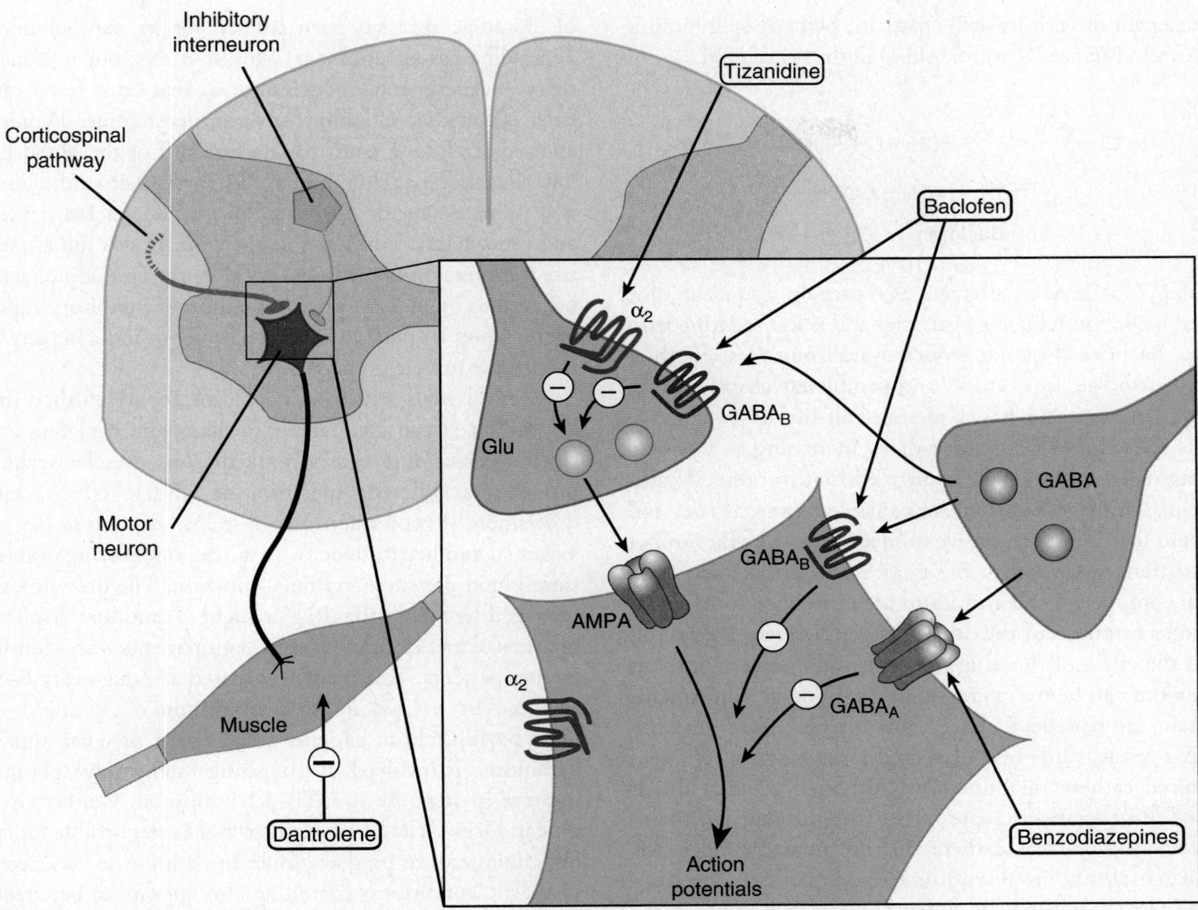

FIGURE 27–10 Postulated sites of spasmolytic action of tizanidine (α_2), benzodiazepines ($GABA_A$), and baclofen ($GABA_B$) in the spinal cord. Tizanidine may also have a postsynaptic inhibitory effect. Dantrolene acts on the sarcoplasmic reticulum in skeletal muscle. Glu, glutamatergic neuron.

A variety of pharmacologic agents described as depressants of the spinal "polysynaptic" reflex arc (eg, barbiturates [phenobarbital] and glycerol ethers [mephenesin]) have been used to treat these conditions of excess skeletal muscle tone. However, as illustrated in Figure 27–10, nonspecific depression of synapses involved in the stretch reflex could reduce the desired GABAergic inhibitory activity, as well as the excitatory glutamatergic transmission. Currently available drugs can provide significant relief from painful muscle spasms, but they are less effective in improving meaningful function (eg, mobility and return to work).

Diazepam

As described in Chapter 22, benzodiazepines facilitate the action of GABA in the CNS. Diazepam acts at $GABA_A$ synapses, and its action in reducing spasticity is at least partly mediated in the spinal cord because it is somewhat effective in patients with cord transection. Although diazepam can be used in patients with muscle spasm of almost any origin (including local muscle trauma), it also produces sedation at the doses required to reduce muscle tone. The initial dosage is 4 mg/d, and it is gradually increased to a maximum of 60 mg/d. Other benzodiazepines have been used as spasmolytics (eg, midazolam), but clinical experience with them is limited.

Meprobamate and carisoprodol are sedatives that have been used as central muscle relaxants, although evidence for their efficacy without sedation is lacking. Carisoprodol is a schedule IV drug; it is metabolized to meprobamate, which is also a schedule IV drug. Withdrawal of carisoprodol and meprobamate after extensive use elicits physical withdrawal, with anxiety, tremors, muscle twitching, insomnia, and auditory and visual hallucinations.

Baclofen

Baclofen (*p*-chlorophenyl-GABA) was designed to be an orally active GABA-mimetic agent and is an agonist at $GABA_B$ receptors. Activation of these receptors by baclofen results in hyperpolarization by three distinct actions: (1) closure of presynaptic calcium channels, (2) increased postsynaptic K^+ conductance, and (3) inhibition of dendritic calcium influx channels. Through reduced release of excitatory transmitters in both the brain and the spinal cord, baclofen suppresses activity of Ia sensory afferents, spinal interneurons, and motor neurons (see Figure 27–10). Baclofen may also reduce pain in patients with spasticity, perhaps by inhibiting the release of substance P (neurokinin 1) in the spinal cord.

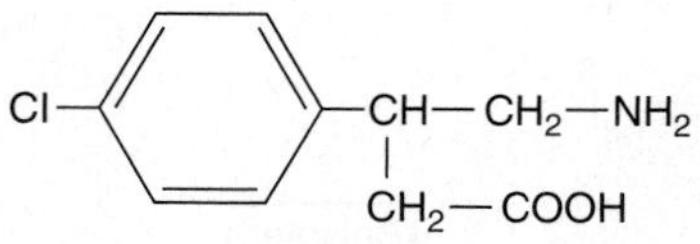

Cl— C_6H_4 —CH— CH_2—NH_2
|
CH_2—COOH

Baclofen

Baclofen is at least as effective as diazepam and tizanidine (discussed below) in reducing spasticity and is less sedating than diazepam. Baclofen does not reduce overall muscle strength as much as dantrolene. It is rapidly and completely absorbed after oral administration and has a plasma half-life of 3–4 hours. Dosage is started at 15 mg twice daily, increasing as tolerated to 100 mg daily. Studies have confirmed that intrathecal catheter administration of baclofen can control severe spasticity and muscle pain that is not responsive to medication by other routes of administration. Owing to the poor egress of baclofen from the spinal cord, peripheral symptoms are rare. Therefore, higher central concentrations of the drug may be tolerated. Partial tolerance to the effect of the drug may occur after several months of therapy but can be overcome by upward dosage adjustments to maintain the beneficial effect. This tolerance was not confirmed in a recent study and decreased response may represent unrecognized catheter malfunctions. Although a major disadvantage of this therapeutic approach is the difficulty of maintaining the drug delivery catheter in the subarachnoid space, risking an acute withdrawal syndrome upon treatment interruption, long-term intrathecal baclofen therapy can improve the quality of life for patients with severe spastic disorders. Adverse effects of high-dose baclofen include excessive somnolence, respiratory depression, and coma. Patients can become tolerant to the sedative effect with chronic administration. Increased seizure activity has been reported in epileptic patients. Withdrawal from baclofen must be done very slowly. Baclofen should be used with caution during pregnancy; although there are no reports of baclofen directly causing human fetal malformations, animal studies using high doses show that it causes impaired sternal ossification and omphalocele.

Oral baclofen has been studied in many other medical conditions, including patients with intractable low back pain, stiff person syndrome, trigeminal neuralgia, cluster headache, intractable hiccups, tic disorder, gastroesophageal reflux disease, and cravings for alcohol, nicotine, and cocaine (see Chapter 32). Efficacy of oral baclofen has not been established in patients with stroke, Parkinson disease, or cerebral palsy.

TIZANIDINE

As noted in Chapter 11, α_2-adrenoceptor agonists such as clonidine and other imidazoline compounds have a variety of effects on the CNS that are not fully understood. Among these effects is the ability to reduce muscle spasm. Tizanidine is a congener of clonidine that has been studied for its spasmolytic actions. Tizanidine has significant α_2-agonist effects, but it reduces spasticity in experimental models at doses that cause fewer cardiovascular effects than clonidine or dexmedetomidine. Tizanidine has approximately one tenth to one fifteenth of the blood pressure-lowering effects of clonidine. Neurophysiologic studies in animals and humans suggest that tizanidine reinforces both presynaptic and postsynaptic inhibition in the cord. It also inhibits nociceptive transmission in the spinal dorsal horn. Tizanidine's actions are believed to be mediated via restoration of inhibitory suppression of the group II spinal interneurons without inducing any changes in intrinsic muscle properties.

Clinical trials with oral tizanidine report efficacy in relieving muscle spasm comparable to diazepam, baclofen, and dantrolene. Tizanidine causes markedly less muscle weakness but produces a different spectrum of adverse effects, including drowsiness, hypotension in 16–33%, dizziness, dry mouth, asthenia, and hepatotoxicity, requiring monitoring of liver function, blood pressure, and renal function. The drowsiness can be managed by taking the drug at night. Tizanidine displays linear pharmacokinetics, and dosage requirements vary considerably among patients. Treatment is initiated at 2 mg every 6–8 hours and can be titrated up to a maximum of 36 mg/d. Dosage must be adjusted in patients with hepatic or renal impairment. Tizanidine is involved in drug-drug interactions; plasma levels increase in response to CYP1A2 inhibition. Conversely, tizanidine induces CYP11A1 activity, which is responsible for converting cholesterol to pregnenolone. In addition to its effectiveness in spastic conditions, tizanidine also appears to be effective for management of chronic migraine. Abrupt withdrawal should be avoided because it results in rebound hypertension, tachycardia, and increased spasms.

OTHER CENTRALLY ACTING SPASMOLYTIC DRUGS

Gabapentin is an antiepileptic drug (see Chapter 24) that has shown considerable promise as a spasmolytic agent in several studies involving patients with multiple sclerosis. Pregabalin is a newer analog of gabapentin that may also prove useful in relieving painful disorders that involve a muscle spasm component. Progabide and glycine have also been found in preliminary studies to reduce spasticity. Progabide is a $GABA_A$ and $GABA_B$ agonist and has active metabolites, including GABA itself. Glycine is another inhibitory amino acid neurotransmitter (see Chapter 21) that appears to possess pharmacologic activity when given orally and readily passes the blood-brain barrier. Idrocilamide and riluzole are newer drugs for the treatment of amyotrophic lateral sclerosis (ALS) that appear to have spasm-reducing effects, possibly through inhibition of glutamatergic transmission in the CNS, although several other mechanisms have been proposed—such as stabilizing the inactivated state of voltage-dependent sodium channels.

BOTULINUM TOXIN

The therapeutic use of botulinum toxin (BoNT) for ophthalmic purposes and for local muscle spasm was mentioned in Chapter 6. This neurotoxin produces chemodenervation and local paralysis when injected into a muscle. Seven immunologically distinct toxins share homologous subunits. The single-chain polypeptide BoNT has little activity until it is cleaved into a heavy chain (100 kDa) and a light chain (50 kDa). The light chain, a zinc-dependent protease, prevents release of acetylcholine by interfering with vesicle fusion, through proteolytically cleaving SNAP*-25 (BoNT-A, BoNT-E) or synaptobrevin-2 (BoNT-B, BoNT-D, BoNT-F). Local facial injections of botulinum toxin are widely used for the short-term treatment (1–3 months per treatment) of wrinkles associated with aging around the eyes and mouth. Local injection of botulinum toxin has also become a useful treatment for generalized spastic disorders (eg, cerebral palsy). Most clinical studies to date have involved administration in one or two limbs, and the benefits appear to persist for weeks to several months after a single treatment. BoNT has virtually replaced anticholinergic medications used in the treatment of dystonia. More recently, FDA approval was granted for treatment of incontinence due to overactive bladder and for chronic migraine. Most studies have used several formulations of type A BoNT, but type B is also available.

Adverse effects include respiratory tract infections, muscle weakness, urinary incontinence, falls, fever, and pain. While immunogenicity is currently of much less concern than in the past, experts still recommend that injections not be administered more frequently than every 3 months. Studies to determine safety of more frequent administration are underway. Besides occasional complications, a major limitation of BoNT treatment is its high cost. In addition, post-marketing reports of systemic and potentially fatal effects from spread of the toxin, generated a black box warning. The risk is greatest for children treated for spasticity, but toxicity can occur in adults as well.

DANTROLENE

Dantrolene is a hydantoin derivative related to phenytoin that has a unique mechanism of spasmolytic activity. In contrast to the centrally acting drugs, dantrolene reduces skeletal muscle strength by interfering with excitation-contraction coupling in the muscle fibers. The normal contractile response involves release of calcium from its stores in the sarcoplasmic reticulum (see Figures 13–1 and 27–10). This activator calcium brings about the tension-generating interaction of actin with myosin. Calcium is released from the sarcoplasmic reticulum via a calcium channel, called the **ryanodine receptor (RyR) channel** because the plant alkaloid ryanodine combines with a receptor on the channel protein. In the case of the skeletal muscle RyR1 channel, ryanodine facilitates the open configuration.

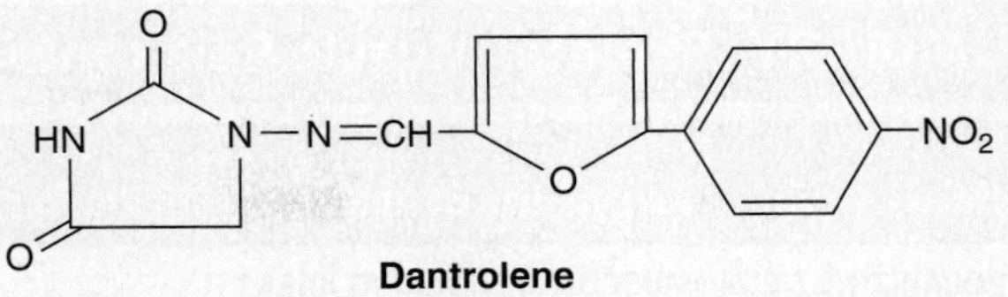

Dantrolene

Dantrolene interferes with the release of activator calcium through this sarcoplasmic reticulum calcium channel by binding to the RyR1 and blocking the opening of the channel. Motor units that contract rapidly are more sensitive to the drug's effects than are slower-responding units. Cardiac muscle and smooth muscle are minimally depressed because the release of calcium from their sarcoplasmic reticulum involves a different RyR channel (RyR2).

Treatment with dantrolene is usually initiated with 25 mg daily as a single dose, increasing to a maximum of 100 mg four times daily as tolerated. Only about one-third of an oral dose of dantrolene is absorbed, and the elimination half-life of the drug is approximately 8 hours. Major adverse effects are generalized muscle weakness, sedation, and occasionally hepatitis.

A special application of dantrolene is in the treatment of **malignant hyperthermia,** a rare heritable disorder that can be triggered by a variety of stimuli, including general anesthetics (eg, volatile anesthetics) and neuromuscular blocking drugs (eg, succinylcholine; see also Chapter 16). Patients at risk for this condition have a hereditary alteration in Ca^{2+}-induced Ca^{2+} release via the RyR1 channel or impairment in the ability of the sarcoplasmic reticulum to sequester calcium via the Ca^{2+} transporter (see Figure 27–10). Several mutations associated with this risk have been identified. After administration of one of the triggering agents, there is a sudden and prolonged release of calcium, with massive muscle contraction, lactic acid production, and increased body temperature. Prompt treatment is essential to control acidosis and body temperature and to reduce calcium release. The latter is accomplished by administering intravenous dantrolene, starting with a dose of 1 mg/kg IV, and repeating as necessary to a maximum dose of 10 mg/kg.

ANTISPASMODICS: DRUGS USED TO TREAT ACUTE LOCAL MUSCLE SPASM

A large number of less well-studied, centrally active drugs (eg, **carisoprodol, chlorzoxazone, cyclobenzaprine, metaxalone, methocarbamol,** and **orphenadrine**) are promoted for the relief of acute muscle spasm caused by local tissue trauma or muscle strains. It has been suggested that these drugs act primarily at the level of the brainstem. Cyclobenzaprine may be regarded as the prototype of the group. Cyclobenzaprine is structurally related to the tricyclic antidepressants and produces antimuscarinic side effects. It is ineffective in treating muscle spasm due to cerebral palsy or spinal cord injury. As a result of its strong antimuscarinic actions, cyclobenzaprine may cause significant sedation, as well as confusion and transient visual hallucinations. The dosage of cyclobenzaprine for acute injury-related muscle spasm is 20–40 mg/d orally in divided doses. This drug class carries risks of significant adverse events and abuse potential.

SUMMARY Skeletal Muscle Relaxants

Subclass, Drug	Mechanism of Action	Effects	Clinical Applications	Pharmacokinetics, Toxicities, Interactions
DEPOLARIZING NEUROMUSCULAR BLOCKING AGENT				
• Succinylcholine	Agonist at nicotinic acetylcholine (ACh) receptors, especially at neuromuscular junctions • depolarizes • may stimulate ganglionic nicotinic ACh and cardiac muscarinic ACh receptors	Initial depolarization causes transient contractions, followed by prolonged flaccid paralysis • depolarization is then followed by repolarization that is also accompanied by paralysis	Placement of endotracheal tube at start of anesthetic procedure • rarely, control of muscle contractions in status epilepticus	Rapid metabolism by plasma cholinesterase • normal duration ~5 min • *Toxicities:* Arrhythmias • hyperkalemia • transient increased intra-abdominal, intraocular pressure • postoperative muscle pain
NONDEPOLARIZING NEUROMUSCULAR BLOCKING AGENTS				
• *d*-Tubocurarine	Competitive antagonist at nACh receptors, especially at neuromuscular junctions	Prevents depolarization by ACh, causes flaccid paralysis • can cause histamine release with hypotension • weak block of cardiac muscarinic ACh receptors	Prolonged relaxation for surgical procedures • superseded by newer nondepolarizing agents	Renal excretion • duration, ~40–60 min • *Toxicities:* Histamine release • hypotension • prolonged apnea
• Cisatracurium	Similar to tubocurarine	Like tubocurarine but lacks histamine release and antimuscarinic effects	Prolonged relaxation for surgical procedures • relaxation of respiratory muscles to facilitate mechanical ventilation in intensive care unit	Not dependent on renal or hepatic function • duration ~25–45 min • *Toxicities:* Prolonged apnea but less toxic than atracurium
• Rocuronium	Similar to cisatracurium	Like cisatracurium but slight antimuscarinic effect	Like cisatracurium • useful in patients with renal impairment	Hepatic metabolism • duration ~20–35 min • *Toxicities:* Like cisatracurium
• *Vecuronium: Intermediate duration; metabolized in liver*				
CENTRALLY ACTING SPASMOLYTIC DRUGS				
• Baclofen	$GABA_B$ agonist, facilitates spinal inhibition of motor neurons	Pre- and postsynaptic inhibition of motor output	Severe spasticity due to cerebral palsy, multiple sclerosis, stroke	Oral, intrathecal • *Toxicities:* Sedation, weakness; rebound spasticity upon abrupt withdrawal
• Diazepam	Facilitates GABAergic transmission in central nervous system (see Chapter 22)	Increases interneuron inhibition of primary motor afferents in spinal cord • central sedation	Chronic spasm due to cerebral palsy, stroke, spinal cord injury • acute spasm due to muscle injury	Hepatic metabolism • duration ~12–24 h • *Toxicities:* See Chapter 22
• Tizanidine	α_2-Adrenoceptor agonist in the spinal cord	Pre- and postsynaptic inhibition of reflex motor output	Spasm due to multiple sclerosis, stroke, amyotrophic lateral sclerosis	Oral • renal and hepatic elimination • duration 3–6 h • *Toxicities:* Weakness, sedation, hypotension, hepatotoxicity (rare), rebound hypertension upon abrupt withdrawal
CENTRALLY ACTING ANTISPASMODIC DRUGS				
• Cyclobenzaprine	Poorly understood inhibition of muscle stretch reflex in spinal cord	Reduction in hyperactive muscle reflexes • antimuscarinic effects	Acute spasm due to muscle injury • inflammation	Hepatic metabolism • duration, ~4–6 h • *Toxicities:* Strong antimuscarinic effects
• *Methocarbamol, orphenadrine, others: Like cyclobenzaprine with varying degrees of antimuscarinic effect. Class side effect: strong central nervous system depression; note carisoprodol is a schedule IV drug.*				
DIRECT-ACTING MUSCLE RELAXANTS				
• Dantrolene	Blocks RyR1 Ca^{2+}-release channels in the sarcoplasmic reticulum of skeletal muscle	Reduces actin-myosin interaction • weakens skeletal muscle contraction	IV: Malignant hyperthermia • Oral: Spasm due to cerebral palsy, spinal cord injury, multiple sclerosis	IV, oral • duration 4–6 h • *Toxicities:* Muscle weakness • Black box warning: hepatotoxicity
• Botulinum toxin	Inhibits synaptic exocytosis through clipping of vesicle fusion proteins in presynaptic nerve terminal	Flaccid paralysis	Upper and lower limb spasm due to cerebral palsy, multiple sclerosis; cervical dystonia, overactive bladder, migraine, hyperhidrosis	Direct injection into muscle • duration 2–3 months • *Toxicities*: Muscle weakness, falls • Black box warning: potential spread of toxin leading to excessive weakness reported after use for cerebral palsy with spasticity

PREPARATIONS AVAILABLE

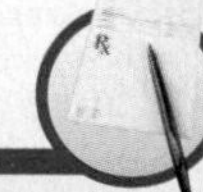

GENERIC NAME	AVAILABLE AS
NEUROMUSCULAR BLOCKING DRUGS	
Atracurium	Generic
Cisatracurium	Generic, Nimbex
Pancuronium	Generic
Rocuronium	Generic, Zemuron
Succinylcholine	Generic, Anectine, Quelicin
Tubocurarine	Generic
Vecuronium	Generic, Norcuron
REVERSAL AGENTS	
Neostigmine	Generic
Edrophonium	Generic
Sugammadex	Bridion
SPASMOLYTICS, ANTISPASMODICS	
Baclofen	Generic, Gablofen, Lioresal
Botulinum toxin type A	Botox, Dysport, Xeomin
Botulinum toxin type B	Myobloc
Carisoprodol	Generic, Soma
Chlorzoxazone	Generic
Cyclobenzaprine	Generic, Amrix, Fexmid, Flexeril
Dantrolene	Generic, Dantrium, Revonto
Diazepam	Generic, Valium, Diastat
Gabapentin	Generic, Fanatrex FusePaq, Gabarone, Gralise, Neurontin
Note: This drug is labeled for use only in epilepsy and postherpetic neuralgia.	
Metaxalone	Generic, Skelaxin
Methocarbamol	Generic, Robaxin
Orphenadrine	Generic, Antiflex, Banflex, Norflex, Flexoject, Flexon, Mio-Rel, Myolin, Norflex Injectable, Orfro, Orphenate
Riluzole	Generic, Rilutek, Tiglutik
Note: This drug is labeled only for use in amyotrophic lateral sclerosis.	
Tizanidine	Generic, Zanaflex

REFERENCES

Neuromuscular Blockers

Belmont MR et al: Clinical pharmacology of GW280430A in humans. Anesthesiology 2004;100:768.

Brull SJ, Murphy GS: Residual neuromuscular block: Lessons unlearned. Part II: Methods to reduce the risk of residual weakness. Anesth Analg 2010;111:129.

Bryson HM, Fulton B, Benfield P: Riluzole. A review of its pharmacodynamic and pharmacokinetic properties and therapeutic potential in amyotrophic lateral sclerosis. Drugs 1996;52:549.

Cammu G et al: Dialysability of sugammadex and its complex with rocuronium in intensive care patients with severe renal impairment. Br J Anaes 2012;109:382.

De Boer HD et al: Reversal of rocuronium-induced (1.2 mg/kg) profound neuromuscular blockade by sugammadex. Anesthesiology 2007;107:239.

Gibb AJ, Marshall IG: Pre- and postjunctional effects of tubocurarine and other nicotinic antagonists during repetitive stimulation in the rat. J Physiol 1984;351:275.

Hemmerling TM, Russo G, Bracco D: Neuromuscular blockade in cardiac surgery: An update for clinicians. Ann Card Anaesth 2008;11:80.

Hirsch NP: Neuromuscular junction in health and disease. Br J Anaesth 2007; 99:132.

Kampe S et al: Muscle relaxants. Best Prac Res Clin Anesthesiol 2003;17:137.

Lee C: Structure, conformation, and action of neuromuscular blocking drugs. Br J Anaesth 2001;87:755.

Lee C et al: Reversal of profound neuromuscular block by sugammadex administered three minutes after rocuronium. Anesthesiology 2009;110:1020.

Lien CA et al: Fumarates: Unique nondepolarizing neuromuscular blocking agents that are antagonized by cysteine. J Crit Care 2009;24:50.

Llauradó S et al: Sugammadex ideal body weight dose adjusted by level of neuromuscular blockade in laparoscopic bariatric surgery. Anesthesiology 2012; 117:93.

Mace SE: Challenges and advances in intubation: Rapid sequence intubation. Emerg Med Clin North Am 2008;26:1043.

Marshall CG, Ogden DC, Colquhoun D: The actions of suxamethonium (succinyldicholine) as an agonist and channel blocker at the nicotinic receptor of frog muscle. J Physiol (Lond) 1990;428:155.

Martyn JA: Neuromuscular physiology and pharmacology. In: Miller RD (editor): *Anesthesia*, 7th ed. Churchill Livingstone, 2010.

Meakin GH: Recent advances in myorelaxant therapy. Paed Anaesthesia 2001;11:523.

Murphy GS, Brull SJ: Residual neuromuscular block: Lessons unlearned. Part I: Definitions, incidence, and adverse physiologic effects of residual neuromuscular block. Anesth Analg 2010;111:120.

Naguib M: Sugammadex: Another milestone in clinical neuromuscular pharmacology. Anesth Analg 2007;104:575.

Naguib M, Brull SJ: Update on neuromuscular pharmacology. Curr Opin Anaesthesiol 2009;22:483.

Naguib M, Kopman AF, Ensor JE: Neuromuscular monitoring and postoperative residual curarisation: A meta-analysis. Br J Anaesth 2007;98:302.

Naguib M et al: Advances in neurobiology of the neuromuscular junction: Implications for the anesthesiologist. Anesthesiology 2002;96:202.

Nicholson WT, Sprung J, Jankowski CJ: Sugammadex: A novel agent for the reversal of neuromuscular blockade. Pharmacotherapy 2007;27:1181.

Pavlin JD, Kent CD: Recovery after ambulatory anesthesia. Curr Opin Anaesthesiol 2008;21:729.

Puhringer FK et al: Reversal of profound, high-dose rocuronium-induced neuromuscular blockade by sugammadex at two different time points. Anesthesiology 2008;109:188.

Sacan O, Klein K, White PF: Sugammadex reversal of rocuronium-induced neuromuscular blockade: A comparison with neostigmine-glycopyrrolate and edrophonium-atropine. Anesth Analg 2007;104:569.

Savarese JJ et al: Preclinical pharmacology of GW280430A (AV430A) in the rhesus monkey and in the cat: A comparison with mivacurium. Anesthesiology 2004;100:835.

Sine SM: End-plate acetylcholine receptor: Structure, mechanism, pharmacology, and disease. Physiol Rev 2012;92:1189.

Staals LM et al: Reduced clearance of rocuronium and sugammadex in patients with severe to end-stage renal failure: A pharmacokinetic study. Br J Anaesth 2010;104:31.

Sugammadex: BRIDION (sugammadex) Injection, for intravenous use initial U.S. Approval: 2015. http://www.accessdata.fda.gov/drugsatfda_docs/label/2015/022225lbl.pdf.

Sunaga H et al: Gantacurium and CW002 do not potentiate muscarinic receptor-mediated airway smooth muscle constriction in guinea pigs. Anesthesiology 2010;112:892.

Viby-Mogensen J: Neuromuscular monitoring. In: Miller RD (editor): *Anesthesia*, 5th ed. Churchill Livingstone, 2000.

Spasmolytics

BOTOX (onabotulinumtoxinA) for injection, for intramuscular, intradetrusor, or intradermal use. https://www.accessdata.fda.gov/drugsatfda_docs/label/2011/103000s5232lbl.pdf

Caron E, Morgan R, Wheless JW: An unusual cause of flaccid paralysis and coma: Baclofen overdose. J Child Neurol 2014;29:555.

Corcia P, Meininger V: Management of amyotrophic lateral sclerosis. Drugs 2008;68:1037.

Cutter NC et al: Gabapentin effect on spasticity in multiple sclerosis: A placebo-controlled, randomized trial. Arch Phys Med Rehabil 2000; 81:164.

Draulans N et al: Intrathecal baclofen in multiple sclerosis and spinal cord injury: Complications and long-term dosage evolution. Clin Rehabil 2013;27:1137.

Gracies JM, Singer BJ, Dunne JW: The role of botulinum toxin injections in the management of muscle overactivity of the lower limb. Disabil Rehabil 2007;29:1789.

Groves L, Shellenberger MK, Davis CS: Tizanidine treatment of spasticity: A meta-analysis of controlled, double-blind, comparative studies with baclofen and diazepam. Adv Ther 1998;15:241.

Jankovic J: Medical treatment of dystonia. Mov Disord 2013;28:1001.

Kheder A, Nair KPS: Spasticity: Pathophysiology, evaluation and management. Pract Neurol 2012;12:289.

Krause T et al: Dantrolene—A review of its pharmacology, therapeutic use and new developments. Anaesthesia 2004;59:364.

Lopez JR et al: Effects of dantrolene on myoplasmic free [Ca^{2+}] measured in vivo in patients susceptible to malignant hyperthermia. Anesthesiology 1992;76:711.

Lovell BV, Marmura MJ: New therapeutic developments in chronic migraine. Curr Opin Neurol 2010;23:254.

Malanga G, Reiter RD, Garay E: Update on tizanidine for muscle spasticity and emerging indications. Expert Opin Pharmacother 2008;9:2209.

Mast N, Linger M, Pikuleva IA: Inhibition and stimulation of activity of purified recombinant CYP11A1 by therapeutic agents. Mol Cell Endocrinol 2013;371:100.

Mirbagheri MM, Chen D, Rymer WZ: Quantification of the effects of an alpha-2 adrenergic agonist on reflex properties in spinal cord injury using a system identification technique. J Neuroeng Rehabil 2010;7:29.

Neuvonen PJ: Towards safer and more predictable drug treatment—Reflections from studies of the First BCPT Prize awardee. Basic Clin Pharmacol Toxicol 2012;110:207.

Nolan KW, Cole LL, Liptak GS: Use of botulinum toxin type A in children with cerebral palsy. Phys Ther 2006;86:573.

Reeves RR, Burke RS: Carisoprodol: Abuse potential and withdrawal syndrome. Curr Drug Abuse Rev 2010;3:33.

Ronan S, Gold JT: Nonoperative management of spasticity in children. Childs Nerv Syst 2007;23:943.

Ross JC et al: Acute intrathecal baclofen withdrawal: A brief review of treatment options. Neurocrit Care 2011;14:103.

Vakhapova V, Auriel E, Karni A: Nightly sublingual tizanidine HCl in multiple sclerosis: Clinical efficacy and safety. Clin Neuropharmacol 2010;33:151.

Verrotti A et al: Pharmacotherapy of spasticity in children with cerebral palsy. Pediatr Neurol 2006;34:1.

Ward AB: Spasticity treatment with botulinum toxins. J Neural Transm 2008;115:607.

Zanaflex Capsules™ Package insert. Prescribing information. Acorda Therapeutics, 2006.

CASE STUDY ANSWER

This patient presents problems that make her management more difficult than the average. She is at higher risk of difficulty with airway management because of obesity, and both obesity and diabetes raise the risk of aspiration. Therefore, the decision to use an endotracheal tube for her airway management is reasonable.

As the case progresses, you are experiencing difficulty with mask ventilation, and the decision to abort the procedure and awaken the patient is probably the best response. In order to do so, the neuromuscular blockade must be fully reversed so she will be able to breathe on her own once awakened.

There are two options for reversal of neuromuscular blockade with rocuronium (and with vecuronium): sugammadex, or neostigmine combined with glycopyrrolate. Sugammadex would be the most appropriate agent. As described in Chapter 7, neostigmine works to increase the level of acetylcholine at the neuromuscular junction by inhibiting the enzymatic breakdown of acetylcholine. Glycopyrrolate (Chapter 8) is given to block the bradycardia associated with increased cholinergic activity. However, if the patient is still fully relaxed with rocuronium, neostigmine will not sufficiently increase acetylcholine to allow full reversal. In contrast, sugammadex actively binds rocuronium and removes it from the neuromuscular junction. In order to fully reverse an intubating dose of rocuronium, a sugammadex dose of 16 mg/kg should be administered. This will reverse the effect of rocuronium within 1.5–3.0 minutes. Sugammadex is renally cleared, so it should not be used in patients in renal failure (creatinine clearance less than 30 mL/min) unless absolutely necessary. This patient has insulin-dependent diabetes, so her creatinine clearance may be abnormally low. If this were the case, the benefit of sugammadex would still outweigh its potential risk. In addition, some studies have found that sugammadex may be dialyzable, and could therefore be removed by that method if needed. This patient is also taking an oral contraceptive agent, and it would be necessary to counsel her that sugammadex may interfere with the efficacy of that agent and the FDA recommends use of another method of contraception for the following 7 days. Other issues that may occur with sugammadex use include anaphylaxis, especially when using the maximum dose of 16 mg/kg, marked bradycardia, hypotension, nausea and vomiting, and headache.

CHAPTER

28

Pharmacologic Management of Parkinsonism & Other Movement Disorders

Michael J. Aminoff, MD, DSc, FRCP

CASE STUDY

A 76-year-old retired banker complains of a shuffling gait with occasional falls over the last year. He has developed a stooped posture, drags his left leg when walking, and is unsteady on turning. He remains independent in all activities of daily living, but he has become more forgetful and occasionally sees his long-deceased father in his bedroom. Examination reveals hypomimia, hypophonia, a slight rest tremor of the right hand and chin, mild rigidity, and impaired rapid alternating movements in all limbs. Neurologic and general examinations are otherwise normal. What is the likely diagnosis and prognosis?

The patient is started on a dopamine agonist, and the dose is gradually built up to the therapeutic range. Was this a good choice of medications?

Six months later, the patient and his wife return for follow-up. It now becomes apparent that he is falling asleep at inappropriate times, such as at the dinner table, and when awake, he spends much of the time in arranging and rearranging the table cutlery or in picking at his clothes. To what is his condition due, and how should it be managed? Would you recommend surgical treatment?

Several types of abnormal movement are recognized. **Tremor** consists of a rhythmic oscillatory movement around a joint and is best characterized by its relation to activity. Tremor at rest is characteristic of parkinsonism, when it is often associated with rigidity and an impairment of voluntary activity. Tremor may occur during maintenance of sustained posture (postural tremor) or during movement (intention tremor). A conspicuous postural tremor is the cardinal feature of benign essential or familial tremor. Intention tremor occurs in patients with a lesion of the brainstem or cerebellum, especially when the superior cerebellar peduncle is involved; it may also occur as a manifestation of toxicity from alcohol or certain other drugs.

Chorea consists of irregular, unpredictable, involuntary muscle jerks that occur in different parts of the body and impair voluntary activity. In some instances, the proximal muscles of the limbs are most severely affected, and because the abnormal movements are then particularly violent, the term *ballismus* has been used to describe them. Chorea may be hereditary or acquired and may occur as a complication of a number of general medical disorders and of therapy with certain drugs.

Abnormal movements may be slow and writhing in character **(athetosis)** and, in some instances, are so sustained that they are more properly regarded as abnormal postures **(dystonia).** Athetosis or dystonia may occur with perinatal brain damage, with focal or generalized cerebral lesions, as an acute complication of certain drugs, as an accompaniment of diverse neurologic disorders, or as an isolated inherited phenomenon of uncertain cause known as isolated generalized torsion dystonia or dystonia musculorum deformans. Various genetic loci have been reported depending on the age of onset, mode of inheritance, and response to dopaminergic therapy. The physiologic basis is uncertain, and treatment is unsatisfactory. Patients with dystonia commonly have psychiatric complications, such as depression, that affect the quality of life. These may be secondary to the dystonia or a nonmotor manifestation of the underlying disorder.

Tics are sudden coordinated abnormal movements that tend to occur repetitively, particularly about the face and head, especially in children, and can be suppressed voluntarily for short periods of time. Common tics include repetitive sniffing or shoulder shrugging. Tics may be single or multiple and transient or chronic. Gilles de la Tourette syndrome is characterized by chronic multiple tics; its pharmacologic management is discussed at the end of this chapter.

Many of the movement disorders have been attributed to disturbances of the basal ganglia. The basic circuitry of the basal ganglia involves three interacting neuronal loops that include the cortex and thalamus as well as the basal ganglia themselves (Figure 28–1). However, the precise function of these anatomic structures is not yet fully understood, and it is not possible to relate individual symptoms to involvement at specific sites.

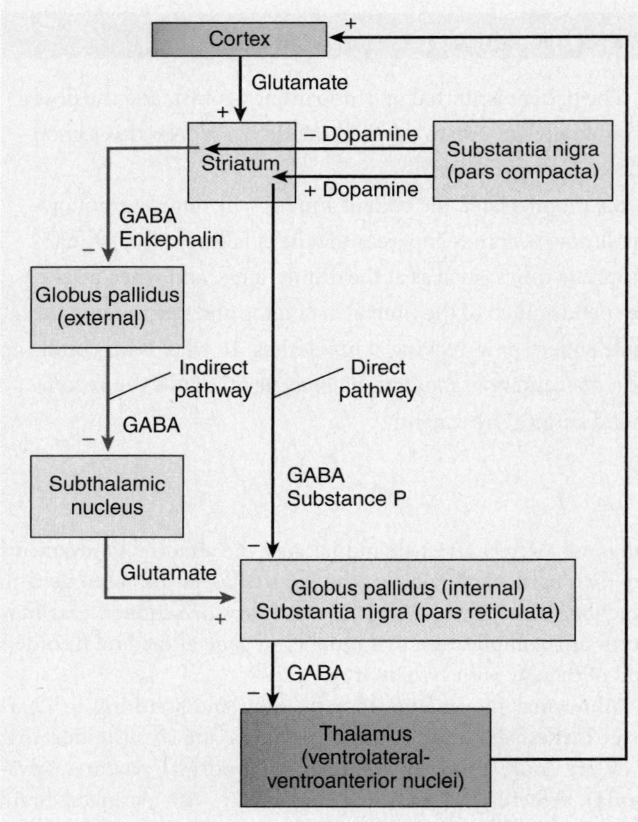

FIGURE 28–1 Functional circuitry between the cortex, basal ganglia, and thalamus. The major neurotransmitters are indicated. In Parkinson disease, there is degeneration of the pars compacta of the substantia nigra, leading to overactivity in the indirect pathway (red) and increased glutamatergic activity by the subthalamic nucleus.

PARKINSONISM & PARKINSON DISEASE

Parkinsonism is characterized by a combination of rigidity, bradykinesia, tremor, and postural instability that can occur for a variety of reasons but is usually idiopathic (Parkinson disease or paralysis agitans). Bradykinesia should be present before a diagnosis of Parkinson disease is made. Focal dystonic features may be present. Cognitive decline occurs in many patients as the disease advances. Other nonmotor symptoms include affective disorders (anxiety or depression); confusion, cognitive impairment, or personality changes; apathy; fatigue; abnormalities of autonomic function (eg, sphincter or sexual dysfunction, dysphagia and choking, sweating abnormalities, sialorrhea, or disturbances of blood pressure regulation); sleep disorders; and sensory complaints or pain. The disease is incurable, is generally progressive, and leads to increasing disability with time, but pharmacologic treatment may relieve motor symptoms and improve the quality of life for many years. Patients with Parkinson disease may develop hyposmia, constipation, depression, anxiety, or rapid-eye-movement (REM) sleep behavior disorder in a preclinical phase before onset of the motor disturbance.

Parkinsonism may also have a hereditary basis, may follow exposure to various toxins (eg, manganese dusts, carbon disulfide, carbon monoxide), may develop after multiple subcortical white-matter infarcts or recurrent head injury (as in boxers), and may occur in association with other neurologic disorders.

Pathogenesis

The pathogenesis of Parkinson disease seems to relate to a combination of impaired degradation of proteins, intracellular protein accumulation and aggregation, oxidative stress, mitochondrial damage, inflammatory cascades, and apoptosis. Studies in twins suggest that genetic factors are important, especially when the disease occurs in patients under age 50. Recognized genetic abnormalities account for 10–15% of cases. Mutations of the α-synuclein gene at 4q21 or duplication and triplication of the normal synuclein gene are associated with Parkinson disease, which is now widely recognized as a *synucleinopathy*. Mutations of the leucine-rich repeat kinase 2 (*LRRK2*) gene at 12cen, and the *UCHL1* gene may also cause autosomal dominant parkinsonism. Mutations in the *parkin* gene (6q25.2–q27) cause early-onset, autosomal recessive, familial parkinsonism, or sporadic juvenile-onset parkinsonism. Several other genes or chromosomal regions have been associated with familial forms of the disease. Environmental or endogenous toxins may also be important in the etiology of the disease. Epidemiologic studies reveal that cigarette smoking, coffee, anti-inflammatory drug use, and high serum uric acid levels are protective, whereas the incidence of the disease is increased in those working in teaching, health care, or farming, and in those with lead or manganese exposure or with vitamin D deficiency.

The finding of Lewy bodies (intracellular inclusion bodies containing α-synuclein) in fetal dopaminergic cells transplanted into the brain of parkinsonian patients some years previously has provided some support for suggestions that Parkinson disease may represent a prion disease.

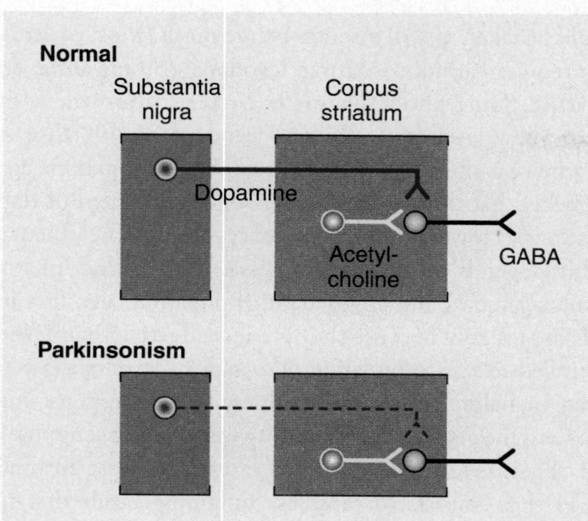

FIGURE 28–2 Schematic representation of the sequence of neurons involved in parkinsonism. A simplified version of the involved circuitry is shown. **Top:** Dopaminergic neurons (red) originating in the substantia nigra normally inhibit the GABAergic output from the striatum, whereas cholinergic neurons (green) exert an excitatory effect. **Bottom:** In parkinsonism, there is a selective loss of dopaminergic neurons (dashed, red).

Staining for α-synuclein has revealed that pathology is more widespread than previously recognized, developing initially in the olfactory nucleus and the medulla or lower brainstem (stage 1 of Braak scale), then higher in the medulla and the pons of the brainstem (stage 2), extending to the midbrain and in particular the substantia nigra (stage 3), the mesocortex and thalamus (stage 4), the neocortex (stage 5), and then spreading more extensively in the neocortex (stage 6). The motor features of Parkinson disease develop at stage 3 on the Braak scale.

The normally high concentration of dopamine in the basal ganglia of the brain is reduced in parkinsonism, and pharmacologic attempts to restore dopaminergic activity with levodopa and dopamine agonists alleviate many of the motor features of the disorder. An alternative but complementary approach has been to restore the normal balance of cholinergic and dopaminergic influences on the basal ganglia with antimuscarinic drugs. The pathophysiologic basis for these therapies is that in idiopathic parkinsonism, there is a loss of dopaminergic neurons in the substantia nigra that normally inhibit the output of GABAergic cells in the corpus striatum (Figure 28–2). Drugs that induce parkinsonian syndromes either are dopamine receptor antagonists (eg, antipsychotic agents; see Chapter 29) or lead to the destruction of the dopaminergic nigrostriatal neurons (eg, 1-methyl-4-phenyl-1,2,3,6-tetrahydropyridine [MPTP]; see below). Various other neurotransmitters, such as norepinephrine, are also depleted in the brain in parkinsonism, but these deficiencies are of uncertain clinical relevance.

LEVODOPA

Dopamine does not cross the blood-brain barrier and if given into the peripheral circulation has no therapeutic effect in parkinsonism. However, (–)-3-(3,4-dihydroxyphenyl)-L-alanine (levodopa), the immediate metabolic precursor of dopamine, does enter the brain (via an L-amino acid transporter, LAT), where it is decarboxylated to dopamine (see Figure 6–5). Several noncatecholamine dopamine receptor agonists have also been developed and may lead to clinical benefit, as discussed in the text that follows.

Dopamine receptors are discussed in detail in Chapters 21 and 29. They exist in five subtypes. D_1 and D_5 receptors are classified as the D_1 receptor family based on genetic and biochemical factors; D_2, D_3, and D_4 are grouped as belonging to the D_2 receptor family. Dopamine receptors of the D_1 type are located in the pars compacta of the substantia nigra and presynaptically on striatal axons coming from cortical neurons and from dopaminergic cells in the substantia nigra. The D_2 receptors are located postsynaptically on striatal neurons and presynaptically on axons in the substantia nigra belonging to neurons in the basal ganglia. The benefits of dopaminergic antiparkinsonism drugs appear to depend mostly on stimulation of the D_2 receptors. However, D_1-receptor stimulation may also be required for maximal benefit, and one of the newer drugs is D_3 selective. Dopamine agonist or partial agonist ergot derivatives such as lergotrile and bromocriptine that are powerful stimulators of the D_2 receptors have antiparkinsonism properties, whereas certain dopamine blockers that are selective D_2 antagonists can induce parkinsonism.

Chemistry

Dopa is the amino acid precursor of dopamine and norepinephrine (discussed in Chapter 6). Its structure is shown in Figure 28–3. Levodopa is the levorotatory stereoisomer of dopa.

Pharmacokinetics

Levodopa is rapidly absorbed from the small intestine, but its absorption depends on the rate of gastric emptying and the pH of the gastric contents. Ingestion of food delays the appearance of levodopa in the plasma. Moreover, certain amino acids from ingested food can compete with the drug for absorption from the gut and for transport from the blood to the brain. Plasma concentrations usually peak between 1 and 2 hours after an oral dose, and the plasma half-life is usually between 1 and 3 hours, although it varies considerably among individuals. About two-thirds of the dose appears in the urine as metabolites within 8 hours of an oral dose, the main metabolic products being 3-methoxy-4-hydroxyphenyl acetic acid (homovanillic acid, HVA) and dihydroxyphenylacetic acid (DOPAC). Unfortunately, only about 1–3% of administered levodopa actually enters the brain unaltered; the remainder is metabolized extracerebrally, predominantly by decarboxylation to dopamine, which does not penetrate the blood-brain barrier. Accordingly, levodopa must be given in large amounts when used alone. However, when given in combination with a dopa decarboxylase inhibitor that does not penetrate the blood-brain barrier, the peripheral metabolism of levodopa is reduced, plasma levels of levodopa are higher, plasma half-life is longer, and more dopa is available for entry into the brain (Figure 28–4). Indeed, concomitant administration of a peripheral dopa decarboxylase inhibitor such as carbidopa may reduce the daily requirements of levodopa by approximately 75%.

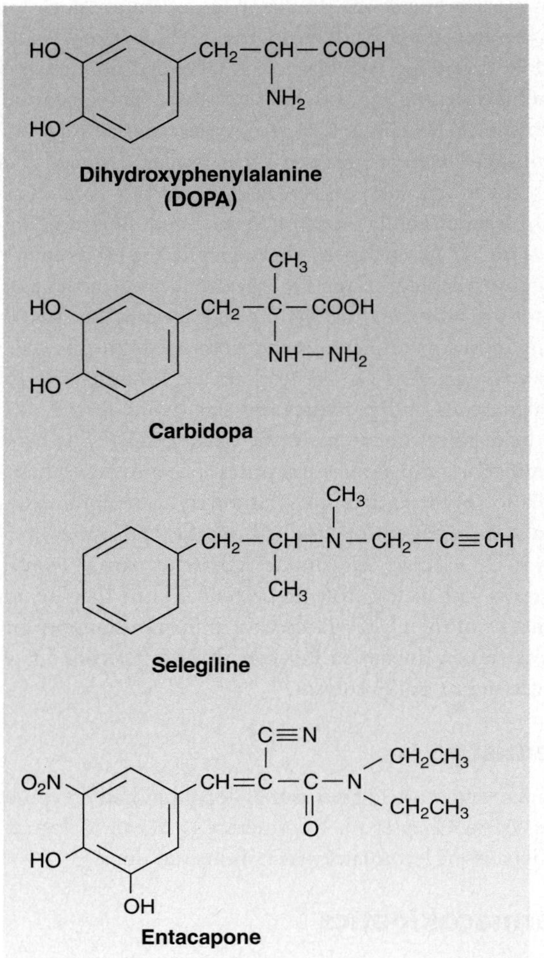

Dihydroxyphenylalanine (DOPA)

Carbidopa

Selegiline

Entacapone

FIGURE 28–3 Some drugs used in the treatment of parkinsonism.

Clinical Use

The best results of levodopa treatment are obtained in the first few years of treatment. This is sometimes because the daily dose of levodopa must be reduced over time to avoid adverse effects at doses that were well tolerated initially. Some patients become less responsive to levodopa, perhaps because of loss of dopaminergic nigrostriatal nerve terminals or some pathologic process directly involving striatal dopamine receptors. For such reasons, the benefits of levodopa treatment often begin to diminish after about 3 or 4 years of therapy, regardless of the initial therapeutic response. Although levodopa therapy does not stop the progression of parkinsonism, its early initiation lowers the mortality rate. However, long-term therapy may lead to a number of problems in management such as the on-off phenomenon discussed below. The most appropriate time to introduce levodopa therapy must therefore be determined individually.

When levodopa is used, it is generally given in combination with **carbidopa** (see Figure 28–3), a peripheral dopa decarboxylase inhibitor, which reduces peripheral conversion to dopamine. Combination treatment is started with a small dose, eg, carbidopa 25 mg, levodopa 100 mg three times daily, and gradually increased. It should be taken 30–60 minutes before meals. Most patients ultimately require carbidopa 25 mg, levodopa 250 mg three or four times daily. Some physicians prefer to keep treatment with this agent at a low level (eg, carbidopa-levodopa 25/100 three times daily) when possible, and if necessary, to add a dopamine agonist, in the belief that this reduces the risk of development of response fluctuations. However, the occurrence of response fluctuations probably depends on disease progression rather than pharmacologic management, and any benefit of dopamine agonists in this regards is probably because they are less effective than levodopa. A controlled-release formulation of carbidopa-levodopa is available and may be helpful in patients with established response fluctuations or as a means of reducing dosing frequency. Even more helpful for response fluctuations is an extended-release formulation **(Rytary)** that consists of capsules containing beads that release carbidopa and levodopa (present in a 1:4 ratio) at different rates over a prolonged time as they dissolve in the stomach. It is substituted for the regular (immediate-release) formulation using dosing guidelines provided by its manufacturer (Table 28–1).

A formulation of carbidopa-levodopa (10/100, 25/100, 25/250) that disintegrates in the mouth and is swallowed with the saliva **(Parcopa)** is available commercially and is best taken about 1 hour before meals. The combination **(Stalevo)** of levodopa, carbidopa, and a catechol-*O*-methyltransferase (COMT) inhibitor (entacapone) is discussed in a later section. Finally, therapy by *infusion* of carbidopa-levodopa into the duodenum or upper jejunum appears to be safe and is superior to a number of oral combination therapies in patients with advanced levodopa-responsive parkinsonism with response fluctuations. A permanent access tube is inserted via a percutaneous endoscopic gastrostomy in patients who have responded well to carbidopa-levodopa gel administered through a nasoduodenal tube. A morning bolus (100–300 mg of levodopa) is delivered via a portable infusion pump, followed by a continuous maintenance dose (40–120 mg/h), with supplemental bolus doses as required.

Levodopa can ameliorate many of the clinical motor features of parkinsonism, but it is particularly effective in relieving bradykinesia and any disabilities resulting from it. When it is first introduced, about one third of patients respond very well and one third less well. Most of the remainder either are unable to tolerate the medication or simply do not respond at all, especially if they do not have classic Parkinson disease.

Adverse Effects

A. Gastrointestinal Effects

When levodopa is given without a peripheral decarboxylase inhibitor, anorexia and nausea and vomiting occur in about 80% of patients. These adverse effects can be minimized by taking the drug in divided doses, with or immediately after meals, and by increasing the total daily dose very slowly. Antacids taken 30–60 minutes before levodopa may also be beneficial. The vomiting has been attributed to stimulation of the chemoreceptor trigger zone located in the brainstem but outside the blood-brain barrier. Fortunately, tolerance to this emetic effect develops in many patients. If not, an additional dose of carbidopa (Lodosyn; 25 mg) taken

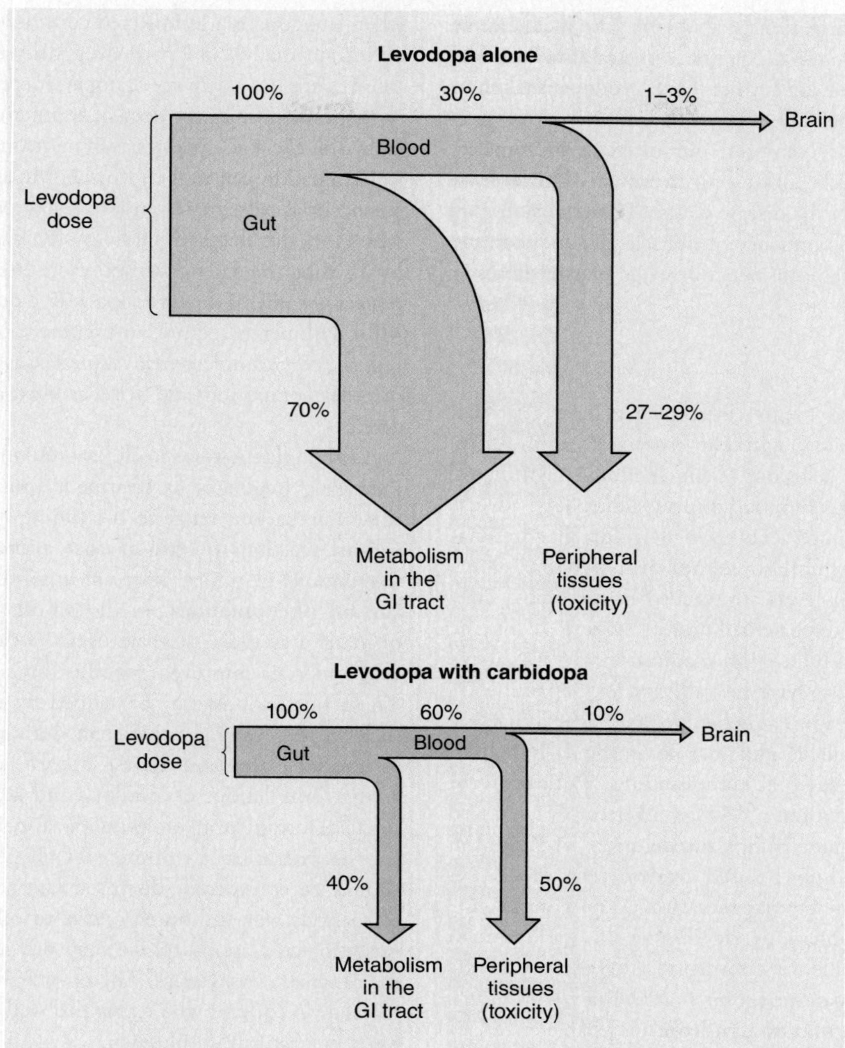

FIGURE 28–4 Fate of orally administered levodopa and the effect of carbidopa, estimated from animal data. The width of each pathway indicates the absolute amount of the drug at each site, whereas the percentages shown denote the relative proportion of the administered dose. The benefits of co-administration of carbidopa include reduction of the amount of levodopa required for benefit and of the absolute amount diverted to peripheral tissues and an increase in the fraction of the dose that reaches the brain. GI, gastrointestinal. (Data from Nutt JG, Fellman JH: Pharmacokinetics of levodopa. Clin Neuropharmacol 1984;7(1):35-49.)

TABLE 28-1 Substitution of Rytary for immediate-release carbidopa/levodopa.

Current Levodopa Total Daily Dose (mg)	Rytary Dose (Carbidopa/Levodopa) (mg)[1]
Zero	23.75/95, 1 cap TID
400–549	23.75/95, 3 caps TID
550–749	23.75/95, 4 caps QID
750–949	36.25/145, 3 caps TID
950–1249	48.75/195, 3 caps TID
1250 or more	48.75/195, 4 caps TID or 61.25/245, 3 caps TID

[1]Dose levels recommended by the manufacturers.

with the regular carbidopa-levodopa dose is often helpful, even though the usual maximum requirement of carbidopa is 75 mg daily. Domperidone (not available in the USA) may also relieve persistent nausea, as may ondansetron. Antiemetics such as phenothiazines should be avoided because they reduce the antiparkinsonism effects of levodopa and may exacerbate the disease.

When levodopa is given in combination with carbidopa, adverse gastrointestinal effects are much less frequent and troublesome, occurring in less than 20% of cases, so that patients can tolerate proportionately higher doses.

B. Cardiovascular Effects

A variety of cardiac arrhythmias have been described in patients receiving levodopa, including tachycardia, ventricular extrasystoles, and rarely, atrial fibrillation. This effect has been attributed to increased catecholamine formation peripherally. The incidence of such arrhythmias is low, even in the presence of established cardiac disease, and may be reduced still further if the levodopa is taken in combination with a peripheral decarboxylase inhibitor.

Postural hypotension is common, but often asymptomatic, and tends to diminish with continuing treatment. However, it sometimes develops later in the disease course. Hypertension may also occur, especially in the presence of nonselective monoamine oxidase inhibitors or sympathomimetics or when massive doses of levodopa are being taken.

C. Behavioral Effects

A wide variety of adverse mental effects have been reported, including depression, anxiety, agitation, insomnia, somnolence, sleep attacks, confusion, delusions, hallucinations, nightmares, euphoria, and other changes in mood or personality. Such adverse effects are more common in patients taking levodopa in combination with a decarboxylase inhibitor rather than levodopa alone, presumably because higher levels are reached in the brain. They may be precipitated by intercurrent illness or surgery. It may be necessary to reduce or withdraw the medication. Several atypical antipsychotic agents that have low affinity for dopamine D_2 receptors (clozapine, olanzapine, quetiapine, and risperidone; see Chapter 29) are now available and may be particularly helpful in counteracting such behavioral complications. **Pimavanserin** (34 mg daily), a selective serotonin 5-HT_{2A} inverse agonist, is also helpful for treating the hallucinations and delusions of Parkinson disease psychosis. It should not be used for dementia-related psychosis and should be avoided in patients with QT prolongation.

Confusion and hallucinations developing in parkinsonian patients is more likely due to treatment with anticholinergic agents, amantadine, or dopamine agonists rather than to levodopa.

The **dopamine dysregulation syndrome** is characterized by compulsive overuse of dopaminergic medication as well as by other impulsive behaviors; such impulse control disorders are more common with dopamine agonists than levodopa and are discussed later. Management involves the close regulation of dopaminergic intake.

Punding designates the performance of stereotyped, complex, but purposeless motor activity, such as sorting or lining up various objects or repetitive grooming behavior. It responds to reduction in dose of dopaminergic agents or to atypical antipsychotic agents.

D. Dyskinesias and Response Fluctuations

Dyskinesias occur in up to 80% of patients receiving levodopa therapy for more than 10 years. The character of dopa dyskinesias varies between patients but tends to remain constant in individual patients. Choreoathetosis of the face and distal extremities is the most common presentation. The development of dyskinesias is dose related, but there is considerable individual variation in the dose required to produce them. Their pathogenesis is unclear, but they may relate to an unequal distribution of striatal dopamine. Dopaminergic denervation plus chronic pulsatile stimulation of dopamine receptors with levodopa has been associated with development of dyskinesias. A lower incidence of dyskinesias occurs when levodopa is administered continuously (eg, intraduodenally or intrajejunally) and with drug delivery systems that enable a more continuous delivery of dopaminergic medication. Reduction of levodopa dose or the dose of adjunctive medications (discussed later) will alleviate dyskinesias in many instances, but motor symptoms of parkinsonism then worsen. Much less commonly, dyskinesias occur as patients respond to levodopa and again as the benefit wears off, and these "diphasic dyskinesias" may be best managed by dividing the daily dose into more frequent smaller doses or by replacing some of the levodopa with a dopamine receptor agonist. Mild dyskinesias require no treatment. Amantadine may help to reduce more troublesome dyskinesias, as may clozapine; a number of other compounds are being studied as possible antidyskinetic agents.

Certain fluctuations in clinical response to levodopa occur with increasing frequency as treatment continues. In some patients, these fluctuations relate to the timing of levodopa intake (**wearing-off** reactions or **end-of-dose akinesia**). In other instances, fluctuations in clinical state are unrelated to the timing of doses **(on-off phenomenon)**. In the on-off phenomenon, off-periods of marked akinesia alternate over the course of a few hours with on-periods of improved mobility but often marked dyskinesia. These fluctuations may be helped by talking the main protein meal in the evening rather than during the day, by adjustments to levodopa dose and dosing interval, and by the use of longer-acting formulations of levodopa and adjunctive medications. An inhaled formulation of levodopa also is available commercially for the intermittent treatment of off-periods. Surgical treatment should be considered (discussed later). For patients with severe off-periods who are unresponsive to other measures, subcutaneously injected apomorphine may provide temporary benefit but may increase dyskinesias. The on-off phenomenon is most likely to occur in patients who responded well to treatment initially. The exact mechanism is unknown.

E. Miscellaneous Adverse Effects

Mydriasis may occur and may precipitate an attack of acute glaucoma in some patients. Other reported but rare adverse effects include various blood dyscrasias; a positive Coombs' test with evidence of hemolysis; hot flushes; aggravation or precipitation of gout; abnormalities of smell or taste; brownish discoloration of saliva, urine, or vaginal secretions; priapism; and mild—usually transient—elevations of blood urea nitrogen and of serum transaminases, alkaline phosphatase, and bilirubin.

Drug Holidays

A drug holiday (discontinuance of the drug for 3–21 days) may temporarily improve responsiveness to levodopa and alleviate some of its adverse effects but is usually of little help in the management of the on-off phenomenon. Furthermore, a drug holiday carries the risks of aspiration pneumonia, venous thrombosis, pulmonary embolism, and depression resulting from the immobility accompanying severe parkinsonism. For these reasons and because of the temporary nature of any benefit, drug holidays are not recommended.

Drug Interactions

Pharmacologic doses of pyridoxine (vitamin B_6) enhance the extracerebral metabolism of levodopa and may therefore prevent its therapeutic effect unless a peripheral decarboxylase inhibitor is also taken. Levodopa should not be given to patients taking monoamine oxidase A inhibitors or within 2 weeks of their discontinuance because such a combination can lead to hypertensive crises.

Contraindications

Levodopa should not be given to psychotic patients because it may exacerbate the mental disturbance. It is also contraindicated in patients with angle-closure glaucoma, but those with chronic open-angle glaucoma may be given levodopa if intraocular pressure is well controlled and can be monitored. When combined with carbidopa, the risk of cardiac dysrhythmia is slight, even in patients with cardiac disease. Patients with active peptic ulcer must be managed carefully, since gastrointestinal bleeding has occasionally occurred with levodopa. Because levodopa is a precursor of skin melanin and conceivably may activate malignant melanoma, it should be used with particular care in patients with a history of melanoma or with suspicious undiagnosed skin lesions; such patients should be monitored regularly by a dermatologist.

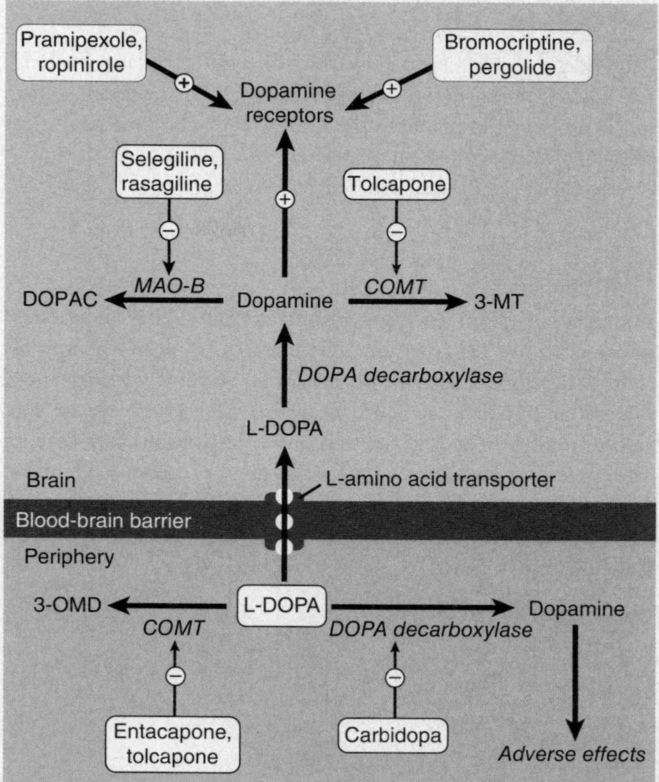

FIGURE 28–5 Pharmacologic strategies for dopaminergic therapy of Parkinson disease. Drugs and their effects are indicated (see text). COMT, catechol-*O*-methyltransferase; DOPAC, dihydroxyphenylacetic acid; L-DOPA, levodopa; MAO, monoamine oxidase; 3-MT, 3-methoxytyramine; 3-OMD, 3-*O*-methyldopa.

DOPAMINE RECEPTOR AGONISTS

Drugs acting directly on postsynaptic dopamine receptors may have a beneficial effect in addition to that of levodopa (Figure 28–5). Unlike levodopa, they do not require enzymatic conversion to an active metabolite, act directly on the postsynaptic dopamine receptors, have no potentially toxic metabolites, and do not compete with other substances for active transport into the blood and across the blood-brain barrier. Moreover, drugs selectively affecting certain (but not all) dopamine receptors may have more limited adverse effects than levodopa. Several dopamine agonists have antiparkinsonism activity. The older dopamine agonists (bromocriptine and pergolide) are ergot (ergoline) derivatives (see Chapter 16) and are rarely—if ever—used to treat parkinsonism. Their side effects are of more concern than those of the newer agents (pramipexole and ropinirole).

There is no evidence that one agonist is superior to another; individual patients, however, may respond to one but not another of these agents. Moreover, their duration of action varies and is lengthened by extended-release preparations. Apomorphine is a potent dopamine agonist but is discussed separately in a later section in this chapter because it is used primarily as a rescue drug for patients with disabling response fluctuations to levodopa.

Dopamine agonists have been used as first-line therapy for Parkinson disease, and their use is associated with a lower incidence of the response fluctuations and dyskinesias that occur with long-term levodopa therapy. Dopaminergic therapy is therefore often initiated with a dopamine agonist, although, compared with levodopa, the agonists generally provide less symptomatic benefit and are more likely to cause mental side effects, somnolence, and edema. In other instances, a low dose of carbidopa plus levodopa (eg, Sinemet, 25/100 three times daily) is introduced, and a dopamine agonist is then added. In either case, the dose of the dopamine agonist is built up gradually depending on response and tolerance. Dopamine agonists may also be given to patients with parkinsonism who are taking levodopa and who have end-of-dose akinesia or on-off phenomenon or are becoming resistant to treatment with levodopa. In such circumstances, it is generally necessary to lower the dose of levodopa to prevent intolerable adverse effects. The response to a dopamine agonist is generally disappointing in patients who have never responded to levodopa.

Bromocriptine

Bromocriptine is a D_2 agonist; its structure is shown in Table 16–7. This drug has been widely used to treat Parkinson disease in the past but is now rarely used for this purpose. The usual daily dose of bromocriptine for parkinsonism varies between 7.5 and 30 mg. To minimize adverse effects, the dose is built up slowly over 2 or 3 months depending on response or the development of adverse reactions.

Pergolide

Pergolide, another ergot derivative, directly stimulates both D_1 and D_2 receptors. It too has been widely used for parkinsonism but is no longer available in the United States because its use has been associated with the development of valvular heart disease. It is nevertheless still used in some countries.

Pramipexole

Pramipexole is not an ergot derivative, but it has preferential affinity for the D_3 receptor. It is effective as monotherapy for mild parkinsonism and is also helpful in patients with advanced disease, permitting the dose of levodopa to be reduced and smoothing out response fluctuations. Pramipexole may ameliorate affective symptoms. A possible neuroprotective effect has been suggested by its ability to scavenge hydrogen peroxide and enhance neurotrophic activity in mesencephalic dopaminergic cell cultures.

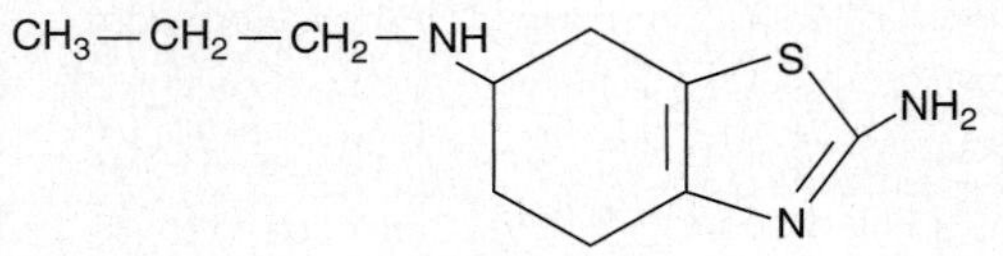

Pramipexole

Pramipexole is rapidly absorbed after oral administration, reaching peak plasma concentrations in approximately 2 hours, and is excreted largely unchanged in the urine. It is started at a dosage of 0.125 mg three times daily, doubled after 1 week, and again after another week. Further increments in the daily dose are by 0.75 mg at weekly intervals, depending on response and tolerance. Most patients require between 0.5 and 1.5 mg three times daily. Renal insufficiency may necessitate dosage adjustment. An extended-release preparation is now available and is taken once daily at a dose equivalent to the total daily dose of standard pramipexole. The extended-release preparation is generally more convenient for patients and avoids swings in blood levels of the drug over the day.

Ropinirole

Another nonergoline derivative, ropinirole (now available in a generic preparation) is a relatively pure D_2 receptor agonist that is effective as monotherapy in patients with mild disease and as a means of smoothing the response to levodopa in patients with more advanced disease and response fluctuations. It is introduced at 0.25 mg three times daily, and the total daily dose is then increased by 0.75 mg at weekly intervals until the fourth week and by 1.5 mg thereafter. In most instances, a dosage between 2 and 8 mg three times daily is necessary. Ropinirole is metabolized by CYP1A2; other drugs metabolized by this isoform may significantly reduce its clearance. A prolonged-release preparation taken once daily is available.

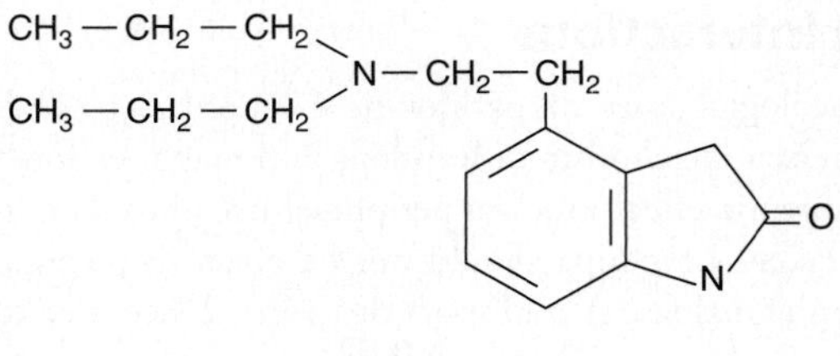

Ropinirole

Rotigotine

The dopamine agonist rotigotine, delivered daily through a skin patch, is approved for treatment of early Parkinson disease. It supposedly provides more continuous dopaminergic stimulation than oral medication in early parkinsonism; its efficacy in more advanced disease is less clear. Benefits and side effects are similar to those of other dopamine agonists but reactions may also occur at the application site and are sometimes serious. Treatment is usually started with the 2 mg/24 hours patch and titrated weekly as necessary by increasing the patch size to 4 mg/24 hours and then to 6 mg/24 hours.

Adverse Effects of Dopamine Agonists

A. Gastrointestinal Effects

Anorexia and nausea and vomiting may occur when a dopamine agonist is introduced and can be minimized by taking the medication with meals. Constipation, dyspepsia, and symptoms of reflux esophagitis may also occur. Bleeding from peptic ulceration has been reported.

B. Cardiovascular Effects

Postural hypotension may occur, particularly at the initiation of therapy. Painless digital vasospasm is a dose-related complication of long-term treatment with the ergot derivatives (bromocriptine or pergolide). When cardiac arrhythmias occur, they are an indication for discontinuing treatment. Peripheral edema is sometimes problematic. Cardiac valvulopathy may occur with pergolide.

C. Dyskinesias

Abnormal movements similar to those introduced by levodopa may occur and are reversed by reducing the total dose of dopaminergic drugs being taken.

D. Mental Disturbances

Confusion, hallucinations, delusions, and other psychiatric reactions may develop as a feature of Parkinson disease or as complications of dopaminergic treatment and are more common and severe with dopamine receptor agonists than with levodopa. They tend to occur earlier in older patients and become more common as the disease advances. There appears to be no difference between the various dopamine agonists in their ability to induce these disorders. They may respond to atypical antipsychotic agents such as clozapine, olanzapine, quetiapine, and risperidone or to pimavanserin.

Disorders of impulse control may occur either as an exaggeration of a previous tendency or as a new phenomenon and may lead to compulsive gambling, shopping, betting, sexual activity, and other behaviors (see Chapter 32). Their prevalence varies in different reports but may be as high as 45% in parkinsonian patients treated with dopamine agonists. They relate to activation of D_2 or D_3 dopamine receptors in the mesocorticolimbic system, may occur with one dopamine agonist and not another, and may occur at any time after the initiation of treatment. They have been associated with increasing dose and duration of treatment; in some patients, a dose reduction may ameliorate them. They resolve on withdrawal of the offending medication. Impulse control disorders are generally under-reported by patients and their families and often unrecognized by health care professionals. Risk factors include an impulsive personality, a history of drug use or other addictive behaviors, and a family history of gambling disorders.

A withdrawal syndrome develops in occasional patients tapered off a dopamine agonist. It consists of a combination of distressing physical and psychological symptoms that are refractory to levodopa and other dopaminergic medications, that may persist for months or longer, and for which no other cause can be found. Anxiety, agitation, panic attacks, depression, suicidal ideation, irritability, fatigue, postural hypotension, nausea, vomiting, diaphoresis, and drug cravings may occur. Risk factors include impulse control behavior disorders and higher dopamine agonist dosage. There is no effective treatment. The dopamine agonist should be reintroduced and tapered more gradually if possible.

Treatment with dopamine agonists should not be stopped abruptly, because doing so may rarely lead to an akinetic (parkinsonian) crisis or to a syndrome resembling neuroleptic malignant syndrome (discussed later).

E. Miscellaneous

Headache, nasal congestion, increased arousal, pulmonary infiltrates, pleural and retroperitoneal fibrosis, and erythromelalgia are other reported adverse effects of the ergot-derived dopamine agonists. Erythromelalgia consists of red, tender, painful, swollen feet and, occasionally, hands, at times associated with arthralgia; symptoms and signs clear within a few days of withdrawal of the causal drug. In rare instances, an uncontrollable tendency to fall asleep at inappropriate times has occurred, particularly in patients receiving pramipexole or ropinirole; this requires discontinuation of the medication.

Contraindications

Dopamine agonists are contraindicated in patients with a history of psychotic illness or recent myocardial infarction, or with active peptic ulceration. The ergot-derived agonists are best avoided in patients with peripheral vascular disease.

MONOAMINE OXIDASE INHIBITORS

Two types of monoamine oxidase have been distinguished in the nervous system. Monoamine oxidase A metabolizes norepinephrine, serotonin, and dopamine; monoamine oxidase B metabolizes dopamine selectively. **Selegiline** (deprenyl) (see Figure 28–3), a selective irreversible inhibitor of monoamine oxidase B at normal doses (at higher doses it inhibits monoamine oxidase A as well), retards the breakdown of dopamine (see Figure 28–5); in consequence, it enhances and prolongs the antiparkinsonism effect of levodopa (thereby allowing the dose of levodopa to be reduced) and may reduce mild on-off or wearing-off phenomena. It is therefore used as adjunctive therapy for patients with a declining or fluctuating response to levodopa. The standard dose of selegiline is 5 mg with breakfast and 5 mg with lunch. Selegiline may cause insomnia when taken later during the day.

Selegiline has only a minor therapeutic effect on parkinsonism when given alone. Studies in animals suggest that it may reduce disease progression, but trials to test the effect of selegiline on the progression of parkinsonism in humans have yielded ambiguous results. The findings in a large multicenter study were taken to suggest a beneficial effect in slowing disease progression but may simply have reflected a symptomatic response.

Rasagiline, another monoamine oxidase B inhibitor, is more potent than selegiline in preventing MPTP-induced parkinsonism and is being used as monotherapy for early treatment in patients with mild symptoms. The standard dosage is 1 mg/d. Rasagiline is also used as adjunctive therapy at a dosage of 0.5 or 1 mg/d to prolong the effects of carbidopa-levodopa in patients with advanced disease and response fluctuations. A large double-blind, placebo-controlled, delayed-start study (the ADAGIO trial) to evaluate whether it had neuroprotective benefit (ie, slowed the disease course) yielded unclear results: a daily dose of 1 mg met all the end points of the study and did seem to slow disease progression, but a 2-mg dose failed to do so. These findings are difficult to explain, and the decision to use rasagiline for neuroprotective purposes therefore remains an individual one.

A third monoamine oxidase B inhibitor, **safinamide,** has been used to reduce response fluctuations in patients taking carbidopa-levodopa, diminishing off-periods in patients with wearing-off effect or on-off phenomena. It is not effective as monotherapy for Parkinson disease. The starting dose is 50 mg orally once daily, increased after 2 weeks to 100 mg once daily.

Monoamine oxidase B inhibitors should not be taken by patients receiving meperidine, tramadol, methadone, propoxyphene, cyclobenzaprine, or St. John's wort. The antitussive dextromethorphan should also be avoided by patients taking one of the monoamine oxidase B inhibitors; indeed, it is wise to advise patients to avoid all over-the-counter cold preparations. Rasagiline, selegiline, or safinamide should not be taken with other monoamine oxidase inhibitors and should be used with care in patients receiving tricyclic antidepressants or serotonin reuptake inhibitors because of the theoretical risk of acute toxic interactions of the serotonin syndrome type (see Chapter 16), but this is rarely encountered in practice. The adverse effects of levodopa, especially dyskinesias, mental changes, nausea, and sleep disorders, may be increased by these drugs. Hypertension may be precipitated or aggravated.

The combined administration of levodopa and an inhibitor of both forms of monoamine oxidase (ie, a nonselective inhibitor) must be avoided, because it may lead to hypertensive crises, probably due to the peripheral accumulation of norepinephrine.

CATECHOL-*O*-METHYLTRANSFERASE INHIBITORS

Inhibition of dopa decarboxylase is associated with compensatory activation of other pathways of levodopa metabolism, especially catechol-*O*-methyltransferase (COMT), and this increases plasma levels of 3-*O*-methyldopa (3-OMD). Elevated levels of 3-OMD have been associated with a poor therapeutic response to levodopa, perhaps in part because 3-OMD competes with levodopa for an active carrier mechanism that governs its transport across the intestinal mucosa and the blood-brain barrier. Selective COMT inhibitors such as **tolcapone** and **entacapone** also prolong the action of levodopa by diminishing its peripheral metabolism (see Figure 28–5). Levodopa clearance is decreased, and relative bioavailability of levodopa is thus increased. Neither the time to reach peak concentration nor the maximal concentration of levodopa is increased. These agents may be helpful in patients receiving levodopa who have developed response fluctuations, leading to a smoother response, more prolonged on-time, and the option of reducing total daily levodopa dose. There is no benefit in taking a COMT inhibitor either alone or with levodopa as initial therapy for parkinsonism.

Tolcapone and entacapone are both widely available, but entacapone is generally preferred because it has not been associated with hepatotoxicity. The pharmacologic effects of tolcapone and entacapone are similar, and both are rapidly absorbed, bound to plasma proteins, and metabolized before excretion. However, tolcapone has both central and peripheral effects, whereas the effect of entacapone is peripheral. The half-life of both drugs is approximately 2 hours, but tolcapone is slightly more potent and has a longer duration of action. Tolcapone is taken in a standard dosage of 100 mg three times daily; some patients require a daily dose of twice that amount. By contrast, entacapone (200 mg) needs to be taken with each dose of levodopa, up to six times daily.

Opicapone (Ongentys) is a newer long-acting, peripherally selective, catechol-*O*-methyl transferase inhibitor that is taken once daily at bedtime, in a 50-mg dose. As with the other COMT inhibitors, it decreases the duration of daily off-periods and increases on-time in patients with a fluctuating response to levodopa.

Adverse effects of the COMT inhibitors relate in part to increased levodopa exposure and include dyskinesias, nausea, and confusion. It is often necessary to lower the daily dose of levodopa by about 30% in the first 48 hours to avoid or reverse such complications. Other adverse effects include diarrhea, abdominal pain, orthostatic hypotension, sleep disturbances, and an orange discoloration of the urine. Tolcapone may cause an increase in liver enzyme levels and has been associated rarely with death from acute hepatic failure; accordingly, it should not be used in patients with abnormal liver function test results. Its use in the USA requires signed patient consent (as provided in the product labeling) plus monitoring of liver function tests every 2–4 weeks during the first 6 months and periodically but less frequently thereafter. The medication should be withdrawn and not reintroduced if hepatic damage becomes evident. No such toxicity has been reported with entacapone.

The commercial preparation named **Stalevo** consists of a combination of levodopa with both carbidopa and entacapone. It is available in three strengths: Stalevo 50 (50 mg levodopa plus 12.5 mg carbidopa and 200 mg entacapone), Stalevo 100 (100 mg, 25 mg, and 200 mg, respectively), and Stalevo 150 (150 mg, 37.5 mg, and 200 mg, respectively). Use of this preparation simplifies the drug regimen and requires the consumption of fewer tablets than otherwise. The combination agent may provide greater symptomatic benefit than carbidopa-levodopa alone. However, despite the convenience of a single combination preparation, use of Stalevo rather than carbidopa-levodopa has been associated with earlier occurrence and increased frequency of dyskinesia. There is no evidence that the use of Stalevo is associated with an increased risk for cardiovascular events (myocardial infarction, stroke, cardiovascular death).

APOMORPHINE

Subcutaneous injection of apomorphine hydrochloride **(Apokyn),** a potent nonergoline dopamine agonist that interacts with postsynaptic D_2 receptors in the caudate nucleus and putamen, is effective for the temporary relief ("rescue") of off-periods of akinesia in patients on optimized dopaminergic therapy. It is rapidly taken up in the blood and then the brain, leading to clinical benefit that begins within about 10 minutes of injection and persists for up to 2 hours. The optimal dose is identified by administering increasing test doses until adequate benefit is achieved or a maximum of 0.6 mL (6 mg) is reached, with the supine and standing blood pressures monitored before injection and then every 20 minutes for an hour after it. Most patients require a dose of 0.3–0.6 mL (3–6 mg), and this should be given usually no more than about three times daily, but occasionally up to five times daily. Apomorphine can also be given as continuous therapy by infusion to reduce off-time and response fluctuations.

Nausea is often troublesome, especially at the initiation of apomorphine treatment; accordingly, oral pretreatment with the antiemetic trimethobenzamide (300 mg three times daily) for 3 days is recommended before apomorphine is introduced and is then continued for at least 1 month, if not indefinitely. Other adverse effects include dyskinesias, drowsiness, insomnia, chest pain, sweating, hypotension, syncope, constipation, diarrhea, mental or behavioral disturbances, panniculitis, and bruising at the injection site. Apomorphine should be prescribed only by physicians familiar with its potential complications and interactions. It should not be used in patients taking serotonin 5-HT_3 antagonists because severe hypotension may result.

AMANTADINE

Amantadine, an antiviral agent, was by chance found to have relatively weak antiparkinsonism properties. Its mode of action in parkinsonism is unclear, but it may potentiate dopaminergic function by influencing the synthesis, release, or reuptake of dopamine. It has been reported to antagonize the effects of adenosine at adenosine A_{2A} receptors, which may inhibit D_2 receptor function.

Release of catecholamines from peripheral stores has also been documented. Amantadine is an antagonist of the NMDA-type glutamate receptor, suggesting an antidyskinetic effect. It is available in an immediate-release formulation (**Symmetrel;** standard dose, 100 mg orally two or three times daily) and extended-release formulations (**Gocovri,** once daily at bedtime; **Osmolex,** 129–322 mg once daily in the morning).

Pharmacokinetics

Peak plasma concentrations of amantadine are reached 1–4 hours after an oral dose of the immediate-release preparation. The plasma half-life is between 2 and 4 hours, with most of the drug being excreted unchanged in the urine.

Clinical Use

Amantadine is less efficacious than levodopa, and its benefits may be short-lived, often disappearing after only a few weeks of treatment. Nevertheless, during that time it may favorably influence the bradykinesia, rigidity, and tremor of parkinsonism. Amantadine may also help in reducing iatrogenic dyskinesias in patients with advanced disease.

Adverse Effects

Amantadine has several undesirable central nervous system effects, all of which can be reversed by stopping the drug. These include restlessness, depression, suicidal ideation, irritability, impulse-control disorders, somnolence, insomnia, agitation, excitement, hallucinations, confusion, and psychosis. Overdosage may produce an acute toxic psychosis. With doses several times higher than recommended, convulsions have occurred.

Livedo reticularis sometimes occurs in patients taking amantadine and usually clears within 1 month after the drug is withdrawn. Other dermatologic reactions have also been described. Peripheral edema, another well-recognized complication, is not accompanied by signs of cardiac, hepatic, or renal disease and responds to diuretics. Other adverse reactions to amantadine include headache, heart failure, postural hypotension, urinary retention, and gastrointestinal disturbances (eg, anorexia, nausea, constipation, and dry mouth).

Amantadine should be used with caution in patients with a history of seizures, heart failure, or moderate or severe renal disease. Discontinuation of the medication should be gradual, as abrupt withdrawal may lead to an acute confusional state, hyperpyrexia, and abrupt worsening of parkinsonism.

ISTRADEFYLLINE

Istradefylline is an analog of caffeine and a selective antagonist of the adenosine A_{2A} receptor. It can be taken orally (20 or 40 mg daily) to reduce off-periods and improve motor function in patients taking carbidopa-levodopa. Side effects include dyskinesias, dizziness, constipation, nausea, hallucinations, and sleeplessness. Hallucinations, psychoses, or impulsive or compulsive behaviors may necessitate dose reductions or discontinuation of the drug.

TABLE 28-2 Some drugs with antimuscarinic properties used in parkinsonism.

Drug	Usual Daily Dose (mg)
Benztropine mesylate	1–6
Biperiden	2–12
Orphenadrine	150–400
Procyclidine	7.5–30
Trihexyphenidyl	6–20

ACETYLCHOLINE-BLOCKING DRUGS

Several centrally acting antimuscarinic preparations are available that differ in their potency and in their efficacy in different patients. Some of these drugs were discussed in Chapter 8. These agents may improve the tremor and rigidity of parkinsonism but have little effect on bradykinesia. They are more effective than placebo. Some of the more commonly used drugs are listed in Table 28–2.

Clinical Use

Treatment is started with a low dose of one of the drugs in this category, the dosage gradually being increased until benefit occurs or until adverse effects limit further increments. If patients do not respond to one drug, a trial with another member of the drug class is warranted and may be successful.

Adverse Effects

Antimuscarinic drugs have several undesirable central nervous system and peripheral effects (see Chapter 8) and are poorly tolerated by the elderly or cognitively impaired. Dyskinesias occur in rare cases. Acute suppurative parotitis sometimes occurs as a complication of dryness of the mouth.

If medication is to be withdrawn, this should be accomplished gradually rather than abruptly to prevent acute exacerbation of parkinsonism. For contraindications to the use of antimuscarinic drugs, see Chapter 8.

SURGICAL PROCEDURES

Ablative surgical procedures for parkinsonism have generally been replaced by functional, reversible lesions induced by high-frequency deep brain stimulation, which has a lower morbidity.

Stimulation of the subthalamic nucleus or globus pallidus by an implanted electrode and stimulator has yielded good results for the management of the clinical fluctuations or the dyskinesias occurring in moderate parkinsonism. The anatomic substrate for such therapy is indicated in Figure 28–1. Such procedures are contraindicated in patients with secondary or atypical parkinsonism, dementia, or failure to respond to dopaminergic medication. The level of antiparkinsonian medication can often be reduced in patients undergoing deep brain stimulation, and this may help to ameliorate dose-related adverse effects of medication. Patients with medically refractory tremor-predominant parkinsonism who are reluctant to undergo surgery may respond to focused ultrasound thalamotomy.

In a controlled trial of the transplantation of dopaminergic tissue (fetal substantia nigra tissue), symptomatic benefit occurred in younger (less than 60 years old) but not older parkinsonian patients. In another trial, benefits were inconsequential. Furthermore, uncontrollable dyskinesias occurred in some patients in both studies, perhaps from a relative excess of dopamine from continued fiber outgrowth from the transplant. Additional basic studies are required before further trials of cellular therapies—in particular, stem cell therapies—are undertaken, and such approaches therefore remain investigational.

NEUROPROTECTIVE THERAPY

Among the compounds that have been investigated as potential neuroprotective agents to slow disease progression are antioxidants, antiapoptotic agents, glutamate antagonists, intraparenchymally administered glial-derived neurotrophic factor, and anti-inflammatory drugs. None of these agents has been shown to be effective in this context, however, and their use for therapeutic purposes is not indicated at this time. Specifically, coenzyme Q10, creatine, pramipexole, and pioglitazone have not been found to be effective despite early hopes to the contrary. The urate precursor inosine, and isradipine, a dihydropyridine calcium-channel blocker with relatively high affinity for $C_{av}1.3$ channels, also failed to show benefit in randomized controlled trials. The possibility that rasagiline has a protective effect was discussed earlier.

Other agents currently being studied as disease-modifying agents include deferiprone (a potent iron chelator) and exenatide, a glucagon-like peptide-1 (GLP-1) receptor agonist (see Chapter 41) that affects various cellular processes likely to be involved in the etiology of Parkinson disease.

Active and passive immunization against α-synuclein or an α-synuclein-mimicking peptide is also being explored. The procedures are generally well-tolerated, without treatment-associated adverse events other than mild injection-site reactions, and lead to generation of antibodies against α-synuclein.

Recent work suggests that an assay for misfolded α-synuclein in the spinal fluid has high sensitivity and specificity in distinguishing Parkinson disease from healthy controls and may serve as a useful biomarker of the disease, even before it becomes manifest clinically. If confirmed, this would permit those at risk of the disease to start protective treatment before they become symptomatic.

GENE THERAPY

Several phase 1 (safety) or phase 2 trials of gene therapy for Parkinson disease have been completed in the USA. All trials involved infusion into the striatum of adeno-associated virus type 2 as the vector for the gene. The genes were for glutamic acid decarboxylase (GAD, to facilitate synthesis of GABA, an inhibitory neurotransmitter), infused into the subthalamic nucleus to cause inhibition; for aromatic acid decarboxylase (AADC), infused into the putamen to increase metabolism of levodopa to dopamine; and for neurturin (a growth factor that may enhance the survival of dopaminergic neurons), infused into the putamen. All agents were deemed safe. A phase 2 study of the GAD gene has been completed and the results are encouraging, but one for neurturin infused into the substantia nigra as well as the putamen was disappointing. In a phase 1b trial of AADC in moderately advanced disease, motor function and quality of life stabilized or improved, and medication requirements were reduced in some patients. The results of a European study involving bilateral intrastriatal delivery of ProSavin, a lentiviral vector-based gene therapy with three genes (decarboxylase, tyrosine hydroxylase, and GTP-cyclohydrolase 1) aimed at restoring local and continuous dopamine production in patients with advanced Parkinson disease, have also been encouraging.

THERAPY FOR NONMOTOR MANIFESTATIONS

Persons with cognitive decline may respond to rivastigmine (1.5–6 mg twice daily), memantine (5–10 mg daily), or donepezil (5–10 mg daily) (see Chapter 60); with affective disorders to antidepressants or anxiolytic agents (see Chapter 30); with psychosis to atypical antipsychotic agents or pimavanserin; with excessive daytime sleepiness to modafinil (100–400 mg in the morning) (see Chapter 9); and with bladder and bowel disorders to appropriate symptomatic therapy (see Chapter 8).

GENERAL COMMENTS ON DRUG MANAGEMENT OF PATIENTS WITH PARKINSONISM

Parkinson disease generally follows a progressive course. Moreover, the benefits of levodopa therapy often diminish as the disease advances, and serious adverse effects may complicate long-term levodopa treatment. Nevertheless, dopaminergic therapy at a relatively early stage may be most effective in alleviating motor symptoms of parkinsonism and may also favorably affect the mortality rate due to the disease. Therefore, several strategies have evolved for optimizing dopaminergic therapy, as summarized in Figure 28–5. Symptomatic treatment of mild parkinsonism is probably best avoided until there is some degree of disability or functional limitation or until symptoms begin to impact the patient's lifestyle or cause significant social impairment.

When symptomatic treatment becomes necessary, a trial of rasagiline, selegiline, amantadine, or an antimuscarinic drug (in young patients) may be worthwhile. With disease progression, dopaminergic therapy becomes necessary. This can conveniently be initiated with either carbidopa-levodopa therapy or a dopamine agonist, either alone or in combination, although an agonist is best avoided in patients older than 70 or when risk factors for impulse control disorders are present. Carbidopa-levodopa is the most effective symptomatic treatment of the motor disturbances of parkinsonism. Physical therapy is helpful in improving mobility. In patients with severe parkinsonism and long-term complications of levodopa therapy such as the on-off phenomenon, a trial of treatment with the newer extended-release formulation of carbidopa-levodopa (Rytary), a COMT inhibitor, or rasagiline may be helpful. Regulation of dietary protein intake may also improve response fluctuations. Deep brain stimulation is often helpful in patients with response fluctuations or dyskinesias who fail to respond adequately to these measures. Treating patients who are young or have mild parkinsonism with rasagiline may delay disease progression and merits consideration, although evidence of benefit is incomplete.

DRUG-INDUCED PARKINSONISM

Reserpine and the related drugs tetrabenazine, deutetrabenazine, and valbenazine deplete biogenic monoamines from their storage sites, whereas haloperidol, metoclopramide, and the phenothiazines block dopamine receptors. These drugs may therefore produce a parkinsonian syndrome, usually within 3 or 4 months after introduction. The disorder tends to be symmetric, with inconspicuous tremor, but this is not always the case. The syndrome is related to high dosage and clears over several weeks or months after withdrawal. If treatment is necessary, antimuscarinic agents are preferred. Levodopa is of no help if neuroleptic drugs are continued and may in fact aggravate the mental disorder for which antipsychotic drugs were prescribed originally.

In 1983, a drug-induced form of parkinsonism was discovered in individuals who attempted to synthesize and use a narcotic drug related to meperidine but actually synthesized and self-administered MPTP, as discussed in the Box: MPTP & Parkinsonism.

ATYPICAL PARKINSONISM SYNDROMES

Several disorders characterized by parkinsonism differ from classic Parkinson disease because of inconspicuous tremor, symmetry of the neurologic findings, and the presence of additional findings (eg, dysautonomia, cerebellar deficits, eye movement abnormalities, or early cognitive and behavioral changes). These disorders include **multisystem atrophy, progressive supranuclear palsy, corticobasal degeneration** (in which parkinsonism may be markedly asymmetric), and **diffuse Lewy body disease**. The prognosis is worse than for Parkinson disease, and the response to antiparkinsonian treatment may be limited. Treatment is symptomatic.

OTHER MOVEMENT DISORDERS

Tremor

Tremor consists of rhythmic oscillatory movements. Physiologic postural tremor, which is a normal phenomenon, is enhanced in amplitude by anxiety, fatigue, thyrotoxicosis, and intravenous epinephrine or isoproterenol. **Propranolol** reduces its amplitude and, if administered intra-arterially, prevents the response to isoproterenol in the perfused limb, presumably through some peripheral action. Certain drugs—especially the bronchodilators, valproate, tricyclic antidepressants, and lithium—may produce a dose-dependent exaggeration of the normal physiologic tremor that is reversed by discontinuing the drug. Although the tremor produced by sympathomimetics such as terbutaline (a bronchodilator) is blocked by propranolol, which antagonizes both β_1 and β_2 receptors, it is not blocked by metoprolol, a β_1-selective antagonist; this suggests that such tremor is mediated mainly by the β_2 receptors.

Essential tremor is a postural tremor, sometimes familial with autosomal dominant inheritance, which is clinically similar to physiologic tremor. Dysfunction of β_1 receptors has been implicated in some instances, since the tremor may respond dramatically to standard doses of metoprolol as well as to propranolol. The tremor may involve the hands, head, voice, and—much less commonly—the legs. Patients may become functionally limited or socially withdrawn, quality of life is affected, and some patients report being seriously disabled by the tremor.

The most useful therapeutic approach is with propranolol, but whether the response depends on a central or peripheral action is unclear. The pharmacokinetics, pharmacologic effects, and adverse reactions of propranolol are discussed in Chapter 10. Total daily doses of propranolol on the order of 120 mg or more (range, 60–320 mg) are usually required, divided into two doses; reported adverse effects have been few. Propranolol should be used with caution in patients with heart failure, heart block, asthma, depression, or hypoglycemia. Other adverse effects include fatigue, malaise, lightheadedness, and impotence. Patients can be instructed to take their own pulse and call the physician if significant bradycardia develops. Long-acting propranolol is also effective and is preferred by many patients because of its convenience. Some patients prefer to take a single dose of propranolol when they anticipate their tremor is likely to be exacerbated, for example, by social situations. Metoprolol is sometimes useful in treating tremor when patients have concomitant pulmonary disease that contraindicates use of propranolol.

Drugs potentiating $GABA_A$ receptors in the central nervous system (such as phenobarbital, primidone, topiramate, and benzodiazepines) also improve tremor, but phenobarbital is not used clinically because of its sedating effect. **Primidone** (an antiepileptic drug; see Chapter 24), in gradually increasing doses up to 250 mg three times daily, is also effective in providing symptomatic control in some cases. Patients with tremor are very sensitive to primidone and often cannot tolerate the doses used to treat seizures; they should be started on 50 mg once daily and the daily dose increased by 50 mg every 2 weeks depending on response. In many instances, a dose of 125 mg two or three times daily is sufficient.

MPTP & Parkinsonism

Reports in the early 1980s of a rapidly progressive form of parkinsonism in young persons opened a new area of research in the etiology and treatment of parkinsonism. The initial report described apparently healthy young people who attempted to support their opioid habit with a meperidine analog synthesized by an amateur chemist. They unwittingly self-administered 1-methyl-4-phenyl-1,2,3,6-tetrahydropyridine (MPTP) and subsequently developed a very severe form of parkinsonism.

MPTP is a protoxin that is converted by monoamine oxidase B to *N*-methyl-4-phenylpyridinium (MPP^+). MPP^+ is selectively taken up by cells in the substantia nigra through an active mechanism normally responsible for dopamine reuptake. MPP^+ inhibits mitochondrial complex I, thereby inhibiting oxidative phosphorylation. The interaction of MPP^+ with complex I probably leads to cell death and thus to striatal dopamine depletion and parkinsonism.

Recognition of the effects of MPTP suggested that spontaneously occurring Parkinson disease may result from exposure to an environmental toxin that is similarly selective in its target. However, no such toxin has yet been identified. It also suggested a successful means of producing an experimental model of Parkinson disease in animals, especially nonhuman primates. This model is useful in the development of new antiparkinsonism drugs. Pretreatment of exposed animals with a monoamine oxidase B inhibitor such as selegiline prevents the conversion of MPTP to MPP^+ and thus protects against the occurrence of parkinsonism. This observation has provided one reason to believe that selegiline or rasagiline may retard the progression of Parkinson disease in humans.

Topiramate, another antiepileptic drug, may also be helpful in a dose of 400 mg daily, built up gradually. **Alprazolam** (in doses up to 3 mg daily) or **gabapentin** (100–2400 mg/d; typically 1200 mg/d) is helpful in some patients. Gabapentin binds to the $\alpha 2\delta$ subunit of calcium channels. It produces less consistent relief of tremor but is associated with fewer side effects than primidone. Other patients are helped by intramuscular injections of botulinum toxin, but dose-dependent weakness may complicate symptomatic benefit. Thalamic stimulation by an implanted electrode and stimulator is worthwhile in advanced cases refractory to pharmacotherapy. Thalamotomy by magnetic resonance imaging-guided focused ultrasound or stereotactic radiosurgery is also effective in reducing upper-extremity tremor. Diazepam, chlordiazepoxide, mephenesin, and antiparkinsonism agents have been advocated in the past but are generally of little benefit. Small quantities of alcohol may suppress essential tremor for a short time but should not be recommended as a treatment strategy because of possible behavioral and other complications of alcohol.

Intention tremor is present during movement but not at rest; sometimes it occurs as a toxic manifestation of alcohol or drugs such as phenytoin. Withdrawal or reduction in dosage provides dramatic relief. There is no satisfactory pharmacologic treatment for intention tremor due to other neurologic disorders.

Rest tremor is usually due to parkinsonism.

Huntington Disease

Huntington disease is an autosomal dominant inherited disorder caused by an abnormality (expansion of a CAG trinucleotide repeat that codes for a polyglutamine tract) of the *huntingtin* gene on chromosome 4. An autosomal recessive form may also occur. Huntington disease-like (HDL) disorders are not associated with an abnormal CAG trinucleotide repeat number of the *huntingtin* gene. Autosomal dominant (*HDL1*, 20pter-p12; *HDL2*, 16q24.3) and recessive forms (*HDL3*, 4p15.3) occur.

Huntington disease is characterized by progressive chorea and dementia that usually begin in adulthood. The development of chorea seems to be related to an imbalance of dopamine, acetylcholine, GABA, and perhaps other neurotransmitters in the basal ganglia (Figure 28–6). Pharmacologic studies indicate that chorea results from functional overactivity in dopaminergic nigrostriatal pathways, perhaps because of increased responsiveness of postsynaptic dopamine receptors or deficiency of a neurotransmitter that normally antagonizes dopamine. Drugs that impair dopaminergic neurotransmission, either by depleting central monoamines (eg, reserpine, tetrabenazine, deutetrabenazine, valbenazine) or

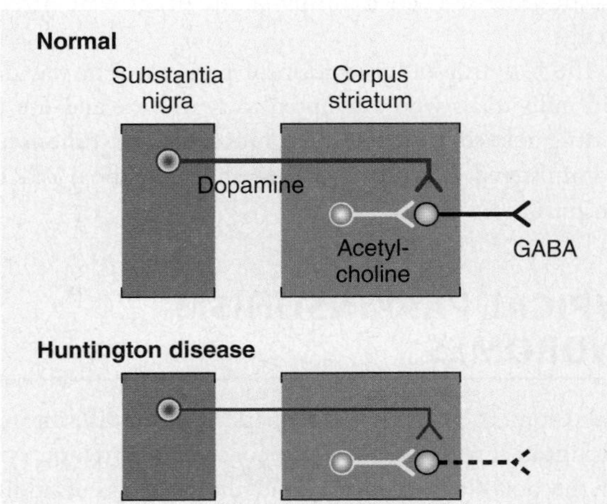

FIGURE 28–6 Schematic representation of the sequence of neurons involved in Huntington chorea. The complex anatomic circuitry has been simplified. **Top:** Dopaminergic neurons (red) originating in the substantia nigra normally inhibit the output of the spiny GABAergic neurons from the striatum, whereas cholinergic neurons (green) exert an excitatory effect. **Bottom:** In Huntington chorea, some cholinergic neurons may be lost, but even more GABAergic neurons (black) degenerate.

by blocking dopamine receptors (eg, phenothiazines, butyrophenones), often alleviate chorea, whereas dopamine-like drugs such as levodopa tend to exacerbate it.

Both GABA and the enzyme (glutamic acid decarboxylase) concerned with its synthesis are markedly reduced in the basal ganglia of patients with Huntington disease, and GABA receptors are usually implicated in inhibitory pathways. There is also a significant decline in concentration of choline acetyltransferase, the enzyme responsible for synthesizing acetylcholine, in the basal ganglia of these patients. These findings may be of pathophysiologic significance and have led to attempts to alleviate chorea by enhancing central GABA or acetylcholine activity, but with disappointing results. Consequently, the most commonly used drugs for controlling dyskinesia in patients with Huntington disease are still those that interfere with dopamine activity. With all the latter drugs, however, reduction of abnormal movements may be associated with iatrogenic parkinsonism.

Tetrabenazine (12.5–50 mg orally three times daily) depletes cerebral dopamine and reduces the severity of chorea. It has less troublesome adverse effects than reserpine, which has also been used for this purpose. Tetrabenazine is metabolized by cytochrome P450 (CYP2D6), and genotyping has therefore been recommended to determine metabolizer status (CYP2D6 expression) in patients needing doses exceeding 50 mg/d. For poor metabolizers, the maximum recommended dose is 50 mg daily (25 mg/dose); otherwise, a maximum dose of 100 mg daily can be used. Treatment with postsynaptic dopamine receptor blockers such as phenothiazines and butyrophenones may also be helpful. **Haloperidol** is started in a small dose, eg, 1 mg twice daily, and increased every 4 days depending on the response. If haloperidol is not helpful, treatment with increasing doses of **fluphenazine** in a similar dose, eg, 1 mg twice daily, sometimes helps. Several recent reports suggest that **olanzapine** may also be useful; the dose varies with the patient, but 10 mg daily is often sufficient, although doses as high as 30 mg daily are sometimes required. The pharmacokinetics and clinical properties of these drugs are considered in greater detail elsewhere in this book. Selective serotonin reuptake inhibitors may reduce depression, aggression, and agitation. However, strong CYP2D6 inhibitors should be used with caution, as it may be necessary to decrease the dose of tetrabenazine taken concurrently.

Deutetrabenazine is a selective inhibitor of the vesicular monoamine 2 transporter (VMAT2) that modulates dopamine stores. It seems as effective as tetrabenazine for treating the chorea of Huntington disease and improving overall motor function, and may have fewer side effects. The dose is built up weekly from 6 mg daily to a maximum of 24 mg twice daily with food (18 mg twice daily in poor CYP2DG metabolizers). It may cause agitation, restlessness, and parkinsonism. Other adverse effects are sedation, dry mouth, diarrhea, insomnia, and fatigue. QT prolongation may occur. Deutetrabenazine is contraindicated in patients on monoamine oxidase inhibitors, reserpine, or tetrabenazine, and in those who are severely depressed or suicidal. **Valbenazine**, discussed later, is also now approved for treating chorea in patients with Huntington disease.

Other important aspects of management include genetic counseling, speech therapy, physical and occupational therapy, dysphagia precautions, and provision of social services.

Other Forms of Chorea

Benign hereditary chorea is inherited (usually autosomal dominant; possibly also autosomal recessive) or arises spontaneously. Chorea develops in early childhood and does not progress during adult life; dementia does not occur. In patients with *TITF-1* gene mutations, thyroid and pulmonary abnormalities may also be present (brain-thyroid-lung syndrome). Familial chorea may also occur as part of the chorea-acanthocytosis syndrome, together with orolingual tics, vocalizations, cognitive changes, seizures, peripheral neuropathy, and muscle atrophy; serum β-lipoproteins are normal. Mutations of the gene encoding chorein at 9q21 may be causal. Treatment of these hereditary disorders is symptomatic. Tetrabenazine (0.5 mg/kg/d for children and 37.5 mg/d for adults) may improve chorea in some instances. The efficacy in this context of the newer selective VMAT2 blockers deutetrabenazine and valbenazine is unclear.

Treatment is directed at the underlying cause when chorea occurs as a complication of general medical disorders such as thyrotoxicosis, polycythemia vera rubra, systemic lupus erythematosus, hypocalcemia, and hepatic cirrhosis. Drug-induced chorea is managed by withdrawal of the offending substance, which may be levodopa, an antimuscarinic drug, amphetamine, lithium, phenytoin, or an oral contraceptive. Neuroleptic drugs may also produce an acute or tardive dyskinesia (discussed below). Sydenham's chorea is temporary and usually so mild that pharmacologic management of the dyskinesia is unnecessary, but dopamine-blocking drugs are effective in suppressing it.

Ballismus

The biochemical basis of ballismus is unknown, but the pharmacologic approach to management is the same as for chorea. Treatment with tetrabenazine, haloperidol, perphenazine, or other dopamine-blocking drugs may be helpful.

Athetosis & Dystonia

The physiologic basis of these disorders is unknown, and there is no satisfactory medical treatment for them. A subset of patients respond well to levodopa medication (dopa-responsive dystonia), which is therefore worthy of trial. Occasional patients with dystonia may respond to diazepam, amantadine, antimuscarinic drugs (in high dosage), carbamazepine, baclofen, haloperidol, or phenothiazines. A trial of these pharmacologic approaches is worthwhile, though often not successful. Patients with focal dystonias such as blepharospasm or torticollis often benefit from injection of botulinum toxin into the overactive muscles. Deep brain stimulation may be helpful in medically intractable cases. The role of repetitive transcranial magnetic stimulation and transcranial direct current stimulation to induce plastic changes in the brain is being explored.

Tics

The pathophysiologic basis of tics is unknown. Chronic multiple tics **(Gilles de la Tourette syndrome)** may require symptomatic treatment if the disorder is severe or is having a significant impact on the patient's life. Education of patients, family, and teachers is important. Comprehensive behavioral intervention may help adults with Tourette syndrome. Pharmacologic therapy may be necessary when tics interfere with social life or otherwise impair activities of daily living.

Treatment is with drugs that block dopamine receptors or deplete dopamine stores, such as fluphenazine, pimozide, and tetrabenazine. These drugs reduce the frequency and intensity of tics by about 60%. **Pimozide,** a dopamine receptor antagonist, may be helpful in patients as a first-line treatment or in those who are either unresponsive to or intolerant of the other agents mentioned. Treatment is started at 1 mg/d, and the dosage is increased by 1 mg every 5 days; most patients require 7–16 mg/d. It has similar side effects to haloperidol but may cause irregularities of cardiac rhythm. **Haloperidol** has been used for many years to treat tic disorders. Patients are better able to tolerate this drug if treatment is started with a small dosage (eg, 0.25 or 0.5 mg daily) and then increased gradually (eg, by 0.25 mg every 4 or 5 days) over the following weeks depending on response and tolerance. Most patients ultimately require a total daily dose of 3–8 mg. Adverse effects include extrapyramidal movement disorders, sedation, dryness of the mouth, blurred vision, and gastrointestinal disturbances. **Deutetrabenazine** and **aripiprazole** (see Chapter 29) have also been found effective in treating tics. **Valbenazine** has failed to provide significant benefit compared to placebo. **Ecopipam,** a novel dopamine D_1 receptor blocker, produced significant reduction in tic severity in children with Tourette syndrome in a phase 2b randomized controlled clinical trial. The drug was well tolerated and further studies are planned.

Although not approved by the US Food and Drug Administration (FDA) for the treatment of tics or Tourette syndrome, certain α_2-adrenergic agonists may be preferred as an initial treatment because they are less likely to cause extrapyramidal side effects than neuroleptic agents. **Clonidine** reduces motor or vocal tics in about 50% of children so treated. It may act by reducing activity in noradrenergic neurons in the locus coeruleus. It is introduced at a dose of 2–3 mcg/kg/d, increasing after 2 weeks to 4 mcg/kg/d and then, if required, to 5 mcg/kg/d. It may cause an initial transient fall in blood pressure. The most common adverse effect is sedation; other adverse effects include reduced or excessive salivation and diarrhea. **Guanfacine,** another α_2-adrenergic agonist, has also been used. Both of these drugs may be particularly helpful for behavioral symptoms, such as impulse control disorders.

Atypical antipsychotics, such as risperidone and aripiprazole, may be especially worthwhile in patients with significant behavioral problems. Clonazepam, baclofen, topiramate, and carbamazepine have also been used to treat tics in preference to dopamine receptor blockers with their potential side effects. The pharmacologic properties of these drugs are discussed elsewhere in this book.

Injection of botulinum toxin A at the site of problematic tics is sometimes helpful when these are focal simple tics. Treatment of any associated attention deficit disorder (eg, with clonidine patch, guanfacine, pemoline, methylphenidate, or dextroamphetamine) or obsessive-compulsive disorder (with selective serotonin reuptake inhibitors or clomipramine) may be required.

Deep brain stimulation is sometimes worthwhile in otherwise intractable cases.

Drug-Induced Dyskinesias

Levodopa or dopamine agonists produce diverse dyskinesias as a dose-related phenomenon in patients with Parkinson disease; dose reduction reverses them. Chorea may also develop in patients receiving phenytoin, carbamazepine, amphetamines, lithium, and oral contraceptives, and it resolves with discontinuance of the offending medication. Dystonia has resulted from administration of dopaminergic agents, lithium, serotonin reuptake inhibitors, carbamazepine, and metoclopramide; and postural tremor from theophylline, caffeine, lithium, valproic acid, thyroid hormone, tricyclic antidepressants, and isoproterenol.

The pharmacologic basis of the acute dyskinesia or dystonia sometimes precipitated by the first few doses of a phenothiazine is not clear. In most instances, parenteral administration of an antimuscarinic drug such as benztropine (2 mg intravenously), diphenhydramine (50 mg intravenously), or biperiden (2–5 mg intravenously or intramuscularly) is helpful, whereas in other instances diazepam (10 mg intravenously) alleviates the abnormal movements.

Tardive dyskinesia, a disorder characterized by a variety of abnormal movements, is a common complication of long-term neuroleptic or metoclopramide drug treatment (see Chapter 29). Its precise pharmacologic basis is unclear. A reduction in dose of the offending medication, a dopamine receptor blocker, commonly worsens the dyskinesia, whereas an increase in dose may suppress it. The drugs most likely to provide immediate symptomatic benefit are those interfering with dopaminergic function, either by depletion (eg, reserpine, tetrabenazine) or receptor blockade (eg, phenothiazines, butyrophenones). Paradoxically, the receptor-blocking drugs are the ones that also cause the dyskinesia.

Deutetrabenazine and **valbenazine** are selective inhibitors of VMAT2, which modulates dopamine release, and both ameliorate tardive dyskinesia. Deutetrabenazine was discussed earlier. Valbenazine is started in a dose of 40 mg once daily for 1 week and then increased to 80 mg once daily. Somnolence and QT prolongation may occur. Adverse effects include anticholinergic effects, impaired balance and falls, headache, akathisia, arthralgia, and nausea and vomiting. Valbenazine should not be used with monoamine oxidase inhibitors; its dose should be reduced in patients receiving a strong inhibitor of CYP2D6 (eg, paroxetine, fluoxetine) or CYP3A4 (eg, carbamazepine, phenytoin).

Tardive dystonia is usually segmental or focal; generalized dystonia is less common and occurs in younger patients. Treatment is the same as for tardive dyskinesia, but anticholinergic drugs may also be helpful; focal dystonias may also respond to local injection of botulinum A toxin. **Tardive akathisia** is treated similarly to drug-induced parkinsonism. **Rabbit syndrome,** another neuroleptic-induced disorder, is manifested by rhythmic vertical movements about the mouth; it may respond to anticholinergic drugs.

Because the tardive syndromes that develop in adults are often irreversible and have no satisfactory treatment, care must be taken to reduce the likelihood of their occurrence. Antipsychotic medication should be prescribed only when necessary and should be withheld periodically to assess the need for continued treatment and to unmask incipient dyskinesia. Thioridazine, a phenothiazine with a piperidine side chain, is an effective antipsychotic agent that seems less likely than most to cause extrapyramidal reactions, perhaps because it has little effect on dopamine receptors in the striatal system. Finally, antimuscarinic drugs should not be prescribed routinely in patients receiving neuroleptics, because the combination may increase the likelihood of dyskinesia.

Neuroleptic malignant syndrome is a rare complication of treatment with neuroleptics and certain antiemetic agents (such as metoclopramide and promethazine). A somewhat similar syndrome may occur with withdrawal of dopaminergic therapy in parkinsonian patients. It is characterized by rigidity, fever, changes in mental status, and autonomic dysfunction (see Table 16–4). Symptoms typically develop over 1–3 days (rather than minutes to hours as in malignant hyperthermia) and may occur at any time during treatment. The serum creatine kinase level is increased to very high levels. Treatment includes withdrawal of antipsychotic drugs, lithium, and anticholinergics; reduction of body temperature; and rehydration. A markedly elevated blood pressure should be lowered. Benzodiazepines (diazepam or lorazepam) help in reducing agitation. Dantrolene, dopamine agonists, levodopa, or amantadine may also be helpful, but there is a high mortality rate (up to 20%) with neuroleptic malignant syndrome.

Restless Legs Syndrome

Restless legs syndrome is characterized by an unpleasant creeping discomfort that seems to arise deep within the legs and occasionally the arms. Symptoms occur particularly when patients are relaxed, especially when they are lying down or sitting, and they lead to an urge to move about. Such symptoms may delay the onset of sleep. A sleep disorder associated with periodic movements during sleep may also occur. The cause is unknown, but the disorder is especially common among pregnant women and also among uremic or diabetic patients with neuropathy. In most patients, no obvious predisposing cause is found, but several genetic loci have been associated with it.

Symptoms may resolve with correction of coexisting iron-deficiency anemia or a low-normal serum ferritin level, or with avoidance of caffeine, sleep deprivation, and various medications that can provoke or exacerbate them, such as serotonergic antidepressants, neuroleptics, metoclopramide, and antihistamines. They often respond to pharmacologic agents. Dopaminergic therapy can be initiated with long-acting dopamine agonists (eg, oral **pramipexole** 0.125–0.75 mg or **ropinirole** 0.25–4.0 mg once daily) or with the rotigotine skin patch to avoid the augmentation that may be associated especially with carbidopa-levodopa (25/100 or 50/200 taken about 1 hour before bedtime). Augmentation refers to the earlier onset or enhancement of symptoms; earlier onset of symptoms at rest; and a briefer response to medication. When augmentation occurs with levodopa, a dopamine agonist should be substituted. If it occurs in patients receiving an agonist, the daily dose should be divided, another agonist tried, or other medications substituted. Dopamine agonist therapy may be associated with development of impulse control disorders.

Gabapentin is effective in reducing the severity of restless legs syndrome and is taken once or twice daily (in the evening and before sleep). The starting dose is 300 mg daily, building up depending on response and tolerance (to approximately 1800 mg daily). Oral gabapentin enacarbil (600 or 1200 mg once daily) or **pregabalin** (150–300 mg daily, in divided doses) may also help. **Clonazepam,** 1 mg daily, is also sometimes worthwhile, especially for those with intermittent symptoms. When **opiates** are required, those with long half-lives or low addictive potential should be used. Oxycodone is often effective; the dose is individualized.

Wilson Disease

A recessively inherited disorder of copper metabolism due to mutations in the copper-transporting gene, *ATP7B*, Wilson disease is characterized biochemically by reduced serum copper and ceruloplasmin concentrations, with increased urinary copper excretion; pathologically by markedly increased concentration of copper in the brain and viscera; and clinically by hepatic, neurologic, and psychiatric dysfunction. Neurologic signs include tremor, choreiform movements, rigidity and hypokinesia (parkinsonism), ataxia, cognitive changes, and dysarthria and dysphagia. Siblings of affected patients should be screened for asymptomatic Wilson disease. Kayser-Fleischer rings, brownish deposits of copper in Descemet membrane in the cornea, are seen in virtually all patients with neurologic abnormalities and in approximately half of those with only hepatic manifestations.

Treatment should start promptly, even in presymptomatic cases, continue indefinitely, and be monitored by laboratory tests and neurologic examination. It involves the removal of excess copper, followed by maintenance of copper balance. Dietary copper should also be kept below 2 mg daily. **Penicillamine** (dimethylcysteine) has been used for many years as the primary agent to remove copper. It is a chelating agent that forms a ring complex with copper (see Chapter 57). It is readily absorbed from the gastrointestinal tract and rapidly excreted in the urine. A common starting dose in adults is 500 mg three or four times daily. After remission occurs, it may be possible to lower the maintenance dose, generally to not less than 1 g daily, which must thereafter be continued indefinitely. Adverse effects include nausea and vomiting, nephrotic syndrome, a lupus-like syndrome, pemphigus, myasthenia, arthropathy, optic neuropathy, and various blood dyscrasias. In about 10% of instances, neurologic worsening occurs with penicillamine. Treatment should be monitored by frequent urinalysis and complete blood counts and serum creatinine determination. Patients receiving penicillamine should also take pyridoxine, 25 mg daily, unless it is part of the penicillamine formulation, to prevent pyridoxine deficiency.

Trientine hydrochloride, another chelating agent, is preferred by many over penicillamine because of the lesser likelihood of drug reactions or neurologic worsening. It may be used in a daily dose of 1–1.5 g. Trientine appears to have few adverse effects other than mild anemia due to iron deficiency in a few patients.

Tetrathiomolybdate may be better than trientine for preserving neurologic function in patients with neurologic involvement and is taken both with and between meals. It is currently undergoing clinical trials (phase 3) and is not yet commercially available or approved by the FDA.

Zinc acetate administered orally increases the fecal excretion of copper and can be used in combination with these other agents. The dose is 50 mg three times a day. Zinc sulfate (200 mg/d orally) has also been used to decrease copper absorption. Zinc blocks copper absorption from the gastrointestinal tract by induction of intestinal cell metallothionein. Its main advantage is its low toxicity compared with that of other anticopper agents, although it may cause gastric irritation when introduced.

Liver transplantation is sometimes necessary to restore hepatic function and ameliorate portal hypertension when medical treatment is inadequate. Its role in the management of patients with primarily neurologic manifestations is unclear. In such patients survival is poorer but transplantation has been proposed as rescue therapy in patients with neurologic involvement resistant to anticopper therapies.

SUMMARY Drugs Used for Selected Movement Disorders

Subclass, Drug	Mechanism of Action	Effects	Clinical Applications	Pharmacokinetics, Toxicities, Interactions
LEVODOPA AND COMBINATIONS				
• Levodopa	Transported into the central nervous system (CNS) and converted to dopamine (which does not enter the CNS); also converted to dopamine in the periphery	Ameliorates all motor symptoms of Parkinson disease and causes significant peripheral dopaminergic effects (see text)	Parkinson disease: Most efficacious therapy but not always used as the first drug due to development of disabling response fluctuations over time	Oral • ~6–8 h effect • *Toxicity:* Gastrointestinal upset, arrhythmias, dyskinesias, on-off and wearing-off phenomena, behavioral disturbances • *Interactions:* Use with carbidopa greatly diminishes required dosage and is now standard • use with COMT or MAO-B inhibitors prolongs duration of effect
• *Levodopa + carbidopa (Sinemet, others): Carbidopa inhibits peripheral metabolism of levodopa to dopamine and reduces required dosage and toxicity; carbidopa does not enter CNS*				
• *Levodopa + carbidopa + entacapone (Stalevo): Entacapone is a catechol-O-methyltransferase (COMT) inhibitor (see below)*				
DOPAMINE AGONISTS				
• Pramipexole	Direct agonist at D_3 receptors, nonergot	Reduces symptoms of parkinsonism • smooths out fluctuations in levodopa response	Parkinson disease: Can be used as initial therapy • also effective in on-off phenomenon	Oral • ~8 h effect • *Toxicity:* Nausea and vomiting, postural hypotension, dyskinesias, confusion, impulse control disorders, sleepiness
• *Ropinirole: Similar to pramipexole; nonergot; relatively pure D_2 agonist*				
• *Bromocriptine: Ergot derivative; potent agonist at D_2 receptors; more toxic than pramipexole or ropinirole; now rarely used for antiparkinsonian effect*				
• *Apomorphine: Nonergot; subcutaneous route useful for rescue treatment in levodopa-induced dyskinesia; high incidence of nausea and vomiting*				
MONOAMINE OXIDASE (MAO) INHIBITORS				
• Rasagiline	Inhibits MAO-B selectively; higher doses also inhibit MAO-A	Increases dopamine stores in neurons; may have neuroprotective effects	Parkinson disease: Adjunctive to levodopa • smooths levodopa response	Oral • *Toxicity & interactions:* May cause serotonin syndrome with meperidine, and theoretically also with selective serotonin reuptake inhibitors, tricyclic antidepressants
• *Selegiline: Like rasagiline, adjunctive use with levodopa; may be less potent than rasagiline*				
• *Safinamide: Also used as adjunct to levodopa in patients with response fluctuations*				
COMT INHIBITORS				
• Entacapone	Inhibits COMT in periphery • does not enter CNS	Reduces metabolism of levodopa and prolongs its action	Parkinson disease	Oral • *Toxicity:* Increased levodopa toxicity • nausea, dyskinesias, confusion
• *Tolcapone: Like entacapone but enters CNS; some evidence of hepatotoxicity, elevation of liver enzymes*				
• *Opicapone: Taken once daily*				
ANTIMUSCARINIC AGENTS				
• Benztropine	Antagonist at M receptors in basal ganglia	Reduces tremor and rigidity • little effect on bradykinesia	Parkinson disease	Oral • *Toxicity:* Typical antimuscarinic effects–sedation, mydriasis, urinary retention, constipation, confusion, dry mouth
• *Biperiden, orphenadrine, procyclidine, trihexyphenidyl: Similar antimuscarinic agents with CNS effects*				

(*continued*)

Subclass, Drug	Mechanism of Action	Effects	Clinical Applications	Pharmacokinetics, Toxicities, Interactions
DRUGS USED IN HUNTINGTON DISEASE				
• Tetrabenazine, deutetrabenazine, reserpine	Deplete amine transmitters, especially dopamine, from nerve endings	Reduce chorea severity	Huntington disease • other applications, see Chapter 11	Oral • *Toxicity:* Hypotension, sedation, depression, diarrhea • deutetrabenazine is the least toxic
• *Haloperidol, fluphenazine, other neuroleptics, olanzapine: Dopamine receptor blockers, sometimes helpful*				
DRUGS USED IN TOURETTE SYNDROME				
• Pimozide, haloperidol	Block central D_2 receptors	Reduce vocal and motor tic frequency, severity	Tourette syndrome • other applications, see Chapter 11	Oral • *Toxicity:* Parkinsonism, other dyskinesias • sedation • blurred vision • dry mouth • gastrointestinal disturbances • pimozide may cause cardiac rhythm disturbances
• *Clonidine, guanfacine: Effective in ~50% of patients; see Chapter 11 for basic pharmacology*				
• *Phenothiazines, atypical antipsychotics, tetrabenazine, deutetrabenazine, clonazepam, carbamazepine, topiramate: Often of value*				

PREPARATIONS AVAILABLE

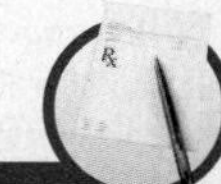

GENERIC NAME	AVAILABLE AS
Amantadine	Generic, Gocovri, Osmolex ER, Symmetrel
Apomorphine	Apokyn
Benztropine	Generic, Cogentin
Biperiden	Akineton
Bromocriptine	Generic, Parlodel
Carbidopa	Lodosyn
Carbidopa/levodopa	Generic, Parcopa, Rytary, Sinemet
Carbidopa/levodopa/entacapone	Generic, Stalevo
Deutetrabenazine	Austedo
Entacapone	Generic, Comtan
Levodopa	Dopar, Inbrija, others
Opicapone	Ongentys
Orphenadrine	Generic, various
Penicillamine	Cuprimine, Depen
Pergolide*	Permax, other
Pramipexole	Generic, Mirapex
Procyclidine	Kemadrin
Rasagiline	Azilect
Ropinirole	Generic, Requip, Requip XL
Safinamide	Xadago
Selegiline (deprenyl)	Emsam
Tetrabenazine	Xenazine
Tolcapone	Tasmar
Trientine	Syprine
Trihexyphenidyl	Generic, Artane, others
Valbenazine	Ingrezza

*Not available in the United States.

REFERENCES

Ahmad A, Torrazza-Perez E, Schilsky ML: Liver transplantation for Wilson disease. Handb Clin Neurol 2017;142:193.

Armstrong MJ, Okun MS: Diagnosis and treatment of Parkinson disease: A review. JAMA 2020;323:548.

Bashir H, Jankovic J: Deutetrabenazine for the treatment of Huntington's chorea. Expert Rev Neurother 2018;18:625.

Bledsoe IO et al: Treatment of dystonia: Medications, neurotoxins, neuromodulation, and rehabilitation. Neurotherapeutics 2020;17:1622.

Bloem BR et al: Parkinson's disease. Lancet 2021;397:2284.

Bond AE et al: Safety and efficacy of focused ultrasound thalamotomy for patients with medication-refractory, tremor-dominant Parkinson disease: A randomized clinical trial. JAMA Neurol 2017;74:1412.

Christine CW et al: Magnetic resonance imaging-guided phase 1 trial of putaminal AADC gene therapy for Parkinson's disease. Ann Neurol 2019;85:704.

Clark LN, Louis ED: Essential tremor. Handb Clin Neurol 2018;147:229.

Corvol JC et al: Longitudinal analysis of impulse control disorders in Parkinson disease. Neurology 2018;91:e189.

Członkowska A, Litwin T: Wilson disease—currently used anticopper therapy. Handb Clin Neurol 2017;142:181.

Dean M, Sung VW: Review of deutetrabenazine: A novel treatment for chorea associated with Huntington's disease. Drug Des Devel Ther 2018;12:313.

Farber RH et al: Clinical development of valbenazine for tics associated with Tourette syndrome. Expert Rev Neurother 2021;21:393.

Ferreira JJ, et al: MDS evidence-based review of treatments for essential tremor. Mov Disord 2019;34:950.

Ghosh R, Tabrizi SJ: Huntington disease. Handb Clin Neurol 2018;147:255.

Gilbert DL et al: Ecopipam, a D1 receptor antagonist, for treatment of Tourette syndrome in children: A randomized, placebo-controlled crossover study. Mov Disord 2018;33:1272.

Gossard TR et al: Restless legs syndrome: Contemporary diagnosis and treatment. Neurotherapeutics 2021;18:140.

Haubenberger D, Hallett M: Essential tremor. N Engl J Med 2018;378:1802.

Hedera P: Wilson's disease: A master of disguise. Parkinsonism Relat Disord 2019;59:140.

Hopfner F, Deuschl G: Managing essential tremor. Neurotherapeutics 2020;17:1603.

Horn S et al: Pimavanserin versus quetiapine for the treatment of psychosis in Parkinson's disease and dementia with Lewy bodies. Parkinsonism Relat Disord 2019;69:119.

Katzenschlager R et al: Apomorphine subcutaneous infusion in patients with Parkinson's disease with persistent motor fluctuations (TOLEDO): A multicentre, double-blind, randomised, placebo-controlled trial. Lancet Neurol 2018;17:749.

Kieburtz K, Reilmann R, Olanow CW: Huntington's disease: Current and future therapeutic prospects. Mov Disord 2018;33:1033.

Kogan M et al: Deep brain stimulation for Parkinson disease. Neurosurg Clin N Am 2019;30:137.

Lorincz MT: Wilson disease and related copper disorders. Handb Clin Neurol 2018;147:279.

Mittur A, Gupta S, Modi NB: Pharmacokinetics of Rytary®, an extended-release capsule formulation of carbidopa-levodopa. Clin Pharmacokinet 2017;56:999.

Paik J: Levodopa inhalation powder: A review in Parkinson's disease. Drugs 2020; 80:821.

Palfi S et al: Long-term follow-up of a phase I/II study of ProSavin, a lentiviral vector gene therapy for Parkinson's disease. Hum Gene Ther Clin Dev 2018;29:148.

Pringsheim T et al: Practice guideline recommendations summary: Treatment of tics in people with Tourette syndrome and chronic tic disorders. Neurology 2019;92:896.

Quezada J, Coffman KA: Current approaches and new developments in the pharmacological management of Tourette syndrome. CNS Drugs 2018;32:33.

Ramirez-Zamora A, Ostrem JL: Globus pallidus interna or subthalamic nucleus deep brain stimulation for Parkinson disease: A review. JAMA Neurol 2018;75:367.

Rodrigues FB et al: Deep brain stimulation for dystonia. Cochrane Database Syst Rev 2019;1:CD012405.

Schaefer SM, Vives Rodriguez A, Louis ED: Brain circuits and neurochemical systems in essential tremor: Insights into current and future pharmacotherapeutic approaches. Expert Rev Neurother 2018;18:101.

Schapira AH et al: Assessment of safety and efficacy of safinamide as a levodopa adjunct in patients with Parkinson disease and motor fluctuations: A randomized clinical trial. JAMA Neurol 2017;74:216.

Scott LJ: Opicapone: A review in Parkinson's disease. CNS Drugs 2021;35:121.

Siderowf A et al: Assessment of heterogeneity among participants in the Parkinson's Progression Markers Initiative cohort using α-synuclein seed amplification: A cross-sectional study. Lancet Neurol 2023;22:407.

Simpson DM et al: Practice guideline update summary: Botulinum neurotoxin for the treatment of blepharospasm, cervical dystonia, adult spasticity, and headache: Report of the Guideline Development Subcommittee of the American Academy of Neurology. Neurology 2016;86:1818.

Singer HS: Tics and Tourette syndrome. Continuum (Minneap Minn) 2019; 25:936.

Stocchi F et al: Initiating levodopa/carbidopa therapy with and without entacapone in early Parkinson disease: The STRIDE-PD study. Ann Neurol 2010;68:18.

Torti M, Vacca L, Stocchi F: Istradefylline for the treatment of Parkinson's disease: Is it a promising strategy? Expert Opin Pharmacother. 2018;19:1821.

Trenkwalder C et al: Comorbidities, treatment, and pathophysiology in restless legs syndrome. Lancet Neurol 2018;17:994.

Van Holst RJ et al: Brain imaging studies in pathological gambling. Curr Psychiatry Rep 2010;12:418.

Vijayakumar D, Jankovic J: Drug-induced dyskinesias (2 parts). Drugs 2016;76:759 and 779.

Volpicelli-Daley L, Brundin P: Prion-like propagation of pathology in Parkinson disease. Handb Clin Neurol 2018;153:321.

Xu W et al: Deep brain stimulation for Tourette's syndrome. Transl Neurodegener 2020;9:4.

Yu XX, Fernandez HH: Dopamine agonist withdrawal syndrome: A comprehensive review. J Neurol Sci 2017;374:53.

Zucconi M et al: An update on the treatment of restless legs syndrome/Willis-Ekbom disease: Prospects and challenges. Expert Rev Neurother 2018;18:705.

CASE STUDY ANSWER

The history is suggestive of parkinsonism, but the inconspicuous tremor and early cognitive changes raise the possibility of atypical parkinsonism rather than classic Parkinson disease. The prognosis of these disorders is worse than that of classic Parkinson disease. Given the cognitive changes and his age, the use of a dopamine agonist was unwise, as these agents are more likely than levodopa to exacerbate or precipitate behavioral and cognitive disturbances. Sleep attacks may occur spontaneously but are especially noted in patients receiving dopamine agonists. The patient has also developed punding, which is a recognized adverse effect of dopaminergic medication. Surgical treatment (deep brain stimulation) is contraindicated in patients with cognitive changes or atypical parkinsonism.

C H A P T E R

29

Antipsychotic Agents & Lithium

Charles DeBattista, MD*

CASE STUDY

A 19-year-old male student is brought into the clinic by his mother, who has been concerned about her son's erratic behavior and strange beliefs. He destroyed a TV because he felt the TV was sending harassing messages to him. In addition, he reports hearing voices telling him that family members are trying to poison his food. As a result, he is not eating. After a diagnosis is made, haloperidol is prescribed at a gradually increasing dose on an outpatient basis. The drug improves the patient's positive symptoms but ultimately causes intolerable adverse effects including severe akathisia. Although more costly, lurasidone is then prescribed, which, over the course of several weeks of treatment, improves his symptoms and is tolerated by the patient. What signs and symptoms would support an initial diagnosis of schizophrenia? In the treatment of schizophrenia, what benefits do the second-generation antipsychotic drugs offer over the traditional agents such as haloperidol? In addition to the management of schizophrenia, what other clinical indications warrant consideration of the use of drugs nominally classified as antipsychotics?

■ ANTIPSYCHOTIC AGENTS

Antipsychotic drugs are able to reduce psychotic symptoms in a wide variety of conditions, including schizophrenia, bipolar disorder, psychotic depression, psychoses associated with dementia, and drug-induced psychoses. They are also able to improve mood and reduce anxiety and sleep disturbances, but they are not the treatment of choice when these symptoms are the primary disturbance in nonpsychotic patients. A **neuroleptic** is a subtype of antipsychotic drug that produces a high incidence of **extrapyramidal side effects (EPS)** at clinically effective doses, or catalepsy in laboratory animals. The **second-generation** or **"atypical" antipsychotic drugs** are now the most widely used type of antipsychotic drug.

*The author thanks Herbert Meltzer, MD, PhD, for his contributions to prior editions of this chapter.

History

Reserpine and chlorpromazine were the first drugs found to be useful to reduce psychotic symptoms in schizophrenia. Reserpine was used only briefly for this purpose and is no longer of interest as an antipsychotic agent. Chlorpromazine is a neuroleptic agent; that is, it produces catalepsy in rodents and EPS in humans. The discovery that its antipsychotic action was related to dopamine (D or DA)-receptor blockade led to the identification of other compounds as antipsychotics between the 1950s and 1970s. The discovery of clozapine in 1959 led to the realization that antipsychotic drugs need not cause EPS in humans at clinically effective doses. Clozapine was called an "atypical" antipsychotic drug because of this dissociation; it produces fewer EPS at equivalent antipsychotic doses in humans and laboratory animals. As a result, there has been a major shift in clinical practice away from typical or first-generation antipsychotic drugs toward the use of an ever-increasing number of atypical or second-generation drugs, which have other advantages as well. The introduction of antipsychotic drugs led to massive changes in disease management, including brief instead of life-long hospitalizations.

These drugs have also proved to be of great value in studying the pathophysiology of schizophrenia and other psychoses. It should be noted that schizophrenia and bipolar disorder are no longer believed by many to be separate disorders but rather to be part of a continuum of brain disorders with psychotic features.

Nature of Psychosis & Schizophrenia

The term *psychosis* denotes a variety of mental disorders that are characterized by the inability to distinguish between what is real and what is not: the presence of delusions (false beliefs); various types of hallucinations, usually auditory or visual, but sometimes tactile or olfactory; and grossly disorganized thinking in a clear sensorium. Schizophrenia is a particular kind of psychosis characterized mainly by a clear sensorium but a marked thinking and perceptual disturbance. Schizophrenia is the most common psychotic disorder, present in about 1% of the population and responsible for approximately half of long-term psychiatric hospitalizations. Psychosis is not unique to schizophrenia and is not present in all patients with schizophrenia at all times.

Schizophrenia is considered to be a neurodevelopmental disorder. This implies that structural and functional changes in the brain are present even in utero in some patients, or that they develop during childhood and adolescence, or both. Twin, adoption, and family studies have established that schizophrenia is a genetic disorder with high heritability. No single gene is involved. Current theories involve multiple genes with common and rare mutations, including large deletions and insertions (copy number variations), combining to produce a very variegated clinical presentation and course.

THE SEROTONIN HYPOTHESIS OF SCHIZOPHRENIA

The discovery that indole hallucinogens such as LSD (lysergic acid diethylamide) and mescaline are serotonin (5-HT) agonists led to the search for endogenous hallucinogens in the urine, blood, and brains of patients with schizophrenia. This proved fruitless, but the identification of many 5-HT-receptor subtypes led to the pivotal discovery that 5-HT_{2A}-receptor and possibly 5-HT_{2C} stimulation was the basis for the hallucinatory effects of these agents.

It has been found that 5-HT_{2A}-receptor blockade is a key factor in the mechanism of action of the main class of second-generation antipsychotic drugs, of which clozapine is the prototype and which includes, in order of their introduction around the world, melperone, risperidone, zotepine, blonanserin, olanzapine, quetiapine, ziprasidone, aripiprazole, sertindole, paliperidone, iloperidone, asenapine, lurasidone, cariprazine, and brexpiprazole. These drugs are *inverse agonists* of the 5-HT_{2A} receptor; that is, they block the constitutive activity of these receptors. These receptors modulate the release of dopamine, norepinephrine, glutamate, GABA, and acetylcholine, among other neurotransmitters in the cortex, limbic region, and striatum. Stimulation of 5-HT_{2A} receptors leads to depolarization of glutamate neurons, but also stabilization of *N*-methyl-D-aspartate (NMDA) receptors on postsynaptic neurons. It has been found that hallucinogens can modulate the stability of a complex consisting of 5-HT_{2A} and NMDA receptors.

5-HT_{2C}-receptor stimulation provides a further means of modulating cortical and limbic dopaminergic activity. Stimulation of 5-HT_{2C} receptors leads to inhibition of cortical and limbic dopamine release. Many atypical antipsychotic drugs, eg, clozapine, asenapine, and olanzapine, are 5-HT_{2C} inverse agonists. 5-HT_{2C} agonists are currently being studied as antipsychotic agents.

THE DOPAMINE HYPOTHESIS OF SCHIZOPHRENIA

The dopamine hypothesis for schizophrenia was the second neurotransmitter-based concept to be developed but is no longer considered adequate to explain all aspects of schizophrenia, especially the cognitive impairment. Nevertheless, it is still highly relevant to understanding the major dimensions of schizophrenia, such as positive (hallucinations, delusions) and negative symptoms (emotional blunting, social withdrawal, lack of motivation), cognitive impairment, and possibly depression. It is also essential to understanding the mechanisms of action of most and probably all antipsychotic drugs.

Several lines of evidence suggest that excessive limbic dopaminergic activity plays a role in psychosis. (1) Many antipsychotic drugs strongly block postsynaptic D_2 receptors in the central nervous system, especially in the mesolimbic and striatal-frontal system; this includes partial dopamine agonists, such as aripiprazole, brexpiprazole, and bifeprunox. (2) Drugs that increase dopaminergic activity, such as levodopa, amphetamines, and bromocriptine and apomorphine, either aggravate schizophrenia psychosis or produce psychosis de novo in some patients. (3) Dopamine-receptor density has been found postmortem to be increased in the brains of schizophrenics who have not been treated with antipsychotic drugs. (4) Some but not all postmortem studies of schizophrenic subjects have reported increased dopamine levels and D_2-receptor density in the nucleus accumbens, caudate, and putamen. (5) Imaging studies have shown increased amphetamine-induced striatal dopamine release, increased baseline occupancy of striatal D_2 receptors by extracellular dopamine, and other measures consistent with increased striatal dopamine synthesis and release.

However, the dopamine hypothesis is far from a complete explanation of all aspects of schizophrenia. *Diminished* cortical or hippocampal dopaminergic activity has been suggested to underlie the cognitive impairment and negative symptoms of schizophrenia. Postmortem and in vivo imaging studies of cortical, limbic, nigral, and striatal dopaminergic neurotransmission in schizophrenic subjects have reported findings consistent with diminished dopaminergic activity in these regions. Decreased dopaminergic innervation in medial temporal cortex, dorsolateral prefrontal cortex, and hippocampus and decreased levels of DOPAC, a metabolite of dopamine, in the anterior cingulate have been reported in postmortem studies. Imaging studies have found increased prefrontal D_1-receptor levels that correlated with working memory impairments.

The fact that several of the atypical antipsychotic drugs have much less effect on D_2 receptors and yet are effective in schizophrenia has redirected attention to the role of other dopamine receptors and to nondopamine receptors. Serotonin receptors—particularly the 5-HT_{2A}-receptor subtype—may mediate synergistic effects or protect against the extrapyramidal consequences of D_2 antagonism. As a result of these considerations, the direction of research has changed to a greater focus on compounds that may act on several transmitter-receptor systems, eg, serotonin and glutamate. The atypical antipsychotic drugs share the property of weak D_2-receptor antagonism and more potent 5-HT_{2A}-receptor blockade.

THE GLUTAMATE HYPOTHESIS OF SCHIZOPHRENIA

Glutamate is the major excitatory neurotransmitter in the brain (see Chapter 21). Phencyclidine (PCP) and ketamine are noncompetitive inhibitors of the NMDA receptor that exacerbate both cognitive impairment and psychosis in patients with schizophrenia. PCP and a related drug, MK-801, increase locomotor activity and, acutely or chronically, a variety of cognitive impairments in rodents and primates. These effects are widely employed as a means to develop novel antipsychotic and cognitive-enhancing drugs. Selective 5-HT_{2A} antagonists, as well as atypical antipsychotic drugs, are much more potent than D_2 antagonists in blocking these effects of PCP and MK-801. This was the starting point for the hypothesis that hypofunction of NMDA receptors, located on GABAergic interneurons, leading to diminished inhibitory influences on neuronal function, contributed to schizophrenia. The diminished GABAergic activity can induce disinhibition of downstream glutamatergic activity, which can lead to hyperstimulation of cortical neurons through non-NMDA receptors. Preliminary evidence suggests that LY2140023, a drug that acts as an agonist of the metabotropic 2/3 glutamate receptor (mGLuR2/3), may be effective in schizophrenia.

The NMDA receptor, an ion channel, requires glycine for full activation. It has been suggested that in patients with schizophrenia, the glycine site of the NMDA receptor is not fully saturated. There have been several trials of high doses of glycine to promote glutamatergic activity, but the results are far from convincing. Currently, glycine transport inhibitors are in development as possible psychotropic agents.

Ampakines are drugs that potentiate currents mediated by AMPA-type glutamate receptors. In behavioral tests, ampakines are effective in correcting behaviors in various animal models of schizophrenia and depression. They protect neurons against neurotoxic insults, in part by mobilizing growth factors such as brain-derived neurotrophic factor (BDNF, see also Chapter 30).

BASIC PHARMACOLOGY OF ANTIPSYCHOTIC AGENTS

Chemical Types

A number of chemical structures have been associated with antipsychotic properties. The drugs can be classified into several groups as shown in Figures 29–1 and 29–2.

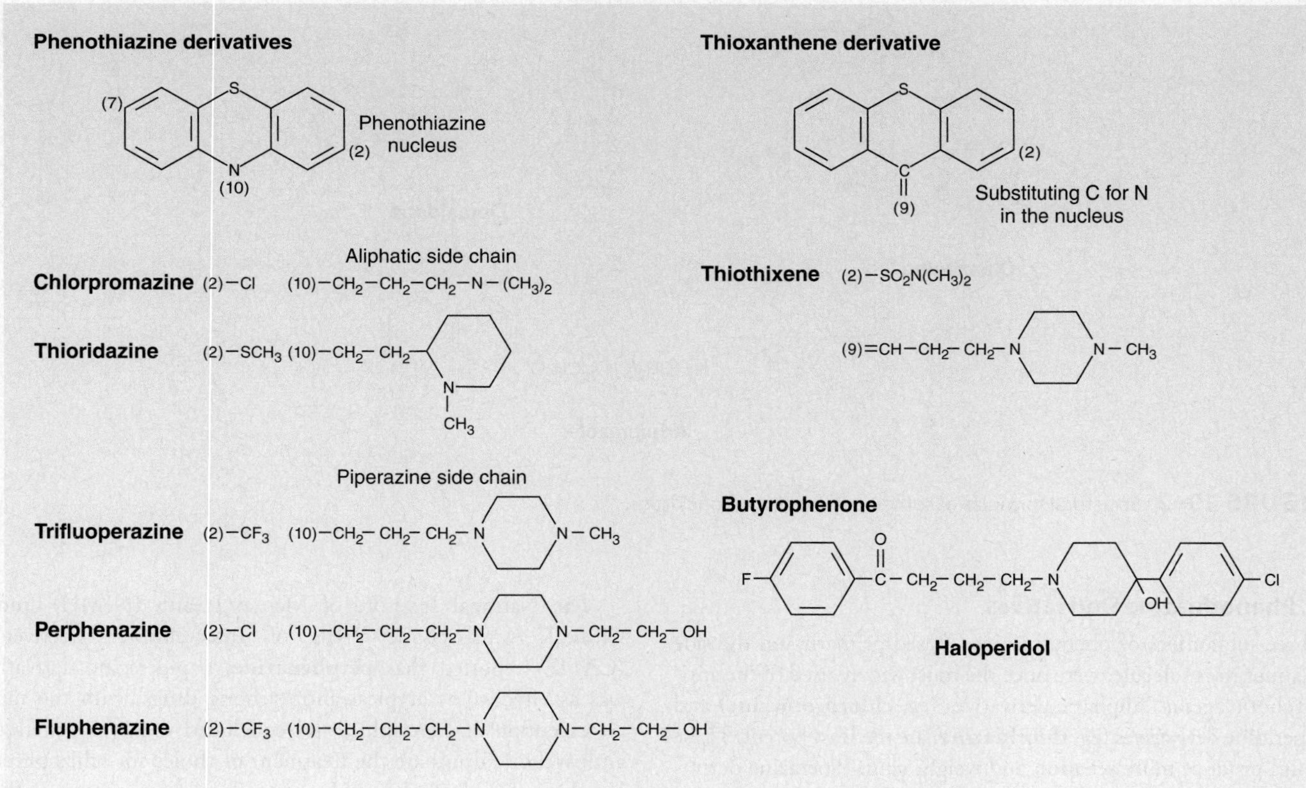

FIGURE 29–1 Structural formulas of some older antipsychotic drugs: phenothiazines, thioxanthenes, and butyrophenones. Only representative members of each type are shown.

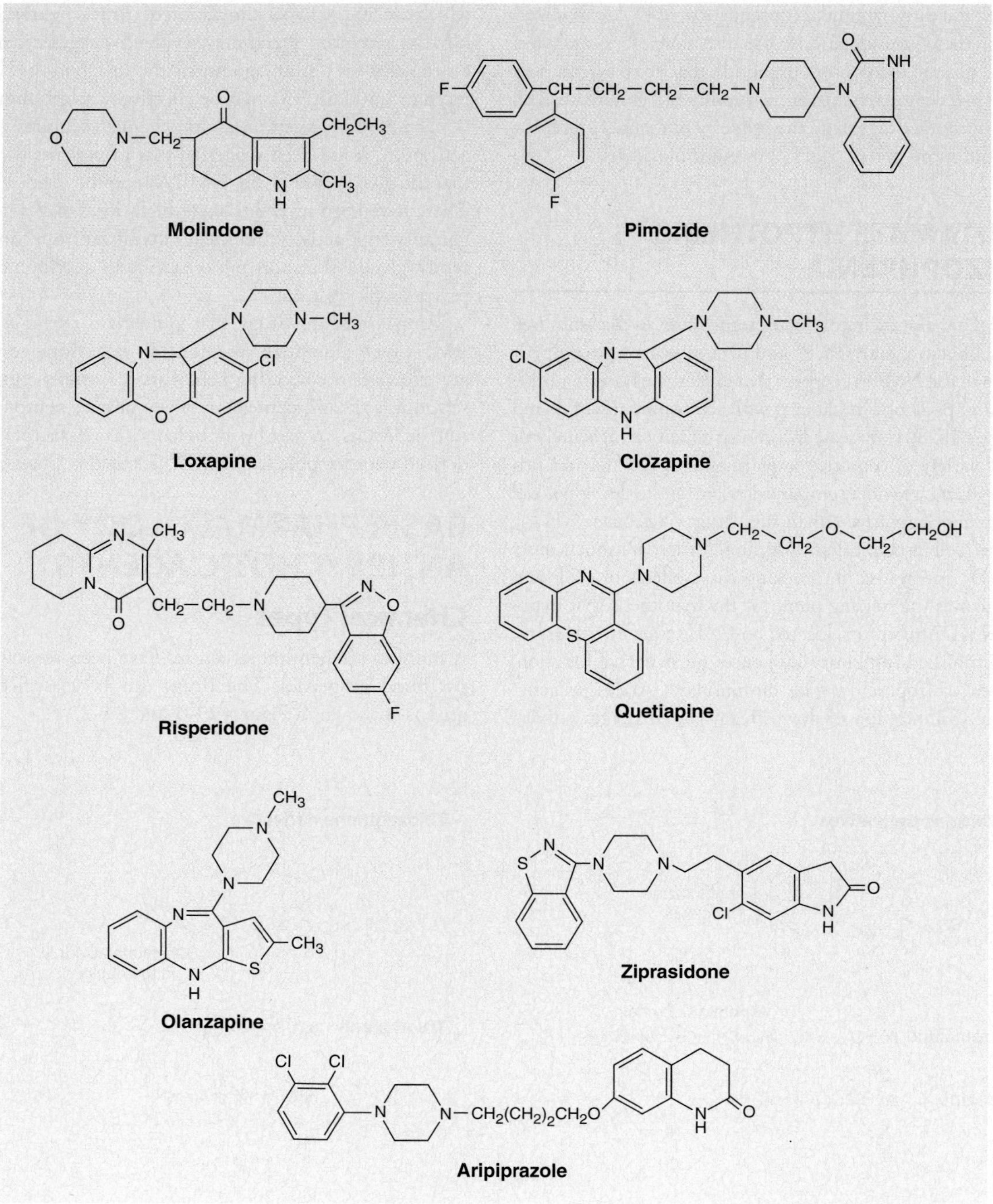

FIGURE 29–2 Structural formulas of some newer antipsychotic drugs.

A. Phenothiazine Derivatives

Three subfamilies of phenothiazines, based primarily on the side chain of the molecule, were once the most widely used of the antipsychotic agents. Aliphatic derivatives (eg, **chlorpromazine**) and piperidine derivatives (eg, **thioridazine**) are the least potent. These drugs produce more sedation and weight gain. Piperazine derivatives are more potent (effective in lower doses) but not necessarily more efficacious. The piperazine derivatives are also more selective in their pharmacologic effects (Table 29–1).

The National Institute of Mental Health (NIMH)-funded Clinical Antipsychotic Trials of Intervention Effectiveness (CATIE) reported that **perphenazine,** a piperazine derivative, was as effective as atypical antipsychotic drugs, with the modest exception of olanzapine, and concluded that first-generation antipsychotic drugs are the treatment of choice for schizophrenia based on their lower cost. However, there were numerous flaws in the design, execution, and analysis of this study, leading to it having only modest impact on clinical practice. In particular, it

TABLE 29–1 Antipsychotic drugs: Relation of chemical structure to potency and toxicities.

Chemical Class	Drug	D_2/5-HT_{2A} Ratio[1]	Clinical Potency	Extrapyramidal Toxicity	Sedative Action	Hypotensive Actions
Phenothiazines						
Aliphatic	Chlorpromazine	High	Low	Medium	High	High
Piperazine	Fluphenazine	High	High	High	Low	Very low
Thioxanthene	Thiothixene	Very high	High	Medium	Medium	Medium
Butyrophenone	Haloperidol	Medium	High	Very high	Low	Very low
Dibenzodiazepine	Clozapine	Very low	Medium	Very low	Low	Medium
Benzisoxazole	Risperidone	Very low	High	Low[2]	Low	Low
Thienobenzodiazepine	Olanzapine	Low	High	Very low	Medium	Low
Dibenzothiazepine	Quetiapine	Low	Low	Very low	Medium	Low to medium
Dihydroindolone	Ziprasidone	Low	Medium	Very low	Low	Very low
Dihydrocarbostyril	Aripiprazole	Medium	High	Very low	Very low	Low

[1]Ratio of affinity for D_2 receptors to affinity for 5-HT_{2A} receptors.

[2]At dosages below 8 mg/d.

failed to consider issues such as dosage of olanzapine, inclusion of treatment resistant patients, encouragement of patients to switch medications inherent in the design, risk for tardive dyskinesia following long-term use of even low-dose typical antipsychotics, and the necessity of large sample sizes in equivalency studies.

B. Thioxanthene Derivatives

This group of drugs is exemplified primarily by **thiothixene.**

C. Butyrophenone Derivatives

This group, of which **haloperidol** is the most widely used, has a very different structure from those of the two preceding groups. Haloperidol, a butyrophenone, is the most widely used first-generation antipsychotic drug, despite its high level of EPS relative to other typical antipsychotic drugs. Diphenylbutylpiperidines are closely related compounds. The butyrophenones and congeners tend to be more potent and to have fewer autonomic effects but greater extrapyramidal effects than phenothiazines (see Table 29–1).

D. Miscellaneous Structures

Pimozide and **molindone** are first-generation antipsychotic drugs. There is no significant difference in efficacy between these newer typical and the older typical antipsychotic drugs.

E. Second-Generation Antipsychotic Drugs

Clozapine, asenapine, olanzapine, quetiapine, paliperidone, risperidone, sertindole, ziprasidone, zotepine, brexpiprazole, cariprazine, lurasidone, and **aripiprazole** are second-generation antipsychotic drugs (some of which are shown in Figure 29–2). Clozapine is the prototype. Paliperidone is 9-hydroxyrisperidone, the active metabolite of risperidone. Risperidone is rapidly converted to 9-hydroxyrisperidone in vivo in most patients, except for about 10% of patients who are poor metabolizers. Sertindole is approved in some European countries but not in the USA.

These drugs have complex pharmacology, but they share a greater ability to alter 5-HT_{2A}-receptor activity than to interfere with D_2-receptor action. In most cases, they act as partial agonists at the 5-HT_{1A} receptor, which produces synergistic effects with 5-HT_{2A} receptor antagonism. Most are also either 5-HT_6 or 5-HT_7 receptor antagonists.

Sulpride and sulpiride constitute another class of atypical agents. They have equivalent potency for D_2 and D_3 receptors, but they are also 5-HT_7 antagonists. They dissociate EPS and antipsychotic efficacy. However, they also produce marked increases in serum prolactin levels and are not as free of the risk of tardive dyskinesia as are drugs such as clozapine and quetiapine. They are not approved in the USA.

Cariprazine represents another type of second-generation agent. In addition to D_2/5-HT_2 antagonism, cariprazine is also a D_3 partial agonist with selectivity for the D_3 receptor. Cariprazine's selectivity for the D_3 receptor may be associated with greater effects on the negative symptoms of schizophrenia. This drug was approved in 2015 in the USA.

F. Glutamatergic Antipsychotics

No glutamate-specific agents are currently approved for the treatment of schizophrenia. However, several agents are in late clinical testing. Among these is **bitopertin,** a glycine transporter 1 (GlyT1) inhibitor. As noted earlier, glycine is a required co-agonist with glutamate at NMDA receptors. Initial phase 2 studies indicated that bitopertin used adjunctively with standard antipsychotics significantly improved negative symptoms of schizophrenia, but subsequent trials have been disappointing. **Sarcosine** (*N*-methylglycine), another GlyT1 inhibitor, in combination with a standard antipsychotic has also shown benefit in improving both negative and positive symptoms of schizophrenia in acutely ill as well as in patients with more chronic schizophrenia.

Another class of investigational antipsychotic agents includes the metabotropic glutamate receptor agonists. Eight metabotropic glutamate receptors are divided into three groups: group I (mGluR1,5), group II (mGluR2,3), and group III (mGluR4,6,7,8). mGluR2,3 inhibits glutamate release presynaptically. Several mGluR2,3 agents are being investigated in the treatment of schizophrenia. One agent, pomaglumetad methionil, showed antipsychotic efficacy in early phase 2 trials, but subsequent trials failed to show benefit in either positive or negative symptoms of schizophrenia. Other metabotropic glutamate receptor agonists are being explored for the treatment of negative and cognitive symptoms of schizophrenia.

Pharmacokinetics

A. Absorption and Distribution

Most antipsychotic drugs are readily but incompletely absorbed. Furthermore, many undergo significant first-pass metabolism. Thus, oral doses of chlorpromazine and thioridazine have systemic availability of 25–35%, whereas haloperidol, which has less first-pass metabolism, has an average systemic availability of about 65%.

Most antipsychotic drugs are highly lipid soluble and protein bound (92–99%). They tend to have large volumes of distribution (usually more than 7 L/kg). They generally have a much longer clinical duration of action than would be estimated from their plasma half-lives. This is paralleled by prolonged occupancy of D_2 dopamine receptors in the brain by the typical antipsychotic drugs.

Metabolites of chlorpromazine may be excreted in the urine weeks after the last dose of chronically administered drug. Long-acting injectable formulations may cause some blockade of D_2 receptors 3–6 months after the last injection. Time to recurrence of psychotic symptoms is highly variable after discontinuation of antipsychotic drugs. The average time for relapse in stable patients with schizophrenia who discontinue their medication is 6 months. Clozapine is an exception in that relapse after discontinuation is usually rapid and severe. Thus, clozapine should never be discontinued abruptly unless clinically needed because of adverse effects such as myocarditis or agranulocytosis, which are true medical emergencies.

B. Metabolism

Most antipsychotic drugs are almost completely metabolized by oxidation or demethylation, catalyzed by liver microsomal cytochrome P450 enzymes. CYP2D6, CYP1A2, and CYP3A4 are the major isoforms involved (see Chapter 4). Drug-drug interactions should be considered when combining antipsychotic drugs with various other psychotropic drugs or drugs—such as ketoconazole—that inhibit various cytochrome P450 enzymes. At the typical clinical doses, antipsychotic drugs do not usually interfere with the metabolism of other drugs.

Pharmacodynamics

The first phenothiazine antipsychotic drugs, with chlorpromazine as the prototype, proved to have a wide variety of central nervous system, autonomic, and endocrine effects. Although efficacy of these drugs is primarily driven by D_2-receptor blockade, their adverse actions were traced to blocking effects at a wide range of receptors including α adrenoceptors and muscarinic, H_1 histaminic, and 5-HT_2 receptors.

A. Dopaminergic Systems

Five dopaminergic systems or pathways are important for understanding schizophrenia and the mechanism of action of antipsychotic drugs. The first pathway—the one most closely related to behavior and psychosis—is the **mesolimbic-mesocortical** pathway, which projects from cell bodies in the ventral tegmentum in separate bundles of axons to the limbic system and neocortex. The second system—the **nigrostriatal** pathway—consists of neurons that project from the substantia nigra to the dorsal striatum, which includes the caudate and putamen; it is involved in the coordination of voluntary movement. Blockade of the D_2 receptors in the nigrostriatal pathway is responsible for EPS. The third pathway—the **tuberoinfundibular** system—arises in the arcuate nuclei and periventricular neurons and releases dopamine into the pituitary portal circulation. Dopamine released by these neurons physiologically inhibits prolactin secretion from the anterior pituitary. The fourth dopaminergic system—the **medullary-periventricular** pathway—consists of neurons in the motor nucleus of the vagus whose projections are not well defined. This system may be involved in eating behavior. The fifth pathway—the **incertohypothalamic** pathway—forms connections from the medial zona incerta to the hypothalamus and the amygdala. It appears to regulate the anticipatory motivational phase of copulatory behavior in rats.

After dopamine was identified as a neurotransmitter in 1959, it was shown that its effects on electrical activity in central synapses and on production of the second messenger cAMP synthesized by adenylyl cyclase could be blocked by antipsychotic drugs such as chlorpromazine, haloperidol, and thiothixene. This evidence led to the conclusion in the early 1960s that these drugs should be considered **dopamine-receptor antagonists** and was a key factor in the development of the dopamine hypothesis of schizophrenia described earlier in this chapter. The antipsychotic action is now thought to be produced (at least in part) by their ability to block the effect of dopamine (D_2 receptors inhibit the activity of adenylyl cyclase in the mesolimbic system).

B. Dopamine Receptors and Their Effects

At present, five dopamine receptors have been described, consisting of two separate families, the D_1-like (D_1, D_5) and D_2-like (D_2, D_3, D_4) receptor groups. The D_1 receptor is coded by a gene on chromosome 5, increases cAMP by G_s-coupled activation of adenylyl cyclase, and is located mainly in the putamen, nucleus accumbens, and olfactory tubercle and cortex. The other member of this family, D_5, is coded by a gene on chromosome 4, also increases cAMP, and is found in the hippocampus and hypothalamus. The therapeutic potency of antipsychotic drugs does not correlate with their affinity for binding to the D_1 receptor (Figure 29–3, top) nor did a selective D_1 antagonist prove to be an effective antipsychotic in patients with schizophrenia. The D_2 receptor is coded on chromosome 11, decreases cAMP (by G_i-coupled inhibition of adenylyl cyclase), and inhibits calcium channels but opens potassium channels. It is found both pre- and postsynaptically on neurons in the caudate-putamen, nucleus accumbens, and olfactory tubercle. A second member of this family, the D_3 receptor, also coded by a gene on chromosome 11, is thought to also decrease cAMP and is located in the frontal cortex, medulla, and midbrain. D_4 receptors also decrease cAMP and are concentrated in the cortex.

The first-generation antipsychotic agents block D_2 receptors stereoselectively for the most part, and their binding affinity is very strongly correlated with clinical antipsychotic and extrapyramidal potency (Figure 29–3, bottom). In vivo imaging studies of D_2-receptor occupancy indicate that for antipsychotic efficacy, the typical antipsychotic drugs must be given in sufficient doses to achieve at least 60% occupancy of striatal D_2 receptors. This is not required for some second-generation antipsychotic drugs such as clozapine and olanzapine, which are effective at lower occupancy levels of 30–50%, most likely because of their concurrent high occupancy of 5-HT_{2A} receptors. The first-generation antipsychotic drugs produce EPS when the occupancy of striatal D_2 receptors reaches 80% or higher.

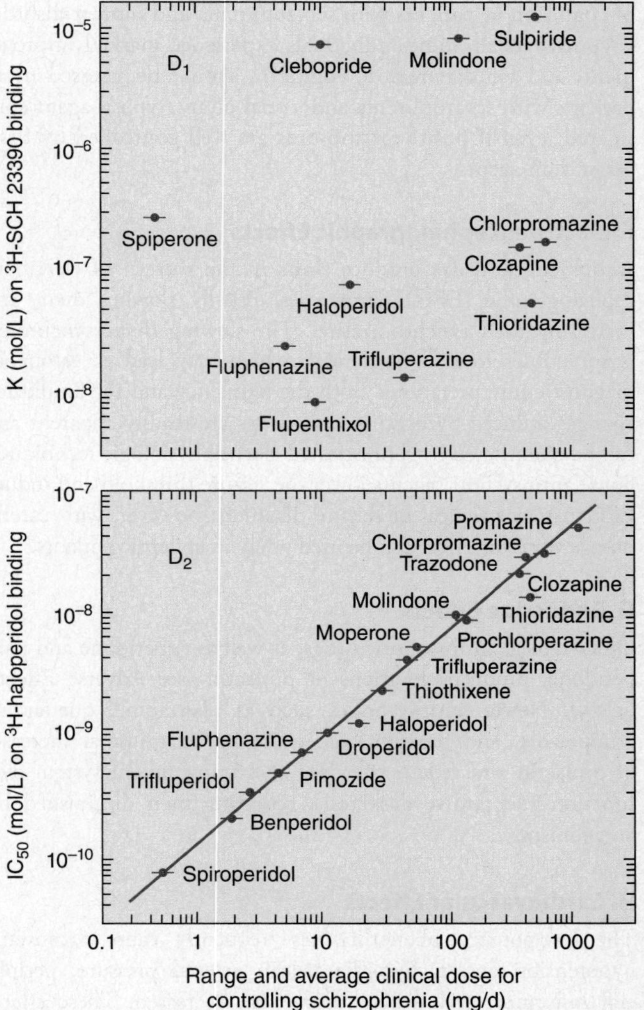

FIGURE 29–3 Correlations between the therapeutic potency of antipsychotic drugs and their affinity for binding to dopamine D_1 (*top*) or D_2 receptors (*bottom*). Potency is indicated on the horizontal axes; it decreases to the right. Binding affinity for D_1 receptors was measured by displacing the selective D_1 ligand SCH 23390; affinity for D_2 receptors was similarly measured by displacing the selective D_2 ligand haloperidol. Binding affinity decreases upward. (Reproduced with permission from Seeman P: Dopamine receptors and the dopamine hypothesis of schizophrenia. Synapse 1987;1(2):133-152.)

Positron emission tomography (PET) studies with aripiprazole show very high occupancy of D_2 receptors, but this drug does not cause EPS because it is a partial D_2-receptor agonist. Aripiprazole also gains therapeutic efficacy through its 5-HT_{2A} antagonism and possibly 5-HT_{1A} partial agonism.

These findings have been incorporated into the dopamine hypothesis of schizophrenia. However, additional factors complicate interpretation of dopamine receptor data. For example, dopamine receptors exist in both high- and low-affinity forms, and it is not known whether schizophrenia or the antipsychotic drugs alter the proportions of receptors in these two forms.

It has not been convincingly demonstrated that antagonism of any dopamine receptor other than the D_2 receptor plays a role in the action of antipsychotic drugs. Selective and relatively specific D_1-, D_3-, and D_4-receptor antagonists have been tested repeatedly with no evidence of antipsychotic action. Most of the newer atypical antipsychotic agents and some of the traditional ones have a higher affinity for the 5-HT_{2A} receptor than for the D_2 receptor (see Table 29–1), suggesting an important role for the serotonin 5-HT system in the etiology of schizophrenia and the action of these drugs.

C. Novel Pharmacodynamic Targets

While currently available antipsychotics predominately act on the D2 receptor, there are at least 2 current agents that appear to have little affinity for the D2 receptor; clozapine and pimavanserin. Pimavanserin is primarily a 5HT2 antagonist approved for the treatment of psychosis in Parkinson's disease while clozapine also is a 5HT2 antagonist with differential effects on D1-D4 receptors. While that available antipsychotics have proven extremetly helpful in mitigating positive psychotic symptoms including hallucinations and delusions that often have intolerable side effects and have not been particularly effective in treating negative and cognitive symptoms. Two drugs in late-stage development with a novel pharmacodynamic profile offer some hope of treating patients for whom the currenly available agents have proven ineffective or too difficult to tolerate. Xenomeline is a muscarine M1/M4 agonist while Ulotaront is a Trace Amine Associated Receptor -1 agonist (TAAR-1). Both of these drugs have shown efficacy in the treatment of schizophrenia and lack the EPS and metabolic side effects of first- and second-generation antipsychotics. In addition, Xenomaline has shown benefit for treating cognitive symptoms of schizophrenia and both drugs may have benefits for treating negative symptoms. Xenomaline is expected to undergo FDA review in 2023 for possible approval while ulotarant has been given a breakthrough designation by the FDA for the treatment of schizophrenia and is expected to seek approval by 2024.

D. Differences among Antipsychotic Drugs

Although almost all effective antipsychotic drugs block D_2 receptors, the degree of this blockade in relation to other actions on receptors varies considerably among drugs. Vast numbers of ligand-receptor binding experiments have been performed in an effort to discover a single receptor action that would best predict antipsychotic efficacy. A summary of the relative receptor-binding affinities of several key agents in such comparisons illustrates the difficulty in drawing simple conclusions from such experiments:

Chlorpromazine: $\alpha_1 = 5\text{-HT}_{2A} > D_2 > D_1$
Haloperidol: $D_2 > \alpha_1 > D_4 > 5\text{-HT}_{2A} > D_1 > H_1$
Clozapine: $D_4 = \alpha_1 > 5\text{-HT}_{2A} > D_2 = D_1$
Olanzapine: $5\text{-HT}_{2A} > H_1 > D_4 > D_2 > \alpha_1 > D_1$
Aripiprazole: $D_2 = 5\text{-HT}_{2A} > D_4 > \alpha_1 = H_1 >> D_1$
Quetiapine: $H_1 > \alpha_1 > M_{1,3} > D_2 > 5\text{-HT}_{2A}$

Thus, most of the second-generation and some first-generation antipsychotic agents are at least as potent in inhibiting 5-HT_2 receptors as they are in inhibiting D_2 receptors. Aripiprazole and brexpiprazole appear to be partial agonists of D_2 receptors. Varying degrees of antagonism of α_2 adrenoceptors are also seen with risperidone, clozapine, olanzapine, quetiapine, and aripiprazole.

Current research is directed toward discovering novel antipsychotic compounds that either are more selective for the mesolimbic system (to reduce their effects on the extrapyramidal system) or have effects on central neurotransmitter receptors—such as those for acetylcholine and excitatory amino acids—that have been proposed as new targets for antipsychotic action.

In contrast to the difficult search for receptors responsible for antipsychotic *efficacy*, the differences in receptor effects of various antipsychotics do explain many of their *toxicities* (Tables 29–1 and 29–2). In particular, extrapyramidal toxicity appears to be consistently associated with high D_2 potency.

TABLE 29–2 Adverse pharmacologic effects of antipsychotic drugs.

Type	Manifestations	Mechanism
Autonomic nervous system	Loss of accommodation, dry mouth, difficulty urinating, constipation	Muscarinic cholinoceptor blockade
	Orthostatic hypotension, impotence, failure to ejaculate	α-Adrenoceptor blockade
Central nervous system	Parkinson syndrome, akathisia, dystonias	Dopamine-receptor blockade
	Tardive dyskinesia	Supersensitivity of dopamine receptors
	Toxic-confusional state	Muscarinic blockade
Endocrine system	Amenorrhea-galactorrhea, infertility, impotence	Dopamine-receptor blockade resulting in hyperprolactinemia
Other	Weight gain	Possibly combined H_1 and 5-HT_2 blockade

E. Psychological Effects

Most antipsychotic drugs cause unpleasant subjective effects in nonpsychotic individuals. The mild to severe EPS, including akathisia, sleepiness, restlessness, and autonomic effects, are unlike any associated with more familiar sedatives or hypnotics. Nevertheless, low doses of some of these drugs, particularly quetiapine, are used to promote sleep onset and maintenance, although there is no approved indication for such usage.

People without psychiatric illness given antipsychotic drugs, even at low doses, experience impaired performance as judged by a number of psychomotor and psychometric tests. Psychotic individuals, however, may actually show improvement in their performance as the psychosis is alleviated. The ability of the second-generation antipsychotic drugs to improve some domains of cognition in patients with schizophrenia and bipolar disorder is controversial. Some individuals experience marked improvement, and for that reason, cognition should be assessed in all patients with schizophrenia and a trial of an atypical agent considered, even if positive symptoms are well controlled by first-generation agents.

F. Electroencephalographic Effects

Antipsychotic drugs produce shifts in the pattern of electroencephalographic (EEG) frequencies, usually slowing them and increasing their synchronization. The slowing (hypersynchrony) is sometimes focal or unilateral, which may lead to erroneous diagnostic interpretations. Both the frequency and the amplitude changes induced by psychotropic drugs are readily apparent and can be quantitated by sophisticated electrophysiologic techniques. Some antipsychotic agents lower the seizure threshold and induce EEG patterns typical of seizure disorders; however, with careful dosage titration, most can be used safely in epileptic patients.

G. Endocrine Effects

Older typical antipsychotic drugs, as well as risperidone and paliperidone, produce elevations of prolactin (see Adverse Effects, below). Newer antipsychotics such as olanzapine, quetiapine, aripiprazole, and brexpiprazole cause no or minimal increases of prolactin and reduce the risks of extrapyramidal system dysfunction and tardive dyskinesia, reflecting their diminished D_2 antagonism.

H. Cardiovascular Effects

The low-potency phenothiazines frequently cause orthostatic hypotension and tachycardia. Mean arterial pressure, peripheral resistance, and stroke volume are decreased. These effects are predictable from the autonomic actions of these agents (see Table 29–2). Abnormal electrocardiograms have been recorded, especially with thioridazine. Changes include prolongation of QT interval and abnormal configurations of the ST segment and T waves. These changes are readily reversed by withdrawing the drug. Since thioridazine is associated with torsades de pointes and an increased risk of sudden death, the branded drug was removed from the market in 2005, and its use currently is as a second-line agent if other drugs have proved intolerable or ineffective.

Among the newest antipsychotics, prolongation of the QT or QT_c interval has received much attention. Because this was believed to indicate an increased risk of dangerous arrhythmias, ziprasidone and quetiapine are accompanied by warnings. There is, however, no evidence that this has actually translated into increased incidence of arrhythmias.

The atypical antipsychotics are also associated with a metabolic syndrome that may increase the risk of coronary artery disease, stroke, and hypertension.

CLINICAL PHARMACOLOGY OF ANTIPSYCHOTIC AGENTS

INDICATIONS

A. Psychiatric Indications

Schizophrenia is the primary indication for antipsychotic agents. However, in the last decade, the use of antipsychotics in the treatment of mood disorders such as type 1 bipolar disorder (BD-1), psychotic depression, and treatment-resistant depression has eclipsed their use in the treatment of schizophrenia.

Catatonic forms of schizophrenia are best managed by intravenous benzodiazepines. Antipsychotic drugs may be needed to treat psychotic components of that form of the illness after catatonia has ended, and they remain the mainstay of treatment for this condition. Unfortunately, many patients show little response, and virtually none shows a complete response.

Antipsychotic drugs are also indicated for **schizoaffective disorders,** which share characteristics of both schizophrenia and affective disorders. No fundamental difference between these two diagnoses has been reliably demonstrated. It is most likely that they are part of a continuum with bipolar psychotic disorder. The psychotic aspects of the illness require treatment with antipsychotic drugs, which may be used with other drugs such as antidepressants, lithium, or valproic acid.

The manic phase in **bipolar affective disorder** often requires treatment with antipsychotic agents, although lithium or valproic acid supplemented with high-potency benzodiazepines (eg, lorazepam or clonazepam) may suffice in milder cases. Controlled trials support the efficacy of monotherapy with second-generation antipsychotics in the acute phase (up to 4 weeks) of mania. In addition, several second-generation antipsychotics are approved in the maintenance treatment of bipolar disorder. They appear more effective in preventing mania than in preventing depression. As mania subsides, the antipsychotic drug may be withdrawn, although maintenance treatment with atypical antipsychotic agents has become more common. Nonmanic excited states may also be managed by antipsychotics, often in combination with benzodiazepines.

An increasingly common use of antipsychotics is in the monotherapy of **acute bipolar depression** and the adjunctive use of antipsychotics with antidepressants in the treatment of **unipolar depression.** Several antipsychotics are now approved by the US Food and Drug Administration (FDA) in the management of bipolar depression including quetiapine, lurasidone, and cariprazine, lumateperone and olanzapine (in a combination formulation with fluoxetine). The antipsychotics appear more consistently effective than antidepressants in the treatment of bipolar depression and also do not increase the risk of inducing mania or increasing the frequency of bipolar cycling. Likewise, several antipsychotics, including aripiprazole, quetiapine, brexpiprazole, and olanzapine (with fluoxetine), are now approved in the adjunctive treatment of unipolar depression. Although many drugs are combined with antidepressants in the adjunctive treatment of major depression, antipsychotic agents are the only class of agents that have been formally evaluated for FDA approval for this purpose. Residual symptoms and partial remission are common, with antipsychotics showing consistent benefit in improving overall antidepressant response.

Some of the intramuscular antipsychotics have been approved for the control of **agitation** associated with bipolar disorder and schizophrenia. Antipsychotics such as haloperidol have long been used in the ICU setting to manage agitation in delirious and postsurgical patients. The intramuscular forms of ziprasidone, olanzapine, and aripiprazole have been shown to improve agitation within 1–2 hours, with fewer extrapyramidal symptoms than typical agents such as haloperidol. An alternative to antipsychotics, also now approved for the management of agitation in bipolar disorder and schizophrenia, is a sublingual analog of etomidate, dexmedetomidate. Etomidate has long been used as an anesthetic, and dexmetetomidate is a sulingual film that that can be given as an alternative or an oral or IM antipsychotic. Dexmetedomidate does not carry the EPS risks of acute antipsychotics. Sedation and dry mouth have been the most common side effects in clinical trials.

Other indications for the use of antipsychotics include **Tourette syndrome** and possibly disturbed behavior in patients with **Alzheimer disease.** However, controlled trials of antipsychotics in the management of behavioral symptoms in dementia patients have generally not demonstrated efficacy. Furthermore, second-generation as well as some first-generation antipsychotics have been associated with increased mortality in these patients. Antipsychotics are not indicated for the treatment of various withdrawal syndromes, eg, opioid withdrawal. In small doses, antipsychotic drugs have been promoted (wrongly) for the relief of anxiety associated with minor emotional disorders. The antianxiety sedatives (see Chapter 22) are preferred in terms of both safety and acceptability to patients.

Psychotic symptoms associated with Parkinson disease represent a clinical challenge. Medications such as levodopa that treat the symptoms of Parkinson disease can also exacerbate psychotic symptoms. Likewise, antipsychotics that can treat the psychotic symptoms can significantly worsen the other symptoms of Parkinson disease. In 2016, a new type of antipsychotic was approved for the treatment of psychosis in Parkinson disease. **Pimavanserin** is a selective serotonin inverse agonist. As such, it has no dopamine antagonist properties and is not associated with EPS. Pimavanserin is currently being investigated as an adjunctive treatment in schizophrenia.

Irritability and behavioral dyscontrol in patients with **autism spectrum disorders (ASD)** can be challenging for care providers and patients alike. Two antipsychotics, risperidone and aripiprazole, are approved to treat irritability in ASD patients.

No medications, however, are known to treat and correct the core symptoms of ASD.

B. Nonpsychiatric Indications

Most older first-generation antipsychotic drugs, with the exception of thioridazine, have a strong **antiemetic** effect. This action is due to dopamine-receptor blockade, both centrally (in the chemoreceptor trigger zone of the medulla) and peripherally (on receptors in the stomach). Some drugs, such as **prochlorperazine** and **benzquinamide,** are promoted solely as antiemetics.

Phenothiazines with shorter side chains have considerable **H_1-receptor-blocking** action and have been used for relief of pruritus or, in the case of **promethazine,** as preoperative sedatives. The butyrophenone **droperidol** is used in combination with the opioid fentanyl in **neuroleptanesthesia.** Droperidol has dose-associated risk of QT prolongation and has been removed from some markets. The use of these drugs in anesthesia practice is described in Chapter 25.

Drug Choice

Choice among antipsychotic drugs is based mainly on differences in adverse effects and possible differences in efficacy. In addition, cost and the availability of a given agent on drug formularies also influence the choice of a specific antipsychotic. Because use of the older drugs is still common, especially for patients treated in the public sector, knowledge of such agents as chlorpromazine and haloperidol remains relevant. Thus, one should be familiar with one member of each of the three subfamilies of phenothiazines, a member of the thioxanthene and butyrophenone group, and all of the newer compounds—clozapine, risperidone, olanzapine, quetiapine, ziprasidone, lurasidone, iloperidone, asenapine, cariprazine, lumateperone, and aripiprazole. Each may have special advantages for selected patients. A representative group of antipsychotic drugs is presented in Table 29–3.

For approximately 70% of patients with schizophrenia, and probably for a similar proportion of patients with bipolar disorder with psychotic features, first- and second-generation antipsychotic drugs are of equal efficacy for treating positive symptoms. However, the evidence favors second-generation drugs for benefit for negative symptoms and cognition, for diminished risk of tardive dyskinesia and other forms of EPS, and for lesser increases in prolactin levels.

Some of the second-generation antipsychotic drugs produce more weight gain and increases in lipids than some first-generation drugs. A small percentage of patients develop diabetes mellitus, most often seen with clozapine and olanzapine. Ziprasidone is the second-generation drug causing the least weight gain. Risperidone, lurasidone, brexpiprazole, paliperidone, and aripiprazole usually produce small increases in weight and lipids. Asenapine and quetiapine have an intermediate effect. Clozapine and olanzapine frequently result in large increases in weight and lipids. Thus, these

TABLE 29–3 Some representative antipsychotic drugs.

Drug Class	Drug	Advantages	Disadvantages
Phenothiazines			
Aliphatic	Chlorpromazine[1]	Generic, inexpensive	Many adverse effects, especially autonomic
Piperidine	Thioridazine[2]	Slight extrapyramidal syndrome; generic	800 mg/d limit; no parenteral form; cardiotoxicity
Piperazine	Fluphenazine[3]	Depot form also available (enanthate, decanoate)	Possible increased tardive dyskinesia
Thioxanthene	Thiothixene	Parenteral form also available; possible decreased tardive dyskinesia	Uncertain
Butyrophenone	Haloperidol	Parenteral form also available; generic	Severe extrapyramidal syndrome
Dibenzoxazepine	Loxapine	Possible no weight gain	Uncertain
Dibenzodiazepine	Clozapine	May benefit treatment-resistant patients; little extrapyramidal toxicity	May cause agranulocytosis in up to 2% of patients; dose-related lowering of seizure threshold
Benzisoxazole	Risperidone	Broad efficacy; little or no extrapyramidal system dysfunction at low doses	Extrapyramidal system dysfunction and hypotension with higher doses
Thienobenzodiazepine	Olanzapine	Effective against negative as well as positive symptoms; little or no extrapyramidal system dysfunction	Weight gain; dose-related lowering of seizure threshold
Dibenzothiazepine	Quetiapine	Similar to olanzapine; perhaps less weight gain	May require high doses if there is associated hypotension; short $t_{1/2}$ and twice-daily dosing
Dihydroindolone	Ziprasidone	Perhaps less weight gain than clozapine, parenteral form available	QT_c prolongation
Dihydrocarbostyril	Aripiprazole	Lower weight gain liability, long half-life, novel mechanism potential	Uncertain, novel toxicities possible

[1]Other aliphatic phenothiazines: promazine, triflupromazine.

[2]Other piperidine phenothiazines: piperacetazine, mesoridazine.

[3]Other piperazine phenothiazines: acetophenazine, perphenazine, carphenazine, prochlorperazine, trifluoperazine.

drugs should be considered as second-line drugs unless there is a specific indication. That is the case with clozapine, which at high doses (300–900 mg/d) is effective in the majority of patients with schizophrenia refractory to other drugs, provided that treatment is continued for up to 6 months. Case reports and several clinical trials suggest that high-dose olanzapine, ie, doses of 30–45 mg/d, may also be efficacious in refractory schizophrenia when given over a 6-month period. Clozapine is the only second-generation antipsychotic drug approved to reduce the risk of suicide in patients with history of schizophrenia. Patients with schizophrenia who have made life-threatening suicide attempts should be seriously evaluated for switching to clozapine.

New antipsychotic drugs have been shown in some trials to be more effective than older ones for treating negative symptoms. The floridly psychotic form of the illness accompanied by uncontrollable behavior probably responds equally well to all potent antipsychotics but is still frequently treated with older drugs that offer intramuscular formulations for acute and chronic treatment. Moreover, the low cost of the older drugs contributes to their widespread use despite their risk of adverse EPS effects. Several of the newer antipsychotics, including clozapine, risperidone, and olanzapine, show superiority over haloperidol in terms of overall response in some controlled trials. More comparative studies with aripiprazole are needed to evaluate its relative efficacy. Moreover, the superior adverse-effect profile of the newer agents and low to absent risk of tardive dyskinesia suggest that these should provide the first line of treatment. Generic forms of many second-generation drugs including clozapine, olanzapine, aripiprazole, risperidone, and quetiapine have become available, and cost of these drugs is much less of a consideration than it once was.

The best guide for selecting a drug for an individual patient is the patient history of past responses to drugs. At present, clozapine is limited to those patients who have failed to respond to substantial doses of conventional antipsychotic drugs. The agranulocytosis and seizures associated with this drug prevent more widespread use. Risperidone's improved adverse-effect profile (compared with that of haloperidol) at dosages of 6 mg/d or less and the apparently lower risk of tardive dyskinesia have contributed to its widespread use. Olanzapine and quetiapine may have even lower risks and have also achieved widespread use. At this writing, aripiprazole is the most commonly prescribed second-generation antipsychotic in the USA due to a relatively favorable side effect profile and aggressive marketing.

Dosage

The range of effective dosages among various antipsychotic agents is broad. Therapeutic margins are substantial. At appropriate dosages, antipsychotics—with the exception of clozapine and perhaps olanzapine—are of equal efficacy in broadly selected groups of patients. However, some patients who fail to respond to one drug may respond to another; for this reason, several drugs may have to be tried to find the one most effective for an individual patient. Patients who have become refractory to two or three antipsychotic agents given in substantial doses become candidates for treatment with clozapine or high-dose olanzapine. Thirty to fifty percent of patients previously refractory to standard doses of other antipsychotic drugs respond to these drugs. In such cases, the increased risk of clozapine can well be justified.

Some dosage relationships between various antipsychotic drugs, as well as possible therapeutic ranges, are shown in Table 29–4.

TABLE 29–4 Dose relationships of antipsychotics.

	Minimum Effective Therapeutic Dose (mg)	Usual Range of Daily Doses (mg)
Chlorpromazine	100	100–1000
Thioridazine	100	100–800
Trifluoperazine	5	5–60
Perphenazine	10	8–64
Fluphenazine	2	2–60
Thiothixene	2	2–120
Haloperidol	2	2–60
Loxapine	10	20–160
Molindone	10	20–200
Clozapine	50	300–600
Cariprazine	1.5	1.5–4.5
Olanzapine	5	10–30
Quetiapine	150	150–800
Risperidone	4	4–16
Ziprasidone	40	80–160
Aripiprazole	10	10–30
Lumateperone	42	42

Parenteral Preparations

Well-tolerated parenteral forms of the high-potency older drugs haloperidol and fluphenazine are available for rapid initiation of treatment as well as for maintenance treatment in noncompliant patients. Since the parenterally administered drugs may have much greater bioavailability than the oral forms, doses should be only a fraction of what might be given orally, and the manufacturer's literature should be consulted. Fluphenazine decanoate and haloperidol decanoate are suitable for long-term parenteral maintenance therapy in patients who cannot or will not take oral medication. In addition, newer long-acting injectable (LAI) second-generation antipsychotics are now available, including formulations of risperidone, olanzapine, aripiprazole, and paliperidone. For some patients, the newer LAI drugs may be better tolerated than the older depot injectables.

Dosage Schedules

Antipsychotic drugs are often given in divided daily doses, titrating to an effective dosage Some others, such as lumateperone are given once a day while many clinicians dose more sedating medications such as quetiapine or olanzapine primarily at night. The low end of the dosage range in Table 29–4 should be tried for at least several weeks. After an effective daily dosage has been defined for an individual patient, doses can be given less frequently. Once-daily doses, usually given at night, are feasible for many patients during chronic maintenance treatment. Simplification of dosage schedules leads to better compliance.

Maintenance Treatment

A very small minority of schizophrenic patients may recover from an acute episode and require no further drug therapy for prolonged periods. In most cases, the choice is between "as needed" increased doses or the addition of other drugs for exacerbations versus continual maintenance treatment with full therapeutic dosage. The choice depends on social factors such as the availability of family or friends familiar with the early symptoms of relapse and ready access to care.

Drug Combinations

Combining antipsychotic drugs confounds evaluation of the efficacy of the drugs being used. Use of combinations, however, is widespread, with more emerging experimental data supporting such practices. Tricyclic antidepressants or, more often, selective serotonin reuptake inhibitors (SSRIs) are often used with antipsychotic agents for symptoms of depression complicating schizophrenia. The evidence for the usefulness of this polypharmacy is minimal. **Electroconvulsive therapy (ECT)** is a useful adjunct for antipsychotic drugs, not only for treating mood symptoms, but for positive symptom control as well. Electroconvulsive therapy can augment clozapine when maximum doses of clozapine are ineffective. In contrast, adding risperidone to clozapine is not beneficial. Lithium or valproic acid is sometimes added to antipsychotic agents with benefit to patients who do not respond to the latter drugs alone. There is some evidence that lamotrigine is more effective than any of the other mood stabilizers for this indication (see below). It is uncertain whether instances of successful combination therapy represent misdiagnosed cases of mania or schizoaffective disorder. Benzodiazepines may be useful for patients with anxiety symptoms or insomnia not controlled by antipsychotics.

Adverse Reactions

Most of the unwanted effects of antipsychotic drugs are extensions of their known pharmacologic actions (see Tables 29–1 and 29–2), but a few effects are allergic in nature, and some are idiosyncratic.

A. Behavioral Effects

The older typical antipsychotic drugs are unpleasant to take. Many patients stop taking these drugs because of the adverse effects, which may be mitigated by giving small doses during the day and the major portion at bedtime. A "pseudodepression" that may be due to drug-induced akinesia usually responds to cautious treatment with antiparkinsonism drugs. Other pseudodepressions may be due to higher doses than needed in a partially remitted patient, in which case decreasing the dose may relieve the symptoms. Toxic-confusional states may occur with very high doses of drugs that have prominent antimuscarinic actions.

B. Neurologic Effects

Extrapyramidal reactions occurring early during treatment with older agents include typical **Parkinson syndrome, akathisia** (uncontrollable restlessness), and **acute dystonic reactions** (spastic retrocollis or torticollis). Parkinsonism can be treated, when necessary, with conventional antiparkinsonism drugs of the antimuscarinic type or, in rare cases, with amantadine. (Levodopa should never be used in these patients.) Parkinsonism may be self-limiting, so an attempt to withdraw antiparkinsonism drugs should be made every 3–4 months. Akathisia and dystonic reactions also respond to such treatment, but many clinicians prefer to use a sedative antihistamine with anticholinergic properties, eg, diphenhydramine, which can be given either parenterally or orally.

Tardive dyskinesia, as the name implies, is a late-occurring syndrome of abnormal choreoathetoid movements. It is the most important unwanted effect of antipsychotic drugs. It has been proposed that it is caused by a relative cholinergic deficiency secondary to supersensitivity of dopamine receptors in the caudate-putamen. The prevalence varies enormously, but tardive dyskinesia is estimated to have occurred in 20–40% of chronically treated patients before the introduction of the newer atypical antipsychotics. Early recognition is important, since advanced cases may be difficult to reverse. Any patient with tardive dyskinesia treated with a first-generation antipsychotic drug or possibly risperidone or paliperidone could be switched to quetiapine or clozapine, the second-generation agents with the least likelihood of causing tardive dyskinesia. Most authorities agree that the first step should be to discontinue or slowly reduce the dose of the current antipsychotic agent or switch to one of the newer atypical agents. A logical second step would be to eliminate all drugs with central anticholinergic action, particularly antiparkinsonism drugs and tricyclic antidepressants. These two steps are often enough to bring about improvement.

In 2017, the first vesicular monoamine transporter type-2 (VMAT-2) inhibitor, **valbenazine,** was approved for the treatment of tardive dyskinesia. It was joined by **deutetrabenazine,** a second VMAT-2 agent in 2018. The VMAT-2 inhibitors selectively bind to the transporter to decrease dopamine to release in a reversible manner. Tardive dyskinesia is thought to be the result of postsynaptic dopamine hypersensitivity, and VMAT-2 inhibitors are more selective for dopamine than other monoamines. In the clinical trials leading to FDA approval, between 40% and 60% of patients were rated to be much or very much improved in their tardive dyskinesia. The most common side effects of valbenazine and deutetrabenazine are fatigue, somnolence, and headaches. Gastrointestinal side effects and akathisia also have been reported with the VMAT-2 inhibitors. Less commonly, QT prolongation also has been reported with both valbenazine and deutetrabenazine.

Seizures, though recognized as a complication of chlorpromazine treatment, were so rare with the high-potency older drugs as to merit little consideration. However, de novo seizures may occur in 2–5% of patients treated with clozapine. Use of an anticonvulsant is able to control seizures in most cases.

C. Autonomic Nervous System Effects

Most patients are able to tolerate the antimuscarinic adverse effects of antipsychotic drugs. Those who are made too uncomfortable or who develop urinary retention or other severe symptoms can be switched to an agent without significant antimuscarinic action. Orthostatic hypotension or impaired ejaculation—common complications of therapy with chlorpromazine or mesoridazine—should be managed by switching to drugs with less marked adrenoceptor-blocking actions.

D. Metabolic and Endocrine Effects

Weight gain is very common, especially with clozapine and olanzapine, and requires monitoring of food intake, especially carbohydrates. Hyperglycemia may develop, but whether secondary to weight gain-associated insulin resistance or to other mechanisms remains to be clarified. Hyperlipidemia may occur. The management of weight gain, insulin resistance, and increased lipids should include monitoring of weight at each visit and measurement of fasting blood sugar and lipids at 3- to 6-month intervals. Measurement of hemoglobin A_{1C} may be useful when it is impossible to be sure of obtaining a fasting blood sugar. Diabetic ketoacidosis has been reported in a few cases. The triglyceride:HDL ratio should be less than 3.5 in fasting samples. Levels higher than that indicate increased risk of atherosclerotic cardiovascular disease.

Hyperprolactinemia in women results in the amenorrhea-galactorrhea syndrome and infertility; in men, loss of libido, impotence, and infertility may result. Hyperprolactinemia may cause osteoporosis, particularly in women. If dose reduction is not indicated, or is ineffective in controlling this pattern, switching to an atypical agent that does not raise prolactin levels, eg, aripiprazole, may be indicated.

E. Toxic or Allergic Reactions

Agranulocytosis, cholestatic jaundice, and skin eruptions occur rarely with the high-potency antipsychotic drugs currently used.

In contrast to other antipsychotic agents, clozapine causes agranulocytosis in a small but significant number of patients—approximately 1–2% of those treated. This serious, potentially fatal effect can develop rapidly, usually between the 6th and 18th weeks of therapy. It is not known whether it represents an immune reaction, but it appears to be reversible upon discontinuance of the drug. *Because of the risk of agranulocytosis, patients receiving clozapine must have weekly blood counts for the first 6 months of treatment and every 3 weeks thereafter.*

F. Ocular Complications

Deposits in the anterior portions of the eye (cornea and lens) are a common complication of chlorpromazine therapy. They may accentuate the normal processes of aging of the lens. Thioridazine is the only antipsychotic drug that causes retinal deposits, which in advanced cases may resemble retinitis pigmentosa. The deposits are usually associated with "browning" of vision. The maximum daily dose of thioridazine has been limited to 800 mg/d to reduce the possibility of this complication.

G. Cardiac Toxicity

Thioridazine in doses exceeding 300 mg daily is almost always associated with minor abnormalities of T waves that are easily reversible. Overdoses of thioridazine are associated with major ventricular arrhythmias, eg, torsades de pointes, cardiac conduction block, and sudden death; it is not certain whether thioridazine can cause these same disorders when used in therapeutic doses. In view of possible additive antimuscarinic and quinidine-like actions with various tricyclic antidepressants, thioridazine should be combined with the latter drugs only with great care. Among the atypical agents, ziprasidone carries the greatest risk of QT prolongation and therefore should not be combined with other drugs that prolong the QT interval, including thioridazine, pimozide, and group 1A or 3 antiarrhythmic drugs. Clozapine is sometimes associated with myocarditis and must be discontinued if myocarditis manifests. Sudden death due to arrhythmias is common in schizophrenia. It is not always drug-related, and there are no studies that definitively show increased risk with particular drugs. Monitoring of QT_c prolongation has proved to be of little use unless the values increase to more than 500 ms and this is manifested in multiple rhythm strips or a Holter monitor study. A 20,000-patient study of ziprasidone versus olanzapine showed minimal or no increased risk of torsades de pointes or sudden death in patients who were randomized to ziprasidone.

H. Use in Pregnancy; Dysmorphogenesis

Although antipsychotic drugs appear to be relatively safe in pregnancy, a small increase in teratogenic risk could be missed. Questions about whether to use these drugs during pregnancy and whether to abort a pregnancy in which the fetus has already been exposed must be decided individually. If a pregnant woman could manage to be free of antipsychotic drugs during pregnancy, this would be desirable because of their effects on the neurotransmitters involved in neurodevelopment.

I. Neuroleptic Malignant Syndrome

This life-threatening disorder occurs in patients who are extremely sensitive to the extrapyramidal effects of antipsychotic agents (see also Chapter 16). The initial symptom is marked muscle rigidity. If sweating is impaired, as it often is during treatment with anticholinergic drugs, fever may ensue, often reaching dangerous levels. The stress leukocytosis and high fever associated with this syndrome may erroneously suggest an infectious process. Autonomic instability, with altered blood pressure and pulse rate, is often present.

Muscle-type creatine kinase levels are usually elevated, reflecting muscle damage. This syndrome is believed to result from an excessively rapid blockade of postsynaptic dopamine receptors. A severe form of extrapyramidal syndrome follows. Early in the course, vigorous treatment of the extrapyramidal syndrome with antiparkinsonism drugs is worthwhile. Muscle relaxants, particularly diazepam, are often useful. Other muscle relaxants, such as dantrolene, or dopamine agonists, such as bromocriptine, have been reported to be helpful. If fever is present, cooling by physical measures should be tried. Various minor forms of this syndrome are now recognized. Switching to an atypical drug after recovery is indicated.

Drug Interactions

Antipsychotics produce more important pharmacodynamic than pharmacokinetic interactions because of their multiple effects. Additive effects may occur when these drugs are combined with others that have sedative effects, α-adrenoceptor-blocking action, anticholinergic effects, and—for thioridazine and ziprasidone—quinidine-like action.

A variety of pharmacokinetic interactions have been reported, but none are of major clinical significance.

Overdoses

Poisonings with antipsychotic agents (unlike tricyclic antidepressants) are rarely fatal, with the exception of those due to mesoridazine and thioridazine (which are no longer available in the USA). In general, drowsiness proceeds to coma, with an intervening period of agitation. Neuromuscular excitability may be increased and proceed to convulsions. Pupils are miotic, and deep tendon reflexes are decreased. Hypotension and hypothermia are the rule, although fever may be present later in the course. The lethal effects of mesoridazine and thioridazine are related to induction of ventricular tachyarrhythmias. Patients should be given the usual "ABCD" treatment for poisonings (see Chapter 58) and treated supportively. Management of overdoses of thioridazine and mesoridazine, which are complicated by cardiac arrhythmias, is similar to that for tricyclic antidepressants (see Chapter 30).

Psychosocial Treatment & Cognitive Remediation

Patients with schizophrenia need psychosocial support based around activities of daily living, including housing, social activities, returning to school, obtaining the optimal level of work they may be capable of, and restoring social interactions. Unfortunately, funding for this crucial component of treatment has been minimized in recent years. Case management and therapy services are a vital part of the treatment program that should be provided to patients with schizophrenia. First-episode patients are particularly needful of this support because they often deny their illness and are noncompliant with medication.

Benefits & Limitations of Drug Treatment

As noted at the beginning of this chapter, antipsychotic drugs have had a major impact on psychiatric treatment. First, they have shifted the vast majority of patients from long-term hospitalization to the community. For many patients, this shift has provided a better life under more humane circumstances and in many cases has made life possible without frequent use of physical restraints. For others, the tragedy of an aimless existence is now being played out in the streets of our communities rather than in mental institutions.

Second, these antipsychotic drugs have markedly shifted psychiatric thinking to a more biologic orientation. Partly because of research stimulated by the effects of these drugs on schizophrenia, we now know much more about central nervous system physiology and pharmacology than was known before the introduction of these agents. However, despite much research, schizophrenia remains a scientific mystery and a personal disaster for the patient. Although most schizophrenic patients obtain some degree of benefit from these drugs—in some cases substantial benefit—none is made well by them.

■ LITHIUM, MOOD-STABILIZING DRUGS, & OTHER TREATMENT FOR BIPOLAR DISORDER

Bipolar disorder, once known as **manic-depressive** illness, was conceived of as a psychotic disorder distinct from schizophrenia at the end of the 19th century. Before that, both of these disorders were considered part of a continuum. The weight of the evidence today indicates that there *is* profound overlap in these disorders. However, there are pathophysiologically important differences, and some drug treatments are differentially effective in these disorders. According to *DSM-IV*, they are separate disease entities while research continues to define the dimensions of these illnesses and their genetic and other biologic markers.

Lithium was the first agent shown to be useful in the treatment of the manic phase of bipolar disorder that was not also an antipsychotic drug. Lithium is sometimes used adjunctively in schizophrenia. Lithium continues to be used for acute-phase illness as well as for prevention of recurrent manic and depressive episodes.

A group of mood-stabilizing drugs that are also anticonvulsant agents has become more widely used than lithium. It includes **carbamazepine** and **valproic acid** for the treatment of acute mania and for prevention of its recurrence. **Lamotrigine** is approved for prevention of recurrence. **Gabapentin, oxcarbazepine,** and **topiramate** are sometimes used to treat bipolar disorder but are not approved by the FDA for this indication. **Aripiprazole, chlorpromazine, olanzapine, quetiapine, risperidone,** and **ziprasidone** are approved by the FDA for treatment of the manic phase of bipolar disorder. Olanzapine plus fluoxetine in combination and quetiapine are approved for treatment of bipolar depression.

Nature of Bipolar Affective Disorder

Bipolar affective disorder occurs in 1–3% of the adult population. It may begin in childhood, but most cases are first diagnosed in the third and fourth decades of life. The key symptoms of bipolar disorder in the manic phase are expansive or irritable mood, hyperactivity, impulsivity, disinhibition, diminished need for sleep, racing thoughts, psychotic symptoms in some (but not all) patients, and cognitive impairment. Depression in bipolar patients is phenomenologically similar to that of major depression, with the key features being depressed mood, diurnal variation, sleep disturbance, anxiety, and sometimes, psychotic symptoms. Mixed manic and depressive symptoms are also seen. Patients with bipolar disorder are at high risk for suicide.

The sequence, number, and intensity of manic and depressive episodes are highly variable. The cause of the mood swings characteristic of bipolar affective disorder is unknown, although a preponderance of catecholamine-related activity may be present. Drugs that increase this activity tend to exacerbate mania, whereas those that reduce activity of dopamine or norepinephrine relieve mania. Acetylcholine or glutamate also may be involved. The nature of the abrupt switch from mania to depression experienced by some patients is uncertain. Bipolar disorder has a strong familial component, and there is abundant evidence that bipolar disorder is genetically determined.

Many of the genes that increase vulnerability to bipolar disorder are common to schizophrenia, but some genes appear to be unique to each disorder. Genome-wide association studies of psychotic bipolar disorder have shown replicated linkage to chromosomes 8p and 13q. Several candidate genes have shown association with bipolar disorder with psychotic features and with schizophrenia. These include genes for dysbindin, *DAOA/G30*, disrupted-in-schizophrenia-1 (*DISC-1*), and neuregulin 1.

BASIC PHARMACOLOGY OF LITHIUM

Lithium was first used therapeutically in the mid-19th century in patients with gout. It was briefly used as a substitute for sodium chloride in hypertensive patients in the 1940s but was banned after it proved too toxic for use without monitoring. In 1949, Cade discovered that lithium was an effective treatment for bipolar disorder, engendering a series of controlled trials that confirmed its efficacy as monotherapy for the manic phase of bipolar disorder.

Pharmacokinetics

Lithium is a small monovalent cation. Its pharmacokinetics are summarized in Table 29–5.

Pharmacodynamics

Despite considerable investigation, the biochemical basis for mood stabilizer therapies including lithium and anticonvulsant mood stabilizers is not clearly understood. Lithium directly inhibits two signal transduction pathways. It both suppresses inositol signaling through depletion of intracellular inositol and inhibits glycogen synthase kinase-3 (GSK-3), a multifunctional protein kinase. GSK-3 is a component of diverse intracellular signaling pathways. These include signaling via insulin/insulin-like growth factor, brain-derived neurotrophic factor (BDNF), and the Wnt pathway. Lithium-induced inhibition of GSK-3 results in reduction of phosphorylation of β-catenin, which allows β-catenin to accumulate and translocate to the nucleus. There, β-catenin facilitates transcription of a variety of proteins. The pathways that are facilitated by the accumulation of β-catenin via GSK-3 inhibition modulate energy metabolism, provide neuroprotection, and increase neuroplasticity.

Studies on the enzyme prolyl oligopeptidase and the sodium myoinositol transporter support an inositol depletion mechanism for the mood-stabilizer action. Valproic acid may indirectly reduce GSK-3 activity and can up-regulate gene expression through inhibition of histone deacetylase. Valproic acid also inhibits inositol signaling through an inositol depletion mechanism. There is no evidence of GSK-3 inhibition by carbamazepine, a second antiepileptic mood stabilizer. In contrast, this drug alters neuronal morphology through an inositol depletion mechanism, as seen with lithium and valproic acid. The mood stabilizers may also have indirect effects on neurotransmitters and their release.

TABLE 29–5 Pharmacokinetics of lithium.

Absorption	Virtually complete within 6–8 hours; peak plasma levels in 30 minutes to 2 hours
Distribution	In total body water; slow entry into intracellular compartment. Initial volume of distribution is 0.5 L/kg, rising to 0.7–0.9 L/kg; some sequestration in bone. No protein binding.
Metabolism	None
Excretion	Virtually entirely in urine. Lithium clearance about 20% of creatinine. Plasma half-life about 20 hours.
Target plasma concentration	0.6–1.4 mEq/L
Dosage	0.5 mEq/kg/d in divided doses

A. Effects on Electrolytes and Ion Transport

Lithium is closely related to sodium in its properties. It can substitute for sodium in generating action potentials and in Na^+-Na^+ exchange across the membrane. At therapeutic concentrations (~1 mEq/L), it does not significantly affect the Na^+-Ca^{2+} exchanger or the Na^+/K^+-ATPase pump.

B. Effects on Second Messengers

Some of the enzymes affected by lithium are listed in Table 29–6. One of the best-defined effects of lithium is its action

TABLE 29–6 Enzymes affected by lithium at therapeutic concentrations.

Enzyme	Enzyme Function; Action of Lithium
Inositol monophosphatase	The rate-limiting enzyme in inositol recycling; inhibited by lithium, resulting in depletion of substrate for IP_3 production (Figure 29–4)
Inositol polyphosphate 1-phosphatase	Another enzyme in inositol recycling; inhibited by lithium, resulting in depletion of substrate for IP_3 production (Figure 29–4)
Bisphosphate nucleotidase	Involved in AMP production; inhibited by lithium; may be target that results in lithium-induced nephrogenic diabetes insipidus
Fructose 1,6-biphosphatase	Involved in gluconeogenesis; inhibition by lithium of unknown relevance
Phosphoglucomutase	Involved in glycogenolysis; inhibition by lithium of unknown relevance
Glycogen synthase kinase-3	Constitutively active enzyme that appears to limit neurotrophic and neuroprotective processes; lithium inhibits

AMP, adenosine monophosphate; IP_3, inositol 1,4,5-trisphosphate.

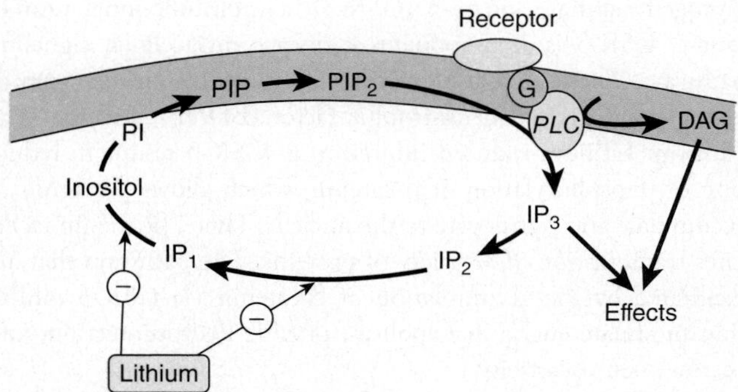

FIGURE 29–4 Effect of lithium on the IP_3 (inositol trisphosphate) and DAG (diacylglycerol) second-messenger system. The schematic diagram shows the synaptic membrane of a neuron. (PI, inorganic phosphate; PIP_2, phosphatidylinositol-4,5-bisphosphate; PLC, phospholipase C; G, coupling protein; Effects, activation of protein kinase C, mobilization of intracellular Ca^{2+}, etc.) Lithium, by inhibiting the recycling of inositol substrates, may cause the depletion of the second-messenger source PIP_2 and therefore reduce the release of IP_3 and DAG. Lithium may also act by other mechanisms (see text).

on inositol phosphates. Early studies of lithium demonstrated changes in brain inositol phosphate levels, but the significance of these changes was not appreciated until the second-messenger roles of inositol-1,4,5-trisphosphate (IP_3) and diacylglycerol (DAG) were discovered. As described in Chapter 2, inositol trisphosphate and diacylglycerol are important second messengers for both α-adrenergic and muscarinic transmission. Lithium inhibits inositol monophosphatase (IMPase) and other important enzymes in the normal recycling of membrane phosphoinositides, including conversion of IP_2 (inositol diphosphate) to IP_1 (inositol monophosphate) and the conversion of IP_1 to inositol (Figure 29–4). This block leads to a depletion of free inositol and ultimately of phosphatidylinositol-4,5-bisphosphate (PIP_2), the membrane precursor of IP_3 and DAG. Over time, the effects of transmitters on the cell diminish in proportion to the amount of activity in the PIP_2-dependent pathways. The activity of these pathways is postulated to be markedly increased during a manic episode. Treatment with lithium would be expected to diminish activity in these circuits.

Studies of noradrenergic effects in isolated brain tissue indicate that lithium can inhibit norepinephrine-sensitive adenylyl cyclase. Such an effect could relate to both its antidepressant and its antimanic effects. The relationship of these effects to lithium's actions on IP_3 mechanisms is currently unknown.

Because lithium affects second-messenger systems involving both activation of adenylyl cyclase and phosphoinositol turnover, it is not surprising that G proteins also are found to be affected. Several studies suggest that lithium may uncouple receptors from their G proteins; indeed, two of lithium's most common side effects, polyuria and subclinical hypothyroidism, may be due to uncoupling of the vasopressin and thyroid-stimulating hormone (TSH) receptors from their G proteins.

The major current working hypothesis for lithium's therapeutic mechanism of action supposes that its effects on phosphoinositol turnover, leading to an early relative reduction of myoinositol in human brain, are part of an initiating cascade of intracellular changes. Effects on specific isoforms of protein kinase C may be most relevant. Alterations of protein kinase C-mediated signaling alter gene expression and the production of proteins implicated in long-term neuroplastic events that could underlie long-term mood stabilization.

CLINICAL PHARMACOLOGY OF LITHIUM

Bipolar Affective Disorder

Until the late 1990s, lithium carbonate was the universally preferred treatment for bipolar disorder, especially in the manic phase. With the approval of valproate, aripiprazole, olanzapine, quetiapine, risperidone, and ziprasidone for this indication, a smaller percentage of bipolar patients now receive lithium. This trend is reinforced by the slow onset of action of lithium, which has often been supplemented with concurrent use of antipsychotic drugs or potent benzodiazepines in severely manic patients. The overall success rate for achieving remission from the manic phase of bipolar disorder can be as high as 80% but lower among patients who require hospitalization. A similar situation applies to maintenance treatment, which is about 60% effective overall but less in severely ill patients. These considerations have led to increased use of combined treatment in severe cases. After mania is controlled, the antipsychotic drug may be stopped and benzodiazepines and lithium continued as maintenance therapy.

The depressive phase of manic-depressive disorder often requires concurrent use of other agents including antipsychotics such as quetiapine or lurasidone. Antidepressants have not shown consistent utility and may be destabilizing. Tricyclic antidepressant agents have been linked to precipitation of mania, with more rapid cycling of mood swings, although most patients do not show this effect. Similarly, selective norepinephrine-serotonin reuptake inhibitor (SNRI) agents (see Chapter 30) have been associated with higher rates of switching to mania than some other antidepressants. Selective serotonin reuptake inhibitors are less likely to induce mania but may have limited efficacy. Bupropion has shown some promise but—like tricyclic antidepressants—may induce mania at higher doses. As shown in recent controlled trials, the anticonvulsant lamotrigine is effective for some patients with bipolar depression, but results have been inconsistent. For some patients, however, one of the older monoamine oxidase inhibitors may be the antidepressant of choice. Quetiapine and the combination of olanzapine plus fluoxetine have been approved for use in bipolar depression.

Unlike antipsychotic or antidepressant drugs, which exert several actions on the central or autonomic nervous system, lithium ion at therapeutic concentrations is devoid of autonomic blocking effects and of activating or sedating effects, although it can produce nausea and tremor. Most important is that the prophylactic use of lithium can prevent both mania and depression. Many experts believe that the aggressive marketing of newer drugs has inappropriately produced a shift to drugs that are less effective than lithium for substantial numbers of patients.

Other Applications

Recurrent depression with a cyclic pattern is controlled by either lithium or imipramine, both of which are superior to placebo. Lithium is also among the better-studied agents used to augment standard antidepressant response in **acute major depression** in those patients who have had inadequate response to monotherapy. For this application, concentrations of lithium at the lower end of the recommended range for bipolar disorder appear to be adequate.

Schizoaffective disorder, another condition with an affective component characterized by a mixture of schizophrenic symptoms and depression or excitement, is treated with antipsychotic drugs alone or combined with lithium. Various antidepressants are added if depression is present.

Lithium alone is rarely successful in treating **schizophrenia,** but adding lithium to an antipsychotic may salvage an otherwise treatment-resistant patient. Carbamazepine may work equally well when added to an antipsychotic drug.

Monitoring Treatment

Clinicians rely on measurements of serum lithium concentrations for assessing both the dosage required for treatment of acute mania and for prophylactic maintenance. These measurements are customarily taken 10–12 hours after the last dose, so all data in the literature pertaining to these concentrations reflect this interval.

An initial determination of serum lithium concentration should be obtained about 5 days after the start of treatment, at which time steady-state conditions should have been attained. If the clinical response suggests a change in dosage, simple arithmetic (new dose equals present dose times desired blood level divided by present blood level) should produce the desired level. The serum concentration attained with the adjusted dosage can be checked after another 5 days. Once the desired concentration has been achieved, levels can be measured at increasing intervals unless the schedule is influenced by intercurrent illness or the introduction of a new drug into the treatment program.

Maintenance Treatment

The decision to use lithium as *prophylactic* treatment depends on many factors: the frequency and severity of previous episodes, a crescendo pattern of appearance, and the degree to which the patient is willing to follow a program of indefinite maintenance therapy. Patients with a history of two or more mood cycles or any clearly defined bipolar I diagnosis are probable candidates for maintenance treatment. It has become increasingly evident that each recurrent cycle of bipolar illness may leave residual damage and worsen the long-term prognosis of the patient. Thus, there is greater consensus among experts that maintenance treatment be started as early as possible to reduce the frequency of recurrence. Although some patients can be maintained with serum levels as low as 0.6 mEq/L, the best results have been obtained with higher levels, such as 0.9 mEq/L.

Drug Interactions

Renal clearance of lithium is reduced about 25% by diuretics (eg, thiazides), and doses may need to be reduced by a similar amount. A similar reduction in lithium clearance has been noted with several of the newer nonsteroidal anti-inflammatory drugs that block synthesis of prostaglandins. This interaction has not been reported for either aspirin or acetaminophen. All neuroleptics tested to date, with the possible exception of clozapine and the newer atypical antipsychotics, may produce more severe extrapyramidal syndromes when combined with lithium.

Adverse Effects & Complications

Many adverse effects associated with lithium treatment occur at varying times after treatment is started. Some are harmless, but it is important to be alert to adverse effects that may signify impending serious toxic reactions.

A. Neurologic and Psychiatric Adverse Effects

Tremor is one of the most common adverse effects of lithium treatment, and it occurs with therapeutic doses. Propranolol and atenolol, which have been reported to be effective in essential tremor, also alleviate lithium-induced tremor. Other reported neurologic abnormalities include choreoathetosis, motor hyperactivity, ataxia, dysarthria, and aphasia. Psychiatric disturbances at toxic concentrations are generally marked by mental confusion and withdrawal. Appearance of any new neurologic or psychiatric symptoms or signs is a clear indication for temporarily stopping treatment with lithium and for close monitoring of serum levels.

B. Decreased Thyroid Function

Lithium probably decreases thyroid function in most patients exposed to the drug, but the effect is reversible or nonprogressive. Few patients develop frank thyroid enlargement, and fewer still show symptoms of hypothyroidism. Although initial thyroid testing followed by regular monitoring of thyroid function has been proposed, such procedures are not cost-effective. Obtaining a serum TSH concentration every 6–12 months, however, is prudent.

C. Nephrogenic Diabetes Insipidus and Other Renal Adverse Effects

Polydipsia and polyuria are common but reversible concomitants of lithium treatment, occurring at therapeutic serum concentrations. The principal physiologic lesion involved is loss of responsiveness to antidiuretic hormone (nephrogenic diabetes insipidus). Lithium-induced diabetes insipidus is resistant to vasopressin but responds to amiloride (see Chapter 15).

Extensive literature has accumulated concerning other forms of renal dysfunction during long-term lithium therapy, including chronic interstitial nephritis and minimal-change glomerulopathy with nephrotic syndrome. Some instances of decreased glomerular filtration rate have been encountered but no instances of marked azotemia or renal failure.

Patients receiving lithium should avoid dehydration and the associated increased concentration of lithium in urine. Periodic tests of renal concentrating ability should be performed to detect changes.

D. Edema

Edema is a common adverse effect of lithium treatment and may be related to some effect of lithium on sodium retention. Although weight gain may be expected in patients who become edematous, water retention does not account for the weight gain observed in up to 30% of patients taking lithium.

E. Cardiac Adverse Effects

The bradycardia-tachycardia ("sick sinus") syndrome is a definite contraindication to the use of lithium because the ion further depresses the sinus node. T-wave flattening is often observed on the electrocardiogram but is of questionable significance.

F. Use during Pregnancy

Renal clearance of lithium increases during pregnancy and reverts to lower levels immediately after delivery. A patient whose serum lithium concentration is in a good therapeutic range during pregnancy may develop toxic levels after delivery. Special care in monitoring lithium levels is needed at these times. Lithium is transferred to nursing infants through breast milk, in which it has a concentration about one third to one half that of serum. Lithium toxicity in newborns is manifested by lethargy, cyanosis, poor suck and Moro reflexes, and perhaps hepatomegaly.

The Issue of lithium-induced dysmorphogenesis is not settled. An earlier report suggested an increase in cardiac anomalies—especially Ebstein anomaly—in lithium babies, and it is listed as such in Table 59–1 in this book. However, more recent data suggest that lithium carries a relatively low risk of teratogenic effects. Further research is needed in this important area.

G. Miscellaneous Adverse Effects

Transient acneiform eruptions have been noted early in lithium treatment. Some of them subside with temporary discontinuance of treatment and do not recur with its resumption. Folliculitis is less dramatic and probably occurs more frequently. Leukocytosis is always present during lithium treatment, probably reflecting a direct effect on leukopoiesis rather than mobilization from the marginal pool. This adverse effect has now become a therapeutic effect in patients with low leukocyte counts.

Overdoses

Therapeutic overdoses of lithium are more common than those due to deliberate or accidental ingestion of the drug. Therapeutic overdoses are usually due to accumulation of lithium resulting from some change in the patient's status, such as diminished serum sodium, use of diuretics, or fluctuating renal function. Since the tissues will have already equilibrated with the blood, the plasma concentrations of lithium may not be excessively high in proportion to the degree of toxicity; any value over 2 mEq/L must be considered as indicating likely toxicity. Because lithium is a small ion, it is dialyzed readily. Both peritoneal dialysis and hemodialysis are effective, although the latter is preferred.

VALPROIC ACID

Valproic acid (valproate), discussed in detail in Chapter 24 as an antiepileptic, has been demonstrated to have antimanic effects and is now being widely used for this indication in the USA. (Gabapentin is not effective, leaving the mechanism of antimanic action of valproate unclear.) Overall, valproic acid shows efficacy equivalent to that of lithium during the early weeks of treatment. It is significant that valproic acid has been effective in some patients who have failed to respond to lithium. For example, mixed states and rapid cycling forms of bipolar disorder may be more responsive to valproate than to lithium. Moreover, its side-effect profile is such that one can rapidly increase the dosage over a few days to produce blood levels in the apparent therapeutic range, with nausea being the only limiting factor in some patients. The starting dosage is 750 mg/d, increasing rapidly to the 1500–2000 mg range with a recommended maximum dosage of 60 mg/kg/d.

Combinations of valproic acid with other psychotropic medications likely to be used in the management of either phase of bipolar illness are generally well tolerated. Valproic acid is an appropriate first-line treatment for mania, although it is not clear that it will be as effective as lithium as a maintenance treatment in all subsets of patients. Many clinicians advocate combining valproic acid and lithium in patients who do not fully respond to either agent alone.

CARBAMAZEPINE

Carbamazepine has been considered to be a reasonable alternative to lithium when the latter is less than optimally efficacious. However, the pharmacokinetic interactions of carbamazepine and its tendency to induce the metabolism of CYP3A4 substrates make it a more difficult drug to use with other standard treatments for bipolar disorder. The mode of action of carbamazepine is unclear, and oxcarbazepine is not effective. Carbamazepine may be used to treat acute mania and also for prophylactic therapy. Adverse effects (discussed in Chapter 24) are generally no greater and sometimes less than those associated with lithium. Carbamazepine may be used alone or, in refractory patients, in combination with lithium or, rarely, valproate.

The use of carbamazepine as a mood stabilizer is similar to its use as an anticonvulsant (see Chapter 24). Dosage usually begins with 200 mg twice daily, with increases as needed. Maintenance dosage is similar to that used for treating epilepsy, ie, 800–1200 mg/d. Plasma concentrations between 3 and 14 mg/L are considered desirable, although the optimal therapeutic range has not been established. Blood dyscrasias have figured prominently in the adverse effects of carbamazepine when it is used as an anticonvulsant, but they have not been a major problem with its use as a mood stabilizer. Overdoses of carbamazepine are a major emergency and should generally be managed like overdoses of tricyclic antidepressants (see Chapter 58).

OTHER DRUGS

Lamotrigine is approved as a maintenance treatment for bipolar disorder. Although not effective in treating acute mania, it appears effective in reducing the frequency of recurrent depressive cycles and may have some utility in the treatment of bipolar depression. A number of novel agents are under investigation for bipolar depression, including riluzole, a neuroprotective agent that is approved for use in amyotrophic lateral sclerosis; ketamine, a noncompetitive NMDA antagonist previously discussed as a drug believed to model schizophrenia but thought to act by producing relative enhancement of AMPA receptor activity; and AMPA receptor potentiators.

SUMMARY Antipsychotic Drugs & Lithium

Subclass, Drug	Mechanism of Action	Effects	Clinical Applications	Pharmacokinetics, Toxicities, Interactions
PHENOTHIAZINES				
• Chlorpromazine • Fluphenazine • Thioridazine **THIOXANTHENE** • Thiothixene	Blockade of D_2 receptors >> 5-HT_{2A} receptors	α-Receptor blockade (fluphenazine least) • muscarinic (M)-receptor blockade (especially chlorpromazine and thioridazine) • H_1-receptor blockade (chlorpromazine, thiothixene) • central nervous system (CNS) depression (sedation) • decreased seizure threshold • QT prolongation (thioridazine)	Psychiatric: schizophrenia (alleviate positive symptoms), bipolar disorder (manic phase) • nonpsychiatric: antiemesis, preoperative sedation (promethazine) • pruritus	Oral and parenteral forms, long half-lives with metabolism-dependent elimination • *Toxicity:* Extensions of effects on α and M receptors • blockade of dopamine receptors may result in akathisia, dystonia, parkinsonian symptoms, tardive dyskinesia, and hyperprolactinemia
BUTYROPHENONE				
• Haloperidol	Blockade of D_2 receptors >> 5-HT_{2A} receptors	Some α blockade, but minimal M-receptor blockade and much less sedation than the phenothiazines	Schizophrenia (alleviates positive symptoms), bipolar disorder (manic phase), Huntington chorea, Tourette syndrome	Oral and parenteral forms with metabolism-dependent elimination • *Toxicity:* Extrapyramidal dysfunction is major adverse effect
SECOND-GENERATION ANTIPSYCHOTICS				
• Aripiprazole • Brexpiprazole • Cariprazine • Clozapine • Lurasidone Lumateperone • Olanzapine • Quetiapine • Risperidone • Ziprasidone	Blockade of 5-HT_{2A} receptors > blockade of D_2 receptors	Some α blockade (clozapine, risperidone, ziprasidone) and M-receptor blockade (clozapine, olanzapine) • variable H_1-receptor blockade (all)	Schizophrenia—improve both positive and negative symptoms • bipolar disorder (olanzapine or risperidone adjunctive with lithium) • agitation in Alzheimer and Parkinson patients (low doses) • major depression (aripiprazole)	*Toxicity:* Agranulocytosis (clozapine), diabetes (clozapine, olanzapine), hypercholesterolemia (clozapine, olanzapine), hyperprolactinemia (risperidone), QT prolongation (ziprasidone), weight gain (clozapine, olanzapine)
LITHIUM	Mechanism of action uncertain • suppresses inositol signaling and inhibits glycogen synthase kinase-3 (GSK-3), a multifunctional protein kinase	No significant antagonistic actions on autonomic nervous system receptors or specific CNS receptors • no sedative effects	Bipolar affective disorder—prophylactic use can prevent mood swings between mania and depression	Oral absorption, renal elimination • half-life 20 h • narrow therapeutic window (monitor blood levels) • *Toxicity:* Tremor, edema, hypothyroidism, renal dysfunction, dysrhythmias • pregnancy category D • *Interactions:* Clearance decreased by thiazides and some NSAIDs
OTHER AGENTS FOR BIPOLAR DISORDER				
• Carbamazepine • Lamotrigine • Valproic acid	Mechanism of action in bipolar disorder unclear (see Chapter 24 for putative actions in seizure disorders)	See Chapter 24	Valproic acid is increasingly used as first choice in acute mania • carbamazepine and lamotrigine are also used both in acute mania and for prophylaxis in depressive phase	Oral absorption • once-daily dosing • carbamazepine forms active metabolite • lamotrigine and valproic acid form conjugates • *Toxicity:* Hematotoxicity and induction of P450 drug metabolism (carbamazepine), rash (lamotrigine), tremor, liver dysfunction, weight gain, inhibition of drug metabolism (valproic acid)

PREPARATIONS AVAILABLE

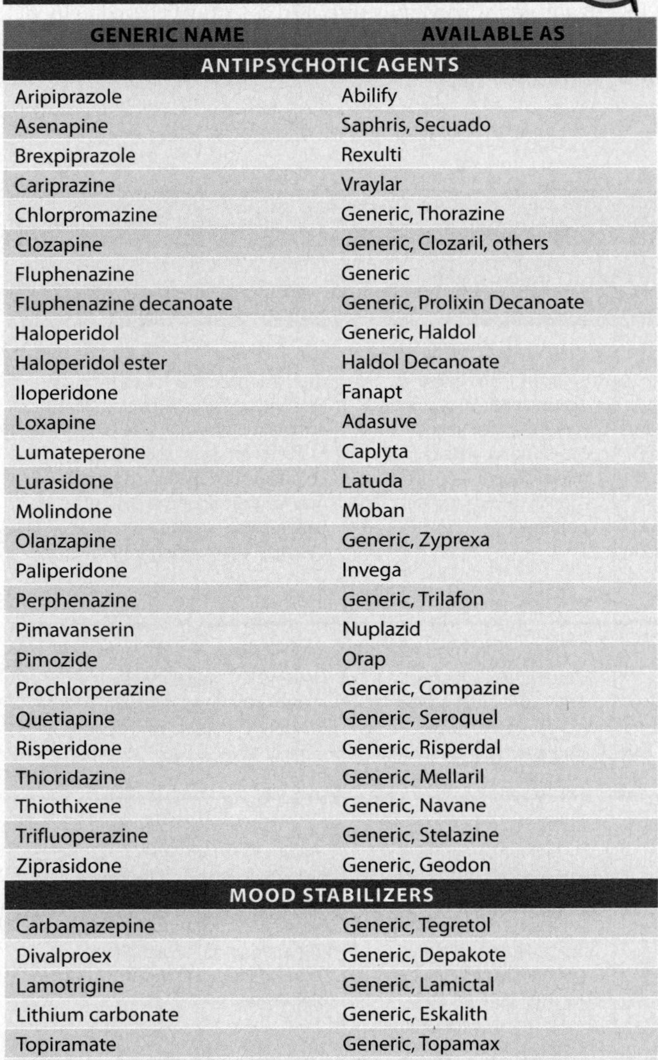

GENERIC NAME	AVAILABLE AS
ANTIPSYCHOTIC AGENTS	
Aripiprazole	Abilify
Asenapine	Saphris, Secuado
Brexpiprazole	Rexulti
Cariprazine	Vraylar
Chlorpromazine	Generic, Thorazine
Clozapine	Generic, Clozaril, others
Fluphenazine	Generic
Fluphenazine decanoate	Generic, Prolixin Decanoate
Haloperidol	Generic, Haldol
Haloperidol ester	Haldol Decanoate
Iloperidone	Fanapt
Loxapine	Adasuve
Lumateperone	Caplyta
Lurasidone	Latuda
Molindone	Moban
Olanzapine	Generic, Zyprexa
Paliperidone	Invega
Perphenazine	Generic, Trilafon
Pimavanserin	Nuplazid
Pimozide	Orap
Prochlorperazine	Generic, Compazine
Quetiapine	Generic, Seroquel
Risperidone	Generic, Risperdal
Thioridazine	Generic, Mellaril
Thiothixene	Generic, Navane
Trifluoperazine	Generic, Stelazine
Ziprasidone	Generic, Geodon
MOOD STABILIZERS	
Carbamazepine	Generic, Tegretol
Divalproex	Generic, Depakote
Lamotrigine	Generic, Lamictal
Lithium carbonate	Generic, Eskalith
Topiramate	Generic, Topamax
Valproic acid	Generic, Depakene

REFERENCES

Antipsychotic Drugs

Bhattacharjee J, El-Sayeh HG: Aripiprazole versus typical antipsychotic drugs for schizophrenia. Cochrane Database Syst Rev 2008;16(3):CD006617.

Blair HA. Lumateperone: First Approval. Drugs. 2020 Mar;80(4):417-423. doi: 10.1007/s40265-020-01271-6. PMID: 32060882.

Caccia S et al: A new generation of antipsychotics: Pharmacology and clinical utility of cariprazine in schizophrenia. Ther Clin Risk Manag 2013;9:319.

Chue P: Glycine reuptake inhibition as a new therapeutic approach in schizophrenia: Focus on the glycine transporter 1 (GlyT1). Curr Pharm Des 2013;19:1311.

Citrome L: A review of the pharmacology, efficacy and tolerability of recently approved and upcoming oral antipsychotics: An evidence-based medicine approach. CNS Drugs 2013;27:879.

Citrome L: Cariprazine: Chemistry, pharmacodynamics, pharmacokinetics, and metabolism, clinical efficacy, safety, and tolerability. Expert Opin Drug Metab Toxicol 2013;9:193.

Citrome L: Cariprazine in bipolar disorder: Clinical efficacy, tolerability, and place in therapy. Adv Ther 2013;30:102.

Citrome L: Cariprazine in schizophrenia: Clinical efficacy, tolerability, and place in therapy. Adv Ther 2013;30:114.

Correll CU et al: Efficacy of brexpiprazole in patients with acute schizophrenia: Review of three randomized, double-blind, placebo-controlled studies. Schizophr Res 2016;174:82.

Coyle JT: Glutamate and schizophrenia: Beyond the dopamine hypothesis. Cell Mol Neurobiol 2006;26:365.

Durgam S et al: An 8-week randomized, double-blind, placebo-controlled evaluation of the safety and efficacy of cariprazine in patients with bipolar I depression. Am J Psychiatry 2016;173:271.

Durgam S et al: Cariprazine in acute exacerbation of schizophrenia: A fixed-dose, phase 3, randomized, double-blind, placebo- and active-controlled trial. J Clin Psychiatry 2015;76:e1574.

Edinoff A, Wu N, deBoisblanc C, Feltner CO, Norder M, Tzoneva V, Kaye AM, Cornett EM, Kaye AD, Viswanath O, Urits I. Lumateperone for the Treatment of Schizophrenia. Psychopharmacol Bull. 2020 Sep 14;50(4):32-59. PMID: 33012872; PMCID: PMC7511146.

Escamilla MA, Zavala JM: Genetics of bipolar disorder. Dialogues Clin Neurosci 2008;10:141.

Fava M et al: Adjunctive brexpiprazole in patients with major depressive disorder and irritability: An exploratory study. J Clin Psychiatry 2016;77:1695.

Fountoulakis KN, Vieta E: Treatment of bipolar disorder: A systematic review of available data and clinical perspectives. Int J Neuropsychopharmacol 2008;11:999.

Freudenreich O, Goff DC: Antipsychotic combination therapy in schizophrenia: A review of efficacy and risks of current combinations. Acta Psychiatr Scand 2002;106:323.

Glassman AH: Schizophrenia, antipsychotic drugs, and cardiovascular disease. J Clin Psychiatry 2005;66(Suppl 6):5.

Grunder G, Nippius H, Carlsson A: The "atypicality" of antipsychotics: A concept re-examined and re-defined. Nat Rev Drug Discov 2009;8:197.

Haddad PM, Anderson IM: Antipsychotic-related QTc prolongation, torsade de pointes and sudden death. Drugs 2002;62:1649.

Harrison PJ, Weinberger DR: Schizophrenia genes, gene expression, and neuropathology: On the matter of their convergence. Mol Psychiatry 2005;10:40.

Hashimoto K et al: Glutamate modulators as potential therapeutic drugs in schizophrenia and affective disorders. Eur Arch Psychiatry Clin Neurosci 2013;263:367.

Herman EJ et al: Metabotropic glutamate receptors for new treatments in schizophrenia. Handb Exp Pharmacol 2012;213:297.

Hermanowicz S, Hermanowicz N: The safety, tolerability and efficacy of pimavanserin tartrate in the treatment of psychosis in Parkinson's disease. Expert Rev Neurother 2016;16:625.

Hovelsø N et al: Therapeutic potential of metabotropic glutamate receptor modulators. Curr Neuropharmacol 2012;10:12.

Javitt DC: Glycine transport inhibitors in the treatment of schizophrenia. Handb Exp Pharmacol 2012;213:367.

Kane JM et al: Overview of short- and long-term tolerability and safety of brexpiprazole in patients with schizophrenia. Schizophr Res 2016;174:93.

Karam CS et al: Signaling pathways in schizophrenia: Emerging targets and therapeutic strategies. Trend Pharmacol Sci 2010;31:381.

Lao KS et al: Tolerability and safety profile of cariprazine in treating psychotic disorders, bipolar disorder and major depressive disorder: A systematic review with meta-analysis of randomized controlled trials. CNS Drugs 2016;30:1043.

Lieberman JA et al: Antipsychotic drugs: Comparison in animal models of efficacy, neurotransmitter regulation, and neuroprotection. Pharmacol Rev 2008;60:358.

Lieberman JA et al: Effectiveness of antipsychotic drugs in patients with chronic schizophrenia. N Engl J Med 2005;353:1209.

McKeage K, Plosker GL: Amisulpride: A review of its use in the management of schizophrenia. CNS Drugs 2004;18:933.

Meltzer HY: Treatment of schizophrenia and spectrum disorders: Pharmacotherapy, psychosocial treatments, and neurotransmitter interactions. Biol Psychiatry 1999;46:1321.

Meltzer HY, Massey BW: The role of serotonin receptors in the action of atypical antipsychotic drugs. Curr Opin Pharmacol 2011;11:59.

Meltzer HY et al: A randomized, double-blind comparison of clozapine and high-dose olanzapine in treatment-resistant patients with schizophrenia. J Clin Psychiatry 2008;69:274.

Newcomer JW, Haupt DW: The metabolic effects of antipsychotic medications. Can J Psychiatry 2006;51:480.

Pimavanserin (Nuplazid) for Parkinson's disease psychosis. Med Lett Drugs Ther 2016;58:74.

Preskorn SH, Zeller S, Citrome L, Finman J, Goldberg JF, Fava M, Kakar R, De Vivo M, Yocca FD, Risinger R. Effect of Sublingual Dexmedetomidine vs Placebo on Acute Agitation Associated With Bipolar Disorder: A Randomized Clinical Trial. JAMA. 2022 Feb 22;327(8):727-736. doi: 10.1001/jama.2022.0799. PMID: 35191924; PMCID: PMC8864508.

Schwarz C et al: Valproate for schizophrenia. Cochrane Database Syst Rev 2008;3:CD004028.

Urichuk L et al: Metabolism of atypical antipsychotics: Involvement of cytochrome p450 enzymes and relevance for drug-drug interactions. Curr Drug Metab 2008;9:410.

Walsh T et al: Rare structural variants disrupt multiple genes in neurodevelopmental pathways in schizophrenia. Science 2008;320:539.

Zhang A et al: Recent progress in development of dopamine receptor subtype-selective agents: Potential therapeutics for neurological and psychiatric disorders. Chem Rev 2007;107:274.

Mood Stabilizers

Baraban JM et al: Second messenger systems and psychoactive drug action: Focus on the phosphoinositide system and lithium. Am J Psychiatry 1989;146:1251.

Bowden CL, Singh V: Valproate in bipolar disorder: 2000 onwards. Acta Psychiatr Scand Suppl 2005;426:13.

Catapano LA, Manji HK: Kinases as drug targets in the treatment of bipolar disorder. Drug Discov Today 2008;13:295.

Fountoulakis KN, Vieta E: Treatment of bipolar disorder: A systematic review of available data and clinical perspectives. Int J Neuropsychopharmacol 2008;11:999.

Jope RS: Anti-bipolar therapy: Mechanism of action of lithium. Mol Psychiatry 1999;4:117.

Mathew SJ et al: Novel drugs and therapeutic targets for severe mood disorders. Neuropsychopharmacology 2008;33:2080.

Quiroz JA et al: Emerging experimental therapeutics for bipolar disorder: Clues from the molecular pathophysiology. Mol Psychiatry 2004;9:756.

Vieta E, Sanchez-Moreno J: Acute and long-term treatment of mania. Dialogues Clin Neurosci 2008;10:165.

Yatham LN et al: Third generation anticonvulsants in bipolar disorder: A review of efficacy and summary of clinical recommendations. J Clin Psychiatry 2002;63:275.

CASE STUDY ANSWER

Schizophrenia is characterized by a disintegration of thought processes and emotional responsiveness. Symptoms commonly include auditory hallucinations, paranoid or bizarre delusions, disorganized thinking and speech, and social and occupational dysfunction. For many patients, first-generation (eg, haloperidol) and second-generation agents (eg, risperidone) are of equal efficacy for treating positive symptoms. Second-generation agents are often more effective for treating negative symptoms and cognitive dysfunction and have lower risk of tardive dyskinesia and hyperprolactinemia. Other indications for the use of selected antipsychotics include bipolar disorder, psychotic depression, Tourette syndrome, disturbed behavior in patients with Alzheimer disease, and, in the case of older drugs (eg, chlorpromazine), treatment of emesis and pruritus.

CHAPTER

30 Antidepressant Agents

Charles DeBattista, MD

CASE STUDY

A 47-year-old woman presents to her primary care physician with a chief complaint of fatigue. She indicates that she was promoted to senior manager in her company approximately 11 months earlier. Although her promotion was welcome and came with a sizable raise in pay, it resulted in her having to move away from an office and group of colleagues she very much enjoyed. In addition, her level of responsibility increased dramatically. The patient reports that for the last 7 weeks, she has been waking up at 3 AM every night and been unable to go back to sleep. She dreads the day and the stresses of the workplace. As a consequence, she is not eating as well as she might and has dropped 7% of her body weight in the last 3 months. She also reports being so stressed that she breaks down crying in the office occasionally and has been calling in sick frequently. When she comes home, she finds she is less motivated to attend to chores around the house and has no motivation, interest, or energy to pursue recreational activities that she once enjoyed such as hiking. She describes herself as "chronically miserable and worried all the time." Her medical history is notable for chronic neck pain from a motor vehicle accident for which she is being treated with tramadol and meperidine. In addition, she is on hydrochlorothiazide and propranolol for hypertension. The patient has a history of one depressive episode after a divorce that was treated successfully with fluoxetine. Medical workup including complete blood cell count, thyroid function tests, and a chemistry panel reveals no abnormalities. She is started on fluoxetine for a presumed major depressive episode and referred for cognitive behavioral psychotherapy. What CYP450 and pharmacodynamic interactions might be associated with fluoxetine use in this patient? Which class of antidepressants would be contraindicated in this patient?

The diagnosis of depression still rests primarily on the clinical interview. Major depressive disorder (MDD) is characterized by depressed mood most of the time for at least 2 weeks or loss of interest or pleasure in most activities, or both. In addition, depression is characterized by disturbances in sleep and appetite as well as deficits in cognition and energy. Thoughts of guilt, worthlessness, and suicide are common. Coronary artery disease, diabetes, and stroke appear to be more common in depressed patients, and depression may considerably worsen the prognosis for patients with a variety of comorbid medical conditions.

According to the Centers for Disease Control and Prevention, antidepressants are consistently among the three most commonly prescribed classes of medications in the USA. The wisdom of such widespread use of antidepressants is debated. However, it is clear that American physicians have been increasingly inclined to use antidepressants to treat a host of conditions and that patients have been increasingly receptive to their use.

The primary indication for antidepressant agents is the treatment of MDD. Major depression, with a lifetime prevalence of around 17% in the USA and a point prevalence of 5%, is associated with substantial morbidity and mortality. MDD represents one of the most common causes of disability in the developed world. In addition, major depression is commonly associated with a variety of medical conditions—from chronic pain to coronary artery disease. When depression coexists with other medical conditions, the patient's disease burden increases, and the quality of life—and often the prognosis for effective treatment—decreases significantly.

Some of the growth in antidepressant use may be related to the broad application of these agents for conditions other than major depression. For example, antidepressants have received US Food and Drug Administration (FDA) approvals for the treatment of panic disorder, generalized anxiety disorder (GAD), post-traumatic stress disorder (PTSD), and obsessive-compulsive disorder (OCD). In addition, antidepressants are commonly used to treat pain disorders such as neuropathic pain and the pain associated with fibromyalgia. Some antidepressants are used for treating premenstrual dysphoric disorder (PMDD), mitigating the vasomotor symptoms of menopause, and treating stress urinary incontinence. Thus, antidepressants have a broad spectrum of use in medical practice. However, their primary use remains the treatment for MDD.

PATHOPHYSIOLOGY OF MAJOR DEPRESSION

There has been a marked shift in the last decade in our understanding of the pathophysiology of major depression. In addition to the older idea that a deficit in function or amount of monoamines (the **monoamine hypothesis**) is central to the biology of depression, there is evidence that neurotrophic and endocrine factors play a major role (the **neurotrophic hypothesis**). Histologic studies, structural and functional brain imaging research, genetic findings, and steroid research all suggest a complex pathophysiology for MDD with important implications for drug treatment.

Neurotrophic Hypothesis

There is substantial evidence that nerve growth factors such as **brain-derived neurotrophic factor (BDNF)** are critical in the regulation of neural plasticity, resilience, and neurogenesis. The evidence suggests that depression is associated with the loss of neurotrophic support and that effective antidepressant therapies increase neurogenesis and synaptic connectivity in cortical areas such as the hippocampus. BDNF is thought to exert its influence on neuronal survival and growth effects by activating the tyrosine kinase receptor B in both neurons and glia (Figure 30–1).

Several lines of evidence support the neurotrophic hypothesis. Animal and human studies indicate that stress and pain are associated with a drop in BDNF levels and that this loss of neurotrophic support contributes to atrophic structural changes in the hippocampus and perhaps other areas such as the medial frontal cortex and anterior cingulate. The hippocampus is known to be important in both contextual memory and regulation of the hypothalamic-pituitary-adrenal (HPA) axis. Likewise, the

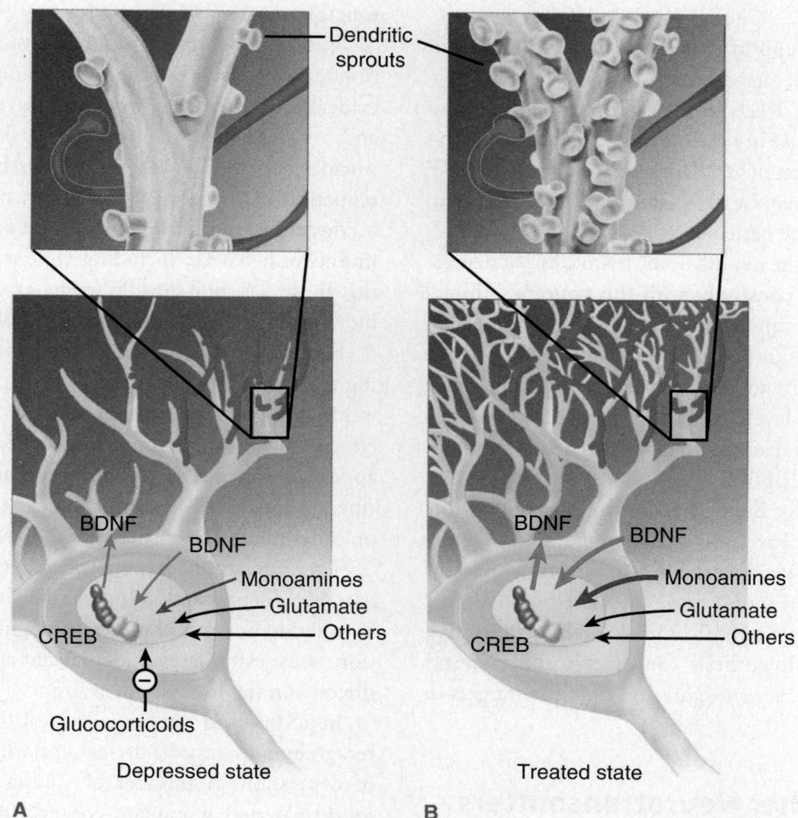

FIGURE 30–1 The neurotrophic hypothesis of major depression. Changes in trophic factors (especially brain-derived neurotrophic factor, BDNF) and hormones appear to play a major role in the development of major depression (**A**). Successful treatment results in changes in these factors (**B**). CREB, cAMP response element-binding (protein); BDNF, brain-derived neurotrophic factor. (Reproduced with permission from Nestler EJ, Barrot M, DiLeone RJ, Eisch AJ, Gold SJ, Monteggia LM. Neurobiology of depression. Neuron 2002 Mar 28;34(1):13-25.)

anterior cingulate plays a role in the integration of emotional stimuli and attention functions, whereas the medial orbital frontal cortex is also thought to play a role in memory, learning, and emotion.

Over 30 structural imaging studies suggest that major depression is associated with a 5–10% loss of volume in the hippocampus, although some studies have not replicated this finding. Depression and chronic stress states have also been associated with a substantial loss of volume in the anterior cingulate and medial orbital frontal cortex. Loss of volume in structures such as the hippocampus also appears to increase as a function of the duration of illness and the amount of time that the depression remains untreated.

Another source of evidence supporting the neurotrophic hypothesis of depression comes from studies of the direct effects of BDNF on emotional regulation. Direct infusion of BDNF into the midbrain, hippocampus, and lateral ventricles of rodents has an antidepressant-like effect in animal models. Moreover, all known classes of antidepressants are associated with an increase in BDNF levels in animal models with chronic (but not acute) administration. This increase in BDNF levels is consistently associated with increased neurogenesis in the hippocampus in these animal models. Other interventions thought to be effective in the treatment of major depression, including electroconvulsive therapy, also appear to robustly stimulate BDNF levels and hippocampus neurogenesis in animal models.

Human studies seem to support the animal data on the role of neurotrophic factors in stress states. Depression appears to be associated with a drop in BDNF levels in the cerebrospinal fluid and serum as well as with a decrease in tyrosine kinase receptor B activity. Conversely, administration of antidepressants increases BDNF levels in clinical trials and may be associated with an increase in hippocampus volume in some patients.

Much evidence supports the neurotrophic hypothesis of depression, but not all evidence is consistent with this concept. Animal studies in BDNF knockout mice have not always suggested an increase in depressive or anxious behaviors that would be expected with a deficiency of BDNF. In addition, some animal studies have found an increase in BDNF levels after some types of social stress and an increase rather than a decrease in depressive behaviors with lateral ventricle injections of BDNF.

A proposed explanation for the discrepant findings on the role of neurotrophic factors in depression is that there are polymorphisms for BDNF that may yield very different effects. Mutations in the *BDNF* gene have been found to be associated with altered anxiety and depressive behavior in both animal and human studies.

Thus, the neurotrophic hypothesis continues to be intensely investigated and has yielded new insights and potential targets in the treatment of MDD.

Monoamines & Other Neurotransmitters

The monoamine hypothesis of depression (Figure 30–2) suggests that depression is related to a deficiency in the amount or function of cortical and limbic serotonin (5-HT), norepinephrine (NE), and dopamine (DA).

Evidence to support the monoamine hypothesis comes from several sources. It has been known for many years that reserpine treatment, which is known to deplete monoamines, is associated with depression in a subset of patients. Similarly, depressed patients who respond to serotonergic antidepressants such as fluoxetine often rapidly suffer relapse when given diets free of tryptophan, a precursor of serotonin synthesis. Patients who respond to noradrenergic antidepressants such as desipramine are less likely to relapse on a tryptophan-free diet. Moreover, depleting catecholamines in depressed patients who have previously responded to noradrenergic agents likewise tends to be associated with relapse. Administration of an inhibitor of norepinephrine synthesis is also associated with a rapid return of depressive symptoms in patients who respond to noradrenergic but not necessarily in patients who had responded to serotonergic antidepressants.

Another line of evidence supporting the monoamine hypothesis comes from genetic studies. A functional polymorphism exists for the promoter region of the serotonin transporter gene, which regulates how much of the transporter protein is available. Subjects who are homozygous for the s (short) allele may be more vulnerable to developing major depression and suicidal behavior in response to stress. In addition, homozygotes for the s allele may also be less likely to respond to and tolerate serotonergic antidepressants. Conversely, subjects with the l (long) allele tend to be more resistant to stress and may be more likely to respond to serotonergic antidepressants.

Studies of depressed patients have sometimes shown an alteration in monoamine function. For example, some studies have found evidence of alteration in serotonin receptor numbers (5-HT_{1A} and 5-HT_{2C}) or norepinephrine (α_2) receptors in depressed and suicidal patients, but these findings have not been consistent. A reduction in the primary serotonin metabolite 5-hydroxyindoleacetic acid in the cerebrospinal fluid is associated with violent and impulsive behavior, including violent suicide attempts. However, this finding is not specific to major depression and is associated more generally with violent and impulsive behavior.

Finally, perhaps the most convincing line of evidence supporting the monoamine hypothesis is the fact that (at the time of this writing) all available antidepressants appear to have significant effects on the monoamine system. All classes of antidepressants appear to enhance the synaptic availability of 5-HT, norepinephrine, or dopamine. Attempts to develop antidepressants that work on other neurotransmitter systems have not been effective to date.

The monoamine hypothesis, like the neurotrophic hypothesis, is at best incomplete. Many studies have not found an alteration in function or levels of monoamines in depressed patients. In addition, some candidate antidepressant agents under study do not act directly on the monoamine system.

In addition to the monoamines, the excitatory neurotransmitter glutamate appears to be important in the pathophysiology of depression. A number of studies of depressed patients have found elevated glutamate content in the cerebrospinal fluid of depressed patients and decreased glutamine/glutamate ratios in their plasma. In addition, postmortem studies have revealed significant increases in the frontal and dorsolateral prefrontal cortex of depressed patients. Likewise, structural neuroimaging

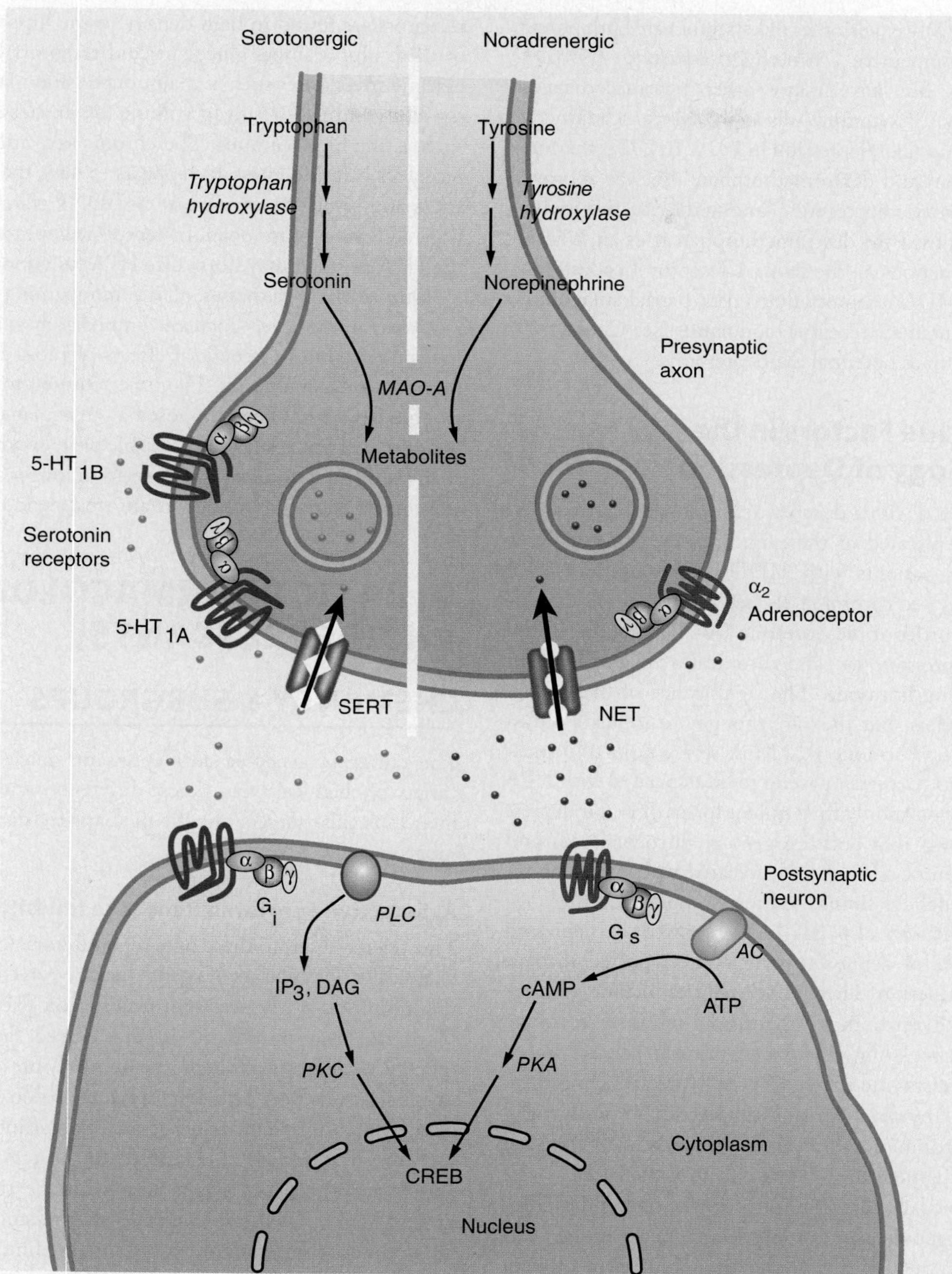

FIGURE 30–2 The amine hypothesis of major depression. Depression appears to be associated with changes in serotonin or norepinephrine signaling in the brain (or both) with significant downstream effects. Most antidepressants cause changes in amine signaling. AC, adenylyl cyclase; CREB, cAMP response element-binding (protein); DAG, diacyl glycerol; 5-HT, serotonin; IP_3, inositol trisphosphate; MAO, monoamine oxidase; NET, norepinephrine transporter; PKC, protein kinase C; PLC, phospholipase C; SERT, serotonin transporter.

studies have consistently found volumetric changes in the brain areas of depressed patients in which glutamate neurons and their connections are most abundant, including the amygdala and hippocampus.

Antidepressants are known to impact glutamate neurotransmission in a variety of ways. For example, chronic antidepressant use is associated with reducing glutamatergic transmission, including the presynaptic release of glutamate in the hippocampus and cortical areas. Similarly, the chronic administration of antidepressants significantly reduces depolarization-evoked release of glutamate in animal models. Stress is known to enhance the release of glutamate in rodents, and antidepressants inhibit stress-induced presynaptic release of glutamate in these models.

Given the effect of antidepressants on the glutamate system, there has been a growing interest in the development of pharmaceutical agents that might modulate the glutamate system. Ketamine and esketamine (the (*S*) + enantiomer of ketamine) are both potent, high-affinity, noncompetitive *N*-methyl-D-aspartate (NMDA) receptor antagonists but have many other pharmacodynamic properties (see below). Esketamine was approved as an adjunctive treatment for resistant major depression in 2019. In 2022, the combination of bupropion and dextromethorphan also was approved for the treatment of major depression. Among the putative mechanisms of action proposed for dextromethorphan is as an NMDA antagonist as well as actions on the sigma-1 receptor. In addition, a number of other NMDA receptor antagonists, partial antagonists, and metabotropic glutamate receptor modulators (see Chapter 29) are under investigation as potential antidepressants.

Neuroendocrine Factors in the Pathophysiology of Depression

Depression is associated with a number of hormonal abnormalities. Among the most replicated of these findings are abnormalities in the HPA axis in patients with MDD. For example, MDD is associated with elevated cortisol levels (see Figure 30–1), nonsuppression of adrenocorticotropic hormone (ACTH) release in the dexamethasone suppression test, and chronically elevated levels of corticotropin-releasing hormone. The significance of these HPA abnormalities is unclear, but they are thought to indicate a dysregulation of the stress hormone axis. More severe types of depression, such as psychotic depression, tend to be associated with HPA abnormalities more commonly than milder forms of major depression. It is well known that both exogenous glucocorticoids and endogenous elevation of cortisol are associated with mood symptoms and cognitive deficits similar to those seen in MDD.

Thyroid dysregulation also has been reported in depressed patients. Up to 25% of depressed patients are reported to have abnormal thyroid function. These abnormalities include a blunting of response of thyrotropin to thyrotropin-releasing hormone and elevations in circulating thyroxine during depressed states. Clinical hypothyroidism often presents with depressive symptoms, which resolve with thyroid hormone supplementation. Thyroid hormones are also commonly used in conjunction with standard antidepressants to augment therapeutic effects of the latter.

Finally, sex steroids also are implicated in the pathophysiology of depression. Estrogen deficiency states, which occur in the postpartum and postmenopausal periods, are thought to play a role in the etiology of depression in some women. Likewise, severe testosterone deficiency in men is sometimes associated with depressive symptoms. Hormone replacement therapy in hypogonadal men and women may be associated with an improvement in mood and depressive symptoms.

Integration of Hypotheses Regarding the Pathophysiology of Depression

The several pathophysiologic hypotheses just described are not mutually exclusive. It is evident that the monoamine, neuroendocrine, and neurotrophic systems are interrelated in important ways. For example, HPA and steroid abnormalities may contribute to suppression of transcription of the *BDNF* gene. Glucocorticoid receptors are found in high density in the hippocampus. Binding of these hippocampal glucocorticoid receptors by cortisol during chronic stress states such as major depression may decrease BDNF synthesis and may result in volume loss in stress-sensitive regions such as the hippocampus. The chronic activation of monoamine receptors by antidepressants appears to have the opposite effect of stress and results in an increase in BDNF transcription. In addition, activation of monoamine receptors appears to down-regulate the HPA axis and may normalize HPA function.

One of the weaknesses of the monoamine hypothesis is the fact that amine levels increase immediately with antidepressant use, but maximum beneficial effects of most antidepressants are not seen for many weeks. The time required to synthesize neurotrophic factors has been proposed as an explanation for this delay of antidepressant effects. Appreciable protein synthesis of products such as BDNF typically takes 2 weeks or longer and coincides with the clinical course of antidepressant treatment.

■ BASIC PHARMACOLOGY OF ANTIDEPRESSANTS

CHEMISTRY & SUBGROUPS

The currently available antidepressants make up a remarkable variety of chemical types. These differences and the differences in their molecular targets provide the basis for distinguishing several subgroups.

A. Selective Serotonin Reuptake Inhibitors

The selective serotonin reuptake inhibitors (SSRIs) represent a chemically diverse class of agents that have as their primary action the inhibition of the serotonin transporter (SERT; Figure 30–3). Fluoxetine was introduced in the United States in 1988 and quickly became one of the most commonly prescribed medications in medical practice. The development of fluoxetine emerged out of the search for chemicals that had high affinity for monoamine receptors but lacked the affinity for histamine, acetylcholine, and α adrenoceptors that is seen with the tricyclic antidepressants (TCAs). There are currently six available SSRIs, and they are the most common antidepressants in clinical use. In addition to their use in major depression, SSRIs have indications in GAD, PTSD, OCD, panic disorder, PMDD, and bulimia. **Fluoxetine, sertraline,** and **citalopram** exist as isomers and are formulated in the racemic forms, whereas **paroxetine** and **fluvoxamine** are not optically active. **Escitalopram** is the (*S*) enantiomer of citalopram. As with all antidepressants, SSRIs are highly lipophilic. The popularity of SSRIs stems largely from their ease of use, safety in overdose, relative tolerability, cost (all are available as generic products), and broad spectrum of uses.

B. Serotonin-Norepinephrine Reuptake Inhibitors

Two classes of antidepressants act as combined serotonin and norepinephrine reuptake inhibitors: selective **serotonin-norepinephrine reuptake inhibitors (SNRIs)** and **TCAs.**

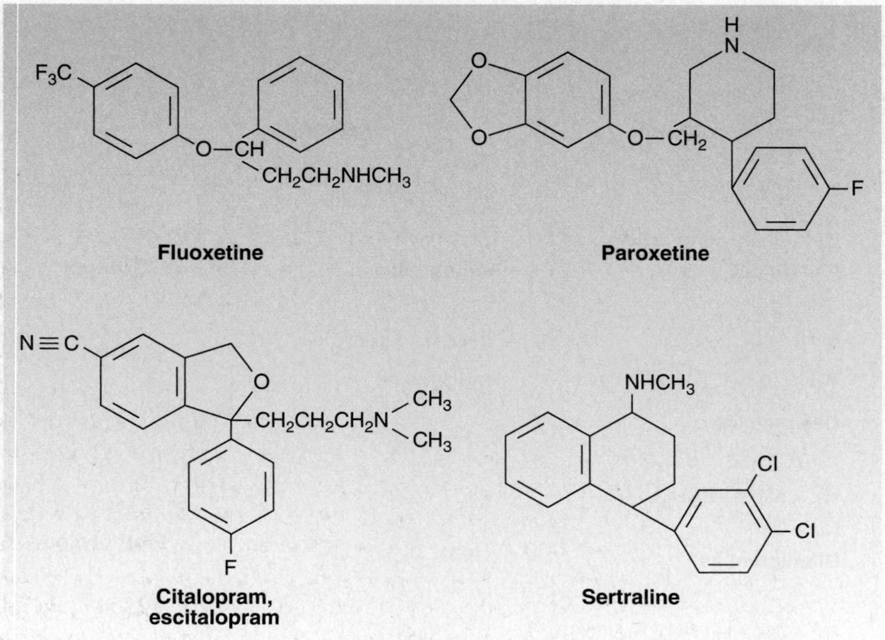

Fluoxetine

Paroxetine

Citalopram, escitalopram

Sertraline

FIGURE 30–3 Structures of several selective serotonin reuptake inhibitors (SSRIs).

1. *Selective serotonin-norepinephrine reuptake inhibitors*— The SNRIs include **venlafaxine,** its metabolite **desvenlafaxine, duloxetine,** and **levomilnacipran.** Levomilnacipran is the active enantiomer of a racemic SNRI, **milnacipran. Milnacipran** has been approved for the treatment of fibromyalgia in the USA and has been used in the treatment of depression in Europe for many years. In addition to their use in major depression, SNRIs have applications in the treatment of pain disorders including neuropathies and fibromyalgia. SNRIs are also used in the treatment of generalized anxiety, stress urinary incontinence, and vasomotor symptoms of menopause.

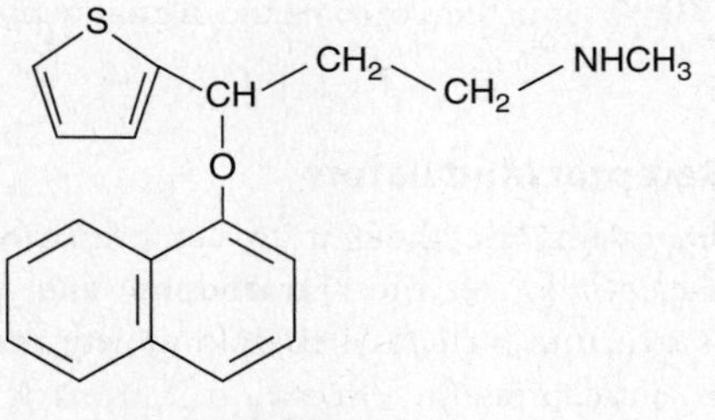

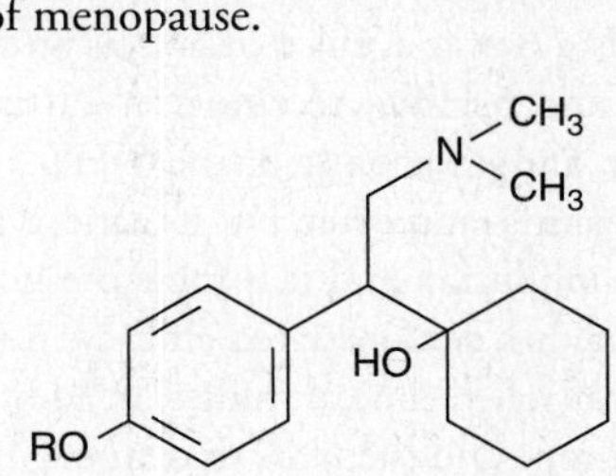

R = CH_3 : **Venlafaxine**
R = H : **Desvenlafaxine**

SNRIs are chemically unrelated to each other. Venlafaxine was discovered in the process of evaluating chemicals that inhibit binding of imipramine. Venlafaxine's in vivo effects are similar to those of imipramine but with a more favorable adverse-effect profile. All SNRIs bind the serotonin (SERT) and norepinephrine (NET) transporters, as do the TCAs. However, unlike the TCAs, the SNRIs do not have much affinity for other receptors. Venlafaxine and desvenlafaxine are bicyclic compounds, whereas duloxetine is a three-ring structure unrelated to the TCAs. Milnacipran contains a cyclopropane ring and is provided as a racemic mixture.

Duloxetine

2. *Tricyclic antidepressants*—The TCAs were the dominant class of antidepressants until the introduction of SSRIs in the 1980s and 1990s. Nine TCAs are available in the USA, and they all have an iminodibenzyl (tricyclic) core (Figure 30–4). The chemical differences between the TCAs are relatively subtle. For example, the prototype TCA **imipramine** and its metabolite, **desipramine,** differ by only a methyl group in the propylamine side chain. However, this minor difference results in a substantial change in their pharmacologic profiles. Imipramine is highly anticholinergic and is a relatively strong serotonin as well as norepinephrine reuptake inhibitor. In contrast, desipramine is much less anticholinergic and is a more potent and somewhat more selective norepinephrine reuptake inhibitor than is imipramine.

At present, the TCAs are used primarily in depression that is unresponsive to more commonly used antidepressants such as the SSRIs or SNRIs. Their loss of popularity stems in large part from relatively poorer tolerability compared with newer agents, difficulty of use, and lethality in overdose. Other uses for TCAs include the treatment of pain conditions, enuresis, and insomnia.

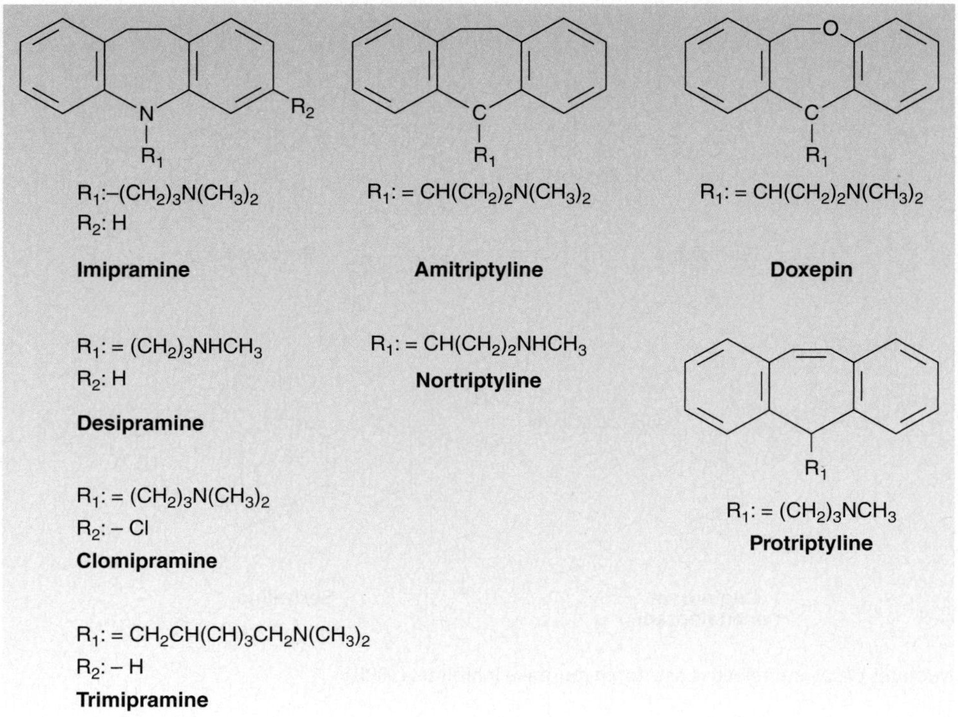

R_1:–$(CH_2)_3N(CH_3)_2$
R_2: H
Imipramine

R_1: = $CH(CH_2)_2N(CH_3)_2$
Amitriptyline

R_1: = $CH(CH_2)_2N(CH_3)_2$
Doxepin

R_1: = $(CH_2)_3NHCH_3$
R_2: H
Desipramine

R_1: = $CH(CH_2)_2NHCH_3$
Nortriptyline

R_1: = $(CH_2)_3N(CH_3)_2$
R_2: – Cl
Clomipramine

R_1: = $(CH_2)_3NCH_3$
Protriptyline

R_1: = $CH_2CH(CH)_3CH_2N(CH_3)_2$
R_2: – H
Trimipramine

FIGURE 30–4 Structures of some tricyclic antidepressants (TCAs).

C. 5-HT_2 Receptor Modulators

Two antidepressants are thought to act primarily as antagonists at the 5-HT_2 receptor: **trazodone** and **nefazodone.** Trazodone's structure includes a triazolo moiety that is thought to impart antidepressant effects. Its primary metabolite, m-chlorophenylpiperazine (m-cpp), is a potent 5-HT_2 antagonist. Trazodone was among the most commonly prescribed antidepressants until it was supplanted by the SSRIs in the late 1980s. The most common use of trazodone in current practice is as an unlabeled hypnotic, since it is highly sedating and not associated with tolerance or dependence.

Nefazodone is chemically related to trazodone. Its primary metabolites, hydroxynefazodone and m-cpp, are both inhibitors of the 5-HT_2 receptor. Nefazodone received an FDA black box warning in 2001 implicating it in hepatotoxicity, including lethal cases of hepatic failure. Although still available generically, nefazodone is no longer commonly prescribed. The primary indications for both nefazodone and trazodone are major depression, although both have also been used in the treatment of anxiety disorders.

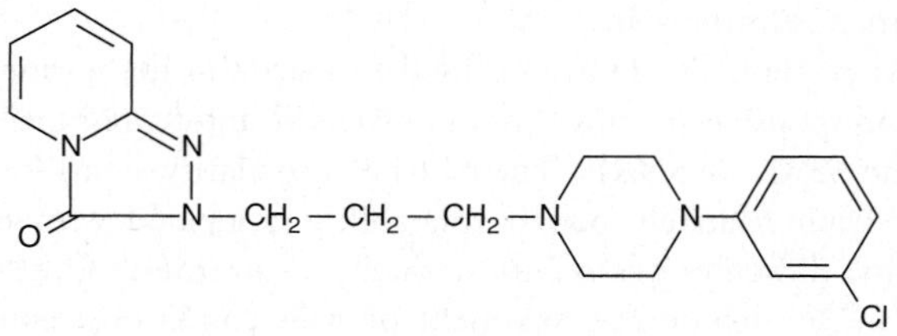

Trazodone

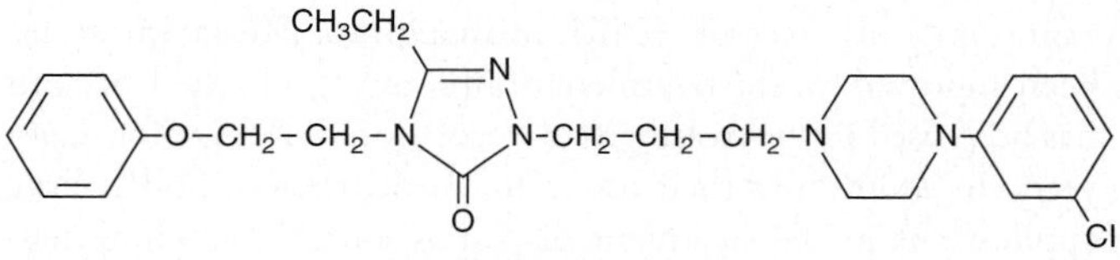

Nefazodone

Vortioxetine is a newer agent that acts as an antagonist of the 5-HT_3, 5-HT_7, and 5-HT_{1D} receptors, a partial agonist of the 5-HT_{1B} receptor, and an agonist of the 5-HT_{1A} receptor. It also inhibits the serotonin transporter, but its actions are not primarily related to SERT inhibition and it is therefore not classified as an SSRI. Vortioxetine has demonstrated efficacy in major depression in a number of controlled clinical studies. In addition, vortioxetine is approved in Europe and the USA to treat cognitive dysfunction associated with depression.

D. Tetracyclic and Unicyclic Antidepressants

A number of antidepressants do not fit neatly into the other classes. Among these are **bupropion, mirtazapine, amoxapine, vilazodone,** and **maprotiline** (Figure 30–5). Bupropion has a unicyclic aminoketone structure. Its unique structure results in a different side-effect profile than most antidepressants (described below). Bupropion somewhat resembles amphetamine in chemical structure and, like the stimulant, has central nervous system (CNS) activating properties.

Mirtazapine was introduced in 1994 and, like bupropion, is one of the few antidepressants not commonly associated with

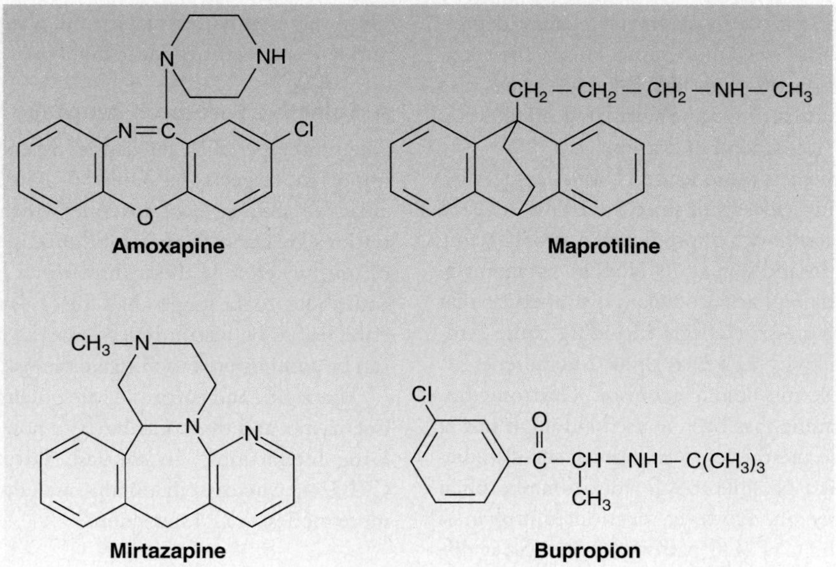

FIGURE 30–5 Structures of the tetracyclics, amoxapine, maprotiline, and mirtazapine and the unicyclic, bupropion.

sexual effects. It has a tetracyclic chemical structure and belongs to the piperazino-azepine group of compounds.

Mirtazapine, amoxapine, and maprotiline have tetracyclic structures. Amoxapine is the *N*-demethylated metabolite of loxapine, an older antipsychotic drug. Amoxapine and maprotiline share structural similarities and side effects comparable to the TCAs. As a result, these tetracyclics are not commonly prescribed in current practice. Their primary use is in MDD that is unresponsive to other agents. Vilazodone has a multi-ring structure that allows it to bind potently to the serotonin transporter but minimally to the dopamine and norepinephrine transporter.

E. Monoamine Oxidase Inhibitors

Arguably the first modern class of antidepressants, monoamine oxidase inhibitors (MAOIs) were introduced in the 1950s but are now rarely used in clinical practice because of toxicity and potentially lethal food and drug interactions. Their primary use now is in the treatment of depression unresponsive to other antidepressants. However, MAOIs have also been used historically to treat anxiety states, including social anxiety and panic disorder. In addition, selegiline is used in the treatment of Parkinson disease (see Chapter 28).

Current MAOIs include the hydrazine derivatives **phenelzine** and **isocarboxazid** and the nonhydrazines **tranylcypromine, selegiline,** and **moclobemide** (the latter is not available in the USA). The hydrazines and tranylcypromine bind irreversibly and nonselectively with MAO-A and B, whereas other MAOIs may have more selective or reversible properties. Some of the MAOIs such as tranylcypromine resemble amphetamine in chemical structure, whereas other MAOIs such as selegiline have amphetamine-like metabolites. As a result, these MAOIs tend to have substantial CNS-stimulating effects.

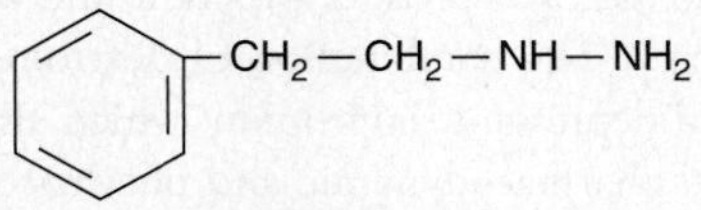

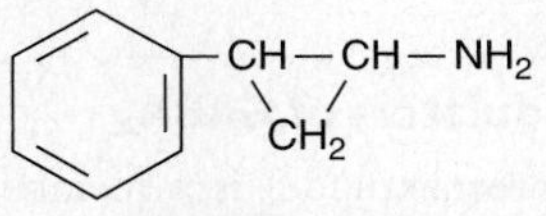

F. NMDA Receptor Antagonists

Esketamine became the first non-monoamine-specific agent approved in the adjunctive treatment of major depression in 2019. Esketamine is the (*S*)-enantiomer of racemic ketamine that has been in use since early 1960s. Ketamine was developed in 1962 as a short-acting analog of phencyclidine. Phencyclidine proved to be unsuitable for use as an anesthetic because of its tendency to produce a prolonged delirium. Thus, phencyclidine never was approved for use in humans although it did become a drug of abuse (PCP, "angel dust").

In contrast to phencyclidine, ketamine has been approved since 1970 in the USA and used in anesthesia and critical care medicine to provide sedation without the degree of cardiorespiratory suppression found in some anesthetics. Observations beginning around 2006 led to an interest in the off-label use of ketamine in treatment-resistant depression. The advantages over existing antidepressants include rapid onset (often within 24 hours) and ketamine's efficacy in patients who had not responded to standard antidepressants. Disadvantages include a short duration of activity (5–7 days), IV route of administration, a tendency to produce dissociative symptoms, and risk of abuse. Esketamine was developed as an intranasal preparation for use in treatment-resistant depression. It may have somewhat fewer dissociative effects than ketamine but has a similar side-effect profile. Esketamine has also been studied as a rapid treatment for acute suicidal ideation and is currently under review for this second indication.

Dextromethorphan, which is a moderate NMDA antagonist, has been available as an antitussive agent since the 1950s. In 2022 it was approved in combination with bupropion as a rapidly acting treatment for depression. In addition to its NMDA antagonism, dextromethorphan has other pharmacodynamic properties that could contribute to antidepressant effects including some serotonin reuptake–blocking activity, as well as alpha-2 noradrenergic, sigma-1, and even modest mu-opioid agonism. Dextromethorphan, like PCP and ketamine, has been abused although not at the levels of the dissociative anesthetics. A number of small studies since 2011 have suggested a possible role for dextromethorphan in the treatment of depression. However, dextromethorphan is rapidly metabolized via the CYP2D6 pathway, rendering it difficult to achieve adequate serum levels. Quinidine is a CYP2D6 inhibitor that has been combined with dextromethorphan and was approved in 2010 for the treatment of pseudobulbar affect. Studies of the combination of quinidine combined with dextromethorphan, including a phase 2 program, did not demonstrate consistent efficacy. The combination of dextromethorphan with an approved antidepressant, bupropion, which also is a CYP2D6 inhibitor, made pharmacodynamic and pharmacodynamic sense. The combination was proven effective in the treatment of depression in both a phase 2 and phase 3 program, leading to FDA approval in 2022.

G. Allosteric Modulators of $GABA_A$

Brexanolone (allopregnanolone) is a member of a new class of neurosteroid antidepressants that are thought to act primarily on the GABA system. Allopregnanolone is a derivative of progesterone and like other $GABA_A$ agents is thought to have anxiolytic and anticonvulsant properties. Brexanolone has been studied as a rapidly acting IV antidepressant in women with postpartum depression and is administered as a 60-hour IV infusion. Like ketamine and esketamine, brexanolone acts rapidly with evidence of response by 60 hours. Unlike ketamine and esketamine, the effect appears durable at least 30 days after infusion and is not associated with dissociative symptoms or risk of abuse. In late 2018, an FDA advisory panel voted to 17 to 1 to support approval of brexanolone as the first drug indicated for the treatment of postpartum depression. Other modulators of $GABA_A$ include zuranolone (Sage 217), which is being evaluated as an oral drug for general major depression and ganaxolone, which is being evaluated in the treatment of PTSD.

PHARMACOKINETICS

The antidepressants share several pharmacokinetic features (Table 30–1). Most have fairly rapid oral absorption, achieve peak plasma levels within 2–3 hours, are tightly bound to plasma proteins, undergo hepatic metabolism, and are renally cleared. However, even within classes, the pharmacokinetics of individual antidepressants varies considerably.

A. Selective Serotonin Reuptake Inhibitors

The prototype SSRI, fluoxetine, differs from other SSRIs in some important respects (see Table 30–1). Fluoxetine is metabolized to an active product, norfluoxetine, which may have plasma concentrations greater than those of fluoxetine. The elimination half-life of norfluoxetine is about three times longer than fluoxetine and contributes to the longest half-life of all the SSRIs. As a result, fluoxetine has to be discontinued 4 weeks or longer before an MAOI can be administered to mitigate the risk of serotonin syndrome.

Fluoxetine and paroxetine are potent inhibitors of the CYP2D6 isoenzyme, and this contributes to potential drug interactions (see Drug Interactions). In contrast, fluvoxamine is an inhibitor of CYP3A4, whereas citalopram, escitalopram, and sertraline have more modest CYP interactions.

B. Serotonin-Norepinephrine Reuptake Inhibitors

1. *Selective serotonin-norepinephrine reuptake inhibitors*— Venlafaxine is extensively metabolized in the liver via the CYP2D6 isoenzyme to *O*-desmethylvenlafaxine (desvenlafaxine). Both have similar half-lives of about 8–11 hours. Despite the relatively short half-lives, both drugs are available in formulations that allow once-daily dosing. Venlafaxine and desvenlafaxine have the lowest protein binding of all antidepressants (27–30%). Unlike most antidepressants, desvenlafaxine is conjugated and does not undergo extensive oxidative metabolism. At least 45% of desvenlafaxine is excreted unchanged in the urine compared with 4–8% of venlafaxine.

Duloxetine is well absorbed and has a half-life of 12–15 hours but is dosed once daily. It is tightly bound to protein (97%) and undergoes extensive oxidative metabolism via CYP2D6 and CYP1A2. Hepatic impairment significantly alters duloxetine levels unlike desvenlafaxine.

Both milnacipran and levomilnacipran are well absorbed after oral dosing. Both have shorter half-lives and lower protein binding than venlafaxine (see Table 30–1). Milnacipran and levomilnacipran are largely excreted unchanged in the urine. Levomilnacipran also undergoes desethylation via 3A3/4.

2. *Tricyclic antidepressants*—The TCAs tend to be well absorbed and have long half-lives (see Table 30–1). As a result, most are dosed once daily at night because of their sedating effects. TCAs undergo extensive metabolism via demethylation, aromatic hydroxylation, and glucuronide conjugation. Only about 5% of TCAs are excreted unchanged in the urine. The TCAs are substrates of the CYP2D6 system, and the serum levels of these agents tend to be substantially influenced by concurrent administration of drugs such as fluoxetine. In addition, genetic polymorphism for CYP2D6 may result in low or extensive metabolism of the TCAs.

The secondary amine TCAs, including desipramine and nortriptyline, lack active metabolites and have fairly linear kinetics. These TCAs have a wide therapeutic window, and serum levels are reliable in predicting response and toxicity.

TABLE 30–1 Pharmacokinetic profiles of selected antidepressants.

Class, Drug	Bioavailability (%)	Plasma $t_{1/2}$ (hours)	Active Metabolite $t_{1/2}$ (hours)	Volume of Distribution (L/kg)	Protein Binding (%)
SSRIs					
Citalopram	80	33–38	ND	15	80
Escitalopram	80	27–32	ND	12–15	80
Fluoxetine	70	48–72	180	12–97	95
Fluvoxamine	90	14–18	14–16	25	80
Paroxetine	50	20–23	ND	28–31	94
Sertraline	45	22–27	62–104	20	98
SNRIs					
Duloxetine	50	12–15	ND	10–14	97
Milnacipran	85–90	6–8	ND	5–6	13
Venlafaxine[1]	45	8–11	9–13	4–10	27
Tricyclics					
Amitriptyline	45	31–46	20–92	5–10	90
Clomipramine	50	19–37	54–77	7–20	97
Imipramine	40	9–24	14–62	15–30	84
5-HT modulators					
Nefazodone	20	2–4	ND	0.5–1	99
Trazodone	95	3–6	ND	1–3	96
Vortioxetine	75	66	ND	ND	98
Tetracyclics and unicyclic					
Amoxapine	ND	7–12	5–30	0.9–1.2	85
Bupropion	70	11–14	15–25	20–30	85
Maprotiline	70	43–45	ND	23–27	88
Mirtazapine	50	20–40	20–40	3–7	85
Vilazodone	72	25	ND	ND	ND
MAOIs					
Phenelzine	ND	11	ND	ND	ND
Selegiline	4	8–10	9–11	8–10	99
NMDA antagonists					
Esketamine	48	7–12	8	709	45
Dextromethorphan + bupropion	20–68	15–22	33–45	ND	60–84
$GABA_A$ modulators					
Brexanolone	100 (IV)	12	ND	3	99

[1]Desvenlafaxine has similar properties but is less completely metabolized.

MAOIs, monoamine oxidase inhibitors; ND, no data found; SNRIs, serotonin-norepinephrine reuptake inhibitors; SSRIs, selective serotonin reuptake inhibitors.

C. 5-HT Receptor Modulators

Trazodone and nefazodone are rapidly absorbed and undergo hepatic metabolism. Both drugs are bound to protein and have limited bioavailability because of extensive metabolism. Because of their short half-lives split dosing is generally required when these drugs are used as antidepressants. However, trazodone is often prescribed as a single dose at night as a hypnotic in lower doses than are used in the treatment of depression. Both trazodone and nefazodone have active metabolites that also exhibit 5-HT_2 antagonism. Nefazodone is a potent inhibitor of the CYP3A4 system and may interact with drugs metabolized by this enzyme (see Drug Interactions). Vortioxetine is not a potent inhibitor of CYP isoenzymes. However, it is extensively metabolized through oxidation by CYP2D6 and other isoenzymes and then undergoes subsequent glucuronic acid conjugation. It is tightly bound to protein and has linear and dose-proportional pharmacokinetics.

D. Tetracyclic and Unicyclic Agents

Bupropion is rapidly absorbed and has a mean protein binding of 85%. It undergoes extensive hepatic metabolism and has a substantial first-pass effect. It has three active metabolites including hydroxybupropion; the latter is being developed as an antidepressant. Bupropion has a biphasic elimination with the first phase lasting about 1 hour and the second phase lasting 14 hours.

Amoxapine is also rapidly absorbed with protein binding of about 85%. The half-life is variable, and the drug is often given in divided doses. Amoxapine undergoes extensive hepatic metabolism. One of the active metabolites, 7-hydroxyamoxapine, is a potent D_2 blocker and is associated with antipsychotic effects. Maprotiline is similarly well absorbed orally and 88% bound to protein. It undergoes extensive hepatic metabolism.

Mirtazapine is demethylated followed by hydroxylation and glucuronide conjugation. Several CYP isozymes are involved in the metabolism of mirtazapine, including 2D6, 3A4, and 1A2. The half-life of mirtazapine is 20–40 hours, and it is usually dosed once in the evening because of its sedating effects.

Vilazodone is well absorbed (see Table 30–1), and absorption is increased when it is given with a fatty meal. It is extensively metabolized by CYP3A4 with minor contributions by CYP2C19 and CYP2D6. Only 1% of vilazodone is excreted unchanged in the urine.

E. Monoamine Oxidase Inhibitors

The different MAOIs are metabolized via different pathways but tend to have extensive first-pass effects that may substantially decrease bioavailability. Tranylcypromine is ring hydroxylated and *N*-acetylated, whereas acetylation appears to be a minor pathway for phenelzine. Selegiline is *N*-demethylated and then hydroxylated. The MAOIs are well absorbed from the gastrointestinal tract.

Because of the prominent first-pass effects and their tendency to inhibit MAO in the gut (resulting in tyramine pressor effects), alternative routes of administration are being developed. For example, selegiline is available in both transdermal and sublingual forms that bypass both gut and liver. These routes decrease the risk of food interactions and provide substantially increased bioavailability.

F. NMDA Receptor Antagonists

The pharmacokinetics of racemic ketamine (usually given IV) and esketamine (intranasal) are similar but differ in part as a function of different routes of administration. Intranasal esketamine is 48% bioavailable, while bioavailability of IV ketamine is complete. Esketamine has a terminal half-life of 7–12 hours while its major metabolite, noresketamine, has a half-life of about 8 hours. IV ketamine has a half-life of approximately 3 hours. The time to reach maximum plasma concentration for intranasal esketamine is 20–40 minutes from the last nasal spray. Less than 1% of esketamine is excreted unchanged, with 78% of all metabolites found in the urine and 2% in feces. Racemic IV ketamine is cleared rapidly (95 L/h/70 kg), with 91% of the dose recovered in urine and 3% in feces.

Bupropion and a putative NMDA antagonist, dextromethorphan, have been combined in an extended-release formulation for the treatment of depression. Bupropion inhibits the metabolism of dextromethorphan via CYP2D6. Peak serum levels are achieved for the combination tablet in 3 hours, and the tablet has a $t_{1/2}$ of 22 hours after 8 days of administration. In CYP2D6 extensive metabolizers, approximately 37–52% of the orally administered dose of dextromethorphan is recovered in the urine. Less than 2% of the administered dose is excreted as unchanged parent drug in the urine. In CYP2D6 poor metabolizers, a higher percentage is recovered in the urine.

G. $GABA_A$ Modulators

IV brexanolone is extensively metabolized by non-CYP450 routes including glucuronidation, sulfation, and ketoreduction. Only 1% of the dose is excreted unchanged, with 47% of the metabolites found in the urine and 42% in the feces. The drug is heavily bound to protein (99%) and is extensively distributed to tissues, with a volume of distribution of 3 L/kg. The terminal half-life of brexanolone is about 9 hours with continuous administration over 60 hours. However, the initial half-life of brexanolone is only about 40 minutes, consistent with its rapid sedating effects.

PHARMACODYNAMICS

As previously noted, all currently available antidepressants enhance monoamine neurotransmission by one of several mechanisms. The most common mechanism is inhibition of the activity of SERT, NET, or both monoamine transporters (Table 30–2). Antidepressants that inhibit SERT, NET, or both include the SSRIs and SNRIs (by definition) and the TCAs. Another mechanism for increasing the availability of monoamines is inhibition of their enzymatic degradation (by the MAOIs). Additional strategies for enhancing monoamine effects include binding presynaptic autoreceptors (mirtazapine) or specific postsynaptic receptors ($5\text{-}HT_2$ antagonists and mirtazapine). Ultimately, the increased availability of monoamines for binding in the synaptic cleft results in a cascade of events that enhance the transcription of some proteins and the inhibition of others. It is the net production of these proteins, including BDNF, glucocorticoid receptors, β adrenoceptors, and other proteins, that appears to determine the benefits as well as the toxicity of a given agent.

A. Selective Serotonin Reuptake Inhibitors

The serotonin transporter (SERT) is a glycoprotein with 12 transmembrane regions embedded in the axon terminal and cell body membranes of serotonergic neurons. When extracellular serotonin binds to receptors on the transporter, conformational changes occur in the transporter and serotonin, Na^+, and Cl^- are moved into the cell. Binding of intracellular K^+ then results in the release of serotonin inside the cell and return of the transporter to its original conformation. SSRIs allosterically inhibit the transporter by binding the SERT receptor at a site other than the serotonin binding site. At therapeutic doses, about 80% of the activity of the transporter is inhibited. Functional polymorphisms exist for SERT that determine the activity of the transporter (see Table 30–2).

SSRIs have modest effects on other neurotransmitters. Unlike TCAs and SNRIs, there is little evidence that SSRIs have

TABLE 30–2 Blocking effects of some antidepressant drugs on several receptors and transporters.

Antidepressant	ACh M	α_1	H_1	$5\text{-}HT_2$	NET	SERT
Amitriptyline	+++	+++	++	0/+	+	++
Amoxapine	+	++	+	+++	++	+
Bupropion	0	0	0	0	0/+	0
Citalopram, escitalopram	0	0	0		0	+++
Clomipramine	+	++	+	+	+	+++
Desipramine	+	+	+	0/+	+++	+
Doxepin	++	+++	+++	0/+	+	+
Fluoxetine	0	0	0	0/+	0	+++
Fluvoxamine	0	0	0	0	0	+++
Imipramine	++	+	+	0/+	+	++
Maprotiline	+	+	++	0/+	++	0
Mirtazapine	0	0	+++	+	+	0
Nefazodone	0	+	0	++	0/+	+
Nortriptyline	+	+	+	+	++	+
Paroxetine	+	0	0	0	+	+++
Protriptyline	+++	+	+	+	+++	+
Sertraline	0	0	0	0	0	+++
Trazodone	0	++	0/+	++	0	+
Trimipramine	++	++	+++	0/+	0	0
Venlafaxine	0	0	0	0	+	++
Vortioxetine[1]	ND	ND	ND	ND	+	+++

[1]Vortioxetine is an agonist or partial agonist at $5\text{-}HT_{1A}$ and $5\text{-}HT_{1B}$ receptors, an antagonist at $5\text{-}HT_3$ and $5\text{-}HT_7$ receptors, and an inhibitor of SERT.

ACh M, acetylcholine muscarinic receptor; α_1, alpha$_1$-adrenoceptor; H_1, histamine$_1$ receptor; $5\text{-}HT_2$, serotonin $5\text{-}HT_2$ receptor; ND, no data found; NET, norepinephrine transporter; SERT, serotonin transporter.

0/+, minimal affinity; +, mild affinity; ++, moderate affinity; +++, high affinity.

prominent effects on β adrenoceptors or the norepinephrine transporter, NET. Binding to the serotonin transporter is associated with tonic inhibition of the dopamine system, although there is substantial interindividual variability in this effect. The SSRIs do not bind aggressively to histamine, muscarinic, or other receptors.

B. Drugs That Block Both Serotonin and Norepinephrine Transporters

A large number of antidepressants have mixed inhibitory effects on both serotonin and norepinephrine transporters. The newer agents in this class (venlafaxine and duloxetine) are termed SNRIs; those in the older group are termed TCAs on the basis of their structures. The NET is structurally very similar to the 5-HT transporter. Like the serotonin transporter, it is a 12-transmembrane domain complex that allosterically binds SNRIs and TCAs. The NET also has a moderate affinity for dopamine.

1. *Serotonin-norepinephrine reuptake inhibitors*—SNRIs bind both the serotonin and the norepinephrine transporters. Venlafaxine is a weak inhibitor of NET, whereas desvenlafaxine, duloxetine, milnacipran, and levomilnacipran are more balanced inhibitors of both SERT and NET. Nonetheless, the affinity of most SNRIs tends to be much greater for SERT than for NET. The SNRIs differ from the TCAs in that they lack the potent antihistamine, α-adrenergic blocking, and anticholinergic effects of the TCAs. As a result, the SNRIs tend to be favored over the TCAs in the treatment of MDD and pain syndromes because of their better tolerability.

2. *Tricyclic antidepressants*—The TCAs resemble the SNRIs in function, and their antidepressant activity is thought to relate primarily to their inhibition of 5-HT and norepinephrine reuptake. Within the TCAs, there is considerable variability in affinity for SERT versus NET. For example, clomipramine has relatively very little affinity for NET but potently binds SERT. This selectivity for the serotonin transporter contributes to clomipramine's known benefits in the treatment of OCD. On the other hand, the secondary amine TCAs, desipramine and nortriptyline, are relatively more selective for NET. Although the tertiary amine TCA imipramine has more serotonin effect initially, its metabolite, desipramine, then balances this effect with more NET inhibition.

Common adverse effects of the TCAs, including dry mouth and constipation, are attributable to the potent antimuscarinic effects of many of these drugs. The TCAs also tend to be potent antagonists of the histamine H_1 receptor. TCAs such as doxepin are sometimes prescribed as hypnotics and used in treatments for pruritus because of their antihistamine properties. The blockade of α adrenoceptors can result in substantial orthostatic hypotension, particularly in older patients.

C. 5-HT Receptor Modulators

The principal action of both nefazodone and trazodone appears to be blockade of the 5-HT_{2A} receptor. Inhibition of this receptor in both animal and human studies is associated with substantial antianxiety, antipsychotic, and antidepressant effects. Conversely, agonists of the 5-HT_{2A} receptor, eg, lysergic acid (LSD) and mescaline, are often hallucinogenic and anxiogenic. The 5-HT_{2A} receptor is a G protein-coupled receptor and is distributed throughout the neocortex.

Nefazodone is a weak inhibitor of both SERT and NET but is a potent antagonist of the postsynaptic 5-HT_{2A} receptor, as are its metabolites. Trazodone is also a weak but selective inhibitor of SERT with little effect on NET. Its primary metabolite, m-cpp, is a potent 5-HT_2 antagonist, and much of trazodone's benefits as an antidepressant might be attributed to this effect. Trazodone also has weak to moderate presynaptic α-adrenergic–blocking properties and is a modest antagonist of the H_1 receptor.

As described above, vortioxetine has multimodal effects on a variety of 5-HT receptors and is an allosteric inhibitor of SERT. It has no known direct activity on norepinephrine or dopamine receptors.

D. Tetracyclic and Unicyclic Antidepressants

The actions of bupropion remain poorly understood. Bupropion and its major metabolite hydroxybupropion are modest to moderate inhibitors of norepinephrine and dopamine reuptake in animal studies. However, these effects seem less than are typically associated with antidepressant benefit. A more significant effect of bupropion is presynaptic release of catecholamines. In animal studies, bupropion appears to substantially increase the presynaptic availability of norepinephrine, and dopamine to a lesser extent. Bupropion has virtually no direct effects on the serotonin system.

Mirtazapine has a complex pharmacology. It is an antagonist of the presynaptic α_2 autoreceptor and enhances the release of both norepinephrine and 5-HT. In addition, mirtazapine is an antagonist of 5-HT_2 and 5-HT_3 receptors. Finally, mirtazapine is a potent H_1 antagonist, which is associated with the drug's sedative effects.

The actions of amoxapine and maprotiline resemble those of TCAs such as desipramine. Both are potent NET inhibitors and less potent SERT inhibitors. In addition, both possess anticholinergic properties. Unlike the TCAs or other antidepressants, amoxapine is a moderate inhibitor of the postsynaptic D_2 receptor. As such, amoxapine possesses some antipsychotic properties.

Vilazodone is a potent serotonin reuptake inhibitor and a partial agonist of the 5-HT_{1A} receptor. Partial agonists of the 5-HT_{1A} receptor such as buspirone are thought to have mild to moderate antidepressant and anxiolytic properties.

E. Monoamine Oxidase Inhibitors

MAOIs act by mitigating the actions of monoamine oxidase in the neuron and increasing monoamine content. There are two forms of monoamine oxidase. MAO-A is present in both dopamine and norepinephrine neurons and is found primarily in the brain, gut, placenta, and liver; its primary substrates are norepinephrine, epinephrine, and serotonin. MAO-B is found primarily in serotonergic and histaminergic neurons and is distributed in the brain, liver, and platelets. MAO-B acts primarily on dopamine, tyramine, phenylethylamine, and benzylamine. Both MAO-A and -B metabolize tryptamine.

MAOIs are classified by their specificity for MAO-A or -B and whether their effects are reversible or irreversible. Phenelzine and tranylcypromine are examples of irreversible, nonselective MAOIs. Moclobemide is a reversible and selective inhibitor of MAO-A but is not available in the USA. Moclobemide can be displaced from MAO-A by tyramine, and this mitigates the risk of food interactions. In contrast, selegiline is an irreversible MAO-B–specific agent at low doses. Selegiline is useful in the treatment of Parkinson disease at these low doses, but at higher doses it becomes a nonselective MAOI similar to other agents.

F. NMDA Receptor Antagonists

While ketamine and esketamine are thought to act primarily as noncompetitive antagonists of the NMDA receptor, these drugs have multiple other pharmacodynamic actions that could contribute to efficacy in depression and other disorders. These include interactions with opioid receptors, monoaminergic receptors, cholinergic receptors, and voltage-sensitive Ca^{2+} channels. Despite its use as an anesthetic, ketamine does not appear to act on GABA receptors.

The effects of ketamine and esketamine on monoamines are not as well established as NMDA effects. Most but not all studies suggest that ketamine can significantly increase dopaminergic activity through dopamine reuptake inhibition. This dopaminergic effect would be consistent with the euphoric and psychotomimetic effects of the drug. In addition, ketamine is thought to enhance the activity of descending serotonergic pathways that may be important in both the antidepressant and analgesic properties of the drug.

G. GABA_A Receptor Modulators

Brexanolone has been proposed to reset dysregulated brain function in depressive episodes through modulation of the GABA_A receptor. GABA_A receptors are ligand-gated, chloride-conducting ion channels (Chapter 22) that have been shown to mediate inhibition of neural networks including those associated with limbic overactivity in major depression. Brexanolone is a positive allosteric modulator of GABA_A receptors both pre- and postsynaptically. As such it induces rapid phasic and tonic inhibition of multiple GABA networks responsible for regulating and maintaining those networks. Brexanolone is also thought to increase tonic inhibition through effects on GABA trafficking to and from neuronal surfaces and laterally between synaptic and extrasynaptic locations. **Zuranolone** (Sage 217) is similar and is in phase 2 trials.

■ CLINICAL PHARMACOLOGY OF ANTIDEPRESSANTS

Clinical Indications

A. Depression

The FDA indication for the use of the antidepressants in the treatment of major depression is fairly broad. Most antidepressants are approved for both acute and long-term treatment of major depression. Acute episodes of MDD tend to last about 6–14 months untreated, but at least 20% of episodes last 2 years or longer.

The goal of acute treatment of MDD is remission of all symptoms. Since antidepressants may not achieve their maximum benefit for 1–2 months or longer, it is not unusual for a trial of therapy to last 8–12 weeks at therapeutic doses. The antidepressants are successful in achieving remission in about 30–40% of patients within a single trial of 8–12 weeks. If an inadequate response is obtained, therapy is often switched to another agent or augmented by addition of another drug. For example, bupropion, an atypical antipsychotic, or mirtazapine might be added to an SSRI or SNRI to augment antidepressant benefit if monotherapy is unsuccessful. Seventy to eighty percent of patients are able to achieve remission with sequenced augmentation or switching strategies. Once an adequate response is achieved, continuation therapy is recommended for a minimum of 6–12 months to reduce the substantial risk of relapse.

Approximately 85% of patients who have a single episode of MDD will have at least one recurrence in a lifetime. Many patients have multiple recurrences, and these recurrences may progress to more serious, chronic, and treatment-resistant episodes. Thus, it is not unusual for patients to require maintenance treatment to prevent recurrences. Although maintenance treatment studies of more than 5 years are uncommon, long-term studies with TCAs, SNRIs, and SSRIs suggest a significant protective benefit when given chronically. Thus, it is commonly recommended that patients be considered for long-term maintenance treatment if they have had two or more serious MDD episodes in the previous 5 years or three or more serious episodes in a lifetime.

It is not clear whether antidepressants are useful for all subtypes of depression. For example, patients with bipolar depression may not benefit much from antidepressants even when added to mood stabilizers. In fact, the antidepressants are sometimes associated with switches into mania or more rapid cycling. There has also been some debate about the overall efficacy of antidepressants in unipolar depression, with some meta-analyses showing large effects and others showing more modest effects. Although this debate is not likely to be settled immediately, there is little debate that antidepressants have important benefits for most patients.

Psychotherapeutic interventions such as cognitive behavioral therapy appear to be as effective as antidepressant treatment for mild to moderate forms of depression. However, cognitive behavioral therapy tends to take longer to be effective and is generally more expensive than antidepressant treatment. Psychotherapy is often combined with antidepressant treatment, and the combination appears more effective than either strategy alone.

B. Anxiety Disorders

After major depression, anxiety disorders represent the most common application of antidepressants. A number of SSRIs and SNRIs have been approved for all the major anxiety disorders, including PTSD, OCD, social anxiety disorder, GAD, and panic disorder. Panic disorder is characterized by recurrent episodes of brief overwhelming anxiety, which often occur without a precipitant. Patients may begin to fear having an attack, or they avoid situations in which they might have an attack. In contrast, GAD is characterized by a chronic, free-floating anxiety and undue worry that tends to be chronic in nature. Although older antidepressants and drugs of the sedative-hypnotic class are still occasionally used for the treatment of anxiety disorders, SSRIs and SNRIs have largely replaced them.

The benzodiazepines (see Chapter 22) provide much more rapid relief of both generalized anxiety and panic than do any of the antidepressants. However, the antidepressants appear to be at least as effective as, and perhaps more effective than, benzodiazepines in the long-term treatment of these anxiety disorders. Furthermore, antidepressants do not carry the risks of dependence and tolerance that may occur with the benzodiazepines.

OCD is known to respond to serotonergic antidepressants. It is characterized by repetitive anxiety-provoking thoughts (obsessions) or repetitive behaviors (compulsions) aimed at reducing anxiety. Clomipramine and several of the SSRIs are approved for the treatment of OCD, and they are moderately effective. Behavior therapy is usually combined with the antidepressant for additional benefits.

Social anxiety disorder is an uncommonly diagnosed but a fairly common condition in which patients experience severe anxiety in social interactions. This anxiety may limit their ability to function adequately in their jobs or interpersonal relationships. Several SSRIs and venlafaxine are approved for the treatment of social anxiety. The efficacy of the SSRIs in the treatment of social anxiety is greater in some studies than their efficacy in the treatment of MDD.

PTSD is manifested when a traumatic or life-threatening event results in intrusive anxiety-provoking thoughts or imagery, hypervigilance, nightmares, and avoidance of situations that remind the patient of the trauma. SSRIs are considered first-line treatment for PTSD and can benefit a number of symptoms including anxious thoughts and hypervigilance. Other treatments, including psychotherapeutic interventions, are usually required in addition to antidepressants.

C. Pain Disorders

Antidepressants possess analgesic properties independent of their mood effects. TCAs have been used in the treatment of neuropathic and other pain conditions since the 1960s. Medications that possess both norepinephrine and 5-HT reuptake blocking properties are often useful in treating pain disorders. Ascending corticospinal monoamine pathways appear to be important in the endogenous analgesic system. In addition, chronic pain conditions are commonly associated with major depression. TCAs continue to be commonly used for some of these conditions, and SNRIs are increasingly used. In 2010, duloxetine was approved for the treatment of chronic joint and muscle pain. As mentioned earlier, milnacipran is approved for the treatment of fibromyalgia in the USA and for MDD in other countries. Other SNRIs, eg, desvenlafaxine, are being investigated for a variety of pain conditions from postherpetic neuralgia to chronic back pain.

D. Premenstrual Dysphoric Disorder

Approximately 5% of women in the child-bearing years will have prominent mood and physical symptoms during the late luteal phase of almost every cycle; these may include anxiety, depressed mood, irritability, insomnia, fatigue, and a variety of other physical symptoms. These symptoms are more severe than those typically seen in premenstrual syndrome (PMS) and can be quite disruptive to vocational and interpersonal activities. The SSRIs are known to be beneficial to many women with PMDD, and fluoxetine and sertraline are approved for this indication. Treating for 2 weeks out of the month in the luteal phase may be as effective as continuous treatment. The rapid effects of SSRIs in PMDD may be associated with rapid increases in pregnenolone levels.

E. Smoking Cessation

Bupropion was approved in 1997 as a treatment for smoking cessation. Approximately twice as many people treated with bupropion as with placebo have a reduced urge to smoke. In addition, patients taking bupropion appear to experience fewer mood symptoms and possibly less weight gain while withdrawing from nicotine dependence. Bupropion appears to be about as effective as nicotine patches in smoking cessation. The mechanism by which bupropion is helpful in this application is unknown, but the drug may mimic nicotine's effects on dopamine and norepinephrine and may inhibit nicotinic receptors. Nicotine is also known to have antidepressant effects in some people, and bupropion may substitute for this effect.

Other antidepressants also may have a role in the treatment of smoking cessation. Nortriptyline has been shown to be helpful in smoking cessation, but the effects have not been as consistent as those seen with bupropion.

F. Eating Disorders

Bulimia nervosa and anorexia nervosa are potentially devastating disorders. Bulimia is characterized by episodic intake of large amounts of food (binges) followed by ritualistic purging through emesis, the use of laxatives, or other methods. Medical complications of the purging, such as hypokalemia, are common and dangerous. Anorexia is a disorder in which reduced food intake results in a loss of weight of 15% or more of ideal body weight, and the person has a morbid fear of gaining weight and a highly distorted body image. Anorexia is often chronic and may be fatal in 10% or more of cases.

Antidepressants appear to be helpful in the treatment of bulimia but not anorexia. Fluoxetine was approved for the treatment of bulimia in 1996, and other antidepressants have shown benefit in reducing the binge-purge cycle. The primary treatment for anorexia at this time is refeeding, family therapy, and cognitive behavioral therapy.

Bupropion may have some benefits in treating obesity. Nondepressed, obese patients treated with bupropion were able to lose somewhat more weight and maintain the loss relative to a similar population treated with placebo. However, the weight loss was not robust, and there appear to be more effective options for weight loss (see Chapter 16).

G. Other Uses for Antidepressants

Antidepressants are used for many other on- and off-label applications. Enuresis in children is an older labeled use for some TCAs, but they are less commonly used now because of their side effects. The SNRI duloxetine is approved in Europe for the treatment of urinary stress incontinence. Many of the serotonergic antidepressants appear to be helpful for treating vasomotor symptoms in perimenopause. Desvenlafaxine is under consideration for FDA approval for the treatment of these vasomotor symptoms, and studies have suggested that SSRIs, venlafaxine, and nefazodone also may provide benefit. Although serotonergic antidepressants are commonly associated with inducing sexual adverse effects, some of these effects might prove useful for some sexual disorders. For example, SSRIs are known to delay orgasm in some patients. For this reason, SSRIs are sometimes used to treat premature ejaculation. In addition, bupropion has been used to treat sexual adverse effects associated with SSRI use, although its efficacy for this use has not been consistently demonstrated in controlled trials.

CHOOSING AN ANTIDEPRESSANT

The choice of an antidepressant depends first on the indication. Not all conditions are equally responsive to all antidepressants. However, in the treatment of MDD, it is difficult to demonstrate that one antidepressant is consistently more effective than another. Thus, the choice of an antidepressant for the treatment of depression rests primarily on practical considerations such as cost, availability, adverse effects, potential drug interactions, the patient's history of response or lack thereof, and patient preference. Other factors such as the patient's age, gender, and medical status also may guide antidepressant selection. For example, older patients are particularly sensitive to the anticholinergic effects of the TCAs. On the other hand, the CYP3A4-inhibiting effects of the SSRI fluvoxamine may make this a problematic choice in some older patients because fluvoxamine may interact with many other medications that an older patient may require. There is some suggestion that female patients may respond to and tolerate serotonergic better than noradrenergic or TCA antidepressants, but the data supporting this gender difference have not been consistent. Patients with narrow-angle glaucoma may have an exacerbation with noradrenergic antidepressants, whereas bupropion and other antidepressants are known to lower the seizure threshold in epilepsy patients.

At present, SSRIs are the most commonly prescribed first-line agents in the treatment of both MDD and anxiety disorders. Their popularity comes from their ease of use, tolerability, and safety in overdose. The starting dose of the SSRIs is usually the same as the therapeutic dose for most patients, and so titration may not be required. In addition, most SSRIs are now generically available and inexpensive. Other agents, including the SNRIs, bupropion, and mirtazapine, also are reasonable first-line agents for the treatment of MDD. Bupropion, mirtazapine, and nefazodone are the antidepressants with the least association with sexual adverse effects and are often prescribed for this reason. However, bupropion is not thought to be effective in the treatment of the anxiety disorders and may be poorly tolerated in anxious patients. The primary indication for bupropion is in the treatment of major depression, including seasonal (winter) depression. Off-label uses of bupropion include the treatment of attention deficit hyperactivity disorder (ADHD), and bupropion is commonly combined with other antidepressants to augment therapeutic response. The primary indication for mirtazapine is in the treatment of major depression. However, its strong antihistamine properties have contributed to its occasional use as a hypnotic and as an adjunctive treatment to more activating antidepressants.

The TCAs and MAOIs are now relegated to second- or third-line treatments for MDD. Both the TCAs and the MAOIs are potentially lethal in overdose, require titration to achieve a therapeutic dose, have serious drug interactions, and have many troublesome adverse effects. As a consequence, their use in the treatment of MDD or anxiety is now reserved for patients who have been unresponsive to other agents. Clearly, there are patients whose depression responds only to MAOIs or TCAs. Thus, TCAs and MAOIs are probably underused in treatment-resistant depressed patients.

The use of antidepressants outside the treatment of MDD tends to require specific agents. For example, the TCAs and SNRIs appear to be useful in the treatment of pain conditions, but other antidepressant classes appear to be far less effective. SSRIs and the highly serotonergic TCA clomipramine are effective in the treatment of OCD, but noradrenergic antidepressants have not proved to be as helpful for this condition. Bupropion and nortriptyline have usefulness in the treatment of smoking cessation, but SSRIs have not been proven useful. Thus, outside the treatment of depression, the choice of antidepressant is primarily dependent on the known benefit of a particular antidepressant or class for a particular indication.

DOSING

The optimal dose of an antidepressant depends on the indication and on the patient. For SSRIs, SNRIs, and a number of newer agents, the starting dose for the treatment of depression is usually a therapeutic dose (Table 30–3). Patients who show little or no benefit after at least 4 weeks of treatment may benefit from a higher dose even though it has been difficult to show a clear advantage for higher doses with SSRIs, SNRIs, and other newer antidepressants. The dose is generally titrated to the maximum dosage recommended or to the highest dosage tolerated if the patient is not responsive to lower doses. Some patients may benefit from doses lower than the usual minimum recommended therapeutic dose. TCAs and MAOIs typically require titration to a therapeutic

TABLE 30–3 Antidepressant dose ranges.

Drug	Usual Therapeutic Dosage (mg/d)
SSRIs	
Citalopram	20–60
Escitalopram	10–30
Fluoxetine	20–60
Fluvoxamine	100–300
Paroxetine	20–60
Sertraline	50–200
SNRIs	
Venlafaxine	75–375
Desvenlafaxine	50–200
Duloxetine	40–120
Milnacipran	100–200
Tricyclics	
Amitriptyline	150–300
Clomipramine	100–250
Desipramine	150–300
Doxepin	150–300
Imipramine	150–300
Nortriptyline	50–150
Protriptyline	15–60
Trimipramine maleate	150–300
5-HT$_2$ antagonists	
Nefazodone	300–500
Trazodone	150–300
Tetracyclics and unicyclics	
Amoxapine	150–400
Bupropion	200–450
Maprotiline	150–225
Mirtazapine	15–45
MAOIs	
Isocarboxazid	30–60
Phenelzine	45–90
Selegiline	20–50
Tranylcypromine	30–60
NMDA antagonists	
Esketamine (intranasal)	56–84
Ketamine (IV)	0.5 mg/kg/h
Dextromethorphan + bupropion	Bup 105 mg/Dex 45 mg BID
GABA$_A$ modulators	
Brexanolone (IV)	30–90 mcg/kg/h

MAOIs, monoamine oxidase inhibitors; SNRIs, serotonin-norepinephrine reuptake inhibitors; SSRIs, selective serotonin reuptake inhibitors.

dosage over several weeks. Dosing of the TCAs may be guided by monitoring TCA serum levels.

Some anxiety disorders may require higher doses of antidepressants than are used in the treatment of major depression. For example, patients treated for OCD often require maximum or somewhat higher than maximum recommended MDD doses to achieve optimal benefits. Likewise, the minimum dose of paroxetine for the effective treatment of panic disorder is higher than the minimum dose required for the effective treatment of depression.

In the treatment of pain disorders, modest doses of TCAs are often sufficient. For example, 25–50 mg/d of imipramine might be beneficial in the treatment of pain associated with a neuropathy, but this would be a subtherapeutic dose in the treatment of MDD. In contrast, SNRIs are usually prescribed in pain disorders at the same doses used in the treatment of depression.

ADVERSE EFFECTS

Although some potential adverse effects are common to all antidepressants, most of their adverse effects are specific to a subclass of agents and to their pharmacodynamic effects. An FDA warning applied to all antidepressants is the risk of increased suicidality in patients younger than 25. The warning suggests that use of antidepressants is associated with suicidal ideation and gestures, but not completed suicides, in up to 4% of patients under 25 who were prescribed antidepressants in clinical trials. This rate is about twice the rate seen with placebo treatment. For those over 25, there is either no increased risk or a reduced risk of suicidal thoughts and gestures on antidepressants, particularly after age 65. Although a small minority of patients may experience a treatment-emergent increase in suicidal ideation with antidepressants, the *absence* of treatment of a major depressive episode in all age groups is a particularly important risk factor in completed suicides.

A. Selective Serotonin Reuptake Inhibitors

The adverse effects of the most commonly prescribed antidepressants—the SSRIs—can be predicted from their potent inhibition of SERT. SSRIs enhance serotonergic tone, not just in the brain but throughout the body. Increased serotonergic activity in the gut is commonly associated with nausea, gastrointestinal upset, diarrhea, and other gastrointestinal symptoms. Gastrointestinal adverse effects usually emerge early in the course of treatment and tend to improve after the first week. Increasing serotonergic tone at the level of the spinal cord and above is associated with diminished sexual function and interest. As a result, at least 30–40% of patients treated with SSRIs report loss of libido, delayed orgasm, or diminished arousal. The sexual effects often persist as long as the patient remains on the antidepressant but may diminish with time.

Other adverse effects related to the serotonergic effects of SSRIs and vortioxetine include an increase in headaches and insomnia or hypersomnia. Some patients gain weight while taking SSRIs, particularly paroxetine. Sudden discontinuation of short half-life SSRIs such as paroxetine and sertraline is associated with a *discontinuation syndrome* in some patients characterized by dizziness, paresthesias, and other symptoms beginning 1 or 2 days after stopping the drug and persisting for 1 week or longer.

Most antidepressants are category C agents by the FDA teratogen classification system. There is an association of paroxetine with cardiac septal defects in first trimester exposures. Thus, paroxetine is a category D agent. Other possible associations of SSRIs with post-birth complications, including pulmonary hypertension, have not been clearly established.

B. Serotonin-Norepinephrine Reuptake Inhibitors and Tricyclic Antidepressants

SNRIs have many of the serotonergic adverse effects associated with SSRIs. In addition, SNRIs may also have noradrenergic effects, including increased blood pressure and heart rate, and CNS activation, such as insomnia, anxiety, and agitation. The hemodynamic effects of SNRIs tend not to be problematic in most patients. A dose-related increase in blood pressure has been seen more commonly with the immediate-release form of venlafaxine than with other SNRIs. Likewise, there are more reports of cardiac toxicity with venlafaxine overdose than with either the other SNRIs or SSRIs. Duloxetine is rarely associated with hepatic toxicity in patients with a history of liver damage. All the SNRIs have been associated with a discontinuation syndrome resembling that seen with SSRI discontinuation.

The primary adverse effects of TCAs have been described in the previous text. Anticholinergic effects are perhaps the most common. These effects include dry mouth, constipation, urinary retention, blurred vision, and confusion. They are more common with tertiary amine TCAs such as amitriptyline and imipramine than with the secondary amine TCAs desipramine and nortriptyline. The potent α-blocking property of TCAs often results in orthostatic hypotension. H_1 antagonism by the TCAs is associated with weight gain and sedation. The TCAs are class 1A antiarrhythmic agents (see Chapter 14) and are arrhythmogenic at higher doses. Sexual effects are common, particularly with highly serotonergic TCAs such as clomipramine. The TCAs have a prominent discontinuation syndrome characterized by cholinergic rebound and flulike symptoms.

C. 5-HT Receptor Modulators

The most common adverse effects associated with the 5-HT_2 antagonists are sedation and gastrointestinal disturbances. Sedative effects, particularly with trazodone, can be quite pronounced. Thus, it is not surprising that the treatment of insomnia is currently the primary application of trazodone. The gastrointestinal effects appear to be dose-related and are less pronounced than those seen with SNRIs or SSRIs. Sexual effects are uncommon with nefazodone or trazodone treatment as a result of the relatively selective serotonergic effects of these drugs on the 5-HT_2 receptor rather than on SERT. However, trazodone has rarely been associated with inducing priapism. Both nefazodone and trazodone are α-blocking agents and may result in a dose-related orthostatic hypotension in some patients. Nefazodone has been associated with hepatotoxicity, including rare fatalities and cases of fulminant hepatic failure requiring transplantation. The rate of serious hepatotoxicity with nefazodone has been estimated at 1 in 250,000 to 1 in 300,000 patient-years of nefazodone treatment.

As with the SSRIs, the most common adverse effects of vortioxetine are serotonergic and include dose-dependent gastrointestinal effects, particularly nausea, as well as sexual dysfunction. Higher doses of vortioxetine tend to increase the rate of GI and sexual side effects. The teratogenic risks of vortioxetine are not known but like most other antidepressants, it is considered a category C agent.

D. Tetracyclics and Unicyclics

Amoxapine is sometimes associated with a parkinsonian syndrome due to its D_2-blocking action. Mirtazapine has significant sedative effect. Maprotiline has a moderately high affinity for NET and may cause TCA-like adverse effects and, rarely, seizures. Bupropion is occasionally associated with agitation, insomnia, and anorexia. Vilazodone may have somewhat higher rates of gastrointestinal upset, including diarrhea and nausea, than the SSRIs.

E. Monoamine Oxidase Inhibitors

The most common adverse effects of the MAOIs leading to discontinuation of these drugs are orthostatic hypotension and weight gain. In addition, the irreversible nonselective MAOIs are associated with the highest rates of sexual effects of all the antidepressants. Anorgasmia is fairly common with therapeutic doses of some MAOIs. The amphetamine-like properties of some MAOIs contribute to activation, insomnia, and restlessness in some patients. Phenelzine tends to be more sedating than either selegiline or tranylcypromine. Confusion is also sometimes associated with higher doses of MAOIs. Because they block metabolism of tyramine and similar ingested amines, MAOIs may cause dangerous interactions with certain foods and with serotonergic drugs (see Interactions). Finally, MAOIs have been associated with a sudden discontinuation syndrome manifested in a delirium-like presentation with psychosis, excitement, and confusion.

F. NMDA Receptor Antagonists

The adverse effects of ketamine and esketamine are consistent with their pharmacologic profile. The short-term adverse effects of these drugs include sedation, dissociation, hypertension, nausea, tachycardia, and cognitive impairment. Most of these effects occur in close proximity to the administration of the drug and usually dissipate in minutes to hours. In the registration trials for esketamine, 8–17% of patients had a systolic blood pressure increase of >40 mm Hg and >25 mm Hg diastolic in the first 1.5 hours after administration. Up to 75% of patients had dissociative symptoms (eg, depersonalization, derealization, out-of-body experiences, distortions of time), although these tended to be most common in the first 2 hours of administration. Therefore, the esketamine prescribing protocol will require that patients be observed in the clinic for at least 2 hours after administration.

Ketamine has been a significant drug of abuse in some parts of the world, notably in parts of China and southeast Asia. Long-term abuse of ketamine has been associated with dependence, psychotomimetic effects (including auditory and visual hallucinations and paranoid delusions), and bladder inflammation and ulcerations. In the long-term depression trials with intranasal esketamine given intermittently (twice weekly for 4 weeks, once weekly for 4 weeks, and once every other week thereafter), there have not been cases of addiction, bladder ulcerations, or other long-term side effects seen in ketamine abusers.

Dextromethorphan has more rarely been abused at higher doses. In clinical trials of the combination pill with bupropion approved for depression, an increase in anxiety was the only side effect that led to discontinuation at rates higher than 1% (2% of trial participants). The most common side effects of the combination pill were dizziness, headaches, dry mouth, and diarrhea.

G. $GABA_A$ Receptor Modulators

The most common adverse effects of IV brexanolone in clinical trials were headaches, dizziness, and somnolence. About 27% of patients in the postpartum depression trials experienced sedation compared with 14% of the placebo-treated patients. Brexanolone has a terminal half-life of about 12 hours, and the sedation did not appear to persist after the infusion stopped. There was a rare adverse effect of syncope and loss of consciousness in 4 patients (1.4%) during the infusion, which resolved with discontinuation of the infusion. Another 4% of patients had excessive sedation or near loss of consciousness relieved by the discontinuation of the infusion. Overall, the rate of adverse events in the brexanolone group was about the same as the rate in the placebo group, and <2% of brexanolone-treated patients discontinued because of side effects. It is anticipated that IV brexanolone will be administered by home health nurses, physicians in the clinic, or infusion centers that will be available for the entire 60-hour infusion to assess for excessive sedation or other side effects.

A number of oral $GABA_A$ receptor modulators are currently in development for the treatment of major depression and anxiety disorders, which would potentially circumvent the need for lengthy IV infusion.

OVERDOSE

Suicide attempts are a common and unfortunate consequence of major depression. The lifetime risk of completing suicide in patients previously hospitalized with MDD may be as high as 15%. Overdose is among the most common methods used in suicide attempts, and antidepressants, especially the TCAs, are frequently involved. Overdose can induce lethal arrhythmias, including ventricular tachycardia and fibrillation. In addition, blood pressure changes and anticholinergic effects including altered mental status and seizures are sometimes seen in TCA overdoses. A 1500-mg dose of imipramine or amitriptyline (less than 7 days' supply at antidepressant doses) is enough to be lethal in many patients. Toddlers taking 100 mg will likely show evidence of toxicity. Treatment typically involves cardiac monitoring, airway support, and gastric lavage. Sodium bicarbonate is often administered to displace the TCA from cardiac sodium channels.

An overdose with an MAOI can produce a variety of effects including autonomic instability, hyperadrenergic symptoms, psychotic symptoms, confusion, delirium, fever, and seizures. Management of MAOI overdoses usually involves cardiac monitoring, vital signs support, and lavage.

Compared with TCAs and MAOIs, the other antidepressants are generally much safer in overdose. Fatalities with SSRI overdose alone are extremely uncommon. Similarly, SNRIs tend to be much safer in overdose than the TCAs. However, venlafaxine has been associated with some cardiac toxicity in overdose and appears to be less safe than SSRIs. Bupropion is associated with seizures in overdose, and mirtazapine may be associated with sedation, disorientation, and tachycardia. With the newer agents, fatal overdoses often involve the combination of the antidepressant with other drugs, including alcohol. Management of overdose with the newer antidepressants usually involves emptying of gastric contents and vital sign support as the initial intervention.

DRUG INTERACTIONS

Antidepressants are commonly prescribed with other psychotropic and nonpsychotropic agents. There is potential for drug interactions with all antidepressants, but the most serious of these involve the MAOIs and, to a lesser extent, the TCAs.

A. Selective Serotonin Reuptake Inhibitors

The most common interactions with SSRIs are pharmacokinetic interactions. For example, paroxetine and fluoxetine are potent CYP2D6 inhibitors (Table 30–4). Thus, administration with 2D6 substrates such as TCAs can lead to dramatic and sometimes unpredictable elevations in the tricyclic drug concentration. The result may be toxicity from the TCA. Similarly, fluvoxamine, a CYP3A4 inhibitor, may elevate the levels of concurrently administered substrates for this enzyme such as diltiazem and induce bradycardia or hypotension. Other SSRIs, such as citalopram and escitalopram, are relatively free of pharmacokinetic interactions. The most serious interactions with the SSRIs are pharmacodynamic interactions with MAOIs that produce a serotonin syndrome (see below).

B. Selective Serotonin-Norepinephrine Reuptake Inhibitors and Tricyclic Antidepressants

The SNRIs have relatively fewer CYP450 interactions than the SSRIs. Venlafaxine is a substrate but not an inhibitor of CYP2D6 or other isoenzymes, whereas desvenlafaxine is a minor substrate for CYP3A4. Duloxetine is a moderate inhibitor of CYP2D6 and so may elevate TCA and levels of other CYP2D6 substrates. Since milnacipran is neither a substrate nor potent inducer of CYP450 isoenzymes, is not tightly protein bound, and is largely excreted unchanged in the urine, it is unlikely to have clinically significant pharmacokinetic drug interactions. On the other hand, levomilnacipran is reported to be a substrate of CYP3A4, and the dosage of the drug should be lowered when combined with potent inhibitors of CYP3A4 such as ketoconazole. Like all serotonergic antidepressants, SNRIs are contraindicated in combination with MAOIs.

Elevated TCA levels may occur when these drugs are combined with CYP2D6 inhibitors or from constitutional factors. About 7% of the Caucasian population in the USA has a CYP2D6 polymorphism that is associated with slow metabolism of TCAs and other 2D6 substrates. Combination of a known CYP2D6 inhibitor and a TCA in a patient who is a slow metabolizer may result in markedly increased effects. Such an interaction has been implicated, though rarely, in cases of TCA toxicity. There may also be additive anticholinergic or antihistamine effects when TCAs are combined with other agents that share these properties such as benztropine or diphenhydramine. Similarly, antihypertensive drugs may exacerbate the orthostatic hypotension induced by TCAs.

C. 5-HT Receptor Modulators

Nefazodone is an inhibitor of the CYP3A4 isoenzyme, so it can raise the level and thus exacerbate adverse effects of many 3A4-dependent drugs. For example, triazolam levels are increased by concurrent administration of nefazodone such that a reduction

TABLE 30–4 Some antidepressant–CYP450 drug interactions.

Enzyme	Substrates	Inhibitors	Inducers
1A2	Tertiary amine tricyclic antidepressants (TCAs), duloxetine, theophylline, phenacetin, TCAs (demethylation), clozapine, diazepam, caffeine	Fluvoxamine, fluoxetine, moclobemide, ramelteon	Tobacco, omeprazole
2C19	TCAs, citalopram (partly), warfarin, tolbutamide, phenytoin, diazepam	Fluoxetine, fluvoxamine, sertraline, imipramine, ketoconazole, omeprazole	Rifampin
2D6	TCAs, benztropine, perphenazine, clozapine, haloperidol, codeine/oxycodone, risperidone, class Ic antiarrhythmics, β blockers, trazodone, paroxetine, maprotiline, amoxapine, duloxetine, mirtazapine (partly), venlafaxine, bupropion	Fluoxetine, paroxetine, duloxetine, hydroxybupropion, methadone, cimetidine, haloperidol, quinidine, ritonavir	Phenobarbital, rifampin
3A4	Citalopram, escitalopram, TCAs, glucocorticoids, androgens/estrogens, carbamazepine, erythromycin, Ca^{2+} channel blockers, levomilnacipran, protease inhibitors, sildenafil, alprazolam, triazolam, vincristine/vinblastine, tamoxifen, zolpidem	Fluvoxamine, nefazodone, sertraline, fluoxetine, cimetidine, fluconazole, erythromycin, protease inhibitors, ketoconazole, verapamil	Barbiturates, glucocorticoids, rifampin, modafinil, carbamazepine

in triazolam dosage by 75% is recommended. Likewise, administration of nefazodone with simvastatin has been associated with 20-fold increase in plasma levels of simvastatin.

Trazodone is a substrate but not a potent inhibitor of CYP3A4. As a result, combining trazodone with potent inhibitors of CYP3A4, such as ritonavir or ketoconazole, may lead to substantial increases in trazodone levels.

Vortioxetine is a substrate of CYP2D6 and 2B6, and it is recommended that the dose be cut in half when it is coadministered with fluoxetine or bupropion. Inducers of CYP isoenzymes such as rifampin, carbamazepine, and phenytoin will lower serum levels of vortioxetine and may require increasing the dose of vortioxetine.

D. Tetracyclic and Unicyclic Antidepressants

Bupropion is metabolized primarily by CYP2B6, and its metabolism may be altered by drugs such as cyclophosphamide, which is a substrate of 2B6. The major metabolite of bupropion, hydroxybupropion, is a moderate inhibitor of CYP2D6 and so can raise desipramine levels. Bupropion should be avoided in patients taking MAOIs.

Mirtazapine is a substrate for several CYP450 enzymes including 2D6, 3A4, and 1A2. Consequently, drugs that inhibit these isozymes may raise mirtazapine levels. However, mirtazapine is not an inhibitor of these enzymes. The sedating effects of mirtazapine may be additive with those of CNS depressants such as alcohol and benzodiazepines.

Amoxapine and maprotiline share most drug interactions common to the TCA group. Both are CYP2D6 substrates and should be used with caution in combination with inhibitors such as fluoxetine. Amoxapine and maprotiline also both have anticholinergic and antihistaminic properties that may be additive with drugs that share a similar profile.

Since vilazodone is primarily a substrate of CYP3A4, strong CYP3A4 inhibitors such as ketoconazole can increase the serum concentration of vilazodone by 50% or more. On the other hand, vilazodone is neither a potent inhibitor nor a strong inducer of any CYP isoenzymes. It may be a mild inducer of CYP2C19.

E. Monoamine Oxidase Inhibitors

MAOIs are associated with two classes of serious drug interactions. The first of these is the pharmacodynamic interaction of MAOIs with serotonergic agents including SSRIs, SNRIs, and most TCAs along with some analgesic agents such as meperidine. These combinations of an MAOI with a serotonergic agent may result in a life-threatening **serotonin syndrome** (see Chapter 16). The serotonin syndrome is thought to be caused by overstimulation of 5-HT receptors in the central gray nuclei and the medulla. Symptoms range from mild to lethal and include a triad of cognitive (delirium, coma), autonomic (hypertension, tachycardia, diaphoresis), and somatic (myoclonus, hyperreflexia, tremor) effects. Most serotonergic antidepressants should be discontinued at least 2 weeks before starting an MAOI. Fluoxetine, because of its long half-life, should be discontinued for 4–5 weeks before an MAOI is initiated. Conversely, an MAOI must be discontinued for at least 2 weeks before starting a serotonergic agent.

The second serious interaction with MAOIs occurs when an MAOI is combined with tyramine in the diet or with sympathomimetic substrates of MAO. An MAOI prevents the breakdown of tyramine in the gut, and this results in high serum levels that enhance peripheral noradrenergic effects, including raising blood pressure dramatically. Patients on an MAOI who ingest large amounts of dietary tyramine may experience malignant hypertension and subsequently a stroke or myocardial infarction. Thus, patients taking MAOIs require a low-tyramine diet and should avoid foods such as aged cheeses, tap beer, soy products, and dried sausages, which contain high amounts of tyramine (see Chapter 9). Similar sympathomimetics also may cause significant hypertension when combined with MAOIs. Thus, over-the-counter cold preparations that contain pseudoephedrine and phenylpropanolamine are contraindicated in patients taking MAOIs.

F. NMDA Receptor Antagonists

Ketamine and esketamine have relatively modest CYP450 interactions but a number of potential pharmacodynamic interactions. Esketamine is a weak inducer of CYP2B6 and CYP3A4. It is not a substrate of p-glycoprotein.

Among the adverse effects of ketamine and esketamine are sedation, hypertension, and tachycardia. CNS depressants such as alcohol, benzodiazepines, and barbiturates can increase the sedation associated with esketamine and ketamine. Stimulants (methylphenidate, dextroamphetamine, modafinil, armodafinil), MAOIs, and sympathomimetics can all increase blood pressure and heart rate when combined with ketamine and esketamine.

Dextromethorphan is metabolized via CYP2D6, as is the major active metabolite of bupropion, hydroxybupropion. Thus, CYP2D6 inhibitors will increase the serum level of both drugs and might increase the adverse effects including seizures, while CYP2D6 inducers will decrease the serum level of combination pill and decrease efficacy. The combination pill is contraindicated with MAOIs because of the risk of a serotonin syndrome or hypertensive crisis.

G. $GABA_A$ Receptor Modulators

Brexanolone is metabolized via multiple alternate pathways and thus is not likely to have significant pharmacokinetic interactions. CYP450 inducers or inhibitors are not expected to have a significant effect on brexanolone levels. Brexanolone appears to be a weak inhibitor of CYP2C9 in vitro, but clinical studies have not demonstrated an effect on the pharmacokinetics of co-administered phenytoin (a CYP2C9 substrate). Brexanolone is expected to be frequently prescribed with other antidepressants; no clinically significant interactions have been noted.

SUMMARY Antidepressants

Subclass, Drug	Mechanism of Action	Effects	Clinical Applications	Pharmacokinetics, Toxicities, Interactions
SELECTIVE SEROTONIN REUPTAKE INHIBITORS (SSRIs)				
• Fluoxetine • Citalopram • Escitalopram • Paroxetine • Sertraline	Highly selective blockade of serotonin transporter (SERT) • little effect on norepinephrine transporter (NET)	Acute increase of serotonergic synaptic activity • slower changes in several signaling pathways and neurotrophic activity	Major depression, anxiety disorders • panic disorder • obsessive-compulsive disorder • post-traumatic stress disorder • perimenopausal vasomotor symptoms • eating disorder (bulimia)	Half-lives from 15 to 75 h • oral activity • *Toxicity:* Well tolerated but cause sexual dysfunction • risk of serotonin syndrome with MAOIs • *Interactions:* Some CYP inhibition (fluoxetine 2D6, 3A4; fluvoxamine 1A2; paroxetine 2D6)
• *Fluvoxamine: Similar to above but approved only for obsessive-compulsive behavior*				
SEROTONIN-NOREPINEPHRINE REUPTAKE INHIBITORS (SNRIs)				
• Duloxetine • Venlafaxine • Levomilnacipran	Moderately selective blockade of NET and SERT	Acute increase in serotonergic and adrenergic synaptic activity • otherwise like SSRIs	Major depression, chronic pain disorders • fibromyalgia, perimenopausal symptoms	*Toxicity:* Anticholinergic, sedation, hypertension (venlafaxine) • *Interactions:* Some CYP2D6 inhibition (duloxetine, desvenlafaxine) • CYP3A4 interactions with levomilnacipran
• *Desvenlafaxine: Desmethyl metabolite of venlafaxine, metabolism is by phase II rather than CYP phase I* • *Milnacipran: Approved only for fibromyalgia in the USA; significantly more selective for NET than SERT; little effect on DAT*				
TRICYCLIC ANTIDEPRESSANTS (TCAs)				
• Imipramine • Many others	Mixed and variable blockade of NET and SERT	Like SNRIs plus significant blockade of autonomic nervous system and histamine receptors	Major depression not responsive to other drugs • chronic pain disorders • incontinence • obsessive-compulsive disorder (clomipramine)	Long half-lives • CYP substrates • active metabolites • *Toxicity:* Anticholinergic, α-blocking effects, sedation, weight gain, arrhythmias, and seizures in overdose • *Interactions:* CYP inducers and inhibitors
5-HT RECEPTOR MODULATORS				
• Nefazodone • Trazodone	Inhibition of 5-HT_{2A} receptor • nefazodone also blocks SERT weakly	Trazodone forms a metabolite (m-cpp) that blocks 5-$HT_{2A,2C}$ receptors	Major depression • sedation and hypnosis (trazodone)	Relatively short half-lives • active metabolites • *Toxicity:* Modest α- and H_1-receptor blockade (trazodone) • *Interactions:* Nefazodone inhibits CYP3A4
• Vortioxetine	Antagonist at 5-HT_3, 5-HT_7, 5-HT_{1D} receptors; partial agonist at 5-HT_{1B} receptor, agonist at 5-HT_{1A} receptor; inhibits SERT	Complex modulation of serotonergic systems	Major depression	Extensively metabolized via CYP2D6 and glucuronic acid conjugation • *Toxicity:* GI disturbances, sexual dysfunction • *Interactions:* Additive with serotonergic agents
TETRACYCLICS, UNICYCLIC				
• Bupropion • Amoxapine • Maprotiline • Mirtazapine	Increased norepinephrine and dopamine activity (bupropion) • NET > SERT inhibition (amoxapine, maprotiline) • increased release of norepinephrine, 5-HT (mirtazapine)	Presynaptic release of catecholamines but no effect on 5-HT (bupropion) • amoxapine and maprotiline resemble TCAs	Major depression • smoking cessation (bupropion) • sedation (mirtazapine) • amoxapine and maprotiline rarely used	Extensive metabolism in liver • *Toxicity:* Lowers seizure threshold (amoxapine, bupropion); sedation and weight gain (mirtazapine) • *Interactions:* CYP2D6 inhibitor (bupropion)

(continued)

Subclass, Drug	Mechanism of Action	Effects	Clinical Applications	Pharmacokinetics, Toxicities, Interactions
MONOAMINE OXIDASE INHIBITORS (MAOIs)				
• Phenelzine • Tranylcypromine • Selegiline	Blockade of MAO-A and MAO-B (phenelzine, nonselective) • MAO-B irreversible selective MAO-B inhibition (low-dose selegiline)	Transdermal formulation of selegiline achieves levels that inhibit MAO-A	Major depression unresponsive to other drugs • Parkinson disease (selegiline)	Very slow elimination • *Toxicity:* Hypotension, insomnia • *Interactions:* Hypertensive crisis with tyramine, other indirect sympathomimetics • serotonin syndrome with serotonergic agents, meperidine
NMDA RECEPTOR ANTAGONISTS				
• Ketamine (off-label) • Esketamine Bupropion + dextromethorphan	Noncompetitive antagonism at the NMDA receptor NE agonist, DA reuptake inhibitor, NMDA antagonist, sigma-1 agonist	Anesthesia; possible increase in serotonergic activity, dopaminergic activity Combination tablet for major depression	Ketamine: anesthesia Esketamine: refractory depression (outside USA: anesthesia)	Ketamine: IV Esketamine: nasal inhalation, rapid onset of action • *Toxicity:* Dissociative symptoms, possible abuse, BP increase
$GABA_A$ RECEPTOR MODULATORS				
• Brexanolone	Positive allosteric modulator of the $GABA_A$ chloride channel, binding site distinct from benzodiazepine site	Unclear: possibly replaces endogenous allopregnanolone, which decreases markedly after delivery	Postpartum depression only	IV infusion over 60 hours • *Toxicity:* Excessive sedation, possible loss of consciousness

PREPARATIONS AVAILABLE

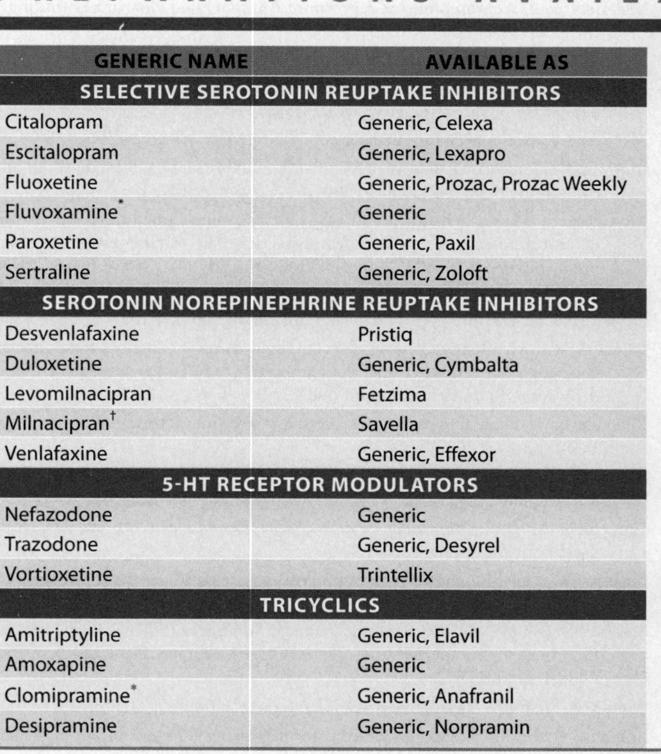

GENERIC NAME	AVAILABLE AS
SELECTIVE SEROTONIN REUPTAKE INHIBITORS	
Citalopram	Generic, Celexa
Escitalopram	Generic, Lexapro
Fluoxetine	Generic, Prozac, Prozac Weekly
Fluvoxamine*	Generic
Paroxetine	Generic, Paxil
Sertraline	Generic, Zoloft
SEROTONIN NOREPINEPHRINE REUPTAKE INHIBITORS	
Desvenlafaxine	Pristiq
Duloxetine	Generic, Cymbalta
Levomilnacipran	Fetzima
Milnacipran†	Savella
Venlafaxine	Generic, Effexor
5-HT RECEPTOR MODULATORS	
Nefazodone	Generic
Trazodone	Generic, Desyrel
Vortioxetine	Trintellix
TRICYCLICS	
Amitriptyline	Generic, Elavil
Amoxapine	Generic
Clomipramine*	Generic, Anafranil
Desipramine	Generic, Norpramin

GENERIC NAME	AVAILABLE AS
Doxepin	Generic, Sinequan
Imipramine	Generic, Tofranil
Nortriptyline	Generic, Pamelor
Protriptyline	Generic, Vivactil
Trimipramine	Surmontil
TETRACYCLIC AND UNICYCLIC AGENTS	
Amoxapine	Generic
Bupropion	Generic, Wellbutrin
Maprotiline	Generic
Mirtazapine	Generic, Remeron
Vilazodone	Viibryd
MONOAMINE OXIDASE INHIBITORS	
Isocarboxazid	Marplan
Phenelzine	Generic, Nardil
Selegiline	Generic, Eldepryl
Tranylcypromine	Generic, Parnate
NMDA RECEPTOR MODULATORS	
Esketamine	Spravato, Ketanest
Bupropion + dextromethorphan	Auvelity
$GABA_A$ RECEPTOR MODULATORS	
Brexanolone‡	Zulresso

*Labeled only for obsessive-compulsive disorder.

†Labeled only for fibromyalgia.

‡Labeled only for postpartum depression.

REFERENCES

Aan Het Rot M et al: Ketamine for depression: Where do we go from here? Biol Psychiatry 2012;72:537.

Alam MY et al: Safety, tolerability, and efficacy of vortioxetine (Lu AA21004) in major depressive disorder: Results of an open-label, flexible-dose, 52-week extension study. Int Clin Psychopharmacol 2014;29:39.

Alessandro S, Kato M: The serotonin transporter gene and effectiveness of SSRIs. Expert Rev Neurother 2008;8(1):111.

Bab I, Yirmiya R: Depression, selective serotonin reuptake inhibitors, and osteoporosis. Curr Osteoporos Rep 2010;8:185.

Barrera AZ, Torres LD, Munoz RF: Prevention of depression: The state of the science at the beginning of the 21st century. Int Rev Psychiatry 2007;19:655.

Bellingham GA, Peng PW: Duloxetine: A review of its pharmacology and use in chronic pain management. Reg Anesth Pain Med 2010;35:294.

Belmaker R, Agam G: Major depressive disorder. N Engl J Med 2008;358:55.

Bockting CL et al: Continuation and maintenance use of antidepressants in recurrent depression. Psychother Psychosom 2008;77:17.

Bonisch H, Bruss M: The norepinephrine transporter in physiology and disease. Handb Exp Pharmacol 2006;175:485.

Castren E, Voikar V, Rantamaki T: Role of neurotrophic factors in depression. Curr Opin Pharmacol 2007;7:18.

Chaki S et al: mGlu2/3 and mGlu5 receptors: Potential targets for novel antidepressants. Neuropharmacology 2013;66:40.

Chappell AS et al: A double-blind, randomized, placebo-controlled study of the efficacy and safety of duloxetine for the treatment of chronic pain due to osteoarthritis of the knee. Pain Pract 2011;11:33.

Chen G et al: Pharmacokinetic drug interactions involving vortioxetine (Lu AA21004), a multimodal antidepressant. Clin Drug Investig 2013; 33:727.

Cipriani A et al: Fluoxetine versus other types of pharmacotherapy for depression. Cochrane Database Syst Rev 2005;4:CD004185.

Cipriani A et al: Metareview on short-term effectiveness and safety of antidepressants for depression: An evidence-based approach to inform clinical practice. Can J Psychiatry 2007;52:553.

Citrome L: Vortioxetine for major depressive disorder: A systematic review of the efficacy and safety profile for this newly approved antidepressant—What is the number needed to treat, number needed to harm and likelihood to be helped or harmed? Int J Clin Pract 2014;68:60.

de Beaurepaire R: Questions raised by the cytokine hypothesis of depression. Brain Behav Immun 2002;16:610.

Dhillon S et al: Escitalopram: A review of its use in the management of anxiety disorders. CNS Drugs 2006;20:763.

Dhillon S et al: Bupropion: A review of its use in the management of major depressive disorder. Drugs 2008;68:653.

Duman RS, Monteggia LM: A neurotrophic model for stress-related mood disorders. Biol Psychiatry 2006;59:1116.

Dvir Y, Smallwood P: Serotonin syndrome: A complex but easily avoidable condition. Gen Hosp Psychiatry 2008;30:284.

Fontenelle LF et al: An update on the pharmacological treatment of obsessive-compulsive disorder. Expert Opin Pharmacother 2007;8:563.

Geisser ME et al: A pooled analysis of two randomized, double-blind, placebo-controlled trials of milnacipran monotherapy in the treatment of fibromyalgia. Pain Pract 2011;11:120.

Gether U et al: Neurotransmitter transporters: Molecular function of important drug targets. Trends Pharmacol Sci 2006;27:375.

Gillespie CF, Nemeroff CB: Hypercortisolemia and depression. Psychosom Med 2005;67(Suppl 1):S26.

Gillman PK: A review of serotonin toxicity data: Implications for the mechanisms of antidepressant drug action. Biol Psychiatry 2006;59:1046.

Gillman PK: Tricyclic antidepressant pharmacology and therapeutic drug interactions updated. Br J Pharmacol 2007;151:737.

Giner L et al: Selective serotonin reuptake inhibitors and the risk for suicidality in adolescents: An update. Int J Adolesc Med Health 2005;17:211.

Guay DR: Vilazodone hydrochloride, a combined SSRI and 5-HT1A receptor agonist for major depressive disorder. Consult Pharm 2012;27:857.

Gundaz-Bruce H et al: Trial of Sage-217 in patients with major depressive disorder. N Engl J Med 2019;381:903.

Gutman DA, Owens MJ: Serotonin and norepinephrine transporter binding profile of SSRIs. Essent Psychopharmacol 2006;7:35.

Tabuteau H et al: Effect of AXS-05 (dextromethorphan-bupropion) in major depressive disorder: a randomized double-blind controlled trial. Am J Psychiatry 2022;179:490.

Harrison J et al: The effects of vortioxetine on cognitive function in patients with major depressive disorder (MDD): A meta-analysis of three randomized controlled trials. Int J Neuropsychopharmacol 2016;19:pyw055.

Hirschfeld RM: Antidepressants in long-term therapy: A review of tricyclic antidepressants and selective serotonin reuptake inhibitors. Acta Psychiatr Scand Suppl 2000;403:35.

Hirschfeld RM: History and evolution of the monoamine hypothesis of depression. J Clin Psychiatry 2000;61(Suppl 6):4.

Holma KM et al: Long-term outcome of major depressive disorder in psychiatric patients is variable. J Clin Psychiatry 2008;69:196.

Jann MW, Slade JH: Antidepressant agents for the treatment of chronic pain and depression. Pharmacotherapy 2007;27:1571.

Kalia M: Neurobiological basis of depression: An update. Metabolism 2005; 54(5 Suppl 1):24.

Kozisek ME et al: Brain-derived neurotrophic factor and its receptor tropomyosin-related kinase B in the mechanism of action of antidepressant therapies. Pharmacol Ther 2008;117:30.

Krystal JH et al: Rapid-acting glutamatergic antidepressants: The path to ketamine and beyond. Biol Psychiatry 2013;73:1133.

Laughren TP et al: Vilazodone: Clinical basis for the US Food and Drug Administration's approval of a new antidepressant. J Clin Psychiatry 2011; 72:1166.

Lesch KP, Gutknecht L: Pharmacogenetics of the serotonin transporter. Prog Neuropsychopharmacol Biol Psychiatry 2005;29:1062.

Majeed A et al: Efficacy of dextromethorphan for the treatment of depression: a systematic review of preclinical and clinical trials. Expert Opin Emerg Drugs 2021;26:63.

Mago R et al: Safety and tolerability of levomilnacipran ER in major depressive disorder: Results from an open-label, 48-week extension study. Clin Drug Investig 2013;33:761.

Maletic V et al: Neurobiology of depression: An integrated view of key findings. Int J Clin Pract 2007;61:2030.

Manji HK et al: The cellular neurobiology of depression. Nat Med 2001;7:541.

Mathews DC, Zarate CA Jr: Current status of ketamine and related compounds for depression. J Clin Psychiatry 2013;74:516.

McCleane G: Antidepressants as analgesics. CNS Drugs 2008;22:139.

McEwen BS: Glucocorticoids, depression, and mood disorders: Structural remodeling in the brain. Metabolism 2005;54(5 Suppl 1):20.

Montgomery SA et al: Efficacy and safety of levomilnacipran sustained release in moderate to severe major depressive disorder: A randomized, double-blind, placebo-controlled, proof-of-concept study. J Clin Psychiatry 2013; 74:363.

Nestler EJ et al: Neurobiology of depression. Neuron 2002;34:13.

Pace TW et al: Cytokine-effects on glucocorticoid receptor function: Relevance to glucocorticoid resistance and the pathophysiology and treatment of major depression. Brain Behav Immun 2007;21:9.

Pilc A et al: Glutamate-based antidepressants: Preclinical psychopharmacology. Biol Psychiatry 2013;73:1125.

Sakinofsky I: Treating suicidality in depressive illness. Part 2: Does treatment cure or cause suicidality? Can J Psychiatry 2007;52(6 Suppl 1):85S.

Schatzberg AF et al: *Manual of Clinical Psychopharmacology*, 6th ed. American Psychiatric Publishing, 2007.

Shapiro JR et al: Bulimia nervosa treatment: A systematic review of randomized controlled trials. Int J Eat Disord 2007;40:321.

Soomro GM et al: Selective serotonin reuptake inhibitors (SSRIs) versus placebo for obsessive compulsive disorder (OCD). Cochrane Database Syst Rev 2008;1:CD001765.

Stein MB, Stein DJ: Social anxiety disorder. Lancet 2008;371(9618):1115.

Stone EA et al: A final common pathway for depression? Progress toward a general conceptual framework. Neurosci Biobehav Rev 2008;32:508.

Thase ME et al: A meta-analysis of randomized, placebo-controlled trials of vortioxetine for the treatment of major depressive disorder in adults. Eur Neuropsychopharmacol 2016;26:979.

Tuccori M et al: Use of selective serotonin reuptake inhibitors during pregnancy and risk of major and cardiovascular malformations: An update. Postgrad Med 2010;122:49.

Warden D et al: The STAR*D Project results: A comprehensive review of findings. Curr Psychiatry Rep 2007;9:449.

Wheeler BW et al: The population impact on incidence of suicide and non-fatal self harm of regulatory action against the use of selective serotonin reuptake inhibitors in under 18s in the United Kingdom: Ecological study. Br Med J 2008;336(7643):542.

Wilson KL et al: Persistent pulmonary hypertension of the newborn is associated with mode of delivery and not with maternal use of selective serotonin reuptake inhibitors. Am J Perinatol 2011;28:19.

Yu S et al: Neuronal actions of glucocorticoids: Focus on depression. J Steroid Biochem Mol Biol 2008;108:300.

CASE STUDY ANSWER

The patient has previously responded to fluoxetine, so this drug is an obvious choice. However, she is taking other drugs and fluoxetine, the prototype SSRI, has a number of pharmacokinetic and pharmacodynamic interactions. Fluoxetine is a CYP450 2D6 inhibitor and thus can inhibit the metabolism of 2D6 substrates such as propranolol and other β blockers; tricyclic antidepressants; tramadol; opioids such as methadone, codeine, and oxycodone; antipsychotics such as haloperidol and thioridazine; and many other drugs. This inhibition of metabolism can result in significantly higher plasma levels of the concurrent drug, and this may lead to an increase in adverse reactions associated with that drug.

As a potent inhibitor of the serotonin transporter, fluoxetine is associated with a number of pharmacodynamic interactions involving serotonergic neurotransmission. The combination of tramadol with fluoxetine has occasionally been associated with a serotonin syndrome, characterized by diaphoresis, autonomic instability, myoclonus, seizures, and coma. The combination of fluoxetine with an MAOI is contraindicated because of the risk of a fatal serotonin syndrome. In addition, meperidine is specifically contraindicated in combination with an MAOI. An interaction with hydrochlorothiazide is not likely.

CHAPTER

31 Opioid Agonists & Antagonists

Mark A. Schumacher, MD, PhD,
Allan I. Basbaum, PhD, & Ramana K. Naidu, MD[*]

CASE STUDY

A 48-year-old man with a body mass index (BMI) of 33 (obesity) and history of obstructive sleep apnea presents to the emergency department with severe back pain following a fall from a ladder. He complains of severe pain without loss of consciousness or focal neurologic deficits. What is the most appropriate immediate treatment for his pain? Are any special precautions needed?

Morphine, the prototypic opioid agonist, has been used throughout history to relieve acute severe pain with remarkable efficacy. The opium poppy is the source of crude opium from which Sertürner in 1803 isolated morphine, the pure alkaloid, naming it after Morpheus, the Greek god of dreams. It remains the standard against which all drugs that have strong analgesic action are compared. These drugs are collectively known as opioids and include not only the natural and semisynthetic alkaloid derivatives from opium but also synthetic surrogates, other opioid-like drugs whose actions are blocked by the nonselective antagonist naloxone, plus several endogenous peptides that interact with the different subtypes of opioid receptors.

■ BASIC PHARMACOLOGY OF THE OPIOIDS

Source

Opium, the source of morphine, is obtained from the poppy, *Papaver somniferum* and *P album*. After incision, the poppy seed pod exudes a white substance that turns into a brown gum that is crude opium. Opium contains many alkaloids, the principal one being morphine, which is present in a concentration of about 10%. Codeine can also be found in opium and is synthesized commercially from morphine.

Classification & Chemistry

The term **opioid** describes all compounds that work at opioid receptors. The term **opiate** specifically describes the naturally occurring alkaloids: morphine, codeine, thebaine, and papaverine. In contrast, **narcotic** was originally used to describe sleep-inducing medications, but in the United States, its usage has shifted into a legal term.

Opioid drugs include full agonists, partial agonists, and antagonists–measures of intrinsic activity or efficacy. Morphine is a full agonist at the **μ (mu)-opioid receptor,** the major analgesic opioid receptor (Table 31–1). Opioids may also differ in receptor-binding affinity. For example, morphine exhibits a greater binding affinity at the μ-opioid receptor than does codeine. Other opioid receptor subtypes include δ **(delta)** and κ **(kappa)** nociception/**opioid-receptor-like subtype 1** (ORL-1) receptors. Simple substitution of an allyl group on the nitrogen of the full *agonist* morphine plus addition of a single hydroxyl group results in naloxone, a strong μ-receptor *antagonist*. The structures of some of these compounds are shown later in this chapter. Some opioids, eg, nalbuphine, a **mixed agonist-antagonist,** are capable of producing an agonist (or partial agonist) effect at one opioid receptor subtype and an antagonist effect at another. The receptor-activating properties and

[*]In memory of Walter (Skip) Way, MD.

TABLE 31–1 Opioid receptor subtypes, their functions, and their endogenous peptide affinities.

Receptor Subtype	Functions	Endogenous Opioid Peptide Affinity
μ(mu)	Supraspinal and spinal analgesia; sedation; inhibition of respiration; slowed gastrointestinal transit; modulation of hormone and neurotransmitter release	Endorphins > enkephalins > dynorphins
δ(delta)	Supraspinal and spinal analgesia; modulation of hormone and neurotransmitter release	Enkephalins > endorphins and dynorphins
κ(kappa)	Supraspinal and spinal analgesia; psychotomimetic effects; slowed gastrointestinal transit	Dynorphins >> endorphins and enkephalins

affinities of opioid analgesics can be manipulated by pharmaceutical chemistry; in addition, certain opioid analgesics are modified in the liver, resulting in compounds with greater analgesic action. Chemically, the opioids derived from opium are phenanthrene derivatives and include four or more fused rings, while most of the synthetic opioids are simpler molecules.

Endogenous Opioid Peptides

Opioid alkaloids (eg, morphine) produce analgesia through actions at central nervous system (CNS) receptors that also respond to certain endogenous peptides with opioid-like pharmacologic properties. The general term currently used for these endogenous substances is **endogenous opioid peptides.**

Three families of endogenous opioid peptides have been described: the **endorphins,** the pentapeptide **enkephalins** (methionine-enkephalin **[met-enkephalin]** and leucine-enkephalin **[leu-enkephalin]**), and the **dynorphins.** These three families of endogenous opioid peptides have overlapping affinities for opioid receptors (see Table 31–1).

The endogenous opioid peptides are derived from three precursor proteins: prepro-opiomelanocortin (POMC), preproenkephalin (proenkephalin A), and preprodynorphin (proenkephalin B). POMC contains the met-enkephalin sequence, β-endorphin, and several nonopioid peptides, including adrenocorticotropic hormone (ACTH), β-lipotropin, and melanocyte-stimulating hormone. Preproenkephalin contains six copies of met-enkephalin and one copy of leu-enkephalin. Leu- and met-enkephalin have slightly higher affinity for the δ (delta) than for the μ-opioid receptor (see Table 31–1). Preprodynorphin yields several active opioid peptides that contain the leu-enkephalin sequence. These are **dynorphin A, dynorphin B,** and α and β **neoendorphins.** Painful stimuli can evoke release of endogenous opioid peptides under the stress associated with pain or the anticipation of pain, and they diminish the perception of pain.

In contrast to the analgesic role of leu- and met-enkephalin, an analgesic action of dynorphin A—through its binding to κ-opioid receptors—remains controversial. Dynorphin A is also found in the dorsal horn of the spinal cord. Increased levels of dynorphin occur in the dorsal horn after tissue injury and inflammation. This elevated dynorphin level is proposed to *increase* pain and induce a state of long-lasting *sensitization* and hyperalgesia. The pronociceptive action of dynorphin in the spinal cord appears to be independent of the opioid receptor system. Beyond their role in pain, κ-opioid receptor agonists can also function as antipruritic agents.

The principal receptor for this novel system is the G protein–coupled **orphanin opioid-receptor–like subtype 1 (ORL1).** Its endogenous ligand has been termed **nociceptin** by one group of investigators and **orphanin FQ** by another group. This ligand-receptor system is currently known as the *N/OFQ* system. Nociceptin is structurally similar to dynorphin except for the absence of an N-terminal tyrosine; it acts only at the ORL1 receptor, now known as **NOP.** The N/OFQ system is widely expressed in the CNS and periphery, reflecting its equally diverse biology and pharmacology. As a result of experiments using highly selective NOP receptor ligands, the N/OFQ system has been implicated in both pro- and antinociceptive activity as well as in the modulation of drug reward, learning, mood, anxiety, and cough processes, and of Parkinsonism.

Pharmacokinetics of Exogenous Opioids

Properties of clinically important opioids are summarized in Table 31–2.

A. Absorption

Most opioid analgesics are well absorbed when given by subcutaneous, intramuscular, and oral routes. However, because of the first-pass effect, the oral dose of the opioid (eg, morphine) to elicit a therapeutic effect may need to be much higher than the parenteral dose. As there is considerable interpatient variability in first-pass opioid metabolism, prediction of an effective oral dose is difficult. Certain analgesics such as codeine and oxycodone are effective orally because they have reduced first-pass metabolism. By avoiding first-pass metabolism, nasal insufflation of certain opioids can rapidly result in therapeutic blood levels. Other routes of opioid administration include oral mucosa via lozenges, and the transdermal route via patches. The latter can provide delivery of potent analgesics over days.

B. Distribution

The uptake of opioids by various organs and tissues is a function of both physiologic and chemical factors. Although all opioids bind to plasma proteins with varying affinity, the drugs rapidly leave the blood compartment and localize in highest concentrations in highly perfused tissues such as the brain, lungs, liver, kidneys, and spleen. Drug concentrations in skeletal muscle may be much lower, but this tissue serves as the main reservoir because of its greater bulk. Even though blood flow to fatty tissue is much lower than to the highly perfused tissues, accumulation can be very important, particularly after frequent high-dose administration or continuous infusion of highly lipophilic opioids that are slowly metabolized, eg, fentanyl.

TABLE 31–2 Common opioid analgesics.

Generic Name	Receptor Effects[1]			Approximately Equivalent Dose (mg)	Oral: Parenteral Potency Ratio	Duration of Analgesia (hours)	Maximum Efficacy
	μ	δ	κ				
Morphine[2]	+++		+	10	Low	4–5	High
Hydromorphone	+++			1.5	Low	4–5	High
Oxymorphone	+++			1.5	Low	3–4	High
Methadone	+++			10[3]	High	4–6	High
Meperidine	+++			60–100	Medium	2–4	High
Fentanyl	+++			0.1	Low	1–1.5	High
Sufentanil	+++	+	+	0.02	Parenteral only	1–1.5	High
Alfentanil	+++			Titrated	Parenteral only	0.25–0.75	High
Remifentanil	+++			Titrated[4]	Parenteral only	0.05[5]	High
Levorphanol	+++			2–3	High	4–5	High
Codeine	±			30–60	High	3–4	Low
Hydrocodone[6]	±			5–10	Medium	4–6	Moderate
Oxycodone[2,7]	++			4.5	Medium	3–4	Mod–High
Pentazocine	±		+	30–50	Medium	3–4	Moderate
Nalbuphine	–		++	10	Parenteral only	3–6	High
Buprenorphine	±	–	–	0.3	Low	4–8	High
Butorphanol	±		+++	2	Parenteral only	3–4	High

[1] +++, +++, +, strong agonist; ±, partial or weak agonist; –, antagonist.

[2] Available in sustained-release forms, morphine (MS Contin); oxycodone (OxyContin).

[3] No consensus—may have higher potency.

[4] Administered as an infusion at 0.025–0.2 mcg/kg/min.

[5] Duration is dependent on a context-sensitive half-time of 3–4 minutes.

[6] Available in tablets containing acetaminophen (Norco, Vicodin, Lortab, others).

[7] Available in tablets containing acetaminophen (Percocet); aspirin (Percodan).

C. Metabolism

The opioids are converted in large part to polar metabolites (mostly glucuronides), which are then readily excreted by the kidneys. For example, morphine, which contains free hydroxyl groups, is primarily conjugated to morphine-3-glucuronide (M3G), a compound with neuroexcitatory properties. The neuroexcitatory effects of M3G do not appear to be mediated by μ receptors and are under further study. In contrast, approximately 10% of morphine is metabolized to morphine-6-glucuronide (M6G), an active metabolite with analgesic potency four to six times that of its parent compound. However, these relatively polar metabolites have limited ability to cross the blood-brain barrier and probably do not contribute significantly to the usual CNS effects of a single dose of morphine. Importantly, accumulation of these metabolites may produce unexpected adverse effects in patients with renal failure or when exceptionally large doses of morphine are administered or high doses are administered over long periods. This can result in M3G-induced CNS excitation (seizures) or enhanced and prolonged opioid action produced by M6G. CNS uptake of M3G and, to a lesser extent, M6G can be enhanced by co-administration of probenecid or of drugs that inhibit the P-glycoprotein drug transporter.

1. *Hepatic P450 metabolism*—Hepatic oxidative metabolism is the primary route of degradation of the phenylpiperidine opioids (fentanyl, meperidine, alfentanil, sufentanil) and eventually leaves only small quantities of the parent compound unchanged for excretion. However, accumulation of a demethylated metabolite of meperidine, normeperidine, may occur in patients with decreased renal function and in those receiving multiple high doses of the drug. In high concentrations, normeperidine may cause seizures. In contrast, no active metabolites of fentanyl have been reported. The P450 isozyme CYP3A4 metabolizes fentanyl by *N*-dealkylation in the liver. CYP3A4 is also present in the mucosa of the small intestine and contributes to the first-pass metabolism of fentanyl when it is taken orally.

Codeine, oxycodone, and hydrocodone undergo metabolism in the liver by P450 isozyme CYP2D6, resulting in the production of metabolites of greater potency. For example, codeine is demethylated to morphine, which is then conjugated. Hydrocodone is metabolized to hydromorphone and, like morphine, hydromorphone is conjugated, yielding hydromorphone-3-glucuronide (H3G), which has CNS excitatory properties. Hydromorphone cannot form a 6-glucuronide metabolite. Similarly, oxycodone is metabolized to oxymorphone, which is then conjugated to oxymorphone-3-glucuronide (O3G).

Genetic polymorphism of CYP2D6 has been documented and linked to the variation in analgesic and adverse responses seen among patients. In contrast, the metabolites of oxycodone and hydrocodone may be of minor consequence; the parent compounds are currently believed to be directly responsible for the majority of their analgesic actions. However, oxycodone and its metabolites can accumulate under conditions of renal failure and have been associated with prolonged action and sedation. In the case of codeine, conversion to morphine may be of greater importance because codeine itself has relatively low affinity for opioid receptors. As a result, some patients (so-called poor metabolizers) may experience no significant analgesic effect. In contrast, there have been case reports of an exaggerated response to codeine due to enhanced metabolic conversion to morphine (ie, ultra-rapid metabolizers; see Chapters 4 and 5) resulting in respiratory depression and death. For this reason, routine use of codeine, especially in pediatric age groups, is now being eliminated in the United States.

The synthetic opioid methadone is metabolized through several CYP450 pathways, in part accounting for its highly variable bioavailability. The most important hepatic pathway for metabolism is CYP2B6.

Although genetic testing of CYP450 pathways is not common, these tests are available and becoming cheaper. Over the next several decades, personalized medicine will help patients who need opioids (and their prescribers) understand which opioids may not be good options for them.

2. *Plasma esterase metabolism*—Esters (eg, heroin, remifentanil) are rapidly hydrolyzed by common plasma and tissue esterases. Heroin (diacetylmorphine) is hydrolyzed to monoacetylmorphine and finally to morphine, which is then conjugated with glucuronic acid.

D. Excretion

Polar metabolites, including glucuronide conjugates of opioid analgesics, are excreted mainly in the urine. Small amounts of unchanged drug may also be found in the urine. In addition, glucuronide conjugates are found in the bile, but enterohepatic circulation represents only a small portion of the excretory process of these polar metabolites. In patients with renal impairment the effects of active polar metabolites should be considered before the administration of potent opioids such as morphine or hydromorphone—especially when given at high doses—due to the risk of sedation and respiratory depression.

Pharmacodynamics

A. Mechanism of Action

Opioid agonists produce analgesia by binding to specific G protein–coupled receptors (GPCRs) that are located in brain and spinal cord regions involved in the transmission and modulation of pain (Figure 31–1). Some effects may be mediated by opioid receptors on peripheral sensory nerve endings.

1. *Receptor types*—As noted previously, three major classes of opioid receptors (μ, δ, and κ) have been identified in various nervous system sites and in other tissues (see Table 31–1). Each of the three major receptors has now been cloned. All are members of the G protein–coupled family of receptors and show significant amino acid sequence homologies. Multiple receptor subtypes have been proposed based on pharmacologic criteria, including μ_1, μ_2; δ_1, δ_2; and κ_1, κ_2, and κ_3. However, genes encoding only one subtype from each of the μ, δ, and κ receptor families have thus far been isolated and characterized. One plausible explanation is that μ-receptor subtypes arise from alternate splice variants of a common gene. This idea has been supported by the identification of receptor splice variants in mice and humans, and a recent report pointed to the selective association of a μ-opioid receptor splice variant (MOR1D) with the induction of itch rather than the suppression of pain.

Since an opioid may function with different potencies as an agonist, partial agonist, or antagonist at more than one receptor class or subtype, it is not surprising that these agents are capable of diverse pharmacologic effects.

2. *Cellular actions*—At the molecular level, opioid receptors form a family of proteins that physically couple to G proteins and through this interaction affect ion channel gating, modulate intracellular Ca^{2+} disposition, and alter protein phosphorylation (see Chapter 2). The opioids have two well-established direct $G_{i/0}$ protein–coupled actions on neurons: (1) they close voltage-gated Ca^{2+} channels on presynaptic nerve terminals and thereby reduce transmitter release, and (2) they open K^+ channels and hyperpolarize and thus inhibit postsynaptic neurons. Figure 31–1 schematically illustrates these effects. The presynaptic action—depressed transmitter release—has been demonstrated for a large number of neurotransmitters, including glutamate, the principal excitatory amino acid released from nociceptive nerve terminals, as well as acetylcholine, norepinephrine, serotonin, and substance P.

3. *Relation of physiologic effects to receptor type*—The majority of currently available opioid analgesics act primarily at the μ-opioid receptor (see Table 31–2). Analgesia and the euphoriant, respiratory depressant, and physical dependence properties of morphine result principally from actions at μ receptors. In fact, the μ receptor was originally defined using the relative potencies for clinical analgesia of a series of opioid alkaloids. However, opioid analgesic effects are complex and include interaction with δ and κ receptors. This is supported in part by the study of genetic knockouts of the μ, δ, and κ genes in mice. The development of μ-receptor–selective agonists could be clinically useful if their side-effect profiles (respiratory depression, risk of dependence) were more favorable than those found with current μ-receptor agonists, such as morphine. Although morphine does act at κ and δ receptor sites, it is unclear to what extent this contributes to its analgesic action. The endogenous opioid peptides differ from most of the alkaloids in their affinity for the δ and κ receptors (see Table 31–1).

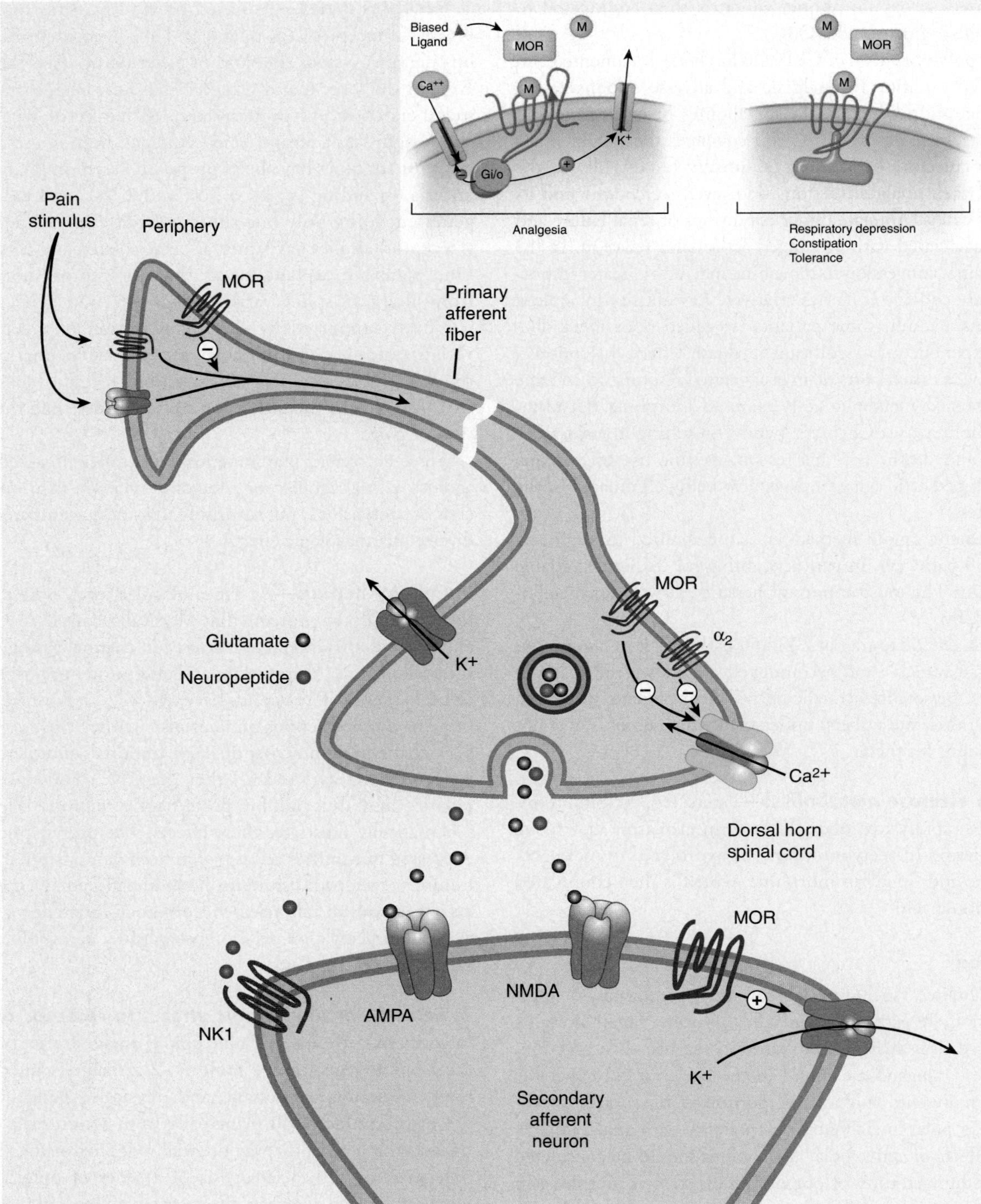

FIGURE 31–1 Potential receptor mechanisms of analgesic drugs. The primary afferent neuron (cell body not shown) originates in the periphery and carries pain signals to the dorsal horn of the spinal cord, where it synapses via glutamate and neuropeptide transmitters with the secondary neuron. Pain stimuli can be attenuated in the periphery (under inflammatory conditions) by opioids acting at μ-opioid receptors (MOR) or blocked in the afferent axon by local anesthetics (not shown). Action potentials reaching the dorsal horn can be attenuated at the presynaptic ending by opioids and calcium blockers (ziconotide), by α_2 agonists, and possibly, by drugs that increase synaptic concentrations of norepinephrine by blocking reuptake (tapentadol). Opioids also inhibit the postsynaptic neuron, as do certain neuropeptide antagonists acting at tachykinin (NK1) and other neuropeptide receptors. Inset: Morphine (M) binds and activates the μ-opioid receptor (MOR) coupling to $G_{i/o}$-mediated calcium channel inhibition and potassium channel activation. Analgesia (left) and β-arrestin–mediated side effects: respiratory depression, constipation, and tolerance (right). Biased ligand (closed triangle) targets a structural aspect of the MOR that facilitates $G_{i/o}$ coupling (analgesia) over β-arrestin (side effects).

In an effort to develop opioid analgesics with a reduced incidence of respiratory depression or propensity for addiction and dependence, compounds that show preference for κ-opioid receptors have been developed. Butorphanol and nalbuphine have shown some clinical success as analgesics, but they can cause dysphoric reactions and have limited potency. It is of interest that butorphanol has also been shown to cause significantly greater analgesia in women than in men. In fact, gender-based differences in analgesia mediated by μ- and δ-receptor activation have been widely reported.

Another approach to improve the therapeutic window of drugs that target opioid receptors is to develop opioid-like molecules that are analgesic but have significantly reduced adverse side effects (respiratory depression, constipation, and dependence). This effort is driven by structural studies of the mu opioid receptor that revealed different amino acid sequences, through which ligand binding to GPCRs influences multiple downstream signaling pathways. For example, morphine exerts its analgesic action via $G_{i/o}$ signaling, but adverse side effects are proposed to occur by engaging the β-arrestin pathway. To avoid the latter pathway, "biased agonists" have been developed that are biased toward G_i signaling (see Figure 31–1, inset). Comparable studies have targeted biased agonist development of kappa opioid receptor agonists that lack the dysphoric effects typical of KOR agonists but retain analgesic efficacy as well as profound anti-pruritogenic effects. Complementary to this approach are the synergistic combinations of opioids that also target peripheral opioid receptors. In light of reports that these biased agonists may, in fact, represent partial agonists, like buprenorphine, caution in interpreting the mechanism of action of these novel opioids is advised.

Another means to reduce opioid side-effects is based on reports of heterodimerization of different opioid receptors, eg, of the mu (MOR) and delta (DOR) opioid receptor. In this case, a hybrid MOR agonist and DOR antagonist retained analgesic action in the tail flick test, but tolerance and dependence were reduced compared to morphine. Other studies have reported heterodimerization between MOR and nonopioid receptors, eg, the nociceptin/orphanin F/Q receptor (NOP). Interestingly, a bifunctional peptide-based hybrid that exerts an agonist action at the MOR and the NOP produced significant analgesic effects with reduced adverse effects. More recently, heterodimers were identified between the MOR and the Gal1 subtype of galanin receptors, contributing a major source of dopamine to nucleus accumbens–mediated reward. Such MOR-GAL1 heterodimers have been implicated in the relatively low-rewarding properties of methadone compared with morphine. The implication is that development of opioid analgesics that preferentially target the MOR-GAL1 heterodimer may provide analgesia with significantly reduced misuse potential.

Of course, an alternative is to identify peripheral or CNS sites where selective targeting can increase the therapeutic window. To this end, recent studies reported that targeting the mu opioid receptor in the lateral habenula can exert significant analgesic actions without reward. Moreover, a rewarding effect only occurred in a pain model, presumably as a consequence of pain relief that may involve regulation of mesolimbic dopaminergic circuitry.

4. Receptor distribution and neural mechanisms of analgesia—Opioid receptor–binding sites have been localized autoradiographically with high-affinity radioligands and with antibodies to unique peptide sequences in each receptor subtype. All three major receptors are present in subregions of the central nervous system including the dorsal horn of the spinal cord. Receptors are present both on spinal cord pain transmission neurons and on the primary afferents that relay the pain message to them (Figure 31–2, sites A and B). Although opioid agonists directly inhibit dorsal horn pain transmission neurons, they also inhibit the release of excitatory transmitters from the primary afferents. Although there are reports that heterodimerization of the μ-opioid and δ-opioid receptors contributes to μ-agonist efficacy (eg, inhibition of presynaptic voltage-gated calcium channel activity), a recent study using a transgenic mouse that expresses a δ-receptor–enhanced green fluorescent protein (eGFP) fusion protein showed little overlap of μ receptor and δ receptor in dorsal root ganglion neurons. Importantly, the μ receptor is associated with TRPV1 and peptide (substance P)-expressing nociceptors, whereas δ-receptor expression predominates in the nonpeptidergic population of nociceptors, including many primary afferents with myelinated axons. This finding is consistent with the action of intrathecal μ-receptor– and δ-receptor–selective ligands

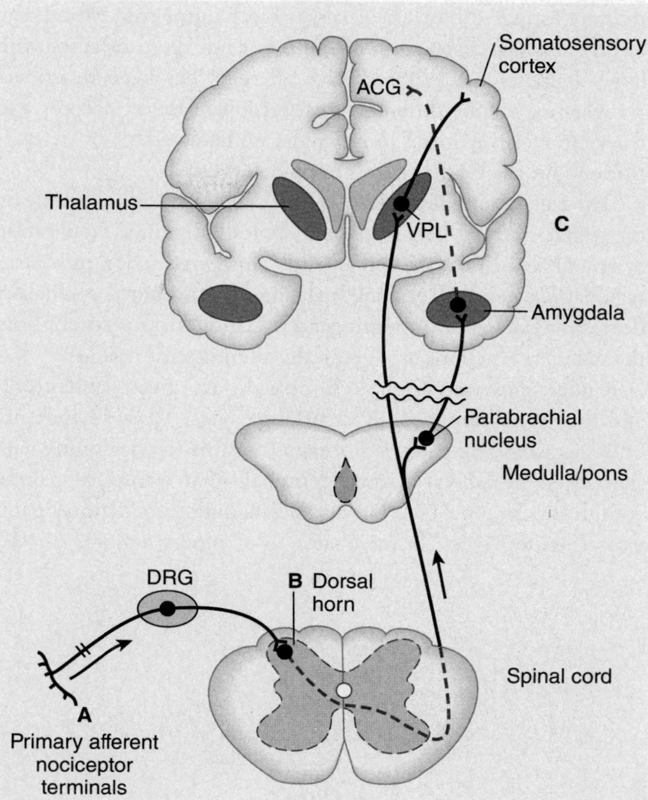

FIGURE 31–2 Putative sites of action of opioid analgesics. Sites of action on the afferent pain transmission pathway from the periphery to the higher centers are shown. **(A)** Direct action of opioids on inflamed or damaged peripheral tissues (see Figure 31–1 for detail). **(B)** Inhibition also occurs in the spinal cord (see Figure 31–1). **(C)** Possible site of action in the amygdala. ACG, anterior cingulate gyrus; DRG, dorsal root ganglion, VPL, ventral posterolateral nucleus of the thalamus.

that are found to block heat versus mechanical pain processing, respectively. An association of the δ but not the μ receptor with large diameter mechanoreceptive afferents has been described. To what extent the differential expression of the μ receptor and δ receptor in the dorsal root ganglia is characteristic of neurons throughout the CNS remains to be determined.

The fact that opioids exert a powerful analgesic effect directly on the spinal cord has been exploited clinically by direct application of opioid agonists to the spinal cord. This *spinal* action provides a regional analgesic effect while reducing the unwanted respiratory depression, nausea and vomiting, and sedation that may occur from the *supraspinal* actions of systemically administered opioids.

Under most circumstances, opioids are given systemically and thus act simultaneously at multiple sites. These include not only the ascending pathways of pain transmission beginning with specialized peripheral sensory terminals that transduce painful stimuli (see Figure 31–2) but also descending (modulatory) pathways (Figure 31–3). At these sites, as at others, opioids directly inhibit neurons; yet this action results in the *activation* of descending inhibitory neurons that send processes to the spinal cord and inhibit pain transmission neurons. This activation has been shown to result from the inhibition of inhibitory neurons in several locations (Figure 31–4). Taken together, interactions at these sites increase the overall analgesic effect of opioid agonists.

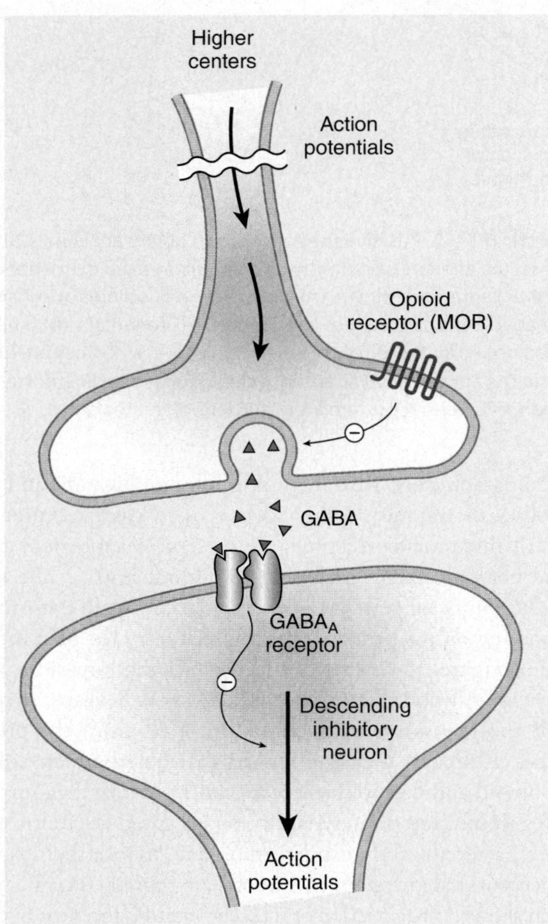

FIGURE 31–3 Brainstem local circuitry underlying the modulating effect of μ-opioid receptor (MOR)–mediated analgesia on descending pathways. The pain-inhibitory neuron is indirectly activated by opioids (exogenous or endogenous), which inhibit an inhibitory (GABAergic) interneuron. This results in *enhanced* inhibition of nociceptive processing in the dorsal horn of the spinal cord (see Figure 31–4).

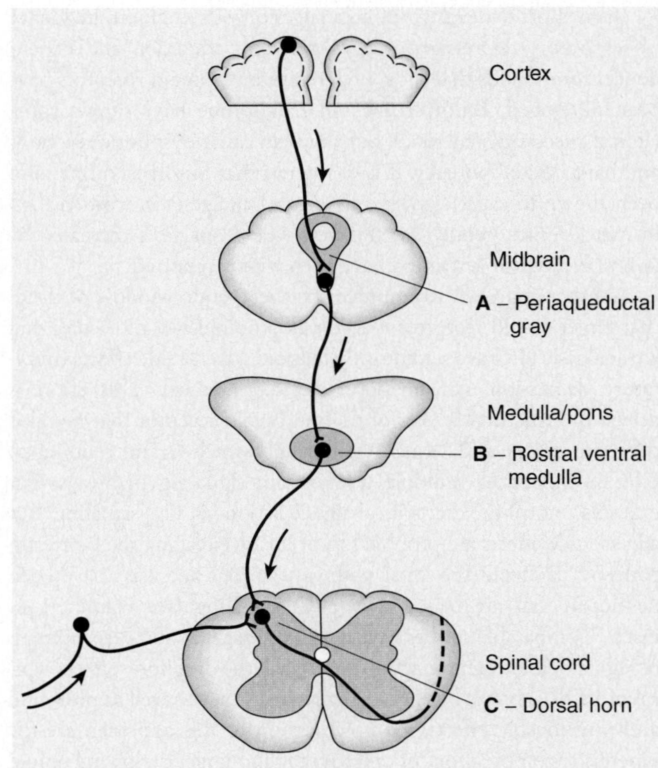

FIGURE 31–4 Opioid analgesic action on the descending inhibitory pathway. Sites of action of opioids on pain-modulating neurons in the midbrain and medulla including the midbrain periaqueductal gray area **(A)**, rostral ventral medulla **(B)**, and the locus coeruleus indirectly control pain transmission pathways by enhancing descending inhibition to the dorsal horn **(C)**.

Moreover, when pain-relieving opioid drugs are given systemically, they presumably act on neuronal circuits normally regulated by endogenous opioids. However, as morphine exerts its action mainly at the mu receptor, while enkephalins engage both mu and delta receptors, it is likely that different analgesia-mediating circuits may be activated by exogenous and endogenous opioids.

Animal and human clinical studies demonstrate that both endogenous and exogenous opioids can also produce analgesia at sites *outside* the CNS. Pain associated with inflammation seems especially sensitive to these peripheral opioid actions. The presence of functional μ receptors on the peripheral terminals of sensory neurons supports this hypothesis. Furthermore, activation of peripheral μ receptors results in a decrease in sensory neuron activity and transmitter release. The endogenous release of β-endorphin produced by immune cells within injured or inflamed tissue represents one source of physiologic peripheral μ-receptor activation. Intra-articular administration of opioids, eg, following arthroscopic knee surgery, has shown some clinical benefit for up to 24 hours. For this reason, opioids selective for a peripheral site of action may be useful adjuncts in the treatment of inflammatory pain (see Box: Ion Channels & Novel Analgesic Targets). Such compounds could have the additional benefit of reducing unwanted effects such as nausea. Also of interest is a recent report that a fentanyl analog that preferentially acts within an acidic environment (namely, diseased colon) can produce analgesia without the typical adverse side effects (constipation and respiratory depression). Interestingly, this compound produces reward that appears to be secondary to its peripheral pain-relieving properties.

5. *Tolerance and dependence*—With frequently repeated therapeutic doses of morphine or its surrogates, there is a gradual loss in effectiveness; this loss of effectiveness is termed tolerance. Attempts to reproduce the original analgesic response require a larger dose to be administered (with variable success). Along with tolerance, physical dependence develops. Physical dependence is defined as a characteristic **withdrawal** or **abstinence syndrome** when a drug is stopped or an antagonist is administered (see also Chapter 32).

The mechanism of development of opioid tolerance and physical dependence is poorly understood, but persistent activation of μ receptors such as occurs with the treatment of severe chronic pain appears to play a primary role in its induction and maintenance. Current concepts have shifted away from tolerance being driven by a simple up-regulation of the cyclic adenosine monophosphate (cAMP) system. Although this process is associated with tolerance, it is not sufficient to explain it. A second hypothesis for the development of opioid tolerance and dependence is based on the concept of **receptor recycling.** Normally, activation of μ receptors by endogenous ligands results in receptor endocytosis followed by resensitization and recycling of the receptor to the plasma membrane (see Chapter 2). However, using genetically modified mice, research now shows that the *failure* of morphine to induce endocytosis of the μ-opioid receptor is an important component of tolerance and dependence. In further support of this idea, methadone, a μ-receptor agonist used for the *treatment* of opioid tolerance and dependence, induces receptor endocytosis. This suggests that maintenance of normal sensitivity of μ receptors requires reactivation by endocytosis and recycling.

The concept of **receptor uncoupling** has also gained prominence. Under this hypothesis, tolerance results from a dysfunction of structural interactions between the μ receptor and G proteins, second-messenger systems, and their target ion channels. Uncoupling and recoupling of μ receptor function are likely linked to receptor recycling. Recent studies demonstrate that receptor internalization of GPCRs is not merely a step in recycling to the membrane or of receptor degradation. Rather, several G protein receptors, after their internalization, can reside and remain functional in cytoplasmic endosomes. This has been demonstrated for pronociceptive ligands (eg, CGRP, substance P, PAR2) and most recently for the delta opioid receptor, which could be engaged by ligands from patient-derived inflamed colon. The NMDA-receptor ion channel complex is also a significant contributor to tolerance development and maintenance. Consistent with this mechanism, NMDA-receptor antagonists such as ketamine can block tolerance development, in part by reducing descending medullary pain facilitatory mechanisms. These studies emphasize that the development of novel NMDA-receptor antagonists or other strategies to recouple μ receptors to their target ion channels provides hope for achieving a clinically effective means to prevent or reverse opioid analgesic tolerance.

Ion Channels & Novel Analgesic Targets

Even the most severe acute pain (lasting hours to days) can usually be controlled—with significant but tolerable adverse effects—using currently available analgesics, especially the opioids. However, chronic pain (lasting months to years) and especially pain arising from neuropathic causes are not very satisfactorily managed with opioids. It is now known that in chronic pain, receptors on sensory nerve terminals in the periphery contribute to increased excitability of these sensory endings (peripheral sensitization). The hyperexcitable sensory neuron bombards the spinal cord, leading to increased excitability and synaptic alterations in the dorsal horn (central sensitization). Such changes are likely important contributors to chronic inflammatory and neuropathic pain states.

In the effort to discover better analgesic drugs for chronic pain, renewed attention is being paid to the molecular basis of peripheral sensory transduction. Potentially important ion channels associated with the primary afferent nociceptor include members of the transient receptor potential family, notably the **capsaicin receptor TRPV1** (which is activated by multiple noxious stimuli such as heat, protons, and products of inflammation) and **TRPA1,** activated by inflammatory mediators, TRPM8, the receptor for menthol-mediated topical analgesia, and **P2X** receptors (which are responsive to purines released from tissue damage). Special subtypes of voltage-gated sodium channels **(Nav 1.7, 1.8, 1.9)** are uniquely associated with nociceptive neurons in dorsal root ganglia. **Lidocaine** and **mexiletine,** which are useful in some chronic pain states, may act by blocking this class of channels. Certain centipede toxins appear to selectively inhibit Nav 1.7 channels and may also be useful in the treatment of chronic pain. Genetic polymorphisms of Nav 1.7 are associated with either absence (congenital insensitivity to pain) or predisposition to pain (erythromelalgia or paroxysmal extreme pain disorder), and there may be a direct link between expressed levels of Nav 1.7 and enkephalin in sensory ganglia. Nav 1.9 is also currently under study as a therapeutic target. Because of the importance of their peripheral sites of action, therapeutic strategies that deliver agents that block peripheral pain transduction or transmission have been introduced in the form of transdermal patches and balms. In addition, products that systemically target peripheral TRPV1, TRPA1, TRPM8, and sodium channel function are in development.

Intrathecal administration of **ziconotide,** a blocker of voltage-gated N-type calcium channels, is approved for producing analgesia in patients with refractory chronic pain. Ziconotide is a synthetic peptide related to the marine snail toxin Ω-conotoxin, which selectively blocks N-type calcium channels. **Gabapentin/pregabalin,** anticonvulsants that act at the α2δ1 subunit of voltage-gated calcium channels, are effective treatments for neuropathic (nerve injury) pain and reduce opioid requirements postoperatively (see Chapter 24). *N*-methyl-D-aspartate (NMDA) receptors appear to play a very important role in central sensitization at both spinal and supraspinal levels. Although certain NMDA antagonists have demonstrated anti-hyperalgesic and analgesic activity (eg, **ketamine**), it has been difficult to find agents with an acceptably low profile of adverse effects or neurotoxicity. However, ketamine infused at very small doses reduces hyperalgesia and can reduce opioid requirements under conditions of opioid tolerance, eg, after major abdominal and spinal surgery. GABA and acetylcholine (through nicotinic receptors) appear to control the central synaptic release of several transmitters involved in nociception. Use of antibodies that bind nerve growth factor (NGF) has been shown to block inflammatory and back pain, but approval of their clinical use may be limited due to safety concerns. Finally, work on cannabinoids and vanilloids and their receptors suggests that **Δ9-tetrahydrocannabinol** (THC) as well as cannabidiol (CBD) and other minor cannabinoids, which act on CB_1 cannabinoid receptors and interact with the TRPV1 capsaicin receptor under certain circumstances, can synergize with μ-receptor agonists to produce analgesia.

As our understanding of peripheral and central pain transduction improves, additional therapeutic targets and strategies will become available. Combined with our present knowledge of opioid analgesics, a "multimodal" approach to pain therapy is paramount. Multimodal analgesia involves the administration of multiple agents (eg, COX-inhibitors or nonsteroidal anti-inflammatory drugs [NSAIDs], gabapentinoids (in select patients), and selective norepinephrine receptor inhibitors with complementary mechanisms of action to provide analgesia that is superior to that provided by an individual compound. Another benefit of multimodal analgesia is reduced opioid requirements with fewer serious adverse effects.

6. *Opioid-induced hyperalgesia (OIH)*—In addition to the development of tolerance, persistent administration of opioid analgesics can *increase* the sensation of pain, resulting in a state of hyperalgesia. This phenomenon can be produced with several opioid analgesics, including morphine, fentanyl, and remifentanil. Some studies have implicated a microglial-expressed opioid receptor or a metabolite of morphine that binds a microglial-expressed TL4 receptor in OIH. In contrast, an earlier report demonstrated that both opioid tolerance and OIH can be prevented by selective deletion of the MOR from primary sensory neurons, not from microglia. Spinal dynorphin and activation of the bradykinin and NMDA receptors have also emerged as important candidates for the mediation of opioid-induced hyperalgesia. This is one more reason why continuously administered opioids for *chronic* noncancer pain has been questioned.

B. Organ System Effects of Morphine and Its Surrogates

The actions described below for morphine, the prototypic opioid agonist, can also be observed with other opioid agonists, partial agonists, and those with mixed receptor effects. Characteristics of specific members of these groups are discussed below.

1. *Central nervous system effects*—The principal effects of opioid analgesics with affinity for μ receptors are on the CNS; the more important ones include analgesia, euphoria, sedation, and respiratory depression. With repeated use, a high degree of tolerance occurs to all of these effects (Table 31–3).

***a. Analgesia*—**Pain consists of both sensory and affective (emotional) components. Opioid analgesics are unique in that they can reduce both aspects of the pain experience. In contrast, nonsteroidal anti-inflammatory analgesic drugs, eg, ibuprofen, have no significant effect on the emotional aspects of pain.

***b. Euphoria*—**Typically, patients or intravenous drug users who receive intravenous morphine experience a pleasant floating sensation with lessened anxiety and distress. However, dysphoria, an unpleasant state characterized by restlessness and malaise, also may occur.

TABLE 31–3 Degrees of tolerance that may develop to some of the effects of the opioids.

High	Moderate	Minimal or None
Analgesia	Bradycardia	Miosis
Euphoria, dysphoria		Constipation
Mental clouding		Convulsions
Sedation		
Respiratory depression		
Antidiuresis		
Nausea and vomiting		
Cough suppression		

c. Sedation—Drowsiness and clouding of mentation are common effects of opioids. There is little or no amnesia. Sleep is induced by opioids more frequently in the elderly than in young, healthy individuals. Ordinarily, the patient can be easily aroused from this sleep. However, the combination of morphine with other central depressant drugs such as the sedative-hypnotics may result in very deep sleep. In standard analgesic doses, morphine (a phenanthrene) disrupts normal rapid eye movement (REM) and non-REM sleep patterns. This disrupting effect is probably characteristic of all opioids. In contrast to humans, a number of other species (cats, horses, cows, pigs) may manifest excitation rather than sedation when given opioids. These paradoxical effects are at least partially dose-dependent.

d. Respiratory depression—All of the opioid analgesics can produce significant respiratory depression by inhibiting brainstem respiratory mechanisms. Alveolar $Paco_2$ may increase, but the most reliable indicator of this depression is a depressed response to a carbon dioxide challenge. The respiratory depression is dose-related and is influenced significantly by the degree of sensory input occurring at the time. For example, it is possible to partially overcome opioid-induced respiratory depression by a variety of stimuli. When strongly painful stimuli that have prevented the depressant action of a large dose of an opioid are relieved, respiratory depression may suddenly become marked. A small to moderate decrease in respiratory function, as measured by $Paco_2$ elevation, may be well tolerated in the patient without prior respiratory impairment. However, in individuals with increased intracranial pressure, asthma, chronic obstructive pulmonary disease, or cor pulmonale, this decrease in respiratory function may not be tolerated. Opioid-induced respiratory depression remains one of the most difficult clinical challenges in the treatment of severe pain. Ongoing research to overcome this problem is focused on μ-receptor pharmacology, serotonin signaling pathways in the brainstem respiratory control centers, and agonist ligands biased toward Gi/o coupling.

e. Cough suppression—Suppression of the cough reflex is a well-recognized action of opioids. Codeine in particular has been used to advantage in persons suffering from pathologic cough. However, cough suppression by opioids may allow accumulation of secretions and thus lead to airway obstruction and atelectasis.

f. Miosis—Constriction of the pupils is seen with virtually all opioid agonists. Miosis is a pharmacologic action to which little or no tolerance develops, even in highly tolerant addicts (see Table 31–3); thus, it is valuable in the diagnosis of opioid overdose. This action, which can be blocked by opioid antagonists, is mediated by parasympathetic pathways, which, in turn, can be blocked by atropine.

g. Truncal rigidity—Several opioids can intensify tone in the large trunk muscles. It was originally believed that truncal rigidity involved a spinal cord action of these drugs, but a supraspinal action is likely. Truncal rigidity reduces thoracic compliance and thus interferes with ventilation. The effect is most apparent when high doses of the highly lipid-soluble opioids (eg, fentanyl, sufentanil, alfentanil, remifentanil) are rapidly administered intravenously. Truncal rigidity may be overcome by administration of an opioid antagonist, which of course will also antagonize the analgesic action of the opioid. Preventing truncal rigidity while preserving analgesia requires the concomitant use of neuromuscular blocking agents.

h. Nausea and vomiting—The opioid analgesics can activate the brainstem chemoreceptor trigger zone to produce nausea and vomiting. As ambulation seems to increase the incidence of nausea and vomiting there may also be a vestibular component in this effect.

i. Temperature—Homeostatic regulation of body temperature is mediated in part by the action of endogenous opioid peptides in the brain. For example, administration of μ-opioid receptor agonists, such as morphine to the anterior hypothalamus produces hyperthermia, whereas administration of κ agonists induces hypothermia.

j. Sleep architecture—Although the mechanism by which opioids interact with circadian rhythm is unclear, they can decrease the percentage of stage 3 and 4 sleep, which may result in fatigue and other sleep disorders, including sleep-disordered breathing and central sleep apnea.

2. Peripheral effects

a. Cardiovascular system—Most opioids have no significant direct effects on the heart and, other than bradycardia, no major effects on cardiac rhythm. Meperidine is an exception to this generalization because its antimuscarinic action can result in tachycardia. Blood pressure is usually well maintained in subjects receiving opioids unless the cardiovascular system is stressed, in which case hypotension may occur. This hypotensive effect is probably due to peripheral arterial and venous dilation, which has been attributed to a number of mechanisms including central depression of vasomotor-stabilizing mechanisms and release of histamine. No consistent effect on cardiac output is seen, and the electrocardiogram is not significantly affected. However, caution should be exercised in patients with decreased blood volume, because the above mechanisms make these patients susceptible to hypotension. Opioid analgesics affect cerebral circulation minimally except when Pco_2 rises as a consequence of respiratory depression. Increased Pco_2 leads to cerebral vasodilation associated with a decrease in cerebral vascular resistance, an increase in cerebral blood flow, and an increase in intracranial pressure.

b. Gastrointestinal tract—Constipation has long been recognized as an effect of opioids, an effect that does not diminish with continued use. That is, tolerance does not develop to opioid-induced constipation (see Table 31–3). Opioid receptors exist in high density in the gastrointestinal tract, and the constipating effects of the opioids are mediated through an action on the enteric nervous system (see Chapter 6) as well as the CNS. In the stomach, motility (rhythmic contraction and relaxation) may decrease but tone (persistent contraction) may increase—particularly in the central portion; gastric secretion of hydrochloric acid is decreased. Small intestine resting tone is increased, with periodic spasms, but the amplitude of nonpropulsive contractions is markedly decreased. In the large intestine, propulsive peristaltic waves are diminished and tone is increased; this delays passage of the fecal mass and allows increased absorption of water, which leads to constipation. The large bowel actions are the basis for the use of opioids in the management of diarrhea, and constipation is a major problem in the use of opioids for control of severe cancer pain. As described later, a new generation of agents designed to block or reverse opioid-induced constipation has been introduced.

c. Biliary tract—The opioids contract biliary smooth muscle, which can result in biliary colic. The sphincter of Oddi may constrict, resulting in reflux of biliary and pancreatic secretions and elevated plasma amylase and lipase levels.

d. Renal—Renal function is depressed by opioids. It is believed that in humans this is chiefly due to decreased renal plasma flow. In addition, μ receptor opioids have an antidiuretic effect in humans. Mechanisms may involve both the CNS and peripheral sites. Opioids also enhance renal tubular sodium reabsorption. The role of opioid-induced changes in antidiuretic hormone (ADH) release is controversial. Ureteral and bladder tone are increased by therapeutic doses of the opioid analgesics. Increased sphincter tone may precipitate urinary retention, especially in postoperative patients. Occasionally, ureteral colic caused by a renal calculus is made worse by opioid-induced increase in ureteral tone.

e. Uterus—The opioid analgesics may prolong labor. Although the mechanism for this action is unclear, both μ- and κ-opioid receptors are expressed in human uterine muscle. Fentanyl and meperidine (pethidine) inhibit uterine contractility but only at supraclinical concentrations; morphine had no reported effects. In contrast, the κ agonist [3H]-D-ala2,L-met5-enkephalinamide (DAMEA) inhibits contractility in human uterine muscle strips.

f. Endocrine—Opioids stimulate the release of ADH, prolactin, and somatotropin but inhibit the release of luteinizing hormone (see Table 31–1). These effects suggest that endogenous opioid peptides, through effects in the hypothalamus, modulate these systems. Patients receiving chronic opioid therapy can have low testosterone resulting in decreased libido, energy, and mood. Women can experience dysmenorrhea or amenorrhea.

g. Pruritus—The opiates, such as morphine and codeine, produce flushing and warming of the skin accompanied sometimes by sweating, urticaria, and itching. Although peripheral histamine release is an important contributor, all opioids can cause pruritus via a central (spinal cord and medullary) action on pruritoceptive neural circuits. When opioids are administered to the neuraxis by the spinal or epidural route, their usefulness may be limited by intense pruritus over the lips and torso. The incidence of opioid-induced pruritus via the neuraxial route is high, estimated at 70–100%. Of interest, the κ agonist/partial μ antagonist nalbuphine and the selective κ agonist nalfurafine have proved effective and in some countries have been approved for the management of itch. Nalfurafine importantly is a highly biased κ agonist that does not produce the dysphoria typical of κ receptor agonists. As to mechanism, a recent preclinical study implicated a κ opioid receptor–expressing medullospinal inhibitory circuit in these controls. On the other hand, with respect to pain regulation, other studies underscore the complex contribution of the κ receptor. Indeed, κ antagonists reportedly can attenuate pain in a preclinical migraine model.

h. Immune—The opioids modulate the immune system by effects on lymphocyte proliferation, antibody production, angioneogenesis, and chemotaxis. In addition, leukocytes migrate to the site of tissue injury and release opioid peptides, which in turn help counter inflammatory pain. However, natural killer cell cytolytic activity and lymphocyte proliferative responses to mitogens are usually inhibited by opioids, which may play a role in tumor progression. Although the mechanisms involved are complex, activation of central opioid receptors could mediate a significant component of the changes observed in peripheral immune function. These effects are mediated by the sympathetic nervous system in the case of acute administration and by the hypothalamic-pituitary-adrenal system in the case of prolonged administration of opioids.

■ CLINICAL PHARMACOLOGY OF THE OPIOID ANALGESICS

Successful management of pain is a challenging task that begins with assessment of and an attempt to understand the source and magnitude of the pain. Pain is an unpleasant sensory and emotional experience with many layers of complexity.

The amount of pain experienced by the patient is often measured by means of a pain numeric rating scale (NRS) or less frequently by marking a line on a 100-mm visual analog scale (VAS, which is more commonly used in research), as well as the verbal rating scale (VRS) with word descriptors ranging from no pain to excruciating pain. In each case, values indicate the magnitude of pain as mild (1–3), moderate (4–6), or severe (7–10). A similar scale can be used with children (Face, Legs, Activity, Cry, Consolability [FLACC] or Wong-Baker scales) and with patients who cannot speak; the Wong-Baker scale depicts five faces ranging from smiling (no pain) to crying (maximum pain). The Brief Pain Inventory is a series of questions regarding the severity of pain. Functional scales include the Oswestry Disability Index or the World Health Organization Disability Assessment Scale 2.0. There are specialized scales for patients with specific conditions including rheumatoid arthritis and dementia. More comprehensive questionnaires such as the McGill Pain Questionnaire address the multiple facets of pain including both the affective and sensory experience.

For a patient in severe acute pain, administration of an opioid analgesic is usually considered a primary part of the overall management plan. Determining the route of administration (oral, parenteral, neuraxial), duration of drug action, ceiling effect (maximal intrinsic activity), duration of therapy, potential for adverse effects, and the patient's past experience with opioids, including their genetics, social history, and family history, all should be addressed. One of the main principles in this process is to establish analgesic treatment goals before initiation of therapy. Just as important is the principle that following delivery of the therapeutic plan, its effectiveness must be monitored and reevaluated frequently, and the plan modified as necessary.

Use of opioid drugs in acute situations should be contrasted with their use in chronic pain management, in which a multitude of other factors must be considered, including the development of tolerance, dependence, and the rarer cases of diversion or misuse.

Clinical Use of Opioid Analgesics

A. Analgesia

Severe, *acute* pain is usually relieved with opioid analgesics having high intrinsic activity (see Table 31–2), whereas sharp, intermittent pain does not appear to be as effectively controlled.

The pain associated with cancer and other terminal illnesses typically involves a combination of mechanisms, must be treated aggressively, and often requires a multidisciplinary approach for effective management. Such conditions may require continuous use of potent opioid analgesics when cancer is active and/or invasive and when the conditions are associated with risk of tolerance and dependence. Importantly, use of multimodal analgesic strategies can reduce these risks. *However, this should not be used as a barrier to providing patients with the best possible care and quality of life.* The World Health Organization Ladder (see http://www.who.int/cancer/palliative/painladder/en/) was created in 1986 to promote awareness of the optimal treatment of pain for individuals with cancer and has helped improve pain care for cancer patients worldwide. Research in the hospice setting has also demonstrated that fixed-interval administration of opioid medication (ie, a regular dose at a scheduled time) is more effective in achieving pain relief than dosing on demand. Dosage forms of opioids that allow slower (sustained) release of the drug are now available, eg, sustained-release forms of morphine (MS Contin) and oxycodone (OxyContin). Their purported advantage is a longer and more stable level of analgesia. However, there is little to no evidence of the superiority of long-term (>3–6 months) use of sustained-release opioids to manage chronic noncancer or chronic low back, hip, or knee pain for 12 months when compared with nonopioid analgesic strategies. Alternately, attempts to control chronic pain with opioids alone may lead to excessive use, dependence and risk of **opioid use disorder (OUD),** overdose, and death (see Box: Educating Opioid Prescribers).

If disturbances of gastrointestinal function prevent the use of oral sustained-release morphine, then a fentanyl transdermal system (fentanyl patch) can be used over long periods. Furthermore, buccal transmucosal fentanyl can be used for short episodes of breakthrough cancer pain (see Alternative Routes of Administration). Administration of strong opioids by nasal insufflation also is efficacious, and nasal preparations are now available in some countries. Opioid analgesics are often used during obstetric labor. Because opioids cross the placental barrier and reach the fetus, care must be taken to minimize neonatal depression. If it occurs, immediate injection of the antagonist naloxone will reverse the depression. The phenylpiperidine drugs (eg, meperidine) appear to produce less depression, particularly respiratory depression, in newborn infants than does morphine; this may justify their use in obstetric practice.

The acute, severe pain of renal and biliary colic often requires a strong agonist opioid for adequate relief. However, the drug-induced increase in smooth muscle tone may cause a paradoxical *increase* in pain secondary to increased spasm.

B. Acute Pulmonary Edema

The relief produced by intravenous morphine in patients with dyspnea from pulmonary edema associated with left ventricular heart failure is remarkable. Proposed mechanisms include reduced anxiety (*perception* of shortness of breath) and reduced cardiac preload (reduced venous tone) and afterload (decreased peripheral resistance). However, if respiratory depression is a problem, a diuretic (furosemide) may be preferred for the treatment of pulmonary edema. On the other hand, morphine can be particularly useful when treating painful myocardial ischemia with pulmonary edema.

C. Cough

Suppression of cough can be obtained at doses lower than those needed for analgesia. However, in recent years, the use of opioid analgesics to allay cough has diminished largely because of the availability of a number of effective synthetic compounds that are neither analgesic nor addictive. These agents are discussed below.

D. Diarrhea

Diarrhea from almost any cause can be controlled with the opioid analgesics, but if diarrhea is associated with infection, such use must not substitute for appropriate treatment. Crude opium preparations (eg, paregoric) were used in the past to control diarrhea, but now synthetic surrogates with more selective gastrointestinal effects and few or no CNS effects, eg, diphenoxylate or loperamide, are used. Several preparations are available specifically for this purpose (see Chapter 62).

E. Shivering

Although all opioid agonists have some propensity to reduce shivering, meperidine is reported to have the most pronounced anti-shivering properties. Meperidine apparently blocks shivering mainly through an action on subtypes of the α_2 adrenoceptor.

F. Applications in Anesthesia

The opioids are frequently used as premedicant drugs before anesthesia and surgery because of their sedative, anxiolytic, and analgesic properties. They are also used intraoperatively as a part of induction, maintenance, and preparation for postoperative analgesia. Opioids are most commonly used in cardiovascular surgery and other types of high-risk surgery in which a primary goal is to minimize cardiovascular depression. In such situations, mechanical respiratory assistance must be provided.

Because of their direct action on the neurons of the superficial dorsal horn of the spinal cord, opioids can also be used as regional analgesics, by administration into the epidural or subarachnoid spaces of the spinal column. A number of studies have demonstrated that long-lasting analgesia with minimal adverse effects can be achieved by epidural administration of 3–5 mg of morphine, followed by slow infusion through a catheter placed in the epidural space. It was initially assumed that the epidural application of opioids might selectively produce analgesia without impairment of motor, autonomic, or sensory functions other than pain. However, respiratory depression can occur after the drug is injected into the epidural space and may require reversal with naloxone. Effects such as pruritus and nausea and vomiting are common after epidural and subarachnoid administration of opioids and may also be reversed with naloxone. The use of epidural opioids in combination with dilute solutions of local anesthetics is common practice for postoperative analgesia following thoracic and abdominal operations and can reduce the amount of systemic opioids, thereby reducing other opioid-related side effects such as sedation or constipation. In rare cases, chronic pain management specialists may elect to implant surgically a programmable infusion pump connected to a spinal catheter for continuous infusion of opioids and/or other analgesic compounds in chronic or cancer pain management.

G. Alternative Routes of Administration

Patient-controlled analgesia (PCA) is widely used for the management of breakthrough pain. With PCA, the patient controls a parenteral (usually intravenous) infusion device by pressing a button to deliver a preprogrammed dose of the desired opioid analgesic, called the **demand dose.** A programmable **lockout interval** prevents administration of another dose for a set period of time. In addition, the pumps can be programmed with a **continuous or basal infusion** (which should generally be avoided due to safety concerns unless directed by an experienced provider) and the **1-hour lockout dose** (the maximum amount of drug that can be delivered in 1 hour). Claims of better patient satisfaction are supported by well-designed clinical trials, making this approach very useful in postoperative pain control. However, healthcare personnel must be very familiar with the use of PCAs to avoid overdosage secondary to misuse or improper programming. There is a proven risk of PCA-associated respiratory depression and hypoxia that requires careful monitoring of vital signs and sedation level, and provision of supplemental oxygen. Continuous pulse oximetry is recommended for patients receiving PCA-administered opioids; this is not a fail-safe method for early detection of hypoventilation or apnea but rather serves as a safety net for an unrecognized adverse event. Monitoring of ventilation is ideal but is often inadequate. The risk of sedation is increased if medications with sedative properties, such as benzodiazepines and certain types of antiemetics, are concurrently prescribed.

Rectal suppositories of morphine and hydromorphone have been used when oral and parenteral routes are undesirable. The **transdermal fentanyl patch** is the most common full opioid agonist in transdermal application and is indicated primarily for the management of persistent unremitting cancer pain. It can provide more consistent blood levels of drug and potentially better pain control while avoiding the need for repeated or continuous parenteral (intravenous) injections. This may be especially important in patients unable to receive opioids via the enteral route due to limited GI function. Because of the complication of fentanyl-induced respiratory depression, the FDA recommends that introduction of a transdermal fentanyl patch (25 mcg/h) be reserved for patients with an established oral morphine requirement of at least 60 mg/d for 1 week or more. Extreme caution must be exercised in any patient initiating therapy or undergoing a dose increase because the peak effects may not be realized until 24–48 hours after patch application. Another alternative to parenteral administration is the **buccal transmucosal** route, which uses a fentanyl citrate lozenge or “lollipop” mounted on a stick for breakthrough cancer pain. The inclusion of the transdermal fentanyl patch for the treatment of chronic noncancer pain is associated with an increased risk of respiratory depression, tolerance, dependence, and opioid use disorder. Evidence is lacking for its superiority over nonopioid analgesic strategies in the treatment of chronic non-cancer pain and is often reserved for patients unable to be administered or absorb enteral opioid analgesics.

The buprenorphine patch (Butrans) is an example of the transdermal delivery of a mixed agonist-antagonist for the treatment of chronic pain in addition to opioid maintenance or detoxification. The **intranasal** route avoids repeated parenteral drug injections and the first-pass metabolism of orally administered drugs. Butorphanol is the only opioid currently available in the USA in a nasal formulation, but more are expected.

Toxicity & Undesired Effects

Direct toxic effects of the opioid analgesics that are extensions of their acute pharmacologic actions include respiratory depression, nausea, vomiting, and constipation (Table 31–4). Tolerance, dependence, diagnosis and treatment of overdosage, and contraindications must be considered.

TABLE 31–4 Adverse effects of the opioid analgesics.

Adverse Effects with Acute Use	Adverse Effects with Chronic Use
Respiratory depression	Hypogonadism
Nausea/vomiting	Immunosuppression
Pruritus	Increased feeding
Urticaria	Increased growth hormone secretion
Constipation	Withdrawal effects
Urinary retention	Tolerance, dependence
Delirium	Abuse, addiction
Sedation	Hyperalgesia
Myoclonus	Impairment while driving
Seizures	

A. Tolerance and Dependence

Drug dependence of the opioid type is marked by a relatively specific withdrawal or abstinence syndrome. Just as there are pharmacologic differences between the various opioids, there are reported differences in psychological dependence and the severity of withdrawal effects. Administration of an opioid *antagonist* to an opioid-dependent person is followed by brief but severe withdrawal symptoms (see antagonist-precipitated withdrawal, below). The potential for physical and psychological dependence of the partial agonist-antagonist opioids appears to be less than that of the strong agonist drugs.

1. *Opioid tolerance*—Opioid tolerance is the phenomenon whereby repeated doses of opioids have a diminishing analgesic effect. Clinically, it has been described as an increasing opioid dose requirement to achieve the analgesia observed at the initiation of opioid administration. Although development of tolerance begins with the first dose of an opioid, tolerance may not become clinically manifest until after 2–3 weeks of frequent exposure to ordinary therapeutic doses. Nevertheless, perioperative and critical care use of ultrapotent opioid analgesics such as remifentanil have been shown to induce opioid tolerance within hours. Tolerance develops most readily when potent opioids are given at short intervals and is minimized by giving small amounts of drug with longer intervals between doses.

Although a high degree of tolerance may develop to the analgesic, sedating, and respiratory depressant effects of opioid agonists (see Table 31–3), it is still possible to produce respiratory arrest in a tolerant (or nontolerant) person with clinically used doses of opioid analgesics—especially if concurrently administered with sedating drugs such as benzodiazepines. Tolerance also develops to the antidiuretic, emetic, and hypotensive effects but not to the miotic, convulsant, and constipating actions. Following discontinuation of opioids, loss of tolerance to the sedating and respiratory effects of opioids is variable and difficult to predict. However, tolerance to the emetic effects may persist for several months after withdrawal of the drug. Therefore, opioid tolerance differs by effect, drug, time, and the individual (genetic-epigenetic factors).

Tolerance also develops to analgesics with mixed receptor effects but to a lesser extent than to the agonists. Adverse effects such as hallucinations, sedation, hypothermia, and respiratory depression are reduced after repeated administration of the mixed receptor drugs. However, tolerance to the latter agents does not generally include cross-tolerance to the agonist opioids. It is also important to note that tolerance does not develop to the antagonist actions of the mixed agents or to those of the pure antagonists.

Cross-tolerance is an extremely important characteristic of the opioids, ie, patients tolerant to morphine often show a reduction in analgesic response to other agonist opioids. This is particularly true of those agents with primarily μ-receptor agonist activity. Morphine and its congeners exhibit cross-tolerance not only with respect to their analgesic actions but also to their euphoriant, sedative, and respiratory effects. However, the cross-tolerance existing among the μ-receptor agonists can often be partial or incomplete. This clinical observation has led to the concept of "opioid rotation," which has been used for many years in the treatment of cancer pain. A patient who is experiencing decreasing effectiveness of one opioid analgesic regimen is "rotated" to a different opioid analgesic (eg, morphine to hydromorphone; hydromorphone to methadone) and typically experiences significantly improved analgesia at a reduced overall equivalent dosage. Another approach is to recouple opioid receptor function as described previously through the use of adjunctive nonopioid agents. NMDA-receptor antagonists (eg, **ketamine**) have shown promise in preventing or reversing opioid-induced hyperalgesia and tolerance in animals and humans. Use of ketamine is increasing because well-controlled studies have shown clinical efficacy in reducing postoperative pain and opioid requirements in opioid-tolerant patients. Agents that independently enhance μ-receptor recycling may also hold promise for improving analgesia in the opioid-tolerant patient.

2. *Dependence*—The development of physical dependence is an invariable accompaniment of tolerance to repeated administration of an opioid of the μ type. Failure to continue administering the drug results in a characteristic withdrawal or abstinence syndrome that reflects an exaggerated rebound from the acute pharmacologic effects of the opioid.

The signs and symptoms of withdrawal include rhinorrhea, lacrimation, yawning, chills, gooseflesh (piloerection), hyperventilation, hyperthermia, mydriasis, muscular aches, vomiting, diarrhea, anxiety, and hostility. The number and intensity of the signs and symptoms are largely dependent on the degree of physical dependence that has developed. Administration of an opioid at this time suppresses abstinence signs and symptoms almost immediately.

The time of onset, intensity, and duration of abstinence syndrome depend on the drug previously used and may be related to its biologic half-life. With fentanyl, heroin, or morphine withdrawal signs may start within 6–10 hours after the last dose. Peak effects are seen at 36–48 hours, after which most of the signs and symptoms gradually subside. By 5 days, most of the effects have disappeared, but some may persist for months. In the case of meperidine, the withdrawal syndrome largely subsides within 24 hours, whereas with methadone several days are required to reach the peak of the abstinence syndrome, and it may last as long as 2 weeks. The slower subsidence of methadone effects is associated with a less intense immediate syndrome, and this is the basis for its use in the detoxification of heroin addicts. However, despite the loss of physical dependence on the opioid, craving for it may persist. In addition to methadone, buprenorphine and the α_2 agonist clonidine are FDA-approved treatments for opioid analgesic detoxification (see Chapter 32).

A transient, explosive abstinence syndrome—**antagonist-precipitated withdrawal**—can be induced in a subject physically dependent on opioids by administering naloxone, another antagonist, or even a partial μ agonist such as buprenorphine. Within seconds to minutes after injection of the antagonist naloxone, signs and symptoms similar to those seen after abrupt discontinuance appear, peaking in 10–20 minutes and largely subsiding after 1 hour. Even in the case of methadone, the antagonist-precipitated abstinence syndrome may be very severe.

In the case of agents with mixed effects, withdrawal signs and symptoms can be induced after repeated administration followed by abrupt discontinuance of pentazocine, cyclazocine, or nalorphine, but the syndrome appears to be somewhat different from that produced by morphine and other agonists. Anxiety, loss of appetite and body weight, tachycardia, chills, increase in body temperature, and abdominal cramps have been noted.

3. *Addiction*—As defined by the American Society of Addiction Medicine, addiction is a primary, chronic disease of brain reward, motivation, memory, and related circuitry. Dysfunction in these circuits leads to characteristic biologic, psychological, and social manifestations. This is reflected in an individual's pathologic pursuit of reward and relief through substance use and other behaviors. Addiction is characterized by inability to abstain, impairment in behavioral control exhibited by a compulsion to use, craving, diminished recognition of significant problems with one's behaviors and interpersonal relationships, use despite consequences, and a dysfunctional emotional response (see Chapter 32).

The risk of inducing dependence and, potentially, addiction is clearly an important consideration in the therapeutic use of opioid drugs. Although opioids administered to treat acute painful conditions such as trauma or surgical intervention are widely accepted as effective, recent reports suggest that even brief periprocedural exposures can increase the risk of long-term use. Therefore, certain principles should be observed by the clinician to minimize the potential harm presented by opioid-induced respiratory depression, dependence, misuse, or abuse:

- Consider using nonopioid analgesics whenever possible. Especially in chronic management, consider using other types of analgesics or compounds exhibiting less pronounced withdrawal symptoms on discontinuance.
- Frequently evaluate continuing analgesic therapy and the patient's need for opioids.
- Establish therapeutic goals before starting opioid therapy. This tends to limit the potential for physical dependence. The patient and his or her family should be included in this process.
- Once an effective dose is established, attempt to limit dosage to this level. This goal is facilitated by use of a written treatment contract that specifically prohibits early refills and having multiple prescribing physicians.
- Discuss the rights, responsibilities, and roles of patients and providers regarding controlled substances. Educate about safe opioid storage and disposal. Difficult decisions may need to be made about availability and use of opioid reversal medication (naloxone) for overdose, the proposed duration of opioid therapy, and the need for tapering or discontinuing opioid therapy.

B. Diagnosis and Treatment of Opioid Overdosage

Intravenous injection of naloxone dramatically reverses coma due to opioid overdose but not that due to other CNS depressants. Use of the antagonist should not, of course, delay the institution of other therapeutic measures, especially respiratory support. (See also The Opioid Antagonists, below, and Chapter 58.) The initial epidemic of prescription opioid overuse has been accompanied by an increase in heroin-related deaths and now an even greater wave of overdose deaths in the United States driven by synthetics such as fentanyl. For this reason, attention is being directed to make naloxone via intranasal and intramuscular routes widely available, including as over-the-counter formulations. With ever-increasing rates of ultrapotent synthetic opioids such as fentanyl-laced products illicitly being distributed in the USA, repeated doses of naloxone may be needed, with 10-fold higher doses, to reverse respiratory depression.

C. Contraindications and Cautions in Therapy

1. *Use of pure agonists with weak partial agonists*—When a weak partial agonist such as pentazocine is given to a patient also receiving a full agonist (eg, morphine), there is a risk of diminishing analgesia or even inducing a state of withdrawal; thus combining a full agonist with partial agonist opioids should be avoided.

2. *Use in patients with head injuries*—Carbon dioxide retention caused by respiratory depression results in cerebral vasodilation. In patients with elevated intracranial pressure, this may lead to lethal alterations in brain function.

3. *Use during pregnancy*—In pregnant women who are chronically using opioids, the fetus may become physically dependent in utero and manifest withdrawal symptoms in the early postpartum period. Daily doses of heroin, fentanyl, and/or polysubstance exposure taken by the mother can result in a withdrawal syndrome in the infant, including irritability, shrill crying, diarrhea, or even seizures. As a result of the opioid epidemic in the USA and other countries, the incidence of these events has dramatically increased. Recognition of the condition known as neonatal abstinence syndrome (NAS) is aided by a careful history, physical examination, and use of validated tools and severity scales. Treatment protocols have evolved and include symptom-based treatment guidelines ranging from increased nonpharmacologic approaches to opioid replacement therapy with morphine or possibly methadone or buprenorphine. Nonopioid adjuncts such as clonidine also have been utilized with positive effect. NAS care plans may also need modification given the possibility of neonatal exposure to multiple nonopioid drugs from the mother.

4. *Use in patients with impaired pulmonary function*—In patients with borderline respiratory reserve, the depressant properties of the opioid analgesics may lead to acute respiratory failure.

5. *Use in patients with impaired hepatic or renal function*—Because morphine and its congeners are metabolized primarily in the liver, their use in patients in prehepatic coma may be questioned. Half-life is prolonged in patients with impaired renal function, and morphine and its active glucuronide metabolite may accumulate; dosage can often be reduced in such patients.

6. *Use in patients with endocrine disease*—Patients with adrenal insufficiency (Addison disease) and those with hypothyroidism (myxedema) may have prolonged and exaggerated responses to opioids.

Drug Interactions

Because seriously ill or hospitalized patients may require a large number of drugs, there is always a possibility of drug interactions

TABLE 31–5 Opioid drug interactions.

Drug Group	Interaction with Opioids
Sedative-hypnotics	Increased central nervous system depression, particularly respiratory depression.
Antipsychotic agents	Increased sedation. Variable effects on respiratory depression. Accentuation of cardiovascular effects (antimuscarinic and α-blocking actions).
Monoamine oxidase inhibitors	Relative contraindication to all opioid analgesics and antitussives because of the high incidence of hyperpyrexic coma; hypertension also has been reported.

when the opioid analgesics are administered. Table 31–5 lists some of these drug interactions and the reasons for not combining the named drugs with opioids.

■ SPECIFIC AGENTS

The following section describes the most important and widely used opioid analgesics, along with features peculiar to specific agents. Data about doses approximately equivalent to 10 mg of intramuscular morphine, oral versus parenteral efficacy, duration of analgesia, and intrinsic activity (maximum efficacy) are presented in Table 31–2.

STRONG AGONISTS

Phenanthrenes

Morphine, hydromorphone, and **oxymorphone** are strong agonists useful in treating severe pain. These prototypic agents have been described in detail above.

Morphine

Heroin (diamorphine, diacetylmorphine) is potent and fast-acting, but its use is prohibited in the USA and Canada. Double-blind studies have not supported the claim that heroin is more effective than morphine in relieving severe pain, at least when given by the intramuscular route.

Phenylheptylamines

Methadone has undergone a dramatic revival as a potent and clinically useful analgesic. It can be administered by the oral, intravenous, subcutaneous and rectal routes. It is well absorbed from the gastrointestinal tract, and its bioavailability, although variable, far exceeds that of oral morphine.

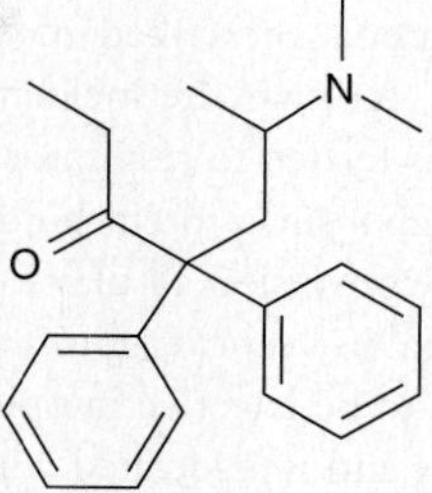

Methadone

Methadone is not only a potent μ-receptor agonist but its racemic mixture of D- and L-methadone isomers can also block both NMDA receptors and monoaminergic reuptake transporters. These nonopioid receptor properties may help explain its ability to relieve difficult-to-treat pain (neuropathic, cancer pain), especially when a previous trial of morphine has failed. In this regard, when analgesic tolerance or intolerable side effects have developed with the use of increasing doses of morphine or hydromorphone in progressive cancer pain, "opioid rotation" to methadone has provided superior analgesia at 10–20% of the morphine-equivalent daily dose. In contrast to its use in suppressing symptoms of opioid withdrawal, use of methadone as an analgesic typically requires administration at more frequent intervals (eg, 8 hours). However, given methadone's highly variable pharmacokinetics and long half-life (~25–52 hours), the initial administration period (loading phase) should be closely monitored to avoid potentially harmful adverse effects, especially respiratory depression. Because methadone is metabolized by CYP2B6 and CYP3A4 isoforms in the liver, inhibition of its metabolic pathway or hepatic dysfunction has also been associated with overdose effects, including respiratory depression or prolonged QT-based cardiac arrhythmias.

Methadone has been widely used in the treatment of opioid use disorders. Tolerance and physical dependence develop more slowly with methadone than with morphine. The withdrawal signs and symptoms occurring after abrupt discontinuance of methadone are often milder, although more prolonged, than those of morphine. In many cases, these properties make methadone a useful drug for detoxification and for maintenance of chronic relapsing opioid use disorder.

For detoxification of a heroin-dependent person, low doses of methadone (5–10 mg orally) have been given two or three times daily for 2 or 3 days to lessen the subsequent withdrawal syndrome.

For maintenance therapy of the opioid recidivist, tolerance to 50–100 mg/d of oral methadone may be deliberately produced; in this state, opioid craving is diminished and there is a cross-tolerance to heroin to limit the addiction-reinforcing effects of heroin. One rationale of maintenance programs is that blocking the reinforcement obtained from illicit opioids removes the drive to obtain them, thereby reducing criminal activity and making the user more amenable to psychiatric and rehabilitative therapy. The pharmacologic basis for the use of methadone in maintenance programs is sound, and the sociologic basis is rational.

The concurrent administration of methadone to heroin addicts known to be recidivists has been questioned because of the increased risk of overdose death secondary to respiratory arrest. As the number of patients prescribed methadone for persistent pain has increased, so, too, has the incidence of accidental overdose and complications related to respiratory depression. Variability in methadone metabolism, protein binding, distribution, and nonlinear opioid dose conversion all play a role in adverse events. Buprenorphine, a partial μ-receptor agonist with long-acting properties, has been found to be effective in opioid detoxification and maintenance programs and is associated with a lower risk of such overdose fatalities. To increase the access of persons with OUD, in the USA, a provider with a controlled substance DEA license may prescribe buprenorphine for OUD.

With the increase in access and legalization of cannabis products in many states in the USA, some authorities have suggested the use of cannabis as a treatment for OUD or to facilitate tapering of opioids. However, there is no strong evidence to support these proposals.

Phenylpiperidines

Fentanyl is one of the most widely used agents in the family of synthetic opioids. The fentanyl subgroup now includes **sufentanil, alfentanil,** and **remifentanil** in addition to the parent compound, fentanyl. An extremely potent analog, **carfentanil,** is used in veterinary medicine for sedating large mammals, eg, elephants. Adulteration of street heroin and counterfeit prescription analgesic pills with fentanyl, carfentanil, or related synthetics has been responsible for a dramatic increase of unintended overdoses and deaths.

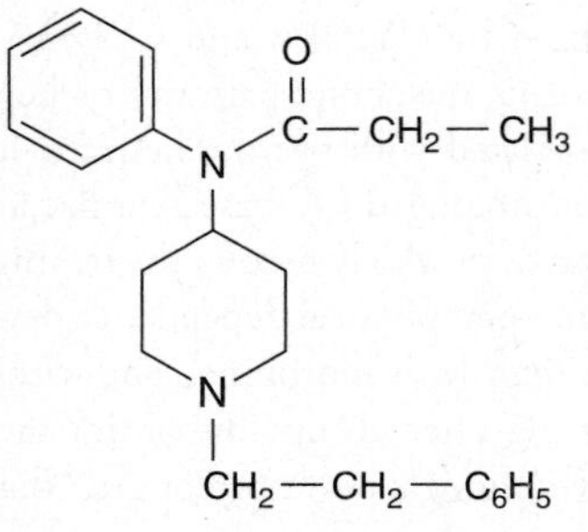

O
C — CH_2 — CH_3
N
N
CH_2 — CH_2 — C_6H_5

Fentanyl

Among the phenylpiperidines, these opioids differ mainly in their potency and biodisposition. Sufentanil is five to seven times more potent than fentanyl. Carfentanil is approximately 100 times more potent than fentanyl. Alfentanil is considerably less potent than fentanyl but acts more rapidly and has a markedly shorter duration of action. Remifentanil is metabolized very rapidly by blood and nonspecific tissue esterases, making its pharmacokinetic and pharmacodynamic half-lives extremely short. Such properties are useful when these compounds are used in anesthesia practice. Although fentanyl is now the predominant analgesic in the phenylpiperidine class, **meperidine** continues to be used. This older opioid has significant antimuscarinic effects, which may be a contraindication if tachycardia would be a problem. Meperidine is also reported to have a negative inotropic action on the heart. In addition, it has the potential for producing seizures secondary to accumulation of its metabolite, normeperidine, in patients receiving high doses or with concurrent renal failure. Given this undesirable profile, use of meperidine as a first-line analgesic is becoming increasingly rare.

Morphinans

Levorphanol is a synthetic opioid analgesic closely resembling morphine and has μ-, δ-, and κ-opioid agonist actions, serotonin-norepinephrine reuptake inhibition, and NMDA receptor antagonist properties.

MILD TO MODERATE AGONISTS

Phenanthrenes

Codeine, dihydrocodeine, and **hydrocodone** have lower binding affinity to μ-opioid receptors than morphine and often have adverse effects that limit the maximum tolerated dose when one attempts to achieve analgesia comparable to that of morphine.

Oxycodone is more potent and is prescribed alone in higher doses as immediate-release or controlled-release forms for the treatment of moderate to severe pain. Combinations of hydrocodone or oxycodone with acetaminophen are the predominant formulations of orally administered analgesics in the United States for the treatment of mild to moderate pain. Since each controlled-release tablet of oxycodone contains a large quantity of oxycodone to allow for prolonged action, those intent on abusing the old formulation have extracted crushed tablets and injected high doses, resulting in misuse and possible fatal overdose. In 2010, the FDA approved a new formulation of the controlled-release form of oxycodone that reportedly prevents the tablets from being cut, broken, chewed, crushed, or dissolved to release more oxycodone. It is hoped that this new formulation will lead to less misuse by snorting or injection. The FDA is now requiring a Risk Evaluation and Mitigation Strategy (REMS) that will include the issuance of a medication guide to patients and a requirement for prescriber education regarding the appropriate use of opioid analgesics in the treatment of pain. (See Box: Educating Opioid Prescribers.)

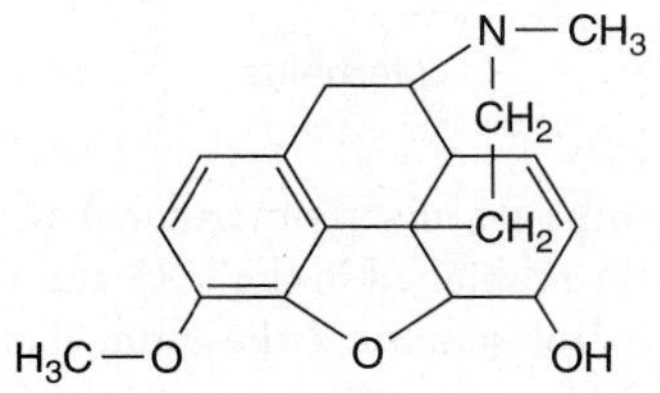

N — CH_3
CH_2
CH_2
H_3C — O
O
OH

Codeine

Phenylheptylamines

Propoxyphene is chemically related to methadone but has extremely low analgesic activity. Its low efficacy makes it unsuitable, even in combination with aspirin, for severe pain.

The increasing incidence of deaths associated with its use and misuse caused it to be withdrawn in the United States.

Phenylpiperidines

Diphenoxylate and its metabolite, **difenoxin,** are not used for analgesia but for the treatment of diarrhea. They are scheduled for minimal control (difenoxin is Schedule IV or V, depending on formulation; diphenoxylate Schedule V; see inside front cover) because the likelihood of their misuse is remote. The poor solubility of the compounds limits their use for parenteral injection. As antidiarrheal drugs, they are used in combination with atropine. The atropine is added in a concentration too low to have a significant antidiarrheal effect but is presumed to further reduce the likelihood of misuse.

Loperamide is a phenylpiperidine derivative used to control diarrhea. Due to action on peripheral μ-opioid receptors and lack of effect on CNS receptors, investigations are ongoing as to whether it could be an effective analgesic. Its potential for misuse is considered very low because of its limited access to the brain. It is therefore available without a prescription.

The usual dose with all of these antidiarrheal agents is two tablets to start and then one tablet after each diarrheal stool.

OPIOIDS WITH MIXED RECEPTOR ACTIONS

Partial agonists may be used in situations where patients may benefit from the profile of the drug compared with full agonists. An example would be for patients who find full μ agonists to be too "strong" and therefore prefer a partial agonist. Care should be taken to administer any partial agonist or drug with mixed opioid receptor actions to patients receiving pure opioid agonists because of the unpredictability of both drugs' effects; reduction of analgesia or precipitation of an explosive abstinence syndrome may result.

Educating Opioid Prescribers—The Opioid Epidemic

The treatment of chronic pain is a difficult biopsychosocial problem, and prescribers of opioids have been caught between a number of competing forces in their attempts to relieve pain and suffering. The USA is the largest user of prescription opioids of any country and continues to experience an epidemic of opioid-related harm and death that has worsened under the SARS- COVID pandemic. Drug overdose is now the leading cause of injury-related deaths in the USA. Following a tidal wave of opioid prescriptions driven by subsequent opioid use disorder (OUD), more than 68,000 died from an opioid overdose in 2020, a leap from nearly 50,000 opioid-related deaths in 2019 and more than 16,000 deaths related to prescription opioids (wonder.cdc.gov). Overall, more than 100,000 deaths from 2020–2021 are attributed to drug overdose with opioids as the primary cause. The line between deaths from illicit versus prescription opioids is blurred since some patients may choose to cross from one opioid to another. In contrast, in several countries the medical use of opioids is prohibited or severely limited, resulting in unmanaged pain after surgery or trauma and near the end of life. Forces that have influenced excessive prescribing of opioids for chronic noncancer pain in the USA include aggressive marketing of opioids, misleading industry-led education on the abuse and addiction potential of opioids, an unjustified assumption of the superiority of opioids over nonopioid therapies for the treatment of chronic noncancer pain, and a paucity of safe, effective, and affordable (covered or reimbursed by insurance) analgesic strategies that have low abuse potential. These findings prompted the Centers for Disease Control (CDC) to create the first Opioid Prescribing Guidelines for Primary Care Prescribers caring for patients with chronic noncancer pain in 2016 that was revised in 2022 (https://www.cdc.gov/mmwr/volumes/71/rr/rr7103a1.htm?s_cid=rr7103a1.htm_w. The US Health and Human Services Interagency Task Force also completed a "Pain Management Best Practices" guide (https://www.hhs.gov/sites/default/files/overview-pmtf-final-report-fact-sheet_508.pdf that integrates input from a comprehensive consortium of governmental and nongovernmental health professional societies. The FDA has also instituted training programs such as a risk evaluation and mitigation strategy (REMS) program for all potent opioid prescribing to help providers better understand potential benefits versus risks of prescription opioids. State medical boards in the USA are establishing their own regulations in addition to creating prescription drug monitoring programs (PDMPs). The US Drug Enforcement Agency has focused efforts on illicit practices and distribution patterns with concerns about diversion. Major efforts to expand research in this domain are now supported through the National Institutes of Health program Helping End Addiction Long Term (HEAL). Litigation of the opioid and drug distribution industry is underway to obtain resources to support prevention and treatment and of OUD in the USA.

Prescribers are advised to learn about the local, state, and national guidelines and laws for the prescribing and monitoring of patients on opioids. A major concern from 2015 to 2019 data has been the number of fentanyl- and heroin-related deaths in persons suffering from OUD. This has resulted from opioids (counterfeit prescription pills, heroin) dealt "on the street" that have been adulterated with the much more potent fentanyl to increase effect. While law-enforcement efforts have been made to reduce supply, it may be more effective to reduce demand. Paramount in such reduction will be the use of multimodal nonopioid strategies in the management of chronic noncancer pain, appropriate opioid tapering, access to opioid maintenance programs, investment in addiction medicine, and development of analgesics without abuse liability.

Phenanthrenes

As noted above, **buprenorphine** is a potent and long-acting phenanthrene derivative that is a partial μ-receptor agonist (low intrinsic activity) and an *antagonist* at the δ and κ receptors and is therefore referred to as a mixed agonist-antagonist. Although buprenorphine is used as an analgesic, it can antagonize the action of more potent μ agonists such as morphine. Buprenorphine also binds to ORL1, the orphanin receptor. Whether this property also participates in opposing μ receptor function is under study. Administration by the sublingual route is preferred to avoid significant first-pass effect. Buprenorphine's long duration of action is due to its slow dissociation from μ receptors. This property renders its effects resistant to naloxone reversal. Buprenorphine was approved by the FDA in 2002 for the management of opioid dependence, and studies suggest it is as effective as methadone for the management of opioid withdrawal and detoxification in programs that include counseling, psychosocial support, and direction by physicians qualified under the Drug Addiction Treatment Act. In the USA, a special Drug Enforcement Administration (DEA) waiver and training were needed to legally prescribe buprenorphine for addiction. In contrast to methadone, high-dose administration of buprenorphine results in a μ-opioid *antagonist* action, limiting its properties of analgesia and respiratory depression. However, buprenorphine formulations can still cause serious respiratory depression and death, particularly when extracted and injected intravenously in combination with benzodiazepines or used with other CNS depressants (ie, sedatives, antipsychotics, or alcohol). Buprenorphine is also available combined with naloxone, a pure μ-opioid antagonist (as Suboxone), to help prevent its diversion for illicit intravenous misuse. A slow-release transdermal patch preparation that releases drug over a 1-week period also is available (Butrans). The FDA has also approved an implanted buprenorphine rod (Probuphine) that lasts for 6 months and is meant to deter misuse. Psychotomimetic effects, with hallucinations, nightmares, and anxiety, have been reported after use of drugs with mixed agonist-antagonist actions.

The management of acute postsurgical pain may be challenging in the patient who is on chronic buprenorphine, as its high affinity for the μ-opioid receptor may render commonly used opioid agonists ineffective for pain management. The current recommendation is for these patients to continue their buprenorphine and employ nonopioid modalities to the greatest degree while educating patients on expectations. In certain cases where the surgical intervention is expected to result in severe postoperative pain not manageable with ongoing buprenorphine, a supervised reduction by tapering the dose may be indicated prior to surgery but rarely if ever should be stopped. Taken together, higher doses of opioids may be needed in situations where pain is severe and concurrent regional anesthetic techniques (nerve blocks) are not available. Patients need to be monitored for risk of relapse and ideally be followed closely by an addiction medicine specialist or counselor.

Kratom, an extract from the leaves of *Mitragyna speciosa*, has come into public view with various claims of its efficacy in opioid tapering or opioid replacement therapy. Although very limited preclinical research on its component alkaloids, mitragynine and 7-hydroxymitragynine, suggests that they can act as partial μ-receptor agonists, a multitude of other effects and harms have been associated with kratom (*Salmonella* bacterial poisoning, hallucinations, seizures, coma, and death). Given the lack of proven benefit and increasing reports of harm, kratom is not considered either safe or effective. Nevertheless, additional studies on kratom may reveal important mechanistic insights useful for future therapeutic development.

Pentazocine (a benzomorphan) and **nalbuphine** are other examples of opioid analgesics with mixed agonist-antagonist properties. Nalbuphine is a strong κ-receptor *agonist* and a partial μ-receptor *antagonist;* it is given parenterally. At higher doses there seems to be a definite ceiling—not noted with morphine—to the respiratory depressant effect. Unfortunately, when respiratory depression does occur, it may be relatively resistant to naloxone reversal due to its greater affinity for the receptor than naloxone. Nalbuphine is equipotent to morphine for analgesia and, at lower doses, can sometimes be effective for pruritus caused by opioids and nonopioids.

Morphinans

Butorphanol produces analgesia equivalent to nalbuphine but appears to produce more sedation at equianalgesic doses. Butorphanol is considered to be predominantly a κ agonist. However, it may also act as a partial agonist or antagonist at the μ receptor.

Benzomorphans

Pentazocine is a κ agonist with weak μ-antagonist or partial agonist properties. It is the oldest mixed agent available. It may be used orally or parenterally. However, because of its irritant properties, the injection of pentazocine subcutaneously is not recommended.

MISCELLANEOUS

Tramadol is a centrally acting analgesic whose mechanism of action is also dependent on the ability of the parent drug and its metabolites to block serotonin and norepinephrine reuptake. Because its analgesic effect is only weakly antagonized by naloxone, it is thought to depend less on its low-affinity binding to the μ receptor for therapeutic activity. The recommended dosage is 50–100 mg orally four times daily; however, its systemic concentration and analgesic effect are dependent on its variable metabolism by CYP2D6 polymorphisms. Toxicity includes association with seizures; the drug is relatively contraindicated in patients with a history of epilepsy and for use with other drugs that lower the seizure threshold. Another serious risk is the development of serotonin syndrome, especially if selective serotonin reuptake inhibitor antidepressants are being administered (see Chapter 16). Other adverse effects include nausea and dizziness, but these symptoms typically abate after several days of therapy. No clinically significant effects on respiration or the cardiovascular system have thus far been reported when used as monotherapy. Given the fact that the analgesic action of tramadol is largely independent of μ-receptor action, tramadol has been considered as an adjunct in the treatment of neuropathic pain; however, this is based on low-quality studies of short duration.

Tapentadol is an analgesic with modest μ-opioid receptor affinity and significant norepinephrine reuptake-inhibiting action. In animal models, its analgesic effects were only moderately reduced by naloxone but strongly reduced by an α_2-adrenoceptor antagonist. Furthermore, its binding to the norepinephrine transporter (NET, see Chapter 6) was stronger than that of tramadol, whereas its binding to the serotonin transporter (SERT) was less than that of tramadol. Tapentadol was approved in 2008 and has been shown to be as effective as oxycodone in the treatment of moderate to severe pain but with a reduced profile of gastrointestinal complaints such as nausea. Clinical studies are ongoing to determine if the lack of active metabolites and lower risk of serotonin syndrome with tapentadol will translate to an improvement in analgesia with reduced adverse effects.

ANTITUSSIVES

The opioid analgesics are among the most effective drugs available for the suppression of cough. This effect is often achieved at doses below those necessary to produce analgesia. The receptors involved in the antitussive effect appear to differ from those associated with the other actions of opioids. For example, the antitussive effect is also produced by stereoisomers of opioid molecules that are devoid of analgesic effects and addiction liability (see below).

The physiologic mechanism of cough is complex, and little is known about the specific mechanism of action of the opioid antitussive drugs. It appears likely that both central and peripheral effects play a role.

The opioid derivatives most commonly used as antitussives are **dextromethorphan, codeine, levopropoxyphene,** and **noscapine** (levopropoxyphene and noscapine are not available in the USA). They should be used with caution in patients taking monoamine oxidase inhibitors (see Table 31–5). Antitussive preparations usually also contain expectorants to thin and liquefy respiratory secretions. Importantly, due to increasing reports of death in young children taking dextromethorphan in formulations of over-the-counter "cold/cough" medications, its use in children younger than 6 years of age has been banned by the FDA. Moreover, because of variations in the metabolism of codeine, its use for any purpose in young children is being reconsidered.

Dextromethorphan is the dextrorotatory stereoisomer of a methylated derivative of levorphanol. It is purported to be free of addictive properties and produces less constipation than codeine. The usual antitussive dose is 15–30 mg three or four times daily. It is available in many over-the-counter products. Dextromethorphan has also been found to enhance the analgesic action of morphine and presumably other μ-receptor agonists. However, misuse of its purified (powdered) form has been reported to lead to serious adverse events including death.

Codeine, as noted, has a useful antitussive action at doses lower than those required for analgesia. Thus, 15 mg is usually sufficient to relieve cough.

Levopropoxyphene is the stereoisomer of the weak opioid agonist dextropropoxyphene. It is devoid of opioid effects, although sedation has been described as a side effect. The usual antitussive dose is 50–100 mg every 4 hours.

THE OPIOID ANTAGONISTS

The pure opioid antagonist drugs **naloxone, naltrexone,** and **nalmefene** are morphine derivatives with bulkier substituents at the N_{17} position. These agents have a relatively high affinity for μ-opioid binding sites. They have lower affinity for the other receptors but can also reverse agonists at δ and κ sites.

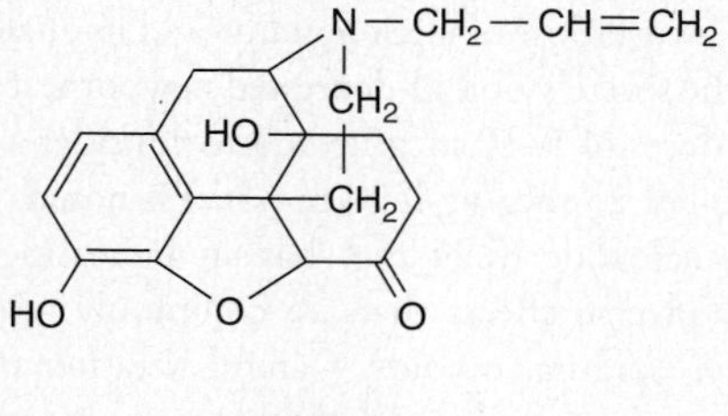

Naloxone

Pharmacokinetics

Naloxone is usually given by injection and has a short duration of action (1–2 hours) when given by this route. Metabolic disposition is chiefly by glucuronide conjugation like that of the agonist opioids with free hydroxyl groups. Naltrexone is well absorbed after oral administration but may undergo rapid first-pass metabolism. It has a half-life of 10 hours, and a single oral dose of 100 mg blocks the effects of injected heroin for up to 48 hours. Nalmefene, the newest of these agents, is a derivative of naltrexone but is available only for intravenous administration. Like naloxone, nalmefene is used for opioid overdose but has a longer half-life (8–10 hours).

Pharmacodynamics

When given in the absence of an agonist drug, these antagonists are almost inert at doses that produce marked antagonism of agonist opioid effects.

When given intravenously to a morphine-treated subject, the antagonist completely and dramatically reverses the opioid effects within 1–3 minutes. In individuals who are acutely depressed by an overdose of an opioid, the antagonist effectively normalizes respiration, level of consciousness, pupil size, bowel activity, and awareness of pain. In dependent subjects who appear normal while taking opioids, naloxone or naltrexone almost instantaneously precipitates an abstinence syndrome.

There is no tolerance to the antagonistic action of these agents, nor does withdrawal after chronic administration precipitate an abstinence syndrome.

Clinical Use

Naloxone is a pure antagonist and is preferred over older weak agonist-antagonist agents that had been used primarily as antagonists, eg, nalorphine and levallorphan.

The major application of naloxone is in the treatment of acute opioid overdose (see also Chapter 58). *It is very important that the relatively short duration of action of naloxone be borne in mind, because a severely depressed patient may recover after a single dose of naloxone and appear normal, only to relapse into coma after 1–2 hours.*

The usual initial dose of naloxone is 0.1–0.4 mg intravenously for life-threatening respiratory and CNS depression. Maintenance is with the same drug, 0.4–0.8 mg given intravenously, and repeated as needed—or provided as a continuous infusion under monitored conditions. Multiple doses of naloxone in excess of 0.8 mg per dose have been required to reverse respiratory depression induced by overdose of illicit fentanyl and its analogs. In using naloxone in the severely opioid-depressed newborn, it is important to start with doses of 5–10 mcg/kg and to consider a second dose of up to a total of 25 mcg/kg if no response is noted.

Low-dose naloxone (0.04 mg) has an increasing role in the treatment of adverse effects that are commonly associated with intravenous or epidural opioids. Careful titration of the naloxone dosage can often eliminate the itching, nausea, and vomiting while sparing the analgesia. For this purpose, oral naloxone, and modified analogs of naloxone and naltrexone, have been approved by the FDA. Analogs include **methylnaltrexone bromide** and **naldemedine** for the treatment of constipation in patients with opioid-induced constipation (OIC) with chronic noncancer pain and late-stage advanced illness—and **naloxegol, naldemedine,** and **alvimopan** for the treatment of postoperative ileus following bowel resection surgery. Methylnaltrexone has a quaternary amine preventing it from crossing the blood-brain barrier. Naloxegol is pegylated naloxone, which limits penetration into the CNS and through peripheral μ-antagonism mitigates constipation. Naldemedine and alvimopan are considered peripheral μ-receptor antagonists. The principal mechanism for the selective therapeutic effect of these agents is peripheral enteric μ-receptor antagonism with minimal CNS penetration.

Because of its long duration of action, naltrexone has been proposed as a maintenance drug for addicts in treatment programs. A single dose given on alternate days blocks virtually all of the effects of a dose of heroin. More recently, a depot formulation of naltrexone has been developed offering extended release over weeks to months. There is evidence that naltrexone decreases the craving for alcohol in chronic alcoholics by increasing baseline β-endorphin release, and it has been approved by the FDA for this purpose (see Chapter 23). Naltrexone also facilitates abstinence from nicotine (cigarette smoking) with reduced weight gain. In fact, a combination of naltrexone plus bupropion (Chapter 16) may also offer an effective and synergistic strategy for weight loss.

SUMMARY Opioids, Opioid Substitutes, and Opioid Antagonists

Subclass, Drug	Mechanism of Action	Effects	Clinical Applications	Pharmacokinetics, Toxicities
OPIOID AGONISTS				
• Morphine • Methadone • Fentanyl	Strong μ-receptor agonists • variable affinity for δ and κ receptors	Analgesia • relief of anxiety • sedation • slowed gastrointestinal transit	Severe pain • adjunct in anesthesia (fentanyl, morphine) • pulmonary edema (morphine only) • maintenance in rehabilitation programs (methadone only)	First-pass effect • duration 1–4 h except methadone, 4–6 h • *Toxicity:* Respiratory depression • severe constipation • addiction liability • convulsions
• *Hydromorphone, oxymorphone: Like morphine in efficacy, but higher potency* • *Meperidine: Strong agonist with anticholinergic effects* • *Oxycodone: Dose-dependent analgesia* • *Sufentanil, alfentanil, remifentanil: Like fentanyl but shorter durations of action* • *Carfentanil: Like fentanyl but much more potent*				
• Codeine • Hydrocodone	Less efficacious than morphine • can antagonize strong agonists	Like strong agonists • weaker effects	Mild-moderate pain • cough (codeine)	Like strong agonists, toxicity dependent on genetic variation of metabolism
MIXED OPIOID AGONIST-ANTAGONISTS				
• Buprenorphine	Partial μ agonist • κ antagonist	Like strong agonists but can antagonize their effects • also reduces craving for alcohol	Moderate pain • some maintenance rehabilitation programs	Long duration of action 4–8 h • may precipitate abstinence syndrome
• Nalbuphine	κ Agonist • μ antagonist	Similar to buprenorphine	Moderate pain	Like buprenorphine
ANTITUSSIVES				
• Dextromethorphan	Poorly understood but strong and partial μ agonists are also effective antitussives	Reduces cough reflex • dextromethorphan, levopropoxyphene not analgesic	Acute debilitating cough	Duration 30–60 min • *Toxicity:* Minimal when taken as directed
• *Codeine, levopropoxyphene: Similar to dextromethorphan in antitussive effect*				

(*continued*)

Subclass, Drug	Mechanism of Action	Effects	Clinical Applications	Pharmacokinetics, Toxicities
OPIOID ANTAGONISTS				
• Naloxone	Antagonist at μ, δ, and κ receptors	Rapidly antagonizes all opioid effects	Opioid overdose	Duration 1–2 h (may have to be repeated when treating overdose) • *Toxicity:* Precipitates abstinence syndrome in dependent users
• *Naltrexone, nalmefene: Like naloxone but longer durations of action (10 h); naltrexone is used in maintenance programs and can block heroin effects for up to 48 h; naltrexone is also used for alcohol and nicotine dependence; when combined with bupropion, may be effective in weight-loss programs*				
• *Alvimopan, methylnaltrexone bromide, naldemedine: Potent μ antagonists with poor entry into the central nervous system; can be used to treat severe opioid-induced constipation without precipitating an abstinence syndrome*				
OTHER ANALGESICS USED IN MODERATE PAIN				
• Tapentadol	Moderate μ agonist, strong NET inhibitor	Analgesia	Moderate pain	Duration 4–6 h • *Toxicity:* Headache; nausea and vomiting; possible dependence
• Tramadol	Mixed effects: weak μ agonist, moderate SERT inhibitor, weak NET inhibitor	Analgesia	Moderate pain • adjunct to opioids in chronic pain syndromes	Duration 4–6 h • *Toxicity:* Seizures • risk of serotonin syndrome

NET, norepinephrine reuptake transporter; SERT, serotonin reuptake transporter.

PREPARATIONS AVAILABLE*

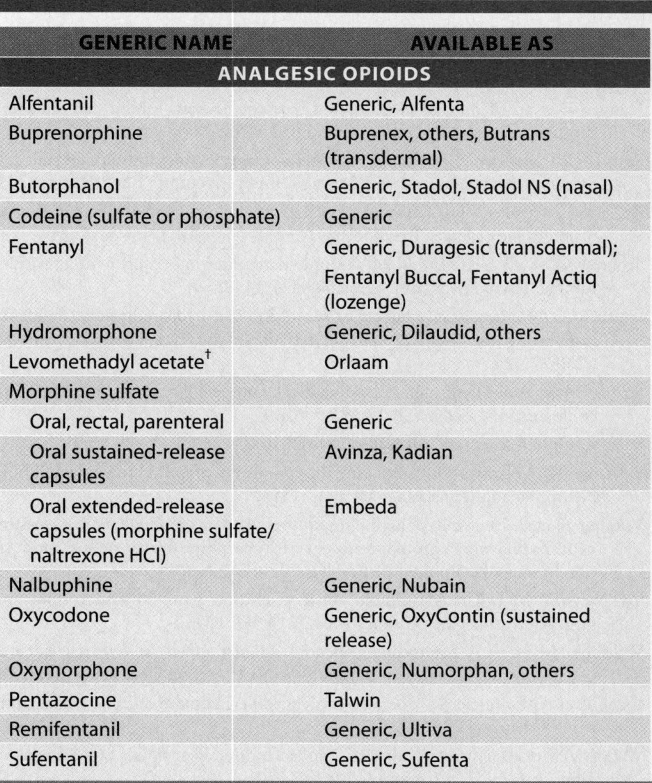

GENERIC NAME	AVAILABLE AS
ANALGESIC OPIOIDS	
Alfentanil	Generic, Alfenta
Buprenorphine	Buprenex, others, Butrans (transdermal)
Butorphanol	Generic, Stadol, Stadol NS (nasal)
Codeine (sulfate or phosphate)	Generic
Fentanyl	Generic, Duragesic (transdermal); Fentanyl Buccal, Fentanyl Actiq (lozenge)
Hydromorphone	Generic, Dilaudid, others
Levomethadyl acetate†	Orlaam
Morphine sulfate	
Oral, rectal, parenteral	Generic
Oral sustained-release capsules	Avinza, Kadian
Oral extended-release capsules (morphine sulfate/naltrexone HCl)	Embeda
Nalbuphine	Generic, Nubain
Oxycodone	Generic, OxyContin (sustained release)
Oxymorphone	Generic, Numorphan, others
Pentazocine	Talwin
Remifentanil	Generic, Ultiva
Sufentanil	Generic, Sufenta

GENERIC NAME	AVAILABLE AS
OTHER ANALGESICS	
Tapentadol	Nucynta
Tramadol	Generic, Ultram, others
Ziconotide	Prialt
ANALGESIC COMBINATIONS‡	
Codeine/acetaminophen	Generic, Tylenol with Codeine, others
Codeine/aspirin	Generic, Empirin Compound, others
Hydrocodone/acetaminophen	Generic, Norco, Vicodin, Lortab, others
Hydrocodone/ibuprofen	Vicoprofen
Oxycodone/acetaminophen	Generic, Percocet, Tylox, others
Oxycodone/aspirin	Generic, Percodan
OPIOID ANTAGONISTS	
Alvimopan	Entereg
Methylnaltrexone	Relistor
Naldemedine	Symproic
Nalmefene	Revex
Naloxone	Generic, Narcan
Naltrexone	Generic, ReVia, Depade, Vivitrol
ANTITUSSIVES	
Codeine	Generic
Dextromethorphan	Generic, Benylin DM, Delsym, others

*Antidiarrheal opioid preparations are listed in Chapter 62.

†Orphan drug approved only for the treatment of narcotic addiction.

‡Dozens of combination products are available; only a few of the most commonly prescribed are listed here. Codeine combination products available in several strengths are usually denoted No. 2 (15 mg codeine), No. 3 (30 mg codeine), and No. 4 (60 mg codeine). Prescribers should be aware of the possible danger of renal and hepatic injury with acetaminophen, aspirin, and nonsteroidal anti-inflammatory drugs contained in these analgesic combinations.

REFERENCES

Anton RF: Naltrexone for the management of alcohol dependence. N Engl J Med 2008;359:715.

Bailly J et al: Targeting morphine-responsive neurons: Generation of a knock-in mouse line expressing Cre-recombinase from the mu-opioid receptor gene locus. eNeuro 2020;7:ENEURO.0433.

Ballantyne JC et al: Refractory dependence on opioid analgesics. Pain 2019;160:2655.

Ballantyne JC, Koob GF: Allostasis theory in opioid tolerance. Pain 2021;162:2315.

Basbaum AI: Pain. In: Kandel ER et al (editors): *Principles of Neural Science*, 6th ed. McGraw Hill, 2021.

Basbaum AI et al: Cellular and molecular mechanisms of pain. Cell 2009;139:267.

Benedetti C, Premuda L: The history of opium and its derivatives. In: Benedetti C et al (editors): *Advances in Pain Research and Therapy*, vol 14. Raven Press, 1990.

Boulos LJ: Mu opioid receptors in the medial habenula contribute to naloxone aversion. Neuropsychopharmacology 2020;45:247.

Brummett CM et al: New persistent opioid use after minor and major surgical procedures in US adults. JAMA Surg 2017;152:e170504.

Brust TF et al: Biased agonists of the kappa opioid receptor suppress pain and itch without causing sedation or dysphoria. Sci Signal 2016;9:ra117.

Colvin LA, Bull F, Hales TG. Perioperative opioid analgesia—when is enough too much? A review of opioid-induced tolerance and hyperalgesia. Lancet 2019;393:1558.

Corder G et al: Loss of μ opioid receptor signaling in nociceptors, but not microglia, abrogates morphine tolerance without disrupting analgesia. Nat Med 2017;23:164.

Darcq E, Kieffer BL: Opioid receptors: drivers to addiction? Nat Rev Neurosci 2018;19:499.

Ding H et al: A novel orvinol analog, BU08028, as a safe opioid analgesic without abuse liability in primates. Proc Natl Acad Sci USA 2016;113:E5511.

Fillingim RB, Gear RW: Sex differences in opioid analgesia: Clinical and experimental findings. Eur J Pain 2004;8:413.

Gillis A et al: Critical assessment of G protein-biased agonism at the μ-opioid receptor. Trends Pharmacol Sci 2020;41:947.

Gomtsian L et al: Morphine effects within the rodent anterior cingulate cortex and rostral ventromedial medulla reveal separable modulation of affective and sensory qualities of acute or chronic pain. Pain 2018;159:2512.

Green JM, Sundman MH, Chou Y-H: Opioid-induced microglia reactivity modulates opioid reward, analgesia, and behavior. Neurosci Biobehav Rev 2022;135:104544.

Grim TW et al: Toward directing opioid receptor signaling to refine opioid therapeutics. Biol Psychiatry 2020;87:15.

Guichard L et al: Opioid-induced hyperalgesia in patients with chronic pain: A systematic review of published cases. Clin J Pain 2022;38:49.

Hall ES et al: A cohort comparison of buprenorphine versus methadone treatment for neonatal abstinence syndrome. J Pediatr 2016;170:39.

Inan S, Cowan A: Antipruritic effects of kappa opioid receptor agonists: Evidence form rodents to humans. Exp Pharmacol 2022;271:275.

Inui S: Nalfurafine hydrochloride for the treatment of pruritus. Expert Opin Pharmacother 2012;13:1507.

Jimenez-Vargas NN et al: Endosomal signaling of delta opioid receptors is an endogenous mechanism and therapeutic target for relief from inflammatory pain. Proc Natl Acad Sci USA 2020;117:15281.

Jiménez-Vargas NN et al: Agonist that activates the μ-opioid receptor in acidified microenvironments inhibits colitis pain without side effects. Gut 2022;71:695.

Joly V et al: Remifentanil-induced postoperative hyperalgesia and its prevention with small-dose ketamine. Anesthesiology 2005;103:147.

Kalso E et al: No pain, no gain: Clinical excellence and scientific rigour—lessons learned from IA morphine. Pain 2002;98:269.

Kharasch ED et al: Methadone pharmacogenetics: CYP2B6 polymorphisms determine plasma concentrations, clearance, and metabolism. Anesthesiology 2015;123:1142.

Kim JA et al: Morphine-induced receptor endocytosis in a novel knockin mouse reduces tolerance and dependence. Curr Biol 2008;18:129.

Krebs EE et al: Effect of opioid vs nonopioid medications on pain-related function in patients with chronic back pain or hip or knee osteoarthritis pain: The SPACE randomized clinical trial. JAMA 2018;319:872.

Kreutzwiser D, Tawfic QA: Expanding role of NMDA receptor antagonists in the management of pain. CNS Drugs 2019;33:347.

Lambert DG: The nociceptin/orphanin FQ receptor: A target with broad therapeutic potential. Nat Rev Drug Discov 2008;7:694.

Lenard NR et al: Absence of conditioned place preference or reinstatement with bivalent ligands containing mu-opioid receptor agonist and delta-opioid receptor antagonist pharmacophores. Eur J Pharmacol 2007;566:75.

Liaw WI et al: Distinct expression of synaptic NR2A and NR2B in the central nervous system and impaired morphine tolerance and physical dependence in mice deficient in postsynaptic density-93 protein. Mol Pain 2008;4:45.

Lilius TO et al: Ketamine coadministration attenuates morphine tolerance and leads to increased brain concentrations of both drugs in the rat. Br J Pharmacol 2015;172:2799.

Liu XY et al: Unidirectional cross-activation of GRPR by MOR1D uncouples itch and analgesia induced by opioids. Cell 2011;147:447.

Manglik A et al: Structure-based discovery of opioid analgesics with reduced side effects. Nature 2016;537:185.

Margolis EB, Fields HL: Mu opioid receptor actions in the lateral habenula. PLoS One 2016;11:e0159097.

Massaly N et al: Uncovering the analgesic effects of a pH-dependent mu-opioid receptor agonist using a model of nonevoked ongoing pain. Pain 2020;161:2798.

McPherson ML et al: Safe and appropriate use of methadone in hospice and palliative care: expert consensus white paper. J Pain Symptom Manage 2019;57:635.

McGaraughty S, Heinricher MM: Microinjection of morphine into various amygdaloid nuclei differentially affects nociceptive responsiveness and RVM neuronal activity. Pain 2002;96:153.

Mercadante S, Arcuri E: Opioids and renal function. J Pain 2004;5:2.

Meunier J et al: The nociceptin (ORL1) receptor: Molecular cloning and functional architecture. Peptides 2000;21:893.

Moreno E et al: Functional mu-opioid-galanin receptor heteromers in the ventral tegmental area. J Neurosci 2017;37:1176.

Navratilova E et al: Pain relief produces negative reinforcement through activation of mesolimbic reward-valuation circuitry. Proc Natl Acad Sci USA 2012;109:20709.

Nguyen E et al: Medullary kappa-opioid receptor neurons inhibit pain and itch through a descending circuit. Brain 2022;145:2586.

Reiss D et al: Mu opioid receptor in microglia contributes to morphine analgesic tolerance, hyperalgesia, and withdrawal in mice. J Neurosci Res 2022;100:203.

Roeckel LA et al: Opioid-induced hyperalgesia: Cellular and molecular mechanisms. Neuroscience 2016;338:160.

Scherrer G et al: Dissociation of the opioid receptor mechanisms that control mechanical and heat pain. Cell 2009;137:1148.

Smith MT: Neuroexcitatory effects of morphine and hydromorphone: Evidence implicating the 3-glucuronide metabolites. Clin Exp Pharmacol Physiol 2000;27:524.

Spahn V et al: A nontoxic pain killer designed by modeling of pathological receptor conformations. Science 2017;355:966.

Stein C: Opioid receptors. Annu Rev Med 2016;67:433.

Valentino RJ, Volkow ND: Untangling the complexity of opioid receptor function. Neuropsychopharmacology 2018;43:2514.

Viisanen H et al: Neurophysiological response properties of medullary pain-control neurons following chronic treatment with morphine or oxycodone: modulation by acute ketamine. J Neurophys 2020;124:790.

Volkow ND, McLellan AT: Opioid abuse in chronic pain: Misconceptions and mitigation strategies. N Engl J Med 2016;374:1253.

Waldhoer M et al: A heterodimer-selective agonist shows in vivo relevance of G protein–coupled receptor dimers. Proc Natl Acad Sci USA 2005;102:9050.

Wang Z et al: Pronociceptive actions of dynorphin maintain chronic neuropathic pain. J Neurosci 2001;21:1779.

Waung MW et al: A diencephalic circuit in rats for opioid analgesia but not positive reinforcement. Nat Commun 2022;13:764.

Wild JE et al: Long-term safety and tolerability of tapentadol extended release for the management of chronic low back pain or osteoarthritis pain. Pain Pract 2010;10:416.

Xie JY et al: Kappa opioid receptor antagonists: A possible new class of therapeutics for migraine prevention. Cephalalgia 2017;37:780.

CASE STUDY ANSWER

In this case of severe pain following a traumatic fall, treatment may require the administration of a potent intravenous opioid analgesic such as morphine, hydromorphone, or fentanyl; however, concurrent use of nonopioid analgesics (such as ketamine) and other nonopioid multimodal analgesic strategies (NSAIDs) often reduce or eliminate opioid requirements and risk of respiratory failure. Given the history of obstructive sleep apnea, before an additional dose of an opioid analgesic is administered, it is expected that the patient will require frequent reevaluation of both the severity of his pain and the presence of potential adverse effects. Reevaluation of his level of consciousness, respiratory rate, fractional oxygen saturation, and other vital parameters can help achieve the goal of pain relief and minimize respiratory depression. Concurrent use of sedative agents such as benzodiazepines should be avoided if possible as they greatly increase the risk of respiratory depression, obstruction, and failure.

CHAPTER

32 Drugs of Abuse

Christian Lüscher, MD

CASE STUDY

A 15-year-old high school student was brought to the emergency department after his parents found him in his room staring at the ceiling and visibly frightened. Earlier that evening, he attended a party but was depressed because his girlfriend just broke up with him. His parents are also worried about a change in his behavior over the last few months. He is failing this year at school and has stopped playing soccer. He has lost interest in school, at times seems depressed, and tells his parents that his pocket money is not sufficient.

When questioned by the intern, he reports that space-cookies were served at the party. He also says that smoking marijuana has become a habit (three to four joints a week) but denies consumption of alcohol and other drugs.

How do you explain the state he was found in? What is the difference between hashish and marijuana? What may be the link to his poor performance at school? Do all drug users necessarily use several drugs?

Drugs are abused (used in ways that are not medically approved) because they cause strong feelings of euphoria. However, repetitive exposure induces widespread adaptive changes in the brain. As a consequence, drug use may become compulsive—the hallmark of addiction.

■ BASIC NEUROBIOLOGY OF DRUG ABUSE

DEPENDENCE VERSUS ADDICTION

There is a conceptual and mechanistic separation of "dependence" and "addiction." The older term "physical dependence" is now denoted as **dependence,** whereas "psychological dependence" is more simply called **addiction.**

Every addictive drug causes its own characteristic spectrum of acute effects, but they all induce strong feelings of euphoria and reward. With repetitive exposure, addictive drugs induce adaptive changes such as tolerance (ie, escalation of dose to maintain effect). Once the abused drug is no longer available, signs of withdrawal become apparent. A combination of such signs, referred to as the **withdrawal syndrome,** defines *dependence*. Dependence is not always a correlate of drug abuse—it can also occur with many classes of nonpsychoactive drugs, eg, sympathomimetic vasoconstrictors and bronchodilators, and organic nitrate vasodilators. *Addiction*, on the other hand, consists of compulsive, relapsing drug use despite negative consequences, at times triggered by cravings that occur in response to contextual cues (see Box: Animal Models in Addiction Research). Although dependence invariably occurs with chronic exposure, only a small percentage of subjects develop a compulsion, lose control, and become addicted. For example, very few patients who receive opioids as analgesics desire the drug after withdrawal. And only one person out of six becomes addicted within 10 years of first use of cocaine. Conversely, relapse is very common in addicts after a successful withdrawal when, by definition, they are no longer dependent.

ADDICTIVE DRUGS INCREASE THE LEVEL OF DOPAMINE (DA): REINFORCEMENT

To understand the long-term changes induced by drugs of abuse, their initial molecular and cellular targets must be identified. A combination of approaches in animals and humans, including functional imaging, has revealed the mesolimbic dopamine system as the prime target of addictive drugs. This system originates in the **ventral tegmental area (VTA),** a tiny structure at the tip of the brainstem, which projects to the **nucleus accumbens (NAc),** the amygdala, the hippocampus, and the prefrontal cortex (Figure 32–1). Most projection neurons of the VTA are dopamine-producing neurons. When the dopamine neurons of the VTA begin to fire in bursts, large quantities of dopamine are released in the nucleus accumbens and the prefrontal cortex. Early animal studies pairing electrical stimulation of the VTA with operant responses (eg, lever pressing) that result in strong reinforcement established the central role of the mesolimbic dopamine system in reward processing. Direct application of drugs into the VTA also acts as a strong reinforcer, and systemic administration of drugs of abuse causes the release of dopamine. Even direct activation of dopamine neurons is sufficient to drive reinforcement and elicit adaptive behavioral changes typically observed with addictive drugs. These very selective interventions use optogenetic methods. Blue light is delivered in a freely moving mouse through light guides to activate channelrhodopsin, a light-gated cation channel that is artificially expressed in dopamine neurons. As a result, mice will "self-administer" light to activate VTA dopamine neurons. After several pairings with a specific environment, a long-lasting place preference is established. Once the light is no longer available, a seeking behavior is observed (but no actual withdrawal syndrome). Finally, some mice will self-stimulate even if they have to endure a punishment (e.g. light electric shock). Conversely, inhibition of VTA dopamine neurons or activation of upstream inhibitory cells causes aversion. Classifying the VTA dopamine neurons based on their activity in response to a rewarding or aversive stimulus suggests distinct groups. The dopamine neurons located in the lateral part of the VTA projecting to the lateral shell of the NAc respond strongly to an unexpected reward and are the prime target of addictive drugs, which also target the medial VTA.

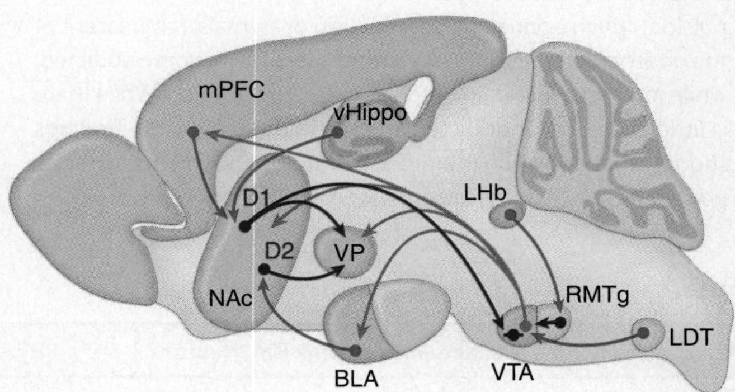

FIGURE 32–1 Major connections of the mesolimbic dopamine system in the brain. Schematic diagram of the brain illustrating that the dopamine projections (red) originate in the ventral tegmental area (VTA) and target the nucleus accumbens (NAc), prefrontal cortex (mPFC), basolateral amygdala (BLA), and ventral pallidum (VP). Neurons in the NAc fall into two classes, one expressing type 1 dopamine receptors (D1s) and the other expressing type 2 receptors (D2s). Both classes contain GABAergic projection neurons (green); the D1R neurons send their axons to both the VP and the VTA (where they target primarily the GABA interneurons), whereas the D2R neurons send their axons selectively to the VP. The NAc is also a site of convergence of excitatory projections from the mPFC, the ventral hippocampus (vHippo), and the BLA. The midbrain dopamine neurons receive a direct excitatory input (blue) from the lateral dorsal tegmentum (LDT), while the GABA neurons of the rostromedial tegmentum (RMTg) at the tail of the VTA are excited by neurons from the lateral habenula (LHb), typically when an aversive stimulus occurs. The projection from the orbitofrontal cortex (OFC) to the dorsal striatum (DS) has been implicated in compulsive drug seeking and taking. The ventral and dorsal parts of the striatum are connected by reciprocal, spiraling connections.

As a general rule, all addictive drugs elicit dopamine transients in the mesolimbic system. Dopamine also peaks in response to unexpected natural rewards and may thus code for the difference between expected and actual rewards. A very appealing hypothesis posits that dopamine constitutes a learning signal and addictive drugs, by their sheer pharmacological power, an excessive learning signal (see Box: The Dopamine Hypothesis of Addiction), which eventually biases decisions in favor of drug consumption, even when associated with major negative consequences.

Each addictive drug activates the mesolimbic system via its specific molecular target, engaging **distinct cellular mechanisms** to increase dopamine levels. The first class of drugs directly stimulates the dopamine neurons. This is the case for nicotine, which binds to excitatory nicotinic receptors expressed on the cell body of dopamine neurons. The second class interferes with the reuptake of dopamine (eg, cocaine) or promotes nonvesicular release (eg, amphetamines). This happens in NAc and the VTA itself because dopamine neurons also express somatodendritic transporters, which normally clear dopamine released by the dendrites. Although drugs of this class also affect transporters of other monoamines (norepinephrine, serotonin), action on the dopamine transporter remains central for addiction. This is consistent with the observations that antidepressants that block serotonin and norepinephrine uptake, but not dopamine uptake, do not cause addiction even after prolonged use. The third mechanism is indirect, whereby the drugs inhibit γ-aminobutyric acid (GABA) neurons that act as local inhibitory interneurons (eg, opioids, cannabis). The three groups also differ by the molecular targets the drug binds to. For example, members of the last group bind to G_{io} protein–coupled receptors, typically of the G_{io} family, that inhibit neurons through postsynaptic hyperpolarization and lower presynaptic transmitter release probability. By contrast, direct activation uses ionotropic receptors or ion channels, and all reuptake blockers interfere with the dopamine transporter (Table 32–1 and Figure 32–2).

Animal Models in Addiction Research

Many of the recent advances in addiction research have been made possible by the use of animal models. Since drugs of abuse are not only rewarding but also reinforcing, an animal will learn a behavior (eg, press a lever) when paired with drug administration. In such a self-administration paradigm, the number of times an animal is willing to press the lever in order to obtain a single dose reflects the strength of reinforcement and is therefore a measure of the motivation of the animal. Observing withdrawal signs specific for rodents (eg, escape jumps or "wet-dog" shakes after abrupt termination of chronic morphine administration) allows the quantification of dependence. When this aversive state is avoided, negative reinforcement may result (ie, the individual takes the drug to avoid withdrawal). Behavioral tests for addiction in rodents certainly do not capture the complexity of the disease. However, it is possible to model *core components* of addiction, for example, by monitoring behavioral sensitization and conditioned place preference. In the first test, an increase in locomotor activity is observed with intermittent drug exposure and may reflect enhanced incentive saliency. The latter tests for the preference of a particular environment associated with drug exposure by measuring the time an animal spends in the compartment where a drug was received compared with the compartment where only saline was injected (conditioned place preference). Both tests have in common that they are sensitive to cue-conditioned effects of addictive drugs. Subsequent exposures to the environment without the drug lead to extinction of the place preference, which can be reinstated with a low dose of the drug or the presentation of a conditioned stimulus. These persistent changes serve as a model of relapse and have been linked to synaptic plasticity of excitatory transmission in the ventral tegmental area, nucleus accumbens, and prefrontal cortex (see also Box: The Dopamine Hypothesis of Addiction). More sophisticated tests rely on self-administration of the drug, in which a rat or a mouse has to press a lever in order to obtain an injection of, for example, cocaine. Once the animal has learned the association with a conditioned stimulus (eg, light or brief sound), the simple presentation of the cue elicits drug seeking. Using an apparatus with two levers, one can demonstrate strong motivation for drug seeking. In this test the animal has to press the lever for a random duration, only after which the second lever is presented that then allows to self-administer the drug. Prolonged self-administration of addictive drugs over weeks, particularly when using intermittent access schedules, elicits behaviors in some rodents that more closely resemble human addiction. Such "addicted" rodents are very strongly motivated to seek cocaine, continue looking for the drug even when no longer available, and self-administer cocaine despite negative consequences, such as punishment in the form of an electric foot shock. The latter is a reflection of compulsion, which occurs only in a fraction of animals, reminiscent of the observation that only some drug users will become addicted, while many can maintain a recreational consumption. While there is little evidence for addicted animals in the wild, these findings suggest that addiction is a disease that does not respect species boundaries once drugs become available.

TABLE 32–1 The mechanistic classification of drugs of abuse.[1]

Name	Main Molecular Target	Pharmacology	Effect on Dopamine (DA) Neurons	RR[2]
Drugs That Activate G Protein–Coupled Receptors				
Opioids	μ-OR (G_{io})	Agonist	Disinhibition	4
Cannabinoids	CB_1R (G_{io})	Agonist	Disinhibition	2
γ-Hydroxybutyric acid (GHB)	$GABA_BR$ (G_{io})	Weak agonist	Disinhibition	?
LSD, mescaline, psilocybin	5-$HT_{2A}R$ (G_q)	Partial agonist	—	1
Drugs That Bind to Ionotropic Receptors and Ion Channels				
Nicotine	nAChR (α4β2)	Agonist	Excitation	4
Alcohol	$GABA_AR$, 5-HT_3R, nAChR, NMDAR, Kir3 channels		Excitation, disinhibition (?)	3
Benzodiazepines	$GABA_AR$	Positive modulator	Disinhibition	3
Phencyclidine, ketamine	NMDAR	Antagonist	—	1
Drugs That Bind to Transporters of Biogenic Amines				
Cocaine	DAT, SERT, NET	Inhibitor	Blocks DA uptake	5
Amphetamine	DAT, NET, SERT, VMAT	Reverses transport	Blocks DA uptake, synaptic depletion	5
Ecstasy	SERT > DAT, NET	Reverses transport	Blocks DA uptake, synaptic depletion	?

5-HT_xR, serotonin receptor; CB_1R, cannabinoid-1 receptor; DAT, dopamine transporter; GABA, γ-aminobutyric acid; Kir3 channels, G protein–coupled inwardly rectifying potassium channels; LSD, lysergic acid diethylamide; μ-OR, μ-opioid receptor; nAChR, nicotinic acetylcholine receptor; NET, norepinephrine transporter; NMDAR, *N*-methyl-D-aspartate receptor; R, receptor; SERT, serotonin transporter; VMAT, vesicular monoamine transporter; ? indicates data not available.

[1]Drugs fall into one of three categories, targeting either G protein–coupled receptors, ionotropic receptors or ion channels, or biogenic amine transporters.

[2]RR, relative risk of addiction; 1 = nonaddictive; 5 = highly addictive.

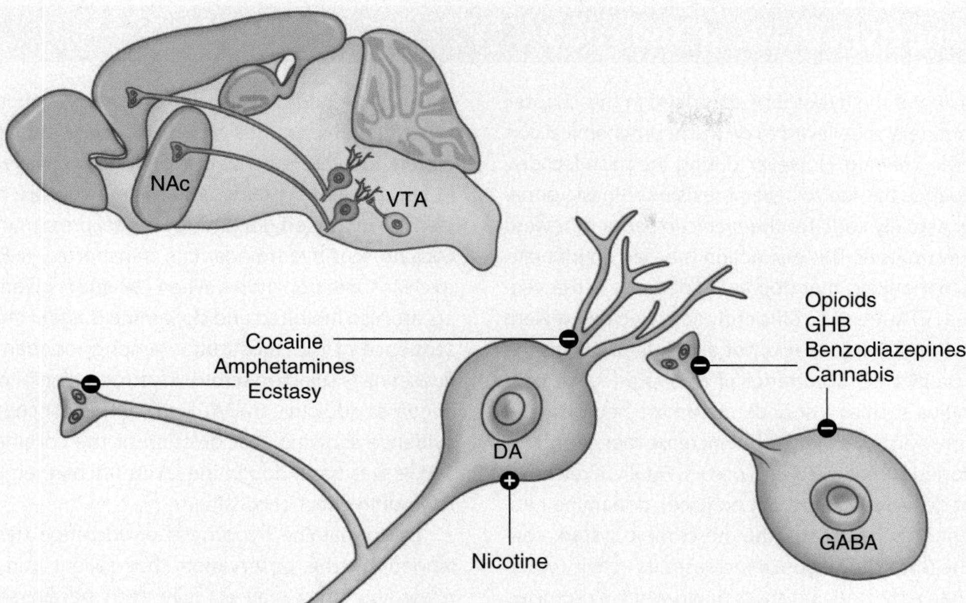

FIGURE 32–2 Neuropharmacological classification of addictive drugs by cellular mechanism engaged (see text and Table 32–1). DA, dopamine; GABA, γ-aminobutyric acid; GHB, γ-hydroxybutyric acid; GPCRs, G protein–coupled receptors; THC, Δ^9-tetrahydrocannabinol.

DEPENDENCE: TOLERANCE & WITHDRAWAL

With chronic exposure to addictive drugs, the brain shows signs of adaptation. For example, if morphine is used at short intervals, the dose has to be progressively increased over the course of several days to maintain rewarding or analgesic effects. This phenomenon is called tolerance. It may become a serious problem because of increasing side effects—eg, respiratory depression—that do not show as much tolerance and may lead to overdose-related fatalities.

Tolerance to opioids may be due to a reduction of the concentration of a drug or a shorter duration of action in a target system (pharmacokinetic tolerance). Alternatively, it may involve changes in μ-opioid receptor function (pharmacodynamic tolerance). Many μ-opioid receptor agonists promote robust receptor phosphorylation that triggers the recruitment of the adaptor protein β-arrestin, causing G proteins to uncouple from the receptor and internalize within minutes (see Chapter 2). Since this decreases signaling, it is tempting to explain tolerance by such a mechanism. However, morphine, which strongly induces tolerance, does not recruit β-arrestins and fails to promote receptor internalization (see Chapter 31).

Conversely, other agonists that drive receptor internalization very efficiently induce only modest tolerance. Based on these observations, it has been hypothesized that desensitization and receptor internalization protect the cell from overstimulation. In this model, morphine, by failing to trigger receptor endocytosis, disproportionally stimulates adaptive processes, which eventually cause tolerance. Although the molecular identity of these processes is still under investigation, they may be similar to the ones involved in withdrawal (see below).

Adaptive changes become fully apparent once drug exposure is terminated. This state is called **withdrawal** and is observed to varying degrees after chronic exposure to most drugs of abuse. Withdrawal from opioids in humans is particularly strong (described below). Studies in rodents have added significantly to our understanding of the neural and molecular mechanisms that underlie dependence. For example, signs of dependence, as well as analgesia and reward (positive reinforcement), are abolished in genome-wide knockout mice lacking the μ-opioid receptor (Chapter 31), but not in mice lacking other opioid receptors (δ, κ). If μ-opioid receptors are selectively deleted on VTA GABA neurons of the VTA, positive reinforcement is lost, but not dependence. Such mice will still show withdrawal upon abrupt termination of opioid exposure, indicating that circuits of dependence are distinct. An input from the periventricular thalamus to the nucleus accumbens, conveying an aversive state during withdrawal, has been implicated. On the molecular level, dependence may involve adaptation of receptor signaling. μ-opioid receptors initially inhibit adenylyl cyclase; this inhibition becomes weaker after several days of repeated exposure. The reduction of the inhibition of adenylyl cyclase is due to a counteradaptation of the enzyme system during exposure to the drug, which results in the overproduction of cAMP during subsequent withdrawal. Several mechanisms exist for this adenylyl cyclase compensatory response, including upregulation of transcription of the enzyme. Increased cAMP concentrations strongly activate the transcription factor cyclic AMP response element binding protein (CREB), leading to the regulation of downstream genes.

The Dopamine Hypothesis of Addiction

In the earliest version of the hypothesis described in this chapter, mesolimbic dopamine was believed to be the neurochemical correlate of pleasure and reward. However, during the past decades, experimental evidence has led to several revisions. Phasic dopamine release may actually code for the *prediction error* of reward rather than the reward itself. This distinction is based on pioneering observations in monkeys that dopamine neurons in the ventral tegmental area (VTA) are most efficiently activated by a reward (eg, a few drops of fruit juice) that is not anticipated. When the animal learns to predict the occurrence of a reward (eg, by pairing it with a stimulus such as a sound), dopamine neurons stop responding to the reward itself (juice), but increase their firing rate when the conditioned stimulus (sound) occurs. Finally, if reward is predicted but not delivered (sound but no juice), dopamine neurons become silent. In other words, the mesolimbic system continuously scans the reward situation. It increases its activity when reward is larger than expected and shuts down when a promised reward is omitted, thus coding for the prediction error of reward. Tonic release of dopamine in turn may reflect motivation.

Under physiologic conditions the phasic mesolimbic dopamine signal could represent a learning signal responsible for reinforcing constructive behavioral adaptation (eg, learning to press a lever for food). Indeed, animals that cannot synthesize dopamine because key enzymes have been ablated genetically show unconditioned reflexes and can execute previously learned behavior, but hardly acquire new responses. Addictive drugs, by directly increasing dopamine, would generate a strong but inappropriate learning signal, thus hijacking the reward system and leading to pathologic reinforcement. As a consequence, over time, through several intermediate steps, behavior may become compulsive in some individuals; that is, decisions are strongly biased in favor of actions to seek and take drugs. This is the hallmark of addiction.

This appealing hypothesis has been challenged by the intriguing observation that mice genetically modified to lack the primary molecular target of cocaine, the dopamine transporter DAT, still self-administer the drug. Only when transporters of other biogenic amines are also knocked out does cocaine completely lose its rewarding properties. However, in $DAT^{-/-}$ mice, in which basal synaptic dopamine levels are high, cocaine still leads to increased dopamine release, presumably because other cocaine-sensitive monoamine transporters (NET, SERT) are able to clear some dopamine. When cocaine is given, these transporters are also inhibited and dopamine is again increased. As a consequence of this substitution among monoamine transporters, fluoxetine (a selective serotonin reuptake inhibitor, see Chapter 30) becomes addictive in $DAT^{-/-}$ mice. This concept is supported by evidence showing that deletion of the cocaine-binding site on DAT leaves basal dopamine levels unchanged but abolishes the rewarding effect of cocaine.

The dopamine hypothesis of addiction has also been challenged by the observation that salient stimuli that are not rewarding (they may actually even be aversive and therefore negative reinforcers) also activate a subpopulation of dopamine neurons in the VTA. The neurons that are activated by aversive stimuli preferentially project to the prefrontal cortex and the tail of the striatum, while the dopamine neurons inhibited by aversive stimuli are those that mostly target the nucleus accumbens. These recent findings suggest that in parallel to the reward system, a system for aversion-learning originates in the VTA.

Regardless of the many roles of dopamine under physiologic conditions, all addictive drugs significantly increase its concentration in target structures of the mesolimbic projection, in particular in the dorsomedial shell of the NAc. This suggests that high levels of dopamine may actually be at the origin of the adaptive changes that underlie dependence and addiction, a concept that is now supported by novel techniques that allow controlling the activity of dopamine neurons in vivo. In fact manipulations that drive sustained activity of VTA dopamine neurons cause the same cellular adaptations and behavioral changes typically observed with addictive drug exposure, including late-stage symptoms such as persistence of self-stimulation during punishment.

ADDICTION: A DISEASE OF MALADAPTIVE LEARNING

Addiction is characterized by a high motivation to obtain and use a drug despite negative consequences. With time, drug use becomes compulsive ("wanting without liking"). Addiction is a recalcitrant, chronic, and stubbornly relapsing disease that is very difficult to treat.

The central problem is that even after successful withdrawal and prolonged drug-free periods, addicted individuals have a high risk of relapsing. Relapse is typically triggered by three conditions: re-exposure to the addictive drug, stress, or a context that recalls prior drug use. It appears that when paired with drug use, a neutral stimulus may undergo a switch and motivate ("trigger") addiction-related behavior. This phenomenon may involve synaptic plasticity in the target nuclei of the mesolimbic projection (eg, projections from the medial prefrontal cortex and the ventral hippocampus to the neurons of the nucleus accumbens that express the D_1 receptors). Several recent studies suggest that the recruitment of circuits in the dorsal striatum is responsible for compulsion. This switch may depend on synaptic plasticity in the nucleus accumbens of the ventral striatum (Figure 32–3), where mesolimbic dopamine afferents converge with glutamatergic afferents to modulate their function. If dopamine release codes for the prediction error of reward (see Box: The Dopamine Hypothesis of Addiction), pharmacologic stimulation of the mesolimbic dopamine system

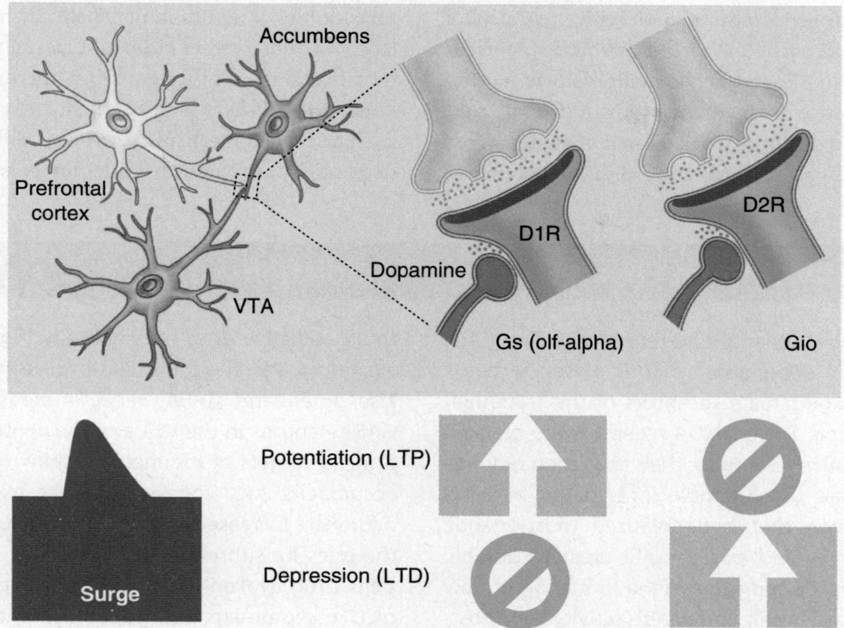

FIGURE 32–3 Rules of synaptic plasticity in the striatum. The tripartite synapse between glutamatergic afferents, the GABAergic medium spiny neurons, and the ascending axons of VTA dopamine neurons can undergo several forms of synaptic plasticity. In cells that express the G_s-coupled D_1 receptor, dopamine favors the appearance of long-term potentiation (LTP), while long-term depression (LTD) is inhibited. Conversely in D_2 receptor-expressing cells, dopamine when released at the same time as glutamate causes LTD and opposes LTP. These rules apply when dopamine is released at the same time as afferent glutamate and may explain the predominant effect of addictive drugs. (Data from Shen W, et al: Dichotomous dopaminergic control of striatal synaptic plasticity, Science 2008;321:848.)

will generate an unusually strong learning signal. Unlike natural rewards, addictive drugs continue to increase dopamine even when reward is expected. Such overriding of the prediction error signal may eventually be responsible for the usurping of memory processes by addictive drugs.

The involvement of learning and memory systems in addiction is also suggested by clinical studies. For example, the role of context in relapse is supported by the fact that soldiers who became addicted to heroin during the Vietnam War had significantly better outcomes when treated after their return home, compared with addicts who remained in the environment where they had taken the drug. In other words, cravings may recur at the presentation of contextual cues (eg, people, places, or drug paraphernalia). Current research therefore focuses on the effects of drugs on associative forms of synaptic plasticity, such as long-term potentiation (LTP), which underlie learning and memory (see Box: Synaptic Plasticity, Altered Circuit Function, & Addiction).

Non-substance-dependent disorders, such as pathologic gambling and compulsive shopping, share many clinical features of addiction. Several lines of arguments suggest that they also share the underlying neurobiological mechanisms. This conclusion is supported by the clinical observation that, as an adverse effect of dopamine agonist medication, patients with Parkinson disease may become pathologic gamblers. Other patients may develop a compulsion for recreational activities, such as shopping, binge eating, or hypersexuality. Although large-scale studies are not yet available, an estimated one in seven parkinsonian patients develops an addiction-like behavior when receiving dopamine agonists (see Chapter 28).

Large individual differences exist also in vulnerability to substance-related addiction. Whereas one person may become "hooked" after a few doses, others may be able to use a drug occasionally during their entire lives without ever having difficulty in stopping. Even in the case of drugs that induce dependence in all subjects, only a percentage of users progress to addiction. For example, a retrospective analysis shows that after several decades of cocaine abuse, only 20% become addicted. With cannabis, the fraction is only 10%, while heroin leads to approximately 30% of users becoming addicts. A similar percentage for cocaine is also observed in rats and mice that have extended access to the drug. With dopamine neuron self-stimulation, the fraction of mice that resist punishment is approximately 50%. Recent studies in rats suggest that impulsivity or excessive anxiety may be crucial traits that represent a risk for addiction. The transition to addiction is determined by a combination of environmental and genetic factors. Heritability of addiction, as determined by comparing monozygotic with dizygotic twins, is relatively modest for cannabinoids but higher for cocaine. It is of interest that the relative risk for addiction (addiction liability) of a drug (see Table 32–1) correlates with its heritability, suggesting that the neurobiologic basis of addiction common to all drugs is what is being inherited. Further genomic analysis indicates that numerous, perhaps even hundreds of alleles need to function in combination to produce the phenotype. However, identification of the genes involved remains elusive. Although some substance-specific candidate genes have been identified (eg, alcohol dehydrogenase, nicotinic acetylcholine receptor subunits), current research focuses on genes implicated in the neurobiologic mechanisms common to all addictive drugs. An appealing idea is the contribution of epigenetics as a determinant of addiction vulnerability. This scenario is supported by the observation that the fraction of transition to compulsion in genetically homogeneous mice is similar to that observed in humans. Cocaine regulates posttranslational modifications of histones, DNA methylation, and signaling via noncoding RNAs, which eventually may have an impact on behavior. The cellular mechanism involved and the relationship to synaptic plasticity are currently under investigation.

Synaptic Plasticity, Altered Circuit Function, & Addiction

Long-term potentiation (LTP) and long-term depression (LTD) are forms of experience-dependent synaptic plasticity that is induced by activating glutamate receptors of the *N*-methyl-D-aspartate (NMDA) type. Since NMDA receptors are blocked by magnesium at negative potentials, their activation requires the concomitant release of glutamate (presynaptic activity) onto a receiving neuron that is depolarized (postsynaptic activity). Correlated pre- and postsynaptic activity durably enhances synaptic efficacy and triggers the formation of new connections. In contrast, weak correlated activity (eg, postsynaptic neurons firing before the presynaptic cell) leads to LTD. Because associativity is a critical component, LTP and LTD have become leading candidate mechanisms underlying learning and memory. They can be elicited at glutamatergic synapses of the mesolimbic reward system and are modulated by dopamine. The dopamine receptors dictate the rules of synaptic plasticity. In D_1R-expressing cells, a surge of dopamine favors LTP of excitatory afferents but blocks LTD. Conversely in D_2R-expressing neurons, dopamine release concomitant to glutamate transmission leads to the depression of the latter and inhibits LTP. Drugs of abuse therefore interfere with LTP and LTD at sites of convergence of dopamine and glutamate projections, leading to drug-evoked synaptic plasticity. Exposure to an addictive drug thus typically triggers a potentiation of excitatory afferents onto D_1R-expressing neurons. Dopamine also potentiates $GABA_A$ receptor-mediated inhibition of the GABA neurons in the VTA and the ventral pallidum (VP), both primary targets of the medium spiny neurons of the nucleus accumbens. As a consequence, the excitability of dopamine neurons is increased, the synaptic calcium sources altered, and the rules for subsequent LTP inverted. In the nucleus accumbens, drug-evoked synaptic plasticity appears with some delay on D_1 receptor-expressing neurons, which are the ones projecting back to the VTA to control the activity of the GABA neurons as well as to the VP. Manipulations in mice that prevent or reverse drug-evoked plasticity in vivo also have effects on persistent changes of drug-associated behavioral sensitization or cue-induced drug seeking, providing more direct evidence for a causal role of synaptic plasticity in drug-adaptive behavior. The strengthening of the projection from the orbitofrontal cortex to the dorsal striatum may be a neural correlate of compulsion in those animals that self-stimulate the VTA dopamine neurons or take a drug even when punished. Together, a circuit model of staged drug-evoked synaptic plasticity is emerging, whereby various symptoms are caused by changes in specific projections, eventually combining into addiction.

NONADDICTIVE DRUGS OF ABUSE

Some drugs of abuse do not lead to addiction. This is the case for substances that alter perception without causing sensations of reward and euphoria, such as psychedelics and dissociative anesthetics (see Table 32–1). Unlike addictive drugs, which primarily target the mesolimbic dopamine system, these agents primarily target cortical and thalamic circuits. Lysergic acid diethylamide (LSD), for example, activates the serotonin 5-HT_{2A} receptor in the prefrontal cortex, acutely enhancing glutamatergic transmission onto pyramidal neurons for the duration of the presence of the drug. These excitatory afferents mainly come from the thalamus and carry sensory information of varied modalities, which may constitute a link to enhanced perception. Phencyclidine (PCP) and ketamine produce a feeling of separation of mind and body (which is why they are called dissociative anesthetics) and, at higher doses, stupor and coma. The principal mechanism of action is a use-dependent inhibition of glutamate receptors of the NMDA type. High doses of dextromethorphan, an over-the-counter cough suppressant, can also elicit a dissociative state. This effect is mediated by a rather nonselective action on serotonin reuptake, and opioid, acetylcholine, and NMDA receptors.

The classification of NMDA antagonists as nonaddictive drugs was based on early assessments, which, in the case of PCP, have recently been questioned. Animal research shows that PCP can increase mesolimbic dopamine concentrations and has some reinforcing properties in rodents. Ketamine also increases dopamine and leads to weak reinforcement but not to long-lasting adaptation, because NMDA receptor blockage precludes the induction of drug-evoked synaptic plasticity. Addiction liability is thus believed to be low, but not zero. Concurrent effects on both thalamocortical and mesolimbic systems also exist for other addictive drugs. Psychosis-like symptoms can be observed with cannabinoids, amphetamines, and cocaine, which may reflect their effects on thalamocortical structures. For example, cannabinoids, in addition to their documented effects on the mesolimbic dopamine system, also enhance excitation in cortical circuits through presynaptic inhibition of GABA release.

Hallucinogens and NMDA antagonists, even if they do not produce dependence or addiction, can still have long-term effects. Flashbacks of altered perception can occur years after LSD use. Moreover, chronic use of PCP may lead to an irreversible schizophrenia-like psychosis.

■ BASIC PHARMACOLOGY OF DRUGS OF ABUSE

Since all addictive drugs increase dopamine concentrations in the target structures of the mesolimbic projections, we classify them based on the underlying cellular mechanism (see Table 32–1 and Figure 32–2). The first group includes **nicotine,** which through its ionotropic receptor stimulates dopamine neurons. The second group comprises **cocaine, amphetamines,** and **ecstasy,** which all bind to monoamine transporters and lead to increased dopamine levels independent of their effect on neuron firing. The third group contains **opioids, cannabinoids, γ-hydroxybutyric acid (GHB),** and **benzodiazepines,** which exert their action through G_{io} protein–coupled receptors and ionotropic receptors and cause disinhibition of dopamine neurons. Alcohol, which has several molecular targets, increases dopamine through a still unknown mechanism. Drugs such as **psychedelics** do not increase dopamine, are not addictive, and are classified based on their molecular target.

DRUGS THAT EXCITE DOPAMINE NEURONS

NICOTINE

In terms of numbers affected, nicotine addiction exceeds all other forms of addiction, touching more than 50% of all adults in some countries. Nicotine exposure occurs primarily through smoking of tobacco, which causes associated diseases that are responsible for many preventable deaths. The chronic use of chewing tobacco and snuff tobacco is also addictive.

Nicotine is a selective agonist of the nicotinic acetylcholine receptor (nAChR) that is normally activated by acetylcholine (see Chapters 6 and 7). Based on nicotine's enhancement of cognitive performance and the association of Alzheimer dementia with a loss of ACh-releasing neurons from the nucleus basalis of Meynert, nAChRs are believed to play an important role in many cognitive processes. The rewarding effect of nicotine requires involvement of the VTA, in which nAChRs are expressed on dopamine neurons. When nicotine excites projection neurons, dopamine is released in the nucleus accumbens and the prefrontal cortex, thus fulfilling the dopamine requirement of addictive drugs. α4β2-containing channels in the VTA are the nAChRs mediating the rewarding effects of nicotine. This statement is based on the observation that knockout mice deficient for the β2 subunit lose interest in self-administering nicotine, and that in these mice, this behavior can be restored through an in vivo transfection of the β2 subunits in neurons of the VTA. Electrophysiologic evidence suggests that homomeric nAChRs made exclusively of α7 subunits also contribute to the reinforcing effects of nicotine. These receptors are mainly expressed on synaptic terminals of excitatory afferents projecting onto the dopamine neurons. They also contribute to nicotine-evoked dopamine release and the long-term changes induced by the drugs related to addiction (eg, long-term synaptic potentiation of excitatory inputs).

Nicotine withdrawal is mild compared with opioid withdrawal and involves irritability and problems sleeping. However, nicotine is among the most addictive drugs (relative risk 4), and relapse after attempted cessation is very common.

Treatment

Treatments for nicotine addiction include nicotine itself in forms that are slowly absorbed and several other drugs. Nicotine that is chewed, inhaled, or transdermally delivered can be substituted for the nicotine in cigarettes, thus slowing the pharmacokinetics and eliminating the many complications associated with the toxic substances found in tobacco smoke. Recently, two partial agonists of α4β2-containing nAChRs have been characterized: the plant-extract **cytisine** and its synthetic derivative **varenicline.** Both work by occupying nAChRs on dopamine neurons of the VTA, thus preventing nicotine from exerting its action. Varenicline may impair the capacity to drive and has been associated with suicidal ideation. The antidepressant **bupropion** is approved for nicotine cessation therapy. It is most effective when combined with behavioral therapies.

Many countries have banned smoking in public places to create smoke-free environments. This important step not only reduces passive smoking and the hazards of secondhand smoke but also the risk that ex-smokers will be exposed to smoke, which as a contextual cue, may trigger relapse.

DRUGS THAT INTERFERE WITH DOPAMINE REUPTAKE

Cocaine

The prevalence of cocaine abuse remains a major public health problem worldwide. Cocaine is highly addictive (relative risk = 5), and its use is associated with a number of complications.

Cocaine is an alkaloid found in the leaves of *Erythroxylum coca*, a shrub indigenous to the Andes. For more than 100 years, it has been extracted and used in clinical medicine, mainly as a local anesthetic and to dilate pupils in ophthalmology. Sigmund Freud famously proposed its use to treat depression and alcohol dependence, but addiction quickly brought an end to these ideas.

Cocaine hydrochloride is a water-soluble salt that can be injected or absorbed by any mucosal membrane (eg, nasal snorting). When heated in an alkaline solution, it is transformed into the free base, "crack cocaine," which can then be smoked. Inhaled crack cocaine is rapidly absorbed in the lungs and penetrates swiftly into the brain, producing an almost instantaneous "rush."

In the peripheral nervous system, cocaine inhibits voltage-gated sodium channels, thus blocking initiation and conduction of action potentials (see Chapter 26). This mechanism, underlying

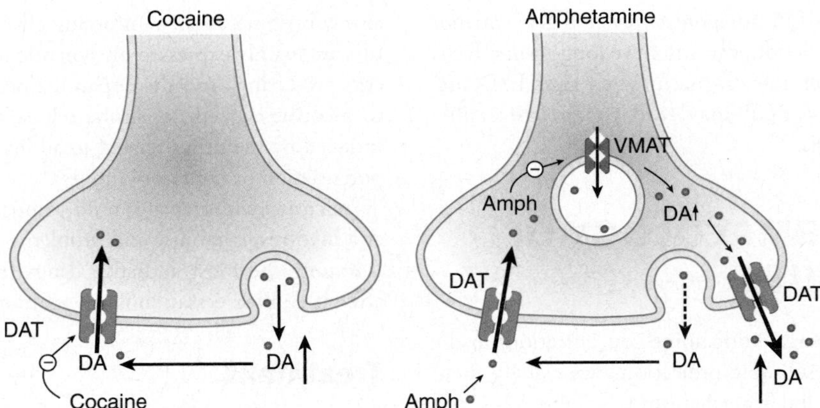

FIGURE 32–4 Mechanism of action of cocaine and amphetamine on synaptic terminal of dopamine (DA) neurons. **Left:** Cocaine inhibits the dopamine transporter (DAT), decreasing DA clearance from the synaptic cleft and causing an increase in extracellular DA concentration. **Right:** Since amphetamine (Amph) is a substrate of the DAT, it competitively inhibits DA transport. In addition, once in the cell, amphetamine interferes with the vesicular monoamine transporter (VMAT) and impedes the filling of synaptic vesicles. As a consequence, vesicles are depleted and cytoplasmic DA increases. This leads to a reversal of DAT direction, strongly increasing nonvesicular release of DA, and further increasing extracellular DA concentrations.

its effect as a local anesthetic, seems responsible for neither the acute rewarding nor the addictive effects. In the central nervous system, cocaine blocks the uptake of dopamine, noradrenaline, and serotonin through their respective transporters. The block of the **dopamine transporter (DAT),** which increases dopamine concentrations in the nucleus accumbens, has been implicated in the rewarding effects of cocaine (Figure 32–4). In fact, the rewarding effects of cocaine are abolished in mutant mice with a cocaine-insensitive DAT. The activation of the sympathetic nervous system results mainly from blockage of the norepinephrine transporter (NET) and leads to an acute increase in arterial pressure, tachycardia, and often, ventricular arrhythmias. Users typically lose their appetite, are hyperactive, and sleep little. Cocaine exposure increases the risk for intracranial hemorrhage, ischemic stroke, myocardial infarction, and seizures. Cocaine overdose may lead to hyperthermia, coma, and death. In the 1970s, when crack-cocaine appeared in the USA, it was suggested that the drug is particularly harmful to the fetus in addicted pregnant women. The term "crack-baby" was used to describe a specific syndrome of the newborn, and the mothers faced harsh legal consequences. The follow-up of the children, now adults, does not confirm a drug-specific handicap in cognitive performance. Moreover, in this population, the percentage of drug-users is comparable to controls matched for socioeconomic environment.

Susceptible individuals may become dependent and addicted after only a few exposures to cocaine. Although a withdrawal syndrome is reported, it is not as strong as that observed with opioids. Tolerance may develop, but in some users, a reverse tolerance is observed; that is, they become sensitized to small doses of cocaine. This behavioral sensitization is in part context-dependent. Cravings are very strong and underlie the very high addiction liability of cocaine. To date, no specific antagonist is available, and the management of intoxication remains supportive. Developing a pharmacologic treatment for cocaine addiction is a top priority.

AMPHETAMINES

Amphetamines are a group of synthetic, indirect-acting sympathomimetic drugs that cause the release of endogenous biogenic amines, such as dopamine and norepinephrine (see Chapters 6 and 9). Amphetamine, methamphetamine, and their many derivatives exert their effects by reversing the action of biogenic amine transporters at the plasma membrane. Amphetamines are substrates of these transporters and are taken up into the cell (see Figure 32–4). Once in the cell, amphetamines interfere with the vesicular monoamine transporter (VMAT; see Figure 6–4), depleting synaptic vesicles of their neurotransmitter content. As a consequence, levels of dopamine (or other transmitter amine) in the cytoplasm increase and quickly become sufficient to cause release into the synapse by reversal of the plasma membrane DAT. Normal vesicular release of dopamine consequently decreases (because synaptic vesicles contain less transmitter), whereas nonvesicular release increases. Similar mechanisms apply for other biogenic amines (serotonin and norepinephrine).

Together with GHB and ecstasy, amphetamines are often referred to as "club drugs" because they are increasingly popular in the club scene. They are often produced in small clandestine laboratories, which makes their precise chemical identification difficult. They differ from ecstasy chiefly in the context of use: intravenous administration and "hard-core" addiction are far more common with amphetamines, especially methamphetamine. In general, amphetamines lead to elevated catecholamine levels that increase arousal and reduce sleep, whereas the effects on the dopamine system mediate euphoria but may also cause abnormal movements and precipitate psychotic episodes. Effects on serotonin transmission may play a role in the hallucinogenic and anorexigenic functions as well as in the hyperthermia often caused by amphetamines.

Unlike many other abused drugs, amphetamines are neurotoxic. The exact mechanism is not known, but neurotoxicity depends on the NMDA receptor and affects mainly serotonin and dopamine neurons.

Amphetamines are typically taken initially in pill form by abusers, but can also be smoked or injected. Heavy users often progress rapidly to intravenous administration. Within hours after oral ingestion, amphetamines increase alertness and cause euphoria, agitation, and confusion. Bruxism (tooth grinding) and skin flushing may occur. Effects on heart rate may be minimal with some compounds (eg, methamphetamine), but with increasing dosage these agents often lead to tachycardia and dysrhythmias. Hypertensive crisis and vasoconstriction may lead to stroke. Spread of HIV and hepatitis infection in inner cities has been closely associated with needle sharing by intravenous users of methamphetamine.

With chronic use, amphetamine tolerance may develop, leading to dose escalation. Withdrawal consists of dysphoria, drowsiness (in some cases, insomnia), and general irritability.

ECSTASY (MDMA)

Ecstasy is the name of a class of drugs that includes a large variety of derivatives of the amphetamine-related compound methylenedioxymethamphetamine (MDMA). MDMA was originally used in some forms of psychotherapy, but no medically useful effects were documented. This is perhaps not surprising, because the main effect of ecstasy appears to be to foster feelings of intimacy and empathy without impairing intellectual capacities. Today, MDMA and its many derivatives are often produced in small quantities in ad hoc laboratories and distributed at parties or "raves," where it is taken orally. Ecstasy therefore is the prototypic **designer drug** and, as such, is increasingly popular.

Similar to the amphetamines, MDMA causes release of biogenic amines by reversing the action of their respective transporters. It has a preferential affinity for the **serotonin transporter (SERT)** and therefore most strongly increases the extracellular concentration of serotonin. This release is so profound that there is a marked intracellular depletion for 24 hours after a single dose. With repetitive administration, serotonin depletion may become permanent, which has triggered a debate on its neurotoxicity. Although direct proof from animal models for neurotoxicity remains weak, several studies report long-term cognitive impairment in heavy users of MDMA.

In contrast, there is a wide consensus that MDMA has several *acute* adverse effects, in particular hyperthermia, which along with dehydration (eg, caused by an all-night dance party) may be fatal. Other complications include serotonin syndrome (mental status change, autonomic hyperactivity, and neuromuscular abnormalities; see Chapter 16) and seizures. Following warnings about the dangers of MDMA, some users have attempted to compensate for hyperthermia by drinking excessive amounts of water, causing water intoxication involving severe hyponatremia, seizures, and even death.

Withdrawal is marked by a mood "offset" characterized by depression lasting up to several weeks. There have also been reports of increased aggression during periods of abstinence in chronic MDMA users.

Taken together, the evidence for irreversible damage to the brain, although not completely convincing, implies that even occasional recreational use of MDMA cannot be considered safe.

■ DRUGS THAT DISINHIBIT DOPAMINE NEURONS

OPIOIDS

Opioids may have been the first drug abused in human history and are still among the most commonly used for nonmedical purposes.

Pharmacology & Clinical Aspects

As described in Chapter 31, opioids comprise a large family of endogenous and exogenous agonists at three G protein–coupled receptors: the μ-, κ-, and δ-opioid receptors. Although all three receptors couple to inhibitory G proteins (ie, they all inhibit adenylyl cyclase and activate K^+ channels), they have distinct, sometimes even opposing effects, mainly because of the cell type-specific expression throughout the brain. In the VTA, for example, μ-opioid receptors are selectively expressed on GABA neurons (which they inhibit), whereas κ-opioid receptors are expressed on and inhibit dopamine neurons. This may explain why μ-opioid agonists cause euphoria, whereas κ agonists induce dysphoria.

In line with the latter observations, the rewarding effects of morphine are absent in knockout mice lacking μ receptors but persist when either of the other opioid receptors are ablated. In the VTA, μ opioids cause an inhibition of GABAergic inhibitory interneurons, which leads to a disinhibition of dopamine neurons, particularly those that project to the medial shell of the nucleus accumbens.

The most commonly abused μ opioids include **morphine, heroin** (diacetylmorphine, which is rapidly metabolized to morphine), **codeine,** and **oxycodone.** The very potent synthetic opioid **fentanyl** (which within minutes saturates opioid receptors at a dose 100× lower than morphine) has become a widely abused drug because of its rapid onset and ease of distribution. Because of its pharmacokinetic properties it is among the most dangerous drugs and accounts for many deaths by overdose. **Meperidine** (also known as **pethidine**) is commonly abused among health professionals. All of these drugs induce strong tolerance and dependence, which increases the risk of transition to addiction by negative reinforcement. Positive and negative reinforcing effects of opioids both depend on μ receptors. In genetically modified mice lacking this receptor, no withdrawal is observed once chronic opioid exposure is terminated. In humans, the withdrawal syndrome may be very severe (except for codeine) and includes intense dysphoria, nausea or vomiting, muscle aches, lacrimation, rhinorrhea, mydriasis, piloerection, sweating, diarrhea, yawning, and fever. Beyond the withdrawal syndrome, which usually lasts no longer than a few days, some individuals who have received opioids as analgesics to treat acute pain develop addiction. Despite this fact, opioid addiction has become a major public health issue in some countries, particularly the USA and Canada. The reason for this epidemic has been identified as careless, widespread chronic prescription of pain killers such as oxycodone to patients, who eventually switched to heroin or other illicit opioids. The relative risk of addiction is 4 out of 5 on a scale of 1 (nonaddictive) to 5 (highly addictive).

Treatment

The opioid antagonist **naloxone** reverses the effects of a dose of morphine or heroin within minutes. This may be lifesaving in the case of an overdose, given typically IV or IM, but also as a nasal spray that can be applied by nonmedical personnel (see Chapters 31 and 58). Naloxone administration also provokes an acute withdrawal (precipitated abstinence) syndrome in a dependent person, which limits compliance. The half-life of naloxone is shorter than morphine (1 h and 2–4 h, respectively), which is why repeated administrations may be necessary.

In treating opioid addiction, a longer-acting opioid (eg, **methadone, buprenorphine, extended-release morphine sulfate**) is often substituted for the shorter-acting, more rewarding opioid (eg, heroin). For substitution therapy, methadone is given orally once daily, facilitating supervised intake. The use of a partial agonist (buprenorphine) and the much longer half-life (methadone, extended-release morphine sulfate, and buprenorphine) may also have some beneficial effects (eg, weaker drug sensitization, which typically requires intermittent exposures), but it is essential to realize that abrupt termination of methadone administration also precipitates a withdrawal syndrome; that is, the subject on substitution therapy remains dependent. Levomethadone, a preparation containing only the active enantiomer, has similar kinetics and effects as methadone, but lower side effects, particularly when cardiac repolarization is perturbed (long QT interval in the electrocardiogram). The use of buprenorphine may be limited by the withdrawal syndrome observed at the beginning of the therapy. Some countries (eg, Canada, Denmark, Netherlands, United Kingdom, Switzerland) allow substitution of medical heroin for street heroin. A follow-up of a cohort of addicts who received heroin injections in a controlled setting and had access to counseling indicates that addicts under heroin substitution have an improved health status and are better integrated in society. The current opioid crisis in the USA has become a leading cause of death in young adults and more than 2 million individuals are dependent.

CANNABINOIDS

Endogenous cannabinoids that act as neurotransmitters include 2-arachidonyl glycerol (2-AG) and anandamide, both of which bind to CB_1 receptors (see also Chapter 63). These very lipid-soluble compounds are released at the postsynaptic somatodendritic membrane, and diffuse through the extracellular space to bind at presynaptic CB_1 receptors, where they inhibit the release of either glutamate or GABA. Because of this backward signaling, endocannabinoids are called retrograde messengers. In the hippocampus, the release of endocannabinoids from pyramidal neurons selectively affects inhibitory transmission and may contribute to the induction of synaptic plasticity during learning and memory formation.

Exogenous cannabinoids, eg, in **marijuana,** which when smoked contains thousands of organic and inorganic chemical compounds, exert their pharmacologic effects through active substances, including **Δ^9-tetra-hydrocannabinol (THC),** a powerful psychoactive substance. Like opioids, THC causes disinhibition of dopamine neurons, mainly by presynaptic inhibition of GABA neurons in the VTA. The half-life of THC is about 4 hours. The onset of effects of THC after smoking marijuana occurs within minutes and reaches a maximum after 1–2 hours. The most prominent effects are euphoria and relaxation. Users also report feelings of well-being, grandiosity, and altered perception of passage of time. Dose-dependent perceptual changes (eg, visual distortions), drowsiness, diminished coordination, and memory impairment may occur. Cannabinoids can also create a dysphoric state and, in rare cases following the use of very high doses, eg, in **hashish,** result in visual hallucinations, depersonalization, and frank psychotic episodes. Additional effects of THC, eg, increased appetite, attenuation of nausea, decreased intraocular pressure, and relief of chronic pain, have led to the use of cannabinoids in medical therapeutics. The justification of medicinal use of marijuana was comprehensively examined more than 20 years ago. Today, medical use of botanical marijuana has been legalized in 25 states and the District of Columbia. Nevertheless this continues to be a controversial issue, mainly because of the fear that cannabinoids may serve as a gateway to the consumption of "hard" drugs or cause schizophrenia in individuals with a predisposition.

Chronic exposure to marijuana leads to dependence, which is revealed by a distinctive, but mild and short-lived withdrawal syndrome that includes restlessness, irritability, mild agitation, insomnia, nausea, and cramping. The relative risk for addiction is 2.

The synthetic Δ^9-THC analog **dronabinol** is a US Food and Drug Administration (FDA)-approved cannabinoid agonist currently marketed in the USA and some European countries. **Nabilone,** an older commercial Δ^9-THC analog, was recently reintroduced in the USA to treat chemotherapy-induced emesis. **Cannabidiol (CBD)** is an active ingredient in marijuana, with low addiction liability, that is legal in all states and most western countries. It may benefit some forms of epilepsy, anxiety, insomnia, and chronic pain. Major side effects include nausea, fatigue, and enhanced blood thinning (particularly in patients receiving anticoagulants). CBD is a low-affinity agonist at CB1/CB2 receptors, but it also binds to other (orphan) GPCRs and can affect serotonin and opioid signaling. **Nabiximols** (trade name Sativex) is a botanical drug obtained by standard extraction. Its active principles are Δ^9-THC and CBD. Initially only marketed in the United Kingdom, it is now widely available to treat symptoms of multiple sclerosis. In the USA, nabiximols is in phase III testing for cancer pain. The cannabinoid system will likely emerge as an essential drug target in the future because of its apparent involvement in several therapeutically desirable effects.

GAMMA-HYDROXYBUTYRIC ACID

Gamma-hydroxybutyric acid (GHB, or sodium oxybate for its salt form) is produced during the metabolism of GABA, but the function of this endogenous agent is unknown at present. The pharmacology of GHB is complex because there are two distinct binding sites. The protein that contains a high-affinity binding site (1 μM) for GHB has been cloned, but its involvement in the cellular effects of GHB at pharmacologic concentrations remains unclear. The low-affinity binding site (1 mM) has been identified as the $GABA_B$ receptor. In mice that lack $GABA_B$ receptors, even very high doses of GHB have no effect; this suggests that $GABA_B$ receptors are the sole mediators of GHB's pharmacologic action.

GHB was first synthesized in 1960 in France and introduced as a general anesthetic. Because of its narrow safety margin and its addictive potential, it is not available in the USA for this purpose. Sodium oxybate (GHB sodium salt) can, however, be prescribed to treat narcolepsy and to decrease daytime sleepiness and episodes of cataplexy through a mechanism unrelated to the reward system. Before causing sedation and coma, GHB causes euphoria, enhanced sensory perceptions, a feeling of social closeness, and amnesia. These properties have made it a popular "club drug" that goes by colorful street names such as "liquid ecstasy," "grievous bodily harm," or "date rape drug." As the latter name suggests, GHB has been used in date rapes because it is odorless and can be readily dissolved in beverages. It is rapidly absorbed after ingestion and reaches a maximal plasma concentration 20–30 minutes after ingestion of a 10–20 mg/kg dose. The elimination half-life is about 30 minutes and leaves the recipient amnesic for events during the drug's duration of action.

Although $GABA_B$ receptors are expressed on all neurons of the VTA, GABA neurons are much more sensitive to GHB than are dopamine neurons (Figure 32–5). This is reflected by the EC_{50}s, which differ by about one order of magnitude, as a result of the difference in coupling efficiency of the $GABA_B$ receptor and the

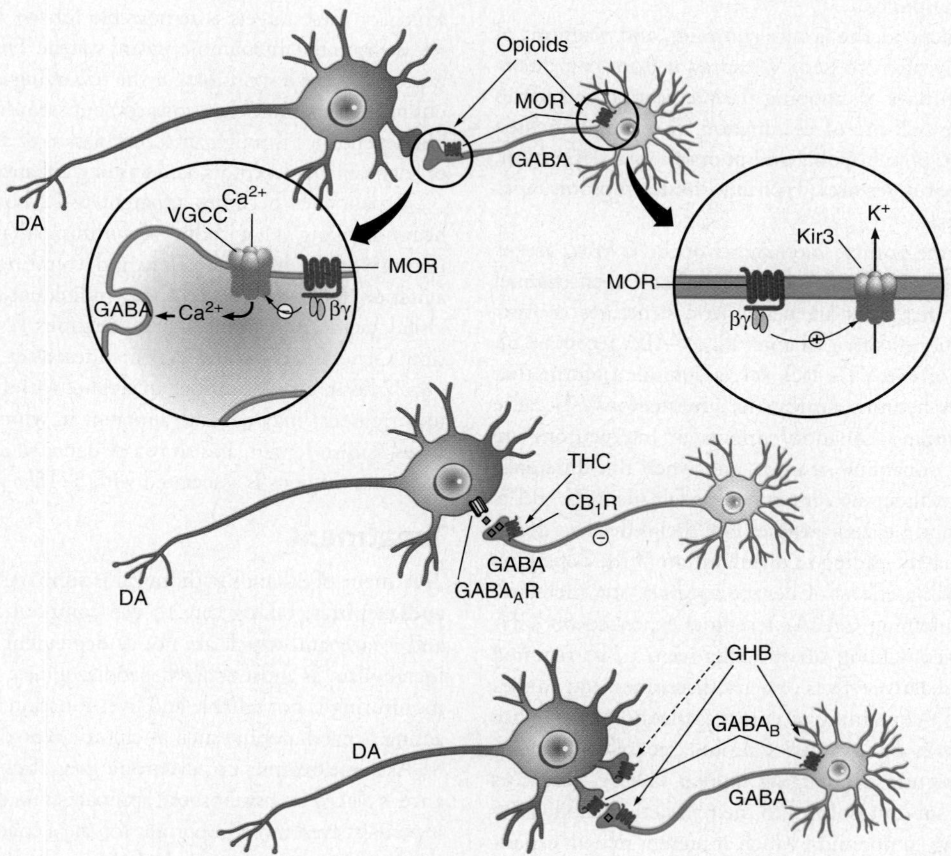

FIGURE 32–5 Disinhibition of dopamine (DA) neurons in the ventral tegmental area (VTA) through drugs that act via G_{io}-coupled receptors. **Top:** Opioids target μ-opioid receptors (MORs) that in the VTA are located exclusively on γ-aminobutyric acid (GABA) neurons. MORs are expressed on the presynaptic terminal of these cells and the somatodendritic compartment of the postsynaptic cells. Each compartment has distinct effectors (*insets*). G protein-βγ-mediated inhibition of voltage-gated calcium channels (VGCC) is the major mechanism in the presynaptic terminal. Conversely, in dendrites MORs activate K channels. Together the pre- and postsynaptic mechanisms reduce transmitter release and suppress activity, ultimately taking away the inhibition by the GABA neurons. **Middle:** Δ^9-tetrahydrocannabinol (THC) and other cannabinoids mainly act through presynaptic inhibition. **Bottom:** Gamma-hydroxybutyric acid (GHB) targets $GABA_B$ receptors, which are located on both cell types. However, GABA neurons are more sensitive to GHB than are DA neurons, leading to disinhibition at concentrations typically obtained with recreational use. CB_1R, cannabinoid receptors.

potassium channels responsible for the hyperpolarization. Because GHB is a weak agonist, only GABA neurons are inhibited at the concentrations typically obtained with recreational use. This feature may underlie the reinforcing effects of GHB and the basis for addiction to the drug. At higher doses, however, GHB also hyperpolarizes dopamine neurons, eventually completely inhibiting dopamine release. Such an inhibition of the VTA may in turn preclude its activation by other addictive drugs and may explain why GHB might have some usefulness as an "anticraving" compound, particularly in the treatment of alcoholism.

BENZODIAZEPINES

Benzodiazepines are commonly prescribed as anxiolytics and sleep medications. They represent a definite risk for abuse, which has to be weighed against their beneficial effects. Some persons abuse benzodiazepines for their euphoriant effects, but most often, abuse occurs concomitant with other drugs, eg, to attenuate anxiety during withdrawal from opioids.

Benzodiazepine dependence is very common, and diagnosis of addiction is probably often missed. Withdrawal from benzodiazepines occurs within days of stopping the medication and varies as a function of the half-life of elimination. Symptoms include irritability, insomnia, phonophobia and photophobia, depression, muscle cramps, and even seizures. Typically, these symptoms taper off within 1–2 weeks.

Benzodiazepines are positive modulators of the $GABA_A$ receptor, increasing both single-channel conductance and open-channel probability. $GABA_A$ receptors are pentameric structures consisting of α, β, and γ subunits (see Chapter 22). GABA receptors on dopamine neurons of the VTA lack $\alpha1$, a subunit isoform that is present in GABA neurons nearby (ie, interneurons). Because of this difference, unitary synaptic currents in interneurons are larger than those in dopamine neurons, and when this difference is amplified by benzodiazepines, interneurons fall silent. GABA is no longer released, and benzodiazepines lose their effect on dopamine neurons, ultimately leading to disinhibition of the dopamine neurons. The rewarding effects of benzodiazepines are, therefore, mediated by $\alpha1$-containing $GABA_A$ receptors expressed on VTA neurons. Receptors containing $\alpha5$ subunits seem to be required for tolerance to the sedative effects of benzodiazepines, and studies in humans link $\alpha2\beta3$-containing receptors to alcohol dependence (the $GABA_A$ receptor is also a target of alcohol; see following text). Taken together, a picture is emerging linking $GABA_A$ receptors that contain the $\alpha1$ subunit isoform to their addiction liability. By extension, $\alpha1$-sparing compounds, which at present remain experimental and are not approved for human use, may eventually be preferred to treat anxiety disorders because of their reduced risk of induced addiction.

Barbiturates, which preceded benzodiazepines as the most commonly abused sedative-hypnotics (after ethanol), are now rarely prescribed to outpatients and therefore constitute a less common prescription drug problem than they did in the past. Street sales of barbiturates, however, continue. Management of barbiturate withdrawal and addiction is similar to that of benzodiazepines.

DRUGS WITH MULTIPLE MECHANISMS OF ACTION

ALCOHOL

Alcohol (ethanol, see Chapter 23) is regularly used by most of the population in many Western countries. Although only a minority becomes dependent and addicted, abuse is a severe public health problem because of the social costs and many diseases associated with alcoholism.

Pharmacology

The pharmacology of alcohol is complex, and no single receptor mediates all of its effects. On the contrary, alcohol alters the function of several receptors and cellular functions, including $GABA_A$ receptors, Kir3/GIRK channels, adenosine reuptake (through the equilibrative nucleoside transporter, ENT1), the glycine receptor, NMDA receptor, and $5\text{-}HT_3$ receptor. They are all, with the exception of ENT1, either ionotropic receptors or ion channels. It is not clear which of these targets is responsible for the increase of dopamine release from the mesolimbic reward system. The inhibition of ENT1 is probably not responsible for the rewarding effects (ENT1 knockout mice drink more than controls) but seems to be involved in alcohol dependence through an accumulation of adenosine, stimulation of adenosine A_2 receptors, and ensuing enhanced CREB signaling.

Dependence becomes apparent 6–12 hours after cessation of heavy drinking as a withdrawal syndrome that may include tremor (mainly of the hands), nausea and vomiting, excessive sweating, agitation, and anxiety. In some individuals, this is followed by visual, tactile, and auditory hallucinations 12–24 hours after cessation. Generalized seizures may manifest after 24–48 hours. Finally, 48–72 hours after cessation, an alcohol withdrawal delirium (delirium tremens) may become apparent in which the person hallucinates, is disoriented, and shows evidence of autonomic instability. Delirium tremens is associated with 5–15% mortality.

Treatment

Treatment of ethanol withdrawal is supportive and relies on **benzodiazepines,** taking care to use compounds such as oxazepam and lorazepam, which are not as dependent on oxidative hepatic metabolism as most other benzodiazepines. In patients in whom monitoring is not reliable and liver function is adequate, a longer-acting benzodiazepine such as chlordiazepoxide is preferred.

As in the treatment of all chronic drug abuse problems, heavy reliance is placed on psychosocial approaches to alcohol addiction. This is perhaps even more important for the alcoholic patient because of the ubiquitous presence of alcohol in many social contexts.

The pharmacologic treatment of alcohol addiction is limited, although several compounds, with different goals, have been used. Therapy is discussed in Chapter 23.

INHALANTS

Inhalant abuse is defined as recreational exposure to chemical vapors, such as **nitrites, ketones,** and aliphatic and aromatic **hydrocarbons.** These substances are present in a variety of household and industrial products that are inhaled by "sniffing," "huffing," or "bagging." Sniffing refers to inhalation from an open container, huffing to the soaking of a cloth in the volatile substance before inhalation, and bagging to breathing in and out of a paper or plastic bag filled with fumes. It is common for novices to start with sniffing and progress to huffing and bagging as addiction develops. Inhalant abuse is particularly prevalent in children and young adults.

The exact mechanism of action of most volatile substances remains unknown. Altered function of ionotropic receptors and ion channels throughout the central nervous system has been demonstrated for a few. Nitrous oxide, for example, binds to NMDA receptors, and fuel additives enhance $GABA_A$ receptor function. Most inhalants produce euphoria; increased excitability of the VTA has been documented for toluene and may underlie its addiction risk. Other substances, such as amyl nitrite ("poppers"), primarily produce smooth muscle relaxation and enhance erection but are not addictive. With chronic exposure to the aromatic hydrocarbons (eg, benzene, toluene), toxic effects can be observed in many organs, including white matter lesions in the central nervous system. Management of overdose remains supportive.

NON-ADDICTIVE DRUGS OF ABUSE

LSD, MESCALINE, & PSILOCYBIN

LSD, mescaline, and psilocybin are commonly called psychedelics because of their ability to alter consciousness, so one senses stimuli that are not present. They induce, often in an unpredictable way, perceptual symptoms, including shape and color distortion. Psychosis-like manifestations (depersonalization, hallucinations, distorted time perception) have led some to classify these drugs as psychotomimetics. They also produce somatic symptoms (dizziness, nausea, paresthesias, and blurred vision). Some users have reported intense reexperiencing of perceptual effects (flashbacks) up to several years after the last drug exposure.

Psychedelics differ from most other drugs described in this chapter in that they induce neither dependence nor addiction. However, repetitive exposure still leads to rapid tolerance (also called tachyphylaxis). Animals do not self-administer hallucinogens, suggesting that they are not rewarding to them. Additional studies show that these drugs also fail to stimulate dopamine release, further supporting the idea that only drugs that activate the mesolimbic dopamine system are addictive. Instead, hallucinogens increase glutamate release in the cortex, presumably by enhancing excitatory afferent input via presynaptic serotonin receptors (eg, $5\text{-HT}_{2A,B}$) from the thalamus. Resolution of the 3D structure of an LSD-bound 5-HT_{2B} receptor reveals an unusual attachment mode, explaining the slow kinetics of the molecule.

LSD is an ergot alkaloid. After synthesis, blotter paper or sugar cubes are sprinkled with the liquid and allowed to dry. When LSD is swallowed, psychoactive effects typically appear after 30 minutes and last 6–12 hours. During this time, subjects have impaired ability to make rational judgments and understand common dangers, which puts them at risk for accidents and personal injury.

In adults, a typical dose is 20–30 mcg. LSD is not considered neurotoxic, but like most ergot alkaloids, it may lead to strong contractions of the uterus that can induce abortion (see Chapter 16).

The main molecular target of LSD and other hallucinogens is the 5-HT_{2A} receptor. This receptor couples to G proteins of the G_q type and generates inositol trisphosphate (IP_3), leading to a release of intracellular calcium. Although hallucinogens, and LSD in particular, have been proposed for several therapeutic indications, efficacy remains elusive pending the outcome of ongoing clinical studies (for historical reasons often being carried out in Switzerland) for cluster headache, depression, and alcohol use disorder.

KETAMINE & PHENCYCLIDINE (PCP)

Ketamine and PCP were developed as general anesthetics (see Chapter 25), but only ketamine is still used for this application, and more recently as an antidepressant (see Chapter 30). Both drugs, along with others, are now classified as "club drugs" and sold under names such as "angel dust," "Hog," and "Special K." They owe their effects to their use-dependent, noncompetitive antagonism of the NMDA receptor. The effects of these substances became apparent when patients undergoing surgery reported unpleasant vivid dreams and hallucinations after anesthesia. Ketamine and PCP are white crystalline powders in their pure forms, but on the street they are also sold as liquids, capsules, or pills, which can be snorted, ingested, injected, or smoked. Psychedelic effects last for about 1 hour and also include increased blood pressure, impaired memory function, and visual alterations. At high doses, unpleasant out-of-body and near-death experiences have been reported. Although ketamine and PCP do not cause dependence and addiction (relative risk = 1), chronic exposure, particularly to the latter, may lead to long-lasting psychosis closely resembling schizophrenia, which may persist beyond drug exposure. Surprisingly, intravenous administration of ketamine can eliminate episodes of depression within hours (see Chapter 30), in strong contrast to selective serotonin reuptake inhibitors and other antidepressants, which usually take weeks to act.

The antidepressive mechanism is believed to involve the antagonism of NMDA receptors. An alternate explanation may involve hydroxynorketamine, a metabolite of ketamine, that targets AMPA receptors to exert the antidepressant effect. Recent findings suggest that ketamine dampens the NMDA receptor dependent burst activity of neurons of the lateral habenula, which leads to a weak disinhibition of the ventral tegmental area. Additional work implicates a disinhibitory circuit in the anterior cingulate cortex. While one ketamine preparation (eg, esketamine, the *S*-enantiomer, introduced in Germany in 1997 as an anesthetic) has received FDA approval to treat depression in adults, a limitation may be the transient nature of the effect, which wears off within days even with repetitive administration.

■ CLINICAL PHARMACOLOGY OF DEPENDENCE & ADDICTION

No single pharmacologic treatment (even in combination with behavioral interventions) efficiently eliminates addiction. This is not to say that addiction is irreversible. Pharmacologic interventions may in fact, be useful at all stages of the disease. This is particularly true in the case of a massive overdose, in which reversal of drug action may be a lifesaving measure. However, FDA-approved antagonists are available only for opioids and benzodiazepines.

Pharmacologic interventions may also alleviate the withdrawal syndrome, particularly after opioid exposure. On the assumption that withdrawal reflects—at least in part—hyperactivity of central adrenergic systems, the α_2-adrenoceptor agonist clonidine (also used as a centrally active antihypertensive drug; see Chapter 11) has been used with some success to attenuate withdrawal. Today, most clinicians prefer to manage opioid withdrawal by very slowly tapering the administration of long-acting opioids.

Another widely accepted treatment is substitution of a legally available agonist that acts at the same receptor as the abused drug. This approach has been approved for opioids and nicotine. For example, heroin addicts may receive methadone to replace heroin; smoking addicts may receive nicotine continuously via a transdermal patch system to replace smoking. In general, a rapid-acting substance is replaced with one that acts or is absorbed more slowly. Some substitution therapies employ a partial agonist (eg, buprenorphine), which, however, may trigger withdrawal. Substitution treatments are largely justified by the benefits of reducing associated health risks, the reduction of drug-associated crime, and better social integration. Although dependence persists, the goal is, with the support of behavioral interventions, to motivate drug users to gradually reduce the dose and become abstinent.

The biggest challenge is the treatment of addiction itself. Several approaches have been proposed, but all remain experimental. One approach is to pharmacologically reduce cravings. The μ-opioid receptor antagonist and partial agonist **naltrexone** is FDA-approved for this indication in opioid and alcohol addiction. Its effect is modest and may involve a modulation of endogenous opioid systems.

Clinical trials are currently being conducted with a number of drugs, including the high-affinity $GABA_B$-receptor agonist **baclofen,** and initial results have shown a significant reduction of craving. This effect may be mediated by the inhibition of the dopamine neurons of the VTA, which is possible at baclofen concentrations obtained by oral administration because of its very high affinity for the $GABA_B$ receptor.

Rimonabant is an inverse agonist of the CB_1 receptor that behaves like an antagonist of cannabinoids. It was developed for smoking cessation and to facilitate weight loss. Because of frequent adverse effects—most notably severe depression carrying a substantial risk of suicide—this drug is no longer used clinically. It was initially used in conjunction with diet and exercise for obese patients (body mass index above 30 kg/m^2). While the cellular mechanism of rimonabant remains to be elucidated, data in rodents convincingly demonstrate that this compound can reduce self-administration in naive as well as drug-experienced animals.

While still experimental, the emergence of a circuit model for addiction has prompted interest in neuromodulatory interventions, such as deep brain stimulation (DBS) or transcranial magnetic stimulation (TMS). Inspired by optogenetic "treatments" in rodent models of addiction, novel protocols have been proposed for DBS in the nucleus accumbens or TMS of the prefrontal cortex. Case studies seem to confirm the potential of such approaches, but controlled clinical studies are lacking.

SUMMARY Drugs Used to Treat Dependence and Addiction

Subclass, Drug	Mechanism of Action	Effects	Clinical Applications	Pharmacokinetics, Toxicities, Interactions
OPIOID RECEPTOR ANTAGONIST				
• Naloxone	Nonselective antagonist of opioid receptors	Reverses the acute effects of opioids; can precipitate severe abstinence syndrome	Opioid overdose	Effect much shorter than morphine (1–2 h); therefore several injections required
• Naltrexone	Antagonist of opioid receptors	Blocks effects of illicit opioids	Treatment of alcoholism, opioid addiction	Half-life 10 h (oral); 5–10 days (depot injection)
SYNTHETIC OPIOID				
• Methadone	Slow-acting agonist of μ-opioid receptor	Acute effects similar to morphine (see text)	Substitution therapy for opioid addicts	High oral bioavailability • half-life highly variable among individuals (range 4–130 h) • *Toxicity:* Respiratory depression, constipation, miosis, tolerance, dependence, arrhythmia, and withdrawal symptoms
• Levomethadone	"Enantiopure" methadone containing only the left-enantiomer of the molecule	Similar to morphine and methadone, but at half the dose of the latter	Substitution therapy	Less toxic compared to racemic methadone, particularly related to cardiac adverse effects (long QT interval)
• Morphine sulphate	A salt containing morphine sulfate pentahydrate	Slow-release version with a longer action than morphine	Substitution therapy	

(continued)

Subclass, Drug	Mechanism of Action	Effects	Clinical Applications	Pharmacokinetics, Toxicities, Interactions
PARTIAL μ-OPIOID RECEPTOR AGONIST				
• Buprenorphine	Partial agonist at μ-opioid receptors	Attenuates acute effects of morphine	Oral substitution therapy for opioid addicts	Long half-life (40 h) • formulated together with naloxone to avoid illicit IV injections
NICOTINIC RECEPTOR PARTIAL AGONIST				
• Varenicline	Partial agonist of nicotinic acetylcholine receptor of the α4β2-type	Occludes "rewarding" effects of smoking • heightened awareness of colors	Smoking cessation	*Toxicity:* Nausea and vomiting, seizures, psychiatric changes
• *Cytisine: Natural analog (extracted from laburnum flowers) of varenicline*				
BENZODIAZEPINES				
• Oxazepam, others	Positive modulators of the $GABA_A$ receptors, increase frequency of channel opening	Enhances GABAergic synaptic transmission; attenuates withdrawal symptoms (tremor, hallucinations, anxiety) in alcoholics • prevents withdrawal seizures	Delirium tremens	Half-life 4–15 h • pharmacokinetics not affected by decreased liver function
• *Lorazepam: Alternate to oxazepam with similar properties*				
***N*-METHYL-D-ASPARTATE (NMDA) ANTAGONIST**				
• Acamprosate	Antagonist of NMDA glutamate receptors	May interfere with forms of synaptic plasticity that depend on NMDA receptors	Treatment of alcoholism • effective only in combination with counseling	*Toxicity:* Allergic reactions, arrhythmia, and low or high blood pressure, headaches, insomnia, and impotence • hallucinations, particularly in elderly patients
CANNABINOID RECEPTOR INVERSE AGONIST				
• Rimonabant	CB_1 receptor inverse agonist	Decreases neurotransmitter release at GABAergic and glutamatergic synapses	Approved in Europe from 2006 to 2008 to treat obesity, then withdrawn because of major side effects • smoking cessation has never been approved, but remains an off-label indication	*Toxicity:* Major depression, including increased risk of suicide

REFERENCES

General

Hancock DB et al: Human genetics of addiction: New insights and future directions. Current Psychiatry Rep 2018;20, doi:10.1007/s11920-018-0873-3.

Lüscher C, Janak PH: Consolidating the circuit model for addiction. Annu Rev Neurosci 2021;44:173.

Lüscher C, Robbins TW, Everitt BJ: The transition to compulsion in addiction. Nat Rev Neurosci 2020;21:247.

Nestler EJ, Lüscher C: The molecular basis of drug addiction: Linking epigenetic to synaptic and circuit mechanisms. Neuron 2019;102:48.

Pascoli V et al: Stochastic synaptic plasticity underlying compulsion in a model of addiction. Nature 2018;564:366.

Redish AD, Jensen S, Johnson A: A unified framework for addiction: Vulnerabilities in the decision process. Behav Brain Sci 2008;31:461.

Pharmacology of Drugs of Abuse

Benowitz NL: Nicotine addiction. N Engl J Med 2010;362:2295.

Corre J et al: Dopamine neurons projecting to medial shell of the nucleus accumbens drive heroin reinforcement. eLife 2018;7:e39945.

Simmler LD et al: Dual action of ketamine confines addiction liability. Nature 2022;608:368.

Maskos U et al: Nicotine reinforcement and cognition restored by targeted expression of nicotinic receptors. Nature 2005;436:103.

Morton J: Ecstasy: Pharmacology and neurotoxicity. Curr Opin Pharmacol 2005;5:79.

Nichols DE: Hallucinogens. Pharmacol Ther 2004;101:131.

Shen W et al: Dichotomous dopaminergic control of striatal synaptic plasticity. Science 2008;321:848.

Snead OC, Gibson KM: Gamma-hydroxybutyric acid. N Engl J Med 2005;352:2721.

Sulzer D et al: Mechanisms of neurotransmitter release by amphetamines: A review. Prog Neurobiol 2005;75:406.

Tan KR et al: Neural basis for addictive properties of benzodiazepines. Nature 2010;463:769.

CASE STUDY ANSWER

When found by his parents, the patient was having visual hallucinations of colorful insects. Hallucinations are often caused by a cannabis overdose, especially when hashish is ingested. The slower kinetics of oral cannabis are more difficult to control compared to smoking marijuana. The poor learning performance may be due to the interference of exogenous cannabis with endocannabinoids that fine-tune synaptic transmission and plasticity. While probably not fulfilling the criteria for addiction at present, the patient is at risk as epidemiologic studies show that drug abuse typically begins in late adolescence. The fact that he is not yet using other drugs is a positive sign.

SECTION VI DRUGS USED TO TREAT DISEASES OF THE BLOOD, INFLAMMATION, & GOUT

CHAPTER 33

Agents Used in Cytopenias; Hematopoietic Growth Factors

James L. Zehnder, MD, & Lacrisha J. Go, DNP, FNP-C*

CASE STUDY

A 25-year-old woman who has been on a strict vegan diet for the past 2 years presents with increasing numbness and paresthesias in her extremities, generalized weakness, a sore tongue, and gastrointestinal discomfort. Physical examination reveals a pale woman with diminished vibration sensation, diminished spinal reflexes, and extensor plantar reflexes (Babinski sign). Examination of her oral cavity reveals atrophic glossitis, in which the tongue appears deep red in color and abnormally smooth and shiny due to atrophy of the lingual papillae. Laboratory testing reveals a macrocytic anemia based on a hematocrit of 30% (normal for women, 37–48%), a hemoglobin concentration of 9.4 g/dL, an erythrocyte mean cell volume (MCV) of 123 fL (normal, 84–99 fL), an erythrocyte mean cell hemoglobin concentration (MCHC) of 34% (normal, 31–36%), and a low reticulocyte count. Further laboratory testing reveals a normal serum folate concentration and a serum vitamin B_{12} (cobalamin) concentration of 98 pg/mL (normal, 250–1100 pg/mL). Once megaloblastic anemia was identified, why was it important to measure serum concentrations of both folic acid and cobalamin? Should this patient be treated with oral or parenteral vitamin B_{12}?

Hematopoiesis, the production from undifferentiated stem cells of circulating erythrocytes, platelets, and leukocytes, is a remarkable process that produces more than 200 billion new blood cells per day in the normal person and even greater numbers of cells in persons with conditions that cause loss or destruction of blood cells. In adults, the hematopoietic machinery resides primarily in the bone marrow and requires a constant supply of three essential nutrients—**iron, vitamin B_{12},** and **folic acid**—as well as the presence of **hematopoietic growth factors,** proteins that regulate

*The authors acknowledge the contributions of the previous author of this chapter, Susan B. Masters, PhD.

the proliferation and differentiation of hematopoietic cells. Inadequate supplies of either the essential nutrients or the growth factors result in deficiency of functional blood cells. **Anemia,** a deficiency in oxygen-carrying erythrocytes, is the most common deficiency and several forms are easily treated. Sickle cell anemia, a condition resulting from a genetic alteration in the hemoglobin molecule, is common but is not easily treated. It is discussed in the Box: Sickle Cell Disease and Hydroxyurea. **Thrombocytopenia** and **neutropenia** are not rare, and some forms are amenable to drug therapy. In this chapter, we first consider the treatment of anemia due to deficiency of iron, vitamin B_{12}, or folic acid; we then turn to the medical use of hematopoietic growth factors to combat anemia, thrombocytopenia, and neutropenia, and to support stem cell transplantation.

■ AGENTS USED IN ANEMIAS

IRON

Basic Pharmacology

Iron deficiency is the most common cause of chronic anemia. Like other forms of chronic anemia, iron deficiency anemia leads to pallor, fatigue, dizziness, exertional dyspnea, and other generalized symptoms of tissue hypoxia. The cardiovascular adaptations to chronic anemia—tachycardia, increased cardiac output, vasodilation—can worsen the condition of patients with underlying cardiovascular disease.

Iron forms the nucleus of the iron-porphyrin heme ring, which together with globin chains forms hemoglobin. Hemoglobin reversibly binds oxygen and provides the critical mechanism for oxygen delivery from the lungs to other tissues. In the absence of adequate iron, small erythrocytes with insufficient hemoglobin are formed, giving rise to **microcytic hypochromic anemia.** Iron-containing heme is also an essential component of myoglobin, cytochromes, and other proteins with diverse biologic functions.

Pharmacokinetics

Free inorganic iron is extremely toxic, but iron is required for essential proteins such as hemoglobin; therefore, evolution has provided an elaborate system for regulating iron absorption, transport, and storage (Figure 33–1). The system uses specialized transport, storage, ferrireductase, and ferroxidase proteins whose concentrations are controlled by the body's demand for hemoglobin synthesis and adequate iron stores (Table 33–1). A peptide called **hepcidin,** produced primarily by liver cells, serves as a key central regulator of the system. Nearly all of the iron used to support hematopoiesis is reclaimed from catalysis of the hemoglobin in senescent or damaged erythrocytes. Normally, only a small amount of iron is lost from the body each day, so dietary requirements are small and easily fulfilled by the iron available in a wide variety of foods. However, in special populations with either increased iron requirements

Sickle Cell Disease and Hydroxyurea

Sickle cell disease is a genetic cause of hemolytic anemia, a form of anemia due to increased erythrocyte *destruction*, instead of the reduced mature erythrocyte *production* seen with iron, folic acid, and vitamin B_{12} deficiency. Patients with sickle cell disease are homozygous for the aberrant β-hemoglobin S (*HbS*) allele (substitution of valine for glutamic acid at amino acid 6 of β-globin) or heterozygous for HbS and a second mutated β-hemoglobin gene such as hemoglobin C (*HbC*) or β-thalassemia. Sickle cell disease has an increased prevalence in individuals of African descent because the heterozygous trait confers resistance to malaria.

In the majority of patients with sickle cell disease, anemia is not the primary presenting problem; the anemia is generally well compensated even though such individuals have a chronically low hematocrit (20–30%), a low serum hemoglobin level (7–10 g/dL), and an elevated reticulocyte count. Instead, the primary problem is that deoxygenated HbS chains form polymeric structures that dramatically change erythrocyte shape, reduce deformability, and elicit membrane permeability changes that further promote hemoglobin polymerization. Abnormal erythrocytes aggregate in the microvasculature—where oxygen tension is low and hemoglobin is deoxygenated—and cause veno-occlusive damage. In the musculoskeletal system, this results in characteristic, extremely severe bone and joint pain. In the cerebral vascular system, it causes ischemic stroke. Damage to the spleen increases the risk of infection, particularly by encapsulated bacteria such as *Streptococcus pneumoniae*. In the pulmonary system, there is an increased risk of infection, and in adults, an increase in embolism and pulmonary hypertension. Supportive treatment includes analgesics, antibiotics, pneumococcal vaccination, and blood transfusions. In addition, the cancer chemotherapeutic drug **hydroxyurea** (hydroxycarbamide) reduces veno-occlusive events. It is approved in the United States for treatment of adults with recurrent sickle cell crises and approved in Europe in adults and children with recurrent vaso-occlusive events. As an anticancer drug used in the treatment of chronic and acute myelogenous leukemia, hydroxyurea inhibits ribonucleotide reductase and thereby depletes deoxynucleoside triphosphate and arrests cells in the S phase of the cell cycle (see Chapter 54). In the treatment of sickle cell disease, hydroxyurea acts through poorly defined pathways to increase the production of fetal hemoglobin γ (HbF), which interferes with the polymerization of HbS. Clinical trials have shown that hydroxyurea decreases painful crises in adults and children with severe sickle cell disease. Its adverse effects include hematopoietic depression, gastrointestinal effects, and teratogenicity in pregnant women. More recently, **voxelotor,** an oral drug that binds HbS and reduces sickling by increasing its affinity for oxygen, has received accelerated approval from the FDA.

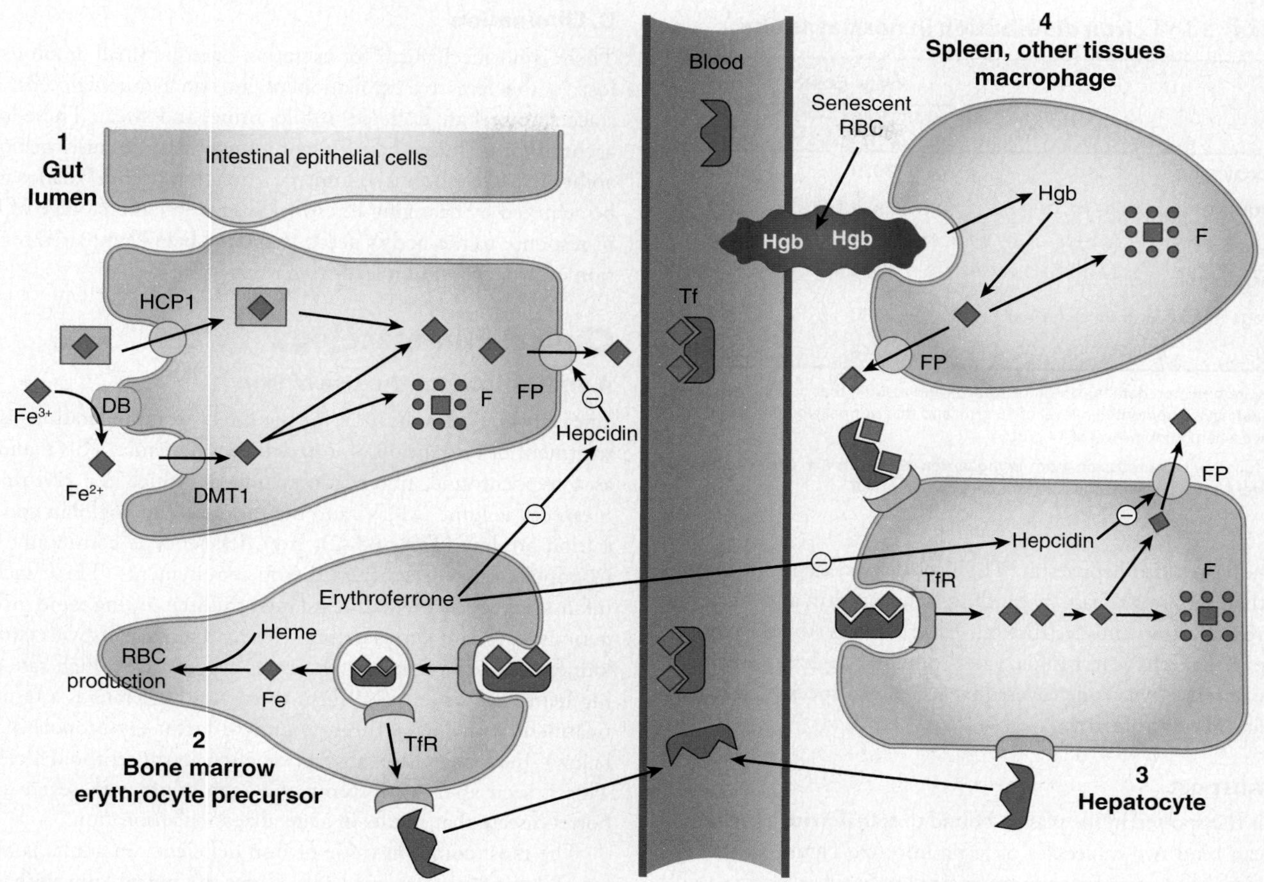

FIGURE 33–1 Absorption, transport, and storage of iron. Intestinal epithelial cells actively absorb inorganic iron via the divalent metal transporter 1 (DMT1) and heme iron via the heme carrier protein 1 (HCP1). Iron that is absorbed or released from absorbed heme iron in the intestine (**1**) is actively transported into the blood by ferroportin (FP) and stored as ferritin (F). In the blood, iron is transported by transferrin (Tf) to erythroid precursors in the bone marrow for synthesis of hemoglobin (Hgb) in red blood cells (RBC) (**2**); or to hepatocytes for storage as ferritin (**3**). The transferrin-iron complex binds to transferrin receptors (TfR) in erythroid precursors and hepatocytes and is internalized. After release of iron, the TfR-Tf complex is recycled to the plasma membrane and Tf is released. Macrophages that phagocytize senescent erythrocytes (RBC) reclaim the iron from the RBC hemoglobin and either export it or store it as ferritin (**4**). Hepatocytes use several mechanisms to take up iron and store the iron as ferritin. High hepatic iron stores increase hepcidin synthesis, and hepcidin inhibits ferroportin; low hepatocyte iron and increased erythroferrone inhibits hepcidin and enhances iron absorption via ferroportin. Ferrous iron (Fe^{2+}), blue diamonds, squares; ferric iron (Fe^{3+}), red; DB, duodenal cytochrome B; F, ferritin. (Modified from Trevor A: *Pharmacology Examination & Board Review*, 9th ed. New York, NY: McGraw Hill; 2010.)

(eg, growing children, pregnant women) or increased losses of iron (eg, menstruating women), iron requirements can exceed normal dietary supplies, and iron deficiency can develop.

A. Absorption

The average American diet contains 10–15 mg of elemental iron daily. A normal individual absorbs 5–10% of this iron, or about 0.5–1 mg daily. Iron is absorbed in the duodenum and proximal jejunum, although the more distal small intestine can absorb iron if necessary. Iron absorption increases in response to low iron stores or increased iron requirements. Total iron absorption increases to 1–2 mg/d in menstruating women and may be as high as 3–4 mg/d in pregnant women.

Iron is available in a wide variety of foods but is especially abundant in meat. The iron in meat protein can be efficiently absorbed, because heme iron in meat hemoglobin and myoglobin can be absorbed intact without first having to be dissociated into elemental iron (see Figure 33–1). Iron in other foods, especially vegetables and grains, is often tightly bound to organic compounds and is much less available for absorption. Nonheme iron in foods and iron in inorganic iron salts and complexes must be reduced by a ferrireductase to ferrous iron (Fe^{2+}) before it can be absorbed by intestinal mucosal cells.

Iron crosses the luminal membrane of the intestinal mucosal cell by two mechanisms: active transport of ferrous iron by the divalent metal transporter DMT1, and absorption of iron complexed with heme (see Figure 33–1). Together with iron split from absorbed heme, the newly absorbed iron can be actively transported into the blood across the basolateral membrane by a transporter known as ferroportin and oxidized to ferric iron (Fe^{3+})

TABLE 33–1 Iron distribution in normal adults.[1]

	Iron Content (mg)	
	Men	Women
Hemoglobin	3050	1700
Myoglobin	430	300
Enzymes	10	8
Transport (transferrin)	8	6
Storage (ferritin and other forms)	750	300
Total	4248	2314

[1]Values are based on data from various sources and assume that normal men weigh 80 kg and have a hemoglobin level of 16 g/dL and that normal women weigh 55 kg and have a hemoglobin level of 14 g/dL.

Reproduced with permission from Wyngaarden JB, Smith LH: *Cecil Textbook of Medicine*, 18th ed. Philadelphia, PA: Saunders/Elsevier; 1988.

by the ferroxidase hephaestin. The liver-derived hepcidin inhibits intestinal cell iron release by binding to ferroportin and triggering its internalization and destruction. Excess iron is stored in intestinal epithelial cells as ferritin, a water-soluble complex consisting of a core of ferric hydroxide covered by a shell of a specialized storage protein called **apoferritin.**

B. Transport

Iron is transported in the plasma bound to **transferrin,** a β-globulin that can bind two molecules of ferric iron (see Figure 33–1). The transferrin-iron complex enters maturing erythroid cells by a specific receptor mechanism. Transferrin receptors—integral membrane glycoproteins present in large numbers on proliferating erythroid cells—bind and internalize the transferrin-iron complex through the process of receptor-mediated endocytosis. In endosomes, the ferric iron is released, reduced to ferrous iron, and transported by DMT1 into the cytoplasm, where it is funneled into hemoglobin synthesis or stored as ferritin. The transferrin-transferrin receptor complex is recycled to the cell membrane, where the transferrin dissociates and returns to the plasma. This process provides an efficient mechanism for supplying the iron required by developing red blood cells.

Increased erythropoiesis is associated with an increase in the number of transferrin receptors on developing erythroid cells and a reduction in hepatic hepcidin release. Iron store depletion and iron deficiency anemia are associated with an increased concentration of serum transferrin.

C. Storage

In addition to the storage of iron in intestinal mucosal cells, iron is also stored, primarily as ferritin, in macrophages in the liver, spleen, and bone, and in parenchymal liver cells (see Figure 33–1). The mobilization of iron from macrophages and hepatocytes is primarily controlled by hepcidin regulation of ferroportin activity. Low hepcidin concentrations result in iron release from these storage sites; high hepcidin concentrations inhibit iron release. Ferritin is detectable in serum. Since the ferritin present in serum is in equilibrium with storage ferritin in reticuloendothelial tissues, the serum ferritin level can be used to estimate total body iron stores.

D. Elimination

There is no mechanism for excretion of iron. Small amounts are lost in the feces by exfoliation of intestinal mucosal cells, and trace amounts are excreted in bile, urine, and sweat. These losses account for no more than 1 mg of iron per day. Because the body's ability to excrete iron is so limited, regulation of iron balance must be achieved by changing intestinal absorption and storage of iron in response to the body's needs. As noted below, impaired regulation of iron absorption leads to serious pathology.

Clinical Pharmacology

A. Indications for the Use of Iron

The only clinical indication for the use of iron preparations is the treatment or prevention of iron deficiency anemia. This manifests as a hypochromic, microcytic anemia in which the erythrocyte mean cell volume (MCV) and the mean cell hemoglobin concentration are low (Table 33–2). Iron deficiency is commonly seen in populations with increased iron requirements. These include infants, especially premature infants; children during rapid growth periods; pregnant and lactating women; and patients with chronic kidney disease who lose erythrocytes at a relatively high rate during hemodialysis and also form them at a high rate as a result of treatment with the erythrocyte growth factor erythropoietin (see below). Inadequate iron absorption also can cause iron deficiency. This is seen after gastrectomy and in patients with severe small bowel disease that results in generalized malabsorption.

The most common cause of iron deficiency in adults is blood loss. Menstruating women lose about 30 mg of iron with each menstrual period; women with heavy menstrual bleeding may lose much more. Thus, many premenopausal women have low iron stores or even iron deficiency. In men and postmenopausal women, the most common site of blood loss is the gastrointestinal tract.

TABLE 33–2 Distinguishing features of the nutritional anemias.

Nutritional Deficiency	Type of Anemia	Laboratory Abnormalities
Iron	Microcytic, hypochromic with MCV <80 fL and MCHC <30%	Low SI <30 mcg/dL with increased TIBC, resulting in a % transferrin saturation (SI/TIBC) of <10%; low serum ferritin level (<20 mcg/L)
Folic acid	Macrocytic, normochromic with MCV >100 fL and normal or elevated MCHC	Low serum folic acid (<4 ng/mL)
Vitamin B_{12}	Same as folic acid deficiency	Low serum cobalamin (<100 pmol/L) accompanied by increased serum homocysteine (>13 μmol/L), and increased serum (>0.4 μmol/L) and urine (>3.6 μmol/mol creatinine) methylmalonic acid

MCV, mean cell volume; MCHC, mean cell hemoglobin concentration; SI, serum iron; TIBC, transferrin iron-binding capacity.

Patients with unexplained iron deficiency anemia should be evaluated for occult gastrointestinal bleeding.

B. Treatment

Iron deficiency anemia is treated with oral or parenteral iron preparations. Oral iron corrects the anemia just as rapidly and completely as parenteral iron in most cases if iron absorption from the gastrointestinal tract is normal. An exception is the high requirement for iron of patients with advanced chronic kidney disease who are undergoing hemodialysis and treatment with erythropoietin; for these patients, parenteral iron administration is preferred.

1. Oral iron therapy—A wide variety of oral iron preparations is available. Because ferrous iron is most efficiently absorbed, ferrous salts should be used. Ferrous sulfate, ferrous gluconate, and ferrous fumarate are all effective and inexpensive and are recommended for the treatment of most patients.

Different iron salts provide different amounts of elemental iron, as shown in Table 33–3. In an iron-deficient individual, about 50–100 mg of iron can be incorporated into hemoglobin daily, and about 25% of oral iron given as ferrous salt can be absorbed. Therefore, 200–400 mg of elemental iron should be given daily to correct iron deficiency most rapidly. Patients unable to tolerate such large doses of iron can be given lower daily doses of iron, which results in slower but still complete correction of iron deficiency. Treatment with oral iron should be continued for 3–6 months after correction of the cause of the iron loss. This corrects the anemia and replenishes iron stores.

Common adverse effects of oral iron therapy include nausea, epigastric discomfort, abdominal cramps, constipation, and diarrhea. These effects are usually dose-related and often can be overcome by lowering the daily dose of iron or by taking the tablets immediately after or with meals, without dairy. Some patients have less severe gastrointestinal adverse effects with one iron salt than another and benefit from changing preparations. Patients taking oral iron commonly develop black stools; this has no clinical significance in itself but may obscure the diagnosis of continued gastrointestinal blood loss.

2. Parenteral iron therapy—Parenteral therapy should be reserved for patients with documented iron deficiency who are unable to tolerate or absorb oral iron and for patients with extensive chronic anemia who cannot be maintained with oral iron alone, or require rapid repletion. This includes patients with advanced chronic renal disease requiring hemodialysis and treatment with erythropoietin, various postgastrectomy conditions and previous small bowel resection, inflammatory bowel disease involving the proximal small bowel, and malabsorption syndromes.

The challenge with parenteral iron therapy is that parenteral administration of inorganic free ferric iron produces serious dose-dependent toxicity, which severely limits the dose that can be administered. However, when the ferric iron is formulated as a colloid containing particles with a core of iron oxyhydroxide surrounded by a core of carbohydrate, bioactive iron is released slowly from the stable colloid particles. In the United States, the three traditional forms of parenteral iron are **iron dextran, sodium ferric gluconate complex,** and **iron sucrose.** Two newer preparations are also available (see below).

Iron dextran is a stable complex of ferric oxyhydroxide and dextran polymers containing 50 mg of elemental iron per milliliter of solution. It can be given by deep intramuscular injection or by intravenous infusion, although the intravenous route is used most commonly. Intravenous administration eliminates the local pain and tissue staining that often occur with the intramuscular route and allows delivery of the entire dose of iron necessary to correct the iron deficiency at one time. Adverse effects of intravenous iron dextran therapy include headache, light-headedness, fever, arthralgias, nausea and vomiting, back pain, flushing, urticaria, bronchospasm, and, rarely, anaphylaxis and death. Owing to the risk of a hypersensitivity reaction, a small test dose of iron dextran should always be given before full intramuscular or intravenous doses are given. Patients with a strong allergy history and patients who have had a prior reaction to parenteral iron are more likely to have hypersensitivity reactions to treatment with parenteral iron dextran. The iron dextran formulations used clinically are distinguishable as high-molecular-weight and low-molecular-weight forms. In the United States, the INFeD preparation is a low-molecular-weight form while Dexferrum is a high-molecular-weight form. Clinical data—primarily from observational studies—indicate that the risk of anaphylaxis is largely associated with high-molecular-weight formulations.

Sodium ferric gluconate complex and **iron-sucrose complex** are alternative parenteral iron preparations. **Ferric carboxymaltose** is a colloidal iron preparation embedded within a carbohydrate polymer. **Ferumoxytol** is a superparamagnetic iron oxide nanoparticle coated with carbohydrate. The carbohydrate shell is removed in the reticuloendothelial system, allowing the iron to be stored as ferritin, or released to transferrin. Ferumoxytol may interfere with magnetic resonance imaging (MRI) studies. Thus if imaging is needed, MRI should be performed prior to ferumoxytol therapy or alternative imaging modality used if needed soon after dosing. The US Food and Drug Administration (FDA) has issued a black box warning about risk of potentially fatal allergic reactions associated with the use of ferumoxytol.

For patients treated chronically with parenteral iron, it is important to monitor iron storage levels to avoid the serious toxicity associated with iron overload. Unlike oral iron therapy, which is subject to the regulatory mechanism provided by the

TABLE 33–3 Some commonly used oral iron preparations.

Preparation	Tablet Size	Elemental Iron per Tablet	Usual Adult Dosage for Treatment of Iron Deficiency (Tablets per Day)
Ferrous sulfate, hydrated	325 mg	65 mg	2–4
Ferrous sulfate, desiccated	200 mg	65 mg	2–4
Ferrous gluconate	325 mg	36 mg	3–4
Ferrous fumarate	325 mg	106 mg	2–3

intestinal uptake system, parenteral administration—which bypasses this regulatory system—can deliver more iron than can be safely stored. Iron stores can be estimated on the basis of serum concentrations of ferritin and the transferrin saturation, which is the ratio of the total serum iron concentration to the total iron-binding capacity (TIBC).

Clinical Toxicity

A. Acute Iron Toxicity

Acute iron toxicity is seen almost exclusively in young children who accidentally ingest iron tablets. As few as 10 tablets of any of the commonly available oral iron preparations can be lethal in young children. Adult patients taking oral iron preparations should be instructed to store tablets in child-proof containers out of the reach of children. Children who are poisoned with oral iron experience necrotizing gastroenteritis with vomiting, abdominal pain, and bloody diarrhea followed by shock, lethargy, and dyspnea. Subsequently, improvement is often noted, but this may be followed by severe metabolic acidosis, coma, and death. Urgent treatment is necessary. **Whole bowel irrigation** (see Chapter 58) should be performed to flush out unabsorbed pills. **Deferoxamine,** a potent iron-chelating compound, can be given intravenously to bind iron that has already been absorbed and to promote its excretion in urine and feces. Activated charcoal, a highly effective adsorbent for most toxins, does ***not*** bind iron and thus is ineffective. Appropriate supportive therapy for gastrointestinal bleeding, metabolic acidosis, and shock must also be provided.

B. Chronic Iron Toxicity

Chronic iron toxicity (iron overload), also known as **hemochromatosis,** results when excess iron is deposited in the heart, liver, pancreas, and other organs. It can lead to organ failure and death. It most commonly occurs in patients with inherited hemochromatosis, a disorder characterized by excessive iron absorption, and in patients who receive many red cell transfusions over a long period of time (eg, individuals with β-thalassemia).

Chronic iron overload in the absence of anemia is most efficiently treated by intermittent phlebotomy. About one unit of blood can be removed every week until all of the excess iron is removed. Iron chelation therapy using parenteral **deferoxamine** or the oral iron chelators **deferasirox** or **deferiprone** (see Chapter 57) is less efficient, and more complicated, expensive, and hazardous, but sometimes the only option for patients with iron overload that cannot be managed by phlebotomy. This is often the case for many individuals with inherited and acquired causes of refractory anemia such as thalassemia major, sickle cell anemia, aplastic anemia, etc. Deferiprone has rarely been associated with agranulocytosis; thus weekly complete blood count monitoring is required.

VITAMIN B_{12}

Vitamin B_{12} (cobalamin) serves as a cofactor for several essential biochemical reactions in humans. Deficiency of vitamin B_{12} leads to megaloblastic anemia (see Table 33–2), gastrointestinal symptoms, and neurologic abnormalities. Although deficiency of vitamin B_{12} due to an inadequate supply in the diet is unusual, deficiency of B_{12} in adults—especially older adults—due to inadequate absorption of dietary vitamin B_{12} is a relatively common and easily treated disorder.

Chemistry

Vitamin B_{12} consists of a porphyrin-like ring with a central cobalt atom attached to a nucleotide. Various organic groups may be covalently bound to the cobalt atom, forming different cobalamins. Deoxyadenosylcobalamin and methylcobalamin are the active forms of the vitamin in humans. **Cyanocobalamin** and **hydroxocobalamin** (both available for therapeutic use) and other cobalamins found in food sources are converted to the active forms. The ultimate source of vitamin B_{12} is from microbial synthesis; the vitamin is not synthesized by animals or plants. The chief dietary source of vitamin B_{12} is microbially derived vitamin B_{12} in meat (especially liver), eggs, and dairy products. Vitamin B_{12} is sometimes called **extrinsic factor** to differentiate it from **intrinsic factor,** a protein secreted by the stomach that is required for gastrointestinal uptake of dietary vitamin B_{12}.

Pharmacokinetics

The average American diet contains 5–30 mcg of vitamin B_{12} daily, 1–5 mcg of which is usually absorbed. The vitamin is avidly stored, primarily in the liver, with an average adult having a total vitamin B_{12} storage pool of 3000–5000 mcg. Only trace amounts of vitamin B_{12} are normally lost in urine and stool. Because the normal daily requirements of vitamin B_{12} are only about 2 mcg, it would take about 5 years for all of the stored vitamin B_{12} to be exhausted and for megaloblastic anemia to develop if B_{12} absorption were stopped. Vitamin B_{12} is absorbed after it complexes with **intrinsic factor,** a glycoprotein secreted by the parietal cells of the gastric mucosa. Intrinsic factor combines with the vitamin B_{12} that is liberated from dietary sources in the stomach and duodenum, and the intrinsic factor-vitamin B_{12} complex is subsequently absorbed in the distal ileum by a highly selective receptor-mediated transport system. Vitamin B_{12} deficiency in humans most often results from malabsorption of vitamin B_{12} due either to lack of intrinsic factor or to loss or malfunction of the absorptive mechanism in the distal ileum. Nutritional deficiency is rare but may be seen in strict vegetarians after many years without meat, eggs, or dairy products.

Once absorbed, vitamin B_{12} is transported to the various cells of the body bound to a family of specialized glycoproteins, transcobalamin I, II, and III. Excess vitamin B_{12} is stored in the liver.

Pharmacodynamics

Two essential enzymatic reactions in humans require vitamin B_{12} (Figure 33–2). In one, methylcobalamin serves as an intermediate in the transfer of a methyl group from N^5-methyltetrahydrofolate to homocysteine, forming methionine (see Figure 33–2A; Figure 33–3, section 1). Without vitamin B_{12}, conversion of the major dietary and storage folate—N^5-methyltetrahydrofolate—to tetrahydrofolate, the precursor of folate cofactors, cannot occur. As a result, vitamin B_{12} deficiency leads to deficiency of folate cofactors necessary for

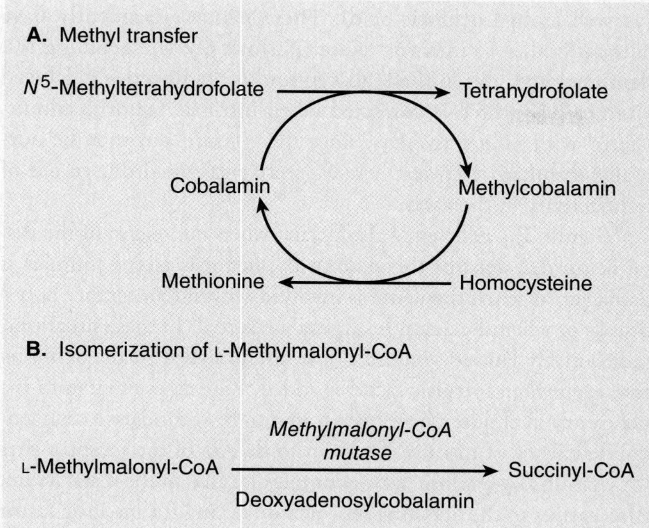

FIGURE 33–2 Enzymatic reactions that use vitamin B_{12}. See text.

several biochemical reactions involving the transfer of one-carbon groups. In particular, the depletion of tetrahydrofolate prevents synthesis of adequate supplies of the deoxythymidylate (dTMP) and purines required for DNA synthesis in rapidly dividing cells, as shown in Figure 33–3, section 2. The accumulation of folate as N^5-methyltetrahydrofolate and the associated depletion of tetrahydrofolate cofactors in vitamin B_{12} deficiency have been referred to as the "methylfolate trap." This is the biochemical step whereby vitamin B_{12} and folic acid metabolism are linked, and it explains why the megaloblastic anemia of vitamin B_{12} deficiency can be partially corrected by ingestion of large amounts of folic acid. Folic acid can be reduced to dihydrofolate by the enzyme dihydrofolate reductase (see Figure 33–3, section 3) and thereby serve as a source of the tetrahydrofolate required for synthesis of the purines and dTMP required for DNA synthesis.

Vitamin B_{12} deficiency causes the accumulation of homocysteine due to reduced formation of methylcobalamin, which is required for the conversion of homocysteine to methionine (see Figure 33–3, section 1). The increase in serum homocysteine can be used to help establish a diagnosis of vitamin B_{12} deficiency (see Table 33–2).

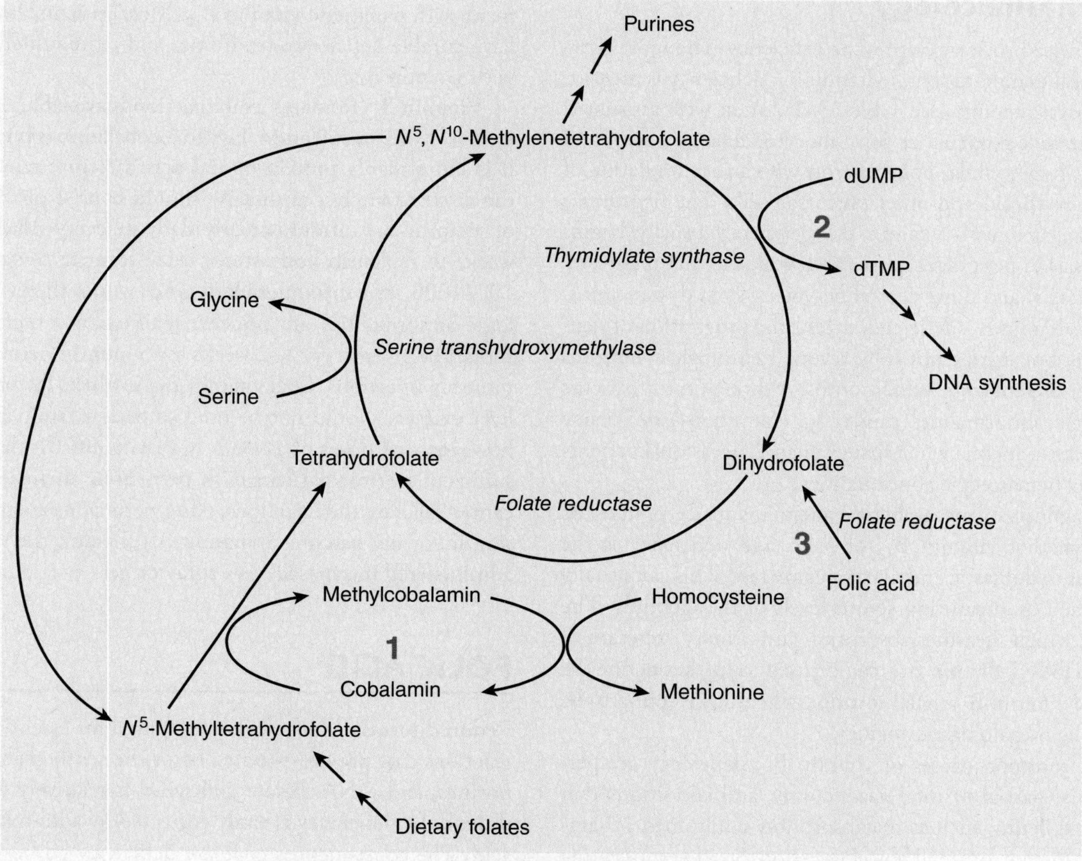

FIGURE 33–3 Enzymatic reactions that use folates. **Section 1** shows the vitamin B_{12}-dependent reaction that allows most dietary folates to enter the tetrahydrofolate cofactor pool and becomes the "folate trap" in vitamin B_{12} deficiency. **Section 2** shows the deoxythymidine monophosphate (dTMP) cycle. **Section 3** shows the pathway by which folic acid enters the tetrahydrofolate cofactor pool. Double arrows indicate pathways with more than one intermediate step. dUMP, deoxyuridine monophosphate.

There is evidence from observational studies that elevated serum homocysteine increases the risk of atherosclerotic cardiovascular disease. However, randomized clinical trials have not shown a definitive reduction in cardiovascular events (myocardial infarction, stroke) in patients receiving vitamin supplementation that lowers serum homocysteine.

The other reaction that requires vitamin B_{12} is isomerization of methylmalonyl-CoA to succinyl-CoA by the enzyme methylmalonyl-CoA mutase (see Figure 33–2B). In vitamin B_{12} deficiency, this conversion cannot take place and the substrate, methylmalonyl-CoA, as well as methylmalonic acid accumulate. The increase in serum and urine concentrations of methylmalonic acid can be used to support a diagnosis of vitamin B_{12} deficiency (see Table 33–2). In the past, it was thought that abnormal accumulation of methylmalonyl-CoA causes the neurologic manifestations of vitamin B_{12} deficiency. However, newer evidence implicates the disruption of the methionine synthesis pathway as the cause of neurologic problems. Whatever the biochemical explanation for neurologic damage, the important point is that administration of folic acid in the setting of vitamin B_{12} deficiency will not prevent neurologic manifestations even though it will largely correct the anemia caused by the vitamin B_{12} deficiency.

Clinical Pharmacology

Vitamin B_{12} is used to treat or prevent deficiency. The most characteristic clinical manifestation of vitamin B_{12} deficiency is megaloblastic, macrocytic anemia (see Table 33–2), often with associated mild or moderate leukopenia or thrombocytopenia (or both), and a characteristic hypercellular bone marrow with an accumulation of megaloblastic erythroid and other precursor cells. The neurologic syndrome associated with vitamin B_{12} deficiency usually begins with paresthesias in peripheral nerves and weakness that progresses to spasticity, ataxia, and other central nervous system dysfunctions. Correction of vitamin B_{12} deficiency arrests the progression of neurologic disease, but it may not fully reverse neurologic symptoms that have been present for several months. Although most patients with neurologic abnormalities caused by vitamin B_{12} deficiency have megaloblastic anemia when first evaluated, occasional patients have few if any hematologic abnormalities.

Once a diagnosis of megaloblastic anemia is made, it must be determined whether vitamin B_{12} or folic acid deficiency is the cause. Other megaloblastic anemia causes are rare. This can usually be accomplished by measuring serum levels of the vitamins. The Schilling test, which measures absorption and urinary excretion of radioactively labeled vitamin B_{12}, can be used to further define the mechanism of vitamin B_{12} malabsorption when this is found to be the cause of the megaloblastic anemia.

The most common causes of vitamin B_{12} deficiency are pernicious anemia, partial or total gastrectomy, and conditions that affect the distal ileum, such as malabsorption syndromes, inflammatory bowel disease, or small bowel resection. Strict vegans eating a diet free of meat and dairy products may become B_{12} deficient.

Pernicious anemia results from defective secretion of intrinsic factor by the gastric mucosal cells. Patients with pernicious anemia have gastric atrophy and fail to secrete intrinsic factor (as well as hydrochloric acid). These patients frequently have autoantibodies to intrinsic factor. Historically, the Schilling test demonstrated diminished absorption of radioactively labeled vitamin B_{12}, which is corrected when intrinsic factor is administered with radioactive B_{12}, since the vitamin can then be normally absorbed. This test is now rarely performed due to use of radioactivity in the assay.

Vitamin B_{12} deficiency also occurs when the region of the distal ileum that absorbs the vitamin B_{12}-intrinsic factor complex is damaged, as when the ileum is involved with inflammatory bowel disease or when the ileum is surgically resected. In these situations, radioactively labeled vitamin B_{12} is not absorbed in the Schilling test, even when intrinsic factor is added. Rare cases of vitamin B_{12} deficiency in children have been found to be secondary to congenital deficiency of intrinsic factor or to defects of the receptor sites for vitamin B_{12}-intrinsic factor complex located in the distal ileum. Alternatives to the Schilling test include testing for intrinsic factor antibodies and testing for elevated homocysteine and methylmalonic acid levels (see Figure 33–2) to make a diagnosis of pernicious anemia with high sensitivity and specificity.

Almost all cases of vitamin B_{12} deficiency are caused by malabsorption of the vitamin; therefore, parenteral injections of vitamin B_{12} are required for therapy. For patients with potentially reversible diseases, the underlying disease should be treated after initial treatment with parenteral vitamin B_{12}. Most patients, however, do not have curable deficiency syndromes and require lifelong treatment with vitamin B_{12}.

Vitamin B_{12} for parenteral injection is available as cyanocobalamin or hydroxocobalamin. Hydroxocobalamin is preferred because it is more highly protein-bound and therefore remains longer in the circulation. Initial therapy should consist of 100–1000 mcg of vitamin B_{12} intramuscularly daily or every other day for 1–2 weeks to replenish body stores. Maintenance therapy consists of 100–1000 mcg intramuscularly once a month for life. If neurologic abnormalities are present, maintenance therapy injections should be given every 1–2 weeks for 6 months before switching to monthly injections. Oral vitamin B_{12}-intrinsic factor mixtures and liver extracts should not be used to treat vitamin B_{12} deficiency; however, oral doses of 1000 mcg of vitamin B_{12} daily are usually sufficient to treat patients with pernicious anemia who refuse or cannot tolerate the injections. After pernicious anemia is in remission following parenteral vitamin B_{12} therapy, the vitamin can be administered intranasally as a spray or gel.

FOLIC ACID

Reduced forms of folic acid are required for essential biochemical reactions that provide precursors for the synthesis of amino acids, purines, and DNA. Folate deficiency is relatively common, even though the deficiency is easily corrected by administration of folic acid. The consequences of folate deficiency go beyond the problem of anemia because folate deficiency is implicated as a cause of congenital malformations in newborns and may play a role in vascular disease (see Box: Folic Acid Supplementation: A Public Health Dilemma).

Folic Acid Supplementation: A Public Health Dilemma

Starting in January 1998, all products made from enriched grains in the United States and Canada were required to be supplemented with folic acid. These rulings were issued to reduce the incidence of congenital neural tube defects (NTDs). Epidemiologic studies show a strong correlation between maternal folic acid deficiency and the incidence of NTDs such as spina bifida and anencephaly. The requirement for folic acid supplementation is a public health measure aimed at the significant number of women who do not receive prenatal care and are not aware of the importance of adequate folic acid ingestion for preventing birth defects in their infants. Observational studies from countries that supplement grains with folic acid have found that supplementation is associated with a significant (20–25%) reduction in NTD rates. Observational studies also suggest that rates of other types of congenital anomalies (heart and orofacial) have fallen since supplementation began.

There may be an added benefit for adults. N^5-Methyltetrahydrofolate is required for the conversion of homocysteine to methionine (Figure 33–2; Figure 33–3, section 1). Impaired synthesis of N^5-methyltetrahydrofolate results in elevated serum concentrations of homocysteine. Data from several sources suggest a positive correlation between elevated serum homocysteine and occlusive vascular diseases such as ischemic heart disease and stroke. Clinical data suggest that the folate supplementation program has improved the folate status and reduced the prevalence of hyperhomocysteinemia in a population of middle-aged and older adults who did not use vitamin supplements. There is also evidence that adequate folic acid protects against several cancers, including colorectal, breast, and cervical cancer.

Although the potential benefits of supplemental folic acid during pregnancy are compelling, the decision to require folic acid in grains was controversial. As described in the text, ingestion of folic acid can partially or totally correct the anemia caused by vitamin B_{12} deficiency. However, folic acid supplementation does not prevent the potentially irreversible neurologic damage caused by vitamin B_{12} deficiency. People with pernicious anemia and other forms of vitamin B_{12} deficiency are usually identified because of signs and symptoms of anemia, which typically occur before neurologic symptoms. Some opponents of folic acid supplementation were concerned that increased folic acid intake in the general population would mask vitamin B_{12} deficiency and increase the prevalence of neurologic disease in the elderly population. To put this in perspective, approximately 4000 pregnancies, including 2500 live births, in the United States each year are affected by NTDs. In contrast, it is estimated that more than 10% of the elderly population in the United States, or several million people, are at risk for the neuropsychiatric complications of vitamin B_{12} deficiency. In acknowledgment of this controversy, the FDA kept its requirements for folic acid supplementation at a somewhat low level. There is also concern based on observational and prospective clinical trials that high folic acid levels can increase the risk of some diseases, such as colorectal cancer, for which folic acid may exhibit a bell-shaped curve. Further research is needed to more accurately define the optimal level of folic acid fortification in food and recommendations for folic acid supplementation in different populations and age groups.

Chemistry

Folic acid (pteroylglutamic acid) is composed of a heterocycle (pteridine), *p*-aminobenzoic acid, and glutamic acid (Figure 33–4). Various numbers of glutamic acid moieties are attached to the pteroyl portion of the molecule, resulting in monoglutamates, triglutamates, or polyglutamates. Folic acid undergoes reduction, catalyzed by the enzyme dihydrofolate reductase ("folate reductase"), to give dihydrofolic acid (see Figure 33–3, section 3). Tetrahydrofolate is subsequently transformed to folate cofactors possessing one-carbon units attached to the 5-nitrogen, to the 10-nitrogen, or to both positions (see Figure 33–3). Folate cofactors are interconvertible by various enzymatic reactions and serve the important biochemical function of donating one-carbon units at various levels of oxidation. In most of these, tetrahydrofolate is regenerated and becomes available for reutilization.

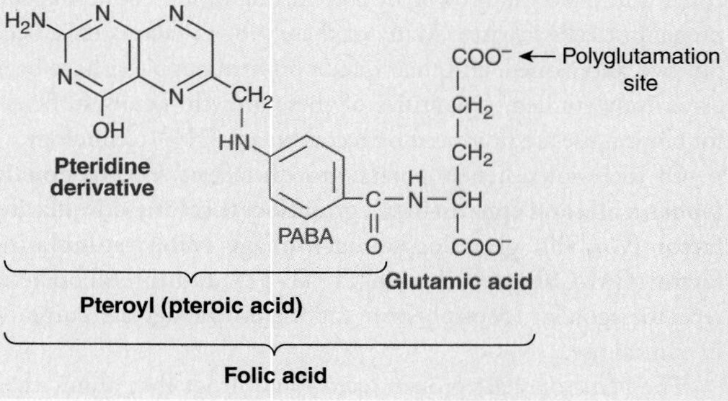

FIGURE 33–4 The structure of folic acid. (Reproduced with permission from Murray RK, Granner DK, Mayes PA, et al: *Harper's Biochemistry*, 24th ed. McGraw Hill, 1996.)

Pharmacokinetics

The average American diet contains 500–700 mcg of folates daily, 50–200 mcg of which is usually absorbed, depending on metabolic requirements. Pregnant women may absorb as much as 300–400 mcg of folic acid daily. Various forms of folic acid are present in a wide variety of plant and animal tissues; the richest sources are yeast, liver, kidney, and green vegetables. Normally, 5–20 mg of folates is stored in the liver and other tissues. Folates are excreted in the urine and stool and are also destroyed by catabolism, so serum levels fall within a few days when intake is diminished. Because body stores of folates are relatively low and daily requirements high, folic acid deficiency and megaloblastic anemia can develop within 1–6 months after the intake of folic acid stops, depending on the patient's nutritional status and the rate of folate utilization.

Unaltered folic acid is readily and completely absorbed in the proximal jejunum. Dietary folates, however, consist primarily of polyglutamate forms of N^5-methyltetrahydrofolate. Before absorption, all but one of the glutamyl residues of the polyglutamates must be hydrolyzed by the enzyme α-1-glutamyl transferase ("conjugase") within the brush border of the intestinal mucosa. The monoglutamate N^5-methyltetrahydrofolate is subsequently transported into the bloodstream by both active and passive transport and is then widely distributed throughout the body. Inside cells, N^5-methyltetrahydrofolate is converted to tetrahydrofolate by the demethylation reaction that requires vitamin B_{12} (see Figure 33–3, section 1).

Pharmacodynamics

Tetrahydrofolate cofactors participate in one-carbon transfer reactions. As described earlier in the discussion of vitamin B_{12}, one of these essential reactions produces the dTMP needed for DNA synthesis. In this reaction, the enzyme thymidylate synthase catalyzes the transfer of the one-carbon unit of N^5, N^{10}-methylenetetrahydrofolate to deoxyuridine monophosphate (dUMP) to form dTMP (see Figure 33–3, section 2). Unlike all the other enzymatic reactions that use folate cofactors, in this reaction the cofactor is oxidized to dihydrofolate, and for each mole of dTMP produced, 1 mole of tetrahydrofolate is consumed. In rapidly proliferating tissues, considerable amounts of tetrahydrofolate are consumed in this reaction, and continued DNA synthesis requires continued regeneration of tetrahydrofolate by reduction of dihydrofolate, catalyzed by the enzyme dihydrofolate reductase. The tetrahydrofolate thus produced can then reform the cofactor N^5, N^{10}-methylenetetrahydrofolate by the action of serine transhydroxymethylase and thus allow for the continued synthesis of dTMP. The combined catalytic activities of dTMP synthase, dihydrofolate reductase, and serine transhydroxymethylase are referred to as the *dTMP synthesis cycle*. Enzymes in the dTMP cycle are the targets of two anticancer drugs: methotrexate inhibits dihydrofolate reductase, and a metabolite of 5-fluorouracil inhibits thymidylate synthase (see Chapter 54).

Cofactors of tetrahydrofolate participate in several other essential reactions. N^5-Methylenetetrahydrofolate is required for the vitamin B_{12}-dependent reaction that generates methionine from homocysteine (see Figure 33–2A; Figure 33–3, section 1). In addition, tetrahydrofolate cofactors donate one-carbon units during the de novo synthesis of essential purines. In these reactions, tetrahydrofolate is regenerated and can reenter the tetrahydrofolate cofactor pool.

Clinical Pharmacology

Folate deficiency results in a megaloblastic anemia that is microscopically indistinguishable from the anemia caused by vitamin B_{12} deficiency (see above). However, folate deficiency does not cause the characteristic neurologic syndrome seen in vitamin B_{12} deficiency. In patients with megaloblastic anemia, folate status is assessed with assays for serum folate or for red blood cell folate. Red blood cell folate levels are often of greater diagnostic value than serum levels, because serum folate levels tend to be labile and do not necessarily reflect tissue levels.

Folic acid deficiency is often caused by inadequate dietary intake of folates. Patients with alcohol dependence and patients with liver disease can develop folic acid deficiency because of poor diet and diminished hepatic storage of folates. Pregnant women and patients with hemolytic anemia have increased folate requirements and may become folic acid-deficient, especially if their diets are marginal. Evidence implicates maternal folic acid deficiency in the occurrence of fetal neural tube defects. (See Box: Folic Acid Supplementation: A Public Health Dilemma.) Patients with malabsorption syndromes also frequently develop folic acid deficiency. Patients who require renal dialysis are at risk of folic acid deficiency because folates are removed from the plasma during the dialysis procedure.

Folic acid deficiency can be caused by drugs. Methotrexate and, to a lesser extent, trimethoprim and pyrimethamine, inhibit dihydrofolate reductase and may result in a deficiency of folate cofactors and ultimately in megaloblastic anemia. Long-term therapy with phenytoin also can cause folate deficiency, but it only rarely causes megaloblastic anemia.

Parenteral administration of folic acid is rarely necessary, since oral folic acid is well absorbed even in patients with malabsorption syndromes. A dose of 1 mg folic acid orally daily is sufficient to reverse megaloblastic anemia, restore normal serum folate levels, and replenish body stores of folates in almost all patients. Therapy should be continued until the underlying cause of the deficiency is removed or corrected. Therapy may be required indefinitely for patients with malabsorption or dietary inadequacy. Folic acid supplementation to prevent folic acid deficiency should be considered in high-risk patients, including pregnant women, patients with alcohol dependence, hemolytic anemia, liver disease, or certain skin diseases, and patients on renal dialysis.

HEMATOPOIETIC GROWTH FACTORS

The hematopoietic growth factors are glycoprotein hormones that regulate the proliferation and differentiation of hematopoietic progenitor cells in the bone marrow. The first growth factors to be identified were called *colony-stimulating factors* because they could stimulate the growth of colonies of various bone marrow progenitor cells in vitro. Many of these growth factors have been purified and cloned, and their effects on hematopoiesis have been extensively studied. Quantities of these growth factors sufficient for clinical use are produced by recombinant DNA technology.

Of the known hematopoietic growth factors, **erythropoietin (epoetin alfa and epoetin beta), granulocyte colony-stimulating factor (G-CSF), granulocyte-macrophage colony-stimulating factor (GM-CSF), interleukin 11 (IL-11),** and thrombopoietin receptor agonists **(romiplostim** and **eltrombopag)** are currently in clinical use.

The hematopoietic growth factors and drugs that mimic their action have complex effects on the function of a wide variety of cell types, including nonhematologic cells. Their usefulness in other areas of medicine, particularly as potential anticancer and anti-inflammatory drugs, is being investigated.

ERYTHROPOIETIN

Chemistry & Pharmacokinetics

Erythropoietin, a 34- to 39-kDa glycoprotein, was the first human hematopoietic growth factor to be isolated. It was originally purified from the urine of patients with severe anemia. Recombinant human erythropoietin (rHuEPO, epoetin alfa) is produced in a mammalian cell expression system. After intravenous administration, erythropoietin has a serum half-life of 4–13 hours in patients with chronic renal failure. It is not cleared by dialysis. It is measured in international units (IU). Darbepoetin alfa is a modified form of erythropoietin that is more heavily glycosylated as a result of changes in amino acids. Darbepoetin alfa has a twofold to threefold longer half-life than epoetin alfa. Methoxy polyethylene glycol-epoetin beta is an isoform of erythropoietin covalently attached to a long polyethylene glycol polymer. This long-lived recombinant product is administered as a single intravenous or subcutaneous dose at 2-week or monthly intervals, whereas epoetin alfa is generally administered three times a week and darbepoetin is administered weekly.

Pharmacodynamics

Erythropoietin stimulates erythroid proliferation and differentiation by interacting with erythropoietin receptors on red cell progenitors. The erythropoietin receptor is a member of the JAK/STAT superfamily of cytokine receptors that use protein phosphorylation and transcription factor activation to regulate cellular function (see Chapter 2). Erythropoietin also induces release of reticulocytes from the bone marrow. Endogenous erythropoietin is produced primarily in the kidney. In response to tissue hypoxia, more erythropoietin is produced through an increased rate of transcription of the erythropoietin gene. This results in correction of the anemia, provided that the bone marrow response is not impaired by red cell nutritional deficiency (especially iron deficiency), primary bone marrow disorders (see below), or bone marrow suppression from drugs or chronic diseases.

Normally, an inverse relationship exists between the hematocrit or hemoglobin level and the serum erythropoietin level. Nonanemic individuals have serum erythropoietin levels of less than 20 IU/L. As the hematocrit and hemoglobin levels fall and anemia becomes more severe, the serum erythropoietin level rises exponentially. Patients with moderately severe anemia usually have erythropoietin levels in the 100–500 IU/L range, and patients with severe anemia may have levels of thousands of IU/L. The most important exception to this inverse relationship is in the anemia of chronic renal failure. In patients with renal disease, erythropoietin levels are usually low because the kidneys cannot produce the growth factor. These are the patients most likely to respond to treatment with exogenous erythropoietin. In most primary bone marrow disorders (aplastic anemia, leukemias, myeloproliferative and myelodysplastic disorders, etc) and most nutritional and secondary anemias, endogenous erythropoietin levels are high, so there is less likelihood of a response to exogenous erythropoietin (but see below).

Clinical Pharmacology

The availability of erythropoiesis-stimulating agents (ESAs) has had a significant positive impact for patients with several types of anemia (Table 33–4). The ESAs consistently improve the hematocrit and hemoglobin level, often eliminate the need for transfusions, and reliably improve quality of life indices. The ESAs are used routinely in patients with anemia secondary to chronic kidney disease. In patients treated with an ESA, an increase in reticulocyte count is usually observed in about 10 days and an increase in hematocrit and hemoglobin levels in 2–6 weeks. Dosages of ESAs are adjusted to maintain a target hemoglobin up to, but not exceeding, 10–12 g/dL. To support the increased erythropoiesis, nearly all patients with chronic kidney disease require oral or parenteral iron supplementation. Folate supplementation may also be necessary in some patients.

TABLE 33–4 Clinical uses of hematopoietic growth factors and agents that mimic their actions.

Hematopoietic Growth Factor	Clinical Condition Being Treated or Prevented	Recipients
Erythropoietin, darbepoetin alfa	Anemia	Patients with chronic renal failure
		HIV-infected patients treated with zidovudine
		Cancer patients treated with myelosuppressive cancer chemotherapy
		Patients scheduled to undergo elective, noncardiac, nonvascular surgery
Granulocyte colony-stimulating factor (G-CSF; filgrastim) and granulocyte-macrophage colony-stimulating factor (GM-CSF; sargramostim)	Neutropenia	Cancer patients treated with myelosuppressive cancer chemotherapy
		Patients with severe chronic neutropenia
		Patients recovering from bone marrow transplantation
	Stem cell or bone marrow transplantation	Patients with nonmyeloid malignancies or other conditions being treated with stem cell or bone marrow transplantation
	Mobilization of peripheral blood progenitor cells (PBPCs)	Donors of stem cells for allogeneic or autologous transplantation
Interleukin-11 (IL-11, oprelvekin)	Thrombocytopenia	Patients with nonmyeloid malignancies who receive myelosuppressive cancer chemotherapy
Romiplostim, eltrombopag	Thrombocytopenia	Patients with idiopathic thrombocytopenic purpura

An alternative approach to treatment of chronic kidney disease anemia may become available in the future as a result of research that led to the Nobel Prize in Physiology or Medicine in 2019. Studies of the response to hypoxia resulted in the identification of a DNA-regulating factor that was named hypoxia-inducible factor (HIF). It was found that HIF was inactivated at normal oxygen levels by a set of enzymes called prolyl hydroxylases (PHDs) and when not inactivated (in hypoxic conditions), increased erythropoiesis. Small molecule PHD inhibitors have been discovered that increase hemoglobin; one such, **roxadustat,** has already been banned by professional sport authorities. This drug is in clinical trials for the treatment of kidney disease anemia.

In selected patients, erythropoietin is also used to reduce the need for red blood cell transfusion in patients undergoing myelosuppressive cancer chemotherapy who have a hemoglobin level of less than 10 g/dL, and for selected patients with low-risk myelodysplastic syndromes and anemia requiring red blood cell transfusion. Patients who have disproportionately low serum erythropoietin levels for their degree of anemia are most likely to respond to treatment. Patients with endogenous erythropoietin levels of less than 100 IU/L have the best chance of response, although patients with erythropoietin levels between 100 and 500 IU/L respond occasionally. Methoxy polyethylene glycol-epoetin beta should not be used for treatment of anemia caused by cancer chemotherapy because a clinical trial found significantly more deaths among patients receiving this form of erythropoietin.

Erythropoietin is one of the drugs commonly used illegally by endurance athletes to enhance performance. Other methods such as autologous transfusion of red cells or use of androgens also have been used to increase hemoglobin. "Blood doping" constitutes a serious health risk to athletes, is considered a form of cheating, and is universally banned and routinely tested for in athletic events.

Toxicity

The most common adverse effects of erythropoietin are hypertension and thrombotic complications. ESAs increase the risk of serious cardiovascular events, thromboembolic events, stroke, and mortality in clinical studies when given to support hemoglobin levels greater than 11 g/dL. In addition, a meta-analysis of 51 placebo-controlled trials of ESAs in cancer patients reported an increased rate of all-cause mortality and venous thrombosis in those receiving an ESA. Based on the accumulated evidence, it is recommended that the hemoglobin level not exceed 11 g/dL in patients with chronic kidney disease receiving an ESA, and that ESAs be used conservatively in cancer patients (eg, when hemoglobin levels are <10 g/dL) and with the lowest dose needed to avoid transfusion. It is further recommended that ESAs not be used when a cancer therapy is being given with curative intent.

Allergic reactions to ESAs have been infrequent. There have been a small number of cases of pure red cell aplasia (PRCA) accompanied by neutralizing antibodies to erythropoietin. PRCA was most commonly seen in dialysis patients treated subcutaneously for a long period with a particular form of epoetin alfa (Eprex with a polysorbate 80 stabilizer rather than human serum albumin) that is not available in the United States. After regulatory agencies required that Eprex be administered intravenously rather than subcutaneously, the rate of ESA-associated PRCA diminished. However, rare cases have still been seen with all ESAs administered subcutaneously for long periods to patients with chronic kidney disease.

MYELOID GROWTH FACTORS

Chemistry & Pharmacokinetics

G-CSF and **GM-CSF,** the two myeloid growth factors currently available for clinical use, were originally purified from cultured human cell lines (see Table 33–4). Recombinant human G-CSF **(rHuG-CSF; filgrastim)** is produced in a bacterial expression system. It is a nonglycosylated peptide of 175 amino acids, with a molecular weight of 18 kDa. **Tbo-filgrastim** is similar to filgrastim, with minor structural differences and equivalent activity. Recombinant human GM-CSF **(rHuGM-CSF; sargramostim)** is produced in a yeast expression system. It is a partially glycosylated peptide of 127 amino acids, comprising three molecular species with molecular weights of 15,500, 15,800, and 19,500. These preparations have serum half-lives of 2–7 hours after intravenous or subcutaneous administration. **Pegfilgrastim,** a covalent conjugation product of filgrastim with a form of polyethylene glycol, has a much longer serum half-life than recombinant G-CSF, and it can be injected once per myelosuppressive chemotherapy cycle instead of daily for several days. **Lenograstim,** used widely in Europe, is a glycosylated form of recombinant G-CSF.

Pharmacodynamics

The myeloid growth factors stimulate proliferation and differentiation by interacting with specific receptors found on myeloid progenitor cells. Like the erythropoietin receptor, these receptors are members of the JAK/STAT superfamily (see Chapter 2). G-CSF stimulates proliferation and differentiation of progenitors already committed to the neutrophil lineage. It also activates the phagocytic activity of mature neutrophils and prolongs their survival in the circulation. G-CSF also has a remarkable ability to mobilize hematopoietic stem cells and increase their concentration in peripheral blood. This biologic effect underlies a major advance in transplantation—the use of **peripheral blood stem cells (PBSCs)** rather than bone marrow stem cells for autologous and allogeneic hematopoietic stem cell transplantation (see below).

GM-CSF has broader biologic actions than G-CSF. It is a multipotential hematopoietic growth factor that stimulates proliferation and differentiation of early and late granulocytic progenitor cells as well as erythroid and megakaryocyte progenitors. Like G-CSF, GM-CSF also stimulates the function of mature neutrophils. GM-CSF acts together with interleukin-2 to stimulate T-cell proliferation and appears to be a locally active factor at the site of inflammation. GM-CSF mobilizes peripheral blood stem cells, but it is significantly less efficacious and more toxic than G-CSF in this regard.

Clinical Pharmacology

A. Cancer Chemotherapy-Induced Neutropenia

Neutropenia is a common adverse effect of the cytotoxic drugs used to treat cancer and increases the risk of serious infection in patients receiving chemotherapy. Unlike the treatment of anemia and thrombocytopenia, transfusion of neutropenic patients with granulocytes collected from donors is rarely performed with limited success. The introduction of G-CSF in 1991 represented a milestone in the treatment of chemotherapy-induced neutropenia. This growth factor dramatically accelerates the rate of neutrophil recovery after dose-intensive myelosuppressive chemotherapy. It reduces the duration of neutropenia and usually raises the nadir count, the lowest neutrophil count seen following a cycle of chemotherapy.

The ability of G-CSF to increase neutrophil counts after myelosuppressive chemotherapy is nearly universal, but its impact on clinical outcomes is more variable. Many, but not all, clinical trials and meta-analyses have shown that G-CSF reduces episodes of febrile neutropenia, requirements for broad-spectrum antibiotics, infections, and days of hospitalization. Clinical trials have not shown improved survival in cancer patients treated with G-CSF. Clinical guidelines for the use of G-CSF after cytotoxic chemotherapy recommend reserving G-CSF for patients at high risk for febrile neutropenia based on age, medical history, and disease characteristics; patients receiving dose-intensive chemotherapy regimens that carry a greater than 20% risk of causing febrile neutropenia; patients with a prior episode of febrile neutropenia after cytotoxic chemotherapy; patients at high risk for febrile neutropenia; and patients who are unlikely to survive an episode of febrile neutropenia. Pegfilgrastim is an alternative to G-CSF for prevention of chemotherapy-induced febrile neutropenia. Pegfilgrastim can be administered once per chemotherapy cycle, and it may shorten the period of severe neutropenia slightly more than G-CSF.

Like G-CSF and pegfilgrastim, GM-CSF also reduces the duration of neutropenia after cytotoxic chemotherapy. It has been more difficult to show that GM-CSF reduces the incidence of febrile neutropenia, probably because GM-CSF itself can induce fever. In the treatment of chemotherapy-induced neutropenia, G-CSF 5 mcg/kg daily or GM-CSF 250 mcg/m^2 daily is usually started within 24–72 hours after completing chemotherapy and is continued until the absolute neutrophil count is greater than 10,000 cells/μL. Pegfilgrastim is given as a single dose of 6 mg.

The utility and safety of the myeloid growth factors in the postchemotherapy supportive care of patients with acute myeloid leukemia (AML) have been the subject of a number of clinical trials. Because leukemic cells arise from progenitors whose proliferation and differentiation are normally regulated by hematopoietic growth factors, including GM-CSF and G-CSF, there was concern that myeloid growth factors could stimulate leukemic cell growth and increase the rate of relapse. The results of randomized clinical trials suggest that both G-CSF and GM-CSF are safe following induction and consolidation treatment of myeloid and lymphoblastic leukemia. There has been no evidence that these growth factors reduce the rate of remission or increase relapse rate. On the contrary, the growth factors accelerate neutrophil recovery and reduce infection rates and days of hospitalization. Both G-CSF and GM-CSF have FDA approval for treatment of patients with AML.

B. Other Applications

G-CSF and GM-CSF have also proved to be effective in treating neutropenia associated with **congenital neutropenia, cyclic neutropenia, myelodysplasia,** and **aplastic anemia.** Many patients with these disorders respond with a prompt and sometimes dramatic increase in neutrophil count. In some cases, this results in a decrease in the frequency of infections. Because neither G-CSF nor GM-CSF stimulates the formation of erythrocytes and platelets, they are sometimes combined with other growth factors for treatment of pancytopenia.

The myeloid growth factors play an important role in **autologous stem cell transplantation** for patients undergoing high-dose chemotherapy. High-dose chemotherapy with autologous stem cell support is increasingly used to treat patients with tumors that are resistant to standard doses of chemotherapeutic drugs. The high-dose regimens produce extreme myelosuppression; the myelosuppression is then counteracted by reinfusion of the patient's own hematopoietic stem cells (which are collected prior to chemotherapy). The administration of G-CSF or GM-CSF early after autologous stem cell transplantation reduces the time to engraftment and to recovery from neutropenia in patients receiving stem cells obtained either from bone marrow or from peripheral blood. These effects are seen in patients being treated for lymphoma or for solid tumors. G-CSF and GM-CSF are also used to support patients who have received allogeneic bone marrow transplantation for treatment of hematologic malignancies or bone marrow failure states. In this setting, the growth factors speed the recovery from neutropenia without increasing the incidence of acute graft-versus-host disease.

Perhaps the most important role of the myeloid growth factors in transplantation is for mobilization of peripheral blood stem cells. Stem cells collected from peripheral blood have nearly replaced bone marrow as the hematopoietic preparation used for autologous and allogeneic transplantation. The cells can be collected in an outpatient setting with a procedure that avoids much of the risk and discomfort of bone marrow collection, including the need for general anesthesia. In addition, there is evidence that PBSC transplantation results in more rapid engraftment of all hematopoietic cell lineages and in reduced rates of graft failure or delayed platelet recovery.

G-CSF is the cytokine most commonly used for PBSC mobilization because of its increased efficacy and reduced toxicity compared with GM-CSF. To mobilize stem cells for autologous transplantation, donors are given 5–10 mcg/kg daily subcutaneously for 4 days. On the fifth day, they undergo leukapheresis. The success of PBSC transplantation depends on transfusion of adequate numbers of stem cells. CD34, an antigen present on early progenitor cells and absent from later, committed, cells, is used as a marker for the requisite stem cells. The goal is to infuse at least 5×10^6 CD34 cells/kg; this number of CD34 cells usually results in prompt and durable engraftment of all cell lineages. It may take several separate leukaphereses to collect enough CD34 cells, especially from older patients and patients who have been exposed to radiation therapy or chemotherapy.

For patients with multiple myeloma or non-Hodgkin lymphoma who respond suboptimally to G-CSF alone, the novel hematopoietic stem cell mobilizer **plerixafor** can be added to G-CSF. Plerixafor is a bicyclam molecule originally developed as an anti-HIV drug because of its ability to inhibit the CXC chemokine receptor 4 (CXCR4), a co-receptor for HIV entry into

CD4+ T lymphocytes (see Chapter 49). Early clinical trials of plerixafor revealed a remarkable ability to increase CD34 cells in peripheral blood. Plerixafor mobilizes CD34 cells by preventing chemokine stromal cell-derived factor-1α (CXCL12) from binding to CXCR4 and directing the CD34 cells to "home" to the bone marrow. Plerixafor is administered by subcutaneous injection after 4 days of G-CSF treatment and 11 hours prior to leukapheresis; it can be used with G-CSF for up to 4 continuous days. Plerixafor is eliminated primarily by the renal route and must be dose-adjusted for patients with renal impairment. The drug is well tolerated; the most common adverse effects associated with its use are injection site reactions, gastrointestinal disturbances, dizziness, fatigue, and headache.

Toxicity

Although the three growth factors have similar effects on neutrophil counts, G-CSF and pegfilgrastim are used more frequently than GM-CSF because they are better tolerated. G-CSF and pegfilgrastim can cause bone pain, which clears when the drugs are discontinued. GM-CSF can cause more severe side effects, particularly at higher doses. These include fever, malaise, arthralgias, myalgias, and a capillary leak syndrome characterized by peripheral edema and pleural or pericardial effusions. Allergic reactions may occur but are infrequent. Splenic rupture is a rare but serious complication of the use of G-CSF for PBSC mobilization.

MEGAKARYOCYTE GROWTH FACTORS

Patients with thrombocytopenia have a high risk of hemorrhage. Although platelet transfusion is commonly used to treat thrombocytopenia, this procedure can cause adverse reactions in the recipient; furthermore, a significant number of patients fail to exhibit the expected increase in platelet count. **Thrombopoietin (TPO)** and **IL-11** both appear to be key endogenous regulators of platelet production. A recombinant form of IL-11 was the first agent to gain FDA approval for treatment of thrombocytopenia. Recombinant human thrombopoietin and a pegylated form of a shortened human thrombopoietin protein underwent extensive clinical investigation in the 1990s. However, further development was abandoned after autoantibodies to the native thrombopoietin formed in healthy human subjects and caused thrombocytopenia. Efforts shifted to investigation of novel, nonimmunogenic agonists of the thrombopoietin receptor, which is known as **MPL**. Three thrombopoietin agonists (romiplostim, eltrombopag, and avatrombopag) are approved for treatment of thrombocytopenia. Fostamatinib is a tyrosine kinase inhibitor prodrug. The active metabolite targets the SYK kinase in the signaling pathway downstream from the B cell receptor and the Fc receptor in the reticuloendothelial system.

Chemistry, Pharmacokinetics, & Pharmacodynamics

Interleukin-11 is a 65- to 85-kDa protein produced by fibroblasts and stromal cells in the bone marrow. **Oprelvekin,** the recombinant form of IL-11 approved for clinical use (see Table 33–4), is produced by expression in *Escherichia coli*. The half-life of IL-11 is 7–8 hours when the drug is injected subcutaneously. Interleukin-11 acts through a specific cell surface cytokine receptor to stimulate the growth of multiple lymphoid and myeloid cells. It acts synergistically with other growth factors to stimulate the growth of primitive megakaryocytic progenitors and, most importantly, increases the number of peripheral platelets and neutrophils.

Romiplostim is a thrombopoietin agonist peptide covalently linked to antibody fragments that serve to extend the peptide's half-life. The MPL-binding peptide has no sequence homology with human thrombopoietin, and there is no evidence in animal or human studies that the MPL-binding peptide or romiplostim induces antibodies to thrombopoietin. After subcutaneous administration, romiplostim is eliminated by the reticuloendothelial system with an average half-life of 3–4 days. Its half-life is inversely related to the serum platelet count; it has a longer half-life in patients with thrombocytopenia and a shorter half-life in patients whose platelet counts have recovered to normal levels. Romiplostim is approved for therapy of patients with chronic immune thrombocytopenia who have had an inadequate response to other therapies. Romiplostim has high affinity for the human MPL receptor and results in a dose-dependent increase in platelet count. Romiplostim is administered once weekly by subcutaneous injection.

Eltrombopag is an orally active small nonpeptide thrombopoietin agonist molecule approved for therapy of patients with chronic immune thrombocytopenia who have had an inadequate response to other therapies, and for treatment of thrombocytopenia in patients with hepatitis C to allow initiation of interferon therapy. Following oral administration, peak eltrombopag levels are observed in 2–6 hours and the half-life is 26–35 hours. Eltrombopag is excreted primarily in the feces. Eltrombopag interacts with the transmembrane domain of the MPL receptor and, similarly to romiplostim, results a dose-dependent increase in platelet count.

Avatrombopag is an orally active thrombopoietin agonist approved for treatment of thrombocytopenia in adult patients with chronic liver disease to increase platelet count to greater than 50,000 prior to procedures, and to treat patients with chronic immune thrombocytopenia who have had an inadequate response to other therapies. The dose in liver disease is 60 mg orally/d for 5 days in patients with a platelet count of less than 40k, and 50 mg/d for 5 days for patients with a platelet count of 40 to less than 50k, 10–13 days prior to the procedure. In clinical studies, the platelet count increased beginning on day 4 post-dose, peaking day 10–13, and returning to baseline values by 4–5 weeks. For patients with immune thrombocytopenia with inadequate response to prior therapy, the starting dose is 20 mg/d.

Fostamatinib is an orally active prodrug approved for use in patients with chronic immune thrombocytopenia who have had an inadequate response to other therapies. The active metabolite, R406, is an SYK tyrosine kinase inhibitor which blocks B-cell activation Fc signaling pathways, decreasing antibody-mediated platelet removal from circulation. R406 is metabolized by CYP3A4, and strong CYP3A4 inhibitors such as ketoconazole increase drug effect. The starting dose is 100 mg twice daily.

Clinical Pharmacology

Interleukin-11 is approved for the secondary prevention of thrombocytopenia in patients receiving cytotoxic chemotherapy for treatment of nonmyeloid cancers. Clinical trials show that it reduces the number of platelet transfusions required by patients who experience severe thrombocytopenia after a previous cycle of chemotherapy. Although IL-11 has broad stimulatory effects on hematopoietic cell lineages in vitro, it does not appear to have significant effects on the leukopenia caused by myelosuppressive chemotherapy. Interleukin-11 is given by subcutaneous injection at a dose of 50 mcg/kg daily. It is started 6–24 hours after completion of chemotherapy and continued for 14–21 days or until the platelet count passes the nadir and rises to more than 50,000/μL.

In patients with chronic immune thrombocytopenia who failed to respond adequately to previous treatment with steroids, immunoglobulins, or splenectomy, romiplostim, eltrombopag, avatrombopag, or fostamatinib can be used to significantly increase platelet count in most patients. All drugs are used at the minimal dose required to maintain platelet counts of greater than 50,000/μL.

Toxicity

The most common adverse effects of IL-11 are fatigue, headache, dizziness, and cardiovascular effects. The cardiovascular effects include anemia (due to hemodilution), dyspnea (due to fluid accumulation in the lungs), and transient atrial arrhythmias. Hypokalemia also has been seen in some patients. All of these adverse effects appear to be reversible.

Eltrombopag is potentially hepatotoxic and liver function must be monitored, particularly when used in patients with hepatitis C. Portal vein thrombosis also has been reported with eltrombopag, romiplostim, and avatrombopag in the setting of chronic liver disease. In patients with myelodysplastic syndromes, romiplostim increases the blast count and risk of progression to acute myeloid leukemia. Marrow fibrosis has been observed with thrombopoietin agonists but is generally reversible when the drug is discontinued. Rebound thrombocytopenia has been observed following discontinuation of TPO agonists. Reported toxicities with fostamatinib include diarrhea, hypertension, hepatic toxicity, and neutropenia.

SUMMARY Agents Used in Anemias and Hematopoietic Growth Factors

Subclass, Drug	Mechanism of Action	Effects	Clinical Applications	Pharmacokinetics, Toxicities, Interactions
IRON				
• Ferrous sulfate	Required for biosynthesis of heme and heme-containing proteins, including hemoglobin and myoglobin	Adequate supplies required for normal heme synthesis • deficiency results in inadequate heme production	Iron deficiency, which manifests as microcytic anemia • oral preparation	Complicated endogenous system for absorbing, storing, and transporting iron • *Toxicity:* Acute overdose results in necrotizing gastroenteritis, abdominal pain, bloody diarrhea, shock, lethargy, and dyspnea • chronic iron overload results in hemochromatosis, with damage to the heart, liver, pancreas, and other organs • organ failure and death can ensue
• *Ferrous gluconate and ferrous fumarate: Oral iron preparations*				
• *Iron dextran, iron sucrose complex, sodium ferric gluconate complex, ferric carboxymaltose, and ferumoxytol: Parenteral preparations can cause pain, hypersensitivity reactions*				
IRON CHELATORS				
• Deferoxamine (see also Chapters 57 and 58)	Chelates excess iron	Reduces toxicity associated with acute or chronic iron overload	Acute iron poisoning; inherited or acquired hemochromatosis	Preferred route of administration is IM or SC • *Toxicity:* Rapid IV administration may cause hypotension • neurotoxicity and increased susceptibility to certain infections have occurred with long-term use
• *Deferasirox: Orally administered iron chelator for treatment of hemochromatosis*				
VITAMIN B_{12}				
• Cyanocobalamin • Hydroxocobalamin	Cofactor required for essential enzymatic reactions that form tetrahydrofolate, convert homocysteine to methionine, and metabolize L-methylmalonyl-CoA	Adequate supplies required for amino acid and fatty acid metabolism, and DNA synthesis	Vitamin B_{12} deficiency, which manifests as megaloblastic anemia and is the basis of pernicious anemia; hydroxocobalamin is also used as a cyanide antidote (see Chapter 58)	Parenteral vitamin B_{12} is required for pernicious anemia and other malabsorption syndromes • *Toxicity:* No toxicity associated with excess vitamin B_{12}

(continued)

Subclass, Drug	Mechanism of Action	Effects	Clinical Applications	Pharmacokinetics, Toxicities, Interactions
FOLIC ACID				
• Folacin (pteroylglutamic acid)	Precursor of an essential donor of methyl groups used for synthesis of amino acids, purines, and deoxynucleotide	Adequate supplies required for essential biochemical reactions involving amino acid metabolism, and purine and DNA synthesis	Folic acid deficiency, which manifests as megaloblastic anemia, and prevention of congenital neural tube defects	Oral; well-absorbed; need for parenteral administration is rare • *Toxicity:* Folic acid is not toxic in overdose, but large amounts can partially compensate for vitamin B_{12} deficiency and put people with unrecognized B_{12} deficiency at risk of neurologic consequences of vitamin B_{12} deficiency, which are not compensated by folic acid
ERYTHROCYTE-STIMULATING AGENTS				
• Epoetin alfa	Agonist of erythropoietin receptors expressed by red cell progenitors	Stimulates erythroid proliferation and differentiation, and induces the release of reticulocytes from the bone marrow	Anemia, especially anemia associated with chronic renal failure, HIV infection, cancer, and prematurity • prevention of the need for transfusion in patients undergoing certain types of elective surgery	IV or SC administration 1–3 times per week • *Toxicity:* Hypertension, thrombotic complications, and, very rarely, pure red cell aplasia • to reduce the risk of serious cerebrovascular events, hemoglobin levels should be maintained <12 g/dL
• *Darbepoetin alfa: Long-acting glycosylated form administered weekly*				
• *Methoxy polyethylene glycol-epoetin beta: Long-acting form administered 1–2 times per month*				
MYELOID GROWTH FACTORS				
• Granulocyte colony-stimulating factor (G-CSF; filgrastim)	Stimulates G-CSF receptors expressed on mature neutrophils and their progenitors	Stimulates neutrophil progenitor proliferation and differentiation • activates phagocytic activity of mature neutrophils and extends their survival • mobilizes hematopoietic stem cells	Neutropenia associated with congenital neutropenia, cyclic neutropenia, myelodysplasia, and aplastic anemia • secondary prevention of neutropenia in patients undergoing cytotoxic chemotherapy • mobilization of peripheral blood cells in preparation for autologous and allogeneic stem cell transplantation	Daily SC administration • *Toxicity:* Bone pain • rarely, splenic rupture
• *Pegfilgrastim: Long-acting form of filgrastim that is covalently linked to a type of polyethylene glycol*				
• *Tbo-filgrastim: Similar to filgrastim*				
• *GM-CSF (sargramostim): Myeloid growth factor that acts through a distinct GM-CSF receptor to stimulate proliferation and differentiation of early and late granulocytic progenitor cells, and erythroid and megakaryocyte progenitors; clinical uses are similar to those of G-CSF, but it is more likely than G-CSF to cause fever, arthralgia, myalgia, and capillary leak syndrome*				
• *Plerixafor: Antagonist of CXCR4 used in combination with G-CSF for mobilization of peripheral blood cells prior to autologous transplantation in patients with multiple myeloma or non-Hodgkin lymphoma who responded suboptimally to G-CSF alone*				
MEGAKARYOCYTE GROWTH FACTORS				
• Oprelvekin (interleukin-11; IL-11)	Recombinant form of an endogenous cytokine • activates IL-11 receptors	Stimulates growth of multiple lymphoid and myeloid cells, including megakaryocyte progenitors • increases the number of circulating platelets and neutrophils	Secondary prevention of thrombocytopenia in patients undergoing cytotoxic chemotherapy for nonmyeloid cancers	Daily SC injection • *Toxicity:* Fatigue, headache, dizziness, anemia, fluid accumulation in the lungs, and transient atrial arrhythmias
• *Romiplostim: Subcutaneously administered thrombopoietin agonist approved for treatment of chronic immune thrombocytopenia with insufficient response to corticosteroids, intravenous immunoglobulin, or splenectomy*				
• *Eltrombopag: Orally active thrombopoietin agonist approved for treatment of chronic immune thrombocytopenia with insufficient response to corticosteroids, intravenous immunoglobulin, or splenectomy; and for treatment of thrombocytopenia in hepatitis C to allow the use of interferon-based therapies*				
• *Avatrombopag: Orally active thrombopoietin agonist approved for treatment of chronic immune thrombocytopenia with insufficient response to corticosteroids, intravenous immunoglobulin, or splenectomy; and for treatment of thrombocytopenia in patients with chronic liver disease to increase platelet count prior to procedures*				
KINASE INHIBITOR				
• *Fostamatinib: Orally active tyrosine kinase inhibitor, decreases signaling though Fc and B cell receptors; results in decreased antibody-mediated platelet destruction*				

PREPARATIONS AVAILABLE

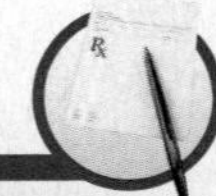

GENERIC NAME	AVAILABLE AS
Avatrombopag	Doptelet
Darbepoetin alfa	Aranesp
Deferasirox	Exjade
Deferoxamine	Generic, Desferal
Eltrombopag	Promacta
Epoetin alfa	Erythropoietin (EPO), Epogen, Procrit
Epoetin beta (Methoxy polyethylene glycol-epoetin beta)	Mircera
Filgrastim (G-CSF)	Neupogen, Granix
Folic acid (folacin, pteroylglutamic acid)	Generic
Iron	
Oral: See Table 33–3.	
Iron dextran (parenteral)	INFeD, Dexferrum
Sodium ferric gluconate complex (parenteral)	Ferrlecit
Iron sucrose (parenteral)	Venofer
Ferric carboxymaltose (parenteral)	Injectafer
Ferumoxytol (parenteral)	Feraheme
Oprelvekin (IL-11)	Neumega
Pegfilgrastim	Neulasta
Plerixafor	Mozobil
Romiplostim	Nplate
Sargramostim (GM-CSF)	Leukine
Vitamin B_{12}	
Oral, parenteral	Generic cyanocobalamin or hydroxocobalamin
Nasal	Nascobal, CaloMist

REFERENCES

Aapro MS et al, European Organisation for Research and Treatment of Cancer: 2010 update of EORTC guidelines for the use of granulocyte-colony stimulating factor to reduce the incidence of chemotherapy-induced febrile neutropenia in adult patients with lymphoproliferative disorders and solid tumours. Eur J Cancer 2011;47:8.

Albaramki J et al: Parenteral versus oral iron therapy for adults and children with chronic kidney disease. Cochrane Database Syst Rev 2012;1:CD007857.

Auerbach M, Al Talib K: Low-molecular weight iron dextran and iron sucrose have similar comparative safety profiles in chronic kidney disease. Kidney Int 2008;73:528.

Barzi A, Sekeres MA: Myelodysplastic syndromes: A practical approach to diagnosis and treatment. Cleve Clin J Med 2010;77:37.

Brittenham GM: Iron-chelating therapy for transfusional iron overload. N Engl J Med 2011;364:146.

Clark SF: Iron deficiency anemia: Diagnosis and management. Curr Opin Gastroenterol 2009;25:122.

Darshan D, Fraer DM, Anderson GJ: Molecular basis of iron-loading disorders. Expert Rev Mol Med 2010;12:e36.

Gertz MA: Current status of stem cell mobilization. Br J Haematol 2010;150:647.

Kessans MR, Gatesman ML, Kockler DR: Plerixafor: A peripheral blood stem cell mobilizer. Pharmacotherapy 2010;30:485.

McKoy JM et al: Epoetin-associated pure red cell aplasia: Past, present, and future considerations. Transfusion 2008;48:1754.

Rees DC, Williams TN, Gladwin MT: Sickle-cell disease. Lancet 2010;376:2018.

Rizzo JD et al: American Society of Clinical Oncology/American Society of Hematology clinical practice guideline update on the use of epoetin and darbepoetin in adult patients with cancer. J Clin Oncol 2010;28:4996.

Sauer J, Mason JB, Choi SW: Too much folate: A risk factor for cancer and cardiovascular disease? Curr Opin Clin Nutr Metab Care 2009;12:30.

Solomon LR: Disorders of cobalamin (vitamin B12) metabolism: Emerging concepts in pathophysiology, diagnosis and treatment. Blood Rev 2007;21:113.

Stasi R et al: Thrombopoietic agents. Blood Rev 2010;24:179.

Wolff T et al: Folic acid supplementation for the prevention of neural tube defects: An update of the evidence for the U.S. Preventive Services Task Force. Ann Intern Med 2009;150:632.

Vichinsky E et al: A phase 3 randomized trial of voxelotor in sickle cell disease. N Engl J Med 2019;381:509.

Zhang D-L et al: Erythrocytic ferroportin reduces intracellular iron accumulation, hemolysis, and malaria risk. Science 2018;359:1520.

CASE STUDY ANSWER

This patient's megaloblastic anemia appears to be due to vitamin B_{12} (cobalamin) deficiency secondary to inadequate dietary B_{12}. It is important to measure serum concentrations of both folic acid and cobalamin because megaloblastic anemia can result from deficiency of either nutrient. It is especially important to diagnose vitamin B_{12} deficiency because this deficiency, if untreated, can lead to irreversible neurologic damage. Folate supplementation, which can compensate for vitamin B_{12}-derived anemia, does not prevent B_{12}-deficiency neurologic damage. To correct this patient's vitamin B_{12} deficiency, she would probably be treated parenterally with cobalamin because of her neurologic symptoms, followed by oral supplementation to maintain her body stores of vitamin B_{12}.

CHAPTER

34 Drugs Used in Disorders of Coagulation

James L. Zehnder, MD

CASE STUDY

A 25-year-old woman presents to the emergency department complaining of acute onset of shortness of breath and pleuritic pain. She had been in her usual state of health until 2 days prior when she noted that her left leg was swollen and red. Her only medication was oral contraceptives. Family history was significant for a history of "blood clots" in multiple members of the maternal side of her family. Physical examination demonstrates an anxious woman with stable vital signs. The left lower extremity demonstrates erythema and edema and is tender to touch. Oxygen saturation by fingertip pulse oximeter while breathing room air is 87% (normal >90%). Ultrasound reveals a deep vein thrombosis in the left lower extremity; chest computed tomography scan confirms the presence of pulmonary emboli. Laboratory blood tests indicate elevated D-dimer levels. What therapy is indicated acutely? What are the long-term therapy options? How long should she be treated? Should this individual use oral contraceptives?

Hemostasis refers to the finely regulated dynamic process of maintaining fluidity of the blood, repairing vascular injury, and limiting blood loss while avoiding vessel occlusion (thrombosis) and inadequate perfusion of vital organs. Either extreme—excessive bleeding or thrombosis—represents a breakdown of the hemostatic mechanism. Common causes of dysregulated hemostasis include hereditary or acquired defects in the clotting mechanism and secondary effects of infection or cancer. Atrial fibrillation is associated with stasis of blood in the atria, formation of clots, and increased risk of occlusive stroke. Because of the high prevalence of chronic atrial fibrillation, especially in the older population, use of anticoagulants is common. Guidelines for the use of oral anticoagulants (**CHA_2DS_2-VASC** score, see January C et al reference) are based on various risk factors (**c**ongestive **h**eart failure, **h**ypertension, **a**ge, **d**iabetes, history of **s**troke, **vasc**ular disease, and sex). The drugs used to inhibit thrombosis and to limit abnormal bleeding are the subjects of this chapter.

MECHANISMS OF BLOOD COAGULATION

The vascular endothelial cell layer lining blood vessels has an anticoagulant phenotype, and circulating blood platelets and clotting factors do not normally adhere to it to an appreciable extent. In the setting of vascular injury, the endothelial cell layer rapidly undergoes a series of changes resulting in a more procoagulant phenotype. Injury exposes reactive subendothelial matrix proteins such as collagen and von Willebrand factor, which results in platelet adherence and activation, and secretion and synthesis of vasoconstrictors and platelet-recruiting and activating molecules. Thus, **thromboxane A_2 (TXA_2)** is synthesized from arachidonic acid within platelets and is a platelet activator and potent vasoconstrictor. Products secreted from platelet granules include **adenosine diphosphate (ADP),** a powerful inducer of platelet aggregation, and **serotonin (5-HT),** which stimulates aggregation and vasoconstriction. Activation of platelets results in a conformational change in the $\alpha_{IIb}\beta_{III}$ integrin (IIb/IIIa) receptor, enabling it to bind fibrinogen, which cross-links adjacent platelets, resulting in aggregation and formation of a platelet plug (Figure 34–1). Simultaneously, the coagulation system cascade is activated, resulting in thrombin generation and a fibrin clot, which stabilizes the platelet plug (see below). Knowledge of the hemostatic mechanism is important for diagnosis of bleeding disorders. Patients with defects in the formation of the primary platelet plug (defects in primary hemostasis, eg, platelet function defects, von Willebrand disease) typically bleed from surface sites (gingiva, skin, heavy menses)

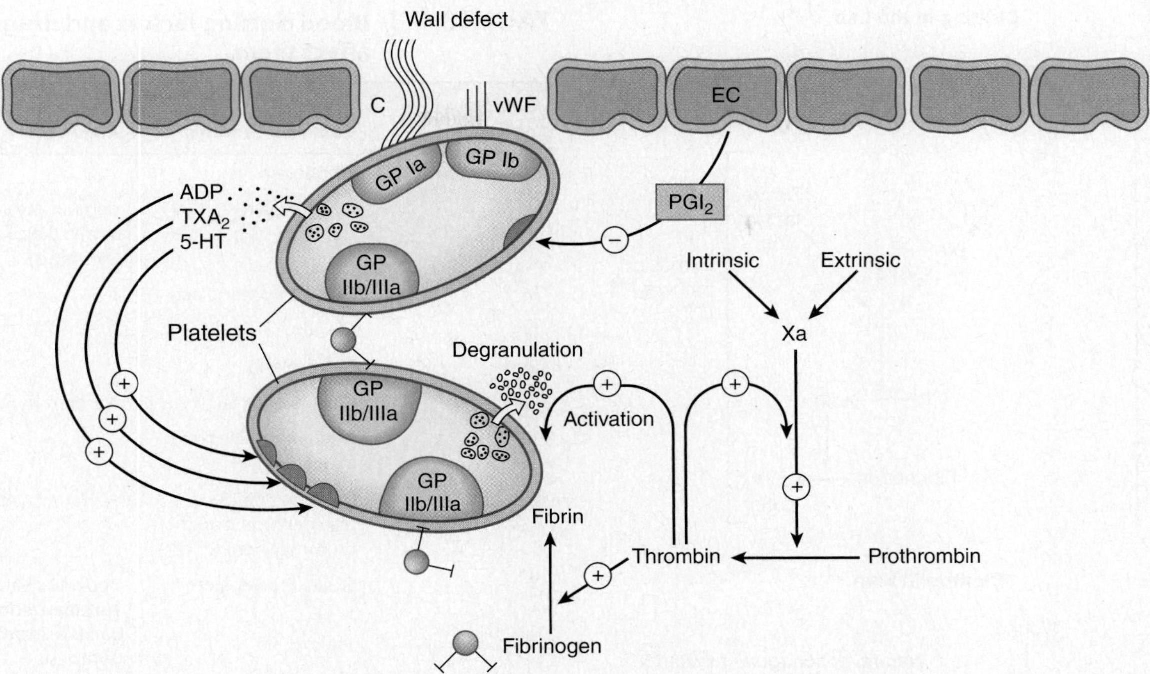

FIGURE 34–1 Thrombus formation at the site of the damaged vascular wall (EC, endothelial cell) and the role of platelets and clotting factors. Platelet membrane receptors include the glycoprotein (GP) Ia receptor, binding to collagen (C); GP Ib receptor, binding von Willebrand factor (vWF); and GP IIb/IIIa, which binds fibrinogen and other macromolecules. Antiplatelet prostacyclin (PGI_2) is released from the endothelium. Aggregating substances released from the degranulating platelet include adenosine diphosphate (ADP), thromboxane A_2 (TXA_2), and serotonin (5-HT). Production of factor Xa by intrinsic and extrinsic pathways is detailed in Figure 34–2.

with injury. In contrast, patients with defects in the clotting mechanism (secondary hemostasis, eg, hemophilia A) tend to bleed into deep tissues (joints, muscle, retroperitoneum), often with no apparent inciting event, and bleeding may recur unpredictably.

The platelet is central to normal hemostasis and thromboembolic disease, and is the target of many therapies discussed in this chapter. Platelet-rich thrombi **(white thrombi)** form in the high flow rate and high shear force environment of arteries. Occlusive arterial thrombi cause serious disease by producing downstream ischemia of extremities or vital organs, and they can result in limb amputation or organ failure. Venous clots tend to be more fibrin-rich, contain large numbers of trapped red blood cells, and are recognized pathologically as **red thrombi.** Deep venous thrombi (DVT) can cause severe swelling and pain of the affected extremity, but the most feared consequence is pulmonary embolism (PE). This occurs when part or all of the clot breaks off from its location in the deep venous system and travels as an embolus through the right side of the heart and into the pulmonary arterial circulation. Occlusion of a large pulmonary artery by an embolic clot can precipitate acute right heart failure and sudden death. In addition lung ischemia or infarction will occur distal to the occluded pulmonary arterial segment. Such emboli usually arise from the deep venous system of the proximal lower extremities or pelvis. Although all thrombi are mixed, the platelet nidus dominates the arterial thrombus and the fibrin tail dominates the venous thrombus.

BLOOD COAGULATION CASCADE

Blood coagulates due to the transformation of soluble fibrinogen into insoluble fibrin by the enzyme thrombin. Several circulating proteins interact in a cascading series of limited proteolytic reactions (Figure 34–2). At each step, a clotting factor zymogen undergoes limited proteolysis and becomes an active protease (eg, factor VII is converted to factor VIIa). Each protease factor activates the next clotting factor in the sequence, culminating in the formation of thrombin (factor IIa). Several of these factors are targets for drug therapy (Table 34–1).

Thrombin has a central role in hemostasis and has many functions. In clotting, thrombin proteolytically cleaves small peptides from fibrinogen, allowing fibrinogen to polymerize and form a fibrin clot. Thrombin also activates many upstream clotting factors, leading to more thrombin generation, and activates factor XIII, a transaminase that cross-links the fibrin polymer and stabilizes the clot. Thrombin is a potent platelet activator and mitogen. Thrombin also exerts *anti*coagulant effects by activating the protein C pathway, which attenuates the clotting response (see Figure 34–2). It should therefore be apparent that the response to vascular injury is a complex and precisely modulated process that ensures that under normal circumstances, repair of vascular injury occurs without thrombosis and downstream ischemia—that is, the response is proportionate and reversible. Eventually vascular remodeling and repair occur with reversion to the quiescent resting anticoagulant endothelial cell phenotype.

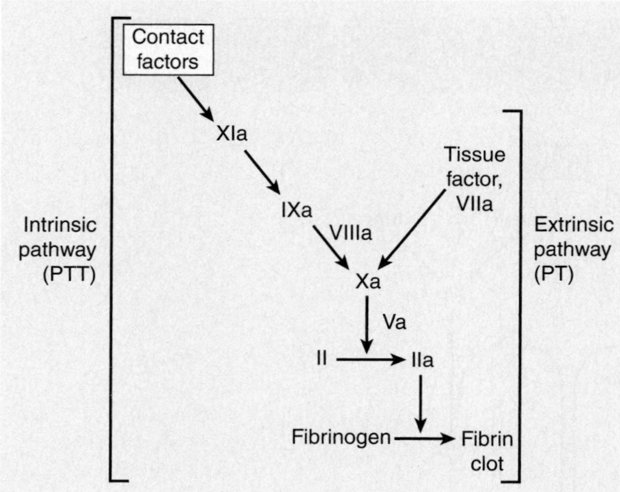

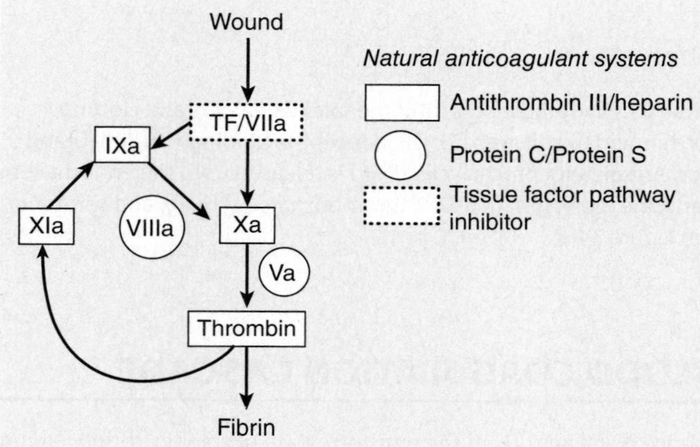

FIGURE 34–2 A model of blood coagulation. With tissue factor (TF), factor VII forms an activated complex (VIIa-TF) that catalyzes the activation of factor IX to factor IXa. Activated factor XIa also catalyzes this reaction. Tissue factor pathway inhibitor inhibits the catalytic action of the VIIa-TF complex. The cascade proceeds as shown, resulting ultimately in the conversion of fibrinogen to fibrin, an essential component of a functional clot. The two major anticoagulant drugs, heparin and warfarin, have very different actions. Heparin, acting in the blood, directly activates anticlotting factors, specifically antithrombin, which inactivates the factors enclosed in rectangles. Warfarin, acting in the liver, inhibits the synthesis of the factors enclosed in circles. Proteins C and S exert anticlotting effects by inactivating activated factors Va and VIIIa.

TABLE 34–1 Blood clotting factors and drugs that affect them.[1]

Component or Factor	Common Synonym	Target for the Action of:
I	Fibrinogen	
II	Prothrombin	Heparin, dabigatran (IIa); warfarin (synthesis)
III	Tissue thromboplastin	
IV	Calcium	
V	Proaccelerin	
VII	Proconvertin	Warfarin (synthesis)
VIII	Antihemophilic factor (AHF)	
IX	Christmas factor, plasma thromboplastin component (PTC)	Warfarin (synthesis)
X	Stuart-Prower factor	Heparin, rivaroxaban, apixaban, edoxaban (Xa); warfarin (synthesis)
XI	Plasma thromboplastin antecedent (PTA)	
XII	Hageman factor	
XIII	Fibrin-stabilizing factor	
Proteins C and S		Warfarin (synthesis)
Plasminogen		Thrombolytic enzymes, aminocaproic acid

[1]See Figure 34–2 and text for additional details.

Initiation of Clotting: The Tissue Factor-VIIa Complex

The main initiator of blood coagulation in vivo is the tissue factor (TF) VIIa pathway (see Figure 34–2). Tissue factor is a transmembrane protein ubiquitously expressed outside the vasculature but not normally expressed in an active form within vessels. The exposure of TF on damaged endothelium or to blood that has extravasated into tissue binds TF to factor VIIa. This complex, in turn, activates factors X and IX. Factor Xa along with factor Va forms the prothrombinase complex on activated cell surfaces, which catalyzes the conversion of prothrombin (factor II) to thrombin (factor IIa). Thrombin, in turn, activates upstream clotting factors, primarily factors V, VIII, and XI, resulting in amplification of thrombin generation. The TF-factor VIIa-catalyzed activation of factor Xa is regulated by tissue factor pathway inhibitor (TFPI). Thus after initial activation of factor X to Xa by TF-VIIa, further propagation of the clot occurs by feedback amplification of thrombin through the intrinsic pathway factors VIII and IX. (This provides an explanation for why patients with deficiency of factor VIII or IX—hemophilia A and hemophilia B, respectively—have a severe bleeding disorder.)

It is also important to note that the coagulation mechanism in vivo does not occur in solution, but is localized to activated *cell surfaces* expressing anionic phospholipids such as phosphatidylserine, and is mediated by Ca^{2+} bridging between the anionic phospholipids and γ-carboxyglutamic acid residues of the clotting factors. This is the basis for using calcium chelators such as ethylenediamine tetraacetic acid (EDTA) or citrate to prevent blood from clotting in a test tube.

Antithrombin (AT) is an endogenous anticoagulant and a member of the serine protease inhibitor (serpin) family; it inactivates the serine proteases IIa, IXa, Xa, XIa, and XIIa. The endogenous anticoagulants **protein C** and **protein S** attenuate the blood clotting cascade by proteolysis of the two cofactors Va and VIIIa. From an evolutionary perspective, it is of interest that factors V and VIII have an identical overall domain structure and considerable homology, consistent with a common ancestor gene; likewise the serine proteases are descendants of a trypsin-like common ancestor. Thus, the TF-VIIa initiating complex, serine proteases, and cofactors each have their own lineage-specific attenuation mechanism (see Figure 34–2). Defects in natural anticoagulants result in an increased risk of venous thrombosis. The most common defect in the natural anticoagulant system is a mutation in factor V (factor V Leiden), which results in resistance to inactivation by the protein C/protein S mechanism.

Fibrinolysis

Fibrinolysis refers to the process of fibrin digestion by the fibrin-specific protease, plasmin. The fibrinolytic system is similar to the coagulation system in that the precursor form of the serine protease plasmin circulates in an inactive form as plasminogen. In response to injury, endothelial cells synthesize and release tissue plasminogen activator (t-PA), which converts plasminogen to plasmin (Figure 34–3). Plasmin remodels the thrombus and limits its extension by proteolytic digestion of fibrin.

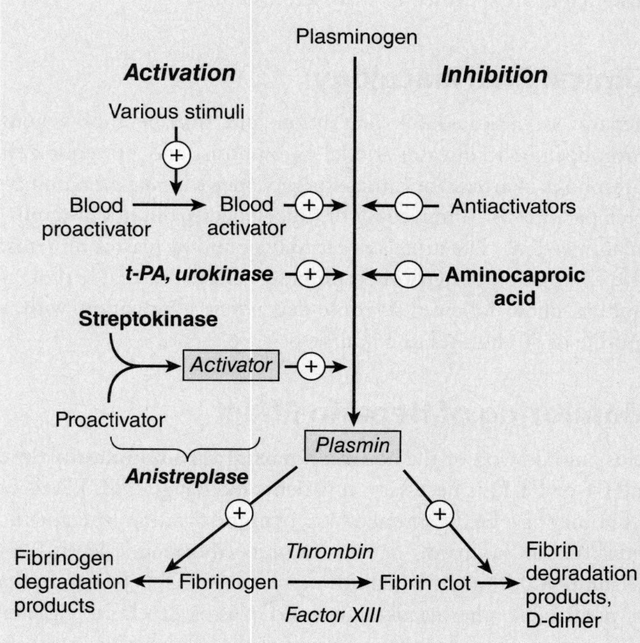

FIGURE 34–3 Schematic representation of the fibrinolytic system. Plasmin is the active fibrinolytic enzyme. Several clinically useful activators are shown on the left in bold. Anistreplase is a combination of streptokinase and the proactivator plasminogen. Aminocaproic acid (*right*) inhibits the activation of plasminogen to plasmin and is useful in some bleeding disorders. t-PA, tissue plasminogen activator.

Both plasminogen and plasmin have specialized protein domains (kringles) that bind to exposed lysines on the fibrin clot and impart clot specificity to the fibrinolytic process. It should be noted that this clot specificity is only observed at *physiologic* levels of t-PA. At the *pharmacologic* levels of t-PA used in thrombolytic therapy, clot specificity is lost and a systemic lytic state is created, with attendant increase in bleeding risk. As in the coagulation cascade, there are negative regulators of fibrinolysis: endothelial cells synthesize and release plasminogen activator inhibitor (PAI), which inhibits t-PA; in addition α_2 antiplasmin circulates in the blood at high concentrations and under physiologic conditions will rapidly inactivate any plasmin that is not clot-bound. However, this regulatory system is overwhelmed by therapeutic doses of plasminogen activators.

If the coagulation and fibrinolytic systems are pathologically activated, the hemostatic system may careen out of control, leading to generalized intravascular clotting and bleeding. This process is called **disseminated intravascular coagulation (DIC)** and may follow massive tissue injury, advanced cancers, obstetric emergencies such as abruptio placentae or retained products of conception, or bacterial sepsis. The treatment of DIC is to control the underlying disease process; if this is not possible, DIC is often fatal.

Regulation of the fibrinolytic system is useful in therapeutics. Increased fibrinolysis is effective therapy for thrombotic disease. **Tissue plasminogen activator, urokinase,** and **streptokinase** all activate the fibrinolytic system (see Figure 34–3). Conversely, decreased fibrinolysis protects clots from lysis and reduces the bleeding of hemostatic failure. **Aminocaproic acid** is a clinically useful inhibitor of fibrinolysis. Heparin and the oral anticoagulant drugs do not affect the fibrinolytic mechanism.

■ BASIC PHARMACOLOGY OF THE ANTICOAGULANT DRUGS

The ideal anticoagulant drug would prevent pathologic thrombosis and limit reperfusion injury yet allow a normal response to vascular injury and limit bleeding. Theoretically this could be accomplished by preservation of the TF-VIIa initiation phase of the clotting mechanism with attenuation of the secondary intrinsic pathway propagation phase of clot development. At this time such a drug does not exist; all anticoagulants and fibrinolytic drugs have an increased bleeding risk as their principal toxicity.

INDIRECT THROMBIN INHIBITORS

The indirect thrombin inhibitors are so-named because their antithrombotic effect is exerted by their interaction with a separate protein, antithrombin. **Unfractionated heparin (UFH),** also known as **high-molecular-weight (HMW) heparin, low-molecular-weight (LMW) heparin,** and the synthetic pentasaccharide **fondaparinux** bind to antithrombin and enhance its inactivation of factor Xa (Figure 34–4). Unfractionated heparin and to a lesser extent LMW heparin also enhance antithrombin's inactivation of thrombin.

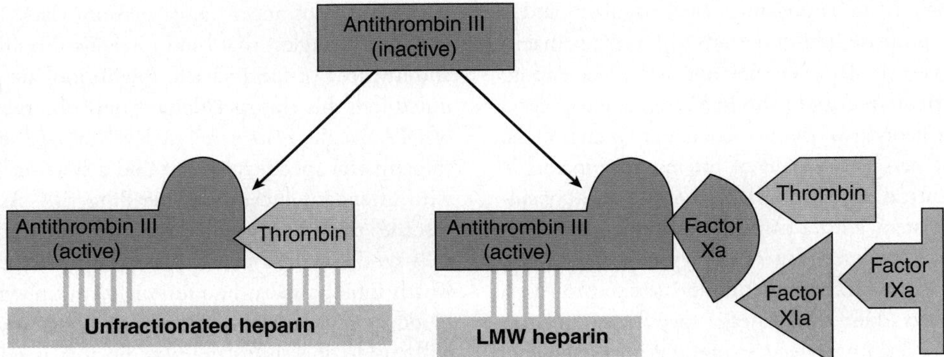

FIGURE 34–4 Differences between low-molecular-weight (LMW) heparins and high-molecular-weight heparin (unfractionated heparin). Fondaparinux is a small pentasaccharide fragment of heparin. Activated antithrombin III (AT III) degrades thrombin, factor X, and several other factors. Binding of these drugs to AT III can increase the catalytic action of AT III 1000-fold. The combination of AT III with unfractionated heparin increases degradation of both factor Xa and thrombin. Combination with fondaparinux or LMW heparin more selectively increases degradation of Xa.

HEPARIN

Chemistry & Mechanism of Action

Heparin is a heterogeneous mixture of sulfated mucopolysaccharides. It binds to endothelial cell surfaces and a variety of plasma proteins. Its biologic activity is dependent upon the endogenous anticoagulant **antithrombin.** Antithrombin inhibits clotting factor proteases, especially thrombin (IIa), IXa, and Xa, by forming equimolar stable complexes with them. In the absence of heparin, these reactions are slow; in the presence of heparin, they are accelerated 1000-fold. Only about a third of the molecules in commercial heparin preparations have an accelerating effect because the remainder lack the unique pentasaccharide sequence needed for high-affinity binding to antithrombin. The active heparin molecules bind tightly to antithrombin and cause a conformational change in this inhibitor. The conformational change of antithrombin exposes its active site for more rapid interaction with the proteases (the activated clotting factors). Heparin functions as a cofactor for the antithrombin-protease reaction without being consumed. Once the antithrombin-protease complex is formed, heparin is released intact for renewed binding to more antithrombin.

The antithrombin binding region of commercial unfractionated heparin consists of repeating sulfated disaccharide units composed of D-glucosamine-L-iduronic acid and D-glucosamine-D-glucuronic acid. High-molecular-weight fractions of heparin with high affinity for antithrombin markedly inhibit blood coagulation by inhibiting all three factors, especially thrombin and factor Xa. Unfractionated heparin has a molecular weight range of 5000–30,000 Da. In contrast, the shorter-chain, low-molecular-weight fractions of heparin inhibit activated factor X but have less effect on thrombin than the HMW species. Nevertheless, numerous studies have demonstrated that LMW heparins such as **enoxaparin, dalteparin,** and **tinzaparin** are effective in several thromboembolic conditions. In fact, these LMW heparins—in comparison with UFH—have equal efficacy, increased bioavailability from the subcutaneous site of injection, and less frequent dosing requirements (once or twice daily is sufficient).

USP heparin is harmonized to the World Health Organization International Standard (IS) unit dose. Enoxaparin is obtained from the same sources as regular UFH, but doses are specified in milligrams. Fondaparinux also is specified in milligrams. Dalteparin, tinzaparin, and danaparoid (an LMW heparinoid containing heparan sulfate, dermatan sulfate, and chondroitin sulfate), on the other hand, are specified in anti-factor Xa units.

Clinical Pharmacology

Heparin is indicated for prevention and treatment of venous thromboembolic disease, arterial thrombosis, and prevention of thrombosis in arterial or cardiac surgery. Heparin may be administered parenterally (intravenous or subcutaneous, but not intramuscular injection). The drug is extensively bound by plasma proteins. The elimination of heparin is complex, with the saturable protein binding phase followed by dose-dependent elimination with a half-life of 30 minutes to 2 hours.

Monitoring of Heparin Effect

Close monitoring of the **activated partial thromboplastin time (aPTT** or **PTT)** is necessary in patients receiving UFH. Levels of UFH may also be determined by protamine titration (therapeutic levels 0.2–0.4 unit/mL) or anti-Xa units (therapeutic levels 0.3–0.7 unit/mL). Weight-based dosing of the LMW heparins results in predictable pharmacokinetics and plasma levels in patients with normal renal function. Therefore, LMW heparin levels are not generally measured except in the setting of renal insufficiency, obesity, and pregnancy. LMW heparin levels can be determined by anti-Xa units. For enoxaparin, peak therapeutic levels should be 0.5–1 unit/mL for twice-daily dosing, determined 4 hours after administration, and approximately 1.5 units/mL for once-daily dosing.

Toxicity

A. Bleeding and Miscellaneous Effects

The major adverse effect of heparin is bleeding. This risk can be decreased by scrupulous patient selection, careful control of dosage, and close monitoring. Elderly women and patients with renal failure are more prone to hemorrhage. Heparin is of animal origin and should be used cautiously in patients with allergy. Increased loss of hair and reversible alopecia have been reported. Long-term heparin therapy is associated with osteoporosis and spontaneous fractures. Heparin accelerates the clearing of postprandial lipemia by causing the release of lipoprotein lipase from tissues, and long-term use is associated with mineralocorticoid deficiency.

B. Heparin-Induced Thrombocytopenia

Heparin-induced thrombocytopenia (HIT) is a systemic hypercoagulable state that occurs in 1–4% of individuals treated with UFH. Surgical patients are at greatest risk. The reported incidence of HIT is lower in pediatric populations outside the critical care setting; it is relatively rare in pregnant women. The risk of HIT may be higher in individuals treated with UFH of bovine origin compared with porcine heparin and is lower in those treated exclusively with LMW heparin.

Morbidity and mortality in HIT are related to thrombotic events. Venous thrombosis occurs most commonly, but occlusion of peripheral or central arteries is not infrequent. If an indwelling catheter is present, the risk of thrombosis is increased in that extremity. Skin necrosis has been described, particularly in individuals treated with warfarin in the absence of a direct thrombin inhibitor, presumably due to acute depletion of the vitamin K–dependent anticoagulant protein C occurring in the presence of high levels of procoagulant proteins and an active hypercoagulable state.

The following points should be considered in all patients receiving heparin: Platelet counts should be performed frequently; thrombocytopenia appearing in a time frame consistent with an immune response to heparin should be considered suspicious for HIT; and any new thrombus occurring in a patient receiving heparin therapy should raise suspicion of HIT. Patients who develop HIT are treated by discontinuance of heparin and administration of the direct thrombin inhibitor argatroban.

Contraindications

Heparin is contraindicated in patients with HIT, hypersensitivity to the drug, active bleeding, hemophilia, significant thrombocytopenia, purpura, severe hypertension, intracranial hemorrhage, infective endocarditis, active tuberculosis, ulcerative lesions of the gastrointestinal tract, threatened abortion, visceral carcinoma, or advanced hepatic or renal disease. Heparin should be avoided in patients who have recently had surgery of the brain, spinal cord, or eye; and in patients who are undergoing lumbar puncture or regional anesthetic block. Despite the apparent lack of placental transfer, heparin should be used in pregnant women only when clearly indicated.

Administration & Dosage

The indications for the use of heparin are described in the section on clinical pharmacology. A plasma concentration of heparin of 0.2–0.4 unit/mL (by protamine titration) or 0.3–0.7 unit/mL (anti-Xa units) is considered to be the therapeutic range for treatment of venous thromboembolic disease. This concentration generally corresponds to a PTT of 1.5–2.5 times baseline. However, the use of the PTT for heparin monitoring is problematic. There is no standardization scheme for the PTT as there is for the prothrombin time (PT) and its international normalized ratio (INR) in warfarin monitoring. The PTT in seconds for a given heparin concentration varies between different reagent/instrument systems. Thus, if the PTT is used for monitoring, the laboratory should determine the clotting time that corresponds to the therapeutic range by protamine titration or anti-Xa activity, as listed above.

In addition, some patients have a prolonged baseline PTT due to factor deficiency or inhibitors (which could increase bleeding risk) or lupus anticoagulant (which is generally not associated with bleeding risk but may be associated with thrombosis risk). Using the PTT to assess heparin effect in such patients is problematic. An alternative is to use anti-Xa activity to assess heparin concentration, a test now widely available on automated coagulation instruments. This approach measures heparin concentration; however, it does not provide the global assessment of intrinsic pathway integrity of the PTT.

The following strategy is recommended: prior to initiating anticoagulant therapy of any type, the integrity of the patient's hemostatic system should be assessed by a careful history of prior bleeding events, as well as baseline PT and PTT. If there is a prolonged clotting time, the cause of this (deficiency or inhibitor) should be determined prior to initiating therapy, and treatment goals stratified to a risk-benefit assessment. In high-risk patients measuring both the PTT and anti-Xa activity may be useful. When *intermittent* heparin administration is used, the aPTT or anti-Xa activity should be measured 6 hours after the administered dose to maintain prolongation of the aPTT to 2–2.5 times that of the control value. However, LMW heparin therapy is the preferred option in this case, as no monitoring is required in most patients.

Continuous intravenous administration of heparin is accomplished via an infusion pump. After an initial bolus injection of 80–100 units/kg, a continuous infusion of about 15–22 units/kg per hour is required to maintain the anti-Xa activity in the range of 0.3–0.7 units/mL. Low-dose prophylaxis is achieved with subcutaneous administration of heparin, 5000 units every 8–12 hours. Because of the danger of hematoma formation at the injection site, heparin must never be administered intramuscularly.

Prophylactic enoxaparin is given subcutaneously in a dosage of 30 mg twice daily or 40 mg once daily. Full-dose enoxaparin therapy is 1 mg/kg subcutaneously every 12 hours. This corresponds to a therapeutic anti-factor Xa level of 0.5–1 unit/mL. Selected patients may be treated with enoxaparin 1.5 mg/kg once a day, with a target anti-Xa level of 1.5 units/mL. The prophylactic dosage of dalteparin is 5000 units subcutaneously once a day; therapeutic dosing is 200 units/kg once a day for venous disease or 120 units/kg every 12 hours for acute coronary syndrome. LMW heparin should be used with caution in patients with renal insufficiency or body weight greater than 150 kg. Measurement of the anti-Xa level is useful to guide dosing in these individuals.

The synthetic pentasaccharide molecule **fondaparinux** avidly binds antithrombin with high specific activity, resulting in efficient inactivation of factor Xa. Fondaparinux has a long half-life of 15 hours, allowing for once-daily dosing by subcutaneous administration. Fondaparinux is effective in the prevention and treatment of venous thromboembolism and does not appear to cross-react with pathologic HIT antibodies in most individuals.

Reversal of Heparin Action

Excessive anticoagulant action of heparin is treated by discontinuance of the drug. If bleeding occurs, administration of a specific antagonist such as **protamine sulfate** is indicated. Protamine is a highly basic, positively charged peptide that combines with negatively charged heparin as an ion pair to form a stable complex devoid of anticoagulant activity. For every 100 units of heparin remaining in the patient, 1 mg of protamine sulfate is given intravenously; the rate of infusion should not exceed 50 mg in any 10-minute period. Excess protamine must be avoided; it also has an anticoagulant effect. Neutralization of LMW heparin by protamine is incomplete. Limited experience suggests that 1 mg of protamine sulfate may be used to partially neutralize 1 mg of enoxaparin. Protamine will not reverse the activity of fondaparinux. Excess danaparoid can be removed by plasmapheresis.

WARFARIN & OTHER COUMARIN ANTICOAGULANTS

Chemistry & Pharmacokinetics

The clinical use of the coumarin anticoagulants began with the discovery of an anticoagulant substance formed in spoiled sweet clover silage, which caused hemorrhagic disease in cattle. At the behest of local farmers, a chemist at the University of Wisconsin identified the toxic agent as bishydroxycoumarin. Dicumarol, a synthesized derivative, and its congeners, most notably warfarin (**W**isconsin **A**lumni **R**esearch **F**oundation, with "-arin" from coumarin added; Figure 34–5), were initially used as rodenticides. In the 1950s, warfarin (under the brand name Coumadin) was introduced as an antithrombotic agent in humans. Warfarin is one of the most commonly prescribed drugs.

Warfarin is generally administered as the sodium salt and has 100% oral bioavailability. Over 99% of racemic warfarin is bound to plasma albumin, which may contribute to its small volume of distribution (the albumin space), its long half-life in plasma (36 hours), and the lack of urinary excretion of unchanged drug. Warfarin used clinically is a racemic mixture composed of equal amounts of two enantiomorphs. The levorotatory *S*-warfarin is four times more potent than the dextrorotatory *R*-warfarin. This observation is useful in understanding the stereoselective nature of several drug interactions involving warfarin.

Mechanism of Action

Coumarin anticoagulants block the γ-carboxylation of several glutamate residues in prothrombin and factors VII, IX, and X as well as

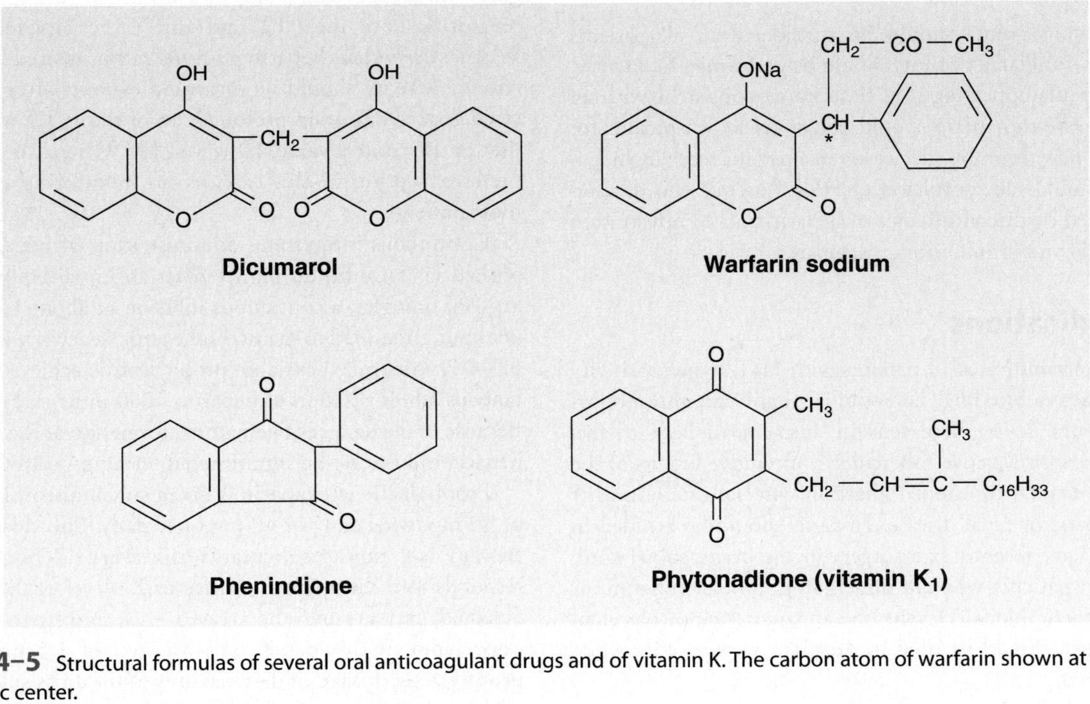

FIGURE 34–5 Structural formulas of several oral anticoagulant drugs and of vitamin K. The carbon atom of warfarin shown at the asterisk is an asymmetric center.

the endogenous anticoagulant proteins C and S (see Figure 34–2 and Table 34–1). The blockade results in incomplete coagulation factor molecules that are biologically inactive. The protein carboxylation reaction is coupled to the oxidation of vitamin K. The vitamin must then be reduced to reactivate it. Warfarin prevents reductive metabolism of the inactive vitamin K epoxide back to its active hydroquinone form (Figure 34–6). Mutational change of the gene for the responsible enzyme, vitamin K epoxide reductase (*VKORC1*), can give rise to genetic resistance to warfarin in humans and rodents.

There is an 8- to 12-hour delay in the action of warfarin. Its anticoagulant effect results from a balance between partially inhibited synthesis and unaltered degradation of the four vitamin K–dependent clotting factors. The resulting inhibition of coagulation is dependent on their degradation half-lives in the circulation. These half-lives are 6, 24, 40, and 60 hours for factors VII, IX, X, and II, respectively. Importantly, protein C has a short half-life similar to factor VIIa. Thus the immediate effect of warfarin is to deplete the procoagulant factor VII and anticoagulant protein C, which can paradoxically create a transient hypercoagulable state due to residual activity of the longer half-life procoagulants in the face of protein C depletion (see below). For this reason in patients with active hypercoagulable states, such as acute DVT or PE, UFH or LMW heparin is always used to achieve immediate anticoagulation until adequate warfarin-induced depletion of the procoagulant clotting factors is achieved. The duration of this overlapping therapy is generally 5–7 days.

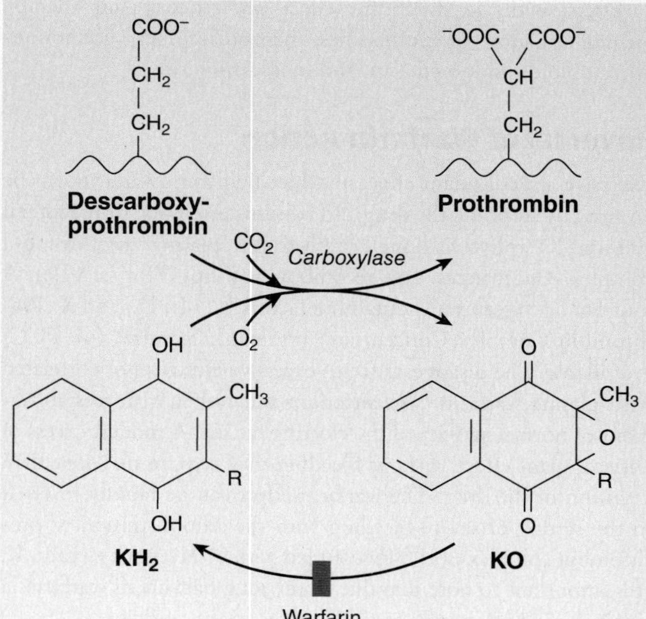

FIGURE 34–6 Vitamin K cycle–metabolic interconversions of vitamin K associated with the synthesis of vitamin K–dependent clotting factors. Vitamin K_1 or K_2 is activated by reduction to the hydroquinone form (KH_2). Stepwise oxidation to vitamin K epoxide (KO) is coupled to prothrombin carboxylation by the enzyme carboxylase. The reactivation of vitamin K epoxide is the warfarin-sensitive step (warfarin). The R on the vitamin K molecule represents a 20-carbon phytyl side chain in vitamin K_1 and a 30- to 65-carbon polyprenyl side chain in vitamin K_2.

Toxicity

Warfarin crosses the placenta readily and can cause a hemorrhagic disorder in the fetus. Furthermore, fetal proteins with γ-carboxyglutamate residues found in bone and blood may be affected by warfarin; the drug can cause a serious birth defect characterized by abnormal bone formation. Thus, warfarin should never be administered during pregnancy. Cutaneous necrosis with reduced activity of protein C sometimes occurs during the first weeks of therapy in patients who have inherited deficiency of protein C. Rarely, the same process causes frank infarction of the breast, fatty tissues, intestine, and extremities. The pathologic lesion associated with the hemorrhagic infarction is venous thrombosis, consistent with a hypercoagulable state due to warfarin-induced depletion of protein C.

Administration & Dosage

Treatment with warfarin should be initiated with standard doses of 5–10 mg. The initial adjustment of the prothrombin time takes about 1 week, which usually results in a maintenance dosage of 5–7 mg/d. The **prothrombin time (PT)** should be increased to a level representing a reduction of prothrombin activity to 25% of normal and maintained there for long-term therapy. When the activity is less than 20%, the warfarin dosage should be reduced or omitted until the activity rises above 20%. Inherited polymorphisms in *2CYP2C9* and *VKORC1* have significant effects on warfarin dosing; however, algorithms incorporating genomic information to predict initial warfarin dosing were no better than standard clinical algorithms in two of three large randomized trials examining this issue (see Chapter 5).

The therapeutic range for oral anticoagulant therapy is defined in terms of an international normalized ratio (INR). The INR is the prothrombin time ratio (patient prothrombin time/mean of normal prothrombin time for lab)^{ISI}, where the ISI exponent refers to the International Sensitivity Index and is dependent on the specific reagents and instruments used for the determination. The ISI serves to relate measured prothrombin times to a World Health Organization reference standard thromboplastin; thus the prothrombin times performed on different properly calibrated instruments with a variety of thromboplastin reagents should give the same INR results for a given sample. For most reagent and instrument combinations in current use, the ISI is close to 1, making the INR roughly the ratio of the patient prothrombin time to the mean normal prothrombin time. The recommended INR for prophylaxis and treatment of thrombotic disease is 2–3. Patients with some types of artificial heart valves (eg, tilting disk) or other medical conditions increasing thrombotic risk have a recommended range of 2.5–3.5. While a prolonged INR is widely used as an indication of integrity of the coagulation system in liver disease and other disorders, it has been validated only in patients in steady state on chronic warfarin therapy.

Occasionally patients exhibit warfarin resistance, defined as progression or recurrence of a thrombotic event while in the therapeutic range. These individuals may have their INR target raised (which is accompanied by an increase in bleeding risk) or be changed to an alternative form of anticoagulation (eg, daily injections of LMW heparin or one of the newer oral anticoagulants). Warfarin resistance is most commonly seen in patients with advanced cancers, typically of gastrointestinal origin (Trousseau syndrome). LMW heparin is superior to warfarin in preventing recurrent venous thromboembolism in patients with cancer.

Drug Interactions

The coumarin anticoagulants often interact with other drugs and with disease states. These interactions can be broadly divided into pharmacokinetic and pharmacodynamic effects (Table 34–2). Pharmacokinetic mechanisms for drug interaction with warfarin mainly involve cytochrome P450 CYP2C9 enzyme induction, enzyme inhibition, and reduced plasma protein binding. Pharmacodynamic mechanisms for interactions with warfarin are synergism (impaired hemostasis, reduced clotting factor synthesis, as in hepatic disease), competitive antagonism (vitamin K), and an altered physiologic control loop for vitamin K (hereditary resistance to oral anticoagulants).

The most serious interactions with warfarin are those that increase the anticoagulant effect and the risk of bleeding. The most dangerous of these interactions are the pharmacokinetic interactions with the mostly obsolete pyrazolones phenylbutazone and sulfinpyrazone. These drugs not only augment the hypoprothrombinemia but also inhibit platelet function and may induce peptic ulcer disease (see Chapter 36). The mechanisms for their hypoprothrombinemic interaction are a stereoselective inhibition of oxidative metabolic transformation of *S*-warfarin (the more potent isomer) and displacement of albumin-bound warfarin, increasing the free fraction. For this and other reasons, neither phenylbutazone nor sulfinpyrazone is in common use in the United States. Metronidazole, fluconazole, and trimethoprim-sulfamethoxazole also stereoselectively inhibit the metabolic transformation of *S*-warfarin, whereas amiodarone, disulfiram, and cimetidine inhibit metabolism of both enantiomorphs of warfarin (see Chapter 4). Aspirin, hepatic disease, and hyperthyroidism augment warfarin's effects—aspirin by its effect on platelet function and the latter two by increasing the turnover rate of clotting factors. The third-generation cephalosporins eliminate the bacteria in the intestinal tract that produce vitamin K and, like warfarin, also directly inhibit vitamin K epoxide reductase.

Barbiturates and rifampin cause a marked *decrease* of the anticoagulant effect by induction of the hepatic enzymes that transform racemic warfarin. Cholestyramine binds warfarin in the intestine and reduces its absorption and bioavailability.

Pharmacodynamic reductions of anticoagulant effect occur with increased vitamin K intake (increased synthesis of clotting factors), the diuretics chlorthalidone and spironolactone (clotting factor concentration), hereditary resistance (mutation of vitamin K reactivation cycle molecules), and hypothyroidism (decreased turnover rate of clotting factors).

Drugs with *no* significant effect on anticoagulant therapy include ethanol, phenothiazines, benzodiazepines, acetaminophen, opioids, indomethacin, and most antibiotics.

TABLE 34–2 Pharmacokinetic and pharmacodynamic drug and body interactions with oral anticoagulants.

Increased Prothrombin Time	Decreased Prothrombin Time
Pharmacokinetic	***Pharmacokinetic***
Amiodarone	Barbiturates
Cimetidine	Cholestyramine
Disulfiram	Rifampin
Fluconazole[1]	
Metronidazole[1]	
Phenylbutazone[1]	
Sulfinpyrazone[1]	
Trimethoprim-sulfamethoxazole	
Pharmacodynamic	***Pharmacodynamic***
Drugs	**Drugs**
Aspirin (high doses)	Diuretics
Cephalosporins, third-generation	Vitamin K
Heparin, argatroban, dabigatran, rivaroxaban, apixaban	
Body factors	**Body factors**
Hepatic disease	Hereditary resistance
Hyperthyroidism	Hypothyroidism

[1]Stereoselectively inhibits the oxidative metabolism of the *S*-warfarin enantiomorph of racemic warfarin.

Reversal of Warfarin Action

Excessive anticoagulant effect and bleeding from warfarin can be reversed by stopping the drug and administering oral or parenteral vitamin K_1 (phytonadione), fresh-frozen plasma, prothrombin complex concentrates, and recombinant factor VIIa (rFVIIa). A four-factor concentrate containing factors II, VII, IX, and X (Prothrombin Complex Concentrate, [Human]; Kcentra) (4F PCC) is available. The disappearance of excessive effect is not correlated with plasma warfarin concentrations but rather with reestablishment of normal activity of the clotting factors. A modest excess of anticoagulant effect without bleeding may require no more than cessation of the drug. The warfarin effect can be rapidly reversed in the setting of severe bleeding with the administration of prothrombin complex or rFVIIa coupled with intravenous vitamin K. It is important to note that due to the long half-life of warfarin, a single dose of vitamin K or rFVIIa may not be sufficient.

ORAL DIRECT FACTOR Xa INHIBITORS

Oral Xa inhibitors, including **rivaroxaban, apixaban, edoxaban,** and **betrixaban,** represent a newer class of oral anticoagulant drugs that require no monitoring. Along with oral direct thrombin inhibitors (discussed below) this class of direct oral anticoagulant (DOAC) drugs is increasingly used in antithrombotic pharmacotherapy.

Pharmacology

Rivaroxaban, apixaban, edoxaban, and betrixaban inhibit factor Xa in the final common pathway of clotting (see Figure 34–2). These drugs are given as fixed doses and do not require monitoring. They have a rapid onset of action and shorter half-lives than warfarin.

Rivaroxaban has high oral bioavailability when taken with food. Following an oral dose, the peak plasma level is achieved within 2–4 hours; the drug is extensively protein-bound. It is a substrate for the cytochrome P450 system and the P-glycoprotein transporter. Drugs inhibiting both CYP3A4 and P-glycoprotein (eg, ketoconazole) result in increased rivaroxaban effect. One third of the drug is excreted unchanged in the urine and the remainder is metabolized and excreted in the urine and feces. The drug half-life is 5–9 hours in patients age 20–45 years and is increased in the elderly and in those with impaired renal or hepatic function.

Apixaban has an oral bioavailability of 50% and prolonged absorption, resulting in a half-life of 12 hours with chronic dosing. The drug is a substrate of the cytochrome P450 system and P-glycoprotein and is excreted in the urine and feces. As with rivaroxaban, drugs inhibiting both CYP3A4 and P-glycoprotein, as well as impairment of renal or hepatic function, result in increased drug effect.

Edoxaban is a once-daily Xa inhibitor with a 62% oral bioavailability. Peak drug concentrations occur 1–2 hours after dosage and are not affected by food. The drug half-life is 10–14 hours. Edoxaban does not induce CYP450 enzymes. No dose reduction is required with concurrent use of P-glycoprotein inhibitors. Edoxaban is primarily excreted unchanged in the urine.

Betrixaban is also a once daily Xa inhibitor with oral bioavailability of 34% and half-life of 19–27 hours; peak levels are achieved in 3–4 hours, and are reduced up to 70% if taken with food. Dose reduction is required if used with P-glycoprotein inhibitors and in renal failure. The drug is primarily excreted by the liver and should be used with caution in patients with liver disease.

Indications & Dosage

Rivaroxaban is approved for prevention of embolic stroke in patients with atrial fibrillation without valvular heart disease; prevention of venous thromboembolism following hip or knee surgery or acutely ill medical patients at risk for VTE; treatment of venous thromboembolic disease (VTE); risk reduction of cardiovascular events (MI, stroke, cardiovascular death) in patients with coronary artery disease (CAD); and risk reduction of thrombotic events in patients with peripheral arterial disease (PAD). The prophylactic dosage is 10 mg orally per day for 35 days for hip replacement or 12 days for knee replacement. For treatment of DVT/PE the dosage is 15 mg twice daily for 3 weeks followed by 20 mg/d. The dose for risk reduction of cardiovascular events in CAD and PAD is 2.5 mg twice daily, along with aspirin, 70–100 mg daily. Depending on clinical presentation and risk factors, patients with VTE are treated for 3–6 months; rivaroxaban is also approved for extended therapy (10 mg once daily) in selected patients to reduce recurrence risk at the treatment dose. Pediatric dosing is weight-based. Dose reduction is recommended for creatine clearance of 15–50 mL/min in AF, and use avoided in patients with creatinine clearance of <15 mL/min. Combined use of P-glycoprotein inhibitors and CYP3A inhibitors increases drug exposure; combined use of p-glycoprotein and CYP3A diminishes drug effect. **Apixaban** is approved for prevention of stroke in nonvalvular atrial fibrillation, for prevention of VTE following hip or knee surgery, and for treatment and long-term prevention of VTE. The dosage for atrial fibrillation is 5 mg twice daily; the dose for VTE is 10 mg twice a day for the first week, followed by 5 mg twice a day. The prophylactic dose for prevention of VTE following hip or knee surgery or long-term prevention of VTE following initial therapy is 2.5 mg twice a day. The recommended duration of therapy in hip and knee replacement is the same as for rivaroxaban. Combined use of P-glycoprotein inhibitors and CYP3A inhibitors increases drug exposure; combined use of p-glycoprotein and CYP3A diminishes drug effect. **Edoxaban** is approved for prevention of stroke in nonvalvular atrial fibrillation, and to treat VTE following treatment with heparin or LMWH for 5–10 days. The dose for atrial fibrillation and VTE treatment is 60 mg once daily. For patients with creatinine clearance of 15–50 mL/min, the dose is 30 mg once daily. Edoxaban is contraindicated in patients with atrial fibrillation and creatinine clearance >95 mL/min, due to the increased rate of ischemic stroke in this group compared with patients taking warfarin. **Betrixaban** is approved for prophylaxis of VTE. The recommended dosage is an initial single dose of 160 mg, followed by 80 mg once daily, taken at the same time each day with food (with dose reductions for severe renal impairment or concomitant P-glycoprotein inhibitor use). The recommended duration of treatment is 35 to 42 days.

Assessment of and Reversal of Anti-Xa Drug Effect

Measurement of anti-Xa drug effect is not needed in most situations but can be accomplished by anti-Xa assays calibrated for the drug in question. **Andexanet alfa** is a factor Xa "decoy" molecule without procoagulant activity that competes for binding to anti-Xa drugs. In clinical trials involving apixaban and rivaroxaban, andexanet given by IV infusion results in rapid decrease in anti-Xa effect. The drug was FDA-approved in 2018 for reversal of life-threatening bleeding in patients treated with apixaban or rivaroxaban. The dosing strategy takes into account the dose of apixaban or rivaroxaban used, and time since the last dose. Low dose is 400 mg IV at a rate of 30 mg/min, followed by 4 mg/min for up to 120 min; high dose is 800 mg bolus given at 30 mg/min followed by 8 mg/min for up to 120 minutes. Thrombotic complications have been reported, as well as cardiac arrest and sudden death. Four-factor concentrate may be considered as an alternative approach to life-threatening bleeding on anti-Xa drugs.

DIRECT THROMBIN INHIBITORS

The direct thrombin inhibitors (DTIs) exert their anticoagulant effect by directly binding to the active site of thrombin, thereby inhibiting thrombin's downstream effects. This is in contrast to indirect thrombin inhibitors such as heparin and LMW heparin (see above), which act through antithrombin. **Hirudin** and **bivalirudin** are large, bivalent DTIs that bind at the catalytic or active site of thrombin as well as at a substrate recognition site. **Argatroban** and **melagatran** are small molecules that bind only at the thrombin active site. One oral thrombin inhibitor **(dabigatran)** is available.

PARENTERAL DIRECT THROMBIN INHIBITORS

Leeches have been used for bloodletting since the age of Hippocrates. More recently, surgeons have used medicinal leeches (*Hirudo medicinalis*) to prevent thrombosis in the fine vessels of reattached digits. **Hirudin** is a specific, irreversible thrombin inhibitor from leech saliva that for a time was available in recombinant form as **lepirudin.** Its action is independent of antithrombin, which means it can reach and inactivate fibrin-bound thrombin in thrombi. Lepirudin has little effect on platelets or the bleeding time. Like heparin, it must be administered parenterally and is monitored by aPTT. Lepirudin was approved by the US Food and Drug Administration (FDA) for use in patients with thrombosis related to heparin-induced thrombocytopenia (HIT). Lepirudin is excreted by the kidney and should be used with great caution in patients with renal insufficiency as no antidote exists. Up to 40% of patients who receive long-term infusions develop an antibody directed against the thrombin-lepirudin complex. These antigen-antibody complexes are not cleared by the kidney and may result in an enhanced anticoagulant effect. Some patients re-exposed to the drug developed life-threatening anaphylactic reactions. Lepirudin production was discontinued by the manufacturer in 2012.

Bivalirudin, another bivalent inhibitor of thrombin, is administered intravenously, with a rapid onset and offset of action. The drug has a short half-life with clearance that is 20% renal and the remainder metabolic. Bivalirudin is FDA-approved for use in percutaneous coronary angioplasty and in patients with heparin-induced thrombocytopenia (HIT) who require coronary interventions.

Argatroban is a small molecule thrombin inhibitor that is FDA-approved for use in patients with HIT with or without thrombosis and coronary angioplasty in patients with HIT. It, too, has a short half-life, is given by continuous intravenous infusion, and is monitored by aPTT. Its clearance is not affected by renal disease but is dependent on liver function; dose reduction is required in patients with liver disease. Patients on argatroban will demonstrate elevated INRs, rendering the transition to warfarin challenging (ie, the INR will reflect contributions from both warfarin and argatroban). (INR is discussed in detail in the section on warfarin administration.) A nomogram is supplied by the manufacturer to assist in this transition.

ORAL DIRECT THROMBIN INHIBITOR

Advantages of oral direct thrombin inhibition include predictable pharmacokinetics and bioavailability, which allow for fixed dosing and predictable anticoagulant response and make routine coagulation monitoring unnecessary. Similar to the direct oral anti-Xa drugs described above, the rapid onset and offset of action of these agents allow for immediate anticoagulation.

Dabigatran etexilate mesylate is the only FDA-approved oral direct thrombin inhibitor. Dabigatran is approved for reduction in risk of stroke and systemic embolism with nonvalvular atrial fibrillation, treatment of VTE following 5–7 days of initial heparin or LMWH therapy, reduction of the risk of recurrent VTE, and VTE prophylaxis following hip or knee replacement surgery.

Pharmacology

Dabigatran and its metabolites are direct thrombin inhibitors. Following oral administration, dabigatran etexilate mesylate, a prodrug, is converted to dabigatran. The oral bioavailability is 3–7% in normal volunteers. The drug is a substrate for the P-glycoprotein efflux pump; P-glycoprotein inhibitors such as ketoconazole should be avoided in patients with impaired renal function. The half-life of the drug in normal volunteers is 12–17 hours. Renal impairment results in prolonged drug clearance.

Administration & Dosage

For prevention of stroke and systemic embolism in nonvalvular atrial fibrillation, the dosage is 150 mg twice daily for patients with creatinine clearance greater than 30 mL/min. For decreased creatinine clearance of 15–30 mL/min, the dosage is 75 mg twice daily. No monitoring is required.

Assessment of & Reversal of Antithrombin Drug Effect

As with any anticoagulant drug, the primary toxicity of dabigatran is bleeding. Dabigatran will prolong the PTT, thrombin time, and ecarin clotting time, which can be used to estimate drug effect if necessary. (The ecarin clotting time [ECT] is another clotting test based on the use of a protein isolated from viper venom.) **Idarucizumab** is a humanized monoclonal antibody Fab fragment that binds to dabigatran and reverses the anticoagulant effect. This reversing drug is approved for use in situations requiring emergent surgery or for life-threatening bleeding. The recommended dose is 5 g given intravenously. If bleeding recurs, a second dose may be given. The drug is primarily excreted by the kidneys. The half-life in patients with normal renal function is approximately 1 hour. As discussed above for reversing anti-Xa therapy, reversal of dabigatran exposes patients to the underlying thrombotic disease they are being treated for, and use should be restricted to those with life-threatening bleeding or surgery.

Summary of the Direct Oral Anticoagulant Drugs

The direct oral anticoagulant drugs have consistently shown equivalent antithrombotic efficacy and lower bleeding rates when compared with traditional warfarin therapy. In addition, these drugs offer the advantages of rapid therapeutic effect, no monitoring requirement, and fewer drug interactions in comparison with warfarin, which has a narrow therapeutic window, is affected by diet and many drugs, and requires monitoring for dosage optimization. However, the short half-life of the newer anticoagulants has the important consequence that patient noncompliance will quickly lead to loss of anticoagulant effect and risk of thromboembolism. Given the convenience of once- or twice-daily oral dosing, lack of a monitoring requirement, and fewer drug and dietary interactions documented thus far, the new direct oral anticoagulants represent a significant advance in the prevention and therapy of thrombotic disease.

■ BASIC PHARMACOLOGY OF THE FIBRINOLYTIC DRUGS

Fibrinolytic drugs rapidly lyse thrombi by catalyzing the formation of the serine protease **plasmin** from its precursor zymogen, plasminogen (see Figure 34–3). These drugs create a generalized lytic state when administered intravenously. Thus, both protective hemostatic thrombi and target thromboemboli are broken down. The Box: Thrombolytic Drugs for Acute Myocardial Infarction describes the use of these drugs in one major application.

Pharmacology

Streptokinase is a protein (but not an enzyme in itself) synthesized by streptococci that combines with the proactivator plasminogen. This enzymatic complex catalyzes the conversion of inactive plasminogen to active plasmin. **Urokinase** is a human enzyme synthesized by the kidney that directly converts plasminogen to active plasmin. Plasmin itself cannot be used because naturally occurring inhibitors (antiplasmins) in plasma prevent its effects. However, the absence of inhibitors for urokinase and the streptokinase-proactivator complex permits their use clinically. Plasmin formed inside a thrombus by these activators is protected from plasma antiplasmins; this allows it to lyse the thrombus from within.

Plasminogen can also be activated endogenously by **tissue plasminogen activators (t-PAs).** These activators preferentially activate plasminogen that is bound to fibrin, which (in theory) confines fibrinolysis to the formed thrombus and avoids systemic activation. Recombinant human t-PA is manufactured as **alteplase. Reteplase** is another recombinant human t-PA from which several amino acid sequences have been deleted, and it has a longer half-life. **Tenecteplase** is a genetically engineered form of t-PA that has increased fibrin-binding affinity and a longer half-life, and it can be given as a single intravenous bolus. Reteplase and tenecteplase are as effective as alteplase and have simpler dosing schemes because of their longer half-lives.

Indications & Dosage

Administration of fibrinolytic drugs by the intravenous route is indicated in cases of **pulmonary embolism with hemodynamic instability,** severe **deep venous thrombosis** such as the superior vena caval syndrome, and **ascending thrombophlebitis** of the iliofemoral vein with severe lower extremity edema. These drugs are also given intra-arterially, especially for peripheral vascular disease.

Thrombolytic therapy in the management of **acute myocardial infarction** requires careful patient selection, the use of a specific thrombolytic agent, and the benefit of adjuvant therapy. Streptokinase is administered by intravenous infusion of a loading dose of 250,000 units, followed by 100,000 units/h for 24–72 hours. Patients with antistreptococcal antibodies can develop fever, allergic reactions, and therapeutic resistance. Urokinase requires a loading dose of 300,000 units given over 10 minutes and a maintenance dose of 300,000 units/h for 12 hours. Alteplase (t-PA) is given as a 15-mg bolus followed by 0.75 mg/kg (up to 50 mg) over 30 minutes and then 0.5 mg/kg (up to 35 mg) over 60 minutes. Reteplase is given as two 10-unit bolus injections, the second administered 30 minutes after the first injection. Tenecteplase is given as a single intravenous bolus ranging from 30 to 50 mg depending on body weight. Alteplase has also been approved for use in acute ischemic stroke within 3 hours of symptom onset. In patients without hemorrhagic infarct or other contraindications, this therapy has been demonstrated to provide better outcomes in several randomized clinical trials. The recommended dose is 0.9 mg/kg, not to exceed 90 mg, with 10% given as a bolus and the remainder during a 1-hour infusion. Streptokinase has been associated with increased bleeding risk in acute ischemic stroke when given at a dose of 1.5 million units, and its use is not recommended in this setting.

■ BASIC PHARMACOLOGY OF ANTIPLATELET AGENTS

Platelet function is regulated by three categories of substances. The first group consists of agents generated outside the platelet that interact with platelet membrane receptors, eg, catecholamines, collagen, thrombin, and prostacyclin. The second category contains agents generated within the platelet that interact with membrane receptors, eg, ADP, prostaglandin D_2, prostaglandin E_2, and serotonin. A third group comprises agents generated within the platelet that act within the platelet, eg, prostaglandin endoperoxides and thromboxane A_2, the cyclic nucleotides cAMP and cGMP, and calcium ion. From this list of agents, several targets for platelet inhibitory drugs have been identified (see Figure 34–1): inhibition of prostaglandin synthesis (aspirin), inhibition of ADP-induced platelet aggregation (clopidogrel, prasugrel, ticlopidine), and blockade of glycoprotein IIb/IIIa (GP IIb/IIIa) receptors on platelets (abciximab, tirofiban, and eptifibatide). Dipyridamole and cilostazol are additional antiplatelet drugs.

ASPIRIN

The prostaglandin **thromboxane A_2** is an arachidonate product that causes platelets to change shape, release their granules, and aggregate (see Chapter 18). Drugs that antagonize this pathway interfere with platelet aggregation in vitro and prolong the bleeding time in vivo. Aspirin is the prototype of this class of drugs.

As described in Chapter 18, aspirin inhibits the synthesis of thromboxane A_2 by irreversible acetylation of the enzyme cyclooxygenase. Other salicylates and nonsteroidal anti-inflammatory drugs also inhibit cyclooxygenase but have a shorter duration of inhibitory action because they cannot acetylate cyclooxygenase; that is, their action is reversible.

In 2014, following a review of the available data, the FDA reversed course and concluded that aspirin for *primary* prophylaxis (patients without a history of myocardial infarction or stroke) was not supported by the available data but did carry significant bleeding risk. A 2019 recommendation by the American College of Cardiology and American Heart Association recommended low

Thrombolytic Drugs for Acute Myocardial Infarction

The paradigm shift in 1980 on the causation of acute myocardial infarction to acute coronary occlusion by a thrombus created the rationale for thrombolytic therapy of this common lethal disease. At that time—and for the first time—intravenous thrombolytic therapy for acute myocardial infarction in the European Cooperative Study Group trial was found to reduce mortality. Later studies, with thousands of patients in each trial, provided enough statistical power for the 20% reduction in mortality to be considered statistically significant. Although the standard of care in areas with adequate facilities and experience in percutaneous coronary intervention (PCI) now favors catheterization and placement of a stent, thrombolytic therapy is still very important where PCI is not readily available.

The proper selection of patients for thrombolytic therapy is critical. The diagnosis of acute myocardial infarction is made clinically and is confirmed by electrocardiography. Patients with ST-segment elevation and bundle branch block on electrocardiography have the best outcomes. All trials to date show the greatest benefit for thrombolytic therapy *when it is given early, within 6 hours* after symptomatic onset of acute myocardial infarction.

Thrombolytic drugs reduce the mortality of acute myocardial infarction. The early and appropriate use of any thrombolytic drug probably transcends possible advantages of a particular drug.

dose aspirin (75–100 mg/d) be considered for primary prevention in adults 40–70 years of age with high risk of atherosclerotic cardiovascular disease and no increased bleeding risk. In contrast, meta-analysis of many published trials of aspirin and other antiplatelet agents have demonstrated the utility of aspirin in the *secondary* prevention of vascular events among patients with a history of vascular events.

THIENOPYRIDINES: TICLOPIDINE, CLOPIDOGREL, & PRASUGREL

Ticlopidine, clopidogrel, and prasugrel reduce platelet aggregation by inhibiting the ADP pathway of platelets. These drugs irreversibly block the ADP $P2Y_{12}$ receptor on platelets. Unlike aspirin, these drugs have no effect on prostaglandin metabolism. Use of ticlopidine, clopidogrel, or prasugrel to prevent thrombosis is now considered standard practice in patients undergoing placement of a coronary stent. As the indications and adverse effects of these drugs are different, they will be considered individually.

Ticlopidine is approved for prevention of stroke in patients with a history of a transient ischemic attack (TIA) or thrombotic stroke, and in combination with aspirin for prevention of coronary stent thrombosis. Adverse effects of ticlopidine include nausea, dyspepsia, and diarrhea in up to 20% of patients, hemorrhage in 5%, and, most seriously, leukopenia in 1%. The leukopenia is detected by regular monitoring of the white blood cell count during the first 3 months of treatment. Development of thrombotic thrombocytopenic purpura has also been associated with the ingestion of ticlopidine. The dosage of ticlopidine is 250 mg twice daily orally. Because of the significant side effect profile, the use of ticlopidine for stroke prevention should be restricted to those who are intolerant of or have failed aspirin therapy. Dosages of ticlopidine less than 500 mg/d may be efficacious with fewer adverse effects.

Clopidogrel is approved for patients with unstable angina or non-ST-elevation acute myocardial infarction (NSTEMI) in combination with aspirin; for patients with ST-elevation myocardial infarction (STEMI); or recent myocardial infarction, stroke, or established peripheral arterial disease. For NSTEMI, the dosage is a 300-mg loading dose orally followed by 75 mg daily of clopidogrel, with a daily aspirin dosage of 75–325 mg. For patients with STEMI, the dosage is 75 mg daily of clopidogrel orally, in association with aspirin as above; and for recent myocardial infarction, stroke, or peripheral vascular disease, the dosage is 75 mg/d.

Clopidogrel has fewer adverse effects than ticlopidine and is rarely associated with neutropenia. Thrombotic thrombocytopenic purpura has been reported. Because of its superior adverse effect profile and dosing requirements, clopidogrel is frequently preferred over ticlopidine. The antithrombotic effects of clopidogrel are dose-dependent; within 5 hours after an oral loading dose of 300 mg, 80% of platelet activity will be inhibited. The maintenance dosage of clopidogrel is 75 mg/d, which achieves maximum platelet inhibition. The duration of the antiplatelet effect is 7–10 days. Clopidogrel is a prodrug that requires activation via the cytochrome P450 enzyme isoform CYP2C19. Depending on the single nucleotide polymorphism (SNP) inheritance pattern in CYP2C19, individuals may be poor metabolizers of clopidogrel, and these patients may be at increased risk of cardiovascular events due to inadequate drug effect. The FDA has recommended CYP2C19 genotyping to identify such patients and advises prescribers to consider alternative therapies in poor metabolizers (see Chapter 5). Drugs that impair CYP2C19 function, such as omeprazole, should be used with caution.

Prasugrel, similar to clopidogrel, is approved for patients with acute coronary syndromes. The drug is given orally as a 60-mg loading dose and then 10 mg/d in combination with aspirin as outlined for clopidogrel. The Trial to Assess Improvement in Therapeutic Outcomes by Optimizing Platelet Inhibition with Prasugrel (TRITON-TIMI38) compared prasugrel with clopidogrel in a randomized, double-blind trial with aspirin and other standard therapies managed with percutaneous coronary interventions. This trial showed a reduction in the primary composite cardiovascular endpoint (cardiovascular death, nonfatal stroke, or nonfatal myocardial infarction) for prasugrel in comparison with clopidogrel. However, the major and minor bleeding risk was increased with prasugrel. Prasugrel is contraindicated in patients with history of TIA or stroke because of increased bleeding risk. In contrast to clopidogrel, cytochrome P450 genotype status is not an important factor in prasugrel pharmacology.

Ticagrelor is a newer type of ADP inhibitor (cyclopentyl triazolopyrimidine) and is also approved for oral use in combination with aspirin in patients with acute coronary syndromes. **Cangrelor** is a *parenteral* P2Y$_{12}$ inhibitor approved for IV use in coronary interventions in patients without previous ADP P2Y$_{12}$ inhibitor therapy.

Vorapaxar is a platelet protease receptor 1 (PAR-1) antagonist indicated for reduction of recurrent events in patients with history of MI or peripheral arterial disease. Vorapaxar has a long half-life with 50% inhibition of platelet aggregation remaining 1 month after cessation of therapy. Dosing is 2.08 mg orally daily. Peak concentrations occur 1–2 hours following a 2.08 mg dose.

Aspirin & Clopidogrel Resistance

The reported incidence of resistance to these drugs varies greatly, from less than 5% to 75%. In part this variation reflects the definition of resistance (recurrent thrombosis while on antiplatelet therapy versus in vitro testing), methods by which drug response is measured, and patient compliance. Several methods for testing aspirin and clopidogrel resistance in vitro are now FDA-approved. However, the measures of drug resistance vary considerably by testing method. These tests may be useful in selected patients to assess compliance or identify patients at increased risk of recurrent thrombotic events. However, their utility in routine clinical decision making outside of clinical trials remains controversial. A randomized prospective trial found no benefit over standard therapy when information obtained from monitoring antiplatelet drug effect was used to alter therapy.

BLOCKADE OF PLATELET GLYCOPROTEIN IIB/IIIa RECEPTORS

The platelet GP IIb/IIIa (integrin $\alpha_{IIb}\beta_{III}$) receptor functions as a receptor mainly for fibrinogen and vitronectin but also for fibronectin and von Willebrand factor. Activation of this receptor complex is the final common pathway for platelet aggregation. Ligands for GP IIb/IIIa contain an Arg-Gly-Asp (RGD) sequence motif important for ligand binding, and thus RGD constitutes a therapeutic target. There are approximately 50,000 copies of this complex on the surface of each platelet. Persons lacking this receptor have a bleeding disorder, Glanzmann's thrombasthenia.

The GP IIb/IIIa antagonists are used in patients with acute coronary syndromes. These drugs target the platelet GP IIb/IIIa receptor complex shown in Figure 34–1. **Abciximab**, a chimeric monoclonal antibody that binds to and blocks the IIb/IIIa and vitronectin (integrin $\alpha_v\beta_{III}$) receptors in a non-RGD-dependent manner, was the first agent approved in this class of drugs. It has been approved for use in percutaneous coronary interventions in combination with aspirin and heparin. **Eptifibatide** is a cyclic peptide derived from rattlesnake venom that contains a variation of the RGD motif (KGD) and is approved for use in acute coronary syndromes and percutaneous interventions in combination with aspirin and heparin. **Tirofiban** is a peptidomimetic inhibitor with the RGD sequence motif approved for use in non-ST-elevation acute coronary syndromes. Eptifibatide and tirofiban inhibit ligand binding to the IIb/IIIa receptor by their occupancy of the receptor but do not block the vitronectin receptor. Because of their short half-lives, they must be given by continuous infusion.

ADDITIONAL ANTIPLATELET-DIRECTED DRUGS

Dipyridamole is a vasodilator that also inhibits platelet function by inhibiting adenosine uptake and cGMP phosphodiesterase activity. Dipyridamole by itself has little or no beneficial effect. Therefore, therapeutic use of this agent is primarily in combination with aspirin to prevent cerebrovascular ischemia. It may also be used in combination with warfarin for primary prophylaxis of thromboemboli in patients with prosthetic heart valves. A combination of dipyridamole complexed with 25 mg of aspirin is now available for secondary prophylaxis of cerebrovascular disease.

Cilostazol is a phosphodiesterase inhibitor that promotes vasodilation and inhibition of platelet aggregation. Cilostazol is used primarily to treat intermittent claudication.

■ CLINICAL PHARMACOLOGY OF DRUGS USED TO PREVENT CLOTTING

VENOUS THROMBOSIS

Risk Factors

A. Inherited Disorders

The inherited disorders characterized by a tendency to form thrombi (thrombophilia) derive from either quantitative or qualitative abnormalities of the natural anticoagulant system. Deficiencies (loss of function mutations) in the natural anticoagulants antithrombin, protein C, and protein S account for approximately 15% of selected patients with juvenile or recurrent thrombosis and 5–10% of unselected cases of acute venous thrombosis. Additional causes of thrombophilia include gain of function mutations such as the factor V Leiden mutation and the prothrombin 20210 mutation, elevated clotting factor and cofactor levels, and hyperhomocysteinemia that together account for the greater number of hypercoagulable patients. Although loss of function mutations are less common, they are associated with the greatest thrombosis risk. Some patients have multiple inherited risk factors or combinations of inherited and acquired risk factors as discussed below. These individuals are at higher risk for recurrent thrombotic events and are often considered candidates for lifelong therapy.

B. Acquired Disease

The increased risk of thromboembolism associated with atrial fibrillation and with the placement of mechanical heart valves has long been recognized. Similarly, prolonged bed rest, high-risk surgical procedures, and the presence of cancer are clearly associated with an increased incidence of deep venous thrombosis and embolism. Antiphospholipid antibody syndrome is another important acquired risk factor. Drugs may function as synergistic risk factors in concert with inherited risk factors. For example, women who have the factor V Leiden mutation and take oral contraceptives have a synergistic increase in risk.

Antithrombotic Management

A. Prevention

Primary prevention of venous thrombosis reduces the incidence of and mortality rate from pulmonary emboli. Heparin and warfarin may be used to prevent venous thrombosis. Subcutaneous administration of low-dose unfractionated heparin, LMW heparin, or fondaparinux provides effective prophylaxis. Warfarin is also effective but requires laboratory monitoring of the prothrombin time.

B. Treatment of Established Disease

Treatment for established venous thrombosis may be initiated with direct oral anticoagulants alone. Alternatively, patients may be treated with unfractionated or LMW heparin for the first 5–7 days, with an overlap with warfarin. Once therapeutic effects of warfarin have been established, therapy with warfarin is continued for 6 weeks to 6 months or longer, depending on the clinical presentation of the patient. In general, patients who have a provoked event (eg, VTE in the postoperative setting with no other risk factors) would be treated on the shorter end of the spectrum, whereas an individual with recurrent VTE or multiple risk factors might be treated indefinitely. Superficial thrombi confined to the calf veins respond well to short courses of LMW heparin.

Warfarin readily crosses the placenta. It can cause hemorrhage at any time during pregnancy as well as developmental defects in the fetus when administered during the first trimester. Therefore, venous thromboembolic disease in pregnant women is generally treated with heparin, best administered by subcutaneous injection.

ARTERIAL THROMBOSIS

Activation of platelets is considered an essential process for arterial thrombosis. Thus, treatment with platelet-inhibiting drugs such as aspirin and clopidogrel or ticlopidine is indicated in patients with TIAs and strokes or unstable angina and acute myocardial infarction. As discussed above, prasugrel and ticagrelor are alternatives to clopidogrel for patients with acute coronary syndromes managed with percutaneous coronary interventions. In angina and infarction, these drugs are often used in conjunction with β blockers, calcium channel blockers, and fibrinolytic drugs.

■ DRUGS USED IN BLEEDING DISORDERS

VITAMIN K

Vitamin K confers biologic activity upon prothrombin and factors VII, IX, and X by participating in their postribosomal modification. Vitamin K is a fat-soluble substance found primarily in leafy green vegetables. The dietary requirement is low because the vitamin is additionally synthesized by bacteria that colonize the human intestine. Two natural forms exist: vitamins K_1 and K_2. Vitamin K_1 (phytonadione; see Figure 34–5) is found in food. Vitamin K_2 (menaquinone) is found in human tissues and is synthesized by intestinal bacteria.

Vitamins K_1 and K_2 require bile salts for absorption from the intestinal tract. Vitamin K_1 is available clinically in oral and parenteral forms. Onset of effect is delayed for 6 hours but the effect is complete by 24 hours when treating depression of prothrombin activity caused by excess warfarin or vitamin K deficiency. Intravenous administration of vitamin K_1 should be slow, as rapid infusion can produce dyspnea, chest and back pain, and even death. Vitamin K repletion is best achieved with intravenous or oral administration because its bioavailability after subcutaneous administration is erratic. Vitamin K_1 is currently administered to all newborns to prevent the hemorrhagic disease of vitamin K deficiency, which is especially common in premature infants.

The water-soluble salt of vitamin K_3 (menadione) should never be used in therapeutics. It is particularly ineffective in the treatment of warfarin overdosage. Vitamin K deficiency frequently occurs in hospitalized patients in intensive care units because of poor diet, parenteral nutrition, recent surgery, multiple antibiotic therapy, and uremia. Severe hepatic failure results in diminished protein synthesis and a hemorrhagic diathesis that is unresponsive to vitamin K.

PLASMA FRACTIONS

Sources & Preparations

Deficiencies in plasma coagulation factors can cause bleeding (Table 34–3). Spontaneous bleeding occurs when factor activity is less than 5–10% of normal. Factor VIII deficiency (**classic hemophilia,** or **hemophilia A**) and factor IX deficiency (**Christmas disease,** or **hemophilia B**) account for most of the heritable coagulation defects. Concentrated plasma fractions and recombinant protein preparations are available for the treatment of these deficiencies. Administration of plasma-derived, heat- or detergent-treated factor concentrates and recombinant factor concentrates are the standard treatments for prevention and treatment of bleeding associated with hemophilia. Lyophilized factor VIII concentrates are prepared from large pools of plasma. Transmission of viral diseases such as hepatitis B and C and HIV is reduced or eliminated by pasteurization and by extraction of plasma with solvents and detergents. However, this treatment does not remove other potential causes of transmissible diseases such as prions. For this reason, recombinant clotting factor preparations are recommended whenever possible for factor replacement. The best use of these therapeutic materials requires diagnostic specificity of the deficient factor and quantitation of its activity in plasma. Recently, several longer-acting factor VIII and IX preparations have been developed. **Eloctate** is a factor VIII-Fc domain conjugate that prolongs the factor VIII half-life and allows twice-weekly dosing in many cases. **Idelvion** is a factor IX-albumin conjugate with a half-life of 100 hours (native factor IX has a half-life of 16 hours) and is FDA-approved for prophylaxis or treatment of bleeding in hemophilia B patients, offering the possibility of once-weekly dosing in the case of Idelvion. Intermediate purity

TABLE 34–3 Therapeutic products for the treatment of coagulation disorders.[1]

Factor	Deficiency State	Hemostatic Levels	Half-Life of Infused Factor	Replacement Source
I	Hypofibrinogenemia	1 g/dL	4 days	Cryoprecipitate, FFP
II	Prothrombin deficiency	30–40%	3 days	Prothrombin complex concentrates (intermediate purity factor IX concentrates)
V	Factor V deficiency	20%	1 day	FFP
VII	Factor VII deficiency	30%	4–6 hours	FFP
				Prothrombin complex concentrates (intermediate purity factor IX concentrates), Recombinant factor VIIa
VIII	Hemophilia A	30–50%	12 hours	Recombinant factor VIII products
		100% for major bleeding or trauma		Plasma-derived high purity concentrates
				Cryoprecipitate[2]
				Some patients with mild deficiency will respond to DDAVP
IX	Hemophilia B	30–50%	24 hours	Recombinant factor IX products
	Christmas disease	100% for major bleeding or trauma		Plasma-derived high purity concentrates
X	Stuart-Prower defect	25%	36 hours	FFP
				Prothrombin complex concentrates
XI	Hemophilia C	30–50%	3 days	FFP
XII	Hageman defect	Not required		Treatment not necessary
von Willebrand	von Willebrand disease	30%	Approximately 10 hours	Intermediate purity factor VIII concentrates that contain von Willebrand factor
				Type I patients respond to DDAVP
				Cryoprecipitate[2]
XIII	Factor XIII deficiency	5%	6 days	FFP
				Cryoprecipitate

FFP, fresh frozen plasma; DDAVP, 1-deamino-8-D-arginine vasopressin.

[1]For warfarin overdose or coumarin rodenticide poisoning, a four-factor concentrate (II, VII, IX, X) is available. Antithrombin concentrates are available for patients with thrombosis in the setting of antithrombin deficiency. Activated protein C concentrates were approved for treatment of sepsis but withdrawn from the market in 2011 following publication of a study demonstrating no benefit in sepsis and increased bleeding risk.

[2]Cryoprecipitate should be used to treat bleeding in the setting of factor VIII deficiency and von Willebrand disease only in an emergency in which pathogen-inactivated products are not available.

factor VIII concentrates (as opposed to recombinant or high purity concentrates) contain significant amounts of von Willebrand factor. **Humate-P** is a factor VIII concentrate that is approved by the FDA for the treatment of bleeding associated with von Willebrand disease. **Vonicog alfa** is a recombinant von Willebrand factor product approved for treatment and control of bleeding in adults with von Willebrand disease. Fresh frozen plasma is used for factor deficiencies for which no recombinant form of the protein is available. A four-factor plasma replacement preparation containing vitamin K–dependent factors II, VII, IX, and X (**4F PCC,** Kcentra) is available for rapid reversal of warfarin in bleeding patients.

Clinical Uses

Hemophilia A and B patients are given factor VIII and IX replacement, respectively, as prophylaxis to prevent bleeding, and in higher doses to treat bleeding events or to prepare for surgery.

Desmopressin acetate increases the factor VIII activity of patients with mild hemophilia A or von Willebrand disease. It can be used in preparation for minor surgery such as tooth extraction without any requirement for infusion of clotting factors if the patient has a documented adequate response. High-dose intranasal desmopressin (see Chapter 37) is available and has been shown to be efficacious and well tolerated by patients.

Freeze-dried concentrates of plasma containing prothrombin, factors IX and X, and varied amounts of factor VII (Proplex, etc) are commercially available for treating deficiencies of these factors (see Table 34–3). Each unit of factor IX per kilogram of body weight raises its activity in plasma 1.5%. Heparin is often added to inhibit coagulation factors activated by the manufacturing process. However, addition of heparin does not eliminate all thromboembolic risk.

Some preparations of factor IX concentrate contain *activated* clotting factors, which has led to their use in treating patients with inhibitors or antibodies to factor VIII or factor IX. Two products are available expressly for this purpose: **Autoplex** (with factor VIII correctional activity) and **FEIBA** (**F**actor **E**ight **I**nhibitor **B**ypass **A**ctivity). These products are not uniformly successful in arresting hemorrhage, and the factor IX inhibitor titers often rise after treatment with them. Acquired inhibitors of coagulation factors may also be treated with porcine factor VIII (for factor VIII inhibitors) and recombinant activated factor VII. Recombinant activated factor VII **(NovoSeven)** increasingly is being used to treat coagulopathy associated with liver disease and major blood loss in trauma and surgery. These recombinant and plasma-derived factor concentrates are very expensive, and the indications for them are very precise. Therefore, close consultation with a hematologist knowledgeable in this area is essential.

Cryoprecipitate is a plasma protein fraction obtainable from whole blood. It is used to treat deficiencies or qualitative abnormalities of fibrinogen, such as that which occurs with disseminated intravascular coagulation and liver disease. A single unit of cryoprecipitate contains 300 mg of fibrinogen.

Cryoprecipitate may also be used for patients with factor VIII deficiency and von Willebrand disease if desmopressin is not indicated and a pathogen-inactivated, recombinant, or plasma-derived product is not available. The concentration of factor VIII and von Willebrand factor in cryoprecipitate is not as great as that found in the concentrated plasma fractions. Moreover, cryoprecipitate is not treated in any manner to decrease the risk of viral exposure. For infusion, the frozen cryoprecipitate unit is thawed and dissolved in a small volume of sterile citrate-saline solution and pooled with other units. Rh-negative women with potential for childbearing should receive only Rh-negative cryoprecipitate because of possible contamination of the product with Rh-positive blood cells.

RECOMBINANT FACTOR VIIa

Recombinant factor VIIa is approved for treatment of inherited or acquired hemophilia A or B with inhibitors, treatment of bleeding associated with invasive procedures in congenital or acquired hemophilia, or factor VII deficiency. In the European Union, the drug is also approved for treatment of Glanzmann thrombasthenia.

Factor VIIa initiates activation of the clotting pathway by activating factor IX and factor X in association with tissue factor (see Figure 34–2). The drug is given by bolus injection. For hemophilia A or B with inhibitors and bleeding, the dosage is 90 mg/kg every 2 hours until hemostasis is achieved, and then continued at 3- to 6-hour intervals until stable. For congenital factor VII deficiency, the recommended dosage is 15–30 mg/kg every 4–6 hours until hemostasis is achieved.

Factor VIIa has been widely used for off-label indications, including bleeding with trauma, surgery, intracerebral hemorrhage, and warfarin toxicity. A major concern of off-label use has been the possibility that thrombotic events may be increased. A recent study examined rates of thromboembolic events in 35 placebo-controlled trials where factor VIIa was administered for nonapproved indications. This study found an increase in arterial, but not venous, thrombotic events, particularly among elderly individuals.

ORPHAN DRUGS FOR TREATMENT OF RARE HEREDITARY COAGULATION DISORDERS

Orphan drug status is a designation given by the FDA to promote development of therapies for rare disorders (see Chapter 1).

Factor XIII is a transaminase that crosslinks fibrin within a clot, thereby stabilizing it. Congenital factor XIII deficiency is a rare bleeding disorder. **Recombinant factor XIII A-subunit** is FDA-approved for prevention of bleeding in patients with factor XIII deficiency.

Factor X concentrate is a plasma-derived factor X preparation that is FDA-approved for control of bleeding in patients with factor X deficiency and for perioperative management of patients with mild factor X deficiency.

Protein C concentrate is a plasma-derived protein C preparation approved for treatment of life-threatening thrombosis or purpura fulminans, a life-threatening disorder involving thrombosis in skin and systemic circulation.

Recombinant antithrombin is FDA-approved for prevention of perioperative and peripartum thromboembolic events in patients with hereditary antithrombin deficiency.

Emicizumab is a novel bispecific monoclonal antibody to factor IXa and factor X that replaces the function of factor VIII. Clinical studies have shown a dramatic reduction in bleeding events in hemophilia patients with or without Factor VIII inhibitors. The drug is FDA-approved to prevent or reduce the frequency of bleeding episodes in adult and pediatric patients with hemophilia A (congenital factor VIII deficiency) with or without factor VIII inhibitors. The dose is 3 mg/kg subcutaneously daily for 1 week (loading dose), followed by 1.5 mg/kg every week, 3 mg/kg biweekly or 6 mg/kg monthly. The bioavailability is 80–90% after subcutaneous injection, and the half-life is approximately 27 days. Thrombosis has been reported in patients also receiving prothrombin complex concentrates. Emicizumab will interfere with standard PTT and PTT-based factor assays. Chromogenic factor VIII assays using bovine components are available to assess endogenous factor VIII levels in patient treated with emicizumab.

FIBRINOLYTIC INHIBITORS: AMINOCAPROIC ACID

Aminocaproic acid (EACA), which is chemically similar to the amino acid lysine, is a synthetic inhibitor of fibrinolysis. It competitively inhibits plasminogen activation (see Figure 34–3). It is rapidly absorbed orally and is cleared from the body by the kidney. The usual oral dosage of EACA is 6 g four times a day. When the drug is administered intravenously, a 5-g loading dose should be infused over 30 minutes to avoid hypotension. **Tranexamic acid** is an analog of aminocaproic acid and has the same properties. It is administered orally with a 15-mg/kg loading dose followed by 30 mg/kg every 6 hours.

Clinical uses of EACA are as adjunctive therapy in hemophilia, as therapy for bleeding from fibrinolytic therapy, and as prophylaxis for rebleeding from intracranial aneurysms. Treatment success has also been reported in patients with postsurgical gastrointestinal bleeding and postprostatectomy bleeding and bladder hemorrhage secondary to radiation- and drug-induced cystitis. Adverse effects of the drug include intravascular thrombosis from inhibition of plasminogen activator, hypotension, myopathy, abdominal discomfort, diarrhea, and nasal stuffiness. The drug should not be used in patients with disseminated intravascular coagulation or genitourinary bleeding of the upper tract, eg, kidney and ureters, because of the potential for excessive clotting.

DRUGS REMOVED FROM MARKET FOR LACK OF EFFICACY OR SAFETY: APROTININ & ACTIVATED PROTEIN C

Aprotinin is a serine protease inhibitor (serpin) that inhibits fibrinolysis by free plasmin and may have other antihemorrhagic effects as well. It also inhibits the plasmin-streptokinase complex in patients who have received that thrombolytic agent. Aprotinin was shown to reduce bleeding—by as much as 50%—from many types of surgery, especially that involving extracorporeal circulation for open-heart procedures and liver transplantation. However, clinical trials and internal data from the manufacturer suggested that use of the drug was associated with an increased risk of renal failure, heart attack, and stroke. A prospective trial was initiated in Canada but halted early because of concerns that use of the drug was associated with increased mortality. The drug was removed from the market in 2007.

Drotrecogin alfa is a recombinant form of activated protein C that was initially approved by the FDA in 2001 for reduction of mortality in adults with sepsis associated with acute organ dysfunction and high mortality. The drug was voluntarily withdrawn from the market in 2011 after a follow-up study showed no survival benefit in sepsis.

PREPARATIONS AVAILABLE

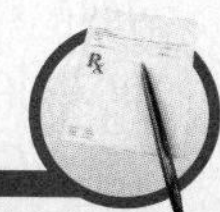

GENERIC NAME	AVAILABLE AS
Abciximab	ReoPro
Alteplase recombinant [t-PA]	Activase
Aminocaproic acid	Generic, Amicar
Anisindione	Miradon (outside the USA)
Antihemophilic factor [factor VIII, AHF]	Alphanate, Bioclate, Helixate, Hemofil M, Koate-HP, Kogenate, Monoclate, Recombinate, others
Anti-inhibitor coagulant complex	Autoplex T, Feiba VH Immuno
Antithrombin III	ATryn, Thrombate III
Apixaban	Eliquis
Argatroban	Generic
Betrixaban	Bevyxxa
Bivalirudin	Generic, Angiomax
Cilostazol	Generic, Pletal
Clopidogrel	Generic, Plavix
Coagulation factor VIIa recombinant	NovoSeven
Dabigatran	Pradaxa
Dalteparin	Fragmin
Danaparoid	Orgaran
Desirudin	Iprivask
Dipyridamole	Generic, Persantine
Edoxaban	Sayvasa
Emicizumab	Hemlibra
Enoxaparin (low-molecular-weight heparin)	Generic, Lovenox
Eptifibatide	Integrilin
Factor VIIa: see Coagulation factor VIIa recombinant	
Factor VIII: see Antihemophilic factor	
Factor IX complex, human	AlphaNine SD, Bebulin VH, BeneFix, Konyne 80, Mononine, Profilnine SD, Proplex T, Proplex SX-T
Factor X complex, human	Coagadex
Four-factor prothrombin complex concentrate (II, VII, IX, X)	Kcentra
Fondaparinux	Generic, Arixtra
Heparin sodium	Generic, Liquaemin
Prasugrel	Effient
Protamine	Generic
Reteplase	Retavase
Rivaroxaban	Xarelto
Streptokinase	Streptase
Tenecteplase	TNKase
Ticlopidine	Generic, Ticlid
Tinzaparin	Innohep
Tirofiban	Aggrastat
Tranexamic acid	Generic, Cyklokapron, Lysteda
Urokinase	Abbokinase, Kinlytic
Vitamin K	Generic, various
Vorapaxar	Zontivity
Warfarin	Generic, Coumadin

REFERENCES

Direct Oral Anticoagulants

Li A, Lopes RD, Garcia DA: Use of direct oral anticoagulants in special populations. Hematol Oncol Clin North Am 2016;30:1053.

Samuelson BT, Cuker A: Measurement and reversal of the direct oral anticoagulants. Blood Rev 2016;31:77.

Yasuda S et al: Antithrombotic therapy for atrial fibrillation with stable coronary disease. N Engl J Med 2019;381:1103.

Blood Coagulation & Bleeding Disorders

Callaghan MU, Sidonio R, Pipe SW: Novel therapeutics for hemophilia and other bleeding disorders. Blood 2018;132:23.

Drugs Used in Thrombotic Disorder

Arnett DK et al: 2019 ACC/AHA Guideline on the Primary Prevention of Cardiovascular Disease: A Report of the American College of Cardiology/American Heart Association Task Force on Clinical Practice Guidelines. Circulation 2019;140:e596.

Kearon C et al: Antithrombotic therapy for VTE disease: Chest guideline and expert panel report. Chest 2016;149:315.

CASE STUDY ANSWER

This patient has pulmonary embolism secondary to a deep venous thrombosis. Options for treating this patient include unfractionated heparin or low-molecular-weight heparin followed by warfarin, with INR goal of 2–3; parenteral anticoagulation for 5–7 days followed by edoxaban or dabigatran; or rivaroxaban, apixaban, or edoxaban alone without monitoring. As this situation can be considered a provoked event given the history of oral contraceptive use, the recommended duration of therapy would be 3–6 months depending on individual risk factors and preferences. The patient should be counseled to use an alternative form of contraception.

CHAPTER

35

Agents Used in Dyslipidemia

Mary J. Malloy, MD, & John P. Kane, MD, PhD

CASE STUDY

A 52-year-old woman was told at age 19 that her "cholesterol" was elevated. Diet and exercise were advised, but she had gained weight, she did no regular exercise, and her diet was high in fat and simple CHO. At her first visit, her direct LDL was 155 mg/dL, triglycerides 458, and HDL 40. Her Lp(a) was not elevated. BMI 30, A1c 6.4, free T4 normal, and ALT about twice the normal. She had no symptoms of coronary or peripheral vascular disease, but a coronary calcium score was greater than zero. Physical examination was normal aside from her obesity that was mostly abdominal. Specific dietary and exercise advice were given. Her mother has T2D and is overweight. Her father survived an MI at age 47. He had no apparent risk factors other than "high cholesterol." Both parents take a statin. At the end of the visit, 20 mg of rosuvastatin and marine omega 3 fatty acids were prescribed. The patient returned after 3 months. She had lost 6 pounds, was fully compliant with diet, and was gradually increasing her exercise. Her LDL was 97, triglycerides 340, HDL 45, A1c 5.8, and ALT unchanged. How would you manage this patient?

Plasma lipids are transported in complexes called **lipoproteins.** Metabolic disorders that involve elevations in any lipoprotein species are termed **hyperlipoproteinemia** or **hyperlipidemia. Hyperlipemia** denotes increased levels of triglycerides.

The major clinical sequelae of hyperlipidemia are acute pancreatitis and atherosclerosis. The former occurs in patients with marked hyperlipemia. Control of triglycerides can prevent recurrent attacks of this life-threatening disease.

Atherosclerosis is the leading cause of death for both genders in the USA and other Western countries. Lipoproteins that contain **apolipoprotein (apo) B-100** convey lipids into the artery wall. These are **low-density (LDL), intermediate-density (IDL), very-low-density (VLDL),** and **lipoprotein(a) (Lp[a]).** Remnant lipoproteins formed during the catabolism of chylomicrons that contain the B-48 protein (apo B-48) can also enter the artery wall, contributing to atherosclerosis.

Cellular components in atherosclerotic plaques (atheromas) include foam cells, which are transformed macrophages, and smooth muscle cells filled with **cholesteryl esters.** These cellular alterations result from endocytosis of modified lipoproteins via at least four species of **scavenger receptors.** Chemical modifications of lipoproteins by free radicals create ligands for these receptors. The atheroma grows with the accumulation of foam cells, collagen, fibrin, and calcium. Whereas such lesions can slowly occlude coronary vessels, clinical symptoms are more frequently precipitated by rupture of unstable atheromatous plaques, leading to activation of platelets and formation of occlusive thrombi.

Although treatment of hyperlipidemia can cause slow physical regression of plaques, the well-documented reduction in acute coronary events that follows vigorous lipid-lowering treatment is attributable chiefly to mitigation of the inflammatory activity of macrophages and is evident within 2–3 months after starting therapy.

High-density lipoproteins (HDL) exert several *anti*atherogenic effects. They participate in retrieval of cholesterol from the artery wall and inhibit the oxidation of atherogenic lipoproteins. Low levels of HDL (hypoalphalipoproteinemia) are associated with atherosclerotic disease and thus are a potential target for intervention.

Cigarette smoking is a major risk factor for coronary disease. It is associated with reduced levels of HDL, impairment of cholesterol retrieval, cytotoxic effects on the endothelium, increased oxidation of lipoproteins, and stimulation of thrombogenesis. Diabetes, also a major risk factor, is another source of oxidative stress. Hypertension contributes significantly to atherosclerotic vascular disease.

Normal coronary arteries can dilate in response to ischemia, increasing delivery of oxygen to the myocardium. This process is mediated by nitric oxide, acting on smooth muscle cells of the arterial media. The release of nitric oxide from the vascular endothelium is impaired by atherogenic lipoproteins, thus aggravating ischemia. Reducing levels of atherogenic lipoproteins and inhibiting their oxidation restores endothelial function.

Because atherogenesis, a dynamic process, is multifactorial, therapy should be directed toward all modifiable risk factors. Quantitative angiographic trials have demonstrated net regression of plaques during aggressive lipid-lowering therapy. Primary and secondary prevention trials have shown significant reduction in mortality from new coronary events and in all-cause mortality.

■ PATHOPHYSIOLOGY OF HYPERLIPOPROTEINEMIA

NORMAL LIPOPROTEIN METABOLISM

Structure

Lipoproteins have hydrophobic core regions containing cholesteryl esters and triglycerides surrounded by unesterified cholesterol, phospholipids, and apoproteins. Certain lipoproteins contain very high-molecular-weight B proteins that exist in two forms: **B-48,** formed in the intestine and found in chylomicrons and their remnants; and **B-100,** synthesized in liver and found in **VLDL, VLDL remnants (IDL), LDL** (formed from VLDL), and **Lp(a) lipoproteins.** HDL consist of at least 20 discrete molecular species containing apolipoprotein A-I (apo A-I). About 100 other proteins are known to be distributed variously among the HDL species, exhibiting antioxidant, antimicrobial, anti-inflammatory, and molecular signaling activities. They also transport microRNAs. Twelve HDL species are recognized in the ovary and six in cerebrospinal fluid.

ACRONYMS

Apo	Apolipoprotein
CETP	Cholesteryl ester transfer protein
CK	Creatine kinase
HDL	High-density lipoproteins
HMG-CoA	3-Hydroxy-3-methylglutaryl-coenzyme A
IDL	Intermediate-density lipoproteins
LCAT	Lecithin:cholesterol acyltransferase
LDL	Low-density lipoproteins
Lp(a)	Lipoprotein(a)
LPL	Lipoprotein lipase
PCSK9	Proprotein convertase subtilisin/kexin type 9
PPAR	Peroxisome proliferator-activated receptor
VLDL	Very-low-density lipoproteins

Synthesis & Catabolism

A. Chylomicrons

Chylomicrons are formed in the intestine and carry **triglycerides** of dietary origin, **unesterified cholesterol,** and **cholesteryl esters.** They transit the thoracic duct to the bloodstream.

Triglycerides are removed from the chylomicrons in extrahepatic tissues through a pathway shared with VLDL that involves hydrolysis by the **lipoprotein lipase (LPL)** system. Decrease in particle diameter occurs as triglycerides are depleted. Surface lipids and small apoproteins are transferred to HDL. The resultant chylomicron remnants are taken up by receptor-mediated endocytosis into hepatocytes.

B. Very-Low-Density Lipoproteins

VLDL are secreted by liver and export triglycerides to peripheral tissues (Figure 35–1). VLDL triglycerides are hydrolyzed by LPL, yielding free fatty acids for storage in adipose tissue and for oxidation in tissues such as cardiac and skeletal muscle. Depletion of triglycerides produces remnants (IDL), some of which undergo endocytosis directly into hepatocytes. The remainder are converted to LDL by further removal of triglycerides mediated by hepatic lipase. This process explains the "beta shift" phenomenon, the increase of LDL (beta-lipoprotein) in serum as hypertriglyceridemia subsides. Increased levels of LDL can also result from increased secretion of VLDL and from decreased LDL catabolism.

C. Low-Density Lipoproteins

LDL are catabolized chiefly in hepatocytes and other cells after receptor-mediated endocytosis. Cholesteryl esters from LDL are hydrolyzed, yielding free cholesterol for the synthesis of cell membranes. Cells also obtain cholesterol by synthesis via a pathway involving the formation of mevalonic acid by HMG-CoA reductase. Production of this enzyme and of LDL receptors is transcriptionally regulated by the content of cholesterol in the cell. Normally, about 70% of LDL is removed from plasma by hepatocytes. Even more cholesterol is delivered to the liver via IDL and chylomicrons. Unlike other cells, hepatocytes can eliminate cholesterol by secretion in bile and by conversion to bile acids.

D. Lp(a) Lipoprotein

Lp(a) is formed from LDL and the (a) protein, linked by a disulfide bridge. The (a) protein is highly homologous with plasminogen but is not activated by tissue plasminogen activator. It occurs in a number of isoforms of different molecular weights. Levels of Lp(a) vary from nil to over 2000 nM/L and are determined chiefly by genetic factors. Lp(a) is found in atherosclerotic plaques and also contributes to coronary disease by inhibiting thrombolysis. It is associated with aortic stenosis. Levels are elevated in certain inflammatory states. The risk of coronary disease is strongly related to the level of Lp(a) and is partially mitigated by aspirin. A common variant (14399M) in the coding region is associated with elevated levels.

E. High-Density Lipoproteins

The apoproteins of HDL are secreted largely by the liver and intestine. Much of the lipid comes from the surface monolayers of

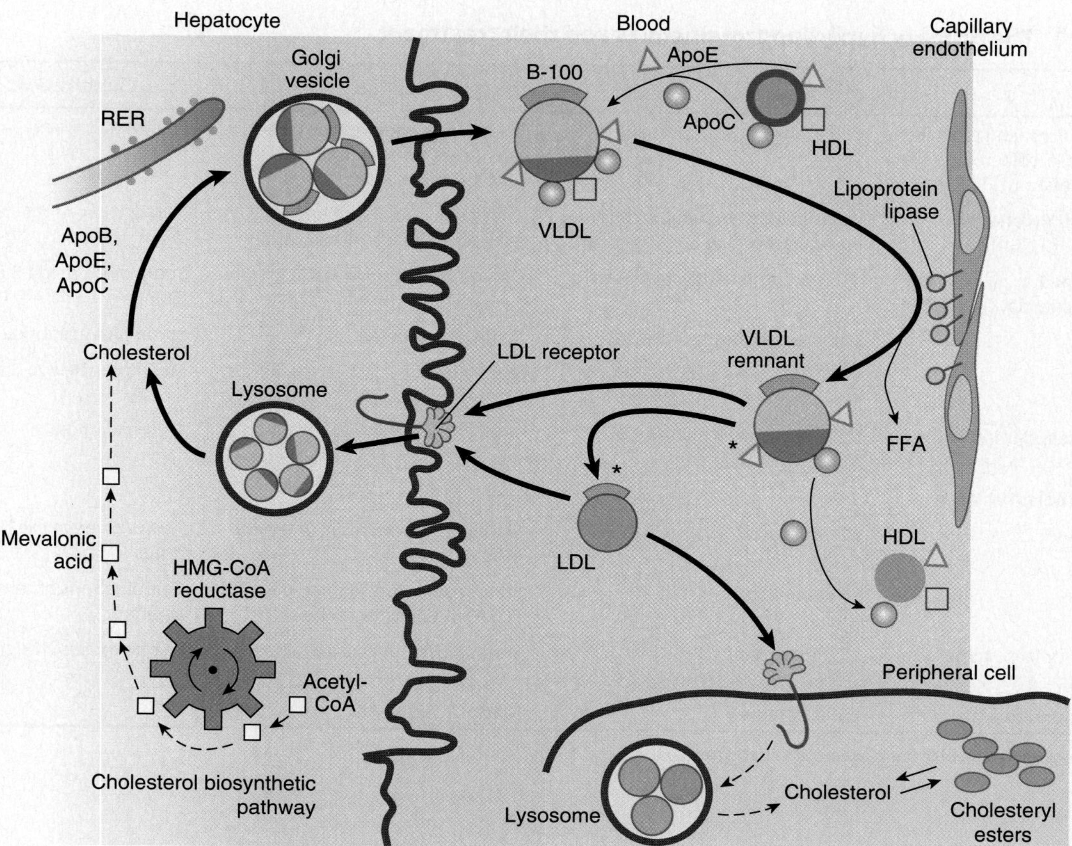

FIGURE 35–1 Metabolism of lipoproteins of hepatic origin. The heavy arrows show the primary pathways. Nascent VLDL are secreted via the Golgi apparatus. They acquire additional apo C lipoproteins and apo E from HDL. Very-low-density lipoproteins (VLDL) are converted to VLDL remnants (IDL) by lipolysis via lipoprotein lipase in the vessels of peripheral tissues. In the process, C apolipoproteins and a portion of the apo E are given back to high-density lipoproteins (HDL). Some of the VLDL remnants are converted to LDL by further loss of triglycerides and loss of apo E. A major pathway for LDL degradation involves the endocytosis of LDL by LDL receptors in the liver and the peripheral tissues, for which apo B-100 is the ligand. Dark color denotes cholesteryl esters; light color denotes triglycerides; the asterisk denotes a functional ligand for LDL receptors; triangles indicate apo E; circles and squares represent C apolipoproteins. FFA, free fatty acid; RER, rough endoplasmic reticulum. (Adapted with permission from Rosenberg RN, Prusiner S, DiMauro S, et al: *The Molecular and Genetic Basis of Neurological Disease*, 2nd ed. Philadelphia, PA: Butterworth-Heinemann; 1997.)

chylomicrons and VLDL during lipolysis. HDL also acquires cholesterol from peripheral tissues, protecting the cholesterol homeostasis of cells. Free cholesterol is chiefly exported from the cell membrane by a transporter, ABCA1, acquired by a small particle termed prebeta-1 HDL, and then esterified by lecithin:cholesterol acyltransferase (LCAT), leading to the formation of larger HDL species. Cholesterol is also exported by the ABCG1 transporter and the scavenger receptor, SR-BI, to large HDL particles. The cholesteryl esters are transferred to VLDL, IDL, LDL, and chylomicron remnants with the aid of cholesteryl ester transfer protein (CETP). Much of the cholesteryl ester thus transferred is ultimately delivered to the liver by endocytosis of the acceptor lipoproteins. HDL can also deliver cholesteryl esters directly to the liver via SR-BI that does not involve endocytosis of the lipoproteins. At the population level, HDL cholesterol (HDL-C) levels relate inversely to atherosclerosis risk. Among individuals, the capacity to accept exported cholesterol can vary widely at identical levels of HDL-C. The ability of peripheral tissues to export cholesterol via the transporter mechanism and the acceptor capacity of HDL are emerging as major determinants of coronary atherosclerosis.

LIPOPROTEIN DISORDERS

Lipoprotein disorders are detected by measuring lipids in serum after a 10-hour fast. Risk of heart disease increases with concentrations of the atherogenic lipoproteins, is inversely related to levels of HDL-C, and is modified by other risk factors. Evidence from clinical trials suggests that an LDL cholesterol (LDL-C) of about 50 mg/dL is optimal for patients with coronary or peripheral arterial disease. Ideally, triglycerides should be below 120 mg/dL. Although LDL-C is still the primary target of treatment, reducing the levels of VLDL and IDL also is important. The lipoproteins involved in each disorder are shown in Table 35–1. Diagnosis of a primary disorder usually requires further clinical and genetic data as well as ruling out secondary hyperlipidemias (Table 35–2). Because measurement of plasma triglycerides commonly focuses

TABLE 35–1 The primary hyperlipoproteinemias and their treatment.

Disorder	Manifestations	Diet + Single Drug	Drug Combination
Primary chylomicronemia (familial lipoprotein lipase, cofactor deficiency; others)	Chylomicrons, VLDL increased	Dietary management; omega-3 fatty acids, fibrate, or niacin (Apo C-III antisense)	Fibrate plus niacin
Familial hypertriglyceridemia	VLDL increased; chylomicrons may be increased	Dietary management; omega-3 fatty acids, fibrate, niacin, statin	Two or three of the individual drugs
Familial combined hyperlipoproteinemia	VLDL predominantly increased	Omega-3 fatty acids, statin, fibrate	Statin plus omega-3 fatty acids or Fibrate
	LDL predominantly increased	Statin or ezetimibe	Statin plus ezetimibe
	VLDL, LDL increased	Statin, omega-3 fatty acids, fibrate	Statin plus omega-3 fatty acids or Fibrate
Familial dysbetalipoproteinemia	VLDL remnants, chylomicron remnants increased	Statin, fibrate	Statin plus fibrate[1]
Familial hypercholesterolemia			
Heterozygous	LDL increased	Statin, ezetimibe, resin, or PCSK9 MAB	Two or three of the individual drugs
Homozygous	LDL increased	Statin, ezetimibe, lomitapide, PCSK9 MAB, evinacumab	Combinations of several single agents
Familial ligand-defective apo B-100	LDL increased	Statin, PCSK9 MAB, ezetimibe	Two or three of the single agents
Lp(a) hyperlipoproteinemia	Lp(a) increased	Niacin, PCSK9 MAB	

[1]Select pharmacologically compatible statin or bempedoic acid (see text).

on constituent glycerol, patients with a rare condition, glycerol kinase deficiency, can be erroneously identified as having hypertriglyceridemia. This can be excluded by ultracentrifugation.

Phenotypes of abnormal lipoprotein distribution are described in this section. Drugs mentioned for use in these conditions are described in the following section on basic and clinical pharmacology.

TABLE 35–2 Secondary causes of hyperlipoproteinemia.

Hypertriglyceridemia	Hypercholesterolemia
Diabetes mellitus	Hypothyroidism
Alcohol ingestion	Early nephrosis
Severe nephrosis	Resolving lipemia
Estrogens	Immunoglobulin-lipoprotein complex disorders
Uremia	Anorexia nervosa
HIV infection	Cholestasis
Myxedema	Hypopituitarism
Glycogen storage disease	Corticosteroid excess
Hypopituitarism	Androgen overdose
Acromegaly	
Immunoglobulin-lipoprotein complex disorders	
Lipodystrophy	
Protease inhibitors, tacrolimus, sirolimus, other drugs	

THE PRIMARY HYPERTRIGLYCERIDEMIAS

Hypertriglyceridemia is associated with increased risk of coronary disease. Chylomicrons, VLDL, and IDL are found in atherosclerotic plaques. These patients tend to have cholesterol-rich VLDL of small particle diameter and small, dense LDL. Hypertriglyceridemic patients with coronary disease or risk equivalents should be treated aggressively. Patients with triglycerides above 700 mg/dL should be treated to prevent acute pancreatitis because the LPL clearance mechanism is saturated at about this level.

Hypertriglyceridemia is an important component of the **metabolic syndrome,** which also includes insulin resistance, hypertension, and abdominal obesity. Reduced levels of HDL-C are usually observed due to transfer of cholesteryl esters to triglyceride-rich lipoproteins. Hyperuricemia is frequently present. Insulin resistance occurs in most patients. Management frequently requires the use of metformin, another antidiabetic agent, or both (see Chapter 41). The severity of hypertriglyceridemia of any cause is increased in the presence of the metabolic syndrome, type 2 diabetes, or the ingestion of alcohol.

Primary Chylomicronemia (Familial Chylomicronemia Syndrome)

Chylomicrons are not present in the serum of normal individuals who have fasted 10 hours. The recessive traits of genetically compromised LPL, its cofactor Apo C-II, and the LMF1, CREB3L3, or GPIHBP1 proteins are usually associated with severe lipemia (1000 mg/dL of triglycerides or higher when the patient is consuming a typical American diet). Mutations in Apo A-V can impair lipolysis in both the homozygous and heterozygous states. Familial chylomicronemia might not be diagnosed until an attack of acute pancreatitis occurs or a woman becomes pregnant. Patients may have eruptive xanthomas, hepatosplenomegaly, hypersplenism, lipemia retinalis, and lipid-laden foam cells in bone marrow, liver, and spleen. The lipemia is increased by estrogens because they stimulate VLDL production. Although these patients have a predominant chylomicronemia, they may also have elevated VLDL, presenting with a pattern called *mixed lipemia*. Deficiency of lipolytic activity can be diagnosed after intravenous injection of heparin. A presumptive diagnosis is made by demonstrating a pronounced decrease in triglycerides 72 hours after elimination of dietary fat. Marked restriction of dietary fat, weight control, exercise, and abstention from alcohol are the basis of effective long-term treatment of chylomicronemia and all hypertriglyceridemias. A fibrate, niacin, or marine omega-3 fatty acids may be of some benefit if VLDL levels are increased. Apo C-III antisense, available in Europe as volanesorsen, is a potential adjunct to therapy. Plasmapheresis may contribute to the rapid reduction of triglycerides in the setting of acute pancreatitis.

Familial Hypertriglyceridemia

The primary hypertriglyceridemias probably reflect a variety of genetic determinants. Variants in a large number of genes have been implicated as causative in patients with hypertriglyceridemia, for which a polygenic risk score has been developed. Many patients have central obesity with insulin resistance. Impaired removal of triglyceride-rich lipoproteins with overproduction of VLDL can result in mixed lipemia. Eruptive xanthomas, lipemia retinalis, epigastric pain, and pancreatitis are variably present depending on the severity of the lipemia. Treatment is primarily dietary. Marine omega-3 fatty acids, especially EPA only, may be helpful for patients with coronary artery disease or who are at high risk. Some patients require treatment with a statin if LDL is elevated, and a fibrate may be needed if triglycerides are consistently greater than 500 mg/dL. If insulin resistance is not present, niacin may be helpful. Metformin is useful in patients with insulin resistance.

Familial Combined Hyperlipoproteinemia (FCH)

The genetic basis of FCH is undetermined but probably involves multiple loci. In this very common disorder, which is associated with an increased incidence of coronary disease, individuals may have elevated levels of VLDL, LDL, or both, and the pattern may change with time. An elevated level of Apo B-100 is a constant feature. FCH involves an approximate doubling in VLDL secretion and appears to be transmitted as a dominant trait. Triglycerides can be increased by factors noted above. Elevations of cholesterol and triglycerides are generally moderate. Diet alone does not normalize lipid levels. A statin alone, or in combination with niacin or fenofibrate, is often required to treat these patients. When fenofibrate is combined with a statin, either pravastatin or rosuvastatin is recommended because neither is metabolized via CYP3A4. Marine omega-3 fatty acids may be useful.

Familial Dysbetalipoproteinemia

In this disorder, remnants of chylomicrons and VLDL accumulate and levels of LDL are decreased. Because remnants are rich in cholesteryl esters, the level of total cholesterol may be as high as that of triglycerides. Diagnosis is confirmed by the absence of the ε3 and ε4 alleles of apo E, the ε2/ε2 genotype. Other rare apo E isoforms that lack receptor ligand properties can also be associated with this disorder. Patients often develop tuberous or tuberoeruptive xanthomas, or characteristic planar xanthomas of the palmar creases. They tend to be obese, and some have impaired glucose tolerance. These factors, as well as hypothyroidism, can increase the lipemia. Coronary and peripheral atherosclerosis occurs with increased frequency. Weight loss, together with decreased fat, cholesterol, and alcohol consumption, may be sufficient. Statins are often effective because they increase hepatic LDL receptors that participate in remnant removal. A fibrate is sometimes needed to control the condition.

THE PRIMARY HYPERCHOLESTEROLEMIAS

LDL Receptor-Deficient Familial Hypercholesterolemia (FH)

This is a common autosomal dominant trait. Although levels of LDL tend to increase throughout childhood, the diagnosis can often be made on the basis of elevated umbilical cord blood cholesterol. In most heterozygotes, cholesterol levels range from 260 to 400 mg/dL. Triglycerides are usually normal. Tendon xanthomas are often present. Arcus corneae and xanthelasma may also be present. Coronary disease tends to occur prematurely. In homozygous FH, which can lead to coronary disease in childhood, levels of cholesterol can range from 500 to over 1000 mg/dL. Early tuberous, tendinous, and planar xanthomas occur, and aortic stenosis is common.

Some individuals have combined heterozygosity for alleles producing nonfunctional and kinetically impaired LDL receptors. In heterozygous patients, LDL can be normalized with reductase inhibitors or combined drug regimens (Figure 35–2). Homozygotes and those with combined heterozygosity whose receptors retain even minimal function may partially respond to combinations of niacin, ezetimibe, and reductase inhibitors. Lomitapide, a small molecule inhibitor of microsomal triglyceride transfer protein (MTP), and monoclonal antibodies directed at PCSK9 also have some effectiveness. Evinacumab, a monoclonal antibody against ANGPTL3, is very effective because its mechanism of action does not depend on LDL receptor function. LDL apheresis is a definitive treatment in medication-refractory patients.

Familial Ligand-Defective Apolipoprotein B-100

Defects in the domain of apo B-100 that binds to the LDL receptor impair the endocytosis of LDL, leading to hypercholesterolemia of

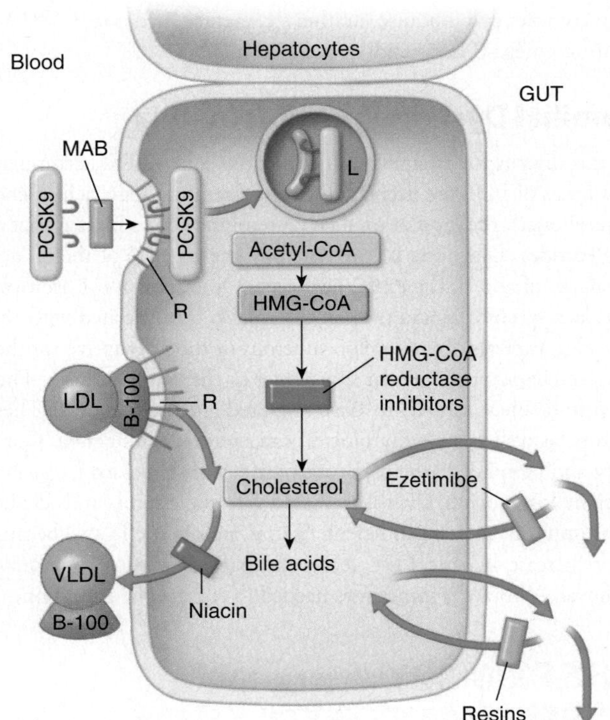

FIGURE 35–2 Sites of action of HMG-CoA reductase inhibitors, PCSK9 MAB, niacin, ezetimibe, and resins used in treating hyperlipidemias. Low-density lipoprotein (LDL) receptors are increased by treatment with resins and HMG-CoA reductase inhibitors. PCSK9 MAB decreases destruction of LDL receptors by PCSK9. VLDL, very-low-density lipoproteins; R, LDL receptor; L, lysosome.

moderate severity. Tendon xanthomas may occur. Response to reductase inhibitors is variable. Upregulation of LDL receptors in liver does not increase uptake of ligand-defective LDL particles. Fibrates or niacin may have beneficial effects by reducing VLDL production.

PCSK9 Gain of Function

The receptor chaperone PCSK9 normally conducts the receptor to the lysosome for degradation (see Figure 35-2). Gain-of-function mutations in PCSK9 are associated with elevated levels of LDL-C and are managed with a PCSK9 antibody.

LDLRAP1 Variants (Autosomal Recessive Hypercholesterolemia)

The RAP1 gene product facilitates the uptake in hepatocytes of the LDL receptor and its associated LDL particle, enhancing the removal of LDL from plasma. Rare defective variants lead to increased LDL, clinically resembling homozygous FH. Statins and bile acid sequestrants may be effective. A similar mechanism for an Apolipoprotein E variant (Leu 167 del) has been described.

CYP7a Deficiency

Decreased catabolism of cholesterol to bile acids and accumulation of cholesterol in hepatocytes result from loss of function mutations in CYP7a. LDL in plasma is increased with downregulation of LDL receptors. LDL is moderately elevated in heterozygous patients. Homozygous patients have higher LDL levels, sometimes elevated triglycerides, early coronary disease, increased risk of gallstones, and are resistant to statins. The addition of niacin to a statin results in a significant reduction in lipid levels.

Familial Combined Hyperlipoproteinemia (FCH)

As described above, some persons with FCH have only an elevation in LDL necessitating treatment with a statin.

Lp(a) Hyperlipoproteinemia

This genetic disorder, which is associated with increased atherogenesis and arterial thrombus formation, is determined chiefly by alleles that dictate increased production of the (a) protein moiety. Lp(a) can be secondarily elevated in patients with severe nephrosis and certain other inflammatory states. Niacin reduces levels of Lp(a) in many patients, and an (a) antisense will be available soon. Reduction of levels of LDL-C below 100 mg/dL decreases the risk of atherosclerosis attributable to Lp(a), and the administration of low-dose aspirin may reduce the risk of thrombus. PCSK9 MABs also reduce levels of Lp(a) by about 25%.

Cholesteryl Ester Storage Disease

Individuals lacking activity of lysosomal acid lipase (LAL) accumulate cholesteryl esters in liver and macrophages leading to hepatomegaly with subsequent fibrosis, and atherosclerosis. They have elevated levels of LDL-C, low levels of HDL-C, and often modest hypertriglyceridemia. Rarely, a fatal totally ablative form, Wolman disease, occurs in infancy. A recombinant replacement enzyme therapy, **sebelipase alfa** given intravenously weekly or every other week, effectively restores the hydrolysis of cholesteryl esters in liver, normalizing plasma lipoprotein levels.

Phytosterolemia

The ABCG5 and ABCG8 half-transporters act together in enterocytes and hepatocytes to export phytosterols into the intestinal lumen and bile, respectively. Homozygous or combined heterozygous ablative mutations in either transporter result in elevated levels of LDL enriched in phytosterols, tendon and tuberous xanthomas, and accelerated atherosclerosis. Many techniques for quantitation of cholesterol include phytosterols and can misdiagnose this disorder. Ezetimibe is the specific therapeutic.

HDL DEFICIENCY

Rare genetic disorders, including Tangier disease and LCAT (lecithin:cholesterol acyltransferase) deficiency, are associated with extremely low levels of HDL. Familial hypoalphalipoproteinemia is a more common disorder with levels of HDL usually below 35 mg/dL in men and 45 mg/dL in women, most commonly attributable to mutations in the *ABCA1* gene. These patients tend to have premature atherosclerosis, and the low HDL may be the only identified risk factor. Paradoxically, HDL levels above 90 mg/dL are associated with increased atherosclerotic vascular disease in population studies. This risk relationship is associated in some cases with variants in the SCARB-1 gene.

Management of HDL deficiency includes special attention to avoidance or treatment of other risk factors. Niacin increases HDL in many of these patients but the effect on clinical outcome is unknown. Reductase inhibitors and fibric acid derivatives exert lesser effects. Aggressive reduction of LDL and VLDL is indicated.

In the presence of hypertriglyceridemia, HDL is low because of exchange of cholesteryl esters from HDL into triglyceride-rich lipoproteins. Treatment of hypertriglyceridemia increases HDL.

SECONDARY HYPERLIPOPROTEINEMIA

Before primary disorders can be diagnosed, secondary causes of the lipid phenotype must be considered. The more common conditions are summarized in Table 35–2. The lipoprotein abnormality usually resolves if the underlying disorder can be treated successfully. These secondary entities can also amplify a primary genetic disorder.

■ DIETARY MANAGEMENT OF HYPERLIPOPROTEINEMIA

Dietary measures are initiated first, unless the patient has evident coronary or peripheral vascular disease, and may obviate the need for drugs. Patients with genetic hypercholesterolemias always require drug therapy in addition to diet. Cholesterol, and saturated and *trans*-fats are the principal factors that increase LDL.

Total fat, sucrose, and, especially, fructose increase VLDL. Alcohol can cause significant hypertriglyceridemia by increasing hepatic secretion of VLDL. Synthesis and secretion of VLDL are increased by excess calories. During weight loss, LDL and VLDL levels may be much lower than can be maintained during neutral caloric balance. The conclusion that diet suffices for management can be made only after weight has stabilized for at least 1 month.

General recommendations include limiting total calories from fat to 20–25% of daily intake, saturated fats to less than 7%, and cholesterol to less than 200 mg/d. Reductions in serum cholesterol range from 10% to 20% on this regimen. Complex carbohydrates and fiber are recommended, and *cis*-monounsaturated fats should predominate. Weight reduction, caloric restriction, and avoidance of alcohol are especially important for patients with elevated triglycerides.

The effect of dietary fats on hypertriglyceridemia is dependent on the disposition of double bonds in the fatty acids. Omega-3 fatty acids found in fish oils activate peroxisome proliferator-activated receptor-alpha (PPAR-α) and can induce profound reduction of triglycerides in some patients. They also have anti-inflammatory and antithrombotic activities. Omega-3 fatty acids are available as a prescription medication containing both docosahexaenoic acid (DHA) and eicosapentaenoic acid (EPA) from marine sources (Lovaza). An EPA-only prescription preparation (icosapent ethyl, Vascepa) is also available and has been shown to reduce elevated triglycerides and remnant lipoproteins, and cardiovascular events. It reduces levels of apolipoprotein C-III, which is an inhibitor of lipoprotein lipase.

Patients with primary chylomicronemia and some with mixed lipemia must consume a diet severely restricted in total fat (10–20 g/d, of which 5 g should be vegetable oils rich in essential fatty acids), and fat-soluble vitamins should be given.

Homocysteine, which initiates proatherogenic changes in endothelium, can be reduced in many patients by restriction of total protein intake to the amount required for amino acid replacement. Supplementation with folic acid plus other B vitamins, and administration of betaine, a methyl donor, is indicated in severe homocysteinemia. Reduction of high levels of homocysteine is especially important in individuals with elevated levels of Lp(a). It liberates the (a) protein from ApoB-100, increasing thrombosis. Consumption of red meat should be minimized to reduce the production by the intestinal biome of trimethyl amine oxide, a compound injurious to arteries.

■ BASIC & CLINICAL PHARMACOLOGY OF DRUGS USED IN HYPERLIPIDEMIA

The decision to use drug therapy for hyperlipidemia is based on the specific metabolic defect and its potential for causing atherosclerosis or pancreatitis. Suggested regimens for the principal lipoprotein disorders are presented in Table 35–1. Experience to date suggests that the available hypolipidemic drugs can be used in various combinations with appropriate safety monitoring. Diet should be continued to achieve the full potential of the drug regimen. These drugs generally should be avoided in pregnant and lactating women and those likely to become pregnant. All drugs that alter plasma lipoprotein concentrations potentially require adjustment of doses of anticoagulants. Children with heterozygous FH may be treated with a resin or reductase inhibitor, the latter usually after about 8 years of age when myelination of the central nervous system is essentially complete. The decision to treat a child should be based on levels of LDL and other atherogenic lipoproteins, other risk factors including the family history, and the child's age. Children with homozygous FH or chylomicronemia syndrome must be treated at the time of diagnosis.

REDUCTASE INHIBITORS: "STATINS"

These compounds are structural analogs of HMG-CoA (3-hydroxy-3-methylglutaryl-coenzyme A, Figure 35–3). **Lovastatin, atorvastatin, fluvastatin, pravastatin, simvastatin, rosuvastatin,** and **pitavastatin** belong to this class. Their principal effect is the reduction of LDL. Other effects include decreased oxidative stress and vascular inflammation with increased stability of atherosclerotic lesions. Emerging effects include inhibition of

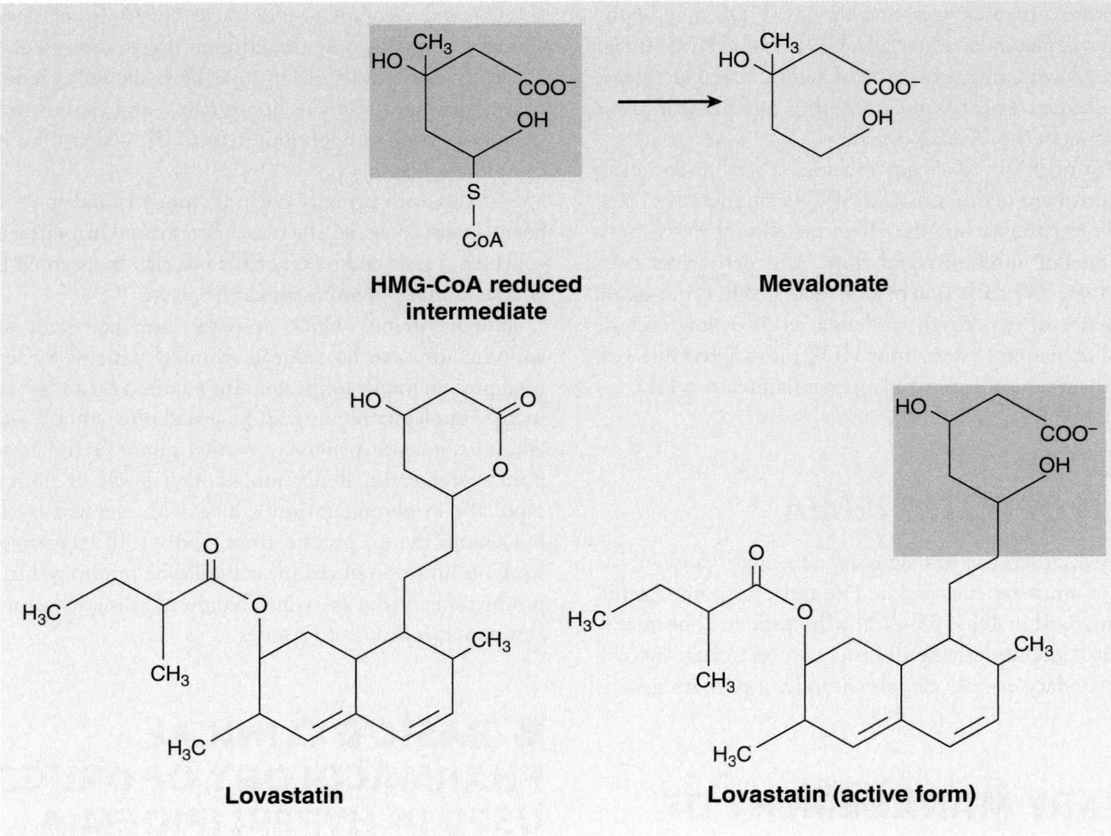

FIGURE 35–3 Inhibition of HMG-CoA reductase. **Top:** The HMG-CoA intermediate that is the immediate precursor of mevalonate, a critical compound in the synthesis of cholesterol. **Bottom:** The structure of lovastatin and its active form, showing the similarity to the normal HMG-CoA intermediate (shaded areas).

certain viruses, mitigation of NAFLD and irritable bowel disease, and retardation of the replication of cancer cells in hepatocellular carcinoma. It has become standard practice to initiate high-dose statin therapy immediately after acute coronary syndromes, regardless of lipid levels.

Chemistry & Pharmacokinetics

Lovastatin and simvastatin are inactive lactone prodrugs that are hydrolyzed in the gastrointestinal tract to the active β-hydroxyl derivatives, whereas pravastatin has an open, active lactone ring. Atorvastatin, fluvastatin, and rosuvastatin are fluorine-containing congeners that are active as given. Absorption of the ingested doses of the reductase inhibitors varies from 40% to 75% with the exception of fluvastatin, which is almost completely absorbed. All have high first-pass extraction by the liver. Most of the absorbed dose is excreted in the bile; 5–20% is excreted in the urine. Plasma half-lives of these drugs range from 1 to 3 hours except for atorvastatin (14 hours), pitavastatin (12 hours), and rosuvastatin (19 hours).

Mechanism of Action

HMG-CoA reductase mediates the first committed step in sterol biosynthesis. The active forms of the reductase inhibitors are structural analogs of the HMG-CoA intermediate (see Figure 35–3) that is formed by HMG-CoA reductase in the synthesis of mevalonate. These analogs cause partial inhibition of the enzyme and thus may impair the synthesis of isoprenoids such as ubiquinone and dolichol, and the prenylation of proteins. It is not known whether this has biologic significance. However, statins clearly induce an increase in high-affinity LDL receptors. This effect increases both the fractional catabolic rate of LDL and the liver's extraction of LDL precursors (VLDL remnants) from the blood, thus reducing LDL (see Figure 35–2). Because of marked first-pass hepatic extraction, the major effect is on the liver. Preferential activity in liver of some congeners appears to be attributable to tissue-specific differences in uptake. Modest decreases in plasma triglycerides and small increases in HDL also occur.

Clinical trials involving many of the statins have demonstrated significant reduction of new coronary events and atherothrombotic stroke. Mechanisms other than reduction of lipoprotein levels also appear to be involved. The availability of isoprenyl groups from the HMG-CoA pathway for prenylation of proteins is reduced by statins, resulting in reduced prenylation of Rho and Rab proteins. Prenylated Rho activates Rho kinase, which mediates a number of mechanisms in vascular biology. The observation that reduction in new coronary events occurs more rapidly than changes in morphology of arterial plaques suggests that these pleiotropic effects may be important. Likewise, decreased prenylation of Rab reduces the accumulation of Aβ protein in neurons, possibly mitigating the manifestations of Alzheimer disease.

Therapeutic Uses & Dosage

Statins are useful alone or in combinations with ezetimibe, PCSK9 MABs, resins, niacin, or bempedoic acid in reducing levels of LDL. If VLDL levels are also elevated, a fibrate may be useful.

Because cholesterol synthesis occurs predominantly at night, reductase inhibitors—except atorvastatin, rosuvastatin, and pitavastatin—should be given in the evening. Absorption generally (with the exception of pravastatin and pitavastatin) is enhanced by food. Daily doses of lovastatin vary from 10 to 80 mg. Pravastatin is nearly as potent on a mass basis as lovastatin with a maximum recommended daily dose of 80 mg. Simvastatin is twice as potent and is given in doses of 5–80 mg daily. Because of increased risk of myopathy with the 80-mg/d dose, the US Food and Drug Administration (FDA) issued labeling for scaled dosing of simvastatin and combined ezetimibe/simvastatin. Pitavastatin is given in doses of 1–4 mg daily. Fluvastatin appears to be about half as potent as lovastatin on a mass basis and is given in doses of 10–80 mg daily. Atorvastatin is given in doses of 10–80 mg/d, and rosuvastatin at 5–40 mg/d. The dose-response curves of pravastatin and especially of fluvastatin tend to level off in the upper part of the dosage range in patients with moderate to severe hypercholesterolemia. Those of other statins are somewhat more linear. Starting doses should be lower in patients of North Asian ancestry.

Toxicity

Elevations of serum aminotransferase (AST/ALT) activity (up to three times normal) occur in some patients. This is often intermittent and usually not associated with other evidence of hepatic toxicity. Therapy may be continued in such patients in the absence of symptoms if AST and ALT are monitored and stable. In some patients, who may have underlying liver disease or a history of alcohol abuse, levels may exceed three times normal. This finding portends more severe hepatic toxicity. These patients may present with malaise, anorexia, and precipitous decreases in LDL. Medication should be discontinued immediately, and also in asymptomatic patients whose AST/ALT activity is persistently elevated to more than three times normal. These agents should be used with caution and in reduced dosage in patients with hepatic parenchymal disease. Severe hepatic disease may preclude their use. In general, AST and ALT activity should be measured at baseline, at 1–2 months, and then every 12 months (if stable). Monitoring of liver enzymes should be more frequent if the patient is taking other drugs that have potential interactions with the statin. Excess intake of alcohol tends to increase hepatotoxic effects of statins.

Fasting plasma glucose levels tend to increase minimally with statin treatment in some patients. A relatively small number develop insulin resistance of varying degree that responds to conventional treatment. Long-term studies have shown a small but significant increase in the incidence of type 2 diabetes in statin-treated patients, many of whom had findings of prediabetes before treatment.

Minor increases in creatine kinase (CK) activity in plasma are observed in some patients receiving statins, frequently associated with heavy physical activity. Rarely, patients may have marked elevations in CK activity, often accompanied by generalized discomfort or weakness in skeletal muscles. If the drug is not discontinued, rhabdomyolysis with myoglobinuria can occur, leading to renal injury. Myopathy may occur with monotherapy, but there is an increased incidence in patients also receiving certain other drugs. Genetic variation in an anion transporter (OATP1B1 protein) is associated with severe myopathy and rhabdomyolysis induced by statins. Variants in the gene (*SLCO1B1*) coding for this protein, which is involved in metabolism of statins can be assessed to identify some individuals intolerant of the drug (see Chapter 5).

The catabolism of lovastatin, simvastatin, and atorvastatin proceeds chiefly through CYP3A4, whereas that of fluvastatin and rosuvastatin, and to a lesser extent pitavastatin, is mediated by CYP2C9. Pravastatin is catabolized through other pathways, including sulfation. The 3A4-dependent reductase inhibitors tend to accumulate in plasma in the presence of drugs that inhibit or compete for the 3A4 cytochrome. These include the macrolide antibiotics, cyclosporine, ketoconazole and its congeners, some HIV protease inhibitors, tacrolimus, nefazodone, fibrates, paroxetine, venlafaxine, and others (see Chapters 4 and 67). Concomitant use of reductase inhibitors with amiodarone or verapamil also increases risk of myopathy.

Drugs such as phenytoin, griseofulvin, barbiturates, rifampin, and thiazolidinediones increase expression of CYP3A4 and can reduce the plasma concentrations of the 3A4-dependent reductase inhibitors. Inhibitors of CYP2C9 such as ketoconazole and its congeners, metronidazole, sulfinpyrazone, amiodarone, and cimetidine may increase plasma levels of fluvastatin and rosuvastatin. Pravastatin and rosuvastatin appear to be the statins of choice for use with verapamil, the ketoconazole group of antifungal agents, macrolides, and cyclosporine. Doses should be kept low and the patient monitored frequently. Plasma levels of lovastatin, simvastatin, and atorvastatin may be elevated in patients ingesting large amounts of grapefruit juice daily.

All statins undergo glycosylation, thus creating a potential interaction with gemfibrozil. Fenofibrate is preferred in combination with a statin.

Creatine kinase activity should be measured in patients receiving potentially interacting drug combinations. If muscle pain or weakness appears, CK should be measured immediately and the drug discontinued if activity is elevated significantly over baseline. The myopathy usually reverses promptly upon cessation of therapy. If the association is unclear, the patient can be rechallenged under close surveillance. Myopathy in the absence of elevated CK can occur. Rarely, hypersensitivity syndromes have been reported that include a lupus-like disorder, dermatomyositis, peripheral neuropathy, and autoimmune myopathy. The latter presents as severe pain and weakness in proximal muscles that does not remit when the statin is discontinued. It is HMG-CoA reductase antibody positive and requires immunosuppressive treatment.

Statins may be temporarily discontinued in the event of serious illness, trauma, or major surgery to minimize the potential for liver and muscle toxicity.

Use of **red yeast rice,** a fermentation product that contains statin activity, is not recommended because the statin content is variable and some preparations contain a nephrotoxin, citrinin.

FIBRIC ACID DERIVATIVES (FIBRATES)

Gemfibrozil and **fenofibrate** decrease levels of VLDL and, in some patients, LDL as well. Another fibrate, **bezafibrate,** is not available in the USA.

Chemistry & Pharmacokinetics

Gemfibrozil is absorbed quantitatively from the intestine and is tightly bound to plasma proteins. It undergoes enterohepatic circulation and readily passes the placenta. The plasma half-life is 1.5 hours. Seventy percent is eliminated through the kidneys, mostly unmodified. The liver modifies some of the drug to hydroxymethyl, carboxyl, or quinol derivatives. Fenofibrate is an isopropyl ester that is hydrolyzed completely in the intestine. Its plasma half-life is 20 hours. Sixty percent is excreted in the urine as the glucuronide, and about 25% in feces.

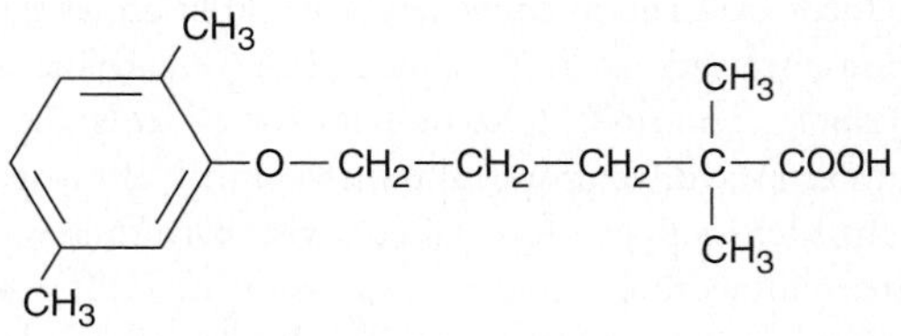

Gemfibrozil

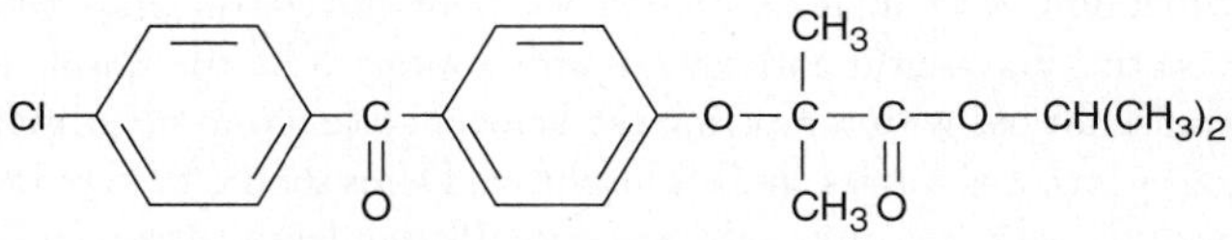

Fenofibrate

Mechanism of Action

Fibrates function primarily as ligands for the nuclear transcription receptor PPAR-α. They transcriptionally up-regulate LPL, apo A-I, and apo A-II, and they down-regulate apo C-III, an inhibitor of lipolysis. A major effect is an increase in oxidation of fatty acids in liver and striated muscle (Figure 35–4). They increase lipolysis of lipoprotein triglyceride via LPL. Intracellular lipolysis in adipose tissue is decreased. Levels of VLDL decrease, in part as a result of decreased secretion by the liver. Only modest reductions of LDL occur in most patients. In others, especially those with combined hyperlipidemia, LDL often increases as triglycerides are reduced. HDL cholesterol increases moderately. Part of this apparent increase is a consequence of lower triglyceride in plasma, resulting in reduction in the exchange of triglycerides into HDL in place of cholesteryl esters.

Therapeutic Uses & Dosage

Fibrates are useful to prevent pancreatitis in severe hypertriglyceridemias in which VLDL predominates, and in dysbetalipoproteinemia. They also may be of benefit in treating the hypertriglyceridemia that results from treatment with antiviral protease inhibitors. The usual dose of gemfibrozil is 600 mg orally once or twice daily. The dosage of fenofibrate as Tricor is one to three 48-mg tablets (or a single 145-mg tablet) daily. Dosages of other preparations vary. Absorption of gemfibrozil is improved when the drug is taken with food. Although useful to reduce triglycerides, the data on their ability to mitigate cardiovascular disease are varied, but increasingly positive in the presence of T2D and the metabolic syndrome. Fibrates can be used in combination with other lipid-lowering agents. Fenofibrate is the fibrate of choice for use in combination with a statin.

Toxicity

Rare adverse effects of fibrates include rashes, gastrointestinal symptoms, myopathy, arrhythmias, hypokalemia, and high blood levels of aminotransferases or alkaline phosphatase. A few patients show decreases in white blood count or hematocrit. Both fibrates may potentiate the action of anticoagulants, and their doses should be adjusted. Rhabdomyolysis has occurred rarely. Fibrates should be avoided in patients with hepatic or renal dysfunction. However, they may have therapeutic value in patients with non-alcoholic fatty liver disease. There appears to be a modest increase in the risk of cholesterol gallstones, reflecting an increase in the cholesterol content of bile. Therefore, fibrates should be used with caution in patients with biliary tract disease or in those at higher risk such as women, obese patients, and Native Americans.

NIACIN (NICOTINIC ACID)

Historically, combination therapy including niacin has been associated with regression of atherosclerotic coronary lesions in three angiographic trials and with extension of lifespan in one large trial in which patients received niacin alone. Response to niacin is individual and highly variable.

Chemistry & Pharmacokinetics

In its role as a vitamin, niacin (vitamin B_3) is converted in the body to the amide, which is incorporated into niacinamide adenine dinucleotide (NAD), which in turn has a critical role in energy metabolism. In pharmacologic doses, it has important effects on lipid metabolism, including mitochondrial activity. It is excreted in the urine unmodified and as several metabolites. One, *N*-methyl nicotinamide, creates a draft on methyl groups that can occasionally result in erythrocyte macrocytosis, similar to deficiency of folate or vitamin B_{12}.

Mechanism of Action

Niacin inhibits VLDL secretion, in turn decreasing production of LDL (see Figure 35–2). It increases clearance of VLDL via the LPL pathway. Excretion of neutral sterols is increased acutely as cholesterol is mobilized from tissue pools. The catabolic rate for HDL is decreased. Fibrinogen levels are reduced, and levels of tissue plasminogen activator appear to increase. Niacin inhibits the intracellular lipase of adipose tissue via receptor-mediated signaling, possibly reducing VLDL production by decreasing the flux of free fatty acids to the liver.

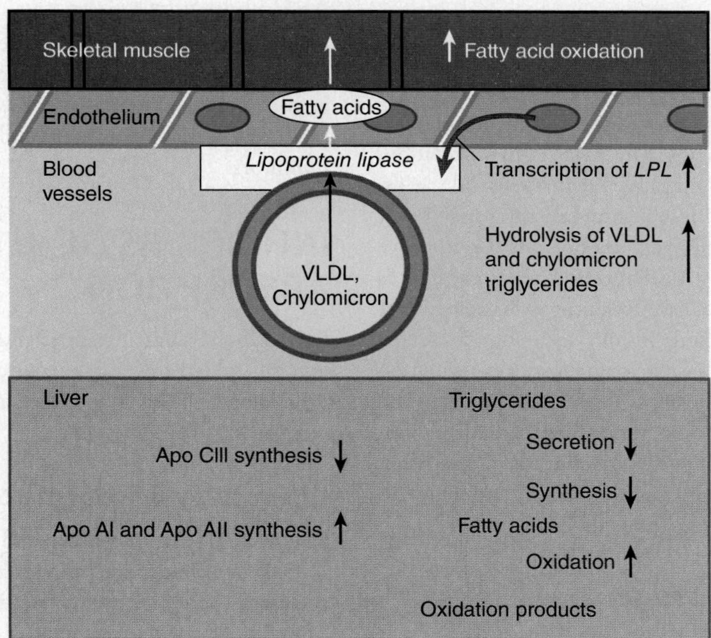

FIGURE 35–4 Hepatic and peripheral effects of fibrates. These effects are mediated by activation of peroxisome proliferator-activated receptor-α, which decreases the secretion of VLDL and increases its peripheral metabolism. LPL, lipoprotein lipase; VLDL, very-low-density lipoproteins.

Therapeutic Uses & Dosage

In combination with a resin and/or reductase inhibitor, niacin can contribute to further reduction of LDL cholesterol. These combinations are also indicated in some cases of nephrosis. In severe mixed lipemia, niacin often produces marked reduction of triglycerides, an effect enhanced by marine omega-3 fatty acids. It is useful in some patients with combined hyperlipidemia and in those with dysbetalipoproteinemia. Niacin is clearly the most effective agent for increasing HDL and reduces Lp(a) in many patients.

For treatment of heterozygous FH, 2–4 g of niacin daily is usually required; more than this should not be given. For other types of hypercholesterolemia and for hypertriglyceridemia, 1.5–3.5 g daily is often sufficient. Crystalline niacin should be given in divided doses with meals, starting with 100 mg two or three times daily and increasing gradually. Several extended-release niacin preparations are available.

Toxicity

Most persons experience a harmless cutaneous vasodilation and sensation of warmth after each dose when niacin is started or the dose increased. Taking 81–325 mg of aspirin 30 minutes beforehand blunts this prostaglandin-mediated effect. Tachyphylaxis to flushing usually occurs within a few days at doses of 1.5–3 g daily. Patients should be warned to expect the flush and understand that it is a harmless side effect. Pruritus, rashes, dry skin or mucous membranes, and acanthosis nigricans have been reported. The latter requires the discontinuance of niacin because of its association with insulin resistance. Some patients experience nausea and abdominal discomfort. Many can continue the drug at reduced dosage, with antacids not containing aluminum. Niacin should be avoided in patients with significant peptic disease.

Reversible elevations in aminotransferases up to twice normal may occur, usually not associated with liver toxicity. However, liver function should be monitored at baseline and at appropriate intervals. Rarely, true hepatotoxicity may occur, and the drug should be discontinued. The association of severe hepatic dysfunction, including acute necrosis, with the use of over-the-counter sustained-release preparations of niacin has been reported. Carbohydrate tolerance may be moderately impaired, especially in obese patients, and insulin resistance may increase. Hyperuricemia occurs in some patients and occasionally precipitates gout. Red cell macrocytosis can occur and is usually not an indication for discontinuing treatment. Significant platelet deficiency occurs rarely and is reversible. Rarely, niacin is associated with arrhythmias, mostly atrial, and with macular edema, both requiring cessation of treatment. Patients should be instructed to report blurring of distance vision. Niacin may potentiate the action of antihypertensive agents, requiring adjustment of their dosages. Birth defects have been reported in offspring of animals given very high doses.

BILE ACID–BINDING RESINS

Colestipol, cholestyramine, and **colesevelam** are useful only for isolated increases in LDL. In patients who also have hypertriglyceridemia, VLDL levels may be further increased during treatment with resins.

Chemistry & Pharmacokinetics

The bile acid-binding agents are large polymeric cationic exchange resins that are insoluble in water. They bind bile acids in the intestinal lumen and prevent their reabsorption. The resin itself is not absorbed.

Mechanism of Action

Bile acids, metabolites of cholesterol, are normally efficiently reabsorbed in the jejunum and ileum (see Figure 35–2). Excretion is increased up to tenfold when resins are given, resulting in enhanced conversion of cholesterol to bile acids in liver via 7α-hydroxylation, which is normally controlled by negative feedback by bile acids. Decreased activation of the FXR receptor by bile acids may result in a modest increase in plasma triglycerides but can also improve glucose metabolism in patients with diabetes. The latter effect is due to increased secretion of the incretin glucagon-like peptide-1 from the intestine, thus increasing insulin secretion. Increased uptake of LDL and IDL from plasma results from up-regulation of LDL receptors, particularly in liver. Therefore, the resins are without effect in patients with homozygous familial hypercholesterolemia who have no functioning receptors but may be useful in those with some residual receptor function and in patients with receptor-defective combined heterozygous states.

Therapeutic Uses & Dosage

The resins are used in treatment of patients with primary hypercholesterolemia, producing approximately 20% reduction in LDL cholesterol in maximal dosage. If resins are used to treat LDL elevations in persons with combined hyperlipidemia, they may cause an increase in VLDL, requiring the addition of a second agent such as a fibrate or niacin. Resins are also used in combination with other drugs to achieve further hypocholesterolemic effect (see below). They may be helpful in relieving pruritus in patients who have cholestasis and bile salt accumulation. Because the resins bind digitalis glycosides, they may be useful in digitalis toxicity.

Colestipol and cholestyramine are available as granular preparations. A gradual increase of dosage from 4 or 5 g/d to 20 g/d is recommended. Total dosages of 30–32 g/d may be needed for maximum effect. The usual dosage for a child is 10–20 g/d. Granular resins are mixed with juice or water and allowed to hydrate for 1 minute. Colestipol is also available in 1-g tablets that must be swallowed whole, with a maximum dose of 16 g daily. Colesevelam is available in 625-mg tablets and as a suspension (1875-mg or 3750-mg packets). The maximum dose is six tablets or 3750 mg as suspension, daily. Resins should be taken in two or three doses with meals.

Toxicity

Common complaints are constipation and bloating, usually relieved by increasing dietary fiber. Resins should be avoided in patients with diverticulitis. Gastric discomfort and diarrhea are occasionally reported. In patients who have preexisting bowel disease or cholestasis, steatorrhea may occur. Malabsorption of vitamin K occurs rarely, leading to hypoprothrombinemia. Prothrombin time should be measured frequently in patients who are taking resins and anticoagulants. Malabsorption of folic acid has been reported rarely. Increased formation of gallstones, particularly in obese persons, was an anticipated adverse effect but has rarely occurred in practice.

Absorption of certain drugs, including those with neutral or cationic charge as well as anions, may be impaired by the resins. These include digitalis glycosides, thiazides, warfarin, tetracycline, thyroxine, iron salts, pravastatin, fluvastatin, ezetimibe, folic acid, phenylbutazone, aspirin, and ascorbic acid, among others. In general, additional medication (except niacin) should be given 1 hour before or at least 2 hours after the resin to ensure adequate absorption. Colesevelam does not bind digoxin, warfarin, or reductase inhibitors.

INHIBITORS OF INTESTINAL STEROL ABSORPTION

Ezetimibe inhibits intestinal absorption of phytosterols and cholesterol. Added to statin therapy, it provides an additional effect, decreasing LDL levels and further reducing the dimensions of atherosclerotic plaques.

Chemistry & Pharmacokinetics

Ezetimibe is readily absorbed and conjugated in the intestine to an active glucuronide, reaching peak blood levels in 12–14 hours. It undergoes enterohepatic circulation, and its half-life is 22 hours. Approximately 80% of the drug is excreted in feces. Plasma concentrations are substantially increased when it is administered with fibrates and reduced when it is given with cholestyramine. Other resins may also decrease its absorption. There are no significant interactions with warfarin or digoxin.

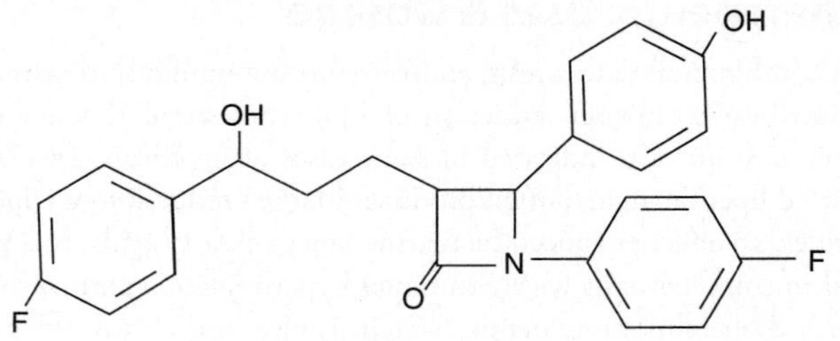

OH OH F O N F

Ezetimibe

Mechanism of Action

Ezetimibe selectively inhibits intestinal absorption of cholesterol and phytosterols. A transport protein, NPC1L1, is the target of the drug. It is effective in the absence of dietary cholesterol because it also inhibits reabsorption of cholesterol excreted in the bile.

Therapeutic Uses & Dosage

A daily dose of 10 mg is used. Average reduction in LDL cholesterol with ezetimibe alone in patients with primary hypercholesterolemia is about 18%, with minimal increases in HDL cholesterol. It is the drug of choice for patients with phytosterolemia. Ezetimibe is synergistic with reductase inhibitors, producing decrements as great as 25% in LDL cholesterol beyond that achieved with the reductase inhibitor alone.

Toxicity

Ezetimibe does not appear to be a substrate for cytochrome P450 enzymes. Experience to date reveals a low incidence of reversible impaired hepatic function with a small increase in incidence when given with a reductase inhibitor. Myositis has been reported rarely.

INHIBITION OF MICROSOMAL TRIGLYCERIDE TRANSFER PROTEIN

Microsomal triglyceride transfer protein (MTP) plays an essential role in the addition of triglycerides to nascent VLDL in liver, and to chylomicrons in the intestine. Its inhibition decreases VLDL secretion and consequently the accumulation of LDL in plasma. An MTP inhibitor, **lomitapide,** is available but is restricted to patients with homozygous FH. It causes accumulation of triglycerides in the liver in some individuals. Elevations in transaminases can occur. Patients must maintain a low-fat diet to avoid steatorrhea and should take steps to minimize deficiency of essential fat-soluble nutrients. Lomitapide is given orally in gradually increasing doses of 5 to 60 mg once daily 2 hours after the evening meal. No more than 30 mg should be given with a 3A4 inhibitor. It is available only through a restricted risk evaluation and mitigation strategy (REMS) program.

PCSK9 INHIBITION

Development of inhibitors of proprotein convertase subtilisin/kexin type 9 (PCSK9) followed on the observation that loss of function mutations result in very low levels of LDL and no apparent morbidity.

Pharmacokinetics and Mode of Action

The PCSK9 protein binds the LDL receptor at the hepatic cell surface, conducting it to destruction in the lysosome (see Figure 35–2). The binding is dependent on heparan sulfate proteoglycans, providing a potential venue for small molecule inhibition of PCSK9 activity by heparan analogs. Humanized antibodies to PCSK9 **(evolocumab, alirocumab)** block interaction with the LDL receptor, allowing the receptor to recycle to the cell surface. LDL reductions of up to 70% at the highest doses have been achieved with these agents. Triglycerides and apo B-100 are reduced, and Lp(a) levels decrease by about 25%.

Therapeutic Uses and Dosage

Use of these agents is restricted to patients who have familial hypercholesterolemia or clinical atherosclerotic cardiovascular disease who require additional reduction of LDL. Outcome data have documented significant reduction of LDL, and of coronary and cerebrovascular disease. They are given alone, or with a statin, bempedoic acid, and/or ezetimibe if needed to reach the patient's LDL goal.

Both are given as subcutaneous injections. Evolocumab is given as 140 mg every 14 days or 420 mg monthly. Alirocumab is given as 75 or 150 mg every 14 days or 300 mg monthly.

Toxicity

Rarely, hypersensitivity reactions have occurred. Local reactions at the injection site, as well as upper respiratory and flu-like symptoms, have been observed.

RNAi INHIBITOR of PCSK9

Inclisiran, a small siRNA now approved, reduces LDL-C about 50% and reduces plasma levels of PCSK9. It is given twice yearly.

ATP CITRATE LYASE INHIBITION

Bempedoic acid, an oral inhibitor of ATP citrate lyase, inhibits cholesterol synthesis in the liver in the HMG-CoA reductase pathway at a site proximal to that of statins. It acts alone, and contributes additional reduction of LDL synthesis when given with a statin. Because its activity is restricted to liver, it is not expected to cause myopathy. Potential side effects include hyperuricemia and tendon rupture.

ANGIOPOIETIN-LIKE-3 INHIBITOR

A monoclonal antibody, evinacumab, binds to angiopoietin-like-3, an inhibitor of lipoprotein lipase and endothelial lipase. Restricted to patients with homozygous familial hypercholesterolemia, it reduces LDL an additional 49% on average when added to other treatments for this disease.

AGENTS UNDER DEVELOPMENT

Antisense Oligonucleotide Inhibitors of Lp(a)

A significant dose-dependent reduction of the Lp(a) lipoprotein and its burden of oxidized lipids is achieved with an antisense oligonucleotide **(pelacarsen).** Reduction of Lp(a) decreases proinflammatory activation of circulating monocytes. Very few side effects have been observed to date. Clinical trials are proceeding. Another antisense and an siRNA targeting Lp(a) are also in development.

Antisense Oligonucleotide Inhibitor of Apo C-III

This agent **(volanesorsen)** is approved in the European Union but not in the USA. It exerts a significant reduction of the very high levels of triglycerides in patients with familial chylomicronemia syndrome. Thrombocytopenia was observed in some patients.

CETP Inhibitor

Inhibition of CETP leads to accumulation of mature HDL particles and diminution of the transport of cholesteryl esters to liver. The accumulation of large HDL particles does not have the anticipated cardioprotective effect. Thus far no drug in this class has been approved.

TREATMENT WITH DRUG COMBINATIONS

Combined drug therapy is useful when LDL and VLDL levels are both elevated, and when levels of either are not at goal with a single agent. The lowest effective doses should be used in combination therapy and the patient monitored more closely for evidence of toxicity. In combinations that include resins, the other agent (with the exception of niacin) should be separated temporally to ensure absorption.

SUMMARY Drugs Used in Dyslipidemia

Subclass, Drug	Mechanism of Action	Effects	Clinical Applications	Pharmacokinetics, Toxicities, Interactions
STATINS				
• Atorvastatin, simvastatin, rosuvastatin, pitavastatin	Inhibit HMG-CoA reductase	Reduce cholesterol synthesis and up-regulate low-density lipoprotein (LDL) receptors on hepatocytes • modest reduction in triglycerides	Elevated LDL • atherosclerotic vascular disease (primary and secondary prevention) • acute coronary syndromes	Oral • duration 12–24 h • *Toxicity:* Myopathy, hepatic dysfunction • *Interactions:* CYP-dependent metabolism (3A4, 2C9) interacts with CYP inhibitors/competitors
• *Fluvastatin, pravastatin, lovastatin: Similar but somewhat less efficacious*				
FIBRATES				
• Fenofibrate, gemfibrozil	Peroxisome proliferator-activated receptor-alpha (PPAR-α) agonists	Decrease secretion of very-low-density lipoproteins (VLDL) • increase lipoprotein lipase activity • increase high-density lipoproteins (HDL)	Hypertriglyceridemia	Oral • duration 3–24 h • *Toxicity:* Low incidence of myopathy, hepatic dysfunction
BILE ACID SEQUESTRANTS				
• Colestipol	Binds bile acids in gut • prevents reabsorption • increases cholesterol catabolism • up-regulates LDL receptors	Decreases LDL	Elevated LDL, digitalis toxicity, pruritus	Oral • taken with meals • not absorbed • *Toxicity:* Constipation, bloating • interferes with absorption of some drugs and vitamins
• *Cholestyramine, colesevelam: Similar to colestipol*				
STEROL ABSORPTION INHIBITOR				
• Ezetimibe	Blocks sterol transporter NPC1L1 in intestine brush border	Inhibits reabsorption of cholesterol excreted in bile • decreases LDL and phytosterols	Elevated LDL, phytosterolemia	Oral • duration 24 h • *Toxicity:* Low incidence of hepatic dysfunction, myositis
NIACIN				
	Decreases catabolism of apo AI • reduces VLDL secretion from liver	Increases HDL • decreases lipoprotein(a) [Lp(a)], LDL	Elevated VLDL, Lp(a)	Oral • large doses • *Toxicity:* Gastric irritation, flushing, low incidence of hepatic toxicity • may reduce glucose tolerance, may induce elevated uric acid, thrombocytopenia Rarely macular edema
• *Extended-release niacin: Similar to regular niacin*				
• *Sustained-release niacin (not the same as extended-release product): hepatic toxicity more likely*				
PCSK9 HUMANIZED MONOCLONAL ANTIBODIES				
• Evolocumab	Complexes PCSK9	Inhibits catabolism of LDL receptor	Familial hypercholesterolemia • incomplete response to other drug therapy	Parenteral • *Toxicity:* injection site reactions, Uncommon nasopharyngitis, flu-like symptoms, rarely myalgia
• *Alirocumab: Similar to evolocumab*				
• Bempedoic Acid	Inhibits cholesterol biosynthesis in liver	Reduces cholesterol synthesis, upregulates LDL receptors	Elevated LDL	Oral • duration 20 h; *Toxicity:* hyperuricemia, tendon rupture

PREPARATIONS AVAILABLE

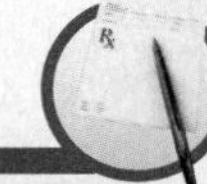

GENERIC NAME	TRADE NAMES
Alirocumab	Praluent
Atorvastatin	Generic, Lipitor
Bempedoic acid	Nexletol
Cholestyramine	Generic, Prevalite, Questran
Colesevelam	Welchol
Colestipol	Generic, Colestid
Evolocumab	Repatha
Evinacumab	Evkeeza
Ezetimibe	Generic, Zetia
Fenofibrate	Generic, Antara, Lofibra, Tricor
Fluvastatin	Generic, Lescol, Lescol XL
Gemfibrozil	Generic, Lopid
Inclisiran	Leqvio
Lomitapide	Juxtapid
Lovastatin	Generic, Altoprev, Mevacor
Niacin, nicotinic acid, vitamin B_3	Generic only
Omega-3 fatty acids–marine	Lovaza, Vascepa
Pitavastatin	Livalo
Pravastatin	Generic, Pravachol
Rosuvastatin	Generic, Crestor
Simvastatin	Generic, Zocor
COMBINATION TABLETS	
Ezetimibe/simvastatin	Vytorin
Bempedoic acid/ezetimibe	Nexlizet
Rosuvastatin/ezetimibe	Roszet

REFERENCES

Burton BK et al: Sebelipase alfa in children and adults with lysosomal acid lipase deficiency. Final results of the ARISE study. J Hepatol 2022;76:587.

Cai T et al: Associations between statins and adverse events in primary prevention of cardiovascular disease: systematic review with pairwise, network, and dose-response meta-analysis. BMJ 2021;14:374.

Cheeley MK et al: NLA scientific statement on statin intolerance: a new definition and key considerations for ASVD risk reduction in the statin intolerant patient. J Clin Lipidol 2020;16:361.

Gaba P et al: Benefits of icosapent ethyl for enhancing residual cardiovascular risk reduction: A review of key findings from REDUCE-IT. J Clin Lipidol 2022;16:389.

Gencer B et al: Efficacy of evolocumab on cardiovascular outcomes in patients with recent myocardial infarctions: a prespecified secondary analysis from the Fourier trial. JAMA Cardiol 2020;5:952.

Ginsberg H et al: Triglyceride-rich lipoproteins and their remnants: Metabolic insights, role in atherosclerotic cardiovascular disease, and emerging therapeutic strategies—a consensus statement for The European Atherosclerosis Society. Eur Heart J 2021;42:4791.

Graham DF, Raal F: Management of familial hypercholesterolemia in pregnancy. Curr Opin Lipidol 2021;32:370.

Guber K et al: Statins and higher diabetes mellitus risk: Incidence, proposed mechanisms, and clinical implication. Cardiol Rev 2021;29:314.

Hardy J et al: A critical review of the efficacy and safety of inclisiran. Am J Cardiovasc Drugs 2021;21:629.

Hashimoto T et al: Lower levels of low-density lipoprotein cholesterol are associated with a lower prevalence of thin-cap fibroatheroma in statin-treated patients with coronary artery disease. J Clin Lipidol 2022;16:104.

Lohia P et al: Association between antecedent statin use and severe disease outcomes in COVID-19: A retrospective study with propensity score matching. J Clin Lipidol 2021;15:451.

Maher LL et al: Roundtable: Global think tank on lipoprotein (a). J Clin Lipidol 2021;15:387.

Marrache MK, Rockkey DC: Statins for treatment of chronic liver disease. Curr Opin Gastroenterol 2021;37:200.

Newman CB et al: Statin safety and associated adverse events: A scientific statement from the American Heart Association. Arterioscler Thromb Vasc Biol 2019;39:e38.

Pastori D et al: Statin liver safety in non-alcoholic fatty liver disease, a systematic review and metanalysis. Br J Pharmacol 2022;88:441.

Sanz-Cuesta BE, Saver JL: Lipid-lowering therapy and hemorrhagic stroke: Comparative meta-analysis of statins and PCSK9 inhibitors. Stroke 2021;52:3142.

Schwartz GG et al: Clinical efficiency and safety of alirocumab after acute coronary syndrome according to achieved level of low-density lipoprotein cholesterol: A propensity score-matched analysis of the ODYSSEY OUTCOMES trial. Circulation 2021;143:1109.

Susekov AV et al: Bempedoic acid in the treatment of patients with dyslipidemia and statin intolerance. Cardiovasc Drugs Ther 2021;35:841.

Thompson GR: Use of apheresis in the age of new therapies for familial hypercholesterolemia. Curr Opin Lipidol 2021;32:363.

Warden BA, Duell PB: Inclisiran: A novel agent for lowering apolipoprotein B-containing lipoproteins: J Cardiovasc Pharmacol 2021;78:157.

CASE STUDY ANSWER

It is likely that her diagnosis is familial combined hyperlipidemia (FCH), with elevations in LDL and VLDL each contributing to risk of CVD, as are her obesity and prediabetes. It is likely that she also has hepatic steatosis based on her elevated ALT and features of the metabolic syndrome. Because of the evidence of early structural coronary disease (elevated calcium score), her FCH diagnosis, her low HDL, and her father's premature CAD, her goal LDL is in the 50-mg/dL range. She opted to add ezetimibe rather than increase the statin dose. After 2 months, her LDL was 58, and triglycerides were 305 mg/dL. Fenofibrate was added, resulting after 3 months in triglycerides of 95, LDL 53, and HDL 49 mg/dL. Four months later, her triglycerides are 92 and LDL 54 mg/dL. Continued diet, exercise, and weight reduction have reduced her A1c to 5.6 and ALT is normal. If her A1c increases, metformin should be considered. She will pause her fibrate and monitor her triglycerides.

CHAPTER

36 Nonsteroidal Anti-Inflammatory Drugs, Disease-Modifying Antirheumatic Drugs, Nonopioid Analgesics, & Drugs Used in Gout

T. Kevin Kafaja, BA, Sana Anwar, MD, & Daniel E. Furst, MD

CASE STUDY

A 48-year-old man presents with complaints of bilateral morning stiffness in his wrists and knees and pain in these joints on exercise. On physical examination, the joints are slightly swollen. The rest of the examination is unremarkable. His laboratory findings are also negative except for slight anemia, elevated erythrocyte sedimentation rate, and positive rheumatoid factor. With the diagnosis of rheumatoid arthritis, he is started on a regimen of naproxen, 220 mg twice daily (bid). After 1 week, the dosage is increased to 440 mg bid. His symptoms are reduced at this dosage, but he complains of significant heartburn that is not controlled by antacids. He is then switched to celecoxib, 200 mg bid, and on this regimen his joint symptoms and heartburn resolve. Two years later, he returns with increased joint symptoms. His hands, wrists, elbows, feet, and knees are all now involved and appear swollen, warm, and tender. He is given oral methotrexate weekly and his disease decreases by about 20%, but he continues to have multiple tender and swollen joints and morning stiffness that lasts 2 hours. What therapeutic options should be considered at this time? What are the possible complications?

ACRONYMS

AS	Ankylosing spondylitis
CAPS	Cryopyrin-associated periodic syndrome
COX	Cyclooxygenase
DMS/PMS	Dermatomyositis/polymyositis
DMARD	Disease-modifying antirheumatic drug
GPA	Granulomatous polyangiitis
IL	Interleukin
JAK	Janus kinase
JIA	Juvenile idiopathic arthritis
NSAID	Nonsteroidal anti-inflammatory drug
OA	Osteoarthritis
PsA	Psoriatic arthritis
PJIA	Polyarticular juvenile idiopathic arthritis
RA	Rheumatoid arthritis
SJIA	Systemic juvenile idiopathic arthritis
SLE	Systemic lupus erythematosus
SSC	Systemic sclerosis
TNF	Tumor necrosis factor

THE IMMUNE RESPONSE

The immune response occurs when immunologically competent cells are activated in response to foreign organisms or antigenic substances liberated during the acute or chronic inflammatory response. The chronic inflammation involves the release of eicosanoids, lipoxygenases, leukotrienes, multiple cytokines and chemokines, and a very complex interplay of immunoactive cells including eosinophils, neutrophils, dendritic cells, lymphocytes and their subsets, and macrophages. These are further elucidated in Chapters 18 and 55.

The whole range of autoimmune diseases (eg, RA, vasculitis, SLE) and inflammatory conditions (eg, gout) derive from abnormalities in this cascade.

The cell damage associated with inflammation acts on cell membranes to release leukocyte lysosomal enzymes; arachidonic acid is then liberated from precursor compounds, and various eicosanoids are synthesized (see Chapter 18). The lipoxygenase pathway of arachidonate metabolism yields leukotrienes, which have a powerful chemotactic effect on eosinophils, neutrophils, and macrophages and promote bronchoconstriction and alterations in vascular permeability. During inflammation, stimulation of the neutrophil membranes produces oxygen-derived free radicals and other reactive molecules such as hydrogen peroxide and hydroxyl radicals. The interaction of these substances with arachidonic acid results in the generation of chemotactic substances, thus perpetuating the inflammatory process.

THERAPEUTIC STRATEGIES

The treatment of patients with inflammation involves two primary goals: first, the relief of symptoms and the maintenance of function, which are usually the major continuing complaints of the patient. For this first goal, both NSAIDs and disease-modifying drugs (DMARDs) are needed. For a second goal, slowing or arrest of the tissue-damaging processes is desirable. For the second goal, DMARDs are absolutely necessary.

To monitor the effects of these medications in RA, SLE, vasculitis, JIA, PMS/DMS, AS, PSA, gout, etc., multiple validated combined indices have been developed and are used to define response. Examples include the Disease Activity Score in 28 joints (DAS28) in RA, SLE Disease Activity Index 2K (SLEDAI-2K) in SLE, Ankylosing Spondylitis Disease Activity Score (ASDAS) in ankylosing spondylitis, etc. These indices often combine measures of joint and muscle tenderness and swelling, patient response, and laboratory data.

■ NONSTEROIDAL ANTI-INFLAMMATORY DRUGS (NSAIDs)

Salicylates and other similar agents used to treat rheumatic disease share the capacity to suppress the signs and symptoms of inflammation including pain. These drugs also exert antipyretic effects.

Since aspirin, the original NSAID, has a number of adverse effects, many other NSAIDs have been developed to improve aspirin's efficacy profile and decrease its toxicity.

Chemistry & Pharmacokinetics

The NSAIDs are grouped in several chemical classes, as shown in Figure 36–1. This chemical diversity yields a broad range of pharmacokinetic characteristics (Table 36–1). Although there are many differences in the kinetics of NSAIDs, they have some general properties in common. All but one of the NSAIDs are weak organic acids as given; the exception, nabumetone, is a ketone prodrug that is metabolized to the acidic active drug.

Most of these drugs are well absorbed, and food does not substantially change their bioavailability. Most of the NSAIDs are highly metabolized, some by phase I followed by phase II mechanisms and others by direct glucuronidation (phase II) alone. NSAID metabolism proceeds, in large part, by way of the CYP3A or CYP2C families of P450 enzymes in the liver (see Chapter 4). While renal excretion is the most important route for final elimination, nearly all undergo varying degrees of biliary excretion and reabsorption (enterohepatic circulation). In fact, the degree of lower gastrointestinal (GI) tract irritation correlates with the amount of enterohepatic circulation. Most of the NSAIDs are highly protein-bound (~98%), usually to albumin. Most of the NSAIDs (eg, ibuprofen, ketoprofen) are racemic mixtures, while one, naproxen, is provided as a single enantiomer and a few have no chiral center (eg, diclofenac).

All NSAIDs can be found in synovial fluid after repeated dosing. Drugs with short half-lives remain in the joints longer than would be predicted from their serum half-lives, while drugs with longer half-lives disappear from the synovial fluid at a rate proportionate to their serum half-lives.

Pharmacodynamics

NSAID anti-inflammatory activity is mediated chiefly through inhibition of prostaglandin biosynthesis (Figure 36–2). Various NSAIDs have additional possible mechanisms of action, including inhibition of chemotaxis, downregulation of IL-1 production, decreased production of free radicals and superoxide, and interference with calcium-mediated intracellular events. Aspirin irreversibly acetylates and blocks platelet COX, while the non-COX-selective NSAIDs are reversible inhibitors.

Selectivity for COX-1 versus COX-2 is variable and incomplete for the older NSAIDs, but drugs that are selective in vitro COX-2 inhibitors have been synthesized. The selective COX-2 inhibitors do not affect platelet function at their usual doses. The in vivo efficacy of COX-2-selective drugs equals that of the older NSAIDs, while GI safety may be improved. On the other hand, selective COX-2 inhibitors increase the incidence of edema, hypertension, and possibly myocardial infarction.

The NSAIDs decrease the sensitivity of vessels to bradykinin and histamine, affect lymphokine production from T lymphocytes, and reverse the vasodilation of inflammation. To varying degrees, all newer NSAIDs are analgesic, anti-inflammatory, and

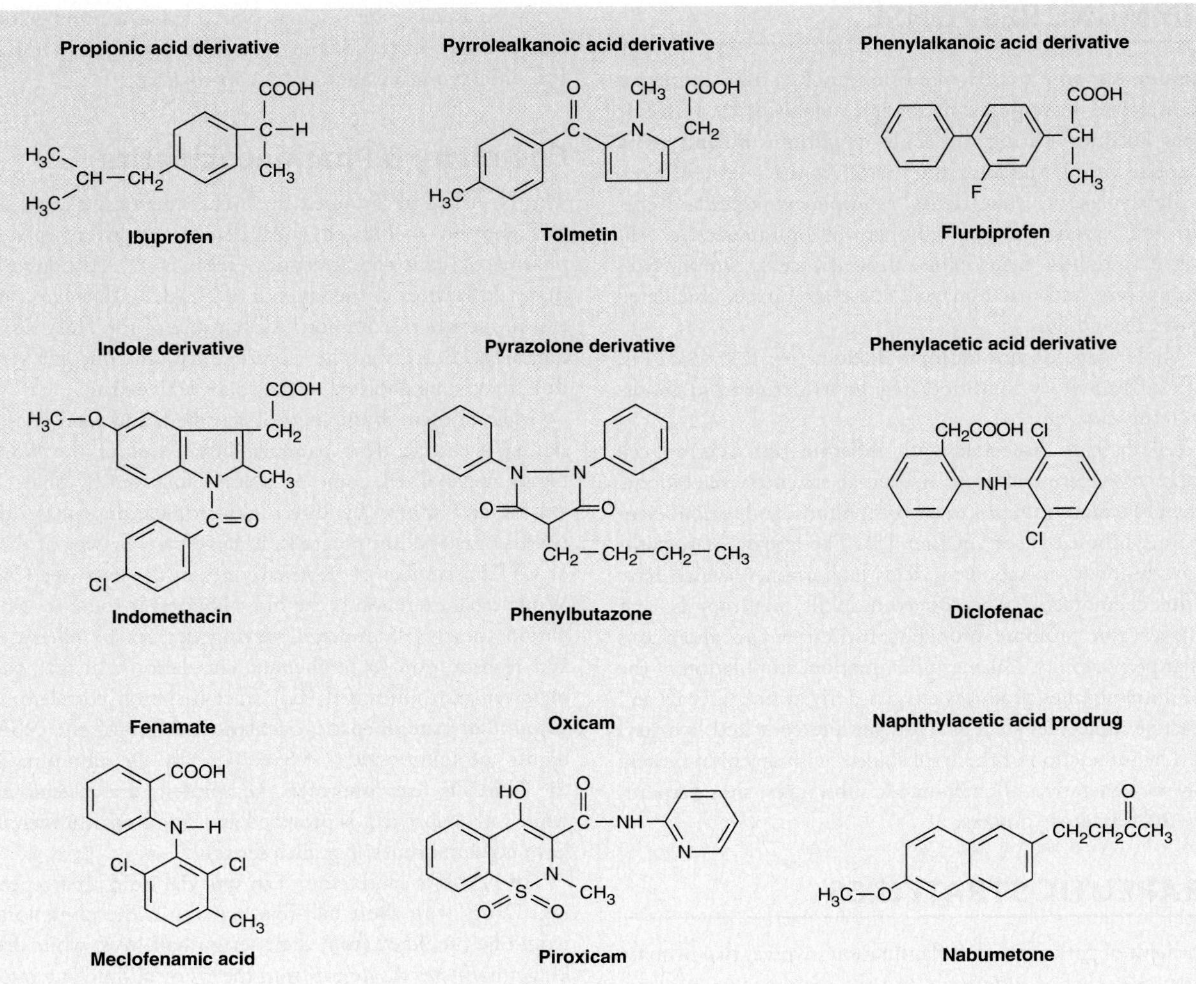

FIGURE 36–1 Chemical structures of some NSAIDs.

antipyretic, and all (except the COX-2-selective agents and the nonacetylated salicylates) inhibit platelet aggregation. NSAIDs are all gastric irritants and can be associated with GI ulcers and bleeding as well, although as a group, the newer agents tend to cause less GI irritation than aspirin. Nephrotoxicity, reported for all NSAIDs, is due in part to interference with the autoregulation of renal blood flow, which is modulated by prostaglandins. Hepatotoxicity also can occur with any NSAID.

Although these drugs effectively inhibit inflammation, there is no evidence that—in contrast to drugs such as methotrexate, biologics, and other DMARDs—they alter the course of any arthritic disorder. Several NSAIDs (including aspirin) reduce the incidence of colon cancer when taken chronically. Several large epidemiologic studies have shown a 50% reduction in relative risk for this neoplasm when the drugs are taken for 5 years or longer.

Although not all NSAIDs are approved by the FDA for the whole range of rheumatic diseases, most are probably effective in RA, seronegative spondyloarthropathies (SpAs—eg, PsA, arthritis associated with inflammatory bowel disease), OA, localized musculoskeletal syndromes (eg, sprains and strains, low back pain), and gout (except tolmetin, which appears to be ineffective in gout).

Adverse effects are generally quite similar for all of the NSAIDs:

1. **Central nervous system:** Headaches, tinnitus, dizziness, and rarely aseptic meningitis.
2. **Cardiovascular:** Fluid retention, hypertension, edema, and rarely myocardial infarction and congestive heart failure (CHF).
3. **Gastrointestinal:** Abdominal pain, dyspepsia, nausea, vomiting, and rarely ulcers or bleeding.
4. **Hematologic:** Rare thrombocytopenia, neutropenia, or even aplastic anemia.
5. **Hepatic:** Abnormal liver function test results and rare liver failure.
6. **Pulmonary:** Asthma.
7. **Skin:** Rashes, all types, pruritus.
8. **Renal:** Renal insufficiency, renal failure, hyperkalemia, and proteinuria.

TABLE 36–1 Pharmacokinetic properties of some nonsteroidal anti-inflammatory drugs.

Drug	Half-Life (hours)	CYP Metabolism	Recommended Anti-inflammatory Dosage
Aspirin[1]	0.25	Yes[a]	1200–1500 mg tid
Salicylic Acid[2]	1.9–12	Yes[b,c,d,e,f,g]	See footnote[2]
Celecoxib	11.2	Yes[c,b]	100–200 mg bid
Diclofenac	1.9–2.3	Yes[b,c,g]	50–75 mg bid
Diflunisal	8–12	No	250–500 mg bid
Etodolac	6.4	No	300–500 mg bid
Flurbiprofen	3.8	Yes[c]	300 mg tid
Ibuprofen	2	Yes[c]	600 mg qid
Indomethacin	4–5	Yes[i]	25–50 mg tid
Ketoprofen	2.1 ± 1.2	No	75 mg tid
Meloxicam	20	Yes[c,g]	7.5–15 mg qd
Nabumetone[3]	22.5–29.8	Yes[j]	1000–2000 mg qd
Naproxen	12–17	Yes[c,j]	375–750 mg bid
Oxaprozin	54.9	No	1200–1800 mg qd
Piroxicam	50	Yes[c]	20 mg qd
Sulindac[4]	16.4	Yes	150–200 mg bid
Tolmetin	1–2	No	200–600 mg tid

bid, twice daily; tid three times daily; qd, once daily; qid, four times daily.

[1]Aspirin is rapidly hydrolyzed to salicylic acid and is undetectable 1–2 hours after dosing.

[2]Major anti-inflammatory metabolite of aspirin; $t_{1/2}$ is dose-dependent.

[3]Nabumetone is a prodrug; half-life, protein binding, T_{max}, clearance, and urinary excretion are for its active metabolite, 6MNA.

[4]Sulindac is a prodrug; half-life, protein binding, T_{max}, and urinary excretion are for its active sulfide metabolite.

[a]CYP2C19 inducer; [b]CYP2C8 substrate; [c]CYP2C9 substrate; [d]CYP2C19 substrate; [e]CYP2D6 substrate; [f]CYP2E1 substrate; [g]CYP3A4 substrate; [h]CYP2D6 inhibitor; [i]CYP2C19 inhibitor; [j]CYP1A2 substrate; [k]CYP1A1 inducer.

ASPIRIN

Aspirin is now rarely used as an anti-inflammatory medication and will be reviewed only in terms of its antiplatelet effects (ie, doses of 81–325 mg once daily, qd). **Mechanism of Action:** Aspirin irreversibly inhibits platelet COX such that aspirin's antiplatelet effect lasts 8–10 days (the life of the platelet). **Pharmacokinetics:** Salicylic acid is a simple organic acid with a pK_a of 3.0. Aspirin (acetylsalicylic acid; ASA) has a pK_a of 3.5 (see Table 1–3). Aspirin is absorbed as such and is rapidly hydrolyzed (serum half-life 15 minutes) to acetic acid and salicylate by esterases in tissue and blood (Figure 36–3, Table 36–1). Salicylate is nonlinearly bound to albumin. Alkalinization of the urine increases the rate of excretion of free salicylate and its water-soluble conjugates. **Clinical Use and Dosing:** Aspirin decreases the incidence of transient ischemic attacks, unstable angina, coronary artery thrombosis with myocardial infarction, and thrombosis after coronary bypass grafting (see Chapter 34). Ticagrelor and aspirin are similar in efficacy in reducing risk for MI, stroke, and cardiovascular death. Coadministration of 2.5 mg bid rivaroxaban and 100 mg qd aspirin may also be effective in reducing MI, stroke, and cardiovascular death compared to aspirin alone. However, it is associated with a greater risk for major bleeding. Coadministration of 75 mg clopidogrel (initial dose of 300 mg) and 75 mg aspirin may be more effective in reducing recurrent ischemic stroke compared to aspirin alone, but it is associated with a higher risk for major hemorrhage (1% rising to 5%). Low-dose aspirin is efficacious in preventing preterm preeclampsia and is recommended by the American College of Obstetricians and Gynecologists for women with a history of preeclampsia. **Adverse Effects:** In addition to the common side effects listed above, aspirin's main adverse effects at antithrombotic doses are gastric upset (intolerance) and gastric and duodenal ulcers. Hepatotoxicity, asthma, rashes, GI bleeding, and renal toxicity rarely if ever occur at antithrombotic doses. The antiplatelet action of aspirin contraindicates its use by patients with hemophilia. Long-term low-dose aspirin usage in patients with type 2 diabetes increases risk for GI bleeding.

NONACETYLATED SALICYLATES

These drugs include magnesium choline salicylate, sodium salicylate, and salicyl salicylate. All nonacetylated salicylates are effective anti-inflammatory drugs, and they do not inhibit platelet aggregation. Although rarely used, they may be preferable when COX inhibition is undesirable such as in patients with asthma, those with bleeding tendencies, and even (under close supervision) those with renal dysfunction.

The nonacetylated salicylates are administered in doses up to 3–4 g of salicylate a day and can be monitored using serum salicylate measurements.

COX-2 SELECTIVE INHIBITORS

COX-2 selective inhibitors, or coxibs, were developed in an attempt to inhibit prostaglandin synthesis by the COX-2 isozyme induced at sites of inflammation without affecting the action of the constitutively active "housekeeping" COX-1 isozyme found in the GI tract, kidneys, and platelets. COX-2 inhibitors at usual doses have no impact on platelet aggregation, which is mediated by thromboxane produced by the COX-1 isozyme. In contrast, they do inhibit COX-2-mediated prostacyclin synthesis in the vascular endothelium and so are not cardioprotective. Recommended doses of COX-2 inhibitors cause renal toxicities similar to those associated with traditional NSAIDs.

Celecoxib

Mechanism of Action: Celecoxib, a benzenesulfonamide, is a selective COX-2 inhibitor, about 10–20 times more selective for COX-2 than COX-1. **Pharmacokinetics:** Refer to Table 36–1. **Indications and Dosage:** Celecoxib is indicated for the treatment of OA, RA, JRA, and AS. The usual dosage is 100–200 mg bid. Celecoxib at 400 mg/d has also shown efficacy as an adjunctive therapy for improving schizophrenic symptoms, most likely due

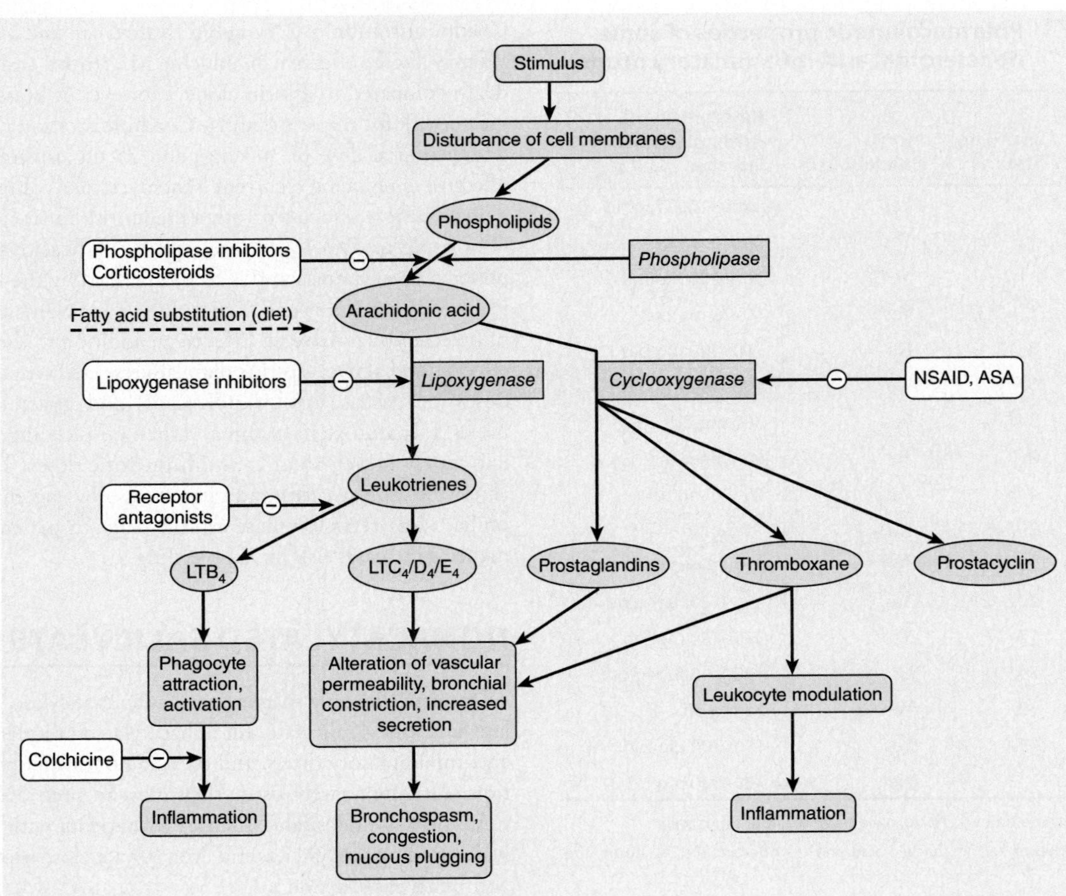

FIGURE 36–2 Prostanoid mediators derived from arachidonic acid and sites of drug action. ASA, acetylsalicylic acid (aspirin); LT, leukotriene; NSAID, nonsteroidal anti-inflammatory drug.

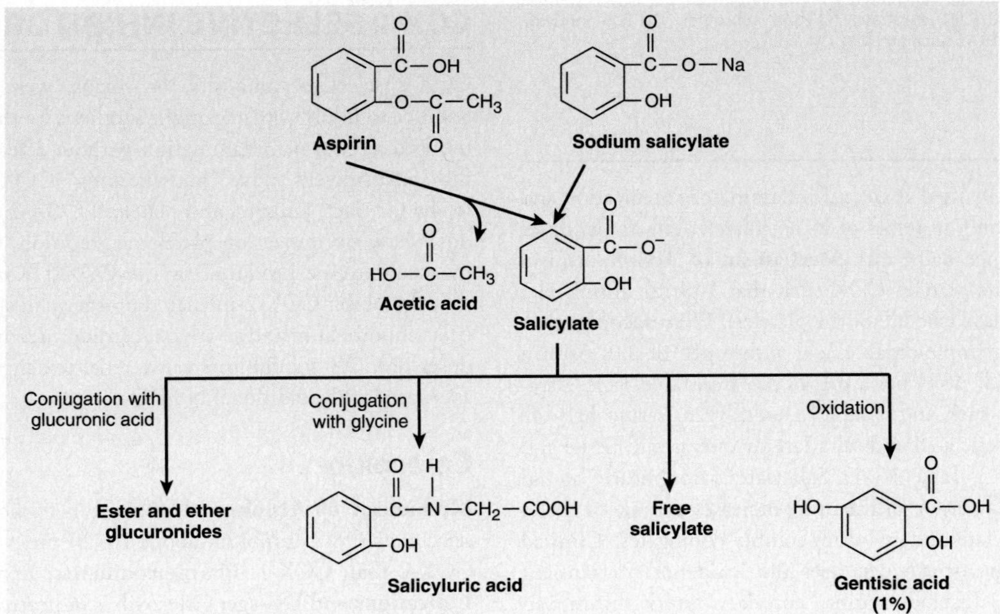

FIGURE 36–3 Structure and metabolism of the salicylates. (Reproduced with permission from Meyers FH, Jawetz E, Goldfien A: *Review of Medical Pharmacology*, 7th ed. McGraw Hill, 1980.)

to suspected neuroinflammation in the disorder. **Adverse Effects:** Celecoxib at usual doses is associated with fewer endoscopic ulcers than most other NSAIDs and is noninferior to naproxen and ibuprofen for most toxicities. It may have a minor effect on platelet aggregation. It interacts occasionally with warfarin and also increases plasma concentrations of both lithium and fluconazole, as would be expected of a drug metabolized by CYP2C9.

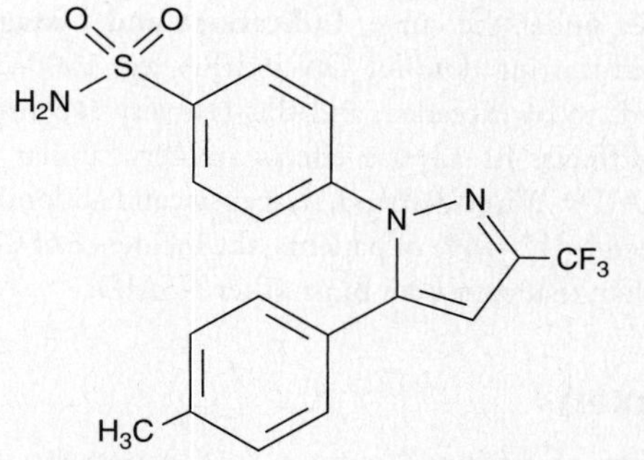

Celecoxib

Etodolac

Mechanism of Action: Etodolac is a racemic acetic acid derivative whose mechanism of action has been described as relatively COX-2 selective. **Pharmacokinetics:** Etodolac has an intermediate half-life and is metabolized principally through glucuronidation as well as inhibiting the WnT pathway (see Table 36–1). **Indications and Dosage:** Etodolac is indicated for the treatment of OA, RA, and JRA. The recommended dosage is 300 mg bid–tid or 500 mg bid initially, then 600 mg/d. **Adverse Effects:** Etodolac may be associated with fewer clinical GI symptoms than nonselective NSAIDs. One report associates etodolac with an increased incidence of acute pancreatitis. Otherwise, this drug has the same spectrum of adverse events as other NSAIDs (see above).

Meloxicam

Mechanism of Action: Meloxicam is an enolcarboxamide related to piroxicam and is a relatively selective COX-2 inhibitor, particularly at 7.5 mg/d. Similarly, while meloxicam inhibits synthesis of thromboxane A2, even at subtherapeutic doses, its blockade of thromboxane A2 does not reach levels that result in decreased in vivo platelet function (see common adverse effects listed above). **Pharmacokinetics:** Refer to Table 36–1. **Indications and Dosage:** The drug is indicated in OA, RA, and JRA patients. Dosage is 7.5–15 mg/d. **Adverse Effects:** Meloxicam is associated with fewer clinical GI symptoms and complications than piroxicam, diclofenac, and naproxen. Other adverse effects are listed above.

NONSELECTIVE COX INHIBITORS

Diclofenac

Mechanism of Action: Diclofenac is a phenylacetic acid derivative that is a relatively nonselective COX inhibitor. **Pharmacokinetics:** See Table 36–1. Coadministration of voriconazole may increase the toxicity of diclofenac, as voriconazole is a CYP2C9 inhibitor. **Indications and Dosage:** See Table 36–1 for dosing information. Diclofenac is indicated for OA, RA, and AS. Off-label use has included biliary colic, corneal abrasions, gout, migraine, and post-episiotomy pain. It is available as sodium, potassium, and epolamine salts, as well as combined in preparations with misoprostol and omeprazole—both of which decrease GI injury. Other preparations include a 0.1% ophthalmic solution, a 1% topical gel, a 3% topical gel, and a rectal suppository form. The 1% gel is available over the counter and is indicated for OA pain and muscular pain, given as 2 g applied locally every 4–6 hours. In Europe, diclofenac is also available as an oral mouthwash and for intramuscular administration. **Adverse Effects:** GI ulceration may occur less frequently than with some other NSAIDs. Elevation of serum aminotransferases occurs more commonly with this drug than with other NSAIDs. Adverse effects are the common toxicities listed above.

Diflunisal

Mechanism of Action: Diflunisal is a difluorophenyl derivative of salicylic acid and is a nonselective COX inhibitor. It is rarely used today. **Pharmacokinetics:** Like salicylic acid, diflunisal is subject to capacity-limited metabolism. Although diflunisal is derived from salicylic acid, it is not metabolized to salicylic acid or salicylate and retains the fluorine atoms, resulting in its longer half-life (see Table 36–1). It undergoes enterohepatic recycling. **Indications and Dosage:** Diflunisal is indicated for OA, RA, and pain at the usual dosage of 500 mg bid. **Adverse Effects:** Diflunisal at 1000 mg bid inhibits platelet aggregation and may cause fecal blood loss but has no effect on bleeding time. Its antiplatelet effect is also reversible and minimal in comparison to those induced by aspirin and piroxicam. Common adverse effects are listed above.

Flurbiprofen

Mechanism of Action: Flurbiprofen is a propionic acid derivative whose (*S*)(+) enantiomer inhibits COX nonselectively. **Pharmacokinetics:** See Table 36–1. It demonstrates enterohepatic circulation with extensive hepatic metabolism. Its (*S*)(+) and (*R*)(–) enantiomers are metabolized differently and undergo minimal chiral conversion, unlike other propionic acid derivatives. **Indications and Dosage:** See Table 36–1 for dosing. Flurbiprofen is approved for OA and RA; it is also used for postoperative analgesia and ophthalmic indications. Flurbiprofen is available orally and as a sodium salt in topical ophthalmic formulation for inhibition of intraoperative miosis. Intravenous flurbiprofen, lozenge, and oral spray are available in Europe. **Adverse Effects:** Although its adverse effect profile is similar to that of other NSAIDs in most ways, flurbiprofen is also rarely associated with cogwheel rigidity, ataxia, tremor, and myoclonus.

Ibuprofen

Mechanism of Action: Ibuprofen is a simple phenylpropionic acid derivative and a nonselective COX inhibitor (see Figure 36–1).

Pharmacokinetics: Refer to Table 36–1. It is available in oral, topical, and intravenous forms. **Indications and Dosage:** Oral ibuprofen is indicated for OA, RA, and JRA. It is available over the counter as 200-mg tablets. In doses of 2400 mg/d, ibuprofen is equivalent to 4 g of aspirin in anti-inflammatory effect. At ≤1600 mg/d, it is analgesic but not anti-inflammatory. Oral and IV ibuprofen are effective in closing patent ductus arteriosus in preterm infants, with much the same efficacy and safety as indomethacin—but it may cause higher bilirubin levels. Pre-emptive 400–600 mg ibuprofen can effectively manage postoperative pain, decrease TNF-α and IL-1β, and reduce opioid consumption. A topical cream preparation is absorbed into fascia and muscle. It can cause "compensated hypogonadism" with decreased testosterone production and secondary increased LH/FSH, resulting in normal testosterone levels but a stressed system, hypothetically resulting in long-term effects (not proven). **Adverse Effects:** In comparison to indomethacin, ibuprofen decreases urine output less and also causes less fluid retention. The drug is relatively contraindicated in individuals with nasal polyps, angioedema, and bronchospastic reactivity to aspirin. Aseptic meningitis, particularly in patients with SLE, has been reported. Rare hematologic effects include agranulocytosis and aplastic anemia. The concomitant administration of ibuprofen and aspirin antagonizes the irreversible platelet inhibition induced by aspirin, limiting the cardioprotective effect of aspirin. Common adverse effects are listed above.

Indomethacin

Mechanism of Action: Indomethacin, introduced in 1963, is an indole derivative (see Figure 36–1) and a potent nonselective COX inhibitor that may also inhibit phospholipase A and C, reduce neutrophil migration, and decrease T-cell and B-cell proliferation. **Pharmacokinetics:** Refer to Table 36–1. **Indications and Dosage:** See Table 36–1 for dosing information. The drug is recommended for OA, RA, AS., bursitis/tendonitis, and acute gouty arthritis. Dosage of 50–70 mg tid may be increased by 25 mg or 50 mg, up to 200 mg/d. Indomethacin accelerates closure of patent ductus arteriosus. Indomethacin has been tried in reactive arthritis, Sweet syndrome, JRA, pleurisy, nephrotic syndrome, tocolysis, diabetes insipidus, urticarial vasculitis, post-episiotomy pain, prophylaxis of heterotopic ossification in arthroplasty, and COVID-19. An ophthalmic preparation is available in Canada and is efficacious for conjunctival inflammation and to reduce pain after traumatic corneal abrasion. Gingival inflammation is reduced after administration of indomethacin oral rinse. Epidural injections produce a degree of pain relief similar to that achieved with methylprednisone in postlaminectomy syndrome. Indomethacin is also available in a rectal formulation. New low-dose indomethacin (20 and 40 mg) capsules containing submicroscopic particles provides analgesic efficacy in acute postoperative pain. **Adverse Effects:** At usual dosages, indomethacin has the common adverse effects listed above. The GI effects may include obstruction, ulcerative colitis, and regional ileitis. Headache is experienced by 11.7% of patients. Indomethacin can aggravate depression, epilepsy, and parkinsonism. It is rarely associated with corneal deposits and retinal disturbances decrease it.

Nabumetone

Mechanism of Action: Nabumetone is the only nonacid NSAID in current use and resembles naproxen in structure (see Figure 36–1). It is a nonselective COX inhibitor. **Pharmacokinetics:** See Table 36–1. Nabumetone is given as a ketone prodrug; 35% of a 1000-mg dose is converted to its active naphthylacetic acid metabolite. Renal impairment results in a doubling of its half-life and a 30% increase in the area under the curve. **Indications and Dosage:** The recommended starting dose for OA and RA (eg, 1500–2000 mg/d) often needs to be exceeded, and this is a very expensive NSAID. **Adverse Effects:** Its adverse effects are very similar to those of other NSAIDs. While diarrhea, dyspepsia, and abdominal pain are experienced by 12–14% of patients, the incidence of GI ulceration is lower than that seen with most other NSAIDs.

Naproxen

Mechanism of Action: Naproxen is a naphthyl-propionic acid derivative and is a nonselective COX inhibitor. **Pharmacokinetics:** see Table 36–1. Naproxen is the only NSAID marketed as a single enantiomer. Naproxen's free fraction is significantly higher in women than in men, but half-life is similar in both sexes (see Table 36–1). **Indications and Dosage:** See Table 36–1 for dosing information. Naproxen is effective for OA, RA, AS, pain, and bursitis/tendonitis. It is also used to treat JIA, acute gout, and migraine. It is available as a slow-release formulation, oral suspension, over the counter (as 220-mg tablets), with sumatriptan (for migraine), as a topical preparation, and as an ophthalmic solution. **Adverse Effects:** Common adverse effects include pressure sensations, nausea, dizziness, and somnolence. The incidence of upper GI bleeding in over-the-counter use is low but still double that of over-the-counter ibuprofen (perhaps due to a dose effect). On the other hand, naproxen has a more favorable cardiovascular risk profile than ibuprofen. Rare cases of allergic pneumonitis, leukocytoclastic vasculitis, and pseudoporphyria as well as the common NSAID-associated adverse effects have been noted. It is contraindicated in patients with hepatic impairment.

Oxaprozin

Mechanism of Action: Oxaprozin, another propionic acid–derivative NSAID, is a nonselective COX inhibitor. **Pharmacokinetics:** Oxaprozin has a long half-life of 50–60 hours and is given once daily (see Table 36–1) and does not reach peak plasma levels for 3 hours despite not undergoing significant enterohepatic circulation. **Indications and Dosage:** See Table 36–1 for dosing information. It is used to treat OA, RA, and JRA. **Adverse Effects:** Its adverse effect profile is like that of other propionic acid derivatives.

Piroxicam

Mechanism of Action: Piroxicam, an enolcarboxamide derivative (see Figure 36–1), is a nonselective COX inhibitor that at high concentration also inhibits polymorphonuclear leukocyte migration, decreases oxygen radical production, and inhibits lymphocyte function. **Pharmacokinetics:** Piroxicam undergoes extensive enterohepatic circulation as indicated by its long half-life of 57 hours, so once-daily dosing is appropriate (see Table 36–1). Steady-state levels are reached within 7–12 days. **Indications and Dosage:** The recommended dosage for OA and RA is 20 mg qd. **Adverse Effects:** At dosages higher than 20 mg/d, piroxicam increases the incidence of peptic ulcer and bleeding (relative risk up to 9.5). See common adverse effects listed above.

Sulindac

Mechanism of Action: Sulindac is a sulfoxide nonselective prodrug whose active metabolite is a nonselective COX inhibitor. **Pharmacokinetics:** Sulindac is reversibly metabolized to the active sulfide metabolite and has enterohepatic cycling; this prolongs the duration of action to 12–16 hours (see Table 36–1). Its metabolite has less effect on renal prostaglandins and thus has been used when renal function is somewhat compromised. **Indications and Dosage:** See Table 36–1 for dosing information. It is used to treat OA, RA, AS, bursitis/tendonitis, and acute gouty arthritis. Sulindac may suppress familial intestinal polyposis. **Adverse Effects:** Sulindac shares the usual NSAID adverse effect profile. As noted above, it is sometimes used in the face of moderate renal compromise. Rare severe adverse reactions include thrombocytopenia, agranulocytosis, and nephrotic syndrome. It is sometimes associated with cholestatic liver damage, pancreatitis, and aseptic meningitis in patients with SLE and mixed connective tissue disease. Coadministration of dimethyl sulfoxide (DMSO) may cause peripheral neuropathy.

Tolmetin

Mechanism of Action: Tolmetin is a pyrrole alkanoic acid derivative (see Figure 36–1) and a nonselective COX inhibitor. It is rarely used today. **Pharmacokinetics:** It has a short half-life of 1–2 hours and reaches peak plasma concentrations within 0.5–1 hour. Refer to Table 36–1. **Indications and Dosage:** See Table 36–1 for dosing information. Tolmetin is indicated for OA, RA, and JRA and is apparently not effective in gout. **Adverse Effects:** Nausea occurs in 11% of patients, and acute interstitial nephritis has been observed. Common adverse effects are listed above.

Other NSAIDs

Meclofenamate and **tenoxicam** are rarely used and are not reviewed here.

CHOICE OF NSAID

All NSAIDs, including aspirin, are about equally efficacious with a few exceptions—tolmetin seems not to be effective for gout, and aspirin is less effective than other NSAIDs (eg, indomethacin) for AS. Therefore, NSAIDs tend to be differentiated on the basis of toxicity and cost-effectiveness. For example, some surveys suggest that indomethacin and tolmetin are the NSAIDs associated with the greatest toxicity, while salsalate, aspirin, and ibuprofen are least toxic. The selective COX-2 inhibitors were not included in these surveys.

For patients with renal insufficiency, nonacetylated salicylates may be best. Diclofenac and sulindac are associated with more liver function test abnormalities than other NSAIDs. The relatively expensive selective COX-2 inhibitor celecoxib is probably safest for patients at high risk for GI bleeding but may have a higher risk of cardiovascular toxicity. Celecoxib or a nonselective NSAID plus omeprazole or misoprostol may be appropriate in patients at highest risk for GI bleeding; in this subpopulation of patients, they are cost-effective despite their high acquisition costs.

The choice of an NSAID thus requires a balance of efficacy, cost-effectiveness, safety, and numerous personal factors (eg, other drugs also being used, concurrent illness, compliance, medical insurance coverage), so that there is no best NSAID for all patients. There may, however, be one or two best NSAIDs for a specific person.

■ DISEASE-MODIFYING ANTIRHEUMATIC DRUGS

RA is a progressive immunologic disease that causes significant systemic effects, shortens life, and reduces mobility and quality of life. Interest has centered on finding treatments that might arrest—or at least slow—this progression by modifying the disease itself. The effects of disease-modifying therapies may take 2 weeks to 6 months to become clinically evident. These therapies include conventional synthetic (cs) and biologic (b) disease-modifying antirheumatic drugs (recently designated **csDMARDs** and **bDMARDs,** respectively). The conventional synthetic agents include small molecule drugs such as methotrexate, azathioprine, chloroquine and hydroxychloroquine, cyclophosphamide, cyclosporine, leflunomide, mycophenolate mofetil, and sulfasalazine. Tofacitinib, although marketed as a biologic, is actually a small molecule targeted synthetic DMARD (tsDMARD). Gold salts, which were once extensively used, are no longer recommended because of their significant toxicities and questionable efficacy. Nevertheless, they have found limited use for RA in Canada. Biologics are large molecule therapeutic agents, usually proteins, that are often produced by recombinant DNA technology. The bDMARDs approved for RA include a T-cell–modulating biologic (abatacept), a B-cell cytotoxic agent (rituximab), anti–IL-6 receptor antibodies (tocilizumab and sarilumab), IL-1–inhibiting agents (anakinra, rilonacept, canakinumab), and the TNF-α–blocking agents (five drugs). bDMARDs are further divided into biological original (or legacy) products and biosimilar DMARDs (boDMARDs and bsDMARDs, respectively).

The small-molecule DMARDs and biologics are discussed alphabetically, independent of origin.

ABATACEPT

Mechanism of Action: Abatacept is a soluble fusion protein composed of the Fc region of human immunoglobulin G1 (IgG1) fused to the extracellular domain of human cytotoxic T-lymphocyte-associated antigen 4 (CTLA-4). Abatacept is designed to inhibit

T-cell activation by binding to ligands CD80 and CD86 on antigen-presenting cells (APCs), ultimately blocking CD80 and CD86 interaction with CD28 on T cells. **Pharmacokinetics:** Abatacept is given by subcutaneous or intravenous administration. The bioavailability of abatacept following subcutaneous administration relative to intravenous administration was 79%. Mean estimates for systemic clearance were 0.28 mL/h/kg, volume of distribution was 0.11 L/kg, and terminal half-life was 14.3 days, with comparability between subcutaneous and intravenous administration. **Indications and Dosage:** Abatacept can be used as monotherapy or in combination with methotrexate or another csDMARD in rheumatoid arthritis, PsA, and polyarthritic JIA in patients 2 years of age and older, plus for the prophylaxis of acute graft-versus-host disease (aGVHD), in combination with a calcineurin inhibitor and methotrexate, and in adults and pediatric patients (≥2 years of age) undergoing hematopoietic stem cell transplantation (HSCT). Abatacept has also been used in SLE, primary Sjögren syndrome, type 1 diabetes, inflammatory bowel disease, Takayasu arteritis, psoriasis vulgaris, and dermatomyositis. Dosing for abatacept is weight adjusted. Intravenous doses are 500 mg monthly if ≤25 to 59 kg, going from 500 mg and maximizing at 1000 mg for those weighing 100 kg. Subcutaneous doses are also weight based, ranging from 50 mg SC weekly (if 10 to <25 kg) kg and maximizing at 125 mg for those weighing 50 kg or more. Methotrexate plus abatacept in early rapidly progressive RA was superior to methotrexate alone to achieve minimal disease activity as early as 2 months, significantly inhibiting radiographic progression at 1 and 2 years. By Bysome measures, abatacept prevented patients from progressing from undifferentiated inflammatory arthritis to rheumatoid arthritis. Abatacept has been associated with a decreased risk of cardiovascular disease and increased HDL compared to TNF inhibitors in RA patients. **Adverse Effects:** There is an increased risk of infection (as with other biologics), predominantly of the upper respiratory and urinary tract, as well as headache, nasopharyngitis, and nausea. Concomitant use with TNF inhibitors or other biologics is probably associated with increased serious infections. All patients should be screened for latent tuberculosis and viral hepatitis before starting, although the risk of latent tuberculosis activation may be slightly less with this drug than with other biologics. Live vaccines should be avoided for up to 3 months after discontinuation of abatacept. Infusion-related reactions, hypersensitivity reactions, and anaphylaxis are reported rarely. Anti-abatacept antibody formation is <5% and does not appear to affect clinical outcomes. There is controversy about whether abatacept increases cancer risk overall, but the weight of evidence is against this association except for a possible increased risk of lymphomas.

ANIFROLUMAB

Mechanism of action: Anifrolumab is a humanized IgG1k monoclonal antibody that binds to subunit 1 of the type 1 IFN receptor, IFNAR, and inhibits formation of the IFN/IFNAR complex. Anifrolumab antagonizes the receptor responsible for cellular signaling induced by IFN-α (predominant in SLE pathogenesis), IFN-β, IFN-ε, IFN-κ, and IFN-ω. Anifrolumab corrects defects in the innate and adaptive immune system by altering protein expression, reversal of cytopenias, and normalization of immune cell population, especially in patients with high type 1 IFN gene-dominant disease, such as is probably true for SLE. **Pharmacokinetics:** Anifrolumab can be administered SC and IV. Anifrolumab serum half-life was 18.5 days for the 300 mg dose and serum concentration dropped below the in vitro effective threshold by 84 days post-dose. Clearance was mostly through the RES system. **Indication and Dosage:** Anifrolumab is one of the three anti–type-1 interferon agents under investigation for the potential treatment for SLE. The US Food and Drug Administration (FDA) approved the drug for nonrenal lupus in June 2021. Phase 2 studies in renal lupus were equivocal, but further studies are ongoing. The anifrolumab dose is 150–300 mg IV every 4 weeks, as higher doses (eg, 1000 mg) resulted in more infections. **Adverse Effects:** The most common adverse effects included upper respiratory tract infection, bronchitis, sinusitis, arthralgia, nasopharyngitis, infusion-related reactions, and UTI. Long-term adverse effects are still under investigation.

APREMILAST

Mechanism of Action: Apremilast is a selective small molecule inhibitor of the enzyme phosphodiesterase 4 (PDE4), hindering the conversion of cyclic AMP to AMP. The inhibition of PDE4 leads to increased intracellular cAMP and decreased production of proinflammatory cytokines including CXCL9 and CXCL10, IFN-γ, TNF-α, and IL-2, -8, -12, and -23. **Pharmacokinetics:** The bioavailability of apremilast is 73%, and its terminal half-life is approximately 6–9 hours. It is 70% metabolized by CYP3A4, thus leading to many potential drug–drug interactions. Elimination is 58% by the kidneys and 39% by the feces, and dose adjustments are recommended if creatinine clearance (CrCl) is ≤30 mL/min. **Indications and Dosage:** Apremilast is given orally, gradually increasing the dose over the first 5 days until the recommended dose of 30 mg bid is reached. It is indicated for plaque psoriasis (in candidates for phototherapy or systemic therapy), psoriatic arthritis, and oral ulcers associated with Behçet disease. **Adverse Effects:** Apremilast's principal adverse effects are gastrointestinal (diarrhea, nausea), but upper abdominal pain, vomiting, upper respiratory tract infections, arthralgia, weight loss, headaches, mood disorders, and suicidal ideation are reported rarely.

AZATHIOPRINE

Mechanism of Action: Azathioprine is a csDMARD and is metabolized to 6-MP and then to its major active metabolite, 6-thioguanine (6-TG). 6-TG suppresses inosinic acid synthesis, ultimately suppressing B- and T-cell function, immunoglobulin production, and IL-2 secretion (see Chapter 55). **Pharmacokinetics:** Azathioprine can be given orally or subcutaneously. Its metabolism is bimodal in humans, with rapid metabolizers clearing the drug four times faster than slow metabolizers. **Indications and Dosage:** Azathioprine is approved for active rheumatoid arthritis (2 mg/kg/day orally).

It is used to prevent kidney transplant rejection in combination with other immunosuppressives. Controlled or open trials show efficacy in psoriatic arthritis, reactive arthritis, polymyositis, SLE (including nephritis), autoimmune hepatitis, maintenance of remission in vasculitis, Behçet disease, IgG4-related disease, and inflammatory myopathies. **Adverse Effects:** Azathioprine suppresses the bone marrow, causes GI disturbances, is carcinogenic, and increases infection risk. Polymorphism of *NUDT15* is strongly associated with azathioprine-induced leukopenia, as is TPMT homozygosity (0.3% of the population).

BARICITINIB

Mechanism of Action: Baricitinib is an anti-inflammatory, targeted, synthetic small molecule (tsDMARD) that in vitro, selectively, and reversibly inhibits JAK1 and JAK3 more than JAK2 and also inhibits the JAK-STAT signaling pathway **Pharmacokinetics:** Baricitinib has an absolute bioavailability of 79%. The elimination half-life is approximately 12 hours. About 10% is metabolized via CYP3A4, so drug interactions are not usually significant. It is excreted mainly by the kidneys, so it should be used cautiously if at all in patients whose glomerular filtration rate is <60 mL/min/1.73 m^2. **Indications and Dosage:** Baricitinib is approved for RA in TNF-α inadequate responders. In a randomized controlled trial, baricitinib was more effective than adalimumab for ACR20 response at 12 weeks. The FDA-approved dose of baricitinib for RA is 2 mg daily in the USA, and its efficacy at this dose is controversial; in Europe, 2 and 4 mg daily are used. It can be used as monotherapy or in combination with methotrexate or other csDMARDs (eg, leflunomide, hydroxychloroquine). A recent phase 2 trial demonstrated efficacy of baricitinib 4 mg daily for patients with active, drug-resistant SLE. It has also been approved in alopecia areata and used in atopic dermatitis and psoriasis. **Adverse Effects:** Baricitinib increases the risk of infection and of herpes virus reactivation. It falls under the FDA "black box" warning for VTE, DVT, and PE, although the data are not strong. Patients should be screened for active and latent tuberculosis prior to initiation of treatment. Lymphoma and other malignancies have been observed. A large study of patients receiving baricitinib found no association with major cardiovascular events, arterial thrombotic events, or congestive heart failure. Gastrointestinal perforations also have been reported, and baricitinib should be used with caution in patients with a history of diverticulitis. Neutropenia, lymphopenia, anemia, liver enzyme elevation, and lipid elevation also have been associated with baricitinib.

BELIMUMAB

Mechanism of Action: Belimumab is a fully human IgG1 monoclonal antibody that selectively inhibits soluble B-lymphocyte stimulator protein (BLyS) from binding to B cells. **Pharmacokinetics:** Belimumab has a distribution half-life of 1.75 days and a terminal half-life of 19.4 days. **Indications and Dosage:** Belimumab is indicated for the treatment of patients aged ≥5 years with SLE or adult active lupus nephritis on background standard of care (SOC) therapy. A recent trial of rituximab followed by belimumab in refractory SLE demonstrated decreased neutrophil extracellular traps (NET), decreased ANA, and improved lupus disease activity states. It has not been tested in combination with other bDMARDs or cyclophosphamide. Belimumab is administered as an intravenous infusion of 10 mg/kg at weeks 0, 2, and 4, and every 4 weeks thereafter or 200 mg SC weekly. **Adverse Effects:** The most common adverse effects of belimumab are nausea, diarrhea, pyrexia, insomnia, extremity pain, migraine, and respiratory tract infections. As with other bDMARDs, there is an increase in serious infection risk. Importantly, depression and suicide have been reported. Infusion reactions occur, including rare anaphylaxis.

RISANKIZUMAB

Mechanism of action: Risankizumab is a humanized Ig G1 monoclonal antibody that selectively targets and binds to the p19 subunit of the IL-23 receptor complex and subsequently inhibits the IL-23-dependent proinflammatory effect. **Pharmacokinetics:** Risankizumab can be administered subcutaneously and intravenously. Risankizumab exhibits linear pharmacokinetics when administered intravenously (0.01 mg/kg to 1200 mg) or subcutaneously (0.25 mg/kg 300 mg), with a long terminal half-life of 28 days. Peak plasma concentration after SC dosing was reached 3–14 days after dosing, with an estimated bioavailability of 89%. **Indication and Dosage:** Risankizumab is approved for the treatment of moderate to severe plaque psoriasis at a dose of 150 mg administered subcutaneously at weeks 0 and 4, and every 12 weeks thereafter. It is also approved for PsA. **Adverse Effects:** The most common side effects include fatigue, arthralgia, nasopharyngitis, headache, skin rashes, and local injection reactions; less common adverse effects include severe infections, reactivation of tuberculosis, and skin cancer.

CALCINEURIN INHIBITORS: CYCLOSPORINE, TACROLIMUS, AND VOCLOSPORIN

Mechanism of Action: Cyclosporine (CSA) and voclosporin (VOCLO) act by binding to cyclophilin-1 while tacrolimus (TAC) binds FK506 binding protein (FKBP), all of which result in inhibition of calcineurin. This selective inhibition impairs the transcription of TNF-α, IL-2, IL-3, IL-4, CD40L, granulocyte-macrophage colony-stimulating factor, interferon-γ, and other cytokines in T-cells. Thus, these drugs interfere with T-cell activation, proliferation, and differentiation. Voclosporin also inhibits p-glycoprotein as well as organic anion transporting polypeptides 1B1 and 1B3 (see Chapter 55). **Pharmacokinetics:** Cyclosporine and tacrolimus absorption are low and erratic (~3–5%), as is that of voclosporin (about 8%), although a microemulsion formulation of cyclosporine provides 20–30% bioavailability. CSA and TOC are available for oral and IV use. Voclosporin is only oral.

All are metabolized by CYP3A4 and therefore are subject to a large number of potential drug interactions (see Chapters 55 and 67). Grapefruit juice increases cyclosporine bioavailability by as much as 62%. The mean terminal half-lives are approximately 30 hours (24.9–36.5 hours). VOCLO has nonlinear kinetics at low doses so that it produces calcineurin inhibition at one-tenth the usual dose of cyclosporine. This means lower tissue concentrations and lower renal and cardiac toxicity, while cyclosporine may be more effective in diseases like psoriasis (in which it reaches higher tissue concentrations). **Indications and Dosage:** Cyclosporine 3–5 mg/kg/day in two divided doses and TAC 2–4 mg qd are clinically active and retard bony erosions in severe and active RA. VOCLO is indicated for SLE nephritis at doses of 23.7 mg bid (tabs are 7.9 mg so three tabs bid) with mycophenolate and/or steroids. CSA and TAC may also be useful in SLE (including nephritis), plaque psoriasis, allogenic post–organ transplant rejection, polymyositis, dermatomyositis, clinically amyopathic dermatomyositis, granulomatous polyangiitis, adult-onset Still disease, JIA, steroid-refractory ulcerative colitis, and refractory eye involvement in Behçet disease. **Adverse Effects:** Leukopenia, thrombocytopenia, and anemia are predictable. High doses can be cardiotoxic, neurotoxic, and nephrotoxic, and they can induce hypertension. Voclosporin may be less reno- and cardiotoxic than CSA. Metabolic abnormalities, hepatotoxicity, life-threatening bacterial, viral, and fungal infections, and malignancies can occur for all three. Bladder cancer is very rare (not reported for VOCLO) but must be looked for, up to 5 years after usage. Sterility has been reported.

CHLOROQUINE AND HYDROXYCHLOROQUINE

Mechanism of Action: Chloroquine and hydroxychloroquine are nonbiologic drugs used for malaria (see Chapter 52) and in rheumatic diseases. They suppress T-lymphocyte responses to mitogens, inhibit leukocyte chemotaxis, stabilize lysosomal enzyme processing by Fc receptor, inhibit DNA and RNA synthesis, and interfere with type 1 IFN through effects on TLR7 and 9. **Pharmacokinetics:** Antimalarials are rapidly absorbed and 50% plasma protein bound, but they are extensively tissue bound, particularly to melanin-containing tissue such as the retina. The drugs are deaminated in the liver and have long and variable plasma elimination half-lives (40–50 days) because of a high volume of distribution, an extended mean residence time (HCQ 1300 hours and CQ 900 hours), and renal clearance. **Indications and Dosage:** Antimalarials are approved for RA (not very effective), systemic lupus erythematosus, chronic discoid lupus erythematosus, JIA, and Sjögren syndrome. They do not alter erosions at their usual dose, and it takes 3–6 months to obtain a clinical response. Antimalarials are used commonly in SLE as they decrease mortality, skin manifestations, serositis, and joint pain in this disease. They have been used in Sjögren syndrome. Based on systematic literature reviews and population-based cohorts, antimalarials reduce the risk of cardiovascular disease in rheumatic disease patients. Although their efficacy in thrombophlebitis in SLE is unclear, they do improve the lipid profile in RA and SLE and prolong pregnancy in threatened preterm delivery. **Adverse Effects:** Dosing was ≤6 mg/kg/d for hydroxychloroquine or ≤2.5 mg/kg/d for chloroquine. At these doses, retinopathy is <1% for up to 5 years and <2% for up to 10 years, and 1% per year thereafter. A baseline ophthalmologic exam and annual screenings after 5 years are recommended, using ocular CT imaging. Other toxicities include dyspepsia, nausea, vomiting, abdominal pain, rashes, weakness from myopathy, cardiomyopathy, cardiac conduction defects, neuromyotoxicity, cytopenias, nightmares, and conduction disorders. These drugs are relatively safe in pregnancy.

CYCLOPHOSPHAMIDE (CYC)

Mechanism of Action: Cyclophosphamide is a csDMARD. Its major metabolite, phosphoramide mustard, cross-links DNA to prevent cell replication (see Chapter 54). It thereby suppresses T- and B-cell function by 30–40%. T-cell suppression correlates with clinical response in the rheumatic diseases. Its pharmacokinetics and toxicities are discussed in Chapter 54. **Indications and Dosage:** Cyclophosphamide is available for oral and intravenous use. It is indicated principally for systemic lupus erythematosus (nephritis and central nervous system lupus), vasculitis, ssc, and possibly myositis. Oral dosing is 2 mg/kg/day while IV monthly CYC is 0.5 (low dose) to 1.0 (high dose) g/m^2. A meta-analysis of seven randomized controlled studies showed equal remission rates after low-dose IV compared to high-dose IV cyclophosphamide, with lower infection rates (in SLE nephritis). The Scleroderma Lung Study (SLS) demonstrated a modest but significant benefit for cyclophosphamide in forced vital capacity dyspnea, skin thickening, and health-related quality of life at 18–24 months. **Adverse Effects:** The most common adverse effects include dyspepsia, nausea, vomiting, neutropenia, thrombocytopenia, infections, and sterility—and in the long term, both skin and bladder cancers.

INTERLEUKIN-1 INHIBITORS

Introduction: IL-1α plays a major role in the pathogenesis of several inflammatory and autoimmune diseases including RA. IL-1α, IL-1β, and IL-1 receptor antagonist (IL-1RA) are other members of the IL-1 family. Three IL-1 inhibitor drugs are marketed.

Anakinra

Mechanism of Action: Anakinra is the oldest drug in this family. Anakinra is a recombinant form of human interleukin 1 (IL-1) receptor antagonist (IL-1Ra). It blocks the effect of IL-1α and IL-1β on IL-1 receptors, hence decreasing the immune response in inflammatory diseases. **Pharmacokinetics:** Anakinra's absolute bioavailability is 95%, and its median (range) half-life is 5.7 (3.1–28.2) hours and is given SC daily. **Indications and Dosage:** See Table 36–2A. Although anakinra is approved for the treatment of active RA, it is rarely used for RA. The recommended dose in the treatment of RA is 100 mg qd; for CAPS it is weight based and maximizes at 8 mg/kg per day. Reduction to every-other-day dosing is recommended if CrCl <30 mL/min. Multiple trials and a meta-analysis showed that anakinra, by targeting hyperinflammation, reduces mortality risk of hospitalized non-intubated patients with COVID-19 without increasing the risk of adverse effects. **Adverse Events:** See below.

Canakinumab

Mechanism of Action: Canakinumab is a human IgG_1/κ monoclonal antibody against IL-1β. It forms a complex with IL-1β, preventing its binding to IL-1 receptors. **Pharmacokinetics:** Canakinumab given subcutaneously has a bioavailability of 66% (less than anakinra) and a 26-day mean terminal half-life. **Indications and Dosage:** see Table 36–2B. In a 10,061-patient, randomized, double-blind trial of canakinumab versus placebo in patients with previous myocardial infarction and elevated CRP, canakinumab lowered recurrent MIs, decreased the incidence and deaths from lung cancer, and improved osteoarthritis pain (all statistically significant). The recommended dose for patients with SJIA who weigh more than 7.5 kg is 4 mg/kg every 4 weeks. There is a weight-adjusted algorithm for treating CAPS.

Rilonacept

Mechanism of Action: Rilonacept is a recombinant form of the ligand-binding domain of the IL-1 receptor. It binds mainly to IL-1β and with lower affinity to IL-1 and a 23-fold lower affinity for IL-1RA. Rilonacept thus neutralizes IL-1β and prevents its attachment to IL-1 receptors. **Pharmacokinetics:** Rilonacept bioavailability is 50% (less than anakinra), and it has an approximate elimination half-life of 1 week (154–184 hours). **Indications and Dosage:** see Table 36–2B. Rilonacept is approved to treat the familial cold autoinflammatory syndrome (FCAS) and Muckle-Wells syndrome (MWS), which are CAPS subtypes, in patients 12 years or older. Rilonacept is also used to treat gout and has been shown to treat recurrent pericarditis. The subcutaneous dose of rilonacept for CAPS is age dependent. **Adverse Effects:** see below.

Adverse Effects of Interleukin 1 Inhibitors

The most common adverse effects of the above IL-1 inhibitors are injection-site reactions (up to 40%) and upper respiratory tract infections. Serious infections including TBC and opportunistic or fungal infections occur very rarely. Headache, abdominal pain, nausea, diarrhea, arthralgia, and flu-like illness all have been reported, as have hypersensitivity reactions. Patients taking IL-1 inhibitors may experience neutrophilia, a physiologic result of inhibiting IL-1 and not an AE; rare transient neutropenia requires neutrophil monitoring.

GUSELKUMAB

Mechanism of Action: Guselkumab is a fully human monoclonal IgG1λ antibody that selectively binds to the p19 subunit of IL-23 with high affinity and inhibits its interaction with the IL-23 receptor, secondarily reducing C-reactive protein (CRP), serum amyloid A (SAA), IL-6, and Th17 effector cytokines (IL-17A, IL-17F and IL-22) in active psoriatic arthritis. **Pharmacokinetics:**

TABLE 36–2A FDA-approved and off-label use of H1 inhibitors ("cases only" denote case reports; rest are studies of varying credibility).

	FDA Approved	Off Label Uses	Off-Label Uses
Anakinra	Deficiency of IL-1 RA antagonist Rheumatoid arthritis	Adult Onset Still's Disease	Hyper IgD (cases only)
		Auto-inflammatory Hearing Loss (cases only)	Kawasaki Syndrome (cases only)
		Behcet's Syndrome (cases only)	Myocarditis (cases only)
		CAPS (FACS, Mukel-Wells, NOMID)	Osteoarthritis
		Congestive Heart Failure	Pericardtis
		CVA (subarachnoid hemorr; Cerebral Thromobsus- a few cases)	Pulmonary Silicosis (cases only)
		Dilated Cardiomyopathy (cases only)	Pyogenic arthritis, pyoderma gangernosum Acne (PAPA) (cases only)
		Dry Eye Syndrome (Topical)	Pustular Psoriasis
		Giant cell Arteritis (cases only)	Pyoderma Gangrenosum
		Gout	Schnitzler Syndrome (cases only)
		Hidradenitis Suppurativa	Systemic Onset JIA
			Takayasu Arteritis (cases only)
			TRAPS (cases only)

CAPS, Cryopyrin-Associated Periodic Syndromes; CHF, congestive heart failure; DM, diabetes mellitus; EMA, European Registration Authority; FACS, Familial cold auto-inflammatory syndrome; IgD, Immunoglobulin D; JIA, Juvenile Inflammatory Arthritis; MAS, Macrophage Activation Syndrome; MI, Myocardial Infarction; NOMID, Neonatal Onset Multisystem Inflammatory Disease; TRAPS, TNF-receptor associated periodic syndrome

TABLE 36–2B FDA-approved and off-label use of H1 inhibitors.

	FDA Approved	Off Label Uses
Canakinumab	CAPS (FACS and Mukel-Wells)	Adult Onset Still's Disease
	TRAPS	DIRAC
	FMF	Gout (USA)
	Gout (EMA only)	Hidradenitis Suppurativa
	Hyper IgD	Osteoarthritis
	Systemic Onset JIA	PAPA
		Psoriasis
		Pyoderma Gangrenosum
		Recurrent MI
		Schnitzler Syndrome
Rilonacept	CAPS (FACS and Mukel-Wells) Pericarditis	FMF
		Gout
		Systemic onset JIA

CAPS, Cryopyrin-Associated Periodic Syndromes; DM, diabetes mellitus; EMA, European Registration Authority; FACS, Familial cold auto-inflammatory syndrome; FMF, Familal Mediterranean Fever; IgD, Immunoglobulin D; JIA, Juvenile Inflammatory Arthritis; MI, Myocardial Infarction; PAPA, Pyogenic Arthritis Pyoderma Gangrenosum Acne

Guselkumab reaches maximum concentration in approximately 5.5 days (Tmax) after a single 100-mg subcutaneous injection. The bioavailability is 49% after a single 100-mg subcutaneous injection with a volume distribution of 7–10 L. The exact metabolic pathway is unknown. The mean elimination half-life is 15–18 days with a mean systemic clearance of 0.516 L/day. It can be administered alone or in combination with a conventional DMARD for patients with psoriatic arthritis. **Indications and Dosage:** Guselkumab is indicated for the treatment of adult active plaque psoriasis patients at 100 mg, by subcutaneous injection at 0 and 4 weeks, and every 8 weeks thereafter. **Adverse Effects:** The most common side effect of guselkumab is upper respiratory infections (nasopharyngitis). Other side effects include headaches, injection-site reactions, arthralgia, diarrhea, and gastroenteritis. Evaluation for tuberculosis prior to starting treatment with guselkumab is needed.

IXEKIZUMAB

Mechanism of Action: Ixekizumab is a human IgG4-κ monoclonal antibody that binds to the IL-17A cytokine (found particularly in psoriasis and psoriatic arthritis) and IL17A/F heterodimers. **Pharmacokinetics:** Ixekizumab is given subcutaneously. Its peak plasma concentration is reached 4 days after the dose. The mean elimination half-life is 13 days. **Indications and Dosage:** Ixekizumab is indicated for adults with moderate to severe plaque psoriasis and adults with PsA. The loading dose for psoriasis is 160 mg subcutaneously followed by 80 mg every 2 weeks to week 12, then 80 mg every 4 weeks. For adults with psoriatic arthritis the recommended dose is 160 mg at week 0, followed by 80 mg every 4 weeks. It can be administered alone or in combination with a csDMARD. Randomized controlled trials have shown efficacy of ixekizumab for radiographic axial spondyloarthritis. **Adverse Effects:** Infection is a common side effect, with upper respiratory tract infections being the most common. Tuberculosis should be evaluated prior to starting therapy. Ixekizumab may cause or exacerbate inflammatory bowel disease.

JANUS KINASE INHIBITORS

While Janus kinase and tyrosine kinase inhibitors (specifically baricitinib, tofacitinib, and upadacitinib) are part of a family of medications, there are some differences amongst them. This will be an overview of the commonalities among these drugs, while specific differences will be discussed for each medication. **Mechanism of Action**: these drugs, at concentrations related to their clinical indications used doses in rheumatic diseases, have some apparent differences in mechanisms of action (see Table 36–3). It should be noted that the effect of these drugs in the tissues, where concentrations may be very different, cannot automatically be extrapolated from these apparent differences in serum concentration–derived mechanisms. **Pharmacokinetics**: These three drugs have a number of similarities (see Table 36–3) and a few differences. The differences will be mentioned within the specific sections below. **Indications and Uses**: The FDA-approved uses of baricitinib, tofacitinib, and upadacitinib are listed in Table 36–3, as are the published off-label uses of these drugs. **Adverse Effects**: For all these medications, there is an increase in infections, particularly upper respiratory infections with cough, headache, fever, etc. Headache and cough are also found without infection. Herpes zoster, particularly, is increased when using JAK inhibitors, although it is rarely disseminated. While there are no data specifically associated with tuberculous, fungal, or opportunistic infections when using JAK inhibitors, these may occur in this patient population independent of these drugs. It is not known whether this propensity is related to the JAK inhibitors, disease activity, or concomitant medications. Nevertheless, all patients should be screened for latent tuberculosis before starting therapy. JAK inhibitors are associated with dose-dependent increases in total cholesterol and LDL, although the relevance to ASCVD is unclear. Lipid levels should be carefully followed and, when appropriate, treated. All JAK inhibitors have a "black box warning" from the FDA relating to increased venous thrombotic events (VTEs), deep-vein thrombosis (DVT), pulmonary emboli (PE), major adverse cardiovascular events (MACE), and cancer. These basically originated from a large, FDA-mandated postmarketing study using tofacitinib in patients with high cardiovascular risk. This study was interpreted as showing an increased risk for these events after tofacitinib at all doses. Upon closer examination, this was a dose-response effect, with 10 mg BID being associated while 5 mg BID was not. Rare events of these sorts had been found in the registration studies, and a few such events were also found for baricitinib and upadacitinib. One can speculate that the rear events in the preregistration studies resulted in the "black box" warning. When using these drugs, one should observe high-risk patients closely, but an appropriate clinical decision with patient input is more appropriate than complete prohibition. GI perforations, initially thought associated with JAK inhibitors, were found principally in patients with a history of diverticulitis, and on corticosteroids. Nevertheless, caution should be exercised in those with histories of diverticulitis. While animal studies indicated teratogenicity and possible infertility, these animal findings used markedly supertherapeutic dosing, and no increased teratogenicity or infertility in humans has thus far been found. Elevated liver function tests, rare lymphomas, and rare neutropenia, lymphopenia, and anemia have been documented for all three JAK inhibitors.

Baricitinib

Mechanism of Action: Baricitinib is an anti-inflammatory, targeted, synthetic small molecule (tsDMARD) that, in vitro, selectively and reversibly inhibits JAK1 and JAK3 more than JAK2 and also inhibits the JAK-STAT signaling pathway **Pharmacokinetics:** See Table 36–3. Only about 10% of baricitinib is metabolized via CYP3A4, so drug interactions are not usually significant. It is excreted mainly by the kidneys, so it should be used cautiously if at all in patients whose glomerular filtration rate is <60 mL/min/1.73 m^2. **Indications and Dosage:** see Table 36–3. In a randomized controlled trial, baricitinib was more effective than adalimumab for ACR20 response at 12 weeks. The FDA-approved dose of baricitinib for RA is 2 mg daily in the USA, and its efficacy at this dose is controversial; in Europe, 2 and 4 mg daily are used. It can be used as monotherapy or in combination with methotrexate or other csDMARDs (eg, leflunomide, hydroxychloroquine). **Adverse Effects:** See introduction. A large study of patients receiving baricitinib found no association with major cardiovascular events, arterial thrombotic events, or congestive heart failure.

Tofacitinib

Mechanism of Action: Tofacitinib is a targeted synthetic small molecule (tsDMARD) that selectively inhibits all members of the Janus kinase (JAK; see Chapter 2) family to varying degrees. At therapeutic doses, tofacitinib exerts its effect mainly by inhibiting JAK 1, 2, and 3, hence interrupting the JAK-STAT signaling pathway. This pathway plays a major role in the pathogenesis of autoimmune diseases including RA. The JAK3/JAK1 complex is responsible for signal transduction from the common chain receptor (IL-2RG) for IL-2, -4, -7, -9, -15, and -21, which subsequently blocks phosphorylation, as well as transcription of several genes that are crucial for the differentiation, proliferation, and function of NK cells and T and B lymphocytes. In addition, JAK1 (in combination with other JAKs) controls signal transduction from IL-6 and interferon receptors. RA patients receiving tofacitinib rapidly reduce C-reactive protein concentrations. **Pharmacokinetics:** Patients taking CYP enzyme inhibitors and those with moderate hepatic or renal impairment require dose reduction to 5 mg once daily. Tofacitinib demonstrates high protein binding compared with the other JAK inhibitors indicates that dialysis may be less effective than for Baricitinib or upadacitinib. It should not be given to patients with severe hepatic disease. **Indications and Dosage**: See introduction to this section and Table 36–3. Tofacitinib can be used as monotherapy or in combination with other csDMARDs, including methotrexate. The recommended dose of tofacitinib in the treatment of RA and PsA is 5 mg twice daily (not 10 mg bid). In 2016, the FDA approved extended-release (XR) tofacitinib citrate 11-mg tablets for once-daily treatment. Its use at 10 mg bid in ulcerative colitis is being reconsidered. **Adverse Effects**: See introduction. Tofacitinib has thus far not been used with potent immunosuppressants (eg, azathioprine, cyclosporine) or biologic bDMARDs (except in one small case series). Tofacitinib increases the risk of EBV in renal transplant patients. particularly in combination with prednisone. A ~5000-patient study in RA patients at risk for cardiac disease demonstrated that, compared to TNF inhibitors, 10-mg bid dosing increased risk for cardiac events, thromboses, pulmonary emboli, and nonmelanotic skin cancers, while 5 mg bid did not demonstrate any of these risks except for nonmelanotic skin cancers. Lymphoma and other malignancies have been reported.

Upadacitinib

Mechanism of Action: Upadacitinib is a small, second-generation Janus kinase selective inhibitor inhibiting JAK 1 and 2 > 3 at usual therapeutic doses, thereby blocking the processes that lead to inflammation in RA and other immune-mediated inflammatory diseases.

Pharmacokinetics: See Table 36–3. Upadacitinib is 79% excreted unchanged in the urine and feces. With little CYP metabolism, drug interactions are unlikely. **Indications and Dosage**: See Table 36–3. The recommended daily dosage is 15 mg. One RCT indicated that it was more effective than abatacept. **Adverse Effects**: See Table 36–3. Serious infections can be seen in patients administered 30 mg in randomized controlled trials. The use of upadacitinib with biologic DMARDs is not recommended, and it should be discontinued before administration of a live attenuated vaccine.

LEFLUNOMIDE

Mechanism of Action: Leflunomide, another csDMARD, is rapidly converted to its active metabolite, A77 1726, in the intestines and plasma. A77 1726 inhibits dihydroorotate dehydrogenase, leading to decreased ribonuclease synthesis and arrest of cells in the G_1 phase of cell growth. Leflunomide therefore inhibits T-cell proliferation, reduces B-cell antibody production, increases IL-10 receptor mRNA, decreases IL-8 receptor mRNA, and decreases TNF-α–dependent NFKβ activation. **Pharmacokinetics:** Leflunomide oral tablets are 80% absorbed with a mean plasma half-life of 19 days for both parent drug and its active metabolite. It undergoes enterohepatic recirculation. Cholestyramine decreases half-life to about 1 day. **Indications and Dosage:** Leflunomide equals methotrexate in efficacy in RA, including inhibition of bony erosions. Methotrexate plus leflunomide more than doubled the ACR 20 response in patients receiving methotrexate alone

TABLE 36–3 Janus kinase inhibitors.

	Baricitinib	Tofacitinib	Upadacitinib
Bioavailability(%)	79	94	76%(ER vs IR)
Metabolism(%)	CYP3A4-10	CYP3A4-70	Unchanged-79%; CYP3A4-<13%
Excretion(%)	Urine-75; Feces-20	Urine-80; Feces-14	Urine-20; Feces-85
Protein Binding(%)	50	94	52
Terminal T ½(hrs)	12.5	3	9-14
FDA Approved	Alopecia areata, Rheumatoid Arthritis(1)	Ankylosing Spondylitis Alopecia areaata Juvenile Inflamm. Arthritis Psoriatic Arthritis Rheumatoid Arthritis(2) Ulcerative Colitis	Ankylosing Spndylitis Atopic Dermatitis Psoriatic Arthritis Rheumatoid Arthritis(2) Ulcerative Colitis
Used	Atopic dermatitis, (COVID19) Systemic Lupus Erythem. psoriasis	Systemic Lupus Erythem.	Alopecia areata

CYYP, liver metabolizing enzyme classification; T ½, terminal half life in serum-~ (1) -in TNFa and methotrexate incomplete resondersresisten; t(2) as in (1) plus conventional synthetic DMARD incomplete responders/resisistent

ER, extended release; IR, immediate release.

(46.2% versus 19.5%). In lupus nephritis, cyclophosphamide and leflunomide were comparably effective, and leflunomide was relatively safe. Leflunomide has been used in giant cell arteritis, Takayasu arteritis, dermatomyositis, and myasthenia gravis. **Adverse Effects:** Diarrhea occurs in 25%, although only 3–5% discontinue the drug secondary to diarrhea. Diarrhea and liver function test abnormalities are reduced by decreasing the leflunomide dose. Mitochondrial dysfunction may be responsible for leflunomide's hepatotoxicity. Leukopenia and thrombocytopenia occur rarely. Mild alopecia, weight gain, and increased blood pressure occur. A meta-analysis found no evidence of the previously reported increased in respiratory adverse events, either infectious or noninfectious.

MESALAMINE

Mechanism of Action: Mesalamine, an aminosalicylate (5-aminosalycylic acid), is hypothesized to have a topical anti-inflammatory effect on colonic epithelial cells, decreasing the synthesis of prostaglandins and leukotrienes. Other potential mechanisms include reducing the activity of NF-κB, and inhibition of TNF, thereby inhibiting the cellular functions of mucosal lymphocytes, macrophages, and natural killer cells. **Pharmacokinetics:** Mesalamine is rapidly metabolized in the intestinal mucosal wall and the liver with an absorption of 20–30% and metabolism to inactive metabolites. Mesalamine's mean elimination half-life is ~25 hours. **Indications and Dosage:** Mesalamine is indicated for the treatment of ulcerative colitis. It has been used, off label, in Crohn disease. Mesalamine can be supplemented with other drugs such as topical or oral glucocorticoids, oral 5-ASA, budesonide multimatrix, or a TNFα inhibitor. **Adverse Effects:** The most common effects are diarrhea, headache, nausea, abdominal pain, dyspepsia, vomiting, and rash. Renal impairment, including interstitial nephritis, nephrotic syndrome, and renal failure, can be seen and must be carefully monitored.

METHOTREXATE (MTX)

Methotrexate is a very important csDMARD used in a wide variety of conditions (see Chapters 54 and 55). **Mechanism of Action:** Low-dose methotrexate inhibits amino-imidazole-carboxamide-ribonucleotide (AICAR) transformylase and thymidylate synthetase. This ultimately leads to extracellular AMP accumulation, which inhibits inflammation, suppressing neutrophil, macrophage, dendritic cell, and lymphocyte function. It secondarily affects polymorphonuclear chemotaxis. MTX directly inhibits proliferation and stimulates apoptosis while its effects on dihydrofolate reductase are relatively minor at rheumatic disease doses. **Pharmacokinetics:** Methotrexate is administered orally, subcutaneously, or intramuscularly. It is approximately 70% absorbed after oral administration. MTX and a less active metabolite are polyglutamated and then retained in cells for prolonged periods. MTX serum half-life is 6–9 hours, although hydroxychloroquine can reduce methotrexate clearance. Methotrexate is excreted principally in the urine but up to 30% may be excreted in the bile. **Indications and Dosage:** Methotrexate oral treatment begins with 7.5 mg weekly and is increased to 15–25 mg weekly. While there is an increased effect up to 30–35 mg weekly, there is also increased toxicity. It decreases the rate of appearance of new erosions in RA. It effectively decreases skin involvement in SSC. Some evidence supports its use in JIA, psoriasis, psoriatic arthritis, peripheral joint disease in AS (not axial disease), granulomatosis with polyangiitis (formerly Wegener granulomatosis), polymyositis, giant cell arteritis, SLE, and vasculitis. Response in RA is predicted by seronegativity, high baseline disease activity, high anxiety scores, and genetic factors. **Adverse Effects:** Nausea and stomatitis are the most common toxicities. Other side effects such as leukopenia, anemia, GI ulceration, and alopecia result from inhibiting cellular proliferation. Dose-related liver enzyme elevations occur frequently. Stomatitis and GI and liver function test abnormalities can be reduced by leucovorin or folic acid, although this may decrease methotrexate efficacy by 10–18%. Methotrexate toxicity in RA is increased in patients who have increased mutations in cytochrome P450 genes (*CYP20A1*, *CYP39A1*), solute carrier genes (*SLC22A2*, *SLC7A7*), and the mitochondrial aldehyde dehydrogenase gene (*ALDH2*). Methotrexate is contraindicated in pregnancy.

MYCOPHENOLATE MOFETIL

Mechanism of Action: Mycophenolate mofetil (MMF), a csDMARD, is converted to mycophenolic acid (MPA), the active form of the drug. The active product inhibits inosine monophosphate dehydrogenase (IMPDH), leading to suppression of T- and B-lymphocyte proliferation. Downstream, it interferes with leukocyte adhesion to endothelial cells through inhibition of E-selectin, P-selectin, and intercellular adhesion molecule. **Pharmacokinetics:** MMF's pharmacokinetics and toxicities are discussed in Chapter 55. **Indications and Dosage:** MMF is indicated in renal and nonrenal SLE (possibly including neuropsychiatric manifestations). It is supplied as 500-mg tablets when used as mycophenolate mofetil and 375 mg as mycophenolic acid; 375 mg of the acid is equivalent to 500 mg of mycophenolate mofetil. As mycophenolate mofetil, dosing is 1000–1500 mg bid and is effective for interstitial lung disease and skin thickening in scleroderma. It has been used in vasculitis, Takayasu arteritis, granulomatous polyangiitis, polymyositis, and dermatomyositis. There is no convincing evidence that MMF is effective in RA. **Adverse Effects:** MMF is associated with GI symptoms (nausea, dyspepsia, abdominal pain), hepatotoxicity, hematologic effects (leukopenia, thrombocytopenia, anemia), and serious infections. It is very rarely associated with malignancy. It is contraindicated in pregnancy.

RITUXIMAB (RTX)

Mechanism of Action: Rituximab is a chimeric monoclonal antibody biologic agent (bDMARD) that targets CD20 B-lymphocytes (see Chapter 55) through cell-mediated and complement-dependent cytotoxicity and stimulation of cell apoptosis. Depletion of B lymphocytes reduces inflammation by decreasing the presentation of antigens to T-lymphocytes and inhibiting the secretion of proinflammatory cytokines. Rituximab rapidly depletes peripheral B-cells (uncorrelated with efficacy or toxicity) and synovial tissue B-cell counts, which do correlate with response in RA. **Pharmacokinetics:** For rheumatoid arthritis, rituximab is given as two intravenous infusions of 1000 mg, separated by 2 weeks. Repeated courses remain effective. For induction therapy in GPA and microscopic polyangiitis, it is given IV, 375 mg/m^2 once weekly for 4 doses. Pretreatment with acetaminophen, an antihistamine, and an H_2 blocker, given 30 minutes prior to infusion decreases the incidence and severity of infusion reactions. **Indications and Dosage:** RTX plus methotrexate treats RA, and RTX with glucocorticoids is approved for GPA and microscopic polyangiitis. In the rheumatic diseases (although different from oncologic practice), RTX is given as 1000 mg with 100 mg methylprednisone infused over several hours. A single course consists of two doses given 2 weeks apart, and courses are given every 6 months, although spacing of doses has varied from every 4 months to every 9 months (or even longer when disease control is achieved). Trials have used single doses and lower doses (as low as 200 mg) after remission was achieved in RA. RA-interstitial lung disease (ILD) was stabilized or improved in an observational study. It has been used for CD20-positive B-cell non-Hodgkin lymphoma (NHL), chronic lymphocytic leukemia (CLL), pemphigus vulgaris, refractory lupus nephritis, Sjögren syndrome, idiopathic inflammatory myositis (including with ILD), IgG4-related disease, and systemic sclerosis. **Adverse Effects:** About 30% of patients develop rash (usually not requiring discontinuation) with the first RTX dose, but rash incidence progressively decreases with each course of therapy thereafter. Urticaria or anaphylactic reactions can occur, as can fatal Stevens-Johnson syndrome. Very low IgG/IgM concentrations may be associated with infection, and IgG/IgM concentrations should be monitored. Serious and even fatal bacterial, fungal, and viral infections have been reported rarely. Rituximab is associated with reactivation of hepatitis B, so ongoing treatment of hepatitis B is appropriate and monitoring for several months after treatment termination is necessary. Rituximab has not been associated with activation of tuberculosis or the de novo occurrence of lymphoma or other tumors (see Chapter 55).

SARILUMAB

Mechanism of Action: IL-6 is a proinflammatory cytokine active in the pathogenesis of RA. Sarilumab is an IL-6 receptor antagonist bDMARD that binds to both soluble and membrane-bound IL-6 receptors, thus inhibiting IL-6-mediated signaling. **Pharmacokinetics:** Sarilumab has a concentration-dependent half-life of 8–10 days with an estimated absolute bioavailability of 80%. **Indications and Dosage:** Sarilumab is effective in rheumatoid arthritis, either as monotherapy or in combination with methotrexate or other csDMARDs. Sarilumab monotherapy appears to be superior to adalimumab monotherapy in RA patients. The recommended dosage is 200 mg once every 2 weeks, administered subcutaneously. **Adverse Effects:** The most common adverse effect of sarilumab is infection. Sarilumab may result in neutropenia, thrombocytopenia, and anemia. Transaminitis >1.5 times higher than normal can occur and should be monitored. Elevated triglycerides and LDL have been reported, and lipids should be tested regularly and treated if abnormal. Perforation with diverticulitis has been reported, although careful studies attribute most of this adverse event to the concomitant use of corticosteroids. Nevertheless, patients with diverticulitis should not be given sarilumab. Malignancies have been observed.

SECUKINUMAB

Mechanism of Action: Secukinumab is a human IgG_1 monoclonal antibody bDMARD that selectively binds to the IL-17A cytokine, inhibiting its interaction with the IL-17A receptor. IL-17A is involved in normal inflammatory and immune responses. **Pharmacokinetics:** Secukinumab is available as a prefilled SC injection or as lyophilized powder for SC injection. Pharmacokinetics are linear, and elimination half-life is 22–31 days. Bioavailability ranged from 55% to 77% following the SC dose of 150 or 300 mg. **Indications and Dosage:** Secukinumab is indicated for moderate to severe plaque psoriasis, or, psoriatic arthritis, ankylosing spondylitis, and nonradiographic axial spondyloarthritis (nr-axSpA) and has been shown to be effective in Ra. An initial loading dose is weekly 300 mg SC for weeks 0–4, followed by 150–300 mg SC monthly. Sarilumab can be used with or without MTX. **Adverse Effects:** As for any of these biologics, infection is a common side effect (28.7%). Nasopharyngitis occurs in about 12%. TB status should be evaluated prior to therapy. Secukinumab may cause or exacerbate inflammatory bowel disease.

SULFASALAZINE

Mechanism of Action: Sulfasalazine, a csDMARD, is metabolized to sulfapyridine (which may be its active moiety in RA) and 5- aminosalicylic acid (see Chapter 62 and Figure 62–8). Some authorities believe that the parent compound, sulfasalazine, also has an effect. 5-aminosalicylic acid is thought to be the active moiety in inflammatory bowel disease, acting by inhibiting the proinflammatory NK-KBs signaling pathway and inhibiting T-cell response to concanavalin and B-cell proliferation, secondarily suppressing the production of IgM and IgG in vitro. Production and release of sulfasalazine and its metabolites also inhibits inflammatory cytokine monocytes/macrophages (eg, IL-1, -6, -8, -11, -12), growth-related gene protein and TNF in vitro. **Pharmacokinetics:** Only 5–13% of orally administered sulfasalazine is absorbed. Sulfasalazine undergoes enterohepatic recirculation. Sulfapyridine is nearly completely absorbed, and its inherited slow acetylator phenotype accounts for most of sulfasalazine's toxicity. Lack of intact colon or use of antibiotics will increase its toxicity, and genetic phenotype can help guide therapy. 5-aminosalicylic acid remains unabsorbed. Some sulfasalazine is excreted unchanged in the urine, whereas sulfapyridine is excreted after hepatic acetylation and hydroxylation. Sulfasalazine's half-life is 6–17 hours. **Indications and Dosage:** Sulfasalazine, 2–3 g/day, is effective in RA and reduces radiologic disease progression. It has also been used in reactive arthritis, JIA, inflammatory bowel disease (FDA approved for ulcerative colitis but not for Crohn disease), gastrointestinal Behçet disease, and HLA-B27–positive anterior uveitis with AS. It decreases platelet aggregation. **Adverse Effects:** Approximately 30% of patients using sulfasalazine discontinue the drug because of toxicity. Common adverse effects include nausea, vomiting, headache, and rash. The most serious skin hypersensitivity reaction is toxic epidermal necrosis. Hemolytic anemia and methemoglobinemia also occur rarely, Neutropenia occurs in 1–5% of patients, and even agranulocytosis has been documented (particularly in HLA-B 08.01 and HLA-AN 31.01 patients). Pulmonary toxicity and positive double-stranded DNA (dsDNA) are occasionally seen, but drug-induced lupus is rare. Reversible infertility occurs in men, but sulfasalazine does not affect fertility in women. The drug appears relatively safe in pregnancy.

TNF-α–BLOCKING AGENTS

TNF-α appears to be particularly important in the inflammatory process associated with rheumatoid arthritis. TNF-α affects cellular function via activation of specific membrane-bound TNF receptors ($TNFR_1$, $TNFR_2$). Five legacy bDMARDs interfering with TNF-α have been approved for the treatment of RA and other rheumatic diseases (Figure 36–4). Biosimilar biologics (bsDMARDs) with lower costs are available in many countries and, at least hypothetically, should decrease cost. The efficacy, toxicity, and immunogenicity of the biosimilars have been found to be equivalent to those of the legacy compounds. TNF-α inhibitors have many adverse effects in common, and these will be treated similarly, with comments for exceptions (see below).

Adalimumab

Mechanism of Action: Adalimumab is a fully human, IgG, anti-TNF monoclonal antibody. This compound complexes with both soluble and membrane-bound TNF and prevents interaction with p55 and p775 cell surface TNF receptors, downregulating macrophage and T-cell function. **Pharmacokinetics:** Adalimumab SC has a half-life of 10–20 days. Absolute bioavailability is 64%. MTX inhibits adalimumab clearance. **Indications and Dosage:** The compound is approved for RA, AS, PsA, JIA, uveitis, hidradenitis suppurativa, plaque psoriasis, Crohn disease, and ulcerative colitis. It decreases the rate of formation of new erosions in RA in both reports and case series. Adalimumab has also been used in Behçet disease, sarcoidosis, and noninfectious uveitis. The usual dose in RA, PsA, and AS is 40 mg every other week, but it is frequently increased to 40 mg weekly (despite the increased cost). In psoriasis, 80 mg is given at week 0, 40 mg at week 1, and then 40 mg every 20 weeks. The initial dose in inflammatory bowel disease is higher: patients receive 160 mg at week 0, 80 mg 2 weeks later, and 40-mg maintenance treatment beyond 8 weeks if they are in remission by that time. Adalimumab dosage depends on body weight in patients with JIA or uveitis. **Adverse Effects:** Adalimumab increases the risk of serious infections—in particular latent TB reactivation, deep fungal infections, worsening or initiation of multiple sclerosis/neurologic diseases, and heart failure. Other uncommon to rare adverse effects include headache, rash, possibly lymphoma, and lupus-like syndrome.

Certolizumab

Mechanism of Action: Certolizumab is a recombinant, humanized antibody Fab fragment conjugated to polyethylene glycol (PEG) with specificity for human TNF-α. Certolizumab neutralizes membrane-bound and soluble TNF-α in a dose-dependent

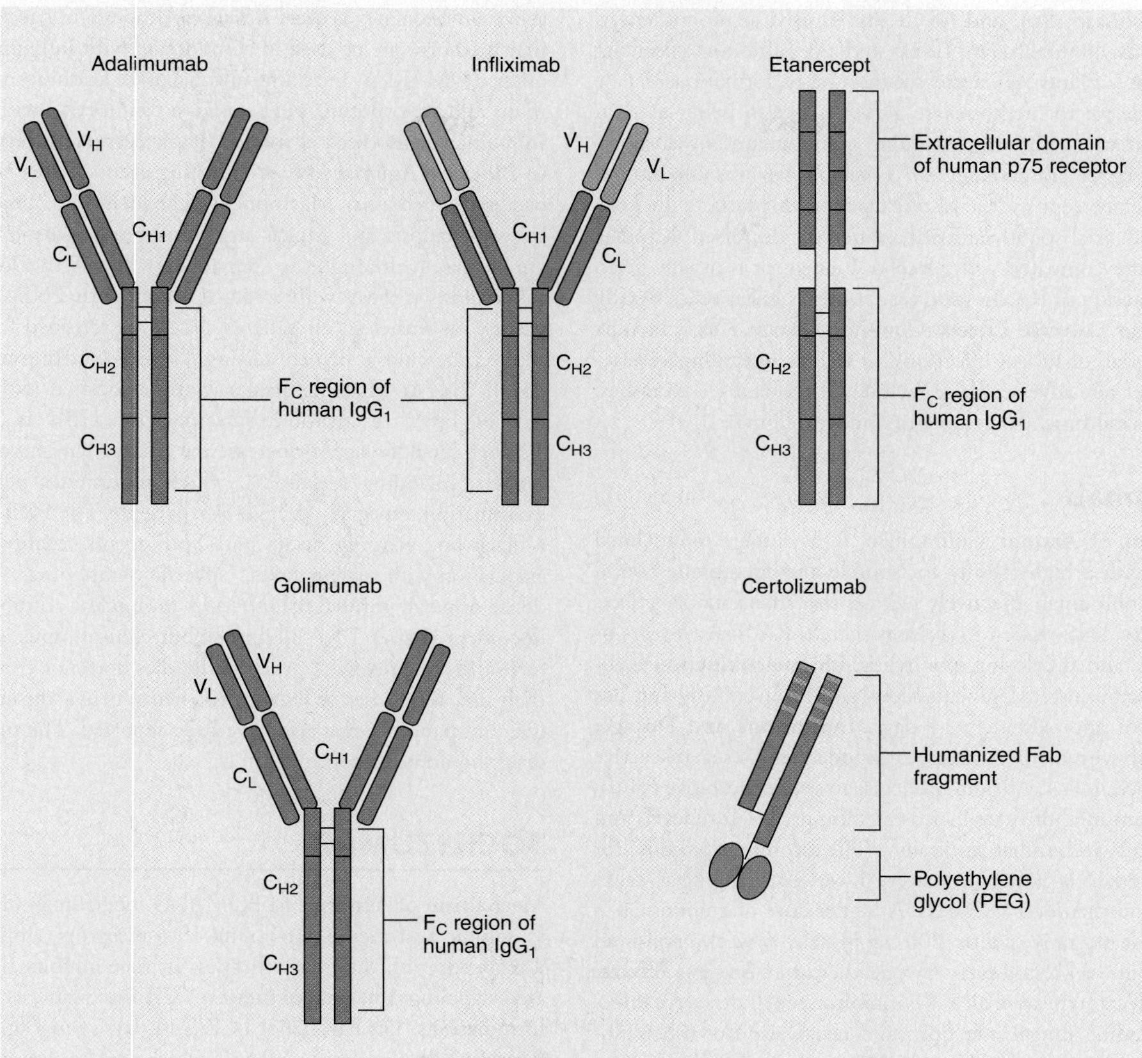

FIGURE 36–4 Structures of TNF-α antagonists used in rheumatoid arthritis. C_H, constant heavy chain; C_L, constant light chain; F_c, complex immunoglobulin region; V_H, variable heavy chain; V_L, variable light chain. Red regions, human derived; blue regions, mouse derived; green regions, polyethylene glycol (PEG).

manner. Additionally, certolizumab does not contain an F_c region and does not fix complement or cause antibody-dependent cell-mediated cytotoxicity in vitro. **Pharmacokinetics:** Certolizumab is given subcutaneously and has a half-life of 14 days. Methotrexate decreases the appearance of anti-certolizumab antibodies. To a very large degree, it does not cross into breast milk or cross the placenta. **Indications and Dosage:** Certolizumab is FDA approved in RA, Crohn disease, plaque psoriasis, PsA, and AS as well as in nonradiographic axial spondyloarthritis. It can be used as monotherapy or in combination with csDMARDs. A trial in moderate to severe MTX-incomplete-responder RA patients comparing adalimumab plus MTX to certolizumab plus MTX showed ACR20 responses at 3 months and achievement of low disease activity at 2 years that were comparable for both treatments. Unfortunately, confounding factors prevent definitive conclusions from this trial. Certolizumab has no to minimal placental transfer from mothers to the fetus, thus suggesting it as a good TNF inhibitor during pregnancy. It also has low to minimal transfer from plasma to breast milk. The usual dose for RA is 400 mg initially and at weeks 2 and 4, followed by 200 mg every other week, or 400 mg every 4 weeks.

Etanercept

Mechanism of action: Etanercept is a recombinant fusion protein consisting of two soluble TNF p75 receptor moieties linked to the F portion of human IgG (see Figure 36-4); it binds TNF and molecules and also inhibits lymphotoxin. **Pharmacokinetics**: After subcutaneous administration, the drug is slowly absorbed, with peak concentrations at 72 hours. **Indications and Dosage**: Etanercept is approved for the treatment of RA, juvenile chronic arthritis, psoriasis, PsA, and AS. It can be used as monotherapy. However, ustekinumab (an IL-12 and 23 inhibitor) receiving methotrexate. Etanercept decreases the rate of formation of new erosions relative to methotrexate alone. It is also being used in other rheumatic syndromes including granulomatosis with polyangiitis (Wegner granulomatosis). Ustekinumab was superior to high-dose etanercept over a 12-week period in psoriasis. In nonradiographic axial spondylarthritis, etanercept decreased sacroiliac MRI erosions compared with placebo. Etanercept is usually given as 50 mg weekly in RA. In psoriasis, 50 mg is given twice weekly for 12 weeks. **Adverse Effects:** Common adverse effects include viral, bacterial, or fungal infections, as well as injection-site reactions. Other rare adverse effects include GI problems, skin rashes, lupus-like syndrome, pancytopenia, and lymphoma.

Golimumab

Mechanism of Action: Golimumab is a human monoclonal antibody with a high affinity for soluble and membrane-bound TNF-α. Golimumab effectively reduces the inflammatory effects produced by TNF-α seen in diseases such as RA, PsA (2 years or older), UC, and ankylosing spondylitis. **Pharmacokinetics:** Golimumab is administered subcutaneously or intravenously and has a half-life of approximately 14 days. **Indications and Dosage:** Golimumab with methotrexate treats moderately to severely active RA. It is used in PsA, AS, and moderate to severe ulcerative colitis. Concomitant methotrexate increases golimumab serum levels and decreases anti-golimumab antibodies. The recommended dose for RA, PsA, and AS is 50 mg given every 4 weeks or 2 mg/kg at weeks 0 and 4, and then every 8 weeks. A higher dose of golimumab is used to treat ulcerative colitis: 200 mg initially at week 0 followed by 100 mg at week 2 and every 4 weeks thereafter. **Adverse Effects:** Adverse effects (typical of all TNF inhibitors) include severe infections (including fungal infections and reactivation of tuberculosis), new onset or exacerbation of CHF, lupus-like syndrome, and worsening or new-onset demyelinated disorders.

Infliximab

Mechanism of Action: Infliximab (see Figure 36–4) is a *E. coli*–derived chimeric (25% mouse, 75% human) IgG monoclonal antibody that binds and inhibits membrane-bound TNF. Its mechanism of action is probably the same as that of adalimumab. **Pharmacokinetics:** The terminal half-life of infliximab is 9–12 days. After intermittent therapy, infliximab elicits human antichimeric antibodies in up to 62% of patients. Concurrent therapy with methotrexate markedly decreases the prevalence of human antichimeric antibodies by 29% at 10 mg. Infliximab treats RA, AS, PsA, Crohn disease, ulcerative colitis, pediatric inflammatory bowel disease, and psoriasis. It is being used off-label in other diseases, including granulomatosis with polyangiitis (Wegener granulomatosis), giant cell arteritis, Behçet disease, and uveitis sarcoidosis. In RA, infliximab plus methotrexate decreases the rate of formation of new erosions. Infliximab is given as an intravenous infusion with induction at 0, 2, and 6 weeks and maintenance infusions every 8 weeks thereafter. Dose range is 3–5 mg/kg, and the usual frequency is every 8 weeks. Although it is recommended that methotrexate be used in conjunction with infliximab, several other csDMARDS, including antimalarials, azathioprine, leflunomide, and cyclosporine, can be used in conjunction with this drug. Infliximab is also used as monotherapy. **Adverse Effects of TNF-α–Blocking Agents:** TNF-α–blocking agents increase the risk of bacterial infections. Macrophage-dependent infections (including tuberculosis and fungal and other opportunistic infections) are increased, although they remain very low. Activation of latent tuberculosis is lower with etanercept than with TNF-α–blocking agents. Nevertheless, all patients should be screened for latent or active tuberculosis before starting TNF-α–blocking agents. The use of TNF-α–blocking agents is also associated with increased risk of HBV reactivation; screening for HBV is important. TNF-α–blocking agents increase the risk for lymphoma and skin cancers, including melanoma, which necessitates periodic skin examination, especially in high-risk patients. The FDA has placed a black box warning on all anti-TNF agents regarding possible association with malignancies, especially lymphomas. A low incidence of newly formed dsDNA and antinuclear antibodies is well documented after TNF inhibitors, but clinical lupus is extremely rare, and the presence of such antibodies does not contraindicate their use. Rare cases of leukopenia, neutropenia, thrombocytopenia, and pancytopenia also have been reported. The precipitating drug should be discontinued.

TOCILIZUMAB

Mechanism of Action: The bDMARD tocilizumab (TCZ) binds to soluble and membrane-bound IL-6 receptors, similar to sarilumab but with different affinities. It, too, inhibits IL-6– mediated signaling. **Pharmacokinetics:** TCZ is available as IV and SC formulations. The half-life of TCZ is 11 days (4 mg/kg) to 13 days (8 mg/kg). It stimulates CYP 450, which may be clinically relevant for drugs such as cyclosporine or warfarin, and dosage adjustment of these medications may be needed. **Indications and Dosage:** TCZ is available for rheumatoid arthritis, systemic sclerosis–associated interstitial lung disease, and giant cell arteritis (GCA) as well as active systemic JIA in patients >2 years old. TCZ can be used in combination with csDMARDs or as monotherapy in RA. It is clinically superior to adalimumab in methotrexate incomplete responders. In GCA, TCZ 162 mg subcutaneously every 1–2 weeks, combined with a 26-week prednisone taper, was effective to sustain glucocorticoid-free remission. In a phase 3 trial in patients with systemic sclerosis–associated interstitial lung disease, TCZ 162 mg was administered SC once every week. In the USA, RA dosing starts at 4 mg/kg IV and may be increased up to 8 mg/kg (maximum 800 mg). A clinical study successfully treated adult patients with COVID-19 pneumonia at a dose of 8 mg/kg IV. In Europe, the starting dose is 8 mg/kg with the same maximum dose. Subcutaneous dosing is 162 mg every 1–2 weeks. **Adverse Effects:** The most common adverse reactions are upper respiratory tract infections, headache, hypertension, and elevated liver enzymes. Serious infections including tuberculosis (prescreening requirement) and fungal, viral, and other opportunistic infections and thrombocytopenia occur occasionally, and lipids should be monitored. GI perforation has been reported when using tocilizumab or TNF inhibitors in patients with diverticulitis, although this is probably associated with glucocorticoid use, rather than TCZ per se. The manufacturer recommends discontinuing tocilizumab therapy if the ALT or AST reach 5 times the ULN, ANC <500 cells/mm^3, or platelets <50,000 cells/mm^3 (more closely associated with corticosteroids than TCZ or TNF inhibitors). Demyelinating disorders including multiple sclerosis are rarely associated with tocilizumab use. Fewer than 1% of patients treated with tocilizumab develop anaphylactic reactions. Anti-tocilizumab antibodies develop in 2% of the patients, and these can be associated with hypersensitivity reactions requiring discontinuation.

USTEKINUMAB

Mechanism of Action: Ustekinumab is a fully human IgG monoclonal IL-12 and IL-23 antagonist at the p-40 protein subunit. Ustekinumab prevents the binding of the p40 subunit of both IL-12 and IL-23 to IL-12RBI, which is found on the surface of CD4 T cells and NK cells and suppresses the formation of proinflammatory TH1 and TH17 cells. **Pharmacokinetics:** Ustekinumab's bioavailability is 57% following SC injection; time to peak plasma concentration is 7–13.5 days and elimination half-life is 21 days. **Indications and Dosage:** Ustekinumab is indicated for treatment of adult patients with PsA as monotherapy or in combination with methotrexate. Other indications include plaque psoriasis, UC, and Crohn disease. It is used as an off-label treatment for giant cell arteritis, Behçet disease, SLE, pyoderma gangrenosum, Takayasu arteritis, lichen planus, synovitis, pustulosis, and atopic dermatitis. Ustekinumab was not effective in axial spondylarthritis. Ustekinumab is used at 45 or 90 mg >100 kg at 0 and 4 weeks and is followed by maintenance doses of 45–90 mg once every 12 weeks. IV infusion as a 260- to 520-mg initial dose followed by 90 mg SC is available for Crohn disease and UC. **Adverse Effects:** Upper respiratory tract infection is the most common side effect, but rare severe infection, malignancy, cryptogenic organizing pneumonia, interstitial or eosinophilic pneumonia, and reversible posterior leukoencephalopathy syndrome have been reported. Ustekinumab should be discontinued ≥15 weeks before live vaccines are administered and can be resumed 2 weeks after.

COMBINATION THERAPY WITH DMARDs

The 2015 ACR guidelines for the treatment of rheumatoid arthritis strongly recommend the use of combination traditional DMARDs (eg, methotrexate, hydroxychloroquine, azathioprine) or addition of TNF inhibitors, non-TNF biologics, or small molecules for patients with RA and moderate or high disease activity refractory to DMARD monotherapy. Combinations of DMARDs can be designed rationally on the basis of complementary mechanisms of action, nonoverlapping pharmacokinetics, and nonoverlapping toxicities. When added to methotrexate background therapy, cyclosporine, chloroquine, hydroxychloroquine, leflunomide, infliximab, adalimumab, rituximab, and etanercept have all shown improved efficacy. Triple therapy with methotrexate, sulfasalazine, and hydroxychloroquine appears to be as effective, clinically, as etanercept and methotrexate, but radiologic outcomes may not be as good. In contrast, azathioprine or sulfasalazine plus methotrexate results in no additional therapeutic benefit. Other combinations have occasionally been used. While it might be anticipated that combination therapy could result in more toxicity, this is often not the case. Combination therapy for patients not responding adequately to monotherapy is now the rule in the treatment of RA.

BIOSIMILARS

Biosimilars are biologic medications that are very similar in properties and actions to existing biologic medications, ie, they are designed to be generic versions of the original biologic molecule. These drugs offer a potential reduction in cost of bDMARDs thereby improving accessibility of these medications to patients. Thus far, these drugs appear to have the same efficacy and toxicity as the legacy compounds and the same degree of immunogenicity.

GLUCOCORTICOID DRUGS (LIMITED TO RHEUMATIC DISEASES)

The general pharmacology of corticosteroids, including mechanism of action, pharmacokinetics, and other applications, as discussed in Chapter 39. **Indications:** Corticosteroids are chronically used in 30–70% of RA patients. Their effects are prompt and dramatic, and they are capable of slowing the appearance of new bone erosions. Corticosteroids may be administered for certain serious extra-articular manifestations of RA such as pericarditis or eye involvement or during periods of exacerbation. When prednisone is required for long-term therapy of RA, the dosage should not exceed 7.5 mg daily, and gradual reduction of the dose should be encouraged. Even doses as low as 2.8 mg prednisone daily over more than 5 years are associated with severe infections. Alternate-day corticosteroid therapy is usually unsuccessful in RA. Other rheumatic diseases in which the corticosteroids' potent anti-inflammatory effects may be useful include vasculitis, SLE, polyangiitis with granulomatosis, PA, giant cell arteritis, sarcoidosis, and gout. Intra-articular corticosteroids are often helpful to alleviate painful symptoms for up to several months. A recent approach uses delayed-release prednisone for the treatment of early morning stiffness and pain in RA. By releasing a pulse of prednisone between 2:00 AM and 4:00 AM, the circadian inflammatory cytokine are decreased. At low doses of 3–5 mg prednisone, the adrenal-pituitary axis does not seem to be impacted. Adrenal function generally recovers by the slow tapering of glucocorticoids, although symptoms independent of adrenal insufficiency may occur at dose as low as 1 mg daily prednisone. **Adverse Effects:** Adverse effect seen are both dose- and time-dependent: weight gain and epistaxis at >5 mg daily; glaucoma, depression, and hypertension at

>7.8 mg daily. Prolonged use of corticosteroids leads to serious and disabling toxic effects as described in Chapter 39. Many of these adverse effects occur at doses below 7.5 mg prednisone equivalent daily, and some data show 3 mg or fewer daily. Prednisone can cause effects when used over prolonged periods. Most common adverse effect on long-term glucocorticoids include osteoporosis, myopathy, osteonecrosis, hyperglycemia, Cushing syndrome, life-threatening infections, fluid retention, impaired wound healing, skin thinning and atrophy, increased risk of cataract, glaucoma, gastric ulcer, and depression.

■ OTHER ANALGESICS

Acetaminophen (also known as **paracetamol**) is one of the most important drugs used in the treatment of mild to moderate pain when an anti-inflammatory effect is not necessary. **Phenacetin** (acetophenetidin), a prodrug that is metabolized to acetaminophen, is more toxic and should not be used.

ACETAMINOPHEN

Mechanism of Action: Acetaminophen is the active metabolite of phenacetin and is responsible for its analgesic effect. It is a weak COX-1 and COX-2 inhibitor in peripheral tissues. Its antinociceptive effects are also due to interactions with the endogenous opioid, cannabinoid, and serotonergic systems. Acetaminophen is antipyretic but possesses no significant anti-inflammatory effects. **Pharmacokinetics:** Acetaminophen is administered orally and is also available for IV injection. After oral administration peak blood concentrations are usually reached in 30–60 minutes. Acetaminophen is poorly bound to plasma proteins and is partially metabolized by hepatic microsomal enzymes to the inactive sulfate and glucuronide (see Figure 4–5). Less than 5% is excreted unchanged. In large doses, a minor but highly reactive metabolite (*N*-acetyl-*p*-benzoquinone) is important because it is toxic to both liver and kidney (see Chapter 4). The half-life of acetaminophen is 2–3 hours and is relatively unaffected by renal function. With toxic doses or liver disease, the half-life may be increased twofold or more.

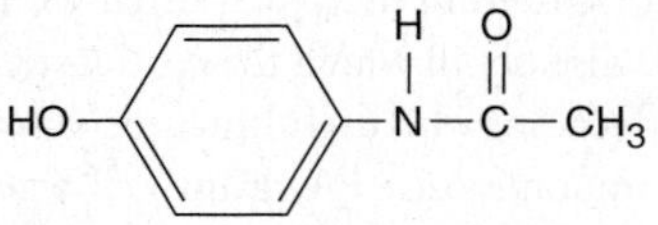

$$HO-C_6H_4-N(H)-C(=O)-CH_3$$

Indications and Dosage: Acetaminophen is said to be equivalent to aspirin as an analgesic and antipyretic agent. It does not affect uric acid levels and lacks platelet-inhibiting effects. The drug is useful in mild to moderate pain such as headache, myalgia, postpartum pain, and other circumstances in which aspirin is an effective analgesic. Acetaminophen alone is inadequate therapy for inflammatory conditions such as RA. For mild analgesia, acetaminophen is the preferred drug in patients allergic to aspirin, when salicylates are poorly tolerated. It is preferable to aspirin in patients with hemophilia, in those with a history of peptic ulcer, and in those in whom bronchospasm is precipitated by aspirin. Unlike aspirin, acetaminophen does not antagonize the effects of uricosuric agents. Recently, acetaminophen has been combined with an NSAID for better pain management; however, this can potentiate the gastrointestinal toxicity of the NSAID. Acute pain and fever may be effectively treated with 325–500 mg four times daily and proportionately less for children. Dosing in adults is recommended not to exceed 4 g/d in most cases. **Adverse Effects:** In therapeutic doses, a mild reversible increase in hepatic enzymes may occasionally occur. With larger doses, dizziness, excitement, and disorientation may occur. Ingestion of 15 g of acetaminophen may be fatal, death being caused by severe hepatotoxicity with centrilobular necrosis, sometimes associated with acute renal tubular necrosis (see Chapters 4 and 58). Present data indicate that even 4 g acetaminophen is associated with increased liver function test abnormalities. Early symptoms of hepatic damage include nausea, vomiting, diarrhea, and abdominal pain. Cases of renal damage without hepatic damage have occurred, even after usual doses of acetaminophen. High doses of acetaminophen can promote oxidative stress and damage cells in the brain. For overdose, in addition to supportive therapy, one should provide sulfhydryl groups in the form of acetylcysteine to neutralize the toxic metabolites (see Chapter 58). Hemolytic anemia, methemoglobinemia, anaphylaxis, and serious skin reactions are very rare adverse events. Interstitial nephritis and papillary necrosis—serious complications of phenacetin—have *not* occurred. Caution is necessary in patients with any type of liver disease, significant alcohol consumption, or malnutrition (prolonged fasting, anorexia).

KETOROLAC

Mechanism of Action: Ketorolac is an analgesic NSAID that decreases inflammation by inhibiting the cyclooxygenase (COX) enzyme; unlike the NSAIDs discussed earlier, it is used almost exclusively as an analgesic. **Pharmacokinetics:** It can be administered intravenously, intramuscularly, intranasally, orally, or as an ophthalmic; it has a half-life of 5–6 hours. Ketorolac is partly metabolized by the liver and about 90% is excreted by the kidneys, with 60% unchanged. **Indications and Dosage:** It can be used as an adjuvant with opioids, other nonopioid analgesics, local anesthetics, and other NSAIDs for pain relief. The recommended initial dose is 30 mg IV, 60 mg IM, or one 15.75-mg spray in each nostril, then 15–30 mg given every 6–8 hours and a maximum daily dose of 120 mg. The initial dose should not be administered orally; an IV or IM dose should be given first, then 10 mg PO every 6 hours. All doses should be halved in those older than 65, with a body mass less than 50 kg, or with renal impairment. **Adverse Effects:** Toxicities are similar to those of other NSAIDs (see page 676), although renal toxicity is more common with chronic use. It has less toxicity than morphine, but its use should not exceed 5 days.

TRAMADOL

Mechanism of Action: Tramadol is a centrally acting synthetic analgesic with a weak affinity for μ-opioid receptors (see Chapter 31). It also acts on serotonin (5-HT) and norepinephrine receptors by reuptake inhibition. **Indications and Dosage**: Tramadol is used in the treatment of acute and chronic pain but does not have significant anti-inflammatory effects. The dose is up to 300mg a day with an elimination half-life of about 6 hours. **Adverse Effects**: Tramadol has fewer side effects and lower addiction potential than classic opioids. Tramadol's most common side effects include nausea, vomiting, vertigo, dizziness, tiredness, sedation, dry mouth, constipation and sweating which tends to occur during the initial treatment period. Other adverse effects include serotonin syndrome, seizures, exacerbated anticoagulant effect, and angioedema.

DRUGS USED IN GOUT

Gout is a metabolic disease characterized by recurrent episodes of acute arthritis due to deposits of monosodium urate in joints and cartilage. Uric acid renal calculi, tophi, and interstitial nephritis also may occur. Adverse cardiovascular outcomes are becoming more evident as well. Gout is usually associated with a high serum uric acid level (hyperuricemia), a poorly soluble substance that is the major end product of purine metabolism. In most mammals, uricase converts acid to the more soluble allantoin; uricase is absent in humans. While clinical gouty episodes are associated with hyperuricemia, most individuals with hyperuricemia never develop a clinical event from urate crystal deposition.

The treatment of gout aims to relieve acute gouty attacks and prevent recurrent gouty episodes and urate lithiasis. Therapies for acute gout are based on our current understanding of the pathophysiologic events that occur in this disease (Figure 36–5). Clinical gout is dependent on a macromolecular complex of proteins, called NLRP3, which regulates the activation of IL-1. Urate crystals activate NLRP3, resulting in release of prostaglandins and lysosomal enzymes by synoviocytes. Attracted by these chemotactic mediators, polymorphonuclear leukocytes migrate into the joint space

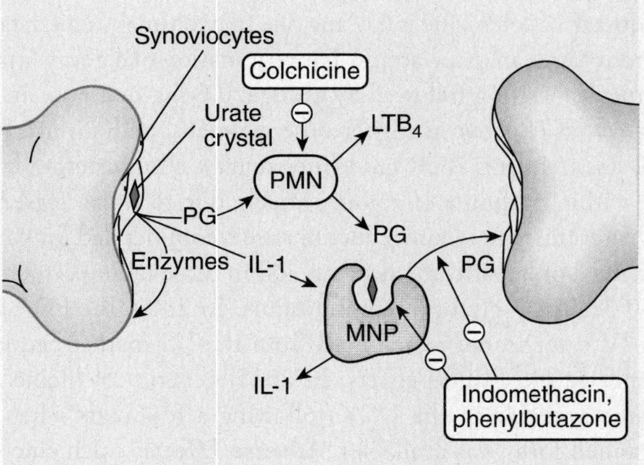

FIGURE 36–5 Pathophysiologic events in a gouty joint. Synoviocytes phagocytose urate crystals and then secrete inflammatory mediators, which attract and activate polymorphonuclear leukocytes (PMN) and mononuclear phagocytes (MNP) (macrophages). Drugs active in gout inhibit crystal phagocytosis and polymorphonuclear leukocyte and macrophage release of inflammatory mediators. PG, prostaglandin; IL-1, interleukin-1; LTB_4, leukotriene B_4.

and amplify the ongoing inflammatory process. In the later phases of the attack, increased numbers of mononuclear phagocytes (macrophages) appear, ingest the urate crystals, and release more inflammatory mediators.

Before starting chronic urate-lowering therapy for gout, patients in whom hyperuricemia is associated with gout and urate lithiasis must be clearly distinguished from individuals with only hyperuricemia. The efficacy of long-term drug treatment in an asymptomatic hyperuricemic person is unproven. Although there are data suggesting a clear relationship between the degree of uric acid elevation and the likelihood of clinical gout, in some individuals, uric acid levels may be elevated up to two standard deviations above the mean for a lifetime without adverse consequences. Many different agents have been used for the treatment of acute and chronic gout. However, nonadherence to these drugs is exceedingly common; adherence has been documented to be 18–26% in younger patients. Providers should be aware of compliance as an important issue.

ALLOPURINOL

Mechanism of Action: Xanthine oxidase is responsible for the conversion of xanthine and hypoxanthine to uric acid. Allopurinol is a purine analogue that inhibits this enzyme, resulting in a fall in the plasma urate level and a decrease in the overall urate burden. The result of xanthine oxidase inhibition is a build-up of its substrates, the more soluble xanthine and hypoxanthine. **Pharmacokinetics**: The structure of allopurinol, an isomer of hypoxanthine, is shown in Figure 36–7. Allopurinol is approximately 80% absorbed after oral administration and has a terminal serum half-life of 1–2 hours. Allopurinol is metabolized by xanthine oxidase to alloxanthine (oxypurinol) with a half-life of 15 hours, which also inhibits xanthine oxidase; its duration of action is >24 hours so that allopurinol is given only once a day. It is renally cleared. **Indications and Dosage**: Allopurinol is often the first-line agent for the treatment of chronic gout in the period between attacks, and it tends to prolong the intercritical period. Therapy is continued for years if not for life. When initiating allopurinol, colchicine or an NSAID should be used until steady state serum uric acid is normalized or decreased to <6 mg/dL in patients with gout and <5 mg/dL in patients with tophaceous gout, and an NSAID or colchicine should be continued for 6 months or longer. Thereafter, colchicine or the NSAID can be cautiously stopped while continuing allopurinol therapy. The recommended initial dosage of allopurinol is 100 mg/d. It should be titrated upward by 100 mg/d every 2–5 weeks until serum uric acid <6 mg/dL or 800 mg/d is reached. For those with chronic kidney disease, the initial dose should not be >50 mg/d and the titrations should be of 50 mg/d. **Adverse Effects**: In addition to precipitating gout (the reason for concomitant use of colchicine or NSAID), GI intolerance (including nausea, vomiting, and diarrhea), peripheral neuritis, necrotizing vasculitis, bone marrow suppression, and aplastic anemia may rarely occur. Hepatic toxicity and interstitial nephritis have been reported. A current tenant allergic skin reaction characterized by pruritic lesions occurs in 3% of patients. Isolated cases of exfoliative dermatitis have been reported. In very rare cases, allopurinol has become bound to the lens, resulting in cataracts. Allopurinol hypersensitivity syndrome (AHS) is very rare but can be lethal. AHS is characterized by Stevens-Johnson syndrome and toxic epidermal necrolysis, eosinophils leukocytes, fever, hepatitis, and renal failure. These symptoms typically occur within 2–4 weeks after starting therapy, and the FDA recommends allopurinol to be stopped at the first sign of a rash. Factors that increase the risk for AHAS are higher starting doses; renal dysfunction; concomitant use of diuretics, amoxicillin, or ampicillin; and HLA-B 5801 genotype. The FDA recommends that patients of Han Chinese, Korean, or Thai descent should be screened for the HLA-B 5801 genotype (because of the high prevalence in these populations), and allopurinol should not be used with a positive test. When chemotherapeutic purines (eg, azathioprine) are given concomitantly with allopurinol, dosage must be reduced by 75%. Allopurinol may also increase the effect of cyclophosphamide. Allopurinol inhibits the metabolism of probenecid and oral anticoagulants and may increase hepatic iron concentration. Allopurinol should not be stopped during flare since it may worsen the attack recovery and may take longer. Safety in children and during pregnancy has not been established.

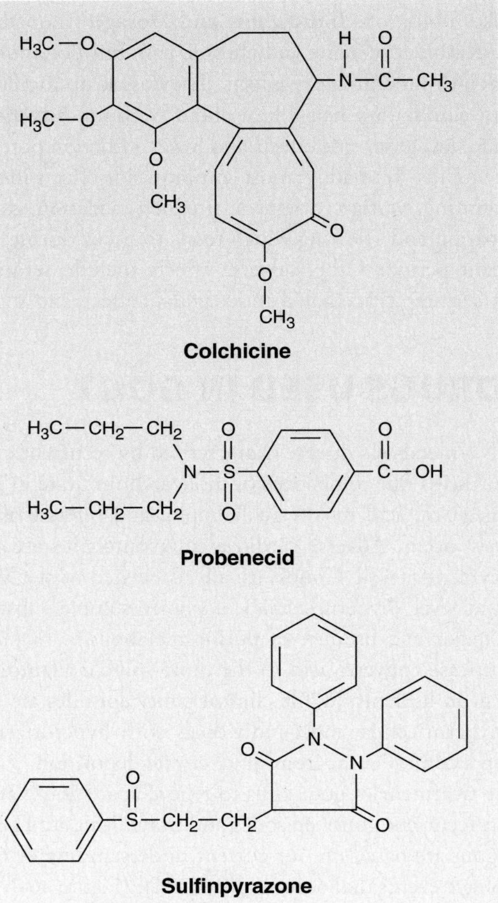

COLCHICINE

Although NSAIDs, corticosteroids, or colchicine are now first-line drugs for acute gout, colchicine was the primary treatment for many years. It can be taken with or without food and is sometimes given in combination with NSAIDs. Colchicine is an alkaloid isolated from the autumn crocus, *Colchicum autumnale*. Its structure is shown in Figure 36–6. **Mechanism of Action**: Colchicine relieves the pain and inflammation of gouty arthritis in 12–24 hours without altering urate metabolism or excretion and without other analgesic effects. By binding to the intracellular protein tubulin, it prevents polymerization into microtubules, resulting in inhibition of leukocyte migration and phagocytosis. It also disrupts the function of caspase-1-activating cryopyrin inflammasome (thus decreasing the formation of IL-1β and IL-18), inhibits the formation of leukotriene B_4, decreases the levels of IFN-α and IL-6, and decreases TNF-α receptor expression on macrophages. Several of colchicine's adverse effects are produced by its inhibition of tubulin polymerization and cell mitosis. **Pharmacokinetics:** Colchicine is absorbed readily after oral administration, reaches peak plasma levels within 2 hours, and is eliminated with a serum half-life of 9 hours. It is not removed by hemodialysis because it is extensively bound to tissues (and has a large volume of distribution); thus, dose reduction in these gout patients is recommended. **Indications and Dosage**: Colchicine is indicated for acute gout and is also used between attacks (the "intercritical period") for prolonged prophylaxis (at low doses) of flares during urate-lowering treatment initiation. It prevents attacks of acute Mediterranean fever and may have a mild beneficial effect in sarcoid arthritis and in hepatic cirrhosis. Colchicine is also used to treat pseudogout, Behçet disease, epidermolysis bullosa acquisita, leukocytoclastic vasculitis, Sweet syndrome, pericarditis, pleurisy, and coronary

FIGURE 36–6 Colchicine and uricosuric drugs.

artery disease, probably due to its anti-inflammatory effect. It is no longer used intravenously. In prophylaxis (the most common use), the dosage of colchicine is 0.6. mg one to two times a daily, starting 12 hours after an acute attack. For termination of a gouty attack, a regimen of 1.2 mg followed by a single 0.6-mg oral dose an hour later was as effective as higher-dose regimens, and adverse events were less frequent. ACR guidelines suggest administering colchicine within 36 hours of a gouty attack, due to its decreased efficacy after this time. Dose reductions are recommended for patients with renal or hepatic impairment, and in those taking cytochrome P450 3A4 or P-glycoprotein inhibitors. In 2009, the FDA asked that IV cytochrome be removed from the US market because of possible severe adverse effects. In 2015, generic colchicine again became available in the USA (following a few years when only a branded form was available). **Adverse Effects:** colchicine often causes diarrhea and may occasionally cause nausea, vomiting, and abdominal pain. CNS symptoms such as fatigue and headache also are observed. Hepatic necrosis, increase in LFTs, pharyngolaryngeal pain, acute renal failure, disseminated intravascular coagulation, and seizures also have been observed. Colchicine may rarely cause hair loss and bone marrow depression, as well as peripheral neuritis, myopathy, rhabdomyolysis, and even death. The more severe adverse events have been associated with the intravenous administration of colchicine, although these effects can also occur (very rarely) after oral use.

FEBUXOSTAT

Mechanism of Action: Febuxostat is a potent and selective non-purine inhibitor of xanthine oxidase (Figure 36–7), thereby reducing the formation of xanthine and uric acid without affecting other enzymes in the purine or pyrimidine metabolic pathway. **Pharmacokinetics:** Febuxostat is more than 80% absorbed following oral administration. Maximum concentration is achieved in approximately 1 hour, and although it has a half-life of 4–8 hours, once-daily dosing is effective. Febuxostat is extensively metabolized in the liver. The drug and its inactive metabolites appear in the urine, with <5% appearing as unchanged drug. **Indications and Dosage:** Febuxostat is approved at doses of 40 or 80 mg daily to treat chronic hyperuricemia in gout patients, with a target of serum uric acid level of <6.0 mg/dL. Although 80–120 mg was more effective than 300 mg daily allopurinol as urate-lowering therapy, 300 mg allopurinol daily does not reflect the actual dosing regimens used in clinical practice. The urate-lowering effect is similar to that of allopurinol, regardless of the cause of hyperuricemia (overproduction or underexcretion). Febuxostat and allopurinol both appear renoprotective over long treatment periods, although adherence issues cloud most results. Febuxostat may be tried in patients with a prior hypersensitivity reaction to allopurinol; however, a reaction with febuxostat may still occur. Unlike allopurinol, febuxostat appears safe in patients with moderate chronic kidney disease. However, there are no data for the safety of febuxostat in patients with severe renal impairment. It is primarily considered an alternative for those who are intolerant or did not respond to allopurinol. Because there was concern for cardiovascular events in the original phase 3 trials, the FDA approved only 40-mg and 80-mg daily doses (not the 120-mg dose used in some trials). **Adverse Effects:** Initial concerns about increased MACE when using febuxostat have not been born out. As with allopurinol, prophylactic treatment with colchicine or NSAIDs should be started at the beginning of therapy to avoid gout flares. The most frequent treatment-related adverse events are liver function abnormalities, diarrhea, headache, and nausea. Febuxostat is well tolerated in patients with a history of allopurinol intolerance. Rashes can occur but are dose dependent.

NSAIDs IN GOUT

Mechanism of Action: In addition to inhibiting prostaglandin synthase, NSAIDs inhibit urate crystal phagocytosis and reduce inflammation and pain in acute gout flare. **Pharmacokinetics:** Aspirin is not used because it causes renal retention of uric acid at lower doses (≤2.6 g/d); it is uricosuric at doses >3.6 g/d. **Indications and Dosage:** All NSAIDs except aspirin, salicylates, and tolmetin have been successfully used to treat acute gouty episodes. Oxaprozin, which also lowers serum uric acid, is hypothetically a good choice and all NSAIDs appear to be as effective and safe as the older drugs like indomethacin. **Adverse Effects:** Side effects associated with NSAID use include gastrointestinal, cardiovascular, and renal events. Selective COX-2 inhibitors have been associated with fewer adverse effects than other NSAIDs.

PEGLOTICASE

Mechanism of Action: Pegloticase is a recombinant mammalian urate oxidase (uricase) that is covalently attached to a methoxy polyethylene glycol (mPEG) to prolong the circulating half-life

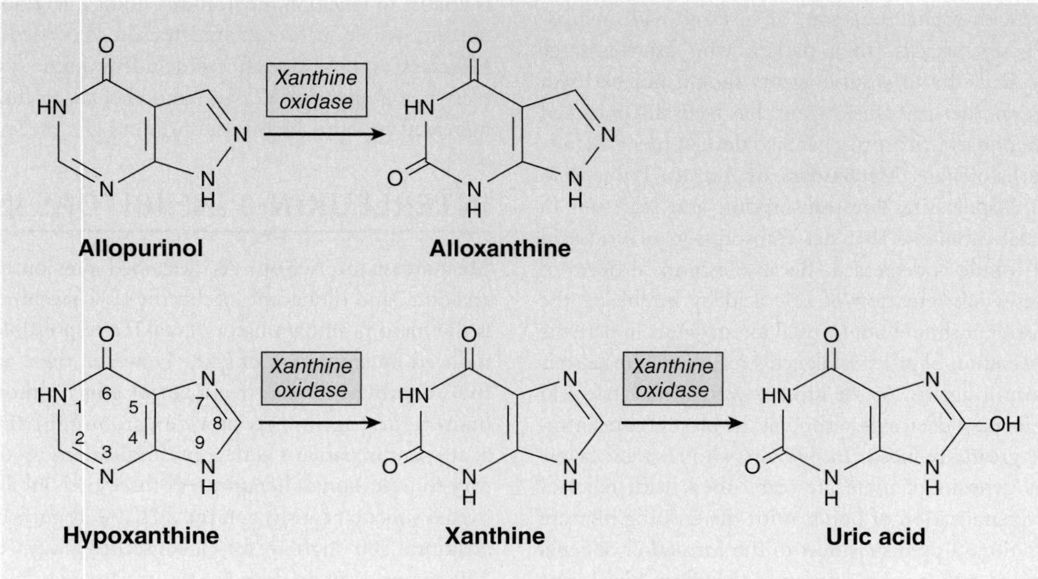

FIGURE 36–7 Inhibition of uric acid synthesis by allopurinol occurs because allopurinol and alloxanthine inhibit xanthine oxidase. (Reproduced with permission from Meyers FH, Jawetz E, Goldfien A: *Review of Medical Pharmacology*, 7th ed. McGraw Hill, 1980.)

and diminish immunogenic responses. Urate oxidase enzyme, absent in humans and some higher primates, converts uric acid to allantoin. Allantoin is highly soluble and can be easily eliminated by the kidneys. **Pharmacokinetics:** It is a rapidly acting drug, achieving a peak effect (decline in uric acid level) within 24–72 hours. The serum half-life ranges from 6 to 14 days. Several studies have shown earlier clearance of PEG-uricase (mean of 11 days vs 16 days) due to antibody production. **Indications and Dosage:** Pegloticase monotherapy and with methotrexate are FDA approved as urate-lowering therapy in symptomatic gout and effectively decrease tophi. Pegloticase lowers urate levels for up to 21 days after a single IV infusion at doses of 4–12 mg, allowing for IV dosing every 2 weeks. Pegloticase should not be used for asymptomatic hyperuricemia. The recommended dose for pegloticase is 8 mg IV every 2 weeks. To prevent infusion reactions, patients should be premedicated with a corticosteroid and antihistamine. **Adverse Effects:** Gout flare can occur during treatment with pegloticase, especially during the first 3–6 months of treatment, requiring prophylaxis with NSAIDs or colchicine. When used with methotrexate, most allergic reactions are abrogated, and efficacy is increased. Mycophenolate mofetil has also been used for the same purpose. Nephrolithiasis, arthralgia, muscle spasm, headache, anemia, and nausea may occur. Other less frequent side effects include upper respiratory tract infection, urinary tract infection, peripheral edema, and diarrhea. There is some concern for hemolytic anemia in patients with glucose-6-phosphate dehydrogenase deficiency because the formation of hydrogen peroxide by uricase is feared; therefore, pegloticase should be avoided in these patients.

PROBENECID AND LESINURAD

Probenecid and **lesinurad** (the latter withdrawn in the USA in 2019) are uricosuric drugs employed to decrease the body pool of urate in patients with tophaceous gout or in those with increasingly frequent gouty attacks. In a patient who excretes large amounts of uric acid, the uricosuric agents should not be used. **Sulfinpyrazone,** another uricosuric agent, has been discontinued in the USA. Other novel uricosuric agents in development include verinurad and arhalofenate. **Mechanism of Action:** Probenecid inhibits active transport sites for reabsorption and secretion in the proximal renal tubule so that net reabsorption of uric acid in the proximal tubule is decreased. Because aspirin in doses of <2.6 g daily causes net retention of uric acid by inhibiting the secretory transporter, it should not be used for analgesia in patients with gout. The secretion of other weak acids (eg, penicillin) also is reduced by uricosuric agents. As the urinary excretion of uric acid increases, the urate pool decreases, although the plasma concentration may not be greatly reduced. In patients who respond favorably, tophaceous deposits of urate are reabsorbed, with relief of arthritis and remineralization of bone. With the ensuing increase in uric acid excretion, a predisposition to the formation of renal stones is augmented rather than decreased; therefore, high urine volume should be maintained and at least early in treatment, the urine pH should be kept above 6.0 by the administration of alkali.

Pharmacokinetics: Probenecid is an organic acid (see Figure 36–6) and acts at the anion transport sites of the renal tubule (see Chapter 15). Probenecid is completely reabsorbed by the renal tubules and is metabolized slowly with a terminal serum half-life of 5–8 hours. **Indications and Dosage:** Uricosuric therapy should be initiated in gouty patients with underexcretion of uric acid when allopurinol or febuxostat is contraindicated or when tophi are present. Therapy should not be started until 2–3 weeks after an acute attack. Probenecid can be used as monotherapy or in combination with a xanthine oxidase inhibitor (eg, allopurinol or febuxostat). Probenecid is usually started at a dosage of 0.5 g orally daily in divided doses, progressing to 1 g daily after 1 week. It is essential to maintain a large urine volume to minimize the possibility of stone formation. **Adverse Effects:** Organic acids cause GI irritation. A rash may appear after the use of probenecid, as may nephrotic syndrome. Probenecid may rarely cause aplastic anemia.

GLUCOCORTICOIDS IN GOUT

Mechanism of Action: As described in Chapter 39, corticosteroids decrease activation, proliferation, and survival of various inflammatory cells. Additionally, they decrease the migration of neutrophils, and they inhibit prostaglandins and proinflammatory cytokines such as IL-1β. **Indications and Dosage:** Corticosteroids are a good alternative for patients in whom NSAIDs or colchicine are contraindicated and in those with renal impairment or chronic kidney disease. Corticosteroids are sometimes used in the treatment of severe symptomatic gout by oral, intra-articular, systemic, or subcutaneous routes. The most commonly used oral corticosteroid is prednisone. The recommended oral dose is 30–50 mg/d for 1–2 days, tapered over 7–10 days; a methylprednisolone dose pack also may be prescribed. Intra-articular injection of 10 mg (small joints), 30 mg (wrist, ankle, elbow), and 40 mg (knee) of triamcinolone acetonide or methylprednisolone can be given if the patient is unable to take oral medications. Joint infection should be ruled out, if possible, before administration of corticosteroids. **Adverse Effects:** Common side effects include immune system suppression (very rare if given for <7 days), mood changes, fluid retention, and increased appetite, blood pressure, and glucose levels.

INTERLEUKIN-1 INHIBITORS IN GOUT

Mechanism of Action: As described previously, canakinumab, anakinra, and rilonacept inhibit the IL-1 receptor pathway. IL-1β is the main proinflammatory cytokine responsible for the crystal-induced inflammation of gout. However, these agents are not yet FDA approved for the treatment of gout. Although the data are limited, these agents may provide a promising treatment option for acute gout in patients with contraindications to, or who are refractory to, traditional therapies. All three IL-1 inhibitors are administered subcutaneously, and the 2012 ACR guidelines recommend anakinra 100 mg/day for 3 consecutive days or canakinumab 150 mg as a single dose for the treatment of acute gout. These medications are also being evaluated as therapies for prevention of gout flares while initiating urate-lowering therapy.

PREPARATIONS AVAILABLE

GENERIC NAME	AVAILABLE AS
NONSTEROIDAL ANTI-INFLAMMATORY DRUGS	
Aspirin, acetylsalicylic acid	Generic, others
Bromfenac	Various
Celecoxib	Generic, Celebrex
Choline salicylate	Various
Diclofenac	Generic, Voltaren, others
Diflunisal	Generic, others
Etodolac	Generic, others
Fenoprofen	Generic, others
Flurbiprofen	Generic, others, Ocufen (ophthalmic)
Ibuprofen	Generic, Advil (OTC), Nuprin (OTC), others
Indomethacin	Generic, Indocin
Ketoprofen	Generic, others
Magnesium salicylate	Doan's Pills, Magan, Mobidin
Meclofenamate sodium	Generic
Mefenamic acid	Generic, others
Meloxicam	Generic, others
Nabumetone	Generic
Naproxen	Generic (OTC), others, Aleve (OTC)
Oxaprozin	Generic, others
Piroxicam	Generic, others
Salicylsalicylic acid	Generic, others
Sodium salicylate	Generic
Sodium thiosalicylate	Generic, others
Sulindac	Generic, others
Tolmetin	Generic, others
DISEASE-MODIFYING ANTIRHEUMATIC DRUGS	
Abatacept	Orencia
Adalimumab	Humira
Anakinra	Kineret
Auranofin	Ridaura
Aurothioglucose	Solganal
Baricitinib	Olumiant
Belimumab	Benlysta
Canakinumab	Ilaris
Certolizumab	Cimzia
Cyclophosphamide	Generic, Cytoxan
Cyclosporine	Generic, Sandimmune
Etanercept	Enbrel
Gold sodium thiomalate	Generic, Aurolate
Golimumab	Simponi
Infliximab	Remicade
Leflunomide	Generic, Arava
Methotrexate	Generic, Rheumatrex
Mycophenolate mofetil	Generic, Cellcept
Rituximab	Rituxan
Sarilumab	Kevzara
Sulfasalazine	Generic, Azulfidine
Tocilizumab	Actemra
Tofacitinib	Xeljanz
Ustekinumab	Stelara
ACETAMINOPHEN AND OTHER ANALGESICS	
Acetaminophen	Generic, Tylenol, Tempra, Panadol, Acephen, others
Ketorolac tromethamine	Generic, Toradol
Tramadol	Generic, Ultram
DRUGS USED IN GOUT	
Allopurinol	Generic, Zyloprim
Colchicine	Generic,* Colchrys, Colcrys
Febuxostat	Uloric
Pegloticase	Krystexxa
Probenecid	Generic
Sulfinpyrazone*	Generic, Anturane

*Outside the United States.

REFERENCES

NSAIDs

Chan FK et al: Celecoxib versus diclofenac and omeprazole in reducing the risk of recurrent ulcer bleeding in patients with arthritis. N Engl J Med 2002;347:2104.

Clevers H: Colon cancer—understanding how NSAIDs work. N Engl J Med 2006;354:761.

Edwards CJ et al: Apremilast, an oral phosphodiesterase 4 inhibitor, in patients with psoriatic arthritis and current skin involvement: a phase III, randomised, controlled trial (PALACE 3). Ann Rheum Dis 2016;75:1065.

Kristensen DM et al: Ibuprofen alters human testicular physiology to produce a state of compensated hypogonadism. Proc Natl Acad Sci USA 2018; 115:e715.

Lago P et al: Safety and efficacy of ibuprofen versus indomethacin in preterm infants treated for patent ductus arteriosus: A randomized controlled trial. Eur J Pediatr 2002;161:202.

Nissen SE et al: Cardiovascular safety of celecoxib, naproxen, or ibuprofen for arthritis. N Engl J Med 2016;375:2519.

Ravichandran R et al: An open label randomized clinical trial of indomethacin for mild and moderate hospitalised Covid-19 patients. Sci Rep 2022;12:6413.

Roberts JS et al: R-etodolac is a more potent Wnt signaling inhibitor than enantiomer, S-etodolac. Biochem Biophys Rep 2022;30:101231.

Solomon DH et al: The risk of major NSAID toxicity with celecoxib, ibuprofen, or naproxen: A secondary analysis of the PRECISION trial. Am J Med 2017;130:1415.

U.S. Food and Drug Administration: FDA Drug Safety Communication: FDA strengthens warning that non-aspirin nonsteroidal anti-inflammatory drugs (NSAIDs) can cause heart attacks or strokes. www.fda.gov/Drugs/DrugSafety/ucm451800.htm.

Zheng W et al: Adjunctive celecoxib for schizophrenia: A meta-analysis of randomized, double-blind, placebo-controlled trials. J Psychiatr Res 2017;92:139.

Disease-Modifying Antirheumatic Drugs & Glucocorticoids

Aboobacker S, Kurn H, Al Aboud AM: *Secukinumab*. StatPearls Publishing, 2022. https://www.ncbi.nlm.nih.gov/books/NBK537091/

Bannwarth B et al: A pharmacokinetic and clinical assessment of tofacitinib for the treatment of rheumatoid arthritis. Expert Opin Drug Metab Toxicol 2013;9:6.

Benson JM et al: Discovery and mechanism of ustekinumab: a human monoclonal antibody targeting interleukin-12 and interleukin-23 for treatment of immune-mediated disorders. MAbs 2011;3:535.

Brunner HI, Ruperto N: Therapeutics: biologics and small molecules. In: Petty RE (editor): *Textbook of Pediatric Rheumatology*, 8th ed. Elsevier, 2021. https://www.clinicalkey.com/#!/content/book/3-s2.0-B9780323636520000148.

Cavalli G, Dinarello G: Anakinra therapy for non-cancer inflammatory diseases. Front Pharmacol 2018;9:1157.

Cronstein B: How does methotrexate suppress inflammation? Clin Exp Rheumatol 2010:28:S21.

Davis JC Jr et al: Recombinant human tumor necrosis factor receptor (etanercept) for treating ankylosing spondylitis: a randomized, controlled trial. Arthritis Rheum 2003;48:3230.

Emery P et al: The impact of T-cell co-stimulation modulation in patients with undifferentiated inflammatory arthritis or very early rheumatoid arthritis: A clinical and imaging study of abatacept. Ann Rheum Dis 2010;69:510.

Feagan BG et al: The effects of infliximab therapy on health-related quality of life in ulcerative colitis patients. Am J Gastroenterol 2007;102:4.

Gabay C et al: Tocilizumab monotherapy versus adalimumab monotherapy for treatment of rheumatoid arthritis (ADACTA): A randomised, double-blind, controlled phase 4 trial. Lancet 2013;4:381.

Giachi A et al: Disease modifying antirheumatic drugs improve the cardiovascular profile in patients with rheumatoid arthritis. Frontiers in cardiovascular medicine. 2022. 9:1012661. DOI 10. 3389/FCVM. 2022. 1012661.

Godfrey MS, Friedman LN: Tuberculosis and biologic therapies: anti-tumor necrosis factor-αand beyond. Clin Chest Med 2019;40:721.

Hanif N, Anwer F. *Rituximab*. StatPearls, 2022. https://www.ncbi.nlm.nih.gov/books/NBK564374/

Harris KM et al: Effect of costimulatory blockade with abatacept after ustekinumab withdrawal in patients with moderate to severe plaque psoriasis: The PAUSE randomized clinical trial. JAMA Dermatol 2021;157:1306.

Huscher D et al: Dose-related patterns of glucocorticoid-induced side effects. Ann Rheum Dis 2009;68:1119.

Igel TF et al: Drugs in the pipeline. In: Schlesinger N, Lipsky PE (editors): *Gout*. Elsevier, 2019.

Kaegi C et al: Systematic review of safety and efficacy of belimumab in treating immune-mediated disorders. Allergy 2021;76:2673.

Khanna D et al: Safety and efficacy of subcutaneous tocilizumab in adults with systemic sclerosis (faSScinate): A phase 2, randomised, controlled trial. Lancet 2016;387:2630.

Kharazmi AB et al: A randomized controlled clinical trial on efficacy and safety of anakinra in patients with severe COVID-19. Immun Inflamm Dis 2022;10:201.

Klotz U: Clinical pharmacology of sulfasalazine and its metabolites. Clin Pharmacokinet 1985;10:285.

Klünder B et al: Population pharmacokinetics of upadacitinib using the immediate-release and extended-release formulations in healthy subjects and subjects with rheumatoid arthritis: analyses of phase I-III clinical trials. Clin Pharmacokinet 2019;58:1045.

Kristensen DM et al: Ibuprofen alters human testicular physiology to produce a state of compensated hypogonadism. Proc Natl Acad Sci USA 2018;115:e715.

Lamb YN: Guselkumab in psoriatic arthritis: a profile of its use. Drugs Ther Perspect 2021;37:285.

Landewé R et al: Efficacy of certolizumab pegol on signs and symptoms of axial spondyloarthritis including ankylosing spondylitis: 24-week results of a double-blind randomised placebo-controlled Phase 3 study. Ann Rheum Dis 2014;73:1.

Lichtenstien GR: Highlights from the new ACG Guideline on Crohn's Disease Management. Gastroenterol Hepatol (NY) 2018;14:482.

LiverTox: Clinical and Research Information on Drug-Induced Liver Injury. National Institute of Diabetes and Digestive and Kidney Diseases, 2012. https://www.ncbi.nlm.nih.gov/books/NBK548442/.

Mariette X et al: Malignancies associated with tumour necrosis factor inhibitors in registries and prospective observational studies: a systematic review and meta-analysis. Ann Rheum Dis 2011;70:1895.

Marzan KA: Role of adalimumab in the management of children and adolescents with juvenile idiopathic arthritis and other rheumatic conditions. Adolesc Health Med Ther 2012;3:85.

McDermott MF: Rilonacept in the treatment of chronic inflammatory diseases. Drugs Today 2009;45:423.

Mease PJ: Adalimumab in the treatment of arthritis. Ther Clin Risk Manag 2007;3:133.

Mease PJ et al: Effect of certolizumab pegol on signs and symptoms in patients with psoriatic arthritis: 24-week results of a phase 3 double-blind randomised placebo-controlled study (RAPID-PsA). Ann Rheum Dis 2014;73:1.

Nakashima J, Preuss CV: Mesalamine (USAN). StatPearls, 2022.

Nassim D, Alajmi A, Jfri A, Pehr K: Apremilast in dermatology: A review of literature. Dermatol Ther 2020;33:e14261.

Padda IS et al: Apremilast. StatPearls, 2022. https://www.ncbi.nlm.nih.gov/books/NBK572078/.

Pang Y et al: Clinical pharmacokinetics and pharmacodynamics of risankizumab in psoriasis patients. Clin Pharmacokinet 2020;59:311.

Papoutsaki M et al: Infliximab in psoriasis and psoriatic arthritis. BioDrugs 2013;27:13.

Peng L et al: Molecular basis for antagonistic activity of anifrolumab, an anti-interferon-α receptor 1 antibody. MAbs 2015;7:428.

Plosker G, Croom K: Sulfasalazine: A review of its use in the management of rheumatoid arthritis. Drugs 2006;65:1825.

Quiles Tsimaratos N, Groupe de recherche sur le psoriasis de la Société française de dermatologie: [Apremilast]. Ann Dermatol Venereol 2019;146:470.

Riese RJ et al: Inhibition of JAK kinases in patients with rheumatoid arthritis: Scientific rationale and clinical outcomes. Best Pract Res Clin Rheumatol 2010;24:4.

Safarini OA et al: Calcineurin inhibitors. StatPearls, 2022. https://www.ncbi.nlm.nih.gov/books/NBK558995/.

Salama C et al: Tocilizumab in patients hospitalized with Covid-19 pneumonia. N Engl J Med 2021;384:20.

Siebert S et al: Guselkumab induces sustained reduction in acute phase proteins and Th17 effector cytokines in active psoriatic arthritis in two phase-3 clinical trials (DISCOVER-1 and DISCOVER-2). Ann Rheum Dis 2020;79:144.

Spies CM et al: Prednisone chronotherapy. Clin Exp Rheumatol 2011;29:5.

Stokkermans TJ et al: Chloroquine and hydroxychloroquine toxicity. StatPearls, 2022. https://www.accessdata.fda.gov/drugsatfda_docs/label/2021/009768s053lbl.pdf.

Tanaka T et al: Tocilizumab for the treatment of rheumatoid arthritis. Expert Rev Clin Immunol 2010;6:6.

Torres T: Selective interleukin-23 p19 inhibition: another game changer in psoriasis? Focus on risankizumab. Drugs 2017;77:1493.

Tracey D et al: Tumor necrosis factor antagonist mechanisms of action: a comprehensive review. Pharmacol Ther 2008;117:244.

Tummala R et al: Safety, tolerability and pharmacokinetics of subcutaneous and intravenous anifrolumab in healthy volunteers. Lupus Sci Med 2018;5:e000252.

Turner D: Severe acute ulcerative colitis: The pediatric perspective. Dig Dis 2009;27:3

Warren RB et al: Efficacy and safety of risankizumab vs. secukinumab in patients with moderate-to-severe plaque psoriasis (IMMerge): results from a phase III, randomized, open-label, efficacy-assessor-blinded clinical trial. Br J Dermatol 2021;184:50.

Weinblatt ME et al: Head-to-head comparison of subcutaneous abatacept versus adalimumab for rheumatoid arthritis: Findings of a phase IIIb, multinational, prospective, randomized study. Arthritis Rheum 2013;65:1.

Westhovens R et al: Disease remission is achieved within two years in over half of methotrexate naive patients with early erosive rheumatoid arthritis (RA) treated with abatacept plus MTX: Results from the AGREE trial (abstract 638). Arthritis Rheum 2009;60:S239.

Xu C et al: Population pharmacokinetics of sarilumab in patients with rheumatoid arthritis. Clin Pharmacokinet 2019;58:1455.

Zerilli T, Ocheretyaner E: Apremilast (Otezla): A new oral treatment for adults with psoriasis and psoriatic arthritis. P T 2015;40:495.

Zouali M, Uy EA: Belimumab therapy in systemic lupus erythematosus. BioDrugs 2013;27:3.

Other Analgesics

Bravo L et al: Discovery and development of tramadol for the treatment of pain. Expert Opinion Drug Discov 12:1281, 2017.

Langley PC et al: Adverse event profile of tramadol in recent clinical studies of chronic osteoarthritis pain. Curr Med Res Opin 2010; 26:2395.

Xu M et al: Physiologically based pharmacokinetic modeling of tramadol to inform dose adjustment and drug-drug interactions according to CYP2D6 phenotypes. Pharmacotherapy 2021;41:277.

Drugs Used in Gout

Abhishek A: New urate-lowering therapies. Curr Opin Rheumatol 2018;30:177.

Becker MA et al: Febuxostat compared with allopurinol in patients with hyperuricemia and gout. N Engl J Med 2005;353:2450.

Chenra YE et al: Cyclooxygenase 2 selective NSAID (etodolac, meloxicam, celecoxib, rofecoxib, etoricoxib, valdecoxib and lumiracoxib) for OA and RA: A systematic review and economic evaluation. Health Technol Assoc 2008;12:1.

Cronberg S et al: Effect on platelet aggregation of oral administration of 10 nonsteroidal analgesics to humans. Scand J Haematol 1984;33:155.

Dalbeth N et al: Gout. Lancet 2016;388:2039.

Davies GD et al: Effects of diflunisal on platelet function and fecal blood loss. Clin Pharmacol Ther 1981;30:378.

Drugs and Lactation Database (LactMed): Colchicine. NIH, 2006.

Khanna D et al: 2012 American College of Rheumatology guidelines for management of gout. Part 1: systematic nonpharmacologic and pharmacologic therapeutic approaches to hyperuricemia. Arthritis Care Res (Hoboken) 2012;64:1431.

Liao KF et al: Etodolac and the risk of acute pancreatitis. Biomedicine (Taipei) 2017;7:4.

Pascual E et al: Severe gout: Strategies and innovations for effective management. Joint Bone Spine 2017;84:541.

So A et al: A pilot study of IL-1 inhibition by anakinra in acute gout. Arthritis Res Ther 2007;9:R28.

Socking R et al: Updates on the treatment of gout, including a review of updated treatment guidelines and use of small molecule therapies for difficult-to-treat gout and gout flares. Expert Opin Pharmacother 18:1115, 2017.

Zhu Y et al: Comparison of the pharmacokinetics of subcutaneous ustekinumab between Chinese and non-Chinese healthy male subjects across two phase 1 Studies. Clin Drug Investig 2013;22:291.

CASE STUDY ANSWER

This patient had good control of his symptoms for 1 year but now has a prolonged flare, probably denoting worsening disease (not just a temporary flare). In addition to physical findings and measurement of acute-phase reactants such as sedimentation rate or C-reactive protein, it would be wise to get hand and feet radiographs to document whether he has developed joint damage. Assuming such damage is found, the appropriate approach would be either a combination of nonbiologic DMARDs (eg, adding sulfasalazine and hydroxychloroquine) or adding a biologic medication, usually a TNF inhibitor followed by non-TNF biologics or JAK inhibitors. Follow-up should be every 1–3 months to gauge response and toxicity. Adverse events requiring caution are an increased risk of infection, possible appearance of lymphoma, and rare liver function test or hematologic abnormalities. Importantly, close follow-up should ensue, including changing medications every 3–6 months if needed, until full disease control is achieved.

CHAPTER 37

Hypothalamic & Pituitary Hormones

Roger K. Long, MD, & Hakan Cakmak, MD

CASE STUDY

A 10-year-old girl (height 126 cm, 3rd percentile; weight 36 kg, approximately 65th percentile) presents with short stature. Review of her growth chart demonstrates normal birth weight and length and growth velocity until a markedly decreased growth velocity over the past 2 years, resulting in a decrease in height percentile from the 50th to the 3rd. Review of history reveals headaches, increased urination and drinking, and dizziness with febrile illnesses. Physical examination demonstrates short stature, mild generalized obesity, a bitemporal visual field defect, and no breast development. The patient is diagnosed with a suprasellar craniopharyngioma. After complete surgical resection, laboratory evaluations demonstrate growth hormone (GH) deficiency and a delayed bone age of 18 months. The patient is treated with recombinant human GH at a dose of 40 mcg/kg per day subcutaneously. After 1 year of treatment, her height velocity has increased from 4 cm/year to 10 cm/year. How does GH stimulate growth in children? What other hormone deficiencies are suggested by the patient's history and physical examination? What other hormone replacements will this patient likely require?

The control of metabolism, growth, and reproduction is mediated by a combination of neural and endocrine systems located in the hypothalamus and pituitary gland. The pituitary weighs about 0.6 g and rests at the base of the brain in the bony sella turcica near the optic chiasm and the cavernous sinuses. The pituitary consists of an anterior lobe (adenohypophysis) and a posterior lobe (neurohypophysis) (Figure 37–1). It is connected to the overlying hypothalamus by a stalk of neurosecretory fibers and blood vessels, including a portal venous system that drains the hypothalamus and perfuses the anterior pituitary. The portal venous system carries small regulatory hormones (Figure 37–1, Table 37–1) from the hypothalamus to the anterior pituitary.

The posterior lobe hormones are synthesized in the hypothalamus and transported via the neurosecretory fibers in the stalk of

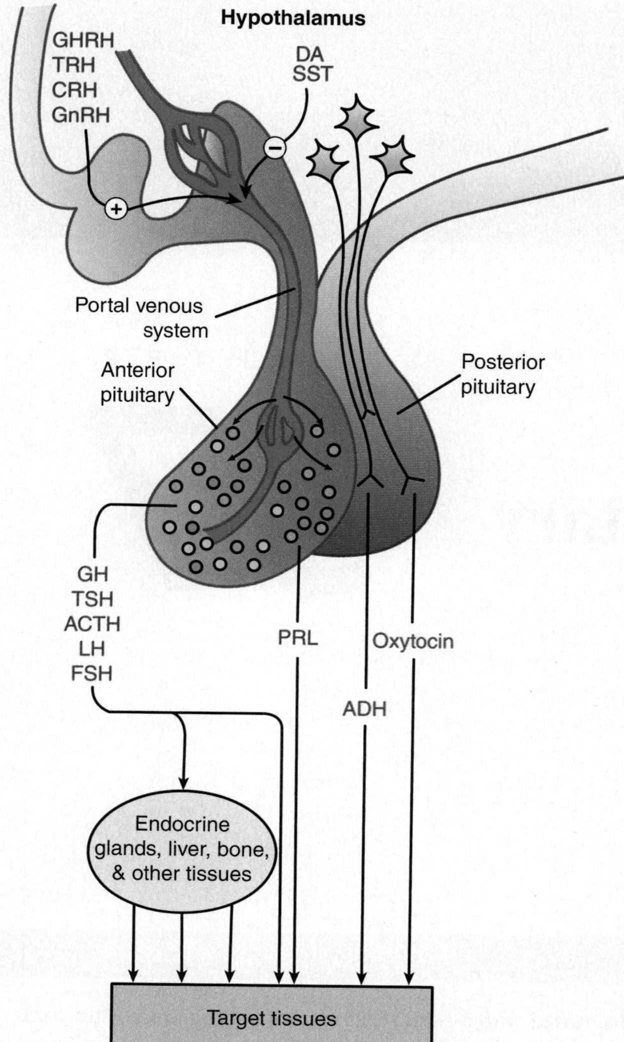

FIGURE 37–1 The hypothalamic-pituitary endocrine system. Hormones released from the anterior pituitary stimulate the production of hormones by a peripheral endocrine gland, the liver, or other tissues, or act directly on target tissues. Prolactin and the hormones released from the posterior pituitary (vasopressin and oxytocin) act directly on target tissues. Hypothalamic factors regulate the release of anterior pituitary hormones. ACTH, adrenocorticotropin; ADH, antidiuretic hormone [vasopressin]; CRH, corticotropin-releasing hormone; DA, dopamine; FSH, follicle-stimulating hormone; GH, growth hormone; GHRH, growth hormone-releasing hormone; GnRH, gonadotropin-releasing hormone; LH, luteinizing hormone; PRL, prolactin; SST, somatostatin; TRH, thyrotropin-releasing hormone; TSH, thyroid-stimulating hormone.

the pituitary to the posterior lobe; from there they are released into the circulation.

Drugs that mimic or block the effects of hypothalamic and pituitary hormones have pharmacologic applications in three primary areas: (1) as replacement therapy for hormone deficiency states; (2) as antagonists for diseases caused by excess production of pituitary hormones; and (3) as diagnostic tools for identifying endocrine abnormalities.

■ ANTERIOR PITUITARY HORMONES & THEIR HYPOTHALAMIC REGULATORS

All the hormones produced by the anterior pituitary except prolactin are key participants in hormonal systems in which they regulate the production of hormones and autocrine-paracrine factors by endocrine glands and other peripheral tissues. In these systems, the secretion of the pituitary hormone is under the control of one or more hypothalamic hormones. Each hypothalamic-pituitary-endocrine gland system or axis provides multiple opportunities for complex neuroendocrine regulation of growth and development, metabolism, and reproductive function.

ANTERIOR PITUITARY & HYPOTHALAMIC HORMONE RECEPTORS

The anterior pituitary hormones can be classified according to hormone structure and the types of receptors that they activate. **Growth hormone (GH)** and **prolactin (PRL),** single-chain protein hormones with significant homology, form one group. Both hormones activate receptors of the JAK/STAT superfamily (see Chapter 2). Three pituitary hormones—**thyroid-stimulating hormone (TSH, thyrotropin), follicle-stimulating hormone (FSH),** and **luteinizing hormone** (LH)—are dimeric proteins that activate G protein-coupled receptors (see Chapter 2). TSH, FSH, and LH share a common α subunit. Their β subunits, though somewhat similar to each other, differ enough to confer receptor specificity. Finally, **adrenocorticotropic hormone (ACTH),** a peptide cleaved from a larger precursor, proopiomelanocortin (POMC), represents a third category. POMC can be cleaved into various other biologically active peptides like

ACRONYMS

ACTH	Adrenocorticotropic hormone (corticotropin)
ADH	Antidiuretic hormone (vasopressin)
CRH	Corticotropin-releasing hormone
FSH	Follicle-stimulating hormone
GH	Growth hormone
GHRH	Growth hormone–releasing hormone
GnRH	Gonadotropin-releasing hormone
hCG	Human chorionic gonadotropin
hMG	Human menopausal gonadotropin
IGF	Insulin-like growth factor
LH	Luteinizing hormone
PRL	Prolactin
rhGH	Recombinant human growth hormone
SST	Somatostatin
TRH	Thyrotropin-releasing hormone
TSH	Thyroid-stimulating hormone (thyrotropin)

TABLE 37–1 Links between hypothalamic, anterior pituitary, and target organ hormone or mediator.[1]

Anterior Pituitary Hormone	Hypothalamic Hormone	Target Organ	Primary Target Organ Hormone or Mediator
Growth hormone (GH, somatotropin)	Growth hormone-releasing hormone (GHRH) (+), Somatostatin (–)	Liver, bone, muscle, kidney, and others	Insulin-like growth factor-I (IGF-I)
Thyroid-stimulating hormone (TSH)	Thyrotropin-releasing hormone (TRH) (+)	Thyroid	Thyroxine, triiodothyronine
Adrenocorticotropin (ACTH)	Corticotropin-releasing hormone (CRH) (+)	Adrenal cortex	Cortisol
Follicle-stimulating hormone (FSH) Luteinizing hormone (LH)	Gonadotropin-releasing hormone (GnRH) (+)[2]	Gonads	Estrogen, progesterone, testosterone
Prolactin (PRL)	Dopamine (–)	Breast	—

[1]All of these hormones act through G protein-coupled receptors except GH and PRL, which act through JAK/STAT receptors.

[2]Endogenous GnRH, which is released in pulses, stimulates LH and FSH release. When administered continuously as a drug, GnRH and its analogs inhibit LH and FSH release through down-regulation of GnRH receptors.

(+), stimulant; (–), inhibitor.

α-melanocyte-stimulating hormone (MSH) and β-endorphin (see Chapter 31). Like TSH, LH, and FSH, ACTH acts through a G protein-coupled receptor. A unique feature of the ACTH receptor (also known as the melanocortin 2 receptor) is that a transmembrane protein, melanocortin 2 receptor accessory protein, is essential for normal ACTH receptor trafficking and signaling.

TSH, FSH, LH, and ACTH share similarities in the regulation of their release from the pituitary. Each is under the control of a distinctive hypothalamic peptide that stimulates their production by acting on G protein-coupled receptors (see Table 37–1). TSH release is regulated by **thyrotropin-releasing hormone (TRH),** whereas the release of LH and FSH (known collectively as gonadotropins) is stimulated by pulses of **gonadotropin-releasing hormone (GnRH).** ACTH release is stimulated by **corticotropin-releasing hormone (CRH).** An important regulatory feature shared by these four structurally related hormones is that they and their hypothalamic releasing factors are subject to feedback inhibitory regulation by the hormones whose production they control. TSH and TRH production are inhibited by the two key thyroid hormones, thyroxine and triiodothyronine (see Chapter 38). Gonadotropin and GnRH production is inhibited in women by estrogen and progesterone, and in men by testosterone and other androgens. ACTH and CRH production are inhibited by cortisol. Feedback regulation is critical to the physiologic control of thyroid, adrenal cortical, and gonadal function and is also important in pharmacologic treatments that affect these systems.

The hypothalamic hormonal control of GH and prolactin differs from the regulatory systems for TSH, FSH, LH, and ACTH. The hypothalamus secretes two hormones that regulate GH; **growth hormone-releasing hormone (GHRH)** stimulates GH production, whereas the peptide **somatostatin (SST)** inhibits GH production. GH and its primary peripheral mediator, **insulin-like growth factor I (IGF-I),** also provide feedback to inhibit GH release. Prolactin production is inhibited by the catecholamine dopamine acting through the D_2 subtype of dopamine receptors. The hypothalamus does not produce a hormone that specifically stimulates prolactin secretion, although TRH can stimulate prolactin release, particularly when TRH concentrations are high in the setting of primary hypothyroidism.

Whereas all the pituitary and hypothalamic hormones described previously are available for use in humans, only a few are of major clinical importance. Because of the greater ease of administration of target endocrine gland hormones or their synthetic analogs, the related hypothalamic and pituitary hormones are used infrequently as treatments. However, many of them (TRH, TSH, CRH, ACTH, GnRH, GHRH) are used for specialized diagnostic testing. These agents are described in Tables 37–2 and 37–3 and are not discussed further in this chapter. In contrast, GH, SST,

TABLE 37–2 Clinical uses of hypothalamic hormones and their analogs.

Hypothalamic Hormone	Clinical Uses
Growth hormone-releasing hormone (GHRH)	Used rarely as a diagnostic test for GH and GHRH sufficiency
Thyrotropin-releasing- hormone (TRH, protirelin)	May be used to diagnose TRH or TSH deficiencies; not currently available for clinical use in the United States
Corticotropin-releasing hormone (CRH)	Used rarely to distinguish Cushing disease from ectopic ACTH secretion
Gonadotropin-releasing hormone (GnRH)	May be used in a single dose to assess initiation of puberty (pubertal gonadotropin response)
	May be used in pulses to treat infertility caused by GnRH deficiency
	Analogs used in long-acting formulations to inhibit gonadal function in children with precocious puberty, in some transgender/gender variant early pubertal adolescents (to block endogenous puberty), in men with prostate cancer and women undergoing assisted reproductive technology (ART) or women who require ovarian suppression for a gynecologic disorder
Dopamine	Dopamine agonists (eg, bromocriptine, cabergoline) used for treatment of hyperprolactinemia

TABLE 37–3 Diagnostic uses of thyroid-stimulating hormone and adrenocorticotropin.

Hormone	Diagnostic Use
Thyroid-stimulating-hormone (TSH; thyrotropin)	In patients who have been treated surgically for thyroid carcinoma, to test for cancer recurrence by assessing TSH-stimulated radioactive iodine uptake and serum thyroglobulin level (see Chapter 38)
Adrenocorticotropin (ACTH)	In patients suspected of adrenal insufficiency, either central (CRH/ACTH deficiency) or peripheral (cortisol deficiency), in particular in suspected cases of congenital adrenal hyperplasia (see Figure 39–1 and Chapter 39)

LH, FSH, GnRH, and dopamine or analogs of these hormones are commonly used and are described in the following text.

GROWTH HORMONE (SOMATOTROPIN)

Growth hormone, an anterior pituitary hormone, is required during childhood and adolescence for attainment of normal adult size and has important effects throughout postnatal life on lipid and carbohydrate metabolism, and on lean body mass and bone density. Its growth-promoting effects are primarily mediated via IGF-I (also known as somatomedin C). Individuals with congenital or acquired deficiency of GH during childhood or early adolescence have an adult height potential significantly lower than their mid-parental target adult height and have disproportionately increased body fat and decreased muscle mass. Adults with GH deficiency also have disproportionately low lean body mass, as well as bone mineral density and perceive a lower quality of life.

Chemistry & Pharmacokinetics

A. Structure

Growth hormone is a 191-amino-acid peptide with two sulfhydryl bridges. Its structure closely resembles that of prolactin. In the past, medicinal GH was isolated from the pituitaries of human cadavers. However, this form of GH was found to be contaminated with prions that could cause Creutzfeldt-Jakob disease. For this reason, it is no longer used. Somatropin, the recombinant form of GH, has a 191-amino-acid sequence that is identical with the predominant native form of human GH.

B. Absorption, Metabolism, and Excretion

Circulating endogenous GH has a half-life of approximately 20 minutes and is predominantly cleared by the liver. Recombinant human GH (rhGH) is administered subcutaneously six to seven times per week. Peak levels occur in 2–4 hours, and active blood levels persist for approximately 36 hours. Weekly subcutaneous dosing with efficacy comparable to daily administration is available with recombinant human GH derivatives that are modified to extend duration action with an added albumin-binding moiety or a transiently linked inert protective carrier.

Pharmacodynamics

Growth hormone mediates its effects via cell surface receptors of the JAK/STAT cytokine receptor superfamily. The hormone has two distinct GH receptor binding sites. Dimerization of two GH receptors is stimulated by a single GH molecule and activates signaling cascades mediated by receptor-associated JAK tyrosine kinases and STATs (see Chapter 2). The hormone has complex effects on growth, body composition, and carbohydrate, protein, and lipid metabolism. The growth-promoting effects are mediated principally, but not solely, through an increase in the production of IGF-I. Much of the circulating IGF-I is produced by the liver. Growth hormone also stimulates production of IGF-I in bone, cartilage, muscle, kidney, and other tissues, where it has autocrine or paracrine roles. It stimulates longitudinal bone growth until the epiphyseal plates fuse—near the end of puberty. In both children and adults, GH has anabolic effects in muscle and catabolic effects in adipose cells that shift the balance of body mass to an increase in muscle mass and a reduction in adiposity. The direct and indirect effects of GH on carbohydrate metabolism are mixed, in part because GH and IGF-I have opposite effects on insulin sensitivity. Growth hormone reduces insulin sensitivity, which results in mild hyperinsulinemia and increased blood glucose levels, whereas IGF-I has insulin-like effects on glucose transport. In patients who are unable to respond to growth hormone because of severe resistance (caused by GH receptor mutations, post-receptor signaling mutations, or GH antibodies), the administration of recombinant human IGF-I may cause hypoglycemia because of its insulin-like effects.

Clinical Pharmacology

A. Growth Hormone Deficiency

Growth hormone deficiency can have a genetic basis, be associated with midline developmental defect syndromes (eg, septo-optic dysplasia), or be acquired as a result of damage to the pituitary or hypothalamus by a traumatic event (including breech or traumatic delivery), intracranial tumors, infection, infiltrative or hemorrhagic processes, or irradiation. Neonates with isolated GH deficiency are typically of normal size at birth because prenatal growth is not GH-dependent. In contrast, IGF-I is essential for normal prenatal and postnatal growth. Through poorly understood mechanisms, IGF-I expression and postnatal growth become GH-dependent during the first year of life. In childhood, GH deficiency typically presents as short stature, often with mild adiposity. Another early sign of GH deficiency is hypoglycemia due to the loss of the counter-regulatory hormonal response of GH to hypoglycemia; young children are at a greater risk for this condition due to their high sensitivity to insulin. Criteria for diagnosis of GH deficiency usually include (1) a subnormal height velocity for age and (2) a subnormal serum GH response following provocative testing with at least two GH secretagogues. Clonidine (α_2-adrenergic agonist), levodopa (dopaminergic agonist), and exercise are factors that increase GHRH levels. Arginine and insulin-induced hypoglycemia cause diminished SST, which increases GH release. The mechanisms by which glucagon stimulates GH secretion remain unclear. Macimorelin, an orally administered ghrelin receptor agonist, is approved for GH stimulation testing in adults. If therapy with rhGH is initiated at an early age, many children with short stature due to GH deficiency will achieve an adult height within their midparental target height range.

In the past, it was believed that adults with GH deficiency do not exhibit a significant syndrome. However, more detailed studies suggest that adults with GH deficiency often have generalized obesity, reduced muscle mass, asthenia, diminished bone mineral density, dyslipidemia, lower quality-of-life assessments, and reduced cardiac output. Growth hormone–deficient adults who have been treated with GH experience reversal of many of these manifestations.

B. Growth Hormone Treatment of Pediatric Patients with Short Stature

Although the greatest improvement in growth occurs in patients with GH deficiency, exogenous GH has some effect on height in children with short stature caused by conditions other than GH deficiency. Growth hormone has been approved for several conditions (Table 37–4) and has been used experimentally or off-label in many others. Prader-Willi syndrome is an autosomal dominant genetic disease associated with growth failure, obesity, and carbohydrate intolerance. In children with Prader-Willi syndrome and growth failure, GH treatment decreases body fat and increases lean body mass, linear growth, and energy expenditure.

TABLE 37–4 Clinical uses of recombinant human growth hormone.

Primary Therapeutic Objective	Clinical Condition
Growth	Growth failure in pediatric patients associated with: Growth hormone deficiency Chronic renal insufficiency pre-transplant Noonan syndrome Prader-Willi syndrome Short stature homeobox-containing gene (SHOX) deficiency Turner syndrome Small-for-gestational-age with failure to catch up by age 2 years Idiopathic short stature
Improved metabolic state, increased lean body mass, sense of well-being	Growth hormone deficiency in adults
Increased lean body mass, weight, and physical endurance	Wasting in patients with HIV infection
Improved gastrointestinal function	Short bowel syndrome in patients who are also receiving specialized nutritional support

Growth hormone treatment has also been shown to have a strong beneficial effect on final height of girls with Turner syndrome (45 X karyotype and variants). In clinical trials, GH treatment has been shown to increase adult height in girls with Turner syndrome by 10–15 cm (4–6 inches). Because girls with Turner syndrome also have either absent or rudimentary ovaries, GH must be judiciously combined with gonadal steroids to achieve maximal height. Other conditions of pediatric growth failure for which GH treatment is approved include chronic renal insufficiency pre-transplant, and small-for-gestational-age at birth with failure of catch-up growth, in which the child's height remains more than 2 standard deviations below normal at 2 years of age.

A controversial but approved use of GH is for children with idiopathic short stature (ISS). This is a heterogeneous population that has in common no identifiable cause of the short stature. ISS is clinically defined as having a height at least 2.25 standard deviations below normal for children of the same age and a predicted adult height that is <2.25 standard deviations below the mean (<59 inches in females, and <63 inches in males). In this group of children, many years of GH therapy result in an average increase in adult height of 4–7 cm (1.57–2.76 inches) at a cost of $5000–$40,000 per year. The complex issues involved in the cost-risk-benefit relationship of this use of GH are important because an estimated 400,000 children in the United States fit the diagnostic criteria for ISS.

Treatment of children with short stature should be carried out by specialists experienced in GH administration. Dose requirements vary with the condition being treated, with GH-deficient children typically being most responsive. Children must be observed closely for slowing of growth velocity, which could indicate a need to increase the dosage or the possibility of epiphyseal plate fusion or intercurrent problems such as hypothyroidism or malnutrition.

Other Uses of Growth Hormone

Growth hormone affects many organ systems and also has a net anabolic effect. It has been tested in a number of conditions that are associated with a severe catabolic state and is approved for the treatment of wasting in patients with AIDS. In 2004, GH was approved for treatment of patients with short bowel syndrome who are dependent on total parenteral nutrition (TPN). After intestinal resection or bypass, the remaining functional intestine in many patients undergoes extensive adaptation that allows it to adequately absorb nutrients. However, other patients fail to adequately adapt and develop a malabsorption syndrome. Growth hormone has been shown to increase intestinal growth and improve its function in experimental animals. Benefits of GH treatment for patients with short bowel syndrome and dependence on TPN have mostly been short-lived in the clinical studies that have been published to date.

Growth hormone is a popular component of "anti-aging" programs. Serum levels of GH normally decline with aging; anti-aging programs claim that injection of GH or administration of drugs purported to increase GH release are effective anti-aging remedies. These claims are largely unsubstantiated. In contrast, studies in mice and the nematode *Caenorhabditis elegans* have clearly demonstrated that analogs of human GH and IGF-I consistently *shorten* life span and that loss-of-function mutations in the signaling pathways for the GH and IGF-I analogs lengthen life span. Another use of GH is by athletes for a purported increase in muscle mass and athletic performance. Growth hormone is one of the drugs banned by the International Olympic Committee.

Toxicity & Contraindications

Children generally tolerate growth hormone treatment well. Adverse events are rare and include pseudotumor cerebri, slipped capital femoral epiphysis, progression of scoliosis, edema, hyperglycemia, and increased risk of asphyxiation in severely obese patients with Prader-Willi syndrome and upper airway obstruction or sleep apnea. Patients with Turner syndrome have an increased risk of otitis media while taking GH. In children with GH deficiency, periodic evaluation of the other anterior pituitary hormones may reveal concurrent deficiencies, which also require treatment (ie, with hydrocortisone, levothyroxine, or gonadal hormones). Pancreatitis, gynecomastia, and nevus growth have occurred in patients receiving GH. Adults tend to have more adverse effects from GH therapy. Peripheral edema, myalgias, and arthralgias (especially in the hands and wrists) occur commonly but remit with dosage reduction. Carpal tunnel syndrome can occur. Growth hormone treatment increases the activity of cytochrome P450 isoforms, which may reduce the serum levels of drugs metabolized by that enzyme system (see Chapter 4). There has been no increased incidence of malignancy among patients receiving GH therapy, but such treatment is contraindicated in a patient with a known active malignancy. Growth hormone treatment does not increase mortality rate in children. However, mortality rates are elevated for children with history of prior malignancy or serious non-GH-deficient medical conditions, and doubled in critically ill patients. The long-term health effects of GH treatment in childhood are unknown. The results from the Safety and Appropriateness of GH in Europe (SAGHE) study are inconsistent. A higher all-cause mortality (mostly due to cardiovascular disease) was found in the GH treatment group in the French arm of the study, but no long-term risks of GH treatment were observed in the study arm from other regions of Europe—including no increased mortality in Sweden when adjusting for birth parameters. A large, prospective, postmarketing observational study (GeNeSIS) revealed no increased risk of mortality or primary cancer.

MECASERMIN

A small number of children with growth failure have severe IGF-I deficiency that is not responsive to exogenous GH. Causes include mutations in the GH receptor and in the GH receptor signaling pathway, neutralizing antibodies to GH, and IGF-I gene defects. In 2005, the US Food and Drug Administration (FDA) approved two forms of recombinant human IGF-I (rhIGF-I) for treatment of severe IGF-I deficiency that is not responsive to GH: mecasermin and mecasermin rinfabate. Mecasermin is rhIGF-I alone, while mecasermin rinfabate is a complex of rhIGF-I and recombinant human insulin-like growth factor–binding protein-3 (rhIGFBP-3). This binding protein significantly increases the circulating half-life of rhIGF-I. Normally, the great majority of the circulating IGF-I is bound to IGFBP-3, which is produced principally by the liver under the control of GH. Due to a patent settlement, mecasermin rinfabate is not available for short stature-related indications. Mecasermin is administered subcutaneously twice daily at a low starting dosage and increased weekly as tolerated up to a maximum twice-daily dose. The growth response rate to rhIGF-I is lower than that observed during GH treatment of GH-deficient children: a growth velocity of 8–9 cm per year compared with 9–14 cm per year, respectively. During the first year of rhIGF-I treatment, height velocity increases by approximately 4–5 cm per year and height standard deviation score (SDS) increases by only 0.5 after 2 years of treatment.

The most important adverse effect observed with mecasermin is hypoglycemia. To avoid hypoglycemia, the prescribing instructions require consumption of a carbohydrate-containing meal or snack within 20 minutes of mecasermin administration. Cases of intracranial hypertension, adenotonsillar hypertrophy, lipohypertrophy, and asymptomatic elevation of liver enzymes have been reported.

GROWTH HORMONE ANTAGONISTS

Antagonists of GH are used to reverse the effects of GH-producing cells (somatotrophs) in the anterior pituitary that form GH-secreting tumors. Hormone-secreting pituitary adenomas occur most commonly in adults. In adults, GH-secreting adenomas cause acromegaly, which is characterized by abnormal growth of cartilage and bone tissue, and many organs including skin, muscle, heart, liver, and the gastrointestinal tract. When a GH-secreting adenoma occurs before the long bone epiphyses close, it leads to a rare condition, gigantism. Larger pituitary adenomas produce greater amounts of GH and also can impair visual and central nervous system function by encroaching on nearby brain structures, ie, optic nerve chiasm. The initial therapy of choice for GH-secreting adenomas is endoscopic transsphenoidal surgery. Medical therapy with GH antagonists is indicated when surgical resection is not possible or GH hypersecretion persists after surgery as determined by elevated IGF-I levels or GH not suppressible to <1 mcg/L. These agents include somatostatin analogs and dopamine receptor agonists, which reduce the production of GH, and the GH receptor antagonist pegvisomant, which prevents GH from activating GH signaling pathways. Radiation therapy is reserved for patients with inadequate response to surgical and medical therapies.

Somatostatin Analogs

Somatostatin, a 14-amino-acid peptide (Figure 37–2), is found in the hypothalamus, other parts of the central nervous system, the pancreas, and other sites in the gastrointestinal tract. It functions primarily as an inhibitory paracrine factor and inhibits the release of GH, TSH, glucagon, insulin, and gastrin. Somatostatin is rapidly cleared from the circulation, with a half-life of 1–3 minutes.

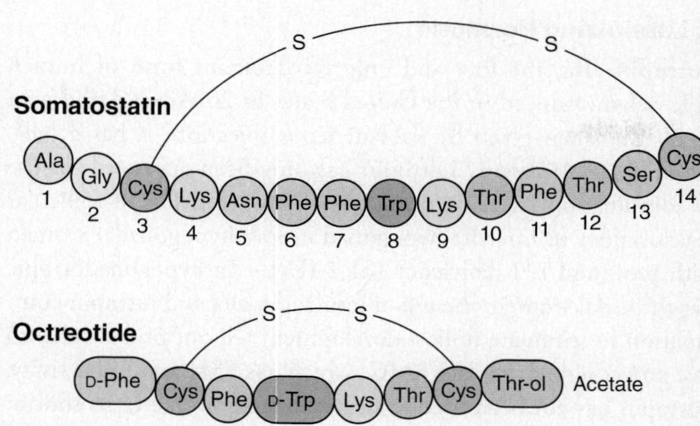

FIGURE 37–2 **Above:** Amino acid sequence of somatostatin. **Below:** Sequence of the synthetic analog, octreotide.

The kidney appears to play an important role in its metabolism and excretion.

Somatostatin has limited therapeutic usefulness because of its short duration of action and multiple effects in many secretory systems. A series of longer-acting somatostatin analogs that retain biologic activity have been developed. Octreotide, the most widely used somatostatin analog (see Figure 37–2), is 45 times more potent than somatostatin in inhibiting GH release but only twice as potent in reducing insulin secretion. Because of this relatively reduced effect on pancreatic beta cells, hyperglycemia rarely occurs during treatment. The plasma elimination half-life of subcutaneous octreotide is about 80 minutes, 30 times longer than that of somatostatin.

Octreotide, 50–200 mcg given subcutaneously every 8 hours, reduces symptoms caused by a variety of hormone-secreting tumors: acromegaly, carcinoid tumor, gastrinoma, glucagonoma, insulinoma, VIPoma, and ACTH-secreting tumor. Other therapeutic use indications include diarrhea—secretory, HIV associated, diabetic, chemotherapy, or radiation induced—and portal hypertension. Somatostatin receptor scintigraphy, using radiolabeled octreotide, is useful in localizing neuroendocrine tumors having somatostatin receptors and helps predict the response to octreotide therapy. Octreotide is also useful for the acute control of bleeding from esophageal varices.

Octreotide acetate injectable long-acting suspension is a slow-release microsphere formulation. It may be instituted after a brief course of shorter-acting octreotide has been demonstrated to be effective and tolerated. Injections into alternate gluteal muscles are repeated at 4-week intervals in doses of 10–40 mg.

Adverse effects of octreotide therapy include nausea, vomiting, abdominal cramps, flatulence, and steatorrhea with bulky bowel movements. Biliary sludge and gallstones may occur after 1 year of use in 20–30% of patients, up to 50% at 5 years of therapy. However, the yearly incidence of symptomatic gallstones is about 1%. Cardiac effects include sinus bradycardia (25%) and conduction disturbances (10%). Pain at the site of injection is common, especially with the long-acting octreotide suspension. Vitamin B_{12} deficiency may occur with long-term use of octreotide.

A long-acting formulation of lanreotide, another octapeptide somatostatin analog, is approved for treatment of acromegaly. Lanreotide appears to have effects comparable to those of octreotide in reducing GH levels and normalizing IGF-I concentrations. Pasireotide is a somatostatin analog with greater affinity for the somatostatin receptor 5 than the other analogs. After 12 months of treatment with a long-acting formulation of pasireotide, there was greater biochemical control of acromegaly than with long-acting octreotide (31.3% versus 19.2%). However, submaximal dosing of the octreotide may have impacted the comparison. Long-acting somatostatin analogs may cause shrinkage of GH-secreting pituitary adenomas in some patients. An oral formulation of octreotide may be used for long-term maintenance treatment in those patients who tolerated and responded to long-acting somatostatin analogs.

Pegvisomant

Pegvisomant is a GH receptor antagonist used to treat acromegaly. It is the polyethylene glycol (PEG) derivative of a mutant GH, B2036. Pegylation reduces its clearance and improves its overall clinical effectiveness. Like native GH, pegvisomant has two GH receptor binding sites. However, one of its GH receptor binding sites has increased affinity for the GH receptor, whereas its second GH receptor binding site has reduced affinity. This differential receptor affinity blocks native GH bindings as it allows the initial step (GH receptor dimerization) but prevents the conformational changes required for signal transduction. In clinical trials, pegvisomant was administered subcutaneously to patients with acromegaly; daily treatment for 12 months or longer reduced serum levels of IGF-I into the normal range in 97%. Pegvisomant does not inhibit GH secretion and may lead to increased GH levels and possible adenoma growth, so monitoring includes measurements of IGF-I and yearly MRIs of the pituitary. No serious problems have been observed; however, increases in liver enzymes without liver failure have been reported.

THE GONADOTROPINS (FOLLICLE-STIMULATING HORMONE & LUTEINIZING HORMONE) & HUMAN CHORIONIC GONADOTROPIN

The gonadotropins are produced by gonadotroph cells, which constitute 7–15% of the cells in the pituitary. These hormones serve complementary functions in the reproductive process. In women, the principal function of FSH is to stimulate ovarian follicle development. Both FSH and LH are needed for ovarian steroidogenesis. In the ovary, LH stimulates androgen production by theca cells in the follicular stage of the menstrual cycle, whereas FSH stimulates the conversion of androgens to estrogens by granulosa cells. In the luteal phase of the menstrual cycle, estrogen and progesterone production is primarily under the control first of LH and then, if pregnancy occurs, under the control of human chorionic gonadotropin (hCG). Human chorionic gonadotropin is a placental glycoprotein nearly identical with LH; its actions are mediated through LH receptors.

In men, FSH is the primary regulator of spermatogenesis, whereas LH is the main stimulus for testosterone synthesis in Leydig cells. FSH helps maintain high local androgen concentrations in the vicinity of developing sperm by stimulating the production of androgen-binding protein in Sertoli cells. FSH also stimulates the conversion by Sertoli cells of testosterone to estrogen that is also required for spermatogenesis.

FSH and hCG are available in several pharmaceutical forms. They are used in states of infertility to stimulate spermatogenesis in men and to induce follicle development and ovulation in women. Their most common clinical use is for the controlled ovarian stimulation that is the cornerstone of assisted reproductive technologies such as in vitro fertilization (IVF, see below).

Chemistry & Pharmacokinetics

All three hormones—FSH, LH, and hCG—are heterodimers that share an identical α subunit in addition to a distinct β subunit that confers receptor specificity. The β subunits of hCG and LH are nearly identical, and hCG is typically used to obtain LH activity due to its longer half-life. All the gonadotropin preparations are administered by subcutaneous or intramuscular injection, usually on a daily basis. Half-lives vary by preparation and route of injection from 10 to 40 hours.

A. Menotropins

The first commercial gonadotropin product containing both FSH and LH was extracted from the urine of postmenopausal women. This purified extract of FSH and LH is known as **menotropin,** or human menopausal gonadotropin **(hMG).** From the early 1960s, these preparations were used for the stimulation of follicle development in women. The early extraction techniques were very crude, requiring around 30 L of urine to manufacture enough hMG needed for a single treatment cycle. These initial preparations were also contaminated with other proteins; less than 5% of the proteins present were bioactive. The FSH-to-LH bioactivity ratio of these early preparations was 1:1. As purity improved, it was necessary to add hCG in order to maintain this ratio of bioactivity.

B. Follicle-Stimulating Hormone

Three forms of purified FSH are available. **Urofollitropin,** also known as uFSH, is a purified preparation of human FSH extracted from the urine of postmenopausal women. Virtually all the LH activity has been removed through a form of immune-affinity chromatography that uses anti-hCG antibodies. Urofollitropin was withdrawn from the United States market in 2015. Two recombinant forms of FSH **(rFSH)** are also available: **follitropin alfa** and **follitropin beta.** The amino acid sequences of these two products are identical to that of human FSH. They differ from each other and urofollitropin in the composition of carbohydrate side chains. The rFSH preparations have a shorter half-life than preparations derived from human urine but stimulate estrogen secretion and follicle development at least as efficiently and, in some studies, more efficiently. Compared with urine-derived gonadotropins, rFSH preparations have little protein contamination and much less batch-to-batch variability, and they may cause less local tissue reaction. The rFSH preparations are considerably more expensive.

C. Luteinizing Hormone

Lutropin alfa, the first and only recombinant form of human LH, was introduced in the United States in 2004 but withdrawn in 2012. When given by subcutaneous injection, it has a half-life of about 10 hours. Lutropin has only been approved for use in combination with follitropin alfa for stimulation of follicular development in infertile hypogonadotropic hypogonadal women with profound LH deficiency (<1.2 IU/L). In hypogonadotropic hypogonadal women, the use of follitropin alfa and lutropin combination to stimulate follicle development fell out of favor due to cost and could not replace hMG, which has FSH and LH activity. Lutropin has not been used to induce ovulation due to its shorter half-life.

D. Human Chorionic Gonadotropin

Human chorionic gonadotropin is produced by the human placenta and excreted into the urine, whence it can be extracted and purified. It is a glycoprotein consisting of a 92-amino-acid α subunit virtually identical to that of FSH, LH, and TSH, and a β subunit of 145 amino acids that resembles that of LH except for the presence of a carboxyl terminal sequence of 30 amino acids not present in LH. **Choriogonadotropin alfa** (rhCG) is a recombinant form of hCG. Because of its greater consistency in biologic activity, rhCG is packaged and dosed on the basis of weight rather than units of activity. All of the other gonadotropins, including rFSH, are packaged and dosed on the basis of units of activity. Both the hCG preparation that is purified from human urine and rhCG can be administered by subcutaneous or intramuscular injection.

Pharmacodynamics

The gonadotropins and hCG exert their effects through G protein-coupled receptors. LH and FSH have complex effects on reproductive tissues in both sexes. In women, these effects change over the time course of a menstrual cycle as a result of a complex interplay among concentration-dependent effects of the gonadotropins, cross-talk of LH, FSH, and gonadal steroids, and the influence of other ovarian hormones. A coordinated pattern of FSH and LH secretion during the menstrual cycle (see Figure 40–1) is required for normal follicle development, ovulation, and pregnancy.

During the first 8 weeks of pregnancy, the progesterone and estrogen required to maintain pregnancy are produced by the ovarian corpus luteum. For the first few days after ovulation, the corpus luteum is maintained by maternal LH. However, as maternal LH concentration falls owing to increasing concentrations of progesterone and estrogen, the corpus luteum will continue to function only if the role of maternal LH is taken over by hCG produced by syncytiotrophoblast cells in the placenta.

Clinical Pharmacology

A. Ovulation Induction

The gonadotropins are used to induce follicle development and ovulation in women with anovulation that is secondary to hypogonadotropic hypogonadism, polycystic ovary syndrome, and other causes. Because of the high cost of gonadotropins and the need for close monitoring during their administration, they are generally reserved for anovulatory women who fail to respond to other less complicated forms of treatment (eg, clomiphene; see Chapter 40). Gonadotropins are also used for **controlled ovarian stimulation** in assisted reproductive technology procedures. Currently, a number of different protocols use gonadotropins in ovulation induction and controlled ovulation stimulation, and new protocols are continually being developed to improve the rates of success and to decrease the two primary risks of ovulation induction: multiple pregnancies and the **ovarian hyperstimulation syndrome** (**OHSS**; see below).

Although the details differ, all of these protocols are based on the complex physiology that underlies a normal menstrual cycle. Like a menstrual cycle, controlled ovulation stimulation is discussed in relation to a cycle that begins on the first day of a menstrual bleed (Figure 37–3). Shortly after the first day (usually on day 2), daily injections with one of the FSH preparations (hMG or rFSH) are begun and continued for approximately 9–12 days. In women with hypogonadotropic hypogonadism, follicle development requires treatment with a combination of FSH and LH because these women do not produce the basal level of LH that is required for normal follicle development. The dose and duration of gonadotropin treatment are based on the response as measured by the serum estradiol concentration and by ultrasound evaluation of ovarian follicle development. When exogenous gonadotropins are used to stimulate follicle development, there is risk of a premature endogenous surge in LH owing to the rapidly increasing serum estradiol levels. To prevent this, gonadotropins are almost always administered in conjunction with a drug that blocks the effects of endogenous GnRH—either continuous administration of a GnRH agonist, which down-regulates GnRH receptors, or a GnRH receptor antagonist (see below and Figure 37–3).

When appropriate follicular growth has occurred, the gonadotropin and the GnRH agonist or GnRH antagonist injections are discontinued and hCG (3300–10,000 IU) is administered subcutaneously to induce final oocyte maturation and, in ovulation induction protocols, ovulation. The hCG administration is followed by timed intercourse or intrauterine insemination in ovulation induction and by oocyte retrieval in assisted reproductive technology procedures. Because use of GnRH agonists or antagonists during the follicular phase of ovulation induction suppresses endogenous LH production, it is important to provide exogenous hormonal support of the luteal phase. In clinical trials, exogenous progesterone, hCG, or a combination of the two have been effective at providing adequate luteal support. However, progesterone is preferred for luteal support because hCG carries a higher risk of OHSS in patients with high follicular response to gonadotropins.

B. Male Infertility

Most of the signs and symptoms of hypogonadism in males (eg, delayed puberty, retention of prepubertal secondary sex characteristics after puberty) can be adequately treated with exogenous androgen; however, treatment of infertility in hypogonadal men requires the activity of both LH and FSH. For many years, conventional therapy has consisted of initial treatment for 8–12 weeks with injections of 1000–2500 IU hCG several times per week. After the initial phase, hMG is injected at a dose of 75–150 IU three times per week. In men with hypogonadal hypogonadism, it takes an average of 4–6 months of such treatment for sperm to appear in the ejaculate in up to 90% of patients, but often not at normal levels. Even if pregnancy does not occur spontaneously, the number of sperm is often sufficient that pregnancy can be achieved by insemination with the patient's semen (intrauterine insemination) or with the help of an assisted reproductive technique such

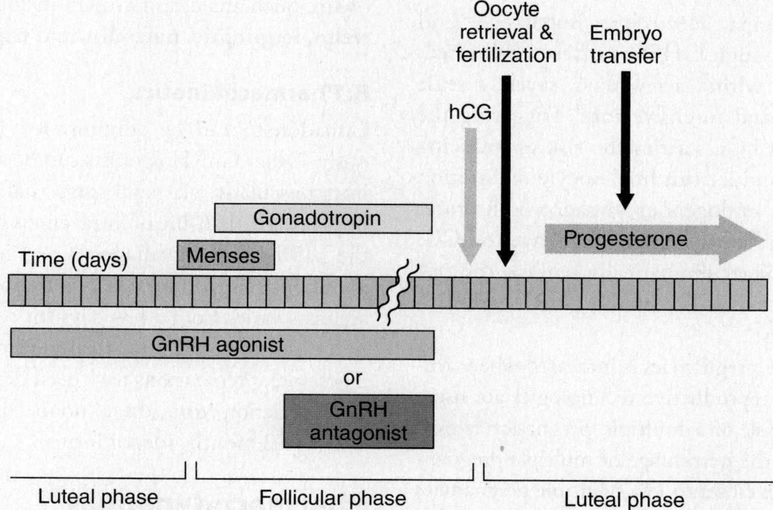

FIGURE 37–3 Controlled ovarian stimulation in preparation for an assisted reproductive technology such as in vitro fertilization. Follicular phase: Follicle development is stimulated with gonadotropin injections that begin about 2 days after menses begin. When the follicles are ready, as assessed by ultrasound measurement of follicle size, final oocyte maturation is induced by an injection of hCG. Luteal phase: Shortly thereafter oocytes are retrieved and fertilized in vitro. The recipient's luteal phase is supported with injections of progesterone. To prevent a premature luteinizing-hormone surge, endogenous LH secretion is inhibited with either a GnRH agonist or a GnRH antagonist. In most protocols, the GnRH agonist is started midway through the preceding luteal cycle.

as in vitro fertilization with or without intracytoplasmic sperm injection (ICSI), in which a single sperm is injected directly into a mature oocyte that has been retrieved after controlled ovarian stimulation of a female partner. With the advent of ICSI, the minimum threshold of spermatogenesis required for pregnancy is greatly lowered.

C. Outdated Uses

Chorionic gonadotropin is approved for the treatment of prepubertal cryptorchidism. Prepubertal boys were treated with intramuscular injections of hCG for 2–6 weeks. However, this clinical use is no longer supported because the long-term efficacy of hormonal treatment of cryptorchidism (~20%) is much lower than the long-term efficacy of surgical treatment (>95%), and because of concerns that early childhood treatment with hCG treatment has a negative impact on germ cells in addition to increasing the risk of precocious puberty.

In the United States, chorionic gonadotropin has a black box warning against its use for increasing weight loss. The use of hCG plus severe calorie restriction for weight loss was popularized by a publication in the 1950s claiming that the hCG selectively mobilizes body fat stores. This practice continues today, despite a preponderance of scientific evidence from placebo-controlled trials that hCG does not provide any weight loss benefit beyond the weight loss associated with severe calorie restriction alone.

Toxicity & Contraindications

In women treated with gonadotropins and hCG, the two most serious complications are **OHSS** and **multiple pregnancies.** Stimulation of the ovary during ovulation induction often leads to uncomplicated ovarian enlargement that usually resolves spontaneously. However, OHSS may occur and can be associated with ovarian enlargement, hypovolemia, ascites, liver dysfunction, pulmonary edema, electrolyte imbalance, and thromboembolic events. Although OHSS is often self-limited, with spontaneous resolution within a few days, severe disease may require hospitalization and intensive care. Triggering the final oocyte maturation with hCG carries the risk of inducing OHSS. GnRH agonists also induce this final oocyte maturation by promoting the release of endogenous gonadotropin stores from the hypophysis and can be used as an alternative to hCG. Use of the GnRH agonist trigger dramatically reduces the risk of OHSS, owing to the short half-life of the GnRH agonist–induced endogenous LH surge.

The probability of multiple pregnancies is increased when ovulation induction and assisted reproductive technologies are used. In ovulation induction, the risk of a multiple pregnancy is estimated to be 5–10%, whereas the percentage of multiple pregnancies in the general population is closer to 1%. Multiple pregnancies carry an increased risk of complications, such as gestational diabetes, preeclampsia, preterm labor, and premature birth. For in vitro fertilization procedures, the risk of a multiple pregnancy is determined primarily by the number of embryos transferred to the patient. A strong trend in recent years has been to transfer single embryos to avoid multiple pregnancy.

Other reported adverse effects of gonadotropin treatment are headache, depression, edema, precocious puberty, and (rarely) production of antibodies to hCG. In men treated with gonadotropins, the risk of gynecomastia is directly correlated with the level of testosterone produced in response to treatment.

GONADOTROPIN-RELEASING HORMONE & ITS ANALOGS

Gonadotropin-releasing hormone is secreted by neurons in the hypothalamus. It travels through the hypothalamic-pituitary venous portal plexus to the anterior pituitary, where it binds to G protein-coupled receptors on the plasma membranes of gonadotrophs. *Pulsatile* GnRH secretion is required to stimulate the gonadotrophs to produce and release LH and FSH.

Sustained *nonpulsatile* administration of GnRH or GnRH analogs *inhibits* the release of FSH and LH by the pituitary in both women and men, resulting in hypogonadotropic hypogonadism. GnRH agonists are used to induce gonadal suppression in children with central precocious puberty, in early adolescents who are transgender or gender diverse, and in men with prostate cancer. They are also used in women who are undergoing assisted reproductive technology procedures or who have a gynecologic problem (like endometriosis) that is benefited by ovarian suppression.

Chemistry & Pharmacokinetics

A. Structure

GnRH is a decapeptide found in all mammals. **Gonadorelin** is an acetate salt of synthetic human GnRH. Substitution of amino acids at the 6 position or replacement of the C-terminal glycine-amide produces synthetic agonists. Both modifications make them more potent and longer-lasting than native GnRH and gonadorelin. Such analogs of GnRH include **goserelin, buserelin, histrelin, leuprolide, nafarelin,** and **triptorelin.**

B. Pharmacokinetics

Gonadorelin can be administered intravenously or subcutaneously. Other GnRH agonists can be administered subcutaneously, intramuscularly, via nasal spray (nafarelin), or as a subcutaneous implant. The half-life of intravenous gonadorelin is 4 minutes, and the half-lives of subcutaneous and intranasal GnRH analogs are approximately 3 hours. The duration of clinical uses of GnRH agonists varies from a few days for controlled ovarian stimulation to a number of years for treatment of metastatic prostate cancer. Therefore, preparations have been developed with a range of durations of action from several hours (for daily administration) to 1, 3, 6, or 12 months (depot forms).

Pharmacodynamics

The physiologic actions of GnRH exhibit complex dose-response relationships that change dramatically from the fetal period through the end of puberty. This is not surprising in view of the complex role that GnRH plays in normal reproduction, particularly in female reproduction. Pulsatile GnRH release occurs and is responsible for stimulating LH and FSH production during the fetal and neonatal period. Subsequently, from the age of 2 years until the onset of puberty, GnRH secretion falls off and the pituitary simultaneously exhibits very low sensitivity to GnRH. Just before puberty, an increase in the frequency and amplitude of GnRH release occurs and then, in early puberty, pituitary sensitivity to GnRH increases, which is due in part to the effect of increasing concentrations of gonadal steroids. In females, it usually takes several months to a year after the onset of puberty for the hypothalamic-pituitary system to produce an LH surge and ovulation. By the end of puberty, the system is well established so that menstrual cycles proceed at relatively constant intervals. The amplitude and frequency of GnRH pulses vary in a regular pattern through the menstrual cycle with the highest amplitudes occurring during the luteal phase and the highest frequency occurring late in the follicular phase. Lower pulse frequencies favor FSH secretion, whereas higher pulse frequencies favor LH secretion. Gonadal steroids as well as the peptide hormones activin, inhibin, and follistatin have complex modulatory effects on the gonadotropin response to GnRH.

In the pharmacologic use of GnRH and its analogs, pulsatile intravenous administration of gonadorelin every 1–4 hours stimulates FSH and LH secretion. Continuous administration of gonadorelin or its longer-acting analogs produces a biphasic response. During the first 7–10 days, an agonist effect results in increased concentrations of gonadal hormones in males and females; this initial phase is referred to as a *flare*. After this period, the continued presence of GnRH results in an inhibitory action that manifests as a drop in the concentration of gonadotropins and gonadal steroids (ie, hypogonadotropic hypogonadal state). The inhibitory action is due to a combination of receptor down-regulation and changes in the signaling pathways activated by GnRH.

Clinical Pharmacology

The GnRH agonists are occasionally used for stimulation of gonadotropin production. They are used far more commonly for suppression of gonadotropin release.

A. Stimulation

1. *Female infertility*—In the current era of widespread availability of gonadotropins and assisted reproductive technology, the use of pulsatile GnRH administration to treat infertility is uncommon. Although pulsatile GnRH is less likely than gonadotropins to cause multiple pregnancies and OHSS, the inconvenience and cost associated with continuous use of an intravenous pump and difficulties obtaining native GnRH (gonadorelin) are barriers to pulsatile GnRH. When this approach is used, a portable battery-powered programmable pump and intravenous tubing deliver pulses of gonadorelin every 90 minutes.

Gonadorelin or a GnRH agonist analog (eg, leuprolide) can be used to initiate an LH surge and ovulation in women with infertility who are undergoing ovulation induction with gonadotropins. Traditionally, hCG has been used to initiate ovulation in this situation. However, gonadorelin or a GnRH agonist is less likely to cause OHSS compared with hCG.

2. *Male infertility*—It is possible to use pulsatile gonadorelin for infertility in men with hypothalamic hypogonadotropic hypogonadism. A portable pump infuses gonadorelin intravenously every 90 minutes. Serum testosterone levels and semen analyses must be done regularly. At least 3–6 months of pulsatile infusions are required before significant numbers of sperm are seen. As described above, treatment of hypogonadotropic hypogonadism is more commonly done with hCG and hMG or their recombinant equivalents.

3. *Diagnosis of LH responsiveness*—GnRH may be useful in determining whether delayed puberty in a hypogonadotropic adolescent is due to constitutional delay or to hypogonadotropic hypogonadism. The LH response (but not the FSH response) to a single dose of GnRH may distinguish between these two conditions; however, there can be significant individual overlap in the LH response between the two groups. Serum LH levels are measured before and at several times after an intravenous or subcutaneous bolus of GnRH. An increase in serum LH with a peak that is >5–8 mIU/mL suggests early pubertal status. An impaired LH response suggests hypogonadotropic hypogonadism due to either pituitary or hypothalamic disease, but it does not rule out constitutional delay of puberty.

B. Suppression of Gonadotropin Production

1. *Controlled ovarian stimulation*—In the controlled ovarian stimulation that provides multiple mature oocytes for assisted reproductive technologies such as in vitro fertilization, it is critical to suppress an endogenous LH surge that could prematurely trigger ovulation. This suppression is achieved by daily subcutaneous injections of leuprolide or daily nasal applications of nafarelin. For leuprolide, treatment is commonly initiated with 1 mg daily for about 10 days until menstrual bleeding occurs. At that point, the dose is reduced to 0.5 mg daily until hCG is administered (see Figure 37–3). For nafarelin, the beginning dosage is generally 400 mcg twice a day, which is decreased to 200 mcg when menstrual bleeding occurs.

2. *Endometriosis*—Endometriosis is defined as the presence of estrogen-sensitive endometrium outside the uterus that results in cyclical abdominal pain in premenopausal women. The pain of endometriosis is often reduced by abolishing exposure to the cyclical changes in the concentrations of estrogen and progesterone that are a normal part of the menstrual cycle. The ovarian suppression induced by continuous treatment with a GnRH agonist greatly reduces estrogen and progesterone concentrations and prevents cyclical changes. The preferred duration of treatment with a GnRH agonist is limited to 6 months because ovarian suppression beyond this period can result in decreased bone mineral density. When relief of pain from treatment with a GnRH agonist supports continued therapy for more than 6 months, the addition of add-back therapy (estrogen or progestins) reduces or eliminates GnRH agonist-induced bone mineral loss and provides symptomatic relief without reducing the efficacy of pain relief. Leuprolide and goserelin are administered as depot preparations that provide 1 or 3 months of continuous

GnRH agonist activity. Nafarelin is administered twice daily as a nasal spray at a dose of 0.2 mg per spray.

3. *Uterine leiomyomata (uterine fibroids)*—Uterine leiomyomata are benign, estrogen-sensitive, smooth muscle tumors in the uterus that can cause menorrhagia, with associated anemia and pelvic pain. Treatment for 3–6 months with a GnRH agonist reduces fibroid size and, when combined with supplemental iron, improves anemia. The effects of GnRH agonists are temporary, with gradual recurrent growth of leiomyomas to previous size within several months after cessation of treatment. GnRH agonists have been used widely for preoperative treatment of uterine leiomyomas, for both myomectomy and hysterectomy. GnRH agonists have been shown to improve hematologic parameters, shorten hospital stay, and decrease blood loss, operating time, and postoperative pain when given for 3 months preoperatively.

4. *Prostate cancer*—Androgen deprivation therapy is the primary medical therapy for prostate cancer. Combined antiandrogen therapy with continuous GnRH agonist and an androgen receptor antagonist is as effective as surgical castration in reducing serum testosterone concentrations and effects. Leuprolide, goserelin, histrelin, buserelin, and triptorelin are approved for this indication. The preferred formulation is one of the long-acting depot forms that provide 1, 3, 4, 6, or 12 months of active drug therapy. During the first 7–10 days of GnRH analog therapy, serum testosterone levels increase because of the agonist action of the drug; this can precipitate pain in patients with bone metastases, and tumor growth and neurologic symptoms in patients with vertebral metastases. It can also temporarily worsen symptoms of urinary obstruction. Such tumor flares can usually be avoided with the concomitant administration of an androgen receptor antagonist (flutamide, bicalutamide, or nilutamide) (see Chapter 40). Within about 2 weeks, serum testosterone levels fall to the hypogonadal range.

5. *Central precocious puberty*—Continuous administration of a GnRH agonist is indicated for treatment of central precocious puberty (onset of secondary sex characteristics before 7–8 years in girls or 9 years in boys). Before embarking on treatment with a GnRH agonist, one must confirm central precocious puberty by demonstrating a pubertal gonadotropin response to GnRH or a "test dose" of a GnRH analog. Treatment is indicated in a child whose final height would be otherwise significantly compromised (as evidenced by a significantly advanced bone age) or in whom the early development of pubertal secondary sexual characteristics or menses causes significant emotional distress. While central precocious puberty is most often idiopathic, it is important to rule out central nervous system pathology with MRI imaging of the hypothalamic-pituitary area.

Treatment is most commonly carried out with either every-month or every-3-months intramuscular or every-6-months subcutaneous depot injection of leuprolide acetate or with a once-yearly implant of histrelin acetate. Daily subcutaneous regimens and multiple daily nasal spray regimens of GnRH agonists also are available but are not recommended due to poor adherence. Treatment with a GnRH agonist is generally continued long enough to optimize adult height and allow pubertal development that is concurrent with peers. Typically, treatment is continued until age 11 in females and age 12 in males.

6. *Other*—The gonadal suppression provided by continuous GnRH agonist treatment is used in the management of advanced breast and ovarian cancer. In addition, clinical practice guidelines recommend the use of continuous GnRH agonist administration in early pubertal transgender adolescents to block endogenous puberty prior to subsequent treatment with cross-gender gonadal hormones.

Toxicity

Gonadorelin can cause headache, light-headedness, nausea, and flushing. Local swelling often occurs at subcutaneous injection sites. Generalized hypersensitivity dermatitis has occurred after long-term subcutaneous administration. Rare acute hypersensitivity reactions include bronchospasm and anaphylaxis. Sudden pituitary apoplexy and blindness have been reported following administration of GnRH to a patient with a gonadotropin-secreting pituitary tumor.

Continuous treatment of women with a GnRH analog (leuprolide, nafarelin, goserelin) causes the typical symptoms of menopause, which include hot flushes, sweats, and headaches. Depression, diminished libido, generalized pain, vaginal dryness, and breast atrophy also may occur. Ovarian cysts may develop within the first month of therapy due to its flare effect on gonadotropin secretion and generally resolve after an additional 6 weeks. Reduced bone mineral density and osteoporosis may occur with prolonged use, so patients should be monitored with bone densitometry before repeated treatment courses. Depending on the condition being treated with the GnRH agonist, it may be possible to ameliorate the signs and symptoms of the hypoestrogenic state without losing clinical efficacy by adding back a small dose of a progestin alone or in combination with a low dose of an estrogen. Contraindications to the use of GnRH agonists in women include pregnancy and breast-feeding.

In men treated with continuous GnRH agonist administration, adverse effects include hot flushes and sweats, edema, gynecomastia, decreased libido, decreased hematocrit, reduced bone density, asthenia, and injection site reactions. GnRH analog treatment of children is generally well tolerated. However, temporary exacerbation of precocious puberty may occur during the first few weeks of therapy. Nafarelin nasal spray may cause or aggravate sinusitis.

GnRH RECEPTOR ANTAGONISTS

Four synthetic decapeptides that function as competitive antagonists of GnRH receptors are available for clinical use. **Ganirelix, cetrorelix, abarelix,** and **degarelix** inhibit the secretion of FSH and LH in a dose-dependent manner. Ganirelix and cetrorelix are approved for use in controlled ovarian stimulation procedures, whereas degarelix and abarelix are approved for men with advanced prostate cancer. More recently, orally active nonpeptide

GnRH-receptor antagonists (eg, **elagolix, relugolix, linzagolix**) were introduced to clinical practice for the management of moderate to severe pain associated with endometriosis and of moderate to severe pain/abnormal uterine bleeding symptoms of uterine fibroids in women of reproductive age.

Pharmacokinetics

Ganirelix and cetrorelix are absorbed rapidly after subcutaneous injection. Administration of 0.25 mg daily maintains GnRH antagonism. Alternatively, a single 3.0-mg dose of cetrorelix suppresses LH secretion for 96 hours. Degarelix therapy is initiated with 240 mg administered as two subcutaneous injections. Maintenance dosing is with an 80-mg subcutaneous injection every 28 days. Elagolix rapidly suppressed LH, FSH, estradiol, and progesterone in a dose-dependent manner when administered orally at doses of 150 mg once daily or 100–400 mg twice daily in premenopausal women.

Clinical Pharmacology

A. Suppression of Gonadotropin Production

1. *Controlled ovarian stimulation*

Ganirelix and cetrorelix are approved for preventing the LH surge during controlled ovarian stimulation. They offer several advantages over continuous treatment with a GnRH agonist. Because GnRH antagonists produce an immediate antagonist effect, their use can be delayed until day 6–8 of the in vitro fertilization cycle (see Figure 37–3), and thus the duration of administration is shorter. They also appear to have a less suppressive effect on the ovarian response to gonadotropin stimulation, which permits a decrease in the total duration and dose of gonadotropin. On the other hand, because their antagonist effects reverse more quickly after their discontinuation, adherence to the treatment regimen is critical.

2. *Endometriosis and uterine leiomyoma*

In 2018, the FDA approved elagolix tablets for the management of moderate to severe pain associated with endometriosis. Elagolix and other non-peptide GnRH-receptor antagonist with and without low-dose hormone add-back therapy are undergoing phase III clinical trial for heavy menstrual bleeding and pain associated with uterine leiomyoma.

3. *Advanced prostate cancer*

Degarelix and abarelix are approved for the treatment of symptomatic advanced prostate cancer. These GnRH antagonists reduce concentrations of gonadotropins and androgens more rapidly than GnRH agonists and avoid the testosterone surge seen with GnRH agonist therapy.

Toxicity

When used for controlled ovarian stimulation, ganirelix and cetrorelix are well tolerated. The most common adverse effects are nausea and headache. Elagolix is also well tolerated in women with endometriosis or uterine leiomyoma with most adverse effects (eg, hot flush, night sweats, headache, mood swings) being of mild to moderate severity. During the treatment of men with prostate cancer, degarelix causes injection-site reactions and increases in liver enzymes. Like continuous treatment with a GnRH agonist, degarelix and abarelix lead to signs and symptoms of androgen deprivation, including hot flushes and weight gain.

PROLACTIN

Prolactin is a 198-amino-acid peptide hormone produced in the anterior pituitary. Its structure resembles that of GH. Prolactin is the principal hormone responsible for lactation. Milk production is stimulated by prolactin when appropriate circulating levels of estrogens, progestins, corticosteroids, and insulin are present. A deficiency of prolactin—which can occur in rare states of pituitary deficiency—is manifested by failure to lactate. No preparation of prolactin is available for use in prolactin-deficient patients.

In pituitary stalk section from surgery or head trauma, stalk compression due to a sellar mass, or rare cases of hypothalamic destruction, prolactin levels may be elevated as a result of impaired transport of dopamine (prolactin-inhibiting hormone) to the pituitary. Much more commonly, prolactin is elevated as a result of prolactin-secreting adenomas. In addition, a number of drugs elevate prolactin levels. These include antipsychotic and gastrointestinal motility drugs that are known dopamine receptor antagonists, estrogens, and opiates. Hyperprolactinemia causes hypogonadism, which manifests with infertility, oligomenorrhea or amenorrhea, and galactorrhea in premenopausal women, and with loss of libido, erectile dysfunction, and infertility in men. In the case of large tumors (macroadenomas), hyperprolactinemia can be associated with symptoms of a pituitary mass, including visual changes due to compression of the optic nerves. The hypogonadism and infertility associated with hyperprolactinemia result from inhibition of GnRH release. For patients with symptomatic hyperprolactinemia, inhibition of prolactin secretion can be achieved with dopamine agonists, which act in the pituitary to inhibit prolactin release.

DOPAMINE AGONISTS

Adenomas that secrete excess prolactin usually retain the sensitivity to inhibition by dopamine exhibited by normal pituitary lactotrophs, prolactin secreting cells. Bromocriptine and cabergoline are ergot derivatives (see Chapters 16 and 28) with a high affinity for dopamine D_2 receptors. Quinagolide, a drug approved in Europe, is a nonergot agent with similarly high D_2 receptor affinity. The chemical structure and pharmacokinetic features of ergot alkaloids are presented in Chapter 16.

Dopamine agonists suppress prolactin release very effectively in patients with hyperprolactinemia and GH release is reduced in patients with acromegaly, although not as effectively as somatostatin analogs. Bromocriptine has also been used in Parkinson disease to improve motor function and reduce levodopa requirements (see Chapter 28). Newer, nonergot D_2 agonists used in Parkinson disease (pramipexole and ropinirole; see Chapter 28) have been reported to interfere with lactation, but they are not approved for use in hyperprolactinemia.

Pharmacokinetics

All available dopamine agonists are active as oral preparations, and all are eliminated by metabolism. They can also be absorbed systemically after vaginal insertion of tablets to avoid nausea due to oral administration. Cabergoline, with a half-life of approximately 65 hours, has the longest duration of action. Quinagolide has a half-life of about 20 hours, whereas the half-life of bromocriptine is about 7 hours. After vaginal administration, serum levels peak more slowly.

Clinical Pharmacology

A. Hyperprolactinemia

A dopamine agonist is the standard first-line treatment for hyperprolactinemia. These drugs shrink pituitary prolactin-secreting tumors, lower circulating prolactin levels, and restore ovulation in approximately 70% of women with microadenomas and 30% of women with macroadenomas (Figure 37–4). Cabergoline is initiated at 0.25 mg twice weekly orally or vaginally. It can be increased gradually, according to serum prolactin determinations, up to a maximum of 1 mg twice weekly. Bromocriptine is generally taken daily after the evening meal at the initial dose of 1.25 mg; the dose is then increased as tolerated. Most patients require 2.5–7.5 mg daily. Long-acting oral bromocriptine formulations (Parlodel SRO) and intramuscular formulations (Parlodel LAR) are available outside the United States.

B. Physiologic Lactation

Dopamine agonists were used in the past to prevent breast engorgement when breast-feeding was not desired. Their use for this purpose has been discouraged because of toxicity (see Toxicity & Contraindications).

C. Acromegaly

A dopamine agonist alone or in combination with pituitary surgery, radiation therapy, or somatostatin analog administration can be used to treat acromegaly. The doses required are higher than those used to treat hyperprolactinemia. For example, patients with acromegaly require 20–30 mg/d of bromocriptine and seldom respond adequately to bromocriptine alone unless the pituitary tumor secretes prolactin as well as GH.

Toxicity & Contraindications

Dopamine agonists can cause nausea, headache, light-headedness, orthostatic hypotension, and fatigue. Psychiatric manifestations occasionally occur, even at lower doses, and may take months to resolve. Erythromelalgia occurs rarely. High dosages of ergot-derived preparations can cause cold-induced peripheral digital vasospasm. Pulmonary infiltrates have occurred with chronic high-dosage therapy. Cabergoline treatment at high doses for Parkinson disease is associated with higher risk of valvular heart disease, but probably not at the lower dose used for hyperprolactinemia. Cabergoline appears to cause nausea less often than bromocriptine. Vaginal administration can reduce nausea, but may cause local irritation.

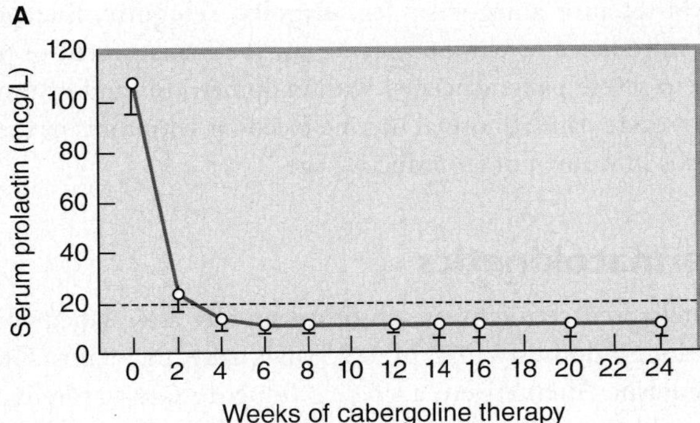

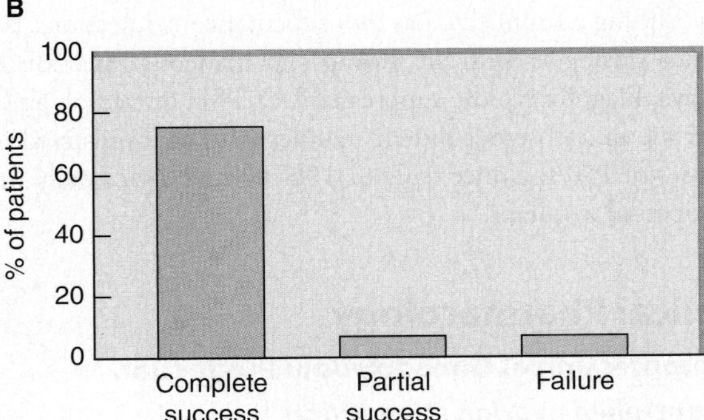

FIGURE 37–4 Results from a clinical trial of cabergoline in women with hyperprolactinemia and anovulation. **(A)** The dashed line indicates the upper limit of normal serum prolactin concentrations. **(B)** Complete success was defined as pregnancy or at least two consecutive menses with evidence of ovulation at least once. Partial success was two menstrual cycles without evidence of ovulation or just one ovulatory cycle. The most common reasons for withdrawal from the trial were nausea, headache, dizziness, abdominal pain, and fatigue. (Data from Webster J, Piscitelli G, Polli A, Ferrari CI, Ismail I, Scanlon MF: A comparison of cabergoline and bromocriptine in the treatment of hyperprolactinemic amenorrhea. Cabergoline Comparative Study Group, N Engl J Med 1994 Oct 6;331(14):904-909.)

Dopamine agonist therapy during the early weeks of pregnancy has not been associated with an increased risk of spontaneous abortion or congenital malformations. Although there has been a longer experience with the safety of bromocriptine during early pregnancy, there is growing evidence that cabergoline is also safe in women with macroadenomas who must continue a dopamine agonist during pregnancy. In patients with small pituitary adenomas, dopamine agonist therapy is discontinued upon conception because the risk of growth of microadenomas during pregnancy is low (2.7%). Patients with macroadenomas require vigilance, as the risk for tumor progression is high (22.9%) and such patients often require a dopamine agonist throughout pregnancy. There have been rare reports of stroke or coronary thrombosis in postpartum women taking bromocriptine to suppress postpartum lactation.

POSTERIOR PITUITARY HORMONES

The two posterior pituitary hormones—vasopressin and oxytocin—are synthesized in neuronal cell bodies in the hypothalamus and transported via their axons to the posterior pituitary, where they are stored and then released into the circulation. Each has limited but important clinical uses.

OXYTOCIN

Oxytocin is a peptide hormone secreted by the posterior pituitary. Oxytocin stimulates muscular contractions in the uterus and myoepithelial contractions in the breast. Thus, it is involved in parturition and the letdown of milk. During the second half of pregnancy, uterine smooth muscle shows an increase in the expression of oxytocin receptors and becomes increasingly sensitive to the stimulant action of endogenous oxytocin.

Chemistry & Pharmacokinetics

A. Structure

Oxytocin is a 9-amino-acid peptide with an intrapeptide disulfide cross-link (Figure 37–5). Its amino acid sequence differs from that of vasopressin at positions 3 and 8.

B. Absorption, Metabolism, and Excretion

Oxytocin is administered intravenously for initiation and augmentation of labor. It also can be administered intramuscularly for control of postpartum bleeding. Oxytocin is not bound to plasma proteins and is rapidly eliminated by the kidneys and liver, with a circulating half-life of 5 minutes.

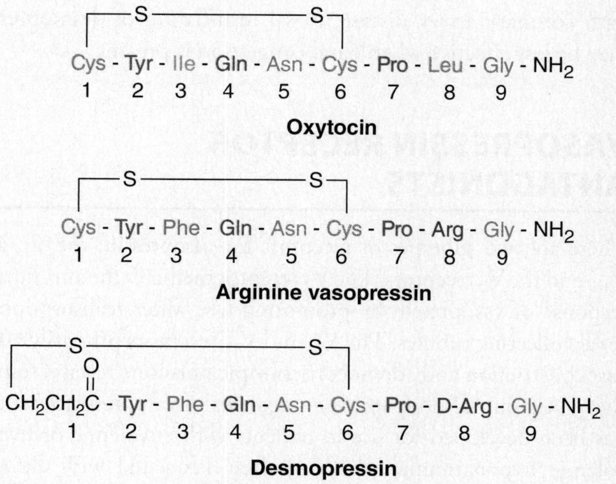

S—S (disulfide bridge between positions 1 and 6)

Cys - Tyr - Ile - Gln - Asn - Cys - Pro - Leu - Gly - NH_2
1 2 3 4 5 6 7 8 9

Oxytocin

S—S (disulfide bridge between positions 1 and 6)

Cys - Tyr - Phe - Gln - Asn - Cys - Pro - Arg - Gly - NH_2
1 2 3 4 5 6 7 8 9

Arginine vasopressin

S—S (disulfide bridge between positions 1 and 6)

$CH_2CH_2C(=O)$ - Tyr - Phe - Gln - Asn - Cys - Pro - D-Arg - Gly - NH_2
1 2 3 4 5 6 7 8 9

Desmopressin

FIGURE 37–5 Posterior pituitary hormones and desmopressin. (Reproduced with permission from Ganong WF: *Review of Medical Physiology*, 21st ed. New York, NY: McGraw Hill; 2003.)

Pharmacodynamics

Oxytocin acts through G protein-coupled receptors and the phosphoinositide-calcium second-messenger system to contract uterine smooth muscle. Oxytocin also stimulates the release of prostaglandins and leukotrienes that augment uterine contraction. In small doses oxytocin increases both the frequency and the force of uterine contractions. At higher doses, it produces sustained contraction.

Oxytocin also causes contraction of myoepithelial cells surrounding mammary alveoli, which leads to milk letdown. Without oxytocin-induced contraction, normal lactation cannot occur. At high concentrations, oxytocin has weak antidiuretic and pressor activity due to activation of vasopressin receptors.

Clinical Pharmacology

Oxytocin is used to induce labor for conditions requiring expedited vaginal delivery such as uncontrolled maternal diabetes, worsening preeclampsia, intrauterine infection, or ruptured membranes after 34 gestational weeks. It is also used to augment protracted labor. Oxytocin can also be used in the immediate postpartum period to stop vaginal bleeding due to uterine atony.

Before delivery, oxytocin is usually administered intravenously via an infusion pump with appropriate fetal and maternal monitoring. For induction of labor, an initial infusion rate of 0.5–2 mU/min is increased every 30–60 minutes until a physiologic contraction pattern is established. The maximum infusion rate is 20 mU/min. For postpartum uterine bleeding, 10–40 units are added to 1 L of 5% dextrose, and the infusion rate is titrated to control uterine atony. Alternatively, 10 units of oxytocin can be administered by intramuscular injection.

During the antepartum period, oxytocin induces uterine contractions that transiently reduce placental blood flow to the fetus. The oxytocin challenge test measures the fetal heart rate response to a standardized oxytocin infusion and provides information about placental circulatory reserve. An abnormal response, seen as late decelerations in the fetal heart rate, may indicate fetal hypoxia and may warrant immediate cesarean delivery.

Toxicity & Contraindications

When oxytocin is used judiciously, serious toxicity is rare. The toxicity that does occur is due either to excessive stimulation of uterine contractions or to inadvertent activation of vasopressin receptors. Excessive stimulation of uterine contractions before delivery can cause fetal distress, placental abruption, or uterine rupture. These complications can be detected early by means of standard fetal monitoring. High concentrations of oxytocin with activation of vasopressin receptors can cause excessive fluid retention, or water intoxication, leading to hyponatremia, heart failure, seizures, and death. Bolus injections of oxytocin can cause hypotension. To avoid hypotension, oxytocin is administered intravenously as dilute solutions at a controlled rate.

Contraindications to oxytocin include fetal distress, fetal malpresentation, placental abruption, and other predispositions for uterine rupture, including previous extensive uterine surgery.

OXYTOCIN ANTAGONIST

Atosiban is an antagonist of the oxytocin receptor that has been approved outside the United States as a treatment (tocolysis) for preterm labor. Atosiban is a modified form of oxytocin that is administered by intravenous infusion for 2–48 hours. In a small number of published clinical trials, atosiban appears to be as effective as β-adrenoceptor-agonist tocolytics and to produce fewer adverse effects. In 1998, however, the FDA decided not to approve atosiban based on concerns about efficacy and safety.

VASOPRESSIN (ANTIDIURETIC HORMONE, ADH)

Vasopressin is a peptide hormone released by the posterior pituitary in response to rising plasma tonicity or falling blood pressure. It possesses antidiuretic and vasopressor properties. A deficiency of this hormone results in central diabetes insipidus (DI) (see Chapters 15 and 17). Central DI is caused by a variety of acquired conditions, including tumors, trauma, and neurosurgical procedures, as well as congenital conditions that result in decreased neurons of the hypothalamic/posterior pituitary axis and loss of vasopressin secretion.

Chemistry & Pharmacokinetics

A. Structure

Vasopressin is a nonapeptide with a 6-amino-acid ring and a 3-amino-acid side chain. The residue at position 8 is arginine in humans and in most other mammals except pigs and related species, whose vasopressin contains lysine at position 8 (see Figure 37–5). Desmopressin acetate (DDAVP, 1-desamino-8-D-arginine vasopressin) is a long-acting synthetic analog of vasopressin with minimal pressor activity and an antidiuretic-to-pressor ratio 4000 times that of vasopressin. Desmopressin is modified at position 1 and contains a D-amino acid at position 8. Like vasopressin and oxytocin, desmopressin has a disulfide linkage between positions 1 and 6.

B. Absorption, Metabolism, and Excretion

Vasopressin is administered by intravenous or intramuscular injection. The half-life of circulating vasopressin is approximately 15 minutes, with renal and hepatic metabolism via reduction of the disulfide bond and peptide cleavage.

Desmopressin can be administered intravenously, subcutaneously, intranasally, or orally. The half-life of circulating desmopressin is 1.5–2.5 hours. Nasal desmopressin is available as a unit dose spray that delivers 10 mcg per spray; it is also available with a calibrated nasal tube that can be used to deliver a more precise dose. Nasal bioavailability of desmopressin is 3–4%, whereas oral bioavailability is less than 1%.

Pharmacodynamics

Vasopressin activates two subtypes of G protein-coupled receptors (see Chapter 17). V_1 receptors are found on vascular smooth muscle cells and mediate vasoconstriction via the coupling protein G_q and phospholipase C. V_2 receptors are found on renal tubule cells and reduce diuresis through increased water permeability and water resorption in the collecting tubules via G_s and adenylyl cyclase. Extrarenal V_2-like receptors regulate the release of coagulation factor VIII and von Willebrand factor, which increases platelet aggregation.

Clinical Pharmacology

Desmopressin is the treatment of choice for pituitary diabetes insipidus. The dosage of desmopressin is 10–40 mcg in two to three divided doses as a nasal spray or, as an oral tablet, 0.1–0.2 mg two to three times daily. Enteral absorption of desmopressin is decreased by 50% when taken with meals, so fasting administration may be required if there is poor response to oral dosing. The dosage by subcutaneous injection is 1–4 mcg every 12–24 hours as needed for polyuria, polydipsia, or hypernatremia. Vasopressin as intermittent subcutaneous injection or low-dose infusion may be used to treat diabetes insipidus with close monitoring of urine output for dose adjustments. Vasopressin infusion is effective in some cases of esophageal variceal bleeding and colonic diverticular bleeding and may be used as a second-line agent in refractory vasodilatory shock. Bedtime desmopressin therapy, by intranasal, oral, or sublingual administration, ameliorates nocturnal enuresis by decreasing nocturnal urine production. Desmopressin is also used for the treatment of coagulopathy in uremia, hemophilia A, and von Willebrand disease (see Chapter 34).

Toxicity & Contraindications

Headache, nausea, abdominal cramps, agitation, and allergic reactions occur rarely with use. Overdosage may cause water intoxication due to impaired ability to excrete free water from the kidneys, which results in hyponatremia that can progress to coma and/or seizures. Vasopressin, but not desmopressin, can cause vasoconstriction and ischemia and should be used cautiously in patients with coronary artery disease. Nasal insufflation of desmopressin may be less effective when nasal congestion is present.

VASOPRESSIN RECEPTOR ANTAGONISTS

There are two subtypes of receptors for vasopressin: the V_{1a} and V_{1b}, and the V_2 receptors. The V_2 receptor mediates the antidiuretic response of vasopressin by promoting free water reabsorption in renal collecting tubules. The V_{1a} and V_{1b} receptors primarily affect vasoconstriction and adrenocorticotropic hormone release, respectively. A group of nonpeptide antagonists of vasopressin receptors has been developed for use in patients with euvolemic or hypervolemic hyponatremia, which is often associated with elevated concentrations of vasopressin. Conivaptan has high affinity for both V_{1a} and V_2 receptors. Tolvaptan has a 30-fold higher affinity for V_2 than for V_1 receptors. In several clinical trials, both agents promote the excretion of free water, restoration of serum sodium concentration, relieve symptoms, and reduce objective signs of hyponatremia and heart failure. Conivaptan, administered intravenously, and tolvaptan, given orally, are approved by the FDA for treatment of persistent hyponatremia that cannot be maintained above 120 mEq/L or in patients with persistent neurologic symptoms. Tolvaptan treatment duration is limited to 30 days due to risk of hepatotoxicity, including life-threatening liver failure, and requires regular monitoring of ALT, AST, and bilirubins. Several other selective nonpeptide vasopressin receptor antagonists are being investigated for hyponatremia, ascites, and autosomal dominant polycystic kidney disease indications.

SUMMARY Hypothalamic & Pituitary Hormones[1]

Subclass, Drug	Mechanism of Action	Effects	Clinical Applications	Pharmacokinetics, Toxicities, Interactions
GROWTH HORMONE (GH)				
• Somatropin	Recombinant form of human GH • acts through GH receptors to increase production of IGF-I	Restores normal growth and metabolic GH effects in GH-deficient individuals • increases final adult height in some children with short stature not due to GH deficiency	Replacement in GH deficiency • increased final adult height in children with certain conditions associated with short stature (see Table 37–4) • wasting in HIV infection • short bowel syndrome	SC injection • *Toxicity:* Pseudotumor cerebri, slipped capital femoral epiphysis, edema, hyperglycemia, progression of scoliosis, risk of asphyxia in severely obese patients with Prader-Willi syndrome and upper airway obstruction or sleep apnea
• *Somapacitan, lonapegsomatropin: weekly formulation of somatropin*				
IGF-I AGONIST				
• Mecasermin	Recombinant form of IGF-I that stimulates IGF-I receptors	Improves growth and metabolic IGF-I effects in individuals with IGF-I deficiency due to severe GH resistance	Replacement in IGF-I deficiency that is not responsive to exogenous GH	SC injection • *Toxicity:* Hypoglycemia, intracranial hypertension, lipohypertrophy, tonsillar hypertrophy, increased liver enzymes
SOMATOSTATIN ANALOGS				
• Octreotide	Agonist at somatostatin receptors	Inhibits production of GH and, to a lesser extent, of TSH, glucagon, insulin, and gastrin	Acromegaly and several other hormone-secreting tumors • acute control of bleeding from esophageal varices • refractory diarrhea	SC or IV injection • oral • long-acting formulation injected IM monthly • *Toxicity:* Transient gastrointestinal disturbances, gallstones, bradycardia, cardiac conduction problems
• *Lanreotide: Similar to octreotide; available as a monthly SC injection formulation for acromegaly*				
• *Pasireotide: available as a monthly IM injection for acromegaly and Cushing disease (also SC dosing); frequent hyperglycemia*				
GH RECEPTOR ANTAGONIST				
• Pegvisomant	Blocks GH receptors	Ameliorates effects of excess GH production	Acromegaly	SC injection • *Toxicity:* Increased liver enzymes • need to monitor for pituitary adenoma growth
GONADOTROPINS: FOLLICLE-STIMULATING HORMONE (FSH) ANALOGS				
• Follitropin alfa	Activates FSH receptors	Mimics effects of endogenous FSH	Controlled ovarian stimulation • infertility due to hypogonadotropic hypogonadism in men	SC injection • *Toxicity:* Ovarian hyperstimulation syndrome and multiple pregnancies in women • gynecomastia in men • headache, depression, edema in both sexes
• *Follitropin beta: A recombinant product with the same peptide sequence as follitropin alfa but differs in its carbohydrate side chains*				
• *Urofollitropin: Human FSH purified from the urine of postmenopausal women*				
• *Menotropins (hMG): Extract of the urine of postmenopausal women; contains both FSH and LH activity*				

(continued)

Subclass, Drug	Mechanism of Action	Effects	Clinical Applications	Pharmacokinetics, Toxicities, Interactions
GONADOTROPINS: LUTEINIZING HORMONE (LH) ANALOGS				
• Human chorionic gonadotropin (hCG)	Agonist at LH receptors	Mimics effects of endogenous LH	Initiation of final oocyte maturation and ovulation during controlled ovarian stimulation • male hypogonadotropic hypogonadism	IM or SC injection • *Toxicity:* Ovarian hyperstimulation syndrome • headache, depression, edema in both sexes
• *Choriogonadotropin alfa: Recombinant form of hCG*				
• *Lutropin: Recombinant form of human LH*				
• *Menotropins (hMG): Extract of the urine of postmenopausal women that contains both FSH and LH activity*				
GONADOTROPIN-RELEASING HORMONE (GnRH) ANALOGS				
• Leuprolide	Agonist at GnRH receptors	Increased LH and FSH secretion with intermittent administration • reduced LH and FSH secretion with prolonged continuous administration	Ovarian suppression • controlled ovarian stimulation • central precocious puberty • block of endogenous puberty in some transgender/gender variant early pubertal adolescents • advanced prostate cancer	Administered IV, SC, IM, or intranasally • depot formulations are available • *Toxicity:* Headache, light-headedness, nausea, injection site reactions • symptoms of hypogonadism with continuous treatment
• *Gonadorelin: Synthetic human GnRH*				
• *Other GnRH analogs: Goserelin, buserelin, histrelin, nafarelin, and triptorelin*				
GONADOTROPIN-RELEASING HORMONE (GnRH) RECEPTOR ANTAGONISTS				
• Ganirelix	Blocks GnRH receptors	Reduces endogenous production of LH and FSH	Prevention of premature LH surge during controlled ovarian stimulation	SC injection • *Toxicity:* Nausea, headache
• *Cetrorelix: Similar to ganirelix, approved for controlled ovarian stimulation*				
• *Elagolix: Approved for the management of moderate to severe pain associated with endometriosis.*				
• *Degarelix and abarelix: Approved for advanced prostate cancer*				
DOPAMINE AGONISTS				
• Bromocriptine	Activates dopamine D_2 receptors	Suppresses pituitary secretion of prolactin and, less effectively, GH • dopaminergic effects on CNS motor control and behavior	Treatment of hyperprolactinemia • acromegaly • Parkinson disease (see Chapter 28)	Administered orally or, for hyperprolactinemia, vaginally • *Toxicity:* Gastrointestinal disturbances, orthostatic hypotension, headache, psychiatric disturbances, vasospasm and pulmonary infiltrates in high doses
• *Cabergoline: Another ergot derivative with similar effects*				
OXYTOCIN	Activates oxytocin receptors	Increased uterine contractions	Induction and augmentation of labor • control of uterine hemorrhage after delivery	IV infusion or IM injection • *Toxicity:* Fetal distress, placental abruption, uterine rupture, fluid retention, hypotension
OXYTOCIN RECEPTOR ANTAGONIST				
• Atosiban	Blocks oxytocin receptors	Decreased uterine contractions	Tocolysis for preterm labor (not available in the USA)	IV infusion • *Toxicity:* Concern about increased rates of infant death; not FDA approved
VASOPRESSIN RECEPTOR AGONISTS				
• Desmopressin	Relatively selective vasopressin V_2 receptor agonist	Acts in the kidney collecting duct cells to decrease the excretion of water • acts on extrarenal V_2 receptors to increase factor VIII and von Willebrand factor	Central diabetes insipidus • primary nocturnal enuresis • hemophilia A and von Willebrand disease	Oral, IV, SC, sublingual, or intranasal • *Toxicity:* Gastrointestinal disturbances, headache, hyponatremia, allergic reactions
• *Vasopressin: Available for treatment of diabetes insipidus and sometimes used to control bleeding from esophageal varices*				

(*continued*)

Subclass, Drug	Mechanism of Action	Effects	Clinical Applications	Pharmacokinetics, Toxicities, Interactions
VASOPRESSIN RECEPTOR ANTAGONIST				
• Conivaptan	Antagonist of vasopressin V_{1a} and V_2 receptors	Increased renal excretion of water in conditions associated with increased vasopressin	Hyponatremia in hospitalized patients	IV infusion • *Toxicity:* Infusion site reactions
• *Tolvaptan: Similar but more selective for vasopressin V_2 receptors; oral administration; indications: autosomal dominant polycystic kidney disease and hyponatremia; treatment course initiated in the hospital and limited to 30 days due to risk of hepatotoxicity*				

[1]See Tables 37–2 and 37–3 for summaries of the clinical uses of the rarely used hypothalamic and pituitary hormones not described in this table.

PREPARATIONS AVAILABLE

GENERIC NAME	AVAILABLE AS
GROWTH FACTOR AGONISTS & ANTAGONISTS	
Lanreotide acetate	Somatuline Depot
Lonapegsomatropin	Skytrofa
Mecasermin	Increlex
Octreotide acetate	Bynfezia, Mycapssa, Sandostatin, Sandostatin LAR Depot
Pasireotide	Signifor, Signifor LAR
Pegvisomant	Somavert
Somapacitan	Sogroya
Somatropin	Genotropin, Humatrope, Norditropin, Nutropin, Omnitrope, Saizen, Serostim, Zomacton, Zorbtive
GONADOTROPIN AGONISTS & ANTAGONISTS	
Abarelix	Plenaxis*
Cetrorelix acetate	Cetrotide
Choriogonadotropin alfa (rhCG)	Ovidrel
Chorionic gonadotropin (hCG)	Pregnyl, Novarel
Degarelix	Firmagon
Elagolix	Orilissa
Follitropin alfa (rFSH)	Gonal-f
Follitropin beta (rFSH)	Follistim
Ganirelix acetate	Antagon, Fyremadel
Gonadorelin hydrochloride (GnRH)	Factrel
Goserelin acetate	Zoladex
Histrelin acetate	Supprelin LA, Vantas
Leuprolide acetate	Eligard, Lupron, Fensolvi
Menotropins (hMG)	Menopur
Nafarelin acetate	Synarel
Triptorelin pamoate	Trelstar, Trelstar LA, Trelstar Depot, Triptodur
PROLACTIN ANTAGONISTS (DOPAMINE AGONISTS)	
Bromocriptine mesylate	Parlodel, Cycloset
Cabergoline	Dostinex
OXYTOCIN	
Oxytocin	Pitocin
VASOPRESSIN AGONISTS AND ANTAGONISTS	
Conivaptan HCl	Vaprisol
Desmopressin acetate	DDAVP, Nocdurna, Noctiva, Stimate
Tolvaptan	Samsca, Jynarque
Vasopressin	Pitressin
OTHER	
Corticorelin ovine triflutate	Acthrel
Corticotropin	H.P. Acthar Gel
ACTH	Cortrosyn, Cosyntropin
Thyrotropin alfa	Thyrogen

*Withdrawn from the USA.

REFERENCES

Abramovici A et al: Tocolytic therapy for acute preterm labor. Obstet Gynecol Clin North Am 2012;39:77.

Al-Inany HG et al: Gonadotrophin-releasing hormone antagonists for assisted reproductive technology. Cochrane Database Syst Rev 2016;(4):CD001750.

Albertsson-Wikland K et al: Mortality is not increased in recombinant human growth hormone-treated patients when adjusting for birth characteristics. J Clin Endocrinol Metab 2016;101:2149.

Bang P et al: Effectiveness and safety of rhIGF-1 therapy in children: The European Increlex Growth Forum Database Experience. Horm Res Paed 2015;83:345.

Bayne AP, Skoog SJ: Nocturnal enuresis: An approach to assessment and treatment. Pediatr Rev 2014;35:327.

Beall SA, DeCherney A: History and challenges surrounding ovarian stimulation in the treatment of infertility. Fertil Steril 2012;97:795.

Bergan-Roller HE, Sheridan MA: The growth hormone signaling system: Insights into coordinating the anabolic and catabolic actions of growth hormone. Gen Comp Endo 2018;258:119.

Bhandari S et al: A systematic review of known interventions for the treatment of chronic nonhypovolaemic hypotonic hyponatraemia and a meta-analysis of the vaptans. Clin Endocrinol 2017;86:761.

Carel JC et al: Long-term mortality after recombinant growth hormone treatment for isolated growth hormone deficiency or childhood short stature: Preliminary report of the French SAGhE study. J Clin Endocrinol Metab 2012;97:416.

Child CJ et al: Safety outcomes during pediatric GH therapy: Final results from the prospective GeNeSIS observational program. J Clin Endocrinol Metab 2019;104:379.

Colao et al: Pasireotide versus octreotide in acromegaly: a head-to-head superiority study. J Clin Endocrinol Metab 2014;99:791.

Deodati A, Cianfarani S: The rationale for growth hormone therapy in children with short stature. J Clin Res Ped Endo 2017;9:23.

Dreicer R et al: New data, new paradigms for treating prostate cancer patients—VI: Novel hormonal therapy approaches. Urology 2011;78(5 Suppl):S494.

Drube J et al: Clinical practice recommendations for growth hormone treatment in children with chronic kidney disease. Nat Rev Nephro 2019;15:577.

Gabe SG et al: Obstetrics: *Normal and Problem Pregnancies*, 6th ed. Churchill Livingstone, 2012.

Garrahy A et al: Diagnosis and management of central diabetes insipidus in adults. Clin Endocrinol 2019;90:23.

Giustina A et al: Multidisciplinary management of acromegaly: a consensus. Rev Endocr Metab Disord 2020;21:667.

Guo M et al: Growth hormone for intestinal adaptation in patients with short bowel syndrome: systematic review and meta-analysis of randomized controlled trials. Curr Ther Res Clin Exp 2011;72:109.

Klein KO, Lee PA: Gonadotropin-releasing hormone (GnRHa) therapy for central precocious puberty (CPP): Review of nuances in assessment of height, hormonal suppression, psychosocial issues, and weight gain, with patient examples. Ped Endo Rev 2018;15:298.

Lamb YN: Elagolix: First global approval. Drugs 2018;78:1501.

Long RK, Rosenthal SM: Endocrine disorders of the hypothalamus and pituitary. In: Swaiman KF et al (editors): *Swaiman's Pediatric Neurology*, 6th ed. Mosby (Elsevier), 2017.

Niederberger C et al: Forty years of IVF. Fertil Steril 2018;110:185.

Melmed S et al (eds): *Williams Textbook of Endocrinology*, 14th ed. Elsevier, 2019.

Papatsonis DN et al: Maintenance therapy with oxytocin antagonists for inhibiting preterm birth after threatened preterm labour. Cochrane Database Syst Rev 2013;(10):CD005938.

Penson D et al: Effectiveness of hormonal and surgical therapies for cryptorchidism: A systematic review. Pediatrics 2013;131:e1897.

Pfaffle R et al: Growth hormone treatment for short stature in the USA, Germany and France: 15 years of surveillance in the Genetics and Neuroendocrinology of Short-Stature International Study. Horm Res Paediatr 2018;90:169.

Prencipe N et al: Biliary adverse events in acromegaly during somatostatin receptor ligands: predictors of onset and response to ursodeoxycholic acid treatment. Pituitary 2021;24:242.

Quigley CA et al: Mortality in children receiving growth hormone treatment of growth disorders: Data from Genetics and Neuroendocrinology of Short Stature International Study. J Clin Endocrinol Metab 2017;102:3195.

Salati JA et al: Prophylactic oxytocin for the third stage of labour to prevent postpartum haemorrhage. Cochrane Database Syst Rev 2019;(4):CD001808.

Sävendahl L et al: Long-term mortality and causes of death in isolated GHD, ISS, and SGA patients treated with recombinant growth hormone during childhood in Belgium, The Netherlands, and Sweden: Preliminary report of 3 countries participating in the EU SAGhE study. J Clin Endocrinol Metab 2012;97:E213.

Strauss JF, Barbieri RL: *Yen & Jaffe's Reproductive Endocrinology*, 8th ed. Elsevier, 2018.

Surrey ES: Gonadotropin-releasing hormone agonist and add-back therapy: What do the data show? Curr Opin Obstet Gynecol 2010;22:283.

Taylor HS et al: *Speroff's Clinical Gynecologic Endocrinology and Infertility*, 9th ed. Lippincott Williams & Wilkins, 2019.

Van Den Berghe G: On the neuroendocrinopathy of critical illness. Perspectives for feeding and novel treatments. Am J Respir Crit Care Med 2016:194:1337.

Vroonen L et al: Epidemiology and management challenges in prolactinomas. Neuroendocrinology 2019;109:20.

Yuen KCJ et al: American Association of Clinical Endocrinologists and American College of Endocrinology guidelines for management of growth hormone deficiency in adults and patients transitioning from pediatric to adult care. Endocr Pract 2019;25:1191.

Youssef MA et al: Gonadotropin-releasing hormone agonist versus HCG for oocyte triggering in antagonist assisted reproductive technology cycles. Cochrane Database Syst Rev 2014;(10):CD008046.

CASE STUDY ANSWER

While growth hormone (GH) may have some direct growth-promoting effects, it is thought to mediate skeletal growth principally through production of insulin-like growth factor I (IGF-I) at the epiphyseal plate, which acts mainly in an autocrine/paracrine manner. IGF-I may also promote statural growth through endocrine mechanisms. This patient is at risk for multiple hypothalamic/pituitary deficiencies due to the location of her tumor and effects of treatments on the hypothalamus and pituitary. She may have ACTH/cortisol and TSH/thyroid hormone deficiencies and thus may require supplementation with hydrocortisone and levothyroxine, in addition to supplementation with GH. She should be evaluated for the presence of central diabetes insipidus in light of her increased urination and fluid intake and, if present, treated with desmopressin, a V_2 vasopressin receptor–selective analog. The patient likely has gonadotropin deficiency and will not initiate puberty spontaneously. She should be evaluated if she manifests delayed puberty in the future and provided increasing doses of estradiol to mimic puberty.

C H A P T E R

38

Thyroid & Antithyroid Drugs*

Betty J. Dong, PharmD, FASHP, FCSHP, FCCP, FAPHA

CASE STUDY

JP is a 33-year-old woman who presents with complaints of fatigue requiring daytime naps, weight gain, cold intolerance, and muscle weakness for the last few months. These complaints are new since she used to always feel "hot," noted difficulty sleeping, and could eat anything that she wanted without gaining weight. She also would like to become pregnant in the near future. Because of poor medication adherence to methimazole and propranolol, she received radioactive iodine (RAI) therapy, developed hypothyroidism, and was started on levothyroxine 100 mcg daily. Other medications include calcium carbonate three times daily to "protect her bones" and omeprazole for "heartburn." On physical examination, her blood pressure is 130/89 mm Hg with a pulse of 50 bpm. Her weight is 136 lb (61.8 kg), an increase of 10 lb (4.5 kg) in the last year. Her thyroid gland is not palpable and her reflexes are delayed. Laboratory findings include a thyroid-stimulating hormone (TSH) level of 24.9 μIU/mL (normal 0.45–4.12 μIU/mL) and a free thyroxine level of 8 pmol/L (normal 10–18 pmol/L). Evaluate the management of her past history of hyperthyroidism and assess her current thyroid status. Identify your treatment recommendations to maximize control of her current thyroid status.

THYROID PHYSIOLOGY

The normal thyroid gland secretes sufficient amounts of the thyroid hormones—**triiodothyronine (T_3)** and **tetraiodothyronine (T_4, thyroxine)**—to normalize growth and development, body temperature, and energy levels. These hormones contain 59% and 65% (respectively) iodine as an essential part of the molecule. Calcitonin, the second type of thyroid hormone, is important in the regulation of calcium metabolism and is discussed in Chapter 42.

Iodide Metabolism

The recommended daily adult iodide (I^-)† intake is 150 mcg (200 mcg during pregnancy and lactation and up to 250 mcg for children).

Iodide, ingested from food, water, or medication, is rapidly absorbed and enters an extracellular fluid pool. The thyroid gland removes about 75 mcg a day from this pool for hormone synthesis, and the balance is excreted in the urine. If iodide intake is increased, the fractional iodine uptake by the thyroid is diminished.

Biosynthesis of Thyroid Hormones

Once taken up by the thyroid gland, iodide undergoes a series of enzymatic reactions that incorporate it into active thyroid hormone (see Figure 38–1). The first step is the transport of iodide into the thyroid gland by an intrinsic follicle cell basement membrane protein called the sodium/iodide symporter (NIS). This can be inhibited by large doses of iodides as well as anions—eg, thiocyanate (SCN^-), pertechnetate (TcO_4^-), and perchlorate (ClO_4^-). At the apical cell membrane a second I^- transport enzyme called pendrin controls the flow of iodide across the membrane. Pendrin is also found in the cochlea of the inner ear. If pendrin is deficient or absent (SLC26A4 mutation), a hereditary syndrome of goiter and deafness, called **Pendred syndrome (PDS),** ensues. At the apical cell membrane,

*This chapter is dedicated to Dr. Francis S. Greenspan, co-author, mentor, colleague, and friend who will be sorely missed by his many colleagues and by his patients for his kindness, generosity, and expert care as chief of the UCSF Thyroid Clinic.

†In this chapter, the term *iodine* denotes all forms of the element; the term *iodide* denotes only the ionic form, I^-.

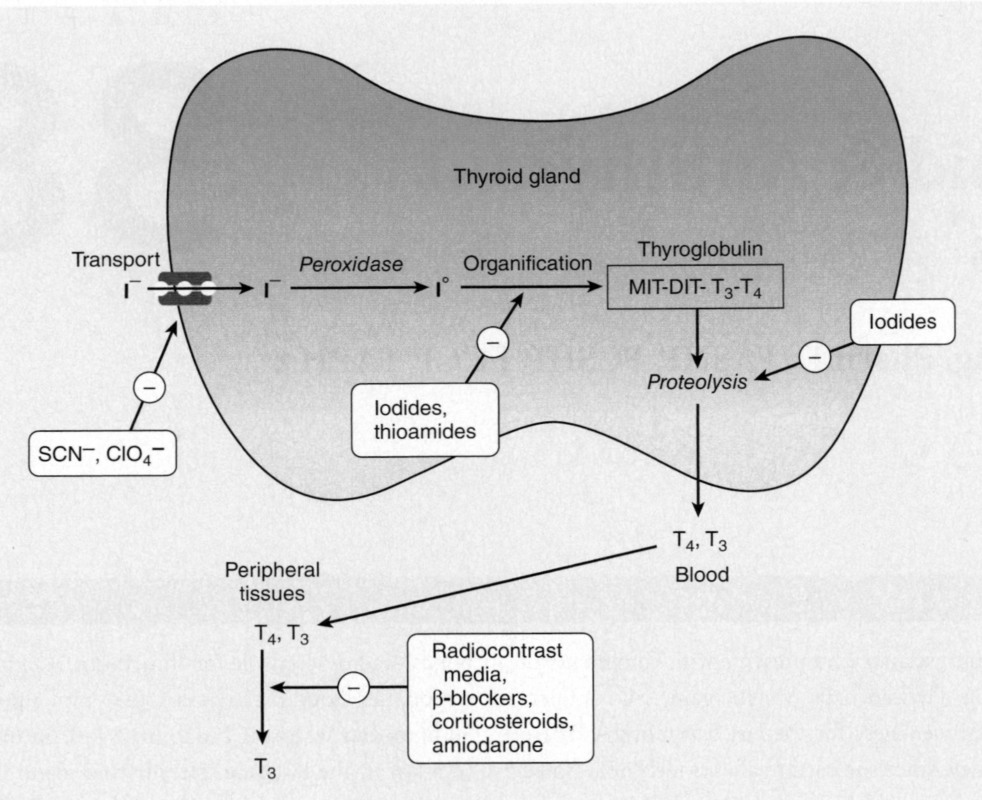

FIGURE 38–1 Biosynthesis of thyroid hormones. The sites of action of various drugs that interfere with thyroid hormone biosynthesis are shown. (Reproduced with permission from Gardner DG, Shoback D: Greenspan's Basic & Clinical Endocrinology, 8th ed. New York, NY: McGraw Hill; 2007.)

iodide is oxidized by thyroidal peroxidase (TPO) to iodine, in which form it rapidly iodinates tyrosine residues within the thyroglobulin molecule to form **monoiodotyrosine (MIT)** and **diiodotyrosine (DIT).** This process is called **iodide organification.** Thyroidal peroxidase is transiently blocked by high levels of intrathyroidal iodide and more persistently blocked by thioamide drugs. Gene expression of TPO is stimulated by thyroid-stimulating hormone (TSH).

Two molecules of DIT combine within the thyroglobulin molecule to form L-thyroxine (T_4). One molecule of MIT and one molecule of DIT combine to form T_3. In addition to thyroglobulin, other proteins within the gland may be iodinated, but these iodoproteins do not have hormonal activity. Thyroxine, T_3, MIT, and DIT are released from thyroglobulin by exocytosis and proteolysis of thyroglobulin at the apical colloid border. The MIT and DIT are then deiodinated within the gland, and the iodine is reutilized. This process of proteolysis is also blocked by high levels of intrathyroidal iodide. The ratio of T_4 to T_3 within thyroglobulin is approximately 5:1, so that most of the hormone released is thyroxine. Eighty percent of T_3 circulating in the blood is derived from peripheral metabolism of thyroxine and the rest from direct thyroid secretion (see below, Figure 38–2).

Transport of Thyroid Hormones

Thyroxine and T_3 in plasma are reversibly bound to protein, primarily thyroxine-binding globulin (TBG). Only about 0.04% of total T_4 and 0.4% of T_3 exist in the free form (as FT_4 and FT_3). Many physiologic and pathologic states and drugs affect T_4, T_3, and thyroid transport. However, the actual levels of free hormone generally remain normal, reflecting feedback control.

Peripheral Metabolism of Thyroid Hormones

The primary pathway for the peripheral metabolism of thyroxine is deiodination by three 5′-deiodinase enzymes (D1, D2, D3). Deiodination of T_4 may occur by monodeiodination of the outer ring, producing 3,5,3′-triiodothyronine (T_3), which is three to four times more potent than T_4. The D1 enzyme is responsible for about 24% of the circulating T_3 while 64% of peripheral T_3 is generated by D2, which also regulates T_3 levels in the brain and pituitary. D3 deiodination produces metabolically inactive 3,3′,5′-triiodothyronine (reverse T_3 [rT_3]) (see Figure 38–2). The low serum levels of T_3 and rT_3 in normal individuals are due to the high metabolic clearances of these two compounds.

Drugs such as amiodarone, iodinated contrast media, β blockers, and corticosteroids, as well as severe illness or starvation, inhibit the 5′-deiodinase necessary for the conversion of T_4 to T_3, resulting in low T_3 and high rT_3 levels in the serum. A polymorphism in the D2 gene can reduce T_3 activation and impair thyroid hormone response. The pharmacokinetics of thyroid hormones are listed in Table 38–1.

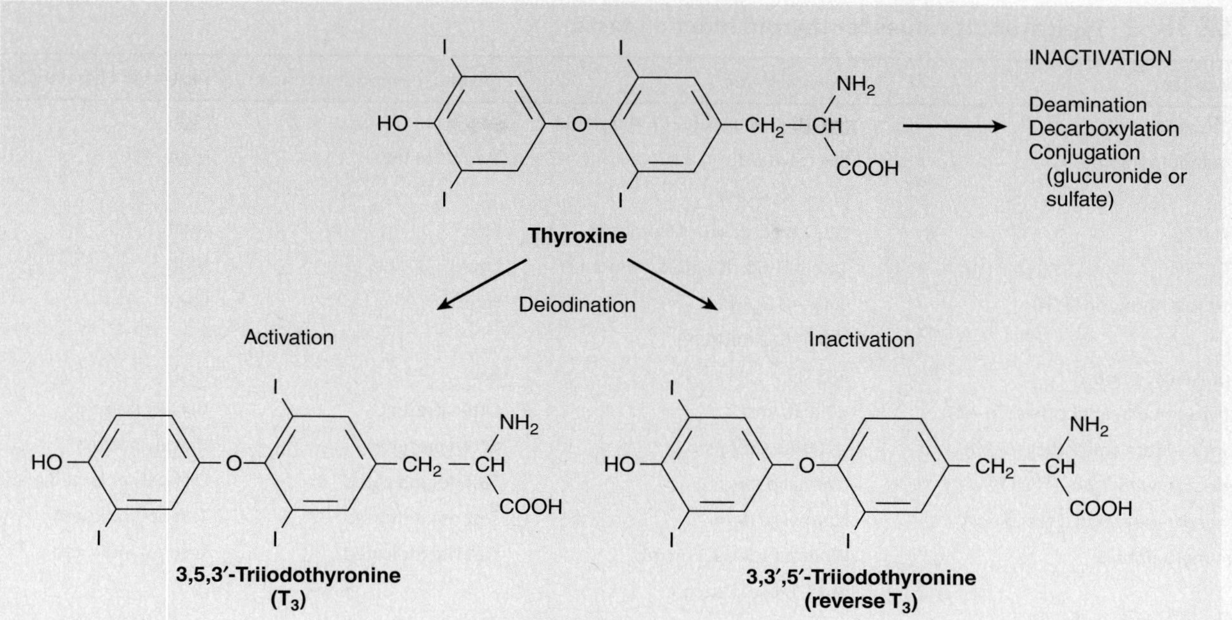

FIGURE 38–2 Peripheral metabolism of thyroxine. (Reproduced with permission from Gardner DG, Shoback D: Greenspan's Basic & Clinical Endocrinology, 8th ed. New York, NY: McGraw Hill; 2007.)

Evaluation of Thyroid Function

Tests used to evaluate thyroid function are listed in Table 38–2.

A. Thyroid-Pituitary Relationships

Control of thyroid function via thyroid-pituitary feedback is also discussed in Chapter 37. Hypothalamic cells secrete thyrotropin-releasing hormone (TRH) (Figure 38–3). TRH is secreted into capillaries of the pituitary portal venous system, and in the pituitary gland, TRH stimulates the synthesis and release of thyrotropin (thyroid-stimulating hormone, TSH). TSH in turn stimulates an adenylyl cyclase–mediated mechanism in the thyroid cell to increase the synthesis and release of T_4 and T_3. T_3, the more active of the two hormones, acts in a negative feedback fashion in the pituitary to block the action of TSH and in the hypothalamus to inhibit the synthesis and secretion of TRH. Other hormones or drugs may also affect the release of TRH or TSH.

TABLE 38–1 Summary of thyroid hormone kinetics.

Variable	T_4	T_3
Volume of distribution	10 L	40 L
Extrathyroidal pool	800 mcg	54 mcg
Daily production	75 mcg	25 mcg
Fractional turnover per day	10%	60%
Metabolic clearance per day	1.1 L	24 L
Half-life (biologic)	7 days	1 day
Serum levels		
Total	4.8–10.4 mcg/dL	59–156 ng/dL
	(62–134 nmol/L)	(09–2.4 nmol/L)
Free	0.8–1.4 ng/dL	169–371 pg/dL
	(10–18 pmol/L)	(2.6–5.7 pmol/L)
Amount bound	99.96%	99.6%
Biologic potency	1	4
Oral absorption	70%	95%

B. Autoregulation of the Thyroid Gland

The thyroid gland also regulates its uptake of iodide and thyroid hormone synthesis by intrathyroidal mechanisms that are independent of TSH. These mechanisms are primarily related to the level of iodine in the blood. Large doses of iodine inhibit iodide organification (Wolff-Chaikoff block; see Figure 38–1). In certain disease states (eg, Hashimoto thyroiditis), this can inhibit thyroid hormone synthesis and result in hypothyroidism. Hyperthyroidism can result from the loss of the Wolff-Chaikoff block in susceptible individuals (eg, multinodular goiter).

C. Abnormal Thyroid Stimulators

In Graves disease (see below), lymphocytes secrete a TSH receptor–stimulating antibody (TSH-R Ab [stim]), also known as thyroid-stimulating immunoglobulin (TSI). This immunoglobulin binds to the TSH receptor and stimulates the gland in the same fashion as TSH itself. The duration of its effect, however, is much longer than that of TSH. TSH receptors, stimulated by high levels of TSH-R Ab [stim], and insulin-like growth factor 1 receptor (IGF-1R) are also found in orbital fibrocytes, and can cause ophthalmopathy.

TABLE 38–2 Typical adult values for thyroid function tests.

Name of Test	Normal Value[1]	Results in Hypothyroidism	Results in Hyperthyroidism
Total thyroxine (T_4)	4.8–10.4 mcg/dL (62–134 nmol/L)	Low	High
Total triiodothyronine (T_3)	59–156 ng/dL (0.9–2.4 nmol/L)	Normal or low	High
Free T_4 (FT_4)	0.8–1.4 ng/dL (10–18 pmol/L)	Low	High
Free T_3 (FT_3)	169–371 ng/dL (2.6–5.7 pmol/L)	Low	High
Thyrotropic hormone (TSH)	0.45–4.12 μIU/mL (0.45–4.12 mIU/L)	High[2]	Low
^{123}I uptake at 24 hours	5–35%	Low	High
Antithyroglobulin antibodies (Tg-Ab)	<200 IU/mL	Often present	Usually present
Thyroperoxidase antibodies (ATPO)	≤100 WHO units	Often present	Usually present
Isotope scan with ^{123}I or $^{99m}TcO_4$	Normal pattern	Test not indicated	Diffusely enlarged gland
Fine-needle aspiration (FNA) biopsy	Normal pattern	Test not indicated	Test not indicated
Serum thyroglobulin	Women: 1.5–38.5 mcg/L Men: 1.4–29.2 mcg/L	Test not indicated	Test not indicated
TSH receptor-stimulating antibody or thyroid-stimulating immunoglobulin (TSI)	Negative <140% of baseline	Test not indicated	Elevated in Graves disease

[1]Results may vary with different laboratories.

[2]Exception is central hypothyroidism.

■ BASIC PHARMACOLOGY OF THYROID & ANTITHYROID DRUGS

THYROID HORMONES

Chemistry

The structural formulas of thyroxine and triiodothyronine as well as reverse triiodothyronine (rT_3) are shown in Figure 38–2. All of these naturally occurring molecules are levo (L) isomers. The synthetic dextro (D) isomer of thyroxine, dextrothyroxine, has approximately 4% of the biologic activity of the L-isomer as evidenced by its lesser ability to suppress TSH secretion and correct hypothyroidism.

Pharmacokinetics

Thyroxine is absorbed best in the duodenum and ileum; its absorption is modified by intraluminal factors such as food, drugs, gastric acidity, and intestinal flora. Oral bioavailability of current tablet preparations of L-thyroxine averages 70–80% (see Table 38–1) and is improved with the Tirosint formulations (see below). In contrast, T_3 is almost completely absorbed (95%). T_4 and T_3 absorption appear unaffected by mild hypothyroidism but may be impaired in severe myxedema with ileus. These factors are important in switching from oral to parenteral therapy. For parenteral use, the intravenous route is preferred for both hormones.

In patients with hyperthyroidism, the metabolic clearances of T_4 and T_3 are increased and the half-lives decreased; the opposite is true in patients with hypothyroidism. Drugs that induce hepatic microsomal enzymes (eg, rifampin, phenobarbital, carbamazepine, phenytoin, tyrosine kinase inhibitors, HIV protease inhibitors) increase the metabolism of both T_4 and T_3 (Table 38–3). Despite this change in clearance, the normal hormone concentration is maintained in the majority of euthyroid patients due to compensatory hyperfunction of the thyroid. However, patients dependent on T_4 replacement medication may require higher dosages to maintain clinical effectiveness. A similar compensation occurs when changes in binding sites occur. When TBG sites are increased by pregnancy, estrogens, or oral contraceptives, levels of bound hormones increase initially, causing reductions in its rate of elimination until the normal free to bound hormone concentration is restored. Thus, the concentration of total and bound hormone will increase, but the concentration of free hormone and the steady-state elimination will remain normal. The reverse occurs when reduced thyroid binding sites occur.

Mechanism of Action

A model of thyroid hormone action is depicted in Figure 38–4, which shows the free forms of thyroid hormones, T_4 and T_3, dissociated from thyroid-binding proteins, entering the cell by the active transporters (eg, monocarboxylate transporter 8 [MCT8], MCT10, and organic anion transporting polypeptide [OATP1C1]). Transporter mutations can result in a clinical syndrome of mental retardation, myopathy, and low serum T_4 levels (Allan-Herndon-Dudley syndrome). Within the cell, T_4 is converted to T_3 by 5′-deiodinase, and the T_3 enters the nucleus, where T_3 binds to a specific T_3 thyroid receptor protein, a member of the *c-erb* oncogene family. (This family also includes the steroid hormone receptors and receptors for vitamins A and D.) The T_3 receptor exists in two forms, α and β. Differing concentrations of

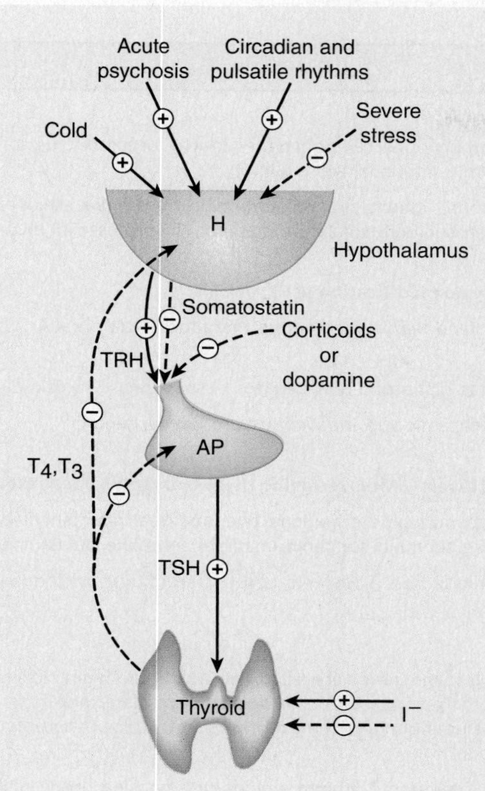

FIGURE 38–3 The hypothalamic-pituitary-thyroid axis. Acute psychosis or prolonged exposure to cold may activate the axis. Hypothalamic thyroid-releasing hormone (TRH) stimulates pituitary thyroid-stimulating hormone (TSH) release, while somatostatin and dopamine inhibit it. TSH stimulates T_4 and T_3 synthesis and release from the thyroid, and they in turn inhibit both TRH and TSH synthesis and release. Small amounts of iodide are necessary for hormone production, but large amounts inhibit T_3 and T_4 production and release. Solid arrows, stimulatory influence; dashed arrows, inhibitory influence. H, hypothalamus; AP, anterior pituitary.

receptors in different tissues (eg, α receptors in the brain and β receptors in the liver) may account for variations in T_3 effect on these tissues. Mutations in both α and β genes have been associated with generalized thyroid hormone resistance. Cigarette smoking and environmental agents (eg, polychlorinated biphenyls) also may interfere with receptor action.

Most of the effects of thyroid on metabolic processes appear to be mediated by activation of nuclear receptors that lead to increased formation of RNA and subsequent protein synthesis, eg, increased formation of Na+/K+-ATPase. This is consistent with the observation that the action of thyroid is evident in vivo with a time lag of hours or days after its administration.

Large numbers of thyroid hormone receptors are found in the most hormone-responsive tissues (pituitary, liver, kidney, heart, skeletal muscle, lung, and intestine), while few receptor sites occur in hormone-unresponsive tissues (spleen, testes). The brain, which lacks an anabolic response to T_3, contains an intermediate number of receptors. In congruence with their biologic potencies, the affinity of the receptor site for T_4 is about 10 times lower than that for T_3. Under some conditions, the number of nuclear receptors may be altered to preserve body homeostasis. For example, starvation lowers both circulating T_3 hormone and cellular T_3 receptors.

Effects of Thyroid Hormones

The thyroid hormones are responsible for optimal growth, development, function, and maintenance of all body tissues. Excess or inadequate amounts result in the signs and symptoms of hyperthyroidism or hypothyroidism, respectively (Table 38–4). Since T_3 and T_4 are qualitatively similar, they may be considered as one hormone in the discussion that follows.

Thyroid hormone is critical for the development and functioning of nervous, skeletal, and reproductive tissues. Its effects depend on protein synthesis as well as potentiation of the secretion and action of growth hormone. Thyroid deprivation in early life results in irreversible mental retardation and dwarfism—typical of congenital cretinism.

Effects on growth and calorigenesis are accompanied by a pervasive influence on metabolism of drugs as well as carbohydrates, fats, proteins, and vitamins. Many of these changes are dependent upon or modified by activity of other hormones. Conversely, the secretion and degradation rates of virtually all other hormones, including catecholamines, cortisol, estrogens, testosterone, and insulin, are affected by thyroid status.

Many of the manifestations of thyroid hyperactivity resemble sympathetic nervous system overactivity (especially in the cardiovascular system), although catecholamine levels are not increased. Changes in catecholamine-stimulated adenylyl cyclase activity as measured by cAMP are found with changes in thyroid activity. Thyroid hormone increases the numbers of β receptors and enhances amplification of the β-receptor signal. Other clinical symptoms reminiscent of excessive epinephrine activity (and partially alleviated by adrenoceptor antagonists) include lid lag and retraction, tremor, excessive sweating, anxiety, and nervousness. The opposite constellation of effects appears in hypothyroidism (see Table 38–4).

Thyroid Preparations

See the Preparations Available section at the end of this chapter for a list of available preparations. These preparations may be synthetic (levothyroxine, liothyronine, liotrix) or of animal origin (desiccated thyroid).

Thyroid hormones are not effective and can be detrimental in the management of obesity, abnormal vaginal bleeding, or depression if thyroid hormone levels are normal. A review of T_3 co-administered with antidepressants showed some promising depression benefits only when combined with tricyclics, but further confirmation of its optimal use is required.

Synthetic levothyroxine (T_4) is the preparation of choice for thyroid replacement and suppression therapy because of its stability, content uniformity, low cost, lack of allergenic foreign protein, easy laboratory measurement of serum levels, long half-life (7 days) permitting once-daily to weekly administration, and long term safety. Generic T_4 preparations provide comparable efficacy and are more cost-effective than branded preparations. Although some

TABLE 38–3 Drug effects and thyroid function.

Drug Effect	Drugs
Change in thyroid hormone synthesis	
Inhibition of TRH or TSH secretion without induction of hypothyroidism or hyperthyroidism	Bexarotene, dopamine, bromocriptine, cabergoline, levodopa, corticosteroids, somatostatin, octreotide, metformin, interleukin-6, heroin
Inhibition of thyroid hormone synthesis or release with the induction of hypothyroidism (or occasionally hyperthyroidism)	Iodides (including amiodarone), lithium, aminoglutethimide, thioamides, ethionamide, tyrosine kinase inhibitors (eg, sunitinib, sorafenib, imatinib), HIV protease inhibitors
Alteration of thyroid hormone transport and serum total T_3 and T_4 levels, but usually no modification of FT_4 or TSH	
Increased TBG	Estrogens, tamoxifen, raloxifene, heroin, methadone, mitotane, 5-fluorouracil, perphenazine
Decreased TBG	Androgens, anabolic steroids, glucocorticoids, danazol, L-asparaginase, nicotinic acid
Displacement of T_3 and T_4 from TBG with transient hyperthyroxinemia	Salicylates, fenclofenac, mefenamic acid, intravenous furosemide, heparin
Alteration of T_4 and T_3 metabolism with modified serum T_3 and T_4 levels but not TSH levels (unless receiving thyroxine replacement therapy)	
Increased hepatic metabolism, enhanced degradation of thyroid hormone	Nicardipine, phenytoin, carbamazepine, primidone, phenobarbital, rifampin, rifabutin, tyrosine kinase inhibitors (eg, sunitinib, sorafenib, imatinib), sertraline, quetiapine
Inhibition of 5′-deiodinase with decreased T_3, increased rT_3	Iopanoic acid, ipodate, amiodarone, β blockers, corticosteroids, propylthiouracil, flavonoids, interleukin-6
Other interactions	
Interference with T_4 absorption from the gut	Oral bisphosphonates, cholestyramine, colesevelam, colestipol, chromium picolinate, charcoal, ciprofloxacin, proton pump inhibitors, sucralfate, Kayexalate, raloxifene, sevelamer hydrochloride, aluminum hydroxide, ferrous sulfate, calcium carbonate, bran/fiber, soy, coffee, orlistat
Induction of autoimmune thyroid disease with hypothyroidism or hyperthyroidism	Interferon-α, interleukin-2, interferon-β, lithium, amiodarone, tyrosine kinase inhibitors (eg, sunitinib, sorafenib, imatinib), immune checkpoint inhibitors (eg, ipilimumab, nivolumab, pembrolizumab, atezolizumab, cemiplimab, avelumab, durvalumab)
Effect of thyroid function on drug effects	
Anticoagulation	Lower doses of warfarin required in hyperthyroidism, higher doses in hypothyroidism
Glucose control	Increased hepatic glucose production and glucose intolerance in hyperthyroidism; impaired insulin action and glucose disposal in hypothyroidism
Cardiac drugs	Higher doses of digoxin required in hyperthyroidism; lower doses in hypothyroidism
Sedatives; analgesics	Increased sedative and respiratory depressant effects from sedatives and opioids in hypothyroidism; converse in hyperthyroidism

recommend that patients remain on a consistent T_4 preparation between refills to avoid changes in bioavailability, a recent study between generics found otherwise. In addition, generic T_4 preparations are FDA approved with the expectation that they are substitutable. Compared with the tablet formulation, a branded soft gel capsule and solution (Tirosint, Tirosint-SOL) provided faster, more complete dissolution; provided 98% bioavailability; was less affected by gastric pH or coffee; and produced lower TSH levels. According to the American Thyroid Association guidelines, these newer formulations may be considered in persons allergic to tablet excipients.

Although liothyronine (T_3) is three to four times more potent than levothyroxine, it is not generally recommended for routine replacement therapy because of its shorter half-life (24 hours,) necessitating multiple daily doses, and difficulty in monitoring its adequacy of replacement by conventional laboratory tests. In addition, T_4 is converted intracellularly to T_3 by deiodinase enzymes producing both hormones so that T_3 administration is usually unnecessary. However, emerging evidence suggests that genetic defects/polymorphisms in D2 enzymes (Thr92Ala-DIO2) in some hypothyroid patients produce insufficient T_3 levels on T_4 alone, leading to continued hypothyroid symptoms. Use T_3 cautiously in persons with cardiac disease due to risk of cardiotoxicity from significant elevations in peak T_3 levels. T_3 is best reserved for short-term TSH suppression or combined with levothyroxine in those with confirmed unresponsiveness to T_4 alone.

The use of desiccated thyroid (DTE) versus synthetic preparations is never justified due to disadvantages of protein antigenicity, product instability, variable hormone concentrations, limited FDA oversight, and difficulty in laboratory monitoring despite its lower cost. DTE treatment results in a much higher serum T3/T4 ratio, and the potential for toxic peak T3 levels. Nevertheless, one randomized, double-blind study found no difference in hormone levels achieved between Armour DTE, T_4, or T_3, with some patients preferring T_3. Similarly, another large study also found that patients were more satisfied with DTE rather than T_4 or T_4 plus T_3. Significant amounts of T_3 found in some thyroid extracts may produce significant and toxic elevations in T_3 levels. Exact equi-effective doses have not been determined. Approximate

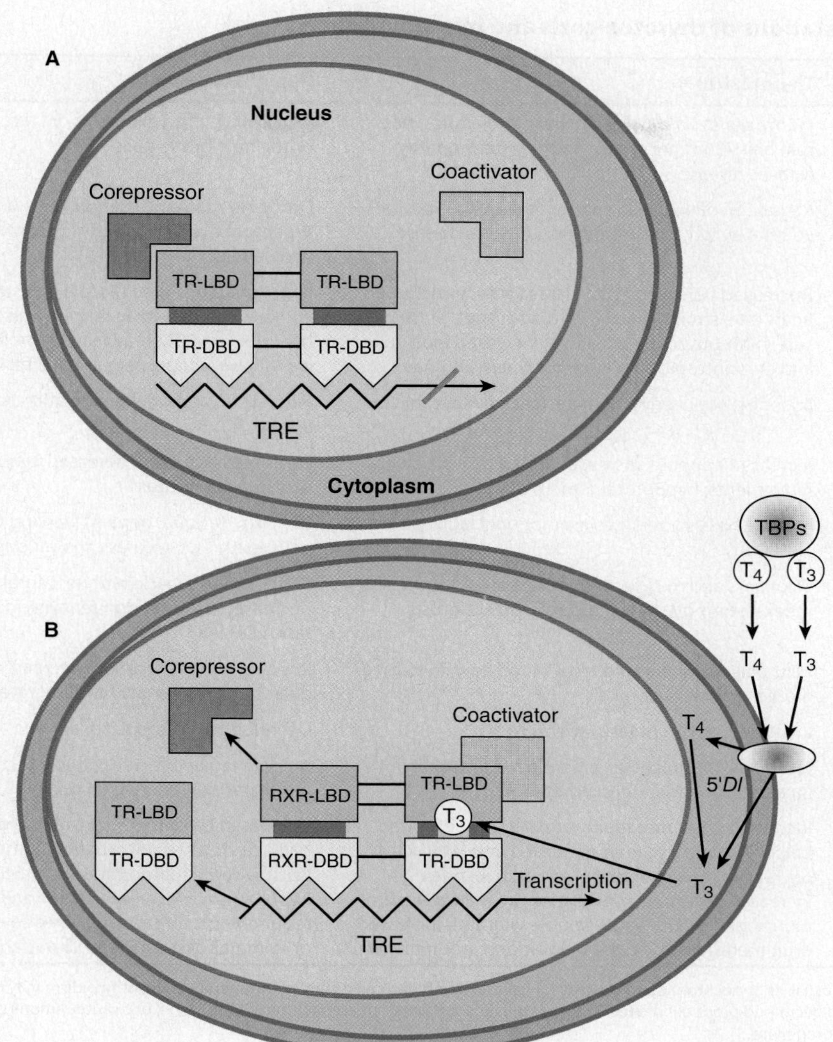

FIGURE 38–4 Model of the interaction of T_3 with the T_3 receptor. **(A)** *Inactive phase*—the unliganded T_3 receptor dimer bound to the thyroid hormone response element (TRE) along with corepressors acts as a suppressor of gene transcription. **(B)** *Active phase*—T_3 and T_4 circulate bound to thyroid-binding proteins (TBPs). The free hormones are transported into the cell by a specific transport system. Within the cytoplasm, T_4 is converted to T_3 by 5′-deiodinase (5′DI); T_3 then moves into the nucleus. There it binds to the ligand-binding domain of the thyroid receptor (TR) monomer. This promotes disruption of the TR homodimer and heterodimerization with retinoid X receptor (RXR) on the TRE, displacement of corepressors, and binding of coactivators. The TR-coactivator complex activates gene transcription, which leads to alteration in protein synthesis and cellular phenotype. TR-LBD, T_3 receptor ligand-binding domain; TR-DBD, T_3 receptor DNA-binding domain; RXR-LBD, retinoid X receptor ligand-binding domain; RXR-DBD, retinoid X receptor DNA-binding domain; T_3, triiodothyronine; T_4, tetraiodothyronine, L-thyroxine. (Reproduced with permission from Gardner DG, Shoback D: Greenspan's Basic & Clinical Endocrinology, 8th ed. New York, NY: McGraw Hill; 2007.)

equivalences suggested between preparations are desiccated thyroid 60 mg (1 grain) to 80–100 mcg of levothyroxine, and to 37.5 mcg of liothyronine. Any dosage conversions should be re-titrated based on laboratory and clinical response.

A consensus statement that provides guidance on adding T_3, desiccated thyroid, or the more expensive fixed-dose combination of T_4 plus T_3 therapy (Liotrix) is available.

The shelf life of synthetic hormone preparations is about 2 years, particularly if they are stored in dark bottles to minimize spontaneous deiodination. The shelf life of desiccated thyroid is unknown with certainty, but its potency is better preserved if it is kept dry.

ANTITHYROID AGENTS

Reduction of thyroid activity and hormone effects is accomplished by agents that interfere with the production of thyroid hormones, modify the tissue response to thyroid hormones, or cause glandular destruction by radiation or surgery. Goitrogens are agents that suppress secretion of T_3 and T_4 to subnormal levels and thereby increase TSH, which in turn produces glandular enlargement (goiter). The antithyroid compounds used clinically include the thioamides, iodides, and radioactive iodine.

TABLE 38–4 Manifestations of thyrotoxicosis and hypothyroidism.

System	Thyrotoxicosis	Hypothyroidism
Skin and appendages	Warm, moist skin; sweating; heat intolerance; fine, thin hair; Plummer's nails; pretibial dermopathy (Graves disease)	Pale, cool, puffy, yellowish skin, face, and hands; dry and brittle hair; brittle nails
Eyes, face	Retraction of upper lid with wide stare; periorbital edema; exophthalmos; diplopia (Graves disease)	Drooping of eyelids; periorbital edema; loss of temporal aspects of eyebrows; puffy, nonpitting facies; large tongue, hoarseness
Cardiovascular system	Decreased peripheral vascular resistance; increased heart rate, stroke volume, cardiac output, pulse pressure; high-output heart failure; increased inotropic and chronotropic effects; arrhythmias; angina	Increased peripheral vascular resistance; decreased heart rate, stroke volume, cardiac output, pulse pressure; low-output heart failure; ECG: bradycardia, prolonged PR interval, flat T wave, low voltage; pericardial effusion
Respiratory system	Dyspnea; hypoventilation; decreased vital capacity	Pleural effusions; hypoventilation and CO_2 retention; sleep apnea
Gastrointestinal system	Increased appetite; increased frequency of bowel movements; hypoproteinemia	Decreased appetite; decreased frequency of bowel movements, constipation; ascites
Central nervous system	Nervousness; hyperkinesia; emotional lability, agitation	Lethargy/fatigue; general slowing of mental processes; neuropathies; weakness and muscle cramps
Musculoskeletal system	Weakness and muscle fatigue; increased deep tendon reflexes; tremors; hypercalcemia; osteoporosis	Stiffness and muscle fatigue; carpal tunnel syndrome; decreased deep tendon reflexes; increased alkaline phosphatase, LDH, AST
Renal system	Mild polyuria; increased renal blood flow; increased glomerular filtration rate	Impaired water excretion; decreased renal blood flow; decreased glomerular filtration rate
Hematopoietic system	Increased erythropoiesis; anemia[1]	Decreased erythropoiesis; anemia[1]
Reproductive system	Menstrual irregularities; amenorrhea; infertility; increased gonadal steroid metabolism	Menorrhagia; infertility; decreased libido; impotence; oligospermia; decreased gonadal steroid metabolism
Metabolic system	Increased basal metabolic rate; negative nitrogen balance; hyperglycemia; increased free fatty acids; decreased total cholesterol and triglycerides; increased hormone degradation; increased requirements for fat- and water-soluble vitamins; increased drug metabolism; decreased warfarin requirement	Decreased basal metabolic rate; slight positive nitrogen balance; delayed degradation of insulin with increased sensitivity; increased total cholesterol and triglycerides; hyponatremia; decreased hormone degradation; decreased requirements for fat- and water-soluble vitamins; decreased drug metabolism; increased warfarin requirement

[1]The anemia of hyperthyroidism is usually normochromic and caused by increased red blood cell turnover. The anemia of hypothyroidism may be normochromic, hyperchromic, or hypochromic and may be due to decreased production rate, decreased iron absorption, decreased folic acid absorption, or to autoimmune pernicious anemia. AST, aspartate aminotransferase; LDH, lactic dehydrogenase.

THIOAMIDES

The thioamides **methimazole** and **propylthiouracil** are major drugs for treatment of thyrotoxicosis. In the United Kingdom, **carbimazole,** which is converted to methimazole in vivo, is widely used. Methimazole is about 10 times more potent than propylthiouracil and is the drug of choice in adults and children. Due to a black box warning about severe hepatitis, propylthiouracil should be reserved for use only during the first trimester of pregnancy, in thyroid storm, and in those experiencing adverse reactions to methimazole (not agranulocytosis or hepatitis). The chemical structures of these compounds are shown in Figure 38–5. The thiocarbamide group is essential for antithyroid activity.

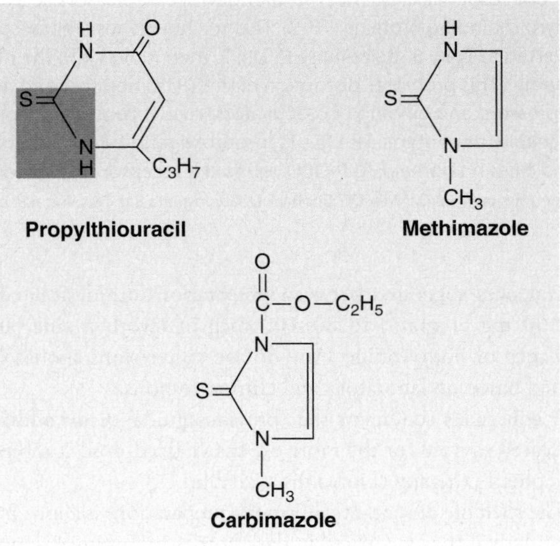

Pharmacokinetics

Methimazole is completely absorbed but at variable rates. It is readily concentrated by the thyroid gland and has a volume of distribution similar to that of propylthiouracil. Excretion is slower

Propylthiouracil

Methimazole

Carbimazole

FIGURE 38–5 Structure of thioamides. The thiocarbamide moiety is shaded in color.

than with propylthiouracil; 65–70% of a dose is recovered in the urine in 48 hours.

In contrast, propylthiouracil is rapidly absorbed, reaching peak serum levels after 1 hour. The bioavailability of 50–80% may be due to incomplete absorption or a large first-pass effect in the liver. The volume of distribution approximates total body water with accumulation in the thyroid gland. The majority of propylthiouracil is excreted within 24 hours by the kidney as the inactive glucuronide.

The short plasma half-life of these agents (1.5 hours for propylthiouracil and 6 hours for methimazole) has little influence on the duration of the antithyroid action or the dosing interval because both agents are concentrated in the thyroid gland. For propylthiouracil, giving the drug every 6–8 hours is reasonable since a single 100 mg dose can inhibit iodine organification by 60% for 7 hours. A single 30-mg dose of methimazole exerts an antithyroid effect for longer than 24 hours, so a single daily dose is effective in the management of mild to severe hyperthyroidism.

Both thioamides cross the placental barrier into the fetal thyroid, so caution is required when using these drugs in pregnancy. Both thioamides are classified by the FDA as pregnancy category D (see Chapter 59) due to the risk of fetal hypothyroidism. Propylthiouracil is preferable during the first trimester of pregnancy because it is more strongly protein-bound and, therefore, crosses the placenta less readily. In addition, methimazole has been, albeit rarely, associated with congenital malformations. Low concentrations of both thioamides found in breast milk are considered safe to use in the nursing infant.

Pharmacodynamics

The thioamides act by multiple mechanisms. The major action is to prevent hormone synthesis by inhibiting the thyroid peroxidase-catalyzed reactions and blocking iodine organification. In addition, they block coupling of the iodotyrosines. They do not block uptake of iodide by the gland. Propylthiouracil, but not methimazole, also inhibits the peripheral deiodination of T_4 and T_3 (see Figure 38–1). Since the synthesis rather than the release of hormones is affected, the onset of these agents is slow, often requiring 3–4 weeks before T_4 stores are depleted.

Toxicity

Adverse reactions to the thioamides occur in 3–12% of treated patients. Most reactions occur early, especially nausea and gastrointestinal distress. An altered sense of taste or smell may occur with methimazole. The most common adverse effect is a maculopapular pruritic rash (4–6%), at times accompanied by systemic signs such as fever. Rare adverse effects include an urticarial rash, vasculitis, a lupus-like reaction, lymphadenopathy, hypoprothrombinemia, exfoliative dermatitis, polyserositis, and acute arthralgia. An increased risk of severe hepatitis, sometimes fatal, is reported with propylthiouracil (black box warning), so it should be avoided in children and adults unless no other options are available. Cholestatic jaundice is more common with methimazole than propylthiouracil. Asymptomatic elevations in transaminase levels can also occur.

The most dangerous complication is agranulocytosis (granulocyte count <500 cells/mm^3), an infrequent but potentially fatal adverse reaction. It occurs in 0.1–0.5% of patients taking thioamides, but the risk appears increased in older patients and usually within the first 90 days in those receiving more than 40 mg/d of methimazole. The reaction is usually rapidly reversible when the drug is discontinued, but broad-spectrum antibiotic therapy may be necessary for complicating infections. Colony-stimulating factors (eg, G-CSF; see Chapter 33) may hasten recovery of the granulocytes. The cross-sensitivity between propylthiouracil and methimazole is about 50%; therefore, switching drugs in patients with severe reactions should be avoided.

ANION INHIBITORS

Monovalent anions such as perchlorate (ClO_4^-), pertechnetate (TcO_4^-), and thiocyanate (SCN^-) can block uptake of iodide by the gland through competitive inhibition of the iodide transport mechanism. Since these effects are overcome by large doses of iodides, their effectiveness is somewhat unpredictable.

The major clinical use for potassium perchlorate is to block thyroidal reuptake of I^- in patients with iodide-induced hyperthyroidism (eg, amiodarone-induced hyperthyroidism). However, potassium perchlorate is rarely used clinically because due to risk of aplastic anemia.

IODIDES

Prior to the introduction of the thioamides in the 1940s, iodides were the major antithyroid agents; today they are rarely used alone.

Pharmacodynamics

Iodides have several actions on the thyroid. They inhibit organification and hormone release, and they decrease the size and vascularity of the hyperplastic gland. In susceptible individuals, iodides can induce hyperthyroidism (Jod-Basedow phenomenon) or precipitate hypothyroidism.

In pharmacologic doses (>6 mg/d), the major action of iodides is to inhibit hormone release, possibly through inhibition of thyroglobulin proteolysis. Improvement in thyrotoxic symptoms occurs rapidly—within 2–7 days—hence the value of iodide therapy in thyroid storm. In addition, iodides decrease the vascularity, size, and fragility of a hyperplastic gland, making the drugs valuable as preoperative preparation for surgery.

Clinical Use of Iodide

Disadvantages of iodide therapy include an increase in intraglandular stores of iodine, which can delay onset of thioamide therapy or prevent use of radioactive iodine therapy for several weeks thereafter. Therefore, avoid iodides if radioactive iodine treatment seems likely and do not administer unless thioamide have begun. If iodides are administered alone, the gland can escape from the iodide block in 2–8 weeks, causing severe exacerbation of thyrotoxicosis in an iodine-enriched gland. Avoid chronic use of iodides in pregnancy due to placenta passage and the risk of fetal goiter. In radiation emergencies involving release of radioactive iodine isotopes, the thyroid-blocking effects of potassium iodide can protect the gland from subsequent damage if administered before radiation exposure.

Toxicity

Adverse reactions to iodine (iodism) are uncommon and in most cases reversible upon discontinuance. They include acneiform rash (similar to that of bromism), swollen salivary glands, mucous membrane ulcerations, conjunctivitis, rhinorrhea, drug fever, metallic taste, bleeding disorders, and rarely, anaphylactoid reactions.

RADIOACTIVE IODINE

^{131}I is the only isotope used for treatment of thyrotoxicosis. (Others are used for diagnosis.) Administered orally in solution as sodium ^{131}I, it is rapidly absorbed, concentrated by the thyroid, and incorporated into storage follicles. Its therapeutic effect depends on emission of β rays with an effective half-life of 5 days and a penetration range of 400–2000 μm. Within a few weeks after administration, destruction of thyroid parenchyma is evident by epithelial swelling and necrosis, follicular disruption, edema, and leukocyte infiltration. Advantages of radioiodine include easy administration, effectiveness, low expense, and absence of pain. Fears of radiation-induced genetic damage, leukemia, and neoplasia have not materialized after more than 50 years of clinical experience with radioiodine therapy for hyperthyroidism. Avoid radioactive iodine in pregnant women or nursing mothers, since it crosses the placenta to destroy the fetal thyroid gland and is secreted in breast milk.

ADRENOCEPTOR-BLOCKING AGENTS

Beta blockers without intrinsic sympathomimetic activity (eg, metoprolol, propranolol, atenolol) are effective therapeutic adjuncts in the management of thyrotoxicosis since many of these symptoms mimic those associated with sympathetic stimulation. Propranolol has been the β blocker most widely studied and used in the therapy of thyrotoxicosis. Beta blockers cause clinical improvement of hyperthyroid symptoms but do not typically alter thyroid hormone levels. Propranolol at doses greater than 160 mg/d may also reduce T_3 levels approximately 20% by inhibiting the peripheral conversion of T_4 to T_3.

■ CLINICAL PHARMACOLOGY OF THYROID & ANTITHYROID DRUGS

HYPOTHYROIDISM

Hypothyroidism is a syndrome resulting from deficiency of thyroid hormones and a reversible slowing of all body functions (see Table 38–4). In infants and children, there is striking retardation of growth and development that results in dwarfism and irreversible mental retardation.

The etiology and pathogenesis of hypothyroidism are summarized in Table 38–5. Hypothyroidism can occur with or without thyroid enlargement (goiter). The laboratory diagnosis of hypothyroidism in the adult is easily confirmed by findings of a low free thyroxine and elevated serum TSH levels (see Table 38–2).

The most common cause of hypothyroidism in the United States at this time is probably Hashimoto thyroiditis, an immunologic disorder in genetically predisposed individuals. In this condition, there is evidence of humoral immunity in the presence of antithyroid antibodies and lymphocyte sensitization to thyroid antigens. Genetic mutations as discussed previously and certain medications also can cause hypothyroidism (see Table 38–5).

TABLE 38–5 Etiology and pathogenesis of hypothyroidism.

Cause	Pathogenesis	Goiter	Degree of Hypothyroidism
Hashimoto thyroiditis	Autoimmune destruction of thyroid	Present early, absent later	Mild to severe
Drug-induced[1]	Blocked hormone formation[2]	Present	Mild to moderate
Dyshormonogenesis	Impaired synthesis of T_4 due to enzyme deficiency	Present	Mild to severe
Radiation, ^{131}I, X-ray, thyroidectomy	Destruction or removal of gland	Absent	Severe
Congenital (cretinism)	Athyreosis or ectopic thyroid, iodine deficiency; TSH receptor-blocking antibodies	Absent or present	Severe
Secondary (TSH deficit)	Pituitary or hypothalamic disease	Absent	Mild

[1]Iodides, lithium, fluoride, thioamides, aminosalicylic acid, phenylbutazone, amiodarone, perchlorate, ethionamide, thiocyanate, cytokines (interferons, interleukins), bexarotene, tyrosine kinase inhibitors, etc. See Table 38–3.

[2]See Table 38–3 for specific pathogenesis.

MANAGEMENT OF HYPOTHYROIDISM

Except for drug-induced hypothyroidism, which is managed in some cases by simply removing the offending agent, the general strategy of replacement therapy is appropriate. The most satisfactory preparation is levothyroxine, administered as either a branded or less costly generic preparation. Switching among three generics in a large claims database in persons with residual thyroid function was not associated with clinically significant changes in TSH level. Multiple trials have documented that combination levothyroxine plus liothyronine is not superior to levothyroxine alone, although some patients remain symptomatic on thyroxine alone. Genetic variations in deiodinases or hormone transporters may account for some of this lack of efficacy.

There is some variability in the absorption of thyroxine; dosage will also vary depending on age and weight. Infants and children require more T_4 per kilogram of body weight than adults. The average dosage for an infant aged 1–6 months old is 10–15 mcg/kg per day, whereas the average adult dosage is about 1.7 mcg/kg per day (0.8 mcg/lb per day) or 125 mcg/d. Older adults (>65 years of age) may require less thyroxine (1.6 mcg/kg or 0.7 mcg/lb per day) for replacement as body mass declines. In patients requiring post-thyroidectomy suppression therapy for thyroid cancer, the average daily dosage of T_4 is 2.2 mcg/kg or 1 mcg/lb. Higher thyroxine requirements have also been reported in persons following bariatric surgery and with other malabsorptive disorders (eg, atrophic gastritis, *Helicobacter pylori* gastritis, celiac disease, lactose intolerance); thyroxine doses may be reduced following treatment of these disorders.

Since interactions with certain foods (eg, bran, soy, coffee) and drugs (see Table 38–3) can impair its absorption, thyroxine is optimally administered on an empty stomach (eg, 30–60 minutes before meals, 4 hours after meals, or at bedtime) to maintain TSH within an therapeutic range of 0.5–2.5 mIU/L. Its long half-life of 7 days permits once-daily dosing. Children require monitoring for normal growth and development. Measure serum TSH and free thyroxine levels before any dosage changes to avoid transient serum alterations. Steady-state thyroxine levels in the bloodstream are not achieved until 6–8 weeks after a consistent dose of thyroxine. Thus, dosage changes need to be adjusted slowly.

In younger patients or those with very mild disease, full replacement therapy can be started immediately. In older patients (>50 years) without cardiac disease, levothyroxine can be started at a dosage of 50 mcg/d. In long-standing hypothyroidism and in older patients with underlying cardiac disease, it is imperative to start with smaller dosages of levothyroxine, 12.5–25 mcg/d for 2 weeks, before increasing by 12.5–25 mcg/d every 2 weeks until euthyroidism or drug toxicity occurs. In cardiac patients, the heart is very sensitive to the level of circulating thyroxine, and if angina pectoris or cardiac arrhythmia develops, it is essential to stop or reduce the thyroxine dosage immediately.

Thyroxine toxicity correlates with the hormone level. In children, restlessness, insomnia, and accelerated bone maturation and growth may be signs of thyroxine toxicity. In adults, increased nervousness, heat intolerance, episodes of palpitation and tachycardia, or unexplained weight loss may be the presenting symptoms. If these symptoms are present, it is important to monitor serum TSH and FT_4 levels (see Table 38–2), which will determine whether the symptoms are due to excess thyroxine blood levels. Chronic overtreatment with T_4, particularly in elderly patients, can increase the risk of atrial fibrillation and accelerated osteoporosis.

Special Problems in Management of Hypothyroidism

A. Myxedema and Coronary Artery Disease

Since myxedema frequently occurs in older persons, it is often associated with underlying coronary artery disease. In this situation, the low levels of circulating thyroid hormone actually protect the heart against increasing demands that could result in angina pectoris, atrial fibrillation, or myocardial infarction. Correction of myxedema must be done cautiously to avoid provoking these cardiac events. If coronary artery surgery is indicated, it should be done first, prior to correction of the myxedema by thyroxine administration.

B. Myxedema Coma

Myxedema coma is an end state of untreated hypothyroidism. It is associated with progressive weakness, stupor, hypothermia, hypoventilation, hypoglycemia, hyponatremia, water intoxication, shock, and death.

Myxedema coma is a medical emergency. The patient should be treated in the intensive care unit, since tracheal intubation and mechanical ventilation may be required. Associated illnesses such as infection or heart failure must be managed with appropriate therapy. It is important to give all preparations intravenously, because patients with myxedema coma absorb drugs poorly from other routes. Administer intravenous fluids cautiously to avoid excessive water intake. These patients have large pools of empty T_3 and T_4 binding sites that must be filled before there is adequate free thyroxine to affect tissue metabolism. Accordingly, the treatment of choice in myxedema coma is to give a loading dose of levothyroxine intravenously—usually 300–400 mcg initially, followed by 50–100 mcg daily. Intravenous T_3 5–20 mcg initially, followed by 2.5–10 mcg every 8 hours, also can be added but may be more cardiotoxic and more difficult to monitor. Lower T_4 and T_3 doses can be considered for smaller or older patients, or those with concomitant cardiac disease or arrhythmias. Intravenous hydrocortisone is indicated if there is associated adrenal or pituitary insufficiency but is probably not necessary in most patients with primary myxedema. Use opioids and sedatives with extreme caution.

C. Hypothyroidism and Pregnancy

Hypothyroid women frequently have anovulatory cycles and are therefore relatively infertile until restoration of the euthyroid state. This has led to the widespread use of thyroid hormone for infertility, although there is no evidence for its usefulness in infertile euthyroid patients. In a pregnant hypothyroid patient receiving thyroxine, it is extremely important that the daily dose of thyroxine is adequate because early development of the fetal brain depends on maternal thyroxine. In many hypothyroid patients, an increase in the thyroxine dose (about 25–30%) is required to normalize the serum TSH level during pregnancy. It is reasonable to counsel women to take one extra dose of their current thyroxine tablet twice a week separated by several days as soon as they are pregnant. Administer thyroxine apart from prenatal vitamins and calcium by at least 4 hours to avoid reducing T4 absorption. Because the elevated maternal TBG levels result in elevated total T_4 levels, adequate maternal thyroxine dosages warrant maintenance of TSH between 0.1 and 3.0 mIU/L (eg, first trimester, 0.1–2.5 mIU/L; second trimester, 0.2–3.0 mIU/L; third trimester, 0.3–3.0 mIU/L) and the total T_4 at or above the upper range of normal.

D. Subclinical Hypothyroidism

Subclinical hypothyroidism, defined as an elevated TSH level and normal thyroid hormone levels, occurs in 4–10% of the general population and up to 20% in women older than age 50. Levothyroxine administration should be individualized based on the risks and benefits of treatment. The consensus of most expert thyroid organizations concluded that thyroid hormone therapy might be considered for patients with TSH levels >10 mIU/L despite conflicting beneficial outcomes, while close TSH monitoring is appropriate for those with lower TSH elevations.

E. Drug-Induced Hypothyroidism

Drug-induced hypothyroidism (see Table 38–3) is satisfactorily managed with levothyroxine therapy if the offending agent cannot be stopped. In the case of amiodarone-induced hypothyroidism, levothyroxine therapy may be necessary even after its discontinuance due to amiodarone's very long half-life.

HYPERTHYROIDISM

Hyperthyroidism (thyrotoxicosis) is the clinical syndrome that occurs when tissues are exposed to high levels of thyroid hormone (see Table 38–4).

GRAVES DISEASE

The most common form of hyperthyroidism is Graves disease, or diffuse toxic goiter. The presenting signs and symptoms of Graves disease are set forth in Table 38–4.

Pathophysiology

Graves disease is an autoimmune disorder in which a defect in suppressor T lymphocytes stimulates B lymphocytes to synthesize antibodies (TSH-R Ab [stim]) to thyroidal antigens. The TSH-R Ab [stim] binds and activates the TSH receptor in the thyroid cell membrane and stimulates growth and biosynthetic activity of the thyroid cell. Genetics, the postpartum state, cigarette smoking, and physical and emotional stress increase TSH-R Ab [stim] development. A genetic predisposition is suggested by a high frequency of HLA-B8 and HLA-DR3 in Caucasians, HLA-Bw46 and HLA-B5 in Chinese, and HLA-B17 in African Americans. Spontaneous remission is rare, so some patients require years of antithyroid therapy.

Laboratory Diagnosis

In most patients with hyperthyroidism, T_3, T_4, FT_4, and FT_3 are elevated and TSH is suppressed (see Table 38–2). Radioiodine uptake is typically markedly elevated as well. Antithyroglobulin, thyroid peroxidase, and TSH-R Ab [stim] antibodies are usually present.

Management of Graves Disease

The three primary methods for controlling hyperthyroidism include antithyroid drug therapy, destruction of the gland with radioactive iodine, and surgical thyroidectomy. None of these methods alters the underlying pathogenesis of the disease.

A. Antithyroid Drug Therapy

Drug therapy is most useful in young patients with small glands and mild disease. Methimazole (preferred) or propylthiouracil administration is continued until spontaneous remission occurs. This is the only therapy that leaves the thyroid gland intact, often requiring a long period of treatment and observation (12–18 months). However, once therapy is stopped, a high rate (50–60%) of relapse may occur.

Methimazole is preferable to propylthiouracil (except in pregnancy and thyroid storm) because it has a lower risk of serious liver injury and can be administered once daily, improving adherence. Antithyroid drug therapy is usually begun with divided doses, shifting to maintenance therapy with single daily doses when the patient becomes clinically euthyroid. However, mild to moderately severe thyrotoxicosis can often be controlled with an initial single dose of 20–40 mg of methimazole administered for 4–8 weeks to normalize hormone levels. Maintenance therapy requires 5–15 mg once daily. Alternatively, administer propylthiouracil 100–150 mg every 6 or 8 hours until the patient is euthyroid, then follow with gradual reduction of the dose to the maintenance level of 50–150 mg once daily. In addition to inhibiting iodine organification, propylthiouracil also inhibits the conversion of T_4 to T_3, so it brings the level of activated thyroid hormone down more quickly than does methimazole. The best clinical guide to remission is reduction in the size of the goiter. Laboratory tests most useful in monitoring the course of therapy are serum FT_3, FT_4, and TSH levels.

Adverse reactions to antithyroid drugs have been described above. A minor rash without systemic symptoms can often be controlled by antihistamine therapy. Because the more severe reaction of agranulocytosis is often preceded by sore throat and a high fever, patients receiving antithyroid drugs must be instructed to discontinue the drug and seek immediate medical attention if these symptoms develop and persist. White blood cell counts with a differential and a throat culture are indicated in such cases, followed by appropriate antibiotic therapy. Stop therapy if significant elevations in transaminases (two to three times the upper limit of normal) occur.

B. Thyroidectomy

A near-total thyroidectomy is the treatment of choice for patients with very large glands or multinodular goiters. Patients are treated with antithyroid drugs until euthyroid (about 6 weeks).

In addition, for 10–14 days prior to surgery, they receive saturated solution of potassium iodide, 5 drops twice daily, to diminish vascularity of the gland and simplify surgery. About 80–90% of patients will require thyroid supplementation following near-total thyroidectomy.

C. Radioactive Iodine

Radioiodine therapy (RAI) utilizing ^{131}I is the preferred treatment for most patients over 21 years of age. In patients without heart disease, the therapeutic dose can be given immediately in a range of 80–120 μCi/g of estimated thyroid weight corrected for uptake. In patients with underlying heart disease or severe thyrotoxicosis and in elderly patients, it is desirable to treat with antithyroid drugs (preferably methimazole) until the patient is euthyroid. Stop the methimazole for 2–3 days before RAI is administered so as not to interfere with RAI retention, but it can be restarted 3–5 days later and then gradually tapered over 4–6 weeks as thyroid function normalizes. Iodides should be avoided to ensure maximal ^{131}I uptake. Six to 12 weeks following the administration of RAI, the gland will shrink in size and the patient will usually become euthyroid or hypothyroid. A second dose may be required 3 months post-RAI if there is insufficient response. Hypothyroidism occurs in about 80% of patients following RAI. Serum FT_4 and TSH levels should be monitored regularly. When hypothyroidism develops, prompt replacement with oral levothyroxine, 50–150 mcg daily, should be started.

D. Adjuncts to Antithyroid Therapy

During the acute phase of thyrotoxicosis, β-adrenoceptor–blocking agents without intrinsic sympathomimetic activity are appropriate additions in symptomatic patients aged 60 years or older, in those with heart rates >90 beats/min, and in those with cardiovascular disease. Propranolol, 20–40 mg orally every 6 hours, or metoprolol, 25–50 mg orally every 6–8 hours, will control tachycardia, hypertension, and atrial fibrillation. Beta-adrenoceptor–blocking agents are gradually withdrawn as serum thyroxine levels return to normal. Diltiazem, 90–120 mg three or four times daily, can be used to control tachycardia in patients in whom β blockers are contraindicated, eg, those with asthma. Dihydropyridine calcium channel blockers may not be as effective as diltiazem or verapamil. Adequate nutrition and vitamin supplements are essential. Barbiturates accelerate T_4 breakdown (by hepatic enzyme induction) and may be helpful both as sedatives and to lower T_4 levels. Bile acid sequestrants (eg, cholestyramine) can also rapidly lower T_4 levels by increasing the fecal excretion of T_4.

TOXIC UNINODULAR GOITER & TOXIC MULTINODULAR GOITER

These forms of hyperthyroidism occur often in older women with nodular goiters. Free thyroxine is moderately elevated or occasionally normal, but FT_3 or T_3 is strikingly elevated. Single toxic adenomas can be managed either with surgical excision of the adenoma or with radioiodine therapy. Toxic multinodular goiter is usually associated with a large goiter and is best treated by preparation with methimazole (preferable) or propylthiouracil followed by subtotal thyroidectomy.

SUBACUTE THYROIDITIS

During the acute phase of a viral infection of the thyroid gland, there is destruction of thyroid parenchyma with transient release of stored thyroid hormones. A similar state may occur in patients with Hashimoto thyroiditis and with some drug-induced dysfunction (eg, immune checkpoint inhibitors, amiodarone) before the onset of hypothyroidism. These episodes of transient thyrotoxicosis have been termed *spontaneously resolving hyperthyroidism*. Supportive therapy is usually all that is necessary, such as β-adrenoceptor–blocking agents without intrinsic sympathomimetic activity (eg, propranolol) for tachycardia and aspirin or nonsteroidal anti-inflammatory drugs to control local pain and fever. Corticosteroids may be necessary in severe cases to control the inflammation.

SPECIAL PROBLEMS

Thyroid Storm

Thyroid storm, or thyrotoxic crisis, is sudden acute exacerbation of all of the symptoms of thyrotoxicosis, presenting as a life-threatening syndrome. Vigorous management is mandatory. Propranolol, 60–80 mg orally every 4 hours, or intravenous propranolol, 1–2 mg slowly every 5–10 minutes to a total of 10 mg, or esmolol, 50–100 mg/kg per min, is helpful to control the severe cardiovascular manifestations. If β blockers are contraindicated by the presence of severe heart failure or asthma, hypertension and tachycardia may be controlled with diltiazem, 90–120 mg orally three or four times daily or 5–10 mg/h by intravenous infusion (asthmatic patients only). Release of thyroid hormones from the gland is blocked by the administration of saturated solution of potassium iodide, 5 drops orally every 6 hours starting 1 hour after giving thioamides. Hormone synthesis is reduced by the administration of propylthiouracil, 500–1000 mg as a loading dose, followed by 250 mg orally every 4 hours. If the patient is unable to take propylthiouracil by mouth, a rectal formulation* can be prepared and administered in a dosage of 400 mg every 6 hours as a retention enema. Methimazole may also be prepared for rectal administration in a dose of 60–80 mg daily. Hydrocortisone, 50 mg intravenously every 6 hours, will protect the patient against shock and will block the conversion of T_4 to T_3, rapidly reducing the level of thyroactive material in the blood.

Supportive therapy is essential to control fever, heart failure, and any underlying disease process that may have precipitated the acute storm. In rare situations, where the above methods are not adequate to control the problem, oral bile acid sequestrants (eg, cholestyramine), plasmapheresis, or peritoneal dialysis has been used to lower the levels of circulating thyroxine.

*To prepare a water suspension propylthiouracil enema, grind eight 50-mg tablets and suspend the powder in 90 mL of sterile water.

Ophthalmopathy

Ophthalmopathy is attributed to the presence of TSH receptors and insulin-like growth factor 1 receptor (IGF-1R) in orbital fibrocytes. Although severe ophthalmopathy is rare, it is difficult to treat. A 15–20% risk of aggravating severe eye disease may occur following RAI, especially in those who smoke. Management requires effective treatment of the thyroid disease, usually by total surgical excision or ^{131}I ablation of the gland plus anti-inflammatory therapies (see below). In addition, local therapy may be necessary, eg, elevation of the head to diminish periorbital edema and artificial tears to relieve corneal drying due to exophthalmos. Smoking cessation is necessary to prevent progression of the ophthalmopathy. For severe, acute inflammatory reaction, prednisone, 60–100 mg orally daily for about a week and then 60–100 mg every other day, tapering the dose over 6–12 weeks, may be effective. Teprotumumab (Tepezza), a monoclonal antibody given once every three weeks for total of eight IV infusions, significantly reduces eye bulges, pain and swelling, and double vision. If the aforementioned therapy fails or is contraindicated, irradiation of the posterior orbit, using well-collimated high-energy X-ray therapy, will frequently result in marked improvement of the acute process. Threatened loss of vision is an indication for surgical decompression of the orbit. Eyelid or eye muscle surgery may be necessary to correct residual problems after the acute process has subsided.

Dermopathy

Dermopathy or pretibial myxedema will often respond to topical corticosteroids applied to the involved area and covered with an occlusive dressing.

Thyrotoxicosis during Pregnancy

Ideally, women in the childbearing period with severe disease should have definitive therapy with ^{131}I or subtotal thyroidectomy *prior* to pregnancy in order to avoid an acute exacerbation of the disease during pregnancy or following delivery. If thyrotoxicosis does develop during pregnancy, RAI is contraindicated due to its placenta passage and injury to the fetal thyroid. During the first trimester, propylthiouracil (lower teratogenic risks than methimazole) is given but to avoid the risk of liver damage, PTU is changed to methimazole for the remainder of the pregnancy. Propylthiouracil must be kept to the minimum dosage necessary for control of the disease (ie, <300 mg/d) to avoid inhibiting the function of the fetal thyroid gland. Alternatively, a subtotal thyroidectomy can be safely performed during the mid-trimester. It is essential to give the patient a thyroid supplement during the balance of the pregnancy.

Neonatal Graves Disease

Graves disease may occur in the newborn infant, due either to passage of maternal TSH-R Ab [stim] through the placenta, stimulating the thyroid gland of the neonate, or to genetic transmission of the trait to the fetus. Laboratory studies reveal an elevated free T_4, a markedly elevated T_3, and a low TSH—in contrast to the normal infant, in whom TSH is elevated at birth. TSH-R Ab [stim] is usually found in the serum of both the child and the mother.

If caused by maternal TSH-R Ab [stim], the disease is usually self-limited and subsides over a period of 4–12 weeks, coinciding with the fall in the infant's TSH-R Ab [stim] level. However, treatment is necessary because of the severe metabolic stress the infant experiences. Therapy includes propylthiouracil at a dosage of 5–10 mg/kg daily in divided doses at 8-hour intervals; Lugol solution (8 mg of iodide per drop), one drop every 8 hours; and propranolol, 2 mg/kg daily in divided doses. Careful supportive therapy is essential. If the infant is very ill, oral prednisone, 2 mg/kg daily in divided doses, will help block conversion of T_4 to T_3. These medications are gradually reduced as the clinical picture improves and can be discontinued by 6–12 weeks.

SUBCLINICAL HYPERTHYROIDISM

Subclinical hyperthyroidism is defined as a suppressed TSH level (below the normal range) in conjunction with normal thyroid hormone levels. Cardiac toxicity (eg, atrial fibrillation), especially in older persons and those with underlying cardiac disease, is of greatest concern. The consensus of thyroid experts agree that hyperthyroidism treatment is appropriate in those with TSH less than 0.1 mIU/L, while close monitoring of the TSH level is appropriate for those with less TSH suppression.

Amiodarone-Induced Thyrotoxicosis

In addition to those patients who develop hypothyroidism caused by amiodarone, approximately 3% of patients receiving this drug will develop hyperthyroidism instead. Two types of amiodarone-induced thyrotoxicosis have been reported: iodine-induced (type I), which often occurs in persons with underlying thyroid disease (eg, multinodular goiter, Graves disease); and an inflammatory thyroiditis (type II) that occurs in patients without thyroid disease due to leakage of thyroid hormone into the circulation. Treatment of type I requires therapy with thioamides, while type II responds best to glucocorticoids. Since it is not always possible to differentiate between the two types, thioamides and glucocorticoids are often co-administered together. Even if amiodarone is stopped, rapid improvement does not occur due to its long half-life.

NONTOXIC GOITER

Nontoxic goiter is a syndrome of thyroid enlargement without excessive thyroid hormone production. Enlargement of the thyroid gland is often due to TSH stimulation from inadequate thyroid hormone synthesis. The most common cause of nontoxic goiter worldwide is iodide deficiency, but in the United States, it is Hashimoto thyroiditis. Other causes include germ-line or acquired mutations in genes involved in hormone synthesis, dietary goitrogens, and neoplasms (see below).

Goiter due to iodide deficiency is best managed by prophylactic administration of iodide. The optimal daily iodide intake is 150–200 mcg. Iodized salt and iodate used as preservatives in flour and bread are excellent sources of iodine in the diet. In areas where it is difficult to introduce iodized salt or iodate preservatives, a solution of iodized poppy-seed oil has been administered intramuscularly to provide a long-term source of inorganic iodine.

Goiter due to ingestion of dietary goitrogens is treated by elimination of the goitrogen or by adding sufficient thyroxine to shut off TSH stimulation. Similarly, in Hashimoto thyroiditis and dyshormonogenesis, adequate thyroxine therapy—150–200 mcg/d orally—will suppress pituitary TSH and result in slow regression of the goiter as well as correction of hypothyroidism.

THYROID NEOPLASMS

Neoplasms of the thyroid gland may be benign (adenomas) or malignant. The primary diagnostic test is a fine-needle aspiration biopsy and cytologic examination. Benign lesions may be monitored for growth or symptoms of local obstruction, which would mandate surgical excision. Levothyroxine therapy is not recommended for the suppression of benign nodules, especially in iodine-sufficient areas. Management of thyroid carcinoma requires a total thyroidectomy, postoperative radioiodine therapy in selected instances, and lifetime replacement with levothyroxine. The evaluation for recurrence of some thyroid malignancies often involves withdrawal of thyroxine replacement for 4–6 weeks—accompanied by the development of hypothyroidism. Tumor recurrence is likely if there is a rise in serum thyroglobulin (ie, a tumor marker) or a positive ^{131}I scan when TSH is elevated. Alternatively, administration of recombinant human TSH (Thyrogen) can produce comparable TSH elevations without discontinuing thyroxine and avoiding hypothyroidism. Recombinant human TSH is administered intramuscularly once daily for 2 days. A rise in serum thyroglobulin or a positive ^{131}I scan will indicate a recurrence of the thyroid cancer.

SUMMARY Drugs Used in the Management of Thyroid Disease

Subclass, Drug	Mechanism of Action and Effects	Indications	Pharmacokinetics, Toxicities, Interactions
THYROID PREPARATIONS			
• Levothyroxine (T_4) • Liothyronine (T_3)	Activation of nuclear receptors results in gene expression with RNA formation and protein synthesis	Hypothyroidism	See Table 38–1 • maximum effect seen after 6–8 weeks of therapy • *Toxicity:* See Table 38–4 for symptoms of thyroid excess
ANTITHYROID AGENTS			
THIOAMIDES			
• Methimazole • Propylthiouracil (PTU)	Inhibit thyroid peroxidase reactions • block iodine organification • inhibit peripheral deiodination of T_4 to T_3 (primarily PTU)	Hyperthyroidism	Oral • duration of action: 24 h (methimazole), 6–8 h (PTU) • delayed onset of action • *Toxicity:* Nausea, gastrointestinal distress, rash, agranulocytosis, hepatitis (PTU black box), hypothyroidism, teratogenicity (methimazole > PTU)
IODIDES			
• Lugol solution • Potassium iodide	Inhibit organification and hormone release • reduce the size and vascularity of the gland	Preparation for surgical thyroidectomy	Oral • acute onset within 2–7 days • *Toxicity:* Rare (see text)
BETA BLOCKERS			
• Propranolol, other β blockers lacking partial agonist activity	Inhibition of β adrenoreceptors • inhibit T_4 to T_3 conversion (only propranolol)	Hyperthyroidism, especially thyroid storm • adjunct to control tachycardia, hypertension, and atrial fibrillation	Onset within hours • duration of 4–6 h (oral propranolol) • *Toxicity:* bronchospasm, AV blockade, hypotension, bradycardia
MONOCLONAL ANTIBODY			
• Teprotumumab	Inhibits insulin-like growth factor receptor type 1 (IGF-1R)	Proptosis, redness, swelling, double vision, from thyroid-associated ophthalmopathy	• Onset before completion of eight total infusions • T1/2 20 days • *Toxicity:* infusion reactions, muscle cramps, nausea, alopecia, diarrhea, transient hyperglycemia, hearing loss
RADIOACTIVE IODINE ^{131}I (RAI)			
	Radiation destruction of thyroid parenchyma	Hyperthyroidism • patients should be euthyroid or on β blockers before RAI • avoid in pregnancy and in nursing mothers	Oral • half-life 5 days • onset in 6–12 weeks • maximum effect in 3–6 months • *Toxicity:* Sore throat, sialitis, hypothyroidism

PREPARATIONS AVAILABLE

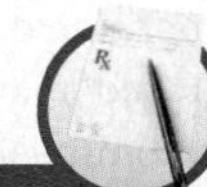

GENERIC NAME	AVAILABLE AS
THYROID AGENTS	
Oral levothyroxine (T_4)	Generic (also IV), Eltroxin, Euthyrox, Levoxyl, Levo-T, Levolet*, Novothyrox, Synthroid (IV also), Thyquidity, Tirosint, Tirosint-SOL, Unithroid
Oral liothyronine (T_3)	Generic, Cytomel, Triostat (IV)
Oral Liotrix (a 4:1 ratio of T_4:T_3)	Thyrolar
Oral Thyroid desiccated (USP)	Generic, Armour, Nature-Throid, Westhroid
ANTITHYROID AGENTS	
Radioactive iodine (^{131}I) sodium	Iodotope, Sodium Iodide I 131 Therapeutic
Oral methimazole	Generic, Northyx, Tapazole
Potassium iodide	
Oral solution (SSKI)	ThyroShield
Oral solution (Lugol solution)	Lugol solution
Oral potassium iodide tablets	IOSAT, Pima, Thyro-Block, ThyroSafe
Oral propylthiouracil [PTU]	Generic
Teprotumumab	Tepezza (IV)
DIAGNOSTIC AGENT	
Thyrotropin; recombinant human TSH	Thyrogen

*Not available in the United States.

REFERENCES

General

American Thyroid Association: Professional Guidelines. www.thyroid.org/professionals/ata-professional-guidelines/.

American Thyroid Association Task Force on Radiation Safety et al: Radiation safety in the treatment of patients with thyroid diseases by radioiodine ^{131}I: Practice recommendations of the American Thyroid Association. Thyroid 2011;21:335.

Cooper DS, Ladenson PW: The thyroid gland. In: Gardner DG et al (editors): *Greenspan's Basic & Clinical Endocrinology*, 10th ed. McGraw Hill, 2018.

Rugge JB, Bougatsos C, Chou R: Screening and treatment of thyroid dysfunction: An evidence review for the U.S. Preventive Services Task Force. Ann Intern Med 2015;162:35.

U.S. Department of Health and Human Services: Potassium iodide as a thyroid blocking agent in radiation emergencies. www.fda.gov/downloads/Drugs/GuidanceComplianceRegulatoryInformation/Guidances/UCM080542.pdf.

Thyroid Hormone Action

Aranda A: MicroRNAs and thyroid hormone action. Mol Cell Endocrinol 2021;525:111175.

Braun D, Schweizer U: Thyroid hormone transport and transporters. Vitam Horm 2018;106:19.

Mallya M, Ogilvy-Stuart AL: Thyrotropic hormones. Best Pract Res Clin Endocrinol Metab 2018;32:17.

Paragliola RM et al: Iodothyronine deiodinases and reduced sensitivity to thyroid hormones. Front Biosci (Landmark Ed). 2020;25:201.

Tedeschi L et al: Main factors involved in thyroid hormone action. Molecules 2021;26:7337.

Management of Hypothyroidism

Brito JP et al: Association between generic-to-generic levothyroxine switching and thyrotropin levels among US adults. JAMA Intern Med 2022;182:418.

Caron P et al: Factors influencing the levothyroxine dose in the hormone replacement therapy of primary hypothyroidism in adults. Rev Endocr Metab Disord 2022;23:463.

Chaker L et al: Hypothyroidism. Nat Rev Dis Primers 2022;8:30.

Cherella C, Wassner AJ: Update on congenital hypothyroidism. Curr Opin Endocrinol Diabetes Obes 2020:27:63.

Ettleson MD, Bianco AC: Individualized therapy for hypothyroidism: Is T4 enough for everyone? J Clin Endocrinol Metab 2020;105:e3090.

Idrees T et al: Liothyronine and desiccated thyroid extract in the treatment of hypothyroidism. Thyroid 2020;30:1399.

Jonklaas J: Optimal thyroid hormone replacement. Endocr Rev 2022;43:366.

Jonklaas J et al: Evidence-based use of levothyroxine/liothyronine combinations in treating hypothyroidism: a consensus document. Thyroid 2021;31:156.

Shakir MKM et al: Comparative effectiveness of levothyroxine, desiccated thyroid extract, and levothyroxine+liothyronine in hypothyroidism. J Clin Endocrinol Metab 2021;106:e4400.

Subclinical Hypothyroidism and Hyperthyroidism

Leng O, Razvi S: Treatment of subclinical hypothyroidism: assessing when treatment is likely to be beneficial. Expert Rev Endocrinol Metab 2021;16:73.

Tsai K, Leung AM: Subclinical hyperthyroidism: a review of the clinical literature. Endocr Pract 2021;27:254.

Wildisen L et al: Effect of levothyroxine therapy on the development of depressive symptoms in older adults with subclinical hypothyroidism: an ancillary study of a randomized clinical trial. JAMA Netw Open 2021;4e2036645.

Antithyroid Agents and Management of Hyperthyroidism

Azizi F et al: Long-term thioamide antithyroid treatment of Graves' disease. Best Pract Res Clin Endocrinol Metab 2023;37:101631.

Antonelli A et al: Graves' disease: Epidemiology, genetic and environmental risk factors and viruses. Best Pract Res Clin Endocrinol Metab 2020;34:101387.

Burch HB, Cooper DS: Antithyroid drug therapy: 70 years later. Eur J Endocrinol 2018;179:R261.

Davies TF et al: Graves' disease. Nat Rev Dis Primers 2020;6:52.

Douglas RS et al: Teprotumumab efficacy, safety, and durability in longer duration thyroid eye disease and retreatment: Optic-X Study. Ophthalmopathy 2022;129:438.

Douglas RS et al: Teprotumumab for the treatment of active thyroid eye disease. N Engl J Med 2020;382:341.

Kahaly GJ Management of Graves thyroidal and extrathyroidal disease. An update. J Clin Endocrinol Metab 2020;105:3704.

Lane LC et al: New therapeutic horizons for Graves' hyperthyroidism. Endocr Rev 2020;41:873.

Sisson JC et al: Radiation safety in the treatment of patients with thyroid diseases by radioiodine 131I: practice recommendations of the American Thyroid Association. Thyroid 2011;21:335.

Pregnancy

Amino N, Arata N: Thyroid dysfunction following pregnancy and implications for breastfeeding. Best Pract Res Clin Endocrinol Metab 2020;34:101438.

Andersen SL, Knøsgaard L: Management of thyrotoxicosis during pregnancy. Best Pract Res Clin Endocrinol Metab 2020;34:101414.

Ilias I, Milionis C, Koukkou E: Further understanding of thyroid function in pregnant women. Expert Rev Endocrinol Metab 2022;17:365.

The Effects of Drugs on Thyroid Function

Basolo A et al: Effects of tyrosine kinase inhibitors on thyroid function and thyroid hormone metabolism. Semin Cancer Biol 2022;79:197.

Bhattacharya S et al: Anticancer drug-induced thyroid dysfunction. Eur Endocrinol 2020;16:32.

Bednarczuk T et al: 2021 European Thyroid Association guidelines for the management of iodine-based contrast media-induced thyroid dysfunction. Eur Thyroid J 2021;10:269.

Iwama S et al: Immune checkpoint inhibitor-related thyroid dysfunction. Best Pract Res Clin Endocrinol Metab 2022;36:101660.

Rochtus AM et al: Antiseizure medications and thyroid hormone homeostasis: Literature review and practical recommendations. Epilepsia 2022;63:259.

Ylli D, Wartofsky L, Burman KD: Evaluation and treatment of amiodarone-induced thyroid disorders. J Clin Endocrinol Metab 2021;106:226.

Zhan L et al: Immune checkpoint inhibitors-related thyroid dysfunction: epidemiology, clinical presentation, possible pathogenesis, and management. Front Endocrinol (Lausanne) 2021;12:649863.

CASE STUDY ANSWER

The initial methimazole treatment was appropriate and preferable to propylthiouracil because of its longer duration of action allowing once-daily dosing and its improved safety profile. JP presents with the typical signs and symptoms of hypothyroidism following RAI despite levothyroxine replacement. Either radioactive iodine or thyroidectomy are reasonable and effective strategies for definitive treatment of her hyperthyroidism, especially before becoming pregnant to avoid an acute hyperthyroid exacerbation during pregnancy or following delivery. Her hypothyroid symptoms should have been easily corrected by the addition of levothyroxine dosed correctly at 1.7 mcg/kg/day or 100 mcg daily. Because she is young and has no cardiac disease, full replacement doses were appropriate to start. However, her elevated TSH level indicates inadequate levothyroxine replacement which may be related to nonadherence, or concomitant calcium and omeprazole co-administration. For optimal absorption, levothyroxine should be taken orally 30–60 minutes before meals (eg, empty stomach) or at bedtime, and separated by 4 hours from her calcium administration. Lower thyroxine doses may also be sufficient if her omeprazole is stopped. Once-weekly thyroxine injections may be effective in those with ongoing nonadherence. Thyroid function tests should be monitored after 6–8 weeks of therapy, obtained before thyroxine administration to avoid transient hormone alterations, and the dosage adjusted to achieve a normal TSH level and resolution of hypothyroid symptoms.

CHAPTER

39 Adrenocorticosteroids & Adrenocortical Antagonists

George P. Chrousos, MD

CASE STUDY

A 19-year-old man complains of anorexia, fatigue, dizziness, and weight loss of 8 months' duration. The examining physician discovers postural hypotension and moderate vitiligo (depigmented areas of skin) and obtains routine blood tests. She finds hyponatremia, hyperkalemia, and acidosis and suspects Addison disease. She performs a standard ACTH 1–24 stimulation test, which reveals an insufficient plasma cortisol response, which is compatible with primary adrenal insufficiency. The diagnosis of autoimmune Addison disease is made, and the patient must start replacement of the hormones he cannot produce himself. How should this patient be treated? What precautions should he take?

The natural adrenocortical hormones are steroid molecules produced and released by the adrenal cortex. Deficiency of the adrenocortical hormones results in the signs and symptoms of **Addison disease.** Excess production causes **Cushing syndrome.** Both natural and synthetic corticosteroids are used for the diagnosis and treatment of disorders of adrenal function. They are also used—more often and in much larger doses—for treatment of a variety of inflammatory, immunologic, and hematologic disorders.

Secretion of adrenocortical steroids, especially the glucocorticoids, is controlled by the pituitary release of **corticotropin (ACTH)** (see Chapter 37). Corticotropin is derived from a larger protein synthesized in the pituitary, **pro-opiomelanocortin (POMC).** Secretion of the salt-retaining hormone aldosterone is primarily under the influence of circulating angiotensin and potassium. Corticotropin has some actions that do not depend on its effect on adrenocortical secretion. However, its pharmacologic value as an anti-inflammatory agent and its use in testing adrenal function depend on its secretory action. Its pharmacology is reviewed only briefly here.

Inhibitors of the synthesis or antagonists of the action of the adrenocortical steroids are important in the treatment of several conditions. These agents are described at the end of this chapter.

■ ADRENOCORTICOSTEROIDS

The adrenal cortex releases a large number of steroids into the circulation. Some have minimal biologic activity and function primarily as precursors, and there are some for which no function has been established. The hormonal steroids may be classified as those having important effects on intermediary metabolism and immune function **(glucocorticoids),** those having principally salt-retaining activity **(mineralocorticoids),** and those having **androgenic** or **estrogenic** activity (see Chapter 40). In humans, the major glucocorticoid is **cortisol** and the most important mineralocorticoid is **aldosterone.** Quantitatively, dehydroepiandrosterone (DHEA) in its sulfated form (DHEAS) is the major adrenal androgen. However, DHEA and two other adrenal androgens, androstenedione and androstenediol, are weak androgens and androstenediol is a potent estrogen. Androstenedione can be converted to testosterone and estradiol in extra-adrenal tissues (Figure 39–1). Adrenal androgens constitute the major endogenous precursors of estrogen in women after menopause and in younger patients in whom ovarian function is deficient or absent.

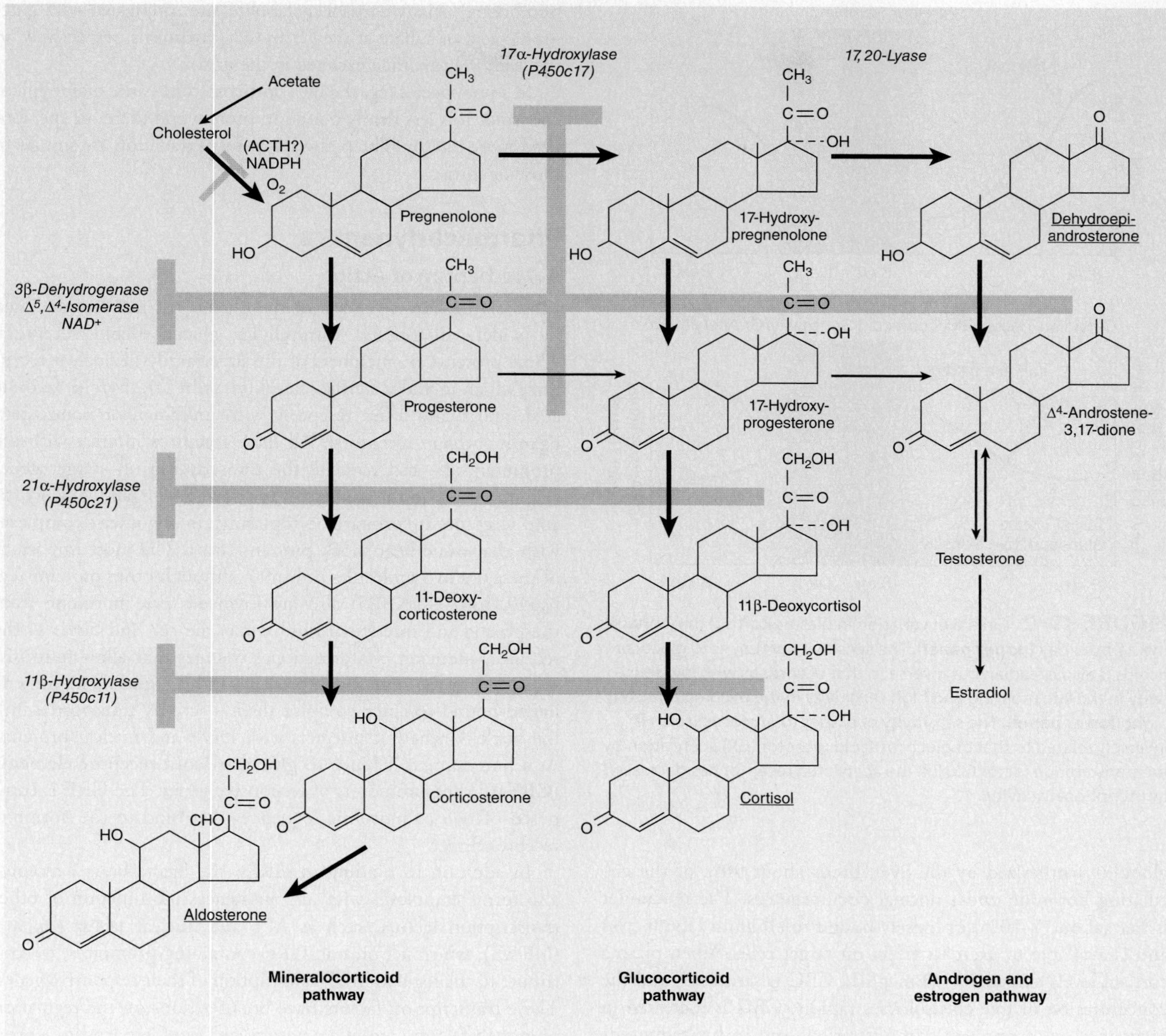

FIGURE 39–1 Outline of major pathways in adrenocortical hormone biosynthesis. The major secretory products are underlined. Pregnenolone is the major precursor of corticosterone and aldosterone, and 17-hydroxypregnenolone is the major precursor of cortisol. The enzymes and cofactors for the reactions progressing down each column are shown on the left and across columns at the top of the figure. When a particular enzyme is deficient, hormone production is blocked at the points indicated by the shaded bars. (Reproduced with permission from Ganong WF: *Review of Medical Physiology*, 22nd ed. New York, NY: McGraw Hill; 2005.)

THE NATURALLY OCCURRING GLUCOCORTICOIDS; CORTISOL (HYDROCORTISONE)

Pharmacokinetics

Cortisol (also called hydrocortisone, compound F) exerts a wide range of physiologic effects, including regulation of intermediary metabolism, cardiovascular function, growth, and immunity. Its synthesis and secretion are tightly regulated by the central nervous system, which is very sensitive to negative feedback by the circulating cortisol and exogenous (synthetic) glucocorticoids. Cortisol is synthesized from cholesterol (as shown in Figure 39–1). The mechanisms controlling its secretion are discussed in Chapter 37.

The rate of secretion follows a circadian rhythm (Figure 39–2) governed by pulses of ACTH that peak in the early morning hours and after meals. In plasma, cortisol is bound to circulating proteins. **Corticosteroid-binding globulin (CBG),** an α_2

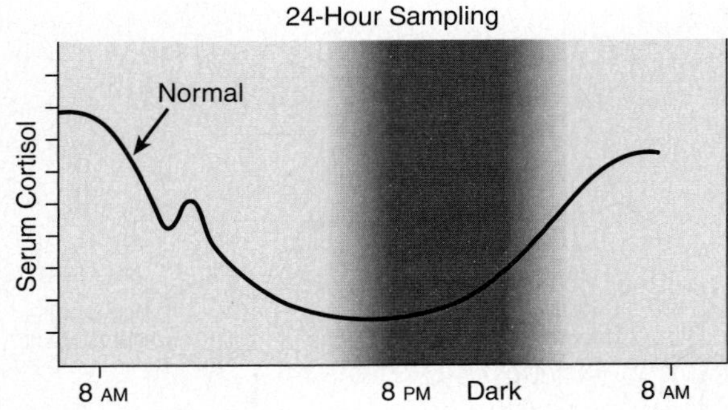

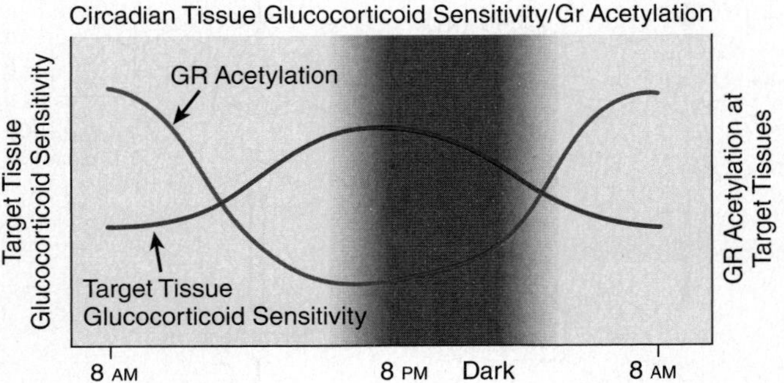

FIGURE 39–2 Circadian variation in plasma cortisol throughout the 24-hour day **(upper panel).** The sensitivity of tissues to glucocorticoids is also circadian but inverse to that of cortisol, with low sensitivity in the late morning and high sensitivity in the evening and early night **(lower panel).** The sensitivity of tissues to glucocorticoids is inversely related to that of glucocorticoid receptor (GR) acetylation by the transcription factor CLOCK; the acetylated receptor has decreased transcriptional activity.

globulin synthesized by the liver, binds about 90% of the circulating hormone under normal circumstances. The remainder is free (about 5–10%) or loosely bound to albumin (about 5%) and is available to exert its effect on target cells. When plasma cortisol levels exceed 20–30 mcg/dL, CBG is saturated, and the concentration of free cortisol rises rapidly. CBG is increased in pregnancy, with estrogen administration, and in hyperthyroidism. It is decreased by hypothyroidism, genetic defects in synthesis, and protein deficiency states. Albumin has a large capacity but low affinity for cortisol, and for practical purposes albumin-bound cortisol should be considered free. Synthetic corticosteroids such as dexamethasone are largely bound to albumin rather than CBG.

The half-life of cortisol in the circulation is normally about 60–90 minutes; it may be increased when hydrocortisone (the pharmaceutical preparation of cortisol) is administered in large amounts or when stress, hypothyroidism, or liver disease is present. Only 1% of cortisol is excreted unchanged in the urine as free cortisol; about 20% of cortisol is converted to cortisone by 11-hydroxysteroid dehydrogenase in the kidney and other tissues with mineralocorticoid receptors (see below) before reaching the liver. Most cortisol is metabolized in the liver. About one-third of the cortisol produced daily is excreted in the urine as dihydroxy ketone metabolites and is measured as 17-hydroxysteroids (see Figure 39–3 for carbon numbering). Many cortisol metabolites are conjugated with glucuronic acid or sulfate at the C_3 and C_{21} hydroxyls, respectively, in the liver; they are then excreted in the urine.

In some species (eg, the rat), corticosterone is the major glucocorticoid. It is less firmly bound to protein and therefore metabolized more rapidly. The pathways of its degradation are similar to those of cortisol.

Pharmacodynamics

A. Mechanism of Action

Most of the known effects of the glucocorticoids are mediated by widely distributed intracellular glucocorticoid receptors. These proteins are members of the superfamily of nuclear receptors, which includes steroid, sterol (vitamin D), thyroid, retinoic acid, and many other receptors with unknown or nonexistent ligands (orphan receptors). All these receptors interact with the promoters of—and regulate the transcription of—target genes (Figure 39–4). In the absence of the hormonal ligand, glucocorticoid receptors are primarily cytoplasmic, in oligomeric complexes with chaperone heat-shock proteins (hsp). The most important of these are two molecules of hsp90, although other proteins (eg, hsp40, hsp70, FKBP5) also are involved. Free hormone from the plasma and interstitial fluid enters the cell and binds to the receptor, inducing conformational changes that allow it to dissociate from the heat shock proteins and dimerize. The dimeric ligand-bound receptor complex then is actively transported into the nucleus, where it interacts with DNA and nuclear proteins. As a homodimer, it binds to **glucocorticoid receptor elements (GREs)** in the promoters of responsive genes. The GRE is composed of two palindromic sequences that bind to the hormone receptor dimer.

In addition to binding to GREs, the ligand-bound receptor also forms complexes with and influences the function of other transcription factors, such as AP1 and nuclear factor kappa-B (NF-κB), which act on non-GRE-containing promoters, to contribute to the regulation of transcription of their responsive genes. These transcription factors have broad actions on the regulation of growth factors, proinflammatory cytokines, etc, and to a great extent mediate the anti-growth, anti-inflammatory, and immunosuppressive effects of glucocorticoids.

Two genes for the corticoid receptor have been identified: one encoding the classic glucocorticoid receptor **(GR)** and the other encoding the mineralocorticoid receptor **(MR).** Alternative splicing of human glucocorticoid receptor pre-mRNA generates two highly homologous isoforms termed hGRα and hGRβ. Human GRα is the classic ligand-activated glucocorticoid receptor, which, in the hormone-bound state, modulates the expression of glucocorticoid-responsive genes. In contrast, hGRβ does not bind glucocorticoids and is transcriptionally inactive. However, hGRβ is able to inhibit the effects of hormone-activated hGRα on glucocorticoid-responsive genes, playing the role of a physiologically relevant endogenous inhibitor of glucocorticoid action. It was recently shown that the two hGR alternative transcripts have eight distinct translation initiation sites—ie, in a human cell there may be up to 16 GRα and GRβ isoforms, which may form

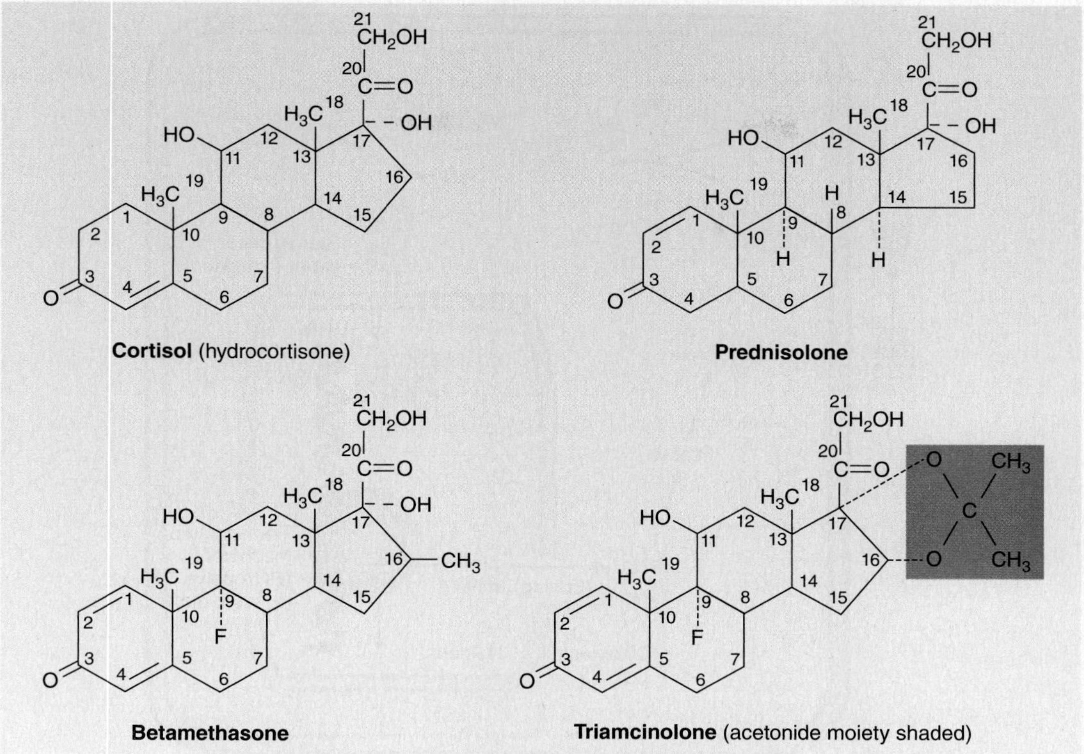

Cortisol (hydrocortisone)

Prednisolone

Betamethasone

Triamcinolone (acetonide moiety shaded)

FIGURE 39–3 Chemical structures of several glucocorticoids. The acetonide-substituted derivatives (eg, triamcinolone acetonide) have increased surface activity and are useful in dermatology. Dexamethasone is identical to betamethasone except for the configuration of the methyl group at C_{16}: in betamethasone it is beta (projecting *up* from the plane of the rings); in dexamethasone it is alpha.

up to 256 homodimers and heterodimers with different transcriptional and possibly nontranscriptional activities. This variability suggests that this important class of steroid receptors has complex stochastic activities. In addition, rare mutations in hGR may result in partial glucocorticoid resistance. Affected individuals have increased ACTH secretion because of reduced pituitary feedback and additional endocrine abnormalities (see below).

The prototype GR isoform is composed of about 800 amino acids and can be divided into three functional domains (see Figure 2–6). The glucocorticoid-binding domain is located at the carboxyl terminal of the molecule. The DNA-binding domain is located in the middle of the protein and contains nine cysteine residues. This region folds into a "two-finger" structure stabilized by zinc ions connected to cysteines to form two tetrahedrons. This part of the molecule binds to the GREs that regulate glucocorticoid action on glucocorticoid-regulated genes. The zinc fingers represent the basic structure by which the DNA-binding domain recognizes specific nucleic acid sequences. The amino terminal domain is involved in the transactivation activity of the receptor and increases its specificity.

The interaction of glucocorticoid receptors with GREs or other transcription factors is facilitated or inhibited by several families of proteins called steroid receptor *coregulators*, divided into *coactivators* and *corepressors*. The coregulators do this by serving as bridges between the receptors and other nuclear proteins and by expressing enzymatic activities such as histone acetylase or deacetylase, which alter the conformation of nucleosomes and the transcribability of genes.

Between 10% and 20% of expressed genes in a cell are regulated by glucocorticoids. The number and affinity of receptors for the hormone, the complement of transcription factors and coregulators, and post-transcription events determine the relative specificity of these hormones' actions in various cells. The effects of glucocorticoids are due mainly to proteins synthesized from mRNA transcribed from their target genes.

Some of the effects of glucocorticoids can be attributed to their binding to mineralocorticoid receptors. Indeed, MRs bind aldosterone and cortisol with similar affinity. A mineralocorticoid effect of the higher levels of cortisol is avoided in some tissues (eg, kidney, colon, salivary glands) by expression of 11β-hydroxysteroid dehydrogenase type 2, the enzyme responsible for biotransformation to its 11-keto derivative (cortisone), which has minimal action on aldosterone receptors.

The GR also interacts with other regulators of cell function. One such molecule is CLOCK/BMAL-1, a transcription factor dimer expressed in all tissues and generating the circadian rhythm of cortisol secretion (see Figure 39–2) at the suprachiasmatic nucleus of the hypothalamus. CLOCK is an acetyltransferase that acetylates the hinge region of the GR, neutralizing its transcriptional activity and thus rendering target tissues resist ant to glucocorticoids. As shown in Figure 39–2, lower panel, the glucocorticoid target tissue sensitivity rhythm generated is in reverse phase to that

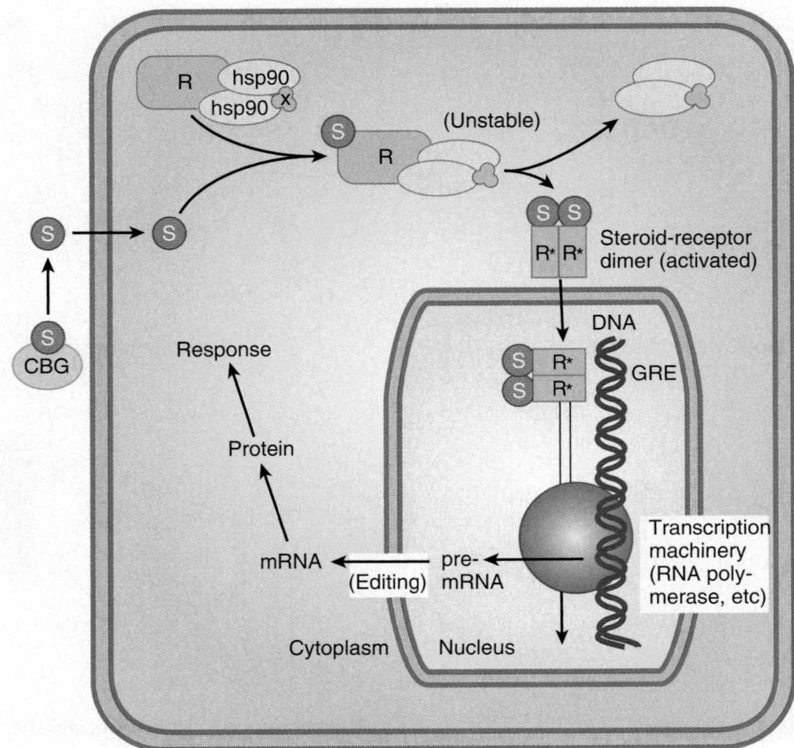

FIGURE 39–4 A model of the interaction of a steroid, S (eg, cortisol), and its receptor, R, and the subsequent events in a target cell. The steroid is present in the blood in bound form on the corticosteroid-binding globulin (CBG) but enters the cell as the free molecule. The intracellular receptor is bound to stabilizing proteins, including two molecules of heat-shock protein 90 (hsp90) and several others including FKBP5, denoted as "X" in the figure. This receptor complex is incapable of activating transcription. When the complex binds a molecule of cortisol, an unstable complex is created and the hsp90 and associated molecules are released. The steroid-receptor complex is now able to dimerize, enter the nucleus, bind to a glucocorticoid response element (GRE) on the regulatory region of the gene, and regulate transcription by RNA polymerase II and associated transcription factors. A variety of regulatory factors (not shown) may participate in facilitating (coactivators) or inhibiting (corepressors) the steroid response. The resulting mRNA is edited and exported to the cytoplasm for the production of protein that brings about the final hormone response. An alternative to the steroid-receptor complex interaction with a GRE is an interaction with and altering the function of other transcription factors, such as NF-κB in the nucleus of cells.

of circulating cortisol concentrations, explaining the increased sensitivity of the organism to evening administration of glucocorticoids. The activated GR also interacts with NF-κB, a regulator of production of cytokines and other molecules involved in inflammation. This explains the circadian variability of the inflammatory reaction, which is enhanced in the evening and early night and suppressed in the morning.

Prompt effects such as initial feedback suppression of pituitary ACTH occur in minutes and are too rapid to be explained on the basis of gene transcription and protein synthesis. It is not known how these effects are mediated. Among the proposed mechanisms are direct effects on cell membrane receptors for the hormone or nongenomic effects of the classic hormone-bound glucocorticoid receptor. The putative membrane receptors might be entirely different from the known intracellular receptors. For example, recent studies implicate G protein-coupled membrane receptors in the response of glutamatergic neurons to glucocorticoids in rats. Furthermore, all steroid receptors (except the MRs) have been shown to have palmitoylation motifs that allow enzymatic addition of palmitate and increased localization of the receptors in the vicinity of plasma membranes. Such receptors are available for direct interactions with, and effects on, various membrane-associated or cytoplasmic proteins without the need for entry into the nucleus and induction of transcriptional actions.

B. Physiologic Effects

The glucocorticoids have widespread effects because they influence the function of most cells in the body. The major metabolic consequences of glucocorticoid secretion or administration are due to direct actions of these hormones in the cell. However, some important effects are the result of homeostatic responses by insulin and glucagon. Although many of the effects of glucocorticoids are dose-related and become magnified when large amounts are administered for therapeutic purposes, there are also other effects—called *permissive* effects—without which many normal functions become deficient. For example, the response of vascular and bronchial smooth muscle to catecholamines is diminished in the absence of cortisol and restored by physiologic amounts of this glucocorticoid. Similarly, the lipolytic responses of fat cells to catecholamines, ACTH, and growth hormone are attenuated in the absence of glucocorticoids.

C. Metabolic Effects

The glucocorticoids have important dose-related effects on carbohydrate, protein, and fat metabolism. The same effects are responsible for some of the serious adverse effects associated with their use in therapeutic doses. Glucocorticoids stimulate and are required for gluconeogenesis and glycogen synthesis in the fasting state. They stimulate phosphoenolpyruvate carboxykinase, glucose-6-phosphatase, and glycogen synthase and the release of amino acids in the course of muscle catabolism.

Glucocorticoids increase serum glucose levels and thus stimulate insulin release but inhibit the uptake of glucose by muscle cells, while they stimulate hormone-sensitive lipase and thus lipolysis. The increased insulin secretion stimulates lipogenesis and to a lesser degree inhibits lipolysis, leading to a net increase in fat deposition combined with increased release of fatty acids and glycerol into the circulation.

The net results of these actions are most apparent in the fasting state, when the supply of glucose from gluconeogenesis, the release of amino acids from muscle catabolism, the inhibition of peripheral glucose uptake, and the stimulation of lipolysis all contribute to maintenance of an adequate glucose supply to the brain.

D. Catabolic and Antianabolic Effects

Although glucocorticoids stimulate RNA and protein synthesis in the liver, they have catabolic and antianabolic effects in lymphoid and connective tissue, muscle, peripheral fat, and skin. Supraphysiologic amounts of glucocorticoids lead to decreased muscle mass and weakness, and thinning of the skin. Catabolic and antianabolic effects on bone are the cause of osteoporosis in Cushing syndrome and impose a major limitation in the long-term therapeutic use of glucocorticoids. In children, glucocorticoids reduce growth. This effect may be partially prevented by administration of growth hormone in high doses, but this use of growth hormone is not recommended except in extreme situations.

E. Anti-Inflammatory and Immunosuppressive Effects

Glucocorticoids dramatically reduce the manifestations of inflammation. This is due to their profound effects on the concentration, distribution, and function of peripheral leukocytes and to their suppressive effects on inflammatory cytokines and chemokines, and on other small molecule mediators of inflammation. Inflammation, regardless of its cause, is characterized by the extravasation and infiltration of leukocytes into the affected tissue. These events are mediated by a complex series of interactions of white cell adhesion molecules with those on endothelial cells and are inhibited by glucocorticoids. After a single dose of a short-acting glucocorticoid, the concentration of neutrophils in the circulation increases while the lymphocytes (T and B cells), monocytes, eosinophils, and basophils decrease. The changes are maximal at 6 hours and are dissipated in 24 hours. The increase in neutrophils is due both to increased influx into the blood from the bone marrow and to decreased migration from the blood vessels, leading to a reduction in the number of cells at the site of inflammation. The reduction in circulating lymphocytes, monocytes, eosinophils, and basophils is primarily the result of their movement from the vascular bed to lymphoid tissue.

Glucocorticoids also inhibit the functions of tissue macrophages as well as dendritic and other antigen-presenting cells. The ability of these cells to respond to antigens and mitogens is reduced. The effect on macrophages is particularly marked and limits their ability to phagocytose and kill microorganisms and to produce tumor necrosis factor α, interleukin 1, metalloproteinases, and plasminogen activator. Both macrophages and lymphocytes produce less interleukin 12 and interferon-γ, important inducers of TH1 cell activity, and cellular immunity.

In addition to their effects on leukocyte function, glucocorticoids influence the inflammatory response by inhibiting phospholipase A_2 and thus reduce the synthesis of arachidonic acid, the precursor of prostaglandins and leukotrienes, and of platelet-activating factor. Finally, glucocorticoids reduce expression of cyclooxygenase 2, the inducible form of this enzyme, in inflammatory cells, thus reducing the amount of enzyme available to produce prostaglandins (see Chapters 18 and 36).

Glucocorticoids cause vasoconstriction when applied directly to the skin, possibly by suppressing mast cell degranulation. They also decrease capillary permeability by reducing the amount of histamine released by basophils and mast cells.

The anti-inflammatory and immunosuppressive effects of glucocorticoids are largely due to the actions described above. In humans, complement activation is unaltered, but its effects are inhibited. Antibody production can be reduced by large doses of steroids, although it is unaffected by moderate doses (eg, 20 mg/d of prednisone).

The anti-inflammatory and immunosuppressive effects of these agents are widely useful therapeutically but are also responsible for some of their most serious adverse effects (see text that follows).

F. Other Effects

Glucocorticoids have important effects on the nervous system. Adrenal insufficiency causes marked slowing of the alpha rhythm of the electroencephalogram and is associated with depression. Increased amounts of glucocorticoids often produce behavioral disturbances in humans: initially insomnia and euphoria and subsequently depression. Large doses of glucocorticoids may increase intracranial pressure (pseudotumor cerebri).

Glucocorticoids given chronically suppress the pituitary release of ACTH, growth hormone, thyroid-stimulating hormone, and luteinizing hormone.

Large doses of glucocorticoids have been associated with the development of peptic ulcer, possibly by suppressing the local immune response against *Helicobacter pylori*. They also promote fat redistribution in the body, with increase of visceral, facial, nuchal, and supraclavicular fat, and they appear to antagonize the effect of vitamin D on calcium absorption. The glucocorticoids also have important effects on the hematopoietic system. In addition to their effects on leukocytes, they increase the number of platelets and red blood cells.

Cortisol deficiency results in impaired renal function (particularly glomerular filtration), augmented vasopressin secretion, and diminished ability to excrete a water load.

Glucocorticoids have important effects on the development of the fetal lungs. Indeed, the structural and functional changes in the lungs near term, including the production of pulmonary surface-active material required for air breathing (surfactant), are stimulated by glucocorticoids.

Recently, glucocorticoids were found to have direct effects on the epigenetic regulation of specific target genes by altering the activities of DNA methyltransferases and other enzymes participating in epigenesis. This is of particular importance in the prenatal treatment of pregnant mothers or treatment of young infants and children, when the epigenetic effects of glucocorticoids may be long term or even permanent. These effects may predispose these patients to behavioral or somatic disorders, such as depression or obesity and metabolic syndrome.

SYNTHETIC CORTICOSTEROIDS

Glucocorticoids have become important agents for use in the treatment of many inflammatory, immunologic, hematologic, and other disorders. This has stimulated the development of many synthetic steroids with anti-inflammatory and immunosuppressive activity.

PHARMACOKINETICS

Pharmaceutical steroids are usually synthesized from cholic acid obtained from cattle or steroid sapogenins found in plants. Further modifications of these steroids have led to the marketing of a large group of synthetic steroids with special characteristics that are pharmacologically and therapeutically important (Table 39–1; see Figure 39–3).

The metabolism of the naturally occurring adrenal steroids has been discussed above. The synthetic corticosteroids (see Table 39–1) are in most cases rapidly and almost completely absorbed when given by mouth. Although they are transported and metabolized in a fashion similar to that of the endogenous steroids, important differences exist.

Alterations in the glucocorticoid molecule influence its affinity for glucocorticoid and mineralocorticoid receptors as well as its protein-binding affinity, side chain stability, rate of elimination, and metabolic products. Halogenation at the 9 position, unsaturation of the Δ1–2 bond of the A ring, and methylation at the 2 or 16 position prolong the half-life by more than 50%. The Δ1 compounds are excreted in the free form. In some cases, the agent given is a prodrug; for example, prednisone is rapidly converted to the active product prednisolone in the body.

TABLE 39–1 Some commonly used natural and synthetic corticosteroids for general use. (See Table 61-4 for dermatologic corticosteroids.)

Agent	Activity[1]			Equivalent Oral Dose (mg)	Forms Available
	Anti-Inflammatory	*Topical*	*Salt-Retaining*		
Short- to medium-acting glucocorticoids					
Hydrocortisone (cortisol)	1	1	1	20	Oral, injectable, topical
Cortisone	0.8	0	0.8	25	Oral
Prednisone	4	0	0.3	5	Oral
Prednisolone	5	4	0.3	5	Oral, injectable
Methylprednisolone	5	5	0.25	4	Oral, injectable
Meprednisone[2]	5		0	4	Oral, injectable
Intermediate-acting glucocorticoids					
Triamcinolone	5	5[3]	0	4	Oral, injectable, topical
Paramethasone[2]	10		0	2	Oral, injectable
Fluprednisolone[2]	15	7	0	1.5	Oral
Long-acting glucocorticoids					
Betamethasone	25–40	10	0	0.6	Oral, injectable, topical
Dexamethasone	30	10	0	0.75	Oral, injectable, topical
Mineralocorticoids					
Fludrocortisone	10	0	250	2	Oral
Desoxycorticosterone acetate[2]	0	0	20		Injectable, pellets

[1]Potency relative to hydrocortisone.

[2]Outside the United States.

[3]Triamcinolone acetonide: Up to 100.

PHARMACODYNAMICS

The actions of the synthetic steroids are similar to those of cortisol (see above). They bind to the specific intracellular receptor proteins and produce the same effects but have different ratios of glucocorticoid to mineralocorticoid potency (Table 39–1).

CLINICAL PHARMACOLOGY

A. Diagnosis and Treatment of Disturbed Adrenal Function

1. *Adrenocortical insufficiency*

***a.* Chronic (Addison disease)**—Chronic adrenocortical insufficiency is characterized by weakness, fatigue, weight loss, hypotension, hyperpigmentation, and inability to maintain the blood glucose level during fasting. In such individuals, minor noxious, traumatic, or infectious stimuli may produce acute adrenal insufficiency with circulatory shock and even death.

In primary adrenal insufficiency, about 20–30 mg of hydrocortisone must be given daily, with increased amounts during periods of stress. Although hydrocortisone has some mineralocorticoid activity, this must be supplemented by an appropriate amount of a salt-retaining hormone such as fludrocortisone. Synthetic glucocorticoids that are long-acting and devoid of salt-retaining activity should not be administered as hormone substitution to these patients.

***b.* Acute**—When acute adrenocortical insufficiency is suspected, treatment must be instituted immediately. Therapy consists of large amounts of parenteral hydrocortisone in addition to correction of fluid and electrolyte abnormalities and treatment of precipitating factors.

Hydrocortisone sodium succinate or phosphate in doses of 100 mg intravenously is given every 8 hours until the patient is stable. The dose is then gradually reduced, achieving maintenance dosage within 5 days.

The administration of salt-retaining hormone is resumed when the total hydrocortisone dosage has been reduced to less than 50 mg/d.

2. *Adrenocortical hypo- and hyperfunction*

***a.* Congenital adrenal hyperplasia**—This group of disorders is characterized by specific defects in the synthesis of cortisol. In pregnancies at high risk for congenital adrenal hyperplasia, fetuses can be protected from genital abnormalities by administration of dexamethasone to the mother.

The most common defect is a decrease in or lack of P450c21 (21α-hydroxylase) activity.* As can be seen in Figure 39–1, this would lead to a reduction in cortisol synthesis and secretion and thus produce a compensatory increase in ACTH release. The adrenal becomes hyperplastic and produces abnormally large amounts of precursors such as 17-hydroxyprogesterone that can be diverted to the androgen pathway, which leads to virilization and can result in ambiguous genitalia in the female fetus. Metabolism of this compound in the liver leads to pregnanetriol, which is characteristically excreted into the urine in large amounts in this disorder and can be used to make the diagnosis and to monitor efficacy of glucocorticoid substitution. However, the most reliable method of detecting this disorder is the increased response of plasma 17-hydroxyprogesterone to ACTH stimulation.

If the defect is in 11-hydroxylation, large amounts of deoxycorticosterone are produced, and because this steroid has mineralocorticoid activity, hypertension with or without hypokalemic alkalosis may ensue. When 17-hydroxylation is defective in the adrenals and gonads, hypogonadism also is present. However, increased amounts of 11-deoxycorticosterone are formed, and the signs and symptoms associated with mineralocorticoid excess—such as hypertension and hypokalemia—also are observed.

When first seen, the infant with congenital adrenal hyperplasia may be in acute adrenal crisis and should be treated as described above, using appropriate electrolyte solutions and an intravenous preparation of hydrocortisone in stress doses. Once the patient is stabilized, oral hydrocortisone, 12–18 mg/m^2 per day in two unequally divided doses (two thirds in the morning, one third in late afternoon) is begun. The dosage is adjusted to allow normal growth and bone maturation and to prevent androgen excess. Alternate-day therapy with prednisone has also been used to achieve greater ACTH suppression without increasing growth inhibition. Fludrocortisone, 0.05–0.2 mg/d, should also be administered by mouth, with added salt to maintain normal blood pressure, plasma renin activity, and electrolytes.

***b.* Cushing syndrome**—Cushing syndrome is usually the result of bilateral adrenal hyperplasia secondary to an ACTH-secreting pituitary adenoma (Cushing disease) but occasionally is due to tumors or nodular hyperplasia of the adrenal gland or ectopic production of ACTH by other nonadrenocortical tumors. The manifestations are those associated with the chronic presence of excessive glucocorticoids. When glucocorticoid hypersecretion is marked and prolonged, a rounded, plethoric face and trunk obesity are striking in appearance. Protein loss may be significant and includes muscle wasting; thinning, purple striae, and easy bruising of the skin; poor wound healing; and osteoporosis. Other serious disturbances include mental disorders, hypertension, and diabetes. This disorder is treated by surgical removal of the tumor producing ACTH or cortisol, irradiation of the pituitary tumor, or resection of one or both adrenals. These patients must receive large doses of cortisol during and after the surgical procedure. Doses of up to 300 mg of soluble hydrocortisone may be given as a continuous intravenous infusion on the day of surgery. The dose must be reduced slowly to normal replacement levels, since rapid reduction in dose may produce withdrawal symptoms, including nausea, vomiting, fever, and joint pain. If adrenalectomy has been performed, long-term maintenance is similar to that outlined above for adrenal insufficiency.

---

*Names for the adrenal steroid synthetic enzymes include the following: P450c11 (11β-hydroxylase), P450c17 (17α-hydroxylase), and P450c21 (21α-hydroxylase).

***c.* Primary generalized glucocorticoid resistance (Chrousos syndrome)**—This rare sporadic or familial genetic condition is usually due to inactivating mutations of the glucocorticoid receptor gene. The hypothalamic-pituitary-adrenal (HPA) axis hyperfunctions in an attempt to compensate for the defect, and the increased production of ACTH leads to high circulating levels of cortisol and cortisol precursors such as corticosterone and 11-deoxycorticosterone with mineralocorticoid activity, as well as of adrenal androgens. These increased levels may result in hypertension with or without hypokalemic alkalosis and hyperandrogenism expressed as virilization and precocious puberty in children and acne, hirsutism, male pattern baldness, and menstrual irregularities (mostly oligo-amenorrhea and hypofertility) in women. The therapy of this syndrome is high doses of synthetic glucocorticoids such as dexamethasone with no inherent mineralocorticoid activity. These doses are titrated to normalize the production of cortisol, cortisol precursors, and adrenal androgens.

***d.* Aldosteronism**—Primary aldosteronism usually results from the excessive production of aldosterone by an adrenal adenoma. However, it may also result from abnormal secretion by hyperplastic glands or from a malignant adrenal tumor. The clinical findings of hypertension, weakness, and tetany are related to the continued renal loss of potassium, which leads to hypokalemia, alkalosis, and elevation of serum sodium concentrations. Recently, aldosteronism was found to be a more frequent cause of hypertension than originally thought, with a rate higher than 20%. This syndrome can also be produced in disorders of adrenal steroid biosynthesis by excessive secretion of deoxycorticosterone, corticosterone, or 18-hydroxycorticosterone—all compounds with inherent mineralocorticoid activity.

In contrast to patients with secondary aldosteronism (see text that follows), these patients have low (suppressed) levels of plasma renin activity and angiotensin II. When treated with fludrocortisone (0.2 mg twice daily orally for 3 days) or deoxycorticosterone acetate (20 mg/d intramuscularly for 3 days—but not available in the United States), patients fail to retain sodium and the secretion of aldosterone is not significantly reduced. When the disorder is mild, it may escape detection if only serum potassium levels are used for screening. However, it may be detected by an increased ratio of plasma aldosterone to renin. Patients generally improve when treated with spironolactone or eplerenone, steroidal aldosterone receptor-blocking agents, and the response to these agents is of diagnostic and therapeutic value. Recently, nonsteroidal compounds with aldosterone receptor-mediated antagonist activity were added to our armamentarium. One of these, finerenone is already in the market.

3. *Use of glucocorticoids for diagnostic purposes*—It is sometimes necessary to suppress the production of ACTH to identify the source of a particular hormone or to establish whether its production is influenced by the secretion of ACTH. In these circumstances, it is advantageous to use a very potent substance such as dexamethasone because the use of small quantities reduces the possibility of confusion in the interpretation of hormone assays in blood or urine. For example, if complete suppression is achieved by the use of 50 mg of cortisol, the urinary 17-hydroxycorticosteroids will be 15–18 mg/24 h, since one-third of the dose given will be recovered in urine as 17-hydroxycorticosteroid. If an equivalent dose of 1.5 mg of dexamethasone is used, suppression will again be complete but the urinary excretion will be only 0.5 mg/24 h and blood levels will be low.

The **dexamethasone suppression test** is used for the diagnosis of Cushing syndrome and has also been used in the differential diagnosis of depressive psychiatric states. As a screening test, 1 mg dexamethasone is given orally at 11 PM, and a plasma sample is obtained the following morning. In normal individuals, the morning cortisol concentration is usually <2 mcg/dL, whereas in Cushing syndrome the level is usually >5 mcg/dL. The results are not reliable in the patient with depression, anxiety, concurrent illness, and other stressful conditions or in the patient who is receiving a medication that enhances the catabolism of dexamethasone in the liver. To distinguish between hypercortisolism due to anxiety, depression, and alcoholism (pseudo-Cushing syndrome) and bona fide Cushing syndrome, a combined test is carried out, consisting of dexamethasone (0.5 mg orally every 6 hours for 2 days) followed by a standard corticotropin-releasing hormone (CRH) test (1 mg/kg given as a bolus intravenous infusion 2 hours after the last dose of dexamethasone).

In patients in whom the diagnosis of Cushing syndrome has been established clinically and confirmed by a finding of elevated free cortisol in the urine, suppression with large doses of dexamethasone will help to distinguish patients with Cushing disease from those with steroid-producing tumors of the adrenal cortex or with the ectopic ACTH syndrome. Dexamethasone is given in a dosage of 0.5 mg orally every 6 hours for 2 days, followed by 2 mg orally every 6 hours for 2 days, and the urine is then assayed for cortisol or its metabolites (Liddle test); or dexamethasone is given as a single dose of 8 mg at 11 PM, and the plasma cortisol is measured at 8 AM the following day. In patients with Cushing disease, the suppressant effect of dexamethasone usually produces a 50% reduction in hormone levels. In patients in whom suppression does not occur, the ACTH level will be low in the presence of a cortisol-producing adrenal tumor and elevated in patients with an ectopic ACTH-producing tumor.

B. Corticosteroids and Stimulation of Lung Maturation in the Fetus

Lung maturation in the fetus is regulated by the fetal secretion of cortisol. Treatment of the mother with large doses of glucocorticoid reduces the incidence of respiratory distress syndrome in infants delivered prematurely. When delivery is anticipated before 34 weeks of gestation, intramuscular betamethasone, 12 mg, followed by an additional dose of 12 mg 18–24 hours later, is commonly used. Betamethasone is chosen because maternal protein binding and placental metabolism of this corticosteroid is less than that of cortisol, allowing increased transfer across the placenta to the fetus. A study of more than 10,000 infants born at 23–25 weeks of gestation indicated that exposure to exogenous corticosteroids before birth reduced the death rate and evidence of neurodevelopmental impairment.

TABLE 39–2 Some therapeutic indications for the use of glucocorticoids in nonadrenal disorders.

Disorder	Examples
Allergic reactions	Angioneurotic edema, asthma, bee stings, contact dermatitis, drug reactions, allergic rhinitis, serum sickness, urticaria
Collagen-vascular disorders	Giant cell arteritis, lupus erythematosus, scleroderma, mixed connective tissue syndromes, polymyositis, rheumatoid arthritis, temporal arteritis
Eye diseases	Acute uveitis, allergic conjunctivitis, choroiditis, optic neuritis
Gastrointestinal diseases	Inflammatory bowel disease, nontropical sprue, subacute hepatic necrosis
Hematologic disorders	Acquired hemolytic anemia, acute allergic purpura, leukemia, lymphoma, autoimmune hemolytic anemia, idiopathic thrombocytopenic purpura, multiple myeloma
Systemic inflammation	Acute respiratory distress syndrome (sustained therapy with moderate dosage accelerates recovery and decreases mortality)
Infections	Acute respiratory distress syndrome, sepsis, COVID-19
Inflammatory conditions of bones and joints	Arthritis, bursitis, tenosynovitis
Nausea and vomiting	A large dose of dexamethasone reduces emetic effects of chemotherapy and general anesthesia
Neurologic disorders	Cerebral edema (large doses of dexamethasone are given to patients following brain surgery to minimize cerebral edema in the postoperative period), multiple sclerosis
Organ transplants	Prevention and treatment of rejection (immunosuppression)
Pulmonary diseases	Aspiration pneumonia, bronchial asthma, prenatal prevention of infant respiratory distress syndrome, sarcoidosis
Renal disorders	Nephrotic syndrome
Skin diseases	Atopic dermatitis, dermatoses, lichen simplex chronicus (localized neurodermatitis), mycosis fungoides, pemphigus, psoriasis, seborrheic dermatitis, xerosis
Thyroid diseases	Malignant exophthalmos, subacute thyroiditis
Miscellaneous	Hypercalcemia, mountain sickness

C. Corticosteroids and Nonadrenal Disorders

The synthetic analogs of cortisol are useful in the treatment of a diverse group of diseases generally unrelated to any known disturbance of adrenal function (Table 39–2). The usefulness of corticosteroids in these disorders is a function of their ability to suppress inflammatory and immune responses and to alter leukocyte function, as previously described (see also Chapter 55). These agents are useful in disorders in which host response is the cause of the major manifestations of the disease. A good example of this is the therapy of patients with severe COVID-19, in whom high doses of a synthetic glucocorticoid decreased mortality by approximately 30%. In instances in which the inflammatory or immune response is important in controlling the pathologic process, therapy with corticosteroids may be dangerous but justified to prevent irreparable damage from an inflammatory response—if used in conjunction with specific therapy for the disease process.

Since corticosteroids are not usually curative, the pathologic process may progress while clinical manifestations are suppressed. Therefore, chronic systemic therapy with these drugs should be undertaken with great care and only when the seriousness of the disorder warrants their use and when less hazardous measures have been exhausted.

In general, attempts should be made to bring the disease process under control using medium- to intermediate-acting glucocorticoids such as prednisone and prednisolone (Table 39–1), as well as all ancillary measures possible to keep the dose low. Where possible, alternate-day therapy should be used (see the following text). Therapy should not be decreased or stopped abruptly. When prolonged therapy is anticipated, it is helpful to obtain chest x-rays and a tuberculin test, since glucocorticoid therapy can reactivate dormant tuberculosis. The presence of diabetes, peptic ulcer, osteoporosis, and psychological disturbances should be taken into consideration, and cardiovascular function should be assessed.

Treatment for transplant rejection is a very important application of glucocorticoids. The efficacy of these agents is based on their ability to reduce antigen expression from the grafted tissue, delay revascularization, and interfere with the sensitization of cytotoxic T lymphocytes and the generation of primary antibody-forming cells.

Toxicity

The benefits obtained from glucocorticoids vary considerably. Use of these drugs must be carefully weighed in each patient against their widespread effects. The major undesirable effects of glucocorticoids are the result of their hormonal actions, which lead to the clinical picture of iatrogenic Cushing syndrome (see later in text).

When glucocorticoids are used for short periods (<2 weeks), it is unusual to see serious adverse effects even with moderately large doses. However, insomnia, behavioral changes (primarily hypomania), and acute peptic ulcers are occasionally observed even after only a few days of treatment. Acute pancreatitis is a rare but serious acute adverse effect of high-dose glucocorticoids.

A. Metabolic Effects

Most patients who are given daily doses of 100 mg of hydrocortisone or more (or the equivalent amount of synthetic steroid) for longer than 2 weeks undergo a series of changes that have been termed **iatrogenic Cushing syndrome.** The rate of development is a function of the dosage and the genetic background of the patient. In the face, rounding, puffiness, fat deposition, and plethora usually appear (moon facies). Similarly, fat tends to be redistributed from the extremities to the trunk, the back of the neck, and the supraclavicular fossae. There is an increased growth of fine hair over the face, thighs, and trunk. Steroid-induced punctate acne may appear, and insomnia and increased appetite are noted. In the treatment of dangerous or disabling disorders, these changes may not require cessation of therapy. However, the underlying metabolic changes accompanying them can be very serious by the time they become obvious. The continuing breakdown of protein and diversion of amino acids to glucose production increase the need for insulin and over time result in weight gain; visceral fat deposition; myopathy and muscle wasting; thinning of the skin, with striae and bruising; hyperglycemia; and eventually osteoporosis, diabetes, and aseptic necrosis of the hip. Wound healing also is impaired under these circumstances. When diabetes occurs, it is treated with diet and insulin. These patients are often resistant to insulin but rarely develop ketoacidosis. In general, patients treated with corticosteroids should be on high-protein and potassium-enriched diets and should receive adequate doses of vitamin D.

B. Other Complications

Other serious adverse effects of glucocorticoids include peptic ulcers and their consequences. The clinical findings associated with certain disorders, particularly bacterial and mycotic infections, may be masked by the corticosteroids, and patients must be carefully monitored to avoid serious mishap when large doses are used. Severe myopathy is more frequent in patients treated with long-acting glucocorticoids. The administration of such compounds has been associated with nausea, dizziness, and weight *loss* in some patients. These effects are treated by changing drugs, reducing dosage, and increasing potassium and protein intake.

Hypomania or acute psychosis may occur, particularly in patients receiving very large doses of corticosteroids. Long-term therapy with intermediate- and long-acting steroids is associated with depression and the development of posterior subcapsular cataracts. Psychiatric follow-up and periodic slit-lamp examination are indicated in such patients. Increased intraocular pressure is common, and glaucoma may be induced. Benign intracranial hypertension also occurs. In dosages of 45 mg/m^2 per day or more of hydrocortisone equivalent, growth retardation occurs in children. Medium-, intermediate-, and long-acting glucocorticoids have greater growth-suppressing potency than the natural steroid at equivalent doses.

When given in larger than physiologic amounts, steroids such as cortisone and hydrocortisone, which have mineralocorticoid effects in addition to glucocorticoid effects, cause some sodium and fluid retention and loss of potassium. In patients with normal cardiovascular and renal function, this leads to a hypokalemic, hypochloremic alkalosis and eventually to a rise in blood pressure. In patients with hypoproteinemia, renal disease, or liver disease, edema also may occur. In patients with heart disease, even small degrees of sodium retention may lead to heart failure. These effects can be minimized by using synthetic non-salt-retaining steroids, sodium restriction, and judicious amounts of potassium supplements.

C. Adrenal Suppression

When corticosteroids are administered for more than 2 weeks, adrenal suppression may occur. If treatment extends over weeks to months, the patient should be given appropriate supplementary therapy at times of minor stress (twofold dosage increases for 24–48 hours) or severe stress (up to tenfold dosage increases for 48–72 hours) such as accidental trauma or major surgery. If corticosteroid dosage is to be reduced, it should be tapered slowly. If therapy is to be stopped, the reduction process should be quite slow when the dose reaches replacement levels. It may take 2–12 months for the hypothalamic-pituitary-adrenal axis to function acceptably, and cortisol levels may not return to normal for another 6–9 months. The glucocorticoid-induced suppression is not a pituitary problem, and treatment with ACTH does not reduce the time required for the return of normal function.

If the dosage is reduced too rapidly in patients receiving glucocorticoids for a certain disorder, the symptoms of the disorder may reappear or increase in intensity. However, patients without an underlying disorder (eg, patients cured surgically of Cushing disease) also develop symptoms with rapid reductions in corticosteroid levels. These symptoms include anorexia, nausea or vomiting, weight loss, lethargy, headache, fever, joint or muscle pain, and postural hypotension. Although many of these symptoms may reflect true glucocorticoid deficiency, they may also occur in the presence of normal or even elevated plasma cortisol levels, suggesting glucocorticoid dependence.

Contraindications & Cautions

A. Special Precautions

Patients receiving glucocorticoids must be monitored carefully for the development of hyperglycemia, glycosuria, sodium retention with edema or hypertension, hypokalemia, peptic ulcer, osteoporosis, and hidden infections.

The dosage should be kept as low as possible, and intermittent administration (eg, alternate-day) should be used when satisfactory therapeutic results can be obtained on this schedule. Even patients maintained on relatively low doses of corticosteroids may require supplementary therapy at times of stress, such as when surgical procedures are performed or intercurrent illnesses or accidents occur.

B. Contraindications

Glucocorticoids must be used with great caution in patients with peptic ulcer, heart disease or hypertension with heart failure, certain infectious illnesses such as varicella and tuberculosis, psychoses, diabetes, osteoporosis, or glaucoma.

Selection of Drug & Dosage Schedule

Glucocorticoid preparations differ with respect to relative anti-inflammatory and mineralocorticoid effect, duration of action, cost, and dosage forms available (Table 39–1), and these factors should be taken into account in selecting the drug to be used.

A. ACTH versus Adrenocortical Steroids

In patients with normal adrenals, ACTH was used in the past to induce the endogenous production of cortisol to obtain similar effects. However, except when an increase in androgens is desirable, the use of ACTH as a therapeutic agent has been abandoned. Instances in which ACTH was claimed to be more effective than glucocorticoids were probably due to the administration of smaller amounts of corticosteroids than were produced by the dosage of ACTH.

B. Dosage

In determining the dosage regimen to be used, the physician must consider the seriousness of the disease, the amount of drug likely to be required to obtain the desired effect, and the duration of therapy. In some diseases, the amount required for maintenance of the desired therapeutic effect is less than the dose needed to obtain the initial effect, and the lowest possible dosage for the needed effect should be determined by gradually lowering the dose until a small increase in signs or symptoms is noted.

When it is necessary to maintain continuously elevated plasma corticosteroid levels to suppress ACTH, a slowly absorbed parenteral preparation or small oral doses at frequent intervals are required. The opposite situation exists with respect to the use of corticosteroids in the treatment of inflammatory and allergic disorders. The same total quantity given in a few doses may be more effective than that given in many smaller doses or in a slowly absorbed parenteral form.

Severe autoimmune conditions involving vital organs must be treated aggressively, and undertreatment is as dangerous as overtreatment. To minimize the deposition of immune complexes and the influx of leukocytes and macrophages, 1 mg/kg per day of prednisone in divided doses is required initially. This dosage is maintained until the serious manifestations respond. The dosage can then be gradually reduced.

When large doses are required for prolonged periods of time, alternate-day administration of the compound may be tried. When used in this manner, very large amounts (eg, 100 mg of prednisone) can sometimes be administered with less marked adverse effects because there is a recovery period between each dose. The transition to an alternate-day schedule can be made after the disease process is under control. It should be done gradually and with additional supportive measures between doses.

When selecting a drug for use in large doses, a medium- or intermediate-acting synthetic steroid with no or little mineralocorticoid effect is advisable. If possible, it should be given as a single morning dose.

C. Special Dosage Forms

Local therapy, such as topical preparations for skin disease, ophthalmic forms for eye disease, intra-articular injections for joint disease, inhaled steroids for asthma, and hydrocortisone enemas for ulcerative colitis, provides a means of delivering large amounts of steroid to the diseased tissue with reduced systemic effects.

Beclomethasone dipropionate and several other glucocorticoids—primarily budesonide, flunisolide, and mometasone furoate, administered as inhaled aerosols—have been found to be extremely useful in the treatment of asthma (see Chapter 20).

Beclomethasone dipropionate, triamcinolone acetonide, budesonide, flunisolide, fluticasone, and others are available as nasal sprays for the topical treatment of allergic rhinitis. They are effective at doses (one or two sprays one, two, or three times daily) that in most patients result in plasma levels that are too low to influence adrenal function or have any other systemic effects.

Corticosteroids incorporated in ointments, creams, lotions, and sprays are used extensively in dermatology. These preparations are discussed in more detail in Chapter 61.

Recently, new timed-release hydrocortisone tablets were developed for the replacement treatment of Addisonian and congenital adrenal hyperplasia patients. These tablets produce plasma cortisol levels that are similar to those secreted normally in a circadian fashion.

For therapeutic reasons, new timed-release prednisone tablets were developed for the therapy of patients with rheumatoid arthritis.

MINERALOCORTICOIDS (ALDOSTERONE, DEOXYCORTICOSTERONE, FLUDROCORTISONE)

The most important mineralocorticoid in humans is aldosterone. However, small amounts of 11-deoxycorticosterone (11-DOC) also are formed and released. Although the amount is normally insignificant, 11-DOC was of some importance therapeutically in the past. Its actions, effects, and metabolism are qualitatively similar to those described below for aldosterone. Fludrocortisone, a synthetic corticosteroid, is the most commonly prescribed salt-retaining hormone.

Aldosterone

Aldosterone is synthesized mainly in the zona glomerulosa of the adrenal cortex. Its structure and synthesis are illustrated in Figure 39–1. The rate of aldosterone secretion is subject to several influences. ACTH produces a moderate stimulation of its release, but this effect is not sustained for more than a few days in the normal individual. The quantities of aldosterone produced by the adrenal cortex and its plasma concentrations are insufficient to participate in any significant feedback control of ACTH secretion.

Without ACTH, aldosterone secretion falls to about half the normal rate, indicating that other factors, eg, angiotensin, are able to maintain and perhaps regulate its secretion (see Chapter 17). Independent variations between cortisol and aldosterone secretion can also be demonstrated by means of lesions in the nervous system such as decerebration, which decreases the secretion of cortisol while increasing the secretion of aldosterone.

A. Physiologic and Pharmacologic Effects

Aldosterone and other steroids with mineralocorticoid properties promote the reabsorption of sodium from the distal part of the distal convoluted renal tubule and from the cortical collecting tubules, loosely coupled to the excretion of potassium and hydrogen ion. Sodium reabsorption in the sweat and salivary glands, in the gastrointestinal mucosa, and across cell membranes in general also is increased. Excessive levels of aldosterone produced by tumors or overdosage with synthetic mineralocorticoids lead to hypokalemia, metabolic alkalosis, increased plasma volume, and hypertension.

Mineralocorticoids act by binding to the mineralocorticoid receptor in the cytoplasm of target cells, especially principal cells of the distal convoluted and collecting tubules of the kidney. The drug-receptor complex activates a series of events similar to those described above for the glucocorticoids and illustrated in Figure 39–4. It is of interest that this receptor has the same affinity for cortisol, which is present in much higher concentrations in the extracellular fluid. The specificity for mineralocorticoids in the kidney appears to be conferred, at least in part, by the presence—in the kidney—of the enzyme 11β-hydroxysteroid dehydrogenase type 2, which converts cortisol to cortisone. The latter has low affinity for the receptor and is inactive as a mineralocorticoid or glucocorticoid in the kidney. The major effect of activation of the aldosterone receptor is increased expression of Na^+/K^+-ATPase and the epithelial sodium channel (ENaC).

B. Metabolism

Aldosterone is secreted at the rate of 100–200 mcg/d in normal individuals with a moderate dietary salt intake. The plasma level in men (resting supine) is about 0.007 mcg/dL. The half-life of aldosterone injected in tracer quantities is 15–20 minutes, and it does not appear to be firmly bound to serum proteins.

The metabolism of aldosterone is similar to that of cortisol, about 50 mcg/24 h appearing in the urine as conjugated tetrahydroaldosterone. Approximately 5–15 mcg/24 h is excreted free or as the 3-oxo glucuronide.

11-Deoxycorticosterone (11-DOC)

11-DOC, which also serves as a precursor of aldosterone (see Figure 39–1), is normally secreted in amounts of about 200 mcg/d. Its half-life when injected into the human circulation is about 70 minutes. Estimates of its concentration in plasma are approximately 0.03 mcg/dL. The control of its secretion differs from that of aldosterone in that the secretion of 11-DOC is primarily under the control of ACTH. Although the response to ACTH is enhanced by dietary sodium restriction, due to adaptations, a low-salt diet does not increase 11-DOC secretion. The secretion of DOC may be markedly increased in abnormal conditions such as adrenocortical carcinoma and congenital adrenal hyperplasia with reduced P450c11 or P450c17 activity.

Fludrocortisone

This compound, a potent steroid with both glucocorticoid and mineralocorticoid activity, is the most widely used mineralocorticoid. Oral doses of 0.1 mg two to seven times weekly have potent salt-retaining activity and are used in the treatment of adrenocortical insufficiency associated with mineralocorticoid deficiency. These dosages are too small to have important anti-inflammatory or antigrowth effects.

ADRENAL ANDROGENS

The adrenal cortex secretes large amounts of DHEA and smaller amounts of androstenedione and testosterone. Although these androgens are thought to contribute to the normal maturation process, they do not stimulate or support major androgen-dependent pubertal changes in humans. Studies suggest that DHEA and its sulfate might have other important physiologic actions. If that is correct, these results are probably due to the peripheral conversion of DHEA to more potent androgens or to estrogens and interaction with androgen and estrogen receptors, respectively. Additional effects may be exerted through an interaction with the $GABA_A$ and glutamate receptors in the brain or with a nuclear receptor in several central and peripheral sites. The therapeutic use of DHEA in humans has been explored, but the substance has already been adopted with uncritical enthusiasm by members of the sports drug and the vitamin and food supplement cultures.

The results of a placebo-controlled trial of DHEA in patients with systemic lupus erythematosus have been reported as well as those of a study of DHEA replacement in women with adrenal insufficiency. In both studies a small beneficial effect was seen, with some improvement of the disease in the former and an added sense of well-being in the latter. The androgenic or estrogenic actions of DHEA could explain the effects of the compound in both situations. In contrast, there is no evidence to support DHEA use to increase muscle strength or improve memory.

■ ANTAGONISTS OF ADRENOCORTICAL AGENTS

SYNTHESIS INHIBITORS & GLUCOCORTICOID ANTAGONISTS

Inhibitors of steroid synthesis act at several different steps, and one glucocorticoid antagonist acts at the receptor level.

AMINOGLUTETHIMIDE

Aminoglutethimide (Figure 39–5) blocks the conversion of cholesterol to pregnenolone (see Figure 39–1) and causes a reduction in the synthesis of all hormonally active steroids. It has been used in conjunction with dexamethasone or hydrocortisone to reduce or eliminate estrogen production in patients with carcinoma of the breast. In a dosage of 1 g/d it was well tolerated; however, with higher dosages, lethargy and skin rash were common effects. The use of aminoglutethimide in breast

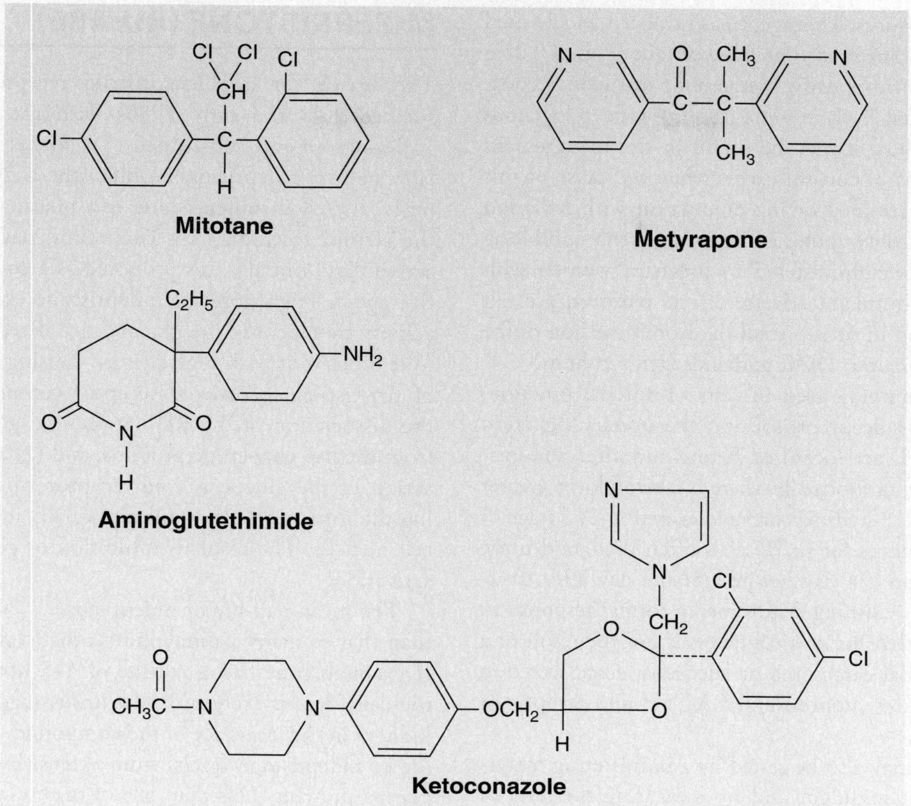

Mitotane

Metyrapone

Aminoglutethimide

Ketoconazole

FIGURE 39–5 Some adrenocortical blockers. Because of their toxicity, some of these compounds are no longer available in the United States.

cancer patients has now been supplanted by tamoxifen or by another class of drugs, the aromatase inhibitors (see Chapters 40 and 54). Aminoglutethimide can be used in conjunction with metyrapone or ketoconazole to reduce steroid secretion in patients with Cushing syndrome due to adrenocortical cancer who do not respond to mitotane.

Aminoglutethimide also apparently increases the clearance of some steroids. It has been shown to enhance the metabolism of dexamethasone, reducing its half-life from 4–5 hours to 2 hours.

KETOCONAZOLE

Ketoconazole, an antifungal imidazole derivative (see Chapter 48), is a potent and rather nonselective inhibitor of adrenal and gonadal steroid synthesis. This compound inhibits the cholesterol side-chain cleavage, P450c17, C17,20-lyase, 3β-hydroxysteroid dehydrogenase, and P450c11 enzymes required for steroid hormone synthesis. The sensitivity of the P450 enzymes to this compound in mammalian tissues is much lower than that needed to treat fungal infections, so that its inhibitory effects on steroid biosynthesis are seen only at high doses.

Ketoconazole has been used in the treatment of patients with Cushing syndrome due to several causes. Dosages of 200–1200 mg/d have caused a reduction in hormone levels and clinical improvement in some patients. This drug has some hepatotoxicity and should be started at 200 mg/d and slowly increased by 200 mg/d every 2–3 days up to a total daily dose of 1000 mg.

ETOMIDATE

Etomidate [R-1-(1-ethylphenyl)imidazole-5-ethyl ester] is used for induction of general anesthesia and sedation. At subhypnotic doses of 0.1 mg/kg per hour this drug inhibits adrenal steroidogenesis at the level of 11β-hydroxylase and has been used as the only parenteral medication available in the treatment of severe Cushing syndrome.

METYRAPONE

Metyrapone (see Figure 39–5) is a relatively selective inhibitor of steroid 11-hydroxylation, interfering with cortisol and corticosterone synthesis. In the presence of a normal pituitary gland, there is a compensatory increase in pituitary ACTH release and adrenal 11-deoxycortisol secretion. This response is a measure of the capacity of the anterior pituitary to produce ACTH and has been adapted for clinical use as a diagnostic test. Although the toxicity of metyrapone is much lower than that of mitotane (see text that follows), the drug may produce transient dizziness and gastrointestinal disturbances. This agent has not been widely used in the treatment of Cushing syndrome. However, in doses of 0.25 g twice daily to 1 g four times daily, metyrapone can reduce cortisol production to normal levels in some patients with endogenous Cushing syndrome. Thus, it may be useful in the management of severe manifestations of cortisol excess while the cause of this condition is being determined or in conjunction with radiation or surgical treatment. Metyrapone is the only adrenal-inhibiting medication that can be administered to pregnant women with Cushing syndrome. The major adverse effects observed are salt and water retention and hirsutism resulting from diversion of the 11-deoxycortisol precursor to DOC and androgen synthesis.

Metyrapone is commonly used in tests of adrenal function. The blood levels of 11-deoxycortisol and the urinary excretion of 17-hydroxycorticoids are measured before and after administration of the compound. Normally, there is a twofold or greater increase in the urinary 17-hydroxycorticoid excretion. A dosage of 300–500 mg every 4 hours for six doses is often used, and urine collections are made on the day before and the day after treatment. In patients with Cushing syndrome, a normal response to metyrapone indicates that the cortisol excess is not the result of a cortisol-secreting adrenal carcinoma or adenoma, since secretion by such tumors produces suppression of ACTH and atrophy of normal adrenal cortex.

Pituitary function may also be tested by administering metyrapone, 2–3 g orally at midnight and by measuring the level of ACTH or 11-deoxycortisol in blood drawn at 8 AM or by comparing the excretion of 17-hydroxycorticosteroids in the urine during the 24-hour periods preceding and following administration of the drug. In patients with suspected or known lesions of the pituitary, this procedure is a means of estimating the ability of the gland to produce ACTH. Metyrapone has been withdrawn from the market in the United States but is available on a compassionate basis.

TRILOSTANE

Trilostane is a 3β-17 hydroxysteroid dehydrogenase inhibitor that interferes with the synthesis of adrenal and gonadal hormones and is comparable to aminoglutethimide. Trilostane's adverse effects are predominantly gastrointestinal; adverse effects occur in about 50% of patients with both trilostane and aminoglutethimide. There is no cross-resistance or crossover of side effects between these compounds. Trilostane is not available in the United States.

ABIRATERONE

Abiraterone is the newest of the steroid synthesis inhibitors to be approved. It blocks 17α-hydroxylase (P450c17) and 17,20-lyase (see Figure 39–1), and it predictably reduces synthesis of cortisol in the adrenal and gonadal steroids in the gonads. A compensatory increase occurs in ACTH and aldosterone synthesis, but this can be prevented by concomitant administration of dexamethasone. Abiraterone is an orally active steroid prodrug and is approved for the treatment of refractory prostate cancer.

MIFEPRISTONE (RU-486)

The search for a glucocorticoid receptor antagonist finally succeeded in the early 1980s with the development of the 11β-aminophenyl-substituted 19-norsteroid called RU-486, later named mifepristone. Unlike the enzyme inhibitors previously discussed, mifepristone is a pharmacologic antagonist at the steroid receptor. This compound has strong antiprogestin activity and initially was proposed as a contraceptive-contragestive agent. High doses of mifepristone exert antiglucocorticoid activity by blocking the glucocorticoid receptor, since mifepristone binds to it with high affinity, causing (1) some stabilization of the hsp-glucocorticoid receptor complex and inhibition of the dissociation of the RU-486–bound glucocorticoid receptor from the hsp chaperone proteins; and (2) alteration of the interaction of the glucocorticoid receptor with coregulators, favoring the formation of a transcriptionally inactive complex in the cell nucleus. The result is inhibition of glucocorticoid receptor activation.

The mean half-life of mifepristone is 20 hours. This is longer than that of many natural and synthetic glucocorticoid agonists. (Dexamethasone has a half-life of 4–5 hours.) Less than 1% of the daily dose is excreted in the urine, suggesting a minor role of kidneys in the clearance of the compound. The long plasma half-life of mifepristone results from extensive and strong binding to plasma proteins. Less than 5% of the compound is found in the free form when plasma is analyzed by equilibrium dialysis. Mifepristone can bind to albumin and α_1-acid glycoprotein, but it has no affinity for corticosteroid-binding globulin.

In humans, mifepristone causes generalized glucocorticoid resistance. Given orally to several patients with Cushing syndrome due to ectopic ACTH production or adrenal carcinoma, it was able to reverse the cushingoid phenotype, eliminate carbohydrate intolerance, normalize blood pressure, correct thyroid and gonadal hormone suppression, and ameliorate the psychological sequelae of hypercortisolism in these patients. At present, this use of mifepristone can only be recommended for inoperable patients with ectopic ACTH secretion or adrenal carcinoma who have failed to respond to other therapeutic manipulations. Its pharmacology and use in women as a progesterone antagonist are discussed in Chapter 40.

MITOTANE

Mitotane (see Figure 39–5), a drug related to the DDT class of insecticides, has a nonselective cytotoxic action on the adrenal cortex in dogs and to a lesser extent in humans. This drug is administered orally in divided doses up to 12 g daily. About one third of patients with adrenal carcinoma show a reduction in tumor mass. In 80% of patients, the toxic effects are sufficiently severe to require dose reduction. These include diarrhea, nausea, vomiting, depression, somnolence, and skin rashes. The drug has been withdrawn from the market in the United States but is available on a compassionate basis.

MINERALOCORTICOID ANTAGONISTS

In addition to agents that interfere with aldosterone synthesis (see above), there are steroids that compete with aldosterone for its receptor and decrease its effect peripherally. Progesterone is mildly active in this respect.

Spironolactone is a 7α-acetylthiospirolactone. Its onset of action is slow, and the effects last for 2–3 days after the drug is discontinued. It is used in the treatment of primary aldosteronism in dosages of 50–100 mg/d. This agent reverses many of the manifestations of aldosteronism. It has been useful in establishing the diagnosis in some patients and in ameliorating the signs and symptoms when surgical removal of an adenoma is delayed. When used diagnostically for the detection of aldosteronism in hypokalemic patients with hypertension, dosages of 400–500 mg/d for 4–8 days—with an adequate intake of sodium and potassium—restore potassium levels to or toward normal. Spironolactone is also useful in preparing these patients for surgery. Dosages of 300–400 mg/d for 2 weeks are used for this purpose and may reduce the incidence of cardiac arrhythmias.

Spironolactone

Spironolactone is also an androgen antagonist and as such is sometimes used in the treatment of hirsutism and acne in women. Dosages of 50–200 mg/d cause a reduction in the density, diameter, and rate of growth of facial hair in patients with idiopathic hirsutism or hirsutism secondary to androgen excess. The effect can usually be seen in 2 months and becomes maximal in about 6 months.

Spironolactone as a diuretic is discussed in Chapter 15. The drug has benefits in heart failure greater than those predicted from its diuretic effects alone (see Chapter 13). Adverse effects reported for spironolactone include hyperkalemia, cardiac arrhythmia, menstrual abnormalities, gynecomastia, sedation, headache, gastrointestinal disturbances, and skin rashes.

Eplerenone, another aldosterone antagonist, is approved for the treatment of hypertension and heart failure (see Chapters 11, 13, and 15). Like spironolactone, eplerenone has also been found to reduce mortality in heart failure. This aldosterone receptor antagonist is somewhat more selective than spironolactone and has no reported effects on androgen receptors. The standard dosage in hypertension is 50–100 mg/d. The most common toxicity is hyperkalemia, but this is usually mild.

Drospirenone, a progestin, is an oral contraceptive (see Chapter 40) and also antagonizes the effects of aldosterone.

Finerenone, a novel nonsteroidal aldosterone antagonist, is approved for the treatment of hypertension and heart failure. It differs from both steroidal agents with respect to physicochemical, pharmacodynamic, and pharmacokinetic properties. It has beneficial anti-inflammatory, anti-remodeling, and antifibrotic properties in the kidneys, heart, and vasculature. At this time, there are several nonsteroidal MRAs under development and clinical assessment; of these, only esaxerenone and finerenone are approved for treatment globally. Compared with steroidal compounds, finerenone more potently inhibits MR co-regulator recruitment and fibrosis and distributes more evenly between the heart and kidneys.

PREPARATIONS AVAILABLE

GENERIC NAME	AVAILABLE AS
GLUCOCORTICOIDS FOR ORAL & PARENTERAL USE*	
Betamethasone	Celestone
Betamethasone sodium phosphate	Generic, Celestone Phosphate
Budesonide	Generic, Entocort EC
Cortisone	Generic
Dexamethasone	Generic, Decadron
Dexamethasone sodium phosphate	Generic
Hydrocortisone (cortisol)	Generic, Cortef
Hydrocortisone acetate	Generic
Hydrocortisone sodium phosphate	Hydrocortone
Hydrocortisone sodium succinate	Generic, Solu-Cortef, others
Methylprednisolone	Generic, Medrol
Methylprednisolone acetate	Generic, Depo-Medrol
Methylprednisolone sodium succinate	Generic, Solu-Medrol, others
Prednisolone	Generic, Prelone, others
Prednisolone acetate	Generic, Flo-Pred
Prednisolone sodium phosphate	Generic, Hydeltrasol
Prednisone	Generic, Deltasone, Prednicot
Triamcinolone acetonide	Generic, Kenalog, Azmacort
Triamcinolone hexacetonide	Aristospan
MINERALOCORTICOIDS	
Fludrocortisone acetate	Generic, Florinef Acetate, Cortineff Acetate
ADRENAL STEROID INHIBITORS	
Abiraterone	Zytiga
Ketoconazole	Generic, Nizoral
Etomidate	Amidate
Mifepristone	Mifeprex, Korlym
Mitotane	Lysodren

*Glucocorticoids for respiratory use: See Chapter 20. Glucocorticoids for dermatologic use: See Chapter 61. Glucocorticoids for gastrointestinal use: See Chapter 62.

REFERENCES

Agorastos A, Chrousos GP: The neuroendocrinology of stress: the stress-related continuum of chronic disease development. Mol Psychiatry 2022;27:502.

Alesci S et al: Glucocorticoid-induced osteoporosis: From basic mechanisms to clinical aspects. Neuroimmunomodulation 2005;12:1.

Alexopoulos A, Chrousos GP: Stress-related skin disorders. Rev Endocr Metab Disord 2016;17:295.

Charmandari E et al: Peripheral CLOCK regulates target-tissue glucocorticoid receptor transcriptional activity in a circadian fashion in man. PLoS One 2011;6:e25612.

Charmandari E, Kino T: Chrousos syndrome: A seminal report, a phylogenetic enigma and the clinical implications of glucocorticoid signaling changes. Eur J Clin Invest 2010;40:932.

Charmandari E et al: Adrenal insufficiency. Lancet 2014;383:2152.

Christaki EV et al: Stress, inflammation and metabolic biomarkers are associated with body composition measures in lean, overweight, and obese children and adolescents. Children (Basel) 2022;9:291.

Chrousos GP: Stress and disorders of the stress system. Nat Rev Endocrinol 2009;5:374.

Chrousos GP, Kino T: Glucocorticoid signaling in the cell: Expanding clinical implications to complex human behavioral and somatic disorders. Ann N Y Acad Sci 2009;1179:153.

Chrousos GP, Meduri GU: Critical COVID-19 disease, homeostasis, and the "surprise" of effective glucocorticoid therapy. Clin Immunol 2020; 219:108550.

Cutolo M et al: Special issue on glucocorticoid therapy in rheumatic diseases. Neuroimmunomodulation 2015;22:3.

Dikranian AH et al: Switching from immediate-release to delayed-release prednisone in moderate to severe rheumatoid arthritis: a practice-based clinical study. Rheumatol Ther 2017;4:363.

Elenkov IJ, Chrousos GP: Stress hormones, TH1/TH2 patterns, pro/anti-inflammatory cytokines and susceptibility to disease. Trends Endocrinol Metab 1999;10:359.

Elenkov IJ et al: Cytokine dysregulation, inflammation, and wellbeing. Neuroimmunomodulation 2005;12:255.

Franchimont D et al: Glucocorticoids and inflammation revisited: The state of the art. Neuroimmunomodulation 2002;10:247.

Georgianos PI, Agarwal R: The non-steroidal MRA finerenone in cardiorenal medicine: a state-of-the-art review of the literature. Am J Hypertens 2023; 36:135.

Graber AL et al: Natural history of pituitary-adrenal recovery following long-term suppression with corticosteroids. J Clin Endocrinol Metab 1965;25:11.

Hochberg Z et al: Endocrine withdrawal syndromes. Endocr Rev 2003;24:523.

Koch CA, Chrousos GP (editors): Endocrine hypertension: Underlying mechanisms and therapy. In: *Contemporary Endocrinology*, vol XIII. Springer, 2013.

Koch CA et al: The molecular pathogenesis of hereditary and sporadic adrenocortical and adrenomedullary tumors. J Clin Endocrinol Metab 2002;87:5367.

Mao J et al: Molecular mechanism of RU 486 action: A review. Mol Cellular Biochem 1992;109:1.

Marik PE et al: Clinical practice guidelines for the diagnosis and management of corticosteroid insufficiency in critical illness: Recommendations of an international task force. Crit Care Med 2008;36:1937.

Markou A et al: Stress-induced aldosterone hyper-secretion in a substantial subset of patients with essential hypertension. J Clin Endocrinol Metab 2015;100:2857.

Markou A et al: Enhanced performance of a modified diagnostic test of primary aldosteronism in patients with adrenal adenomas. Eur J Endocrinol 2022;186:265.

Mavrogeni S et al: Cardiac remodeling in hypertension: clinical impact on brain, heart, and kidney function. Horm Metab Res 2022;54:273.

Meduri GU, Chrousos GP: General adaptation in critical illness: glucocorticoid receptor-alpha master regulator of homeostatic corrections. Front Endocrinol (Lausanne) 2020;11:161.

Meduri GU et al: Activation and regulation of systemic inflammation in ARDS: Rationale for prolonged glucocorticoid therapy. Chest 2009;136:1631.

Merke DP et al: Future directions in the study and management of congenital adrenal hyperplasia due to 21-hydroxylase deficiency. Ann Intern Med 2002;136:320.

Nader N et al: Interactions of the circadian CLOCK system and the HPA axis. Trends Endocrinol Metab 2010;21:277.

Preda VA et al: Etomidate in the management of hypercortisolaemia in Cushing's syndrome: A review. Eur J Endocrinol 2012;167:137.

Stefanaki C et al: Chronic stress and body composition disorders: Implications for health and disease. Hormones (Athens) 2018;17:33.

Stewart PM: Modified-release hydrocortisone: is it time to change clinical practice? J Endocr Soc 2019;3:1150.

Tsigos C, Chrousos GP: Differential diagnosis and management of Cushing's syndrome. Annu Rev Med 1996;47:443.

Tyfoxylou E et al: High prevalence of primary aldosteronism in patients with type 2 diabetes mellitus and hypertension. Biomedicines 2022;10:2308.

Voulgaris N et al: Prevalence of primary aldosteronism across the stages of hypertension based on a new combined overnight test. Horm Metab Res 2021;53:461.

Wahrborg P et al: The physiology of stress and stress recovery. In: van der Bosch M, Bird W (editors): *Oxford Text book of Nature and Public Health: The Role of Nature in Improving the Health of a Population.* Oxford Univ Press, 2018:33–39.

Whitaker MJ et al: An oral multiparticulate, modified-release, hydrocortisone replacement therapy that provides physiological cortisol exposure. Clin Endocrinol (Oxf) 2014;80:554.

Zannas AS, Chrousos GP: Epigenetic programming by stress and glucocorticoids along the human lifespan. Mol Psychiatry 2017;22:640.

CASE STUDY ANSWER

The patient should be placed on replacement oral hydrocortisone at 10 mg/m^2 per day and fludrocortisone at 75 mcg/d. He should be given a MedicAlert bracelet and instructions for increased treatment at two times standard glucocorticoid dosage for 24 hours for minor stress and 10 times replacement of hydrocortisone for major stress over 48 hours.

CHAPTER

40

The Gonadal Hormones & Inhibitors

George P. Chrousos, MD

CASE STUDY

A 25-year-old woman with menarche at 13 years and menstrual periods until about 1 year ago complains of hot flushes, skin and vaginal dryness, weakness, poor sleep, and scanty and infrequent menstrual periods of a year's duration. She visits her gynecologist, who obtains plasma levels of follicle-stimulating hormone and luteinizing hormone, both of which are moderately elevated. She is diagnosed with premature ovarian failure, and estrogen and progesterone replacement therapy is recommended. A dual-energy absorptiometry scan (DEXA) reveals a bone density t-score of <2.5 SD, ie, frank osteoporosis. How should the ovarian hormones she lacks be replaced? What extra measures should she take for her osteoporosis while receiving treatment?

■ THE OVARY (ESTROGENS, PROGESTINS, OTHER OVARIAN HORMONES, ORAL CONTRACEPTIVES, INHIBITORS & ANTAGONISTS, & OVULATION-INDUCING AGENTS)

The ovary has important gametogenic functions that are integrated with its hormonal activity. In the human female, the gonad is relatively quiescent during childhood, the period of rapid growth and maturation. At puberty, the ovary begins a 30- to 40-year period of cyclic function called the **menstrual cycle** because of the regular episodes of bleeding that are its most obvious manifestation. It then fails to respond to gonadotropins secreted by the anterior pituitary gland, and the cessation of cyclic bleeding that occurs is called **menopause.**

The mechanism responsible for the onset of ovarian function at the time of puberty is thought to be neural in origin, because the immature gonad can be stimulated by gonadotropins already present in the pituitary and because the pituitary is responsive to exogenous **hypothalamic gonadotropin-releasing hormone (GnRH).** Despite extensive research in the field, the mechanism of puberty initiation still remains an enigma. Pulsatile pituitary gonadotropin secretion under the guidance of GnRH definitely constitutes a *sine qua non* for pubertal onset. However, the secretion of GnRH in the human hypothalamus is regulated by kisspeptin and its receptor, as well as by permissive or opposing signals mediated by neurokinin B and dynorphin acting on their respective receptors. These three supra-GnRH regulators compose the **Kisspeptin, Neurokinin B, and Dynorphin neuron (KNDy) system,** a key player in pubertal onset and progression. Recently, makorin ring finger protein 3 (MKRN3) was also implicated in pubertal onset by contributing to the regulation of the KNDy system. However, the inhibitory (gamma-amino butyric acid, neuropeptide Y, and RFamide-related peptide-3) and stimulatory (glutamate) signals acting upstream of KNDy call into question the primary role of MKRN3 as the gatekeeper of puberty. Recently, epigenetic mechanisms involving derepression of genes, such as that of kisspeptin, have been implicated in pubertal onset. Ultimately, withdrawal of a childhood-related inhibitory effect upon hypothalamic arcuate nucleus neurons allows these neurons to produce GnRH in pulses with the appropriate amplitude, which stimulate the release of **follicle-stimulating hormone (FSH)** and **luteinizing hormone (LH)** (see Chapter 37). At first, small amounts of the latter two

ACRONYMS

CBG	Corticosteroid-binding globulin (transcortin)
DHEA	Dehydroepiandrosterone
DHEAS	Dehydroepiandrosterone sulfate
ERE	Estrogen response element
FSH	Follicle-stimulating hormone
GnRH	Gonadotropin-releasing hormone
HDL	High-density lipoprotein
HRT	Hormone replacement therapy (also called HT)
LDL	Low-density lipoprotein
LH	Luteinizing hormone
PRE	Progesterone response element
SERM	Selective estrogen receptor modulator
SHBG	Sex hormone-binding globulin
TBG	Thyroxine-binding globulin

hormones are released during the night, and the limited quantities of ovarian estrogen secreted in response start to cause breast development. Subsequently, FSH and LH are secreted throughout the day and night, causing secretion of higher amounts of estrogen and leading to further breast enlargement, alterations in fat distribution, and a growth spurt that culminates in epiphyseal closure in the long bones. The change of ovarian function at puberty is called **gonadarche.**

A year or so after gonadarche, sufficient estrogen is produced to induce endometrial changes and periodic bleeding **(menarche).** After the first few irregular cycles, which may be anovulatory, normal cyclic function is established.

At the beginning of each cycle, a variable number of follicles (vesicular follicles), each containing an ovum, begin to enlarge in response to FSH. After 5 or 6 days, one follicle, called the dominant follicle, begins to develop more rapidly. The outer theca and inner granulosa cells of this follicle multiply and, under the influence of LH, synthesize and release estrogens at an increasing rate. The estrogens appear to inhibit FSH release and may lead to regression of the smaller, less mature follicles. The mature dominant ovarian follicle consists of an ovum surrounded by a fluid-filled antrum lined by granulosa and theca cells. The estrogen secretion reaches a peak just before midcycle, and the granulosa cells begin to secrete progesterone. These changes stimulate the brief surge in LH and FSH release that precedes and causes ovulation. When the follicle ruptures, the ovum is released into the abdominal cavity near the opening of the uterine tube.

Following the above events, the cavity of the ruptured follicle fills with blood (corpus hemorrhagicum), and the luteinized theca and granulosa cells proliferate and replace the blood to form the corpus luteum. The cells of this structure produce estrogens and progesterone for the remainder of the cycle, or longer if pregnancy occurs.

If pregnancy does not occur, the corpus luteum begins to degenerate and ceases hormone production, eventually becoming a corpus albicans. The endometrium, which proliferated during

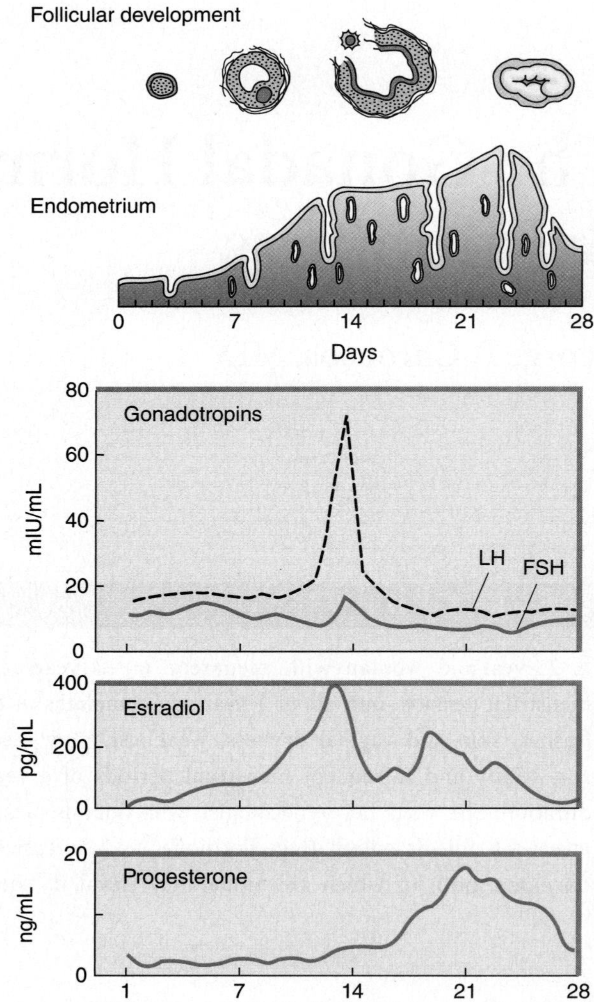

FIGURE 40–1 The menstrual cycle, showing plasma levels of pituitary and ovarian hormones and histologic changes.

the follicular phase and developed its glandular function during the luteal phase, is shed in the process of menstruation. These events are summarized in Figure 40–1.

The ovary normally ceases its gametogenic and endocrine function with time. This change is accompanied by a cessation in uterine bleeding (menopause) and occurs at a mean age of 52 years in the United States. Although the ovary ceases to secrete estrogen, significant levels of estrogen persist in many women as a result of conversion of adrenal and ovarian steroids such as androstenedione to estrone and estradiol in adipose and possibly other nonendocrine tissues.

Disturbances in Ovarian Function

Disturbances of cyclic function are common even during the peak years of reproduction. A minority of these result from inflammatory or neoplastic processes that influence the functions of the uterus, ovaries, or pituitary. Many of the minor disturbances leading to periods of amenorrhea or anovulatory cycles are self-limited.

They are often associated with emotional or physical stress and reflect temporary alterations in the stress centers in the brain that control the secretion of GnRH. Anovulatory cycles are also associated with eating disorders (bulimia, anorexia nervosa) and with severe exercise such as distance running and swimming. Among the more common organic causes of persistent ovulatory disturbances are pituitary prolactinomas and syndromes and tumors characterized by excessive ovarian or adrenal androgen production. Normal ovarian function can be modified by androgens produced by the adrenal cortex or tumors arising from it. The ovary also gives rise to androgen-producing neoplasms such as arrhenoblastomas, as well as to estrogen-producing granulosa cell tumors.

THE ESTROGENS

Estrogenic activity is shared by a large number of chemical substances. In addition to the variety of steroidal estrogens derived from animal sources, numerous nonsteroidal estrogens have been synthesized. Many phenols are estrogenic, and estrogenic activity has been identified in diverse forms of life including those found in ocean sediments. Estrogen-mimetic compounds (flavonoids) are found in many plants, including saw palmetto, and soybeans and other foods. A diet rich in these plant products may cause slight estrogenic effects. Additionally, some compounds used in the manufacture of plastics (bisphenols, alkylphenols, phthalate phenols) have been found to be estrogenic. It has been proposed that these agents are associated with an increased breast cancer incidence in both women and men in the industrialized world.

Natural Estrogens

The major estrogens produced by women are **estradiol** (17β-estradiol, E_2), **estrone** (E_1), and **estriol** (E_3) (Figure 40–2). Estradiol is the major secretory product of the ovary. Although some estrone is produced in the ovary, most estrone and estriol are formed in the liver from estradiol or in peripheral tissues from androstenedione and other androgens (see Figure 39–1). As noted above, during the first part of the menstrual cycle estrogens are produced in the ovarian follicle by the theca and granulosa cells. After ovulation, the estrogens as well as progesterone are synthesized by the luteinized granulosa and theca cells of the corpus luteum, and the pathways of biosynthesis are slightly different.

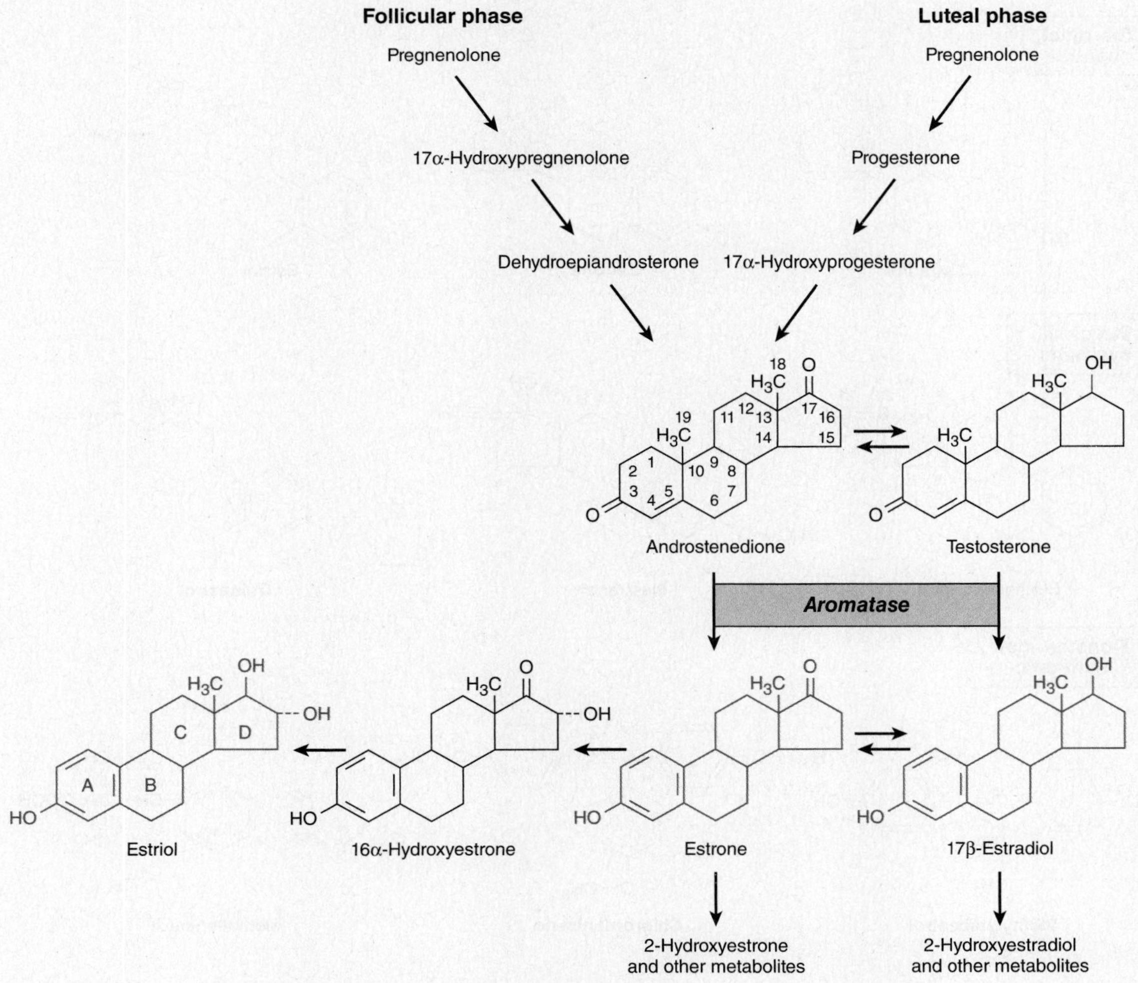

FIGURE 40–2 Biosynthesis and metabolism of estrogens and testosterone.

During pregnancy, a large amount of estrogen is synthesized by the fetoplacental unit—consisting of the fetal adrenal zone, secreting androgen precursor, and the placenta, which aromatizes it into estrogen. The estriol synthesized by the fetoplacental unit is released into the maternal circulation and excreted into the urine. Repeated assay of maternal urinary estriol excretion has been used in the assessment of fetal well-being.

One of the most prolific natural sources of estrogenic substances is the stallion, which liberates more of these hormones than the pregnant mare or pregnant woman. The equine estrogens—equilenin and equilin—and their congeners are unsaturated in the B as well as the A ring and are excreted in large quantities in urine, from which they can be recovered and used for medicinal purposes.

In normal women, estradiol is produced at a rate that varies during the menstrual cycle, resulting in plasma levels as low as 50 pg/mL in the early follicular phase to as high as 350–850 pg/mL at the time of the preovulatory peak (see Figure 40–1).

Synthetic Estrogens

A variety of chemical alterations have been applied to the natural estrogens. The most important effect of these alterations has been to increase their oral effectiveness. Some structures are shown in Figure 40–3. Those with therapeutic use are listed in Table 40–1.

In addition to the steroidal estrogens, a variety of nonsteroidal compounds with estrogenic activity have been synthesized and used clinically. These include dienestrol, diethylstilbestrol, benzestrol, hexestrol, methestrol, methallenestril, and chlorotrianisene.

Pharmacokinetics

When released into the circulation, estradiol binds strongly to an α_2 globulin (sex hormone–binding globulin [SHBG]) and with lower affinity to albumin. Bound estrogen is relatively unavailable for diffusion into cells, and it is the free fraction that is physiologically active. Estradiol is converted by the liver and other tissues to estrone and estriol (see Figure 40–2) and their 2-hydroxylated derivatives and conjugated metabolites (which are too insoluble in lipid to cross the cell membrane readily) and excreted in the bile. Estrone and estriol have low affinity for the estrogen receptor. However, the conjugates may be hydrolyzed in the intestine to active, reabsorbable compounds. Estrogens are also excreted in small amounts in the breast milk of nursing mothers.

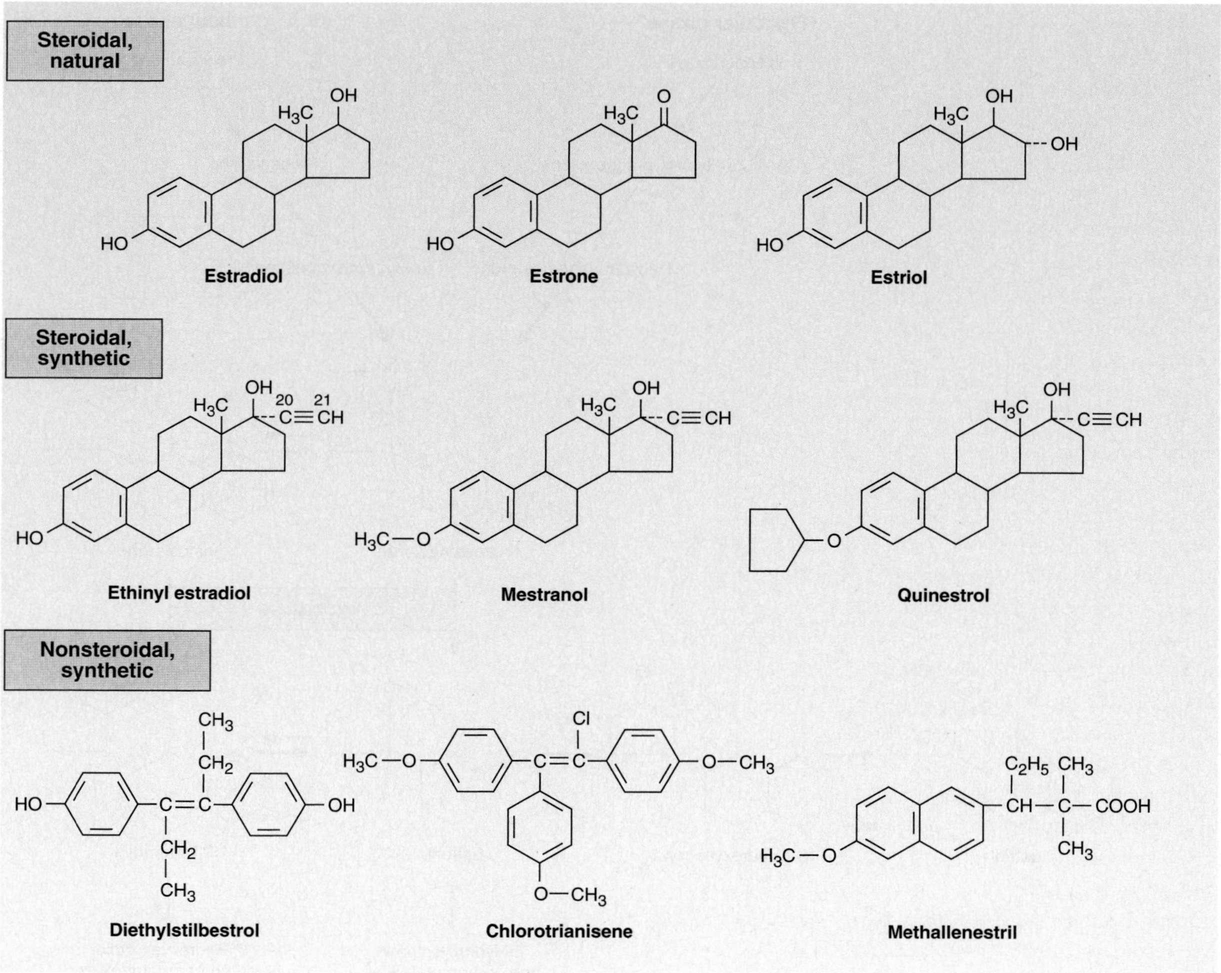

FIGURE 40–3 Compounds with estrogenic activity.

TABLE 40–1 Commonly used estrogens.

Preparation	Average Replacement Dosage
Ethinyl estradiol	0.005–0.02 mg/d
Micronized estradiol	1–2 mg/d
Estradiol cypionate	2–5 mg every 3–4 weeks
Estradiol valerate	2–20 mg every other week
Estropipate	1.25–2.5 mg/d
Conjugated, esterified, or mixed estrogenic substances:	
Oral	0.3–1.25 mg/d
Injectable	0.2–2 mg/d
Transdermal	Patch
Quinestrol	0.1–0.2 mg/week
Chlorotrianisene	12–25 mg/d
Methallenestril	3–9 mg/d

Because significant amounts of estrogens and their active metabolites are excreted in the bile and reabsorbed from the intestine, the resulting enterohepatic circulation ensures that orally administered estrogens will have a high ratio of hepatic to peripheral effects. As noted below, the hepatic effects are thought to be responsible for some undesirable actions such as increased synthesis of clotting factors and plasma renin substrate. The hepatic effects of estrogen can be minimized by routes that avoid first-pass liver exposure, ie, vaginal, transdermal, or by injection.

Physiologic Effects

A. Mechanism

Estrogens in the blood and interstitial fluid are bound to SHBG, from which they dissociate to cross the cell membrane, enter the nucleus, and bind to their receptor. Two genes code for two estrogen receptor isoforms, α and β, which are members of the superfamily of steroid, sterol, retinoic acid, and thyroid receptors. Unlike glucocorticoid receptors, estrogen receptors are found predominantly in the nucleus, where they are bound to heat shock proteins that stabilize them (see Figure 39–4).

Binding of the hormone to its receptor alters the receptor's conformation and releases it from the stabilizing proteins (predominantly Hsp90). The receptor-hormone complex forms dimers (usually ERα-ERα, ERβ-ERβ, or ERα-ERβ) that bind to a specific sequence of nucleotides, called **estrogen response elements (EREs),** in the regulatory regions of various genes and regulate their transcription. The ERE is composed of two half-sites arranged as a palindrome separated by a small group of nucleotides called the spacer. The interaction of a receptor dimer with the ERE also involves a number of nuclear proteins, the coregulators, as well as components of the transcription machinery. Complex interactions with various coregulators appear to be responsible for some of the tissue-specific effects that govern the actions of **selective estrogen receptor modulators** (**SERMs,** see below). The receptor may also bind to other transcription factors to influence the effects of these factors on their responsive genes. Interestingly, although ERβ has its own separate actions from ERα, it also acts as a dominant negative inhibitor of ERα. Thus, while ERα has many growth-promoting properties, ERβ has antigrowth effects. Many phytoestrogens act via the ERβ protecting cells from the pro-growth effects of ERα.

The relative concentrations and types of receptors, receptor coregulators, and transcription factors confer the cell specificity of the hormone's actions. The genomic effects of estrogens are mainly due to proteins synthesized by translation of RNA transcribed from a responsive gene. Some of the effects of estrogens are indirect, mediated by the autocrine and paracrine actions of autacoids such as growth factors, lipids, glycolipids, and cytokines produced by the target cells in response to estrogen.

Rapid estrogen-induced effects such as granulosa cell Ca^{2+} uptake and increased uterine blood flow do not require gene activation. These appear to be mediated by nongenomic effects of the classic estrogen receptor-estrogen complex, influencing several intracellular signaling pathways.

Recently, all steroid receptors except the mineralocorticoid receptors were shown to have palmitoylation motifs that allow enzymatic addition of palmitate and increased localization of the receptors in the vicinity of plasma membranes. Such receptors are available for direct interactions with, and effects on, various membrane-associated or cytoplasmic proteins without the need for entry into the nucleus and induction of transcriptional actions.

B. Female Maturation

Estrogens are required for the normal sexual maturation and growth of the female. They stimulate the development of the vagina, uterus, and uterine tubes as well as the secondary sex characteristics. They stimulate stromal development and ductal growth in the breast and are responsible for the accelerated growth phase and the closing of the epiphyses of the long bones that occur at puberty. They contribute to the growth of axillary and pubic hair and alter the distribution of body fat to produce typical female body contours. Larger quantities also stimulate development of pigmentation in the skin, most prominent in the region of the nipples and areolae and in the genital region.

C. Endometrial Effects

In addition to its growth effects on uterine muscle, estrogen plays an important role in the development of the endometrial lining. When estrogen production is properly coordinated with the production of progesterone during the normal human menstrual cycle, regular periodic bleeding and shedding of the endometrial lining occur. Continuous exposure to estrogens for prolonged periods leads to hyperplasia of the endometrium that is usually associated with abnormal bleeding patterns.

D. Metabolic and Cardiovascular Effects

Estrogens have a number of important metabolic and cardiovascular effects. They seem to be partially responsible for maintenance of the normal structure and function of the skin and blood vessels in women. Estrogens also decrease the rate of resorption of bone by promoting the apoptosis of osteoclasts and by antagonizing the osteoclastogenic and pro-osteoclastic effects of parathyroid hormone and interleukin 6. Estrogens also stimulate adipose tissue production of leptin and are in part responsible for the higher levels of this hormone in women than in men.

In addition to stimulating the synthesis of enzymes and growth factors leading to uterine and breast growth and differentiation, estrogens alter the production and activity of many other proteins in the body. Metabolic alterations in the liver are especially important, so that there is a higher circulating level of proteins such as transcortin (corticosteroid-binding globulin [CBG]), thyroxine-binding globulin (TBG), SHBG, transferrin, renin substrate, and fibrinogen. This leads to increased circulating levels of thyroxine, estrogen, testosterone, iron, copper, and other substances.

Alterations in the composition of the plasma lipids caused by estrogens are characterized by an increase in the high-density lipoproteins (HDL), a slight reduction in the low-density lipoproteins (LDL), and a reduction in total plasma cholesterol levels. Plasma triglyceride levels are increased. Estrogens decrease hepatic oxidation of adipose tissue lipid to ketones and increase synthesis of triglycerides.

E. Effects on Blood Coagulation

Estrogens enhance the coagulability of blood. Many changes in factors influencing coagulation have been reported, including increased circulating levels of factors II, VII, IX, and X and decreased antithrombin III, partially as a result of the hepatic effects mentioned above. Increased plasminogen levels and decreased platelet adhesiveness have also been found (see Hormonal Contraception, below).

F. Other Effects

Estrogens induce the synthesis of progesterone receptors. They are responsible for estrous behavior in animals and may influence behavior and libido in humans. Administration of estrogens stimulates central components of the stress system, including the production of corticotropin-releasing hormone and the activity of the sympathetic system, and promotes a sense of well-being when given to women who are estrogen-deficient. They also facilitate the loss of intravascular fluid into the extracellular space, producing edema. The resulting decrease in plasma volume causes a compensatory retention of sodium and water by the kidney. Estrogens also modulate sympathetic nervous system control of smooth muscle function.

Clinical Uses*

A. Primary Hypogonadism

Estrogens have been used extensively for replacement therapy in estrogen-deficient patients. The estrogen deficiency may be due to primary failure of development of the ovaries, premature menopause, castration, or menopause.

Treatment of primary hypogonadism is usually begun at 11–13 years of age in order to stimulate the development of secondary sex characteristics and menses, to stimulate optimal growth, to prevent osteoporosis, and to avoid the psychological consequences of delayed puberty and estrogen deficiency. Treatment attempts to mimic the physiology of puberty. It is initiated with small doses of estrogen (0.3 mg conjugated estrogens or 5–10 mcg ethinyl estradiol) on days 1–21 each month and is slowly increased to adult doses and then maintained until the age of menopause (approximately 51 years of age). A progestin is added after the first uterine bleeding. When growth is completed, chronic therapy consists mainly of the administration of adult doses of both estrogens and progestins, as described below.

B. Postmenopausal Hormonal Therapy

In addition to the signs and symptoms that follow closely upon the cessation of normal ovarian function—such as loss of menstrual periods, vasomotor symptoms, sleep disturbances, and genital atrophy—there are longer-lasting changes that influence the health and well-being of postmenopausal women. These include an acceleration of bone loss, which in susceptible women may lead to vertebral, hip, and wrist fractures; and lipid changes, which may contribute to the acceleration of atherosclerotic cardiovascular disease noted in postmenopausal women. The effects of estrogens on bone have been extensively studied, and the effects of hormone withdrawal have been well characterized. However, the role of estrogens and progestins in the cause and prevention of cardiovascular disease, which is responsible for 350,000 deaths per year, and breast cancer, which causes 35,000 deaths per year, is less well understood.

When normal ovulatory function ceases and the estrogen levels fall after menopause, oophorectomy, or premature ovarian failure, there is an accelerated rise in plasma cholesterol and LDL concentrations, while LDL receptors decline. HDL is not much affected, and levels remain higher than in men. Very-low-density lipoprotein and triglyceride levels are also relatively unaffected. Since cardiovascular disorders account for most deaths in this age group, the risk for these disorders constitutes a major consideration in deciding whether hormonal "replacement" therapy (HRT, also correctly called HT) is indicated and influences the selection of hormones to be administered. Estrogen replacement therapy has a beneficial effect on circulating lipids and lipoproteins, and this was earlier thought to be accompanied by a reduction in myocardial infarction by about 50% and of fatal strokes by as much as 40%. These findings, however, have been disputed by the results of a large study from the Women's Health Initiative (WHI) project showing no cardiovascular benefit from estrogen plus progestin replacement therapy in perimenopausal or older postmenopausal patients. In fact, there may be a small increase in cardiovascular problems as well as breast cancer in women who received the replacement therapy. Interestingly, a small protective effect against colon cancer was observed. Although current clinical guidelines do not recommend routine hormone therapy in postmenopausal women, the validity of the WHI report has been questioned. In any case, there is no increased risk for breast cancer if therapy is given immediately after menopause and for the first 7 years, while the cardiovascular risk depends on the degree of atherosclerosis at the onset of therapy. Transdermal or vaginal administration of estrogen may be associated with decreased cardiovascular risk because it bypasses the liver circulation. Women with premature menopause should definitely receive hormone replacement therapy.

*The use of estrogens in contraception is discussed later in this chapter.

In some studies, a protective effect of estrogen replacement therapy against Alzheimer disease was observed. However, several other studies have not supported these results.

Progestins antagonize estrogen's effects on LDL and HDL to a variable extent. However, one large study has shown that the addition of a progestin to estrogen replacement therapy does not influence the cardiovascular risk.

Optimal management of the postmenopausal patient requires careful assessment of her symptoms as well as consideration of her age and the presence of (or risks for) cardiovascular disease, osteoporosis, breast cancer, and endometrial cancer. Bearing in mind the effects of the gonadal hormones on each of these disorders, the goals of therapy can then be defined and the risks of therapy assessed and discussed with the patient.

If the main indication for therapy is hot flushes and sleep disturbances, therapy with the lowest dose of estrogen required for symptomatic relief is recommended. Treatment may be required for only a limited period of time and the possible increased risk for breast cancer is avoided. In women who have undergone hysterectomy, estrogens alone can be given 5 days per week or continuously, since progestins are not required to reduce the risk for endometrial hyperplasia and cancer. Hot flushes, sweating, insomnia, and atrophic vaginitis are generally relieved by estrogens; many patients experience some increased sense of well-being; and climacteric depression and other psychopathologic states are improved. Recently, neurokinin 3 receptor antagonists have completed phase 3 studies for prevention of menopausal or estrogen deficiency-related hot flushes.

The role of estrogens in the prevention and treatment of osteoporosis has been carefully studied (see Chapter 42). The amount of bone present in the body is maximal in the young active adult in the third decade of life and begins to decline more rapidly in middle age in both men and women. The development of osteoporosis also depends on the amount of bone present at the start of this process, on vitamin D and calcium intake, and on the degree of physical activity. The risk of osteoporosis is highest in smokers who are thin, Caucasian, and inactive and have a low calcium intake and a strong family history of osteoporosis. Depression also is a major risk factor for development of osteoporosis in women.

Estrogens should be used in the smallest dosage consistent with relief of symptoms. In women who have not undergone hysterectomy, it is most convenient to prescribe estrogen on the first 21–25 days of each month. The recommended dosages of estrogen are 0.3–1.25 mg/d of conjugated estrogen or 0.01–0.02 mg/d of ethinyl estradiol. Dosages in the middle of these ranges have been shown to be maximally effective in preventing the decrease in bone density occurring at menopause. From this point of view, it is important to begin therapy as soon as possible after the menopause for maximum effect. In these patients and others not taking estrogen, calcium supplements that bring the total daily calcium intake up to 1500 mg are useful.

Patients at low risk of developing osteoporosis who manifest only mild atrophic vaginitis can be treated with topical preparations. The vaginal route of application is also useful in the treatment of urinary tract symptoms in these patients. It is important to realize, however, that although locally administered estrogens escape the first-pass effect (so that some undesirable hepatic effects are reduced), they are almost completely absorbed into the circulation, and these preparations should be given cyclically.

As noted below, the administration of estrogen is associated with an increased risk of endometrial carcinoma. The administration of a progestational agent with the estrogen prevents endometrial hyperplasia and markedly reduces the risk of this cancer. When estrogen is given for the first 25 days of the month and the progestin medroxyprogesterone (10 mg/d) is added during the last 10–14 days, the risk is only half of that in women not receiving hormone replacement therapy. On this regimen, some women will experience a return of symptoms during the period off estrogen administration. In these patients, the estrogen can be given continuously. If the progestin produces sedation or other undesirable effects, its dose can be reduced to 2.5–5 mg/d for the last 10 days of the cycle with a slight increase in the risk for endometrial hyperplasia. These regimens are usually accompanied by bleeding at the end of each cycle. Some women experience migraine headaches during the last few days of the cycle. The use of a continuous estrogen regimen will often prevent their occurrence. Women who object to the cyclic bleeding associated with sequential therapy can also consider continuous therapy. Daily therapy with 0.625 mg of conjugated equine estrogens and 2.5–5 mg of medroxyprogesterone will eliminate cyclic bleeding, control vasomotor symptoms, prevent genital atrophy, maintain bone density, and show a favorable lipid profile with a small decrease in LDL and an increase in HDL concentrations. These women have endometrial atrophy on biopsy. About half of these patients experience breakthrough bleeding during the first few months of therapy. About 70–80% become amenorrheic after the first 4 months, and most remain so. The main disadvantage of continuous therapy is the need for uterine biopsy if bleeding occurs after the first few months.

As noted above, estrogens may also be administered vaginally or transdermally. When estrogens are given by these routes, the liver is bypassed on the first circulation, and the ratio of the liver effects to peripheral effects is reduced.

In patients in whom estrogen replacement therapy is contraindicated, such as those with estrogen-sensitive tumors, relief of vasomotor symptoms may be obtained by the use of clonidine.

C. Other Uses

Estrogens combined with progestins can be used to suppress ovulation in patients with intractable dysmenorrhea or when suppression of ovarian function is used in the treatment of hirsutism and amenorrhea due to excessive secretion of androgens by the ovary. Under these circumstances, greater suppression may be needed, and oral contraceptives containing 50 mcg of estrogen or a combination of a low-estrogen pill with GnRH suppression may be required.

Adverse Effects

Adverse effects of variable severity have been reported with the therapeutic use of estrogens. Many other effects reported in conjunction with hormonal contraceptives may be related to their estrogen content. These are discussed below.

A. Uterine Bleeding

Estrogen therapy is a major cause of postmenopausal uterine bleeding. Unfortunately, vaginal bleeding at this time of life may also be due to carcinoma of the endometrium. To avoid confusion, patients should be treated with the smallest amount of estrogen possible. It should be given cyclically so that bleeding, if it occurs, will be more likely to occur during the withdrawal period. As noted above, endometrial hyperplasia can be prevented by administration of a progestational agent with estrogen in each cycle.

B. Cancer

The relation of estrogen therapy to cancer continues to be the subject of active investigation. Although no adverse effect of short-term estrogen therapy on the incidence of breast cancer has been demonstrated, a small increase in the incidence of this tumor may occur with prolonged therapy. Although the risk factor is small (1.25), the impact may be great since this tumor occurs in 10% of women, and addition of progesterone does not confer a protective effect. Studies indicate that following unilateral excision of breast cancer, women receiving tamoxifen (an estrogen partial agonist, see below) show a 35% decrease in contralateral breast cancer compared with controls. These studies also demonstrate that tamoxifen is well tolerated by most patients, produces estrogen-like alterations in plasma lipid levels, and stabilizes bone mineral loss. Studies bearing on the possible efficacy of tamoxifen and raloxifene in postmenopausal women at high risk for breast cancer show decreases of risk for at least 5 years, but of unknown further duration. Another study showed that postmenopausal hormone replacement therapy with estrogens plus progestins was associated with greater breast epithelial cell proliferation and breast epithelial cell density than estrogens alone or no replacement therapy. Furthermore, with estrogens plus progestins, breast proliferation was localized to the terminal duct-lobular unit of the breast, which is the main site of development of breast cancer. Thus, further studies are needed to conclusively assess the possible association between progestins and breast cancer risk.

Many studies show an increased risk of endometrial carcinoma in patients taking estrogens alone. The risk seems to vary with the dose and duration of treatment: 15 times greater in patients taking large doses of estrogen for 5 or more years, in contrast with 2 to 4 times greater in patients receiving lower doses for short periods. However, as noted above, the concomitant use of a progestin prevents this increased risk and may in fact reduce the incidence of endometrial cancer to less than that in the general population.

There have been a number of reports of adenocarcinoma of the vagina in young women whose mothers were treated with large doses of diethylstilbestrol early in pregnancy. These cancers are most common in young women (ages 14–44). The incidence is less than 1 per 1000 women exposed—too low to establish a cause-and-effect relationship with certainty. However, the risks for infertility, ectopic pregnancy, and premature delivery also are increased. It is now recognized that there is no indication for the use of diethylstilbestrol during pregnancy, and it should be avoided. It is not known whether other estrogens have a similar effect or whether the observed phenomena are peculiar to diethylstilbestrol. This agent should be used only in the treatment of cancer (eg, of the prostate) or as a "morning after" contraceptive (see page 761).

C. Other Effects

Nausea and breast tenderness are common and can be minimized by using the smallest effective dose of estrogen. Hyperpigmentation also occurs. Estrogen therapy is associated with an increase in frequency of migraine headaches as well as cholestasis, gallbladder disease, and hypertension.

Contraindications

Estrogens should not be used in patients with estrogen-dependent neoplasms such as carcinoma of the endometrium or in those with—or at high risk for—carcinoma of the breast. They should be avoided in patients with undiagnosed genital bleeding, liver disease, or a history of thromboembolic disorder. In addition, the use of estrogens should be avoided by heavy smokers.

Preparations & Dosages

The dosages of commonly used natural and synthetic preparations are listed in Table 40–1. Although all of the estrogens produce almost the same hormonal effects, their potencies vary both between agents and depending on the route of administration. As noted above, estradiol is the most active endogenous estrogen, and it has the highest affinity for the estrogen receptor. However, its metabolites estrone and estriol have weak uterine effects.

For a given level of gonadotropin suppression, oral estrogen preparations have more effect on the circulating levels of CBG, SHBG, and a host of other liver proteins, including angiotensinogen, than do transdermal preparations. The oral route of administration allows greater concentrations of hormone to reach the liver, thus increasing the synthesis of these proteins. Transdermal preparations were developed to avoid this effect. When administered transdermally, 50–100 mcg of estradiol has effects similar to those of 0.625–1.25 mg of conjugated oral estrogens on gonadotropin concentrations, endometrium, and vaginal epithelium. Furthermore, the transdermal estrogen preparations do not significantly increase the concentrations of renin substrate, CBG, and TBG and do not produce the characteristic changes in serum lipids. Combined oral preparations containing 0.625 mg of conjugated estrogens and 2.5 mg of medroxyprogesterone acetate are available for menopausal replacement therapy. Tablets containing 0.625 mg of conjugated estrogens and 5 mg of medroxyprogesterone acetate are available to be used in conjunction with conjugated estrogens in a sequential fashion. Estrogens alone are taken on days 1–14 and the combination on days 15–28.

THE PROGESTINS

Natural Progestins: Progesterone

Progesterone is the most important progestin in humans. In addition to having important hormonal effects, it serves as a precursor to the estrogens, androgens, and adrenocortical steroids.

It is synthesized in the ovary, testis, and adrenal cortex from circulating cholesterol. Large amounts are also synthesized and released by the placenta during pregnancy.

In the ovary, progesterone is produced primarily by the corpus luteum. Normal males appear to secrete 1–5 mg of progesterone daily, resulting in plasma levels of about 0.03 mcg/dL. The level is only slightly higher in the female during the follicular phase of the cycle, when only a few milligrams per day of progesterone are secreted. During the luteal phase, plasma levels range from 0.5 mcg/dL to more than 2 mcg/dL (see Figure 40–1). Plasma levels of progesterone are further elevated and reach their peak levels in the third trimester of pregnancy.

Synthetic Progestins

A variety of progestational compounds have been synthesized. Some are active when given by mouth. They are not a uniform group of compounds, and all of them differ from progesterone in one or more respects. Table 40–2 lists some of these compounds and their effects. In general, the 21-carbon compounds (hydroxyprogesterone, medroxyprogesterone, megestrol, and dimethisterone) are the most closely related, pharmacologically as well as chemically, to progesterone. A new group of third-generation synthetic progestins has been introduced, principally as components of oral contraceptives. These "19-nor, 13-ethyl" steroid compounds include desogestrel (see Figure 40–4), gestodene, and norgestimate. They are claimed to have lower androgenic activity than older synthetic progestins.

Pharmacokinetics

Progesterone is rapidly absorbed following administration by any route. Its half-life in the plasma is approximately 5 minutes, and small amounts are stored temporarily in body fat. It is almost completely metabolized in one passage through the liver, and for that reason it is quite ineffective when the usual formulation is administered orally. However, high-dose oral micronized progesterone preparations have been developed that provide adequate progestational effect.

In the liver, progesterone is metabolized to pregnanediol and conjugated with glucuronic acid. It is excreted into the urine as pregnanediol glucuronide. The amount of pregnanediol in the urine has been used as an index of progesterone secretion. This measure has been very useful despite the fact that the proportion of secreted progesterone converted to this compound varies from day to day and from individual to individual. In addition to progesterone, 20α- and 20β-hydroxyprogesterone (20α- and 20β-hydroxy-4-pregnene-3-one) also are found. These compounds have about one fifth the progestational activity of progesterone in humans and other species. Little is known of their physiologic role, but 20α-hydroxyprogesterone is produced in large amounts in some species and may be of some importance biologically.

The usual routes of administration and durations of action of the synthetic progestins are listed in Table 40–2. Most of these agents are extensively metabolized to inactive products that are excreted mainly in the urine.

TABLE 40–2 Properties of some progestational agents.

			Activities[1]				
	Route	**Duration of Action**	***Estrogenic***	***Androgenic***	***Antiestrogenic***	***Antiandrogenic***	***Anabolic***
Progesterone and derivatives							
Progesterone	IM	1 day	–	–	+	–	–
Hydroxyprogesterone caproate	IM	8–14 days	sl	sl	–	–	–
Medroxyprogesterone acetate	IM, PO	Tabs: 1–3 days; injection: 4–12 weeks	–	+	+	–	–
Megestrol acetate	PO	1–3 days	–	+	–	+	–
17-Ethinyl testosterone derivatives							
Dimethisterone	PO	1–3 days	–	–	sl	–	–
19-Nortestosterone derivatives							
Desogestrel	PO	1–3 days	–	–	–	–	–
Norethynodrel	PO	1–3 days	+	–	–	–	–
Lynestrenol[2]	PO	1–3 days	+	+	–	–	+
Norethindrone	PO	1–3 days	sl	+	+	–	+
Norethindrone acetate	PO	1–3 days	sl	+	+	–	+
Ethynodiol diacetate	PO	1–3 days	sl	+	+	–	–
L-Norgestrel[2]	PO	1–3 days	–	+	+	–	+

[1]*Interpretation:* + = active; – = inactive; sl = slightly active. Activities have been reported in various species using various end points and may not apply to humans.

[2]Not available in the USA.

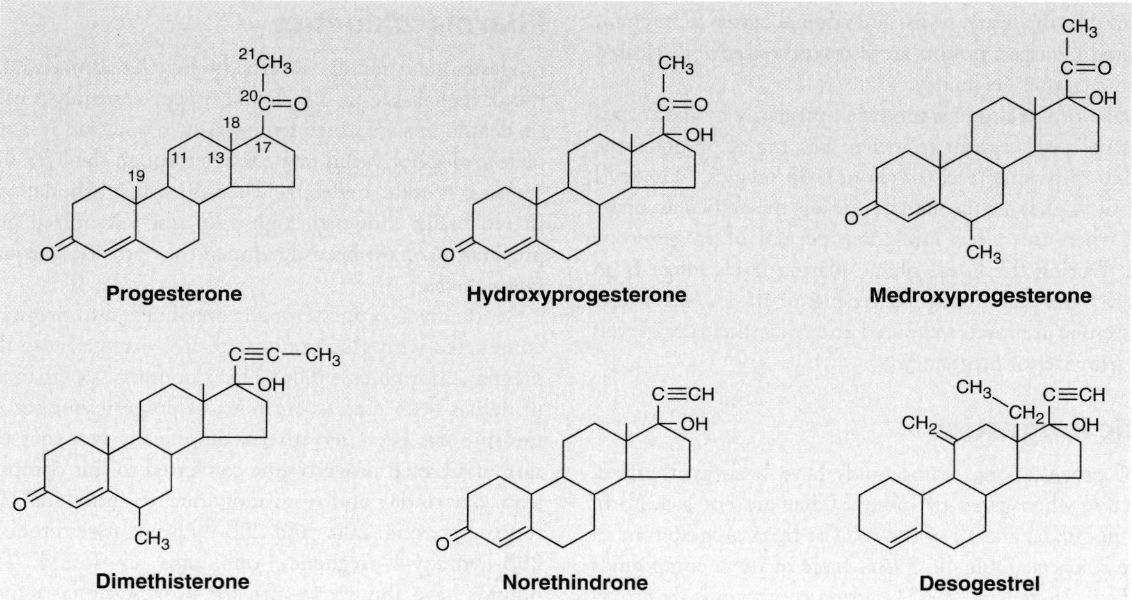

FIGURE 40–4 Progesterone and some progestational agents in clinical use.

Physiologic Effects

A. Mechanism

The mechanism of action of progesterone—described in more detail above—is similar to that of other steroid hormones. Progestins enter the cell and bind to progesterone receptors that are distributed in the nucleus and the cytoplasm. The ligand-receptor complex binds to a progesterone response element (PRE) to activate gene transcription. The response element for progesterone appears to be similar to the corticosteroid response element, and the specificity of the response depends upon which receptor is present in the cell as well as upon other cell-specific receptor coregulators and interacting transcription factors. The progesterone-receptor complex forms a dimer before binding to DNA. Like the estrogen receptor, it can form heterodimers as well as homodimers between two isoforms, A and B. These isoforms are produced by alternative splicing of the same gene.

B. Effects of Progesterone

Progesterone has little effect on protein metabolism. It stimulates lipoprotein lipase activity and seems to favor fat deposition. The effects on carbohydrate metabolism are more marked. Progesterone increases basal insulin levels and the insulin response to glucose. There is usually no manifest change in carbohydrate tolerance. In the liver, progesterone promotes glycogen storage, possibly by facilitating the effect of insulin. Progesterone also promotes ketogenesis.

Progesterone can compete with aldosterone for the mineralocorticoid receptor of the renal tubule, causing a decrease in Na^+ reabsorption. This leads to an increased secretion of aldosterone by the adrenal cortex (eg, in pregnancy). Progesterone increases body temperature in humans. The mechanism of this effect is not known, but an alteration of the temperature-regulating centers in the hypothalamus has been suggested. Progesterone also alters the function of the respiratory centers. The ventilatory response to CO_2 is increased by progesterone but synthetic progestins with an ethinyl group do not have respiratory effects. This leads to a measurable reduction in arterial and alveolar P_{CO_2} during pregnancy and in the luteal phase of the menstrual cycle. Progesterone and related steroids also have depressant and hypnotic effects on the brain.

Progesterone is responsible for the alveolobular development of the secretory apparatus in the breast. It also participates in the preovulatory LH surge and causes the maturation and secretory changes in the endometrium that are seen following ovulation (see Figure 40–1).

Progesterone decreases the plasma levels of many amino acids and leads to increased urinary nitrogen excretion. It induces changes in the structure and function of smooth endoplasmic reticulum in experimental animals.

Other effects of progesterone and its analogs are noted below in the section, Hormonal Contraception.

C. Synthetic Progestins

The 21-carbon progesterone analogs antagonize aldosterone-induced sodium retention (see above). The remaining compounds ("19-nortestosterone" third-generation agents) produce a decidual change in the endometrial stroma, do not support pregnancy in test animals, are more effective gonadotropin inhibitors, and may have minimal estrogenic and androgenic or anabolic activity (Table 40–2; see Figure 40–4). They are sometimes referred to as "impeded androgens." Progestins without androgenic activity include desogestrel, norgestimate, and gestodene. The first two of these compounds are dispensed in combination with ethinyl estradiol for oral contraception (Table 40–3) in the United States. Oral contraceptives containing the progestin cyproterone acetate

TABLE 40–3 Some oral and implantable contraceptive agents in use.[1]

	Estrogen (mg)		Progestin (mg)	
Monophasic Combination Tablets				
Aviane, Falmina, Lessina, Lutera, Orsythia, Sronyx	Ethinyl estradiol	0.02	L-Norgestrel	0.1
Beyaz, Gianvi, Loryna, Yaz, Vestura	Ethinyl estradiol	0.02	Drospirone	3
Gildess 1/20, Junel, Loestrin, Microgestin, Minastrin	Ethinyl estradiol	0.02	Norethindrone	1
Apri, Desogen, Ortho-Cept, Reclipsen, Solia	Ethinyl estradiol	0.03	Desonorgestrel	0.15
Altavera, Chateal, Introvate, Jolessa, Kurvelo, Levora, Marlissa, Portia	Ethinyl estradiol	0.03	L-Norgestrel	0.15
Cryselle, Elinest, Low-Ogestrel	Ethinyl estradiol	0.03	Norgestrel	0.30
Ocella, Safyral, Syeda, Yasmin, Zarah	Ethinyl estradiol	0.03	Drospirenone	3
Gildess, Junel, Loestrin, Microgestin	Ethinyl estradiol	0.03	Norethindrone	1.5
Cyclafem 1/35, Necon 1/35, Norinyl 1/35	Ethinyl estradiol	0.035	Norethindrone	1
Estarylla, MonoNessa, Ortho-Cyclen, Previfem, Sprintec	Ethinyl estradiol	0.035	Norgestimate	0.25
Alyacen 1/35; Cyclafem 1/35, Dasetta 1/35, Necon 1/35, Norinyl 1+35, Nortrel 1/35, Ortho-Novum 1/35, Pirmella 1/35	Ethinyl estradiol	0.035	Norethindrone	1
Brevicon, Modicon, Necon 0.5/35, Nortrel 0.5/35, Wera	Ethinyl estradiol	0.035	Norethindrone	0.5
Ovcon-35, Femcon Fe, Balziva, Briellyn, Gildagia, others	Ethinyl estradiol	0.035	Norethindrone	0.4
Ogestrel 0.5/50	Ethinyl estradiol	0.05	D,L-Norgestrel	0.5
Norinyl 1+50, Necon 1/50	Mestranol	0.05	Norethindrone	1
Biphasic Combination Tablets				
Azurette, Kariva, Mircette, Viorele				
Days 1–21	Ethinyl estradiol	0.02	Desogestrel	0.15
Days 22–27	Ethinyl estradiol	0.01	None	
Necon 10/11				
Days 1–10	Ethinyl estradiol	0.035	Norethindrone	0.5
Days 11–21	Ethinyl estradiol	0.035	Norethindrone	1.0
Triphasic Combination Tablets				
Enpresse, Levonest, Myzilra, Triphasil, Tri-Levlen, Trivora				
Days 1–6	Ethinyl estradiol	0.03	L-Norgestrel	0.05
Days 7–11	Ethinyl estradiol	0.04	L-Norgestrel	0.075
Days 12–21	Ethinyl estradiol	0.03	L-Norgestrel	0.125
Casiant, Cyclessa, Cesia, Velivet				
Days 1–6	Ethinyl estradiol	0.025	Desogestrel	0.1
Days 7–14	Ethinyl estradiol	0.025	Desogestrel	0.125
Days 15–21	Ethinyl estradiol	0.025	Desogestrel	0.15
Alyacen 7/7/7, Cyclafem 7/7/7, Dasetta 7/7/7, Ortho-Novum 7/7/7, Necon 7/7/7, Nortrel 7/7/7, Pirmella 7/7/7				
Days 1–7	Ethinyl estradiol	0.035	Norethindrone	0.5
Days 8–14	Ethinyl estradiol	0.035	Norethindrone	0.75
Days 15–21	Ethinyl estradiol	0.035	Norethindrone	1.0
Ortho-Tri-Cyclen				
Days 1–7	Ethinyl estradiol	0.035	Norgestimate	0.18
Days 8–14	Ethinyl estradiol	0.035	Norgestimate	0.215
Days 15–21	Ethinyl estradiol	0.035	Norgestimate	0.25

(continued)

TABLE 40–3 Some oral and implantable contraceptive agents in use.[1] (Continued)

	Estrogen (mg)		Progestin (mg)	
4-Phasic Combination Tablet				
Natazia				
Days 1–2	Estradiol valerate	3	None	—
Days 3–8	Estradiol valerate	2	Dienogest	2
Days 9–25	Estradiol valerate	2	Dienogest	3
Day 26–27	Estradiol valerate	1	None	—
Daily Progestin Tablets				
Camila, Errin, Heather, Jencycla, Jolivette, Lyza, Nora-BE, Nor-QD, Ortho Micronor	None	—	Norethindrone	0.35
Contraceptive Transdermal Patch (Apply 1 Patch per Week)				
Ortho Evra	Ethinyl estradiol	0.02/24 h	Norgestromin	0.150/24 h
Implantable Progestin Preparation				
Implanon, Nexplanon	None		Etonogestrel (one tube of 68 mg)	

[1]The estrogen-containing compounds are arranged in order of increasing content of estrogen. Other preparations are available. (Ethinyl estradiol and mestranol have similar potencies.)

(also an antiandrogen) in combination with ethinyl estradiol are investigational in the United States.

Clinical Uses

A. Therapeutic Applications

The major uses of progestational hormones are for hormone replacement therapy (see above) and hormonal contraception (see below). In addition, they are useful in producing long-term ovarian suppression for other purposes. When used alone in large doses parenterally (eg, medroxyprogesterone acetate, 150 mg intramuscularly every 90 days), prolonged anovulation and amenorrhea result. This therapy has been employed in the treatment of dysmenorrhea, endometriosis, and bleeding disorders when estrogens are contraindicated, and for contraception. The major problem with this regimen is the prolonged time required in some patients for ovulatory function to return after cessation of therapy. It should not be used for patients planning a pregnancy in the near future. Similar regimens will relieve hot flushes in some menopausal women and can be used if estrogen therapy is contraindicated.

Medroxyprogesterone acetate, 10–20 mg orally twice weekly—or intramuscularly in doses of 100 mg/m^2 every 1–2 weeks—will prevent menstruation, but it will not arrest accelerated bone maturation in children with precocious puberty.

Progestins do not appear to have any place in the therapy of threatened or habitual abortion. Early reports of the usefulness of these agents resulted from the unwarranted assumption that after several abortions the likelihood of repeated abortions was over 90%. When progestational agents were administered to patients with previous abortions, a salvage rate of 80% was achieved. It is now recognized that similar patients abort only 20% of the time even when untreated. On the other hand, progesterone was given experimentally to delay premature labor with encouraging results.

Progesterone and medroxyprogesterone have been used in the treatment of women who have difficulty in conceiving and who demonstrate a slow rise in basal body temperature. There is no convincing evidence that this treatment is effective.

Preparations of progesterone and medroxyprogesterone have been used to treat premenstrual syndrome. Controlled studies have not confirmed the effectiveness of such therapy except when doses sufficient to suppress ovulation have been used.

B. Diagnostic Uses

Progesterone can be used as a test of estrogen secretion. The administration of progesterone, 150 mg/d, or medroxyprogesterone, 10 mg/d, for 5–7 days, is followed by withdrawal bleeding in amenorrheic patients only when the endometrium has been stimulated by estrogens. A combination of estrogen and progestin can be given to test the responsiveness of the endometrium in patients with amenorrhea.

Contraindications, Cautions, & Adverse Effects

Studies of progestational compounds alone and with combination oral contraceptives indicate that the progestin in these agents may increase blood pressure in some patients. The more androgenic progestins also reduce plasma HDL levels in women. (See section Hormonal Contraception.) Two recent studies suggest that combined progestin plus estrogen replacement therapy in postmenopausal women may increase breast cancer risk significantly compared with the risk in women taking estrogen alone. These findings require careful examination and if confirmed will lead to important changes in postmenopausal hormone replacement practice.

OTHER OVARIAN HORMONES

The normal ovary produces small amounts of **androgens,** including testosterone, androstenedione, and dehydroepiandrosterone. Of these, only testosterone has a significant amount of biologic activity, although androstenedione can be converted to testosterone or estrone in peripheral tissues. The normal woman produces less than 200 mcg of testosterone in 24 hours, and about one-third of this is probably formed in the ovary directly. The physiologic significance of these small amounts of androgens is not established, but they may be partly responsible for normal hair growth at puberty, for stimulation of female libido, and, possibly, for metabolic effects. Androgen production by the ovary may be markedly increased in some abnormal states, usually in association with hirsutism and amenorrhea as noted above.

The ovary also produces **inhibin** and **activin.** These peptides consist of several combinations of α and β subunits and are described in greater detail later. The $\alpha\beta$ dimer (inhibin) inhibits FSH secretion while the $\beta\beta$ dimer (activin) increases FSH secretion. Studies in primates indicate that inhibin has no direct effect on ovarian steroidogenesis but that activin modulates the response to LH and FSH. For example, simultaneous treatment with activin and human FSH enhances FSH stimulation of progesterone synthesis and aromatase activity in granulosa cells. When combined with LH, activin suppressed the LH-induced progesterone response by 50% but markedly enhanced basal and LH-stimulated aromatase activity. Activin may also act as a growth factor in other tissues. The physiologic roles of these modulators are not fully understood.

Relaxin is another peptide that can be extracted from the ovary. The three-dimensional structure of relaxin is related to that of growth-promoting peptides and is similar to that of insulin. Although the amino acid sequence differs from that of insulin, this hormone, like insulin, consists of two chains linked by disulfide bonds, cleaved from a prohormone. It is found in the ovary, placenta, uterus, and blood. Relaxin synthesis has been demonstrated in luteinized granulosa cells of the corpus luteum. It has been shown to increase glycogen synthesis and water uptake by the myometrium and to decrease uterine contractility. In some species, it changes the mechanical properties of the cervix and pubic ligaments, facilitating delivery.

In women, relaxin has been measured by immunoassay. Levels were highest immediately after the LH surge and during menstruation. A physiologic role for this peptide has not been established.

Clinical trials with relaxin have been conducted in patients with dysmenorrhea. Relaxin has also been administered to patients in premature labor and during prolonged labor. When applied to the cervix of a woman at term, it facilitates dilation and shortens labor.

Several other nonsteroidal substances such as corticotropin-releasing hormone, follistatin, and prostaglandins are produced by the ovary. These probably have paracrine effects within the ovary.

■ HORMONAL CONTRACEPTION (ORAL, PARENTERAL, & IMPLANTED CONTRACEPTIVES)

A large number of oral contraceptives containing estrogens or progestins (or both) are now available for clinical use (see Table 40–3). These preparations vary chemically and pharmacologically and have many properties in common as well as definite differences important for the correct selection of the optimum agent.

Two types of preparations are used for oral contraception: (1) combinations of estrogens and progestins and (2) continuous progestin therapy without concomitant administration of estrogens. The combination agents are further d ivided into **monophasic** forms (constant dosage of both components during the cycle) and **multiphasic** forms (dosage of one or both components is changed once or more during the cycle). The preparations for oral use are all adequately absorbed, and in combination preparations the pharmacokinetics of neither drug is significantly altered by the other.

Only one implantable contraceptive preparation is available at present in the USA. Etonogestrel, also used in some oral contraceptives, is available in the subcutaneous implant form listed in Table 40–3. Several hormonal contraceptives are available as vaginal rings or intrauterine devices. Intramuscular injection of large doses of medroxyprogesterone also provides contraception of long duration.

Pharmacologic Effects

A. Mechanism of Action

The combinations of estrogens and progestins exert their contraceptive effect largely through selective inhibition of pituitary function that results in inhibition of ovulation. The combination agents also produce a change in the cervical mucus, in the uterine endometrium, and in motility and secretion in the uterine tubes, all of which decrease the likelihood of conception and implantation. The continuous use of progestins alone does not always inhibit ovulation. The other factors mentioned, therefore, play a major role in the prevention of pregnancy when these agents are used.

B. Effects on the Ovary

Chronic use of combination agents depresses ovarian function. Follicular development is minimal, and corpora lutea, larger follicles, stromal edema, and other morphologic features normally seen in ovulating women are absent. The ovaries usually become smaller even if enlarged before therapy.

The great majority of patients return to normal menstrual patterns when these drugs are discontinued. About 75% will ovulate in the first posttreatment cycle and 97% by the third posttreatment cycle. About 2% of patients remain amenorrheic for periods of up to several years after administration is stopped.

The cytologic findings on vaginal smears vary depending on the preparation used. However, with almost all of the combined drugs, a low maturation index is found because of the presence of progestational agents.

C. Effects on the Uterus

After prolonged use, the cervix may show some hypertrophy and polyp formation. There are also important effects on the cervical mucus, making it more like postovulation mucus, ie, thicker and less copious.

Agents containing both estrogens and progestins produce further morphologic and biochemical changes of the endometrial stroma under the influence of the progestin, which also stimulates glandular secretion throughout the luteal phase. The agents containing "19-nor" progestins—particularly those with the smaller amounts of estrogen—tend to produce more glandular atrophy and usually less bleeding.

D. Effects on the Breast

Stimulation of the breasts occurs in most patients receiving estrogen-containing agents. Some enlargement is generally noted. The administration of estrogens and combinations of estrogens and progestins tends to suppress lactation, but when the doses are small, the effects on breast-feeding are not appreciable. Studies of the transport of the oral contraceptives into breast milk suggest that only small amounts of these compounds cross into the milk, and they have not been considered to be of importance.

E. Other Effects of Oral Contraceptives

1. *Effects on the central nervous system*—The central nervous system effects of the oral contraceptives have not been well studied in humans. A variety of effects of estrogen and progesterone have been noted in animals. Estrogens tend to increase excitability in the brain, whereas progesterone tends to decrease it. The thermogenic action of progesterone and some of the synthetic progestins is also thought to occur in the central nervous system.

It is very difficult to evaluate any behavioral or emotional effects of these compounds in humans. Although the incidence of pronounced changes in mood, affect, and behavior appears to be low, milder changes are commonly reported, and estrogens are being successfully employed in the therapy of premenstrual tension syndrome, postpartum depression, and climacteric depression.

2. *Effects on endocrine function*—The inhibition of pituitary gonadotropin secretion has been mentioned. Estrogens also alter adrenal structure and function. Estrogens given orally or at high doses increase the plasma concentration of the α_2 globulin that binds cortisol (corticosteroid-binding globulin). Plasma concentrations may be more than double the levels found in untreated individuals, and urinary excretion of free cortisol is elevated.

These preparations cause alterations in the renin-angiotensin-aldosterone system. Plasma renin activity has been found to increase, and there is an increase in aldosterone secretion.

Thyroxine-binding globulin is increased. As a result, total plasma thyroxine (T_4) levels are increased to those commonly seen during pregnancy. Since more of the thyroxine is bound, the free thyroxine level in these patients is normal. Estrogens also increase the plasma level of SHBG and decrease plasma levels of free androgens by increasing their binding; large amounts of estrogen may decrease androgens by gonadotropin suppression.

3. *Effects on blood*—Serious thromboembolic phenomena occurring in women taking oral contraceptives gave rise to a great many studies of the effects of these compounds on blood coagulation. A clear picture of such effects has not yet emerged. The oral contraceptives do not consistently alter bleeding or clotting times. The changes that have been observed are similar to those reported in pregnancy. There is an increase in factors VII, VIII, IX, and X and a decrease in antithrombin III. Increased amounts of coumarin anticoagulants may be required to prolong prothrombin time in patients taking oral contraceptives.

There is an increase in serum iron and total iron-binding capacity similar to that reported in patients with hepatitis.

Significant alterations in the cellular components of blood have not been reported with any consistency. A number of patients have been reported to develop folic acid deficiency anemias.

4. *Effects on the liver*—These hormones also have profound effects on the function of the liver. Some of these effects are deleterious and will be considered below in the section on adverse effects. The effects on serum proteins result from the effects of the estrogens on the synthesis of the various α_2 globulins and fibrinogen. Serum haptoglobins produced in the liver are depressed rather than increased by estrogen. Some of the effects on carbohydrate and lipid metabolism are probably influenced by changes in liver metabolism (see below).

Important alterations in hepatic drug excretion and metabolism also occur. Estrogens in the amounts seen during pregnancy or used in oral contraceptive agents delay the clearance of sulfobromophthalein and reduce the flow of bile. The proportion of cholic acid in bile acids is increased while the proportion of chenodeoxycholic acid is decreased. These changes may be responsible for the observed increase in cholelithiasis associated with the use of these agents.

5. *Effects on lipid metabolism*—As noted above, estrogens increase serum triglycerides and free and esterified cholesterol. Phospholipids are also increased, as are HDL; levels of LDL usually decrease. Although the effects are marked with doses of 100 mcg of mestranol or ethinyl estradiol, doses of 50 mcg or less have minimal effects. The progestins (particularly the "19-nortestosterone" derivatives) tend to antagonize these effects of estrogen. Preparations containing small amounts of estrogen and a progestin may slightly decrease triglycerides and HDL.

6. *Effects on carbohydrate metabolism*—The administration of oral contraceptives produces alterations in carbohydrate metabolism similar to those observed in pregnancy. There is a reduction in the rate of absorption of carbohydrates from the gastrointestinal tract. Progesterone increases the basal insulin level and the rise in insulin induced by carbohydrate ingestion. Preparations with more potent progestins such as norgestrel may cause progressive decreases in carbohydrate tolerance over several years. However, the changes in glucose tolerance are reversible on discontinuing medication.

7. *Effects on the cardiovascular system*—These agents cause small increases in cardiac output associated with higher systolic and diastolic blood pressure and heart rate. The pressure returns to pretreatment levels when treatment is terminated. Although the magnitude of the pressure change is small in most patients, it is marked in a few. It is important that blood pressure be followed in each patient. An increase in blood pressure has been reported to occur in a few postmenopausal women treated with estrogens alone.

8. *Effects on the skin*—The oral contraceptives have been noted to increase pigmentation of the skin (chloasma). This effect seems to be enhanced in women with dark complexions and by exposure to ultraviolet light. Some of the androgen-like progestins might increase the production of sebum, causing acne in some patients. However, since ovarian androgen is suppressed, many patients note decreased sebum production, acne, and terminal hair growth. The sequential oral contraceptive preparations as well as estrogens alone often decrease sebum production.

Clinical Uses

The most important use of combined estrogens and progestins is for oral contraception. A large number of preparations are available for this specific purpose, some of which are listed in Table 40–3. They are specially packaged for ease of administration. In general, they are very effective; when these agents are taken according to directions, the risk of conception is extremely small. The pregnancy rate with combination agents is estimated to be about 5–12 per 100 woman-years at risk. (Under conditions of perfect adherence, the pregnancy rate would be 0.5–1 per 100 woman-years.) Contraceptive failure has been observed in some patients when one or more doses are missed, if phenytoin is also being used (which may increase catabolism of the compounds), or if antibiotics are taken that alter enterohepatic cycling of metabolites.

Progestins and estrogens are also useful in the treatment of endometriosis. When severe dysmenorrhea is the major symptom, the suppression of ovulation with estrogen alone may be followed by painless periods. However, in most patients this approach is inadequate. The long-term administration of large doses of progestins or combinations of progestins and estrogens prevents the periodic breakdown of the endometrial tissue and in some cases will lead to endometrial fibrosis and prevent the reactivation of implants for prolonged periods.

As is true with most hormonal preparations, many of the undesired effects are physiologic or pharmacologic actions that are objectionable only because they are not pertinent to the situation for which they are being used. Therefore, the product containing the smallest effective amounts of hormones should be selected for use.

Adverse Effects

The incidence of serious known toxicities associated with the use of these drugs is low—far lower than the risks associated with pregnancy. There are a number of reversible changes in intermediary metabolism. Minor adverse effects are frequent, but most are mild and many are transient. Continuing problems may respond to simple changes in pill formulation. Although it is not often necessary to discontinue medication for these reasons, as many as one-third of all patients started on oral contraception discontinue use for reasons other than a desire to become pregnant.

A. Mild Adverse Effects

1. Nausea, mastalgia, breakthrough bleeding, and edema are related to the amount of estrogen in the preparation. These effects can often be alleviated by a shift to a preparation containing smaller amounts of estrogen or to agents containing progestins with more androgenic effects.
2. Changes in serum proteins and other effects on endocrine function (see above) must be taken into account when thyroid, adrenal, or pituitary function is being evaluated. Increases in sedimentation rate are thought to be due to increased levels of fibrinogen.
3. Headache is mild and often transient. However, migraine is often made worse and has been reported to be associated with an increased frequency of cerebrovascular accidents. When this occurs or when migraine has its onset during therapy with these agents, treatment should be discontinued.
4. Withdrawal bleeding sometimes fails to occur—most often with combination preparations—and may cause confusion with regard to pregnancy. If this is disturbing to the patient, a different preparation may be tried or other methods of contraception used.

B. Moderate Adverse Effects

Any of the following may require discontinuance of oral contraceptives:

1. Breakthrough bleeding is the most common problem in using progestational agents alone for contraception. It occurs in as many as 25% of patients. It is more frequently encountered in patients taking low-dose preparations than in those taking combination pills with higher levels of progestin and estrogen. The biphasic and triphasic oral contraceptives (see Table 40–3) decrease breakthrough bleeding without increasing the total hormone content.
2. Weight gain is more common with the combination agents containing androgen-like progestins. It can usually be controlled by shifting to preparations with less progestin effect or by dieting.
3. Increased skin pigmentation may occur, especially in dark-skinned women. It tends to increase with time, the incidence being about 5% at the end of the first year and about 40% after 8 years. It is thought to be exacerbated by vitamin B deficiency. It is often reversible upon discontinuance of medication but may disappear very slowly.
4. Acne may be exacerbated by agents containing androgen-like progestins (see Table 40–2), whereas agents containing large amounts of estrogen usually cause marked improvement in acne.

5. Hirsutism may also be aggravated by the "19-nortestosterone" derivatives, and combinations containing nonandrogenic progestins are preferred in these patients.
6. Ureteral dilation similar to that observed in pregnancy has been reported, and bacteriuria is more frequent.
7. Vaginal infections are more common and more difficult to treat in patients who are using oral contraceptives.
8. Amenorrhea occurs in some patients. Following cessation of administration of oral contraceptives, 95% of patients with normal menstrual histories resume normal periods and all but a few resume normal cycles during the next few months. However, some patients remain amenorrheic for several years. Many of these patients also have galactorrhea. Patients who have had menstrual irregularities before taking oral contraceptives are particularly susceptible to prolonged amenorrhea when the agents are discontinued. Prolactin levels should be measured in these patients, since many have prolactinomas.

C. Severe Adverse Effects

1. *Vascular disorders*—Thromboembolism was one of the earliest of the serious unanticipated effects to be reported and has been the most thoroughly studied.

***a.* VENOUS THROMBOEMBOLIC DISEASE—**Superficial or deep thromboembolic disease in women not taking oral contraceptives occurs in about 1 patient per 1000 woman years. The overall incidence of these disorders in patients taking low-dose oral contraceptives is about threefold higher. The risk for this disorder is increased during the first month of contraceptive use and remains constant for several years or more. The risk returns to normal within a month when use is discontinued. The risk of venous thrombosis or pulmonary embolism is increased among women with predisposing conditions such as stasis, altered clotting factors such as antithrombin III, increased levels of homocysteine, or injury. Genetic disorders, including mutations in the genes governing the production of protein C (factor V Leiden), protein S, hepatic cofactor II, and others, markedly increase the risk of venous thromboembolism. The incidence of these disorders is too low for cost-effective screening by current methods, but prior episodes or a family history may be helpful in identifying patients with increased risk.

The incidence of venous thromboembolism appears to be related to the estrogen but not the progestin content of oral contraceptives and is not related to age, parity, mild obesity, or cigarette smoking. Decreased venous blood flow, endothelial proliferation in veins and arteries, and increased coagulability of blood resulting from changes in platelet functions and fibrinolytic systems contribute to the increased incidence of thrombosis. The major plasma inhibitor of thrombin, antithrombin III, is substantially decreased during oral contraceptive use. This change occurs in the first month of treatment and lasts as long as treatment persists, reversing within a month thereafter.

***b.* MYOCARDIAL INFARCTION—**The use of oral contraceptives is associated with a slightly higher risk of myocardial infarction in women who are obese, have a history of preeclampsia or hypertension, or have hyperlipoproteinemia or diabetes. There is a much higher risk in women who smoke. The risk attributable to oral contraceptives in women 30–40 years of age who do not smoke is about 4 cases per 100,000 users per year, as compared with 185 cases per 100,000 among women 40–44 who smoke heavily. The association with myocardial infarction is thought to involve acceleration of atherogenesis because of decreased glucose tolerance, decreased levels of HDL, increased levels of LDL, and increased platelet aggregation. In addition, facilitation of coronary arterial spasm may play a role in some of these patients. The progestational component of oral contraceptives decreases HDL cholesterol levels, in proportion to the androgenic activity of the progestin. The net effect, therefore, will depend on the specific composition of the pill used and the patient's susceptibility to the particular effects. Recent studies suggest that risk of infarction is not increased in past users who have discontinued oral contraceptives.

***c.* CEREBROVASCULAR DISEASE—**The risk of stroke is concentrated in women over age 35. It is increased in current users of oral contraceptives but not in past users. However, subarachnoid hemorrhages have been found to be increased among both current and past users and may increase with time. The risk of thrombotic or hemorrhagic stroke attributable to oral contraceptives (based on older, higher-dose preparations) has been estimated at about 37 cases per 100,000 users per year.

In summary, available data indicate that oral contraceptives increase the risk of various cardiovascular disorders at all ages and among both smokers and nonsmokers. However, this risk appears to be concentrated in women 35 years of age or older who are heavy smokers. It is clear that these risk factors must be considered in each individual patient for whom oral contraceptives are being considered. Some experts have suggested that screening for coagulopathy should be performed before starting oral contraception.

2. *Gastrointestinal disorders*—Many cases of cholestatic jaundice have been reported in patients taking progestin-containing drugs. The differences in incidence of these disorders from one population to another suggest that genetic factors may be involved. The jaundice caused by these agents is similar to that produced by other 17-alkyl-substituted steroids. It is most often observed in the first three cycles and is particularly common in women with a history of cholestatic jaundice during pregnancy. Jaundice and pruritus disappear 1–8 weeks after the drug is discontinued.

These agents have also been found to increase the incidence of symptomatic gallbladder disease, including cholecystitis and cholangitis. This is probably the result of the alterations responsible for jaundice and bile acid changes described above.

It also appears that the incidence of hepatic adenomas is increased in women taking oral contraceptives. Ischemic bowel disease secondary to thrombosis of the celiac and superior and inferior mesenteric arteries and veins has also been reported in women using these drugs.

3. *Depression*—Depression of sufficient degree to require cessation of therapy occurs in about 6% of patients treated with some preparations.

4. *Cancer*—The occurrence of malignant tumors in patients taking oral contraceptives has been studied extensively. It is now clear that these compounds *reduce* the risk of endometrial and ovarian cancer. The lifetime risk of breast cancer in the population as a whole does not seem to be affected by oral contraceptive use. Some studies have shown an increased risk in younger women, and it is possible that tumors that develop in younger women become clinically apparent sooner. The relation of risk of cervical cancer to oral contraceptive use is still controversial. It should be noted that a number of recent studies associate the use of oral contraceptives by women who are infected with human papillomavirus with an increased risk of cervical cancer.

5. *Other*—In addition to the above effects, a number of other adverse reactions have been reported for which a causal relation has not been established. These include alopecia, erythema multiforme, erythema nodosum, and other skin disorders.

Contraindications & Cautions

These drugs are contraindicated in patients with thrombophlebitis, thromboembolic phenomena, and cardiovascular and cerebrovascular disorders or a past history of these conditions. They should not be used to treat vaginal bleeding when the cause is unknown. They should be avoided in patients with known or suspected tumors of the breast or other estrogen-dependent neoplasms. Since these preparations have caused aggravation of preexisting disorders, they should be avoided or used with caution in patients with liver disease, asthma, eczema, migraine, diabetes, hypertension, optic neuritis, retrobulbar neuritis, or convulsive disorders.

The oral contraceptives may produce edema, and for that reason they should be used with great caution in patients in heart failure or in whom edema is otherwise undesirable or dangerous.

Estrogens may increase the rate of growth of fibroids. Therefore, for women with these tumors, agents with the smallest amounts of estrogen and the most androgenic progestins should be selected. The use of progestational agents alone for contraception might be especially useful in such patients (see below).

These agents are contraindicated in adolescents in whom epiphyseal closure has not yet been completed.

Women using oral contraceptives must be made aware of an important interaction that occurs with antimicrobial drugs. Because the normal gastrointestinal flora increase the enterohepatic cycling (and bioavailability) of estrogens, antimicrobial drugs that interfere with these organisms may reduce the efficacy of oral contraceptives. Additionally, coadministration with potent inducers of the hepatic microsomal metabolizing enzymes, such as rifampin, may increase liver catabolism of estrogens or progestins and diminish the efficacy of oral contraceptives.

Contraception with Progestins Alone

Small doses of progestins administered orally or by implantation under the skin can be used for contraception. They are particularly suited for use in patients for whom estrogen administration is undesirable. They are about as effective as intrauterine devices or combination pills containing 20–30 mcg of ethinyl estradiol. There is a high incidence of abnormal bleeding.

Effective contraception can also be achieved by injecting 150 mg of depot medroxyprogesterone acetate (DMPA) every 3 months. After a 150-mg dose, ovulation is inhibited for at least 14 weeks. Almost all users experience episodes of unpredictable spotting and bleeding, particularly during the first year of use. Spotting and bleeding decrease with time, and amenorrhea is common. This preparation is not desirable for women planning a pregnancy soon after cessation of therapy because ovulation suppression can sometimes persist for as long as 18 months after the last injection. Long-term DMPA use reduces menstrual blood loss and is associated with a decreased risk of endometrial cancer. Suppression of endogenous estrogen secretion may be associated with a reversible reduction in bone density, and changes in plasma lipids are associated with an increased risk of atherosclerosis.

The progestin implant method utilizes the subcutaneous implantation of capsules containing etonogestrel. These capsules release one fifth to one-third as much steroid as oral agents, are extremely effective, and last for 2–4 years. The low levels of hormone have little effect on lipoprotein and carbohydrate metabolism or blood pressure. The disadvantages include the need for surgical insertion and removal of capsules and some irregular bleeding rather than predictable menses. An association of intracranial hypertension with an earlier type of implant utilizing norgestrel was observed in a small number of women. Patients experiencing headache or visual disturbances should be checked for papilledema.

Contraception with progestins is useful in patients with hepatic disease, hypertension, psychosis or mental retardation, or prior thromboembolism. The side effects include headache, dizziness, bloating and weight gain of 1–2 kg, and a reversible reduction of glucose tolerance.

A. Postcoital Contraceptives

Pregnancy can be prevented following coitus by the administration of estrogens alone, progestin alone, or in combination (**morning after** contraception). When treatment is begun within 72 hours, it is effective 99% of the time. Some effective schedules are shown in Table 40–4. The hormones are often administered with antiemetics, since 40% of patients have nausea or vomiting. Other adverse effects include headache, dizziness, breast tenderness, and abdominal and leg cramps. Considerable controversy has accompanied the proposal to make these agents available without a prescription in the United States.

Mifepristone, an antagonist at progesterone and glucocorticoid receptors, has a luteolytic effect and is effective as a postcoital contraceptive. When combined with a prostaglandin it is also an effective abortifacient.

TABLE 40–4 Schedules for use of postcoital contraceptives.

Conjugated estrogens: 10 mg three times daily for 5 days
Ethinyl estradiol: 2.5 mg twice daily for 5 days
Diethylstilbestrol: 50 mg daily for 5 days
Mifepristone: 600 mg once with misoprostol, 400 mcg once[1]
L-Norgestrel: 1.5 mg once (Plan B One-Step[2])
L-Norgestrel: 0.75 mg twice daily for 1 day (eg, Plan B[2])
Norgestrel, 0.5 mg, with ethinyl estradiol, 0.05 mg (eg, Ovral, Preven[2]): Two tablets and then two in 12 hours

[1]Mifepristone given on day 1, misoprostol on day 3.
[2]Sold as emergency contraceptive kits.

Beneficial Effects of Oral Contraceptives

It has become apparent that reduction in the dose of the constituents of oral contraceptives has markedly reduced mild and severe adverse effects, providing a relatively safe and convenient method of contraception for many young women. Treatment with oral contraceptives has also been shown to be associated with many benefits unrelated to contraception. These include a reduced risk of ovarian cysts, ovarian and endometrial cancer, and benign breast disease. There is a lower incidence of ectopic pregnancy. Iron deficiency and rheumatoid arthritis are less common, and premenstrual symptoms, dysmenorrhea, endometriosis, acne, and hirsutism may be ameliorated with their use.

ESTROGEN & PROGESTERONE INHIBITORS & ANTAGONISTS

TAMOXIFEN & RELATED PARTIAL AGONIST ESTROGENS

Tamoxifen, a competitive partial agonist inhibitor of estradiol at the estrogen receptor (Figure 40–5), was the first **selective estrogen receptor modulator (SERM)** to be introduced. The mechanism of its mixed agonist/antagonist relations to the estrogen receptor has been intensively studied but is still not completely understood. Proposals include recruitment of different coregulators to the estrogen receptor when it binds tamoxifen rather than estrogen, differential activation of heterodimers (ERα-ERβ) versus homodimers, competition of ERα by ERβ and others. Tamoxifen is extensively used in the palliative treatment of breast cancer in postmenopausal women and is approved for chemoprevention of breast cancer in high-risk women (see Chapter 54). It is a nonsteroidal agent (see structure below) that is given orally. Peak plasma levels are reached in a few hours. Tamoxifen has an initial half-life of 7–14 hours in the circulation and is predominantly excreted by the liver. One of its metabolites via CYP2D6 is 4-hydroxytamoxifen (endoxifen), a more potent SERM. Therefore, strong inhibitors of 2D6 should be avoided in patients receiving tamoxifen. It is used in doses of 10–20 mg twice daily. Hot flushes and nausea and vomiting occur in 25% of patients, and many other minor adverse effects are observed. Studies of patients treated with tamoxifen as adjuvant therapy for early breast cancer have shown a 35% decrease in contralateral breast cancer. However, adjuvant therapy extended beyond 5 years in patients with breast cancer has shown no further improvement in outcome. In fact, resistant lines of tumor cells may recognize tamoxifen as an agonist rather than an antagonist, perhaps due to changes in the coregulators that interact with the estrogen receptor. **Toremifene** is a structurally similar compound with very similar properties, indications, and toxicities.

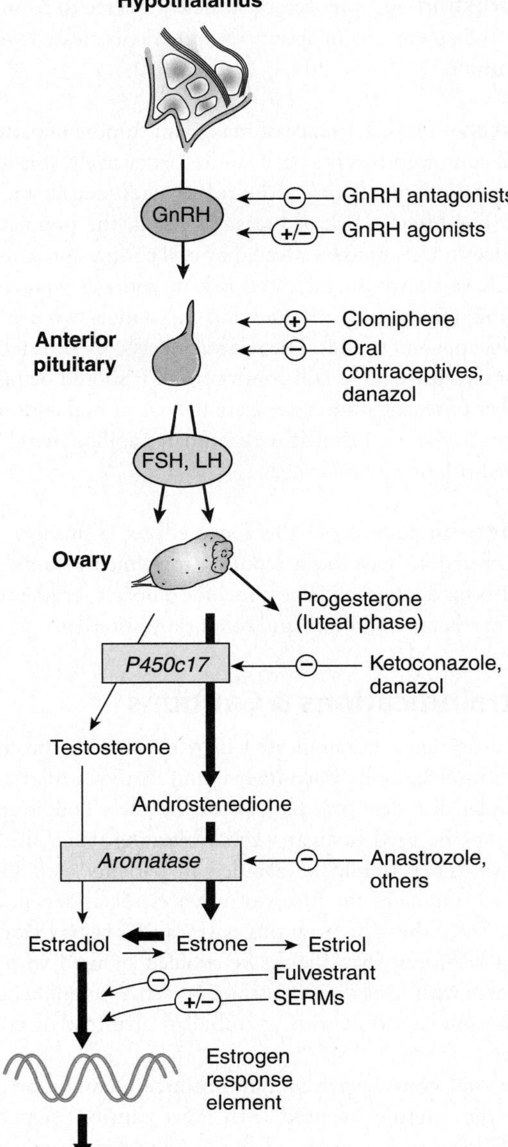

FIGURE 40–5 Control of ovarian secretion and the actions of its hormones. In the follicular phase the ovary produces mainly estrogens; in the luteal phase it produces estrogens and progesterone. SERMs, selective estrogen receptor modulators. See text.

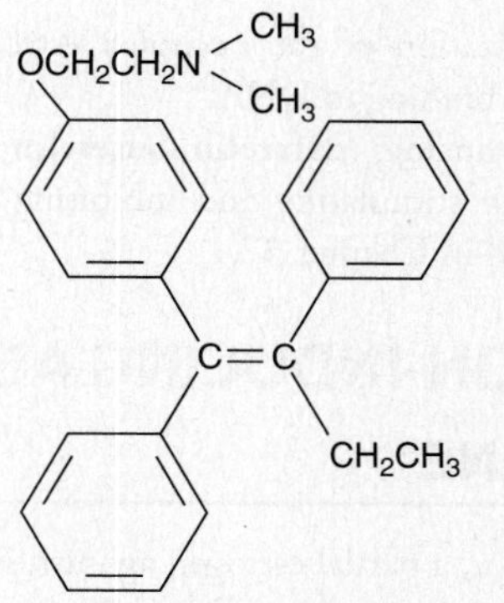

Tamoxifen

Prevention of the expected loss of lumbar spine bone density and plasma lipid changes consistent with a reduction in the risk for atherosclerosis have also been reported in tamoxifen-treated patients following spontaneous or surgical menopause. However, this agonist activity also affects the uterus and may increase the risk of endometrial cancer.

Raloxifene is another partial estrogen agonist-antagonist at some but not all target tissues. It has estrogenic effects on lipids and bone but appears not to stimulate the endometrium or breast. Although subject to a high first-pass effect, raloxifene has a very large volume of distribution and a long half-life (>24 hours), so it can be taken once a day. Raloxifene has been approved in the United States for the prevention of postmenopausal osteoporosis and prophylaxis of breast cancer in women with risk factors. Newer SERMs have been developed and one, **bazedoxifene,** in combination with conjugated estrogens, is approved for treatment of menopausal symptoms and prophylaxis of postmenopausal osteoporosis.

Clomiphene is an older partial agonist, a weak estrogen that also acts as a competitive inhibitor of endogenous estrogens (see Figure 40–5). It has found use as an ovulation-inducing agent (see below).

MIFEPRISTONE (RU-486)

Mifepristone is a "19-norsteroid" that binds strongly to the progesterone and glucocorticoid receptors and inhibits the activity of progesterone and that of glucocorticoids (see Chapter 39). The drug has luteolytic properties in 80% of women when given in the midluteal period. The mechanism of this effect is unknown, but it may provide the basis for using mifepristone as a contraceptive (as opposed to an abortifacient). However, because the compound has a long half-life of 20–40 hours, large doses may prolong the follicular phase of the subsequent cycle and so make it difficult to use continuously for this purpose. A single dose of 600 mg is an effective emergency postcoital contraceptive, though it may result in delayed ovulation in the following cycle. As noted in Chapter 39, the drug also binds to and acts as an antagonist at the glucocorticoid receptor. Limited clinical studies suggest that mifepristone or other analogs with similar properties may be useful in the treatment of endometriosis, Cushing syndrome, breast cancer, and possibly other neoplasms such as meningiomas that contain glucocorticoid or progesterone receptors.

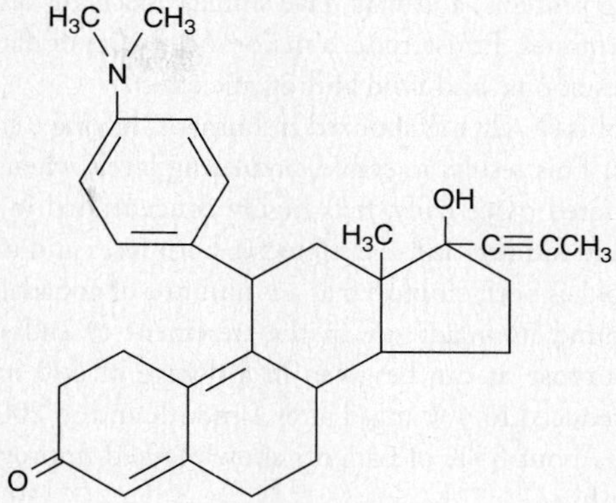

Mifepristone

Mifepristone's major use thus far has been to terminate early pregnancies. Doses of 400–600 mg/d for 4 days or 800 mg/d for 2 days successfully terminated pregnancy in >85% of the women studied. The major adverse effect was prolonged bleeding that on most occasions did not require treatment. The combination of a single oral dose of 600 mg of mifepristone and a vaginal pessary containing 1 mg of prostaglandin E_1 or oral misoprostol has been found to effectively terminate pregnancy in over 95% of patients treated during the first 7 weeks after conception. The adverse effects of the medications included vomiting, diarrhea, and abdominal or pelvic pain. As many as 5% of patients have vaginal bleeding requiring intervention. Because of these adverse effects, mifepristone is administered only by physicians at family planning centers. *Note:* In a very small number of cases, use of a vaginal tablet for the prostaglandin dose has been associated with sepsis, so it is recommended that *both* drugs be given by mouth in all patients.

ZK 98734 (lilopristone) is a potent experimental progesterone inhibitor and abortifacient in doses of 25 mg twice daily. Like mifepristone, it also appears to have antiglucocorticoid activity.

DANAZOL

Danazol, an isoxazole derivative of ethisterone (17α-ethinyltestosterone) with weak progestational, androgenic, and glucocorticoid activities, is used to suppress ovarian function. Danazol inhibits the midcycle surge of LH and FSH and can prevent the compensatory increase in LH and FSH following castration in animals, but it does not significantly lower or suppress basal LH or FSH levels in normal women (see Figure 40–5). Danazol binds to androgen, progesterone, and glucocorticoid receptors and can translocate the androgen receptor into the nucleus to initiate androgen-specific RNA synthesis. It does not bind to intracellular estrogen receptors, but it does bind to sex hormone–binding and corticosteroid-binding globulins. It inhibits P450scc (the cholesterol side chain–cleaving enzyme), 3β-hydroxysteroid dehydrogenase, 17α-hydroxysteroid dehydrogenase, P450c17 (17α-hydroxylase), P450c11 (11β-hydroxylase), and P450c21 (21β-hydroxylase). However, it does not inhibit aromatase, the enzyme required for estrogen synthesis. It increases the mean clearance of progesterone, probably by competing with the hormone for binding proteins, and may have similar effects on other active steroid hormones. Ethisterone, a major metabolite of danazol, has both progestational and mild androgenic effects.

Danazol is slowly metabolized in humans, having a half-life of >15 hours. This results in stable circulating levels when the drug is administered twice daily. It is highly concentrated in the liver, adrenals, and kidneys and is excreted in both feces and urine.

Danazol has been employed as an inhibitor of gonadal function and has found its major use in the treatment of endometriosis. For this purpose, it can be given in a dosage of 600 mg/d. The dosage is reduced to 400 mg/d after 1 month and to 200 mg/d in 2 months. About 85% of patients show marked improvement in 3–12 months.

Danazol has also been used in the treatment of fibrocystic disease of the breast and hematologic or allergic disorders, including hemophilia, Christmas disease, idiopathic thrombocytopenic purpura, and angioneurotic edema.

The major adverse effects are weight gain, edema, decreased breast size, acne and oily skin, increased hair growth, deepening of the voice, headache, hot flushes, changes in libido, and muscle cramps. Although mild adverse effects are very common, it is seldom necessary to discontinue the drug because of them. Occasionally, because of its inherent glucocorticoid activity, danazol may cause adrenal suppression.

Danazol should be used with great caution in patients with hepatic dysfunction, since it has been reported to produce mild to moderate hepatocellular damage in some patients, as evidenced by enzyme changes. It is also contraindicated during pregnancy and breast-feeding, as it may produce urogenital abnormalities in the offspring.

OTHER INHIBITORS

Anastrozole, a selective nonsteroidal inhibitor of aromatase (the enzyme required for estrogen synthesis; see Figures 40–2 and 40–5), is effective in some women whose breast tumors have become resistant to tamoxifen (see Chapter 54). **Letrozole** is similar. **Exemestane,** a steroid molecule, is an irreversible inhibitor of aromatase. Like anastrozole and letrozole, it is approved for use in women with advanced breast cancer (see Chapter 54).

Several other aromatase inhibitors are undergoing clinical trials in patients with breast cancer. **Fadrozole** is an oral nonsteroidal (triazole) inhibitor of aromatase activity. These compounds appear to be as effective as tamoxifen. In addition to their use in breast cancer, aromatase inhibitors have been successfully employed as adjuncts to androgen antagonists in the treatment of precocious puberty and as primary treatment in the excessive aromatase syndrome.

Fulvestrant is a pure estrogen receptor antagonist that has been somewhat more effective than those with partial agonist effects in some patients who have become resistant to tamoxifen. Fulvestrant is approved for use in breast cancer patients who have become resistant to tamoxifen. ICI 164,384 is a newer antagonist; it inhibits dimerization of the occupied estrogen receptor and interferes with its binding to DNA.

GnRH and its analogs (**nafarelin, buserelin,** etc) have become important in both stimulating and inhibiting ovarian function. They are discussed in Chapter 37.

OVULATION-INDUCING AGENTS

CLOMIPHENE

Clomiphene citrate, a partial estrogen agonist, is closely related to the estrogen chlorotrianisene (see Figure 40–3). This compound is well absorbed when taken orally. It has a half-life of 5–7 days and is excreted primarily in the urine. It exhibits significant protein binding and enterohepatic circulation and is distributed to adipose tissues.

Pharmacologic Effects

A. Mechanisms of Action

Clomiphene is a partial agonist at estrogen receptors. The estrogenic agonist effects are best demonstrated in animals with marked gonadal deficiency. Clomiphene has also been shown to effectively inhibit the action of stronger estrogens. In humans it leads to an increase in the secretion of gonadotropins and estrogens by inhibiting estradiol's negative feedback effect on the release of gonadotropins (see Figure 40–5).

B. Effects

The pharmacologic importance of clomiphene rests on its ability to stimulate ovulation in women with oligomenorrhea or amenorrhea and ovulatory dysfunction. The majority of patients suffer from polycystic ovary syndrome, a common disorder affecting about 7% of women of reproductive age. The syndrome is characterized by gonadotropin-dependent ovarian hyperandrogenism associated with anovulation and infertility. The disorder is frequently accompanied by adrenal hyperandrogenism. Clomiphene probably blocks the feedback inhibitory influence of estrogens on the hypothalamus, causing a surge of gonadotropins, which leads to ovulation.

Clinical Use

Clomiphene is used in the treatment of disorders of ovulation in patients who wish to become pregnant. Usually, a single ovulation is induced by a single course of therapy, and the patient must be treated repeatedly until pregnancy is achieved, since normal cyclic ovulatory function does not usually resume. The compound is of no value in patients with ovarian or pituitary failure.

When clomiphene is administered in a dosage of 100 mg/d for 5 days, a rise in plasma LH and FSH is observed after several days. In patients who ovulate, the initial rise is followed by a second rise of gonadotropin levels just prior to ovulation.

Adverse Effects

The most common adverse effects in patients treated with this drug are hot flushes, which resemble those experienced by menopausal patients. They tend to be mild, and disappear when the drug is discontinued. There have been occasional reports of eye symptoms due to intensification and prolongation of afterimages. These are generally of short duration. Headache, constipation, allergic skin reactions, and reversible hair loss have been reported occasionally.

The effective use of clomiphene is associated with some stimulation of the ovaries and usually with ovarian enlargement. The degree of enlargement tends to be greater and its incidence higher in patients who have enlarged ovaries at the beginning of therapy.

A variety of other symptoms such as nausea and vomiting, increased nervous tension, depression, fatigue, breast soreness, weight gain, urinary frequency, and heavy menses have also been reported. However, these appear to result from the hormonal changes associated with an ovulatory menstrual cycle rather than from the medication. The incidence of multiple pregnancy is approximately 10%. Clomiphene has not been shown to have an adverse effect when inadvertently given to women who are already pregnant.

Contraindications & Cautions

Special precautions should be observed in patients with enlarged ovaries. These women are thought to be more sensitive to this drug and should receive small doses. Any patient who complains of abdominal symptoms should be examined carefully. Maximum ovarian enlargement occurs after the 5-day course has been completed, and many patients can be shown to have a palpable increase in ovarian size by the seventh to tenth days. Treatment with clomiphene for more than a year may be associated with an increased risk of low-grade ovarian cancer; however, the evidence for this effect is not conclusive.

Special precautions must also be taken in patients who have visual symptoms associated with clomiphene therapy, since these symptoms may make activities such as driving more hazardous.

OTHER DRUGS USED IN OVULATORY DISORDERS

In addition to clomiphene, a variety of other hormonal and nonhormonal agents are used in treating anovulatory disorders. They are discussed in Chapter 37.

■ THE TESTIS (ANDROGENS & ANABOLIC STEROIDS, ANTIANDROGENS, & MALE CONTRACEPTION)

The testis, like the ovary, has both gametogenic and endocrine functions. The onset of gametogenic function of the testes is controlled largely by the secretion of FSH by the pituitary. High concentrations of testosterone locally are also required for continuing sperm production in the seminiferous tubules. The Sertoli cells in the seminiferous tubules may be the source of the estradiol produced in the testes via aromatization of locally produced testosterone. With LH stimulation, testosterone is produced by the interstitial or Leydig cells found in the spaces between the seminiferous tubules.

The Sertoli cells in the testis synthesize and secrete a variety of active proteins, including müllerian duct inhibitory factor, inhibin, and activin. As in the ovary, inhibin and activin appear to be the product of three genes that produce a common α subunit and two β subunits, A and B. Activin is composed of the two β subunits ($\beta_A\beta_B$). There are two inhibins (A and B), which contain the α subunit and one of the β subunits. Activin stimulates pituitary FSH release and is structurally similar to transforming growth factor-β, which also increases FSH. The inhibins in conjunction with testosterone and dihydrotestosterone are responsible for the feedback inhibition of pituitary FSH secretion.

ANDROGENS & ANABOLIC STEROIDS

In humans, the most important androgen secreted by the testis is testosterone. The pathways of synthesis of testosterone in the testes are similar to those previously described for the adrenal gland and ovary (see Figures 39–1 and 40–2).

In men, approximately 8 mg of testosterone is produced daily. About 95% is produced by the Leydig cells and only 5% by the adrenals. The testis also secretes small amounts of another potent androgen, dihydrotestosterone, as well as androstenedione and dehydroepiandrosterone, which are weak androgens. Pregnenolone and progesterone and their 17-hydroxylated derivatives are also released in small amounts. Plasma levels of testosterone in males are about 0.6 mcg/dL after puberty and appear to decline after age 50. Testosterone is also present in the plasma of women in concentrations of approximately 0.03 mcg/dL and is derived in approximately equal parts from the ovaries and adrenals and by the peripheral conversion of other hormones.

About 65% of circulating testosterone is bound to sex hormone-binding globulin. SHBG is increased in plasma by estrogen, by thyroid hormone, and in patients with cirrhosis of the liver. It is decreased by androgen and growth hormone and is lower in obese individuals. Most of the remaining testosterone is bound to albumin. Approximately 2% remains free and available to enter cells and bind to intracellular receptors.

Metabolism

In many target tissues, testosterone is converted to dihydrotestosterone by 5α-reductase. In these tissues, dihydrotestosterone is the major active androgen. The conversion of testosterone to estradiol by P450 aromatase also occurs in some tissues, including adipose tissue, liver, and the hypothalamus, where it may be of importance in regulating gonadal function.

The major pathway for the degradation of testosterone in humans occurs in the liver, with the reduction of the double bond and ketone in the A ring, as is seen in other steroids with a Δ^4-ketone configuration in the A ring. This leads to the production of inactive substances such as androsterone and etiocholanolone that are then conjugated and excreted in the urine.

Androstenedione, dehydroepiandrosterone (DHEA), and dehydroepiandrosterone sulfate (DHEAS) are also produced in significant amounts in humans, although largely in the adrenal gland rather than in the testes. They contribute slightly to the normal maturation process supporting other androgen-dependent pubertal changes in the human, primarily development of pubic and axillary hair and bone maturation. As noted in Chapter 39, some studies suggest that DHEA and DHEAS may have other central nervous system and metabolic effects and may prolong life in rabbits. In men they may improve the sense of well-being and inhibit atherosclerosis. In a placebo-controlled clinical trial in patients with systemic lupus erythematosus, DHEA demonstrated some beneficial effects (see Adrenal Androgens, Chapter 39). Adrenal androgens are to a large extent metabolized in the same fashion as testosterone. Both steroids—but particularly androstenedione—can be converted by peripheral tissues to estrone in very small amounts (1–5%). The P450 aromatase enzyme responsible for this conversion is also found in the brain and is thought to play an important role in development.

Physiologic Effects

In the normal male, testosterone or its active metabolite 5α-dihydrotestosterone is responsible for the many changes that occur in puberty. In addition to the general growth-promoting properties of androgens on body tissues, these hormones are responsible for penile and scrotal growth. Changes in the skin include the appearance of pubic, axillary, and beard hair. The sebaceous glands become more active, and the skin tends to become thicker and oilier. The larynx grows and the vocal cords become thicker, leading to a lower-pitched voice. Skeletal growth is stimulated and epiphyseal closure accelerated. Other effects include growth of the prostate and seminal vesicles, darkening of the skin, and increased skin circulation. Androgens play an important role in stimulating and maintaining sexual function in men. Androgens increase lean body mass and stimulate body hair growth and sebum secretion. Metabolic effects include the reduction of hormone binding and other carrier proteins and increased liver synthesis of clotting factors, triglyceride lipase, α_1-antitrypsin, haptoglobin, and sialic acid. They also stimulate renal erythropoietin secretion and decrease HDL levels.

Synthetic Steroids with Androgenic & Anabolic Action

Testosterone, when administered by mouth, is rapidly absorbed. However, it is largely converted to inactive metabolites, and only about one sixth of the dose administered is available in active form. Testosterone can be administered parenterally, but it has a more prolonged absorption time and greater activity in the propionate, enanthate, undecanoate, or cypionate ester forms. These derivatives are hydrolyzed to release free testosterone at the site of injection. Testosterone derivatives alkylated at the 17 position, eg, methyltestosterone and fluoxymesterone, are active when given by mouth.

Testosterone and its derivatives have been used for their anabolic effects as well as in the treatment of testosterone deficiency.

TABLE 40–5 Androgens: Preparations available and relative androgenic:anabolic activity in animals.

Drug	Androgenic:Anabolic Activity
Testosterone	1:1
Testosterone cypionate	1:1
Testosterone enanthate	1:1
Methyltestosterone	1:1
Fluoxymesterone	1:2
Oxymetholone	1:3
Oxandrolone	1:3–1:13
Nandrolone decanoate	1:2.5–1:4

Although testosterone and other known active steroids can be isolated in pure form and measured by weight, biologic assays are still used in the investigation of new compounds. In some of these studies in animals, the anabolic effects of the compound as measured by trophic effects on muscles or the reduction of nitrogen excretion may be dissociated from the other androgenic effects. This has led to the marketing of compounds claimed to have anabolic activity associated with only weak androgenic effects. Unfortunately, this dissociation is less marked in humans than in the animals used for testing (Table 40–5), and all are potent androgens.

Pharmacologic Effects

A. Mechanism of Action

Like other steroids, testosterone acts intracellularly in target cells. In skin, prostate, seminal vesicles, and epididymis, it is converted to 5α-dihydrotestosterone by 5α-reductase. In these tissues, dihydrotestosterone is the dominant androgen. The distribution of this enzyme in the fetus is different and has important developmental implications.

Testosterone and dihydrotestosterone bind to the intracellular androgen receptor, initiating a series of events similar to those described above for estradiol and progesterone, leading to growth, differentiation, and synthesis of a variety of enzymes and other functional proteins.

B. Effects

In the male at puberty, androgens cause development of the secondary sex characteristics (see above). In the adult male, large doses of testosterone—when given alone—or its derivatives suppress the secretion of gonadotropins and result in some atrophy of the interstitial tissue and the tubules of the testes. Since fairly large doses of androgens are required to suppress gonadotropin secretion, it has been postulated that inhibin, in combination with androgens, is responsible for the feedback control of secretion. In women, androgens are capable of producing changes similar to those observed in the prepubertal male. These include growth of facial and body hair, deepening of the voice, enlargement of the clitoris, frontal baldness, and prominent musculature. The natural androgens stimulate erythrocyte production.

The administration of androgens reduces the excretion of nitrogen into the urine, indicating an increase in protein synthesis or a decrease in protein breakdown within the body. This effect is much more pronounced in women and children than in normal men.

Clinical Uses

A. Androgen Replacement Therapy in Men

Androgens are used to replace or augment endogenous androgen secretion in hypogonadal men (Table 40–6). Even in the presence of pituitary deficiency, androgens are used rather than gonadotropins except when normal spermatogenesis is to be achieved. In patients with hypopituitarism, androgens are not added to the treatment regimen until puberty, at which time they are instituted in gradually increasing doses to achieve the growth spurt and the development of secondary sex characteristics. In these patients, therapy should be started with long-acting agents such as testosterone enanthate or cypionate in doses of 50 mg intramuscularly, initially every 4, then every 3, and finally every 2 weeks, with each change taking place at 3-month intervals. The dose is then doubled to 100 mg every 2 weeks until maturation is complete. Finally, it is changed to the adult replacement dose of 200 mg at 2-week intervals.

Testosterone propionate, though potent, has a short duration of action and is not practical for long-term use. Testosterone undecanoate can be given orally, administering large amounts of the steroid twice daily (eg, 40 mg/d); however, this is not recommended because oral testosterone administration has been associated with liver tumors. Testosterone can also be administered transdermally; skin patches or gels are available for scrotal or other skin area application. Two applications daily are usually required for replacement therapy. Implanted pellets and other longer-acting preparations are under study. The development of polycythemia or hypertension may require some reduction in dose.

B. Gynecologic Disorders

Androgens are used occasionally in the treatment of certain gynecologic disorders, but the undesirable effects in women are such that they must be used with great caution. Androgens have been used to reduce breast engorgement during the postpartum period, usually in conjunction with estrogens. The weak androgen danazol is used in the treatment of endometriosis (see above).

Androgens are sometimes given in combination with estrogens for replacement therapy in the postmenopausal period in an attempt to eliminate the endometrial bleeding that may occur when only estrogens are used and to enhance libido. They have been used for chemotherapy of breast tumors in premenopausal women.

TABLE 40–6 Androgen preparations for replacement therapy.

Drug	Route of Administration	Dosage
Methyltestosterone	Oral	25–50 mg/d
	Sublingual (buccal)	5–10 mg/d
Fluoxymesterone	Oral	2–10 mg/d
Testosterone enanthate	Intramuscular	See text
Testosterone cypionate	Intramuscular	See text
Testosterone	Transdermal	2.5–10 mg/d
	Topical gel (1%)	5–10 g/d

C. Use as Protein Anabolic Agents

Androgens and anabolic steroids have been used in conjunction with dietary measures and exercises in an attempt to reverse protein loss after trauma, surgery, or prolonged immobilization and in patients with debilitating diseases. Evidence to support this use of androgens is poor except when hypogonadism is also present.

D. Anemia

In the past, large doses of androgens were employed in the treatment of refractory anemias such as aplastic anemia, Fanconi anemia, sickle cell anemia, myelofibrosis, and hemolytic anemias. Recombinant erythropoietin has largely replaced androgens for this purpose.

E. Osteoporosis

Androgens and anabolic agents have been used in the treatment of osteoporosis, either alone or in conjunction with estrogens. With the exception of substitution therapy in hypogonadism, bisphosphonates have largely replaced androgen use for this purpose.

F. Use as Growth Stimulators

These agents have been used to stimulate growth in boys with delayed puberty. If the drugs are used carefully, these children will probably achieve their expected adult height. If treatment is too vigorous, the patient may grow rapidly at first but will not achieve full predicted final stature because epiphyseal closure is accelerated. It is difficult to control this type of therapy adequately even with frequent x-ray examination of the epiphyses, since the action of the hormones on epiphyseal centers may continue for many months after therapy is discontinued.

G. Anabolic Steroid and Androgen Abuse in Sports

The use of anabolic steroids by athletes has received worldwide attention. Many athletes and their coaches believe that anabolic steroids—in doses 10–200 times larger than the daily normal physiologic production—increase strength and aggressiveness, thereby improving competitive performance. Such effects have been unequivocally demonstrated only in women. Furthermore, the adverse effects of these drugs clearly make their use inadvisable. As a result, most sports organizations have developed extremely sensitive assays, conduct random testing, and apply strong penalties if drugs are detected.

H. Aging Men

Androgen production falls with age in men and may contribute to a decline in muscle mass, strength, and libido. Testosterone levels decline gradually with advancing age after peaking in the second and third decades of life, and genetic factors, obesity and its comorbid conditions, and generally, the gradual age-dependent worsening of the so-called "chronic noncommunicable diseases," influence the trajectory of age-related decline in testosterone levels. About 10% of middle-aged and older men have low morning fasting total testosterone (<250 ng/dL). Such men usually have low or inappropriately normal luteinizing hormone level, ie, secondary hypogonadism, while a smaller fraction has elevated luteinizing hormone, ie, primary hypogonadism. Age-related secondary hypogonadism is usually associated with presence of chronic noncommunicable diseases, while primary hypogonadism is mainly associated with age.

The majority of testosterone prescriptions today are written for middle aged and older men, even though testosterone is not approved by the US Food and Drug Administration (FDA) for age-related decline in testosterone levels. As experts have debated whether older men with testosterone deficiency might indeed benefit from testosterone treatment, several recent randomized controlled trials have provided important information on the efficacy and short-term safety of testosterone treatment in older men. Studies of androgen replacement in aging males with low testosterone levels show an increase in lean body mass and hematocrit and a decrease in bone turnover. Sense of well-being may improve, and increased energy and muscle strength are reported. To date, it does not seem that there is an association of this treatment with an increase in prostate cancer diagnosis. It is important to recommend, however, that the pros and the cons for an aging man's decision to receive testosterone therapy should be discussed with an expert physician, the risk for prostate cancer should be taken into account, and careful monitoring of the patient should take place.

Adverse Effects

The adverse effects of these compounds are due largely to their masculinizing actions and are most noticeable in women and prepubertal children. In women, the administration of more than 200–300 mg of testosterone per month is usually associated with hirsutism, acne, amenorrhea, clitoral enlargement, and deepening of the voice. These effects may occur with even smaller doses in some women. Some of the androgenic steroids exert progestational activity, leading to endometrial bleeding upon discontinuation. These hormones also alter serum lipids and could conceivably increase susceptibility to atherosclerotic disease in women.

Except under the most unusual circumstances, androgens should not be used in infants. Recent studies in animals suggest that administration of androgens in early life may have profound effects on maturation of central nervous system centers governing sexual development, particularly in the female. Administration of these drugs to pregnant women may lead to masculinization or undermasculinization of the external genitalia in the female and male fetus, respectively. Although the above-mentioned effects may be less marked with the anabolic agents, they do occur.

Sodium retention and edema are not common but must be carefully watched for in patients with heart and kidney disease.

Most of the synthetic androgens and anabolic agents are 17-alkyl-substituted steroids. Administration of drugs with this structure is often associated with evidence of hepatic dysfunction. Hepatic dysfunction usually occurs early in the course of treatment, and the degree is proportionate to the dose. Bilirubin levels may increase until clinical jaundice is apparent. The cholestatic jaundice is reversible upon cessation of therapy, and permanent changes do not occur. In older males, prostatic hyperplasia may develop, causing urinary retention.

Replacement therapy in men may cause acne, sleep apnea, erythrocytosis, gynecomastia, and azoospermia. Supraphysiologic doses of androgens produce azoospermia and decrease in testicular size, both of which may take months to recover after cessation of therapy. The alkylated androgens in high doses can produce peliosis hepatis, cholestasis, and hepatic failure. They lower plasma HDL and may increase LDL. Hepatic adenomas and carcinomas have also been reported. Behavioral effects include psychological dependence, increased aggressiveness, and psychotic symptoms.

Contraindications & Cautions

The use of androgenic steroids is contraindicated in pregnant women or women who may become pregnant during the course of therapy.

Androgens should not be administered to male patients with carcinoma of the prostate or breast. Until more is known about the effects of these hormones on the central nervous system in developing children, they should be avoided in infants and young children.

Special caution is required in giving these drugs to children to produce a growth spurt. In most patients, the use of somatotropin is more appropriate (see Chapter 37).

Care should be exercised in the administration of these drugs to patients with renal or cardiac disease predisposed to edema. If sodium and water retention occurs, it will respond to diuretic therapy.

Methyltestosterone therapy is associated with creatinuria, but the significance of this finding is not known.

Caution: Several cases of hepatocellular carcinoma have been reported in patients with aplastic anemia treated with androgen anabolic therapy. Erythropoietin and colony-stimulating factors (see Chapter 33) should be used instead.

ANDROGEN SUPPRESSION & ANTIANDROGENS

ANDROGEN SUPPRESSION

In contrast to the lack of strong indications for the use of androgen supplementation (except in the case of hypogonadism), the use of inhibitors of androgen synthesis and of androgen antagonists has several well-documented applications. The treatment of advanced prostatic carcinoma often requires orchiectomy or large doses of estrogens to reduce available endogenous androgen.

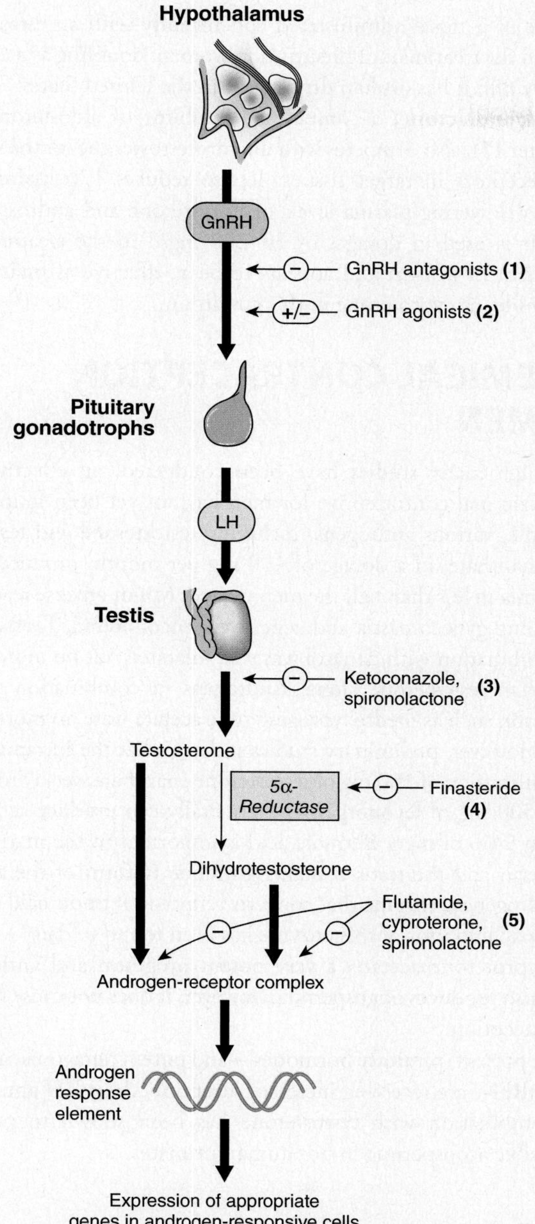

FIGURE 40–6 Control of androgen secretion and activity and some sites of action of antiandrogens: (**1**) competitive inhibition of GnRH receptors; (**2**) stimulation (+, pulsatile administration) or inhibition via desensitization of GnRH receptors (–, continuous administration); (**3**) decreased synthesis of testosterone in the testis; (**4**) decreased synthesis of dihydrotestosterone by inhibition of 5α-reductase; (**5**) competition for binding to cytosol androgen receptors.

The psychological effects of the former and gynecomastia produced by the latter make these approaches undesirable. As noted in Chapter 37, the GnRH analogs, such as goserelin, nafarelin, buserelin, and leuprolide acetate, produce effective gonadal suppression when blood levels are continuous rather than pulsatile (see Chapter 37 and Figure 40–6).

ANTIANDROGENS

The potential usefulness of antiandrogens in the treatment of patients producing excessive amounts of testosterone has led to the search for effective drugs that can be used for this purpose. Several approaches to the problem, especially inhibition of synthesis and receptor antagonism, have met with some success.

Steroid Synthesis Inhibitors

Ketoconazole, used primarily in the treatment of fungal disease, is an inhibitor of adrenal and gonadal steroid synthesis, as described in Chapter 39. It does not affect ovarian aromatase, but it reduces human placental aromatase activity. It displaces estradiol and dihydrotestosterone from sex hormone-binding protein in vitro and increases the estradiol:testosterone ratio in plasma in vivo by a different mechanism. However, it does not appear to be clinically useful in women with increased androgen levels because of the toxicity associated with prolonged use of the 400–800 mg/d required. The drug has also been used experimentally to treat prostatic carcinoma, but the results have not been encouraging. Men treated with ketoconazole often develop reversible gynecomastia during therapy; this may be due to the demonstrated increase in the estradiol:testosterone ratio.

Inhibition of Conversion of Steroid Precursors to Androgens

Several compounds have been developed that inhibit the 17-hydroxylation of progesterone or pregnenolone, thereby preventing the action of the side chain-splitting enzyme and the further transformation of these steroid precursors to active androgens. A few of these compounds have been tested clinically but have been too toxic for prolonged use. As noted in Chapter 39, **abiraterone,** a newer 17α-hydroxylase inhibitor, has been approved for use in metastatic prostate cancer.

Since dihydrotestosterone—not testosterone—appears to be the essential androgen in the prostate, androgen effects in this and similar dihydrotestosterone-dependent tissues can be reduced by an inhibitor of 5α-reductase (see Figure 40–6). **Finasteride,** a steroid-like inhibitor of this enzyme, is orally active and causes a reduction in dihydrotestosterone levels that begins within 8 hours after administration and lasts for about 24 hours. The half-life is about 8 hours (longer in elderly individuals). About 40–50% of the dose is metabolized; more than half is excreted in the feces. Finasteride has been reported to be moderately effective in reducing prostate size in men with benign prostatic hyperplasia and is approved for this use in the United States. The dosage is 5 mg/d. **Dutasteride** is a similar orally active steroid derivative with a slow onset of action and a much longer half-life than finasteride. It is approved for treatment of benign prostatic hyperplasia at a dosage of 0.5 mg daily. These drugs are not approved for use in women or children, although finasteride has been used successfully in the treatment of hirsutism in women and is approved for treatment of early male pattern baldness in men (1 mg/d). Toxicity includes decreased libido and possible erectile and ejaculatory dysfunction.

A recent study suggested that, compared to antimuscarinic agents (tamsulosin), use of 5α-reductase inhibitors may increase the risk of type 2 diabetes.

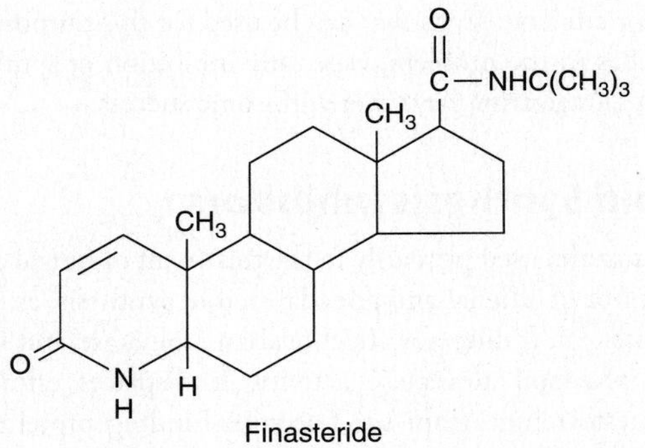

Finasteride

Receptor Inhibitors

Flutamide, a substituted anilide, is a potent antiandrogen that has been used in the treatment of prostatic carcinoma. Although not a steroid, it behaves like a competitive antagonist at the androgen receptor. It is rapidly metabolized in humans. It frequently causes mild gynecomastia (probably by increasing testicular estrogen production) and occasionally causes mild reversible hepatic toxicity. Administration of this compound causes some improvement in most patients with prostatic carcinoma who have not had prior endocrine therapy. Preliminary studies indicate that flutamide is also useful in the management of excess androgen effect in women.

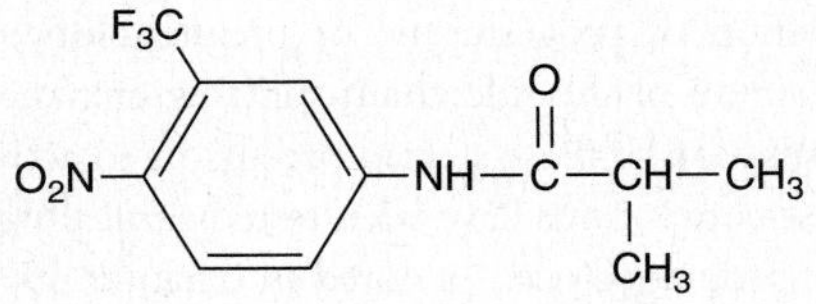

Flutamide

Bicalutamide, nilutamide, and **enzalutamide** are potent orally active antiandrogens that can be administered as a single daily dose and are used in patients with metastatic carcinoma of the prostate. Studies in patients with carcinoma of the prostate indicate that these agents are well tolerated. Bicalutamide is recommended (to reduce tumor flare) for use in combination with a GnRH analog and may have fewer gastrointestinal side effects than flutamide. A dosage of 150–200 mg/d (when used alone) is required to reduce prostate-specific antigen levels to those achieved by castration, but, in combination with a GnRH analog, 50 mg/d may be adequate. Nilutamide is administered in a dosage of 300 mg/d for 30 days followed by 150 mg/d. The dosage of enzalutamide is 160 mg/d orally.

Cyproterone and **cyproterone acetate** are effective antiandrogens that inhibit the action of androgens at the target organ. The acetate form has a marked progestational effect that suppresses the feedback enhancement of LH and FSH, leading to a more effective antiandrogen effect. These compounds have been used in women to treat hirsutism and in men to decrease excessive sexual drive and are being studied in other conditions in which the reduction of androgenic effects would be useful. Cyproterone acetate in a dosage of 2 mg/d administered concurrently with an estrogen is used in the treatment of hirsutism in women, doubling as a contraceptive pill; it has orphan drug status in the United States.

Spironolactone, a competitive inhibitor of aldosterone (see Chapter 15), also competes with dihydrotestosterone for the androgen receptors in target tissues. It also reduces 17α-hydroxylase activity, lowering plasma levels of testosterone and androstenedione. It is used in dosages of 50–200 mg/d in the treatment of hirsutism in women and appears to be as effective as finasteride, flutamide, or cyproterone in this condition.

CHEMICAL CONTRACEPTION IN MEN

Although many studies have been conducted, an effective and nontoxic oral contraceptive for men has not yet been found. For example, various androgens, including testosterone and testosterone enanthate, in a dosage of 400 mg per month, produced azoospermia in less than half the men treated. Minor adverse reactions, including gynecomastia and acne, were encountered. Testosterone in combination with danazol was well tolerated but no more effective than testosterone alone. Androgens in combination with a progestin such as medroxyprogesterone acetate were no more effective. However, preliminary studies indicate that the intramuscular administration of 100 mg of testosterone enanthate weekly together with 500 mg of levonorgestrel daily orally can produce azoospermia in 94% of men. Retinoic acid is important in the maturation of sperm and the testis contains a unique isoform of the alcohol dehydrogenase enzyme that converts retinol to retinoic acid but no nontoxic inhibitor of this enzyme has been found to date.

Cyproterone acetate, a very potent progestin and antiandrogen, also produces oligospermia; however, it does not cause reliable contraception.

At present, pituitary hormones—and potent antagonist analogs of GnRH—are receiving increased attention. A GnRH antagonist in combination with testosterone has been shown to produce reversible azoospermia in nonhuman primates.

GOSSYPOL

Extensive trials of this cottonseed derivative have been conducted in China. This compound destroys elements of the seminiferous epithelium but does not significantly alter the endocrine function of the testis.

In Chinese studies, large numbers of men were treated with 20 mg/d of gossypol or gossypol acetic acid for 2 months, followed by a maintenance dosage of 60 mg/week. On this regimen, 99% of men developed sperm counts below 4 million/mL. Preliminary data indicate that recovery (return of normal sperm count) following discontinuance of gossypol administration is more apt to occur in men whose counts do not fall to extremely low levels and when administration is not continued for more than 2 years. Hypokalemia is the major adverse effect and may lead to transient paralysis. Because of low efficacy and significant toxicity, gossypol has been abandoned as a candidate male contraceptive.

PREPARATIONS AVAILABLE*

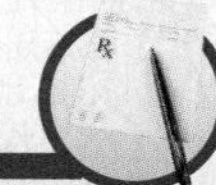

GENERIC NAME	AVAILABLE AS
ESTROGENS	
Conjugated estrogens (equine)	Premarin
Diethylstilbestrol†	Generic, DES, Stilphostrol
Esterified estrogens	Cenestin, Enjuvia, Menest
Estradiol	Generic, Estrace, others
Estradiol cypionate in oil	Depo-Estradiol, others
Estradiol transdermal	Generic, Estraderm, Estrasorb, Estrogel, others
Estradiol valerate in oil	Generic, Delestrogen
Estropipate	Generic, Ogen
PROGESTINS	
Levonorgestrel	Generic, Plan B, others
Medroxyprogesterone acetate	Generic, Provera
Megestrol acetate	Generic, Megace
Norethindrone acetate	Generic, Aygestin
Progesterone	Generic, Prometrium, others
ANDROGENS & ANABOLIC STEROIDS	
Fluoxymesterone	Androxy
Methyltestosterone	Android, others
Nandrolone decanoate	Generic, Deca Durabolin, others
Oxandrolone	Generic, Oxandrin
Oxymetholone	Androl-50
Testosterone	Generic
Testosterone cypionate in oil	Generic, Depo-testosterone
Testosterone enanthate in oil	Generic, Delatestryl
Testosterone transdermal system	Androderm, AndroGel
Testosterone pellets	Testopel
ANTAGONISTS & INHIBITORS	
(See also Chapter 37)	
Abiraterone	Zytiga
Anastrozole	Generic, Arimidex
Bazedoxifene (in combination with conjugated equine estrogens)	Duavee
Bicalutamide	Generic, Casodex
Clomiphene	Generic, Clomid, Serophene, Milophene
Danazol	Generic, Danocrine
Dutasteride	Avodart
Enzalutamide	Xtandi
Exemestane	Generic, Aromasin
Finasteride	Generic, Propecia, Proscar
Flutamide	Generic, Eulexin
Fulvestrant	Faslodex
Letrozole	Generic, Femara
Mifepristone	Mifeprex, Korlym
Nilutamide	Nilandron
Raloxifene	Evista
Tamoxifen	Generic, Nolvadex
Toremifene	Fareston

*Oral contraceptives are listed in Table 40–3.

†Withdrawn in the United States.

REFERENCES

Acconcia F et al: Palmitoylation-dependent estrogen receptor alpha membrane localization: Regulation by 17beta-estradiol. Mol Biol Cell 2005;16:231.

Anderson GL et al for the Women's Health Initiative Steering Committee: Effects of conjugated equine estrogen in postmenopausal women with hysterectomy. JAMA 2004;291:1701.

Bacopoulou F, Greydanus DE, Chrousos GP: Reproductive and contraceptive issues in chronically ill adolescents. Eur J Contracept Reprod Health Care 2010;15:389.

Bhasin S: Testosterone replacement in aging men: an evidence-based patient-centric perspective J Clin Invest 2021;131:e146607.

Basaria S et al: Adverse events associated with testosterone administration. N Engl J Med 2010;363:109.

Baulieu E-E: Contragestion and other clinical applications of RU 486, an antiprogesterone at the receptor. Science 1989;245:1351.

Bechlioulis A et al: Endothelial function, but not carotid intima-media thickness, is affected early in menopause and is associated with severity of hot flushes. J Clin Endocrinol Metab 2010;95:1199.

Bhupathiraju SN et al: Exogenous hormone use: Oral contraceptives, postmenopausal hormone therapy, and health outcomes in the Nurses' Health Study. Am J Pub Health 2016;106:1631.

Binkhorst L et al: Augmentation of endoxifen exposure in tamoxifen-treated women following SSRI switch. Clin Pharmacokin 2016;55:259.

Böttner M, Thelen P, Jarry H: Estrogen receptor beta: Tissue distribution and the still largely enigmatic physiological function. J Steroid Biochem Mol Biol 2014;139:245.

Burkman R, Schlesselman JJ, Zieman M: Safety concerns and health benefits associated with oral contraception. Am J Obstet Gynecol 2004;190(Suppl 4):S5.

Chlebowski RT et al: Estrogen plus progestin and breast cancer incidence and mortality in postmenopausal women. JAMA 2010;304:1684.

Chrousos GP: Perspective: Stress and sex versus immunity and inflammation. Sci Signal 2010;3:pe36.

Chrousos GP, Torpy DJ, Gold PW: Interactions between the hypothalamic-pituitary-adrenal axis and the female reproductive system: Clinical implications. Ann Intern Med 1998;129:229.

Coomarasamy A et al: A randomized trial of progesterone in women with recurrent miscarriages. N Engl J Med 2015;373:2141.

Cui J, Shen Y, Li R: Estrogen synthesis and signaling pathways during aging: From periphery to brain. Trends Mol Med 2013;19:197.

Cuzick J et al: SERM Chemoprevention of Breast Cancer Overview Group: Selective oestrogen receptor modulators in prevention of breast cancer: An updated meta-analysis of individual participant data. Lancet 2013;381:1827.

Diamanti-Kandarakis E et al: Pathophysiology and types of dyslipidemia in PCOS. Trends Endocrinol Metab 2007;18:280.

Finkelstein JS et al: Gonadal steroids and body composition, strength, and sexual function in men. N Engl J Med 2013;369:1011.

Fuqua SAW, Schiff R: Mechanisms of action of selective estrogen receptor modulators and down regulators. UpToDate 2016; topic 762.

Geronikolou SA et al: Polycystic ovary syndrome revisited: An interactions network approach. Eur J Clin Invest. 2021;51:e13578.

Gomes MPV, Deitcher SR: Risk of venous thromboembolic disease associated with hormonal contraceptives and hormone replacement therapy: A clinical review. Arch Intern Med 2004;164:1965.

Hall JM, McDonnell DP, Korach KS: Allosteric regulation of estrogen receptor structure, function, and co-activator recruitment by different estrogen response elements. Mol Endocrinol 2002;16:469.

Harman SM et al: Longitudinal effects of aging on serum total and free testosterone levels in healthy men: Baltimore Longitudinal Study of Aging. J Clin Endocrinol Metab 2001;86:724.

Imai Y et al: Nuclear receptors in bone physiology and diseases. Physiol Rev 2013;93:481.

Kalantaridou S, Chrousos GP: Monogenic disorders of puberty. J Clin Endocrinol Metab 2002;87:2481.

Kalantaridou S et al: Premature ovarian failure, endothelial dysfunction, and estrogen-progesterone replacement. Trends Endocrinol Metab 2006;17:101.

Kalantaridou SN et al: Impaired endothelial function in young women with premature ovarian failure: Normalization with hormone therapy. J Clin Endocrinol Metab 2004;89:3907.

Kanaka-Gantenbein C et al: Assisted reproduction and its neuroendocrine impact on the offspring. Prog Brain Res 2010;182C:161.

Lidegaard Ø et al: Thrombotic stroke and myocardial infarction with hormonal contraception. N Engl J Med 2012;366:2257.

Livadas S, Chrousos GP: Control of the onset of puberty. Curr Opin Pediatr 2016;28:551.

Manson JE et al: Estrogen plus progestin and the risk of coronary heart disease. N Engl J Med 2003;349:523.

Martin KA, Barbieri RL: Menopausal hormone therapy: Benefits and risks. UpToDate 2016.

McDonnell DP, Wardell SE: The molecular mechanisms underlying the pharmacological actions of ER modulators: Implications for new drug discovery in breast cancer. Curr Opin Pharmacol 2010;10:620.

Merke DP et al: Future directions in the study and management of congenital adrenal hyperplasia due to 21-hydroxylase deficiency. Ann Intern Med 2002; 136:320.

Naka KK et al: Effect of the insulin sensitizers metformin and pioglitazone on endothelial function in young women with polycystic ovary syndrome: A prospective randomized study. Fertil Steril 2011;95:203.

Nelson HD et al: Use of medication to reduce risk for primary breast cancer: A systematic review for the U.S. Preventive Services Task Force. Ann Intern Med 2013;158:604.

Paulmurugan R et al: In vitro and in vivo molecular imaging of estrogen receptor α and β homo- and heterodimerization: Exploration of new modes of receptor regulation. Mol Endocrinol 2011;25:2029.

Prague JK et al: Neurokinin 3 receptor antagonism as a novel treatment for menopausal hot flushes: A phase 2, randomised, double-blind, placebo-controlled trial. Lancet 2017;389:1809.

Price VH: Treatment of hair loss. N Engl J Med 1999;341:964.

Rossouw JE et al: Risks and benefits of estrogen plus progestin in healthy postmenopausal women: Principal results from the Women's Health Initiative randomized controlled trial. JAMA 2002;288:321.

Scher HI et al: Increased survival with enzalutamide in prostate cancer after chemotherapy. N Engl J Med 2012;367:1187.

Smith RE: A review of selective estrogen receptor modulators in national surgical adjuvant breast and bowel project clinical trials. Semin Oncol 2003;30(Suppl 16):4.

Snyder PJ et al: Effect of testosterone replacement in hypogonadal men. J Clin Endocrinol Metab 2000;85:2670.

Stegeman BH et al: Different combined oral contraceptives and the risk of venous thrombosis: Systematic review and network meta-analysis. Brit Med J 2013;347:f5298.

U.S. Preventive Services Task Force: Hormone therapy for the prevention of chronic conditions in postmenopausal women. Ann Intern Med 2005;142:855.

Valsamakis G et al: In pregnancy increased maternal STAI trait stress score shows decreased insulin sensitivity and increased stress hormones. Psychoneuroendocrinology 2017;84:11.

Wehrmacher WH, Messmore H: Women's Health Initiative is fundamentally flawed. Gend Med 2005;2:4.

Zandi PP et al: Hormone replacement therapy and incidence of Alzheimer's disease in older women. JAMA 2002;288:2123.

CASE STUDY ANSWER

The patient should be advised to start daily transdermal estradiol therapy (100 mcg/d) along with oral natural progesterone (200 mg/d) for the last 12 days of each 28-day cycle. On this regimen, her symptoms should disappear and normal monthly uterine bleeding resume. She should also be advised to get adequate exercise and increase her calcium and vitamin D intake as treatment for her osteoporosis.

CHAPTER

41

Pancreatic Hormones & Glucose-Lowering Drugs

Umesh Masharani, MBBS, MRCP (UK), & Lisa Kroon, PharmD, CDCES

CASE STUDY

A 66-year-old obese Caucasian man presented to an academic Diabetes Center for advice regarding his diabetes treatment. His diabetes was diagnosed 10 years previously on routine testing. He was initially given metformin but when he was no longer achieving his glycemic targets, the metformin was stopped and insulin treatment initiated. The patient was taking 50 units of insulin glargine and an average of 25 units of insulin aspart pre-meals. He had never seen a diabetes educator or a dietitian. He was checking his glucose levels four times a day and smoking half a pack of cigarettes a day. On examination, his weight was 132 kg (BMI 39.5) and blood pressure 145/71, and signs of mild peripheral neuropathy were present. Laboratory tests noted an HbA_{1c} value of 8.1% (normal <5.7%), urine albumin 3007 mg/g creatinine (normal <30), serum creatinine 0.86 mg/dL, estimated GFR >69 mL/min/1.73 m^2, total cholesterol 128 mg/dL, triglycerides 86 mg/dL, HDL cholesterol 38 mg/dL, and LDL cholesterol 73 mg/dL (on atorvastatin 40 mg daily). How would you treat this patient?

■ THE ENDOCRINE PANCREAS

The endocrine pancreas in the adult human consists of approximately 1 million islets of Langerhans interspersed throughout the pancreatic gland. Within the islets, at least four hormone-producing cells are present (Table 41–1). Their hormone products include **insulin,** the storage and anabolic hormone of the body; **islet amyloid polypeptide (IAPP, or amylin),** which modulates appetite, gastric emptying, and glucagon and insulin secretion; **glucagon,** the hyperglycemic factor that mobilizes glycogen stores; **somatostatin,** a universal inhibitor of secretory cells; **pancreatic peptide,** a small protein that facilitates digestive processes by a mechanism not yet clarified; and **ghrelin,** a peptide known to increase pituitary growth hormone release.

■ INSULIN

Chemistry

Human insulin is a small protein with a molecular weight of 5808 that contains 51 amino acids arranged in two chains (A and B) linked by disulfide bridges. There are species differences in the amino acids of both chains. Proinsulin, a long single-chain protein molecule, is processed within the Golgi apparatus of beta cells and packaged into granules, where it is hydrolyzed into insulin and a residual connecting segment called C-peptide by removal of four amino acids (Figure 41–1).

Insulin and C-peptide are secreted in equimolar amounts in response to all insulin secretagogues; a small quantity of

TABLE 41–1 Pancreatic islet cells and their secretory products.

Cell Types[1]	Approximate Percent of Islet Mass	Secretory Products
Alpha (A) cell	20	Glucagon, proglucagon
Beta (B) cell	75	Insulin, C-peptide, proinsulin, amylin
Delta (D) cell	3–5	Somatostatin
Epsilon cell	<1	Ghrelin

[1]Within pancreatic polypeptide-rich lobules of adult islets, located only in the posterior portion of the head of the human pancreas, glucagon cells are scarce (<0.5%) and F cells make up as much as 80% of the cells.

unprocessed or partially hydrolyzed proinsulin is released as well. Although proinsulin may have some mild hypoglycemic action, C-peptide has no known physiologic function. Granules within the beta cells store the insulin in the form of hexameric crystals consisting of two atoms of zinc and six molecules of insulin. The entire human pancreas contains up to 8 mg of insulin, representing approximately 200 biologic units. Originally, the unit was defined on the basis of the hypoglycemic activity of insulin in rabbits. With improved purification techniques, the unit is presently defined on the basis of weight, and present insulin standards used for assay purposes contain 28 units per milligram.

Insulin Secretion

Insulin is released from pancreatic beta cells at a low basal rate and at a much higher stimulated rate in response to a variety of stimuli, especially glucose. Other stimulants such as other sugars (eg, mannose), amino acids (especially gluconeogenic amino acids, eg, leucine, arginine), hormones such as glucagon-like polypeptide 1 (GLP-1), glucose-dependent insulinotropic polypeptide (GIP), glucagon, cholecystokinin, high concentrations of fatty acids, and β-adrenergic sympathetic activity are recognized. Stimulatory drugs include sulfonylureas, meglitinides, D-phenylalanine derivatives, isoproterenol, and acetylcholine. Inhibitory signals are hormones including insulin itself, islet amyloid polypeptide, somatostatin, and leptin; α-adrenergic sympathetic activity; chronically elevated glucose; and low concentrations of fatty acids. Inhibitory drugs include diazoxide, phenytoin, vinblastine, clonidine, verapamil, and colchicine.

One mechanism of stimulated insulin release is diagrammed in Figure 41–2. As shown in the figure, glucose is taken up by the beta cell through the transporter, GLUT2. Hyperglycemia results in increased intracellular ATP levels, which close ATP-dependent potassium channels. Decreased outward potassium efflux results in depolarization of the beta cell and opening of voltage-gated calcium channels. The resulting increased intracellular calcium triggers secretion of the hormone. The insulin secretagogue drug group (sulfonylureas, meglitinides, and D-phenylalanine derivatives) exhibit their glucose lowering effects through parts of this mechanism.

Insulin Degradation

The liver and kidney are the two main organs that remove insulin from the circulation. The liver normally clears the blood of approximately 60% of the insulin released from the pancreas by virtue of its location as the terminal site of portal vein blood flow, with the kidney removing 35–40% of the endogenous hormone. However, in insulin-treated diabetics receiving subcutaneous insulin injections, this ratio is reversed, with as much as 60% of exogenous insulin being cleared by the kidney and the liver removing no more than 30–40%. The half-life of circulating insulin is 3–5 minutes.

Circulating Insulin

Basal serum insulin values of 5–15 μU/mL (30–90 pmol/L) are found in normal humans, with a peak rise to 60–90 μU/mL (360–540 pmol/L) during meals.

The Insulin Receptor

After insulin has entered the circulation, it diffuses into tissues, where it is bound by specialized receptors that are found on the membranes of most tissues. The biologic responses promoted by

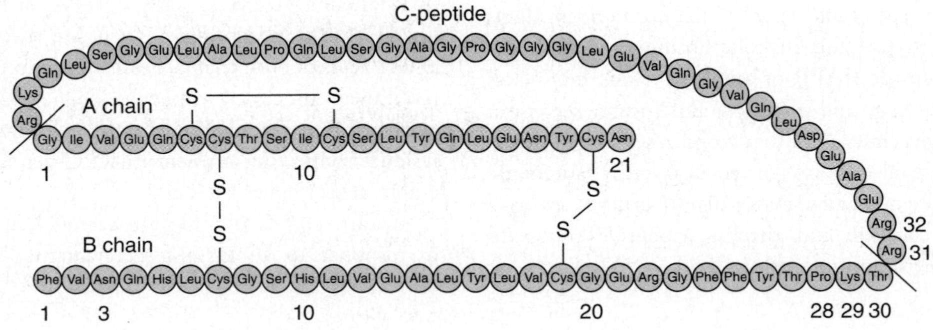

FIGURE 41–1 Structure of human proinsulin (C-peptide plus A and B chains of insulin). Insulin is shown as the shaded (orange color) peptide chains, A and B. Differences in the A and B chains and amino acid modifications for the rapid-acting insulin analogs (aspart, lispro, and glulisine) and long-acting insulin analogs (degludec, detemir, and glargine) are discussed in the text. (Reproduced with permission from Gardner DG, Shoback D: *Greenspan's Basic & Clinical Endocrinology*, 9th ed. New York, NY: McGraw Hill; 2011.)

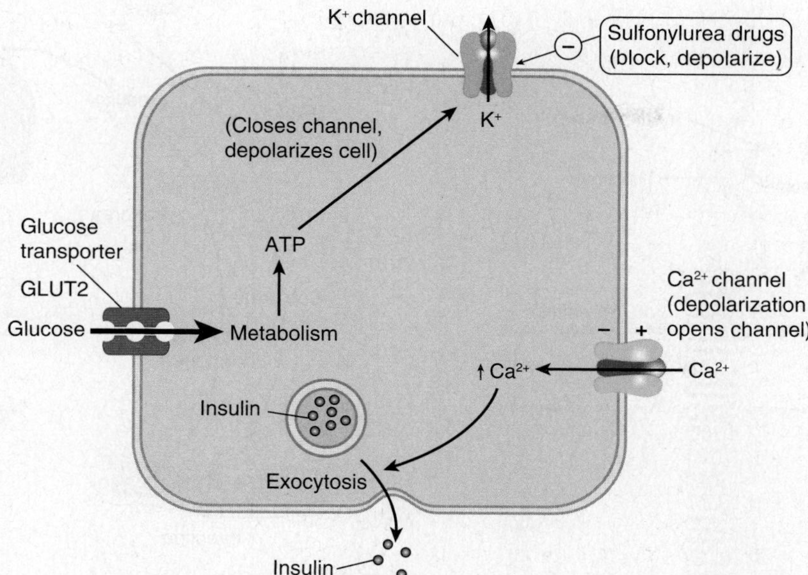

FIGURE 41–2 One model of control of insulin release from the pancreatic beta cell by glucose and by sulfonylurea drugs. In the resting cell with normal (low) ATP levels, potassium diffuses down its concentration gradient through ATP-gated potassium channels, maintaining the intracellular potential at a fully polarized, negative level. Insulin release is minimal. If glucose concentration rises, ATP production increases, potassium channels close, and depolarization of the cell results. As in muscle and nerve, voltage-gated calcium channels open in response to depolarization, allowing more calcium to enter the cell. Increased intracellular calcium results in increased insulin secretion. Insulin secretagogues close the ATP-dependent potassium channel, thereby depolarizing the membrane and causing increased insulin release by the same mechanism.

these insulin-receptor complexes have been identified in the primary target tissues regulating energy metabolism, ie, liver, muscle, and adipose tissue. The receptors bind insulin with high specificity and affinity in the picomolar range. The full insulin receptor consists of two covalently linked heterodimers, each containing an α subunit, which is entirely extracellular and constitutes the recognition site, and a β subunit that spans the membrane (Figure 41–3). The β subunit contains a tyrosine kinase. The binding of an insulin molecule to the α subunits at the outside surface of the cell activates the receptor and through a conformational change brings the catalytic loops of the opposing cytoplasmic β subunits into closer proximity. This facilitates mutual phosphorylation of tyrosine residues on the β subunits and tyrosine kinase activity directed at cytoplasmic proteins.

The first proteins to be phosphorylated by the activated receptor tyrosine kinases are the docking proteins: insulin receptor substrates (IRS). After tyrosine phosphorylation at several critical sites, the IRS molecules bind to and activate other kinases subserving energy metabolism—most significantly phosphatidylinositol-3-kinase—which produce further phosphorylations. Alternatively, they may stimulate a mitogenic pathway and bind to an adaptor protein such as growth factor receptor–binding protein 2, which translates the insulin signal to a guanine nucleotide-releasing factor that ultimately activates the GTP binding protein, Ras, and the mitogen-activated protein kinase (MAPK) system. The particular IRS-phosphorylated tyrosine kinases have binding specificity with downstream molecules based on their surrounding 4–5 amino acid sequences or motifs that recognize specific Src homology 2 (SH2) domains on the other protein. This network of phosphorylations within the cell represents insulin's second message and results in multiple effects, including translocation of glucose transporters (especially GLUT 4, Table 41–2) to the cell membrane with a resultant increase in glucose uptake; increased glycogen synthase activity and increased glycogen formation; multiple effects on protein synthesis, lipolysis, and lipogenesis; and activation of transcription factors that enhance DNA synthesis and cell growth and division.

Various hormonal agents (eg, glucocorticoids) lower the affinity of insulin receptors for insulin; growth hormone in excess increases this affinity slightly. Aberrant serine and threonine phosphorylation of the insulin receptor β subunits or IRS molecules may result in insulin resistance and functional receptor down-regulation.

Effects of Insulin on Its Targets

Insulin promotes the storage of fat as well as glucose (both sources of energy) within specialized target cells (Figure 41–4) and influences cell growth and the metabolic functions of a wide variety of tissues (Table 41–3).

■ GLUCAGON

Chemistry & Metabolism

Glucagon is synthesized in the alpha cells of the pancreatic islets of Langerhans (see Table 41–1). Glucagon is a peptide—identical in all mammals—consisting of a single chain of 29 amino acids, with a molecular weight of 3485. Selective proteolytic cleavage converts a large precursor molecule of approximately 18,000

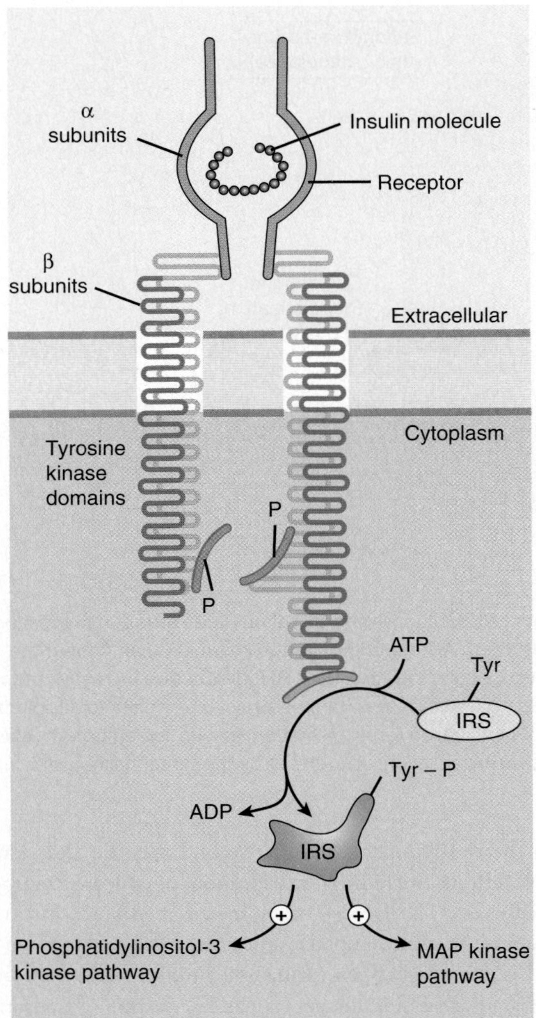

FIGURE 41–3 Schematic diagram of the insulin receptor heterodimer in the activated state. IRS, insulin receptor substrate; MAP, mitogen-activated protein; P, phosphate; Tyr, tyrosine.

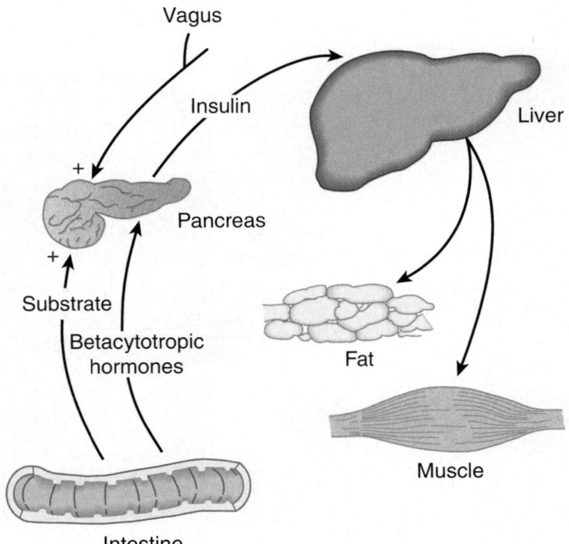

FIGURE 41–4 Insulin promotes synthesis (from circulating nutrients) and storage of glycogen, triglycerides, and protein in its major target tissues: liver, fat, and muscle. The release of insulin from the pancreas is stimulated by increased blood glucose, incretins, vagal nerve stimulation, and other factors (see text).

MW to glucagon. One of the precursor intermediates consists of a 69-amino-acid peptide called **glicentin,** which contains the glucagon sequence interposed between peptide extensions.

Glucagon is extensively degraded in the liver and kidney as well as in plasma and at its tissue receptor sites. Its half-life in plasma is between 3 and 6 minutes, which is similar to that of insulin.

Pharmacologic Effects of Glucagon

The first six amino acids at the amino terminal of the glucagon molecule bind to specific G_s protein-coupled receptors on liver cells. This leads to an increase in cAMP, which facilitates catabolism of stored glycogen and increases gluconeogenesis and ketogenesis. The immediate pharmacological result of glucagon infusion is to raise blood glucose by using stored hepatic glycogen. There is no effect on skeletal muscle glycogen, presumably because of the lack of glucagon receptors on skeletal muscle. Pharmacological amounts of glucagon cause release of insulin from normal pancreatic beta cells, catecholamines from pheochromocytoma, and calcitonin from medullary carcinoma cells.

Glucagon has a potent inotropic and chronotropic effect on the heart, mediated by the cAMP mechanism described above. Thus, it produces an effect very similar to that of β-adrenoceptor agonists without requiring functioning β receptors.

Large doses of glucagon produce profound relaxation of the intestine. In contrast to the above effects of the peptide, this action

TABLE 41–2 Glucose transporters.

Transporter	Tissues	Glucose K_m (mmol/L)	Function
GLUT 1	All tissues, especially red cells, brain	1–2	Basal uptake of glucose; transport across the blood-brain barrier
GLUT 2	Beta cells of pancreas; liver, kidney; gut	15–20	Regulation of insulin release, other aspects of glucose homeostasis
GLUT 3	Brain, placenta	<1	Uptake into neurons, other tissues
GLUT 4	Muscle, adipose	~5	Insulin-mediated uptake of glucose
GLUT 5	Gut, kidney	1–2	Absorption of fructose

TABLE 41–3 Endocrine effects of insulin.

Effect on liver:
Reversal of catabolic features of insulin deficiency
Inhibits glycogenolysis
Inhibits conversion of fatty acids and amino acids to keto acids
Inhibits conversion of amino acids to glucose
Anabolic action
Promotes glucose storage as glycogen (induces glucokinase and glycogen synthase, inhibits phosphorylase)
Increases triglyceride synthesis and very-low-density lipoprotein formation
Effect on muscle:
Increased protein synthesis
Increases amino acid transport
Increases ribosomal protein synthesis
Increased glycogen synthesis
Increases glucose transport
Induces glycogen synthase and inhibits phosphorylase
Effect on adipose tissue:
Increased triglyceride storage
Lipoprotein lipase is induced and activated by insulin to hydrolyze triglycerides from lipoproteins
Glucose transport into cell provides glycerol phosphate to permit esterification of fatty acids supplied by lipoprotein transport
Intracellular lipase is inhibited by insulin

on the intestine may be due to mechanisms other than adenylyl cyclase activation.

Clinical Uses

The major clinical use of glucagon is for emergency treatment of severe hypoglycemic reactions due to insulin therapy when a person is unable to self-treat with oral glucose (eg, unconsciousness) and intravenous glucose treatment is not possible. Recombinant glucagon is currently available in a 1-mg vial for parenteral (IV, IM, or SC) use; a single-dose 0.5-mg (for pediatric patients) or 1-mg (for adults) pen or prefilled syringe for subcutaneous injection; and a 3-mg dose of a nasal powder for inhalation. The main adverse effect is transient nausea and occasional vomiting. It is therefore important to place unconscious patients on their side after administering the drug.

Intravenous glucagon is commonly used in the endoscopic retrograde cholangiopancreatography procedure to facilitate the relaxation of the sphincter of Oddi. Glucagon is sometimes used in the treatment of beta blocker overdose because of the drug's ability to increase cAMP production in the heart independent of β-receptor function.

Glucagon should not be given to patients with pheochromocytoma in whom it can cause release of catecholamines and increase blood pressure; it also should not be given to patients with insulinoma where it can cause rebound hypoglycemia.

DIABETES MELLITUS

Diabetes mellitus is defined as an elevated blood glucose associated with absent or inadequate pancreatic insulin secretion, with or without concurrent impairment of insulin action. The disease states underlying the diagnosis of diabetes mellitus are now classified into four categories: **type 1, type 2, other specific types,** and **gestational diabetes mellitus.**

Type 1 Diabetes Mellitus

The hallmark of type 1 diabetes is selective beta cell destruction and *severe* or *absolute* insulin deficiency. Type 1 diabetes is further subdivided into immune-mediated (type 1a) and idiopathic causes (type 1b). The immune form is the most common form of type 1 diabetes. Although most patients are younger than 30 years of age at the time of diagnosis, the onset can occur at any age. Type 1 diabetes is found in all ethnic groups, but the highest incidence is in people from northern Europe and from Sardinia. Susceptibility appears to involve a multifactorial genetic linkage, but only 10–15% of patients have a positive family history. Most patients with type 1 diabetes have one or more circulating antibodies, including antibodies to glutamic acid decarboxylase 65 (GAD 65), insulin autoantibody, tyrosine phosphatase IA2 (ICA 512), and zinc transporter 8 (ZnT8) at the time of diagnosis. These antibodies facilitate the diagnosis of type 1a diabetes and can also be used to screen family members at risk for developing the disease. Most type 1 diabetes patients with acute symptomatic presentation have significant beta cell loss and insulin therapy is essential to control glucose levels and to prevent ketosis.

Some patients have a more indolent autoimmune process and initially retain enough beta cell function to avoid ketosis. They can be treated at first with oral glucose-lowering agents but then need insulin as their beta cell function declines. Antibody studies in northern Europeans indicate that up to 10–15% of "type 2" patients may actually have this milder form of type 1 diabetes (latent autoimmune diabetes of adulthood; LADA).

The CD3 complex is the major signal-transducing element of the T-cell receptor, and anti-CD3 antibodies have been shown to modulate the autoimmune response in persons with type 1 diabetes. **Teplizumab-mzwv,** a humanized monoclonal antibody against CD3, has been approved for use in individuals at high risk for type 1 diabetes (two positive antibodies and impaired glucose tolerance [stage 2 type 1 diabetes]) age 8 and older. The drug is infused daily for 14 days. The treatment delays the time to onset of overt type 1 diabetes (ie, stage 3 type 1 diabetes) by 25 months. Common adverse reactions include transient decreases in white cell and lymphocyte counts, rash, and headache.

Type 2 Diabetes Mellitus

Type 2 diabetes is a heterogenous group of conditions characterized by tissue resistance to the action of insulin combined with a *relative* deficiency in insulin secretion. A given individual may have more insulin resistance or more beta cell deficiency, and the glucose abnormalities may be mild or severe. Although the circulating endogenous insulin is sufficient to prevent ketoacidosis, it is inadequate to prevent hyperglycemia. Patients with type 2 diabetes can initially be controlled with diet, exercise, and non-insulin glucose-lowering drugs (oral and injectable). Some patients have progressive beta cell failure and eventually may also need insulin therapy.

Other Specific Types of Diabetes Mellitus

The "other" designation refers to multiple *other* specific causes of an elevated blood glucose: pancreatectomy, pancreatitis, nonpancreatic diseases, drug therapy, etc. For a detailed list the reader is referred to the American Diabetes Association report, 2014.

Gestational Diabetes Mellitus

Gestational diabetes (GDM) is defined as any abnormality in glucose levels noted for the first time during pregnancy. Gestational diabetes is diagnosed in approximately 7% of all pregnancies in the United States. During pregnancy, the placenta and placental hormones create an insulin resistance that is most pronounced in the last trimester. Risk assessment for diabetes is suggested starting at the first prenatal visit. High-risk women should be screened immediately. Screening may be deferred in lower-risk women until the 24th to 28th week of gestation.

Laboratory Findings

A. Plasma or Serum Glucose

A plasma glucose level of 126 mg/dL (7 mmol/L) or higher on more than one occasion after at least 8 hours of fasting is diagnostic of diabetes mellitus (see Table 41–4). Fasting plasma glucose levels of 100–125 mg/dL (5.6–6.9 mmol/L) are associated with increased risk of diabetes (impaired fasting glucose tolerance).

B. Hemoglobin A_{1c} Measurements

When plasma glucose levels are in the normal range, about 4–6% of hemoglobin A has one or both of the N terminal valines of their beta chains irreversibly glycated by glucose—referred to as hemoglobin$_{1c}$ (HbA_{1c}). The HbA_{1c} fraction is abnormally elevated in people with diabetes with chronic hyperglycemia. Since red blood cells have a lifespan of up to 120 days, the HbA_{1c} value reflects plasma glucose levels over the preceding 8–12 weeks.

In patients who monitor their glucose levels, the HbA_{1c} value provides a valuable check on the accuracy of their monitoring. In patients who do not monitor their glucose levels, HbA_{1c} measurements are essential for adjusting treatment. The American Diabetes Association has endorsed the use of HbA_{1c} as a diagnostic test for diabetes. A cutoff value of 6.5% was chosen because the risk of retinopathy increases substantially above this value. Less than 5.7% is normal, and patients with levels of 5.7–6.4% are considered at high risk for developing diabetes (see Table 41–4).

C. Oral Glucose Tolerance Test

If either the HbA_{1c} level is less than 6.5% or the fasting plasma glucose level is less than 126 mg/dL (7 mMol/L) but diabetes is nonetheless suspected, then a standardized oral glucose tolerance test may be done (see Table 41–4). The patient should eat nothing after midnight prior to the test day. On the morning of the test, adults are then given 75 g of glucose in 300 mL of water; children are given 1.75 g of glucose per kilogram of ideal body weight. The glucose load is consumed within 5 minutes. Patients should not smoke or be active during the test. Blood samples for plasma glucose are obtained at 0 and 120 minutes after ingestion of glucose. An oral glucose tolerance test is normal if the fasting venous plasma glucose value is less than 100 mg/dL (5.6 mmol/L) and the 2-hour value falls below 140 mg/dL (7.8 mmol/L). A fasting value of 126 mg/dL (7 mmol/L) or higher or a 2-hour value of greater than 200 mg/dL (11.1 mmol/L) is diagnostic of diabetes mellitus. Patients with 2-hour value of 140–199 mg/dL (7.8–11.1 mmol/L) have impaired glucose tolerance.

D. Urine or Blood Ketones

Qualitative detection of ketone bodies can be accomplished by nitroprusside tests (Acetest or Ketostix). Although these tests do not detect beta-hydroxybutyric acid, which lacks a ketone group, the semiquantitative estimation of ketonuria thus obtained is nonetheless usually adequate for clinical purposes. Many laboratories now measure beta-hydroxybutyric acid, and meters are available (FORA meters; Nova Max Plus) for patient use that measure beta-hydroxybutyric acid levels in capillary blood glucose samples.

TABLE 41–4 Diagnostic criteria for diabetes.

	Normal Glucose Tolerance, mg/dL (mMol/L)	Prediabetes	Diabetes Mellitus[2]
Fasting plasma glucose mg/dL (mmol/L)	<100 (5.6)	100–125 (5.6–6.9) (impaired fasting glucose)	≥126 (7.0)
Two hours after glucose load[1] mg/dL (mmol/L)	<140 (7.8)	≥140.199 (7.8–11.0) (impaired glucose tolerance)	≥200 (11.1)
HbA_{1c} (%) (ADA criteria)	<5.7	5.7–6.4	≥6.5

[1]Give 75 g of glucose dissolved in 300 mL of water after an overnight fast in persons who have been receiving at least 150–200 g of carbohydrate daily for 3 days before the test.

[2]A fasting plasma glucose ≥126 mg/dL (7.0 mmol) or HbA_{1c} ≥6.5% is diagnostic of diabetes if confirmed by repeat testing.

Symptoms and random glucose level >200 mg/dL (11.1 mmol/L) are diagnostic, and there is no need to do additional testing.

Beta-hydroxybutyrate levels >0.6 mmol/L require evaluation. A level >3.0 mmol/L, which is equivalent to very high urinary ketones, will require hospitalization.

E. Self-Monitoring of Capillary Blood Glucose

Many blood glucose meters are available for measuring glucose from capillary blood samples. All are accurate, but they vary with regard to speed, convenience, size of blood samples required, reporting capability, and cost. Some meters are designed to communicate with an insulin pump. Providers and patients should be aware of the limitations of the blood glucose monitoring (BGM) systems. BGM strips have expiration dates; expired strips should not be used. Improper storage of strips (high temperature; open bottle) can affect their function. Conditions that impair the circulation to the fingers can artificially lower blood glucose measurements. When capillary glucose levels are measured at alternate sites such as the forearm, there can be a 5- to 20-minute lag in glucose response on the arm with respect to the glucose response on the finger. For this reason, alternate-site testing should not be used when the glucose is rapidly changing (eg, postprandial or if hypoglycemia is suspected).

F. Continuous Glucose Monitors

These systems utilize a subcutaneous sensor that measures glucose concentrations in the interstitial fluid for 10–14 days. Studies show that pediatric and adult patients with type 1 diabetes who use continuous glucose monitoring (CGM) devices have improved glucose control without an increased incidence of hypoglycemia. The glucose data are transmitted wirelessly to smart phones and the screens of insulin pumps. There are directional arrows that indicate rate and direction of change of glucose levels, and alerts can be set for high and low glucose levels. The data from these CGM devices can be used to automatically deliver insulin by continuous subcutaneous insulin infusion pump (closed loop systems).

■ MEDICATIONS FOR HYPERGLYCEMIA

Insulin Preparations

Human insulin is dispensed as regular (R) and neutral protamine hagedorn (NPH) formulations. There are also six analogs of human insulin. Three of the analogs are rapidly acting: insulin lispro, insulin aspart, and insulin glulisine; and three are long acting: insulin glargine, insulin detemir, and insulin degludec. Animal insulins are not available in the United States. Pork and beef preparations (isophane, neutral, 70/30, and lente) are still available in other parts of the world. Most insulins in the United States are available in a concentration of 100 units/mL (U100) and dispensed as 10-mL vials or 0.3-mL cartridges or prefilled disposable pens. Several insulins are also available at higher concentrations in the prefilled disposable pen form: insulin glargine 300 units/mL (U300); insulin degludec 200 units/mL (U200); insulin lispro 200 units/mL (U200); and regular insulin 500 units/mL (U500) (Tables 41–5, 41–6).

A. Short-Acting Insulin Preparations (Tables 41–5, 41–6)

The short-acting preparations include regular human insulin and the three rapid-acting insulin analogs. All are clear solutions at neutral pH. The insulin molecules exist as dimers that assemble into hexamers in the presence of two zinc ions. The hexamers are further stabilized by phenolic compounds such as phenol and meta-Cresol. The mutations engineered into the rapidly acting insulin analogs are designed to disrupt the stabilizing intermolecular interactions of the dimers and hexamers, leading to more rapid absorption into the circulation after subcutaneous injection.

1. *Regular insulin*—Regular insulin is a short-acting, soluble crystalline zinc insulin whose hypoglycemic effect appears within 30 minutes after subcutaneous injection, peaks at about 2 hours, and lasts for 5–7 hours when usual quantities (ie, 5–15 U) are administered. For very insulin-resistant subjects who would otherwise require large volumes of insulin solution, a U500 preparation of human regular insulin is available both in a vial and a disposable pen. A U500 insulin syringe should be used to measure the dose when using the vial. If a U100 insulin syringe or tuberculin syringe is used, then the clinician should carefully note the dose in both units and volume to avoid overdosage. The disposable pen avoids this conversion issue and dispenses the regular U500 insulin in 5-unit increments. U-500 regular insulin, a concentrated insulin, has a different time action profile than U-100 regular insulin; it is similar to NPH insulin.

When intravenous insulin is needed (eg, inpatient setting), regular insulin is used; it is particularly useful in the treatment

TABLE 41–5 Summary of bioavailability characteristics of the insulins.

Insulin Preparations	Onset of Action	Peak Action	Effective Duration
Insulins lispro, aspart, glulisine	5–15 min	1–1.5 h	3–4 h
Human regular	30–60 min	2 h	6–8 h
Technosphere inhaled insulin	5–15 min	1 h	3 h
Human NPH	2–4 h	6–7 h	10–20 h
Insulin glargine	0.5–1 h	Flat	~24 h
Insulin detemir	0.5–1 h	Flat	17 h
Insulin degludec	0.5–1.5 h	Flat	>42 h

TABLE 41–6 Some insulin preparations available in the United States.

Preparation	Species Source	Concentration
Short-acting insulins		
Insulin lispro (Humalog, Lyumjev, Lilly; Admelog, sanofi-aventis)	Human analog	U100
		U200 (Humalog and Lyumjev only)
Insulin aspart, insulin aspart niacinamide (Novolog, Fiasp, Novo Nordisk)	Human analog	U100
Insulin glulisine (Apidra, sanofi-aventis)	Human analog	U100
Regular insulin (Humulin R, Lilly; Novolin R, Novo Nordisk)	Human	U100
		U500 (Humulin R only)
Regular insulin inhaled (MannKind)	Human	—
Long-acting insulins		
NPH insulin (Humulin N, Lilly; Novolin N, Novo Nordisk)	Human	U100
Insulin glargine (Lantus, Toujeo, sanofi-aventis; Basaglar, Rezvoglar, Lilly; Semglee,[1] Mylan)	Human analog	U100
		U300 (Toujeo only)
Insulin detemir (Levemir, Novo Nordisk)	Human analog	U100
Insulin degludec (Tresiba, Novo Nordisk)	Human analog	U100, U200
Premixed insulins		
70 NPH/30 regular (Novolin, Novo Nordisk; Humulin, Lilly)	Human	U100
75/25 NPL, Lispro (Humalog mix 75/25, Lilly)	Human analog	U100
50/50 NPL, Lispro (Humalog mix 50/50, Lilly)	Human analog	U100
70/30 NPA, Aspart (Novolog mix 70/30, Novo Nordisk)	Human analog	U100
70/30 Degludec/Aspart (Ryzodeg, Novo Nordisk)	Human analog	U100

All insulins are now made by recombinant technology; they should be refrigerated and brought to room temperature just before injection.

NPA, neutral protamine aspart; NPL, neutral protamine lispro.

[1]Semglee and Rezvoglar are interchangeable (biosimilar) insulins with Lantus.

of diabetic ketoacidosis and during perioperative glucose management.

2. *Rapidly acting insulin analogs*—Insulin lispro (Humalog) is an insulin analog in which the proline at position B28 is reversed with the lysine at B29. Insulin aspart (Novolog, Admelog, FiAsp) is a single substitution of proline by aspartic acid at position B28. Insulin glulisine (Apidra) differs from human insulin in that the amino acid asparagine at position B3 is replaced by lysine and the lysine in position B29 by glutamic acid. When injected subcutaneously, these three analogs quickly dissociate into monomers and are absorbed very rapidly, reaching peak serum values in as little as 1 hour. The amino acid changes in these analogs do not interfere with their binding to the insulin receptor, with the circulating half-life, or with their immunogenicity, which are all identical to those of human regular insulin. An insulin aspart formulation (FiAsp) that contains niacinamide (Vitamin B_3) has a more rapid absorption and its onset of action is about 10 minutes faster than the standard insulin aspart formulation. Similarly, there is an insulin lispro formulation (Lyumjev) whose onset of action is 11 minutes faster than the insulin lispro formulation. This formulation contains citrate and treprostinil. The former increases vascular permeability and the latter induces vasodilatation, thus increasing the subcutaneous absorption speed.

Clinical trials have demonstrated that the optimal times of preprandial rapidly acting insulin analogs and regular human insulin are 15 minutes and 45 minutes before the meal, respectively. The rapidly acting insulins are more convenient as patients can inject immediately before eating and do not have to wait as with regular insulin. It is important that patients ingest adequate carbohydrate early in the meal to avoid hypoglycemia during the meal. These analogs also have lowest variability of absorption: approximately 5% variation, compared to 25% for regular insulin. Another desirable feature of rapidly acting insulin analogs is that their duration of action is consistently about 4 hours for most commonly used dosages. This contrasts with regular insulin, whose duration of action is significantly prolonged when larger doses are used.

The rapidly acting analogs are the insulin of choice for insulin pumps. In a double-blind crossover study comparing insulin lispro with regular insulin in insulin pumps, patients using insulin lispro had lower HbA_{1c} values and improved postprandial glucose control with the same frequency of hypoglycemia.

B. Long-Acting Insulin Preparations (Tables 41–5, 41–6)

1. *NPH (neutral protamine Hagedorn, or isophane) insulin*—NPH insulin is an intermediate-acting insulin whose absorption and onset of action are delayed by combining appropriate amounts of insulin and protamine so that neither is present in an uncomplexed form ("isophane"). After subcutaneous

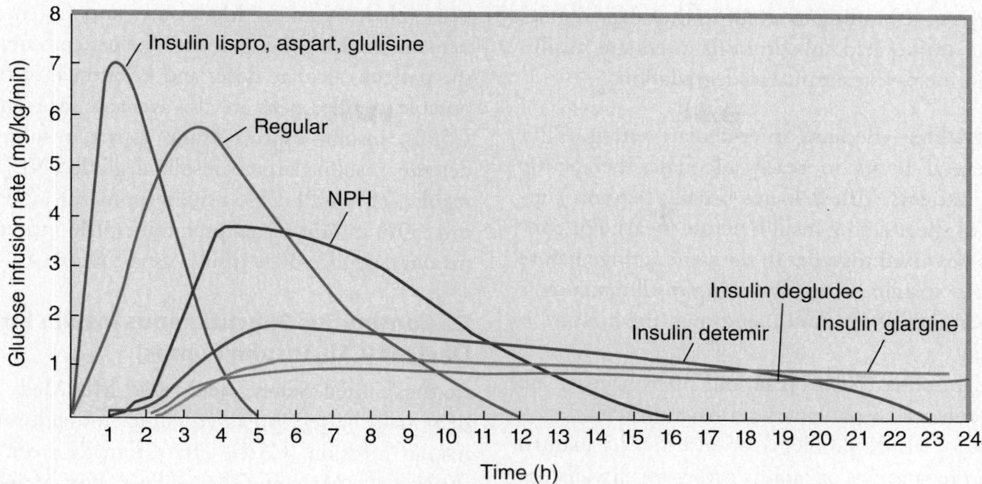

FIGURE 41–5 Extent and duration of action of various types of insulin as indicated by the glucose infusion rates (mg/kg/min) required to maintain a constant glucose concentration. The durations of action shown are typical of an average dose of 0.2–0.3 U/kg. The durations of regular and NPH insulin increase considerably when dosage is increased.

injection, proteolytic tissue enzymes degrade the protamine to permit absorption of insulin. NPH insulin has an onset of approximately 2–4 hours, peak action 6-7 hours and duration of 10–20 hours (Figure 41–5); it is usually mixed with regular, lispro, aspart, or glulisine insulin and given two to four times daily for insulin replacement. The dose regulates the action profile; specifically, small doses have lower, earlier peaks and a short duration of action with the converse true for large doses.

2. *Insulin glargine*—Insulin glargine is a soluble, "peakless" (ie, having a broad plasma concentration plateau), long-acting insulin analog. The attachment of two arginine molecules to the B-chain carboxyl terminal and substitution of a glycine for asparagine at the A21 position created an analog that is soluble in an acidic solution but precipitates in the more neutral body pH after subcutaneous injection. Individual insulin molecules slowly dissolve away from the crystalline depot and provide a low, continuous level of circulating insulin. Insulin glargine has a slow onset of action (0.5–1 hours) and the effective duration of action is approximately 24 hours. Glargine is usually given once daily, although some very insulin-sensitive individuals (requiring small doses, less than about 20 units daily) or insulin-resistant individuals (requiring very large doses) benefit from split (twice a day) dosing. To maintain solubility, the formulation is unusually acidic (pH 4.0), and insulin glargine should not be mixed with other insulins. If administered via a syringe, a separate syringe must be used to minimize the risk of contamination and subsequent loss of efficacy. The absorption pattern of insulin glargine appears to be independent of the anatomic site of injection, and this drug is associated with less immunogenicity than human insulin in animal studies. Glargine's interaction with the insulin receptor is similar to that of native insulin and shows no increase in mitogenic activity in vitro. It has sixfold to sevenfold greater binding than native insulin to the insulin-like growth factor 1 (IGF-1) receptor, but the clinical significance of this is unclear.

3. *Insulin detemir*—In this insulin, the terminal threonine is dropped from the B30 position and myristic acid (a C-14 fatty acid chain) is attached to the B29 lysine. These modifications prolong the availability of the injected analog by increasing both self-aggregation in subcutaneous tissue and reversible albumin binding. The affinity of insulin detemir is four- to five-fold lower than that of human soluble insulin and, therefore, the U100 formulation of insulin detemir has a concentration of 2400 nmol/mL compared with 600 nmol/mL for NPH. The duration of action for insulin detemir is about 17 hours at therapeutically relevant doses. It is recommended that the insulin be injected once or twice a day to achieve a stable basal coverage. This insulin has been reported to have lower within-subject pharmacodynamic variability compared with NPH insulin and insulin glargine.

4. *Insulin degludec*—In this insulin analog, the threonine at position B30 has been removed and the lysine at position B29 is conjugated to hexadecanoic acid via a gamma-L-glutamyl spacer. In solution and in the presence of phenol and zinc, the insulin is in the form of dihexamers; however, when injected subcutaneously, it self-associates into large multihexameric chains consisting of thousands of dihexamers. The chains slowly dissolve in the subcutaneous tissue, and insulin monomers are steadily released into the systemic circulation. The half-life of the insulin is 25 hours. Its onset of action is in 30–90 minutes, and its duration of action is more than 42 hours. Degludec is generally injected once a day to achieve a stable basal coverage. Insulin degludec is available in two concentrations, U100 and U200, and in prefilled disposable pens.

5. *Insulin icodec*—This is a basal insulin analog that is given once a week. The lysine at B29 of the insulin is conjugated to 1,20-icosanedioic acid (C20). There are three aminoacid substitutions (A14E, B16H and B25H). The C20 diacid group results in strong, reversible binding to albumin thus delaying SC absorption, and the amino acid substitutions attenuate insulin receptor affinity and increase resistance to degradation.

6. *Mixtures of insulins*—Because intermediate-acting NPH insulins require several hours to reach adequate therapeutic levels, their use in patients with diabetes usually requires supplements of rapid- or short-acting insulin before meals. For convenience, these can be mixed together in the same syringe before injection. The regular insulin or rapidly acting insulin analog is withdrawn first, then the NPH insulin, and then the mixture is injected immediately.

Stable premixed insulins (70% NPH and 30% regular) are available as a convenience to patients who have difficulty mixing insulin because of visual problems or insufficient manual dexterity. Premixed preparations of rapidly acting insulin analogs (lispro, aspart) and NPH are not stable because of exchange of the rapidly acting insulin analog for the human regular insulin in the protamine complex. Consequently, over time, the soluble component becomes a mixture of regular and rapidly acting insulin analog at varying ratios. To remedy this problem, intermediate insulins composed of isophane complexes of protamine with the rapidly acting insulin analogs were developed (neutral protamine lispro [NPL]; aspart protamine). Premixed combinations of NPL and insulin lispro are now available for clinical use (Humalog Mix 75/25 and Humalog Mix 50/50). These mixtures have a more rapid onset of glucose-lowering activity compared with 70% NPH/30% regular human insulin mixture and can be given within 15 minutes before or after starting a meal. A similar 70% insulin aspart protamine/30% insulin aspart (NovoLog Mix 70/30) is now available. The main advantages of these new mixtures are that (1) they can be given within 15 minutes of starting a meal and (2) they are more effective in achieving glucose targets with the postprandial glucose rise after a carbohydrate-rich meal. Insulin glargine and insulin detemir cannot be mixed in the same syringe with other insulins.

Insulin Delivery Systems

A. Insulin Syringes and Needles

Disposable plastic syringes with needles attached are available in 1-mL (100 units), 0.5-mL (50 units), and 0.3-mL (30 units) sizes. The "low-dose" 0.3-mL syringes are popular because many patients with diabetes do not take more than 30 units of insulin in a single injection and the markings are easier to read. They are also available in half-unit markings. Three lengths of needles are available; longer needles are preferable in overweight/obese patients to ensure insulin absorption. If the skin is clean, it is not necessary to use alcohol. Rotation of sites is recommended to avoid problems with absorption due to lipohypertrophy from overuse of injection sites.

B. Insulin Pens

The pens eliminate the need for carrying insulin vials and syringes. Cartridges of insulin aspart and lispro are available for reusable pens (Novo Nordisk, Medtronic, and Owen Mumford). Smart pens are available that pair with the patient's smart phone and help the patient calculate doses and keep track of the injections. Disposable prefilled pens are also available for regular insulin (U100, U500), insulin lispro, insulin aspart, insulin glulisine, insulin detemir, insulin glargine, insulin degludec, NPH, 70% NPH/30% regular, 75% NPL/25% insulin lispro, 50% NPL/50% insulin lispro, 70% insulin aspart protamine/30% insulin aspart, and 70% insulin degludec/30% insulin aspart (Table 41–6).

C. Continuous Subcutaneous Insulin Infusion Devices (CSII, Insulin Pumps)

In the United States, Medtronic MiniMed, Insulet, and Tandem make battery-operated pumps for continuous subcutaneous insulin infusion (CSII). The externally worn pumps are about the size of a pager and they deliver short-acting insulin throughout the day and night. The catheter connecting the insulin reservoir to the subcutaneous cannula can be disconnected, allowing the patient to remove the pump temporarily (eg, for bathing). Omnipod (Insulet Corporation) is a disposable waterproof electronic patch pump in which the insulin reservoir and infusion set are integrated into one unit (pod), so there is no catheter. The pod, placed on the skin, delivers subcutaneous basal and bolus insulin based on wirelessly transmitted instructions from a personal digital assistant.

A major advantage of an insulin pump is that it allows for establishment of a basal profile tailored to the patient allowing for better overnight, between-meals glucose control, and management of glycemic excursions that occur with exercise. Software assists the patient in calculating boluses based on glucose reading and carbohydrates to be consumed. The insulin pumps keep track of the time elapsed since the last insulin bolus and reduce the risk of overcorrecting and subsequent hypoglycemia.

CSII therapy is appropriate for patients with type 1 diabetes who are motivated, mechanically inclined, educated about diabetes (diet, insulin action, treatment of hypoglycemia and hyperglycemia), and willing to monitor their blood glucose four to six times a day. Known complications of CSII include ketoacidosis, which can occur when insulin delivery is interrupted, and skin infections. Another disadvantage is its cost and the additional time needed by the clinician and staff to initiate therapy. Almost all patients use rapidly acting insulin analogs in their pumps.

V-Go (MannKind) is a wearable patch pump designed specifically for people with type 2 diabetes who use a basal/bolus insulin regimen. The device uses rapid-acting insulin and is preset to deliver one of three fixed and flat basal rates (0.83 units/h [20 units], 1.25 units/h [30 units], or 1.67 units/h [40 units]) for 24 hours (at which point the device must be replaced). It can also deliver 2-unit increments (up to 36 units) by pressing a button, for meal coverage and high sugar correction. CeQur Simplicity (CeQur) is a 3-day wearable patch device that holds 200 units of rapid-acting insulin and delivers 2-unit increments of rapid-acting insulin by squeezing two buttons for meal coverage and high sugar correction.

D. Closed-Loop Systems

Algorithms have been devised to use glucose data from the CGM systems to automatically deliver insulin by CSII pump. These closed-loop systems ("artificial pancreas") have been shown to reduce nighttime hypoglycemia and lower HbA1c levels. The MiniMed 770 G closed loop uses glucose data from a sensor to automatically adjust basal insulin doses every 5 minutes, targeting a sensor glucose level of 120 mg/dL (6.7 mmol/L). Insulin delivery is suspended when the sensor glucose level falls below or is predicted to fall below target level. The Tandem Control-IQ targets a sensor glucose level of 112.5 mg/dL (6.25 mmol/L). The Omnipod 5 targets a user-programmed glucose value between 100 and 150 mg/dL. The patient is still responsible for bolusing insulin for meals and snacks. Communities of patients with type 1 diabetes have also developed open source algorithms for smart phone that use glucose data from CGM systems to automatically adjust insulin delivery by their pumps (open artificial pancreas, open APS). One such system, called the "Loop," uses the Dexcom G6 sensor, the iPhone, and the Omnipod insulin pump. The "Loop" controller is downloaded on to the iPhone and it uses the Dexcom G6 sensor glucose measurements (also on the iPhone) to automatically adjust basal insulin delivery on the Omnipod pump. These open APS systems have not been approved for use by the FDA.

E. Inhaled Insulin

A dry powder formulation of regular human insulin (technosphere insulin, Afrezza) is approved for use in adults with diabetes. It consists of 2- to 2.5-μm crystals of the excipient, fumaryl diketopiperazine, that provide a large surface area for adsorption of proteins like insulin. After inhalation from the small, single-use device, pharmacokinetic studies show that peak levels are reached in 12–15 minutes and decline to baseline in 3 hours, significantly faster in onset and shorter in duration than subcutaneous insulin. Pharmacodynamic studies show that median time to maximum effect with inhaled insulin is approximately 1 hour and declines to baseline by about 3 hours. In contrast, the median time to maximum effect with subcutaneous insulin lispro is about 2 hours and declines to baseline by 4 hours. In trials, inhaled insulin combined with injected basal insulin was as effective in lowering glucose as injected rapid-acting insulin combined with basal insulin. It is formulated as a single-use color-coded cartridge delivering 4, 8, or 12 units immediately before the meal. The manufacturer provides a dose conversion table; patients injecting up to 4 units of rapid-acting insulin analog should use the 4-unit cartridge. Those injecting 5–8 units should use the 8-unit cartridge. For a dose of 9–12 units of rapid-acting insulin pre-meal, one 4-unit cartridge and one 8-unit cartridge or one 12-unit cartridge should be used. The most common adverse effect of inhaled insulin was cough, affecting 27% of trial patients. A small decrease in pulmonary function (forced expiratory volume in 1 second [FEV_1]) was seen in the first 3 months of use, which persisted over 2 years of follow-up. Inhaled insulin is contraindicated in persons who smoke or those with chronic lung disease, such as asthma and chronic obstructive pulmonary disease. Spirometry should be performed to identify potential lung disease prior to initiating therapy. During the clinical trials, there were two cases of lung cancer in patients who were taking inhaled insulin and none in the comparator-treated patients.

Immunopathology of Insulin Therapy

At least five molecular classes of insulin antibodies may be produced in patients during the course of insulin therapy: IgA, IgD, IgE, IgG, and IgM. There are two major types of immune disorders in these patients:

1. *Insulin allergy*—Insulin allergy, an immediate type hypersensitivity, is a rare condition in which local or systemic urticaria results from histamine release from tissue mast cells sensitized by anti-insulin IgE antibodies. In severe cases, anaphylaxis results. Because sensitivity is often to non-insulin protein contaminants, the human and analog insulins have markedly reduced the incidence of insulin allergy, especially local reactions.

2. *Immune insulin resistance*—A low titer of circulating IgG anti-insulin antibodies that neutralize the action of insulin to a negligible extent develops in most insulin-treated patients. Rarely, the titer of insulin antibodies leads to insulin resistance and may be associated with other systemic autoimmune processes such as lupus erythematosus.

Lipodystrophy at Injection Sites

Injection of animal insulin preparations sometimes led to atrophy of subcutaneous fatty tissue at the site of injection. Since the development of human and analog insulin preparations of neutral pH, this type of immune complication is almost never seen. Injection of these newer preparations directly into the atrophic area often results in restoration of normal contours.

Hypertrophy of subcutaneous fatty tissue remains a problem if insulin is injected repeatedly at the same site. However, this may be corrected by avoiding the specific injection site.

■ MEDICATIONS FOR TREATMENT OF TYPE 2 DIABETES

Several categories of glucose-lowering agents are available for patients with type 2 diabetes: (1) agents that bind to the sulfonylurea receptor and stimulate insulin secretion (sulfonylureas, meglitinides, D-phenylalanine derivatives); (2) agents that lower glucose levels by their actions on liver, muscle, and adipose tissue (biguanides, thiazolidinediones); (3) agents that principally slow the intestinal absorption of glucose (α-glucosidase inhibitors); (4) agents that mimic incretin effect or prolong incretin action (GLP-1 receptor agonists, glucose-dependent insulinotropic polypeptide [GIP]/GLP-1 receptor agonists, dipeptidyl peptidase 4 [DPP-4] inhibitors); (5) agents that inhibit the reabsorption of glucose in the kidney (sodium-glucose co-transporter inhibitors [SGLTs]); and (6) agents that act by other or ill-defined mechanisms (pramlintide, bromocriptine, colesevelam).

DRUGS THAT PRIMARILY STIMULATE INSULIN RELEASE BY BINDING TO THE SULFONYLUREA RECEPTOR

SULFONYLUREAS

Mechanism of Action

The major action of sulfonylureas is to increase insulin release from the pancreas (Table 41–7). They bind to a 140-kDa high-affinity sulfonylurea receptor that is associated with a beta-cell inward rectifier ATP-sensitive potassium channel (see Figure 41–2). Binding of a sulfonylurea inhibits the efflux of potassium ions through the channel and results in depolarization. Depolarization opens a voltage-gated calcium channel and results in calcium influx and the release of preformed insulin.

Efficacy & Safety of the Sulfonylureas

Sulfonylureas are metabolized by the liver and, with the exception of acetohexamide, the metabolites are either weakly active or inactive. The metabolites are excreted by the kidney and, in the case of the second-generation sulfonylureas, partly excreted in the bile. Idiosyncratic reactions are rare, with skin rashes or hematologic toxicity (leukopenia, thrombocytopenia) occurring in less than 0.1% of cases. The second-generation sulfonylureas have greater affinity for their receptor compared with the first-generation agents. The correspondingly lower effective doses and plasma levels of the second-generation drugs therefore lower the risk of drug-drug interactions based on competition for plasma binding sites or hepatic enzyme action.

In 1970, the University Group Diabetes Program (UGDP) in the United States reported that the number of deaths due to cardiovascular disease in patients with type 2 diabetes treated with tolbutamide was excessive compared with either insulin-treated patients or those receiving placebos. Owing to design flaws, this study and its conclusions were not generally accepted. In the United Kingdom, the United Kingdom Prospective Diabetes Study (UKPDS) did not find an untoward cardiovascular effect of sulfonylurea usage in their large, long-term study. The sulfonylureas continue to be widely prescribed, and three are available in the United States.

TABLE 41–7 Regulation of insulin release in humans.

Regulation of insulin release
Stimulants of insulin release
Humoral: Glucose, mannose, leucine, arginine, other amino acids, fatty acids (high concentrations)
Hormonal: Glucagon, glucagon-like peptide 1 (7–37), glucose-dependent insulinotropic polypeptide, cholecystokinin, gastrin
Neural: β-Adrenergic stimulation, vagal stimulation
Drugs: Sulfonylureas, meglitinide, nateglinide, isoproterenol, acetylcholine
Inhibitors of insulin release
Hormonal: Somatostatin, insulin, leptin
Neural: α-Sympathomimetic effect of catecholamines
Drugs: Diazoxide, phenytoin, vinblastine, colchicine

Reproduced with permission from Greenspan FS, Gardner DG: *Basic & Clinical Endocrinology*, 6th ed. New York, NY: McGraw Hill; 2001.

FIRST-GENERATION SULFONYLUREAS

Tolbutamide is well absorbed but rapidly metabolized in the liver. Its duration of effect is relatively short (6–10 hours), with an elimination half-life of 4–5 hours, and it is best administered in divided doses (eg, 500 mg before each meal). Some patients only need one or two tablets daily. The maximum dosage is 3000 mg daily. Because of its short half-life and inactivation by the liver, it is relatively safe in the elderly and in patients with renal impairment.

Chlorpropamide, tolazamide, and acetohexamide (no longer available in the US) are now rarely used in clinical practice and are not further discussed. Drug label information for tolazamide can be found at https://dailymed.nlm.nih.gov/dailymed/.

SECOND-GENERATION SULFONYLUREAS

Glyburide, glipizide, gliclazide, and glimepiride are 100–200 times more potent than tolbutamide. They should be used with caution in patients with cardiovascular disease or in elderly patients, in whom hypoglycemia would be especially dangerous.

Glyburide (also named glibenclamide outside the USA) is metabolized in the liver into products with low hypoglycemic activity. The usual starting dosage is 2.5 mg/d or less, and the average maintenance dosage is 5–10 mg/d given as a single morning dose; maintenance dosages higher than 20 mg/d are not recommended. A formulation of "micronized" glyburide (Glynase PresTab) is available in a variety of tablet sizes. However, there is some question as to its bioequivalence with non-micronized formulations, and the FDA recommends careful monitoring to re-titrate dosage when switching from standard glyburide doses or from other sulfonylurea drugs.

Glyburide is metabolized in the liver and the metabolic products of glyburide have hypoglycemic activity. This explains why assays specific for the unmetabolized compound suggest a plasma half-life of only 1–2 hours, yet the biologic effects of glyburide are clearly persistent 24 hours after a single morning dose in patients with diabetes. Glyburide is unique among sulfonylureas in that it not only binds to the pancreatic B cell membrane sulfonylurea receptor but also becomes sequestered within the B cell. This may also contribute to its prolonged biologic effect despite its relatively short circulating half-life.

Glyburide should not be used in patients with liver failure and chronic kidney disease because of an increased risk of hypoglycemia. Elderly patients are at particular risk for hypoglycemia.

Glipizide has the shortest half-life (2–4 hours) of the more potent sulfonylureas. Food can delay the absorption of this drug and if possible, the patient should wait 30 minutes before eating. With chronic use, the clinical significance of this recommendation is less clear and the drug is effective even if it is taken immediately before the meal. The recommended starting dosage is 5 mg/d, with up to 15 mg/d given as a single dose. When higher daily dosages are required, they should be divided and given before meals. The maximum total daily dosage recommended by the manufacturer is 40 mg/d, although some studies indicate that the maximum therapeutic effect is achieved by 15–20 mg of the drug. An extended-release preparation (Glucotrol XL) provides 24-hour action after a once-daily morning dose (maximum of 20 mg/d). However, this formulation appears to have sacrificed its lower propensity for severe hypoglycemia compared with longer-acting glyburide without showing any demonstrable therapeutic advantages over the latter (which can be obtained as a generic drug). At least 90% of glipizide is metabolized in the liver to inactive products, and the remainder is excreted unchanged in the urine. Glipizide therapy is therefore contraindicated in patients with significant hepatic impairment. Because of its shorter duration of action and completely inactive metabolites, it is preferable to glyburide in the elderly and for those patients with renal impairment.

Glimepiride is use as monotherapy or as combination therapy and taken once daily. Glimepiride achieves blood glucose lowering with the lowest dosage of any sulfonylurea compound. A single daily dose of 1 mg has been shown to be effective, and the recommended maximal daily dosage is 8 mg. Glimepiride's half-life under multidose conditions is 5–9 hours. It is completely metabolized by the liver to metabolites with weak or no activity.

Gliclazide (not available in the United States) has a half-life of 10 hours. The recommended starting dosage is 40–80 mg daily with a maximum dosage of 320 mg daily. Higher dosages are usually divided and given twice a day. It is completely metabolized by the liver to inactive metabolites.

Hypoglycemia and weight gain are the most common adverse effects of the sulfonylureas. Some sulfonamides (sulfisoxazole) and oral azole antifungal medications can inhibit metabolism of tolbutamide and result in prolonged hypoglycemia. Glyburide can occasionally cause flushing after ethanol ingestion, and this compound slightly enhances free water clearance.

MEGLITINIDE ANALOGS

Repaglinide is the first member of the meglitinide group of insulin secretagogues. These drugs modulate beta cell insulin release by regulating potassium efflux through the potassium channels previously discussed. There is overlap with the sulfonylureas in their molecular sites of action because the meglitinides have two binding sites in common with the sulfonylureas and one unique binding site.

Repaglinide has a fast onset of action, with a peak concentration and peak effect within approximately 1 hour after ingestion, but the duration of action is 4–7 hours. It is cleared by hepatic CYP3A4 with a plasma half-life of 1 hour. Because of its rapid onset, repaglinide is indicated for use in controlling postprandial glucose excursions. The drug should be taken just before each meal in doses of 0.25–4 mg (maximum 16 mg/d); hypoglycemia is a risk if the meal is delayed or skipped or contains inadequate carbohydrate. It can be used in patients with renal impairment and in the elderly. Repaglinide is used as monotherapy or as combination therapy. There is no sulfur in its structure, so repaglinide may be used in patients with type 2 diabetes with a severe sulfur or sulfonylurea allergy.

Mitiglinide (not available in the United States) is a benzylsuccinic acid derivative that binds to the sulfonylurea receptor and is similar to repaglinide in its clinical effects. It is available for use in Japan.

D-PHENYLALANINE DERIVATIVE

Nateglinide is a D-phenylalanine derivative and stimulates rapid and transient release of insulin from beta cells through closure of the ATP-sensitive K^+ channel. It is absorbed within 20 minutes after oral administration with a time to peak concentration of less than 1 hour and is metabolized in the liver by CYP2C9 and CYP3A4 with a half-life of about 1 hour. The overall duration of action is about 4 hours. It is taken before the meal and reduces the postprandial rise in blood glucose levels. It is available as 60- and 120-mg tablets. The lower dose is used in patients with mild elevations in HbA_{1c}. Nateglinide is efficacious when given alone or in combination with non-secretagogue oral agents (such as metformin). Hypoglycemia is the main adverse effect. It can be used in patients with renal impairment and in the elderly.

DRUGS THAT PRIMARILY LOWER GLUCOSE LEVELS BY THEIR ACTIONS ON THE LIVER, MUSCLE, & ADIPOSE TISSUE

BIGUANIDES

The structure of **metformin** is shown below.

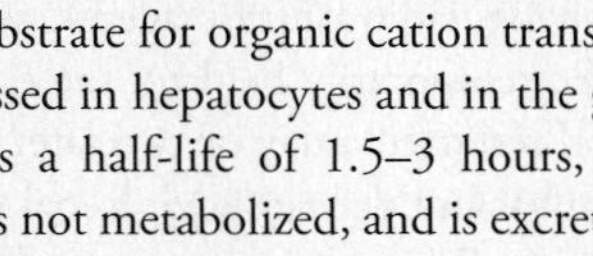

Metformin

Metformin's therapeutic effects primarily derive from increasing hepatic adenosine monophosphate–activated protein kinase activity, which reduces hepatic gluconeogenesis and lipogenesis. Metformin is a substrate for organic cation transporter 1, which is abundantly expressed in hepatocytes and in the gut.

Metformin has a half-life of 1.5–3 hours, is not bound to plasma proteins, is not metabolized, and is excreted by the kidneys as the active compound. As a consequence of metformin's blockade of gluconeogenesis, the drug may impair the hepatic metabolism of lactic acid. In patients with renal insufficiency, the biguanide accumulates and thereby increases the risk of lactic acidosis, which appears to be a dose-related complication. Metformin can be safely used in patients with estimated glomerular filtration rates (eGFR) between 60 and 45 mL/min per 1.73 m^2. It can be used cautiously in patients with stable eGFR between 45 and 30 mL/min per 1.73 m^2. It is contraindicated if the eGFR is less than 30 mL/min per 1.73 m^2. Patients with decompensated liver failure should do not take metformin because of the increased risk of lactic acidosis.

The current recommendation is to start metformin at diagnosis of type 2 diabetes. The United Kingdom Prospective Diabetes Study reported that in the obese patients with type 2 diabetes, metformin decreased the risk for cardiovascular disease as well as microvascular disease. Metformin is also used in combination with non-insulin agents (oral and injectable) and insulin in patients with type 2 diabetes in whom monotherapy is inadequate. Metformin is useful in the prevention of type 2 diabetes; the landmark Diabetes Prevention Program concluded that metformin is efficacious in preventing the new onset of type 2 diabetes in middle-aged, obese persons with impaired glucose tolerance and fasting hyperglycemia. Epidemiologic studies suggest that metformin use may reduce the risk of some cancers.

Although the recommended maximal dosage is 2550 mg daily, little benefit is seen above a total dosage of 2000 mg daily. Treatment is typically initiated at 500 mg daily with a meal and increased gradually in divided doses. Common dosing schedules are 500 mg once or twice daily increased to 1000 mg twice daily. The maximal dosage is 850 mg three times a day.

The most common adverse effects of metformin are gastrointestinal (anorexia, nausea, vomiting, abdominal discomfort, and diarrhea), occurring in up to 20% of patients. They are dose-related, tend to occur at the onset of therapy, and are often transient. Taking metformin with food or use of an extended-release formulation can ameliorate the symptoms. However, in 3–5% of patients, therapy may have to be discontinued because of persistent diarrhea.

Metformin interferes with the calcium-dependent absorption of vitamin B_{12}-intrinsic factor complex in the terminal ileum, and vitamin B_{12} deficiency can occur after many years of metformin use. Periodic screening for vitamin B_{12} deficiency should be considered, especially in patients with peripheral neuropathy or macrocytic anemia. Increased intake of calcium may prevent the metformin-induced B_{12} malabsorption.

Lactic acidosis can rarely occur with metformin therapy. It is more likely to occur in conditions of tissue hypoxia when there is increased production of lactic acid and in renal failure when there is decreased clearance of metformin. Almost all reported cases have involved patients with associated risk factors that should have contraindicated its use (kidney, liver, or cardiorespiratory insufficiency; alcoholism). Acute kidney failure can occur rarely in certain patients receiving radiocontrast agents. Metformin therapy should therefore be temporarily held on the day of radiocontrast administration and restarted a day or two later after confirmation that renal function has not deteriorated. Renal function should be checked at least annually in patients on metformin therapy, and lower doses (eg, 500 mg twice a day) should be used in the elderly who may have limited renal reserve and in those with eGFR between 30 and 45 mL/min per 1.73 m^2.

THIAZOLIDINEDIONES

The thiazolidinediones are ligands of **peroxisome proliferator-activated receptor gamma (PPAR-γ),** members of the steroid and thyroid superfamily of nuclear receptors. These PPAR receptors are found in muscle, fat, and liver. PPAR-γ receptors modulate the expression of the genes involved in lipid and glucose metabolism, insulin signal transduction, and adipocyte and other tissue differentiation. Observed effects of the thiazolidinediones include increased glucose transporter expression (GLUT 1 and GLUT 4), decreased free fatty acid levels, decreased hepatic glucose output, increased adiponectin and decreased release of resistin from adipocytes, and increased differentiation of preadipocytes to adipocytes. Thiazolidinediones have also been shown to decrease levels of plasminogen activator inhibitor type 1, matrix metalloproteinase 9, C-reactive protein, and interleukin 6. Two thiazolidinediones are currently available: pioglitazone and rosiglitazone. Rosiglitazone is no longer available in the United States and Europe Their clinical effect is to lower insulin requirements (improve insulin sensitivity)

Pioglitazone has some PPAR-α as well as PPAR-γ activity. It is absorbed within 2 hours of ingestion; although food may delay uptake, total bioavailability is not affected. Absorption is decreased with concomitant use of bile acid sequestrants. Pioglitazone is metabolized by CYP2C8 and CYP3A4 to active metabolites. The bioavailability of numerous other drugs also degraded by these enzymes may be affected by pioglitazone therapy, including estrogen-containing oral contraceptives; additional methods of contraception are advised. Pioglitazone may be taken once daily; the usual starting dosage is 15–30 mg/d, and the maximum is 45 mg/d.

Rosiglitazone is rapidly absorbed and highly protein bound. It is metabolized in the liver to minimally active metabolites, predominantly by CYP2C8 and to a lesser extent by CYP2C9. It is administered once or twice daily; 2–8 mg is the usual total dosage.

Both pioglitazone and rosiglitazone are effective as monontherapy and combination therapy.

These drugs also have some additional effects apart from glucose lowering. Pioglitazone lowers triglycerides and increases high-density lipoprotein (HDL) cholesterol without affecting total cholesterol and low-density lipoprotein (LDL) cholesterol. Rosiglitazone increases total cholesterol, HDL cholesterol, and LDL cholesterol but does not have significant effect on triglycerides. These drugs have been shown to improve the biochemical and histologic features of nonalcoholic fatty liver disease. They seem to have a positive effect on endothelial function: pioglitazone reduces neointimal proliferation after coronary stent placement, and rosiglitazone has been shown to reduce microalbuminuria. In nondiabetic insulin-resistant patients who had a recent history of ischemic stroke or transient ischemic attack, pioglitazone therapy reduced the risk of subsequent stroke or myocardial infarction.

Safety concerns and troublesome side effects have significantly reduced the use of this class of drugs. A meta-analysis of randomized clinical trials with rosiglitazone suggested an increased risk of angina pectoris or myocardial infarction. As a result, rosiglitazone was suspended in Europe and severely restricted in the United States. A subsequent large prospective clinical trial (the RECORD study) failed to confirm the meta-analysis findings. While the US lifted restrictions, rosiglitazone (Avandia) has been discontinued by the manufacturer. The drug remains unavailable in Europe and several other countries.

Fluid retention occurs in about 3–4% of patients on thiazolidinedione monotherapy and occurs more frequently (10–15%) in patients on concomitant insulin therapy. Heart failure can occur, and the drugs are contraindicated in patients with New York Heart Association class III and IV cardiac status (see Chapter 13). Macular edema is a rare adverse effect that improves when the drug is discontinued. Loss of bone mineral density and increased atypical extremity bone fractures in women are described for both drugs; this is postulated to be due to decreased osteoblast formation. Other adverse effects include anemia, which might be due to a dilutional effect of increased plasma volume rather than a reduction in red blood cell mass. Weight gain occurs, especially when used in combination with a sulfonylurea or insulin. Some of the weight gain is fluid retention but there is also an increase in total fat mass. In preclinical trials, bladder tumors were observed in male rats on pioglitazone. Initial clinical reports indicated that this might also be true in humans. A 10-year observational cohort study of patients taking pioglitazone, however, failed to find an association with bladder cancer. A large multi-population pooled analysis (1.01 million persons over 5.9 million person-years) also failed to find an association between cumulative exposure of pioglitazone or rosiglitazone and incidence of bladder cancer. Another population-based study generating 689,616 person-years of follow-up did find that pioglitazone but not rosiglitazone was associated with an increased risk of bladder cancer.

Troglitazone, the first medication in this class, was withdrawn because of cases of fatal liver failure. Although rosiglitazone and pioglitazone have not been reported to cause liver injury, the drugs are not recommended for use in patients with active liver disease or pretreatment elevation of alanine aminotransferase (ALT) 2.5 times greater than normal. Liver function tests should be performed prior to initiation of treatment and periodically thereafter.

DRUGS THAT AFFECT ABSORPTION OF GLUCOSE

The **α-glucosidase inhibitors** competitively inhibit the intestinal α-glucosidase enzymes and reduce post-meal glucose excursions by delaying the digestion and absorption of starch and disaccharides. **Acarbose** and **miglitol** are available in the United States. **Voglibose** is available in Japan, Korea, and India. Acarbose and miglitol are potent inhibitors of glucoamylase, α-amylase, and sucrase but have less effect on isomaltase and hardly any on trehalase and lactase. Acarbose has the molecular mass and structural features of a tetrasaccharide and very little is absorbed. In contrast, miglitol has structural similarity to glucose and is absorbed.

Acarbose is initiated at a dosage of 50 mg twice daily just before the meal, with gradual increase to 100 mg three times a day. It lowers postprandial glucose levels by 30–50%. Miglitol therapy is initiated at a dosage of 25 mg three times a day. The usual maintenance dosage is 50 mg three times a day, but some patients may need 100 mg three times a day. The drug is not metabolized and is cleared by the kidney. It should not be used in renal failure.

Prominent adverse effects of α-glucosidase inhibitors include flatulence, diarrhea, and abdominal pain and result from the appearance of undigested carbohydrate in the colon that is then fermented into short-chain fatty acids, releasing gas. These adverse effects tend to diminish with ongoing use because chronic exposure to carbohydrate induces the expression of α-glucosidase in the jejunum and ileum, increasing distal small intestine glucose absorption and minimizing the passage of carbohydrate into the colon. Although not a problem with monotherapy or combination therapy with a biguanide, hypoglycemia may occur with concurrent insulin secretagogue treatment. Hypoglycemia should be treated with glucose (dextrose) and not sucrose, whose breakdown may be blocked. An increase in hepatic aminotransferases has been noted in clinical trials with acarbose, especially with dosages greater than 300 mg/d. The abnormalities resolve on stopping the drug.

These drugs are infrequently prescribed in the United States because of their prominent gastrointestinal adverse effects and relatively modest glucose-lowering benefit.

DRUGS THAT MIMIC INCRETIN EFFECT OR PROLONG INCRETIN ACTION

An oral glucose load provokes a higher insulin response compared with an equivalent dose of glucose given intravenously. This is because the oral glucose causes a release of gut hormones ("incretins"), principally GLP-1 and glucose-dependent insulinotropic peptide (GIP), that amplify the glucose-induced insulin secretion. When GLP-1 is infused in patients with type 2 diabetes, it stimulates insulin release and lowers glucose levels. The GLP-1 effect is glucose-dependent in that the insulin release is more pronounced when glucose levels are elevated but less pronounced when glucose levels are normal. For this reason, GLP-1 has a lower risk for hypoglycemia than the sulfonylureas. In addition to its insulin stimulatory effect, GLP-1 has a number of other biologic effects. It suppresses glucagon secretion, delays gastric emptying, and reduces apoptosis of human islets in culture. In animals, GLP-1 inhibits feeding by a central nervous system mechanism. Patients with type 2 diabetes on GLP-1 therapy are less hungry. It is unclear whether this is mainly related to the deceleration of gastric emptying or whether there is a central nervous system effect as well. GIP, like GLP-1, potentiates glucose-dependent insulin secretion.

GLP-1 is rapidly degraded by dipeptidyl peptidase 4 (DPP-4) and by other enzymes such as endopeptidase 24.11 and is also cleared by the kidney. The native peptide therefore cannot be used therapeutically. One approach to this problem was to develop metabolically stable analogs or derivatives of GLP-1 that are not subject to the same enzymatic degradation or renal clearance. Five GLP-1 receptor agonists—dulaglutide, exenatide (and exenatide XR), liraglutide, lixisenatide, and semaglutide—are available for clinical use.The other approach was to develop inhibitors of DPP-4 and prolong the action of endogenously released GLP-1 and GIP. Three oral DPP-4 inhibitors, alogliptin, linagliptin, and sitagliptin are available in the

United States. Saxagliptin was recently removed from the market. An additional inhibitor, vildagliptin, is available in Europe. Other DPP-4 inhibitors—gemigliptin, anagliptin, teneligliptin, trelagliptin, omarigliptin, evogliptin, and gosogliptin—have been approved outside the United States and European Union (Korea, India, Thailand, Japan, Russia, and several South American countries).

GLUCAGON-LIKE PEPTIDE-1 (GLP-1) RECEPTOR AGONISTS

Exenatide, a derivative of the exendin-4 peptide in Gila monster venom, has a 53% homology with native GLP-1 and a glycine substitution to reduce degradation by DPP-4. It is available in fixed-dose pens (5 mcg and 10 mcg). It is injected subcutaneously within 60 minutes before breakfast and dinner. It reaches a peak concentration in approximately 2 hours with a duration of action of up to 10 hours. Therapy is initiated at 5 mcg twice daily for the first month and if tolerated can be increased to 10 mcg twice daily. Exenatide extended-release is a once-weekly pen preparation that is dispensed as a powder (2 mg). It is suspended in the provided diluent just prior to injection. When exenatide is added to preexisting sulfonylurea therapy, the sulfonylurea dosage may need to be decreased to prevent hypoglycemia. Exenatide monotherapy and combination therapy results in HbA_{1c} reductions of 0.2–1.2%. Weight loss in the range of 2–3 kg occurs and contributes to the improvement of glucose control. In comparative trials the extended-release formulation lowers the HbA_{1c} level a little more than the twice-daily preparation. Exenatide undergoes glomerular filtration, and the drug is not approved for use in patients with estimated GFR of less than 30 mL/min per 1.73 m^2.

High-titer antibodies against exenatide develop in about 6% of patients, and in half of these patients an attenuation of glycemic response has been seen.

Liraglutide is a soluble fatty acid-acylated GLP-1 analog. Lysine is replaced with arginine at position 34 and a C16 acyl chain is attached to a lysine at position 26. The fatty-acyl GLP-1 retains affinity for GLP-1 receptors but the addition of the C16 acyl chain allows for noncovalent binding to albumin, both hindering DPP-4 access to the molecule and contributing to a prolonged half-life (approximately 12 hours) and duration of action. The half-life permits once-daily dosing. Treatment is initiated at 0.6 mg and increased after 1 week to 1.2 mg daily. If needed, the dosage can be increased to 1.8 mg daily. In clinical trials liraglutide results in a reduction of HbA_{1c} of 0.8–1.5%; weight loss ranges from none to 3.2 kg. Liraglutide at a dose of 3 mg daily is approved for weight loss in patients without diabetes.

In a postmarketing multinational study of 9340 patients with type 2 diabetes with known cardiovascular disease, the addition of liraglutide was associated with a lower primary composite outcome of death from cardiovascular causes, nonfatal myocardial infarction, or nonfatal stroke (hazard ratio 0.87, P = 0.01). Patients taking liraglutide had lower HbA_{1c} levels, weight loss of more than 2 kg, lower systolic blood pressure, and fewer episodes of severe hypoglycemia.

Dulaglutide consists of two GLP-1 analog molecules covalently linked to an Fc fragment of human IgG4. The GLP-1 moiety has amino acid substitutions that resist DPP-4 degradation. The half-life of dulaglutide is about 5 days. The usual dose is 0.75 mg weekly by subcutaneous injection. The maximum recommended dose is 4.5 mg weekly. **Lixisenatide** is a synthetic analog of exendin-4 (deletion of a proline and addition of 6 lysines to the C-terminal region) with a half-life of 3 hours. It is available in two fixed-dose pens (10 mcg and 20 mcg). The 10-mcg dose is injected once daily before breakfast for the first 2 weeks, and if tolerated, the dose is then increased to 20 mcg daily. Its clinical effect is about the same as exenatide with HbA_{1c} lowering in the 0.4–0.6% range. Weight loss ranges from 1 to 3 kg. Antibodies to lixisenatide occur frequently (70%) and about 2.4% of patients with the highest antibody titers have attenuated glycemic response.

Semaglutide is a synthetic analog of GLP-1 with a half-life of about 1 week. It has an alpha-aminoisobutyric acid substitution at position 8 that makes the molecule resistant to DPP-4 degradation and a C-18 fatty diacid chain attached to lysine at position 26 that binds to albumin, which accounts for the drug's long half-life. The low dose pen delivers 0.25 mg or 0.5 mg and the higher dose pens delivers 1 and 2 mg. The recommendation is to start at 0.25 mg dose for the first 4 weeks and if tolerated increase the dose to 0.5 mg weekly; the dose can be further titrated to 2 mg dose after being on 1 mg dose for 4 weeks for additional glucose lowering. Semaglutide monotherapy and combination therapy lowers HbA_{1c} from 1.5% to 1.8%. An increase in diabetic retinopathy was observed in the semaglutide treated group in one of the clinical trials. It is thought that this might have been secondary to the rapid glucose lowering with the drug. Semaglutide at a dose of 2.4 mg daily is approved for weight loss in patients without diabetes.

Semaglutide coformulated with sodium N-[8(2-hydroxybenzoyl) amino] caprylate (SNAC) results in a complex that is lipophilic and resistant to proteolysis. It can therefore be given orally. The oral bioavailability is only 0.4% to 1%; thus oral semaglutide must be taken fasting with a glass of water and the patient must wait half an hour to eat or drink or take other medicines. The recommended starting dose is 3 mg daily for the first month and then increased to 7 mg daily. A dose of 14 mg daily can be used for additional glucose lowering.

The most frequent adverse reactions of the GLP-1 receptor agonists are nausea (11–40%), vomiting (4–13%), and diarrhea (9–17%). The reactions are more frequent at the higher doses. All of the GLP-1 receptor agonists may increase the risk of pancreatitis. Patients on these drugs should be counseled to seek immediate medical care if they experience unexplained persistent severe abdominal pain. Cases of renal impairment and acute renal injury have been reported in patients taking exenatide. Some of these patients had preexisting kidney disease or other risk factors for renal injury. A number of them reported having nausea, vomiting, and diarrhea and it is possible that volume depletion contributed to the development of renal injury. Both exenatide and liraglutide stimulate thyroidal C-cell (parafollicular) tumors in rodents. Human thyroidal C cells express very few GLP-1 receptors, and the relevance to human therapy is unclear. The drugs, however, should not be used in persons with a past medical or family history of medullary thyroid cancer or multiple endocrine neoplasia (MEN) syndrome type 2.

DUAL GLUCOSE-DEPENDENT INSULINOTROPIC POLYPEPTIDE (GIP) AND GLUCAGON-LIKE PEPTIDE-1 (GLP-1) RECEPTOR AGONIST

Tirzepatide is a dual GIP/GLP-1 receptor agonist. It is an analog of the GIP hormone with a 1,20-eicosanedioic acid linked to the lysine residue at position 20. The peptide sequence also contains two non-coded amino acid residues (alpha amino isobutyric acid) at positions 2 and 13, and the c-terminus is amidated. The acylation results in albumin binding, allowing for prolonged action and once-weekly dosing. The recommend starting dose is a 2.5-mg subcutaneous injection weekly. The dose is increased to 5 mg weekly after 4 weeks. If additional glucose lowering is needed, the dose can be increased by increments of 2.5 mg every 4 weeks to a maximum dose of 15 mg. Treatment with tirzepatide resulted in dose-dependent HbA1c reductions of 1.9% to 2.6%. The average weight loss ranged from 6.2 to 12.9 kg. Beneficial effects were observed on lipid profile, blood pressure lowering, and fatty liver. The safety profile is the same as with the GLP-1 receptor agonists. Gastrointestinal side effects (nausea, vomiting, diarrhea) occurred more frequently at the higher doses. In the clinical trials, there was a slightly higher rate of pancreatitis in the treated group compared with the comparator-treated group (0.23 vs 0.11 patients per 100 years of exposure).

DIPEPTIDYL PEPTIDASE 4 (DPP-4) INHIBITORS

Sitagliptin is given orally as 100 mg once daily, has an oral bioavailability of over 85%, achieves peak concentrations within 1–4 hours, and has a half-life of approximately 12 hours. It is primarily excreted in the urine, in part by active tubular secretion of the drug. Hepatic metabolism is limited and mediated largely by the cytochrome CYP3A4 isoform and, to a lesser degree, by CYP2C8. The metabolites have insignificant activity. Dosage should be reduced in patients with impaired renal function (50 mg if estimated GFR is 30–50 mL/min per 1.73 m^2 and 25 mg if <30 mL/min per 1.73 m^2). Therapy with sitagliptin has resulted in HbA_{1c} reductions of 0.5–1.0%.

Saxagliptin (not available in the United States) is given orally as 2.5–5 mg daily. The drug reaches maximal concentrations within 2 hours (4 hours for its active metabolite). It is minimally protein bound and undergoes hepatic metabolism by CYP3A4/5. The major metabolite is active, and excretion is by both renal and hepatic pathways. The terminal plasma half-life is 2.5 hours for saxagliptin and 3.1 hours for its active metabolite. Dosage adjustment is recommended for individuals with renal impairment and concurrent use of strong inhibitors or inducers of CYP3A4/5 such as ketoconazole, some anticonvulsants, rifampin, and rifabutin.

Linagliptin lowers HbA_{1c} by 0.4–0.6% when added to metformin, sulfonylurea, or pioglitazone. The dosage is 5 mg daily orally and, since it is primarily excreted via the bile, no dosage adjustment is needed in renal failure. **Alogliptin** lowers HbA_{1c} by about 0.5–0.6% when added to metformin, sulfonylurea, or pioglitazone. The usual dose is 25 mg orally daily. The 12.5-mg dose is used in patients with calculated creatinine clearance of 30 to 60 mL/min; the dose is 6.25 mg for clearance <30 mL/min. **Vildagliptin** (not available in the United States) lowers HbA_{1c} levels by 01% when added to the therapeutic regimen of patients with type 2 diabetes. The dosage is 50 mg orally once or twice daily.

The main adverse effect of DPP-4 inhibitors appears to be a predisposition to nasopharyngitis or upper respiratory tract infection. Hypersensitivity reactions including anaphylaxis, angioedema, and exfoliative skin conditions such as Stevens-Johnson syndrome have been reported. The frequency of pancreatitis is unclear. In clinical trials, of 5902 patients on alogliptin, pancreatitis occurred in 11 (0.2%) and in 5 of 5183 patients receiving all comparators (less than 0.1%). Cases of hepatic failure have been reported with the use of alogliptin, but it is uncertain if alogliptin was the cause. The medication, however, should be discontinued in the event of liver failure. Rare cases of hepatic dysfunction, including hepatitis, have been reported with the use of vildagliptin; and liver biochemical testing is recommended quarterly during the first year of use and periodically thereafter. Saxagliptin may increase the risk of heart failure (hazard ratio 1.27 found in a post-marketing study). In a large postmarketing study, alogliptin, was associated with a slightly increased rate of heart failure. The FDA has issued a warning that the DPP-4 inhibitors can occasionally cause joint pains that resolve after stopping the drug.

SODIUM-GLUCOSE CO-TRANSPORTER 2 (SGLT2) INHIBITORS

Glucose is freely filtered by the renal glomeruli and is reabsorbed in the proximal tubules by the action of sodium-glucose transporters (SGLTs). Sodium-glucose transporter 2 (SGLT2) accounts for 90% of glucose reabsorption, and its inhibition causes glycosuria and lowers glucose levels in patients with type 2 diabetes. The SGLT2 inhibitors **canagliflozin, dapagliflozin, empagliflozin,** and **ertugliflozin** are approved for clinical use in the United States. These agents reduce the threshold for glycosuria from a plasma glucose threshold of ~180 mg/dL to ~40 mg/dL, and lower HbA_{1c} by 0.5–1% when used alone or in combination with other oral agents or insulin. The efficacy is greater at higher HbA_{1c} levels when more glucose is excreted as a result of SGLT2 inhibition. The loss of calories results in modest weight loss of 2–5 kg.

The usual dose of canagliflozin is 100 mg daily but up to 300 mg daily can be used in patients with normal kidney function. The dose of dapagliflozin is 10 mg daily but 5 mg daily is the recommended initial dose in patients with hepatic failure. The usual dose of empagliflozin is 10 mg daily but a higher dose of 25 mg daily can be used. The recommended starting dose of ertugliflozin is 5 mg but the dose can be increased to 15 mg daily if additional glucose lowering is needed.

In a large postmarketing study of patients with type 2 diabetes with known cardiovascular disease, the addition of empagliflozin was associated with a significantly lower primary composite outcome of death from cardiovascular causes, nonfatal myocardial infarction, or nonfatal stroke. The mechanisms regarding the benefit remain unclear. Weight loss, lower blood pressure, and diuresis may have played a role since there were fewer deaths from heart failure in the treated group, whereas the rates of myocardial infarction were unaltered. A similar large multinational study was performed with canagliflozin in patients with type 2 diabetes with known or increased risk for cardiovascular disease. The canagliflozin-treated group had a lower primary composite outcome of death from cardiovascular causes, nonfatal myocardial infarction, or nonfatal stroke (hazard ratio 0.86, P = 0.02). In a heart failure study of 4744 patients with NYHA class II, III, IV heart failure and ejection fraction of <40%, dapagliflozin reduced the cumulative incidence of worsening heart failure or cardiovascular death (hazard ratio, 0.74; p <0.001). In all, 42% of the patients had diabetes; the findings in patients with and without diabetes were the same.

The SGLT2 inhibitors have also shown benefit in reducing the progression of albuminuria. In a study of patients with type 2 diabetes with stage 2 to 3 chronic kidney disease (eGFR 30 to less than 90 mg/kg/1.73 m^2) and urine albumin excretion ranging from 300–5000 mcg albumin/g creatinine, and on an ACE inhibitor or ARB, canagliflozin reduced the risk of end stage renal disease, the risk of doubling of serum creatinine, and the risk of renal death. In a multinational study of 4304 patients with chronic kidney disease, dapagliflozin reduced the risk of end-stage renal disease or death from renal and cardiovascular causes. A third of the patients in the study did not have diabetes and had benefit.

As might be expected, the efficacy of the SGLT2 inhibitors is reduced in chronic kidney disease. They can also increase creatinine and decrease eGFR, especially in patients with kidney impairment. Their use is generally not recommended in patients with eGFR less than 45 mL/min/1.73 m^2 (for glycemic control) and are contraindicated in patients with eGFR less than 30 mL/min/1.73 m^2. The study of dapagliflozin in chronic kidney disease noted that the drug was safe and beneficial in patients with eGFR as low as 25 mL/min/1.73 m2 (for the renal benefits).

The major adverse effects are increased incidence of genital mycotic infections and urinary tract infections affecting ~8–9% of patients. There have also been reports of cases of pyelonephritis and septicemia requiring hospitalization. Cases of necrotizing fasciitis of the perineum (Fournier gangrene) have been reported. The glycosuria can cause intravascular volume contraction and hypotension.

Canagliflozin and empagliflozin caused a modest increase in LDL cholesterol levels (4–8%). In clinical trials patients taking dapagliflozin had higher rates of breast cancer (nine cases versus none in comparator arms) and bladder cancer (nine cases versus one in placebo arm). These cancer rates exceeded the expected rates in an age-matched reference diabetes population. Canagliflozin has been reported to cause a decrease in bone mineral density at the lumbar spine and the hip. In a pooled analysis of eight clinical trials (mean duration 68 weeks), an increase in fractures by about 30% was observed in patients on canagliflozin. It is likely that the effect on the bones is a class effect and not restricted to canagliflozin. A modest increase in upper limb fractures was observed with canagliflozin therapy. It is not known if this is due to an effect on bone strength or related to falls due to hypotension. One multinational study of canagliflozin showed an increase in risk of amputations, especially of the toes. This finding has not been observed in other studies using this drug or with the other SGLT2 inhibitors.

Cases of euglycemic diabetic ketoacidosis have been reported with off-label use of SGLT2 inhibitors in patients with type 1 diabetes. Patients with type 1 diabetes are taught to give less insulin if their glucose levels are not elevated. Because patients with type 1 taking an SGLT2 inhibitor may have normal glucose levels, they may either withhold or reduce their insulin doses to such a degree as to induce ketoacidosis. Therefore, SGLT2 inhibitors should not be used in patients with type 1 diabetes and in those patients labelled as having type 2 diabetes but who are very insulin deficient and prone to ketosis.

OTHER GLUCOSE-LOWERING DRUGS

Pramlintide is an islet amyloid polypeptide (IAPP, amylin) analog. IAPP is a 37-amino-acid peptide present in insulin secretory granules and secreted with insulin. It has approximately 46% homology with the calcitonin gene-related peptide (CGRP; see Chapter 17) and physiologically acts as a negative feedback on insulin secretion. At pharmacologic doses, IAPP reduces glucagon secretion, slows gastric emptying by a vagally mediated mechanism, and centrally decreases appetite. Pramlintide is an IAPP analog with substitutions of proline at positions 25, 28, and 29. These modifications make pramlintide soluble, non-self-aggregating, and suitable for pharmacologic use. Pramlintide is approved for use in insulin-treated type 1 and type 2 patients. It is rapidly absorbed after subcutaneous administration; levels peak within 20 minutes, and the duration of action is not more than 150 minutes. It is metabolized and excreted by the kidney, but even at low creatinine clearance there is no significant change in bioavailability. It has not been evaluated in dialysis patients.

Pramlintide is injected immediately before eating; doses range from 15 to 60 mcg subcutaneously for type 1 patients and from 60 to 120 mcg for type 2 patients. Therapy with this agent should be initiated at the lowest dosage and titrated upward. Because of the risk of hypoglycemia, concurrent rapid- or short-acting mealtime insulin dosages should be decreased by 50% or more at initiation. Pramlintide should be injected using a separate syringe because it cannot be mixed with insulin. The major adverse effects of pramlintide are hypoglycemia and gastrointestinal symptoms, including nausea, vomiting, and anorexia. Since the drug slows gastric emptying, recovery from hypoglycemia can be problematic because of the delay in absorption of fast-acting carbohydrates.

Selected patients with type 1 diabetes who have problems with postprandial hyperglycemia can use pramlintide effectively to control the glucose rise especially in the setting of a high-carbohydrate meal. The drug is not very useful in type 2 patients who can instead use the GLP-1 receptor agonists or SGLT2 inhibitors.

Colesevelam hydrochloride, the bile acid sequestrant and cholesterol-lowering drug, is approved as an antihyperglycemic agent for patients with type 2 diabetes who are taking other glucose-lowering medications or have not achieved adequate control with diet and exercise. The mechanism of action is unknown but presumed to involve an interruption of the enterohepatic circulation and a decrease in farnesoid X receptor (FXR) activation. FXR is a nuclear receptor with multiple effects on cholesterol, glucose, and bile acid metabolism. Bile acids are natural ligands of the FXR. Additionally, the drug may impair glucose absorption. In clinical trials, it lowered the HbA_{1c} concentration 0.3–0.5%. Adverse effects include gastrointestinal complaints (constipation, indigestion, flatulence). It can also exacerbate the hypertriglyceridemia that commonly occurs in patients with type 2 diabetes.

Bromocriptine, a dopamine agonist, in randomized placebo-controlled studies lowered HbA_{1c} by 0–0.2% compared with baseline and by 0.4–0.5% compared with placebo. The mechanism by which it lowers glucose levels is not known. The main adverse events are nausea, fatigue, dizziness, vomiting, and headache.

Colesevelam and bromocriptine have very modest efficacy in lowering glucose levels, and their use in diabetes is questionable.

MANAGEMENT OF THE PATIENT WITH DIABETES

Diet

A well-balanced, nutritious diet remains a fundamental element of therapy for diabetes. It is recommended that the macronutrient proportions (carbohydrate, protein, and fat) be individualized based on the patient's eating patterns, preferences, and goals. Generally most patients with diabetes consume about 45% of their calories as carbohydrates, 25–35% fats, and 10–35% proteins. Limiting the carbohydrate intake and substituting some of the calories with monounsaturated fats, such as olive oil, rapeseed (canola) oil, or the oils in nuts and avocados, can lower triglycerides and increase HDL cholesterol. A Mediterranean-style eating pattern (a diet supplemented with walnuts, almonds, hazelnuts, and olive oil) has been shown to improve glycemic control and lower combined endpoints for cardiovascular events and stroke. Caloric restriction and weight loss are important goals for the obese patient with type 2 diabetes.

Education

Education of the patient and family is a critical component of care. The patient should be informed about the kind of diabetes he or she has and the rationale for achieving target glucose levels (see Box: Benefits of Tight Glycemic Control in Diabetes). Glucose monitoring (CGM or BGM) should be emphasized, especially if the patient is on insulin or oral secretagogues that can cause hypoglycemia. The patient on insulin therapy should understand the time action profile of the insulins. He or she should know how to determine if the basal insulin dose is correct and how to adjust the rapidly acting insulin dose for carbohydrate content of meals. Insulin adjustments for exercise and infections should be discussed. The patient and family members also should be informed about the signs and symptoms of hypoglycemia.

Glycemic Targets

The American Diabetes Association criteria for acceptable control include an HbA_{1c} of less than 7% (53 mmol/mol), pre-meal glucose levels of 90–130 mg/dL (5–7.2 mmol/L), and peak postprandial glucose of less than 180 mg/dL (10 mmol/L). While the HbA_{1c} target is appropriate for individuals treated with lifestyle interventions and euglycemic therapy, it may need to be modified for individuals treated with insulin or insulin secretagogues due to their increased risk of hypoglycemia. Less stringent glycemic control also is appropriate for children as well as patients with a history of severe hypoglycemia, significant microvascular and macrovascular disease, other co-morbidities (eg, coronary heart disease), and limited life expectancy. For the elderly, frail patient an HbA_{1c} close to 8% may be appropriate. More stringent glycemic control is appropriate for adult patients with newly diagnosed diabetes, limited comorbidities, and a long life-expectancy. For patients using CGM, the TIR and GMI are used to tailor the diabetes management plan, in addition to the $HbA_{1c.}$

Treatment

Treatment must be individualized based on the type of diabetes and specific needs of each patient.

A. Type 1 Diabetes

In patients with type 1 diabetes, a combination of rapid-acting insulin analogs and long-acting insulin analogs allow for more physiologic insulin replacement. A newly diagnosed patient may require minimal doses of basal and bolus insulins because they still have endogenous insulin production. In patients with longer duration of diabetes, the 24-hour basal insulin needs are usually based on age and body weight. An adolescent might need as much as 0.4 unit/kg/day; young adult (less than 25 years), 0.35 unit/kg/day; and older adults, 0.25 unit/kg/day. The meal bolus varies based on the time of day and the patient's age. Adolescents and young adults usually require 1 unit per 10 g of carbohydrate. Older adults usually require about 1 unit for 15 g of carbohydrate. The correction factor—how much insulin is needed to lower glucose levels by 50 mg/dL—can be calculated from the insulin-to-carbohydrate ratios. For example, if 1 unit is required for 15 g of carbohydrate, then 1 unit will lower glucose levels by 50 mg/dL. If 1.5 units of insulin is required for 15 g of carbohydrate (that is, 1 unit for 10 g carbohydrate), then 1.5 units of insulin will lower glucose levels by 50 mg/dL and 1 unit will lower glucose level by 33 mg/dL. These are approximate values and should be individualized.

Table 41–8 illustrates regimens of rapidly acting insulin analogs and basal analogs that might be appropriate for a 70-kg person with type 1 diabetes. If the patient is on an insulin pump, he or she may require a basal infusion rate of 0.6 units per hour throughout the 24 hours with the exception of 4:00 AM to 8:00 AM, when 0.7 units per hour might be appropriate (dawn phenomenon). The ratios might be one unit for 12 g carbohydrate plus one unit for 50 mg/dL (2.8 mmol/L) of blood glucose above a target value of 120 mg/dL (6.7 mmol/L).

The currently available closed-loop systems enable patients to better achieve glycemic targets with reduced rates of hypoglycemia. These systems should be offered to most patients with type 1 diabetes.

TABLE 41–8 Examples of intensive insulin regimens using rapid-acting insulin analogs (insulin lispro, aspart, or glulisine) and NPH, or insulin detemir, glargine, or degludec in a 70-kg man with type 1 diabetes.[1–3]

	Prebreakfast	Prelunch	Predinner	Bedtime
Rapid-acting insulin analog	5 U	4 U	6 U	—
NPH insulin	3 U	3 U	2 U	8–9 U
or				
Rapid-acting insulin analog	5 U	4 U	6 U	—
Insulin glargine or degludec	—	—	—	15–16 U
Insulin detemir	6–7 U	—	—	8–9 U

[1]Assumes that patient is consuming approximately 75 g carbohydrate at breakfast, 60 g at lunch, and 90 g at dinner.

[2]The dose of rapid-acting insulin analogs can be raised by 1 or 2 U if extra carbohydrate (15–30 g) is ingested or if premeal blood glucose is >170 mg/dL. The rapid-acting insulin analogs can be mixed in the same syringe with NPH insulin.

[3]Insulin glargine or insulin detemir must be given as a separate injection.

Benefits of Tight Glycemic Control in Diabetes

A long-term randomized prospective study involving 1441 type 1 patients in 29 medical centers reported in 1993 that "near normalization" of blood glucose resulted in a delay in onset and a major slowing of progression of microvascular and neuropathic complications of diabetes during follow-up periods of up to 10 years (Diabetes Control and Complications Trial [DCCT] Research Group, 1993). In the intensively treated group, mean glycated hemoglobin (HbA_{1c}) of 7.2% (normal <6%) and mean blood glucose of 155 mg/dL were achieved, whereas in the conventionally treated group, HbA_{1c} averaged 8.9% with mean blood glucose of 225 mg/dL. Over the study period, which averaged 7 years, a reduction of approximately 60% in risk of diabetic retinopathy, nephropathy, and neuropathy was noted in the tight control group compared with the standard control group.

The DCCT study, in addition, introduced the concept of *glycemic memory*, which comprises the long-term benefits of any significant period of glycemic control. During a 6-year follow-up period, both the intensively and conventionally treated groups had similar levels of glycemic control, and both had progression of carotid intimal-medial thickness. However, the intensively treated cohort had significantly less progression of intimal thickness.

The United Kingdom Prospective Diabetes Study (UKPDS) was a very large randomized prospective study carried out to study the effects of intensive glycemic control with several types of therapies and the effects of blood pressure control in patients with type 2 diabetes. A total of 3867 newly diagnosed patients with type 2 diabetes were studied over 10 years. A significant fraction of these were overweight and hypertensive. Patients were given dietary treatment alone or intensive therapy with insulin, chlorpropamide, glyburide, or glipizide. Metformin was an option for patients with inadequate response to other therapies. Tight control of blood pressure was added as a variable, with an angiotensin-converting enzyme inhibitor, a β blocker, or in some cases, a calcium channel blocker available for this purpose.

Tight control of diabetes, with reduction of HbA_{1c} from 9.1% to 7%, was shown to reduce the risk of microvascular complications overall compared with that achieved with conventional therapy (mostly diet alone, which decreased HbA_{1c} to 7.9%). Cardiovascular complications were not noted for any particular therapy; metformin treatment alone reduced the risk of macrovascular disease (myocardial infarction, stroke). Epidemiologic analysis of the study suggested that every 1% decrease in the HbA_{1c} achieved an estimated risk reduction of 37% for microvascular complications, 21% for any diabetes-related end point and death related to diabetes, and 14% for myocardial infarction.

Tight control of hypertension also had a surprisingly significant effect on microvascular disease (as well as more conventional hypertension-related sequelae) in these patients. Epidemiologic analysis of the results suggested that every 10-mm Hg decrease in the systolic pressure achieved an estimated risk reduction of 13% for diabetic microvascular complications, 12% for any diabetes-related complication, 15% for death related to diabetes, and 11% for myocardial infarction.

Post-study monitoring showed that 5 years after the closure of the UKPDS, the benefits of intensive management on diabetic end points were maintained and the risk reduction for a myocardial infarction became significant. The benefits of metformin therapy were maintained.

These studies show that tight glycemic control benefits both type 1 and type 2 diabetes patients.

B. Type 2 Diabetes

Normalization of glucose levels can occur with weight loss and improved insulin sensitivity in the obese patient with type 2 diabetes. A combination of caloric restriction and increased exercise is necessary if a weight reduction program is to be successful. Understanding the long-term consequences of poorly controlled diabetes may motivate some patients to lose weight. For selected patients, medical or surgical options should be considered. Orlistat, phentermine/topiramate, lorcaserin (removed from US market in February 2020 due to increased occurrence of cancer), naltrexone plus extended-release bupropion, high-dose liraglutide, and semaglutide are approved weight loss medications for use in combination with diet and exercise. Bariatric surgery (Roux-en-Y, gastric banding, gastric sleeve, biliopancreatic diversion/duodenal switch) typically results in significant weight loss and can result in remission of the diabetes.

Nonobese patients with type 2 diabetes frequently have increased visceral adiposity—the so-called metabolically obese, normal weight patient. There is less emphasis on weight loss in such patients, but exercise is important.

Multiple medications may be required to achieve glycemic control (Figure 41–6) in patients with type 2 diabetes. Unless there is a contraindication, medical therapy should be initiated with intensive lifestyle interventions (diet and exercise), diabetes self-management education, and metformin. If glycemic targets are no longer achieved with metformin monotherapy, a second agent is added. Options include sulfonylureas, repaglinide or nateglinide, pioglitazone, GLP-1 receptor agonists, dual GIP/GLP1 receptor agonist, DPP-4 inhibitors, SGLT2 inhibitors, and insulin. In the choice of the second agent, consideration should be given to efficacy of the agent, hypoglycemic risk, effect on weight, presence of cardiovascular disease or renal disease, adverse effects, and cost. The DPP-4 inhibitors and SGLT2 inhibitors are of moderate efficacy and all other agents are of high efficacy. Sulfonylureas and insulins have increased risk of hypoglycemia. Sulfonylureas, insulin, and pioglitazone cause weight gain. Metformin and DPP-4 inhibitors are weight neutral, whereas GLP-1 and GIP/GLP1 receptor agonists and SGLT2 inhibitors cause weight loss. The GLP-1 receptor agonists, the SGLT2 inhibitors, and pioglitazone have cardiovascular benefits and the SGLT2 inhibitors delay progression of diabetic nephropathy. The major risk factors include lactic acidosis with metformin; fracture risk, heart failure, and possible bladder cancer with pioglitazone; GI side effects and pancreatitis with GLP-1 receptor agonists; nasopharyngitis, joint pains, and allergic reactions with DPP-4 inhibitors; genital infection, urinary tract infections, and ketoacidosis with SGLT2 inhibitors. All the agents are expensive except for metformin and sulfonylureas. In patients who experience hyperglycemia after a carbohydrate-rich meal, a short-acting secretagogue before that meal may suffice to control the glucose levels. Patients with severe insulin resistance may be candidates for pioglitazone. Patients who are very concerned about weight gain may benefit from a trial of a GLP-1, a GIP/GLP1 receptor agonist, or an SGLT2 inhibitor, which cause weight loss, or a DPP-4 inhibitor, which is weight neutral. Presence of cardiovascular disease should be considered; liraglutide, empagliflozin, and canagliflozin have been shown to have improved cardiovascular outcomes. The SGLT2 inhibitors should be considered as second choice in those patients with diabetic nephropathy or heart failure. If two agents are inadequate, a third agent is added, although data regarding efficacy of such combined therapy are limited.

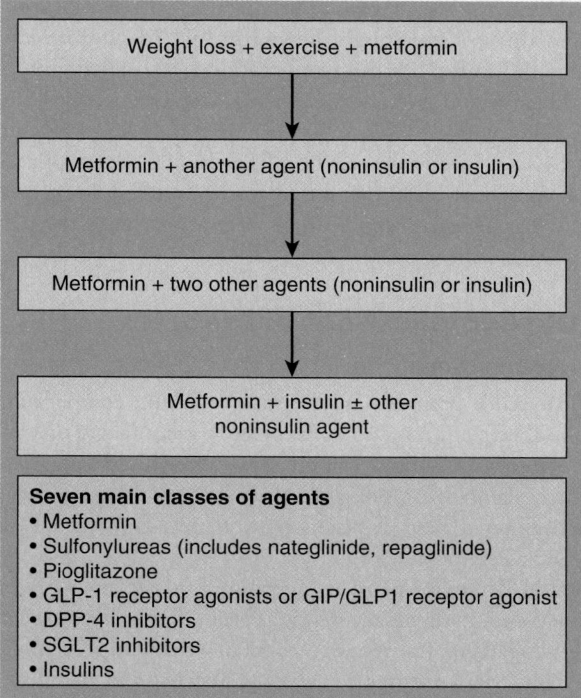

FIGURE 41–6 Suggested algorithm for the treatment of type 2 diabetes. The seven main classes of agents are metformin, sulfonylureas (includes nateglinide, repaglinide), pioglitazone, GLP-1 receptor agonists or dual GIP/GLP1 receptor agonist, DPP-4 inhibitors, SGLT2 inhibitors, insulins. Take into account efficacy, hypoglycemic risk, effect on weight, cardiovascular and renal benefits, major side effects, and cost. α-Glucosidase inhibitors, colesevelam, pramlintide, and bromocriptine not included because of limited efficacy and significant adverse reactions. (Data from Davies MJ, D'Alessio DA, Fradkin J, et al. Management of hyperglycaemia in type 2 diabetes, 2018. A consensus report by the American Diabetes Association (ADA) and the European Association for the Study of Diabetes (EASD), Diabetologia 2018 Dec;61(12):2461-2498.)

When the combination of non-insulin agents (oral medications and injectable GLP-1 or GIP/GLP1 receptor agonists) fail to adequately control glucose levels, insulin therapy should be instituted. Various insulin regimens may be effective. Simply adding nighttime intermediate- or long-acting insulin to the medication regimen may lead to improved fasting glucose levels and adequate control during the day. If daytime glucose levels are problematic, premixed insulins before breakfast and dinner may help. If such a regimen does not achieve adequate control or leads to unacceptable rates of hypoglycemia, a more intensive basal bolus insulin regimen (long-acting basal insulin) combined with rapid-acting analog before meals can be instituted.

Metformin has been shown to be effective when combined with insulin therapy and should be continued. Pioglitazone can be used with insulin, but this combination is associated with more weight gain and peripheral and macular edema. Continuing with sulfonylureas, GLP-1 receptor agonists, DPP-4 inhibitors, and SGLT2 inhibitors can be of benefit in selected patients. Cost, complexity, and risk for adverse events should be considered when deciding which drugs to continue once the patient starts on insulin therapy.

Acute Complications of Diabetes

A. Hypoglycemia

Hypoglycemic reactions are the most common complication of insulin therapy. It can also occur in any patient taking oral agents that stimulate insulin secretion (eg, sulfonylureas, meglitinide, D-phenylalanine analogs), particularly if the patient is elderly, has renal or liver disease. It occurs more frequently with the use of long-acting sulfonylureas.

Rapid development of hypoglycemia in persons with intact hypoglycemic awareness causes signs of autonomic hyperactivity—both sympathetic (tachycardia, palpitations, sweating, tremulousness) and parasympathetic (nausea, hunger)—and may progress to convulsions and coma if untreated. In patients exposed to frequent hypoglycemic episodes during tight glycemic control, autonomic warning signals of hypoglycemia are less common or even absent. This dangerous acquired condition is termed *hypoglycemic unawareness*. When patients lack the early warning signs of low blood glucose, they may not take corrective measures in time. In patients with persistent, untreated hypoglycemia, the manifestations of insulin excess may develop—confusion, weakness, bizarre behavior, coma, seizures—at which point they may not be able to procure or safely swallow glucose-containing foods. Hypoglycemic awareness may be restored by preventing frequent hypoglycemic episodes. An identification bracelet, necklace, or card in the wallet or purse, as well as some form of rapidly absorbed glucose, should be carried by every diabetic person who is receiving hypoglycemic drug therapy.

All the manifestations of hypoglycemia are relieved by glucose administration. To expedite absorption, simple sugar or glucose should be given, preferably in liquid form. To treat mild hypoglycemia in a patient who is conscious and able to swallow, dextrose tablets, glucose gel, or any sugar-containing beverage or food may be given. If more severe hypoglycemia has produced unconsciousness or stupor, the treatment of choice is 1 mg of glucagon injected either subcutaneously or intramuscularly or 3 mg of intranasal glucagon for adults. This may restore consciousness within 15 minutes to permit ingestion of sugar. Emergency medical services should be called in the event of loss of consciousness. The emergency personnel can restore consciousness by giving 20–50 mL of 50% glucose solution by intravenous bolus over a period of 2–3 minutes.

B. Diabetic Coma

1. *Diabetic ketoacidosis*—Diabetic ketoacidosis (DKA) is a life-threatening medical emergency caused by inadequate or absent insulin replacement, which occurs in people with type 1 diabetes and infrequently in those with type 2 diabetes. It typically occurs in newly diagnosed type 1 patients or in those who have experienced interrupted insulin replacement, and rarely in people with type 2 diabetes who have concurrent unusually stressful conditions such as sepsis or pancreatitis or are on high-dose steroid therapy. DKA occurs more frequently in patients on insulin pumps. Poor adherence—either for psychological reasons or because of inadequate education—is one of the most common causes of DKA, particularly when episodes are recurrent. Cases of euglycemic diabetic ketoacidosis have been reported with the off-label use of SGLT2 inhibitors in patients with type 1 diabetes and in type 2 patients who are probably quite insulin deficient.

Signs and symptoms include nausea, vomiting, abdominal pain, deep slow (Kussmaul) breathing, change in mental status (including coma), elevated blood and urinary ketones and glucose, an arterial blood pH lower than 7.3, and low bicarbonate (15 mmol/L).

The fundamental treatment for DKA includes aggressive intravenous hydration and insulin therapy and maintenance of potassium and other electrolyte levels. Fluid and insulin therapy is based on the patient's individual needs and requires frequent reevaluation and modification. Close attention must be given to hydration and renal status, sodium and potassium levels, and the rate of correction of plasma glucose and plasma osmolality. Fluid therapy generally begins with normal saline. Regular human insulin should be used for intravenous therapy with a usual starting dosage of about 0.1 U/kg/h.

2. *Hyperosmolar hyperglycemic syndrome*—Hyperosmolar hyperglycemic syndrome (HHS) is diagnosed in persons with type 2 diabetes and is characterized by profound hyperglycemia and dehydration. It is associated with inadequate oral hydration, especially in elderly patients; with other illnesses; with the use of medication that elevates the blood sugar or causes dehydration, such as phenytoin, steroids, diuretics, and calcium channel blockers; and with peritoneal dialysis and hemodialysis. The diagnostic hallmarks are declining mental status and even seizures, a plasma glucose >600 mg/dL, and a calculated serum osmolality >320 mmol/L. Persons with HHS are not acidotic unless DKA is also present.

The treatment of HHS centers around aggressive rehydration and restoration of glucose and electrolyte homeostasis; the rate of correction of these variables must be monitored closely. Low-dose insulin therapy may be required.

Chronic Complications of Diabetes

Late clinical manifestations of diabetes mellitus include a number of pathologic changes that involve small and large blood vessels, cranial and peripheral nerves, the skin, and the eye. These lesions lead to hypertension, end-stage chronic kidney disease, blindness, autonomic and peripheral neuropathy, amputations of the lower extremities, myocardial infarction, and cerebrovascular accidents. These late manifestations correlate with the duration of the diabetic state after the onset of puberty and glycemic control. In type 1 diabetes, end-stage chronic kidney disease develops in up to 40%

of patients, compared with less than 20% of patients with type 2 diabetes. Proliferative retinopathy ultimately develops in both types of diabetes but has a slightly higher prevalence in type 1 patients (25% after 15 years' duration). In patients with type 1 diabetes, complications from end-stage chronic kidney disease are a major cause of death, whereas patients with type 2 diabetes are more likely to have macrovascular diseases leading to myocardial infarction and stroke as the main causes of death. Tobacco use adds significantly to the risk of both microvascular and macrovascular complications inpatients with diabetes.

SUMMARY Drugs Used for Diabetes

Subclass, Drug	Mechanism of Action	Effects	Clinical Applications	Pharmacokinetics, Adverse Effects
INSULINS				
• Rapid-acting: Lispro, aspart, glulisine, inhaled, lispro + tresprostinil & citrate regular, aspart + niacinamide • Short-acting: Regular • Intermediate-acting: NPH • Long-acting: Detemir, glargine, degludec, icodec	Activate insulin receptor	Reduce circulating glucose	Type 1 and type 2 diabetes	Parenteral (SC or IV [regular]) • duration varies (see text) • *Adverse effects:* Hypoglycemia, weight gain, lipodystrophy (rare)
SULFONYLUREAS				
• Glipizide • Glyburide • Glimepiride • Gliclazide[1]	Insulin secretagogues: Close K^+ channels in beta cells • increase insulin release	Reduce circulating glucose in patients with functioning beta cells	Type 2 diabetes	Oral • duration 10–24 h • *Adverse effects:* Hypoglycemia, weight gain
• *Tolazamide, tolbutamide, chlorpropamide, acetohexamide: Older sulfonylureas, lower potency, greater toxicity; rarely used*				
MEGLITINIDE ANALOGS; D-PHENYLANALINE DERIVATIVE				
• Repaglinide, nateglinide • Mitiglinide[1]	Insulin secretagogue: Similar to sulfonylureas with some overlap in binding sites	In patients with functioning beta cells, reduce circulating glucose	Type 2 diabetes	Oral • very fast onset of action • duration 5–8 h, nateglinide • 4 h • *Adverse effects:* Hypoglycemia
BIGUANIDES				
• Metformin	Activates AMP kinase • reduces hepatic and renal gluconeogenesis	Decreases circulating glucose	Type 2 diabetes	Oral • maximal plasma concentration in 2–3 h • *Adverse effects:* Gastrointestinal symptoms, lactic acidosis (rare) • cannot use if impaired renal/hepatic function • heart failure (HF), hypoxic/acidotic states, alcoholism
ALPHA-GLUCOSIDASE INHIBITORS				
• Acarbose, miglitol • Voglibose[1]	Inhibit intestinal α-glucosidases	Reduce conversion of starch and disaccharides to monosaccharides • reduce postprandial hyperglycemia	Type 2 diabetes	Oral • rapid onset • *Adverse effects:* Gastrointestinal symptoms • cannot use if impaired renal/hepatic function, intestinal disorders
THIAZOLIDINEDIONES				
• Pioglitazone, rosiglitazone[1]	Regulate gene expression by binding to PPAR-γ and PPAR-α	Reduce insulin resistance	Type 2 diabetes	Oral • long-acting (>24 h) • *Adverse effects:* Fluid retention, edema, anemia, weight gain, macular edema, bone fractures, especially in women • cannot use if HF, hepatic disease
GLUCAGON-LIKE POLYPEPTIDE-1 (GLP-1) RECEPTOR AGONISTS				
• Dulaglutide, exenatide (and exenatide ER), liraglutide, lixisenatide[1], semaglutide	Analogs of GLP-1: Bind to GLP-1 receptors	Reduce post-meal glucose excursions: Increase glucose-mediated insulin release, lower glucagon levels, slow gastric emptying, decrease appetite	Type 2 diabetes, liraglutide only: obesity	Parenteral (SubC), (Oral: semaglutide only) • *Adverse effects:* Nausea, headache, vomiting, anorexia, mild weight loss, pancreatitis, C-cell tumors in rodents

(*continued*)

Subclass, Drug	Mechanism of Action	Effects	Clinical Applications	Pharmacokinetics, Adverse Effects
DUAL GIP/GLP1 RECEPTOR AGONIST-4				
• Tirzepatide	Analog of GIP: Binds to GIP and GLP1 receptors	Reduces post-meal glucose excursions: Increases glucose-mediated insulin release, lowers glucagon levels, slows gastric emptying, decreases appetite	Type 2 diabetes	Parental (SC) • *Adverse effects:* Nausea, vomiting, diarrhea, anorexia, weight loss, pancreatitis, C-cell tumor in rodents
DIPEPTIDYL PEPTIDASE-4 (DPP-4) INHIBITORS				
• Alogliptin, linagliptin, saxagliptin[1], sitagliptin, vildagliptin[1]	Block degradation of GLP-1, raise circulating GLP-1 levels	Reduces post-meal glucose excursions: Increases glucose-mediated insulin release, lowers glucagon levels, slows gastric emptying, decreases appetite	Type 2 diabetes	Oral • half-life ~12 h • 24–h duration of action • *Adverse effects:* Rhinitis, upper respiratory infections, headaches, joint pain, pancreatitis, rare allergic reactions
SODIUM-GLUCOSE CO-TRANSPORTER 2 (SGLT2) INHIBITORS				
• Canagliflozin, dapagliflozin, empagliflozin, ertugliflozin	Block renal glucose resorption	Increase glucosuria, lower plasma glucose levels	Type 2 diabetes	Oral • half-life ~10–14 h • *Adverse effects:* Genital and urinary tract infections, polyuria, pruritus, thirst, osmotic diuresis, constipation
ISLET AMYLOID POLYPEPETIDE ANALOG				
• Pramlintide	Analog of amylin: Binds to amylin receptors	Reduces post-meal glucose excursions: Lowers glucagon levels, slows gastric emptying, decreases appetite	Type 1 and type 2 diabetes	Parenteral (SC) • rapid onset • half-life ~48 min • *Adverse effects:* Nausea, anorexia, hypoglycemia, headache
BILE ACID SEQUESTRANT				
• Colesevelam hydrochloride	Bile acid binder: Lowers glucose through unknown mechanisms	Reduces glucose levels	Type 2 diabetes	Oral • 24-h duration of action • *Adverse effects:* Constipation, indigestion, flatulence
DOPAMINE AGONIST				
• Bromocriptine	D_2 receptor agonist: Lowers glucose through unknown mechanism	Reduces glucose levels	Type 2 diabetes	Oral • 24-h action • *Adverse effects:* Nausea, vomiting, dizziness, headache

[1]Not available in the United States.

PREPARATIONS AVAILABLE*

GENERIC NAME	AVAILABLE IN US AS
SULFONYLUREAS	
Glimepiride	Generic, Amaryl
Glipizide	Generic, Glucotrol XL
Glyburide	Generic, Glynase
MEGLITINIDES	
Repaglinide	Generic (formerly available as Prandin)
D-PHENYLALANINE DERIVATIVE	
Nateglinide	Generic (formerly available as Starlix)
BIGUANIDE	
Metformin	Generic, Glutmetza (extended release), Riomet (solution), Riomet XR (solution) (formerly available as Glucophage)
METFORMIN COMBINATIONS	
Glipizide plus metformin	Generic
Glyburide plus metformin	Generic
Pioglitazone plus metformin	Generic, ACTOplus Met, ACTOplus Met XR
Saxagliptin plus metformin	Kombiglyze XR
Sitagliptin plus metformin	Janumet, Janumet XR
Linagliptin plus metformin	Jentadueto, Jentadueto XR
Alogliptin plus metformin	Generic, Kazano
Dapagliflozin plus metformin	Xigduo XR
Canagliflozin plus metformin	Invokamet
Empagliflozin plus metformin	Synjardy, Synjardy XR
Ertugliflozin plus metformin	Segluromet
THIAZOLIDINEDIONE DERIVATIVE	
Pioglitazone	Generic, Actos
THIAZOLIDINEDIONE COMBINATION	
Pioglitazone plus glimepiride	Generic, Duetact
Alogliptin plus pioglitazone	Generic, Oseni
ALPHA-GLUCOSIDASE INHIBITORS	
Acarbose	Generic, Precose
Miglitol	Generic, Glyset
GLUCAGON-LIKE POLYPEPTIDE-1 RECEPTOR AGONISTS	
Exenatide	Byetta, Bydureon
Liraglutide	Victoza
Dulaglutide	Trulicity
Lixisenatide	Adlyxin
Semaglutide	Ozempic, Rybelsus (oral)
GLP-1 RECEPTOR AGONIST INHIBITORS COMBINATION	
Lixisenatide plus insulin glargine	Soliqua
DUAL GIP/GLP1 RECEPTOR AGONIST	
Tirzepatide	Mounjaro
DIPEPTIDYL PEPTIDASE-4 INHIBITORS	
Linagliptin	Tradjenta
Saxagliptin	Onglyza
Sitagliptin	Januvia
Alogliptin	Nesina
SODIUM GLUCOSE CO-TRANSPORTER 2 INHIBITORS	
Canagliflozin	Invokana
Dapagliflozin	Farxiga
Empagliflozin	Jardiance
Ertugliflozin	Steglatro
SODIUM GLUCOSE CO-TRANSPORTER INHIBITORS COMBINATION	
Dapagliflozin plus saxagliptin	Qtern
Empagliflozin plus linagliptin	Glyxambi
Empagliflozin plus linagliptin plus metformin	Trijardy XR
Ertuglifozin plus sitagliptin	Staglujan
MISCELLANEOUS DRUGS	
ISLET AMYLOID POLYPEPTIDE ANALOG	
Pramlintide	Symlin
BILE ACID SEQUESTRANT	
Colesevelam hydrochloride	Welchol
DOPAMINE RECEPTOR AGONIST	
Bromocriptine	Generic, Parlodel, Cycloset
GLUCAGON	
Glucagon	Generic

*See Table 41–5 for insulin preparations.

REFERENCES

Action to Control Cardiovascular Risks in Diabetes Study Group: Effects of intensive glucose lowering in type 2 diabetes. N Engl J Med 2008;358:2545.

Adler AI et al: Association of systolic blood pressure with macrovascular and microvascular complications of type 2 diabetes (UKPDS 36): Prospective observational study. Br Med J 2000;321:412.

ADVANCE Collaborative Group: Intensive blood glucose control and vascular outcomes in patients with type 2 diabetes. N Engl J Med 2008;358:2560.

American Diabetes Association: Diagnosis and classification of diabetes mellitus. Diabetes Care 2014;37:S81.

American Diabetes Association: Classification and diagnosis of diabetes: standards of care in diabetes—2023. Diabetes Care 2023;46:S19.

Bailey CJ, Day C.: The future of new drugs for diabetes management. Diabetes Res Clin Pract 2019;155:107785.

Bekiari E et al: Artificial pancreas treatment for outpatients with type 1 diabetes: Systematic review and meta-analysis. BMJ 2018;361:k1310.

Davies MJ et al: Management of hyperglycaemia in type 2 diabetes, 2018: A consensus report by the American Diabetes Association (ADA) and the European Association for the Study of Diabetes (EASD). Diabetologia 2018;61:2461.

DeFronzo RA et al: Pioglitazone: The forgotten, cost-effective cardioprotective drug for type 2 diabetes. Diab Vasc Dis Res 2019;16:133.

Diabetes Prevention Program Research Group: Reduction in the incidence of type 2 diabetes with lifestyle intervention or metformin. N Engl J Med 2002;346:393.

Gaede P et al: Effect of a multifactorial intervention on mortality in type 2 diabetes. N Engl J Med 2008;358:580.

Firas JP et al: Tirzepatide versus semaglutide once weekly in patients with type 2 diabetes. N Engl J Med 2021;385:503.

Herold KC et al: An anti-CD3 antibody, teplizumab, in relatives at risk for type 1 diabetes. N Eng J Med 2019;381:603.

Kitabchi A et al: Thirty years of personal experience in hyperglycemic crises: Diabetic ketoacidosis and hyperglycemic hyperosmolar state. J Clin Endocrinol Metab 2008;93:1541.

Miyazaki Y, DeFronzo RA: Rosiglitazone and pioglitazone similarly improve insulin sensitivity and secretion, glucose tolerance and adipocytokines in type 2 diabetic patients. Diabetes Obes Metab 2008;10:1204.

Nauck M: Incretin therapies: Highlighting common features and differences in the modes of action of glucagon-like peptide-1 receptor agonists and dipeptidyl peptidase-4 inhibitors. Diabetes Obes Metab 2016;18:203.

Perkovic V et al: Canagliflozin and renal outcomes in type 2 diabetes and nephropathy. N Engl J Med 2019;380:2295.

Reitman ML et al: Pharmacogenetics of metformin response: A step in the path toward personalized medicine. J Clin Invest 2007;117:1226.

Ripamonti E et al. A systematic review of observational studies of the association between pioglitazone use and bladder cancer. Diabet Med 2019;36:22.

Rosenstock J, Ferrannini E: Euglycemic diabetic ketoacidosis: A predictable, detectable, and preventable safety concern with SGLT2 inhibitors. Diabetes Care 2015;38:1638.

Switzer SM et al: Intensive insulin therapy in patients with type 1 diabetes mellitus. Endocrinol Metab Clin North Am 2012;41:89.

United Kingdom Prospective Diabetes Study (UKPDS) Group: Glycemic control with diet, sulfonylurea, metformin, or insulin in patients with type 2 diabetes mellitus: Progressive requirement for multiple therapies: UKPDS 49. JAMA 1999;281:2005.

United Kingdom Prospective Diabetes Study (UKPDS) Group: Tight blood pressure control and risk of macrovascular and microvascular complications in type 2 diabetes: UKPDS 38. BMJ 1998;317:703.

Zelniker TA et al. SGLT2 inhibitors for primary and secondary prevention of cardiovascular and renal outcomes in type 2 diabetes: A systematic review and meta-analysis of cardiovascular outcome trials. Lancet 2019;393:31.

CASE STUDY ANSWER

This patient had significant insulin resistance, taking about 125 units of insulin daily (approximately 1 unit per kilogram). He had received limited education on how to manage his diabetes. He had peripheral neuropathy, proteinuria, low HDL-cholesterol levels, and hypertension. The patient underwent multifactorial intervention targeting his weight, glucose levels, and blood pressure. He was advised to stop smoking and provided counseling support and smoking cessation medications. He attended structured diabetes classes and received individualized instruction from a diabetes educator and a dietitian. Metformin therapy was reinitiated and his insulin doses were reduced. The patient was then given the GLP-1 receptor agonist, exenatide. The patient lost about 8 kg in weight over the next 3 years and was able to stop his insulin. He had excellent control with an HbA_{1c} of 6.5 % on a combination of metformin, exenatide, and glimepiride. The patient, however, regained some of the weight and his HbA_{1c} increased. The glimepiride dose was reduced and SGLT2 inhibitor therapy instituted because of the diabetic nephropathy. His antihypertensive therapy was optimized and his urine albumin excretion declined to 1569 mg/g creatinine. This case illustrates the importance of weight loss in achieving target glucose levels in the obese patient with type 2 diabetes. It also shows that simply increasing the insulin dose is not always effective. Combining metformin with other oral agents and non-insulin injectables may be a better option.

CHAPTER

42

Agents That Affect Bone Mineral Homeostasis

Daniel D. Bikle, MD, PhD

CASE STUDY

A 65-year-old man is referred to you from his primary care physician (PCP) for evaluation and management of possible osteoporosis. He saw his PCP for evaluation of low back pain. X-rays of the spine showed some degenerative changes in the lumbar spine plus several wedge deformities in the thoracic spine. The patient is a long-time smoker (up to two packs per day) and has two to four glasses of wine with dinner, more on the weekends. He has chronic bronchitis, presumably from smoking, and has been treated on numerous occasions with oral prednisone for exacerbations of bronchitis. He is currently on 10 mg/d prednisone. Examination shows kyphosis of the thoracic spine, with some tenderness to fist percussion over the thoracic spine. The dual-energy x-ray absorptiometry (DEXA) measurement of the lumbar spine is "within the normal limits," but the radiologist noted that the reading may be misleading because of degenerative changes. The hip measurement shows a T score (number of standard deviations by which the patient's measured bone density differs from that of a normal young adult) in the femoral neck of –2.2. What further workup should be considered, and what therapy should be initiated?

■ BASIC PHARMACOLOGY

Calcium and phosphate, the major mineral constituents of bone, are also two of the most important minerals for general cellular function. Accordingly, the body has evolved complex mechanisms to carefully maintain calcium and phosphate homeostasis (Figure 42–1). Approximately 98% of the 1–2 kg of calcium and 85% of the 1 kg of phosphorus in the human adult are found in bone, the principal reservoir for these minerals. This reservoir is dynamic, with constant remodeling of bone and ready exchange of bone mineral with that in the extracellular fluid. Bone also serves as the principal structural support for the body and provides the space for hematopoiesis. This relationship is more than fortuitous, as elements of the bone marrow affect skeletal processes just as skeletal elements affect hematopoietic processes. During aging and in nutritional diseases such as anorexia nervosa and obesity, fat accumulates in the marrow, suggesting a dynamic interaction between marrow fat and bone. Furthermore, bone has been implicated as an endocrine tissue with release of osteocalcin, which in its uncarboxylated form stimulates insulin secretion, testicular function, and muscle endurance. Abnormalities in bone mineral homeostasis can lead to a wide variety of cellular dysfunctions (eg, tetany, coma, muscle weakness), disturbances in structural support of the body (eg, osteoporosis with fractures), and loss of hematopoietic capacity (eg, infantile osteopetrosis).

Calcium and phosphate enter the body from the intestine. The average American diet provides 600–1000 mg of calcium per day, of which approximately 100–250 mg is absorbed. This amount represents net absorption, because both absorption and secretion occur. Although the duodenum is the site of the highest rate of calcium absorption, the long dwell time of intestinal contents in the ileum makes it the site of the greatest amount of calcium absorption. The quantity of phosphorus in the American diet is about the same as that of calcium. However, the efficiency of absorption (principally in the jejunum) is greater, ranging from 70% to 90%, depending on intake. In the steady state, renal excretion of calcium and phosphate balances intestinal absorption. In general, more than 98% of filtered calcium and 85% of filtered phosphate are reabsorbed by the kidney. The movement of calcium and phosphate across the

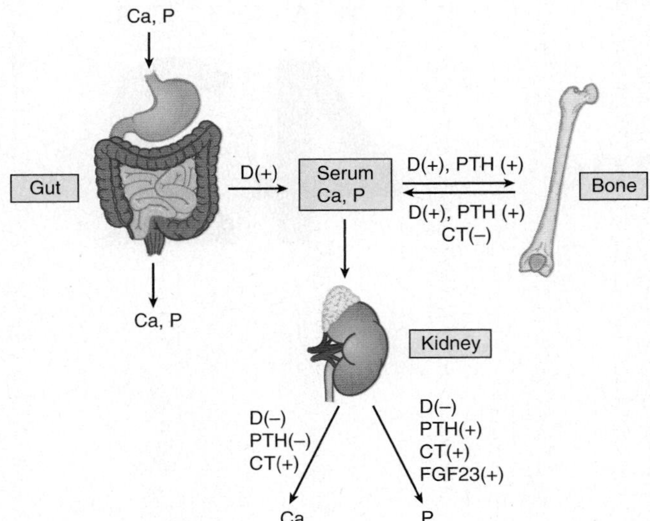

FIGURE 42–1 Mechanisms contributing to bone mineral homeostasis. Serum calcium (Ca) and phosphorus (P) concentrations are controlled principally by three hormones, 1,25-dihydroxyvitamin D (D), fibroblast growth factor 23 (FGF23), and parathyroid hormone (PTH), through their action on absorption from the gut and from bone and on renal excretion. PTH and 1,25(OH)$_2$D increase the input of calcium and phosphorus from bone into the serum and stimulate bone formation. 1,25(OH)$_2$D also increases calcium and phosphate absorption from the gut. In the kidney, 1,25(OH)$_2$D decreases excretion of both calcium and phosphorus, whereas PTH reduces calcium but increases phosphorus excretion. FGF23 stimulates renal excretion of phosphate. Calcitonin (CT) is a less critical regulator of calcium homeostasis, but in pharmacologic concentrations can reduce serum calcium and phosphorus by inhibiting bone resorption and stimulating their renal excretion. Feedback may alter the effects shown; for example, 1,25(OH)$_2$D increases urinary calcium excretion indirectly through increased calcium absorption from the gut and inhibition of PTH secretion and may increase urinary phosphate excretion because of increased phosphate absorption from the gut and stimulation of FGF23 production.

intestinal and renal epithelia is closely regulated. Dysfunction of the intestine (eg, nontropical sprue) or kidney (eg, chronic renal failure) can disrupt bone mineral homeostasis.

Three hormones serve as the principal regulators of calcium and phosphate homeostasis: **parathyroid hormone (PTH), fibroblast growth factor 23 (FGF23),** and **vitamin D** via its active metabolite **1,25-dihydroxyvitamin D (1,25[OH]$_2$D)** (Figure 42–2). The role of **calcitonin** (CT) is less critical during adult life but may play a greater role during pregnancy and lactation. The term *vitamin D*, when used without a subscript, refers to both vitamin D$_2$ (ergocalciferol) and vitamin D$_3$ (cholecalciferol). This applies also to the metabolites of vitamin D$_2$ and D$_3$. Vitamin D$_2$ and its metabolites differ from vitamin D$_3$ and its metabolites only in the side chain where they contain a double bond between C-22–23 and a methyl group at C-24 (Figure 42–3). Vitamin D is considered a prohormone because it must be further metabolized to gain biologic activity (see Figure 42–3). Vitamin D$_3$ is produced in the skin under ultraviolet B (UVB) radiation (eg, in sunlight) from its precursor, 7-dehydrocholesterol (7-DHC). The initial product, pre-vitamin D$_3$, undergoes a temperature-sensitive isomerization to vitamin D$_3$. 7-DHC is on the pathway to cholesterol, a step controlled by the enzyme 7-dehydrocholesterol reductase (DHCR7). Levels and regulation of DHCR7 control the levels of 7-DHC in the skin and thus the amount of substrate available for vitamin D production. The precursor of vitamin D$_2$ is ergosterol, found in plants and fungi (mushrooms). It undergoes a similar transformation to vitamin D$_2$ with UVB radiation. Vitamin D$_2$ thus comes only from the diet, whereas vitamin D$_3$ comes from the skin or the diet, or both. The subsequent metabolism of these two forms of vitamin D is essentially the same and follows the illustration for vitamin D$_3$ metabolism in Figure 42–3. The first step is the 25-hydroxylation of vitamin D to 25-hydroxyvitamin D (25[OH]D). A number of enzymes in the liver and other tissues perform this function, of which CYP2R1 is the most important at least in the liver. 25(OH)D is then metabolized to the active hormone 1,25-dihydroxyvitamin D (1,25[OH]$_2$D) in the kidney and elsewhere. PTH stimulates the production of 1,25(OH)$_2$D in the kidney, whereas FGF23 is inhibitory. Elevated levels of blood phosphate and calcium also inhibit 1,25(OH)$_2$D production in part by their effects on FGF23 (high phosphate stimulates FGF23 production) and PTH (high calcium inhibits PTH production). 1,25(OH)$_2$D regulates its own levels by stimulating the enzyme 24-hydroxyase (CYP24A1), which begins the catabolism of 1,25(OH)$_2$D, by suppressing PTH production, and by stimulating FGF23 production, all of which combine to reduce 1,25(OH)$_2$D levels. Other tissues also produce 1,25(OH)$_2$D; the control of this production differs from that in the kidney, as will be discussed subsequently. The complex interplay among PTH, FGF23, and 1,25(OH)$_2$D is discussed in detail later.

To summarize: 1,25(OH)$_2$D suppresses the production of PTH, as does calcium, but stimulates the production of FGF23. Phosphate stimulates both PTH and FGF23 secretion. In turn PTH stimulates 1,25(OH)$_2$D production, whereas FGF23 is inhibitory. 1,25(OH)$_2$D stimulates the intestinal absorption of calcium and phosphate. 1,25(OH)$_2$D and PTH promote both bone formation and resorption in part by stimulating the proliferation and differentiation of osteoblasts and osteoclasts. Both PTH and 1,25(OH)$_2$D enhance renal retention of calcium, but PTH promotes renal phosphate excretion, as does FGF23, whereas 1,25(OH)$_2$D promotes renal reabsorption of phosphate. These feedback loops combine to maintain calcium and phosphate homeostasis.

Other hormones—calcitonin, prolactin, growth hormone, insulin, insulin-like growth factors, thyroid hormone, glucocorticoids, and sex steroids—influence calcium and phosphate homeostasis under certain physiologic circumstances and can be considered secondary regulators. Deficiency or excess of these secondary regulators within a physiologic range does not produce the disturbance of calcium and phosphate homeostasis that is observed in situations of deficiency or excess of PTH, FGF23, and vitamin D. However, certain of these secondary regulators—especially calcitonin, glucocorticoids, and estrogens—are useful therapeutically and are discussed in subsequent sections.

In addition to these hormonal regulators, calcium and phosphate themselves, other ions such as sodium and fluoride, and a variety of drugs (bisphosphonates, anticonvulsants, various anti-HIV drugs, and diuretics) also alter calcium and phosphate homeostasis.

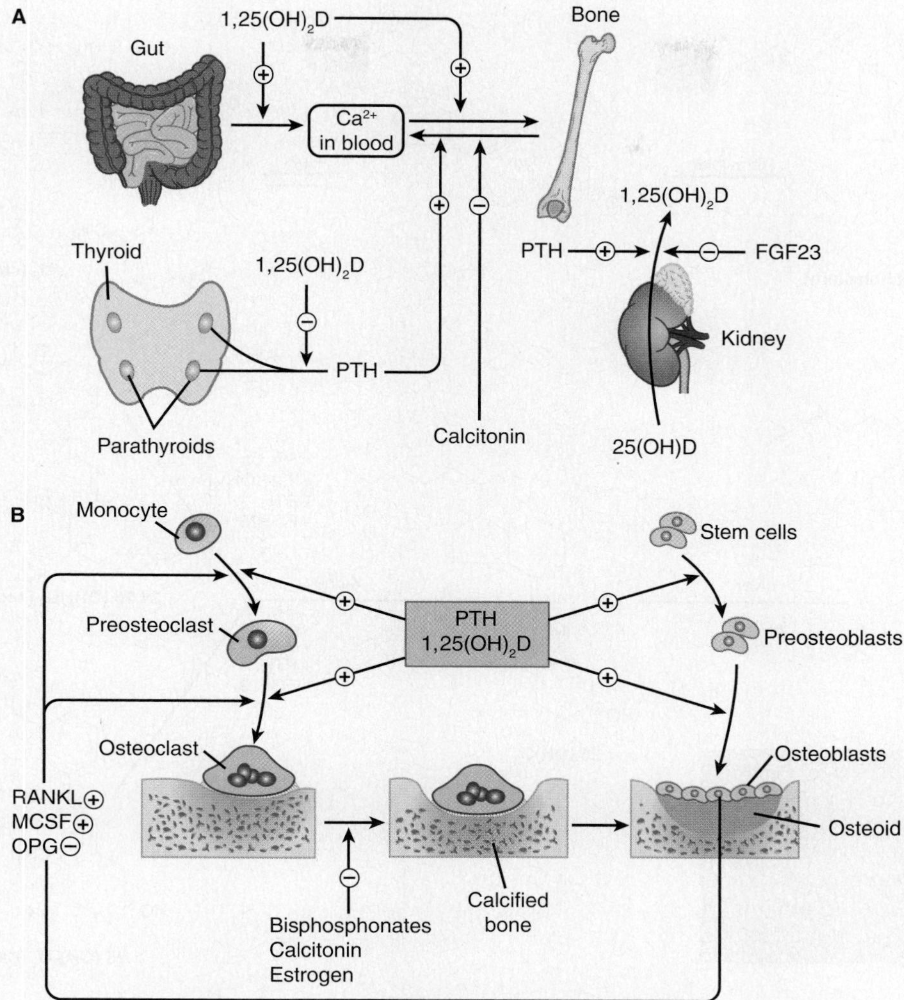

FIGURE 42–2 The hormonal interactions controlling bone mineral homeostasis. In the body **(A)**, 1,25-dihydroxyvitamin D (1,25[OH]$_2$D) is produced by the kidney under the control of parathyroid hormone (PTH), which stimulates its production, and fibroblast growth factor 23 (FGF23), which inhibits its production. 1,25(OH)$_2$D in turn inhibits the production of PTH by the parathyroid glands and stimulates FGF23 release from bone. 1,25(OH)$_2$D is the principal regulator of intestinal calcium and phosphate absorption. At the level of the bone **(B)**, both PTH and 1,25(OH)$_2$D regulate bone formation and resorption, with each capable of stimulating both processes. This is accomplished by their stimulation of preosteoblast proliferation and differentiation into osteoblasts, the bone-forming cell. PTH also stimulates osteoblast formation indirectly by inhibiting the osteocyte's production of sclerostin, a protein that blocks osteoblast proliferation by inhibiting the wnt pathway (not shown). PTH and 1,25(OH)$_2$D stimulate the expression of RANKL by the osteoblast, which, with MCSF, stimulates the differentiation and subsequent activation of osteoclasts, the bone-resorbing cell. OPG blocks RANKL action, and may be inhibited by PTH and 1,25(OH)$_2$D. FGF23 in excess leads to osteomalacia indirectly by inhibiting 1,25(OH)$_2$D production and lowering phosphate levels. MCSF, macrophage colony-stimulating factor; OPG, osteoprotegerin; RANKL, ligand for receptor for activation of nuclear factor-κB.

PRINCIPAL HORMONAL REGULATORS OF BONE MINERAL HOMEOSTASIS

PARATHYROID HORMONE

Parathyroid hormone (PTH) is a single-chain peptide hormone composed of 84 amino acids. It is produced in the parathyroid gland in a precursor form of 115 amino acids, the excess 31 amino terminal amino acids being cleaved off before secretion. Within the gland is a calcium-sensitive protease capable of cleaving the intact hormone into fragments, thereby providing one mechanism by which calcium limits the production of PTH. A second mechanism involves the calcium-sensing receptor (CaSR) which, when stimulated by calcium, reduces PTH production and secretion. The parathyroid gland also contains the vitamin D receptor (VDR) and the enzyme, CYP27B1, that produces 1,25(OH)$_2$D, thus enabling circulating or endogenously produced 1,25(OH)$_2$D to suppress PTH production. 1,25(OH)$_2$D also induces the CaSR, making the parathyroid gland more sensitive to suppression by calcium. Biologic activity resides in the amino terminal region of PTH such that

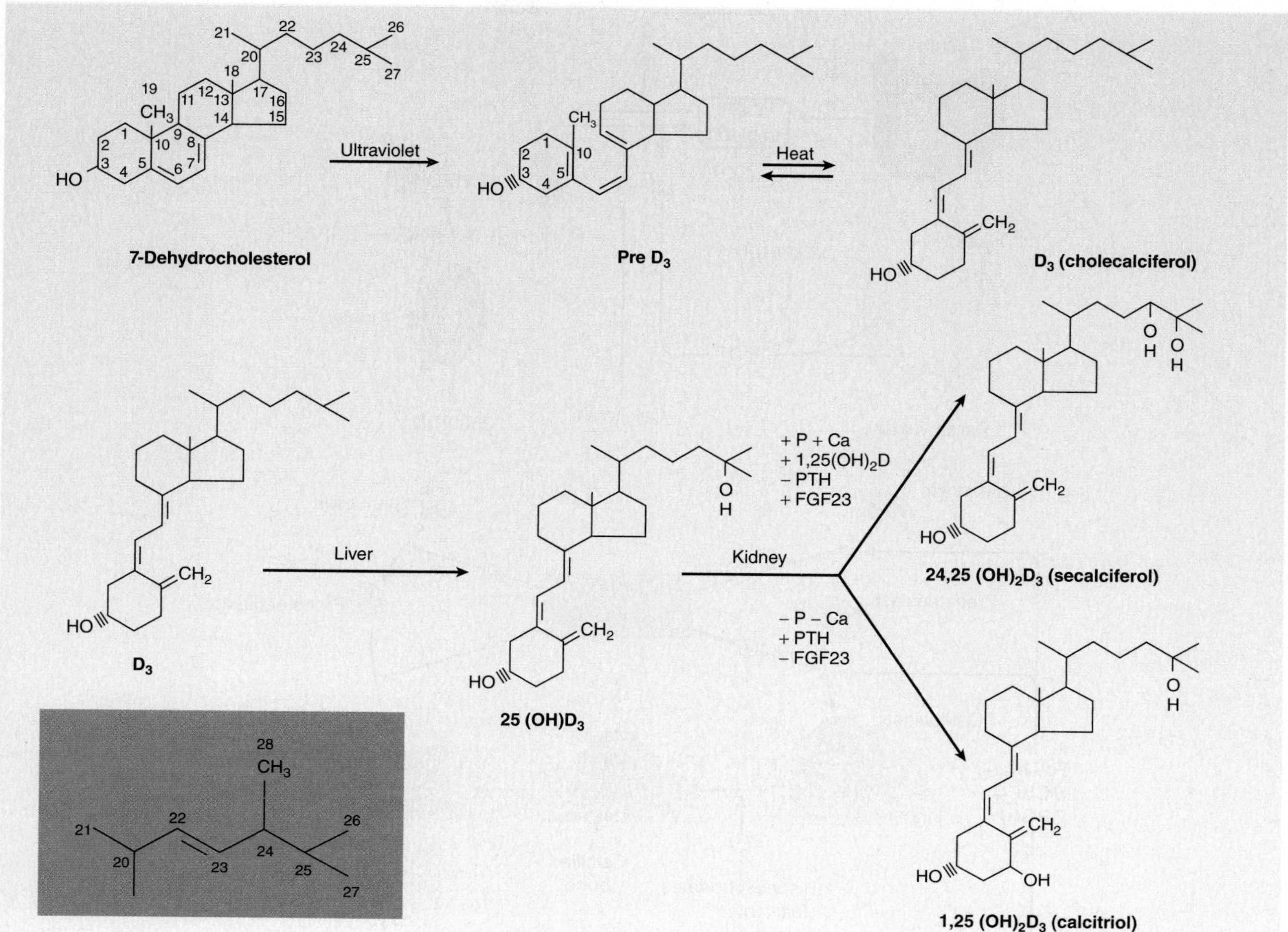

FIGURE 42–3 Conversion of 7-dehydrocholesterol to vitamin D_3 in the skin and its subsequent metabolism to 25-hydroxyvitamin D_3 (25[OH]D_3) in the liver and to 1,25-dihydroxyvitamin D_3 (1,25[OH]$_2D_3$) and 24,25-dihydroxyvitamin D_3 (24,25[OH]$_2D_3$) in the kidney. Control of vitamin D metabolism is exerted primarily at the level of the kidney, where high concentrations of serum phosphorus (P) and calcium (Ca) as well as fibroblast growth factor 23 (FGF23) inhibit production of 1,25(OH)$_2D_3$ (indicated by a minus [–] sign), but promote that of 24,25(OH)$_2D_3$ (indicated by a plus [+] sign). Parathyroid hormone (PTH), on the other hand, stimulates 1,25(OH)$_2D_3$ production but inhibits 24,25(OH)$_2D_3$ production. The insert (shaded) shows the side chain for ergosterol, vitamin D_2, and the active vitamin D_2 metabolites. Ergosterol is converted to vitamin D_2 (ergocalciferol) by UV radiation similar to the conversion of 7-dehydrocholesterol to vitamin D_3. Vitamin D_2, in turn, is metabolized to 25-hydroxyvitamin D_2, 1,25-dihydroxyvitamin D_2, and 24,25-dihydroxyvitamin D_2 via the same enzymes that metabolize vitamin D_3. In humans, corresponding D_2 and D_3 metabolites have equivalent biologic effects, although they differ in pharmacokinetics. +, facilitation; –, inhibition; P, phosphorus; Ca, calcium; PTH, parathyroid hormone; FGF23, fibroblast growth factor 23.

synthetic PTH 1-34 (available as teriparatide) is fully active and used in the treatment of osteoporosis However, a full length form of PTH (rhPTH 1-84, **Natpara**) has been approved for treatment of hypoparathyroidism. In addition, an analog of PTHrP **(abaloparatide)** that functions much like teriparatide has recently been approved for the treatment of osteoporosis. Other analogs of PTH are currently in development. Loss of the first two amino terminal amino acids eliminates most biologic activity.

The metabolic clearance of intact PTH is rapid, with a half-time of disappearance measured in minutes. Most of the clearance occurs in the liver and kidney. The inactive carboxyl terminal fragments produced by metabolism of the intact hormone have a much lower clearance, especially in renal failure. In the past, this accounted for the very high PTH values observed in patients with renal failure when the hormone was measured by radioimmunoassays directed against the carboxyl terminal region. Currently, most PTH assays differentiate between intact PTH 1-34 and large inactive fragments, so that it is possible to more accurately evaluate biologically active PTH status in patients with renal failure. That said, in renal failure biologically inactive fragments of PTH detected by the newer "intact" PTH assays still complicate the measurement.

PTH regulates calcium and phosphate flux across cellular membranes in bone and kidney, resulting in increased serum calcium and decreased serum phosphate (see Figure 42–1). In bone, PTH increases the activity of osteoblasts, the bone-forming cells, as well as the activity and number of osteoclasts, the cells responsible for bone resorption (see Figure 42–2). However, this stimulation of osteoclasts is not a direct effect. Rather, PTH acts on the osteoblast to induce membrane-bound and secreted soluble forms of a protein called **RANK ligand (RANKL).** RANKL acts on osteoclasts and osteoclast precursors to increase both the numbers and activity of osteoclasts. This action increases bone remodeling, a specific sequence of cellular events initiated by osteoclastic bone resorption and followed by osteoblastic bone formation. **Denosumab,** an antibody that inhibits the action of RANKL, has been developed for the treatment of excess bone resorption in patients with osteoporosis and certain cancers. PTH also inhibits the production and secretion of sclerostin from osteocytes. Sclerostin is one of several proteins that block osteoblast proliferation by inhibiting the wnt pathway. Antibodies against sclerostin (eg, **romosozumab**) have recently been approved for the treatment of osteoporosis. Unlike PTH, romosozumab does not stimulate osteoclast activity, but rather suppresses it, at least initially. Thus, PTH directly and indirectly increases proliferation of osteoblasts, the cells responsible for bone formation. Although both bone resorption and bone formation are enhanced by PTH, the net effect of excess endogenous PTH is to increase bone resorption. However, administration of exogenous PTH in low and intermittent doses increases bone formation without first stimulating bone resorption. This net anabolic action may be indirect, involving other growth factors such as insulin-like growth factor 1 (IGF1) as well as inhibition of sclerostin as noted above. These anabolic actions have led to the approval of recombinant PTH 1-34 and its PTHrP analog **teriparatide** and **abaloparatide,** respectively, for the treatment of osteoporosis. In the kidney, PTH stimulates 1,25(OH)$_2$D production, and increases tubular reabsorption of calcium and magnesium, but reduces reabsorption of phosphate, amino acids, bicarbonate, sodium, chloride, and sulfate. As mentioned earlier, full-length PTH **(rhPTH 1-84, Natpara)** has been approved in part for these renal effects, which otherwise limit standard calcium and calcitriol treatment of hypoparathyroidism.

VITAMIN D

Vitamin D is a secosteroid produced in the skin from 7-dehydrocholesterol under the influence of ultraviolet radiation. Vitamin D is also found in certain foods and is used to supplement dairy products and other foods. Both the natural form (vitamin D$_3$, cholecalciferol) and the plant-derived form (vitamin D$_2$, ergocalciferol) are present in the diet. As discussed earlier these forms differ in that ergocalciferol contains a double bond and an additional methyl group in the side chain (see Figure 42–3). Ergocalciferol and its metabolites bind less well than cholecalciferol and its metabolites to vitamin D–binding protein (DBP), the major transport protein of these compounds in blood, and have a somewhat different path of catabolism. As a result, their half-lives are shorter than those of the cholecalciferol metabolites. This influences treatment strategies, as will be discussed. However, the key steps in metabolism and biologic activities of the active metabolites are comparable, so with this exception the following comments apply equally well to both forms of vitamin D.

Vitamin D is a precursor to a number of biologically active metabolites (see Figure 42–3). Vitamin D is first hydroxylated in the liver and other tissues to form 25(OH)D (calcifediol). As noted earlier, there are a number of enzymes with 25-hydroxylase activity. This metabolite is further converted in the kidney to a number of other forms, the best studied of which are 1,25(OH)$_2$D (calcitriol) and 24,25-dihydroxyvitamin D (secalciferol, 24,25[OH]$_2$D), by the enzymes CYP27B1 and CYP24A1, respectively. The regulation of vitamin D metabolism is complex, involving calcium, phosphate, and a variety of hormones, the most important of which are PTH, which stimulates, and FGF23, which inhibits the production of 1,25(OH)$_2$D by the kidney while reciprocally inhibiting or promoting the production of 24,25(OH)$_2$D. The importance of CYP24A1, the enzyme that 24-hydroxylates 25(OH)D and 1,25(OH)$_2$D, is well demonstrated in children and adults with inactivating mutations of this enzyme who develop high levels of calcium and 1,25(OH)$_2$D resulting in kidney damage from nephrocalcinosis and stones. Of the natural metabolites, vitamin D, 25(OH)D **(calcifediol)** and 1,25(OH)$_2$D (as **calcitriol**) are available for clinical use (Table 42–1). A number of analogs of 1,25(OH)$_2$D have been synthesized to extend the usefulness of this metabolite to a variety of nonclassic conditions. **Calcipotriene** (calcipotriol), for example, is being used to treat psoriasis, a hyperproliferative skin disorder (see Chapter 61). **Doxercalciferol** and **paricalcitol** are approved for the treatment of secondary hyperparathyroidism in patients with chronic kidney disease. **Eldecalcitol** is approved in Japan for the treatment of osteoporosis. Other analogs are being investigated for the treatment of various malignancies.

Vitamin D and its metabolites circulate in plasma tightly bound to the DBP. This α-globulin binds 25(OH)D and 24,25(OH)$_2$D with comparable high affinity and vitamin D and 1,25(OH)$_2$D with lower affinity. There is increasing evidence that it is the free or unbound forms of these metabolites that have biologic activity. This is of clinical importance because patients with liver disease or nephrotic syndrome have lower levels of DBP, whereas DBP levels are increased with estrogen therapy and during the later stages of pregnancy. Furthermore, there are several different forms of DBP in the population with different affinities for the vitamin D

TABLE 42–1 Vitamin D and its major metabolites and analogs.

Chemical and Generic Names	Abbreviation
Vitamin D$_3$; cholecalciferol	D$_3$
Vitamin D$_2$; ergocalciferol	D$_2$
25-Hydroxyvitamin D$_3$; calcifediol	25(OH)D$_3$
1,25-Dihydroxyvitamin D$_3$; calcitriol	1,25(OH)$_2$D$_3$
24,25-Dihydroxyvitamin D$_3$; secalciferol	24,25(OH)$_2$D$_3$
Dihydrotachysterol	DHT
Calcipotriene (calcipotriol)	None
1α-Hydroxyvitamin D$_2$; doxercalciferol	1α(OH)D$_2$
19-nor-1,25-Dihydroxyvitamin D$_2$; paricalcitol	19-nor-1,25(OH)D$_2$

metabolites, and, as noted earlier, the affinity of DBP for the D_2 metabolites is less than that for the D_3 metabolites. Thus individuals can vary with respect to the fraction of free metabolite available, so that measuring only the total metabolite concentration may be misleading with respect to assessing vitamin D status. In normal subjects, the terminal half-life of injected calcifediol (25[OH]D) is around 23 days, whereas in anephric subjects it is around 42 days. The half-life of 24,25$(OH)_2$D is probably similar. Tracer studies with vitamin D have shown a rapid clearance from the blood. The liver appears to be the principal organ for clearance. Excess vitamin D is stored in adipose tissue. The metabolic clearance of calcitriol (1,25$[OH]_2$D) in humans likewise indicates a rapid turnover, with a terminal half-life measured in hours. Several of the 1,25$(OH)_2$D analogs are bound poorly by DBP. As a result, their clearance is very rapid, with a terminal half-life of minutes. Such analogs have less hypercalcemic, hypercalciuric effect than calcitriol, an important aspect of their use in the management of conditions such as psoriasis and secondary hyperparathyroidism.

The mechanism of action of the vitamin D metabolites remains under active investigation. However, 1,25$(OH)_2$D is well established as the most potent stimulant of intestinal calcium and phosphate transport and bone resorption. 1,25$(OH)_2$D appears to act on the intestine both by induction of new protein synthesis (eg, calcium-binding protein and TRPV6, an intestinal calcium channel) and by modulation of calcium flux across the brush border and basolateral membranes by processes that do not all require new protein synthesis. The molecular action of 1,25$(OH)_2$D on bone is more complex and controversial as it is both direct and indirect. Much of the skeletal effect is attributed to the provision of adequate calcium and phosphate from the diet by stimulation of their intestinal absorption. However, like PTH, 1,25$(OH)_2$D can induce RANKL in osteoblasts to regulate osteoclast activity and proteins such as osteocalcin and alkaline phosphatase, which may regulate the mineralization process by osteoblasts. The metabolites 25(OH)D and 24,25$(OH)_2$D are far less potent stimulators of intestinal calcium and phosphate transport or bone resorption.

Specific receptors for 1,25$(OH)_2$D (VDR) exist in nearly all tissues, not just intestine, bone, and kidney. As a result much effort has been made to develop analogs of 1,25$(OH)_2$D that will target these nonclassic target tissues without increasing serum calcium. These nonclassic actions include regulation of the secretion of PTH, insulin, and renin; regulation of innate and adaptive immune function through actions on dendritic cell and T-cell differentiation; enhanced muscle function; and proliferation and differentiation of a number of cancer cells. Thus, the potential clinical utility of 1,25$(OH)_2$D and its analogs is expanding. A different receptor has recently been found for 24,25$(OH)_2$D. However, the physiologic role of this receptor is not yet fully understood.

FIBROBLAST GROWTH FACTOR 23

Fibroblast growth factor 23 (FGF23) is a single-chain protein with 251 amino acids, including a 24-amino-acid leader sequence. It inhibits 1,25$(OH)_2$D production and phosphate reabsorption (via the sodium phosphate cotransporters NaPi 2a and 2c) in the kidney and can lead to both hypophosphatemia and inappropriately low levels of circulating 1,25$(OH)_2$D. Whereas FGF23 was originally identified in certain mesenchymal tumors, osteoblasts and osteocytes in bone appear to be its primary site of production. Other tissues can also produce FGF23, though at lower levels. FGF23 requires *O*-glycosylation for its secretion, a glycosylation mediated by the glycosyl transferase GALNT3. Mutations in GALNT3 result in abnormal deposition of calcium phosphate in periarticular tissues (tumoral calcinosis) with elevated phosphate and 1,25$(OH)_2$D. FGF23 is normally inactivated by cleavage at an RXXR site (amino acids 176–179). Mutations of the arginines (R) in this site lead to excess FGF23, the underlying problem in autosomal dominant hypophosphatemic rickets. A similar disease, X-linked hypophosphatemic rickets (XLH), is due to mutations in PHEX, an endopeptidase, which initially was thought to cleave FGF23. However, this concept has been shown to be invalid, and the mechanism by which PHEX mutations lead to increased FGF23 levels remains obscure. FGF23 binds to FGF receptors (FGFR) 1 and 3c in the presence of the accessory receptor Klotho-α. Both Klotho and the FGFR must be present for signaling in most tissues, although high levels of FGF23 appear to affect cardiomyocytes lacking Klotho. Mutations in Klotho disrupt FGF23 signaling, resulting in elevated phosphate and 1,25$(OH)_2$D levels, a phenotype quite similar to inactivating mutations in FGF23 or GALNT3. FGF23 production is stimulated by 1,25$(OH)_2$D and phosphate and directly or indirectly inhibited by the dentin matrix protein DMP1 found in osteocytes. Mutations in DMP1 lead to increased FGF23 levels and osteomalacia. Recently an antibody to FGF23, **burosumab,** has been approved for the treatment of XLH, an approval likely to extend to other diseases marked by high FGF23 levels.

INTERACTION OF PTH, FGF23, & VITAMIN D

A summary of the principal actions of PTH, FGF23, and vitamin D on the three main target tissues—intestine, kidney, and bone—is presented in Table 42–2. The net effect of PTH is to raise serum calcium, reduce serum phosphate, and increase 1,25$(OH)_2$D; the net effect of FGF23 is to decrease serum phosphate and 1,25$(OH)_2$D; the net effect of vitamin D is to raise both calcium and phosphate while decreasing PTH and increasing FGF23. Regulation of calcium and phosphate homeostasis is achieved through important feedback loops. Calcium is one of two principal regulators of PTH secretion. It binds to a novel ion recognition site that is part of a G_q protein-coupled receptor called the calcium-sensing receptor (CaSR) that employs the phosphoinositide second messenger system to link changes in the extracellular calcium concentration to changes in the intracellular free calcium. As serum calcium levels rise and activate this receptor, intracellular calcium levels increase and inhibit PTH secretion. This inhibition by calcium of PTH secretion, along with inhibition of renin and atrial natriuretic peptide secretion, is the opposite of the effect of calcium in other tissues such as the beta cell of the pancreas, in which calcium stimulates secretion. Phosphate regulates PTH

TABLE 42–2 Actions of parathyroid hormone (PTH), vitamin D, and FGF23 on gut, bone, and kidney.

	PTH	Vitamin D	FGF23
Intestine	Increased calcium and phosphate absorption (by increased 1,25[OH]$_2$D production)	Increased calcium and phosphate absorption by 1,25(OH)$_2$D	Decreased calcium and phosphate absorption by decreased 1,25(OH)$_2$ production
Kidney	Decreased calcium excretion, increased phosphate excretion, stimulation of 1,25(OH)$_2$D production	Calcium and phosphate excretion may be decreased by 25(OH)D and 1,25(OH)$_2$D[1]	Increased phosphate excretion, decreased 1,25(OH)$_2$D production
Bone	Calcium and phosphate resorption increased by high doses. Low doses increase bone formation.	Increased calcium and phosphate resorption by 1,25(OH)$_2$D; bone formation may be increased by 1,25(OH)$_2$D	Decreased mineralization due to hypophosphatemia and low 1,25(OH)$_2$D levels
Net effect on serum levels	Serum calcium increased, serum phosphate decreased	Serum calcium and phosphate both increased	Decreased serum phosphate

[1]Direct effect. Vitamin D also indirectly increases urine calcium owing to increased calcium absorption from the intestine and decreased PTH.

secretion directly and indirectly. Its indirect actions are the result of forming complexes with calcium in the serum. Because it is the ionized free concentration of extracellular calcium that is detected by the parathyroid gland, increases in serum phosphate levels reduce the ionized calcium levels, leading to enhanced PTH secretion. Whether the parathyroid gland expresses phosphate receptors that mediate the direct action of phosphate on PTH secretion remains unclear. Such feedback regulation is appropriate to the net effect of PTH to raise serum calcium and reduce serum phosphate levels. Likewise, both calcium and phosphate at high levels reduce the amount of 1,25(OH)$_2$D produced by the kidney and increase the amount of 24,25(OH)$_2$D produced.

High serum calcium works directly and indirectly by reducing PTH secretion. High serum phosphate works directly and indirectly by increasing FGF23 levels. Since 1,25(OH)$_2$D raises serum calcium and phosphate, whereas 24,25(OH)$_2$D has less effect, such feedback regulation is again appropriate. 1,25(OH)$_2$D directly inhibits PTH secretion (independent of its effect on serum calcium) by a direct inhibitory effect on PTH gene transcription. The parathyroid gland expresses both the VDR and CYP27B1, so that endogenous production of 1,25(OH)$_2$D within the parathyroid gland may be more important for the regulation of PTH secretion than serum levels of 1,25(OH)$_2$D. This provides yet another negative feedback loop. In patients with chronic renal failure who frequently are deficient in producing 1,25(OH)$_2$D due in part to elevated FGF23 levels, loss of this 1,25(OH)$_2$D-mediated feedback loop coupled with impaired phosphate excretion and intestinal calcium absorption leads to secondary hyperparathyroidism. The ability of 1,25(OH)$_2$D to inhibit PTH secretion directly is being exploited with calcitriol analogs that have less effect on serum calcium because of their lesser effect on intestinal calcium absorption. Such drugs are proving useful in the management of secondary hyperparathyroidism accompanying chronic kidney disease and may be useful in selected cases of primary hyperparathyroidism. 1,25(OH)$_2$D also stimulates the production of FGF23. This completes the negative feedback loop in that FGF23 inhibits 1,25(OH)$_2$D production while promoting hypophosphatemia, which in turn inhibits FGF23 production and stimulates 1,25(OH)$_2$D production. However, the rise in FGF23 in the early stages of renal failure remains unexplained and is not due to increases in either 1,25OH)$_2$D or phosphate, and appears not to be under the same feedback control as operates under normal physiologic conditions. The interaction between FGF23 and PTH is less clear. FGF23 has been found to suppress PTH secretion, although it appears to enhance PTH actions on the kidney, at least with respect to phosphate excretion. PTH, on the other hand, has been reported to promote FGF23 production in bone.

SECONDARY HORMONAL REGULATORS OF BONE MINERAL HOMEOSTASIS

A number of hormones modulate the actions of PTH, FGF23, and vitamin D in regulating bone mineral homeostasis. Compared with that of PTH, FGF23, and vitamin D, the physiologic impact of such secondary regulation on bone mineral homeostasis is minor. However, in pharmacologic amounts, several of these hormones, including calcitonin, glucocorticoids, and estrogens, have actions on bone mineral homeostatic mechanisms that can be exploited therapeutically.

CALCITONIN

The calcitonin secreted by the parafollicular cells of the mammalian thyroid is a single-chain peptide hormone with 32 amino acids and a molecular weight of 3600. A disulfide bond between positions 1 and 7 is essential for biologic activity. Calcitonin is produced from a precursor with a molecular weight of 15,000. The circulating forms of calcitonin are multiple, ranging in size from the monomer (molecular weight 3600) to forms with an apparent molecular weight of 60,000. Whether such heterogeneity includes precursor forms or covalently linked oligomers is not known. Because of its chemical heterogeneity, calcitonin preparations are standardized by bioassay in rats. Activity is compared to a standard maintained by the British Medical Research Council (MRC) and expressed as MRC units.

Human calcitonin monomer has a half-life of about 10 minutes. Salmon calcitonin has a longer half-life of 40–50 minutes, making it more attractive as a therapeutic agent. Much of the clearance occurs in the kidney by metabolism; little intact calcitonin appears in the urine.

The principal effects of calcitonin are to lower serum calcium and phosphate by actions on bone and kidney. Calcitonin inhibits osteoclastic bone resorption. Although bone formation is not impaired at first after calcitonin administration, with time both formation and resorption of bone are reduced. In the kidney, calcitonin reduces both calcium and phosphate reabsorption as well as reabsorption of other ions, including sodium, potassium, and magnesium. Tissues other than bone and kidney are also affected by calcitonin. Calcitonin in pharmacologic amounts decreases gastrin secretion and reduces gastric acid output while increasing secretion of sodium, potassium, chloride, and water in the gut. Pentagastrin is a potent stimulator of calcitonin secretion (as is hypercalcemia), suggesting a possible physiologic relationship between gastrin and calcitonin. In the adult human, no readily demonstrable problem develops in cases of calcitonin deficiency (thyroidectomy) or excess (medullary carcinoma of the thyroid). However, the ability of calcitonin to block bone resorption and lower serum calcium makes it a useful drug for the treatment of Paget disease, hypercalcemia, and osteoporosis, albeit a less efficacious drug than other available agents such as the bisphosphonates.

GLUCOCORTICOIDS

Glucocorticoid hormones alter bone mineral homeostasis by antagonizing vitamin D-stimulated intestinal calcium transport, stimulating renal calcium excretion, blocking bone formation, and at least initially stimulating bone resorption. Although these observations underscore the negative impact of glucocorticoids on bone mineral homeostasis, these hormones have proved useful in reversing the hypercalcemia associated with lymphomas and granulomatous diseases such as sarcoidosis in which unregulated ectopic production of $1,25[OH]_2D$ occurs or in cases of vitamin D intoxication. Prolonged administration of glucocorticoids is a common cause of osteoporosis in adults and can cause stunted skeletal development in children (see Chapter 39).

ESTROGENS

Estrogens can prevent accelerated bone loss during the immediate postmenopausal period and at least transiently increase bone in postmenopausal women.

The prevailing hypothesis advanced to explain these observations is that estrogens reduce the bone-resorbing action of PTH. Estrogen administration leads to an increased $1,25(OH)_2D$ level in blood, but estrogens have no direct effect on $1,25(OH)_2D$ production in vitro. The increased $1,25(OH)_2D$ levels in vivo following estrogen treatment may result from decreased serum calcium and phosphate and increased PTH. However, estrogens also increase DBP production by the liver, which increases the total concentrations of the vitamin D metabolites in circulation without necessarily increasing the free levels. Estrogen receptors have been found in bone, and estrogen has direct effects on bone remodeling. Case reports of men who lack the estrogen receptor or who are unable to produce estrogen because of aromatase deficiency noted marked osteopenia and failure to close epiphyses. This further substantiates the role of estrogen in bone development, even in men. The principal therapeutic application for estrogen administration in disorders of bone mineral homeostasis is the treatment or prevention of postmenopausal osteoporosis. However, long-term use of estrogen has fallen out of favor due to concern about adverse effects. Selective estrogen receptor modulators (SERMs) have been developed to retain the beneficial effects on bone while minimizing deleterious effects on breast, uterus, and the cardiovascular system (see Box: Therapies for Osteoporosis and Chapter 40).

Therapies for Osteoporosis

Bone undergoes a continuous remodeling process involving resorption and formation. Any process that disrupts this balance by increasing bone resorption relative to formation results in osteoporosis. Inadequate gonadal hormone production is a major cause of osteoporosis in men and women. Estrogen replacement therapy at menopause is a well-established means of preventing osteoporosis in the female, but many women fear its adverse effects, particularly the increased risk of breast cancer from continued estrogen use (the well-demonstrated increased risk of endometrial cancer is prevented by combining the estrogen with a progestin) and do not like the persistence of menstrual bleeding that often accompanies this form of therapy. Medical enthusiasm for this treatment has waned with the demonstration that it does not protect against and may increase the risk of heart disease. Raloxifene was the first of the selective estrogen receptor modulators (SERMs; see Chapter 40) to be approved for the prevention of osteoporosis. Raloxifene shares some of the beneficial effects of estrogen on bone without increasing the risk of breast or endometrial cancer (it may actually reduce the risk of breast cancer). Although not as effective as estrogen in increasing bone density, raloxifene has been shown to reduce vertebral fractures.

Nonhormonal forms of therapy for osteoporosis have been developed with proven efficacy in reducing fracture risk. Bisphosphonates such as alendronate, risedronate, ibandronate, and zoledronate have been conclusively shown to increase bone density and reduce fractures over at least 5 years when used continuously at a dosage of 10 mg/d or 70 mg/week for alendronate; 5 mg/d or 35 mg/week for risedronate; 2.5 mg/d or 150 mg/month for ibandronate; and 5 mg annually for intravenous zoledronate.

Side-by-side trials between alendronate and calcitonin (another approved nonestrogen drug for osteoporosis) indicated a greater efficacy of alendronate. Bisphosphonates are poorly absorbed and must be given on an empty stomach or infused intravenously. At the higher oral doses used in the treatment of Paget disease, alendronate causes gastric irritation, but this is not a significant problem at the doses recommended for osteoporosis when patients are instructed to take the drug with a glass of water and remain upright. Denosumab is a human monoclonal antibody directed against RANKL, and it is very effective in inhibiting osteoclastogenesis and activity. Denosumab is given in 60-mg doses subcutaneously every 6 months. Unlike the bisphosphonates, when denosumab treatment is discontinued there is often a surge of bone resorption that is only partially prevented with antiresorptive agents like zoledronate. However, recent trials indicate that denosumab treatment continues to increase bone mineral density up to 10 years, unlike the plateau seen with bisphosphonates after a couple of years. All of these drugs inhibit bone resorption with secondary effects to inhibit bone formation. On the other hand, teriparatide, the recombinant form of PTH 1-34 and abaloparatide, an analog of PTHrP, directly stimulate bone formation as well as bone resorption. However, teriparatide and abaloparatide are given daily by subcutaneous injection. Their efficacy in preventing fractures is at least as great as that of the bisphosphonates. More recently, antibodies to sclerostin, an inhibitor of bone formation that is produced in osteocytes, have been developed. **Romosozumab** is now approved for the treatment of osteoporosis. Romosozumab is injected monthly subcutaneously in 210-mg doses for one year. No renal adjustment is required. However, it carries a black box warning indicating it should not be used in patients with risks of stroke or coronary vascular disease. It is important that following the one year treatment patients are started on an antiresorptive to maintain the bone that was gained. In all cases, adequate intake of calcium and vitamin D needs to be maintained.

Furthermore, there are several other forms of therapy used in other countries but not available in the United States. In Europe, **strontium ranelate,** a drug that appears to stimulate bone formation and inhibit bone resorption, has been used for several years with favorable results in large clinical trials. However, approval for its use in the United States has not been achieved. In Japan, **eldecalcitol,** an analog of $1,25(OH)_2D$, has been approved for the treatment of osteoporosis with minimal effects on serum calcium. It is not yet available in the United States.

NONHORMONAL AGENTS AFFECTING BONE MINERAL HOMEOSTASIS

BISPHOSPHONATES

The bisphosphonates are analogs of pyrophosphate in which the P-O-P bond has been replaced with a nonhydrolyzable P-C-P bond (Figure 42–4). Currently available bisphosphonates include **etidronate, pamidronate, alendronate, risedronate, tiludronate, ibandronate,** and **zoledronate.** With the development of the more potent bisphosphonates, etidronate is seldom used.

Results from animal and clinical studies indicate that less than 10% of an oral dose of these drugs is absorbed. Food reduces absorption even further, necessitating their administration on an empty stomach. A major adverse effect of oral forms of the bisphosphonates (risedronate, alendronate, ibandronate) is esophageal and gastric irritation, which limits the use of this route by patients with upper gastrointestinal disorders. This complication can be circumvented with infusions of pamidronate, zoledronate, and ibandronate. Intravenous dosing also allows a larger amount of drug to enter the body and markedly reduces the frequency of administration (eg, zoledronate is infused once per year). Nearly half of the absorbed drug accumulates in bone; the remainder is excreted unchanged in the urine. Decreased renal function dictates a reduction in dosage. The portion of drug retained in bone depends on the rate of bone turnover; drug in bone often is retained for months to years.

The bisphosphonates exert multiple effects on bone mineral homeostasis, which make them useful for the treatment of hypercalcemia associated with malignancy, for Paget disease, and for osteoporosis (see Box: Therapies for Osteoporosis). They owe at

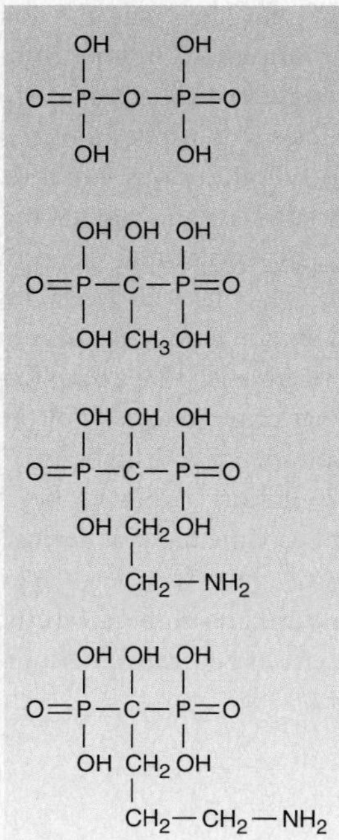

Inorganic pyrophosphoric acid

Etidronate: ethane-1-hydroxy-1, 1-bisphosphonate

Pamidronate: 3-Amino-1-hydroxy-propylidene bisphosphonate

Alendronate: 4-Amino-1-hydroxy-butylidene bisphosphonate

FIGURE 42–4 The structure of pyrophosphate and of the first three bisphosphonates—etidronate, pamidronate, and alendronate—that were approved for use in the United States.

least part of their clinical usefulness and toxicity to their ability to retard formation and dissolution of hydroxyapatite crystals within and outside the skeletal system as well as inhibiting osteoclast activity. Some of the newer bisphosphonates appear to increase bone mineral density well beyond the 2-year period predicted for a drug whose effects are limited to slowing bone resorption. This may be due to their other cellular effects, which include inhibition of 1,25$(OH)_2D$ production, inhibition of intestinal calcium transport, metabolic changes in bone cells such as inhibition of glycolysis, inhibition of cell growth, and changes in acid and alkaline phosphatase activity.

Amino bisphosphonates such as alendronate and risedronate inhibit farnesyl pyrophosphate synthase, an enzyme in the mevalonate pathway that appears to be critical for osteoclast survival. The cholesterol-lowering statin drugs (eg, lovastatin), which block mevalonate synthesis (see Chapter 35), stimulate bone formation, at least in animal studies. Thus, the mevalonate pathway appears to be important in bone cell function and provides new targets for drug development. The mevalonate pathway effects vary depending on the bisphosphonate used (only amino bisphosphonates have this property) and may account for some of the clinical differences observed in the effects of the various bisphosphonates on bone mineral homeostasis.

With the exception of the induction of a mineralization defect by higher than approved doses of etidronate and gastric and esophageal irritation by the oral bisphosphonates, these drugs have proved to be remarkably free of adverse effects when used at the doses recommended for the treatment of osteoporosis. Esophageal irritation can be minimized by taking the drug with a full glass of water and remaining upright for 30 minutes or by using the intravenous forms of these compounds. The initial infusion of zoledronate is commonly associated with several days of a flu-like syndrome that generally does not recur with subsequent infusions. Of other complications, osteonecrosis of the jaw has received considerable attention but is rare in patients receiving usual doses of bisphosphonates (perhaps 1/100,000 patient-years). This complication is more frequent when high intravenous doses of zoledronate are used to control bone metastases and cancer-induced hypercalcemia. Concern has also been raised about over-suppressing bone turnover. This may underlie the occurrence of subtrochanteric femur fractures in patients on long-term bisphosphonate treatment. This complication appears to be rare, comparable to that of osteonecrosis of the jaw, but has led some authorities to recommend a "drug holiday" after 5 years of treatment if the clinical condition warrants it (ie, if the fracture risk of discontinuing the bisphosphonate is not deemed high). Impetus to reevaluate the results of antiresorptive therapy after 5 years of treatment (3 years for zoledronate) comes from the observation that these relatively rare side effects become more common as treatment extends beyond 5 years.

DENOSUMAB

Denosumab is a fully humanized monoclonal antibody that binds to and prevents the action of RANKL. As described earlier, RANKL is produced by osteoblasts and other cells, including T lymphocytes. It stimulates osteoclastogenesis via RANK, the receptor for RANKL that is present on osteoclasts and osteoclast precursors. By interfering with RANKL function, denosumab inhibits osteoclast formation and activity. It is at least as effective as the potent bisphosphonates in inhibiting bone resorption and has been approved for treatment of postmenopausal osteoporosis and some cancers (prostate and breast). The latter application is to limit the development of bone metastases or bone loss resulting from the use of drugs that suppress gonadal function. Denosumab is administered subcutaneously every 6 months. The drug appears to be well tolerated, but four concerns remain. First, a number of cells in the immune system also express RANKL, suggesting that there could be an increased risk of infection associated with the use of denosumab. Second, because the suppression of bone turnover with denosumab is similar to that of the potent bisphosphonates, the potential risk of osteonecrosis of the jaw and subtrochanteric fractures is comparable. Third, denosumab can lead to transient hypocalcemia, especially in patients with marked bone loss (and bone hunger) or compromised calcium regulatory mechanisms, including chronic kidney disease and vitamin D deficiency. That said, denosumab can be used in patients with advanced renal disease, unlike the bisphosphonates, as it is not cleared by the kidney, and it has the advantage over bisphosphonates in that it is readily reversible because it does not deposit in bone. However, when used in patients with renal failure, careful attention to serum calcium levels is necessary. Fourth, denosumab does not result in the death of osteoclasts, unlike the bisphosphonates, so that if denosumab therapy is interrupted a surge of bone resorption can occur putting the patient at risk for new fractures. Efforts to prevent this surge of bone resorption with potent antiresorptives like zoledronate are only partially effective.

SCLEROSTIN ANTIBODIES

Sclerostin is a protein produced by osteocytes that blocks the action of the wnt receptor in osteoblasts. The wnt receptor when activated by selected wnts promotes beta-catenin signaling increasing the proliferation of osteoblasts. Sclerostin blocks wnt activation, suppressing bone formation. Antibodies to sclerostin have been developed, of which only **romosozumab** has been FDA approved for the treatment of osteoporosis. This form of therapy promotes bone formation and inhibits bone resorption, although the mechanism for its effects on osteoclasts is not well understood. The use of romosozumab is limited to one year after which it is recommended that patients be switched to an antiresorptive to prevent loss of the bone gained. In some of the trials with this drug there appeared to be an increased risk of myocardial infarction (MI), stroke, and cardiovascular death, thus generating a black box warning contraindicating its use in patients with a previous MI or stroke within the past year.

CALCIMIMETICS

Cinacalcet is the first representative of a new class of drugs that activates the calcium-sensing receptor (CaSR) described above. **Etelcalcetide** is a more recently approved and somewhat more potent calcimimetic that currently is approved only for secondary hyperparathyroidism in CKD patients on dialysis. CaSR is widely distributed but has its greatest concentration in the parathyroid gland. By activating the parathyroid gland CaSR, these drugs inhibit PTH secretion. These drugs are approved for the treatment of secondary hyperparathyroidism in chronic kidney disease (CKD), and cinacalcet is also approved for the treatment of parathyroid carcinoma and severe primary hyperparathyroidism. In CKD patients requiring dialysis, hypocalcemia can occur with the use of these drugs, and nausea is often a limiting factor. CaSR antagonists are also being developed and may be useful in conditions of hypoparathyroidism or as a means to stimulate intermittent PTH secretion in the treatment of osteoporosis.

THIAZIDE DIURETICS

The chemistry and pharmacology of the thiazide family of drugs are discussed in Chapter 15. The principal application of thiazides in the treatment of bone mineral disorders is in reducing renal calcium excretion. Thiazides may increase the effectiveness of PTH in stimulating reabsorption of calcium by the renal tubules or may act on calcium reabsorption secondarily by increasing sodium reabsorption in the proximal tubule. In the distal tubule, thiazides block sodium reabsorption at the luminal surface, increasing the calcium-sodium exchange at the basolateral membrane and thus enhancing calcium reabsorption into the blood at this site (see Figure 15–4). Thiazides have proved to be useful in reducing the hypercalciuria and incidence of urinary stone formation in subjects with idiopathic hypercalciuria. Part of their efficacy in reducing stone formation may lie in their ability to decrease urine oxalate excretion and increase urine magnesium and zinc levels, both of which inhibit calcium oxalate stone formation. By reducing urine calcium losses, these drugs may also support treatment of osteoporosis.

FLUORIDE

Fluoride is well established as effective for the prophylaxis of dental caries and has previously been investigated for the treatment of osteoporosis. Both therapeutic applications originated from epidemiologic observations that subjects living in areas with naturally fluoridated water (1–2 ppm) had fewer dental caries and fewer vertebral compression fractures than subjects living in nonfluoridated water areas. Fluoride accumulates in bones and teeth, where it may stabilize the hydroxyapatite crystal. Such a mechanism may explain the effectiveness of fluoride in increasing the resistance of teeth to dental caries, but it does not explain its ability to promote new bone growth.

Fluoride in drinking water appears to be most effective in preventing dental caries if consumed before the eruption of the permanent teeth. The optimum concentration in drinking water supplies is 0.5–1 ppm. Topical application is most effective if done just as the teeth erupt. There is little further benefit to giving fluoride after the permanent teeth are fully formed. Excess fluoride in drinking water leads to mottling of the enamel proportionate to the concentration above 1 ppm.

Fluoride has also been evaluated for the treatment of osteoporosis. Results of earlier studies indicated that fluoride alone, without adequate calcium supplementation, produced osteomalacia. Subsequent studies in which calcium supplementation has been adequate demonstrated an improvement in calcium balance, an increase in bone mineral, and an increase in trabecular bone volume. Despite these promising effects of fluoride on bone mass, clinical studies have failed to demonstrate a reliable reduction in fractures, and some studies showed an increase in fracture rate. At present, fluoride is not approved by the US. Food and Drug Administration (FDA) for treatment or prevention of osteoporosis, and it is unlikely to be.

Adverse effects observed—at the higher doses used for testing fluoride's effect on bone—include nausea and vomiting, gastrointestinal blood loss, arthralgias, and arthritis in a substantial proportion of patients. Such effects are usually responsive to reduction of the dose or giving fluoride with meals (or both).

STRONTIUM RANELATE

Strontium ranelate is composed of two atoms of strontium bound to an organic ion, ranelic acid. Although not approved for use in the United States, this drug is used in Europe for the treatment of osteoporosis. Strontium ranelate appears to block differentiation of osteoclasts while promoting their apoptosis, thus inhibiting bone resorption. At the same time, strontium ranelate appears to promote bone formation. Unlike bisphosphonates, denosumab, or teriparatide, but similar to romosozumab, strontium ranelate increases bone formation markers while inhibiting bone resorption markers. Large clinical trials have demonstrated its efficacy in increasing bone mineral density and decreasing fractures in the spine and hip. Toxicities reported thus far are similar to placebo.

■ CLINICAL PHARMACOLOGY

Individuals with disorders of bone mineral homeostasis usually present with abnormalities in serum or urine calcium levels (or both), often accompanied by abnormal serum phosphate levels. These abnormal mineral concentrations may themselves cause symptoms requiring immediate treatment (eg, coma in malignant hypercalcemia, tetany in hypocalcemia). More commonly, they serve as clues to an underlying disorder in hormonal regulators (eg, primary hyperparathyroidism, vitamin D deficiency), target tissue response (eg, chronic kidney disease), or drug misuse (eg, vitamin D intoxication). In such cases, treatment of the underlying disorder is of prime importance.

Since bone, intestine, and kidney play central roles in bone mineral homeostasis, conditions that alter bone mineral homeostasis usually affect one or more of these tissues secondarily. Effects on bone can result in osteoporosis (abnormal loss of bone; remaining bone histologically normal), osteomalacia (abnormal bone formation due to inadequate mineralization), or osteitis fibrosa (excessive bone resorption with fibrotic replacement of resorption cavities and marrow). Biochemical markers of skeletal involvement include changes in serum levels of the skeletal isoenzyme of alkaline phosphatase, osteocalcin, and N- and C-terminal propeptides of type I collagen (reflecting osteoblastic activity), and serum and urine levels of tartrate-resistant acid phosphatase and collagen breakdown products (reflecting osteoclastic activity). The kidney becomes involved when the calcium × phosphate product in serum rises above the point at which ectopic calcification occurs (nephrocalcinosis) or when the calcium × oxalate (or phosphate) product in urine exceeds saturation, leading to nephrolithiasis. Subtle early indicators of such renal involvement include polyuria, nocturia, and hyposthenuria. Radiologic evidence of nephrocalcinosis and stones is not generally observed until later. The degree of the ensuing renal failure is best followed by monitoring the decline in creatinine clearance. On the other hand, chronic kidney disease can be a primary cause of bone disease because of altered handling of calcium and phosphate, decreased $1,25(OH)_2D$ production, increased FGF23 levels, and secondary hyperparathyroidism. As the intestine is the source of calcium and phosphate as well as dietary vitamin D for the body, numerous intestinal diseases and surgical procedures lead to their malabsorption, secondarily leading to skeletal disease such as osteoporosis and osteomalacia.

ABNORMAL SERUM CALCIUM & PHOSPHATE LEVELS

HYPERCALCEMIA

Hypercalcemia causes central nervous system depression, including coma, and is potentially lethal. Its major causes (other than thiazide therapy) are hyperparathyroidism and cancer, with or without bone metastases. Less common causes are hypervitaminosis D, sarcoidosis, thyrotoxicosis, milk-alkali syndrome, adrenal insufficiency, and immobilization. With the possible exception of hypervitaminosis D, the latter disorders seldom require emergency lowering of serum calcium. A number of approaches are used to manage the hypercalcemic crisis.

Saline Diuresis

In hypercalcemia of sufficient severity to produce symptoms, rapid reduction of serum calcium is required. The first steps include rehydration with saline and diuresis with furosemide, although the efficacy of furosemide in this setting has not been proved. Most patients presenting with severe hypercalcemia have a substantial component of prerenal azotemia owing to dehydration, which prevents the kidney from compensating for the rise in serum calcium by excreting more calcium in the urine. Therefore, the initial infusion of 500–1000 mL/h of saline to reverse the dehydration and restore urine flow can by itself substantially lower serum calcium. The addition of a loop diuretic such as furosemide following rehydration enhances urine flow and also inhibits calcium reabsorption in the ascending limb of the loop of Henle (see Chapter 15). Monitoring of central venous pressure is important to forestall the development of heart failure and pulmonary edema in predisposed subjects. In many subjects, saline diuresis suffices to reduce serum calcium to a point at which more definitive diagnosis and treatment of the underlying condition can be achieved. If this is not the case or if more prolonged medical treatment of hypercalcemia is required, the following agents are available (discussed in order of preference).

Bisphosphonates

Pamidronate, 60–90 mg, infused over 2–4 hours, and **zoledronate,** 4 mg, infused over at least 15 minutes, have been approved for the treatment of hypercalcemia of malignancy and have replaced the less effective etidronate for this indication. The bisphosphonate effects generally persist for weeks, but treatment can be repeated after a 7-day interval if necessary and if renal function is not impaired. Some patients experience a self-limited flu-like syndrome after the initial infusion, but subsequent infusions generally do not have this adverse effect. Repeated doses of these drugs have been linked to renal deterioration, atypical subtrochanteric fractures of the femur, and osteonecrosis of the jaw, but these adverse effects are rare.

Calcitonin

Calcitonin has proved useful as ancillary treatment in some patients. Calcitonin by itself seldom restores serum calcium to normal, and refractoriness frequently develops. However, its lack of toxicity permits frequent administration at high doses (200 MRC units or more). An effect on serum calcium is observed within 4–6 hours and lasts for 6–10 hours. **Calcimar** (salmon calcitonin) is available for parenteral and nasal administration.

Gallium Nitrate

Gallium nitrate is approved by the FDA for the management of hypercalcemia of malignancy. This drug inhibits bone resorption. At a dosage of 200 mg/m^2 body surface area per day given as a continuous intravenous infusion in 5% dextrose for 5 days, gallium nitrate proved superior to calcitonin in reducing serum calcium in cancer patients. Because of potential nephrotoxicity, patients should be well hydrated and have good renal output before starting the infusion. However, because of its toxicity it is seldom used, especially as better and safer means of reducing calcium levels are available.

Phosphate

Intravenous phosphate administration is probably the fastest and surest way to reduce serum calcium, but it is a hazardous procedure if not done properly. Intravenous phosphate should be used only after other methods of treatment (bisphosphonates, calcitonin, and saline diuresis) have failed to control symptomatic hypercalcemia. Phosphate must be given slowly (50 mmol or 1.5 g elemental phosphorus over 6–8 hours) and the patient switched to oral phosphate (1–2 g/d elemental phosphorus, as one of the salts indicated below) as soon as symptoms of hypercalcemia have cleared. The risks of intravenous phosphate therapy include sudden hypocalcemia, ectopic calcification, acute renal failure, and hypotension. Oral phosphate can also lead to ectopic calcification and renal failure if serum calcium and phosphate levels are not carefully monitored, but the risk is less and the time of onset much longer. Phosphate is available in oral and intravenous forms as sodium or potassium salts. Amounts required to provide 1 g of elemental phosphorus are as follows:

Intravenous:
In-Phos, 40 mL; or Hyper-Phos-K, 15 mL

Oral:
Fleet Phospho-Soda, 6.2 mL; or Neutra-Phos, 300 mL; or K-Phos-Neutral, 4 tablets

Glucocorticoids

Glucocorticoids have no clear role in the immediate treatment of hypercalcemia. However, the chronic hypercalcemia of sarcoidosis, vitamin D intoxication, and certain cancers may respond within several days to glucocorticoid therapy. Prednisone in oral doses of 30–60 mg daily is generally used, although equivalent doses of other glucocorticoids are effective. The rationale for the use of glucocorticoids in these diseases differs, however. The hypercalcemia of sarcoidosis and other granulomatous diseases is secondary to increased production of $1,25(OH)_2D$ by the abnormal tissue itself. Glucocorticoid therapy directed at the reduction of the granulomatous tissue results in restoration of normal serum calcium and $1,25(OH)_2D$ levels. The treatment of hypervitaminosis D with glucocorticoids probably does not alter vitamin D metabolism significantly but is thought to reduce vitamin D–mediated intestinal calcium transport and increase renal excretion of calcium. An action of glucocorticoids to reduce vitamin D–mediated bone resorption has not been excluded, however. The effect of glucocorticoids on the hypercalcemia of cancer is probably twofold. The malignancies responding best to glucocorticoids (ie, multiple myeloma and related lymphoproliferative diseases) are sensitive to the lytic action of glucocorticoids. Therefore, part of the effect may be related to decreased tumor mass and activity. Glucocorticoids have also been shown to inhibit the secretion or effectiveness of cytokines elaborated by multiple myeloma and related cancers that stimulate osteoclastic bone resorption. Other causes of hypercalcemia—particularly primary hyperparathyroidism—do not respond to glucocorticoid therapy.

HYPOCALCEMIA

The main features of hypocalcemia are neuromuscular: tetany, paresthesias, laryngospasm, muscle cramps, and seizures. The major causes of hypocalcemia in the adult are hypoparathyroidism, vitamin D deficiency, chronic kidney disease, and malabsorption. Magnesium deficiency is another important cause of hypocalcemia because of its inhibitory impact on both PTH secretion and tissue response. Acute magnesium deficiency can follow binge drinking in alcoholics. Hypocalcemia can also accompany the infusion of potent bisphosphonates and denosumab for the treatment of osteoporosis, but this is seldom of clinical significance unless the patient is already hypocalcemic at the onset of the infusion or has a disease such as chronic kidney failure that prevents normal regulation of calcium homeostasis. Neonatal hypocalcemia is a common disorder that usually resolves without therapy. The roles of PTH, vitamin D, and calcitonin in the neonatal syndrome are under investigation. Large infusions of citrated blood can produce hypocalcemia secondary to the formation of citrate-calcium complexes. Calcium and vitamin D (or its metabolites) form the mainstay of treatment of hypocalcemia. However, in patients with hypoparathyroidism, teriparatide or Natpara may prove useful (only Natpara has been FDA approved for this condition).

Calcium

A number of calcium preparations are available for intravenous, intramuscular, and oral use. Calcium gluceptate (0.9 mEq calcium/mL), calcium gluconate (0.45 mEq calcium/mL), and calcium chloride (0.68–1.36 mEq calcium/mL) are available for intravenous therapy. Calcium gluconate is preferred because it is less irritating to veins. Oral preparations include calcium carbonate (40% calcium), calcium lactate (13% calcium), calcium phosphate (25% calcium), and calcium citrate (21% calcium). Calcium carbonate is often the preparation of choice because of its high percentage of calcium, ready availability (eg, Tums), low cost, and antacid properties. In achlorhydric patients, calcium carbonate should be given with meals to increase absorption, or the patient should be switched to calcium citrate, which is somewhat better absorbed. Combinations of vitamin D and calcium are available, but treatment must be tailored to the individual patient and the individual disease, a flexibility lost by fixed-dosage combinations.

Treatment of severe symptomatic hypocalcemia can be accomplished with slow infusion of 5–20 mL of 10% calcium gluconate. Rapid infusion can lead to cardiac arrhythmias. Less severe hypocalcemia is best treated with oral forms sufficient to provide approximately 1000–1500 mg of elemental calcium per day. Dosage must be adjusted to avoid hypercalcemia and hypercalciuria.

Vitamin D

When rapidity of action is required, $1,25(OH)_2D_3$ (calcitriol), 0.25–1 mcg daily, is the vitamin D metabolite of choice because it is capable of raising serum calcium within 24–48 hours. Calcitriol also raises serum phosphate, although this action is usually not observed early in treatment. The combined effects of calcitriol and all other vitamin D metabolites and analogs on both calcium and phosphate make careful monitoring of these mineral levels especially important to prevent ectopic calcification secondary to an abnormally high serum calcium × phosphate product. Since the choice of the appropriate vitamin D metabolite or analog for long-term treatment of hypocalcemia depends on the nature of the underlying disease, further discussion of vitamin D treatment is found under the headings of the specific diseases.

HYPERPHOSPHATEMIA

Hyperphosphatemia is a common complication of renal failure and is also found in all types of hypoparathyroidism (idiopathic, surgical, and pseudohypoparathyroidism), vitamin D intoxication, and the rare syndrome of tumoral calcinosis (usually due to insufficient bioactive FGF23). Emergency treatment of hyperphosphatemia is seldom necessary but can be achieved by dialysis or glucose and insulin infusions. In general, control of hyperphosphatemia involves restriction of dietary phosphate plus phosphate-binding gels such as **sevelamer**, or **lanthanum carbonate** and calcium supplements. Because of their potential to induce aluminum-associated bone disease, aluminum-containing antacids should be used sparingly and only when other measures fail to control the hyperphosphatemia. In patients with chronic kidney disease, enthusiasm for the use of large doses of calcium to control hyperphosphatemia has waned because of the risk of ectopic calcification.

HYPOPHOSPHATEMIA

Hypophosphatemia is associated with a variety of conditions, including primary hyperparathyroidism, vitamin D deficiency, idiopathic hypercalciuria, conditions associated with increased bioactive FGF23 (eg, X-linked and autosomal dominant hypophosphatemic rickets and tumor-induced osteomalacia), other forms of renal phosphate wasting (eg, Fanconi syndrome), overzealous use of phosphate binders, and parenteral nutrition with inadequate phosphate content. Acute hypophosphatemia may cause a reduction in the intracellular levels of high-energy organic phosphates (eg, ATP), interfere with normal hemoglobin-to-tissue oxygen transfer by decreasing red cell 2,3-diphosphoglycerate levels, and lead to rhabdomyolysis. However, clinically significant acute effects of hypophosphatemia are seldom seen, and emergency treatment is generally not indicated. The long-term effects include proximal muscle weakness and abnormal bone mineralization (osteomalacia). Therefore, hypophosphatemia should be avoided when using forms of therapy that can lead to it (eg, phosphate binders, certain types of parenteral nutrition) and treated in conditions that cause it, such as the various forms of hypophosphatemic rickets. Oral forms of phosphate are listed above.

SPECIFIC DISORDERS INVOLVING BONE MINERAL–REGULATING HORMONES

PRIMARY HYPERPARATHYROIDISM

This rather common disease, if associated with symptoms, significant hypercalcemia, and hypercalciuria, osteoporosis, and kidney disease, is best treated surgically. Oral phosphate and bisphosphonates have been tried but cannot be recommended. That said, bisphosphonates can protect the bone, although they do not correct the hyperparathyroidism, hypercalcemia, or hypercalciuria. A substantial proportion of asymptomatic patients with mild disease do not get worse and may be followed without treatment, although a number of such patients do end up requiring surgery. The calcimimetic agents **cinacalcet** and **etelcalceteide,** discussed previously, have been approved for secondary hyperparathyroidism (both), parathyroid carcinoma (cinacalcet), and primary hyperparathyroidism (cinacalcet) in patients with severe hypercalcemia who are not surgical candidates. Cinacalcet is usually started at 30 mg given daily orally, a dose that can be increased to 90 mg as tolerated and necessary to bring the PTH and calcium levels into an acceptable range. Etelcalcetide is approved for dialysis patients and given IV at the time of dialysis in a range of 2.5–15 mg as tolerated and needed to control the secondary hyperparathyroidism. Primary hyperparathyroidism is often associated with low levels of 25(OH)D, suggesting that mild vitamin D deficiency may be contributing to the elevated PTH levels, although this could also be due to the stimulation by PTH of $1{,}25(OH)_2D$ production that in turn induces CYP24A1, which will increase 25(OH)D (and $1{,}25(OH)_2D$) catabolism. Vitamin D supplementation in such situations has proved safe with respect to further elevations of serum and urine calcium levels, but calcium should be monitored nevertheless when vitamin D supplementation is provided. Familial hypocalciuric hypercalcemia (FHH) is a condition that can be mistaken for primary hyperparathyroidism. This generally benign condition can present with mildly elevated PTH and calcium levels. However, urinary calcium excretion is low, with calcium/creatinine clearance ratio almost always below 0.02. However, this low level of calcium/creatinine clearance can overlap with similar findings in some patients with primary hyperparathyroidism making the distinction difficult when primary hyperparathyroidism is mild. A long-standing history of hypercalcemia and a family history of such are important clues to making the diagnosis of FHH. The key point is to avoid surgery on these individuals as the condition will not be corrected unless all parathyroid glands are removed, thus inducing hypoparathyroidism.

HYPOPARATHYROIDISM

In PTH deficiency (idiopathic or surgical hypoparathyroidism) or an abnormal target tissue response to PTH (pseudohypoparathyroidism), serum calcium falls and serum phosphate rises. In such patients, $1{,}25(OH)_2D$ levels are usually low, presumably reflecting the lack of stimulation by PTH of $1{,}25(OH)_2D$ production. The skeletons of patients with idiopathic or surgical hypoparathyroidism have normal bone mineral densities but with a slow turnover rate and poorer quality of bone that could increase fracture risk. A number of patients with pseudohypoparathyroidism appear to have osteitis fibrosa, suggesting that the normal or high PTH levels found in such patients are capable of acting on bone but not on the kidney. The distinction between pseudohypoparathyroidism and idiopathic hypoparathyroidism is made on the basis of normal or high PTH levels but deficient renal response (ie, diminished excretion of cAMP or phosphate) in patients with pseudohypoparathyroidism.

The principal therapeutic goal for patients with hypoparathyroidism is to restore normocalcemia and normophosphatemia. Standard therapy involves the use of calcitriol and dietary calcium supplements. However, many patients develop hypercalciuria with this regimen, which limits the ability to correct the hypocalcemia. Full-length PTH (rhPTH 1-84, **Natpara**) is approved for the treatment of hypoparathyroidism and reduces the need for large doses of calcium and calcitriol with less risk of hypercalciuria.

NUTRITIONAL VITAMIN D DEFICIENCY OR INSUFFICIENCY

The level of vitamin D thought to be necessary for good health is somewhat controversial. Vitamin D acts on a large number of cell types beyond those responsible for bone and mineral metabolism, but the optimal levels are uncertain for these nonskeletal tissues and remain controversial even for skeletal health, for which most data have been generated. A level of 25(OH)D above 12 ng/mL is necessary for preventing rickets or osteomalacia. However, substantial epidemiologic and some prospective trial data indicate that a higher level, such as 20–30 ng/mL, is required to optimize intestinal calcium absorption, optimize the accrual and maintenance of bone mass, reduce falls and fractures, and prevent a wide variety of diseases including diabetes mellitus, hyperparathyroidism, autoimmune diseases, and cancer. An expert panel for the National Academy of Medicine (NAM) has recommended that a level of 20 ng/mL (50 nM) was sufficient, although up to 50 ng/mL (125 nM) was considered safe. For individuals between the ages of 1 and 70 years, 600 IU/d vitamin D was thought to be sufficient to meet these goals, although up to 4000 IU was considered safe. These recommendations are based primarily on data from randomized placebo-controlled clinical trials (RCTs) that evaluated falls and fractures; data supporting the nonskeletal effects of vitamin D were considered too preliminary to be used in their recommendations because of lack of RCTs for these other actions. The lower end of these recommendations has been considered too low and the upper end too restrictive by a number of vitamin D experts, and the Endocrine Society has published a different set of recommendations suggesting that 30 ng/mL for 25(OH)D levels was a more appropriate lower limit. Since the initial NAM report a number of large RCTs have been completed, generally in subject populations with adequate vitamin D status (mean levels of 25(OH)D around 30 ng/mL). These studies indicate that individuals with sufficient vitamin D levels (ie, 25[OH]D levels around 30 ng/mL) do not further benefit from vitamin D supplementation with respect to lowering the risk of fractures or falls, cardiovascular disease, cancer, or diabetes mellitus at least over the time frame (5 years or less) of the study. Whether subjects with 25(OH)D levels below 20 ng/mL or studied for longer time frames will receive benefit seems plausible but has not been adequately documented by RCTs of sufficient size and duration. However, this subject remains controversial. The NAM guidelines—at least with respect to the lower recommended levels of vitamin D supplementation—are unlikely to correct vitamin D deficiency in individuals with obesity, dark complexions, limited capacity for sunlight exposure, or malabsorption. Vitamin D deficiency or insufficiency can be treated by higher dosages (either D_2 or D_3, 1000–4000 IU/d or 50,000 IU/week for several weeks). No other vitamin D metabolite is indicated, although extended release capsules with 30 mcg of calcifediol (25[OH]D) are available and appear to be at least as efficacious as vitamin D in restoring adequate 25(OH)D levels. Because the half-life of vitamin D_3 metabolites in blood is greater than that of vitamin D_2, there are advantages to using vitamin D_3 rather than vitamin D_2 supplements, although when administered on a daily or weekly schedule these differences may be moot. The diet should also contain adequate amounts of calcium as several studies indicate a synergism between calcium and vitamin D with respect to a number of their actions.

CHRONIC KIDNEY DISEASE

The major sequelae of chronic kidney disease (CKD) that impact bone mineral homeostasis are deficient $1,25(OH)_2D$ production, retention of phosphate with an associated reduction in ionized calcium levels, and the secondary hyperparathyroidism that results from the parathyroid gland response to lowered serum ionized calcium and low $1,25(OH)_2D$. FGF23 levels rise early in this disorder for unclear reasons, and this can further reduce $1,25(OH)_2D$ production by the kidney. Moreover, the increase in FGF23 is associated with increased morbidity and mortality in CKD in part due to its impact on the heart. Antibodies to FGF23 in the early stages of renal failure result in normalization of $1,25(OH)_2D$ levels, but inhibition of FGF23 may further the rise in serum phosphate with the potential for increased vascular calcification, a major issue in CKD, and are not approved for this disease. With impaired $1,25(OH)_2D$ production, less calcium is absorbed from the intestine, and less bone is resorbed under the influence of PTH. As a result hypocalcemia usually develops, furthering the development of secondary hyperparathyroidism. The bones show a mixture of osteomalacia and osteitis fibrosa.

In contrast to the hypocalcemia that is more often associated with chronic kidney disease, some patients may become hypercalcemic from overzealous treatment with calcium. However, the most common cause of hypercalcemia is the development of severe secondary (sometimes referred to as tertiary) hyperparathyroidism. In such cases, the PTH level in blood is very high. Serum alkaline phosphatase levels also tend to be high. Treatment often requires parathyroidectomy. A less common circumstance leading to hypercalcemia is development of a form of bone disease characterized by a profound decrease in bone cell activity and loss of the calcium buffering action of bone (adynamic bone disease). In the absence of kidney function, any calcium absorbed from the intestine accumulates in the blood. Such patients are very sensitive to the hypercalcemic action of $1,25(OH)_2D$. These individuals generally have a high serum calcium but nearly normal alkaline phosphatase and PTH levels. The bone in such patients may have a high aluminum content, especially in the mineralization front, which blocks normal bone mineralization, although with the use of deionized water during dialysis this complication has nearly vanished. Nevertheless, adynamic bone remains a problem. These patients do not respond favorably to parathyroidectomy. Deferoxamine, an agent used to chelate iron (see Chapter 57), also binds aluminum and is being used to treat this disorder in patients with presumed aluminum or iron overload. However, with the reduction in use of aluminum-containing phosphate binders and use of deionized water during dialysis, most cases of adynamic bone disease are not associated with aluminum deposition but are attributed in some cases to overzealous suppression of PTH secretion.

Vitamin D Preparations

The choice of vitamin D preparation to be used in the setting of chronic kidney disease depends on the type and extent of bone disease and hyperparathyroidism. Individuals with vitamin D deficiency or insufficiency should first have their 25(OH)D levels restored to normal (20–30 ng/mL) with vitamin D. Calcifediol or $1,25(OH)_2D_3$ **(calcitriol)** rapidly corrects hypocalcemia and at least partially reverses secondary hyperparathyroidism and osteitis fibrosa. Many patients with muscle weakness and bone pain gain an improved sense of well-being.

Two analogs of calcitriol—**doxercalciferol** and **paricalcitol**—are approved in the United States for the treatment of secondary hyperparathyroidism of chronic kidney disease. (In Japan, maxacalcitol [22-oxa-calcitriol] and falecalcitriol [26,27 F_6-$1,25(OH)_2D_3$] are approved for this purpose.) Their principal advantage is that they are less likely than calcitriol to induce hypercalcemia for any given reduction in PTH (less true for falecalcitriol). Their greatest impact is in patients in whom the use of calcitriol may lead to unacceptably high serum calcium levels.

Regardless of the drug used, careful attention to serum calcium and phosphate levels is required. A calcium × phosphate product (in mg/dL units) less than 55 is desired with both calcium and phosphate in the normal range. Calcium adjustments in the diet and dialysis bath and phosphate restriction (dietary and with oral ingestion of phosphate binders) should be used along with vitamin D metabolites. Monitoring of serum PTH and alkaline phosphatase levels is useful in determining whether therapy is correcting or preventing secondary hyperparathyroidism. In patients on dialysis, a PTH value of approximately twice the upper limits of normal is considered desirable to prevent adynamic bone disease. Although not generally available, percutaneous bone biopsies for quantitative histomorphometry may help in choosing appropriate therapy and following the effectiveness of such therapy, especially in suspected cases of adynamic bone disease. Unlike the rapid changes in serum values, changes in bone morphology require months to years. Monitoring of serum vitamin D metabolite levels is useful for determining adherence, absorption, and metabolism.

INTESTINAL OSTEODYSTROPHY

A number of gastrointestinal and hepatic diseases cause disordered calcium and phosphate homeostasis, which ultimately leads to bone disease. As bariatric surgery becomes more common, this problem is likely to increase. The bones in such patients show a combination of osteoporosis and osteomalacia. Osteitis fibrosa does not occur, in contrast to renal osteodystrophy. The important common feature in this group of diseases appears to be malabsorption of calcium and vitamin D. Liver disease may, in addition, reduce the production of 25(OH)D from vitamin D, although its importance in patients other than those with terminal liver failure remains in dispute. Recent evidence suggests that in obesity, the liver enzyme CYP2R1, which 25-hydroxylates vitamin D to 25(OH)D, is reduced, contributing to the reduction of 25(OH)D levels in this condition. That said, the major explanation for the low 25(OH)D levels in patients with liver disease is the reduction in vitamin D-binding protein production, the major carrier of vitamin D metabolites in the blood. Free 25(OH)D is generally normal in patients with liver disease. The malabsorption of vitamin D is probably not limited to exogenous vitamin D as the liver secretes into bile a substantial number of vitamin D metabolites and conjugates that are normally reabsorbed in the distal jejunum and ileum. Interference with this process could deplete the body of endogenous vitamin D metabolites in addition to limiting absorption of dietary vitamin D.

In mild forms of malabsorption, high doses of vitamin D (25,000–50,000 IU one to three times per week) should suffice to raise serum levels of 25(OH)D into the normal range. Many patients with severe disease do not respond to vitamin D. Clinical experience with the other metabolites is limited, but both calcitriol and calcifediol have been used successfully in doses similar to those recommended for treatment of renal osteodystrophy. Theoretically, calcifediol should be the drug of choice under these conditions, because no impairment of the renal metabolism of 25(OH)D to $1,25(OH)_2D$ and $24,25(OH)_2D$ exists in these patients. However, calcifediol is only approved in the United States for use in chronic kidney disease and secondary hyperparathyroidism. Both calcitriol and $24,25(OH)_2D$ may be of importance in reversing the bone disease. Intramuscular injections of vitamin D would be an alternative form of therapy, but there are currently no FDA-approved intramuscular preparations available in the United States. The skin remains a good source of vitamin D production, although care is needed to prevent UVB overexposure (ie, by avoiding sunburn) to reduce the risk of photoaging and skin cancer.

As in the other diseases discussed, treatment of intestinal osteodystrophy with vitamin D and its metabolites should be accompanied by appropriate dietary calcium supplementation and monitoring of serum calcium and phosphate levels.

OSTEOPOROSIS

Osteoporosis is defined as abnormal loss of bone predisposing to fractures. It is most common in postmenopausal women but also occurs in men. The annual direct medical cost of fractures in older women and men in the United States is estimated to be at least $20 billion per year and is increasing as the population ages. Osteoporosis is most commonly associated with loss of gonadal function as in menopause or antiandrogen therapy as in prostate cancer treatment, but may also occur as an adverse effect of long-term administration of glucocorticoids or other drugs, including those that inhibit sex steroid production; as a manifestation of endocrine

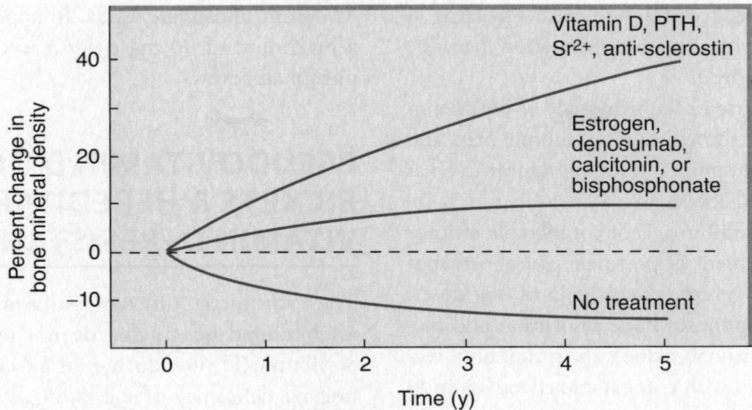

FIGURE 42–5 Typical changes in bone mineral density with time after the onset of menopause, with and without treatment. In the untreated condition, bone is lost during aging in both men and women. Strontium (Sr^{2+}), parathyroid hormone (PTH), and vitamin D promote bone formation and can increase bone mineral density in subjects who respond to them throughout the period of treatment, although PTH and vitamin D in high doses also activate bone resorption. Sclerostin antibodies provide a pure anabolic action in the treatment of osteoporosis by promoting bone formation and inhibiting bone resorption. In contrast, estrogen, calcitonin, denosumab, and bisphosphonates block bone resorption. This leads to a transient increase in bone mineral density because bone formation is not initially decreased. However, with time, both bone formation and bone resorption decrease with these pure antiresorptive agents, and bone mineral density reaches a new plateau.

disease such as thyrotoxicosis or hyperparathyroidism; as a feature of malabsorption syndrome; as a consequence of alcohol abuse and cigarette smoking; or without obvious cause (idiopathic). The ability of some agents to reverse the bone loss of osteoporosis is shown in Figure 42–5 and discussed earlier in the box labelled Treatment of Osteoporosis. The postmenopausal form of osteoporosis may be accompanied by lower $1,25(OH)_2D$ levels and reduced intestinal calcium transport. This form of osteoporosis is due to reduced estrogen production and can be treated with estrogen (combined with a progestin in women with a uterus to prevent endometrial carcinoma). However, concern that estrogen increases the risk of breast cancer and fails to reduce or may actually increase the development of heart disease has reduced enthusiasm for this form of therapy, at least in older individuals.

Bisphosphonates are potent inhibitors of bone resorption. They increase bone density and reduce the risk of fractures in the hip, spine, and other locations. **Alendronate, risedronate, ibandronate,** and **zoledronate** are approved for the treatment of osteoporosis, using daily dosing schedules of alendronate, 10 mg/d, risedronate, 5 mg/d, or ibandronate, 2.5 mg/d; or weekly schedules of alendronate, 70 mg/week, or risedronate, 35 mg/week; or monthly schedules of ibandronate, 150 mg/month; or quarterly (every 3 months) injections of ibandronate, 3 mg; or annual infusions of zoledronate, 5 mg. These drugs are effective in men as well as women and for various causes of osteoporosis.

As previously noted, estrogen-like SERMs (selective estrogen receptor modulators, Chapter 40) have been developed that prevent the increased risk of breast and uterine cancer associated with estrogen while maintaining the benefit to bone. The SERM **raloxifene** is approved for treatment of osteoporosis. Like tamoxifen, raloxifene reduces the risk of breast cancer. It protects against spine fractures but not hip fractures—unlike bisphosphonates, denosumab, and teriparatide, which protect against both. Raloxifene does not prevent hot flushes and imposes the same increased risk of venous thromboembolism as estrogen. To counter the reduced intestinal calcium transport associated with osteoporosis, vitamin D therapy should be used in combination with dietary calcium supplementation. In several large studies, vitamin D supplementation (800 IU/d) with calcium has been shown to improve bone density, reduce falls, and prevent fractures, although calcium and vitamin D are generally used as supplements with other drugs in the treatment of osteoporosis. Calcitriol and its analog, $1\alpha(OH)D_3$, have also been shown to increase bone mass and reduce fractures. Use of these agents for osteoporosis is not FDA approved, although they are used for this purpose in other countries. The $1,25(OH)_2D$ analog eldecalcitol is approved for use in Japan, largely replacing the use of $1\alpha(OH)D_3$ in that country.

Teriparatide, the recombinant form of PTH 1-34, is approved for treatment of osteoporosis. It is given in a dosage of 20 mcg subcutaneously daily. Teriparatide stimulates new bone formation, but unlike fluoride, this new bone appears structurally normal and is associated with a substantial reduction in the incidence of fractures. The drug is approved for only 2 years of use. Current recommendations are to follow teriparatide treatment with an antiresorptive drug. More recently the PTHrP analog **abaloparatide** has been approved for osteoporosis. This drug has efficacy at least comparable to teriparitide in increasing BMD and preventing fractures. Like teriparatide it is administered subcutaneously daily but in 80 mcg doses. Other delivery systems such as a transepidermal needle patch are being tested. Like teriparatide, abaloparatide is approved for 2 years of use, again with the recommendation to follow its use with an antiresorptive agent.

Romosozumab, a sclerostin antibody, has recently been approved for osteoporosis. It is given monthly in 210-mg doses by subcutaneous injection. Romosozumab has a strong effect on BMD, as it both stimulates bone formation and inhibits bone resorption, and substantially reduces fracture risk. The drug is approved for 1 year treatment with the recommendation that it be followed with an antiresorptive drug.

Calcitonin is approved for use in the treatment of postmenopausal osteoporosis. It has been shown to increase bone mass and reduce fractures, but only in the spine. It does not appear to be as effective as the other drugs listed above.

Denosumab, the RANKL inhibitor, is of comparable efficacy to bisphosphonates in the treatment of postmenopausal osteoporosis. It is given subcutaneously every 6 months in 60-mg doses. Like the bisphosphonates it suppresses bone resorption and secondarily bone formation. Denosumab reduces the risk of both vertebral and nonvertebral fractures with comparable effectiveness to the potent bisphosphonates.

Strontium ranelate has not been approved in the United States for the treatment of osteoporosis but is being used in Europe, generally at a dose of 2 g/d.

X-LINKED & AUTOSOMAL DOMINANT HYPOPHOSPHATEMIA & RELATED DISEASES

These disorders usually manifest in childhood as rickets and hypophosphatemia, although they may first present in adults. In both X-linked and autosomal dominant hypophosphatemia, biologically active FGF23 accumulates, leading to phosphate wasting in the urine and hypophosphatemia. In autosomal dominant hypophosphatemia, mutations in the FGF23 gene replace an arginine required for proteolysis and result in increased FGF23 stability. X-linked hypophosphatemia is caused by mutations in the gene encoding the PHEX protein, an endopeptidase. Initially, it was thought that FGF23 was a direct substrate for PHEX, but this no longer appears to be the case. Tumor-induced osteomalacia is a phenotypically similar but acquired syndrome in adults that results from overexpression of FGF23 in tumor cells. The current concept for all of these diseases is that FGF23 blocks the renal uptake of phosphate and blocks 1,25$(OH)_2$D production, leading to rickets in children and osteomalacia in adults. Phosphate is critical to normal bone mineralization; when phosphate stores are deficient, a clinical and pathologic picture resembling vitamin D–dependent rickets develops. However, affected children fail to respond to the standard doses of vitamin D used in the treatment of nutritional rickets. A defect in 1,25$(OH)_2$D production by the kidney contributes to the phenotype as 1,25$(OH)_2$D levels are low relative to the degree of hypophosphatemia observed. This combination of low serum phosphate and low or low-normal serum 1,25$(OH)_2$D provides the rationale for treating these patients with oral phosphate (1–3 g daily) and calcitriol (0.25–2 mcg daily). Reports of such combination therapy are encouraging in this otherwise debilitating disease, although prolonged treatment often leads to secondary hyperparathyroidism. More recently the FGF23 antibody burosumab has been approved for children and adults with X-linked hypophosphatemic (XLH) rickets. In children the dose ranges from 0.8 to 2 mg/kg every 2 weeks by subcutaneous injection based on serum phosphate levels. In adults the dose is 1 mg/kg up to a maximum of 90 mg every 4 weeks, adjusted based on serum phosphate levels.

PSEUDOVITAMIN D DEFICIENCY RICKETS & HEREDITARY VITAMIN D–RESISTANT RICKETS

These distinctly different autosomal recessive diseases present as childhood rickets that do not respond to conventional doses of vitamin D. Pseudovitamin D–deficiency rickets is due to an isolated deficiency of 1,25$(OH)_2$D production caused by mutations in 25(OH)-D-1α-hydroxylase (CYP27B1). This condition is treated with calcitriol (0.25–0.5 mcg daily). Hereditary vitamin D–resistant rickets (HVDRR) is caused by mutations in the gene for the vitamin D receptor. The serum levels of 1,25$(OH)_2$D are very high in HVDRR, whereas they are inappropriately low for the level of calcium in pseudovitamin D–deficient rickets. Treatment with large doses of calcitriol has been claimed to be effective in restoring normocalcemia in some HVDRR patients, presumably those with a partially functional vitamin D receptor, although many patients are completely resistant to all forms of vitamin D. Calcium and phosphate infusions have been shown to correct the rickets in some children, similar to studies in mice in which the *VDR* gene has been deleted. Following puberty the requirements for treatment are often less and may no longer exist. These diseases are rare.

IDIOPATHIC INFANTILE HYPERCALCEMIA

Mutations in CYP24A1, the enzyme catabolizing 25(OH)D and 1,25$(OH)_2$D, have recently been found to account for a number of cases of idiopathic infantile hypercalcemia. However, these mutations have also been described in adults with previously unexplained hypercalcemia and elevated 1,25$(OH)_2$D levels. In some women symptoms develop during pregnancy as 1,25$(OH)_2$D levels increase. At this point no definitive therapy has been established, but vitamin D supplementation needs to be avoided. The diagnosis can be made by finding a reduced ratio of 24,25$(OH)_2$D to 25(OH)D in the blood.

NEPHROTIC SYNDROME

Patients with nephrotic syndrome can lose vitamin D metabolites in the urine, presumably by loss of the vitamin D–binding protein. Such patients may have very low 25(OH)D levels. Some of them develop bone disease. It is not yet clear what value vitamin D therapy has in such patients, because therapeutic trials with vitamin D (or any vitamin D metabolite) have not yet been carried out. Because the problem is not related to vitamin D metabolism, one would not anticipate any advantage in using the more expensive vitamin D metabolites in place of vitamin D.

IDIOPATHIC HYPERCALCIURIA

Individuals with idiopathic hypercalciuria, characterized by hypercalciuria and nephrolithiasis with normal serum calcium and PTH levels, have been divided into three groups: (1) hyperabsorbers, patients with increased intestinal absorption of calcium, resulting in high-normal serum calcium, low-normal PTH, and a secondary increase in urine calcium; (2) renal calcium leakers, patients with a primary decrease in renal reabsorption of filtered calcium, leading to low-normal serum calcium and high-normal serum PTH; and (3) renal phosphate leakers, patients with a primary decrease in renal reabsorption of phosphate, leading to increased $1,25(OH)_2D$ production, increased intestinal calcium absorption, increased ionized serum calcium, low-normal PTH levels, and a secondary increase in urine calcium. There is some disagreement about this classification, and many patients are not readily categorized. Many such patients present with mild hypophosphatemia, and oral phosphate has been used with some success in reducing stone formation. However, a clear role for phosphate in the treatment of this disorder has not been established and it is not recommended.

Therapy with hydrochlorothiazide, up to 50 mg twice daily, or chlorthalidone, 50–100 mg daily, is recommended. Loop diuretics such as furosemide and ethacrynic acid should not be used because they increase urinary calcium excretion. The major toxicity of thiazide diuretics, besides hypokalemia, hypomagnesemia, and hyperglycemia, is hypercalcemia. This is seldom more than a biochemical observation unless the patient has a disease such as hyperparathyroidism in which bone turnover is accelerated. Accordingly, one should screen patients for such disorders before starting thiazide therapy and monitor serum and urine calcium when therapy has begun.

An alternative to thiazides is allopurinol. Some studies indicate that hyperuricosuria is associated with idiopathic hypercalciuria and that a small nidus of urate crystals could lead to the calcium oxalate stone formation characteristic of idiopathic hypercalciuria. Allopurinol, 100–300 mg daily, may reduce stone formation by reducing uric acid excretion.

OTHER DISORDERS OF BONE MINERAL HOMEOSTASIS

PAGET DISEASE OF BONE

Paget disease is a localized bone disorder characterized by uncontrolled osteoclastic bone resorption with secondary increases in poorly organized bone formation. The cause of Paget disease is obscure, although some studies suggest that a measles-related virus may be involved. The disease is fairly common, although symptomatic bone disease is less common. Recent studies indicate that this infection may produce a factor that increases the stimulation of bone resorption by $1,25(OH)_2D$. The biochemical parameters of elevated serum alkaline phosphatase and urinary hydroxyproline are useful for diagnosis. Along with the characteristic radiologic and bone scan findings, these biochemical determinations provide good markers by which to follow therapy.

The goal of treatment is to reduce bone pain and stabilize or prevent other problems such as progressive deformity, fractures, hearing loss, high-output cardiac failure, and immobilization hypercalcemia. Calcitonin and bisphosphonates are the first-line agents for this disease. Calcitonin is administered subcutaneously or intramuscularly in doses of 50–100 MRC (Medical Research Council) units every day or every other day. Nasal inhalation at 200–400 units/d is also effective. Higher or more frequent doses have been advocated when this initial regimen is ineffective. Improvement in bone pain and reduction in serum alkaline phosphatase and urine hydroxyproline levels require weeks to months. Often a patient who responds well initially loses the response to calcitonin. This refractoriness is not correlated with the development of antibodies.

Sodium etidronate, alendronate, risedronate, tiludronate, and zoledronate are the bisphosphonates currently approved for clinical use in Paget disease of bone in the United States, although etidronate is seldom used anymore as the other bisphosphonates are more effective. Other bisphosphonates, including pamidronate, are being used in other countries. The recommended doses of bisphosphonates are etidronate, 5 mg/kg per day; alendronate, 40 mg/d; risedronate, 30 mg/d; and tiludronate, 400 mg/d. These doses are higher than the doses used for osteoporosis. Zoledronate is given as a 5 mg infusion, and if the alkaline phosphatase is still elevated after several months the infusion can be repeated. Long-term remission (months to years) may be expected in patients who respond to a bisphosphonate. Treatment should not exceed 6 months per course but can be repeated after 6 months if necessary. The principal toxicity of etidronate is the development of osteomalacia and an increased incidence of fractures when the dosage is raised substantially above 5 mg/kg per day. The newer bisphosphonates such as risedronate and alendronate do not share this adverse effect. Some patients treated with etidronate develop bone pain similar in nature to the bone pain of osteomalacia. This subsides after stopping the drug. The principal adverse effect of alendronate and the newer bisphosphonates is gastric irritation when used at these high doses. This is reversible on cessation of the drug.

ENTERIC OXALURIA

Patients with short bowel syndromes and associated fat malabsorption can present with renal stones composed of calcium and oxalate. Such patients characteristically have normal or low urine calcium levels but elevated urine oxalate levels. The reasons for the development of oxaluria in such patients are thought to be twofold: first, in the intestinal lumen, calcium (which is now bound to fat) fails to bind oxalate and no longer prevents its absorption; second, enteric flora, acting on the increased supply of nutrients reaching the colon, produce larger amounts of oxalate. Although one would ordinarily avoid treating a patient with calcium oxalate stones with calcium supplementation, this is precisely what is done in patients with enteric oxaluria. The increased intestinal calcium binds the excess oxalate and prevents its absorption. Calcium carbonate (1–2 g) can be given daily in divided doses, with careful monitoring of urinary calcium and oxalate to be certain that urinary oxalate falls without a dangerous increase in urinary calcium.

SUMMARY Major Drugs Used in Diseases of Bone Mineral Homeostasis

Subclass, Drug	Mechanism of Action	Effects	Clinical Applications	Toxicities
VITAMIN D, METABOLITES, ANALOGS				
• Cholecalciferol (D_3) • Ergocalciferol (D_2) • Calcitriol • Calcifediol • Doxercalciferol • Paricalcitol • Calcipotriene	Regulate gene transcription via the vitamin D receptor	Stimulate intestinal calcium absorption, bone resorption, renal calcium and phosphate reabsorption • decrease parathyroid hormone (PTH) • promote innate immunity • inhibit adaptive immunity	Osteoporosis, osteomalacia, renal failure, malabsorption, psoriasis	Hypercalcemia, hypercalciuria • the vitamin D preparations have much longer half-lives than the metabolites and analogs
BISPHOSPHONATES				
• Alendronate • Risedronate • Ibandronate • Pamidronate • Zoledronate	Suppress the activity of osteoclasts in part via inhibition of farnesyl pyrophosphate synthesis	Inhibit bone resorption	Osteoporosis, bone metastases, hypercalcemia	Adynamic bone, possible renal failure, rare osteonecrosis of the jaw, rare subtrochanteric (femur) fractures
HORMONES				
• Teriparatide • Abaloparatide • Calcitonin • rhPTH1-84 (Natpara)	These hormones act via their cognate G protein-coupled receptors • teriparatide, abaloparatide, and Natpara all share the same receptor	Teriparatide, abaloparatide, and Natpara stimulate bone turnover, increase $1,25(OH)_2D$ production, increase RANKL, decrease sclerostin, enhance calcium reabsorption from the kidney • calcitonin suppresses bone resorption and increases renal calcium excretion	Teriparatide and abaloparatide are used in osteoporosis • calcitonin is used for hypercalcemia and Paget disease, Natpara is used in hypoparathyroidism	Teriparatide, abaloparatide, Natpara may cause hypercalcemia and hypercalciuria
SELECTIVE ESTROGEN RECEPTOR MODULATORS (SERMS)				
• Raloxifene	Interacts selectively with estrogen receptors	Inhibits bone resorption without stimulating breast or endometrial hyperplasia	Osteoporosis	Does not prevent hot flashes • increased risk of venous thromboembolism
RANK LIGAND (RANKL) INHIBITOR				
• Denosumab	Monoclonal antibody • binds to RANKL and prevents it from stimulating osteoclast differentiation and function	Blocks bone resorption	Osteoporosis	May increase risk of infections; when discontinued bone resorption increases and may increase fracture risk
CALCIUM RECEPTOR AGONIST				
• Cinacalcet • Etelcalcetide	Activates the calcium-sensing receptor	Inhibits PTH secretion	Hyperparathyroidism, primary and secondary	Nausea, hypocalcemia in CKD patients
MINERALS				
• Calcium, phosphate • Strontium	Multiple physiologic actions through regulation of multiple enzymatic pathways	Strontium suppresses bone resorption and increases bone formation • calcium and phosphate required for bone mineralization	Osteoporosis • osteomalacia • deficiencies in calcium or phosphate	Ectopic calcification, renal stones, hypercalcemia
SCLEROSTIN ANTIBODY				
• Romosozumab	Inhibits sclerostin	Stimulates bone formation	Osteoporosis	Possible increased risk of cardiovascular events and strokes
FGF23 ANTIBODY				
• Burosumab	Blocks FGF23 binding	Increases serum phosphate and $1,25(OH)_2D$ levels by decreasing the inhibition by FGF23 on renal phosphate excretion and $1,25(OH)_2D$ production	XLH	Nephrocalcinosis, hyperphosphatemia

PREPARATIONS AVAILABLE

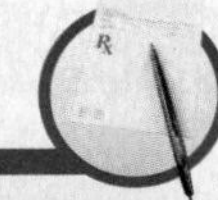

GENERIC NAME	AVAILABLE AS
VITAMIN D, METABOLITES, AND ANALOGS	
Calcifediol (25(OH)D3)	Rayaldee
Calcitriol	
Oral	Generic, Rocaltrol
Parenteral	Calcijex
Cholecalciferol (D_3) (vitamin D_3)	Generic, Delta-D
Doxercalciferol	Generic, Hectorol
Ergocalciferol (D_2) (vitamin D_2, calciferol)	Generic, Drisdol, others
Paricalcitol	Generic, Zemplar
CALCIUM	
Calcium acetate (25% calcium)	Generic, PhosLo
Calcium carbonate (40% calcium)	Generic, Tums, Cal-Sup, Os-Cal 500
Calcium chloride (27% calcium)	Generic
Calcium citrate (21% calcium)	Generic, Cal-C-Caps, Cal-Cee
Calcium glubionate (6.5% calcium)	Neo-Calglucon, Calcionate, Calciquid
Calcium gluceptate (8% calcium)	Generic
Calcium gluconate (9% calcium)	Generic
Calcium lactate (13% calcium)	Generic
Tricalcium phosphate (39% calcium)	Posture

GENERIC NAME	AVAILABLE AS
PHOSPHATE AND PHOSPHATE BINDER	
Phosphate	
Oral: solution	Fleet Phospho-soda, K-Phos-Neutral, Neutra-Phos, Neutra-Phos-K
Sevelamer carbonate or HCl	Renagel, Renvela
Lanthanum carbonate	Fosrenol
BISPHOSPHONATES	
Alendronate sodium	Generic, Fosamax
Etidronate disodium	Generic, Didronel
Ibandronate sodium	Generic, Boniva
Pamidronate disodium	Generic, Aredia
Risedronate sodium	Actonel, Atelvia
Tiludronate disodium	Skelid
Zoledronic acid	Zometa, Reclast
OTHER DRUGS	
Abaloparatide	Tymlos
Burosumab	Crysvita
Calcitonin-salmon	Miacalcin, Calcimar, Salmonine
Cinacalcet	Sensipar
Denosumab	Prolia, Xgeva
Etelcalcetide	Parsabiv
Gallium nitrate	Ganite
Recombinant human PTH 1-84	Natpara
Romosozumab	Evenity
Sodium fluoride	Generic
Teriparatide (1-34 active segment of PTH)	Forteo

REFERENCES

Bär L et al: Regulation of fibroblast growth factor 23 (FGF23) in health and disease. FEBS Lett 2019;593:1879.

Bikle DD: Extraskeletal actions of vitamin D. Ann NY Acad Sci 2016; 1376:29.

Bikle DD, Schwartz J: Vitamin D binding protein, total and free vitamin D levels in different physiological and pathophysiological conditions. Front Endocrinol (Lausanne) 2019;10:317.

Bikle DD: Vitamin D: newer concepts of its metabolism and function at the basic and clinical level. J Endo Soc 2020;4:bvz038.

Bouillon R: Comparative analysis of nutritional guidelines for vitamin D. Nat Rev Endocrinol 2017;13:466.

Compston JE, McClung MR, Leslie WD: Osteoporosis. Lancet 2019;393:364.

Hagino H: Eldecalcitol: Newly developed active vitamin D(3) analog for the treatment of osteoporosis. Expert Opin Pharmacother 2013;14:817.

Holick MF et al: Evaluation, treatment, and prevention of vitamin D deficiency: An Endocrine Society Clinical Practice Guideline. J Clin Endocrinol Metab 2011;96:1911.

Karsenty G: Update on the biology of osteocalcin. Endocr Pract 2017;23:1270.

Imel EA, White KE: Pharmacological management of X-linked hypophosphataemia. Br J Clin Pharmacol 2019;85:1188.

LeBoff MS et al: Supplemental vitamin D and incident fractures in midlife and older adults. N Engl J Med 2022;387:299.

Manson JE et al: VITAL Research Group. Vitamin D supplements and prevention of cancer and cardiovascular disease. N Engl J Med 2019;380:33.

Martin A, David V, Quarles LD: Regulation and function of the FGF23/Klotho endocrine pathways. Physiol Rev 2012;92:131.

Martineau C et al: Optimal bone fracture repair requires 24R,25-dihydroxyvitamin D3 and its effector molecule FAM57B2. J Clin Invest 2018;128:3546.

McClung MR: Romosozumab for the treatment of osteoporosis. Osteoporos Sarcopenia 2018;4:11.

Mirrakhimov AE: Hypercalcemia of malignancy: An update on pathogenesis and management. N Am J Med Sci 2015;7:483.

Mosekilde L, Vestergaard P, Rejnmark L: The pathogenesis, treatment, and prevention of osteoporosis in men. Drugs 2013;73:15.

Nigwekar SU, Tamez H, Thadhani RI: Vitamin D and chronic kidney disease–mineral bone disease (CKD–MBD). Bonekey Rep 2014;3:498.

Palmer SC et al: Comparative effectiveness of calcimimetic agents for secondary hyperparathyroidism in adults: a systemic review. Am J Kidney Dis 2020;76:321.

Pittas AG et al: D2d Research Group. Vitamin D supplementation and prevention of type 2 diabetes. N Engl J Med 2019;381:520.

Ross AC et al: The 2011 report on dietary reference intakes for calcium and vitamin D from the Institute of Medicine: What clinicians need to know. J Clin Endocrinol Metab 2011;96:53.

Tay Y-K D, Tabaccco G, Bilezikian J: Bone quality in hypoparathyroidism. Minerva Endocrinol 2021;46:325.

Thandrayen K, Pettifor JM: The roles of vitamin D and dietary calcium in nutritional rickets. Bone Rep 2018;8:81.

Zwolak P, Dudek AZ: Antineoplastic activity of zoledronic acid and denosumab. Anticancer Res 2013;33:2981.

CASE STUDY ANSWER

There are multiple reasons for this patient's osteoporosis, including a heavy smoking history, possible alcoholism, and chronic inflammatory disease treated with glucocorticoids. High levels of cytokines from the chronic inflammation activate osteoclasts. Glucocorticoids increase urinary losses of calcium, suppress bone formation, and inhibit intestinal calcium absorption as well as decreasing gonadotropin production, leading to hypogonadism. Management should include measurement of serum testosterone, calcium, 25(OH)D, and the 24-hour urine calcium and creatinine levels (to verify completeness of collection), with treatment as appropriate for these secondary causes, plus initiation of bisphosphonate or denosumab therapy as primary treatment.

SECTION VIII CHEMOTHERAPEUTIC DRUGS

INTRODUCTION TO ANTIMICROBIAL AGENTS

Antimicrobial agents provide some of the most dramatic examples of the advances of modern medicine. Many infectious diseases once considered incurable and potentially lethal can now be treated effectively with antibiotics. The remarkably powerful and specific activity of antimicrobial drugs is due to their selectivity for targets that are either unique to prokaryote and fungal microorganisms or much more important in these organisms than in humans. Among these targets are bacterial and fungal cell wall-synthesizing enzymes (Chapters 43 and 48), the bacterial ribosome (Chapters 44 and 45), the enzymes required for nucleotide synthesis and DNA replication (Chapter 46), and the machinery of viral replication (Chapter 49). The special group of drugs used in mycobacterial infections is discussed in Chapter 47. Antiseptics and disinfectants are discussed in Chapter 50. The clinical uses of many antimicrobial agents are summarized in Chapter 51.

The major problem threatening the continued success of antimicrobial drugs is the development of resistant organisms. Antibiotic resistance mechanisms existed long before the clinical use of antibiotics. Because resistance mechanisms are already present in nature, an inevitable consequence of antimicrobial use is the selection of resistant microorganisms. Since the start of the antibiotic era, antibiotic use in patients and animals has fueled a major increase in the prevalence of drug-resistant pathogens. In recent years, highly resistant gram-negative organisms with novel mechanisms of resistance have developed. Some of these strains have spread widely as a result of patients seeking medical care in different countries.

Much attention has been focused on eliminating the misuse of antibiotics to slow the tide of resistance. Antibiotics are misused in a variety of ways, including use in patients who are unlikely to have bacterial infections, use over unnecessarily prolonged periods, and use of multiple agents or broad-spectrum agents when not needed. Large quantities of antibiotics have been used in agriculture to stimulate growth and prevent infection in livestock, and this has added to the selection pressure that results in resistant organisms. Since 2017, the USA has not allowed antibiotics that are medically important to be used for growth promotion in livestock. Both the United Nations and the World Health Organization have programs aimed at promoting antimicrobial stewardship and combating antibiotic resistance. However, even if these programs are successful, it will take years before the benefits are apparent.

Antibiotic resistance has many negative consequences. The prevalence of resistant organisms drives the use of antibiotics that may be broader-spectrum, less efficacious, more toxic, or more expensive. Not surprisingly, infections caused by antibiotic-resistant pathogens are associated with increased costs, morbidity, and mortality. The Centers for Disease Control and Prevention estimates that every year in the United States more than 2.8 million people acquire infections due to and 35,000 people die from infections caused by resistant bacteria.

Unfortunately, as the need has grown in recent years, development of novel antibiotics has not kept pace. While a number of new antimicrobial agents have been approved in the last decade, most are similar to older drugs. Pending the identification and development of new targets and compounds, we will have to rely on currently available families of drugs. In the face of continuing development of resistance, considerable effort will be required to maintain the effectiveness of these drug groups.

In the chapters that follow, reference will be made to drugs that are "effective against susceptible organisms." This indicates that some strains of a specified bacterial species have acquired resistance but other strains have not; the latter strains are still susceptible to the drug. In many infections, especially those that are serious, susceptibility testing is important.

CHAPTER

43 Beta-Lactam & Other Cell Wall- & Membrane-Active Antibiotics

Camille E. Beauduy, PharmD, & Lisa G. Winston, MD*

CASE STUDY

A 45-year-old man is brought to the local hospital emergency department by ambulance. His wife reports that he had been in his normal state of health until 3 days ago when he developed a fever and a productive cough. During the last 24 hours, he has complained of a headache and is increasingly confused. His wife reports that his medical history is significant only for hypertension, for which he takes hydrochlorothiazide and lisinopril, and that he is allergic to amoxicillin. She says that he developed a rash many years ago when prescribed amoxicillin for bronchitis. In the emergency department, the man is febrile (38.7°C [101.7°F]), hypotensive (90/54 mm Hg), tachypneic (36/min), and tachycardic (110/min). He has no signs of meningismus but is oriented only to person. A stat chest x-ray shows a left lower lung consolidation consistent with pneumonia. A CT scan of the head is not concerning for lesions or elevated intracranial pressure. The plan is to start empiric antibiotics and perform a lumbar puncture to rule out bacterial meningitis. What antibiotic regimen should be prescribed to treat both pneumonia and meningitis? Does the history of amoxicillin rash affect the antibiotic choice? Why or why not?

■ BETA-LACTAM COMPOUNDS

PENICILLINS

The penicillins share features of chemistry, mechanism of action, pharmacology, and immunologic characteristics with cephalosporins, monobactams, carbapenems, and β-lactamase inhibitors. All are β-lactam compounds, so named because of their four-membered lactam ring.

Chemistry

All penicillins have the basic structure shown in Figure 43–1. A thiazolidine ring (A) is attached to a β-lactam ring (B) that carries a secondary amino group (RNH–). Substituents (R; examples shown in Figure 43–2) can be attached to the amino group. Structural integrity of the 6-aminopenicillanic acid nucleus (rings A plus B) is essential for the biologic activity of these compounds. Hydrolysis of the β-lactam ring by bacterial β-lactamases yields penicilloic acid, which lacks antibacterial activity.

A. Classification

Substituents of the 6-aminopenicillanic acid moiety determine the essential pharmacologic and antibacterial properties of the resulting molecules. Penicillins can be assigned to one of three groups (below). Within each of these groups are compounds that are relatively stable to gastric acid and suitable for oral administration, eg, penicillin V, dicloxacillin, and amoxicillin. The side chains of some representatives of each group are shown in Figure 43–2.

*The authors thank Dr. Henry F. Chambers and Dr. Daniel Deck for their contributions to this chapter in previous editions.

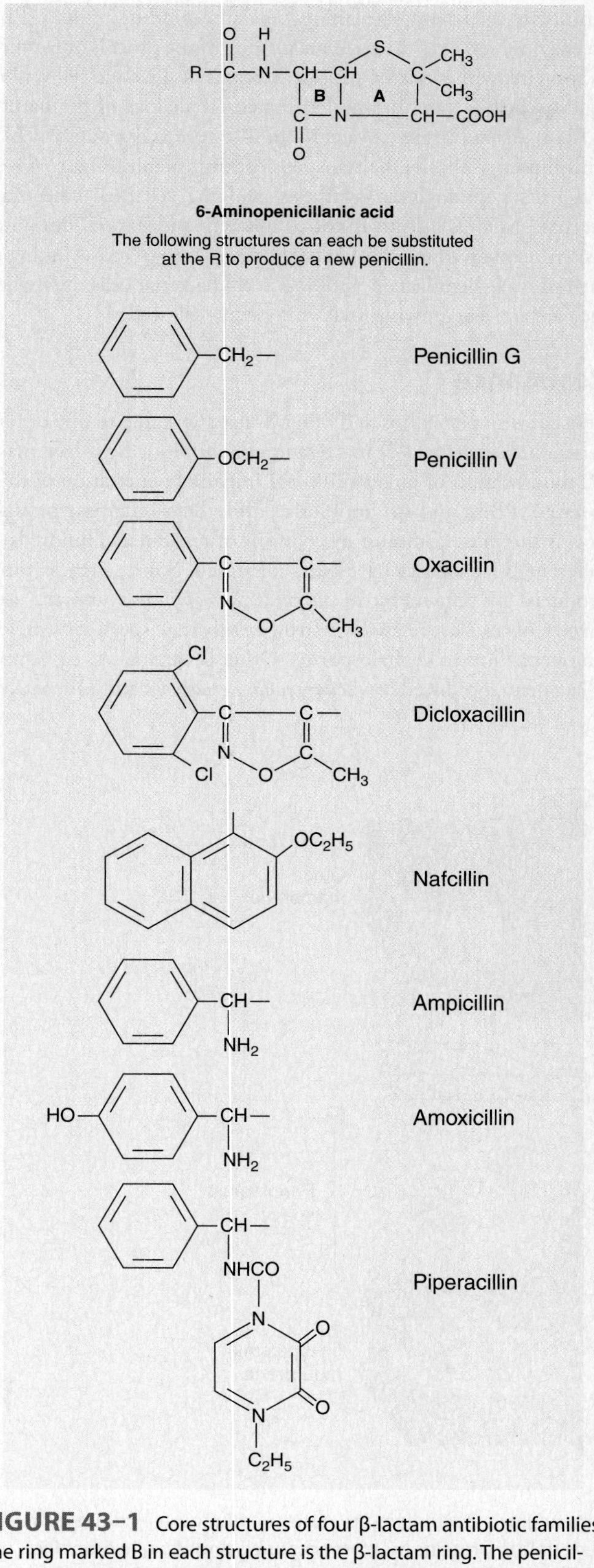

6-Aminopenicillanic acid

The following structures can each be substituted at the R to produce a new penicillin.

Penicillin G

Penicillin V

Oxacillin

Dicloxacillin

Nafcillin

Ampicillin

Amoxicillin

Piperacillin

FIGURE 43–1 Core structures of four β-lactam antibiotic families. The ring marked B in each structure is the β-lactam ring. The penicillins are susceptible to inactivation by amidases and lactamases at the points shown. Note that the carbapenems have a different stereochemical configuration in the lactam ring that imparts resistance to most common β-lactamases. Substituents for the penicillin and cephalosporin families are shown in Figures 43–2 and 43–6, respectively.

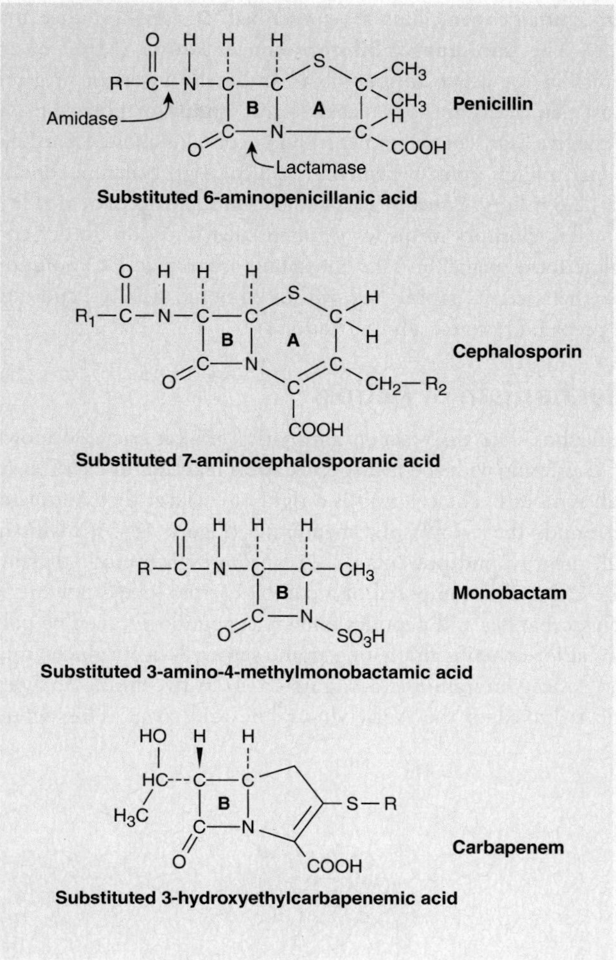

Amidase — Lactamase — Penicillin

Substituted 6-aminopenicillanic acid

Cephalosporin

Substituted 7-aminocephalosporanic acid

Monobactam

Substituted 3-amino-4-methylmonobactamic acid

Carbapenem

Substituted 3-hydroxyethylcarbapenemic acid

FIGURE 43–2 Side chains of some penicillins (R groups).

1. *Penicillins (eg, penicillin G)*—These have greatest activity against gram-positive organisms, gram-negative cocci, and non-β-lactamase-producing anaerobes. However, they have little activity against gram-negative rods, and they are susceptible to hydrolysis by β-lactamases.

2. *Antistaphylococcal penicillins (eg, nafcillin)*—These penicillins are resistant to staphylococcal β-lactamases. They are active against staphylococci and streptococci but not against enterococci, anaerobic bacteria, and gram-negative cocci and rods.

3. *Extended-spectrum penicillins (aminopenicillins and antipseudomonal penicillins)*—These drugs retain the antibacterial spectrum of penicillin and have improved activity against gram-negative rods. Like penicillin, however, they are relatively susceptible to hydrolysis by β-lactamases.

B. Penicillin Units and Formulations

The activity of penicillin G was originally defined in units. Crystalline sodium penicillin G contains approximately 1600 units per mg (1 unit = 0.6 mcg; 1 million units of penicillin = 0.6 g).

Semisynthetic penicillins are prescribed by weight rather than units. The **minimum inhibitory concentration (MIC)** of any penicillin (or other antimicrobial) is usually given in mcg/mL. Most penicillins are formulated as the sodium or potassium salt of the free acid. Potassium penicillin G contains about 1.7 mEq of K^+ per million units of penicillin (2.8 mEq/g). Nafcillin contains Na^+, 2.8 mEq/g. Procaine salts and benzathine salts of penicillin G provide repository forms for intramuscular injection. In dry crystalline form, penicillin salts are stable for years at 4°C. Solutions lose their activity rapidly (eg, within 24 hours at 20°C) and must be prepared fresh for administration.

Mechanism of Action

Penicillins, like all β-lactam antibiotics, inhibit bacterial growth by interfering with the **transpeptidation reaction** of bacterial cell wall synthesis. The cell wall is a rigid outer layer that completely surrounds the cytoplasmic membrane (Figure 43–3), maintains cell integrity, and prevents cell lysis from high osmotic pressure. The cell wall is composed of a complex, cross-linked polymer of polysaccharides and peptides known as peptidoglycan. The polysaccharide contains alternating amino sugars, *N*-acetylglucosamine and *N*-acetylmuramic acid (Figure 43–4). A five-amino-acid peptide is linked to the *N*-acetylmuramic acid sugar. This peptide terminates in D-alanyl-D-alanine. Penicillin-binding protein (PBP, an enzyme) removes the terminal alanine in the process of forming a cross-link with a nearby peptide. Cross-links give the cell wall its rigidity. Beta-lactam antibiotics, structural analogs of the natural D-Ala-D-Ala substrate, covalently bind to the active site of PBPs. This binding inhibits the transpeptidation reaction (Figure 43–5) and halts peptidoglycan synthesis, and the cell dies. The exact mechanism of cell death is not completely understood, but autolysins are involved in addition to the disruption of cross-linking of the cell wall. Beta-lactam antibiotics kill bacterial cells only when they are actively growing and synthesizing cell wall.

Resistance

Resistance to penicillins and other β-lactams is due to one of four general mechanisms: (1) inactivation of antibiotic by β-lactamase, (2) modification of target PBPs, (3) impaired penetration of drug to target PBPs, and (4) antibiotic efflux. Beta-lactamase production is the most common mechanism of resistance. Hundreds of different β-lactamases have been identified. Some, such as those produced by *Staphylococcus aureus*, *Haemophilus influenzae*, and *Escherichia coli*, are relatively narrow in substrate specificity, preferring penicillins to cephalosporins. Other β-lactamases, eg, AmpC β-lactamase produced by *Pseudomonas aeruginosa* and *Enterobacter*

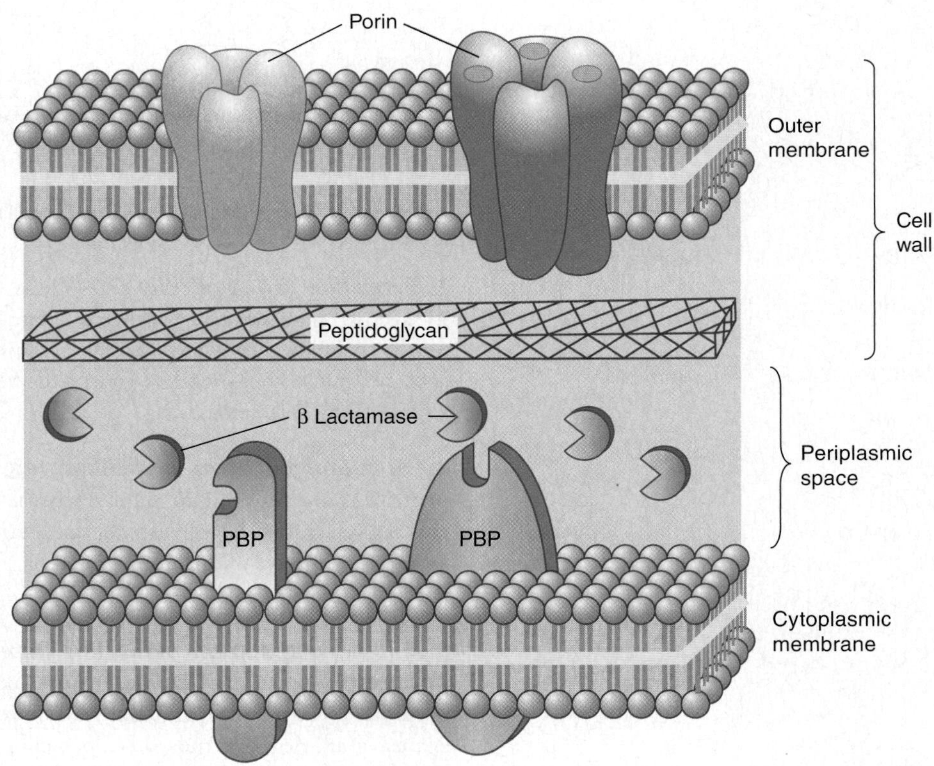

FIGURE 43–3 A highly simplified diagram of the cell envelope of a gram-negative bacterium. The outer membrane, a lipid bilayer, is present in gram-negative but not gram-positive organisms. It is penetrated by porins, proteins that form channels providing hydrophilic access to the cytoplasmic membrane. The peptidoglycan layer is unique to bacteria and is much thicker in gram-positive organisms than in gram-negative ones. Together, the outer membrane and the peptidoglycan layer constitute the cell wall. Penicillin-binding proteins (PBPs) are membrane proteins that cross-link peptidoglycan. Beta-lactamases, if present, reside in the periplasmic space or on the outer surface of the cytoplasmic membrane, where they may destroy β-lactam antibiotics that penetrate the outer membrane.

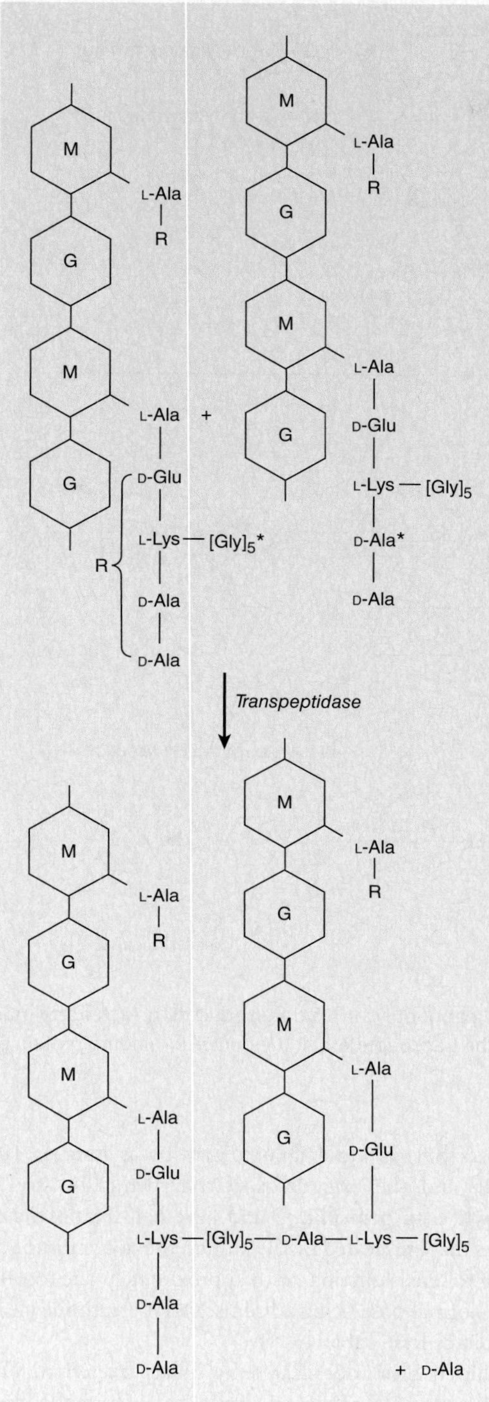

FIGURE 43–4 The transpeptidation reaction in *Staphylococcus aureus* that is inhibited by β-lactam antibiotics. The cell wall of gram-positive bacteria is made up of long peptidoglycan polymer chains consisting of the alternating aminohexoses *N*-acetylglucosamine (G) and *N*-acetylmuramic acid (M) with pentapeptide side chains linked (in *S aureus*) by pentaglycine bridges. The exact composition of the side chains varies among species. The diagram illustrates small segments of two such polymer chains and their amino acid side chains. These linear polymers must be cross-linked by transpeptidation of the side chains at the points indicated by the asterisk to achieve the strength necessary for cell viability.

sp and extended-spectrum β-lactamases (ESBLs) in Enterbacterales, hydrolyze both cephalosporins and penicillins. Carbapenems are highly resistant to hydrolysis by penicillinases and cephalosporinases, but they are hydrolyzed by metallo-β-lactamases and other carbapenemases.

Altered target PBPs are the basis of methicillin resistance in staphylococci and of penicillin resistance in pneumococci and most resistant enterococci. These resistant organisms produce PBPs that have low affinity for binding β-lactam antibiotics, and they are not inhibited except at relatively high, often clinically unachievable, drug concentrations.

Resistance due to impaired penetration of antibiotic occurs only in gram-negative species because of the impermeable outer membrane of their cell wall, which is absent in gram-positive bacteria. Beta-lactam antibiotics cross the outer membrane and enter gram-negative organisms via outer membrane protein channels called porins. Absence of the proper channel or down-regulation of its production can greatly impair drug entry into the cell. Poor penetration alone is usually not sufficient to confer resistance because enough antibiotic eventually enters the cell to inhibit growth. However, this barrier can become important in the presence of a β-lactamase, even a relatively inefficient one, as long as it can hydrolyze drug faster than it enters the cell. Gram-negative organisms also may produce an efflux pump, which consists of cytoplasmic and periplasmic protein components that efficiently transport some β-lactam antibiotics from the periplasm back across the cell wall outer membrane.

Pharmacokinetics

Absorption of orally administered drug differs greatly for individual penicillins, depending in part on their acid stability and protein binding. Gastrointestinal absorption of nafcillin is erratic, so it is not suitable for oral administration. Dicloxacillin, ampicillin, and amoxicillin are acid-stable and relatively well absorbed, producing serum concentrations in the range of 4–8 mcg/mL after a 500-mg oral dose. Absorption of most oral penicillins (amoxicillin being an exception) is impaired by food, and the drugs should be administered at least 1–2 hours before or after a meal.

Intravenous administration of penicillin G is preferred to the intramuscular route because of irritation and local pain from intramuscular injection of large doses. Serum concentrations 30 minutes after an intravenous injection of 1 g of penicillin G (equivalent to approximately 1.6 million units) are 20–50 mcg/mL. Only a fraction of the total drug in serum is present as free drug, the concentration of which is determined by protein binding. Highly protein-bound penicillins (eg, nafcillin) generally achieve lower free-drug concentrations in serum than less protein-bound penicillins (eg, penicillin G or ampicillin). Penicillins are widely distributed in body fluids and tissues with a few exceptions. They are polar molecules, so intracellular concentrations are well below those found in extracellular fluids.

Benzathine and procaine penicillins are formulated to delay absorption, resulting in prolonged blood and tissue concentrations. A single intramuscular injection of 1.2 million units of benzathine penicillin maintains serum levels above 0.02 mcg/mL

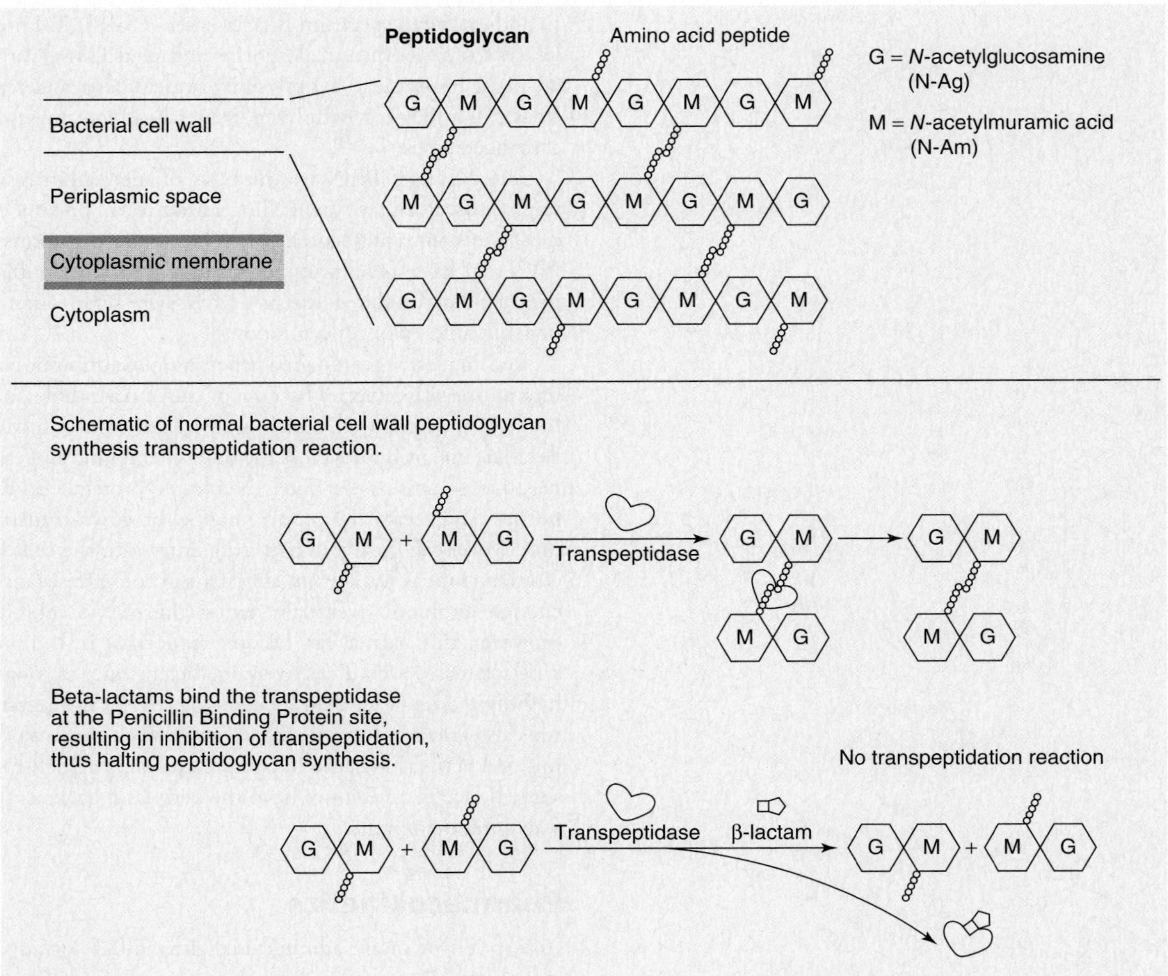

FIGURE 43–5 Schematic of a bacterial cell wall and normal synthesis of cell wall peptidoglycan via transpeptidation; M, *N*-acetylmuramic acid; Glc, glucose; NAcGlc or G, *N*-acetylglucosamine. Beta-lactams work by binding the transpeptidase at the penicillin-binding protein site, resulting in inhibition of transpeptidation, thus halting peptidoglycan synthesis.

for 10 days, sufficient to treat β-hemolytic streptococcal infections. After 3 weeks, levels still exceed 0.003 mcg/mL, which is enough to prevent most β-hemolytic streptococcal infections. A 600,000-unit dose of procaine penicillin yields peak concentrations of 1–2 mcg/mL and clinically useful concentrations for 12–24 hours after a single intramuscular injection.

Penicillin concentrations in most tissues are equal to those in serum. Penicillin is also excreted into sputum and breast milk to levels 3–15% of those in the serum. Penetration into the eye, the prostate, and the central nervous system is poor. However, with active inflammation of the meninges, as in bacterial meningitis, penicillin concentrations of 1–5 mcg/mL can be achieved with a daily parenteral dose of 18–24 million units. These concentrations are sufficient to kill susceptible strains of pneumococci and meningococci.

Penicillin is rapidly excreted by the kidneys; small amounts are excreted by other routes. Tubular secretion accounts for about 90% of renal excretion, and glomerular filtration accounts for the remainder. The normal half-life of penicillin G is approximately 30 minutes but, in renal failure, may be as long as 10 hours. Ampicillin and the extended-spectrum penicillins are secreted more slowly than penicillin G and have half-lives of 1 hour. For penicillins that are cleared by the kidney, the dose must be adjusted according to renal function, with approximately one fourth to one third the normal dose being administered if creatinine clearance is 10 mL/min or less (Table 43–1).

Nafcillin is primarily cleared by biliary excretion. Oxacillin, dicloxacillin, and cloxacillin are eliminated by both the kidney and biliary excretion, and no dosage adjustment is required for these drugs in patients in renal failure. Because clearance of penicillins is less efficient in the newborn, doses adjusted for weight alone result in higher systemic concentrations for longer periods than in the adult.

Clinical Uses

Except for amoxicillin, oral penicillins should be given 1–2 hours before or after a meal; they should not be given with food to

TABLE 43–1 Guidelines for dosing of some commonly used penicillins.

Antibiotic (Route of Administration)	Adult Dose	Pediatric Dose[1]	Neonatal Dose[2]	Adjusted Dose as a Percentage of Normal Dose for Renal Failure Based on Creatinine Clearance (Cl_{cr})	
				Cl_{cr} Approx 50 mL/min	Cl_{cr} Approx 10 mL/min
Penicillins					
Penicillin G (IV)	1–4 × 10^6 units q4–6h	100,000–400,000 units/kg/d in 4–6 doses	100,000–150,000 units/kg/d in 2 or 3 doses	50–75%	25%
Penicillin V (PO)	0.25–0.5 g qid	25–75 mg/kg/d in 4 doses		None	None
Antistaphylococcal penicillins					
Cloxacillin, dicloxacillin (PO)	0.25–0.5 g qid	25–100 mg/kg/d in 4 doses		100%	100%
Nafcillin (IV)	1–2 g q4–6h	100–200 mg/kg/d in 4–6 doses	50–200 mg/kg/d in 2 or 3 doses	100%	100%
Oxacillin (IV)	1–2 g q4–6h	50–200 mg/kg/d in 4–6 doses	50–200 mg/kg/d in 2 or 3 doses	100%	100%
Extended-spectrum penicillins					
Amoxicillin (PO)	0.25–0.5 g tid	20–40 mg/kg/d in 3 doses		66%	33%
Amoxicillin/potassium clavulanate (PO)	500/125 mg tid–875/125 mg bid	20–40 mg/kg/d in 3 doses		66%	33%
Piperacillin/ tazobactam (IV)	3.375–4.5 g q4–6h	240–300 mg/kg/d in 3–4 doses[3]	160–300 mg/kg/d in 2–4 doses[3]	50–75%	25–33%

[1]The total dose should not exceed the adult dose.

[2]The lower dosage range should be used for neonates ≤7 days old and/or weighing <2 kg. After the first month of life, pediatric doses may be used.

[3]Dose is based on piperacillin component.

minimize binding to food proteins and acid inactivation. Amoxicillin may be given without regard to meals. Blood levels of all penicillins can be raised by simultaneous administration of probenecid, 0.5 g (10 mg/kg in children) every 6 hours orally, which impairs renal tubular secretion of weak acids such as β-lactam compounds. Penicillins, like all antibacterial antibiotics, should never be used for viral infections and should be prescribed only when there is reasonable suspicion of, or documented infection with, susceptible organisms.

A. Penicillin

Penicillin G is a drug of choice for infections caused by streptococci, meningococci, some enterococci, penicillin-susceptible pneumococci, staphylococci confirmed to be non-β-lactamase-producing, *Treponema pallidum* and certain other spirochetes, some *Clostridium* species, *Actinomyces* and certain other gram-positive rods, and non-β-lactamase-producing gram-negative anaerobic organisms. Depending on the organism, the site, and the severity of infection, effective doses range between 4 and 24 million units per day administered intravenously in four to six divided doses. High-dose penicillin G can also be given as a continuous intravenous infusion.

Penicillin V, the oral form of penicillin, is indicated only in minor infections because of its relatively poor bioavailability, the need for dosing four times a day, and its narrow antibacterial spectrum. Amoxicillin (see below) is often used instead.

Benzathine penicillin and procaine penicillin G for intramuscular injection yield low but prolonged drug levels. A single intramuscular injection of benzathine penicillin, 1.2 million units, is effective treatment for β-hemolytic streptococcal pharyngitis. Given intramuscularly once every 3–4 weeks, it prevents reinfection. Benzathine penicillin G, 2.4 million units intramuscularly once a week for 1–3 weeks, is effective in the treatment of syphilis. Procaine penicillin G was once a commonly used treatment for pneumococcal pneumonia and gonorrhea; however, it is rarely used now because many gonococcal strains are penicillin-resistant, and many pneumococci require higher doses of penicillin G or the use of more potent β-lactams.

B. Penicillins Resistant to Staphylococcal Beta-Lactamase (Methicillin, Nafcillin, Oxacillin, and Isoxazolyl Penicillins)

These semisynthetic penicillins are indicated for infections caused by β-lactamase-producing staphylococci, although penicillin-susceptible strains of streptococci and pneumococci also are susceptible to these agents. *Listeria monocytogenes*, enterococci, and methicillin-resistant strains of staphylococci are resistant. The empiric use of these drugs has decreased substantially because of increasing rates of methicillin resistance in staphylococci. However, for infections caused by methicillin-susceptible and penicillin-resistant strains of staphylococci, these are considered drugs of choice.

An isoxazolyl penicillin such as dicloxacillin, 0.25–0.5 g orally every 4–6 hours (25–100 mg/kg/d for children), is suitable for treatment of mild to moderate localized staphylococcal infections. These drugs are relatively acid-stable and have reasonable bioavailability. However, food interferes with absorption, and the drugs should be administered 1 hour before or after meals.

Methicillin, the first antistaphylococcal penicillin to be developed, is no longer used clinically due to high rates of adverse effects. Oxacillin and nafcillin, 8–12 g/d, given by intermittent intravenous infusion of 1–2 g every 4–6 hours (50–200 mg/kg/d for children), are considered drugs of choice for serious staphylococcal infections such as endocarditis.

C. Extended-Spectrum Penicillins (Aminopenicillins, Carboxypenicillins, and Ureidopenicillins)

These drugs have greater activity than penicillin against gram-negative bacteria because of their enhanced ability to penetrate the gram-negative outer membrane. Like penicillin G, they are inactivated by many β-lactamases.

The aminopenicillins, ampicillin and amoxicillin, have very similar spectrums of activity, but amoxicillin is better absorbed orally. Amoxicillin, 250–500 mg three times daily, is equivalent to the same amount of ampicillin given four times daily. Amoxicillin is given orally to treat otitis and lower respiratory tract infections. Ampicillin and amoxicillin are the most active of the oral β-lactam antibiotics against pneumococci with elevated MICs to penicillin and are the preferred β-lactam antibiotics for treating infections suspected to be caused by these strains. Ampicillin is effective against susceptible strains of *Shigella*, but amoxicillin appears to be less effective. Ampicillin, at dosages of 4–12 g/d intravenously, is useful for treating serious infections caused by susceptible organisms, including anaerobes, enterococci, *L monocytogenes*, and β-lactamase-negative strains of gram-negative cocci and bacilli such as *E coli*, and *Salmonella* sp. Non-β-lactamase-producing strains of *H influenzae* are generally susceptible, but strains that are resistant because of altered PBPs are emerging. Due to production of β-lactamases by gram-negative bacilli, ampicillin can no longer be used for empiric therapy of urinary tract infections and typhoid fever. Ampicillin is not active against *Klebsiella* sp, *Enterobacter* sp, *P aeruginosa*, *Citrobacter* sp, *Serratia marcescens*, indole-positive *Proteus* species, and other gram-negative aerobes that are commonly encountered in hospital-acquired infections. These organisms intrinsically produce β-lactamases that inactivate ampicillin.

The carboxypenicillins, carbenicillin and ticarcillin, were developed to broaden the spectrum of penicillins against gram-negative pathogens, including *P aeruginosa*; however, neither agent is available in the USA. The ureidopenicillin piperacillin is active against many gram-negative bacilli, such as *Klebsiella pneumoniae* and *P aeruginosa*. Piperacillin is available only as a co-formulation with the β-lactamase inhibitor tazobactam. Due to the propensity of *P aeruginosa* to develop resistance during therapy, there has been interest in using an antipseudomonal β-lactam in combination with an aminoglycoside or fluoroquinolone, particularly in infections outside the urinary tract; however, most clinical data do not support combination therapy over single-drug therapy once cultures and susceptibilities are available.

Ampicillin, amoxicillin, and piperacillin are available in combination with one of several β-lactamase inhibitors: **sulbactam, clavulanic acid,** or **tazobactam.** The addition of a β-lactamase inhibitor extends the activity of these penicillins to include β-lactamase-producing strains of *S aureus* as well as some β-lactamase-producing gram-negative bacteria (see Beta-Lactamase Inhibitors).

Adverse Reactions

The penicillins are generally well tolerated, and, unfortunately, this may encourage inappropriate use, a major cause of development of resistance. Most of the serious adverse effects are due to hypersensitivity. The antigenic determinants are degradation products of penicillins, particularly penicilloic acid and products of alkaline hydrolysis bound to host protein. A patient's history of a penicillin reaction is often unreliable. About 5–8% of people report a penicillin allergy, but only a small number of these will have a serious reaction when given penicillin. Less than 1% of persons who previously received penicillin without incident will have an allergic reaction when given penicillin. Because of the potential for anaphylaxis, however, penicillin should be administered with caution or a substitute drug given if the person has a history of serious penicillin allergy. Penicillin skin testing may also be used to evaluate type I hypersensitivity. If skin testing is negative, most patients can safely receive penicillin.

Allergic reactions include anaphylactic shock (very rare—0.05% of recipients); serum sickness–type reactions (now rare—urticaria, fever, joint swelling, angioedema, pruritus, and respiratory compromise occurring 7–12 days after exposure); and a variety of skin rashes. Oral lesions, fever, interstitial nephritis (an autoimmune reaction to a penicillin-protein complex), eosinophilia, hemolytic anemia and other hematologic disturbances, and vasculitis also may occur. Most patients allergic to penicillins can be treated with alternative drugs. However, if necessary (eg, treatment of enterococcal endocarditis or neurosyphilis), desensitization can be accomplished with gradually increasing doses of penicillin in patients with type 1 hypersensitivity.

In patients with renal failure, penicillin in high doses can cause seizures. Nafcillin is associated with neutropenia and interstitial nephritis, oxacillin can cause hepatitis, and methicillin commonly caused interstitial nephritis (and is no longer used for this reason). Large doses of penicillins given orally may lead to gastrointestinal upset, particularly nausea, vomiting, and diarrhea. Penicillins, along with many other antibiotics, are associated with the development of colitis due to *Clostridioides* (formerly *Clostridium*) *difficile* infection. Secondary candidal infections in the oropharynx (thrush) and vagina may occur. Ampicillin and amoxicillin can be associated with skin rashes when prescribed in the setting of viral illnesses, particularly noted during acute Epstein-Barr virus infection, but the incidence of rash may be lower than originally reported. Piperacillin-tazobactam when combined with vancomycin has been associated with greater incidence of acute kidney injury compared to alternate β-lactam agents in combination with vancomycin.

■ CEPHALOSPORINS & CEPHAMYCINS

Cephalosporins are similar to penicillins but are more stable to many bacterial β-lactamases and, therefore, have a broader spectrum of activity. However, strains of *E coli* and *Klebsiella* sp expressing extended-spectrum β-lactamases that can hydrolyze most cephalosporins are a growing clinical concern. Cephalosporins are not active against *L monocytogenes,* and of the available cephalosporins, only ceftaroline has some activity against enterococci when given as a single drug.

Chemistry

The nucleus of the cephalosporins, 7-aminocephalosporanic acid (Figure 43–6), bears a close resemblance to 6-aminopenicillanic acid (see Figure 43–1). The intrinsic antimicrobial activity of natural cephalosporins is low, but the attachment of various R_1 and R_2 groups has yielded hundreds of potent compounds, many with low toxicity. Cephalosporins traditionally have been classified into four major groups or generations, depending mainly on the spectrum of antimicrobial activity. Several cephalosporins developed more recently do not fit the traditional classification groups. Their unique characteristics and spectra of activity are outlined below.

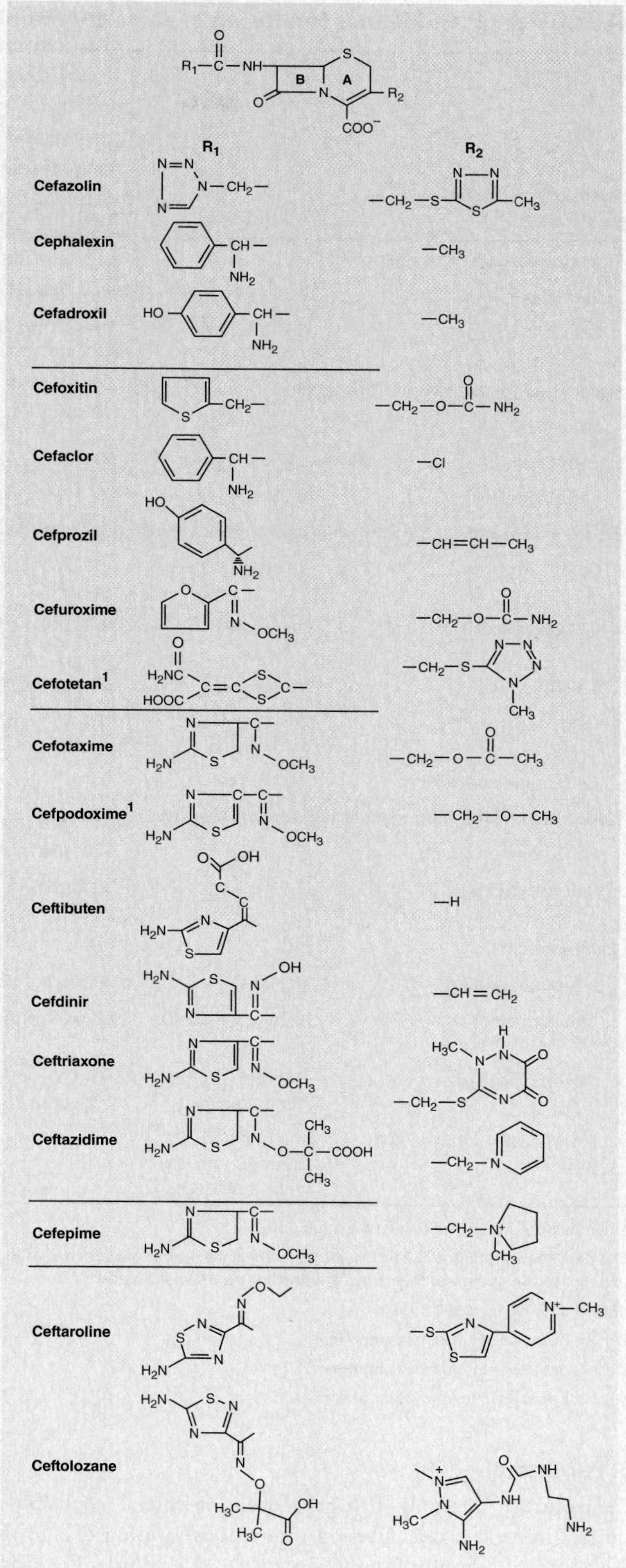

FIGURE 43–6 Structures of some cephalosporins. R_1 and R_2 structures are substituents on the 7-aminocephalosporanic acid nucleus pictured at the top. [1]These structures contain additional substituents that are not shown.

FIRST-GENERATION CEPHALOSPORINS

First-generation cephalosporins include **cefazolin, cefadroxil, cephalexin, cephalothin, cephapirin,** and **cephradine.** Cefazolin and cephalexin are the only two available in the USA. These drugs are very active against gram-positive cocci, such as streptococci and staphylococci. Traditional cephalosporins are not active against methicillin-resistant strains of staphylococci; however, new compounds have been developed that have activity against methicillin-resistant strains (see below). *E coli, K pneumoniae,* and *Proteus mirabilis* are often sensitive to first-generation cephalosporins, but activity against *P aeruginosa,* indole-positive *Proteus* species, *Enterobacter* sp, *S marcescens, Citrobacter* sp, and *Acinetobacter* sp is poor. Gram-positive anaerobic cocci (eg, peptococci, peptostreptococci) are usually sensitive, but *Bacteroides fragilis* is not.

Pharmacokinetics & Dosage

A. Oral

Cephalexin is the oral first-generation agent widely used in the USA. After oral doses of 500 mg, peak serum levels are 15–20 mcg/mL. Urine concentration is usually very high, but in most tissues levels are variable and generally lower than in serum. Cephalexin typically is given in oral dosages of 0.25–0.5 g four times daily (25–100 mg/kg/d in pediatrics). Excretion is mainly by glomerular filtration and tubular secretion into the urine. Drugs that block tubular secretion, eg, probenecid, may increase serum levels substantially. In patients with impaired renal function, dosage must be reduced (Table 43–2).

TABLE 43–2 Guidelines for dosing of some commonly used cephalosporins and carbapenems.

Antibiotic (Route of Administration)	Adult Dose	Pediatric Dose[1]	Neonatal Dose[2]	Adjusted Dose as a Percentage of Normal Dose for Renal Failure Based on Creatinine Clearance (Cl_{cr})	
				Cl_{cr} Approx 50 mL/min	Cl_{cr} Approx 10 mL/min
First-generation cephalosporins					
Cephalexin (PO)	0.25–0.5 g qid	50–100 mg/kg/d in 4 doses		50%	25%
Cefazolin (IV)	0.5–2 g q8h	50–150 mg/kg/d in 3 or 4 doses	50–150 mg/kg/d in 2 or 3 doses	50%	25%
Second-generation cephalosporins					
Cefoxitin (IV)	1–2 g q6–8h	75–150 mg/kg/d in 3 or 4 doses		50–75%	25%
Cefotetan (IV)	1–2 g q12h	60–100 mg/kg/d in 2 doses		50%	25%
Cefuroxime (IV)	0.75–1.5 g q8h	50–100 mg/kg/d in 3 or 4 doses		66%	25–33%
Third- and fourth-generation cephalosporins including ceftaroline fosamil					
Cefotaxime (IV)	1–2 g q6–12h	100–200 mg/kg/d in 4–6 doses	100–200 mg/kg/d in 2 doses	50%	25%
Ceftazidime (IV)	1–2 g q8–12h	100–300 mg/kg/d in 3 doses	100–150 mg/kg/d in 2 or 3 doses	50%	25%
Ceftriaxone (IV)	1–4 g q24h	50–100 mg/kg/d in 1 or 2 doses	50 mg/kg/d qd	None	None
Cefepime (IV)	0.5–2 g q8-12h	100–150 mg/kg/d in 2 or 3 divided doses	60–150 mg/kg/d in 2 or 3 doses	50%	25%
Ceftaroline fosamil (IV)	600 mg q8-12h			50–66%	33%
Cephalosporin–β-lactamase inhibitor combinations					
Ceftazidime-avibactam (IV)	2.5 g q8h	120–150 mg/kg/d in 3 doses[4]		25–50%	6.25–12.5%
Ceftolozane-tazobactam (IV)	1.5 g q8h	60 mg/kg/d in 3 doses[5]	60 mg/kg/d in 3 doses[5]	25–50%	Not studied
Carbapenems					
Ertapenem (IM or IV)	1 g q24h	30 mg/kg/d in 2 doses		100%[3]	50%
Imipenem (IV)	0.25–0.5 g q6–8h	60–100 mg/kg/d in 3 or 4 doses	50–75 mg/kg/d in 2 or 3 doses	75%	50%
Meropenem (IV)	1 g q8h (2 g q8h for meningitis)	60–120 mg/kg/d in 3 doses (maximum of 2 g q8h)	40–90 mg/kg/d in 2 or 3 doses	66%	50%
Meropenem-vaborbactam (IV)	4 g q8h (2 g meropenem, 2 g vaborbactam)			50%	16%

[1]The total dose should not exceed the adult dose.

[2]The dose shown is during the first week of life. The daily dose should be increased by approximately 33–50% after the first week of life. The lower dosage range should be used for neonates weighing less than 2 kg. After the first month of life, pediatric doses may be used.

[3]50% of dose for Cl_{cr} < 30 mL/min.

[4]Dose is based on ceftazidime component.

[5]Dose is based on ceftolozane component.

[6]Dose is based on imipenem component.

B. Parenteral

Cefazolin is the only first-generation parenteral cephalosporin still in general use. After an intravenous infusion of 1 g, the peak level of cefazolin is approximately 185 mcg/mL. The usual intravenous dosage of cefazolin for adults is 0.5–2 g intravenously every 8 hours. Cefazolin can also be administered intramuscularly. Excretion is via the kidney, and dose adjustments must be made for impaired renal function.

Clinical Uses

Oral drugs may be used for the treatment of urinary tract infections and staphylococcal or streptococcal infections, including cellulitis or soft tissue abscess. However, oral cephalosporins should not be relied on in serious systemic infections.

Cefazolin penetrates well into most tissues. It is a drug of choice for surgical prophylaxis and for many streptococcal and staphylococcal infections requiring intravenous therapy. Cefazolin may be used for infections due to *E coli* or *K pneumoniae* when the organism has been documented to be susceptible. Cefazolin does not penetrate the central nervous system and cannot be used to treat meningitis. Cefazolin is better tolerated than antistaphylococcal penicillins, and it has been shown to be effective for serious staphylococcal infections, eg, bacteremia. It can also be used in patients with mild penicillin allergy other than immediate hypersensitivity.

SECOND-GENERATION CEPHALOSPORINS

Members of the second-generation cephalosporins include **cefaclor, cefamandole, cefonicid, cefuroxime, cefprozil, loracarbef,** and **ceforanide**—of which **cefaclor, cefuroxime,** and **cefprozil** are available in the USA—and the structurally related cephamycins **cefoxitin** and **cefotetan,** which have activity against anaerobes. This is a heterogeneous group with differences in activity, pharmacokinetics, and toxicity. In general, second-generation cephalosporins are relatively active against organisms inhibited by first-generation drugs, but, in addition, they have extended gram-negative coverage. *Klebsiella* sp (including those resistant to first-generation cephalosporins) are usually sensitive. Cefuroxime and cefaclor are active against *H influenzae* but not against *Serratia* or *B fragilis*. In contrast, cefoxitin and cefotetan are active against *B fragilis* and some *Serratia* strains but are less active against *H influenzae*. As with first-generation agents, no member of this group is active against enterococci or *P aeruginosa*. Compared with other cephalosporins, cefoxitin shows improved stability in the presence of extended-spectrum β-lactamases produced by *E coli* and *Klebsiella* sp. Clinical data are limited, but it may offer an alternative to carbapenems in treating certain infections due to these organisms. Second-generation cephalosporins may exhibit in vitro activity against *Enterobacter* sp, but resistant mutants that express a chromosomal β-lactamase that hydrolyzes these compounds (and third-generation cephalosporins) are readily selected; these drugs should not be used to treat *Enterobacter* infections.

Pharmacokinetics & Dosage

A. Oral

Cefuroxime axetil is commonly used in the USA. The usual dosage for adults is 250–500 mg orally twice daily; children should be given 20–40 mg/kg/d up to a maximum of 1 g/d. These drugs are not predictably active against penicillin-non-susceptible pneumococci.

B. Parenteral

After a 1-g intravenous infusion, serum levels are 75–125 mcg/mL for most second-generation cephalosporins. Intramuscular administration is painful and should be avoided. Doses and dosing intervals vary depending on the specific agent (see Table 43–2). There are differences in half-life, protein binding, and interval between doses. All are renally cleared and require dosage adjustment in renal failure.

Clinical Uses

The oral second-generation cephalosporins are active against β-lactamase-producing *H influenzae* or *Moraxella catarrhalis* and have been used primarily to treat sinusitis, otitis, and lower respiratory tract infections. Because of their activity against anaerobes (including many *B fragilis* strains), cefoxitin and cefotetan can be used to treat mixed anaerobic infections such as peritonitis, diverticulitis, and pelvic inflammatory disease. Cefuroxime is sometimes used to treat community-acquired pneumonia because it is active against β-lactamase-producing *H influenzae* and also many pneumococci. Although cefuroxime crosses the blood-brain barrier, it is less effective in treatment of meningitis than ceftriaxone or cefotaxime and should not be used.

THIRD-GENERATION CEPHALOSPORINS

Third-generation agents include **cefoperazone, cefotaxime, ceftazidime, ceftizoxime, ceftriaxone, cefixime, cefpodoxime proxetil, cefdinir, cefditoren pivoxil, ceftibuten,** and **moxalactam. Cefoperazone, ceftizoxime, cefditoren,** and **moxalactam** are no longer commercially available in the USA.

Antimicrobial Activity

Compared with second-generation agents, these drugs have expanded gram-negative coverage, and some are able to cross the blood-brain barrier. Third-generation drugs may be active against *Citrobacter*, *S marcescens*, and *Providencia*. They are also effective against β-lactamase-producing strains of *Haemophilus* and *Neisseria*. Ceftazidime is the only agent with useful activity against *P aeruginosa*. Like the second-generation drugs, third-generation cephalosporins are hydrolyzed by AmpC β-lactamase, and they are not reliably active against *Enterobacter* species, which commonly have inducible AmpC β-lactamase production. *Serratia*, *Providencia*, *Acinetobacter*, and *Citrobacter* also produce a chromosomally encoded cephalosporinase that, when constitutively expressed, can confer resistance to third-generation cephalosporins. Cefixime, cefdinir, ceftibuten, and cefpodoxime proxetil are oral agents possessing similar activity except that cefixime and ceftibuten are much less active against pneumococci and have poor activity against *S aureus*.

Pharmacokinetics & Dosage

Intravenous infusion of 1 g of a parenteral cephalosporin produces serum levels of 60–140 mcg/mL. Third-generation cephalosporins penetrate body fluids and tissues well, and when administered intravenously achieve levels in the cerebrospinal fluid sufficient to inhibit most susceptible pathogens.

The half-lives of these drugs and the necessary dosing intervals vary greatly: ceftriaxone (half-life 7–8 hours) can be injected once every 24 hours at a dosage of 15–50 mg/kg/d. A single daily 1-g dose is sufficient for most serious infections, with 2 g every 12 hours recommended for treatment of meningitis and 2 g every 24 hours recommended for endocarditis or osteomyelitis. The remaining drugs in the group (half-life 1–1.7 hours) can be infused every 6–8 hours in dosages between 2 and 12 g/d, depending on the severity of infection. Cefixime can be given orally (200 mg twice daily or 400 mg once daily) for urinary tract infections. Due to increasing resistance, cefixime is no longer recommended for the treatment of uncomplicated gonococcal urethritis and cervicitis. Intramuscular ceftriaxone is the regimen of choice for treating gonococcal infections. The adult dose for cefpodoxime proxetil is 200–400 mg twice daily; for ceftibuten, 400 mg once daily; and for cefdinir, 300 mg/12 h. Ceftriaxone excretion is mainly through the biliary tract, and no dosage adjustment is required for renal impairment. The other third-generation cephalosporins are excreted by the kidney and therefore require dosage adjustment in renal insufficiency.

Clinical Uses

Third-generation cephalosporins are used to treat a wide variety of serious infections caused by organisms that are resistant to many other drugs. Strains expressing extended-spectrum β-lactamases, however, are not susceptible. Third-generation cephalosporins should be avoided in treatment of *Enterobacter* infections—even if the clinical isolate appears susceptible in vitro—because of emergence of resistance. Ceftriaxone and cefotaxime are approved for treatment of meningitis, including meningitis caused by pneumococci, meningococci, *H influenzae*, and susceptible enteric gram-negative rods, but not by *L monocytogenes*. Ceftriaxone and cefotaxime are the most active cephalosporins against penicillin-non-susceptible strains of pneumococci and are recommended for empiric therapy of serious infections that may be caused by these strains. Meningitis caused by strains of pneumococci with penicillin MICs >1 mcg/mL may not respond even to these agents, and addition of vancomycin is recommended. Other potential indications include empiric therapy of sepsis in both the immunocompetent and the immunocompromised patient and treatment of infections for which a cephalosporin is the least toxic drug available.

FOURTH-GENERATION CEPHALOSPORINS

Cefepime is the only available fourth-generation cephalosporin. It is more resistant to hydrolysis by chromosomal β-lactamases (eg, those produced by *Enterobacter*). However, like the third-generation compounds, it is hydrolyzed by extended-spectrum β-lactamases. Cefepime has good activity against *P aeruginosa*, Enterbacterales, methicillin-susceptible *S aureus*, and *S pneumoniae*. It is highly active against *Haemophilus* and *Neisseria* sp. It penetrates well into cerebrospinal fluid. It is cleared by the kidneys and has a half-life of 2 hours, and its pharmacokinetic properties are very similar to those of ceftazidime. Unlike ceftazidime, however, cefepime has good activity against most penicillin-non-susceptible strains of streptococci, and it is useful in treatment of *Enterobacter* infections. The standard dose for cefepime is 1–2 g infused every 12 hours; however, when treating more complicated infections due to *P aeruginosa* or in the setting of immunocompromise, doses are typically increased to 2 g every 8 hours. Because of its broad-spectrum activity, cefepime is commonly used empirically in patients presenting with febrile neutropenia, in combination with other agents.

Cephalosporins Active Against Methicillin-Resistant Staphylococci

Beta-lactam antibiotics with activity against methicillin-resistant staphylococci have now been developed. **Ceftaroline fosamil,** the prodrug of the active metabolite ceftaroline, is the first such drug to be approved for clinical use in the USA. Ceftaroline has increased binding to penicillin-binding protein 2a, which mediates methicillin resistance in staphylococci, resulting in bactericidal activity against these strains. It has some in vitro activity against enterococci and a broad gram-negative spectrum similar to ceftriaxone. It is not active against AmpC or extended-spectrum β-lactamase-producing organisms. Ceftaroline is currently approved for the treatment of skin and soft tissue infections and community-acquired pneumonia at a dose of 600 mg infused every 12 hours. It has been used off-label to treat complicated infections such as bacteremia, endocarditis, and osteomyelitis, sometimes in combination with other agents and often at an increased dose of 600 mg every 8 hours. The normal half-life is about 2.7 hours; ceftaroline is primarily excreted renally and requires dose adjustment in renal impairment.

Cephalosporins Combined with β-lactamase Inhibitors

Novel cephalosporin-β-lactamase inhibitor combinations have been developed to combat resistant gram-negative infections; see the subsequent section for more information on β-lactamase inhibitors. Ceftolozane-tazobactam and ceftazidime-avibactam are both FDA-approved for the treatment of complicated intra-abdominal infections, complicated urinary tract infections, and hospital-acquired and ventilator-associated bacterial pneumonia. Both agents have potent in vitro activity against gram-negative organisms, including *P aeruginosa* and AmpC and extended-spectrum β-lactamase-producing Enterobacterales. While neither agent is active against organisms producing metallo-β-lactamases, ceftazidime-avibactam may be an option for carbapenemase-producing organisms. Due to limited activity against anaerobic pathogens, both should be combined with metronidazole when treating complicated intra-abdominal infections. Both agents have short half-lives of 2–3 hours and are dosed every 8 hours. Both are primarily renally excreted and require dose adjustment in patients with impaired renal clearance.

Siderophore Cephalosporin

A novel cephalosporin called **cefiderocol** is available for treatment of resistant β-lactamase-producing gram-negative organisms. Cefiderocol, like other cephalosporins, works by binding penicillin binding proteins, thus inhibiting cell wall synthesis.

It differs from other β-lactams, which rely on passive transport across porin channels in a bacterial cell wall, in that cefiderocol is bound by active iron transporters and pumped into the bacterial cell at high concentration. In addition to this active transport, cefiderocol is stable in the presence of all types of β-lactamases, including those responsible for multidrug resistance, such as metallo-β-lactamases. Because of these unique characteristics, cefiderocol has potent in vitro activity against aerobic gram-negative organisms, including drug-resistant Enterobacterales, *Pseudomonas aeruginosa*, and *Acinetobacter baumannii*. However, cefiderocol does carry a warning that it is associated with increased mortality in patients with carbapenem-resistant gram-negative infections based on results in one clinical trial. Thus, the drug label indicates that cefiderocol should be reserved for circumstances in which there are limited or no alternative treatment options. It is not expected to have activity against gram-positive or anaerobic organisms.

ADVERSE EFFECTS OF CEPHALOSPORINS

A. Allergy

Like penicillins, cephalosporins may elicit a variety of hypersensitivity reactions, including anaphylaxis, fever, skin rashes, nephritis, granulocytopenia, and hemolytic anemia. Patients with documented penicillin anaphylaxis have an increased risk of reacting to cephalosporins compared with patients without a history of penicillin allergy. However, the chemical nucleus of cephalosporins is sufficiently different from that of penicillins such that many individuals with a history of penicillin allergy tolerate cephalosporins. Overall, the frequency of cross-allergenicity between the two groups of drugs is low (~1%). Cross-allergenicity appears to be most common among penicillin, aminopenicillins, and early-generation cephalosporins, which share similar R-1 side chains. Patients with a history of anaphylaxis to penicillins should not receive first- or second-generation cephalosporins, while third- and fourth-generation cephalosporins should be administered with caution, preferably in a monitored setting.

B. Toxicity

Local irritation can produce pain after intramuscular injection and thrombophlebitis after intravenous injection. Renal toxicity, including interstitial nephritis and tubular necrosis, may occur uncommonly.

Cephalosporins that contain a methylthiotetrazole group may cause hypoprothrombinemia and bleeding disorders. Historically, this group included cefamandole, cefmetazole, and cefoperazone; however, cefotetan is the only methylthiotetrazole-containing agent used in the USA. Oral administration of vitamin K, 10 mg twice weekly, can prevent this uncommon problem. Drugs with the methylthiotetrazole ring can also cause severe disulfiram-like reactions; consequently, alcohol and alcohol-containing medications must be avoided.

OTHER BETA-LACTAM DRUGS

MONOBACTAMS

Monobactams are drugs with a monocyclic β-lactam ring (see Figure 43–1). Their spectrum of activity is limited to aerobic gram-negative organisms (including *P aeruginosa*). Unlike other β-lactam antibiotics, they have no activity against gram-positive bacteria or anaerobes. **Aztreonam** is the only monobactam available in the USA. It has structural similarities to ceftazidime, and its gram-negative spectrum is similar to that of the third-generation cephalosporins. It is stable to many β-lactamases, with notable exceptions being AmpC β-lactamases and extended-spectrum β-lactamases. It penetrates well into the cerebrospinal fluid. Aztreonam is given intravenously every 8 hours in a dose of 1–2 g, providing peak serum levels of 100 mcg/mL. The half-life is 1–2 hours and is greatly prolonged in renal failure.

Penicillin-allergic patients tolerate aztreonam without reaction. Notably, because of its structural similarity to ceftazidime, there is potential for cross-reactivity; aztreonam should be used with caution in the case of documented severe allergies to ceftazidime. Occasional skin rashes and elevations of serum aminotransferases occur during administration of aztreonam, but major toxicity is uncommon. In patients with a history of penicillin anaphylaxis, aztreonam may be used to treat serious infections such as pneumonia, meningitis, and sepsis caused by susceptible gram-negative pathogens.

BETA-LACTAMASE INHIBITORS (CLAVULANIC ACID, SULBACTAM, TAZOBACTAM, AVIBACTAM, & VABORBACTAM)

Traditional β-lactamase inhibitors (clavulanic acid, sulbactam, and tazobactam) resemble β-lactam molecules (Figure 43–7), but they have very weak antibacterial action. They are potent inhibitors of many but not all bacterial β-lactamases and can protect hydrolyzable penicillins from inactivation by these enzymes. The traditional β-lactamase inhibitors are most active against Ambler class A β-lactamases (plasmid-encoded transposable element [TEM] β-lactamases in particular), such as those produced by staphylococci, *H influenzae*, *N gonorrhoeae*, *Salmonella*, *Shigella*, *E coli*, and *K pneumoniae*. They are not good inhibitors of class C β-lactamases produced by *Enterobacter* sp, *Citrobacter* sp, *S marcescens*, and *P aeruginosa*, which typically are chromosomally encoded and may be inducible. However, they do inhibit chromosomal β-lactamases of *B fragilis* and *M catarrhalis*. The novel non-β-lactam β-lactamase inhibitors avibactam and vaborbactam are active against Ambler class A and Ambler class C β-lactamases. Avibactam has activity against some Ambler class D β-lactamases, such as OXA-48, which can confer carbapenem resistance and has been identified in highly resistant *Klebsiella pneumoniae* isolates. **Relebactam** is another β-lactamase inhibitor and is approved for use in a fixed-dose combination with the carbapenem imipenem-cilastatin; it is expected to have activity similar to avibactam.

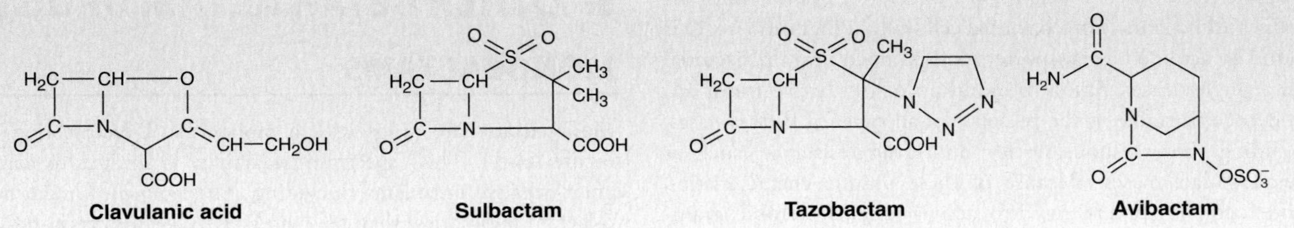

FIGURE 43–7 Beta-lactamase inhibitors.

Beta-lactamase inhibitors are available only in fixed combinations with specific penicillins and cephalosporins. (The fixed combinations available in the USA are listed in Preparations Available.) An inhibitor extends the spectrum of its companion β-lactam provided that the inactivity against a particular organism is due to destruction by a β-lactamase and that the inhibitor is active against the β-lactamase that is produced. Thus, ampicillin-sulbactam is active against β-lactamase-producing *S aureus* and *H influenzae* but not against *Serratia*, which produces a β-lactamase that is not inhibited by sulbactam. Similarly, if a strain of *P aeruginosa* is resistant to piperacillin, it is also resistant to piperacillin-tazobactam because tazobactam does not inhibit the chromosomal β-lactamase produced by *P aeruginosa*.

Beta-lactam–β-lactamase inhibitor combinations are frequently used as empiric therapy for infections caused by a wide range of potential pathogens in both immunocompromised and immunocompetent patients. Adjustments for renal insufficiency are made based on the β-lactam component.

CARBAPENEMS

The carbapenems are structurally related to other β-lactam antibiotics (see Figure 43–1). **Ertapenem, imipenem,** and **meropenem** are licensed for use; doripenem was similar in spectrum to imipenem and meropenem but is no longer available in the USA. Imipenem, the first drug of this class, has a wide spectrum with good activity against most gram-negative rods, including *P aeruginosa*, gram-positive organisms, and anaerobes. It is resistant to most β-lactamases but not serine carbapenemases nor metallo-β-lactamases. *Enterococcus faecium*, methicillin-resistant strains of staphylococci, *Clostridioides difficile*, *Burkholderia cepacia*, and *Stenotrophomonas maltophilia* are resistant. Imipenem is inactivated by dehydropeptidases in renal tubules. Consequently, it is administered together with an inhibitor of renal dehydropeptidase, **cilastatin,** for clinical use. Doripenem and meropenem are similar to imipenem but have slightly greater activity against gram-negative aerobes and slightly less activity against gram-positives. They are not significantly degraded by renal dehydropeptidase and do not require an inhibitor. Despite their broad-spectrum activity, the carbapenems can be degraded by highly resistant organisms, such as carbapenemase-producing gram-negative pathogens, frequently carbapenem-resistant Enterbacterales, or CRE. As a result, novel combination products have been developed. The first to gain FDA approval was meropenem-vaborbactam, which can restore meropenem's activity against certain β-lactamase producers. A fixed-dose combination of imipenem and relebactam also retains activity against these highly drug-resistant organisms. Unlike the other carbapenems, ertapenem does not have appreciable activity against *P aeruginosa* and *Acinetobacter* species. It is not degraded by renal dehydropeptidase.

Carbapenems penetrate body tissues and fluids well, including the cerebrospinal fluid for all but ertapenem; data are limited regarding CNS penetration of meropenem-vaborbactam. All carbapenems are cleared renally, and the dose must be reduced in patients with renal insufficiency. The usual dosage of imipenem is 0.25–0.5 g given intravenously every 6–8 hours (half-life 1 hour). The usual adult dosage of meropenem is 0.5–1 g intravenously every 8 hours; when combined with vaborbactam, the usual dose is 4 g (2 g meropenem and 2 g of vaborbactam) administered as a 3-hour infusion every 8 hours. The usual adult dosage of doripenem is 0.5 g administered as a 1- or 4-hour infusion every 8 hours. Ertapenem has the longest half-life (4 hours) and is administered as a once-daily dose of 1 g intravenously or intramuscularly. Intramuscular ertapenem is irritating, and the drug can be mixed with 1% lidocaine for administration by this route.

A carbapenem is indicated for infections caused by susceptible organisms that are resistant to other available drugs, eg, *P aeruginosa*, and for treatment of mixed aerobic and anaerobic infections. Carbapenems are active against many penicillin-non-susceptible strains of pneumococci. Carbapenems are highly active in the treatment of *Enterobacter* infections because they are resistant to destruction by the β-lactamase produced by these organisms. Clinical experience and data suggest that carbapenems are also the treatment of choice for serious infections caused by extended-spectrum β-lactamase-producing gram-negative bacteria. Ertapenem is not sufficiently active against *P aeruginosa* and should not be used to treat infections caused by this organism. Imipenem, meropenem, or doripenem, with or without an aminoglycoside, may be effective treatment for patients with febrile neutropenia.

The most common adverse effects of carbapenems—which tend to be more common with imipenem—are nausea, vomiting, diarrhea, skin rashes, and reactions at the infusion sites. Excessive levels of imipenem in patients with renal failure may lead to seizures. Meropenem and ertapenem are much less likely to cause seizures than imipenem. Patients allergic to penicillins may be allergic to carbapenems, but the incidence of cross-reactivity is thought to be less than 1%.

Tebipenem pivoxil hydrobromide is an orally bioavailable carbapenem under study in clinical trials. If approved in the USA, it would be the first oral option in the carbapenem class. Due to its broad gram-negative spectrum, it would likely play a role in treating urinary tract infections caused by organisms resistant to other oral antibiotics. It may also be useful in treating infections due to drug-resistant *Shigella* and typhoidal *Salmonella*.

GLYCOPEPTIDE ANTIBIOTICS

VANCOMYCIN

Vancomycin is an antibiotic isolated from the bacterium now known as *Amycolatopsis orientalis.* It is active primarily against gram-positive bacteria due to its large molecular weight and lack of penetration through gram-negative cell membranes. The intravenous product is water soluble and stable for 14 days in the refrigerator following reconstitution.

Mechanisms of Action & Basis of Resistance

Vancomycin inhibits cell wall synthesis by binding firmly to the D-Ala-D-Ala terminus of nascent peptidoglycan pentapeptide (Figure 43–8). This inhibits the transglycosylase, preventing further elongation of peptidoglycan and cross-linking. The peptidoglycan is thus weakened, and the cell becomes susceptible to lysis. The cell membrane also is damaged, which contributes to the antibacterial effect.

Resistance to vancomycin in enterococci is due to modification of the D-Ala-D-Ala binding site of the peptidoglycan building

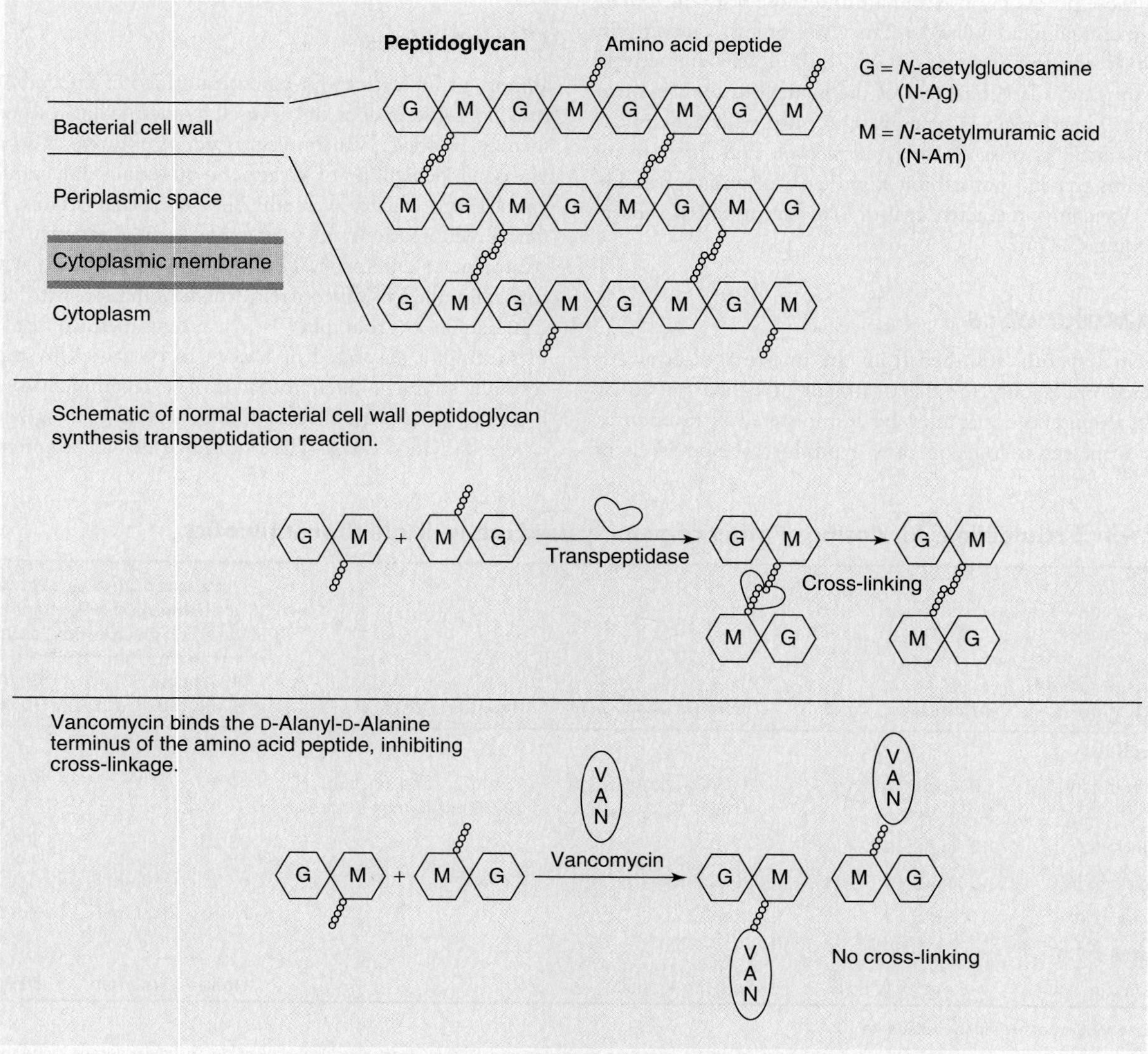

FIGURE 43–8 Schematic of a bacterial cell wall and normal synthesis of cell wall peptidoglycan via transpeptidation; M, *N*-acetylmuramic acid; Glc, glucose; NAcGlc or G, *N*-acetylglucosamine. Vancomycin binds the D-Alanine (D-Ala D-Ala) terminus of the amino acid peptide, inhibiting cross-linkage of the cell wall.

block in which the terminal D-Ala is replaced by D-lactate. This results in the loss of a critical hydrogen bond that facilitates high-affinity binding of vancomycin to its target and loss of activity. This mechanism is also present in rare vancomycin-resistant *S aureus* strains (MIC ≥16 mcg/mL), which have acquired the enterococcal resistance determinants. The underlying mechanism for reduced vancomycin susceptibility in vancomycin-intermediate strains (MIC = 4–8 mcg/mL) of *S aureus* is not fully known. However, these strains have altered cell wall metabolism that results in a thickened cell wall with increased numbers of D-Ala-D-Ala residues, which serve as dead-end binding sites for vancomycin. Vancomycin is sequestered within the cell wall by these false targets and may be unable to reach its site of action.

Antibacterial Activity

Vancomycin is bactericidal for gram-positive bacteria in concentrations of 0.5–10 mcg/mL. Most pathogenic staphylococci, including those producing β-lactamase and those resistant to nafcillin and methicillin, are killed by 2 mcg/mL or less. Vancomycin kills staphylococci relatively slowly and only if cells are actively dividing; the rate is less than that of the penicillins both in vitro and in vivo. Vancomycin is synergistic in vitro with gentamicin and streptomycin against *Enterococcus faecium* and *Enterococcus faecalis* strains that do not exhibit high levels of aminoglycoside resistance. Vancomycin is active against many gram-positive anaerobes including *C difficile*.

Pharmacokinetics

Vancomycin is poorly absorbed from the intestinal tract and is administered orally only for the treatment of colitis caused by *C difficile*. Parenteral doses must be administered intravenously. A 1-hour intravenous infusion of 1 g produces blood levels of 15–30 mcg/mL for 1–2 hours. The drug is widely distributed in the body, including adipose tissue. Cerebrospinal fluid levels 7–30% of simultaneous serum concentrations are achieved if there is meningeal inflammation. Ninety percent of the drug is excreted by glomerular filtration. In the presence of renal insufficiency, striking accumulation may occur (Table 43–3). In functionally anephric patients, the half-life of vancomycin is 6–10 days. A significant amount of vancomycin is removed during a standard hemodialysis run using a high-flux membrane. Traditionally, clinicians and institutions have employed therapeutic-drug monitoring by monitoring trough levels. However, the pharmacokinetic target that has been associated with clinical efficacy has been an AUC:MIC ratio of ≥400 mg-h/L. This has been difficult to measure in clinical practice; however, more tools such as online calculators or pharmacokinetic software have become available. Guidelines suggest that AUC monitoring may be preferred to optimize the time at appropriate targets while decreasing likelihood of developing nephrotoxicity (see Table 43-3).

Clinical Uses

Important indications for parenteral vancomycin are bloodstream infections and endocarditis caused by methicillin-resistant staphylococci. However, vancomycin is not as effective as an antistaphylococcal penicillin for treatment of serious infections such as endocarditis caused by methicillin-susceptible strains. Vancomycin in combination with gentamicin is an alternative regimen for treatment of enterococcal endocarditis in a patient with serious penicillin allergy. Vancomycin (in combination with cefotaxime, ceftriaxone, or rifampin) is also recommended for treatment of meningitis suspected or known to be caused by a penicillin-resistant strain of pneumococcus. The recommended dosage in a patient with normal renal function is 30–60 mg/kg/d in two or three divided doses. The traditional dosing regimen in adults

TABLE 43–3 Guidelines for dosing of other commonly used cell-wall inhibitor antibiotics.

				Adjusted Dose as a Percentage of Normal Dose for Renal Failure Based on Creatinine Clearance (Cl_{cr})	
Antibiotic (Route of Administration)	**Adult Dose**	**Pediatric Dose**[1]	**Neonatal Dose**[2]	**Cl_{cr} Approx 50 mL/min**	**Cl_{cr} Approx 10 mL/min**
Glycopeptides					
Vancomycin (IV)[3]	30–60 mg/kg/d in 2–3 doses	40–60 mg/kg/d in 3 or 4 doses	15 mg/kg load, then 20–30 mg/kg/d in 2 doses	40%	10%
Telavancin (IV)	10 mg/kg daily			75%	50%
Dalbavancin (IV)	1500 mg × 1	18–22.5 mg/kg × 1	22.5 mg/kg × 1	None >30 mL/min	75%
Oritavancin (IV)	1200 mg × 1			None >30 mL/min	Not studied
Lipopeptides (IV)					
Daptomycin	4–6 mg/kg IV daily[4]	4–10 mg/kg daily		None >30 mL/min	50%

[1]The total dose should not exceed the adult dose.

[2]The dose shown is during the first week of life. The daily dose should be increased by approximately 33–50% after the first week of life. The lower dosage range should be used for neonates weighing less than 2 kg. After the first month of life, pediatric doses may be used.

[3]Dose varies based on achievement of pharmacokinetic targets, such as trough concentration or AUC:MIC ratio.

[4]Doses used in clinical practice are often higher; typically 8–10 mg/kg daily, sometimes as high as 12 mg/kg daily.

with normal renal function is 1 g every 12 hours (~30 mg/kg/d); however, this dose typically will not achieve the trough concentrations or AUC:MIC ratio recommended for serious infections. For serious infections (see below), a starting dose of 45–60 mg/kg/d should be given with titration of the dose to achieve trough levels of 15–20 mcg/mL or AUC:MIC ratio of 400–600 mcg*h/mL. The dosage in children is 40–60 mg/kg/d in three or four divided doses. Clearance of vancomycin is directly proportional to creatinine clearance, and the dosage is reduced accordingly in patients with renal insufficiency. For patients receiving hemodialysis, a common dosing regimen is a 1-g loading dose followed by 500 mg after each dialysis session, but this may adjusted based on serum trough concentrations.

Oral vancomycin, 0.125–0.5 g every 6 hours, is used to treat colitis caused by *C difficile* but recent guidelines express a preference for fidaxomicin due to lower rates of relapse.

Adverse Reactions

Adverse reactions with parenteral administration of vancomycin are encountered fairly frequently. Most reactions are relatively minor and reversible. Vancomycin is irritating to tissue, resulting in phlebitis at the site of injection. Chills and fever may occur. Ototoxicity is rare, but nephrotoxicity is still encountered regularly with current preparations, especially with high trough levels. Administration with another ototoxic or nephrotoxic drug, such as an aminoglycoside, increases the risk of these toxicities. Ototoxicity can be minimized by maintaining peak serum concentrations below 60 mcg/mL. Among the more common reactions is infusion-related flushing caused by release of histamine. It can be largely prevented by prolonging the infusion period to 1–2 hours (preferred) or pretreatment with an antihistamine such as diphenhydramine.

TEICOPLANIN

Teicoplanin is a glycopeptide antibiotic that is very similar to vancomycin in mechanism of action and antibacterial spectrum. Unlike vancomycin, it can be given intramuscularly as well as intravenously. Teicoplanin has a long half-life (45–70 hours), permitting once-daily dosing. This drug is available in Europe but has not been approved for use in the USA.

TELAVANCIN

Telavancin is a semisynthetic lipoglycopeptide derived from vancomycin. Telavancin is active versus gram-positive bacteria and has in vitro activity against many strains with reduced susceptibility to vancomycin. Telavancin has two mechanisms of action. Like vancomycin, telavancin inhibits cell wall synthesis by binding to the D-Ala-D-Ala terminus of peptidoglycan in the growing cell wall. In addition, it increases membrane permeability and disrupts the bacterial cell membrane potential. The half-life of telavancin is approximately 8 hours, which supports once-daily intravenous dosing. The drug is approved for treatment of complicated skin and soft tissue infections and hospital-acquired pneumonia at a dose of 10 mg/kg IV daily. Unlike vancomycin therapy, monitoring of serum telavancin levels is not required. In clinical trials, telavancin was associated with substantial nephrotoxicity and concern for increased mortality associated with renal impairment, leading to boxed warnings. It is potentially teratogenic, so administration to pregnant women must be avoided.

DALBAVANCIN AND ORITAVANCIN

Dalbavancin and oritavancin are semisynthetic lipoglycopeptides derived from teicoplanin. Dalbavancin and oritavancin inhibit cell wall synthesis via the same mechanism of action as vancomycin and teicoplanin; oritavancin works by additional mechanisms, including disruption of cell membrane permeability and inhibition of RNA synthesis. Compared with vancomycin, both agents have lower MICs against many gram-positive bacteria including methicillin-resistant and vancomycin-intermediate *S aureus*. Dalbavancin is not active against most strains of vancomycin-resistant enterococci (VRE). Oritavancin has in vitro activity against VRE, but its clinical utility in treating VRE infections remains unclear. Both agents have extremely long half-lives of greater than 10 days, which allows for once-weekly intravenous administration. Dalbavancin and oritavancin have been approved for the treatment of skin and soft tissue infections. Limited clinical data support the use of dalbavancin for uncomplicated catheter-associated bloodstream infections, although it is not FDA-approved for this indication. Dalbavancin was originally approved as a two-dose, once-weekly intravenous regimen (1000 mg infused on day 1 and 500 mg infused on day 8), but a subsequent phase 3 study comparing the two-dose regimen with a single, 1500-mg intravenous dose showed that the single-dose regimen is noninferior. The results of this study allowed for updated labeling, making both dalbavancin and oritavancin appropriate for single-dose treatments for complicated skin and soft tissue infections. Dalbavancin has been studied for the treatment of osteomyelitis, including one trial in which patients received two weekly intravenous doses of 1500 mg and achieved a 97% cure rate. A practical difference between the two is the infusion time: dalbavancin can be administered over 30 minutes, while oritavancin must be infused over 3 hours. Neither requires dose adjustment in mild to moderate renal or hepatic impairment, and neither is removed by dialysis.

■ OTHER CELL WALL- OR MEMBRANE-ACTIVE AGENTS

DAPTOMYCIN

Daptomycin is a novel cyclic lipopeptide fermentation product of *Streptomyces roseosporus* (Figure 43–9). Its spectrum of activity is similar to that of vancomycin except that it may be active against vancomycin-resistant strains of enterococci and *S aureus*. In vitro, it has more rapid bactericidal activity than vancomycin. The precise mechanism of action is not fully understood, but it is known

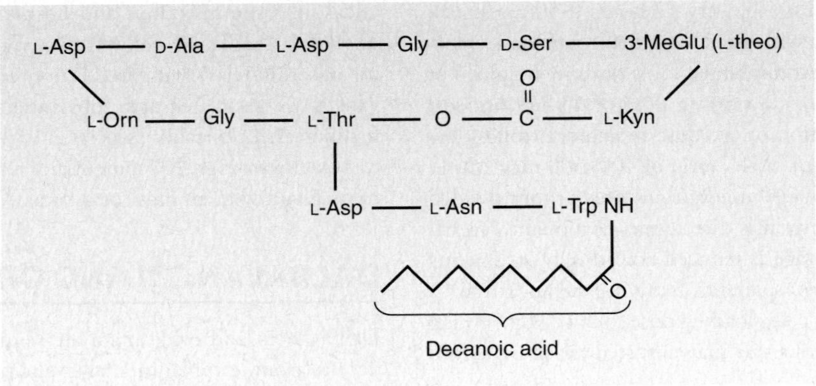

L-Asp — D-Ala — L-Asp — Gly — D-Ser — 3-MeGlu (L-theo)

L-Orn — Gly — L-Thr — O — C(=O) — L-Kyn

L-Asp — L-Asn — L-Trp NH

Decanoic acid

FIGURE 43–9 Structure of daptomycin. (Kyn, deaminated tryptophan.)

to bind to the cell membrane via calcium-dependent insertion of its lipid tail. This results in depolarization of the cell membrane with potassium efflux and rapid cell death (Figure 43–10). Daptomycin is cleared renally. The approved doses are 4 mg/kg/dose for treatment of skin and soft tissue infections and 6 mg/kg/dose for treatment of bacteremia and endocarditis once daily in patients with normal renal function and every other day in patients with creatinine clearance of less than 30 mL/min. For serious infections, many experts recommend using 8–10 mg/kg/dose. These higher doses appear to be safe and well tolerated, although evidence supporting increased efficacy is lacking. In clinical trials, daptomycin was noninferior in efficacy to vancomycin. It can cause myopathy, and creatine phosphokinase levels should be monitored weekly. Pulmonary surfactant antagonizes daptomycin, and it should not be used to treat pneumonia. Daptomycin can also cause an allergic pneumonitis in patients receiving prolonged therapy (>2 weeks). Treatment failures have been reported in association with an increase in daptomycin MIC during therapy. Daptomycin is often an effective alternative to vancomycin, sometimes as monotherapy, or it may be combined with a second antibacterial, such as a β-lactam.

FOSFOMYCIN

Fosfomycin trometamol, a stable salt of fosfomycin (phosphonomycin), inhibits a very early stage of bacterial cell wall synthesis. An analog of phosphoenolpyruvate, it is structurally unrelated to any other antimicrobial agent. It inhibits the cytoplasmic enzyme enolpyruvate transferase by covalently binding to the cysteine

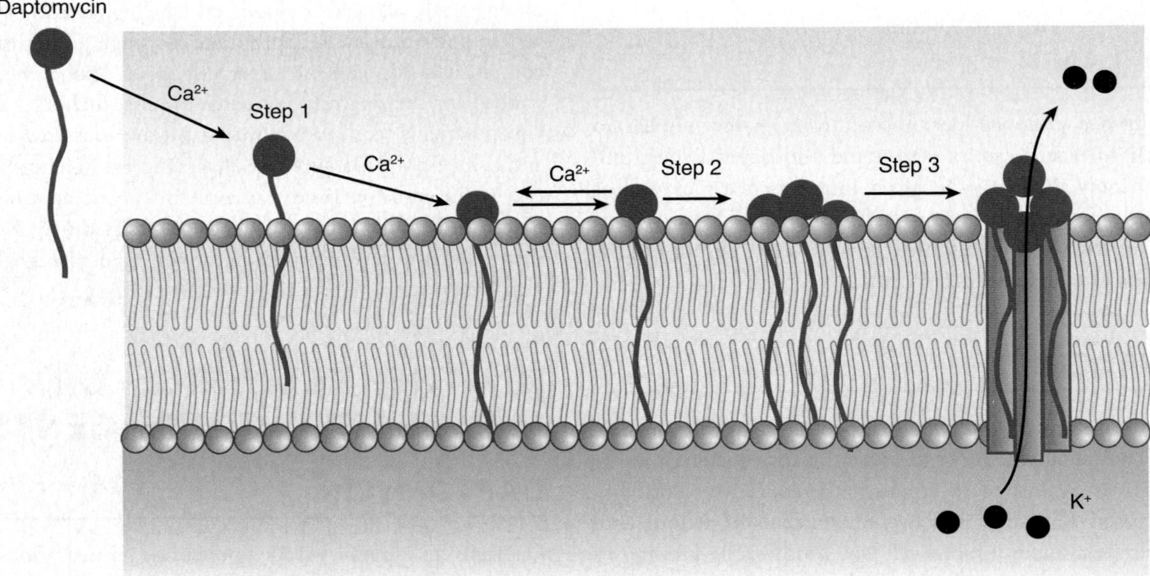

FIGURE 43–10 Proposed mechanism of action of daptomycin. Daptomycin first binds to the cytoplasmic membrane (step 1) and then forms complexes in a calcium-dependent manner (steps 2 and 3). Complex formation causes a rapid loss of cellular potassium, possibly by pore formation, and membrane depolarization. This is followed by arrest of DNA, RNA, and protein synthesis resulting in cell death. Cell lysis does not occur.

residue of the active site and blocking the addition of phosphoenolpyruvate to UDP-*N*-acetylglucosamine. This reaction is the first step in the formation of UDP-*N*-acetylmuramic acid, the precursor of *N*-acetylmuramic acid, which is found only in bacterial cell walls. The drug is transported into the bacterial cell by glycerophosphate or glucose 6-phosphate transport systems. Resistance is due to inadequate transport of drug into the cell.

Fosfomycin is active against both gram-positive and gram-negative organisms at concentrations ≥125 mcg/mL. Susceptibility tests should be performed in growth medium supplemented with glucose 6-phosphate to minimize false-positive indications of resistance. In vitro synergism occurs when fosfomycin is combined with β-lactam antibiotics, aminoglycosides, or fluoroquinolones.

Fosfomycin trometamol is available in both oral and parenteral formulations. Currently, only the oral preparation is approved for use in the USA. Oral bioavailability is approximately 40%. Peak serum concentrations are 10 mcg/mL and 30 mcg/mL following a 2-g or 4-g oral dose, respectively. The half-life is approximately 4 hours. The active drug is excreted by the kidney, with urinary concentrations exceeding MICs for most urinary tract pathogens.

Fosfomycin is approved for use as a single 3-g dose for treatment of uncomplicated lower urinary tract infections (UTI) in women. Limited data in case reports have suggested efficacy in males with UTI and prostatitis; in these cases, a 3-g dose has been given every 3 days for 9 days when treating UTI or 21 days for prostatitis. There is a lack of data to support using oral fosfomycin to treat pyelonephritis. The drug appears to be safe for use in pregnancy.

BACITRACIN

Bacitracin is a cyclic peptide mixture first obtained from the Tracy strain of *Bacillus subtilis* in 1943. It is active against gram-positive microorganisms. Bacitracin inhibits cell wall formation by interfering with dephosphorylation in cycling of the lipid carrier that transfers peptidoglycan subunits to the growing cell wall. There is no cross-resistance between bacitracin and other antimicrobial drugs.

Bacitracin is highly nephrotoxic when administered systemically and is only used topically (Chapter 61). Bacitracin is poorly absorbed, and topical application results in local antibacterial activity. Bacitracin, 500 units/g in an ointment base (often combined with polymyxin or neomycin), is used for the treatment of infections due to mixed bacterial flora in surface lesions of the skin or on mucous membranes. Bacitracin is commonly associated with hypersensitivity and should not be applied to wounds for the purpose of preventing infection.

CYCLOSERINE

Cycloserine is an antibiotic produced by *Streptomyces orchidaceous*. It is water soluble and very unstable at acid pH. Cycloserine inhibits many gram-positive and gram-negative organisms, but it is used almost exclusively to treat tuberculosis caused by strains of *Mycobacterium tuberculosis* resistant to first-line agents (see Chapter 47). Cycloserine is a structural analog of D-alanine and inhibits the incorporation of D-alanine into peptidoglycan pentapeptide by inhibiting alanine racemase, which converts L-alanine to D-alanine, and D-alanyl-D-alanine ligase. After ingestion of 0.25 g of cycloserine, blood levels reach 20–30 mcg/mL—sufficient to inhibit many strains of mycobacteria and gram-negative bacteria. The drug is widely distributed in tissues. Most of the drug is excreted in active form into the urine. The dosage for treating tuberculosis is 0.5 to 1 g/d in two or three divided doses.

Cycloserine causes serious, dose-related central nervous system toxicity with headaches, tremors, acute psychosis, and convulsions. If oral dosages are maintained below 0.75 g/d, such effects can usually be avoided.

SUMMARY Beta-Lactam & Other Cell Wall- & Membrane-Active Antibiotics

Subclass, Drug	Mechanism of Action	Effects	Clinical Applications	Pharmacokinetics, Toxicities, Interactions
PENICILLINS				
• Penicillin G	Prevents bacterial cell wall synthesis by binding to and inhibiting cell wall transpeptidases	Rapid bactericidal activity against susceptible bacteria	Streptococcal infections, meningococcal infections, neurosyphilis	IV administration • rapid renal clearance (half-life 30 min, so requires dosing every 4 h) • *Toxicity:* Immediate hypersensitivity, rash, seizures

- *Penicillin V: Oral, low systemic levels limit widespread use*
- *Benzathine penicillin, procaine penicillin: Intramuscular, long-acting formulations*
- *Nafcillin, oxacillin: Intravenous, added stability to staphylococcal β-lactamase, biliary clearance*
- *Ampicillin, amoxicillin, piperacillin: Greater activity versus gram-negative bacteria; addition of β-lactamase inhibitor restores activity against many -lactamase-producing bacteria*

(continued)

Subclass, Drug	Mechanism of Action	Effects	Clinical Applications	Pharmacokinetics, Toxicities, Interactions
CEPHALOSPORINS				
• Cefazolin	Prevents bacterial cell wall synthesis by binding to and inhibiting cell wall transpeptidases	Rapid bactericidal activity against susceptible bacteria	Skin and soft tissue infections, urinary tract infections, surgical prophylaxis	IV administration • renal clearance (half-life 1.5 h) • given every 8 h • poor penetration into the central nervous system (CNS) • *Toxicity:* Rash, drug fever
• *Cephalexin: Oral, first-generation drug used for treating skin and soft tissue infections and urinary tract infections* • *Cefuroxime: Oral and intravenous, second-generation drug, improved activity versus pneumococcus and* Haemophilus influenzae • *Cefotetan, cefoxitin: Intravenous, second-generation drugs, activity versus* Bacteroides fragilis *allows for use in abdominal/pelvic infections* • *Ceftriaxone: Intravenous, third-generation drug, mixed clearance with long half-life (6 hours), good CNS penetration, many uses including pneumonia, meningitis, pyelonephritis, and gonorrhea* • *Cefotaxime: Intravenous, third-generation, similar to ceftriaxone; however, clearance is renal and half-life is 1 hour* • *Ceftazidime: Intravenous, third-generation drug, poor gram-positive activity, good activity versus* Pseudomonas aeruginosa • *Cefepime: Intravenous, fourth-generation drug, broad activity with improved stability to chromosomal β-lactamases* • *Ceftaroline: Intravenous, active against methicillin-resistant staphylococci, broad gram-negative activity not including* Pseudomonas aeruginosa • *Ceftazidime-avibactam, ceftolozane-tazobactam: Intravenous, cephalosporin-β-lactamase inhibitor combination drugs, broad activity with improved stability to chromosomal β-lactamase and some extended-spectrum β-lactamases*				
CARBAPENEMS				
• Imipenem-cilastatin	Prevents bacterial cell wall synthesis by binding to and inhibiting cell wall transpeptidases	Rapid bactericidal activity against susceptible bacteria	Serious infections such as pneumonia and sepsis	IV administration • renal clearance (half-life 1 h), dosed every 6–8 h, cilastatin added to prevent hydrolysis by renal dehydropeptidase • *Toxicity:* Seizures especially in renal failure or with high doses (>2 g/d)
• *Meropenem, meropenem-vaborbactam: Intravenous, similar activity to imipenem; stable to renal dehydropeptidase, lower incidence of seizures* • *Ertapenem: Intravenous, longer half-life allows for once-daily dosing, lacks activity versus* Pseudomonas aeruginosa *and* Acinetobacter				
MONOBACTAMS				
• Aztreonam	Prevents bacterial cell wall synthesis by binding to and inhibiting cell wall transpeptidases	Rapid bactericidal activity against susceptible bacteria	Infections caused by aerobic, gram-negative bacteria in patients with immediate hypersensitivity to penicillins	IV administration • renal clearance half-life 1.5 h • dosed every 8 h • *Toxicity:* No cross-allergenicity with penicillins
GLYCOPEPTIDE				
• Vancomycin	Inhibits cell wall synthesis by binding to the d-Ala-d-Ala terminus of nascent peptidoglycan	Bactericidal activity against susceptible bacteria, slower kill than -lactam antibiotics	Infections caused by gram-positive bacteria including sepsis, endocarditis, and meningitis • *C difficile* colitis (oral formulation)	Oral, IV administration • renal clearance (half-life 6 h) • starting dose of 30 mg/kg/d in two or three divided doses in patients with normal renal function • trough concentrations of 10–15 mcg/mL sufficient for most infections • *Toxicity:* "Red man" syndrome • nephrotoxicity
• *Teicoplanin: Intravenous, similar to vancomycin except that long half-life (45–70 h) permits once-daily dosing* • *Dalbavancin: Intravenous, very long half-life (>10 days) permits once-weekly dosing* • *Oritavancin: Intravenous, very long half-life (>10 days) permits once-weekly dosing* • *Telavancin: Intravenous, once-daily dosing*				
LIPOPEPTIDE				
• Daptomycin	Binds to cell membrane, causing depolarization and rapid cell death	Bactericidal activity against susceptible bacteria • more rapidly bactericidal than vancomycin	Infections caused by gram-positive bacteria including sepsis and endocarditis	IV administration • renal clearance (half-life 8 h) • dosed once daily • inactivated by pulmonary surfactant so cannot be used to treat pneumonia • *Toxicity:* Myopathy • monitoring of weekly creatine phosphokinase levels recommended

PREPARATIONS AVAILABLE

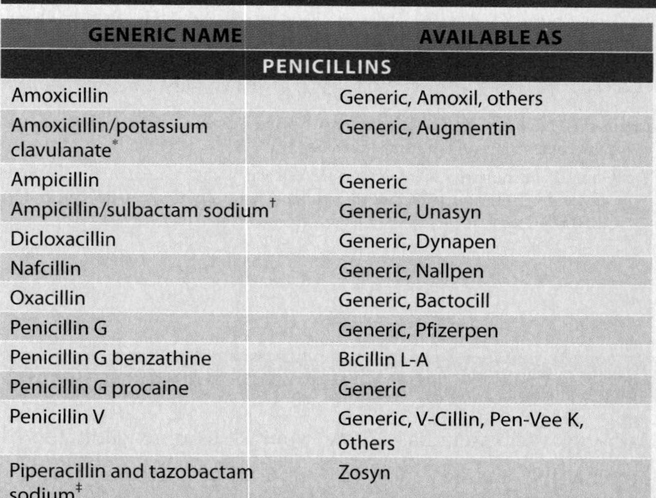

GENERIC NAME	AVAILABLE AS
PENICILLINS	
Amoxicillin	Generic, Amoxil, others
Amoxicillin/potassium clavulanate*	Generic, Augmentin
Ampicillin	Generic
Ampicillin/sulbactam sodium†	Generic, Unasyn
Dicloxacillin	Generic, Dynapen
Nafcillin	Generic, Nallpen
Oxacillin	Generic, Bactocill
Penicillin G	Generic, Pfizerpen
Penicillin G benzathine	Bicillin L-A
Penicillin G procaine	Generic
Penicillin V	Generic, V-Cillin, Pen-Vee K, others
Piperacillin and tazobactam sodium‡	Zosyn
CEPHALOSPORINS & OTHER BETA-LACTAM DRUGS	
Narrow-spectrum (first-generation) cephalosporins	
Cefadroxil	Generic
Cefazolin	Generic, Ancef, Kefzol
Cephalexin	Generic, Keflex, others
Intermediate-spectrum (second-generation) cephalosporins	
Cefaclor	Generic
Cefotetan	Generic, Cefotan
Cefoxitin	Generic
Cefprozil	Generic
Cefuroxime	Generic, Ceftin, Zinacef
Broad-spectrum (third- & fourth-generation) cephalosporins	
Cefdinir	Generic
Cefepime	Generic, Maxipime
Cefixime	Suprax
Cefotaxime	Generic, Claforan
Cefpodoxime proxetil	Generic
Ceftaroline fosamil	Teflaro
Ceftazidime	Generic, Fortaz, Tazicef
Ceftazidime/avibactam§	Avycaz
Ceftibuten	Generic, Cedax
Ceftolozane/tazobactam‖	Zerbaxa
Ceftriaxone	Generic, Rocephin
Monobactam & Carbapenems	
Aztreonam	Generic, Azactam, Cayston
Ertapenem	Generic, Invanz
Imipenem/cilastatin	Generic, Primaxin IM, Primaxin IV
Imipenem/cilastatin-relebactam	Recarbrio
Meropenem	Generic, Merrem IV
Meropenem-vaborbactam±	Vabomere IV
OTHER DRUGS DISCUSSED IN THIS CHAPTER	
Cycloserine	Generic
Dalbavancin	Dalvance
Daptomycin	Generic, Cubicin
Fosfomycin	Monurol
Oritavancin	Orbactiv
Telavancin	Vibativ
Vancomycin	Generic, Vancocin

*Clavulanate content varies with the formulation; see package insert.

†Sulbactam content is half the ampicillin content.

‡Tazobactam content is 12.5% of the piperacillin content.

§Avibactam content is 25% of the ceftazidime content.

‖Tazobactam content is half the ceftolozane content.

±Vaborbactam content is equal to the meropenem content.

REFERENCES

Biek D et al: Ceftaroline fosamil: A novel broad-spectrum cephalosporin with expanded gram-positive activity. J Antimicrob Chemother 2010; 65(Suppl 4):iv9.

Billeter M et al: Dalbavancin: A novel once-weekly lipoglycopeptide antibiotic. Clin Infect Dis 2008;46:577.

Boucher HW et al: Once-weekly dalbavancin versus daily conventional therapy for skin infection. N Engl J Med 2014;370:2169.

Carpenter CF, Chambers HF: Daptomycin: Another novel agent for treating infections due to drug-resistant gram-positive pathogens. Clin Infect Dis 2004;38:994.

Castells M et al: Penicillin allergy. N Engl J Med 2019;381:2338.

Centers for Disease Control and Prevention (CDC): Antibiotic resistance threats in the United States, 2019. https://www.cdc.gov/drugresistance/biggest-threats.html.

Chang C et al: Overview of penicillin allergy. Clinic Rev Allerg Immunol 2012;43:84.

Chovel-Sella A et al: The incidence of rash after amoxicillin treatment in children with infectious mononucleosis. Pediatrics 2013;131:1424.

Corey GR et al: Single-dose oritavancin versus 7-10 days of vancomycin in the treatment of gram-positive acute bacterial skin and skin structure infections: The SOLO II noninferiority study. Clin Infect Dis 2015; 60:254.

DePestel DD et al: Cephalosporin use in treatment of patients with penicillin allergies. J Am Pharm Assoc 2008;48:530.

Fowler VG et al: Daptomycin versus standard therapy for bacteremia and endocarditis caused by *Staphylococcus aureus*. N Engl J Med 2006;355:653.

Jacoby GA, Munoz-Price LS: The new beta-lactamases. N Engl J Med 2005; 352:380.

Johnson S et al: Clinical Practice Guideline by the Infectious Diseases Society of America and Society for Healthcare Epidemiology of America: 2021 Focused Update Guidelines on Management of *Clostridioides difficile* Infection in Adults. Clin Infect Dis 2021;73:e1029.

Keating GM, Perry CM: Ertapenem: A review of its use in the treatment of bacterial infections. Drugs 2005;65:2151.

Kerneis S et al: Cefoxitin as a carbapenem-sparing antibiotic for infections caused by extended-spectrum beta-lactamase producing *Escherichia coli* and *Klebsiella pneumoniae*. Infect Dis 2015;47:789.

Leonard SN, Rybak MJ: Telavancin: An antimicrobial with a multifunctional mechanism of action for the treatment of serious gram-positive infections. Pharmacotherapy 2008;28:458.

Marston HD et al: Antimicrobial resistance. JAMA 2016;316:1193.

Noskin GA et al: National trends in *Staphylococcus aureus* infection rates: Impact on economic burden and mortality over a 6-year period. Clin Infect Dis 2007;45:1132.

Portsmouth S et al: Cefiderocol versus imipenem-cilastatin for the treatment of complicated urinary tract infections caused by Gram-negative uropathogens: A phase 2, randomised, double-blind, non-inferiority trial. Lancet Infect Dis 2018;18:1319.

Rappo U et al: Dalbavancin for the treatment of osteomyelitis in adult patients: A randomized clinical trial of efficacy and safety. Open Forum Infect Dis 2018;6:ofy331.

Rybak M et al: Therapeutic monitoring of vancomycin for serious methicillin-resistant *Staphylococcus aureus* infections: A revised consensus guideline and review of the American Society of Health-System Pharmacists, the Infectious Diseases Society of America, the Pediatric Infectious Diseases Society, and the Society of Infectious Diseases Pharmacists. Am J Health Syst Pharm 2020;77:835.

Sievart DM et al: Vancomycin-resistant Staphylococcus aureus in the United States, 2002-2006. Clin Infect Dis 2008;46:668.

Tamma PD et al: The use of cefepime for treating AmpC β-lactamase-producing enterobacteriaceae. Clin Infect Dis 2013;57:781.

Van Duin D and Bonomo RA: Ceftazidime/avibactam and ceftolozane/tazobactam: Second-generation β-lactam/β-lactamase combinations. Clin Infect Dis 2016;63;234.

CASE STUDY ANSWER

An intravenous third-generation cephalosporin (ceftriaxone or cefotaxime) with adequate penetration into inflamed meninges that is active against the common bacteria that cause community-acquired pneumonia and meningitis in middle-aged adults (pneumococcus and meningococcus) should be ordered. Vancomycin also should be administered until culture and sensitivity results are available in case the patient is infected with a resistant pneumococcus. Although the patient has a history of rash to amoxicillin, the presentation was not consistent with an anaphylactic reaction. The aminopenicillins are frequently associated with rashes that are not caused by type I hypersensitivity. In this instance, cross-reactivity with a cephalosporin is unlikely—particularly with a third-generation drug—and the patient presents with life-threatening illness necessitating appropriate and proven antibiotic coverage.

CHAPTER

44

Tetracyclines, Macrolides, Clindamycin, Chloramphenicol, Streptogramins, Oxazolidinones, & Pleuromutilins

Camille E. Beauduy, PharmD, & Lisa G. Winston, MD*

CASE STUDY

A 22-year-old woman presents to her college medical clinic complaining of a 2-week history of vaginal discharge. She has not had fever or abdominal pain. She has had vaginal intercourse with two men in the last 6 months and used condoms intermittently. A pelvic examination is performed and is positive for mucopurulent discharge from the endocervical canal. No cervical motion tenderness is present. A first-catch urine specimen is obtained for chlamydia and gonorrhea nucleic acid amplification testing. A pregnancy test is also ordered, and the patient reports she "missed her last period." Pending these results, the decision is made to treat her presumptively for chlamydial cervicitis. What are potential treatment options for her possible chlamydial infection? How would pregnancy affect the treatment decision?

The drugs described in this chapter inhibit bacterial protein synthesis by binding to and interfering with ribosomes. Most are bacteriostatic, but a few are bactericidal against certain organisms. Resistance to the older tetracyclines and to macrolides is common. Except for tigecycline, eravacycline, and the streptogramins, these antibiotics may be administered orally.

■ TETRACYCLINES

All of the tetracyclines have the basic structure shown on the next page:

Free tetracyclines are crystalline amphoteric substances of low solubility. They are available as hydrochlorides, which are

*The authors thank Henry F. Chambers, MD, and Daniel H. Deck, PharmD, for their contributions to previous editions.

	R_7	R_6	R_5	R_9
Tetracycline	—H	$—CH_3$	—H	—H
Demeclocycline	—Cl	—H	—H	—H
Doxycycline	—H	$—CH_3$*	—OH	—H
Minocycline	$—N(CH_3)_2$	—H*	—H	—H
Tigecycline	$—N(CH_3)_2$	—H	—H	$—NH—C(=O)—CH_2—NH—C(CH_3)_3$
Eravacycline	—F	—H	—H	$—NH—C(=O)—CH_2—N(CH_2)_4$ (pyrrolidinyl)
Omadacycline	$—N(CH_3)_2$	—H	—H	$—CH_2—NH—CH_2—C(CH_3)_3$

*There is no —OH at position 6 on doxycycline, and minocycline

more soluble. Such solutions are acidic and fairly stable. Tetracyclines chelate divalent metal ions, which can interfere with their absorption and activity. Tigecycline is a glycylcycline and a semisynthetic derivative of minocycline, omadacycline is a synthetic aminomethylcycline derivative of minocycline, and eravacycline is a structural analog of tigecycline classified as a fluorocycline.

Mechanism of Action & Antimicrobial Activity

Tetracyclines are broad-spectrum bacteriostatic antibiotics that inhibit protein synthesis. Tetracyclines enter microorganisms in part by passive diffusion and in part by an energy-dependent process of active transport. Susceptible organisms concentrate the drug intracellularly. Once inside the cell, tetracyclines bind reversibly to the 30S subunit of the bacterial ribosome, blocking the binding of aminoacyl-tRNA to the acceptor site on the mRNA-ribosome complex (Figure 44–1). This prevents addition of amino acids to the growing peptide.

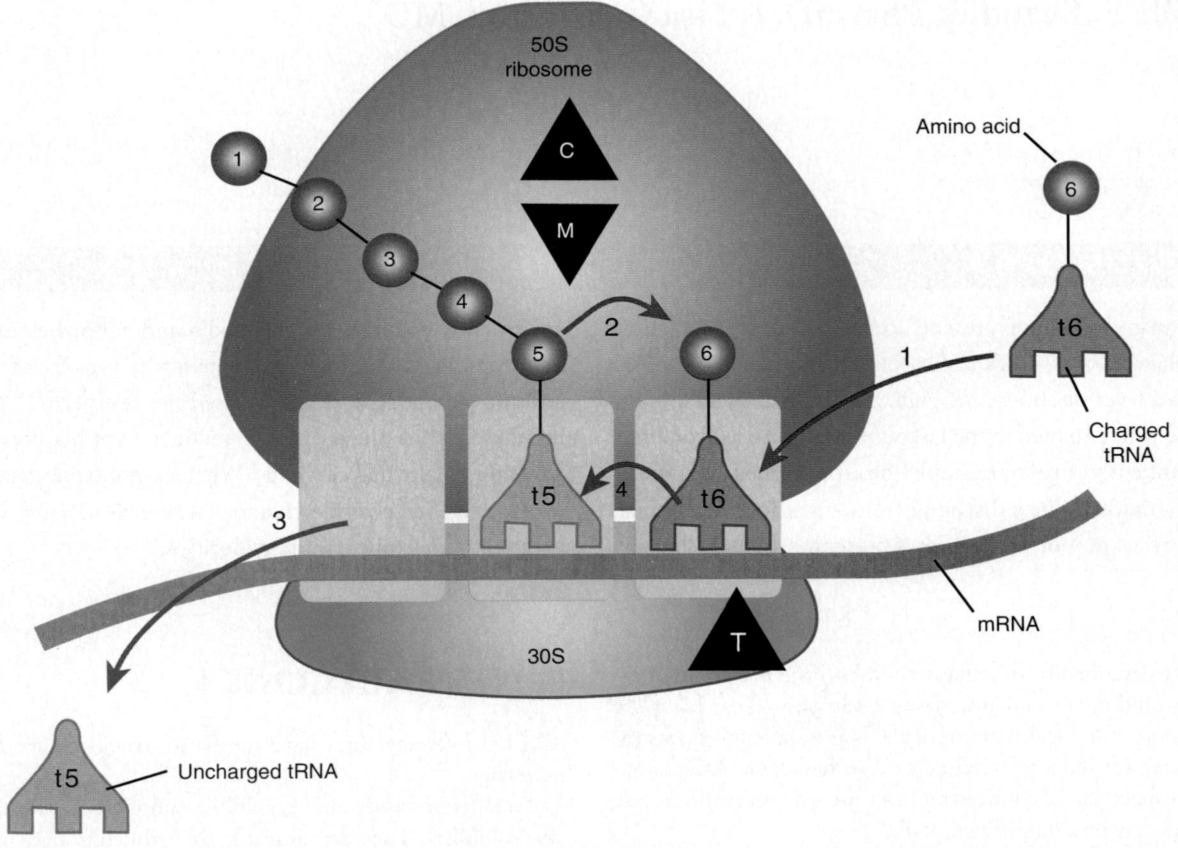

FIGURE 44–1 Steps in bacterial protein synthesis and targets of several antibiotics. Amino acids are shown as numbered circles. The 70S ribosomal mRNA complex is shown with its 50S and 30S subunits. In step 1, the charged tRNA unit carrying amino acid 6 binds to the acceptor site on the 70S ribosome. The peptidyl tRNA at the donor site, with amino acids 1 through 5, then binds the growing amino acid chain to amino acid 6 (peptide bond formation, step 2). The uncharged tRNA left at the donor site is released (step 3), and the new 6-amino acid chain with its tRNA shifts to the peptidyl site (translocation, step 4). The antibiotic binding sites are shown schematically as triangles. Chloramphenicol (C) and macrolides (M) bind to the 50S subunit and block peptide bond formation (step 2). The tetracyclines (T) bind to the 30S subunit and prevent binding of the incoming charged tRNA unit (step 1).

Tetracyclines are active against many gram-positive and gram-negative bacteria, including certain anaerobes, rickettsiae, chlamydiae, and mycoplasmas. For susceptible organisms, differences in clinical efficacy may be attributable to features of absorption, distribution, and excretion of individual drugs. Tetracycline-resistant strains may be susceptible to doxycycline and minocycline, which are poor substrates for the efflux pump, when that is the mechanism of resistance. Similarly, the broader-spectrum drugs, tigecycline, eravacycline, and omadacycline, retain activity against tetracycline-resistant strains, whether the mechanism of resistance is due to ribosomal protection or drug efflux.

Resistance

Three mechanisms of resistance to tetracycline analogs have been described: (1) impaired influx or increased efflux by an active transport protein pump; (2) ribosome protection due to production of proteins that interfere with tetracycline binding to the ribosome; and (3) enzymatic inactivation. The most important of these are production of an efflux pump and ribosomal protection. Tet(AE) efflux pump–expressing gram-negative species are resistant to the older tetracyclines, doxycycline, and minocycline. They are susceptible, however, to tigecycline, eravacycline, and omadacycline, which are not substrates of these pumps. Similarly, a different pump [Tet(K)] of staphylococci confers resistance to tetracycline but not to doxycycline, minocycline, tigecycline, eravacycline, or omadacycline, none of which is a pump substrate. The Tet(M) ribosomal protection protein expressed by gram-positives produces resistance to tetracycline, doxycycline, and minocycline, but not to tigecycline, eravacycline, or omadacycline—which, because of bulky substituents, have a steric hindering effect on Tet(M) binding to the ribosome. Tigecycline, eravacycline, and omadacycline are substrates of the chromosomally encoded multidrug efflux pumps of *Proteus* sp and *Pseudomonas aeruginosa*, accounting for the intrinsic resistance of these organisms, and their resistance to all other tetracyclines.

Pharmacokinetics

Tetracyclines differ in their absorption after oral administration and in their elimination. Absorption after oral administration is approximately 60–70% for tetracycline and demeclocycline (not typically used as an antibiotic; see below) and 95–100% for doxycycline and minocycline. Tigecycline and eravacycline are poorly absorbed orally and must be administered intravenously. Omadacycline bioavailability is approximately 35%, so the oral formulation is three times the intravenous dose. A portion of an orally administered dose of tetracycline remains in the gut lumen, alters intestinal flora, and is excreted in the feces. Absorption occurs mainly in the upper small intestine and is impaired by multivalent cations (Ca^{2+}, Mg^{2+}, Fe^{2+}, Al^{3+}); by dairy products and antacids, which contain multivalent cations; and by alkaline pH. Tetracycline, demeclocycline, and omadacycline should be administered on an empty stomach, while doxycycline and minocycline absorption is not impaired by food. Specially buffered doxycycline and minocycline solutions are formulated for intravenous administration.

Tetracyclines are 40–80% bound by serum proteins, with the exception of omadacycline, which is only 20% protein-bound. Oral dosages of 500 mg every 6 hours of tetracycline hydrochloride produce peak blood levels of 4–6 mcg/mL. Peak levels of 2–4 mcg/mL are achieved with a 200-mg dose of doxycycline or minocycline. The following are the steady-state peak serum concentrations after standard dosages of other tetracyclines: tigecycline 0.6 mcg/mL; eravacycline 1.8 mcg/mL; and omadacycline 2 mcg/mL for intravenous and 0.9 mcg/mL for oral administration. Tetracyclines are distributed widely to tissues and body fluids except for cerebrospinal fluid, where concentrations are 10–25% of those in serum. Tetracyclines cross the placenta and are also excreted in breast milk. As a result of chelation with calcium, tetracyclines bind to—and damage—growing bones and teeth. Carbamazepine, phenytoin, barbiturates, and chronic alcohol ingestion may shorten the half-life of tetracycline, doxycycline, and eravacycline by 50% due to induction of hepatic enzymes that metabolize the drugs.

Tetracyclines are excreted mainly in bile and urine. Concentrations in bile exceed those in serum 10-fold. Some of the drug excreted in bile is reabsorbed from the intestine (enterohepatic circulation) and may contribute to maintenance of serum levels. Ten to fifty percent of various tetracyclines is excreted into the urine, mainly by glomerular filtration. Ten to forty percent of the drug is excreted in feces. Doxycycline and tigecycline, in contrast to other tetracyclines, are eliminated by nonrenal mechanisms and do not accumulate significantly in renal failure, requiring no dosage adjustment.

The older tetracyclines have been classified as short-acting (tetracycline, as well as the agricultural agents chlortetracycline and oxytetracycline), intermediate-acting (demeclocycline), or long-acting (doxycycline and minocycline) based on serum half-lives of 6–8 hours, 12 hours, and 16–18 hours, respectively. Tigecycline, eravacycline, and omadacycline have long half-lives of 36, 20, and 16 hours, respectively. Despite these prolonged half-lives, tigecycline and eravacycline require twice-daily dosing to maintain adequate serum concentrations; however, omadacycline can be dosed once daily after an initial loading dose. The almost complete absorption and slow excretion of doxycycline and minocycline allow for once-daily dosing for certain indications, but, by convention, these two drugs are usually dosed twice daily.

Clinical Uses

A tetracycline is the drug of choice in the treatment of most infections caused by rickettsiae and *Borrelia* sp, including Rocky Mountain spotted fever and Lyme disease. Tetracyclines are used preferentially to treat *Anaplasma phagocytophilum* and *Ehrlichia* sp. Tetracyclines are also excellent drugs for the treatment of *Mycoplasma pneumoniae*, chlamydiae, and some spirochetes. They are used in combination regimens to treat gastric and duodenal ulcer disease caused by *Helicobacter pylori*. They may be used in various gram-positive and gram-negative bacterial infections, including vibrio infections, provided the organism is not resistant. In susceptible cholera, tetracyclines rapidly stop the shedding of vibrios, but tetracycline resistance is a problem. Tetracyclines remain effective in chlamydial infections, including sexually transmitted infections. **Doxycycline** is also an alternative agent recommended by the Centers for Disease Control and Prevention for primary and secondary syphilis in patients with penicillin allergy. A tetracycline—in combination with other antibiotics—is indicated for plague, tularemia, brucellosis, and bartonellosis. Tetracyclines are sometimes used in the treatment or prophylaxis of protozoal infections, eg, those due to *Plasmodium falciparum* (see Chapter 52). Other uses include treatment of acne, exacerbations of bronchitis, community-acquired pneumonia, leptospirosis, and some nontuberculous mycobacterial infections (eg, *Mycobacterium marinum*). Tetracyclines formerly were used for a variety of common infections, including bacterial gastroenteritis and urinary tract infections. However, many strains of bacteria causing these infections are now resistant, and other agents have largely supplanted tetracyclines.

Minocycline, 100 mg orally twice daily for 5 days, can eradicate the meningococcal carrier state, but, because of side effects and resistance of many meningococcal strains, ciprofloxacin or rifampin is preferred. **Demeclocycline** is rarely used as an antibacterial, but it has been used off-label in the treatment of inappropriate secretion of antidiuretic hormone because of its inhibition of antidiuretic hormone in the renal tubule (see Chapter 15).

Tigecycline, the first glycylcycline to reach clinical practice, and the subsequently developed analogs **eravacycline** and **omadacycline** have several unique features that warrant their consideration apart from the older tetracyclines. Their spectra of activity are very broad, and many tetracycline-resistant strains are susceptible because they are not affected by the common resistance determinants. Susceptible organisms include coagulase-negative staphylococci and *Staphylococcus aureus*, including methicillin-resistant, vancomycin-intermediate, and vancomycin-resistant strains; streptococci, penicillin-susceptible and resistant; enterococci, including vancomycin-resistant strains; gram-positive rods; Enterobacterales; multidrug-resistant strains of *Acinetobacter* sp; anaerobes, both gram-positive and gram-negative; rickettsiae, *Chlamydia* sp, and *Legionella pneumophila*; and rapidly growing mycobacteria. *Proteus* and *Providencia* sp and *P aeruginosa*, however, are intrinsically resistant.

Tigecycline, formulated for intravenous administration only, is given as a 100-mg loading dose, then 50 mg every 12 hours. Eravacycline is available only for intravenous use. It is given as a 1-mg/kg dose every 12 hours; it must be adjusted to 1.5 mg/kg every 12 hours when coadministered with potent CYP3A inducers, such as rifampin. Omadacycline is available in both intravenous and oral formulations; the intravenous form should be given as 100 mg twice daily on the first day, then once daily thereafter. The oral form can be given as 450 mg once daily on Days 1 and 2, then 300 mg daily thereafter. As with all tetracyclines, tissue and intracellular penetration with these agents is excellent; consequently, the volume of distribution is quite large and peak serum concentrations are low. Elimination is primarily biliary, and no dosage adjustment is needed for patients with renal insufficiency. In addition to the tetracycline class effects, the chief adverse effect of tigecycline is nausea, which occurs in up to one-third of patients, and occasionally vomiting; nausea has been the most commonly reported adverse effect for eravacycline and omadacycline as well, but it appears to be less common.

Tigecycline is approved for treatment of skin and skin-structure infection, intra-abdominal infections, and community-acquired pneumonia. However, in a meta-analysis of clinical trials, tigecycline was associated with a small but significant increase in the risk of death compared with other antibiotics used to treat these infections. The increased risk was most apparent in hospital-acquired and ventilator-associated pneumonia but was also seen in other infections. This led the US Food and Drug Administration (FDA) to issue a black box warning that tigecycline should be reserved for situations where alternative treatments are not suitable. Because active drug concentrations in the urine and serum are relatively low, tigecycline may not be effective for urinary tract infections or primary bacteremia. Tigecycline has in vitro activity against a wide variety of multidrug-resistant pathogens (eg, methicillin-resistant *S aureus*, extended-spectrum β-lactamase-producing gram-negatives, and *Acinetobacter* sp); however, its clinical efficacy in infections with multidrug-resistant organisms, compared with other agents, is unclear.

Eravacycline is approved for the treatment of complicated intra-abdominal infections based on two phase 3 trials showing noninferiority to comparators (ertapenem in one study, meropenem in the other) for this indication. Like tigecycline, it retains activity against many multidrug-resistant organisms. In vitro studies suggest that it may be two to four times more potent than tigecycline, but clinical studies are not complete. Of note, eravacycline should not be used to treat urinary tract infections because it failed to show noninferiority to comparator agents (levofloxacin or ertapenem) in two separate phase 3 trials.

Omadacycline is approved for the treatment of community-acquired bacterial pneumonia and acute bacterial skin and skin structure infections based on two different phase 3 trials showing noninferiority to comparators (moxifloxacin and linezolid, respectively). Similar to tigecycline and eravacycline, omadacycline is not affected by the most common resistance mechanisms; thus, it retains activity against a broad array of pathogens resistant to older drugs. It differs from tigecycline and eravacycline in its much lower protein-binding and its availability as an oral formulation. Of note, coadministration with any food leads to substantial decreases in absorption of the oral form, so omadacycline must be administered at least 4 hours after and 2 hours before any food or liquid other than water. Like other tetracyclines, its absorption is decreased by coadministration of calcium and other metal cations, so supplements such as antacids or multivitamins must be given at least 4 hours before or after omadacycline.

A. Oral Dosage

The oral dosage for tetracycline hydrochloride is 0.25–0.5 g four times daily for adults and 25–50 mg/kg/d for children (8 years of age and older). For severe systemic infections, the higher dosage is indicated, at least for the first few days. The dosage for doxycycline is 100 mg once or twice daily; the minocycline dose is 100 mg twice daily; the omadacycline maintenance dose is 300 mg once daily. Doxycycline is the oral tetracycline of choice for most indications because it is generally well tolerated, it can be given twice daily, and its absorption is not significantly affected by food. All tetracyclines chelate with metals and should not be administered orally with milk, antacids, or ferrous sulfate. To avoid deposition in growing bones or teeth, tetracyclines should be avoided in pregnant women and children younger than 8 years except in unusual circumstances, eg, treatment of suspected Rocky Mountain spotted fever.

B. Parenteral Dosage

Doxycycline and minocycline are available for intravenous injection and are given at the same doses as the oral formulations; omadacycline's intravenous maintenance dose is 100 mg daily, which is lower than the oral dose due to limited oral bioavailability. As described previously, tigecycline and eravacycline are available only as intravenous injectable forms. Intramuscular injection is not recommended because of pain and inflammation at the injection site.

Adverse Reactions

Hypersensitivity reactions (drug fever, skin rashes) to tetracyclines are uncommon. Most adverse effects are due to direct toxicity of the drug or to alteration of microbial flora.

A. Gastrointestinal Adverse Effects

Nausea, vomiting, and diarrhea are the most common reasons for discontinuing tetracyclines. These effects are attributable to direct local irritation of the intestinal tract. Oral tetracyclines can rarely cause esophageal ulceration, so patients should be instructed to take them with 8 ounces of water and remain upright for at least 30 minutes after each dose.

Tetracyclines alter the normal gastrointestinal flora, with suppression of susceptible coliform organisms and overgrowth of *Pseudomonas*, *Proteus*, staphylococci, resistant coliforms, clostridia, and *Candida*. This can result in intestinal functional disturbances, anal pruritus, vaginal or oral candidiasis, or *Clostridioides difficile* colitis. However, the risk of *C difficile* colitis may be lower with tetracyclines than with other antibiotics.

B. Bony Structures and Teeth

Tetracyclines are readily bound to calcium deposited in newly formed bone or teeth in young children. When a tetracycline is given during pregnancy, it can be deposited in the fetal teeth, leading to fluorescence, discoloration, and enamel dysplasia. It can also be deposited in bone, where it may cause deformity or growth inhibition. Because of these effects, tetracyclines are generally avoided in pregnancy. If the drug is given for long periods to children younger than 8 years, similar changes can result.

C. Other Toxicities

Tetracyclines can impair hepatic function, especially during pregnancy, in patients with preexisting liver disease, and when high doses are given intravenously. Hepatic necrosis has been reported with daily doses of 4 g or more intravenously. Renal tubular acidosis and Fanconi syndrome have been attributed to the administration of outdated tetracycline preparations. Tetracyclines given along with diuretics may cause nephrotoxicity. Tetracycline and minocycline may accumulate to toxic levels in patients with impaired kidney function. Intravenous injection can lead to venous thrombosis. Intramuscular injection produces painful local irritation and should be avoided. Systemically administered tetracyclines commonly induce sensitivity to sunlight or ultraviolet light, particularly in fair-skinned persons. Dizziness, vertigo, and tinnitus have been noted, particularly with high doses or prolonged administration of minocycline. These symptoms may also occur with higher doses of doxycycline.

■ MACROLIDES

The macrolides are a group of closely related compounds characterized by a macrocyclic lactone ring (usually containing 14 or 16 atoms) to which deoxy sugars are attached. The prototype drug, erythromycin, which consists of two sugar moieties attached to a 14-atom lactone ring, was obtained in 1952 from *Streptomyces erythreus*, now called *Saccharopolyspora erythraea*. Clarithromycin and azithromycin are semisynthetic derivatives of erythromycin.

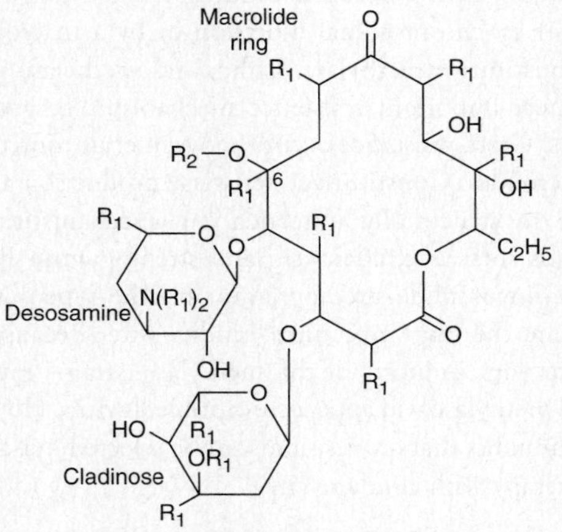

Erythromycin ($R_1 = CH_3$, $R_2 = H$)
Clarithromycin (R_1, $R_2 = CH_3$)

ERYTHROMYCIN

Chemistry

The general structure of erythromycin is shown with the macrolide ring and the sugars desosamine and cladinose. It is poorly soluble in water (0.1%) but dissolves readily in organic solvents. Solutions are fairly stable at 4°C but lose activity rapidly at 20°C and at acid pH. Erythromycins are usually dispensed as esters and salts.

Mechanism of Action & Antimicrobial Activity

The antibacterial action of erythromycin and other macrolides may be inhibitory or bactericidal, particularly at higher concentrations, for susceptible organisms. Activity is enhanced at alkaline pH.

Inhibition of protein synthesis occurs via binding to the 50S ribosomal RNA. The binding site is near the peptidyltransferase center, and peptide chain elongation (ie, transpeptidation) is prevented by blocking of the polypeptide exit tunnel. As a result, peptidyl-tRNA is dissociated from the ribosome. Erythromycin also inhibits the formation of the 50S ribosomal subunit (see Figure 44–1).

Erythromycin is active against susceptible strains of gram-positive organisms, especially pneumococci, streptococci, staphylococci, and corynebacteria. *Mycoplasma pneumoniae*, *L pneumophila*, *Chlamydia trachomatis*, *Chlamydophila psittaci*, *Chlamydophila pneumoniae*, *H pylori*, *Listeria monocytogenes*, and certain mycobacteria *(Mycobacterium kansasii*, *Mycobacterium scrofulaceum)* also are susceptible. Gram-negative organisms such as *Neisseria* sp, *Bordetella pertussis*, *Bartonella henselae*, and *Bartonella quintana* as well as some *Rickettsia* species, *Treponema pallidum*, and *Campylobacter* species are susceptible. *Haemophilus influenzae* is somewhat less susceptible.

Resistance to erythromycin is usually plasmid-encoded. Three general mechanisms have been identified: (1) reduced permeability of the cell membrane or active efflux; (2) production (by Enterobacteriales) of esterases that hydrolyze macrolides; and (3) modification of the ribosomal binding site (so-called ribosomal protection) by chromosomal mutation or by a macrolide-inducible or constitutive methylase. Efflux and methylase production are the most important resistance mechanisms in gram-positive organisms. Cross-resistance occurs between erythromycin and the other macrolides. Constitutive methylase production also confers resistance to structurally unrelated but mechanistically similar compounds such as clindamycin and streptogramin B (so-called macrolide-lincosamide-streptogramin, or MLS-type B, resistance), which share the same ribosomal binding site. Because nonmacrolides are poor inducers of the methylase, strains expressing an inducible methylase will appear susceptible in vitro. However, constitutive mutants that are resistant can be selected out and emerge during therapy with clindamycin.

Pharmacokinetics

Erythromycin base is destroyed by stomach acid and must be administered with enteric coating. Food interferes with absorption. The stearate and ethylsuccinate formulations are fairly acid-resistant and somewhat better absorbed. A 500-mg intravenous dose of erythromycin lactobionate produces serum concentrations of 10 mcg/mL 1 hour after dosing. The serum half-life is approximately 1.5 hours normally and 5 hours in patients with anuria. Adjustment for renal failure is not necessary. Erythromycin is not removed by dialysis. Large amounts of an administered dose are excreted in the bile, and only 5% is excreted in the urine. Absorbed drug is distributed widely except to the brain and cerebrospinal fluid. Erythromycin is taken up by polymorphonuclear leukocytes and macrophages. It traverses the placenta and reaches the fetus.

Clinical Uses

Erythromycin has been a traditional drug of choice in certain corynebacterial infections (eg, diphtheria and erythrasma) and in respiratory, neonatal, ocular, or genital chlamydial infections. While it was used in treatment of community-acquired pneumonia because its spectrum of activity includes the pneumococcus, *M pneumoniae*, and *L pneumophila*, newer macrolides are better tolerated and more commonly selected. Macrolide resistance is increasing in pneumococci and *M pneumoniae*. Erythromycin had also been useful as a penicillin substitute in penicillin-allergic individuals with infections caused by staphylococci and streptococci. Emergence of erythromycin resistance in staphylococci and in strains of group A streptococci has made macrolides less attractive as first-line agents for treatment of pharyngitis and skin and soft tissue infections. Erythromycin has been studied as prophylaxis against endocarditis during dental procedures in individuals with valvular heart disease who are unable to tolerate the first-line amoxicillin, but other better tolerated agents are recommended, such as cephalexin, azithromycin, clarithromycin, or doxycycline.

The oral dosage of erythromycin base or stearate is 0.25–0.5 g every 6 hours (for children, 40 mg/kg/d). The dosage of erythromycin ethylsuccinate is 0.4–0.8 g every 6 hours. Oral erythromycin base (1 g) is sometimes combined with oral neomycin or kanamycin for preoperative preparation of the colon. The intravenous dosage of erythromycin lactobionate is 0.5–1.0 g every 6 hours for adults and 15–20 mg/kg/d divided every 6 hours for children. The higher dosage is recommended when treating pneumonia caused by *L pneumophila*.

Adverse Reactions

Anorexia, nausea, vomiting, and diarrhea are common. Gastrointestinal intolerance, which is due to a direct stimulation of gut motility, is a common reason for selecting an alternative to erythromycin. This side effect may actually be desirable in some circumstances, leading to the off-label use of erythromycin to treat patients with gastroparesis.

Erythromycins, particularly the older estolate formulation, can produce acute cholestatic hepatitis (fever, jaundice, impaired liver function), probably as a hypersensitivity reaction. Other allergic reactions include fever, eosinophilia, and rashes.

Erythromycin metabolites inhibit cytochrome P450 enzymes and, thus, increase the serum concentrations of numerous drugs, including azole antifungal agents, direct-acting anticoagulants, warfarin, cyclosporine, and methylprednisolone. Erythromycin increases serum concentrations of oral digoxin by increasing its bioavailability.

CLARITHROMYCIN

Clarithromycin is derived from erythromycin by addition of a methyl group and has improved acid stability and oral absorption compared with erythromycin. Its mechanism of action is the same as that of erythromycin. Clarithromycin is available only as an oral preparation. Clarithromycin and erythromycin are similar with respect to antibacterial activity except that clarithromycin is more active against *Mycobacterium avium* complex (see Chapter 47). Clarithromycin also has activity against *Mycobacterium leprae*, *Toxoplasma gondii*, and *H influenzae*. Erythromycin-resistant streptococci and staphylococci are also resistant to clarithromycin.

A 500-mg dose of clarithromycin produces serum concentrations of 2–3 mcg/mL. The longer half-life of clarithromycin (6 hours) compared with erythromycin permits twice-daily dosing. The recommended dosage is 250–500 mg orally twice daily or 1000 mg of the extended-release formulation once daily. Clarithromycin penetrates most tissues well, with concentrations equal to or exceeding serum concentrations.

Clarithromycin is metabolized in the liver and is partially eliminated in the urine. The major metabolite, 14-hydroxyclarithromycin, also has antibacterial activity and is eliminated in the urine. Dosage reduction (eg, a 500-mg loading dose, then 250 mg once or twice daily) is recommended for patients with creatinine clearances less than 30 mL/min. Clarithromycin has drug interactions similar to those described for erythromycin.

The advantages of clarithromycin compared with erythromycin are lower incidence of gastrointestinal intolerance and less frequent dosing.

AZITHROMYCIN

Azithromycin, a 15-atom lactone macrolide ring compound, is derived from erythromycin by addition of a methylated nitrogen into the lactone ring. Its spectrum of activity, mechanism of action, and clinical uses are similar to those of clarithromycin. Azithromycin can be administered orally or intravenously. Azithromycin is active against *M avium* complex and *T gondii*. Azithromycin is slightly less active than erythromycin and clarithromycin against staphylococci and streptococci and slightly more active against *H influenzae*. Azithromycin is highly active against *Chlamydia* sp.

Azithromycin differs from erythromycin and clarithromycin mainly in pharmacokinetic properties. A 500-mg dose of azithromycin produces relatively low serum concentrations of approximately 0.4 mcg/mL. However, azithromycin penetrates into most tissues (except cerebrospinal fluid) and phagocytic cells extremely well, with tissue concentrations exceeding serum concentrations by 10- to 100-fold. The drug is slowly released from tissues (tissue half-life of 2–4 days) to produce an elimination half-life approaching 3 days. These unique properties permit once-daily dosing and shortening of the duration of treatment in many cases. For example, a single 1-g dose of azithromycin is as an alternative option for treatment of chlamydial cervicitis and urethritis (the preferred option is a 7-day course of doxycycline). Azithromycin, as a 500-mg loading dose, followed by a 250-mg single daily dose for the next 4 days, is commonly used alone or in combination with a beta-lactam antibiotic to treat community-acquired pneumonia.

Azithromycin is rapidly absorbed and well tolerated orally. Aluminum and magnesium antacids do not alter bioavailability but delay absorption and reduce peak serum concentrations. Because it has a 15-member (not 14-member) lactone ring, azithromycin does not inactivate cytochrome P450 enzymes and, therefore, is free of the drug interactions that occur with erythromycin and clarithromycin.

Macrolide antibiotics prolong the electrocardiographic QT interval due to an effect on potassium channels. Prolongation of the QT interval can lead to the torsades de pointes arrhythmia. Recent studies have suggested that azithromycin may be associated with a small increased risk of cardiac death.

FIDAXOMICIN

Fidaxomicin, a minimally absorbed macrolide used to treat *Clostridioides difficile* (formerly *Clostridium difficile*) infections, is discussed in Chapter 50.

KETOLIDES

Ketolides are semisynthetic, 14-membered ring macrolides, differing from erythromycin by substitution of a 3-keto group for the neutral sugar L-cladinose. **Telithromycin** was approved for community-acquired bacterial pneumonia, but it is no longer available in the USA. It is active in vitro against *Streptococcus pyogenes*, *S pneumoniae*, *S aureus*, *H influenzae*, *Moraxella catarrhalis*, *Mycoplasma* sp, *L pneumophila*, *Chlamydia* sp, *H pylori*, *Neisseria gonorrhoeae*, *B fragilis*, *T gondii*, and certain nontuberculous mycobacteria. Many macrolide-resistant strains are susceptible to ketolides because the structural modification of these compounds renders them poor substrates for efflux pump–mediated resistance, and they bind to ribosomes of some bacterial species with higher affinity than macrolides.

Oral bioavailability of telithromycin is 57%, and tissue and intracellular penetration is generally good. Telithromycin is metabolized in the liver and eliminated by a combination of biliary and urinary routes of excretion. It is administered as a once-daily dose of 800 mg, which results in peak serum concentrations of approximately 2 mcg/mL. It is a reversible inhibitor of the CYP3A4 enzyme system and may slightly prolong the QT_c interval. In the USA, telithromycin was indicated only for treatment of community-acquired bacterial pneumonia after it was recognized that telithromycin can cause hepatitis and liver failure. Telithromycin is also contraindicated in patients with myasthenia gravis because it may exacerbate this condition.

Solithromycin is a non-FDA-approved, novel fluoroketolide that was studied in two phase 3 clinical trials and showed noninferiority when compared with moxifloxacin in the treatment of community-acquired pneumonia. The dosage used was a loading dose of 800 mg orally or intravenously, followed by 400 mg daily for a total of 5 days. The intravenous formulation was associated with higher rates of infusion-related reactions compared with moxifloxacin. Similar to telithromycin, solithromycin maintains in vitro activity against macrolide-resistant bacteria, including *S pneumoniae*, staphylococci, enterococci, *Chlamydia trachomatis*, and *Neisseria gonorrhoeae*. Its chemical structure lacks the pyridine-imidazole side chain group, which is thought to contribute to telithromycin's hepatotoxicity. While severe hepatotoxicity was not seen in phase 2 or 3 clinical trials, the FDA review panel expressed concerns that this potential adverse effect was inadequately studied in clinical trials and solithromycin's approval for community-acquired pneumonia was declined until further safety analyses have been completed. There has been additional interest in solithromycin's efficacy in treating sexually transmitted infections; however, results of a phase 3 trial in patients with infections caused by *Neisseria gonorrhoeae* with or without concomitant *C trachomatis* failed to show noninferiority against the standard regimen of ceftriaxone with azithromycin. Solithromycin's future place in therapy is unclear.

■ CLINDAMYCIN

Clindamycin is a chlorine-substituted derivative of **lincomycin,** an antibiotic that is elaborated by *Streptomyces lincolnensis.*

Clindamycin

Mechanism of Action & Antibacterial Activity

Clindamycin, like erythromycin, inhibits protein synthesis by interfering with the formation of initiation complexes and with aminoacyl translocation reactions. The binding site for clindamycin on the 50S subunit of the bacterial ribosome is identical with that for erythromycin. Streptococci, staphylococci, and pneumococci are inhibited by clindamycin at a concentration of 0.5–5 mcg/mL. Enterococci and gram-negative aerobic organisms are resistant. *Bacteroides* sp and other anaerobes are often susceptible, although resistance rates may be increasing, particularly in gram-negative anaerobes. Resistance to clindamycin, which generally confers cross-resistance to macrolides, is due to (1) mutation of the ribosomal receptor site; (2) modification of the receptor by a constitutively expressed methylase (see section on erythromycin resistance, above); and (3) enzymatic inactivation of clindamycin. Gram-negative aerobic species are intrinsically resistant because of poor permeability of the outer membrane.

Pharmacokinetics

Oral dosages of clindamycin, 0.15–0.3 g every 8 hours (10–20 mg/kg/d for children), yield serum levels of 2–3 mcg/mL. When administered intravenously, 600 mg of clindamycin every 8 hours gives levels of 5–15 mcg/mL. The drug is about 90% protein-bound. Clindamycin penetrates well into most tissues, with brain and cerebrospinal fluid being important exceptions. It penetrates well into abscesses and is actively taken up and concentrated by phagocytic cells. Clindamycin is metabolized by the liver, and both active drug and active metabolites are excreted in bile and urine. The half-life is about 3 hours in adults, increasing to 6 hours in patients with anuria. No dosage adjustment is required for renal failure.

Clinical Use

Clindamycin is indicated for the treatment of skin and soft-tissue infections caused by streptococci and staphylococci. It may be active against community-acquired strains of methicillin-resistant *S aureus*, although resistance has been increasing. Many strains of group B streptococci have developed resistance, and resistance is also increasing among group A streptococci. It is commonly used in conjunction with a beta-lactam antibiotic to treat toxic shock syndrome or necrotizing fasciitis caused by group A *Streptococcus.* In this setting, clindamycin use is typically limited to the initial 48-72 hours of treatment for the purpose of inhibiting toxin production. Clindamycin is also indicated for treatment of infections caused by susceptible *Bacteroides* sp and other anaerobes. Clindamycin, sometimes in combination with an aminoglycoside or cephalosporin, is used to treat penetrating wounds of the abdomen and the gut; infections originating in the female genital tract, eg, septic abortion, pelvic abscesses, or pelvic inflammatory disease; and lung and periodontal abscesses. Clindamycin was historically recommended for prophylaxis of endocarditis in patients with specific valvular heart disease who are undergoing certain dental procedures and have significant penicillin allergies; however, it was removed from guidelines due to its association with *C difficile* infection. Clindamycin plus primaquine is an effective alternative to trimethoprim-sulfamethoxazole for moderate to moderately severe *Pneumocystis jiroveci* pneumonia in patients with acquired immunodeficiency syndrome (AIDS). It is also used in combination with pyrimethamine for AIDS-related toxoplasmosis of the brain.

Adverse Effects

Common adverse effects are diarrhea, nausea, and skin rashes. Impaired liver function (with or without jaundice) and neutropenia sometimes occur. Administration of clindamycin is a risk factor for diarrhea and colitis due to *C difficile*.

■ STREPTOGRAMINS

MECHANISM OF ACTION & ANTIBACTERIAL ACTIVITY

Quinupristin-dalfopristin is a combination of two streptogramins—quinupristin, a streptogramin B, and dalfopristin, a streptogramin A—in a 30:70 ratio. The streptogramins share the same ribosomal binding site as the macrolides and clindamycin and thus inhibit protein synthesis in an identical manner. Quinupristin-dalfopristin is rapidly bactericidal for most susceptible organisms except *Enterococcus faecium*, which is killed slowly. Quinupristin-dalfopristin is active against gram-positive cocci, including multidrug-resistant strains of streptococci, penicillin-resistant strains of *S pneumoniae*, methicillin-susceptible and resistant strains of staphylococci, and *E faecium* (but not *Enterococcus faecalis*). Resistance is due to modification of the quinupristin binding site (MLS-B type resistance), enzymatic inactivation of dalfopristin, or efflux.

Pharmacokinetics

Quinupristin-dalfopristin is administered intravenously at a dosage of 7.5 mg/kg every 8–12 hours. Peak serum concentrations following an infusion of 7.5 mg/kg over 60 minutes are 3 mcg/mL for quinupristin and 7 mcg/mL for dalfopristin. Quinupristin and dalfopristin are rapidly metabolized, with half-lives of 0.85 and 0.7 hours, respectively. Elimination is principally by the fecal route. Dose adjustment is not necessary for renal failure, peritoneal dialysis, or hemodialysis. Patients with hepatic insufficiency may not tolerate the drug at usual doses, however, because of increased area under the concentration curve of both parent drugs and metabolites. This may necessitate a dose reduction to 7.5 mg/kg every 12 hours or 5 mg/kg every 8 hours. Quinupristin and dalfopristin significantly inhibit CYP3A4, which metabolizes warfarin, diazepam, quetiapine, simvastatin, and cyclosporine, among many others. Dosage reduction of agents with narrow therapeutic windows, such as cyclosporine or tacrolimus, may be necessary.

Clinical Uses & Adverse Effects

Quinupristin-dalfopristin is approved for treatment of infections caused by staphylococci or streptococci. It is also active against vancomycin-resistant strains of *E faecium*, but not *E faecalis*, which is intrinsically resistant, probably because of an efflux-type resistance mechanism. The principal toxicities are infusion-related events, such as pain at the infusion site, and an arthralgia-myalgia syndrome. Quinupristin-dalfopristin is used to a limited extent in the USA due to the availability of better-tolerated alternatives.

CHLORAMPHENICOL

Crystalline chloramphenicol is a neutral, stable compound with the following structure:

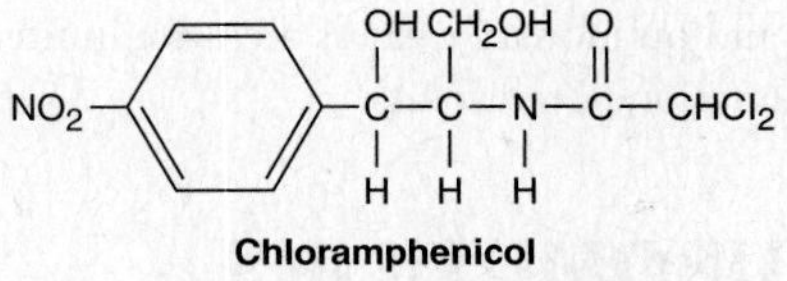

Chloramphenicol

It is soluble in alcohol but poorly soluble in water. Chloramphenicol succinate, which is used for parenteral administration, is highly water-soluble. It is hydrolyzed in vivo with liberation of free chloramphenicol.

Mechanism of Action & Antimicrobial Activity

Chloramphenicol is an inhibitor of microbial protein synthesis and is bacteriostatic against most susceptible organisms. It binds reversibly to the 50S subunit of the bacterial ribosome (see Figure 44–1) and inhibits peptide bond formation (step 2). Chloramphenicol is a broad-spectrum antibiotic that is active against both aerobic and anaerobic gram-positive and gram-negative organisms. It is active also against rickettsiae. Most gram-positive bacteria are inhibited at concentrations of 1–10 mcg/mL, and many gram-negative bacteria are inhibited by concentrations of 0.2–5 mcg/mL. *H influenzae*, *Neisseria meningitidis*, and some strains of *Bacteroides* are highly susceptible; for these organisms, chloramphenicol may be bactericidal.

Low-level resistance to chloramphenicol may emerge from large populations of chloramphenicol-susceptible cells by selection of mutants that are less permeable to the drug. Clinically significant resistance is due to production of chloramphenicol acetyltransferase, a plasmid-encoded enzyme that inactivates the drug.

Pharmacokinetics

The usual dosage of chloramphenicol is 50–100 mg/kg/d divided every 6 hours. It is no longer available in the USA as an oral formulation, and the intravenous product is rarely used. The parenteral formulation is a prodrug, chloramphenicol succinate, which is hydrolyzed to yield free chloramphenicol, giving blood levels somewhat lower than those achieved with orally administered drug. Chloramphenicol is widely distributed to virtually all tissues and body fluids, including the central nervous system and cerebrospinal fluid, such that the concentration of chloramphenicol in brain tissue may be equal to that in serum. The drug penetrates cell membranes readily.

Most of the drug is inactivated either by conjugation with glucuronic acid (principally in the liver) or by reduction to inactive aryl amines. Active chloramphenicol, about 10% of the total dose administered, and its inactive degradation products are eliminated in the urine. A small amount of active drug is excreted into bile and feces. There are no specific dosage adjustments recommended in renal or hepatic insufficiency; however, the drug will accumulate and should be used with extra caution in these situations. Newborns less than a week old and premature infants also clear chloramphenicol inefficiently, and the dosage should be reduced to 25 mg/kg/d.

Clinical Uses

Because of potential toxicity, bacterial resistance, and the availability of many other effective alternatives, chloramphenicol has been used rarely in the United States for many years. It may be considered for treatment of serious rickettsial infections such as typhus and Rocky Mountain spotted fever. It is an alternative to a β-lactam antibiotic for treatment of bacterial meningitis occurring in patients who have major hypersensitivity reactions to penicillin.

Adverse Reactions

Adults occasionally develop gastrointestinal disturbances, including nausea, vomiting, and diarrhea. These symptoms are rare in children. Oral or vaginal candidiasis may occur as a result of alteration of normal microbial flora.

Chloramphenicol commonly causes a dose-related reversible suppression of red cell production at dosages exceeding 50 mg/kg/d after 1–2 weeks. Aplastic anemia, a rare consequence (1 in 24,000-40,000 courses of therapy) of chloramphenicol administration by any route, is an idiosyncratic reaction unrelated to dose, although it occurs more frequently with prolonged use.

Aplastic anemia tends to be irreversible and can be fatal, although it may respond to bone marrow transplantation or immunosuppressive therapy. Due to the severity of this reaction, a boxed warning is included in its US labeling.

Newborn infants lack an effective glucuronic acid conjugation mechanism for the degradation and detoxification of chloramphenicol. Consequently, when infants are given dosages above 50 mg/kg/d, the drug may accumulate, resulting in the **gray baby syndrome,** with vomiting, flaccidity, hypothermia, gray color, shock, and vascular collapse. To avoid this toxic effect, chloramphenicol should be used with caution in infants and the dosage limited to 50 mg/kg/d (or less during the first week of life) in full-term infants and 25 mg/kg/d in premature infants.

Chloramphenicol inhibits hepatic microsomal enzymes that metabolize several drugs. Half-lives of these drugs are prolonged, and the serum concentrations of phenytoin, tolbutamide, chlorpropamide, and warfarin are increased.

■ OXAZOLIDINONES

MECHANISM OF ACTION & ANTIMICROBIAL ACTIVITY

Linezolid is a member of the oxazolidinone class of synthetic antimicrobials. It is active against gram-positive organisms including staphylococci, streptococci, enterococci, gram-positive anaerobic cocci, and gram-positive rods such as corynebacteria, *Nocardia* sp, and *L monocytogenes.* It is primarily a bacteriostatic agent but is bactericidal against streptococci. It is also active against *Mycobacterium tuberculosis.*

Linezolid inhibits protein synthesis by preventing formation of the ribosome complex that initiates protein synthesis. Its unique binding site, located on 23S ribosomal RNA of the 50S subunit, results in no cross-resistance with other drug classes. Resistance is caused by mutation of the linezolid binding site on 23S ribosomal RNA.

Pharmacokinetics

Linezolid is 100% bioavailable after oral administration and has a half-life of 4–6 hours. It is metabolized by oxidative metabolism, yielding two inactive metabolites. It is neither an inducer nor an inhibitor of cytochrome P450 enzymes. Peak serum concentrations average 18 mcg/mL following a 600-mg oral dose; cerebrospinal fluid (CSF) concentrations reach approximately 60–70% of the serum level. The recommended dosage for most indications is 600 mg twice daily, either orally or intravenously.

Clinical Uses

Linezolid is approved for vancomycin-resistant *E faecium* infections, health care–associated pneumonia, community-acquired pneumonia, and both complicated and uncomplicated skin and soft tissue infections caused by susceptible gram-positive bacteria. Off-label uses of linezolid include treatment of multidrug-resistant tuberculosis and *Nocardia* infections.

Adverse Effects

The principal toxicity of linezolid is hematologic; the effects are reversible and generally mild. Thrombocytopenia is the most common manifestation (seen in approximately 3% of treatment courses), particularly when the drug is administered for longer than 2 weeks. Anemia and neutropenia also may occur, most commonly in patients with a predisposition to or underlying bone marrow suppression. Cases of optic and peripheral neuropathy and lactic acidosis have been reported with prolonged courses of linezolid. These side effects are thought to be related to linezolid-induced inhibition of mitochondrial protein synthesis. There are case reports of serotonin syndrome (see Chapter 16) occurring when linezolid is coadministered with serotonergic drugs, most frequently selective serotonin reuptake inhibitor antidepressants. The FDA has issued a warning regarding the use of the drug with serotonergic agents.

Tedizolid is the active moiety of the prodrug tedizolid phosphate, a next-generation oxazolidinone, with high potency against gram-positive bacteria, including methicillin-resistant *S aureus,* vancomycin-resistant enterococci, streptococci, and gram-positive anaerobes. It has 91% oral bioavailability and is FDA-approved at a dose of 200 mg orally or intravenously once daily for 6 days for the treatment of skin and soft tissue infection. Potential advantages over linezolid include increased potency against staphylococci and a longer half-life of 12 hours, allowing once-daily dosing. There is no need for dose adjustment in renal or hepatic impairment. Although the randomized trials are limited to 6 days of therapy, evidence from case reports and case series suggest a decreased risk of bone marrow suppression with a prolonged duration of therapy. It is thought to have a lower risk of serotonergic toxicity, but concomitant use with serotonin reuptake inhibitors has not been formally evaluated. Tedizolid is more highly protein-bound (70–90%) than linezolid (31%). Plasma concentrations are a good indicator for tissue concentrations as it penetrates well into muscle, adipose, and pulmonary tissues; there are limited data regarding CSF penetration of tedizolid.

■ PLEUROMUTILINS

Lefamulin is a novel antibacterial agent approved in 2019 for the treatment of pneumonia; it is the first systemic agent available in the pleuromutilin class for human use. The pleuromutilin class was discovered in the 1950s, but previously it was used only in veterinary medicine.

MECHANISM OF ACTION & ANTIBACTERIAL ACTIVITY

Lefamulin works by binding the 50S ribosome, thus inhibiting bacterial protein synthesis. Its mechanism is unique in that it causes the binding pocket to close around the drug molecule, preventing bacterial transfer RNA from binding appropriately. It has bactericidal activity against organisms commonly seen in lower respiratory tract infections such as *Streptococcus pneumoniae*, *Haemophilus influenzae*, and atypical pathogens such as *Legionella pneumophila*, *Mycoplasma pneumoniae*, and *Chlamydophila pneumoniae*. It also has in vitro activity against most aerobic gram-positive organisms, including *S pyogenes*, *Staphylococcus aureus*, and *Enterococcus faecium*. It may also have activity against certain organisms causing sexually transmitted infections, such as *Mycoplasma genitalium*, *Neisseria gonorrhoeae*, and *Chlamydia trachomatis*. Notably, lefamulin lacks activity against *Enterococcus faecalis*, *Pseudomonas aeruginosa*, *Acinetobacter baumannii*, and the Enterobacterales group of gram-negative organisms.

Resistance

Thus far, the risk for inducing bacterial resistance mutations with lefamulin appears to be low, but resistance mutations have been observed in vitro. It is unclear how common clinical resistance will be, but some potential mechanisms for resistance include ribosomal target site alteration and active efflux from the site of action.

Pharmacokinetics and Adverse Effects

Lefamulin is available as both intravenous and oral formulations. It is 25% bioavailable, so a 600-mg oral dose is roughly equivalent to 150 mg given intravenously, with optimal absorption in an unfed state (at least 1 hour before or 2 hours after a meal). It is 95–97% protein-bound and is excreted primarily through hepatic metabolism via the CYP3A4 enzyme pathway. The elimination half-life is about 8 hours, so the standard dose is administered twice daily; the dose may require adjustment for severe hepatic impairment. Common adverse effects seen in clinical trials included infusion-site reactions for the intravenous formulation and gastrointestinal disturbances, particularly nausea and diarrhea, for the oral formulation. Lefamulin should be avoided in pregnancy because animal studies show increased risk of congenital malformations. It has not been studied in pregnant humans to date.

Clinical Use

At the time of writing, lefamulin is approved only for the treatment of adult patients with community-acquired pneumonia, based on results of two randomized clinical trials in which lefamulin was deemed noninferior to moxifloxacin. There is interest in its potential use for other indications, such as skin and skin-structure infections or sexually transmitted infections based on in vitro activity and some success in phase 2 trials.

SUMMARY Tetracyclines, Macrolides, Clindamycin, Chloramphenicol, Streptogramins, Oxazolidinones, & Pleuromutilins

Subclass, Drug	Mechanism of Action	Effects	Clinical Applications	Pharmacokinetics, Toxicities, Interactions
TETRACYCLINES				
• Tetracycline	Prevents bacterial protein synthesis by binding to the 30S ribosomal subunit	Bacteriostatic activity against susceptible bacteria	Infections caused by mycoplasma, chlamydiae, rickettsiae, some spirochetes • malaria • *H pylori* • acne	Oral • mixed clearance (half-life 8 h) • dosed every 6 h • divalent cations impair oral absorption • *Toxicity:* Gastrointestinal upset, hepatotoxicity, photosensitivity, deposition in bone and teeth
• *Doxycycline: Oral and IV; longer half-life (18 h) so dosed twice daily; nonrenal elimination; absorption is minimally affected by divalent cations; used to treat community-acquired pneumonia and exacerbations of bronchitis*				
• *Minocycline: Oral and IV; longer half-life (16 h) so dosed twice daily; frequently causes reversible vestibular toxicity*				
• *Tigecycline: IV; dosed twice daily; unaffected by common tetracycline resistance mechanisms; very broad spectrum of activity against gram-positive, gram-negative, and anaerobic bacteria; nausea and vomiting are the primary toxicities*				
• *Eravacycline: IV; dosed twice daily; unaffected by common tetracycline resistance mechanisms; very broad spectrum of activity against gram-positive, gram-negative, and anaerobic bacteria; nausea and vomiting are the primary toxicities*				
• *Omadacycline: Oral and IV; dosed once daily after initial loading dose; oral absorption impeded by food, cations, must be administered on empty stomach; unaffected by common tetracycline resistance mechanisms; very broad spectrum of activity against gram-positive, gram-negative, and anaerobic bacteria; nausea and vomiting are the primary toxicities but thought to be lower than with other new tetracyclines*				
MACROLIDES				
• Erythromycin	Prevents bacterial protein synthesis by binding to the 50S ribosomal subunit	Bacteriostatic activity against susceptible bacteria	Community-acquired pneumonia • pertussis • corynebacterial and chlamydial infections	Oral, IV • hepatic clearance (half-life 1.5 h) • dosed every 6 h • cytochrome P450 inhibitor • *Toxicity:* Gastrointestinal upset, hepatotoxicity, QT_c prolongation
• *Clarithromycin: Oral; longer half-life (6 h) so dosed twice daily; added activity versus M avium complex, toxoplasma, and M leprae*				
• *Azithromycin: Oral, IV; very long half-life (68 h) allows for once-daily dosing and 5-day course of therapy of community-acquired pneumonia; does not inhibit cytochrome P450 enzymes*				
LINCOSAMIDE				
• Clindamycin	Prevents bacterial protein synthesis by binding to the 50S ribosomal subunit	Bacteriostatic activity against susceptible bacteria	Skin and soft tissue infections • anaerobic infections	Oral, IV • hepatic clearance (half-life 2.5 h) • dosed every 6–8 h • *Toxicity:* Gastrointestinal upset, colitis

(continued)

Subclass, Drug	Mechanism of Action	Effects	Clinical Applications	Pharmacokinetics, Toxicities, Interactions
STREPTOGRAMINS				
• Quinupristin-dalfopristin	Prevents bacterial protein synthesis by binding to the 50S ribosomal subunit	Rapid bactericidal activity against most susceptible bacteria	Infections caused by staphylococci or vancomycin-resistant strains of enterococci	IV • hepatic clearance • dosed every 8–12 h • cytochrome P450 inhibitor • *Toxicity:* Severe infusion-related myalgias and arthralgias
CHLORAMPHENICOL				
	Prevents bacterial protein synthesis by binding to the 50S ribosomal subunit	Bacteriostatic activity against susceptible bacteria	Use is rare in the developed world because of serious toxicities	IV • hepatic clearance (half-life 2.5 h) • dosage is 50–100 mg/kg/d in four divided doses • *Toxicity:* Dose-related anemia, idiosyncratic aplastic anemia, gray baby syndrome
OXAZOLIDINONES				
• Linezolid	Prevents bacterial protein synthesis by binding to the 23S ribosomal RNA of 50S subunit	Bacteriostatic activity against susceptible bacteria	Infections caused by methicillin-resistant staphylococci and vancomycin-resistant enterococci	Oral, IV • hepatic clearance (half-life 6 h) • dosed twice-daily • *Toxicity:* Duration-dependent bone marrow suppression, neuropathy, and optic neuritis • serotonin syndrome may occur when coadministered with other serotonergic drugs (eg, selective serotonin reuptake inhibitors)
Tedizolid: Oral and IV; longer half-life (12 h) so dosed once daily; increased efficacy versus staphylococci; approved for use in skin and soft tissue infections.				
PLEUROMUTILINS				
• Lefamulin	Prevents bacterial protein synthesis by binding to the 50S ribosomal subunit	Bactericidal activity against most susceptible bacteria; bacteriostatic against some	Community-acquired pneumonia	Oral, IV • hepatic clearance (half-life 8 h) • dosed twice daily • cytochrome P450 3A4 substrate • *Toxicity:* Infusion-related reactions and gastrointestinal disturbances

PREPARATIONS AVAILABLE

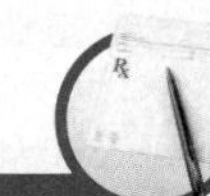

GENERIC NAME	AVAILABLE AS
Chloramphenicol	Generic, Chloromycetin
TETRACYCLINES	
Demeclocycline	Generic, Declomycin
Doxycycline	Generic, Vibramycin, others
Minocycline	Generic, Minocin, others
Tetracycline	Generic, others
Tigecycline	Generic, Tygacil
Eravacycline	Xerava
Omadacycline	Nuzyra
MACROLIDES	
Azithromycin	Generic, Zithromax
Clarithromycin	Generic, Biaxin
Erythromycin	Generic, others
LINCOMYCIN	
Clindamycin	Generic, Cleocin
STREPTOGRAMINS	
Quinupristin and dalfopristin	Synercid
OXAZOLIDINONES	
Linezolid	Generic, Zyvox
Tedizolid	Sivextro
PLEUROMUTILIN	
Lefamulin	Xenleta

REFERENCES

Barrera CM et al: Efficacy and safety of oral solithromycin versus oral moxifloxacin for treatment of community-acquired bacterial pneumonia: A global, double-blind, multicenter, randomized, active-controlled, non-inferiority trial (SOLITAIRE-ORAL). Lancet 2016;16:421.

Benavent E et al: Long-term use of tedizolid in osteoarticular infections: benefits among oxazolidinone drugs. Antibiotics 2021;10:53.

Chopra I, Roberts M: Tetracycline antibiotics: Mode of action, applications, molecular biology, and epidemiology of bacterial resistance. Microbiol Mol Biol Rev 2001;65:232.

De Vriese AS et al: Linezolid-induced inhibition of mitochondrial protein synthesis. Clin Infect Dis 2006;42:1111.

Dryden MS: Linezolid pharmacokinetics and pharmacodynamics in clinical treatment. J Antimicrob Chemother. 2011;66(Suppl 4):S7.

File Jr. TM et al: SOLITAIRE-IV: A randomized, double-blind, multicenter study comparing the efficacy and safety of intravenous-to-oral solithromycin to intravenous-to-oral moxifloxacin for treatment of community-acquired bacterial pneumonia. Clin Infect Dis 2016;63:1007.

Hancock RE: Mechanisms of action of newer antibiotics for gram-positive pathogens. Lancet Infect Dis 2005;5:209.

Leclerq R: Mechanisms of resistance to macrolides and lincosamides: Nature of the resistance elements and their clinical implications. Clin Infect Dis 2002;34:482.

Lee M et al: Linezolid for treatment of chronic extensively drug-resistant tuberculosis. N Engl J Med 2012;367:1508.

Livermore DM: Tigecycline: What is it, and where should it be used? J Antimicrob Chemother 2005;56:611.

Moran GJ et al: Methicillin-resistant *S aureus* infections among patients in the emergency department. N Engl J Med 2006;355:666.

Moran GJ et al: Tedizolid for 6 days versus linezolid for 10 days for acute bacterial skin and skin-structure infections (ESTABLISH-2): A randomized, double-blind, phase 3, non-inferiority trial. Lancet 2014;14:696.

O'Riordan W et al: Omadacycline for acute bacterial skin and skin structure infections. N Engl J Med 2019;380:528.

Prokocimer P et al: Tedizolid phosphate vs linezolid for treatment of acute bacterial skin and skin structure infections. JAMA 2013;309:559.

Solomkin J et al: Assessing the efficacy and safety of eravacycline vs ertapenem in complicated intra-abdominal infections in the Investigating Gram-Negative Infections Treated with Eravacycline (IGNITE 1) Trial: A Randomized Clinical Trial. JAMA Surg 2017;152:224.

Solomkin J et al: IGNITE4: Results of a phase 3, randomized, multicenter, prospective trial of eravacycline vs. meropenem in the treatment of complicated intra-abdominal infections. Clin Infect Dis 2019;69:921.

Stets R et al: Omadacycline for community-acquired bacterial pneumonia. N Engl J Med 2019;380:517.

Tasina E et al: Efficacy and safety of tigecycline for the treatment of infectious diseases: A meta-analysis. Lancet Infect Dis 2011;11:834.

Van Bambeke F: Renaissance of antibiotics against difficult infections: Focus on oritavancin and new ketolides and quinolones. Ann Med 2014;46:512.

Veve M, Wagner J: Lefamulin: Review of a promising novel pleuromutilin antibiotic. Pharmacother 2018;38:935.

Wayne RA et al: Azithromycin and risk of cardiovascular death. N Engl J Med 2012;366:1881.

Wilson WR et al: Prevention of viridans group streptococcal infective endocarditis: a scientific statement from the American Heart Association. Circulation 2021;143:e963.

Woytowish MR, Rowe AS: Clinical relevance of linezolid-associated serotonin toxicity. Ann Pharmacother 2013;47:388.

Zuckerman JM: Macrolides and ketolides: Azithromycin, clarithromycin, telithromycin. Infect Dis Clin North Am 2004;18:621.

CASE STUDY ANSWER

Doxycycline at a dose of 100 mg PO bid for 7 days is the preferred treatment for chlamydia cervicitis. Azithromycin as a single 1-g dose is an alternative treatment. If the patient is pregnant, then tetracyclines would be contraindicated and she should receive azithromycin, which is safe in pregnancy.

CHAPTER

45

Aminoglycosides & Spectinomycin

Camille E. Beauduy, PharmD, & Lisa G. Winston, MD*

CASE STUDY

A 45-year-old man with no significant medical history was admitted to the intensive care unit (ICU) 10 days ago after suffering third-degree burns over 40% of his body. He had been relatively stable until the last 24 hours. Now, he is febrile (39.5°C [103.1°F]), and his white blood cell count has risen from 8500 to 20,000/mm^3. He has also had an episode of hypotension (86/50 mmHg) that responded to a fluid bolus. Blood cultures were obtained at the time of his fever, and results are pending. The ICU attending physician is concerned about a bloodstream infection and decides to treat with empiric combination therapy directed against *Pseudomonas aeruginosa*. The combination therapy includes tobramycin. The patient weighs 70 kg (154 lb) and has an estimated creatinine clearance of 90 mL/min. How should tobramycin be dosed using once-daily and traditional dosing strategies? How should each regimen be monitored for efficacy and toxicity?

The drugs described in this chapter are bactericidal inhibitors of protein synthesis that interfere with ribosomal function. These agents are useful mainly against aerobic gram-negative microorganisms.

■ AMINOGLYCOSIDES

The aminoglycosides include **streptomycin, neomycin, kanamycin, amikacin, gentamicin, tobramycin, sisomicin, netilmicin, plazomicin**, and others. They are used most widely in combination with other agents to treat drug-resistant organisms; for example, they are used with a β-lactam antibiotic in serious infections with gram-negative bacteria, with a β-lactam antibiotic or vancomycin for gram-positive endocarditis, and with one or several other agents for treatment of mycobacterial infections such as tuberculosis.

General Properties of Aminoglycosides

A. Physical and Chemical Properties

Aminoglycosides have a hexose ring, either streptidine (in streptomycin) or 2-deoxystreptamine (in other aminoglycosides), to which various amino sugars are attached by glycosidic linkages (Figures 45–1 and 45–2). They are water-soluble, stable in solution, and more active at alkaline than at acid pH.

B. Mechanism of Action

The mode of action of streptomycin has been studied more closely than that of other aminoglycosides, but all aminoglycosides are thought to act similarly. Aminoglycosides are irreversible inhibitors of protein synthesis. The initial event is passive diffusion via porin channels across the outer membrane (Figure 43–3). Drug is then actively transported across the cell membrane into the cytoplasm by an oxygen-dependent process. The transmembrane electrochemical gradient supplies the energy for this process, and transport is coupled to a proton pump. Low extracellular pH and anaerobic conditions inhibit transport by reducing the gradient. Transport may be enhanced by cell wall–active drugs such as penicillin or vancomycin; this

*The authors thank Henry F. Chambers, MD, and Daniel H. Deck, PharmD, for their contributions to previous editions.

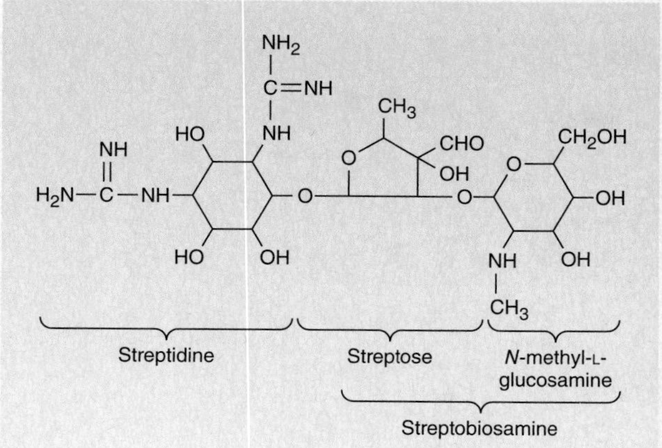

FIGURE 45–1 Structure of streptomycin.

enhancement may be the basis of the synergy of those antibiotics with aminoglycosides.

Inside the cell, aminoglycosides bind to 30S-subunit ribosomal proteins. Protein synthesis is inhibited by aminoglycosides in at least three ways (see Figure 45–3): (1) interference with the initiation complex of peptide formation; (2) misreading of mRNA, which causes incorporation of incorrect amino acids into the peptide and results in a nonfunctional protein; and (3) breakup of polysomes into nonfunctional monosomes. These activities occur more or less simultaneously, and the overall effect is irreversible and leads to cell death.

C. Mechanisms of Resistance

Three principal mechanisms of resistance have been established: (1) production of a transferase enzyme that inactivates the

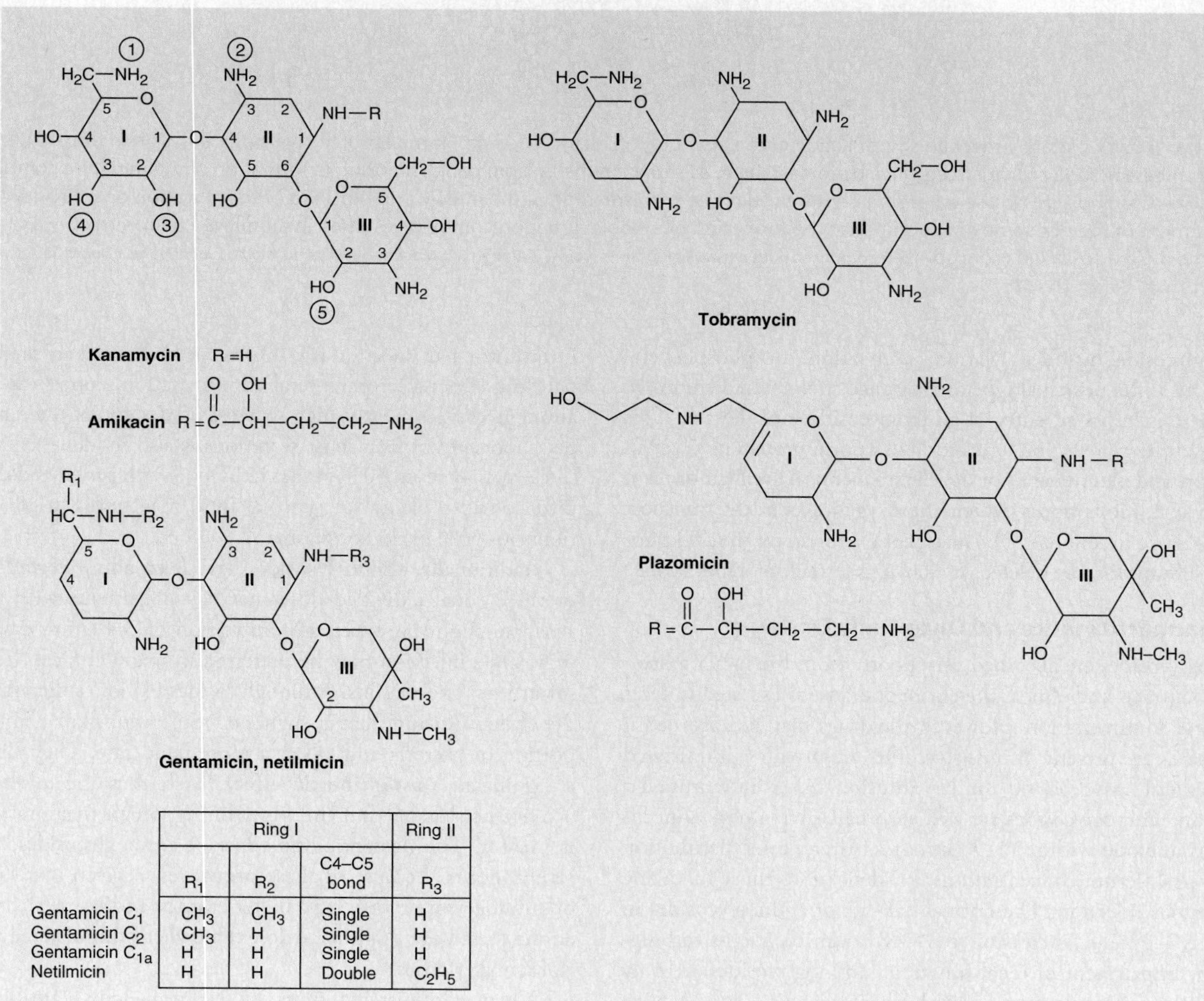

	Ring I			Ring II
	R_1	R_2	C4–C5 bond	R_3
Gentamicin C_1	CH_3	CH_3	Single	H
Gentamicin C_2	CH_3	H	Single	H
Gentamicin C_{1a}	H	H	Single	H
Netilmicin	H	H	Double	C_2H_5

FIGURE 45–2 Structures of several aminoglycoside antibiotics. Ring II is 2-deoxystreptamine. The resemblance between kanamycin and amikacin and between gentamicin, netilmicin, and tobramycin can be seen. Plazomicin's ring II and III are similar to the other structures; it shares the same hydroxyl-aminobutyric acid R group as amikacin. Its ring I differs from amikacin in that it is unsaturated. The circled numerals on the kanamycin molecule indicate points of attack of plasmid-mediated bacterial transferase enzymes that can inactivate this drug. ①, ②, and ③, acetyltransferase; ④, phosphotransferase; ⑤, adenylyltransferase. Amikacin is resistant to modification at ②, ③, ④, and ⑤, whereas plazomicin is resistant to modification at ①, ②, ④, and ⑤.

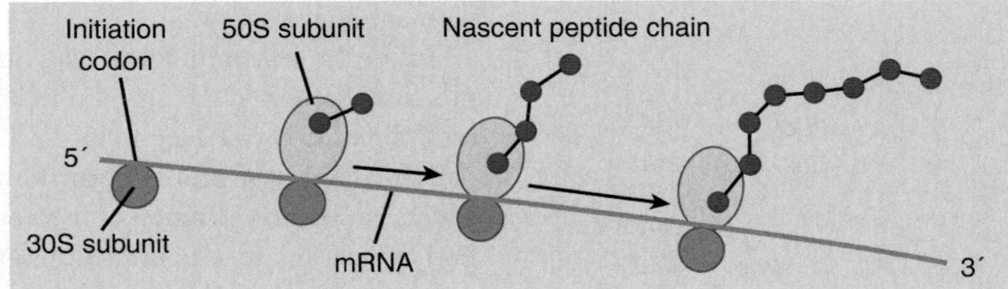

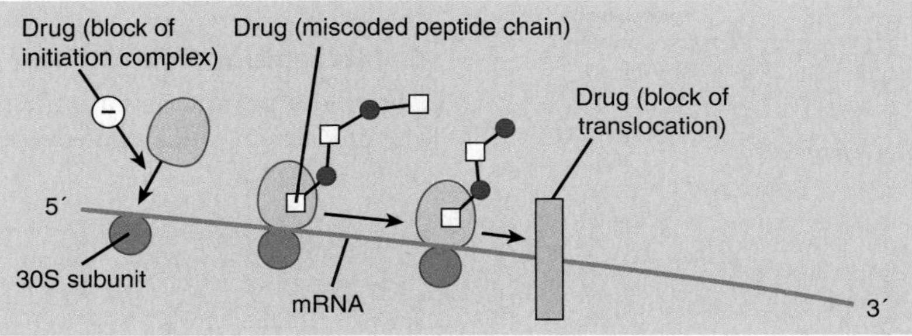

FIGURE 45–3 Putative mechanisms of action of the aminoglycosides in bacteria. Normal protein synthesis is shown in the top panel. At least three aminoglycoside effects have been described, as shown in the bottom panel: blocking of formation of the initiation complex; miscoding of amino acids in the emerging peptide chain due to misreading of the mRNA; and blocking of translocation on mRNA. Blocking of movement of the ribosome may occur after the formation of a single initiation complex, resulting in an mRNA chain with only a single ribosome on it, a so-called monosome. (Reproduced with permission from Trevor AT, Katzung BG, Masters SB: *Pharmacology: Examination & Board Review*, 6th ed. New York, NY: McGraw Hill; 2002.)

aminoglycoside by adenylylation, acetylation, or phosphorylation. This is the principal type of resistance encountered clinically. (2) There is impaired entry of aminoglycoside into the cell. This may result from mutation or deletion of a porin protein involved in transport and maintenance of the electrochemical gradient or from growth conditions under which the oxygen-dependent transport process is not functional. (3) The receptor protein on the 30S ribosomal subunit may be deleted or altered as a result of a mutation.

D. Pharmacokinetics and Once-Daily Dosing

Aminoglycosides are absorbed very poorly from the intact gastrointestinal tract, and almost the entire oral dose is excreted in feces after oral administration. However, the drugs may be absorbed if ulcerations are present. Aminoglycosides are usually administered intravenously as a 30–60 minute infusion. After intramuscular injection, aminoglycosides are well absorbed, giving peak concentrations in blood within 30–90 minutes. After a brief distribution phase, peak serum concentrations are identical to those following intravenous injection. The normal half-life of aminoglycosides in serum is 2–3 hours, increasing to 24–48 hours in patients with significant impairment of renal function. Aminoglycosides are only partially and irregularly removed by hemodialysis—eg, 40–60% for gentamicin—and even less effectively by peritoneal dialysis. Aminoglycosides are highly polar compounds that do not enter cells readily. They are largely excluded from the central nervous system and the eye. In the presence of active inflammation, however, cerebrospinal fluid levels reach 20% of plasma levels, and, in neonatal meningitis, the levels may be higher. Intrathecal or intraventricular injection is required for high levels in cerebrospinal fluid. Even after parenteral administration, concentrations of aminoglycosides are not high in most tissues except the renal cortex. Concentration in most secretions is also modest; in the bile, the level may reach 30% of that in blood. With prolonged therapy, diffusion into pleural or synovial fluid may result in concentrations 50–90% of that of plasma.

Traditionally, aminoglycosides have been administered in two or three equally divided doses per day in patients with normal renal function. However, administration of the entire daily dose in a single injection may be preferred in many clinical situations for at least two reasons. Aminoglycosides exhibit **concentration-dependent killing;** that is, higher concentrations kill a larger proportion of bacteria and kill at a more rapid rate. They also have a significant **postantibiotic effect**, such that the antibacterial activity persists beyond the time during which measurable drug is present. The postantibiotic effect of aminoglycosides can last several hours. Because of these properties, a given total amount of aminoglycoside may have better efficacy and less toxicity when administered as a single large dose than when administered as multiple smaller doses.

When administered with a cell wall–active antibiotic (a β-lactam or vancomycin), aminoglycosides may exhibit **synergistic killing** against certain bacteria. The effect of the drugs in combination is greater than the anticipated effect of each individual drug; ie, the killing effect of the combination is more than additive. This synergy may be important in certain clinical situations, such as endocarditis.

Adverse effects from aminoglycosides are both time- and concentration-dependent. Toxicity is unlikely to occur until a certain threshold concentration is reached, but, once that concentration is achieved, the time beyond this threshold becomes critical. This threshold is not precisely defined, but a trough concentration above 2 mcg/mL is predictive of toxicity. At clinically relevant doses, the total time above this threshold is greater with multiple smaller doses of drug than with a single large dose.

Numerous clinical studies demonstrate that a single daily dose of aminoglycoside is just as effective—and probably less toxic—than multiple smaller doses. Therefore, many authorities recommend that aminoglycosides be administered as a single daily dose in most clinical situations. However, the efficacy of once-daily aminoglycoside dosing in combination therapy of enterococcal endocarditis and staphylococcal endocarditis in patients with a prosthetic valve remains to be defined, and administration of lower doses two or three times daily is still recommended. In contrast, limited data do support once-daily dosing in streptococcal endocarditis. The role of once-daily dosing in pregnancy, obesity, and in neonates also is not well defined.

Once-daily dosing has potential practical advantages. For example, repeated determinations of serum concentrations are unnecessary unless an aminoglycoside is given for more than 3 days. A drug administered once a day rather than three times a day is less labor intensive. And once-a-day dosing is more feasible for outpatient therapy.

Aminoglycosides are cleared by the kidney, and excretion is directly proportional to creatinine clearance. To avoid accumulation and toxic levels, once-daily dosing of aminoglycosides is generally avoided if renal function is impaired. Rapidly changing renal function, which may occur with acute kidney injury, must also be monitored to avoid overdosing or underdosing. Provided these pitfalls are avoided, once-daily aminoglycoside dosing is safe and effective. If the creatinine clearance is >60 mL/min, then a single daily dose of 5–7 mg/kg of gentamicin or tobramycin is recommended (15 mg/kg for amikacin and plazomicin). For patients with creatinine clearance <60 mL/min, traditional dosing as described below is recommended. Of note, plazomicin has been studied using only the extended or once-daily dosing strategy; specific information on dosing and therapeutic drug monitoring is outlined in the plazomicin section that follows. With once-daily dosing, serum concentrations need not be routinely checked until the second or third day of therapy, depending on the stability of renal function and the anticipated duration of therapy. In most circumstances, it is unnecessary to check peak concentrations; an exception may be when ensuring adequately high peak concentrations for treating infections caused by drug-resistant pathogens. The goal is to administer drug so that concentrations of <1 mcg/mL are present between 18 and 24 hours after dosing. This provides sufficient time for washout of drug to occur before the next dose is given. Several nomograms have been developed and validated to assist clinicians with once-daily dosing (eg, Freeman reference, Hartford nomogram).

With traditional dosing, adjustments must be made to prevent accumulation of drug and toxicity in patients with renal insufficiency. Either the dose of drug is kept constant and the interval between doses is increased, or the interval is kept constant and the dose is reduced. Nomograms and formulas have been constructed relating serum creatinine levels to adjustments in traditional treatment regimens. For a traditional twice- or thrice-daily dosing regimen, peak serum concentrations should be determined from a blood sample obtained 30–60 minutes after a dose, and trough concentrations from a sample obtained just before the next dose. Doses of gentamicin and tobramycin should be adjusted to maintain peak levels between 5 and 10 mcg/mL (typically between 8 and 10 mcg/mL in more serious infections) and trough levels <2 mcg/mL (<1 mcg/mL is optimal).

E. Adverse Effects

All aminoglycosides are ototoxic and nephrotoxic. Ototoxicity and nephrotoxicity are more likely to be encountered when therapy is continued for more than 5 days, at higher doses, in the elderly, and in the setting of renal insufficiency. Concurrent use with loop diuretics (eg, furosemide, bumetanide, or ethacrynic acid) or other nephrotoxic antimicrobial agents (eg, vancomycin or amphotericin) can potentiate nephrotoxicity and should be avoided if possible. Ototoxicity can manifest either as auditory damage, resulting in tinnitus and high-frequency hearing loss initially, or as vestibular damage with vertigo, ataxia, and loss of balance. Nephrotoxicity can be identified by rising serum creatinine levels or reduced estimated glomerular filtration rate, although the earliest indication can be an increase in trough serum aminoglycoside concentrations. Neomycin, kanamycin, and amikacin are the agents most likely to cause auditory damage. Streptomycin and gentamicin are the most vestibulotoxic. Neomycin, tobramycin, and gentamicin are the most nephrotoxic. Plazomicin may be associated with lower rates of ototoxicity and nephrotoxicity compared to older aminoglycosides; however, as the newest aminoglycoside, clinical experience is limited.

In very high doses, aminoglycosides can produce a curare-like effect with neuromuscular blockade that results in respiratory paralysis. This paralysis is usually reversible by calcium gluconate, when given promptly, or neostigmine. Hypersensitivity occurs infrequently.

F. Clinical Uses

Aminoglycosides are mostly used against aerobic gram-negative bacteria, especially when there is concern for drug-resistant pathogens or in critically ill patients. Tobramycin and gentamicin are almost always used in combination with a β-lactam antibiotic to extend empiric coverage and to take advantage of the potential synergy between these two classes of drugs. Amikacin and streptomycin are frequently given in combination with other antibacterials for the treatment of mycobacterial infections. It remains unclear whether plazomicin will be given alone or in combination with other agents. Penicillin-aminoglycoside combinations have also been used to achieve bactericidal activity in treatment of enterococcal endocarditis and to shorten duration of therapy for viridans streptococcal endocarditis. Due to toxicity, these combinations are used less frequently when alternate regimens are available. For example, in the case of enterococcal endocarditis, studies suggest that the combination of ampicillin and ceftriaxone is an effective regimen with less risk for nephrotoxicity. When aminoglycosides are used, the selection of agent and dose depends on the infection being treated and the susceptibility of the isolate.

STREPTOMYCIN

Streptomycin (see Figure 45–1) was isolated from a strain of *Streptomyces griseus.* The antimicrobial activity of streptomycin is typical of that of other aminoglycosides, as are the mechanisms of resistance. Resistance has emerged in most species, restricting the current usefulness of streptomycin, with the exceptions listed below. Ribosomal resistance to streptomycin develops readily, limiting its role as a single agent.

Clinical Uses

A. Mycobacterial Infections

Streptomycin is mainly used as a second-line agent for treatment of tuberculosis. The dosage is 15 mg/kg/d with a maximum of 1 g/d (20–40 mg/kg/d for children), and it may be given intramuscularly or intravenously. It should be used only in combination with other agents to prevent emergence of resistance. See Chapter 47 for additional information regarding the use of streptomycin in mycobacterial infections.

B. Nontuberculous Infections

In plague, tularemia, and (sometimes) brucellosis, streptomycin, 1 g twice daily (15 mg/kg twice daily for children), may be given intramuscularly in combination with an oral tetracycline.

Penicillin plus streptomycin is effective for enterococcal endocarditis and for 2-week treatment of viridans streptococcal endocarditis; however, for susceptible strains, gentamicin is used more commonly when an aminoglycoside is selected as adjunct therapy. Streptomycin retains activity against some enterococcal species that are resistant to gentamicin (and therefore also resistant to netilmicin, tobramycin, and amikacin), so streptomycin remains a potential alternate agent for treating gentamicin-nonsusceptible enterococcal infections.

Adverse Reactions

Fever, skin rashes, and other allergic manifestations may result from hypersensitivity to streptomycin. This occurs most frequently with a prolonged course of treatment (eg, for tuberculosis).

Pain at the injection site is common but usually not severe. The most serious toxic effect with streptomycin is disturbance of vestibular function—vertigo and loss of balance. The frequency and severity of this disturbance are in proportion to the age of the patient, the blood levels of the drug, and the duration of administration. Vestibular dysfunction may follow a few weeks of unusually high blood levels (eg, in individuals with impaired renal function) or months of relatively low blood levels. Vestibular toxicity tends to be irreversible. Streptomycin given during pregnancy can cause deafness in the newborn.

GENTAMICIN

Gentamicin is a mixture of three closely related constituents, C_1, C_{1a}, and C_2 (see Figure 45–2) isolated from *Micromonospora purpurea.* It is active against both gram-positive and gram-negative organisms, and many of its properties resemble those of other aminoglycosides.

Antimicrobial Activity

Gentamicin sulfate, 2–10 mcg/mL, inhibits in vitro many strains of staphylococci and gram-negative bacteria, including *P aeruginosa* and Enterobacterales. Like all aminoglycosides, it has no activity against anaerobes.

Resistance

Streptococci and enterococci are relatively resistant to gentamicin owing to failure of the drug to penetrate into the cell. However, gentamicin in combination with some penicillins or vancomycin produces a potent bactericidal effect, which in part is due to enhanced uptake of drug that occurs with inhibition of cell wall synthesis. Resistance to gentamicin rapidly emerges in staphylococci during monotherapy owing to selection of permeability mutants. Ribosomal resistance is rare. Among gram-negative bacteria, resistance is most commonly due to plasmid-encoded aminoglycoside-modifying enzymes. Gram-negative bacteria that are gentamicin-resistant usually are susceptible to amikacin, which is much more resistant to modifying enzyme activity. The enterococcal enzyme that modifies gentamicin is a bifunctional enzyme that also inactivates amikacin, netilmicin, and tobramycin but not streptomycin; the latter is modified by a different enzyme. For this reason, some gentamicin-resistant enterococci are susceptible to streptomycin.

Clinical Uses

A. Intramuscular or Intravenous Administration

Gentamicin is used mainly in severe infections caused by gram-negative bacteria that are likely to be resistant to other drugs, especially *P aeruginosa*, *Enterobacter* sp, *Serratia marcescens*, *Proteus* sp, *Acinetobacter* sp, and *Klebsiella* sp. It usually is used in combination with a second agent because an aminoglycoside alone may not be effective for infections outside the urinary tract. Aminoglycosides should not be used as single agents for therapy of pneumonia because penetration of infected lung tissue is poor and local conditions of low pH and low oxygen tension contribute to limited activity. Gentamicin 5–7 mg/kg/d traditionally is given intravenously in three equal doses, but once-daily administration is just as effective for some organisms and less toxic (see above).

Gentamicin, in combination with a cell wall–active antibiotic, may also be indicated in the treatment of endocarditis caused by gram-positive bacteria (streptococci, staphylococci, and enterococci) as discussed earlier.

B. Topical and Ocular Administration

Creams, ointments, and solutions containing 0.1–0.3% gentamicin sulfate have been used for the treatment of infected burns, wounds, or skin lesions and in attempts to prevent intravenous catheter infections. The effectiveness of topical preparations for these indications is unclear. Topical gentamicin is partly inactivated by purulent exudates. Gentamicin can be injected intraocularly for treatment of certain eye infections.

C. Intrathecal Administration

Meningitis caused by gram-negative bacteria has been treated by the intrathecal injection of gentamicin sulfate, 1–10 mg/d. However, neither intrathecal nor intraventricular gentamicin was beneficial in neonates with meningitis, and intraventricular gentamicin was toxic, raising questions about the usefulness of this form of therapy. Moreover, the availability of third-generation cephalosporins for gram-negative meningitis has rendered this therapy obsolete in most cases. It may be used in cases of drug-resistant or treatment-refractory meningitis or severe β-lactam allergy.

Adverse Reactions

Nephrotoxicity is usually reversible upon drug discontinuation. It occurs in 5–25% of patients receiving gentamicin for longer than 3–5 days. Such toxicity requires, at the very least, adjustment of the dosing regimen and should prompt reconsideration of the need for the drug if there is a less toxic alternative agent. Measurement of gentamicin serum levels is essential. Ototoxicity, which tends to be irreversible, manifests mainly as vestibular dysfunction. Hearing loss also can occur. Ototoxicity is in part genetically determined, having been linked to point mutations in mitochondrial DNA, and occurs in 1–5% for patients receiving gentamicin for more than 5 days. Hypersensitivity reactions to gentamicin are uncommon.

TOBRAMYCIN

This aminoglycoside (see Figure 45–2) has an antibacterial spectrum similar to that of gentamicin. Although there is some cross-resistance between gentamicin and tobramycin, it is unpredictable in individual strains. Separate laboratory susceptibility tests are, therefore, necessary.

A. Intramuscular or Intravenous Administration

The pharmacokinetic properties of tobramycin are virtually identical with those of gentamicin. The daily dose of tobramycin is 5–7 mg/kg intramuscularly or intravenously, traditionally divided into three equal amounts and given every 8 hours but now often given as a single daily dose. Monitoring blood levels in renal insufficiency is an essential guide to proper dosing.

Tobramycin has almost the same antibacterial spectrum as gentamicin with a few exceptions. Gentamicin is slightly more active against *S marcescens*; tobramycin is slightly more active against *P aeruginosa*; *Enterococcus faecalis* is susceptible to both gentamicin and tobramycin, but *E faecium* is resistant to tobramycin. Gentamicin and tobramycin are otherwise interchangeable clinically.

Like other aminoglycosides, tobramycin is ototoxic and nephrotoxic. Nephrotoxicity of tobramycin may be slightly less than that of gentamicin.

B. Inhaled and Ophthalmic Administration

Tobramycin is formulated in solution (300 mg in 5 mL) for inhalation for treatment of *P aeruginosa* lower respiratory tract infections complicating cystic fibrosis. The drug is recommended as a 300-mg dose regardless of the patient's age or weight for administration twice daily in repeated cycles of 28 days on therapy, followed by 28 days off therapy. Serum concentrations 1 hour after inhalation average 1 mcg/mL; consequently, nephrotoxicity and ototoxicity rarely occur. Caution should be used when administering tobramycin to patients with preexisting renal, vestibular, or hearing disorders. Tobramycin is also available as 0.3% ophthalmic ointment and drops for the treatment of superficial eye infections. These formulations result in minimal systemic absorption and are unlikely to cause systemic adverse effects.

AMIKACIN

Amikacin is a semisynthetic derivative of kanamycin; it is less toxic than the parent molecule (see Figure 45–2). It is resistant to many enzymes that inactivate gentamicin and tobramycin, and, therefore, can be used against some microorganisms resistant to the latter drugs. Many gram-negative bacteria, including many strains of *Proteus*, *Pseudomonas*, *Enterobacter*, and *Serratia*, are inhibited by 1–20 mcg/mL amikacin in vitro. After injection of 500 mg of amikacin every 12 hours (15 mg/kg/d) intramuscularly, peak levels in serum are 10–30 mcg/mL.

Strains of multidrug-resistant *Mycobacterium tuberculosis*, including streptomycin-resistant strains, are usually susceptible to amikacin. Kanamycin-resistant strains may be cross-resistant to amikacin. The dosage of amikacin for tuberculosis is 10–15 mg/kg/d as a once-daily or twice- or thrice-weekly injection and always in combination with other drugs to which the isolate is susceptible.

Like all aminoglycosides, amikacin is nephrotoxic and ototoxic (particularly for the auditory portion of the eighth nerve). Serum concentrations should be monitored. Target peak serum concentrations for an every-12-hours dosing regimen are 20–40 mcg/mL, and trough levels should be maintained between 4 and 8 mcg/mL.

NETILMICIN

Netilmicin shares many characteristics with gentamicin and tobramycin. However, the addition of an ethyl group to the 1-amino position of the 2-deoxystreptamine ring (ring II, see Figure 45–2) sterically protects the netilmicin molecule from enzymatic degradation at the 3-amino (ring II) and 2-hydroxyl (ring III) positions. Consequently, netilmicin may be active against some gentamicin-resistant and tobramycin-resistant bacteria.

The dosage (5–7 mg/kg/d) and the routes of administration are the same as for gentamicin. Netilmicin is largely interchangeable with gentamicin or tobramycin but is no longer available in the United States.

NEOMYCIN, KANAMYCIN, & PAROMOMYCIN

Neomycin, kanamycin, and **paromomycin** have similar pharmacologic properties.

Antimicrobial Activity & Resistance

Drugs of the neomycin group are active against gram-positive and gram-negative bacteria and some mycobacteria. *P aeruginosa* and streptococci are generally resistant. Mechanisms of antibacterial action and resistance are the same as with other aminoglycosides. The former widespread use of these drugs in bowel preparation for elective surgery contributed to the selection of resistant organisms. Cross-resistance between kanamycin and neomycin is complete and may result in amikacin cross-resistance.

Pharmacokinetics

Like all aminoglycosides, drugs of the neomycin group are poorly absorbed from the gastrointestinal tract. After oral administration, the susceptible intestinal flora is suppressed, and the drug is excreted in the feces. Excretion of any absorbed drug is mainly through glomerular filtration into the urine.

Clinical Uses

Neomycin is generally limited to topical and oral use due to toxicity associated with parenteral use and higher resistance rates compared to other aminoglycosides. Kanamycin use is limited to treatment of multidrug-resistant tuberculosis, although alternate agents, such as amikacin, may be preferred. It is no longer available in the USA. Paromomycin has been shown to be effective against visceral leishmaniasis when given parenterally (see Chapter 52) and can be used topically for cutaneous leishmaniasis. Paromomycin can be used for intestinal *Entamoeba histolytica* infection and is sometimes used for intestinal infections with other parasites.

A. Topical Administration

Solutions containing 1–5 mg/mL neomycin have been used on infected surfaces or injected into joints, the pleural cavity, tissue spaces, or abscess cavities where infection is present. The total amount of drug given in this fashion must be limited to 15 mg/kg/d because at higher doses enough drug may be absorbed to produce systemic toxicity. However, the effectiveness of topical application in this manner has not been demonstrated. Ointments, often formulated as a neomycin-polymyxin-bacitracin combination, can be applied to infected skin lesions or in the nares for suppression of staphylococci, but they are largely ineffective.

B. Oral Administration

In preparation for elective bowel surgery, 1 g of neomycin may be given orally every 6–8 hours for 1–2 days, often combined with 1 g of erythromycin base. This reduces the aerobic bowel flora with little effect on anaerobes. In hepatic encephalopathy, coliform flora can be suppressed by giving 1 g every 6–8 hours together with reduced protein intake, thus reducing ammonia production. Use of neomycin for hepatic encephalopathy has been largely supplanted by lactulose and other medications that are less toxic. Use of paromomycin in the treatment of protozoal infections is discussed in Chapter 52.

C. Intravenous and Intramuscular Administration

When used intravenously, the standard dose for kanamycin is 15 mg/kg/day in two to three divided doses, whereas for treatment of tuberculosis, 15 mg/kg is usually given intramuscularly as a single daily dose. In the case of once-daily administration, kanamycin peak concentrations are typically between 35 and 45 mcg/mL, while trough concentrations should be undetectable.

Adverse Reactions

All members of the neomycin group have significant nephrotoxicity and ototoxicity. Auditory function is affected more than vestibular function. Deafness may occur, especially in adults with impaired renal function and prolonged elevation of drug levels.

The sudden absorption of postoperatively instilled kanamycin from the peritoneal cavity (3–5 g) has resulted in curare-like neuromuscular blockade and respiratory arrest. Calcium gluconate and neostigmine can act as antidotes.

Application of neomycin-containing ointments to skin and eyes can result in irritation or allergic reactions.

PLAZOMICIN

Plazomicin is the newest aminoglycoside to gain FDA approval for treatment of complicated urinary tract infections (cUTI). It is a synthetic molecule derived from sisomicin, an aminoglycoside no longer available. Various structural modifications have yielded a compound less susceptible to most aminoglycoside-modifying enzymes, thus retaining activity against aminoglycoside-resistant pathogens. It appears to have similarly potent in vitro activity against Enterobacterales and displays two- to fourfold lower MICs against nonfermenting gram-negative bacilli (eg, *P aeruginosa*) when compared with gentamicin, tobramycin, and amikacin. It has activity similar to gentamicin against staphylococci. A 15-mg/kg dose yields mean peak and trough concentrations of 113 mcg/mL and 0.43 mcg/mL, respectively. The half-life is 3–4 hours, and it is given as a single daily 15-mg/kg intravenous dose, infused over 30–60 minutes. Traditional twice- or thrice-daily regimens are not recommended, even in patients with impaired renal function. As such, therapeutic drug monitoring is more straightforward, requiring monitoring of trough levels only, rather than peak and trough. The target trough level is <3 mcg/ mL to prevent nephrotoxicity, which appears to be more common when trough levels exceed that value. Patients with impaired renal function are likely to require dose adjustments when estimated creatinine clearance is <60 mL/min. These monitoring parameters are most applicable when treating the FDA-approved indication of complicated urinary tract infections. Due to limited experience, it remains unclear whether modified pharmacokinetic targets will be necessary for treatment of off-label indications.

A key phase 3 trial of plazomicin showed clinical noninferiority when plazomicin was compared to meropenem for the treatment of cUTI, including pyelonephritis. Approximately 30% of participants had organisms resistant to at least one agent in at least three different antibacterial classes. An additional small phase 3 clinical trial compared plazomicin to colistin, in combination regimens for various infections caused by carbapenem-resistant Enterobacterales (CRE). The primary outcome, a composite of death and disease-related complications at 28 days, occurred in fewer patients who had received plazomicin (4 of 17, or 24%) compared to colistin (10 of 20, or 50%). There were also lower rates of acute kidney injury with plazomicin compared to colistin. While these data are extremely limited, they do suggest that plazomicin may be a useful alternative for patients with few antibacterial treatment options due to drug resistance.

Due to limited clinical experience, it is unclear whether the toxicity profile of plazomicin will be similar to other aminoglycosides. However, no ototoxicity or nephrotoxicity was observed in early trials. In a phase 3 trial, there were higher rates of renal-related adverse effects in the group receiving plazomicin compared to meropenem (3.6% and 1.3%, respectively), but most participants with nephrotoxicity had full renal recovery at the time of the final follow-up visit.

SPECTINOMYCIN

Spectinomycin is an aminocyclitol antibiotic that is structurally related to aminoglycosides. It lacks amino sugars and glycosidic bonds.

Spectinomycin

Spectinomycin is active in vitro against many gram-positive and gram-negative organisms, but it is used almost solely as an alternative treatment for drug-resistant gonorrhea or gonorrhea in penicillin-allergic patients. The majority of gonococcal isolates are inhibited by 6 mcg/mL of spectinomycin. Strains of gonococci may be resistant to spectinomycin, but there is no cross-resistance with other drugs used in gonorrhea. Notably, it is not recommended for treatment of pharyngeal gonococcal infections due to high failure rates regardless of in vitro susceptibility. Spectinomycin is rapidly absorbed after intramuscular injection. The standard regimen is a single dose of 2–4 g/d (40 mg/kg in children). Pain at the injection site is common, and fever and nausea occasionally occur. Nephrotoxicity and anemia have been observed rarely. Spectinomycin is no longer available for use in the USA.

SUMMARY Aminoglycosides

Subclass, Drug	Mechanism of Action	Effects	Clinical Applications	Pharmacokinetics, Toxicities, Interactions
AMINOGLYCOSIDES & SPECTINOMYCIN				
• Gentamicin	Prevents bacterial protein synthesis by binding to the 30S ribosomal subunit	Bactericidal activity against susceptible bacteria • synergistic effects against gram-positive bacteria when combined with β-lactams or vancomycin • concentration-dependent killing and a significant post-antibiotic effect	Sepsis caused by aerobic gram-negative bacteria • synergistic activity in endocarditis caused by streptococci, staphylococci, and enterococci	IV • renal clearance (half-life 2.5 h) • conventional dosing 1.3–1.7 mg/kg q8h with goal peak levels 5–8 mcg/mL • trough levels <2 mcg/mL • once-daily dosing at 5–7 mg/kg as effective and may have less toxicity than conventional dosing • *Toxicity:* Nephrotoxicity (reversible), ototoxicity (irreversible), neuromuscular blockade

- *Tobramycin: Intravenous; more active than gentamicin versus* Pseudomonas; *may also have less nephrotoxicity*
- *Amikacin: Intravenous; resistant to many enzymes that inactivate gentamicin and tobramycin; higher doses and target peaks and troughs than gentamicin and tobramycin*
- *Plazomicin: Intravenous; resistant to many enzymes that inactivate gentamicin and tobramycin; more active versus CRE; once-daily dosing only; no target peak levels; higher target trough levels acceptable*
- *Streptomycin: Intramuscular, widespread resistance limits use to specific indications such as tuberculosis and enterococcal endocarditis*
- *Neomycin: Oral or topical, poor bioavailability; used before bowel surgery to decrease aerobic flora*
- *Spectinomycin: Intramuscular; sole use is for treatment of antibiotic-resistant gonococcal infections or gonococcal infections in penicillin-allergic patients; not available in the USA*

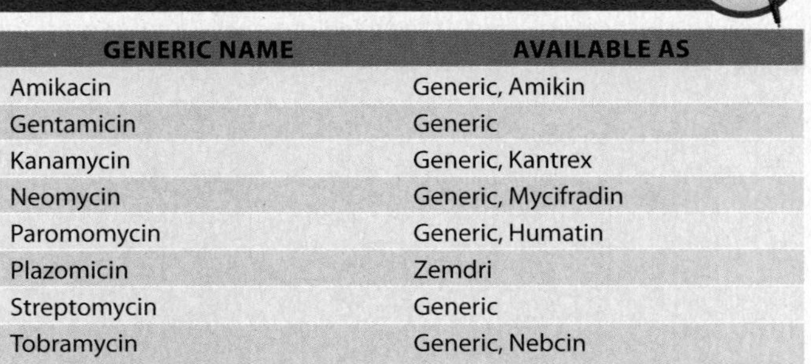

PREPARATIONS AVAILABLE

GENERIC NAME	AVAILABLE AS
Amikacin	Generic, Amikin
Gentamicin	Generic
Kanamycin	Generic, Kantrex
Neomycin	Generic, Mycifradin
Paromomycin	Generic, Humatin
Plazomicin	Zemdri
Streptomycin	Generic
Tobramycin	Generic, Nebcin

REFERENCES

Baddour L et al: Infective endocarditis in adults: Diagnosis, antimicrobial therapy, and management of complications. Circulation 2015;132:1435.

Busse H-J et al: The bactericidal action of streptomycin: Membrane permeabilization caused by the insertion of mistranslated proteins into the cytoplasmic membrane of *Escherichia coli* and subsequent caging of the antibiotic inside the cells due to degradation of these proteins. J Gen Microbiol 1992; 138:551.

Cheer SM et al: Inhaled tobramycin (TOBI): A review of its use in the management of *Pseudomonas aeruginosa* infections in patients with cystic fibrosis. Drugs 2003;63:2501.

Freeman CD et al: Once-daily dosing of aminoglycosides: Review and recommendations for clinical practice. J Antimicrob Chemother 1997;39:677.

Jackson J et al: Aminoglycosides: How should we use them in the 21st century? Curr Opin Infect Dis 2013;26:516.

Le T, Bayer AS: Combination antibiotic therapy for infective endocarditis. Clin Infect Dis 2003;36:615.

McKinnell JA et al: Plazomicin for infections caused by carbapenem-resistant enterobacteriaceae. N Engl J Med 2019;380:791.

Olsen KM et al: Effect of once-daily dosing vs. multiple daily dosing of tobramycin on enzyme markers of nephrotoxicity. Crit Care Med 2004;32:1678.

Paul M et al: Beta-lactam monotherapy versus beta-lactam-aminoglycoside combination therapy in cancer patients with neutropenia. Cochrane Database Syst Rev 2013 Jun 29;6:CD003038.

Peña C et al: Effect of adequate single-drug versus combination antimicrobial therapy on mortality in *Pseudomonas aeruginosa* bloodstream infections. Clin Infect Dis 2013;57:208.

Poole K: Aminoglycoside resistance in *Pseudomonas aeruginosa*. Antimicrob Agents Chemother 2005;49:479.

Shaeer KM et al: Plazomicin: A next-generation aminoglycoside. Pharmacotherapy 2019;39:77.

Wagenlehner FME et al: Once-daily plazomicin for complicated urinary tract infections. N Engl J Med 2019;380:729.

Zhanel G et al: Comparison of the next generation aminoglycoside plazomicin to gentamicin, tobramycin, and amikacin. Expert Rev Anti Infect Ther 2012;10:459.

CASE STUDY ANSWER

The patient has normal renal function and, thus, qualifies for once-daily dosing. Tobramycin could be administered as a single once-daily injection at a dose of 350–490 mg (5–7 mg/kg). A serum level between 1.5 and 6 mcg/mL measured 8 hours after infusion correlates with an appropriate trough level. Alternatively, the same total daily dose could be divided and administered every 8 hours, as a traditional dosing strategy. With traditional dosing, peak and trough concentrations should be monitored with the target peak concentration of 5–10 mcg/mL and the target trough concentration of <2 mcg/mL

CHAPTER

46

Sulfonamides, Trimethoprim, & Quinolones

Camille E. Beauduy, PharmD, & Lisa G. Winston, MD*

CASE STUDY

A 59-year-old woman presents to an urgent care clinic with a 4-day history of frequent and painful urination. She has had fevers, chills, and flank pain for the past 2 days. Her physician advised her to come immediately to the clinic for evaluation. In the clinic, she is febrile (38.5°C [101.3°F]) but otherwise stable and states she is not experiencing any nausea or vomiting. Her urine dipstick test is positive for leukocyte esterase. Urinalysis and urine culture are ordered. Her past medical history is significant for three urinary tract infections in the past year. Each episode was uncomplicated, treated with trimethoprim-sulfamethoxazole, and promptly resolved. She also has osteoporosis for which she takes a daily calcium supplement. The decision is made to treat her with oral antibiotics for a complicated urinary tract infection with close follow-up. Given her history, what would be a reasonable empiric antibiotic choice? Depending on the antibiotic choice, are there potential drug interactions?

■ ANTIFOLATE DRUGS

SULFONAMIDES

Chemistry

The basic formulas of the sulfonamides and their structural similarity to *p*-aminobenzoic acid (PABA) are shown in Figure 46–1. Sulfonamides with varying physical, chemical, pharmacologic, and antibacterial properties are produced by attaching substituents to the amido group (—SO_2—NH—R) or the amino group (—NH_2) of the sulfanilamide nucleus. Sulfonamides tend to be much more soluble at alkaline than at acid pH. Most can be prepared as sodium salts, which are used for intravenous administration.

Mechanism of Action & Antimicrobial Activity

Sulfonamide-susceptible organisms, unlike mammals, cannot use exogenous folate but must synthesize it from PABA. This pathway (Figure 46–2) is thus essential for production of purines and nucleic acid synthesis. As structural analogs of PABA, sulfonamides inhibit dihydropteroate synthase and folate production. Sulfonamides inhibit both gram-positive bacteria, such as *Staphylococcus* sp, and gram-negative enteric bacteria, such as *Escherichia coli*, *Klebsiella pneumoniae*, *Salmonella*, *Shigella*, and *Enterobacter* sp, as well as *Nocardia* sp, *Chlamydia trachomatis*, and some protozoa. Rickettsiae are not inhibited by sulfonamides but instead may be stimulated in their growth. Activity is poor against anaerobes. *Pseudomonas aeruginosa* is intrinsically resistant to sulfonamide antibiotics.

Combination of a sulfonamide with an inhibitor of dihydrofolate reductase (trimethoprim or pyrimethamine) provides synergistic activity because of sequential inhibition of folate synthesis (see Figure 46–2).

*The authors thank Henry F. Chambers, MD, and Daniel H. Deck, PharmD, for their contributions to previous editions.

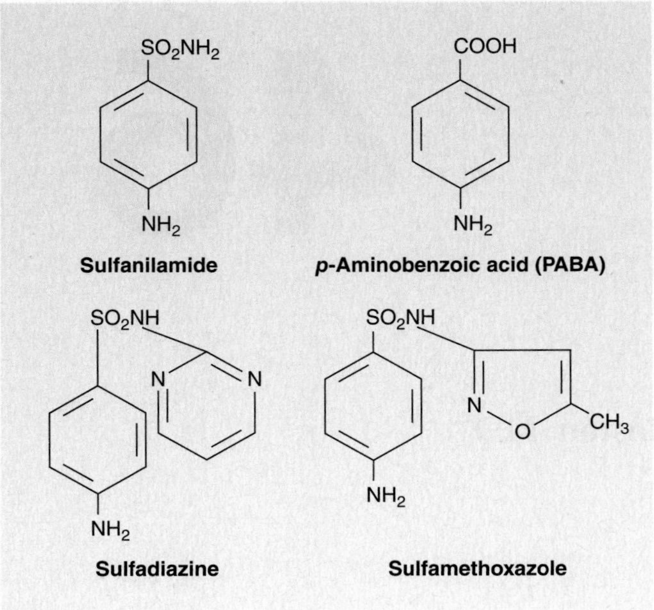

Sulfanilamide

p-Aminobenzoic acid (PABA)

Sulfadiazine

Sulfamethoxazole

FIGURE 46–1 Structures of some sulfonamides and *p*-aminobenzoic acid.

Resistance

Some bacteria lack the enzymes required for folate synthesis from PABA and, like mammals, depend on exogenous sources of folate; therefore, they are not susceptible to sulfonamides. Sulfonamide resistance may also occur as a result of mutations that (1) cause overproduction of PABA, (2) cause production of a folic acid-synthesizing enzyme that has low affinity for sulfonamides, or (3) impair permeability to the sulfonamide. Dihydropteroate synthase with low sulfonamide affinity is often encoded on a plasmid that is transmissible and can disseminate rapidly and widely. Sulfonamide-resistant dihydropteroate synthase mutants also can emerge under selective pressure.

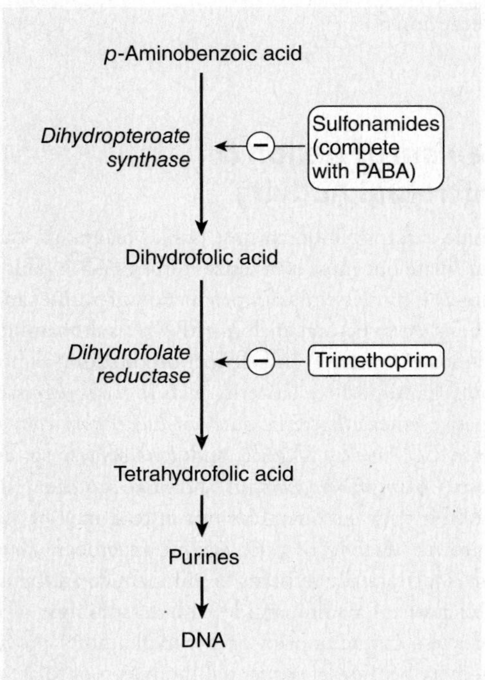

FIGURE 46–2 Actions of sulfonamides and trimethoprim.

Pharmacokinetics

Sulfonamides can be divided into three major groups: (1) oral, absorbable; (2) oral, nonabsorbable; and (3) topical. Oral absorbable sulfonamides are absorbed from the stomach and small intestine and distributed widely to tissues and body fluids (including the central nervous system and cerebrospinal fluid), placenta, and fetus. Protein binding varies from 20% to over 90%. Therapeutic concentrations are in the range of 40–100 mcg/mL of blood. Blood levels generally peak 2–6 hours after oral administration.

A portion of absorbed drug is acetylated or glucuronidated in the liver. Sulfonamides and inactive metabolites are then excreted in the urine, mainly by glomerular filtration. The dosage of sulfonamides must be reduced in patients with significant renal failure.

Clinical Uses

Sulfonamides are infrequently used as single agents. Many strains of formerly susceptible species, including meningococci, pneumococci, streptococci, staphylococci, and gonococci, are now resistant. The fixed-drug combination of trimethoprim-sulfamethoxazole is the drug of choice for infections such as *Pneumocystis jirovecii* (formerly *P carinii*) pneumonia, toxoplasmosis, and nocardiosis.

A. Oral Absorbable Agents

Sulfamethoxazole is a commonly used absorbable agent; however, in the USA, it is available only as the fixed-dosed combination **trimethoprim-sulfamethoxazole.** Typical dosing and indications are discussed below.

Administration of **sulfadiazine** with pyrimethamine is first-line therapy for treatment of acute toxoplasmosis. Using sulfadiazine plus pyrimethamine, a potent inhibitor of dihydrofolate reductase, is synergistic because these drugs block sequential steps in the folate synthesis pathway (see Figure 46–2). However, there have been periodic challenges with manufacturing, supply, and pricing of pyrimethamine in the USA. In some cases, clinicians have obtained a compounded product through specialty pharmacies or prescribed alternate agents, such as trimethoprim-sulfamethoxazole. **Sulfadoxine** is a long-acting sulfonamide that is coformulated with pyrimethamine **(Fansidar).** This combination is no longer commercially available in the USA but may be found in other parts of the world where it has been used as a second-line treatment for malaria (see Chapter 52).

B. Oral Nonabsorbable Agents

Sulfasalazine (salicylazosulfapyridine) is used in the treatment of inflammatory bowel disease (see Chapter 62).

C. Topical Agents

Sodium **sulfacetamide** ophthalmic solution or ointment is effective in the treatment of bacterial conjunctivitis but is considered a second-line agent due to the potential for allergic reactions. Another sulfonamide, **mafenide acetate,** is available for topical use but can be absorbed from burn sites. The drug and its primary metabolite inhibit carbonic anhydrase and can cause metabolic acidosis, a side effect that limits its usefulness. **Silver sulfadiazine** is a less toxic topical sulfonamide that has been widely used for prevention of infection of burn wounds; however, it may slow wound healing, and non-silver-containing products may be preferred.

Adverse Reactions

Historically, drugs containing a sulfonamide moiety, including antimicrobial sulfas, diuretics, diazoxide, and the sulfonylurea hypoglycemic agents, were considered to be cross-allergenic. However, more recent evidence suggests cross-reactivity is uncommon and many patients who are allergic to nonantibiotic sulfonamides tolerate sulfonamide antibiotics. The most common adverse effects are fever, skin rashes, exfoliative dermatitis, photosensitivity, urticaria, nausea, vomiting, diarrhea, and difficulties referable to the urinary tract (see below). Stevens-Johnson syndrome, although relatively uncommon (<1% of treatment courses), is a particularly serious and potentially fatal type of skin and mucous membrane eruption associated with sulfonamide use. Other adverse effects include stomatitis, conjunctivitis, arthritis, hematopoietic disturbances (see below), hepatitis, and, rarely, polyarteritis nodosa and psychosis.

A. Urinary Tract Disturbances

Sulfonamides may precipitate in urine, especially at neutral or acid pH, producing crystalluria, hematuria, or even obstruction. This is rarely a problem with the more soluble sulfonamides (eg, sulfisoxazole). Sulfadiazine and sulfamethoxazole are relatively insoluble in acidic urine and can cause crystalluria, particularly when given in large doses or if fluid intake is poor. Crystalluria is treated by administration of sodium bicarbonate to alkalinize the urine and fluids to increase urine flow. Sulfonamides have also been implicated in allergic nephritis and other renal disorders.

B. Hematopoietic Disturbances

Sulfonamides can cause hemolytic or aplastic anemia, granulocytopenia, thrombocytopenia, or leukemoid reactions. Sulfonamides may provoke hemolytic reactions in patients with glucose-6-phosphate dehydrogenase deficiency. Sulfonamides taken near the end of pregnancy increase the risk of kernicterus in newborns.

TRIMETHOPRIM & TRIMETHOPRIM-SULFAMETHOXAZOLE MIXTURES

Mechanism of Action

Trimethoprim, a trimethoxybenzylpyrimidine, selectively inhibits bacterial dihydrofolic acid reductase, which converts dihydrofolic acid to tetrahydrofolic acid, a step leading to the synthesis of purines and ultimately to DNA (see Figure 46–2). Trimethoprim is a much less efficient inhibitor of mammalian dihydrofolic acid reductase. The combination of trimethoprim and sulfamethoxazole is often bactericidal, compared with the bacteriostatic activity of a sulfonamide alone.

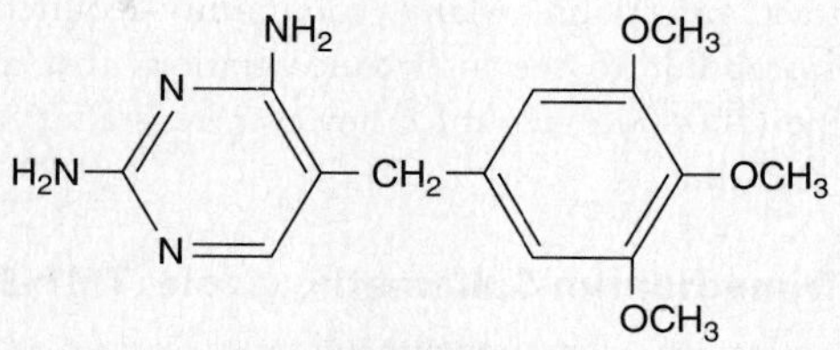

Trimethoprim

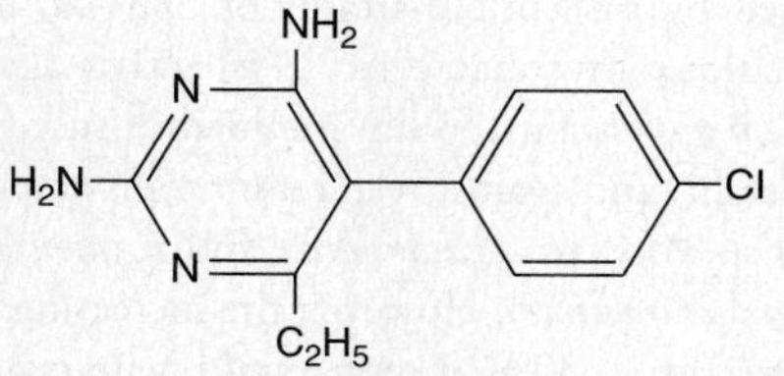

Pyrimethamine

Resistance

Resistance to trimethoprim can result from reduced cell permeability, overproduction of dihydrofolate reductase, or production of an altered reductase with reduced drug binding. Resistance can emerge by mutation, although more commonly it is due to plasmid-encoded trimethoprim-resistant dihydrofolate reductases. These resistant enzymes may be coded within transposons on conjugative plasmids that exhibit a broad host range, accounting for rapid and widespread dissemination of trimethoprim resistance among numerous bacterial species.

Pharmacokinetics

Trimethoprim is usually given orally, alone or in combination with sulfamethoxazole, which has a similar half-life. Trimethoprim-sulfamethoxazole can also be given intravenously. Trimethoprim is well absorbed from the gut and distributed widely in body fluids and tissues, including cerebrospinal fluid.

Because trimethoprim is more lipid-soluble than sulfamethoxazole, it has a larger volume of distribution than the latter drug. Therefore, when 1 part of trimethoprim is given with 5 parts of sulfamethoxazole (the ratio in the formulation), the peak plasma concentrations are in the ratio of 1:20, which is optimal for the combined effects of these drugs in vitro. About 30–50% of the sulfonamide and 50–60% of the trimethoprim (or their respective metabolites) are excreted in the urine within 24 hours. The dose should be reduced by half for patients with creatinine clearances of 15–30 mL/min.

Trimethoprim (a weak base) concentrates in prostatic fluid and in vaginal fluid, which are more acidic than plasma. Therefore, it has more antibacterial activity in prostatic and vaginal fluids than many other antimicrobial drugs.

Clinical Uses

A. Oral Trimethoprim

Trimethoprim can be given alone (100 mg twice daily) in acute urinary tract infections. Many community-acquired organisms are susceptible to the high concentrations that are found in the urine (200–600 mcg/mL); however, resistance rates have increased over time.

B. Oral Trimethoprim-Sulfamethoxazole (TMP-SMZ)

A combination of trimethoprim-sulfamethoxazole is effective treatment for a wide variety of infections including *P jirovecii* pneumonia, urinary tract infections, prostatitis, and some infections caused by susceptible strains of *Shigella, Salmonella*, and nontuberculous mycobacteria. It is active against most *Staphylococcus aureus* strains, both methicillin-susceptible and methicillin-resistant, and against respiratory tract pathogens such as *Haemophilus* sp, *Moraxella catarrhalis*, and *K pneumoniae* (but not *Mycoplasma pneumoniae*). However, the increasing prevalence of strains of *E coli* (up to 30% or more) and pneumococci that are resistant to trimethoprim-sulfamethoxazole must be considered before using this combination for empiric therapy of upper urinary tract infections or pneumonia. Trimethoprim-sulfamethoxazole is commonly used for the treatment of uncomplicated skin and soft tissue infections.

One double-strength tablet (each tablet contains trimethoprim 160 mg plus sulfamethoxazole 800 mg) given every 12 hours is effective treatment for urinary tract infections, prostatitis, uncomplicated skin and soft tissue infections, and infections caused by susceptible strains of *Shigella* and *Salmonella*. Bone and joint infections caused by *S aureus* can be effectively treated, typically at doses of 8–10 mg/kg per day of the trimethoprim component. One single-strength tablet (containing trimethoprim 80 mg plus sulfamethoxazole 400 mg) given three times weekly may serve as prophylaxis in recurrent urinary tract infections of some women. The dosage for children treated for shigellosis, urinary tract infection, or otitis media is trimethoprim 8 mg/kg per day and sulfamethoxazole 40 mg/kg per day divided every 12 hours.

Infections with *P jirovecii* and some other pathogens, such as *Nocardia* or *Stenotrophomonas maltophilia*, can be treated with high doses of either the oral or intravenous combination (dosed on the basis of the trimethoprim component at 15–20 mg/kg/d). *P jirovecii* can be prevented in immunosuppressed patients by a number of low-dose regimens such as one double-strength tablet daily or three times weekly.

C. Intravenous Trimethoprim-Sulfamethoxazole

A solution of the mixture containing 80 mg trimethoprim plus 400 mg sulfamethoxazole per 5 mL diluted in 125 mL of 5% dextrose in water can be administered by intravenous infusion over 60–90 minutes. It is the agent of choice for moderately severe to severe *Pneumocystis* pneumonia. Trimethoprim-sulfamethoxazole can also be used to treat gram-negative bacteremia caused by susceptible organisms. It may be an effective alternative for infections caused by some multidrug-resistant species such as *Enterobacter* and *Serratia*; shigellosis; or typhoid. It is the preferred alternate therapy for serious *Listeria* infections in patients unable to tolerate ampicillin. The dosage is 10–20 mg/kg/d of the trimethoprim component.

D. Oral Pyrimethamine with Sulfonamide

Pyrimethamine and sulfadiazine are used in the treatment of toxoplasmosis. The dosage of sulfadiazine is 1–1.5 g four times daily, with pyrimethamine given as a 200-mg loading dose followed by a once-daily dose of 50–75 mg. Leucovorin, also known as folinic acid, 10 mg orally each day, should be administered to minimize bone marrow suppression seen with pyrimethamine. Some clinicians recommend using trimethoprim-sulfamethoxazole as an alternate option if pyrimethamine is not available.

In falciparum malaria, the combination of pyrimethamine with sulfadoxine (Fansidar) has been used (see Chapter 52), but resistance has emerged in many parts of the world; it is no longer commercially available in the USA.

Adverse Effects

Trimethoprim produces the predictable adverse effects of an antifolate drug, especially megaloblastic anemia, leukopenia, and granulocytopenia. The combination trimethoprim-sulfamethoxazole may cause all of the untoward reactions associated with sulfonamides. Nausea and vomiting, drug fever, vasculitis, renal damage, and central nervous system disturbances occasionally occur. Patients with AIDS and pneumocystis pneumonia have a particularly high frequency of untoward reactions to trimethoprim-sulfamethoxazole, especially fever, rashes, leukopenia, diarrhea, elevations of hepatic aminotransferases, hyperkalemia, and hyponatremia. Trimethoprim inhibits secretion of creatinine at the distal renal tubule, resulting in mild elevation of serum creatinine without impairment of glomerular filtration rate. This nontoxic effect is important to distinguish from true nephrotoxicity that may be caused by sulfonamides.

DNA GYRASE INHIBITORS

FLUOROQUINOLONES

The clinically relevant quinolones are synthetic fluorinated analogs of nalidixic acid (Figure 46–3). They are active against a variety of gram-positive and gram-negative bacteria.

Mechanism of Action

Quinolones block bacterial DNA synthesis by inhibiting bacterial topoisomerase II (DNA gyrase) and topoisomerase IV. Inhibition of DNA gyrase prevents the relaxation of positively supercoiled DNA

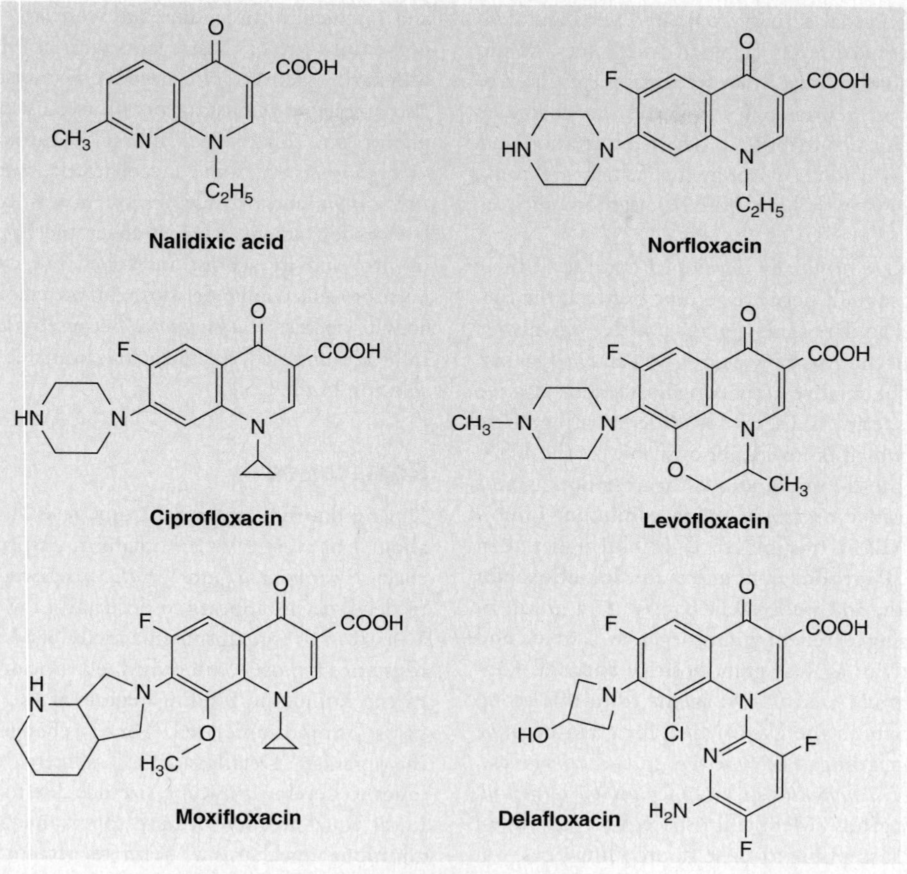

FIGURE 46–3 Structures of nalidixic acid and some fluoroquinolones.

that is required for normal transcription and replication. Inhibition of topoisomerase IV interferes with separation of replicated chromosomal DNA into the respective daughter cells during cell division. While all quinolones have activity at both target sites, most have higher affinity for one or the other. This can explain differences in spectra of activity since DNA gyrase is the primary target for gram-negative and topoisomerase IV is the primary target for gram-positive organisms. Delafloxacin has a uniquely balanced affinity for both target sites, which may contribute to its broader spectrum of activity and reduced likelihood for induction of resistance, both of which are discussed in further detail later in the chapter.

Antibacterial Activity

Earlier quinolones such as nalidixic acid did not achieve systemic antibacterial levels and were useful only in the treatment of lower urinary tract infections. Fluorinated derivatives (ciprofloxacin, levofloxacin, and others; Figure 46–3 and Table 46–1) have

TABLE 46–1 Pharmacokinetic properties of some fluoroquinolones.

Drug	Half-Life (h)	Oral Bioavailability (%)	Peak Serum Concentration (mcg/mL)	Oral Dose (mg)	Primary Route of Excretion
Ciprofloxacin	3–5	70	2.4	500 twice daily	Renal
Delafloxacin	4–8	59	7.5	450 twice daily	Renal and nonrenal
Gemifloxacin	8	70	1.6	320 once daily	Renal and nonrenal
Levofloxacin	5–7	95	5.7	500 once daily	Renal
Moxifloxacin	9–10	>85	3.1	400 once daily	Nonrenal
Norfloxacin	3.5–5	80	1.5	400 twice daily	Renal
Ofloxacin	5–7	95	2.9	400 twice daily	Renal

greatly improved antibacterial activity compared with nalidixic acid and achieve bactericidal levels in blood and tissues. While most of the fluoroquinolones exist in zwitterionic forms in vivo, delafloxacin is anionic at neutral pH and carries no charge at acidic pH. This appears to contribute to better penetration and more potent activity in acidic environments, which are commonly seen in infections with high bacterial burden, such as abscess fluid.

Fluoroquinolones were originally developed because of their excellent activity against gram-negative aerobic bacteria; the earliest agents had limited activity against gram-positive organisms. Subsequent members of the group have improved activity against gram-positive cocci. The relative activity against gram-negative versus gram-positive species is useful for differentiating these agents. **Norfloxacin,** which is no longer available in the USA, is the least active of the fluoroquinolones against both gram-negative and gram-positive organisms, with minimum inhibitory concentrations (MICs) fourfold to eightfold higher than those of ciprofloxacin. **Ciprofloxacin, enoxacin, lomefloxacin, levofloxacin, ofloxacin,** and **pefloxacin** constitute a group of similar agents possessing excellent gram-negative activity and moderate to good activity against gram-positive bacteria. Ciprofloxacin and levofloxacin are the two agents from this group that are used systemically in the USA. MICs for gram-negative cocci and bacilli, including *Enterobacter* sp, *P aeruginosa*, *Neisseria meningitidis*, *Haemophilus* sp, and *Campylobacter jejuni*, typically are ≤1–2 mcg/mL. Methicillin-susceptible strains of *S aureus* generally are susceptible to these fluoroquinolones, but methicillin-resistant strains of staphylococci are often resistant. When treating staphylococcal infections, fluoroquinolones typically are used in combination with a second active agent, such as rifampin, to prevent emergence of resistance while on therapy. Enterococci tend to be less susceptible than staphylococci, limiting the efficacy of fluoroquinolones in infections caused by these organisms. Ciprofloxacin is the most active agent of this group against gram-negative organisms, particularly *P aeruginosa.* Levofloxacin, the L-isomer of ofloxacin, has greater activity than ciprofloxacin against gram-positive organisms, especially *Streptococcus pneumoniae.* In addition to its potent activity against gram-positive organisms, discussed below, delafloxacin has similar activity to ciprofloxacin against gram-negative organisms, including *P aeruginosa*.

Gatifloxacin, gemifloxacin, moxifloxacin, and **delafloxacin** make up a group of fluoroquinolones with improved activity against gram-positive organisms, particularly *S pneumoniae* and some staphylococci. Moxifloxacin and delafloxacin are the only two with systemic preparations available in the USA. Although MICs of these agents for staphylococci are lower than those of ciprofloxacin (and the other compounds mentioned in the paragraph above), it is not known whether the enhanced activity is sufficient to permit use of this group of antibiotics for treatment of infections caused by ciprofloxacin-resistant strains. When compared to other fluoroquinolones, delafloxacin has three- to fivefold more potent in vitro activity against most gram-positive organisms including pneumococci, beta-hemolytic streptococci, and methicillin-susceptible and -resistant *S aureus.* Delafloxacin is the only one of these agents with activity comparable to ciprofloxacin against gram-negative organisms. Fluoroquinolones also are active against agents of atypical pneumonia (eg, mycoplasmas and chlamydiae) and against intracellular pathogens such as *Legionella* and some mycobacteria, including *Mycobacterium tuberculosis* and *Mycobacterium avium* complex. Moxifloxacin has modest activity against anaerobic bacteria; delafloxacin has in vitro activity against anaerobes, but clinical efficacy has not been proven. Unlike delafloxacin, moxifloxacin lacks appreciable activity against *P aeruginosa.* Because of toxicity when systemically administered, gatifloxacin is available only as an ophthalmic solution in the USA.

Resistance

During fluoroquinolone therapy, resistant organisms emerge in about 1 of every 10^7–10^9 organisms, especially among staphylococci, *P aeruginosa*, and *Serratia marcescens.* Emergent resistance to delafloxacin appears to occur at a lower rate, approximately 1 in 10^9–10^{11} organisms in a study of MRSA strains. Emerging resistance is most commonly due to one or more point mutations in the quinolone binding region of the target enzyme (DNA gyrase or topoisomerase IV) or to a change in the permeability of the organism. Delafloxacin is less likely than other fluoroquinolones to develop clinical resistance due to point mutations since it has equal affinity for both topoisomerase enzymes. However, additional mechanisms seem to account for the relative ease with which resistance develops in highly susceptible bacteria. Two types of plasmid-mediated resistance have been described. The first type utilizes Qnr proteins, which protect DNA gyrase from the fluoroquinolones. The second is a variant of an aminoglycoside acetyltransferase capable of modifying ciprofloxacin. Both mechanisms confer low-level resistance that may facilitate the point mutations that confer high-level resistance and also may be associated with resistance to other antibacterial drug classes. These modes of plasmid-mediated resistance have been described for all modern fluoroquinolones, including delafloxacin in vitro; given limited experience, it is unclear how it will contribute to clinical outcomes with delafloxacin. Resistance to one fluoroquinolone, particularly if it is high-level resistance, generally confers cross-resistance to all other members of this class; the key exception appears to be delafloxacin, which retains activity against fluoroquinolone-resistant gram-positive organisms. There are reports of emergent resistance to delafloxacin, however, so susceptibility should be confirmed when treating serious infections, especially in patients with prior fluoroquinolone-resistantant infections or extensive prior exposure to antibacterials.

Pharmacokinetics

After oral administration, the fluoroquinolones are well absorbed. Most have bioavailability between 80% and 95%. Delafloxacin is only 59% bioavailable; the oral dose (450 mg) is higher than the IV (300 mg). All fluoroquinolones are widely distributed in body fluids and tissues (see Table 46–1). Serum half-lives range from 3 to 10 hours. The relatively long half-lives of levofloxacin, gemifloxacin, and moxifloxacin permit once-daily dosing. Oral absorption is impaired by divalent and trivalent cations, including those in antacids. Therefore, oral fluoroquinolones should be taken 2 hours before or 4–6 hours after any products containing these cations. Serum concentrations of intravenously administered drug are similar to those of orally administered drug. Most fluoroquinolones, moxifloxacin being an important exception, are eliminated by renal mechanisms, either tubular secretion or glomerular filtration (see Table 46–1). Dosage adjustment is required for patients with creatinine clearances <50 mL/min, the exact adjustment depending on the degree of renal impairment and the specific fluoroquinolone being used. Delafloxacin requires renal dose adjustment for the IV formulation only when creatinine clearance is <30 mL/min; neither the IV nor oral forms are recommended in end-stage renal failure (creatinine clearance <15 mL/min or hemodialysis). Dosage adjustment for renal failure is not necessary for moxifloxacin since it is metabolized in the liver; it should be used with caution in patients with hepatic failure.

Clinical Uses

Fluoroquinolones (other than moxifloxacin, which achieves relatively low urinary levels) are effective in urinary tract infections caused by many organisms, including *P aeruginosa*. These agents are also effective for bacterial diarrhea caused by *Shigella*, *Salmonella*, toxigenic *E coli*, and *Campylobacter*. Fluoroquinolones (except norfloxacin, which does not achieve adequate systemic concentrations) are used in infections of soft tissues, bones, and joints and in intra-abdominal and respiratory tract infections, including those caused by multidrug-resistant organisms such as *Pseudomonas* and *Enterobacter*. Ciprofloxacin is a drug of choice for prophylaxis and treatment of anthrax; the newer fluoroquinolones are active in vitro, and levofloxacin is also approved by the US Food and Drug Administration (FDA) for anthrax prophylaxis.

Ciprofloxacin and levofloxacin are no longer recommended for the treatment of gonococcal infection in the USA, as resistance is now common. Gemifloxacin is no longer recommended as alternate therapy due to limited availability. Delafloxacin initially appeared promising in vitro against ciprofloxacin-resistant gonococcal strains; however, in clinical trials it failed to show activity comparable to the standard treatment, ceftriaxone. Levofloxacin is recommended by the US Centers for Disease Control and Prevention as an alternative treatment options for chlamydial urethritis or cervicitis. Ciprofloxacin, levofloxacin, or moxifloxacin is occasionally used as part of a treatment regimen for tuberculosis and nontuberculous mycobacterial infections. Clinical data for delafloxacin against mycobacteria are lacking, but it shows promising in vitro activity. These agents are suitable for eradication of meningococci from carriers and for prophylaxis of bacterial infection in patients with neutropenia due to cancer therapy.

With their enhanced gram-positive activity and activity against atypical pneumonia agents (chlamydiae, *Mycoplasma*, and *Legionella*), levofloxacin, gemifloxacin, and moxifloxacin—so-called respiratory fluoroquinolones—are effective for treatment of lower respiratory tract infections. Delafloxacin is also FDA-approved for this indication, and it has similar or more potent activity against these atypical organisms.

Adverse Effects

The most common adverse effects of fluoroquinolones are nausea, vomiting, and diarrhea. Occasionally, headache, dizziness, insomnia, skin rash, or abnormal liver function tests develop. Photosensitivity has been reported with lomefloxacin and pefloxacin. Prolongation of the QT_c interval may occur with gatifloxacin, levofloxacin, gemifloxacin, and moxifloxacin; these drugs should be avoided or used with caution in patients with known QT_c interval prolongation or uncorrected hypokalemia; in those receiving class 1A (eg, procainamide) or class 3 antiarrhythmic agents (sotalol, ibutilide, amiodarone); and in patients receiving other agents known to increase the QT_c interval (eg, erythromycin, tricyclic antidepressants). Gatifloxacin has been associated with hyperglycemia in diabetic patients and with hypoglycemia in patients also receiving oral hypoglycemic agents. Because of these serious effects (including some fatalities), gatifloxacin was withdrawn from sale in the USA in 2006.

In animal models, fluoroquinolones may damage growing cartilage and cause an arthropathy. Thus, these drugs have not been recommended as first-line agents for patients under 18 years of age. However, there is consensus that fluoroquinolones may be used in children if needed (eg, for treatment of pseudomonal infections in patients with cystic fibrosis). Tendinitis, a complication in adults, can be serious because of the risk of tendon rupture. Risk factors for tendinitis include advanced age, renal insufficiency, and concurrent steroid use. Fluoroquinolones should be avoided during pregnancy in the absence of specific data documenting their safety. They have rarely been associated with aortic dissection or rupture, particularly in patients with atherosclerosis or hypertension. Oral or intravenously administered fluoroquinolones have also been associated with peripheral neuropathy and central neurotoxicities, such as agitation or impaired memory or attention. These neurotoxicities can occur at any time during treatment with fluoroquinolones and may persist after the drug is stopped. In some cases, neurotoxicity may be permanent. Although many of the listed adverse effects are uncommon, the FDA requires inclusion of safety warnings for all fluoroquinolones, stating that these agents should be reserved for patients who do not have alternative options, particularly in less severe infections such as upper respiratory infections or uncomplicated cystitis.

SUMMARY Sulfonamides, Trimethoprim, and Fluoroquinolones

Subclass, Drug	Mechanism of Action	Effects	Clinical Applications	Pharmacokinetics, Toxicities, Interactions
FOLATE ANTAGONISTS				
• Trimethoprim-sulfamethoxazole	Synergistic combination of folate antagonists blocks purine production and nucleic acid synthesis	Bactericidal activity against susceptible bacteria	Urinary tract infections • soft tissue infections • bone and joint infections • *P jirovecii* pneumonia • toxoplasmosis • nocardiosis	Oral, IV • renal clearance (half-life 8 h) • dosed every 8–12 h • formulated in a 5:1 ratio of sulfamethoxazole to trimethoprim • *Toxicity:* Rash, fever, bone marrow suppression, hyperkalemia, nephrotoxicity
• *Sulfadiazine: Oral; first-line therapy for toxoplasmosis when combined with pyrimethamine*				
• *Trimethoprim: Oral; used alone only for lower urinary tract infections; may be safely prescribed to patients with sulfonamide allergy*				
• *Pyrimethamine: Oral; first-line therapy for toxoplasmosis when combined with sulfadiazine; coadminister with leucovorin to limit bone marrow toxicity*				
• *Pyrimethamine-sulfadoxine: Oral; some activity against malaria but resistance limits use*				
FLUOROQUINOLONES				
• Ciprofloxacin	Inhibits DNA replication by binding to DNA gyrase and topoisomerase IV	Bactericidal activity against susceptible bacteria	Urinary tract infections • gastroenteritis • osteomyelitis • anthrax	Oral, IV • mixed clearance (half-life 4 h) • dosed every 12 h • divalent and trivalent cations impair oral absorption • *Toxicity:* Gastrointestinal upset, neurotoxicity, tendinitis
• *Levofloxacin: Oral, IV; L-isomer of ofloxacin; once-daily dosing; renal clearance; "respiratory" fluoroquinolone with improved activity versus pneumococcus*				
• *Moxifloxacin: Oral, IV; "respiratory" fluoroquinolone; once-daily dosing; improved activity versus anaerobes and* M tuberculosis*; hepatic clearance results in lower urinary levels so use in urinary tract infections is not recommended*				
• *Delafloxacin: Oral, IV; "next-generation" fluoroquinolone; more potent activity versus gram-positive organisms including pneumococcus and staphylococcus; similar activity to ciprofloxacin versus gram-negative organisms, including* P aeruginosa				

PREPARATIONS AVAILABLE

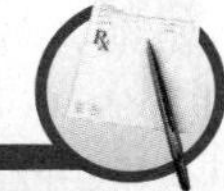

GENERIC NAME	AVAILABLE AS
GENERAL-PURPOSE SULFONAMIDES	
Sulfadiazine	Generic
SULFONAMIDES FOR SPECIAL APPLICATIONS	
Mafenide	Generic, Sulfamylon
Silver sulfadiazine	Generic, Silvadene
Sulfacetamide sodium (ophthalmic)	Generic
TRIMETHOPRIM	
Trimethoprim	Generic, Proloprim, Trimpex
Trimethoprim-sulfamethoxazole (co-trimoxazole, TMP-SMZ)	Generic, Bactrim, Septra, others
PYRIMETHAMINE	
Pyrimethamine	Generic, Daraprim
Pyrimethamine-sulfadoxine	Generic, Fansidar
FLUOROQUINOLONES	
Ciprofloxacin	Generic, Cipro, Cipro I.V., Ciloxan (ophthalmic)
Delafloxacin	Baxdela
Levofloxacin	Levaquin, Quixin (ophthalmic)
Moxifloxacin	Generic, Avelox, others
Norfloxacin	Noroxin
Ofloxacin	Generic, Floxin, Ocuflox (ophthalmic), Floxin Otic (otic)

REFERENCES

Briasoulis A et al: QT prolongation and torsade de pointes induced by fluoroquinolones: Infrequent side effects from commonly used medications. Cardiology 2011;120:103.

Cohen JS: Peripheral neuropathy associated with fluoroquinolones. Ann Pharmacother 2001;35:1540.

Davidson R et al: Resistance to levofloxacin and failure of treatment of pneumococcal pneumonia. N Engl J Med 2002;346:747.

Gupta K et al: International clinical practice guidelines for the treatment of acute uncomplicated cystitis and pyelonephritis in women. Clin Infect Dis 2011;52:103.

Iregui A et al: Emergence of delafloxacin-resistant *Staphylococcus aureus* in Brooklyn, New York. Clin Infect Dis 2020;70:1758.

Jorgensen SCJ et al: Delafloxacin: Place in therapy and review of microbiologic, clinical, and pharmacologic properties. Infect Dis Ther 2018;7:197.

Keating GM, Scott LJ: Moxifloxacin: A review of its use in the management of bacterial infections. Drugs 2004;64:2347.

Metlay JP et al: Diagnosis and treatment of adults with community-acquired pneumonia. An official clinical practice guideline of the American Thoracic Society and Infectious Diseases Society of America. Am J Respir Crit Care Med 2019;200:e45.

Mwenya DM et al: Impact of cotrimoxazole on carriage and antibiotic resistance of *Streptococcus pneumoniae* and *Haemophilus influenzae* in HIV-infected children in Zambia. Antimicrob Agents Chemother 2010;54:3756.

Nouira S et al: Standard versus newer antibacterial agents in the treatment of severe acute exacerbation of chronic obstructive pulmonary disease: A randomized trial of trimethoprim-sulfamethoxazole versus ciprofloxacin. Clin Infect Dis 2010;51:143.

Rodriguez-Martinez JM et al: Plasmid-mediated quinolone resistance: An update. J Infect Chemother 2011;17:149.

Scheld WM: Maintaining fluoroquinolone class efficacy: Review of influencing factors. Emerg Infect Dis 2003;9:1.

Schmitz GR et al: Randomized controlled trial of trimethoprim-sulfamethoxazole for uncomplicated skin abscesses in patients at risk for community-associated methicillin-resistant *Staphylococcus aureus* infection. Ann Emerg Med 2010; 56:283.

Strom BL et al: Absence of cross-reactivity between sulfonamide antibiotics and sulfonamide nonantibiotics. N Engl J Med 2003;349:1628.

Talan DA et al: Prevalence of and risk factor analysis of trimethoprim-sulfamethoxazole- and fluoroquinolone-resistant *E. coli* infection among emergency department patients with pyelonephritis. Clin Infect Dis 2008; 47:1150.

Workowski KA et al: Sexually transmitted diseases treatment guidelines, 2015. MMWR Recomm Rep 2015;64(RR-03):1.

Ziganshina LE et al: Fluoroquinolones for treating tuberculosis (presumed drug sensitive). Cochrane Database Syst Rev 2013;(6):CD004795.

CASE STUDY ANSWER

A fluoroquinolone that achieves good urinary and systemic levels (ciprofloxacin or levofloxacin) would be a reasonable choice for empiric treatment of this patient's complicated urinary tract infection. Given the possibility of a fluoroquinolone-resistant organism, one dose of a parenteral agent such as ceftriaxone (given IV or IM) would be reasonable pending culture results confirming fluoroquinolone susceptibility. Her recent exposure to multiple courses of trimethoprim-sulfamethoxazole increases her chances of having a urinary tract infection with an isolate that is resistant to this antibiotic. The patient should be told to take the oral fluoroquinolone 2 hours before or 4 hours after her calcium supplement, as divalent and trivalent cations can significantly impair the absorption of oral fluoroquinolones.

CHAPTER

47 Antimycobacterial Drugs

Camille E. Beauduy, PharmD, & Lisa G. Winston, MD*

CASE STUDY

A 60-year-old man presents to the emergency department with a 2-month history of fatigue, weight loss (10 kg), fevers, night sweats, and a productive cough. He is currently living with friends and has been intermittently without housing, spending time in shelters. He reports drinking about six beers per day. In the emergency department, a chest x-ray shows a right apical infiltrate. Given the high suspicion for pulmonary tuberculosis, the patient is placed in respiratory isolation. His first sputum smear shows many acid-fast bacilli, and an HIV test returns with a positive result. What drugs should be started for treatment of presumptive pulmonary tuberculosis? Does the patient have a heightened risk of developing medication toxicity? If so, which medication(s) would be likely to cause toxicity?

Mycobacteria are intrinsically resistant to most antibiotics. Because they grow more slowly than other bacteria, antibiotics that are most active against rapidly growing cells are relatively ineffective. Mycobacterial cells can also be dormant and, thus, resistant to many drugs or killed only very slowly. The lipid-rich mycobacterial cell wall is impermeable to many agents. Mycobacterial species are intracellular pathogens, and organisms residing within macrophages are inaccessible to drugs that penetrate these cells poorly. Finally, mycobacteria are notorious for their ability to develop resistance. Combinations of two or more drugs are required to overcome these obstacles and to prevent emergence of resistance during the course of therapy. The response of mycobacterial infections to chemotherapy is slow, and treatment must be administered for months to years, depending on which drugs are used. The drugs used to treat tuberculosis, atypical mycobacterial infections, and leprosy are described in this chapter.

■ DRUGS USED IN TUBERCULOSIS

Isoniazid (INH), rifampin (or other **rifamycin**), **pyrazinamide,** and **ethambutol** together make up the traditional first-line 6- to 9-month treatment regimen for drug-susceptible tuberculosis. **Rifapentine, moxifloxacin, isoniazid**, and **pyrazinamide** make up the newer 4-month treatment regimen (Table 47–1). In the traditional regimen, isoniazid and rifampin are the most active drugs. An isoniazid-rifampin combination administered for 9 months will cure 95–98% of cases of tuberculosis caused by susceptible strains. An initial intensive phase of treatment is recommended for the first 2 months of both the traditional and new regimens due to the prevalence of resistant strains. The addition of pyrazinamide during this intensive phase allows the total duration of therapy to be reduced. In practice, therapy is usually initiated with a four-drug regimen of either isoniazid, rifampin, pyrazinamide, and ethambutol or rifapentine, moxifloxacin, isoniazid, and pyrazinamide until susceptibility of the clinical isolate has been determined. In susceptible isolates, the continuation phase consists of an additional 4 months with isoniazid and rifampin or an additional 2 months of rifapentine, moxifloxacin, and isoniazid (Table 47–2). Neither ethambutol nor other drugs adds substantially to the overall activity of the regimen (ie, the duration of treatment cannot be further reduced if another drug is used), but the fourth drug is included in the traditional regimen in case the isolate proves to be resistant to isoniazid, rifampin, or both. If traditional therapy is initiated after the isolate is known to be susceptible to isoniazid and rifampin, ethambutol does not need to be added. The prevalence of isoniazid resistance among clinical isolates in the USA is approximately 10%. Prevalence of resistance to both isoniazid and rifampin (termed multidrug resistance) was 1.9% in the USA in 2017, and it has remained stable for approximately 20 years.

*The authors thank Henry F. Chambers, MD, and Daniel H. Deck, PharmD, for their contributions to previous editions.

TABLE 47–1 Antimicrobials used in the treatment of tuberculosis.

Drug	Typical Adult Dosage[1]
First-line agents	
Ethambutol	15–25 mg/kg/d
Isoniazid	300 mg/d
Moxifloxacin	400 mg/d
Pyrazinamide	25 mg/kg/d
Rifampin	600 mg/d
Rifapentine	1200 mg once daily
Second-line agents	
Amikacin	15 mg/kg/d
Aminosalicylic acid	8–12 g/d
Bedaquiline	400 mg/d
Capreomycin	15 mg/kg/d
Clofazimine	200 mg/d
Cycloserine	500–1000 mg/d, divided
Ethionamide	500–750 mg/d
Levofloxacin	500–750 mg/d
Linezolid	600 mg/d
Pretomanid	200 mg/d
Rifabutin[2]	300 mg/d
Streptomycin	15 mg/kg/d

[1]Assuming normal renal function.

[2]150 mg/d if used concurrently with a protease inhibitor or cobicistat; 600 mg/d with efavirenz.

Multidrug resistance is much more prevalent in many other parts of the world. Resistance to rifampin alone is uncommon.

ISONIAZID

Isoniazid is the most active drug for the treatment of tuberculosis caused by susceptible strains. It is a small molecule (molecular weight 137) that is freely soluble in water. The structural similarity to pyridoxine is shown below.

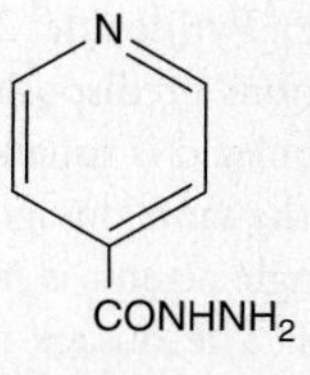

N
$CONHNH_2$

Isoniazid

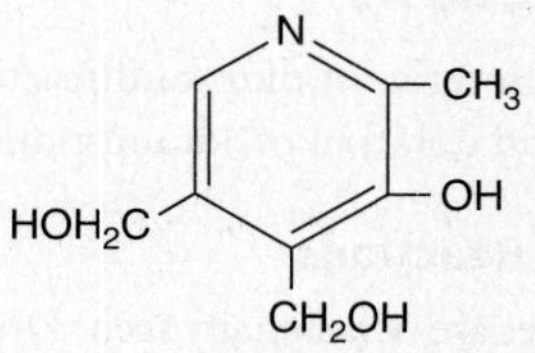

N
CH_3
OH
HOH_2C
CH_2OH

Pyridoxine

In vitro, isoniazid inhibits most tubercle bacilli at a concentration of 0.2 mcg/mL or less and is bactericidal for actively growing tubercle bacilli. It is less effective against nontuberculous mycobacteria. Isoniazid penetrates into macrophages and is active against both extracellular and intracellular organisms.

Mechanism of Action & Basis of Resistance

Isoniazid inhibits synthesis of mycolic acids, which are essential components of mycobacterial cell walls. Isoniazid is a prodrug that is activated by KatG, the mycobacterial catalase-peroxidase. The activated form of isoniazid forms a covalent complex with an acyl carrier protein (AcpM) and KasA, a beta-ketoacyl carrier protein synthetase, which blocks mycolic acid synthesis. Resistance to isoniazid is associated with mutations resulting in overexpression of *inhA*, which encodes an NADH-dependent acyl carrier protein reductase; mutation or deletion of the *katG* gene; promoter mutations resulting in overexpression of *ahpC*, a gene involved in protection of the cell from oxidative stress; and mutations in *kasA*. Overproducers of *inhA* express low-level isoniazid resistance and cross-resistance to ethionamide. *KatG* mutants express high-level isoniazid resistance and often are not cross-resistant to ethionamide.

Drug-resistant mutants are normally present in susceptible mycobacterial populations at about 1 bacillus in 10^6. Since tuberculous lesions often contain more than 10^8 tubercle bacilli, resistant mutants are readily selected if isoniazid or any other drug is given as a single agent. The use of two independently acting drugs in combination is much more effective. The probability that a bacillus is initially resistant to both drugs is approximately 1 in $10^6 \times 10^6$, or 1 in 10^{12}, several orders of magnitude greater than the number of infecting organisms. Thus, at least two (or more in certain cases) active agents should always be used to treat active tuberculosis to prevent emergence of resistance during therapy.

Pharmacokinetics

Isoniazid is readily absorbed from the gastrointestinal tract, optimally on an empty stomach; peak concentrations may be decreased by up to 50% when taken with a fatty meal. A 300-mg oral dose (5 mg/kg in children) achieves peak plasma concentrations of 3–5 mcg/mL within 1–2 hours. Isoniazid diffuses readily into all body fluids and tissues. The concentration in the central nervous system and cerebrospinal fluid ranges between 20% and 100% of simultaneous serum concentrations.

Metabolism of isoniazid, especially acetylation by liver *N*-acetyltransferase, is genetically determined (see Chapter 4). The average plasma concentration of isoniazid in rapid acetylators is about one third to one half of that in slow acetylators, and average half-lives are less than 1 hour and 3 hours, respectively. More rapid clearance of isoniazid by rapid acetylators is usually of no therapeutic consequence when appropriate doses are administered daily, but subtherapeutic concentrations may occur if drug is administered as a once-weekly dose or if there is malabsorption.

Isoniazid metabolites and a small amount of unchanged drug are excreted in the urine. The dosage need not be adjusted in renal

TABLE 47–2 Recommended treatment for drug-susceptible tuberculosis.

	Intensive Phase (duration = 8 weeks)		Continuation Phase (duration = 9 weeks)		
4-Month Regimen	**Drugs**	**Dosing Interval**	**Drugs**	**Dosing Interval**	**Comments**
1	RPT MOX INH PZA	7 days per week	RPT MOX INH	7 days per week	Noninferior to standard 6-month regimen for drug-susceptible pulmonary tuberculosis in persons age 12 and older who weigh at least 40 kg.

	Intensive Phase (min duration = 8 weeks)		Continuation Phase (min duration = 18 weeks)[1]		
6-9-Month Regimen (in order of preference)	**Drugs**	**Dosing Interval**	**Drugs**	**Dosing Interval**	**Comments**
1	INH RIF PZA EMB	7 days per week[2]	INH RIF	7 days per week[2]	Preferred regimen.
2	INH RIF PZA EMB	7 days per week[2]	INH RIF	3 days per week	Preferred alternative if less frequent DOT is needed.
3	INH RIF PZA EMB	3 days per week	INH RIF	3 days per week	Caution in patients with HIV and/or cavitary disease due to concerns for treatment failure, relapse, drug resistance.
4	INH RIF PZA EMB	7 days per week × 2 weeks, then 2 days per week × 6 weeks	INH RIF	2 days per week	Avoid in patients with HIV or those with smear-positive and/or cavitary disease.

[1]Experts recommend prolonged continuation phase (31 weeks) for patients with cavitation on initial chest radiograph and positive cultures at the end of the intensive treatment phase.

[2]May consider 5 days per week if needed for DOT. No studies compare 5 versus 7 doses per week, but extensive experience suggests efficacy of this regimen.

DOT, directly observed therapy; EMB, ethambutol; HIV, human immunodeficiency virus; INH, isoniazid; PZA, pyrazinamide; RIF, rifampin.

failure. Dose adjustment is not well defined in patients with severe preexisting hepatic insufficiency and should be guided by serum concentrations if a reduction in dose is contemplated. Isoniazid inhibits several cytochrome P450 enzymes, leading to increased concentrations of such medications as phenytoin, carbamazepine, and benzodiazepines. However, when used in combination with rifampin, a potent CYP enzyme inducer, the concentrations of these medications are usually decreased.

Clinical Uses

The typical dosage of isoniazid is 5 mg/kg/d; a typical adult dose is 300 mg given once daily. Up to 10 mg/kg/d may be used for serious infections or if malabsorption is a problem. A 15-mg/kg dose, or 900 mg, may be used in a twice to three times-weekly dosing regimen in combination with a second antituberculous agent (eg, rifampin, 600 mg). Pyridoxine, 25–50 mg/d, is recommended for those with conditions predisposing to neuropathy, an adverse effect of isoniazid. Isoniazid is usually given by mouth but can be given parenterally in the same dosage.

Isoniazid as a single agent is also indicated for treatment of latent tuberculosis. The dosage is 300 mg/d (5 mg/kg/d) or 900 mg twice weekly, and the duration is usually 9 months.

Adverse Reactions

The incidence and severity of untoward reactions to isoniazid are related to dosage and duration of administration.

A. Immunologic Reactions

Fever and skin rashes are occasionally seen. Drug-induced systemic lupus erythematosus has been reported.

B. Direct Toxicity

Isoniazid-induced hepatitis is the most common major toxic effect. This is distinct from the minor increases in liver aminotransferases (up to three or four times normal), which do not require cessation of the drug and which are seen in 10–20% of patients, who usually are asymptomatic. Clinical hepatitis with loss of appetite, nausea, vomiting, jaundice, and right upper quadrant pain occurs in 1% of isoniazid recipients and can be fatal, particularly if the drug is not discontinued promptly. Isoniazid-induced hepatitis is associated with histologic evidence of hepatocellular damage and necrosis. The risk of hepatitis depends on age. It occurs rarely under age 20, in 0.3% of those age 21–35, 1.2% of those age 36–50, and 2.3% in those age 50 and above. The risk of hepatitis is greater in individuals with alcohol use disorders and possibly during pregnancy and the postpartum period. Development of isoniazid hepatitis contraindicates further use of the drug.

Peripheral neuropathy is observed in 10–20% of patients given dosages >5 mg/kg/d, but it is infrequently seen with the standard 300-mg adult dose. Peripheral neuropathy is more likely to occur in slow acetylators and patients with predisposing conditions such as malnutrition, alcohol use disorder, diabetes, AIDS, and end-stage renal disease. Neuropathy is due to a relative pyridoxine deficiency. Isoniazid promotes excretion of pyridoxine, and this toxicity is readily reversed by administration of pyridoxine in a dosage as low as 10 mg/d. Central nervous system toxicity, which is less common, includes memory loss, psychosis, ataxia, and seizures. These effects may also respond to pyridoxine.

Miscellaneous other reactions include hematologic abnormalities, provocation of pyridoxine deficiency anemia, tinnitus, and gastrointestinal discomfort.

RIFAMPIN

Rifampin is a semisynthetic derivative of rifamycin, an antibiotic produced by *Amycolatopsis rifamycinica*, which has several former names including *Streptomyces mediterranei*. It is active in vitro against gram-positive organisms, some gram-negative organisms, such as *Neisseria* and *Haemophilus* species, mycobacteria, and chlamydiae. Susceptible organisms are inhibited by <1 mcg/mL. Resistant mutants are present in all microbial populations at approximately 1 in 106 organisms and are rapidly selected out if rifampin is used as a single drug, especially in a patient with active infection. There is no cross-resistance to other classes of antimicrobial drugs, but there is cross-resistance to other rifamycin derivatives, eg, rifabutin and rifapentine.

Mechanism of Action, Resistance, & Pharmacokinetics

Rifampin binds to the β subunit of bacterial DNA-dependent RNA polymerase and thereby inhibits RNA synthesis. Resistance results from any one of several possible point mutations in *rpoB*, the gene for the β subunit of RNA polymerase. These mutations result in reduced binding of rifampin to RNA polymerase. Human RNA polymerase does not bind rifampin and is not inhibited by it. Rifampin is bactericidal for mycobacteria. It readily penetrates most tissues and penetrates into phagocytic cells. It can kill organisms that are poorly accessible to many other drugs, such as intracellular organisms and those sequestered in abscesses and lung cavities.

Rifampin is well absorbed after oral administration and excreted mainly through the liver into bile. It then undergoes enterohepatic recirculation, with the bulk excreted as a deacylated metabolite in feces and a small amount excreted in the urine. Dosage adjustment for renal or hepatic insufficiency is not necessary. Usual doses result in serum levels of 5–7 mcg/mL. Rifampin is distributed widely in body fluids and tissues. The drug is relatively highly protein-bound, and adequate cerebrospinal fluid concentrations are achieved only in the presence of meningeal inflammation.

Rifampin strongly induces most cytochrome P450 isoforms (CYP1A2, 2C9, 2C19, 2D6, and 3A4), which increases the elimination of numerous other drugs including methadone, anticoagulants, cyclosporine, some anticonvulsants, protease inhibitors, some nonnucleoside reverse transcriptase inhibitors, integrase strand transfer inhibitors, contraceptives, and a host of others (see Chapters 4 and 67). Coadministration of rifampin results in significantly lower serum levels of these drugs.

Clinical Uses

A. Mycobacterial Infections

Rifampin, usually 600 mg/d (10 mg/kg/d) orally, must be administered with isoniazid or other antituberculous drugs to patients with active tuberculosis to prevent emergence of drug-resistant mycobacteria. In some courses of therapy, 600 mg of rifampin is given twice weekly. Rifampin, 600 mg daily or twice weekly for 6 months, is also effective in combination with other agents in some atypical mycobacterial infections and in leprosy. Rifampin, 600 mg daily for 4 months as a single drug, is an effective and preferred treatment for latent tuberculosis.

B. Other Indications

Rifampin has other uses in bacterial infections. An oral dosage of 600 mg twice daily for 2 days can eliminate meningococcal carriage. Rifampin, 20 mg/kg (maximum 600 mg) once daily for 4 days, is used as prophylaxis in contacts of children with *Haemophilus influenzae* type b disease. Rifampin combination therapy is also used for treatment of serious staphylococcal infections such as osteomyelitis, prosthetic joint infections, and prosthetic valve endocarditis.

Adverse Reactions

Rifampin imparts a harmless orange color to urine, sweat, and tears. (Soft contact lenses may be permanently stained.) Adverse effects include rashes, thrombocytopenia, and nephritis. Rifampin may cause cholestatic jaundice and occasionally hepatitis, and it commonly causes light-chain proteinuria. If administered less often than twice weekly, rifampin may cause an influenza-like syndrome characterized by fever, chills, myalgias, anemia, and thrombocytopenia. Its use has been associated with acute tubular necrosis.

RIFAPENTINE

Rifapentine is an analog of rifampin. It is active against both *M tuberculosis* and MAC. As with all rifamycins, it is a bacterial RNA polymerase inhibitor, and cross-resistance between rifampin and rifapentine is complete. Like rifampin, rifapentine is a potent inducer of cytochrome P450 enzymes, and it has the same drug interaction profile; however, when rifapentine is administered intermittently, induction of metabolism of other medications is less pronounced compared with rifampin. Toxicity is similar to that of rifampin. Rifapentine and its microbiologically active metabolite, 25-desacetylrifapentine, have an elimination half-life of 13 hours. Rifapentine can now be used as part of a 4-month treatment regimen for drug-susceptible pulmonary tuberculosis. It should be administered at a dose of 1200 mg once daily in combination with isoniazid, pyrazinamide, and moxifloxacin. This regimen was found to be noninferior to the standard 6-month treatment in patients aged 12 years and older who weigh at least 40 kg, including those with HIV receiving or planned to initiate efavirenz-based antiretroviral therapy. This study was published after the most recent 2016 CDC treatment guidelines, but it will be incorporated in the next revision and is the basis for interim guidance published in 2022. Intermittently dosed rifapentine, when given as 600 mg (10 mg/kg) once or twice weekly, has been used for treatment of tuberculosis caused by rifampin-susceptible strains during the continuation phase (ie, after the first 2 months of therapy and, ideally, after conversion of sputum cultures to negative); however, this regimen has decreased efficacy compared with the standard rifampin-based regimen. Current treatment guidelines recommend against it. In particular, its use should be avoided in patients at higher risk of failure, including those with positive cultures at the end of the intensive treatment phase and those with evidence of cavitation on chest radiographs or in patients with HIV infection because of an unacceptably high relapse rate with rifampin-resistant organisms. Rifapentine in combination with isoniazid, typically both dosed at 900 mg once weekly for 3 months (12 doses each in total), is an effective short-course treatment for latent tuberculosis infection (LTBI). Rifapentine combined with isoniazid, both dosed daily for 1 month, has shown efficacy against LTBI in patients with HIV. Special caution must be taken to avoid drug-drug interactions since coadministration of rifapentine can lead to subtherapeutic levels of numerous antiretroviral agents.

ETHAMBUTOL

Ethambutol is a synthetic, water-soluble, heat-stable compound, the dextro-isomer of the structure shown below, dispensed as the dihydrochloride salt.

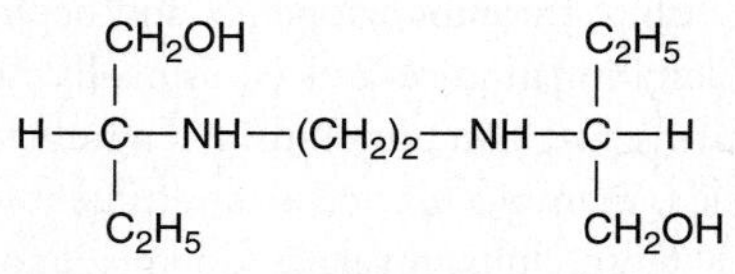

```
     CH2OH                      C2H5
       |                          |
   H—C—NH—(CH2)2—NH—C—H
       |                          |
     C2H5                       CH2OH
```

Ethambutol

Mechanism of Action & Clinical Uses

Ethambutol inhibits mycobacterial arabinosyl transferases, which are encoded by the *embCAB* operon. Arabinosyl transferases are involved in the polymerization reaction of arabinoglycan, an essential component of the mycobacterial cell wall. Resistance to ethambutol is due to mutations resulting in overexpression of *emb* gene products or within the *embB* structural gene. Susceptible strains of *Mycobacterium tuberculosis* and other mycobacteria are inhibited in vitro by ethambutol, 1–5 mcg/mL.

Ethambutol is well absorbed from the gut. After ingestion of 25 mg/kg, a blood level peak of 2–5 mcg/mL is reached in 2–4 hours. About 20% of the drug is excreted in feces and 50% in urine in unchanged form. Ethambutol accumulates in renal failure, and the dose should be reduced from daily to three times weekly if creatinine clearance is <30 mL/min. Ethambutol crosses the blood-brain barrier only when the meninges are inflamed. Concentrations in cerebrospinal fluid are highly variable, ranging from 4% to 64% of serum levels in the setting of meningeal inflammation.

As with all antituberculous drugs, resistance to ethambutol emerges rapidly when the drug is used alone. Therefore, ethambutol is always given in combination with other antituberculous drugs. Ethambutol hydrochloride, 15–25 mg/kg, is usually given as a single daily dose in combination with isoniazid, rifampin, and pyrazinamide during the initial intensive phase of active tuberculosis treatment. The higher dose may be used for treatment of tuberculous meningitis. Higher doses have been used with intermittent dosing regimens for directly observed therapy—for example, 25–30 mg/kg three times weekly or 50 mg/kg administered twice weekly. Ethambutol is also used in combination with other agents for the treatment of nontuberculous mycobacterial infections, such as *Mycobacterium avium complex* (MAC) or *M kansasii*; the typical dose for these infections is 15 mg/kg once daily.

Adverse Reactions

Hypersensitivity to ethambutol is rare. The most common serious adverse event is retrobulbar neuritis, resulting in loss of visual acuity and red-green color blindness. This dose-related adverse effect is more likely to occur at dosages of 25 mg/kg/d continued for several months. At 15 mg/kg/d or less, visual disturbances occur in approximately 2% of patients, typically after at least 1 month of treatment. Experts recommend baseline and monthly visual acuity and color discrimination testing, with particular attention to patients on higher doses or with impaired renal function. Ethambutol is relatively contraindicated in children too young to permit assessment of visual acuity and red-green color discrimination.

PYRAZINAMIDE

Pyrazinamide (PZA) is a relative of nicotinamide, and it is used only for treatment of tuberculosis. It is stable and slightly soluble in water. It is inactive at neutral pH, but at pH 5.5 it inhibits tubercle bacilli at concentrations of approximately 20 mcg/mL.

The drug is taken up by macrophages and exerts its activity against mycobacteria residing within the acidic environment of lysosomes.

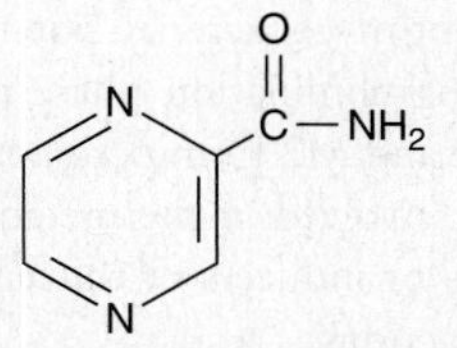

Pyrazinamide (PZA)

Mechanism of Action & Clinical Uses

Pyrazinamide is converted to pyrazinoic acid—the active form of the drug—by mycobacterial pyrazinamidase, which is encoded by *pncA*. Pyrazinoic acid disrupts mycobacterial cell membrane metabolism and transport functions. Resistance may be due to impaired uptake of pyrazinamide or mutations in *pncA* that impair conversion of PZA to its active form.

Serum concentrations of 30–50 mcg/mL at 1–2 hours after oral administration are achieved with dosages of 25 mg/kg/d. Pyrazinamide is well absorbed from the gastrointestinal tract and widely distributed in body tissues, including inflamed meninges. The half-life is 8–11 hours. The parent compound is metabolized by the liver, but metabolites are renally cleared; therefore, PZA should be administered at 25–35 mg/kg three times weekly (not daily) in hemodialysis patients and those in whom the creatinine clearance is <30 mL/min. In patients with normal renal function, a dose of 30–50 mg/kg is used for thrice-weekly or twice-weekly treatment regimens.

Pyrazinamide is an important front-line drug used in conjunction with isoniazid and rifampin in short-course (ie, 6-months or fewer) regimens as a "sterilizing" agent active against residual intracellular organisms that may cause relapse. Tubercle bacilli develop resistance to pyrazinamide fairly readily, but there is no cross-resistance with isoniazid or other antimycobacterial drugs.

Adverse Reactions

Major adverse effects of PZA include hepatotoxicity (in 1–5% of patients), nausea, vomiting, drug fever, photosensitivity, and hyperuricemia. The latter occurs uniformly and is not a reason to halt therapy if patients are asymptomatic.

Fluoroquinolones

In addition to their activity against many gram-positive and gram-negative bacteria (discussed in Chapter 46), ciprofloxacin, levofloxacin, gatifloxacin, and moxifloxacin inhibit strains of *M tuberculosis* at concentrations <2 mcg/mL. They are also active against atypical mycobacteria. Moxifloxacin is the most active against *M tuberculosis* in vitro. Levofloxacin tends to be slightly more active than ciprofloxacin against *M tuberculosis*, whereas ciprofloxacin is slightly more active against atypical mycobacteria. Clinical data are lacking with regard to delafloxacin; however, its in vitro activity against mycobacteria appears to be greater than that of levofloxacin.

Fluoroquinolones are an important addition to the drugs available for tuberculosis. They have traditionally been reserved for strains that are resistant to or for patients intolerant of first-line agents, but moxifloxacin may be used more frequently as initial therapy following recent data showing noninferiority of a 4-month treatment regimen (moxifloxacin, rifapentine, isoniazid, and pyrazinamide) when compared to standard therapy for drug-susceptible pulmonary tuberculosis. Resistance, which may result from one of several single point mutations in the gyrase A subunit, develops rapidly if a fluoroquinolone is used as a single agent; thus, the drug must be used in combination with two or more additional active agents. Typically, resistance to one fluoroquinolone indicates class resistance. However, moxifloxacin may retain some activity in strains resistant to ofloxacin. The dosage of levofloxacin is 500–750 mg once a day, and some clinicians increase to 1000 mg daily if tolerated. The dosage of moxifloxacin is 400 mg once a day. Some experts recommend checking peak serum concentrations. Expected levels at about 2 hours post-dose are 8–12 mcg/mL for levofloxacin and 3–5 mcg/mL for moxifloxacin.

SECOND-LINE DRUGS FOR TUBERCULOSIS

The alternative drugs listed below are usually considered only (1) in case of resistance to first-line agents; (2) in case of failure of clinical response to conventional therapy; and (3) in case of serious treatment-limiting adverse drug reactions. However, linezolid may be selected as an alternative to a first-line drug due to a more favorable toxicity profile in a particular patient. Expert guidance is desirable if therapy with second-line drugs is required. For many drugs listed in the following text, the dosage, emergence of resistance, and long-term toxicity have not been fully established.

Linezolid

Linezolid (discussed in Chapter 44) inhibits strains of *M tuberculosis* in vitro at concentrations of 4–8 mcg/mL. It achieves good intracellular concentrations, and it is active in murine models of tuberculosis. Linezolid has been used in combination with other second- and third-line drugs to treat patients with tuberculosis caused by multidrug-resistant strains. Most recently, it is recommended for use in combination with bedaquiline and pretomanid for multidrug-resistant pulmonary tuberculosis at a dosage of 1200 mg once daily for 6 months. Significant adverse effects, including bone marrow suppression and irreversible peripheral and optic neuropathy, have been reported with prolonged courses, so some experts favor using a lower 600-mg daily dose, or adjusting the dose based on therapeutic drug levels. Some data suggest the 600-mg dose is sufficient and may limit the occurrence of these adverse effects. Experts recommend supplemental pyridoxine for patients treated with linezolid. Linezolid is generally avoided in patients on concomitant serotonergic agents due to concern for serotonin syndrome.

Rifabutin

Rifabutin is derived from rifamycin and is related to rifampin. It has significant activity against *M tuberculosis*, MAC, and *Mycobacterium fortuitum* (see below). Its activity is similar to that of rifampin, and cross-resistance with rifampin is virtually complete. Some rifampin-resistant strains may appear susceptible to rifabutin in vitro, but a clinical response is unlikely because the molecular basis of resistance, *rpoB* mutation, is the same. Rifabutin is both a substrate and inducer of cytochrome P450 enzymes. Because it is a less potent inducer, rifabutin is often used in place of rifampin for treatment of tuberculosis in patients with HIV infection who are receiving antiretroviral therapy with a protease inhibitor, a nonnucleoside reverse transcriptase inhibitor (eg, efavirenz), or an integrase strand transfer inhibitor (eg dolutegravir), drugs that also are cytochrome P450 or UDP glucuronosyltransferase (UGT) substrates.

The typical dosage of rifabutin is 300 mg/d unless the patient is receiving a protease inhibitor, in which case the dosage should be reduced, typically by half. If efavirenz (a cytochrome P450 inducer) is used, the recommended dosage of rifabutin is 600 mg/d. Rifabutin may accumulate in severe renal impairment, and the dose should be reduced by half if creatinine clearance is <30 mL/min. Rifabutin is associated with similar rates of hepatotoxicity or rash compared to rifampin; it can also cause leukopenia, thrombocytopenia, and optic neuritis.

Bedaquiline

When approved by the US Food and Drug Administration (FDA) in 2012, bedaquiline, a diarylquinoline, was the first drug with a novel mechanism of action against *M tuberculosis* to be approved since 1971. Bedaquiline inhibits adenosine 5′-triphosphate (ATP) synthase in mycobacteria, has in vitro activity against both replicating and nonreplicating bacilli, and has bactericidal and sterilizing activity in the murine model of tuberculosis. Cross-resistance has been reported between bedaquiline and clofazimine, likely via upregulation of the multisubstrate efflux pump, MmpL5.

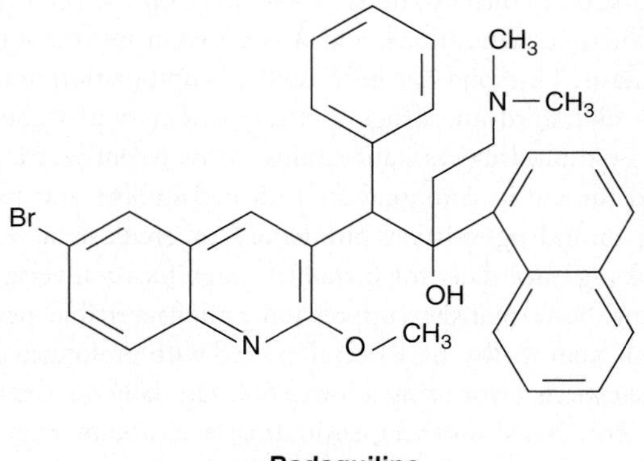

Bedaquiline

Peak plasma concentration and plasma exposure to bedaquiline increase approximately twofold when administered with high-fat food. Bedaquiline is highly protein-bound (>99%), is metabolized chiefly through the cytochrome P450 system, and is excreted primarily via the feces. The mean terminal half-life of bedaquiline and its major metabolite (M2), which is four to six times less active in terms of antimycobacterial potency, is approximately 5.5 months. This long elimination phase probably reflects slow release of bedaquiline and M2 from peripheral tissues. CYP3A4 is the major isoenzyme involved in the metabolism of bedaquiline, and potent inhibitors or inducers of this enzyme cause clinically significant drug interactions.

Current recommendations state that bedaquiline should be included in treatment regimens for patients with pulmonary multidrug-resistant tuberculosis based on meta-analyses that showed improved likelihood of treatment success and lower risk of death in patients who received bedaquiline. The recommended dosage for bedaquiline is 400 mg once daily orally for 2 weeks, followed by 200 mg three times a week for 22 weeks taken orally with food in order to maximize absorption. The most common adverse effects, occurring at rates of 25% or more, are nausea, arthralgia, and headache. Bedaquiline has been associated with both hepatotoxicity and cardiac toxicity. The FDA has issued a black-box warning related to the risk of QTc prolongation and associated mortality. It should be reserved for patients who do not have preferable treatment options and used with caution in patients with other risk factors for cardiac conduction abnormalities.

Pretomanid

Approved by the FDA in 2019, pretomanid is a nitroimidazooxazine compound and a member of the nitroimidazole class. It is related to **delamanid**, a drug approved in a number of countries, but not currently in the USA, for the treatment of multidrug-resistant tuberculosis. Nitroimidazoles require chemical reduction to be active, and selective activation in microorganisms is responsible for the relative lack of toxicity to host cells. *M tuberculosis* appears to reduce pretomanid under both aerobic and anaerobic conditions, and pretomanid has activity against both actively replicating and latent *M tuberculosis*. When the organism is actively replicating under aerobic conditions, pretomanid inhibits production of the cell wall by blocking mycolic acid synthesis. When *M tuberculosis* is not replicating under anaerobic conditions, killing seems to be mediated by the release of nitric oxide, which has multiple potential toxic effects on intracellular mycobacteria. Pretomanid is dosed orally at 200 mg daily with a half-life of approximately 16 hours. It is metabolized by multiple pathways, in part by CYP3A4; coadministration with potent CYP3A4 inducers should be avoided due to risk of subtherapeutic levels. Pretomanid is excreted in both the urine and the feces.

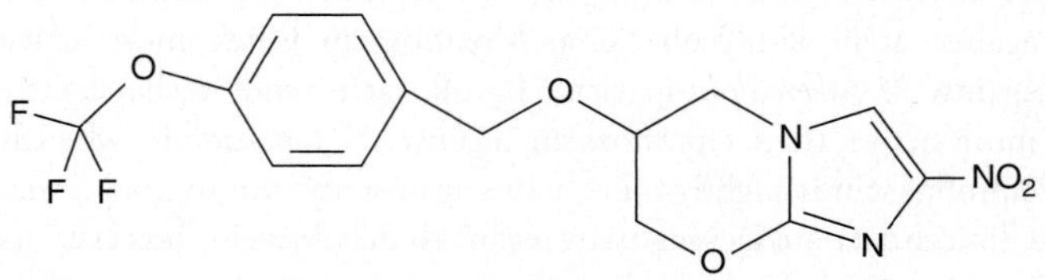

Pretomanid

Pretomanid was developed specifically to treat drug-resistant tuberculosis. It is recommended by the CDC to treat extensively drug-resistant, pre-extensively drug-resistant, or treatment-nonresponsive multidrug-resistant pulmonary tuberculosis when given in combination with linezolid and bedaquiline for 6 months. When administered as a single drug to healthy volunteers, pretomanid seemed to be well tolerated, with headache and gastrointestinal side effects occurring most commonly. When administered in combination with bedaquiline and linezolid, adverse events included neuropathy, headache, acne, anemia, gastrointestinal symptoms, elevated liver enzymes, rash, and hyperamylasemia. Linezolid was thought to account for many of these effects; however, pretomanid also has been associated with elevated liver enzymes, and routine monitoring is recommended during therapy. QT prolongation has been observed with this regimen and is a known effect of bedaquiline, so routine ECG monitoring is recommended. Other toxicities that were reported in less than 5% of study participants include pancreatitis, elevated creatine phosphokinase, electrolyte disturbances, and seizures.

Streptomycin

The mechanism of action and other pharmacologic features of streptomycin, an aminoglycoside, are discussed in Chapter 45. The typical adult dosage is 1 g/d (15 mg/kg/d). If the creatinine clearance is <30 mL/min or the patient is on hemodialysis, the dosage is 15 mg/kg two or three times per week. Most tubercle bacilli are inhibited by streptomycin, 1–10 mcg/mL, in vitro. Nontuberculous species of mycobacteria other than *Mycobacterium avium* complex (MAC) and *Mycobacterium kansasii* are resistant. All large populations of tubercle bacilli contain some streptomycin-resistant mutants. On average, 1 in 108 tubercle bacilli can be expected to be resistant to streptomycin at levels of 10–100 mcg/mL. Resistance may be due to a point mutation in either the *rpsL* gene encoding the S12 ribosomal protein or the *rrs* gene encoding 16S ribosomal RNA, which alters the ribosomal binding site.

Streptomycin penetrates into cells poorly and is active mainly against extracellular tubercle bacilli. The drug crosses the blood-brain barrier and achieves therapeutic concentrations with inflamed meninges.

A. Clinical Use in Tuberculosis

Streptomycin sulfate is used when an injectable drug is needed and in the treatment of infections resistant to other drugs. The usual dosage is 15 mg/kg/d intramuscularly or intravenously daily for adults (20–40 mg/kg/d for children, not to exceed 1 g) for several weeks, followed by 15 mg/kg two or three times weekly for several months. Serum concentrations of approximately 40 mcg/mL are achieved 30–60 minutes after intramuscular injection of a 15-mg/kg dose. Other drugs are always given in combination to prevent emergence of resistance.

B. Adverse Reactions

Streptomycin is ototoxic and nephrotoxic. Vertigo and hearing loss are the most common adverse effects and may be permanent. Toxicity is dose-related, and the risk is increased in the elderly. As with all aminoglycosides, the dose must be adjusted according to renal function (see Chapter 45). Toxicity can be reduced by limiting therapy to no more than 6 months whenever possible.

Kanamycin & Amikacin

The aminoglycoside antibiotics are discussed in Chapter 45. Kanamycin had been used for treatment of tuberculosis caused by streptomycin-resistant strains, but it is no longer available in the USA, and less toxic alternatives (eg, capreomycin, amikacin) have taken its place.

Amikacin has a significant role in the treatment of tuberculosis due to the prevalence of multidrug-resistant strains. Prevalence of amikacin-resistant strains is low, and most multidrug-resistant strains remain amikacin-susceptible. *M tuberculosis* is inhibited at concentrations of 1 mcg/mL or less. Amikacin is also active against atypical mycobacteria. There is no cross-resistance between streptomycin and amikacin, but kanamycin resistance often indicates resistance to amikacin as well. Peak serum concentrations of 30–45 mcg/mL are achieved 30–60 minutes after a 15-mg/kg intravenous infusion or intramuscular injection. Amikacin is indicated for treatment of tuberculosis suspected or known to be caused by streptomycin-resistant or multidrug-resistant strains. This drug must be used in combination with at least one and preferably two or three other drugs to which the isolate is susceptible for treatment of drug-resistant cases. The recommended dosage is 15 mg/kg once daily initially, followed by intermittent dosing two or three times per week.

Ethionamide

Ethionamide is chemically related to isoniazid and similarly blocks the synthesis of mycolic acids. It is poorly water soluble and available only for oral use. It is metabolized by the liver.

Ethionamide

Most tubercle bacilli are inhibited in vitro by ethionamide, 2.5 mcg/mL or less. Some other species of mycobacteria also are inhibited by ethionamide, 10 mcg/mL. Serum concentrations in plasma and tissues of approximately 1–5 mcg/mL are achieved by a dosage of 1 g/d. Cerebrospinal fluid concentrations are equal to those in serum.

Ethionamide is administered at an initial dose of 250 mg once daily, which is increased in 250-mg increments to the recommended dosage of 1 g/d (or 15 mg/kg/d), if possible. The 1-g/d dosage, although theoretically desirable, is poorly tolerated because of gastric irritation and neurologic symptoms, often limiting the tolerable daily dose to 500–750 mg. Ethionamide is also hepatotoxic. Neurologic symptoms may be alleviated by pyridoxine.

Resistance to ethionamide as a single agent develops rapidly in vitro and in vivo. There can be low-level cross-resistance between isoniazid and ethionamide.

Capreomycin

Capreomycin is a peptide protein synthesis inhibitor antibiotic produced by *Streptomyces capreolus*. Daily injection of 15 mg/kg intramuscularly results in peak serum levels of 35–45 mcg/mL 2 hours after a dose. Such concentrations in vitro are inhibitory for many mycobacteria, including multidrug-resistant strains of *M tuberculosis*.

Capreomycin (15 mg/kg/d) is a potential injectable agent for treatment of drug-resistant tuberculosis. Strains of *M tuberculosis* that are resistant to streptomycin usually are susceptible to capreomycin, although some data suggest cross-resistance with strains resistant to amikacin and kanamycin. Resistance to capreomycin, when it occurs, has been associated with *rrs*, *eis*, or *tlyA* gene mutations.

Capreomycin is nephrotoxic and ototoxic. Tinnitus, deafness, and vestibular disturbances occur. The injection causes significant local pain, and sterile abscesses may develop.

Typical dosing of capreomycin is 15 mg/kg/day initially, which is then reduced to two or three times weekly after an initial response has been achieved with a daily dosing schedule. The intermittent dosing regimen may minimize risk of toxicity.

Cycloserine

Cycloserine—a structural analog of D-alanine—inhibits cell wall synthesis, as discussed in Chapter 43. Concentrations of 15–20 mcg/mL inhibit many strains of *M tuberculosis*. The usual dosage of cycloserine in tuberculosis is 0.5–1 g/d in two divided oral doses. The drug is widely distributed to tissues, including the central nervous system. This drug is cleared renally, and the dose should be reduced by half if creatinine clearance is <50 mL/min. Alternatively, it may be reduced to 500 mg three times weekly.

The most serious toxic effects are peripheral neuropathy and central nervous system dysfunction, including depression and psychoses. Pyridoxine, 100 mg or more per day, should be given with cycloserine because this ameliorates neurologic toxicity. Adverse effects, which are most common during the first 2 weeks of therapy, occur in 25% or more of patients, especially at higher doses leading to peak concentrations >35 mcg/mL. Adverse effects can be minimized by monitoring peak serum concentrations. The peak concentration is reached 2–4 hours after dosing. The recommended range of peak concentrations is 20–35 mcg/mL.

Aminosalicylic Acid (PAS)

Aminosalicylic acid is a folate synthesis antagonist that is active almost exclusively against *M tuberculosis*. It is structurally similar to *p*-amino-benzoic acid (PABA) and is thought to have a similar mechanism of action to the sulfonamides (see Chapter 46). In the USA, PAS is commercially available as a 4-g packet of delayed-release granules. In order to protect the integrity of the delayed-release coating, the granules must be administered sprinkled over applesauce or yogurt or swirled in fruit juice and swallowed whole.

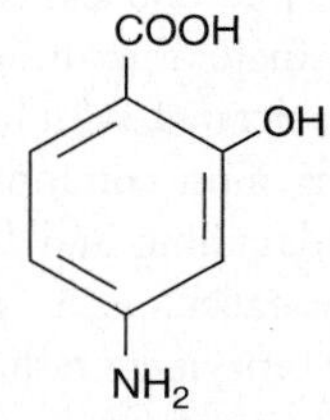

Aminosalicylic acid (PAS)

Tubercle bacilli are usually inhibited in vitro by aminosalicylic acid, 1–5 mcg/mL. The granule formulation of aminosalicylic acid results in improved absorption from the gastrointestinal tract. Peak serum levels are expected to be 20–60 mcg/mL 6 hours after a 4 g oral dose. The dosage is 8–12 g/d orally for adults and 300 mg/kg/d for children, administered in two or three divided doses. The drug is widely distributed in tissues and body fluids except the cerebrospinal fluid. Aminosalicylic acid is rapidly excreted in the urine, in part as active PAS and in part as the acetylated compound and other metabolic products. To avoid accumulation in renal impairment, the maximum dose is 4 g twice daily when creatinine clearance is <30 mL/min. Very high concentrations of aminosalicylic acid are reached in the urine, which can result in crystalluria.

Aminosalicylic acid is used infrequently in the USA because other oral drugs are better tolerated. Gastrointestinal symptoms are common but occur less frequently with the delayed-release granules; they may be diminished by giving the drug with meals and with antacids. Peptic ulceration and hemorrhage may occur. Hypersensitivity reactions manifested by fever, joint pains, skin rashes, hepatosplenomegaly, hepatitis, adenopathy, and granulocytopenia often occur after 3–8 weeks of PAS therapy, making it necessary to stop administration temporarily or permanently.

■ DRUGS ACTIVE AGAINST NONTUBERCULOUS MYCOBACTERIA

Many mycobacterial infections seen in clinical practice in the USA are caused by nontuberculous mycobacteria (NTM), formerly known as "atypical mycobacteria." These organisms have distinctive laboratory characteristics, are present in the environment, and are generally not communicable from person to person. As a rule, these mycobacterial species are less susceptible than *M tuberculosis* to antituberculous drugs. Agents such as macrolides, sulfonamides, and tetracyclines, which are not active against *M tuberculosis*, may be effective for infections caused by NTM. Emergence of resistance during therapy is also a problem with these mycobacterial species, and active infection should be treated

TABLE 47–3 Clinical features and treatment options for infections with atypical mycobacteria.

Species	Clinical Features	Treatment Options
M kansasii	Resembles tuberculosis	Amikacin, clarithromycin, ethambutol, isoniazid, moxifloxacin, rifampin, streptomycin, trimethoprim-sulfamethoxazole
M marinum	Granulomatous cutaneous disease	Amikacin, clarithromycin, ethambutol, doxycycline, levofloxacin, minocycline, rifampin, trimethoprim-sulfamethoxazole
M scrofulaceum	Cervical adenitis in children	Amikacin, erythromycin (or other macrolide), rifampin, streptomycin (Surgical excision is often curative and the treatment of choice.)
M avium complex (MAC)	Pulmonary disease in patients with chronic lung disease; disseminated infection in AIDS	Amikacin, azithromycin, clarithromycin, ethambutol, moxifloxacin, rifabutin
M chelonae	Abscess, sinus tract, ulcer; bone, joint, tendon infection	Amikacin, doxycycline, imipenem, linezolid, macrolides, tobramycin
M fortuitum	Abscess, sinus tract, ulcer; bone, joint, tendon infection	Amikacin, cefoxitin, ciprofloxacin, doxycycline, imipenem, minocycline, moxifloxacin, ofloxacin, trimethoprim-sulfamethoxazole
M ulcerans	Skin ulcers	Clarithromycin, isoniazid, streptomycin, rifampin, minocycline, moxifloxacin (Surgical excision may be effective.)

with combinations of drugs. A few representative pathogens, with the clinical presentation and the drugs to which they are often susceptible, are given in Table 47–3. *M kansasii* is susceptible to rifampin and ethambutol, partially susceptible to isoniazid, and completely resistant to pyrazinamide. A three-drug combination of isoniazid, rifampin, and ethambutol is the conventional treatment for *M kansasii* infection.

M avium complex (MAC), which includes both *M avium* and *M intracellulare,* causes disseminated disease in late stages of AIDS (CD4 counts <50/μL). MAC is much less susceptible than *M tuberculosis* to most antituberculous drugs. Combinations of agents are required to suppress the infection. Azithromycin, 500–600 mg once daily, or clarithromycin, 500 mg twice daily, plus ethambutol, 15 mg/kg/d, is an effective regimen for treatment of disseminated disease. Some authorities recommend use of a third agent, especially rifabutin, 300 mg once daily. Other agents that may be useful are listed in Table 47–3. Azithromycin and clarithromycin are the prophylactic drugs of choice for preventing disseminated MAC in patients with AIDS and CD4 cell counts <50/μL if the CD4 count is not expected to rise quickly with antiretroviral therapy. Rifabutin in a single daily dose of 300 mg has been shown to reduce the incidence of MAC bacteremia but is less effective than macrolides. MAC also causes pulmonary disease, which is more common in older people, with a higher prevalence in women. Not all persons from whom MAC is isolated require treatment, and treatment is generally offered when specific clinical and radiographic criteria are met. When the organism is susceptible to macrolides, a combination of azithromycin (or clarithromycin) plus rifampin and ethambutol is commonly used.

DRUGS USED IN LEPROSY

Mycobacterium leprae has never been grown in vitro, but animal models, such as growth in injected mouse footpads, have permitted laboratory evaluation of drugs. Only those drugs with the widest clinical use are presented here.

DAPSONE & OTHER SULFONES

Several drugs closely related to the sulfonamides have been used effectively in the long-term treatment of leprosy. The most widely used is dapsone (diaminodiphenylsulfone). Like the sulfonamides, it inhibits folate synthesis. Resistance can emerge in large populations of *M leprae*, eg, in lepromatous leprosy, particularly if low doses are given. Therefore, the combination of dapsone, rifampin, and clofazimine is recommended for initial therapy of lepromatous leprosy. A combination of dapsone plus rifampin is commonly used for leprosy with a lower organism burden. Dapsone may also be used to prevent and treat *Pneumocystis jiroveci* pneumonia in persons with AIDS and other types of immunocompromise.

NH_2–C$_6$H$_4$–SO_2–C$_6$H$_4$–NH_2

Dapsone

Sulfones are well absorbed from the gut and widely distributed throughout body fluids and tissues. Dapsone's half-life is 1–2 days, and drug tends to be retained in skin, muscle, liver, and kidney. Skin heavily infected with *M leprae* may contain several times more drug than normal skin. Sulfones are excreted into bile and reabsorbed in the intestine. Excretion into urine is variable, and most excreted drug is acetylated. In renal failure, the dose may have to be adjusted. The usual adult dosage in leprosy is 100 mg daily. For children, the dose is proportionately less, depending on weight.

Dapsone is usually well tolerated. Many patients develop some hemolysis, particularly if they have glucose-6-phosphate dehydrogenase deficiency. Methemoglobinemia is common but usually is not clinically significant. Gastrointestinal intolerance, fever, pruritus, and rash may occur. During dapsone therapy of lepromatous leprosy, erythema nodosum leprosum, an immune-mediated inflammatory reaction, often develops. It is sometimes difficult to distinguish reactions to dapsone from manifestations of the underlying illness. Erythema nodosum leprosum may be suppressed by **thalidomide** (see Chapter 55).

RIFAMPIN

Rifampin (see earlier discussion) in a dosage of 600 mg daily is highly effective in leprosy and is given with at least one other drug to prevent emergence of resistance. Even a dose of 600 mg per month may be beneficial in combination therapy.

CLOFAZIMINE

Clofazimine is a phenazine dye used in the treatment of multibacillary leprosy, which is defined as having a positive smear from any site of infection. Its mechanism of action has not been clearly established. Absorption of clofazimine from the gut is variable, and a major portion of the drug is excreted in feces. Clofazimine is stored widely in reticuloendothelial tissues and skin, and its crystals can be seen inside phagocytic reticuloendothelial cells. It is slowly released from these deposits, so the serum half-life may be 2 months. A common dosage of clofazimine is 100–200 mg/d orally. The most prominent adverse effect is discoloration of the skin and conjunctivae. Gastrointestinal side effects are common. This medication is no longer commercially available, but it can be obtained through established programs. For example, an investigational new drug (IND) program is established in the USA through the National Hansen's Disease Program. For other infections, providers must contact the FDA to request an individual IND. Internationally, ministries of health can make requests directly to the World Health Organization.

SUMMARY Traditional First-Line Antituberculous Drugs

Subclass, Drug	Mechanism of Action	Effects	Clinical Applications	Pharmacokinetics, Toxicities, Interactions
ISONIAZID	Inhibits synthesis of mycolic acids, an essential component of mycobacterial cell walls	Bactericidal activity against susceptible strains of *M tuberculosis*	First-line agent for tuberculosis • treatment of latent infection • less active against nontuberculous mycobacteria	Oral, IV • hepatic clearance (half-life 1 h) • reduces levels of phenytoin • *Toxicity:* Hepatotoxic, peripheral neuropathy (give pyridoxine to prevent)
RIFAMYCINS				
• Rifampin	Inhibits DNA-dependent RNA polymerase, thereby blocking production of RNA	Bactericidal activity against susceptible bacteria and mycobacteria • resistance rapidly emerges when used as a single drug in the treatment of active infection	First-line agent for tuberculosis • nontuberculous mycobacterial infections • eradication of meningococcal colonization, staphylococcal infections	Oral, IV • hepatic clearance (half-life 3.5 h) • potent cytochrome P450 inducer • turns body fluids orange color • *Toxicity:* Rash, nephritis, thrombocytopenia, cholestasis, influenza-like syndrome with intermittent dosing
• *Rifabutin: Oral; similar to rifampin but less cytochrome P450 induction and fewer drug interactions*				
• *Rifapentine: Oral; long-acting analog of rifampin that may be given once daily as part of a 4-month treatment of tuberculosis; it may be given weekly in select cases during the continuation phase of tuberculosis treatment or for treatment of latent tuberculosis*				
PYRAZINAMIDE	Not fully understood; see text • pyrazinamide is converted to the active pyrazinoic acid under acidic conditions in macrophage lysosomes	Bacteriostatic activity against susceptible strains of *M tuberculosis* • may be bactericidal against actively dividing organisms	"Sterilizing" agent used during first 2 months of therapy • allows total duration of therapy to be shortened to 6 months	Oral • hepatic clearance (half-life 9 h), but metabolites are renally cleared so use three doses weekly if creatinine clearance <30 mL/min • *Toxicity:* Hepatotoxic, hyperuricemia
ETHAMBUTOL	Inhibits mycobacterial arabinosyl transferases, which are involved in the polymerization reaction of arabinoglycan, an essential component of the mycobacterial cell wall	Bacteriostatic activity against susceptible mycobacteria	Given in four-drug initial combination therapy for tuberculosis until drug sensitivities are known • also used for nontuberculous mycobacterial infections	Oral • mixed clearance (half-life 4 h) • dose must be reduced in renal failure • *Toxicity:* Retrobulbar neuritis

PREPARATIONS AVAILABLE*

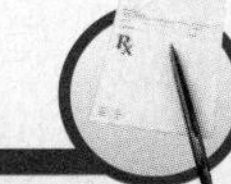

GENERIC NAME	AVAILABLE AS
DRUGS USED IN TUBERCULOSIS	
Aminosalicylic acid	Paser
Bedaquiline fumarate	Sirturo
Capreomycin	Capastat
Ethambutol	Generic, Myambutol
Ethionamide	Trecator, Trecator-SC
Isoniazid	Generic
Moxifloxacin	Generic
Pretomanid	Generic, Dovprela
Pyrazinamide	Generic
Rifabutin	Generic, Mycobutin
Rifampin	Generic, Rifadin, Rimactane
Rifapentine	Priftin
Streptomycin	Generic
DRUGS USED IN LEPROSY	
Clofazimine	Lamprene
Dapsone	Generic

*Drugs used against nontuberculous mycobacteria are listed in Chapters 43–46.

REFERENCES

Carr W et al: Interim guidance: 4-month rifapentine-moxifloxacin regimen for the treatment of drug-susceptible pulmonary tuberculosis – United States 2022. MMWR Morb Mortal Wkly Rep 2022;71:285.

Centers for Disease Control and Prevention (CDC): Provisional CDC Guidance for the Use of Pretomanid as part of a regimen [Bedaquiline, Pretomanid, and Linezolid (BPaL)] to treat drug-resistant Tuberculosis Disease. https://www.cdc.gov/tb/topic/drtb/bpal/default.htm. Accessed August 3, 2022.

Centers for Disease Control and Prevention (CDC): Provisional CDC Guidelines for the use and safety monitoring of bedaquiline fumarate (Sirturo) for the treatment of multidrug-resistant tuberculosis. MMWR Morb Mortal Wkly Rep 2013;62:1.

Centers for Disease Control and Prevention (CDC): Recommendations for use of an isoniazid-rifapentine regimen with direct observation to treat latent *Mycobacterium tuberculosis* infection. MMWR Morb Mortal Wkly Rep 2011; 60:1650.

Centers for Disease Control and Prevention (CDC): Update: Adverse event data and revised American Thoracic Society/CDC recommendations against the use of rifampin and pyrazinamide for treatment of latent tuberculosis infection—United States, 2003. MMWR Morb Mortal Wkly Rep 2003; 52:735.

Curry International Tuberculosis Center and California Department of Public Health, 2016: Drug-Resistant Tuberculosis: A Survival Guide for Clinicians, Third Edition [1-305].

Gillespie SH et al: Early bactericidal activity of a moxifloxacin and isoniazid combination in smear-positive pulmonary tuberculosis. J Antimicrob Chemother 2005;56:1169.

Griffith DE et al: An official ATS/IDSA statement: Diagnosis, treatment, and prevention of nontuberculous mycobacterial disease. Am J Respir Crit Care Med 2007;175:367.

Hugonnet J-E et al: Meropenem-clavulanate is effective against extensively drug-resistant *Mycobacterium tuberculosis*. Science 2009;323:1215.

Jasmer RM et al: Latent tuberculosis infection. N Engl J Med 2002;347: 1860.

Kinzig-Schippers M et al: Should we use N-acetyltransferase type 2 genotyping to personalize isoniazid doses? Antimicrob Agents Chemother 2005; 49:1733.

Lee M et al: Linezolid for treatment of chronic extensively drug-resistant tuberculosis. N Engl J Med 2012;367:1508.

Nahid P et al: Official American Thoracic Society/Centers for Disease Control and Prevention/Infectious Diseases Society of America Clinical Practice Guidelines: Treatment of Drug-Susceptible Tuberculosis. Clin Infect Dis 2016;63:e147.

Nahid P et al: Treatment of drug-resistant tuberculosis. An official ATS/CDC/ERS/IDSA Clinical Guideline. Am J Respir Crit Care Med 2019; 200:e93.

Sulochana S et al: In vitro activity of fluoroquinolones against *Mycobacterium tuberculosis*. J Chemother 2005;17:169.

Targeted tuberculin testing and treatment of latent tuberculosis infection. Am J Respir Crit Care Med 2000;161(4 Part 2):S221.

Zhang Y, Yew WW: Mechanisms of drug resistance in *Mycobacterium tuberculosis*. Int J Tuberc Lung Dis 2009;13:1320.

Zumla A et al: Current concepts—tuberculosis. N Engl J Med 2013;368:745.

CASE STUDY ANSWER

The patient should be started on four-drug therapy with one of two regimens: rifampin, isoniazid, pyrazinamide, and ethambutol or rifapentine, isoniazid, pyrazinamide, and moxifloxacin. He should also be started on antiretroviral therapy (ART) for HIV. If the latter antituberculous regimen is chosen, he should be started on efavirenz-based ART. For any other ART, the patient should receive rifampin, isoniazid, pyrazinamide, and ethambutol. If a protease inhibitor–based antiretroviral regimen is used to treat his HIV, rifabutin should replace rifampin because of the drug-drug interactions between rifampin and protease inhibitors. If dolutegravir is chosen, it must be administered twice daily due to the interaction with rifampin; alternatively, rifabutin can be used in place of rifampin, and dolutegravir can be dosed once daily. The patient is at increased risk of developing hepatotoxicity from both isoniazid and pyrazinamide given his history of alcohol use.

CHAPTER

48 Antifungal Agents

Theora Canonica, PharmD, Jennifer S. Mulliken, MD, Harry W. Lampiris, MD, & Daniel S. Maddix, PharmD*

CASE STUDY

The patient is a 37-year-old African-American man who lives in San Jose, California. He was recently incarcerated near Bakersfield, California and returned to Oakland about 3 months ago. He is currently experiencing 1 month of severe headache and double vision. He has a temperature of 38.6°C (101.5°F), and the physical examination reveals nuchal rigidity and right-sided sixth cranial nerve palsy. MRI of his brain is normal, and lumbar puncture reveals 330 WBC with 20% eosinophils, protein 75, and glucose 20. HIV test is negative, TB skin test is negative, CSF cryptococcal antigen is negative, and CSF gram stain is negative. Patient receives empiric therapy for bacterial meningitis with vancomycin and ceftriaxone, and he is unimproved after 72 hours of treatment. After 3 days, a white mold is identified growing from his CSF culture. What medical therapy would be most appropriate now?

Human fungal infections have increased dramatically in incidence and severity in recent years, owing mainly to advances in surgery, cancer treatment, treatment of patients with solid organ and bone marrow transplantation, the HIV epidemic, and increasing use of broad-spectrum antimicrobial therapy in critically ill patients. These changes have resulted in increased numbers of patients at risk for fungal infections.

For many years, **amphotericin B** was the only efficacious antifungal drug available for systemic use. While highly effective in many serious infections, it is also quite toxic. In the last several decades, pharmacotherapy of fungal disease has been revolutionized by the introduction of the relatively nontoxic **azole** drugs (both oral and parenteral formulations) and the **echinocandins** (available only for parenteral administration). The new agents in these classes offer more targeted, less toxic therapy than older agents such as amphotericin B for patients with serious systemic fungal infections. Combination therapy is being reconsidered, and new formulations of old agents are becoming available. Unfortunately, the appearance of azole-resistant and echinocandin-resistant organisms, as well as the rise in the number of patients at risk for mycotic infections, has created new challenges.

The antifungal drugs presently available fall into the following categories: systemic drugs (oral or parenteral) for systemic infections, oral systemic drugs for mucocutaneous infections, and topical drugs for mucocutaneous infections.

■ SYSTEMIC ANTIFUNGAL DRUGS FOR SYSTEMIC INFECTIONS

AMPHOTERICIN B

Amphotericin A and B are antifungal antibiotics produced by *Streptomyces nodosus.* Amphotericin A is not in clinical use.

Chemistry & Pharmacokinetics

Amphotericin B is an amphoteric polyene macrolide (polyene = containing many double bonds; macrolide = containing a large lactone ring of 12 or more atoms). It is nearly insoluble in water and is therefore prepared as a colloidal suspension of amphotericin B and sodium deoxycholate for intravenous injection. Several formulations have been developed in which amphotericin B is

*In memoriam, 1962—2020.

TABLE 48–1 Properties of conventional amphotericin B and some lipid formulations.[1]

Drug	Physical Form	Dosing (mg/kg/d)	C_{max}	Clearance	Nephrotoxicity	Infusional Toxicity	Daily Cost ($)
Conventional formulation							
Fungizone	Micelles	1	—	—	—	—	24
Lipid formulations							
AmBisome	Spheres	3–5	↑	↓	↓	↓	1300
Amphotec	Disks	5	↓	↑	↓	↑(?)	660
Abelcet	Ribbons	5	↓	↑	↓	↓(?)	570

[1]Changes in C_{max} (peak plasma concentration), clearance, nephrotoxicity, and infusional toxicity are relative to conventional amphotericin B.

packaged in a lipid-associated delivery system (Table 48–1 and Box: Lipid Formulation of Amphotericin B).

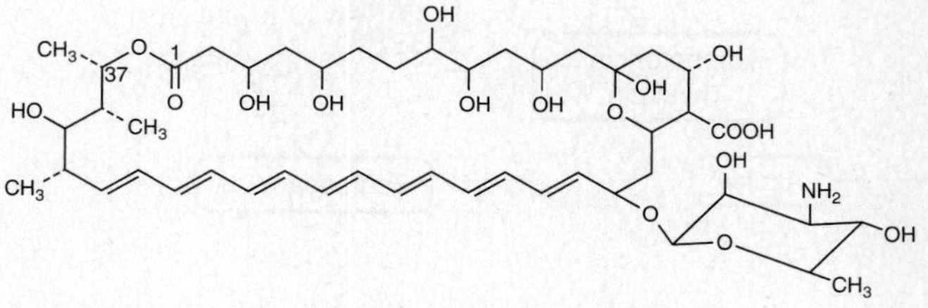

Amphotericin B

Amphotericin B is poorly absorbed from the gastrointestinal tract. Oral amphotericin B is thus effective only on fungi within the lumen of the tract and cannot be used for treatment of systemic disease. The intravenous injection of 0.6 mg/kg/d of amphotericin B results in average blood levels of 0.3–1 mcg/mL; the drug is >90% bound by serum proteins. Although it is mostly metabolized, some amphotericin B is excreted slowly in the urine over a period of several days. The serum half-life is approximately 15 days. Hepatic impairment, renal impairment, and dialysis have little impact on drug concentrations, and therefore no dose adjustment is required. The drug is widely distributed in most tissues, but only 2–3% of the blood level is reached in cerebrospinal fluid, thus occasionally necessitating intrathecal therapy for certain types of fungal meningitis.

Mechanisms of Action & Resistance

Amphotericin B is selective in its fungicidal effect because it exploits the difference in lipid composition of fungal and mammalian cell membranes. **Ergosterol,** a cell membrane sterol, is found in the cell membrane of fungi, whereas the predominant sterol of bacteria and human cells is **cholesterol.** Amphotericin B binds to ergosterol and alters the permeability of the cell by forming amphotericin B–associated pores in the cell membrane (Figure 48–1). As suggested by its chemistry, amphotericin B combines avidly with lipids (ergosterol) along the double-bond-rich side of its structure and associates with water molecules along the hydroxyl-rich side. This amphipathic characteristic facilitates pore formation by multiple amphotericin molecules, with the lipophilic portions around the outside of the pore and the hydrophilic regions lining the inside. The pore allows the leakage of intracellular ions and macromolecules, eventually leading to cell death.

Lipid Formulation of Amphotericin B

Therapy with amphotericin B is often limited by toxicity, especially drug-induced renal impairment. This has led to the development of lipid drug formulations on the assumption that lipid-packaged drug binds to the mammalian membrane less readily, permitting the use of effective doses of the drug with lower toxicity. Liposomal amphotericin preparations package the active drug in lipid delivery vehicles, in contrast to the colloidal suspensions, which were previously the only available forms. Amphotericin binds to the lipids in these vehicles with an affinity between that for fungal ergosterol and that for human cholesterol. The lipid vehicle then serves as an amphotericin reservoir, reducing nonspecific binding to human cell membranes. This preferential binding allows for a reduction of toxicity without sacrificing efficacy and permits use of larger doses. Furthermore, some fungi contain lipases that may liberate free amphotericin B directly at the site of infection.

Three such formulations are now available and have differing pharmacologic properties as summarized in Table 48–1. Although clinical trials have demonstrated different renal and infusion-related toxicities for these preparations compared with regular amphotericin B, there are no trials comparing the different formulations with each other. Limited studies have suggested at best a moderate improvement in the clinical efficacy of the lipid formulations compared with conventional amphotericin B. In resource-limited settings, lipid amphotericin preparations may not be available because of cost, and use of amphotericin B products has decreased because of the availability of the echinocandins and mold-active azole agents, which are extremely effective and better tolerated, especially in patients receiving cancer chemotherapy, and in patients who have received organ or bone marrow transplantation.

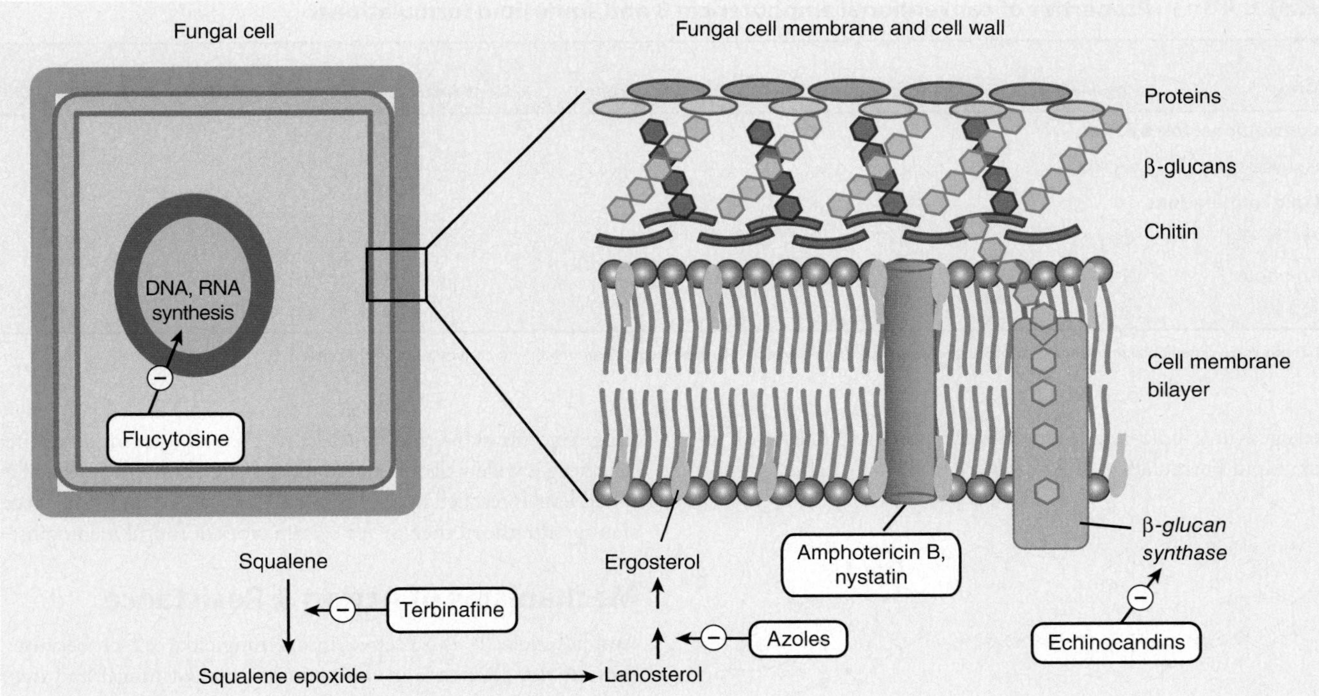

FIGURE 48–1 Targets of antifungal drugs. Except for flucytosine (and possibly griseofulvin, not shown), all currently available antifungals target the fungal cell membrane or cell wall.

Some binding to human membrane sterols does occur, probably accounting for the drug's prominent toxicity.

Resistance to amphotericin B occurs if ergosterol binding is impaired, either by decreasing the membrane concentration of ergosterol or by modifying the sterol target molecule to reduce its affinity for the drug.

Antifungal Activity & Clinical Uses

Amphotericin B remains the antifungal agent with the broadest spectrum of action. It has activity against the clinically significant yeasts, including *Candida albicans* and *Cryptococcus neoformans*; the organisms causing endemic mycoses, including *Histoplasma capsulatum*, *Blastomyces dermatitidis*, and *Coccidioides immitis*; and the pathogenic molds, such as *Aspergillus fumigatus* and the agents of mucormycosis. Some fungal organisms such as *Candida lusitaniae* and *Pseudallescheria boydii* display intrinsic amphotericin B resistance.

Owing to its broad spectrum of activity and fungicidal action, amphotericin B remains a useful agent for nearly all life-threatening mycotic infections, although newer, less toxic agents have largely replaced it for most conditions. Amphotericin B is often used as the initial induction regimen to rapidly reduce fungal burden and then replaced by one of the newer azole drugs (described below) for chronic therapy or prevention of relapse. Such induction therapy is especially important for immunosuppressed patients and those with severe fungal pneumonia, severe cryptococcal meningitis, or disseminated infections with one of the endemic mycoses such as histoplasmosis or coccidioidomycosis. Once a clinical response has been elicited, these patients then often continue maintenance therapy with an azole; therapy may be lifelong in patients at high risk for disease relapse. For treatment of systemic fungal disease, amphotericin B is given by slow intravenous infusion at a dosage of 0.5–1 mg/kg/d. Intrathecal therapy for fungal meningitis is poorly tolerated and fraught with difficulties related to maintaining cerebrospinal fluid access. Thus, intrathecal therapy with amphotericin B is being increasingly supplanted by other therapies but remains an option in cases of fungal central nervous system infections that have not responded to other agents.

Local or topical administration of amphotericin B has been used with success. Mycotic corneal ulcers and keratitis can be cured with topical drops as well as by direct subconjunctival injection. Fungal arthritis has been treated with adjunctive local injection directly into the joint. Candiduria responds to bladder irrigation with amphotericin B, and this route has been shown to produce no significant systemic toxicity.

Adverse Effects

The toxicity of amphotericin B can be divided into two broad categories: immediate reactions, related to the infusion of the drug, and those occurring more slowly.

A. Infusion-Related Toxicity

Infusion-related reactions are nearly universal and consist of fever, chills, muscle spasms, vomiting, headache, and hypotension. They can be ameliorated by slowing the infusion rate or decreasing the daily dose. Premedication with antipyretics, antihistamines, meperidine, or corticosteroids can be helpful. When starting therapy, many clinicians administer a test dose of 1 mg intravenously to gauge the severity of the reaction. This can serve as a guide to an initial dosing regimen and premedication strategy.

B. Cumulative Toxicity

Renal damage is the most significant toxic reaction. Renal impairment occurs in nearly all patients treated with clinically significant doses of amphotericin. The degree of azotemia is variable and often stabilizes during therapy, but it can be serious enough to necessitate dialysis. A reversible component is associated with decreased renal perfusion and represents a form of prerenal renal failure. An irreversible component results from renal tubular injury and subsequent dysfunction. The irreversible form of amphotericin nephrotoxicity usually occurs in the setting of prolonged administration (>4 g cumulative dose). Renal toxicity commonly manifests as renal tubular acidosis and severe potassium and magnesium wasting. There is some evidence that the prerenal component can be attenuated with sodium loading, and it is common practice to administer normal saline infusions with the daily doses of amphotericin B.

Abnormalities of liver function tests are occasionally seen, as is a varying degree of anemia due to reduced erythropoietin production by damaged renal tubular cells. After intrathecal therapy with amphotericin, seizures and a chemical arachnoiditis may develop, often with serious neurologic sequelae.

FLUCYTOSINE

Chemistry & Pharmacokinetics

Flucytosine (5-FC) was discovered in 1957 during a search for novel antineoplastic agents. Though devoid of anticancer properties, it became apparent that it is a potent antifungal agent. Flucytosine is a water-soluble pyrimidine analog related to the chemotherapeutic agent 5-fluorouracil (5-FU). Its spectrum of action is much narrower than that of amphotericin B.

Flucytosine

Flucytosine is currently available in North America only in an oral formulation. The dosage is 100 mg/kg/d in divided doses in patients with normal renal function. It is well absorbed (>90%), with serum concentrations peaking 1–2 hours after an oral dose. It is poorly protein-bound and penetrates well into all body fluid compartments, including the cerebrospinal fluid. It is eliminated by glomerular filtration with a half-life of 3–4 hours and is removed by hemodialysis. Levels rise rapidly with renal impairment and can lead to toxicity. Toxicity is more likely to occur in patients with AIDS and those with renal insufficiency. Peak serum concentrations should be measured periodically in patients with renal insufficiency and maintained between 50 and 100 mcg/mL.

Mechanisms of Action & Resistance

Flucytosine is taken up by fungal cells via the enzyme cytosine permease. It is converted intracellularly first to 5-FU and then to 5-fluorodeoxyuridine monophosphate (FdUMP) and fluorouridine triphosphate (FUTP), which inhibit DNA and RNA synthesis, respectively (see Figure 48–1). Human cells are unable to convert the parent drug to its active metabolites, resulting in selective toxicity.

Synergy with amphotericin B has been demonstrated in vitro and in vivo. It may be related to enhanced penetration of the flucytosine through amphotericin-damaged fungal cell membranes. In vitro synergy with azole drugs also has been seen, although the mechanism is unclear.

Resistance is thought to be mediated through altered metabolism of flucytosine, and, although uncommon in primary isolates, it develops rapidly in the course of flucytosine monotherapy.

Clinical Uses & Adverse Effects

The spectrum of activity of flucytosine is restricted to *C neoformans*, some *Candida* sp, and the dematiaceous molds that cause chromoblastomycosis. Flucytosine is rarely used as a single agent because of its demonstrated synergy with other agents and to avoid the development of secondary resistance. At present clinical use is confined to combination therapy with amphotericin B for cryptococcal meningitis, or with itraconazole for chromoblastomycosis. Flucytosine also has limited utility as monotherapy for fluconazole-resistant candidal urinary tract infections.

The adverse effects of flucytosine result from metabolism (possibly by intestinal flora) to the toxic antineoplastic compound fluorouracil. Bone marrow toxicity with anemia, leukopenia, and thrombocytopenia are the most common adverse effects, with derangement of liver enzymes occurring less frequently. A form of toxic enterocolitis can occur. There seems to be a narrow therapeutic window, with an increased risk of toxicity at higher drug levels and resistance developing rapidly at subtherapeutic concentrations. The use of drug concentration measurements may be helpful in reducing the incidence of toxic reactions, especially when flucytosine is combined with nephrotoxic agents such as amphotericin B.

AZOLES

Chemistry & Pharmacokinetics

Azoles are synthetic compounds that can be classified as either imidazoles or triazoles according to the number of nitrogen atoms in the five-membered azole ring, as indicated below. The imidazoles consist of ketoconazole, miconazole, and clotrimazole (Figure 48–2). The latter two drugs are now used only in topical therapy. The triazoles include itraconazole, fluconazole, voriconazole, isavuconazole, and posaconazole. Other triazoles are currently under investigation.

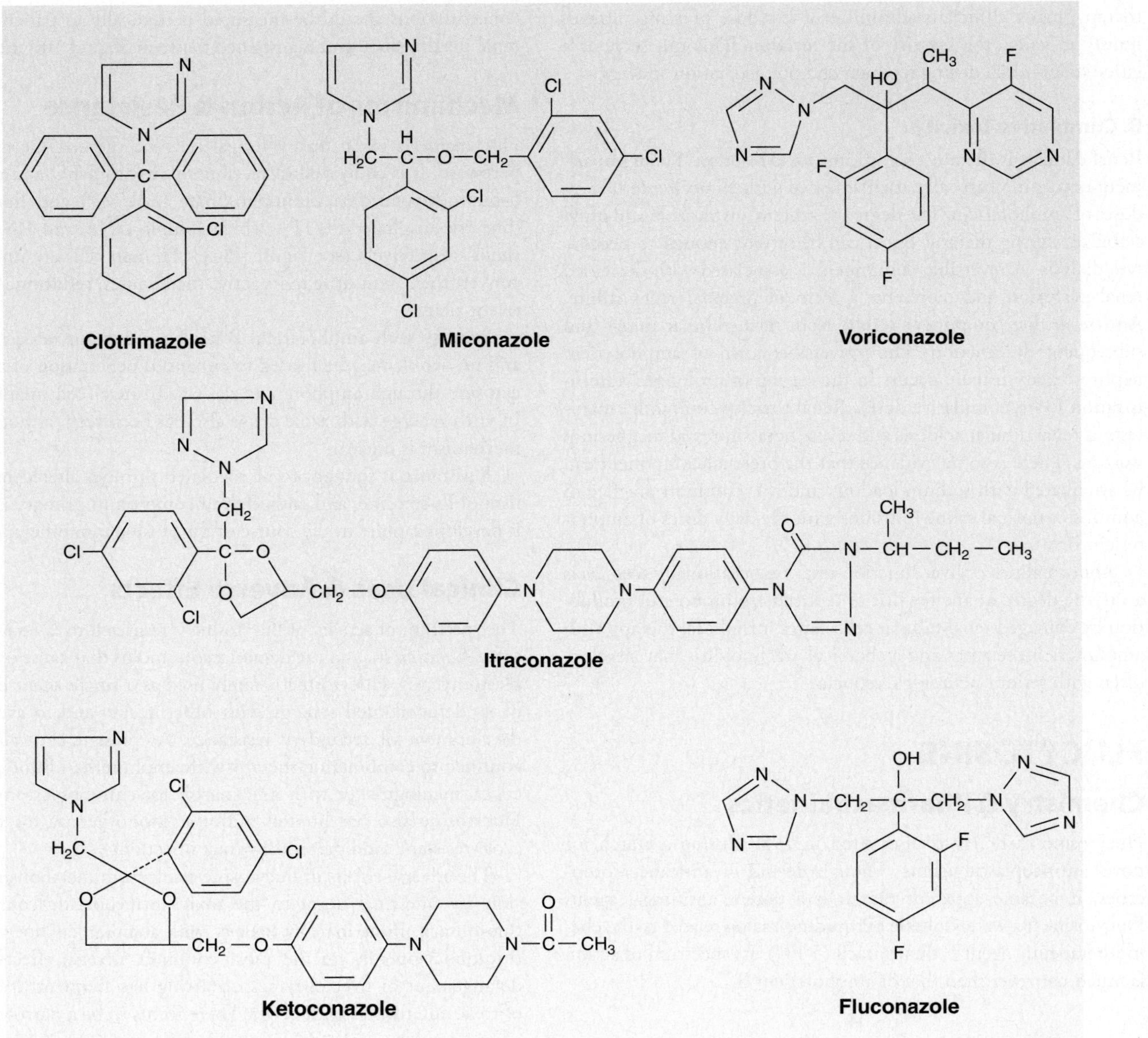

Clotrimazole Miconazole Voriconazole

Itraconazole

Ketoconazole Fluconazole

FIGURE 48–2 Structural formulas of some antifungal azoles.

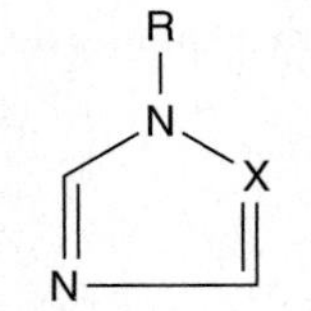

X = C, imidazole
X = N, triazole

Azole nucleus

The pharmacology of each of the azoles is unique and accounts for some of the variations in clinical use. Table 48–2 summarizes the differences among six of the azoles.

Mechanisms of Action & Resistance

The antifungal activity of azole drugs results from the reduction of ergosterol synthesis by inhibition of fungal cytochrome P450 enzymes (see Figure 48–1). The selective toxicity of azole drugs results from their greater affinity for fungal than for human cytochrome P450 enzymes. Imidazoles exhibit a lesser degree of selectivity than the triazoles, accounting for their higher incidence of drug interactions and adverse effects.

Resistance to azoles occurs via multiple mechanisms. Once rare, increasing numbers of resistant strains are being reported, suggesting that increasing use of these agents for prophylaxis and therapy may be selecting for clinical drug resistance in certain settings.

Clinical Uses, Adverse Effects, & Drug Interactions

The spectrum of action of azole medications is broad, including many species of *Candida*, *C neoformans*, the endemic mycoses

TABLE 48–2 Pharmacologic properties of seven systemic azole drugs.

	Water Solubility	Absorption	CSF: Serum Concentration Ratio	$t_{1/2}$ (hours)	Elimination	Formulations
Ketoconazole	Low	Variable	<0.1	7–10	Hepatic	Oral
Itraconazole	Low	Variable	<0.01	24–42	Hepatic	Oral, IV
Fluconazole	High	High	>0.7	22–31	Renal	Oral, IV
Voriconazole	High	High	>0.21	6	Hepatic	Oral, IV
Posaconazole	Low	High	—	25	Hepatic	Oral, IV
Isavuconazole	High	High	—	130	Hepatic	Oral, IV
Oteseconazole	Low	High	—	3,312	Fecal	Oral

(blastomycosis, coccidioidomycosis, histoplasmosis), the dermatophytes, and, in the case of itraconazole, posaconazole, isavuconazole, and voriconazole, even *Aspergillus* infections. They are also useful in the treatment of intrinsically amphotericin-resistant organisms such as *P boydii.*

As a group, the azoles are relatively nontoxic. The most common adverse reaction is relatively minor gastrointestinal upset. All azoles have been reported to cause abnormalities in liver enzymes and, very rarely, clinical hepatitis. Adverse effects specific to individual agents are discussed below.

All azole drugs are prone to drug interactions because they affect the mammalian cytochrome P450 enzyme system to some extent. The most significant reactions are indicated below.

KETOCONAZOLE

Ketoconazole was the first oral azole introduced into clinical use. It is distinguished from triazoles by its greater propensity to inhibit mammalian cytochrome P450 enzymes; that is, it is less selective for fungal P450 than are the newer azoles. As a result, systemic ketoconazole has fallen out of clinical use in the USA and is not discussed in any detail here. It is no longer recommended for the treatment of fungal nail or skin infections.

ITRACONAZOLE

Itraconazole is available in oral and intravenous formulations and is used at a dosage of 100–400 mg/d. Drug absorption from capsules is increased by food and by low gastric pH. Like other lipid-soluble azoles, it interacts with hepatic microsomal enzymes, though to a lesser degree than ketoconazole. An important drug interaction is reduced bioavailability of itraconazole when taken with rifamycins (rifampin, rifabutin, rifapentine). It does not affect mammalian steroid synthesis, and its effects on the metabolism of other hepatically cleared medications are much less than those of ketoconazole. While itraconazole displays potent antifungal activity, effectiveness can be limited by reduced bioavailability. Newer formulations, including an oral liquid and an intravenous preparation, have utilized cyclodextrin as a carrier molecule to enhance solubility and bioavailability. Like ketoconazole, itraconazole penetrates poorly into the cerebrospinal fluid. Itraconazole is the azole of choice for treatment of disease due to the dimorphic fungi *Histoplasma*, *Blastomyces*, and *Sporothrix*. Itraconazole has activity against *Aspergillus* sp, but it has been replaced by voriconazole as the azole of choice for aspergillosis. Itraconazole is used extensively in the treatment of dermatophytoses and onychomycosis.

FLUCONAZOLE

Fluconazole displays a high degree of water solubility and good cerebrospinal fluid penetration. Unlike ketoconazole and itraconazole, its oral bioavailability is high. Drug interactions are also less common because fluconazole has the least effect of all the azoles on hepatic microsomal enzymes. Because of fewer hepatic enzyme interactions and better gastrointestinal tolerance, fluconazole has the widest therapeutic index of the azoles, permitting more aggressive dosing in a variety of fungal infections. The drug is available in oral and intravenous formulations and is used at a dosage of 100–800 mg/d.

Fluconazole is the azole of choice in the treatment and secondary prophylaxis of cryptococcal meningitis. Intravenous fluconazole has been shown to be equivalent to amphotericin B in treatment of candidemia in ICU patients with normal white blood cell counts, although echinocandins may have superior activity for this indication. Fluconazole is the agent most commonly used for the treatment of mucocutaneous candidiasis. Activity against the dimorphic fungi is mainly limited to coccidioidal disease, and in particular for meningitis, where high doses of fluconazole often obviate the need for intrathecal amphotericin B. Fluconazole displays no activity against *Aspergillus* or other filamentous fungi.

Prophylactic use of fluconazole has been demonstrated to reduce fungal disease in bone marrow transplant recipients and AIDS patients, but the emergence of fluconazole-resistant fungi has raised concerns about this indication.

VORICONAZOLE

Voriconazole is available in intravenous and oral formulations. The recommended dosage is 400 mg/d. The drug is well absorbed orally, with a bioavailability exceeding 90%, and it exhibits less protein binding than itraconazole. Metabolism is predominantly hepatic. Voriconazole is a clinically relevant inhibitor of mammalian

Candida auris, an Emerging Multidrug-Resistant Nosocomial Pathogen

Candida auris is an emerging multidrug-resistant (MDR) pathogen that has caused severe infections including candidemia and other invasive candidal infections and is associated with nosocomial outbreaks worldwide, including East and South Asia, South America, Southern Africa, the United Kingdom, and the USA. The organism can persist in the environment, and patients may continue to harbor the organism on their skin for long periods of time after acquisition (perhaps indefinitely), making containment of outbreaks (often in intensive care units) challenging. The organism is typically resistant to all azole agents; many isolates are also resistant to amphotericin B. The treatment of choice of serious *Candida auris* infections is an echinocandin, although resistance to echinocandins has been described.

CYP3A4, and dose reduction of a number of medications is required when voriconazole is started. These include cyclosporine, tacrolimus, and HMG-CoA reductase inhibitors. Observed toxicities include rash and elevated hepatic enzymes. Visual disturbances are common, occurring in up to 30% of patients receiving intravenous voriconazole, and include blurring and changes in color vision or brightness. These visual changes usually occur immediately after a dose of voriconazole and resolve within 30 minutes. Photosensitivity dermatitis is commonly observed in patients, and skin cancers have been reported in patients receiving chronic oral therapy. Rare toxicities include fluorosis (painful bone inflammation associated with elevated blood fluoride levels).

Voriconazole is similar to itraconazole in its spectrum of action, having excellent activity against *Candida* sp (including some fluconazole-resistant species such as *Candida krusei*) and the dimorphic fungi. Voriconazole is less toxic than amphotericin B and is the treatment of choice for invasive aspergillosis and some environmental molds. Measurement of voriconazole levels may predict toxicity and clinical efficacy, especially in immunocompromised patients. Therapeutic trough levels should be between 1 and 5 mcg/mL.

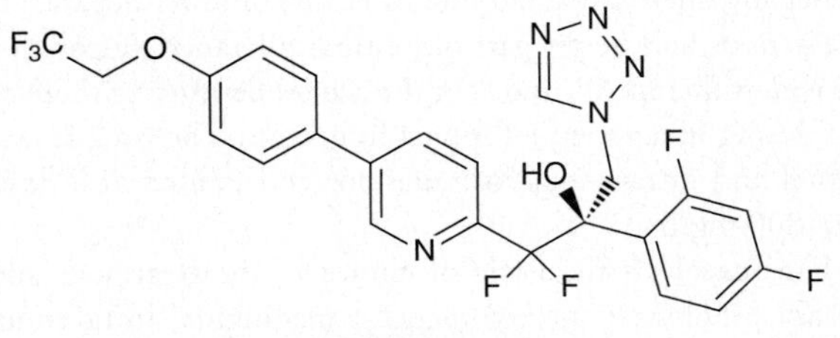

Oteseconazole

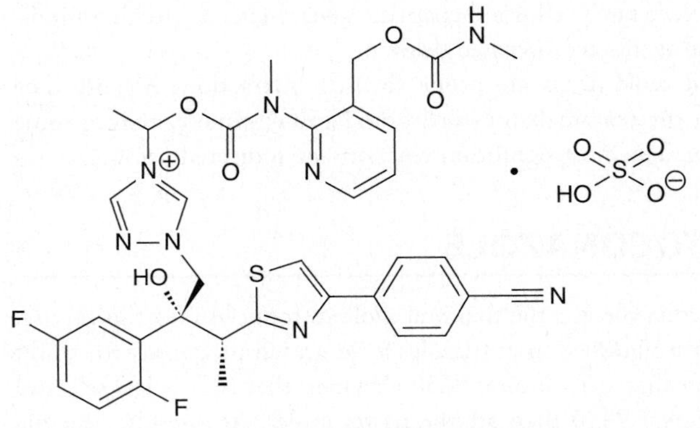

Isavuconazonium Sulfate

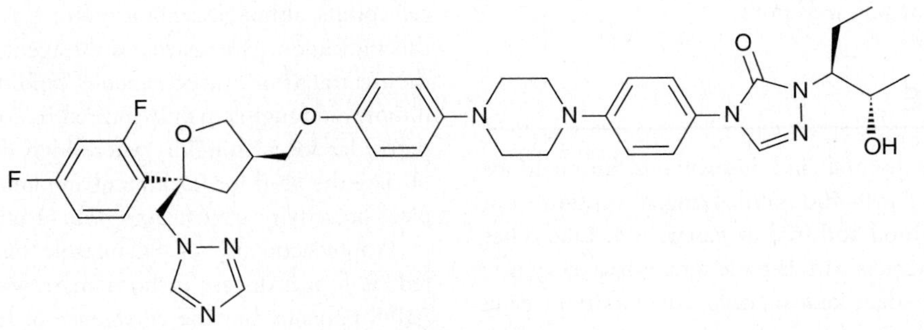

Posaconazole

POSACONAZOLE

Posaconazole was originally available only in a liquid oral formulation and is used at a dosage of 800 mg/d, divided into two or four doses. Absorption is improved when taken with meals high in fat. An intravenous form of posaconazole and a sustained-acting tablet form with higher bioavailability are now available. Posaconazole is rapidly distributed to the tissues, resulting in high tissue levels but relatively low blood levels. Measurement of posaconazole levels is recommended in patients with serious invasive fungal infections (especially mold infections); steady-state posaconazole levels should be between 0.5 and 1.5 mcg/mL. Drug interactions with increased levels of CYP3A4 substrates such as tacrolimus and cyclosporine have been documented.

Posaconazole is the broadest-spectrum member of the azole family, with activity against most species of *Candida* and *Aspergillus*. It is the first azole with significant activity against the agents of mucormycosis. It is currently licensed for salvage therapy in invasive aspergillosis, as well as prophylaxis of fungal infections during induction chemotherapy for leukemia, and for allogeneic bone marrow transplant patients with graft-versus-host disease. A rare side effect of posaconazole is hyperaldosteronism, which can cause hypertension and hypokalemia.

ISAVUCONAZOLE (ISAVUCONAZONIUM SULFATE)

Isavuconazonium sulfate is a prodrug of the newest triazole, isavuconazole; 186 mg of the water-soluble prodrug is equivalent to 100 mg of isavuconazole. It is available as highly bioavailable oral capsules and an intravenous formulation. Following a 2-day loading dose of 372 mg administered every 8 hours, isavuconazonium sulfate is given as a single 372-mg daily dose. Food does not significantly impact the oral absorption of isavuconazonium sulfate. Measurement of isavuconazole levels has not been demonstrated to be of benefit. Coadministration with strong 3A4 inhibitors (eg, ritonavir) or inducers (eg, rifampin) is not recommended.

Isavuconazole has an antifungal spectrum similar to that of posaconazole. It is currently licensed for the treatment of invasive aspergillosis and invasive mucormycosis. Data from published clinical trials are limited. Preliminary evidence indicates that it is better tolerated than voriconazole.

OTESECONAZOLE

Oteseconazole is a tetrazole antifungal with activity most *Candida* species, including fluconazole-resistant strains such as *Candida glabrata* and *Candida krusei*. Oteseconazole is available as a 150-mg oral tablet. The half life is approximately 138 days. It does not undergo significant metabolism, and approximately 56% is eliminated in feces through biliary excretion with another 26% eliminated in urine.

Similar to other azole drugs, oteseconazole inhibits fungal cytochrome P450 enzymes, which leads to reduced ergosterol synthesis and accumulation of 14-methylated sterols, some of which are toxic to fungi. Oteseconazole has much lower affinity for human CYP enzymes than triazole antifungals, leading to reduced potential for toxicity and associated adverse effects.

Oteseconazole was granted FDA approval for the treatment of recurrent vulvovaginal candidiasis in females who are not of reproductive potential. Recurrent vulvovaginal candiasis is defined in clinical studies as ≥3 episodes of vulvovaginal candidiasis in a 12-month period. Of note, oteseconazole is contraindicated in pregnant and lactating females because of potential risks to a fetus or breastfed infant based on animal studies.

For qualifying patients with a history of recurrent vulvovaginal candidiasis, two different regimens have been approved for use (oteseconazole only or oteseconazole/fluconazole). For the oteseconazole-only regimen, oteseconazole is administered as 600 mg on day 1, 450 mg on day 2, and 150 mg once weekly for 11 weeks (weeks 2 through 12). For the fluconazole/otseconazole regimen, fluconazole 150 mg is administered on days 1, 4, and 7, followed by oteseconazole 150 mg daily on days 14 through 20, followed by oteseconazole 150 mg weekly for 11 weeks (weeks 4 through 14). In the three clinical trials leading to FDA approval, both of these regimens were shown to be effective in treating recurrent vulvovaginal candiasisis and preventing future episodes during the post-treatment follow-up period (through week 48).

Overall, oteseconazole is very well tolerated. The most common adverse reactions among patients treated with oteseconazole include headache and nausea. In less than 2% of patients, transient elevations in blood creatinine phosphokinase (≥10 times the upper limit of normal) have been noted. Oteseconazole is a BRCP (breast cancer resistance protein) inhibitor. Concomitant use of otececonazole with BRCP substrates (eg, rosuvastatin) may increase the risk of adverse reactions associated with these medications.

ECHINOCANDINS

Chemistry & Pharmacokinetics

Echinocandins are large cyclic peptides linked to a long-chain fatty acid. **Caspofungin, micafungin,** and **anidulafungin** are the only licensed agents in this category of antifungals, although other drugs are under active investigation. These agents are active against *Candida* and *Aspergillus*, but not *C neoformans* or the agents of zygomycosis and mucormycosis.

Echinocandins are available only in intravenous formulations. Caspofungin is administered as a single loading dose of 70 mg, followed by a daily dose of 50 mg. Caspofungin is water soluble and highly protein-bound. The half-life is 9–11 hours, and the metabolites are excreted by the kidneys and gastrointestinal tract. Dosage adjustments are required only in the presence of severe hepatic insufficiency. Micafungin displays similar properties with a half-life of 11–15 hours and is used at a dose of 150 mg/d for treatment of esophageal candidiasis, 100 mg/d for treatment of candidemia, and 50 mg/d for prophylaxis of fungal infections. Anidulafungin has a half-life of 24–48 hours. For esophageal candidiasis, it is administered intravenously at 100 mg on the first day and 50 mg/d thereafter for 14 days. For candidemia, a loading dose of 200 mg is recommended with 100 mg/d thereafter for at least 14 days after the last positive blood culture.

Mechanism of Action

Echinocandins act at the level of the fungal cell wall by inhibiting the synthesis of β(1–3)-glucan (see Figure 48–1). This results in disruption of the fungal cell wall and cell death.

Clinical Uses & Adverse Effects

Caspofungin is currently licensed for disseminated and mucocutaneous candidal infections, as well as for empiric antifungal

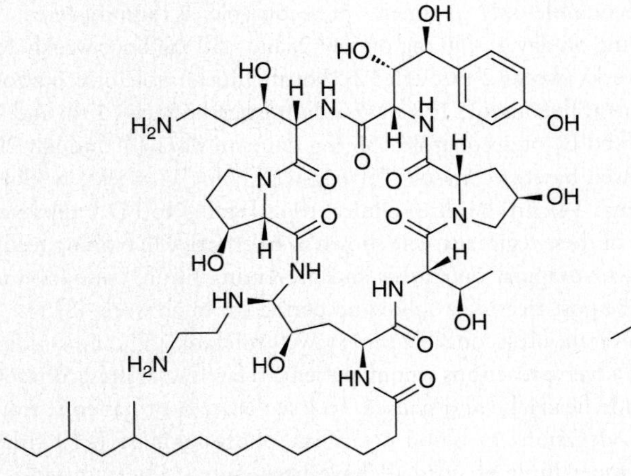

Caspofungin

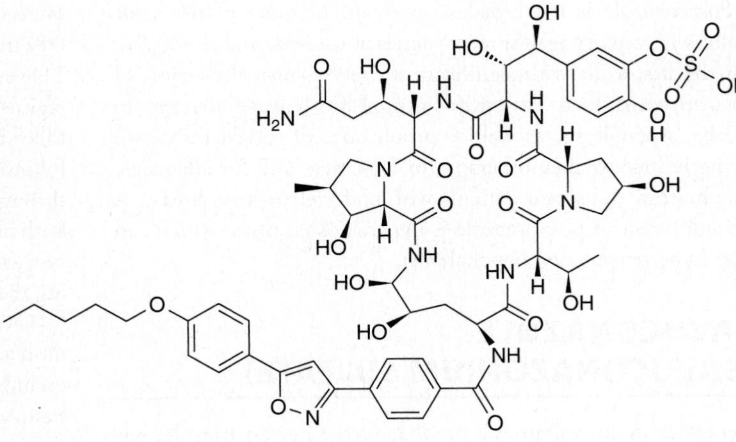

Micafungin

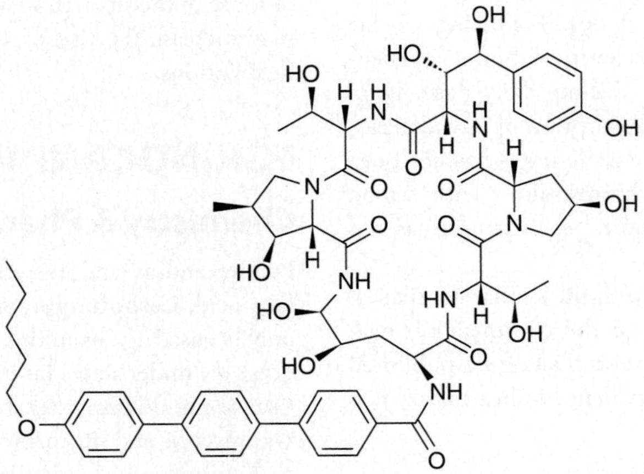

Anidulafungin

therapy during febrile neutropenia, and has largely replaced amphotericin B for the latter indication. Of note, caspofungin is licensed for use in invasive aspergillosis only as salvage therapy in patients who have failed to respond to amphotericin B, and not as primary therapy. Micafungin is licensed for mucocutaneous candidiasis, candidemia, and prophylaxis of candidal infections in bone marrow transplant patients. Anidulafungin is approved for use in esophageal candidiasis and invasive candidiasis, including candidemia.

Echinocandin agents are extremely well tolerated, with minor gastrointestinal side effects and flushing reported infrequently. Elevated liver enzymes have been noted in several patients receiving caspofungin in combination with cyclosporine, and this combination should be avoided. Micafungin has been shown to increase levels of nifedipine, cyclosporine, and sirolimus. Anidulafungin does not seem to have significant drug interactions, but histamine release may occur during intravenous infusion. Clinically significant echinocandin resistance is an emerging concern especially with invasive *Candida glabrata* infections in immunocompromised patients.

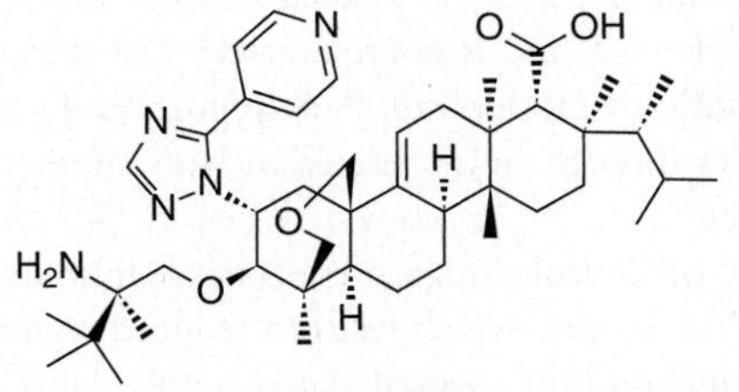

Ibrexafungerp

TRITERPENOIDS

Chemistry & Pharmacokinetics

Triterpenoids are a newly developed class of antifungal agents. The first and only antifungal in this class is **ibrexafungerp**. This agent demonstrates concentration-dependent fungicidal activity against most *Candida* species including azole-resistant isolates. Additionally, ibrexafungerp demonstrates in vitro activity against *Aspergillus* species. Ibrexafungerp is available as a 150-mg oral tablet. The half-life is approximately 20 hours. Metabolism occurs via hydroxylation by CYP3A4, followed by glucuronidation and sulfation of a hydroxylated inactive metabolite. The metabolites are primarily excreted via feces with 51% excreted as unchanged drug.

Mechanism of Action

Similar to echinocandins, triterpenoids inhibit the synthesis of β(1–3)-glucan in the fungal cell wall, which destabilizes the fungal cell wall resulting in cell death (see Figure 48–1).

Clinical Uses & Advese Effects

Ibrexafungerp was granted FDA approval for the treatment of vulvovaginal candidiasis in adult and postmenarche pediatric females. For this indication, ibrexafungerp is administered at a dose of 300 mg by mouth twice daily for a total of two doses. Of note, the use of ibrexafungerp is contraindicated in pregnant patients as it may cause fetal harm based on the results of animal studies. Due to lack of sufficient data at this time, it is advised to verify the pregnancy status of female patients with reproductive potential prior to starting ibrexafungerp.

Overall ibrexafungerp is very well tolerated. The most common side effects include diarrhea, nausea, vomiting, abdominal pain, and dizziness. Due to CYP3A4 metabolism, ibrexafungerp is impacted by CYP3A4-mediated drug-drug interactions. It cannot be co-administered with moderate to strong CYP34 inducers such as rifampin and requires dose adjustment if co-administered with CYP3A inhibitors.

NEW SYSTEMIC ANTIFUNGAL DRUGS UNDER INVESTIGATION

The following drugs are in early preclinical or clinical trials. **ATI-2307**, a novel arylamidine, is in preclinical studies. **Fosmanogepix,** a prodrug of **manogepix,** and **encochleated amphotericin B**, an oral formulation of amphotericin B, are in phase 2 clinical trials. **Rezafungin**, a new very long-acting echinocandin agent, **olorofim**, a novel pyrimidine synthesis inhibitor, and **opelconazole**, an inhaled triazole, are currently undergoing phase 3 clinical trials.

■ ORAL SYSTEMIC ANTIFUNGAL DRUGS FOR MUCOCUTANEOUS INFECTIONS

GRISEOFULVIN

Griseofulvin is a very insoluble fungistatic drug derived from a species of penicillium. Its only use is in the systemic treatment of dermatophytosis (see Chapter 61). It is administered in a microcrystalline oral form at a dosage of up to 1 g/d. Absorption is improved when it is given with fatty foods. Griseofulvin's mechanism of action at the cellular level is unclear, but it is deposited in newly forming skin where it binds to keratin, protecting the skin from new infection. Because its action is to prevent infection of these new skin structures, griseofulvin must be administered for 2–6 weeks for skin and hair infections to allow the replacement of infected keratin by the resistant structures. Nail infections may require therapy for months to allow regrowth of the new protected nail and is often followed by relapse. Adverse effects include an allergic syndrome much like serum sickness, serious skin reactions, a lupus-like syndrome, hepatotoxicity, and drug interactions with warfarin and phenobarbital. Griseofulvin has been largely replaced by newer antifungal medications such as itraconazole and terbinafine.

TERBINAFINE

Terbinafine is a synthetic allylamine that is available in an oral formulation and is used at a dosage of 250 mg/d. It is used in the treatment of dermatophytoses, especially onychomycosis (see Chapter 61). Like griseofulvin, terbinafine is a keratophilic medication, but unlike griseofulvin, it is fungicidal. Like the azole drugs, it interferes with ergosterol biosynthesis, but rather than interacting with the P450 system, terbinafine inhibits the fungal enzyme squalene epoxidase (see Figure 48–1). This leads to the accumulation of the sterol squalene, which is toxic to the organism. One 250-mg tablet given daily for 12 weeks achieves a cure rate of up to 90% for onychomycosis and is more effective than griseofulvin or itraconazole. Adverse effects are rare, consisting primarily of gastrointestinal upset and headache, but serious hepatotoxicity has been reported. Terbinafine does not seem to affect the P450 system and has demonstrated no significant drug interactions to date.

■ TOPICAL ANTIFUNGAL THERAPY

NYSTATIN

Nystatin is a polyene macrolide much like amphotericin B. It is too toxic for parenteral administration and is used only topically. Nystatin is currently available in creams, ointments, suppositories, and other forms for application to skin and mucous membranes. It is not absorbed to a significant degree from skin, mucous membranes, or the gastrointestinal tract. As a result, nystatin has little toxicity, although oral use is often limited by the unpleasant taste.

Nystatin is active against most *Candida* sp and is most commonly used for suppression of local candidal infections. Some common indications include oropharyngeal thrush, vaginal candidiasis, and intertriginous candidal infections.

TOPICAL AZOLES

The two azoles most commonly used topically are clotrimazole and miconazole; several others are available (see Preparations Available). Both are available over the counter and are often used for vulvovaginal candidiasis. Oral clotrimazole troches are available for treatment of oral thrush and are a pleasant-tasting alternative to nystatin. In cream form, both agents are useful for dermatophytic infections, including tinea corporis, tinea pedis, and tinea cruris. Absorption is negligible, and adverse effects are rare.

Topical and shampoo forms of ketoconazole are also available and useful in the treatment of seborrheic dermatitis and pityriasis versicolor. Several other azoles are available for topical use (see Preparations Available).

TOPICAL ALLYLAMINES

Terbinafine and naftifine are allylamines available as topical creams (see Chapter 61). Both are effective for treatment of tinea cruris and tinea corporis. Terbinafine is available without prescription; naftifine is a prescription drug in the USA.

SUMMARY Antifungal Drugs

Subclass, Drug	Mechanism of Action	Effects	Clinical Applications	Pharmacokinetics, Toxicities, Interactions
POLYENE MACROLIDE				
• Amphotericin B	Forms pores in fungal membranes (which contain ergosterol) but not in mammalian (cholesterol-containing) membranes	Loss of intracellular contents through pores is fungicidal • broad spectrum of action	Localized and systemic candidemia • *Cryptococcus* • *Histoplasma* • *Blastomyces* • *Coccidioides* • *Aspergillus*	Oral form is not absorbed • IV for systemic use • intrathecal for fungal meningitis • topical for ocular and bladder infections • duration, days • *Toxicity:* Infusion reactions • renal impairment • *Interactions:* Additive with other renal toxic drugs
• *Lipid formulations: Lower toxicity, higher doses can be used*				
PYRIMIDINE ANALOG				
• Flucytosine	Interferes with DNA and RNA synthesis selectively in fungi	Synergistic with amphotericin • systemic toxicity in host due to DNA and RNA effects	*Cryptococcus* and chromoblastomycosis infections	Oral • duration, hours • renal excretion • *Toxicity:* Myelosuppression
AZOLES				
• Ketoconazole	Blocks fungal P450 enzymes and interferes with ergosterol synthesis	Poorly selective • also interferes with mammalian P450 function	Broad spectrum but toxicity restricts use to topical therapy	Oral, topical • *Toxicity and interactions:* Interferes with steroid hormone synthesis and phase I drug metabolism
• Itraconazole	Same as for ketoconazole	Much more selective than ketoconazole	Broad spectrum: *Candida*, *Cryptococcus*, blastomycosis, coccidioidomycosis, histoplasmosis	Oral and IV • duration, 1–2 d • poor entry into central nervous system (CNS) • *Toxicity and interactions:* Low toxicity
• *Fluconazole, voriconazole, posaconazole, isavuconazole, oteseconazole: Fluconazole has excellent CNS penetration, used in fungal meningitis*				
ECHINOCANDINS				
• Caspofungin	Blocks β-glucan synthase	Prevents synthesis of fungal cell wall	Fungicidal *Candida* sp • also used in aspergillosis	IV only • duration, 11–15 h • *Toxicity:* Minor gastrointestinal effects, flushing • *Interactions:* Increases cyclosporine levels (avoid combination)
• *Micafungin, anidulafungin: Micafungin increases levels of nifedipine, cyclosporine, sirolimus; anidulafungin is relatively free of this interaction*				
ALLYLAMINE				
• Terbinafine	Inhibits epoxidation of squalene in fungi • increased levels are toxic to fungi	Reduces ergosterol • prevents synthesis of fungal cell membrane	Mucocutaneous fungal infections	Oral • duration, days • *Toxicity:* Gastrointestinal upset, headache, hepatotoxicity • *Interactions:* None reported
TRITERPENOIDS				
• Ibrexafungerp	Blocks β-glucan synthase	Prevents synthesis of fungal cell wall	Fungicidal *Candida* sp • In vivo activity against *Aspergillosis* sp.	Oral only • duration, days • *Toxicity:* Fetal toxicity (avoid during pregancny), gastrointestinal upset, and dizziness • *Interactions:* Avoid moderate to strong CYP34 inducers

PREPARATIONS AVAILABLE

GENERIC NAME	AVAILABLE AS
Amphotericin B	
Conventional formulation	Generic
Lipid formulations	Abelcet, AmBisome
Anidulafungin	Eraxis
Butenafine	Mentax
Butoconazole	Gynazole-1
Caspofungin	Cancidas
Clotrimazole	Generic, Lotrimin, Mycelex, others
Econazole	Generic, Ecoza
Fluconazole	Generic, Diflucan
Flucytosine	Generic, Ancobon
Griseofulvin	Grifulvin, Gris-Peg
Ibrexafungerp	Brexafemme
Itraconazole	Generic, Sporanox, Onmel
Ketoconazole	Generic, Nizoral, others
Micafungin	Mycamine
Miconazole	Generic, Oravig, Micatin
Naftifine	Naftin
Natamycin	Natacyn
Nystatin	Generic
Oteseconazole	Vivjoa
Oxiconazole	Generic, Oxistat, others
Posaconazole	Noxafil
Sulconazole	Exelderm
Terbinafine	Generic, Lamisil
Terconazole	Generic, Terazol 3, Terazol 7
Tioconazole	Vagistat 1, Monistat 1
Tolnaftate	Generic, Aftate, Tinactin, others
Voriconazole	Generic, Vfend

REFERENCES

Ashbee HR et al: Therapeutic drug monitoring (TDM) of antifungal agents: Guidelines from the British Society for Medical Mycology. J Antimicrob Chemother 2014;69:1162.

Cornely OA et al: Posaconazole vs. fluconazole or itraconazole prophylaxis in patients with neutropenia. N Engl J Med 2007;356:348.

Diekema DJ et al: Activities of caspofungin, itraconazole, posaconazole, ravuconazole, voriconazole, and amphotericin B against 448 recent clinical isolates of filamentous fungi. J Clin Microbiol 2003;41:3623.

Eyre DW et al: A *Candida auris* outbreak and its control in an intensive care setting. N Engl J Med 2018;379:1322.

Felton T et al: Tissue penetration of antifungal agents. Clin Microbiol Rev 2014:27:68.

Herbrecht R et al: Voriconazole versus amphotericin B for primary therapy of invasive aspergillosis. N Engl J Med 2002;347:408.

Jallow S, Govender N: Ibrexafungerp: a first-in-class oral triterpenoid glucan synthase inhibitor. J Fungi (Basel) 2021;7:163.

Lamoth F, Lewis RE, Dimitrios PK: Investigational antifungal agents for invasive mycoses: a clinical perspective. Clin Infect Dis 2022;75:534.

Lewis RE: Current concepts in antifungal pharmacology. Mayo Clin Proc 2011;86:805.

Maertens JA et al: Isavuconazole versus voriconazole for primary treatment of invasive mold disease caused by *Aspergillus* and other filamentous fungi. Lancet 2016;387:760.

McCarty TP, Pappas PG: Antifungal pipeline. Front Cell Infect Microbiol 2021;11:732223.

Nett JE, Andes DR: Antifungal agents: Spectrum of activity, pharmacology, and clinical indications. Infect Dis Clin North Am 2016;30:51.

Pasqualotto AC, Denning DW: New and emerging treatments for fungal infection. J Antimicrob Chemother 2008;61:i19.

Perlin DS: Echinocandin resistance, susceptibility testing and prophylaxis: Implications for patient management. Drugs 2014;74:1573.

Rogers TR: Treatment of zygomycosis: Current and new options. J Antimicrob Chemother 2008;61:i35.

Van Daele R et al: Antifungal drugs: What brings the future? Med Mycol 2019;57:S328.

Wong-Beringer A et al: Lipid formulations of amphotericin B: Clinical efficacy and toxicities. Clin Infect Dis 1998;27:603.

CASE STUDY ANSWER

The mold subsequently isolated from the patient's CSF was identified as Coccidioides immitis. Patients of African-American and Southeast Asian descent as well as immunocompromised patients are at an increased risk for developing chronic forms of coccidioidomycosis such as meningitis. C immitis is a dimorphic fungus that grows in the soil of the San Joaquin Valley in California, while closely related C posadasii is found elsewhere in desert regions of the southwest USA, parts of Mexico, and Central and South America. Oral therapy with fluconazole was initiated at a dose of 800 mg/day, and patient's headache, fever, and double vision resolved within 7 days. Patients experiencing treatment failure with fluconazole may require treatment with intrathecal amphotericin B. Generally, coccidioidal meningitis requires lifelong therapy because of a high incidence of disease relapse with treatment discontinuation, and it is 100% fatal without antifungal treatment.

CHAPTER

49 Antiviral Agents

Sharon Safrin, MD

CASE STUDY

A 35-year-old white woman who recently tested seropositive for both HIV and hepatitis B virus surface antigen is referred for evaluation. She is feeling well overall but reports a 25-pack-year smoking history. She drinks 3–4 beers per week and has no known medication allergies. She has a history of heroin use and is currently receiving methadone. Physical examination reveals normal vital signs and no abnormalities. White blood cell count is 5800 cells/mm^3 with a normal differential, hemoglobin is 11.8 g/dL, all liver tests are within normal limits, CD4 cell count is 278 cells/mm^3, and viral load (HIV RNA) is 110,000 copies/mL. What other laboratory tests should be ordered? Which antiretroviral medications would you begin?

Viruses are obligate intracellular parasites; their replication depends primarily on synthetic processes of the host cell. Therefore, to be effective, antiviral agents must either block viral entry into or exit from the cell or be active inside the host cell. As a corollary, nonselective inhibitors of virus replication may interfere with host cell function and result in toxicity.

Progress in antiviral chemotherapy began in the early 1950s, when the search for anti-cancer drugs generated several new compounds capable of inhibiting viral DNA synthesis. The two first-generation antiviral agents, 5-iododeoxyuridine and trifluorothymidine, had poor specificity (ie, they inhibited host cell DNA as well as viral DNA) that rendered them too toxic for systemic use. However, both agents are effective when used topically for the treatment of herpes keratitis.

Knowledge of the mechanisms of viral replication has provided insights into critical steps in the viral life cycle that can serve as potential targets for antiviral therapy. Recent research has focused on identifying agents with greater selectivity, higher potency, in vivo stability, and reduced toxicity. Antiviral therapy is now available for herpes simplex virus (HSV), cytomegalovirus (CMV), varicella zoster virus (VZV), hepatitis C virus (HCV), hepatitis B virus (HBV), influenza, human immunodeficiency virus (HIV), and respiratory syncytial virus (RSV). Antiviral drugs share the common property of being virustatic; they are active only against replicating viruses and do not affect latent virus. Whereas some infections require monotherapy for brief periods of time (eg, HSV, influenza), others require multiple drug therapy for indefinite periods (HIV). In chronic illnesses such as viral hepatitis and HIV infection, potent inhibition of viral replication is crucial in limiting the extent of systemic damage.

Viral replication requires several steps (Figure 49–1). Antiviral agents can potentially target any of these steps.

ACRONYMS & OTHER NAMES

3TC	Lamivudine
AZT	Zidovudine (previously azidothymidine)
CMV	Cytomegalovirus
CYP	Cytochrome P450
d4T	Stavudine
ddC	Zalcitabine
ddI	Didanosine
EBV	Epstein-Barr virus
FTC	Emtricitabine
HBeAg	Hepatitis e antigen
HBV, HCV	Hepatitis B virus, C virus
HHV-6, -8	Human herpesvirus-6, human herpesvirus-8
HIV	Human immunodeficiency virus
HSV	Herpes simplex virus
INSTI	Integrase strand transfer inhibitor
NNRTI	Nonnucleoside reverse transcriptase inhibitor
NRTI	Nucleoside/nucleotide reverse transcriptase inhibitor
PI	Protease inhibitor
RSV	Respiratory syncytial virus
SVR	Sustained viral response
UGT1A1	UDP-glucuronosyltransferase 1A1
VZV	Varicella-zoster virus

AGENTS TO TREAT HERPES SIMPLEX VIRUS (HSV) & VARICELLA-ZOSTER VIRUS (VZV) INFECTIONS

Three oral nucleoside analogs are licensed for the treatment of HSV and VZV infections: acyclovir, valacyclovir, and famciclovir. They have similar mechanisms of action and comparable indications for clinical use (Table 49–1); all are well tolerated.

Comparative trials have demonstrated similar efficacies of these three agents for the treatment of HSV. In first episodes of genital herpes, treatment shortens the duration of symptoms by approximately 2 days, time to lesion healing by 4 days, and duration of viral shedding by 7 days. In recurrent genital herpes, treatment shortens the overall time course by 1–2 days. Treatment of first-episode genital herpes does not alter the frequency or severity of recurrent outbreaks. Long-term suppression with antiherpes agents in patients with frequent recurrences of genital herpes decreases the frequency of symptomatic recurrences and of asymptomatic viral shedding, thus decreasing the rate of sexual transmission. However, outbreaks may resume upon discontinuation of suppression. The efficacy of the antiherpes agents in orolabial herpes is generally less than that in anogenital herpes.

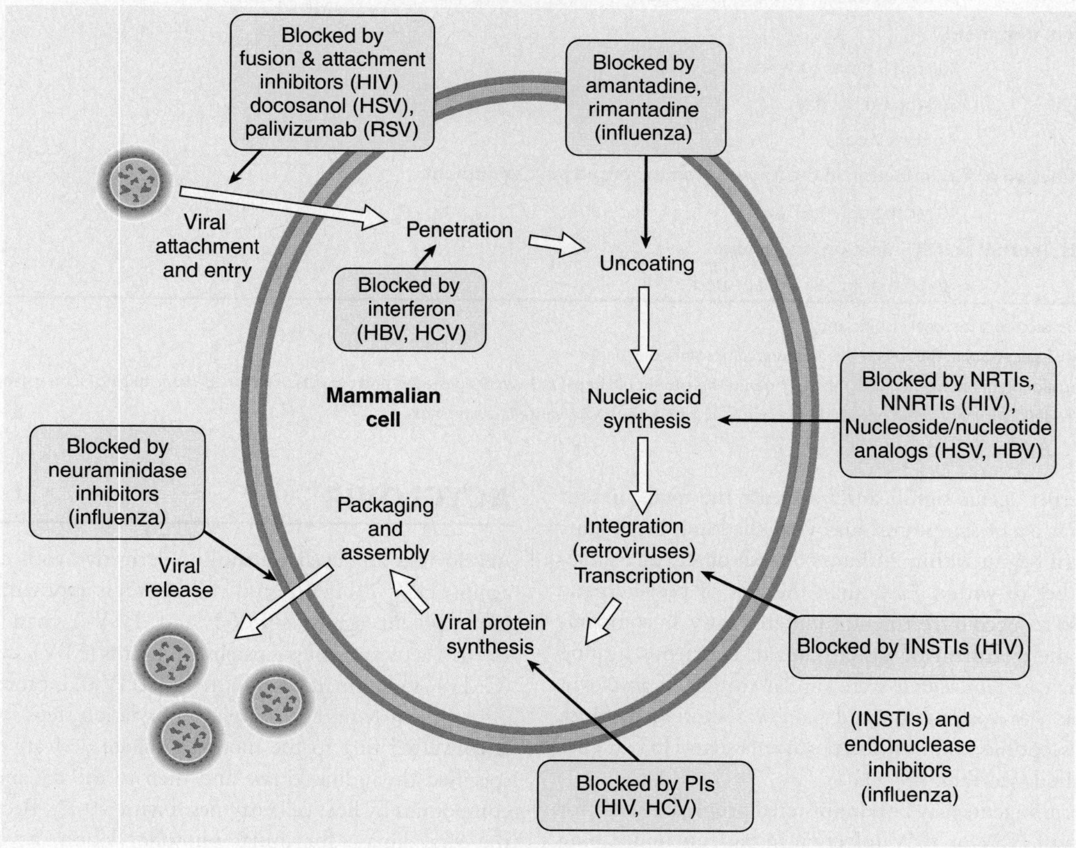

FIGURE 49–1 The major sites of antiviral drug action. *Note:* Interferon alfas are speculated to have multiple sites of action. (Reproduced with permission, from Trevor AJ, Katzung BG, Masters SB: *Pharmacology: Examination & Board Review*, 9th ed. NY McGraw-Hill, 2010.)

TABLE 49–1 Agents to treat or prevent herpes simplex virus (HSV) and varicella-zoster virus (VZV) infections.

Agent	Treatment of First Episode	Treatment of Recurrent Episodes	Suppression
Genital Herpes			
Acyclovir, oral[1]	400 mg tid × 7–10 days	800 mg tid × 2 days or 800 mg bid × 5 days × 5 days	400 mg bid[2,3]
Famciclovir, oral[1]	250 mg tid × 7–10 days	1000 mg bid × 1 day or 125 mg bid × 5 days or 500 mg once then 250 mg bid × 2 days[2]	250 mg bid[2,3]
Valacyclovir, oral[1]	1000 mg bid × 7-10 days	500 mg bid × 3 days or 1 g qd × 5 days	500–1000 mg[2]
Orolabial herpes			
Acyclovir, oral[1]	400 mg tid × 7–10 days or 200 mg 5 times daily	400 mg tid × 5 days	400 mg bid[2]
Famciclovir, oral[1]	250 mg tid or 500 mg bid × 7–10 days	1500 mg once or 750 mg bid × 1 day	500 mg bid
Valacyclovir, oral[1]	1 g bid × 7–10 days	2 g bid × 1 day	500–1000 mg qd
Severe HSV infection, treatment			
Acyclovir, IV[1]	5–10 mg/kg q8h × 7–14 days		
Herpes encephalitis, treatment			
Acyclovir, IV[1]	10 mg/kg q8h × 14–21 days		
Neonatal HSV infection, treatment			
Acyclovir, IV[1]	20 mg/kg q8h × 14–21 days		
Varicella infection, treatment			
Acyclovir, oral[1]	20 mg/kg (maximum 800 mg) qid × 5 days		
Valacyclovir, oral[1]	20 mg/kg (maximum, 1 g) tid × 5 days		
Zoster infection, treatment			
Acyclovir, oral[1]	800 mg 5 times daily × 7 days		
Famciclovir, oral[1]	500 mg tid × 7 days		
Valacyclovir, oral[1]	1 g tid × 7 days		
Severe VZV infection or VZV infection in the immunocompromised host, treatment			
Acyclovir, IV[1]	10 mg/kg q8h × ≥7 days		
Acyclovir-resistant HSV or VZV infection, treatment			
Foscarnet, IV[1]	40–60 mg/kg q8h until healed[2]		

[1]Dose adjustment is necessary for renal insufficiency.

[2]Higher doses may be necessary in HIV-infected or immunocompromised patients.

[3]Suppressive therapy for pregnant women with recurrent genital herpes should begin at 36 weeks gestation and consists of either acyclovir 400 mg TID or valacyclovir 500 mg bid.

HIV, human immunodeficiency virus; HSV, herpes simplex virus; IV, intravenous; VZV, varicella-zoster virus.

The antiherpes agents significantly decrease the total number of lesions, duration of symptoms, and viral shedding in patients with varicella (if begun within 24 hours of rash onset) or cutaneous zoster (if begun within 72 hours); the risk of post-herpetic neuralgia is also reduced if treatment is initiated early. In comparative trials for the treatment of zoster, rates of cutaneous healing with valacyclovir or famciclovir were similar to that of acyclovir, but the duration of zoster-associated pain was shortened. Since VZV is less susceptible to the antiherpes agents than HSV, higher doses are required (see Table 49–1).

The antiherpes agents may be administered prophylactically for the prevention of HSV or VZV infection in patients undergoing organ transplantation, as well as for the treatment of these infections should they occur.

ACYCLOVIR

Acyclovir is an acyclic guanosine derivative with clinical activity against HSV-1, HSV-2, and VZV, but it is approximately 10 times more potent against HSV-1 and HSV-2 than against VZV. In vitro activity against Epstein-Barr virus (EBV), cytomegalovirus (CMV), and human herpesvirus-6 (HHV-6) is present but weaker.

Acyclovir requires three phosphorylation steps for activation. It is converted first to the monophosphate derivative by the virus-specified thymidine kinase and then to the di- and triphosphate compounds by host cell enzymes (Figure 49–2). Because it requires the viral kinase for initial phosphorylation, acyclovir is selectively activated and accumulates only in infected cells. Acyclovir triphosphate inhibits viral DNA synthesis by two mechanisms:

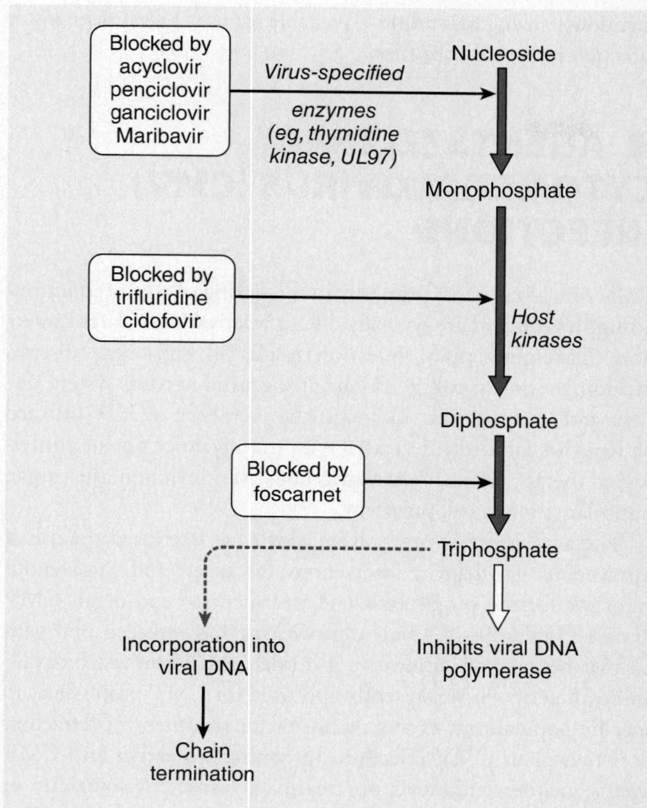

FIGURE 49–2 Mechanism of action of antiherpes agents.

competition with deoxyGTP for the viral DNA polymerase, resulting in binding to the DNA template as an irreversible complex; and chain termination following incorporation into the viral DNA.

The bioavailability of oral acyclovir is low (15–20%) and is unaffected by food. Topical formulations produce high intralesional concentrations but undetectable systemic concentrations.

Acyclovir is cleared primarily by glomerular filtration and tubular secretion. The half-life is 2.5–3 hours in patients with normal renal function and 20 hours in patients with anuria. Acyclovir diffuses readily into most tissues and body fluids. Cerebrospinal fluid concentrations are 20–50% of serum values.

Acyclovir is the only one of the three antiherpes agents that is available for intravenous use in the United States. Intravenous acyclovir is the treatment of choice for herpes simplex encephalitis, neonatal HSV infection, and serious HSV or VZV infections (see Table 49–1). In neonates with central nervous system HSV, oral acyclovir suppression for 6 months following acute treatment improves neurodevelopmental outcomes. In immunocompromised patients with VZV infection, intravenous acyclovir reduces the incidence of cutaneous and visceral dissemination.

Resistance to acyclovir can develop in HSV or VZV through alteration in either the viral thymidine kinase or the DNA polymerase. Although rare in the immunocompetent host, clinically resistant infections have been reported in up to 10% of immunocompromised hosts. Most clinical isolates are resistant on the basis of mutations in the UL23 gene that encodes the viral thymidine kinase and thus are cross-resistant to valacyclovir, famciclovir, and ganciclovir. Agents such as foscarnet, cidofovir, and trifluridine do not require activation by viral thymidine kinase and therefore have preserved activity against the most prevalent acyclovir-resistant strains (see Figure 49–2).

Acyclovir is generally well tolerated, although nausea, diarrhea, and headache may occur. Intravenous infusion may be associated with reversible renal toxicity (ie, crystalline nephropathy or interstitial nephritis), neurologic effects (eg, tremors, delirium, seizures), and reversible dose-dependent neutropenia. However, these are uncommon with adequate hydration and avoidance of rapid infusion rates. High doses of acyclovir cause chromosomal damage and testicular atrophy in rats, but there has been no evidence of teratogenicity, reduction in sperm production, or cytogenetic alterations in peripheral blood lymphocytes in patients receiving daily suppression of genital herpes for more than 10 years. Initiation of suppressive acyclovir therapy beginning at 36 weeks gestation in pregnant women with recurrent genital herpes is recommended to reduce the risk of recurrence at delivery and possibly the need for cesarean section.

Concurrent use of nephrotoxic agents may enhance the potential for nephrotoxicity. Probenecid and cimetidine decrease acyclovir clearance and increase exposure. Somnolence and lethargy may occur in patients receiving concomitant zidovudine and acyclovir.

VALACYCLOVIR

Valacyclovir is the L-valyl ester of acyclovir. It is rapidly converted to acyclovir after oral administration via first-pass enzymatic hydrolysis in the liver and intestine, resulting in serum levels that are three to five times greater than those achieved with oral acyclovir and approximate those achieved with intravenous acyclovir. Oral bioavailability is 54–70%, and cerebrospinal fluid levels are about 50% of those in serum. Elimination half-life is 2.5–3.3 hours.

Valacyclovir is generally well tolerated, although nausea, headache, vomiting, or rash may occur. At high doses, confusion, hallucinations, and seizures have been reported. AIDS patients who received high-dosage valacyclovir chronically (ie, 8 g/d) had increased gastrointestinal intolerance as well as thrombotic thrombocytopenic purpura/hemolytic uremic syndrome; this dose has also been associated with confusion and hallucinations in transplant patients.

Suppressive therapy with valacyclovir is recommended beginning at 36 weeks gestation in pregnant women with recurrent genital herpes.

FAMCICLOVIR

Famciclovir is the diacetyl ester prodrug of 6-deoxypenciclovir, an acyclic guanosine analog. After oral administration, famciclovir is rapidly deacetylated and oxidized by first-pass metabolism to penciclovir. It is active in vitro against HSV-1, HSV-2, VZV, EBV, and HBV. As with acyclovir, activation by phosphorylation is catalyzed by the virus-specified thymidine kinase in infected cells, followed by competitive inhibition of the viral DNA polymerase to block DNA synthesis. Unlike acyclovir, however, penciclovir does not cause chain termination. Penciclovir triphosphate has lower affinity for the viral DNA polymerase than acyclovir triphosphate, but it achieves higher intracellular concentrations. The most commonly encountered clinical mutants of HSV are thymidine kinase-deficient; these are cross-resistant to acyclovir and famciclovir.

The bioavailability of penciclovir from orally administered famciclovir is 70%. The intracellular half-life of penciclovir triphosphate is prolonged, at 7–20 hours. Penciclovir is excreted primarily in the urine.

Oral famciclovir is generally well tolerated, although headache, nausea, or diarrhea may occur. As with acyclovir, testicular toxicity has been demonstrated in animals receiving repeated doses. However, men receiving daily famciclovir (250 mg every 12 hours) for 18 weeks had no changes in sperm morphology or motility. In one study, there was no evidence of increased birth defects in infants exposed to famciclovir during the first trimester. The incidence of mammary adenocarcinoma was increased in female rats receiving famciclovir for 2 years.

TOPICAL AGENTS

Topical agents, including acyclovir 5% cream, acyclovir mucoadhesive buccal tablets, penciclovir 1% cream, and docosanol 10% cream, are available but provide only marginal benefit in the treatment of orolabial herpes; they lack efficacy in genital herpes. There are case reports of successful treatment of acyclovir-resistant cutaneous herpes using topical 5% imiquimod.

INVESTIGATIONAL AGENTS

Two compounds (**pritelivir** and **amenamevir**) belong to the new class of helicase-primase inhibitors and are under development for HSV infection and VZV infection, respectively. The oral thymidine analog **brivudine** is available for use to treatment zoster infection in several countries.

AGENTS TO TREAT CYTOMEGALOVIRUS (CMV) INFECTIONS

CMV infections occur primarily in the setting of advanced immunosuppression and are typically due to reactivation of latent infection. Dissemination of infection results in end-organ disease, including retinitis, colitis, esophagitis, central nervous system disease, and pneumonitis. Although the incidence in HIV-infected patients has markedly decreased with the advent of potent antiretroviral therapy, clinical reactivation of CMV infection after organ transplantation is still prevalent.

The availability of oral valganciclovir has decreased the use of intravenous ganciclovir, intravenous foscarnet, and intravenous cidofovir for the prophylaxis and treatment of end-organ CMV disease (Table 49–2). Oral valganciclovir has replaced oral ganciclovir because of its lower pill burden and improved bioavailability. Letermovir was recently approved for CMV prophylaxis in specific populations, as was maribavir for treatment of refractory post-transplant CMV infection. In contrast to earlier anti-CMV agents, neither letermovir nor maribavir cause myelotoxicity or nephrotoxicity.

GANCICLOVIR

Ganciclovir is an acyclic guanosine analog that requires activation by triphosphorylation before inhibiting the viral DNA polymerase. Initial phosphorylation is catalyzed by the virus-specified protein kinase phosphotransferase UL97 in CMV-infected cells. The activated compound competitively inhibits viral DNA polymerase and

TABLE 49–2 Agents to treat cytomegalovirus (CMV) infection.

Agent	Route of Administration	Use	Recommended Adult Dosage
Valganciclovir[1]	Oral	CMV retinitis treatment	Induction: 900 mg bid × 21 days
			Maintenance: 900 mg daily
	Oral	CMV prophylaxis (transplant patients)	900 mg daily
Letermovir	Oral, intravenous	CMV prophylaxis (transplant patients)	480 mg once daily orally or IV over 1 hour
Maribavir	Oral	Treatment of refractory CMV disease (transplant patients)	400 mg twice daily
Ganciclovir[1]	Intravenous	CMV retinitis treatment	Induction: 5 mg/kg q12h × 14–21 days
			Maintenance: 5 mg/kg/d or 6 mg/kg five times per week
Foscarnet[1]	Intravenous	CMV retinitis treatment	Induction: 60 mg/kg q8h or 90 mg/kg q12h × 14–21 days
			Maintenance: 90–120 mg/kg/d
Cidofovir[1]	Intravenous	CMV retinitis treatment	Induction: 5 mg/kg/week × 2 weeks
			Maintenance: 5 mg/kg every week

[1]Dosage must be reduced in patients with renal insufficiency.

causes termination of viral DNA elongation (see Figure 49–2). Ganciclovir has in vitro activity against CMV, HSV, VZV, EBV, HHV-6, and HHV-8. Its activity against CMV is up to 100 times greater than that of acyclovir.

Ganciclovir is administered intravenously. The bioavailability of oral ganciclovir is poor, and it is no longer available in the USA. Ganciclovir gel is available for the treatment of acute herpetic keratitis. Cerebrospinal fluid concentrations are approximately 50% of serum concentrations. The elimination half-life is 4 hours, and the intracellular half-life is prolonged at 16–24 hours. Clearance of the drug is linearly related to creatinine clearance. Ganciclovir is readily cleared by hemodialysis.

Intravenous ganciclovir has been shown to delay progression of CMV retinitis in immunocompromised patients. Dual therapy with foscarnet and ganciclovir is more effective in delaying progression of retinitis than either drug alone in patients with AIDS (see Foscarnet), although adverse effects are compounded. Intravenous ganciclovir is also used to treat CMV colitis, esophagitis, and pneumonitis (the latter often in combination with intravenous cytomegalovirus immunoglobulin) in immunocompromised patients. Intravenous ganciclovir, followed by either oral valganciclovir or high-dose oral acyclovir, reduces the risk of CMV infection in transplant recipients. Limited data in infants with symptomatic congenital neurologic CMV disease suggest that treatment with IV ganciclovir may reduce hearing loss. The risk of Kaposi's sarcoma is reduced in AIDS patients receiving long-term ganciclovir, presumably because of activity against HHV-8.

Intravitreal injections of ganciclovir may be used to treat CMV retinitis. Concurrent therapy with a systemic anti-CMV agent is necessary to prevent other sites of end-organ CMV disease.

Resistance to ganciclovir increases with duration of use. The more common UL97 mutation results in decreased levels of the triphosphorylated (ie, active) form of ganciclovir. The less common UL54 mutation in DNA polymerase results in higher levels of resistance and potential cross-resistance with cidofovir and foscarnet. Antiviral susceptibility testing is recommended in patients in whom resistance is suspected clinically.

The most common adverse effect of intravenous ganciclovir treatment is myelosuppression, which may be dose-limiting. Other potential adverse effects are nausea, diarrhea, fever, rash, headache, insomnia, and peripheral neuropathy. Central nervous system toxicity (confusion, seizures, psychiatric disturbance) and hepatotoxicity have rarely been reported. Intravitreal ganciclovir has been associated with vitreous hemorrhage and retinal detachment. Ganciclovir is mutagenic in mammalian cells and carcinogenic and embryotoxic at high doses in animals and causes aspermatogenesis; the clinical significance of these preclinical data is unclear.

Levels of ganciclovir may rise in patients concurrently taking probenecid or trimethoprim.

VALGANCICLOVIR

Valganciclovir is an L-valyl ester prodrug of ganciclovir that exists as a mixture of two diastereomers. After oral administration, both diastereomers are rapidly hydrolyzed to ganciclovir by esterases in the intestinal wall and liver.

Valganciclovir has a bioavailability of 60% and should be taken with food. The AUC_{0-24h} resulting from oral valganciclovir (900 mg once daily) is similar to that after 5 mg/kg once daily of intravenous ganciclovir and approximately 1.65 times that of oral ganciclovir. The major route of elimination is renal, through glomerular filtration and active tubular secretion. Plasma concentrations of valganciclovir are reduced ~50% by hemodialysis.

Valganciclovir is as effective as intravenous ganciclovir for the treatment of CMV retinitis and is also indicated for the prevention of CMV disease in high-risk solid organ and bone marrow transplant recipients. Adverse effects, drug interactions, and resistance patterns are the same as those associated with ganciclovir.

FOSCARNET

Foscarnet (phosphonoformic acid) is an inorganic pyrophosphate analog that inhibits herpesvirus DNA polymerase, RNA polymerase, and HIV reverse transcriptase directly without requiring activation by phosphorylation. Foscarnet blocks the pyrophosphate binding site of these enzymes and inhibits cleavage of pyrophosphate from deoxynucleotide triphosphates. It has in vitro activity against HSV, VZV, CMV, EBV, HHV-6, HHV-8, HIV-1, and HIV-2.

Foscarnet is available in an intravenous formulation only; poor oral bioavailability and gastrointestinal intolerance preclude oral use. Cerebrospinal fluid concentrations are 43–67% of steady-state serum concentrations. Although the mean plasma half-life is 3–7 hours, up to 30% of foscarnet may be deposited in bone, with a half-life of several months. The clinical repercussions of this are unknown. Clearance of foscarnet is primarily renal and is directly proportional to creatinine clearance. Serum drug concentrations are reduced ~50% by hemodialysis.

Foscarnet is effective in the treatment of end-organ CMV disease (ie, retinitis, colitis, and esophagitis), including ganciclovir-resistant disease; it is also effective against acyclovir-resistant HSV and VZV infections. The dosage of foscarnet must be titrated according to the patient's calculated creatinine clearance before each infusion. Use of an infusion pump to control the rate of infusion is important to prevent toxicity, and large volumes of fluid are required because of the drug's poor solubility. The combination of ganciclovir and foscarnet is synergistic in vitro against CMV and has been shown to be superior to either agent alone in delaying progression of retinitis; however, toxicity is also increased when these agents are administered concurrently. As with ganciclovir, a decrease in the incidence of Kaposi's sarcoma has been observed in patients who have received long-term foscarnet.

Foscarnet has been administered intravitreally for the treatment of CMV retinitis in patients with AIDS, but data regarding efficacy and safety are incomplete.

Resistance to foscarnet in HSV and CMV isolates is due to point mutations in the DNA polymerase gene and is typically associated with prolonged or repeated exposure to the drug. Mutations in the HIV-1 reverse transcriptase gene have also been described. Although foscarnet-resistant CMV isolates are typically cross-resistant to ganciclovir, foscarnet activity is usually maintained against ganciclovir- and cidofovir-resistant isolates of CMV.

Potential adverse effects of foscarnet include renal impairment, hypo- or hypercalcemia, hypo- or hyperphosphatemia, hypokalemia, and hypomagnesemia. Saline preloading helps prevent nephrotoxicity, as does avoidance of concomitant administration of drugs with nephrotoxic potential (eg, amphotericin B, pentamidine, aminoglycosides). The risk of severe hypocalcemia, caused by chelation of divalent cations, is increased with concomitant use of pentamidine. Genital ulcerations associated with foscarnet therapy may be due to high levels of ionized drug in the urine. Nausea, vomiting, anemia, elevation of liver enzymes, and fatigue have been reported; the risk of anemia may be additive in patients receiving concurrent zidovudine. Central nervous system toxicity includes headache, hallucinations, and seizures; the risk of seizures may be increased with concurrent use of imipenem. Foscarnet caused chromosomal damage in preclinical studies.

CIDOFOVIR

Cidofovir is an acyclic cytosine nucleotide analog with in vitro activity against CMV, HSV-1, HSV-2, VZV, EBV, HHV-6, HHV-8, adenovirus, poxviruses, polyomaviruses, and human papillomavirus. In contrast to ganciclovir, phosphorylation of cidofovir to the active diphosphate is independent of viral enzymes (see Figure 49–2); thus, activity is maintained against thymidine kinase-deficient or -altered strains of CMV or HSV. Cidofovir diphosphate acts both as a potent inhibitor of and as an alternative substrate for viral DNA polymerase, competitively inhibiting DNA synthesis and becoming incorporated into the viral DNA chain. Cidofovir-resistant isolates tend to be cross-resistant with ganciclovir but retain susceptibility to foscarnet.

Although the terminal half-life of cidofovir is approximately 2.6 hours, the active metabolite cidofovir diphosphate has a prolonged intracellular half-life of 17–65 hours, thus allowing infrequent dosing. A separate metabolite, cidofovir phosphocholine, has a half-life of at least 87 hours and may serve as an intracellular reservoir of active drug. Cerebrospinal fluid penetration is poor. Elimination is by active renal tubular secretion; over 80% of the drug is excreted unchanged in the urine within 24 hours.

Intravenous cidofovir is effective for the treatment of CMV retinitis and is used experimentally to treat adenovirus, human papillomavirus, BK polyomavirus, vaccinia, and poxvirus infections. Intravenous cidofovir must be administered with high-dose probenecid (2 g at 3 hours before the infusion and 1 g at 2 and 8 hours after), which blocks active tubular secretion, decreases nephrotoxicity, and may result in the doubling of serum concentrations. Before each infusion, cidofovir dosage must be adjusted according to the calculated creatinine clearance or the presence of urine protein, and aggressive adjunctive hydration is required. Initiation of cidofovir therapy is contraindicated in patients with existing renal insufficiency. Direct intravitreal administration of cidofovir is not recommended due to ocular toxicity.

The primary adverse effect of intravenous cidofovir is a dose-dependent proximal tubular nephrotoxicity, which may be reduced with normal saline prehydration. Proteinuria, azotemia, metabolic acidosis, and Fanconi syndrome may occur. Concurrent administration of other potentially nephrotoxic agents (eg, amphotericin B, aminoglycosides, nonsteroidal anti-inflammatory drugs, pentamidine, foscarnet) should be avoided. Prior administration of foscarnet may increase the risk of nephrotoxicity. Other potential adverse effects include uveitis, ocular hypotony, and neutropenia (15–24%). Probenecid may cause nausea or rash and/or may result in drug-drug interactions (see Chapter 36). Cidofovir is mutagenic, gonadotoxic, and embryotoxic and causes hypospermia and mammary adenocarcinomas in animals.

LETERMOVIR

Letermovir is indicated for CMV prophylaxis in adult CMV-seropositive recipients of an allogenic hematopoietic stem cell transplant. It is available in both oral and intravenous formulations. It has a novel mechanism of action, inhibiting the CMV DNA terminase subunit pUL56 required for DNA packaging and processing and thus replication; this component of the terminase subunit has no equivalent target enzyme in the human body. Letermovir's antiviral activity is highly specific to CMV and is currently the most active molecule against CMV, with preserved activity against CMV isolates that are resistant to other antiviral agents. However, letermovir-resistant isolates with the UL56 mutation have been reported during treatment.

The most commonly reported side effects are nausea, diarrhea, vomiting, peripheral edema, cough, headache, fatigue, and abdominal pain; tachycardia and atrial fibrillation also have been reported.

Since it is a moderate CYP3A4 and OATP1B1/3 inhibitor, an inducer of CYP2C9, and a substrate of OATP1B1/3, there are multiple potential drug-drug interactions. Co-administration with drugs that are inhibitors of OATP1B1/3 transporters may result in increases in letermovir plasma concentrations, while co-administration with OATP1B1/3 substrates may result in clinically relevant increases in the concentrations of these agents. Letermovir increases cyclosporine, tacrolimus, and sirolimus exposure while decreasing exposure to voriconazole. Concomitant administration with pimozide and ergot alkaloids is contraindicated.

MARIBAVIR

Maribavir is indicated for the treatment of post-transplant CMV infection that is refractory to treatment with other anti-CMV agents. It works through inhibition of the UL97 protein kinase and impairment of viral DNA assembly. Its activity is specific for CMV.

Maribavir is taken orally, 400 mg twice daily, without regard to food. It is 98% protein-bound. The mean half-life in transplant patients is 4.32 hours. The main route of metabolism is hepatic; however use in patients with severe hepatic insufficiency has not been studied.

The most commonly reported side effects are dysgeusia, nausea, diarrhea, and fatigue; however, these are not generally dose-limiting.

Maribavir is metabolized by the CYP3A4 system, resulting in potential drug-drug interactions. Since both maribavir and ganciclovir requires activation by the CMV UL97 protein kinase, concurrent use of maribavir results in antagonism of ganciclovir's or valganciclovir's antiviral activity such that co-administration is contraindicated. Maribavir levels may be decreased when co-administered with carbamazepine, phenobarbital, phenytoin, rifampin, rifabutin, or St. John's wort. Digoxin, rosuvastatin, cyclosporine, sirolimus, tacrolimus, and everolimus levels may be increased when co-administered with maribavir.

EXPERIMENTAL AGENTS

Brincidofovir is a nucleoside agent with activity against HSV, CMV, adenovirus, BK virus, ebolavirus, and poxvirus. As a lipophilic prodrug of cidofovir, it has a similar mechanism of action. There is lesser nephrotoxicity; however, gastrointestinal tract toxicity may limit its use. It is currently also under evaluation for the treatment of monkeypox and adenoviremia.

■ ANTIRETROVIRAL AGENTS

Substantial advances have been made in antiretroviral therapy since the introduction of the first agent, zidovudine, in 1987. Classes of antiretroviral agents now available for use include nucleoside/nucleotide reverse transcriptase inhibitors (NRTIs), non-nucleoside reverse transcriptase inhibitors (NNRTIs), protease inhibitors (PIs), integrase strand transfer inhibitors (INSTIs), fusion inhibitors, CCR5 co-receptor antagonists, CD4 T lymphocyte post-attachment inhibitors, gp120 attachment inhibitors, and capsid inhibitors (Table 49–3). These agents inhibit HIV replication at different parts of the cycle (Figure 49–3). In addition, two drugs, ritonavir and cobicistat, are used as enhancers (or boosters) to improve the pharmacokinetic profiles of anti-HIV agents such as the PIs, tenofovir alafenamide, and elvitegravir; ritonavir is also used in combination with nirmatrelvir for COVID-19.

Knowledge of viral dynamics through the use of viral load and resistance testing has made it clear that combination therapy with maximally potent agents will reduce viral replication to the lowest possible level, thereby reducing the number of cumulative mutations and decreasing the likelihood of emergence of resistance. Thus, administration of combination antiretroviral therapy has become the standard of care. Viral susceptibility to specific agents varies among patients and may change with time. Therefore, such combinations must be chosen with care and tailored to the individual, as must changes to a given regimen. In addition to potency and susceptibility, important factors in the selection of agents for any given patient are tolerability, convenience, and optimization of adherence. New drugs with high potency, low toxicity, and good tolerability increase the feasibility of early, lifelong treatment. As new agents have become available, several older ones have had diminished usage, because of suboptimal safety, inferior efficacy, high pill burden, or pharmacologic concerns, including fosamprenavir, delavirdine, didanosine (ddI), indinavir, nelfinavir, nevirapine, saquinavir, stavudine (d4T), and tipranavir. Zalcitabine (ddC; dideoxycytidine) is no longer marketed. Therefore, these agents have been omitted from this chapter.

Decrease of the circulating viral load by antiretroviral therapy is correlated with enhanced survival as well as decreased morbidity. Also, the use of antiretroviral therapy strongly reduces the risk for HIV transmission.

Discussion of antiretroviral agents in this chapter is specific to HIV-1. Patterns of susceptibility of HIV-2 to these agents may vary; however, there is innate resistance to the NNRTIs and enfuvirtide as well as a lower barrier of resistance to NRTIs and PIs.

NUCLEOSIDE & NUCLEOTIDE REVERSE TRANSCRIPTASE INHIBITORS (NRTIs)

The NRTIs act by competitive inhibition of HIV-1 reverse transcriptase; incorporation into the growing viral DNA chain causes chain termination due to inhibition of binding with the incoming nucleotide (see Figure 49–3). Each agent requires intracytoplasmic activation via phosphorylation by cellular enzymes to the triphosphate form.

Typical resistance mutations include M184V, K65R/K, and L74V. Lamivudine or emtricitabine therapy tends to select rapidly for the M184I/V mutation in regimens that are not fully suppressive; this mutation is also frequently found in patients receiving abacavir. While the M184V mutation confers reduced susceptibility to lamivudine and emtricitabine; its presence may restore phenotypic susceptibility to tenofovir and zidovudine. K65R/N andK70E/G/Q are typical mutations in patients with tenofovir resistance.

All NRTIs may be associated with mitochondrial toxicity, which may manifest as peripheral neuropathy, pancreatitis, lipoatrophy, or hepatic steatosis. Less commonly, lactic acidosis may occur, which can be fatal. NRTI treatment should be suspended in the setting of rapidly rising aminotransferase levels, progressive hepatomegaly, or metabolic acidosis of unknown cause. Lipoatrophy and insulin resistance may occur most frequently with use of the thymidine analogs (eg, zidovudine), and least frequently with use of tenofovir, lamivudine, emtricitabine, and abacavir. Immune reconstitution syndrome has also been described in association with the NRTIs.

ABACAVIR

Abacavir is a guanosine analog that is well absorbed following oral administration (83%) and is unaffected by food. The serum half-life is 1.5 hours. The drug undergoes hepatic glucuronidation and carboxylation. Dosage reduction is recommended in mild hepatic impairment; use is not recommended in patients

TABLE 49–3 Currently available antiretroviral agents.

Agent	Class of Agent	Recommended Adult Dosage	Administration Recommendation	Characteristic Adverse Effects	Comments
Abacavir	NRTI[1]	300 mg bid or 600 mg qd	Test to rule out the presence of the HLA-B5701 allele prior to initiation of therapy.	Rash, hypersensitivity reaction, nausea; possible increase in myocardial infarction	Avoid alcohol.
Atazanavir	PI[2]	400 mg qd alone; 300 mg qd with ritonavir 100 mg qd or cobicistat 150 mg qd; adjust dose in hepatic insufficiency	Take with food. Avoid concomitant antacids. Separate dosing acid-reducing agents by ≥10 h.	Nausea, rash, indirect hyperbilirubinemia, diarrhea, ↑ liver enzymes, prolonged PR interval	See footnote 4. Avoid elvitegravir/cobicistat, etravirine. Avoid in severe hepatic insufficiency. The oral powder contains phenylalanine.
Bictegravir	INSTI	In a fixed-dose combination tablet qd: bictegravir 50 mg/TAF 25 mg/emtricitabine 200 mg/d	Separate dosing from antacids by ≥2 h.	Nausea, diarrhea, headache, rash ↑ total bilirubin and serum creatinine	See footnote 4.
Cabotegravir	INSTI	In a fixed-dose combination: 30 mg cabotegravir/25 mg rilpivirine qd orally or 400 mg IM q month/rilpivirine 600 m IM q month	Avoid concomitant antacids.		See footnote 4.
Darunavir	PI[2]	Treatment-naïve: 800 mg qd with ritonavir 100 mg qd or cobicistat 150 mg qd Treatment-experienced: 600 mg bid with ritonavir 100 mg bid	Take with food.	Diarrhea, headache, nausea, rash, hyperlipidemia, ↑ liver enzymes, ↑ serum amylase	See footnote 4. Avoid elvitegravir/cobicistat and simeprevir. Avoid in patients with sulfa allergy.
Dolutegravir	INSTI	INSTI-naïve: 50 mg qd If co-administered with efavirenz or rifampin or if certain INSTI mutations: 50 mg bid	Separate dosing from antacids and polyvalent cations by ≥2 h.	Insomnia, headache, hypersensitivity reaction, ↑ liver enzymes	Avoid carbamazepine, dofetilide, phenobarbital, phenytoin.
Doravirine	NNRTI	100 mg qd		Headache, nausea, diarrhea, rash, ↑ liver enzymes	See footnote 4
Efavirenz	NNRTI	600 mg qd	Take on an empty stomach, at bedtime.	Neuropsychiatric symptoms, rash, ↑ liver enzymes, headache, nausea	See footnote 4. Avoid elvitegravir/cobicistat, etravirine, simeprevir. Teratogenic in primates.
Elvitegravir	INSTI	150 mg qd with cobicistat 150, emtricitabine 200, and 10 mg alafenamide or 300 mg tenofovir disoproxil tenofovir[3]	Take with food. Separate dosing from antacids by ≥2 h.	Diarrhea, rash, ↑ liver enzymes	See footnote 4. Avoid efavirenz.
Emtricitabine	NRTI[1]	200 mg qd[3]		Headache, diarrhea, nausea, rash, hyperpigmentation	Avoid concurrent lamivudine.

Enfuvirtide	Fusion inhibitor	90 mg subcutaneously bid		Injection site reactions, hypersensitivity reaction, insomnia, headache, dizziness, nausea, eosinophilia; possible increased bacterial pneumonia	
Etravirine	NNRTI	200 mg bid	Take with food.	Rash, nausea, diarrhea	See footnote 4. Avoid atazanavir, efavirenz, elvitegravir/cobicistat, unboosted protease inhibitors.
Fostemsavir	Gp120 attachment inhibitor	600 mg bid		Nausea, liver enzyme elevations in patients with HBV or HCV infection and QT prolongation	See footnote 4.
Ibalizumab	CD4 post-attachment inhibitor	Single loading dose of 2000 mg IV then 800 mg every 2 weeks		Diarrhea, dizziness, nausea, and rash	
Lamivudine	NRTI[1]	150 mg bid or 300 mg qd[3]		Nausea, headache, dizziness, fatigue	Do not administer with emtricitabine.
Lenacapavir	Capsid inhibitor	600 mg Day 1, 2 then 300 mg Day 8 then 927 mg subcutaneously every 6 months		Injection site reactions, nausea	See footnote 4.
Lopinavir/ritonavir	PI/PI[2]	400/100 mg bid or 800/200 mg qd		Diarrhea, nausea, hypertriglyceridemia, ↑ liver enzymes, ↑cholesterol.	See footnote 4. Avoid disulfiram and metronidazole with oral solution.
Maraviroc	CCR5 inhibitor	300 mg bid; 150 bid with CYP3A inhibitors; 600 mg bid with CYP3A inducers		Cough, muscle pain, diarrhea, sleep disturbance, ↑ liver enzymes; possible increase in myocardial infarction	See footnote 4. Do not administer in patients with severe renal dysfunction.
Raltegravir	INSTI	400 mg bid or 1200 mg once daily		Nausea, headache, fatigue, muscle aches, ↑ amylase levels, ↑ liver enzymes	The chewable tablets contain phenylalanine.
Rilpivirine	NNRTI	25 mg qd	Take with food. Separate dosing from antacids or H_2 blockers by ≥4 h.	Headache, insomnia, depression, rash, ↑ liver enzymes	See footnote 4.

(continued)

TABLE 49–3 Currently available antiretroviral agents. (Continued)

Agent	Class of Agent	Recommended Adult Dosage	Administration Recommendation	Characteristic Adverse Effects	Comments
Tenofovir alafenamide (TAF)	NRTI[1]	10–25 mg/d in fixed dose combinations with other antiretrovirals		Gastrointestinal symptoms, headache, ↑ creatinine, proteinuria, bone loss	Avoid inducers of p-glycoprotein (rifampin, rifabutin, phenytoin, phenobarbital, St John's wort). Avoid in severe renal insufficiency. Co-administration with adefovir is contraindicated.
Tenofovir disoproxil fumarate	NRTI[1]	300 mg qd[3]		Nausea, diarrhea, vomiting, flatulence, headache, renal insufficiency, bone loss	Avoid atazanavir, probenecid. Co-administration with adefovir is contraindicated.
Zidovudine	NRTI[1]	200 mg tid or 300 mg bid[3]		Macrocytic anemia, neutropenia, nausea, headache, insomnia, myopathy	Avoid concurrent myelosuppressive drugs (eg, ganciclovir, ribavirin).

[1]All NRTI agents carry the risk of lactic acidosis with hepatic steatosis as a potential adverse event.

[2]All PI agents carry the risk of hyperlipidemia, fat maldistribution, hyperglycemia, and insulin resistance as potential adverse events.

[3]Adjust dose in renal insufficiency.

[4]Because of altered systemic exposures, concurrent drugs that interact with the CYP3A4 system should be used with caution, including alfuzosin, amiodarone, aprepitant, artemether/lumefantrine, astemizole, atovaquone, benzodiazepines (diazepam, midazolam, triazolam), bexarotene, bepridil, bosentan, bupropion, calcium channel blockers (diltiazem, felodipine, nifedipine, nimodipine, verapamil), carbamazepine, ceritinib, cimetidine, cisapride, clopidogrel, colchicine, conivaptan, corticosteroids, cyclosporine, dabrafenib, dapsone, desipramine, direct Factor Xa inhibitors (apixaban, rivaroxaban), disopyramide, dofetilide, dronedarone, enzalutamide, ergot alkaloid derivatives, ethinyl estradiol/norethindrone acetate, flecainide, fluticasone, gestodene, idelalisib, irinotecan, ivacaftor, levodopa, lidocaine, lumacaftor, lurasidone, macrolide agents (clarithromycin, telithromycin), methadone, mitotane, nafcillin, PDE5 inhibitors, phenobarbital, phenytoin, pimozide, primidone, propafenone, protein pump inhibitors, quinidine, ranolazine, rifabutin, salmeterol, spironolactone, statin agents, St. John's wort, tacrolimus, triazole antifungal agents (itraconazole, ketoconazole, posaconazole, voriconazole), terfenadine, and warfarin.

HBV, hepatitis B virus; HCV, hepatitis C virus; INSTI, integrase strand transfer inhibitor; IV, intravenous; NNRTI, nonnucleoside reverse transcriptase inhibitor; NRTI, nucleoside/nucleotide reverse transcriptase inhibitor; PI, protease inhibitor; TAF, tenofovir alafenamide.

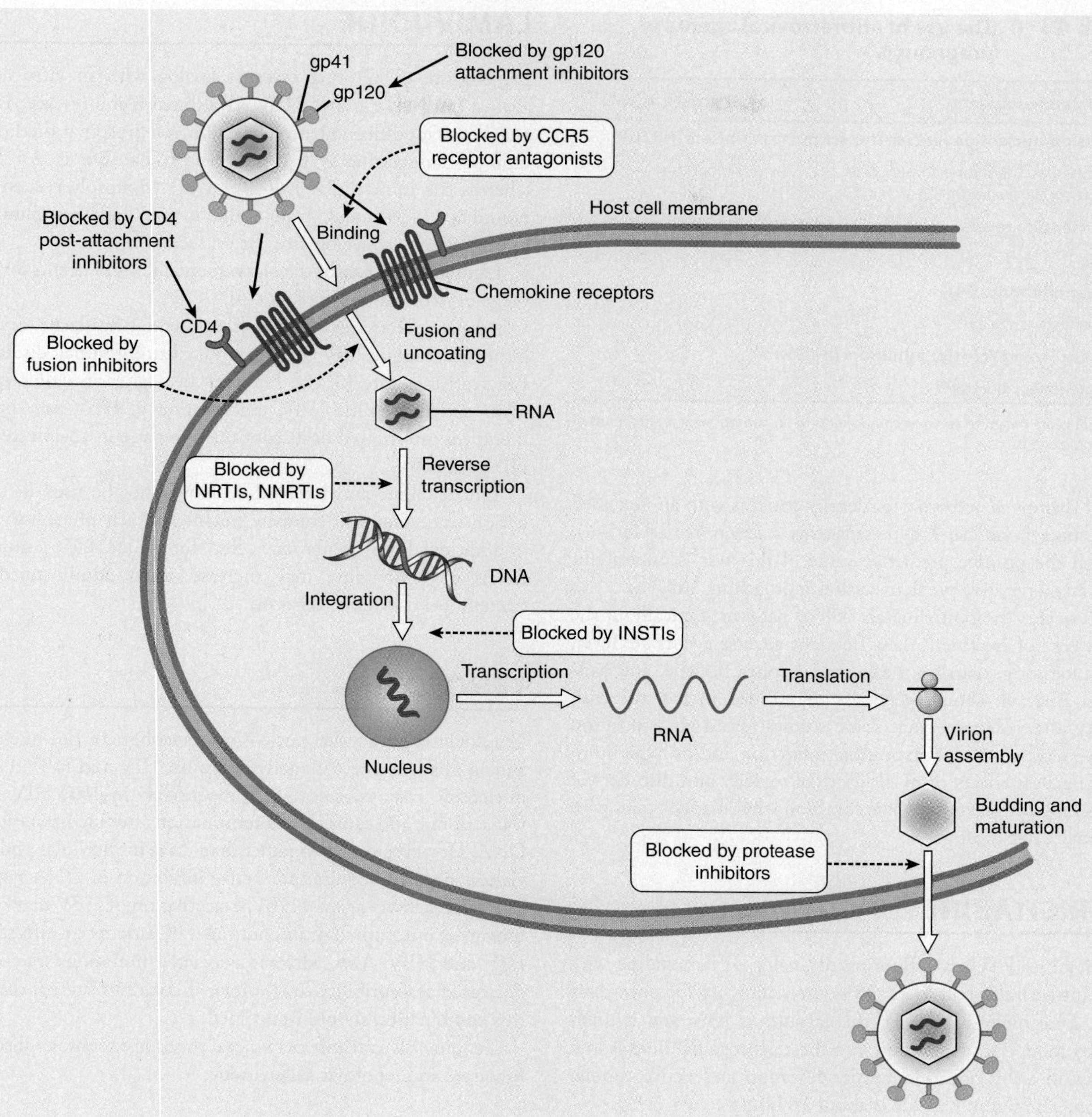

FIGURE 49–3 Life cycle of HIV. Binding of viral glycoproteins to host cell CD4 and chemokine receptors leads to fusion of the viral and host cell membranes via gp41 and entry of the virion into the cell. After uncoating, reverse transcription copies the single-stranded HIV RNA genome into double-stranded DNA, which is integrated into the host cell genome. Gene transcription by host cell enzymes produces messenger RNA, which is translated into proteins that assemble into immature noninfectious virions that bud from the host cell membrane. Maturation into fully infectious virions is through proteolytic cleavage. NNRTIs, nonnucleoside reverse transcriptase inhibitors; NRTIs, nucleoside/nucleotide reverse transcriptase inhibitors.

with moderate or severe liver disease. Since the drug is metabolized by alcohol dehydrogenase, serum levels of abacavir may be increased with concurrent alcohol (ie, ethanol) ingestion. Cerebrospinal fluid levels are approximately one-third those of plasma. Abacavir is one of the NRTI agents recommended for use in pregnancy (Table 49–4).

Concurrent administration with atazanavir or lopinavir may decrease abacavir serum levels to a clinically significant degree.

Hypersensitivity reactions, occasionally fatal, have been reported in up to 8% of patients receiving abacavir and may be more severe with once-daily dosing. Symptoms, which generally occur within the first 6 weeks of therapy, include fever, fatigue, nausea, vomiting, diarrhea, and abdominal pain. Dyspnea, pharyngitis, cough, and elevations in serum aminotransferase or creatine kinase levels may also be present, with skin rash in ~50% of patients. Rechallenge is contraindicated. Screening for HLA-B*5701 before initiation of

TABLE 49–4 The use of antiretroviral agents in pregnancy.

Recommended Agents[1]	Alternate Agents[1]
Nucleoside/nucleotide reverse transcriptase inhibitors (NRTIs)	
Abacavir, emtricitabine, lamivudine, tenofovir alafenamide, tenofovir disoproxil	Zidovudine
Nonnucleoside reverse transcriptase inhibitors (NNRTIs)	
None	Efavirenz, rilpivirine
Protease inhibitors (PIs)	
Atazanavir, darunavir	
Integrase Strand Transfer inhibitors (INSTIs)	
Dolutegravir, raltegravir	

[1]These agents are meant to serve as components in an antiretroviral regimen rather than as single agents.

abacavir therapy is necessary to identify patients with an increased risk for abacavir-associated hypersensitivity reaction (see Table 5–4). Although the positive predictive value of this test is only about 50%, it has a negative predictive value approaching 100%.

Rash occurs in approximately 5% of patients, typically in the first 6 weeks of treatment. Less frequent adverse events are fever, nausea, vomiting, diarrhea, headache, dyspnea, fatigue, and pancreatitis. Abacavir should generally be avoided in patients with coronary artery disease, since some studies found an association with an increased risk of myocardial infarction and/or hyperlipidemia. The class effects of mitochondrial toxicity and disorders of lipid metabolism seem to be less common with abacavir than with other nucleoside analogs.

EMTRICITABINE

Emtricitabine (FTC) is a fluorinated analog of lamivudine with a long intracellular half-life (>24 hours), allowing for once-daily dosing. Oral bioavailability of the capsules is 93% and is unaffected by food, but penetration into the cerebrospinal fluid is low. Elimination is by both glomerular filtration and active tubular secretion. The serum half-life is about 10 hours.

Emtricitabine is one of the NRTI agents recommended for use in pregnancy (see Table 49–4). The combination of emtricitabine and tenofovir disoproxil fumarate is the only FDA-approved formulation for pre-exposure prophylaxis to reduce HIV acquisition in high-risk persons.

The most common adverse effects observed in patients receiving emtricitabine are headache, diarrhea, nausea, and rash. Hyperpigmentation of the palms or soles may occur (~2%), particularly in African Americans (up to 13%). Clinically significant drug-drug interactions involving emtricitabine have not been identified. Due to its activity against HBV, exacerbation of HBV may occur if therapy is interrupted or discontinued in patients co-infected with HIV.

Emtricitabine and lamivudine should not be used in combination since they will compete for intracellular phosphorylation; in addition, both agents may select for the M184V/I mutation.

LAMIVUDINE

Lamivudine (3TC) is a cytosine analog with in vitro activity against both HIV-1 and HBV. Oral bioavailability exceeds 80% and is not food-dependent. The mean cerebrospinal fluid:plasma ratio of lamivudine is 0.1–0.2. Serum half-life is 2.5 hours, whereas the intracellular half-life of the triphosphorylated compound is 11–14 hours. Lamivudine is predominantly eliminated in the urine by active organic cation secretion.

Lamivudine is one of the recommended NRTI agents for use in pregnant women (see Table 49–4).

Adverse effects are uncommon but include headache, dizziness, insomnia, fatigue, dry mouth, and gastrointestinal discomfort. Pancreatitis is rare (0.3%) but may be higher in children. Due to its activity against HBV, exacerbation of HBV may occur if therapy is interrupted or discontinued in patients co-infected with HIV and HBV.

Emtricitabine and lamivudine should not be used in combination since they will compete for intracellular phosphorylation; in addition, both agents may select for the M184V/I mutation. Levels of lamivudine may increase when administered with trimethoprim-sulfamethoxazole.

TENOFOVIR

Tenofovir is an acyclic nucleoside phosphonate (ie, nucleotide) analog of adenosine with activity against HIV and HBV. Like the nucleoside analogs, tenofovir competitively inhibits HIV reverse transcriptase and causes chain termination after incorporation into DNA. However, only two rather than three intracellular phosphorylation steps are required for active inhibition of DNA synthesis. Due to its activity against HBV, exacerbation of HBV may occur if therapy is interrupted or discontinued in patients co-infected with HIV and HBV. Also, adefovir-associated mutations may lead to decreased susceptibility to tenofovir if co-administered; therefore, this combination should be avoided.

Tenofovir is available as two oral prodrugs: tenofovir disoproxil fumarate and tenofovir alafenamide.

TENOFOVIR DISOPROXIL FUMARATE

Tenofovir disoproxil fumarate is a water-soluble prodrug of active tenofovir. The prolonged serum (12–17 hours) and intracellular half-lives allow once-daily dosing. Elimination occurs by both glomerular filtration and active tubular secretion, and dosage adjustment in patients with renal insufficiency is recommended.

Tenofovir disoproxil fumarate is one of the NRTI agents recommended for use in pregnancy (see Table 49–4). The combination of tenofovir disoproxil and emtricitabine is the only FDA-approved formulation for pre-exposure prophylaxis to reduce HIV acquisition in high-risk persons.

Gastrointestinal complaints (eg, nausea, diarrhea, vomiting, flatulence) are the most common adverse effects but rarely require discontinuation. Since tenofovir is formulated with lactose, these may occur more frequently in patients with lactose intolerance. Cumulative loss of renal function has been observed, possibly increased with concurrent use of boosted PI regimens, in patients with pre-existing renal disease or in patients receiving concurrent nephrotoxic agents. Acute renal failure, Fanconi syndrome, and nephrogenic diabetes insipidus also have been reported. For this reason, tenofovir should be used with caution in patients at risk for renal dysfunction. Serum creatinine levels should be monitored during therapy and tenofovir discontinued for new proteinuria, glycosuria, or a ≥25% decline in calculated creatinine clearance to <60 mL/min. Tenofovir-associated proximal renal tubulopathy causes excessive renal phosphate and calcium losses and 1-hydroxylation defects of vitamin D; since loss of bone mineral density and osteomalacia have been reported, tenofovir is not recommended in individuals with or at risk for bone demineralization.

Tenofovir may compete with other drugs that are actively secreted by the kidneys, such as cidofovir, acyclovir, and ganciclovir. Concurrent use of probenecid is contraindicated. Tenofovir disoproxil levels may increase when co-administered with atazanavir or lopinavir/ritonavir.

TENOFOVIR ALAFENAMIDE

Tenofovir alafenamide is a phosphonoamidate prodrug of tenofovir that is currently available only in co-formulation with other antiretroviral or pharmacokinetic boosting agents (eg, emtricitabine, elvitegravir, rilpivirine, cobicistat, ritonavir). Tenofovir alafenamide achieves similar antiviral efficacy to tenofovir disoproxil at much lower plasma concentrations of tenofovir (approximately 90% lower), since metabolism occurs in lymphocytes and macrophages (as well as hepatocytes and some other cells) rather than blood.

Tenofovir alafenamide has less renal and bone toxicity than tenofovir disoproxil fumarate but may cause greater weight gain or lipid elevation. It does not require dose adjustment in patients with creatinine clearance >30 mL/min.

Adverse effects appear to be uncommon but may include gastrointestinal symptoms or headache. Tenofovir alafenamide has also been approved for treatment of HBV infection.

Tenofovir alafenamide is one of the agents recommended for use in pregnant women (see Table 49–4).

Because of differences in drug transporters involved in tenofovir alafenamide versus tenofovir disoproxil absorption, potential drug-drug interactions differ. Inhibition of intestinal P-glycoprotein by cobicistat or ritonavir necessitates lowering of the tenofovir alafenamide dose due to higher plasma levels. Lopinavir may increase the serum concentration of tenofovir disoproxil and thus enhance the nephrotoxic effect. Conversely, darunavir, rifampin, rifabutin, and St. John's wort can decrease tenofovir concentrations.

ZIDOVUDINE

Zidovudine (azidothymidine; AZT) is a deoxythymidine analog that is well absorbed (63%) and distributed to most body tissues and fluids, including the cerebrospinal fluid, where drug levels are 60–65% of those in serum. Although the serum half-life averages 1 hour, the intracellular half-life of the phosphorylated compound is 3–4 hours, allowing twice-daily dosing. Zidovudine is eliminated primarily by renal excretion following glucuronidation in the liver.

Zidovudine was the first antiretroviral agent to be approved and has been well studied. Studies evaluating the use of zidovudine during pregnancy, labor, and postpartum showed significant reductions in the rate of vertical transmission, and zidovudine is one of the NRTI agents recommended as an alternative component of an antiretroviral regimen during pregnancy (see Table 49–4). Zidovudine is also recommended as an option for postexposure prophylaxis in individuals exposed to HIV.

The most common adverse effects of zidovudine are macrocytic anemia (1–4%) and neutropenia (2–8%). Gastrointestinal intolerance, headaches, nausea, and insomnia may occur but tend to resolve during therapy. A symptomatic myopathy may occur with prolonged use. Lipoatrophy appears to be more common in patients receiving zidovudine or other thymidine analogs. High doses can cause anxiety, confusion, and tremulousness.

Induction or inhibition of glucuronidation may alter serum levels of zidovudine when co-administered with atovaquone, lopinavir/ritonavir, probenecid, or valproic acid.

NONNUCLEOSIDE REVERSE TRANSCRIPTASE INHIBITORS (NNRTIs)

The NNRTIs bind directly to HIV-1 reverse transcriptase (see Figure 49–3), resulting in allosteric inhibition of RNA- and DNA-dependent DNA polymerase activity. The binding site of NNRTIs is near to but distinct from that of NRTIs. Unlike the NRTI agents, NNRTIs neither compete with nucleoside triphosphates nor require phosphorylation to be active.

Oral NNRTIs have a long plasma half-life, typically >24 hours in adults, with the exception of doravirine, which has a half-life of 15–21 hours. The long half-life allows NNRTIs to be administered once daily. The second-generation NNRTIs (doravirine, etravirine, rilpivirine) tend to have higher potency, longer half-lives, reduced side-effect profiles, and a higher barrier to resistance than the older NNRTIs (delavirdine, efavirenz, nevirapine).

Baseline genotypic testing is recommended prior to initiating NNRTI treatment since primary resistance rates range from ~2% to 8%. NNRTI resistance occurs rapidly with monotherapy and can result from a single mutation. The K103N and Y181C mutations confer resistance to the first-generation NNRTIs, but typically not to etravirine or rilpivirine. Other mutations (eg, L100I, Y188C, G190A) may also confer cross-resistance among the NNRTI class. However, there is no cross-resistance between the NNRTIs and the NRTIs; in fact, some nucleoside-resistant viruses display hypersusceptibility to NNRTIs (and vice versa).

As a class, NNRTI agents tend to be associated with varying degrees of gastrointestinal intolerance and skin rash, the latter of which may infrequently be serious (eg, Stevens-Johnson syndrome).

A further limitation to use of NNRTI agents as a component of antiretroviral therapy is their metabolism by the CYP450 system, leading to innumerable potential drug-drug interactions (see Tables 49–3 and 49–4). All NNRTI agents are substrates for CYP3A4 and can act as inducers (nevirapine) or mixed inducers and inhibitors (efavirenz, etravirine). Given the large number of non-HIV medications that are also metabolized by this pathway (see Chapter 4), drug-drug interactions must be expected and looked for; dosage adjustments are frequently required and some combinations are contraindicated.

DORAVIRINE

The pyridinone doravirine may be taken with or without food. The absolute bioavailability of doravirine is 64% with a T_{max} of 2 hours; it is 76% protein-bound and the half-life is 15 hours.

Doravirine has a unique resistance pathway, with the majority of mutants in clinical trials having V106 or F227 substitutions rather than the more typical E138K or K103N in this class of agents. However, most of these mutants have shown low replication capacity to date. Also, mutants containing the F27C substitution are hypersusceptible to some NRTIs (zidovudine, tenofovir, lamivudine).

The most common adverse effects are headache, nausea, diarrhea, and rash. Doravirine is associated with fewer central nervous system side effects and fewer negative effects on lipids than efavirenz and darunavir.

Inducers of CYP450 3A such as rifampin, rifapentine, efavirenz, carbamazepine, phenobarbital, phenytoin, and St. John's wort may substantially decrease doravirine concentrations and are contraindicated. Levels of doravirine may decrease when co-administered with efavirenz. The dosage of doravirine must be increased if co-administered with rifabutin.

EFAVIRENZ

Efavirenz is moderately well absorbed following oral administration (45%); the elimination half-life of a single dose is 52–76 hours. Due to increased bioavailability after a high-fat meal, efavirenz should be taken on an empty stomach. Efavirenz is principally metabolized by CYP3A4 and CYP2B6 to inactive hydroxylated metabolites; the remainder is eliminated in the feces as unchanged drug. It is highly bound to albumin (~ 99%), and cerebrospinal fluid levels range from 0.3% to 1.2% of plasma levels.

The principal adverse effects of efavirenz involve the central nervous system. Dizziness, drowsiness, insomnia, nightmares, and headache tend to diminish with continued therapy; dosing on an empty stomach to lessen absorption and/or bedtime administration may be helpful. Higher rates are observed in African-American patients due to a genetically determined slower metabolism of the medication. Psychiatric symptoms such as depression, mania, psychosis, and suicidality are more common in the first weeks following initiation of therapy but may persist. Skin rash has been reported early in therapy in up to 28% of patients; the rash is usually mild to moderate in severity and typically resolves despite continuation. Rarely, rash has been severe or life-threatening. Other potential adverse reactions are moderate to severe liver disease, QT prolongation, nausea, vomiting, diarrhea, crystalluria, and hyperlipidemia. High rates of fetal abnormalities, such as neural tube defects, occurred in pregnant monkeys exposed to efavirenz; however, this toxicity has not been observed in meta-analyses of humans receiving efavirenz.

Efavirenz is recommended as an alternative component of an antiretroviral regimen during pregnancy (see Table 49–4).

As both an inducer and an inhibitor of CYP3A4, efavirenz induces its own metabolism and interacts with the metabolism of many other drugs (see Table 49–3). Co-administration with doravirine, elvitegravir/cobicistat, elbasvir/grazoprevir, etravirine, itraconazole, ketoconazole, sofosbuvir/velpatasvir, and St. John's wort is contraindicated. Levels of efavirenz may be reduced by concomitant phenobarbital and phenytoin and increased by darunavir or doravirine. Levels of atazanavir, bictegravir, cabotegravir, darunavir, dolutegravir, doravirine, elvitegravir, etravirine, lopinavir/ritonavir, maraviroc, methadone, raltegravir, rifabutin, and the statin agents may be reduced when administered with efavirenz.

ETRAVIRINE

Etravirine, a diarylpyrimidine, was designed to be effective against strains of HIV that had developed resistance to first-generation NNRTIs due to mutations such as K103N and Y181C. Although etravirine has a higher genetic barrier to resistance than the other NNRTIs, mutations selected by etravirine usually are associated with resistance to efavirenz.

Etravirine should be taken with a meal to increase systemic exposure, since absorption is increased by 50% with food. It is highly protein-bound and is primarily metabolized by the liver. Mean terminal half-life is estimated at 41 hours.

The most common adverse effects of etravirine are rash, nausea, and diarrhea. The rash is typically mild and usually resolves after 1–2 weeks without discontinuation of therapy. Rarely, rash has been severe or life-threatening. Laboratory abnormalities include elevations in serum cholesterol, triglyceride, glucose, and hepatic aminotransferase levels. Aminotransferase elevations are more common in patients with HBV or HCV co-infection.

Etravirine is a substrate as well as an inducer of CYP3A4 and an inhibitor of CYP2C9 and CYP2C19 and thus has potential for numerous drug-drug interactions (see Table 49–3). Some of the interactions are difficult to predict. For example, etravirine may decrease itraconazole and ketoconazole concentrations but increase voriconazole concentrations. Etravirine should not be given with atazanavir, carbamazepine, phenytoin, phenobarbital, clopidogrel, efavirenz, elvitegravir/cobicistat, rifampin, rifapentine, St. John's wort, unboosted protease inhibitors, and several of the anti–hepatitis C agents. Levels of etravirine are decreased with concurrent darunavir or efavirenz. Co-administration with clarithromycin, statin agents, or the antimalarial agent artemether/lumefantrine should be avoided if possible.

RILPIVIRINE

Rilpivirine, a diarylpyrimidine, must be administered with a meal (preferably high fat or >400 kcal). Its oral bioavailability is dependent on an acid gastric environment for optimal absorption; thus, antacids and H_2-receptor antagonists should be separated in time and proton pump inhibitors are contraindicated. The drug is highly protein-bound, and the terminal elimination half-life is 50 hours. Rilpivirine is also available in an injectable formulation that must be used with cabotegravir.

Rilpivirine is recommended as an alternative component of an antiretroviral regimen during pregnancy (see Table 49–4).

The most common adverse effects associated with rilpivirine therapy are rash, depression, headache, insomnia, and increased serum aminotransferases. Increased serum cholesterol and fat redistribution syndrome have also been reported. Neurologic and psychiatric side effects are less common than with efavirenz. Since high doses have been associated with QT prolongation, administration with agents that may prolong the QT interval or in patients with long QT syndrome is to be avoided. Inhibition of renal tubular secretion of creatinine causes a reversible elevation in serum creatinine, but glomerular filtration rate is not affected.

Rilpivirine is primarily metabolized by CYP3A4, and drugs that induce or inhibit CYP3A4 may thus affect the clearance of rilpivirine (see Table 49–3). Co-administration of rifampin or rifabutin is contraindicated.

PROTEASE INHIBITORS (PIs)

During the later stages of the HIV growth cycle, the *gag* and *gag-pol* gene products are translated into polyproteins, which become immature budding particles. The HIV protease is responsible for cleaving these precursor molecules to produce the final structural proteins of the mature virion core. By preventing post-translational cleavage of the Gag-Pol polyprotein, protease inhibitors (PIs) prevent the processing of viral proteins into functional conformations, resulting in the production of immature, noninfectious viral particles (see Figure 49–3). Unlike the NRTIs, PIs do not need intracellular activation.

PIs are typically administered with a boosting agent, either cobicistat or low-dose (100–200 mg) ritonavir. These agents increase the concentration of the PI by inhibiting the hepatic microsomal enzyme CYP3A4. In contrast to ritonavir, cobicistat has no antiviral activity.

Pharmacologically boosted PIs achieve high serum concentrations and have a high genetic barrier to resistance; therefore, decreased drug susceptibility generally requires the accumulation of multiple mutations and is uncommon.

As a class, PIs are associated with gastrointestinal intolerance, which may be dose-limiting, and lipodystrophy, which includes both metabolic (hyperglycemia, hyperlipidemia, insulin resistance) and morphologic (lipoatrophy, fat deposition) derangements. A syndrome of redistribution and accumulation of body fat that results in central obesity, dorsocervical fat enlargement (buffalo hump), peripheral and facial wasting, breast enlargement, and a cushingoid appearance has been observed, least commonly with atazanavir. PIs may be associated with cardiac conduction abnormalities, including PR and QT interval prolongation. A baseline electrocardiogram and avoidance of other agents causing prolonged PR or QT intervals should be considered. Abacavir and lopinavir/ritonavir have been associated with an increased risk of cardiovascular disease in some, but not all, studies. Drug-induced hepatitis and rare severe hepatotoxicity have been reported to varying degrees with all PIs; the frequency of hepatic events is higher with tipranavir/ritonavir than with other PIs. Unconjugated hyperbilirubinemia may occur with atazanavir. Whether PI agents are associated with bone loss and osteoporosis after long-term use is under investigation. PIs have been associated with increased spontaneous bleeding in patients with hemophilia A or B; an increased risk of intracranial hemorrhage has been reported in patients receiving tipranavir/ritonavir. Darunavir is a sulfonamide; caution should be used in patients with a history of sulfa allergy.

All of the antiretroviral PIs are extensively metabolized by CYP3A4. Some PI agents, such as ritonavir, are also inducers of specific CYP isoforms. As a result, there is enormous potential for drug-drug interactions with other antiretroviral agents and other commonly used medications (see Table 49–3 and the section on anti–hepatitis C virus agents for a description of drug-drug interactions with protease inhibitors). It is noteworthy that the potent CYP3A4 inhibitory properties of ritonavir and cobicistat are used to clinical advantage by having them "boost" the levels of other PI agents when given in combination, thus acting as a pharmacokinetic enhancer rather than an antiretroviral agent. Boosting increases drug exposure, thereby prolonging the drug's half-life and allowing reduction in frequency; in addition, the genetic barrier to resistance is raised.

Several older PIs are no longer administered or are rarely used because of poor efficacy and/or toxicity. Such agents include indinavir, fosamprenavir, nelfinavir, saquinavir, and tipranavir. Therefore, they have been omitted from this chapter.

ATAZANAVIR

Atazanavir is an azapeptide PI with a pharmacokinetic profile that allows once-daily dosing. Atazanavir requires an acidic medium for absorption and has pH-dependent aqueous solubility; therefore, it should be taken with meals. Separation of ingestion from acid-reducing agents is recommended and concurrent proton pump inhibitors are contraindicated. Atazanavir is able to penetrate both the cerebrospinal and seminal fluids. The plasma half-life is 7–8 hours, which increases to 9–18 hours when co-administered with a boosting agent The primary route of elimination is biliary; atazanavir should not be given to patients with severe hepatic insufficiency.

Boosted atazanavir (ie, atazanavir plus ritonavir or cobicistat) is one of the recommended PI agents for use in pregnant women (see Table 49–4).

Atazanavir has better gastrointestinal tolerance than the other PIs and is not associated with insulin resistance or an increased risk of cardiovascular disease. The most common adverse effects in patients receiving atazanavir are diarrhea and nausea; vomiting, abdominal pain, headache, and peripheral neuropathy may also occur. Skin rash, reported in ~20% of patients, is generally mild; however severe rash and Stevens Johnson syndrome have been reported. Indirect hyperbilirubinemia with overt jaundice may occur in ~10% of patients, owing to inhibition of the UGT1A1 glucuronidation enzyme; this is reversible upon discontinuation of atazanavir. Elevation of serum aminotransferases has separately been observed, usually in patients with underlying HBV or HCV co-infection. Kidney stones, proximal tubular dysfunction, interstitial nephritis, gallstones, PR prolongation, and decreased bone mineral density also have been reported. The oral powder contains phenylalanine, which can be harmful to patients with phenylketonuria.

As an inhibitor of CYP3A4, CYP2C9, and UGT1A1, the potential for drug-drug interactions with atazanavir is great (see Table 49–3). Concurrent administration with lopinavir may increase atazanavir serum levels to a clinically significant degree whereas co-administration with efavirenz, elvitegravir, etravirine, or tenofovir may decrease atazanavir levels. Due to decreased atazanavir levels, unboosted atazanavir should not be administered with cisapride, ergotamine, etravirine, or proton pump inhibitors. In addition, co-administration of atazanavir with other drugs that inhibit UGT1A1, such as irinotecan, may increase its levels. Atovaquone, lopinavir, and voriconazole levels may be decreased with co-administration, and levels of bictegravir, etravirine, maraviroc, ranolazine, and raltegravir may be increased.

DARUNAVIR

Darunavir must be co-administered with ritonavir or cobicistat. Darunavir should be taken with meals to improve bioavailability, since absorption is increased by ~40% with food. It is highly protein-bound and primarily metabolized by the liver. Elimination half-life is ~15 hours. The dose may vary according to which drug-resistance mutations are present.

Boosted darunavir is one of the PI agents recommended for use in pregnancy (see Table 49–4).

Darunavir is one of the most well-tolerated PI agents. Adverse effects include diarrhea, nausea, headache, and increases in amylase and hepatic aminotransferase levels. Rash occurs in 2–7% of patients and may occasionally be severe. Liver toxicity, including severe hepatitis, has been reported, such that liver function tests should be monitored; the risk may be higher for persons with HBV, HCV, or other chronic liver disease. Darunavir contains a sulfonamide moiety and may cause a hypersensitivity reaction, particularly in patients with sulfa allergy.

Darunavir both inhibits and is metabolized by the CYP3A enzyme system, conferring many possible drug-drug interactions (see Table 49–3). In addition, co-administered ritonavir and/or cobicistat are potent inhibitors of CYP3A and CYP2D6, resulting in further drug-drug interactions. Darunavir levels may be increased when co-administered with tenofovir and may be decreased with concurrent efavirenz or lopinavir/ritonavir. Levels of clarithromycin, colchicine, cyclophosphamide, and digoxin may be increased when administered with darunavir, and levels of paroxetine and sertraline may be decreased.

LOPINAVIR

Lopinavir is available only in combination with low-dose ritonavir as a pharmacologic "booster" via inhibition of its CYP3A-mediated metabolism, resulting in increased exposure and a reduced pill burden.

Lopinavir is highly protein-bound (98–99%), and its half-life is 5–6 hours. It is extensively metabolized by CYP3A, which is inhibited by ritonavir and cobicistat.

The most common adverse effects of lopinavir are diarrhea, nausea, vomiting, increased serum lipids, and increased serum aminotransferases (more common in patients with HBV or HCV co-infection). Prolongation of the PR and/or QT interval may occur. In some studies but not in others, lopinavir/ritonavir has been associated with a higher risk of myocardial infarction. Pancreatitis has rarely been reported. Boosted lopinavir may be more commonly associated with gastrointestinal adverse effects than other PIs. Lopinavir/ritonavir has been associated with an increased risk of preterm birth and is therefore not recommended as a component of antiretroviral therapy in pregnant women.

Potential drug-drug interactions are extensive (see Table 49–3). Lopinavir may increase the serum concentration of atazanavir and may also result in PR prolongation when co-administered. Conversely, atazanavir may decrease the serum concentration of lopinavir. Lopinavir levels may also be decreased with concurrent efavirenz or etravirine and increased when co-administered with darunavir. Levels of lamotrigine and methadone may be reduced with co-administration, and levels of bosentan may be increased. Concurrent use of darunavir is contraindicated. Since the oral solution of lopinavir/ritonavir contains alcohol, concurrent disulfiram and metronidazole are contraindicated. The oral solution also contains propylene glycol, contraindicating the co-administration of other drugs containing propylene glycol.

RITONAVIR

Ritonavir has a high bioavailability (~75%) that increases with food. It is 98% protein-bound and has a serum half-life of 3–5 hours. Metabolism to an active metabolite occurs via the CYP3A and CYP2D6 isoforms; excretion is primarily in the feces.

Adverse effects of full-dose ritonavir include asthenia, gastrointestinal disturbances, and hepatitis; these are greatly reduced with the lower doses (100–200 mg bid) used for boosting. Dose escalation over 1–2 weeks decreases these side effects. Other potential adverse effects include altered taste, paresthesias (circumoral or peripheral), elevated serum aminotransferase and lipid levels, headache, elevations in serum creatine kinase, and pancreatitis. Inhibition of renal tubular secretion of creatinine causes a reversible elevation in serum creatinine, but glomerular filtration rate is not affected.

Ritonavir is a potent inhibitor of CYP3A4, a characteristic that has been used to great advantage in combination with any of the other PI agents, to permit lower or less frequent dosing (or both) with greater tolerability as well as the potential for greater efficacy against resistant virus. Therapeutic levels of digoxin and theophylline should be monitored when co-administered with ritonavir.

Cobicistat

Cobicistat acts as a pharmacokinetic enhancer (ie, booster) when co-administered with atazanavir or darunavir, resulting increased systemic exposure of these agents. The dose is 150 mg once daily. It is highly protein-bound, with a terminal half-life of 3–4 hours. Unlike ritonavir, it does not have antiviral activity of its own.

Potential adverse effects include increased serum creatine kinase, rash, and hyperlipidemia. Concurrent use with nephrotoxic agents is contraindicated. Cobicistat is a strong CYP34A inhibitor and thus may engender drug-drug interactions of its own. As with low-dose ritonavir, however, this characteristic is important in increasing the serum concentrations of co-administered atazanavir or darunavir.

INTEGRASE STRAND TRANSFER INHIBITORS (INSTIs)

This class of agents binds integrase, a viral enzyme essential to the replication of both HIV-1 and HIV-2. By doing so, they inhibit strand transfer, the third and final step of provirus integration, thus terminating the integration of reverse-transcribed HIV DNA into the chromosomes of host cells (see Figure 49–3). As a class, these agents tend to be well tolerated, with headache and gastrointestinal effects the most commonly reported adverse events. They are a good option for patients with coronary artery disease or abnormal lipid profiles, since adverse effects in these categories are infrequent. Regimens containing dolutegravir or bictegravir have a higher genetic barrier to resistance and lower pill burden than the first-generation INSTIs, making them frequent choices as part of first-line regimens. However, their use in co-formulated antiretroviral regimens (eg, bictegravir with tenofovir alafenamide and emtricitabine) or with cobicistat (ie, elvitegravir) means that additional adverse events and/or drug-drug interactions need to be considered. Rare severe events include systemic hypersensitivity reactions and rhabdomyolysis.

BICTEGRAVIR

This agent is available as a co-formulated tablet with tenofovir alafenamide and emtricitabine, administered as a single pill to be taken once daily. Polyvalent cations (eg, antacids) may interfere with gastrointestinal absorption of bictegravir and should thus be separated by at least 2 hours from ingestion of bictegravir.

The most common adverse effects are nausea, diarrhea, and headache. Bictegravir carries a genetically high barrier to resistance.

Bictegravir is a substrate of both CYP3A4 and UGT1A1 and is thus subject to many potential drug-drug interactions (see Table 49–3). Efavirenz, rifampin, rifapentine, carbamazepine, phenytoin, phenobarbital, and St. John's wort are among the drugs that may decrease bictegravir plasma levels. Atazanavir may greatly increase bictegravir plasma levels. Bictegravir also inhibits the renal transporters organic cation transporter 2 (OCT2) and multidrug and toxin extrusion transporter 1 (MATE1) and may increase levels of drugs that are substrates of these transporters, such as metformin.

CABOTEGRAVIR

Cabotegravir is a long-acting INSTI administered in combination with the NNRTI rilpivirine; it is available in both oral and injectable formulations. The oral preparation had been used as a lead-in to injectable therapy for one month to assess tolerability; however, this is no longer recommended. Intramuscular cabotegravir/rilpivirine is administered every 4–8 weeks in treatment-experienced patients. In addition, monotherapy with intramuscular cabotegravir every 4–8 weeks has shown effectiveness as pre-exposure prophylaxis to prevent sexual HIV transmission.

Cabotegravir is highly protein-bound. Absorption of oral cabotegravir is decreased by antacids. Terminal half-life of the oral formulation is 41 hours and of the injectable, 5.6–11.5 weeks. Residual concentrations of both cabotegravir and rilpivirine may remain in the systemic circulation of patients for prolonged periods (up to 12 months or longer); however, the clinical significance of this is unclear.

The most common adverse reactions are injection-site reactions, pyrexia, fatigue, headache, musculoskeletal pain, nausea, sleep disorders, dizziness, and rash. Hypersensitivity reactions and post-injection reactions may cause discontinuation. Hepatotoxicity also has been reported and may be increased in patients with underlying liver disease. Depressive disorders, including suicidality, may occur. Rilpivirine may cause prolongation of the QT interval.

Cabotegravir is primarily metabolized by UGT1A1 with some contribution from UGT1A9, whereas rilpivirine is metabolized by CYP3A4. Drugs that induce UGT1A1 may decrease the plasma concentrations of the components of cabotegravir and are contraindicated, including carbamazepine, phenobarbital, phenytoin, rifabutin, rifampin, rifapentine, dexamethasone, and St. John's wort. Co-administration with lopinavir may increase cabotegravir levels, whereas concurrent efavirenz may decrease its levels.

DOLUTEGRAVIR

The frequency of dosing of dolutegravir depends on the presence or absence of integrase inhibitor–associated resistance mutations and the concurrent use of efavirenz or rifampin (see Table 49–3). Dolutegravir should be taken 2 hours before or 6 hours after cation-containing antacids or laxatives, sucralfate, oral iron supplements, oral calcium supplements, or buffered medications. Peak plasma concentrations occur within 2–3 hours of ingestion. Dolutegravir is highly protein-bound (99%). The terminal half-life is ~14 hours. Serum levels may be reduced in patients with severe renal insufficiency.

Adverse effects of dolutegravir are infrequent but may include insomnia, headache, increased serum aminotransferase levels, and rarely, rash. A hypersensitivity reaction, including rash and systemic symptoms, has been reported; the drug should be discontinued immediately if this occurs and not restarted. Dolutegravir increases serum creatinine by inhibiting tubular secretion of creatinine but has no effect on actual glomerular filtration rate. Dolutegravir may be associated with more central nervous side effects (eg, insomnia, dizziness) than other INSTIs, particularly in women and in patients older than 60 years. There is some evidence of an increased rate of neural tube defects in patients receiving dolutegravir, but the absolute risk is felt to be low.

Dolutegravir is one of the agents recommended for treatment of pregnant women with HIV (see Table 49-4). In addition, it is used for nonoccupational post-exposure prophylaxis.

Since dolutegravir is primarily metabolized via UGT1A1 with some contribution from CYP3A, plasma concentrations may be affected when co-administered with drugs that inhibit or induce these pathways (see Table 49–3). Levels of dolutegravir may decrease when co-administered with efavirenz, etravirine, rifampin, or rifapentine, in some instances necessitating increased doses of dolutegravir or boosting or both. Co-administration with phenytoin, phenobarbital, carbamazepine, and St. John's wort should be avoided. Dolutegravir inhibits the renal organic cation transporter OCT2, thereby increasing plasma concentrations of drugs eliminated via OCT2 such as dofetilide and metformin.

ELVITEGRAVIR

Elvitegravir is available only in fixed-dose combination with emtricitabine, cobicistat, and either tenofovir alafenamide or tenofovir disoproxil. Elvitegravir should be taken with food, and it should be taken 2 hours before or 6 hours after cation-containing antacids or laxatives, sucralfate, oral iron supplements, oral calcium supplements, or buffered medications. Peak levels occur within 4 hours of ingestion; elvitegravir is highly protein-bound (>98%). Cobicistat inhibits renal tubular secretion of creatinine; therefore, fixed-dose combinations need to be adjusted for renal function. It is contraindicated in patients with severe renal or hepatic insufficiency.

There appear to be few adverse effects associated with elvitegravir, but they may include nausea, diarrhea, rash, and elevation in serum aminotransferases.

Elvitegravir is primarily metabolized by CYP3A enzymes, so drugs that induce or inhibit the action of CYP3A may affect its serum levels (see Table 49–3). In addition, cobicistat strongly inhibits CYP3A. Elvitegravir levels may be lowered by concurrent efavirenz, rifampin, rifabutin, carbamazepine, phenytoin, or St. John's wort and may be increased when co-administered with atazanavir, darunavir, or lopinavir/ritonavir. Concurrent use of azole antifungal drugs is contraindicated due to a potential increase in elvitegravir levels; rifabutin levels may also be increased by concurrent elvitegravir. Elvitegravir also induces CYP2D9 and may lower concentrations of substrates of this enzyme. With the fixed-dose combination, concurrent alfuzosin, atazanavir, cisapride, darunavir, efavirenz, etravirine, ledipasvir, lopinavir/ritonavir, methylprednisolone, midazolam, pimozide, prednisolone, rifampin, and rifabutin are contraindicated. Since elvitegravir has a lower barrier to resistance than the newer INSTIs such as dolutegravir and bictegravir, as well as a higher risk for drug-drug interactions due to its CYP450 metabolism, it is not as frequently recommended in a first-line regimen.

Standard elvitegravir and cobicistat dosing during the second and third trimesters of pregnancy results in significantly lower exposure, which may increase the risk of virologic failure and mother-to-child transmission; therefore, it is not recommended for use in pregnant women.

RALTEGRAVIR

Raltegravir may be taken without regard to meals. Terminal half-life is ~9 hours. Since raltegravir has a lower barrier to resistance than the newer INSTIs such as dolutegravir and bictegravir, it is not as frequently recommended in a first-line regimen.

Raltegravir is one of the agents recommended as a treatment for pregnant women with HIV infection (see Table 49–4).

Adverse effects of raltegravir are uncommon but include nausea, headache, fatigue, dizziness, muscle aches, and increased aminotransferase, serum amylase, and serum creatine kinase levels. Raltegravir may enhance the myopathic (rhabdomyolytic) effect of zidovudine. Severe, potentially life-threatening and fatal skin reactions have been reported, including Stevens-Johnson syndrome, hypersensitivity reaction, and toxic epidermal necrolysis.

Raltegravir levels may be increased when co-administered with atazanavir and decreased with concurrent etravirine. Raltegravir does not interact with the CYP450 system but is metabolized by glucuronidation, particularly UGT1A1. Therefore, concurrent use of inducers or inhibitors of UGT1A1 such as rifampin and rifapentine may necessitate dosage adjustment of raltegravir. The chewable tablets contain phenylalanine, which can be harmful to patients with phenylketonuria.

FUSION INHIBITORS

The process of HIV-1 entry into host cells is complex; each step presents a potential target for inhibition. Viral attachment to the host cell entails binding of the viral envelope glycoprotein complex gp160 (consisting of gp120 and gp41) to its cellular receptor CD4. This binding induces conformational changes in gp120 that enable access to the chemokine receptors CCR5 or CXCR4. Chemokine receptor binding induces further conformational changes in gp120, allowing exposure to gp41 and leading to fusion of the viral envelope with the host cell membrane and subsequent entry of the viral core into the cellular cytoplasm.

ENFUVIRTIDE

Enfuvirtide is a synthetic 36-amino-acid peptide fusion inhibitor that blocks HIV entry into the cell (see Figure 49–3). Enfuvirtide binds to the gp41 subunit of the viral envelope glycoprotein, preventing the conformational changes required for the fusion of the viral and cellular membranes.

Enfuvirtide is administered by twice-daily subcutaneous injection. Metabolism appears to be by proteolytic hydrolysis without involvement of the CYP450 system. The drug is 92% protein-bound, and elimination half-life is 3.8 hours. Median time to peak plasma concentration is 8 hours. The drug does not penetrate into the cerebrospinal fluid.

Resistance to enfuvirtide can result from mutations in gp41; the frequency and significance of this are being investigated. However, enfuvirtide lacks cross-resistance with the other currently approved antiretroviral drug classes.

The most common adverse effects are local injection site reactions, consisting of painful erythematous nodules. Although frequent, these are typically mild-to-moderate in severity and rarely lead to discontinuation. Other potential side effects include insomnia, headache, dizziness, and nausea. Hypersensitivity reactions may rarely occur, are of varying severity, and may recur on rechallenge. Eosinophilia is the primary laboratory abnormality seen with enfuvirtide administration. In Phase 3 studies, bacterial pneumonia was seen at a higher rate in patients who received enfuvirtide than in those who did not receive enfuvirtide.

No drug-drug interactions have been identified that would require the alteration of the dosage of concomitant antiretroviral or other drugs.

CCR5 CO-RECPTOR ANTAGONISTS

MARAVIROC

Maraviroc is approved for use in combination with other antiretroviral agents in adult patients who are infected only with CCR5-tropic HIV-1. Maraviroc binds specifically and selectively to the host protein CCR5, one of two chemokine receptors necessary for entrance of HIV into CD4+ cells. Since maraviroc is active against HIV that uses the CCR5 co-receptor exclusively, and not against HIV strains with CXCR4, dual, or mixed tropism, co-receptor tropism should be determined by specific testing before maraviroc is started. Substantial proportions of patients, particularly those with advanced HIV infection, are likely to have virus that is not exclusively CCR5-tropic.

The absorption of maraviroc is rapid but variable, with the time to maximum absorption generally 1–4 hours after ingestion of the drug. Most of the drug (≥75%) is excreted in the feces, whereas approximately 20% is excreted in urine. Elimination half-life is 14–18 hours. The recommended dose of maraviroc varies according to the concomitant use of CYP3A inducers or inhibitors (see Table 49–3). Maraviroc is contraindicated in patients with severe renal impairment and caution is advised when used in patients with preexisting hepatic impairment and in those co-infected with HBV or HCV. Maraviroc has excellent penetration into the cervicovaginal fluid, with levels almost four times higher than the corresponding concentrations in blood plasma.

Resistance to maraviroc is associated with one or more mutations in the V3 loop of gp120. However, emergence of CXCR4 virus (either previously undetected or newly developed) appears to be a more common cause of virologic failure than the development of resistance mutations. There is no cross-resistance with drugs from any other class.

Potential adverse effects of maraviroc include upper respiratory tract infection, cough, pyrexia, rash, dizziness, muscle and joint pain, diarrhea, sleep disturbance, and elevations in serum aminotransferases. Hepatotoxicity has been reported, which may be preceded by a systemic allergic reaction (ie, pruritic rash, eosinophilia, or elevated IgE); discontinuation of maraviroc should be prompt if this constellation occurs. Myocardial ischemia and infarction have been observed in patients receiving maraviroc; therefore, caution is advised in patients at increased cardiovascular risk. There is an increased risk of postural hypotension in patients with severe renal impairment.

There has been concern that blockade of the chemokine CCR5 receptor—a human protein—may result in decreased immune surveillance, with a subsequent increased risk of malignancy or infection. To date, however, there has been no evidence of an increased risk of either malignancy or infection in patients receiving maraviroc.

Maraviroc is a substrate for CYP3A4 and therefore requires adjustment in the presence of drugs that interact with these enzymes (see Table 49–3). It is also a substrate for P-glycoprotein, which limits intracellular concentrations of the drug. The dosage of maraviroc must be decreased if it is co-administered with strong CYP3A inhibitors (eg, ketoconazole, itraconazole, clarithromycin, or any protease inhibitor) and must be increased if co-administered with CYP3A inducers (eg, efavirenz, etravirine, carbamazepine, phenytoin, or St. John's wort). Co-administration of atazanavir, darunavir, or lopinavir/ritonavir may increase maraviroc levels. Concurrent use of rifampin is contraindicated.

CD4 POST-ATTACHMENT INHIBITORS

IBALIZUMAB

Ibalizumab (also known as ibalizumab-uiyk) is a monoclonal antibody that binds the CD4 receptor and blocks HIV entry to CD4 cells. It is indicated for use in patients with multidrug-resistant HIV who are on a failing antiretroviral regimen and is active against both CCR5- and CXCR4-tropic HIV isolates.

Ibalizumab is administered intravenously every 2 weeks. The half-life is estimated at 3–3.5 days. The most common side effects are diarrhea, dizziness, nausea, and rash. Hypersensitivity reactions including infusion-related reactions and anaphylactic reactions have been reported. Drug-drug interactions are not expected.

Based on animal data, ibalizumab may cause reversible immunosuppression (CD4+ T cell and B cell lymphocytopenia) in infants born to mothers exposed to ibalizumab during pregnancy; caution is advised.

GP120 ATTACHMENT INHIBITORS

Fostemsavir

Fostemsavir, a first-in-class attachment inhibitor, is a prodrug that is converted to the active metabolite temsavir. Temsavir binds directly to the HIV-1 envelope glycoprotein gp120 and prevents viral attachment and subsequent entry of virus into host T cells. Fostemsavir is indicated for the treatment of HIV-1 infection in heavily treatment-experienced adults with multidrug-resistant HIV-1 infection, in combination with other antiretroviral(s). It is active regardless of viral tropism, and there is no cross-resistance to other antiretroviral agents.

Following oral administration, fostemsavir levels were not detectable in plasma; increases in temsavir exposure were dose-proportional and not dependent on food. The drug is 88% protein-bound. The metabolic pathways of elimination are hydrolysis and oxidation (CYP3A4); half-life is 11 hours.

Potential adverse reactions include nausea, liver enzyme elevations in patients with hepatitis B or C infection, and QT prolongation. Autoimmune disorders also have been reported.

Temsavir is a substrate of CYP3A, esterases, P-gp, and BCRP as well as an inhibitor of OATP1B1 and OATP1B3. Co-administration with strong CYP3A inducers may cause significant decreases in temsavir plasma concentrations and are contraindicated: carbamazepine, phenytoin, rifabutin, St. John's wort as well as enzalutamide and mitotane. Temsavir may increase plasma concentrations of grazoprevir or voxilaprevir to a clinically relevant extent due to OATP1B1/3 inhibition and may also increase the concentrations of ethinyl estradiol when co-administered with oral contraceptives and/or statin agents.

CAPSID INHIBITORS

Lenacapavir is a long-acting first-in-class capsid inhibitor for people with multidrug-resistant HIV infection; treatment is initiated orally and then subcutaneously every 6 months. Following oral administration, absolute bioavailability is low (6–10%), T_{max} is ~4 hours, and median half-life is 10–12 days. Following subcutaneous administration, lenacapavir is slowly released but completely absorbed, with peak plasma concentrations occurring at 84 days post-dose and median half-life 8–12 weeks.

The most common adverse reactions are injection site reactions and nausea.

Lenacapavir is a moderate CYP3A inhibitor; concomitant administration is contraindicated with strong CYP3A inducers, since they may decrease plasma concentrations of lenacapavir. Since residual concentrations of lenacapavir may remain in the systemic circulation of patients for up to 12 months or longer, increased exposure and potential adverse reactions may persist.

There is no known cross-resistance to other existing drug classes.

EXPERIMENTAL AGENTS

Islatravir is a first-in-class oral nucleoside reverse transcriptase translocation inhibitor with multiple mechanisms of action that is being investigated for both HIV prevention and treatment. **Albuvirtide** is a novel fusion inhibitor that binds to the gp41 envelope protein; it is administered subcutaneously once weekly.

■ ANTIHEPATITIS AGENTS

The development of effective nucleoside/nucleotide analogs for the treatment of hepatitis has greatly diminished the use of interferon therapy, due to fewer adverse effects and once-daily oral administration. Although interferon agents have no known resistance, they must be administered by injection, are costlier than oral agents, and have multiple potential adverse effects. Additionally, a number of relative and absolute contraindications to the use of interferon exist, including the presence of decompensated cirrhosis and hypersplenism, thyroid disease, autoimmune diseases, severe coronary artery disease, renal transplant disease, pregnancy, seizures, psychiatric illness, concomitant use of certain drugs, retinopathy, thrombocytopenia, and leukopenia. The interferons cannot be used in infants less than 1 year old and in pregnant women.

INTERFERON ALFA

Interferons are host cytokines that exert complex antiviral, immunomodulatory, and antiproliferative actions (see Chapter 55). Interferon alfa appears to function by induction of intracellular signals following binding to specific cell membrane receptors, resulting in inhibition of viral penetration, translation, transcription, protein processing, maturation, and release, as well as increased host expression of major histocompatibility complex antigens, enhanced phagocytic activity of macrophages, and augmentation of the proliferation and survival of cytotoxic T cells.

Pegylation (the attachment of polyethylene glycol to a protein) reduces the rate of absorption following subcutaneous injection, reduces renal and cellular clearance, and decreases the immunogenicity of the protein, resulting in a longer half-life, steadier plasma concentrations, and the ability to administer injections once weekly. Therefore, pegylated interferons have replaced standard interferon for the treatment of patients with hepatitis. Renal elimination of pegylated interferon alfa-2a accounts for about 30% of clearance; dose must be adjusted in renal insufficiency due to impaired clearance. The polyethylene glycol moiety is a nontoxic polymer that is readily excreted in the urine.

Pegylated interferon alfa-2a is licensed to treat chronic HBV and HCV infection. However, the availability of newer and highly effective antiviral agents for HCV infection has greatly diminished the use of the interferons for this indication.

The adverse effects of interferon alfa include a flu-like syndrome (ie, headache, fevers, chills, myalgias, and malaise) that occurs within 6 hours after dosing in more than 30% of patients; it tends to resolve upon continued administration. Transient hepatic enzyme elevations to at least twofold at baseline occur in 30–50% of patients, presumably due to immune-mediated lysis of infected hepatocytes; this may be transient and appears to be more common in responders. Potential adverse effects during chronic therapy include neurotoxicities (mood disorders, depression, somnolence, confusion, seizures), myelosuppression, profound fatigue, weight loss, rash, cough, myalgia, alopecia, tinnitus, reversible hearing loss, retinopathy, pneumonitis, and possibly cardiotoxicity. Induction of autoantibodies may occur, causing exacerbation or unmasking of autoimmune disease (particularly thyroiditis). Pegylated interferon alfa-2b has been associated with uveitis.

Contraindications to interferon alfa therapy include decompensated liver disease, compensated cirrhosis, autoimmune disease, and history of cardiac arrhythmia. Caution is advised in the setting of psychiatric disease, epilepsy, thyroid disease, ischemic cardiac disease, severe renal insufficiency, and cytopenia. Alfa interferons are abortifacient in primates and should not be administered in pregnancy. Potential drug-drug interactions include increased theophylline and methadone levels. Co-administration with zidovudine may exacerbate cytopenias.

TREATMENT OF HEPATITIS B VIRUS INFECTION

No specific treatment is available for the treatment of acute hepatitis B infection, which is most often treated supportively.

The decision to treat patients with chronic HBV is based on a number of factors, including the presence or absence of cirrhosis, the serum aminotransferase level, HBV DNA level, HBe antigen positivity, and comorbidities such as malignancy, HCV or HIV co-infection, and pregnancy.

The goals of chronic HBV therapy are the suppression of HBV DNA to undetectable levels, seroconversion of HBeAg (or more rarely, HBsAg) from positive to negative, and reduction in elevated serum aminotransferase levels. These endpoints are correlated with improvement in necroinflammatory disease, a decreased risk of cirrhosis and hepatocellular carcinoma, and a decreased need for liver transplantation. All of the currently licensed therapies achieve these goals. In contrast to the treatment of HCV infection (see below), cure is rare. In addition, because current therapies suppress HBV replication without eradicating the virus, initial responses may not be durable. The covalently closed circular (ccc) viral DNA exists in stable form indefinitely within the cell, serving as a reservoir for HBV throughout the life of the cell and resulting in the capacity to reactivate. Relapse is more common in patients co-infected with hepatitis D virus.

As of 2022, five oral nucleoside/nucleotide analogs (lamivudine, adefovir dipivoxil, tenofovir disoproxil, tenofovir alafenamide, entecavir) and two injectable interferon drugs (interferon alfa-2b, pegylated interferon alfa-2a) are licensed for the treatment of patients with chronic HBV infection (Table 49–5). Telbivudine has been discontinued by the manufacturer and is omitted from this chapter. Combination therapies may reduce the development of resistance. The optimal duration of therapy is variable, and is influenced by HBeAg status, duration of HBV DNA suppression, and presence of cirrhosis and/or decompensation.

TABLE 49–5 Nucleoside and nucleotide drugs used to treat chronic hepatitis B virus infection.

Agent	Recommended Adult Dosage	Potential Adverse Effects
Preferred		
Entecavir[1]	500 or 1000 mg qd orally	Headache, fatigue, upper abdominal pain, lactic acidosis
Tenofovir alafenamide fumarate	25 mg qd orally	Nausea, abdominal pain, diarrhea, dizziness, fatigue, nephropathy, lactic acidosis
Tenofovir disoproxil[1]	300 mg qd orally	Nausea, abdominal pain, diarrhea, nephropathy, Fanconi syndrome, osteomalacia, lactic acidosis
Non-preferred		
Adefovir dipivoxil[1]	10 mg qd orally	Renal dysfunction, Fanconi syndrome, lactic acidosis
Lamivudine[1]	100 mg qd orally	Headache, nausea, diarrhea, dizziness, myalgia, pancreatitis, lactic acidosis

[1]Dose must be reduced in patients with renal insufficiency.

Several anti-HBV agents have anti-HIV activity as well, including tenofovir disoproxil, tenofovir alafenamide, lamivudine, and adefovir dipivoxil. Although agents with dual HBV and HIV activity are particularly useful as part of a first-line regimen in co-infected patients, it is important to note that acute exacerbation of hepatitis may occur upon discontinuation or interruption of these agents; this may be severe or even fatal.

Advantages of interferon treatment for patients with chronic HBV infection include a finite treatment duration, higher rates of HBsAg and HBeAg seroconversion compared with the same duration of nucleoside/nucleotide treatment, and lack of drug resistance. However, the disadvantage is a greater incidence of adverse effects. Assessment of off-treatment response is important with interferon treatment, since loss of HBeAg and HBsAg, as well as seroconversion to hepatitis B e antibody and hepatitis B surface antibody negativity, may be delayed.

ADEFOVIR DIPIVOXIL

Although initially and abortively developed for treatment of HIV infection, adefovir dipivoxil gained approval, at lower and less toxic doses, for treatment of HBV infection. Adefovir dipivoxil is the diester prodrug of adefovir, an acyclic phosphonated adenine nucleotide analog. It is phosphorylated by cellular kinases to the active diphosphate metabolite and then competitively inhibits HBV DNA polymerase to cause chain termination after incorporation into viral DNA. Adefovir is active in vitro against a wide range of DNA and RNA viruses, including HBV, HIV, and herpesviruses.

Oral bioavailability of adefovir dipivoxil is ~59% and is unaffected by meals; it is rapidly and completely hydrolyzed to the parent compound by intestinal and blood esterases. Protein binding is low (<5%). The intracellular half-life of the diphosphate ranges from 5 to 18 hours in various cells; this makes once-daily dosing feasible. Adefovir is excreted by both glomerular filtration and active tubular secretion and requires dose adjustment for renal dysfunction; however, it may be administered to patients with decompensated liver disease.

Of the oral agents, adefovir may be slower to suppress HBV DNA levels and least likely to induce HBeAg seroconversion. Emergence of resistance is up to 29% after 5 years of use. Since there is no cross-resistance between adefovir and either lamivudine or entecavir, adefovir treatment is particularly useful in patients with HBV that is resistant to these agents. However, tenofovir may also be used in this setting, and it is more potent and effective as monotherapy.

Adefovir is well tolerated at doses used to treat HBV infection. A reversible increase in serum creatinine has been reported in 3–9% of patients after 4–5 years of treatment. Other potential adverse effects are headache, diarrhea, asthenia, and abdominal pain. As with other NRTI agents, lactic acidosis and hepatic steatosis are a risk owing to mitochondrial dysfunction. Pivalic acid, a by-product of adefovir metabolism, can esterify free carnitine and result in decreased carnitine levels. However, it is not necessary to administer carnitine supplementation with the low doses used to treat patients with HBV (10 mg/d). Adefovir is embryotoxic in rats at high doses and is genotoxic in preclinical studies.

ENTECAVIR

Entecavir is an orally administered cyclopentyl guanosine nucleoside analog that competitively inhibits all three functions of HBV DNA polymerase, including base priming, reverse transcription of the negative strand, and synthesis of the positive strand of HBV DNA. Oral bioavailability approaches 100% but is decreased by food; therefore, entecavir should be taken on an empty stomach. The intracellular half-life of the active phosphorylated compound is 15 hours and plasma half-life is prolonged at 128–149 hours, allowing once-daily dosing. It is excreted by the kidney, undergoing both glomerular filtration and net tubular secretion, and dosage should be adjusted in the setting of renal insufficiency.

Suppression of HBV DNA levels was greater with entecavir than with lamivudine or adefovir in comparative trials. Entecavir appears to have a higher barrier to the emergence of resistance than lamivudine. Although selection of resistant isolates with the S202G mutation has been documented during therapy, clinical resistance is rare (<1% at 5 years). However, resistance is more frequent in lamivudine-refractory patients (~50% at 5 years). Entecavir has weak anti-HIV activity and can induce development of the M184V variant in HBV/HIV co-infected patients, resulting in resistance to emtricitabine and lamivudine.

Entecavir is well tolerated. Potential adverse events are headache, fatigue, dizziness, nausea, cough, and upper abdominal pain. Co-administration of entecavir with drugs that reduce renal function or compete for active tubular secretion may increase serum concentrations of either entecavir or the co-administered drug. Severe lactic acidosis was reported in a case series of entecavir; thus, caution is advised in the setting of severe hepatic decompensation. Lung adenomas and hepatocellular carcinomas in mice as well as brain gliomas in rats have been observed at varying exposures, although there has not been evidence of an increased incidence of malignancy in patients on entecavir followed for up to 10 years.

LAMIVUDINE

The pharmacokinetics of lamivudine, which also has antiretroviral activity, are described earlier in this chapter (see Nucleoside and Nucleotide Reverse Transcriptase Inhibitors). The more prolonged intracellular half-life in HBV-infected cell lines (17–19 hours) than in HIV-infected cell lines (10.5–15.5 hours) allows for lower doses and less frequent administration. Dose reduction is required for renal insufficiency, but lamivudine can be safely administered to patients with decompensated liver disease. Prolonged treatment has been shown to decrease clinical progression of HBV, as well as development of hepatocellular cancer by approximately 50%. Also, lamivudine has been effective in preventing vertical transmission of HBV from mother to newborn when given in the last 4 weeks of gestation.

Lamivudine inhibits HBV DNA polymerase and HIV reverse transcriptase by competing with deoxycytidine triphosphate for incorporation into the viral DNA, resulting in chain termination. Although lamivudine results in rapid and potent virus suppression, chronic therapy is limited by the emergence of lamivudine-resistant HBV isolates (L180M or M204I/V), estimated to occur in 15–30% of patients at 1 year and in up to 65% after 5 years of therapy. Resistance has been associated with flares of hepatitis and progressive liver disease. Cross-resistance between lamivudine and emtricitabine or entecavir may occur; however, adefovir and tenofovir maintain activity against lamivudine-resistant strains of HBV.

In the doses used for HBV infection, lamivudine has an excellent safety profile. Headache, nausea, diarrhea, dizziness, myalgia, and malaise are rare. Co-infection with HIV may increase the risk of pancreatitis.

TENOFOVIR DISOPROXIL & TENOFOVIR ALAFENAMIDE

Tenofovir, a nucleotide analog of adenosine in use as an antiretroviral agent, has potent activity against HBV. The characteristics of tenofovir disoproxil and tenofovir alafenamide are described earlier in this chapter (see Nucleoside & Nucleotide Reverse Transcriptase Inhibitors). Tenofovir maintains activity against lamivudine- and entecavir-resistant hepatitis virus isolates. Comparative trials show a higher rate of virologic response and histologic improvement with tenofovir than with adefovir, as well as a lower rate of emergence of resistance in patients with chronic HBV infection. Resistance to tenofovir has not been documented in clinical trials, even among patients who have been treated with tenofovir for up to 8 years. However, efficacy is lower in patients who have resistance to adefovir and double mutations (A181T/V and N236T).

Tenofovir alafenamide is more stable than tenofovir disoproxil in plasma and delivers the active metabolite to hepatocytes more efficiently, allowing a lower dose to be used with similar antiviral activity and less systemic exposure (see Table 49-5).

The most common adverse effects of tenofovir in patients with HBV infection are nausea, abdominal pain, diarrhea, dizziness, and fatigue. Proximal tubulopathy with ensuing renal insufficiency as well as decreased bone mineral density are potential side effects of tenofovir therapy. In comparative trials, tenofovir alafenamide was associated with less renal and bone toxicity compared with tenofovir disoproxil.

EXPERIMENTAL AGENTS

The subcutaneously delivered lipopeptide **bulevirtide** (formerly known as myrcludex B) is being evaluated for treatment of hepatitis D. Bulevirtide is a peptide derived from the hepatitis B surface antigen. **Lonafarnib** is an oral inhibitor of farnesyl transferase that is also under evaluation for the treatment of hepatitis D, either as monotherapy or in combination with interferon-alfa or ritonavir. **Bepirovirsen**, an antisense oligonucleotide that targets all HBV mRNAs and acts to decrease levels of viral proteins, is under evaluation in patients with chronic HBV infection.

TREATMENT OF HEPATITIS C INFECTION

In contrast to the treatment of patients with chronic HBV infection, the primary goal of treatment in patients with HCV infection is viral eradication. In clinical trials, the primary efficacy endpoint is typically achievement of sustained viral response (SVR), defined as the absence of detectable viremia 12 weeks after completion of therapy. SVR is associated with improvement in liver histology, reduction in risk of end-stage liver disease and hepatocellular carcinoma, and, occasionally, with regression of cirrhosis. Additionally, SVR is associated with a 97–100% chance of being HCV RNA negative during long-term follow-up and is therefore considered a cure.

In acute hepatitis C, the rate of clearance of the virus without therapy is estimated at 20–35%. Therefore, most practitioners choose to delay therapy for a minimum of 6 months after the initial infection. If treatment is initiated thereafter due to persistent HCV RNA viremia, the regimens are the same as those administered for chronic HCV infection.

The advent of the first-generation direct-acting antiviral agents (DAAs) boceprevir and telaprevir dramatically altered the landscape for the optimal treatment of chronic HCV infection. Until 2011, a combination of pegylated interferon and ribavirin was the standard treatment for patients with HCV. As noted above, interferon has multiple potential side effects and must be administered parenterally; additionally, ribavirin has its own set of potential adverse effects and drug-drug interactions. Therefore, they have effectively been replaced by combination regimens of oral DAAs (see Table 49–6). The first-generation HCV protease inhibitors (ie, boceprevir, telaprevir) have been replaced by newer DAAs over the past several years, with improved efficacy and tolerability, improved dosing schedules, lesser genotype specificity, and fewer potential drug-drug interactions. Boceprevir, daclatasvir, dasabuvir, ombitasvir, paritaprevir, simeprevir, and telaprevir have been discontinued by the manufacturer and are omitted from this chapter.

There are four current classes of DAAs, which are defined by their mechanism of action and therapeutic target: nonstructural protein (NS)5A inhibitors, NS5B nucleoside polymerase inhibitors, NS5B non-nucleoside polymerase inhibitors (none available currently), and NS 3/4A protease inhibitors. The main targets of the DAAs are the HCV-encoded proteins that are vital to the replication of the virus (see Figure 49–1).

The safety profiles of all the combination regimens (see Table 49–6) are generally excellent, with adverse events of mild severity and very low rates of discontinuation in the absence of concurrent ribavirin use. All patients should be tested for current or prior HBV infection prior to the initiation of DAAs for HCV, since HBV reactivation has been reported in HCV/HBV co-infected patients during DAA therapy. Some cases have resulted in fulminant hepatitis, hepatic failure, and death.

The choice of treatment regimen is determined by several factors, including HCV genotype (see Table 49–6), HIV and/or HBV co-infection, the presence of renal insufficiency, treatment history, and the presence of cirrhosis.

TABLE 49–6 Direct-acting antiviral combination regimens for the treatment of chronic hepatitis C infection in adult patients without cirrhosis.[1]

Regimen	Class of Agent(s)	HCV Genotype(s)
Elbasvir 50 mg/grazoprevir 100 mg once daily[2,3]	NS5A inhibitor/NS 3/4 A protease inhibitor	1a, 1b, 4
Ledipasvir 90 mg/sofosbuvir 400 mg once daily	NS5A inhibitor/NS5B polymerase inhibitor	1a, 1b, 4, 5, 6
Sofosbuvir 400 mg once daily plus weight-based ribavirin	NS5B polymerase inhibitor plus guanosine analog	2, 3
Glecaprevir 300 mg/pibrentasvir 120 mg once daily	NS 3/4 A protease inhibitor/NS5A inhibitor	1a, 1b, 2, 3, 4, 5, 6
Velpatasvir 100 mg/sofosbuvir 400 mg once daily[3]	NS5A inhibitor/NS5B polymerase inhibitor	1a, 1b, 2, 3, 4, 5, 6
Voxilaprevir 100 mg/sofosbuvir 400 mg/velpatasvir 100 mg once daily	NS 3/4 A protease inhibitor/NS5B polymerase inhibitor/ NS5A inhibitor	1, 2, 3, 4, 5, 6

[1]Regimens may differ in the presence of cirrhosis.

[2]As an alternative regimen, elbasvir 50 mg/grazoprevir 100 mg once daily may be given in combination with weight-based ribavirin for 16 weeks.

[3]Dose adjustment may be required if co-administered with a CYP3A substrate.

NS5A INHIBITORS

The NS5A protein plays a role in both viral replication and the assembly of HCV; however, the exact mechanism of action of the HCV NS5A replication complex inhibitors remains unclear.

The presence of baseline NS5A resistance-associated variants (RAVs) significantly reduces rates of SVR at 12 weeks; they have perhaps the greatest impact on treatment response in patients with genotype 1a or 3 infections. Since 10–15% of patients without prior exposure will have NS5A RAVs, baseline testing should be considered prior initiation of therapy.

Elbasvir

Elbasvir is only available as a fixed-dose combination with grazoprevir, recommended for treatment of HCV genotypes 1a, 1b, and 4 (see Table 49–6).

Absorption is not food-dependent. Peak concentrations after ingestion occur at a median of 3 hours. Elbasvir is extensively bound to plasma proteins (>99.9%), partially eliminated by oxidative metabolism, and primarily excreted in the feces. Elbasvir/grazoprevir should not be administered to patients with moderate or severe hepatic impairment or in conjunction with organic anion transporting polypeptides 1B1/3 (OATP1B1/3) inhibitors or strong inducers or inhibitors of CYP3A. Elbasvir/grazoprevir should not be co-administered with cobicistat, efavirenz, etravirine, or any of the HIV protease inhibitors.

The most common side effects during therapy with elbasvir/grazoprevir are fatigue, headache, nausea, and elevations in serum aminotransferases.

Ledipasvir

Ledipasvir was the first NS5A inhibitor to be available in the United States. It is available in a fixed-dose combination with sofosbuvir for the treatment of HCV genotype 1a, 1b, 4, 5, and 6 (Table 49–6).

Ledipasvir is not affected by food intake. Concurrent antacids may decrease absorption of ledipasvir. Median peak plasma concentrations occur 4–4.5 hours after oral administration of ledipasvir/sofosbuvir. It is highly bound (>99.8%) to plasma proteins; unchanged ledipasvir is the major species present in feces. The median terminal half-life of ledipasvir following administration of ledipasvir/sofosbuvir is 47 hours. No dose adjustment is required in the setting of mild or moderate renal insufficiency or mild, moderate or severe hepatic insufficiency. The dose in patients with severe renal insufficiency has not yet been determined.

The most common adverse reactions in patients receiving ledipasvir/sofosbuvir are fatigue, headache, nausea, and insomnia. Serious symptomatic bradycardia has been reported in patients receiving ledipasvir in combination with sofosbuvir and amiodarone.

Ledipasvir is an inhibitor of the drug transporters P-gp and BCRP and may increase intestinal absorption of co-administered substrates for these transporters. Additionally, co-administration of P-gp inducers (e.g., rifampin or St. John's wort) with ledipasvir/sofosbuvir may decrease plasma concentrations of both of these agents.

Renal function should be monitored in patients receiving ledipasvir/sofosbuvir in combination with tenofovir disoproxil; this combination should be avoided in patients with creatinine clearance <60 mL/min.

Pibrentasvir

Pibrentasvir is available only in a fixed-dose combination table with glecaprevir, an NS3/4a protease inhibitor, given once daily. The two antivirals have synergistic activity in vitro with a high barrier to resistance and potent activity against common polymorphisms. Both components are pangenotypic (Table 49–6). It is not recommended in patients with moderate hepatic impairment and is contraindicated in patients with severe hepatic impairment. The major route of excretion is biliary; renal excretion is negligible.

The most common adverse reactions are headache, fatigue, and nausea.

Glecaprevir and pibrentasvir are inhibitors of P-gp, BCRP, OATP 1B1/3, UGT1A1, CYP3A, and CYP1A2. Therefore, there is substantial potential for drug-drug interactions. Concurrent use of atazanavir or rifampin is contraindicated. Carbamazepine, efavirenz, and St. John's wort may significantly decrease plasma concentrations of glecaprevir and pibrentasvir; conversely their concentrations may increase when co-administered with darunavir, lopinavir, ritonavir, or cyclosporine. Serum levels of digoxin, dabigatran, and the statin agents may increase when co-administered with glecaprevir/pibrentasvir.

Velpatasvir

Velpatasvir is available only in a fixed-dose combination with the NS5B polymerase inhibitor sofosbuvir. It is the first once-daily single-tablet regimen with pangenotypic activity (Table 49–6). No dose adjustment is required for patients with mild or moderate renal insufficiency, or any degree of hepatic impairment. Sofosbuvir exposure is increased in patients with severe renal impairment, including those on dialysis.

Velpatasvir is administered without regard to food; peak plasma concentrations are observed at 3 hours post-dose. Since increased gastric pH levels decrease velpatasvir absorption, co-administration with proton pump inhibitors is contraindicated. Velpatasvir is >99% bound to plasma proteins. Its median terminal half-life is 15 hours.

The most common adverse events in patients receiving velpatasvir/sofosbuvir are headache, fatigue, nausea, asthenia, and insomnia.

Velpatasvir is metabolized by CYP2B6 CYP2C8, and CYP3A4. Velpatasvir and sofosbuvir are substrates of P-gp and BCRP; velpatasvir is also transported by OATP1B1 and OATP1B3. Inducers of P-gp and/or moderate or potent inducers of CYP2B6, CYP2C8, or CYP3A4 (eg, rifampin, St. John's wort, carbamazepine) may decrease plasma concentrations of velpatasvir and/or sofosbuvir; co-administration with drugs that inhibit P-gp and/or BCRP may increase velpatasvir and/or sofosbuvir concentrations and drugs that inhibit CYP2B6, CYP2C8, or CYP3A4 may increase plasma concentration of velpatasvir. Therefore, co-administration with rifampin, rifabutin, phenytoin, carbamazepine, and efavirenz is contraindicated. Renal function should be monitored in patients receiving velpatasvir-containing regimens concurrently with tenofovir disoproxil due to increased serum concentrations of the latter agent; this combination should be avoided in patients with creatinine clearance <60 mL/min.

Virologic failure has been associated with emergence of the Y93N/H mutation in the NS5A gene in genotypes 1 and 3 virus. Therefore, baseline testing for NS5a RAS is recommended in patients with genotype 3 and cirrhosis; if Y93H RAS is present, a different regimen should be chosen.

NS5B RNA POLYMERASE INHIBITORS

NS5B is an RNA-dependent RNA polymerase involved in post-translational processing that is necessary for replication of HCV. The enzyme has a catalytic site for nucleoside binding and at least four other sites at which a non-nucleoside compound can bind and cause allosteric alteration. The enzyme's structure is highly conserved across all HCV genotypes, giving agents that inhibit NS5B efficacy against all six genotypes.

Sofosbuvir

The nucleotide analog sofosbuvir is administered in combination with several other anti-HCV medications, including velpatasvir, ledipasvir, peginterferon-alfa plus ribavirin, or ribavirin alone. It is also available in a fixed-dose combination with ledipasvir for treatment of HCV genotypes 1, 4, 5, and 6 (Table 49–6).

Sofosbuvir is a prodrug that is rapidly converted after ingestion to GS-331007, which is efficiently taken up by hepatocytes and converted by cellular kinase to its pharmacologically active uridine analog 5'-triphosphate form GS-461203. The triphosphate is incorporated by the HCV RNA polymerase into the elongating RNA primer strand, resulting in chain termination.

Sofosbuvir is administered without regard to food; peak plasma concentrations are observed at 0.5–1 hours post-dose. It is 61–65% bound to plasma proteins and is metabolized in the liver. Renal clearance is the major elimination pathway for GS-331007. The median terminal half-lives of sofosbuvir and GS-331007 are 0.4 and 27 hours, respectively. No dose adjustment is required for patients with mild or moderate renal insufficiency, or any degree of hepatic impairment. Sofosbuvir exposure is increased in patients with severe renal impairment, including those on dialysis.

Sofosbuvir is generally well tolerated. Drug-specific adverse effects are difficult to discern since it is always administered with other antiviral agents. In patients receiving sofosbuvir with ledipasvir, the most commonly reported adverse effects were fatigue, headache, and asthenia. Rare cases of symptomatic bradycardia have been reported patients taking sofosbuvir and amiodarone in combination with another DAAs, particularly in patients also receiving beta blockers, or in those with underlying cardiac comorbidities and/or advanced liver disease. There have been reports of severe cutaneous reactions in patients receiving sofosbuvir-containing regimens.

Sofosbuvir is a substrate of drug transporter P-gp; therefore, potent P-gp inducers in the intestine may decrease sofosbuvir concentrations and should not be co-administered. Sofosbuvir/velpatasvir should not be used with efavirenz, etravirine, or ritonavir-boosted atazanavir. Renal function should be monitored in patients receiving concurrent sofosbuvir/velpatasvir with tenofovir disoproxil; this combination should be avoided in patients with creatinine clearance <60 mL/min.

NS3/4A PROTEASE INHIBITORS

NS3/4A protease inhibitors are inhibitors of the NS3/4A serine protease, an enzyme involved in post-translational processing and replication of HCV (Figure 49–4).

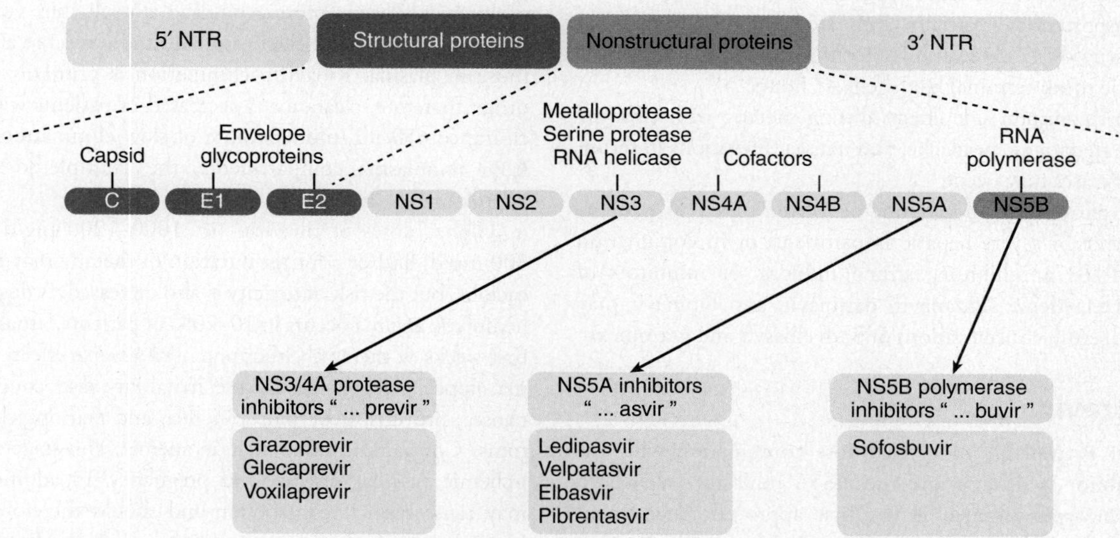

FIGURE 49–4 HCV genome and potential targets of drug action. C, E1, E2, etc, protein products of specific genes; Nucs, nucleoside inhibitors; Non-Nucs, nonnucleoside inhibitors. (Adapted with permission from Asselah T, Marcellin P: Direct-acting antivirals for the treatment of chronic hepatitis C: One pill a day for tomorrow. Liver Int. 2012;32 Suppl 1:88–102.)

Glecaprevir

Glecaprevir is available only in a fixed-dose combination table with pibrentasvir, an NS5A inhibitor, for the treatment of HCV genotypes 1a, 1b, 2, 3, 4, 5, and 6 (Table 49–6). It is not recommended in patients with moderate hepatic impairment and is contraindicated in patients with severe hepatic impairment. The major route of excretion is biliary.

The most common adverse reactions are headache, fatigue, and nausea.

Glecaprevir and pibrentasvir are inhibitors of P-gp, BCRP, OATP 1B1/3, UGT1A1, CYP3A, and CYP1A2. Therefore, there are substantial potential for drug-drug interactions. Concurrent use of atazanavir or rifampin is contraindicated. Carbamazepine, efavirenz, and St. John's wort may significantly decrease plasma concentrations of glecaprevir and pibrentasvir; conversely their concentrations may increase when co-administered with darunavir, lopinavir, ritonavir, or cyclosporine. Serum levels of digoxin, dabigatran, and the statin agents may increase when co-administered with glecaprevir/pibrentasvir.

Grazoprevir

Grazoprevir is a potent protease inhibitor, reversibly binding to HCV NS3/4A protease. It is distinct from earlier-generation protease inhibitors due to its pangenotypic activity, as well as activity against some of the major resistance-associated variants (R155K and D168Y) that resulted in failure with first-generation protease inhibitors. It is only available in combination with elbasvir for treatment of HCV genotypes 1 and 4 (Table 49–6).

Grazoprevir can be taken without regard to food. Oral exposures are ~2-fold greater in HCV-infected subjects than in healthy subjects. Peak plasma concentrations are reached at a median of 2 hours after ingestion. Grazoprevir is extensively bound to plasma proteins (98.8%) and distributes predominantly to the liver, likely facilitated by active transport through the OATP1B1/3 liver uptake transporter. It is partially eliminated by oxidative metabolism, primarily by CYP3A, and is mostly eliminated in the feces. Its geometric mean terminal half-life is 31 hours.

The most common side effects during therapy with elbasvir/grazoprevir are fatigue, headache, and nausea. Elevations in serum aminotransferases may occur.

Elbasvir/grazoprevir should not be administered to patients with moderate or severe hepatic impairment, or in conjunction with OATP1B1/3 inhibitors, strong inducers or inhibitors of CYP3A, or efavirenz. Atazanavir, darunavir, and lopinavir may increase the serum concentrations of both elbasvir and grazoprevir.

Voxilaprevir

Voxilaprevir is available in a fixed-dose combination with the NS5B inhibitor sofosbuvir and the NS5A inhibitor velpatasvir. This pangenotypic regimen is the first approved re-treatment option for patients that have previously received, and failed, a regimen containing an NS5A inhibitor for treatment of chronic HCV infection or for patients with genotypes 1a or 3 infection that have previously been treated with an HCV regimen containing sofosbuvir without an NS5A inhibitor. However, it is not to be used in treatment-experienced patients who have moderate or severe liver disease or cirrhosis.

The combination is generally well tolerated; the most common adverse effects are headache, fatigue, diarrhea, and nausea.

When administered in combination with sofosbuvir and velpatasvir, Cmax of voxilaprevir is reached in 4 hours. It is >99% protein-bound and is primarily eliminated by biliary excretion; half-life is 33 hours. Voxilaprevir is primarily metabolized by CYP3A4 and to a lesser extent by CYP2C8 and CYP1A, such that the potential for drug-drug interactions is large. Serious symptomatic bradycardia has been reported in patients receiving voxilaprevir/sofosbuvir/velpatasvir and amiodarone. Concurrent use with P-gp inducers and/or moderate to potent inducers of CYP2B6, CYP2C8 or CYP3A4 (eg, St. John's wort, carbamazepine) is contraindicated due to the potential for lowered serum levels of sofosbuvir, velpatasvir, and/or voxilaprevir. Also contraindicated are concurrent phenytoin, phenobarbital, oxcarbazepine, rifampin, rifabutin, rifapentine, atazanavir, lopinavir, efavirenz, rosuvastatin, pitavastatin, and cyclosporine.

RIBAVIRIN

Ribavirin is a guanosine analog that is phosphorylated intracellularly by host cell enzymes. Although its mechanism of action has not been fully elucidated, it appears to interfere with the synthesis of guanosine triphosphate, to inhibit capping of viral messenger RNA, and to inhibit the viral RNA–dependent polymerase of certain viruses. Ribavirin triphosphate inhibits the replication of a wide range of DNA and RNA viruses, including influenza A and B, parainfluenza, respiratory syncytial virus, paramyxoviruses, HCV, and HIV-1.

The absolute oral bioavailability of ribavirin is 45–64%, increases with high-fat meals, and decreases with co-administration of antacids. Plasma protein binding is negligible, volume of distribution is large, and cerebrospinal fluid levels are about 70% of those in plasma. Ribavirin elimination is primarily through the urine; therefore, clearance is decreased in patients with creatinine clearance <50 mL/min. Because of slow elimination of ribavirin from nonplasma compartments, the multiple-dose half-life is approximately 298 hours.

Higher doses of ribavirin (ie, 1000–1200 mg/d rather than 800 mg/d) and/or a longer duration of therapy may be more efficacious, but the risk of toxicity is also increased. A dose-dependent hemolytic anemia occurs in 10–20% of patients, usually within the first weeks of therapy. Other potential adverse effects are leukopenia, alopecia, depression, fatigue, irritability, rash, cough, insomnia, nausea, pruritus, hyperbilirubinemia, and neuropsychiatric symptoms. Contraindications include anemia, end-stage renal failure, ischemic vascular disease, and pregnancy. In addition, ribavirin may cause bronchoconstriction and should therefore be avoided in patients with chronic obstructive pulmonary disease. Ribavirin is teratogenic and embryotoxic in animals as well as mutagenic in mammalian cells. Therefore, two effective forms of contraception should be used by both sexual partners during treatment.

Female patients who receive ribavirin should avoid pregnancy for 9 months after completion of treatment, and female partners of men who receive ribavirin should avoid pregnancy for 6 months.

The co-administration of ribavirin with azathioprine or zidovudine may result in additive myelotoxicity.

EXPERIMENTAL AGENTS

Ravidasvir is an investigational NS5A inhibitor in clinical trials for the treatment of patients with chronic HCV genotype 4.

■ AGENTS TO TREAT COVID-19

The antiviral agents nirmatrelvir/ritonavir, molnupiravir, and remdesivir have all been shown to reduce the risk of hospitalization when given early in the course of COVID-19. Nirmatrelvir/ritonavir is approved, and molnupiravir has Emergency Use Authorization, in nonhospitalized patients with mild to moderate COVID-19 infection who are at high risk of developing severe disease. However, nirmatrelvir/ritonavir has been found to be substantially more effective against hospitalization and death than molnupiravir. Remdesivir has FDA approval for treatment of COVID-19 in hospitalized patients and in nonhospitalized patients with mild-to-moderate illness who are at high risk for progression to severe disease or death.

Several immune modulators have also gained approval for treatment of COVID-19, including anakinra, baricitinib, tocilizumab, and vilobelimab (see below). Most have been previously approved for treatment of rheumatoid arthritis and other hyperinflammatory states.

NIRMATRELVIR

Nirmatrelvir is an orally bioavailable protease inhibitor that is active against M^{PRO}, a viral protease that plays an essential role in viral replication by cleaving the two viral polyproteins. Since it is metabolized mainly by CYP3A4, co-administration with low-dose ritonavir, a protease inhibitor and strong CYP3A4 inhibitor, is required to increase nirmatrelvir concentrations to the target therapeutic range and prolong its half-life to 6 hours. The median time to maximum serum concentration of nirmatrelvir when administered with ritonavir is 3 hours. Steady state is achieved on day 2 with an approximately 2-fold accumulation.

Treatment with nirmatrelvir (300 mg)/ritonavir (100 mg) orally every 12 hours for 5 days in nonhospitalized unvaccinated adults with mild to moderate COVID-19 who were at high risk for progression resulted in a rate of COVID-related hospitalization or death at day 28 that was 89% lower than in patients treated with placebo, as well as a decreased viral load by day 5. Treatment should be initiated within 5 days of symptom onset or COVID-19 diagnosis. The major route of elimination is renal; the dose should be reduced in patients with moderate renal impairment (GFR ≥30 to <60 mL/min). Nirmatrelvir is not recommended in patients with severe renal or hepatic impairment.

Potential adverse events include elevated serum aminotransferases, dysgeusia, metallic taste, and diarrhea.

Since both nirmatrelvir and ritonavir are CYP3A substrates, there are multiple potential drug-drug interactions in treated patients. Nirmatrelvir/ritonavir is contraindicated in combination with drugs that are highly dependent on CYP3A for clearance (eg, alfuzosin, pethidine, propoxyphene, ranolazine, amiodarone, flecainide, propafenone, quinidine, colchicine, clozapine, pimozide, ergotamine, lovastatin, simvastatin, sildenafil, triazolam, midazolam, voriconazole, rivaroxaban, salmeterol) due to the potential for elevated serum concentrations, or with drugs that are potent CYP3A inducers (carbamazepine, phenobarbital, phenytoin, St. John's wort, rifampin), due to the potential for reduced serum concentrations. Moreover, there may be increased plasma concentrations of medications that are metabolized by CYP3A.

There have been recent reports of COVID-19 rebound occurring between 2 and 8 days after initial recovery in patients treated with nirmatrelvir/ritonavir; this is characterized by a recurrence of COVID-19 symptoms and/or a new positive viral test after having tested negative. The etiology is unclear.

MOLNUPIRAVIR

Molnupiravir is the oral prodrug of beta-D-N4-hydroxycytidine (NHC), a ribonucleoside that has broad antiviral activity against RNA viruses. NHC uptake in the triphosphate form by viral RNA-dependent RNA polymerases results in viral mutations and lethal mutagenesis of SARS-CoV-2.

Molnupiravir (800 mg) should be taken orally every 12 hours for 5 days, within 5 days of symptom onset or COVID-19 diagnosis. This regimen, in patients with mild to moderate COVID-19 who were at risk for progression, reduced the rate of hospitalization or death by 30% compared with placebo in the key clinical trial. No dosage adjustment is required in patients with renal or hepatic insufficiency. NHC is eliminated by metabolism to uridine and/or cytidine; elimination half-life is 3.3 hours.

The most common adverse reactions in patients treated with molnupiravir are diarrhea, nausea, and dizziness. No drug interactions have been identified. Due to developmental toxicities in animal studies, use during pregnancy or lactation is contraindicated; in addition, due to potential adverse effects on bone and cartilage growth, molnupiravir should not be used in patients less than 18 years of age.

REMDESIVIR

Remdesivir is an adenosine nucleotide prodrug that is phosphorylated into the triphosphate form by cellular kinases, competing with high selectivity over the natural ATP substrate for incorporation into nascent RNA chains by the SARS-CoV-2 RNA-dependent RNA polymerase, resulting in chain termination. Time to maximum serum concentration is 0.67 hours, and the parent drug is ~90% protein-bound. Elimination half-life is 1–1.3 hours.

Remdesivir is administered by IV infusion over 30–120 minutes, at a dose of 200 mg on day 1, followed by 100 mg once daily for a total of 3–10 days, in nonhospitalized patients with mild-to-moderate disease who are at high risk of progression or in hospitalized patients with COVID-19. A total of 3 days is administered to nonhospitalized patients; hospitalized patients receive at least 5 days of treatment with extension to 10 days in the absence of substantial improvement. Remdesivir is often co-administered with dexamethasone in hospitalized patients.

Although shortening of the time to clinical improvement and length of hospitalization appear to result in hospitalized patients with COVID-19 who are treated with remdesivir, no mortality benefit has been observed in trials to date. Moreover, the emergence of remdesivir resistance during treatment of an immunocompromised patient with COVID19 has been reported.

Potential adverse reactions include hypersensitivity reactions (including anaphylaxis), elevated serum aminotransferases, nausea, bradycardia, and hypotension.

Although remdesivir is a substrate for CYP3A4, OATP1B1, and P-gp transporters, no adjustment for potential drug-drug interactions is recommended. However, co-administration of remdesivir with chloroquine or hydroxychloroquine is contraindicated based on in vitro data demonstrating potential antagonism.

NEUTRALIZING MONOCLONAL ANTIBODIES

There are several monoclonal antibodies targeting the spike protein of SARS-CoV-2 that have gained approval in the USA for the treatment of patients with COVID-19. These agents require parenteral administration, have limited availability, and must be given early in the course of illness. There is an increased risk for serious infections and/or hypersensitivity reactions in patients with COVID-19 who are receiving these agents.

The activity of the available monoclonal antibodies against the subtypes of the Omicron variant of COVID-19 varies greatly. The use of tixagevimab/cilgavimab, sotrovimab, bamlanivimab, casirivimab/imdevimab and bebtelovimab has been discontinued due to lack of activity against certain SARS-CoV-2 Omicron variants.

Baricitinib, an oral Janus kinase (JAK) inhibitor, was the first immunomodulatory treatment for COVID-19 to receive FDA approval. Baricitinib is administered orally (4 mg/d for 14 days) in hospitalized patients with COVID-19 who require supplemental oxygen or mechanical ventilation. The dose must be modified in patients with renal insufficiency or severe hepatic insufficiency.

The absolute bioavailability of baricitinib is approximately 80%, and it is ~50% protein-bound. Renal elimination is the principal clearance mechanism for baricitinib through filtration and active secretion. The half-life is 10.8 hours.

Potential adverse effects include serious venous thrombosis, serious infection, and increased risk of cardiovascular events and malignancies. Other potential adverse effects include increased serum aminotransferases, neutropenia, thrombocytosis, and increased creatine kinase. Although CYP3A4 is the main metabolizing enzyme, few clinically significant drug-drug interactions have been identified. However, baricitinib exposure is increased when co-administered with strong OAT3 inhibitors (such as probenecid).

Tocilizumab, a recombinant humanized interleukin-6 receptor antagonist, is approved for the treatment of COVID-19 in hospitalized adults receiving systemic corticosteroids who require supplemental oxygen, mechanical ventilation, or extracorporeal membrane oxygenation. Tocilizumab is administered intravenously as a single dose (8 mg/kg); no dose adjustment is necessary for renal or hepatic impairment. Initiation in patients with neutropenia, thrombocytopenia, or serum aminotransferases elevated more than tenfold is contraindicated.

Potential adverse reactions include constipation, anxiety, diarrhea, insomnia, hypertension, nausea, neutropenia, thrombocytopenia, and elevated serum aminotransferases; gastrointestinal perforation has been reported in patients receiving tocilizumab for rheumatoid arthritis.

There is a potential for increased metabolism of drugs that are CYP450 substrates, causing decreased effectiveness when co-administered.

Anakinra, a recombinant interleukin (IL)-1 receptor antagonist, is authorized for treatment of COVID-19 in hospitalized adults who require supplemental oxygen, are at risk of progressing to severe respiratory failure, and are likely to have an elevated plasma soluble urokinase plasminogen activator receptor.

The recommended dose is 100 mg/d by subcutaneous injection for 10 days; decreased dosage should be considered in patients with decreased renal clearance. In subjects with rheumatoid arthritis, maximum plasma concentrations occurred 3-7 hours after subcutaneous administration; the terminal half- life ranged from 4 to 6 hours.

The most common adverse reactions are elevated serum aminotransferases, neutropenia, rash, and injection site reactions.

Vilobelimab, an anti-C5a monoclonal antibody, is authorized for the treatment of COVID-19 in hospitalized adults when initiated within 48 hours of receiving invasive mechanical ventilation or extracorporeal membrane oxygenation. The recommended dose is 800 mg IV, for a maximum of 6 doses.

Cmax increases dose proportionally while AUC increases more than dose proportionally. The elimination half-life is 95 hours.

Venous thrombosis, increased serum aminotransferases, constipation, thrombocytopenia, and rash have been reported as adverse reactions.

INVESTIGATIONAL AGENTS

VV116 is a chemically-modified version of remdesivir with oral bioavailability. In comparative clinical trials in adults with mild-to-moderate COVID-19 who were at risk for progression, VV116 was noninferior to nirmatrelvir–ritonavir with fewer safety concerns. **Ensitrelvir** is an oral 3CL protease inhibitor under evaluation for patients with mild-to-moderate COVID-19 infection.

ANTI-INFLUENZA AGENTS

Influenza virus strains are classified by their core proteins (ie, A, B, or C), species of origin (eg, avian, swine), and geographic site of isolation. Influenza A, the only strain that causes pandemics, is classified into 16 H (hemagglutinin) and 9 N (neuraminidase) subtypes based on surface proteins. Although influenza B viruses usually infect only people, influenza A viruses can infect a variety of animal hosts, including birds, providing an extensive reservoir. Current influenza A subtypes that are circulating among worldwide populations include H1N1, H1N2, and H3N2. Although avian influenza subtypes are typically highly species-specific, they have on rare occasions crossed the species barrier to infect humans and cats. Viruses of the H5 and H7 subtypes (eg, H5N1, H7N9) may rapidly mutate within poultry flocks from a low to high pathogenic form and have recently expanded their host range to cause both avian and human disease. However, person-to-person spread of these avian viruses to date has been rare, limited, and unsustained.

Until 2018, there were five anti-influenza drugs approved for use in the United States: three neuraminidase inhibitors (oral oseltamivir, inhaled zanamivir, IV peramivir) and two adamantanes (amantadine, rimantadine). The recent availabilities of oral baloxavir, a selective inhibitor of influenza cap-dependent endonuclease, and IV zanamivir offer additional options for the treatment of influenza (Table 49–7). The advent of the neuraminidase and endonuclease inhibitors caused the adamantanes to fall into disuse, due to their activity against both influenza A and influenza B (compared with activity against influenza A only by the adamantanes), as well as a low level of resistance (vs >99% resistance to the adamantanes among recent circulating influenza viruses). Although the rates of resistance to oseltamivir, zanamivir, and peramivir are currently low, the emergence of more widespread resistance remains a threat. Baloxavir retains in vitro activity against neuraminidase inhibitor–resistant viruses, as well as highly pathogenic avian influenza viruses.

BALOXAVIR MARBOXIL

Baloxavir marboxil is a first-in-class prodrug that is converted by hydrolysis to the active baloxavir, a cap-dependent endonuclease inhibitor which interferes with viral RNA transcription and blocks virus replication of both influenza A and influenza B. Thus, it acts earlier in the viral replication cycle than does oseltamivir. Since it binds to a different part of the virus than the neuraminidase inhibitors, enhanced efficacy with combinations of these agents is a possibility and is under study.

Due to its long half-life of 80 hours, baloxavir is given orally as a single-dose treatment (40 mg or 80 mg, depending on body weight). Treatment should be initiated within 48 hours of the onset of symptoms. Baloxavir may also be used in the same dose as post-exposure prophylaxis.

Use of baloxavir resulted in a decreased duration of symptoms by a median of 24–29 hours compared with placebo in two clinical trials. When compared with oseltamivir, there was a similar time to alleviation of symptoms but superior reduction in viral load at 1 day by baloxavir. Baloxavir was well tolerated.

Viral mutations conferring reduced susceptibility to baloxavir were detected in 2–10% of patients in clinical trials, but the

TABLE 49–7 Anti-influenza agents.[1]

Antiviral Agent	Class of Agent	Dose	Most Common Adverse Effects	Comments
Oral oseltamivir[2]	Neuraminidase inhibitor	Treatment: 75 mg twice daily × 5 days Prophylaxis: 75 mg once daily × 7 days	Nausea, vomiting, headache	
Inhaled zanamivir[3]	Neuraminidase inhibitor	Treatment: 10 mg twice daily × 5 days Prophylaxis: 10 mg once daily × 7 days	Cough, bronchospasm, throat discomfort	Contraindicated in patients with underlying airway disease
Intravenous peramivir	Neuraminidase inhibitor	Treatment: 600 mg once[2,4]	Diarrhea; hypersensitivity reaction	Not recommended for prophylaxis due to lack of data
Oral baloxavir	Endonuclease inhibitor	Treatment or prophylaxis: 40–80 mg once[5]		Avoid concurrent antacids or dairy products; contraindicated in immunocompromised patients due to unknown risk of resistance and in pregnant patients due to lack of data

[1]All listed agents have activity against both influenza A and influenza B.

[2]Dose reduction recommended in patients with renal insufficiency.

[3]Zanamivir is also available in a parenteral formulation for use in patients with severe influenza; dose reduction is necessary in patients with renal insufficiency.

[4]May be administered for up to 5 days in patients with severe influenza.

[5]Dose is dependent on body weight.

clinical significance is not yet known. However, given concern for the emergence of resistance, baloxavir should not be used in immunocompromised patients. Baloxavir remains effective against oseltamivir-resistant viruses, and conversely, oseltamivir is effective against baloxavir-resistant viruses.

Baloxavir can be taken with or without food; it is 93% bound to plasma proteins. The drug is metabolized via UGT1A3 with a minor contribution from CYP3A4. Co-administration of baloxavir with polyvalent cation-containing products (eg, laxatives, antacids, calcium supplements) or dairy products is contraindicated due to a resultant decrease in baloxavir plasma concentrations. Baloxavir is not recommended for use in pregnant women due to lack of data.

OSELTAMIVIR & ZANAMIVIR

The neuraminidase inhibitors oseltamivir and zanamivir, analogs of sialic acid, interfere with release of progeny influenza A and B virus from infected host cells, thus halting the spread of infection within the respiratory tract. These agents competitively and reversibly interact with the active enzyme site to inhibit viral neuraminidase activity at low nanomolar concentrations, resulting in clumping of newly released influenza virions to each other and to the membrane of the infected cell. Early administration is crucial because replication of influenza virus peaks at 24–72 hours after the onset of illness. Although resistance to oseltamivir and zanamivir may emerge during therapy and be transmissible, only a small number of influenza isolates tested in 2019–2021 by the Centers for Disease Control were resistant, and the prevalence of resistance is stable.

Oseltamivir is an orally administered prodrug that is activated by hepatic esterases and widely distributed throughout the body. Oral bioavailability is ~80%, plasma protein binding is low, and concentrations in the middle ear and sinus fluid are similar to those in plasma. The half-life of oseltamivir is 6–10 hours, and excretion is by glomerular filtration and tubular secretion. Probenecid reduces renal clearance by 50%.

Initiation of a 5-day course of therapy within 48 hours after the onset of illness (75 mg twice daily) decreased the time to first alleviation of symptoms by ~17 hours, as well as duration of viral shedding and viral titer; some studies have also shown a decrease in the incidence of complications. Once-daily prophylaxis (75 mg once daily) is 70–90% effective in preventing disease after exposure.

Serum concentrations of oseltamivir carboxylate, the active metabolite of oseltamivir, increase with declining renal function; therefore, dosage should be adjusted in patients with renal insufficiency. Potential adverse effects include nausea, vomiting, and headache. Taking oseltamivir with food does not interfere with absorption and may decrease nausea and vomiting. Fatigue and diarrhea have also been reported and appear to be more common with prophylactic use. Rash is rare. Neuropsychiatric events (self-injury or delirium) have been reported, particularly in adolescents and adults living in Japan.

Zanamivir is administered directly to the respiratory tract via inhalation, twice daily. Approximately 10–20% reaches the lungs; the remainder is deposited in the oropharynx. The concentration of the drug in the respiratory tract is estimated to be more than 1000 times the 50% inhibitory concentration for neuraminidase, and the pulmonary half-life is 2.8 hours. Of the total dose (10 mg twice daily for 5 days for treatment or 10 mg once daily for prevention), 5–15% is absorbed and excreted in the urine with minimal metabolism. Zanamivir reduced the time to first alleviation of symptoms by ~14 hours. Potential adverse effects include cough, bronchospasm (occasionally severe), reversible decrease in pulmonary function, and transient nasal and throat discomfort. Zanamivir administration is not recommended for patients with underlying airway disease.

Zanamivir is also available in a parenteral formulation for use in patients with severe influenza; dose adjustment is necessary in the setting of renal insufficiency.

PERAMIVIR

The neuraminidase inhibitor peramivir, a cyclopentane analog, has activity against both influenza A and B viruses, and is approved as a single 600-mg IV dose for the treatment of acute uncomplicated influenza in adults, although it may be administered for up to 5 days in patients with severe influenza. As with the other neuraminidase inhibitors, early treatment is optimal (ie, within 48 hours).

Less than 30% of peramivir is protein-bound. Peramivir is not significantly metabolized in humans and the major route of elimination is the kidney. Dose adjustment is recommended for renal insufficiency. The elimination half-life following IV administration is ~20 hours.

The main potential side effect is diarrhea, although serious skin or hypersensitivity reactions (e.g., Stevens-Johnson syndrome, erythema multiforme) have been rarely reported. In addition, as with the other neuraminidase inhibitors, an increased risk of hallucinations, delirium, and abnormal behavior in patients with influenza receiving peramivir has been reported.

AMANTADINE & RIMANTADINE

Amantadine (1-aminoadamantane hydrochloride) and its α-methyl derivative, rimantadine, are tricyclic amines of the adamantane family that block the M2 proton ion channel of the virus particle and inhibit uncoating of the viral RNA within infected host cells, thus preventing its replication. They are active against influenza A only. Rimantadine is four to ten times more active than amantadine in vitro. Amantadine is well absorbed and 67% protein-bound, with a plasma half-life of 12–18 hours that varies by creatinine clearance. Rimantadine is about 40% protein-bound and has a half-life of 24–36 hours. Nasal mucus concentrations of rimantadine average 50% higher than those in plasma, and cerebrospinal fluid levels are 52–96% of those in the serum. Amantadine is excreted unchanged in the urine, whereas rimantadine undergoes extensive metabolism by hydroxylation, conjugation, and glucuronidation before urinary excretion. Dose reductions are required for both agents in the elderly and in patients with renal insufficiency, and for rimantadine in patients with severe hepatic insufficiency.

In the absence of resistance, both amantadine and rimantadine are 70–90% protective in the prevention of clinical illness when initiated before exposure and limit the duration of clinical illness by 1–2 days when administered as treatment. However, due to high rates of resistance in both H1N1 and H3N2 viruses, these agents are no longer recommended for the prevention or treatment of influenza.

The most common adverse effects are gastrointestinal (nausea, anorexia) and central nervous system (nervousness, difficulty in concentrating, insomnia, lightheadedness). More serious side effects (eg, marked behavioral changes, delirium, hallucinations, agitation, and seizures) may be due to alteration of dopamine neurotransmission (see Chapter 28); are less frequent with rimantadine than with amantadine; are associated with high plasma concentrations; may occur more frequently in patients with renal insufficiency, seizure disorders, or advanced age; and may increase with concomitant antihistamines, anticholinergic drugs, hydrochlorothiazide, and trimethoprim-sulfamethoxazole. Clinical manifestations of anticholinergic activity are typically present in acute amantadine overdose. Both agents are teratogenic and embryotoxic in rodents, and birth defects have been reported after exposure during pregnancy.

INVESTIGATIONAL AGENTS

The long-acting neuraminidase inhibitor **laninamivir** is administered intranasally and may retain activity against oseltamivir-resistant virus. **DAS181** is a host-directed antiviral agent with activity against influenza and parainfluenza that acts by removing the virus receptor, sialic acid, from adjacent glycan structures.

■ AGENTS TO TREAT MONKEYPOX

Monkeypox, caused by an orthopoxvirus similar to smallpox (variola), is endemic to Central and West Africa. The first clinical cases were reported in 1970. Since early May 2022, however, an increasing number of clinical cases have been reported in Europe, Australia, Canada, and the United States.

TECOVIRIMAT

The antiviral tecovirimat (also known as TPOXX) is an inhibitor of viral p37, blocking the ability of virus particles to be released from infected cells. It was approved for the treatment of smallpox in 2018 and is available under an Expanded Access Investigational Drug protocol in the USA for monkeypox. The potential efficacy of tecovirimat for monkeypox was initially based on in vitro and animal data showing decreased mortality when administered early in the course of disease; a recent small study also supports its efficacy in the treatment of human monkeypox infection.

Tecovirimat is available in both oral and intravenous formulations. Dosage is weight-based and duration of treatment is 14 days. Drug absorption of the oral formulation is dependent on concurrent intake of a full, fatty meal, with absorption increased by 40–50%. It is approximately 80% protein-bound and reaches maximum serum concentrations in 4–6 hours. Tecovirimat is metabolized by hydrolysis of the amide bond and glucuronidation. The terminal half-life is 19.3 hours. Although no dose adjustment of the oral formulation is necessary in patients with renal insufficiency, IV tecovirimat should be administered with caution in patients with mild or moderate renal impairment and is contraindicated in patients with several renal insufficiency (CCl <30 mL/min).

Potential adverse effects of oral tecovirimat include fatigue, headache, nausea, vomiting, and abdominal pain. Prolongation of the QT interval has been reported, such that co-administration with drugs that have the same potential should be avoided. Administration of IV tecovirimat may result in infusion site reactions and/or headache. In addition, tecovirimat has a low barrier to viral resistance.

Tecovirimat is an inducer of CYP3A, an inhibitor of CYP2C8 and 2C19, and inhibits BCRP. Clinically significant drug-drug interactions reported to date include co-administration of repaglinide (hypoglycemia) and midazolam (decreased effectiveness of midazolam).

BRINCIDOFOVIR

Brincidofovir is a long-acting lipid-conjugated prodrug that is converted intracellularly to cidofovir, a nucleotide analog DNA polymerase inhibitor (see section on Cytomegalovirus). Brincidofovir was approved for treatment of smallpox in the USA in 1996. Its potential efficacy against monkeypox is based on data from in vitro and animal studies. Oral brincidofovir is administered once weekly (200 mg) for two consecutive doses.

Brincidofovir is converted intracellularly to cidofovir, which is subsequently phosphorylated to cidofovir diphosphate, the active antiviral moiety. The metabolite cidofovir diphosphate reaches maximum concentration at 47 hours; terminal half-life is 19.3 hours.

Potential adverse effects include elevated serum aminotransferases and/or bilirubin, diarrhea, nausea, vomiting, and abdominal pain. Although it may have less renal toxicity than the parent cidofovir molecule, elevated liver enzymes caused termination of treatment in three patients with monkeypox. Monitoring of hepatic enzymes before and during treatment with brincidofovir is recommended.

Animal data showed embryo-fetal toxicity and structural malformations; therefore, administration during pregnancy is contraindicated. In addition, squamous cell carcinoma, mammary adenocarcinoma, and testicular toxicity were noted in rats.

Brincidofovir is a direct and reversible inhibitor of several CYP enzymes and BRCP. Concomitant use with OATP1B1 and OATP1B3 inhibitors (eg, clarithromycin, cyclosporine, erythromycin, gemfibrozil, HIV and HCV protease inhibitors, rifampin) increase brincidofovir exposure, which may increase adverse reactions.

OTHER ANTIVIRAL AGENTS

INTERFERONS

Interferons have been studied for numerous clinical indications. In addition to HBV and HCV infections (see Antihepatitis Agents), intralesional injection of interferon alfa-2b or interferon alfa-n3 may be used for treatment of condylomata acuminata (see Chapter 61).

RIBAVIRIN

In addition to oral administration for HCV infection in combination with interferon (see Antihepatitis Agents), aerosolized ribavirin is administered by nebulizer (20 mg/mL for 12–18 hours continuously per day) to children and infants with severe RSV bronchiolitis or pneumonia to reduce the severity and duration of illness. However, its efficacy has not been clearly proven. Systemic absorption is low (<1%). Aerosolized ribavirin may cause conjunctival or bronchial irritation, and the aerosolized drug may precipitate on contact lenses. Ribavirin is teratogenic and embryotoxic. Health care workers and pregnant women should be protected against extended inhalation exposure.

Ribavirin has in vitro activity against a number of viruses other than RSV, including Lassa, West Nile, measles, influenza, and parainfluenza. However, clinical data regarding effectiveness are lacking.

PALIVIZUMAB

Palivizumab is a humanized monoclonal antibody directed against an epitope in the A antigen site on the F surface protein of RSV. It is licensed for the prevention of RSV infection in high-risk infants and children, such as premature infants requiring supplemental oxygen and those with bronchopulmonary dysplasia or congenital heart disease. It is dosed at 15 mg/kg of body weight intramuscularly for up to 5 consecutive months. The elimination half-life is 24.5 days.

A placebo-controlled trial using this regimen beginning at the start of the RSV season demonstrated a statistically significant decrease in RSV hospitalizations, fewer ICU admissions, and fewer days in the hospital. Resistant strains have been isolated in the laboratory and, rarely, from patients who have been treated with palivizumab.

Palivizumab is generally well tolerated; potential adverse effects include fever, rash, diarrhea, vomiting, cough, and elevation in serum aminotransferase levels. Acute hypersensitivity reactions have been reported.

Agents under investigation for the treatment or prophylaxis of patients with RSV infection include small molecule inhibitors that interfere with RSV fusion through interaction with the F protein of RSV, anti-RSV monoclonal antibodies, nonfusion replication inhibitors of RSV, and nucleoside analogs.

IMIQUIMOD

Imiquimod is an immune response modifier shown to be effective in the topical treatment of external genital and perianal warts (ie, condyloma acuminatum; see Chapter 61). The 5% cream is applied three times weekly and washed off 6–10 hours after each application. Recurrences appear to be less common than after ablative therapies. Imiquimod may also be effective against molluscum contagiosum. Local skin reactions are the most common adverse effect; these tend to resolve within weeks after therapy. However, pigmentary skin changes may persist. Systemic adverse effects such as fatigue and influenza-like syndrome have occasionally been reported.

PREPARATIONS AVAILABLE

GENERIC NAME	AVAILABLE AS
Abacavir	Generic, Ziagen
Abacavir/lamivudine	Epzicom
Abacavir/lamivudine/zidovudine	Trizivir
Acyclovir	Generic, Zovirax
Adefovir	Generic, Hepsera
Amantadine	Generic, Symmetrel
Atazanavir	Reyataz
Boceprevir	Victrelis
Cidofovir	Generic, Vistide
Darunavir	Prezista (must be taken with ritonavir)
Delavirdine	Rescriptor
Didanosine (dideoxyinosine, ddI)	Generic, Videx, Videx-EC
Docosanol	Abreva (over-the-counter)
Efavirenz	Sustiva

GENERIC NAME	AVAILABLE AS
Emtricitabine	Emtriva
Emtricitabine/tenofovir	Truvada
Emtricitabine/tenofovir/efavirenz	Atripla
Enfuvirtide	Fuzeon
Entecavir	Baraclude
Etravirine	Intelence
Famciclovir	Generic, Famvir
Fosamprenavir	Lexiva
Foscarnet	Generic, Foscavir
Ganciclovir	Generic, Cytovene
Imiquimod	Generic, Aldara, others
Indinavir	Crixivan
Interferon alfa-2a	Roferon-A
Interferon alfa-2b	Intron-A

GENERIC NAME	AVAILABLE AS
Interferon alfa-2b/ribavirin	Rebetron
Interferon alfa-n3	Alferon N
Interferon alfacon-1	Infergen
Lamivudine	Generic, Epivir, Epivir-HBV
Lamivudine/zidovudine	Combivir
Lamivudine/abacavir/zidovudine	Trizivir
Lopinavir/ritonavir	Kaletra
Maraviroc	Selzentry
Nelfinavir	Viracept
Nevirapine	Generic, Viramune
Oseltamivir	Tamiflu
Palivizumab	Synagis
Peginterferon alfa-2a (pegylated interferon alfa-2a)	Pegasys
Peginterferon alfa-2b (pegylated interferon alfa-2b)	PEG-Intron
Penciclovir	Denavir
Raltegravir	Isentress
Ribavirin	Generic, Rebetol
Ribavirin/interferon alfa-2b	Rebetron
Ribavirin Aerosol	Virazole
Rilpivirine	Edurant
Rilpivirine/emtricitabine/-tenofovir	Complera
Rimantadine	Generic, Flumadine
Ritonavir	Norvir
Saquinavir	Invirase
Sofosbuvir	Sovaldi
Stavudine	Generic, Zerit, Zerit XR
Telaprevir	Incivek
Telbivudine	Tyzeka
Tenofovir	Viread
Tipranavir	Aptivus
Trifluridine	Generic, Viroptic
Valacyclovir	Generic, Valtrex
Valganciclovir	Valcyte
Zalcitabine (dideoxycytidine, ddC)	Hivid (withdrawn)
Zanamivir	Relenza
Zidovudine (azidothymidine, AZT)	Generic, Retrovir
Zidovudine/lamivudine	Combivir
Zidovudine/lamivudine/abacavir	Trizivir

REFERENCES

American Association for the Study of Liver Diseases (AASLD)-Infectious Diseases Society of America (IDSA): HCV Guidance: Recommendations for testing, managing, and treating hepatitis C. www.hcvguidelines.org.

Department of Health and Human Services: Guidelines for the Use of Antiretroviral Agents in Adults and Adolescents with HIV. clinicalinfo.hiv.gov/sites/default/files/guidelines/documents/adult-adolescent-arv/guidelines-adult-adolescent-arv.pdf.

Guarner J et al: Monkeypox in 2022—what clinicians need to know. JAMA 2022;328:139.

Infectious Diseases Society of America: IDSA Guidelines on the Treatment and Management of Patients with COVID-19. www.idsociety.org/practice-guideline/covid-19-guideline-treatment-and-management/.

Panel on Treatment of HIV During Pregnancy and Prevention of Perinatal Transmission: Recommendations for the Use of Antiretroviral Drugs During Pregnancy and Interventions to Reduce Perinatal HIV Transmission in the United States. clinicalinfo.hiv.gov/en/guidelines/perinatal/whats-new.

Terrault NA et al: Update on prevention, diagnosis, and treatment of chronic hepatitis B: AASLD 2018 hepatitis B guidance. Hepatology 2018;67:1560.

RELEVANT WEBSITES

www.hiv-druginteractions.org

www.iasusa.org

www.hepatitisc.uw.edu/page/treatment/drugs

CASE STUDY ANSWER

Combination antiviral therapy against both HIV and hepatitis B virus (HBV) is indicated in this patient, given the high viral load and low CD4 cell count. However, the use of methadone and possibly excessive alcohol consumption necessitate caution. Tenofovir alafenamide plus emtricitabine (two nucleoside/nucleotide reverse transcriptase inhibitors) would be excellent choices as the NRTI "backbone" of a fully suppressive regimen, since both are active against HIV-1 and HBV, do not interact with methadone, and are available in a once-daily, fixed-dose combination. An integrase strand inhibitor such as bictegravir, raltegravir, or dolutegravir could be added. There are other alternatives as well. Prior to initiation of this regimen, renal and liver function should be checked, HBV DNA level should be assessed, the patient should be screened for Hepatitis A and HCV infection, and a bone mineral density test should be considered. Pregnancy should be ruled out. Avoidance of alcohol should be recommended. The potential for lowered methadone levels with darunavir, if used, necessitates close monitoring and possibly an increased dose of methadone. Finally, the patient should be made aware that abrupt cessation of these medications may precipitate an acute flare of hepatitis.

CHAPTER

50 Miscellaneous Antimicrobial Agents; Disinfectants, Antiseptics, & Sterilants

Camille E. Beauduy, PharmD, & Lisa G. Winston, MD*

CASE STUDY

A 56-year-old man is admitted to the intensive care unit of a hospital for treatment of community-acquired pneumonia. He receives ceftriaxone and azithromycin upon admission, rapidly improves, and is transferred to a semi-private ward room. On day 7 of his hospitalization, he develops copious diarrhea with eight bowel movements but is otherwise clinically stable. *Clostridioides difficile* infection is confirmed by stool testing. What is an acceptable treatment for the patient's diarrhea? The patient is transferred to a single-bed room. The housekeeping staff asks what product should be used to clean the patient's old room.

■ METRONIDAZOLE, FIDAXOMYCIN, RIFAXIMIN, MUPIROCIN, POLYMYXINS, & URINARY ANTISEPTICS

METRONIDAZOLE

Metronidazole is a nitroimidazole antiprotozoal drug (see Chapter 52) that also has potent antibacterial activity against anaerobes, including *Bacteroides* and *Clostridioides* (formerly *Clostridium*) species. Metronidazole is selectively absorbed by anaerobic bacteria and sensitive protozoa. Once taken up by anaerobes, it is nonenzymatically reduced by reacting with reduced ferredoxin. This reduction results in products that accumulate in and are toxic to anaerobic cells. The metabolites of metronidazole are taken up into bacterial DNA, forming unstable molecules. This action occurs only when metronidazole is partially reduced, and, because this reduction usually happens only in anaerobic cells, it has relatively little effect on human cells or aerobic bacteria.

Metronidazole is well absorbed after oral administration, is widely distributed in tissues, and reaches serum levels of 4–6 mcg/mL after a 250-mg oral dose. It can also be given intravenously. The drug penetrates well into the cerebrospinal fluid and brain, reaching levels similar to those in serum. Metronidazole is metabolized in the liver and may accumulate in hepatic insufficiency.

Metronidazole is indicated for treatment of anaerobic or mixed intra-abdominal infections and pelvic inflammatory disease (in combination with other agents with activity against aerobic organisms), vaginitis (trichomonas infection, bacterial vaginosis), and brain abscess. While it is no longer a first-line treatment for *Clostridioides difficile* infection when administered alone, it may be given intravenously, combined with oral vancomycin, to patients with fulminant *C difficile* infection. The typical dosage for most indications is 500 mg three times daily orally or intravenously

*The authors thank Henry F. Chambers, MD, and Daniel H. Deck, PharmD, for their contributions to previous editions.

(30 mg/kg/d). Vaginitis may respond to a single 2-g dose. A vaginal gel is available for topical use.

Adverse effects include nausea, diarrhea, stomatitis, and peripheral neuropathy with prolonged use. It had been thought that metronidazole has a disulfiram-like effect necessitating the avoidance of alchol, but re-evaluation of available data suggests that this is not the case. Although teratogenic in some animals, metronidazole has not been associated with this effect in humans. Other properties of metronidazole are discussed in Chapter 52.

A structurally similar agent, **tinidazole**, is a once-daily drug approved for treatment of trichomonas infection, giardiasis, amebiasis, and bacterial vaginosis. It also is active against anaerobic bacteria, but is not approved in the USA for treatment of anaerobic infections.

FIDAXOMICIN

Fidaxomicin is a narrow-spectrum, macrocyclic antibiotic that is active against gram-positive aerobes and anaerobes but lacks activity against gram-negative bacteria (Figure 50–1). Fidaxomicin inhibits bacterial protein synthesis by binding to the sigma subunit of RNA polymerase. When administered orally, systemic absorption is negligible but fecal concentrations are high, so it is not associated with many systemic toxicities and should only be used to treat infections confined to the gastrointestinal tract. Fidaxomicin has been approved for the treatment for *C difficile* infection in adults. It is as effective as oral vancomycin and is recommended as the preferred first-line agent for treatment of *C difficile* given its lower rates of relapsing disease compared to oral vancomycin.

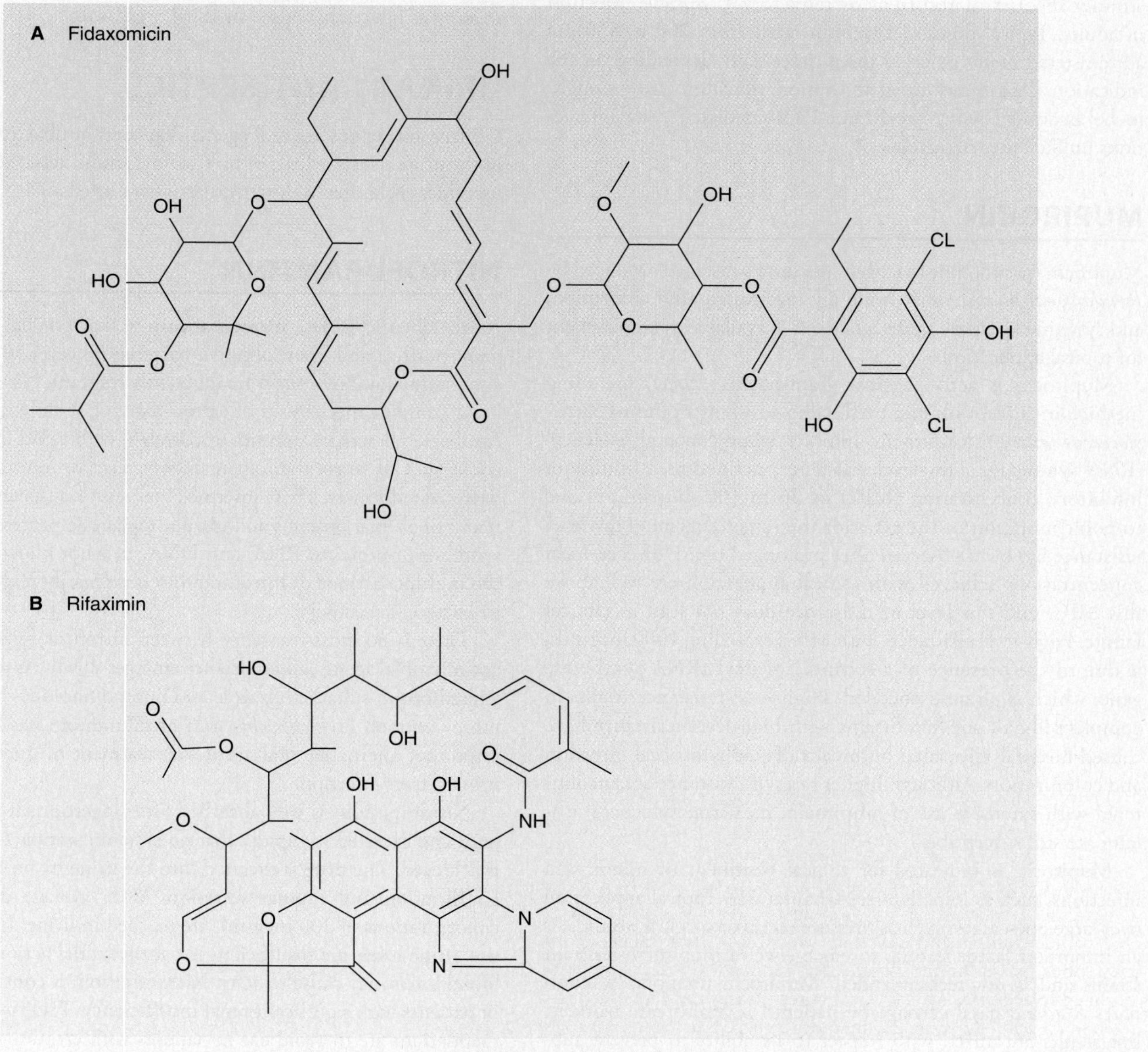

A Fidaxomicin

B Rifaximin

FIGURE 50–1 Examples of poorly absorbed antibacterial agents include fidaxomicin (panel **A**) and rifaximin (panel **B**). Both agents have high molecular weight and poor water solubility that contribute to their minimal systemic absorption. This results in high drug concentrations in the gastrointestinal lumen, allowing for therapeutic efficacy in local gastrointestinal infections.

Fidaxomicin is administered orally as a 200-mg tablet twice daily for 10 days.

RIFAXIMIN

Rifaximin is a derivative of rifampin (see Figure 50–1). It is active against gram-positive and gram-negative aerobes and anaerobes. Rifaximin inhibits bacterial protein synthesis by binding to the beta subunit of DNA-dependent RNA polymerase. When administered orally, systemic absorption is <0.5%, but fecal concentrations are high; following a 3-day course for travelers' diarrhea, the fecal concentrations were 8000 mcg/g. Rifaximin was originally approved by the FDA for the treatment of travelers' diarrhea, and it is now used in the management of hepatic encephalopathy, irritable bowel syndrome with diarrhea, and, occasionally, as an adjunct in cases of recurrent or refractory *C difficile* infection in adults. Typical doses of rifaximin range from 200 to 550 mg administered orally twice to three times daily depending on the indication. Due to its limited absorption, rifaximin is not thought to be associated with cytochrome-P450-mediated drug interactions unlike other rifamycins.

MUPIROCIN

Mupirocin (pseudomonic acid) is a natural substance produced by *Pseudomonas fluorescens*. It is rapidly inactivated after absorption, and systemic levels are undetectable. It is available as an ointment for topical application.

Mupirocin is active against gram-positive cocci, including methicillin-susceptible and methicillin-resistant strains of *Staphylococcus aureus*. Mupirocin inhibits staphylococcal isoleucyl tRNA synthetase. Low-level resistance, defined as a minimum inhibitory concentration (MIC) of up to 100 mcg/mL, is due to point mutation in the gene for the target enzyme. Low-level resistance has been observed after prolonged use. However, local concentrations achieved with topical application are well above this MIC, and this level of resistance does not lead to clinical failure. High-level resistance, with MICs exceeding 1000 mcg/mL, is due to the presence of a second isoleucyl tRNA synthetase gene, which is plasmid-encoded. High-level resistance results in complete loss of activity. Strains with high-level resistance have caused hospital-associated outbreaks of staphylococcal infection and colonization. Although higher rates of resistance are encountered with extensive use of mupirocin, most staphylococcal isolates are still susceptible.

Mupirocin is indicated for topical treatment of minor skin infections, such as impetigo (see Chapter 61). Topical application over large open areas, such as pressure ulcers or surgical wounds, is an important factor leading to emergence of mupirocin-resistant strains and is not recommended. Mupirocin temporarily eliminates *S aureus* nasal carriage by patients or health care workers, but results are mixed with respect to its ability to prevent subsequent staphylococcal infection. Patients most likely to benefit from decolonization are those undergoing orthopedic or cardiothoracic procedures.

POLYMYXINS

The polymyxins are a group of basic peptides active against gram-negative bacteria and include **polymyxin B** and **polymyxin E (colistin).** Polymyxins act as cationic detergents. They attach to and disrupt bacterial cell membranes. They also bind and inactivate endotoxin. Gram-positive organisms, *Proteus* sp, and *Neisseria* sp are resistant.

Owing to their significant toxicity with systemic administration (especially nephrotoxicity), polymyxins were historically largely restricted to topical use. Ointments containing polymyxin B, 5000 units/g, in mixtures with bacitracin or neomycin (or both) are commonly applied to infected superficial skin lesions. Emergence of strains of *Acinetobacter baumannii, Pseudomonas aeruginosa*, and Enterobacteriaceae that are resistant to all other agents has renewed interest in polymyxins as parenteral agents for salvage therapy of infections caused by these organisms.

URINARY ANTISEPTICS

Urinary antiseptics are oral agents that exert antibacterial activity in the urine but have little or no systemic antibacterial effect. Their usefulness is limited to lower urinary tract infections.

NITROFURANTOIN

At therapeutic doses, **nitrofurantoin** is bactericidal for many gram-positive and gram-negative bacteria; however, *P aeruginosa* and many strains of *Proteus* are inherently resistant. Nitrofurantoin has a complex mechanism of action that is not fully understood. Antibacterial activity appears to correlate with rapid intracellular conversion of nitrofurantoin to highly reactive intermediates by bacterial reductases. These intermediates react nonspecifically with many ribosomal proteins and disrupt metabolic processes and the synthesis of proteins, RNA, and DNA. It is not known which of the multiple actions of nitrofurantoin is primarily responsible for its bactericidal activity.

There is no cross-resistance between nitrofurantoin and other antimicrobial agents, and resistance emerges slowly. As resistance to trimethoprim-sulfamethoxazole and fluoroquinolones has become more common in *Escherichia coli*, nitrofurantoin has become an important alternative oral agent for treatment of uncomplicated urinary tract infection.

Nitrofurantoin is well absorbed after ingestion. It is metabolized and excreted so rapidly that no systemic antibacterial action is achieved. The drug is excreted into the urine by both glomerular filtration and tubular secretion. With average daily doses, concentrations of 200 mcg/mL are reached in urine. In renal failure, urine levels are insufficient for antibacterial action, but high blood levels may cause toxicity. Nitrofurantoin is contraindicated in patients with significant renal insufficiency. Traditional recommendations are to avoid use in patients with creatinine clearance <60 mL/min; however, some data suggest short-term nitrofurantoin treatment is acceptable in patients with creatinine clearance >30 mL/min.

The dosage for urinary tract infection in adults is 100 mg orally taken four times daily. A long-acting formulation **(Macrobid)** can be taken twice daily. Each long-acting capsule contains two forms of nitrofurantoin. Macrocrystalline nitrofurantoin, which has slower dissolution and absorption than nitrofurantoin monohydrate, constitutes 25%. The remaining 75% is nitrofurantoin monohydrate contained in a powder blend, which, upon exposure to gastric and intestinal fluids, forms a gel matrix that releases nitrofurantoin over time.

The drug should not be used to treat upper urinary tract infection due to inadequate drug levels. It is desirable to keep urinary pH below 5.5, which greatly enhances drug activity. A single daily dose of nitrofurantoin, 100 mg, can prevent recurrent urinary tract infections in some women.

Anorexia, nausea, and vomiting are the principal side effects of nitrofurantoin. Neuropathies and pulmonary toxicities may occur, particularly with prolonged use or in patients with renal impairment. Hemolytic anemia can occur in patients with glucose-6-phosphate dehydrogenase deficiency. Nitrofurantoin antagonizes the action of nalidixic acid and possibly some older fluoroquinolones, such as norfloxacin and ciprofloxacin. Rashes, pulmonary infiltration and fibrosis, and other hypersensitivity reactions have been reported.

METHENAMINE MANDELATE & METHENAMINE HIPPURATE

Methenamine mandelate is the salt of mandelic acid and methenamine and possesses properties of both of these urinary antiseptics. Methenamine hippurate is the salt of hippuric acid and methenamine. Below pH 5.5, methenamine releases formaldehyde, which is antibacterial (see the section Aldehydes). Oral mandelic acid or hippuric acid is absorbed and excreted unchanged in the urine. These drugs are bactericidal for some gram-negative bacteria when urine pH is less than 5.5.

Methenamine mandelate, 1 g four times daily, or methenamine hippurate, 1 g twice daily by mouth (in children age 6–12 years, 500 mg four times daily or twice daily, respectively), is used only as a urinary antiseptic to prevent, not treat, symptomatic urinary tract infection. Acidifying agents (eg, ascorbic acid, 4–12 g/d) may be given to lower urinary pH below 5.5. Sulfonamides should not be given at the same time because they may form an insoluble compound with the formaldehyde released by methenamine. Persons taking methenamine mandelate may exhibit falsely elevated tests for catecholamine metabolites.

■ DISINFECTANTS, ANTISEPTICS, & STERILANTS

Disinfectants are chemical agents or physical procedures that inhibit or kill microorganisms (Table 50–1). Antiseptics are disinfecting chemical agents with sufficiently low toxicity for host cells that they can be used directly on skin, mucous membranes, or wounds. Sterilants kill both vegetative cells and spores when applied to materials for appropriate times and temperatures. Some of the terms used in this context are defined in Table 50–2.

Disinfection prevents infection by reducing the number of potentially infective organisms by killing, removing, or diluting them. Disinfection can be accomplished by application of chemical agents or use of physical agents such as ionizing radiation, dry or moist heat, or superheated steam (autoclave, 120°C) to kill microorganisms. Often a combination of agents is used, eg, water and moderate heat over time (pasteurization); ethylene oxide and moist heat (a sterilant); or addition of disinfectant to a detergent. Prevention of infection also can be achieved by washing, which dilutes the potentially infectious organism.

Hand hygiene is probably the most important means of preventing transmission of infectious agents from person to person or from regions of high microbial load, eg, mouth, nose, or gut, to

TABLE 50–1 Activities of disinfectants.

	Bacteria			Viruses			Other		
	Gram-Positive	*Gram-Negative*	*Acid-Fast*	*Spores*	*Lipophilic*	*Hydrophilic*	*Fungi*	*Amebic Cysts*	*Prions*
Alcohols (isopropanol, ethanol)	HS	HS	S	R	S	V	—	—	R
Aldehydes (glutaraldehyde, formaldehyde)	HS	HS	MS	S (slow)	S	MS	S	—	R
Chlorhexidine gluconate	HS	MS	R	R	V	R	—	—	R
Sodium hypochlorite, chlorine dioxide	HS	HS	MS	S (pH 7.6)	S	S (at high conc)	MS	S	MS (at high conc)
Hexachlorophene	S (slow)	R	R	R	R	R	R	R	R
Povidone, iodine	HS	HS	S	S (at high conc)	S	R	S	S	R
Phenols, quaternary ammonium compounds	HS	HS	MS	R	S	R	S	—	R

conc, concentration; HS, highly susceptible; MS, moderately susceptible; —, no data; R, resistant; S, susceptible; V, variable.

TABLE 50–2 Commonly used terms related to chemical and physical killing of microorganisms.

Antisepsis	Application of an agent to living tissue for the purpose of preventing infection
Decontamination	Process that produces marked reduction in number or activity of microorganisms
Disinfection	Chemical or physical treatment that destroys most vegetative microbes and viruses, but not spores, in or on inanimate surfaces
Sanitization	Reduction of microbial load on an inanimate surface to a level considered acceptable for public health purposes
Sterilization	A process intended to kill or remove all types of microorganisms, including spores, and usually including viruses, with an acceptably low probability of their survival
Pasteurization	A process that kills nonsporulating microorganisms by hot water or steam at 65–100°C

potential sites of infection. Alcohol-based hand rubs and soap and warm water are used to kill or remove bacteria. Skin disinfectants along with detergent and water are usually used preoperatively as a surgical scrub for the hands and arms of surgical team members.

Evaluation of effectiveness of antiseptics, disinfectants, and sterilants, although seemingly simple in principle, is very complex. Factors in any evaluation include the intrinsic resistance of the microorganism, the number of microorganisms present, mixed populations of organisms, amount of organic material present (eg, blood, feces, tissue), concentration and stability of disinfectant or sterilant, time and temperature of exposure, pH, and hydration and binding of the agent to surfaces. Specific, standardized assays of activity are defined for each use. Toxicity for humans also must be evaluated. In the USA, the Environmental Protection Agency (EPA) regulates disinfectants and sterilants and the FDA regulates antiseptics.

Users of antiseptics, disinfectants, and sterilants need to consider their short-term and long-term toxicity because they may have general biocidal activity and may accumulate in the environment or in the body. Disinfectants and antiseptics may also become contaminated by resistant microorganisms—eg, spores, *P aeruginosa*, or *Serratia marcescens*—and actually transmit infection. Most topical antiseptics interfere with wound healing to some degree. Cleansing of wounds with soap and water may be less damaging than the application of antiseptics.

Some of the chemical classes of antiseptics, disinfectants, and sterilants are described briefly in the text that follows. The reader is referred to the general references for descriptions of physical disinfection and sterilization methods.

ALCOHOLS

The two alcohols most frequently used for antisepsis and disinfection are **ethanol** and **isopropyl alcohol (isopropanol).** They are rapidly active, killing vegetative bacteria, *Mycobacterium tuberculosis*, and many fungi, and inactivating lipophilic viruses. The optimum bactericidal concentration is 60–90% by volume in water. They probably act by denaturation of proteins. They are not used as sterilants because they are not sporicidal, do not penetrate protein-containing organic material, and may not be active against hydrophilic viruses. Their skin-drying effect can be alleviated by addition of emollients to the formulation. Use of alcohol-based hand rubs has been shown to reduce transmission of health care–associated pathogens including SARS-CoV-2 and is recommended by the Centers for Disease Control and Prevention (CDC) as the preferred method of hand decontamination in health care settings. Alcohol-based hand rubs are ineffective against spores of *C difficile*, and handwashing with soap and water is required for decontamination after caring for a patient with *C difficile* infection.

Alcohols are flammable and must be stored in cool, well-ventilated areas. They must be allowed to evaporate before cautery, electrosurgery, or laser surgery. Alcohols may be damaging if applied directly to corneal tissue. Therefore, instruments such as tonometers that have been disinfected in alcohol should be rinsed with sterile water, or the alcohol should be allowed to evaporate before they are used.

CHLORHEXIDINE

Chlorhexidine is a cationic biguanide with very low water solubility. Water-soluble chlorhexidine digluconate is used in water-based formulations as an antiseptic. It is active against vegetative bacteria and mycobacteria and has variable activity against fungi and viruses. It strongly adsorbs to bacterial membranes, causing leakage of small molecules and precipitation of cytoplasmic proteins. It is active at pH 5.5–7.0. Chlorhexidine gluconate is slower in its action than alcohols, but, because of its persistence, it has residual activity, producing bactericidal action equivalent to alcohols. It is most effective against gram-positive cocci and less active against gram-positive and gram-negative rods. Spore germination is inhibited by chlorhexidine. Chlorhexidine digluconate is resistant to inhibition by blood and organic materials. However, anionic and nonionic agents in moisturizers, neutral soaps, and surfactants may neutralize its action. Chlorhexidine digluconate formulations of 4% concentration have slightly greater antibacterial activity than 2% formulations. The combination of chlorhexidine gluconate in 70% alcohol, available in some countries including the USA, is the preferred agent for skin antisepsis in many surgical and percutaneous procedures. The advantage of this combination over povidone-iodine may derive from its more rapid action after application, its retained activity after exposure to body fluids, and its persistent activity on the skin. Chlorhexidine has a very low skin-sensitizing or irritating capacity. Oral toxicity is low because it is poorly absorbed from the alimentary tract. Chlorhexidine must not be used during surgery on the middle ear because it causes sensorineural deafness. Similar neural toxicity may be encountered during neurosurgery.

HALOGENS

Iodine

Iodine in a 1:20,000 solution is bactericidal in 1 minute and kills spores in 15 minutes. Tincture of iodine USP contains 2% iodine and 2.4% sodium iodide in alcohol. It is the most active antiseptic for intact skin. It is not commonly used due to serious hypersensitivity reactions and staining of clothing and dressings.

Iodophors

Iodophors are complexes of iodine with a surface-active agent such as **polyvinyl pyrrolidone (PVP; povidone-iodine).** Iodophors retain the activity of iodine. They kill vegetative bacteria, mycobacteria, fungi, and lipid-containing viruses. They may be sporicidal with prolonged exposure. Iodophors can be used as antiseptics or disinfectants, the latter containing more iodine. The amount of free iodine is low, but it is released as the solution is diluted. An iodophor solution must be diluted according to the manufacturer's directions to obtain full activity.

Iodophors are less irritating and less likely to produce skin hypersensitivity than tincture of iodine. They require drying time on skin before becoming active, which can be a disadvantage. Although iodophors have a somewhat broader spectrum of activity than chlorhexidine, including sporicidal action, they lack its persistent activity on skin.

Chlorine

Chlorine is a strong oxidizing agent and universal disinfectant that is commonly provided as a 5.25% **sodium hypochlorite** solution, a typical formulation for **household bleach.** Because formulations may vary, the exact concentration should be verified on the label. A 1:10 dilution of household bleach (producing a 0.525% concentration) provides 5000 ppm of available chlorine. The CDC recommends this concentration for disinfection of blood spills. Less than 5 ppm kills vegetative bacteria, whereas up to 5000 ppm is necessary to kill bacterial spores. A concentration of 1000–10,000 ppm is tuberculocidal. One hundred ppm kills vegetative fungal cells in 1 hour, but fungal spores require 500 ppm. Viruses are inactivated by 200–500 ppm. Dilutions of sodium hypochlorite made up in pH 7.5–8.0 tap water retain their activity for months when kept in tightly closed, opaque containers. Frequent opening and closing of the container reduces the activity markedly.

Because chlorine is inactivated by blood, serum, feces, and protein-containing materials, surfaces should be cleaned before chlorine disinfectant is applied. Undissociated hypochlorous acid (HOCl) is the active biocidal agent. When pH is increased, the less active hypochlorite ion, OCl^-, is formed. When hypochlorite solutions contact formaldehyde, the carcinogen bis(chloromethyl) is formed. Rapid evolution of irritating chlorine gas occurs when hypochlorite solutions are mixed with acid and urine. Solutions are corrosive to aluminum, silver, and stainless steel.

Alternative chlorine-releasing compounds include **chlorine dioxide** and **chloramine-T.** These agents have a prolonged bactericidal action.

PHENOLICS

Phenol itself (perhaps the oldest of the surgical antiseptics) is no longer used even as a disinfectant because of its corrosive effect on tissues, its toxicity when absorbed, and its carcinogenic effect. These adverse actions are diminished by forming derivatives in which a functional group replaces a hydrogen atom in the aromatic ring. The phenolic agents most commonly used are ***o*-phenylphenol**, ***o*-benzyl-*p*-chlorophenol**, and ***p*-tertiary amylphenol.** Mixtures of phenolic derivatives may be used. Some of these are derived from coal tar distillates, eg, cresols and xylenols. Skin absorption and skin irritation still occur with these derivatives, and appropriate care is necessary in their use. Detergents are often added to formulations to clean and remove organic material that may decrease the activity of a phenolic compound.

Phenolic compounds disrupt cell walls and membranes, precipitate proteins, and inactivate enzymes. They are bactericidal (including mycobacteria) and fungicidal and are capable of inactivating lipophilic viruses. They are not sporicidal. Dilution and time of exposure recommendations of the manufacturer must be followed.

Phenolic disinfectants have been used for hard surface decontamination in hospitals and laboratories, eg, floors, beds, and counter or bench tops. They are not recommended for use in nurseries and especially near infants, where their use has been associated with hyperbilirubinemia. Use of **hexachlorophene** as a skin disinfectant has caused cerebral edema and seizures in premature infants and, occasionally, in adults. It is no longer available in the United States.

QUATERNARY AMMONIUM COMPOUNDS

The quaternary ammonium compounds ("quats") are cationic surface-active detergents. The active cation has at least one long water-repellent hydrocarbon chain, which causes the molecules to concentrate as an oriented layer on the surface of solutions and colloidal or suspended particles. The charged nitrogen portion of the cation has high affinity for water and prevents separation out of solution. The bactericidal action of quaternary compounds has been attributed to inactivation of energy-producing enzymes, denaturation of proteins, and disruption of the cell membrane. These agents are fungistatic and sporistatic and also inhibit algae. They are bactericidal for gram-positive bacteria and moderately active against gram-negative bacteria. Lipophilic viruses are inactivated. They are not tuberculocidal or sporicidal, and they do not inactivate hydrophilic viruses. Quaternary ammonium compounds bind to the surface of colloidal protein in blood, serum, and milk and to the fibers in cotton, mops, cloths, and paper towels used to apply them, which can cause inactivation of the agent by removing it from solution. They are inactivated by anionic detergents (soaps), by many nonionic detergents, and by calcium, magnesium, ferric, and aluminum ions.

Quaternary compounds are used for sanitation of noncritical surfaces (floors, bench tops, etc). Their low toxicity has led to their use as sanitizers in food production facilities. Quaternary ammonium compounds such as **benzalkonium chloride** are not recommended for use as antiseptics because outbreaks of infections have occurred that were due to growth of *Pseudomonas* and other gram-negative bacteria in quaternary ammonium antiseptic solutions.

ALDEHYDES

Formaldehyde and **glutaraldehyde** are used for disinfection or sterilization of instruments such as fiberoptic endoscopes, respiratory therapy equipment, hemodialyzers, and dental instruments that cannot withstand exposure to the high temperatures of steam sterilization. They are not corrosive for metal, plastic, or rubber. These agents have a broad spectrum of activity against microorganisms. They act by alkylation of chemical groups in proteins and nucleic acids. Failures of disinfection or sterilization can occur as a result of dilution below the known effective concentration, the presence of organic material, and the failure of liquid to penetrate into small channels in the instruments. Automatic circulating baths increase penetration of aldehyde solution into the instrument while decreasing exposure of the operator to irritating fumes.

Formaldehyde is available as a 40% weight per volume solution in water (100% **formalin**). An 8% formaldehyde solution in water has a broad spectrum of activity against bacteria, fungi, and viruses. Sporicidal activity may take as long as 18 hours. Rapidity of action is increased by solution in 70% isopropanol. Formaldehyde solutions are used for high-level disinfection of hemodialyzers, preparation of vaccines, and preservation and embalming of tissues. The 4% formaldehyde (10% formalin) solutions used for fixation of tissues and embalming may not be mycobactericidal.

Glutaraldehyde is a dialdehyde (1,5-pentanedial). Solutions of 2% weight per volume glutaraldehyde are most commonly used. The solution must be alkalinized to pH 7.4–8.5 for activation. Activated solutions are bactericidal, sporicidal, fungicidal, and viricidal for both lipophilic and hydrophilic viruses. Glutaraldehyde has greater sporicidal activity than formaldehyde, but it may have less tuberculocidal activity. Lethal action against mycobacteria and spores may require prolonged exposure. Once activated, solutions have a shelf life of 14 days, after which polymerization reduces activity. Other means of activation and stabilization can increase the shelf life. Because glutaraldehyde solutions are frequently reused, the most common reason for loss of activity is dilution and exposure to organic material. Test strips to measure residual activity are recommended.

Formaldehyde has a characteristic pungent odor and is highly irritating to respiratory mucous membranes and eyes at concentrations of 2–5 ppm. The US Occupational Safety and Health Administration (OSHA) has declared that formaldehyde is a potential carcinogen and has established a standard that limits employee exposure. Protection of health care workers from exposure to glutaraldehyde concentrations greater than 0.2 ppm is advisable. Increased air exchange, enclosure in hoods with exhausts, tight-fitting lids on exposure devices, and use of protective personal equipment such as goggles, respirators, and gloves may be necessary to limit exposure.

Ortho-phthalaldehyde (OPA) is a phenolic dialdehyde chemical sterilant with a spectrum of activity comparable to glutaraldehyde, although it is several times more rapidly bactericidal. OPA solution typically contains 0.55% OPA. High-level disinfection can be achieved more rapidly than with glutaraldehyde. Unlike glutaraldehyde, OPA requires no activation, is less irritating to mucous membranes, and does not require exposure monitoring. It has good materials compatibility and an acceptable environmental safety profile. OPA is useful for disinfection or sterilization of endoscopes, surgical instruments, and other medical devices.

SUPEROXIDIZED WATER

Electrolysis of saline yields a mixture of oxidants, primarily hypochlorous acid and chlorine, with potent disinfectant and sterilant properties. The solution generated by the process, which has been commercialized and marketed as **Sterilox** for disinfection of endoscopes and dental materials, is rapidly bactericidal, fungicidal, tuberculocidal, and sporicidal. High-level disinfection is achieved with a contact time of 10 minutes. The solution is nontoxic and nonirritating and requires no special disposal precautions.

PEROXYGEN COMPOUNDS

The peroxygen compounds, **hydrogen peroxide** and **peracetic acid**, have high killing activity and a broad spectrum against bacteria, spores, viruses, and fungi when used in appropriate concentration. They have the advantage that their decomposition products are not toxic and do not injure the environment. They are powerful oxidizers that are used primarily as disinfectants and sterilants.

Hydrogen peroxide is a very effective disinfectant when used for inanimate objects or materials with low organic content. Systems that produce hydrogen peroxide vapor or dry mist are now available for room decontamination in healthcare facilities. Organisms that produce the enzymes catalase and peroxidase rapidly degrade hydrogen peroxide. The innocuous degradation products are oxygen and water. Concentrated solutions containing 90% weight per volume H_2O_2 are prepared electrochemically. When diluted in high-quality deionized water to 6% and 3% and put into clean containers, the products remain stable. Concentrations of 10–25% hydrogen peroxide are sporicidal. Vapor-phase hydrogen peroxide (VPHP) is a cold gaseous sterilant that has advantages over the toxic or carcinogenic gases ethylene oxide and formaldehyde. VPHP does not require a pressurized chamber and is active at temperatures as low as 4°C and concentrations as low as 4 mg/L. It is incompatible with liquids and cellulose products. It penetrates the surface of some plastics. Automated equipment using vaporized hydrogen peroxide or hydrogen peroxide mixed with formic acid is available for sterilizing endoscopes.

Peracetic acid (CH_3COOOH) is prepared commercially from hydrogen peroxide, acetic acid, and a catalyst such as sulfuric acid. It is explosive in the pure form. It is usually used in dilute solution and transported in containers with vented caps to prevent increased pressure as oxygen is released. Peracetic acid is more active than hydrogen peroxide as a bactericidal and sporicidal agent. Concentrations of 250–500 ppm are effective against a broad range of bacteria in 5 minutes at pH 7.0 at 20°C. Bacterial spores are inactivated by 500–30,000 ppm peracetic acid. Only slightly increased concentrations are necessary in the presence of organic matter. Viruses require variable exposures. Enteroviruses require 2000 ppm for 15–30 minutes for inactivation.

An automated machine that uses buffered peracetic acid liquid of 0.1–0.5% concentration can be used for sterilization of medical, surgical, and dental instruments. Peracetic acid sterilization systems have also been adopted for hemodialyzers. The food processing and beverage industries use peracetic acid extensively because the breakdown products in high dilution do not produce objectionable odor, taste, or toxicity, and rinsing is not necessary.

Peracetic acid is a potent tumor promoter but a weak carcinogen. It is not mutagenic in the Ames test.

ULTRAVIOLET IRRADIATION

Ultraviolet irradiation is used in some health care facilities as an alternate mode of disinfection for patient care areas. It is typically deployed via an automated system, allowing for less staff exposure to decontamination products. It has rapid cidal activity against numerous pathogens, providing effective decontamination for most vegetative bacteria in less than 25 minutes and against *C difficile* in less than 1 hour.

HEAVY METALS

Heavy metals, principally mercury and silver, are now rarely used as disinfectants. Mercury is an environmental hazard, and some pathogenic bacteria have developed plasmid-mediated resistance to mercurials. Hypersensitivity to thimerosal is common, possibly in up to 40% of the population. These compounds are absorbed from solution by rubber and plastic closures. **Thimerosal** 0.001–0.004% is used safely as a preservative of certain vaccines, antitoxins, and immune sera.

Inorganic silver salts are strongly bactericidal. **Silver nitrate**, 1:1000, had been most commonly used, particularly as a preventive for gonococcal ophthalmitis in newborns. Antibiotic ointments have replaced silver nitrate for this indication. **Silver sulfadiazine** slowly releases silver and has been used to suppress bacterial growth in burn wounds (see Chapter 46).

STERILANTS

For many years, pressurized **steam (autoclaving)** at 120°C for 30 minutes has been the basic method for sterilizing instruments and other heat-resistant materials. When autoclaving is not possible, as with lensed instruments and materials containing plastic and rubber, **ethylene oxide**—diluted with either fluorocarbon or carbon dioxide to diminish explosive hazard—has been used at 440–1200 mg/L at 45–60°C with 30–60% relative humidity. The higher concentrations increase penetration.

Ethylene oxide is classified as a mutagen and carcinogen. The OSHA permissible exposure limit (PEL) for ethylene oxide is 1 ppm calculated as a time-weighted average. Alternative sterilants now being used include vapor-phase hydrogen peroxide, peracetic acid, ozone, gas plasma, chlorine dioxide, formaldehyde, and propylene oxide. Each of these sterilants has potential advantages and problems. Automated peracetic acid systems are used commonly for high-level decontamination and sterilization of endoscopes and hemodialyzers because of their effectiveness, automated features, and the low toxicity of the residual products of sterilization.

PRESERVATIVES

Disinfectants are used as preservatives to prevent the overgrowth of bacteria and fungi in pharmaceutical products, laboratory sera and reagents, cosmetic products, and contact lenses. Multi-use vials of medication that may be reentered through a rubber diaphragm, eye drops, and nose drops require preservatives. Preservatives should not be irritating or toxic to tissues to which they will be applied, they must be effective in preventing growth of microorganisms likely to contaminate solutions, and they must have sufficient solubility and stability to remain active.

Commonly used preservative agents include organic acids such as **benzoic acid** and salts, the **parabens** (alkyl esters of *p*-hydroxybenzoic acid), sorbic acid and salts, phenolic compounds, quaternary ammonium compounds, alcohols, and mercurials such as thimerosal in 0.001–0.004% concentration.

SUMMARY Miscellaneous Antimicrobials

Subclass, Drug	Mechanism of Action	Effects	Clinical Applications	Pharmacokinetics, Toxicities, Interactions
NITROIMIDAZOLE				
• Metronidazole	Disruption of electron transport chain	Bactericidal activity against susceptible anaerobic bacteria and protozoa	Anaerobic infections • vaginitis • *C difficile* colitis	Oral or IV • hepatic clearance ($t_{1/2}$ 8 h) • *Toxicity:* Gastrointestinal upset • metallic taste • neuropathy • seizures
• *Tinidazole: Oral; similar to metronidazole but dosed once daily; approved for trichomonas, giardiasis, and amebiasis*				
MACROLIDE				
• Fidaxomicin	Inhibits bacterial RNA polymerase	Bactericidal in gram-positive bacteria	*C difficile* colitis	Oral • blood levels negligible • *Toxicity:* Nonspecific gastrointestinal upset
RIFAMYCIN				
• Rifaximin	Inhibits bacterial RNA polymerase	Bactericidal activity in gram-positive and gram-negative bacteria	Travelers' diarrhea, hepatic encephalopathy, irritable bowel syndrome	Oral • blood levels negligible • *Toxicity:* Nausea
URINARY ANTISEPTICS				
• Nitrofurantoin	Not fully understood • disrupts protein synthesis and inhibits multiple bacterial enzyme systems	Bacteriostatic or bactericidal activity against susceptible bacteria	Uncomplicated urinary tract infections • long-term prophylaxis	Oral • rapid renal clearance ($t_{1/2}$ 0.5 h) • blood levels are negligible • contraindicated in renal failure • *Toxicity:* Gastrointestinal upset • neuropathies • hypersensitivity pneumonitis
• *Methenamine hippurate and methenamine mandelate: Oral; release formaldehyde at acidic pH in the urine; used only for prophylaxis, not treatment, of urinary tract infections*				

PREPARATIONS AVAILABLE

GENERIC NAME	AVAILABLE AS
MISCELLANEOUS ANTIMICROBIAL DRUGS	
Colistimethate sodium	Generic, Coly-Mycin M
Fidaxomicin	Dificid
Methenamine hippurate	Generic, Hiprex
Methenamine mandelate	Generic, Mandelamine
Metronidazole	Generic, Flagyl, Metro
Mupirocin	Generic, Bactroban, Centany
Nitrofurantoin	Generic, Macrodantin, Macrobid
Polymyxin B (Polymyxin B sulfate)	Generic
Rifaximin	Xifaxan

GENERIC NAME	AVAILABLE AS
DISINFECTANTS, ANTISEPTICS, & STERILANTS	
Benzalkonium	Generic, Zephiran
Benzoyl peroxide	Generic
Chlorhexidine gluconate topical	Generic, Hibiclens, Betasept, others
Chlorhexidine gluconate, oral rinse: 0.12%	Peridex, Periogard
Glutaraldehyde	Cidex
Iodine aqueous	Generic, Lugol's Solution
Iodine tincture	Generic
Nitrofurazone	Generic, Furacin
Ortho-phthalaldehyde	Cidex OPA
Povidone-iodine	Generic, Betadine
Silver nitrate	Generic
Thimerosal	Generic, Mersol

REFERENCES

Bischoff WE et al: Handwashing compliance by health care workers: The impact of introducing an accessible, alcohol-based hand antiseptic. Arch Intern Med 2000;160:1017.

Gordin FM et al: Reduction in nosocomial transmission of drug-resistant bacteria after introduction of an alcohol-based hand-rub. Infect Control Hosp Epidemiol 2005;26:650.

Hoonmo LK, DuPont HL: Rifaximin: A unique gastrointestinal-selective antibiotic for enteric diseases. Curr Opin Gastroenterol 2010;26:17.

Humphreys PN: Testing standards for sporicides. J Hosp Infect 2011;77:193.

Johnson S et al: Clinical Practice Guideline by the Infectious Diseases Society of America (IDSA) and Society for Healthcare Epidemiology of America (SHEA): 2021 Focused Update Guidelines on Management of *Clostridioides difficile* Infection in Adults. Clin Infect Dis 2021;73:e1029.

Leslie RA et al: Inactivation of SARS-CoV-2 by commercially available alcohol-based hand sanitizers. Am J Infect Control 2021;49:401.

Louie TJ et al: Fidaxomicin versus vancomycin for *Clostridium difficile* infection. N Engl J Med 2011;364:422.

Medical Letter: Tinidazole (Tindamax)—a new anti-protozoal drug. Med Lett Drugs Ther 2004;46:70.

Meyer GW: Endoscope disinfection. UpToDate 2019. www.uptodate.com/contents/endoscope-disinfection.

Noorani A et al: Systematic review and meta-analysis of preoperative antisepsis with chlorhexidine versus povidone-iodine in clean-contaminated surgery. Br J Surg 2010;97:1614.

Rutala WA, Weber DJ: Disinfection and sterilization in health care facilities: An overview and current issues. Infect Dis Clin N Am 2016;30:609.

Rutala WA, Weber DJ: New disinfection and sterilization methods. Emerg Infect Dis 2001;7:348.

Widmer AF, Frei R: Decontamination, disinfection, and sterilization. In: Murray PR et al (editors): *Manual of Clinical Microbiology*, 7th ed. American Society for Microbiology, 1999.

Workowski KA et al: Sexually Transmitted Infections Treatment Guidelines, 2021. MMWR Recomm Rep 2021;70:1.

CASE STUDY ANSWER

The patient may be treated with oral fidaxomicin, which is the preferred first-line drug for *C difficile* infection. Oral vancomycin is the alternate first-line agent and may be used preferentially due to lower cost compared to fidaxomicin. Metronidazole has shown clinical inferiority to oral vancomycin, and it should be reserved for mild cases of *C difficile* infection in patients who are unable to tolerate the preferred options or as an additional agent in fulmnant *C difficile* infection. The room should be cleaned with a bleach solution (5000 ppm) because it is sporicidal. Other sporicidal disinfectants also may be effective.

C H A P T E R

51 Clinical Use of Antimicrobial Agents

Saman Nematollahi, MD, Harry W. Lampiris, MD, & Daniel S. Maddix, PharmD*

CASE STUDY

A 65-year-old man undergoes percutaneous nephrostomy for acute nephrolithiasis and urosepsis while travelling in India. He receives systemic antimicrobial therapy with ciprofloxacin for 7 days and completely recovers. Two weeks later he returns to the USA and presents to the emergency department with confusion, dysuria, and chills. Physical examination reveals a blood pressure of 90/50, pulse 120, temperature 38.5°C, and respiratory rate 24. The patient is disoriented, but the physical examination is otherwise unremarkable. Laboratory test shows WBC 24,000/mm^3 and elevated serum lactate; urinalysis shows 300 WBC per high power field and 4+ bacteria. What possible organisms are likely to be responsible for the patient's symptoms? What antibiotic(s) would you choose for initial therapy of this potentially life-threatening infection?

The development of antimicrobial drugs represents one of the most important advances in therapeutics, both in the control or cure of serious infections and in the prevention and treatment of infectious complications of other therapeutic modalities such as cancer chemotherapy, immunosuppression, and surgery. However, evidence is overwhelming that antimicrobial agents are vastly overprescribed in outpatient settings in the USA, and the availability of antimicrobial agents without prescription in many developing countries has—by facilitating the development of resistance—already severely limited therapeutic options in the treatment of life-threatening infections.

The threat of antimicrobial resistance and its impact on treatment of severe infections is urgent. Antibiotic-resistant bacteria, especially the "ESKAPE" pathogens (*Enterococcus faecium, Staphylococcus aureus, Klebsiella pneumoniae, Acinetobacter baumannii, Pseudomonas aeruginosa,* and *Enterobacter* species) have been identified as specific MDR (multidrug-resistant) pathogens by the US Centers for Disease Control and Prevention (CDC) and the World Health Organization. Additionally, organisms classified by the CDC as urgent health threats include *Candida auris*, carbapenem-resistant Enterobacterales, carbapenem-resistant *Acinetobacter*, *Clostridioides difficile*, and drug-resistant *Neisseria gonorrhoeae*. The Infectious Disease Society of America had launched the "10 × '20 initiative" encouraging the development of 10 novel, efficacious, and safe systemically administered antibacterial agents by 2020. As of 2020, 14 antibacterials received FDA approval, 3 of which are novel agents, and dozens are in clinical development. Table 51–1 shows some of the novel agents and their spectrum of activity, such as anti-MRSA cephalosporin (ceftaroline), siderophore cephalosporin (cefiderocol), cephalosporin/β-lactamase inhibitor combinations (ceftazidime-avibactam and ceftolozane-tazobactam), carbapenem/β-lactamase inhibitor combinations (imipenem-cilastatin-relebactam and meropenem-vaborbactam), tetracycline (eravacycline), and aminoglycoside (plazomicin).

With the rise in antimicrobial resistance, the clinician should first determine whether antimicrobial therapy is warranted for a given patient. The specific questions one should ask include the following:

1. Is an antimicrobial agent indicated on the basis of clinical findings? Or is it prudent to wait until such clinical findings become apparent?

*In memoriam, 1962—2020.

TABLE 51–1 Novel antibacterials and spectrum of activity.

Agent	MRSA	Enterobacteriaceae				*Pseudomonas aeruginosa*	*Acinetobacter baumannii*
		ESBL	KPC	NDM	OXA-48		
Ceftaroline	+	–	–	–	–	–	–
Cefiderocol	–	+	+	+	+	+	+
Ceftazidime-avibactam	–	+	+	–	+	±	–
Ceftolozane-tazobactam	–	+	–	–	–	+	–
Imipenem-cilastatin-relebactam	–	+	+	–	–	+	–
Meropenem-vaborbactam	–	+	+	–	–	±	–
Eravacycline	+	+	+	+	+	–	+
Plazomicin	–	+	+	–	+	±	±

MRSA, methicillin-resistant *Staphylococcus aureus*; ESBL, extended-spectrum β-lactamase; KPC, *Klebsiella pneumoniae* carbapenemase; NDM, New Delhi metallo-β-lactamase; OXA-48, oxacillin carbapenemase number 48.

2. Have appropriate clinical specimens been obtained to establish a microbiologic diagnosis?
3. What are the likely etiologic agents for the patient's illness?
4. What measures should be taken to protect individuals exposed to the index case to prevent secondary cases, and what measures should be implemented to prevent further exposure?
5. Is there clinical evidence (eg, from well-executed clinical trials) that antimicrobial therapy will confer clinical benefit for the patient?

Once a specific cause is identified based on specific microbiologic tests, the following further questions should be considered:

1. If a specific microbial pathogen is identified, can a narrower-spectrum agent be substituted for the initial empiric drug?
2. Is one agent or a combination of agents necessary?
3. What is the optimal dose, route of administration, and duration of therapy?
4. What specific tests (eg, susceptibility testing) should be undertaken to identify patients who will not respond to treatment?
5. What adjunctive measures can be undertaken to eradicate the infection? For example, is surgery feasible for removal of devitalized tissue or foreign bodies—or drainage of an abscess—into which antimicrobial agents may be unable to penetrate? Is it possible to decrease the dosage of immunosuppressive therapy in patients who have undergone organ transplantation? Is it possible to reduce morbidity or mortality due to the infection by reducing host immunologic response to the infection (eg, using corticosteroids for the treatment of severe *Pneumocystis jirovecii* pneumonia or meningitis due to *Streptococcus pneumoniae*)?

EMPIRIC ANTIMICROBIAL THERAPY

Antimicrobial agents are frequently used before the pathogen responsible for a particular illness or the susceptibility to a particular antimicrobial agent is known. This use of antimicrobial agents is called empiric (or presumptive) therapy and is based on experience with a particular clinical entity. The usual justification for empiric therapy is the hope that early intervention will improve the outcome; in the best cases, this has been established by placebo-controlled, double-blind, prospective clinical trials. For example, treatment of febrile episodes in neutropenic cancer patients with empiric antimicrobial therapy has been demonstrated to have impressive morbidity and mortality benefits even though the specific bacterial agent responsible for fever is determined for only a minority of such episodes.

Finally, there are many clinical entities, such as certain episodes of community-acquired pneumonia, in which it is difficult to identify a specific pathogen. In such cases, a clinical response to empiric therapy may be an important clue to the likely pathogen.

Frequently, the signs and symptoms of infection diminish as a result of empiric therapy, and microbiologic test results become available to establish a specific microbiologic diagnosis. At the time that the pathogenic organism responsible for the illness is identified, empiric therapy is optimally modified to **definitive therapy,** which is typically narrower in coverage and is given for an appropriate duration based on the results of clinical trials, or experience when clinical trial data are not available.

Approach to Empiric Therapy

Initiation of empiric therapy should follow a specific and systematic approach.

A. Formulate a Clinical Diagnosis of Microbial Infection

Using all available data, the clinician should determine that there is a clinical syndrome compatible with infection (eg, pneumonia, cellulitis, sinusitis).

B. Obtain Specimens for Laboratory Examination

Examination of stained specimens by microscopy or simple examination of an uncentrifuged sample of urine for white blood cells and bacteria may provide important immediate etiologic clues. Cultures of selected anatomic sites (blood, sputum, urine, cerebrospinal fluid, and stool) and nonculture methods (antigen testing, polymerase chain reaction, and serology) also may confirm specific etiologic agents.

C. Formulate a Microbiologic Diagnosis

The history, physical examination, and immediately available laboratory results (eg, Gram stain of urine or sputum) may provide highly specific information. For example, in a young man with urethritis and a Gram-stained smear from the urethral meatus demonstrating intracellular Gram-negative diplococci, the most likely pathogen is *Neisseria gonorrhoeae*. In the latter instance, however, the clinician should be aware that a significant number of patients with gonococcal urethritis have negative Gram stains for the organism and that a significant number of patients with gonococcal urethritis harbor concurrent chlamydial infection that is not demonstrated on the Gram-stained smear.

D. Determine the Necessity for Empiric Therapy

Whether to initiate empiric therapy is an important clinical decision based partly on experience and partly on data from clinical trials. Empiric therapy is indicated when there is a significant risk of serious morbidity or mortality if therapy is withheld until a specific pathogen is detected by the clinical laboratory.

In other settings, empiric therapy may be indicated for public health reasons rather than for demonstrated superior outcome of therapy in a specific patient. For example, urethritis in a young sexually active man usually requires treatment for *N gonorrhoeae* and *Chlamydia trachomatis* despite the absence of microbiologic confirmation at the time of diagnosis. Because the risk of noncompliance with follow-up visits in this patient population may lead to further transmission of these sexually transmitted pathogens, empiric therapy is warranted.

E. Institute Treatment

Selection of empiric therapy may be based on the microbiologic diagnosis or a clinical diagnosis without available microbiologic clues. If no microbiologic information is available, the antimicrobial spectrum of the agent or agents chosen must necessarily be broader, taking into account the most likely pathogens responsible for the patient's illness.

Choice of Antimicrobial Agent

Selection from among several drugs depends on **host factors** that include the following: (1) concomitant disease states (eg, advanced HIV, neutropenia due to the use of cytotoxic chemotherapy, organ transplantation, severe chronic liver or kidney disease) or the use of immunosuppressive medications; (2) prior adverse drug effects; (3) impaired elimination or detoxification of the drug (may be genetically predetermined but more frequently is associated with impaired renal or hepatic function due to underlying disease); (4) age of the patient; (5) pregnancy status; and (6) epidemiologic exposure (eg, exposure to a sick family member or pet, recent hospitalization, recent travel, occupational exposure, or new sexual partner).

Pharmacologic factors include (1) the kinetics of absorption, distribution, and elimination; (2) the ability of the drug to be delivered to the site of infection; (3) the potential toxicity of an agent; and (4) pharmacokinetic or pharmacodynamic interactions with other drugs.

Knowledge of the **susceptibility** of an organism to a specific agent in a hospital or community setting is important in the selection of empiric therapy. Pharmacokinetic differences among agents with similar antimicrobial spectrums may be exploited to reduce the frequency of dosing (eg, ceftriaxone, ertapenem, or daptomycin may be conveniently given once every 24 hours). Finally, increasing consideration is being given to the cost of antimicrobial therapy, especially when multiple agents with comparable efficacy and toxicity are available for a specific infection. Changing from intravenous to oral antibiotics for prolonged administration can be particularly cost-effective.

Brief guides to empiric therapy based on presumptive microbial diagnosis and site of infection are given in Tables 51–2 and 51–3.

TABLE 51–2 Empiric antimicrobial therapy based on microbiologic etiology.

Suspected or Proven Disease or Pathogen	Drugs of First Choice	Alternative Drugs
Gram-negative cocci (aerobic)		
Moraxella (Branhamella) catarrhalis	TMP-SMZ,[1] cephalosporin (second- or third-generation)[2], amoxicillin-clavulanate	Quinolone,[3] macrolide[4]
Neisseria gonorrhoeae	Ceftriaxone, cefixime	Gentamicin + azithromycin
Neisseria meningitidis	Penicillin G, ceftriaxone	Chloramphenicol, ampicillin, cefotaxime
Gram-negative rods (aerobic)		
E coli, Klebsiella, Proteus	Cephalosporin (first- or second-generation),[2] TMP-SMZ[1]	Quinolone,[3] aminoglycoside[5]
Enterobacter, Citrobacter, Serratia	TMP-SMZ,[1] quinolone,[3] carbapenem[6]	Antipseudomonal penicillin,[7] aminoglycoside,[5] cefepime

(*continued*)

TABLE 51–2 Empiric antimicrobial therapy based on microbiologic etiology. (Continued)

Suspected or Proven Disease or Pathogen	Drugs of First Choice	Alternative Drugs
Shigella	Quinolone[3]	TMP-SMZ,[1] ampicillin, azithromycin, ceftriaxone
Salmonella	Quinolone,[3] ceftriaxone	Chloramphenicol, ampicillin, TMP-SMZ[1]
Campylobacter jejuni	Erythromycin or azithromycin	Doxycycline, quinolone[3]
Brucella species	Doxycycline + rifampin or aminoglycoside[5]	Chloramphenicol + aminoglycoside[5] or TMP-SMZ[1]
Helicobacter pylori	Proton pump inhibitor + amoxicillin + clarithromycin	Bismuth + metronidazole + tetracycline + proton pump inhibitor
Vibrio species	Doxycycline	Quinolone,[3] TMP-SMZ[1]
Pseudomonas aeruginosa	Antipseudomonal penicillin, cefepime	Antipseudomonal penicillin ± quinolone,[3] ceftazidime, antipseudomonal carbapenem,[6] or aztreonam, tobramycin
Burkholderia cepacia (formerly *Pseudomonas cepacia*)	TMP-SMZ[1]	Ceftazidime, chloramphenicol
Stenotrophomonas maltophilia (formerly *Xanthomonas maltophilia*)	TMP-SMZ[1]	Minocycline, ticarcillin-clavulanate, tigecycline, ceftazidime, quinolone[3]
Legionella species	Azithromycin, quinolone[3]	Clarithromycin, erythromycin
Gram-positive cocci (aerobic)		
Streptococcus pneumoniae	Penicillin[8]	Doxycycline, ceftriaxone, antipneumococcal quinolone,[3] macrolide,[4] linezolid
Streptococcus pyogenes (group A)	Penicillin, clindamycin	Erythromycin, aminopenicillin, cephalosporin (first-generation)[2]
Streptococcus agalactiae (group B)	Penicillin (± aminoglycoside[5])	Vancomycin
Viridans streptococci	Penicillin	Cephalosporin (first- or third-generation),[2] vancomycin
Staphylococcus aureus		
β-Lactamase negative	Penicillin	Cephalosporin (first-generation),[2] vancomycin
β-Lactamase positive	Penicillinase-resistant penicillin[9]	As above
Methicillin-resistant	Vancomycin	TMP-SMZ,[1] minocycline, linezolid, daptomycin, tigecycline
Enterococcus (ampicillin/penicillin susceptible)	Penicillin, ampicillin	Ampicillin + aminoglycoside[5]/ceftriaxone (for endocarditis), vancomycin
Enterococcus (ampicillin-resistant, vancomycin susceptible)	Vancomycin	Linezolid, daptomycin
Enterococcus (ampicillin- and vancomycin-resistant)[10]	Linezolid, daptomycin	Tigecycline, quinupristin/dalfopristin (E faecium only)
Gram-positive rods (aerobic)		
Bacillus species (non-*anthracis*)	Vancomycin	Imipenem, quinolone,[3] clindamycin
Listeria species	Ampicillin (± aminoglycoside[5])	TMP-SMZ[1], meropenem
Nocardia species	Sulfadiazine, TMP-SMZ[1]	Minocycline, imipenem, amikacin, linezolid
Anaerobic bacteria		
Gram-positive *(clostridia, Peptococcus, Actinomyces, Peptostreptococcus)*	Penicillin, clindamycin	Vancomycin, carbapenem,[6] chloramphenicol
Clostridioides difficile	Vancomycin (oral), fidaxomicin	Metronidazole
Bacteroides fragilis	Metronidazole	Chloramphenicol, carbapenem,[6] β-lactam–β-lactamase-inhibitor combinations, clindamycin, tigecycline
Fusobacterium, Prevotella, Porphyromonas	Metronidazole	As for *B fragilis*

(continued)

TABLE 51–2 Empiric antimicrobial therapy based on microbiologic etiology. (Continued)

Suspected or Proven Disease or Pathogen	Drugs of First Choice	Alternative Drugs
Mycobacteria		
Mycobacterium tuberculosis	Isoniazid + rifampin + ethambutol + pyrazinamide	Streptomycin, capreomycin, moxifloxacin, amikacin, ethionamide, cycloserine, PAS, linezolid, bedaquiline
Mycobacterium leprae		
Multibacillary	Dapsone + rifampin + clofazimine	
Paucibacillary	Dapsone + rifampin	
Mycoplasma pneumoniae	Doxycycline, azithromycin	Erythromycin, clarithromycin, quinolone[3]
Chlamydia		
C trachomatis	Doxycycline	Azithromycin, ofloxacin, levofloxacin
C pneumoniae	Doxycycline, erythromycin	Clarithromycin, azithromycin, levofloxacin, moxifloxacin
C psittaci	Doxycycline	Azithromycin
Spirochetes		
Borrelia recurrentis	Doxycycline	Erythromycin, chloramphenicol, penicillin
Borrelia burgdorferi		
Early	Doxycycline, amoxicillin	Cefuroxime axetil, azithromycin
Late	Ceftriaxone	Doxycycline
Leptospira species	Penicillin, ceftriaxone	Doxycycline
Treponema species	Penicillin	Doxycycline, ceftriaxone
Fungi		
Aspergillus species	Voriconazole	Amphotericin B, itraconazole, posaconazole, isavuconazole
Blastomyces species	Amphotericin B (severe infection)	Itraconazole
Candida species	Amphotericin B, echinocandin[11]	Fluconazole, itraconazole, voriconazole, otesecon-azole, ibrexafungerp
Cryptococcus neoformans	Amphotericin B ± flucytosine (5-FC)	Fluconazole, voriconazole
Coccidioides immitis/posadasii	Amphotericin B (severe infection)	Fluconazole, itraconazole, voriconazole, posacon-azole, isavuconazole
Fusarium solani	Voriconazole	Amphotericin B, posaconazole, isavuconazole
Histoplasma capsulatum	Amphotericin B (severe infection)	Itraconazole, posaconazole, isavuconazole
Mucorales (Rhizopus, Mucor)	Amphotericin B	Posaconazole, isavuconazole
Sporothrix schenckii	Amphotericin B (severe infection)	Itraconazole

[1]Trimethoprim-sulfamethoxazole (TMP-SMZ) is a mixture of one part trimethoprim plus five parts sulfamethoxazole.

[2]First-generation cephalosporins: cefazolin for parenteral administration; cefadroxil or cephalexin for oral administration. Second-generation cephalosporins: cefuroxime for parenteral administration; cefaclor, cefuroxime axetil, cefprozil for oral administration. Third-generation cephalosporins: ceftazidime, cefotaxime, ceftriaxone for parenteral administration; cefixime, cefpodoxime, ceftibuten, cefdinir, cefditoren for oral administration. Fourth-generation cephalosporin: cefepime for parenteral administration. Cephamycins: cefoxitin and cefotetan for parenteral administration.

[3]Quinolones: ciprofloxacin, gemifloxacin, levofloxacin, moxifloxacin, norfloxacin, ofloxacin. Norfloxacin is not effective for the treatment of systemic infections. Gemifloxacin, levofloxacin, and moxifloxacin have excellent activity against pneumococci. Ciprofloxacin and levofloxacin have good activity against *Pseudomonas aeruginosa*. Moxifloxacin, levofloxacin, and gemifloxacin are used as the respiratory quinolones.

[4]Macrolides: azithromycin, clarithromycin, dirithromycin, erythromycin.

[5]Generally, streptomycin and gentamicin are used to treat infections with gram-positive organisms, whereas gentamicin, tobramycin, and amikacin are used to treat infections with gram-negatives.

[6]Carbapenems: doripenem, ertapenem, imipenem, meropenem. Ertapenem lacks activity against enterococci, *Acinetobacter*, and *P aeruginosa*.

[7]Antipseudomonal penicillin: piperacillin, piperacillin-tazobactam, ticarcillin-clavulanic acid.

[8]See footnote 3 in Table 51–2 for guidelines on the treatment of penicillin-resistant pneumococcal meningitis.

[9]Parenteral nafcillin or oxacillin; oral dicloxacillin.

[10]There is no regimen that is reliably bactericidal for vancomycin-resistant enterococcus for which there is extensive clinical experience; daptomycin has bactericidal activity in vitro. Regimens that have been reported to be efficacious include nitrofurantoin (for urinary tract infection); potential regimens for bacteremia include daptomycin, linezolid, and quinupristin/dalfopristin.

[11]Echinocandins: anidulafungin, caspofungin, micafungin.

TABLE 51–3 Empiric antimicrobial therapy based on site of infection.

Presumed Site of Infection	Common Pathogens	Drugs of First Choice	Alternative Drugs
Bacterial endocarditis			
Acute	*Staphylococcus aureus*	Vancomycin + ceftriaxone	Penicillinase-resistant penicillin[1] + gentamicin
Subacute	Viridans *streptococci*, enterococci	Penicillin + gentamicin	Vancomycin + gentamicin
Septic arthritis			
Child	*Haemophilus influenzae, S aureus*, β-hemolytic streptococci	Vancomycin + ceftriaxone	Vancomycin + ampicillin-sulbactam or ertapenem
Adult	*S aureus*, Enterobacteriaceae, *Neisseria gonorrhoeae*	Vancomycin + ceftriaxone	Vancomycin + ertapenem, or quinolone
Acute otitis media, sinusitis	*H influenzae, Streptococcus pneumoniae, Moraxella catarrhalis*	Amoxicillin	Amoxicillin-clavulanate, cefuroxime axetil, cefpodoxime
Meningitis			
Neonate	Group B streptococcus, *Escherichia coli, Listeria monocytogenes*	Ampicillin + cephalosporin (third-generation)	Ampicillin + aminoglycoside, chloramphenicol, meropenem
Child	*H influenzae, S pneumoniae, N meningitidis*	Ceftriaxone ± vancomycin[3]	Chloramphenicol, meropenem
Adult (18–50 years)	*S pneumoniae, N meningitidis*	Ceftriaxone	Vancomycin + ceftriaxone[2]
Adult (>50 years) or immunocompromised	*S pneumoniae, N meningitidis, Listeria monocytogenes*	Ceftriaxone + ampicillin	Vancomycin + ceftriaxone + ampicillin[2]
Peritonitis due to ruptured viscus; intraabdominal infection	Coliforms, *Bacteroides fragilis*, Enterococci, viridans *Streptococci*	Metronidazole + cephalosporin (third-generation), piperacillin-tazobactam	Carbapenem, tigecycline, metronidazole + levofloxacin/ciprofloxacin
Pneumonia			
Neonate	As in neonatal meningitis		
Child	*S pneumoniae, S aureus, H influenzae*	Ceftriaxone, cefuroxime, cefotaxime	Ampicillin-sulbactam
Adult (community-acquired)	*S pneumoniae, Mycoplasma pneumoniae, Legionella pneumophila, H influenzae, S aureus, Chlamydia pneumoniae*	**Outpatient, healthy/no recent antibiotic exposure:** Macrolide,[3] amoxicillin, doxycycline **Outpatient, comorbidities/recent antibiotic exposure:** Respiratory quinolne;[4] amoxicillin-clavulanate or cefuroxime or cefpodoxime + macrolide[3] or doxycycline	
		Inpatient: Macrolide[3] or doxycycline + cefotaxime, ceftriaxone, ertapenem, or ampicillin; respiratory quinolone[4]	
Adult (hospital-acquired)	*S aureus, Pseudomonas aeruginosa*, Enterobacterales	Vancomycin or linezolid (if concern for MRSA) + piperacillin-tazobactam or cefepime or antipseudomonal carbapenem ± aminoglycoside or respiratory quinolone[5] (depending on local antibiogram and illness severity)	
Skin/soft tissue infection	*Streptococcus pyogenes* (group A), *S aureus*	**Nonpustular, no MRSA**: First-generation cephalosporin, penicillinase-resistant penicillin	
		Pustular, MRSA: TMP-SMZ, doxycycline, linezolid, vancomycin, daptomycin	
Skin/soft tissue infection (diabetic foot)	Above, plus Enterobacterales, *Bacteroides fragilis*, enterococci	Ceftriaxone or cefepime or levofloxacin or ciprofloxacin + metronidazole, ampicillin-sulbactam, piperacillin-tazobactam, carbapenem, ± vancomycin or linezolid (depending on MRSA risk factors)	
Septicemia	Any	Vancomycin + cephalosporin (third-generation) or piperacillin-tazobactam or imipenem or meropenem	
Septicemia with granulocytopenia	Any	Antipseudomonal penicillin + aminoglycoside; ceftazidime; cefepime; imipenem or meropenem; consider vancomycin if concern for catheter-related infection or severe mucositis; consider addition of systemic antifungal therapy if fever persists beyond 5-7 days of empiric therapy	
Urinary tract infection (uncomplicated)	*E coli, Klebsiella pneumoniae, Proteus mirabilis, Staphylococcus saprophyticus*, enterococci	TMP-SMZ, fosfomycin, nitrofurantoin	
Urinary tract infection (complicated or pyelonephritis)	Above	**Community**: Ceftriaxone, levofloxacin, ciprofloxacin, ertapenem	
	Above, plus *Enterobacter* species, *Pseudomonas aeruginosa*	**Nosocomial:** Cefepime, piperacillin-tazobactam, antipseudomonal carbapenem	

[1]See footnote 9, Table 51–2.

[2]When meningitis with penicillin-resistant pneumococcus is suspected, empiric therapy with this regimen is recommended.

[3]Clarithromycin or azithromycin (an azalide) may be used. Can be used as outpatient monotherapy if local pneumococcal resistance to macrolides is <25%.

[4]Quinolones used to treat pneumococcal infections include levofloxacin, moxifloxacin, and gemifloxacin.

ANTIMICROBIAL THERAPY OF INFECTIONS WITH KNOWN ETIOLOGY

INTERPRETATION OF CULTURE RESULTS

Properly obtained and processed specimens for culture frequently yield reliable information about the cause of infection. The lack of a confirmatory microbiologic diagnosis may be due to the following:

1. Sample error, eg, obtaining cultures after antimicrobial agents have been administered, inadequate volume or quantity of specimen obtained, or contamination of specimens sent for culture
2. Noncultivable or slow-growing organisms (*Histoplasma capsulatum*, *Bartonella* or *Brucella* species), in which cultures are often discarded before sufficient growth has occurred for detection
3. Requesting *bacterial* cultures when infection is due to other organisms
4. Not recognizing the need for special media or isolation techniques (eg, charcoal yeast extract agar for isolation of *Legionella* species, shell-vial tissue culture system for rapid isolation of cytomegalovirus)

Even in the setting of a classic infectious disease for which isolation techniques have been established for decades (eg, pneumococcal pneumonia, pulmonary tuberculosis, streptococcal pharyngitis), the sensitivity of the culture technique may be inadequate to identify all cases of the disease.

GUIDING ANTIMICROBIAL THERAPY OF ESTABLISHED INFECTIONS

Susceptibility Testing

Testing bacterial pathogens in vitro for their susceptibility to antimicrobial agents is extremely valuable in confirming susceptibility, ideally to a narrow-spectrum nontoxic antimicrobial drug. Tests measure the concentration of drug required to inhibit growth of the organism **(minimal inhibitory concentration [MIC])** or to kill the organism **(minimal bactericidal concentration [MBC])**. The results of these tests can then be correlated with known drug concentrations in various body compartments. Only MICs are routinely measured in most infections, whereas in infections in which bactericidal therapy is required for eradication of infection (eg, meningitis, endocarditis, sepsis in the granulocytopenic host), MBC measurements occasionally may be useful.

Specialized Assay Methods

A. Beta-Lactamase Assay

For some bacteria (eg, *Haemophilus* species), the susceptibility patterns of strains are similar except for the production of β lactamase. In these cases, extensive susceptibility testing may not be required, and a direct test for β lactamase using a chromogenic β-lactam substrate (nitrocefin disk) may be substituted.

B. Synergy Studies

Synergy studies are in vitro tests that attempt to measure synergistic, additive, indifferent, or antagonistic drug interactions. In general, these tests have not been standardized and have not correlated well with clinical outcome. (See section Antimicrobial Drug Combinations for details.)

MONITORING THERAPEUTIC RESPONSE: DURATION OF THERAPY

The therapeutic response may be monitored microbiologically or clinically. Cultures of specimens taken from infected sites should eventually become sterile or demonstrate eradication of the pathogen and are useful for documenting recurrence or relapse. Follow-up cultures may also be useful for detecting superinfections or the development of resistance. Clinically, the patient's systemic manifestations of infection (malaise, fever, leukocytosis) should abate, and the clinical findings should improve (eg, as shown by clearing of radiographic infiltrates or lessening hypoxemia in pneumonia).

The duration of definitive therapy required for cure depends on the pathogen, the site of infection, and host factors (immunocompromised patients generally require longer courses of treatment). Precise data on duration of therapy exist for some infections (eg, streptococcal pharyngitis, syphilis, gonorrhea, tuberculosis, and cryptococcal meningitis). In many other situations, duration of therapy is determined empirically. Minimizing duration of antimicrobial therapy for specific infections is an intervention that may help prevent the development of antimicrobial resistance. Recent studies have shown that shorter durations are as effective as prolonged therapies for syndromes such as pneumonia, cellulitis, pyelonephritis, and uncomplicated Gram-negative bacteremia. For many infections, a combined medical-surgical approach may be required for clinical cure.

Clinical Failure of Antimicrobial Therapy

When the patient has an inadequate clinical or microbiologic response to antimicrobial therapy selected by in vitro susceptibility testing, systematic investigation should be undertaken to determine the cause of failure. Errors in susceptibility testing are rare, but the original results should be confirmed by repeat testing. Drug dosing and absorption should be scrutinized and tested directly using serum measurements, pill counting, or directly observed therapy.

The clinical data should be reviewed to determine whether the patient's immune function is adequate and, if not, what can be done to maximize it. For example, are adequate numbers of granulocytes present and is undiagnosed immunodeficiency, malignancy, or malnutrition present? The presence of abscesses or foreign bodies should also be considered. Finally, culture and susceptibility testing should be repeated to determine whether superinfection has occurred with another organism or whether the original pathogen has developed drug resistance.

ANTIMICROBIAL PHARMACODYNAMICS

The time course of drug concentration is closely related to the antimicrobial effect at the site of infection and to any toxic effects. Pharmacodynamic factors include pathogen susceptibility testing, drug bactericidal versus bacteriostatic activity, drug synergism, antagonism, and post-antibiotic effects. Together with pharmacokinetics, pharmacodynamic information permits the selection of optimal antimicrobial dosage regimens.

Bacteriostatic Versus Bactericidal Activity

Antibacterial agents may be classified as bacteriostatic or bactericidal (Table 51–4). For agents that are primarily bacteriostatic, inhibitory drug concentrations are much lower than bactericidal drug concentrations. In general, cell wall-active agents are bactericidal, and drugs that inhibit protein synthesis are bacteriostatic.

The classification of antibacterial agents as bactericidal or bacteriostatic has limitations. Some agents that are considered to be bacteriostatic may be bactericidal against selected organisms. On the other hand, enterococci are inhibited but not killed by vancomycin, penicillin, or ampicillin used as single agents.

Bacteriostatic and bactericidal agents are equivalent for the treatment of most infectious diseases in immunocompetent hosts. Bactericidal agents should be selected over bacteriostatic ones in circumstances in which local or systemic host defenses are impaired. Bactericidal agents are required for treatment of endocarditis and other endovascular infections, meningitis, and infections in neutropenic patients.

Bactericidal agents can be divided into two groups: agents that exhibit **concentration-dependent killing** (eg, aminoglycosides and quinolones) and agents that exhibit **time-dependent killing** (eg, β-lactams and vancomycin). For drugs whose killing action is concentration-dependent, the rate and extent of killing increase with increasing drug concentrations. Concentration-dependent killing is one of the pharmacodynamic factors responsible for the efficacy of once-daily dosing of aminoglycosides. For drugs whose killing action is time-dependent, bactericidal activity continues as long as serum concentrations are greater than the MBC.

TABLE 51–4 Bactericidal and bacteriostatic antibacterial agents.

Bactericidal Agents	Bacteriostatic Agents
Aminoglycosides	Chloramphenicol
Bacitracin	Clindamycin
β-Lactam antibiotics	Ethambutol
Daptomycin	Macrolides
Fosfomycin	Nitrofurantoin
Glycopeptide antibiotics	Novobiocin
Isoniazid	Oxazolidinones
Ketolides	Sulfonamides
Metronidazole	Tetracyclines
Polymyxins	Tigecycline
Pyrazinamide	Trimethoprim
Quinolones	
Rifampin	
Streptogramins	

Post-Antibiotic Effect

Persistent suppression of bacterial growth after limited exposure to an antimicrobial agent is known as the post-antibiotic effect (PAE). The PAE can be expressed mathematically as follows:

$$PAE = T - C$$

where T is the time required for the viable count in the test (in vitro) culture to increase 10-fold above the count observed immediately before drug removal and C is the time required for the count in an untreated culture to increase 10-fold above the count observed immediately after completion of the same procedure used on the test culture. The PAE reflects the time required for bacteria to return to logarithmic growth.

Proposed mechanisms include (1) slow recovery after reversible nonlethal damage to cell structures; (2) persistence of the drug at a binding site or within the periplasmic space; and (3) the need to synthesize new enzymes before growth can resume. Most antimicrobials possess significant in vitro PAEs (≥1.5 hours) against susceptible Gram-positive cocci (Table 51–5). Antimicrobials with significant PAEs against susceptible Gram-negative bacilli are limited to carbapenems and agents that inhibit protein or DNA synthesis.

TABLE 51–5 Antibacterial agents with in vitro post-antibiotic effects ≥1.5 hours.

Against Gram-Positive Cocci	Against Gram-Negative Bacilli
Aminoglycosides	Aminoglycosides
Carbapenems	Carbapenems
Cephalosporins	Chloramphenicol
Chloramphenicol	Quinolones
Clindamycin	Rifampin
Daptomycin	Tetracyclines
Glycopeptide antibiotics	Tigecycline
Ketolides	
Macrolides	
Oxazolidinones	
Penicillins	
Quinolones	
Rifampin	
Streptogramins	
Sulfonamides	
Tetracyclines	
Tigecycline	
Trimethoprim	

In vivo PAEs are usually much longer than in vitro PAEs. This is thought to be due to **post-antibiotic leukocyte enhancement (PALE)** and exposure of bacteria to subinhibitory antibiotic concentrations. The efficacy of once-daily dosing regimens is in part due to the PAE. Aminoglycosides and quinolones possess concentration-dependent PAEs; thus, high doses of aminoglycosides given once daily result in enhanced bactericidal activity and extended PAEs. This combination of pharmacodynamic effects allows aminoglycoside serum concentrations that are below the MICs of target organisms to remain effective for extended periods of time.

PHARMACOKINETIC CONSIDERATIONS

Route of Administration

Many antimicrobial agents have similar pharmacokinetic properties when given orally or parenterally (eg, tetracyclines, trimethoprim-sulfamethoxazole, quinolones, metronidazole, clindamycin, rifampin, linezolid, and fluconazole). In most cases, oral therapy with these drugs is equally effective, is less costly, and results in fewer complications than parenteral therapy.

The intravenous route is preferred in the following situations: (1) for critically ill patients; (2) for patients with bacterial meningitis or endocarditis (at least initially); (3) for patients with lack of source control; (4) for patients with nausea, vomiting, gastrectomy, ileus, or diseases that may impair oral absorption; and (5) when giving antimicrobials that are poorly absorbed following oral administration. There is now accumulating evidence that oral antibacterials can be used for osteomyelitis, endocarditis, and bacteremias.

Conditions That Alter Antimicrobial Pharmacokinetics

Various diseases and physiologic states alter the pharmacokinetics of antimicrobial agents. Impairment of renal or hepatic function may result in decreased elimination. Table 51–6 lists drugs that require dosage reduction in patients with renal or hepatic insufficiency. Failure to reduce antimicrobial agent dosage in such patients may cause toxic effects. Conversely, patients with burns, cystic fibrosis, or trauma may have increased dosage requirements for selected agents. The pharmacokinetics of antimicrobials is also altered in the elderly (see Chapter 60), in neonates (see Chapter 59), and in pregnancy.

Drug Concentrations in Body Fluids

Most antimicrobial agents are well distributed to most body tissues and fluids. Penetration into the cerebrospinal fluid is an exception. Most do not penetrate uninflamed meninges to an appreciable extent. In the presence of meningitis, however, the cerebrospinal fluid concentrations of many antimicrobials increase (Table 51–7).

TABLE 51–7 Cerebrospinal fluid (CSF) penetration of selected antimicrobials.

Antimicrobial Agent	CSF Concentration (Uninflamed Meninges) as % of Serum Concentration	CSF Concentration (Inflamed Meninges) as % of Serum Concentration
Ampicillin	2–3	2–100
Aztreonam	2	5
Cefepime	0–2	4–12
Cefotaxime	22.5	27–36
Ceftazidime	0.7	20–40
Ceftriaxone	0.8–1.6	16
Cefuroxime	20	17–88
Ciprofloxacin	6–27	26–37
Imipenem	3.1	11–41
Meropenem	0–7	1–52
Nafcillin	2–15	5–27
Penicillin G	1–2	8–18
Sulfamethoxazole	40	12–47
Trimethoprim	<41	12–69
Vancomycin	0	1–53

TABLE 51–6 Antimicrobial agents that require dosage adjustment or are contraindicated in patients with renal or hepatic impairment.

Dosage Adjustment Needed in Renal Impairment	Contraindicated in Renal Impairment	Dosage Adjustment Needed in Hepatic Impairment
Acyclovir, amantadine, aminoglycosides, aztreonam, carbapenems, cephalosporins,[1] clarithromycin, colistin, cycloserine, dalbavancin, daptomycin, didanosine, emtricitabine, ethambutol, ethionamide, famciclovir, fluconazole, flucytosine, foscarnet, ganciclovir, lamivudine, oseltamivir, penicillins,[2] peramivir, polymyxin B, pyrazinamide, quinolones,[3] ribavirin, rifabutin, rimantadine, stavudine, telavancin, telbivudine, telithromycin, tenofovir, terbinafine, trimethoprim-sulfamethoxazole, valacyclovir, vancomycin, zidovudine	Cidofovir, methenamine, nalidixic acid, nitrofurantoin, sulfonamides (long-acting), tetracyclines[4]	Abacavir, atazanavir, caspofungin, chloramphenicol, clindamycin, erythromycin, fosamprenavir, indinavir, metronidazole, rimantadine, tigecycline

[1]Except ceftriaxone.

[2]Except antistaphylococcal penicillins (eg, nafcillin and dicloxacillin).

[3]Except moxifloxacin.

[4]Except doxycycline and minocycline.

Monitoring Serum Concentrations of Antimicrobial Agents

For most antimicrobial agents, the relation between dose and therapeutic outcome is well established, and serum concentration monitoring is unnecessary for these drugs. To justify routine serum concentration monitoring, it should be established (1) that a direct relationship exists between drug concentrations and efficacy or toxicity; (2) that substantial interpatient variability exists in serum concentrations on standard doses; (3) that a small difference exists between therapeutic and toxic serum concentrations; (4) that the clinical efficacy or toxicity of the drug is delayed or difficult to measure; and (5) that an accurate assay is available.

In clinical practice, serum concentration monitoring is routinely performed on patients receiving azoles, aminoglycosides, or vancomycin. Flucytosine serum concentration monitoring has been shown to reduce toxicity when doses are adjusted to maintain peak concentrations below 100 mcg/mL.

MANAGEMENT OF ANTIMICROBIAL DRUG TOXICITY

Owing to the large number of antimicrobials available, it is usually possible to select an effective alternative in patients who develop serious drug toxicity (see Table 51–2). However, for some infections there are no effective alternatives to the drug of choice. For example, in patients with neurosyphilis who have a history of anaphylaxis to penicillin, it is necessary to perform skin testing and desensitization to penicillin. It is important to obtain a clear history of drug allergy and other adverse drug reactions. A patient with a documented antimicrobial allergy should carry a card with the name of the drug and a description of the reaction. Cross-reactivity between penicillins and cephalosporins is less than 10%. Cephalosporins may be administered to patients with penicillin-induced maculopapular rashes but should be avoided in patients with a history of penicillin-induced immediate hypersensitivity reactions. On the other hand, aztreonam does not cross-react with penicillins and can be safely administered to patients with a history of penicillin-induced anaphylaxis. For mild reactions, it may be possible to continue therapy with use of adjunctive agents or dosage reduction.

Adverse reactions to antimicrobials occur with increased frequency in several groups, including neonates, geriatric patients, renal failure patients, and patients with advanced HIV. Dosage adjustment of the drugs listed in Table 51–6 is essential for the prevention of adverse effects in patients with renal failure. In addition, several agents are contraindicated in patients with renal impairment because of increased rates of serious toxicity (see Table 51–6). See the preceding chapters for discussions of specific drugs.

ANTIMICROBIAL DRUG COMBINATIONS

RATIONALE FOR COMBINATION ANTIMICROBIAL THERAPY

Most infections should be treated with a single antimicrobial agent. Although indications for combination therapy exist, antimicrobial combinations are often overused in clinical practice. The unnecessary use of antimicrobial combinations increases toxicity and costs and may occasionally result in reduced efficacy due to antagonism of one drug by another. Antimicrobial combinations should be selected for one or more of the following reasons:

1. To provide broad-spectrum empiric therapy in seriously ill patients.
2. To treat polymicrobial infections (such as intra-abdominal abscesses, which typically are due to a combination of anaerobic and aerobic Gram-negative organisms, and enterococci). The antimicrobial combination chosen should cover the most commonly known or suspected pathogens but need not cover all possible pathogens. The availability of antimicrobials with excellent polymicrobial coverage (eg, β-lactamase inhibitor combinations or carbapenems) may reduce the need for combination therapy in the setting of polymicrobial infections.
3. To decrease the emergence of resistant strains. The value of combination therapy in this setting has been clearly demonstrated for tuberculosis.
4. To decrease dose-related toxicity by using reduced doses of one or more components of the drug regimen. The use of flucytosine in combination with amphotericin B for the treatment of cryptococcal meningitis in non-HIV-infected patients allows for a reduction in amphotericin B dosage with decreased amphotericin B–induced nephrotoxicity.
5. To obtain enhanced inhibition or killing. This use of antimicrobial combinations is discussed in the paragraphs that follow.

SYNERGISM & ANTAGONISM

When the inhibitory or killing effects of two or more antimicrobials used together are significantly greater than expected from their effects when used individually, synergism is said to result. Synergism is marked by a fourfold or greater reduction in the MIC or MBC of each drug when used in combination versus when used alone. Antagonism occurs when the combined inhibitory or killing effects of two or more antimicrobial drugs are significantly less than observed when the drugs are used individually.

Mechanisms of Synergistic Action

The need for synergistic combinations of antimicrobials has been clearly established for the treatment of enterococcal endocarditis. Bactericidal activity is essential for the optimal management of bacterial endocarditis. Penicillin or ampicillin in combination with gentamicin/streptomycin or ceftriaxone is superior to monotherapy with a penicillin or vancomycin. When tested alone, penicillins and vancomycin are only bacteriostatic against susceptible enterococcal isolates. When these agents are combined with an aminoglycoside, however, bactericidal activity results. The addition of gentamicin or streptomycin to penicillin allows for a reduction in the duration of therapy for selected patients with viridans streptococcal endocarditis.

Other synergistic antimicrobial combinations have been shown to be more effective than monotherapy with individual components. Trimethoprim-sulfamethoxazole has been successfully used in the treatment of bacterial infections and *P jirovecii* (*carinii*) pneumonia.[†] β-Lactamase inhibitors restore the activity of intrinsically active but hydrolyzable β lactams against organisms such as *Staphylococcus aureus* and *Bacteroides fragilis*. Three major mechanisms of antimicrobial synergism have been established:

1. **Blockade of sequential steps in a metabolic sequence:** Trimethoprim-sulfamethoxazole is the best-known example of this mechanism of synergy (see Chapter 46). Blockade of the two sequential steps in the folic acid pathway by trimethoprim-sulfamethoxazole results in a much more complete inhibition of growth than achieved by either component alone.
2. **Inhibition of enzymatic inactivation:** Enzymatic inactivation of β-lactam antibiotics is a major mechanism of antibiotic resistance. Inhibition of β lactamase by β-lactamase inhibitor drugs (eg, sulbactam) results in synergism.
3. **Enhancement of antimicrobial agent uptake:** Penicillins and other cell wall-active agents can increase the uptake of aminoglycosides by a number of bacteria, including staphylococci, enterococci, streptococci, and *P aeruginosa*. Enterococci are thought to be intrinsically resistant to aminoglycosides because of permeability barriers. Similarly, amphotericin B is thought to enhance the uptake of flucytosine by fungi.

Mechanisms of Antagonistic Action

There are few clinically relevant examples of antimicrobial antagonism. The most striking example was reported in a study of patients with pneumococcal meningitis. Patients who were treated with the combination of penicillin and chlortetracycline had a mortality rate of 79% compared with a mortality rate of 21% in patients who received penicillin monotherapy (illustrating the first mechanism set forth below).

The use of an antagonistic antimicrobial combination does not preclude other potential beneficial interactions. For example, rifampin may antagonize the action of anti-staphylococcal penicillins or vancomycin against staphylococci. However, the aforementioned antimicrobials may prevent the emergence of resistance to rifampin.

[†] *Pneumocystis jirovecii* is a fungal organism found in humans (*P carinii* infects animals) that responds to antiprotozoal drugs. See Chapter 52.

Two major mechanisms of antimicrobial antagonism have been established:

1. **Inhibition of cidal activity by static agents:** Bacteriostatic agents such as tetracyclines and chloramphenicol can antagonize the action of bactericidal cell wall-active agents because cell wall-active agents require that the bacteria be actively growing and dividing.
2. **Induction of enzymatic inactivation:** Some Gram-negative bacilli, including *Enterobacter* species, *P aeruginosa*, *Serratia marcescens*, and *Citrobacter freundii*, possess inducible β-lactamases. β-Lactam antibiotics such as imipenem, cefoxitin, and ampicillin are potent inducers of β-lactamase production. If an inducing agent is combined with an intrinsically active but hydrolyzable β-lactam such as piperacillin, antagonism may result.

■ ANTIMICROBIAL PROPHYLAXIS

Antimicrobial agents are effective in preventing infections in many settings. Antimicrobial prophylaxis should be used in circumstances in which efficacy has been demonstrated and benefits outweigh the risks of prophylaxis. Antimicrobial prophylaxis may be divided into surgical prophylaxis and nonsurgical prophylaxis.

Surgical Prophylaxis

Surgical wound infections are a major category of nosocomial infections. The estimated annual cost of surgical wound infections in the USA is more than $1.5 billion.

The National Research Council (NRC) Wound Classification Criteria have served as the basis for recommending antimicrobial prophylaxis. NRC criteria consist of four classes (see Box: National Research Council [NRC] Wound Classification Criteria).

The Study of the Efficacy of Nosocomial Infection Control (SENIC) identified four independent risk factors for postoperative wound infections: operations on the abdomen, operations lasting more than 2 hours, contaminated or dirty wound classification, and at least three medical diagnoses. Patients with at least two SENIC risk factors who undergo clean surgical procedures have an increased risk of developing surgical wound infections and should receive antimicrobial prophylaxis.

Surgical procedures that necessitate the use of antimicrobial prophylaxis include contaminated and clean-contaminated operations, selected operations in which postoperative infection may be catastrophic such as open-heart surgery, clean procedures that involve placement of prosthetic materials, and any procedure in an immunocompromised host. The operation should carry a significant risk of postoperative site infection or cause significant bacterial contamination.

National Research Council (NRC) Wound Classification Criteria

Clean: Elective, primarily closed procedure; respiratory, gastrointestinal, biliary, genitourinary, or oropharyngeal tract not entered; no acute inflammation and no break in technique; expected infection rate ≤2%.

Clean contaminated: Urgent or emergency case that is otherwise clean; elective, controlled opening of respiratory, gastrointestinal, biliary, or oropharyngeal tract; minimal spillage or minor break in technique; expected infection rate ≤10%.

Contaminated: Acute nonpurulent inflammation; major technique break or major spill from hollow organ; penetrating trauma less than 4 hours old; chronic open wounds to be grafted or covered; expected infection rate about 20%.

Dirty: Purulence or abscess; preoperative perforation of respiratory, gastrointestinal, biliary, or oropharyngeal tract; penetrating trauma more than 4 hours old; expected infection rate about 40%.

General principles of antimicrobial surgical prophylaxis include the following:

1. The antibiotic should be active against common surgical wound pathogens; unnecessarily broad coverage should be avoided.
2. The antibiotic should have proved efficacy in clinical trials.
3. The antibiotic must achieve concentrations greater than the MIC of suspected pathogens, and these concentrations must be present at the time of incision.
4. The shortest possible course—ideally a single dose—of the most effective and least toxic antibiotic should be used.
5. The newer broad-spectrum antibiotics should be reserved for therapy of resistant infections.
6. If all other factors are equal, the least expensive agent should be used.

The proper selection and administration of antimicrobial prophylaxis are of utmost importance. Common indications for surgical prophylaxis are shown in Table 51–8. Cefazolin is the prophylactic agent of choice for head and neck, gastroduodenal, biliary tract, gynecologic, and clean procedures. Local wound infection patterns should be considered when selecting antimicrobial prophylaxis. The selection of vancomycin over cefazolin may be necessary in hospitals with high rates of methicillin-resistant *S aureus* or *S epidermidis* infections. The antibiotic should be present in adequate concentrations at the operative site before incision and throughout the procedure; initial dosing is dependent on the volume of distribution, peak levels, clearance, protein binding, and bioavailability. Parenteral agents should be administered during the interval beginning 60 minutes before incision. In cesarean section, the antibiotic is administered after umbilical cord clamping. For many antimicrobial agents, doses should be repeated if the procedure exceeds 2–6 hours in duration. Single-dose prophylaxis is effective for most procedures and results in decreased toxicity and antimicrobial resistance.

Improper administration of antimicrobial prophylaxis leads to excessive surgical wound infection rates. Common errors in

TABLE 51–8 Recommendations for surgical antimicrobial prophylaxis.

Type of Operation	Common Pathogens	Drug of Choice
Cardiac (with median sternotomy)	Staphylococci, enteric gram-negative rods	Cefazolin
Noncardiac, thoracic	Staphylococci, streptococci, enteric gram-negative rods	Cefazolin
Vascular (abdominal and lower extremity)	Staphylococci, enteric gram-negative rods	Cefazolin
Neurosurgical (craniotomy)	Staphylococci	Cefazolin
Orthopedic (with hardware insertion)	Staphylococci	Cefazolin
Head and neck (with entry into the oropharynx)	*Staphylococcus aureus*, oral flora	Cefazolin + metronidazole
Gastroduodenal	*S aureus*, oral flora, enteric gram-negative rods	Cefazolin
Biliary tract	*S aureus*, enterococci, enteric gram-negative rods	Cefazolin
Colorectal (elective surgery)	Enteric gram-negative rods, anaerobes	Oral erythromycin + neomycin[1]
Colorectal (emergency surgery or obstruction)	Enteric gram-negative rods, anaerobes	Cefoxitin, cefotetan, ertapenem, or cefazolin + metronidazole
Appendectomy, nonperforated	Enteric gram-negative rods, anaerobes	Cefoxitin, cefotetan, or cefazolin + metronidazole
Hysterectomy	Enteric gram-negative rods, anaerobes, enterococci, group B streptococci	Cefazolin, cefotetan, or cefoxitin
Cesarean section	Enteric gram-negative rods, anaerobes, enterococci, group B streptococci	Cefazolin

[1]In conjunction with mechanical bowel preparation.

antibiotic prophylaxis include selection of the wrong antibiotic, administering the first dose too early or too late, failure to repeat doses during prolonged procedures, excessive duration of prophylaxis, and inappropriate use of broad-spectrum antibiotics.

Nonsurgical Prophylaxis

Nonsurgical prophylaxis includes the administration of antimicrobials to prevent colonization or asymptomatic infection as well as the administration of drugs following colonization by or inoculation of pathogens but before the development of disease. Nonsurgical prophylaxis is indicated in individuals who are at high risk for temporary exposure to selected virulent pathogens and in patients who are at increased risk for developing infection because of underlying disease (eg, immunocompromised hosts). Prophylaxis is most effective when directed against organisms that are predictably susceptible to antimicrobial agents. Common indications and drugs for nonsurgical prophylaxis are listed in Table 51–9.

TABLE 51–9 Recommendations for nonsurgical antimicrobial prophylaxis.

Infection to Be Prevented	Indication(s)	Drug of Choice	Efficacy
Anthrax	Suspected exposure	Ciprofloxacin or doxycycline	Proposed effective
Candida species	High-risk patients (eg, leukemia, neutropenia, transplant)	Fluconazole, posaconazole, echinocandin	Excellent
Cytomegalovirus	High-risk patients (eg, leukemia, transplant)	Valganciclovir, letermovir	Excellent
Diphtheria	Unimmunized contacts	Penicillin or erythromycin	Proposed effective
Endocarditis	Dental, oral, or upper respiratory tract procedures[1] in at-risk patients[2]	Amoxicillin, cephalexin, clindamycin	Proposed effective
Genital herpes simplex	Recurrent infection (≥4 episodes per year)	Acyclovir, valacyclovir	Excellent
Herpes simplex type 1/2 infection	Mothers with primary HSV or frequent recurrent genital HSV; high-risk patients (eg, leukemia, transplant)	Acyclovir, valacyclovir	Excellent
Group B streptococcal (GBS) infection	Mothers with cervical or vaginal GBS colonization and their newborns with one or more of the following: (a) onset of labor or membrane rupture before 37 weeks' gestation, (b) prolonged rupture of membranes (>18 hours), (c) maternal intrapartum fever, (d) GBS bacteriuria during pregnancy, (e) mothers who have given birth to infants who had early GBS disease or with a history of streptococcal bacteriuria during pregnancy	Ampicillin or penicillin	Excellent
Haemophilus influenzae type B infection	Index case, close contacts of a case in incompletely immunized children (<48 months old), <18 years old and immunocompromised, childcare attendees if >2 invasive cases within 60-day period, asplenia	Rifampin	Excellent
HIV infection	Health care workers exposed to blood after needle-stick injury	Tenofovir/emtricitabine and raltegravir or dolutegravir	Good
	Pregnant HIV-infected women; newborns of HIV-infected women for the first 6 weeks of life, beginning 6–12 hours after birth	ART[3]	Excellent
Influenza A and B	Unvaccinated geriatric patients, immunocompromised hosts, and health care workers during outbreaks	Oseltamivir	Good
Malaria	Travelers to areas endemic for chloroquine-susceptible disease	Chloroquine	Excellent
	Travelers to areas endemic for chloroquine-resistant disease	Mefloquine, doxycycline, atovaquone/proguanil, tafenoquine,[4] primaquine[4]	Excellent
Meningococcal infection	Close contacts of a case, asplenia	Rifampin, ciprofloxacin, or ceftriaxone	Excellent
Mycobacterium avium complex	HIV-infected patients with CD4 count <50/μL and not on ART[3]	Azithromycin, clarithromycin, or rifabutin	Excellent
Otitis media	Recurrent infection	Amoxicillin	Good

(continued)

TABLE 51–9 Recommendations for nonsurgical antimicrobial prophylaxis. (Continued)

Infection to Be Prevented	Indication(s)	Drug of Choice	Efficacy
Pertussis	Close contacts of a case	Azithromycin	Excellent
Plague	Close contacts of a case	Doxycycline, ciprofloxacin, levofloxacin	Excellent
Pneumococcemia	Children with sickle cell disease, asplenia	Penicillin	Excellent
Pneumocystis jirovecii pneumonia (PJP)	High-risk patients (eg, advanced HIV, leukemia, transplant, high dose systemic corticosteroids)	Trimethoprim-sulfamethoxazole, dapsone,[4] atovaquone, pentamidine	Excellent
Rheumatic fever	History of rheumatic fever or known rheumatic heart disease	Benzathine penicillin	Excellent
Toxoplasmosis	HIV-infected patients with IgG antibody to *Toxoplasma* and CD4 count <100/μL; transplant	Trimethoprim-sulfamethoxazole	Good
Tuberculosis	Persons with positive tuberculin skin test or interferon-γ release assay without active tuberculosis	Isoniazid or rifampin or isoniazid + rifapentine or isoniazid + rifampin	Excellent
Urinary tract infections	Recurrent infection	Trimethoprim-sulfamethoxazole, nitrofurantoin	Excellent

[1]Prophylaxis is recommended for the following: dental procedures that involve manipulation of gingival tissue or the periapical region of teeth or perforation of the oral mucosa, and invasive procedure of the respiratory tract that involves incision or biopsy of the respiratory mucosa, such as tonsillectomy and adenoidectomy.

[2]Prophylaxis should be targeted to those with the following risk factors: prosthetic heart valves, previous bacterial endocarditis, congenital cardiac malformations, cardiac transplantation patients who develop cardiac valvulopathy.

[3]Antiretroviral therapy. See aidsinfo.nih.gov/ for updated guidelines.

[4]Check G6PD before starting therapy due to risk of hemolytic anemia

REFERENCES

Baddour LM et al: Infective endocarditis: Diagnosis, antimicrobial therapy, and management of complications. Circulation 2015;132:1435.

Baron EJ et al: Guide to utilization of the microbiology laboratory for diagnosis of infectious diseases: 2013 recommendations by the Infectious Diseases Society of America (IDSA) and the American Society for Microbiology (ASM). Clin Infect Dis 2013;57:e22.

Bratzler DW et al: Clinical practice guidelines for antimicrobial prophylaxis in surgery. Am J Health Syst Pharm 2013;70:195.

Chow AW et al: IDSA clinical practice guideline for acute bacterial rhinosinusitis in children and adults. Clin Infect Dis 2012;54:e72.

Elbadawi LI et al: Carbapenem-resistant Enterobacteriaceae transmission in health care facilities - Wisconsin, February-May 2015. MMWR Morb Mortal Wkly Rep 2016;65:906.

Holmes AH et al: Understanding the mechanisms and drivers of antimicrobial resistance. Lancet 2016;387:176.

Kalil AC et al: Management of adults with hospital-acquired and ventilator-associated pneumonia: 2016 Clinical practice guidelines by the Infectious Disease Society of America and the American Thoracic Society. Clin Infect Dis 2016;63:e61.

Kaye KS, Kaye D: Antibacterial therapy and newer agents. Infect Dis Clin North Am 2009;23:757.

Lee RA Et al: Short-course antibiotics for common infections: what do we know and where do we go from here? Clin Microbiol Infect 2023;29:150.

Mandell LA et al: Infectious Diseases Society of America/American Thoracic Society Consensus guidelines on the management of community-acquired pneumonia in adults. Clin Infect Dis 2007;44:S27.

Martin RF: Surgical infections. Surg Clin North Am 2014;94:1135.

Nahid P et al: Official American Thoracic Society/Centers for Disease Control and Prevention/Infectious Diseases Society of America Clinical Practice Guidelines: Treatment of drug-susceptible tuberculosis. Clin Infect Dis 2016;63:e147.

National Nosocomial Infections Surveillance System: National Nosocomial Infections Surveillance (NNIS) System Report, Data Summary from January 1992–June 2004, issued October 2004. Am J Infect Control 2004;32:470.

Panel on Opportunistic Infections in HIV-Infected Adults and Adolescents: Guidelines for the prevention and treatment of opportunistic infections in HIV-infected adults and adolescents: Recommendations from the Centers for Disease Control and Prevention, the National Institutes of Health, and the HIV Medicine Association of the Infectious Diseases Society of America. Available at: https://aidsinfo.nih.gov/contentfiles/lvguidelines/adult_oi.pdf.

Peleg AY et al: Hospital-acquired infections due to gram negative bacteria. N Engl J Med 2010;362:1804.

Simons FE: Anaphylaxis. J Allergy Clin Immunol 2010;125(Suppl 2):S161.

Shenoy ES: Evaluation and management of penicillin allergy: A review. JAMA 2019:321:188.

Spellberg B et al: The future of antibiotics and resistance. N Engl J Med 2013;368:299.

Talbot GH et al: The Infectious Disease Society of America's 10 × '20 Initiative (10 new systemic antibacterial agents US Food and Drug Administration approved by 2020): Is 20 × '20 a possibility? Clin Infect Dis 2019; 69:1.

Tamma PD et al: Infectious Diseases Society of America 2022 Guidance on the Treatment of Extended-Spectrum β-lactamase Producing Enterobacterales (ESBL-E), Carbapenem-Resistant Enterobacterales (CRE), and *Pseudomonas aeruginosa* with Difficult-to-Treat Resistance (DTR-*P. aeruginosa*). Clin Infect Dis 2022;75:187.

Tamma PD, Hsu AJ: Defining the role of novel β-lactam agents that target carbapenem-resistant gram-negative organisms. J Pediatric Infect Dis Soc: 2019;8:251.

Tunkel AR et al: Practice guidelines for the management of bacterial meningitis. Clin Infect Dis 2004;39:1267.

Wald-Dickler N et al: Oral is the new IV. Challenging decades of blood and bone infection dogma: a systematic review. Am J Med 2022;135:369.

Wilson W et al: Prevention of infective endocarditis: Guidelines from the American Heart Association. Circulation 2007;116:1736.

Workowski KA, Bolan GA: Sexually transmitted diseases treatment guidelines 2015. Centers for Disease Control and Prevention. MMWR Morb Mortal Wkly Rep 2015;64(RR-3):1.

CASE STUDY ANSWER

This patient is experiencing a health care-associated urinary tract infection that may have resulted from recurrent nephrolithiasis despite his initial treatment in India. It is likely that the patient is experiencing a sepsis-like syndrome and has a systemic infection with a uropathogen that is resistant to the antibiotic that he has received. Possible bacteria that may be responsible for the patient's symptoms are methicillin-resistant *Staphylococcus aureus*, *Enterococcus* sp, and enteric Gram-negative rods that are resistant to ciprofloxacin such as ESBL-positive *E coli* or *Klebsiella pneumoniae*, carbapenemase-producing carbapenem-resistant Enterobacteriaceae (CPCRE), or other hospital-acquired Gram-negative organisms such as *Pseudomonas aeruginosa*. The patient was treated with vancomycin and meropenem, and blood and urine cultures were both positive for ESBL-positive *E coli* that was resistant to ciprofloxacin. The patient defervesced and hemodynamically stabilized over the subsequent 48 hours. ESBL-positive *E coli* is an emerging urinary tract pathogen that may be acquired in the outpatient setting, and oral antibiotic therapy may not reliably be effective; empiric therapy with a carbapenem (ertapenem, doripenem, meropenem, imipenem) is recommended for serious infections due to this organism. Unfortunately, isolates of *E coli* and *Klebsiella pneumoniae* that are resistant to carbapenems (CPCRE) have also caused infection in association with international travel and occasionally cause severe infections in hospitalized patients.

CHAPTER

52

Antiprotozoal Drugs

Philip J. Rosenthal, MD

CASE STUDY

A 5-year-old American girl presents with a 1-week history of intermittent chills, fever, and sweats. She had returned home 2 weeks earlier after leaving the USA for the first time to spend 3 weeks with her grandparents in Nigeria. She received all standard childhood immunizations, but no additional treatment before travel, since her parents have returned to their native Nigeria frequently without medical consequences. Three days ago, the child was seen in an outpatient clinic and diagnosed with a viral syndrome. Examination reveals a lethargic child, with a temperature of 39.8°C (103.6°F) and splenomegaly. She has no skin rash or lymphadenopathy. Initial laboratory studies are remarkable for hematocrit 29.8%, platelets 45,000/mm^3, creatinine 2.5 mg/dL (220 μmol/L), and mildly elevated bilirubin and transaminases. A blood smear shows ring forms of *Plasmodium falciparum* at 1.5% parasitemia. What treatment should be started?

■ MALARIA

Malaria is the most important parasitic disease of humans and causes hundreds of millions of illnesses and about half a million deaths per year. Four species of plasmodium typically cause human malaria: *Plasmodium falciparum*, *P vivax*, *P malariae*, and *P ovale*. A fifth species, *P knowlesi*, is primarily a pathogen of monkeys but can cause illness, including severe disease, in humans in Southeast Asia. Although all of the species may cause significant illness, *P falciparum* is responsible for the majority of serious complications and deaths. Drug resistance is an important therapeutic problem, most notably with *P falciparum*.

PARASITE LIFE CYCLE

An anopheline mosquito inoculates plasmodium sporozoites to initiate human infection (Figure 52–1). Circulating sporozoites rapidly invade liver cells, and exoerythrocytic stage tissue schizonts mature in the liver. Merozoites are subsequently released from the liver and invade erythrocytes. Only erythrocytic parasites cause clinical illness. Repeated cycles of infection can lead to the infection of many erythrocytes and serious disease. Sexual stage gametocytes also develop in erythrocytes before being taken up by mosquitoes, where they develop into infective sporozoites.

In *P falciparum* and *P malariae* infection, only one cycle of liver cell invasion and multiplication occurs, and liver infection ceases spontaneously in less than 4 weeks. Thus, treatment that eliminates erythrocytic parasites will cure these infections. In *P vivax* and *P ovale* infections, a dormant hepatic stage, the hypnozoite, is not eradicated by most drugs, and relapses can occur after therapy directed against erythrocytic parasites. Eradication of both erythrocytic and hepatic parasites is required to cure these infections.

DRUG CLASSIFICATION

Several classes of antimalarial drugs are available (Table 52–1 and Figure 52–2). Drugs that eliminate developing or dormant liver forms are called **tissue schizonticides;** those that act on erythrocytic parasites are **blood schizonticides;** and those that kill sexual stages and prevent transmission to mosquitoes are **gametocides.** No single available agent can reliably effect a **radical cure,** ie, eliminate both hepatic and erythrocytic stages. Few available agents are **causal prophylactic drugs,** ie, capable of preventing erythrocytic infection. However, all effective chemoprophylactic agents kill erythrocytic parasites before they increase sufficiently in number to cause clinical disease.

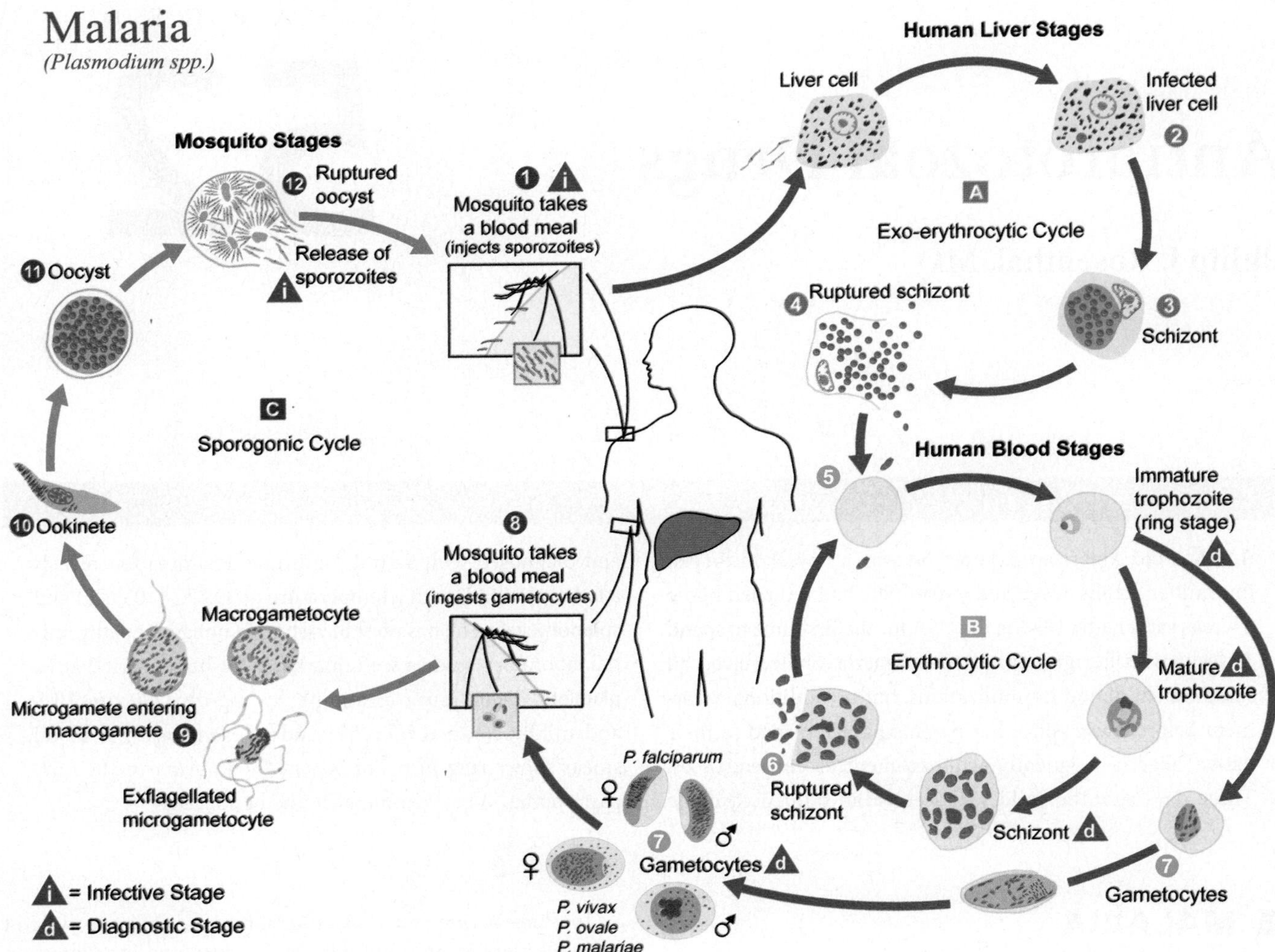

FIGURE 52–1 Life cycle of malaria parasites. Only the asexual erythrocytic stage of infection causes clinical malaria. All effective antimalarial treatments are blood schizonticides that kill this stage. (CDC/Alexander J. da Silva, PhD; Melanie Moser.)

CHEMOPROPHYLAXIS & TREATMENT

When patients are counseled on the prevention of malaria, it is imperative to emphasize measures to prevent mosquito bites (eg, with insect repellents, insecticides, and bed nets), because parasites are increasingly resistant to multiple drugs and no chemoprophylactic regimen is fully protective. Current recommendations from the US Centers for Disease Control and Prevention (CDC) include the use of chloroquine for chemoprophylaxis in the few areas infested by only chloroquine-sensitive malaria parasites (principally Hispaniola and Central America west of the Panama Canal), and Malarone,* mefloquine, or doxycycline for most other malarious areas (Table 52–2). Alternative chemoprophylactic drugs are primaquine and tafenoquine. CDC recommendations should be checked regularly (Phone: 770-488-7788; after hours 770-488-7100; e-mail: malaria@cdc.gov; Internet: www.cdc.gov/malaria), because these may change in response to changing resistance patterns and increasing experience with new drugs. In some circumstances, it may be appropriate for travelers to carry supplies of drugs with them in case they develop a febrile illness when medical attention is unavailable. Regimens for self-treatment include new artemisinin-based combination therapies (see below), which are widely available internationally (and, in the case of Coartem, in the USA); Malarone; mefloquine; and quinine. Most authorities do not recommend routine terminal chemoprophylaxis with primaquine or tafenoquine to eradicate dormant hepatic stages of *P vivax* and *P ovale* after travel, but this may be appropriate in some circumstances, especially for travelers with major exposure to these parasites.

Multiple drugs are available for the treatment of malaria that presents in the USA (Table 52–3). Most nonfalciparum infections and falciparum malaria from areas without known resistance should be treated with chloroquine. For vivax malaria from areas

*Malarone is a proprietary formulation of atovaquone plus proguanil.

TABLE 52–1 Major antimalarial drugs.

Drug	Class	Use
Chloroquine	4-Aminoquinoline	Treatment and chemoprophylaxis of infection with sensitive parasites
Amodiaquine[1]	4-Aminoquinoline	Treatment of infection with some chloroquine-resistant *P falciparum* strains and in fixed combination with artesunate
Piperaquine[1]	Bisquinoline	Treatment of *P falciparum* infection in fixed combination with dihydroartemisinin
Quinine	Quinoline methanol	Oral and intravenous[1] treatment of *P falciparum* infections
Mefloquine	Quinoline methanol	Chemoprophylaxis and treatment of infections with *P falciparum*
Primaquine	8-Aminoquinoline	Radical cure and terminal prophylaxis of infections with *P vivax* and *P ovale*; alternative chemoprophylaxis for all species
Tafenoquine	8-Aminoquinoline	Radical cure and terminal prophylaxis of infections with *P vivax* and *P ovale*; alternative chemoprophylaxis for all species
Sulfadoxine-pyrimethamine (Fansidar)	Folate antagonist combination	Treatment of infections with some chloroquine-resistant *P falciparum*, including combination with artesunate; intermittent preventive therapy in endemic areas
Atovaquone-proguanil (Malarone)	Quinone-folate antagonist combination	Treatment and chemoprophylaxis of *P falciparum* infection
Doxycycline	Tetracycline	Treatment (with quinine) of infections with *P falciparum*; chemoprophylaxis
Lumefantrine[2]	Amyl alcohol	Treatment of *P falciparum* malaria in fixed combination with artemether (Coartem)
Pyronaridine	Mannich base acridine	Treatment of *P falciparum* malaria in fixed combination with artesunate (Pyramax)
Artemisinins (artesunate, artemether,[2] dihydroartemisinin[1])	Sesquiterpene lactone endoperoxides	Treatment of *P falciparum* infections; oral combination therapies for uncomplicated disease; intravenous artesunate for severe disease

[1]Not available in the USA.

[2]Available in the USA only as the fixed combination Coartem.

with suspected chloroquine resistance, including Indonesia and Papua New Guinea, other therapies effective against falciparum malaria may be used. Vivax and ovale malaria should subsequently be treated with primaquine or tafenoquine to eradicate liver forms. Uncomplicated falciparum malaria from most areas is most often treated in the USA with Coartem or Malarone; other artemisinin-based combinations are used internationally. Other agents that are generally effective against resistant falciparum malaria include mefloquine and quinine, which have toxicity concerns at treatment dosages. Severe falciparum malaria is treated with intravenous artesunate.

CHLOROQUINE

Chloroquine has been a drug of choice for both treatment and chemoprophylaxis of malaria since the 1940s, but its usefulness against *P falciparum* has been seriously compromised by drug resistance. It remains the drug of choice in the treatment of sensitive *P falciparum* and other species of human malaria parasites.

Chemistry & Pharmacokinetics

Chloroquine is a synthetic 4-aminoquinoline (see Figure 52–2) formulated as the phosphate salt for oral use. It is rapidly and almost completely absorbed from the gastrointestinal tract, reaches maximum plasma concentrations in about 3 hours, and is rapidly distributed to the tissues. It has a very large apparent volume of distribution of 100–1000 L/kg and is slowly released from tissues and metabolized. Chloroquine is principally excreted in the urine with an initial half-life of 3–5 days but a much longer terminal elimination half-life of 1–2 months.

Antimalarial Action & Resistance

When not limited by resistance, chloroquine is a highly effective blood schizonticide. Chloroquine is not reliably active against liver stage parasites or gametocytes. The drug probably acts by concentrating in parasite food vacuoles, preventing the biocrystallization of the hemoglobin breakdown product, heme, into hemozoin, and thus eliciting parasite toxicity due to the buildup of free heme.

Resistance to chloroquine is now very common among strains of *P falciparum* and uncommon but increasing for *P vivax*. In *P falciparum*, mutations in a putative transporter, PfCRT, are the primary mediators of resistance. Chloroquine resistance can be reversed by certain agents, including verapamil, desipramine, and chlorpheniramine, but the clinical value of resistance-reversing drugs is not established.

Clinical Uses

1. *Treatment*—Chloroquine is the drug of choice in the treatment of uncomplicated nonfalciparum and sensitive falciparum malaria. It rapidly terminates fever (usually in 24–48 hours) and clears parasitemia (in 48–72 hours) caused by sensitive parasites. Chloroquine has been replaced by other drugs, principally artemisinin-based combination therapies, as the standard therapy

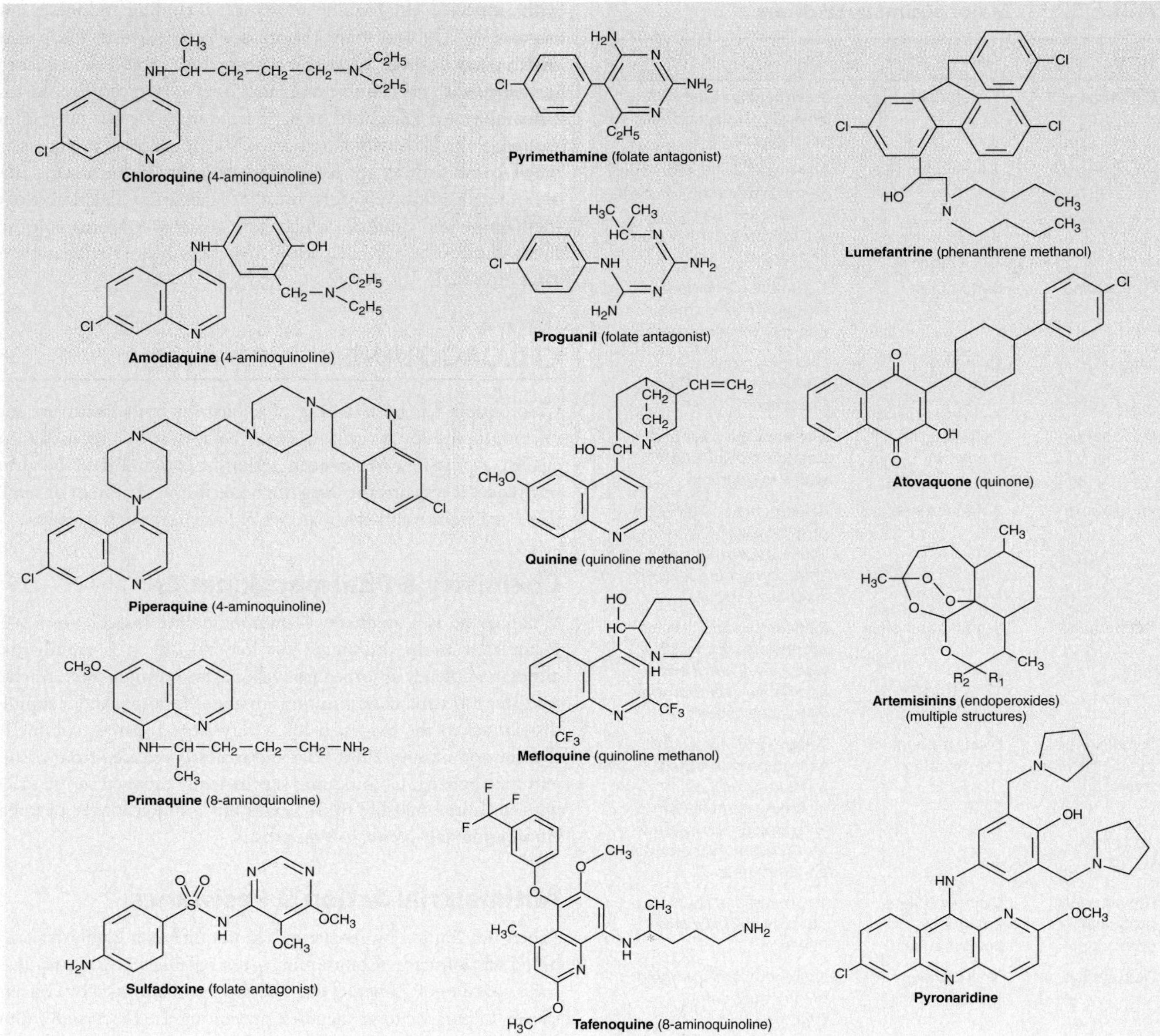

FIGURE 52–2 Structural formulas of some antimalarial drugs.

to treat falciparum malaria in most endemic countries. Chloroquine does not eliminate dormant liver forms of *P vivax* and *P ovale*, and for that reason primaquine or tafenoquine must be added for the radical cure of these species.

2. *Chemoprophylaxis*—Chloroquine is the preferred chemoprophylactic agent in malarious regions without resistant falciparum malaria. Eradication of *P vivax* and *P ovale* requires a course of primaquine to clear hepatic stages.

3. *Amebic liver abscess*—Chloroquine reaches high liver concentrations and may be used for amebic abscesses that fail initial therapy with metronidazole (see below).

Adverse Effects

Chloroquine is usually very well tolerated, even with prolonged use. Pruritus is common, primarily in Africans. Nausea, vomiting, abdominal pain, headache, anorexia, malaise, blurring of vision, and urticaria are uncommon. Dosing after meals may reduce some adverse effects. Rare reactions include hemolysis in glucose-6-phosphate dehydrogenase (G6PD)-deficient persons, impaired hearing, confusion, psychosis, seizures, agranulocytosis, exfoliative dermatitis, alopecia, bleaching of hair, hypotension, and electrocardiographic changes. The long-term administration of high doses of chloroquine for rheumatologic diseases (see Chapter 36) can result in irreversible ototoxicity, retinopathy, myopathy, and

TABLE 52–2 Drugs for the prevention of malaria in travelers.[1]

Drug	Use[2]	Adult Dosage[3]
Chloroquine	Areas without resistant *P falciparum*	500 mg weekly
Malarone	Areas with chloroquine-resistant *P falciparum*	1 tablet (250 mg atovaquone/100 mg proguanil) daily
Mefloquine	Areas with chloroquine-resistant *P falciparum*	250 mg weekly
Doxycycline	Areas with multidrug-resistant *P falciparum*	100 mg daily
Primaquine[4]	Terminal prophylaxis of *P vivax* and *P ovale* infections; alternative for primary prevention	52.6 mg (30 mg base) daily for 14 days after travel; for primary prevention 52.6 mg (30 mg base) daily
Tafenoquine[4]	Terminal prophylaxis of *P vivax* and *P ovale* infections; alternative for primary prevention	200 mg once daily for 3 days and then weekly until 1 week after last exposure

[1]Recommendations may change, as resistance to all available drugs is increasing. See text for additional information on toxicities and cautions. For additional details and pediatric dosing, see CDC guidelines (phone: 877-FYI-TRIP; www.cdc.gov). Travelers to remote areas should consider carrying effective therapy (see text) for use if they develop a febrile illness and cannot reach medical attention quickly.

[2]Areas without known chloroquine-resistant *P falciparum* are Central America west of the Panama Canal, Haiti, Dominican Republic, Egypt, and most malarious countries of the Middle East. Malarone or mefloquine are currently recommended for other malarious areas except for border areas of Thailand, where doxycycline is recommended.

[3]For drugs other than primaquine, begin 1–2 weeks before departure (except 2 days before for doxycycline and Malarone) and continue for 4 weeks after leaving the endemic area (except 1 week for Malarone). All dosages refer to salts.

[4]Screen for glucose-6-phosphate dehydrogenase (G6PD) deficiency before using primaquine or tafenoquine.

TABLE 52–3 Treatment of malaria.

Clinical Setting	Drug Therapy[1]	Alternative Drugs
Chloroquine-sensitive *P falciparum* and *P malariae* infections	Chloroquine phosphate, 1 g, followed by 500 mg at 6, 24, and 48 hours *or* Chloroquine phosphate, 1 g at 0 and 24 hours, then 0.5 g at 48 hours	
P vivax and *P ovale* infections	Chloroquine (as above), then (if G6PD normal) primaquine, 52.6 mg (30 mg base) for 14 days or tafenoquine 300 mg once	For infections from Indonesia, Papua New Guinea, and other areas with suspected resistance: therapies listed for uncomplicated chloroquine-resistant *P falciparum* plus primaquine
Uncomplicated infections with chloroquine-resistant *P falciparum*	Coartem (artemether, 20 mg, plus lumefantrine, 120 mg), four tablets twice daily for 3 days	Malarone, four tablets (total of 1 g atovaquone, 400 mg proguanil) daily for 3 days *or* Mefloquine, 15 mg/kg once or 750 mg, then 500 mg in 6–8 hours *or* Quinine sulfate, 650 mg 3 times daily for 3 days, plus doxycycline, 100 mg twice daily for 7 days, or clindamycin, 600 mg twice daily for 7 days *or* Other artemisinin-based combination regimens (see Table 52–4)
Severe or complicated infections with *P falciparum*	Artesunate,[2] 2.4 mg/kg IV, every 12 hours for 1 day, then daily for 2 additional days; follow with 7-day oral course of doxycycline or clindamycin or full treatment course of Coartem, Malarone, or mefloquine	Artemether,[3] 3.2 mg/kg IM, then 1.6 mg/kg/d IM; follow with oral therapy as for artesunate *or* Quinine dihydrochloride,[3–5] 20 mg/kg IV, then 10 mg/kg every 8 hours

[1]All dosages are oral and refer to salts unless otherwise indicated. See text for additional information on all agents, including toxicities and cautions. See CDC guidelines (phone: 770-488-7788; www.cdc.gov) for additional information and pediatric dosing.

[2]Approved by the FDA in 2020 for use in the USA.

[3]Not available in the USA.

[4]Cardiac monitoring should be in place during intravenous administration of quinine. Change to an oral regimen as soon as the patient can tolerate it.

[5]Avoid loading doses in persons who have received quinine, or mefloquine in the prior 24 hours.

G6PD, glucose-6-phosphate dehydrogenase.

TABLE 52–4 WHO recommendations for the treatment of falciparum malaria.

Regimen	Notes
Artemether-lumefantrine (Coartem, Riamet)	Co-formulated; first-line therapy in many countries; approved in the USA
Artesunate-amodiaquine (ASAQ, Arsucam, Coarsucam)	Co-formulated; first-line therapy in many African countries
Artesunate-mefloquine	Co-formulated; first-line therapy in parts of Southeast Asia and South America
Dihydroartemisinin-piperaquine (Artekin, Duocotecxin)	Co-formulated; first-line therapy in some countries in Southeast Asia
Artesunate-pyronaridine (Pyramax)	Co-formulated; efficacy similar to that of other leading ACTs
Artesunate-sulfadoxine-pyrimethamine	First-line therapy in some countries, but efficacy lower than other regimens in most areas

Data from World Health Organization: Guidelines for the Treatment of Malaria, 3rd ed. World Health Organization. Geneva; 2015.

peripheral neuropathy, but these are rarely seen with standard-dose weekly chemoprophylaxis. Intramuscular injections or intravenous infusions of chloroquine hydrochloride can result in severe hypotension and respiratory and cardiac arrest, and should be avoided.

Contraindications & Cautions

Chloroquine is contraindicated in patients with psoriasis or porphyria. It should generally not be used in those with retinal or visual field abnormalities or myopathy, and should be used with caution in patients with liver, neurologic, or hematologic disorders. The antidiarrheal agent kaolin and calcium- and magnesium-containing antacids interfere with the absorption of chloroquine and should not be coadministered. Chloroquine is considered safe in pregnancy and for young children.

OTHER 4-AMINOQUINOLINES

Amodiaquine is closely related to chloroquine, and it probably shares mechanisms of action and resistance. Amodiaquine was widely used to treat malaria because of its low cost, limited toxicity, and, in some areas, effectiveness against chloroquine-resistant strains of *P falciparum*, but toxicities, including agranulocytosis, aplastic anemia, and hepatotoxicity, have limited its use. However, recent reevaluation has shown that serious toxicity from amodiaquine is uncommon. The most important current use of amodiaquine is in combination therapy. The World Health Organization (WHO) lists artesunate plus amodiaquine as a recommended therapy for falciparum malaria (Table 52–4). This combination is now available as a single tablet (ASAQ, Arsucam, Coarsucam) and is the first-line therapy for the treatment of uncomplicated falciparum malaria in many countries in Africa. Long-term chemoprophylaxis with amodiaquine is best avoided because of its apparent increased toxicity with long-term use, but short-term seasonal malaria chemoprevention with amodiaquine plus sulfadoxine-pyrimethamine (monthly treatment doses for 3–4 months during the transmission season) is now recommended by the WHO for the Sahel sub-region of Africa.

Piperaquine is a bisquinoline that was used widely to treat chloroquine-resistant falciparum malaria in China in the 1970s–1980s, but its use waned after resistance became widespread. Subsequently, piperaquine combined with dihydroartemisinin (Artekin, Duocotecxin) showed excellent efficacy and safety for the treatment of falciparum malaria, although decreased efficacy has been seen recently in Southeast Asia, linked to decreased activity of both components of the combination. Piperaquine has a longer half-life (~28 days) than amodiaquine (~14 days), mefloquine (~14 days), or lumefantrine (~4 days), leading to a longer period of post-treatment prophylaxis with dihydroartemisinin-piperaquine than with the other leading artemisinin-based combinations; this feature should be particularly advantageous in high-transmission areas. Dihydroartemisinin-piperaquine is now the first-line therapy for the treatment of uncomplicated falciparum malaria in some countries in Asia. As dihydroartemisinin-piperaquine offers extended protection against malaria, there is interest in chemoprevention with monthly dosing of the drug, which has shown excellent efficacy in children and pregnant women in Africa.

ARTEMISININ & ITS DERIVATIVES

Artemisinin (**qinghaosu**) is a sesquiterpene lactone endoperoxide (see Figure 52–2), the active component of an herbal medicine that has been used as an antipyretic in China for more than 2000 years. Artemisinin is insoluble and can only be used orally. Analogs have been synthesized to increase solubility and improve antimalarial efficacy. The most important of these analogs are **artesunate** (water-soluble; oral, intravenous, intramuscular, and rectal administration), **artemether** (lipid-soluble; oral, intramuscular, and rectal administration), and **dihydroartemisinin** (water-soluble; oral administration).

Chemistry & Pharmacokinetics

Artemisinin and its analogs are complex 3- and 4-ring structures (see Figure 52–2). They are rapidly absorbed, with peak plasma levels occurring promptly. Half-lives after oral administration are 30–60 minutes for artesunate and dihydroartemisinin, and 2–3 hours for artemether. Artemisinin, artesunate, and artemether are rapidly metabolized to the active metabolite dihydroartemisinin. Drug levels appear to decrease after a number of days of therapy.

Antimalarial Action & Resistance

The artemisinins are now widely available, but monotherapy for the treatment of uncomplicated malaria is strongly *discouraged*. Rather, co-formulated artemisinin-based combination therapies are recommended to improve efficacy and prevent the selection of artemisinin-resistant parasites. The oral combination regimen Coartem (artemether-lumefantrine) was approved by the US Food and Drug Administration (FDA) in 2009, and it can be considered the first-line therapy in the USA for uncomplicated falciparum malaria, although it may not be widely available. Intravenous artesunate was recently approved by the FDA, and it is the standard of care to treat severe malaria.

Artemisinin and its analogs are very rapidly acting blood schizonticides against all human malaria parasites. Artemisinins have no effect on hepatic stages. They are active against young, but not mature gametocytes. The antimalarial activity of artemisinins appears to result from the production of free radicals that follows the iron-catalyzed cleavage of the artemisinin endoperoxide bridge. Delayed clearance of *P falciparum* infections after treatment with artemisinins and decreased treatment efficacy of some artemisinin-based combination regimens in parts of Southeast Asia demonstrate a worrisome focus of resistance. Delayed clearance, mediated by the same mechanisms as in Asia, has recently been identified in East Africa, raising concern about resistance to first-line therapies in the region with the greatest malaria problem.

Clinical Uses

Artemisinin-based combination therapy is now the standard of care for treatment of uncomplicated falciparum malaria in nearly all endemic areas. The leading regimens are highly efficacious, safe, and well tolerated. These regimens were developed because the short plasma half-lives of the artemisinins led to unacceptably high recrudescence rates after short-course therapy, which were reversed by inclusion of longer-acting drugs. Combination therapy also helps to protect against the selection of artemisinin resistance. However, with completion of dosing after 3 days, the artemisinin components are rapidly eliminated, and so selection of resistance to partner drugs is of concern.

The WHO recommends several artemisinin-based combinations for the treatment of uncomplicated falciparum malaria; all are available in combined formulations (see Table 52–4). Either artemether-lumefantrine or artesunate-amodiaquine is the standard treatment for uncomplicated falciparum malaria in most countries in Africa and some additional countries on other continents. Artesunate-mefloquine is highly effective in Southeast Asia, where resistance to many antimalarials is common; it is the first-line therapy in some countries in Southeast Asia and South America. This regimen is less practical for other areas, particularly Africa, because of its relatively poor tolerability. Dihydroartemisinin-piperaquine has shown excellent efficacy and is a first-line therapy for falciparum malaria in some countries. Of concern, increased failure rates for artesunate-mefloquine and dihydroartemisinin-piperaquine have been reported recently in parts of Southeast Asia, in the setting of decreased activity of both components of the regimens. Artesunate-pyronaridine (Pyramax) appears to offer efficacy similar to that of other combinations, but data are limited. Artesunate-sulfadoxine-pyrimethamine is not recommended in many areas owing to unacceptable levels of resistance to sulfadoxine-pyrimethamine, but it is the first-line therapy in some countries.

Artemisinins also have outstanding efficacy in the treatment of complicated falciparum malaria. Large randomized trials and meta-analyses have shown that intramuscular artemether has an efficacy equivalent to that of quinine and that intravenous artesunate is superior to intravenous quinine in terms of parasite clearance time and—most important—patient survival. Intravenous artesunate also has a superior side-effect profile when compared with intravenous quinine (or quinidine, now obsolete). Thus, intravenous artesunate has replaced quinine as the standard of care for the treatment of severe falciparum malaria. Artesunate and artemether have also been effective in the treatment of severe malaria when administered rectally, offering a valuable treatment modality when parenteral therapy is not available.

Adverse Effects & Cautions

Artemisinins are generally very well tolerated. The most commonly reported adverse effects are nausea, vomiting, diarrhea, and dizziness, and these may often be due to underlying malaria rather than the medications. Rare serious toxicities include neutropenia, anemia, hemolysis, elevated liver enzymes, and allergic reactions. In addition, delayed hemolysis after artemisinins for severe malaria appears to be quite common (estimated in 13% of cases), typically beginning 2–3 weeks after therapy, with 73% of identified cases requiring transfusion. Irreversible neurotoxicity has been seen in animals, but only after doses much higher than those used to treat malaria. Artemisinins have been embryotoxic in animal studies, but rates of congenital abnormalities, stillbirths, and abortions were not elevated in women who received artemisinins during pregnancy, compared with those of controls. Based on this information and the significant risk of malaria during pregnancy, the WHO recommends artemisinin-based combination therapies for the treatment of uncomplicated falciparum malaria during the second and third trimesters of pregnancy (quinine plus clindamycin or mefloquine is recommended during the first trimester), and intravenous artesunate for the treatment of severe malaria during all stages of pregnancy.

QUININE

Quinine remains an important therapy for falciparum malaria—especially severe disease—although toxicity may complicate therapy.

Chemistry & Pharmacokinetics

Quinine is derived from the bark of the cinchona tree, a traditional remedy for intermittent fevers from South America. The alkaloid quinine was purified in 1820 and has been used in the treatment and prevention of malaria since that time. Quinidine, the dextrorotatory stereoisomer of quinine, is at least as effective as parenteral quinine in the treatment of severe falciparum malaria, but is no longer used. After oral administration, quinine is rapidly absorbed, reaches peak plasma levels in 1–3 hours, and is widely distributed in body tissues. The use of a loading dose in severe malaria allows the achievement of peak levels within a few hours. Individuals with malaria develop higher plasma levels of quinine than healthy controls, but toxicity is not increased, apparently because of increased protein binding. The half-life of quinine also is longer in those with severe malaria (18 hours) than in healthy controls (11 hours). Quinidine has a shorter half-life than quinine, mostly as a result of decreased protein binding. Quinine is primarily metabolized in the liver and excreted in the urine.

Antimalarial Action & Resistance

Quinine is a rapid-acting, highly effective blood schizonticide against the four species of human malaria parasites. The drug is gametocidal against *P vivax* and *P ovale* but not *P falciparum*. It is not active against liver stage parasites. The mechanism of action of quinine is unknown. Resistance to quinine is common in some areas of Southeast Asia, especially border areas of Thailand, where the drug may fail if used alone to treat falciparum malaria. However, quinine still provides at least a partial therapeutic effect in most patients.

Clinical Uses

1. *Parenteral treatment of severe falciparum malaria*— For many years quinine dihydrochloride or quinidine gluconate were the treatments of choice for severe falciparum malaria, although intravenous artesunate is now preferred. Quinine can be administered slowly intravenously or, in a dilute solution, intramuscularly, but parenteral preparations are not available in the USA. Quinidine availability in the USA ended in 2019. Therapy should be changed to an effective oral agent as soon as the patient has improved sufficiently.

2. *Oral treatment of falciparum malaria*—Quinine sulfate is appropriate therapy for uncomplicated falciparum malaria except when the infection was transmitted in an area without documented chloroquine resistance. Quinine is commonly used with a second drug (most often doxycycline or, in children, clindamycin) to shorten the duration of use (usually to 3 days) and limit toxicity. Quinine is not generally used to treat nonfalciparum malaria.

3. *Babesiosis*—Quinine is first-line therapy, in combination with clindamycin, in the treatment of infection with *Babesia microti* or other human babesial infections.

Adverse Effects

Therapeutic dosages of quinine (and quinidine) commonly cause tinnitus, headache, nausea, dizziness, flushing, and visual disturbances, a constellation of symptoms termed **cinchonism**. Mild symptoms of cinchonism do not warrant the discontinuation of therapy. More severe findings, often after prolonged therapy, include more marked visual and auditory abnormalities, vomiting, diarrhea, and abdominal pain. Hypersensitivity reactions include skin rashes, urticaria, angioedema, and bronchospasm. Hematologic abnormalities include hemolysis (especially with G6PD deficiency), leukopenia, agranulocytosis, and thrombocytopenia. Therapeutic doses may cause hypoglycemia through stimulation of insulin release; this is a particular problem in severe infections and in pregnant patients, who may have increased sensitivity to insulin. Quinine can stimulate uterine contractions, especially in the third trimester. However, this effect is mild, and quinine remains appropriate for treatment of severe falciparum malaria during pregnancy. Intravenous infusions of the drug may cause thrombophlebitis.

Severe hypotension can follow too-rapid intravenous infusions of quinine (or quinidine). Electrocardiographic abnormalities (QT interval prolongation) are fairly common with intravenous quinidine, but dangerous arrhythmias are uncommon when the drug is administered appropriately in a monitored setting.

Blackwater fever is a rare severe illness that includes marked hemolysis and hemoglobinuria in the setting of quinine therapy for malaria. It appears to be due to a hypersensitivity reaction to the drug, although its pathogenesis is uncertain.

Contraindications & Cautions

Quinine should be discontinued if signs of severe cinchonism, hemolysis, or hypersensitivity occur. It should be avoided if possible in patients with underlying visual or auditory problems. It must be used with great caution in those with underlying cardiac abnormalities. Quinine should not be given concurrently with mefloquine and should be used with caution in a patient with malaria who has recently received mefloquine. Absorption may be blocked by aluminum-containing antacids. Quinine can raise plasma levels of warfarin and digoxin. Dosage must be reduced in renal insufficiency.

MEFLOQUINE

Mefloquine is effective therapy for many chloroquine-resistant strains of *P falciparum* and against other species. Although toxicity is a concern, mefloquine is one of the recommended chemoprophylactic drugs for use in most malaria-endemic regions with chloroquine-resistant strains.

Chemistry & Pharmacokinetics

Mefloquine hydrochloride is a synthetic 4-quinoline methanol that is chemically related to quinine. It can only be given orally because severe local irritation occurs with parenteral use. It is well absorbed, and peak plasma concentrations are reached in about 18 hours. Mefloquine is highly protein-bound, extensively distributed in tissues, and eliminated slowly, allowing a single-dose treatment regimen. The terminal elimination half-life is about 20 days, allowing weekly dosing for chemoprophylaxis. With weekly dosing, steady-state drug levels are reached over a number of weeks. Mefloquine and its metabolites are slowly excreted, mainly in the feces.

Antimalarial Action & Resistance

Mefloquine has strong blood schizonticidal activity against *P falciparum* and *P vivax*, but it is not active against hepatic stages or gametocytes. The mechanism of action is unknown. Sporadic resistance to mefloquine has been reported from many areas, but resistance appears to be uncommon except in regions of Southeast Asia with high rates of multidrug resistance. Mefloquine resistance does not appear to be associated with resistance to chloroquine.

Clinical Uses

1. *Chemoprophylaxis*—Mefloquine is effective in prophylaxis against most strains of *P falciparum* and probably all other human malarial species. Mefloquine is therefore among the drugs recommended by the CDC for chemoprophylaxis in all malarious areas except those with no chloroquine resistance (where chloroquine is preferred) and some rural areas of Southeast Asia with a high prevalence of mefloquine resistance. As with chloroquine, eradication of *P vivax* and *P ovale* requires a course of primaquine.

2. *Treatment*—Mefloquine is effective in treating uncomplicated falciparum malaria. The drug is not appropriate for treating individuals with severe or complicated malaria, since quinine and artemisinins are more rapidly active, and since drug resistance is less likely with those agents. The combination of artesunate plus mefloquine is one of the combination therapies recommended by the WHO and is first-line in some countries for the treatment of uncomplicated falciparum malaria (see Table 52–4).

Adverse Effects

Weekly dosing with mefloquine for chemoprophylaxis may cause nausea, vomiting, dizziness, sleep and behavioral disturbances, epigastric pain, diarrhea, abdominal pain, headache, rash, and dizziness. Neuropsychiatric toxicities have received a good deal of publicity, but despite frequent anecdotal reports of seizures and psychosis, a number of controlled studies have found the frequency of serious adverse effects from mefloquine to be similar to that with other common antimalarial chemoprophylactic regimens. However, concern about reported long-term effects of short-term use of mefloquine led in 2013 to the FDA adding a black box warning regarding potential neurologic and psychiatric toxicities. Leukocytosis, thrombocytopenia, and aminotransferase elevations have also been reported.

Adverse effects are more common with the higher dosages of mefloquine required for treatment. These effects may be lessened by administering the drug in two doses separated by 6–8 hours. The incidence of neuropsychiatric symptoms appears to be about 10 times greater than with chemoprophylactic dosing, with widely varying frequencies of up to about 50% reported. Serious neuropsychiatric toxicities (depression, confusion, acute psychosis, or seizures) have been reported in less than 1 in 1000 treatments, but some authorities believe that these toxicities are actually more common. Mefloquine can also alter cardiac conduction, and arrhythmias and bradycardia have been reported.

Contraindications & Cautions

Mefloquine is contraindicated in a patient with a history of epilepsy, psychiatric disorders, arrhythmia, cardiac conduction defects, or sensitivity to related drugs. It should not be coadministered with quinine, quinidine, or halofantrine, and caution is required if quinine is used to treat malaria after mefloquine chemoprophylaxis. The CDC no longer advises against mefloquine use in patients receiving β-adrenoceptor antagonists. Mefloquine is also now considered safe in young children, and it is the only chemoprophylactic other than chloroquine approved for children weighing less than 5 kg and for pregnant women. Available data suggest that mefloquine is safe throughout pregnancy. An older recommendation to avoid mefloquine use in those requiring fine motor skills (eg, airline pilots) is controversial. Mefloquine chemoprophylaxis should be discontinued if significant neuropsychiatric symptoms develop.

PRIMAQUINE AND TAFENOQUINE

Primaquine is the drug of choice for the eradication of dormant liver forms of *P vivax* and *P ovale* and can also be used for chemoprophylaxis against all malarial species. Tafenoquine, which has the same indications and simplified dosing, was approved by the FDA in 2018. Tafenoquine is available in different dosing formulations for eradication of liver forms (Krintafel) and chemoprophylaxis (Arakoda). Primaquine and tafenoquine are contraindicated in those with G6PD deficiency.

Chemistry & Pharmacokinetics

These drugs are related 8-aminoquinolines (see Figure 52–2). Primaquine is well absorbed orally, reaching peak plasma levels in 1–2 hours. The plasma half-life is 3–8 hours. Primaquine is widely distributed to the tissues, but only a small amount is bound there. It is rapidly metabolized and excreted in the urine. Tafenoquine is slowly absorbed, with maximum concentrations reached in 12–15 hours; coadministration with food increases exposure. The half-life is approximately 2 weeks. Tafenoquine is slowly excreted in the urine.

Antimalarial Action & Resistance

Primaquine and tafenoquine are active against hepatic stages of all human malaria parasites, including dormant hypnozoite stages of *P vivax* and *P ovale*. The drugs are also gametocidal and have modest activity against asexual erythrocytic stage parasites. The mechanisms of antimalarial action are unknown.

Some strains of *P vivax* appear to be relatively resistant to primaquine, and repeated therapy may be required to eliminate hypnozoites.

Clinical Uses

1. *Therapy (radical cure) of acute vivax and ovale malaria*—Standard therapy for these infections includes chloroquine to eradicate erythrocytic forms and primaquine or tafenoquine to eradicate liver hypnozoites and prevent a subsequent relapse. Chloroquine (or another antimalarial) is given acutely, and therapy with primaquine or tafenoquine is withheld until the G6PD status of the patient is known. If the G6PD level is normal, a 14-day course of primaquine or a single dose of tafenoquine is given. Prompt evaluation of the G6PD level is helpful, since primaquine appears to be most effective when instituted before completion of dosing with chloroquine.

2. *Terminal prophylaxis of vivax and ovale malaria*—Standard chemoprophylaxis does not prevent a relapse of vivax or ovale malaria, because the hypnozoite forms of these parasites are not eradicated by available blood schizonticides. To diminish the likelihood of relapse, some authorities advocate the use of primaquine after the completion of travel to an endemic area.

3. *Chemoprophylaxis of malaria*—Daily treatment with 30 mg (0.5 mg/kg) of primaquine base provided good protection against falciparum and vivax malaria, and the drug is now listed as an alternative chemoprophylactic regimen by the CDC. Tafenoquine was approved in 2018 as another chemoprophylactic regimen, with simplified dosing (200 mg daily for 3 days and then weekly).

4. *Gametocidal action*—Primaquine renders *P falciparum* gametocytes noninfective to mosquitoes. Including primaquine with treatment for falciparum malaria is used in some areas to decrease transmission, and routine inclusion of single low doses of primaquine (which may be safe without testing for G6PD deficiency) is under study, and recommended in some regions.

5. *Pneumocystis jirovecii infection*—The combination of clindamycin and primaquine is an alternative regimen in the treatment of pneumocystosis, particularly mild to moderate disease. This regimen offers improved tolerance compared with high-dose trimethoprim-sulfamethoxazole or pentamidine, although its efficacy against severe pneumocystis pneumonia is not well studied.

Adverse Effects

Primaquine in recommended doses is generally well tolerated. It infrequently causes nausea, epigastric pain, abdominal cramps, and headache, and these symptoms are more common with higher dosages and when the drug is taken on an empty stomach. More serious but rare adverse effects are leukopenia, agranulocytosis, leukocytosis, and cardiac arrhythmias. Tafenoquine is also well tolerated; reported adverse effects include headache, diarrhea, dizziness, nausea, and vomiting. Standard doses of primaquine or tafenoquine may cause hemolysis or methemoglobinemia (manifested by cyanosis), especially in persons with G6PD deficiency or other hereditary metabolic defects.

Contraindications & Cautions

Primaquine and tafenoquine should be avoided in patients with a history of granulocytopenia or methemoglobinemia, in those receiving potentially myelosuppressive drugs, and in those with disorders that commonly include myelosuppression.

Patients should be tested for G6PD deficiency before primaquine or tafenoquine is prescribed. When a patient is deficient in G6PD, tafenoquine should be avoided (its long half-life increases potential risks) and treatment strategies for primaquine may include withholding therapy and treating subsequent relapses, if they occur, with chloroquine; treating patients with standard dosing, paying close attention to their hematologic status; or treating with weekly primaquine (45 mg base) for 8 weeks. G6PD-deficient individuals of Mediterranean and Asian ancestry are most likely to have severe deficiency, whereas those of African ancestry usually have a milder biochemical defect. This difference can be taken into consideration in choosing a treatment strategy. In any event, primaquine and tafenoquine should be discontinued if there is evidence of hemolysis or anemia. Primaquine and tafenoquine should be avoided in pregnancy because the fetus is relatively G6PD-deficient and thus at risk of hemolysis.

ATOVAQUONE

Atovaquone, a hydroxynaphthoquinone (see Figure 52–2), is a component of **Malarone,** which is recommended for the treatment and prevention of malaria. Atovaquone has also been approved by the FDA for the treatment of mild to moderate *P jirovecii* pneumonia.

The drug is only administered orally. Its bioavailability is low and erratic, but absorption is increased by fatty food. The drug is heavily protein-bound, has a half-life of 2–3 days, and is mostly eliminated unchanged in the feces. Atovaquone acts against plasmodia by disrupting mitochondrial electron transport. It is active against tissue and erythrocytic schizonts, allowing chemoprophylaxis to be discontinued only 1 week after the end of exposure (compared with 4 weeks for mefloquine or doxycycline, which lack activity against tissue schizonts).

Initial use of atovaquone to treat malaria led to disappointing results, with frequent failures due to the selection of resistant parasites during therapy. In contrast, Malarone, a fixed combination of atovaquone (250 mg) and proguanil (100 mg), is highly effective for both the treatment and chemoprophylaxis of falciparum malaria, and it is now approved for both indications in the USA. For chemoprophylaxis, Malarone must be taken daily (see Table 52–2). It has an advantage over mefloquine and doxycycline in requiring shorter periods of treatment before and after the period at risk for malaria transmission, but it is more expensive than the other agents. It should be taken with food.

Atovaquone is an alternative therapy for *P jirovecii* infection, although its efficacy is lower than that of trimethoprim-sulfamethoxazole. Standard dosing is 750 mg taken with food twice daily for 21 days. Atovaquone has also been effective in small numbers of immunocompromised patients with toxoplasmosis unresponsive to other agents.

Malarone is generally well tolerated. Adverse effects include abdominal pain, nausea, vomiting, diarrhea, headache, insomnia, and rash, and these are more common with the higher dosage required for treatment. Reversible elevations in liver enzymes have been reported. The safety of atovaquone in pregnancy is unknown, and its use is not advised in pregnant women. It is considered safe for use in children with body weight above 5 kg. Plasma concentrations of atovaquone are decreased about 50% by coadministration of tetracycline or rifampin.

INHIBITORS OF FOLATE SYNTHESIS

Inhibitors of enzymes involved in folate metabolism are used, generally in combination regimens, in the treatment and prevention of malaria.

Chemistry & Pharmacokinetics

Pyrimethamine is a 2,4-diaminopyrimidine related to trimethoprim (see Chapter 46). **Proguanil** is a biguanide derivative (see Figure 52–2). Both drugs are slowly but adequately absorbed from the gastrointestinal tract. Pyrimethamine reaches peak plasma levels 2–6 hours after an oral dose, is bound to plasma proteins, and has an elimination half-life of about 3.5 days. Proguanil reaches peak plasma levels about 5 hours after an oral dose and has an elimination half-life of about 16 hours. Therefore, proguanil must be administered daily for chemoprophylaxis, whereas pyrimethamine can be given once a week. Pyrimethamine is extensively metabolized before excretion. Proguanil is a prodrug for its active triazine metabolite, cycloguanil. **Fansidar,** a fixed combination of the sulfonamide **sulfadoxine** (500 mg per tablet) and **pyrimethamine** (25 mg per tablet), is well absorbed. Its components display peak plasma levels within 2–8 hours and are excreted mainly by the kidneys. The average half-life of sulfadoxine is about 170 hours.

Antimalarial Action & Resistance

Pyrimethamine and proguanil act slowly against erythrocytic forms of susceptible strains of all four human malaria species. Proguanil also has activity against hepatic forms. Neither drug is adequately gametocidal or effective against hypnozoites of *P vivax* or *P ovale*. Sulfonamides and sulfones are weakly active against erythrocytic schizonts but not against liver stages or gametocytes.

Pyrimethamine and proguanil inhibit plasmodial dihydrofolate reductase, a key enzyme in the pathway for synthesis of folate. Sulfonamides and sulfones inhibit another enzyme in the folate pathway, dihydropteroate synthase. As described in Chapter 46, inhibitors of these two enzymes provide synergistic activity (see Figure 46–2).

Resistance of *P falciparum* to folate antagonists and sulfonamides is common in many areas. Resistance is due primarily to mutations in dihydrofolate reductase and dihydropteroate synthase, with increasing numbers of mutations leading to increasing levels of resistance. Resistance seriously limits the efficacy of sulfadoxine-pyrimethamine for the treatment of malaria in most areas, but in Africa most parasites exhibit an intermediate level of resistance, such that antifolates may continue to offer some preventive efficacy.

Clinical Uses

1. *Chemoprophylaxis*—Chemoprophylaxis with single folate antagonists is not recommended because of frequent resistance. However, the antifolate combination trimethoprim-sulfamethoxazole is commonly used as a daily prophylactic therapy for HIV-infected patients, offering partial preventive efficacy against malaria in Africa.

2. *Intermittent preventive therapy*—A strategy for malaria control is intermittent preventive therapy, in which high-risk patients receive intermittent treatment for malaria, regardless of their infection status. In pregnancy, three or more (up to monthly) doses of sulfadoxine-pyrimethamine after the first trimester is now standard policy in Africa, although efficacy is limited by resistance. In children, intermittent preventive therapy has not been widely accepted, but the WHO recommends seasonal malaria chemoprevention with amodiaquine plus sulfadoxine-pyrimethamine in the Sahel sub-region of Africa, where malaria is highly seasonal and high-level resistance to antifolates is uncommon. In most other areas drug resistance seriously limits the preventive efficacy of antifolates.

3. *Treatment of chloroquine-resistant falciparum malaria*—Fansidar is no longer a recommended therapy for malaria, and in particular it should not be used for severe malaria, since it is slower-acting than other available agents. Fansidar is also not reliably effective in vivax malaria, and its usefulness against *P ovale* and *P malariae* has not been adequately studied. Artesunate plus sulfadoxine-pyrimethamine is listed by the WHO to treat falciparum malaria (see Table 52–4), but other artemisinin-based combinations are generally preferred.

4. *Toxoplasmosis*—Pyrimethamine, in combination with sulfadiazine, is first-line therapy in the treatment of toxoplasmosis, including acute infection, congenital infection, and disease in immunocompromised patients. For immunocompromised patients, high-dose therapy is required followed by chronic suppressive therapy. Folinic acid is included to limit myelosuppression. The replacement of sulfadiazine with clindamycin provides an effective alternative regimen. Recent problems with pricing and availability of pyrimethamine in the USA made the use of this drug more difficult.

5. *Pneumocystosis*—*P jirovecii* is the cause of human pneumocystosis and is now recognized to be a fungus, but this organism is discussed in this chapter because it responds to antiprotozoal drugs, not antifungals. First-line therapy of pneumocystosis is trimethoprim plus sulfamethoxazole (see also Chapter 46). Standard treatment includes high-dose intravenous or oral therapy (15 mg/kg trimethoprim and 75 mg/kg sulfamethoxazole per day in three or four divided doses) for 21 days. High-dose therapy entails significant toxicity, especially in patients with AIDS. Important toxicities include nausea, vomiting, fever, rash, leukopenia, hyponatremia, elevated hepatic enzymes, azotemia, anemia, and thrombocytopenia. Less common effects include severe skin reactions, mental status changes, pancreatitis, and hypocalcemia. Trimethoprim-sulfamethoxazole is also the standard chemoprophylactic drug for the prevention of *P jirovecii* infection in immunocompromised individuals. Dosing is one double-strength tablet daily or three times per week. The chemoprophylactic dosing schedule is much better tolerated than high-dose therapy, but rash, fever, leukopenia, or hepatitis may necessitate changing to another drug.

Adverse Effects & Cautions

Most patients tolerate pyrimethamine and proguanil well. Gastrointestinal symptoms, skin rashes, and itching are rare. Mouth ulcers and alopecia have been described with proguanil. Fansidar uncommonly causes severe cutaneous reactions, including erythema multiforme, Stevens-Johnson syndrome, and toxic epidermal necrolysis. Severe reactions appear to be much less common with single-dose or intermittent therapy, compared to regular chemoprophylaxis, and use of the drug has been justified by the risks associated with falciparum malaria.

Rare adverse effects with Fansidar are those associated with other sulfonamides, including hematologic, gastrointestinal, central nervous system, dermatologic, and renal toxicity. Folate antagonists should be used cautiously in the presence of renal or hepatic dysfunction. Although pyrimethamine is teratogenic in animals, Fansidar has been safely used in pregnancy. Proguanil is considered safe in pregnancy. In pregnant women receiving Fansidar preventive therapy, high-dose folate supplementation (eg, 5 mg daily) should be replaced by the standard recommended dosage (0.4–0.6 mg daily) to avoid potential loss of protective efficacy.

ANTIBIOTICS

A number of antibiotics are modestly active antimalarials. Bacterial protein synthesis inhibitors appear to act against malaria parasites by inhibiting protein synthesis in a plasmodial prokaryote-like organelle, the apicoplast. None of the antibiotics should be used as single agents in the treatment of malaria because their action is much slower than that of standard antimalarials.

Tetracycline and doxycycline (see Chapter 44) are active against erythrocytic schizonts of all human malaria parasites. They are not active against liver stages. Doxycycline is used in the treatment of falciparum malaria in conjunction with quinine, allowing a shorter and better-tolerated course of that drug. Doxycycline has also become a standard chemoprophylactic drug, especially for use in areas of Southeast Asia with high rates of resistance to other antimalarials, including mefloquine. Doxycycline adverse effects include gastrointestinal symptoms, esophagitis, candidal vaginitis, and photosensitivity. Clindamycin (see Chapter 44) is slowly active against erythrocytic schizonts and can replace doxycycline in children and pregnant women. Antimalarial activity of azithromycin and fluoroquinolones has also been demonstrated, but efficacy for the therapy or chemoprophylaxis of malaria has been suboptimal.

Antibiotics are also active against other protozoans. Tetracycline and erythromycin are alternative therapies for the treatment of intestinal amebiasis. Clindamycin, in combination with other agents, is effective therapy for toxoplasmosis, pneumocystosis, and babesiosis. Spiramycin is a macrolide antibiotic that is used to treat primary toxoplasmosis acquired during pregnancy. Treatment lowers the risk of the development of congenital toxoplasmosis.

LUMEFANTRINE & PYRONARIDINE

Lumefantrine, an aryl alcohol, is available only as a fixed-dose combination with artemether (Coartem, Riamet), which is now the first-line therapy for uncomplicated falciparum malaria in many endemic countries. In addition, Coartem is approved in many nonendemic countries, including the USA. The half-life of lumefantrine, when used in combination, is 3–4 days. Drug levels may be altered by interactions with other drugs, including those that affect CYP3A4 metabolism. Oral absorption is variable and improved when the drug is taken with food. Coartem should be administered with fatty food to maximize antimalarial efficacy. Coartem is very well tolerated. The most commonly reported adverse events have been gastrointestinal disturbances, headache, dizziness, rash, and pruritus, and in many cases these toxicities may have been due to underlying malaria or concomitant medications rather than to Coartem. Coartem can cause minor prolongation of the QT interval, but this appears to be clinically insignificant.

Pyronaridine, a Mannich base acridine, has been studied as an antimalarial for many years and used as monotherapy in China. It is now available in combination with artesunate as Pyramax. Pyronaridine is well absorbed orally without important food effects. It has a half-life of about 8 days, with primarily renal elimination. Artesunate-pyronaridine has generally demonstrated excellent efficacy against falciparum and vivax malaria and been well tolerated. Adverse events have included eosinophilia and transaminitis. Recent studies suggest that artesunate-pyronaridine is as safe and efficacious as other leading artemisinin-based combinations for treating falciparum malaria.

■ AMEBIASIS

Amebiasis is infection with *Entamoeba histolytica*. This organism can cause asymptomatic intestinal infection, mild to moderate colitis, severe intestinal infection (dysentery), ameboma, liver abscess, and other extraintestinal infections. The choice of drugs for amebiasis depends on the clinical presentation (Table 52–5).

Treatment of Specific Forms of Amebiasis

1. *Asymptomatic intestinal infection*—Asymptomatic carriers generally are not treated in endemic areas, but in nonendemic areas they are treated with a luminal amebicide. A tissue amebicidal drug is unnecessary. Standard luminal amebicides are diloxanide furoate, iodoquinol, and paromomycin. Each drug eradicates carriage in about 80–90% of patients. Therapy with a luminal amebicide is also required in the treatment of all other forms of amebiasis.

2. *Amebic colitis*—Metronidazole plus a luminal amebicide is the treatment of choice for amebic colitis and dysentery. Tetracyclines and erythromycin are alternative drugs for moderate colitis but are not effective against extraintestinal disease.

3. *Extraintestinal infections*—The treatment of choice for extraintestinal infections is metronidazole plus a luminal amebicide. A 10-day course of metronidazole cures over 95% of uncomplicated liver abscesses. For unusual cases in which initial

TABLE 52–5 Treatment of amebiasis. Not all preparations are available in the USA.[1]

Clinical Setting	Drugs of Choice and Adult Dosage	Alternative Drugs and Adult Dosage
Asymptomatic intestinal infection	Luminal agent: Paromomycin, 10 mg/kg 3 times daily for 7 days *or* Diloxanide furoate,[2] 500 mg 3 times daily for 10 days *or* Iodoquinol, 650 mg 3 times daily for 21 days	
Mild to moderate intestinal infection	Metronidazole, 750 mg 3 times daily (or 500 mg IV every 6 hours) for 10 days *or* Tinidazole, 2 g daily for 3 days *plus* Luminal agent (see above)	Luminal agent (see above) *plus either* Tetracycline, 250 mg 3 times daily for 10 days *or* Erythromycin, 500 mg 4 times daily for 10 days
Severe intestinal infection	Metronidazole, 750 mg 3 times daily (or 500 mg IV every 6 hours) for 10 days *or* Tinidazole, 2 g daily for 3 days *plus* Luminal agent (see above)	Luminal agent (see above) *plus* Tetracycline, 250 mg 3 times daily for 10 days
Hepatic abscess, ameboma, and other extraintestinal disease	Metronidazole, 750 mg 3 times daily (or 500 mg IV every 6 hours) for 10 days *or* Tinidazole, 2 g daily for 5 days *plus* Luminal agent (see above)	Chloroquine, 500 mg twice daily for 2 days, then 500 mg daily for 21 days *plus* Luminal agent (see above)

[1]Route is oral unless otherwise indicated. See text for additional details and cautions.

[2]Not available in the USA.

therapy with metronidazole has failed, aspiration of the abscess and the addition of chloroquine to a repeat course of metronidazole should be considered.

METRONIDAZOLE & TINIDAZOLE

The nitroimidazoles metronidazole and tinidazole (Figure 52–3) are the drugs of choice in the treatment of extraluminal amebiasis. They kill trophozoites but not cysts of *E histolytica* and effectively eradicate intestinal and extraintestinal tissue infections. Tinidazole appears to have similar activity and a better toxicity profile compared to metronidazole; it offers simpler dosing and can be substituted for the indications listed below.

Pharmacokinetics & Mechanism of Action

Oral metronidazole and tinidazole are readily absorbed and permeate all tissues by simple diffusion. Intracellular concentrations rapidly approach extracellular levels. Peak plasma concentrations are reached in 1–3 hours. Protein binding of both drugs is low (10–20%); the half-life of unchanged drug is 7.5 hours for metronidazole and 12–14 hours for tinidazole. Metronidazole and its metabolites are excreted mainly in the urine. Plasma clearance of metronidazole is decreased in patients with impaired liver function. The nitro group of metronidazole is chemically reduced in anaerobic bacteria and sensitive protozoans. Reactive reduction products appear to be responsible for antiprotozoal and antibacterial activity. The mechanism of tinidazole is assumed to be the same.

Clinical Uses

1. *Amebiasis*—Metronidazole or tinidazole is the drug of choice in the treatment of all tissue infections with *E histolytica*. Neither drug is reliably effective against luminal parasites and so must be used with a luminal amebicide to ensure eradication of the infection.

2. *Giardiasis*—Metronidazole is the treatment of choice for giardiasis. The dosage for giardiasis is much lower than that for amebiasis, and the drug is thus better tolerated. Efficacy after a single treatment is about 90%. Tinidazole is at least equally effective, and can be used as a single dose.

3. *Trichomoniasis*—Metronidazole is the treatment of choice. A single dose of 2 g is effective. Metronidazole-resistant organisms can lead to treatment failures. Tinidazole may be effective against some of these resistant organisms.

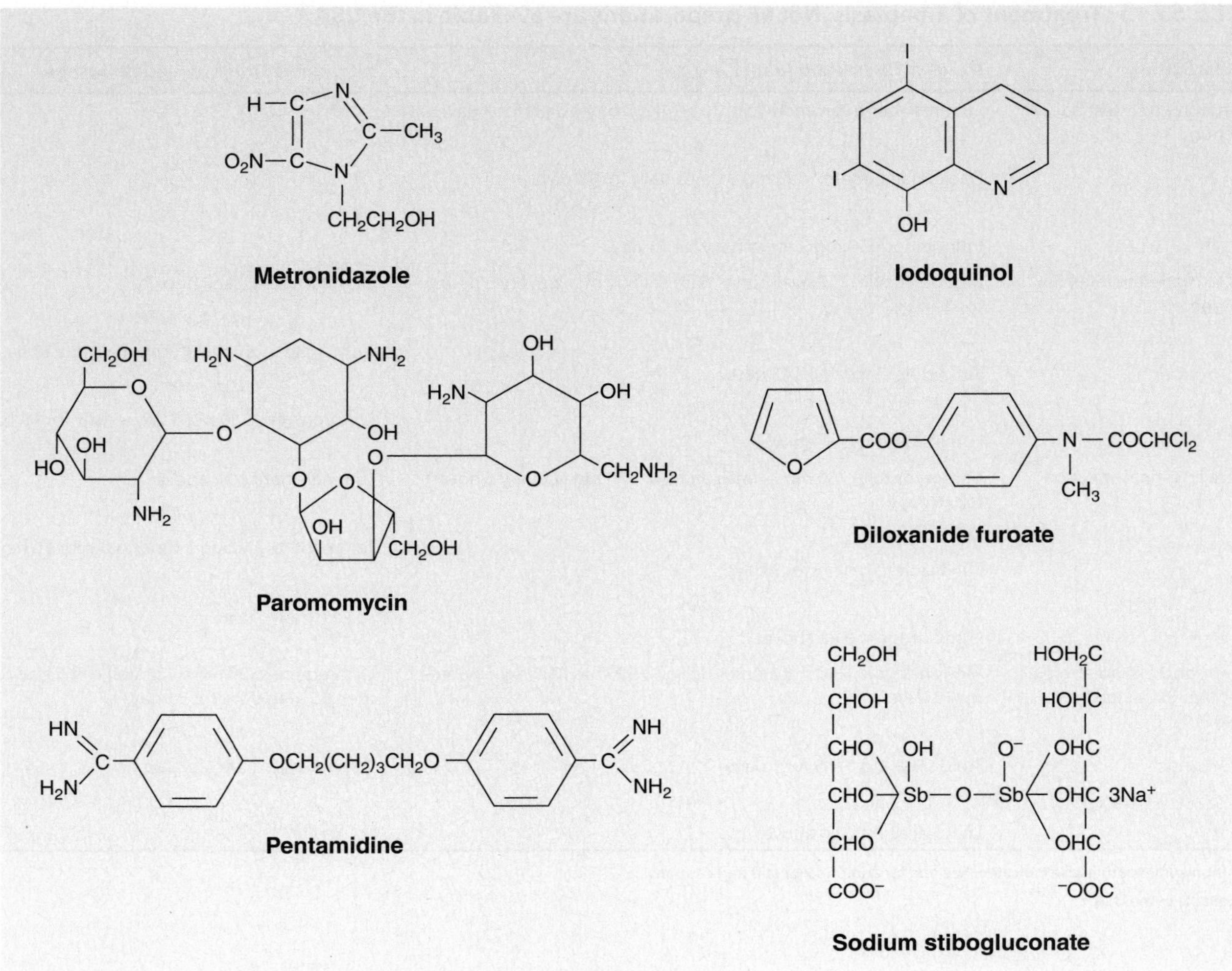

FIGURE 52–3 Structural formulas of other antiprotozoal drugs.

Adverse Effects & Cautions

With metronidazole, nausea, headache, dry mouth, and a metallic taste in the mouth occur commonly. Infrequent adverse effects include vomiting, diarrhea, insomnia, weakness, dizziness, thrush, rash, dysuria, dark urine, vertigo, paresthesias, encephalopathy, and neutropenia. Taking the drug with meals lessens gastrointestinal irritation. Pancreatitis and severe central nervous system toxicity (ataxia, encephalopathy, seizures) are rare. Metronidazole has a disulfiram-like effect, so that nausea and vomiting can occur if alcohol is ingested during therapy. The drug should be used with caution in patients with central nervous system disease. Intravenous infusions have rarely caused seizures or peripheral neuropathy. The dosage should be adjusted for patients with severe liver or renal disease. Tinidazole has a similar adverse-effect profile, although it appears to be somewhat better tolerated than metronidazole.

Metronidazole has been reported to potentiate the anticoagulant effect of coumarin-type anticoagulants. Phenytoin and phenobarbital may accelerate elimination of the drug, whereas cimetidine may decrease plasma clearance. Lithium toxicity may occur when the drug is used with metronidazole. Metronidazole and its metabolites are mutagenic in bacteria and tumorigenic in mice. Data on teratogenicity are inconsistent. Metronidazole is thus best avoided in pregnant or nursing women, although congenital abnormalities have not clearly been associated with use in humans.

PAROMOMYCIN SULFATE

Paromomycin sulfate is an aminoglycoside antibiotic (see also Chapter 45) that is not significantly absorbed from the gastrointestinal tract. It is used as a luminal amebicide and has no effect against extraintestinal organisms. The small amount absorbed is slowly excreted unchanged, mainly by glomerular filtration. However, the drug may accumulate with renal insufficiency and contribute to renal toxicity. Paromomycin appears to have similar efficacy and less toxicity than other luminal agents; in one study it was superior to diloxanide furoate in clearing asymptomatic infections. As it is readily available, paromomycin can be considered the antiamebic luminal agent of choice in the USA. Adverse effects include occasional abdominal distress and diarrhea. Parenteral paromomycin is now used to treat visceral leishmaniasis and is discussed separately in the text that follows.

IODOQUINOL

Iodoquinol (diiodohydroxyquin), a halogenated hydroxyquinoline, is an effective luminal amebicide. Pharmacokinetic data are incomplete but 90% of the drug is retained in the intestine and excreted in the feces. The remainder enters the circulation, has a half-life of 11–14 hours, and is excreted in the urine as glucuronides. Iodoquinol is effective against organisms in the bowel lumen but not against trophozoites. Infrequent adverse effects include diarrhea, anorexia, nausea, vomiting, abdominal pain, headache, rash, and pruritus. Iodoquinol should be taken with meals to limit gastrointestinal toxicity. It should be used with caution in patients with optic neuropathy, renal or thyroid disease, or nonamebic hepatic disease. The drug should be discontinued if it produces persistent diarrhea or signs of iodine toxicity (dermatitis, urticaria, pruritus, fever). It is contraindicated in patients with intolerance to iodine.

DILOXANIDE FUROATE

Diloxanide furoate is a dichloroacetamide derivative. It is an effective luminal amebicide but is not active against trophozoites. In the gut, diloxanide furoate is split into diloxanide and furoic acid; about 90% of the diloxanide is rapidly absorbed and then conjugated to form the glucuronide, which is promptly excreted in the urine. The unabsorbed diloxanide is the active antiamebic substance. Diloxanide furoate is not available commercially in the USA but can be obtained from some compounding pharmacies. It does not produce serious adverse effects. Flatulence is common, but nausea and abdominal cramps are infrequent and rashes are rare. The drug is not recommended in pregnancy.

■ LEISHMANIASIS

Infection with many different species of *Leishmania* can cause visceral leishmaniasis, which is typically fatal without therapy; cutaneous leishmaniasis, which entails chronic ulcers at the site of sand fly bites; and mucocutaneous leishmaniasis, in which skin ulcers are followed by destructive oral and nasal lesions (Table 52–6).

SODIUM STIBOGLUCONATE

Pentavalent antimonials, including sodium stibogluconate (pentostam; see Figure 52–3) and meglumine antimoniate, are first-line agents for cutaneous and visceral leishmaniasis, but they have been replaced by other agents in some regions, especially India, where efficacy has diminished greatly. The drugs are rapidly absorbed and distributed after intravenous (preferred) or intramuscular administration and eliminated in two phases, with a short initial (about 2-hour) half-life and a much longer terminal (>24-hour) half-life. Treatment is given at a dosage of 20 mg/kg once daily intravenously or intramuscularly for 20 days in cutaneous leishmaniasis and 28 days in visceral and mucocutaneous disease.

Few adverse effects occur initially, but the toxicity of stibogluconate increases over the course of therapy. Most common are gastrointestinal symptoms, fever, headache, myalgias, arthralgias, and rash. Intramuscular injections can be very painful and lead to sterile abscesses. Electrocardiographic changes may occur, most commonly T-wave changes and QT prolongation. These changes are generally reversible, but continued therapy may lead to dangerous arrhythmias. Thus, the electrocardiogram should be monitored during therapy. Hemolytic anemia and serious liver, renal, and cardiac effects are rare.

AMPHOTERICIN

This important antifungal drug (see Chapter 48) is an alternative therapy for visceral leishmaniasis, and has become the preferred treatment in India, where there is high-level resistance to sodium stibogluconate. Liposomal amphotericin has shown excellent efficacy in various regimens, including 3 mg/kg/d intravenously on days 1 through 5, 14, and 21; 4 doses of 5 mg/kg over 4–10 days; and, remarkably, a single dose of 10 mg/kg. Single-dose therapy has recently become standard in India, but efficacy has been lower in other regions, in particular Africa, and multiple-dose regimens may be required in these areas and for other forms of leishmaniasis. Other formulations of amphotericin B are also effective, including lipid emulsions and amphotericin B deoxycholate.

MILTEFOSINE

Miltefosine is an alkylphosphocholine analog that is the first effective oral drug for visceral leishmaniasis. It has shown excellent efficacy in the treatment of visceral leishmaniasis in India, where it is administered orally (2.5 mg/kg/d with varied dosing schedules) for 28 days. It was also recently shown to be effective in regimens including a single dose of liposomal amphotericin followed by 7–14 days of miltefosine; combination therapy with longer courses of both drugs has shown good efficacy against African visceral leishmaniasis. A 28-day course of miltefosine (2.5 mg/kg/d) was also effective for the treatment of New World cutaneous leishmaniasis. Vomiting and diarrhea are common but generally short-lived toxicities. Transient elevations in liver enzymes and nephrotoxicity are also seen. The drug should be avoided in pregnancy (and in women who may become pregnant within 2 months of treatment) because of its teratogenic effects. Resistance to miltefosine develops readily in vitro, and resistance may limit the role of this drug, especially as monotherapy.

PAROMOMYCIN

Paromomycin sulfate, an aminoglycoside antibiotic that is an effective luminal amebicide when provided orally, has been developed as a parenteral treatment of visceral leishmaniasis. It is much

TABLE 52–6 Treatment of other protozoal infections. Not all preparations are available in the USA.[1]

Organism or Clinical Setting	Drugs of Choice[2]	Alternative Drugs
Babesia species	Clindamycin, 600 mg 3 times daily for 7 days *plus* Quinine, 650 mg 3 times daily for 7 days (preferred for severe disease)	Atovaquone, 750 mg twice daily for 7 days *plus* Azithromycin, 600 mg once daily for 7 days (preferred for mild disease)
Balantidium coli	Tetracycline, 500 mg 4 times daily for 10 days	Metronidazole, 750 mg 3 times daily for 5 days
Cryptosporidium species	Paromomycin, 500–750 mg 3 or 4 times daily for 10 days	Azithromycin, 500 mg daily for 21 days
Cyclospora cayetanensis	Trimethoprim-sulfamethoxazole, one double-strength tablet 4 times daily for 7–14 days	
Dientamoeba fragilis	Iodoquinol, 650 mg 3 times daily for 20 days	Tetracycline, 500 mg 4 times daily for 10 days *or* Paromomycin, 500 mg 3 times daily for 7 days
Giardia lamblia	Metronidazole, 250 mg 3 times daily or 500 mg twice daily for 5 days *or* Tinidazole, 2 g once	Furazolidone, 100 mg 4 times daily for 7 days *or* Albendazole, 400 mg daily for 5 days
Isospora belli	Trimethoprim-sulfamethoxazole, one double-strength tablet 4 times daily for 10 days, then twice daily for 21 days	Pyrimethamine, 75 mg daily for 14 days *plus* Folinic acid, 10 mg daily for 14 days
Microsporidia	Albendazole, 400 mg twice daily for 20–30 days	
Leishmaniasis[3]		
Visceral *(L donovani, L chagasi, L infantum)* or mucosal *(L braziliensis)*	Sodium stibogluconate, 20 mg/kg/d IV or IM for 28 days *or* Amphotericin (liposomal preparations preferred [3 mg/kg/d IV on days 1–5, 14, and 21]); various other dosing regimens, including single dose *or* Miltefosine, 2.5 mg/kg/d for 28 days *or* Paromomycin,15 mg/kg for 21 days	Meglumine antimoniate *or* Pentamidine, 2–4 mg/kg IM daily or every other day for up to 15 doses *or* Combinations of listed drugs
Cutaneous *(L major, L tropica, L mexicana, L braziliensis)*	Sodium stibogluconate, 20 mg/kg/d IV or IM for 20 days	Meglumine antimoniate *or* Miltefosine *or* Topical or intralesional therapies
Pneumocystis jirovecii, P carinii[4]	Trimethoprim-sulfamethoxazole, 15–20 mg trimethoprim component/kg/d IV, or two double-strength tablets every 8 hours for 21 days	Pentamidine *or* Trimethoprim-dapsone *or* Clindamycin *plus* primaquine *or* Atovaquone

(continued)

TABLE 52–6 Treatment of other protozoal infections. Not all preparations are available in the USA.[1] (Continued)

Organism or Clinical Setting	Drugs of Choice[2]	Alternative Drugs
Toxoplasma gondii		
Acute, congenital, immunocompromised	Pyrimethamine *plus* clindamycin *plus* folinic acid	Pyrimethamine *plus* sulfadiazine *plus* folinic acid
Pregnancy	Spiramycin, 3 g daily until delivery	
Trichomonas vaginalis	Metronidazole, 2 g once or 250 mg 3 times daily for 7 days or Tinidazole, 2 g once	
Trypanosoma cruzi	Nifurtimox or Benznidazole	

[1]Additional information may be obtained from the Parasitic Disease Drug Service, Parasitic Diseases Branch, CDC, Atlanta, Georgia (phone: 404-639-3670; www.cdc.gov/laboratory/drugservice/).

[2]Established, relatively simple dosing regimens are provided. Route is oral unless otherwise indicated. See text for additional information, toxicities, cautions, and discussions of dosing for the more rarely used drugs, many of which are highly toxic.

[3]Specific recommendations for leishmaniasis vary geographically. Combination regimens are increasingly used.

[4]*P jirovecii* (*carinii* in animals) has traditionally been considered a protozoan because of its morphology and drug sensitivity, but molecular analyses have shown it to be most closely related to fungi.

less expensive than amphotericin or miltefosine. A trial in India showed excellent efficacy, with a daily intramuscular dosage of 11 mg/kg for 21 days yielding a 95% cure rate, and noninferiority compared with amphotericin. However, a trial showed poorer efficacy in Africa, with the cure rate for paromomycin significantly inferior to that with sodium stibogluconate. In initial studies, paromomycin was well tolerated, with common mild injection pain, uncommon ototoxicity, reversible liver enzyme elevations, and no nephrotoxicity. Paromomycin has also shown good efficacy when topically applied, alone or with gentamicin, for the treatment of cutaneous leishmaniasis.

Drug Combinations Used in the Treatment of Visceral Leishmaniasis

The use of drug combinations to improve treatment efficacy, shorten treatment courses, and reduce the selection of resistant parasites has been an active area of research. In a recent trial in India, compared to a standard 30-day (treatment on alternate days) course of amphotericin, noninferior efficacy and decreased adverse events were seen with a single dose of liposomal amphotericin plus a 7-day course of miltefosine, a single dose of liposomal amphotericin plus a 10-day course of paromomycin, or a 10-day course of miltefosine plus paromomycin. The combination regimens may not be needed in India, where single-dose liposomal amphotericin shows excellent efficacy, but they may have important roles elsewhere, where the efficacy of liposomal amphotericin is lower. A combination of sodium stibogluconate (20 mg/kg/d IV) plus paromomycin (15 mg/kg/d IM) for 17 days was shown to be safe and effective for visceral leishmaniasis in East Africa.

AFRICAN TRYPANOSOMIASIS

West and East African trypanosomiases, caused by related organisms, cause progressive systemic and neurological illnesses that are commonly fatal. Treatment differs for the two syndromes and for non-neurological illness and infections that have advanced to the CNS (Table 52–7).

PENTAMIDINE

Pentamidine has activity against trypanosomatid protozoans and against *P jirovecii*, but toxicity is significant.

TABLE 52–7 Treatment of African trypanosomiasis.

Disease	Stage	First-Line Drugs	Alternative Drugs
West African	Early	Pentamidine	Suramin,[1] eflornithine,[1] fexinidazole
	CNS involvement	Eflornithine[1]	Melarsoprol,[1] eflornithine-nifurtimox,[1] fexinidazole
East African	Early	Suramin[1]	Pentamidine
	CNS involvement	Melarsoprol[1]	

[1]Available in the USA from the Drug Service, CDC, Atlanta, Georgia (phone: 404-639-3670; www.cdc.gov/laboratory/drugservice/).

Chemistry & Pharmacokinetics

Pentamidine is an aromatic diamidine (see Figure 52–3) formulated as an isethionate salt. The drug is administered parenterally. It leaves the circulation rapidly, with an initial half-life of about 6 hours, but is bound avidly by tissues. Pentamidine thus accumulates and is eliminated very slowly, with a terminal elimination half-life of about 12 days. Only trace amounts of pentamidine appear in the central nervous system, so it is not effective against CNS African trypanosomiasis. The mechanism of action of pentamidine is unknown.

Clinical Uses

1. *Pneumocystosis*—Pentamidine is a well-established alternative therapy for pulmonary and extrapulmonary disease caused by *P jirovecii*. The drug has somewhat lower efficacy and greater toxicity than trimethoprim-sulfamethoxazole. The standard dosage is 3 mg/kg/d intravenously for 21 days. Significant adverse reactions are common, and with multiple regimens now available to treat *P jirovecii* infection, pentamidine is best reserved for patients with severe disease who cannot tolerate or fail other drugs.

Pentamidine is also an alternative agent for primary or secondary prophylaxis against pneumocystosis in immunocompromised individuals, including patients with advanced AIDS. For this indication, pentamidine is administered as an inhaled aerosol (300 mg inhaled monthly). The drug is well tolerated in this form. Its efficacy is good, but less than that of daily trimethoprim-sulfamethoxazole.

2. *African trypanosomiasis (sleeping sickness)*—Pentamidine has been used since 1940 and is the drug of choice to treat the early hemolymphatic stage of disease caused by *Trypanosoma brucei gambiense* (West African sleeping sickness). The drug is inferior to suramin for the treatment of early East African sleeping sickness. Pentamidine should not be used to treat late trypanosomiasis with central nervous system involvement. A number of dosing regimens have been described, generally providing 2–4 mg/kg daily or on alternate days for a total of 10–15 doses. Pentamidine has also been used for chemoprophylaxis against African trypanosomiasis, with dosing of 4 mg/kg every 3–6 months.

3. *Leishmaniasis*—Pentamidine is an alternative to sodium stibogluconate and newer agents for the treatment of visceral leishmaniasis. The drug has been successful in some cases that have failed therapy with antimonials. The dosage is 2–4 mg/kg intramuscularly daily or every other day for up to 15 doses, and a second course may be necessary. Pentamidine has also shown success against cutaneous leishmaniasis, but it is not routinely used for this purpose.

Adverse Effects & Cautions

Pentamidine is a highly toxic drug, with adverse effects noted in about 50% of patients receiving 4 mg/kg/d. Rapid intravenous administration can lead to severe hypotension, tachycardia, dizziness, and dyspnea, so the drug should be administered slowly (over 2 hours), and patients should be recumbent and monitored closely during treatment. With intramuscular administration, pain at the injection site is common, and sterile abscesses may develop.

Pancreatic toxicity is common. Hypoglycemia due to inappropriate insulin release often appears 5–7 days after onset of treatment, can persist for days to several weeks, and may be followed by hyperglycemia. Reversible renal insufficiency is also common. Other adverse effects include rash, metallic taste, fever, gastrointestinal symptoms, abnormal liver function tests, acute pancreatitis, hypocalcemia, thrombocytopenia, hallucinations, and cardiac arrhythmias. Inhaled pentamidine is generally well tolerated but may cause cough, dyspnea, and bronchospasm.

SURAMIN

Suramin is a sulfated naphthylamine that was introduced in the 1920s. It is the first-line therapy for early hemolymphatic East African trypanosomiasis (*T brucei rhodesiense* infection), but because it does not enter the central nervous system, it is not effective against advanced disease. Suramin is less effective than pentamidine for early West African trypanosomiasis. The drug's mechanism of action is unknown. It is administered intravenously and displays complex pharmacokinetics with very tight protein binding. Suramin has a short initial half-life but a terminal elimination half-life of about 50 days. The drug is slowly cleared by renal excretion.

Suramin is administered after a 200-mg intravenous test dose. Regimens that have been used include 1 g on days 1, 3, 7, 14, and 21 or 1 g each week for 5 weeks. Combination therapy with pentamidine may improve efficacy. Suramin can also be used for chemoprophylaxis against African trypanosomiasis. Adverse effects are common. Immediate reactions can include fatigue, nausea, vomiting, and, more rarely, seizures, shock, and death. Later reactions include fever, rash, headache, paresthesias, neuropathies, renal abnormalities including proteinuria, chronic diarrhea, hemolytic anemia, and agranulocytosis.

MELARSOPROL

Melarsoprol is a trivalent arsenical that has been available since 1949 and is first-line therapy for advanced CNS East African trypanosomiasis, and second-line therapy (after eflornithine) for advanced West African trypanosomiasis. After intravenous administration it is excreted rapidly, but clinically relevant concentrations accumulate in the CNS within 4 days. Melarsoprol is administered in propylene glycol by slow intravenous infusion at a dosage of 3.6 mg/kg/d for 3–4 days, with repeated courses at weekly intervals, if needed. A regimen of 2.2 mg/kg daily for 10 days had efficacy and toxicity similar to that of three courses over 26 days. Melarsoprol is extremely toxic. The use of such a toxic drug is justified only by the severity of advanced trypanosomiasis and the lack of alternatives. Immediate adverse effects include fever, vomiting, abdominal pain, and arthralgias. The most important toxicity is a reactive encephalopathy that generally appears within the first week of therapy (in 5–10% of patients) and is probably due to disruption of trypanosomes in the central nervous system. Coadministration of corticosteroids may decrease the likelihood of encephalopathy. Common consequences of the encephalopathy include cerebral edema, seizures, coma, and death. Other serious toxicities include renal and cardiac disease and hypersensitivity reactions. Failure rates with melarsoprol appear to have increased recently in parts of Africa, suggesting drug resistance.

EFLORNITHINE

Eflornithine (difluoromethylornithine), an inhibitor of ornithine decarboxylase, is the first-line drug for advanced West African trypanosomiasis, usually in combination with nifurtimox, but it is not effective for East African disease. Eflornithine is administered intravenously, and good CNS drug levels are achieved. The elimination half-life is about 3 hours. The usual regimen is 100 mg/kg intravenously every 6 hours for 7–14 days (14 days was superior for a newly diagnosed infection). Eflornithine appears to be as effective as melarsoprol against advanced West African trypanosomiasis, but its efficacy against East African disease is limited by drug resistance. Combining eflornithine with a 10-day course of nifurtimox afforded efficacy against West African trypanosomiasis similar to a 14-day regimen of eflornithine alone, with simpler and shorter treatment (injections every 12 hours for 7 days). Toxicity from eflornithine is significant, but considerably less than that from melarsoprol. Adverse effects include diarrhea, vomiting, anemia, thrombocytopenia, leukopenia, and seizures. These effects are generally reversible.

FEXINIDAZOLE

Fexinidazole is a DNA synthesis inhibitor that was approved by the European Medicines Agency in 2018 for the treatment of early and advanced (CNS) West African trypanosomiasis in patients aged ≥6 years and weighing ≥20 kg. This drug offers the first oral therapy for trypanosomiasis. It is administered once daily for 10 days. Fexinidazole is rapidly absorbed, with exposure increased when administered with food. Elimination is via nonrenal routes, with a terminal elimination half-life of 9–15 hours. Fexinidazole has demonstrated equivalent efficacy to eflornithine plus nifurtimox for the treatment of advanced disease, with success in over 90% of treated subjects. The drug has an acceptable safety profile, in particular compared to older therapies, but adverse events include headache, nausea, vomiting, insomnia, anxiety, weakness, tremor, and decreased appetite. Fexinidazole is likely to play an important role in simplifying the treatment of West African trypanosomiasis.

■ AMERICAN TRYPANOSOMIASIS

American trypanosomiasis (Chagas disease) is endemic in a large part of South and Central America and causes generally mild acute illness followed years later by severe smooth and cardiac muscle abnormalities.

BENZNIDAZOLE

Benznidazole is an orally administered nitroimidazole that probably has improved efficacy and safety compared to nifurtimox. These drugs can eliminate parasites and prevent progression when used to treat acute infection, but activity against chronic Chagas disease is suboptimal. In a recent randomized trial, treatment of Chagas cardiomyopathy with benznidazole did not offer clinical benefit. Standard dosage is 5 mg/kg/d in two or three divided doses for 60 days, given with meals. Important toxicities, which are generally reversible, include rash (in 20–30% of those treated), peripheral neuropathy, gastrointestinal symptoms, and myelosuppression.

NIFURTIMOX

Nifurtimox, a nitrofuran, is a standard drug for Chagas disease and is also used in the treatment of West African trypanosomiasis in combination with eflornithine. Nifurtimox is well absorbed after oral administration and eliminated with a plasma half-life of about 3 hours. The drug is administered at a dosage of 8–10 mg/kg/d in three divided doses with meals for 60–90 days. Toxicity related to nifurtimox is common. Adverse effects include nausea, vomiting, abdominal pain, fever, rash, headache, restlessness, insomnia, neuropathies, and seizures. These effects are generally reversible but often lead to cessation of therapy before completion of a standard course.

■ TREATMENT OF GIARDIASIS AND CRYPTOSPORIDIOSIS

Giardiasis is treated with metronidazole, tinidazole (see above), or nitazoxanide. Cryptosporidiosis responds poorly to therapy, especially in immunocompromised hosts, but nitazoxanide is approved for this purpose.

NITAZOXANIDE

Nitazoxanide is a nitrothiazolyl-salicylamide prodrug. It is approved in the USA for use against *Giardia lamblia* and *Cryptosporidium parvum*. It is rapidly absorbed and converted to tizoxanide and tizoxanide conjugates, which are subsequently excreted in both urine and feces. The active metabolite, tizoxanide, inhibits the pyruvate-ferredoxin oxidoreductase pathway. Nitazoxanide appears to have activity against metronidazole-resistant protozoal strains and is well tolerated. Unlike metronidazole, nitazoxanide and its metabolites appear to be free of mutagenic effects. Other organisms that may be susceptible to nitazoxanide include *E histolytica, Helicobacter pylori, Ascaris lumbricoides*, several tapeworms, and *Fasciola hepatica*. The recommended adult dosage is 500 mg twice daily for 3 days.

PREPARATIONS AVAILABLE

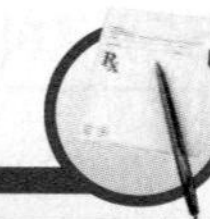

GENERIC NAME	AVAILABLE AS
Artemether/lumefantrine	Coartem, Riamet
Artesunate (intravenous)	
Artesunate-amodiaquine	ASAQ, Arsucam, Coarsucam
Artesunate-mefloquine	ASMQ
Artesunate-pyronaridine†	Pyramax
Atovaquone	Generic, Mepron
Atovaquone-proguanil	Malarone
Benznidazole	
Chloroquine	Generic, Aralen
Clindamycin	Generic, Cleocin
Doxycycline	Generic, Vibramycin
Eflornithine*	Vaniqa, Ornidyl
Fexinidazole†	Generic
Iodoquinol	Diquinol, Yodoxin
Mefloquine	Generic, Lariam
Melarsoprol*	Mel B
Metronidazole	Generic, Flagyl
Nifurtimox	Lampit
Nitazoxanide	Alinia
Paromomycin	Generic, Humatin
Pentamidine	Pentam 300, Pentacarinat, pentamidine isethionate, Nebupent (aerosol)
Primaquine	Generic
Pyrimethamine	Daraprim
Quinine	Generic
Sodium stibogluconate*	Pentostam
Sulfadoxine-pyrimethamine	Fansidar
Suramin*	Various
Tafenoquine	Krintafel, Arakoda
Tinidazole	Generic, Tindamax

*Available in the USA only from the Drug Service, CDC, Atlanta, Georgia (phone: 404-639-3670; www.cdc.gov/laboratory/drugservice/).

†Not available in the USA.

REFERENCES

Malaria

Amaratunga C et al: Dihydroartemisinin-piperaquine resistance in *Plasmodium falciparum* malaria in Cambodia: A multisite prospective cohort study. Lancet Infect Dis 2016;16:357.

Ashley EA et al: Tracking Resistance to Artemisinin Collaboration (TRAC): Spread of artemisinin resistance in *Plasmodium falciparum* malaria. N Engl J Med 2014;371:411.

Ashley EA, Pyae Phyo A, Woodrow CJ: Malaria. Lancet 2018;391:1608.

Baird JK: 8-Aminoquinoline therapy for latent malaria. Clin Microbiol Rev 2019;32:e00011.

Balikagala B et al: Evidence of artemisinin-resistant malaria in Africa. N Engl J Med 2021;385:1163.

Conrad MD, Rosenthal PJ: Antimalarial drug resistance in Africa: The calm before the storm? Lancet Infect Dis 2019;19:e338.

D'Alessandro U et al: Treatment of uncomplicated and severe malaria during pregnancy. Lancet Infect Dis 2018;18:e133.

Desai M et al: Prevention of malaria in pregnancy. Lancet Infect Dis 2018;18:e119.

Dondorp AM et al: Artesunate versus quinine in the treatment of severe falciparum malaria in African children (AQUAMAT): An open-label, randomised trial. Lancet 2010;376:1647.

Efferth T, Kaina B: Toxicity of the antimalarial artemisinin and its derivatives. Crit Rev Toxicol 2010;40:405.

Frampton JE: Tafenoquine: First global approval. Drugs 2018;78:1517.

German PI, Aweeka FT: Clinical pharmacology of artemisinin-based combination therapies. Clin Pharmacokinet 2008;47:91.

McGready R et al: Adverse effects of falciparum and vivax malaria and the safety of antimalarial treatment in early pregnancy: A population-based study. Lancet Infect Dis 2012;12:388.

Moore BR, Davis TME: Pharmacotherapy for the prevention of malaria in pregnant women: Currently available drugs and challenges. Expert Opin Pharmacother 2018;19:1779.

Morris CA et al: Review of the clinical pharmacokinetics of artesunate and its active metabolite dihydroartemisinin following intravenous, intramuscular, oral or rectal administration. Malar J 2011;10:263.

Rehman K et al: Haemolysis associated with the treatment of malaria with artemisinin derivatives: A systematic review of current evidence. Int J Infect Dis 2014;29:268.

Rosenthal PJ: Artesunate for the treatment of severe falciparum malaria. N Engl J Med 2008;358:1829.

Rosenthal PJ: The interplay between drug resistance and fitness in malaria parasites. Mol Microbiol 2013;89:1025.

Saito M et al: Antimalarial drugs for treating and preventing malaria in pregnant and lactating women. Expert Opin Drug Saf 2018;17:1129.

Stepniewska K, White NJ: Pharmacokinetic determinants of the window of selection for antimalarial drug resistance. Antimicrob Agents Chemother 2008;52:1589.

Tilley L et al: Artemisinin action and resistance in *Plasmodium falciparum*. Trends Parasitol 2016;32:682.

Uwimana A et al: Association of *Plasmodium falciparum* kelch13 R561H genotypes with delayed parasite clearance in Rwanda: an open-label, single-arm, multicentre, therapeutic efficacy study. Lancet Infect Dis 2021;21:1120.

West African Network for Clinical Trials of Antimalarial Drugs (WANECAM): Pyronaridine-artesunate or dihydroartemisinin-piperaquine versus current first-line therapies for repeated treatment of uncomplicated malaria: A randomised, multicentre, open-label, longitudinal, controlled, phase 3b/4 trial. Lancet 2018;391:1378.

World Health Organization: Guidelines for the treatment of malaria. Geneva. 2015. www.who.int/malaria/publications/atoz/9789241549127/en/.

Intestinal Protozoal Infections

Granados CE et al: Drugs for treating giardiasis. Cochrane Database Syst Rev 2012;12:CD007787.

Marcos LA, Gotuzzo E: Intestinal protozoan infections in the immunocompromised host. Curr Opin Infect Dis 2013;26:295.

Pasupuleti V et al: Efficacy of 5-nitroimidazoles for the treatment of giardiasis: A systematic review of randomized controlled trials. PLoS Negl Trop Dis 2014;8:e2733.

Shirley DT et al: A review of the global burden, new diagnostics, and current therapeutics for amebiasis. Open Forum Infect Dis 2018;5:ofy161.

Trypanosomiasis & Leishmaniasis

Aronson N et al: Diagnosis and treatment of leishmaniasis: Clinical practice guidelines by the Infectious Diseases Society of America (IDSA) and the American Society of Tropical Medicine and Hygiene (ASTMH). Clin Infect Dis 2016;63:1539.

Ben Salah A et al: Topical paromomycin with or without gentamicin for cutaneous leishmaniasis. N Engl J Med 2013;368:524.

Berman J: Liposomal amphotericin B treatment and the leishmaniases. Am J Trop Med Hyg 2019;101:727.

Bern C: Chagas' disease. N Engl J Med 2015;373:456.

Burza S et al: Five-year field results and long-term effectiveness of 20 mg/kg liposomal amphotericin B (Ambisome) for visceral leishmaniasis in Bihar, India. PLoS Negl Trop Dis 2014;8:e2603.

Burza S et al: Leishmaniasis. Lancet 2018;392:951.

Büscher P et al: Human African trypanosomiasis. Lancet 2017;390:2397.

Deeks ED: Fexinidazole: First global approval. Drugs 2019;79:215.

Diro E et al: A randomized trial of AmBisome monotherapy and AmBisome and miltefosine combination to treat visceral leishmaniasis in HIV co-infected patients in Ethiopia. PLoS Negl Trop Dis 2019;13:e0006988.

Jackson Y et al: Tolerance and safety of nifurtimox in patients with chronic Chagas disease. Clin Infect Dis 2010;51:e69.

Kimutai R et al: Safety and effectiveness of sodium stibogluconate and paromomycin combination for the treatment of visceral leishmaniasis in eastern Africa: Results from a pharmacovigilance programme. Clin Drug Investig 2017;37:259.

Mesu VKBK et al: Oral fexinidazole for late-stage African *Trypanosoma brucei gambiense* trypanosomiasis: A pivotal multicentre, randomised, non-inferiority trial. Lancet 2018;391:144.

Morillo CA et al: Randomized trial of benznidazole for chronic Chagas' cardiomyopathy. N Engl J Med 2015;373:1295.

Musa A et al: Sodium stibogluconate (SSG) & paromomycin combination compared to SSG for visceral leishmaniasis in East Africa: A randomised controlled trial. PLoS Negl Trop Dis 2012;6:e1674.

Pérez-Molina JA, Molina I: Chagas disease. Lancet 2018; 391:82.

Ponte-Sucre A et al: Drug resistance and treatment failure in leishmaniasis: A 21st century challenge. PLoS Negl Trop Dis 2017;11:e0006052.

Priotto G et al: Nifurtimox-eflornithine combination therapy for second-stage African *Trypanosoma brucei gambiense* trypanosomiasis: A multicentre, randomised, phase III, non-inferiority trial. Lancet 2009;374:56.

Rubiano LC et al: Noninferiority of miltefosine versus meglumine antimoniate for cutaneous leishmaniasis in children. J Infect Dis 2012;205:684.

Sundar S, Singh A: Recent developments and future prospects in the treatment of visceral leishmaniasis. Ther Adv Infect Dis 2016;3:98.

Sundar S et al: Comparison of short-course multidrug treatment with standard therapy for visceral leishmaniasis in India: An open-label, non-inferiority, randomised controlled trial. Lancet 2011;377:477.

Sundar S et al: Efficacy and safety of amphotericin B emulsion versus liposomal formulation in Indian patients with visceral leishmaniasis: A randomized, open-label study. PLoS Negl Trop Dis 2014;8:e3169.

Sundar S et al: Efficacy of miltefosine in the treatment of visceral leishmaniasis in India after a decade of use. Clin Infect Dis 2012;55:543.

Sundar S et al: Single-dose liposomal amphotericin B for visceral leishmaniasis in India. N Engl J Med 2010;362:504.

van Griensven J et al: Combination therapy for visceral leishmaniasis. Lancet Infect Dis 2010;10:184.

Vélez I et al: Efficacy of miltefosine for the treatment of American cutaneous leishmaniasis. Am J Trop Med Hyg 2010;83:351.

CASE STUDY ANSWER

This child has acute falciparum malaria, and her lethargy and abnormal laboratory tests are consistent with progression to severe disease. She should be hospitalized and treated urgently with intravenous artesunate. She should be followed closely for progression of severe malaria, in particular neurologic, renal, or pulmonary complications.

CHAPTER

53 Pharmacology of the Antihelminthic Drugs

Philip J. Rosenthal, MD

CASE STUDY

A 29-year-old Peruvian man presents with the incidental finding of a 10 × 8 × 8-cm liver cyst on an abdominal computed tomography (CT) scan. The patient had noted 2 days of abdominal pain and fever, and his clinical evaluation and CT scan were consistent with appendicitis. His clinical findings resolved after laparoscopic appendectomy. The patient immigrated to the USA 10 years ago from a rural area of Peru where his family trades in sheepskins. His father and sister have undergone resection of abdominal masses, but details of their diagnoses are unavailable. What is your differential diagnosis? What are your diagnostic and therapeutic plans?

CHEMOTHERAPY OF HELMINTHIC INFECTIONS

Helminths (worms) are multicellular organisms that infect very large numbers of humans and cause a broad range of diseases. More than 1 billion people are infected with intestinal nematodes, and many millions are infected with filarial nematodes, flukes, and tapeworms. Many drugs, directed against a number of different targets, are available to treat helminthic infections. In many cases, especially in the developing world, the goal is control of infection, with elimination of most parasites, alleviating disease symptoms, and decreasing the transmission of infection. In other cases, complete elimination of parasites is the goal of therapy, although this goal can be challenging with certain helminthic infections, because of both limited efficacy of drugs and frequent reinfection after therapy in endemic areas.

Table 53–1 lists the major helminthic infections and provides a guide to the drug of choice and alternative drugs for each infection. In the text that follows, these drugs are arranged alphabetically. In general, parasites should be identified before treatment is started.

ALBENDAZOLE

Albendazole, a broad-spectrum oral antihelminthic, is the drug of choice and is approved in the USA for treatment of hydatid disease and cysticercosis. It is also used in the treatment of pinworm and hookworm infections, ascariasis, trichuriasis, and strongyloidiasis.

Basic Pharmacology

Albendazole is a benzimidazole carbamate. After oral administration, it is erratically absorbed (increased with a fatty meal) and then rapidly undergoes first-pass metabolism in the liver to the active metabolite albendazole sulfoxide. It reaches variable maximum plasma concentrations about 3 hours after a 400-mg oral dose, and its plasma half-life is 8–12 hours. The sulfoxide is mostly protein-bound, distributes well to tissues, and enters bile, cerebrospinal fluid, and hydatid cysts. Albendazole metabolites are excreted in the urine.

Benzimidazoles are thought to act against nematodes by inhibiting microtubule synthesis. Albendazole also has larvicidal effects in hydatid disease, cysticercosis, ascariasis, and hookworm infection and ovicidal effects in ascariasis, ancylostomiasis, and trichuriasis.

TABLE 53–1 Drugs for the treatment of helminthic infections.[1]

Infecting Organism	Drug of Choice	Alternative Drugs
Roundworms (nematodes)		
Ascaris lumbricoides (roundworm)	Albendazole or pyrantel pamoate or mebendazole	Ivermectin, piperazine
Trichuris trichiura (whipworm)	Mebendazole or albendazole	Ivermectin, oxantel pamoate, drug combinations
Necator americanus (hookworm); *Ancylostoma duodenale* (hookworm)	Albendazole or mebendazole or pyrantel pamoate	
Strongyloides stercoralis (threadworm)	Ivermectin	Albendazole or thiabendazole
Enterobius vermicularis (pinworm)	Mebendazole or pyrantel pamoate	Albendazole
Trichinella spiralis (trichinosis)	Mebendazole or albendazole; add corticosteroids for severe infection	
Trichostrongylus species	Pyrantel pamoate or mebendazole	Albendazole
Cutaneous larva migrans (creeping eruption)	Albendazole or ivermectin	Thiabendazole (topical)
Visceral larva migrans	Albendazole	Mebendazole
Angiostrongylus cantonensis	Albendazole or mebendazole	
Wuchereria bancrofti (filariasis); *Brugia malayi* (filariasis); tropical eosinophilia; *Loa loa* (loiasis)	Diethylcarbamazine	Ivermectin
Onchocerca volvulus (onchocerciasis)	Ivermectin	Moxidectin
Dracunculus medinensis (guinea worm)	Metronidazole	Thiabendazole or mebendazole
Capillaria philippinensis (intestinal capillariasis)	Albendazole	Mebendazole
Flukes (trematodes)		
Schistosoma haematobium (bilharziasis)	Praziquantel	Metrifonate
Schistosoma mansoni	Praziquantel	Oxamniquine
Schistosoma japonicum	Praziquantel	
Clonorchis sinensis (liver fluke); *Opisthorchis* species	Praziquantel	Albendazole
Paragonimus westermani (lung fluke)	Praziquantel	Bithionol
Fasciola hepatica (sheep liver fluke)	Triclabendazole	Bithionol
Fasciolopsis buski (large intestinal fluke)	Praziquantel or niclosamide	
Heterophyes heterophyes; Metagonimus yokogawai (small intestinal flukes)	Praziquantel or niclosamide	
Tapeworms (cestodes)		
Taenia saginata (beef tapeworm)	Praziquantel or niclosamide	Mebendazole
Diphyllobothrium latum (fish tapeworm)	Praziquantel or niclosamide	
Taenia solium (pork tapeworm)	Praziquantel or niclosamide	
Cysticercosis (pork tapeworm larval stage)	Albendazole	Praziquantel
Hymenolepis nana (dwarf tapeworm)	Praziquantel	Niclosamide, nitazoxanide
Echinococcus granulosus (hydatid disease); *Echinococcus multilocularis*	Albendazole	

[1]Additional information may be obtained from the Parasitic Disease Drug Service, Parasitic Diseases Branch, Centers for Disease Control and Prevention, Atlanta, Georgia, 30333. Telephone: (404) 639-3670. Some of the drugs listed are not generally available in the USA.

Clinical Uses

Albendazole is administered on an empty stomach when used against intraluminal parasites but with a fatty meal when used against tissue parasites.

1. Ascariasis, trichuriasis, and hookworm and pinworm infections—For adults and children older than 2 years with ascariasis and pinworm infections, the treatment for ascariasis is a single dose of 400 mg orally (repeated daily for 2–3 days for heavy infections and in 2 weeks for pinworm infections). These treatments typically achieve good cure rates and marked reduction in egg counts in those not cured. For hookworm infections and trichuriasis, albendazole at 400 mg orally once daily for 3 days is now recommended, with albendazole showing improved efficacy over mebendazole. For trichuriasis, combination of either mebendazole or albendazole with ivermectin and combination of albendazole with oxantel pamoate markedly improved treatment outcomes.

2. Hydatid disease—Albendazole is the treatment of choice for medical therapy and is a useful adjunct to surgical removal or aspiration of cysts. It is more active against *Echinococcus granulosus* than against *Echinococcus multilocularis*. Dosing is 400 mg twice daily with meals for 1 month or longer. Daily therapy for up to 6 months has been well tolerated. One reported therapeutic strategy is to treat with albendazole and praziquantel, to assess response after 1 month or more, and, depending on the response, to then manage the patient with continued chemotherapy or combined surgical and drug therapy.

3. Neurocysticercosis—Indications for medical therapy for neurocysticercosis are controversial, since antihelminthic therapy is not clearly superior to therapy with corticosteroids alone and may exacerbate neurologic disease. Therapy is probably most appropriate for symptomatic parenchymal or intraventricular cysts. Corticosteroids are usually given with the antihelminthic drug to decrease inflammation caused by dying organisms. Albendazole is now generally considered the drug of choice over praziquantel because of its shorter course, lower cost, improved penetration into the subarachnoid space, and increased drug levels (as opposed to decreased levels of praziquantel) when administered with corticosteroids. Albendazole is given in a dosage of 400 mg twice daily for up to 21 days. Albendazole combined with praziquantel improves efficacy in patients with multiple brain cysts.

4. Other infections—Albendazole is the drug of choice in the treatment of cutaneous larva migrans (400 mg daily for 3 days), visceral larva migrans (400 mg twice daily for 5 days), intestinal capillariasis (400 mg daily for 10 days), microsporidial infections (400 mg twice daily for 2 weeks or longer), and gnathostomiasis (400 mg twice daily for 3 weeks). It also has activity against taeniasis (400 mg daily for 3 days), trichinosis (400 mg twice daily for 1–2 weeks), and clonorchiasis (400 mg twice daily for 1 week). There have been reports of effectiveness in treatment of opisthorchiasis, toxocariasis, and loiasis. Albendazole is included in programs to control lymphatic filariasis. It appears to be less active than diethylcarbamazine or ivermectin for this purpose, but it is included in combination with either of those drugs in control programs. Albendazole has been recommended as empiric therapy to treat those who return from the tropics with persistent unexplained eosinophilia. Albendazole has activity against giardiasis, but with decreased efficacy compared to tinidazole.

Adverse Reactions, Contraindications, & Cautions

When used for 1–3 days, albendazole is nearly free of significant adverse effects. Mild and transient epigastric distress, diarrhea, headache, nausea, dizziness, lassitude, and insomnia can occur. In long-term use for hydatid disease, albendazole is well tolerated, but it can cause abdominal distress, headaches, fever, fatigue, alopecia, increases in liver enzymes, and pancytopenia.

Blood counts and liver function should be monitored during long-term therapy. The drug should not be given to patients with known hypersensitivity to other benzimidazole drugs or to those with cirrhosis. The safety of albendazole in pregnancy and in children younger than 2 years has not been established. Exposure to albendazole is increased by dexamethasone, praziquantel, and cimetidine, and decreased by phenytoin, phenobarbital, carbamazepine, and ritonavir.

BITHIONOL

Bithionol is an alternative to triclabendazole for the treatment of fascioliasis (sheep liver fluke) and an alternative to praziquantel for the treatment of paragonimiasis.

Basic Pharmacology & Clinical Uses

After ingestion, bithionol reaches peak blood levels in 4–8 hours. Excretion appears to be mainly via the kidney.

For treatment of paragonimiasis and fascioliasis, the dosage of bithionol is 30–50 mg/kg in two or three divided doses, given orally after meals on alternate days for 10–15 doses. For pulmonary paragonimiasis, cure rates are over 90%. For cerebral paragonimiasis, repeat courses may be necessary.

Adverse Reactions, Contraindications, & Cautions

Adverse effects, which occur in up to 40% of patients, are generally mild and transient, but occasionally their severity requires interruption of therapy. These problems include diarrhea, abdominal cramps, anorexia, nausea, vomiting, dizziness, and headache. Skin rashes may occur after a week or more of therapy, suggesting a reaction to antigens released from dying worms. Bithionol should be used with caution in children younger than 8 years because there has been limited experience in this age group.

DIETHYLCARBAMAZINE CITRATE

Diethylcarbamazine is a drug of choice in the treatment of filariasis, loiasis, and tropical eosinophilia. It has been replaced by ivermectin for the treatment of onchocerciasis.

Basic Pharmacology

Diethylcarbamazine, a synthetic piperazine derivative, is rapidly absorbed from the gastrointestinal tract; after a dose of 0.5 mg/kg, peak plasma levels are reached within 1–2 hours. The plasma half-life is 2–3 hours in the presence of acidic urine but about 10 hours if the urine is alkaline, a Henderson-Hasselbalch trapping effect (see Chapter 1). The drug rapidly equilibrates with all tissues except fat. It is excreted, principally in the urine, as unchanged drug and the *N*-oxide metabolite. Dosage should be reduced in patients with renal impairment.

Diethylcarbamazine immobilizes microfilariae and alters their surface structure, displacing them from tissues and making them more susceptible to destruction by host defense mechanisms. The mode of action against adult worms is unknown.

Clinical Uses

The drug should be taken after meals.

1. Wuchereria bancrofti, Brugia malayi, Brugia timori, and Loa loa**—**Diethylcarbamazine is the drug of choice for treatment of infections with these parasites because of its efficacy and lack of serious toxicity. Microfilariae of all species are rapidly killed; adult parasites are killed more slowly, often requiring several courses of treatment. Lymphatic filariasis is treated with 2 mg/kg three times a day for 12 days, and loiasis is treated with the same regimen for 2–3 weeks. Antihistamines may be given for the first few days of therapy to limit allergic reactions, and corticosteroids should be started and doses of diethylcarbamazine lowered or interrupted if severe reactions occur. Cures may require several courses of treatment. For lymphatic filariasis, recent trials have shown that a single dose of a triple drug combination of diethylcarbamazine, albendazole, and ivermectin offers outstanding efficacy in clearance of microfilaremia. For patients with high *L loa* worm burdens (more than 2500 circulating parasites/mL), strategies to decrease risks of severe toxicity include (1) apheresis, if available, to remove microfilariae before treatment with diethylcarbamazine, or (2) therapy with albendazole, which is slower acting and better tolerated, followed by therapy with diethylcarbamazine or ivermectin. Diethylcarbamazine may also be used for chemoprophylaxis against filarial infections (300 mg weekly or 300 mg on 3 successive days each month for loiasis; 50 mg monthly for bancroftian and Malayan filariasis).

2. Other uses**—**For tropical eosinophilia, diethylcarbamazine is given orally at a dosage of 2 mg/kg three times daily for 2–3 weeks. Diethylcarbamazine is effective in *Mansonella streptocerca* infections, since it kills both adults and microfilariae. Limited information suggests that the drug is not effective, however, against adult *Mansonella ozzardi* or *Mansonella perstans* and that it has limited activity against microfilariae of these parasites. An important application of diethylcarbamazine has been mass treatment to reduce the prevalence of *W bancrofti* infection, generally in combination with ivermectin or albendazole. This strategy has led to excellent progress in disease control in a number of countries.

Adverse Reactions, Contraindications, & Cautions

Reactions to diethylcarbamazine, which are generally mild and transient, include headache, malaise, anorexia, weakness, nausea, vomiting, and dizziness. Adverse effects also occur as a result of the release of proteins from dying microfilariae or adult worms. Reactions can be particularly severe with onchocerciasis, but diethylcarbamazine is no longer commonly used for this infection because ivermectin is equally efficacious and less toxic. Reactions to dying microfilariae are usually mild in *W bancrofti*, more intense in *B malayi*, and occasionally severe in *L loa* infections. Reactions include fever, malaise, papular rash, headache, gastrointestinal symptoms, cough, chest pain, and muscle or joint pain. Leukocytosis is common, and eosinophilia may increase with treatment. Proteinuria also may occur. Symptoms are most likely to occur in patients with heavy loads of microfilariae. Retinal hemorrhages and, rarely, encephalopathy have been described. Local reactions may occur in the vicinity of dying adult or immature worms. These include lymphangitis with localized swellings in *W bancrofti* and *B malayi*, small wheals in the skin in *L loa*, and flat papules in *M streptocerca* infections. Patients with attacks of lymphangitis due to *W bancrofti* or *B malayi* should be treated during a quiescent period between attacks. Caution is advised when using diethylcarbamazine in patients with hypertension or renal disease.

DOXYCYCLINE

This tetracycline antibiotic is described in more detail in Chapter 44. Doxycycline has recently been shown to have significant macrofilaricidal activity against *W bancrofti*, suggesting better activity than any other available drug against adult worms. Activity is also seen against onchocerciasis. Doxycycline acts indirectly, by killing *Wolbachia*, an intracellular bacterial symbiont of filarial parasites. It may prove to be an important drug for filariasis and onchocerciasis, both for treatment of active disease and in mass chemotherapy campaigns.

IVERMECTIN

Ivermectin is the drug of choice in strongyloidiasis and onchocerciasis. It is also an alternative drug for a number of other helminthic infections (see Table 53–1).

Basic Pharmacology

Ivermectin, a semisynthetic macrocyclic lactone derived from the soil actinomycete *Streptomyces avermitilis*, is a mixture of avermectin B_{1a} and B_{1b}. Ivermectin is available only for oral administration in humans. The drug is rapidly absorbed, reaching maximum plasma concentrations 4 hours after a 12-mg dose. Ivermectin has a wide tissue distribution and a volume of distribution of about 50 L. Its half-life is about 16 hours. Excretion of the drug and its metabolites is almost exclusively in the feces.

Ivermectin appears to paralyze nematodes and arthropods by intensifying γ-aminobutyric acid (GABA)-mediated transmission of signals in peripheral nerves. In onchocerciasis, ivermectin is microfilaricidal. It does not effectively kill adult worms but blocks the release of microfilariae for some months after therapy. After a single standard dose, microfilariae in the skin diminish rapidly within 2–3 days, remain low for months, and then gradually increase; microfilariae in the anterior chamber of the eye decrease slowly over months, eventually clear, and then gradually return. With repeated doses of ivermectin, the drug appears to have a low-level macrofilaricidal action and to permanently reduce microfilarial production.

Clinical Uses

1. Onchocerciasis**—**Treatment is with a single oral dose of ivermectin, 150 mcg/kg, with water on an empty stomach. After acute therapy, treatment is repeated at 12-month intervals until the adult worms die, which may take 10 years or longer. With the first treatment only, patients with microfilariae in the cornea or anterior chamber may be treated with corticosteroids to avoid inflammatory eye reactions.

Ivermectin also now plays a key role in onchocerciasis control. Annual mass treatments have led to major reductions in disease transmission. However, evidence of diminished responsiveness after mass administration of ivermectin has raised concern regarding selection of drug-resistant parasites.

2. Strongyloidiasis**—**Treatment consists of 200 mcg/kg once daily for 2 days. In immunosuppressed patients with disseminated infection, repeated treatment is often needed, and cure may not be possible. In this case, suppressive therapy—ie, once monthly—may be helpful.

3. Other parasites**—**Ivermectin reduces microfilariae in *B malayi* and *M ozzardi* infections but not in *M perstans* infections. It has been used with diethylcarbamazine and albendazole for the control of *W bancrofti*, but it does not kill adult worms. In loiasis, although the drug reduces microfilaria concentrations, it can occasionally induce severe reactions and appears to be more dangerous in this regard than diethylcarbamazine. Ivermectin is also effective in controlling scabies, lice, and cutaneous larva migrans and in eliminating a large proportion of ascarid worms. Ivermectin is under study for the control of malaria transmission due to activity against mosquitoes feeding on treated subjects.

Adverse Reactions, Contraindications, & Cautions

In strongyloidiasis treatment, infrequent adverse effects of ivermectin include fatigue, dizziness, nausea, vomiting, abdominal pain, and rashes. In onchocerciasis treatment, adverse effects are principally from the killing of microfilariae and can include fever, headache, dizziness, somnolence, weakness, rash, increased pruritus, diarrhea, joint and muscle pains, hypotension, tachycardia, lymphadenitis, lymphangitis, and peripheral edema. This reaction starts on the first day and peaks on the second day after treatment. It occurs in 5–30% of persons and is generally mild, but it may be more frequent and more severe in individuals who are not long-term residents of onchocerciasis-endemic areas. A more intense reaction occurs in 1–3% of persons and a severe reaction in 0.1%, including high fever, hypotension, and bronchospasm. Corticosteroids are indicated in these cases, at times for several days. Toxicity diminishes with repeated dosing. Swellings and abscesses occasionally occur at 1–3 weeks, presumably at sites of adult worms. Some patients develop corneal opacities and other eye lesions several days after treatment. These are rarely severe and generally resolve without corticosteroid treatment. It is best to avoid concomitant use of ivermectin with other drugs that enhance GABA activity, eg, barbiturates, benzodiazepines, and valproic acid. Ivermectin should not be used during pregnancy. Safety in children younger than 5 years has not been established.

MEBENDAZOLE

Mebendazole is a synthetic benzimidazole that has a wide spectrum of antihelminthic activity and a low incidence of adverse effects.

Basic Pharmacology

Less than 10% of orally administered mebendazole is absorbed. The absorbed drug is protein-bound (>90%), is rapidly converted to inactive metabolites (primarily during its first pass in the liver), and has a half-life of 2–6 hours. It is excreted mostly in the urine, principally as decarboxylated derivatives, as well as in the bile. Absorption is increased if the drug is ingested with a fatty meal.

Mebendazole probably acts by inhibiting microtubule synthesis; the parent drug appears to be the active form. Efficacy of the drug varies with gastrointestinal transit time, with intensity of infection, and perhaps with the strain of parasite. The drug kills hookworm, *Ascaris*, and *Trichuris* eggs.

Clinical Uses

Mebendazole is indicated for use in ascariasis, trichuriasis, hookworm and pinworm infections, and certain other helminthic infections. It can be taken before or after meals; the tablets should be chewed before swallowing. For pinworm infection, the dose is 100 mg once, repeated at 2 weeks. For ascariasis, trichuriasis, hookworm, and *Trichostrongylus* infections, a dosage of 100 mg twice daily for 3 days is used for adults and for children older than 2 years. Cure rates are good for pinworm infections and ascariasis but have been disappointing in recent studies of trichuriasis, although efficacy for trichuriasis is better than that of albendazole. Cure rates are also low for hookworm infections, but a marked reduction in the worm burden occurs in those not cured. For intestinal capillariasis, mebendazole is used at a dosage of 200 mg twice daily for 21 or more days. In trichinosis, limited reports suggest efficacy against adult worms in the intestinal tract and tissue larvae. Treatment is three times daily, with fatty foods, at 200–400 mg per dose for 3 days and then 400–500 mg per dose for 10 days; corticosteroids should be coadministered for severe infections.

Adverse Reactions, Contraindications, & Cautions

Short-term mebendazole therapy for intestinal nematodes is nearly free of adverse effects. Mild nausea, vomiting, diarrhea, and abdominal pain have been reported infrequently. Rare side effects, usually with high-dose therapy, are hypersensitivity reactions (rash, urticaria), agranulocytosis, alopecia, and elevation of liver enzymes.

Mebendazole is teratogenic in animals and therefore contraindicated in pregnancy. It should be used with caution in children younger than 2 years because of limited experience and rare reports of convulsions in this age group. Plasma levels may be decreased by concomitant use of carbamazepine, phenytoin, or ritonavir, and increased by cimetidine. Mebendazole should be used with caution in patients with cirrhosis.

METRIFONATE (TRICHLORFON)

Metrifonate is a safe, low-cost alternative drug for the treatment of *Schistosoma haematobium* infections. It is not active against *Schistosoma mansoni* or *Schistosoma japonicum*. It is not available in the USA.

Basic Pharmacology

Metrifonate, an organophosphate, is rapidly absorbed after oral administration. After the standard oral dose, peak blood levels are reached in 1–2 hours; the half-life is about 1.5 hours. Clearance appears to be through nonenzymatic transformation to dichlorvos, its active metabolite. Metrifonate and dichlorvos are well distributed to the tissues and are completely eliminated in 24–48 hours.

The mode of action is thought to be cholinesterase inhibition, temporarily paralyzing adult worms, resulting in their transit from bladder vasculature to small arterioles in the lungs, where they are killed. The drug is not effective against *S haematobium* eggs; live eggs continue to pass in the urine for several months after all adult worms have been killed.

Clinical Uses

In the treatment of *S haematobium*, an oral dose of 7.5–10 mg/kg is given three times at 14-day intervals. Cure rates on this schedule are 44–93%, with marked reductions in egg counts in those not cured. Metrifonate was also effective as a prophylactic agent when given monthly to children in a highly endemic area, and it has been used in mass treatment programs. In mixed infections with *S haematobium* and *S mansoni*, metrifonate has been successfully combined with oxamniquine.

Adverse Reactions, Contraindications, & Cautions

Some studies note mild and transient cholinergic symptoms, including nausea and vomiting, diarrhea, abdominal pain, bronchospasm, headache, sweating, fatigue, weakness, dizziness, and vertigo. Metrifonate should not be used after recent exposure to insecticides or drugs that might potentiate cholinesterase inhibition. It is contraindicated in pregnancy.

MOXIDECTIN

Moxidectin, a macrocyclic lactone, was approved by the FDA in 2018 for the treatment of onchocerciasis in persons ≥12 years old. The drug has also demonstrated activity for strongyloidiasis and trichuriasis, although it was not superior to standard treatments for these infections. The dosage for onchocerciasis is 8 mg orally taken once. After oral administration the drug has a half-life of 3–4 weeks. In a recent trial for treatment of onchocerciasis, moxidectin decreased skin microfilarial loads more effectively than did ivermectin, suggesting an improved impact on disease transmission. Adverse events with moxidectin in those with onchocerciasis have included pruritus, musculoskeletal pain, headache, tachycardia, and rash.

NICLOSAMIDE

Niclosamide is a second-line drug for the treatment of most tapeworm infections, but it is not available in the USA.

Basic Pharmacology

Niclosamide is a salicylamide derivative. It appears to be minimally absorbed from the gastrointestinal tract—neither the drug nor its metabolites have been recovered from the blood or urine. Adult worms (but not ova) are rapidly killed, presumably due to inhibition of oxidative phosphorylation or stimulation of ATPase activity.

Clinical Uses

The adult dose of niclosamide is 2 g once, given in the morning on an empty stomach. The tablets must be chewed thoroughly and then swallowed with water.

1. Taenia saginata (beef tapeworm), Taenia solium (pork tapeworm), and Diphyllobothrium latum (fish tapeworm)—A single 2-g dose of niclosamide results in cure rates of >85% for *D latum* and about 95% for *T saginata*. It is probably equally effective against *T solium*. Cysticercosis can theoretically occur after treatment of *T solium* infections, because viable ova are released into the gut lumen after digestion of segments, but no such cases have been reported.

2. Other tapeworms—Most patients treated with niclosamide for *Hymenolepis diminuta* and *Dipylidium caninum* infections are cured with a 7-day course of treatment; a few require a second course. Praziquantel is superior for *Hymenolepis nana* (dwarf tapeworm) infection. Niclosamide is not effective against cysticercosis or hydatid disease.

3. Intestinal fluke infections—Niclosamide can be used as an alternative drug in the treatment of *Fasciolopsis buski*, *Heterophyes heterophyes*, and *Metagonimus yokogawai* infections. The standard dose is given every other day for three doses.

Adverse Reactions, Contraindications, & Cautions

Infrequent, mild, and transitory adverse events include nausea, vomiting, diarrhea, and abdominal discomfort. Alcohol should not be consumed during or for 1 day after treatment. Safety has not been established in pregnancy or for children younger than 2 years.

OXAMNIQUINE

Oxamniquine is an alternative to praziquantel for the treatment of *S mansoni* infections. It has also been used extensively for mass treatment. It is not effective against *S haematobium* or *S japonicum*. It is not available in the USA.

Basic Pharmacology

Oxamniquine, a semisynthetic tetrahydroquinoline, is readily absorbed orally; it should be taken with food. Its plasma half-life is about 2.5 hours. The drug is extensively metabolized to inactive metabolites and excreted in the urine—up to 75% in the first 24 hours. Intersubject variations in serum concentration have been noted, which may explain some treatment failures.

Oxamniquine is active against both mature and immature stages of *S mansoni* but does not appear to be cercaricidal. The mechanism of action is unknown. Contraction and paralysis of the worms results in detachment from terminal venules in the mesentery and transit to the liver, where many die; surviving females return to the mesenteric vessels but cease to lay eggs. Strains of *S mansoni* in different parts of the world vary in susceptibility. Oxamniquine has been effective in instances of praziquantel resistance.

Clinical Uses

Oxamniquine is safe and effective in all stages of *S mansoni* disease, including advanced hepatosplenomegaly. The drug is generally less effective in children, who require higher doses than adults. It is better tolerated with food.

Optimal dosage schedules vary for different regions of the world. In the western hemisphere and western Africa, the adult oxamniquine dosage is 12–15 mg/kg given once. In northern and southern Africa, standard schedules are 15 mg/kg twice daily for 2 days. In eastern Africa and the Arabian peninsula, standard dosage is 15–20 mg/kg twice in 1 day. Cure rates are 70–95%, with marked reduction in egg excretion in those not cured. In mixed schistosome infections, oxamniquine has been successfully used in combination with metrifonate.

Adverse Reactions, Contraindications, & Cautions

Mild symptoms occur in more than one-third of patients receiving oxamniquine. Central nervous system symptoms (dizziness, headache, drowsiness) are most common; nausea and vomiting, diarrhea, colic, pruritus, and urticaria also occur. Infrequent adverse effects are low-grade fever, an orange to red discoloration of the urine, proteinuria, microscopic hematuria, and transient leukopenia. Seizures have been reported rarely.

Since the drug makes many patients dizzy or drowsy, it should be used with caution in patients whose work or activity requires mental alertness (eg, no driving for 24 hours). It should be used with caution in those with a history of epilepsy. Oxamniquine is contraindicated in pregnancy.

PIPERAZINE

Piperazine is an alternative for the treatment of ascariasis, with cure rates over 90% when taken for 2 days, but it is not recommended for other helminth infections. Piperazine is available as the hexahydrate and as a variety of salts. It is readily absorbed, and maximum plasma levels are reached in 2–4 hours. Most of the drug is excreted unchanged in the urine in 2–6 hours, and excretion is complete within 24 hours. Piperazine causes paralysis of ascaris by blocking acetylcholine at the myoneural junction; live worms are expelled by peristalsis.

For ascariasis, the dosage of piperazine (as the hexahydrate) is 75 mg/kg (maximum dose, 3.5 g) orally once daily for 2 days. For heavy infections, treatment should be continued for 3–4 days or repeated after 1 week.

Occasional mild adverse effects include nausea, vomiting, diarrhea, abdominal pain, dizziness, and headache. Neurotoxicity and allergic reactions are rare. Piperazine should not be given to pregnant women, patients with impaired renal or hepatic function, or those with a history of epilepsy or chronic neurologic disease.

PRAZIQUANTEL

Praziquantel is effective in the treatment of schistosome infections of all species and most other trematode and cestode infections, including cysticercosis. The drug's safety and effectiveness as a single oral dose have also made it useful in mass treatment of several infections.

Basic Pharmacology

Praziquantel is a synthetic isoquinoline-pyrazine derivative. It is rapidly absorbed, with a bioavailability of about 80% after oral administration. Peak serum concentrations are reached 1–3 hours after a therapeutic dose. Cerebrospinal fluid concentrations of praziquantel reach 14–20% of the drug's plasma concentration. About 80% of the drug is bound to plasma proteins. Most of the drug is rapidly metabolized to inactive mono- and polyhydroxylated products after a first pass in the liver. The half-life is 0.8–1.5 hours. Excretion is mainly via the kidneys (60–80%) and bile (15–35%). Plasma concentrations of praziquantel increase when the drug is taken with a high-carbohydrate meal or with cimetidine; bioavailability is markedly reduced by phenytoin, carbamazepine, or corticosteroids.

Praziquantel appears to increase the permeability of trematode and cestode cell membranes to calcium, resulting in paralysis, dislodgement, and death. In schistosome infections of experimental animals, praziquantel is effective against adult worms and immature stages, and it has a prophylactic effect against cercarial infection.

Clinical Uses

Praziquantel tablets are taken with liquid after a meal; they should be swallowed without chewing because their bitter taste can induce retching and vomiting.

1. Schistosomiasis—Praziquantel is the drug of choice for all forms of schistosomiasis. The dosage is 20 mg/kg per dose for two (*S mansoni* and *S haematobium*) or three (*S japonicum* and *S mekongi*) doses at intervals of 4–6 hours. High cure rates (75–95%) are achieved when patients are evaluated at 3–6 months; there is marked reduction in egg counts in those not cured. The drug is effective in adults and children and is generally well tolerated by patients in the hepatosplenic stage of advanced disease. There is no standard regimen for acute schistosomiasis (Katayama syndrome), but standard doses as described above, often with corticosteroids to limit inflammation from the acute immune response and dying worms, are recommended. Increasing evidence indicates rare *S mansoni* drug resistance, which may be countered with extended courses of therapy (eg, 3–6 days at standard dosing) or treatment with oxamniquine. Effectiveness of praziquantel for chemoprophylaxis has not been established.

2. Clonorchiasis, opisthorchiasis, and paragonimiasis—Standard dosing is 25 mg/kg three times daily for 2 days for each of these fluke infections.

3. Taeniasis and diphyllobothriasis—A single dose of praziquantel, 5–10 mg/kg, results in nearly 100% cure rates for *T saginata*, *T solium*, and *D latum* infections. Because praziquantel does not kill eggs, it is theoretically possible that larvae of *T solium* released from eggs in the large bowel could penetrate the intestinal wall and give rise to cysticercosis, but this hazard is probably minimal.

4. Neurocysticercosis—Albendazole is now the preferred drug, but when it is not appropriate or available, praziquantel has similar efficacy. Indications for praziquantel are similar to those for albendazole. The praziquantel dosage is 100 mg/kg/d in three divided doses for 1 day, then 50 mg/kg/d to complete a 2- to 4-week course. Praziquantel—but not albendazole—has diminished bioavailability when taken concurrently with a corticosteroid. A combination of albendazole plus praziquantel increases parasiticidal effects in patients with multiple brain cysts. Recommendations on use of both antihelminthics and corticosteroids in neurocysticercosis vary.

5. Hymenolepis nana—Praziquantel is the drug of choice for *H nana* infections and the first drug to be highly effective. A single dose of 25 mg/kg is taken initially and repeated in 1 week.

6. Hydatid disease—In hydatid disease, praziquantel kills protoscoleces but does not affect the germinal membrane. Praziquantel may be used as an adjunct with albendazole pre- and post-surgery. In addition to its direct action, praziquantel enhances the plasma concentration of albendazole.

7. Other parasites—Limited trials showed effectiveness of praziquantel at a dosage of 25 mg/kg three times daily for 1–2 days against fasciolopsiasis, metagonimiasis, and other forms of heterophyiasis. Praziquantel was not effective for fascioliasis, however, even at dosages as high as 25 mg/kg three times daily for 3–7 days.

Adverse Reactions, Contraindications, & Cautions

Mild and transient adverse effects are common. They begin within hours after ingestion of praziquantel and may persist for about 1 day. Most common are headache, dizziness, drowsiness, and lassitude; others include nausea, vomiting, abdominal pain, loose stools, pruritus, urticaria, arthralgia, myalgia, and low-grade fever. Mild and transient elevations of liver enzymes have been reported. Several days after starting praziquantel, low-grade fever, pruritus, and skin rashes (macular and urticarial), sometimes associated with worsened eosinophilia, may occur, probably due to the release of proteins from dying worms rather than direct drug toxicity. The intensity and frequency of adverse effects increase with dosage such that they occur in up to 50% of patients who receive 25 mg/kg three times daily.

In neurocysticercosis, neurologic abnormalities may be exacerbated by inflammatory reactions around dying parasites. Common findings in patients who do not receive corticosteroids, usually presenting during or shortly after therapy, are headache, meningismus, nausea, vomiting, mental changes, and seizures (often accompanied by increased cerebrospinal fluid pleocytosis). More serious reactions, including arachnoiditis, hyperthermia, and intracranial hypertension, also may occur. Corticosteroids are commonly used with praziquantel in the treatment of neurocysticercosis to decrease the inflammatory response, but this is controversial and complicated by knowledge that corticosteroids decrease the plasma level of praziquantel up to 50%. Praziquantel is contraindicated in ocular cysticercosis because parasite destruction in the eye may cause irreparable damage. Some workers also caution against use of the drug in spinal neurocysticercosis.

Praziquantel is safe and well tolerated in children. Recent data suggest that the drug can be given safely during pregnancy. Because praziquantel induces dizziness and drowsiness, patients should not drive during therapy and should be warned regarding activities requiring particular physical coordination or alertness.

PYRANTEL PAMOATE

Pyrantel pamoate is a broad-spectrum antihelminthic highly effective for the treatment of pinworm, ascaris, and *Trichostrongylus orientalis* infections. It is moderately effective against both species of hookworm. It is not effective in trichuriasis or strongyloidiasis. Oxantel pamoate, an analog of pyrantel not available in the USA, has shown better efficacy against trichuriasis than any other single agent and promising activity in combination with albendazole or ivermectin for this indication. Pyrantel/oxantel pamoate combinations are widely used in veterinary medicine and have been studied for some human indications.

Basic Pharmacology

Pyrantel pamoate is a tetrahydropyrimidine derivative. It is poorly absorbed from the gastrointestinal tract and active mainly against luminal organisms. Peak plasma levels are reached in 1–3 hours. Over half of the administered dose is recovered unchanged in the feces. Pyrantel is effective against mature and immature forms of susceptible helminths within the intestinal tract but not against migratory stages in the tissues or against ova. The drug is a neuromuscular blocking agent that causes release of acetylcholine and inhibition of cholinesterase; this results in paralysis of worms, followed by expulsion.

Clinical Uses

The standard dose is 11 mg (base)/kg (maximum, 1 g), given orally once with or without food. For pinworm, the dose is repeated in 2 weeks, and cure rates are >95%. The drug is available in the USA without prescription for this indication. For ascariasis, a single dose yields cure rates of 85–100%. Treatment should be repeated if eggs are found 2 weeks after treatment. For hookworm infections, a single dose is effective against light infections; for heavy infections, especially with *Necator americanus*, a 3-day course is necessary to achieve 90% cure rates. A course of treatment can be repeated in 2 weeks. The triple combination of albendazole, pyrantel pamoate, and oxantel pamoate appears to be superior to two-drug regimens for the treatment of hookworm infections.

Adverse Reactions, Contraindications, & Cautions

Pyrantel's adverse effects are infrequent, mild, and transient. They may include nausea, vomiting, diarrhea, abdominal cramps, dizziness, drowsiness, headache, insomnia, rash, fever, and weakness. Pyrantel should be used with caution in patients with liver dysfunction, as transient aminotransferase elevations have been noted. Experience with the drug in pregnant women and children younger than 2 years is limited.

THIABENDAZOLE

Thiabendazole is an alternative to ivermectin or albendazole for the treatment of strongyloidiasis and cutaneous larva migrans.

Basic Pharmacology

Thiabendazole is a benzimidazole compound. Although it is a chelating agent that forms stable complexes with a number of metals, including iron, it does not bind calcium. Thiabendazole is rapidly absorbed after ingestion. With a standard dose, drug concentrations in plasma peak within 1–2 hours; the half-life is 1.2 hours. The drug is almost completely metabolized in the liver to the 5-hydroxy form; 90% is excreted in the urine in 48 hours, largely as the glucuronide or sulfonate conjugate. Thiabendazole can also be absorbed from the skin. The mechanism of action of thiabendazole is probably the same as that of other benzimidazoles (inhibition of microtubule synthesis). The drug has ovicidal effects against some parasites.

Clinical Uses

The standard dosage, 25 mg/kg (maximum, 1.5 g) twice daily, should be given after meals. Tablets should be chewed. For *Strongyloides* infection, treatment is for 2 days. Cure rates are reportedly 93%. A course can be repeated in 1 week if indicated. In patients with hyperinfection syndrome, the standard dose is continued twice daily for 5–7 days. For cutaneous larva migrans, thiabendazole cream can be applied topically, or the oral drug can be given for 2 days (although albendazole is less toxic and therefore preferred).

Adverse Reactions, Contraindications, & Cautions

Thiabendazole is much more toxic than other benzimidazoles and more toxic than ivermectin, so other agents are now preferred for most indications. Common adverse effects include dizziness, anorexia, nausea, and vomiting. Less common problems are epigastric pain, abdominal cramps, diarrhea, pruritus, headache, drowsiness, and neuropsychiatric symptoms. Irreversible liver failure and fatal Stevens-Johnson syndrome have been reported. Experience with thiabendazole is limited in children weighing less than 15 kg. The drug should not be used in pregnancy or in the presence of hepatic or renal disease.

TRICLABENDAZOLE

The benzimidazole triclabendazole has been the drug of choice to treat fascioliasis for many years, and it was approved by the FDA in 2019 for this purpose in persons ≥6 years of age. Triclabendazole is also an alternative therapy for paragonimiasis. The drug is well absorbed orally, with a half-life of about 8 hours and excretion primarily in the feces. The recommended regimen is two 10-mg/kg doses with food 12 hours apart. The most common adverse reactions have been abdominal pain, hyperhidrosis, vertigo, nausea, urticaria, vomiting, and headache. The drug may prolong the QT interval. Triclabendazole has been heavily used to treat livestock, and the emergence of resistance in this context threatens efficacy for human disease.

PREPARATIONS AVAILABLE

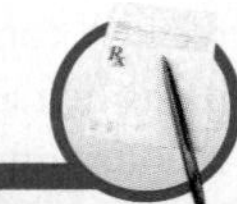

GENERIC NAME	AVAILABLE AS
Albendazole	Albenza
Bithionol	Bitin
Diethylcarbamazine	Hetrazan
Ivermectin	Mectizan, Stromectol
Mebendazole	Generic, Vermox
Metrifonate	Trichlorfon, Bilarcil
Moxidectin	Various
Niclosamide	Niclocide
Oxamniquine	Vansil, Mansil
Oxantel pamoate	Quantrel
Oxantel/pyrantel pamoate	Telopar
Piperazine	Generic, Vermizine
Praziquantel	Biltricide; others outside the USA
Pyrantel pamoate	Ascarel, Pamix, Pin Rid, Pin-X
Thiabendazole	Mintezol
Triclabendazole	Egaten

REFERENCES

Bagheri H et al: Adverse drug reactions to anthelmintics. Ann Pharmacother 2004;38:383.

Barda B et al: Efficacy of moxidectin versus ivermectin against *Strongyloides stercoralis* infections: A randomized, controlled noninferiority trial. Clin Infect Dis 2017;65:276.

Colley DG et al: Human schistosomiasis. Lancet 2014;383:2253.

Debrah AY et al: Doxycycline leads to sterility and enhanced killing of female *Onchocerca volvulus* worms in an area with persistent microfilaridermia after repeated ivermectin treatment: A randomized, placebo-controlled, double-blind trial. Clin Infect Dis 2015;61:517.

Del Brutto OH: Clinical management of neurocysticercosis. Expert Rev Neurother 2014;14:389.

Fürst T et al: Manifestation, diagnosis, and management of foodborne trematodiasis. BMJ 2012;344:e4093.

Garcia HH et al: Cysticidal efficacy of combined treatment with praziquantel and albendazole for parenchymal brain cysticercosis. Clin Infect Dis 2016;62:1375.

Garcia HH et al: Efficacy of combined antiparasitic therapy with praziquantel and albendazole for neurocysticercosis: A double-blind, randomised controlled trial. Lancet Infect Dis 2014;14:687.

Henriquez-Camacho C et al: Ivermectin versus albendazole or thiabendazole for *Strongyloides stercoralis* infection. Cochrane Database Syst Rev 2016:CD007745.

Jourdan PM et al: Soil-transmitted helminth infections. Lancet 2018;391:252.

King CL et al: A trial of a triple-drug treatment for lymphatic filariasis. N Engl J Med 2018;379:1801.

Levecke B et al: Assessment of anthelmintic efficacy of mebendazole in school children in six countries where soil-transmitted helminths are endemic. PLoS Negl Trop Dis 2014;8:e3204.

Mejia R, Nutman TB: Screening, prevention, and treatment for hyperinfection syndrome and disseminated infections caused by *Strongyloides stercoralis*. Curr Opin Infect Dis 2012;25:458.

Metzger WG, Mordmüller B: *Loa loa*-does it deserve to be neglected? Lancet Infect Dis 2014;14:353.

Moser W et al: Efficacy and safety of oxantel pamoate in school-aged children infected with *Trichuris trichiura* on Pemba Island, Tanzania: A parallel, randomised, controlled, dose-ranging study. Lancet Infect Dis 2016;16:53.

Moser W et al: Efficacy and tolerability of triple drug therapy with albendazole, pyrantel pamoate, and oxantel pamoate compared with albendazole plus oxantel pamoate, pyrantel pamoate plus oxantel pamoate, and mebendazole plus pyrantel pamoate and oxantel pamoate against hookworm infections in school-aged children in Laos: A randomised, single-blind trial. Lancet Infect Dis 2018;18:729.

Moser W et al: Efficacy of recommended drugs against soil transmitted helminths: Systematic review and network meta-analysis. BMJ 2017;358:j4307.

Nash TE, Garcia HH: Diagnosis and treatment of neurocysticercosis. Nat Rev Neurol 2011;7:584.

Olveda RM et al: Efficacy and safety of praziquantel for the treatment of human schistosomiasis during pregnancy: A phase 2, randomised, double-blind, placebo-controlled trial. Lancet Infect Dis 2016;16:199.

Opoku NO et al: Single dose moxidectin versus ivermectin for *Onchocerca volvulus* infection in Ghana, Liberia, and the Democratic Republic of the Congo: A randomised, controlled, double-blind phase 3 trial. Lancet 2018;392:1207.

Palmeirim MS et al: Efficacy and safety of co-administered ivermectin plus albendazole for treating soil-transmitted helminths: A systematic review, meta-analysis and individual patient data analysis. PLoS Negl Trop Dis 2018;12:e0006458.

Pawluk SA et al: A review of pharmacokinetic drug-drug interactions with the anthelmintic medications albendazole and mebendazole. Clin Pharmacokinet 2015;54:371.

Soukhathammavong PA et al: Low efficacy of single-dose albendazole and mebendazole against hookworm and effect on concomitant helminth infection in Lao PDR. PLoS Negl Trop Dis 2012;6:e1417.

Speich B et al: Efficacy and safety of albendazole plus ivermectin, albendazole plus mebendazole, albendazole plus oxantel pamoate, and mebendazole alone against *Trichuris trichiura* and concomitant soil-transmitted helminth infections: A four-arm, randomised controlled trial. Lancet Infect Dis 2015;15:277.

Speich B et al: Oxantel pamoate-albendazole for *Trichuris trichiura* infection. N Engl J Med 2014;370:610.

Steinmann P et al: Efficacy of single-dose and triple-dose albendazole and mebendazole against soil-transmitted helminths and *Taenia* spp.: A randomized controlled trial. PLoS One 2011;6:e25003.

Tamarozzi F et al: Acceptance of standardized ultrasound classification, use of albendazole, and long-term follow-up in clinical management of cystic echinococcosis: A systematic review. Curr Opin Infect Dis 2014;27:425.

White AC et al: Diagnosis and treatment of Neurocysticercosis: 2017 clinical practice guidelines by the Infectious Diseases Society of America (IDSA) and the American Society of Tropical Medicine and Hygiene (ASTMH). Am J Trop Med Hyg 2018;98:945.

Zwang J, Olliaro PL: Clinical efficacy and tolerability of praziquantel for intestinal and urinary schistosomiasis: A meta-analysis of comparative and noncomparative clinical trials. PLoS Negl Trop Dis 2014;8:e3286.

CASE STUDY ANSWER

The presentation is highly suggestive of cystic hydatid disease (infection with *Echinococcus granulosus*), which is transmitted by eggs from the feces of dogs in contact with livestock. Other causes of liver fluid collections include amebic and pyogenic abscesses, but these are usually not cystic in appearance. For echinococcosis, a typical cystic lesion and positive serology support the diagnosis, and treatment generally entails albendazole in conjunction with cautious surgery or percutaneous aspiration. One approach is treatment with albendazole followed by aspiration to confirm the diagnosis and, if it is confirmed, aspiration of the infecting worms.

CHAPTER

54 Cancer Chemotherapy

Edward Chu, MD

CASE STUDY

A 55-year-old man presents with increasing fatigue, 15-pound weight loss, and a microcytic anemia. Colonoscopy identifies a mass in the ascending colon, and biopsy specimens reveal well-differentiated colorectal cancer (CRC). He undergoes surgical resection and is found to have high-risk stage III CRC with five positive lymph nodes. After surgery, he feels entirely well with no symptoms. Of note, he has no other illnesses. What is this patient's overall prognosis? Based on his prognosis, what are the possible benefits of adjuvant chemotherapy? How long should he receive adjuvant chemotherapy? The patient receives a combination of 5-fluorouracil (5-FU), leucovorin, and oxaliplatin (FOLFOX) as adjuvant therapy. One week after receiving the first cycle of therapy, he experiences significant toxicity in the form of myelosuppression, diarrhea, and altered mental status. What is the most likely explanation for this increased toxicity? Is there any role for genetic testing to determine the etiology of the increased toxicity?

In 2023, approximately 1.9 million new cancer cases will be diagnosed in the USA, and nearly 609,000 individuals are expected to die from this disease. Cancer is the second most common cause of death in the USA, accounting for 1 in 4 deaths. It is a disease characterized by a defect in the normal control mechanisms that govern cell survival, proliferation, and differentiation. Cells that have undergone neoplastic transformation usually express cell surface antigens that may be of normal fetal type, and they may display other signs of apparent immaturity. They may exhibit qualitative or quantitative chromosomal abnormalities, including various translocations, fusions, and the appearance of amplified gene sequences. It is well established that a small subpopulation of cells, referred to as *tumor stem cells*, reside within a tumor mass. They retain the ability to undergo repeated cycles of proliferation as well as to migrate to distant sites in the body to colonize various organs in the process called *metastasis*. Such tumor stem cells have clonogenic (colony-forming) capability, and they are characterized by chromosome abnormalities reflecting their genetic instability, which leads to progressive selection of subclones that can survive more readily in the multicellular environment of the host. This genetic instability provides cancer cells with the ability to become resistant to radiotherapy and to systemic therapies, including cytotoxic chemotherapy, targeted therapy, and immunotherapy. The invasive and metastatic processes as well as a series of metabolic abnormalities associated with the cancer result in tumor-related symptoms and eventual death of the patient unless the neoplasm can be eradicated with treatment.

CAUSES OF CANCER

The incidence, geographic distribution, and behavior of specific types of cancer are related to multiple factors, including sex, age, race, genetic predisposition, and exposure to environmental carcinogens. Of these factors, **environmental exposure** is probably most important, although it is clear that the interplay between genetic alterations and environment plays a critical role in the development of cancer. Exposure to ionizing radiation has been shown to be a significant risk factor for several cancers, including acute leukemias, thyroid cancer, breast cancer, lung cancer, soft tissue sarcoma, and basal cell and squamous cell skin cancers. Chemical carcinogens (particularly those in tobacco smoke) as well as azo dyes, aflatoxins, asbestos, benzene, and radon all have been associated with a wide range of human cancers, including lung cancer and bladder cancer.

Several **viruses** have been implicated in the etiology of various human cancers. For example, chronic infection with hepatitis B (HBV) and hepatitis C (HCV) leads to the development of

ACRONYMS

ABVD	Doxorubicin (Adriamycin, hydroxydaunorubicin), bleomycin, vinblastine, dacarbazine
ALL	Acute lymphoblastic leukemia
AML	Acute myelogenous leukemia
BCMA	B-cell maturation agent
BCNU	Carmustine
CAPOX	Capecitabine, oxaliplatin
CCNU	Lomustine
CLL	Chronic lymphocytic leukemia
CHOP	Cyclophosphamide, doxorubicin (Adriamycin, hydroxydaunorubicin), vincristine (Oncovin), prednisone
CMF	Cyclophosphamide, methotrexate, fluorouracil
CML	Chronic myelogenous leukemia
COP	Cyclophosphamide, vincristine (Oncovin), prednisone
CRC	Colorectal cancer
FAC	5-Fluorouracil, doxorubicin (Adriamycin, hydroxydaunorubicin), cyclophosphamide
FEC	5-Fluorouracil, epirubicin, cyclophosphamide
5-FU	5-Fluorouracil
FOLFIRI	5-Fluorouracil, leucovorin, irinotecan
FOLFOX	5-Fluorouracil, leucovorin, oxaliplatin
MP	Melphalan, prednisone
6-MP	6-Mercaptopurine
MOPP	Mechlorethamine, vincristine (Oncovin), procarbazine, prednisone
MTX	Methotrexate
NSCLC	Non-small cell lung cancer
PCV	Procarbazine, lomustine, vincristine
PEB	Cisplatin (platinum), etoposide, bleomycin
6-TG	6-Thioguanine
SCLC	Small cell lung cancer
VAD	Vincristine, doxorubicin (Adriamycin, hydroxydaunorubicin), dexamethasone
VEGF	Vascular endothelial growth factor

hepatocellular cancer; HIV is associated with Hodgkin and non-Hodgkin lymphomas as well as several other solid tumors, including anal cancer; human papillomavirus (HPV) is associated with cervical cancer, anal and penile cancers, and oropharyngeal head and neck cancer; Epstein-Barr virus (EBV), also known as human herpesvirus 4 (HHV-4), is associated with nasopharyngeal cancer, Burkitt lymphoma, and Hodgkin lymphoma; and Merkel cell polyomavirus (MCV) causes Merkel cell cancer, a rare but aggressive form of skin cancer. The development of virus-induced cancers depends on additional host and environmental factors that modulate the transformation process. Cellular genes are known that are homologous to the transforming genes of the retroviruses, a family of RNA viruses, and induce oncogenic transformation. These mammalian cellular genes are referred to as **oncogenes,** and they code for specific growth factors and their corresponding receptors. These genes may be amplified with an increased number of gene copies or be mutated, both of which can lead to constitutive overexpression in malignant cells. The *Bcl*-2 family of genes represents a series of prosurvival genes that promotes tumor cell survival by directly inhibiting apoptosis, a key pathway of programmed cell death.

Tumor suppressor genes prevent the development of cancer, but when deleted or mutated, their protein products are either absent or dysfunctional, which then gives rise to the neoplastic phenotype. The *p53* gene is the best-established tumor suppressor gene identified to date, and the normal wild-type protein encoded by this gene plays a critical role in suppressing malignant transformation. Of note, *p53* is mutated in up to 50% of all human solid tumors, including liver, breast, colon, lung, cervix, bladder, prostate, and skin.

CANCER TREATMENT MODALITIES

With present methods of treatment, when the tumor remains localized at the time of diagnosis, about one-third of patients are cured with local treatment strategies, such as surgery or radiotherapy. In the remaining cases, however, early micrometastasis is a characteristic feature, indicating that a systemic approach with chemotherapy is required for effective cancer management. In patients with locally advanced disease, chemotherapy is often combined with radiotherapy to allow for subsequent surgical resection to take place, and such a combined modality approach has led to improved clinical outcomes. At present, about 50% of patients who are initially diagnosed with cancer can be cured. In contrast, chemotherapy alone is able to cure less than 10% of all cancer patients when the tumor is diagnosed at an advanced stage.

Chemotherapy is presently used in three main clinical settings: (1) primary induction treatment for advanced disease or for cancers for which there are no other effective treatment approaches, (2) neoadjuvant treatment for patients who present with localized disease, for whom local forms of therapy such as surgery or radiation, or both, are inadequate by themselves, and (3) adjuvant treatment to local modalities of treatment, including surgery, radiation therapy, or both.

Primary chemotherapy refers to chemotherapy administered as the primary treatment in patients who present with advanced cancer for which no alternative treatment exists. This has been the main approach in treating patients with metastatic disease. In most cases, the goals of therapy are to relieve tumor-related symptoms, improve overall quality of life, and prolong time to tumor progression. Studies in a wide range of solid tumors have shown that chemotherapy in patients with advanced disease confers survival benefit when compared with supportive care, providing sound rationale for the early initiation of drug treatment. However, cancer chemotherapy is curative in only a small subset of patients who present with advanced disease. In adults, these curable cancers include Hodgkin and non-Hodgkin lymphoma, acute myelogenous leukemia, germ cell cancer, and choriocarcinoma, while the curable childhood cancers include acute lymphoblastic leukemia, Burkitt lymphoma, Wilms tumor, and embryonal rhabdomyosarcoma.

Neoadjuvant chemotherapy refers to the use of chemotherapy in patients who present with localized cancer for which alternative local therapies, such as surgery, exist but which have been shown to be less than completely effective. At present, neoadjuvant therapy is most often administered in the treatment of anal cancer, bladder cancer, breast cancer, gastroesophageal cancer, laryngeal cancer, locally advanced non-small cell lung cancer (NSCLC), osteogenic sarcoma, and locally advanced rectal cancer. For diseases such as anal cancer, gastroesophageal cancer, laryngeal cancer, NSCLC, and rectal cancer, optimal clinical benefit is derived when chemotherapy is administered with radiation therapy either concurrently or sequentially. The goal of the neoadjuvant approach is to reduce the size of the primary tumor so that surgical resection can be made easier and more effective. In addition, with rectal cancer and laryngeal cancer, the administration of combined modality therapy prior to surgery can result in sparing of vital normal organs, such as the rectum or larynx. In general, additional chemotherapy is given for a defined period of time, usually on the order of 3–4 months, after surgery has been performed.

One of the most important roles for cancer chemotherapy is as an adjuvant to local treatment modalities such as surgery, and this has been termed **adjuvant chemotherapy.** In this setting, chemotherapy is administered after surgical resection, and the goal of chemotherapy is to reduce the incidence of both local and systemic recurrence and to improve the overall survival of patients. In general, chemotherapy regimens with clinical activity against advanced disease may have curative potential following surgical resection of the primary tumor, provided the appropriate dose and schedule are administered. Adjuvant chemotherapy is effective in prolonging both disease-free survival (DFS) and overall survival (OS) in patients with breast cancer, colon cancer, gastric cancer, NSCLC, Wilms tumor, anaplastic astrocytoma, and osteogenic sarcoma. Patients with primary malignant melanoma at high risk of local or systemic recurrence derive clinical benefit from adjuvant treatment with the immune checkpoint inhibitors nivolumab or pembrolizumab. Finally, the antihormonal agents tamoxifen, anastrozole, and letrozole are effective in the adjuvant therapy of postmenopausal women with early-stage breast cancer whose breast tumors express the estrogen receptor (see Chapter 40 for additional details). However, because these agents are cytostatic rather than cytocidal, they must be administered for a prolonged period of time, with the standard recommendation being 5 years' duration.

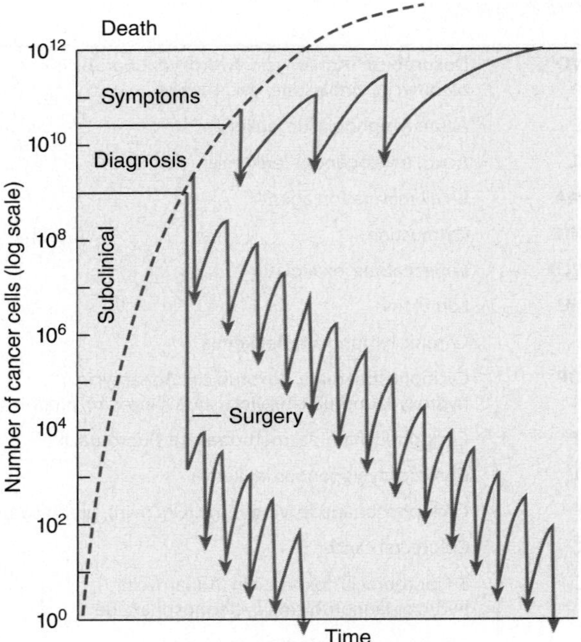

FIGURE 54–1 Log-kill hypothesis: relationship of tumor cell number to time of diagnosis, symptoms, treatment, and survival. Three alternative approaches to drug treatment are shown for comparison with the course of tumor growth when no treatment is given *(dashed line)*. In the protocol diagrammed at top, treatment (indicated by the arrows) is given infrequently, and the result is manifested as prolongation of survival but with recurrence of symptoms between courses of treatment and eventual death of the patient. The combination chemotherapy treatment diagrammed in the middle section is begun earlier, and multiple cycles are administered at consistent intervals. Tumor cell kill exceeds regrowth, drug resistance does not develop, and "cure" results. In this example, treatment has been continued until there is no longer clinical evidence of cancer. This approach has been established as effective in the treatment of childhood acute leukemia, testicular cancer, and Hodgkin lymphoma. In the treatment diagrammed near the bottom of the graph, early surgery has been employed to remove the primary tumor and intense adjuvant chemotherapy has been administered long enough to eradicate the remaining tumor cells that comprise the occult micrometastases.

ROLE OF CELL CYCLE KINETICS & ANTICANCER EFFECT

The principles of cell cycle kinetics were initially developed using the murine L1210 leukemia as the experimental model system (Figure 54–1). However, drug treatment of human cancers requires a clear understanding of the differences between the characteristics of this rodent leukemia and of human cancers, as well as an understanding of the differences in growth rates of normal target tissues between mice and humans. For example, L1210 is a rapidly growing leukemia with a high percentage of cells synthesizing DNA, as measured by the uptake of tritiated thymidine (the labeling index). Because L1210 leukemia has a growth fraction approaching 100% (ie, all its cells are actively progressing through the cell cycle), its life cycle is consistent and predictable. The murine L1210 model predicts that the cytotoxic effects of anticancer drugs follow log cell-kill kinetics. As such, a given agent would be predicted to kill a constant fraction of cells as opposed to a constant number.

If a particular dose of an individual drug leads to a 3-log kill of cancer cells and reduces the tumor burden from 10^{10} to 10^7 cells, the same dose used at a tumor burden of 10^5 cells reduces the tumor mass to 10^2 cells. Cell kill is, therefore, proportional, regardless of tumor burden. The cardinal rule of chemotherapy—the invariable inverse relation between cell number and curability—was established with the murine L1210 leukemia model, and this relationship is clearly applicable to rapidly growing hematologic malignancies, such as acute leukemias and lymphomas.

Although growth of murine leukemias simulates exponential cell kinetics, mathematical modeling suggest that the large majority of human solid tumors do not grow in such an exponential manner.

Rather, the experimental data in human solid cancers support a Gompertzian model of tumor growth and regression. The critical distinction between Gompertzian and exponential growth is that the growth fraction of the tumor is not constant with Gompertzian kinetics but instead decreases exponentially with time (exponential growth is matched by exponential retardation of growth, due to blood supply limitations and other factors). The growth fraction peaks when the tumor is approximately one-third its maximum size. According to the Gompertzian model, when a patient with advanced cancer is treated, the tumor mass is larger, its growth fraction is low, and the fraction of cells killed is, therefore, small. An important feature of Gompertzian growth is that response to chemotherapy in drug-sensitive tumors depends, in large measure, on where the tumor is in its particular growth curve.

Information on cell and population kinetics of cancer cells explains, in part, the limited effectiveness of most available anticancer drugs. A schematic summary of cell cycle kinetics is presented in Figure 54–2. This information is relevant to the mode of action, indications, and scheduling of cell cycle–specific (CCS) and cell cycle–nonspecific (CCNS) drugs. Agents falling into these two major classes are summarized in Table 54–1.

The Role of Combination Chemotherapy

With rare exceptions (eg, choriocarcinoma and Burkitt lymphoma), single drugs are unable to cure cancers when they are in an advanced stage. In the 1960s and early 1970s, drug combination regimens were developed based on the known biochemical actions of available anticancer drugs rather than on their clinical efficacy. Such regimens were, however, largely ineffective. The era of effective combination chemotherapy began when a number of active drugs from different classes became available for use in combination in the treatment of the acute leukemias and lymphomas. Following this initial success with hematologic malignancies, combination chemotherapy was extended to the treatment of solid tumors.

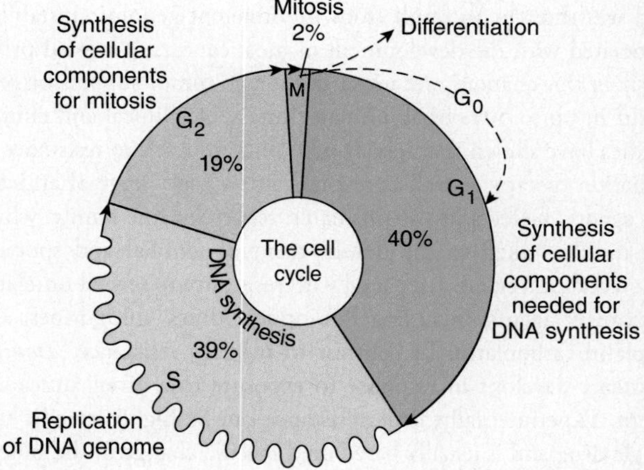

FIGURE 54–2 Cell cycle and cancer. The percentages given represent the approximate percentage of time spent in each phase by both normal cells and neoplastic cells. The duration of G_1, however, can vary markedly. Many of the effective anticancer drugs exert their action on cells traversing the cell cycle and are called cell cycle–specific (CCS) drugs (see Table 54–1). A second group of agents called cell cycle–nonspecific (CCNS) drugs can kill tumor cells whether they are cycling or resting in the G_0 compartment. CCNS drugs can kill both G_0 and cycling cells (although cycling cells are more sensitive).

TABLE 54–1 Cell cycle effects of major classes of anticancer drugs.

Cell Cycle–Specific (CCS) Agents	Cell Cycle–Nonspecific (CCNS) Agents
Antimetabolites (S phase)	**Alkylating agents**
Capecitabine	Altretamine
Cladribine	Bendamustine
Clofarabine	Busulfan
Cytarabine (ara-C)	Carmustine
Fludarabine	Chlorambucil
5-Fluorouracil (5-FU)	Cyclophosphamide
Gemcitabine	Dacarbazine
6-Mercaptopurine (6-MP)	Lomustine
Methotrexate (MTX)	Lurbinectedin
Nelarabine	Mechlorethamine
Pralatrexate	Melphalan
TAS-102	Temozolomide
6-Thioguanine (6-TG)	Thiotepa
Topoisomerase II inhibitor (G_1–S phase)	Trabectedin
	Antitumor antibiotics
Etoposide	Dactinomycin
Topoisomerase I inhibitors (Camptothecins, G_2-M)	Mitomycin
	Platinum analogs
Deruxtecan (DXd)	Carboplatin
Govitecan (SN-38)	Cisplatin
Irinotecan (CPT-11)	Oxaliplatin
Topotecan	**Anthracyclines**
Taxanes (M phase)	Daunorubicin
Albumin-bound paclitaxel (nab-paclitaxel)	Doxorubicin
Cabazitaxel	Epirubicin
Docetaxel	Idarubicin
Paclitaxel	Mitoxantrone
Vinca alkaloids (M phase)	
Vinblastine	
Vincristine	
Vinorelbine	
Antimicrotubule inhibitor (M phase)	
Ixabepilone	
Eribulin	
Antitumor antibiotics (G_2-M phase)	
Bleomycin	

The use of combination chemotherapy is important for several reasons. First, it provides maximal cell kill within the range of toxicity tolerated by the host for each drug as long as dosing is not compromised. Second, it provides a broader range of interaction between drugs and tumor cells with different genetic abnormalities in a heterogeneous tumor population. Finally, it may prevent or slow the subsequent development of cellular drug resistance. Of note, these same concepts apply to the therapy of chronic infections, such as HIV and tuberculosis.

Certain principles have guided the selection of drugs in the most effective drug combinations, and they provide a paradigm for the development of new drug therapeutic programs.

1. **Efficacy:** Only drugs known to have some degree of clinical efficacy when used alone against a given tumor should be selected for use in combination. When available, drugs that produce complete remission in some fraction of patients are preferred to those that produce only partial responses.
2. **Toxicity:** When several drugs of a given class are available and are equally effective, a drug should be selected on the basis of toxicity that does not overlap with the toxicity of other drugs in the combination. Although such selection leads to a wider range of adverse effects, it minimizes the risk of a lethal effect caused by multiple insults to the same organ system by different drugs and allows dose intensity to be maximized.
3. **Optimum scheduling:** Drugs should be used in their optimal dose and schedule, and drug combinations should be administered at consistent intervals. Because long intervals between cycles negatively affect dose intensity, the treatment-free interval between cycles should be the shortest time necessary for recovery of the most sensitive normal target tissue, which is usually the bone marrow.
4. **Mechanism of interaction:** There should be a clear understanding of the biochemical, molecular, and/or pharmacokinetic mechanisms of interaction between the individual drugs in a given combination, to allow for maximal antitumor effect. Omission of a drug from a combination may allow overgrowth by a tumor clone sensitive to that drug alone and resistant to other drugs in the combination.
5. **Avoidance of arbitrary dose changes:** An arbitrary reduction in the dose of an effective drug in order to add other less effective drugs may reduce the dose of the most effective agent below the threshold of effectiveness and destroy the ability of the combination to cure disease in a given patient.

Dose Intensity

Dose intensity is one of the main factors limiting the ability of chemotherapy or radiation therapy to achieve cure. As described in Chapter 2, the dose-response curve in biologic systems is usually sigmoidal in shape, with a threshold, a linear phase, and a plateau phase. For chemotherapy, therapeutic selectivity is dependent on the difference between the dose-response curves of normal and tumor tissues. In experimental animal models, the dose-response curve is usually steep in the linear phase, and a reduction in dose when the tumor is in the linear phase of the dose-response curve almost always results in a loss in the capacity to cure the tumor effectively before a reduction in the antitumor activity is observed. Although complete remissions may continue to be observed with dose reductions down to as low as 20% of the optimal dose, residual tumor cells may not be entirely eliminated, thereby allowing for eventual relapse. It is often appealing for clinicians to prevent acute toxicity by simply reducing the dose or by increasing the time interval between each cycle of treatment (or both). However, such empiric modifications in dose represent a major cause of treatment failure, especially in patients with drug-sensitive tumors.

A positive relationship between dose intensity and clinical efficacy has been documented in several solid tumors, including advanced ovarian, breast, lung, and colon cancers, as well as in hematologic malignancies, such as the lymphomas. At present, there are three main approaches to dose-intense delivery of chemotherapy. The first approach, **dose escalation,** involves increasing the doses of the respective anticancer agents. The second strategy is administration of anticancer agents in a dose-intense manner by **reducing the interval** between treatment cycles, while the third approach involves **sequential scheduling** of either single agents or combination regimens. Each of these strategies is presently being applied to the treatment of a wide range of solid cancers, including breast, colorectal, and NSCLC. In general, such dose-intense regimens have significantly improved clinical outcomes.

DRUG RESISTANCE

A fundamental challenge to the efficacy of cancer chemotherapy is the development of cellular drug resistance. *Primary* or *inherent resistance* refers to drug resistance in the absence of prior exposure to available standard agents. The concept of inherent drug resistance was first proposed by Goldie and Coleman in the early 1980s and was thought to result from the inherent genomic instability associated with the development of most cancers. As noted previously in this chapter, mutations in the *p53* tumor suppressor gene occur in up to 50% of all human tumors. Preclinical and clinical studies have shown that loss of *p53* function leads to resistance to radiation therapy as well as resistance to a wide range of anticancer agents. Defects in the mismatch repair enzyme family, which are tightly linked to the development of familial and sporadic colorectal cancer, are associated with resistance to several unrelated anticancer agents, including fluoropyrimidines, thiopurines, and cisplatin/carboplatin. In contrast to primary resistance, *acquired resistance* develops in response to exposure to a given anticancer agent. Experimentally, drug resistance can be highly specific to a single drug and is usually based on a specific change in the genetic machinery of a given tumor cell with amplification or increased expression of one or more genes. In other instances, a multidrug-resistant phenotype occurs, associated with increased expression of the *MDR1* gene, which encodes a cell surface transporter glycoprotein (P-glycoprotein, see Chapter 5). This form of drug resistance leads to enhanced drug efflux and reduced intracellular accumulation of a broad range of structurally unrelated anticancer agents, including the anthracyclines, vinca alkaloids, taxanes, camptothecins, epipodophyllotoxins, and even small molecule inhibitors, such as imatinib.

BASIC PHARMACOLOGY OF CANCER CHEMOTHERAPEUTIC DRUGS

ALKYLATING AGENTS

The major clinically useful alkylating agents (Figure 54–3) have a structure containing a bis(chloroethyl)amine, ethyleneimine, or nitrosourea moiety, and they are classified in six different groups. Among the bis(chloroethyl)amines, cyclophosphamide, mechlorethamine, melphalan, and chlorambucil are the most useful. Ifosfamide is closely related to cyclophosphamide but has a somewhat different spectrum of activity and toxicity. Thiotepa and busulfan are used to treat breast and ovarian cancer, and chronic myeloid leukemia, respectively. The major nitrosoureas are carmustine (BCNU) and lomustine (CCNU), and they have activity in brain cancers and hematologic malignancies. The tetrahydroisoquinolines lurbinectedin and trabectedin are the newest class of alkylating agents. Lurbinectedin is approved for the treatment of metastatic small cell lung cancer, while trabectedin is approved for unresectable or metastatic liposarcoma or leiomyosarcoma.

Mechanism of Action

As a class, the alkylating agents exert their cytotoxic effects via transfer of their alkyl groups to various cellular constituents. Alkylation of DNA within the nucleus probably represents the major interaction leading to cell death. However, these drugs react chemically with sulfhydryl, amino, hydroxyl, carboxyl, and phosphate groups of other cellular nucleophiles as well. The general mechanism of action of these drugs involves intramolecular cyclization to form an ethyleneimonium ion that may directly or through formation of a carbonium ion transfer an alkyl group to a cellular constituent. In addition to alkylation, a secondary mechanism that occurs with nitrosoureas involves carbamoylation of lysine residues of proteins through formation of isocyanates.

The major site of alkylation within DNA is the N7 position of guanine; however, other sites are also alkylated albeit to lesser degrees, including N1 and N3 of adenine, N3 of cytosine, and O6 of guanine. These interactions can occur on a single strand or on

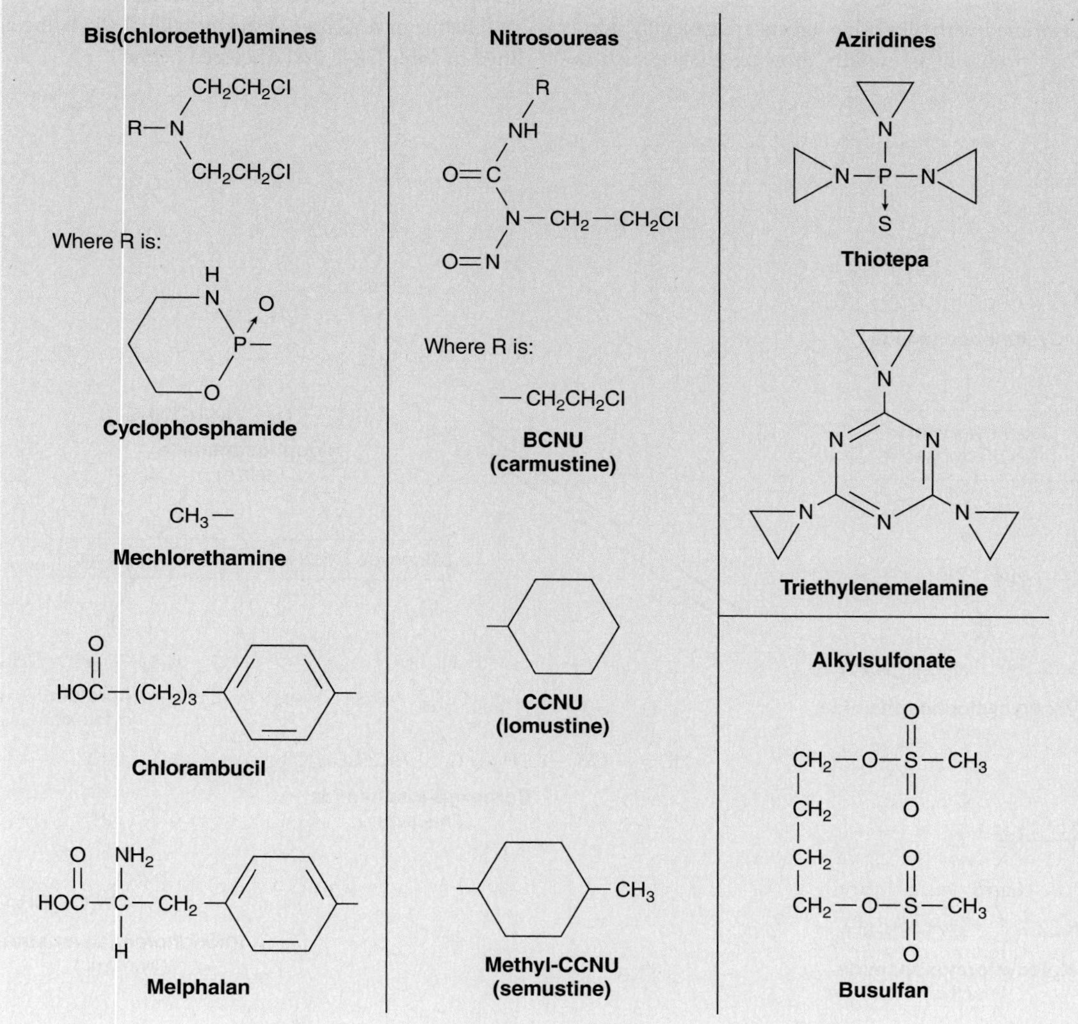

FIGURE 54–3 Structures of major classes of alkylating agents.

both strands of DNA through cross-linking, as most major alkylating agents are bifunctional, with two reactive groups. Alkylation of guanine can result in miscoding through abnormal base pairing with thymine or in depurination by excision of guanine residues. The latter effect leads to DNA strand breakage through scission of the sugar-phosphate backbone of DNA. Cross-linking of DNA appears to play a key role in the cytotoxic action of alkylating agents, and replicating cells are most susceptible to these drugs. Although alkylating agents are not cell cycle–specific, cancer cells are most susceptible to this class of drugs in late G_1 and S phases of the cell cycle.

Resistance

The mechanism of acquired resistance to alkylating agents may involve increased capability to repair DNA lesions through increased expression and activity of DNA repair enzymes, decreased cellular transport of the alkylating drug, and increased expression or activity of glutathione and glutathione-associated proteins, which are needed to conjugate the alkylating agent, or increased glutathione *S*-transferase activity, which catalyzes the conjugation.

Adverse Effects

The toxicities associated with alkylating agents are generally dose-related and occur primarily in rapidly growing tissues such as bone marrow (myelosuppression), gastrointestinal tract (diarrhea, mucositis), and reproductive system (infertility, sterility, and loss of menses). Nausea and vomiting can also be a serious issue with a number of these agents. In addition, they are potent vesicants and can damage tissues at the site of administration as well as produce systemic toxicity. Alkylating agents are carcinogenic in nature, and there is an increased risk of secondary malignancies, specifically acute myelogenous leukemia (AML).

Cyclophosphamide is one of the most widely used alkylating agents. One significant advantage of this compound relates to its high oral bioavailability. As a result, it can be administered via the oral and intravenous routes with equal clinical efficacy. It is inactive in its parent form and must be activated to cytotoxic metabolites by liver microsomal enzymes (Figure 54–4). The cytochrome P450 mixed-function oxidase system converts cyclophosphamide to 4-hydroxycyclophosphamide, which is in equilibrium with aldophosphamide. These active metabolites are delivered to both tumor and normal tissue, where nonenzymatic cleavage of aldophosphamide to the cytotoxic forms—phosphoramide mustard and acrolein—occurs. The liver appears to be protected through the enzymatic formation of the inactive metabolites 4-ketocyclophosphamide and carboxyphosphamide.

The major toxicities of the individual alkylating agents are outlined in Table 54–2 and discussed below.

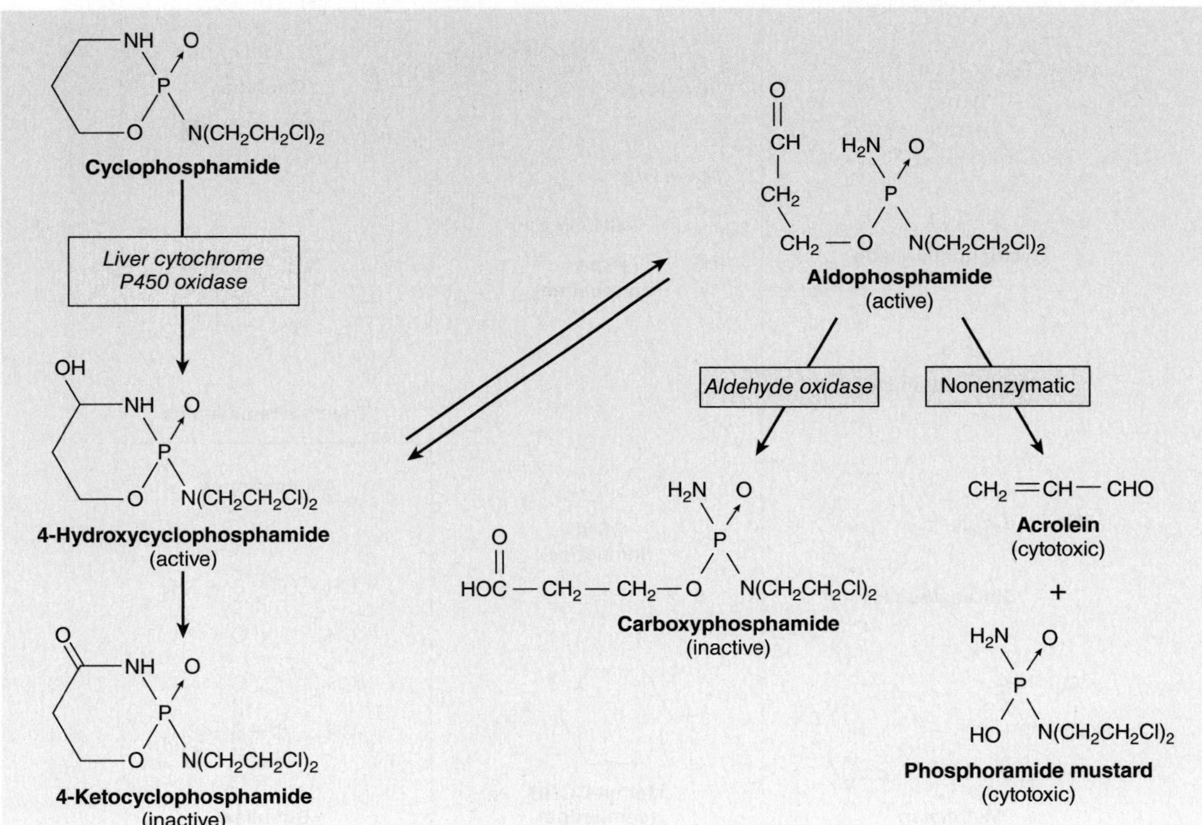

FIGURE 54–4 Cyclophosphamide metabolism.

TABLE 54–2 Alkylating agents and platinum analogs: Clinical activity and toxicities.

Alkylating Agent	Mechanism of Action	Clinical Applications	Acute Toxicity	Delayed Toxicity
Mechlorethamine	Forms DNA cross-links, resulting in inhibition of DNA synthesis and function	Hodgkin and non-Hodgkin lymphoma	Nausea and vomiting	Moderate depression of peripheral blood count; excessive doses produce severe bone marrow depression with leukopenia, thrombocytopenia, and bleeding
Chlorambucil	Same as above	CLL and non-Hodgkin lymphoma	Nausea and vomiting	
Cyclophosphamide	Same as above	Breast cancer, ovarian cancer, non-Hodgkin lymphoma, CLL, soft tissue sarcoma, neuroblastoma, Wilms tumor, rhabdomyosarcoma	Nausea and vomiting	Alopecia and hemorrhagic cystitis occasionally occur. Cystitis can be prevented with adequate hydration
Bendamustine	Same as above	CLL and non-Hodgkin lymphoma	Nausea and vomiting	
Melphalan	Same as above	Multiple myeloma, breast cancer, ovarian cancer	Nausea and vomiting	
Thiotepa	Same as above	Breast cancer, ovarian cancer, superficial bladder cancer	Nausea and vomiting	
Busulfan	Same as above	CML	Nausea and vomiting	Associated with skin pigmentation, pulmonary fibrosis, and adrenal insufficiency
Carmustine	Same as above	Brain cancer, Hodgkin and non-Hodgkin lymphoma	Nausea and vomiting	Myelosuppression; rarely interstitial lung disease (ILD) and interstitial nephritis
Lomustine	Same as above	Brain cancer	Nausea and vomiting	
Altretamine	Same as above	Ovarian cancer	Nausea and vomiting	Myelosuppression, peripheral neuropathy, flu-like syndrome
Lurbinectedin	Same as above	Small cell lung cancer	Nausea and vomiting	Myelosuppression, hepatotoxicity
Trabectedin	Same as above	Liposarcoma, leiomyosarcoma	Diarrhea, mucositis	Cardiac toxicity, pulmonary toxicity with ILD, skin rash and dermatitis
Temozolomide	Methylates DNA and inhibits DNA synthesis and function	Brain cancer, melanoma	Nausea and vomiting, headache and fatigue	Myelosuppression, mild elevation in liver function tests, photosensitivity
Procarbazine	Methylates DNA and inhibits DNA synthesis and function	Hodgkin and non-Hodgkin lymphoma, brain tumors	Central nervous system depression	Myelosuppression, hypersensitivity reactions
Dacarbazine	Methylates DNA and inhibits DNA synthesis and function	Hodgkin lymphoma, melanoma, soft tissue sarcoma	Nausea and vomiting	Myelosuppression, central nervous system toxicity with neuropathy, ataxia, lethargy, and confusion
Cisplatin	Forms intrastrand and interstrand DNA cross-links; binding to nuclear and cytoplasmic proteins	Non-small cell and small cell lung cancer, breast cancer, bladder cancer, cholangiocarcinoma, gastroesophageal cancer, head and neck cancer, ovarian cancer, germ cell cancer	Nausea and vomiting	Nephrotoxicity, peripheral sensory neuropathy, ototoxicity, nerve dysfunction
Carboplatin	Same as cisplatin	Non-small cell and small cell lung cancer, breast cancer, bladder cancer, head and neck cancer, ovarian cancer; non-Hodgkin lymphoma	Nausea and vomiting	Myelosuppression; rarely peripheral neuropathy, renal toxicity, hepatic dysfunction
Oxaliplatin	Same as cisplatin	Colorectal cancer, gastroesophageal cancer, pancreatic cancer, non-Hodgkin lymphoma	Nausea and vomiting, laryngopharyngeal dysesthesias	Myelosuppression, peripheral sensory neuropathy, GI toxicity with diarrhea and/or mucositis

CLL, chronic lymphocytic leukemia; CML, chronic myelogenous leukemia.

NITROSOUREAS

The nitrosoureas are generally non-cross-resistant with other alkylating agents, and all require biotransformation, which occurs by non-enzymatic decomposition, to metabolites with both alkylating and carbamoylating activities. The nitrosoureas are highly lipid-soluble and are able to readily cross the blood-brain barrier, making them effective in the treatment of brain tumors. Although the majority of alkylations by the nitrosoureas are on the N7 position of guanine in DNA, the critical alkylation responsible for cytotoxicity appears to be on the O6 position of guanine, which leads to G-C crosslinks in DNA. After oral administration of lomustine, peak plasma levels of metabolites appear within 1–4 hours; central nervous system concentrations reach 30–40% of the activity present in the plasma. Urinary excretion appears to be the major route of elimination from the body.

NONCLASSIC ALKYLATING AGENTS

Several other compounds have mechanisms of action that involve DNA alkylation as their cytotoxic mechanism of action. These agents include procarbazine, dacarbazine, and bendamustine. Their clinical activities and toxicities are listed in Table 54–2.

Procarbazine

Procarbazine is an orally active methylhydrazine derivative, and is used in combination regimens for Hodgkin and non-Hodgkin lymphoma as well as for brain tumors.

The precise mechanism of action of procarbazine has not been well-characterized; it inhibits DNA, RNA, and protein biosynthesis; prolongs interphase; and produces chromosome breaks. Oxidative metabolism of this drug by microsomal enzymes generates azoprocarbazine and H_2O_2, which may be responsible for DNA strand scission. Several other drug metabolites are formed that may be cytotoxic. One metabolite is a weak monoamine oxidase (MAO) inhibitor, and adverse events can occur when procarbazine is given with other MAO inhibitors as well as with sympathomimetic agents, tricyclic antidepressants, antihistamines, central nervous system depressants, antidiabetic agents, alcohol, and tyramine-containing foods.

As with classic alkylating agents, procarbazine is associated with an increased risk of secondary cancers in the form of AML. Moreover, its carcinogenic potential is thought to be higher than that of other alkylating agents.

Dacarbazine

Dacarbazine is a synthetic compound that functions as an alkylating agent following metabolic activation in the liver by oxidative *N*-demethylation to the monomethyl derivative. This metabolite spontaneously decomposes to diazomethane, which generates a methyl carbonium ion that is believed to be the key cytotoxic species. Dacarbazine is administered parenterally and is used in the treatment of Hodgkin lymphoma, soft tissue sarcomas, and neuroblastoma. The main dose-limiting toxicity is myelosuppression, but nausea and vomiting can be severe in some cases. This agent is a potent vesicant, and care must be taken to avoid extravasation during drug administration.

Bendamustine

Bendamustine is a bifunctional alkylating agent consisting of a purine benzimidazole ring and a nitrogen mustard moiety. It forms cross-links with DNA resulting in single- and double-stranded breaks, leading to inhibition of DNA synthesis and function. This agent also inhibits mitotic checkpoints and induces mitotic catastrophe, which then leads to cell death. Of note, the cross-resistance between bendamustine and other alkylating agents is only partial, thereby providing a rationale for its clinical activity despite the development of resistance to other alkylating agents. This agent is used to treat chronic lymphocytic leukemia, and clinical activity is also observed in Hodgkin and non-Hodgkin lymphoma, multiple myeloma, and breast cancer. The main dose-limiting toxicities include myelosuppression and mild nausea and vomiting. Hypersensitivity infusion reactions, skin rash, and other skin reactions occur rarely.

PLATINUM ANALOGS

Three platinum analogs are currently used in clinical practice: cisplatin, carboplatin, and oxaliplatin. Cisplatin is an inorganic metal complex that was initially discovered through a serendipitous observation that neutral platinum complexes inhibited division and filamentous growth of *Escherichia coli*. It is well-established that the platinum analogs exert their cytotoxic effects in the same manner as alkylating agents. As such, they kill tumor cells in all stages of the cell cycle and bind DNA through the formation of intrastrand and interstrand cross-links, thereby leading to inhibition of DNA synthesis and function. The primary binding site on DNA is the N7 position of guanine, but covalent interaction with the N3 position of adenine and O6 position of cytosine also can occur. In addition to targeting DNA, the platinum analogs are able to bind to both cytoplasmic and nuclear proteins, which may also contribute to their antitumor effects. The platinum analogs appear to synergize with certain other anticancer drugs, including alkylating agents, fluoropyrimidines, and taxanes. The major toxicities of the individual platinum analogs are outlined in Table 54–2.

H_3N Cl
Pt
H_3N Cl

Cisplatin

Cisplatin has major antitumor activity in a broad range of solid tumors, including non-small cell and small cell lung cancer, esophageal and gastric cancer, cholangiocarcinoma, head and neck cancer, and genitourinary cancers, particularly testicular, ovarian, and bladder cancer. When used in combination regimens, cisplatin-based therapy has led to the cure of non-seminomatous testicular cancer. Cisplatin and the other platinum analogs are eliminated by the kidneys and excreted in the urine. As a result, dose modification is required in patients with renal dysfunction.

Carboplatin is a second-generation platinum analog whose mechanisms of cytotoxic action, mechanisms of resistance, and clinical pharmacology are identical to those described for cisplatin. As with cisplatin, carboplatin has broad-spectrum activity against a wide range of solid tumors. However, in contrast to cisplatin, its main dose-limiting toxicity is myelosuppression with significantly less renal and gastrointestinal toxicity. It has been widely used in transplant regimens to treat refractory hematologic malignancies. Moreover, since vigorous intravenous hydration is not required for carboplatin therapy, carboplatin is viewed as an easier agent to administer to patients. As such, it has replaced cisplatin in a wide range of combination chemotherapy regimens.

Oxaliplatin is a third-generation diaminocyclohexane platinum analog, and its mechanism of action and clinical pharmacology are identical to those of cisplatin and carboplatin. However, tumors that are resistant to cisplatin or carboplatin on the basis of mismatch repair defects are not cross-resistant to oxaliplatin, and this finding may explain the clinical activity of this platinum compound in colorectal cancer (CRC). Oxaliplatin was initially approved for use as second-line therapy in combination with 5-fluorouracil (5-FU) and leucovorin, termed the FOLFOX regimen, for metastatic CRC. There are various iterations of the FOLFOX regimen, which has now become the most widely used combination in the first-line treatment of metastatic CRC. This regimen also plays a major role in the adjuvant therapy of stage III colon cancer and high-risk stage II colon cancer. Oxaliplatin-based regimens have shown clinical activity in other gastrointestinal cancers, such as pancreatic, gastroesophageal, and hepatocellular cancer. Neurotoxicity is the main dose-limiting toxicity, and it is manifested by a peripheral sensory neuropathy. There are two forms of neurotoxicity, an acute form that is often triggered and worsened by exposure to cold, and a chronic form that is dose-dependent. Although the chronic form of oxaliplatin toxicity is dependent on the cumulative dose of drug administered, it tends to be more readily reversible than the neuropathy observed with cisplatin-induced neurotoxicity.

ANTIMETABOLITES

The antimetabolites represent an important class of agents that were rationally designed and synthesized based on an understanding of the critical cellular processes involved in DNA biosynthesis. The individual antimetabolites and their respective clinical spectrum and toxicities are presented in Table 54–3 and are discussed below.

ANTIFOLATES

Methotrexate

Methotrexate (MTX) is a folic acid analog that binds with high affinity to the active catalytic site of dihydrofolate reductase (DHFR). This results in inhibition of synthesis of tetrahydrofolate (THF), the key one-carbon carrier for enzymatic processes involved in de novo synthesis of thymidylate, purine nucleotides, and the amino acids serine and methionine. Inhibition of these metabolic processes interferes with the formation of DNA, RNA, and key cellular proteins (see Figure 33–3). Intracellular formation of polyglutamate metabolites, with the addition of up to 5–7 glutamate residues, is critically important for the therapeutic action of MTX, and this process is catalyzed by the enzyme folylpolyglutamate synthase (FPGS). MTX polyglutamates are selectively retained within cancer cells, and they display increased inhibitory effects on enzymes involved in de novo purine nucleotide and thymidylate biosynthesis, making them important determinants of MTX's cytotoxic action.

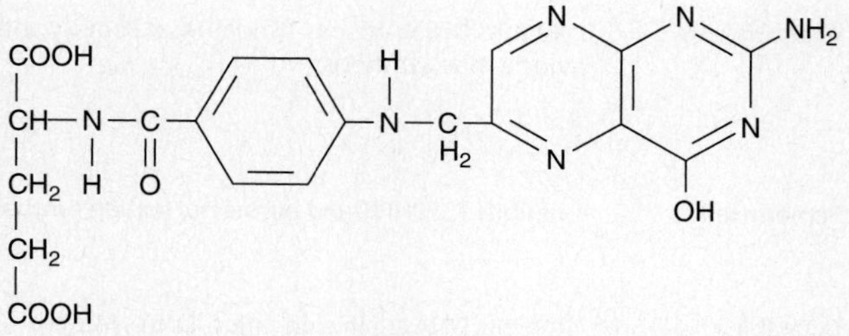

Folic acid

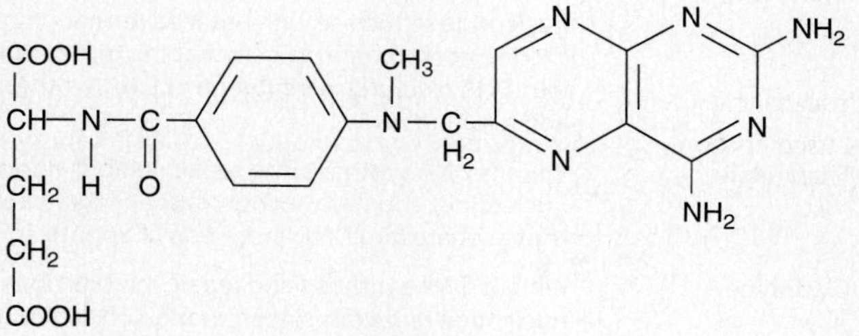

Methotrexate

Several resistance mechanisms to MTX have been identified, and they include (1) decreased drug transport via the reduced folate carrier (RFC) or folate receptor protein (FRP), (2) decreased formation of cytotoxic MTX polyglutamates, (3) increased levels of the target enzyme DHFR through gene amplification and other genetic mechanisms, and (4) altered DHFR protein with reduced affinity for MTX. Recent studies have suggested that decreased accumulation of drug through activation of the multidrug resistance transporter P170 glycoprotein also may result in drug resistance.

MTX is administered by the intravenous, intrathecal, or oral route. However, oral bioavailability is saturable and erratic at doses greater than 25 mg/m^2. Renal excretion is the main route of elimination and is mediated by glomerular filtration and tubular secretion. As a result, dose modification is required in patients with renal dysfunction. Caution must also be taken when MTX is used in the presence of drugs such as aspirin, nonsteroidal anti-inflammatory agents, penicillin, and cephalosporins, as these agents inhibit the renal excretion of MTX. The biologic effects of MTX can be reversed by administration of the reduced folate leucovorin (5-formyltetrahydrofolate) or by L-leucovorin, which is the active

TABLE 54–3 Antimetabolites: Clinical activity and toxicities.

Drug	Mechanism of Action	Clinical Applications	Toxicity
Capecitabine	Inhibits TS; incorporation of FUTP into RNA resulting in alteration in RNA processing; incorporation of FdUTP into DNA resulting in inhibition of DNA synthesis and function	Breast cancer, colorectal cancer, gastroesophageal cancer, hepatocellular cancer, pancreatic cancer	Diarrhea, hand-foot syndrome, myelosuppression, nausea and vomiting
5-Fluorouracil	Inhibits TS; incorporation of FUTP into RNA resulting in alteration in RNA processing; incorporation of FdUTP into DNA resulting in inhibition of DNA synthesis and function	Colorectal cancer, anal cancer, breast cancer, gastroesophageal cancer, head and neck cancer, hepatocellular cancer	Nausea, mucositis, diarrhea, myelosuppression, neurotoxicity
TAS-102	Inhibits TS; incorporation of trifluridine triphosphate into DNA, resulting in inhibition of DNA synthesis and function	Colorectal cancer, gastric or gastroesophageal cancer	Myelosuppression, diarrhea, fatigue, anorexia, asthenia
Methotrexate	Inhibits DHFR; inhibits TS; inhibits de novo purine nucleotide synthesis	Breast cancer, head and neck cancer, osteogenic sarcoma, primary central nervous system lymphoma, non-Hodgkin lymphoma, bladder cancer, choriocarcinoma	Mucositis, diarrhea, myelosuppression with neutropenia and thrombocytopenia
Pemetrexed	Inhibits TS, DHFR, and purine nucleotide synthesis	Mesothelioma, non-small cell lung cancer	Myelosuppression, skin rash, mucositis, diarrhea, fatigue, hand-foot syndrome
Cytarabine	Inhibits DNA chain elongation, DNA synthesis and repair; inhibits ribonucleotide reductase with reduced formation of dNTPs; incorporation of cytarabine triphosphate into DNA	AML, ALL, CML in blast crisis	Nausea and vomiting, myelosuppression with neutropenia and thrombocytopenia, cerebellar ataxia
Gemcitabine	Inhibits DNA synthesis and repair; inhibits ribonucleotide reductase with reduced formation of dNTPs; incorporation of gemcitabine triphosphate into DNA resulting in inhibition of DNA synthesis and function	Pancreatic cancer, bladder cancer, breast cancer, non-small cell lung cancer, ovarian cancer, non-Hodgkin lymphoma, soft tissue sarcoma	Nausea, vomiting, diarrhea, myelosuppression
Fludarabine	Inhibits DNA synthesis and repair; inhibits ribonucleotide reductase; incorporation of fludarabine triphosphate into DNA; induction of apoptosis	Non-Hodgkin lymphoma, CLL	Myelosuppression, immunosuppression, nausea and vomiting, fever, myalgias, arthralgias
Cladribine	Inhibits DNA synthesis and repair; inhibits ribonucleotide reductase; incorporation of cladribine triphosphate into DNA; induction of apoptosis	Hairy cell leukemia, CLL, non-Hodgkin lymphoma	Myelosuppression, nausea and vomiting, and immunosuppression
6-Mercaptopurine (6-MP)	Inhibits de novo purine nucleotide synthesis; incorporation of triphosphate into RNA; incorporation of triphosphate into DNA	AML	Myelosuppression, immunosuppression, and hepatotoxicity
6-Thioguanine	Same as 6-MP	ALL, AML	Same as 6-MP

ALL, acute lymphoblastic leukemia; AML, acute myelogenous leukemia; CLL, chronic lymphocytic leukemia; CML, chronic myelogenous leukemia; DHFR, dihydrofolate reductase; dNTP, deoxyribonucleotide triphosphate; FdUTP, 5-fluorodeoxyuridine-5′-triphosphate; FUTP, 5-fluorouridine-5′-triphosphate; TS, thymidylate synthase.

enantiomer. Leucovorin rescue is typically used in conjunction with high-dose MTX therapy to rescue normal cells from undue toxicity, and it has also been used in cases of accidental drug overdose. The main adverse effects of MTX are listed in Table 54–3.

Pemetrexed

Pemetrexed is a pyrrolopyrimidine antifolate analog with activity in the S phase of the cell cycle. As with MTX, it is transported into the cell via the RFC and requires activation by FPGS to yield higher polyglutamate forms. While this agent targets DHFR and enzymes involved in de novo purine nucleotide biosynthesis, its main mechanism of action is inhibition of thymidylate synthase (TS). Pemetrexed is currently approved for use in combination with cisplatin in the treatment of mesothelioma, as a single agent in the second-line therapy of NSCLC, in combination with cisplatin for the first-line treatment of NSCLC, and most recently, as maintenance therapy in patients with NSCLC whose disease has not progressed after four cycles of platinum-based chemotherapy. As with all antifolates, pemetrexed is excreted mainly in urine, and dose modification is required in patients with renal dysfunction. The main adverse effects include myelosuppression, skin rash, mucositis, diarrhea, fatigue, and hand-foot syndrome. Of note, vitamin supplementation with folic acid and vitamin B_{12} significantly reduces the toxicities associated with pemetrexed, while not interfering with clinical efficacy. The hand-foot syndrome is manifested by painful erythema and swelling of the hands and feet, and treatment with the steroid dexamethasone is effective in reducing the incidence and severity of this skin toxicity.

Pralatrexate

Pralatrexate is a 10-deaza-aminopterin antifolate analog, is transported into the cell via the RFC, and requires activation by FPGS to yield higher polyglutamate forms. This molecule was rationally designed to be a more potent substrate for the RFC-1 carrier protein and to serve as an improved substrate for FPGS. This agent inhibits DHFR, inhibits enzymes involved in de novo purine nucleotide biosynthesis, and also inhibits TS. Pralatrexate is approved for use in the treatment of relapsed or refractory peripheral T-cell lymphoma. As with other antifolate analogs, pralatrexate is excreted mainly in urine, and dose modification is required in the setting of renal dysfunction. The main toxicities include myelosuppression, skin rash, mucositis, diarrhea, and fatigue. As with pemetrexed, vitamin supplementation with folic acid and vitamin B_{12} appears to reduce the toxicities associated with pralatrexate, without interfering with clinical efficacy.

FLUOROPYRIMIDINES

5-Fluorouracil

5-Fluorouracil (5-FU) is inactive in its parent form and requires activation via a complex series of enzymatic reactions to ribosyl and deoxyribosyl nucleotide metabolites. One of these metabolites, 5-fluoro-2′-deoxyuridine-5′-monophosphate (FdUMP), forms a covalently bound ternary complex with the enzyme TS and the reduced folate 5,10-methylenetetrahydrofolate, a reaction critical for the de novo synthesis of thymidylate. Formation of this ternary complex results in inhibition of DNA synthesis through "thymineless death." 5-FU is converted to 5-fluorouridine-5′-triphosphate (FUTP), which is then incorporated into RNA, where it interferes with RNA processing and mRNA translation. 5-FU is also converted to 5-fluorodeoxyuridine-5′-triphosphate (FdUTP), which is subsequently incorporated into cellular DNA, resulting in inhibition of DNA synthesis and function. Thus, the cytotoxicity of 5-FU is thought to be mediated by the combined effects of both DNA- and RNA-mediated events. In addition, 5-FU and all other fluoropyrimidines exert their cytotoxic effects in the S-phase of the cell cycle.

5-FU is only administered via the IV route because of the rapid breakdown of drug by the catabolic enzyme dihydropyrimidine dehydrogenase (DPD) in the GI tract. Because of its extremely short half-life in peripheral blood, on the order of 10–15 minutes, infusion administration schedules are now favored over bolus schedules as longer administration times are associated with improved clinical efficacy and reduced toxicity. Up to 80–85% of an administered dose of 5-FU is catabolized by the DPD enzyme. There is an autosomal recessive pharmacogenetic syndrome involving partial or complete deficiency of the DPD enzyme that is seen in up to 5% of cancer patients. In this setting, severe, excessive toxicity is observed with the classic triad of myelosuppression, GI toxicity in the form of diarrhea, mucositis or both, and neurotoxicity. However, DPD deficiency does not always present with this classic triad, and patients can present with only one of these major toxicities.

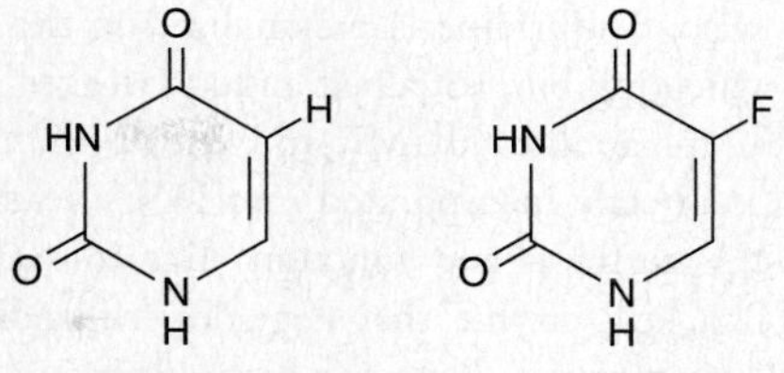

Uracil 5-FU

5-FU remains the most widely used agent in the treatment of CRC, both as adjuvant therapy and for advanced disease. It also has activity against a wide range of solid tumors, including cancers of the breast, stomach, pancreas, esophagus, liver, head and neck, and anus. Major toxicities include myelosuppression, gastrointestinal toxicity in the form of mucositis and diarrhea, skin toxicity manifested by the hand-foot syndrome, and neurotoxicity. Cardiac toxicity, in the form of ischemic heart disease, also has been observed.

Capecitabine

Capecitabine is a fluoropyrimidine carbamate prodrug with 70–80% oral bioavailability. As with 5-FU, capecitabine is inactive in its parent form and undergoes extensive metabolism in the liver by the enzyme carboxylesterase to an intermediate, 5′-deoxy-5-fluorocytidine. This metabolite is then converted to 5′-deoxy-5-fluorouridine by the enzyme cytidine deaminase. These two initial steps occur mainly in the liver. The 5′-deoxy-5-fluorouridine metabolite is finally hydrolyzed by thymidine phosphorylase to 5-FU directly in the tumor. The expression of thymidine phosphorylase has been shown to be significantly higher in a broad range of solid tumors than in corresponding normal tissue, particularly in breast cancer and colorectal cancer.

Capecitabine was initially approved for the treatment of metastatic breast cancer either as a single agent or in combination with other anticancer agents, including docetaxel, paclitaxel, lapatinib, ixabepilone, and trastuzumab. It is also approved for use in the adjuvant therapy of stage II and stage III colon cancer, and used in the treatment of metastatic CRC as monotherapy or in combination with other active cytotoxic agents, including irinotecan and oxaliplatin. The capecitabine/oxaliplatin (CAPOX) regimen is now widely used for the first-line treatment of metastatic CRC as well as in the adjuvant setting for patients with stage III and high-risk stage II colon cancer. The main toxicities of capecitabine include diarrhea and the hand-foot syndrome. While myelosuppression, nausea and vomiting, mucositis, and alopecia are observed with capecitabine, their incidence is much less than that observed with intravenous 5-FU.

TAS-102

TAS-102 is an oral fluoropyrimidine analog approved for the treatment of refractory, metastatic CRC. As with 5-FU, TAS-102 is inactive in its parent form. It is made up of two main components: trifluridine, a fluorinated pyrimidine nucleoside analog, and tipiracil, a thymidine phosphorylase (TP) inhibitor, combined in a

1:0.5 molar ratio. Trifluridine is metabolized to the monophosphate form, which inhibits TS, albeit a much weaker TS inhibitor than the 5-FU metabolite FdUMP, and also to the triphosphate form, which is directly incorporated into DNA, leading to inhibition of DNA synthesis and function. The role of tipiracil is to inhibit TP, a key enzyme that degrades trifluridine to inactive forms. Thus, tipiracil allows for higher levels of trifluridine, which can then be metabolized to the active nucleotide metabolite forms. The advantages of TAS-102 are that it retains clinical activity in 5-FU-resistant tumors and has similar clinical activity in the setting of wild-type and mutant *RAS* colorectal cancer. The main dose-limiting toxicity is myelosuppression, with neutropenia more commonly observed than anemia and thrombocytopenia. The other adverse effects commonly observed with this oral fluoropyrimidine are GI toxicity with diarrhea and nausea/vomiting, fatigue, and anorexia.

DEOXYCYTIDINE ANALOGS

Cytarabine

Cytarabine (ara-C) is an S phase–specific antimetabolite that is converted by deoxycytidine kinase to the 5′-mononucleotide (ara-CMP). Ara-CMP is further metabolized to the diphosphate and triphosphate metabolites, and the ara-CTP triphosphate is thought to be the main cytotoxic metabolite. Ara-CTP competitively inhibits DNA polymerase-α and DNA polymerase-β, thereby resulting in blockade of DNA synthesis and DNA repair, respectively. This metabolite is also incorporated into RNA and DNA. Incorporation into DNA leads to interference with chain elongation and defective ligation of fragments of newly synthesized DNA. The cellular retention of ara-CTP appears to correlate with its cytotoxicity in malignant cells.

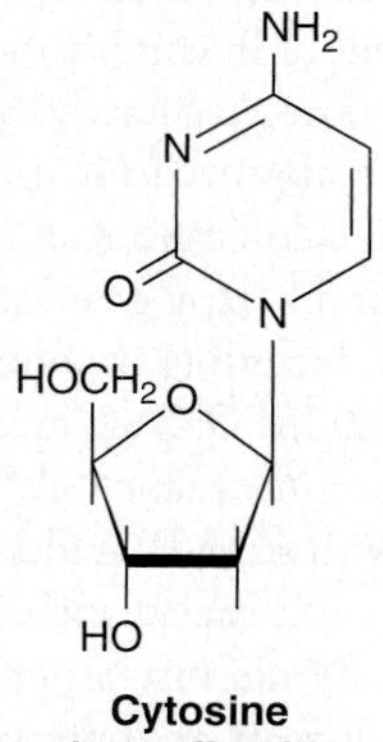

Cytosine deoxyriboside 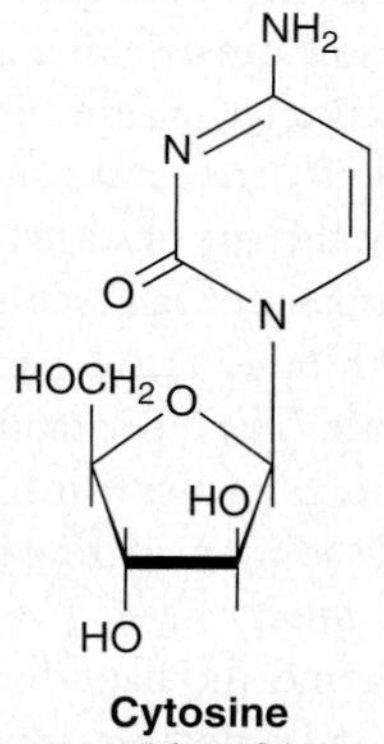 **Cytosine arabinoside (cytarabine)**

After IV administration, cytarabine is cleared rapidly, with the major portion of an administered dose being deaminated to inactive metabolites. The stoichiometric balance between the level of activation and catabolism of cytarabine is critical in determining its eventual cytotoxicity. The clinical activity of cytarabine is highly schedule-dependent and, because of its rapid degradation, it is usually administered via continuous infusion over a 5- to 7-day period. Its activity is limited exclusively to hematologic malignancies, including acute myelogenous leukemia and non-Hodgkin lymphoma. This agent has absolutely no activity in solid tumors. The main adverse effects associated with cytarabine therapy include myelosuppression, mucositis, nausea and vomiting, and neurotoxicity when high-dose therapy is administered.

Gemcitabine

Gemcitabine is a fluorine-substituted deoxycytidine analog that is phosphorylated initially by the enzyme deoxycytidine kinase to the monophosphate form and then by other nucleoside kinases to the diphosphate and triphosphate nucleotide forms. The antitumor effect is considered to result from several mechanisms: inhibition of ribonucleotide reductase by gemcitabine diphosphate, which reduces the level of deoxyribonucleoside triphosphates required for DNA synthesis; inhibition by gemcitabine triphosphate of DNA polymerase-α and DNA polymerase-β, thereby resulting in blockade of DNA synthesis and DNA repair; and incorporation of gemcitabine triphosphate into DNA, leading to inhibition of DNA synthesis and function.

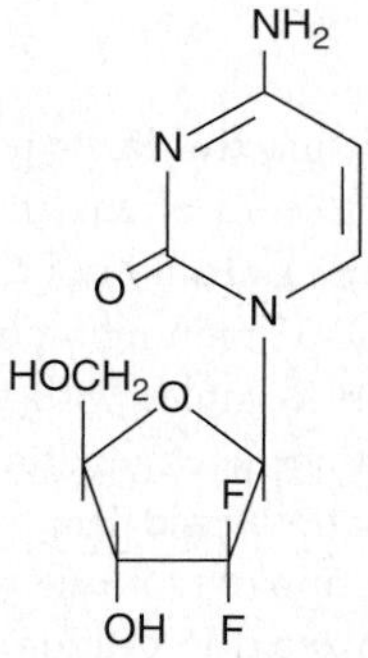

Gemcitabine

In contrast to cytarabine, which has no activity in solid tumors, gemcitabine has broad-spectrum activity against both solid tumors and hematologic malignancies. This nucleoside analog was initially approved for use in advanced pancreatic cancer and is now widely used to treat a broad range of malignancies, including NSCLC, bladder cancer, ovarian cancer, soft tissue sarcoma, and non-Hodgkin lymphoma. Myelosuppression in the form of neutropenia is the principal dose-limiting toxicity. Nausea and vomiting occur in 70% of patients, and a flu-like syndrome also has been observed. In rare cases, renal microangiopathy syndromes, including hemolytic-uremic syndrome (HUS) and thrombotic thrombocytopenic purpura (TTP), have been reported.

PURINE ANTAGONISTS

6-Thiopurines

6-Mercaptopurine (6-MP) was the first of the thiopurine analogs found to have clinical efficacy in cancer therapy. This agent is used primarily in the treatment of childhood acute leukemia, and a closely related analog, azathioprine, is used as an immunosuppressive agent (see Chapter 55). As with other thiopurines, 6-MP is inactive in its parent form and must be metabolized by hypoxanthine-guanine phosphoribosyl transferase (HGPRT) to form the monophosphate nucleotide 6-thioinosinic acid, which in turn, inhibits several enzymes of de novo purine nucleotide synthesis. The monophosphate form is eventually metabolized to the triphosphate form, which can then be incorporated into both RNA and DNA. Significant levels of thioguanylic acid and 6-methylmercaptopurine ribotide (MMPR) also are formed from 6-MP. These metabolites may contribute to its cytotoxic action.

6-Thioguanine (6-TG) also inhibits several enzymes in the de novo purine nucleotide biosynthetic pathway. Various metabolic lesions result, including inhibition of purine nucleotide interconversion; decrease in intracellular levels of guanine nucleotides, which leads to inhibition of glycoprotein synthesis; interference with the formation of DNA and RNA; and incorporation of thiopurine nucleotides into both DNA and RNA. 6-TG has a synergistic action when used together with cytarabine in the treatment of adult acute leukemia.

6-MP is converted to an inactive metabolite (6-thiouric acid) by an oxidation reaction catalyzed by xanthine oxidase, whereas 6-TG undergoes deamination. This is an important distinction because the purine analog allopurinol, a potent xanthine oxidase inhibitor, is frequently used as a supportive care measure in the treatment of acute leukemias to prevent the development of hyperuricemia that often occurs with tumor cell lysis. Because allopurinol inhibits xanthine oxidase, simultaneous therapy with allopurinol and 6-MP leads to increased levels of 6-MP, thereby leading to excessive toxicity. In this setting, the dose of 6-MP must be reduced by 50–75%. In contrast, such a drug-drug interaction does not occur with 6-TG, which can be used in full doses with allopurinol.

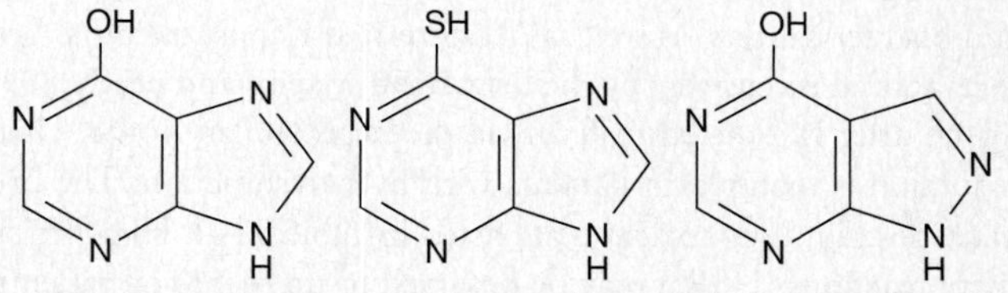

Hypoxanthine **6-Mercaptopurine** **Allopurinol**

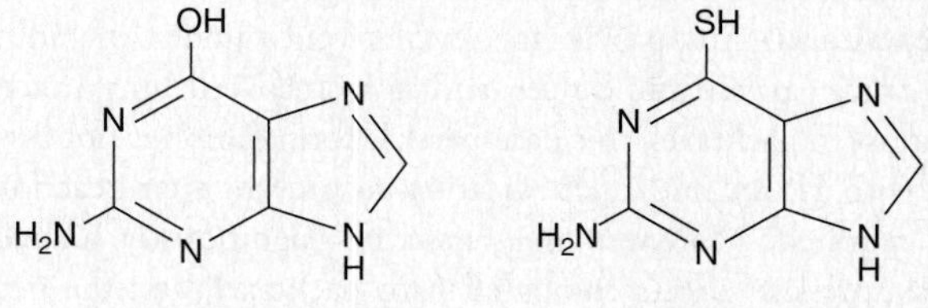

Guanine **6-Thioguanine**

The thiopurines are also metabolized by the enzyme thiopurine methyltransferase (TPMT), in which a methyl group is attached to the thiopurine ring. There is an autosomal recessive pharmacogenetic syndrome that results in partial or complete deficiency of this enzyme. These patients are at increased risk for developing severe toxicities in the form of myelosuppression and gastrointestinal toxicity with mucositis and diarrhea. Unfortunately, these patients do not manifest a phenotype until they are treated with a thiopurine.

Fludarabine

Fludarabine phosphate is rapidly dephosphorylated to 2-fluoro-arabinofuranosyladenosine and then phosphorylated intracellularly by deoxycytidine kinase to the monophosphate, which is eventually converted to the triphosphate. Fludarabine triphosphate interferes with the processes of DNA synthesis and DNA repair through inhibition of DNA polymerase-α and DNA polymerase-β. The triphosphate form can also be directly incorporated into DNA, resulting in inhibition of DNA synthesis and function. The diphosphate metabolite of fludarabine inhibits ribonucleotide reductase, leading to inhibition of essential deoxyribonucleotide triphosphates. Finally, fludarabine induces apoptosis in susceptible cells through as yet undetermined mechanisms. This purine nucleotide analog is used mainly in the treatment of low-grade non-Hodgkin lymphoma and chronic lymphocytic leukemia (CLL). It is given parenterally, and up to 25–30% of parent drug is excreted in the urine. The main dose-limiting toxicity is myelosuppression. This agent is a potent immunosuppressant with inhibitory effects on CD4 and CD8 T cells. Patients are at increased risk for opportunistic infections, including fungus, herpes, and *Pneumocystis jirovecii* pneumonia (PJP). Patients should receive PJP prophylaxis with trimethoprim-sulfamethoxazole (double-strength) at least three times a week, and this should continue for up to 1 year even after termination of fludarabine therapy.

Cladribine

Cladribine (2-chlorodeoxyadenosine) is a purine nucleoside analog with high specificity for lymphoid cells. Inactive in its parent form, it is initially phosphorylated by deoxycytidine kinase to the monophosphate form and eventually metabolized to the triphosphate form, which can then be incorporated into DNA. The triphosphate metabolite can also interfere with DNA synthesis and DNA repair by inhibiting DNA polymerase-α and DNA polymerase-β, respectively. Cladribine is indicated for the treatment of hairy cell leukemia, with activity in other low-grade lymphoid malignancies such as CLL and low-grade non-Hodgkin lymphoma. This agent is normally administered as a single continuous 7-day infusion, and under these conditions, it has a very manageable safety profile with the main toxicity consisting of transient myelosuppression. As with other purine nucleoside analogs, it has immunosuppressive effects, and a decrease in CD4 and CD8 T cells, lasting for >1 year, is observed.

NATURAL PRODUCT CANCER CHEMOTHERAPY DRUGS

VINCA ALKALOIDS

The vinca alkaloids inhibit the process of tubulin polymerization, which disrupts assembly of microtubules, especially those involved in the mitotic spindle apparatus. This inhibitory effect results in mitotic arrest in metaphase, bringing cell division to a halt, which then leads to cell death. Thus, the vinca alkaloids exert their main cytotoxic effect in the M phase of the cell cycle. Microtubules also play an important role in maintaining cell shape and cellular motility, and they facilitate the intracellular transport of cellular proteins. Inhibition of microtubule formation has important consequences that can lead to cell death.

Vinblastine

Vinblastine is an alkaloid derived from the periwinkle plant *Vinca rosea*. Vinblastine and other vinca alkaloids are metabolized by the liver P450 system, and the majority of the drug is excreted in feces via the hepatobiliary system. As such, dose modification is required in patients with liver dysfunction. The main adverse effects are outlined in Table 54–4, and they include nausea and vomiting, bone marrow suppression, and alopecia. This agent is also a potent vesicant, and care must be taken in its administration. It has clinical activity in the treatment of Hodgkin and non-Hodgkin lymphomas, breast cancer, and germ cell cancer.

Vincristine

Vincristine is another alkaloid derivative of *Vinca rosea* and is closely related in structure to vinblastine. Its mechanism of action, mechanism of resistance, and clinical pharmacology are identical to those of vinblastine. Despite these similarities to vinblastine, vincristine has a strikingly different spectrum of clinical activity and safety profile, which results, in large part, from its higher affinity for axonal microtubules.

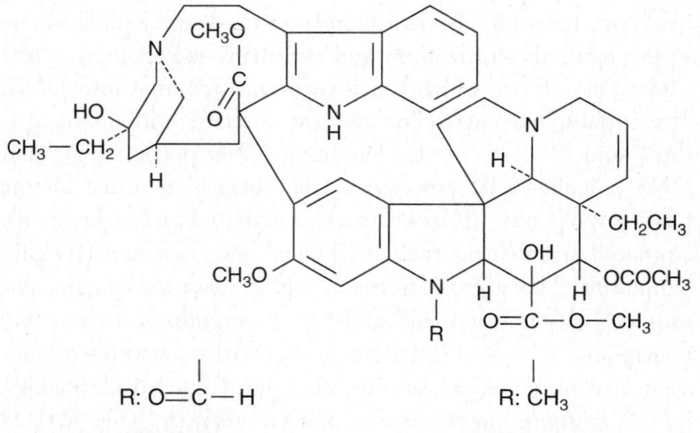

R: O=C—H | R: CH_3

Vincristine | **Vinblastine**

Vincristine has been effectively combined with prednisone for remission induction in acute lymphoblastic leukemia in children. It is also active in various hematologic malignancies such as Hodgkin and non-Hodgkin lymphomas, and multiple myeloma, and in several pediatric tumors including rhabdomyosarcoma, neuroblastoma, Ewing sarcoma, and Wilms tumor.

The main dose-limiting toxicity is neurotoxicity, usually manifested as a peripheral sensory neuropathy, although autonomic nervous system dysfunction with orthostatic hypotension, urinary retention, and paralytic ileus or constipation, cranial nerve palsies, ataxia, seizures, and coma have been observed. While myelosuppression occurs, it is generally milder and much less significant than with vinblastine. The other adverse effect that may develop is the syndrome of inappropriate secretion of antidiuretic hormone (SIADH), which can also be observed with the other vinca alkaloids.

Vinorelbine

Vinorelbine is a semisynthetic derivative of vinblastine whose mechanism of action is identical to that of vinblastine and vincristine, ie, inhibition of mitosis of cells in the M phase. This agent has activity in NSCLC, breast cancer, and ovarian cancer. Myelosuppression with neutropenia is the dose-limiting toxicity, but other adverse effects include nausea and vomiting, transient elevations in liver function tests, and SIADH.

TAXANES & OTHER ANTI-MICROTUBULE DRUGS

Paclitaxel is an alkaloid ester derived from the Pacific yew (*Taxus brevifolia*) and the European yew (*Taxus baccata*). It is a mitotic spindle poison that acts through high-affinity binding to microtubules with enhancement of tubulin polymerization. This promotion of microtubule assembly by paclitaxel results in inhibition of mitosis and cell division. Therefore, paclitaxel and the other taxanes are active in the M phase of the cell cycle.

Paclitaxel has significant activity in a broad range of solid tumors, including ovarian, advanced breast, NSCLC and small cell lung cancer (SCLC), head and neck, esophageal, prostate, and bladder cancers, as well as AIDS-related Kaposi sarcoma. It is metabolized extensively by the liver P450 system, and nearly 80% of the drug is excreted in feces via the hepatobiliary route. Dose reduction is required in patients with liver dysfunction. The primary dose-limiting toxicities are listed in Table 54–4. Hypersensitivity reactions (HSRs) may be observed in up to 5% of patients, but the incidence is significantly reduced by premedication with dexamethasone, diphenhydramine, and an H_2 blocker.

An **albumin-bound paclitaxel nanoparticle formulation (nab-paclitaxel)** is approved for several solid tumors, including breast cancer, pancreatic cancer, and non-small cell lung cancer. In contrast to paclitaxel, this nanoparticle formulation is not associated with HSRs, and premedication to prevent such reactions is not required. Moreover, this agent has significantly reduced myelosuppressive effects compared with paclitaxel, and the neurotoxicity that results appears to be more readily reversible than is typically observed with paclitaxel.

Docetaxel is a semisynthetic taxane derived from the European yew tree that appears to be more potent than paclitaxel. Its mechanism of action, metabolism, elimination, and mechanisms of resistance are identical to those of paclitaxel. It is approved for use as second-line therapy in advanced breast cancer and NSCLC, and it also has major activity in head and neck cancer, small cell lung cancer, gastric cancer, advanced platinum-refractory ovarian cancer, and bladder cancer. Its major toxicities are listed in Table 54–4.

TABLE 54–4 Natural product cancer chemotherapy drugs: Clinical activity and toxicities.

Drug	Mechanism of Action	Clinical Applications	Acute Toxicity	Delayed Toxicity
Bleomycin	Oxygen free radicals bind to DNA causing single- and double-strand DNA breaks	Hodgkin and non-Hodgkin lymphoma, germ cell cancer, head and neck cancer	Allergic reactions, fever, hypotension	Skin toxicity, pulmonary fibrosis, mucositis, alopecia
Daunorubicin	Oxygen free radicals bind to DNA causing single- and double-strand DNA breaks; inhibits topoisomerase II; intercalates into DNA	AML, ALL	Nausea and vomiting, fever, red urine (not hematuria)	Cardiotoxicity (see text), alopecia, myelosuppression
Docetaxel	Inhibits mitosis	Breast cancer, non-small cell lung cancer, prostate cancer, gastric cancer, head and neck cancer, ovarian cancer, bladder cancer	Hypersensitivity	Neurotoxicity, fluid retention, myelosuppression with neutropenia
Doxorubicin	Oxygen free radicals bind to DNA causing single- and double-strand DNA breaks; inhibits topoisomerase II; intercalates into DNA	Breast cancer, Hodgkin and non-Hodgkin lymphoma, soft tissue sarcoma, ovarian cancer, non-small cell and small cell lung cancer, thyroid cancer, Wilms tumor, neuroblastoma	Nausea, red urine (not hematuria)	Cardiotoxicity (see text), alopecia, myelosuppression, stomatitis
Etoposide	Inhibits topoisomerase II	Non-small cell and small cell lung cancer; non-Hodgkin lymphoma, gastric cancer	Nausea, vomiting, hypotension	Alopecia, myelosuppression
Idarubicin	Oxygen free radicals bind to DNA causing single- and double-strand DNA breaks; inhibits topoisomerase II; intercalates into DNA	AML, ALL, CML in blast crisis	Nausea and vomiting	Myelosuppression, mucositis, cardiotoxicity
Irinotecan	Inhibits topoisomerase I	Colorectal cancer, gastroesophageal cancer, non-small cell and small cell lung cancer	Diarrhea, nausea, vomiting	Diarrhea, myelosuppression, nausea and vomiting
Mitomycin	Acts as an alkylating agent and forms cross-links with DNA; formation of oxygen free radicals, which target DNA	Superficial bladder cancer, gastric cancer, breast cancer, non-small cell lung cancer, head and neck cancer (in combination with radiotherapy)	Nausea and vomiting	Myelosuppression, mucositis, anorexia and fatigue, hemolytic-uremic syndrome
Paclitaxel	Inhibits mitosis	Breast cancer, non-small cell and small cell lung cancer, ovarian cancer, gastroesophageal cancer, prostate cancer, bladder cancer, head and neck cancer	Nausea, vomiting, hypotension, arrhythmias, hypersensitivity	Myelosuppression, peripheral sensory neuropathy
Topotecan	Inhibits topoisomerase I	Small cell lung cancer, ovarian cancer	Nausea and vomiting	Myelosuppression
Vinblastine	Inhibits mitosis	Hodgkin and non-Hodgkin lymphoma, germ cell cancer, breast cancer, Kaposi sarcoma	Nausea and vomiting	Myelosuppression, mucositis, alopecia, syndrome of inappropriate secretion of antidiuretic hormone (SIADH), vascular events
Vincristine	Inhibits mitosis	ALL, Hodgkin and non-Hodgkin lymphoma, rhabdomyosarcoma, neuroblastoma, Wilms tumor	None	Neurotoxicity with peripheral neuropathy, paralytic ileus, myelosuppression, alopecia, SIADH
Vinorelbine	Inhibits mitosis	Non-small cell lung cancer, breast cancer, ovarian cancer	Nausea and vomiting	Myelosuppression, constipation, SIADH

ALL, acute lymphoblastic leukemia; AML, acute myelogenous leukemia; CML, chronic myelogenous leukemia.

Cabazitaxel is another semisynthetic taxane and its mechanism of action, metabolism, and elimination are identical to those of the other taxanes. However, unlike other taxanes, cabazitaxel is a poor substrate for the multidrug resistance P-glycoprotein efflux pump and may, therefore, be useful for treating multidrug-resistant tumors. It is approved for use in combination with prednisone in the second-line therapy of hormone-refractory metastatic prostate cancer previously treated with a docetaxel-containing regimen. Its major toxicities include myelosuppression, neurotoxicity, and allergic reactions.

Ixabepilone is an epothilone B analog and, like the taxanes, functions as a microtubule inhibitor and binds directly to β-tubulin subunits on microtubules, leading to inhibition of normal microtubule dynamics. As such, it is active in the M phase of the cell cycle. This agent is presently approved for metastatic breast cancer in combination with the oral fluoropyrimidine capecitabine or as monotherapy. Of note, this agent has activity in drug-resistant tumors that overexpress P-glycoprotein or tubulin mutations. The main adverse effects include myelosuppression, HSRs, and neurotoxicity in the form of peripheral sensory neuropathy.

Eribulin is a synthetic analog of halichondrin B, and it inhibits microtubule function, leading to a block in the G_2-M phase of the cell cycle. This agent appears to be less sensitive to the multidrug resistance–mediated P-glycoprotein efflux pump, and one of its advantages is that it has activity in drug-resistant tumors that overexpress P-glycoprotein. It is approved for the treatment of patients with metastatic breast cancer and unresectable or metastatic liposarcoma.

EPIPODOPHYLLOTOXINS

Etoposide is a semisynthetic derivative of podophyllotoxin, which is extracted from the mayapple root (*Podophyllum peltatum*). Intravenous and oral formulations of etoposide are approved for clinical use in the USA. Oral bioavailability is about 50%, requiring oral dosage to be twice that of IV dosage. Up to 30–50% of an administered dose of drug is excreted in the urine, and dose reduction is required in patients with renal dysfunction. Etoposide forms a complex with topoisomerase II, the enzyme responsible for cutting and religating double stranded DNA, and DNA, leading to inhibition of the functional activity of topoisomerase II with inhibition of DNA synthesis and function. Etoposide has clinical activity in germ cell cancer, small cell and NSCLC, Hodgkin and non-Hodgkin lymphomas, and gastric cancer. Major toxicities are listed in Table 54–4.

CAMPTOTHECINS

The camptothecins are natural products derived from the *Camptotheca acuminata* tree originally found in China; they inhibit the activity of topoisomerase I (topo I), the key enzyme responsible for cutting and religating single DNA strands. Inhibition of this enzyme results in DNA damage. **Irinotecan, topotecan, deruxtecan,** and **govitecan** are the camptothecin analogs used in clinical practice in the USA. Although they inhibit the same molecular target, their spectrum of clinical activity is quite different.

Irinotecan is a prodrug that is converted mainly in the liver by the carboxylesterase enzyme to **govitecan**, the **SN-38** metabolite that is 1000-fold more potent as an inhibitor of topo I than the parent compound. Irinotecan and SN-38 are mainly eliminated in bile and feces, and dose reduction is required in the setting of liver dysfunction. Irinotecan was originally approved as second-line monotherapy in patients with metastatic colorectal cancer who had failed fluorouracil-based therapy. It is approved as first-line therapy when used in combination with 5-FU and leucovorin, and this combination is known as FOLFIRI. Myelosuppression and diarrhea are the two most common adverse events (see Table 54–4). There are two forms of diarrhea: an early form that occurs within 24 hours after administration, which is thought to be a cholinergic event effectively treated with atropine, and a late form that usually occurs 2–10 days after treatment. The late diarrhea may be severe, leading to significant electrolyte imbalance and dehydration in some cases.

Liposomal irinotecan is approved in combination with 5-FU and leucovorin for the treatment of metastatic adenocarcinoma of the pancreas after disease progression following gemcitabine-based therapy. The main toxicities associated with the liposomal formulation are myelosuppression and GI toxicity with diarrhea and nausea/vomiting. Relatively little is known about the clinical pharmacology and metabolism of this liposomal formulation of irinotecan.

Topotecan is indicated for the treatment of advanced ovarian cancer as second-line therapy following initial treatment with platinum-based chemotherapy. It is also approved as second-line therapy of small cell lung cancer. In contrast to irinotecan, the main route of elimination for topotecan is renal excretion, and dosage must be adjusted in patients with renal impairment.

Deruxtecan is a 10-fold more potent inhibitor of topo I than SN-38, the active metabolite, and it is conjugated with trastuzumab to form an antibody-drug conjugate (ADC). The activity of this molecule is dependent on HER expression and not on HER2 gene amplification, which is in contrast to other anti-HER2 inhibitors.

ANTITUMOR ANTIBIOTICS

Screening of microbial products led to the discovery of a number of growth-inhibiting compounds that have proved to be clinically useful in cancer chemotherapy. Many of these antibiotics bind to DNA through intercalation between specific bases and block the synthesis of RNA, DNA, or both; cause DNA strand scission; and interfere with cell replication. All of the anticancer antibiotics used in everyday clinical practice are products of various strains of the soil microbe *Streptomyces*, and these include several anthracyclines, bleomycin, and mitomycin.

ANTHRACYCLINES

The anthracycline antibiotics, isolated from *Streptomyces peucetius* var *caesius*, are among the most widely used cytotoxic anticancer drugs. The structures of the two original anthracyclines, **doxorubicin** and **daunorubicin,** are shown below. Several other anthracycline analogs have entered clinical practice, including **idarubicin, epirubicin,** and **mitoxantrone.** The anthracyclines exert their cytotoxic action through four major mechanisms: (1) inhibition of topoisomerase II; (2) generation of semiquinone free radicals and oxygen free radicals through an iron-dependent, enzyme-mediated reductive process; (3) high-affinity binding to DNA through intercalation, with consequent blockade of the synthesis of DNA and RNA, and DNA strand scission; and (4) binding to cellular membranes to alter fluidity and ion transport. While the precise mechanisms by which the anthracyclines exert their cytotoxic effects remain to be defined in the clinical setting, the free radical mechanism is well-established to be the cause of the cardiotoxicity associated with the anthracyclines (see Table 54–4).

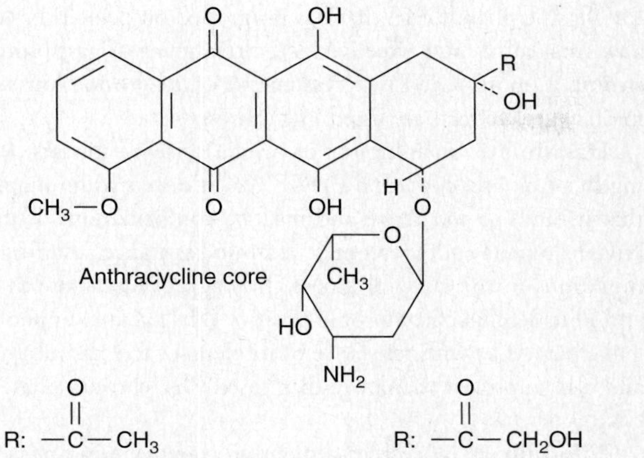

Anthracycline core

R: $-C(=O)-CH_3$ **Daunorubicin**

R: $-C(=O)-CH_2OH$ **Doxorubicin**

Anthracyclines are administered via the intravenous route. They are metabolized extensively in the liver, with reduction and hydrolysis of the ring substituents. The hydroxylated metabolite is an active species, whereas the aglycone is inactive. Up to 50% of drug is eliminated in the feces via biliary excretion, and dose reduction is required in patients with liver dysfunction. Although anthracyclines are usually administered on an every-3-week schedule, alternative schedules such as low-dose weekly or 72- to 96-hour continuous infusions have been shown to yield equivalent clinical efficacy with reduced toxicity.

Doxorubicin is one of the most important anticancer drugs in clinical practice, with major clinical activity in cancers of the breast, endometrium, ovary, testicle, thyroid, stomach, bladder, liver, and lung; in soft tissue sarcomas; and in several childhood cancers, including neuroblastoma, Ewing sarcoma, osteosarcoma, and rhabdomyosarcoma. It also has clinical activity in hematologic malignancies, including acute lymphoblastic leukemia, multiple myeloma, and Hodgkin and non-Hodgkin lymphomas. It is generally used in combination with other anticancer agents (eg, cyclophosphamide, cisplatin, and 5-FU), and clinical activity is enhanced when used in combination regimens as opposed to monotherapy.

Daunorubicin was the first agent in this class to be isolated, and it is still used in combination with cytarabine for the treatment of AML. Compared to doxorubicin, its efficacy in solid tumors is limited.

Idarubicin is a semisynthetic anthracycline glycoside analog of daunorubicin, and it is approved for use in combination with cytarabine for induction therapy of acute myeloid leukemia. When combined with cytarabine, idarubicin appears to be more active than daunorubicin in producing complete remissions and in improving survival in patients with AML.

Epirubicin is an anthracycline analog whose mechanism of action and clinical pharmacology are identical to those of all other anthracyclines. It was initially approved for use as a component of adjuvant therapy in early-stage, node-positive breast cancer but is also used in the treatment of metastatic breast cancer and metastatic gastric and gastroesophageal cancer.

Mitoxantrone (dihydroxyanthracenedione) is an anthracene compound whose structure resembles the anthracycline ring. It binds to DNA to produce strand breakage and inhibits both DNA and RNA synthesis. It is used in the treatment of advanced, hormone-refractory prostate cancer and low-grade non-Hodgkin lymphoma. It is also indicated in breast cancer and in pediatric and adult acute myeloid leukemias. Myelosuppression with leukopenia is the dose-limiting toxicity, and mild nausea and vomiting, mucositis, and alopecia also occur. Although the drug is thought to be less cardiotoxic than doxorubicin, both acute and chronic cardiac toxicities are observed. A blue discoloration of the fingernails, sclera, and urine is observed 1–2 days after drug administration.

The main dose-limiting toxicity of the anthracyclines is myelosuppression, with neutropenia more commonly observed than thrombocytopenia. In some cases, mucositis is dose-limiting. Two forms of cardiotoxicity are observed. The acute form occurs within the first 2–3 days and presents as arrhythmias and conduction abnormalities, other electrocardiographic changes, pericarditis, and myocarditis. This acute toxicity is usually transient and in most cases is asymptomatic. The chronic form is a dose-dependent, dilated cardiomyopathy associated with heart failure. The chronic cardiac toxicity appears to result from increased production of oxygen free radicals within the myocardium. This effect is rarely seen at total doxorubicin dosages below 400–450 mg/m^2. Use of lower weekly doses or continuous infusions of doxorubicin appear to reduce the incidence of cardiac toxicity. In addition, treatment with the iron-chelating agent **dexrazoxane** (ICRF-187) is approved to prevent or reduce anthracycline-induced cardiotoxicity in women with metastatic breast cancer who have received a total cumulative dose of doxorubicin of 300 mg/m^2. The anthracyclines are also associated with a "radiation recall reaction," with erythema and desquamation of the skin observed at sites of prior radiation therapy.

MITOMYCIN

Mitomycin (mitomycin C) is an antibiotic isolated from *Streptomyces caespitosus*. It undergoes metabolic activation through an enzyme-mediated reduction to generate an alkylating agent that cross-links DNA. Hypoxic tumor stem cells of solid tumors exist in an environment conducive to reductive reactions and are more sensitive to the cytotoxic effects of mitomycin than normal cells and oxygenated tumor cells. This agent is active in all phases of the cell cycle and is the best available drug for use in combination with radiation therapy to attack hypoxic tumor cells. Its clinical use is mainly limited to the treatment of squamous cell cancer of the anus in combination with 5-FU and radiation therapy. One special application of mitomycin has been in the intravesical treatment of superficial bladder cancer. Because virtually none of the agent is absorbed, there is little or no systemic toxicity when mitomycin is administered via the intravesical route.

The common adverse events of mitomycin are outlined in Table 54–4. Hemolytic-uremic syndrome, manifested as microangiopathic hemolytic anemia, thrombocytopenia, and renal failure, as well as occasional instances of interstitial pneumonitis have been reported.

BLEOMYCIN

Bleomycin is a small peptide that contains a DNA-binding region and an iron-binding domain at opposite ends of the molecule. It binds to DNA, which results in single- and double-strand breaks following free radical formation, and inhibition of DNA biosynthesis. The fragmentation of DNA is due to oxidation of a DNA-bleomycin-Fe(II) complex and leads to chromosomal aberrations. Bleomycin is a cell cycle–specific drug that causes accumulation of cells in the G_2 phase of the cell cycle.

Bleomycin is indicated for the treatment of Hodgkin and non-Hodgkin lymphomas, germ cell tumor, head and neck cancer, and squamous cell cancer of the skin, cervix, and vulva. One advantage of this agent is that it can be administered subcutaneously, intramuscularly, or intravenously. Elimination of bleomycin is mainly via renal excretion, and dose modification is recommended in patients with renal dysfunction. Another potential advantage of this agent is that it can be safely combined with other cytotoxic agents that are myelosuppressive, given its relatively minimal effects on the bone marrow.

Pulmonary toxicity is dose-limiting for bleomycin and usually presents as pneumonitis with cough, dyspnea, dry inspiratory crackles on physical examination, and infiltrates on chest x-ray. The incidence of pulmonary toxicity is increased in patients older than 70 years of age, in those who receive cumulative doses greater than 400 units, in those with underlying pulmonary disease, and in those who have received prior mediastinal or chest irradiation. In rare cases, pulmonary toxicity can be fatal. Other toxicities are listed in Table 54–4.

MISCELLANEOUS ANTICANCER DRUGS

There is now a growing list of anticancer drugs that have been approved for clinical use and that do not fit traditional categories; some of these agents are listed in Table 54–5.

BCR-ABL TYROSINE KINASE INHIBITORS (TKIs)

Imatinib is an inhibitor of the tyrosine kinase domain of the Bcr-Abl oncoprotein and prevents phosphorylation of the kinase substrate by ATP. It is indicated for the treatment of chronic myelogenous leukemia (CML), a pluripotent hematopoietic stem cell disorder characterized by the t(9:22) Philadelphia chromosomal translocation. This translocation results in the Bcr-Abl fusion protein, the causative agent in CML, and is present in up to 95% of patients with this disease. This agent also inhibits other receptor tyrosine kinases for platelet-derived growth factor receptor (PDGFR) and c-kit.

Imatinib is well absorbed orally, and it is metabolized in the liver, with elimination of metabolites occurring mainly in feces via biliary excretion. This agent is approved for use as first-line therapy in chronic phase CML, in blast crisis, and as second-line therapy for chronic phase CML that has progressed on prior IFN-α therapy. Imatinib is also effective in the treatment of gastrointestinal stromal tumors (GIST) expressing the c-kit tyrosine kinase. The main adverse effects are listed in Table 54–5.

Dasatinib is an inhibitor of several tyrosine kinases, including Bcr-Abl, Src, c-kit, and PDGFR-α. It differs from imatinib in that it binds to the active and inactive conformations of the Abl kinase domain and overcomes imatinib resistance resulting from mutations in the Bcr-Abl kinase. It is approved for use in CML and Philadelphia chromosome-positive (Ph+) acute lymphoblastic leukemia (ALL) with resistance or intolerance to imatinib therapy, and also approved for newly diagnosed Ph+ chronic phase (CP) CML.

Nilotinib is a second-generation phenylamino-pyrimidine molecule that inhibits Bcr-Abl, c-kit, and PDGFR-β tyrosine kinases. It has a higher binding affinity (up to 20- to 50-fold) for the Abl kinase when compared with imatinib, and it overcomes imatinib resistance resulting from Bcr-Abl mutations. It was originally approved for chronic phase and accelerated phase CML with resistance or intolerance to prior therapy that included imatinib and now also approved as first-line therapy of Ph+ chronic phase CML.

Bosutinib is a potent inhibitor of the Bcr-Abl tyrosine kinase, and it retains activity in 16 of 18 imatinib-resistant Bcr-Abl mutations. However, it is not effective against T315I and V299L mutations, which reside within the ATP-binding domain of the Abl tyrosine kinase. It is approved for the treatment of adult patients with chronic, accelerated, or blast phase Ph+ CML with resistance or intolerance to prior therapy.

Ponatinib is a potent inhibitor of the Bcr-Abl tyrosine kinase, and it inhibits all known mutant forms of BCR-ABL, including the gatekeeper mutation T315I. This agent has a much broader spectrum of biological activity and inhibits a wide range of tyrosine kinases, including members of VEGF-R, PDGF, FGF, Flt3, TIE-2, Src family kinases, Kit, TET, and EPH. This agent is FDA-approved for adult patients with chronic, accelerated, or blast phase CML that is resistant or intolerant to prior TKI therapy and for Ph+ ALL that is resistant or intolerant to prior TKI therapy.

All of the Bcr-Abl TKIs are metabolized in the liver, mainly by the CYP3A4 liver microsomal enzymes and then eliminated in feces via the hepatobiliary route. It is also important to review the patient's current list of prescription and non-prescription drugs because these agents have potential drug-drug interactions, especially with those that are also metabolized by the CYP3A4 system. In addition, patients should avoid grapefruit products, starfruit, and pomelos while on therapy, as these food products may inhibit the metabolism of these small molecule inhibitors, leading to increased drug levels and toxicity (see Chapter 4).

Asciminib is a small molecule allosteric inhibitor that targets the myristoyl pocket of Bcr-Abl, and it induces and stabilizes an inactive conformation of the kinase. It is different than other conventional TKIs that bind to the catalytic ATP-binding site, and it is associated with significantly less off-target activity. This agent is approved for adult patients with Ph+ CP CML and in Ph+ CP CML with the T315I mutation. As with the other Bcr-Abl TKIs, asciminib is metabolized mainly in the liver by CYP3A4

TABLE 54–5 Miscellaneous anticancer drugs: Clinical activity and toxicities.

Drug	Mechanism of Action[1]	Clinical Applications[1]	Acute Toxicity	Delayed Toxicity
Bortezomib	Inhibitor of the 26S proteosome; results in down-regulation of the NF-κB signaling pathway	Multiple myeloma, mantle cell lymphoma	Nausea and vomiting, fever	Peripheral sensory neuropathy, diarrhea, orthostatic hypotension, fever, pulmonary toxicity, reversible posterior leukoencephalopathy (RPLS), congestive heart failure (CHF), rare cases of QT prolongation
Carfilzomib	Inhibitor of the 26S proteosome; results in down-regulation of the NF-κB signaling pathway; maintains activity in bortezomib-resistant tumors	Multiple myeloma	Fever	Fatigue, cardiac toxicity with CHF and myocardial infarction, myelosuppression, pulmonary toxicity, hepatotoxicity, orthostatic hypotension
Ixazomib	Inhibitor of the 26S proteosome; results in down-regulation of the NF-κB signaling pathway; maintains activity in bortezomib-resistant tumors	Multiple myeloma	Fatigue	Myelosuppression, neurologic toxicity with peripheral sensory neuropathy, diarrhea, hepatotoxicity, skin rash
Erlotinib	Inhibits EGFR exon 19 deletion or exon 21 (L858R) substitution mutations; also inhibits wild-type EGFR tyrosine kinase leading to inhibition of EGFR signaling	Non-small cell lung cancer, pancreatic cancer	Diarrhea	Skin rash, diarrhea, anorexia, interstitial lung disease
Afatinib	Inhibits kinase domains of EGFR, HER2, and HER4, leading to inhibition of downstream ErbB signaling	Non-small cell lung cancer	Diarrhea	Skin rash, anorexia, interstitial lung disease, hepatotoxicity, keratitis
Osimertinib	Inhibits specific mutant forms of EGFR, including exon 19 deletion or exon 21 (T790M, L858R) substitution mutations	Non-small cell lung cancer	Diarrhea	Skin rash, fatigue, anorexia, pulmonary toxicity in the form of interstitial lung disease (ILD), cardiomyopathy and CHF, QT prolongation
Imatinib	Inhibits Bcr-Abl tyrosine kinase and other receptor tyrosine kinases, including PDGFR and c-kit	CML, gastrointestinal stromal tumor (GIST), Philadelphia chromosome–positive (Ph+) ALL	Nausea and vomiting	Fluid retention with ankle and periorbital edema, diarrhea, myalgias, congestive heart failure
Dasatinib	Inhibits Bcr-Abl tyrosine kinase and Src family of kinases	CML, Ph+ ALL	Fatigue and anorexia	Bleeding complications, myelosuppression, fluid retention, diarrhea, congestive heart failure, hepatotoxicity, QT prolongation
Nilotinib	Inhibits Bcr-Abl tyrosine kinase and other receptor tyrosine kinases, including PDGFR and c-kit	CML	Fatigue and anorexia	Myelosuppression, QT prolongation, electrolyte abnormalities with hypophosphatemia, hypokalemia, hypocalcemia, and hyponatremia, and hepatotoxicity
Bosutinib	Inhibits Bcr-Abl tyrosine kinase and retains activity in imatinib-resistant Bcr-Abl mutations except for the T315I and V299L mutations. Inhibits Src family tyrosine kinases	CML	Nausea and vomiting	Diarrhea, fluid retention, myelosuppression, skin rash hepatotoxicity
Ponatinib	Inhibits Bcr-Abl tyrosine kinase and retains activity in imatinib-resistant Bcr-Abl mutations including the T315I gatekeeper mutation; inhibits other tyrosine kinases, including VEGFR, PDGFR, FGFR, Flt3, Src family kinases, Kit, Ret, and EPH	CML, Ph+ ALL	Hypertension	Hepatotoxicity, bleeding complications, arterial thromboembolic events, cardiac arrhythmias, fluid retention, gastrointestinal perforation, wound healing complications, skin rash
Asciminib	Inhibits Bcr-Abl tyrosine kinase by targeting the myristoyl pocket. Reduced off-target activity as inactive against other tyrosine kinases, including SRC	CML, Ph+ ALL	Hypertension	Myelosuppression, pancreatitis, hepatotoxicity, cardiovascular toxicity
Cetuximab	IgG1 antibody binds to EGFR and inhibits downstream EGFR signaling; enhances response to chemotherapy and radiotherapy	Colorectal cancer, head and neck cancer (used in combination with radiotherapy), non-small cell lung cancer	Infusion reaction	Skin rash, hypomagnesemia, fatigue, interstitial lung disease

(*continued*)

TABLE 54–5 Miscellaneous anticancer drugs: Clinical activity and toxicities. (Continued)

Drug	Mechanism of Action[1]	Clinical Applications[1]	Acute Toxicity	Delayed Toxicity
Panitumumab	IgG2 antibody binds to EGFR and inhibits downstream EGFR signaling; enhances response to chemotherapy and radiotherapy	Colorectal cancer	Infusion reaction (rarely)	Skin rash, hypomagnesemia, fatigue, interstitial lung disease
Necitumumab	IgG1 antibody binds to EGFR and inhibits downstream EGFR signaling; enhances response to chemotherapy and radiotherapy	Non-small cell lung cancer (squamous)	Infusion reaction	Skin rash, hypomagnesemia, fatigue, interstitial lung disease, venous and arterial thromboembolic events
Trastuzumab	IgG1 antibody binds to extracellular domain (subdomain IV) of the HER2 growth factor receptor and inhibits HER2 intracellular signaling	Breast cancer, gastric and gastroesophageal cancer	Infusion reaction	Cardiotoxicity with reduced LV function leading to CHF, mild GI toxicity with nausea/vomiting and diarrhea, and rare cases of pulmonary toxicity
Pertuzumab	IgG1 antibody binds to extracellular domain (subdomain II) of the HER2 growth factor receptor and inhibits HER2 intracellular signaling	Breast cancer	Infusion reaction	Cardiotoxicity with reduced LV function leading to CHF, mild GI toxicity with nausea/vomiting and diarrhea, and fatigue
Ado-trastuzumab emtansine	Antibody-drug conjugate made up of anti-HER2 IgG1 antibody and microtubule inhibitor DM1	Breast cancer	Infusion reaction	Cardiotoxicity with reduced LV function leading to CHF, hepatotoxicity, myelosuppression, nausea/vomiting, and rare cases of pulmonary toxicity
Trastuzumab deruxtecan	Antibody-drug conjugate made up of anti-HER2 IgG1 antibody and topo I inhibitor deruxtecan	Breast cancer, gastric and gastroesophageal cancer, NSCLC, and CRC	Infusion reaction	Pulmonary toxicity, cardiotoxicity with reduced LV function, myelosuppression, nausea/vomiting, and fatigue
Sacituzumab govitecan	Antibody-drug conjugate made up of anti-Trop-2 antibody and topo I inhibitor SN38	Breast cancer	Diarrhea, infusion reaction	Myelosuppression, fatigue and anorexia, nausea/vomiting
Lapatinib	Small molecule inhibitor of tyrosine kinases associated with EGFR and HER2 resulting in inhibition of intracellular ErbB signaling	Breast cancer	Diarrhea	Cardiac toxicity with LV dysfunction, myelosuppression, fatigue and anorexia, hepatotoxicity, hand-foot syndrome, and skin rash
Neratinib	Small molecule inhibitor of tyrosine kinases associated with EGFR, HER2, and HER4 resulting in inhibition of intracellular ErbB signaling	Breast cancer	Diarrhea	Hepatotoxicity, fatigue and anorexia, skin rash, muscle spasms
Tucatinib	Small molecule inhibitor of tyrosine kinases associated with HER2 resulting in inhibition of intracellular ErbB signaling	Breast cancer	Diarrhea	Hepatotoxicity, fatigue and anorexia, skin rash, muscle weakness
Bevacizumab	Inhibits binding of VEGF-A to VEGFR leading to inhibition of VEGF signaling; inhibits tumor vascular permeability; enhances tumor blood flow and drug delivery	Colorectal cancer, breast cancer, non-small cell lung cancer, renal cell cancer, glioblastoma multiforme	Hypertension, infusion reaction	Arterial thromboembolic events, gastrointestinal perforation, wound healing complications, bleeding complications, proteinuria
Ziv-aflibercept	Inhibits binding of VEGF-A, VEGF-B, and PlGF to VEGFR leading to inhibition of VEGF signaling; inhibits tumor vascular permeability; enhances tumor blood flow and drug delivery	Colorectal cancer	Hypertension	Arterial thromboembolic events, gastrointestinal perforation, wound healing complications, bleeding complications, diarrhea, mucositis, proteinuria
Ramucirumab	IgG1 antibody directed against VEGFR-2 and prevents binding of VEGF-A, VEGF-C, and VEGF-D ligands to the target VEGFR-2; inhibits tumor vascular permeability; enhances tumor blood flow and drug delivery	Colorectal cancer, gastric or gastroesophageal cancer, non-small cell lung cancer	Hypertension	Arterial thromboembolic events, gastrointestinal perforation, wound healing complications, bleeding complications, diarrhea, mucositis, proteinuria
Sorafenib	Inhibits multiple RTKs, including raf kinase, VEGF-R2, VEGF-R3, and PDGFR-β leading to inhibition of angiogenesis, invasion, and metastasis	Renal cell cancer, hepatocellular cancer	Nausea, hypertension	Skin rash, fatigue and asthenia, bleeding complications, hypophosphatemia
Sunitinib, pazopanib	Inhibits multiple RTKs, including VEGF-R1, VEGF-R2, VEGF-R3, PDGFR-α, and PDGFR-β leading to inhibition of angiogenesis, invasion, and metastasis	Renal cell cancer, GIST	Hypertension	Skin rash, fatigue and asthenia, bleeding complications, cardiac toxicity leading to congestive heart failure in rare cases

[1]See text for acronyms.

and also via glucuronidation by UGT2B7 and UGT2B17, with elimination of drug and metabolites mainly in feces (80%). No dose adjustment is required for patients with mild to severe hepatic and/or renal impairment. The main side effects include myelosuppression, pancreatitis, hypertension, mild nausea and vomiting, fatigue, and musculoskeletal pain.

GROWTH FACTOR RECEPTOR INHIBITORS

Epidermal Growth Factor Receptor

The epidermal growth factor receptor **(EGFR)** is a member of the erb-B family of growth factor receptors, and it is overexpressed in different solid tumors, including CRC, head and neck cancer, NSCLC, and pancreatic cancer. Activation of the EGFR signaling pathway results in downstream activation of several key cellular events involved in cellular growth and proliferation, invasion and metastasis, and angiogenesis. In addition, this pathway inhibits the cytotoxic activity of various anticancer agents and radiation therapy, presumably through suppression of key apoptotic mechanisms, thereby leading to the development of cellular drug resistance.

Cetuximab is a chimeric IgG1 monoclonal antibody directed against the extracellular domain of the EGFR, and it is approved for use in combination with irinotecan for metastatic CRC in the refractory setting or as monotherapy in patients who are deemed to be irinotecan-refractory. Because cetuximab is of the G_1 isotype, its antitumor activity may also be mediated, in part, by immunologic-mediated mechanisms. Cetuximab can be effectively and safely combined with irinotecan- and oxaliplatin-based chemotherapy in the first-line treatment of metastatic CRC as well. Of note, the efficacy of cetuximab is restricted to only those patients whose tumors express the wild-type *RAS* gene, which includes *KRAS* and *NRAS*. Combination regimens of cetuximab with cytotoxic chemotherapy may be of particular benefit in the neoadjuvant therapy of patients with liver-limited disease. Although this antibody was initially approved to be administered on a weekly schedule, pharmacokinetic studies have shown that an every-2-week schedule provides the same level of clinical activity as the weekly schedule. This agent is also approved for use in combination with radiation therapy in patients with locally advanced head and neck cancer. Cetuximab is well tolerated, with the main adverse effects being an acneiform skin rash, hypersensitivity infusion reaction, and hypomagnesemia. However, when cetuximab is combined with radiation therapy for head and neck cancer, there is a very low but real increased risk (1%) of sudden death, which has resulted in a black-box warning for the drug.

Panitumumab is a fully human monoclonal antibody directed against the EGFR and works through inhibition of the EGFR signaling pathway. In contrast to cetuximab, this antibody is of the G_2 isotype and, as such, is not expected to exert any immunologic-mediated effects. Panitumumab was originally approved for patients with refractory metastatic CRC. However, it is now also approved for use in combination with FOLFOX chemotherapy in the first-line treatment of metastatic CRC. As with cetuximab, this antibody is only effective in patients whose tumors express wild-type *RAS*. Recent clinical studies have shown that this antibody can also be effectively and safely combined with irinotecan-based chemotherapy in the second-line treatment of metastatic CRC. Acneiform skin rash and hypomagnesemia are the two main adverse effects associated with its use. Despite being a fully human antibody, infusion-related reactions may still be observed, although much less commonly than seen with cetuximab.

Necitumumab is a fully human IgG1 monoclonal antibody directed against EGFR. Like cetuximab and panitumumab, it works through inhibition of the EGFR signaling pathway. Necitumumab is of the G_1 isotype, and its antitumor activity may also be mediated, at least in part, through immunologically mediated mechanisms. Its clinical activity is different from the other anti-EGFR antibodies, and it is approved for use in combination with gemcitabine and cisplatin chemotherapy for the treatment of metastatic squamous NSCLC. The main adverse effects are what have been previously described for other anti-EGFR antibodies. However, in contrast to the other anti-EGFR antibodies approved in the USA, this agent is associated with an increased risk for both venothrombolic and arterioembolic events.

Erlotinib is a small molecule inhibitor of the tyrosine kinase domain associated with the EGFR. It is approved as first-line treatment of metastatic NSCLC in patients whose tumors have EGFR exon 19 deletions or exon 21 (L858R) mutations and are refractory to at least one prior chemotherapy regimen. It is also approved for maintenance therapy of patients with metastatic NSCLC whose disease has not progressed after four cycles of platinum-based chemotherapy. Patients who are nonsmokers and who have a bronchoalveolar histologic subtype appear to be more responsive to these agents. In addition, erlotinib has been approved for use in combination with gemcitabine for the treatment of advanced pancreatic cancer. It is metabolized in the liver by the CYP3A4 enzyme system, and elimination is mainly hepatic with excretion in feces. Caution must be taken when using erlotinib with drugs that also are metabolized by the liver CYP3A4 system, such as phenytoin and warfarin, and the use of grapefruit products should be avoided. An acneiform skin rash, diarrhea, and anorexia and fatigue are the most common adverse effects observed with these small molecules (see Table 54–5).

Afatinib is a small molecule inhibitor of the tyrosine kinase domains associated with EGFR, HER2, and HER4, and causes inhibition of downstream ErbB signaling. It is approved for the first-line treatment of metastatic NSCLC with EGFR exon 19 deletions or exon 21 L858R mutations. The toxicities associated with this agent are similar to those seen with erlotinib.

Osimertinib is a small molecule inhibitor initially approved for the treatment of metastatic EGFR T790M mutant NSCLC following progression on or after EGFR tyrosine kinase inhibitor therapy. In addition to targeting the T790M mutant, this agent targets the exon 21 L858R and exon 19 EGFR mutations, and it is approved for first-line treatment of patients with metastatic NSCLC whose tumors have epidermal growth factor receptor (EGFR) exon 19 deletions or exon 21 L858R mutations. It is also approved as adjuvant therapy for patients with NSCLC who have undergone surgical resection and whose tumors have EGFR exon

19 deletions or exon 21 L858R mutations. The side effect profile is similar to erlotinib and afatinib, but unique cardiac toxicities are associated with osimertinib, including QT_c prolongation and cardiomyopathy.

Vascular Endothelial Growth Factor

Vascular endothelial growth factor **(VEGF)** is one of the most important angiogenic growth factors. The growth of both primary and metastatic solid tumors requires an intact vasculature; thus, the VEGF signaling pathway represents an attractive target for chemotherapy. Several approaches have been taken to inhibit VEGF signaling; they include inhibition of VEGF interactions with its receptor by targeting either the VEGF ligand with antibodies or soluble chimeric decoy receptors, or by direct inhibition of VEGF receptor–associated tyrosine kinase activity by small molecule inhibitors.

Bevacizumab (BV) is a recombinant humanized monoclonal antibody that targets all forms of the VEGF-A ligand. This antibody binds to and prevents VEGF-A ligand from interacting with the target VEGF receptors. BV can be safely and effectively combined with 5-FU-, irinotecan-, and oxaliplatin-based chemotherapy in the treatment of metastatic CRC. BV is FDA-approved for several solid tumors in the advanced, metastatic disease setting, including CRC, NSCLC, glioblastoma, renal cell cancer, cervical cancer, and ovarian cancer, fallopian tube, or primary peritoneal cancer. One potential advantage of BV is that it does not appear to exacerbate the toxicities typically observed with cytotoxic chemotherapy. The main safety concerns associated with BV include hypertension, an increased incidence of arterial thromboembolic events (transient ischemic attack, stroke, angina, and myocardial infarction), wound healing complications, gastrointestinal perforations, and proteinuria.

Ziv-aflibercept is a recombinant fusion protein made up of portions of the extracellular domains of human VEGF receptors (VEGFR) 1 and 2 fused to the Fc portion of the human IgG1 molecule. This molecule serves as a soluble receptor to VEGF-A, VEGF-B, and placental growth factor (PlGF), and it binds with significantly higher affinity to VEGF-A ligand than bevacizumab. Presumably, binding of the VEGF ligands prevents their subsequent interactions with the target VEGF receptors, which then results in inhibition of downstream VEGFR signaling. This agent is FDA-approved in combination with the FOLFIRI regimen for patients with metastatic CRC that has progressed on oxaliplatin-based chemotherapy. The main adverse effects are similar to those observed with BV.

Ramucirumab is an IgG1 antibody that directly targets the VEGF-R2 receptor, which is considered to be the main VEGF receptor that mediates tumor angiogenesis. This antibody inhibits binding of the VEGF ligands VEGF-A, VEGF-C, and VEGF-D to the VEGF-R2 receptor, which then results in inhibition of downstream VEGFR signaling. This agent is FDA-approved for advanced gastric or gastroesophageal junction adenocarcinoma, metastatic NSCLC, metastatic CRC, and hepatocellular cancer. The main adverse events are similar to those observed with BV and other anti-VEGF inhibitors.

Sorafenib is a small molecule that inhibits multiple receptor tyrosine kinases (RTKs), especially VEGF-R2 and VEGF-R3, platelet-derived growth factor β (PDGFR-β), and raf kinase. It was initially approved for advanced renal cell cancer and is now also approved for advanced hepatocellular cancer.

Sunitinib is similar to sorafenib in that it inhibits multiple RTKs, although the specific types are somewhat different. They include PDGFR-α and PDGFR-β, VEGF-R1, VEGF-R2, VEGF-R3, and c-kit. It is approved for the treatment of advanced renal cell cancer and for the treatment of gastrointestinal stromal tumors after disease progression on or with intolerance to imatinib.

Pazopanib is a small molecule that inhibits multiple RTKs, especially VEGF-R2 and VEGF-R3, PDGFR-β, and raf kinase. This oral agent is approved for the treatment of advanced renal cell cancer.

Sorafenib, sunitinib, and pazopanib are metabolized in the liver by the CYP3A4 system, and elimination is primarily hepatic with excretion in feces. Therefore, each of these agents has potential interactions with drugs that are also metabolized by the CYP3A4 system, especially warfarin. In addition, patients should avoid grapefruit products, starfruit, pomelos, and St. John's Wort, as they may alter the metabolism of these agents. Hypertension, bleeding complications, and fatigue are the most common adverse effects seen with these drugs. With respect to sorafenib, skin rash and the hand-foot syndrome are observed in up to 30–50% of patients. For sunitinib, there is also an increased risk of cardiac dysfunction, which in some cases can lead to congestive heart failure.

■ CANCER CHEMOTHERAPEUTIC DRUGS AND THEIR USE IN HUMAN CANCERS

The use of specific cytotoxic and biologic agents for each of the main cancers is discussed in the following sections.

THE LEUKEMIAS

ACUTE LEUKEMIA

Childhood Leukemia

Acute lymphoblastic leukemia (ALL) is the main leukemia in childhood, and it is the most common cancer in children. Children with this disease now have a relatively good prognosis. A subset of patients with neoplastic lymphocytes expressing surface antigenic features of T lymphocytes has a poor prognosis (see Chapter 55). A cytoplasmic enzyme expressed by normal thymocytes, terminal deoxycytidyl transferase (terminal transferase), is also expressed in many cases of ALL. T-cell ALL also expresses high levels of the enzyme adenosine deaminase (ADA). This led to interest in the use of the ADA inhibitor pentostatin (deoxycoformycin) for treatment of such T-cell cases. Until 1948, the median length of survival in ALL was 3 months. With the advent of MTX, the length of survival was greatly increased. Corticosteroids, 6-mercaptopurine, cyclophosphamide, vincristine, daunorubicin, and asparaginase also are active against this disease. A combination of vincristine and prednisone plus other agents is currently used to induce remission. More than 90% of children enter complete remission with this therapy with only minimal toxicity. However, circulating leukemic cells often migrate to sanctuary sites located in the brain and testes. The value of prophylactic intrathecal methotrexate therapy for prevention of central nervous system leukemia (a major mechanism of relapse) has been clearly demonstrated. Intrathecal therapy with MTX should therefore be considered as a standard component of the induction regimen for children with ALL. For patients with B-cell precursor ALL that is refractory to first-line therapy or in second or later relapse, tisagenlecleucel is a potential treatment option. This is a CD19-directed genetically modified autologous T-cell immunotherapy **(CAR T-cell therapy)** that binds to CD19-expressing tumor cells. As part of this treatment, patients are treated with a lymphocyte-depleting regimen with cyclophosphamide and fludarabine, which results in increased systemic levels of IL-15 and other pro-inflammatory cytokines and chemokines ("cytokine storm") that enhance CAR T-cell activity. The conditioning regimen may also reduce the number of immunosuppressive regulatory T cells, activate antigen-presenting cells, and induce pro-inflammatory tumor cell damage.

Adult Leukemia

Acute myelogenous leukemia (AML) is the most common leukemia in adults. The single most active agent for AML is cytarabine. However, it is best used in combination with an anthracycline, which leads to complete remissions in about 70% of patients. While there are several anthracyclines that can be effectively combined with cytarabine, idarubicin is preferred. An alternative approach for newly diagnosed AML is to administer a liposomal formulation that contains daunorubicin and cytarabine in a fixed 1:5 molar ratio. Once remission of AML is achieved, consolidation chemotherapy is required to maintain a durable remission and to induce cure.

CHRONIC MYELOGENOUS LEUKEMIA

Chronic myelogenous leukemia (CML) arises from a chromosomally abnormal hematopoietic stem cell in which a balanced translocation between the long arms of chromosomes 9 and 22, t(9:22), is observed in 90–95% of cases. This translocation results in constitutive expression of the Bcr-Abl fusion oncoprotein with a molecular weight of 210 kDa. The clinical symptoms and course are related to the white blood cell count and its rate of increase. Most patients with white cell counts greater than 50,000/μL should be treated. Since it was first developed, the TKI imatinib has been considered as standard first-line therapy in previously untreated patients with CP CML. Nearly all patients treated with imatinib exhibit a complete hematologic response, and up to 40–50% of patients show a complete cytogenetic response. This drug is generally well tolerated and is associated with relatively minor adverse effects. Initially, dasatinib and nilotinib were approved for patients who were intolerant or resistant to imatinib and are now also indicated as first-line treatment of chronic phase CML. Bosutinib and ponatinib are used only in the refractory disease setting, with ponatinib retaining activity against all known Bcr-Abl mutations, including the T315I gatekeeper mutation. Asciminib is the newest kinase inhibitor approved for Ph+ CP CML previously treated with two or more TKIs and in Ph+ CP CML with the T315I mutation.

HODGKIN & NON-HODGKIN LYMPHOMAS

HODGKIN LYMPHOMA

The treatment of Hodgkin lymphoma has undergone dramatic evolution over the last 50 years. This lymphoma is now widely recognized as a B-cell neoplasm in which the malignant Reed-Sternberg cells have rearranged *VH* genes. In addition, the Epstein-Barr virus genome has been identified in up to 80% of tumor specimens.

Complete staging evaluation is required before a definitive treatment plan can be made. For patients with stage I and stage IIA disease, there has been a significant change in the treatment approach. Initially, these patients were treated with extended-field radiation therapy. However, given the well-documented late effects of radiation therapy, which include hypothyroidism, an increased risk of secondary cancers, and coronary artery disease, combined-modality therapy with a brief course of combination chemotherapy and involved field radiation therapy is now the recommended approach. The main advance for patients with advanced stage III and IV Hodgkin lymphoma came with the development of MOPP (mechlorethamine, vincristine, procarbazine, and prednisone) chemotherapy in the 1960s. This regimen resulted initially in high complete response rates, on the order of 80–90%, with cures in up to 60% of patients. More recently, the anthracycline-containing regimen termed ABVD (doxorubicin, bleomycin, vinblastine, and dacarbazine) has been shown to be more effective and less toxic than MOPP, especially with regard to the incidence of infertility and secondary malignancies. In general, four cycles of ABVD are given to patients. An alternative regimen, termed Stanford V, utilizes a 12-week course of combination chemotherapy (doxorubicin, vinblastine, mechlorethamine, vincristine, bleomycin, etoposide, and prednisone), followed by involved radiation therapy.

With all of these regimens, more than 80% of previously untreated patients with advanced Hodgkin lymphoma (stages III and IV) are expected to go into complete remission, with disappearance of all disease-related symptoms and objective evidence of disease. In general, approximately 50–60% of all patients with Hodgkin lymphoma are cured of their disease.

For patients with refractory disease, the immune checkpoint inhibitors nivolumab and pembrolizumab have been approved. Each of these agents targets the programmed cell death 1 (PD-1) receptor expressed on T cells, which then leads to enhanced T-cell immune responses with activation and proliferation of T cells in the tumor microenvironment.

NON-HODGKIN LYMPHOMA

Non-Hodgkin lymphoma (NHL) is a heterogeneous disease, and the clinical characteristics of NHL subsets are related to the underlying histopathologic features and the extent of disease involvement. In general, the nodular (or follicular) lymphomas have a far better prognosis, with a median survival up to 7 years, compared with the diffuse lymphomas, which have a median survival of only about 1–2 years.

Combination chemotherapy is the treatment standard for patients with diffuse NHL. The anthracycline-containing regimen CHOP (cyclophosphamide, doxorubicin, vincristine, and prednisone) has been considered the best treatment in terms of initial therapy. Randomized phase III clinical studies have shown that the combination of CHOP with the anti-CD20 antibody rituximab results in improved response rates, disease-free survival, and overall survival compared with CHOP chemotherapy alone. For relapsed or refractory diffuse large B-cell lymphoma that has progressed after two or more lines of systemic therapy, the CAR T-cell therapies tisagenlecleucel and axicabtagene ciloleucel, both of which target CD19-expressing lymphoma cells, are approved given their significant clinical activity in this disease.

The nodular follicular lymphomas are low-grade, relatively slow-growing tumors that tend to present in an advanced stage and are usually confined to lymph nodes, bone marrow, and spleen. This NHL subset, when presenting at an advanced stage, is considered incurable, and treatment is generally palliative. To date, there is no evidence that immediate treatment with combination chemotherapy offers clinical benefit over close observation and "watchful waiting" with initiation of chemotherapy at the onset of disease symptoms.

MULTIPLE MYELOMA

Multiple myeloma is one of the models of neoplastic disease in humans, as it arises from a single tumor stem cell. It typically involves the bone marrow and bone, causing bone pain, lytic lesions, bone fractures, and anemia as well as an increased susceptibility to infection. Most patients with multiple myeloma are symptomatic at the time of initial diagnosis and require treatment with systemic therapy. For more than 30 years, the combination of the alkylating agent melphalan and prednisone (MP) was considered standard first-line treatment for this disease. However, over the past 10–15 years, a dramatic evolution has taken place in the treatment of this disease with an explosion of new drugs that have significant clinical activity. The proteasome inhibitors and immunomodulatory analogs (IMiDs) now play a major role in first-line treatment. Currently, the most active treatments are a triplet regimen that includes a proteasome inhibitor plus an IMiD, usually lenalidomide, and dexamethasone, or a doublet regimen of a proteasome inhibitor plus dexamethasone.

Bortezomib was first approved for use in relapsing or refractory multiple myeloma and is now widely used as first-line therapy. This agent is thought to exert its main cytotoxic effects through inhibition of the 26S proteosome, resulting in down-regulation of the nuclear factor kappa B (NF-κB) signaling pathway, which appears to be a major signaling pathway for this disease. Of note, inhibition of NF-κB has also been shown to restore chemosensitivity. One potential advantage of bortezomib is that it can be administered by the intravenous or subcutaneous route. **Carfilzomib** is an epoxyketone 26S proteosome inhibitor that is approved for patients with multiple myeloma who have received at least two prior therapies, including bortezomib and an immunomodulatory agent. This agent is important because it is able to overcome resistance to bortezomib, and preclinical and clinical studies suggest that it has broad-spectrum activity in hematologic malignancies and solid tumors. **Ixazomib** is the newest proteosome inhibitor to be approved for multiple myeloma, and in contrast to the other proteosome inhibitors, it is orally administered with good oral bioavailability. This agent can cause peripheral sensory neuropathy, and it is also associated with GI toxicity in the form of diarrhea and nausea and vomiting, thrombocytopenia, and hepatotoxicity.

Thalidomide is a well-established agent for treating refractory or relapsed disease, and about 30% of patients will achieve a response to this therapy. Thalidomide has been used in combination with dexamethasone, resulting in response rates approaching 65%. **Lenalidomide** and **pomalidomide** are two newer-generation immunomodulatory analogs (IMiDs) of thalidomide. Lenalidomide was initially approved in combination with dexamethasone for multiple myeloma patients who have received at least one prior therapy, but it is now widely used as part of various combination regimens in first-line therapy. Pomalidomide is the most recent IMiD to receive approval, and one of the potential advantages of this drug is that it appears to overcome resistance to thalidomide and lenalidomide. The side-effect profiles of these IMiDs are similar, although neurotoxicity is observed more commonly with thalidomide, somewhat less often with pomalidomide, and rarely with lenalidomide.

Daratumumab is an IgG1 human monoclonal antibody directed against CD38, a cell surface glycoprotein that is highly expressed on multiple myeloma cells. This antibody is approved as monotherapy and in various combination regimens for patients who have received one or more prior therapies. For patients with relapsed or refractory multiple myeloma after four or more lines of therapy, the CAR T-cell therapy **idecabtagene vicleucel** (ide-cel), which targets the B-cell maturation antigen (BCMA) expressed on malignant plasma cells, has been recently approved. While significant clinical activity has been observed, ide-cel is associated with a serious adverse events, including cytokine release syndrome (CRS), neurologic toxicities, prolonged cytopenias, and the hemophagocytic lymphohistiocytosis/macrophage activation syndrome (HLH/MAS).

BREAST CANCER

STAGE II DISEASE

The management of primary breast cancer has undergone a remarkable evolution as a result of major efforts at early diagnosis (through encouragement of self-examination as well as through the use of cancer detection centers) and the implementation of combined modality approaches incorporating systemic chemotherapy as an adjuvant to surgery and radiation therapy.

Women with node-positive disease have a high risk of both local and systemic recurrence. Lymph node positivity directly indicates the risk of occult distant micrometastasis. In this setting, postoperative use of systemic adjuvant chemotherapy with six cycles of cyclophosphamide, methotrexate, and fluorouracil (CMF) or of fluorouracil, doxorubicin, and cyclophosphamide (FAC) has been shown to significantly reduce the relapse rate and prolong survival. Alternative regimens with equivalent clinical benefit include four cycles of doxorubicin and cyclophosphamide and six cycles of fluorouracil, epirubicin, and cyclophosphamide (FEC). Each of these chemotherapy regimens has benefited women with stage II breast cancer with one to three involved lymph nodes. Women with four or more involved nodes have had limited benefit thus far from adjuvant chemotherapy. Long-term analysis has shown improved survival rates in node-positive premenopausal women who have been treated aggressively with multiagent combination chemotherapy. The results from randomized clinical trials clearly show that the addition of **trastuzumab,** a monoclonal antibody directed against the HER2 receptor, to anthracycline- and taxane-containing adjuvant chemotherapy benefits women with HER2-overexpressing breast cancer with respect to disease-free and overall survival. Neratinib is a small molecule inhibitor of the tyrosine kinases associated with EGFR, HER2, and HER4, and this agent is approved for the extended adjuvant therapy of patients with early-stage HER2-overexpressed breast cancer following adjuvant trastuzumab-based therapy.

Breast cancer was the first neoplasm shown to be responsive to hormonal manipulation. **Tamoxifen** is beneficial in postmenopausal women when used alone or in combination with cytotoxic chemotherapy. The present recommendation is to administer tamoxifen for 5 years of continuous therapy after surgical resection. Longer durations of tamoxifen therapy do not appear to offer additional clinical benefit. Postmenopausal women who complete 5 years of tamoxifen therapy should be placed on an aromatase inhibitor such as **anastrozole** for at least 2.5 years, although the optimal duration is unknown. In women who have completed 2–3 years of tamoxifen therapy, treatment with an aromatase inhibitor for a total of 5 years of hormonal therapy is now recommended (see Chapter 40).

STAGE III & STAGE IV DISEASE

The approach to women with advanced breast cancer remains a major challenge, as current treatment options are only palliative. Combination chemotherapy, endocrine therapy, or a combination of both results in overall response rates of 40–50%, but only a 10–20% complete response rate. Breast cancers expressing estrogen receptors (ER) or progesterone receptors (PR) retain intrinsic hormonal sensitivities of the normal breast—including the growth-stimulatory response to ovarian, adrenal, and pituitary hormones. Patients who show improvement with hormonal ablative procedures also respond to the addition of tamoxifen. The aromatase inhibitors anastrozole and letrozole are now approved as first-line therapy in women with advanced breast cancer whose tumors are hormone receptor–positive. **Fulvestrant** is an ER antagonist indicated for the treatment of hormone receptor (HR)-positive, HER2-negative advanced breast cancer in postmenopausal women not previously treated with endocrine therapy. Cyclin-dependent kinase (CDK) 4/6 inhibitors, including **palbociclib, ribociclib,** and **abemaciclib,** improve clinical activity when combined with fulvestrant as first-line or subsequent therapies.

Patients with significant visceral involvement of the lung, liver, or brain or those with rapidly progressive disease rarely benefit from hormonal therapies. In this setting, systemic chemotherapy is usually indicated. For the 25–30% of patients whose tumors express the HER2 growth factor receptor, trastuzumab is available for therapeutic use alone or in combination with cytotoxic chemotherapy. There are several other agents that target HER2 signaling, which include **pertuzumab**, **ado-trastuzumab emtansine**, **trastuzumab deruxtecan**, and **sacituzumab govitecan** and the small molecule TKIs **lapatinib, neratinib,** and **tucatinib. Pertuzumab** is a humanized IgG1 antibody that targets a different epitope on the HER2 receptor than trastuzumab, and this antibody inhibits heterodimerization of HER2 with other HER family members, including EGFR, HER3, and HER4. This drug is used in combination with trastuzumab and docetaxel for HER2-positive metastatic breast cancer in patients who have not previously received anti-HER2 chemotherapy for metastatic disease. **Ado-trastuzumab emtansine** is an antibody-drug conjugate (ADC) composed of trastuzumab and the small molecule microtubule inhibitor DM1. **Trastuzumab deruxtecan** is an ADC composed of **trastuzumab** and the topo I inhibitor **deruxtecan** (DXd), which is a 10-fold more potent inhibitor of topo I than SN-38, the active metabolite of irinotecan. **Sacituzumab govitecan** is an ADC made up of the humanized IgG1 antibody sacituzumab directed against Trop-2 conjugated to the topo I inhibitor SN-38. This newest ADC is approved for women with metastatic triple-negative breast cancer who have received at least two prior therapies.

With respect to the small molecules targeting HER2, **lapatinib** represents the first-generation TKI, and it inhibits the tyrosine kinases associated with EGFR (ErbB1) and HER2 (ErbB2). This agent is used in combination with the oral fluoropyrimidine capecitabine for metastatic breast cancer whose tumors overexpress HER2 and who have received prior therapy with an anthracycline, a taxane, and trastuzumab. **Tucatinib** is a potent and selective inhibitor of the tyrosine kinase associated with HER2, and it is approved in combination with trastuzumab and capecitabine for metastatic HER-positive breast cancer, including brain metastases. **Neratinib** has much broader biological activity than lapatinib and tucatinib, as it is a potent irreversible small molecule inhibitor of the tyrosine kinases associated with EGFR, HER2, and HER4. It is approved as monotherapy in the adjuvant setting of patients following surgical resection of early-stage HER2-positive disease and also in combination with capecitabine for metastatic HER2-positive breast cancer in the metastatic disease setting.

About 50–60% of patients with metastatic disease respond to initial chemotherapy. A broad range of anticancer agents have activity in this disease, including the anthracyclines (doxorubicin, mitoxantrone, and epirubicin) and the taxanes (docetaxel, paclitaxel, and nab-paclitaxel), along with the microtubule inhibitor ixabepilone, navelbine, capecitabine, gemcitabine, cyclophosphamide, methotrexate, and cisplatin. The anthracyclines and the taxanes are two of the most active classes of cytotoxic drugs for metastatic breast cancer. Combination chemotherapy has been found to induce higher and more durable remissions in up to 50–80% of patients, and anthracycline-containing regimens are now considered the standard of care in first-line therapy. With most combination regimens, partial remissions have a median duration of about 10 months and complete remissions have a duration of about 15 months. Unfortunately, only 10–20% of patients achieve complete remissions with any of these regimens, and as noted, complete remissions are usually not long-lasting.

PROSTATE CANCER

Prostate cancer was the second cancer shown to be responsive to hormonal manipulation. The treatment of choice for patients with metastatic prostate cancer is elimination of testosterone production by the testes through either surgical or chemical castration. Bilateral orchiectomy or estrogen therapy in the form of diethylstilbestrol was previously used as first-line therapy. Presently, the use of luteinizing hormone-releasing hormone (LHRH) agonists—including **leuprolide** and **goserelin** agonists, alone or in combination with an antiandrogen (eg, **flutamide, bicalutamide, enzalutamide,** or **nilutamide**)—is the preferred approach (see Chapter 40). There appears to be no survival advantage of total androgen blockade using a combination of LHRH agonist and antiandrogen agent compared with single-agent therapy. **Abiraterone,** an inhibitor of steroid synthesis (see Chapter 39), is approved in combination with prednisone for metastatic, high-risk, castration-sensitive prostate cancer and also in the setting of metastatic, castration-resistant prostate cancer following prior chemotherapy containing docetaxel. Hormonal treatment reduces symptoms—especially bone pain—in 70–80% of patients and may cause a significant reduction in the prostate-specific antigen (PSA) level, which is now widely accepted as a surrogate marker for response to treatment in prostate cancer. Although initial hormonal manipulation is able to control symptoms for up to 2 years, patients usually develop progressive disease. Second-line hormonal therapies include aminoglutethimide plus hydrocortisone, the antifungal agent ketoconazole plus hydrocortisone, or hydrocortisone alone. **Apalutamide** is a nonsteroidal antiandrogen agent that binds to the androgen receptor (AR) and inhibits AR-mediated transcription. This agent is approved for non-metastatic castration-resistant prostate cancer.

Nearly all patients with advanced prostate cancer eventually become refractory to hormone therapy. A regimen of mitoxantrone and prednisone is approved in patients with hormone-refractory prostate cancer because it provides effective palliation in those who experience significant bone pain. **Estramustine** is an antimicrotubule agent that produces an almost 20% response rate as a single agent. However, when used in combination with either etoposide or a taxane such as docetaxel or paclitaxel, response rates are more than doubled to 40–50%. The combination of docetaxel and prednisone was recently shown to confer survival advantage when compared with the mitoxantrone-prednisone regimen, and this combination has now become the standard of care for hormone-refractory prostate cancer.

Sipuleucel-T is a dendritic cell vaccine that is approved for patients with minimally symptomatic metastatic chemotherapy-resistant or castration-resistant prostate cancer (CRPC). This vaccine is prepared from peripheral blood mononuclear cells (PBMCs) obtained by leukapheresis, and the PBMCs are then exposed ex vivo to a novel recombinant protein immunogen, which consists of prostatic acid phosphatase (PAP) fused to human granulocyte-macrophage colony-stimulating factor (GM-CSF). These activated cells are then infused back into the patient approximately 3 days after the original harvesting. Its use is restricted to patients with slowly progressive disease, where a relatively rapid response to treatment is not required.

GASTROINTESTINAL CANCERS

Colorectal cancer (CRC) is the most common gastrointestinal malignancy. Nearly 150,000 new cases are diagnosed each year in the USA; worldwide, nearly 1.2 million cases are diagnosed annually. At the time of initial presentation, only about 40% of patients are potentially curable with surgery. Patients presenting with high-risk stage II disease and stage III disease are candidates for adjuvant chemotherapy with an oxaliplatin-based regimen in combination with 5-FU plus leucovorin (FOLFOX) or with oral capecitabine (CAPOX) and are generally treated for 6 months following surgical resection. Recent data from several large randomized clinical trials suggest that 3 months of adjuvant therapy may be as effective as 6 months of therapy. Treatment with these oxaliplatin-based combination regimens reduces the recurrence rate after surgery by 35% and clearly improves overall patient survival compared with surgery alone.

Significant advances have been made over the past 10–15 years with respect to treatment of metastatic CRC (mCRC). Five active cytotoxic agents have been approved during this time period—5-FU, the oral fluoropyrimidine analogs **capecitabine** and **TAS-102**, **oxaliplatin**, and **irinotecan**. In addition, five novel biologic agents and one small molecule inhibitor have been approved, including the anti-VEGF antibody **bevacizumab**; the recombinant fusion protein **ziv-aflibercept**, which targets VEGF-A, VEGF-B, and PlGF; the anti-VEGF-R2 antibody **ramucirumab**, which inhibits binding of the VEGF ligands VEGF-A, VEGF-C, and VEGF-D; the two anti-EGFR antibodies **cetuximab** and **panitumumab**; and the small molecule TKI inhibitor **regorafenib**. In the setting of microsatellite instability-high (MSI-H) metastatic CRC, the immune checkpoint inhibitors **pembrolizumab** and **nivolumab** have been approved. For patients who can tolerate more aggressive treatment, the combination of **nivolumab** plus **ipilimumab,** an antibody that targets the cytotoxic T-lymphocyte–associated antigen 4 (CTLA-4) expressed on CD4 and CD8 T cells, is approved given its improved clinical activity when compared to single-agent nivolumab.

In general, a fluoropyrimidine—either intravenous 5-FU or oral capecitabine—serves as the main foundation of cytotoxic chemotherapy regimens for mCRC. For patients whose tumors express wild-type *KRAS*/*NRAS*, FOLFOX/FOLFIRI regimens in combination with the anti-VEGF antibody bevacizumab or with the anti-EGFR antibodies cetuximab or panitumumab provide significantly improved clinical efficacy when compared to cytotoxic chemotherapy. In order for patients to derive maximal benefit from systemic therapy, they should be treated with each of these active agents in a continuum-of-care approach. **Regorafenib** and **TAS-102** are approved for the metastatic chemorefractory disease setting, but unfortunately, each drug is associated with only limited clinical efficacy, low overall response rates, and significant toxicities, especially in the older patient population. Given all of the available treatment regimens, median overall survival for metastatic CRC is now in the 30-plus month range and, in some cases, approaches or even exceeds 3 years.

Hepatocellular cancer (HCC) has been a relatively difficult tumor to treat as it frequently occurs in the context of chronic liver disease and cirrhosis. It is usually diagnosed late in the course of chronic liver disease, and a large majority of patients have underlying poor liver function with limited hepatic reserve. This disease has been considered to be relatively resistant to chemotherapy, and as such, palliative chemotherapy is usually not recommended as first-line therapy in patients with unresectable or advanced HCC. Since its original approval in 2008, sorafenib therapy had been the sole agent used in the first-line treatment of advanced or unresectable HCC. However, over the past few years, significant advances have been made in the treatment of this disease. The small molecule TKI **lenvatinib** is considered a reasonable treatment for patients who are unable to tolerate sorafenib in the front-line setting. The combination regimen of **atezolizumab** plus **bevacizumab** is now considered standard first-line therapy for patients who can tolerate more aggressive treatment. In the second-line setting, patients with good performance status and intact liver function can be treated with the multikinase inhibitors **regorafenib** or **cabozantinib**. The immune checkpoint inhibitors **pembrolizumab** and **nivolumab** are also appropriate second-line treatment options. For patients with Child-Pugh A liver disease and an alpha-fetoprotein level >400 ng/mL, the anti-VEGF-R2 antibody **ramucirumab** is an appropriate second-line therapy.

LUNG CANCER

Lung cancer is divided into two main histopathologic subtypes, non-small cell and small cell. Non-small cell lung cancer (NSCLC) makes up about 75–80% of all cases of lung cancer, and this group includes adenocarcinoma, squamous cell cancer, and large cell cancer, while small cell lung cancer (SCLC) makes up the remaining 20–25%. When NSCLC is diagnosed in an advanced stage with metastatic disease and left untreated, the prognosis is extremely poor, with a median survival of about 8 months. It is clear that prevention (primarily through avoidance of cigarette smoking) and early detection remain the most important means of control. When diagnosed at an early stage, surgical resection results in patient cure. Moreover, recent studies have shown that adjuvant platinum-based chemotherapy provides a survival benefit in patients with pathologic stage IB, II, and IIIA disease. However, in most cases, distant metastases have occurred at the time of diagnosis. In certain instances, radiation therapy can be offered for palliation of pain, airway obstruction, or bleeding and to treat patients whose performance status would not allow for more aggressive treatments.

In patients with advanced disease, systemic chemotherapy is generally recommended. Combination regimens that include a platinum agent ("platinum doublets") appear superior to non-platinum doublets, and either cisplatin or carboplatin are appropriate platinum agents for such regimens. Paclitaxel and vinorelbine appear to have activity independent of histology when used as the second drug, while the antifolate pemetrexed should be used for non-squamous cell cancer, and gemcitabine for squamous cell cancer. For patients with good performance status and those with non-squamous histology, the combination of the anti-VEGF antibody bevacizumab with carboplatin and paclitaxel is a standard treatment option. In patients deemed not to be appropriate candidates for bevacizumab therapy and those with squamous cell histology, a platinum-based chemotherapy regimen in combination with the anti-EGFR antibody cetuximab is a reasonable treatment strategy. Maintenance chemotherapy with pemetrexed is now used in patients with non-squamous NSCLC whose disease has remained stable after four cycles of platinum-based first-line chemotherapy. In patients with metastatic non-squamous NSCLC and in the absence of EGFR or ALK genomic tumor alterations, combination treatment with pemetrexed and platinum chemotherapy with the immune checkpoint inhibitor **pembrolizumab** is now approved as first-line treatment.

All patients with metastatic NSCLC should have molecular testing of their tumor. Patients whose tumors contain an actionable mutation should then be treated with an agent that is specifically directed at that molecular target. For example, first-line therapy with **erlotinib** significantly improves outcomes in advanced NSCLC patients with sensitizing EGFR mutations, which include exon 19 deletions or exon 21 (L858R) substitution mutations. **Afatinib** is a small molecule inhibitor of EGFR, HER2, and HER4, and it is approved for the first-line treatment of metastatic NSCLC whose tumors have EGFR exon 19 deletions or exon 21 mutations. **Osimertinib** was originally approved for the treatment of metastatic EGFR T790M-mutant NSCLC following progression on or after EGFR TKI therapy, but it is now approved for the first-line treatment of metastatic NSCLC with sensitizing EGFR mutations, which include exon 19 deletions or exon 21 (L858R) substitution mutations. This agent is able to overcome the resistance that arises from the emergence of the T790M gatekeeper mutation either de novo or following previous EGFR TKI therapy. When compared to other TKIs, however, osimertinib is associated with higher rates of cardiotoxicity, which include atrial fibrillation, QT prolongation, and congestive heart failure.

In NSCLC with an ALK mutation, five small molecule drugs are available: **crizotinib, ceritinib, alectinib, brigatinib,** and **lorlatinib.** Crizotinib is the first-generation ALK inhibitor, while ceritinib, alectinib, brigatinib, and lorlatinib have clinical efficacy in patients whose disease has progressed on or who have become intolerant to crizotinib. Of note, **lorlatinib** has significant clinical activity in ROS1-positive NSCLC. In addition, it has impressive intracranial activity, regardless of prior crizotinib exposure, as more than half the patients will exhibit a significant and durable intracranial response to lorlatinib therapy.

Squamous cell NSCLC makes up approximately 30% of NSCLC. This NSCLC subtype is responsive to platinum-based chemotherapy with either cisplatin or carboplatin in combination with gemcitabine. Recent studies have shown superior clinical activity when cisplatin and gemcitabine are combined with the anti-EGFR antibody necitumumab when compared to the cisplatin-gemcitabine combination in the first-line treatment of metastatic disease. The immune checkpoint inhibitor nivolumab is approved to treat metastatic squamous cell NSCLC whose cancer has progressed during or after standard platinum-based chemotherapy. This agent binds to the PD-1 receptor and inhibits the PD-1 immune signaling pathway, which then leads to activation and proliferation of T cells as well as inhibition of T-regulatory cells. The combination of **pembrolizumab** plus carboplatin and either paclitaxel or nab-paclitaxel has shown significant clinical activity in the first-line setting. For this reason, this combination is approved as first-line treatment of patients with metastatic squamous NSCLC.

Small cell lung cancer (SCLC) is the most aggressive form of lung cancer. It is usually exquisitely sensitive, at least initially, to platinum-based combination regimens, including cisplatin and etoposide or cisplatin and irinotecan. The combination of carboplatin plus etoposide with the anti-PD-L1 inhibitor **atezolizumab** has significant clinical activity against extensive-stage SCLC, and this regimen is approved for use as first-line therapy. Unfortunately, drug resistance eventually develops in nearly all patients with extensive disease. When diagnosed at an early stage, this disease is potentially curable using combined chemotherapy and radiation therapy. The topo I inhibitor topotecan and the alkylating agent **lurbinectedin** are considered standard second-line options for patients who have failed a platinum-based regimen. However, given the increased toxicities associated with topotecan, lurbinectedin is considered the more appropriate option in the second-line setting. The anti-PD1 inhibitor **nivolumab** is an alternative treatment for patients who have progressed on front-line therapy.

OVARIAN CANCER

In the majority of patients, ovarian cancer remains occult and becomes symptomatic only after it has already metastasized to the peritoneal cavity. At this stage, it usually presents with malignant ascites. It is important to accurately stage this cancer with laparoscopy, ultrasound, and CT scanning. Patients with stage I disease appear to benefit from whole-abdomen radiotherapy and may receive additional benefit from combination chemotherapy with cisplatin and cyclophosphamide.

Combination chemotherapy is the standard approach to stage III and stage IV disease. Randomized clinical studies have shown that the combination of paclitaxel and cisplatin provides survival benefit compared with the previous standard combination of cisplatin plus cyclophosphamide. More recently, carboplatin plus paclitaxel has become the treatment of choice. In patients who present with recurrent disease, topotecan, altretamine, or liposomal doxorubicin are used as single-agent monotherapy.

Olaparib, niraparib, and **rucaparib** are small molecule inhibitors of poly (ADP-ribose) polymerase (PARP) enzymes, including PARP1, PARP2, and PARP3, and these agents display enhanced antitumor activity in tumors that are *BRCA*-deficient. Therefore, they are approved for the treatment of deleterious germline BRCA-deficient-mutated advanced ovarian cancer following treatment with previous lines of cytotoxic chemotherapy. They are also approved for maintenance therapy of recurrent epithelial ovarian cancer in complete or partial response to platinum-based chemotherapy.

TESTICULAR CANCER

The introduction of platinum-based combination chemotherapy gave rise to the curative treatment of patients with advanced testicular cancer. Presently, chemotherapy is recommended for patients with stage IIC or stage III seminomas and non-seminomatous disease. Over 90% of patients respond to chemotherapy, and, depending upon the extent and severity of disease, complete remissions are observed in 70–80% of patients. More than 50% of patients achieving complete remission are cured with chemotherapy. In patients with good risk features, three cycles of cisplatin, etoposide, and bleomycin (PEB protocol) or four cycles of cisplatin and etoposide yield virtually identical results. In patients with high-risk disease, the combination of cisplatin, etoposide, and ifosfamide is used as well as etoposide and bleomycin with high-dose cisplatin.

MALIGNANT MELANOMA

Malignant melanoma is curable with surgical resection when it presents locally (see also Chapter 61). For nearly 25 years, high-dose interferon α (IFN-α) was the only option for adjuvant treatment of high-risk melanoma following surgical resection. The development of immune checkpoint inhibitors has changed the entire approach to adjuvant therapy of high-risk melanoma, and currently, the immune checkpoint inhibitors **nivolumab, pembrolizumab,** and **ipilimumab** are approved as single agents in this setting. For patients with BRAFV600E or BRAFV600K mutant early-stage melanoma with lymph node involvement, the combination of two targeted agents, **dabrafenib** plus **trametinib,** is indicated.

Historically, once metastatic disease was diagnosed, malignant melanoma was considered to be one of the most difficult cancers to treat. However, the treatment landscape has significantly changed with the development of effective immunotherapies and targeted agents. While dacarbazine, temozolomide, and cisplatin remain the most active cytotoxic agents for this disease, the overall response rates to these agents remain dismally low, and their use has dramatically declined. Biologic agents, including **IFN-α** and **interleukin 2** (**IL-2**), have greater activity than traditional cytotoxic agents, and treatment with high-dose IL-2 has led to cures, albeit in a relatively small subset of patients. **Ipilimumab** binds to cytotoxic T-lymphocyte–associated antigen 4 (CTLA-4), which is expressed on the surface of activated CD4 and CD8 T cells, and inhibition of CTLA-4 signaling leads to enhanced T-cell immune responses with T-cell activation and proliferation. This agent is approved for the treatment of metastatic melanoma. **Nivolumab** and **pembrolizumab** are IgG4 antibodies that bind to the PD-1 receptor, which is expressed on T cells, and they inhibit the interaction between PD-L1 and PD-L2 ligands and the PD-1 receptor. The PD-1 signaling pathway mediates an immune escape mechanism, and inhibition of this pathway enhances T-cell immune response, leading to T-cell activation and proliferation. Each of these agents is approved for unresectable or metastatic melanoma as monotherapy. Nivolumab is also approved in combination with ipilimumab for unresectable or metastatic melanoma.

BRAF mutations are present in up to 50–60% of melanomas, and the vast majority are V600E mutations. This mutation results in constitutive activation of BRAF kinase, which then leads to activation of downstream signaling pathways involved in cell growth and proliferation. Three oral and highly selective small molecule inhibitors of BRAF V600E and V600K are approved for metastatic melanoma: **vemurafenib, dabrafenib,** and **encorafenib.** Studies are ongoing to determine their activity in combination with other cytotoxic and biologic agents for metastatic melanoma as well as their potential role in the adjuvant and neoadjuvant therapy of early-stage melanoma.

Trametinib, cobimetinib, and **binimetinib** are reversible inhibitors of mitogen-activated extracellular signal-regulated kinase 1 (MEK1) and kinase 2 (MEK2). In combination with a BRAF inhibitor, they are approved for patients with metastatic melanoma whose tumors express the BRAF V600E or V600K mutation. While these agents have clinical activity as monotherapies, clinical studies suggest that the most promising clinical activity is seen when they are used in combination with a BRAF inhibitor.

BRAIN CANCER

In general, chemotherapy has had only limited efficacy in the treatment of malignant gliomas. Because of their ability to cross the blood-brain barrier, the nitrosoureas have historically been the most active agents in this disease. Carmustine (BCNU) has been used as a single agent, and lomustine (CCNU) is used in combination with procarbazine and vincristine (PCV regimen). The alkylating agent **temozolomide** is active when combined with radiotherapy. It is also used in patients with newly diagnosed glioblastoma multiforme (GBM) as well as in those with recurrent disease. The histopathologic subtype oligodendroglioma has been shown to be especially chemosensitive, and the PCV combination regimen is the treatment of choice for this disease. It is now well-established that the anti-VEGF antibody bevacizumab alone or in combination with chemotherapy has documented clinical activity in adult GBM. The anti-VEGF antibody bevacizumab is presently approved as a single agent for adult GBM in the setting of progressive disease following first-line chemotherapy.

SECONDARY MALIGNANCIES & CANCER CHEMOTHERAPY

The development of secondary malignancies is a late complication of the alkylating agents and the epipodophyllotoxin etoposide. For both drug classes, the most frequent secondary malignancy is acute myelogenous leukemia (AML). AML develops in up to 15% of patients with Hodgkin lymphoma who have received radiotherapy plus MOPP chemotherapy and in patients with multiple myeloma, ovarian carcinoma, or breast carcinoma treated with melphalan. The increased risk of AML is observed as early as 2–4 years after the initiation of chemotherapy and typically peaks at 5 and 9 years. With improvements in the clinical efficacy of various combination chemotherapy regimens resulting in prolonged survival and in some cases actual cure of cancer, the issue of how second cancers may affect long-term survival assumes greater importance. Certain alkylating agents (eg, cyclophosphamide) may be less carcinogenic than others, such as melphalan. In addition to AML, other secondary malignancies have been well described, including non-Hodgkin lymphoma and bladder cancer, the latter most typically associated with cyclophosphamide therapy. Etoposide can give rise to an 11:23 translocation, which has been associated with the development of the M4 and M5 AML histologic subtypes.

Myelodysplastic syndrome (MDS) and secondary AML have also been reported in patients receiving PARP inhibitors, including **olaparib, rucaparib, niraparib,** and **talazoparib.** A potential confounding factor is that most of these patients had previously been treated with platinum-based chemotherapy or other DNA damaging agents. In addition, most of the cases of MDS and AML occurred in the setting of mutations in the *BRCA* gene. Finally, secondary squamous cell skin cancers and keratoacanthomas have been observed with treatment with the BRAF inhibitors vemurafenib, dabrafenib, and encorafenib.

SUMMARY Anticancer Drugs

See Tables 54–2, to 54–5.

PREPARATIONS AVAILABLE

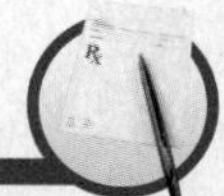

The reader is referred to the Internet and manufacturers' literature for the most recent information on preparations available.

REFERENCES

Books & Monographs

Blaney SM et al: *Pizzo and Poplack's Principles and Practice of Pediatric Oncology*, 8th ed. Wolters Kluwer, 2020.

Chabner BA, Longo DL: *Cancer Chemotherapy and Biotherapy: Principles and Practice*, 6th ed. Lippincott Williams & Wilkins, 2018.

Chu E, DeVita VT Jr: *Cancer Chemotherapy Drug Manual 2023*, 21st ed. Jones & Bartlett, 2023.

DeVita VT Jr et al: *Cancer: Principles and Practice of Oncology*, 12th ed. Wolters Kluwer, 2023.

DeVita VT Jr et al: *Cancer: Principles and Practice of Oncology Primer of Molecular Biology in Cancer*, 3rd ed. Wolters Kluwer, 2020.

Harris JR et al: *Diseases of the Breast*, 5th ed. Wolters Kluwer, 2014.

Niederhuber J et al: *Abeloff's Clinical Oncology*, 6th ed. Elsevier, 2019.

Pass HI et al: *Thoracic Oncology*, 2nd ed. Elsevier, 2017.

Articles & Reviews

DeVita VT, Chu E: The history of cancer chemotherapy. Cancer Res 2008;68:8643.

Pan ST et al: Molecular mechanisms for tumour resistance to cancer chemotherapy. Clin Exp Pharmacol Physiol 2016;43:723.

Schoenfeld AJ, Hellmann MD: Acquired resistance to immune checkpoint inhibitors. Cancer Cell 2020;37:443-455.

CASE STUDY ANSWER

The 5-year survival rate for patients with high-risk stage III colon cancer is on the order of 25–30%. Because the patient has no symptoms after surgery and has no comorbid illnesses, he would be an appropriate candidate to receive aggressive adjuvant chemotherapy. Adjuvant chemotherapy is usually begun 4–6 weeks after surgery to allow sufficient time for the surgical wound to heal. The usual recommendation would be to administer 6 months of oxaliplatin-based chemotherapy using either intravenous 5-FU or oral capecitabine as the fluoropyrimidine base in combination with oxaliplatin. It is now well established that 3 months of oxaliplatin-based chemotherapy may provide the same level of clinical benefit as 6 months of therapy in patients with stage III colon cancer. However, in this patient with high-risk stage III colon cancer (5 positive lymph nodes), the recommendation would be to treat for a total of 6 months.

Patients with partial or complete deficiency in the enzyme dihydropyrimidine dehydrogenase (DPD) experience an increased incidence of severe toxicity to fluoropyrimidines in the form of myelosuppression, gastrointestinal toxicity with mucositis and diarrhea, and neurotoxicity. This is an autosomal recessive pharmacogenetic syndrome that is present in up to 10% of the North American population (see Chapter 5). Although mutations in DPD can be identified in peripheral blood mononuclear cells, nearly 50% of patients who exhibit severe 5-FU toxicity do not have a defined mutation in the *DPD* gene. In addition, mutations in the *DPD* gene may not result in reduced expression of the DPD protein or in altered enzymatic activity. For this reason, genetic testing is not recommended at this time as part of routine clinical practice. There is an immunoassay that measures 5-FU drug levels in the peripheral blood that can help guide 5-FU dosing even in the setting of DPD deficiency.

CHAPTER 55

Immunopharmacology

Douglas F. Lake, PhD, & Adrienne D. Briggs, MD

CASE STUDY

A 59-year-old woman with myelodysplastic syndrome undergoes high-dose chemotherapy followed by an allogeneic stem cell transplant from an unrelated donor. She receives tacrolimus and low-dose methotrexate as prophylaxis for graft-versus-host disease (GVHD). One month after blood count recovery, she develops a skin rash despite ongoing tacrolimus therapy. A skin biopsy confirms grade II acute GVHD. She is placed on 1 mg/kg/d of prednisone, but 1 week later her rash is worse. Her liver enzymes are elevated, and she is having voluminous bloody diarrhea. Endoscopic biopsy of upper and lower gut shows grade IV acute GVHD. The patient is put on high-dose methylprednisolone for 5 days without symptom improvement. What is the next step in managing this complex patient?

Agents that suppress the immune system play an important role in preventing the rejection of organ or tissue grafts and in the treatment of certain diseases that arise from dysregulation of the immune response. While precise details of the mechanisms of action of a number of these agents are still obscure, knowledge of the elements of the immune system is useful in understanding their effects. Agents that augment the immune response or selectively alter the balance of various components of the immune system are also becoming important in the management of certain diseases such as cancer, AIDS, and autoimmune or inflammatory diseases. A growing number of other conditions (infections, cardiovascular diseases, organ transplantation) also are areas for immune manipulation.

■ ELEMENTS OF THE IMMUNE SYSTEM

NORMAL IMMUNE RESPONSES

The immune system has evolved to protect the host from invading pathogens and to eliminate disease. When functioning at its best, the immune system is exquisitely responsive to invading pathogens while retaining the capacity to recognize self tissues and antigens to which it is tolerant. Protection from infection and disease is provided by the collaborative efforts of the innate and the adaptive immune systems.

The Innate Immune System

The innate immune system is the first line of defense against invading pathogens (eg, bacteria, viruses, fungi, parasites) and consists of mechanical, biochemical, and cellular components. Mechanical components include skin/epidermis and mucus; biochemical components include antimicrobial peptides and proteins (eg, defensins), complement, enzymes (eg, lysozyme, acid hydrolases), interferons, acidic pH, and free radicals (eg, hydrogen peroxide, superoxide anions); cellular components include neutrophils, monocytes, macrophages, natural killer (NK) cells, and natural killer-T (NKT) cells. Unlike adaptive immunity, the innate immune response exists prior to infection, is not enhanced by repeated infection, and is generally not antigen-specific. An intact skin or mucosa is the first barrier to infection. When this barrier is breached, an immediate innate immune response, referred to as "inflammation," is provoked and ultimately leads to destruction of the pathogen. The process of pathogen destruction can be accomplished, for example, by biochemical components such as lysozyme (which breaks down bacterial peptidoglycan cell walls) and complement activation. Complement components (Figure 55–1) enhance macrophage and neutrophil phagocytosis by acting as opsonins (C3b) and chemoattractants (C3a, C5a), which recruit

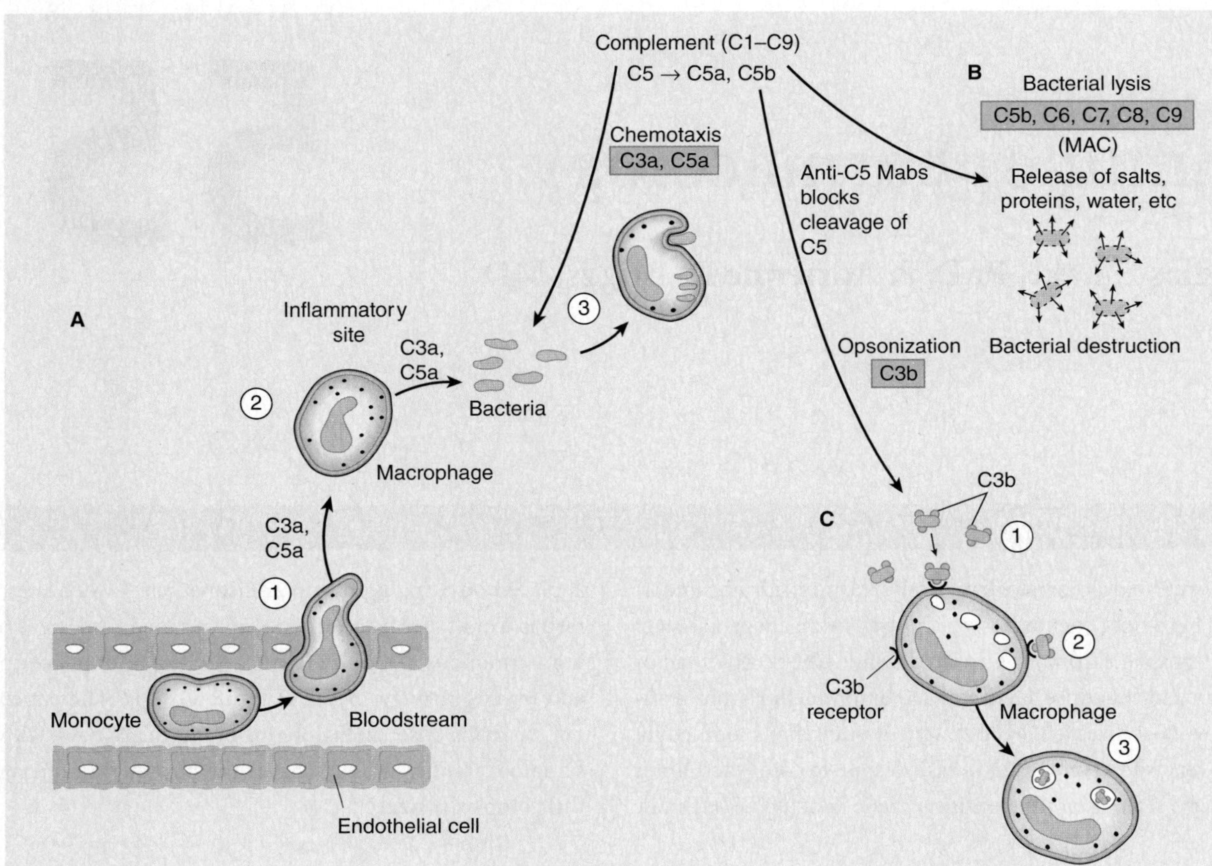

FIGURE 55–1 Role of complement in innate immunity. Complement is made up of nine proteins (C1–C9), which are split into fragments during activation. **(A)** Complement components (C3a, C5a) attract phagocytes (1) to inflammatory sites (2), where the phagocytes ingest and degrade pathogens (3). **(B)** Complement components C5b, C6, C7, C8, and C9 associate to form a membrane attack complex (MAC) that lyses bacteria, causing their destruction. Eculizumab and ravulizumab are monoclonal antibodies that block cleavage of C5. **(C)** Complement component C3b is an opsonin that coats bacteria (1) and facilitates their ingestion (2) and digestion (3) by phagocytes.

immune cells from the bloodstream to the site of infection. The activation of complement eventually leads to pathogen lysis via the generation of a membrane attack complex that creates holes in the pathogen membrane, killing it. Although the complement cascade helps eliminate invading pathogens from the host, in some individuals with complement inhibitor deficiency, complement may lyse host red blood cells and cause a disease called paroxysmal nocturnal hemoglobinuria (PNH). These patients can be treated with a **monoclonal antibody (Mab)** that binds the C5 component of complement (see Mab section below), disrupting the lytic cascade. However, patients taking a C5 inhibitor are at risk of life-threatening meningococcal infections.

During the inflammatory response triggered by infection, neutrophils and monocytes enter the tissue sites from the peripheral circulation. This cellular influx is mediated by the action of **chemoattractant cytokines (chemokines)** (eg, interleukin 8 [IL-8; CXCL8], macrophage chemotactic protein 1 [MCP-1; CCL2], and macrophage inflammatory protein 1α [MIP-1α; CCL3]) released from activated endothelial cells and immune cells (mostly tissue macrophages) at the inflammatory site. Egress of the immune cells from blood vessels into the inflammatory site is mediated by adhesive interactions between cell surface receptors (eg, L-selectin, integrins) on the immune cells and ligands (eg, sialyl-Lewis x, intercellular adhesion molecule-1 [ICAM-1]) on the activated endothelial cell surface. The tissue macrophages as well as dendritic cells express pattern recognition receptors (PRRs) that include Toll-like receptors (TLRs), nucleotide-binding oligomerization domain-like receptors (NLRs), scavenger receptors, mannose receptors, and lipopolysaccharide (LPS)-binding protein, which recognize key evolutionarily conserved pathogen components referred to as pathogen-associated molecular patterns (PAMPs). Examples of PAMPs include microbe-derived unmethylated CpG DNA, flagellin, double-stranded RNA, peptidoglycan, and LPS. The PRRs recognize PAMPs in various components of pathogens and stimulate the release of proinflammatory cytokines, chemokines, and interferons. If the innate immune response is successfully executed, the invading pathogen is ingested, degraded, and eliminated, and disease either is prevented or is of short duration.

In addition to monocytes and neutrophils, NK, NKT, and gamma-delta T (γδ T) cells recruited to the inflammatory site contribute to the innate response by secreting interferon gamma (IFN-γ)

ACRONYMS

ADA	Adenosine deaminase
ADC	Antibody-drug conjugate
ALG	Antilymphocyte globulin
APC	Antigen-presenting cell
ATG	Antithymocyte globulin
CD	Cluster of differentiation
CSF	Colony-stimulating factor
CTL	Cytotoxic T lymphocyte
DC	Dendritic cell
DTH	Delayed-type hypersensitivity
FKBP	FK-binding protein
GVHD	Graft-versus-host disease
HAMA	Human antimouse antibody
HLA	Human leukocyte antigen
IFN	Interferon
IGIV, IVIG	Immune globulin intravenous, intravenous immune globulin
IL	Interleukin
LFA	Leukocyte function-associated antigen
Mab	Monoclonal antibody
MHC	Major histocompatibility complex
NK cell	Natural killer cell
SCID	Severe combined immunodeficiency disease
TCR	T-cell receptor
TGF-β	Transforming growth factor beta
TH1, TH2	T helper cell types 1 and 2
TNF	Tumor necrosis factor

and interleukin 17 (IL-17),* which activate resident tissue macrophages and dendritic cells and recruit neutrophils, respectively, to successfully eliminate invading pathogens. NK cells are so called because they are able to recognize and destroy virus-infected normal cells as well as tumor cells without prior stimulation. This activity is regulated by "killer cell immunoglobulin-like receptors" (KIRs) on the NK cell surface that are specific for major histocompatibility complex (MHC) class I molecules. When NK cells bind self MHC class I proteins (expressed on all nucleated cells), these receptors deliver inhibitory signals, preventing them from killing normal host cells. Tumor cells or virus-infected cells that have down-regulated MHC class I expression do not engage these KIRs, resulting in activation of NK cells and subsequent destruction of the target cell. NK cells kill target cells by releasing cytotoxic granules such as perforins and granzymes that induce programmed cell death.

NKT cells express T-cell receptors as well as receptors commonly found on NK cells. NKT cells recognize microbial lipid antigens presented by a unique class of MHC-like molecules known as CD1 and have been implicated in host defense against microbial agents, autoimmune diseases, and tumors.

*Interferons and interleukins are cytokines, which are discussed later in this chapter.

The Adaptive Immune System

The adaptive immune system is mobilized by cues from the innate response when the innate processes are incapable of coping with an infection. The adaptive immune system has a number of characteristics that contribute to its success in eliminating pathogens. These include the ability to (1) respond to a variety of antigens, each in a specific manner; (2) discriminate between foreign ("non-self") antigens (pathogens) and self antigens of the host; and (3) respond to a previously encountered antigen in a learned way by initiating a vigorous memory response. This adaptive response culminates in the production of **antibodies,** which are the effectors of **humoral immunity,** and the activation of **T lymphocytes,** which are the effectors of **cell-mediated immunity.**

The induction of specific adaptive immunity requires the participation of professional **antigen-presenting cells (APCs),** which include dendritic cells (DCs), macrophages, and B lymphocytes. These cells play pivotal roles in the induction of an adaptive immune response because of their capacity to phagocytize particulate antigens (eg, pathogens) or endocytose protein antigens, and enzymatically digest them to generate peptides, which are then loaded onto class I or class II MHC proteins and "presented" to the cell surface T-cell receptor (TCR) (Figure 55–2). CD8 T cells recognize class I–MHC peptide complexes while CD4 T cells recognize class II–MHC peptide complexes. At least two signals are necessary for the activation of T cells. The first signal is delivered following engagement of the TCR with peptide-bound MHC molecules. In the absence of a second signal, the T cells become unresponsive (anergic) or undergo apoptosis. The second signal involves binding of costimulatory molecules (CD40, CD80 [also known as B7-1],

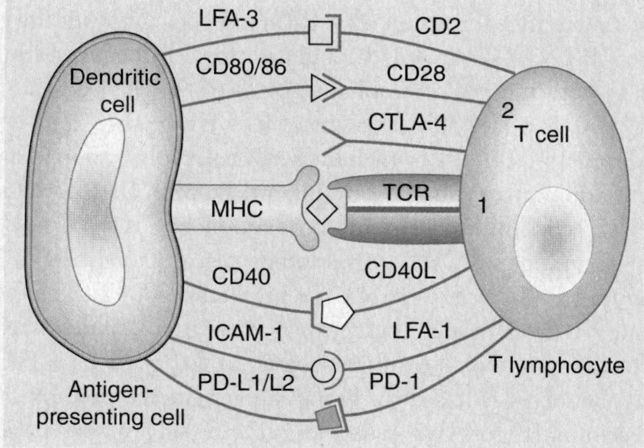

FIGURE 55–2 T-cell activation by an antigen-presenting cell requires engagement of the T-cell receptor by the MHC-peptide complex (signal 1) and binding of the costimulatory molecules (CD80, CD86) on the dendritic cell to CD28 on the T cell (signal 2). The activation signals are strengthened by CD40/CD40L and ICAM-1/LFA-1 interactions. In a normal immune response, T-cell activation is regulated by T-cell–derived CTLA-4 and PD-1. CTLA-4 binds to CD80 or CD86 with higher affinity than CD28 and sends inhibitory signals to the nucleus of the T cell, while ligation of PD-1 by PD-L1 or -L2 also inhibits T cell proliferation.

and CD86 [also known as B7-2]) on the APC to their respective ligands (CD40L for CD40, CD28 for CD80 or CD86). Activation of T cells is regulated via a negative feedback loop involving another molecule known as T-lymphocyte–associated antigen 4 (CTLA-4). Following engagement of CD28 with CD80 or CD86, CTLA-4 in the cytoplasm is mobilized to the cell surface where, because of its higher affinity of binding to CD80 and CD86, it outcompetes or displaces CD28 resulting in suppression of T-cell activation and proliferation. This property of CTLA-4 has been exploited as a strategy for sustaining a desirable immune response such as that directed against cancer. A recombinant humanized antibody (ipilimumab) that binds CTLA-4 prevents its association with CD80/CD86. In so doing, the activated state of T cells is sustained. Programmed cell death protein 1 (PD-1) is another negative regulator of T cells. Ligation of PD-1 with its ligands (PD-L1 or PD-L2) suppresses T-cell activity. Like CTLA-4, Mabs have been developed to block the interaction of PD-1 with PD-L1, having the effect of sustained T cell activation. Mabs to CTLA-4 and PD-1/PD-L1 are **immune checkpoint inhibitors**. They have been associated in some patients with the development of autoimmune toxicity that subsides upon discontinuation of Mab therapy.

T lymphocytes develop and learn to recognize self and non-self antigens in the thymus; those T cells that bind with high affinity to self antigens in the thymus undergo apoptosis (negative selection), while those that are capable of recognizing foreign antigens in the presence of self MHC molecules are retained and expanded (positive selection) for export to the periphery (lymph nodes, spleen, mucosa-associated lymphoid tissue, peripheral blood), where they become activated after encountering MHC-presented peptides (Figures 55–2 and 55–3).

Studies have demonstrated the presence of two subsets of T helper lymphocytes (**TH1** and **TH2)** based on the cytokines they secrete after activation. The TH1 subset characteristically produces IFN-γ, IL-2, and IL-12 and induces cell-mediated immunity by activation of macrophages, cytotoxic T cells (CTLs), and NK cells. The TH2 subset produces IL-4, IL-5, IL-6, and IL-10 (and sometimes IL-13), which induce B-cell proliferation and differentiation into antibody-secreting plasma cells. IL-10 produced by TH2 cells inhibits cytokine production by TH1 cells via the downregulation of MHC expression by APCs. Conversely, IFN-γ produced by TH1 cells inhibits the proliferation of TH2 cells (see Figure 55–3). Although these subsets have been well described in vitro, the nature of the antigenic challenge that elicits a TH1 or TH2 phenotype is less clear. Extracellular bacteria typically cause the elaboration of TH2 cytokines, culminating in the production of neutralizing or opsonic antibodies. In contrast, intracellular organisms (eg, mycobacteria) elicit the production of TH1 cytokines, which lead to the activation of effector cells such as macrophages.

Another subset of CD4 T cells that secrete IL-17 (TH17) is important in leukocyte recruitment to sites of bacterial and fungal pathogens. TH17 cells also contribute to the pathogenesis of autoimmune diseases such as **psoriasis, inflammatory bowel disease, rheumatoid arthritis,** and **multiple sclerosis.** In fact, new Mabs for some of these diseases that neutralize IL-17 by binding to the cytokine itself or to its receptor (see Mab section below) have recently been FDA approved.

Regulatory T (Treg) cells constitute a population of CD4 T cells that is essential for preventing autoimmunity and allergy as well as maintaining homeostasis and tolerance to self antigens. This cell population exists as natural Treg (nTreg), derived directly from the thymus, and induced (adaptive) Treg (iTreg), generated from naïve CD4 T cells in the periphery. Both populations have also been shown to inhibit antitumor immune responses and are implicated in fostering tumor growth and progression. Development of Tregs is controlled by a transcription factor called Foxp3.

CD8 T lymphocytes recognize endogenously processed peptides presented by virus-infected cells or tumor cells. These peptides are usually nine-amino-acid fragments derived from virus or protein tumor antigens in the cytoplasm and are loaded onto MHC class I molecules (see Figure 55–2) in the endoplasmic reticulum. In contrast, class II MHC molecules present peptides (usually 11–22 amino acids) derived from extracellular (exogenous) pathogens to CD4 T helper cells. In some instances, exogenous antigens, upon ingestion by APCs, can be presented on class I MHC molecules to CD8 T cells. This phenomenon, referred to as "cross-presentation," involves retro-translocation of antigens from the endosome to the cytosol for peptide generation in the proteosome and is thought to be useful in generating effective immune responses against infected host cells that are incapable of priming T lymphocytes. Upon activation, CD8 T cells induce target cell death via lytic granule enzymes ("granzymes"), perforin, and the Fas-Fas ligand (Fas-FasL) apoptosis pathways.

B lymphocytes undergo selection in the bone marrow, during which self-reactive B lymphocytes are clonally deleted while B-cell clones specific for foreign antigens are retained and expanded. The repertoire of antigen specificities by B cells and T cells is genetically determined and arises from *immunoglobulin* and *T-cell receptor* gene rearrangements. These specificities occur prior to encounters with antigen. Upon an encounter with antigen, a mature B cell binds the antigen, internalizes and processes it, and presents its peptide—bound to class II MHC—to CD4 helper cells, which in turn secrete IL-4 and IL-5. These interleukins stimulate B-cell proliferation and differentiation into memory B cells and antibody-secreting plasma cells. The primary antibody response consists mostly of IgM-class immunoglobulins. Subsequent antigenic stimulation results in a vigorous "booster" response accompanied by class (isotype) switching to produce IgG, IgA, and IgE antibodies with diverse effector functions (see Figure 55–3). These antibodies also undergo affinity maturation, which allows them to bind more efficiently to the antigen. With the passage of time, this results in accelerated elimination of microorganisms in subsequent infections. Antibodies mediate their functions by acting as opsonins to enhance phagocytosis and cellular cytotoxicity, by activating complement to elicit an inflammatory response and induce bacterial lysis and by Fc engagement by either phagocytic cells or NK cells via Fc receptors (Figure 55–4). Antibody engineering techniques can replace certain amino acids in the Fc portion of IgG molecules such that antibody-dependent cellular cytotoxicity and complement-dependent lysis are either enhanced or suppressed.

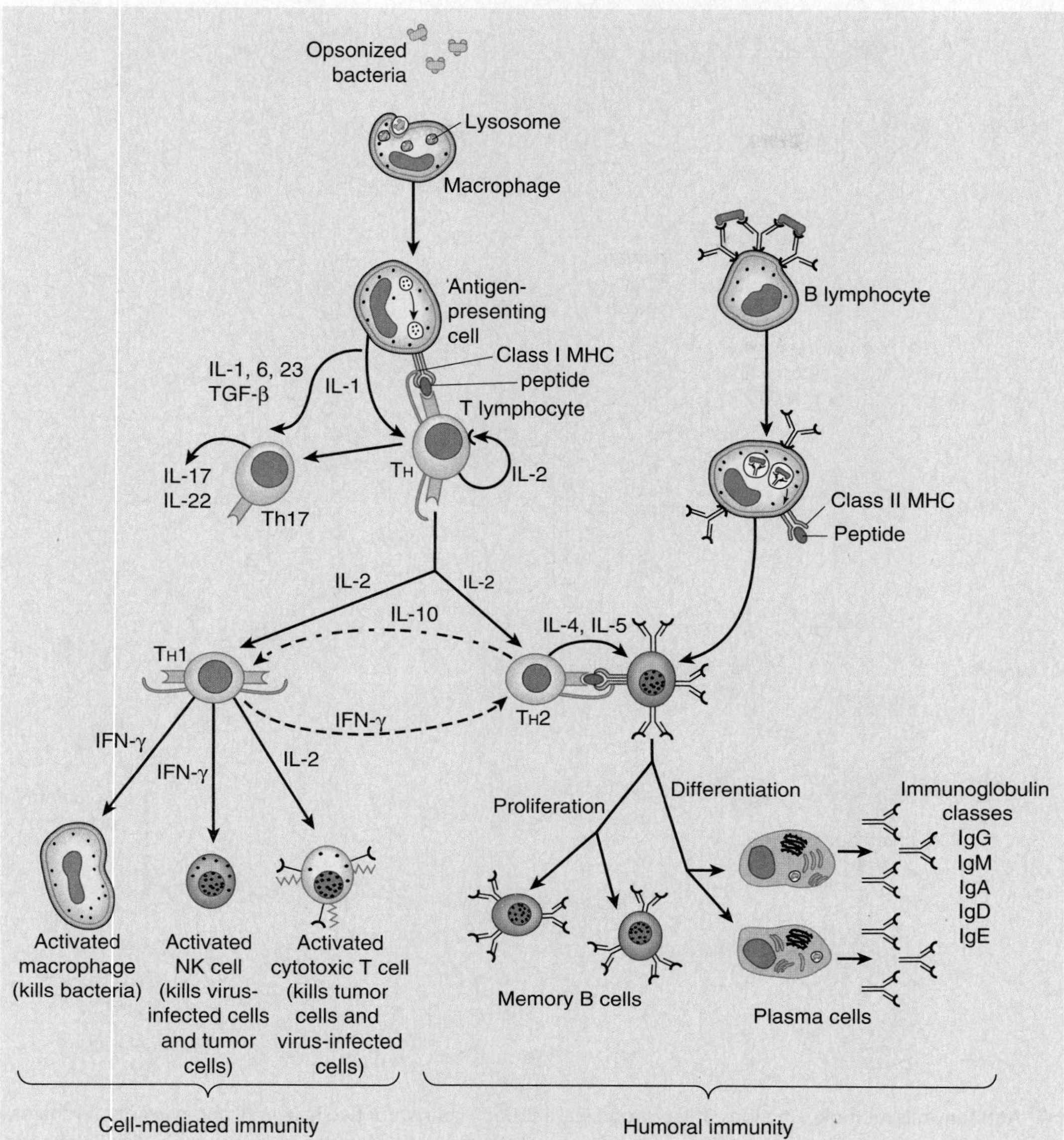

FIGURE 55–3 Scheme of cellular interactions during the generation of cell-mediated and humoral immune responses (see text). The cell-mediated arm of the immune response involves the ingestion and digestion of antigen by antigen-presenting cells such as macrophages. Activated TH cells secrete IL-2, which causes proliferation and activation of cytotoxic T lymphocytes as well as TH1 and TH2 cell subsets. TH1 cells also produce IFN-γ and IL-2 which can directly activate macrophages and NK cells. TH17 cells may be induced by IL-1, -6, -23, or TGF-β secretion by antigen-presenting cells; TH17 cells are inflammatory and secrete IL-17 and -22. The humoral response is triggered when B lymphocytes bind antigen via their surface immunoglobulin. They are then induced by TH2-derived IL-4 and IL-5 to proliferate and differentiate into memory cells and antibody-secreting plasma cells. Interaction of CD40L on TH2 cells with CD40 on B cells (not shown for clarity reasons) causes them to switch from producing IgM to IgG. Regulatory cytokines such as IFN-γ and IL-10 down-regulate TH2 and TH1 responses, respectively (*dashed arrows*).

ABNORMAL IMMUNE RESPONSES

Whereas the normally functioning immune response can successfully neutralize toxins, inactivate viruses, destroy transformed cells, and eliminate pathogens, inappropriate responses can lead to extensive tissue damage (hypersensitivity) or reactivity against self antigens (autoimmunity); conversely, impaired reactivity to appropriate targets (immunodeficiency) may occur and abrogate essential defense mechanisms.

Hypersensitivity

Hypersensitivity can be classified as antibody-mediated or cell-mediated. Three types of hypersensitivity are antibody-mediated (types I–III), while the fourth is cell-mediated (type IV). Hypersensitivity occurs in two phases: the sensitization phase and the effector phase. Sensitization occurs upon initial encounter with an antigen; the effector phase involves immunologic memory and often results in tissue damage upon a subsequent encounter with that antigen.

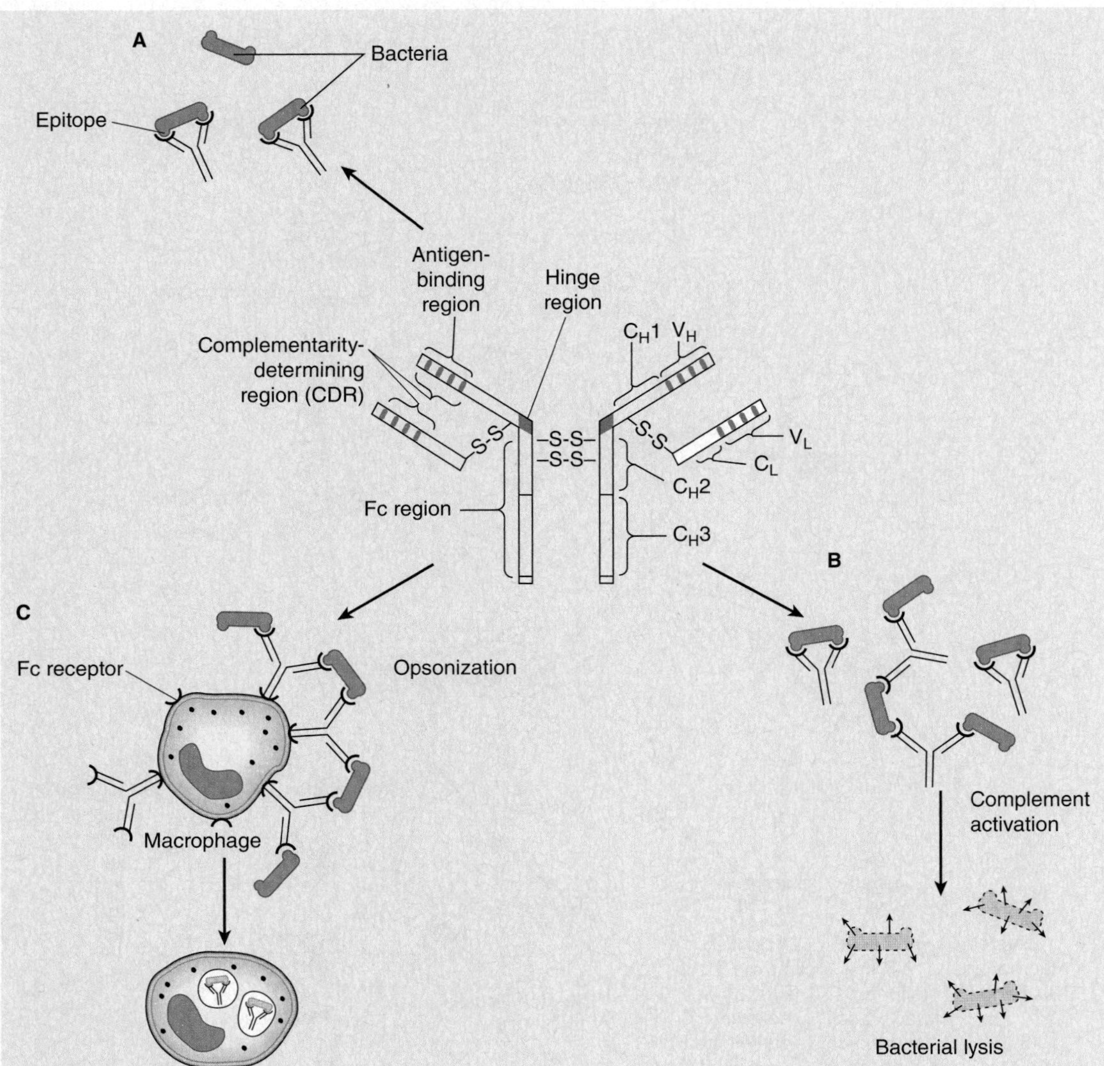

FIGURE 55–4 Antibody has multiple functions. The prototypical antibody consists of two heavy (H) and two light (L) chains, each subdivided into constant (C_L, C_H) and variable (V_L, V_H) domains. The structure is held together by intra- and interchain disulfide bonds. **(A)** The complementarity-determining region (CDR) of the antigen-binding portion of the antibody engages the antigenic determinant (epitope) in a lock-and-key fashion. **(B)** Antigen-antibody complexes activate and split complement components that cause bacterial lysis. **(C)** The Fc portion of antibodies binds to Fc receptors on phagocytes (eg, macrophages, neutrophils) and facilitates uptake of bacteria (opsonization).

1. *Type I*—Immediate, or type I, hypersensitivity is IgE-mediated, with symptoms usually occurring within minutes following the patient's reencounter with antigen. Type I hypersensitivity results from cross-linking of membrane-bound IgE on blood basophils or tissue mast cells by antigen. This cross-linking causes cells to degranulate, releasing substances such as histamine, leukotrienes, and eosinophil chemotactic factor, which induce anaphylaxis, asthma, hay fever, or urticaria (hives) in affected individuals (Figure 55–5). A severe type I hypersensitivity reaction such as systemic anaphylaxis (eg, from insect envenomation, ingestion of certain foods, or drug hypersensitivity) requires immediate medical intervention.

2. *Type II*—Type II hypersensitivity results from the formation of antigen-antibody complexes between foreign antigen and IgM or IgG immunoglobulins. One example of this type of hypersensitivity is a blood transfusion reaction that can occur if blood is not cross-matched properly. Preformed antibodies in the recipient bind to red blood cell membrane antigens that activate the complement cascade, generating a membrane attack complex that lyses the transfused red blood cells. In hemolytic disease of the newborn, anti-Rh IgG antibodies produced by an Rh-negative mother cross the placenta, bind to red blood cells of an Rh-positive fetus, and damage them. The disease is prevented by the administration of anti-Rh antibodies to the mother at week 28 of pregnancy and again to the mother within 72 hours after birth if the child is Rh+ (see Immunosuppressive Antibodies, below). Type II hypersensitivity can also be drug-induced and may occur during the administration of penicillin (for example)

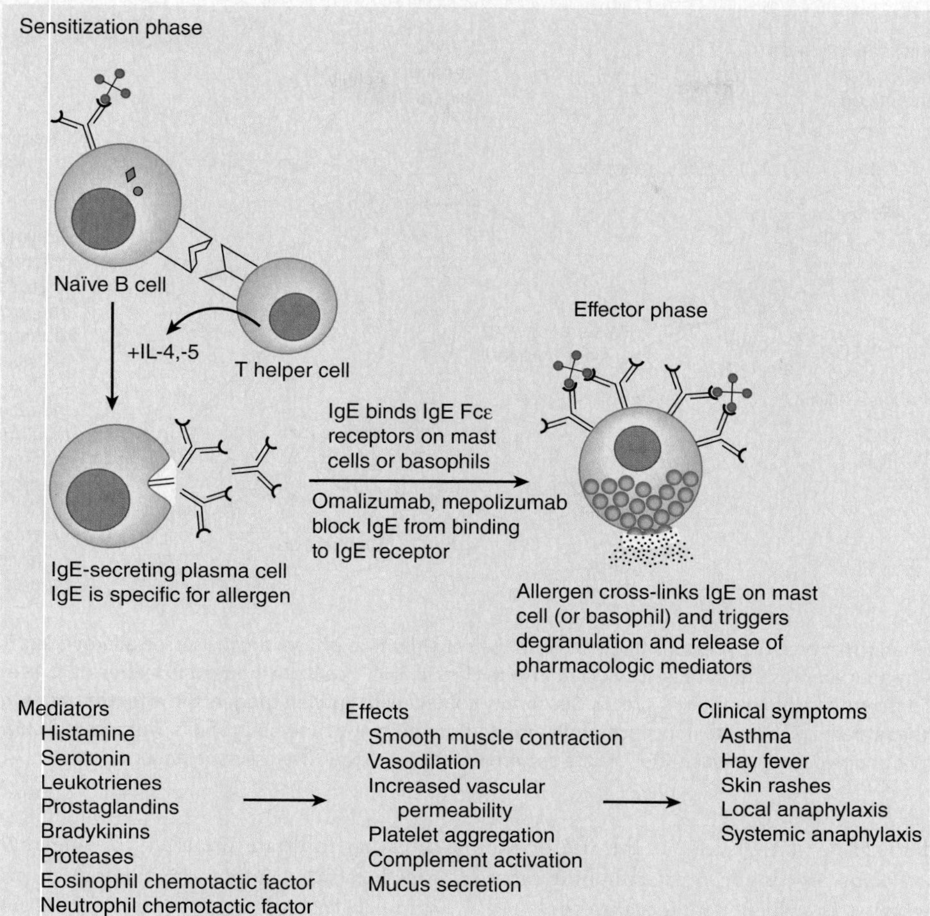

FIGURE 55–5 Mechanism of type I hypersensitivity. Initial exposure to allergen **(sensitization phase)** leads to production of IgE by plasma cells differentiated from allergen-specific B cells (not shown). The secreted IgE binds IgE-specific receptors (FcεR) on blood basophils and tissue mast cells. Re-exposure to allergen leads to cross-linking of membrane-bound IgE **(effector phase)**. This cross-linking causes degranulation of cytoplasmic granules and release of mediators that induce vasodilation, smooth muscle contraction, and increased vascular permeability. These effects lead to the clinical symptoms characteristic of type I hypersensitivity. Omalizumab prevents IgE from binding to IgE receptors on mast cells and basophils, preventing degranulation.

to allergic patients. In these patients, penicillin binds to red blood cells or other host tissue to form a neoantigen that evokes production of antibodies capable of inducing complement-mediated red cell lysis. In some circumstances, subsequent administration of the drug can lead to systemic anaphylaxis (type I hypersensitivity).

3. *Type III*—Type III hypersensitivity is due to the presence of elevated levels of antigen-antibody complexes in the circulation that ultimately deposit on basement membranes in tissues and vessels. Immune complex deposition activates complement to produce components with anaphylatoxic and chemotactic activities (C5a, C3a, C4a) that increase vascular permeability and recruit neutrophils to the site of complex deposition. Complex deposition and the action of lytic enzymes released by neutrophils can cause skin rashes, glomerulonephritis, and arthritis in these individuals. If patients have type III hypersensitivity against a particular antigen, clinical symptoms usually occur 3–4 days after exposure to the antigen.

4. *Type IV: Delayed-type hypersensitivity*—Unlike type I, II, and III hypersensitivities, delayed-type hypersensitivity (DTH) is cell-mediated, and responses occur 2–3 days after exposure to the sensitizing antigen. DTH is caused by antigen-specific DTH TH1 cells and induces a local inflammatory response that causes tissue damage characterized by the influx of antigen-*non*-specific inflammatory cells, especially macrophages. These cells are recruited under the influence of TH1-produced cytokines (Figure 55–6), which chemoattract circulating monocytes and neutrophils, induce myelopoiesis, and activate macrophages. The activated macrophages are primarily responsible for the tissue damage associated with DTH. Although widely considered to be deleterious, DTH responses are very effective in eliminating infections caused by intracellular pathogens such as *Mycobacterium tuberculosis* and *Leishmania* species. Clinical manifestations of DTH include **tuberculin** and **contact hypersensitivities.** Tuberculosis exposure is determined using a DTH skin test. Positive responses show erythema and induration caused by accumulation

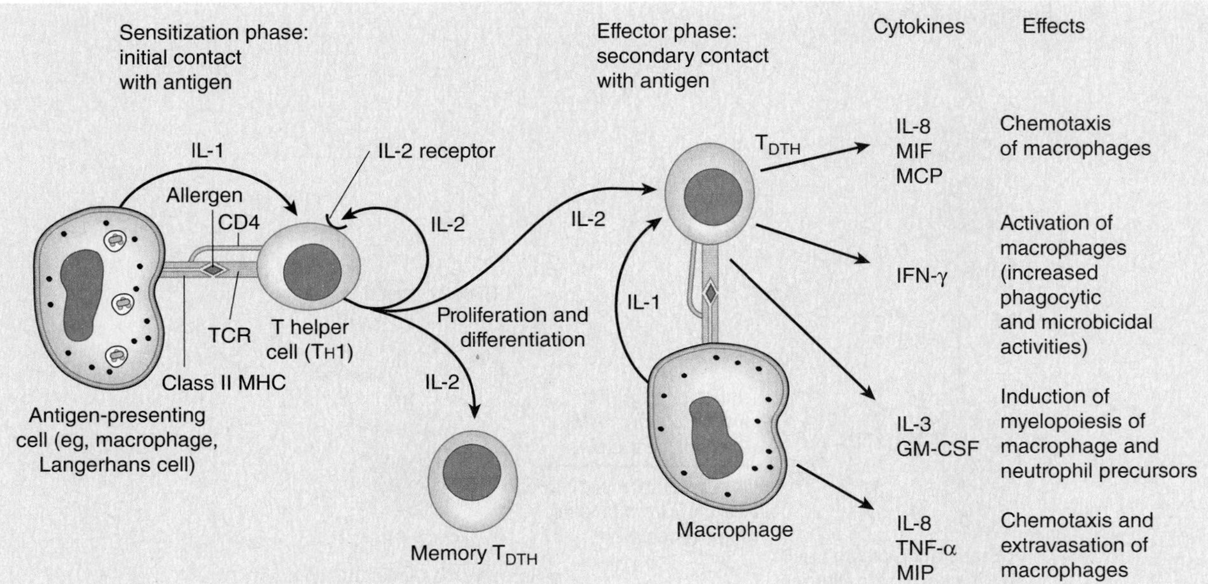

FIGURE 55–6 Mechanism of type IV hypersensitivity (DTH). In the **sensitization phase,** the processed allergen (eg, from poison ivy) is presented to CD4 TH1 cells by antigen-presenting cells in association with class II MHC. T cells are induced to express IL-2 receptors and are stimulated to proliferate and differentiate into memory T_{DTH} cells. Secondary contact with antigen triggers the **effector phase,** in which memory T_{DTH} cells release cytokines that attract and activate nonspecific inflammatory macrophages and neutrophils. These cells display increased phagocytic and microbicidal activities and release large quantities of lytic enzymes that cause extensive tissue damage.

of macrophages and DTH T (T_{DTH}) cells at the site of the tuberculin injection. **Poison ivy** is the most common cause of contact hypersensitivity, in which pentadecacatechol, the lipophilic chemical in poison ivy, modifies cellular tissue and results in a DTH T-cell response.

Autoimmunity

Autoimmune disease arises when the body mounts an immune response against itself due to failure to distinguish self tissues and cells from foreign (non-self) antigens or loss of tolerance to self. This phenomenon derives from the activation of self-reactive T and B lymphocytes that generate cell-mediated or humoral immune responses directed against self antigens. The pathologic consequences of this reactivity constitute several types of autoimmune diseases. Autoimmune diseases are highly complex due to MHC genetics, environmental conditions, infectious entities, and dysfunctional immune regulation. Examples of such diseases include rheumatoid arthritis, psoriasis, systemic lupus erythematosus, multiple sclerosis, and insulin-dependent diabetes mellitus (type 1 diabetes). In rheumatoid arthritis, IgM antibodies (rheumatoid factors) are produced that react with the Fc portion of IgG and may form immune complexes that activate the complement cascade, causing chronic inflammation of the joints and kidneys. In systemic lupus erythematosus, antibodies are made against DNA, histones, red blood cells, platelets, and other cellular components. In multiple sclerosis and type 1 diabetes, cell-mediated autoimmune attack destroys myelin surrounding nerve cells and insulin-producing islet beta cells of the pancreas, respectively. In type 1 diabetes, activated CD4 T_{DTH} cells that infiltrate the islets of Langerhans and recognize self islet beta cell peptides are thought to produce cytokines that stimulate macrophages to produce lytic enzymes, which destroy islet beta cells. Autoantibodies directed against the islet beta cell antigens are produced but do not contribute significantly to disease.

Immunodeficiency Diseases

Immunodeficiency diseases result from inadequate function in the immune system; the consequences include increased susceptibility to infections and prolonged duration and severity of disease. Immunodeficiency diseases either are congenital or arise from extrinsic factors such as bacterial or viral infections or drug treatment. Affected individuals frequently succumb to infections caused by opportunistic organisms of low pathogenicity for the immunocompetent host. Examples of congenitally acquired immunodeficiency diseases include X-linked agammaglobulinemia, DiGeorge syndrome, and severe combined immunodeficiency disease (SCID) due to adenosine deaminase (ADA) deficiency.

X-linked agammaglobulinemia is a disease affecting males that is characterized by a failure of immature B lymphocytes to mature into antibody-producing plasma cells. These individuals are susceptible to recurrent bacterial infections, although the cell-mediated responses directed against viruses and fungi are preserved. DiGeorge syndrome is due to failure of the thymus to develop, resulting in diminished T-cell responses (T_{DTH}, CTL), while the humoral response remains functional but does not benefit from T-cell help.

The ADA enzyme normally prevents the accumulation of toxic deoxy-ATP in cells. Deoxy-ATP is particularly toxic to lymphocytes, and it leads to death of T and B cells. Absence of the enzyme therefore results in SCID. Infusion of the purified enzyme (**pegademase,** from bovine sources) and transfer of ADA gene-modified lymphocytes have both been used successfully to treat this disease.

AIDS represents the classic example of immunodeficiency disease caused by extrinsic viral infection, in this instance the human immunodeficiency virus (HIV). This virus exhibits a strong tropism for CD4 T helper cells; these become depleted, giving rise to increased frequency of opportunistic infections and malignancies in infected individuals. AIDS is also characterized by an imbalance in TH1 and TH2 cells, and the ratios of cells and their functions are skewed toward TH2. This results in loss of cytotoxic T-lymphocyte activity, loss of delayed hypersensitivity, and hypergammaglobulinemia.

IMMUNOSUPPRESSIVE THERAPY

Immunosuppressive agents have proved very useful in minimizing the occurrence or impact of deleterious effects of exaggerated or inappropriate immune responses. Unfortunately, these agents also have the potential to cause disease and to increase the risk of infection and malignancies.

GLUCOCORTICOIDS

Glucocorticoids (corticosteroids) were the first hormonal agents recognized as having lympholytic properties. Administration of any glucocorticoid reduces the size and lymphoid content of the lymph nodes and spleen, although it has no toxic effect on proliferating myeloid or erythroid stem cells in the bone marrow.

Glucocorticoids are thought to interfere with the cell cycle of activated lymphoid cells. The mechanism of their action is described in Chapter 39. Glucocorticoids are quite cytotoxic to certain subsets of T cells, but their immunologic effects are probably due to their ability to modify cellular functions rather than to direct cytotoxicity. Although cellular immunity is more affected than humoral immunity, antibody responses can be diminished. Additionally, continuous administration of corticosteroid increases the fractional catabolic rate of IgG, the major class of antibody immunoglobulins, thus lowering the effective concentration of specific antibodies. Contact hypersensitivity mediated by DTH T cells, for example, is usually abrogated by glucocorticoid therapy.

Glucocorticoids are used in a wide variety of conditions (Table 55–1). It is thought that the immunosuppressive and anti-inflammatory properties of corticosteroids account for their beneficial effects in diseases like idiopathic thrombocytopenic purpura and rheumatoid arthritis. Glucocorticoids modulate allergic reactions and are useful in the treatment of diseases like asthma or as premedication for other agents (eg, blood products, chemotherapy) that might cause undesirable immune responses. Glucocorticoids are first-line immunosuppressive therapy for both solid organ and hematopoietic stem cell transplant recipients, with variable results. The toxicities of long-term glucocorticoid therapy can be severe and are discussed in Chapter 39.

CALCINEURIN INHIBITORS

Cyclosporine

Cyclosporine (cyclosporin A, CSA) is an immunosuppressive agent with efficacy in human organ transplantation, in the treatment of graft-versus-host (GVH) disease after hematopoietic stem cell transplantation, and in the treatment of selected autoimmune disorders. Cyclosporine is a peptide antibiotic that appears to act at an early stage in the antigen receptor–induced differentiation of T cells and blocks their activation. Cyclosporine binds to cyclophilin, a member of a class of intracellular proteins called immunophilins. Cyclosporine and cyclophilin form a complex that inhibits the cytoplasmic phosphatase, calcineurin, which is necessary for the activation of a T cell–specific transcription factor. This transcription factor, NF-AT, is involved in the synthesis of interleukins (eg, IL-2) by activated T cells. In vitro studies have indicated that cyclosporine inhibits the gene transcription of IL-2, IL-3, IFN-γ, and other factors produced by antigen-stimulated T cells, but it does not block the effect of such factors on primed T cells nor does it block interaction with antigen.

Cyclosporine may be given intravenously or orally, although it is slowly and incompletely absorbed (20–50%). The absorbed drug is primarily metabolized by the P450 3A enzyme system in the liver with resultant multiple drug interactions. This propensity for drug interactions contributes to significant interpatient variability in bioavailability, such that cyclosporine requires individual patient dosage adjustments based on steady-state blood levels and the desired therapeutic ranges for the drug. Cyclosporine ophthalmic solution is now available for severe dry eye syndrome, as well as ocular GVH disease. Inhaled cyclosporine is being investigated for use in lung transplantation.

Toxicities are numerous and include nephrotoxicity, hypertension, hyperglycemia, liver dysfunction, hyperkalemia, altered mental status, seizures, and hirsutism. Cyclosporine causes very little bone marrow toxicity. While an increased incidence of lymphoma and other cancers (Kaposi sarcoma, skin cancer) have been observed in transplant recipients receiving cyclosporine, other immunosuppressive agents also may predispose recipients to cancer. Some evidence suggests that tumors may arise after cyclosporine treatment because the drug induces TGF-β, which promotes tumor invasion and metastasis.

Cyclosporine may be used alone or in combination with other immunosuppressants, particularly glucocorticoids. It has been used successfully as the sole immunosuppressant for cadaveric transplantation of the kidney, pancreas, and liver, and it has proved extremely useful in cardiac transplantation as well. In combination with methotrexate, cyclosporine is a standard prophylactic regimen to prevent GVH disease after allogeneic stem cell transplantation. Cyclosporine has also proved useful in a variety of autoimmune

TABLE 55–1 Clinical uses of immunosuppressive agents.

Source	Immunopharmacologic Agents Used	Response
Autoimmune diseases		
Idiopathic thrombocytopenic purpura (ITP)	Prednisone,[1] vincristine, occasionally cyclophosphamide, mercaptopurine, or azathioprine; commonly high-dose gamma globulin, plasma immunoadsorption or plasma exchange	Usually good
Autoimmune hemolytic anemia	Prednisone,[1] cyclophosphamide, chlorambucil, mercaptopurine, azathioprine, high-dose gamma globulin	Usually good
Acute glomerulonephritis	Prednisone,[1] mercaptopurine, cyclophosphamide	Usually good
Acquired factor XIII antibodies	Cyclophosphamide plus factor XIII	Usually good
Autoreactive tissue disorders (autoimmune diseases)[2]	Prednisone, cyclophosphamide, methotrexate, interferon-α and -β, azathioprine, cyclosporine, infliximab, etanercept, adalimumab	Often good, variable
Isoimmune disease		
Hemolytic disease of the newborn	Rh_o(D) immune globulin	Excellent
Organ transplantation		
Renal	Cyclosporine, azathioprine, prednisone, ALG, OKT3, tacrolimus, basiliximab,[3] daclizumab,[3] sirolimus	Very good
Heart	Cyclosporine, azathioprine, prednisone, ALG, OKT3, tacrolimus, basiliximab,[3] daclizumab,[3] sirolimus	Good
Liver	Cyclosporine, prednisone, azathioprine, tacrolimus, sirolimus	Fair
Bone marrow	Cyclosporine, cyclophosphamide, prednisone, methotrexate, ALG	Good
Prevention of cell proliferation		
Coronary stents	Sirolimus (impregnated stent)	Good
Neovascular macular degeneration	Ranibizumab (labeled), bevacizumab (off-label)	Fair

[1]Drug of choice.

[2]Including systemic lupus erythematosus, rheumatoid arthritis, scleroderma, dermatomyositis, mixed tissue disorder, multiple sclerosis, Wegener's granulomatosis, chronic active hepatitis, lipoid nephrosis, and inflammatory bowel disease.

[3]Basiliximab and daclizumab are approved for renal transplant only.

disorders, including uveitis, rheumatoid arthritis, psoriasis, and asthma. Its combination with newer agents is showing considerable efficacy in clinical and experimental settings where effective and less toxic immunosuppression is needed. Newer formulations of cyclosporine are improving patient compliance (smaller, better-tasting pills) and increasing bioavailability.

Tacrolimus

Tacrolimus (FK 506) is an immunosuppressant macrolide antibiotic produced by *Streptomyces tsukubaensis*. It is not chemically related to cyclosporine, but their mechanisms of action are similar. Both drugs bind to cytoplasmic peptidylprolyl isomerases that are abundant in all tissues. While cyclosporine binds to cyclophilin, tacrolimus binds to the immunophilin FK-binding protein (FKBP). Both complexes inhibit calcineurin, which is necessary for the activation of the T cell–specific transcription factor NF-AT.

On a weight basis, tacrolimus is 10–100 times more potent than cyclosporine in inhibiting immune responses. Tacrolimus is utilized for the same indications as cyclosporine, particularly in organ and stem cell transplantation. Multicenter studies in the USA and in Europe indicate that both graft and patient survival are similar for the two drugs. Tacrolimus has proven to be effective therapy for preventing rejection in solid organ transplant patients even after failure of standard rejection therapy, including anti–T-cell antibodies. It is now considered a standard prophylactic agent (usually in combination with methotrexate or mycophenolate mofetil) for GVH disease.

Tacrolimus can be administered orally or intravenously. The half-life of the intravenous form is approximately 9–12 hours. Like cyclosporine, tacrolimus is metabolized primarily by P450 enzymes in the liver, and there is potential for drug interactions. The dosage is determined by trough blood level at steady state. Its toxic effects are similar to those of cyclosporine and include nephrotoxicity, neurotoxicity, hyperglycemia, hypertension, hyperkalemia, and gastrointestinal complaints.

Because of the effectiveness of systemic tacrolimus in some dermatologic diseases, a topical preparation is now available. Tacrolimus ointment is currently used in the therapy of atopic dermatitis and psoriasis.

PROLIFERATION SIGNAL INHIBITORS

A newer class of immunosuppressive agents called proliferation-signal inhibitors (PSIs) includes **sirolimus** (rapamycin) and its derivative **everolimus.** The mechanism of action of PSIs differs from that of the calcineurin inhibitors. PSIs bind the circulating immunophilin FK506-binding protein 12, resulting in an active complex that blocks the molecular target of rapamycin (mTOR).

The mTOR is a key component of a complex intracellular signaling pathway involved in cellular processes such as cell growth and proliferation, angiogenesis, and metabolism. Thus, blockade of mTOR ultimately can lead to inhibition of interleukin-driven T-cell proliferation. Both everolimus and sirolimus also may inhibit B-cell proliferation and immunoglobulin production.

Sirolimus is available only as an oral drug. Its half-life is about 60 hours, while that of everolimus is about 43 hours. Both drugs are rapidly absorbed and elimination is similar to that of cyclosporine and tacrolimus, being substrates for both cytochrome P450 3A and P-glycoprotein. Hence, significant drug interactions can occur. For example, use with cyclosporine can increase the plasma levels of both sirolimus and everolimus such that drug levels need to be monitored. Target dose-ranges of these drugs vary depending on clinical use.

Sirolimus has been used effectively alone and in combination with other immunosuppressants (corticosteroids, cyclosporine, tacrolimus, and mycophenolate mofetil) to prevent rejection of solid organ allografts. It is used as prophylaxis and as therapy for steroid-refractory acute and chronic GVH disease in hematopoietic stem cell transplant recipients. Topical sirolimus is also used in some dermatologic disorders and, in combination with cyclosporine, in the management of uveoretinitis. Recently, sirolimus-eluting coronary stents have been shown to reduce restenosis and additional adverse cardiac events in patients with severe coronary artery disease, due to the drug's antiproliferative effects. Everolimus is a newer drug that has shown clinical efficacy similar to sirolimus in solid organ transplant recipients; it is under investigation as an additional therapeutic agent for the treatment of chronic cardiac allograft vasculopathy.

Toxicities of the PSIs can include profound myelosuppression (especially thrombocytopenia), hepatotoxicity, diarrhea, hypertriglyceridemia, pneumonitis, and headache. Because nephrotoxicity is of major concern when administering calcineurin inhibitors, and since renal toxicity is less common with PSIs, there is interest in increased early use of the latter agents. However, increased use in stem cell transplantation regimens as GVH disease prophylaxis, particularly when combined with tacrolimus, has revealed an increased incidence of hemolytic-uremic syndrome.

Tofacitinib (Xeljanz) inhibits JAK enzymes that stimulate hematopoiesis and immune cell function in response to cytokine or growth factor signaling. Tofacitinib reduces circulating NK cells, serum immunoglobulins, and C-reactive protein. It is approved for adults with moderate to severe RA. It has a black box warning for serious infections and malignancies, similar to anti–TNF-α Mabs (see below).

MYCOPHENOLATE MOFETIL

Mycophenolate mofetil (MMF) is a semisynthetic derivative of mycophenolic acid, isolated from the mold *Penicillium glaucus*. In vitro, it inhibits T- and B-lymphocyte responses, including mitogen and mixed lymphocyte responses, probably by inhibition of de novo synthesis of purines. Mycophenolate mofetil is hydrolyzed to mycophenolic acid, the active immunosuppressive moiety; it is synthesized and administered as MMF to enhance bioavailability.

Mycophenolate mofetil is available in both oral and intravenous forms. The oral form is rapidly metabolized to mycophenolic acid. Although the cytochrome P450 3A system is not involved, some drug interactions still occur. Plasma drug levels should be monitored frequently.

Mycophenolate mofetil is used in solid organ transplant patients for refractory rejection and, in combination with prednisone, as an alternative to cyclosporine or tacrolimus in patients who do not tolerate those drugs. Its antiproliferative properties make it the first-line drug for preventing or reducing chronic allograft vasculopathy in cardiac transplant recipients. Mycophenolate mofetil is used as prophylaxis for and treatment of both acute and chronic GVH disease in hematopoietic stem cell transplant patients. Newer immunosuppressant applications for MMF include lupus nephritis, rheumatoid arthritis, inflammatory bowel disease, and some dermatologic disorders.

Toxicities include gastrointestinal disturbances (nausea and vomiting, diarrhea, abdominal pain), headache, hypertension, and reversible myelosuppression (primarily neutropenia).

THALIDOMIDE

Thalidomide is an oral sedative drug that was withdrawn from the market in the 1960s because of disastrous teratogenic effects when used during pregnancy. Nevertheless, it has significant immunomodulatory actions and is currently in active use or in clinical trials for more than 40 different illnesses. Thalidomide inhibits angiogenesis and has anti-inflammatory and immunomodulatory effects. It inhibits tumor necrosis factor-alpha (TNF-α), reduces phagocytosis by neutrophils, increases production of IL-10, alters adhesion molecule expression, and enhances cell-mediated immunity via interactions with T cells. The complex actions of thalidomide continue to be studied as its clinical use evolves.

Thalidomide is currently used in the treatment of multiple myeloma at initial diagnosis and for relapsed-refractory disease (see Chapter 54). Patients generally show signs of response within 2–3 months of starting the drug, with response rates of 20–70%. When combined with dexamethasone, the response rates in myeloma are 90% or more in some studies. Many patients have durable responses—up to 12–18 months in refractory disease and even longer in some patients treated at diagnosis. The success of thalidomide in myeloma has led to numerous clinical trials in other diseases such as myelodysplastic syndrome, acute myelogenous leukemia, and GVH disease, as well as in solid tumors like colon cancer, renal cell carcinoma, melanoma, and prostate cancer, with variable results to date. Thalidomide has been used for many years in the treatment of some manifestations of leprosy and has been reintroduced in the USA for erythema nodosum leprosum; it is also useful in management of the skin manifestations of lupus erythematosus.

The adverse-effect profile of thalidomide is extensive. The most important toxicity is teratogenesis. Because of this effect, thalidomide prescription and use is closely regulated by the manufacturer.

Other adverse effects of thalidomide include peripheral neuropathy, constipation, rash, fatigue, hypothyroidism, and increased risk of deep-vein thrombosis. Thrombosis is sufficiently frequent, particularly in the hematologic malignancy population, that most patients are placed on some type of anticoagulant when thalidomide treatment is initiated.

Owing to thalidomide's serious toxicity profile, considerable effort has been expended in the development of analogs. Immunomodulatory derivatives of thalidomide are termed **IMiDs.** Some IMiDs are much more potent than thalidomide in regulating cytokines and affecting T-cell proliferation. **Lenalidomide** is an oral IMiD that in animal and in vitro studies has been shown to be similar to thalidomide in action, but with less toxicity, especially teratogenicity. Lenalidomide was approved by the FDA when trials showed its effectiveness in the treatment of the myelodysplastic syndrome with the chromosome 5q31 deletion. Clinical trials using lenalidomide to treat multiple myeloma showed similar efficacy, leading to approval for both primary and relapsed/refractory myeloma. **Pomalidomide** (originally called CC-4047) is a newer oral IMiD that is FDA approved. Like the other IMiDs, it has numerous mechanisms of actions including antiangiogenic activity, inhibition of TNF-α, and stimulation of apoptosis and cytotoxic T-cell activity. Most clinical trials of pomalidomide have targeted patients with relapsed/refractory multiple myeloma, for which the FDA approved the drug in 2013. Both lenalidomide and pomalidomide have side-effect profiles similar to that of thalidomide.

CYTOTOXIC AGENTS

Azathioprine

Azathioprine is a prodrug of mercaptopurine and, like mercaptopurine, functions as an antimetabolite (see Chapter 54). Although its action is presumably mediated by conversion to mercaptopurine and further metabolites, it has been more widely used than mercaptopurine for immunosuppression in humans. These agents represent prototypes of the antimetabolite group of cytotoxic immunosuppressive drugs. Many other agents that kill proliferative cells appear to work at a similar level in the immune response.

Azathioprine is well absorbed from the gastrointestinal tract and is metabolized primarily to mercaptopurine. Xanthine oxidase converts much of the active material to 6-thiouric acid prior to excretion in the urine. After administration of azathioprine, small amounts of unchanged drug and mercaptopurine are also excreted by the kidney, and as much as a twofold increase in toxicity may occur in anephric or anuric patients. Since much of the drug's inactivation depends on xanthine oxidase, patients who are also receiving allopurinol (see Chapters 36 and 54) for control of hyperuricemia should have the dose of azathioprine reduced to one fourth to one third the usual amount to prevent excessive toxicity.

Azathioprine and mercaptopurine appear to produce immunosuppression by interfering with purine nucleic acid metabolism at steps that are required for the wave of lymphoid cell proliferation that follows antigenic stimulation. The purine analogs are thus cytotoxic agents that destroy stimulated lymphoid cells. Although continued messenger RNA synthesis is necessary for sustained antibody synthesis by plasma cells, these analogs appear to have less effect on this process than on nucleic acid synthesis in proliferating cells. Cellular immunity as well as primary and secondary serum antibody responses can be blocked by these agents.

Azathioprine and mercaptopurine appear to be of definite benefit in maintaining renal allografts and may be of value in transplantation of other tissues. These antimetabolites have also been used with some success in the management of acute glomerulonephritis, in the renal component of systemic lupus erythematosus, and in some cases of rheumatoid arthritis, Crohn's disease, and multiple sclerosis. The drugs have been of occasional use in prednisone-resistant antibody-mediated idiopathic thrombocytopenic purpura and autoimmune hemolytic anemias.

The chief toxic effect of azathioprine and mercaptopurine is bone marrow suppression, usually manifested as leukopenia, although anemia and thrombocytopenia may occur. Skin rashes, fever, nausea and vomiting, and sometimes diarrhea occur, with the gastrointestinal symptoms seen mainly at higher dosages. Hepatic dysfunction, manifested by very high serum alkaline phosphatase levels and mild jaundice, occurs occasionally, particularly in patients with preexisting hepatic dysfunction.

Cyclophosphamide

The alkylating agent cyclophosphamide is one of the most efficacious immunosuppressive drugs available. Cyclophosphamide destroys proliferating lymphoid cells (see Chapter 54) but also appears to alkylate some resting cells. It has been observed that very large doses (eg, >120 mg/kg intravenously over several days) may induce an apparent specific tolerance to a new antigen if the drug is administered simultaneously with, or shortly after, the antigen. In smaller doses, it has been effective against autoimmune disorders (including systemic lupus erythematosus) and in patients with acquired factor XIII antibodies and bleeding syndromes, autoimmune hemolytic anemia, antibody-induced pure red cell aplasia, and Wegener granulomatosis.

Treatment with large doses of cyclophosphamide carries considerable risk of pancytopenia and therefore is generally combined with stem cell rescue (transplant) procedures. Although cyclophosphamide appears to induce tolerance for marrow or immune cell grafting, its use does not prevent the subsequent GVH syndrome, which may be serious or lethal if the donor is a poor histocompatibility match (despite the severe immunosuppression induced by high doses of cyclophosphamide). The drug may also cause hemorrhagic cystitis, which can be prevented or treated with **mesna.** Other adverse effects of cyclophosphamide include nausea, vomiting, cardiac toxicity, and electrolyte disturbances.

Pyrimidine Synthesis Inhibitors

Leflunomide is a prodrug of an inhibitor of pyrimidine synthesis. **Teriflunomide** is the principal active metabolite of leflunomide. They both reversibly inhibit the mitochondrial enzyme dihydroorotate dehydrogenase, which is involved in pyrimidine synthesis; they ultimately result in decreased lymphocyte activation. They have anti-inflammatory activity in addition to immunomodulatory properties.

Leflunomide is orally active, and the active metabolite has a long half-life of several weeks. Thus, the drug should be started with a loading dose, but it can be taken once daily after reaching steady state. It is approved only for rheumatoid arthritis at present, although studies are underway combining leflunomide with mycophenolate mofetil for a variety of autoimmune and inflammatory skin disorders, as well as preservation of allografts in solid organ transplantation. Leflunomide also appears (from murine data) to have antiviral activity. Toxicities include elevation of liver enzymes with some risk of liver damage and renal impairment. Patients with severe liver disease should not receive leflunomide. This drug is teratogenic and contraindicated in pregnancy. A low frequency of cardiovascular effects (angina, tachycardia) has been reported.

Teriflunomide is FDA approved for the treatment of **relapsing-remitting multiple sclerosis.** Although immunomodulatory, its exact mechanism of action in the treatment of multiple sclerosis is unclear. It is hypothesized to decrease the number of activated lymphocytes in the central nervous system. It is a once-daily oral drug that, unlike leflunomide, does not require a loading dose. Teriflunomide's side-effect profile is similar to that of leflunomide, and it is contraindicated in pregnancy and severe liver disease. The incidence of neutropenia in patients taking the drug is 15%, and 10% of patients have a decrease in platelet counts.

Hydroxychloroquine

Hydroxychloroquine is an antimalarial agent with immunosuppressant properties. It is thought to suppress intracellular antigen processing and loading of peptides onto MHC class II molecules by increasing the pH of lysosomal and endosomal compartments, thereby decreasing T-cell activation.

Because of these immunosuppressant activities, hydroxychloroquine is used to treat some autoimmune disorders (see Chapter 36), eg, rheumatoid arthritis and systemic lupus erythematosus. It has also been used to both treat and prevent GVH disease after allogeneic stem cell transplantation. Hydroxychloroquine has not been shown to benefit COVID-19.

Other Cytotoxic Agents

Other cytotoxic agents, including **methotrexate, vincristine,** and **cytarabine** (see Chapter 54), also have immunosuppressive properties. Methotrexate has been used extensively in rheumatoid arthritis (see Chapter 36) and in the treatment of GVH disease. Although the other agents can be used for immunosuppression, their use has not been as widespread as the purine antagonists, and their indications for immunosuppression are less certain. The use of methotrexate (which can be given orally) appears reasonable in patients with idiosyncratic reactions to purine antagonists. The antibiotic dactinomycin has also been used with some success at the time of impending renal transplant rejection. **Vincristine** appears to be quite useful in idiopathic thrombocytopenic purpura refractory to prednisone. The related vinca alkaloid **vinblastine** has been shown to prevent mast cell degranulation in vitro by binding to microtubule units within the cell and to prevent release of histamine and other vasoactive compounds.

Pentostatin is an adenosine deaminase inhibitor that has been used mainly as an antineoplastic agent for lymphoid malignancies; it produces a profound lymphopenia. It is now frequently used for steroid-resistant GVH disease after allogeneic stem cell transplantation, as well as in preparative regimens prior to those transplants to provide severe immunosuppression to prevent allograft rejection.

Miscellaneous Agents

Three other FDA-approved immunomodulators are used exclusively in the treatment of relapsing-remitting multiple sclerosis.

Dimethyl fumarate (DMF) is the methyl ester of fumaric acid. Its exact mechanism of action is unknown, but it appears to activate the nuclear factor (erythroid-derived 2)-like 2 (NRF-2) transcriptional pathway. Activation of the NRF-2 pathway results in reduction of the oxidative stress that contributes to demyelination; it also appears to help protect the nerve cells from inflammation. DMF is given orally. Lymphopenia may be significant, so blood counts must be monitored regularly and the drug may be withheld if active infection is present. Flushing is common with treatment initiation and usually improves with time. Other less common adverse effects include nausea, diarrhea, abdominal pain, increased hepatic enzymes, and eosinophilia.

Glatiramer acetate (GA) is a mixture of synthetic polypeptides and four amino acids (L-glutamic acid, L-alanine, L-lysine, and L-tyrosine) in a fixed molar ratio. Its mechanism of immunomodulation in multiple sclerosis is unknown. Studies suggest that GA downregulates the immune response to myelin antigens by induction and activation of suppressive T cells that migrate to the central nervous system. It is given as a subcutaneous injection (not intravenously) in variable dosages and schedules. Toxicities include skin hypersensitivity and, rarely, lipoatrophy and skin necrosis at the injection site. Other adverse effects include flushing, chest pain, dyspnea, throat constriction, and palpitations, all of which are usually mild and self-limited.

Fingolimod hydrochloride (FH) is an orally active sphingosine 1-phosphate (S1P) receptor modulator that is derived from the fungal metabolite myriocin. The S1P receptor (subtype 1) controls the release of lymphocytes from lymph nodes and the thymus. FH is metabolized to fingolimod phosphate, which subsequently binds the S1P receptor and ultimately decreases circulating lymphocyte numbers in the periphery and central nervous system. S1P receptors are also expressed on neurons, such that FH may also be affecting neurodegeneration, gliosis, and endogenous repair mechanisms as well as resulting in lymphopenia to modify disease activity in multiple sclerosis. FH can cause serious cardiac toxicity including bradycardia, prolongation of the QT interval, and other abnormalities. Because of these potential complications, the drug requires cardiac monitoring for 6 hours after the first dose is given. FH is contraindicated in patients with preexisting conditions such as type II or III heart block, prolonged QTc, recent myocardial infarction, or heart failure. Less common adverse effects include macular edema, elevated hepatic enzymes, headache, diarrhea, and cough. The drug is metabolized primarily by the cytochrome P450 system; thus caution is needed when it is used in combination with other drugs metabolized in the same manner.

Siponimod is a new oral agent for the treatment of secondary progressive multiple sclerosis (SPMS). It binds to sphingosine-1-phosphate receptors, which are found on lymphocytes and other cell types, and inhibits the migration of lymphocytes into the CNS.

IMMUNOSUPPRESSIVE ANTIBODIES

The development of hybridoma technology by Milstein and Köhler in 1975 revolutionized the antibody field and radically increased the purity and specificity of antibodies used in the clinic and for diagnostic tests in the laboratory. Hybridomas are B cells fused to immortal plasmacytoma cells that secrete monoclonal antibodies specific for a target antigen. Large-scale hybridoma culture facilities are employed by the pharmaceutical industry to produce diagnostic and clinical-grade monoclonal antibodies.

More recently, molecular biology has been used to develop monoclonal antibodies. Combinatorial libraries of cDNAs encoding immunoglobulin heavy and light chains expressed on bacteriophage surfaces are screened against purified antigens. The result is an antibody fragment with specificity and high affinity for the antigen of interest. This technique has been used to develop antibodies specific for viruses (eg, HIV), bacterial proteins, tumor antigens, and even cytokines. Many antibodies developed in this manner are FDA approved for use in humans.

Other genetic engineering techniques involve production of chimeric and humanized versions of murine monoclonal antibodies in order to reduce their antigenicity and increase the half-life of the antibody in the patient. Murine antibodies administered as such to human patients elicit production of human antimouse antibodies (HAMAs), which clear the original murine proteins very rapidly. Humanization involves replacing most of the murine antibody with equivalent human regions while keeping only the variable, antigen-specific regions intact. Chimeric mouse-human antibodies have similar properties with less complete replacement of the murine components. *The current naming convention for these engineered substances uses the suffix "-umab" or "-zumab" for humanized antibodies, and "-imab" or "-ximab" for chimeric products.* These molecular engineering procedures have been successful in reducing or preventing HAMA production for many of the antibodies discussed below.

Antilymphocyte & Antithymocyte Antibodies & Chimeric Molecules

Antisera directed against lymphocytes have been prepared sporadically for over 100 years. With the advent of human organ transplantation as a realistic therapeutic option, heterologous antilymphocyte globulin (ALG) took on new importance. ALG and antithymocyte globulin (ATG) are now in clinical use in many medical centers, especially in transplantation programs. The antiserum is usually obtained by immunization of horses, sheep, or rabbits with human lymphoid cells.

ALG acts primarily on the small, long-lived peripheral lymphocytes that circulate between the blood and lymph. With continued administration, "thymus-dependent" (T) lymphocytes from lymphoid follicles also are depleted, as they normally participate in the recirculating pool. As a result of the destruction or inactivation of T cells, an impairment of delayed hypersensitivity and cellular immunity occurs while humoral antibody formation remains relatively intact. ALG and ATG are useful for suppressing certain major compartments (ie, T cells) of the immune system and play a definite role in the management of solid organ and bone marrow transplantation.

Monoclonal antibodies directed against specific cell surface proteins such as CD2, CD3, CD25, or cytokine receptors and various integrins much more selectively influence T-cell subset function. The high specificity of these antibodies improves selectivity and reduces toxicity of the therapy, altering the disease course in several different autoimmune disorders.

In the management of transplants, ALG and monoclonal antibodies can be used in the induction of immunosuppression, in the treatment of initial rejection, and in the treatment of steroid-resistant rejection. There has been some success in the use of ALG and ATG plus cyclosporine to prepare recipients for bone marrow transplantation. In this procedure, the recipient is treated with ALG or ATG in large doses for 7–10 days prior to transplantation of bone marrow cells from the donor. ALG appears to destroy the T cells in the donor marrow graft, and the probability of severe GVH disease is reduced.

The adverse effects of ALG are mostly those associated with injection of a foreign protein. Local pain and erythema often occur at the injection site (type III hypersensitivity). Since the humoral antibody response remains active in the recipient, skin-reactive and precipitating antibodies may be formed against the foreign ALG. Similar reactions occur with monoclonal antibodies of murine origin caused by the release of cytokines by T cells and monocytes.

Anaphylactic and serum sickness reactions to ALG and murine monoclonal antibodies have been observed and usually require cessation of therapy. Complexes of host antibodies with horse ALG may precipitate and localize in the glomeruli of the kidneys, causing kidney damage.

Immune Globulin Intravenous (IGIV)

A different approach to immunomodulation is the intravenous use of polyclonal human immunoglobulin. This immunoglobulin preparation (usually IgG) is prepared from pools of thousands of healthy donors, and no single, specific antigen is the target of the "therapeutic antibody." Rather, one expects that the pool of different antibodies will have a normalizing effect upon the patient's immune networks.

IGIV in high doses (2 g/kg) has proved effective in a variety of applications ranging from immunoglobulin deficiencies to autoimmune disorders to HIV disease to bone marrow transplantation. In patients with Kawasaki disease, it has been shown to be safe and effective, reducing systemic inflammation and preventing coronary artery aneurysms. It has also brought about good clinical responses in systemic lupus erythematosus and refractory idiopathic thrombocytopenic purpura. Possible mechanisms of action of IGIV include a reduction of T helper cells, increase of regulatory T cells, decreased spontaneous immunoglobulin production, Fc receptor blockade, increased antibody catabolism, and idiotypic–anti-idiotypic interactions with "pathologic antibodies." Although its precise mechanism of action is still unknown, IGIV brings undeniable clinical benefit to many patients with a variety of immune syndromes.

Rh_o(D) Immune Globulin

One of the earliest major advances in immunopharmacology was the development of a technique for preventing Rh hemolytic disease of the newborn. The technique is based on the observation that a *primary* antibody response to a foreign antigen can be blocked if specific antibody to that antigen is administered passively at the time of exposure to antigen. Rh_o(D) immune globulin is a concentrated (15%) solution of human IgG containing high-titer antibodies against the Rh_o(D) antigen of the red cell.

Sensitization of Rh-negative mothers to the D antigen occurs usually at the time of birth of an Rh_o(D)-positive or D^u-positive infant, when fetal red cells leak into the mother's bloodstream. Sensitization might also occur occasionally with miscarriages or ectopic pregnancies. In subsequent pregnancies, maternal antibody against Rh-positive cells is transferred to the fetus during the third trimester, leading to the development of erythroblastosis fetalis (hemolytic disease of the newborn).

If an injection of Rh_o(D) antibody is administered to the Rh-negative mother within 24–72 hours after the birth of an Rh-positive infant, the mother's own antibody response to the foreign Rh_o(D)-positive cells is suppressed because the infant's red cells are cleared from circulation before the mother can generate a B-cell response against Rh_o(D). Therefore, she has no memory B cells that can activate upon subsequent pregnancies with an Rh_o(D)-positive fetus.

When the mother has been treated in this fashion, Rh hemolytic disease of the newborn has not been observed in subsequent pregnancies. For this prophylactic treatment to be successful, the mother must be Rh_o(D)-negative and D^u-negative and must not already be immunized to the Rh_o(D) factor. Treatment is also often advised for Rh-negative mothers antepartum at 26–28 weeks' gestation who have had miscarriages, ectopic pregnancies, or abortions, when the blood type of the fetus is unknown. *Note: Rh_o(D) immune globulin is administered to the mother and must not be given to the infant.*

The usual dose of Rh_o(D) immune globulin is 2 mL intramuscularly, containing approximately 300 mcg anti-Rh_o(D) IgG. Adverse reactions are infrequent and consist of local discomfort at the injection site or, rarely, a slight temperature elevation.

Hyperimmune Immunoglobulins

Hyperimmune immunoglobulins are IGIV preparations made from pools of selected human or animal donors with high titers of antibodies against particular agents of interest such as viruses or toxins (see also Appendix). Various hyperimmune IGIVs are available for treatment of **respiratory syncytial virus, cytomegalovirus, varicella zoster, human herpesvirus 3, hepatitis B virus, rabies, tetanus,** and **digoxin overdose.** Intravenous administration of the hyperimmune globulins is a passive transfer of high-titer antibodies that either reduces risk or reduces the severity of infection. Rabies hyperimmune globulin is injected around the wound and given intravenously. Tetanus hyperimmune globulin is administered intravenously when indicated for prophylaxis. **Rattlesnake** and **coral snake** hyperimmune globulins (antivenoms) are of equine or ovine origin and are effective for North and South American rattlesnakes and some coral snakes (but not Arizona coral snake). Equine and ovine antivenoms are available for rattlesnake envenomations, but only equine antivenom is available for coral snake bite. An **Arizona bark scorpion** antivenom is also available as equine (Fab)′2. This preparation prevents neurologic manifestations of scorpion envenomation and is generally used in young children and infants.

MONOCLONAL ANTIBODIES (Mabs)

Advances in the ability to select human memory B cells, and to genetically isolate and synthesize immunoglobulin genes, have resulted in the development of fully human, humanized and chimeric monoclonal antibodies directed against a wide array of therapeutic targets. As described above, the only murine portions of humanized monoclonal antibodies are the complementarity-determining regions in the variable domains of immunoglobulin heavy and light chains. Complementarity-determining regions are primarily responsible for the antigen-binding capacity of antibodies. Chimeric antibodies typically contain antigen-binding murine variable regions and human constant regions. The newest fully human antibodies are the result of the ability to select memory B cells from peripheral blood using a target antigen and then genetically isolate the variable heavy and light chains. Interestingly, some Mabs initially developed for certain types of leukemias may also be used in autoimmune diseases such as multiple sclerosis. Mabs are discussed below by the molecular target they recognize.

Miscellaneous Mabs

Alemtuzumab is a humanized IgG_1 that binds to CD52. CD52 is found on normal and malignant B and T lymphocytes, NK cells, monocytes, macrophages, and a small population of granulocytes. Alemtuzumab was first approved for the treatment of B-cell chronic leukemias. Currently, alemtuzumab is approved for the treatment of patients diagnosed with relapsing remitting multiple sclerosis, for which alemtuzumab depletes autoimmune inflammatory T and B cells by direct antibody-dependent lysis. Repopulating lymphocytes appear to temporarily rebalance the immune system. Patients receiving this antibody become lymphopenic and may also become neutropenic, anemic, and thrombocytopenic. As a result, patients should be closely monitored for opportunistic infections and hematologic toxicity.

Daratumumab and isatuximab bind to CD38, which is over-expressed on myeloma cells. Binding of these Mabs to CD38 on myeloma cells likely induces cell death by apoptosis, complement-dependent cytotoxicity, or antibody-dependent cytotoxicity. They are approved by the FDA for use in multiple myeloma patients who are refractory to standard treatments either alone or in combination with other myeloma drugs such as dexamethasone, pomalidomide, and various proteasome inhibitors. **Elotuzumab** is FDA approved for the treatment of relapsed multiple myeloma in combination with other myeloma drugs. This Mab binds signaling lymphocytic activation molecule F7 (SLAMF7) on myeloma cells. It enables killing of multiple myeloma tumor cells by antibody-dependent cell-mediated cytotoxicity (ADCC).

Teclistamab is a bispecific Mab with one arm of the IgG binding B cell maturation antigen (BCMA) on multiple myeloma cells and the other arm binding CD3. These types of antibodies are called bispecific T cell engagers, or BiTEs, as they bring T cells in close proximity to tumor cells for enhanced antitumor activity.

Dinutuximab and **naxitamab** are ganglioside D2 (GD2)-binding Mabs approved for pediatric or adult patients with high-risk neuroblastoma in combination with granulocyte-macrophage colony-stimulating factor (GM-CSF), interleukin 2 (IL-2), and 13-cis-retinoic acid (RA) who achieve at least a partial response to prior first-line multiagent, multimodality therapy. Dinutuximab has a black box warning for serious infusion reactions and neurotoxicity in the majority of patients, while naxitamab has a shorter outpatient infusion time.

Anti–Vascular Endothelial Growth Factor (VEGF) and VEGF Receptor (R) Mabs

Anti-VEGF and VEGFR Mabs are anti-angiogenic drugs that inhibit VEGF from binding to its receptor, especially on endothelial cells, thereby inhibiting growth of blood vessels (angiogenesis). **Bevacizumab** is a humanized IgG_1 monoclonal antibody that is used for first- and second-line treatment of multiple cancers. It is approved for patients with metastatic colorectal cancer in combination with appropriate chemotherapy. It is also approved for treatment of non-squamous non-small cell lung cancer, glioblastoma multiforme that has progressed after prior treatment, metastatic kidney cancer when used with IFN-α, persistent, recurrent, or metastatic cervical cancer, and also ovarian, fallopian tube, or primary peritoneal cancer of epithelial origin in combination with appropriate chemotherapy. Since bevacizumab is antiangiogenic, it should not be administered until patients heal from surgery. Patients taking the drug should be watched for hemorrhage, gastrointestinal perforations, and wound healing problems. Bevacizumab has also been used off label by intravitreal injection to slow progression of neovascular macular degeneration (see ranibizumab, below).

Brolucizumab, faricimab, and **ranibizumab** are engineered humanized antibody fragments that bind to VEGF-A. They are approved for intravitreal injection in patients with neovascular age-related macular degeneration and diabetic macular edema. **Pegaptanib** is a pegylated oligonucleotide that binds extracellular VEGF and is also given by intravitreal injection to slow macular degeneration.

Ramucirumab is a human Mab that binds to VEGF receptor 2 on tumor cells as a receptor antagonist, blocking the binding of VEGF to VEGFR2. It is FDA approved for the following indications: metastatic colon cancer in combination with a FOLFIRI chemotherapy regimen (folinic acid, fluorouracil, and irinotecan), platinum-resistant metastatic small cell lung cancer in combination with docetaxel, advanced gastric or gastroesophageal junction adenocarcinoma with or without paclitaxel, and hepatocellular carcinoma as a single agent in patients with an alpha fetoprotein (AFP) >400 ng/mL who have been treated with sorafenib.

Anti–Epidermal Growth Factor Receptor (EGFR) Mabs

Cetuximab is a human-mouse chimeric monoclonal antibody that blocks EGF ligands from binding to EGFR. It inhibits tumor cell growth by a variety of mechanisms, including decreases in kinase activity, matrix metalloproteinase activity, and growth factor production, as well as increased apoptosis. It is approved for use in patients with EGFR-positive head and neck squamous cell carcinoma in combination with radiotherapy or appropriate chemotherapy. It is also approved for treatment of KRAS-negative, EGFR-positive metastatic colorectal cancer in combination with radiotherapy or appropriate chemotherapy, or as a single agent in patients who cannot tolerate certain chemotherapies. Cetuximab may be administered in combination with irinotecan or alone in patients who cannot tolerate irinotecan. HAMAs are generated by about 4% of patients being treated with cetuximab.

Necitumumab is another EGFR-targeted Mab indicated for use in patients with metastatic squamous non-small cell lung cancer in combination with gemcitabine and cisplatin. Unlike cetuximab, it is a fully human monoclonal antibody with the same mechanism of action and similar toxicities including hypomagnesemia in 83% of patients receiving the drug and cardiopulmonary arrest in 3% of patients. Although dermatologic and infusion-related toxicities are common, the distinct advantage over cetuximab is that it is fully human (ie, does not elicit HAMAs) and thus has an extended half-life in the circulation.

Panitumumab is another fully human IgG_2 Mab. It is approved for the treatment of EGFR-expressing metastatic colorectal carcinoma in patients whose disease has progressed while taking or following fluoropyrimidine-, oxaliplatin-, and irinotecan-containing chemotherapy regimens. Like other anti-EGFR Mabs, it inhibits cell growth, induces apoptosis, decreases vascular growth factor production, and suppresses internalization of the EGFR. This was the first FDA-approved monoclonal antibody produced from transgenic mice expressing the human immunoglobulin gene loci.

Amivantamab is a genetically engineered human IgG1 bispecific Mab. One arm of the antibody binds to EGFR and the other arm binds to mesenchymal-epithelial transition factor (MET) to inhibit MET-ligand binding, further suppressing tumor signaling and growth. It is approved for the treatment of patients with locally advanced or metastatic non-small cell lung cancer with EGFR exon 20 insertion mutations.

Immune Checkpoint Inhibitor Mabs

Immune checkpoint inhibitor Mabs have changed the treatment of many cancers. They have surpassed cytotoxic drugs and are now considered first-line treatment options for many cancers. Once antitumor T cells are activated, immune checkpoint inhibitor Mabs prevent these T cells from being suppressed or de-activated by tumors or regulatory cells. This allows them to more completely destroy tumors, but it can also lead to **cytokine release syndrome,** which can be life-threatening depending on severity.

Ipilimumab and **tremelimumab** bind to CTLA-4 on T cells, preventing CD80/86 from delivering a suppressive signal to T cells. This has the effect of maintaining T-cell activation. It is approved for the treatment of adult and pediatric patients (>12 years) with unresectable or metastatic melanoma, cutaneous melanoma with regional nodes in the adjuvant surgical setting, renal cell carcinoma in combination with nivolumab, and colorectal cancer patients whose tumors have DNA repair defects. Tremelimumab is approved in combination with durvalumab for the treatment of patients with unresectable hepatocellular carcinoma.

Nivolumab, pembrolizumab, cemiplimab, and **dostarlimab** are anti-PD-1 Mabs. They allow potential antitumor T cells to remain activated by blocking the interaction of PD-1 on T-cells with PD-ligand 1 (PD-L1) on tumor cells. Blocking this interaction allows T cells to remain activated. Nivolumab is approved for Hodgkin lymphoma, renal cell carcinoma, non-small cell lung cancer (NSCLC), melanoma, recurrent or metastatic squamous cell carcinoma of the head and neck, metastatic urothelial cell carcinoma, hepatocellular carcinoma after progression on sorafenib, and metastatic colorectal cancer in patients who have DNA repair mutations and progressed on other antineoplastic agents. Similar to nivolumab, pembrolizumab is approved for the treatment of head and neck cancer, NSCLC, small cell lung cancer (SCLC), Hodgkin lymphoma, melanoma, Merkel cell carcinoma, primary mediastinal large B-cell lymphoma, urothelial cell carcinoma, renal cell carcinoma, esophageal, gastric and cervical cancers, hepatocellular carcinoma, and patients whose tumors have DNA repair defects. More recently, cemiplimab was approved for patients with locally advanced and metastatic basal cell carcinoma. Dostarlimab is approved for recurrent or advanced solid tumors in adult patients with mismatch repair deficiency.

Relatlimab is a Mab directed against lymphocyte activation gene 3 (LAG-3) that is approved for treatment of adult and pediatric patients (≥12 years old) with metastatic melanoma only in combination with nivolumab.

Atezolizumab, avelumab, and durvalumab bind to PD-L1 on tumor cells, also interfering with suppressive PD-1 signaling in T cells. Atezolizumab, a humanized IgG1 anti-PD-L1 Mab, is approved for urothelial carcinoma, NSCLC, SCLC, and metastatic triple negative breast cancer. Avelumab is approved for adult and pediatric patients (≥12 years old) with Merkel cell carcinoma and locally advanced or metastatic urothelial carcinoma whose disease progressed on platinum-based therapy. It is also approved for first-line treatment in combination with axitinib for patients with advanced renal cell carcinoma. Durvalumab (anti-PD-L1) is approved for treatment of patients with locally advanced or metastatic urothelial carcinoma who have progressed on platinum-based therapy. It is also approved for patients with unresectable stage III NSCLC whose disease has not progressed on platinum-based or radiation therapy.

Margetuximab, pertuzumab, and trastuzumab are approved for the treatment of patients with HER-2/*neu*-positive breast cancer with high risk of occurrence in combination with antineoplastic chemotherapy. These antibodies are antagonists for HER-2/*neu* and suppress tumor growth by preventing heterodimerization of the human epidermal growth factor receptor HER-2/*neu* with other HER family members, thus inhibiting ligand-mediated intracellular signaling through MAP kinase and PI3 kinase pathways. They also mediate antibody-dependent cell-mediated cytotoxicity (ADCC) on HER-2/*neu*-positive tumor cells. Trastuzumab is approved for first-line treatment along with paclitaxel of HER-2/*neu*-positive tumors in patients with breast cancer and for patients with metastatic gastric or gastroesophageal junction adenocarcinoma. As a single agent it induces remission in 15–20% of breast cancer patients; in combination with chemotherapy, it increases response rates and duration as well as 1-year survival. Another formulation of trastuzumab includes hyaluronidase (Herceptin Hylecta), which can be administered subcutaneously, unlike trastuzumab alone (which must be given IV). Patients should be monitored for potential cardiomyopathy while taking these drugs.

Rituximab is a chimeric murine-human monoclonal IgG_1 (human Fc) that binds to the CD20 molecule on normal and malignant B lymphocytes. It was one of the first Mabs approved for treatment of cancer. It is approved for the therapy of patients with CD20-positive non-Hodgkin lymphoma, as a single agent or in combination with appropriate chemotherapy and for treatment of chronic lymphocytic leukemia (CLL) in combination with chemotherapy. Rituximab is also approved for the treatment of rheumatoid arthritis in combination with methotrexate in patients for whom anti-TNF-α therapy has failed. Recent indications for rituximab are for the treatment of Wegener granulomatosis and microscopic polyangiitis, and moderate to severe pemphigus vulgaris. The mechanism of action includes complement-mediated lysis, antibody-dependent cellular cytotoxicity, and induction of apoptosis in malignant lymphoma cells and in B cells involved in the pathogenesis of rheumatoid arthritis and granulomatosis and polyangiitis. In lymphoma, this drug appears to be synergistic with chemotherapy (eg, fludarabine, CHOP; see Chapter 54). A large number of adverse reactions are associated with rituximab treatment depending on the patient population.

Obinutuzumab and **ofatumumab** are humanized/human IgG Mabs directed against CD20 on B lymphocytes. Obinutuzumab is approved for treatment of previously untreated patients with CLL in combination with chlorambucil. It is also approved for treatment of patients with follicular lymphoma who (1) are refractory to a rituximab-containing regimen, (2) achieved a partial remission with chemotherapy, or (3) have previously untreated stage II bulky, III, or IV disease. Ofatumumab is approved for patients with CLL who are refractory to fludarabine and alemtuzumab. Like rituximab and obinutuzumab, ofatumumab binds to all B cells including B-CLL. It is thought to lyse B-CLL cells in the presence of complement and to mediate antibody-dependent cellular cytotoxicity. Ofatumumab also appears to have significant benefits in relapsing multiple sclerosis. There is a slight risk of hepatitis B virus reactivation in patients taking obinutuzumab and ofatumumab.

Ocrelizumab is a humanized IgG Mab targeting CD20 on B lymphocytes. It is indicated for treatment of adults with relapsing or primary progressing multiple sclerosis. Ocrelizumab works by binding CD20 on B and pre-B lymphocytes followed by antibody-dependent cellular cytotoxicity and complement-mediated lysis of CD20+ cells. Since this is a B cell–depleting Mab, patients should be monitored for increased risk of infection including upper respiratory tract infections. Immunoglobulin replacement therapy should be used when patients become hypogammaglobulinemic.

Tafasitamab is an anti-CD19 Mab that has a genetically engineered hybrid IgG1/2 human Fc. It is directly cytotoxic to CD19-bearing B cells and also mediates ADCC. It is approved for treatment of adults with relapsed or refractory diffuse large B-cell lymphoma who are not eligible for autologous stem cell transplant.

Blinatumomab is a bispecific CD19-directed CD3 T cell engager (BiTE) that is approved for children and adults with treatment-refractory or relapsed B-cell precursor acute lymphoblastic leukemia (ALL). It is also approved for adults and children who are in remission from ALL, but with minimal residual disease of 0.1% or greater. The strategy of BiTE therapy is to bring CD3+ T cells and CD19+ leukemia cells in close proximity so that T cells can kill ALL cells. Patients should be monitored for cytokine release syndrome (CRS), neurologic toxicities, and infections.

Mabs Used to Deliver Isotopes & Toxins (Antibody Drug Conjugate, ADC) to Tumors

Ado-trastuzumab emtansine and fam-trastuzumab deruxtecan are antibody-drug conjugates in which the anti-HER-2/*neu* antibody trastuzumab (see above) is chemically linked to the cytotoxic agent mertansine, a microtubule disruptor (emtansine) or topoisomerase inhibitor (deruxtecan). Ado-trastuzumab emtansine is approved for patients with HER-2/*neu*-positive breast cancer who have previously received trastuzumab and a taxane separately or in combination, and whose disease recurred or progressed during prior treatment. Toxicities include those of trastuzumab alone as well as hepatotoxicity due to emtansine. Fam trastuzumab deruxtecan is approved for patients with unresectable or metastatic breast, NSCLC, or gastric or gastroesophageal junction adenocarcinoma who have received prior trastuzumab-based treatment.

Arcitumomab is a murine Fab fragment from an anti-carcinoembryonic antigen (CEA) antibody labeled with technetium 99m (^{99m}Tc) that is used for imaging patients with metastatic colorectal carcinoma (immunoscintigraphy) to determine extent of disease. CEA is often up-regulated in patients with gastrointestinal carcinomas. The use of the Fab fragment decreases the immunogenicity of the agent so that it can be given more than once; intact murine monoclonal antibodies would elicit stronger HAMA.

Belantamab mafodotin is a humanized IgG1 Mab coupled to a microtubule inhibitor. Its target is B-cell maturation antigen (BCMA) on multiple myeloma cells. When internalized, the microtubule inhibitor is cleaved from the Mab and induces apoptosis. Belantamab mafodotin may also kill multiple myeloma cells by ADCC. It is approved for patients who have been previously treated with an anti-CD38 Mab who are refractory to treatment. There is a boxed warning for this Mab because it has ocular toxicity—specifically it may damage the corneal epithelium, resulting in vision changes or even vision loss.

Brentuximab vedotin is an antibody-drug conjugate that binds CD30, a cell surface marker in the TNF receptor superfamily that is expressed on anaplastic large T-cell lymphomas and on Reed-Sternberg cells in Hodgkin lymphoma; it may also be expressed on normal activated leukocytes. Brentuximab vedotin consists of a chimeric (mouse-human) IgG_1 linked to monomethylauristatin E (MMAE), a microtubule-disrupting agent that induces cell cycle arrest and apoptosis. When this ADC binds CD30 on the cell surface, the complex is internalized followed by proteolytic cleavage of MMAE, a microtubule disrupting agent from the IgG. Brentuximab is approved for treatment of patients with Hodgkin lymphoma after failure of autologous stem cell transplantation or after failure of at least two previous chemotherapy regimens. It is also approved for patients with systemic anaplastic large cell lymphoma after failure of at least one previous multiagent chemotherapy regimen. Patients taking brentuximab vedotin should be monitored primarily for neutropenia and peripheral sensory neuropathy.

Capromab pendetide is a murine monoclonal antibody specific for prostate-specific membrane antigen. It is coupled to isotopic indium (^{111}In) and is used in immunoscintigraphy for patients with biopsy-confirmed prostate cancer and post-prostatectomy in patients with rising prostate-specific antibody level to determine extent of disease.

Ibritumomab tiuxetan is an anti-CD20 murine monoclonal antibody labeled with isotopic yttrium (^{90}Y) or ^{111}In. The radiation of the isotope coupled to the antibody provides the major antitumor activity of this drug. Ibritumomab is approved for use in patients with relapsed or refractory low-grade, follicular, or B-cell non-Hodgkin lymphoma, including patients with rituximab-refractory follicular disease. It is used in conjunction with rituximab in a two-step therapeutic regimen.

Inotuzumab ozogamicin is an antibody-drug conjugate (ADC) directed against CD22. It is intended for use in adults with relapsing or treatment-refractory acute B-cell lymphoblastic leukemia (B-ALL). When the ADC binds to CD22 on leukemic (and nonmalignant) CD22+ B cells, it is internalized into an acidic vesicle where N-acetyl-gamma-calicheamicin is cleaved from the Mab—after which calicheamicin causes double-strand breaks in DNA that result in cell death.

Loncastuximab tesirine is a humanized anti-CD19 IgG1 ADC coupled to an alkylating agent. It is approved for treatment of patients with relapsed or treatment refractory large and diffuse large B-cell lymphomas. Upon binding to CD19, the ADC is internalized and the Mab and alkylating agent are separated by proteolysis followed by the alkylating agent causing inter-strand DNA cross-links resulting in cell death.

Moxetumomab pasudotox is another anti-CD22 ADC; it is indicated for the treatment of adult patients with relapsed or refractory hairy cell leukemia who received two previous systemic therapies including a purine nucleoside analog. When the pasudotox is released from the Mab, it ADP-ribosylates elongation factor 2 in the cell, inhibiting protein synthesis and causing apoptotic cell death.

Polatuzumab vedotin is a human IgG ADC that targets CD79b on actively dividing B cells. It is approved for use in adult patients with relapsed or treatment-refractory diffuse large B-cell lymphomas (DLBCL) in combination with bendamustine and a rituximab product. Once internalized by the B cell, it kills the cell in the same manner as brentuximab vedotin (microtubule-disrupting agent).

Enfortumab vedotin is a human IgG1 ADC that targets the cell surface adhesion protein nectin 4. It is approved for patients with locally advanced or metastatic urothelial cancer who previously received anti-PD-1, anti-PD-L1, and platinum-containing chemotherapy or who are ineligible for cisplatin-based therapies.

Sacituzumab govitecan is a humanized IgG1 ADC that binds to trophoblast cell surface antigen (Trop-2). It is coupled to a topoisomerase inhibitor that is cleaved from the Mab upon cellular internalization. It is approved for patients who have metastatic or locally advanced triple-negative breast cancer who have received two or more prior systemic therapies. It is also approved for patients with locally advanced or metastatic urothelial cancer who previously received a platinum-based therapy or an anti-PD-1 Mab therapy.

Tisotumab vedotin is an ADC directed against tissue factor (TF). It is approved for treatment of patients with recurrent or metastatic cervical cancer with disease progression during or after chemotherapy. Boxed warnings include ocular toxicities.

Mabs and Fusion Proteins Used as Immunomodulatory & Anti-Inflammatory Agents

Adalimumab, certolizumab pegol, etanercept, golimumab, and **infliximab** are antibodies that bind and neutralize the biologic activity of TNF-α, a proinflammatory cytokine that is important in adult and juvenile rheumatoid arthritis and similar inflammatory diseases such as plaque psoriasis, psoriatic arthritis, ankylosing spondylitis, Crohn's's disease, and ulcerative colitis. Patients taking anti-TNF-α drugs should be monitored for past infection, as well as reactivation of TB, valley fever, and lymphoma. Patients should not receive live vaccines while taking anti-TNF-α drugs.

Abatacept and **belatacept** are recombinant fusion proteins composed of the extracellular domain of cytotoxic T-lymphocyte-associated antigen 4 (CTLA-4) fused to the Fc domains of human IgG_1 (Figure 55–7). Abatacept is approved for use in rheumatoid and other forms of arthritis and is discussed in Chapter 36. Belatacept is approved to help prevent rejection in kidney transplants. Both fusion proteins block the activation of T cells by binding CD80, blocking the CD28 activation signal in T cells.

Anakinra is a recombinant form of the naturally occurring IL-1 receptor antagonist that prevents IL-1 from binding to its receptor, stemming the cascade of cytokines that would otherwise

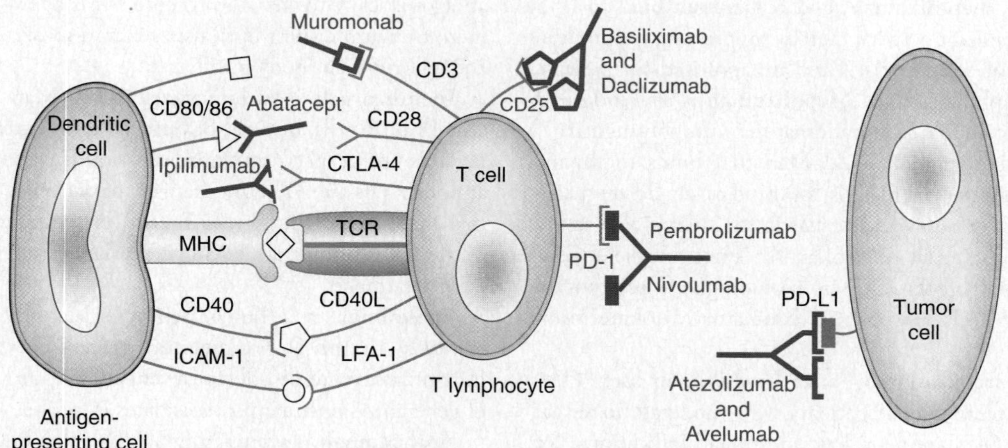

FIGURE 55–7 Actions of some monoclonal antibodies (*shown in red*). CTLA-4-IgFc fusion protein (CTLA-4-Ig, abatacept) binds to CD80/86 on DC and inhibits T-cell costimulation. Muromonab blocks T-cell function by binding to CD3. It may also facilitate removal of T cells via ADCC. Basiliximab blocks IL-2 from binding to the IL-2 receptor (CD25) on T cells, preventing activation; CD25 is also important for the survival of T regulatory cells. T-cell activation can be maintained or restored if CTLA-4 interaction with CD80/86 is blocked using an anti–CTLA-4 antibody (ipilimumab); ipilimumab inhibits CTLA-4 signaling and prolongs activation. Pembrolizumab and nivolumab bind to PD-1, while atezolizumab, avelumab, and durvalumab bind to PD-L1. Anti-PD-1 and anti-PD-L1 Mabs inhibit the negative signal delivery by PD-1, also prolonging T-cell activation.

be released. Anakinra is approved for use in adult rheumatoid arthritis patients who have failed treatment with one or more disease-modifying antirheumatic drugs. It is also indicated for patients with cryopyrin-associated periodic syndrome (CAPS). **Rilonacept** is a dimeric fusion protein consisting of the ligand-binding domains of the extracellular portions of the human interleukin 1 receptor component (IL-1RI) and IL-1 receptor accessory protein (IL-1RAcP) fused to the Fc portion of human IgG_1. It is indicated for treatment of CAPS, familial cold autoinflammatory syndrome (FCAS), and Muckle-Wells syndrome (MWS) in children >12 years old and adults. These diseases are caused by mutations in a gene (*NLRP-3*) that encodes cryopyrin, an important component of the inflammasome. *NLRP-3* mutations cause excessive release of IL-1β, causing autoimmune inflammation resulting in fever, urticaria-like rash, arthralgia, myalgia, fatigue, and conjunctivitis.

Canakinumab is a human IgG Mab that prevents IL-1β from binding to its receptor. It is approved for adults and children 4 years old and older with CAPS. It is also approved for treatment of systemic juvenile idiopathic arthritis in children ≥2 years old and for TNF receptor–associated periodic syndrome (TRAPS), hyperimmunoglobulin D syndrome (HIDS)/mevalonate kinase deficiency (MKD), and familial Mediterranean fever (FMF) in adult and pediatric patients.

Dupilumab is a human Mab that binds to the IL-4 receptor alpha chain. Since both IL-4 and IL-13 share the same alpha chain receptor, dupilumab inhibits binding of both IL-4 and IL-13 to their receptors on a variety of cells including mast cells, eosinophils, macrophages, epithelial cells, and goblet cells. Dupilumab is indicated for moderate to severe atopic dermatitis in patients >12 years old and as an add-on maintenance treatment for patients suffering from moderate to severe eosinophilic asthma or inadequately controlled chronic rhinosinusitis with nasal polyposis.

Benralizumab, mepolizumab, and **reslizumab** bind to IL-5 and neutralize its biologic activity, thereby suppressing the production and survival of eosinophils. They are approved for patients with severe eosinophilic asthma. **Mepolizumab** is also indicated for patients with eosinophilic granulomatosis with polyangiitis.

Tezepelumab is a human IgG2 Mab that binds to thymic stromal lymphopoietin (TSLP). It is approved as an add-on maintenance treatment for adult and pediatric (≥12 years old) severe asthma. Although the mechanism of action is not completely elucidated, Tezepelumab blocks TSLP from binding to its receptor on epithelial cells and limits upstream inflammatory cytokines from being produced.

Ixekizumab, secukinumab, and **brodalumab** are FDA approved for the treatment of patients with moderate to severe plaque psoriasis. Secukinumab has additional indications for patients with psoriatic arthritis and ankylosing spondylitis. Ixekizumab and secukinumab bind the IL-17 cytokine and prevent it from binding to its receptor, while brodalumab blocks IL-17 by binding to the IL-17 receptor itself.

Guselkumab, risankizumab, and **tildrakizumab** are approved for treatment of adults with moderate to severe plaque psoriasis. These Mabs target IL-23 and block it from binding to the IL-23 receptor. Like ixekizumab and secukinumab, administration is injected subcutaneously and patients may self-administer the Mab after training. Patients receiving Mabs that neutralize the activities of IL-17 and IL-23 should be evaluated for active or previous TB infection prior to treatment. Live vaccines should be avoided during treatment.

Tralokinumab is a human IgG4 Mab that binds to IL-13, preventing it from binding to the IL-13 receptor complex. It is approved for the treatment of moderate to severe atopic dermatitis in adults whose disease has not been controlled with topical cortical steroids. Treatment of patients with tralokinumab suppresses the production of pro-inflammatory cytokines and chemokines in skin lesions.

Siltuximab is a chimeric Mab that binds to and prevents IL-6 from binding to its cellular receptor. It is approved for the treatment of patients with multicentric Castleman disease who are HIV-negative and HHV-8-negative.

Tocilizumab is a recombinant humanized IgG_1 that binds to soluble and membrane-associated IL-6 receptors. It inhibits IL-6-mediated signaling on lymphocytes, suppressing inflammatory processes. Similar to anti-TNF-α Mabs, patients receiving tocilizumab should be closely monitored for infectious diseases such as tuberculosis and other invasive bacterial, fungal, and viral infections. Tocilizumab is also commonly used off-label to treat cytokine release syndrome that results from immune checkpoint therapy or CAR T-cell immunotherapy (see below). Interestingly, for biologics, tocilizumab is available in both injectable and oral formulations.

Sarilumab is a human IgG1 Mab that also binds antagonistically to the IL-6 receptor. It is approved for patients with moderate to severe active rheumatoid arthritis who have not responded to disease modifying antirheumatic drugs. It must be used with caution in patients with certain infectious diseases, similar to tocilizumab.

Satralizumab is another humanized IgG2 Mab that also binds antagonistically to the IL-6 receptor. It is approved for the treatment of neuromyelitis optica spectrum disorder in adults who are aquaphorin-4 antibody positive.

Inebilizumab is a humanized IgG1 Mab directed against CD-19 on B cells, but is also approved for the treatment of neuromyelitis optica spectrum disorder in adults who are aquaphorin-4 antibody positive. The mechanism of action is not known, but this Mab is cytolytic toward B cells. Patients should be screened for hepatitis B infection and active or latent tuberculosis infection prior treatment.

Spesolimab is a humanized IgG1Mab that binds antagonistically to the IL-36 receptor, preventing downstream pro-inflammatory and pro-fibrotic events. It is approved the treatment of generalized pustular psoriasis flares in adults.

Anifrolumab is a human IgG1 Mab that binds to the IFN-α receptor, preventing IFN-α from binding. It is approved for patients with moderate to severe systemic lupus erythematosus (SLE) who are also receiving standard therapy. Because it blocks IFN-α from binding to its receptor, IFN-α-mediated inflammatory signals are blocked at the cellular level.

Emapalumab is a human IgG1 Mab that binds and neutralizes IFN-γ. It is approved for use in pediatric (including infants) and adult patients with hemophagocytic lymphohistiocytosis (HLH). HLH is a rare genetic disease in which too many activated lymphocytes are present and secreting cytokines aberrantly. Since IFN-γ stimulates the release of many other cytokines and chemokines, neutralizing the activity of IFN-γ provides some therapeutic benefit.

Basiliximab is a chimeric mouse-human IgG_1 that binds to CD25, the IL-2 receptor α chain on activated lymphocytes. It functions as an IL-2 antagonist, blocking IL-2 from binding to activated lymphocytes, and is therefore immunosuppressive. It is indicated for prophylaxis of acute organ rejection in renal transplant patients and may be used as part of an immunosuppressive regimen that also includes glucocorticoids and cyclosporine.

Belimumab is a Mab that inhibits B cell activating factor, also known as B lymphocyte stimulator, preventing B cells from being stimulated. It is approved for patients >5 years old with active, autoantibody-positive systemic lupus erythematosus (SLE) who are also receiving standard therapy.

Mogamulizumab is a humanized IgG Mab that binds to chemokine (CC) receptor type 4 (CCR4). It is approved for adult patients with relapsed or refractory mycosis fungoides or Sezary syndrome. This Mab mediates ADCC on T cells expressing CCR4.

Omalizumab is an anti-IgE recombinant humanized Mab that is approved for the treatment of allergic asthma in adult and adolescent patients whose symptoms are refractory to inhaled corticosteroids (see Chapter 20). The Mab is also approved for chronic urticaria. The antibody blocks the binding of IgE to the high-affinity Fcε receptor on basophils and mast cells, which suppresses IgE-mediated release of type I allergy mediators such as histamine and leukotrienes. Total serum IgE levels may remain elevated in patients for up to 1 year after administration of omalizumab.

Guselkumab and **ustekinumab** are human IgG_1 monoclonal antibodies that bind IL-23 and are approved for patients with moderate to severe plaque psoriasis. Guselkumab binds to the p19 subunit of IL-23, preventing it from binding to its receptor and reducing levels of inflammatory cytokines IL-17 and IL-22. Ustekinumab binds to the p40 subunit of IL-12 and IL-23 cytokines. It blocks IL-12 and IL-23 from binding to their receptors, thereby inhibiting receptor-mediated signaling in lymphocytes. Ustekinumab is indicated for adult and pediatric patients (≥12 years old) with moderate to severe plaque psoriasis, patients with active psoriatic arthritis either alone or with methotrexate, and patients with moderate to severe Crohn's's disease who have failed anti-TNF-α drugs. The advantage of ustekinumab over anti-TNF-α drugs for psoriasis is faster and longer-term improvement in symptoms along with very infrequent dosing.

Natalizumab is a humanized IgG_4 monoclonal antibody that binds to the α4-subunit of α4β1 and α4β7 integrins expressed on the surfaces of all leukocytes except neutrophils. It inhibits the α4-mediated adhesion of leukocytes to their cognate receptor. It is indicated for patients with multiple sclerosis and Crohn's disease who have not tolerated or had inadequate responses to conventional treatments. Natalizumab should not be used with any of the anti-TNF-α drugs listed above. Natalizumab increases risk of progressive multifocal leukoencephalopathy.

Vedolizumab is a humanized monoclonal antibody that targets the α4β7 integrin in the gastrointestinal tract. It does not appear to induce systemic immunosuppression of other α4β7 integrin-binding antibodies such as natalizumab because it does not bind to the majority of α4β7 integrin on lymphocytes. It has been recommended for approval for the treatment of adults with Crohn's disease and ulcerative colitis.

Other Mabs

Burosumab is a human Mab that neutralizes the activity of fibroblast growth factor 23 (FGF23; see Chapter 42) and is approved for pediatric and adult patients with X-linked hypophosphatemia (XLH). XLH is caused by production of excess FGF23, which suppresses renal tubular phosphate reabsorption and production of 1,25 dihydroxy vitamin D by the kidney. Treatment with burosumab has the effect of restoring renal phosphate reabsorption and increasing levels of 1,25 dihydroxy vitamin D.

Caplacizumab is an engineered single-domain antibody fragment that targets von Willebrand factor (vWF) and inhibits the interaction between vWF and platelets. It is FDA approved for adults with acquired thrombotic thrombocytopenic purpura (aTTP) in combination with plasma exchange and immunosuppressive therapy.

Crizanlizumab is a humanized IgG Mab directed against P-selectin on activated endothelium and platelets. It blocks interactions between endothelial cells, platelets, red blood cells, and leukocytes. It is FDA approved to reduce the occurrence of vaso-occlusive disease in adult and pediatric patients (>16 years) with sickle cell disease.

Eptinezumab, erenumab, fremanezumab, and **galcanezumab** are humanized Mabs used to treat patients with frequent migraine headaches (see Chapter 16). Erenumab binds the calcitonin gene-related peptide (CGRP) receptor and prevents activation. Fremanezumab and galcanezumab bind to the peptide (CGRP) ligand, inhibiting its binding to the receptor. These Mabs are self-administered subcutaneously to prevent migraine headaches.

Idarucizumab is a Fab fragment whose target is the thrombin inhibitor dabigatran, a small molecule. It is used in patients taking dabigatran who are at risk for bleeding due to excessive anticoagulant activity of dabigatran.

Ibalizumab is a humanized IgG4 Mab whose target is CD4. It is used in patients with multidrug-resistant HIV infection in combination with other anti-retroviral drugs (see Chapter 49). It blocks entry of HIV into CD4 T cells without causing immunosuppression or interfering with normal function of helper T cells.

Muromonab CD3 was the first Mab approved for human use by the FDA. It is a murine Mab approved for treatment of acute renal, steroid-resistant cardiac, or steroid-resistant hepatic allograft rejection. Muromonab CD3 suppresses T-cell function. Because the Mab is of murine origin, patients are usually pre-treated with immune suppressants prior to muromonab CD3 therapy.

Abciximab is a Fab fragment of a murine-human monoclonal antibody that binds to the integrin GPIIb/IIIa receptor on activated platelets and inhibits fibrinogen, von Willebrand factor, and other adhesion molecules from binding to activated platelets, thus preventing their aggregation. It is indicated as an adjunct to percutaneous coronary intervention in combination with aspirin and heparin for the prevention of cardiac ischemic complications. See Chapter 34 for additional details.

Alirocumab, evolocumab, and **evinacumab** are anticholesterol Mabs (see Chapter 35). Alirocumab and evolocumab lower LDL levels by blocking proprotein convertase subtilisin/kexin type 9 (PCSK9) from binding to LDL receptors (LDRL) and causing LDL receptor degradation. Therefore, these Mabs have the effect of increasing LDLR on hepatocytes, which lowers LDL levels in circulation. Evinacumab is an angiopoietin-like 3 inhibitor, but it also has the effect of lowering LDL by promoting LDL processing and clearance upstream of LDL formation. These human Mabs are approved as an adjunct to diet and maximally tolerated statin therapy in adults with homo- or heterozygous familial hypercholesterolemia or atherosclerotic cardiovascular disease who require additional lowering of LDL-C.

Denosumab is a human IgG_2 monoclonal antibody specific for human RANKL (receptor activator of nuclear factor kappa-B ligand; see Chapter 42). By binding RANKL it inhibits the maturation of osteoclasts, the cells responsible for bone resorption. Denosumab is indicated for treatment of postmenopausal women with osteoporosis at high risk for fracture. It is also indicated in men and women at high risk for bone fracture as a result of glucocorticoid-induced osteoporosis, androgen deprivation therapy (men), and aromatase inhibitor therapy for breast cancer. Before starting denosumab, patients must be evaluated to be sure they are not hypocalcemic. During treatment, patients should receive supplements of calcium and vitamin D.

Eculizumab and **ravulizumab** are humanized IgG Mabs that bind the C5 complement component, inhibiting its cleavage into C5a and C5b thereby inhibiting the terminal pore-forming lytic activity of complement. Eculizumab is approved for patients with paroxysmal nocturnal hemoglobinuria (PNH) and atypical hemolytic uremic syndrome (aHUS). It dramatically reduces the need for red blood cell transfusions. It prevents PNH symptoms of anemia, fatigue, thrombosis, and hemoglobinemia by inhibiting intravascular hemolysis. Similarly in aHUS, eculizumab prevents complement-mediated thrombotic microangiopathy. Patients should be immunized or boosted with meningococcal vaccines prior to receiving these Mabs because complement C5 is a key innate immune factor for neutralizing meningococcal bacteria. Ravulizumab is similar with a longer duration of action.

Lanadelumab binds to plasma kallikrein and inhibits its proteolytic activity. This Mab is approved for prevention of hereditary angioedema (HAE) in patients ≥12 years old. In patients with HAE, plasma kallikrein levels are unregulated due to the absence of C1-inhibitor (see Chapter 17). Plasma kallikrein cleaves high–molecular–weight kininogen, which leads to increased levels of bradykinin resulting in swelling and pain observed in patients with HAE. After training, patients can self-administer this drug subcutaneously.

Sutimlimab is a humanized IgG4 Mab that inhibits the classic complement cascade by binding to C1s, preventing it from cleaving C4 and thereby lysing red blood cells in patients with cold agglutinin disease. It is approved to reduce complement-mediated hemolysis of red blood cells in pediatric and adult patients with cold agglutinin disease.

Aducanumab is a human IgG1 that bind to amyloid beta protein and is approved for the treatment of patients with Alzheimer's disease. It is thought to reduce the number of amyloid beta plaques in the brains of patients with Alzheimer's disease. This Mab is not without controversy because some of the side effects are Alzheimer's disease-like.

Palivizumab is a humanized IgG_1 monoclonal antibody that binds to the fusion protein of respiratory syncytial virus (RSV), preventing serious lower respiratory tract disease. It is used in neonates at risk for this viral infection and reduces the frequency of infection and hospitalization by about 50% (see Chapter 49).

Ansuvimab is a human IgG1 Mab that binds to Zaire Ebola virus surface glycoprotein (GP1,2), blocking the virus from binding to its cellular receptor. **Atoltivimab, maftivimab, and odesivimab** constitute a Mab cocktail that also neutralizes Zaire Ebola infection. It is approved for adult and pediatric patients infected with Zaire Ebola. Patients who have been treated with ansuvimab or the Mab cocktail should not receive the Ebola vaccine for several months to avoid reducing efficacy of the vaccine.

Obiltoxaximab and **raxibacumab** are FDA-approved Mabs for treatment of patients after inhalation exposure to *Bacillus anthracis* spores. Both Mabs block the binding of *B anthracis* "protective antigen" to its cellular receptor, preventing entry of anthrax lethal and edema factors into cells. They are approved for the treatment or prophylaxis of adults and children with inhalational anthrax in combination with appropriate antibacterial drugs. Interestingly, these Mabs were not tested in humans because exposing a control cohort to inhalational anthrax is unethical and there are too few living naturally infected persons to conduct a proper clinical trial.

Teprotumumab is a human IgG1 Mab. It binds to insulin-like growth factor 1 receptor and is FDA approved for treatment of patients with thyroid eye disease.

CELLULAR IMMUNOTHERAPIES: CHIMERIC ANTIGEN RECEPTOR T CELLS (CAR T CELLS)

CAR T cells are living drugs composed of T cells that have been "re-targeted" toward a desired cell surface antigen on tumor cells. Although research is moving toward "off-the-shelf" CAR T cells, they currently require peripheral blood leukocytes (PBL) from each patient. After T cells are purified from PBL, they are transduced with a lentivirus (retrovirus) engineered to express heavy and light chain antibody variable regions that are genetically fused to T cell intracellular signaling domains that activate the T cell when the antibody variable regions bind to the target antigen. Once the T cells are transduced, they are expanded in number and finally infused back into the same patient (an autologous therapy), where they kill cells expressing the intended target.

Six CAR T cell products are currently approved for B-cell malignancies. Four of them target CD19 and are approved for various B-cell leukemias and B-cell lymphomas (**axicabtagene ciloleucel, tisagenlecleucel, brexucabtagene autoleucel, and**

lisocabtagene maraleucel), and two target BCMA on multiple myeloma cells (**idecabtagene vicleucel and ciltacabtagene autoleucel**). Tisagenlecleucel is the only CAR T cell product approved for children and young adults with B-cell acute lymphoblastic leukemia (B-ALL).

Patients are often pre-treated with cyclophosphamide prior to CAR T cell therapy to accommodate large numbers of T cells in the infusion. Administration of these autologous CAR T-cell therapies can result in cytokine release syndrome (CRS), which is life-threatening. CRS may be treated with tocilizumab with or without corticosteroids. Neurologic toxicities also may occur; treatment is supportive. Prolonged hypogammaglobulinemia may occur due to B-cell destruction by anti-CD19 CAR T cells. Treatment for this hypogammaglobulinemia is IGIV. CAR T cells have become a very active area of research, and many groups are continuing to develop new CAR T cell therapies, especially for solid tumors.

■ CLINICAL USES OF IMMUNOSUPPRESSIVE DRUGS

Immunosuppressive agents are commonly used in two clinical circumstances: transplantation and autoimmune disorders. The agents used differ somewhat for the specific disorders treated (see specific agents and Table 55–1), as do administration schedules. Because autoimmune disorders are very complex, optimal treatment schedules have yet to be established in many of them.

SOLID ORGAN & BONE MARROW TRANSPLANTATION

In organ transplantation, tissue typing—based on donor and recipient histocompatibility matching with the human leukocyte antigen (HLA) haplotype system—is required. Close histocompatibility matching reduces the likelihood of graft rejection and may also reduce the requirements for intensive immunosuppressive therapy. Prior to transplant, patients may receive an immunosuppressive regimen, including antithymocyte globulin, or basiliximab. Four types of rejection can occur in a solid organ transplant recipient: **hyperacute, accelerated, acute,** and **chronic.** Hyperacute rejection is due to preformed antibodies against the donor organ, such as anti–blood group antibodies. Hyperacute rejection occurs within hours of the transplant and cannot be stopped with immunosuppressive drugs. It results in rapid necrosis and failure of the transplanted organ. Accelerated rejection is mediated by both antibodies and T cells, and it also cannot be stopped by immunosuppressive drugs. Acute rejection of an organ occurs within days to months and involves mainly cellular immunity. Reversal of acute rejection is usually possible with general immunosuppressive drugs such as azathioprine, mycophenolate mofetil, cyclosporine, tacrolimus, glucocorticoids, cyclophosphamide, methotrexate, and sirolimus. Recently, biologic agents such as anti-CD3 monoclonal antibodies have been used to stem acute rejection. Chronic rejection usually occurs months or even years after transplantation. It is characterized by thickening and fibrosis of the vasculature of the transplanted organ, involving both cellular and humoral immunity. Chronic rejection is treated with the same drugs as those used for acute rejection.

Allogeneic hematopoietic stem cell transplantation is a well-established treatment for many malignant and nonmalignant diseases. An HLA-matched donor, usually a family member, is located, patients are conditioned with high-dose chemotherapy and/or radiation therapy, and then donor stem cells are infused. The conditioning regimen is used not only to kill cancer cells in the case of malignant disease, but also to totally suppress the immune system so that the patient does not reject the donor stem cells. As patients' blood counts recover (after reduction by the conditioning regimen), they develop a new immune system that is created from the donor stem cells. Rejection of donor stem cells is uncommon and can be treated only by infusion of more stem cells from the donor.

GVH disease, however, is very common, occurring in the majority of patients who receive an allogeneic transplant. GVH disease occurs because donor T cells fail to recognize the patient's skin, liver, and gut (usually) as self and attack those tissues. Although patients are given immunosuppressive therapy (cyclosporine, methotrexate, and others) early in the transplant course to help prevent this development, it often occurs despite these medications. Acute GVH disease occurs within the first 100 days and is usually manifested as a skin rash, severe diarrhea, or hepatotoxicity. Additional medications are added, invariably starting with high-dose corticosteroids and adding drugs such as mycophenolate mofetil, sirolimus, tacrolimus, daclizumab, and others, with variable success rates. Patients generally progress to chronic GVH disease (after 100 days) and require therapy for variable periods thereafter. Unlike solid-organ transplant patients, however, most stem cell transplant patients are able to eventually discontinue immunosuppressive drugs as GVH disease resolves (usually 1–2 years after their transplant).

AUTOIMMUNE DISORDERS

The effectiveness of immunosuppressive drugs in autoimmune disorders varies widely. Nonetheless, with immunosuppressive therapy, remissions can be obtained in many instances of autoimmune hemolytic anemia, idiopathic thrombocytopenic purpura, type 1 diabetes, Hashimoto thyroiditis, and temporal arteritis. Improvement is also often seen in patients with systemic lupus erythematosus, acute glomerulonephritis, acquired factor VIII inhibitors (antibodies), rheumatoid arthritis, inflammatory myopathy, scleroderma, and certain other autoimmune states. Multiple sclerosis is an important autoimmune disease that responds variably to drugs in this class (see Box: Treatment of Multiple Sclerosis).

Immunosuppressive therapy is also utilized in chronic severe asthma, where cyclosporine is often effective and sirolimus is another alternative (see Chapter 20). Omalizumab (anti-IgE antibody) has been approved for the treatment of severe asthma (see previous section). Tacrolimus is currently under clinical investigation for the management of autoimmune chronic active hepatitis and of multiple sclerosis, where IFN-β has a definitive role.

Treatment of Multiple Sclerosis

Multiple sclerosis (MS) is a demyelinating autoimmune disease that affects the central nervous system. Three general types of MS are recognized: relapsing-remitting, secondary progressive, and primary progressive. For unknown reasons, the incidence of MS is higher in populations that live north of the 37th parallel than in populations living south of this parallel, and it is twice as common in women as in men. MS is caused by CD4-positive T cells (TH1 and TH17) reacting with myelin and secreting cytokines that attract inflammatory cells such as macrophages around the nerves, spinal cord, and brain. Patients may demonstrate weakness, paralysis, double vision, balance and bladder problems, and peripheral neuropathies. There is no cure for MS, but approved treatments to prevent or lengthen the time between attacks/episodes of relapsing-remitting MS are available. They are listed below and mentioned in the sections covering relevant drugs. Many drugs in addition to ofatumumab may be used off-label for MS due to its refractory nature.

Infused Drugs	Injectable Drugs	Oral Drugs
Alemtuzumab	Interferon β-1a and pegylated interferon β-1a	High-dose prednisone
Mitoxantrone	Glatiramer acetate	Teriflunomide
Ocrelizumab	Ofatumumab (off-label)	Fingolimod
Natalizumab		Cladribine
		Siponimod
		Dimethyl fumarate
		Diroximel fumarate

IMMUNOMODULATION THERAPY

The development of agents that modulate the immune response rather than suppress it has become an important area of pharmacology. The rationale underlying this approach is that such drugs may *increase* the immune responsiveness of patients who have either selective or generalized immunodeficiency. The major potential uses are in immunodeficiency disorders, chronic infectious diseases, and cancer. The AIDS epidemic has greatly increased interest in developing more effective immunomodulating drugs.

CYTOKINES

The cytokines are a large and heterogeneous group of proteins with diverse functions. Some are immunoregulatory proteins synthesized by leukocytes and play numerous interacting roles in the function of the immune system and in the control of hematopoiesis. The cytokines that have been clearly identified are summarized in Table 55–2. In most instances, cytokines mediate their effects through receptors on relevant target cells and appear to act in a manner similar to the mechanism of action of hormones. In other instances, cytokines may have antiproliferative, antimicrobial, and antitumor effects.

The first group of cytokines discovered, the interferons (IFNs), were followed by the colony-stimulating factors (CSFs, discussed in Chapter 33). The latter regulate the proliferation and differentiation of bone marrow progenitor cells. Most of the more recently discovered cytokines have been classified as interleukins (ILs) and numbered in the order of their discovery. Pharmaceutical cytokines are produced using gene cloning techniques.

Most cytokines (including TNF-α, IFN-γ, IL-2, G-CSF, and granulocyte-macrophage colony-stimulating factor [GM-CSF]) have very short serum half-lives (minutes). The usual subcutaneous route of administration provides slower release into the circulation and a longer duration of action. Each cytokine has its own unique toxicity, but some toxicities are shared. For example, IFN-α, IFN-β, IFN-γ, IL-2, and TNF-α all induce fever, flu-like symptoms, anorexia, fatigue, and malaise.

Interferons are proteins that are currently grouped into three families: **IFN-α, IFN-β,** and **IFN-γ.** The IFN-α and IFN-β families constitute type I IFNs, ie, acid-stable proteins that bind to the same receptor on target cells. IFN-γ, a type II IFN, is acid-labile and binds to a separate receptor on target cells. Type I IFNs are usually induced by virus infections, with leukocytes producing IFN-α. Fibroblasts and epithelial cells produce IFN-β. IFN-γ is usually the product of activated T lymphocytes.

IFNs interact with cell receptors to produce a wide variety of effects that depend on the cell and IFN types. IFNs, particularly IFN-γ, display immune-enhancing properties, which include increased antigen presentation and macrophage, NK cell, and cytotoxic T-lymphocyte activation. IFNs also inhibit cell proliferation. In this respect, IFN-α and IFN-β are more potent than IFN-γ. Another striking IFN action is increased expression of MHC molecules on cell surfaces. While all three types of IFN induce MHC class I molecules, only IFN-γ induces class II expression. In glial cells, IFN-β antagonizes this effect and may, in fact, decrease antigen presentation within the nervous system.

IFN-α is approved for the treatment of several neoplasms, including hairy cell leukemia, chronic myelogenous leukemia, malignant melanoma, and Kaposi sarcoma, and for treatment of hepatitis B and C infections. It has also shown activity as an anticancer agent in renal cell carcinoma, carcinoid syndrome, and T-cell leukemia. IFN-β is approved for use in relapsing-type multiple sclerosis. IFN-γ is approved for the treatment of chronic granulomatous disease, and IL-2 for metastatic renal cell carcinoma and malignant melanoma. Clinical investigations of other cytokines,

TABLE 55–2 The cytokines.

Cytokine	Properties
Interferon-α (IFN-α)	Antiviral, oncostatic, activates NK cells
Interferon-β (IFN-β)	Antiviral, oncostatic, activates NK cells
Interferon-γ (IFN-γ)	Antiviral, oncostatic, secreted by and activates or up-regulates TH1 cells, NK cells, CTLs, and macrophages
Interleukin-1 (IL-1)	T-cell activation, B-cell proliferation and differentiation
Interleukin-2 (IL-2)	T-cell proliferation, TH1, NK, and LAK cell activation
Interleukin-3 (IL-3)	Hematopoietic precursor proliferation and differentiation
Interleukin-4 (IL-4)	TH2 and CTL activation, B-cell proliferation
Interleukin-5 (IL-5)	Eosinophil proliferation, B-cell proliferation and differentiation
Interleukin-6 (IL-6)	HCF, TH2, CTL, and B-cell proliferation
Interleukin-7 (IL-7)	CTL, NK, LAK, and B-cell proliferation, thymic precursor stimulation
Interleukin-8 (IL-8)	Neutrophil chemotaxis, proinflammatory
Interleukin-9 (IL-9)	T-cell proliferation
Interleukin-10 (IL-10)	TH1 suppression, CTL activation, B-cell proliferation
Interleukin-11 (IL-11)	Megakaryocyte proliferation, B-cell differentiation
Interleukin-12 (IL-12)	TH1 and CTL proliferation and activation
Interleukin-13 (IL-13)	Macrophage function modulation, B-cell proliferation
Interleukin-14 (IL-14)	B-cell proliferation and differentiation
Interleukin-15 (IL-15)	TH1, CTL, and NK/LAK activation, expansion of T-cell memory pools
Interleukin-16 (IL-16)	T-lymphocyte chemotaxis, suppresses HIV replication
Interleukin-17 (IL-17)	Stromal cell cytokine production
Interleukin-18 (IL-18)	Induces TH1 responses
Interleukin-19 (IL-19)	Proinflammatory
Interleukin-20 (IL-20)	Promotes skin differentiation
Interleukin-21 (IL-21)	Promotes proliferation of activated T cells, maturation of NK cells
Interleukin-22 (IL-22)	Regulator of TH2 cells
Interleukin-23 (IL-23)	Promotes proliferation of TH1 memory cells
Interleukin-24 (IL-24)	Induces tumor apoptosis, induces TH1 responses
Interleukin-27 (IL-27)	Stimulates naive CD4 cells to produce IFN-γ
Interleukin-28 and -29 (IL-28, IL-29)	Antiviral, interferon-like properties
Interleukin-30 (IL-30)	p28 subunit of IL-27
Interleukin-31 (IL-31)	Contributes to type I hypersensitivities and TH2 responses
Interleukin-32 (IL-32)	Involved in inflammation
Interleukin-34 (IL-34)	Stimulates monocyte proliferation via the CSF-1 receptor (CSF-1R)
Interleukin-35 (IL-35)	Induces regulatory T cells (iT_R35)
Tumor necrosis factor-α (TNF-α)	Oncostatic, macrophage activation, proinflammatory
Tumor necrosis factor-β (TNF-β)	Oncostatic, proinflammatory, chemotactic
Granulocyte colony-stimulating factor	Granulocyte production
Granulocyte-macrophage colony-stimulating factor	Granulocyte, monocyte, eosinophil production
Macrophage colony-stimulating factor	Monocyte production, activation
Erythropoietin (epoetin, EPO)	Red blood cell production
Thrombopoietin (TPO)	Platelet production

Note: Many interleukin activities overlap and are influenced by each other.

HCF, hematopoietic cofactor; LAK, lymphokine-activated killer cell.

including IL-1, -3, -4, -6, -10, -11, and -12, are ongoing. Toxicities of IFNs, which include fever, chills, malaise, myalgias, myelosuppression, headache, and depression, can severely restrict their clinical use.

TNF-α has been extensively tested in the therapy of various malignancies, but results have been disappointing due to dose-limiting toxicities. One exception is the use of intra-arterial high-dose TNF-α for malignant melanoma and soft tissue sarcoma of the extremities. In these settings, response rates greater than 80% were noted.

Denileukin diftitox is IL-2 fused to diphtheria toxin, used for the treatment of patients with CD25+ cutaneous T-cell lymphomas. IL-12 and GM-CSF have also shown adjuvant effects with vaccines. GM-CSF is of particular interest because it promotes recruitment of professional antigen-presenting cells such as the dendritic cells required for priming naïve antigen-specific T-lymphocyte responses. There are some reports that GM-CSF can itself stimulate an antitumor immune response, resulting in tumor regression in melanoma and prostate cancer.

It is important to emphasize that cytokine interactions with target cells often result in the release of a cascade of different endogenous cytokines, which exert their effects sequentially or simultaneously. For example, IFN-γ exposure increases the number of cell-surface receptors on target cells for TNF-α. Therapy with IL-2 induces the production of TNF-α, while experimental therapy with IL-12 induces the production of IFN-γ.

■ IMMUNOLOGIC REACTIONS TO DRUGS & DRUG ALLERGY

The basic immune mechanism and the ways in which it can be suppressed or stimulated by drugs have been discussed in previous sections of this chapter. Drugs also activate the immune system in undesirable ways that are manifested as adverse drug reactions. These reactions are generally grouped in a broad classification as "drug allergy." Indeed, many drug reactions such as those to penicillin, iodides, phenytoin, and sulfonamides are allergic in nature. These drug reactions are manifested as skin eruptions, edema, anaphylactoid reactions, glomerulonephritis, fever, and eosinophilia.

Drug reactions mediated by immune responses can have several different mechanisms. Thus, any of the four major types of hypersensitivity discussed earlier in this chapter can be associated with allergic drug reactions:

- **Type I:** IgE-mediated acute allergic reactions to stings, pollens, and drugs, including anaphylaxis, urticaria, and angioedema. IgE is fixed to tissue mast cells and blood basophils, and after interaction with antigen the cells release potent mediators.
- **Type II:** Drugs often modify host proteins, thereby eliciting antibody responses to the modified protein. These allergic responses involve IgG or IgM in which the antibody becomes fixed to a host cell, which is then subject to complement-dependent lysis or to antibody-dependent cellular cytotoxicity.
- **Type III:** Drugs may cause serum sickness, which involves immune complexes containing IgG complexed with a foreign antigen and is a multisystem complement-dependent vasculitis that may also result in urticaria.
- **Type IV:** Cell-mediated allergy is the mechanism involved in allergic contact dermatitis from topically applied drugs or induration of the skin at the site of an antigen injected intradermally.

In some drug reactions, several of these hypersensitivity responses may occur simultaneously.

Some adverse reactions to drugs may be mistakenly classified as allergic or immune when they are actually genetic deficiency states or are idiosyncratic and not mediated by immune mechanisms (eg, hemolysis due to primaquine in glucose-6-phosphate dehydrogenase deficiency, or aplastic anemia caused by chloramphenicol). See Figure 55–6.

IMMEDIATE (TYPE I) DRUG ALLERGY

Type I (immediate) sensitivity allergy to certain drugs occurs when the drug, not capable of inducing an immune response by itself, covalently links to a host carrier protein (hapten). When this happens, the immune system detects the drug-hapten conjugate as "modified self" and responds by generating IgE antibodies specific for the drug-hapten. It is not known why some patients mount an IgE response to a drug while others mount IgG responses. Under the influence of IL-4, -5, and -13 secreted by TH2 cells, B cells specific for the drug secrete IgE antibody. The mechanism for IgE-mediated immediate hypersensitivity is diagrammed in Figure 55–5.

Fixation of the IgE antibody to high-affinity Fc receptors (FcεRs) on blood basophils or their tissue equivalent (mast cells) sets the stage for an acute allergic reaction. The most important sites for mast cell distribution are skin, nasal epithelium, lung, and gastrointestinal tract. When the offending drug is reintroduced into the body, it binds and cross-links basophil and mast cell-surface IgE to signal release of the mediators (eg, histamine, leukotrienes; see Chapters 16 and 18) from granules. Mediator release is associated with calcium influx and a fall in intracellular cAMP within the mast cell. Many of the drugs that block mediator release appear to act through the cAMP mechanism (eg, catecholamines, glucocorticoids, theophylline), others block histamine release, and still others block histamine receptors. Other vasoactive substances such as kinins also may be generated during histamine release. These mediators initiate immediate vascular smooth muscle relaxation, increased vascular permeability, hypotension, edema, and bronchoconstriction.

Drug Treatment of Immediate Allergy

One can test an individual for possible sensitivity to a drug by a simple scratch test, ie, by applying an extremely dilute solution of the drug to the skin and making a scratch with the tip of a needle. If allergy is present, an immediate (within 10–15 minutes) wheal (edema) and flare (increased blood flow) will occur. However, skin tests may be negative in spite of IgE hypersensitivity to a hapten or to a metabolic product of the drug, especially if the patient is taking steroids or antihistamines.

Drugs that modify allergic responses act at several links in this chain of events. Prednisone, often used in severe allergic reactions, is immunosuppressive; it blocks proliferation of the IgE-producing clones and inhibits IL-4 production by T helper cells in the IgE response, since glucocorticoids are generally toxic to lymphocytes. In the efferent limb of the allergic response, isoproterenol, epinephrine, and theophylline reduce the release of mediators from mast cells and basophils and produce bronchodilation. Epinephrine opposes histamine; it relaxes bronchiolar smooth muscle and contracts vascular muscle, relieving both bronchospasm and hypotension. *As noted in* Chapter 9, *epinephrine is the drug of choice in anaphylactic reactions.* The antihistamines competitively inhibit histamine, which would otherwise produce bronchoconstriction and increased capillary permeability in end organs. Glucocorticoids may also act to reduce tissue injury and edema in the inflamed tissue, as well as facilitating the actions of catecholamines in cells that may have become refractory to epinephrine or isoproterenol. Several agents directed toward the inhibition of leukotrienes may be useful in acute allergic and inflammatory disorders (see Chapter 20).

Desensitization to Drugs

When reasonable alternatives are not available, certain drugs (eg, penicillin, insulin) must be used for life-threatening illnesses even in the presence of known allergic sensitivity. In such cases, desensitization (also called hyposensitization) can sometimes be accomplished by starting with very small doses of the drug and gradually increasing the dose over a period of hours or days to the full therapeutic range (see Chapter 43). This practice is hazardous and must be performed under direct medical supervision with epinephrine available for immediate injection, as anaphylaxis may occur before desensitization has been achieved. It is thought that slow and progressive administration of the drug gradually binds all available IgE on mast cells, triggering a gradual release of granules. Once all of the IgE on the mast cell surfaces has been bound and the cells have been degranulated, therapeutic doses of the offending drug may be given with minimal further immune reaction. Therefore, a patient is desensitized only during administration of the drug.

AUTOIMMUNE (TYPE II) REACTIONS TO DRUGS

Certain autoimmune syndromes can be induced by drugs. Examples include systemic lupus erythematosus following hydralazine or procainamide therapy, "lupoid hepatitis" due to cathartic sensitivity, autoimmune hemolytic anemia resulting from methyldopa administration, thrombocytopenic purpura due to quinidine, and agranulocytosis due to a variety of drugs. As indicated in other chapters of this book, a number of drugs are associated with type I and type II reactions. In these drug-induced autoimmune states, IgG antibodies bind to drug-modified tissue and are destroyed by the complement system or by phagocytic cells with Fc receptors. Fortunately, autoimmune reactions to drugs usually subside within several months after the offending drug is withdrawn. Immunosuppressive therapy is warranted only when the autoimmune response is unusually severe.

SERUM SICKNESS & VASCULITIC (TYPE III) REACTIONS

Immunologic reactions to drugs resulting in serum sickness are more common than immediate anaphylactic responses, but type II and type III hypersensitivities often overlap. The clinical features of serum sickness include urticarial and erythematous skin eruptions, arthralgia or arthritis, lymphadenopathy, glomerulonephritis, peripheral edema, and fever. The reactions generally last 6–12 days and usually subside once the offending drug is eliminated. Antibodies of the IgM or IgG class are usually involved. The mechanism of tissue injury is immune complex formation and deposition on basement membranes (eg, lung, kidney), followed by complement activation and infiltration of leukocytes, causing tissue destruction. Glucocorticoids are useful in attenuating severe serum sickness reactions to drugs. In severe cases, plasmapheresis can be used to remove the offending drug and immune complexes from circulation.

Immune vasculitis can also be induced by drugs. The sulfonamides, penicillin, thiouracil, anticonvulsants, and iodides all have been implicated in the initiation of hypersensitivity angiitis. Erythema multiforme is a relatively mild vasculitic skin disorder that may be secondary to drug hypersensitivity. Stevens-Johnson syndrome is probably a more severe form of this hypersensitivity reaction and consists of erythema multiforme, arthritis, nephritis, central nervous system abnormalities, and myocarditis. It frequently has been associated with sulfonamide therapy. Administration of nonhuman monoclonal or polyclonal antibodies such as rattlesnake antivenom may cause serum sickness.

CELL-MEDIATED (TYPE IV) REACTIONS

Type IV hypersensitivity occurs 24–48 hours after exposure to the allergen and therefore is called delayed type hypersensitivity (DTH). Like other drug hypersensitivities, the drug may chemically react with host tissue to create a new antigen. Upon first exposure to the allergen (drug), antigen-presenting cells stimulate a T-cell response specific for that allergen. This takes 1–2 weeks. Upon second and all subsequent exposures, tissue-derived antigen-presenting cells that come in contact with the new antigen (allergen-modified host protein) secrete chemokines and cytokines that attract memory T cells to the site of allergen re-exposure. This takes only 24–48 hours. Lymphocytes and antigen-presenting cells such as macrophages accumulate at the site, causing induration, erythema, and swelling. Contact hypersensitivity is a form of DTH and occurs when an allergen elicits DTH on the skin, resulting in spongiosis such as when an ointment containing an allergen is applied to skin.

PREPARATIONS AVAILABLE*

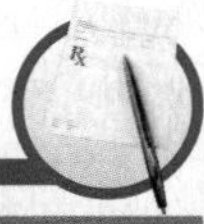

GENERIC NAME	AVAILABLE AS
Abatacept	Orencia
Abciximab	ReoPro
Adalimumab	Humira
Ado-trastuzumab emtansine	Kadcyla
Alemtuzumab	Campath and Lemtrada
Alirocumab	Praluent
Amivantamab, amivantamab	Rybrevant
Anakinra	Kineret
Anifrolumab	Saphnelo
Ansuvimab	Ebanga
Antithymocyte globulin	Thymoglobulin
Arcitumomab	CEA-Scan
Atezolizumab	Tecentriq
Atoltivimab, maftivimab, and odesivimab	Inmazeb
Avelumab	Bavencio
Axicabtagene ciloleucel	Yescarta
Azathioprine	Generic, Imuran
Basiliximab	Simulect
Belantamab mafodotin	Blenrep
Belatacept	Nulojix
Belimumab	Benlysta
Benralizumab	Fasenra
Bevacizumab	Avastin
Blinatumomab	Blincyto
Brentuximab vedotin	Adcetris
Brexucabtagene autoleucel	Tecartus
Brodalumab	Siliq
Brolucizumab	Beovu
Burosumab	Crysvita
Canakinumab	Ilaris
Caplacizumab	Cablivi
Capromab pendetide	ProstaScint
Cemiplimab	Libtayo
Certolizumab pegol	Cimzia
Cetuximab	Erbitux
Ciltacabtagene autoleucel	Carvykti
Crizanlizumab	Adakveo
Cyclophosphamide	Generic
Cyclosporine	Generic, Sandimmune, Restasis
Daratumumab	Darzalex
Denileukin diftitox	Ontak
Denosumab	Prolia
Dimethyl fumarate	Tecfidera
Dinutuximab	Unituxin
Dostarlimab	Jemperli
Dupilumab	Dupixent
Durvalumab	Imfinzi
Eculizumab	Soliris
Elotuzumab	Empliciti
Emapalumab-lzsg	Gamifant
Enfortumab vedotin	Padcev
Eptinezumab	Vyepti

GENERIC NAME	AVAILABLE AS
Erenumab-aooe	Aimovig
Etanercept	Enbrel
Everolimus	Afinitor, Zortress
Evinacumab	Evkeeza
Evolocumab	Repatha
Faricimab	Vabysmo
Fingolimod hydrochloride	Gilenya
Fremanezumab-vfrm	Ajovy
Galcanezumab-gnlm	Emgality
Glatiramer acetate	Copaxone
Golimumab	Simponi
Guselkumab	Tremfya
Ibalizumab	Trogarzo
Ibritumomab tiuxetan	Zevalin
Idarucizumab	Praxbind
Idecabtagene vicleucel	Abecma
Immune globulin intravenous [IGIV]	Various
Inebilizumab	Uplizna
Infliximab	Remicade
Inotuzumab ozogamicin	Elzonris
Interferon alfa-2a	Roferon
Interferon alfa-2b	Intron-A
Interferon beta-1a	Avonex, Rebif
Interferon beta-1b	Betaseron, Extavia
Interferon gamma-1b	Actimmune
Interleukin 2 (IL-2, aldesleukin)	Proleukin
Ipilimumab	Yervoy
Isatuximab	Sarclisa
Ixekizumab	Taltz
Lanadelumab	Takhzyro
Leflunomide	Arava
Lenalidomide	Revlimid
Lisocabtagene maraleucel	Breyanzi
Loncastuximab tesirine	Zynlonta
Lymphocyte immune globulin	Atgam
Margetuximab	Margenza
Mepolizumab	Nucala
Mogamulizumab	Poteligeo
Moxetumomab pasudotox-tdfk	Lumoxiti
Muromonab CD3	OKT3
Mycophenolate mofetil	Generic, CellCept
Natalizumab	Tysabri
Naxitamab	Danyelza
Necitumumab	Portrazza
Nivolumab	Opdivo
Obiltoxaximab	Anthim
Ocrelizumab	Ocrevus
Ofatumumab	Arzerra
Omalizumab	Xolair
Palivizumab	Synagis
Panitumumab	Vectibix
Pegademase bovine (bovine adenosine deaminase)	Adagen

(*continued*)

GENERIC NAME	AVAILABLE AS	GENERIC NAME	AVAILABLE AS
Pegaptanib	Macugen	Siltuximab	Sylvant
Peginterferon alfa-2a	Pegasys	Siplizumab	
Peginterferon alfa-2b	PEG-Intron	Sirolimus	Generic, Rapamune
Pembrolizumab	Keytruda	Spesolimab	Spevigo
Pertuzumab	Perjeta	Sutimlimab	Enjaymo
Polatuzumab vedotin-piiq	Polivy	Tacrolimus (FK 506)	Generic, Prograf, others
Pomalidomide	Pomalyst	Teriflunomide	Aubagio
Ramucirumab	Cyramza	Tafasitamab	Monjuvi
Ranibizumab	Lucentis	Teclistamab	Tecvayli
Ravulizumab	Ultomiris	Teprotumumab	Teprezza
Raxibacumab	ABthrax	Tezepelumab	Tezspire
Relatlimab (relatlimab + nivolumab combo)	Opdualag	Thalidomide	Thalomid
Reslizumab	Cinqair	Tisotumab vedotin	Tivdak
Rh_o(D) immune globulin micro-dose	RhoGAM, others	Tildrakizumab	Ilumya
Rilonacept	Arcalyst	Tisagenlecleucel	Kymriah
Risankizumab-rzaa	Skyrizi	Tocilizumab	Actemra
Rituximab	Rituxan	Trastuzumab	Herceptin
Romosozumab	Evenity	fam-trastuzumab deruxtecan	Enhertu
Sacituzumab govitecan	Trodelvy	Tralokinumab	Adtralza
Satralizumab	Enspryng	Tremelimumab	Imjudo
Scorpion antivenom (equine (Fab)'2)	Anascorp	Ustekinumab	Stelara
Secukinumab	Cosentyx	Vedolizumab	Entyvio

[*]Several drugs discussed in this chapter are available as orphan drugs but are not listed here. Other drugs not listed here will be found in other chapters (see Index).

REFERENCES

General Immunology

Levinson WE: *Review of Medical Microbiology and Immunology*, 17th ed. McGraw Hill, 2022.

Murphy KM et al (editors): *Janeway's Immunobiology*, 10th ed. Garland Science, 2022.

Wei SC et al: Fundamental mechanisms of immune checkpoint blockade therapy. Cancer Discov 2018;8:1069.

Hypersensitivity

Brusselle GG et al: Biologic therapies for severe asthma. N Engl J Med 2022;386:157.

Waldron JL et al: Hypersensitivity and immune-related adverse events in biologic therapy. Clin Rev Allergy Immunol 2022;62:413.

Autoimmunity

Patil S et al: Exploring the role of immunotherapeutic drugs in autoimmune diseases: A comprehensive review. J Oral Biol Craniofac Res 2021; 11:291.

Kaegi C et al: Systematic review of safety and efficacy of second and third-generation CD20-targeting biologics in treating immune-mediated disorders. Front Immunol 2021;12:788.

Immunodeficiency Diseases

Freeman CM et al: Immunoglobulin treatment for B cell immunodeficiencies. J Immunol Methods 2022;509:113336.

Immunosuppressive Agents

Meyer F et al: Safety of biologic treatments in solid organ transplant recipients: A systematic review. Semin Arthritis Rheum 2021;51:1263.

Privitera G et al: Novel trends with biologics in inflammatory bowel disease: sequential and combined approaches. Therap Adv Gastroenterol 2021;14;1.

Hamilton BK: Updates in chronic graft-versus-host disease. Hematology 2021;1:648.

Antilymphocyte Globulin & Monoclonal Antibodies

Panackel C et al: Immunosuppressive drugs in liver transplant: an insight. J Clin Exp Hepatol 2022;12:1557.

Goleva E et al: Our current understanding of checkpoint inhibitor therapy in cancer immunotherapy. Ann Allergy Asthma Immunol 2021;126:630.

Cytokines

Propper DJ, Balkwill FR: Harnessing cytokines and chemokines for cancer therapy. Nat Rev Clin Oncol 2022;19:237.

Tuzlak S et al: Repositioning TH cel polarization from single cytokines to complex help. Nat Immunol 2021;22:1210.

Drug Allergy

Macy E et al: Advances in the understanding of drug hypersensitivity: 2012–2022. J Allergy Clin Immunol Pract 2023;11:805.

Cellular Immunotherapy

Fischer JW, Bhattarai N: CAR-T cell therapy: Mechanism, management and mitigation of inflammatory toxicities. Front Immunol 2021;12:693016.

CASE STUDY ANSWER

This patient has steroid-refractory acute GVHD. Pharmacologic management would include additional immunosuppressive therapy. The standard of care is not established in this very serious condition; multiple ongoing clinical trials are evaluating various therapies. At this time, many centers would initiate therapy for acute steroid-refractory GVHD with infliximab and photopheresis in addition to continuing tacrolimus.

SECTION IX TOXICOLOGY

CHAPTER 56

Introduction to Toxicology: Occupational & Environmental

Alison K. Bauer, PhD*

CASE STUDY

A 6-year-old girl is brought to the emergency department by her parents. She is comatose, tachypneic (25 breaths per minute), and tachycardic (150 bpm), but she appears flushed, and fingertip pulse oximetry is normal (97%) breathing room air. Questioning of her parents reveals that they are homeless and have been living in their car (a small van). The nights have been cold, and they have used a small charcoal burner to keep warm inside the vehicle. What is the most likely diagnosis? What treatment should be instituted immediately? If her mother is pregnant, what additional measures should be taken?

Humans live in a chemical world. They inhale, ingest, and absorb through the skin many of these chemicals. The occupational-environmental toxicologist is primarily concerned with the recognition, prevention, and treatment of adverse effects in humans that may result from exposure to chemicals encountered at work or in the general environment. In clinical practice, the occupational-environmental toxicologist must identify and treat the adverse health effects of these exposures. In addition, the trained occupational-environmental toxicologist will be called upon to assess and identify hazards associated with chemicals used in the workplace or introduced into the human environment, and to develop strategies and procedures to prevent the ill effects of the identified chemical hazards. A major hazard that has changed during the past 10 years that needs our focus is exposures caused by climate change, such as increased air pollution due to wildfires or urban fires that affects both workers and the human environment.

Occupational and environmental (OE) toxicology cases present complex problems. Exposure is rarely limited to a single type

*The author thanks Daniel T. Teitelbaum, MD, emeritus, and the late Gabriel L. Plaa, PhD, the previous author's of this chapter, for their enduring contributions.

of molecule. Most workplace or environmental materials are compounds or mixtures. The ingredients are often poorly described in the documentation available for review. Moreover, although regulatory agencies in many countries have requirements for disclosure of hazardous materials and their health impacts, proprietary information exclusions often make it difficult for those who treat OE-poisoned patients to understand the nature and scope of the presenting illness. Because many of these illnesses have long latency periods before they become manifest, it is often a matter of detective work to uncover and characterize the original processes and causal materials. Monitoring of exposure concentrations both in the workplace and in the general environment has become more common. However, the records of monitoring are often difficult to locate and to relate to an individual or small group of exposed individuals. The records that are available often are inadequate to establish the extent of the person or group's exposure, its duration, and its dose rate. This information may be critical to the clinical and forensic identification of the toxic disorder and its management.

Occupational Toxicology

Occupational toxicology deals with the effects of chemicals found in the workplace. The major emphasis of occupational toxicology is to identify the agents of concern, identify the acute and chronic diseases that they cause, define the conditions under which they may be used safely, and prevent absorption of harmful amounts of these chemicals. The occupational toxicologist will also be called upon to treat the diseases caused by these chemicals if he or she is a physician. Occupational toxicologists may also define and carry out programs for the surveillance of exposed workers and the environment in which they work. They frequently work with occupational hygienists, certified safety professionals, and occupational health nurses in their activities.

Regulatory limits and voluntary guidelines have been elaborated to establish "safe" chemical exposure limits for workers. In the USA these limits are promulgated by the Occupational Safety and Health Administration (OSHA). They are denoted **Permissible Exposure Limits (PELs).** In addition to the PELs that appear in tables in OSHA publications and on the website, OSHA promulgates standards for specific materials of particularly serious toxicity. These standards are developed following extensive scientific study, stakeholder input at hearings, public comment, and other steps such as publication in the *Federal Register*. Such standards have the force of law in the USA, and employers who use these materials are obligated to comply with the standards. Failure to comply with the standards may result in a range of civil penalties. OSHA has no authority to prosecute criminal violations of its rules and standards. OSHA standards may be found in full on the OSHA website at www.osha.gov. Copies of the US Mine Safety and Health Administration (MSHA) standards may be found at www.msha.gov.

Voluntary organizations, such as the American Conference of Governmental Industrial Hygienists (ACGIH), periodically prepare lists of their consensus versions of "safe" **threshold limit values (TLVs)** for many chemicals. These are not enforceable and have legal standing only in limited circumstances. Regulatory imperatives in the United States may be updated from time to time when new information about toxicity becomes available. The process is slow and requires input from many sources except under certain extraordinary circumstances. In those cases, alterations to standards may be made and an emergency temporary standard may be promulgated after appropriate regulatory procedures. The ACGIH TLV guidelines are useful as reference points in the evaluation of potential workplace exposures in the absence of OSHA requirements. Compliance with these voluntary guidelines is not a substitute for compliance with the OSHA regulations in the United States. Current TLV lists may be obtained from the ACGIH at www.acgih.org.

Environmental Toxicology

Environmental toxicology, now often called *ecotoxicology*, deals with the deleterious impact of chemicals, present as *pollutants* in the environment, on living organisms. Ecotoxicology is concerned with the toxic effects of chemical and physical agents on populations and communities of living organisms within defined ecosystems. It includes study of the transfer pathways of those agents and their interactions with the environment. Traditional toxicology is concerned with toxic effects on individual organisms; ecotoxicology is concerned with the impact on populations of living organisms or on ecosystems. Ecotoxicology research has become one of the foremost areas of study for toxicologists.

Changes in the condition of our planet's air and water is the major international concern. Treaties negotiated among many nations designed to control pollutants that impact climate change are in effect. Climate change is the most important priority for environmental scientists. The Paris Climate Accords seek to reduce global greenhouse gas emissions, largely generated by fossil fuels, that have led to increased temperatures and the subsequent effects of those increased temperatures, such as wildfires and artic warming. As of Jan 20, 2021, the USA is again participating in these critical accords. In addition, the current administration supports many climate adaptation and resilience plans to mitigate climate change effects, such as the DOD climate assessment tool (media.defense.gov/2021/Apr/05/2002614579/-1/-1/0/DOD-CLIMATE-ASSESSMENT-TOOL.PDF).

The term *environment* includes all the surroundings of an individual organism, but particularly the air, soil, and water. Although humans are considered a target species of particular interest, other species are of considerable importance as potential ecotoxicologic targets. Scientific study of adverse health effects in in animals often provides early warning of impending human events as a result of ecotoxic impacts and these species are called indicator species, such as most *Mustelidae* (eg, minks) and amphibians (eg, frogs). In the USA, environmental pollution is regulated by the Environmental Protection Agency (EPA). Its agents have police-like powers and may impose both civil and criminal penalties for violations of EPA regulations.

Before now, air pollution was typically considered a product of industrialization, technologic development, and increased urbanization. However, the increased number of recent wildland fires across the country and world changed the sources of air pollutants, for example, particulate matter (PM, see below). In fact, in the US, wildland fires are now the largest source of PM emissions to the atmosphere. Although rare, natural phenomena such as volcanic eruptions may result in air pollution with gases, vapors, or particulates that are harmful to humans. Humans may also be exposed to chemicals used in the agricultural environment as pesticides or in food processing that may persist as residues or ingredients in food products. Air contaminants are regulated in the USA by the EPA based on both health-based (primary) and esthetic (secondary) considerations. The Clean Air Act requires the EPA to have set National Ambient Air Quality Standards (NAAQS), and the six criteria air pollutants are listed in Table 56–1. Additonal tables of primary and secondary regulated air contaminants and other regulatory issues that relate to air contaminants in the USA may be found at www.epa.gov. Many states within the USA also have individual air contaminant regulations that may be more rigorous than those of the EPA, such as California. Many other nations and some supragovernmental organizations regulate air contaminants. In the case of adjoining countries, transborder air and water pollution problems have been of concern in recent years. Particulates, radionuclides, acid rain, and similar problems have resulted in cross-contamination of air and water in different countries. Maritime contamination, too, has raised concern about oceanic pollution and has had an impact on the fisheries of some countries. This type of pollution is now the subject of much research and of new international treaties.

The United Nations Food and Agriculture Organization and the World Health Organization (FAO/WHO) Joint Expert Commission on Food Additives adopted the term *acceptable daily intake (ADI)* to denote the daily intake of a chemical from food that, during an entire lifetime, appears to be without appreciable risk. These guidelines are reevaluated as new information becomes available. In the USA, the Food and Drug Administration (FDA) and the Department of Agriculture are responsible for the regulation of contaminants such as pesticides, drugs, and chemicals in foods. Major international problems have occurred because of traffic among nations in contaminated or adulterated foods from countries whose regulations and enforcement of pure food and drug laws are lax or nonexistent. For example, both human and animal illnesses have resulted from ingestion of products imported from China that contained melamine.

TABLE 56–1 Examples of OSHA standards (permissible exposure limit values [PELs]) and EPA standards of the criteria air pollutants.

	OSHA Standards[1]	EPA NAAQS Standards[3]	
Compound	**PEL[2] (ppm)**	**Averaging Time**	**EPA Primary Standard (1-h level/8-h levels)[4]**
Carbon monoxide	50 ppm	8 h	9 ppm
		1 h	35 ppm
Lead (Pb)[5]	50 ug/m^3	Rolling 3-month average	0.15 mcg/m^3
Nitrogen dioxide	5 ppm	1 h	100 ppb
		1 year	53 ppb
Ozone	0.1 ppm	8 h	0.07 ppm
Particulate matter $(PM)_{2.5}$	By specific type; see OSHA Table Z-1[1]	1 year	12 mcg/m^3
		24 h	35 mcg/m^3
Sulfur dioxide	5 ppm	1 h	75 ppm

[1]These exposure limits can be found at www.osha.gov, 1910.1000, Tables Z-1 and Z-2 (www.osha.gov/laws-regs/regulations/standardnumber/1910/1910.1000TABLEZ1 and www.osha.gov/laws-regs/regulations/standardnumber/1910/1910.1000TABLEZ2). The OSHA standards are updated frequently, and readers are referred to the website for the most current information.

[2]PELs are 8-hour time-weighted average (TWA) values for a normal 8-hour workday to which workers may be repeatedly exposed without adverse effects.

[3]These EPA standards and more details can be found at www.epa.gov/criteria-air-pollutants/naaqs-table.

[4]Primary standard for criteria air pollutants that provides public health protection, including protecting the health of "sensitive" populations (www.epa.gov/criteria-air-pollutants/naaqs-table).

[5]See Chapter 57 for more details about current OSHA blood lead levels.

TOXICOLOGIC TERMS & DEFINITIONS

Hazard & Risk

Hazard is the ability of a chemical agent to cause injury in a given situation or setting; the conditions of use and exposure are primary considerations. To assess hazard, one needs to have knowledge about both the inherent toxicity of the substance and the amounts to which individuals are liable to be exposed. Hazard is often a description based on subjective estimates rather than objective evaluation.

Risk is defined as the expected frequency of the occurrence of an undesirable effect arising from exposure to a chemical or physical agent. Estimation of risk makes use of dose-response data and extrapolation from the observed relationships to the expected responses at doses occurring in actual exposure situations. The quality and suitability of the biologic data used in such estimates are major limiting factors. Risk assessment has become an integral part of the regulatory process in most countries. However, many of the assumptions of risk assessment scientists remain unproven, and only long-term observation of population causes and outcomes will provide the basis for validation of newer risk assessment technologies.

Routes of Exposure

The route of entry for chemicals into the body differs in different exposure situations. In the industrial setting, inhalation is the major route of entry. The transdermal route is also quite important, but oral ingestion is a relatively minor route. Consequently, primary prevention should be designed to reduce or eliminate absorption by inhalation or by topical contact. Atmospheric pollutants gain entry by inhalation and by dermal contact. Water and soil pollutants are absorbed through inhalation, ingestion, and dermal contact.

Quantity, Duration, & Intensity of Exposure

Toxic reactions may differ depending on the quantity of exposure, its duration, and the rate at which the exposure takes place.

An exposure to a toxic substance that is absorbed by the target human or animal results in a dose. Acute exposure indicates a single exposure or multiple exposures that occur over a brief period from seconds to 1–2 days. Intense, rapidly absorbed acute doses of substances that may ordinarily be detoxified by enzymatic mechanisms in small doses may overwhelm the body's ability to detoxify the substance and may result in serious or even fatal toxicity. The same amount of the substance, absorbed slowly, may result in little or no toxicity. This is the case with cyanide exposure. Rhodanese, a mitochondrial enzyme present in humans, effectively detoxifies cyanide to relatively nontoxic thiocyanate when cyanide is presented in small amounts, but the enzyme is overwhelmed (or saturated) by large, rapidly encountered cyanide doses, with lethal effect.

Single or multiple exposures over a longer period of time represent chronic exposure. In the occupational setting, both acute (eg, accidental discharge) and chronic (eg, repetitive handling of a chemical) exposures occur. Exposures to chemicals as air and water pollutants are often chronic. They may cause chronic disease, as in the Minamata Bay, Japan, waterborne industrially generated methyl mercury disaster. Itai-itai disease in Japan, caused by a chronic waterborne industrial pollutant exposure to cadmium, began as far back as 1912 but was only officially recognized as an environmental disease by the Japanese government in 1968. Sudden large chemical releases may result in acute massive population exposure with serious or lethal consequences. The disaster in Bhopal, India in 1984, was such an event. Methyl isocyanate was released into a crowded population area. It caused almost 4000 deaths and more than half a million injuries. The release of dioxin in Seveso, Italy in 1976, contaminated a populated area with a persistent organic chemical and caused both acute and long-term chronic effects. The massive oil spill caused by the explosion of BP's Deepwater Horizon drilling rig in 2010 in the Gulf of Mexico highlighted the potential for long-term ecotoxic impacts on a widespread geographic area. Extensive studies of the effects of this environmental disaster are still underway, and the total environmental consequences remain to be determined; some species, such as the bottlenose dolphin, may have multigenerational adverse effects.

ENVIRONMENTAL CONSIDERATIONS

Certain chemical and physical characteristics are important for the estimation of the potential hazard of environmental toxicants. Data on toxic effects of different organisms, along with knowledge about degradability, bioaccumulation, and transport and biomagnification through food chains, help in this estimation. (See Box: Bioaccumulation & Biomagnification for a classic example involving the Great Lakes.) Poorly degraded chemicals (by abiotic or biotic pathways) exhibit environmental persistence and can accumulate. Such chemicals include the persistent organic pollutants (POPs)—polychlorinated biphenyls, dioxins and furans, and similar substances. Methyl mercury discharges from paper mills in Scandinavia have been responsible for bioaccumulation of mercury compounds in higher marine mammals and fish higher in the food chain. These compounds have been responsible for neurotoxic outcomes in human populations whose diets include these organisms as food sources. Lipophilic substances such as the largely banned or abandoned organochlorine pesticides tend to bioaccumulate in body fat. This results in tissue residues that are slowly released over time. These residues and their metabolites may have chronic adverse effects such as endocrine disruption, neurologic disorders, and carcinogenesis. When a persistent toxicant enters the food chain, biomagnification occurs as one species feeds on others. This concentrates the chemical in organisms higher on the food chain. Humans stand at the apex of the food chain. They may be exposed to highly concentrated pollutant loads as bioaccumulation and biomagnification occur. The pollutants that have the widest environmental impact are poorly degradable; are relatively mobile in air, water, and soil; exhibit bioaccumulation; and also exhibit biomagnification.

Bioaccumulation & Biomagnification

If the intake of a long-lasting contaminant by an organism exceeds the latter's ability to metabolize or excrete the substance, the chemical accumulates within the tissues of the organism. This is called **bioaccumulation.**

Although the concentration of a contaminant may be virtually undetectable in water, it may be magnified hundreds or thousands of times as the contaminant passes up the food chain. This is called **biomagnification.**

The biomagnification of polychlorinated biphenyls (PCBs) in the Great Lakes of North America is illustrated by the following residue values available from a classic *Environment Canada* report published by the Canadian government, and elsewhere.

The biomagnification for this substance in the food chain, beginning with phytoplankton and ending with the herring gull, is nearly 50,000-fold. Domestic animals and humans may eat fish from the Great Lakes, resulting in PCB residues in these species as well.

Source	PCB Concentration (ppm)[1]	Concentration Relative to Phytoplankton
Phytoplankton	0.0025	1
Zooplankton	0.123	49.2
Rainbow smelt	1.04	416
Lake trout	4.83	1932
Herring gull	124	49,600

[1]Data from Environment Canada, *The State of Canada's Environment*, 1991, Government of Canada, Ottawa; and other publications.

SPECIFIC CHEMICALS

AIR POLLUTANTS

Air pollution may result from vapors, aerosols, smoke, particulates, and individual chemicals. There are six EPA priority air pollutants, one of which will be discussed in Chapter 57 (lead). The other five major substances in air pollution are carbon monoxide, sulfur oxides, nitrogen oxides, ozone, and particulate matter. Agriculture, especially industrial-scale farming, contributes a variety of air pollutants: dusts as particulates, pesticidal chemicals, hydrogen sulfide, and others. Sources of pollutants include fossil fuel burning, transportation, manufacturing, other industrial activities, generation of electric power, space heating, refuse disposal, and others. Studies in Helsinki and other cities have shown that uncatalyzed automobile traffic emissions are larger contributors to ground-level air pollution than any other source. The introduction of catalytic converters on automobiles and their mandatory use in many countries has greatly reduced automobile-released air pollution. The ban on tetraethyl lead in gasoline has eliminated a major source of lead contamination and childhood lead poisoning in urban environments. In emerging economies, the use of transport based on two-cycle engines creates heavy ground-level air pollution in very crowded cities. The introduction of "clean, low-sulfur" diesel fuels is helping to reduce urban and highway pollutants such as sulfur oxides. Some cities are also switching to electric buses (both public and school) and taxis to further reduce air pollution, such as Denver, Colorado. Recent intensive studies of a broader range of impacts of air pollutants as varied as nitrogen dioxide, particulate matter, and sulfur dioxide have demonstrated statistically significant adverse effects on pregnancy outcome, increased incidence of pre-eclampsia, poor cardiovascular outcomes, exacerbation of symptoms in chronic obstructive pulmonary disease (COPD), increased mental health issues, and aggravation of symptoms in patients with idiopathic pulmonary fibrosis. Many other meaningful physiologic alterations in humans, especially in children, are suspected as a result of air pollutants. This chapter will not cover the effects of mixtures of these air pollutants, such as TRAP (traffic-related air pollution), but it is notable that mixture effects of these pollutants do lead to significant increases in adverse health effects.

Sulfur dioxide and smoke from incomplete combustion of coal have been associated with acute adverse effects among children, the elderly, and individuals with preexisting cardiac or respiratory disease. Ambient air pollution has been implicated as a cause of cardiac disease, bronchitis, obstructive ventilatory disease, pulmonary emphysema, bronchial asthma, and airway or lung cancer. Extensive basic science and clinical epidemiologic literature on air pollutant toxicology has been published and has led to modifications of regulatory standards for air pollutants. EPA standards for these substances apply to the general environment, and OSHA standards apply to workplace exposure (see Table 56-1 for more details). The AirNow website provides location-specific air pollution data in the USA (www.airnow.gov).

Carbon Monoxide

Carbon monoxide (CO) is a colorless, tasteless, odorless, and nonirritating gas, a byproduct of incomplete combustion. The average concentration of CO in the atmosphere is about 0.1 ppm; in heavy traffic, the concentration may exceed 100 ppm. Current recommended PEL values and EPA standards are shown in Table 56–1 (see also www.osha.gov, Standard Number 1910.1000, Table Z-1).

1. *Mechanism of action*—CO combines tightly but reversibly with the oxygen-binding sites of hemoglobin and has an affinity for hemoglobin that is about 220 times that of oxygen. The product formed—carboxyhemoglobin—cannot transport oxygen. Furthermore, the presence of carboxyhemoglobin interferes with the dissociation of oxygen from the remaining oxyhemoglobin as a result of the Bohr effect. This reduces the transfer of oxygen to tissues. Organs with the highest oxygen demand (the brain, heart, and kidneys) are most seriously affected. Normal nonsmoking adults have carboxyhemoglobin levels of less than 1% saturation (1% of total hemoglobin is in the form of carboxyhemoglobin); this has been attributed to the endogenous formation of CO from heme catabolism. Smokers may exhibit 5–10% CO saturation. The level depends on their smoking habits. A person who breathes air that contains 0.1% CO (1000 ppm) would have a carboxyhemoglobin level of about 50% in a short period of time.

2. *Clinical effects*—The principal signs of CO intoxication are those of hypoxia. They progress in the following sequence: (1) psychomotor impairment; (2) headache and tightness in the temporal area; (3) confusion and loss of visual acuity; (4) tachycardia, tachypnea, syncope, and coma; and (5) deep coma, convulsions, shock, and respiratory failure. There is great variability in individual responses to carboxyhemoglobin concentration. Carboxyhemoglobin levels below 15% may produce headache and malaise; at 25% many workers complain of headache, fatigue, decreased attention span, and loss of fine motor coordination. Collapse and syncope may appear at around 40%; and with levels above 60%, death may ensue as a result of irreversible damage to the brain and myocardium. The clinical effects may be aggravated by heavy labor, high altitudes, and high ambient temperatures. CO intoxication is usually thought of as a form of acute toxicity. There is evidence that chronic exposure to low CO levels may lead to adverse cardiac effects, neurologic disturbance, and emotional disorders. The developing fetus is quite susceptible to the effects of CO exposure. Exposure of a pregnant woman to elevated CO levels at critical periods of fetal development may cause fetal death or serious and irreversible but survivable birth defects. Recent studies on low exposures to carbon monoxide in pregnant women have indicated lower birth weights and less successful pregnancy outcomes when initial prenatal visit carbon monoxide levels are elevated. These levels may be associated with unreported smoking or ambient exposure. The studies suggest CO screening at the first prenatal visit to detect and mitigate this risk.

3. *Treatment*—Patients who have been exposed to CO must be removed from the exposure source immediately. Respiration must be maintained, and high flow and concentration of oxygen—the specific antagonist to CO—should be administered promptly. If respiratory failure is present, mechanical ventilation is required. High concentrations of oxygen may be toxic and may contribute to the development of acute respiratory distress syndrome. Therefore, patients should be treated with high concentrations only for a short period. With room air at 1 atm, the elimination half-time of CO is about 320 minutes; with 100% oxygen, the half-time is about 80 minutes; and with hyperbaric oxygen (2–3 atm), the half-time can be reduced to about 20 minutes. Although some controversy exists about hyperbaric oxygen for CO poisoning, it may be used if it is readily available. It is particularly recommended for the management of pregnant women exposed to CO. Hypothermic therapy to reduce metabolic demand of the brain also has been useful. Cerebral edema that results from CO poisoning does not seem to respond to either mannitol or steroid therapy and may be persistent. Progressive recovery from treated CO poisoning, even of a severe degree, can be complete, but some patients manifest neuropsychological and motor dysfunction for a long time after recovery from acute CO poisoning.

Sulfur Dioxide

Sulfur dioxide (SO_2) is a colorless irritant gas generated primarily by the combustion of sulfur-containing fossil fuels. The current OSHA PEL and EPA standards are given in Table 56–1.

1. *Mechanism of action*—At room temperature, the solubility of SO_2 is approximately 200 g SO_2/L of water. Because of its high solubility, when SO_2 contacts moist membranes, it transiently forms sulfurous acid. This acid has severe irritant effects on the eyes, mucous membranes, and skin. Approximately 90% of inhaled SO_2 is absorbed in the upper respiratory tract, the site of its principal effect. The inhalation of SO_2 causes bronchial constriction and produces profuse bronchorrhea; parasympathetic reflexes and altered smooth muscle tone appear to be involved. The clinical outcome is an acute irritant asthma. Exposure to 5 ppm SO_2 for 10 minutes leads to increased resistance to airflow in most humans. Exposures of 5–10 ppm are reported to cause severe bronchospasm; 10–20% of the healthy young adult population is estimated to be reactive to even lower concentrations. The phenomenon of adaptation to irritating concentrations has been reported in workers. However, current studies have not confirmed this phenomenon. Asthmatic individuals are especially sensitive to SO_2.

2. *Clinical effects and treatment*—The signs and symptoms of intoxication include irritation of the eyes, nose, and throat, reflex bronchoconstriction, and increased bronchial secretions. In asthmatic subjects, exposure to SO_2 may result in an acute asthmatic episode. When a severe acute SO_2 exposure has occurred, delayed-onset pulmonary edema may be observed. Cumulative effects from chronic low-level exposure to SO_2 are not striking, particularly in humans, but these effects have been associated with aggravation of chronic cardiopulmonary disease. When combined exposure to high respirable particulate loads and SO_2 occurs, the mixed irritant load may increase the toxic respiratory response. Treatment is not specific for SO_2 but depends on therapeutic maneuvers used to treat irritation of the respiratory tract and asthma. In some severely polluted urban air basins, elevated SO_2 concentrations combined with elevated particulate loads have led to air pollution emergencies and a marked increase in cases of acute asthmatic bronchitis. Children and the elderly seem to be at greatest risk. In Detroit, an EPA sulfur dioxide non-attainment area, many hospital days and asthma-related respiratory symptom days per year occur in children in disadvantaged populations from sulfur dioxide exposure. The principal source of urban SO_2 is the burning of coal, both for domestic heating and in coal-fired power plants. High-sulfur transportation fuels also contribute. Both also contribute to the respirable fine particulate load and to increased urban cardiorespiratory morbidity and mortality.

Nitrogen Oxides

Nitrogen dioxide (NO_2) is a brownish irritant gas sometimes associated with fires. It is formed also from fresh silage; exposure of farmers to NO_2 in the confines of a silo can lead to silo-filler's disease, a severe and potentially lethal form of acute respiratory distress syndrome (ARDS). The disorder is uncommon today. Miners who are regularly exposed to diesel equipment exhaust have been particularly affected by nitrogen oxide emissions with serious respiratory effects. Today, the most common source of human exposure to oxides of nitrogen, including NO_2, is automobile and truck traffic emissions. Recent air pollution inventories in cities with high traffic congestion have demonstrated the important role that internal combustion engines have in the increasing NO_2 urban air pollution. A variety of disorders of the respiratory system, cardiovascular system, and other problems have been linked to NO_2 exposure.

1. *Mechanism of action*—NO_2 is a relatively insoluble deep lung irritant. It is capable of producing pulmonary edema and acute adult respiratory distress syndrome. Inhalation damages the lung infrastructure that produces the surfactant necessary to allow smooth and low-effort lung alveolar expansion. The type I cells of the alveoli appear to be the cells chiefly affected by acute low to moderate inhalation exposure. At higher exposure, both type I and type II alveolar cells are damaged. If only type I cells are damaged, after an acute period of severe distress, it is likely that treatment with modern ventilation equipment and medications will result in recovery. Some patients develop non-allergic asthma, or "twitchy airway" disease, after such a respiratory insult. If severe damage to the type I and type II alveolar cells occurs, replacement of the type I cells may be impaired; progressive fibrosis may ensue that eventually leads to bronchial ablation and alveolar collapse. This can result in permanent restrictive respiratory disease. In addition to the direct deep lung effect, long-term exposure to lower concentrations of nitrogen dioxide has been linked to cardiovascular disease, increased incidence of stroke, and other chronic disease.

The current PEL for NO_2 and EPA standards are given in Table 56–1. Exposure to 25 ppm of NO_2 is irritating to some individuals; 50 ppm is moderately irritating to the eyes and nose. Exposure for 1 hour to 50 ppm can cause pulmonary edema and perhaps subacute or chronic pulmonary lesions; 100 ppm can cause pulmonary edema and death.

2. *Clinical effects*—The signs and symptoms of acute exposure to NO_2 include irritation of the eyes and nose, cough, mucoid or frothy sputum production, dyspnea, and chest pain. Pulmonary edema may appear within 1–2 hours. In some individuals, the clinical signs may subside in about 2 weeks; the patient may then pass into a second stage of abruptly increasing severity, including recurring pulmonary edema and fibrotic destruction of terminal bronchioles (bronchiolitis obliterans). Chronic exposure of laboratory animals to 10–25 ppm NO_2 has resulted in emphysematous changes; thus, chronic effects in humans are of concern.

3. *Treatment*—There is no specific treatment for acute intoxication by NO_2; therapeutic measures for the management of deep lung irritation and noncardiogenic pulmonary edema are used. These measures include maintenance of gas exchange with adequate oxygenation and alveolar ventilation. Drug therapy may include bronchodilators, sedatives, and antibiotics. New approaches to the management of NO_2-induced ARDS have been developed, and considerable controversy now exists about the precise respiratory protocol to use in any given patient.

Ozone & Other Oxides

Ozone (O_3) is a bluish irritant gas found in the earth's atmosphere (stratosphere), where it is an important absorbent of ultraviolet light at high altitude. At ground level, ozone is an important pollutant. Ground level ozone pollution is derived from photolysis of oxides of nitrogen, volatile organic compounds, and heat and sunlight. These compounds are produced primarily when fossil fuels such as gasoline, oil, or coal are burned or when some chemicals (eg, solvents) evaporate. Nitrogen oxides are emitted from power plants, motor vehicles, and other sources of high-heat combustion. Volatile organic compounds are emitted from motor vehicles, chemical plants, refineries, factories, gas stations, paint, and other sources, such as oil and gas drilling and hydraulic fracturing (fracking) (see www.colorado.gov/airquality/tech_doc_repository.aspx?action=open&file=FRAPPE-NCAR_Final_Report_July2017.pdf). More information on ground-level ozone and its sources and consequences may be found at www.epa.gov/ground-level-ozone-pollution/ground-level-ozone-basics.

Ozone can be generated in the workplace by high-voltage electrical equipment, and around ozone-producing devices used for air and water purification. Agricultural sources of ozone are also important as well, as there are numerous adverse effects to plants (see www.nps.gov/subjects/air/nature-ozone.htm). There is a near-linear gradient between exposure to ozone (1-hour level, 20–100 ppb) and bronchial smooth muscle response. See Table 56–1 for the current PEL and EPA standards for ozone.

1. *Mechanism of action and clinical effects*—Ozone is an irritant of mucous membranes. Mild exposure produces upper respiratory tract irritation. Severe exposure can cause deep lung irritation, with pulmonary edema when inhaled at sufficient concentrations. Ozone penetration in the lung depends on tidal volume; consequently, exercise can increase the amount of ozone reaching the distal lung. Some of the effects of O_3 resemble those seen with radiation, suggesting that O_3 toxicity may result from the formation of reactive free radicals. The gas causes shallow, rapid breathing and a decrease in pulmonary compliance. Enhanced sensitivity of the lung to bronchoconstrictors also is observed. Exposure around 0.1 ppm O_3 for 10–30 minutes causes irritation and dryness of the throat; above 0.1 ppm, one finds changes in visual acuity, substernal pain, and dyspnea. Pulmonary function is impaired at concentrations exceeding 0.8 ppm.

Airway hyperresponsiveness and airway inflammation have been observed in humans. The response of the lung to O_3 is a dynamic one. The morphologic and biochemical changes are the result of both direct injury and secondary responses to the initial damage. Both acute and chronic exposure in animals results in morphologic and functional pulmonary changes; many mechanistic pathways involved have been identified. Chronic bronchitis, bronchiolitis, fibrosis, and emphysematous changes have been reported in a variety of species, including humans, exposed to concentrations above 1 ppm. Increased visits to hospital emergency departments for cardiopulmonary disease during ozone alerts have been reported. Studies in high ozone areas in China have shown a significant loss of years of life and a large economic impact in patients with COPD from chronic elevated ozone levels. The impacts were more significant in cold seasons than in the warmer months. Studies of the basic physiologic responses of humans to ozone exposure and the biomarkers evoked provide useful insight into the fundamental toxicologic impacts of ozone.

2. *Treatment*—There is no specific treatment for acute O_3 exposure. Ozone effects can be mitigated by reducing the time outside during high ozone days, especially for those more susceptible populations such as older adults and children (see www.airnow.gov). Management depends on therapeutic measures used for deep lung irritation and noncardiogenic pulmonary edema that have resulted in ARDS.

Particulate Matter

Particulate matter is a complicated topic due to the fact that there are different sizes of particulates and health effects differ depending on the size (Figure 56–1). PM_{10} is 10 microns and while it does elicit health effects, it is $PM_{2.5}$ or 2.5 microns or smaller, that elicits the most profound effects. While both are inhalable particles, $PM_{2.5}$ can reach deeper regions of the lungs. $PM_{2.5}$ can be emitted from construction sites, industries (smoke stacks), vehicles (eg, diesel exhaust), and fires, but the types of constituents of these particles can differ depending on the source. For example, particulate matter in Grand Rapids Michigan was not the same in toxicity in rats compared to particulate matter collected in Detroit, Michigan due to differences in composition. These particles originate from combinations of acids (eg, nitrates and sulfates), soil, dust, metals,

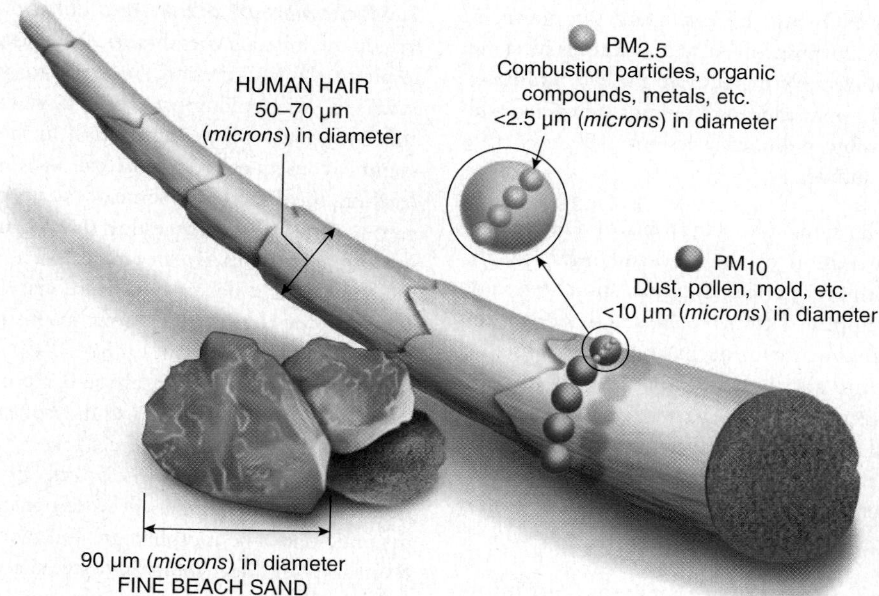

FIGURE 56–1 Particle size comparisons from EPA (www.epa.gov/pm-pollution/particulate-matter-pm-basics#PM).

organic materials (eg, molds and bacteria), and carcinogens, such as polycyclic aromatic hydrocarbons (PAHs). (PAHs will not be covered in detail, but information about PAHs can be found at the following references: www.epa.gov/sites/default/files/2014-03/documents/pahs_factsheet_cdc_2013.pdf; www.atsdr.cdc.gov/csem/polycyclic-aromatic-hydrocarbons/what_are_pahs.html; also see IARC reference.) In addition, these particles can be transported from long distances, which can change their composition and toxicity. For example, in the past 5 years, particulate air pollution from wildfires has spread from the West Coast to East Coast in the USA, and it can spread across oceans as well (see www.nationalgeographic.com/environment/article/wildfire-smoke-blowing-across-country-more-toxic-than-we-thought). Regulations for $PM_{2.5}$ from both OSHA and EPA can be found in Table 56–1, but experts in air pollution strongly hypothesize the current levels are not sufficient.

An emerging concern with air particulates is those that result from plastics that break down into micro- to nanosized particles, called microplastics or nanoplastics. (This topic will not be covered, but more details can be found at blogs.cdc.gov/niosh-science-blog/2020/02/19/microplastics/ and the following references: Amato-Lourenco et al, 2020; Prata et al, 2020.) In addition, these microplastics are also a large concern for water and soil contamination (see www.epa.gov/water-research/microplastics-research for more details).

1. *Mechanism of action and clinical effects*—Coarse particles in the range of 2.5–10 microns (PM_{10}) tend to deposit in the upper thoracic airways; fine particles less than 2.5 microns ($PM_{2.5}$) can deposit in the gas exchange areas. Ultrafine particles, those less than 0.1 micron in size, are suspected to cause serious health effects, although the epidemiologic data are hard to gather as this fraction is not generally sampled in ambient air. $PM_{2.5}$ elicits lung inflammation, in part by oxidative stress; reduces lung function, among other effects that can exacerbate pre-existing pulmonary conditions, such as asthma and chronic obstructive pulmonary disease; and is associated with higher mortality in these patients. There is also biologic evidence that $PM_{2.5}$ is associated with mortality from cardiovascular diseases, such as ventricular arrhythmia, thrombotic processes, increased systemic inflammation/oxidative stress, and hypertension, among others (see Bowe et al, 2019; Shi et al, 2016). Other diseases that are associated with $PM_{2.5}$ include chronic kidney disease and numerous effects on mental health such as Alzheimer disease, suicide, and bipolarity. In addition, during pregnancy, $PM_{2.5}$ exposure can lead to reduced cognition in infants. Ultimately, the challenge is that not all particulate matter is the same (eg, wildfire versus urban traffic) and thus, as noted above, the composition of the PM will matter with regard to cellular and organ toxicity.

2. *Treatment*—Similar to ozone exposures, there are no specific treatments for acute or chronic particulate matter exposures. Mitigation of particulate matter adverse effects consists of reducing time spent outside during high-particulate-matter days, especially for more suspceptible populations such as older adults and children (see www.airnow.gov), wearing an N95 or KN95 mask when outdoors, and using a HEPA-filter air filtration system indoors.

SOLVENTS

Halogenated Aliphatic Hydrocarbons

These "halohydrocarbon" agents once found wide use as industrial solvents, degreasing agents, and cleaning agents. The substances include carbon tetrachloride, chloroform, trichloroethylene, tetrachloroethylene (perchloroethylene), and 1,1,1-trichloroethane (methyl chloroform). Many halogenated aliphatic hydrocarbons are classified as known or probable human carcinogens. Carbon tetrachloride and trichloroethylene have largely been removed from the workplace. Perchloroethylene and trichloroethane are still in use for dry cleaning and solvent degreasing, but it is likely that their use will be very limited in the future. In 2016, the National Institute of Environmental Sciences (NIEHS) listed trichloroethylene as a known carcinogen by all routes of exposure. The EPA considers perchloroethylene a likely human carcinogen. The EPA data sheet may be found at www.epa.gov/haps/health-effects-notebook-hazardous-air-pollutants. Dry cleaning as an occupation is listed as a class 2B carcinogenic activity by the International Agency for Research on Cancer (IARC). The Canadian Center for Occupational Health and Safety lists occupations and exposures to occupational carcinogens at www.ccohs.ca/oshanswers/diseases/cancer/carcinogen_occupation.html.

Fluorinated aliphatics such as the freons and closely related compounds also have been used in the workplace, in consumer goods, and in stationary and mobile air conditioning systems. Because of the severe damage they cause to the ozone layer in the troposphere, their use has been limited or eliminated by international treaty agreements. The common halogenated aliphatic solvents also create serious problems as persistent water pollutants. They are widely found in both groundwater and drinking water as a result of poor disposal practices.

Recommended OSHA PELs for these compounds can be found at www.osha.gov, Table Z-1.

1. *Mechanism of action and clinical effects*—In laboratory animals, the halogenated hydrocarbons cause central nervous system (CNS) depression, liver injury, kidney injury, and some degree of cardiotoxicity. Several are also carcinogenic in animals and are considered probable human carcinogens. Trichloroethylene and tetrachloroethylene are listed as "reasonably anticipated to be a human carcinogen" by the US National Toxicology Program, and as class 2A probable human carcinogens by IARC. These substances are depressants of the CNS in humans. Chronic workplace exposure to halogenated hydrocarbon solvents can cause significant neurotoxicity with impaired memory and peripheral neuropathy. All halohydrocarbon solvents can cause cardiac arrhythmias in humans, particularly in situations involving sympathetic excitation and norepinephrine release.

Hepatotoxicity is also a common toxic effect that can occur in humans after acute or chronic halohydrocarbon exposures. Nephrotoxicity can occur in humans exposed to carbon tetrachloride, chloroform, and trichloroethylene. Chloroform, carbon tetrachloride, trichloroethylene, and tetrachloroethylene carcinogenicity have been observed in lifetime exposure studies performed in rats and mice and in some human epidemiologic studies. Dichloromethane (methylene chloride) is a potent neurotoxin, a generator of CO in humans, and a probable human carcinogen. It has been widely used as a paint stripper, as a plastic glue, and for other purposes. Epidemiologic studies of workers who have been exposed to aliphatic hydrocarbon solvents that include dichloromethane, trichloroethylene, and tetrachloroethylene have found significant associations between the agents and renal, prostate, and testicular cancer. Trichloroethylene is now considered a class 1 known human carcinogen by IARC; renal cancers and non-Hodgkin lymphoma have been reported. Other cancers have increased, but their incidence has not reached statistical significance.

2. *Treatment*—There is no specific treatment for acute intoxication resulting from exposure to halogenated hydrocarbons. Management depends on the organ system involved.

Aromatic Hydrocarbons

Several aromatic hydrocarbons will be discussed here: benzene, toluene, and xylene.

Benzene is used for its solvent properties and as an intermediate in the synthesis of other chemicals. It remains an important component of gasoline. Benzene may be found in premium gasolines at concentrations of about 1.5%. In cold climates such as Alaska, benzene concentrations in gasoline may reach 5% in order to provide an octane boost. It is one of the most widely used industrial chemicals in the world. The current PEL is 1.0 ppm in the air (see www.osha.gov, Table Z-1), and a 5-ppm limit is recommended for skin exposure. The National Institute for Occupational Safety and Health (NIOSH) and others have recommended that the exposure limits for benzene be further reduced to 0.1 ppm because excess blood cancers occur at the current PEL.

The acute toxic effect of benzene is depression of the CNS. Exposure to 7500 ppm for 30 minutes can be fatal. Exposure to concentrations greater than 3000 ppm may cause euphoria, nausea, locomotor problems, and coma. Vertigo, drowsiness, headache, and nausea may occur at concentrations ranging from 250 to 500 ppm. No specific treatment exists for the acute toxic effect of benzene.

Chronic exposure to benzene can result in very serious toxic effects. The most significant effect is bone marrow injury. Aplastic anemia, leukopenia, pancytopenia, and thrombocytopenia occur, as do various blood cancers including acute myelogenous leukemia. Chronic exposure to low levels of benzene has been associated with leukemia of several other types as well as lymphomas, myeloma, and myelodysplastic syndrome. Several studies have shown increased occurrence of leukemia following worker exposures as low as 2 ppm-years. The pluripotent bone marrow stem cells appear to be targets of benzene or its metabolites, and other stem cells also may be targets.

Benzene has long been known to be a potent clastogen, a mutagen that acts by causing chromosomal breakage. Recent studies have suggested specific chromosome reorganization and genomic patterns that are associated with benzene-induced leukemia. Evidence suggests specific gene patterns are specific to benzene exposure. A study examining gene expression response in peripheral blood cells of petroleum workers concluded that gene expression patterns differed significantly between workers exposed to benzene at concentrations well below 0.5 ppm benzene and non-exposed referents (see Jørgensen et al, 2018). Reviews of benzene carcinogenicity provide comprehensive overviews of benzene as a cancer-causing agent. Epidemiologic data confirm the causal association between benzene exposure and leukemia and other bone marrow cancers in workers. IARC classifies benzene as a class 1, known human carcinogen. Most national and international organizations classify benzene as a known human carcinogen.

Toluene (methylbenzene) does not possess the myelotoxic properties of benzene, nor has it been associated with leukemia. It is not carcinogenic and is listed as class 3 by IARC. It is, however, a CNS depressant and a skin and eye irritant. It is also neurotoxic and fetotoxic. See OSHA Tables Z-1 and Z-2 (www.osha.gov) for the PELs. Exposure to 800 ppm can lead to severe fatigue and ataxia; 10,000 ppm can produce rapid loss of consciousness. Chronic effects of long-term toluene exposure are unclear because human studies indicating behavioral effects usually concern exposures to several solvents. In limited occupational studies, however, metabolic interactions and modification of toluene's effects have not been observed in workers also exposed to other solvents. Less refined grades of toluene contain benzene. If technical-grade toluene is to be used where there is human contact or exposure, analysis of the material for benzene content is advisable. If benzene is present, then monitoring should be instituted immediately.

Xylene (dimethylbenzene) has been substituted for benzene in many solvent degreasing operations. Like toluene, the three xylenes do not possess the myelotoxic properties of benzene, nor have they been associated with leukemia. Xylene is a CNS depressant and a skin irritant. Less refined grades of xylene contain benzene. Similar need for monitoring of benzene exposure is indicated if technical-grade xylene is contaminated with benzene. Estimated TLV–time-weighted average and TLV–short-term exposure limit are 100 and 150 ppm, respectively. The current OSHA PELs may be found at www.osha.gov, Table Z-1.

PESTICIDES

Organochlorine Pesticides

These agents are usually classified into four groups: DDT (chlorophenothane) and its analogs, benzene hexachlorides, cyclodienes, and toxaphenes (Table 56–2). They are aryl, carbocyclic, or heterocyclic compounds containing chlorine substituents. The individual compounds differ widely in their biotransformation and capacity for storage in tissues; toxicity and storage are not always correlated. They can be absorbed through the skin as well as by inhalation or oral ingestion. There are, however, important quantitative differences among the various derivatives; DDT in solution is poorly absorbed through the skin, whereas dieldrin absorption from the skin is very efficient. Organochlorine pesticides have largely been abandoned because they cause severe environmental damage. They are now known to be endocrine disrupters in animals and humans. DDT continues to have very restricted use for domestic mosquito elimination in malaria-infested areas of Africa. This use is controversial, but it is very effective and is likely to remain in place for the foreseeable future. Organochlorine pesticide residues in humans, animals, and the environment present long-term problems that are not yet fully understood. A major unresolved concern is the metabolic degradation of fat-stored residues to compounds that are potentially more toxic than the original compound.

1. *Human toxicology*—The acute toxic properties of all the organochlorine pesticides in humans are qualitatively similar. These agents interfere with inactivation of the sodium channel in excitable membranes and cause rapid repetitive firing in most neurons. Calcium ion transport is inhibited. These events affect repolarization and enhance the excitability of neurons. The major effect is CNS stimulation. With DDT, tremor may be the first manifestation, possibly continuing to convulsions, whereas with the other compounds convulsions often appear as the first sign of intoxication. There is no specific treatment for the acute intoxicated state, and management is symptomatic.

The potential carcinogenic properties of organochlorine pesticides have been extensively studied, and results indicate that chronic administration to laboratory animals over long periods results in enhanced carcinogenesis. Endocrine pathway disruption is the postulated mechanism. Numerous mechanisms for xenoestrogen (estrogen-like) carcinogenesis have been postulated.

TABLE 56–2 Organochlorine pesticides.

Chemical Class	Compounds	Toxicity Rating[1]	ADI[2]
DDT and analogs	Dichlorodiphenyltrichloroethane (DDT)	4	0.005
	Methoxychlor	3	0.1
	Tetrachlorodiphenylethane (TDE)	3	—
Benzene hexachlorides	Benzene hexachloride (BHC; hexachlorocyclohexane)	4	0.008
	Lindane	4	0.008
Cyclodienes	Aldrin	5	0.0001
	Chlordane	4	0.0005
	Dieldrin	5	0.0001
	Heptachlor	4	0.0001
Toxaphenes	Toxaphene (camphechlor)	4	—

[1]Toxicity rating: Probable human oral lethal dosage for class 3 = 500–5000 mg/kg, class 4 = 50–500 mg/kg, and class 5 = 5–50 mg/kg. (See Gosselin et al, 1984.)

[2]ADI, acceptable daily intake (mg/kg/d).

To date, however, several large epidemiologic studies in humans have not found a significant association between the risk of cancer and specific compounds or serum levels of organochlorine pesticide metabolites. Several recent studies demonstrate elevated concentrations of organochlorine pesticide metabolites in various human cancer tissues, but causality is uncertain. Various pathways by which these metabolites might initiate or promote human tumors are under study, but no consensus has been reached. The results of a case-control study conducted to investigate the relation between dichlorodiphenyldichloroethylene (DDE, the primary metabolite of DDT) and DDT breast adipose tissue levels and breast cancer risk did not confirm a positive association. In contrast, recent work supports an association between prepubertal exposure to DDT and brain cancer. Recent studies also suggest that the risk of testicular cancer and non-Hodgkin lymphoma is increased in persons with elevated organochlorine levels. Noncancer end points are also of concern. Cryptorchidism and hypospadias in newborns is related to maternal adipose levels of chlordane metabolites. These residues are also linked to testicular cancer.

2. *Environmental toxicology*—The organochlorine pesticides are considered persistent chemicals. Degradation is quite slow when compared with other pesticides, and bioaccumulation, particularly in aquatic ecosystems, is well documented. Their mobility in soil depends on the composition of the soil; the presence of organic matter favors the adsorption of these chemicals onto the soil particles, whereas adsorption is poor in sandy soils. Once adsorbed, they do not readily desorb. These compounds induce significant abnormalities in the endocrine balance of sensitive animal and bird species, in addition to their adverse impact on humans. Since the early 1960s, when Rachel Carson's work and subsequent book, *Silent Spring*, brought attention to the issue, the organochlorine pesticides have been recognized as pernicious environmental toxins. Their use is banned in most jurisdictions.

Organophosphorus (OP) Pesticides

These agents, some of which are listed in Table 56–3, are used to combat a large variety of pests. They are useful pesticides when in direct contact with insects or when used as **plant systemics,** where the agent is translocated within the plant and exerts its effects on insects that feed on the plant. The many varieties currently in use are applied by spray techniques including hand, tractor, and aerial methods. They are often spread widely by wind and weather and are subject to widespread drift. The organophosphate pesticides are based on compounds such as soman, sarin, and tabun, often called the G compounds, which were developed in Germany as insecticides and were later weaponized for use as war gases. Later, British scientists developed VX, a nerve gas that was 20 times more potent than the G series compounds. Many of these compounds were also manufactured in the United States.

Parathion, malathion, azinphos, and other OP compounds that are less toxic than the military-grade compounds are widely used in agriculture throughout the world. In the USA, efforts have been made to reduce the use of OP compounds because of food contamination concerns and occupational health and safety issues. Several laws regulate the use of these chemicals. Their effect has been to reduce overall use of the more toxic OP compounds on food crops in the USA. However, ongoing problems with the cotton boll weevil have required some farmers to rely more heavily on aerially sprayed parathion and its derivatives in recent years. Some of the less toxic organophosphorus compounds are used in human and veterinary medicine as local or systemic antiparasitics (see Chapters 7 and 53). Organophosphates are absorbed by the skin as well as by the respiratory and gastrointestinal tracts. Biotransformation is rapid, particularly when compared with the rates observed with the chlorinated hydrocarbon pesticides. Storm and collaborators have reviewed current and suggested human inhalation occupational exposure limits for 30 organophosphate pesticides (see Pesticide References).

TABLE 56–3 Organophosphorus pesticides.

Compound	Toxicity Rating[1]	ADI[2]
Azinphos-methyl	5	0.005
Chlorfenvinphos	—	0.002
Diazinon	4	0.002
Dichlorvos	—	0.004
Dimethoate	4	0.01
Fenitrothion	—	0.005
Malathion	4	0.02
Parathion	6	0.005
Parathion-methyl	5	0.02
Trichlorfon	4	0.01

[1]Toxicity rating: Probable human oral lethal dosage for class 4 = 50–500 mg/kg, class 5 = 5–50 mg/kg, and class 6 = ≤5 mg/kg; —, data not found. (See Gosselin et al, 1984.)

[2]ADI, acceptable daily intake (mg/kg/d).

1. *Human toxicology*—In mammals as well as insects, the major effect of these agents is inhibition of acetylcholinesterase through phosphorylation of the esteratic site. The signs and symptoms that characterize acute intoxication are due to inhibition of this enzyme and accumulation of acetylcholine; some of the agents also possess direct cholinergic activity. Specific treatment with antidotes and useful antagonists is available. In addition, pretreatment with physostigmine and other short-acting compounds may provide protection against these pesticides or their war gas analogs if used in timely fashion. These effects and their treatment are described in Chapters 7 and 8 of this book. Altered neurologic and cognitive functions, as well as psychological symptoms of variable duration, have been associated with exposure to these pesticides. Furthermore, there is some indication of an association of low arylesterase activity with neurologic symptom complexes in Gulf War veterans.

In addition to—and independently of—inhibition of acetylcholinesterase, some of these agents are capable of phosphorylating another enzyme present in neural tissue, the so-called **neuropathy target esterase (NTE).** This results in progressive demyelination of the longest nerves. Associated with paralysis and axonal degeneration, this lesion is sometimes called organophosphorus ester-induced delayed polyneuropathy (OPIDP). Delayed central and autonomic neuropathy may occur in some poisoned patients. Hens are particularly sensitive to these properties and have proved very useful for studying the pathogenesis of the lesion and for identifying potentially neurotoxic organophosphorus derivatives. There is no specific treatment for NTE toxicity.

In humans, progressive chronic axonal neurotoxicity has been observed with **triorthocresyl phosphate (TOCP),** a noninsecticidal organophosphorus compound. It is also thought to occur with the pesticides dichlorvos, trichlorfon, leptophos, methamidophos, mipafox, trichloronat, and others. The polyneuropathy usually begins as burning and tingling sensations, particularly in the feet, with motor weakness occurring a few days later. Sensory and motor difficulties may extend to the legs and hands. Gait is affected, and ataxia may be present. Central nervous system and autonomic changes may develop still later. There is no specific treatment for this form of delayed neurotoxicity. The long-term prognosis of NTE inhibition is highly variable. Reports of this type of neuropathy (and other toxicities) in pesticide manufacturing workers and in agricultural pesticide applicators have been published.

Recent clinical observation has also defined an intermediate syndrome in severely organophosphate-poisoned patients. This syndrome is characterized by neuromuscular transmission failure, and cardiac failure more typical of nicotinic than muscarinic poisoning. Progressive neuromuscular failure leads to weakness of the respiratory muscles and eventually to death. The physiologic abnormalities are complex but involve a progressive decrement in neuromuscular junction transmission efficiency. Patients who develop this intermediate syndrome are at great risk of cardiorespiratory failure and may require mechanical ventilation. Because organophosphorus poisoning frequently occurs in less developed parts of the world where medical resources are very limited, the development of the intermediate syndrome is frequently a lethal complication. It is not effectively treated with the usual management protocol for organophosphate pesticide poisoning.

2. *Environmental toxicology*—Organophosphorus pesticides are not considered to be persistent pesticides. They are relatively unstable and break down in the environment as a result of hydrolysis and photolysis. As a class they are considered to have a small permanent impact on the environment, in spite of their acute effects on organisms.

Carbamate Pesticides

These compounds (Table 56–4) inhibit acetylcholinesterase by carbamoylation of the esteratic site. Thus, they possess the toxic properties associated with inhibition of this enzyme as described for the organophosphorus pesticides. However, as described in Chapters 7 and 8, the binding is relatively weak, dissociation occurs after minutes to hours, and clinical effects are of shorter duration than those observed with organophosphorus compounds. Spontaneous reactivation of cholinesterase is more rapid after inhibition by the carbamates. The therapeutic index, the ratio of the doses that cause severe toxicity or death to those that result in minor intoxication, is larger with carbamates than with the organophosphorus agents. Although the clinical approach to carbamate poisoning is similar to that for organophosphates, the use of pralidoxime is not recommended.

The carbamates are considered to be nonpersistent pesticides. They exert only a small impact on the environment.

TABLE 56–4 Carbamate pesticides.

Compound	Toxicity Rating[1]	ADI[2]
Aldicarb	6	0.005
Aminocarb	5	—
Carbaryl	4	0.01
Carbofuran	5	0.01
Dimetan	4	—
Dimetilan	4	—
Isolan	5	—
Methomyl	5	—
Propoxur	4	0.02
Pyramat	4	—
Pyrolan	5	—
Zectran	5	—

[1]Toxicity rating: Probable human oral lethal dosage for class 4 = 50–500 mg/kg, class 5 = 5–50 mg/kg, and class 6 = ≤5 mg/kg. (See Gosselin et al, 1984.)

[2]ADI, acceptable daily intake (mg/kg/d); —, data not found.

Botanical Pesticides

Pesticides derived from natural sources include **nicotine, rotenone,** and **pyrethrum.** Nicotine is obtained from the dried leaves of *Nicotiana tabacum* and *N rustica*. It is rapidly absorbed from mucosal surfaces; the free alkaloid, but not the salt, is readily absorbed from the skin. Nicotine reacts with the acetylcholine receptor of the postsynaptic membrane (sympathetic and parasympathetic ganglia, neuromuscular junction), resulting in depolarization of the membrane. Toxic doses cause stimulation rapidly followed by blockade of transmission. These actions are described in Chapter 7. Treatment is directed toward maintenance of vital signs and suppression of convulsions. Nicotine analogs **(neonicotinoids)** have been developed for use as agricultural pesticides and have been implicated in bee colony collapse.

Rotenone (Figure 56–2) is obtained from *Derris elliptica*, *D mallaccensis*, *Lonchocarpus utilis*, and *L urucu*. The oral ingestion of rotenone produces gastrointestinal irritation. Conjunctivitis, dermatitis, pharyngitis, and rhinitis also can occur. Treatment is symptomatic.

Pyrethrum consists of six known insecticidal esters: pyrethrin I (see Figure 56–2), pyrethrin II, cinerin I, cinerin II, jasmolin I, and jasmolin II. Synthetic pyrethroids account for an increasing percentage of worldwide pesticide usage. Pyrethrum may be absorbed after inhalation or ingestion. When absorbed in sufficient quantities, the major site of toxic action is the CNS; excitation, convulsions, and tetanic paralysis can occur. Voltage-gated sodium, calcium, and chloride channels are considered targets,

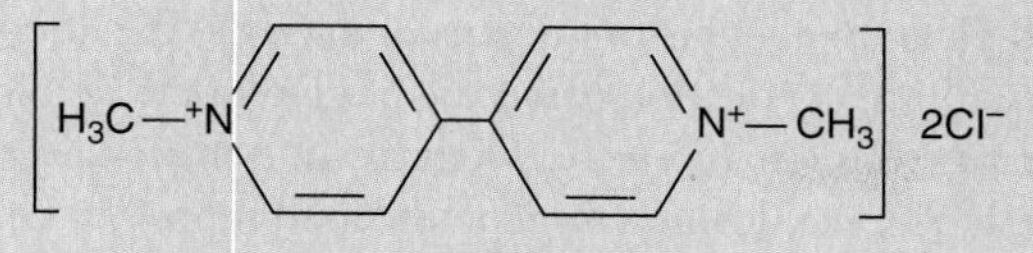

Paraquat dichloride

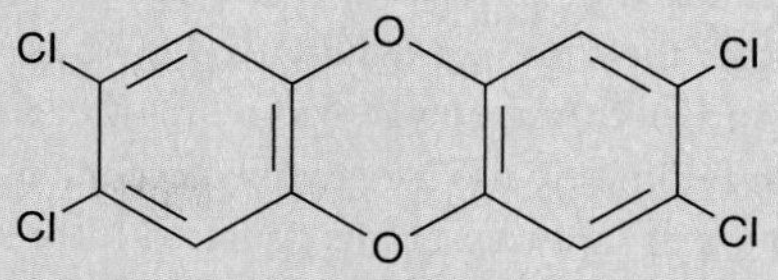

2,3,7,8-Tetrachlorodibenzodioxin (TCDD)

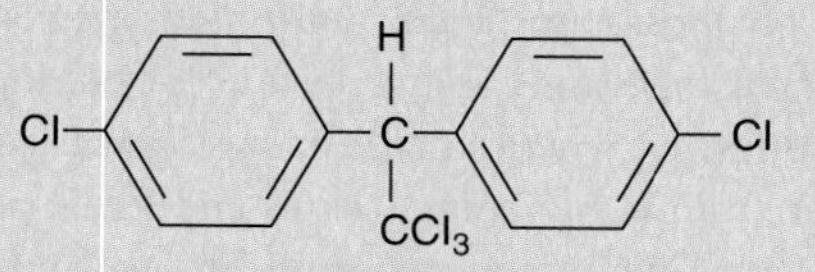

Dichlorodiphenyltrichloroethane (DDT)

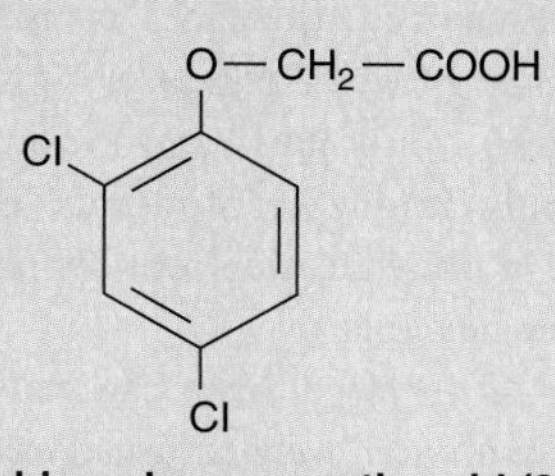

2,4-Dichlorophenoxyacetic acid (2,4-D)

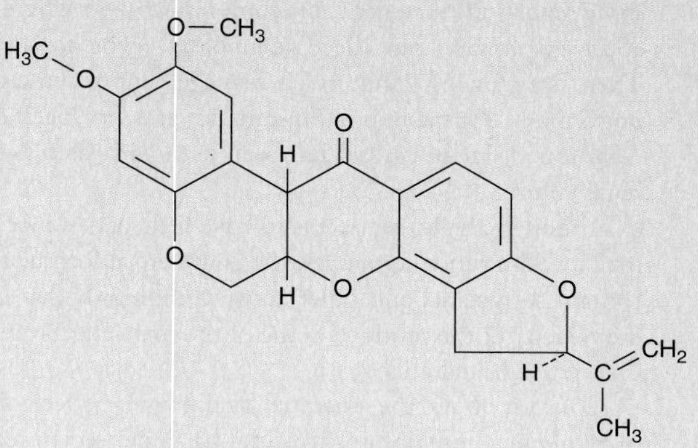

Rotenone

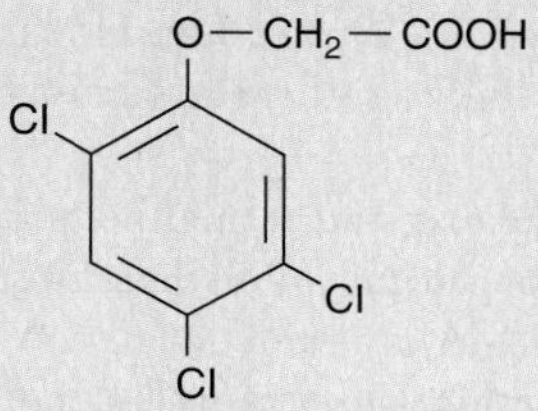

2,4,5-Trichlorophenoxyacetic acid (2,4,5-T)

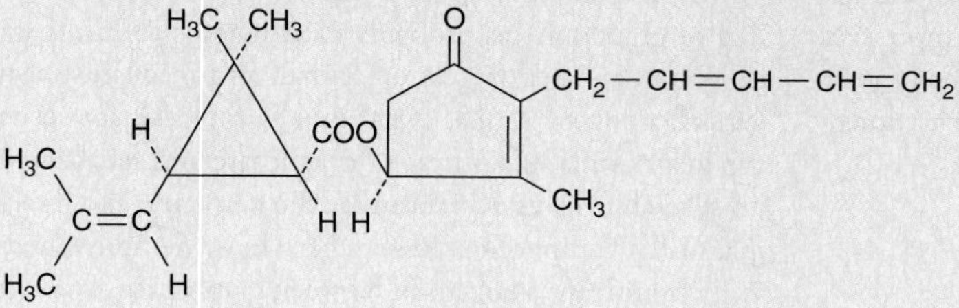

Pyrethrin I

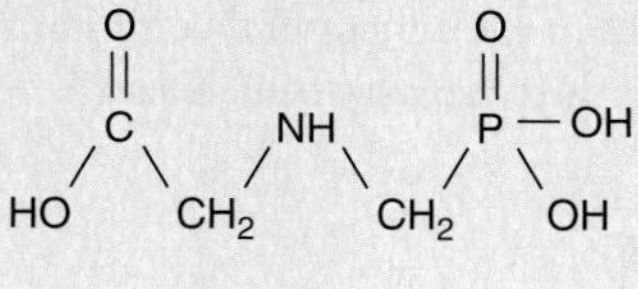

Glyphosate

FIGURE 56–2 Chemical structures of selected herbicides and pesticides.

as are peripheral-type benzodiazepine receptors. Treatment of exposure is usually directed at management of symptoms. Anticonvulsants are not consistently effective. The chloride channel agonist ivermectin is of use, as are pentobarbital and mephenesin. The pyrethroids are highly irritating to the eyes, skin, and respiratory tree. They may cause irritant asthma and, potentially, reactive airways dysfunction syndrome (RADS) and even anaphylaxis. The most common injuries reported in humans result from their allergenic and irritant effects on the airways and skin. Cutaneous paresthesias have been observed in workers spraying synthetic pyrethroids. The use of persistent synthetic pyrethroids to exterminate insects on aircraft has caused respiratory and skin problems as well as some neurologic complaints in flight attendants and other aircraft workers. Severe occupational exposures to synthetic pyrethroids in China resulted in marked effects on the CNS, including convulsions. Other previously unreported toxic manifestations have been observed in pyrethrin-exposed individuals.

HERBICIDES

Chlorophenoxy Herbicides

2,4-Dichlorophenoxyacetic acid (2,4-D), 2,4,5-trichlorophenoxyacetic acid (2,4,5-T), and their salts and esters have been used as herbicides for the destruction of weeds (see Figure 56–2).

These compounds are of relatively low acute human toxicity. However, despite their low acute hazard, they cause serious long-term human and environmental toxicity. 2,4-D remains in wide commercial and domestic use for lawn weed control. 2,4,5-T had similar uses but was infamously incorporated into Agent Orange, used as a defoliant during the Vietnam conflict. Agent Orange was contaminated with 2,3,7,8-tetrachlorodibenzo-*p*-dioxin (a potent animal carcinogen and likely human carcinogen) and other toxic, persistent, and undesirable polychlorinated compounds. When this toxicity was discovered, the US Department of Agriculture canceled the domestic pesticide registrations for trichlorophenoxy herbicides, and these compounds are no longer used. However, other less thoroughly studied compounds, eg, chlorinated xanthenes, are present in both the dichlorophenoxy and trichlorophenoxy herbicides (see below).

In humans, 2,4-D in large doses can cause coma and generalized muscle hypotonia. Rarely, muscle weakness and marked hypotonia may persist for several weeks. In laboratory animals, signs of liver and kidney dysfunction have also been reported with chlorophenoxy herbicides. Several epidemiologic studies performed by the US National Cancer Institute confirmed the causal link between 2,4-D and non-Hodgkin lymphoma. Evidence for a causal link to soft tissue sarcoma, however, is considered equivocal.

The dichlorophenoxy and related herbicides have been found to contain and to generate dimethylnitrosamine (*N*-nitrosodimethylamine; NDMA), a potent human carcinogen, during environmental transformation as well as non-chlorine water disinfection. Studies by Environment Canada and others have questioned the use of this compound because of water contamination. Studies of related nitrosamine-forming herbicidal compounds have raised questions about the suitability of these compounds for general weed control. Because of the extremely high economic value of herbicides to the agricultural community, however, long-term decisions on their use have been delayed.

Glyphosate

Glyphosate (*N*-[phosphonomethyl] glycine; see Figure 56–2) is the principal ingredient in Roundup. Other similar herbicides are manufactured and sold under various trade names. Glyphosate-containing herbicides are now the most widely used herbicides in the world. Glyphosate functions as a contact herbicide. It is absorbed through the leaves and roots of plants. It is generally formulated with surfactant to enhance its intended effect on noxious plants. Because it is nonselective, it may damage important crops and desirable ornamental plants even when used as directed. To reduce the economic impact on valuable plants, genetically modified species such as soybean, corn, and cotton that are glyphosate-resistant have been developed and patented. They are widely grown throughout the world. Almost all soybean crops and many corn crops grown today are of the glyphosate-resistant type. These genetically modified (GMO) crops are grown from patented seeds and have great economic value to growers, contributing to the food supply significantly. However, in some jurisdictions their use is highly controversial. While there is no evidence that genetically modified crops are toxic or dangerous to humans or animals, the long-term agricultural impact of widespread use of glyphosate herbicides on resistant crops remains to be determined. Additionally, the impact of effective weed elimination on the food supply and habitat of critical species—eg, bees, butterflies, and some migrating birds—has been a source of increasing concern.

Because of the widespread availability and use of this herbicide, glyphosate-surfactant poisonings are common. Many of the observed ingestions and reports of poisoning are from developing countries, where suicide by pesticide is common. Many injuries are minor, but some serious and lethal poisonings have been reported. Glyphosate is a significant eye and skin irritant. When ingested it can cause mild to moderate esophageal erosion. It also causes aspiration pneumonia and renal failure. There have been some reports of teratogenic outcomes in workers who handle and apply glyphosate, but the epidemiologic evidence is not clear. There is a growing literature on management of acute glyphosate poisoning. Treatment is symptomatic, and no specific protocol is indicated. Hemodialysis has been used with success in cases of renal failure.

Although glyphosate seems to have little persistence and lower toxicity than other herbicides, the commercial formulations often contain surfactants and other active compounds that complicate the toxicity of the product. Some of the toxic effects are related to the surfactant material.

Concern about the potential carcinogenic effect of exposure to glyphosate-containing herbicides has increased in recent years. Although the scientific evidence both in animals and in humans has been uncertain, various interpretations and reinterpretations of the available animal and human evidence have led to the listing of glyphosate as probably carcinogenic to humans. This classification is based largely on animal and mechanistic studies. The classification of 2A has been used as the basis for several lawsuits against the manufacturers of glyphosate and has been convincing to several juries as evidence that the herbicide was the cause of the plaintiff's lymphoma. Researchers have demonstrated a statistically significant association between glyphosate exposure and non-Hodgkin lymphoma in humans (Zhang et al, 2019). The issue of the carcinogenicity of glyphosate is still under active study (www.epa.gov/ingredients-used-pesticide-products/glyphosate#actions), as is its potential role in diseases such as chronic kidney disease of unknown cause (Johnson et al, 2019).

Bipyridyl Herbicides

Paraquat is the most important agent of this class (see Figure 56–2). Its mechanism of action is said to be similar in plants and animals and involves single-electron reduction of the herbicide to free radical species. Ingestion (accidental or suicidal) is among the most serious and potentially lethal pesticide poisonings. Many serious exposures take place in developing countries where limited treatment resources are available. Paraquat accumulates slowly in the lung by an active process and causes lung edema, alveolitis, and progressive fibrosis. It probably inhibits superoxide dismutase, resulting in intracellular free-radical oxygen toxicity.

In humans, the first signs and symptoms after oral exposure are hematemesis and bloody stools. Within a few days, however, delayed toxicity occurs, with respiratory distress and the development of congestive hemorrhagic pulmonary edema accompanied by widespread cellular proliferation. During the acute period, oxygen should be used cautiously to combat dyspnea or cyanosis, because it may aggravate the pulmonary lesions. Hepatic, renal, or myocardial involvement may develop. The interval between ingestion and death may be several weeks.

Because of the delayed pulmonary toxicity, prompt immobilization of the paraquat to prevent absorption is important. Adsorbents (eg, activated charcoal, Fuller's earth) are routinely given to bind the paraquat and minimize its absorption. Gastric lavage is not recommended, as it may promote aspiration from the stomach into the lungs. Once the paraquat is absorbed, treatment is successful in less than 50% of cases. Monitoring of plasma and urine paraquat concentrations is useful for prognostic assessment. Computed tomography scanning has also been used to follow the pulmonary lesions as they develop and to help with prognosis. The pulmonary proliferative phase begins 1–2 weeks after paraquat ingestion. Although a few reports indicate some success with dialysis, hemodialysis and hemoperfusion rarely change the clinical course. Many approaches have been used to slow or stop the progressive pulmonary fibrosis. Immunosuppression using corticosteroids and cyclophosphamide is widely practiced, but evidence for efficacy is weak. Antioxidants such as acetylcysteine and salicylate might be beneficial through free radical-scavenging, anti-inflammatory, and nuclear factor kappa-B inhibitory actions. However, there are no published human trials. The case fatality rate is high in all centers despite large variations in treatment. Patients require prolonged observation and treatment for respiratory and renal insufficiency if they survive the acute stage of poisoning.

ENVIRONMENTAL POLLUTANTS

Polychlorinated & Polybrominated Biphenyls

Highly halogenated biphenyl compounds, which have desirable properties for insulation, fire retardancy, and many other uses, were manufactured in large quantities during the mid-20th century. The quantities produced and the almost universal dispersion of the materials in which they were incorporated have produced an enormous environmental problem. Both chlorinated and brominated biphenyls are environmentally dangerous and significantly toxic and are now banned from use.

The **polychlorinated biphenyls (PCBs, coplanar biphenyls)** were used as dielectric and heat transfer fluids, lubricating oils, plasticizers, wax extenders, and flame retardants. Their industrial use and manufacture in the USA were terminated by 1977. The chlorinated products used commercially were actually mixtures of PCB isomers and homologs containing 12–68% chlorine. These chemicals are very stable, highly lipophilic, poorly metabolized, and very resistant to environmental degradation; thus they bioaccumulate in food chains.

Food is the major source of PCB residues in humans. Accumulation of PCB in fish species led Canada and the USA to restrict commercial fishing and to limit consumption of fish from the Great Lakes of North America (see Box: Bioaccumulation & Biomagnification, earlier). In addition, large industrial-site contamination, illegal dumping, migration from hazardous waste sites and other large-scale sources, and widespread use of PCBs in electrical transformers have led to multiple localized areas of contamination and human exposure. Leakage of transformer dielectric fluids in neighborhoods and backyards has caused significant numbers of serious but highly localized PCB exposure events.

There are numerous reports of large population exposures to PCBs. A serious exposure to PCBs—lasting several months—occurred in Japan in 1968 as a result of cooking oil contamination with PCB-containing transfer medium (Yusho disease). A similar outbreak called Yucheng disease occurred at about the same time in Taiwan. Effects on the fetus and on the development of the offspring of poisoned women were reported. It is now known that the contaminated cooking oil contained not only PCBs but also polychlorinated dibenzofurans (PCDFs) and polychlorinated quaterphenyls (PCQs). It is likely that the effects initially attributed to the PCBs were actually caused by a mixture of contaminants. Workers occupationally exposed to PCBs develop dermatologic problems that include chloracne, folliculitis, erythema, dryness, rash, hyperkeratosis, and hyperpigmentation. Some hepatic abnormalities have been found in PCB poisoning, and plasma triglycerides are elevated.

Information about the effects of PCBs on reproduction and development is accumulating. The halogenated pesticides are potent endocrine disrupters, and there is widespread concern about the persistent estrogenic effect of these chemicals. Adverse reproductive impacts of PCBs have been found in many animal studies. Direct teratogenic effects in humans have yet to be established: studies in workers and in the general population exposed to moderate or very high levels of PCBs have not been conclusive. Some adverse behavioral effects in infants have been reported. An association between prenatal exposure to PCBs and deficits in childhood intellectual function was described in children born to mothers who had eaten large quantities of contaminated fish. Epidemiologic studies have established increases in various cancers including melanoma, breast, pancreatic, and thyroid cancers. These findings and animal studies provided a sufficient basis for the IARC to classify some coplanar PCBs as class 1, carcinogenic to humans, in volume 100 of the IARC monographs. A comprehensive EPA fact sheet on PCBs may be found at www.epa.gov/pcbs.

The polybrominated biphenyls (PBBs) and their ethers (PBDEs) share many of the toxic and environmentally damaging persistent qualities of PCBs. They were introduced as fire retardants in the 1950s and have been used in massive quantities since that time. The biphenyls are no longer produced and may no longer be used, but the biphenyl ethers remain in use as fire retardants in plastics for bedding and in automobile upholstery. PBB fire-retardant contamination has been extensive in the Great Lakes region, resulting in large exposure to the population. PBBs are considered IARC class 2a: probable human carcinogens. PBDEs are not classified. An EPA technical fact sheet on PBB and PBDEs may be found at www2.epa.gov/fedfac/technical-fact-sheet-polybrominated-diphenyl-ethers-pbdes-and-polybrominated-biphenyls-pbbs.

The **polychlorinated dibenzo-*p*-dioxins (PCDDs),** or ***dioxins,*** are a group of halogenated congeners of which tetrachlorodibenzodioxin **(TCDD)** has been the most carefully studied. There is a large group of dioxin-like compounds, including **polychlorinated dibenzofurans (PCDFs)** and **coplanar biphenyls.** While PCBs were used commercially, PCDDs and PCDFs are unwanted byproducts that appear in the environment and in manufactured products as contaminants because of improperly controlled combustion processes. They are also produced when unexpected heating to temperatures over 600°C occurs as in lightning strikes or electrical fires in PCB-containing transformers. Like PCBs, these chemicals are very stable and highly lipophilic. They are poorly metabolized and very resistant to environmental degradation. Several significant environmental contamination episodes involving dioxins and furans from industrial sites have occurred. Recent publications have demonstrated an elevated incidence of subsequent chronic diseases (eg, diabetes, metabolic syndrome, obesity) in exposed persons. Laboratory studies of the blood concentrations of TCDD and its metabolites have provided insight into the persistence and metabolism of the contaminants.

In laboratory animals, TCDD has produced a variety of toxic effects. Wasting syndrome (severe weight loss accompanied by reduction of muscle mass and adipose tissue), thymic atrophy, epidermal changes, hepatotoxicity, immunotoxicity, effects on reproduction and development, teratogenicity, and carcinogenicity have been produced. The effects observed in workers involved in the manufacture of 2,4,5-T (and therefore presumably exposed to TCDD) consisted of contact dermatitis and chloracne. In severely TCDD-intoxicated patients, discrete chloracne may be the only manifestation.

The presence of TCDD in 2,4,5-T, commercially known as Silvex or Fenoprop, was believed to be responsible for other human toxicities associated with the herbicide. There is epidemiologic evidence for an association between occupational exposure to the phenoxy herbicides and an excess incidence of non-Hodgkin lymphoma. The TCDD contaminant in these herbicides seems to play a role in a number of cancers such as soft tissue sarcomas, lung cancer, Hodgkin lymphomas, and others. TCDD is considered an IARC class 1, known human carcinogen. Other halogenated compounds of this type are not currently classifiable as to carcinogenicity; they are listed as IARC class 3. As noted above, TCDD was part of the herbicide mixture of Agent Orange that many military personnel were exposed to during the Vietnam War. The Veterans Administration (VA) in the USA has added additional adverse effects that are now included in VA disability compensation for those individuals exposed to Agent Orange (bladder cancer, hypothyroidism, parkinsonism), but many other adverse effects have been associated, including the specific cancers noted above and others, type 2 diabetes, ischemic heart disease, peripheral neuropathy, and numerous others (see www.va.gov/disability/eligibility/hazardous-materials-exposure/agent-orange/#am-i-eligible-for-va-disabilit).

Perfluorinated Compounds (PFCs, PFOA)

Fluorinated hydrocarbon chemicals have been of commercial interest since the mid-20th century and are now called "forever chemicals." Their uses have included coolant materials in air conditioning systems; artificial oxygen-carrying substances in experimental clinical studies; and heat-, stain-, and stick-resistant coatings for cookware, fabrics, and other materials. The fluorocarbons were produced in very large quantities and have become widespread in the environment. When it later became apparent that migration of lower-molecular-weight fluorocarbons to the troposphere had a deleterious effect on the protective ozone layer, they were banned from use. The higher-molecular-weight, more highly fluorinated compounds, now called *perfluorinated substances* (eg, Teflon), have remained in broad use. Like the heavily chlorinated and brominated hydrocarbons, their commercial usefulness has been complicated by a recognition of adverse environmental and suspected human toxic impacts that resemble some of the adverse qualities of the other halogenated hydrocarbons. A useful reference is the Centers for Disease Control and Prevention (CDC) fact sheet on PFCs. It is found at www.cdc.gov/biomonitoring/pdf/PFCs_FactSheet.pdf.

1. *Human toxicology*—Concerns about the toxicology of PFCs have centered on their estrogenic properties and accumulation and persistence in humans. Human exposure to perfluoro compounds takes place through ingestion and inhalation. Since these compounds enter the food chain and water sources and are persistent, ingestion of contaminated food and water products is a major source of human accumulation. The human half-life of perfluorooctanoic acid (PFOA) is estimated to be about 3 years. As a persistent chemical and an endocrine disrupter, it is likely that it has some long-term adverse impact on reproductive function, cellular proliferation, and other cellular homeostatic mechanisms. Several PFCs (but not perfluoro compounds derived from PFOA) have been found to act as proliferators of breast cancer cells. However, a large epidemiologic study recently demonstrated a statistically significant association between high and very high serum PFOA levels in workers and kidney cancer, and possibly prostate cancer, ovarian cancer, and non-Hodgkin lymphoma. There also may be modest associations with cholesterol elevation and uric acid abnormalities. Finally, an acute pulmonary disorder, **polymer fume fever,** is caused by the pyrolysis of PFOA. Like metal fume fever, seen in welders as a result of cadmium vaporization, polymer fume fever has an acute onset several hours after exposure to the vaporized PFOA and may cause severe respiratory distress. The onset of symptoms, malaise, chills and fever, and respiratory distress is characteristic of fume fevers. While polymer fume fever is usually mild and self-limited, noncardiogenic pulmonary edema has occurred. Whenever PFOA is heated above 350–400°C, toxic fumes capable of causing polymer fume fever are emitted. Overheated household cookware or burning of coated fabrics present this risk.

Other human effects are not clearly defined, although animal studies have shown toxic effects on immune, liver, and endocrine function, and some increase in tumors and neonatal deaths. A useful American Cancer Society fact sheet on the subject may be found at www.cancer.org/cancer/cancer-causes/teflon-and-perfluorooctanoic-acid-pfoa.html.

2. *Environmental toxicology*—Perfluoro compounds are persistent environmental chemicals having a broad environmental impact. PFOA and related compounds are now found widely in water, soil, and many terrestrial and avian species. Aquatic organisms have accumulated significant loads of PFCs. An extensive risk assessment of the perfluoro chemicals has been carried out by Environment Canada, and guidelines have been developed for the management of PFOA and related compounds. These may be found at www.ec.gc.ca/ese-ees/default.asp?lang=En&n=451C95ED-1.

Concerns about PFOA persistence in water and their transmission to food crops, milk, and other edibles from the water has increased as the widespread persistent compounds have been found in many water supplies. PFOA and PFAS are used in firefighting foams among many other sources (as noted above) and as a result can end up in the ground water near communities. Several studies have now measured significant levels of these PFAS/PFOS in human serum in regions living near air force bases (such as in Colorado Springs), among others.

Endocrine Disruptors

As described above, the potential hazardous effects of some chemicals in the environment are receiving considerable attention because of their estrogen-like or antiandrogenic properties. Compounds that affect thyroid function also are of concern. Since 1998, the process of prioritization, screening, and testing of chemicals for such actions has been undergoing worldwide development. These chemicals mimic, enhance, or inhibit a hormonal action. They include a number of plant constituents (phytoestrogens) and some mycoestrogens as well as industrial chemicals, persistent organochlorine agents (eg, DDT), PCBs, and brominated flame retardants. Concerns exist because of their increasing contamination of the environment, the appearance of bioaccumulation, and their potential for toxicity. In vitro assays alone are unreliable for regulatory purposes, and animal studies are considered indispensable. Modified endocrine responses in reptiles and marine invertebrates have been observed. In humans, however, a causal relation between exposure to a specific environmental agent and an adverse health effect due to endocrine modulation has not been fully established. Epidemiologic studies of populations exposed to higher concentrations of endocrine-disrupting environmental chemicals are underway. There are indications that breast and other reproductive cancers are increased in these patients. Prudence dictates that exposure to environmental chemicals that disrupt endocrine function should be reduced. Lastly, a recent study indicated that infant adiposity and weight were associated with maternal PFAS serum levels, linking these environmental contaminants to adverse effects on children (see Starling et al, 2019).

Cyanotoxins

Cyanotoxins are a large family of cyclic peptides, alkaloids, and lipopolysaccharides; they are products of blue-green algae that are widely distributed in lakes and in salt water where, at warm temperatures, they form blooms. If ingested at high concentrations, cyanotoxins can cause poisoning and rapid death by respiratory failure. At lower concentrations they may cause gastrointestinal or skin conditions, and neurologic, hepatic, and other organ system dysfunction. The cyanobacteria neurotoxin BMAA has been implicated as a cause of neurodegenerative disease.

Asbestos

Asbestos in many of its forms has been widely used in industry for over 100 years. All forms of asbestos have been shown to cause progressive fibrotic lung disease (asbestosis), lung cancer, and mesothelioma. Every form of asbestos, including chrysotile asbestos, causes an increase in lung cancer and mesothelioma. Lung cancer occurs in people exposed at fiber concentrations well below concentrations that produce asbestosis. Very large-scale studies of insulation workers have shown that cigarette smoking and exposure to radon daughters increase the incidence of asbestos-caused lung cancer in a synergistic fashion. Asbestos exposure and smoking is a very hazardous combination.

All forms of asbestos cause mesothelioma of the pleura or peritoneum at very low doses. Other cancers (colon, laryngeal, stomach, and perhaps even lymphoma) are increased in asbestos-exposed patients. The mechanism for asbestos-caused cancer is not yet delineated. Arguments that chrysotile asbestos does not cause mesothelioma are contradicted by many epidemiologic studies of worker populations. Recognition that all forms of asbestos are dangerous and carcinogenic has led many countries to ban all uses of asbestos. Countries such as Canada, Zimbabwe, Russia, Brazil, and others that still produce asbestos argue that asbestos can be used safely with careful workplace environmental controls. However, studies of industrial practice make the "safe use" of asbestos highly improbable. Recent attempts to limit international trade in asbestos have been thwarted by heavy pressure from the asbestos industry and the producing countries. Information on countries that currently ban asbestos and the International Ban Asbestos movement may be found at ibasecretariat.org/alpha_ban_list.php.

METALS

Occupational and environmental poisoning with metals, metalloids, and metal compounds is a major health problem. Toxic metal exposure occurs in many industries, in the home, and elsewhere in the nonoccupational environment. The classic metal poisons (arsenic, lead, and mercury) continue to be widely used. (Treatment of their toxicities is discussed in Chapter 57.) Occupational exposure and poisoning due to **beryllium, cadmium, manganese,** and **uranium** are relatively new occupational problems. In 2016, **cobalt** and cobalt-releasing compounds were listed by the National Institute of Environmental Health Sciences as "reasonably anticipated to be" human carcinogens.

Beryllium

Beryllium (Be) is a light alkaline metal that confers special properties on the alloys and ceramics in which it is incorporated. Beryllium-copper alloys find use as components of computers, in the encasement of the first stage of nuclear weapons, in devices that require hardening such as missile ceramic nose cones, and in heat shield tiles used in space vehicles. Because of the use of beryllium in dental appliances, dentists and dental appliance makers are often exposed to beryllium dust in toxic concentrations and may develop beryllium disease.

Beryllium is highly toxic by inhalation and is classified by the IARC as a class 1, known human carcinogen. Inhalation of beryllium particles produces both acute beryllium disease and chronic disease characterized by progressive pulmonary fibrosis. Skin disease also develops in workers exposed to beryllium. The pulmonary disease is called chronic beryllium disease (CBD) and is a chronic granulomatous pulmonary fibrosis. In the 5–15% of the population that is immunologically sensitive to beryllium, CBD is the result of activation of an autoimmune attack on the skin and lungs. The disease is progressive and may lead to severe disability, cancer, and death. Although some treatment approaches to CBD show promise, the prognosis is poor in most cases.

The current permissible exposure levels for beryllium of 0.01 mcg/m^3 averaged over a 30-day period or 2 mcg/m^3 over an 8-hour period are insufficiently protective to prevent CBD. Both NIOSH and the ACGIH have recommended that the 8-hour PEL and TLV be reduced to 0.05 mcg/m^3. In September 2020, new OSHA regulations reduced the PEL to 0.2 mcg/m^3 over an 8-hour period. Current OSHA information on beryllium appears at www.osha.gov/beryllium.

Environmental beryllium exposure is not generally thought to be a hazard to human health except in the vicinity of industrial sites where air, water, and soil pollution have occurred.

Cadmium

Cadmium (Cd) is a transition metal widely used in industry. Workers are exposed to cadmium in the manufacture of nickel-cadmium batteries, pigments, and low-melting-point eutectic materials; in solder; in television phosphors; and in plating operations. It is also used extensively in semiconductors and in plastics as a stabilizer. Cadmium smelting is often done from residual dust from lead smelting operations, and cadmium smelter workers often face both lead and cadmium toxicity.

Cadmium is toxic by inhalation and by ingestion. When metals that have been plated with cadmium or welded with cadmium-containing materials are vaporized by the heat of torches or cutting implements, the fine dust and fumes released produce an acute respiratory disorder called **cadmium fume fever.** This disorder, common in welders, is usually characterized by shaking chills, cough, fever, and malaise. Although it may produce pneumonia, it is usually transient. However, chronic exposure to cadmium dust produces a far more serious progressive pulmonary fibrosis. Cadmium also causes severe kidney damage, including renal failure if exposure continues. Cadmium is a human carcinogen and is listed as a class 1, known human carcinogen by the IARC.

The current OSHA PEL for cadmium is 5 mcg/m^3 but is insufficiently protective of worker health. The OSHA cadmium standard may be found at www.osha.gov/pls/oshaweb/owadisp.show_document?p_table=STANDARDS&p_id=10036.

Nanomaterials

Nanomaterials are defined as any material, natural or manufactured, that has at least one dimension that lies between 1 and 100 nanometers (nm) in size. The Stanford University Health and Safety Department gives a more precise definition at ehs.stanford.edu/topic/hazardous-materials/nanomaterials. The aspect ratio for the nanomaterial is its longest dimension to shortest dimension.

Nanomaterials have been of increasing commercial interest and are now used for an extraordinary range of purposes. In the pharmaceutical manufacturing industry, nanoparticles are being tested and used to deliver cancer chemotherapeutic and other drugs. Currently produced nanomaterials include gold, silver, cadmium, germanium, ceramic, and aluminum oxide nanowires; carbon, silicon, and germanium nanotubes; zinc oxide nanocrystals; gold nanowafers; and copper oxide nanocubes. The increasing use of nanomaterials has led to release of these nanoscale substances into the workplace and the general environment. Because nanomaterials behave in unique patterns of chemical and physical reactivity, their toxicology is often novel and there is insufficient information on the likely human or environmental impact of dispersal of these manufactured products in the environment. The University of North Carolina laboratory safety and health manual outlines the problems of working with nanomaterials in the laboratory and their safe use at policies.unc.edu/TDClient/2833/Portal/KB/ArticleDet?ID=132030.

1. *Human toxicology*—Inhalation, oral ingestion, dermal absorption, and parenteral administration of nanomaterials have been the sources of human exposure. Because of the unique physicochemical properties of nanomaterials, their toxicity may be similar to or very different from the larger, bulk materials encountered in traditional toxicology studies. The nature of the exposure will impact the likelihood that nanomaterials will reach target organs or cells. Nanomaterials can cross cellular membranes, may penetrate nuclear material and genetic information, and may impact cellular response at a nanoscale. Silica nanoparticles have been demonstrated to produce kidney toxicity in humans, silver nanoparticles are toxic to human and rodent mast cells, and zinc oxide nanoparticles are toxic to human liver cells. Multiwalled carbon nanotubes (MWCNT) have been found to be cytotoxic in human lung cells. Numerous studies have been done to evaluate toxicity of nanomaterials, such as MWCNT. Following extensive animal studies using Mitsui-7 (one form of MWCNT), IARC evaluated and approved MWCNT Mitsui-7 as a group 2B carcinogen (see monographs.iarc.who.int/wp-content/uploads/2018/06/mono111-01.pdf). It is highly likely that other MWCNTs of similar aspect ratio also are carcinogens. Titanium dioxide nanoparticles that are widely used in sunscreens, other cosmetics, pharmaceuticals, and many other products have been noted to be toxic in the lungs and elsewhere.

2. *Environmental toxicology*—Nanomaterials can enter the environment at all stages of their industrial life cycle, including manufacturing, delivery, use, and disposal. When nanomaterials are placed into waste streams they may enter water systems, or be carried by wind or soils, and enter the food chain. An EPA fact sheet on nanomaterials in the environment is available at www.epa.gov/sites/production/files/2014-03/documents/ffrrofactsheet_emergingcontaminant_nanomaterials_jan2014_final.pdf.

The increasing production of nanomaterials and their multiple uses have led to environmental contamination. Many species, including bacteria, small mammals, and fish and other aquatic organisms have been studied in laboratory assessments of nanomaterial toxicity. The ecotoxicology of nanomaterials remains an area of deep concern and ongoing research.

REFERENCES

Air pollution

Alexis NE et al: Low-level ozone exposure induces airways inflammation and modifies cell surface phenotypes in healthy humans. Inhal Toxicol 2010;22:593.

Amato-Lourenco LF et al: An emerging class of air pollutants: Potential effects of microplastics to respiratory human health? Sci Total Environ 2020;749:141676.

Bauer AK, Kleeberger SR: Genetic mechanisms of susceptibility to ozone-induced lung disease. Ann NY Acad Sci 2010;1203:113.

Bowe B et al: Burden of cause-specific mortality associated with PM2.5 air pollution in the United States. JAMA Netw Open 2019;2:e1915834.

Buckley A et al: Hyperbaric oxygen for carbon monoxide poisoning: A systematic review and critical analysis of the evidence. Toxicol Rev 2005;24:75.

Carlsen HK et al: Ozone is associated with cardiopulmonary and stroke emergency hospital visits in Reykjavík, Iceland 2003–2009. Environ Health 2013;12:28.

Dockery DW et al: Effect of air pollution control on mortality and hospital admissions in Ireland. Res Rep Health Eff Inst 2013;176:3.

Fanelli V et al: Acute respiratory distress syndrome: New definition, current and future therapeutic options. J Thorac Dis 2013;5:326.

Goyal P, Mishra D, Kumar A: Vehicular emission inventory of criteria pollutants in Delhi. Springerplus 2013;2:216.

Hatch GE et al: Biomarkers of dose and effect of inhaled ozone in resting versus exercising human subjects: Comparison with resting rats. Biomark Insights 2013;8:53.

Heinrich J et al: Long-term exposure to NO2 and PM10 and all-cause and cause-specific mortality in a prospective cohort of women. Occup Environ Med 2013;70:179.

Hernandez ML et al: Low-level ozone has both respiratory and systemic effects in African American adolescents with asthma despite asthma controller therapy. J Allergy Clin Immunol 2018;142:1974.

Howden R et al: The influence of Nrf2 on cardiac responses to environmental stressors. Oxid Med Cell Longev 2013;2013:901239.

Hwang IY et al: Association of short-term particulate matter exposure with suicide death among major depressive disorder patients: a time-stratified case-crossover analysis. Sci Rep 2022;12:8471.

International Agency for Research on Cancer (IARC): Some non-heterocyclic polycyclic aromatic hydrocarbons and some related exposures. In: *IARC Monographs on the Evaluation of Carcinogenic Risks to Humans*. World Health Organiziation, 2010.

Iglesias-Vazquez L et al: Maternal exposure to air pollution during pregnancy and child's cognitive, language, and motor function: ECLIPSES study. Environ Res 2022;212:113501.

Independent Particulate Matter Review et al: The need for a tighter particulate-matter air-quality standard. N Engl J Med 2020;383:680.

Järvholm B, Reuterwall C: A comparison of occupational and non-occupational exposure to diesel exhausts and its consequences for studying health effects. Occup Environ Med 2012;69:851.

Jerrett M et al: Long-term ozone exposure and mortality. N Engl J Med 2009;360:1085.

Kao JW, Nanagas KA: Carbon monoxide poisoning. Emerg Med Clin North Am 2004;22:985.

Keeler GJ et al: Characterization of urban atmospheres during inhalation exposure studies in Detroit and Grand Rapids, Michigan. Toxicol Pathol 2007;35:15.

Kellogg CA, Griffin DW: Aerobiology and the global transport of desert dust. Trends Ecol Evol 2006;21:638.

Lin J et al: China's international trade and air pollution in the United States. Proc Natl Acad Sci U S A 2014;111:1736.

Mann A, Early GL: Acute respiratory distress syndrome. Mo Med 2012;109:371.

Mehta AJ et al: Long-term exposure to ambient fine particulate matter and renal function in older men: The Veterans Administration Normative Aging Study. Environ Health Perspect 2016;124:1353.

Prata JC et al: Environmental exposure to microplastics: An overview on possible human health effects. Sci Total Environ 2020;702:134455.

Raub JA et al: Carbon monoxide poisoning—a public health perspective. Toxicology 2000;145:1.

Shi L et al: Low-concentration PM2.5 and mortality: Estimating acute and chronic effects in a population-based study. Environ Health Perspect 2016;124:46.

Thurston GD et al: Outdoor air pollution and new-onset airway disease. An official American Thoracic Society Workshop Report. Ann Am Thorac Soc 2020;17:387.

Zhang Y et al: Fine particulate matter (PM2.5) and chronic kidney disease. Rev Environ Contam Toxicol 2021;254:183.

Environmental Pollutants

Barton KE et al: Sociodemographic and behavioral determinants of serum concentrations of per- and polyfluoroalkyl substances in a community highly exposed to aqueous film-forming foam contaminants in drinking water. Int J Hyg Environ Health 2020;223:256.

Booker SM: Dioxin in Vietnam: fighting a legacy of war. Environ Health Perspect 2001;109:A116.

Fucic A et al: Environmental exposure to xenoestrogens and oestrogen related cancers: Reproductive system, breast, lung, kidney, pancreas, and brain. Environ Health 2012;11:S8.

Geusau A et al: Severe 2,3,7,8-tetrachlorodibenzo-*p*-dioxin (TCDD) intoxication: Clinical and laboratory effects. Environ Health Perspect 2001;109:865.

Gosselin RE, Smith RP, Hodge HC: *Clinical Toxicology of Commercial Products*, 5th ed. Williams & Wilkins, 1984.

Hamm JI, Chen CY, Birnbaum LS: A mixture of dioxin, furans, and non-ortho PCBs based upon consensus toxic equivalency factors produces dioxin-like reproductive effects. Toxicol Sci 2003;74:182.

Jacobson JL, Jacobson SW: Association of prenatal exposure to an environmental contaminant with intellectual function in childhood. J Toxicol Clin Toxicol 2002;40:467.

Maras M et al: Estrogen-like properties of fluorotelemer alcohols as revealed by mcg-7 breast cancer cell proliferation. Environ Health Perspect 2006;114:100.

McDonough CA et al: Unsaturated PFOS and other PFASs in human serum and drinking water from an AFFF-impacted community. Environ Sci Technol 2021;55:8139.

Sadasivaiah S, Tozan Y, Breman JG: Dichlorodiphenyltrichloroethane (DDT) for indoor residual spraying in Africa: How can it be used for malaria control? Am J Trop Med Hyg 2007;77:249.

Shusterman DJ: Polymer fume fever and other fluorocarbon pyrolysis-related syndromes. Occup Med 1993;8:519.

Starling AP et al : Prenatal exposure to per- and polyfluoroalkyl substances and infant growth and adiposity: the Healthy Start Study. Environ Int 2019;131:104983.

St Hilaire S et al: Estrogen receptor positive breast cancers and their association with environmental factors. Int J Health Geogr 2011;10:10.

Svirčev Z et al: Global geographical and historical overview of cyanotoxin distribution and cyanobacterial poisonings. Arch Toxicol 2019;93:2429.

United States Environmental Protection Agency, *National Emissions Inventory*. 2022; Available from: https://www.epa.gov/air-emissions-inventories/national-emissions-inventory-nei.

Vieira VM et al: Perfluorooctanoic acid exposure and cancer outcomes in a contaminated community: A geographic analysis. Environ Health Perspect 2013;121:318.

Warner M et al: Diabetes, metabolic syndrome, and obesity in relation to serum dioxin concentrations: The Seveso women's health study. Environ Health Perspect 2013;121:906.

Metals

Cummings KJ et al: A reconsideration of acute beryllium disease. Environ Health Perspect 2009;117:1250.

Kelleher P, Pacheco K, Newman LS: Inorganic dust pneumonias: The metal-related parenchymal disorders. Environ Health Perspect 2000;108:685.

Nanomaterials/Nanotoxicology

Aldossari AA et al: Influence of physicochemical properties of silver nanoparticles on mast cell activation and degranulation. Toxicol In Vitro 2015; 29:195.

Anderson DS et al: Influence of particle size on persistence and clearance of aerosolized silver nanoparticles in the rat lung. Toxicol Sci 2015;144:366.

Johnson RJ, Wesseling C, Newman LS: Chronic kidney disease of unknown cause in agricultural communities. N Engl J Med 2019;380:1843.

Nowack B et al: Analysis of the occupational, consumer and environmental exposure to engineered nanomaterials used in 10 technology sectors. Nanotoxicology 2013;7:1152.

Sargent LM et al: Promotion of lung adenocarcinoma following inhalation exposure to multi-walled carbon nanotubes. Part Fibre Toxicol 2014;11:3.

Siegrist KJ et al: Mitsui-7, heat-treated, and nitrogen-doped multi-walled carbon nanotubes elicit genotoxicity in human lung epithelial cells. Part Fibre Toxicol 2019;16:36.

Sharifi S et al: Toxicity of nanomaterials. Chem Soc Rev 2012;41:2323.

Warheit DB: How to measure hazards/risks following exposures to nanoscale or pigment-grade titanium dioxide particles. Toxicol Lett 2013;220:193.

Pesticides

Brandt A et al: The neonicotinoids thiacloprid, imidacloprid, and clothianidin affect the immunocompetence of honey bees (*Apis mellifera L.*). J Insect Physiol 2016;86:40.

Bräuner EV et al: A prospective study of organochlorines in adipose tissue and risk of non-Hodgkin lymphoma. Environ Health Perspect 2012; 120:105.

Cattani D et al: Mechanisms underlying the neurotoxicity induced by glyphosate-based herbicide in immature rat hippocampus: Involvement of glutamate excitotoxicity. Toxicology 2014;320:34.

Centers for Disease Control and Prevention (CDC): Acute illnesses associated with insecticides used to control bed bugs—seven states, 2003–2010. MMWR Morb Mortal Wkly Rep 2011;60:1269.

Cha YS et al: Pyrethroid poisoning: Features and predictors of atypical presentations. Emerg Med J 2014;31:899.

Gawarammana IB, Buckley NA: Medical management of paraquat ingestion. Br J Clin Pharmacol 2011;72:745.

Gosselin RE, Smith RP, Hodge HC: Clinical Toxicology of Commercial Products, 5th ed. Williams & Wilkins, 1984.

Haley RW et al: Association of low PON1 type Q (type A) arylesterase activity with neurologic symptom complexes in Gulf War veterans. Toxicol Appl Pharmacol 1999;157:227.

Lorenzoni PJ et al: An electrophysiological study of the intermediate syndrome of organophosphate poisoning. J Clin Neurosci 2010;17:1217.

Lotti M, Moretto A: Organophosphate-induced delayed polyneuropathy. Toxicol Rev 2005;24:37.

Mrema EJ et al: Persistent organochlorinated pesticides and mechanisms of their toxicity. Toxicology 2013;307:74.

Ray DE, Fry JR: A reassessment of the neurotoxicity of pyrethroid insecticides. Pharmacol Ther 2006;111:174.

Soderlund DM et al: Mechanisms of pyrethroid neurotoxicity: Implications for cumulative risk assessment. Toxicology 2002;171:3.

Storm JE, Rozman KK, Doull J: Occupational exposure limits for 30 organophosphate pesticides based on inhibition of red blood cell acetylcholinesterase. Toxicology 2000;150:1.

Trabert B et al: Maternal pregnancy levels of trans-nonachlor and oxychlordane and prevalence of cryptorchidism and hypospadias in boys. Environ Health Perspect 2012;120:478.

Wigfield YY, McLenaghan CC: Levels of N-nitrosodimethylamine in nitrogen fertilizers/herbicide mixtures containing 2,4-D present as dimethylamine salt. Bull Environ Contam Toxicol 1990;45:847.

Zhang L et al: Exposure to glyphosate-based herbicides and risk for non-Hodgkin lymphoma: A meta-analysis and supporting evidence. Mutat Res 2019; 781:186.

Solvents

Jørgensen KM et al: Gene expression response in peripheral blood cells of petroleum workers exposed to sub-ppm benzene levels. Int J Environ Res Public Health 2018;15:2385.

Loomis D et al: Carcinogenicity of benzene. Lancet Oncol 2017;18:1574.

Rappaport SM et al: Human benzene metabolism following occupational and environmental exposures. Chem Biol Interact 2010;184:189.

Rusyn I et al: Trichloroethylene: Mechanistic, epidemiologic and other supporting evidence of carcinogenic hazard. Pharmacol Ther 2014;141:55.

Others

Balmes JR.: The changing nature of wildfires: impacts on the health of the public. Clin Chest Med 2020;41:771.

Bayram H et al: Environment, global climate change, and cardiopulmonary health. Am J Respir Crit Care Med 2017;195:718.

De Guise S et al: Long-term immunological alterations in bottlenose dolphin a decade after the Deepwater Horizon oil spill in the Northern Gulf of Mexico: Potential for multigenerational effects. Environ Toxicol Chem 2021;40:1308.

U.S. Department of Health and Human Services, National Institute of Environmental Health Services, National Toxicology Program: 15th Report on Carcinogens. 2021. ntp.niehs.nih.gov/go/roc15.

CASE STUDY ANSWER

The child presents with classic signs (and history) of carbon monoxide (CO) exposure. Pulse oximetry is unreliable in CO poisoning, although newer instruments may distinguish between carboxyhemoglobin (CO-Hgb) and oxyhemoglobin. Institute the ABCDs of poisoning (Chapter 58). Immediate high-flow oxygen is mandatory and should be administered via a tight-fitting face mask or endotracheal catheter. A blood sample for blood gases and carboxyhemoglobin content should be obtained. If the CO-Hgb is greater than 50%, hyperbaric oxygen treatment (if available) may be considered. The electrocardiogram should be continuously monitored for arrhythmias. Anticonvulsant drugs may be required if seizures occur. Neurologic damage due to CO exposure may be subtle and long-lasting; the child should be followed for years if necessary. The fetus is particularly susceptible to hypoxia, and if the mother is pregnant, her blood gases and CO-Hgb should be measured. If the latter is high, hyperbaric oxygen therapy should be considered.

CHAPTER

57

Heavy Metal Intoxication & Chelators

Michael J. Kosnett, MD, MPH

CASE STUDY

Following Sunday morning services, 27 people attended a church social where coffee, baked goods, and sandwiches were served. Within 15–60 minutes, 13 people developed vomiting and abdominal discomfort, accompanied over the next several hours by nonbloody diarrhea. Within 12 hours, seven of these individuals were hospitalized with ongoing gastrointestinal symptoms, hypotension, and anion gap metabolic acidosis. Fluid resuscitation and pressors were accompanied by adequate urine output. What diagnoses should be considered? What tests should be conducted, and what therapy should be considered?

Some metals such as iron are essential for life, whereas others such as lead are present in all organisms but serve no useful biologic purpose. Some of the oldest diseases of humans can be traced to heavy metal poisoning associated with metal mining, refining, and use. Even with the present recognition of the hazards of heavy metals, the incidence of intoxication remains significant, and the need for preventive strategies and effective therapy remains high. Toxic heavy metals interfere with the function of essential cations, cause enzyme inhibition, generate oxidative stress, alter gene expression, and perturb cell signaling. As a result, multisystem signs and symptoms are a hallmark of heavy metal intoxication.

When intoxication occurs, chelator molecules (from *chela* "claw"), or their in vivo biotransformation products, may be used to bind the metal and facilitate its excretion from the body. Chelator drugs are discussed in the second part of this chapter.

■ TOXICOLOGY OF HEAVY METALS

LEAD

Lead poisoning is one of the oldest occupational and environmental diseases in the world. Despite its recognized hazards, lead continues to have widespread commercial application, including production of storage batteries (more than 90% of US consumption), ammunition, metal alloys, solder, glass, plastics, pigments, and ceramics. Corrosion of lead plumbing in older buildings or supply lines may increase the lead concentration of tap water. Environmental lead exposure, ubiquitous by virtue of the anthropogenic distribution of lead to air, water, and food, has declined considerably in the last four decades as a result of the elimination of lead as an additive in gasoline, as well as diminished contact with lead-based paint and other lead-containing consumer products, such as lead solder in cans used as food containers. Legislation in the United States in 2011 further reduced the maximum permissible lead content of children's products to 100 ppm. Lead continues to be used in some formulations of aviation gasoline for piston-engine aircraft. The presence of lead in certain folk medicines (eg, the Mexican remedies azarcon and greta, and certain Ayurvedic preparations) and in cosmetics (eg, kohl utilized around the eyes in certain African and Asian communities) has contributed to lead exposure to children and adults. Although public health measures, together with improved workplace conditions, have decreased the incidence of serious overt lead poisoning, there remains considerable concern over the effects of low-level lead exposure. Extensive evidence indicates that low levels of lead exposure may have subtle subclinical adverse effects on neurocognitive function in children and may contribute to hypertension and cardiovascular disease in adults. Lead serves no useful purpose in the human body. In key target organs such as the developing central nervous system, no level of lead exposure has been shown to be without deleterious effects.

Pharmacokinetics

Inorganic lead is slowly but consistently absorbed via the respiratory and gastrointestinal tracts. It is poorly absorbed through the skin. Absorption of lead dust via the respiratory tract is the most common cause of industrial poisoning. The intestinal tract is the primary route of entry in nonindustrial exposure (Table 57–1). Absorption via the gastrointestinal tract varies with the nature of the lead compound, but in general, adults absorb about 10–15% of the ingested amount, whereas young children absorb up to 50%. Low dietary calcium, iron deficiency, and ingestion on an empty stomach all have been associated with increased lead absorption.

Once absorbed from the respiratory or gastrointestinal tract, lead enters the bloodstream, where approximately 99% is bound to erythrocytes and 1% is present in the plasma. Lead is subsequently distributed to soft tissues such as the bone marrow, brain, kidney, liver, muscle, and gonads; then to the subperiosteal surface of bone; and later to bone matrix. Lead also crosses the placenta and poses a potential hazard to the fetus. The kinetics of lead clearance from the body follows a multicompartment model, composed predominantly of the blood and soft tissues, with a half-life of 1–2 months; and the skeleton, with a half-life of years to decades. Approximately 70% of the lead that is eliminated appears in the urine, with lesser amounts excreted through the bile, skin, hair, nails, sweat, and breast milk. The fraction not undergoing prompt excretion, approximately half of the absorbed lead, may be incorporated into the skeleton, the repository of more than 90% of the body lead burden in most adults. In patients with high bone lead burdens, slow release from the skeleton may elevate blood lead concentrations for years after exposure ceases, and pathologic high bone turnover states such as hyperthyroidism or prolonged immobilization may result in frank lead intoxication. Retained lead bullet fragments, particularly but not exclusively those located in a joint space, pseudocyst, or other fluid-filled cavity or adjacent to bone, have

TABLE 57–1 Toxicology of selected arsenic, lead, and mercury compounds.

	Form Entering Body	Major Route of Absorption	Distribution	Major Clinical Effects	Key Aspects of Mechanism	Metabolism and Elimination
Arsenic	Inorganic arsenic salts	Gastrointestinal, respiratory (all mucosal surfaces)	Predominantly soft tissues (highest in liver, kidney). Avidly bound in skin, hair, nails	Acute cardiovascular: shock, arrhythmias; chronic: coronary heart disease CNS: encephalopathy, peripheral neuropathy. Gastroenteritis; pancytopenia; cancer (many sites)	Inhibits enzymes; interferes with oxidative phosphorylation; alters cell signaling, gene expression	Methylation. Renal (major); sweat and feces (minor)
Lead	Inorganic lead oxides and salts	Gastrointestinal, respiratory	Soft tissues; redistributed to skeleton (>90% of adult body burden)	CNS deficits; peripheral neuropathy; anemia; nephropathy; hypertension and cardiovascular mortality; reproductive toxicity	Inhibits enzymes; interferes with essential cations; alters membrane structure	Renal (major); feces and breast milk (minor)
	Organic (tetraethyl lead)	Skin, gastrointestinal, respiratory	Soft tissues, especially liver, CNS	Encephalopathy	Hepatic dealkylation (fast) → trialkyl metabolites (slow) → dissociation to lead	Urine and feces (major); sweat (minor)
Mercury	Elemental mercury	Respiratory tract	Soft tissues, especially kidney, CNS	CNS: tremor, behavioral (erethism); gingivostomatitis, peripheral neuropathy; acrodynia; pneumonitis (high-dose)	Inhibits enzymes; alters membranes	Elemental Hg converted to Hg^{2+}. Urine (major); feces (minor)
	Inorganic: Hg^{+} (less toxic); Hg^{2+} (more toxic)	Gastrointestinal, skin (minor)	Soft tissues, especially kidney	Acute renal tubular necrosis; gastroenteritis; CNS effects (rare)	Inhibits enzymes; alters membranes	Urine
	Organic: alkyl, aryl	Gastrointestinal, skin, respiratory (minor)	Soft tissues	CNS effects, birth defects	Inhibits enzymes; alters microtubules, neuronal structure	Deacylation. Fecal (alkyl, major); urine (Hg^{2+} after deacylation, minor)

been responsible for the development of lead poisoning signs and symptoms years or decades after an initial gunshot injury. Recently updated biokinetic models relate lead intake to lead concentration in blood and bone over time, including the US Environmental Protection Agency's All-Ages Lead Model, the Leggett+ Model, and the DoD-O'Flaherty Model. These models have utility in the development of public health standards pertaining to permissible lead exposure in the workplace and in the environment.

Pharmacodynamics

Lead exerts multisystemic toxic effects that are mediated by multiple modes of action, including inhibition of enzymatic function; interference with the action of essential cations, particularly calcium, iron, and zinc; generation of oxidative stress; changes in gene expression; alterations in cell signaling; and disruption of the integrity of membranes in cells and intracellular organelles.

A. Nervous System

The developing central nervous system of the fetus and young child is the most sensitive target organ for lead's toxic effect. Epidemiologic studies suggest that blood lead concentrations <5 mcg/dL may result in subclinical deficits in neurocognitive function in lead-exposed young children, with no demonstrable threshold or "no effect" level. The dose response between low blood lead concentrations and cognitive function in young children is nonlinear, such that the decrement in intelligence associated with an increase in blood lead from <1 to 10 mcg/dL (6.2 IQ points) exceeds that associated with a change from 10 to 30 mcg/dL (3.0 IQ points).

Adults are less sensitive to the central nervous system (CNS) effects of lead, but long-term exposure to blood lead concentrations in the range of 10–30 mcg/dL may be associated with subclinical effects on neurocognitive function. At blood lead concentrations higher than 30 mcg/dL, behavioral and neurocognitive signs or symptoms may gradually emerge, including irritability, fatigue, decreased libido, anorexia, sleep disturbance, impaired visual-motor coordination, and slowed reaction time. Headache, arthralgias, and myalgias are also common complaints. Tremor occurs but is less common. Lead encephalopathy, usually occurring at blood lead concentrations higher than 100 mcg/dL, is typically accompanied by increased intracranial pressure and may cause ataxia, stupor, coma, convulsions, and death. Recent epidemiological studies suggest that lead may accentuate an age-related decline in cognitive function in older adults. In experimental animals, developmental lead exposure, possibly acting through epigenetic mechanisms, has been associated with increased expression of beta-amyloid, increased phosphorylated tau protein, oxidative DNA damage, and Alzheimer-type pathology in the aging brain. There is wide interindividual variation in the magnitude of lead exposure required to cause overt lead-related signs and symptoms.

Overt peripheral neuropathy may appear after chronic high-dose lead exposure, usually following months to years of blood lead concentrations higher than 100 mcg/dL. Predominantly motor in character, the neuropathy may present clinically with painless weakness of the extensors, particularly in the upper extremity, resulting in classic wrist-drop. Preclinical signs of lead-induced peripheral nerve dysfunction may be detectable by electrodiagnostic testing.

B. Blood

Lead can induce an anemia that may be either normocytic or microcytic and hypochromic. Lead interferes with heme synthesis by blocking the incorporation of iron into protoporphyrin IX and by inhibiting the function of enzymes in the heme synthesis pathway, including aminolevulinic acid dehydratase and ferrochelatase. Within 2–8 weeks after an elevation in blood lead concentration (generally to 30–50 mcg/dL or greater), increases in heme precursors, notably free erythrocyte protoporphyrin or its zinc chelate, zinc protoporphyrin, may be detectable in whole blood. Lead also contributes to anemia by increasing erythrocyte membrane fragility and decreasing red cell survival time. Frank hemolysis may occur with high exposure. Basophilic stippling on the peripheral blood smear, thought to be a consequence of lead inhibition of the enzyme 3′,5′-pyrimidine nucleotidase, is sometimes a suggestive—albeit insensitive and nonspecific—diagnostic clue to the presence of lead intoxication.

C. Kidneys

Chronic high-dose lead exposure, usually associated with months to years of blood lead concentrations >80 mcg/dL, may result in renal interstitial fibrosis and nephrosclerosis. Lead nephropathy may have a latency period of years. Lead may alter uric acid excretion by the kidney, resulting in recurrent bouts of gouty arthritis ("saturnine gout"). Acute high-dose lead exposure sometimes produces transient azotemia, possibly as a consequence of intrarenal vasoconstriction. Studies conducted in general population samples have documented an association between blood lead concentration and measures of renal function, including serum creatinine and creatinine clearance. The presence of other risk factors for renal insufficiency, including hypertension and diabetes, may increase susceptibility to lead-induced renal dysfunction.

D. Reproductive Organs

High-dose lead exposure is a recognized risk factor for stillbirth or spontaneous abortion. Epidemiologic studies of the impact of low-level lead exposure on reproductive outcome such as low birth weight, preterm delivery, or spontaneous abortion have yielded mixed results. However, a well-designed nested case-control study detected an odds ratio for spontaneous abortion of 1.8 (95% CI 1.1–3.1) for every 5 mcg/dL increase in maternal blood lead across an approximate range of 5–20 mcg/dL. Recent studies have linked prenatal exposure to low levels of lead (eg, maternal blood lead concentrations of 5–15 mcg/dL) to decrements in physical and cognitive development assessed during the neonatal period and early childhood. In males, blood lead concentrations higher than 40 mcg/dL have been associated with diminished or aberrant sperm production.

E. Gastrointestinal Tract

Moderate lead poisoning may cause loss of appetite, constipation, and, less commonly, diarrhea. At high dosage, intermittent bouts of severe colicky abdominal pain ("lead colic") may occur. The mechanism of lead colic is unclear but is believed to involve spasmodic contraction of the smooth muscles of the intestinal wall, mediated by alteration in synaptic transmission at the smooth muscle-neuromuscular junction. In heavily exposed individuals with poor dental hygiene, the reaction of circulating lead with sulfur ions released by microbial action may produce dark deposits of lead sulfide at the gingival margin ("gingival lead lines"). Although frequently mentioned as a diagnostic clue in the past, in recent times this has been a relatively rare sign of lead exposure.

F. Cardiovascular System

Epidemiologic, experimental, and in vitro mechanistic data indicate that lead exposure elevates blood pressure in experimental animals and in susceptible humans. The pressor effect of lead may be mediated by an interaction with calcium-mediated contraction of vascular smooth muscle, as well as generation of oxidative stress and an associated interference in nitric oxide signaling pathways. In populations with environmental or occupational lead exposure, blood lead concentration is linked with increases in systolic and diastolic blood pressure. Studies of middle-aged and elderly men and women have identified relatively low levels of lead exposure sustained by the general population to be an independent risk factor for hypertension. Lead exposure has also been associated with prolongation of the QT_c interval on the electrocardiogram. Epidemiologic findings derived from prospective cohort studies have linked chronic environmental lead exposure associated with population blood lead concentrations in the range of 10–25 mcg/dL to a significantly increased risk of cardiovascular mortality. This is of considerable public health concern because these concentrations were prevalent in the USA prior to the 1980s. Although general population blood lead concentrations have since fallen considerably (see below), exposure associated with blood lead in this range persists in occupational settings worldwide.

Major Forms of Lead Intoxication

A. Inorganic Lead Poisoning (Table 57–1)

1. *Acute*—Acute inorganic lead poisoning is uncommon today. It usually results from industrial inhalation of large quantities of lead oxide fumes or, in small children, from ingestion of a large oral dose of lead in the form of lead-based paint chips; small objects, eg, toys coated or fabricated from lead; or contaminated food or drink. The onset of severe symptoms usually requires several days or weeks of recurrent exposure and manifests as signs and symptoms of encephalopathy or colic. Evidence of hemolytic anemia (or anemia with basophilic stippling if exposure has been subacute) and elevated hepatic aminotransferases may be present.

The diagnosis of acute inorganic lead poisoning may be difficult, and depending on the presenting symptoms, the condition has sometimes been mistaken for appendicitis, peptic ulcer, biliary colic, pancreatitis, or infectious meningitis. Subacute presentation, featuring headache, fatigue, intermittent abdominal cramps, myalgias, and arthralgias, has often been mistaken for a flu-like viral illness. When there has been recent ingestion of lead-containing paint chips, glazes, pellets, or weights, radiopacities may be visible on abdominal radiographs.

2. *Chronic*—The patient with symptomatic chronic lead intoxication typically presents with multisystemic findings, including complaints of anorexia, fatigue, and malaise; neurologic complaints, including headache, difficulty in concentrating, and irritability or depressed mood; weakness, arthralgias, or myalgias; and gastrointestinal symptoms. Lead poisoning should be strongly suspected in any patient presenting with headache, abdominal pain, and anemia; and less commonly with motor neuropathy, gout, and renal insufficiency. Chronic lead intoxication should be considered in any child with neurocognitive deficits, growth retardation, or developmental delay. It is important to recognize that adverse effects of lead that are of considerable public health significance, such as subclinical decrements in neurodevelopment in children and hypertension and other adverse cardiovascular effects in adults, are usually nonspecific and may not come to medical attention.

The diagnosis of lead intoxication is best confirmed by measuring lead in whole blood. Although this test reflects lead currently circulating in blood and soft tissues and is not a reliable marker of either recent or cumulative lead exposure, most patients with lead-related disease have blood lead concentrations higher than the normal range. Average background blood lead concentrations in North America and Europe have declined by >90% in recent decades, and the geometric mean blood lead concentration in the USA in 2017–2018 was estimated to be 0.753 mcg/dL. Though predominantly a research tool, the concentration of lead in bone assessed by noninvasive K X-ray fluorescence measurement of lead has been correlated with long-term cumulative lead exposure, and its relationship to numerous lead-related disorders is the subject of ongoing investigation. Measurement of lead excretion in the urine after a single dose of a chelating agent (sometimes called a "chelation challenge test") primarily reflects the lead content of soft tissues and may not be a reliable marker of long-term lead exposure, remote past exposure, or skeletal lead burden. Accordingly, this test is rarely indicated in clinical practice. Because of the lag time associated with lead-induced elevations in circulating heme precursors, the finding of a blood lead concentration of 30 mcg/dL or more with no concurrent increase in zinc protoporphyrin suggests that the lead exposure was of recent onset.

B. Organolead Poisoning

Poisoning from organolead compounds is now very rare, in large part because of the worldwide phase-out of tetraethyl and tetramethyl lead as antiknock additives in gasoline. However, organolead compounds such as lead stearate or lead naphthenate are still used in certain commercial processes, and lead styphnate is used in ammunition primers and explosives. Because of their volatility or lipid solubility, organolead compounds tend to be well absorbed through either the respiratory tract or the skin. Organolead compounds predominantly target the CNS, producing dose-dependent effects that may include neurocognitive deficits, insomnia, delirium, hallucinations, tremor, convulsions, and death.

Prevention of Lead Poisoning: An Ongoing Effort

Exposure: Sources	Examples of Preventive Measures
Home exposure: The US Consumer Product Safety Commission adopted major restrictions on the use of lead in residential house paint in 1977. Prior to then, thousands of tons of lead pigments were applied in millions of homes. The American Healthy Homes Survey II (2018–2019) estimated that 30% of homes had some lead-based paint and 25% had one or more lead-based paint hazards.	The US Environmental Protection Agency's (EPA) Lead Renovation, Repair, and Painting Rule requires that companies performing renovation, repair, and painting projects that disturb lead-based paint in homes, child care facilities, and preschools built before 1978 have their firm certified by EPA (or an EPA-authorized state), use certified renovators who are trained by EPA-approved training providers, and follow lead-safe work practices. In 2021, EPA issued updated clearance standards for lead in dust following residential lead paint abatement (www.epa.gov/lead/renovation-repair-and-painting-program).
Workplace exposure: The US Occupational Health and Safety Administration (OSHA) estimates that more than 1.6 million workers are potentially exposed to lead. State and federal OSHA programs have established permissible exposure levels for lead in workplace air, as well as medical surveillance requirements for workers that may mandate periodic blood lead monitoring.	Present OSHA rules regarding workplace lead exposure and medical removal protection date from the late 1970s and no longer offer adequate protection. The Occupational Lead Poisoning Prevention Program of the California Department of Public Health offers up-to-date, health protective guidance (www.cdph.ca.gov/Programs/CCDPHP/DEODC/OHB/OLPPP/Pages/OLPPP.aspx). In 2022, OSHA issued an advanced notice of proposed rulemaking signaling an intent to update workplace lead standards (www.osha.gov/lead/rulemaking).
Water: Lead may enter drinking water when service pipes or interior plumbing, fittings, or faucets contain lead, especially when the water has high acidity or low mineral content that corrodes pipes and plumbing fixtures.	Under EPA's Lead and Copper Rule (www.epa.gov/sdwa/use-lead-free-pipes-fittings-fixtures-solder-and-flux-drinking-water), if more than 10% of tap water samples at sites likely to have lead plumbing exceed the lead action level of 15 parts per billion, water systems are required to institute corrosion control and other measures. The Safe Drinking Water Act, amended by the Reduction of Lead in Drinking Water Act of 2011, sets limits on the lead content of new plumbing materials for potable water (www.epa.gov/dwstandardsregulations/use-lead-free-pipes-fittings-fixtures-solder-and-flux-drinking-water). In 2021, EPA announced augmented efforts to inventory and remove lead service lines that transport drinking water from utility water mains to homes.
Children: Because of normal mouthing behavior, children are at special risk of exposure to lead present in toys, jewelry, printed material, and other consumer products.	The US Consumer Product Safety Commission has promulgated rules that limit the amount of lead that can be present in children's products (https://www.cpsc.gov/Business--Manufacturing/Business-Education/Lead/Total-Lead-Content-Business-Guidance-and-Small-Entity-Compliance-Guide www.cpsc.gov/Business--Manufacturing/Business-Education/Lead/Lead-in-Paint).

Production of lead began 6000 years ago, and lead poisoning is one of the oldest known occupational illnesses. Worldwide, lead production has doubled over the past two decades in part because of the growing demand for lead acid storage batteries. Efforts to prevent lead poisoning from multiple industrial, commercial, and environmental sources remain an active focus of public health in the USA.

Treatment

A. Inorganic Lead Poisoning

Treatment of inorganic lead poisoning involves immediate termination of exposure, supportive care, and the judicious use of chelation therapy. (Chelation is discussed later in this chapter.) Lead encephalopathy is a medical emergency that requires intensive supportive care. Cerebral edema may improve with corticosteroids and mannitol or hypertonic saline, and anticonvulsants may be required to treat seizures. Radiopacities on abdominal radiographs may suggest the presence of retained lead objects requiring gastrointestinal decontamination. Adequate urine flow should be maintained, but overhydration should be avoided. Intravenous **edetate calcium disodium ($CaNa_2EDTA$)** is administered at a dosage of 1000–1500 mg/m^2/d (approximately 30–50 mg/kg/d) by continuous infusion for up to 5 days. Some clinicians advocate that chelation treatment for lead encephalopathy be initiated with an intramuscular injection of **dimercaprol,** followed in 4 hours by concurrent administration of dimercaprol and EDTA. Parenteral chelation is limited to 5 or fewer days, at which time oral treatment with another chelator, **succimer (DMSA),** may be instituted. In situations where $CaNa_2EDTA$ has been unavailable, treatment of lead encephalopathy with oral succimer has been successfully initiated via a nasogastric tube. The end point for chelation is usually resolution of symptoms or return of the blood lead concentration to the premorbid range. In patients with chronic exposure, cessation of chelation may be followed by an upward rebound in blood lead concentration as the lead re-equilibrates from bone lead stores.

Although most clinicians support chelation for symptomatic patients with elevated blood lead concentrations, the decision to chelate asymptomatic subjects is more controversial. Since 1991, the Centers for Disease Control and Prevention (CDC) has recommended chelation for all children with blood lead concentrations of 45 mcg/dL or greater. However, a randomized, double-blind, placebo-controlled clinical trial of succimer in children with blood lead concentrations between 25 and 44 mcg/dL found no benefit on neurocognitive function or long-term blood lead reduction. Prophylactic use of chelating agents in the workplace should never be a substitute for reduction or prevention of excessive exposure.

Management of elevated blood lead levels in children and adults should include a conscientious effort to identify and reduce all potential sources of future lead exposure. Many local, state, or national governmental agencies maintain lead poisoning prevention programs that can assist in case management. Blood lead screening of family members or coworkers of a lead poisoning patient is often indicated to assess the scope of the exposure. In 2012, the CDC adopted a new policy that defined as elevated any childhood blood lead concentrations at or exceeding a reference value corresponding to the 97.5th percentile of quadrennial reports of the National Health and Nutrition Examination Survey (NHANES). The blood lead reference value established in 2012 was 5 mcg/dL, and it was revised to 3.5 mcg/dL in 2021. Because there is no blood lead concentration known to be devoid of deleterious effects, the finding of a blood lead concentration exceeding the reference value (ie, elevated in relation to the general population) should prompt clinical and environmental investigation (www.cdc.gov/nceh/lead/acclpp/final_document_030712.pdf). The US Occupational Safety and Health Administration (OSHA) lead regulations introduced in the late 1970s mandate that workers be removed from lead exposure for blood lead levels higher than 50–60 mcg/dL. That regulation is now outdated, and an expert panel in 2007 recommended that removal be initiated for a single blood lead level >30 mcg/dL or when two successive blood lead levels measured over a 4-week interval are 20 mcg/dL or greater (www.ncbi.nlm.nih.gov/pmc/articles/PMC1849937/pdf/ehp0115-000463.pdf). The longer-term goal should be for workers to maintain blood lead levels <10 mcg/dL, and for pregnant women to avoid occupational or avocational exposure that would result in blood lead levels higher than 3.5 mcg/dL. Environmental Protection Agency (EPA) regulations effective since 2010 require that contractors who perform renovation, repair, and painting projects that disturb lead-based paint in pre-1978 residences and child-occupied facilities must be certified and must follow specific work practices to prevent lead contamination (see Box: Prevention of Lead Poisoning: An Ongoing Effort).

B. Organic Lead Poisoning

Initial treatment consists of decontaminating the skin and preventing further exposure. Treatment of seizures requires appropriate use of anticonvulsants. Empiric chelation may be attempted if high blood lead concentrations are present.

ARSENIC

Arsenic is a naturally occurring element in the earth's crust with a long history of use as a constituent of commercial and industrial products, as a component in pharmaceuticals, and as an agent of deliberate poisoning. Recent commercial applications of arsenic include its use in the manufacture of semiconductors, wood preservatives for industrial applications (eg, marine timbers or utility poles), nonferrous alloys, glass, and the turf herbicide monosodium methane arsonate (MSMA). The use of phenylarsenic compounds as feed additives for poultry and swine was terminated in the United States in 2015. In some regions of the world, groundwater may contain high levels of arsenic that has leached from natural mineral deposits. Arsenic in drinking water in the Ganges delta of India and Bangladesh is now recognized as one of the world's most pressing environmental health problems. Environmental risk assessments have suggested that arsenic migrating from coal combustion wastes (eg, coal ash) deposited in unlined landfills may contaminate underlying groundwater. The US Food and Drug Administration (FDA) recently proposed action levels for inorganic arsenic in apple juice of 10 ppb and rice cereals of 100 ppb in an effort to reduce dietary arsenic exposure, particularly to young children (www.fda.gov/food/metals/arsenic-food-and-dietary-supplements). Arsine, an arsenous hydride (AsH_3) gas with potent hemolytic effects, is manufactured predominantly for use in the semiconductor industry but may also be generated accidentally when arsenic-containing ores or scrap gallium arsenide semiconductors come in contact with acidic solutions.

It is of historical interest that Fowler's solution, which contains 1% potassium arsenite, was widely used as a medicine for many conditions from the eighteenth century through the mid-twentieth century. Organic arsenicals were the first pharmaceutical antimicrobials* and were widely used for the first half of the twentieth century until supplanted by sulfonamides and other more effective and less toxic agents.

Other organoarsenicals, most notably lewisite (dichloro-[2-chlorovinyl]arsine), were developed in the early 20th century as chemical warfare agents. Arsenic trioxide was reintroduced into the United States Pharmacopeia in 2000 as an orphan drug for the treatment of relapsed acute promyelocytic leukemia and is finding expanded use in experimental cancer treatment protocols. Melarsoprol, another trivalent arsenical, is used in the treatment of advanced African trypanosomiasis (see Chapter 52).

Pharmacokinetics

Soluble arsenic compounds are well absorbed through the respiratory and gastrointestinal tracts (see Table 57–1). Percutaneous absorption is limited but may be clinically significant after heavy exposure to concentrated arsenic reagents. Most of the absorbed inorganic arsenic undergoes methylation, mainly in the liver, to monomethylarsonic acid and dimethylarsinic acid, which are excreted, along with residual inorganic arsenic, in the urine. When chronic daily absorption is <1000 mcg of soluble inorganic arsenic, approximately two thirds of the absorbed dose is excreted in the urine within 2–3 days. After massive ingestions, the elimination half-life is prolonged. Inhalation of arsenic compounds of low solubility may result in prolonged retention in the lung and may not be reflected by urinary arsenic excretion. Arsenic binds to sulfhydryl groups present in keratinized tissue, and following cessation of exposure, hair, nails, and skin may contain elevated levels after urine values have returned to normal. However, arsenic in hair and nails as a result of external deposition may be indistinguishable from that incorporated after internal absorption.

Pharmacodynamics

Arsenic compounds are thought to exert their toxic effects by several modes of action. Interference with enzyme function may result from sulfhydryl group binding by trivalent arsenic or by substitution for phosphate. Inorganic arsenic or its metabolites may induce oxidative stress, alter gene expression, and interfere with cell signal transduction. Although on a molar basis, inorganic trivalent arsenic (As^{3+}, arsenite) is generally two to ten times more acutely toxic than inorganic pentavalent arsenic (As^{5+}, arsenate), in vivo interconversion is known to occur, and the full spectrum of arsenic toxicity has occurred after sufficient exposure to either form. The trivalent form of the methylated metabolites (eg, monomethylarsonous acid [MMA^{III}]) are more toxic than the inorganic parent compounds. Reduced efficiency in the methylation of MMA to dimethylarsonous acid (DMA), resulting in an elevated percentage of MMA in the urine, has been associated with an increased risk of chronic adverse effects. Arsenic methylation requires *S*-adenosylmethionine, a universal methyl donor in the body, and arsenic-associated perturbations in one-carbon metabolism may underlie some arsenic-induced epigenetic effects such as altered gene expression.

Arsine gas is oxidized in vivo and exerts a potent hemolytic effect associated with alteration of ion flux across the erythrocyte membrane; it also disrupts cellular respiration in other tissues. Arsenic is a recognized human carcinogen and has been associated with cancer of the lung, skin, and bladder. Marine organisms may contain large amounts of a well-absorbed trimethylated organoarsenic, arsenobetaine, as well as a variety of arsenosugars and arsenolipids. Arsenobetaine exerts no known toxic effects when ingested by mammals and is excreted in the urine unchanged; arsenosugars are partially metabolized to dimethylarsinic acid. Thioarsenite compounds that occur as minor metabolites of inorganic arsenic and methylated arsenic compounds in vivo may contribute to toxicity.

Major Forms of Arsenic Intoxication

A. Acute Inorganic Arsenic Poisoning

Within minutes to hours after exposure to high doses (tens to hundreds of milligrams) of soluble inorganic arsenic compounds, many systems are affected. Initial gastrointestinal signs and symptoms include nausea, vomiting, diarrhea, and abdominal pain. Diffuse capillary leak, combined with gastrointestinal fluid loss, may result in hypotension, shock, and death. Cardiopulmonary toxicity, including congestive cardiomyopathy, cardiogenic or noncardiogenic pulmonary edema, and ventricular arrhythmias (particularly in association with QT_c prolongation on the electrocardiogram) may occur promptly or after a delay of several days. Pancytopenia usually develops within 1 week, and basophilic stippling of erythrocytes may be present soon after. Central nervous system effects, including delirium, encephalopathy, and coma, may occur within the first few days of intoxication. An ascending sensorimotor peripheral neuropathy may begin to develop after a delay of 2–6 weeks. This neuropathy may ultimately involve the proximal musculature and result in neuromuscular respiratory failure. Months after an acute poisoning, transverse white striae (Aldrich-Mees lines) may be visible in the nails.

Acute inorganic arsenic poisoning should be considered in an individual presenting with abrupt onset of gastroenteritis in combination with hypotension and metabolic acidosis. Suspicion should be further heightened when these initial findings are followed by cardiac dysfunction, pancytopenia, and peripheral neuropathy. The diagnosis may be confirmed by demonstration of elevated amounts of inorganic arsenic and its metabolites in the urine (typically in the range of several thousand micrograms in the first 2–3 days after acute symptomatic poisoning). Arsenic disappears rapidly from the blood, and except in anuric patients, blood arsenic levels should not be used for diagnostic purposes. Treatment is based on appropriate gut decontamination, intensive supportive care, and prompt chelation with **unithiol,** 3–5 mg/kg intravenously every 4–6 hours, or **dimercaprol,** 3–5 mg/kg intramuscularly every 4–6 hours. In animal studies, the efficacy of

*Paul Ehrlich's "magic bullet" for syphilis (arsphenamine, Salvarsan) was an arsenical.

chelation has been highest when it is administered within minutes to hours after arsenic exposure; therefore, if diagnostic suspicion is high, treatment should not be withheld for the several days to weeks often required to obtain laboratory confirmation.

Succimer has also been effective in animal models and has a higher therapeutic index than dimercaprol. However, because it is available in the United States only for oral administration, its use may not be advisable in the initial treatment of acute arsenic poisoning, when severe gastroenteritis and splanchnic edema may limit absorption by this route.

B. Chronic Inorganic Arsenic Poisoning

Chronic inorganic arsenic poisoning also results in multisystemic signs and symptoms. Overt noncarcinogenic effects may be evident after chronic absorption of more than 0.01 mg/kg/d (~500–1000 mcg/d in adults). The time to appearance of symptoms varies with dose and interindividual tolerance. Constitutional symptoms of fatigue, weight loss, and weakness may be present, along with anemia, nonspecific gastrointestinal complaints, and a sensorimotor peripheral neuropathy, particularly featuring a stocking glove pattern of dysesthesia. Skin changes—among the most characteristic effects—typically develop after years of exposure and include a "raindrop" pattern of hyperpigmentation, and hyperkeratoses involving the hands and feet. Peripheral vascular disease and noncirrhotic portal hypertension may also occur. Epidemiologic studies suggest a possible link to hypertension, cardiovascular disease mortality, diabetes, chronic nonmalignant respiratory disease, and adverse reproductive outcomes. Cancer of the lung, skin, bladder, and possibly other sites, including the kidney and liver, may appear years after exposure to doses of arsenic that are not high enough to elicit other acute or chronic effects. Some studies suggest that tobacco smoking may interact synergistically with arsenic in increasing the risk of certain adverse health outcomes.

Administration of arsenite in cancer chemotherapy regimens, often at a daily dose of 10–20 mg for weeks to a few months, has been associated with prolongation of the QT interval on the electrocardiogram and occasionally has resulted in malignant ventricular arrhythmias such as torsades de pointes.

The diagnosis of chronic arsenic poisoning involves integration of the clinical findings with confirmation of exposure. The urine concentration of the sum of inorganic arsenic and its primary metabolites MMA and DMA is <20 mcg/L in the general population. High urine levels associated with overt adverse effects may return to normal within days to weeks after exposure ceases. Because it may contain large amounts of nontoxic organoarsenic such as arsenobetaine, or arsenosugars that are metabolized to DMA, all seafood should be avoided for at least 3 days before submission of a urine sample for diagnostic purposes. The arsenic content of hair and nails (normally <1 ppm) may sometimes reveal past elevated exposure, but results should be interpreted cautiously in view of the potential for external contamination. Segmental analysis of hair or nails using sensitive methods such as neutron activation analysis or synchrotron radiation sources may sometimes have forensic value for investigation of the temporal pattern of arsenic poisoning.

Management of chronic arsenic poisoning consists primarily of termination of exposure and nonspecific supportive care. Although empiric short-term oral chelation with **unithiol** or **succimer** for symptomatic individuals with elevated urine arsenic concentrations may be considered, it has no proven benefit beyond removal from exposure alone. Preliminary studies suggest that dietary supplementation of folate—thought to be a cofactor in arsenic methylation—might be of value in arsenic-exposed individuals, particularly men, who are also deficient in folate.

C. Arsine Gas Poisoning

Arsine gas poisoning produces a distinctive pattern of intoxication dominated by profound hemolytic effects. After a latent period that may range from 2 to 24 hours postinhalation (depending on the magnitude of exposure), massive intravascular hemolysis may occur. Initial symptoms may include malaise, headache, dyspnea, weakness, nausea, vomiting, abdominal pain, jaundice, and hemoglobinuria. Oliguric renal failure, a consequence of hemoglobin deposition in the renal tubules, often appears within 1–3 days. In massive exposures, lethal effects on cellular respiration may occur before renal failure develops. Urinary arsenic levels are elevated but are seldom available to confirm the diagnosis during the critical period of illness. Intensive supportive care—including exchange transfusion, vigorous hydration, and, in the case of acute renal failure, hemodialysis—is the mainstay of therapy. Currently available chelating agents have not been demonstrated to be of clinical value in arsine poisoning.

MERCURY

Metallic mercury as "quicksilver"—the only metal that is liquid under ordinary conditions—has attracted scholarly and scientific interest from antiquity. The mining of mercury was early recognized as being hazardous to health. As industrial use of mercury became common during the last 200 years, new forms of toxicity were recognized that were found to be associated with various transformations of the metal. In the early 1950s, a mysterious epidemic of birth defects and neurologic disease occurred in the Japanese fishing village of Minamata. The causative agent was determined to be methylmercury in contaminated seafood, traced to industrial discharges into the bay from a nearby factory. In addition to elemental mercury and alkylmercury (including methylmercury), other key mercurials include inorganic mercury salts and aryl mercury compounds, each of which exerts a relatively unique pattern of clinical toxicity.

Mercury is mined predominantly as HgS in cinnabar ore and is then converted commercially to a variety of chemical forms. Recycling enables recovery of mercury from commercial products such as fluorescent lighting, switches, barometers, thermometers, and other products where its use is being phased out. Recent key industrial and commercial applications of mercury have been found in the manufacture of dental amalgam (43% of US domestic use); relays, sensors, and switches (41% of US domestic use), electrolytic production of chlorine and caustic soda; and manufacture of bulbs, lamps and lighting. The widespread use of elemental mercury in artisanal gold production is a problem in many developing countries. Mercury use in pharmaceuticals and in biocides has declined substantially in recent years, but occasional use in antiseptics, folk medicines, and cosmetic skin-lightening creams is still encountered. Thimerosal, an organomercurial preservative that is metabolized in part to ethylmercury, has been removed from almost all the vaccines in which it was formerly present. Environmental releases of mercury from the burning of fossil fuels, which contributes to the bioaccumulation of methylmercury in fish, remains a concern in some regions of the world. Low-level exposure to mercury released from dental amalgam fillings occurs, but systemic toxicity from this source has not been established.

The United States banned the export of elemental mercury in 2013. The international Minamata Convention on Mercury, signed by 137 countries since 2013, called for the phase-out in 2020 of mercury in numerous products including batteries, switches and relays, fluorescent lamps, pesticides, biocides and antiseptics, measuring instruments (eg, thermometers, sphygmomanometers), and manufacturing processes such as chloralkali production (by 2025). Actions to control and reduce mercury emissions from sources such as power plants, smelting operations, and waste incineration and disposal also are required.

Pharmacokinetics

The absorption of mercury varies considerably depending on the chemical form of the metal. Elemental mercury is quite volatile and can be absorbed from the lungs (see Table 57–1). It is poorly absorbed from the intact gastrointestinal tract. Inhaled mercury is the primary source of occupational exposure. Organic short-chain alkylmercury compounds are volatile and potentially harmful by inhalation as well as by ingestion. Percutaneous absorption of metallic mercury and inorganic mercury can be of clinical concern following massive acute or long-term chronic exposure. Alkylmercury compounds appear to be well absorbed through the skin, and acute contact with a few drops of dimethylmercury has resulted in severe, delayed toxicity. After absorption, mercury is distributed to the tissues within a few hours, with the highest concentration occurring in the kidney. Inorganic mercury is excreted through the urine and feces. Excretion of inorganic mercury follows a multicompartment model: most is excreted within weeks to months, but a fraction may be retained in the kidneys and brain for years. After inhalation of elemental mercury vapor, urinary mercury levels decline with a half-life of approximately 1–3 months. Urine mercury concentration is <1.5 mcg/L in most individuals without occupational exposure, and the median general population urine mercury concentration in the 2017–2018 NHANES study was less than the limit of detection of 0.13 mcg/L. Methylmercury, which has a blood and whole-body half-life of approximately 50 days, undergoes biliary excretion and enterohepatic circulation, with more than two-thirds eventually excreted in the feces. The geometric mean total blood mercury concentration in the US population in the 2017–2018 NHANES was 0.643 mcg/L; the 95th percentile was 3.87 mcg/L (~90% present as methylmercury). Mercury binds to sulfhydryl groups in keratinized tissue, and as with lead and arsenic, traces appear in the hair and nails. Mercury in hair has served as a valid biomarker of methylmercury exposure over an interval of weeks to months in epidemiologic studies.

Major Forms of Mercury Intoxication

Mercury interacts with sulfhydryl groups in vivo, inhibiting enzymes and altering cell membranes. The pattern of clinical intoxication from mercury depends to a great extent on the chemical form of the metal and the route and severity of exposure.

A. Acute

Acute inhalation of elemental mercury vapors may cause chemical pneumonitis and noncardiogenic pulmonary edema. Acute gingivostomatitis may occur, and neurologic sequelae (see following text) may also ensue. Acute ingestion of inorganic mercury salts, such as mercuric chloride, can result in a corrosive, potentially life-threatening hemorrhagic gastroenteritis followed within hours to days by acute tubular necrosis and oliguric renal failure.

B. Chronic

Chronic poisoning from inhalation of mercury vapor results in a classic triad of tremor, neuropsychiatric disturbance, and gingivostomatitis. The tremor usually begins as a fine intention tremor of the hands, but the face may also be involved, and progression to choreiform movements of the limbs may occur. Neuropsychiatric manifestations, including memory loss, fatigue, insomnia, and anorexia, are common. There may be an insidious change in mood to shyness, withdrawal, and depression along with explosive anger or blushing (a behavioral pattern referred to as **erethism**). Recent studies suggest that low-dose exposure may produce subclinical neurologic effects. Gingivostomatitis, sometimes accompanied by loosening of the teeth, may be reported after high-dose exposure. Evidence of peripheral nerve damage may be detected on electrodiagnostic testing, but overt peripheral neuropathy is rare. Acrodynia is an uncommon idiosyncratic reaction to subacute or chronic mercury exposure and occurs mainly in children. It is characterized by painful erythema of the extremities and may be associated with hypertension, diaphoresis, anorexia, insomnia, irritability or apathy, and a miliary rash. Chronic exposure to inorganic mercury salts, sometimes via topical application in cosmetic skin-lightening creams, has been associated with neurological symptoms and renal toxicity in case reports and case series. Severe methylmercury intoxication from illicitly produced skin-lightening creams has been reported.

Methylmercury intoxication affects mainly the CNS and results in facial and peripheral paresthesias, ataxia, hearing impairment, dysarthria, neuropsychiatric disturbance, and progressive constriction of the visual fields. Signs and symptoms of methylmercury intoxication may first appear several weeks or months after exposure begins. Methylmercury is a reproductive toxin. High-dose prenatal exposure to methylmercury may produce severe intellectual disability and a cerebral palsy-like syndrome in the offspring. Low-level prenatal exposures to methylmercury have been associated with a risk of subclinical neurodevelopmental deficits.

A 2004 report by the Institute of Medicine's Immunization Safety Review Committee concluded that available evidence favored rejection of a causal relation between thimerosal-containing vaccines and autism. In like manner, a retrospective cohort study and other investigations conducted by or with the CDC did not support a causal association between early prenatal or postnatal exposure to mercury from thimerosal-containing vaccines and neuropsychological functioning later in childhood (www.cdc.gov/vaccinesafety/pdf/cdcstudiesonvaccinesandautism.pdf).

Dimethylmercury is a rarely encountered but extremely neurotoxic form of organomercury that may result in delayed lethality following exposure to minute quantities.

The diagnosis of mercury intoxication involves integration of the history and physical findings with confirmatory laboratory testing or other evidence of exposure. In the absence of occupational exposure, the urine mercury concentration is usually <1.5 mcg/L, and whole blood mercury is <5 mcg/L. In 2013, the American Conference of Governmental Industrial Hygienists (ACGIH) revised its Biological Exposure Index for elemental mercury to a pre-shift urine value of 20 mcg/g creatinine based on neurological and renal toxicity. In the initial diagnostic approach to a patient with potential mercury intoxication, measurement of both urine and whole blood mercury is advisable. To minimize the risk of developmental neurotoxicity from methylmercury, FDA and EPA have advised pregnant women, women who might become pregnant, nursing mothers, and young children to avoid consumption of fish with high mercury levels (eg, swordfish), to limit consumption of canned light tuna to two to three servings per week or of albacore tuna to one serving per week, and to otherwise consume 8–12 ounces of a variety of low-mercury fish per week (see www.fda.gov/food/consumers/advice-about-eating-fish).

Treatment

A. Acute Exposure

In addition to intensive supportive care, prompt chelation with oral or intravenous **unithiol,** intramuscular **dimercaprol,** or oral **succimer** may be of value in diminishing nephrotoxicity after acute overexposure to inorganic mercury salts. Vigorous hydration may help to maintain urine output, but if acute renal failure ensues, days to weeks of hemodialysis or hemodiafiltration in conjunction with chelation may be necessary. Because the efficacy of chelation declines with time since exposure, treatment should not be delayed until the onset of oliguria or other major systemic effects.

B. Chronic Exposure

Unithiol and **succimer** increase urine mercury excretion following acute or chronic elemental mercury inhalation, but the impact of such treatment on clinical outcome is unknown. Dimercaprol has been shown to redistribute mercury to the central nervous system from other tissue sites, and since the brain is a key target organ, dimercaprol should not be used in treatment of chronic exposure to elemental or organic mercury. Limited data suggest that succimer, unithiol, and *N*-acetyl-L-cysteine (NAC) may enhance body clearance of methylmercury.

■ PHARMACOLOGY OF CHELATORS

Chelating agents are drugs used to prevent or reverse the toxic effects of a heavy metal on an enzyme or other cellular target, or to accelerate the elimination of the metal from the body. By forming a complex with the heavy metal, the chelating agent renders the metal unavailable for toxic interactions with functional groups of enzymes or other proteins, coenzymes, cellular nucleophiles, and membranes. Chelating agents contain one or more coordinating atoms, usually oxygen, sulfur, or nitrogen, which donate a pair of electrons to a cationic metal ion to form one or more coordinate-covalent bonds. Depending on the number of metal-ligand bonds, the complex may be referred to as mono-, bi-, or polydentate. Figure 57–1 depicts the hexadentate chelate formed by interaction of edetate (ethylenediaminetetraacetate) with a metal atom, such as lead.

In some cases, the metal-mobilizing effect of a therapeutic chelating agent may not only enhance that metal's excretion—a desired effect—but may also redistribute some of the metal to other vital organs. This has been demonstrated for dimercaprol, which redistributes mercury and arsenic to the brain while also enhancing urinary mercury and arsenic excretion. Although several chelating agents have the capacity to mobilize cadmium, their tendency to redistribute cadmium to the kidney and increase nephrotoxicity has negated their therapeutic value in cadmium intoxication.

In addition to removing the target metal that is exerting toxic effects on the body, some chelating agents may enhance excretion of essential cations, such as zinc in the case of calcium EDTA and diethylenetriaminepentaacetic acid (DTPA), and zinc and copper in the case of succimer. No clinical significance of this effect has been demonstrated, although some animal data suggest the possibility of adverse developmental impact. If prolonged chelation during the prenatal period or early childhood period is necessary, judicious supplementation of the diet with zinc might be considered.

The longer the half-life of a metal in a particular organ, the less effectively it will be removed by chelation. For example, in the case of lead chelation with calcium EDTA or succimer, or of plutonium chelation with DTPA, the metal is more effectively removed from soft tissues than from bone, where incorporation into bone matrix results in prolonged retention.

In most cases, the capacity of chelating agents to prevent or reduce the adverse effects of toxic metals appears to be greatest when such agents are administered very soon after an acute metal exposure. Use of chelating agents days to weeks after an acute metal exposure ends—or their use in the treatment of chronic metal intoxication—may still be associated with increased metal excretion. However, at that point, the capacity of such enhanced

A

B

C

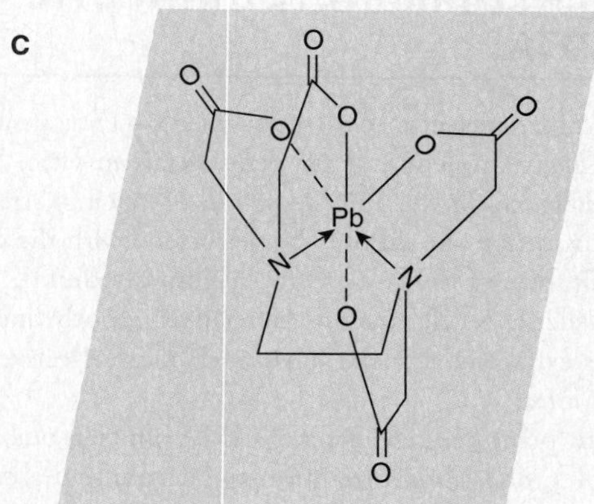

FIGURE 57–1 Salt and chelate formation with edetate (ethylenediaminetetraacetate, EDTA). **(A)** In a solution of the disodium salt of EDTA, the sodium and hydrogen ions are chemically and biologically available. **(B)** In solutions of calcium disodium edetate, calcium is bound by coordinate-covalent bonds with nitrogens as well as by the usual ionic bonds. **(C)** In the lead–edetate chelate, lead is incorporated into five heterocyclic rings. (Reproduced with permission from Meyers FH, Jawetz E, Goldfien A: *Review of Medical Pharmacology*, 7th ed. New York, NY: McGraw Hill; 1980.)

excretion to mitigate the pathologic effect of the metal exposure may be reduced.

The most important chelating agents currently in use in the USA are described below.

DIMERCAPROL (2,3-DIMERCAPTOPROPANOL, BAL)

Dimercaprol (Figure 57–2), an oily, colorless liquid with a strong mercaptan-like odor, was developed in Great Britain during World War II as a therapeutic antidote against poisoning by the arsenic-containing warfare agent lewisite. It thus became known as British anti-lewisite, or BAL. Because aqueous solutions of dimercaprol are unstable and oxidize readily, it is dispensed in 10% solution in peanut oil and must be administered by intramuscular injection, which is often painful.

In animal models, dimercaprol prevents and reverses arsenic-induced inhibition of sulfhydryl-containing enzymes and, if given soon after exposure, may protect against the lethal effects of inorganic and organic arsenicals. Human data indicate that it can increase the rate of excretion of arsenic and lead and may offer therapeutic benefit in the treatment of acute intoxication by arsenic, lead, and mercury.

Indications & Toxicity

Dimercaprol is FDA approved as single-agent treatment of acute poisoning by arsenic and inorganic mercury and for the treatment of severe lead poisoning when used in conjunction with edetate calcium disodium (EDTA; see below). Although studies of its metabolism in humans are limited, intramuscularly administered dimercaprol appears to be readily absorbed, metabolized, and excreted by the kidney within 4–8 hours. Animal models indicate that it may also undergo biliary excretion, but the role of this excretory route in humans and other details of its biotransformation are uncertain.

When used in therapeutic doses, dimercaprol is associated with a high incidence of adverse effects, including hypertension, tachycardia, nausea, vomiting, lacrimation, salivation, fever (particularly

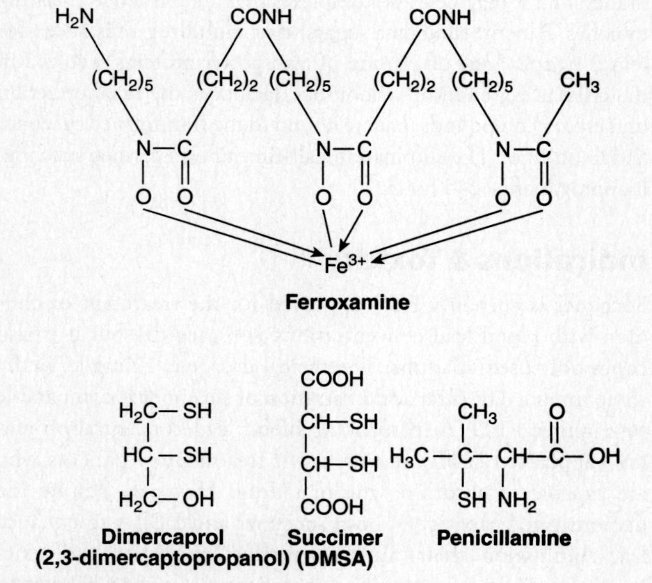

Ferroxamine

Dimercaprol (2,3-dimercaptopropanol) **Succimer (DMSA)** **Penicillamine**

FIGURE 57–2 Chemical structures of several chelators. Ferroxamine (ferrioxamine) without the chelated iron is deferoxamine. It is represented here to show the functional groups; the iron is actually held in a caged system. The structures of the in vivo metal-chelator complexes for dimercaprol, succimer, penicillamine, and unithiol (see text) are not known and may involve the formation of mixed disulfides with amino acids. (Reproduced with permission from Meyers FH, Jawetz E, Goldfien A: *Review of Medical Pharmacology*, 7th ed. New York, NY: McGraw Hill; 1980.)

in children), and pain at the injection site. Its use has also been associated with thrombocytopenia and increased prothrombin time—factors that may limit intramuscular injection because of the risk of hematoma formation at the injection site. Despite its protective effects in acutely intoxicated animals, dimercaprol may redistribute arsenic and mercury to the central nervous system, and it is not advocated for treatment of chronic poisoning. Water-soluble analogs of dimercaprol—unithiol and succimer—have higher therapeutic indices and have replaced dimercaprol in many settings.

SUCCIMER (DIMERCAPTOSUCCINIC ACID, DMSA)

Succimer is a water-soluble analog of dimercaprol, and like that agent it has been shown in animal studies to prevent and reverse metal-induced inhibition of sulfhydryl-containing enzymes and to protect against the acute lethal effects of arsenic. In humans, treatment with succimer is associated with an increase in urinary lead excretion and a decrease in blood lead concentration. It may also decrease the mercury content of the kidney, a key target organ of inorganic mercury salts. In the USA, succimer is formulated exclusively for oral use, but intravenous formulations have been used successfully elsewhere. It is absorbed rapidly but somewhat variably after oral administration. Peak blood levels of succimer occur at approximately 3 hours. The drug binds in vivo to the amino acid cysteine to form 1:1 and 1:2 mixed disulfides, possibly in the kidney, and it may be these complexes that are the active chelating moieties. Experimental data suggest that multidrug-resistance protein 2 (Mrp2), one of a group of transporter proteins involved in the cellular excretion of xenobiotics, facilitates the renal excretion of mercury compounds that are bound to the transformed succimer and to unithiol. The elimination half-time of transformed succimer is approximately 2–4 hours.

Indications & Toxicity

Succimer is currently FDA approved for the treatment of children with blood lead concentrations >45 mcg/dL, but it is also commonly used in adults. The typical dosage is 10 mg/kg orally three times a day. Oral administration of succimer is comparable to parenteral EDTA in reducing blood lead concentration and has supplanted EDTA in outpatient treatment of patients who are capable of absorbing the oral drug. However, despite the demonstrated capacity of both succimer and EDTA to enhance lead elimination, their value in reversing established lead toxicity or in otherwise improving therapeutic outcome has yet to be established by a placebo-controlled clinical trial. In a study in lead-exposed juvenile rats, high-dose succimer did reduce lead-induced neurocognitive impairment when administered to animals with moderate- and high-dose lead exposure. Conversely, when administered to the control group that was not lead exposed, succimer was associated with a decrement in neurocognitive performance. Based on its protective effects against arsenic in animals and its ability to mobilize mercury from the kidney, succimer has also been used in the treatment of arsenic and mercury poisoning.

In limited clinical trials, succimer has been well tolerated. It has a negligible impact on body stores of calcium, iron, and magnesium. It induces a mild increase in urinary excretion of zinc and, less consistently, copper. This effect on trace metal balance has not been associated with overt adverse effects, but its long-term impact on neurodevelopment is uncertain. Gastrointestinal disturbances, including anorexia, nausea, vomiting, and diarrhea, are the most common side effects, occurring in <10% of patients. Rashes, sometimes requiring discontinuation of the medication, have been reported in <5% of patients. Mild, reversible increases in liver aminotransferases have been noted in <5% of patients, and isolated cases of mild to moderate neutropenia have been reported.

EDETATE CALCIUM DISODIUM (ETHYLENEDIAMINETETRAACETIC ACID, EDTA)

Ethylenediaminetetraacetic acid (see Figure 57–1) is an efficient chelator of many divalent and trivalent metals in vitro. To prevent potentially life-threatening depletion of calcium, treatment of metal intoxication should only be performed with the calcium disodium salt form of EDTA (edetate calcium disodium).

EDTA penetrates cell membranes relatively poorly and therefore chelates extracellular metal ions much more effectively than intracellular ions.

The highly polar ionic character of EDTA limits its oral absorption. Moreover, oral administration may increase lead absorption from the gut. Consequently, EDTA should be administered by intravenous infusion. In patients with normal renal function, EDTA is rapidly excreted by glomerular filtration, with 50% of an injected dose appearing in the urine within 1 hour. EDTA mobilizes lead from soft tissues, causing a marked increase in urinary lead excretion and a corresponding decline in blood lead concentration. In patients with renal insufficiency, excretion of the drug—and its metal-mobilizing effects—may be delayed.

Indications & Toxicity

Edetate calcium disodium is indicated chiefly for the chelation of lead, but it may also have usefulness in poisoning by zinc, manganese, and certain heavy radionuclides. A randomized, double-blind, placebo-controlled prospective trial of *edetate disodium* (not edetate calcium disodium) observed a significant decrease in cardiovascular events in a subgroup consisting of diabetic patients with a prior history of myocardial infarction. A follow-up randomized, placebo-controlled trial of *edetate disodium* chelation in a larger cohort of post-MI diabetic subjects is underway.

Because the drug and the mobilized metals are excreted via the urine, the drug is relatively contraindicated in anuric patients. In such instances, the use of low doses of EDTA in combination with high-flux hemodialysis or hemofiltration has been described.

Nephrotoxicity from EDTA has been reported, but in most cases can be prevented by maintenance of adequate urine flow, avoidance of excessive doses, and limitation of a treatment course to 5 or fewer consecutive days. EDTA may result in temporary zinc depletion that is of uncertain clinical significance. Analogs of EDTA, the calcium and zinc disodium salts of DTPA, diethylenetriaminepentaacetate, have been used for removal ("decorporation") of certain transuranic, rare earth, and transition metal radioisotopes, and in 2004 were approved by the FDA for treatment of contamination with plutonium, americium, and curium.

Although calcium EDTA is a generic drug first introduced to the USP formulary in the 1950s, the sole US distributor of 1 g pre-mixed ampoules for injection dramatically raised the average wholesale cost of a 5 ampoule package from approximately $950 to $27,000 in 2014 (see: www.statnews.com/pharmalot/2016/10/11/valeant-drug-prices-lead-poisoning/). Consequently, very few hospital pharmacies in the USA continue to stock pre-mixed ampoules for emergency treatment of severe lead intoxication. As of late 2022, pharmaceutical ampoules of calcium EDTA have been entirely unavailable due to a nationwide drug shortage in the United States.

UNITHIOL (DIMERCAPTOPROPANESULFONIC ACID, DMPS)

Unithiol, a dimercapto chelating agent that is a water-soluble analog of dimercaprol, has been available in the official formularies of Russia and other former Soviet countries since 1958 and in Germany since 1976. It has been legally available from compounding pharmacies in the USA since 1999, and an interim decision was reaffirmed in 2019 when it was included on the 503A Category 1 list of "Bulk Substances Under Evaluation." Unithiol can be administered orally and intravenously. Bioavailability by the oral route is approximately 50%, with peak blood levels occurring in approximately 4 hours. Over 80% of an intravenous dose is excreted in the urine, mainly as cyclic DMPS sulfides. The elimination half-time of total unithiol (parent drug and its transformation products) is approximately 20 hours. Unithiol exhibits protective effects against the toxic action of mercury and arsenic in animal models, and it increases the excretion of mercury, arsenic, and lead in humans. Animal studies and a few case reports suggest that unithiol may also have usefulness in the treatment of poisoning by bismuth compounds.

```
SH     SH     SO2H
|      |      |
CH2 — CH  —  CH2
```

Unithiol

Indications & Toxicity

Unithiol has no FDA-approved indications, but experimental studies and its pharmacologic and pharmacodynamic profile suggest that intravenous unithiol offers advantages over intramuscular dimercaprol or oral succimer in the initial treatment of severe acute poisoning by inorganic mercury or arsenic. Aqueous preparations of unithiol (usually 50 mg/mL in sterile water) can be administered at a dosage of 3–5 mg/kg every 4 hours by slow intravenous infusion over 20 minutes. If a few days of treatment are accompanied by stabilization of the patient's cardiovascular and gastrointestinal status, it may be possible to change to oral administration of 4–8 mg/kg every 6–8 hours. Oral unithiol may also be considered as an alternative to oral succimer in the treatment of lead intoxication. Intravenous unithiol in conjunction with high-flux hemodialysis or hemodiafiltration may be useful in the treatment of patients with anuric renal failure caused by mercury salts and bismuth.

Unithiol has been reported to have a low overall incidence of adverse effects (<4%). Self-limited dermatologic reactions (drug exanthems or urticaria) are the most commonly reported adverse effects, although isolated cases of major allergic reactions, including erythema multiforme and Stevens-Johnson syndrome, have been reported. Because rapid intravenous infusion may cause vasodilation and hypotension, unithiol should be infused slowly over 15–20 minutes.

PENICILLAMINE (D-DIMETHLCYSTEINE)

Penicillamine (see Figure 57–2) is a white, crystalline, water-soluble derivative of penicillin. D-Penicillamine is less toxic than the L-isomer and consequently is the preferred therapeutic form. Penicillamine is readily absorbed from the gut and is resistant to metabolic degradation.

Indications & Toxicity

Penicillamine is used chiefly for treatment of poisoning with copper or to prevent copper accumulation, as in Wilson disease (hepatolenticular degeneration). It is also used occasionally in the treatment of severe rheumatoid arthritis (see Chapter 36). Its ability to increase urinary excretion of lead and mercury had occasioned its use in outpatient treatment for intoxication with these metals, but succimer, with its stronger metal-mobilizing capacity and lower adverse-effect profile, has generally replaced penicillamine for these purposes.

Adverse effects have been seen in up to one third of patients receiving penicillamine. Hypersensitivity reactions include rash, pruritus, and drug fever, and the drug should be used with extreme caution, if at all, in patients with a history of penicillin allergy. Nephrotoxicity with proteinuria has also been reported, and protracted use of the drug may result in renal insufficiency. Pancytopenia has been associated with prolonged drug intake. Pyridoxine deficiency is a frequent toxic effect of other forms of the drug but is rarely seen with the D isomer. An acetylated derivative, *N*-acetylpenicillamine, has been used experimentally in mercury poisoning and may have superior metal-mobilizing capacity, but it is not commercially available.

DEFEROXAMINE

Deferoxamine is isolated from *Streptomyces pilosus*. It binds iron avidly (see Figure 57–2) but binds essential trace metals poorly. Furthermore, though competing for loosely bound iron in iron-carrying proteins (hemosiderin and ferritin), it fails to compete for biologically chelated iron, as in microsomal and mitochondrial cytochromes and hemoproteins. Consequently, it is the parenteral chelator of choice for iron poisoning (see Chapters 33 and 58). A placebo-controlled clinical trial investigating acute deferoxamine treatment in patients with spontaneous intracerebral hemorrhage observed beneficial clinical outcome at 180 days in the subgroup of patients who had moderate-sized hematoma volume at presentation. The mode of action may be reduction in brain iron overload resulting from hemoglobin breakdown. Deferoxamine plus hemodialysis may also be useful in the treatment of aluminum toxicity in renal failure. Deferoxamine is poorly absorbed when administered orally and may increase iron absorption when given by this route. It should therefore be administered intravenously. It is believed to be metabolized, but the pathways are unknown. The iron-chelator complex is excreted in the urine, often turning the urine an orange-red color.

Rapid intravenous administration may result in hypotension. Adverse idiosyncratic responses such as flushing, abdominal discomfort, and rash have also been observed. Pulmonary complications (eg, acute respiratory distress syndrome) have been reported in some patients undergoing deferoxamine infusions lasting longer than 24 hours, and neurotoxicity and increased susceptibility to certain infections (eg, with *Yersinia enterocolitica*) have been described after long-term therapy of iron overload conditions (eg, thalassemia major).

DEFERASIROX & DEFERIPRONE

Deferasirox is a tridentate chelator with a high affinity for iron and low affinity for other metals, eg, zinc and copper. It is orally active and well absorbed. In the circulation, it binds iron, and the complex is excreted in the bile. Deferasirox was approved by the FDA in 2005 for the oral treatment of iron overload caused by blood transfusions, a problem in the treatment of thalassemia and myelodysplastic syndrome. Long-term usage is generally well tolerated, with the most common adverse effects consisting of mild to moderate gastrointestinal disturbances and skin rash. Monitoring of liver and renal function has been advised because renal and liver impairment and failure associated with deferasirox have been reported during treatment of older adults with myelodysplastic syndromes.

Deferiprone, a bidentate iron chelator cleared predominantly via the kidney, was approved by the FDA in 2011 as a second-line oral chelator for patients with transfusional iron overload due to thalassemia. Because neutropenia has occurred in 5–10% of patients, with agranulocytosis in approximately 1%, regular hematologic monitoring is recommended. Deferiprone and deferasirox appear to have similar efficacy in the treatment of transfusion-dependent hemoglobinopathies that require long-term iron chelation.

Magnetic resonance imaging has been increasingly used to evaluate cardiac and hepatic iron burden and to guide iron chelation therapy. Regimens that combine iron-chelating agents have been used in cases when monotherapy has yielded suboptimal results.

PRUSSIAN BLUE (FERRIC HEXACYANOFERRATE)

Ferric hexacyanoferrate (insoluble Prussian blue) is a hydrated crystalline compound in which Fe^{2+} and Fe^{3+} atoms are coordinated with cyanide groups in a cubic lattice structure. Although used as a dark blue commercial pigment for nearly 300 years, it was only three decades ago that its potential usefulness as a pharmaceutical chelator was recognized. Primarily by ion exchange, and secondarily by mechanical trapping or adsorption, the compound has high affinity for certain univalent cations, particularly cesium and thallium. Used as an oral drug, insoluble Prussian blue undergoes minimal gastrointestinal absorption (<1%). Because the complexes it forms with cesium or thallium are nonabsorbable, oral administration of the chelator diminishes intestinal absorption or interrupts enterohepatic and enteroenteric circulation of these cations, thereby accelerating their elimination in the feces. In clinical case series, the use of Prussian blue has been associated with a decline in the biologic half-life (ie, in vivo retention) of radioactive cesium and thallium.

Indications & Toxicity

In 2003, Prussian blue was approved by the FDA for the treatment of contamination with radioactive cesium (^{137}Cs) and intoxication with thallium salts. Approval was prompted by concern over potential widespread human contamination with radioactive cesium caused by terrorist use of a radioactive dispersal device ("dirty bomb"). The drug is part of the Strategic National Stockpile of pharmaceuticals and medical material maintained by the CDC (www.cdc.gov/phpr/stockpile/). (*Note:* Although soluble forms of Prussian blue, such as potassium ferric hexacyanoferrate, may have better utility in thallium poisoning, only the insoluble form is currently available as a pharmaceutical.)

After exposure to ^{137}Cs or thallium salts, the approved adult dosage of Prussian blue is 3 g orally three times a day; the corresponding pediatric dosage (2–12 years of age) is 1 g orally three times a day. Serial monitoring of urine and fecal radioactivity (^{137}Cs) and urinary thallium concentrations can guide the recommended duration of therapy. Adjunctive supportive care for possible acute radiation illness (^{137}Cs) or systemic thallium toxicity should be instituted as needed.

Prussian blue has not been associated with significant adverse effects. Constipation, which may occur in some cases, should be treated with laxatives or increased dietary fiber.

PREPARATIONS AVAILABLE

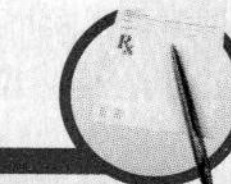

GENERIC NAME	AVAILABLE AS
Deferasirox	Exjade, Jadenu
Deferiprone	Ferriprox
Deferoxamine	Generic, Desferal
Dimercaprol	BAL in Oil
Edetate calcium (calcium EDTA)	Calcium Disodium Versenate
Penicillamine	Cuprimine, Depen
Pentetate calcium trisodium (calcium DTPA) and Pentetate zinc trisodium (zinc DTPA)	Generic
Prussian blue	Radiogardase
Succimer	Chemet, Succicaptal (in Europe)
Unithiol	Dimaval

REFERENCES

Lead

Centers for Disease Control and Prevention (CDC): Advisory Committee on Childhood Lead Poisoning Prevention of the Centers for Disease Control and Prevention: Low Level Lead Exposure Harms Children: A Renewed Call for Primary Prevention. 2012. www.cdc.gov/nceh/lead/ACCLPP/Final_Document_030712.pdf.

Agency for Toxic Substances and Disease Registry (ATSDR). Toxicological Profile for Lead. 2020. www.atsdr.cdc.gov/toxprofiles/tp13.pdf.

Centers for Disease Control and Prevention (CDC): Guidelines for the Identification and Management of Lead Exposure in Pregnant and Lactating Women. 2010. www.cdc.gov/nceh/lead/publications/LeadandPregnancy2010.pdf.

Crump KS et al: A statistical reevaluation of the data used in the Lanphear et al. (2005) pooled-analysis that related low levels of blood lead to intellectual deficits in children. Crit Rev Toxicol 2013;43:785

Environmental Protection Agency: Integrated Science Assessment for Lead. 2013. www.epa.gov/isa/integrated-science-assessment-isa-lead.

Kosnett MJ et al: Recommendations for medical management of adult lead exposure. Environ Health Perspect 2007;115:463.

Kosnett MJ et al: Workplace health and safety necessitates an update to occupational lead standard provisions for medical removal protection, medical surveillance triggers, and the action level and permissible exposure level for lead in workplace air: ACOEM response to OSHA. J Occup Environ Med 2023; 65:e170.

Lanphear BP et al: Low-level environmental lead exposure and children's intellectual development: An international pooled analysis. Environ Health Perspect 2005;113:894.

Reuben A: Childhood lead exposure and adult neurodegenerative disease. J Alzheimers Dis 2018;64:17.

Weisskopf MG et al: Biased exposure-health effect estimates from selection in cohort studies: Are environmental studies at particular risk? Environ Health Perspect 2015;123:1113. [Note: Study reports relationship between bone lead concentration and cardiovascular mortality.]

Arsenic

Baker BA et al: Arsenic exposure, assessment, toxicity, diagnosis and management: Guidance for occupational and environmental physicians. J Occup Env Med 2018;60:e634.

Carlin DJ et al: Arsenic and environmental health: State of the science and future research opportunities. Environ Health Perspect 2016;124:890.

Gurnari C et al: When poisons cure: the case of arsenic in acute promyelocytic leukemia. Chemotherapy 2019;64:238.

James KA et al: Association between lifetime exposure to inorganic arsenic in drinking water and coronary heart disease in Colorado residents. Environ Health Perspect 2015;123:128.

Kononenko M, Frishman WH: Association between arsenic exposure and cardiovascular disease. Cardiol Rev 2021;29:217.

Kuo CC et al: The association of arsenic metabolism with cancer, cardiovascular disease, and diabetes: A systematic review of the epidemiological evidence. Environ Health Perspect 2017;125:087001.

Quansah R et al: Association of arsenic with adverse pregnancy outcomes/infant mortality: A systematic review and meta-analysis. Environ Health Perspect 2015;123:412.

Sanchez TR et al: A meta-analysis of arsenic exposure and lung function: Is there evidence of restrictive or obstructive lung disease? Curr Environ Health Rep 2018;5:244.

Mercury

Agency for Toxic Substances and Disease Registry (ATSDR): Toxicological Profile for Mercury (draft for public comment). 2022. www.atsdr.cdc.gov/toxprofiles/tp46.pdf.

Al-Saleh I: Potential health consequences of applying mercury-containing skin-lightening creams during pregnancy and lactation periods. Int J Hyg Environ Health 2016;219:468.

Beasley DMG et al: Full recovery from a potentially lethal dose of mercuric chloride. J Med Toxicol 2014;10:40.

Bellinger DC et al: Dental amalgam restorations and children's neuropsychological function: The New England Children's Amalgam Trial. Environ Health Perspect 2007;115:440.

Bose-O'Reilly S et al: Signs and symptoms of mercury-exposed gold miners. Int J Occ Med Environ Health 2017;30:249.

Environmental Protection Agency: EPA-FDA advice about eating fish and shellfish. 2019. www.epa.gov/fish-tech/epa-fda-advice-about-eating-fish-and-shellfish.

Grandjean P et al: Adverse effects of methylmercury: Environmental health research implications. Environ Health Perspect 2010;118:1137.

McKean SJ et al: Prenatal mercury exposure, autism, and developmental delay, using pharmacokinetic combination of newborn blood concentrations and questionnaire data: A case control study. Environ Health 2015;14:62.

Yorifuji T et al: Long-term exposure to methylmercury and neurologic signs in Minamata and neighboring communities. Epidemiology 2008;19:3.

Chelating Agents

Bradberry S, Vale A: A comparison of sodium calcium edetate (edetate calcium disodium) and succimer (DMSA) in the treatment of inorganic lead poisoning. Clin Toxicol 2009;47:841.

Dargan PI et al: Case report: Severe mercuric sulphate poisoning treated with 2,3-dimercaptopropane-1-sulphonate and haemodiafiltration. Crit Care 2003;7:R1.

Escolar E et al: The effect of an EDTA-based chelation regimen on patients with diabetes mellitus and prior myocardial infarction in the Trial to Assess Chelation Therapy (TACT). Circ Cardiovasc Qual Outcomes 2014;7(1):15.

Hider RC, Hoffbrand AV: The role of deferiprone in iron chelation. N Engl J Med 2018; 379:2140.

Kosnett MJ: Chelation for heavy metals (arsenic, lead, and mercury): Protective or perilous? Clin Pharmacol Ther 2010;88:412.

Kosnett MJ: The role of chelation in the treatment of arsenic and mercury poisoning. J Med Toxicol 2013;9:347.

Pelclova D et al: Is chelation therapy efficient for the treatment of intravenous metallic mercury intoxication? Basic Clin Pharmacol Toxicol 2017;120:628.

Sakthithasan K et al: A comparative study of edetate calcium disodium and dimercaptosuccinic acid in the treatment of lead poisoning in adults. Clin Toxicol 2018;56:1143.

Thompson DF, Called ED: Soluble or insoluble Prussian blue for radiocesium and thallium poisoning? Ann Pharmacother 2004;38:1509.

Thurtle N et al: Description of 3,180 courses of chelation with dimercaptosuccinic acid in children ≤ 5 y with severe lead poisoning in Zamfara, Northern Nigeria: A retrospective analysis of programme data. PLOS Med 2014;11:e1001739.

Wei C et al: Effect of deferoxamine on outcome according to baseline hematoma volume: a post hoc analysis of the i-DEF trial. Stroke 2022;53:1149.

CASE STUDY ANSWER

Bacterial food poisoning is the most common cause of gastrointestinal signs and symptom appearing in a group of individuals within several hours of a common meal. Consumption of food contaminated with preformed bacterial toxins such as *Staphylococcus* or *Bacillus cereus* toxins can result in vomiting after an incubation interval as short as 1–2 hours. However, the onset of vomiting in some individuals within 15 minutes and the progression to hypotension and metabolic acidosis in several individuals are *not* typical for bacterial food poisoning and are more suggestive of intoxication by certain toxic chemicals or drugs, including inorganic arsenic and mercury salts (eg, sodium arsenite or mercuric chloride). The absence of hematemesis, bloody diarrhea, or renal insufficiency lowered the likelihood that inorganic mercury was responsible. An epidemiologic investigation subsequently revealed that all affected individuals had consumed the deliberately adulterated coffee, which contained 6300 ppm of inorganic arsenic. Analysis of urine for arsenic and mercury and stool and emesis for bacterial pathogens would be reasonable initial diagnostic tests. Pending test results, prompt empiric treatment of this constellation of findings with the chelating agents unithiol, succimer, or dimercaprol would be appropriate. (Based on an actual incident, see: Gensheimer KF et al: Arsenic poisoning caused by intentional contamination of coffee at a church gathering: An epidemiological approach to a forensic investigation. J Forensic Sci 2010;55:1116).

CHAPTER

58

Management of the Poisoned Patient

Craig Smollin, MD, & Stephen Petrou, MD

CASE STUDY

A 62-year-old woman with a history of depression is found in her apartment in a lethargic state. An empty bottle of bupropion is on the bedside table. In the emergency department, she is unresponsive to verbal and painful stimuli. She has a brief generalized seizure, followed by a respiratory arrest. The emergency physician performs endotracheal intubation and administers a drug intravenously, followed by another substance via a nasogastric tube. The patient is admitted to the intensive care unit for continued supportive care and recovers the next morning. What drug might be used intravenously to prevent further seizures? What substance is commonly used to adsorb drugs still present in the gastrointestinal tract?

Over 1 million cases of acute poisoning occur in the USA each year, although only a small number are fatal. Most deaths are due to intentional suicidal overdose by an adolescent or adult. Childhood deaths due to accidental ingestion of a drug or toxic household product have been markedly reduced in the last 50 years as a result of safety packaging and effective poisoning prevention education.

Even with a serious exposure, poisoning is rarely fatal if the victim receives prompt medical attention and good supportive care. Careful management of respiratory failure, hypotension, seizures, and thermoregulatory disturbances has resulted in improved survival of patients who reach the hospital alive.

This chapter reviews the basic principles of poisoning, initial management, and specialized treatment of poisoning, including methods of increasing the elimination of drugs and toxins.

■ TOXICOKINETICS & TOXICODYNAMICS

The term **toxicokinetics** denotes the absorption, distribution, excretion, and metabolism of toxins, toxic doses of therapeutic agents, and their metabolites. The term **toxicodynamics** is used to denote the injurious effects of these substances on body functions. Although many similarities exist between the pharmacokinetics and toxicokinetics of most substances, there are also important differences. The same caution applies to pharmacodynamics and toxicodynamics.

SPECIAL ASPECTS OF TOXICOKINETICS

Volume of Distribution

The volume of distribution (V_d) is defined as the apparent volume into which a substance is distributed in the body (see Chapter 3). It is a mathematical representation that describes, inversely, how much of the drug remains in the vascular system. A large V_d implies that the drug distributes from the blood to other tissues, and is therefore not readily accessible to measures aimed at purifying the blood, such as hemodialysis. A small V_d implies that the drug is retained within the blood or extracellular fluid rather than distributing into tissues. Examples of drugs with large volumes of distribution (>5 L/kg) that are sometimes involved in dangerous overdoses include antidepressants, antipsychotics, antimalarials, opioids, propranolol, and verapamil. Drugs with a relatively small V_d (<1 L/kg) include salicylate, acetaminophen, ethanol, phenobarbital, lithium, valproic acid, and phenytoin (see Table 3–1).

Clearance

Clearance is a measure of the volume of plasma that is cleared of drug per unit time (see Chapter 3). The total clearance for most drugs is the sum of clearances via excretion by the kidneys and metabolism by the liver. In planning a detoxification strategy, it is important to know the contribution of each organ to total clearance. For example, if a drug is 95% cleared by liver metabolism and only 5% cleared by renal excretion, even a dramatic increase in urinary concentration of the drug will have little effect on overall elimination.

Drug overdose can alter the usual pharmacokinetic processes, and must be considered when applying kinetics to poisoned patients. For example, dissolution of tablets or gastric emptying time may be slowed so that absorption and peak toxic effects are delayed. Drugs, especially poisons, may injure the epithelial barrier of the gastrointestinal tract and thereby increase absorption. If the capacity of the liver to metabolize a drug is exceeded, the first-pass effect will be reduced and more drug will be delivered to the circulation. With a dramatic increase in the concentration of drug in the blood, protein-binding capacity may be exceeded, resulting in an increased fraction of free drug and greater toxic effect. At normal dosage, most drugs are eliminated at a rate proportional to the plasma concentration (first-order kinetics). If the plasma concentration is very high and normal metabolism is saturated, the rate of elimination may become fixed (zero-order kinetics). This change in kinetics may markedly prolong the apparent serum half-life and increase toxicity.

SPECIAL ASPECTS OF TOXICODYNAMICS

The general dose-response principles described in Chapter 2 are relevant when estimating the potential severity of an intoxication. When considering dose-response data, both the therapeutic index and the overlap of therapeutic and toxic response curves must be considered. For instance, two drugs may have the same therapeutic index but unequal safe dosing ranges if the slopes of their dose-response curves are not the same. For some drugs, eg, sedative-hypnotics, the major toxic effect is a direct extension of the therapeutic action, as shown by their graded dose-response curve (see Figure 22–1). In the case of a drug with a linear dose-response curve (drug A), lethal effects may occur at 10 times the normal therapeutic dose. In contrast, a drug with a curve that reaches a plateau (drug B) may not be lethal at 100 times the normal dose.

For many drugs, at least part of the toxic effect may be different from the therapeutic action. For example, intoxication with drugs that have atropine-like effects (eg, tricyclic antidepressants) reduces sweating, making it more difficult to dissipate heat. In tricyclic antidepressant intoxication, there may also be increased muscular activity or seizures; the body's production of heat is thus enhanced, and lethal hyperpyrexia may result. Overdoses of drugs that depress the cardiovascular system, eg, β blockers or calcium channel blockers, can profoundly alter not only cardiac function but all functions that are dependent on blood flow. These include renal and hepatic elimination of the toxin and that of any other drugs that may be given.

■ APPROACH TO THE POISONED PATIENT

HOW DOES THE POISONED PATIENT DIE?

An understanding of common mechanisms of death due to poisoning can help prepare the caregiver to treat patients effectively. Many toxins depress the central nervous system (CNS), resulting in obtundation or coma. Comatose patients frequently lose their airway protective reflexes and their respiratory drive. Thus, they may die as a result of airway obstruction by the flaccid tongue, aspiration of gastric contents into the tracheobronchial tree, or respiratory arrest. These are the most common causes of death due to overdoses of narcotics and sedative-hypnotic drugs (eg, barbiturates and alcohol).

Cardiovascular toxicity is also frequently encountered in poisoning. Hypotension may be due to depression of cardiac contractility; hypovolemia resulting from vomiting, diarrhea, or fluid sequestration; peripheral vascular collapse due to blockade of α-adrenoceptor-mediated vascular tone; or cardiac arrhythmias. Hypothermia or hyperthermia due to exposure as well as the temperature-dysregulating effects of many drugs can also produce hypotension. Lethal arrhythmias such as ventricular tachycardia and fibrillation can occur with overdoses of many cardioactive drugs such as ephedrine, amphetamines, cocaine, digitalis, and theophylline; and drugs not usually considered cardioactive, such as tricyclic antidepressants, antihistamines, and some opioid analogs.

Cellular hypoxia may occur despite adequate ventilation and oxygen administration when poisoning is due to cyanide, hydrogen sulfide, carbon monoxide, and other poisons that interfere with transport or utilization of oxygen. Such patients may not be cyanotic, but cellular hypoxia is evident by the development of tachycardia, hypotension, severe lactic acidosis, and signs of ischemia on the electrocardiogram.

Seizures, muscular hyperactivity, and rigidity may result in death. Seizures may cause pulmonary aspiration, hypoxia, and brain damage. Hyperthermia may result from sustained muscular hyperactivity and can lead to muscle breakdown and myoglobinuria, renal failure, lactic acidosis, coagulopathy, and hyperkalemia. Drugs and poisons that often cause seizures include antidepressants, isoniazid (INH), bupropion, diphenhydramine, cocaine, and amphetamines. In addition, withdrawal from certain drugs or medications can also lead to seizures (e.g., ethanol or baclofen).

Other organ system damage may occur after poisoning and is sometimes delayed in onset. Paraquat attacks lung tissue, resulting in pulmonary fibrosis, beginning several days after ingestion. Massive hepatic necrosis due to poisoning by acetaminophen or certain mushrooms results in hepatic encephalopathy and death 48–72 hours or longer after ingestion.

Finally, some patients may die before hospitalization because the behavioral effects of the ingested drug may result in traumatic injury.

Intoxication with alcohol and other sedative-hypnotic drugs is a common contributing factor to motor vehicle accidents. Patients under the influence of hallucinogens such as phencyclidine (PCP) or lysergic acid diethylamide (LSD) may suffer trauma when they become combative or fall from a height.

■ INITIAL MANAGEMENT OF THE POISONED PATIENT

The initial management of a patient with coma, seizures, or otherwise altered mental status should follow the same approach regardless of the poison involved: supportive measures are the basics (**"ABCDs"**) of poisoning treatment.

First, the **airway** should be cleared of vomitus or any other obstruction and an oral airway or endotracheal tube inserted if needed. For many patients, simple positioning in the lateral, left-side-down position or implementation of a "jaw thrust" maneuver is sufficient to move the flaccid tongue out of the airway. **Breathing** should be assessed by observation, pulse oximetry, end tidal carbon dioxide monitoring, and, if in doubt, by measuring arterial blood gases. Patients with respiratory insufficiency should be intubated and mechanically ventilated. The **circulation** should be assessed by continuous monitoring of pulse rate, blood pressure, urinary output, and evaluation of peripheral perfusion. An intravenous line should be placed and blood drawn for serum glucose and other routine determinations.

At this point, every patient with altered mental status should receive a challenge with concentrated **dextrose,** unless a rapid bedside blood glucose test demonstrates that the patient is not hypoglycemic. Adults are given 25 g (50 mL of 50% dextrose solution) intravenously, children 0.5 g/kg (2 mL/kg of 25% dextrose). Hypoglycemic patients may appear to be intoxicated, and there is no rapid and reliable way to distinguish them from poisoned patients. Alcoholic or malnourished patients should also receive 100 mg of thiamine intramuscularly or in the intravenous infusion solution at this time to prevent Wernicke syndrome.

The opioid antagonist **naloxone** may be given in a dose of 0.4–2 mg intravenously. Naloxone reverses respiratory and CNS depression due to all varieties of opioid drugs (see Chapter 31). It is useful to remember that these drugs cause death primarily by respiratory depression; therefore, if airway and breathing assistance have already been instituted, naloxone may not be necessary. Larger doses of naloxone may be needed for patients with overdose involving fentanyl, codeine, and some other opioids. The benzodiazepine antagonist **flumazenil** (see Chapter 22) may be of value in patients with suspected benzodiazepine overdose, but it should not be used if there is a history of chronic benzodiazepine use, tricyclic antidepressant overdose, or a seizure disorder, as it can unmask convulsions in such patients.

History & Physical Examination

Once the essential initial ABCD interventions have been instituted, one can begin a more detailed evaluation to make a specific diagnosis. This includes gathering any available history and performing a toxicologically oriented physical examination. Other causes of coma or seizures such as head trauma, meningitis, or metabolic abnormalities should be sought and treated. Some common intoxications are described under Common Toxic Syndromes.

A. History

Oral statements about the amount and even the type of drug ingested in toxic emergencies may be unreliable. Even so, family members, police, and fire department or paramedical personnel should be asked to describe the environment in which the toxic emergency occurred and should bring to the emergency department any syringes, empty bottles, household products, or over-the-counter medications in the immediate vicinity of the possibly poisoned patient.

B. Physical Examination

A brief examination should be performed, emphasizing those areas most likely to give clues to the toxicologic diagnosis. These include vital signs, eyes and mouth, skin, abdomen, and nervous system.

1. *Vital signs*—Careful evaluation of vital signs (blood pressure, pulse, respirations, and temperature) are essential in all toxicologic emergencies. Hypertension and tachycardia are typical with amphetamines, cocaine, and antimuscarinic (anticholinergic) drugs. Hypotension and bradycardia are characteristic features of overdose with calcium channel blockers, β blockers, clonidine, and sedative-hypnotics. Hypotension with tachycardia is common with tricyclic antidepressants, trazodone, quetiapine, vasodilators, and β agonists. Rapid respirations are typical of salicylates, carbon monoxide, and other toxins that produce metabolic acidosis or cellular asphyxia. Hyperthermia may be associated with sympathomimetics, anticholinergics, salicylates, and drugs producing seizures or muscular rigidity. Hypothermia can be caused by any CNS-depressant drug, especially when accompanied by exposure to a cold environment.

2. *Eyes*—The eyes are a valuable source of toxicologic information. Constriction of the pupils (miosis) is typical of opioids, clonidine, phenothiazines, and cholinesterase inhibitors (eg, organophosphate insecticides), and deep coma due to sedative drugs. Dilation of the pupils (mydriasis) is common with amphetamines, cocaine, LSD, and atropine and other anticholinergic drugs. Horizontal nystagmus is characteristic of intoxication with phenytoin, alcohol, barbiturates, and other sedative drugs. The presence of both vertical and horizontal nystagmus is strongly suggestive of phencyclidine poisoning. Ptosis, sluggish pupils, and ophthalmoplegia are characteristic features of botulism.

3. *Mouth*—The mouth may show signs of burns due to corrosive substances, or soot from smoke inhalation. Typical odors of alcohol, hydrocarbon solvents, or ammonia may be noted. Poisoning due to cyanide can be recognized by some examiners as an odor like bitter almonds.

4. *Skin*—The skin often appears flushed, hot, and dry in poisoning with atropine and other antimuscarinics. Excessive sweating occurs with organophosphates, nicotine, and sympathomimetic drugs. Cyanosis may be caused by hypoxemia or by methemoglobinemia. Icterus may suggest hepatic necrosis due to acetaminophen or *Amanita phalloides* mushroom poisoning.

5. *Abdomen*—Abdominal examination may reveal ileus, which is typical of poisoning with antimuscarinic, opioid, and sedative drugs. Hyperactive bowel sounds, abdominal cramping, and diarrhea are common in poisoning with organophosphates, iron, arsenic, theophylline, *A phalloides*, and *A muscaria*.

6. *Nervous system*—A careful neurologic examination is essential. Focal seizures or motor deficits suggest a structural lesion (eg, intracranial hemorrhage due to trauma) rather than toxic or metabolic encephalopathy. Nystagmus, dysarthria, and ataxia are typical of phenytoin, carbamazepine, alcohol, and other sedative intoxication. Twitching and muscular hyperactivity are common with atropine and other anticholinergic agents, and cocaine and other sympathomimetic drugs. Muscular rigidity can be caused by haloperidol and other antipsychotic agents, and by strychnine or by tetanus. Generalized hypertonicity of muscles and lower extremity clonus are typical of serotonin syndrome. Seizures are often caused by overdose with antidepressants (especially tricyclic antidepressants and bupropion [as in the case study]), cocaine, amphetamines, theophylline, isoniazid, and diphenhydramine. Flaccid coma with absent reflexes and even an isoelectric electroencephalogram may be seen with deep coma due to sedative-hypnotic or other CNS depressant intoxication and may be mistaken for brain death.

Laboratory & Imaging Procedures

A. Blood Gases

Hypoventilation results in an elevated P_{CO_2} (hypercapnia) and a low P_{O_2} (hypoxia). This may be seen in opioid or ethanol toxicity. The P_{O_2} may also be low in a patient with aspiration pneumonia or drug-induced pulmonary edema. Poor tissue oxygenation due to hypoxia, hypotension, or cyanide poisoning will result in metabolic acidosis. The P_{O_2} measures only oxygen dissolved in the plasma and not total blood oxygen content or oxyhemoglobin saturation and may appear normal in patients with severe carbon monoxide poisoning. Pulse oximetry may also give falsely normal results in carbon monoxide intoxication.

B. Electrolytes

Sodium, potassium, chloride, and bicarbonate should be measured. The anion gap is then calculated by subtracting the measured anions from cations:

$$\text{Anion gap} = (Na^+ + K^+) - (HCO_3^- + Cl^-)$$

Normally, the sum of the cations exceeds the sum of the anions by no more than 12–16 mEq/L (or 8–12 mEq/L if the formula used for estimating the anion gap omits the potassium level). A larger than expected anion gap is caused by the presence of unmeasured anions (lactate, etc) accompanying metabolic acidosis. This may occur with numerous conditions, such as diabetic ketoacidosis, renal failure, or shock-induced lactic acidosis. Drugs that may induce an elevated anion gap metabolic acidosis (Table 58–1) include aspirin, metformin, methanol, ethylene glycol, isoniazid, and iron.

TABLE 58–1 Examples of drug-induced anion gap acidosis.

Type of Elevation of the Anion Gap	Agents
Organic acid metabolites	Methanol, ethylene glycol, diethylene glycol, oxoprolinuria (rare complication of acetaminophen)
Lactic acidosis	Cyanide, carbon monoxide, ibuprofen, isoniazid, metformin, salicylates, valproic acid; any drug-induced seizures, hypoxia, or hypotension

Note: The normal anion gap calculated from $(Na^+ + K^+) - (HCO_3^- + Cl^-)$ is 12–16 mEq/L; calculated from $(Na^+) - (HCO_3^- + Cl^-)$, it is 8–12 mEq/L.

Alterations in the serum potassium level are hazardous because they can result in cardiac arrhythmias. Drugs that may cause hyperkalemia despite normal renal function include potassium itself, β blockers, digitalis glycosides, potassium-sparing diuretics, and fluoride. Drugs associated with hypokalemia include barium, β agonists, caffeine, theophylline, and thiazide and loop diuretics.

C. Renal Function Tests

Some toxins have direct nephrotoxic effects; in other cases, renal failure is due to shock or myoglobinuria. Blood urea nitrogen and creatinine levels should be measured and urinalysis performed. Elevated serum creatine kinase (CK) and myoglobin in the urine suggest muscle necrosis due to seizures or muscular rigidity. Oxalate crystals in large numbers in the urine suggest ethylene glycol poisoning.

D. Serum Osmolality

The calculated serum osmolality is dependent mainly on the serum sodium, glucose, and blood urea nitrogen. It can be estimated from the following formula:

$$2 \times Na^+ (\text{mEq/L}) + \frac{\text{Glucose (mg/dL)}}{18} + \frac{\text{BUN (mg/dL)}}{3}$$

This calculated value is normally 280–290 mOsm/L. Ethanol and other alcohols may contribute significantly to the measured serum osmolality but, since they are not included in the calculation, cause an osmol gap:

$$\text{Osmol gap} = \text{Measured osmolality} - \text{Calculated osmolality}$$

Substances that are often associated with an abnormal osmol gap include **acetone, ethanol, ethylene glycol, isopropyl alcohol, methanol,** and **propylene glycol.**

E. Electrocardiogram

Widening of the QRS complex duration (to more than 100 milliseconds) is typical of overdose of tricyclic antidepressants and other drugs that block the sodium channel in cardiac conducting tissue (Figure 58–1). The QT_c interval may be prolonged

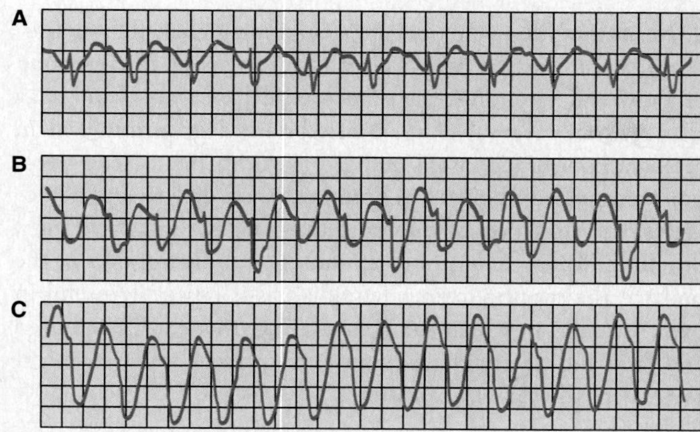

FIGURE 58–1 Changes in the electrocardiogram in tricyclic antidepressant overdosage. **(A)** Slowed intraventricular conduction results in prolonged QRS interval (0.18 seconds; normal, 0.08 seconds). **(B** and **C)** Supraventricular tachycardia with progressive widening of QRS complexes mimics ventricular tachycardia. (Reproduced with permission from Haddad LM, Shannon MW, Winchester JF: *Clinical Management of Poisoning and Drug Overdose*, 3rd ed. Philadelphia, PA: WB Saunders; 1998.)

in many poisonings, including antidepressants and antipsychotics, methadone, lithium, and arsenic (see also https://www.crediblemeds.org/everyone/composite-list-all-qtdrugs/). Variable atrioventricular (AV) block and a variety of atrial and ventricular arrhythmias are common with poisoning by digoxin and other cardiac glycosides. Hypoxemia due to carbon monoxide poisoning may result in ischemic changes on the electrocardiogram.

F. Imaging Findings

A plain film of the abdomen may be useful because some tablets, particularly iron and potassium, may be radiopaque. Chest radiographs may reveal aspiration pneumonia, hydrocarbon pneumonia, or pulmonary edema. When head trauma is suspected, a computed tomography (CT) scan is recommended.

Toxicology Screening Tests

It is a common misconception that a toxicology "screen" is the best way to diagnose and manage an acute poisoning. Unfortunately, rapid urine "drugs of abuse" screens are limited to a few classes of drugs and are subject to many false-positive and false-negative results. More reliable comprehensive toxicology screening is available but is time-consuming and expensive, and results of tests may not be available for days. Moreover, many highly toxic drugs such as calcium channel blockers, β blockers, and isoniazid are not included in the screening process. The clinical examination of the patient and selected routine laboratory tests are usually sufficient to generate a tentative diagnosis and an appropriate treatment plan. Although screening tests (so-called "drugs of abuse" panels) may be helpful in confirming a suspected intoxication, they should not delay needed treatment. Furthermore, they may be indicative of exposure but do not provide information regarding the time of exposure or the quantity of drug present in the patient's body. More formal, comprehensive screening may be necessary in cases of suspected brain death (to rule out drugs as a cause of coma), child abuse, or as part of a postmortem examination.

When a specific antidote or other treatment is under consideration, quantitative laboratory testing may be indicated. For example, determination of the acetaminophen level is useful in assessing the need for antidotal therapy with acetylcysteine. Serum levels of salicylate (aspirin), ethylene glycol, methanol, theophylline, carbamazepine, lithium, valproic acid, and other drugs and poisons may indicate the need for hemodialysis (Table 58–2).

Decontamination

Decontamination procedures should be undertaken simultaneously with initial stabilization, diagnostic assessment, and laboratory evaluation. Decontamination involves removing toxins from the skin or gastrointestinal tract. The provider should always wear appropriate personal protective equipment when performing patient decontamination to avoid inadvertent secondary exposure to potential toxins.

A. Skin

Contaminated clothing should be completely removed and double-bagged to prevent illness in health care providers and for possible laboratory analysis. Wash contaminated skin with soap and water.

B. Gastrointestinal Tract

Controversy remains regarding the efficacy of gastrointestinal decontamination, especially when treatment is initiated more than

TABLE 58–2 Hemodialysis in drug overdose and poisoning.[1]

Hemodialysis may be indicated depending on the severity of poisoning or the blood concentration:
Carbamazepine
Ethylene glycol
Lithium
Methanol
Metformin
Phenobarbital
Salicylate
Theophylline
Valproic acid
Hemodialysis is ineffective or is not useful:
Amphetamines
Antidepressants
Antipsychotic drugs
Benzodiazepines
Calcium channel blockers
Digoxin
Metoprolol and propranolol
Opioids

[1]This listing is not comprehensive.

1 hour after ingestion. For most ingestions, clinical toxicologists recommend simple administration of activated charcoal to bind ingested poisons in the gut before they can be absorbed (as in the case study). In unusual circumstances, gastric lavage or whole bowel irrigation may also be used. Inducing emesis is ineffective, potentially harmful, and no longer recommended.

1. *Gastric lavage*—If the patient is awake or if the airway is protected by an endotracheal tube, gastric lavage may be performed using an orogastric or nasogastric tube—as large a tube as possible. Lavage solutions (usually 0.9% saline) should be at body temperature to prevent hypothermia.

2. *Activated charcoal*—Owing to its large surface area, activated charcoal can adsorb many drugs and poisons. It is most effective if given in a ratio of at least 10:1 of charcoal to estimated dose of toxin by weight. Charcoal does not bind iron, lithium, or potassium, and it binds alcohols and cyanide only poorly. It does not appear to be useful in poisoning due to corrosive mineral acids and alkali. Repeated doses of oral activated charcoal may enhance systemic elimination of some drugs (including carbamazepine, dapsone, and phenobarbital) by a mechanism referred to as "gut dialysis," although the clinical benefit is unproved.

3. *Cathartics*—Administration of a cathartic (laxative) agent may hasten removal of toxins from the gastrointestinal tract and reduce absorption, although no controlled studies have been done. Whole bowel irrigation with a balanced polyethylene glycol-electrolyte solution (GoLYTELY, CoLyte) can enhance gut decontamination after ingestion of iron tablets, enteric-coated medicines, illicit drug-filled packets, and foreign bodies. The solution is administered orally at 1–2 L/h (500 mL/h in children) for several hours until the rectal effluent is clear.

Specific Antidotes

There is a popular misconception that there is an antidote for every poison. Actually, selective antidotes are available for only a few classes of toxins. The major antidotes and their characteristics are listed in Table 58–3.

Methods of Enhancing Elimination of Toxins

After appropriate diagnostic and decontamination procedures and administration of antidotes, it is important to consider whether measures for enhancing elimination, such as hemodialysis or urinary alkalinization, can improve the clinical outcome. Table 58–2 lists intoxications for which dialysis may be beneficial.

A. Dialysis Procedures

1. *Peritoneal dialysis*—Although it is a relatively simple and available technique, peritoneal dialysis is inefficient in removing most drugs.

2. *Hemodialysis*—Hemodialysis is more efficient than peritoneal dialysis and has been well studied. It assists in correction of fluid and electrolyte imbalance, acid-base status, and may also enhance removal of toxic metabolites (eg, formic acid in methanol poisoning; oxalic and glycolic acids in ethylene glycol poisoning). The efficiency of both peritoneal dialysis and hemodialysis is a function of the molecular weight, water solubility, protein binding, endogenous clearance, and distribution in the body of the specific toxin. Hemodialysis is especially useful in overdose cases in which the precipitating drug can be removed and fluid and electrolyte imbalances are present and can be corrected (eg, salicylate intoxication).

B. Forced Diuresis and Urinary pH Manipulation

Previously popular but of unproved value, forced diuresis may cause volume overload and electrolyte abnormalities and is not recommended. Renal elimination of a few toxins can be enhanced by alteration of urinary pH. For example, urinary alkalinization is useful in cases of salicylate overdose. Acidification may increase the urine concentration of drugs such as phencyclidine and amphetamines but is not advised because it may worsen renal complications from rhabdomyolysis, which often accompanies the intoxication.

■ COMMON TOXIC SYNDROMES

ACETAMINOPHEN

Acetaminophen is one of the drugs commonly involved in suicide attempts and accidental poisonings, both as the sole agent and in combination with other drugs. Acute ingestion of more than 150–200 mg/kg (children) or 7 g total (adults) is considered potentially toxic. A highly toxic metabolite is produced in the liver (see Figure 4–5).

Initially, the patient is asymptomatic or has mild gastrointestinal upset (nausea, vomiting). After 24–36 hours, evidence of liver injury appears, with elevated aminotransferase levels and hypoprothrombinemia. Fulminant liver failure may ensue, leading to metabolic acidosis, hypoglycemia, encephalopathy, and death. Renal failure may also occur. With acute massive ingestion and very high serum levels, metabolic acidosis can occur in the absence of liver failure. Rarely, chronic acetaminophen ingestion can cause 5-oxoprolinuria due to glutathione depletion resulting in an anion gap metabolic acidosis.

The severity of poisoning is estimated from a serum acetaminophen concentration measurement. If the level is greater than 150 mg/L approximately 4 hours after ingestion, the patient is at risk for liver injury. Chronic alcoholics or patients taking drugs that enhance P450 production of toxic metabolites may be at risk with lower levels. The antidote acetylcysteine acts as a glutathione substitute, binding the toxic metabolite as it is produced. It is most effective when given early and should be started within 8–10 hours if possible. Liver transplantation may be required for patients with fulminant hepatic failure.

TABLE 58–3 Examples of specific antidotes.

Antidote	Poison(s)	Comments
Acetylcysteine (Acetadote, Mucomyst)	Acetaminophen	Best results if given within 8–10 hours of overdose. Follow liver function tests and acetaminophen blood levels. Acetadote is given intravenously; Mucomyst is given orally.
Atropine	Anticholinesterase intoxication: organophosphates, carbamates	An initial dose of 1–2 mg (for children, 0.05 mg/kg) is given IV, and if there is no response, the dose is doubled every 10–15 minutes, with decreased wheezing and pulmonary secretions as therapeutic end points.
Atropine	Rapid-onset mushroom poisoning with predominant muscarinic excess symptoms	Useful for control of muscarinic symptoms. *Note:* Of no value in delayed-onset mushroom poisoning.
Bicarbonate, sodium	Membrane-depressant cardiotoxic drugs (tricyclic antidepressants, quinidine, etc)	1–2 mEq/kg IV bolus usually reverses cardiotoxic effects (wide QRS, hypotension). Give cautiously in heart failure (avoid sodium overload).
Calcium	Fluoride; calcium channel blockers	Large doses may be needed in severe calcium channel blocker overdose. Start with 15 mg/kg IV.
Deferoxamine	Iron salts	If poisoning is severe, give 15 mg/kg/h IV. 100 mg of deferoxamine binds 8.5 mg of iron.
Digoxin antibodies	Digoxin and related cardiac glycosides	One vial binds 0.5 mg digoxin; indications include serious arrhythmias, hyperkalemia.
Esmolol	Theophylline, caffeine, metaproterenol	Short-acting β blocker. Infuse 25–50 mcg/kg/min IV.
Ethanol	Methanol, ethylene glycol	A loading dose is calculated so as to give a blood level of at least 100 mg/dL (42 g/70 kg in adults). Fomepizole (see below) is easier to use.
Flumazenil	Benzodiazepines	Adult dose is 0.2 mg IV, repeated as necessary to a maximum of 3 mg. *Do not give to patients with seizures, benzodiazepine dependence, or tricyclic overdose.*
Fomepizole	Methanol, ethylene glycol	More convenient than ethanol. Give 15 mg/kg; repeat every 12 hours.
Glucagon	β blockers	5–10 mg IV bolus may reverse hypotension and bradycardia.
Hydroxocobalamin	Cyanide	Adult dose is 5 g IV over 15 minutes. Converts cyanide to cyanocobalamin (vitamin B_{12}).
Naloxone	Narcotic drugs, other opioid derivatives	A specific antagonist of opioids; give 0.4–2 mg initially by IV, IM, or SC injection. Larger doses may be needed to reverse the effects of overdose with propoxyphene, codeine, or fentanyl derivatives. Duration of action (2–3 hours) may be significantly shorter than that of the opioid being antagonized.
Oxygen	Carbon monoxide	Give 100% by high-flow nonrebreathing mask; use of hyperbaric chamber is controversial but often recommended for severe poisoning.
Physostigmine	Suggested for delirium caused by anticholinergic agents	Adult dose is 0.5–1 mg IV slowly. The effects are transient (30–60 minutes), and the lowest effective dose may be repeated when symptoms return. May cause bradycardia, increased bronchial secretions, seizures. Have atropine ready to reverse excess effects. *Do not use for tricyclic antidepressant overdose.*
Pralidoxime (2-PAM)	Organophosphate (OP) cholinesterase inhibitors	Adult dose is 1 g IV, which should be repeated every 3–4 hours as needed or preferably as a constant infusion of 250–400 mg/h. Pediatric dose is approximately 250 mg. No proved benefit in carbamate poisoning; uncertain benefit in established OP poisoning.

AMPHETAMINES & OTHER STIMULANTS

Stimulant drugs commonly abused in the USA include methamphetamine ("crank," "crystal"), methylenedioxymethamphetamine (MDMA, "ecstasy"), and cocaine ("crack") as well as pharmaceuticals such as pseudoephedrine (Sudafed) and ephedrine (as such and in the herbal agent *Ma-huang*) (see Chapter 32). Caffeine is often added to dietary supplements sold as "metabolic enhancers" or "fat burners." Newer synthetic analogs of amphetamines (often sold on the street as "bath salts") and synthetic agonists of the endogenous cannabinoid receptors (sold as "research chemicals", "K2" or "spice") are becoming popular drugs of abuse.

At usual doses, euphoria and wakefulness are accompanied by a sense of power and well-being. At higher doses, restlessness, agitation, and acute psychosis may occur, accompanied by hypertension and tachycardia. Prolonged muscular hyperactivity or seizures may contribute to hyperthermia and rhabdomyolysis. Body temperatures as high as 42°C (107.6°F) have been recorded. Hyperthermia can cause brain damage, hypotension, coagulopathy, and renal failure.

Treatment for stimulant toxicity includes general supportive measures as outlined earlier. There is no specific antidote. Seizures and hyperthermia are the most dangerous manifestations and must be treated aggressively. Seizures are usually managed with intravenous benzodiazepines (eg, lorazepam). Severe hyperthermia is a life-threatening emergency and must be treated rapidly. Temperature is reduced by removing clothing, spraying with tepid water, and encouraging evaporative cooling with fanning or by immersion in ice. For very high body temperatures (eg, >40–41°C [104–105.8°F]), neuromuscular paralysis (eg, with vecuronium) is used to abolish muscle activity quickly. Excess serotonin produced through inhibition of its reuptake or promotion of its release by some stimulants may lead to the serotonin syndrome (see Chapter 16).

ANTICHOLINERGIC AGENTS

A large number of prescription and nonprescription drugs, as well as a variety of plants and mushrooms, can inhibit the effects of acetylcholine at muscarinic receptors. Some drugs used for other purposes (eg, antihistamines) also have anticholinergic effects, in addition to other potentially toxic actions. For example, antihistamines such as diphenhydramine can cause seizures; tricyclic antidepressants, which have anticholinergic, quinidine-like, and α-blocking effects, can cause severe cardiovascular toxicity.

The classic anticholinergic (technically, "antimuscarinic") syndrome is remembered as "red as a beet" (skin flushed), "hot as a hare" (hyperthermia), "dry as a bone" (dry mucous membranes, no sweating), "blind as a bat" (blurred vision, cycloplegia), and "mad as a hatter" (confusion, delirium). Patients usually have sinus tachycardia, and the pupils are usually dilated (see Chapter 8). Agitated delirium or coma may be present. Muscle twitching is common, but seizures are unusual unless the patient has ingested an antihistamine or a tricyclic antidepressant. Urinary retention is common, especially in older men.

Treatment for anticholinergic syndrome is largely supportive. Agitated patients may require sedation with a benzodiazepine or an antipsychotic agent (eg, haloperidol or olanzapine). The specific antidote for peripheral and central anticholinergic syndrome is physostigmine, which has a prompt and dramatic effect and is especially useful for patients who are very agitated. Physostigmine is given in small intravenous doses (0.5–1 mg) with careful monitoring, because it can cause bradycardia and seizures if given too rapidly. Physostigmine should not be given to a patient with serious tricyclic antidepressant overdose because it can aggravate cardiotoxicity, resulting in heart block or asystole. Catheterization of the bladder may be needed to prevent excessive distention.

ANTIDEPRESSANTS

Tricyclic antidepressants (eg, amitriptyline, desipramine, doxepin, many others; see Chapter 30) can cause life-threatening drug overdose. Ingestion of more than 1 g of a tricyclic (or about 15–20 mg/kg) is considered potentially lethal.

Tricyclic antidepressants are competitive antagonists at muscarinic cholinergic receptors, and anticholinergic findings (tachycardia, dilated pupils, dry mouth) are common even at moderate doses. Some tricyclics are also strong α blockers, which can lead to vasodilation. They also contain antihistamine properties and antagonize GABA-A receptors which may lead to seizures. Centrally mediated agitation and seizures may be followed by depression and hypotension. Most important is the fact that tricyclics inhibit the cardiac sodium channel, causing slowed conduction with a wide QRS interval and depressed cardiac contractility. This cardiac toxicity may result in serious arrhythmias (Figure 58–1), including ventricular conduction block and ventricular tachycardia.

Treatment of tricyclic antidepressant overdose includes general supportive care as outlined earlier. Endotracheal intubation and assisted ventilation may be needed. Intravenous fluids are given for hypotension, and dopamine or norepinephrine is added if necessary. Many toxicologists recommend norepinephrine as the initial drug of choice for tricyclic-induced hypotension. The antidote for cardiac toxicity (manifested by a wide QRS complex) is sodium bicarbonate: a bolus of 50–100 mEq (or 1–2 mEq/kg) provides a rapid increase in extracellular sodium that helps overcome sodium channel blockade. Although physostigmine does effectively reverse anticholinergic signs, it can aggravate depression of cardiac conduction and cause seizures and is not recommended.

Monoamine oxidase inhibitors (eg, tranylcypromine, phenelzine) are older antidepressants that are occasionally used for resistant depression. They can cause severe hypertensive reactions when interacting foods or drugs are taken (see Chapters 9 and 30), and they can interact with the selective serotonin reuptake inhibitors (SSRIs).

Newer antidepressants (eg, fluoxetine, paroxetine, citalopram, venlafaxine) are mostly SSRIs and are generally safer than the tricyclic antidepressants and monoamine oxidase inhibitors, although they can cause seizures. SSRIs may interact with each other or especially with monoamine oxidase inhibitors to cause the **serotonin syndrome,** characterized by agitation, muscle hyperactivity, and hyperthermia (see Chapter 16). **Bupropion** (not an SSRI) has caused seizures even in therapeutic doses. Some antidepressants have been associated with QT prolongation and torsades de pointes arrhythmia.

ANTIPSYCHOTICS

Antipsychotic drugs include the older phenothiazines and butyrophenones, as well as newer so-called "atypical" drugs. All of these can cause CNS depression, seizures, and hypotension. Some can cause QT prolongation. The potent dopamine D_2 blockers are also associated with parkinsonian movement disorders (dystonic reactions) and in rare cases with the neuroleptic malignant syndrome, characterized by "lead-pipe" rigidity, hyperthermia, and autonomic instability (see Chapters 16 and 29).

ASPIRIN (SALICYLATE)

Salicylate poisoning (see Chapter 36) is a much less common cause of childhood poisoning deaths since the introduction of child-resistant containers and the reduced use of children's aspirin. It still accounts for numerous suicidal and accidental poisonings.

Acute ingestion of more than 200 mg/kg is likely to produce intoxication. Poisoning can also result from chronic overmedication; this occurs most commonly in elderly patients using salicylates for chronic pain who become confused about their dosing. Poisoning causes uncoupling of oxidative phosphorylation and disruption of normal cellular metabolism.

The first sign of salicylate toxicity is often hyperventilation and respiratory alkalosis due to medullary stimulation. Metabolic acidosis follows, and an increased anion gap results from accumulation of lactate as well as excretion of bicarbonate by the kidney to compensate for respiratory alkalosis. Arterial blood gas testing often reveals a mixed respiratory alkalosis and metabolic acidosis. Body temperature may be elevated owing to uncoupling of oxidative phosphorylation. Severe hyperthermia may occur in serious cases. Vomiting and hyperpnea as well as hyperthermia contribute to fluid loss and dehydration. With very severe poisoning, profound metabolic acidosis, seizures, coma, pulmonary edema, and cardiovascular collapse may occur. Absorption of salicylate and signs of toxicity may be delayed after very large overdoses or ingestion of enteric-coated tablets.

General supportive care is essential. After massive aspirin ingestions (eg, more than 100 tablets), aggressive gut decontamination is advisable, including gastric lavage, repeated doses of activated charcoal, and consideration of whole bowel irrigation. Intravenous fluids are used to replace fluid losses caused by tachypnea, vomiting, and fever. For moderate intoxications, intravenous sodium bicarbonate is given to alkalinize the urine and promote salicylate excretion by trapping the salicylate in its ionized, polar form. For severe poisoning (eg, patients with severe acidosis, coma, and serum salicylate level >90–100 mg/dL), emergency hemodialysis is performed to remove the salicylate more quickly and restore acid-base balance and fluid status.

BETA BLOCKERS

In overdose, β blockers inhibit both β_1 and β_2 adrenoceptors; selectivity, if any, is lost at high dosage. The most toxic β blocker is propranolol. As little as two to three times the therapeutic dose can cause serious toxicity. This may be because propranolol in high doses causes sodium channel-blocking effects similar to those seen with tricyclic antidepressants, and it is lipophilic, allowing it to enter the CNS (see Chapter 10).

Bradycardia and hypotension are the most common manifestations of toxicity. Agents with partial agonist activity (eg, pindolol) can cause tachycardia and hypertension. Seizures and cardiac conduction block (wide QRS complex) may be seen with propranolol overdose.

General supportive care should be provided as outlined earlier. The usual measures used to raise the blood pressure and heart rate, such as intravenous fluids, β-agonist drugs, and atropine, are generally ineffective. Glucagon is a useful antidote that—like β agonists—acts on cardiac cells to raise intracellular cAMP but does so independent of β adrenoceptors. It can improve heart rate and blood pressure when given in high doses (5–10 mg intravenously).

CALCIUM CHANNEL BLOCKERS

Calcium antagonists can cause serious toxicity or death with relatively small overdoses. These channel blockers depress sinus node automaticity and slow AV node conduction (see Chapter 12). They also reduce cardiac output and blood pressure. Overdoses of verapamil and diltiazem are generally more dangerous, resulting in bradycardia, hypotension, and cardiogenic shock. Dihydropyridines (eg, nifedipine and amlodipine) are more selective for vascular calcium channels, resulting in vasodilation, hypotension, and reflex tachycardia. In massive overdose, this selectivity may be lost, and all of the listed cardiovascular effects can occur with any of the calcium channel blockers.

Treatment requires general supportive care. Since most ingested calcium antagonists are in sustained-release form, it may be possible to expel them before they are completely absorbed; initiate whole bowel irrigation and oral activated charcoal as soon as possible, before calcium antagonist-induced ileus intervenes. Calcium, given intravenously in doses of 2–10 g, is a useful antidote for depressed cardiac contractility but less effective for nodal block or peripheral vascular collapse. Other treatments reported to be helpful in managing hypotension associated with calcium channel blocker poisoning include high-dose insulin (0.5–1 unit/kg/h) plus glucose supplementation to maintain euglycemia; glucagon; veno-arterial extracorporeal membrane oxygenation (ECMO-VA); and methylene blue. A few case reports have suggested benefit from administration of lipid emulsion (normally used as an intravenous dietary fat supplement) for severe verapamil overdose.

CARBON MONOXIDE & OTHER TOXIC GASES

Carbon monoxide (CO) is a colorless, odorless gas that is ubiquitous because it is created whenever carbon-containing materials are burned. Most cases of CO poisoning occur in victims of fires, but accidental and suicidal exposures are also common. The diagnosis and treatment of carbon monoxide poisoning are described in Chapter 56. Many other toxic gases are produced in fires or released in industrial accidents (Table 58–4).

CHOLINESTERASE INHIBITORS

Organophosphate and carbamate cholinesterase inhibitors (see Chapter 7) are widely used to kill insects and other pests. Most cases of serious organophosphate or carbamate poisoning result from intentional ingestion in attempted suicide, but poisoning has also occurred at work (pesticide application or packaging), as a result of food contamination, or as a terrorist attack (eg, release of the chemical warfare nerve agent sarin in the Tokyo subway system in 1995).

Stimulation of muscarinic receptors causes abdominal cramps, diarrhea, excessive salivation, sweating, urinary frequency, and increased bronchial secretions (see Chapters 6 and 7). Stimulation of nicotinic receptors causes generalized ganglionic activation,

TABLE 58–4 Characteristics of poisoning with some gases.

Gas	Mechanism of Toxicity	Clinical Features and Treatment
Irritant gases (eg, chlorine, ammonia, sulfur dioxide, nitrogen oxides)	Corrosive effect on upper and lower airways	Cough, stridor, wheezing, pneumonia *Treatment:* Humidified oxygen, bronchodilators
Carbon monoxide	Binds to hemoglobin, reducing oxygen delivery to tissues	Headache, dizziness, nausea, vomiting, seizures, coma *Treatment:* 100% oxygen; consider hyperbaric oxygen
Cyanide	Binds to cytochrome, blocks cellular oxygen use	Headache, nausea, vomiting, syncope, seizures, coma *Treatment:* Conventional antidote kit consists of nitrites to induce methemoglobinemia (which binds cyanide) and thiosulfate (which hastens conversion of cyanide to less toxic thiocyanate); a newer antidote kit (Cyanokit) consists of concentrated hydroxocobalamin, which directly converts cyanide into cyanocobalamin
Hydrogen sulfide	Similar to cyanide	Similar to cyanide. Smell of rotten eggs *Treatment:* No specific antidote; some authorities recommend the nitrite portion of the conventional cyanide antidote kit
Oxidizing agents (eg, nitrogen oxides)	Can cause methemoglobinemia	Dyspnea, cyanosis (due to brown color of methemoglobin), syncope, seizures, coma *Treatment:* Methylene blue (which hastens conversion back to normal hemoglobin)

which can lead to hypertension and either tachycardia or bradycardia. Muscle twitching and fasciculations may progress to weakness and respiratory muscle paralysis. CNS effects include agitation, confusion, and seizures. The mnemonic DUMBELS (diarrhea, urination, miosis and muscle weakness, bronchospasm, excitation, lacrimation, and seizures, sweating, and salivation) helps recall the common findings. Blood testing may be used to document depressed activity of red blood cell (acetylcholinesterase) and plasma (butyrylcholinesterase) enzymes, which provide an indirect estimate of synaptic cholinesterase activity.

General supportive care should be provided as outlined above. Precautions should be taken to ensure that rescuers and health care providers are not poisoned themselves by exposure to contaminated clothing or skin. This is especially critical for the most potent substances such as parathion or nerve gas agents. Antidotal treatment consists of atropine and pralidoxime (see Table 58–3). Atropine is an effective competitive inhibitor at muscarinic sites but has no effect at nicotinic sites. Pralidoxime given early enough may be capable of restoring the cholinesterase activity and is active at both muscarinic and nicotinic sites; however, studies are conflicting regarding its effect on clinical outcome.

CYANIDE

Cyanide (CN^-) salts and hydrogen cyanide (HCN) are highly toxic chemicals used in chemical synthesis, as rodenticides, formerly as a method of execution, and as agents of suicide or homicide. Hydrogen cyanide is formed from the burning of plastics, wool, and many other synthetic and natural products. Cyanide is also released after ingestion of various plants (eg, cassava) and seeds (eg, apple, peach, and apricot).

Cyanide binds readily to the ferric iron (Fe^{3+}) in cytochrome oxidase, inhibiting oxygen utilization within the cell mitochondria and leading to cellular hypoxia and lactic acidosis. Symptoms of cyanide poisoning include shortness of breath, agitation, and tachycardia followed by seizures, coma, hypotension, and death. Severe metabolic acidosis is characteristic. The venous oxygen content may be elevated because oxygen is not being taken up by cells.

Treatment of cyanide poisoning includes rapid oral administration of antidote, activated charcoal (although charcoal binds cyanide poorly, it can reduce absorption), and general supportive care. There are two FDA-approved antidotes for the treatment of cyanide toxicity. Hydroxocobalamin (Cyanokit) is a form of vitamin B_{12} that combines rapidly with CN^- to form nontoxic cyanocobalamin (another form of vitamin B_{12}). Nithiodote is an older cyanide treatment kit containing sodium nitrite and sodium thiosulfate. Sodium nitrite induces methemoglobinemia, which binds CN^-, creating the less toxic cyanomethemoglobin. Sodium thiosulfate is a cofactor in the enzymatic conversion of CN^- to the much less toxic thiocyanate (SCN^-).

DIGOXIN

Digitalis and other cardiac glycosides and cardenolides are found in many plants (see Chapter 13) and in the skin of some toads. Toxicity may occur as a result of acute overdose or from accumulation of digoxin in a patient with renal insufficiency or from taking a drug that interferes with digoxin elimination.

Vomiting is common in patients with digitalis overdose. Hyperkalemia may be caused by acute digitalis overdose or severe poisoning, whereas hypokalemia may be present in patients who are on long-term diuretic treatment and may worsen toxicity

(Digitalis does not cause hypokalemia). A variety of cardiac rhythm disturbances may occur, including sinus bradycardia, AV block, atrial tachycardia with block, accelerated junctional rhythm, premature ventricular beats, bidirectional ventricular tachycardia, and other ventricular arrhythmias.

General supportive care should be provided. Atropine is often effective for bradycardia or AV block. The use of **digoxin antibodies** (see Chapter 13) has revolutionized the treatment of digoxin toxicity; they should be administered intravenously in the dosage indicated in the package insert. Symptoms usually improve within 30–60 minutes after antibody administration. Digoxin antibodies may also be tried in cases of poisoning by other cardiac glycosides (eg, digitoxin, oleander), although larger doses may be needed due to incomplete cross-reactivity.

ETHANOL & SEDATIVE-HYPNOTIC DRUGS

Overdosage with ethanol and sedative-hypnotic drugs (eg, benzodiazepines, barbiturates, γ-hydroxybutyrate [GHB], carisoprodol [Soma]; see Chapters 22 and 23) occurs frequently because of their common availability and use.

Patients with ethanol or other sedative-hypnotic overdose may be euphoric and rowdy ("drunk") or in a state of stupor or coma ("dead drunk"). Comatose patients often have depressed respiratory drive. Depression of protective airway reflexes may result in pulmonary aspiration of gastric contents, leading to pneumonia. Hypothermia may be present because of environmental exposure and depressed shivering. Ethanol blood levels greater than 300 mg/dL usually cause deep coma, but regular users are often tolerant to the effects of ethanol and may be ambulatory despite even higher levels. Patients with GHB overdose are often deeply comatose for 3–4 hours and then awaken fully in a matter of minutes.

General supportive care should be provided. With careful attention to protecting the airway (including endotracheal intubation) and assisting ventilation, most patients recover as the drug effects wear off. Hypotension usually responds to intravenous fluids, body warming if cold, and, if needed, a vasopressor. Patients with isolated benzodiazepine overdose may awaken after intravenous flumazenil, a benzodiazepine antagonist. However, this drug is not widely used as empiric therapy for drug overdose because it may precipitate seizures in patients who are chronically taking benzodiazepines or who have also ingested a convulsant drug (eg, a tricyclic antidepressant). There are no antidotes for ethanol, barbiturates, or most other sedative-hypnotics; supportive care is critical.

ETHYLENE GLYCOL & METHANOL

Ethylene glycol and methanol are alcohols that are important toxins because of their metabolism to highly toxic organic acids (see Chapter 23). They are capable of causing CNS depression and a drunken state similar to ethanol overdose, accompanied by an osmol gap. In addition, their products of metabolism—formic acid (from methanol) or hippuric, oxalic, and glycolic acids (from ethylene glycol)—cause a severe metabolic acidosis and can lead to coma and blindness (in the case of formic acid) or renal failure (from oxalic acid and glycolic acid). Initially, the patient appears drunk, but after a delay of up to several hours, a severe anion gap metabolic acidosis becomes apparent, accompanied by hyperventilation and altered mental status. Patients with methanol poisoning may have visual disturbances ranging from blurred vision to blindness.

Metabolism of ethylene glycol and methanol to their toxic products can be blocked by inhibiting the enzyme alcohol dehydrogenase with a competing drug, such as fomepizole (4-methylpyrazole). Ethanol is also an effective antidote, but it can be difficult to achieve a safe and effective blood level. Hemodialysis can remove both the parent alcohol and the toxic metabolites and is generally indicated in patients with acidosis or signs of end organ dysfunction (coma, renal failure [ethylene glycol] or visual changes [methanol]).

IRON & OTHER METALS

Iron is widely used in over-the-counter vitamin preparations. As few as 10–12 prenatal multivitamins with iron may cause serious illness in a small child. Poisoning with other metals (lead, mercury, arsenic) is also important, especially in industry. See Chapters 33, 56, and 57 for detailed discussions of poisoning by iron and other metals.

MARIJUANA

Tetrahydrocannabinol (THC) is the constituent in marijuana responsible for most of its mood-altering effects (see Chapter 63). Exposure to THC is increasingly common due to legalization for both medical and recreational use. The cannabis industry produces a variety of foods, beverages, and candies containing added THC, which may lead to accidental and childhood exposures. Synthetic cannabinoids marketed as "herbal incense" or "spice" may cause marked stimulant effects, psychosis, and seizures. **Cannabidiol,** another important component of cannabis, appears to be devoid of most of the mood-altering effects of THC. For a detailed discussion on marijuana use, overdose, and treatment, see Chapters 24, 32, and 63.

OPIOIDS

Opioids (opium, morphine, heroin, meperidine, methadone, etc) are common drugs of abuse (see Chapters 31 and 32), and overdose is a common result of using the poorly standardized preparations sold on the street. In recent years, there has been an increase in fentanyl exposures due to adulteration of heroin and methamphetamine, as well as the emergence of fake pills sold underground as "Norco" and "Xanax" to unwitting consumers. See Chapter 31 for a detailed discussion of opioid overdose and its treatment.

RATTLESNAKE ENVENOMATION

In the USA, rattlesnakes are the most common venomous reptiles. Bites are rarely fatal, and 20% do not involve envenomation. However, about 60% of bites cause significant morbidity due to the destructive digestive enzymes found in the venom. Evidence of rattlesnake envenomation includes severe pain, swelling, bruising, hemorrhagic bleb formation, and obvious fang marks. Systemic effects include nausea, vomiting, muscle fasciculations, tingling and metallic taste in the mouth, shock, and systemic coagulopathy with prolonged clotting time and reduced platelet count.

Studies have shown that emergency field remedies such as incision and suction, tourniquets, and ice packs are far more damaging than useful. Avoidance of unnecessary motion, on the other hand, does help to limit the spread of the venom. Definitive therapy relies on intravenous antivenom (also known as antivenin), and this should be started as soon as possible. There are two FDA-approved antivenoms in the United States; Crotalidae polyvalent immune Fab antivenom (Crofab) and Crotalidae equine immune F(ab')2 (Anavip).

THEOPHYLLINE

Although it has been largely replaced by inhaled β agonists, theophylline continues to be used for the treatment of bronchospasm by some patients with asthma and bronchitis (see Chapter 20). A dose of 20–30 tablets can cause serious or fatal poisoning in an adult. Chronic or subacute theophylline poisoning can also occur as a result of accidental overmedication or use of a drug that interferes with theophylline metabolism (eg, cimetidine, ciprofloxacin, erythromycin; see Chapter 4). Caffeine produces similar toxic effects and it is available in several "energy" supplements.

In addition to sinus tachycardia and tremor, vomiting is common after overdose. Hypotension, tachycardia, hypokalemia, and hyperglycemia may occur, probably owing to β_2-adrenergic activation. The cause of this activation is not fully understood, but the effects can be ameliorated by β blockers (see below). Cardiac arrhythmias include atrial tachycardias, premature ventricular contractions, and ventricular tachycardia. In severe poisoning (eg, acute overdose with serum level >100 mg/L), seizures often occur and are usually resistant to common anticonvulsants. Toxicity may be delayed in onset for many hours after ingestion of sustained-release tablet formulations.

General supportive care should be provided. Aggressive gut decontamination should be carried out using repeated doses of activated charcoal and whole bowel irrigation. Propranolol or other β blockers (eg, esmolol) are useful antidotes for β-mediated hypotension and tachycardia. Hemodialysis is indicated for serum concentrations >100 mg/L and for intractable seizures in patients with lower levels.

REFERENCES

Dart RD (editor): *Medical Toxicology*, 3rd ed. Lippincott Williams & Wilkins, 2004.

Nelson LS, Howland MA, Lewin NA, et al (editors): *Goldfrank's Toxicologic Emergencies*, 11th ed. McGraw-Hill, 2019.

Olson KR, Smollin CG, Anderson IB, et al (editors): *Poisoning & Drug Overdose*, 8th ed. McGraw-Hill, 2021.

POISINDEX. (Revised Quarterly.) Thomson/Micromedex.

CASE STUDY ANSWER

Overdose of bupropion can cause seizures that are often recurrent or prolonged. Drug-induced seizures are treated with an intravenous benzodiazepine such as lorazepam or diazepam. If this is not effective, phenobarbital or another more potent central nervous system depressant may be used. To prevent ingested drugs and poisons from being absorbed systemically, a slurry of activated charcoal is often given orally or by nasogastric tube.

CHAPTER

59

Special Aspects of Perinatal & Pediatric Pharmacology

Sean P. Elliott, MD, FAAP, FPIDS,
& Gideon Koren, MD, FRCPC, FACMT

The effects of drugs on the fetus and newborn infant are based on the general principles set forth in Chapters 1–4 of this book. However, the physiologic contexts in which these pharmacologic principles operate are different in pregnant women and in rapidly maturing infants. At present, the unique pharmacokinetic factors operative in these patients are beginning to be understood, whereas information regarding pharmacodynamic differences (eg, receptor characteristics and responses) is still grossly incomplete.

DRUG THERAPY IN PREGNANCY

Pharmacokinetics

Most drugs taken by pregnant women can cross the placenta and expose the developing embryo and fetus to their pharmacologic and teratogenic effects. However, most drugs, despite entering the fetal compartment, do not endanger the fetus when used in recommended doses. Table 59–1 lists teratogenic drugs in humans. Critical factors affecting placental drug transfer and drug effects on the fetus include the following: (1) the physicochemical properties of the drug; (2) the rate at which the drug crosses the placenta and the amount of drug reaching the fetus; (3) the duration of exposure to the drug; (4) distribution characteristics in different fetal tissues; (5) the stage of placental and fetal development at the time of exposure to the drug; and (6) the effects of drugs used in combination.

A. Lipid Solubility

As is true also of other biologic membranes, drug passage across the placenta is dependent on lipid solubility and the degree of drug ionization. Lipophilic drugs tend to diffuse readily across the placenta and enter the fetal circulation. For example, thiopental, a drug commonly used for cesarean sections, crosses the placenta almost immediately and can produce sedation or apnea in the newborn infant. Highly ionized drugs such as succinylcholine and tubocurarine, also used for cesarean sections, cross the placenta slowly and achieve very low concentrations in the fetus. Impermeability of the placenta to polar compounds is relative rather than absolute. If sufficiently high maternal-fetal concentration gradients are achieved, polar compounds also cross the placenta in measurable amounts. Salicylate, which is almost completely ionized at physiologic pH, crosses the placenta readily. This occurs because the small amount of salicylate that is not ionized is highly lipid-soluble.

TABLE 59–1 Drugs with significant teratogenic or other adverse effects on the fetus.

Drug	Trimester	Effect
ACE inhibitors	All, especially second and third	Renal damage, hypocalvaria
Aminopterin	First	Multiple major anomalies
Amphetamines	All	Suspected abnormal developmental patterns, decreased school performance
Androgens	Second and third	Masculinization of female fetus
Antidepressants, tricyclic	Third	Neonatal withdrawal symptoms have been reported in a few cases with clomipramine, desipramine, and imipramine.
Barbiturates	All	Chronic use can lead to neonatal dependence
Busulfan	All	Various major malformations
Carbamazepine	First	Neural tube defects
Chlorpropamide	All	Prolonged symptomatic neonatal hypoglycemia
Clomipramine	Third	Neonatal lethargy, hypotonia, cyanosis, hypothermia
Cocaine	All	Increased risk of spontaneous abortion, abruptio placentae, and premature labor; neonatal cerebral infarction, increased risk for attention deficit hyperactivity disorder
Cyclophosphamide	First	Various major malformations
Cytarabine	First, second	Various major malformations
Diazepam	All	Chronic use may lead to neonatal dependence
Dydrogesterone First		Hypospadias, cardiovascular malformations, spina bifida
Diethylstilbestrol	All	Vaginal adenosis, clear cell vaginal adenocarcinoma
Ethanol	All	Risk of fetal alcohol spectrum disorder
Etretinate	All	High risk of major congenital malformations
Heroin	All	Chronic use leads to neonatal abstinence syndrome.
Iodide	All	Congenital goiter, hypothyroidism
Isotretinoin	All	High risk of CNS, face, ear, and other malformations
Lithium	First, third	Ebstein anomaly and other cardiac malformations, neonatal toxicity after third trimester exposure
Methadone	All	Chronic use may lead to neonatal abstinence syndrome.
Methotrexate	First	Multiple major malformations
Misoprostol	First	Möbius sequence
Mycophenolate mofetil	First	Major malformations of the face, limbs, and other organs
Organic solvents	First	Neurodevelopmental effects, color blindness
Penicillamine	First	Cutis laxa, other congenital malformations
Phencyclidine	All	Abnormal neurologic examination, poor suck reflex and feeding
Phenytoin	All	Fetal hydantoin syndrome
Propylthiouracil	All	Congenital goiter
Serotonin reuptake inhibitors	Third	Neonatal abstinence syndrome, persistent pulmonary hypertension of the newborn
Smoking (constituents of tobacco smoke)	All	Intrauterine growth restriction; prematurity; sudden infant death syndrome; perinatal complications, oral cleft
Tamoxifen	All	Increased risk of spontaneous abortion or fetal damage
Tetracycline	All	Discoloration and defects of teeth and altered bone growth
Thalidomide	First	Phocomelia (shortened or absent long bones of the limbs) and many internal malformations
Trimethadione	All	Multiple major anomalies
Topiramate	First	Oral cleft
Valproic acid	All	Neural tube defects, cardiac and limb malformations; developmental delay; possibly autism
Warfarin	First	Hypoplastic nasal bridge, chondrodysplasia punctata
	Second	CNS malformations
	Third	Risk of bleeding. Discontinue use 1 month before delivery.

B. Molecular Size and pH

The molecular weight of the drug also influences the rate of transfer and the amount of drug transferred across the placenta. Drugs with molecular weights of 250–500 can cross the placenta readily, depending upon their lipid solubility and degree of ionization; those with molecular weights of 500–1000 cross the placenta with more difficulty; and those with molecular weights >1000 cross very poorly. An important clinical application of this property is the choice of heparin as an anticoagulant in pregnant women. Because it is a very large (and polar) molecule, heparin is unable to cross the placenta and this is true also for low molecular weight but polar heparins. Unlike warfarin, which is teratogenic and should be avoided during the first trimester and even beyond (as the brain continues to develop), heparin may be safely given to pregnant women who need anticoagulation. Yet the placenta contains drug transporters, which can carry larger molecules to the fetus. For example, a variety of maternal antibodies cross the placenta and may cause fetal morbidity, as in Rh incompatibility. Starting in the second trimester of pregnancy, the placenta develops transporters that allow immunoglobulins to cross from the mother to the fetus despite their large molecular size. This has important clinical implications, because an increasing number of biological drugs (eg, anti-tumor necrosis factor therapy) have been shown to cross the placenta. In addition to the detection of biologicals in cord blood, risks of such autoimmune disorders as severe neonatal neutropenia, anemia, and thrombocytopenia and cases of fetal dissemination of bacillus Calmette-Guérin (BCG) are reported.

Because maternal blood has a pH of 7.4, whereas the fetal blood is 7.3, basic drugs with a pK_a above 7.4 will be more ionized in the fetal compartment, leading to ion trapping and, hence, to higher fetal levels (see Chapter 1, Ionization of Weak Acids and Weak Bases).

C. Placental Transporters

During the last decade, many drug transporters have been identified in the placenta, with increasing recognition of their effects on drug transfer to the fetus. For example, the P-glycoprotein transporter encoded by the *MDR1* gene pumps back into the maternal circulation a variety of drugs, including cancer drugs (eg, vinblastine, doxorubicin) and other agents. Similarly, viral protease inhibitors, which are substrates to P-glycoprotein, achieve only low fetal concentrations—an effect that may increase the risk of vertical HIV infection from the mother to the fetus. The hypoglycemic drug glyburide has lower plasma levels in the fetus as compared with the mother. Recent work has documented that this agent is effluxed from the fetal circulation by the BCRP transporter as well as by the MRP3 transporter located in the placental brush border membrane. In addition, very high maternal protein binding of glyburide (>98.8%) also contributes to its lower fetal levels as compared with maternal concentrations.

D. Protein Binding

The degree to which a drug is bound to plasma proteins (mostly to albumin) may also affect the rate of transfer and the amount transferred. However, if a compound is very lipid-soluble (eg, some anesthetic gases), it will not be affected greatly by protein binding. Transfer of these more lipid-soluble drugs and their overall rates of equilibration are more dependent on (and proportionate to) placental blood flow. This is because very lipid-soluble drugs diffuse across placental membranes so rapidly that their overall rates of equilibration do not depend on the free drug concentrations becoming equal on both sides. If a drug is poorly lipid-soluble and is ionized, its transfer is slow and will probably be impeded by its binding to maternal plasma proteins. Differential protein binding is also important since some drugs exhibit greater protein binding in maternal plasma than in fetal plasma because of a lower binding affinity of fetal proteins. This has been shown for sulfonamides, barbiturates, phenytoin, and local anesthetic agents.

E. Placental and Fetal Drug Metabolism

Two mechanisms help protect the fetus from drugs in the maternal circulation: (1) The placenta itself plays a role both as a semipermeable barrier and as a site of metabolism of some drugs passing through it. Several different types of aromatic oxidation reactions (eg, hydroxylation, *N*-dealkylation, demethylation) have been shown to occur in placental tissue. Pentobarbital is oxidized in this way. Conversely, it is possible that the metabolic capacity of the placenta may lead to creation of toxic metabolites, and the placenta may therefore augment toxicity (eg, ethanol, benzpyrenes). (2) Because of the ability of the placenta to convert prednisolone to the inactive prednisone, prednisolone can be used in pregnant patients requiring corticosteroid treatment without the risk of fetal exposure to an active corticosteroid. Drugs that have crossed the placenta enter the fetal circulation via the umbilical vein. About 40–60% of umbilical venous blood flow enters the fetal liver; the remainder bypasses the liver and enters the general fetal circulation. A drug that enters the liver may be partially metabolized there before it enters the fetal circulation. In addition, a large proportion of drug present in the umbilical artery (returning to the placenta) may be shunted through the placenta back to the umbilical vein and into the liver again. It should be noted that metabolites of some drugs may be more active than the parent compound and may affect the fetus adversely.

Pharmacodynamics

A. Maternal Drug Actions

The effects of drugs on the reproductive tissues (breast, uterus, etc) of the pregnant woman are sometimes altered by the endocrine environment appropriate for the stage of pregnancy. Drug effects on other maternal tissues (heart, lungs, kidneys, central nervous system, etc) are not changed significantly by pregnancy, although the physiologic context (cardiac output, renal blood flow, etc) may be altered, requiring the use of drugs that are not needed by the same woman when she is not pregnant. For example, cardiac glycosides and diuretics may be needed for heart failure precipitated by the increased cardiac workload of pregnancy, or insulin may be required for control of blood glucose in gestational diabetes.

B. Therapeutic Drug Actions in the Fetus

Fetal therapeutics is an emerging area in perinatal pharmacology. This involves drug administration, mostly to the pregnant woman, with the fetus as the target of the drug. At present, corticosteroids are used to stimulate fetal lung maturation when preterm birth is expected. Phenobarbital, when given to pregnant women near term, can induce fetal hepatic enzymes responsible for the glucuronidation of bilirubin, and the incidence of jaundice is lower in newborns when mothers are given phenobarbital than when phenobarbital is not used. Before phototherapy became the preferred mode of therapy for neonatal indirect hyperbilirubinemia, phenobarbital was used for this indication. Administration of phenobarbital to the mother was suggested historically as a means of decreasing the risk of intracranial bleeding in preterm infants; however, more recent large randomized studies failed to confirm this effect and instead demonstrated an increased need for mechanical ventilation. Antiarrhythmic drugs administered to mothers are a consideration for treatment of fetal cardiac arrhythmias. Although their efficacy has not yet been established by controlled studies, digoxin, flecainide, procainamide, verapamil, and other antiarrhythmic agents have been shown to be effective in case series. Similarly, it has been shown that maternal use of zidovudine and other HIV drugs substantially decreases transmission of HIV from the mother to the fetus, and use of combinations of three antiretroviral agents can eliminate fetal infection almost entirely (see Chapter 49). This effect is demonstrated only if the infant also is treated with antiretroviral agents after birth; thus, the effect of maternal treatment likely is more related to suppression of her HIV viral load than to any specific treatment effect on the fetus.

C. Predictable Toxic Drug Actions in the Fetus

Chronic use of opioids by the mother often produces dependence in the fetus and newborn. This dependence may be manifested after delivery as a neonatal withdrawal syndrome, now known as neonatal abstinence syndrome. A less well understood fetal drug toxicity is caused by the use of angiotensin-converting enzyme inhibitors during late pregnancy. In late pregnancy these drugs can result in significant and irreversible renal damage in the fetus and are therefore contraindicated in the second and third trimesters. Adverse effects may also be delayed, as in the case of female fetuses exposed to diethylstilbestrol, who may be at increased risk for adenocarcinoma of the vagina after puberty.

D. Teratogenic Drug Actions

A single intrauterine exposure to a drug can affect fetal structures undergoing rapid development at the time of exposure. Thalidomide is the classic example of a drug that may profoundly affect the development of the limbs after only brief exposure. This exposure, however, must be at a critical time in the development of the limbs. Thalidomide-induced phocomelia occurs during the fourth through the seventh weeks of gestation because it is during this time that the arms and legs develop (Figure 59–1).

1. *Teratogenic mechanisms*—The mechanisms by which different drugs produce teratogenic effects are poorly understood

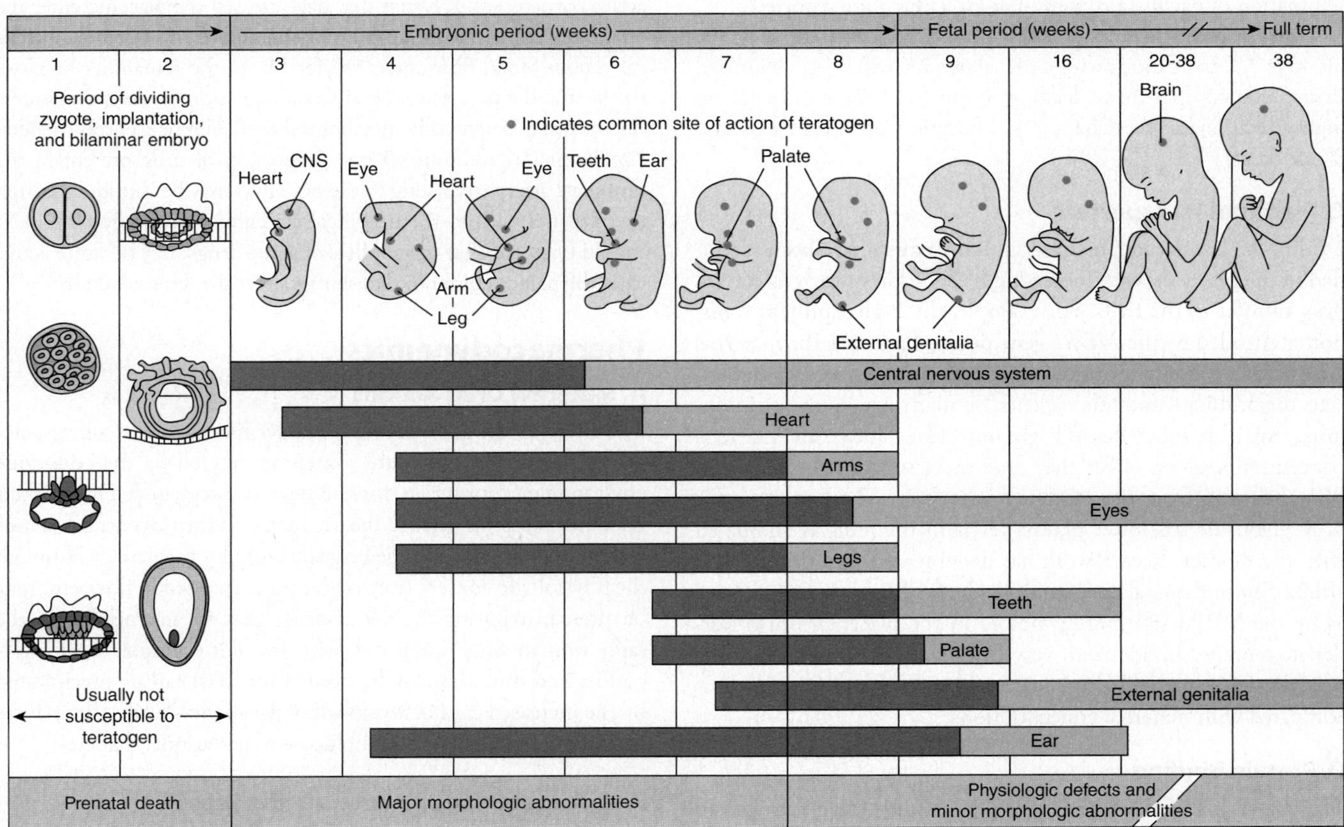

FIGURE 59–1 Schematic diagram of critical periods of human development. (Reproduced with permission from Moore KL: *The Developing Human: Clinically Oriented Embryology*, 4th ed. Philadelphia, PA: Saunders, 1988.)

and are probably multifactorial. For example, drugs may have a direct effect on maternal tissues with secondary or indirect effects on fetal tissues. Drugs may interfere with the passage of oxygen or nutrients through the placenta and therefore have effects on the most rapidly metabolizing tissues of the fetus. Also, drugs may have important direct actions on the processes of differentiation in developing tissues. For example, vitamin A (retinol) has been shown to have important differentiation-directing actions in normal tissues. Several vitamin A analogs (isotretinoin, etretinate) are powerful human teratogens, altering the normal processes of differentiation. Finally, deficiency of a critical substance appears to play a role in some types of abnormalities. For example, folic acid supplementation before and during early pregnancy reduces the incidence of neural tube defects by up to 75% (see Chapter 33 Box, Folic Acid Supplementation).

Continued exposure to a teratogen may produce cumulative effects or may affect several organs going through varying stages of development. Chronic consumption of high doses of ethanol during pregnancy, particularly during the first and second trimesters, may result in the fetal alcohol spectrum disorder (see Chapter 23). In this syndrome, the central nervous system, growth, and facial development are adversely affected.

2. *Defining a teratogen*—To be considered teratogenic, a candidate substance or process should (1) result in a characteristic set of malformations, indicating selectivity for certain target organs; (2) exert its effects at a particular stage of fetal development, eg, during the limited time period of organogenesis of the target organs (see Figure 59–1); and (3) show a dose-dependent incidence. A drug or a pathological process may induce teratogenic effects by adversely affecting placental processes. For example, untreated hypertension of pregnancy has been shown to increase rates of major malformations. Some drugs with known teratogenic or other adverse effects in pregnancy are listed in Table 59–1. Teratogenic effects are not limited to major malformations, but also include intrauterine growth restriction (eg, cigarette smoking), miscarriage (eg, alcohol), stillbirth (eg, cigarette smoke), and neurocognitive delay (eg, alcohol, valproic acid).

In addition to teratogenic drugs, teratogenicity can be induced by a large group of infectious pathogens, including viruses such as rubella, cytomegalovirus, herpes, and recently, Zika virus. Similarly, numerous chemicals, such as heavy metals (eg, mercury, lead) and environmental factors (eg, radiation, hyperthermia) can damage the fetus. It is important to consider these nondrug factors in the differential diagnosis of drug-induced adverse fetal effects.

The FDA implemented new labeling requirements for pregnancy and breastfeeding for all new drug submissions in the United States as of June 30, 2015. The new format removes the letter-based categorization of risk (A, B, C, D, X) (Table 59–2) and provides more complete information pertaining to assessing risk versus benefit of medication use in pregnancy and breastfeeding and in males and females of reproductive potential. Labeling changes for medications submitted on or after June 30, 2001 were phased in gradually. Medications approved prior to June 30, 2001 were required to remove the letter category before June 30, 2018

TABLE 59–2 FDA teratogenic risk categories.[1]

Category	Description
A	Controlled studies in women fail to demonstrate a risk to the fetus in the first trimester (and there is no evidence of a risk in late trimesters), and the possibility of fetal harm appears remote.
B	Either animal-reproduction studies have not demonstrated a fetal risk, but there are no controlled studies in pregnant women, or animal-reproduction studies have shown an adverse effect (other than a decrease in fertility) that was not confirmed in controlled studies in women in the first trimester (and there is no evidence of a risk in later trimesters).
C	Either studies in animals have revealed adverse effects on the fetus (teratogenic or embryocidal or other) and there are no controlled studies in women or studies in women and animals are not available. Drugs should be given only if the potential benefit justifies the potential risk to the fetus.
D	There is positive evidence of human fetal risk, but the benefits from use in pregnant women may be acceptable despite the risk (eg, if the drug is needed in a life-threatening situation or for a serious disease for which safer drugs cannot be used or are ineffective).
X	Studies in animals or human beings have demonstrated fetal abnormalities or there is evidence of fetal risk based on human experience or both, and the risk of the use of the drug in pregnant women clearly outweighs any possible benefit. The drug is contraindicated in women who are or may become pregnant.

[1]This system has been changed as of 2015 by eliminating the A, B, C qualifications and replacing it by specific structured narratives for each drug.

but were not subject to the new narrative labeling requirements. Labeling for nonprescription medications was not affected.

The new format of information includes for the first time data from specific pregnancy exposure registries, which collect and maintain data on approved drugs prescribed for pregnant women. This format consists of Risk Summary, Clinical Considerations, and Data. These are narratives that detail what has been described on fetal and maternal safety, and will be updated as new information emerges. This format is more in line with the form that is used for other adverse drug effects, and thus replaces the old system, where almost three quarters of all drugs were designated as category "C," causing redundancy and lack of clarity. The detailed narratives will allow clinicians to make more specific decisions on prescribing in pregnancy, considering the incidence of specific risks and their clinical meaning.

3. *Counseling women about teratogenic risk*—Since the dramatic demonstration of severe thalidomide teratogenicity, many healthcare providers presume that every drug is a potential human teratogen. Instead, fewer than 30 such drugs have been identified, with hundreds of agents proven safe for the unborn. Owing to high levels of anxiety among pregnant women, and because nearly half of US pregnancies are unplanned, many thousands of women annually need counseling about fetal exposure to drugs, chemicals, and radiation. The ability of appropriate counseling to prevent unnecessary abortions has been documented.

Clinicians who wish to provide such counseling to pregnant women must ensure that their information is up-to-date and evidence-based and that the woman understands that the baseline teratogenic risk in pregnancy (ie, the risk of a neonatal abnormality in the absence of any known teratogenic exposure) is about 3%. It is also critical to address the maternal-fetal risks of the untreated condition if a medication is avoided. Recent studies have shown serious morbidity in women who discontinued selective serotonin reuptake inhibitor therapy for depression in pregnancy due to fears of teratogenicity.

DRUG THERAPY IN INFANTS & CHILDREN

Physiologic processes that influence pharmacokinetic variables in the infant change significantly in the first year of life, particularly during the first few months. Therefore, special attention must be paid to pharmacokinetics in this age group. Pharmacodynamic differences between pediatric and other patients have not been explored in great detail but are probably important for those specific target tissues that mature at birth or immediately thereafter (eg, the ductus arteriosus).

Drug Absorption

Drug absorption in infants and children follows the same general principles as in adults. Unique factors that influence drug absorption include blood flow at the site of administration, as determined by the physiologic status of the infant or child; and, for orally administered drugs, gastrointestinal function, which changes rapidly during the first few days after birth. Age after birth also influences the regulation of drug absorption.

A. Blood Flow at the Site of Administration

Absorption after intramuscular or subcutaneous injection depends mainly, in neonates as in adults, on the rate of blood flow to the muscle or subcutaneous area injected. Physiologic conditions that might reduce blood flow to these areas are cardiovascular shock, vasoconstriction due to sympathomimetic agents, and heart failure. However, sick preterm infants requiring intramuscular injections may have very little muscle mass. This is further complicated by diminished peripheral perfusion to these areas. In such cases, absorption becomes irregular and difficult to predict, because the drug may remain in the muscle and be absorbed more slowly than expected. If perfusion suddenly improves, there can be a sudden and unpredictable increase in the amount of drug entering the circulation, resulting in high and potentially toxic concentrations of drug. Examples of drugs especially hazardous in such situations are cardiac glycosides, aminoglycoside antibiotics, and anticonvulsants.

B. Gastrointestinal Function

Significant biochemical and physiologic changes occur in the neonatal gastrointestinal tract shortly after birth. In full-term infants, gastric acid secretion begins soon after birth and increases gradually over several hours. In preterm infants, the secretion of gastric acid occurs more slowly, with the highest concentrations appearing on the fourth day of life.

TABLE 59–3 Oral drug absorption (bioavailability) of various drugs in the neonate compared with older children and adults.

Drug	Oral Absorption
Acetaminophen	Decreased
Ampicillin	Increased
Diazepam	Normal
Digoxin	Normal
Penicillin G	Increased
Phenobarbital	Decreased
Phenytoin	Decreased
Sulfonamides	Normal

Gastric emptying time is prolonged (up to 6 or 8 hours) in the first days after delivery. Therefore, drugs that are absorbed primarily in the stomach may be absorbed more completely than anticipated. In the case of drugs absorbed in the small intestine, therapeutic effect may be delayed. Peristalsis in the neonate is irregular and may be slow. The fraction of drug absorbed in the small intestine may therefore be unpredictable; more than the usual amount of drug may be absorbed if peristalsis is slowed, and this could result in toxicity from an otherwise standard dose. Table 59–3 summarizes data on oral bioavailability of various drugs in neonates compared with older children and adults. An increase in peristalsis, as in diarrheal conditions, tends to decrease the extent of absorption, because contact time with the large absorptive surface of the intestine is decreased.

Gastrointestinal enzyme activities tend to be lower in the newborn than in the adult. Activities of α-amylase and other pancreatic enzymes in the duodenum are low in infants up to 4 months of age. Neonates also have low concentrations of bile acids and lipase, which may decrease the absorption of lipid-soluble drugs.

Drug Distribution

As body composition changes with development, the distribution volumes of drugs are also changed. The neonate has a higher percentage of its body weight in the form of water (70–75%) than does the adult (50–60%). Differences can also be observed between the full-term neonate (70% of body weight as water) and the small preterm neonate (85% of body weight as water). Similarly, extracellular water is 40% of body weight in the neonate, compared with 20% in the adult. Most neonates will experience diuresis in the first 24–48 hours of life. Since many drugs are distributed throughout the extracellular water space, the size (volume) of the extracellular water compartment may be important in determining the concentration of drug at receptor sites. This is especially important for water-soluble drugs (such as aminoglycosides) and less crucial for lipid-soluble agents.

Preterm infants have much less fat than full-term infants. Total body fat in preterm infants is about 1% of total body weight, compared with 15% in full-term neonates. Therefore, organs that generally accumulate high concentrations of lipid-soluble drugs in adults and older children may accumulate smaller amounts of these agents in less mature infants.

Another major factor determining drug distribution is drug binding to plasma proteins. Albumin is the plasma protein with the greatest binding capacity. In general, protein binding of drugs is reduced in the neonate, as seen with local anesthetic drugs, diazepam, phenytoin, ampicillin, and phenobarbital. Therefore, the concentration of free (unbound) drug in plasma is increased initially. Because the free drug exerts the pharmacologic effect, this can result in greater drug effect or toxicity despite a normal or even low plasma concentration of total drug (bound plus unbound). As an example, consider a therapeutic dose of a drug (eg, diazepam) given to a patient. The concentration of total drug in the plasma is 300 mcg/L. If the drug is 98% protein-bound in an older child or adult, then 6 mcg/L is the concentration of free drug. Assume that this concentration of free drug produces the desired effect in the patient without producing toxicity. However, if this drug is given to a preterm infant in a dosage adjusted for body weight and it produces a total drug concentration of 300 mcg/L—and protein binding is only 90%—then the free drug concentration will be 30 mcg/L, or five times higher. Although the higher free concentration may result in faster elimination (see Chapter 3), this concentration may be quite toxic initially.

Some drugs compete with serum bilirubin for binding to albumin. Drugs given to a neonate with jaundice can displace bilirubin from albumin. Because of the greater permeability of the neonatal blood-brain barrier, substantial amounts of bilirubin may enter the brain and cause kernicterus. This was in fact observed when sulfonamide antibiotics were given to preterm neonates as prophylaxis against sepsis and is the reason why the antibiotic ceftriaxone is avoided completely in infants under 2 months of age. Conversely, as the serum bilirubin rises for physiologic reasons or because of a blood group incompatibility, bilirubin can displace a drug from albumin and substantially raise the free drug concentration. This may occur without altering the total drug concentration and would result in greater therapeutic effect or toxicity at normal concentrations, as has been shown with phenytoin.

Distribution of drugs to the neonatal brain depends on permeability through the blood-brain barrier (BBB). For example, the neonate is substantially more sensitive than older children or adults to the CNS depressive effect of morphine. Recent research has shown that the neonatal BBB has substantially less P-glycoprotein (PgP) transporter, which pumps morphine back out to the systemic circulation. Hence, under similar serum concentrations, the neonatal brain is exposed to substantially more morphine than it will be exposed to 2–3 months later.

Drug Metabolism

The metabolism of most drugs occurs in the liver (see Chapter 4). The drug-metabolizing activities of the cytochrome P450 superfamily and the conjugating enzymes are substantially lower (50–70% of adult values) in early neonatal life than later. The point in development at which enzymatic activity reaches adult levels depends on the specific enzyme system in question. Glucuronide formation reaches adult values (per kilogram body weight) between the third and fourth years of life. Because of the neonate's decreased ability to metabolize drugs, many drugs have slow clearance rates and prolonged elimination half-lives in early life. If drug doses and dosing schedules are not altered appropriately, this immaturity predisposes the neonate to adverse effects from drugs that are metabolized by the liver. Table 59–4 demonstrates how neonatal and adult drug elimination half-lives can differ and how the half-lives of phenobarbital and phenytoin decrease as the neonate grows older. The process of maturation must be considered when administering drugs to this age group, especially in the case of drugs administered over long periods.

TABLE 59–4 Comparison of elimination half-lives of various drugs between neonates and adults.

Drug	Neonatal Age	Neonates $t_{1/2}$ (hours)	Adults $t_{1/2}$ (hours)
Acetaminophen		2.2–5	0.9–2.2
Diazepam		25–100	40–50
Digoxin		60–70	30–60
Phenobarbital	0–5 days	200	64–140
	5–15 days	100	
	1–30 months	50	
Phenytoin	0–2 days	80	12–18
	3–14 days	18	
	14–50 days	6	
Salicylate		4.5–11	10–15
Theophylline	Neonate	13–26	5–10
	Child	3–4	

Another consideration for the neonate is whether or not the mother was receiving drugs (eg, phenobarbital) that can induce early maturation of fetal hepatic enzymes. In this case, the ability of the neonate to metabolize certain drugs will be greater than expected, and one may see less therapeutic effect and lower plasma drug concentrations when the usual neonatal dose is given. During toddlerhood (12–36 months), the metabolic rate of many drugs exceeds adult values, often necessitating larger doses per kilogram than later in life.

Drug Excretion

The glomerular filtration rate is much lower in newborns than in older infants, children, or adults, and this limitation persists during the first few days of life. Calculated on the basis of body surface area, glomerular filtration in the neonate is only 30–40% of the adult value. The glomerular filtration rate is even lower in neonates born before 34 weeks of gestation. Function improves substantially during the first week of life. At the end of the first week, the glomerular filtration rate and renal plasma flow have increased 50% from the first day. By the end of the third week, glomerular filtration is 50–60% of the adult value; by 6–12 months, it reaches adult values (per unit surface area). Subsequently, during toddlerhood, it exceeds adult values, often necessitating larger doses per kilogram than in adults, as described previously for drug-metabolic rate. Therefore, drugs that depend on renal function for elimination are cleared from the body very slowly in the first weeks of life.

Penicillins, for example, are cleared by preterm infants at 17% of the adult rate based on comparable surface area and 34% of the adult rate when adjusted for body weight. The dosage of ampicillin for a neonate less than 7 days old is 50–100 mg/kg/d in two doses at 12-hour intervals. The dosage for a neonate over 7 days old is 100–200 mg/kg/d in three doses at 8-hour intervals. A decreased rate of renal elimination in the neonate has also been observed with aminoglycoside antibiotics (kanamycin, gentamicin, neomycin, and streptomycin). The dosage of gentamicin for a neonate less than 7 days old is 5 mg/kg/d in two doses at 12-hour intervals. The dosage for a neonate over 7 days old is 7.5 mg/kg/d in three doses at 8-hour intervals. Total body clearance of digoxin is directly dependent upon adequate renal function, and accumulation of digoxin can occur when glomerular filtration is decreased. Since renal function in a sick infant may not improve at the predicted rate during the first weeks and months of life, appropriate adjustments in dosage and dosing schedules may be very difficult. In this situation, adjustments are best made on the basis of plasma drug concentrations determined at intervals throughout the course of therapy.

Although great focus is naturally concentrated on the neonate, it is important to remember that toddlers may have *shorter* elimination half-lives of drugs than older children and adults, due to *increased* renal elimination and metabolism. For example, the dose per kilogram of digoxin is much higher in toddlers than in adults. The mechanisms for these developmental changes are still poorly understood.

Special Pharmacodynamic Features in the Neonate

The appropriate use of drugs has made possible the survival of neonates with severe abnormalities who would otherwise die within days or weeks after birth. For example, administration of indomethacin (see Chapter 36) causes the rapid closure of a patent ductus arteriosus, which would otherwise require surgical closure in an infant with a normal heart. Infusion of prostaglandin E_1, on the other hand, causes the ductus to remain open, which can be lifesaving in an infant with transposition of the great vessels or tetralogy of Fallot (see Chapter 18). An unexpected effect of such infusion has been described when the drug caused antral hyperplasia with gastric outlet obstruction as a clinical manifestation in 6 of 74 infants who received it. This phenomenon appears to be dose-dependent. Neonates are also more sensitive to the central depressant effects of opioids than are older children and adults, necessitating extra caution when they are exposed to some narcotics (eg, codeine) through breast milk.

At birth, the function of drug transporters may be very low; for example, P-glycoprotein, which pumps morphine from the blood-brain barrier back to the systemic circulation. As described above, low-level function of P-glycoprotein at birth can explain why neonates are substantially more sensitive than older children to the central nervous system depressant effects of morphine.

PEDIATRIC DOSAGE FORMS & ADHERENCE

The form in which a drug is manufactured and the way in which the parent dispenses the drug to the child determine the actual dose administered. Many drugs prepared for children are in the form of elixirs or suspensions. **Elixirs** are alcoholic solutions in which the drug molecules are dissolved and evenly distributed. No shaking is required, and unless some of the vehicle has evaporated, the first dose from the bottle and the last dose should contain equivalent amounts of drug. **Suspensions** contain undissolved particles of drug that must be distributed throughout the vehicle by shaking. If shaking is not thorough each time a dose is given, the first doses from the bottle may contain less drug than the last doses, with the result that less than the expected plasma concentration or effect of the drug may be achieved early in the course of therapy. Conversely, toxicity may occur late in the course of therapy, when it is not expected. This uneven distribution is a potential cause of inefficacy or toxicity in children taking phenytoin suspensions. It is thus essential that the prescriber know the form in which the drug will be dispensed and provide proper instructions to the pharmacist and patient or parent.

Adherence (formerly called compliance) may be more difficult to achieve in pediatric practice than otherwise, since it involves not only the parent's conscientious effort to follow directions but also such practical matters as measuring errors, spilling, and spitting out. For example, the measured volume of "teaspoons" can vary from 2.5 to 7.8 mL. The parents should obtain a calibrated medicine spoon or syringe from the pharmacy as these devices improve the accuracy of dose measurements and simplify administration of drugs to children.

When evaluating adherence, it is important to ask if an attempt has been made to give a further dose after the child has spilled half of what was offered. The parents may not always be able to say with confidence how much of a dose the child actually received. The parents must be told whether or not to wake the infant for its every-6-hour dose day or night. These matters should be discussed and made clear, and no assumptions should be made about what the parents may or may not do. Nonadherence frequently occurs when antibiotics are prescribed to treat otitis media or urinary tract infections and the child feels well after 4 or 5 days of therapy. The parents may not feel there is any reason to continue giving the medicine even though it was prescribed for 10 or 14 days. This common situation should be anticipated so the parents can be told why it is important to continue giving the medicine for the prescribed period even if the child seems to be "cured."

Practical and convenient dosage forms and dosing schedules should be chosen to the extent possible. The easier it is to administer and take the medicine and the easier the dosing schedule is to follow, the more likely it is that adherence will be achieved. Palatability (taste) also is an important consideration in drug adherence, as many suspensions and elixirs have a bitter or unpalatable taste and children find them difficult to tolerate. Here, the prescriber or pharmacist must get creative in use of flavored additives, juices, applesauce, chocolate sauce, or other tasty substances to hide the taste of the prescribed medication.

Consistent with their ability to comprehend and cooperate, children should also be given some responsibility for their own health care and for taking medications. This should be discussed in appropriate terms both with the child and with the parents. Possible adverse effects and drug interactions with over-the-counter medicines or foods should also be discussed. Whenever a drug does not achieve its therapeutic effect, the possibility of nonadherence should be considered. There is ample evidence that in such cases parents' or children's reports may be grossly inaccurate. Random pill counts and measurement of serum concentrations may help disclose nonadherence. The use of computerized pill containers, which record each lid opening, has been shown to be very effective in measuring adherence.

Because many pediatric doses are calculated—eg, using body weight—rather than simply read from a list, major dosing errors may result from incorrect calculations. Typically, 10-fold errors due to incorrect placement of the decimal point have been described. In the case of digoxin, for example, an intended dose of 0.1 mL containing 5 mcg of drug, when replaced by 1.0 mL—which is still a small volume—can result in a fatal overdose. Different strategies have been developed to prevent these potentially fatal errors. For drugs with narrow therapeutic windows (eg, digoxin, insulin, potassium), independent double-checking of dose and volume calculations is widely practiced. A good rule for avoiding such "decimal point" errors is to use a leading "0" plus decimal point when dealing with doses less than "1" and to avoid using a zero after a decimal point (see Chapter 66). Safe prescribing practices may also call for writing out the dose in addition to the numerical approach. This is especially important in such drugs as penicillin, typically prescribed in thousands or millions of units. An example of this would be "Penicillin G, 200,000 units IV Q 6 hours AKA two hundred thousand units intravenously every 6 hours."

DRUG USE DURING LACTATION

Despite the fact that most drugs are excreted into breast milk in amounts too small to adversely affect neonatal health, thousands of women taking medications do not breast-feed because of fears of harming the baby and misperception of risk. Unfortunately, physicians often contribute to this bias. It is important to remember that, compared with breast-feeding, formula feeding is associated with higher infant morbidity and mortality in all socioeconomic groups.

Most drugs administered to lactating women are detectable in breast milk. Fortunately, the concentration of drugs achieved in breast milk is usually low (Table 59–5). Therefore, for most drugs the total amount the infant would receive in a day is substantially less than what would be considered a "therapeutic dose." There are a limited number of medications where neonatal exposure through breastmilk would be clinically meaningful, including some cases of exposure to lithium, amiodarone, and atenolol. As a rule of thumb, if the dose offered to the suckling infant is less than 10% of maternal weight-corrected dose, the likelihood of neonatal toxicity is negligible. If the nursing mother needs to take medications and the drug is a relatively safe one, she should optimally take it 30–60 minutes after nursing and 3–4 hours before the next feeding. In some cases this may allow time for drugs to be partially cleared from the mother's blood, and the concentrations in breast milk will be relatively low. Most antibiotics taken by nursing mothers can be detected in breast milk. Tetracycline concentrations in breast milk are approximately 70% of maternal serum concentrations and present a risk of permanent tooth staining in the infant. Isoniazid rapidly reaches equilibrium between breast milk and maternal blood. The concentrations achieved in breast milk are sufficiently high so that signs of pyridoxine deficiency may occur in the infant if the mother is not given pyridoxine supplements.

Most sedatives and hypnotics achieve concentrations in breast milk sufficient to produce a pharmacologic effect in some infants. Barbiturates taken in hypnotic doses by the mother can produce lethargy, sedation, and poor suck reflexes in the infant. Chloral hydrate can produce sedation if the infant is fed at peak milk concentrations. Diazepam can have a sedative effect on the nursing infant, but, most importantly, its long half-life can result in significant drug accumulation.

Opioids such as heroin, methadone, and morphine enter breast milk in quantities potentially sufficient to prolong the state of neonatal narcotic dependence if the drug was taken chronically by the mother during pregnancy. If conditions are well controlled and there is a good relationship between the mother and the physician, an infant could be breast-fed while the mother is taking methadone. She should not, however, stop taking the drug abruptly; the infant can be tapered off the methadone as the mother's dose is tapered. The infant should be watched for signs of narcotic withdrawal. Although codeine has been believed to be safe, a case of neonatal death from opioid toxicity revealed that the mother was an ultra-rapid metabolizer of cytochrome 2D6 substrates, producing substantially higher amounts of morphine. Hence, polymorphism in maternal drug metabolism may affect neonatal exposure and safety. A subsequent case-control study has shown that this situation is not rare. The FDA has published a warning to lactating mothers to exert extra caution while using painkillers containing codeine. More recent research has also shown that blood-brain barrier levels of P-glycoprotein are lower at birth, allowing more morphine to penetrate into the brain, than later in infancy and childhood. This can explain sedation in breast-fed neonates even when there is no genetic variability in CYP2D6.

Minimal use of alcohol by the mother has not been reported to harm nursing infants. Excessive amounts of alcohol, however, can produce sedative effects in the infant. Nicotine concentrations in the breast milk of smoking mothers are low and do not produce effects in the infant. Very small amounts of caffeine are excreted in the breast milk of coffee-drinking mothers.

Lithium enters breast milk in concentrations equal to those in maternal serum. Clearance of this drug is almost completely dependent upon renal elimination, and women who are receiving lithium may expose the infant to relatively large amounts of the drug.

TABLE 59–5 Drugs often used during lactation and possible effects on the nursing infant.

Drug	Effect on Infant	Comments
Ampicillin	Minimal	No significant adverse effects; possible occurrence of diarrhea or allergic sensitization.
Aspirin	Minimal	Occasional doses are safe.
Caffeine	Minimal	Caffeine intake in moderation is safe; concentration in breast milk is low.
Chloral hydrate	Significant	May cause drowsiness if infant is fed at peak concentration in milk.
Chloramphenicol	Significant	Concentrations too low to cause gray baby syndrome; possibility of bone marrow suppression does exist; recommend not taking chloramphenicol while breast-feeding.
Chlorothiazide	Minimal	No adverse effects reported.
Chlorpromazine	Minimal	Appears insignificant.
Codeine	Variable, based on genetic polymorphism	Safe in most cases. Neonatal toxicity described when the mother is an ultra rapid 2D6 metabolizer, producing substantially more morphine from codeine.
Dicumarol	Minimal	No adverse side effects reported; may wish to follow infant's prothrombin time.
Digoxin	Minimal	Insignificant quantities enter breast milk.
Ethanol	Moderate	Moderate ingestion by mother unlikely to produce effects in infant; large amounts consumed by mother can produce alcohol effects in infant.
Heroin	Significant	Enters breast milk and can prolong neonatal opioid dependence.
Iodine (radioactive)	Significant	Enters milk in quantities sufficient to cause thyroid suppression in infant.
Isoniazid (INH)	Minimal	Milk concentrations equal maternal plasma concentrations. Possibility of pyridoxine deficiency developing in the infant.
Lithium	Variable	In some cases—but not in others—large amounts enter breast milk.
Methadone	Significant	(See heroin.) Under close physician supervision, breast-feeding can be continued. Signs of opioid withdrawal in the infant may occur if mother stops taking methadone or stops breast-feeding abruptly.
Oral contraceptives	Minimal	May suppress lactation in high doses.
Penicillin	Minimal	Very low concentrations in breast milk.
Phenobarbital	Moderate	Hypnotic doses can cause sedation in the infant.
Phenytoin	Moderate	Amounts entering breast milk are not sufficient to cause adverse effects in infant.
Prednisone	Moderate	Low maternal doses (5 mg/d) probably safe. Doses 2 or more times physiologic amounts (>15 mg/d) should probably be avoided.
Propranolol	Minimal	Very small amounts enter breast milk.
Propylthiouracil	Variable	Rarely may suppress thyroid function in infant.
Radioactive nuclides	Variable	Will expose baby to radioactivity; ensure that the mother has cleared the radioactivity.
Spironolactone	Minimal	Very small amounts enter breast milk.
Tetracycline	Moderate	Possibility of permanent staining of developing teeth in the infant. Should be avoided during lactation.
Theophylline	Moderate	Can enter breast milk in moderate quantities but not likely to produce significant effects.
Thyroxine	Minimal	No adverse effects in therapeutic doses.
Tolbutamide	Minimal	Low concentrations in breast milk.
Warfarin	Minimal	Very small quantities found in breast milk.

Radioactive substances such as iodinated ^{125}I albumin and radioiodine can cause thyroid suppression in infants and may increase the risk of subsequent thyroid cancer as much as 10-fold. Breast-feeding is contraindicated after large doses and should be withheld for days to weeks after small doses. Similarly, breast-feeding should be avoided in mothers receiving cancer chemotherapy or being treated with cytotoxic or immunomodulating agents for collagen diseases such as lupus erythematosus or after organ transplantation.

PEDIATRIC DRUG DOSAGE

Because of differences in pharmacokinetics in infants and children, simple proportionate reduction in the adult dose may not be adequate to determine a safe and effective pediatric dose. The most reliable pediatric dose information is usually that provided by the manufacturer in the package insert. However, such information is not available for the majority of products, even when studies have been published in the medical literature, reflecting the reluctance of manufacturers to label their products for children. Recently, in accordance with the Pediatric Rule (1998) for pediatric testing, the FDA has moved toward more explicit expectations that manufacturers test their new products in infants and children. Still, most drugs in the common formularies, eg, *Physicians' Desk Reference*, are not specifically approved for children, in part because manufacturers often lack the economic incentive to evaluate drugs for use in the pediatric market.

Most drugs approved for use in children have recommended pediatric doses, generally stated as milligrams per kilogram or per pound. In the absence of explicit pediatric dose recommendations, an approximation can be made by any of several methods based on age, weight, or surface area. These rules are not precise and should not be used if the manufacturer provides a pediatric dose. When pediatric doses are calculated (either from one of the methods set forth below or from a manufacturer's dose), the pediatric dose should never exceed the adult dose.

The current epidemic proportions of childhood obesity calls for a fresh and careful look at pediatric drug dosages. Studies in adults indicate that dosing based on per-kilogram body weight may constitute overdosing, because in obese subjects, drugs are distributed based on lean body weight.

Surface Area, Age, & Weight

Calculations of dosage based on age or weight (see below) are conservative and tend to underestimate the required dose. Doses based on surface area (Table 59–6) are more likely to be adequate.

Age (Young's rule):

$$Dose = \text{Adult dose} \times \frac{\text{Age (years)}}{\text{Age} + 12}$$

TABLE 59–6 Determination of drug dosage from surface area.[1]

Weight		Approximate	Surface	Percent of
(kg)	***(lb)***	**Age**	**Area (m^2)**	**Adult Dose**
3	6.6	Newborn	0.2	12
6	13.2	3 months	0.3	18
10	22	1 year	0.45	28
20	44	5.5 years	0.8	48
30	66	9 years	1	60
40	88	12 years	1.3	78
50	110	14 years	1.5	90
60	132	Adult	1.7	102
70	154	Adult	1.76	103

[1]For example, if adult dose is 1 mg/kg, dose for 3-month-old infant would be 0.18 mg/kg or 1.1 mg total.

Reproduced with permission from Silver HK, Kempe CH, Bruyn HB: *Handbook of Pediatrics*, 14th ed. New York, NY: McGraw HIll; 1983.

Weight (somewhat more precise is Clark's rule):

$$Dose = \text{Adult dose} \times \frac{\text{Weight (kg)}}{70}$$

or

$$Dose = \text{Adult dose} \times \frac{\text{Weight (lb)}}{150}$$

Despite these approximations, only by conducting studies in children can safe and effective doses for a given age group and condition be determined.

REFERENCES

Briggs GG, Freeman RK, Yaffe SJ: *Drugs in Pregnancy and Lactation: A Reference Guide to Fetal and Neonatal Risk*, 10th ed. Wolters Kluwer/Lippincott Williams & Wilkins, 2015.

de Wildt SN et al: Ontogeny of midazolam glucuronidation in preterm infants. Eur J Clin Pharmacol 2010;66:165.

Gavin PJ, Yogev R: The role of protease inhibitor therapy in children with HIV infection. Paediatr Drugs 2002;4:581.

Hansten PD, Horn JR: *Drug Interactions, Analysis and Management*. Facts & Comparisons. [Quarterly.]

International Liaison Committee on Resuscitation: The International Liaison Committee on Resuscitation (ILCOR) consensus on science with treatment recommendations for pediatric and neonatal patients: Pediatric basic and advanced life support. Pediatrics 2006;117:e955.

Iqbal MM, Sohhan T, Mahmud SZ: The effects of lithium, valproic acid, and carbamazepine during pregnancy and lactation. J Toxicol Clin Toxicol 2001;39:381.

Ito S: Drug therapy for breast feeding women. N Engl J Med 2000;343:118.

Kearns GL et al: Developmental pharmacology—drug disposition, action and therapy in infants and children. N Engl J Med 2003;349:1157.

Koren G: *Medication Safety during Pregnancy and Breastfeeding: A Clinician's Guide*, 4th ed. McGraw-Hill, 2006.

Koren G, Nordeng H: Antidepressant use during pregnancy: The benefit-risk ratio. Am J Obstet Gynecol 2012;207:157.

Koren G, Pariente G: Pregnancy-associated changes in pharmacokinetics and their clinical implications. Pharm Res 2018;35:61.

Koren G, Pastuszak A: Prevention of unnecessary pregnancy terminations by counseling women on drug, chemical, and radiation exposure during the first trimester. Teratology 1990;41:657.

Koren G, Pastuszak A, Ito E: Drugs in pregnancy. N Engl J Med 1998;338:1128.

Koren G et al: Sex differences in the pharmacokinetics and bioequivalence of the delayed-release combination of doxylamine succinate-pyridoxine hydrochloride: Implications for pharmacotherapy in pregnancy. J Clin Pharmacol 2013;53:1268.

Lam J et al: The ontogeny of P-glycoprotein in the developing human blood-brain barrier: Implication for opioid toxicity in neonates. Pediatr Res 2015;78:417.

Madadi P et al: Pharmacogenetics of neonatal opioid toxicity following maternal use of codeine during breastfeeding: A case control study. Clin Pharmacol Ther 2009;85:31.

Namouz-Haddad S, Koren G: Fetal pharmacotherapy 2: Fetal arrhythmia. J Obstet Gynaecol Can 2013;35:1023.

Pauwels S, Allegaert K: Therapeutic drug monitoring in neonates. Arch Dis Child 2016;101:377.

Peled N et al: Gastric-outlet obstruction induced by prostaglandin therapy in neonates. N Engl J Med 1992;327:505.

SickKids Drug Handbook and Formulary 2015/2016. The Hospital for Sick Children, Toronto.

Tetelbaum M et al: Back to basics: Understanding drugs in children: Pharmacokinetic maturation. Pediatr Rev 2005;26:321.

Van Lingen RA et al: The effects of analgesia in the vulnerable infant during the perinatal period. Clin Perinatol 2002;29:511.

CHAPTER

60 Special Aspects of Geriatric Pharmacology

Bertram G. Katzung, MD, PhD

CASE STUDY

A 77-year-old man comes to your office at his wife's insistence. He has had documented moderate hypertension for 18 years but does not like to take his medications. He says he has no real complaints, but his wife remarks that he has become much more forgetful lately and has almost stopped reading the newspaper and watching television. A Mini-Mental State Examination reveals that he is oriented as to name and place but is unable to give the month or year. He cannot remember the names of his three adult children or three random words (eg, tree, flag, chair) for more than 2 minutes. No cataracts are visible, but he is unable to read standard newsprint without a powerful magnifier. His hearing and comprehension of conversation appear to be limited (he nods and smiles in response to both statements and questions). Why doesn't he take his antihypertensive medications? What therapeutic measures are available for the treatment of Alzheimer disease? How might macular degeneration be treated?

Society has traditionally classified everyone over 65 as "elderly," but most authorities consider the field of geriatrics to apply to persons over 75—even though this too is an arbitrary definition. Furthermore, chronologic age is only an indirect determinant of the changes pertinent to drug therapy that occur in older people. In addition to the chronic diseases of adulthood, the elderly have an increased incidence of many conditions, including Alzheimer disease, Parkinson disease, and vascular dementia; stroke; visual impairment, especially cataracts and macular degeneration; atherosclerosis, coronary and peripheral vascular disease, and heart failure; diabetes; arthritis, osteoporosis and fractures; and cancer. Hearing impairment and urinary incontinence are extremely common. As a result, the need for drug treatment is great in this age group. And as the average life span approaches (and in some countries, already exceeds) 80 years, this need will increase dramatically.

When all confounders are accounted for, age itself is still the strongest risk factor for cardiovascular and neurodegenerative diseases and most forms of cancer. Research into the molecular basis of aging has answered a few questions and opened many more. Unlike mammals, some species of turtles and tortoises (testudines) have little or no evidence of senescence over extremely long lives. It has long been known that caloric restriction alone can prolong the life span of animals, including mammals. Some evidence suggests that calorically restricted mice also remain healthier for a longer time. Drugs that mimic caloric restriction have been shown to increase life span in the nematode *Caenorhabditis elegans*, as well as other species, including mice. **Metformin** and **rapamycin** each increase life span in these species when given alone and appear to have synergistic effects when given together. Sirtuins, a class of endogenous protein deacetylase enzymes, may be linked to life span in some species, but activators (such as resveratrol) of certain sirtuins have not been shown to prolong life in mice. Assuming that safer alternatives to metformin or rapamycin can be found, should everyone over the age of 40 or 60 years take such a drug? Few would maintain that a simple increase in the years of life—life span—is desirable unless accompanied by an increase in the years of healthy life—"health span." Regular exercise is a recognized contributor to longer health span. This appears to be a part of the reason why blood plasma from younger or from exercising older animals has a beneficial effect on cognitive ability in older, sedentary animals. Provocative research suggests that variables such as telomere length on chromosomes may predict prospective life span and that proteins in the blood of young animals may "rejuvenate" older animals, but these studies provide no guidance regarding the current treatment of diseases in older patients.

Important changes in responses to some drugs occur with increasing age in many individuals. For other drugs, age-related changes are minimal, especially in the "healthy old." Drug usage patterns also change as a result of the increasing incidence of disease with age and the tendency to prescribe heavily for patients in nursing homes. General changes in the lives of older people have significant effects on the way drugs are used. Among these changes with advancing age are the increased incidence of several simultaneous diseases, nutritional problems, reduced financial resources, and—in some patients—decreased dosing adherence (also called compliance) for a variety of reasons. The health practitioner should be aware of the changes in pharmacologic responses that may occur in older people and should know how to deal with these changes. Finally, dependent elders are sometimes abused physically or financially by caregivers at home or in nursing homes, and the health practitioner should investigate abuse as a cause of nonadherence, as well as bruises, dehydration, and other morbidities.

PHARMACOLOGIC CHANGES ASSOCIATED WITH AGING

In the general population, measurements of functional capacity of most of the major organ systems show a decline beginning in young adulthood and continuing throughout life. As shown in Figure 60–1, there is no "middle-age plateau" but rather a linear decrease beginning no later than age 45. However, these data reflect the mean and do not apply to every person above a certain age; approximately one third of healthy subjects have no age-related decrease in, for example, creatinine clearance up to the age of 75. Some of these changes result in altered pharmacokinetics. For the pharmacologist and the clinician, the most important of these is the decrease in renal function. Other changes and concurrent diseases may alter the pharmacodynamic characteristics of particular drugs in certain patients.

Pharmacokinetic Changes

A. Absorption

There is little evidence of any major alteration in drug absorption with age. However, conditions associated with age may alter the rate at which some drugs are absorbed. Such conditions include altered nutritional habits, greater consumption of nonprescription drugs (eg, antacids and laxatives), and changes in gastric emptying, which is often slower in older persons, especially in older diabetics.

B. Distribution

Compared with young adults, the elderly have reduced lean body mass, reduced body water, and increased fat as a percentage of body mass. Some of these changes are shown in Table 60–1. There is usually a decrease in serum albumin, which binds many drugs, especially weak acids. There may be a concurrent *increase* in serum orosomucoid (α-acid glycoprotein), a protein that binds many basic drugs. Thus, the ratio of bound to free drug may be significantly altered. As explained in Chapter 3, these

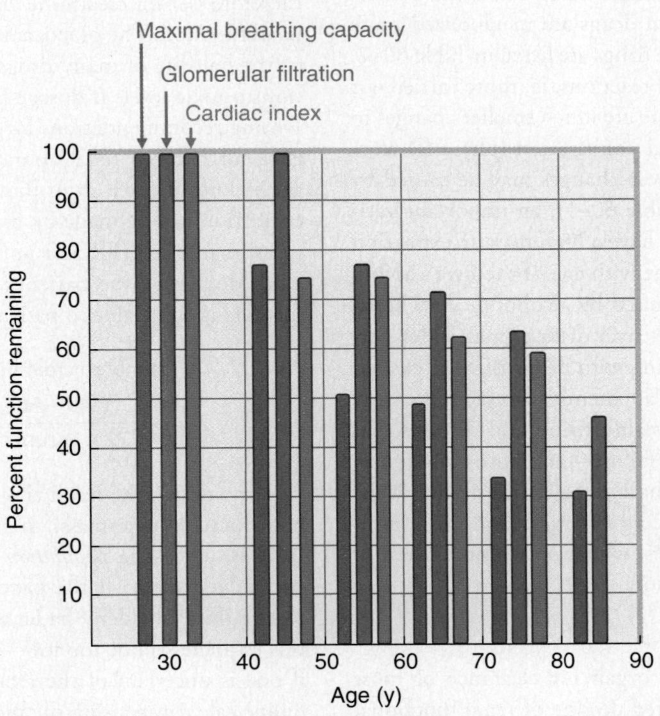

FIGURE 60–1 Effect of age on some physiologic functions.

TABLE 60–1 Some changes related to aging that affect pharmacokinetics of drugs.

Variable	Young Adults (20–30 years)	Older Adults (60–80 years)
Body water (% of body weight)	61	53
Lean body mass (% of body weight)	19	12
Body fat (% of body weight)	26–33 (women)	38–45
	18–20 (men)	36–38
Serum albumin (g/dL)	4.7	3.8
Kidney weight (% of young adult value)	100	80
Hepatic blood flow (% of young adult value)	100	55–60

TABLE 60–2 Effects of age on hepatic clearance of some drugs.

Age-Related Decrease in Hepatic Clearance Found	No Age-Related Difference Found
Alprazolam	Ethanol
Barbiturates	Isoniazid
Carbenoxolone	Lidocaine
Chlordiazepoxide	Lorazepam
Chlormethiazole	Nitrazepam
Clobazam	Oxazepam
Desmethyldiazepam	Prazosin
Diazepam	Salicylate
Flurazepam	Warfarin
Imipramine	
Meperidine	
Nortriptyline	
Phenylbutazone	
Propranolol	
Quinidine, quinine	
Theophylline	
Tolbutamide	

changes may alter the appropriate loading dose of a drug. However, since both the clearance and the receptor-binding effects of drugs are related to the free concentration, the steady-state effects of a maintenance dosage regimen should not be altered by these factors alone. For example, the loading dose of digoxin in an elderly patient with heart failure should be reduced (if used at all) because of the decreased apparent volume of distribution. The maintenance dose may have to be reduced because of reduced clearance of the drug.

C. Metabolism

The capacity of the liver to metabolize drugs declines with age for some, but not all, drugs. Animal studies and some clinical studies have suggested that certain drugs are metabolized more slowly in the elderly; some of these drugs are listed in Table 60–2. The greatest changes are in phase I reactions, ie, those carried out by microsomal P450 systems. There are much smaller changes in the ability of the liver to carry out conjugation (phase II) reactions (see Chapter 4). Some of these changes may be caused by decreased liver blood flow (see Table 60–1), an important variable in the clearance of drugs that have a high hepatic extraction ratio. In addition, there is a decline with age of the liver's ability to recover from injury, eg, that caused by alcohol or viral hepatitis. Therefore, a history of recent liver disease in an older person should lead to caution in dosing with drugs that are cleared primarily by the liver, even after apparently complete recovery from the hepatic insult. Finally, malnutrition and diseases that affect hepatic function—eg, heart failure—are more common in the elderly. Heart failure may dramatically alter the ability of the liver to metabolize drugs by reducing hepatic blood flow. Similarly, severe nutritional deficiencies, which occur more often in old age, may impair hepatic function.

D. Elimination

Because the kidney is the major organ for clearance of most drugs from the body, the age-related decline of renal functional capacity is very important. A decline in creatinine clearance (Cl_{cr})—the usual measure of estimated glomerular filtration rate (eGFR)—occurs with aging in about two thirds of the population. It is important to note that this decline is not reflected in an equivalent rise in serum creatinine because the production of creatinine is also reduced as muscle mass declines with age; therefore, serum creatinine alone is not an adequate measure of renal function. The practical result of this change is prolongation of the half-life of many drugs, and the possibility of accumulation to toxic levels if dosage is not reduced in size or frequency. Dosing recommendations for the elderly often include an allowance for reduced renal clearance. If only the young adult dosage is known for a drug that requires renal clearance, a rough correction can be made by using the **Cockcroft-Gault formula** to estimate the GFR and multiplying the recommended young adult dosage by the patient's eGFR/100. The Cockcroft-Gault formula is applicable to patients age 40 through 80:

$$\text{Estimated creatinine clearance (mL/min)} = \frac{(140 - \text{Age}) \times (\text{Weight in kg})}{72 \times \text{Serum creatinine in mg/dL}}$$

For women, the result should be multiplied by 0.85 (because of reduced muscle mass). It must be emphasized that this estimate is, at best, a *population* estimate and may not apply to a particular patient. If the patient has normal renal function (up to one third of elderly patients), a dose corrected on the basis of this estimate will be too low—but a low dose is initially desirable if one is uncertain of the renal function in any patient. Simple online calculators using the more modern MDRD (Modification of Diet in Renal Disease) formula are available, eg, www.niddk.

nih.gov/health-information/communication-programs/nkdep/laboratory-evaluation/glomerular-filtration-rate-calculators/mdrd-adults-conventional-units.

If a precise measure is needed, a standard 12- or 24-hour creatinine clearance determination should be obtained. As indicated above, nutritional changes alter pharmacokinetic parameters. A patient who is severely dehydrated (not uncommon in patients with stroke or other motor impairment) may have an additional marked reduction in renal drug clearance that is completely reversible by rehydration.

The lungs are important for the excretion of volatile drugs. As a result of reduced respiratory capacity (see Figure 60–1) and the increased prevalence of active pulmonary disease in the elderly, the use of inhalation anesthesia is less common and intravenous agents more common in this age group (see Chapter 25).

Pharmacodynamic Changes

It was long believed that geriatric patients were much more "sensitive" to the action of many drugs, implying a change in the pharmacodynamic interaction of the drugs with their receptors. It is now recognized that many—perhaps most—of these apparent changes result from altered pharmacokinetics or diminished homeostatic responses. Clinical studies have supported the idea that the elderly are more sensitive to *some* sedative-hypnotics and analgesics. In addition, some data from animal studies suggest actual changes with age in the characteristics or numbers of a few receptors. The most extensive studies suggest a *decrease* in responsiveness to β-adrenoceptor agonists. Other examples are discussed below.

Important homeostatic control mechanisms are often blunted in the elderly. Since homeostatic responses are significant contributors to the overall response to many drugs, these physiologic alterations may change the pattern or intensity of drug response. In the cardiovascular system, the cardiac output increment required by mild or moderate exercise is successfully provided until at least age 75 (in individuals without obvious cardiac disease), but the increase is the result primarily of increased stroke volume in the elderly and not tachycardia, as in young adults. Average blood pressure goes up with age (in most Western countries), but the incidence of symptomatic orthostatic *hypotension* also increases markedly. It is thus particularly important to check for orthostatic hypotension (>20 mm Hg drop in systolic blood pressure on standing) on every visit. Similarly, the average 2-hour postprandial blood glucose level increases by about 1 mg/dL for each year of age above 50. Temperature regulation is also impaired, and hypothermia is poorly tolerated by the elderly.

Behavioral & Lifestyle Changes

Major changes in the conditions of daily life accompany the aging process and have an impact on health. Some of these (eg, forgetting to take one's pills) are the result of cognitive changes associated with vascular or other pathology. Hearing impairment is very common, especially in men, and leads to reduced comprehension of conversation (even with hearing aids) and social isolation.

One of the most important changes is the loss of a spouse. Others relate to economic stresses associated with greatly reduced income and, frequently, increased expenses due to illness.

■ MAJOR DRUG GROUPS

CENTRAL NERVOUS SYSTEM DRUGS

Sedative-Hypnotics

The half-lives of many benzodiazepines and barbiturates increase by 50–150% between ages 30 and 70. Much of this change occurs during the decade from 60 to 70. For some of the benzodiazepines, both the parent molecule and its metabolites (produced in the liver) are pharmacologically active (see Chapter 22). The age-related decline in renal function and liver disease, if present, both contribute to the reduction in elimination of these compounds. In addition, an increased volume of distribution has been reported for some of these drugs. Lorazepam and oxazepam may be less affected by these changes than the other benzodiazepines. In addition to these pharmacokinetic factors, it is generally believed that the elderly vary more in their sensitivity to the sedative-hypnotic drugs on a pharmacodynamic basis as well. Among the toxicities of these drugs, ataxia and other stability impairments lead to increased falls and fractures.

Analgesics

The opioid analgesics show variable changes in pharmacokinetics with age. However, the elderly are often markedly more sensitive to the respiratory effects of these agents because of age-related changes in respiratory function. Therefore, this group of drugs should be used with caution until the sensitivity of the particular patient has been evaluated, and the patient should then be dosed appropriately for full effect. Opioids are not as effective in chronic pain syndromes as they are for acute pain, eg, fracture pain (see Chapter 31). Unfortunately, studies show that opioids are consistently *underutilized* in patients who require strong analgesics for chronic severely painful conditions such as cancer. In contrast, opioids have been overprescribed in many countries for poorly documented indications, resulting in the widely reported epidemic of opioid addiction and overdose deaths. Good pain management plans are readily available (see Morrison and Morrison, 2006; Rabow et al, 2021).

Antipsychotic & Antidepressant Drugs

The traditional antipsychotic agents (phenothiazines and haloperidol) have been very heavily used (and often misused) in the management of a variety of psychiatric conditions in the elderly. There is no doubt that they may be useful in the management of schizophrenia in old age, and also in the treatment of some symptoms associated with delirium, dementia, agitation, combativeness, and a paranoid syndrome that occurs in some geriatric patients (see Chapter 29). However, they are not fully satisfactory in these geriatric conditions, and dosage should not be increased on the assumption that full control is possible. There is no evidence that these drugs have any beneficial effects in Alzheimer dementia, and on theoretical grounds the antimuscarinic effects of the phenothiazines might be expected to worsen memory impairment and cognitive dysfunction (see below). **Pimavanserin** is approved for psychosis associated with Parkinson disease; it is under study for behavioral disturbances of Alzheimer disease (see Chapters 28 and 29).

Much of the apparent improvement produced by these drugs in agitated and combative patients may simply reflect their sedative effects. When a sedative antipsychotic is desired, a phenothiazine such as thioridazine is appropriate. If sedation is to be avoided, haloperidol or an atypical antipsychotic is more appropriate. Haloperidol has increased extrapyramidal toxicity, however, and should be avoided in patients with preexisting extrapyramidal disease. The phenothiazines, especially older drugs such as chlorpromazine, often induce orthostatic hypotension because of their α-adrenoceptor-blocking effects. They are even more prone to do so in the elderly. If they must be used, dosage of these drugs should be started at a fraction of that used in young adults. The second generation antipsychotic agents (clozapine, olanzapine, quetiapine, risperidone, aripiprazole) do not appear to be significantly superior to the traditional agents in efficacy although they have fewer autonomic adverse effects. Evidence supporting the benefits of olanzapine is somewhat stronger than that for the other atypical agents.

Lithium is often used in the treatment of mania in the aged. Because it is cleared by the kidneys, dosages must be adjusted appropriately and blood levels monitored. Concurrent use of thiazide diuretics reduces the clearance of lithium and should be accompanied by further reduction in dosage and more frequent measurement of lithium blood levels.

Psychiatric major depressive disorder is thought to be underdiagnosed and undertreated in the elderly. The suicide rate in the over-65 age group (twice the national average) supports this view. Unfortunately, the apathy, flat affect, and social withdrawal of major depression may be mistaken for senile dementia. Clinical evidence suggests that the elderly are as responsive to antidepressants (of all types) as younger patients but are more likely to experience adverse effects. This factor along with the reduced clearance of some of these drugs underlines the importance of careful dosing and monitoring of toxic effects. Some authorities prefer selective serotonin reuptake inhibitors (SSRIs) to tricyclic antidepressants because the SSRIs have fewer autonomic adverse effects. If a tricyclic is to be used, a drug with reduced antimuscarinic effects should be selected, eg, nortriptyline or desipramine (see Table 30–2).

Tremor

Essential tremor is the cause of shaking in many older persons. Both rest and intention tremor may be present and may be so severe as to limit activities of daily living (ADL). Drugs that have been found useful include β-adrenoceptor blockers, eg, propranolol, and some benzodiazepines, eg, alprazolam (see Chapter 28).

Drugs Used in Alzheimer Disease

Alzheimer disease (AD) is characterized by progressive memory impairment, dementia, and cognitive dysfunction, and may lead to a completely vegetative state, resulting in early death. Prevalence increases with age and may be as high as 20% in individuals over 85. The annual cost of dementia in the United States is estimated at $150–$215 billion annually. Both familial and sporadic forms have been identified. Early onset of Alzheimer disease is associated with several gene defects, including trisomy 21 (chromosome 21), a mutation of the gene for presenilin-1 on chromosome 14, and an abnormal allele, ε4, for the lipid-associated protein, ApoE, on chromosome 19. Unlike the common forms (ApoE ε2 and ε3), the ε4 form strongly correlates with the formation of **amyloid beta (Aβ)** deposits (see below). Considerable effort is being made to develop laboratory tests that, at a very early stage, would predict later onset of Alzheimer disease; high sensitivity measurement of serum Aβ is one such test (see Schindler 2019). Recent genetic testing has detected protective genetic variants that may be utilized in the near future to protect cognitive health. Many of the genetic links to Alzheimer's disease converge on the function of the microglia and its response to the pathogenesis of the disease. The microglia will upregulate many of these recently recognized genetic changes in Alzheimer's due to exposed to amyloid plaques.

Pathologic changes include increased deposits of Aβ peptide in the cerebral cortex, which eventually forms extracellular plaques and cerebral vascular lesions, and intra- and interneuronal fibrillary tangles consisting of the **tau protein**. There is a progressive loss of neurons, especially cholinergic neurons, and thinning of the cortex. An inflammatory process involving the NLRP3 inflammasome appears to contribute to this pathology, and anti-inflammatory nonsteroidal anti-inflammatory drugs (NSAIDs), eg, mefenamic acid, reverse some of the markers of Alzheimer disease in animal models. The loss of cholinergic neurons results in a marked decrease in choline acetyltransferase and other markers of cholinergic activity. Patients with Alzheimer disease are often exquisitely sensitive to the central nervous system toxicities of drugs with antimuscarinic effects. Some evidence implicates excess excitation by glutamate as a contributor to neuronal death. Fyn, a protein in the Src kinase family, is activated by Aβ, leading to synaptic dysfunction. Fyn can be inhibited by **saracatinib,** a small molecule drug that was first developed as an anticancer agent. Early studies in mice suggest that saracatinib may improve synaptic function in mice with an Alzheimer pattern of dysfunction. In addition, abnormalities of mitochondrial function may contribute to neuronal death. Recent studies suggest that co-infection with herpes simplex and varicella zoster viruses may trigger the production of tau and Aβ proteins. This raises the possibility of prevention by vaccination against both viruses.

Many methods of treatment of Alzheimer disease have been explored (Table 60–3). Much attention has been focused on the cholinomimetic drugs because of the evidence of loss of cholinergic neurons noted earlier. Monoamine oxidase (MAO)

TABLE 60–3 Some potential strategies for the prevention or treatment of Alzheimer disease.

Therapy	Comment
Cholinesterase inhibitors	Increase cholinergic activity, positive results confirmed; 4 drugs approved
N-methyl-D-aspartate glutamate antagonists	Inhibit glutamate excitotoxicity; 1 drug, memantine, approved
Modifiers of glucose utilization	PPAR-γ agonists
Antilipid drugs	Statins (off-label use)
Retinoid X receptor	Bexarotene transiently reduced Aβ in mice
NSAIDs	Disappointing results with cyclooxygenase (COX)-2 inhibitors but interest continues
Anti-amyloid vaccines	In clinical trials
Anti-amyloid antibodies	Bapineuzumab and solanezumab failed clinical trials but did modify Aβ kinetics; should treatment be started *before* symptoms appear? Aducanumab failed to halt Aβ accumulation in human patients but late results suggest slowing of cognitive decline; approved (see text)
Inhibitors of Aβ synthesis	γ-Secretase modulator studies in progress
Microtubule stabilizers	Drugs that inhibit disassembly of microtubules reduce accumulation of tau protein tangles in mice
Anticytokine antibodies	Anti-IL-12 and 23 antibodies reversed age-related cognitive decline and Aβ accumulation in mice
Anti-FYN drug	Small molecule saracatinib, a kinase inhibitor, shows positive results in mice; further studies needed
Anti-TNFα drugs	Mixed results with thalidomide and with etanercept in clinical trials; further studies needed
Antioxidants	Disappointing results
Nerve growth factor	One very small trial
PERK inhibitor GSK2606414	Preliminary study in mice

Aβ, amyloid beta; IL, interleukin; PERK, protein kinase RNA-like ER kinase; PPAR-γ, peroxisome proliferator-activated receptor-gamma.

type B inhibition with selegiline (L-deprenyl) has been suggested to have some beneficial effects. One drug that inhibits *N*-methyl-D-aspartate (NMDA) glutamate receptors is available (see below), and "ampakines," substances that facilitate synaptic activity at glutamate AMPA receptors, are under intense study. Some evidence suggests that lipid-lowering statins are beneficial. So-called cerebral vasodilators are *not* effective.

Tacrine (tetrahydroaminoacridine, THA), a long-acting cholinesterase inhibitor and muscarinic modulator, was the first drug shown to have any benefit in Alzheimer disease. Because of its hepatic toxicity, tacrine has been replaced in clinical use by newer cholinesterase inhibitors: **donepezil, rivastigmine,** and **galantamine.** These agents are orally active, have adequate penetration into the central nervous system, and are much less toxic than tacrine. Although evidence for the benefit of cholinesterase inhibitors (and memantine; see below) is statistically significant, the amount of benefit is modest, varies markedly among patients, and does not prevent the progression of the disease. The cholinesterase inhibitors cause significant adverse effects, including nausea and vomiting, diarrhea, and other peripheral cholinomimetic effects. These drugs should be used with caution in patients receiving other drugs that inhibit cytochrome P450 enzymes (eg, ketoconazole, quinidine; see Chapter 4). Preparations available are listed in Chapter 7.

Excitotoxic activation of glutamate transmission via NMDA receptors has been postulated to contribute to the pathophysiology of Alzheimer disease. **Memantine** binds to NMDA receptor channels in a use-dependent manner and produces a noncompetitive blockade. Its limited efficacy in moderate-to-severe Alzheimer disease is similar to or smaller than that of the cholinesterase inhibitors. However, this drug may be better tolerated and less toxic than the cholinesterase inhibitors. In contrast, a small study of memantine in Alzheimer disease in persons with Down syndrome found no benefit. Combination therapy with both memantine and one of the cholinesterase inhibitors has produced mixed results. Memantine is available as Namenda in 5- and 10-mg oral tablets and in combination formulations with donepezil. Adverse effects are uncommon, but dizziness or confusion have been reported.

Recent research has focused on amyloid beta, because the characteristic plaques consist mostly of this peptide. Unfortunately, two anti-amyloid antibodies, **solanezumab** and **bapineuzumab,** both failed to improve cognition or slow progression in recent clinical trials. In contrast, late analyses of the results of a trial of **aducanumab,** another Aβ antibody, has suggested that such drugs may indeed have some benefit. The development of this biological was halted when initial results showed failure to halt Aβ accumulation. More recently, follow-up studies confirmed that the drug can reduce brain amyloid levels, but this does not reliably ameliorate the disease. At the highest dosage, the agent modestly slowed cognitive decline and improved memory, orientation, and language functions but only in some patients. These findings resulted in a highly controversial FDA approval. **Donanemab**, a newer Aβ antibody, appears promising. **Verubecestat,** an inhibitor of beta-site amyloid precursor protein cleaving enzyme (BACE1), reduces the production of amyloid β. This drug showed safety in an early clinical trial, but a randomized, controlled phase 3 trial did not show benefit.

Another effort suggests that the accumulation of filamentous tangles of tau protein is a critical component of neuronal damage in Alzheimer and several other neurodegenerative conditions. Accumulation of tau appears to be associated with dissociation from microtubules in neurons, which has stimulated interest in drugs that inhibit microtubule disassembly, such as **epothilone-D.** Failure of so many drugs in clinical trials has been ascribed to the fact that these trials have been carried out in patients who have signs of Alzheimer disease and may therefore already have irreversible changes. It is hoped that improved methods for predicting the condition will permit trials at an earlier stage of the pathology while reversal is still possible. A large-scale, long-term randomised controlled trial in Finland showed that a combined healthy balanced nutrition, physical exercise, cognitive training and social activities, with vascular and metabolic risk management intervention can reduce the risk of cognitive impairment among individuals at risk. The trial showed benefits on cognition that included individuals with genetic susceptibility to Alzheimer's disease.

Studies in transgenic Alzheimer mice indicate that use of phosphodiesterase 5 inhibitors may improve synaptic function. A retrospective survey of users of sildenafil suggested that users had a lower risk of developing Alzheimer disease. This observation requires a randomized double-blind evaluation before any recommendation can be made.

CARDIOVASCULAR DRUGS

Antihypertensive Drugs

Blood pressure, especially systolic pressure, increases with age in Western countries and in most cultures in which salt intake is high. In women, the increase is more marked after age 50. Although often ignored in the past, clinicians now believe that hypertension should be treated in the elderly. In fact, more aggressive treatment of hypertension is one factor that may contribute to the reported decline in the incidence of dementia.

The basic principles of therapy are not different in the geriatric age group from those described in Chapter 11, but the usual cautions regarding altered pharmacokinetics and blunted compensatory mechanisms apply. Because of its safety, nondrug therapy (weight reduction in the obese and moderate salt restriction) should be encouraged. Thiazides are a reasonable first step in drug therapy. The hypokalemia, hyperglycemia, and hyperuricemia caused by these agents are more relevant in the elderly because of the higher prevalence in these patients of arrhythmias, type 2 diabetes, and gout. Thus, use of low antihypertensive doses—rather than maximum diuretic doses—is important. Calcium channel blockers are effective and safe if titrated to the appropriate response. They are especially useful in patients who also have atherosclerotic angina (see Chapter 12). Beta blockers are potentially hazardous in patients with obstructive airway disease and are considered less useful than calcium channel blockers in older patients unless chronic heart failure is present. Angiotensin-converting enzyme inhibitors are also considered less useful in the elderly unless heart failure or diabetes is present. The most powerful drugs, such as minoxidil, are rarely needed. Every patient receiving antihypertensive drugs should be checked regularly for orthostatic hypotension because of the danger of cerebral ischemia and falls.

Positive Inotropic Agents

Heart failure is a common and particularly lethal disease in the elderly. Fear of this condition is one reason why physicians overuse cardiac glycosides in this age group. The toxic effects of digoxin are particularly dangerous in the geriatric population, since the elderly are more susceptible to arrhythmias. The clearance of digoxin is usually decreased in the older age group, and although the volume of distribution is often decreased as well, the half-life of this drug may be increased by 50% or more. Because the drug is cleared mostly by the kidneys, renal function must be considered in designing a dosage regimen. There is no evidence that there is any increase in pharmacodynamic sensitivity to the therapeutic effects of the cardiac glycosides; in fact, animal studies suggest a possible decrease in therapeutic sensitivity. On the other hand, there is probably an increase in sensitivity to the toxic arrhythmogenic actions. Hypokalemia, hypomagnesemia, hypoxemia (from pulmonary disease), and coronary atherosclerosis all contribute to the high incidence of digitalis-induced arrhythmias in geriatric patients. The less common toxicities of digitalis such as delirium, visual changes, and endocrine abnormalities (see Chapter 13) also occur more often in older than in younger patients.

Antiarrhythmic Agents

The treatment of arrhythmias in the elderly is particularly challenging because of the lack of good hemodynamic reserve, the frequency of electrolyte disturbances, and the prevalence of significant coronary disease. The clearances of quinidine and procainamide decrease and their half-lives increase with age. Disopyramide should probably be avoided in the geriatric population because its major toxicities—antimuscarinic action, leading to voiding problems in men; and negative inotropic cardiac effects, leading to heart failure—are particularly undesirable in these patients. The clearance of lidocaine appears to be little changed, but the half-life is increased in the elderly. It is recommended that the loading dose of this drug be reduced in geriatric patients because of their greater sensitivity to its toxic effects.

Recent evidence indicates that many patients with atrial fibrillation—a very common arrhythmia in the elderly—do as well with simple control of ventricular rate as with conversion to normal sinus rhythm. Measures (such as anticoagulant drugs) must be taken to reduce the risk of thromboembolism in chronic atrial fibrillation.

ANTIMICROBIAL THERAPY

Several age-related changes contribute to the high incidence of infections in geriatric patients. A reduction in host defenses in the elderly is manifested in the increase in both serious infections and cancer. This may reflect an alteration in T-lymphocyte function. In the lungs, a major age and tobacco-dependent decrease in mucociliary clearance significantly increases susceptibility to infection. In the urinary tract, the incidence of serious infection is greatly increased by urinary retention and catheterization in men. Preventive immunizations should be maintained: influenza vaccine should be given annually, tetanus toxoid every 10 years, and pneumococcal and zoster vaccines once.

Since 1940, the antimicrobial drugs have contributed more to the prolongation of life than any other drug group because they can compensate to some extent for this deterioration in natural defenses. The basic principles of therapy of the elderly with these agents are no different from those applicable in younger patients and have been presented in Chapter 51. The major pharmacokinetic changes relate to decreased renal function; because most of the β-lactam, aminoglycoside, and fluoroquinolone antibiotics are excreted by this route, important changes in half-life may be expected. This is particularly important in the case of the aminoglycosides, because they cause concentration- and time-dependent toxicity in the kidney and in other organs. The half-lives of gentamicin, kanamycin, and netilmicin are more than doubled. The increase may be less marked for tobramycin.

ANTI-INFLAMMATORY DRUGS

Osteoarthritis is a very common disease of the elderly. Rheumatoid arthritis is less exclusively a geriatric problem, but the same drug therapy is usually applicable to both types of disease. The basic principles laid down in Chapter 36 and the properties of the anti-inflammatory drugs described there apply fully here.

The nonsteroidal anti-inflammatory agents (NSAIDs) must be used with special care in geriatric patients because they cause toxicities to which the elderly are very susceptible. In the case of aspirin, the most important of these is gastrointestinal irritation and bleeding. In the case of the newer NSAIDs, the most important is renal damage, which may be irreversible. Because they are cleared primarily by the kidneys, these drugs accumulate more rapidly in the geriatric patient and especially in the patient whose renal function is already compromised beyond the average range for his or her age. A vicious circle is easily set up in which cumulation of the NSAID causes more renal damage, which causes more cumulation. There is no evidence that the cyclooxygenase (COX)-2 selective NSAIDs are safer with regard to renal function. Elderly patients receiving high doses of any NSAID should be carefully monitored for changes in renal function.

Corticosteroids are extremely useful in elderly patients who cannot tolerate full doses of NSAIDs. However, they consistently cause a dose- and duration-related increase in osteoporosis, an especially hazardous toxic effect in the elderly. It is not certain whether this drug-induced effect can be reduced by increased calcium and vitamin D intake, but it would be prudent to consider these agents (and bisphosphonates if osteoporosis is already present, see Qaseem reference) and to encourage frequent exercise in any patient taking corticosteroids.

OPHTHALMIC DRUGS

Drugs Used in Glaucoma

Glaucoma is more common in the elderly, but its treatment does not differ from that of glaucoma of earlier onset. Management of glaucoma is discussed in Chapter 10.

Macular Degeneration

Age-related macular degeneration (AMD) is the most common cause of blindness in the elderly in the developed world. Two forms of advanced AMD are recognized: the neovascular "wet" form, which is associated with intrusion of new blood vessels in the subretinal space, and a more common "dry" form, which is not associated with abnormal vascularization. Although the cause of AMD is not known, smoking is a documented risk factor, and oxidative stress has long been thought to play a role. On this premise, antioxidants have been used to prevent or delay the onset of AMD. Proprietary oral formulations of vitamins C and E, β-carotene, zinc oxide, and cupric oxide are available. Some include the carotenoids lutein and zeaxanthin, and omega-3 long-chain polyunsaturated fatty acids. Evidence for the efficacy of these antioxidants is modest.

In advanced neovascular AMD, treatment has been moderately successful. This form of AMD can now be treated with laser phototherapy or with antibodies against vascular endothelial growth factor (VEGF). Two antibodies are available—bevacizumab (Avastin, used off-label) and ranibizumab (Lucentis)—as well as aflibercept (Eylea, a decoy protein receptor that binds VEGF) and the oligopeptide pegaptanib (Macugen). Aflibercept is also approved for the treatment of diabetic macular degeneration. These agents are injected into the vitreous for local effect. Ranibizumab is extremely expensive. Other agents that bind VEGF are under study.

■ ADVERSE DRUG REACTIONS IN THE ELDERLY

The relation between the number of drugs taken and the incidence of adverse drug reactions (ADRs) has been well documented. In long-term care facilities, in which a high percentage of the population is elderly, the average number of prescriptions per patient varies between 6 and 8. Studies have shown that the percentage of patients with adverse reactions increases from about 10% when a single drug is being taken to nearly 100% when 10 drugs are taken.

Thus, it may be expected that about half of patients in long-term care facilities will have recognized or unrecognized ADRs at some time. Patients living at home may see several different practitioners for different conditions and accumulate multiple prescriptions for drugs with overlapping actions. It is useful to conduct a "brown bag" analysis in such patients. The brown bag analysis consists of asking the patient to bring to the practitioner a bag containing *all* the medications, supplements, vitamins, etc, that he or she is currently taking. Some prescriptions will be found to be duplicates, and others unnecessary. The total number of medications taken can often be reduced by 30–50%.

The overall incidence of ADRs in geriatric patients is estimated to be at least twice that in the younger population. Reasons for this high incidence include errors in prescribing on the part of the practitioners and errors in drug usage by the patient. Practitioner errors sometimes occur because the physician does not appreciate the importance of changes in pharmacokinetics with age and age-related diseases. Some errors occur because the practitioner is unaware of incompatible drugs prescribed by other practitioners for the same patient. For example, cimetidine, an H_2-blocking drug heavily prescribed (or recommended in its over-the-counter form) to the elderly, causes a higher incidence of untoward effects (eg, confusion, slurred speech) in the geriatric population than in younger patients. It also inhibits the hepatic metabolism of many drugs, including phenytoin, warfarin, β blockers, and other agents. A patient who has been taking one of the latter agents without untoward effect may develop markedly elevated blood levels and severe toxicity if cimetidine is added to the regimen without adjustment of dosage of the other drugs. Additional examples of drugs that inhibit liver microsomal enzymes and lead to adverse reactions are described in Chapters 4 and 67.

Patient errors may result from nonadherence for reasons described below. In addition, they often result from use of nonprescription drugs taken without the knowledge of the physician. As noted in Chapters 64 and 65, many over-the-counter agents and herbal medications contain "hidden ingredients" with potent pharmacologic effects. For example, many antihistamines contained in over-the-counter drugs have significant sedative effects and are inherently more hazardous in patients with impaired cognitive function. Similarly, their antimuscarinic action may precipitate urinary retention in geriatric men or glaucoma in patients with a narrow anterior chamber angle. If the patient is also taking a CYP metabolism inhibitor such as cimetidine, the probability of an adverse reaction is greatly increased. A patient taking an herbal medication containing ginkgo is more likely to experience bleeding while taking low doses of aspirin.

■ PRACTICAL ASPECTS OF GERIATRIC PHARMACOLOGY

The quality of life in elderly patients can be greatly improved and life span can be prolonged by the intelligent use of drugs. However, the prescriber must recognize several practical obstacles to compliance.

The expense of drugs can be a major disincentive in patients receiving marginal retirement incomes who are not covered or inadequately covered by health insurance. The prescriber must be aware of the cost of the prescription and of cheaper alternative therapies. For example, the monthly cost of arthritis therapy with newer NSAIDs may exceed $100, whereas that for generic ibuprofen and naproxen, two older but equally effective NSAIDs, about $20.

Nonadherence may result from forgetfulness or confusion, especially if the patient has several prescriptions and different dosing intervals. A survey carried out in 1986 showed that the population over 65 years of age accounted for 32% of drugs prescribed in the USA, although these patients represented only 11–12% of the population at that time. Since the prescriptions are often written by several different practitioners, there is usually no attempt to design "integrated" regimens that use drugs with similar dosing intervals for the several conditions being treated. Patients may forget instructions regarding the need to complete a fixed duration of therapy when a course of anti-infective drug is being given. The disappearance of symptoms is often regarded as the best reason to halt drug taking, especially if the prescription was expensive.

Nonadherence may also be deliberate. A decision not to take a drug may be based on prior experience with it. There may be excellent reasons for such "intelligent" noncompliance, and the practitioner should try to elicit them. Such efforts may also improve compliance with alternative drug regimens, because enlisting the patient as a participant in therapeutic decisions increases the motivation to succeed.

Some errors in drug taking are caused by physical disabilities. Hearing impairment, arthritis, tremor, and visual problems may all contribute. Comprehension of verbal instructions should be confirmed by having the patient repeat them back to the prescriber; written instructions may be helpful. Liquid medications that are to be measured "by the spoonful" are inappropriate for patients with any type of tremor or motor disability. Use of a dosing syringe is essential in such cases. Because of decreased production of saliva, older patients often have difficulty swallowing large tablets. "Childproof" containers are often "elder-proof" if the patient has arthritis. Cataracts and macular degeneration occur in a large number of patients over 70. Therefore, labels on prescription bottles should be large enough for the patient with diminished vision to read or should be color-coded if the patient can see but can no longer read.

Drug therapy has considerable potential for both helpful and harmful effects in the geriatric patient. The balance may be tipped in the right direction by adherence to a few principles:

1. Take a careful drug history. The disease to be treated may be drug-induced, or drugs being taken may lead to interactions with drugs to be prescribed.
2. Prescribe only for a specific and rational indication. Do not prescribe omeprazole for "dyspepsia." Expert guidelines are published regularly by national organizations and websites such as UpToDate.com.
3. Define the goal of drug therapy. Then start with small doses and titrate to the response desired. Wait at least three half-lives

(adjusted for age) before increasing the dose. If the expected response does not occur at the normal adult dosage, check blood levels. If the expected response does not occur at the appropriate blood level, switch to a different drug.

4. Maintain a high index of suspicion regarding drug reactions and interactions. Know what other drugs the patient is taking, including over-the-counter and botanical (herbal) drugs.
5. Simplify the regimen as much as possible. When multiple drugs are prescribed, try to use drugs that can be taken at the same time of day. Whenever possible, reduce the number of drugs being taken.

REFERENCES

Acosta-Rodriguez V et al: Circadian alignment of early onset caloric restriction promotes longevity in male C57BL/6J mice. Science 2022;376:1192.

American College of Cardiology Foundation Task Force: ACCF/AHA 2011 Expert consensus document on hypertension in the elderly. J Am Coll Cardiol 2011;57:2037.

American Geriatrics Society 2015 Beers Update Expert Panel: American Geriatrics Society 2015 updated Beers criteria for potentially inappropriate medication use in older adults. J Am Geriatr Soc 2015;63:2227.

Ancolli-Israel S, Ayalon L: Diagnosis and treatment of sleep disorders in older adults. Am J Geriatr Psychiatry 2006;14:95.

Andrieu S et al. Effect of long-term omega 3 polyunsaturated fatty acid supplementation with or without multidomain intervention on cognitive function in elderly adults with memory complaints (MAPT): a randomised, placebo-controlled trial. Lancet Neurol 2017;16:377.

Aronow WS: Drug treatment of systolic and diastolic heart failure in elderly persons. J Gerontol A Biol Med Sci 2005;60:1597.

Arvanitakis Z, Shah RC, Bennett DA: Diagnosis and management of dementia: Review. JAMA 2019;322:1589.

Blackburn EH, Epel ES, Liu J: Human telomere biology: A contributory and interactive factor in aging, disease risks, and protection. Science 2015; 350:1193.

Bouton K: *Shouting Won't Help.* Picador, 2013.

Cassel C, Fulmer T: Achieving diagnostic excellence for older patients. JAMA 2022;327:919.

Cockcroft DW, Gault MH: Prediction of creatinine clearance from serum creatinine. Nephron 1976;16:31.

Coleman AL, McLeod SD: Screening for impaired visual acuity in older adults. JAMA 2022;327:2090.

Coupland CAC et al: Anticholinergic drug exposure and the risk of dementia: A nested case-control study. JAMA Intern Med 2019:179:1084.

da Silva R et al: Slow and negligible senescence among testudines challenges evolutionary theories of senescence. Science 2022;376:1466

Dergal JM et al: Potential interactions between herbal medicines and conventional drug therapies used by older adults attending a memory clinic. Drugs Aging 2002;19:879.

Docherty JR: Age-related changes in adrenergic neuroeffector transmission. Auton Neurosci 2002;96:8.

Drugs for cognitive loss and dementia. Treat Guidelines Med Lett 2013;11:95.

Epstein NU et al: Medication for Alzheimer's disease and associated fall hazard: A retrospective cohort study from the Alzheimer's disease neuroimaging initiative. Drugs Aging 2014;31:125.

Fang J et al: Endophenotype-based in silico network medicine discovery combined with insurance record data mining identifies sildenafil as a candidate drug for Alzheimer's disease. Nat Aging 2021;1:1175.

Ferrari AU: Modifications of the cardiovascular system with aging. Am J Geriatr Cardiol 2002;11:30.

Gandy S: Lifelong management of amyloid-beta metabolism to prevent Alzheimer's disease. N Engl J Med 2012;367:864.

Guarente L: Sirtuins, aging, and medicine. N Engl J Med 2011;364:2235.

Hartholt KA et al: Mortality from falls in US adults aged 75 years or older, 2000-2016. JAMA 2019;321:2131.

Horowitz AL et al: Blood factors transfer beneficial effects of exercise on neurogenesis and cognition to the aged brain. Science 2020;369:167.

Hubbard BP, Sinclair DA: Small molecule SIRT1 activators for the treatment of aging and age-related diseases. Trends Pharmacol Sci 2014;35:146.

Jager RD, Mieler WF, Miller JW: Age-related macular degeneration. N Engl J Med 2008;358:2606.

Japp D et al: Mineralocorticoid receptor antagonists in elderly patients with heart failure: A systematic review and meta-analysis. Age Ageing 2017;46:18.

Kaufman AC et al: Fyn inhibition rescues established memory and synapse loss in Alzheimer mice. Ann Neurol 2015;77:953.

Kelly AS, Morrison RS: Palliative care for the seriously ill. N Engl J Med 2015;373:747.

Kennedy BK, Pennypacker JK: Drugs that modulate aging: The promising yet difficult path ahead. Translat Res 2013;163:1.

Kirby J et al: A systematic review of the clinical and cost-effectiveness of memantine in patients with moderately severe to severe Alzheimer's disease. Drugs Aging 2006;23:227.

Lachs MS, Pillemer KA: Elder abuse. N Engl J Med 2015;373:1947.

Lamming DW et al: Rapamycin-induced insulin resistance is mediated by mTORC2 loss and uncoupled from longevity. Science 2012;335:1638.

Levey AS et al: Using standardized serum creatinine values in the modification of diet in renal disease study equation for estimating glomerular filtration rate. Ann Int Med 2006;145:247.

Lipska KJ et al: Polypharmacy in the aging patient. A review of glycemic control in older adults with type 2 diabetes. JAMA 2016;315:1034.

Mangoni AA: Cardiovascular drug therapy in elderly patients: Specific age-related pharmacokinetic, pharmacodynamic and therapeutic considerations. Drugs Aging 2005;22:913.

Marcantonio ER: Delirium in hospitalized older patients. N Engl J Med 2017;377:1456.

Maust DT et al: Prevalence of central nervous system-active polypharmacy among older adults with dementia in the US. JAMA 2021;325:952.

Moreno JA et al: Oral treatment targeting the unfolded protein response prevents neurodegeneration and clinical disease in prion-infected mice. Sci Transl Med 2013;5:206ra138.

Morrison LJ, Morrison RS: Palliative care and pain management. Med Clin N Am 2006;90:983.

Press D, Buss SS: Treatment of Alzheimer disease. Uptodate.com 2022

Qaseem A et al: Treatment of low bone density or osteoporosis to prevent fractures in men and women: A clinical practice guideline update from the American College of Physicians. Ann Int Med 2017; doi: 10.7326/M15-1361.

Qato DM et al: Use of prescription and over-the-counter medications and dietary supplements among older adults in the United States. JAMA 2008; 300:2867.

Rabow MW et al: Palliative care and pain management. In: Papadakis MA, McPhee SJ, Rabow MW (editors): *Current Medical Diagnosis & Treatment 2021.* McGraw-Hill, 2021.

Satizabal CL et al: Incidence of dementia over three decades in the Framingham Heart Study. N Engl J Med 2016;374:523.

Sawhney R, Sehl M, Naeim A: Physiologic aspects of aging: Impact on cancer management and decision making, part I. Cancer J 2005;11:449.

Scheltens P et al: Alzheimer's disease. Lancet 2021;397:1577–90.

Schindler SE et al: High-Precision plasma β-amyloid 42/40 predicts current and future brain amyloidosis. Neurology. 2019;93:e1647.

Staskin DR: Overactive bladder in the elderly: A guide to pharmacological management. Drugs Aging 2005;22:1013.

Teixeira A et al: Management of acute heart failure in elderly patients. Arch Cardiovasc Dis 2016;109:422.

Vaillaint GE: *Aging Well.* Little, Brown, 2002.

Vandenberghe R et al: Bapineuzumab for mild to moderate Alzheimer's disease in two global, randomized, phase 3 trials. Alzheimers Res Ther 2016;8:18.

Vik SA et al: Medication nonadherence and subsequent risk of hospitalisation and mortality among older adults. Drugs Aging 2006;23:345.

Zott B et al: A vicious cycle of β amyloid-dependent neuronal hyperactivation. Science 2019:365:559.

Zuccarello E et al. Development of novel phosphodiesterase 5 inhibitors for the therapy of Alzheimer's disease. Biochem Pharmacol 2020;176: 113818.

CASE STUDY ANSWER

This patient has several conditions that warrant careful treatment. Hypertension is eminently treatable; the steps described in Chapter 11 are appropriate and effective in the elderly as well as in young patients. Patient education is critical in combating his reluctance to take his medications. Because of his hearing impairment, good comprehension must be confirmed. Alzheimer disease may respond to one of the anticholinesterase agents (donepezil, rivastigmine, galantamine). Alternatively, memantine may be tried. Unfortunately, age-related macular degeneration (the most likely cause of his visual difficulties) is not readily treated, but the "wet" (neovascular) variety may respond well to one of the drugs currently available (bevacizumab, ranibizumab, pegaptanib). However, these therapies are expensive.

CHAPTER

61

Dermatologic Pharmacology

Dirk B. Robertson, MD, Howard I. Maibach, MD, & Rebecca M. Law, PharmD

CASE STUDY

A 43-year-old woman presents with a complaint of worsening rosacea. She initially responded to once-daily topical metronidazole 0.75% gel with excellent clearing of the papulopustular component of her acne rosacea. Recently, she has noted increasing persistent facial erythema. What therapeutic options are available?

Diseases of the skin offer special opportunities to the clinician. In particular, the topical administration route is especially appropriate for skin diseases, although some dermatologic diseases respond as well or better to drugs administered systemically.

The general pharmacokinetic principles governing the use of drugs applied to the skin are similar to those involved in other routes of administration (see Chapters 1 and 3). However, human skin is a complex series of diffusion barriers (Figure 61–1). At least 20 factors affect percutaneous flux. Quantitation of the flux of drugs and drug vehicles through these barriers is the basis for pharmacokinetic analysis of dermatologic therapy, and techniques for making such measurements are rapidly increasing in number and sensitivity.

Major factors that determine pharmacologic response to drugs applied to the skin include the following:

1. **Physicochemical properties of the drug:** A drug's particle size/molecular weight (MW), lipophilicity, volatility, pH, pKa, and partition coefficients (oil:water and formulation:skin) may all play a role in drug penetration through skin. For example, most topical drugs are less than or around 500 Da in size/MW with a few exceptions such as calcineurin inhibitors (tacrolimus MW 822 Da and pimecrolimus MW 810 Da). Drugs with larger particle sizes will have difficulty penetrating through skin effectively.
2. **Regional variation in drug penetration:** For example, the scrotum, face, axilla, and scalp are far more permeable than the forearm and may require less drug (or a less potent drug) for equivalent effect. For example, lower-potency corticosteroids are used on face and skin folds whereas high potency corticosteroids may be needed for palms and soles.
3. **Concentration gradient:** Increasing the concentration gradient increases the mass of drug transferred per unit time, just as in the case of diffusion across other barriers (see Chapter 1). Thus, lack of efficacy of topical corticosteroids can sometimes be overcome by use of higher concentrations of drug.
4. **Dosing schedule:** Because of its physical properties, skin acts as a reservoir for many drugs. As a result, the "local half-life" may be long enough to permit once-daily application of drugs with short systemic half-lives. For example, once-daily application of corticosteroids appears to be just as effective as multiple applications in many conditions.
5. **Vehicles and occlusion:** An appropriate vehicle maximizes the ability of the drug to penetrate the outer layers of the skin. In addition, through their physical properties (moistening or drying effects), vehicles may themselves have important therapeutic benefits. Occlusion (application of a plastic wrap to hold the drug and its vehicle in close contact with the skin) is extremely effective in maximizing efficacy. Vehicles have varying degrees of occlusive properties: ointments > creams > lotions, etc. Thus a drug in an ointment base will be more efficacious than a drug in a cream or lotion, at the same drug concentration.

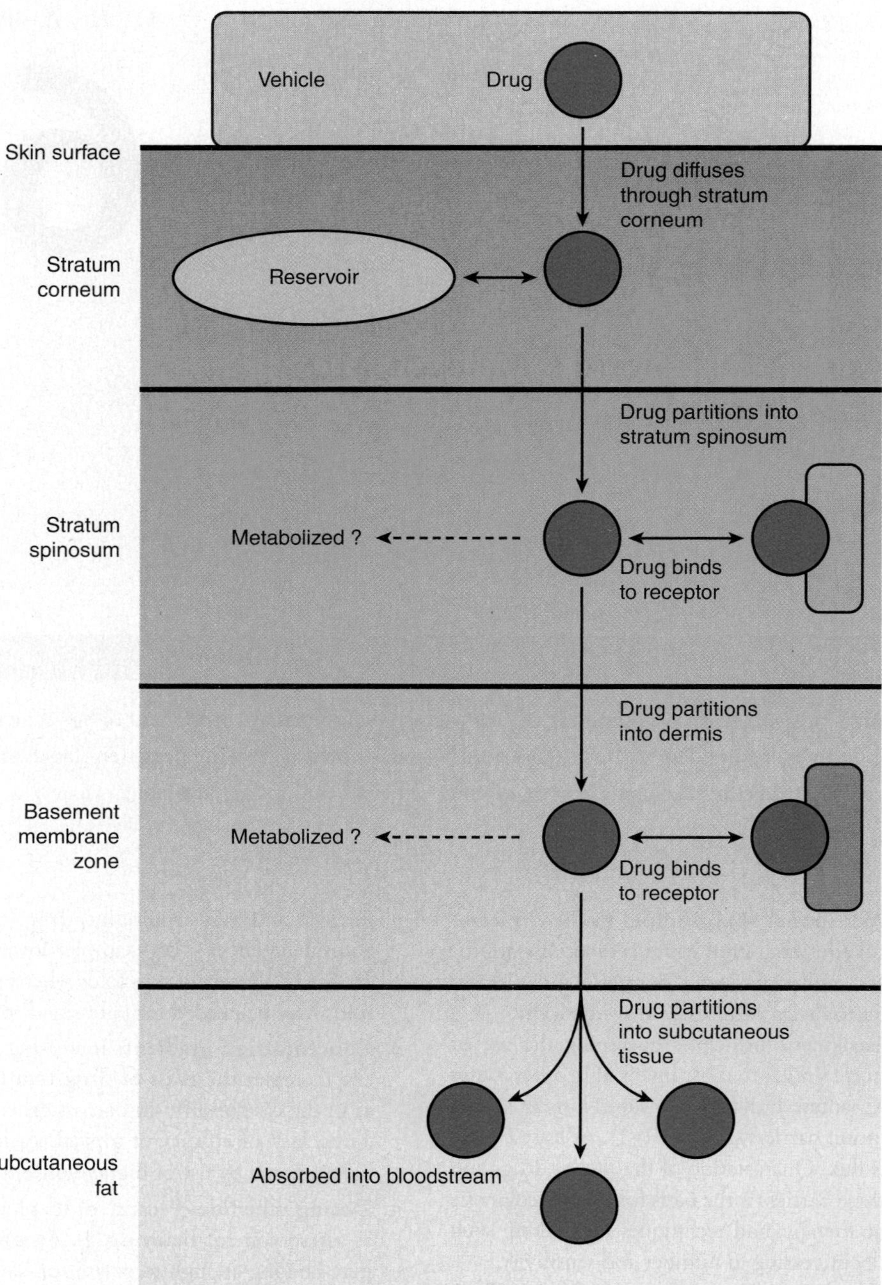

FIGURE 61–1 Schematic diagram of percutaneous absorption. (Reproduced with permission from Orkin M, Maibach HI, Dahl MV: Dermatology. New York, NY: McGraw Hill; 1991.)

This is discussed in greater detail below along with discussions of other vehicle/formulation differences that affect drug penetration.

6. **Skin conditions, skin health, and skin integrity:** Skin hydration, skin pH, skin temperature, skin surface topography, skin trauma, and skin diseases may all affect drug penetration. Skin damage or trauma or clinical disease such as atopic dermatitis may compromise skin integrity, resulting in enhanced drug penetration.

For a discussion of additional factors affecting percutaneous flux, such as lateral spread, substantivity/adherence, binding to skin proteins or other components, rubbing, washing, exfoliation, age, etc, see the General section in References.

■ REACTIONS TO DERMATOLOGIC MEDICATIONS

Skin reacts to many systemic medications with a variety of symptom-generating responses. In addition, some dermatologic medications themselves cause skin reactions. The major types of reactions are summarized in Table 61–1.

TABLE 61–1 Local cutaneous reactions to topical medications.

Reaction Type	Mechanism	Comment
Irritation	Nonallergic	Most common local reaction
Photoirritation	Nonallergic	Phototoxicity; usually requires UVA exposure
Allergic contact dermatitis	Allergic	Type IV delayed hypersensitivity
Photoallergic contact dermatitis	Allergic	Type IV delayed hypersensitivity; usually requires UVA exposure
Immunologic contact urticaria	Allergic	IgE-mediated type I immediate hypersensitivity; may result in anaphylaxis
Nonimmunologic contact urticaria	Nonallergic	Most common contact urticaria; occurs without prior sensitization

DERMATOLOGIC VEHICLES

Topical medications usually consist of active ingredients incorporated in a vehicle that facilitates cutaneous application. Important considerations in vehicle selection include solubility of the active agent in the vehicle; the rate of release of the agent from the vehicle; the ability of the vehicle to hydrate the stratum corneum, thus enhancing penetration; the stability of the therapeutic agent in the vehicle; and interactions, chemical and physical, of the vehicle, stratum corneum, and active agent.

Depending upon the vehicle, dermatologic formulations may be classified as tinctures, wet dressings, lotions, gels, aerosols, powders, pastes, creams, foams, and ointments. The ability of the vehicle to retard evaporation from the surface of the skin increases in this series, being least in tinctures and wet dressings and greatest in ointments. In general, acute inflammation with oozing, vesiculation, and crusting is best treated with drying preparations such as tinctures, wet dressings, and lotions, whereas chronic inflammation with xerosis, scaling, and lichenification is best treated with more lubricating preparations such as creams and ointments. Tinctures, lotions, gels, foams, and aerosols are convenient for application to the scalp and hairy areas. Emulsified vanishing-type creams may be used in intertriginous areas without causing maceration.

Emulsifying agents provide homogeneous, stable preparations when mixtures of immiscible liquids such as oil-in-water creams are compounded. Some patients develop irritation from these agents. Substituting a preparation that does not contain them or using one containing a lower concentration may resolve the problem.

ANTIBACTERIAL AGENTS

TOPICAL ANTIBACTERIAL PREPARATIONS

Topical antibacterial agents may be useful in preventing infections in clean wounds, in the early treatment of infected dermatoses and wounds, in reducing colonization of the nares by staphylococci, in axillary deodorization, and in the management of acne vulgaris. Efficacy of antibiotics in these topical applications is not uniform. The general pharmacology of the antimicrobial drugs is discussed in Chapters 43–51.

Some topical anti-infectives contain corticosteroids in addition to antibiotics. There is no convincing evidence that topical corticosteroids inhibit the antibacterial effect of antibiotics when the two are incorporated in the same preparation. In the treatment of secondarily infected dermatoses, which are usually colonized with streptococci, staphylococci, or both, combination therapy may prove superior to corticosteroid therapy alone. Antibiotic-corticosteroid combinations may be useful in treating diaper dermatitis, otitis externa, and impetiginized eczema.

Selection of a particular antibiotic depends upon the diagnosis and, when appropriate, in vitro culture and sensitivity studies of clinical samples. The pathogens isolated from most infected dermatoses are group A β-hemolytic streptococci, *Staphylococcus aureus*, or both. The pathogens present in surgical wounds will be those resident in the environment. Information about regional patterns of drug resistance is therefore important in selecting a therapeutic agent. Prepackaged topical antibacterial preparations that contain multiple antibiotics are available in fixed dosages well above the therapeutic threshold. These formulations offer the advantages of efficacy in mixed infections, broader coverage for infections due to undetermined pathogens, and delayed microbial resistance to any single component antibiotic.

BACITRACIN & GRAMICIDIN

Bacitracin and gramicidin are peptide antibiotics active against gram-positive organisms such as streptococci, pneumococci, and staphylococci. In addition, most anaerobic cocci, neisseriae, tetanus bacilli, and diphtheria bacilli are sensitive. Bacitracin is compounded in an ointment base alone or in combination with neomycin, polymyxin B, or both. The use of bacitracin in the anterior nares may temporarily decrease colonization by pathogenic staphylococci. Microbial resistance may develop following prolonged use. Bacitracin-induced contact urticaria syndrome, including anaphylaxis, occurs rarely. Allergic contact dermatitis occurs frequently, and immunologic allergic contact urticaria rarely. Bacitracin is poorly absorbed through the skin, so systemic toxicity is rare.

Gramicidin is available only for topical use, in combination with other antibiotics such as neomycin, polymyxin B, bacitracin, and nystatin. Systemic toxicity limits this drug to topical use. The incidence of sensitization following topical application is exceedingly low in therapeutic concentrations.

OZENOXACIN

Ozenoxacin (Xepi) is a novel, non-fluorinated quinolone that has been shown to be bactericidal against *S aureus* and *S pyogenes*, including methicillin-resistant *S aureus* (MRSA). Topical ozenoxacin 1% cream is indicated for the treatment of impetigo caused by *S aureus* or *S pyogenes* in patients 2 months of age and older.

The recommended dosing regimen is twice-daily application to the affected area for 5 days. Topically applied ozenoxacin demonstrates negligible systemic absorption, resulting in minimal adverse effects.

MUPIROCIN

Mupirocin (pseudomonic acid A) is structurally unrelated to other currently available topical antibacterial agents. Most gram-positive aerobic bacteria, including methicillin-resistant *S aureus* (MRSA), are sensitive to mupirocin (see Chapter 50). It is effective in the treatment of impetigo caused by *S aureus* and group A β-hemolytic streptococci. Microbial resistance is increasing.

Intranasal mupirocin ointment for eliminating nasal carriage of *S aureus* may be associated with irritation of mucous membranes caused by the polyethylene glycol vehicle. Dosage forms with benzoyl alcohol should not be used in neonates to avoid potentially fatal "gasping syndrome" if exposed to large amounts. Mupirocin is not appreciably absorbed systemically after topical application to intact skin, but systemic toxicity may occur through large areas of denuded skin.

RETAPAMULIN

Retapamulin (Altabax) is a semisynthetic pleuromutilin derivative effective in the treatment of uncomplicated superficial skin infection caused by group A β-hemolytic streptococci and *S aureus*, excluding MRSA. Topical retapamulin 1% ointment is indicated for use in adult and pediatric patients, 9 months or older, for the treatment of impetigo. Recommended treatment regimen is twice-daily application for 5 days. Retapamulin is well tolerated with only occasional local irritation of the treatment site. Although uncommon, allergic contact dermatitis has been reported.

POLYMYXIN B SULFATE

Polymyxin B is a peptide antibiotic effective against gram-negative organisms, including *Pseudomonas aeruginosa*, *Escherichia coli*, *Enterobacter*, and *Klebsiella*. Most strains of *Proteus* and *Serratia* are resistant, as are all gram-positive organisms. Topical preparations may be compounded in either a solution or ointment base. Numerous prepackaged antibiotic combinations contain polymyxin B. Detectable serum concentrations are difficult to achieve from topical application, but the total daily dose applied to denuded skin or open wounds should not exceed 200 mg in order to reduce the likelihood of neurotoxicity and nephrotoxicity. Allergic contact dermatitis to topically applied polymyxin B sulfate is uncommon.

NEOMYCIN & GENTAMICIN

Neomycin and gentamicin are aminoglycoside antibiotics active against gram-negative organisms, including *E coli*, *Proteus*, *Klebsiella*, and *Enterobacter*. Gentamicin generally shows greater activity against *P aeruginosa* than neomycin. Gentamicin is also more active against staphylococci and group A β-hemolytic streptococci. Widespread topical use of gentamicin, especially in a hospital environment, should be avoided to slow the appearance of gentamicin-resistant organisms.

Neomycin is available in numerous topical formulations, alone and in combination with polymyxin B, bacitracin, and other antibiotics. It is also available as a sterile powder for topical use. Gentamicin is available as an ointment or cream, alone and in combination with betamethasone as cream, ointment, or solution for ophthalmic or otic use.

Topical application of neomycin rarely results in detectable serum concentrations. However, in the case of gentamicin, serum concentrations of 1–18 mcg/mL are possible if the drug is applied in a water-miscible preparation to large areas of denuded skin, as in burned patients. Both drugs are water-soluble and are excreted primarily in the urine. Renal failure may permit the accumulation of these antibiotics, with possible nephrotoxicity, neurotoxicity, and ototoxicity.

Neomycin frequently causes allergic contact dermatitis, particularly if applied to eczematous dermatoses or if compounded in an ointment vehicle. When sensitization occurs, cross-sensitivity to streptomycin, kanamycin, paromomycin, and gentamicin is possible.

TOPICAL ANTIBIOTICS IN ACNE OR ROSACEA

Systemic antibiotics traditionally used in the treatment of acne vulgaris have been shown effective when applied topically. Currently, several antibiotics are used topically for this indication: clindamycin phosphate, erythromycin base, and minocycline. Effectiveness of topical therapy is less than that achieved by its oral administration. Therefore, topical therapy is generally suitable in mild to moderate cases of inflammatory acne. Some topical therapies are suitable for rosacea or acne/rosacea.

Clindamycin

Clindamycin has in vitro activity against *Cutibacterium acnes*; this has been postulated as the mechanism of its beneficial effect in acne therapy. Approximately 10% of an applied dose is absorbed, and rare cases of bloody diarrhea and pseudomembranous colitis have been reported following topical application. The hydroalcoholic vehicle and foam formulation (Evoclin) may cause drying and irritation of the skin, with complaints of burning and stinging. The water-based gel and lotion formulations are well tolerated and less likely to cause irritation. Allergic contact dermatitis is uncommon. Clindamycin is also available in fixed-combination topical gels with benzoyl peroxide (Acanya, BenzaClin, Duac, Neuac, Onexton) and with tretinoin (Veltin, Ziana).

Erythromycin

In topical preparations, erythromycin base rather than a salt is used to facilitate penetration. The mechanism of action of topical erythromycin in inflammatory acne vulgaris primarily due to its inhibitory effects on RNA-dependent protein synthesis in *C acnes*. One complication of topical therapy is the development of antibiotic-resistant strains of organisms, including staphylococci.

If this occurs in association with a clinical infection, topical erythromycin should be discontinued and appropriate systemic antibiotic therapy started. Adverse local reactions to erythromycin solution may include a burning sensation at application time and drying and irritation of the skin (the alcohol component causes skin drying and peeling). The topical water-based gel is less drying and may be better tolerated. However, the topical gel may be flammable. Some dosage forms may include propylene glycol which has potential toxicities if large amounts are used, especially in pediatrics. Allergic contact dermatitis is uncommon. Erythromycin is also available in a fixed combination preparation with benzoyl peroxide (Benzamycin, Aktipak) for topical treatment of acne vulgaris.

Minocycline

Minocycline 4% foam (Amzeeq) is an FDA-approved formulation for the topical treatment of inflammatory lesions of moderate to severe acne vulgaris in adults and pediatric patients 9 years of age and older. Minocycline 1.5% foam (Zilxi) is FDA-approved for topical treatment of inflammatory lesions of rosacea in adults. The mechanism of action of topical minocycline foam for acne or rosacea is unknown. Ideally the foam should be applied once daily to acne-affected areas on the face at least 1 hour before bedtime. If acne is present on other parts of the patient's body such as the neck, shoulders, arms, back, or chest, additional amounts of topical foam should be applied to these areas. The most common side effects with facial use are mild erythema and hyperpigmentation.

Available data with 4% minocycline foam use in pregnant women are insufficient to evaluate for a drug-associated risk of major birth defects, miscarriage, or other adverse maternal or fetal outcomes. Although the amount of systemic minocycline after topical use is less than after oral use, tetracyclines as a class are recommended to be avoided during pregnancy.

Metronidazole

Topical metronidazole is effective in rosacea treatment. The mechanism of action is unknown, but it may relate to the inhibitory effects of metronidazole on *Demodex brevis*; alternatively, the drug may act as an anti-inflammatory agent by direct effect on neutrophil cellular function. No disulfiram-like reactions have been reported after topical application although the drug is detectable systemically. Oral metronidazole crosses both the placenta and appears in breast milk. Oral doses appear in breast milk in similar concentrations as maternal plasma concentrations. It is carcinogenic in susceptible rodent species, and teratogenicity presenting as cleft lip ± cleft palate has been reported in infants after first-trimester exposure. Oral use during the first trimester is not recommended, and caution should be exercised with topical or intravaginal use. For breastfeeding mothers, some manufacturers recommend a decision be made whether to temporarily discontinue breastfeeding or to discontinue metronidazole and use alternative therapy. However, for the treatment of inflammatory lesions and erythema of rosacea topical antibiotics including metronidazole have been considered compatible with breastfeeding (Murase 2014). Use in children under 12 years old is not recommended.

Adverse local effects of the water-based gel formulation (MetroGel) include dryness, burning, and stinging. Less drying formulations may be better tolerated (MetroCream, MetroLotion, and Noritate cream). Caution should be exercised when applying metronidazole near the eyes to avoid excessive tearing.

Ivermectin

Topical ivermectin is available as a 1% cream (Soolantra) for the treatment of inflammatory lesions of rosacea. The mechanism of action is unknown. Oral ivermectin has antiparasitic activity against *Demodex* mites and possibly an anti-inflammatory effect. Topical application is well tolerated with occasional complaints of burning and irritation.

Sodium Sulfacetamide

Topical sulfacetamide is available alone as a 10% lotion (Klaron) and as a 10% wash (Ovace), and in several preparations in combination with sulfur for the treatment of acne vulgaris and acne rosacea. The mechanism of action is thought to be inhibition of *C acnes* by competitive inhibition of *p*-aminobenzoic acid utilization. Approximately 4% of topically applied sulfacetamide is absorbed percutaneously, and its use is therefore contraindicated in patients having a known hypersensitivity to sulfonamides. Dosage forms containing propylene glycol or benzyl alcohol should be used with caution in neonates.

Dapsone

Topical dapsone is available as a 5% and 7.5% gel (Aczone) for the treatment of acne vulgaris. The mechanism of action is unknown. Topical use in patients with glucose-6-phosphate dehydrogenase (G6PD) deficiency has not been shown to cause clinically relevant hemolysis or anemia, but a slight decrease in hemoglobin concentration was noted in patients with G6PD deficiency, suggestive of mild hemolysis. Cases of methemoglobinemia have been reported in association with topical dapsone gel, and its use should be avoided in patients with congenital or idiopathic methemoglobinemia. Adverse local effects include mild dryness, redness, oiliness, and skin peeling. Application of dapsone gel followed by benzoyl peroxide may result in a temporary yellow discoloration of the skin and hair.

■ ANTIFUNGAL AGENTS

The treatment of superficial fungal infections caused by dermatophytic fungi may be accomplished (1) with topical antifungal agents, eg, clotrimazole, efinaconazole, econazole, ketoconazole, luliconazole, miconazole, oxiconazole, sertaconazole, sulconazole, ciclopirox olamine, naftifine, terbinafine, butenafine, and tolnaftate; or (2) with orally administered agents, eg, griseofulvin, terbinafine, fluconazole, and itraconazole. Their mechanisms of action are described in Chapter 48. Superficial infections caused by *Candida* species may be treated with topical applications of clotrimazole, miconazole, econazole, ketoconazole, oxiconazole, ciclopirox olamine, nystatin, or amphotericin B.

TOPICAL ANTIFUNGAL PREPARATIONS

Topical Azole Derivatives

The topical imidazoles, which include clotrimazole, econazole, ketoconazole, luliconazole, miconazole, oxiconazole, sertaconazole, and sulconazole, have a wide range of activity against dermatophytes (*Epidermophyton*, *Microsporum*, and *Trichophyton*) and yeasts, including *Candida albicans* and *Pityrosporum orbiculare* (see Chapter 48). In comparison with nystatin for yeast infections, azoles are more efficacious.

Miconazole (Monistat, Micatin) is available for topical application as a cream or lotion and as vaginal cream or suppositories for use in vulvovaginal candidiasis. Clotrimazole (Lotrimin, Mycelex) is available for topical application to the skin as a cream or lotion and as vaginal cream and tablets for use in vulvovaginal candidiasis.

Efinaconazole (Jublia) is available as a 10% solution for the treatment of onychomycosis of the toenails. Daily application to affected toenails should be continued for 48 weeks. Complete cure rates in clinical trials are between 15% and 18%. Econazole (Spectazole) is available as a cream for topical application. Oxiconazole (Oxistat) is available as a cream and lotion for topical use. Ketoconazole (Nizoral) is available as a cream for topical treatment of dermatophytosis and candidiasis and as a shampoo or foam for the treatment of seborrheic dermatitis. Luliconazole (Luzu) is available as a cream. Sulconazole (Exelderm) is available as a cream or solution. Sertaconazole (Ertaczo) is available as a cream. Topical antifungal-corticosteroid fixed combinations have been introduced on the basis of providing more rapid symptomatic improvement than an antifungal agent alone. Clotrimazole-betamethasone dipropionate cream (Lotrisone) is one such combination.

Once- or twice-daily application to the affected area will generally result in clearing of superficial dermatophyte infections in 2–3 weeks, although the medication should be continued until eradication of the organism is confirmed. Paronychial and intertriginous candidiasis can be treated effectively by any of these agents when applied three or four times daily. Seborrheic dermatitis should be treated with twice-daily applications of ketoconazole until clinical clearing is obtained.

Adverse local reactions to the imidazoles may include stinging, pruritus, erythema, and local irritation. Allergic contact dermatitis is uncommon. Azoles such as miconazole used topically may be absorbed systemically in high enough concentrations to cause systemic adverse effects, such as interaction with warfarin causing an increased INR.

Ciclopirox Olamine

Ciclopirox olamine is a synthetic broad-spectrum antimycotic agent with inhibitory activity against dermatophytes, *Candida* species, and *P orbiculare*. This agent inhibits the uptake of precursors of macromolecular synthesis; the site of action is probably the fungal cell membrane.

Pharmacokinetic studies indicate that 1–2% of the dose is absorbed when applied as a solution on the back under an occlusive dressing. Ciclopirox olamine is available as a 1% cream and lotion (Loprox) for the topical treatment of dermatomycosis, candidiasis, and tinea versicolor. The incidence of adverse reactions has been low. Pruritus and worsening of clinical disease have been reported. The potential for allergic contact dermatitis is small.

Topical 8% ciclopirox olamine (Penlac nail lacquer) is approved for the treatment of mild to moderate onychomycosis of fingernails and toenails. Although well tolerated with minimal side effects, the complete cure rates in clinical trials are between 5.5% and 8.5%.

Tavaborole

Tavaborole is the first oxaborole antifungal drug approved for the topical treatment of toenail onychomycosis. Tavaborole blocks fungal protein synthesis by inhibiting aminoacyl-transfer ribonucleic acid synthetase. Tavaborole is available as a 5% solution (Kerydin) that should be applied to the affected toenails once daily for 48 weeks. Complete cure rates in clinical trials are between 6.5% and 9.1%.

Allylamines: Naftifine & Terbinafine

Naftifine hydrochloride and terbinafine (Lamisil) are allylamines that are highly active against dermatophytes but less active against yeasts. The antifungal activity derives from selective inhibition of squalene epoxidase, a key enzyme for the synthesis of ergosterol (see Figure 48–1).

They are available as 1–2% creams and other forms for the topical treatment of dermatophytosis, to be applied on a once- or twice-daily dosing schedule for 2–4 weeks depending on the site of infection. Adverse reactions include local irritation, burning sensation, and erythema. Contact with mucous membranes should be avoided.

Butenafine

Butenafine hydrochloride (Mentax) is a benzylamine that is structurally related to the allylamines. As with the allylamines, butenafine inhibits the epoxidation of squalene, thus blocking the synthesis of ergosterol, an essential component of fungal cell membranes. Butenafine is available as a 1% cream to be applied usually once daily for 2 weeks for the treatment of superficial dermatophytosis, although other regimens are used for tinea pedis.

Tolnaftate

Tolnaftate is a synthetic antifungal compound effective topically against dermatophyte infections caused by *Epidermophyton*, *Microsporum*, and *Trichophyton*. It is also active against *P orbiculare* but not against *Candida*.

Tolnaftate (Aftate, Tinactin) is available as a cream, solution, powder, or powder aerosol for application twice daily to infected areas. Recurrences following cessation of therapy are common, and infections of the palms, soles, and nails are usually unresponsive to tolnaftate alone. The powder or powder aerosol may be used chronically following initial treatment in patients susceptible to tinea infections. Tolnaftate is generally well tolerated and rarely causes irritation or allergic contact dermatitis. Tolnaftate is usually applied twice daily for 4 weeks as treatment for tinea pedis and corporis, twice daily for 2 weeks for tinea cruris, and once or twice daily as prevention for tinea pedis only.

Nystatin & Amphotericin B

Nystatin and amphotericin B are useful in the topical therapy of *C albicans* infections but ineffective against dermatophytes. Nystatin is limited to topical treatment of cutaneous and mucosal candida infections because of its narrow spectrum and negligible absorption from the gastrointestinal tract following oral administration. Amphotericin B has a broader antifungal spectrum and is used intravenously in the treatment of many systemic mycoses (see Chapter 48) and to a lesser extent in the treatment of cutaneous *Candida* infections.

The recommended dosage for topical preparations of nystatin in treating paronychial and intertriginous candidiasis is application two or three times a day. Oral candidiasis (thrush) is treated by holding 5 mL (infants, 2 mL) of nystatin oral suspension in the mouth for several minutes four times daily before swallowing. An alternative therapy for thrush is to retain a vaginal tablet in the mouth until dissolved four times daily. Recurrent or recalcitrant perianal, vaginal, vulvar, and diaper area candidiasis may respond to oral nystatin, 0.5–1 million units in adults (100,000 units in children) four times daily, in addition to local therapy. Vulvovaginal candidiasis may be treated by insertion of 1 vaginal tablet twice daily for 14 days, then nightly for an additional 14–21 days. (Intravaginal or oral azoles may be more efficacious and require shorter treatment durations—see above and below).

Amphotericin B (Fungizone) is available for topical use in cream and lotion form. The recommended dosage in the treatment of paronychial and intertriginous candidiasis is application two to four times daily to the affected area.

Adverse effects associated with oral administration of nystatin include mild nausea, diarrhea, and occasional vomiting. Topical application is nonirritating, and allergic contact hypersensitivity is exceedingly uncommon. Topical amphotericin B is well tolerated and only occasionally locally irritating. The drug may cause a temporary yellow staining of the skin, especially when the cream vehicle is used.

ORAL ANTIFUNGAL AGENTS

Oral Azole Derivatives

Azole derivatives currently available for oral treatment of candida and dermatophyte infections include fluconazole (Diflucan) and itraconazole (Sporanox). Ketoconazole (another azole) is not indicated for treatment of onychomycosis, cutaneous dermatophyte infections, or Candida infections. As discussed in Chapter 48, imidazole derivatives act by affecting the permeability of the cell membrane of sensitive cells through alterations of the biosynthesis of lipids, especially sterols, in the fungal cell.

Fluconazole and itraconazole are effective in the therapy of cutaneous infections caused by *Epidermophyton*, *Microsporum*, and *Trichophyton* species as well as *Candida*. Tinea versicolor is responsive to short courses of oral azoles.

Fluconazole is well absorbed following oral administration, with a plasma half-life of 30 hours. In view of this long half-life, daily doses of 100 mg are sufficient to treat mucocutaneous candidiasis. Once-weekly doses are sufficient for dermatophyte infections—tinea versicolor is treated for 2 weeks and other tinea infections for 2–6 weeks. Coccidioidomycosis, histoplasmosis, or cryptococcal infections may require longer treatment durations of 6 months to a year or longer. Use of oral fluconazole is not recommended in pregnancy including single doses for vaginal candidiasis. Itraconazole is also contraindicated for treatment of onychomycosis and other fungal infections during pregnancy, and in females planning a pregnancy. The plasma half-life of itraconazole is similar to that of fluconazole, and detectable therapeutic concentrations remain in the stratum corneum for up to 28 days following termination of therapy. Itraconazole is effective for the treatment of onychomycosis in a dosage of 200 mg daily taken with food to ensure maximum absorption. Itraconazole treatment durations are variable and disease specific (7–14 days to 8 weeks to greater than 12 months). Routine evaluation of hepatic function is recommended for patients receiving itraconazole or fluconazole for onychomycosis or other fungal infections requiring prolonged treatment courses. Rare cases of liver failure have occurred. Therefore, use azoles with caution, monitoring closely for signs/symptoms of hepatotoxicity. There are many clinically significant drug-drug interactions for oral azoles, as they are strong inhibitors of CYP3A4 (itraconazole), CYP2C19 and 2C9 (fluconazole), and other interactions. Concomitant use with other drugs may result in clinically serious increased effect/toxicity. Coadministration can cause elevated plasma concentrations of some drugs, leading to QT prolongation and ventricular arrhythmias. Life-threatening cardiac dysrhythmias and sudden death have occurred. Use is contraindicated in patients with evidence of ventricular dysfunction (eg, CHF).

Terbinafine

Terbinafine (described above) is effective given orally for the treatment of onychomycosis. Recommended oral dosage is 250 mg daily for 6 weeks for fingernail infections and 12 weeks for toenail infections. Patients receiving terbinafine for onychomycosis should be monitored closely with periodic laboratory evaluations for possible hepatic dysfunction. Rare cases of liver failure have occurred with the use of oral terbinafine; therefore, its use is not recommended in patients with chronic or active liver disease. In comparison with azoles, the hepatotoxicity risk is significantly less than ketoconazole and less than or similar to other azoles.

Griseofulvin

Griseofulvin, effective orally against dermatophyte infections caused by *Epidermophyton*, *Microsporum*, and *Trichophyton*, is ineffective against *Candida* and *P orbiculare.* Griseofulvin's mechanism of antifungal action is not fully understood, but it is active only against growing cells.

Following oral administration of 1 g of microsize griseofulvin, drug can be detected in the stratum corneum 4–8 hours later. Reducing the particle size of the medication greatly increases drug absorption. Formulations that contain the smallest particle size are labeled "ultramicrosize." Ultramicrosize griseofulvin achieves bioequivalent plasma levels with half the dose of microsize drug. In addition, solubilizing griseofulvin in polyethylene glycol enhances absorption even further. Microsize griseofulvin is available as 250-mg and 500-mg tablets, and ultramicrosize drug as 125-mg, 165-mg, 250-mg, and 330-mg tablets and as 250-mg capsules.

The usual adult dosage of the microsize form of the drug is 500 mg daily in single or divided doses with meals; occasionally, 1 g/d is indicated in the treatment of recalcitrant infections. The pediatric dosage is 10 mg/kg of body weight daily in single or divided doses with meals. An oral suspension is available for use in children. Adult dosage of the ultramicrosize form is 375 mg daily in single or divided doses, with up to 750 mg daily in divided doses for more difficult-to-eradicate infections such as tinea unguium and tinea pedis.

Griseofulvin is most effective in treating tinea infections of the scalp and glabrous (nonhairy) skin. In general, infections of the scalp respond to treatment in 4–6 weeks, and infections of glabrous skin will respond in 3–4 weeks. Dermatophyte infections of the nails respond only to prolonged administration. Fingernails may respond to 6 months of therapy, whereas toenails are recalcitrant to treatment and may require 8–18 months of therapy; relapse almost invariably occurs.

Adverse effects seen with griseofulvin therapy include headaches, nausea, vomiting, diarrhea, photosensitivity, peripheral neuritis, granulocytopenia, hepatotoxicity, and occasionally mental confusion. Griseofulvin is derived from a *Penicillium* mold, and cross-sensitivity with penicillin may occur. It is contraindicated in patients with porphyria or hepatic failure or those who have had hypersensitivity reactions to it in the past. Therefore, in patients undergoing prolonged therapy, routine evaluation of the hepatic, renal, and hematopoietic systems is advisable. Coumarin anticoagulant activity may be altered by griseofulvin, and anticoagulant dosage may require adjustment. It is contraindicated in pregnancy, and use in breastfeeding is not recommended.

■ TOPICAL ANTIVIRAL AGENTS

ACYCLOVIR, VALACYCLOVIR, PENCICLOVIR, & FAMCICLOVIR

Acyclovir, valacyclovir, penciclovir, and famciclovir are synthetic guanine analogs with inhibitory activity against members of the herpesvirus family, including herpes simplex types 1 and 2. Their mechanism of action, indications, and oral use in the treatment of cutaneous infections are discussed in Chapter 49.

Topical acyclovir (Zovirax) is available as a 5% ointment and 50-mg buccal tablet; topical penciclovir (Denavir) is available as a 1% cream for the treatment of recurrent orolabial herpes simplex virus infection in immunocompetent adults. Adverse local reactions to acyclovir and penciclovir may include pruritus and mild pain with transient stinging or burning.

■ IMMUNOMODULATORS

IMIQUIMOD

Imiquimod is available as a 5% cream (Aldara) for the treatment of biopsy-proven primary superficial basal cell carcinomas on the trunk, neck, extremities, and other areas such as the nose. The 3.75% (Zyclara) and 5% creams are indicated for treatment of external genital and perianal warts in adults, and creams with lower concentrations of 2.5% and 3.75% are available for the treatment of face and scalp actinic keratoses. The mechanism of its action is thought to be related to imiquimod's ability to stimulate peripheral mononuclear cells to release interferon alpha and to stimulate macrophages to produce interleukin 1 (IL-1), IL-6, and IL-8, and tumor necrosis factor α (TNF-α).

Imiquimod should be applied to the wart tissue three times per week and left on the skin for 6–10 hours prior to washing off with mild soap and water. Treatment should be continued until eradication of the warts is accomplished, but not for more than a total of 16 weeks. Recommended treatment of actinic keratoses consists of twice-weekly applications of the 5% cream on the contiguous area of involvement or nightly applications of the 2.5% or 3.75% cream. The cream is removed after approximately 8 hours with mild soap and water. Treatment of superficial basal cell carcinoma consists of five-times-per-week application of 5% cream to the tumor and surrounding area, for a 6-week course of therapy. The total tumor treatment area should not exceed 3 cm—ie, a maximum of 2 cm tumor diameter plus a 1-cm margin of surrounding skin.

Percutaneous absorption is minimal, with less than 0.9% absorbed following a single-dose application. Adverse effects consist of local inflammatory reactions, including pruritus, erythema, and superficial erosion.

TACROLIMUS & PIMECROLIMUS

Tacrolimus (as Protopic) and pimecrolimus (as Elidel) are topical calcineurin inhibitors that have been shown to be of significant benefit in the treatment of atopic dermatitis. Both agents inhibit T-lymphocyte activation and prevent the release of inflammatory cytokines and mediators from mast cells in vitro after stimulation by antigen-IgE complexes. Tacrolimus is available as 0.03% and 0.1% ointments, and pimecrolimus is available as a 1% cream. Both are indicated for short-term and intermittent long-term therapy for mild to moderate atopic dermatitis. Tacrolimus 0.03% ointment and pimecrolimus 1% cream are approved for use in children older than 2 years of age, and all strengths are approved for adult use. Recommended dosing of both agents is twice-daily application to affected skin until clearing is noted. Neither medication should be used with occlusive dressings. The most common side effect of both drugs is a burning sensation in the applied area that improves with continued use. The US Food and Drug Administration (FDA) mandates a black box warning regarding the long-term safety of topical tacrolimus and pimecrolimus because of animal tumorigenicity data.

CRISABOROLE (AND APREMILAST)

Crisaborole (Eucrisa) is a benzoxaborole, nonsteroidal, topical, anti-inflammatory phosphodiesterase (PDE) 4 inhibitor approved as a 2% ointment for the treatment of mild to moderate atopic dermatitis in patients 2 years of age and older. It is applied twice daily. The most frequent adverse effect is burning or stinging at the site of application. The specific mechanism of action in atopic dermatitis is unknown. Recent studies have shown a favorable safety profile for the long-term treatment of atopic dermatitis. (Note: Apremilast is an oral PDE-4 inhibitor approved for psoriasis—see below).

JANUS KINASE (JAK) INHIBITORS

Tofacitinib is an oral and topical Janus kinase (JAK) inhibitor. Selective inhibition of JAK1 and JAK3 blocks signaling through common cytokine receptors (IL2, IL4, IL7, IL9, IL15, IL21), and JAK1 inhibition attenuates signaling by pro-inflammatory cytokines (eg, IL6, type 1 interferon). The oral form is FDA approved for psoriasis and psoriatic arthritis and other rheumatic/immunologic conditions such as rheumatoid arthritis and ulcerative colitis. The topical formulation may be useful for psoriasis, alopecia areata, and vitiligo.

Additional JAK inhibitors useful in the treatment of atopic dermatitis include abrocitinib (Cibinqo), upadacitinib (Rinvoq), and ruxolitinib cream (Opzelura).

DUPILUMAB

Dupilumab (Dupixent) is an IL-4 receptor alpha antagonist that binds to and inhibits the receptor for IL-4 and indirectly reduces IL-13 cytokine activity. It is indicated for the treatment of adult patients with moderate to severe atopic dermatitis. It may be used concurrently with topical corticosteroids. The recommended dosing is an initial dose of 600 mg given as two 300-mg injections, followed by 300 mg injected once every other week. The most common adverse effects include injection site reactions as well as conjunctivitis and keratitis. Patients with new onset or worsening of eye symptoms should notify their health care provider. Eosinophilia and vasculitis are rare.

■ ECTOPARASITICIDES

PERMETHRIN

Permethrin is toxic to *Pediculus humanus, Pthirus pubis,* and *Sarcoptes scabiei*. Less than 2% of an applied dose is absorbed percutaneously. Residual drug persists up to 10 days following application. Resistance to permethrin is becoming more widespread.

It is recommended that permethrin 1% cream rinse (Nix) be applied undiluted to affected areas of pediculosis for 10 minutes and then rinsed off with warm water. For the treatment of scabies, a single application of 5% cream (Elimite, Acticin) is applied to the body from the neck down, left on for 8–14 hours, and then washed off. Adverse reactions to permethrin include transient burning, stinging, and pruritus. Cross-sensitization to pyrethrins or chrysanthemums has been alleged but inadequately documented.

SPINOSAD

Spinosad (Natroba) suspension is approved for the topical treatment of head lice in patients 4 years of age and older. Spinosad is derived from the fermentation of a soil *Actinomyces* bacterium and is toxic to *P humanus* with no appreciable absorption from topical application. It is recommended that the 0.9% suspension be applied to the hair and scalp for 10 minutes and then rinsed out. A repeat treatment may be applied 1 week later if live lice are present.

IVERMECTIN

Ivermectin (as Sklice) 0.5% lotion is approved for head lice treatment in patients 6 months of age and older. Ivermectin is toxic to *P humanus*, resulting in paralysis and death of the parasite. The pharmacology of ivermectin is discussed in Chapter 53. The lotion should be applied to the hair and scalp and rinsed out after 10 minutes. Ivermectin is for single use only and should not be repeated without health care provider recommendation.

LINDANE (HEXACHLOROCYCLOHEXANE)

The gamma isomer of hexachlorocyclohexane was commonly called gamma benzene hexachloride, a misnomer, since no benzene ring is present in this compound. Percutaneous absorption studies using a solution of lindane in acetone have shown that almost 10% of a dose applied to the forearm is absorbed, to be subsequently excreted in the urine over a 5-day period. After absorption, lindane is concentrated in fatty tissues, including the brain.

Lindane is available as a 1% shampoo. For pediculosis capitis or pubis, 30 mL of shampoo is applied to dry hair on the scalp or genital area for 4 minutes and then rinsed off. Patients should not use lindane more than one time to treat lice. Lindane is not a drug of first choice. Consider permethrin or crotamiton first.

Concerns about the toxicity of lindane have altered treatment guidelines for its use in scabies; the current recommendation calls for a single 30-mL application to the entire body from the neck down, left on for 8–12 hours, and then washed off. Patients should not use lindane more than one time to treat scabies.

Concerns about neurotoxicity have resulted in warnings that lindane should be used with caution in infants, children, the elderly, individuals with skin conditions, and those who weigh <110 pounds (<50 kg). The current US package insert states that lindane is contraindicated in premature infants and in patients with known uncontrolled seizure disorders. Additionally, lindane should be used only in patients who cannot tolerate or have failed first-line treatment with safer medications for the treatment of either scabies or lice.

CROTAMITON

Crotamiton, *N*-ethyl-*o*-crotonotoluidide, is a scabicide with some antipruritic properties; its mechanism of action is not known. Studies on percutaneous absorption have revealed detectable levels of crotamiton in the urine following a single application on the forearm.

Crotamiton (Crotan, Eurax) is available as a 10% cream or lotion. Suggested guidelines for scabies treatment call for two applications massaged onto the entire body from the chin down to the toes (with special attention to skin folds, creases, and interdigital spaces) at 24-hour intervals, with a cleansing bath 48 hours after the last application. One may re-treat if new lesions appear or itching persists more than 2–4 weeks after initial treatment. Crotamiton is an effective agent that could be tried first before considering lindane due to its safety profile. Allergic contact dermatitis and primary irritation may occur, necessitating discontinuance of therapy. Application to acutely inflamed skin or to the eyes or mucous membranes should be avoided.

SULFUR

Sulfur has a long history as a scabicide. Although it is nonirritating, it has an unpleasant odor, is staining, and is thus disagreeable to use. It has been replaced by more agreeable and effective scabicides in recent years, but it remains a possible alternative drug for use in infants and pregnant women. The usual formulation is 5% precipitated sulfur in petrolatum.

MALATHION

Malathion is an organophosphate cholinesterase inhibitor that is hydrolyzed and inactivated by plasma carboxylesterases much faster in humans than in insects, thereby providing a therapeutic advantage in treating pediculosis (see Chapter 7). Malathion is available as a 0.5% lotion (Ovide) that should be applied to the hair when dry; 4–6 hours later, the hair is combed to remove nits and lice. Shampoo after 8–12 hours. If required, repeat with second application in 7–9 days. Further treatment is generally not necessary.

BENZYL ALCOHOL

Benzyl alcohol (Ulesfia) is available as a 5% lotion for the treatment of head lice in patients older than 6 months. The lotion is applied to dry hair and left on for 10 minutes prior to rinsing off with water. Because the drug is not ovicidal, the treatment must be repeated after 7 days. Eye irritation and allergic contact dermatitis have been reported.

ISOPROPYL MYRISTATE

Isopropyl myristate (Resultz) has been given clearance by the FDA as an over-the-counter, pesticide-free pediculicide rinse containing 50% isopropyl myristate and 50% cyclomethicone. The solution is applied to dry hair and massaged in until the hair is thoroughly wet. After 10 minutes the hair is rinsed with warm water. This treatment is repeated in 7 days to kill any newly hatched lice. This product works by dissolving the wax covering on the exoskeleton of headlice, resulting in dehydration and subsequent death. Since this is a physical mode of action, resistance is unlikely.

■ AGENTS AFFECTING PIGMENTATION

HYDROQUINONE, MONOBENZONE, & MEQUINOL

Hydroquinone, monobenzone (Benoquin, the monobenzyl ether of hydroquinone), and mequinol (the monomethyl ether of hydroquinone) are used to reduce hyperpigmentation of the skin. Topical hydroquinone and mequinol usually result in temporary lightening, whereas monobenzone causes irreversible depigmentation.

The mechanism of action of these compounds appears to involve inhibition of the enzyme tyrosinase, thus interfering with the biosynthesis of melanin. In addition, monobenzone may be toxic to melanocytes, resulting in permanent loss of these cells. Some percutaneous absorption of these compounds takes place, because monobenzone may cause hypopigmentation at sites distant from the area of application. Both hydroquinone and monobenzone may cause local irritation. Allergic contact dermatitis to these compounds can occur. Prescription combinations of hydroquinone, fluocinolone acetonide, and retinoic acid (Tri-Luma) and mequinol and retinoic acid (Solagé) are more effective than their individual components.

RUXOLITINIB

Ruxolitinib (Opzulura) received FDA approval for the treatment of nonsegmental vitiligo in July 2022. (Ruxolitinib has also received FDA approval for atopic dermatitis in September 2021.) This is a Janus kinase inhibitor which should not be used concomitantly with other biologics or potent immunosuppressants. It is approved for adults and children >12 years old. The application area for the treatment of vitiligo should not exceed 10% BSA, with a maximum dose of 60 g per week or 100 g per 2 weeks. There are significant drug interactions with many immunosuppressants (additive immunosuppressive effect), COVID-19 and many other vaccines (immunosuppression affecting vaccine effectiveness), CYP3A4 inhibitors (increasing serum concentration of ruxolitinib), and other drug interactions. Some of these interactions warrant avoidance of concomitant use. Consult drug interaction resources prior to use.

TRIOXSALEN & METHOXSALEN

Trioxsalen and methoxsalen are psoralens used for the repigmentation of vitiligo and psoriasis treatment. With the development of high-intensity long-wave ultraviolet fluorescent lamps, photochemotherapy with oral methoxsalen for psoriasis and with oral trioxsalen for vitiligo has been shown to be effective.

Psoralens must be photoactivated by long-wavelength ultraviolet light in the range of 320–400 nm (ultraviolet A [UVA]) to produce a beneficial effect. Psoralens intercalate with DNA, and with subsequent UVA irradiation, cyclobutane adducts are formed with pyrimidine bases. Both monofunctional and bifunctional adducts may be formed, the latter causing interstrand cross-links. These DNA photoproducts may inhibit DNA synthesis. The major long-term risks of psoralen photochemotherapy are cataracts and skin cancer.

■ SUNSCREENS

Topical sunscreens useful in protecting against sunlight contain either chemical compounds that absorb ultraviolet light or opaque minerals such as titanium dioxide and zinc oxide that reflect light, called sunshades. The three classes of chemical compounds most commonly used in sunscreens are *p*-aminobenzoic acid (PABA) and its esters, the benzophenones, and the dibenzoylmethanes.

Most sunscreen preparations are designed to absorb ultraviolet light in the ultraviolet B (UVB) wavelength range from 280 to 320 nm, which is the range responsible for most of the erythema and sunburn associated with sun exposure and tanning. Chronic exposure to light in this range induces aging of the skin and photocarcinogenesis. Para-aminobenzoic acid and its esters are the most effective available absorbers in the B region, although they do not absorb UVA. In addition, due to their unfavorable safety profile, PABA has been banned from cosmetics in Europe. Ultraviolet in the longer UVA range, 320–400 nm, also is associated with skin aging and cancer. Thus, sunscreen products with UVA and UVB protection and marketed as "broad spectrum" should be selected.

The benzophenones include oxybenzone, dioxybenzone, and sulisobenzone. These compounds provide a broader spectrum of absorption from 250 to 360 nm, but their effectiveness in the UVB erythema range is less than that of PABA. The dibenzoylmethanes include Parsol and Eusolex. These compounds absorb wavelengths throughout the longer UVA range, with maximum absorption at 360 nm. Patients particularly sensitive to UVA wavelengths include individuals with polymorphous light eruption, cutaneous lupus erythematosus, and drug-induced photosensitivity. In these patients, dibenzoylmethane-containing sunscreen may provide improved photoprotection. Ecamsule (Mexoryl) appears to provide greater UVA protection than the dibenzoylmethanes and is less prone to photodegradation.

The sun protection factor (SPF) of a given sunscreen, a measure of its effectiveness in absorbing erythrogenic ultraviolet light, is determined by measuring the minimal erythema dose with and without the sunscreen in a group of normal people. The ratio of the minimal erythema dose with sunscreen to the minimal erythema dose without sunscreen is the SPF.

FDA regulations limit the claimed maximum SPF value on sunscreen labels to 50+ because data are insufficient to show that products with SPF values higher than 50 provide greater protection for users. These regulations require that sunscreens labeled "broad spectrum" pass a standard test comparing the amount of UVA radiation protection in relation to the amount of UVB protection. Broad-spectrum sunscreens with SPF values of 15 or higher help protect against not only sunburn, but also skin cancer and early skin aging when used as directed. Sunscreens with an SPF value between 2 and 14 can only claim that they help prevent sunburn. In addition, products claiming to be water resistant must indicate whether they remain effective for 40 minutes or 80 minutes while swimming or sweating, based on standard testing. These regulations are poorly enforced.

Recent studies showing percutaneous absorption of active ingredients in commercially available sunscreens have prompted the FDA to issue a proposed rule to update regulatory requirements for most sunscreen products in the USA. The FDA recommends continued use of sunscreens while awaiting their evaluation of new safety and effectiveness data.

Environmental studies have demonstrated detrimental effects of sunscreens containing oxybenzone and octinoxate on coral reefs. The use of "reef-friendly" sunscreens containing zinc oxide and titanium dioxide is currently recommended by the US National Park Service to help protect the coral reef ecosystem.

■ ACNE PREPARATIONS

RETINOIC ACID & DERIVATIVES

Retinoic acid, also known as *tretinoin* or all-*trans*-retinoic acid, is the acid form of vitamin A. It is an effective topical treatment for acne vulgaris. Several analogs of vitamin A, eg, 13-*cis*-retinoic acid (isotretinoin), have been shown to be effective in various dermatologic diseases when given orally. Vitamin A alcohol is the physiologic form of vitamin A. The topical therapeutic agent, **retinoic acid,** is formed by the oxidation of the alcohol group, with all four double bonds in the side chain in the *trans* configuration as shown.

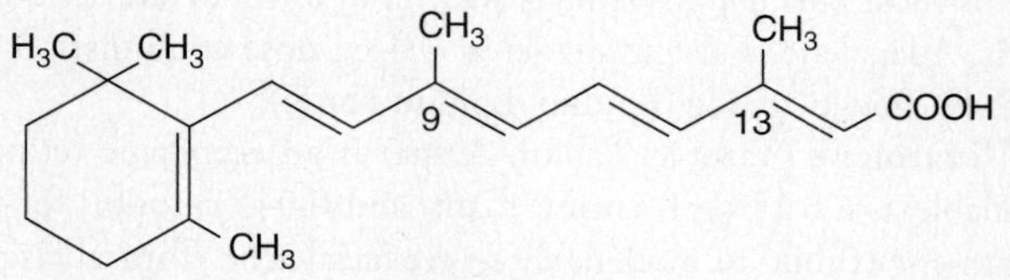

H_3C CH_3 CH_3 CH_3 9 13 COOH CH_3

Retinoic acid

Retinoic acid is insoluble in water but soluble in many organic solvents. Topically applied retinoic acid remains chiefly in the epidermis, with less than 10% absorption into the circulation. The small quantities of retinoic acid absorbed following topical application are metabolized by the liver and excreted in bile and urine.

Retinoic acid has several effects on epithelial tissues. It stabilizes lysosomes, increases ribonucleic acid polymerase activity, increases prostaglandin E_2, cAMP, and cGMP levels, and increases the incorporation of thymidine into DNA. Its action in acne has been attributed to decreased cohesion between epidermal cells and increased epidermal cell turnover. This is thought to result in the expulsion of open comedones and the transformation of closed comedones into open ones.

Topical retinoic acid is applied initially in a concentration sufficient to induce slight erythema with mild peeling. The concentration or frequency of application may be decreased if too much irritation occurs. Topical retinoic acid should be applied to dry skin only, and care should be taken to avoid contact with the corners of the nose, eyes, mouth, and mucous membranes. During the first 4–6 weeks of therapy, comedones not previously evident may appear and give the impression that the acne has been aggravated by the retinoic acid. However, with continued therapy, the lesions will clear, and in 8–12 weeks optimal clinical improvement should occur. A timed-release formulation of tretinoin containing microspheres (Retin-A Micro) delivers the medication over time and may be less irritating for sensitive patients.

The effects of tretinoin on keratinization and desquamation offer benefits for patients with photo-damaged skin. Prolonged use of tretinoin promotes dermal collagen synthesis, new blood vessel formation, and thickening of the epidermis, which helps diminish fine lines and wrinkles. Specially formulated moisturizing 0.05% cream (Renova, Refissa) is marketed for this purpose.

The most common adverse effects of topical retinoic acid are erythema and dryness that occur in the first few weeks of use, but these can be expected to resolve with continued therapy. Animal studies suggest that this drug may increase the tumorigenic potential of ultraviolet radiation. In light of this, patients using retinoic acid should be advised to avoid or minimize sun exposure and use a protective sunscreen. Allergic contact dermatitis to topical retinoic acid is rare.

Adapalene (Differin) is a derivative of naphthoic acid that resembles retinoic acid in structure and effects. It is available for daily application as a 0.1% gel, cream, or lotion and a 0.3% gel. The 0.1% gel has recently been approved by the FDA for over-the-counter sale. Unlike tretinoin, adapalene is photochemically stable and shows little decrease in efficacy when used in combination with benzoyl peroxide. Adapalene is less irritating than tretinoin and is most effective in patients with mild to moderate acne vulgaris. Adapalene is also available in a fixed-dose combination gel with benzoyl peroxide (Epiduo, Epiduo Forte).

Tazarotene (Tazorac, Fabior, Avage) is an acetylenic retinoid available as a 0.1% gel, cream, foam, and 0.045% lotion for the treatment of mild to moderately severe facial acne. Topical tazarotene should be used by women of childbearing age only after contraceptive counseling. It is recommended that tazarotene should not be used by pregnant women.

ISOTRETINOIN

Isotretinoin is a synthetic retinoid currently restricted to the oral treatment of severe cystic acne that is recalcitrant to standard therapies. The precise mechanism of action of isotretinoin in cystic acne is not known, although it appears to act by inhibiting sebaceous gland size and function. The drug is well absorbed, is extensively bound to plasma albumin, and has an elimination half-life of 20–24 hours. A lipid-solubilized formulation, CIP-isotretinoin (as Absorica), provides more consistent absorption and can be taken with or without food.

Start with 0.5 mg/kg/day in two divided doses for 1 month, and then increase to 1 mg/kg/day in two divided doses as tolerated for 4–5 months. Adults with very severe disease/scarring may require up to 2 mg/kg/day. If severe cystic acne persists following this initial treatment, after a period of 2 months, a second course of therapy may be initiated. Common adverse effects resemble hypervitaminosis A and include dryness and itching of the skin and mucous membranes. Less common side effects are headache, corneal opacities, pseudotumor cerebri, inflammatory bowel disease, anorexia, alopecia, and muscle and joint pains. These effects are all reversible on discontinuance of therapy. Skeletal hyperostosis has been observed in patients receiving isotretinoin with premature closure of epiphyses noted in children treated with this medication. Lipid abnormalities (triglycerides, high-density lipoproteins) are frequent, and elevated triglycerides may lead to acute pancreatitis with fatal hemorrhagic pancreatic (rare) reported.

Teratogenicity is a significant risk in patients taking isotretinoin; therefore, the FDA mandates that women of childbearing potential *must* use an effective form of contraception for at least 1 month before, throughout isotretinoin therapy, and for one or more menstrual cycles following discontinuance of treatment. A negative serum pregnancy test *must* be obtained within 2 weeks before starting therapy in these patients, and therapy should be initiated only on the second or third day of the next normal menstrual period. In the USA, health care professionals, pharmacists, and patients must utilize the mandatory iPLEDGE registration and follow-up risk evaluation and mitigation strategy (REMS) program.

BENZOYL PEROXIDE

Benzoyl peroxide, an effective topical agent in acne vulgaris treatment, penetrates the stratum corneum or follicular openings unchanged and is converted metabolically to benzoic acid within the epidermis and dermis. Less than 5% of an applied dose is absorbed from the skin in an 8-hour period. It has been postulated that the mechanism of action of benzoyl peroxide in acne is related to its antimicrobial activity against *P acnes* and to its peeling and comedolytic effects.

To decrease the likelihood of irritation, application should be limited to a low concentration (2.5%) once daily for the first week of therapy and increased in frequency and strength if the preparation is well tolerated. Fixed-combination formulations of 5% benzoyl peroxide with 3% erythromycin base (Benzamycin) or 1% clindamycin (BenzaClin, Duac), 3.75% benzoyl peroxide with 1.2% clindamycin (Onexton), 2.5% benzoyl peroxide with 1.2% clindamycin (Acanya), 2.5% benzoyl peroxide with 0.1% adapalene (Epiduo), and 3% benzoyl peroxide with 0.1% tretinoin (Twyneo) appear to be more effective than individual agents alone.

The FDA has approved a proprietary formulation of 5% benzoyl peroxide cream (Epsolay) for the treatment of inflammatory lesions of rosacea in adults. The benzoyl peroxide is encapsulated within silica-based microcapsules that slowly release the benzoyl peroxide over time, thus providing efficacious treatment with minimal irritation.

Benzoyl peroxide is a potent contact sensitizer in experimental studies, and this adverse effect may occur in up to 1% of acne patients. Care should be taken to avoid contact with the eyes and mucous membranes. Benzoyl peroxide is an oxidant and may rarely cause bleaching of the hair or colored fabrics.

AZELAIC ACID

Azelaic acid is a straight-chain saturated dicarboxylic acid that is effective in the treatment of acne vulgaris (as Azelex) and acne rosacea (as Finacea, Finacea foam). Its mechanism of action has not been fully determined, but preliminary studies demonstrate antimicrobial activity against *P acnes* as well as in vitro inhibitory effects on the conversion of testosterone to dihydrotestosterone. Initial therapy is begun with once-daily applications of the 20% cream, 15% gel, or 15% foam to the affected areas for 1 week and twice-daily applications thereafter. Most patients experience mild irritation with redness and dryness of the skin during the first week of treatment. Clinical improvement is noted in 6–8 weeks of continuous therapy.

BRIMONIDINE & OXYMETAZOLINE

Brimonidine (as Mirvaso), a selective α_2-adrenergic receptor agonist, and oxymetazoline (as Rhofade), a selective α_{1a}-adrenergic receptor agonist, are indicated for the topical treatment of persistent facial erythema of rosacea in adults 18 years of age or older. Daily topical application of brimonidine 0.33% gel or oxymetazoline 1% cream may reduce erythema through direct vasoconstriction. Exacerbation of facial erythema and flushing may occur with brimonidine, ranging from 30 minutes to several hours after application. Alpha-adrenergic agonists may impact blood pressure (see Chapter 11); therefore, brimonidine and oxymetazoline should be used with caution in patients with severe, unstable, or uncontrolled cardiovascular disease.

■ DRUGS FOR PSORIASIS

TAPINAROF

Tapinarof 1% cream (Vtama) was approved by the FDA in 2022 as the first aryl hydrocarbon receptor agonist indicated for the topical treatment of plaque type psoriasis in adults. Tapinarof is a bacteria-derived polyphenol that acts on the aryl hydrocarbon receptor (AHR) and nuclear factor erythroid 2–related factor that protect against inflammatory-induced oxidative damage. This is the first and only steroid-free topical medication in this class.

ACITRETIN

Acitretin (Soriatane), a metabolite of the aromatic retinoid etretinate, is effective in the treatment of psoriasis, especially pustular forms. It is given orally at a dosage of 25–50 mg/d. Adverse effects attributable to acitretin therapy are similar to those seen with isotretinoin and resemble hypervitaminosis A. Elevations in cholesterol and triglycerides may be noted with acitretin, and hepatotoxicity with fatal hepatitis has been reported. Liver enzyme elevations occur in up to one-third of patients and generally require drug discontinuation. Monitor for hepatotoxicity. Acitretin is more teratogenic than isotretinoin in the animal species studied to date, which is of special concern in view of the drug's prolonged elimination time (more than 3 months) after chronic administration. In cases where etretinate is formed by concomitant administration of acitretin and ethanol, etretinate may be found in plasma and subcutaneous fat for many years.

Acitretin must not be used by women who are pregnant or may become pregnant while undergoing treatment or at any time for at least 3 years after treatment is discontinued. Patients must commit to using two effective forms of birth control starting 1 month prior to acitretin treatment and for 3 years after discontinuation. In the USA, prescribers should use the Do Your P.A.R.T. program. Ethanol must be strictly avoided during treatment with acitretin and for 2 months after discontinuing therapy. Patients must not donate blood during treatment and for 3 years after acitretin is stopped.

TAZAROTENE

Tazarotene (Tazorac) is a topical acetylenic retinoid prodrug that is hydrolyzed to its active form by an esterase. The active metabolite, tazarotenic acid, binds to retinoic acid receptors, resulting in modified gene expression. The precise mechanism of action in psoriasis is unknown but may relate to both anti-inflammatory and antiproliferative actions. Tazarotene is absorbed percutaneously, and teratogenic systemic concentrations may be achieved if applied to more than 20% of total body surface area. Women of childbearing potential must therefore be advised of the risk prior to initiating therapy, and adequate birth control measures must be utilized while on therapy.

Treatment of psoriasis should be limited to once-daily application of either 0.05% or 0.1% cream or gel, with the gel not to exceed 20% of total body surface area used in patients 12 years and older. The 0.05% or 0.1% cream is for use in patients 18 years and older. Adverse local effects include a burning or stinging sensation (sensory irritation) and peeling, erythema, and localized edema of the skin (irritant dermatitis). Potentiation of photosensitizing medication may occur, and patients should be cautioned to minimize sunlight exposure and to use sunscreens and protective clothing. Tazarotene is also available in a fixed-drug combination with halobetasol propionate (Duobrii).

CALCIPOTRIENE & CALCITRIOL

Calcipotriene and calcitriol are vitamin D analogs that are considered first-line treatments for mild to moderate psoriasis, especially in pediatric patients. Calcipotriene (as Dovonex, Sorilux) is a synthetic vitamin D_3 derivative (available as a 0.005% ointment, cream, scalp lotion, and foam) that is effective in the treatment of plaque-type psoriasis vulgaris of mild to moderate severity. Improvement of psoriasis is generally noted following 2 weeks of therapy, with continued improvement for up to 8 weeks of treatment. Adverse effects include burning, itching, and mild irritation, with dryness and erythema of the treatment area. Care should be

TABLE 61–2 Biologic agents for psoriasis.

Biologic Agents	Brand Names
TNF-α inhibitors	
Adalimumab	Cyltezo, Humira
Certolizumab	Cimzia
Etanercept	Enbrel, Erelzi
Infliximab	Ixifi, Remicade, Renflexis
IL-17 & IL-17A inhibitors	
Brodalumab	Siliq
Ixekizumab	Taltz
Secukinumab	Cosentyx
IL-23 inhibitors	
Guselkumab	Tremfya
Risankizumab	Skyrizi
Tildrakizumab	Ilumya
IL-12 & IL-23 inhibitors	
Ustekinumab	Stelara

taken to avoid facial contact, which may cause ocular irritation. A once-daily two-compound ointment (as Taclonex) or foam (as Enstilar) containing calcipotriene and betamethasone dipropionate are available. This combination is more effective than its individual ingredients and is well tolerated, with a safety profile similar to betamethasone dipropionate.

Calcitriol (as Vectical) contains 1,25-dihydroxycholecalciferol, the hormonally active form of vitamin D_3. Calcitriol 3-mcg/g ointment is similar in efficacy to calcipotriene 0.005% ointment for the treatment of plaque-type psoriasis on the body and is better tolerated in intertriginous and sensitive areas of the skin. Clinical studies show comparable safety data regarding adverse cutaneous and systemic reactions between topical calcitriol and calcipotriene ointment.

BIOLOGIC AGENTS

Biologic agents useful in treating adult patients with moderate to severe chronic plaque psoriasis include the TNF-α inhibitors adalimumab, etanercept, infliximab, and certolizumab, and various types of cytokine inhibitors including the IL-17 inhibitors ixekizumab, secukinumab, and brodalumab, the IL-12 & IL-23 inhibitor ustekinumab, the IL-23 inhibitors guselkumab, tildrakizumab, and risankizumab (Table 61–2), and other agents on the horizon. The pharmacology of these agents is discussed in Chapters 36 and 55.

SELECTIVE PHOSPHODIESTERASE 4 (PDE-4) INHIBITORS: APREMILAST & CRISABOROLE

Apremilast (as Otezla) is an oral phosphodiesterase 4 (PDE-4) inhibitor that is effective in treating moderate to severe plaque psoriasis, and crisaborole is a topical PDE-4 inhibitor FDA-approved for treatment of mild to moderate atopic dermatitis (AD) in adults and children 3 months of age or older. Cyclic nucleotide PDEs break down cAMP into inactive metabolites. There is increased PDE activity in AD creating a proinflammatory state that results in increased inflammatory mediators. PDE-4 inhibitors inhibit the increased PDE activity. Initial dosage titration of apremilast from day 1 to day 5, intended to reduce the gastrointestinal symptoms associated with starting therapy, is shown in Table 61–3. Following the 5-day titration, a maintenance dose of 30 mg twice daily is started on day 6.

Adverse effects for apremilast include severe diarrhea, nausea, vomiting, depression, suicidal ideation, mood changes, and weight loss, and it should be used with caution in renal impairment with appropriate dose reductions. Patients should have their weight monitored regularly due to possible weight loss associated with therapy. Use of cytochrome P450 enzyme inducers (see Chapter 4) may result in a loss of efficacy and is not recommended. Apremilast is generally well tolerated, with mild gastrointestinal complaints occurring early in the course of treatment and resolving with time.

Crisaborole (Eucrisa) is applied topically twice daily (not for ophthalmic, oral or intravaginal use), and adverse effects are limited to local application site pain and hypersensitivity-type reactions such as urticaria and allergic contact dermatitis.

Roflumilast 0.3% cream (Zoryve) is the first topical PDE-4 inhibitor approved by the FDA for the treatment of mild, moderate, and severe plaque psoriasis for patients age 12 years or older. The cream should be applied once daily to the affected areas with no limitation on the duration of use. This steroid-free cream is particularly useful for the treatment of intertriginous psoriasis.

FUMARIC ACID ESTERS

Fumaric acid esters are licensed in Germany (as Fumaderm) and the EU (as Skilarence) for the oral treatment of psoriasis. They are considered homeopathic treatment in the USA and are not approved or regulated by the FDA for the treatment of psoriasis. Dimethyl fumarate (Tecfidera) and diroximel fumarate (Vumerity) are fumaric acid derivatives approved by the FDA for treatment of multiple sclerosis (see Chapter 55). The mechanism of action of dimethyl fumarate in psoriasis may be due to immunomodulatory

TABLE 61–3 Apremilast dosage titration schedule.

Day 1	Day 2		Day 3		Day 4		Day 5		Day 6 & Thereafter	
AM	AM	PM	AM	PM	AM	PM	AM	PM	AM	PM
10 mg	10 mg	10 mg	10 mg	20 mg	20 mg	20 mg	20 mg	30 mg	30 mg	30 mg

effects on lymphocytes and keratinocytes, resulting in a shift away from a psoriatic cytokine profile. Note that several cases of progressive multifocal leukoencephalopathy have been reported in psoriasis patients treated with fumaric acid esters.

ANTI-INFLAMMATORY AGENTS

TOPICAL CORTICOSTEROIDS

The remarkable efficacy of topical corticosteroids in the treatment of inflammatory dermatoses was noted soon after the introduction of hydrocortisone in 1952. Numerous analogs are now available that offer extensive choices of potencies, concentrations, and vehicles. The therapeutic effectiveness of topical corticosteroids is based primarily on their anti-inflammatory activity. Definitive explanations of the effects of corticosteroids on endogenous mediators of inflammation await further experimental clarification. The antimitotic effects of corticosteroids on human epidermis may account for an additional mechanism of action in psoriasis and other dermatologic diseases associated with increased cell turnover. The general pharmacology of these endocrine agents is discussed in Chapter 39.

Chemistry & Pharmacokinetics

The original topical glucocorticosteroid was hydrocortisone, the natural glucocorticosteroid of the adrenal cortex. The 9α-fluoro derivative of hydrocortisone was active topically, but its salt-retaining properties made it undesirable even for topical use. Prednisolone and methylprednisolone are as active topically as hydrocortisone (Table 61–4). The 9α-fluorinated steroids

TABLE 61–4 Relative efficacy of some topical corticosteroids in various formulations.

Concentration in Commonly Used Preparations	Drug	Concentration in Commonly Used Preparations	Drug
Lowest efficacy		**Intermediate efficacy**	
0.25–2.5%	Hydrocortisone	0.05%	Fluticasone propionate (Cutivate)
0.25%	Methylprednisolone acetate (Medrol)	0.05%	Desonide (Desowen)
0.1%	Dexamethasone[1] (Decaderm)	0.025%	Halcinonide[1] (Halog)
1.0%	Methylprednisolone acetate (Medrol)	0.05%	Desoximetasone[1] (Topicort L.P.)
0.5%	Prednisolone (MetiDerm)	0.05%	Flurandrenolide[1] (Cordran)
0.2%	Betamethasone[1] (Celestone)	0.1%	Triamcinolone acetonide[1]
Low efficacy		0.025%	Fluocinolone acetonide[1]
0.01%	Fluocinolone acetonide[1] (Fluonid, Synalar)	**High efficacy**	
0.01%	Betamethasone valerate[1] (Valisone)	0.05%	Fluocinonide[1] (Lidex)
0.025%	Fluorometholone[1] (Oxylone)	0.05%	Betamethasone dipropionate[1] (Diprosone, Maxivate)
0.05%	Alclometasone dipropionate (Aclovate)	0.1%	Amcinonide[1] (Cyclocort)
0.025%	Triamcinolone acetonide[1] (Aristocort, Kenalog, Triacet)	0.25%	Desoximetasone[1] (Topicort)
0.1%	Clocortolone pivalate[1] (Cloderm)	0.5%	Triamcinolone acetonide[1]
0.03%	Flumethasone pivalate[1] (Locorten)	0.2%	Fluocinolone acetonide[1] (Synalar-HP)
Intermediate efficacy		0.05%	Diflorasone diacetate[1] (Florone, Maxiflor)
0.2%	Hydrocortisone valerate (Westcort)	0.1%	Halcinonide[1] (Halog)
0.1%	Mometasone furoate (Elocon)	**Highest efficacy**	
0.1%	Hydrocortisone butyrate (Locoid)	0.05%	Betamethasone dipropionate in optimized vehicle (Diprolene)[1]
0.1%	Hydrocortisone probutate (Pandel)		
0.025%	Betamethasone benzoate[1] (Uticort)	0.05%	Diflorasone diacetate[1] in optimized vehicle (Psorcon)
0.025%	Flurandrenolide[1] (Cordran)		
0.1%	Betamethasone valerate[1] (Valisone)	0.05%	Halobetasol propionate[1] (Ultravate)
0.1%	Prednicarbate (Dermatop)	0.05%	Clobetasol propionate[1] (Temovate)

[1]Fluorinated steroids.

Other corticosteroid potency tables are available. See under Drugs for Psoriasis references.

dexamethasone and betamethasone did not have any advantage over hydrocortisone. However, triamcinolone and fluocinolone, the acetonide derivatives of the fluorinated steroids, do have a distinct efficacy advantage in topical therapy. Similarly, betamethasone is not very active topically, but attaching a 5-carbon valerate chain to the 17-hydroxyl position results in a compound (betamethasone valerate) more than 300 times as active as hydrocortisone for topical use. Fluocinonide is the 21-acetate derivative of fluocinolone acetonide; the addition of the 21-acetate enhances the topical activity about fivefold. Fluorination of the corticoid is not required for high potency.

Corticosteroids are only minimally absorbed following application to normal skin; for example, approximately 1% of a dose of hydrocortisone solution applied to the ventral forearm is absorbed. Long-term occlusion with an impermeable film such as plastic wrap is an effective method of enhancing penetration, yielding a 10-fold increase in absorption. There is a marked regional anatomic variation in corticosteroid penetration. Compared with the absorption from the forearm, hydrocortisone is absorbed 0.14 times as well through the plantar foot arch, 0.83 times as well through the palm, 3.5 times as well through the scalp, 6 times as well through the forehead, 9 times as well through vulvar skin, and 42 times as well through scrotal skin. Penetration is increased severalfold in the inflamed skin of atopic dermatitis, and in severe exfoliative diseases, such as erythrodermic psoriasis, there appears to be little barrier to penetration.

Experimental studies on the percutaneous absorption of hydrocortisone fail to reveal a significant increase in absorption when applied on a repetitive basis, and a single daily application may be effective in most conditions. Ointment bases tend to give better activity to the corticosteroid than do cream or lotion vehicles. Increasing the concentration of a corticosteroid increases the penetration but not proportionately. For example, approximately 1% of a 0.25% hydrocortisone solution is absorbed from the forearm. A 10-fold increase in concentration causes only a fourfold increase in absorption. Solubility of the corticosteroid in the vehicle is a significant determinant of the percutaneous absorption of a topical steroid. Marked increases in efficacy are noted when optimized vehicles are used, as demonstrated by newer formulations of betamethasone dipropionate and diflorasone diacetate.

Table 61–4 groups topical corticosteroid formulations according to approximate relative efficacy. Table 61–5 lists major dermatologic diseases in order of their responsiveness to these drugs. In the first group of diseases, low- to medium-efficacy corticosteroid preparations often produce clinical remission. In the second group, it is often necessary to use high-efficacy preparations, occlusion therapy, or both. Once a remission has been achieved, every effort should be made to maintain the improvement with a low-efficacy corticosteroid.

The limited penetration of topical corticosteroids can be overcome in certain clinical circumstances by the intralesional injection of relatively insoluble corticosteroids, eg, triamcinolone acetonide, triamcinolone diacetate, triamcinolone hexacetonide, and betamethasone acetate-phosphate. When these agents are injected into the lesion, measurable amounts remain in place and are gradually released for 3–4 weeks. This form of therapy is often effective for the lesions listed in Table 61–5 that are generally unresponsive to topical corticosteroids. The dosage of the triamcinolone salts should be limited to 1 mg per treatment site, ie, 0.1 mL of 10 mg/mL suspension, to decrease the incidence of local atrophy.

TABLE 61–5 Dermatologic disorders responsive to topical corticosteroids ranked in order of sensitivity.

Very responsive
Atopic dermatitis
Seborrheic dermatitis
Lichen simplex chronicus
Pruritus ani
Later phase of allergic contact dermatitis
Later phase of irritant dermatitis
Nummular eczematous dermatitis
Stasis dermatitis
Psoriasis, especially of genitalia and face
Less responsive
Discoid lupus erythematosus
Psoriasis of palms and soles
Necrobiosis lipoidica diabeticorum
Sarcoidosis
Lichen striatus
Pemphigus
Familial benign pemphigus
Pemphigoid
Vitiligo
Granuloma annulare
Least responsive: Intralesional injection required
Keloids
Hypertrophic scars
Hypertrophic lichen planus
Alopecia areata
Acne cysts
Prurigo nodularis
Chondrodermatitis nodularis chronica helicis

Adverse Effects

All absorbable topical corticosteroids possess the potential to suppress the hypothalamic-pituitary-adrenal (HPA) axis (see Chapter 39). Although most patients with HPA-axis suppression demonstrate only a laboratory test abnormality, cases of severely impaired stress response can occur. Iatrogenic Cushing syndrome may occur as a result of protracted use of topical corticosteroids in large quantities. Applying potent corticosteroids to extensive areas of the body for prolonged periods, with or without occlusion, increases the likelihood of systemic effects. Fewer of these factors are required to produce adverse systemic effects in children, and growth retardation is of particular concern in the pediatric age group.

Adverse local effects of topical corticosteroids include the following: atrophy, which may present as depressed, shiny, often wrinkled "cigarette paper"–appearing skin with prominent telangiectases and a tendency to develop purpura and ecchymosis; corticoid rosacea, with persistent erythema, telangiectatic vessels, pustules, and papules in central facial distribution; perioral dermatitis, steroid acne, alterations of cutaneous infections, hypopigmentation, and hypertrichosis; increased intraocular pressure; and allergic contact dermatitis. The latter may be confirmed by patch testing with high concentrations of corticosteroids, ie, 1% in petrolatum, because topical corticosteroids are not irritating. Screening for allergic contact dermatitis potential is performed with tixocortol pivalate, budesonide, and hydrocortisone valerate or butyrate. Topical corticosteroids are contraindicated in individuals who demonstrate hypersensitivity to them. Some sensitized subjects develop a generalized flare when dosed with adrenocorticotropic hormone or oral prednisone. Systemic corticosteroid use is discussed in Chapter 39.

CRISABOROLE

Crisaborole (as Eucrisa) is a benzoxaborole, nonsteroidal, topical, anti-inflammatory PDE4 inhibitor approved as a 2% ointment for the treatment of mild-to-moderate atopic dermatitis in patients 2 years of age and older. The most frequent adverse effect is burning or stinging at the site of application. The specific mechanism of action in atopic dermatitis is unknown. Recent studies have shown a favorable safety profile for the long-term treatment of atopic dermatitis.

TAR COMPOUNDS

Tar preparations are used mainly in the treatment of psoriasis, dermatitis, and lichen simplex chronicus. The phenolic constituents endow these compounds with antipruritic properties, making them particularly valuable in the treatment of chronic lichenified dermatitis. Acute dermatitis with vesiculation and oozing may be irritated by even weak tar preparations, which should be avoided. However, in the subacute and chronic stages of dermatitis and psoriasis, these preparations are quite useful and offer an alternative to the use of topical corticosteroids.

The most common adverse reaction to coal tar compounds is an irritant folliculitis, necessitating discontinuance of therapy to the affected areas for a period of 3–5 days. Photo-irritation and allergic contact dermatitis also may occur. Tar preparations should be avoided in patients who have previously exhibited sensitivity to them.

■ KERATOLYTIC & DESTRUCTIVE AGENTS

SALICYLIC ACID

Salicylic acid has been extensively used in dermatologic therapy as a keratolytic agent. The mechanism by which it produces its keratolytic and other therapeutic effects is poorly understood. The drug may solubilize cell surface proteins that keep the stratum corneum intact, thereby resulting in desquamation of keratotic debris. Salicylic acid is keratolytic in concentrations of 3–6%. In concentrations greater than 6%, it can be destructive to tissues.

COOH
OH

Salicylic acid

Salicylism and death have occurred following topical application. In an adult, 1 g of a topically applied 6% salicylic acid preparation will raise the serum salicylate level not more than 0.5 mg/dL of plasma; the threshold for toxicity is 30–50 mg/dL. Higher serum levels are possible in children, who are therefore at a greater risk for salicylism. In cases of severe intoxication, hemodialysis is the treatment of choice (see Chapter 58). It is advisable to limit both the total amount of salicylic acid applied and the frequency of application. Urticarial, anaphylactic, and erythema multiforme reactions may occur in patients who are allergic to salicylates. Topical use may be associated with local irritation, acute inflammation, and even ulceration with the use of high concentrations of salicylic acid. Particular care must be exercised when using the drug on the extremities of patients with diabetes or peripheral vascular disease.

HYDROGEN PEROXIDE

Hydrogen peroxide 40% topical solution (as Eskata) is approved for the treatment of raised seborrheic keratosis. Because this concentrated solution is caustic, it is to be applied only by health care providers. Direct contact with the eye can result in permanent eye injury including blindness. Treating seborrheic keratosis within the orbital rim is contraindicated. Severe local skin reactions include erosion, ulceration, and scarring. It should not be applied to open or infected seborrheic keratosis.

PROPYLENE GLYCOL

Propylene glycol is used extensively in topical preparations because it is an excellent vehicle for organic compounds. It has been used alone as a keratolytic agent in 40–70% concentrations, with plastic occlusion, or in gel with 6% salicylic acid.

Only minimal amounts of a topically applied dose are absorbed through normal stratum corneum. Percutaneously absorbed propylene glycol is oxidized by the liver to lactic acid and pyruvic acid, with subsequent utilization in general body metabolism. Approximately 12–45% of the absorbed agent is excreted unchanged in the urine.

Propylene glycol is an effective keratolytic agent for the removal of hyperkeratotic debris. It is also an effective humectant and increases the water content of the stratum corneum. The hygroscopic characteristics of propylene glycol may help it to develop an osmotic gradient through the stratum corneum, thereby increasing hydration of the outermost layers by drawing water out from the inner layers of the skin.

Propylene glycol is used under polyethylene occlusion or with 6% salicylic acid for the treatment of ichthyosis, palmar and plantar keratodermas, psoriasis, pityriasis rubra pilaris, keratosis pilaris, and hypertrophic lichen planus.

In concentrations greater than 10%, propylene glycol may act as an irritant in some patients; those with eczematous dermatitis may be more sensitive. Allergic contact dermatitis occurs with propylene glycol, and a 4% aqueous propylene glycol solution is recommended for the purpose of patch testing.

UREA

Urea in a compatible cream vehicle or ointment base has a softening and moisturizing effect on the stratum corneum. It has the ability to make creams and lotions feel less greasy, and this has been utilized in dermatologic preparations to decrease the oily feel of a preparation that otherwise might feel unpleasant. It is a white crystalline powder with a slight ammonia odor when moist.

Urea is absorbed percutaneously, although the amount absorbed is minimal. It is distributed predominantly in the extracellular space and excreted in urine. Urea is a natural product of metabolism, and systemic toxicities with topical application do not occur.

Urea increases the water content of the stratum corneum, presumably as a result of the hygroscopic characteristics of this naturally occurring molecule. Urea is also keratolytic. The mechanism of action appears to involve alterations in prekeratin and keratin, leading to increased solubilization. In addition, urea may break hydrogen bonds that keep the stratum corneum intact.

As a humectant, urea is used in concentrations of 2–20% in creams and lotions. As a keratolytic agent, it is used in 20% concentration in diseases such as ichthyosis vulgaris, hyperkeratosis of palms and soles, xerosis, and keratosis pilaris. Concentrations of 30–50% applied to the nail plate have been useful in softening the nail prior to avulsion.

PODOPHYLLUM RESIN & PODOFILOX

Podophyllum resin (Podocon-25, Podocon), an alcoholic extract of *Podophyllum peltatum*, commonly known as mandrake root or May apple, is used in the treatment of condyloma acuminatum and other verrucae. It is a mixture of podophyllotoxin, α and β peltatin, deoxypodophyllotoxin, dehydropodophyllotoxin, and other compounds. It is soluble in alcohol, ether, chloroform, and compound tincture of benzoin.

Percutaneous absorption of podophyllum resin occurs, particularly in intertriginous areas and from applications to large moist condylomas. It is soluble in lipids and therefore is distributed widely throughout the body, including the central nervous system.

The major use of podophyllum resin is in the treatment of condyloma acuminatum. Podophyllotoxin and its derivatives are active cytotoxic agents with specific affinity for the microtubule protein of the mitotic spindle. Normal assembly of the spindle is prevented, and epidermal mitoses are arrested in metaphase. A 25% concentration of podophyllum resin in compound tincture of benzoin is recommended for the treatment of condyloma acuminatum. Podophyllum resin is currently not recommended by the CDC for treatment of external genital warts due to reports of systemic toxicity if applied incorrectly (safer agents are available). Application should be by physician and restricted to wart tissue only, to limit the total amount of medication used and to prevent severe erosive changes in adjacent tissue. In treating cases of large condylomas, it is advisable to limit application to sections of the affected area to minimize systemic absorption. The patient is instructed to wash off the preparation 30–40 minutes after the initial application to test patient sensitivity, as the irritant reaction is variable. Depending on the individual patient's reaction, this period can be extended to 1–4 hours on subsequent applications. If three to five applications have not resulted in significant resolution, other methods of treatment should be considered. This drug is *not* to be used on bleeding warts, warts with hair growth, or moles and birthmarks.

Toxic symptoms associated with excessively large applications include nausea, vomiting, alterations in sensorium, muscle weakness, neuropathy with diminished tendon reflexes, coma, and even death. Local irritation is common, and inadvertent contact with the eye may cause severe conjunctivitis. Use during pregnancy is contraindicated in view of possible cytotoxic effects on the fetus.

Pure podophyllotoxin (podofilox) is approved for use as either a 0.5% solution or gel (Condylox) for application by the patient in the treatment of genital condylomas. The low concentration of podofilox significantly reduces the potential for systemic toxicity. Most men with penile warts may be treated with less than 70 μL per application. At this dose, podofilox is not routinely detected in the serum. Treatment is self-administered in treatment cycles of twice-daily application for 3 consecutive days followed by a 4-day drug-free period. This cycle may be repeated up to four times until there is no visible wart tissue. Local adverse effects include inflammation, erosions, burning pain, and itching.

SINECATECHINS

Sinecatechins 15% ointment (Veregen) is a prescription botanical drug product of a partially purified fraction of the water extract of green tea leaves from *Camellia sinensis* containing a mixture of catechins. Sinecatechins ointment is indicated for the topical treatment of external genital and perianal warts in immunocompetent patients 18 years and older. The mechanism of action is unknown. Sinecatechins ointment should be applied three times daily to the warts until complete clearance, not to exceed 16 weeks of therapy.

■ DRUGS FOR ACTINIC KERATOSES

FLUOROURACIL

Fluorouracil is a fluorinated pyrimidine antimetabolite that resembles uracil, with a fluorine atom substituted for the 5-methyl group. Its systemic pharmacology is described in Chapter 54. Fluorouracil is used topically for the treatment of multiple actinic or solar keratoses and superficial basal cell carcinoma.

Approximately 6% of a topically applied dose is absorbed—an amount insufficient to produce adverse systemic effects. Most of the absorbed drug is metabolized and excreted as carbon dioxide, urea, and α-fluoro-β-alanine. A small percentage is eliminated unchanged in the urine. Fluorouracil inhibits thymidylate synthetase activity, interfering with the synthesis of DNA and, to a lesser extent, RNA. These effects are most marked in atypical, rapidly proliferating cells.

Fluorouracil is available in multiple formulations containing 0.5%, 1%, 2%, 4%, and 5% concentrations (as Carac, Efudex, Fluoroplex, Tolak). The response to treatment begins with erythema and progresses through vesiculation, erosion, superficial ulceration, necrosis, and finally reepithelialization. Fluorouracil should be continued until the inflammatory reaction reaches the stage of ulceration and necrosis, usually in 3–4 weeks, at which time treatment should be terminated. The healing process may continue for 1–2 months after therapy is discontinued. Local adverse reactions may include pain, pruritus, a burning sensation, tenderness, and residual postinflammatory hyperpigmentation. Excessive exposure to sunlight during treatment may increase the intensity of the reaction and should be avoided. Allergic contact dermatitis to fluorouracil has been reported, and its use is contraindicated in patients with known hypersensitivity or in pregnancy, as birth defects and miscarriage have been reported after topical application to mucous membranes in pregnant women.

TIRBANIBULIN

Tirbanibulin 1% ointment (Klisyri) is a synthetic, first-in-class antiproliferative agent that disrupts Src kinase signaling and inhibits tubulin polymerization. This results in significant activity against keratinocyte growth and offers a new topical field therapy for actinic keratosis. The mechanism of action of tirbanibulin for the topical treatment of actinic keratosis is unknown. Treatment requires once-daily application on face or scalp for 5 consecutive days with a sufficient amount of 1% ointment to cover up to 25 cm^2 of contiguous skin using one single single-dose packet per application. Particular care should be taken to avoid transfer of the drug into the eyes and periocular area during and after application. Patients should be instructed to wash their hands immediately after application. If accidental ocular exposure does occur, patients should immediately flush their eyes with water and seek medical care as soon as possible.

NONSTEROIDAL ANTI-INFLAMMATORY DRUGS

A topical 3% gel formulation of the nonsteroidal anti-inflammatory drug diclofenac (as Solaraze) has shown moderate effectiveness in the treatment of actinic keratoses. The mechanism of action is unknown. As with other NSAIDs, anaphylactoid reactions may occur with diclofenac, and it should be given with caution to patients with known aspirin hypersensitivity (see Chapter 36).

AMINOLEVULINIC ACID

Aminolevulinic acid (ALA) is an endogenous precursor of photosensitizing porphyrin metabolites (Table 61–6). When exogenous ALA is provided to the cell through topical applications, protoporphyrin IX (PpIX) accumulates in the cell. When exposed to light of appropriate wavelength and energy, the accumulated PpIX produces a photodynamic reaction resulting in the formation of cytotoxic superoxide and hydroxyl radicals. The basis for ALA photodynamic therapy is photosensitization of actinic keratoses using either ALA (as Levulan Kerastick) and illumination with a blue light photodynamic therapy illuminator (BLU-U) or ALA nanoemulsion gel (as Ameluz) and illumination with a narrow-band red light photodynamic therapy illuminator (BF-RhodoLED).

Treatment consists of applying ALA 20% topical solution to individual actinic keratoses followed by blue light photodynamic illumination 14–18 hours later. Transient stinging or burning at the treatment site occurs during the period of light exposure. Patients *must* avoid exposure to sunlight or bright indoor lights for at least 40 hours after ALA application. Redness, swelling, and crusting of the actinic keratoses will occur and gradually resolve over a 3- to 4-week time course. Allergic contact dermatitis to methyl ester may occur.

■ ANTIPRURITIC AGENTS

DOXEPIN

Topical doxepin hydrochloride 5% cream (as Zonalon, Prudoxin) may provide significant antipruritic activity when utilized in the treatment of pruritus associated with atopic dermatitis or lichen simplex chronicus. The precise mechanism of action is unknown but may relate to the potent H_1- and H_2-receptor antagonist properties of dibenzoxepin tricyclic compounds. Percutaneous absorption is variable and may result in significant drowsiness in some patients. In view of the anticholinergic effect of doxepin, topical use is contraindicated in patients with untreated narrow-angle glaucoma or a tendency to urinary retention. In view of the fact that doxepin is a tricyclic antidepressant, drug-induced QT prolongation and torsade de pointes are of concern especially in susceptible patients.

TABLE 61–6 Aminolevulinic acid (ALA) formulations.

Name	Formulation	Time between Application and PDT*	PDT Light Color	PDT Duration
Ameluz	10% gel	3 hours	Red (~635 nm)	10 minutes
Levulan Kerastick	20% solution	14–18 hours	Blue (~410 nm)	16.7 minutes

*PDT, photodynamic therapy.

Plasma levels of doxepin similar to those achieved during oral therapy may be obtained with topical application; the usual drug interactions associated with tricyclic antidepressants may occur. Therefore, monoamine oxidase inhibitors must be discontinued at least 2 weeks prior to the initiation of doxepin cream. Topical application of the cream should be performed four times daily for up to 8 days of therapy. The safety and efficacy of chronic dosing have not been established. Adverse local effects include marked burning and stinging of the treatment site, which may necessitate discontinuation of the cream in some patients. Allergic contact dermatitis appears to be frequent, and patients should be monitored for symptoms of hypersensitivity.

PRAMOXINE

Pramoxine hydrochloride is a topical anesthetic that can provide temporary relief from pruritus associated with mild eczematous dermatoses. Pramoxine is available as a 1% cream, lotion, or gel and in combination with hydrocortisone acetate. Application to the affected area two to four times daily may provide short-term relief of pruritus. Local adverse effects include transient burning and stinging. Care should be exercised to avoid contact with the eyes.

■ ANTISEBORRHEA AGENTS

Table 61–7 lists topical formulations for the treatment of seborrheic dermatitis. These are of variable efficacy and may necessitate concomitant treatment with topical corticosteroids for severe cases.

TABLE 61–7 Antiseborrhea agents.

Active Ingredient	Typical Trade Name
Betamethasone valerate foam	Luxiq
Chloroxine shampoo	Capitrol
Coal tar shampoo	Ionil-T, Pentrax, Theraplex-T, T-Gel
Fluocinolone acetonide shampoo	FS Shampoo
Ketoconazole shampoo and gel	Nizoral, Xolegel
Selenium sulfide shampoo	Selsun, Exsel
Zinc pyrithione shampoo	DHS-Zinc, Theraplex-Z

■ TRICHOGENIC & ANTITRICHOGENIC AGENTS

BARICITINIB

Once-daily oral baricitinib (Olumiant) received FDA approval in 2022 as a first-in-disease systemic treatment for adults with severe alopecia areata. Baricitinib is a selective inhibitor of Janus kinase (JAK) JAK1 and JAK2. It is available as 1-mg, 2-mg, and 4-mg tablets. In keeping with the JAK inhibitor class of drugs, baricitinib has a boxed warning for serious infections, malignancy, mortality, adverse cardiovascular events, and thrombosis.

MINOXIDIL

Topical minoxidil (as Rogaine) is effective in reversing the progressive miniaturization of terminal scalp hairs associated with androgenic alopecia. Vertex balding is more responsive to therapy than frontal balding. The mechanism of action of minoxidil on hair follicles is unknown. Chronic dosing studies have demonstrated that the effect of minoxidil is not permanent, and cessation of treatment will lead to hair loss in 4–6 months. Percutaneous absorption of minoxidil in normal scalp is minimal, but possible systemic effects on blood pressure (see Chapter 11) should be monitored in patients with cardiac disease. Adverse effects include transient (weeks to months) hair shedding, which is an indication that minoxidil is stimulating new hair growth and therapy should not be stopped for this reason. Irritant and contact dermatitis may occur.

Topical minoxidil is available as a 2% or 5% solution, with the 5% recommended for men due to greater efficacy; only the 2% lotion is approved for use in women with androgenetic alopecia.

FINASTERIDE

Finasteride (Propecia) is a 5α-reductase inhibitor that blocks the conversion of testosterone to dihydrotestosterone (see Chapter 40), the androgen responsible for androgenic alopecia in genetically predisposed men. Oral finasteride, 1 mg/d, promotes hair growth and prevents further hair loss in a significant proportion of men with androgenic alopecia. Treatment for at least 3–6 months is necessary to see increased hair growth or prevent further hair loss. Continued treatment with finasteride is necessary to sustain benefit. Reported adverse effects include decreased libido, ejaculation disorders, and erectile dysfunction, which resolve in most men who remain on therapy and in all men who discontinue finasteride. Other adverse effects include orthostatic hypotension and dizziness.

There are no data to support the use of finasteride in women with androgenic alopecia. Pregnant women should not be exposed to finasteride either by use or by handling crushed tablets because of the risk of hypospadias developing in a male fetus.

BIMATOPROST

Bimatoprost (as Latisse) is a prostaglandin analog available as a 0.03% ophthalmic solution to treat hypotrichosis of the eyelashes. Mechanism of action is unknown. Treatment consists of nightly application to the skin of the upper eyelid margins at the base of the eyelashes using a separate disposable applicator for each eyelid. Contact lenses should be removed prior to bimatoprost application. Side effects include pruritus, conjunctival hyperemia, skin pigmentation, and erythema of the eyelids. Although iris darkening has not been reported with applications confined to the upper eyelid skin, increased brown iris pigmentation, which is likely to be permanent, has occurred when bimatoprost ophthalmic solution was instilled onto the eye for glaucoma.

EFLORNITHINE

Eflornithine (as Vaniqa) is an irreversible inhibitor of ornithine decarboxylase, which catalyzes the rate-limiting step in the biosynthesis of polyamines. Polyamines are required for cell division and differentiation, and inhibition of ornithine decarboxylase affects the rate of hair growth. Topical eflornithine has been shown effective in reducing facial hair growth in approximately 30% of women when applied twice daily for 6 months of therapy. Hair growth was observed to return to pretreatment levels 8 weeks after discontinuation. Local adverse effects include stinging, burning, and folliculitis.

ANTINEOPLASTIC AGENTS

The treatment of melanoma is discussed in Chapter 54. 5-fluorouracil is discussed under Drugs for Actinic Keratoses.

Alitretinoin (Panretin) is a topical formulation of 9-*cis*-retinoic acid that is approved for the treatment of cutaneous lesions in patients with AIDS-related Kaposi sarcoma. Localized reactions may include intense erythema, edema, and vesiculation necessitating discontinuation of therapy. Patients who are applying alitretinoin should not concurrently use products containing DEET, a common component of insect repellant products.

Bexarotene (as Targretin), a member of a subclass of retinoids that selectively binds and activates retinoid X receptor subtypes, is available both in an oral formulation and as a topical gel for the treatment of cutaneous T-cell lymphoma. Teratogenicity is a significant risk for both systemic and topical treatment with bexarotene, and women of childbearing potential must avoid becoming pregnant throughout therapy and for at least 1 month following discontinuation of the drug. Male patients must use condoms during intercourse during treatment and for at least 1 month after drug discontinuation. Bexarotene may increase levels of triglycerides and cholesterol; therefore, lipid levels must be monitored during treatment.

Vismodegib (Erivedge) and **sonidegib** (Odomzo) are oral hedgehog pathway inhibitors for the treatment of metastatic basal cell carcinoma or locally advanced basal cell carcinoma in adults who are not candidates for surgery or radiation. They are highly effective in patients with basal cell nevus syndrome. The recommended dosage of vismodegib is 150 mg daily and sonidegib is 200 mg daily. Recommended use is to continue daily until disease progress or unacceptable toxicity is seen; if a missed dose occurs, resume dosing with the next scheduled dose. The most common adverse effects include dysgeusia and ageusia, alopecia, fatigue, and muscle spasms.

Obtain baseline serum creatine kinase and creatinine levels prior to initiating therapy and monitoring during treatment may be indicated for significant musculoskeletal symptoms.

Hedgehog pathway inhibitors are embryotoxic, fetotoxic, and teratogenic in animals. Pregnancy status of females of reproductive potential must be verified within 7 days prior to initiating therapy. Exposure may occur through seminal fluid.

Vorinostat (Zolinza) and **romidepsin** (Istodax) are systemic histone deacetylase inhibitors that are approved for the treatment of cutaneous T-cell lymphoma in patients with progressive, persistent, or recurrent disease after prior systemic therapy. Adverse effects include thrombocytopenia, anemia, QT prolongation/ECG changes, serious infections (occasionally fatal), tumor lysis syndrome, and gastrointestinal disturbances. Pulmonary embolism, which has occurred with vorinostat, has not been reported to date with romidepsin.

MISCELLANEOUS MEDICATIONS

Drugs used primarily for other conditions may also find use as therapeutic agents for dermatologic conditions. A few such preparations are listed in Table 61–8.

TABLE 61–8 Miscellaneous medications and the dermatologic conditions in which they are used.

Drug or Group	Conditions	For More Details, See
Antihistamines	Pruritus (any cause), urticarial	Chapter 16
Antimalarials	Lupus erythematosus, photosensitization	Chapters 36, 52
Antimetabolites	Pemphigus, pemphigoid	Chapter 54
Becaplermin	Diabetic neuropathic ulcers	Chapter 41
Belimumab	Systemic lupus erythematosus	Chapters 36, 54
Capsaicin	Postherpetic neuralgia	Chapter 31
Corticosteroids	Pemphigus, pemphigoid, lupus erythematosus, allergic contact dermatoses, and certain other dermatoses	Chapter 39
Cyclosporine	Psoriasis	Chapter 55
Dapsone	Dermatitis herpetiformis, erythema elevatum diutinum, pemphigus, pemphigoid, bullous lupus erythematosus	Chapter 47

(*continued*)

TABLE 61–8 Miscellaneous medications and the dermatologic conditions in which they are used. (Continued)

Drug or Group	Conditions	For More Details, See
Denileukin diftitox	Cutaneous T-cell lymphomas	Chapters 54, 55
Diacerein	Epidermolysis bullosa	
Drospirenone/ethinyl estradiol	Moderate female acne	Chapter 39
Mechlorethamine gel	Cutaneous T-cell lymphoma	Chapter 54
Methotrexate	Psoriasis	Chapter 54
Mycophenolate mofetil	Bullous disease	Chapters 54, 55
Rituximab	Pemphigus vulgaris	Chapter 55
Thalidomide	Erythema nodosum leprosum	Chapters 54, 55
Ubidecarenone	Epidermolysis bullosa	

REFERENCES

General

Dragicevic, N, Maibach HI: *Percutaneous Penetration: Principles and Practices*, 5th ed. Taylor & Francis, 2021.

Law RM, Maibach HI: Lateral spread and percutaneous penetration: an overview. Int J Pharm 2020;588:119765.

Law RM et al: Twenty clinically pertinent factors/observations for percutaneous absorption in humans. Am J Clin Dermatol 2020;21:85.

Lebwohl MG et al: *Treatment of Skin Disease*, 4th ed. Elsevier-Saunders, 2014.

LexiComp Online: online.Lexi.com.

Maibach HI, Gorouhi F: *Evidence-Based Dermatology*, 2nd ed. Peoples Medical Publishing, 2012.

Wakelin S et al: *Systemic Drug Treatment in Dermatology*, 3rd ed. CRC Press, 2022.

Wilhem KP et al: *Marzulli & Maibach Dermatotoxicology*, 8th ed. Informa Healthcare, 2012.

Wolverton S: *Comprehensive Dermatologic Drug Therapy*, 2nd ed. Saunders, 2007.

Antibacterial, Antifungal, & Antiviral Drugs

Spelman D, Baddour LM: Skin abscesses in adults: Treatment. UpToDate July 2023. Accessed August 10, 2023.

James WD: Clinical practice. Acne. N Engl J Med 2005;352:1463.

Ectoparasiticides

Leone PA: Scabies and pediculosis pubis: An update of treatment regimens and general review. Clin Infect Dis 2007;44(Suppl 3):S153.

Agents Affecting Pigmentation

Levitt J: The safety of hydroquinone. J Am Acad Dermatol 2007;57:854.

Stolk LML, Siddiqui AH: Biopharmaceutics, pharmacokinetics, and pharmacology of psoralens. Gen Pharmacol 1988;19:649.

Retinoids & Other Acne Preparations

Shalita AR et al: Tazarotene gel is safe and effective in the treatment of acne vulgaris. A multicenter, double-blind, vehicle-controlled study. Cutis 1999;63:349.

Tzellos T et al: Topical retinoids for the treatment of acne vulgaris. Cochrane Database Syst Rev 2013;8:CD009470.

Anti-Inflammatory Agents

Bowie AC et al: Agreement and correlation between different topical corticosteroid potency classification systems. JAMA Dermatol 2022;158:796.

Brazzini B, Pimpinelli N: New and established topical corticosteroids in dermatology: Clinical pharmacology and therapeutic use. Am J Clin Dermatol 2002;3:47.

Kitzen JM et al: Crisaborole and apremilast: PDE4 inhibitors with similar mechanism of action, different indications for management of inflammatory skin conditions. Pharmacology & Pharmacy 2018;9:357.

Williams JD, Griffiths CE: Cytokine blocking agents in dermatology. Clin Exp Dermatol 2002;27:585.

Drugs for Psoriasis

Drugs for psoriasis. Med Lett Drugs Ther 2019;61:89.

Elmets CA et al: Joint AAD–NPF guidelines of care for the management and treatment of psoriasis with topical therapy and alternative medicine modalities for psoriasis severity measures. J Am Acad Dermatol 2021;84:432.

Feldman SR: Treatment of psoriasis in adults. UpToDate Current through July 2023. Accessed August 10, 2023.

Jeon C et al: Topical treatments. In: Bhutani T et al (editors): *Evidence-Based Psoriasis, Diagnosis and Treatment. Updates in Clinical Dermatology*. Springer, 2018.

Korman NJ: Management of psoriasis as a systemic disease: What is the evidence? Br J Dermatol 2019;182:840.

Law RM, Gulliver WP: Chapter 118Psoriasis. In: DiPiro JT et al (editors): *Pharmacotherapy: A Pathophysiologic Approach*, 12th ed. McGraw-Hill Medical, NY. Pp. 1639-1660, 2023.

Murase JE, Heller MM, Butler DC. Safety of dermatologi medications in pregnancy and lactation: Part I. Pregnancy. J Am Acad Dermatol 2014;70(3):401.

Samarasekera EJ et al: Topical therapies for the treatment of plaque psoriasis: Systematic review and network meta-analyses. Br J Dermatol 2013;168:954.

CASE STUDY ANSWER

Initiation of oral doxycycline therapy was discussed with the patient. She expressed concerns regarding possible adverse effects of prolonged systemic therapy. In light of this, daily morning application of oxymetazoline 1% cream was added to her treatment regimen. The patient noted prompt response with significant improvement of her facial redness.

CHAPTER

62

Drugs Used in the Treatment of Gastrointestinal Diseases

George T. Fantry, MD

CASE STUDY

A 21-year-old woman comes with her parents to discuss therapeutic options for her Crohn disease. She was diagnosed with Crohn disease 2 years ago, and it involves her terminal ileum and proximal colon, as confirmed by colonoscopy and small bowel radiography. She was initially treated with mesalamine and budesonide with good response, but over the last 2 months, she has had a relapse of her symptoms. She is experiencing fatigue, cramping, abdominal pains, and nonbloody diarrhea up to 10 times daily, and she has had a 15-lb weight loss.

She has no other significant medical or surgical history. Her current medications are mesalamine 2.4 g/d and budesonide 9 mg/d. She appears thin and tired. Abdominal examination reveals tenderness without guarding in the right lower quadrant; no masses are palpable. On perianal examination, there is no tenderness, fissure, or fistula. Her laboratory data are notable for anemia and elevated C-reactive protein. What are the options for immediate control of her symptoms and disease? What are the long-term management options?

INTRODUCTION

Many of the drug groups discussed elsewhere in this book have important applications in the treatment of diseases of the gastrointestinal tract and other organs. Other groups are used almost exclusively for their effects on the gut; these are discussed in the following text according to their therapeutic uses.

■ DRUGS USED IN ACID-PEPTIC DISEASES

Acid-peptic diseases include gastroesophageal reflux disease (GERD), peptic ulcer disease (gastric and duodenal ulcers), and stress-related mucosal injury. In all these conditions, mucosal erosions or ulceration arise when the caustic effects of aggressive factors (acid, pepsin, NSAIDs. *H pylori*, bile) overwhelm the defensive factors of the gastrointestinal mucosa (mucus and bicarbonate secretion, prostaglandins, blood flow, and the processes of restitution and regeneration after cellular injury). Symptoms and esophageal mucosal damage in GERD are caused by reflux of normal gastric content, including acid and pepsin, into the esophagus. Over 90% of peptic ulcers are caused by infection with the bacterium *Helicobacter pylori* or by use of nonsteroidal anti-inflammatory drugs (NSAIDs). Drugs used in the treatment of acid-peptic disorders may be divided into two classes: agents that reduce intragastric acidity and agents that promote mucosal defense.

AGENTS THAT REDUCE INTRAGASTRIC ACIDITY

Physiology of Acid Secretion

The parietal cell contains receptors for gastrin (CCK-B), histamine (H_2), and acetylcholine (muscarinic, M_3) (Figure 62–1). When acetylcholine (from vagal postganglionic nerves) and gastrin (released from antral G cells into the blood) bind to the parietal

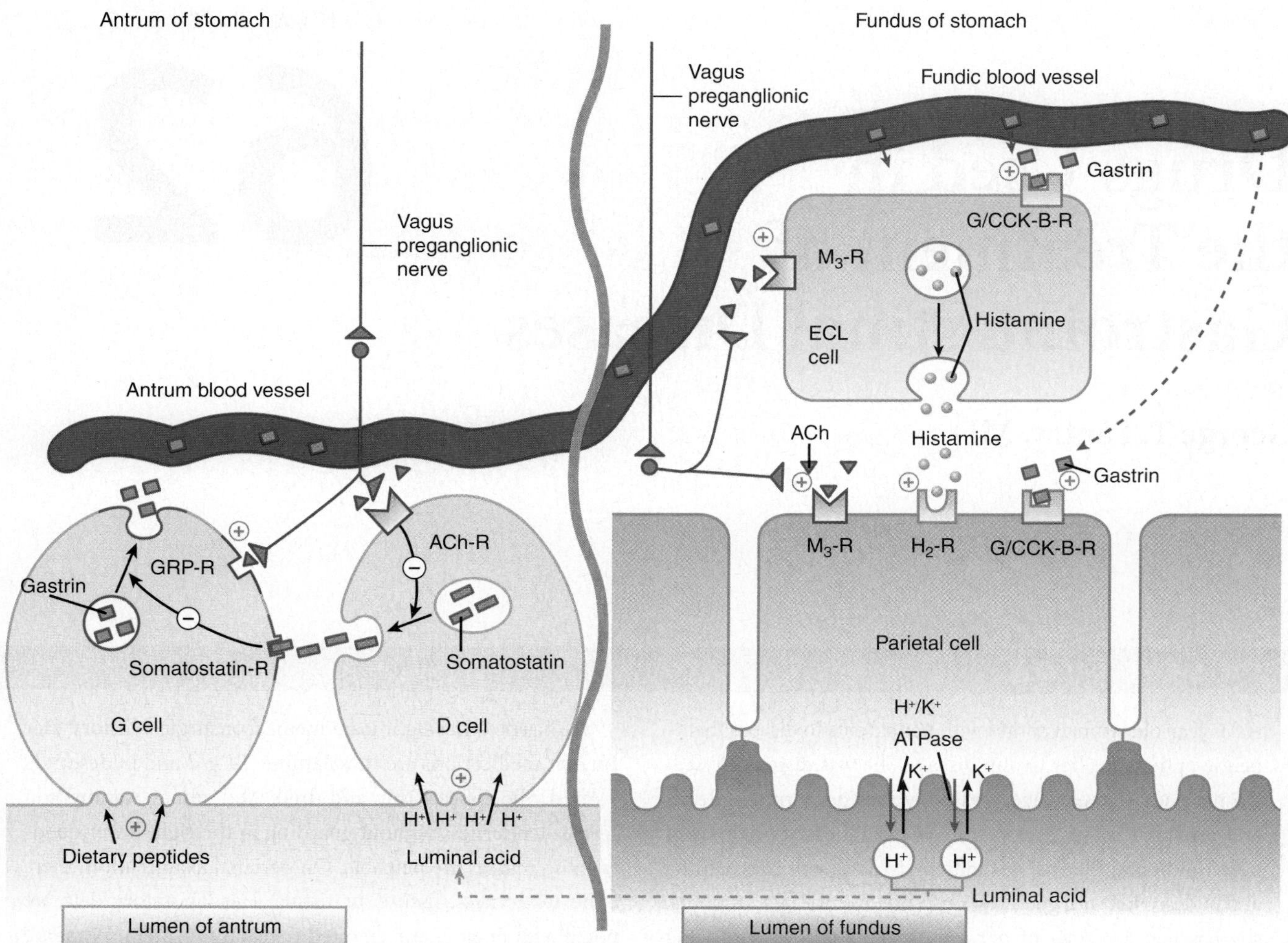

FIGURE 62–1 Schematic model for physiologic control of hydrogen ion (acid) secretion by the parietal cells of the gastric fundic glands. Parietal cells are stimulated to secrete acid (H^+) by gastrin (acting on gastrin/CCK-B receptor), acetylcholine (M_3 receptor), and histamine (H_2 receptor). Acid is secreted across the parietal cell canalicular membrane by the H^+/K^+-ATPase proton pump into the gastric lumen. Gastrin is secreted by antral G cells into blood vessels in response to intraluminal dietary peptides. Within the gastric body, gastrin passes from the blood vessels into the submucosal tissue of the fundic glands, where it binds to gastrin-CCK-B receptors on parietal cells and enterochromaffin-like (ECL) cells. The vagus nerve stimulates postganglionic neurons of the enteric nervous system to release acetylcholine (ACh), which binds to M_3 receptors on parietal cells and ECL cells. Stimulation of ECL cells by gastrin (CCK-B receptor) or acetylcholine (M_3 receptor) stimulates release of histamine. Within the gastric antrum, vagal stimulation of postganglionic enteric neurons enhances gastrin release directly by stimulation of antral G cells (through gastrin-releasing peptide, GRP) and indirectly by inhibition of somatostatin secretion from antral D cells. Acid secretion must eventually be turned off. Antral D cells are stimulated to release somatostatin by the rise in intraluminal H^+ concentration and by CCK that is released into the bloodstream by duodenal I cells in response to proteins and fats (not shown). Binding of somatostatin to receptors on adjacent antral G cells inhibits further gastrin release. ATPase, H^+/K^+-ATPase proton pump; CCK, cholecystokinin; M_3-R, muscarinic receptors.

cell receptors, they cause an increase in cytosolic calcium, which in turn stimulates protein kinases that stimulate acid secretion from a H^+/K^+-ATPase (the proton pump) on the canalicular surface.

In close proximity to the parietal cells are gut endocrine cells called **enterochromaffin-like (ECL) cells.** ECL cells also have receptors for gastrin and acetylcholine, which stimulate histamine release. Histamine binds to the H_2 receptor on the parietal cell, resulting in activation of adenylyl cyclase, which increases intracellular cyclic adenosine monophosphate (cAMP) and activates protein kinases that stimulate acid secretion by the H^+/K^+-ATPase. In humans, it is believed that the major effect of gastrin upon acid secretion is mediated indirectly through the release of histamine from ECL cells rather than through direct parietal cell stimulation. In contrast, acetylcholine provides potent direct parietal cell stimulation.

Antacids

Antacids have been used for centuries in the treatment of patients with dyspepsia and acid-peptic disorders. They were the mainstay of treatment for acid-peptic disorders until the advent of H_2-receptor antagonists and proton-pump inhibitors (PPIs). They continue to be used commonly by patients as nonprescription remedies for the treatment of intermittent heartburn and dyspepsia.

Antacids are weak bases that react with gastric hydrochloric acid to form a salt and water. Their principal mechanism of action is reduction of intragastric acidity. After a meal, approximately 45 mEq/h of hydrochloric acid is secreted. A single dose of 156 mEq of antacid given 1 hour after a meal effectively neutralizes gastric acid for up to 2 hours. However, the acid-neutralization capacity among different proprietary formulations of antacids is highly variable, depending on their rate of dissolution (tablet versus liquid), water solubility, rate of reaction with acid, and rate of gastric emptying.

Sodium bicarbonate (eg, baking soda, Alka Seltzer) reacts rapidly with hydrochloric acid (HCl) to produce carbon dioxide and sodium chloride. Formation of carbon dioxide results in gastric distention and belching. Unreacted alkali is readily absorbed, potentially causing metabolic alkalosis when given in high doses or to patients with renal insufficiency. Sodium chloride absorption may exacerbate fluid retention in patients with heart failure, hypertension, and renal insufficiency. **Calcium carbonate** (eg, Tums, Os-Cal) is less soluble and reacts more slowly than sodium bicarbonate with HCl to form carbon dioxide and calcium chloride ($CaCl_2$). Like sodium bicarbonate, calcium carbonate may cause belching or metabolic alkalosis. Calcium carbonate is used for a number of other indications apart from its antacid properties (see Chapter 42). Excessive doses of either sodium bicarbonate or calcium carbonate with calcium-containing dairy products can lead to hypercalcemia, renal insufficiency, and metabolic alkalosis (milk-alkali syndrome).

Formulations containing **magnesium hydroxide** or **aluminum hydroxide** react slowly with HCl to form magnesium chloride or aluminum chloride and water. Because no gas is generated, belching does not occur. Metabolic alkalosis is also uncommon because of the efficiency of the neutralization reaction. Because unabsorbed magnesium salts may cause an osmotic diarrhea and aluminum salts may cause constipation, these agents are commonly administered together in proprietary formulations (eg, Gelusil, Maalox, Mylanta) to minimize the impact on bowel function. Both magnesium and aluminum are absorbed and excreted by the kidneys. Hence, patients with renal insufficiency should not take these agents for a long term.

All antacids may affect the absorption of other medications by binding the drug (reducing its absorption) or by increasing intragastric pH so that the drug's dissolution or solubility (especially weakly basic or acidic drugs) is altered. Therefore, antacids should not be given within 2 hours of doses of tetracyclines, fluoroquinolones, itraconazole, and iron.

H_2-Receptor Antagonists

From their introduction in the 1970s until the early 1990s, H_2-receptor antagonists (commonly referred to as H_2 blockers) were the most commonly prescribed drugs in the world (see Clinical Uses). With the recognition of the role of *H pylori* in ulcer disease (which may be treated with appropriate antibacterial therapy) and the advent of PPIs, the use of prescription H_2 blockers has declined markedly.

A. Chemistry & Pharmacokinetics

Three H_2 antagonists are in clinical use: **cimetidine, famotidine,** and **nizatidine.** After nearly four decades since its approval, all prescription and over-the-counter ranitidine drugs were withdrawn from the market due to potential health risks related to a contaminant, N-nitrosodimethylamine (NDMA), which is a probable human carcinogen. NDMA was found at unacceptable levels in some ranitidine medications, particularly when stored at higher room temperatures over time. All three agents are rapidly absorbed from the intestine. Cimetidine and famotidine undergo first-pass hepatic metabolism resulting in a bioavailability of approximately 50%. Nizatidine has little first-pass metabolism. The serum half-lives of the three agents range from 1.1 to 4 hours; however, duration of action depends on the dose given (Table 62–1). H_2 antagonists are cleared by a combination of hepatic metabolism, glomerular filtration, and renal tubular secretion. Dose reduction is required in patients with moderate to severe renal (and possibly severe hepatic) insufficiency. In the elderly, there is a decline of up to 50% in drug clearance as well as a significant reduction in volume of distribution.

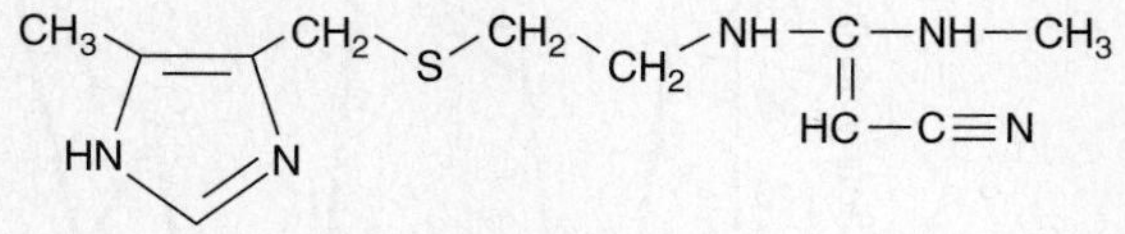

Cimetidine

TABLE 62–1 Clinical comparisons of H_2-receptor blockers.

Drug	Relative Potency	Dose to Achieve >50% Acid Inhibition for 10 Hours	Usual Dose for Acute Duodenal or Gastric Ulcer	Usual Dose for Gastroesophageal Reflux Disease	Usual Dose for Prevention of Stress-Related Bleeding
Cimetidine	1	400–800 mg	800 mg HS or 400 mg bid	800 mg bid	50 mg/h continuous infusion
Nizatidine	4–10	150 mg	300 mg HS or 150 mg bid	150 mg bid	Not available
Famotidine	20–50	20 mg	40 mg HS or 20 mg bid	20 mg bid	20 mg IV every 12 h

bid, twice daily; HS, bedtime.

B. Pharmacodynamics

The H_2 antagonists exhibit competitive inhibition at the parietal cell H_2 receptor and suppress basal and meal-stimulated acid secretion (Figure 62–2) in a linear, dose-dependent manner. They are highly selective and do not affect H_1 or H_3 receptors (see Chapter 16). The volume of gastric secretion and the concentration of pepsin are also reduced.

H_2 antagonists reduce acid secretion stimulated by histamine as well as by gastrin and cholinomimetic agents through two mechanisms. First, histamine released from ECL cells by gastrin or vagal stimulation is blocked from binding to the parietal cell H_2 receptor. Second, direct stimulation of the parietal cell by gastrin or acetylcholine has a diminished effect on acid secretion in the presence of H_2-receptor blockade.

The potencies of the three H_2-receptor antagonists vary over a 50-fold range (see Table 62–1). When given in usual prescription doses, however, all inhibit 60–70% of total 24-hour acid secretion. H_2 antagonists are especially effective at inhibiting nocturnal acid secretion (which depends largely on histamine), but they have a modest impact on meal-stimulated acid secretion (which is stimulated by gastrin and acetylcholine as well as histamine). Therefore, nocturnal and fasting intragastric pH is raised to 4–5, but the impact on the daytime, meal-stimulated pH profile is less. Recommended prescription doses maintain greater than 50% acid inhibition for 10 hours; hence, these drugs are commonly given twice daily. At doses available in over-the-counter formulations, the duration of acid inhibition is 6–10 hours.

C. Clinical Uses

H_2-receptor antagonists continue to be prescribed, but PPIs (see below) are more commonly prescribed than H_2 antagonists for most clinical indications. The over-the-counter preparations of the H_2 antagonists are heavily used by the public.

1. *Gastroesophageal reflux disease (GERD)*—Patients with infrequent heartburn or dyspepsia (fewer than three times per week) may take either antacids or intermittent H_2 antagonists for symptom relief. Because antacids provide rapid acid neutralization, they afford faster symptom relief than H_2 antagonists. However, the effect of antacids is short-lived (1–2 hours) compared with H_2 antagonists (6–10 hours). H_2 antagonists may be taken prophylactically before meals to reduce the likelihood of heartburn. Frequent heartburn is better treated with twice-daily H_2 antagonists (see Table 62–1) or PPIs to prevent heartburn and esophageal mucosal damage. In patients with erosive esophagitis (approximately 50% of patients with GERD), H_2 antagonists afford healing in less than 50% of patients; hence PPIs are preferred because of their superior acid inhibition.

2. *Peptic ulcer disease*—PPIs have largely replaced H_2 antagonists in the treatment of acute peptic ulcer disease. PPIs taken once daily provide faster control of symptoms and higher ulcer healing rates than H2 antagonists due to their stronger acid suppression. The duration of treatment, typically 4–8 weeks, varies based on ulcer characteristics (size, location: gastric vs duodenal), etiology (*H pylori*, NSAIDs), and the presence of complications

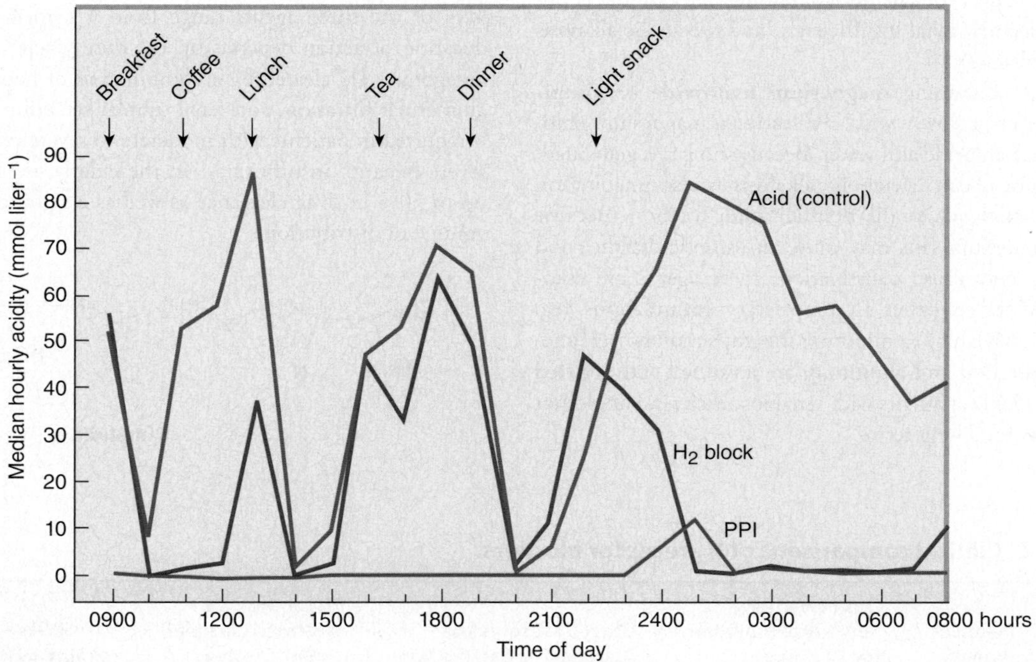

FIGURE 62–2 Twenty-four-hour median intragastric acidity pretreatment (red) and after 1 month of treatment with either ranitidine, 150 mg twice daily (blue, H_2 block), or omeprazole, 20 mg once daily (green, PPI). Note that H_2-receptor antagonists have a marked effect on nocturnal acid secretion but only a modest effect on meal-stimulated secretion. Proton-pump inhibitors (PPIs) markedly suppress meal-stimulated and nocturnal acid secretion. (Reproduced with permission from Lanzon-Miller S, Pounder RE, Hamilton MR, et al. Twenty-four-hour intragastric acidity and plasma gastrin concentration before and during treatment with either ranitidine or omeprazole. Aliment Pharmacol Ther. 1987;1(3):239-251.)

(bleeding, penetration, perforation, gastric outlet obstruction). For patients with ulcers caused by aspirin or other NSAIDs, the NSAID should be discontinued. If the NSAID must be continued for clinical reasons despite active ulceration, a PPI should be given to promote ulcer healing. Patients with acute peptic ulcers caused by *H pylori* should be treated with a 14-day course of therapy including a PPI and two or three antibiotics (see below).

3. *Nonulcer dyspepsia*—H_2 antagonists are commonly used as over-the-counter agents and prescription agents for treatment of intermittent dyspepsia not caused by peptic ulcer. However, benefit compared with placebo has never been convincingly demonstrated.

4. *Prevention of bleeding from stress-related gastritis*— Clinically important bleeding from upper gastrointestinal erosions or ulcers occurs in 1–3% of critically ill patients due to impaired mucosal defense mechanisms caused by poor perfusion. Although most critically ill patients have normal or decreased acid secretion, numerous studies have shown that antisecretory agents (H_2 antagonists or PPIs) that increase intragastric pH reduce the incidence of clinically significant bleeding and should be administered to patients who are at high risk of gastrointestinal bleeding. However, the optimal agent is uncertain. For patients who are able to receive enteral medications, an oral PPI is preferred. For patients who are unable to receive enteral medications, either intravenous H_2 antagonists or PPIs may be administered. Continuous infusions of H_2 antagonists are generally preferred to bolus infusions because they achieve more consistent, sustained elevation of intragastric pH.

D. Adverse Effects

H_2 antagonists are extremely safe drugs. Adverse effects occur in less than 3% of patients and include diarrhea, headache, fatigue, myalgias, and constipation. Some studies suggest that intravenous H_2 antagonists (or PPIs) may increase the risk of nosocomial pneumonia in critically ill patients.

Mental status changes (confusion, hallucinations, agitation) may occur with administration of intravenous H_2 antagonists, especially in patients in the intensive care unit who are elderly or who have renal or hepatic dysfunction. These events may be more common with cimetidine. Mental status changes rarely occur in ambulatory patients.

Cimetidine inhibits binding of dihydrotestosterone to androgen receptors, inhibits metabolism of estradiol, and increases serum prolactin levels. When used long-term or in high doses, it may cause gynecomastia or impotence in men and galactorrhea in women. These effects are specific to cimetidine and do not occur with the other H_2 antagonists.

Although there are no known harmful effects on the fetus, H_2 antagonists cross the placenta. Therefore, they should not be administered to pregnant women unless absolutely necessary. The H_2 antagonists are secreted into breast milk and may therefore affect nursing infants.

H_2 antagonists may rarely cause blood dyscrasias. Blockade of cardiac H_2 receptors may cause bradycardia, but this is rarely of clinical significance. Rapid intravenous infusion may cause bradycardia and hypotension through blockade of cardiac H_2 receptors; therefore, intravenous infusions should be given over 30 minutes. H_2 antagonists rarely cause reversible abnormalities in liver chemistry.

E. Drug Interactions

Cimetidine interferes with several important hepatic cytochrome P450 drug metabolism pathways, including those catalyzed by CYP1A2, CYP2C9, CYP2D6, and CYP3A4 (see Chapter 4). Hence, the half-lives of drugs metabolized by these pathways may be prolonged. Negligible CYP interaction occurs with nizatidine and famotidine.

H_2 antagonists compete with creatinine and certain drugs (eg, procainamide) for renal tubular secretion. All of these agents except famotidine inhibit gastric first-pass metabolism of ethanol, especially in women. Although the importance of this is debated, increased bioavailability of ethanol could lead to increased blood ethanol levels.

Proton-Pump Inhibitors (PPIs)

Since their introduction in the late 1980s, these efficacious acid inhibitory agents have assumed the major role for the treatment of acid-peptic disorders. PPIs are now among the most widely prescribed drugs worldwide.

A. Chemistry & Pharmacokinetics

Six PPIs are available for clinical use: **omeprazole, esomeprazole, lansoprazole, dexlansoprazole, rabeprazole,** and **pantoprazole.** All are substituted benzimidazoles that resemble H_2 antagonists in structure (Figure 62–3) but have a completely different mechanism of action. Omeprazole and lansoprazole are racemic mixtures of *R*- and *S*-isomers. Esomeprazole is the *S*-isomer of omeprazole and dexlansoprazole the *R*-isomer of lansoprazole. All are available in oral formulations. Esomeprazole and pantoprazole are also available in intravenous formulations (Table 62–2).

PPIs are administered as inactive prodrugs. To protect the acid-labile prodrug from rapid destruction within the gastric lumen, oral products are formulated for delayed release as acid-resistant, enteric-coated capsules or tablets. After passing through the stomach into the alkaline intestinal lumen, the enteric coatings dissolve and the prodrug is absorbed. For children or patients with dysphagia or enteral feeding tubes, capsule formulations (but not tablets) may be opened and the microgranules mixed with apple or orange juice or mixed with soft foods (eg, applesauce). Esomeprazole, omeprazole, and pantoprazole are also available as oral suspensions. Lansoprazole is available as a tablet formulation that disintegrates in the mouth, and rabeprazole is available in a formulation that may be sprinkled on food. Omeprazole is also available as a powder formulation (capsule or packet) that contains sodium bicarbonate (1100–1680 mg $NaHCO_3$; 304–460 mg of sodium) to protect the naked (non-enteric-coated) drug from acid degradation. When administered on an empty stomach by mouth or enteral tube, this "immediate-release" suspension results in rapid omeprazole absorption (T_{max} <30 minutes) and onset of acid inhibition.

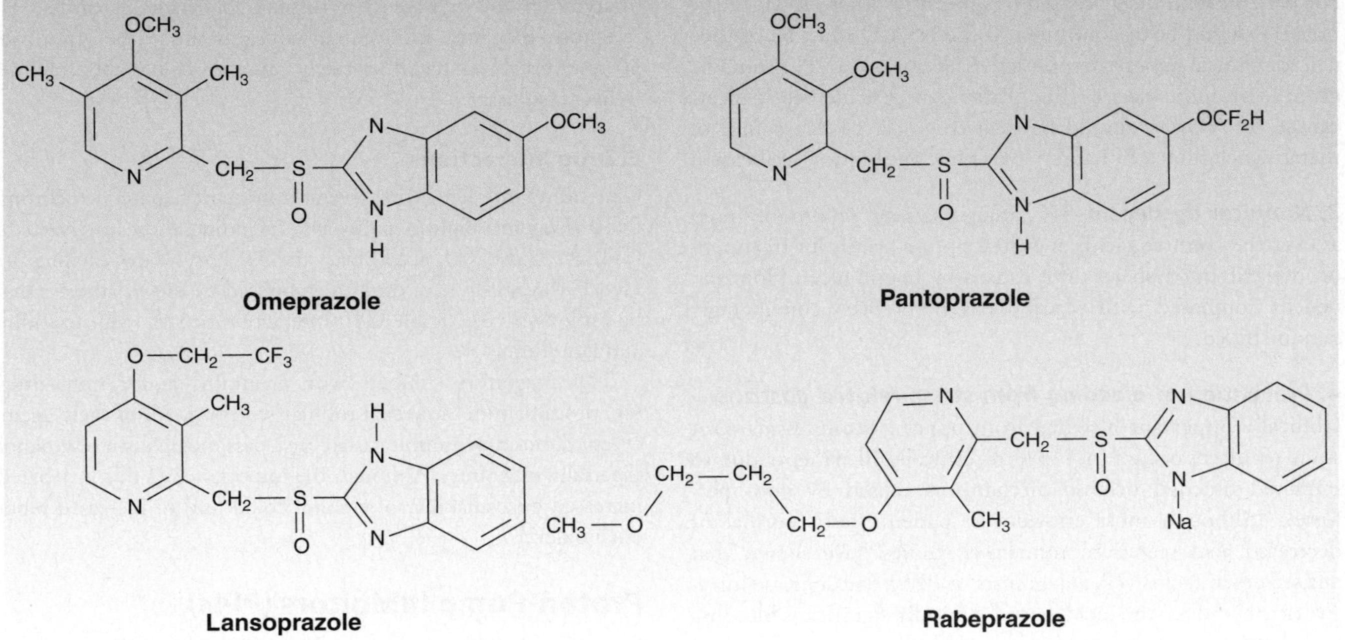

Omeprazole

Pantoprazole

Lansoprazole

Rabeprazole

FIGURE 62–3 Molecular structure of the proton-pump inhibitors: omeprazole, lansoprazole, pantoprazole, and the sodium salt of rabeprazole. Omeprazole and esomeprazole have the same chemical structure (see text).

The PPIs are lipophilic weak bases (pK_a 4–5) and, after intestinal absorption, diffuse readily across lipid membranes into acidified compartments (eg, the parietal cell canaliculus). The prodrug rapidly becomes protonated within the canaliculus and is concentrated more than 1000-fold by Henderson-Hasselbalch trapping (see Chapter 1). There, it rapidly undergoes a molecular conversion to the active form, a reactive thiophilic sulfenamide cation, which forms a covalent disulfide bond with the H^+/K^+-ATPase, irreversibly inactivating the enzyme.

The pharmacokinetics of available PPIs are shown in Table 62–2. Immediate-release omeprazole has a faster onset of acid inhibition than other oral formulations. Although differences in pharmacokinetic profiles may affect speed of onset and duration of acid inhibition in the first few days of therapy, they are of little clinical importance with continued daily administration. The bioavailability of all agents is decreased approximately 50% by food; hence, the drugs should be administered on an empty stomach. In a fasting state, only 10% of proton pumps are actively secreting acid and susceptible to inhibition. PPIs should be administered 30 to 60 minutes before breakfast, so that the peak serum concentration coincides with the maximal activity of proton-pump secretion. The drugs have a short serum half-life of about 1.5 hours, but acid inhibition lasts up to 24 hours owing to the irreversible inactivation of the proton pump. At least 18 hours are required for synthesis of new H^+/K^+-ATPase pump molecules. Because not all proton pumps are inactivated with the first dose of medication, up to 3–4 days of daily medication are required before the full acid-inhibiting potential is reached. Similarly, after stopping the drug, it takes 3–4 days for full acid secretion to return.

TABLE 62–2 Pharmacokinetics of proton pump inhibitors.

Drug	pK_a	Bioavailability (%)	$t_{1/2}$ (h)	T_{max} (h)	Usual Dosage for Peptic Ulcer or GERD
Omeprazole	4	40–65	0.5–1.0	1–3	20–40 mg qd
Esomeprazole	4	>80	1.5	1.6	20–40 mg qd
Lansoprazole	4	>80	1.0–2.0	1.7	30 mg qd
Dexlansoprazole	4	NA	1.0–2.0	5.0	30–60 mg qd
Pantoprazole	3.9	77	1.0–1.9	2.5–4.0	40 mg qd
Rabeprazole	5	52	1.0–2.0	3.1	20 mg qd

GERD, gastroesophageal reflux disease; NA, data not available.

PPIs undergo rapid first-pass and systemic hepatic metabolism and have negligible renal clearance. Dose reduction is not needed for patients with renal insufficiency or mild to moderate liver disease but should be considered in patients with severe liver impairment. Although other proton pumps exist in the body, the H^+/K^+-ATPase appears to exist only in the parietal cell and is distinct structurally and functionally from other H^+-transporting enzymes.

The intravenous formulations of esomeprazole and pantoprazole have characteristics similar to those of the oral drugs. When given to a fasting patient, they inactivate acid pumps that are actively secreting, but they have no effect on pumps in quiescent, nonsecreting vesicles. Because the half-life of a single injection of the intravenous formulation is short, acid secretion returns several hours later as pumps move from the tubulovesicles to the canalicular surface. Thus, to provide maximal inhibition during the first 24–48 hours of treatment, the intravenous formulations must be given as a continuous infusion or as repeated bolus injections. The optimal dosing of intravenous PPIs to achieve maximal blockade in fasting patients is not yet established.

From a pharmacokinetic perspective, PPIs are ideal drugs: they have a short serum half-life, they are concentrated and activated near their site of action, and they have a long duration of action.

B. Pharmacodynamics

In contrast to H_2 antagonists, PPIs inhibit both fasting and meal-stimulated secretion because they block the final common pathway of acid secretion, the proton pump. In standard doses, PPIs inhibit 90–98% of 24-hour acid secretion (see Figure 62–2). When administered at equivalent doses, the different agents show little difference in clinical efficacy. In a crossover study of patients receiving long-term therapy with five PPIs, the mean 24-hour intragastric pH varied from 3.3 (pantoprazole, 40 mg) to 4.0 (esomeprazole, 40 mg), and the mean number of hours the pH was higher than 4 varied from 10.1 (pantoprazole, 40 mg) to 14.0 (esomeprazole, 40 mg). Although dexlansoprazole has a delayed-release formulation that results in a longer T_{max} and greater AUC than other PPIs, it appears comparable to other agents in the ability to suppress acid secretion. This is because acid suppression is more dependent upon irreversible inactivation of the proton pump than the pharmacokinetics of different agents.

C. Clinical Uses

1. *Gastroesophageal reflux disease*—PPIs are the most effective agents for the treatment of erosive reflux disease, esophageal complications of reflux disease (peptic stricture or Barrett esophagus), and extraesophageal manifestations of reflux disease. Once-daily dosing provides effective symptom relief and tissue healing in 85–90% of patients; up to 15% of patients require twice-daily dosing.

GERD symptoms recur in over 80% of patients within 6 months after discontinuation of a PPI. For patients with erosive esophagitis or esophageal complications, long-term daily maintenance therapy with a full-dose or half-dose PPI is usually needed. Many patients with mild nonerosive GERD may be treated successfully with intermittent courses of PPIs or H_2 antagonists taken as needed ("on demand") for recurrent symptoms.

In current clinical practice, many patients with symptomatic GERD are treated empirically with medications without prior endoscopy, ie, without knowledge of whether the patient has erosive or nonerosive reflux disease. Empiric treatment with PPIs provides sustained symptomatic relief in 70–80% of patients, compared with 50–60% with H_2 antagonists. Because of recent cost reductions, PPIs have been used as first-line therapy for patients with symptomatic GERD. However, due to safety concerns associated with long-term PPI use, initial empiric treatment with an H_2 antagonist should be considered, particularly in patients with mild and intermittent symptoms.

Sustained acid suppression with twice-daily PPIs for at least 3 months is used to treat extraesophageal complications of reflux disease (asthma, chronic cough, laryngitis, and noncardiac chest pain).

2. *Peptic ulcer disease*—Compared with H_2 antagonists, PPIs afford more rapid symptom relief and faster ulcer healing for duodenal ulcers and, to a lesser extent, gastric ulcers. All the pump inhibitors heal more than 90% of duodenal ulcers within 4 weeks and a similar percentage of gastric ulcers within 6–8 weeks.

***a.* H *PYLORI*–ASSOCIATED ULCERS—**For *H pylori*–associated ulcers, there are two therapeutic goals: to heal the ulcer and to eradicate the organism. The most effective regimens for *H pylori* eradication are combinations of two antibiotics and a PPI. PPIs promote eradication of *H pylori* through several mechanisms: direct antimicrobial properties (minor) and—by raising intragastric pH—lowering the minimal inhibitory concentrations of antibiotics against *H pylori.* Until recently, the most commonly recommended treatment regimen consisted of a 14-day regimen of "triple therapy": a PPI twice daily; clarithromycin, 500 mg twice daily; and either amoxicillin, 1 g twice daily, or metronidazole, 500 mg twice daily. Due to increasing treatment failures attributable to rising clarithromycin resistance, "quadruple therapy" is now recommended as first-line treatment for patients who likely have clarithromycin resistance due to prior exposure or to residence in regions with high clarithromycin resistance. Two 14-day treatment regimens currently are recommended. Each includes a PPI twice daily with either (a) bismuth subsalicylate 524 mg, metronidazole 500 mg, and tetracycline 500 mg, all given four times daily; or (b) amoxicillin 1 g, clarithromycin 500 mg, and metronidazole 500 mg, all given twice daily. A combination capsule containing bismuth subsalicylate, metronidazole, and tetracycline is commercially available. After completion of antibiotic therapy, the PPI should be continued once daily for a total of 4–6 weeks to ensure complete ulcer healing. Eradication should be confirmed in all patients by a fecal antigen test, urea breath test, or upper endoscopy with biopsy 4 weeks after completion of antibiotic therapy. To reduce the risk of false-negative results, PPI therapy should be discontinued 2 weeks prior to testing.

***b.* NSAID-ASSOCIATED ULCERS—**For patients with ulcers caused by aspirin or other NSAIDs, either H_2 antagonists or PPIs provide rapid ulcer healing so long as the NSAID is discontinued; however, continued use of the NSAID impairs ulcer healing. In patients with NSAID-induced ulcers who require continued

NSAID therapy, treatment with a PPI more reliably promotes ulcer healing.

Asymptomatic peptic ulceration develops in 10–20% of people taking frequent NSAIDs, and ulcer-related complications (bleeding, perforation) develop in 1–2% of persons per year. PPIs taken once daily are effective in reducing the incidence of ulcers and ulcer complications in patients taking aspirin or other NSAIDs.

c. Prevention of rebleeding from peptic ulcers—In patients with acute gastrointestinal bleeding due to peptic ulcers, the risk of rebleeding from ulcers that have a visible vessel or adherent clot is increased. Rebleeding of this subset of high-risk ulcers is reduced significantly with PPIs administered for 3–5 days either as high-dose oral therapy (eg, omeprazole, 40 mg orally twice daily) or as a continuous intravenous infusion. It is believed that an intragastric pH higher than 6 may enhance coagulation and platelet aggregation. The optimal dose of intravenous PPI needed to achieve and maintain this level of near-complete acid inhibition is unknown; however, initial bolus administration of esomeprazole or pantoprazole (80 mg) followed by constant infusion (8 mg/h) is commonly recommended.

3. *Nonulcer dyspepsia*—PPIs have modest efficacy for treatment of nonulcer dyspepsia, benefiting 10–20% more patients than placebo. Despite their use for this indication, superiority to H_2 antagonists (or even placebo) has not been conclusively demonstrated.

4. *Prevention of stress-related mucosal bleeding*—As discussed previously (see H_2-Receptor Antagonists), PPIs (given orally, by nasogastric tube, or by intravenous infusions) may be administered to reduce the risk of clinically significant stress-related mucosal bleeding in critically ill patients. The only PPI approved by the US Food and Drug Administration (FDA) for this indication is an oral immediate-release omeprazole formulation, which is administered by nasogastric tube twice daily on the first day, then once daily. Although not FDA approved for this indication, other PPI suspension formulations (esomeprazole, omeprazole, pantoprazole) also may be used. For patients with nasoenteric tubes, PPI suspensions may be preferred to intravenous H_2 antagonists or PPIs because of comparable efficacy, lower cost, and ease of administration.

For patients without a nasoenteric tube or with significant ileus, intravenous H_2 antagonists may be preferred to intravenous PPIs because of their proven efficacy. Although PPIs are increasingly used, there are no controlled trials demonstrating efficacy or optimal dosing.

5. *Gastrinoma and other hypersecretory conditions*—Patients with isolated gastrinomas are best treated with surgical resection. In patients with metastatic or unresectable gastrinomas, massive acid hypersecretion results in peptic ulceration, erosive esophagitis, and malabsorption. With PPIs, excellent acid suppression can be achieved in all patients. Dosage is titrated to reduce basal acid output to less than 5–10 mEq/h. Typical doses of omeprazole are 60–120 mg/d.

D. Adverse Effects

1. *General*—Although PPIs have been considered to be extremely safe, a number of recent safety concerns have been raised. The studies raising concern are largely of retrospective observational design. Hence, it is difficult to determine whether the modest associations identified are due to a causal relationship or confounding variables and biases. As with most drugs, PPIs should be prescribed at the lowest effective dose and the risks versus benefits of long-term use carefully weighed. Diarrhea, headache, and abdominal pain are reported in 1–5% of patients, although the frequency of these events is only slightly increased compared with placebo. In large observational studies, PPIs have been associated with an increased risk of acute interstitial nephritis and chronic kidney disease compared to nonusers or users of H_2-receptor antagonists. A mechanism by which kidney damage might occur has not been determined. Although some epidemiologic studies have detected an increased risk of dementia in long-term PPI users, a meta-analysis of published studies did not identify an increased risk. PPIs are not teratogenic in animal models; however, safety during pregnancy has not been established.

2. *Nutrition*—Acid is important in releasing vitamin B_{12} from food. A minor reduction in oral cyanocobalamin absorption occurs during proton-pump inhibition, potentially leading to subnormal B_{12} levels with prolonged therapy. Acid also promotes absorption of food-bound minerals (non-heme iron, insoluble calcium salts, magnesium). Meta-analyses of cohort and case-control studies have detected a modest increase in the risk of hip fracture in patients taking long-term PPIs. Although a causal relationship is unproven, PPIs may reduce calcium absorption or inhibit osteoclast function. All PPIs carry an FDA-mandated warning of a possible increased risk of hip, spine, and wrist fractures. Patients who require long-term PPIs—especially those with risk factors for osteoporosis—should have monitoring of bone density and should be provided calcium supplements. The FDA has also issued a warning regarding a risk of life-threatening hypomagnesemia with secondary hypocalcemia, possibly due to decreased intestinal absorption, which normalizes after PPI discontinuation. Monitoring of serum magnesium should be considered in patients on diuretic therapy.

3. *Respiratory and enteric infections*—Gastric acid is an important barrier to colonization and infection of the stomach and intestine from ingested bacteria. Increases in gastric bacterial concentrations are detected in patients taking PPIs, which is of unknown clinical significance. Some studies have reported an increased risk of both community-acquired respiratory infections and nosocomial pneumonia among patients taking PPIs.

There is a two- to threefold increased risk for hospital- and community-acquired *Clostridium difficile* infection in patients taking PPIs. There also is a small increased risk of other enteric infections (eg, *Salmonella, Shigella, Escherichia coli, Campylobacter*), which should be considered particularly when traveling in underdeveloped countries.

4. Potential problems due to increased serum gastrin—Gastrin levels are regulated by intragastric acidity. Acid suppression alters normal feedback inhibition so that median serum gastrin levels rise 1.5- to twofold in patients taking PPIs. Although gastrin levels remain within normal limits in most patients, they exceed 500 pg/mL (normal, <100 pg/mL) in 3%. Upon stopping the drug, the levels normalize within 4 weeks. The rise in serum gastrin levels may stimulate hyperplasia of ECL and parietal cells, which may cause transient rebound acid hypersecretion with increased dyspepsia or heartburn after drug discontinuation, which abate within 2–4 weeks after gastrin and acid secretion normalize. In female rats given PPIs for prolonged periods, hypergastrinemia caused gastric carcinoid tumors that developed in areas of ECL hyperplasia. Although humans who take PPIs for a long time also may exhibit ECL hyperplasia, carcinoid tumor formation has not been documented. At present, routine monitoring of serum gastrin levels is not recommended in patients receiving prolonged PPI therapy.

5. Other potential problems due to decreased gastric acidity—Among patients infected with *H pylori*, long-term acid suppression leads to increased chronic inflammation in the gastric body and decreased inflammation in the antrum. Concerns have been raised that increased gastric inflammation may accelerate gastric gland atrophy (atrophic gastritis) and intestinal metaplasia—known risk factors for gastric adenocarcinoma. A special FDA Gastrointestinal Advisory Committee concluded that there is no evidence that prolonged PPI therapy produces the kind of atrophic gastritis (multifocal atrophic gastritis) or intestinal metaplasia that is associated with increased risk of adenocarcinoma. Routine testing for *H pylori* is not recommended in patients who require long-term PPI therapy. Long-term PPI therapy is associated with the development of small benign gastric fundic-gland polyps in a small number of patients, which may disappear after stopping the drug and are of uncertain clinical significance.

E. Drug Interactions

Decreased gastric acidity may alter absorption of drugs for which intragastric acidity affects drug bioavailability, eg, ketoconazole, itraconazole, digoxin, and atazanavir. All PPIs are metabolized by hepatic P450 cytochromes, including CYP2C19 and CYP3A4. Because of the short half-lives of PPIs, clinically significant drug interactions are rare. Omeprazole may inhibit the metabolism of clopidogrel, warfarin, diazepam, and phenytoin. Esomeprazole may also decrease metabolism of diazepam. Lansoprazole may enhance clearance of theophylline. Rabeprazole and pantoprazole have no significant drug interactions.

The FDA has issued a warning about a potentially important adverse interaction between clopidogrel and PPIs. Clopidogrel is a prodrug that requires activation by the hepatic P450 CYP2C19 isoenzyme, which also is involved to varying degrees in the metabolism of PPIs (especially omeprazole, esomeprazole, lansoprazole, and dexlansoprazole). Thus, PPIs could reduce clopidogrel activation (and its antiplatelet action) in some patients. Several large retrospective studies have reported an increased incidence of serious cardiovascular events in patients taking clopidogrel and a PPI. In contrast, three smaller prospective randomized trials have not detected an increased risk. When PPIs are prescribed to patients taking clopidogrel, agents with minimal CYP2C19 inhibition (pantoprazole or rabeprazole) may be preferred.

MUCOSAL PROTECTIVE AGENTS

The gastroduodenal mucosa has evolved a number of defense mechanisms to protect itself against the noxious effects of acid and pepsin. Both mucus and epithelial cell–cell tight junctions restrict back diffusion of acid and pepsin. Epithelial bicarbonate secretion establishes a pH gradient within the mucous layer in which the pH ranges from 7 at the mucosal surface to 1–2 in the gastric lumen. Blood flow carries bicarbonate and vital nutrients to surface cells. Areas of injured epithelium are quickly repaired by restitution, a process in which migration of cells from gland neck cells seals small erosions to reestablish intact epithelium. Mucosal prostaglandins appear to be important in stimulating mucus and bicarbonate secretion and mucosal blood flow. A number of agents that potentiate these mucosal defense mechanisms are available for the prevention and treatment of acid-peptic disorders.

Sucralfate

A. Chemistry & Pharmacokinetics

Sucralfate is a salt of sucrose complexed to sulfated aluminum hydroxide. In water or acidic solutions it forms a viscous, tenacious paste that binds selectively to ulcers or erosions for up to 6 hours. Sucralfate has limited solubility, breaking down into sucrose sulfate (strongly negatively charged) and an aluminum salt. Less than 3% of intact drug and aluminum is absorbed from the intestinal tract; the remainder is excreted in the feces.

B. Pharmacodynamics

A variety of beneficial effects have been attributed to sucralfate, but the precise mechanism of action is unclear. It is believed that the negatively charged sucrose sulfate binds to positively charged proteins in the base of ulcers or erosion, forming a physical barrier that restricts further caustic damage and stimulates mucosal prostaglandin and bicarbonate secretion.

C. Clinical Uses

Sucralfate is administered in a dosage of 1 g four times daily on an empty stomach (at least 1 hour before meals). At present, its clinical uses are limited. Sucralfate (administered as a slurry through a nasogastric tube) reduces the incidence of clinically significant upper gastrointestinal bleeding in critically ill patients hospitalized in the intensive care unit, although it is slightly less effective than intravenous H_2 antagonists. Sucralfate is still used by many clinicians for prevention of stress-related bleeding because of concerns that acid inhibitory therapies (antacids, H_2 antagonists, and PPIs) may increase the risk of nosocomial pneumonia.

D. Adverse Effects

Because it is not absorbed, sucralfate is virtually devoid of systemic adverse effects. Constipation occurs in 2% of patients due to the aluminum salt. Because a small amount of aluminum is absorbed, it should not be used for prolonged periods in patients with renal insufficiency.

E. Drug Interactions

Sucralfate may bind to other medications, impairing their absorption.

Prostaglandin Analogs

A. Chemistry, Pharmacokinetics, Clinical Uses, & Adverse Effects

The human gastrointestinal mucosa synthesizes a number of prostaglandins (see Chapter 18), primarily prostaglandins E and F. **Misoprostol,** a methyl analog of PGE_1, has been approved for gastrointestinal conditions. After oral administration, it is rapidly absorbed and metabolized to a metabolically active free acid. The serum half-life is less than 30 minutes; hence, it must be administered 3–4 times daily. It is excreted in the urine; however, dose reduction is not needed in patients with renal insufficiency.

Misoprostol has both acid inhibitory and mucosal protective properties. It is believed to stimulate mucus and bicarbonate secretion and enhance mucosal blood flow. Misoprostol can reduce the incidence of NSAID-induced ulcers to less than 3% and the incidence of ulcer complications by 50%. It is approved for prevention of NSAID-induced ulcers in high-risk patients; however, misoprostol has never achieved widespread use owing to its high adverse-effect profile (dose-dependent abdominal pain and diarrhea) and need for multiple daily dosing.

Bismuth Compounds

A. Chemistry & Pharmacokinetics

Two bismuth compounds are available: **bismuth subsalicylate,** a nonprescription formulation containing bismuth and salicylate, and **bismuth subcitrate potassium.** In the USA, bismuth subcitrate is available only as a combination prescription product that also contains metronidazole and tetracycline for the treatment of *H pylori*. Bismuth subsalicylate undergoes rapid dissociation within the stomach, allowing absorption of salicylate. More than 99% of the bismuth appears in the stool. Although minimal (<1%), bismuth is absorbed; it is stored in many tissues and has slow renal excretion. Salicylate (like aspirin) is readily absorbed and excreted in the urine.

B. Pharmacodynamics

The precise mechanisms of action of bismuth are unknown. Bismuth coats ulcers and erosions, creating a protective layer against acid and pepsin. It may also stimulate prostaglandin, mucus, and bicarbonate secretion. Bismuth subsalicylate reduces stool frequency and liquidity in acute infectious diarrhea, due to salicylate inhibition of intestinal prostaglandin and chloride secretion. Bismuth has direct antimicrobial effects and binds enterotoxins, accounting for its benefit in preventing and treating traveler's diarrhea. Bismuth compounds have direct antimicrobial activity against *H pylori*.

C. Clinical Uses

Despite the lack of comparative trials, nonprescription bismuth compounds (eg, Pepto-Bismol, Kaopectate) are widely used by patients for the nonspecific treatment of dyspepsia and acute diarrhea. Bismuth subsalicylate also is used for the prevention of traveler's diarrhea (30 mL or two tablets four times daily).

Bismuth compounds are used in four-drug regimens for the eradication of *H pylori* infection (see earlier discussion of *H pylori*-associated ulcers). One regimen consists of a PPI twice daily combined with bismuth subsalicylate (two tablets; 262 mg each), tetracycline (250–500 mg), and metronidazole (500 mg) four times daily for 10–14 days. Another regimen consists of a PPI twice daily combined with three capsules of a combination prescription formulation (each capsule containing bismuth subcitrate 140 mg, metronidazole 125 mg, and tetracycline 125 mg) taken four times daily for 10–14 days.

D. Adverse Effects

All bismuth formulations have excellent safety profiles. Bismuth causes harmless blackening of the stool, which may be confused with gastrointestinal bleeding. Liquid formulations may cause harmless darkening of the tongue. Bismuth agents should be used for short periods only and should be avoided in patients with renal insufficiency. Prolonged usage of some bismuth compounds may rarely lead to bismuth toxicity, resulting in encephalopathy (ataxia, headaches, confusion, seizures). However, such toxicity is not reported with bismuth subsalicylate or bismuth citrate. High dosages of bismuth subsalicylate may lead to salicylate toxicity.

■ DRUGS STIMULATING GASTROINTESTINAL MOTILITY

Drugs that can selectively stimulate gut motor function (**prokinetic** agents) have significant potential clinical usefulness. Agents that increase lower esophageal sphincter pressures may be useful for GERD. Drugs that improve gastric emptying may be helpful for gastroparesis and postsurgical gastric emptying delay. Agents that stimulate the small intestine may be beneficial for postoperative ileus or chronic intestinal pseudo-obstruction. Finally, agents that enhance colonic transit may be useful in the treatment of constipation. Unfortunately, only a limited number of agents in this group are available for clinical use at this time.

Physiology of the Enteric Nervous System

The enteric nervous system (see also Chapter 6) is composed of interconnected networks of ganglion cells and nerve fibers mainly located in the submucosa (submucosal plexus) and between the circular and longitudinal muscle layers (myenteric plexus). These networks give rise to nerve fibers that connect with the mucosa and muscle. Although extrinsic sympathetic and parasympathetic nerves project onto the submucosal and myenteric plexuses, the enteric nervous system can independently regulate gastrointestinal motility and secretion. Extrinsic primary afferent neurons project via the dorsal root ganglia or vagus nerve to the central nervous system (Figure 62–4). Release of serotonin (5-HT) from intestinal mucosa enterochromaffin (EC) cells stimulates 5-HT_3 receptors on the extrinsic afferent nerves, stimulating nausea, vomiting, or abdominal pain. Serotonin also stimulates submucosal 5-HT_{1P} receptors of the intrinsic primary afferent nerves (IPANs), which contain calcitonin gene-related peptide (CGRP) and acetylcholine and project to myenteric plexus interneurons. 5-HT_4 receptors on the presynaptic terminals of the IPANs appear to enhance release of CGRP or acetylcholine. The myenteric interneurons are important in controlling the peristaltic reflex, promoting release of excitatory mediators proximally and inhibitory mediators distally. Motilin may stimulate excitatory neurons or muscle cells directly. Dopamine acts as an inhibitory neurotransmitter in the

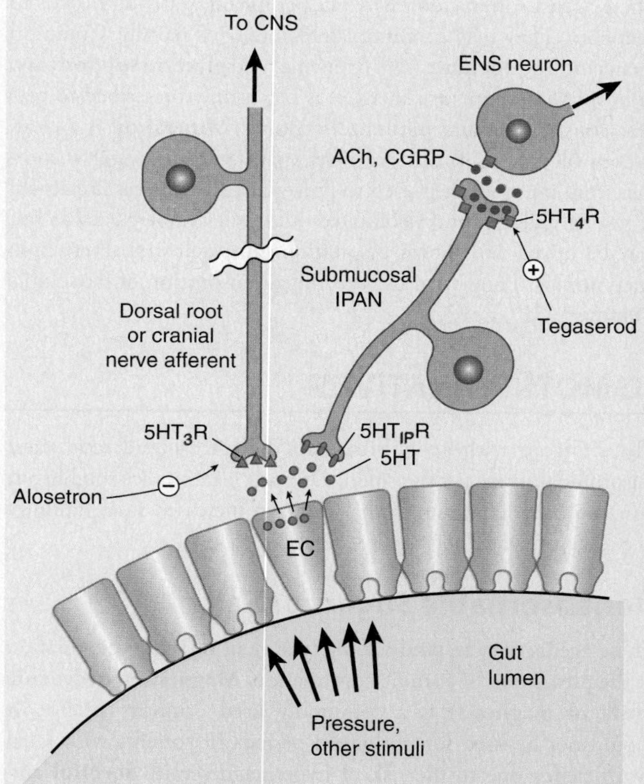

FIGURE 62–4 Release of serotonin (5-HT) by enterochromaffin (EC) cells from gut distention stimulates submucosal intrinsic primary afferent neurons (IPANs) via 5-HT_{1P} receptors and extrinsic primary afferent neurons via 5-HT_3 receptors (5-HT_{1P}R, 5-HT_3R). Submucosal IPANs activate the enteric neurons responsible for peristaltic and secretory reflex activity. Stimulation of 5-HT_4 receptors (5-HT_4R) on presynaptic terminals of IPANs enhances release of acetylcholine (ACh) and calcitonin gene-related peptide (CGRP), promoting reflex activity. CNS, central nervous system; ENS, enteric nervous system. (From Gershon MD. Serotonin and its implication for the management of irritable bowel syndrome. Rev Gastroenterol Disord. 2003;3 Suppl 2:S25-S34. Courtesy of Michael D. Gershon, M.D.)

gastrointestinal tract, decreasing the intensity of esophageal and gastric contractions.

Although there are at least 14 serotonin receptor subtypes, 5-HT drug development for gastrointestinal applications to date has focused on **5-HT_3-receptor antagonists** and **5-HT_4-receptor agonists.** These agents—which have effects on gastrointestinal motility and visceral afferent sensation—are discussed under Drugs Used in the Treatment of Irritable Bowel Syndrome and Antiemetic Agents. Other drugs acting on 5-HT receptors are discussed in Chapters 16, 29, and 30.

CHOLINOMIMETIC AGENTS

Cholinomimetic agonists such as bethanechol stimulate muscarinic M_3 receptors on muscle cells and at myenteric plexus synapses (see Chapter 7). Bethanechol was used in the past for the treatment of GERD and gastroparesis. Owing to multiple cholinergic effects and the advent of less toxic agents, it is now seldom used. The acetylcholinesterase inhibitor neostigmine can enhance gastric, small intestine, and colonic emptying. Intravenous **neostigmine** is used for the treatment of hospitalized patients with acute large bowel distention (known as acute colonic pseudo-obstruction or Ogilvie syndrome). Administration of 2 mg results in prompt colonic evacuation of flatus and feces in the majority of patients. Cholinergic effects include excessive salivation, nausea, vomiting, diarrhea, and bradycardia.

METOCLOPRAMIDE & DOMPERIDONE

Metoclopramide and domperidone are dopamine D_2-receptor antagonists. Within the gastrointestinal tract, activation of dopamine receptors inhibits cholinergic smooth muscle stimulation; blockade of this effect is believed to be the primary prokinetic mechanism of action of these agents. These agents increase esophageal peristaltic amplitude, increase lower esophageal sphincter pressure, and enhance gastric emptying but have no effect on small intestine or colonic motility. Metoclopramide and domperidone also block dopamine D_2 receptors in the chemoreceptor trigger zone of the medulla (area postrema), resulting in potent antinausea and antiemetic action.

Clinical Uses

1. *Gastroesophageal reflux disease*—Metoclopramide is available for clinical use in the USA; domperidone is available in many other countries. These agents are rarely used in the treatment of symptomatic GERD and are not effective in patients with erosive esophagitis. Because of the superior efficacy and safety of antisecretory agents in the treatment of heartburn, prokinetic agents are used mainly in combination with antisecretory agents in patients with persistent regurgitation or refractory heartburn and evidence of delayed gastric emptying.

2. *Impaired gastric emptying*—These agents are widely used as first-line therapy in the treatment of patients with delayed gastric emptying due to postsurgical disorders (vagotomy, antrectomy) and diabetic gastroparesis. Metoclopramide is sometimes administered in hospitalized patients to promote advancement of nasoenteric feeding tubes from the stomach into the duodenum.

3. *Nonulcer dyspepsia*—These agents lead to symptomatic improvement in a small number of patients with chronic dyspepsia. Use is reserved for patients with nonulcer dyspepsia who have failed other therapies.

4. *Prevention of vomiting*—Because of their potent antiemetic action, metoclopramide and domperidone are used for the prevention and treatment of emesis.

5. *Postpartum lactation stimulation*—Domperidone is sometimes recommended to promote postpartum lactation (see also Adverse Effects).

Adverse Effects

The most common adverse effects of metoclopramide involve the central nervous system. Restlessness, drowsiness, insomnia, anxiety, and agitation occur in 10–20% of patients, especially the elderly. Extrapyramidal effects (dystonias, akathisia, parkinsonian features) due to central dopamine receptor blockade occur acutely in 25% of patients given high doses and in 5% of patients receiving long-term therapy. Tardive dyskinesia, sometimes irreversible, has developed in patients treated for a prolonged period with metoclopramide. For this reason, long-term use should be avoided unless absolutely necessary, especially in the elderly. Elevated prolactin levels (caused by both metoclopramide and domperidone) can cause galactorrhea, gynecomastia, impotence, and menstrual disorders.

Domperidone is extremely well tolerated. Because it does not cross the blood-brain barrier to a significant degree, neuropsychiatric and extrapyramidal effects are rare.

MACROLIDES

Macrolide antibiotics such as **erythromycin** directly stimulate motilin receptors on gastrointestinal smooth muscle and promote the onset of a migrating motor complex. Patients with gastroparesis who fail to respond to metoclopramide and domperidone may be treated with a trial of oral erythromycin. However, tolerance rapidly develops, limiting benefits of chronic administration. Intravenous erythromycin (3 mg/kg) is beneficial in some patients with acute exacerbations of gastroparesis. It may be used in patients with acute upper gastrointestinal hemorrhage to promote gastric emptying of blood before endoscopy.

■ LAXATIVES

The overwhelming majority of people do not need laxatives; yet they are self-prescribed by a large portion of the population. For most people, intermittent constipation is best prevented with a high-fiber diet, adequate fluid intake, regular exercise, and the heeding of nature's call. Patients not responding to dietary changes or fiber supplements should undergo medical evaluation before initiating long-term laxative treatment. Laxatives may be classified by their major mechanism of action, but many work through more than one mechanism.

BULK-FORMING LAXATIVES

Bulk-forming laxatives are indigestible, hydrophilic colloids that absorb water, forming a bulky, emollient gel that distends the colon and promotes peristalsis. Common preparations include natural plant products **(psyllium, methylcellulose)** and synthetic fibers **(polycarbophil).** Bacterial digestion of plant fibers within the colon may lead to increased bloating and flatus.

STOOL SURFACTANT AGENTS (SOFTENERS)

These agents soften stool material, permitting water and lipids to penetrate. They may be administered orally or rectally. Common agents include **docusate** (oral or enema) and **glycerin suppository.** In hospitalized patients, docusate is commonly prescribed to prevent constipation and minimize straining. **Mineral oil** is a clear, viscous oil that lubricates fecal material, retarding water absorption from the stool. It is used to prevent and treat fecal impaction in young children and debilitated adults. It is not palatable but may be mixed with juices. Aspiration can result in a severe lipid pneumonitis. Long-term use can impair absorption of fat-soluble vitamins (A, D, E, K).

OSMOTIC LAXATIVES

The colon can neither concentrate nor dilute fecal fluid: fecal water is isotonic throughout the colon. Osmotic laxatives are soluble but nonabsorbable compounds that result in increased stool liquidity due to an obligate increase in fecal fluid.

Nonabsorbable Sugars or Salts

These agents may be used for the treatment of acute constipation or the prevention of chronic constipation. **Magnesium hydroxide (milk of magnesia)** is a commonly used osmotic laxative. It should not be used for prolonged periods in patients with renal insufficiency due to the risk of hypermagnesemia. **Sorbitol** and **lactulose** are nonabsorbable sugars that can be used to prevent or treat chronic constipation. These sugars are metabolized by colonic bacteria, producing flatus and cramps.

High doses of osmotically active agents produce prompt bowel evacuation (purgation) within 1–3 hours. The rapid movement of water into the distal small bowel and colon leads to a high volume of liquid stool followed by bowel evacuation. Several purgatives are available, which may be used for the treatment of acute constipation or to cleanse the bowel prior to medical procedures (eg, colonoscopy). These include **magnesium citrate, sulfate solution,** and a proprietary combination of magnesium oxide, sodium picosulfate, and citrate (Prepopik). When taking these purgatives, it is very important that patients maintain adequate hydration by taking increased oral liquids to compensate for fecal fluid loss. **Sodium phosphate** also is available—by prescription—as a tablet formulation but is infrequently used due to the risk of hyperphosphatemia, hypocalcemia, hypernatremia, and hypokalemia. Although these electrolyte abnormalities are clinically insignificant in most patients, they may lead to cardiac arrhythmias or acute renal failure due to tubular deposition of calcium phosphate (nephrocalcinosis). Sodium phosphate preparations should not be used in patients who are frail or elderly, have renal insufficiency, have significant cardiac disease, or are unable to maintain adequate hydration during bowel preparation.

Balanced Polyethylene Glycol

Lavage solutions containing **polyethylene glycol (PEG)** are commonly used for complete colonic cleansing before gastrointestinal endoscopic procedures. These balanced, isotonic solutions contain an inert, nonabsorbable, osmotically active sugar (PEG) with sodium sulfate, sodium chloride, sodium bicarbonate, and potassium chloride. The solution is designed so that no significant intravascular fluid or electrolyte shifts occur. Therefore, they are safe for all patients. For optimal bowel cleansing, 1–2 L of solution should be ingested rapidly (over 1–2 hours) on the evening before the procedure and again 4–6 hours before the procedure. For treatment or prevention of chronic constipation, smaller doses of PEG powder may be mixed with water or juices (17 g/8 oz) and ingested daily. In contrast to sorbitol or lactulose, PEG does not produce significant cramps or flatus.

STIMULANT LAXATIVES

Stimulant laxatives (cathartics) induce bowel movements through a number of poorly understood mechanisms. These include direct stimulation of the enteric nervous system and colonic electrolyte and fluid secretion. There has been concern that long-term use of cathartics could lead to dependence and destruction of the myenteric plexus, resulting in colonic atony and dilation. More recent research suggests that long-term use of these agents probably is safe in most patients. Cathartics may be required on a long-term basis, especially in patients who are neurologically impaired and in bed-bound patients in long-term care facilities.

Anthraquinone Derivatives

Aloe, senna, and **cascara** occur naturally in plants. These laxatives are poorly absorbed and, after hydrolysis in the colon, produce a bowel movement in 6–12 hours when given orally and within 2 hours when given rectally. Chronic use leads to a characteristic brown pigmentation of the colon known as "melanosis coli." There has been some concern that these agents may be carcinogenic, but epidemiologic studies do not suggest a relation to colorectal cancer.

Diphenylmethane Derivatives

Bisacodyl is available in tablet and suppository formulations for the treatment of acute and chronic constipation. It also is used in conjunction with PEG solutions for colonic cleansing prior to colonoscopy. It induces a bowel movement within 6–10 hours when given orally and 30–60 minutes when taken rectally. It has minimal systemic absorption and appears to be safe for acute and long-term use.

CHLORIDE SECRETION ACTIVATORS

Lubiprostone is a prostanoic acid derivative labeled for use in chronic constipation and irritable bowel syndrome (IBS) with predominant constipation. It acts by stimulating the type 2 chloride channel (ClC-2) in the small intestine. This increases chloride-rich fluid secretion into the intestine, which stimulates intestinal motility and shortens intestinal transit time. More than 50% of patients experience a bowel movement within 24 hours of taking one dose. A dose of 24 mcg orally twice daily is the recommended dose for treatment of chronic constipation. There appears to be no loss of efficacy with long-term therapy. After discontinuation of the drug, constipation may return to its pretreatment severity. Lubiprostone has minimal systemic absorption but is designated category C for pregnancy because of increased fetal loss in guinea pigs. Lubiprostone may cause nausea in up to 30% of patients due to delayed gastric emptying.

Linaclotide and **plecanatide** are minimally absorbed, short amino acid peptides that stimulate intestinal chloride secretion through a different mechanism by binding to and activating guanylate cyclase-C on the luminal surface. This leads to increased intracellular and extracellular cyclic guanosine monophosphate (cGMP) with activation of the cystic fibrosis transmembrane conductance regulator (CFTR), followed by chloride-rich secretion and acceleration of intestinal transit. Both agents are approved for the treatment of chronic constipation (linaclotide 145 mcg orally once daily; plecanatide 3 mg orally once daily); linaclotide is also approved for the treatment of irritable bowel syndrome with constipation (290 mcg orally once daily). These agents result in an average increase of 1–2 bowel movements per week that usually occurs within the first week of treatment. Upon discontinuation of the drug, bowel movement frequency returns to normal within 1 week. The most common side effect is diarrhea, which occurs in up to 20% of patients, leads to discontinuation in 4–5%, and is severe in 0.6–2%. These drugs have negligible absorption at standard doses. Both drugs are contraindicated in pediatric patients because of reports of increased mortality in juvenile mice from dehydration. (**Crofelemer** is a small molecule with the opposite effect: it is an *inhibitor* of the CFTR channel and is approved for the treatment of HIV-drug-induced diarrhea.)

OPIOID RECEPTOR ANTAGONISTS

Acute and chronic therapy with opioids may cause constipation by increasing nonpropulsive colonic contractions, which result in prolonged transit time and increased absorption of fecal water (see Chapter 31). Use of opioids after surgery for treatment of pain as well as endogenous opioids also may prolong the duration of postoperative ileus. These effects are mainly mediated through intestinal mu (μ)-opioid receptors. Four selective antagonists of the μ-opioid receptor are commercially available: **naldemedine, naloxegol, methylnaltrexone bromide,** and **alvimopan.** Because these agents do not readily cross the blood-brain barrier, they inhibit peripheral μ-opioid receptors without impacting analgesic effects within the central nervous system. Naldemedine (0.2 mg orally once daily) and naloxegol (12.5–25 mg orally once daily) are approved for treatment of opioid-induced constipation in patients with chronic noncancer pain with inadequate response to laxatives. In clinical trials, the number of patients able to achieve at least 3 spontaneous bowel movements/week was 42–52% with these agents compared with 30–35% with placebo. Both agents are metabolized by the hepatic CYP3A system, with serum concentrations increased by CYP3A4 inhibitors and reduced by strong CYP3A4 inducers. Methylnaltrexone is approved for the treatment of opioid-induced constipation in patients with chronic noncancer pain and patients receiving palliative care for advanced illness who have had inadequate response to other agents. It is administered either orally (450 mg) or as a subcutaneous injection (0.15 mg/kg) every 1–2 days. A dose reduction is recommended for patients with renal impairment (creatinine clearance [Cl_{cr}] <60 mL/min) and hepatic impairment. It has no significant drug interactions. Adverse events occurring with all three agents include nausea, abdominal pain, and diarrhea. Uncommon events include symptoms of opioid withdrawal and gastrointestinal perforation in the presence of underlying GI disorders. Alvimopan is approved for short-term use to shorten the period of postoperative ileus in hospitalized patients who have undergone small or large bowel resection. Alvimopan (12 mg capsule) is administered orally within 5 hours before surgery and twice daily after surgery until bowel function has recovered, but for no more than 7 days. Because of possible cardiovascular toxicity, alvimopan currently is restricted to short-term use in hospitalized patients only.

SEROTONIN 5-HT$_4$-RECEPTOR AGONISTS

5-HT$_4$ receptors are located throughout the GI tract on smooth muscle cells, the myenteric plexus, and enterochromaffin cells. Activation of the 5-HT$_4$ receptor increases cAMP, which facilitates release of neurotransmitters, including acetylcholine from stimulatory myenteric neurons, nitric oxide from inhibitory myenteric neurons, and calcitonin gene-related peptide and acetylcholine from intrinsic primary afferent neurons (see Figure 62–4). The most important outcome is the enhanced release of acetylcholine, which stimulates motility throughout the GI tract, including the stomach, small intestine, and colon. In the colon, acetylcholine stimulates contraction of the longitudinal muscle layer and relaxation of the circular muscle layer, leading to high-amplitude propagating (peristaltic) contractions (HAPC) of the proximal colon and inhibition of the distal colon, which results in forward propulsion of fecal contents.

Prucalopride is a high-affinity 5-HT$_4$ agonist that is approved for the treatment of chronic constipation at a dose of 2 mg once daily. Prucalopride increases both the strength and number of colonic HAPCs, thereby reducing mean transit time of feces through the colon by 12 hours. In contrast to cisapride and tegaserod (which were removed from the market due to adverse cardiovascular events), it does not appear to have significant affinities for either hERG K^+ channels or 5-HT$_{1B}$ receptors and has no identified cardiovascular risk. In six 12- to 24-week clinical trials of patients with chronic constipation, 19–38% of patients treated with prucalopride experienced at least 3 spontaneous bowel movements per week, which was 5–23% more than placebo. Prucalopride is well absorbed and excreted largely unchanged by the kidneys. A dose reduction to 1 mg/day is recommended in patients with Cl_{cr} <30 ml/min. The most frequent side effects are nausea, abdominal pain, and diarrhea, which lead to drug discontinuation in up to 5%. Prucalopride has no identified clinically significant drug interactions.

ANTIDIARRHEAL AGENTS

Antidiarrheal agents may be used safely in patients with mild to moderate acute diarrhea. However, these agents should not be used in patients with bloody diarrhea, high fever, or systemic toxicity because of the risk of worsening the underlying condition. They should be discontinued in patients whose diarrhea is worsening despite therapy. Antidiarrheals are also used to control chronic diarrhea caused by such conditions as IBS or inflammatory bowel disease (IBD).

OPIOID AGONISTS

As previously noted, opioids have significant constipating effects (see Chapter 31). They increase colonic phasic segmenting activity through inhibition of presynaptic cholinergic nerves in the submucosal and myenteric plexuses and lead to increased colonic transit time and fecal water absorption. They also decrease mass colonic movements and the gastrocolic reflex. Although all opioids have antidiarrheal effects, central nervous system effects and potential for addiction limit the usefulness of most.

Loperamide is a nonprescription opioid agonist that does not cross the blood-brain barrier and has no analgesic properties or potential for addiction. Tolerance to long-term use has not been reported. It is typically administered in doses of 2 mg taken one to four times daily. **Diphenoxylate** is a prescription opioid agonist that has no analgesic properties in standard doses; however, higher doses have central nervous system effects, and prolonged use can lead to opioid dependence. Commercial preparations commonly contain small amounts of atropine to discourage overdosage (2.5 mg diphenoxylate with 0.025 mg atropine). The anticholinergic properties of atropine may contribute to the antidiarrheal action.

Eluxadoline is a prescription opioid agonist with high affinity for the mu receptor (as well as low affinity for the delta receptor). When taken orally, eluxadoline binds to gut opioid receptors, resulting in slower colonic transit and increased fecal fluid absorption. Eluxadoline is approved for the treatment of patients with diarrhea-predominant IBS at a dose of 75–100 mg twice daily. In two randomized placebo-controlled trials, eluxadoline 100 mg twice daily led to significant improvement in abdominal pain and diarrhea in 30% of patients compared with 16% with placebo. Constipation may occur in 8% of patients. Approximately 1% of patients may experience sphincter of Oddi spasm (usually within the first week of therapy) resulting in abdominal pain, pancreatitis, and/or elevated pancreatic or liver enzymes. Eluxadoline should not be used in patients with a history of pancreatitis, alcoholism, or known sphincter of Oddi disease. Caution is advised in patients with prior cholecystectomy, in whom there is up to a 5% risk of complications due to sphincter of Oddi spasm. Eluxadoline 75 mg twice daily is recommended for patients with prior cholecystectomy, mild to moderate liver disease, or side effects at the higher dose.

COLLOIDAL BISMUTH COMPOUNDS

See the section under Mucosal Protective Agents.

BILE SALT-BINDING RESINS

Conjugated bile salts are normally absorbed in the terminal ileum. Disease of the terminal ileum (eg, Crohn disease) or surgical resection leads to malabsorption of bile salts, which may cause colonic secretory diarrhea. The bile salt-binding resins **cholestyramine, colestipol,** or **colesevelam** may decrease diarrhea caused by excess fecal bile acids (see Chapter 35). These products come in a variety of powder and pill formulations that may be taken one to three times daily before meals. Adverse effects include bloating, flatulence, constipation, and fecal impaction. In patients with diminished circulating bile acid pools, further removal of bile acids may lead to an exacerbation of fat malabsorption. Cholestyramine and colestipol bind a number of drugs and reduce their absorption; hence, they should not be given within 2 hours of other drugs. Colesevelam does not appear to have significant effects on absorption of other drugs.

OCTREOTIDE

Somatostatin is a 14-amino-acid peptide that is released in the gastrointestinal tract and pancreas from paracrine cells, D cells, and enteric nerves as well as from the hypothalamus (see Chapter 37). Somatostatin is a key regulatory peptide that has many physiologic effects:

1. It inhibits the secretion of numerous hormones and transmitters, including gastrin, cholecystokinin, glucagon, growth hormone, insulin, secretin, pancreatic polypeptide, vasoactive intestinal peptide, and 5-HT.
2. It reduces intestinal fluid secretion and pancreatic secretion.
3. It slows gastrointestinal motility and inhibits gallbladder contraction.
4. It reduces portal and splanchnic blood flow.
5. It inhibits secretion of some anterior pituitary hormones.

The clinical usefulness of somatostatin is limited by its short half-life in the circulation (3 minutes) when it is administered by intravenous injection. **Octreotide** is a synthetic octapeptide with actions similar to somatostatin. When administered intravenously, it has a serum half-life of 1.5 hours. It also may be administered by subcutaneous injection, resulting in a 6- to 12-hour duration of action. A longer-acting formulation is available for once-monthly depot intramuscular injection.

Clinical Uses

1. *Inhibition of endocrine tumor effects*—Two gastrointestinal neuroendocrine tumors (carcinoid, VIPoma) cause secretory diarrhea and systemic symptoms such as flushing and wheezing. For patients with advanced symptomatic tumors that cannot be completely removed by surgery, octreotide decreases secretory diarrhea and systemic symptoms through inhibition of hormonal secretion and may slow tumor progression.

2. *Other causes of diarrhea*—Octreotide inhibits intestinal secretion and has dose-related effects on bowel motility. In low doses (50 mcg subcutaneously), it stimulates motility, whereas at higher doses (eg, 100–250 mcg subcutaneously), it inhibits motility. Octreotide is effective in higher doses for the treatment of diarrhea due to vagotomy or dumping syndrome as well as for diarrhea caused by short-bowel syndrome or AIDS. Octreotide has been used in low doses (50 mcg subcutaneously) to stimulate small bowel motility in patients with small bowel bacterial overgrowth or intestinal pseudo-obstruction secondary to scleroderma.

3. *Other uses*—Because it inhibits pancreatic secretion, octreotide may be of value in patients with pancreatic fistula. The role of octreotide in the treatment of pituitary tumors (eg, acromegaly) is discussed in Chapter 37. Octreotide is sometimes used in gastrointestinal bleeding (see below).

Adverse Effects

Impaired pancreatic secretion may cause steatorrhea, which can lead to fat-soluble vitamin deficiency. Alterations in gastrointestinal motility cause nausea, abdominal pain, flatulence, and diarrhea. Because of inhibition of gallbladder contractility and alterations in fat absorption, long-term use of octreotide can cause formation of sludge or gallstones in over 50% of patients, which rarely results in the development of acute cholecystitis. Because octreotide alters the balance among insulin, glucagon, and growth hormone, hyperglycemia or, less frequently, hypoglycemia (usually mild) can occur. Prolonged treatment with octreotide may result in hypothyroidism. Octreotide can also cause bradycardia.

■ DRUGS USED IN THE TREATMENT OF IRRITABLE BOWEL SYNDROME

IBS is an idiopathic chronic, relapsing disorder characterized by abdominal discomfort (pain, bloating, distention, or cramps) in association with alterations in bowel habits (diarrhea, constipation, or both). With episodes of abdominal pain or discomfort, patients note a change in the frequency or consistency of their bowel movements.

Pharmacologic therapies for IBS are directed at relieving abdominal pain and discomfort and improving bowel function. For patients with predominant diarrhea, antidiarrheal agents, especially loperamide, are helpful in reducing stool frequency and fecal urgency. For patients with predominant constipation, fiber supplements may lead to softening of stools and reduced straining; however, increased gas production may exacerbate bloating and abdominal discomfort. Consequently, osmotic laxatives (PEG, milk of magnesia) are commonly used to soften stools and promote increased stool frequency.

For chronic abdominal pain, low doses of tricyclic antidepressants (eg, amitriptyline or desipramine, 10–50 mg/d) appear to be helpful (see Chapter 30). At these doses, these agents have no effect on mood but may alter central processing of visceral afferent information. The anticholinergic properties of these agents also may have effects on gastrointestinal motility and secretion, reducing stool frequency and liquidity. Finally, tricyclic antidepressants may alter receptors for enteric neurotransmitters such as serotonin, affecting visceral afferent sensation.

Several other agents are available that are specifically intended for the treatment of IBS.

ANTISPASMODICS (ANTICHOLINERGICS)

Some agents are promoted as providing relief of abdominal pain or discomfort through antispasmodic actions. However, small or large bowel spasm has not been found to be an important cause of symptoms in patients with IBS. Antispasmodics work primarily through anticholinergic activities. Commonly used medications in this class include **dicyclomine** and **hyoscyamine** (see Chapter 8). These drugs inhibit muscarinic cholinergic receptors in the enteric plexus and on smooth muscle. Antispasmodics can provide short-term relief of abdominal pain in patients with IBS, but their long-term efficacy for relief of abdominal symptoms has never been convincingly established. At low doses, they have minimal autonomic effects. However, at higher doses they exhibit significant additional anticholinergic effects, including dry mouth, visual disturbances, urinary retention, and constipation. For these reasons, antispasmodics are infrequently used.

SEROTONIN 5-HT$_3$-RECEPTOR ANTAGONISTS

5-HT$_3$ receptors in the gastrointestinal tract activate visceral afferent pain sensation via extrinsic sensory neurons from the gut to the spinal cord and central nervous system. Inhibition of afferent gastrointestinal 5-HT$_3$ receptors may reduce unpleasant visceral afferent sensation, including nausea, bloating, and pain. Blockade of central 5-HT$_3$ receptors also reduces the central response to visceral afferent stimulation. In addition, 5-HT$_3$-receptor blockade on the terminals of enteric cholinergic neurons inhibits colonic motility, especially in the left colon, increasing total colonic transit time.

Alosetron is a highly potent and selective antagonist of the 5-HT$_3$ receptor. It is approved for the treatment of women with severe IBS in whom diarrhea is the predominant symptom ("diarrhea-predominant IBS"). Its efficacy in men has not been established. (Figure 62–5). Four other 5-HT$_3$ antagonists (ondansetron, granisetron, dolasetron, and palonosetron) have been approved for the prevention and treatment of nausea and vomiting (see Antiemetics); however, their efficacy in the treatment of IBS has not been determined. The differences between these 5-HT$_3$ antagonists that determine their pharmacodynamic effects have not been well studied.

In a dosage of 1 mg once or twice daily, alosetron reduces IBS-related lower abdominal pain, cramps, urgency, and diarrhea. Approximately 50–60% of patients report adequate relief of pain and discomfort with alosetron compared with 30–40% of patients treated with placebo. It also leads to a reduction in the mean number of bowel movements per day and improvement in stool consistency.

In contrast to the excellent safety profile of other 5-HT$_3$-receptor antagonists, alosetron is associated with rare but serious gastrointestinal toxicity. Constipation occurs in up to 30% of patients with diarrhea-predominant IBS, requiring discontinuation of the drug in 10%. Serious complications of constipation requiring hospitalization or surgery have occurred in 1 of every 1000 patients. Episodes of ischemic colitis—some fatal—have been reported in up to 3 per 1000 patients. Given the seriousness of these adverse events, alosetron is restricted to women with severe diarrhea-predominant IBS who have not responded to conventional therapies and who have been educated about the relative risks and benefits.

CHLORIDE CHANNEL ACTIVATORS

As discussed previously, **lubiprostone** is a prostanoic acid derivative that stimulates the type 2 chloride channel (ClC-2) in the small intestine. Lubiprostone is approved for the treatment of women with IBS with predominant constipation. Its efficacy for men with IBS is unproven. The approved dose for IBS is 8 mcg twice daily (compared with 24 mcg twice daily for chronic constipation). In clinical trials, lubiprostone resulted in modest clinical benefit—only 8% more patients than with placebo. Lubiprostone is listed as category C for pregnancy and should be avoided in women of child-bearing age.

Also discussed previously, **linaclotide** and **plecanatide** are guanylyl cyclase-C agonists that lead to activation of the CFTR in the small intestine with stimulation of chloride-rich intestinal secretion. Both are approved for treatment of adults with IBS with constipation: linaclotide at a dose of 290 mcg once daily (compared with 145 mcg once daily for chronic constipation) and plecanatide 3 mg once daily. In clinical trials, up to 25% more patients treated with these agents demonstrated significant clinical improvement compared with placebo. Linaclotide is listed as category C for pregnancy, and both agents are contraindicated for pediatric patients.

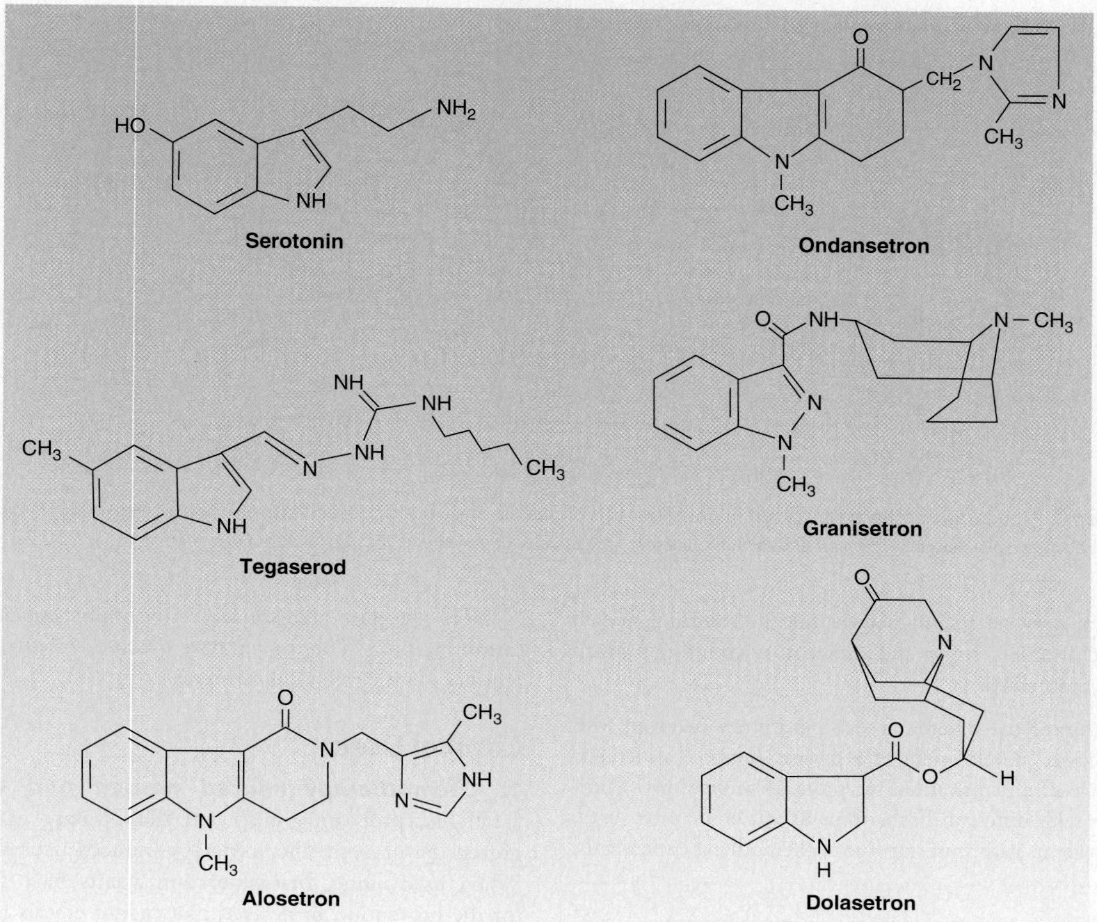

Serotonin

Ondansetron

Granisetron

Tegaserod

Alosetron

Dolasetron

FIGURE 62–5 Chemical structure of serotonin; the 5-HT_3 antagonists ondansetron, granisetron, dolasetron, and alosetron; and the 5-HT_4 partial agonist tegaserod.

Due to their high cost and lack of information about long-term safety and efficacy, the role of these agents in the treatment of IBS with constipation is uncertain. Neither agent has been compared with other less expensive laxatives (eg, milk of magnesia).

ANTIEMETIC AGENTS

Nausea and vomiting may be manifestations of a wide variety of conditions, including adverse effects from medications; systemic disorders or infections; pregnancy; vestibular dysfunction; central nervous system infection or increased pressure; peritonitis; hepatobiliary disorders; radiation or chemotherapy; and gastrointestinal obstruction, dysmotility, or infections.

PATHOPHYSIOLOGY

The brainstem "vomiting center" is a loosely organized neuronal region within the lateral medullary reticular formation and coordinates the complex act of vomiting through interactions with cranial nerves VIII and X and neural networks in the nucleus tractus solitarius that control respiratory, salivatory, and vasomotor centers. High concentrations of muscarinic M_1, histamine H_1, neurokinin 1 (NK_1), and serotonin 5-HT_3 receptors have been identified in the vomiting center (Figure 62–6).

There are four important sources of afferent input to the vomiting center:

1. The "chemoreceptor trigger zone" or area postrema is located at the caudal end of the fourth ventricle. This is outside the blood-brain barrier and is accessible to emetogenic stimuli in the blood or cerebrospinal fluid. The chemoreceptor trigger zone is rich in dopamine D_2 receptors and opioid receptors, and possibly serotonin 5-HT_3 receptors and NK_1 receptors.
2. The vestibular system is important in motion sickness via cranial nerve VIII. It is rich in muscarinic M_1 and histamine H_1 receptors.
3. Vagal and spinal afferent nerves from the gastrointestinal tract are rich in 5-HT_3 receptors. Irritation of the gastrointestinal mucosa by chemotherapy, radiation therapy, distention, or acute infectious gastroenteritis leads to release of mucosal serotonin and activation of these receptors, which stimulate vagal afferent input to the vomiting center and chemoreceptor trigger zone.

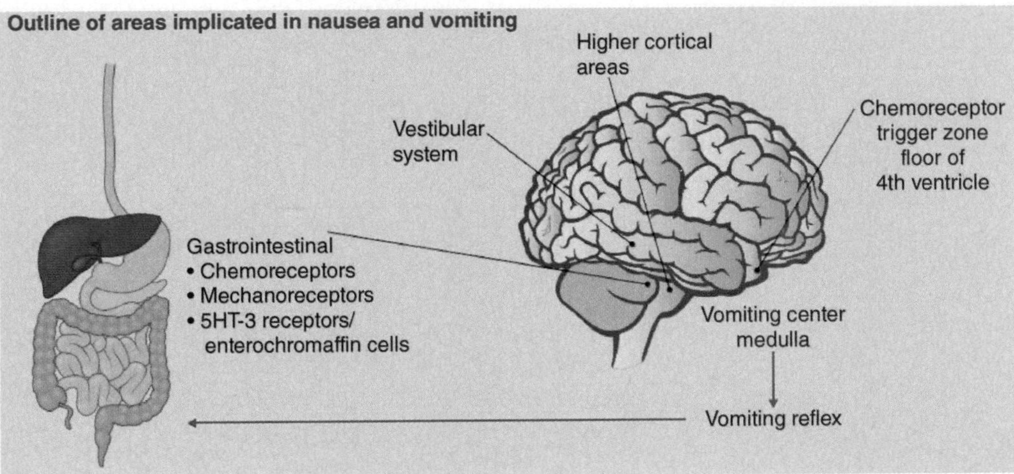

FIGURE 62–6 Neurologic pathways involved in pathogenesis of nausea and vomiting (see text). (Reproduced with permission from Denholm L., Gallagher G. Physiology and pharmacology of nausea and vomiting. Anaesthesia & Intensive Care Medicine. 2021;22(10): 663-666.)

4. The central nervous system plays a role in vomiting due to psychiatric disorders, stress, and anticipatory vomiting prior to cancer chemotherapy.

Identification of the different neurotransmitters involved with emesis has allowed development of a diverse group of antiemetic agents that have affinity for various receptors. Combinations of antiemetic agents with different mechanisms of action are often used, especially in patients with vomiting due to chemotherapeutic agents.

SEROTONIN 5-HT$_3$ ANTAGONISTS

Pharmacokinetics & Pharmacodynamics

Selective 5-HT$_3$-receptor antagonists have potent antiemetic properties that are mediated in part through central 5-HT$_3$-receptor blockade in the vomiting center and chemoreceptor trigger zone but mainly through blockade of peripheral 5-HT$_3$ receptors on extrinsic intestinal vagal and spinal afferent nerves. The antiemetic action of these agents is restricted to emesis attributable to vagal stimulation (eg, postoperative) and chemotherapy; other emetic stimuli such as motion sickness are poorly controlled.

Four agents are available in the USA: **ondansetron, granisetron, dolasetron,** and **palonosetron.** (**Tropisetron** and **ramosetron** are available outside the USA.) The three "first-generation" agents (ondansetron, granisetron, and dolasetron; see Figure 62–5) have a serum half-life of 4–9 hours and have comparable efficacy when administered at equipotent doses. Palonosetron is a "second-generation" agent that has greater affinity for the 5-HT$_3$ receptor and a long serum half-life of 40 hours. All agents except dolasetron are available in oral and intravenous formulations. Granisetron is also available as a transdermal patch. All four drugs undergo extensive hepatic metabolism and are eliminated by renal and hepatic excretion. However, dose reduction is not required in geriatric patients or patients with renal insufficiency. For patients with hepatic insufficiency, dose reduction may be required with ondansetron.

5-HT$_3$-receptor antagonists do not inhibit dopamine or muscarinic receptors. They do not have effects on esophageal or gastric motility but may slow colonic transit.

Clinical Uses

1. *Chemotherapy-induced nausea and vomiting—* 5-HT$_3$-receptor antagonists are the primary agents for the prevention of acute chemotherapy-induced nausea and emesis. When used alone, first-generation agents have little efficacy for the prevention of delayed nausea and emesis (ie, occurring >24 hours after chemotherapy). The second-generation agent palonosetron is more effective than the first-generation agents in the prevention of acute nausea and emesis, and it is also effective in the prevention of delayed nausea and emesis. The drugs are most effective when given as a single dose by intravenous injection 30 minutes prior to administration of chemotherapy in the following doses: ondansetron, 8 mg; granisetron, 1 mg; dolasetron, 100 mg; or palonosetron, 0.25 mg. A single oral dose given 1 hour before chemotherapy may be equally effective in the following regimens: ondansetron 8 mg twice daily; granisetron, 2 mg; dolasetron, 100 mg; or palonosetron 0.5 mg. Although 5-HT$_3$-receptor antagonists are effective as single agents for the prevention of chemotherapy-induced nausea and vomiting, their efficacy is enhanced by combination therapy with a corticosteroid (dexamethasone), NK$_1$-receptor antagonist, and a dopamine D$_2$ antagonist (antipsychotics; see below).

2. *Postoperative and postradiation nausea and vomiting—* 5-HT$_3$-receptor antagonists are used to prevent or treat postoperative nausea and vomiting. Because of adverse effects and increased restrictions on the use of other antiemetic agents, 5-HT$_3$-receptor antagonists are increasingly used for this indication. They are also effective in the prevention and treatment of nausea and vomiting in patients undergoing radiation therapy to the whole body or abdomen.

Adverse Effects

The 5-HT_3-receptor antagonists are well-tolerated agents with excellent safety profiles. The most commonly reported adverse effects are headache, dizziness, and constipation. The first-generation agents cause a small but statistically significant prolongation of the QT interval, but this is most pronounced with dolasetron. The FDA has advised that these agents should not be administered to patients with prolonged QT or in conjunction with other medications that may prolong the QT interval (see Chapter 14). Palonosetron does not appear to cause QT interval prolongation. Serotonin syndrome has been reported in patients taking 5-HT_3-receptor antagonists in combination with other serotonergic drugs (selective serotonin reuptake inhibitors [SSRIs] and serotonin-norepinephrine reuptake inhibitors [SNRIs]; see Chapter 30).

Drug Interactions

No significant drug interactions have been reported with 5-HT_3-receptor antagonists. All four agents undergo some metabolism by the hepatic cytochrome P450 system, but they do not appear to affect the metabolism of other drugs. However, other drugs may reduce hepatic clearance of the 5-HT_3-receptor antagonists, altering their half-life.

CORTICOSTEROIDS

Corticosteroids (dexamethasone, methylprednisolone) have antiemetic properties, but the basis for these effects is unknown. The pharmacology of this class of drugs is discussed in Chapter 39. These agents appear to enhance the efficacy of 5-HT_3-receptor antagonists for prevention of acute and delayed nausea and vomiting in patients receiving moderately to highly emetogenic chemotherapy regimens. Although a number of corticosteroids have been used, dexamethasone, 8–20 mg orally or intravenously before chemotherapy, followed by 8 mg/d orally for 2–4 days, is commonly administered.

NEUROKININ RECEPTOR ANTAGONISTS

Neurokinin 1 (NK_1)-receptor antagonists have antiemetic properties that are mediated through central blockade in the area postrema. **Aprepitant, netupitant,** and **rolapitant** (all oral formulations) are highly selective NK_1-receptor antagonists that cross the blood-brain barrier and occupy brain NK_1 receptors. They have no affinity for serotonin, dopamine, or corticosteroid receptors. Netupitant (300 mg) is available only as a combination product with palonosetron (0.5 mg). **Fosaprepitant** is an intravenous formulation that is converted within 30 minutes after infusion to aprepitant.

Pharmacokinetics

The oral bioavailability of aprepitant is 65%, and the serum half-life is 12 hours. Netupitant and rolapitant have longer half-lives (90 and 180 hours, respectively), allowing single-dose administration. All three agents are metabolized by the liver, primarily by the CYP3A4 pathway.

Clinical Uses

NK_1-receptor antagonists are used in combination with 5-HT_3-receptor antagonists and corticosteroids for the prevention of acute and delayed nausea and vomiting from highly emetogenic chemotherapeutic regimens. Combined therapy with an NK_1-receptor antagonist, a 5-HT_3-receptor antagonist, and dexamethasone prevents acute emesis in 80–90% of patients compared with less than 70% of patients treated without an NK_1 antagonist. Prevention of delayed emesis occurs in more than 70% of patients receiving combined therapy versus 30–50% treated without an NK_1 antagonist. Oral NK_1-receptor antagonists may be administered as follows: aprepitant 125 mg given 1 hour before chemotherapy, followed by oral aprepitant 80 mg/d for 2 days after chemotherapy; rolapitant 180 mg; or netupitant 300 mg/palonosetron 0.5 mg given as a single dose 1–2 hours before chemotherapy. For patients unable to tolerate oral therapy, intravenous fosaprepitant 115 mg or rolapitant 166.5 mg may be given as a single dose 1 hour before chemotherapy. The addition of the antipsychotic agent olanzapine 10 mg on days 1–4 further decreases the incidence of acute and delayed nausea and vomiting with highly emetogenic chemotherapeutic regimens by 15–30%.

Adverse Effects & Drug Interactions

The NK_1-receptor antagonists are well tolerated with a low incidence of fatigue and dizziness. The drugs are metabolized by CYP3A4 and may inhibit the metabolism of other drugs metabolized by the CYP3A4 pathway. Several chemotherapeutic agents are metabolized by CYP3A4, including docetaxel, paclitaxel, etoposide, irinotecan, imatinib, vinblastine, and vincristine, as well as dexamethasone. To date, there is no clinical evidence of prolonged exposure and increased toxicity to the chemotherapeutic agents. The dose of dexamethasone when used in combination with an NK_1-receptor antagonist as part of an antiemetic regimen is commonly reduced. Drugs that inhibit CYP3A4 metabolism may significantly increase aprepitant plasma levels (eg, ketoconazole, ciprofloxacin, clarithromycin, nefazodone, ritonavir, nelfinavir, verapamil, and quinidine). Aprepitant decreases the international normalized ratio (INR) in patients taking warfarin.

ANTIPSYCHOTIC AGENTS AS ANTIEMETICS (PHENOTHIAZINES, BUTYROPHENONES, & THIENOBENZODIAZEPINES)

Several classes of antipsychotic agents can be used for their antiemetic and sedative properties (see Chapter 29). The antiemetic properties of phenothiazines are mediated through inhibition of dopamine and muscarinic receptors. Sedative properties are due to their antihistamine activity. The agents most commonly used as antiemetics are **prochlorperazine, promethazine,** and **thiethylperazine.** The antiemetic properties of **olanzapine** (a thienobenzodiazepine) may be attributable to inhibition of dopamine D_2 and serotonin 5-HT_{1c} and 5-HT_3 receptors.

Antipsychotic butyrophenones also possess antiemetic properties due to their central dopaminergic blockade (see Chapter 29). The main agent used is **droperidol,** which can be given by intramuscular or intravenous injection. In antiemetic doses, droperidol is extremely sedating. Previously, it was used extensively for postoperative nausea and vomiting, in conjunction with opiates and benzodiazepines for sedation for surgical and endoscopic procedures, for neuroleptanalgesia, and for induction and maintenance of general anesthesia. Extrapyramidal effects and hypotension may occur. Droperidol may prolong the QT interval, rarely resulting in fatal episodes of ventricular tachycardia including torsades de pointes. Therefore, droperidol should not be used in patients with QT prolongation and should be used only in patients who have not responded adequately to alternative agents.

SUBSTITUTED BENZAMIDES

Substituted benzamides include **metoclopramide** (discussed previously) and **trimethobenzamide.** Their primary mechanism of antiemetic action is believed to be dopamine-receptor blockade. Trimethobenzamide also has weak antihistaminic activity. For prevention and treatment of nausea and vomiting, metoclopramide may be given in the relatively high dosage of 10–20 mg orally or intravenously every 6 hours. The usual dose of trimethobenzamide is 300 mg orally, or 200 mg by intramuscular injection. The principal adverse effects of these central dopamine antagonists are extrapyramidal: restlessness, dystonias, and parkinsonian symptoms.

H_1 ANTIHISTAMINES & ANTICHOLINERGIC DRUGS

The pharmacology of anticholinergic agents is discussed in Chapter 8 and that of H_1 antihistaminic agents in Chapter 16. As single agents, these drugs have weak antiemetic activity, although they are particularly useful for the prevention or treatment of motion sickness. Their use may be limited by dizziness, sedation, confusion, dry mouth, cycloplegia, and urinary retention. **Diphenhydramine** and one of its salts, **dimenhydrinate,** are first-generation histamine H_1 antagonists that also have significant anticholinergic properties. Because of its sedating properties, diphenhydramine is commonly used in conjunction with other antiemetics for treatment of emesis due to chemothe rapy. **Meclizine** is an H_1 antihistaminic agent with minimal anticholinergic properties that also causes less sedation. It is used for the prevention of motion sickness and the treatment of vertigo due to labyrinth dysfunction.

Hyoscine (scopolamine), a prototypic muscarinic receptor antagonist, is one of the best agents for the prevention of motion sickness. However, it has a very high incidence of anticholinergic effects when given orally or parenterally. It is better tolerated as a transdermal patch. Superiority to dimenhydrinate has not been proved.

BENZODIAZEPINES

Benzodiazepines such as lorazepam or diazepam are used before the initiation of chemotherapy to reduce anticipatory vomiting or vomiting caused by anxiety. The pharmacology of these agents is presented in Chapter 22.

CANNABINOIDS

Dronabinol is Δ^9-tetrahydrocannabinol (THC), the major psychoactive chemical in marijuana (see Chapters 32 and 63). After oral ingestion, the drug is almost completely absorbed but undergoes significant first-pass hepatic metabolism. Its metabolites are excreted slowly over days to weeks in the feces and urine. Like crude marijuana, dronabinol is a psychoactive agent that is used medically as an appetite stimulant and as an antiemetic, but the mechanisms for these effects are not understood. **Nabilone** is a closely related THC analog that has been available in other countries and is now approved for use in the USA.

Adverse effects of cannabinoids include euphoria, dysphoria, sedation, hallucinations, dry mouth, and increased appetite. They have some autonomic effects that may result in tachycardia, conjunctival injection, and orthostatic hypotension. Although there are no significant drug-drug interactions, they may potentiate the clinical effects of other psychoactive agents. Because of the availability of more effective agents, cannabinoids are not commonly prescribed for the prevention of chemotherapy-induced nausea and vomiting, although some patients may utilize medical marijuana.

■ DRUGS USED TO TREAT INFLAMMATORY BOWEL DISEASE (IBD)

IBD comprises two distinct disorders: ulcerative colitis and Crohn disease. The etiology and pathogenesis of these disorders remain unknown. For this reason, pharmacologic treatment of inflammatory bowel disorders often involves drugs that belong to different therapeutic classes and have different but nonspecific mechanisms of anti-inflammatory action. Drugs used in IBD are chosen on the basis of disease severity, responsiveness, and drug toxicity.

AMINOSALICYLATES

Chemistry & Formulations

Drugs that contain **5-aminosalicylic acid (5-ASA)** have been used successfully for decades in the treatment of IBDs (Figure 62–7). 5-ASA differs from salicylic acid only by the addition of an amino group at the 5 (meta) position. Aminosalicylates are believed to

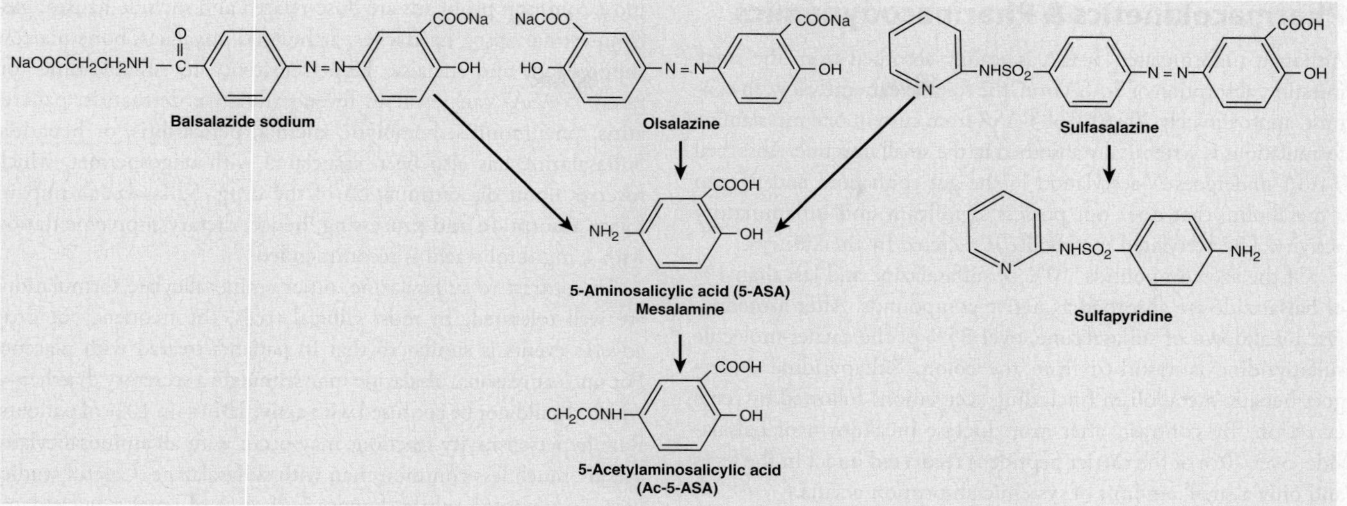

FIGURE 62–7 Chemical structures and metabolism of aminosalicylates. Azo compounds (balsalazide, olsalazine, sulfasalazine) are converted by bacterial azoreductase to 5-aminosalicylic acid (mesalamine), the active therapeutic moiety.

work topically (not systemically) in areas of diseased gastrointestinal mucosa. Up to 80% of unformulated, aqueous 5-ASA is absorbed from the small intestine and does not reach the distal small bowel or colon in appreciable quantities. To overcome the rapid absorption of 5-ASA from the proximal small intestine, a number of formulations have been designed to deliver 5-ASA to various distal segments of the small bowel or the colon. These include **sulfasalazine, olsalazine, balsalazide,** and various forms of **mesalamine.**

1. *Azo compounds*—Sulfasalazine, balsalazide, and olsalazine contain 5-ASA bound by an azo (N=N) bond to an inert compound or to another 5-ASA molecule (see Figure 62–7). In sulfasalazine, 5-ASA is bound to sulfapyridine; in balsalazide, 5-ASA is bound to 4-aminobenzoyl-β-alanine; and in olsalazine, two 5-ASA molecules are bound together. The azo structure markedly reduces absorption of the parent drug from the small intestine. In the terminal ileum and colon, resident bacteria cleave the azo bond by means of an azoreductase enzyme, releasing the active 5-ASA. Consequently, high concentrations of active drug are made available in the terminal ileum or colon.

2. *Mesalamine compounds*—Other proprietary formulations have been designed that package 5-ASA itself in various ways to deliver it to different segments of the small or large bowel. These 5-ASA formulations are known generically as **mesalamine. Pentasa** is a mesalamine formulation that contains timed-release microgranules that release 5-ASA throughout the small intestine (Figure 62–8). **Asacol** and **Apriso** have 5-ASA coated in a pH-sensitive resin that dissolves at pH 6–7 (the pH of the distal ileum and proximal colon). **Lialda** also uses a pH-dependent resin that encases a multimatrix core. On dissolution of the pH-sensitive resin in the colon, water slowly penetrates its hydrophilic and lipophilic core, leading to slow release of mesalamine throughout the colon. 5-ASA also may be delivered in high concentrations to the rectum and sigmoid colon by means of enema formulations **(Rowasa)** or suppositories **(Canasa).**

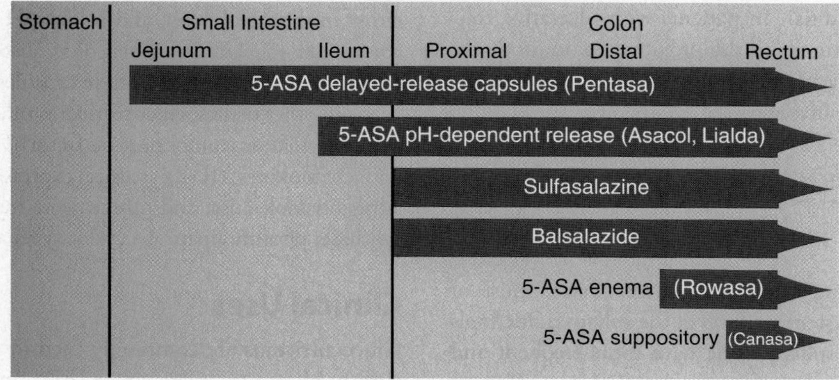

FIGURE 62–8 Sites of 5-aminosalicylic acid (5-ASA) release from different formulations in the small and large intestines.

Pharmacokinetics & Pharmacodynamics

Although unformulated 5-ASA is readily absorbed from the small intestine, absorption of 5-ASA from the colon is extremely low. In contrast, approximately 20–30% of 5-ASA from current oral mesalamine formulations is systemically absorbed in the small intestine. Absorbed 5-ASA undergoes *N*-acetylation in the gut epithelium and liver to a metabolite that does not possess significant anti-inflammatory activity. The acetylated metabolite is excreted by the kidneys.

Of the azo compounds, 10% of sulfasalazine and less than 1% of balsalazide are absorbed as native compounds. After azoreductase breakdown of sulfasalazine, over 85% of the carrier molecule sulfapyridine is absorbed from the colon. Sulfapyridine undergoes hepatic metabolism (including acetylation) followed by renal excretion. By contrast, after azoreductase breakdown of balsalazide, over 70% of the carrier peptide is recovered intact in the feces and only a small amount of systemic absorption occurs.

The mechanism of action of 5-ASA compounds is not certain, but they are thought to act topically. The primary action of salicylate and other NSAIDs is due to systemic blockade of prostaglandin synthesis by inhibition of cyclooxygenase. However, the aminosalicylates have variable effects on prostaglandin production. It is thought that 5-ASA modulates inflammatory mediators derived from both the cyclooxygenase and lipoxygenase pathways. Other potential mechanisms of action of the 5-ASA drugs relate to their ability to interfere with the production of inflammatory cytokines. 5-ASA inhibits the activity of nuclear factor-κB (NF-κB), an important transcription factor for proinflammatory cytokines. 5-ASA may also inhibit cellular functions of natural killer cells, mucosal lymphocytes, and macrophages, and it may scavenge reactive oxygen metabolites.

Clinical Uses

5-ASA drugs induce and maintain remission in ulcerative colitis and are considered to be the first-line agents for treatment of mild to moderate active ulcerative colitis. Their efficacy in Crohn disease is unproven, although many clinicians use 5-ASA agents as first-line therapy for mild to moderate disease involving the colon or distal ileum.

The effectiveness of 5-ASA therapy depends in part on achieving high drug concentration at the site of active disease. Thus, 5-ASA suppositories or enemas are useful in patients with ulcerative colitis or Crohn disease confined to the rectum (proctitis) or distal colon (proctosigmoiditis). In patients with ulcerative colitis or Crohn colitis that extends to the proximal colon, both the azo compounds and mesalamine formulations are useful. For the treatment of Crohn disease involving the small bowel, mesalamine compounds, which release 5-ASA in the small intestine, have a theoretic advantage over the azo compounds.

Adverse Effects

Sulfasalazine has a high incidence of adverse effects, most of which are attributable to systemic effects of the sulfapyridine molecule. Slow acetylators of sulfapyridine have more frequent and more severe adverse effects than fast acetylators. Up to 40% of patients cannot tolerate therapeutic doses of sulfasalazine. The most common problems are dose-related and include nausea, gastrointestinal upset, headaches, arthralgias, myalgias, bone marrow suppression, and malaise. Hypersensitivity to sulfapyridine (or, rarely, 5-ASA) can result in fever, exfoliative dermatitis, pancreatitis, pneumonitis, hemolytic anemia, pericarditis, or hepatitis. Sulfasalazine has also been associated with oligospermia, which reverses upon discontinuation of the drug. Sulfasalazine impairs folate absorption and processing; hence, dietary supplementation with 1 mg/d folic acid is recommended.

In contrast to sulfasalazine, other aminosalicylate formulations are well tolerated. In most clinical trials, the frequency of drug adverse events is similar to that in patients treated with placebo. For unclear reasons, olsalazine may stimulate a secretory diarrhea—which should not be confused with active IBD—in 10% of patients. Rare hypersensitivity reactions may occur with all aminosalicylates but are much less common than with sulfasalazine. Careful studies have documented subtle changes indicative of renal tubular damage in patients receiving high doses of aminosalicylates. Rare cases of interstitial nephritis are reported, particularly in association with high doses of mesalamine formulations; this may be attributable to the higher serum 5-ASA levels attained with these drugs. Sulfasalazine and other aminosalicylates rarely cause worsening of colitis, which may be misinterpreted as refractory colitis.

GLUCOCORTICOIDS

Pharmacokinetics & Pharmacodynamics

In gastrointestinal practice, **prednisone** and **prednisolone** are the most commonly used oral glucocorticoids. These drugs have an intermediate duration of biologic activity allowing once-daily dosing.

Hydrocortisone enemas, foam, or suppositories are used to maximize colonic tissue effects and minimize systemic absorption via topical treatment of active IBD in the rectum and sigmoid colon. Absorption of hydrocortisone is reduced with rectal administration, although 15–30% of the administered dosage is still absorbed.

Budesonide is a potent synthetic analog of prednisolone that has high affinity for the glucocorticoid receptor but is subject to rapid first-pass hepatic metabolism (in part by CYP3A4), resulting in low oral bioavailability. Two pH-controlled delayed-release oral formulations of budesonide are available that release the drug either in the distal ileum and colon (pH >5.5, Entocort) or in the colon (pH >7, Uceris), where it is absorbed. The bioavailability of controlled-release budesonide capsules is approximately 10%.

As in other tissues, glucocorticoids inhibit production of inflammatory cytokines (tumor necrosis factor [TNF]-α, interleukin [IL]-1) and chemokines (IL-8); reduce expression of inflammatory cell adhesion molecules; and inhibit gene transcription of nitric oxide synthase, phospholipase A_2, cyclooxygenase-2, and NF-κB.

Clinical Uses

Glucocorticoids are commonly used in the treatment of patients with moderate to severe active IBD. Active disease is commonly treated with an initial oral dosage of 40–60 mg/d of prednisone or prednisolone. Higher doses have not been shown to be more efficacious but have significantly greater adverse effects. Once a patient responds to initial therapy (usually within 1–2 weeks), the dosage is tapered to minimize development of adverse effects. In severely ill patients, the drugs are usually administered intravenously.

For the treatment of IBD involving the rectum or sigmoid colon, rectally administered glucocorticoids are preferred because of their lower systemic absorption.

The oral controlled-release budesonide (9 mg/d) formulations described above are used in the treatment of mild to moderate Crohn disease involving the ileum and proximal colon (Entocort) and ulcerative colitis (Uceris). They are slightly less effective than prednisolone in achieving clinical remission but have significantly less adverse systemic effects.

Corticosteroids are not useful for maintaining disease remission. Other medications such as aminosalicylates or immunosuppressive agents should be used for this purpose.

Adverse Effects

Oral controlled-release budesonide formulations are metabolized extensively in the liver by CYP3A4. Potent inhibitors of CYP3A4 can increase budesonide plasma levels severalfold, increasing the likelihood of adverse effects. General adverse effects of glucocorticoids are reviewed in Chapter 39.

PURINE ANALOGS: AZATHIOPRINE & 6-MERCAPTOPURINE

Pharmacokinetics & Pharmacodynamics

Azathioprine and 6-mercaptopurine (6-MP) are purine antimetabolites that have immunosuppressive properties (see Chapters 54 and 55).

The bioavailability of azathioprine (80%) is superior to that of 6-MP (50%). After absorption, azathioprine is rapidly converted by a nonenzymatic process to 6-MP. 6-Mercaptopurine subsequently undergoes a complex biotransformation via competing catabolic enzymes (xanthine oxidase and thiopurine methyltransferase) that produce inactive metabolites, and anabolic pathways that produce active thioguanine nucleotides. Azathioprine and 6-MP have a serum half-life of less than 2 hours; however, the active 6-thioguanine nucleotides are concentrated in cells resulting in a prolonged half-life of days. The prolonged kinetics of 6-thioguanine nucleotide results in a median delay of 17 weeks before onset of therapeutic benefit from oral azathioprine or 6-MP is observed in patients with IBD.

Clinical Uses

Azathioprine and 6-MP are important agents in the induction and maintenance of remission of ulcerative colitis and Crohn disease. Although the optimal dose is uncertain, most patients with normal thiopurine-*S*-methyltransferase (TPMT) activity (see below) are treated with 6-MP, 1–1.5 mg/kg/d, or azathioprine, 2–2.5 mg/kg/d. In current clinical practice, they are most commonly used in combination with anti-TNF therapy during acute induction and maintenance therapy of patients with moderate to severe disease. The added benefit of purine analog co-therapy is believed to be due (1) synergistic anti-inflammatory activities that lead to higher rates of remission following acute induction therapy; (2) reduced clearance of the anti-TNF agent, leading to higher serum drug levels; and (3) reduced development of neutralizing antibodies against the anti-TNF agent. Among patients treated with corticosteroids to control active disease, purine analogs are sometimes used as single agents to allow dose reduction or elimination of steroids.

Adverse Effects

Dose-related toxicities of azathioprine or 6-MP include nausea, vomiting, bone marrow depression (leading to leukopenia, macrocytosis, anemia, or thrombocytopenia), and hepatic toxicity. Routine laboratory monitoring with complete blood count and liver function tests is required in all patients. Leukopenia or elevations in liver chemistries usually respond to medication dose reduction. Severe leukopenia may predispose to opportunistic infections; leukopenia may respond to therapy with granulocyte stimulating factor. Catabolism of 6-MP by TPMT is low in 11% and absent in 0.3% of the population, leading to increased production of active 6-thioguanine metabolites and increased risk of bone marrow depression. TPMT levels can be measured before initiating therapy. These drugs should not be administered to patients with no TPMT activity and should be initiated at lower doses in patients with intermediate activity. Hypersensitivity reactions to azathioprine or 6-MP occur in 5% of patients. These include fever, rash, pancreatitis, diarrhea, and hepatitis.

As with transplant recipients receiving long-term 6-MP or azathioprine therapy, there appears to be an increased risk of lymphoma among patients with IBD, some of which may be related to Epstein-Barr virus infection. Long-term use is associated with an increased risk of hepatosplenic T-cell lymphoma, particularly in young men. The drugs are also associated with an increased risk of nonmelanoma skin cancers. These drugs cross the placenta; however, there are many reports of successful pregnancies in women taking these agents, and the risk of teratogenicity appears to be small.

Drug Interactions

Allopurinol markedly reduces xanthine oxide catabolism of the purine analogs, potentially increasing active 6-thioguanine nucleotides that may lead to severe leukopenia. Allopurinol or febuxostat should not be given to patients taking 6-MP or azathioprine except in carefully monitored situations.

ANTI–TUMOR NECROSIS FACTOR THERAPY

Pharmacokinetics & Pharmacodynamics

A dysregulation of the helper T cell type 1 (TH1) response and regulatory T cells (Tregs) is present in IBD, especially Crohn disease. One of the key proinflammatory cytokines in IBD is tumor necrosis factor (TNF). TNF is produced by the innate immune system (eg, dendritic cells, macrophages), the adaptive immune system (especially TH1 cells), and nonimmune cells (fibroblasts, smooth muscle cells). TNF exists in two biologically active forms: soluble TNF and membrane-bound TNF. The biologic activity of soluble and membrane-bound TNF is mediated by binding to TNF receptors (TNFR) that are present on some cells (especially TH1 cells, innate immune cells, and fibroblasts). Binding of TNF to TNFR initially activates components including NF-κB that stimulate transcription, growth, and expansion. Biologic actions ascribed to TNFR activation include release of proinflammatory cytokines from macrophages, T-cell activation and proliferation, fibroblast collagen production, up-regulation of endothelial adhesion molecules responsible for leukocyte migration, and stimulation of hepatic acute phase reactants. Activation of TNFR may later lead to apoptosis (programmed cell death) of activated cells.

Four monoclonal antibodies to human TNF are approved for the treatment of IBD: infliximab, adalimumab, golimumab, and certolizumab (Table 62–3). Infliximab, adalimumab, and golimumab are antibodies of the IgG_1 subclass. Certolizumab is a recombinant antibody that contains an Fab fragment that is conjugated to polyethylene glycol (PEG) but lacks an Fc portion. The Fab portion of infliximab is a chimeric mouse-human antibody, but adalimumab, certolizumab, and golimumab are fully humanized. Infliximab is administered as an intravenous infusion. At therapeutic doses of 5–10 mg/kg, the half-life of infliximab is approximately 8–10 days, resulting in plasma disappearance of antibodies over 8–12 weeks. Adalimumab, golimumab, and certolizumab are administered by subcutaneous injection. Their half-lives are approximately 2 weeks.

All four agents bind to soluble and membrane-bound TNF with high affinity, preventing the cytokine from binding to its receptors. Binding of all three antibodies to membrane-bound TNF also causes reverse signaling that suppresses cytokine release. When infliximab, adalimumab, or golimumab bind to membrane-bound TNF, the Fc portion of the human IgG_1 region promotes antibody-mediated apoptosis, complement activation, and cellular cytotoxicity of activated T lymphocytes and macrophages. Certolizumab, without an Fc portion, lacks these properties.

Clinical Uses

Infliximab, adalimumab, and certolizumab are approved for the acute and chronic treatment of patients with moderate to severe Crohn disease who have had an inadequate response to conventional therapies. Infliximab, adalimumab, and golimumab are approved for the acute and chronic treatment of moderate to severe ulcerative colitis. With induction therapy, these approved agents lead to symptomatic improvement in 60% and disease remission in 30% of patients with moderate to severe Crohn disease, including patients who have been dependent on glucocorticoids or who have not responded to 6-MP or methotrexate. The median time to clinical response is 2 weeks. Induction therapy is generally given as follows: infliximab 5 mg/kg intravenous infusion at 0, 2, and 6 weeks; adalimumab 160 mg (in divided doses) initially and 80 mg subcutaneous injection at 2 weeks; and certolizumab 400 mg subcutaneous injection at 0, 2, and 4 weeks. Patients who respond may be treated with chronic maintenance therapy, as follows: infliximab 5 mg/kg intravenous infusion every 8 weeks; adalimumab 40 mg subcutaneous injection every 2 weeks; certolizumab 400 mg subcutaneous injection every 4 weeks. With chronic, regularly scheduled therapy, clinical response is maintained in more than 60% of patients and disease remission in 40%. However, one-third of patients eventually lose response despite higher doses or more frequent injections. Loss of response in many patients may be due to

TABLE 62–3 Anti-TNF antibodies used in inflammatory bowel disease.

	Infliximab	Adalimumab	Certolizumab	Golimumab
Class	Monoclonal antibody	Monoclonal antibody	Monoclonal antibody	Monoclonal antibody
% Human	75%	100%	95%	100%
Structure	IgG_1	IgG_1	Fab fragment attached to PEG (lacks Fc portion)	IgG_1
Route of administration	Intravenous	Subcutaneous	Subcutaneous	Subcutaneous
Half-life	8–10 days	10–20 days	14 days	14 days
Neutralizes soluble TNF	Yes	Yes	Yes	Yes
Neutralizes membrane-bound TNF	Yes	Yes	Yes	Yes
Induces apoptosis of cells expressing membrane-bound TNF	Yes	Yes	No	Yes
Complement-mediated cytotoxicity of cells expressing membrane-bound TNF	Yes	Yes	No	Yes
Induction dose	5 mg/kg at 0, 2, and 6 weeks	160 mg, 80 mg, and 40 mg at 0, 2, and 4 weeks	400 mg at 0, 2, and 4 weeks	200 mg, 100 mg at 0, 2 weeks
Maintenance dose	5 mg/kg every 8 weeks	40 mg every 2 weeks	400 mg every 4 weeks	100 mg every 4 weeks

TNF, tumor necrosis factor.

the development of antibodies to the TNF antibody or to other mechanisms.

Infliximab is approved for the treatment of patients with moderate to severe ulcerative colitis who have had inadequate response to mesalamine or corticosteroids. After induction therapy of 5–10 mg/week at 0, 2, and 6 weeks, 70% of patients have a clinical response and one third achieve a clinical remission. With continued maintenance infusions every 8 weeks, approximately 50% of patients have continued clinical response. Adalimumab and golimumab also are approved for the treatment of moderate to severe ulcerative colitis but appear to be less effective than intravenous infliximab. After induction therapy, less than 55% of patients have a clinical response and less than 20% achieve remission. The reason why subcutaneous anti-TNF formulations are less effective than intravenous infliximab is uncertain.

Adverse Effects

Serious adverse events occur in up to 6% of patients with anti-TNF therapy. The most important adverse effect of these drugs is infection due to suppression of the TH1 inflammatory response. This may lead to serious infections such as bacterial sepsis, tuberculosis, invasive fungal organisms, reactivation of hepatitis B, listeriosis, and other opportunistic infections. Reactivation of latent tuberculosis, with dissemination, has occurred. Before administering anti-TNF therapy, all patients must undergo testing with tuberculin skin tests or interferon gamma release assays. Prophylactic therapy for tuberculosis is warranted for patients with positive test results before beginning anti-TNF therapy. More common but usually less serious infections include upper respiratory infections (sinusitis, bronchitis, and pneumonia) and cellulitis. The risk of serious infections is increased markedly in patients taking concomitant corticosteroids.

Antibodies to the antibody (ATA) may develop with all four agents. These antibodies may attenuate or eliminate the clinical response and increase the likelihood of developing acute or delayed infusion or injection reactions. Antibody formation is much more likely in patients given episodic anti-TNF therapy than regular scheduled injections. In patients on chronic maintenance therapy, the prevalence of ATA with infliximab is 10%, with certolizumab 8%, and with adalimumab or golimumab 3%. Antibody development also is less likely in patients who receive concomitant therapy with immunomodulators (ie, 6-MP or methotrexate). Concomitant treatment with anti-TNF agents and immunomodulators may increase the risk of lymphoma.

Infliximab intravenous infusions result in acute adverse infusion reactions in up to 10% of patients, but discontinuation of the infusion for severe reactions is required in less than 2%. Infusion reactions are more common with the second or subsequent infusions than with the first. Early mild reactions include fever, headache, dizziness, urticaria, or mild cardiopulmonary symptoms that include chest pain, dyspnea, or hemodynamic instability. Reactions to subsequent infusions may be reduced with prophylactic administration of acetaminophen, diphenhydramine, or corticosteroids. Severe acute reactions include significant hypotension, shortness of breath, muscle spasms, and chest discomfort; such reactions may require treatment with oxygen, epinephrine, and corticosteroids.

A delayed serum sickness–like reaction may occur 1–2 weeks after anti-TNF therapy in 1% of patients. These reactions consist of myalgia, arthralgia, jaw tightness, fever, rash, urticaria, and edema and usually require discontinuation of that agent. Positive antinuclear antibodies and anti-double-stranded DNA develop in a small number of patients. Development of a lupus-like syndrome is rare and resolves after discontinuation of the drug.

Rare but serious adverse effects of all anti-TNF agents also include severe hepatic reactions leading to acute hepatic failure, demyelinating disorders, hematologic reactions, and new or worsened congestive heart failure in patients with underlying heart disease. Anti-TNF agents may cause a variety of psoriatic skin rashes, which usually resolve after drug discontinuation.

Lymphoma appears to be increased in patients with untreated IBD. Anti-TNF agents may further increase the risk of lymphoma in this population, although the relative risk is uncertain. An increased number of cases of hepatosplenic T-cell lymphoma, a rare but usually fatal disease, have been noted in children and young adults, virtually all of whom have been on combined therapy with immunomodulators, anti-TNF agents, or corticosteroids. Anti-TNF agents may also be associated with an increased risk of nonmelanoma skin cancers.

ANTI-INTEGRIN THERAPY

Integrins are a family of adhesion molecules on the surface of leukocytes that may interact with another class of adhesion molecules on the surface of the vascular endothelium known as selectins, allowing circulating leukocytes to adhere to the vascular endothelium and subsequently move through the vessel wall into the tissue. Integrins consist of heterodimers that contain two subunits, alpha and beta. **Natalizumab** is a humanized IgG_4 monoclonal antibody targeted only against the $\alpha4$ subunit; thus, it blocks several integrins on circulating inflammatory cells and prevents binding to the vascular adhesion molecules and subsequent migration into surrounding tissues, including the bowel and central nervous system. Unfortunately, patients treated with natalizumab may develop progressive multifocal leukoencephalopathy (PML) due to central nervous system reactivation of a human polyomavirus (JC virus), which is present in latent form in over 80% of adults. Patients who are positive for JC virus antibody have a mean risk of PML of 3.9 per 1000 patients; however, the risk is markedly increased in patients treated for more than 24 months or receiving other immunosuppressants. With the advent of vedolizumab, natalizumab is almost never used for the treatment of IBD except in patients with multiple sclerosis.

Vedolizumab is a monoclonal antibody with activity directed specifically against the $\alpha4/\beta7$ integrin, thereby blocking interaction of leukocytes with gut vascular endothelial cell adhesion molecules. Because lymphocytes trafficking to the brain are unaffected, the risk of reactivation of JC virus and PML is believed to be extremely low. Vedolizumab is used as a second-line treatment for patients with moderate to severe ulcerative colitis or Crohn disease who cannot take anti-TNF agents due to side effects, lack of efficacy, or loss of response and as first-line therapy in elderly patients in whom the risks of anti-TNF therapy may be increased. After intravenous induction therapy of 300 mg at 0, 2, and 6 weeks, patients with a clinical response are treated with intravenous maintenance therapy every 8 weeks. Vedolizumab appears to have a very low incidence of serious adverse effects. Neutralizing antibodies develop in less than 3% of patients.

ANTI–IL-23 THERAPY

Ustekinumab is a human IgG_1 monoclonal antibody that binds to the p40 subunit of both the IL-12 and IL-23 cytokines, blocking cell signaling, cytokine production, and gene activation with resultant inhibition of TH1 and TH17 cell-mediated responses, which are believed to be important in Crohn disease inflammatory response. Ustekinumab can be used in adults with moderate to severe Crohn disease who are naïve to biologics or have failed standard therapy with corticosteroids, immunomodulators (eg, thiopurine analogs), or anti-TNF agents. Ustekinumab is administered for initial induction therapy as a single body-weight-based intravenous infusion. Thereafter a subcutaneous dose of 90 mg is administered every 8 weeks. Ustekinumab is well tolerated and has a low risk of serious adverse events, including hypersensitivity reactions (anaphylaxis), infections (viral, bacterial, fungal), and reactivation of latent infections (tuberculosis, herpes). Neutralizing antibodies occur in <3% of patients.

Risankizumab is a humanized monoclonal antibody that binds to the p19 subunit of IL-23 and was recently approved for treating moderate to severe Crohn disease and may be used as an alternative to other first-line biologic agents. An intravenous induction dose of 600 mg at 0, 4, and 8 weeks is followed by maintenance dosing of 360 mg subcutaneously at 12 weeks and every 8 weeks thereafter. A reported adverse reaction to risankizumab is drug-induced liver injury. Liver enzymes and bilirubin are evaluated pretreatment, during and after induction therapy, and then every 3 to 6 months.

JANUS KINASE INHIBITORS

Tofacitinib is a nonselective inhibitor of the Janus kinase (JAK) family, especially JAK3 and JAK1, interrupting the JAK-STAT signaling pathway that influences production of several interleukins that regulate synthesis and differentiation of B and T lymphocytes that are involved in mucosal inflammation (see Chapter 36). Tofacitinib is a small molecule that is rapidly absorbed after oral intake and has a short serum half-life of 3 hours. It undergoes both renal excretion and hepatic metabolism, mainly by CYP3A4; hence interaction with drugs that inhibit or induce CYP3A4 should be considered. Dose reduction is recommended in patients with renal or hepatic impairment. Tofacitinib is approved for the treatment of moderate to severe ulcerative colitis in patients who have not responded to or cannot tolerate anti-TNF therapy. The induction dose is 10 mg orally twice daily for 8 weeks, followed by long-term maintenance of 5–10 mg orally twice daily. As with other immunosuppressive agents, tofacitinib may increase the risk of infections (upper respiratory, urinary tract), serious infections, and reactivation of latent infection (tuberculosis). There is a fourfold increased risk of herpes zoster reactivation. When possible, vaccination with inactivated recombinant zoster vaccine (Shingrix) 3–4 weeks before treatment with tofacitinib may be advised. There may be an increase in total cholesterol (both HDL and LDL); hence lipid testing is recommended 8 weeks after drug initiation. **Upadacitinib** is a selective JAK1 inhibitor approved for treatment of patients with moderate to severe ulcerative colitis who have not responded to or cannot tolerate anti-TNF therapy. The induction dose is 45 mg orally once daily for 8 weeks, followed by long-term maintenance of 15 mg orally once daily. The FDA has issued a boxed warning for these JAK inhibitors due to an increased risk of serious heart-related events such as heart attack or stroke, thrombosis, pulmonary embolism, cancer, and death associated with the medications.

SPHINGOSINE-1-PHOSPHATE (S1P) RECEPTOR MODULATOR

Ozanimod is a sphingosine-1-phosphate receptor agonist, an immunomodulatory medication that alters lymphocyte migration, sequestering lymphocytes in lymph nodes and away from sites of chronic inflammation. Ozanimod was recently approved to treat patients with moderate to severe ulcerative colitis. Treatment is initiated with a 7-day titration schedule beginning with 0.23 mg orally once daily for days 1–4, followed by 0.46 mg orally once daily days 5–7, and subsequent maintenance with 0.92 mg orally once daily. Ozanimod is contraindicated in patients with myocardial infarction, unstable angina, stroke, TIA, or heart failure in the last 6 months and in patients with Mobitz type II second- or third-degree atrioventricular block, sick sinus syndrome, or sinoatrial block, unless the patient has a functioning pacemaker. It is also contraindicated in patients with severe untreated sleep apnea and for patients taking a monoamine oxidase inhibitor. Infrequent severe adverse events include infections, bradyarrhythmia, liver injury, and macular edema. Screening with a complete blood count, liver function tests, and an EKG are typically performed prior to initialization of therapy.

■ PANCREATIC ENZYME SUPPLEMENTS

Exocrine pancreatic insufficiency is most commonly caused by cystic fibrosis, chronic pancreatitis, or pancreatic resection. When secretion of pancreatic enzymes falls below 10% of normal, fat and protein digestion is impaired and can lead to steatorrhea, azotorrhea, vitamin malabsorption, and weight loss. Pancreatic enzyme supplements, which contain a mixture of amylase, lipase, and proteases, are the mainstay of treatment for pancreatic enzyme insufficiency. Two major types of preparations in use are **pancreatin** and **pancrelipase.** Pancreatin is an alcohol-derived extract of hog pancreas with relatively low concentrations of lipase and proteolytic enzymes, whereas pancrelipase is an enriched preparation. On a per-weight basis, pancrelipase has approximately 12 times the lipolytic activity and more than 4 times the proteolytic activity of pancreatin. Consequently, pancreatin is no longer in common clinical use. Only pancrelipase is discussed here.

Pancrelipase is available worldwide in both non-enteric-coated and enteric-coated preparations. Formulations are available in sizes containing varying amounts of lipase, amylase, and protease. However, manufacturers' listings of enzyme content do not always reflect true enzymatic activity. Pancrelipase enzymes are rapidly and permanently inactivated by gastric acids. Viokace is a non-enteric-coated tablet that should be given concomitantly with acid suppression therapy (PPI or H_2 antagonist) to reduce acid-mediated destruction within the stomach. Enteric-coated formulations are more commonly used because they do not require concomitant acid suppression therapy. At present, five enteric-coasted, delayed-release formulations are approved for use (Creon, Pancreaze, Zenpep, Ultresa, and Pertyze).

Pancrelipase preparations are administered with each meal and snack. Enzyme activity may be listed in international units (IU) or USP units. One IU is equal to 2–3 USP units. Dosing should be individualized according to the age and weight of the patient, the degree of pancreatic insufficiency, and the amount of dietary fat intake. Therapy is initiated at a dose that provides 60,000–90,000 USP units (20,000–30,000 IU) of lipase activity in the prandial and postprandial period—a level that is sufficient to reduce steatorrhea to a clinically insignificant level in most cases. Suboptimal response to enteric-coated formulations may be due to poor mixing of granules with food or slow dissolution and release of enzymes. Gradual increase of dose, change to a different formulation, or addition of acid suppression therapy may improve response. For patients with feeding tubes, microspheres may be mixed with enteral feeding prior to administration.

Pancreatic enzyme supplements are well tolerated. The capsules should be swallowed, not chewed, because pancreatic enzymes may cause oropharyngeal mucositis. Excessive doses may cause diarrhea and abdominal pain. The high purine content of pancreas extracts may lead to hyperuricosuria and renal stones. Several cases of colonic strictures were reported in patients with cystic fibrosis who received high doses of pancrelipase with high lipase activity. These high-dose formulations have since been removed from the market.

■ GLUCAGON-LIKE PEPTIDE 2 ANALOG FOR SHORT-BOWEL SYNDROME

Extensive surgical resection or disease of the small intestine may result in short-bowel syndrome with malabsorption of nutrients and fluids. Patients with less than 200 cm of small intestine (with or without colon resection) usually are dependent on partial or complete parenteral nutritional support to maintain hydration and nutrition. **Teduglutide** is a glucagon-like peptide 2 analog that binds to enteric neurons and endocrine cells, stimulating release of a number of trophic hormones (including insulin-like growth factor) that stimulate mucosal epithelial growth and enhance fluid absorption. In clinical trials, 54% of patients treated with teduglutide (0.05 mg/kg once daily by subcutaneous injection) reduced their need for parenteral support by at least 1 day/week compared with 23% treated with placebo. Teduglutide may be associated with an increased risk of colorectal and small bowel neoplasia.

■ BILE ACID AGENTS

Ursodiol (ursodeoxycholic acid) is a naturally occurring bile acid that makes up less than 5% of the circulating bile salt pool in humans and a much higher percentage in bears. After oral administration, it is absorbed, conjugated in the liver with glycine or taurine, and excreted in the bile. Conjugated ursodiol undergoes extensive enterohepatic recirculation. The serum half-life is approximately 100 hours. With long-term daily administration, ursodiol constitutes 30–50% of the circulating bile acid pool. A small amount of unabsorbed conjugated or unconjugated ursodiol passes into the colon, where it is either excreted or undergoes dehydroxylation by colonic bacteria to lithocholic acid, a substance with potential hepatic toxicity.

Pharmacodynamics

The solubility of cholesterol in bile is determined by the relative proportions of bile acids, lecithin, and cholesterol. Although prolonged ursodiol therapy expands the bile acid pool, this does not appear to be the principal mechanism of action for dissolution of gallstones. Ursodiol decreases the cholesterol content of bile by reducing hepatic cholesterol secretion. Ursodiol also appears to stabilize hepatocyte canalicular membranes, possibly through a reduction in the concentration of other endogenous bile acids or through inhibition of immune-mediated hepatocyte destruction.

Clinical Use

Ursodiol is used for dissolution of small cholesterol gallstones in patients with symptomatic gallbladder disease who refuse cholecystectomy or who are poor surgical candidates. At a dosage of 10 mg/kg/d orally for 12–24 months, dissolution occurs in up to 50% of patients with small (<5–10 mm) noncalcified gallstones. It is also effective for the prevention of gallstones in obese patients undergoing rapid weight loss therapy.

Ursodiol is also the first-line agent used for the treatment of early primary biliary cirrhosis (PBC). As a nontoxic bile acid, ursodiol is believed to reduce liver injury by replacement of more toxic endogenous bile acids and through anti-inflammatory effects. At a dose of 13–15 mg/kg/d, ursodiol improves liver biochemical abnormalities, slows the rate of clinical and histologic progression, reduces the need for liver transplantation, and improves long-term survival. Approximately 35% of patients with PBC do not respond to ursodiol.

Adverse Effects

Ursodiol is practically free of serious adverse effects. Bile salt-induced diarrhea is uncommon. Unlike its predecessor, chenodeoxycholate, ursodiol has not been associated with hepatotoxicity.

Obeticholic acid is a synthetic derivative of the naturally occurring bile acid chenodeoxycholate. Like ursodiol, it is a non-toxic bile acid and is believed to reduce liver injury by decreasing hepatic concentrations of more toxic endogenous bile acids. It also is a ligand for the nuclear farnesoid X receptor, which modulates hepatic inflammation, fibrosis, gluconeogenesis, lipid synthesis, and insulin sensitivity. Obeticholic acid is approved for the treatment of PBC at a dose of 5–10 mg/d orally in combination with ursodiol in patients who have had an inadequate response to ursodiol monotherapy. In a randomized, double-blind, placebo-controlled, 12-month trial, almost 50% of patients treated with combination therapy had a clinical response compared with 10% treated with ursodiol alone. Obeticholic acid causes severe pruritus in up to 25% of patients (especially at the 10 mg dose), leading to discontinuation in up to 10% of patients. Obeticholic acid is being evaluated for treatment of non-alcoholic steatohepatitis but is not yet FDA approved for this indication. In randomized clinical trials of non-alcoholic steatohepatitis, obeticholic acid 25 mg once daily for 18 months resulted in significant improvement in liver histology, including fibrosis.

■ DRUGS USED TO TREAT VARICEAL HEMORRHAGE

Portal hypertension most commonly occurs as a consequence of chronic liver disease. Portal hypertension is caused by increased blood flow within the portal venous system and increased resistance to portal flow within the liver. Splanchnic blood flow is increased in patients with cirrhosis due to low arteriolar resistance that is mediated by increased circulating vasodilators and decreased vascular sensitivity to vasoconstrictors. Intrahepatic vascular resistance is increased in cirrhosis due to fixed fibrosis within the spaces of Disse and hepatic veins as well as reversible vasoconstriction of hepatic sinusoids and venules. Among the consequences of portal hypertension are ascites, hepatic encephalopathy, and the development of portosystemic collaterals—especially gastric or esophageal varices. Varices can rupture, leading to massive upper gastrointestinal bleeding.

Several drugs are available that reduce portal pressures. These may be used in the short term for the treatment of active variceal hemorrhage or long term to reduce the risk of hemorrhage.

SOMATOSTATIN & OCTREOTIDE

The pharmacology of octreotide is discussed above under Antidiarrheal Agents. In patients with cirrhosis and portal hypertension, intravenous somatostatin (250 mcg/h) or octreotide (50 mcg/h) reduces portal blood flow and variceal pressures; the mechanism by which they do so is poorly understood. They do not appear to induce direct contraction of vascular smooth muscle. Their activity may be mediated through inhibition of release of glucagon and other gut peptides that alter mesenteric blood flow. Although data from clinical trials are conflicting, these agents are probably effective in promoting initial hemostasis from bleeding esophageal varices. They are generally administered for 3–5 days.

VASOPRESSIN & TERLIPRESSIN

Vasopressin (antidiuretic hormone) is a polypeptide hormone secreted by the hypothalamus and stored in the posterior pituitary. Its pharmacology is discussed in Chapters 17 and 37. Although its primary physiologic role is to maintain serum osmolality, it is also a potent arterial vasoconstrictor. When administered intravenously by continuous infusion, vasopressin causes splanchnic arterial vasoconstriction that leads to reduced splanchnic perfusion and lowered portal venous pressures. Before the advent of octreotide, vasopressin was commonly used to treat acute variceal hemorrhage. However, because of its high adverse-effect profile, it is no longer used for this purpose. In contrast, for patients with acute gastrointestinal bleeding from small bowel or large bowel vascular ectasias or diverticulosis, vasopressin may be infused—to promote vasospasm—into one of the branches of the superior or inferior mesenteric artery through an angiographically placed catheter. Adverse effects with systemic vasopressin are common. Systemic and peripheral vasoconstriction can lead to hypertension, myocardial ischemia or infarction, or mesenteric infarction. These effects may be reduced by coadministration of nitroglycerin, which may further reduce portal venous pressures (by reducing portohepatic vascular resistance) and may also reduce the coronary and peripheral vascular vasospasm caused by vasopressin. Other common adverse effects are nausea, abdominal cramps, and diarrhea (due to intestinal hyperactivity). Furthermore, the antidiuretic effects of vasopressin promote retention of free water, which can lead to hyponatremia, fluid retention, and pulmonary edema.

Terlipressin is a vasopressin analog that appears to have similar efficacy to vasopressin with fewer adverse effects. Although this agent is available in other countries, it has not been approved for use in the USA.

BETA-RECEPTOR-BLOCKING DRUGS

The pharmacology of β-receptor-blocking agents is discussed in Chapter 10. Beta-receptor antagonists reduce portal venous pressures via a decrease in portal venous inflow. This decrease is due to a decrease in cardiac output (β_1 blockade) and to splanchnic vasoconstriction (β_2 blockade) caused by the unopposed effect of systemic catecholamines on α receptors. Thus, nonselective β blockers such as propranolol and nadolol are more effective than selective β_1 blockers in reducing portal pressures. Among patients with cirrhosis and esophageal varices who have not previously had an episode of variceal hemorrhage, the incidence of bleeding among patients treated with nonselective β blockers is 15% compared with 25% in control groups. Among patients with a history of variceal hemorrhage, the likelihood of recurrent hemorrhage is 80% within 2 years. Nonselective β blockers significantly reduce the rate of recurrent bleeding, although a reduction in mortality is unproven.

SUMMARY Drugs Used Primarily for Gastrointestinal Conditions

Subclass, Drug	Mechanism of Action	Effects	Clinical Applications	Pharmacokinetics, Toxicities, Interactions
DRUGS USED IN ACID-PEPTIC DISEASES				
• Proton-pump inhibitors (PPIs), eg, omeprazole, lansoprazole	Irreversible blockade of H^+/K^+-ATPase pump in active parietal cells of stomach	Long-lasting reduction of stimulated and nocturnal acid secretion	Peptic ulcer, gastroesophageal reflux disease, erosive gastritis	Half-lives much shorter than duration of action • low toxicity reduction of stomach acid may reduce absorption of some drugs and increase that of others
• *H_2-receptor blockers, eg, cimetidine: Effective reduction of nocturnal acid but less effective against stimulated secretion; very safe, available over the counter (OTC) Cimetidine, but not other H_2 blockers, is a weak antiandrogenic agent and a potent CYP enzyme inhibitor*				
• *Sucralfate: Polymerizes at site of tissue damage (ulcer bed) and protects against further damage; very insoluble with no systemic effects; must be given four times daily*				
• *Antacids: Popular OTC medication for symptomatic relief of heartburn; not as useful as PPI and H_2 blockers in peptic diseases*				
DRUGS STIMULATING MOTILITY				
• Metoclopramide	D_2-receptor blocker • removes inhibition of acetylcholine neurons in enteric nervous system	Increases gastric emptying and intestinal motility	Gastric paresis (eg, in diabetes) • antiemetic (see below)	Parkinsonian symptoms due to block of central nervous system (CNS) D_2 receptors
• *Domperidone: Like metoclopramide, but less CNS effect; not available in the USA*				
• *Cholinomimetics: Neostigmine often used for colonic pseudo-obstruction in hospitalized patients*				
• *Macrolides: Erythromycin useful in diabetic gastroparesis but tolerance develops*				
LAXATIVES				
• Magnesium hydroxide, other nonabsorbable salts and sugars	Osmotic agents increase water content of stool	Usually causes evacuation within 4–6 h, sooner in large doses	Simple constipation; bowel prep for endoscopy (especially polyethylene glycol [PEG] solutions)	Magnesium may be absorbed and cause toxicity in renal impairment
• *Bulk-forming laxatives: Methylcellulose, psyllium, etc: increase volume of colon contents, stimulate evacuation*				
• *Stimulants: Senna, cascara; stimulate activity; prucalopride, 5-HT_4 agonist, stimulates high-amplitude proximal colonic contractions; may cause cramping*				
• *Stool surfactants: Docusate, mineral oil; lubricate stool, ease passage*				
• *Chloride channel activators: Lubiprostone, prostanoic acid derivative, stimulates chloride secretion into intestine, increasing fluid content; linaclotide, plecanatide, guanylyl cyclase-C agonist, stimulates chloride secretion by CFTR*				
• *Opioid receptor antagonists: Alvimopan, methylnaltrexone, naldemedine, naloxegol; block intestinal μ-opioid receptors but do not enter CNS, so analgesia is maintained*				
ANTIDIARRHEAL DRUGS				
• Loperamide	Activates μ-opioid receptors in enteric nervous system	Slows motility in gut with negligible CNS effects	Nonspecific, noninfectious diarrhea	Mild cramping but little or no CNS toxicity
• *Diphenoxylate: Similar to loperamide, but high doses can cause CNS opioid effects and toxicity*				
• *Colloidal bismuth compounds: Subsalicylate and citrate salts available. OTC preparations popular and have some value in travelers' diarrhea due to adsorption of toxins*				
• *Kaolin + pectin: Adsorbent compounds available OTC in some countries*				
DRUGS FOR IRRITABLE BOWEL SYNDROME (IBS)				
• Alosetron	5-HT_3 antagonist of high potency and duration of binding	Reduces smooth muscle activity in gut	Approved for severe diarrhea-predominant IBS in women	Rare but serious constipation • ischemic colitis • infarction
• *Anticholinergics: Nonselective action on gut activity, usually associated with typical antimuscarinic toxicity*				
• *Chloride channel activator: Lubiprostone (see above); useful in constipation-predominant IBS in women; linaclotide (see above): useful in adults with constipation-predominant IBS*				

(continued)

Subclass, Drug	Mechanism of Action	Effects	Clinical Applications	Pharmacokinetics, Toxicities, Interactions
ANTIEMETIC DRUGS				
• Ondansetron, other 5-HT_3 antagonists	5-HT_3 blockade in gut and CNS with shorter duration of binding than alosetron	Extremely effective in preventing chemotherapy-induced and postoperative nausea and vomiting	First-line agents in cancer chemotherapy; also useful for postop emesis	Usually given IV but orally active in prophylaxis • 4–9 h duration of action • very low toxicity but may slow colonic transit
• Aprepitant	NK_1-receptor blocker in CNS	Interferes with vomiting reflex • no effect on 5-HT, dopamine, or steroid receptors	Effective in reducing both early and delayed emesis in cancer chemotherapy	Given orally • IV fosaprepitant available • fatigue, dizziness, diarrhea • CYP interactions
• *Corticosteroids: Mechanism not known but useful in antiemetic IV cocktails*				
• *Antimuscarinics (scopolamine): Effective in emesis due to motion sickness; not other types*				
• *Antihistaminics: Moderate efficacy in motion sickness and chemotherapy-induced emesis*				
• *Phenothiazines: Act primarily through block of D_2 and muscarinic receptors*				
• *Cannabinoids: Dronabinol is available for use in chemotherapy-induced nausea and vomiting, but is associated with CNS marijuana effects*				
DRUGS USED IN INFLAMMATORY BOWEL DISEASE (IBD)				
• 5-Aminosalicylates, eg, mesalamine in many formulations, sulfasalazine	Mechanism uncertain • may be inhibition of eicosanoid inflammatory mediators	Topical therapeutic action • systemic absorption may cause toxicity	Mild to moderately severe Crohn disease and ulcerative colitis	Sulfasalazine causes sulfonamide toxicity and may cause GI upset, myalgias, arthralgias, myelosuppression • other aminosalicylates much less toxic
• Purine analogs and antimetabolites, eg, 6-mercaptopurine	Mechanism uncertain • may promote apoptosis of immune cells	Generalized suppression of immune processes	Moderately severe to severe Crohn disease and ulcerative colitis	GI upset, mucositis • myelosuppression • purine analogs may cause hepatotoxicity
• Anti-TNF antibodies, eg, infliximab, others	Bind tumor necrosis factor and prevent it from binding to its receptors	Suppression of several aspects of immune function, especially TH1 lymphocytes	Infliximab: Moderate to severe Crohn disease and ulcerative colitis • others approved in Crohn disease	Infusion reactions • reactivation of latent tuberculosis • increased risk of dangerous systemic fungal and bacterial infections
• Vedolizumab	Binds leukocyte integrins	Prevents binding to vascular adhesin molecules and leukocyte migration into tissue	Moderate to severe Crohn disease and ulcerative colitis	Upper respiratory infections
• Ustekinumab • Risankizumab	Binds p40 subunit of IL-12 and IL-23 Binds to the p19 subunit of IL-23	Blocks cell signaling and cytokine production, leading to inhibition of TH1 and TH17 inflammatory responses	Moderate to severe Crohn that has failed therapy with immunomodulators or anti-TNF	Infusion reactions, reactivation of latent tuberculosis; increased risk of systemic infections (viral, bacterial, fungal)
• Tofacitinib • Upadacitinib	Nonselective Janus Kinase inhibitor Selective JAK1 inhibitor	Interrupts JAK-STAT signaling pathway, decreasing synthesis and differentiation of B and T cells involved in mucosal inflammation	Moderate to severe ulcerative colitis	Increased risk of Herpes zoster reactivation; increased lipids (LDL and HDL); increased risk of thrombosis and pulmonary embolism
• Ozanimod	Sphingosine-1-phosphate (S1P) receptor Modulator	Alters lymphocyte migration, sequestering lymphocytes in lymph nodes and away from sites of chronic inflammation	Moderate to severe ulcerative colitis	Increased risk of infections, bradyarrhythmia, liver injury, and macular edema
• *Corticosteroids: Generalized anti-inflammatory effect; see Chapter 39*				
PANCREATIC SUPPLEMENTS				
• Pancrelipase	Replacement enzymes from animal pancreatic extracts	Improves digestion of dietary fat, protein, and carbohydrate	Pancreatic insufficiency due to cystic fibrosis, pancreatitis, pancreatectomy	Taken with every meal • may increase incidence of gout
• *Pancreatin: Similar pancreatic extracts but much lower potency; rarely used*				

(continued)

Subclass, Drug	Mechanism of Action	Effects	Clinical Applications	Pharmacokinetics, Toxicities, Interactions
BILE ACID THERAPY FOR GALLSTONES AND PRIMARY BILIARY CIRRHOSIS				
• Ursodiol	Reduces cholesterol secretion into bile and concentration of endogenous hepatocyte bile salts	Dissolves gallstones • reduces hepatic inflammation and fibrosis	Gallstones in patients refusing or not eligible for surgery • early primary biliary cirrhosis	May cause diarrhea
• Obeticholic acid	Binds to hepatocyte nuclear farnesoid X receptor	Reduces hepatic inflammation and fibrosis	Treatment of primary biliary cirrhosis in patients with inadequate response to ursodiol	Severe pruritus
DRUGS USED TO TREAT VARICEAL HEMORRHAGE				
• Octreotide	Somatostatin analog • mechanism not certain	May alter portal blood flow and variceal pressures	Patients with bleeding varices or at high risk of repeat bleeding	Reduced endocrine and exocrine pancreatic activity • other endocrine abnormalities • GI upset
• *Beta blockers: Reduce cardiac output and splanchnic blood flow; see Chapter 10*				

PREPARATIONS AVAILABLE

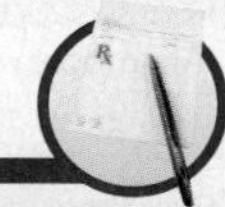

GENERIC NAME	AVAILABLE AS
ANTACIDS	
Aluminum hydroxide gel	Generic, AlternaGEL, others
Calcium carbonate	Generic, Tums, others
Combination aluminum hydroxide and magnesium hydroxide preparations	Generic, Maalox, Mylanta, Gaviscon, Gelusil, others
H_2 HISTAMINE RECEPTOR BLOCKERS	
Cimetidine	Generic, Tagamet, Tagamet HB
Famotidine	Generic, Pepcid, Pepcid AC, Pepcid Complete, Zantac 360
Nizatidine	Generic, Axid, Axid AR
SELECTED ANTICHOLINERGIC DRUGS	
Atropine	Generic
Belladonna alkaloids tincture	Generic
Dicyclomine	Generic, Bentyl, others
Glycopyrrolate	Generic, Robinul
Hyoscyamine	Anaspaz, Levsin, others
Scopolamine	Generic, Transderm Scop
PROTON-PUMP INHIBITORS	
Dexlansoprazole	Dexilant
Esomeprazole magnesium	Nexium
Esomeprazole strontium	
Lansoprazole	Generic, Prevacid
Omeprazole	Generic, Prilosec, Prilosec OTC*
Omeprazole-sodium bicarbonate	Zegerid
Pantoprazole	Generic, Protonix
Rabeprazole	Generic, Aciphex
MUCOSAL PROTECTIVE AGENTS	
Sucralfate	Generic, Carafate
DIGESTIVE ENZYMES	
Pancrelipase	Creon, Pancreaze, Zenpep, Pertyze, Ultresa

GENERIC NAME	AVAILABLE AS
DRUGS FOR MOTILITY DISORDERS & SELECTED ANTIEMETICS	
5-HT_3-RECEPTOR ANTAGONISTS	
Alosetron	Lotronex
Dolasetron	Anzemet
Granisetron	Generic, Kytril
Ondansetron	Generic, Zofran
Palonosetron	Aloxi
OTHER MOTILITY AND ANTIEMETIC AGENTS	
Aprepitant	Emend
Dronabinol	Generic, Marinol
Fosaprepitant	Emend, Emend IV
Metoclopramide	Generic, Reglan, others
Nabilone	Cesamet
Netupitant/palonosetron	Akynzeo
Prochlorperazine	Generic, Compazine
Promethazine	Generic, Phenergan, others
Rolapitant	Varubi
Scopolamine	Transderm Scop
Trimethobenzamide	Generic, Tigan, others
SELECTED ANTI-INFLAMMATORY DRUGS USED IN GASTROINTESTINAL DISEASE (SEE ALSO CHAPTER 55)	
Adalimumab	Humira
Balsalazide	Colazal
Budesonide	Entocort, Uceris
Certolizumab	Cimzia
Golimumab	Simponi
Hydrocortisone	Cortenema, Cortifoam, Proctofoam–HC
Infliximab	Remicade
Mesalamine	5-ASA
Oral:	Asacol, Lialda, Apriso, Pentasa
Rectal:	Rowasa, Canasa
Methylprednisolone	Medrol Enpack

(continued)

GENERIC NAME	AVAILABLE AS
Olsalazine	Dipentum
Ozanimod	Zeposia
Risankizumab	Skyrizi
Sulfasalazine	Generic, Azulfidine
Tofacitinib	Xeljanz
Upadacitinib	Rinvoq
Ustekinumab	Stelara
Vedolizumab	Entyvio
SELECTED ANTIDIARRHEAL DRUGS	
Bismuth subsalicylate	Pepto-Bismol, others
Difenoxin	Motofen
Diphenoxylate	Generic, Lomotil, others
Eluxadoline	Viberzi
Loperamide	Generic, Imodium
BULK-FORMING LAXATIVES	
Methylcellulose	Generic, Citrucel
Psyllium	Generic, Serutan, Metamucil, others
OTHER SELECTED LAXATIVE DRUGS	
Alvimopan	Entereg
Bisacodyl	Generic, Dulcolax, others

GENERIC NAME	AVAILABLE AS
Cascara sagrada	Generic
Docusate	Generic, Colace, others
Lactulose	Generic, Chronulac, Cephulac, others
Linaclotide	Linzess
Lubiprostone	Amitiza
Plecanatide	Trulance
Prucalopride	Motegrity
Magnesium hydroxide (milk of magnesia, Epsom Salt)	Generic
Methylnaltrexone bromide	Relistor
Polycarbophil	Equalactin, Mitrolan, FiberCon, Fiber–Lax
Polyethylene glycol electrolyte solution	CoLyte, GoLYTELY, HalfLytely, Moviprep, others
Senna	Senokot, ExoLax, others
Sodium Phosphate	Fleets Phospho-soda, OsmoPrep, Visicol
DRUGS THAT DISSOLVE GALLSTONES	
Obeticholic acid	Ocaliva
Ursodiol	Generic, Actigall, URSO

*Over-the-counter formulations.

REFERENCES

Acid-Peptic Diseases

Alshamsi F et al: Efficacy and safety of proton pump inhibitors for stress ulcer prophylaxis in critically ill patients: A systematic review and meta-analysis of randomized trials. Crit Care 2016;20:120.

Barletta JF et al: Stress ulcer prophylaxis. Crit Care Med 2016;44:1395.

Chey WD et al: ACG Clinical Guideline: Treatment of *Helicobacter pylori*. Am J Gastroenterol 2017;112:212.

Drugs for GERD and peptic ulcer disease. Med Lett Drugs Ther 2018;60:9.

Fallone CA et al: The Toronto Consensus for the treatment of *Helicobacter pylori* infection in adults. Gastroenterology 2016;151:51.

Ford AC et al: Eradication therapy for peptic ulcer disease in *Helicobacter pylori*-positive people. Cochrane Database Syst Rev 2016;4:CD003840.

Freedberg DE et al: The risks and benefits of long-term use of proton pump inhibitors; expert review and best practice from the American Gastroenterological Association. Gastroenterology 2017;152:706.

Gyawali CP et al: Management of gastroesophageal reflux disease. Gastroenterology 2018;154:302.

Jaynes M et al: The risks of long-term proton pump inhibitors: A critical review. Ther Adv Drug Saf 2019;10:2042098618809927.

Katz PO et al: ACG Clinical Guideline for the diagnosis and management of gastroesophageal reflux disease. Am J Gastroenterol 2022;117:27.

Krag M et al: Pantoprazole in patients at risk for gastrointestinal bleeding in the ICU. N Engl J Med 2018;379:2199.

Lanas A et al: Peptic ulcer disease. Lancet 2017;390:613.

Melcarne L et al: Management of NSAID-associated peptic ulcer disease. Expert Rev Gastroenterol Hepatol 2016;10:723.

Strand DS et al: 25 years of proton pump inhibitors; a comprehensive review. Gut Liver 2017;11:27.

Targownik LE et al: De-prescribing proton pump inhibitors (PPIs). Gastroenterology 2022;162:1334.

Yadlapati R et al: Personalized approach to the evaluation and management of gastroesophageal reflux disease (GERD). Clin Gastro Hep 2022; 20:984.

Motility Disorders

Tack J et al: New developments in the treatment of gastroparesis and functional dyspepsia. Curr Opin Pharmacol 2018;43:111.

Vijayvargiya P et al: Effects of promotility agents on gastric emptying and symptoms: A systematic review and meta-analysis. Gastroenterology 2019;156:1650.

Laxatives

ASGE Standards of Practice Committee: Bowel preparation before colonoscopy. Gastrointest Endosc 2015;81:781.

Bharucha AE et al: Chronic constipation. Mayo Clin Proc 2019;94:2340.

Black CJ et al: Efficacy of secretagogues in patients with irritable bowel syndrome with constipation: Systematic review and meta-analysis. Gastroenterology 2018;155:1753.

Crockett SD et al: American Gastroenterological Association Institute Guideline on the medical management of opioid-induced constipation. Gastroenterology 2019;156:218.

Farmer AD et al: Pathophysiology, diagnosis, and management of opioid-induced constipation. Lancet Gastroenterol Hepatol 2018 2:203.

Hassan C et al: Bowel preparation for colonoscopy: European Society of Gastrointestinal Endoscopy Guideline—Update 2019. Endoscopy 2019;51:775.

Miner PB Jr et al: A randomized phase III clinical trial with plecanatide, a uroguanylin analog in patients with chronic idiopathic constipation. Am J Gastroenterol 2017;112:613.

Murphy JA et al: Evidence based review of pharmacotherapy for opioid-induced constipation in noncancer pain. Ann Pharmacother 2018;52:370.

Nee J et al: Efficacy of treatments for opioid-induced constipation: Systematic review and meta-analysis. Clin Gastroenterol Hepatol 2018;16:1569.

Shah ED et al: Efficacy and tolerability of guanylate cyclase-C agonists for irritable bowel syndrome with constipation and chronic idiopathic constipation: A systematic review and meta-analysis. Am J Gastroenterol 2018;113:329.

Vijayvargiya P et al: Use of prucalopride in adults with chronic constipation. Expert Rev Clin Pharmacol 2019;12:579.

Wald A: Constipation: Advances in diagnosis and treatment. JAMA 2016;315:185.

Waldman SA et al: Guanylate cyclase-C as a therapeutic target in gastrointestinal disorders. Gut 2018;67:1543.

Antidiarrheal Agents

Camilleri M: Bile acid diarrhea: Prevalence, pathogenesis, and therapy. Gut Liver 2015;9:332.

Schiller LR: Antidiarrheal drug therapy. Curr Gastroenterol Rep 2018;19:18.

Schiller LR et al: Chronic diarrhea: Diagnosis and management. Clin Gastroenterol Hepatol 2017;15:182.

Drugs Used for Irritable Bowel Syndrome

Alammar N et al: Irritable bowel syndrome: What therapies really work. Med Clin North Am 2019;103:137.

Black CJ et al: Efficacy of pharmacological therapies in patients with IBS with diarrhea or mixed stool pattern: Systematic review and network meta-analysis. Gut 2020;69:74.

Black CJ et al: Efficacy of secretagogues in patients with irritable bowel syndrome with constipation: Systematic review and network meta-analysis. Gastroenterology 2018;155:1753.

Brenner DM et al: Efficacy and safety of eluxadoline in patients with irritable bowel syndrome with diarrhea who report inadequate symptom control with loperamide: RELIEF phase 4 study. Am J Gastroenterol 2019;114:1502.

Chang L et al: Pharmacological management of irritable bowel syndrome with constipation (IBS-C). Gastroenterology 2022;163:118.

Chang L et al: 2015 James W. Freston Topic Conference: A renaissance in the understanding and management of irritable bowel syndrome. Clin Gastroenterol Hepatol 2016;14:e77.

Ford AC et al: American College of Gastroenterology monograph on management of irritable bowel syndrome. Am J Gastroenterol 2018;113:1.

Ford AC et al: Irritable bowel syndrome. N Engl J Med 2017;376:2566.

Lembo AJ et al: Eluxadoline for irritable bowel syndrome with diarrhea. N Engl J Med 2016;374:242.

Lembo A et al: Pharmacological management of irritable bowel syndrome with diarrhea (IBS-D). Gastroenterology 2022;163:137.

Moayyedi P et al: Canadian Association of Gastroenterology Clinical Practice Guideline for the management of irritable bowel syndrome. J Can Assoc Gastroenterol 2019;2:6.

Munjal A et al: Update on pharmacotherapy for irritable bowel syndrome. Curr Gastroenterol Repub 2019;21:25.

Antiemetic Agents

Canziani BC et al: Clinical practice: Nausea and vomiting in acute gastroenteritis: Physiopathology and management. Eur J Pediatr 2018;177:1.

Gilmore J et al: Recent advances in antiemetics: New formations of 5-HT3-receptor antagonists. Cancer Manag Res 2018;10:1827.

Hasketh PG et al: Antiemetics: American Society of Clinical Oncology clinical practice guideline update. J Clin Oncol 2017;35:3240.

Hendren G et al: Safety and efficacy of commonly used antiemetics. Expert Opin Drug Metab Toxicol 2015;11:1753.

Karthaus M et al: Neurokinin-1 receptor antagonists: Review of their role for the prevention of chemotherapy-induced nausea and vomiting in adults. Expert Rev Clin Pharmacol 2019;12:661.

Kovac AL: Comparative pharmacology and guide to the use of the serotonin 5-HT3 receptor antagonists for postoperative nausea and vomiting. Drugs 2016;76:1719.

Lacy BE et al: Chronic nausea and vomiting: Evaluation and treatment. Am J Gastroenterol 2018;113:647.

McKenzie E et al: Radiation-induced nausea and vomiting: A comparison between MASCC/ESMO, ASCO and NCCN antiemetic guidelines. Support Care Cancer 2019;27:783.

Navarri R et al: Antiemetic prophylaxis for chemotherapy-induced nausea and vomiting. N Engl J Med 2016;374:1356.

Oliver I et al: 2016 Updated MASCC/ESMO Consensus Recommendations: Controlling nausea and vomiting with chemotherapy of low or minimal emetic potential. Support Care Cancer 2018;25:297.

Razvi Y et al: ASCO, NCCN, MASCO/ESMO: A comparison of antiemetic guidelines for the treatment of chemotherapy-induced nausea and vomiting in adult patients. Support Care Cancer 2019;27:87.

Tateosian VS et al: What is new in the battle against postoperative nausea and vomiting? Best Pract Res Clin Anaesthesiol 2018;32:137.

Drugs Used for Inflammatory Bowel Disease

Adedokun OJ et al: Pharmacokinetics and exposure response relationships of ustekinumab in patients with Crohn's disease. Gastroenterology 2018; 154:1660.

Chang JY et al: Thiopurine therapy in patients with inflammatory bowel disease: A focus on metabolism and pharmacogenetics. Dig Dis Sci 2019; 64:2395.

Danese S et al: Upadacitinib as induction and maintenance therapy for moderately to severely active ulcerative colitis: results from three phase 3, multicentre, double-blind, randomised trials. Lancet 2022;399:2113.

De Boer NKH et al: Thiopurines in inflammatory bowel disease: New findings and perspectives. J Crohns Colitis 2018;12:610.

D'Haens G: Risankizumab as induction therapy for Crohn's disease: results from the phase 3 ADVANCE and MOTIVATE induction trials. Lancet 2022;399:2015.

D'Haens G: Systematic review: Second-generation vs. conventional corticosteroids for induction of remission in ulcerative colitis. Aliment Pharmacol Ther 2016;44:1018.

Ferrante M et al: Risankizumab as maintenance therapy for moderately to severely active Crohn's disease: results from the multicentre, randomised, double-blind, placebo-controlled, withdrawal phase 3 FORTIFY maintenance trial. Lancet 2022;399:2031.

Feuerstein JD et al: Medical management of moderate to severe luminal and perianal fistulizing Crohn's disease. Gastroenterology 2021;160:2496.

Hoy SM: Budesonide MMX: A review of its use in patients with mild to moderate colitis. Drugs 2015;75:879.

Kuenzig ME et al: Budesonide for the induction and maintenance of remission in Crohn's disease: Systematic review and meta-analysis for the Cochrane collection. J Can Assoc Gastroenterol 2018;1:159.

Lichenstein GR et al: ACG Clinical Guideline: Management of Crohn's disease in adults. Am J Gastroenterol 2018;113:481.

Löwenberg M et al: Vedolizumab induces endoscopic and histologic remission in patients with Crohn's disease. Gastroenterology 2019;157:997.

Mosli MH et al: Vedolizumab for induction and maintenance of remission in ulcerative colitis: A Cochrane systematic review and meta-analysis. Inflamm Bowel Dis 2015;21:1151.

Nalagatla N et al: Effect of accelerated infliximab induction on short- and long-term outcomes of acute severe ulcerative colitis: A retrospective multicenter study and meta-analysis. Clin Gastroenterol Hepatol 2019;17:502.

Narula N et al: Vedolizumab for ulcerative colitis: Treatment outcomes from the VICTORY consortium. Am J Gastroenterol 2018;113:1345.

Panaccione R et al: Canadian Association of Gastroenterology Clinical Practice Guideline for the management of luminal Crohn's disease. Clin Gastroenterol Hepatol 2019;17:1680.

Peyrin-Biroulet L et al: Loss of response to vedolizumab and ability of dose intensification to restore response in patients with Crohn's disease or ulcerative colitis; a systematic review and meta-analysis. Clin Gastroenterol Hepatol 2019;17:838.

Rubin DT et al: ACG Clinical Guideline: Ulcerative colitis in adults. Am J Gastroenterol 2019;114:384.

Rutgeerts P et al: Efficacy of ustekinumab for inducing endoscopic healing in patients with Crohn's disease. Gastroenterology 2018;155:1045.

Salice M et al: Budesonide MMX: Efficacy and safety profile in the treatment of ulcerative colitis. Expert Rev Gastroenterol Hepatol 2019;13:607.

Sandborn WJ et al: Ozanimod as induction and maintenance therapy for ulcerative colitis. N Engl J Med 2021;385:1280.

Sandborn WJ et al: Safety of tofacitinib for treatment of ulcerative colitis, based on 4.4 years of data from global trials. Clin Gastroenterol Hepatol 2019;17:1541.

Sandborn WJ et al: Tofacitinib as induction and maintenance therapy for ulcerative colitis. N Engl J Med 2017;376:1723.

Shivaji UN et al: Review article: Managing the adverse events caused by anti-TNF therapy in inflammatory bowel disease. Aliment Pharmacol Ther 2019;49:664.

Singh S et al: AGA Technical Review on the management of mild-to-moderate ulcerative colitis. Gastroenterology 2019;156:769.

Singh S et al: Systematic review with network meta-analysis: First- and second-line pharmacotherapy for moderate-severe ulcerative colitis. Aliment Pharmacol 2018;47:162.

Van Gennep S et al: Thiopurine treatment in ulcerative colitis: A critical review of the evidence for current clinical practice. Inflamm Bowel Dis 2017;24:67.

Pancreatic Enzyme Supplements

Dominguez-Munoz JE. Management of pancreatic exocrine insufficiency. Curr Opin Gastroenterol 2019;35:455.

Patel V et al: The management of chronic pancreatitis. Med Clin North Am 2019;103:153.

Bile Acids

Gossard AA et al: Current and promising therapy for primary biliary cholangitis. Expert Opin Pharmacother 2019;20:1161.

Hempfling W et al: Systematic review: Ursodeoxycholic acid—adverse effects and drug interactions. Aliment Pharmacol Ther 2003;18:963.

Neuschwander-Tetri B et al: Farnesoid X nuclear receptor ligand obeticholic acid for non-cirrhotic, non-alcoholic steatohepatitis (FLINT): A multicenter, randomized, placebo-controlled trial. Lancet 2015;385:956.

Nevens F et al: A placebo-controlled trial of obeticholic acid in primary biliary cirrhosis. N Engl J Med 2016;375:631.

Drugs for Portal Hypertension

Baiges A et al: Pharmacologic prevention of variceal bleeding and rebleeding. Hepatol Int 2018;12(Suppl 1):68.

Bhutta AQ et al: The role of medical therapy for variceal bleeding. Gastrointest Endosc Clin N Am 2015;25:479.

Drugs for Short-Bowel Syndrome

Kochar B et al: Teduglutide for the treatment of short bowel syndrome—a safety evaluation. Expert Opin Drug Saf 2018;17:733.

Seidner DL et al: Reduction of parenteral nutrition and hydration support and safety with long-term teduglutide treatment in patients with short bowel syndrome-associated intestinal failure: STEPS-3 study. Nutr Clin Pract 2018;33:520.

CASE STUDY ANSWER

The immediate goals of therapy are to improve this young woman's symptoms of abdominal pain, diarrhea, weight loss, and fatigue. Equally important goals are to reduce the intestinal inflammation in hopes of preventing progression to intestinal stenosis, fistulization, and need for surgery. One option now is to step up her therapy by giving her a slow, tapering course of systemic corticosteroids (eg, prednisone) for 8–12 weeks in order to quickly bring her symptoms and inflammation under control while also initiating therapy with an immunomodulator (eg, azathioprine or mercaptopurine) in hopes of achieving long-term disease remission. If satisfactory disease control is not achieved within 3–6 months, therapy with an anti-TNF agent would then be recommended. Alternatively, patients with moderate to severe Crohn disease who have failed mesalamine may be treated immediately with *both* an anti-TNF agent and immunomodulators, which achieves higher remission rates than either agent alone and may improve long-term outcomes.

CHAPTER

63

Cannabinoid Drugs

Todd W. Vanderah, PhD, &
Tally M. Largent-Milnes, PhD

CASE STUDY

A 42-year-old woman with metastatic breast cancer being treated with a combination of cyclophosphamide, doxorubicin, and fluorouracil (5-FU) complains of pain due to chemotherapy-induced peripheral neuropathy. She has been unwilling to eat due to nausea and vomiting induced by her medications. She is receiving heavy doses of oxycodone for pain, but this has resulted in severe constipation. Upon her visit with the oncologist she shows physical signs of cachexia and reports ongoing pain in her back and hips. Friends suggest medical marijuana as a strategy for controlling her present symptoms. What evidence supports this approach? What might be the unwanted effects of this strategy?

The medical use of cannabinoids and crude marijuana has been controversial, but like many other pharmaceuticals, there is a long history of their use in a variety of illnesses. There are numerous reports of cannabinoids being used for pain relief, nausea, and glaucoma, and for inhibiting excitatory disorders such as epilepsy, Parkinson disease, and Tourette syndrome. In the USA, 38 states have legalized cannabis for medicinal use. Although the use of cannabis remains illegal in the USA under Drug Enforcement Agency (DEA) rules, some of its derivative compounds have been approved by the US Food and Drug Administration (FDA). Medical marijuana contains approximately 50 different cannabinoids termed **phytocannabinoids,** and two of these components have received careful scientific study. The first, **delta-9 tetrahydrocannabinol (THC),** is believed to be the most psychoactive and is responsible for the symptoms of euphoria. The second component, **cannabidiol (CBD),** does not demonstrate psychoactive or euphoric activity, appears to have a complex mechanism of action, and has been reported to be useful for a variety of disorders.

The discovery of cannabinoid receptors has generated interest in the therapeutic potential of marijuana, and the identification of widespread cellular production of endogenous cannabinoids in humans and animals has revitalized the science of medicinal cannabinoids.

CANNABINOID RECEPTORS

Cannabinoid (CB) receptors were identified pharmacologically in the 1980s and confirmed by cloning in 1990. Studies identified two unique G protein–coupled receptors termed CB_1 and CB_2, which demonstrated $G_{i/o}$ coupling and a corresponding decrease in cAMP levels when activated. Despite similar coupling, the receptors have very different expression patterns. CB_1 demonstrates widespread expression in most of the organs of the body as well as high expression on the neurons of the central and peripheral nervous system. CB_2 receptor expression is far less extensive, with demonstrated activity primarily on immune cells (ie, macrophages, monocytes, organ-specific resident immune cells), spleen, lymph nodes, microglia of the CNS, and specialized immune cells such as osteoclasts. Since the discovery of the CB receptors, numerous studies have identified their function in a variety of tissues as well as changes of receptor expression due to diseases, hormone alterations, and sustained activation. However, only a few cannabinoid molecules have been approved by the FDA for medicinal use; possibly due to federal regulations, there has been a lack of pharmaceutical investment in a market that would encounter difficult regulation, market competition with nonmedical marijuana, and unforeseen consequences of side effects and societal stigma.

ENDOGENOUS CANNABINOIDS

In 1992, the discovery of the endogenous cannabinoid system sparked interest in novel medical methods to increase or decrease production of endogenous cannabinoid agonists. Anandamide (AEA) was the first endogenous cannabinoid discovered. Soon thereafter a second endogenous cannabinoid, 2-arachidonoyl glycerol (2-AG), was discovered. 2-AG demonstrated a greater than 200-fold increase in endogenous expression compared with anandamide in the CNS and is thought to be the dominant endocannabinoid. AEA is synthesized from lipids of the cell membrane by the enzyme N-acetyltransferase (NAT) followed by a selective phospholipase-D (NAPE-PLD) enzyme (Figure 63–1).

Likewise, 2-AG is synthesized from lipids of the cell membrane by the enzymes phospholipase C (PLC) and diacylglycerol lipase (DAGL) (see Figure 63–1). DAGL inhibitors are in the early stages of development. In preclinical studies, they have been suggested to be useful in obesity. Both AEA and 2-AG are rapidly metabolized by intracellular enzymes that are potential pharmaceutical targets (to increase endogenous cannabinoids). The enzyme fatty acid amide hydrolase (FAAH) breaks down AEA into arachidonic acid (AA) and ethanolamine, AA being a product that can create inflammation via the cyclooxygenase enzymes (see Chapter 18). The enzymes monoacylglycerol lipase (MAGL) and alpha/beta-hydrolase domain-containing 6 (ABHD6) both metabolize 2-AG into arachidonic acid, which may be further broken down by cyclooxygenase to produce prostaglandins (see Figures 18–1 and 63–1). Several experimental compounds (eg, URB629, MJN110, JZL184, WWL70, PF-06818883, ABX-1431, KT182) have been shown in preclinical studies to block the degradation of endogenous cannabinoids and inhibit pain and inflammation with several of these entering into clinical trials.

CANNABINOID COMPOUNDS

Three cannabinoids are currently approved by the FDA for medicinal use in the USA. The first two, nabilone and dronabinol (Figure 63–2), are schedule II medications and have been approved to treat nausea and vomiting associated with cancer chemotherapy in patients who have taken other medications without relief. Dronabinol is also approved to treat anorexia and weight loss in persons with AIDS. Dronabinol is the synthetic form of THC, whereas nabilone is a synthetic analog of dronabinol (see Figure 63–2). It is used in the USA and elsewhere for chronic pain as well as nausea and vomiting, anorexia, and weight loss. The primary target for both dronabinol and nabilone is the CB_1 receptor.

Dronabinol and nabilone can both produce psychotropic effects and often cause lethargy, drowsiness, ataxia, and dry mouth. More rarely they result in euphoria.

Dronabinol and nabilone are highly lipophilic, and both are available in oral form with approximately 20–30% bioavailability. Both are metabolized by microsomal hydroxylation and oxidation catalyzed by the cytochrome P450 (CYP) complex, mainly the CYP2C isoform, and have half-lives of approximately 2–20 hours due to lipid content that may vary in individuals along with predictive active metabolites. Traces of both compounds can remain in the body for more than 35 hours, with some metabolites being found weeks after a single use. Excretion is mainly by the gastrointestinal tract and kidneys.

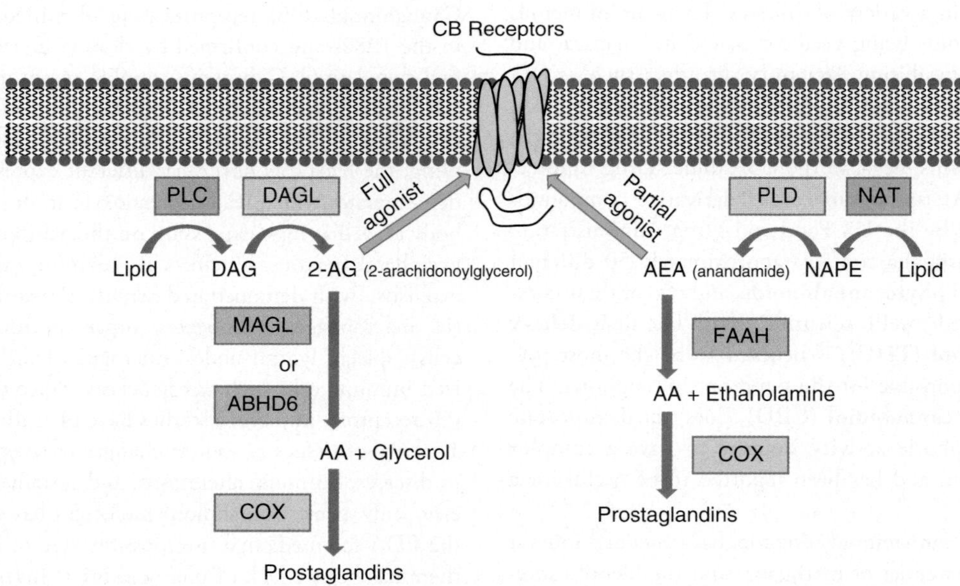

FIGURE 63–1 Pathways of the synthesis and degradation of the endogenous cannabinoids (ECBs). Both AEA and 2-AG are synthesized from membrane lipids by two different enzymes. AEA is degraded by the fatty acid amide hydrolase (FAAH) enzyme, releasing arachidonic acid (AA) and ethanolamine, while 2-AG is degraded by either monoacylglycerol lipase (MAGL) or alpha/beta-hydrolase domain-containing 6 (ABHD6) depending on the cellular expression. Degradation of 2-AG releases arachidonic acid as well as glycerol. 2-AG is more than 200-fold more abundant than AEA, yet both ECBs act at CB1 and CB2 receptors. AEA behaves like a partial agonist, whereas 2-AG is a full agonist.

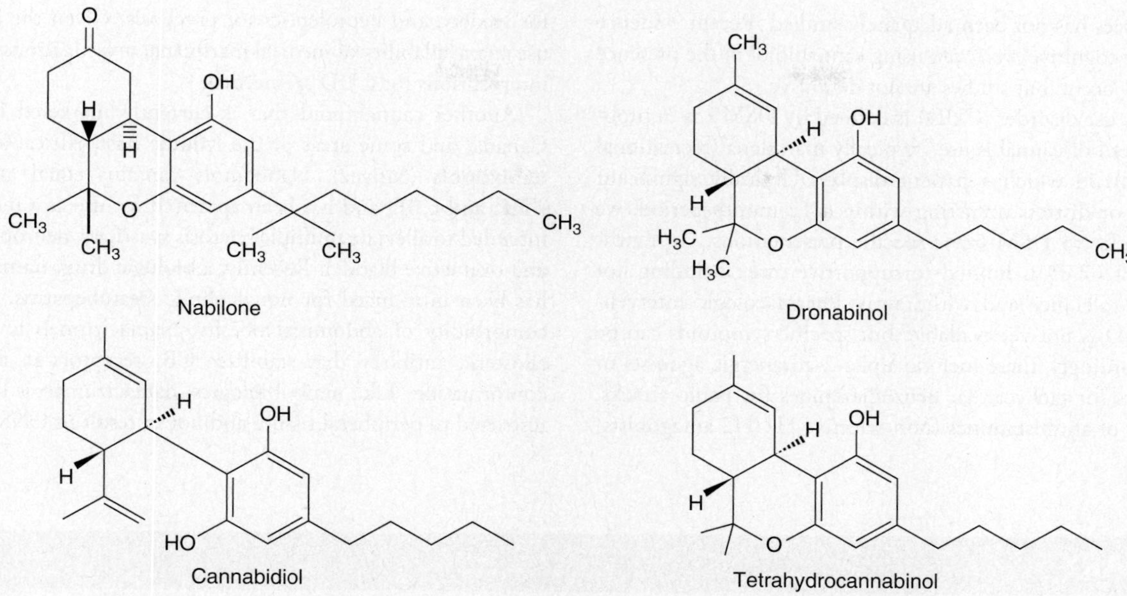

FIGURE 63–2 The chemical structures of the FDA-approved cannabinoids, nabilone, dronabinol, and cannabidiol, and of THC. Dronabinol is the synthetic version of THC, whereas nabilone is an analog of dronabinol.

The third FDA-approved cannabinoid is CBD (see Figure 63–2), a schedule V drug. As discussed in Chapter 24, CBD is approved for seizures associated with Dravet syndrome and Lennox-Gastaut syndrome. Although CBD is classified as a phytocannabinoid, it does not have activity at the CB_1 or the CB_2 receptors. The mechanism of action is therefore unknown at present, leaving many to speculate whether there is an additional cannabinoid receptor or whether CBD is acting at a different, previously identified receptor(s). Recent studies have documented interactions and activity of CBD via a GPR55 receptor (currently classified as an orphan G protein), 5-HT_1 receptors, TRPV1 channels, and interactions with other ion channels including $GABA_A$ and T-type voltage-gated calcium channels ($Ca_{v3.2}$). Several case reports and open-label clinical studies have suggested that CBD reduces pain, inflammation, and anxiety, but proof of clinical efficacy and safety will require randomized, controlled, blind clinical trials. A recent, small, open-label, clinical case study in patients with post-traumatic stress disorder (PTSD) identified CBD as effective in treating PTSD symptoms when added to current therapy. A study in patients with Crohn disease demonstrated that CBD significantly prevented inflammation-induced gastrointestinal hyperpermeability. In addition, some studies suggest efficacy of CBD for its ability to attenuate drug dependence, and clinical trials are ongoing.

Hemp is a distinct strain of *Cannabis sativa* defined as containing <0.3% THC that has been used industrially for its strong fiber content, and it produces much higher concentrations of CBD than does the marijuana strain of *C sativa.* CBD for the most part has been well tolerated and lacks the psychoactive and euphoric effects seen with the CB_1 agonists, as well as medical marijuana, which tends to have higher concentrations of Δ9-THC and lower concentrations of CBD. The oral bioavailability of CBD is approximately 20%, and the half-life is 15–20 hours. CBD is metabolized by liver cytochrome P450s including the CYP2C, CYP1A, and CYP3A families; it is excreted mainly via the feces and urine.

Finally, medical marijuana, which is still currently a schedule I substance and federally illegal within the USA, is nevertheless widely available across the USA and elsewhere in a variety of formulations described below. Medical marijuana contains more than 100 different cannabinoids and acts at CB_1 and CB_2 receptors as well as other unidentified sites including the CBD site(s). Among different strains of medical marijuana, average THC content is reported to be >22% whereas CBD content is more variable (1–16%). In addition, medical marijuana chemovars may contain varying percentages of terpenes (1–10%), which may contribute to therapeutic outcomes (ie, entourage effect). As above, many of the constituent's target CYPs with low bioavailability and active metabolites. A multitude of chemovars (ie, strains) are being prescribed for conditions including pain, glaucoma, stress, PTSD, nausea and vomiting associated with cancer chemotherapy, loss of appetite and weight loss, muscle spasms, and epilepsy, although limited evidence for selective chemovar effect exists to date. Medical marijuana is prescribed in multiple forms including smoking, vaping, edibles, capsules, lozenges, dermal patches, topicals (salves and lotions), and dermal sprays. Medical marijuana is reported to produce several minor to moderate adverse effects including psychoactive effects, tiredness, dizziness, impaired motor coordination, cardiovascular effects (tachycardia, peripheral vasodilation, hypotension), impaired short-term memory, and psychosis at increased doses. Review of the literature on neuropsychological task-based measures of cognition have described impairment—by acute and chronic exposure to cannabis—in verbal learning and memory, as well as attention tasks. Psychomotor function is most affected during acute intoxication, whereas impaired verbal memory, attention, and some executive functions may persist after prolonged use and abstinence. However, cognitive testing with a better selection of pure substances has not been adequately studied. Recent evidence suggests that cognitive *protection* using cannabidiol in the presence of THC may occur, but studies are not definitive.

Cannabis use disorder (CUD) is defined by DSM5 as "a problematic pattern of cannabis use," typically marijuana (recreational and medical), in which a patient displays clinically significant impairment or distress occurring within a 12-month period; we refer the reader to DSM 5 for specific presentations. Currently, treatment for CUD is limited to supportive care, including hot showers for tolerance and withdrawal. Pharmacologic intervention for CUD is not yet available, but specific symptoms can be treated; accordingly, these include alpha-2-adrenergic agonists or beta-blockers for tachycardia, benzodiazepines for panic attacks, off-label use of antihistamines (non-selective H1/H2 antagonists) for anxiety, and neuroleptics for psychosis. Given the increase in use and availability of medical marijuana, investigations evaluating interventions for CUD are needed.

Another cannabinoid that is currently marketed in Europe, Canada, and some areas of the Middle East, Africa, and Asia is **nabiximols** (Sativex). Nabiximols contains equal amounts of THC and CBD and has been approved for use as a mouth spray intended to alleviate multiple sclerosis spasticity, neuropathic pain, and overactive bladder. Recently, a biologic drug, **namacizumab,** has been introduced for nonalcoholic steatohepatitis, a frequent comorbidity of abdominal obesity. Namacizumab is a negative allosteric antibody that stabilizes CB_1 receptors in an inactive conformation. Like many biologics, namacizumab is likely to be restricted to peripheral tissues and not to result in CNS effects.

SUMMARY

Subclass, Drug	Mechanism of Action	Effects	Clinical Applications	Toxicity
Cannabidiol	Uncertain	See Chapter 24	Dravet syndrome, Lennox-Gastaut syndrome	See Chapter 24
Dronabinol, nabilone	Agonism at CB_1, CB_2 receptors		Nausea, vomiting of chemotherapy; anorexia of AIDS	Euphoria, dizziness, vasodilation, hypotension

PREPARATIONS AVAILABLE

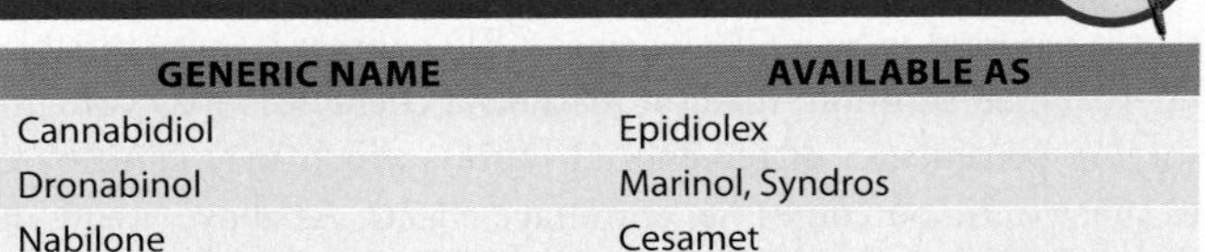

GENERIC NAME	AVAILABLE AS
Cannabidiol	Epidiolex
Dronabinol	Marinol, Syndros
Nabilone	Cesamet

REFERENCES

Bird Rock Bio: Bird Rock Bio Completes Single Ascending Dose Human Clinical Trial for Namacizumab; Generates Safety, Tolerability, and Pharmacokinetics Data; Prepares To Initiate Study in Non-Alcoholic Fatty Liver Disease Patients. PR Newswire, 2017.

Bisogno T et al: A novel fluorophosphonate inhibitor of the biosynthesis of the endocannabinoid 2-arachidonoylglycerol with potential anti-obesity effects. Br J Pharmacol 2013;169:784.

Broyd SJ et al: Acute and chronic effects of cannabinoids on human cognition—a systematic review. Biol Psychiatry 2016;79;557.

Cogan PS: On healthcare by popular appeal: Critical assessment of benefit and risk in cannabidiol based dietary supplements. Expert Rev Clin Pharmacol 2019;12:501.

Costa B et al: The non-psychoactive cannabis constituent cannabidiol is an orally effective therapeutic agent in rat chronic inflammatory and neuropathic pain. Eur J Pharmacol 2007;556:75.

Couch DG et al: Cannabidiol and palmitoylethanolamide are anti-inflammatory in the acutely inflamed human colon. Clin Sci (Lond) 2017;131:2611.

Couch DG et al: Palmitoylethanolamide and cannabidiol prevent inflammation-induced hyperpermeability of the human gut in vitro and in vivo—a randomized, placebo-controlled, double-blind controlled trial. Inflamm Bowel Dis 2019;25:1006.

Devane WA et al: Isolation and structure of a brain constituent that binds to the cannabinoid receptor. Science 1992;258:1946.

Di Marzo V: New approaches and challenges to targeting the endocannabinoid system. Nat Rev Drug Discov 2018;17:623.

Greydanus DE et al: Cannabis: Effective and safe analgesic? J Pain Manag 2014;7:209.

Howlett AC et al: International Union of Pharmacology. XXVII. Classification of cannabinoid receptors. Pharmacol Rev 2002;54:161.

Karst M et al: Role of cannabinoids in the treatment of pain and (painful) spasticity. Drugs 2010;70:2409.

Klein TW et al: The cannabinoid system and immune modulation. J Leukoc Biol 2003;74:486.

Liktor-Busa E et al: Analgesic potential of terpenes derived from *Cannabis sativa*. Pharmacol Rev 2021;73:1269.

Long LE et al: Distinct neurobehavioural effects of cannabidiol in transmembrane domain neuregulin 1 mutant mice. PLoS One 2012;7:e34129.

Lozano-Ondoua AN et al: Disease modification of breast cancer-induced bone remodeling by cannabinoid CB2 receptor agonists. J Bone Miner Res 2013;28:92.

Mechoulam R: The pharmacohistory of *Cannabis sativa.* In: Mechoulam R (editor): *Cannabinoids as Therapeutic Agents.* Boca Raton: CRC Press; 1986.

Pertwee RG: Cannabinoid pharmacology: The first 66 years, Br J Pharmacol 2006;147(Suppl 1):S163.

Russo EB et al: Agonistic properties of cannabidiol at 5-HT1a receptors. Neurochem Res 2005;30(8):1037.

Ryberg E et al: The orphan receptor GPR55 is a novel cannabinoid receptor. Br J Pharmacol 2007;152:1092.

Ulrich Reimann-P et al: Cannabis chemovar nomenclature misrepresents chemical and genetic diversity; survey of variations in chemical profiles and genetic markers in Nevada medical cannabis samples. Cannabis Cannabinoid Res 2020;5:215.

CASE STUDY ANSWER

Medical marijuana might be the best strategy even though one could also prescribe either nabilone or dronabinol. The multiple components of medical marijuana (which contains THC) may help control the patient's cachexia, nausea and vomiting, and pain. The cannabidiol and other cannabinoids in medical marijuana may help with the chemotherapy-induced pain. The patient should be informed of possible adverse effects such as psychotropic effects, dry mouth, dizziness, and drowsiness.

CHAPTER

64 Therapeutic & Toxic Potential of Over-the-Counter Agents

Valerie B. Clinard, PharmD, & Robin L. Corelli, PharmD

CASE STUDY

AH, a 58-year-old male, presents to the emergency department with confusion, abdominal pain, nausea, and complaints of new-onset flu symptoms over the past several days. His past medical history is significant for hyperlipidemia and bilateral knee osteoarthritis. His current medications include Tylenol Arthritis Pain (acetaminophen 650 mg/tablet; two tablets three times daily for pain) and atorvastatin (10 mg daily). AH also reported recent use of several over-the-counter (OTC) medications over the past 3 days to treat the new-onset flu symptoms, including Alka-Seltzer Plus Cold & Flu Day (two gel caps every 4 hours during the day) and Alka-Seltzer Plus Cold & Flu Night (two gel caps at bedtime). His social history is significant for alcohol use (three shots of bourbon/night). His vital signs include the following: temperature 99.8°F, blood pressure 132/64 mm Hg, pulse 78 bpm, and respiratory rate 15/min. On physical examination, he had left upper abdominal tenderness with evidence of hepatomegaly and mild scleral icterus. Laboratory data revealed the following: alanine aminotransferase, 557 IU/L (normal 10–35 IU/L); aspartate aminotransferase, 485 IU/L (normal <35 IU/L); and bilirubin, 2.9 mg/dL (normal 0.1–0.3 mg/dL). What medications do OTC cold and flu pre-parations typically contain? Which of the OTC medications might have contributed to the patient's current symptoms?

In the USA, medications are divided by law into two classes: those restricted to sale by prescription only and those for which directions for safe use by the public can be written. The latter category constitutes the nonprescription, or over-the-counter (OTC), medications. This category does not include supplements (vitamins, minerals, herbals, and botanicals), which are subject to different regulatory requirements (see Chapter 65). In 2022, US consumers spent approximately $41.2 billion on OTC products to self-manage a wide variety of acute and chronic medical conditions.

It is apparent that many OTC medications are comparable products advertised to consumers in ways that suggest significant differences between them. For example, there are more than 100 different systemic analgesic products, almost all of which contain aspirin, acetaminophen, nonsteroidal anti-inflammatory drugs (NSAIDs) such as ibuprofen, or a combination of these agents as primary ingredients. They are made different from one another by the addition of questionable ingredients such as caffeine or antihistamines; by brand names chosen to suggest a specific use or strength (eg, "migraine," "arthritis," "maximum"); or by special dosage formulations (eg, enteric-coated tablets, gel tabs, liquids, orally disintegrating strips and tablets, sustained-release products, powders, seltzers). Generally, a price is attached to all of these features, and in most cases, a less expensive generic product can be equally effective. It is probably safe to assume that consumers are generally overwhelmed and confused by the wide array of products presented and will likely use those that are most heavily advertised.

Since 1976, the US Food and Drug Administration (FDA) has been engaged in a process whereby medications previously available by prescription only have been made available for OTC use because they were judged by expert review panels to be generally

TABLE 64–1 Selected agents switched from prescription to over-the-counter status by the US Food and Drug Administration (2006–2023).

Ingredient	Indication (Pharmacologic Category)	Year Ingredient First Switched	Single-Ingredient Product Examples
Adapalene	Acne (topical retinoid)	2016	Differin Gel
Alcaftadine	Itchy eyes (ophthalmic antihistamine)	2021	Lastacaft
Azelastine	Hay fever/upper respiratory allergies (topical nasal antihistamine)	2021	Astepro Allergy, Children's Astepro Allergy
Brimonidine	Eye redness (topical ophthalmic α_2 agonist)	2017	Lumify
Budesonide	Allergic rhinitis (topical glucocorticoid)	2015	Rhinocort Allergy Spray
Cetirizine	Hay fever/upper respiratory allergies (antihistamine)	2007	Zyrtec
Diclofenac	Arthritis pain (topical nonsteroidal anti-inflammatory)	2020	Voltaren Arthritis Pain
Esomeprazole	Acid reducer (proton-pump inhibitor)	2014	Nexium 24 hour
Fexofenadine	Hay fever/upper respiratory allergies (antihistamine)	2011	Allegra 12 hour, Allegra 24 hour
Fluticasone	Allergic rhinitis (topical glucocorticoid)	2014	Flonase Allergy Relief, Flonase Sensimist Allergy-Relief
Ivermectin	Head lice infestation (lotion)	2020	Sklice
Ketotifen	Itchy eyes (ophthalmic antihistamine)	2006	Alaway, Zaditor
Lansoprazole	Acid reducer (proton-pump inhibitor)	2009	Prevacid 24 hour
Levocetirizine	Hay fever/upper respiratory allergies (antihistamine)	2017	Xyzal
Levonorgestrel	Emergency contraceptive (progestin)	2006	Plan B One-Step
Mometasone	Allergic rhinitis (topical glucocorticoid)	2022	Nasonex 24 hour Allergy
Naloxone	Opioid overdose (nasal opioid antagonist)	2023	Narcan
Norgestrel	Prevention of pregnancy (progestin)	2023	Opill
Olopatadine	Itchy eyes (ophthalmic antihistamine)	2020	Pataday Once Daily, Pataday Twice Daily
Orlistat	Weight loss aid (lipase inhibitor)	2007	Alli
Oxybutynin	Overactive bladder (transdermal anticholinergic)	2013	Oxytrol for Women
Polyethylene glycol	Constipation (osmotic laxative)	2006	MiraLAX
Triamcinolone	Allergic rhinitis (topical glucocorticoid)	2013	Nasacort Allergy 24 hour

safe and effective for consumer use without medical supervision (Table 64–1). This prescription-to-OTC switch process has significantly enhanced and expanded self-care options for US consumers with more than 100 OTC active ingredients or formulations on the market today that were previously available only by prescription. In 2023, two switches with significant public health implications were authorized by the FDA through the approval of naloxone nasal spray for OTC use in the management of known or suspected opioid overdose and norgestrel for OTC use in the prevention of pregnancy. Examples of other prescription medications with the potential for future OTC reclassification include sumatriptan for migraine headache, and nicotine replacement therapy (oral inhaler, nasal spray) and varenicline for smoking cessation. The prescription-to-OTC reclassification process is both costly and rigorous, and only select prescription medications are appropriate candidates for a switch (ie, a consumer can self-diagnose and safely treat the condition). For example, the cholesterol-lowering agents lovastatin and pravastatin were denied OTC status on the basis that these agents could not be used safely and effectively in an OTC setting. The nonprescription drug advisory committee believed that diagnosis and ongoing management by a health care professional was necessary for the management of hyperlipidemia, a chronic, asymptomatic condition with potentially life-threatening consequences. In a similar recommendation, oral acyclovir for OTC use in the treatment of recurrent genital herpes was not approved because of concerns about misdiagnosis and inappropriate use leading to increased viral resistance.

There are three reasons why it is essential for clinicians to be familiar with the OTC class of products. First, many OTC medications are effective in treating common ailments, and it is important to be able to help the patient select a safe, effective product. Because health care insurance practices encourage clinicians to reduce costs, many providers will recommend effective OTC treatments, since these medications are generally not paid for by health plans. Second, many of the active ingredients contained in OTC medications may worsen existing medical conditions or interact with prescription medications (see Chapter 67). Finally, the misuse or abuse of OTC products may actually produce significant medical complications. Phenylpropanolamine, for example, a sympathomimetic previously found in many cold, allergy, and weight control products, was withdrawn from the US market by the FDA based on reports that the drug increased the risk of hemorrhagic stroke. Dextromethorphan, an antitussive found in many cough and cold preparations, is abused in high doses (eg, >5–10 times the recommended antitussive dose) by adolescents as a hallucinogen. Although severe complications associated with dextromethorphan as a single agent in overdose are uncommon, many dextromethorphan-containing products are formulated with other ingredients (acetaminophen, antihistamines, and sympathomimetics) that can be fatal in overdose. Loperamide is sometimes used in large doses to create an opioid-like high or to self-treat opioid withdrawal symptoms and can cause altered mental status, respiratory depression, and ventricular arrhythmias. Pseudoephedrine, a decongestant contained in numerous OTC cold preparations, has been used in the illicit manufacture of methamphetamine and is now available only in locked cabinets or behind the counter with regulations (eg, quantity limits, photo identification to purchase) to control the sale of this agent. A general awareness of these products and their formulations will enable clinicians to more fully appreciate the potential for OTC medication-related problems in their patients.

Table 64–2 lists examples of OTC products that may be used effectively to treat common medical conditions. The selection of one ingredient over another may be important in patients with certain medical conditions or in patients taking multiple medications. These are discussed in detail in other chapters. The recommendations listed in Table 64–2 are based on the efficacy of

TABLE 64–2 Ingredients of known efficacy for selected over-the-counter (OTC) classes.

OTC Category	Generic Name (Brand Example)	Labeled Use	Warnings	Considerations
Acid reducers (H_2 antagonists)	Cimetidine (Tagamet HB) Famotidine (Pepcid AC)	Relief and prevention of heartburn associated with acid indigestion.	Avoid use: in children <12 years of age; if patient has trouble or pain swallowing food, vomiting with blood, or bloody or black stools; with other acid reducers; if symptoms include heartburn with lightheadedness, sweating, dizziness, or chest pain; for treatment durations >14 days. Adverse effects include: nausea, agitation, headache, dizziness, and gynecomastia (cimetidine; rare).	• To prevent symptoms, take before consuming food or beverages that cause heartburn (0–60 minutes; see product instructions) • Cimetidine may increase the serum concentrations of theophylline, warfarin, and phenytoin.
Acid reducers (proton-pump inhibitors [PPIs])	Esomeprazole (Nexium 24 hour) Lansoprazole (Prevacid 24 hour) Omeprazole (Prilosec OTC)	Treatment of frequent heartburn (occurs 2 or more days a week).	Avoid use: in children <18 years of age; if patient has trouble or pain swallowing food, vomiting with blood, or bloody or black stools; if symptoms include heartburn with lightheadedness, sweating, dizziness, or chest pain; for treatment durations >14 days. Adverse effects include: headache, abdominal pain, nausea, and diarrhea.	• Not intended for immediate relief (products take 1–4 days for full effect). • Take with water before eating in the morning. • Patients may repeat a 2-week course of therapy every 4 months. • PPI therapy can increase risk of *Clostridium difficile*-associated diarrhea, pneumonia, and risk of fracture. • Stop use if patient develops a rash or joint pain as new onset or exacerbation of an existing autoimmune disorder may occur. • Esomeprazole, lansoprazole, and omeprazole may interact with warfarin, clopidogrel, cilostazol, antifungal medications, diazepam, digoxin, tacrolimus, theophylline, and HIV antiretrovirals.
Acne	Adapalene (Differin) Benzoyl peroxide (Neutrogena Clear Pore) Salicylic acid (Stridex Essential; Noxzema Anti-blemish Daily Scrub)	Topical treatment of acne vulgaris.	Avoid use: in children <12 years of age (adapalene); on areas with cuts or abrasions; near eyes and mucous membranes. Use with caution in those with sensitive skin. Adverse effects include: erythema, scaling, dryness, burning, pruritis, and excessive drying of skin (benzoyl peroxide and salicylic acid).	• Erythema, dryness, and scaling, burning, and pruritis may occur more often in the first 2–4 weeks of therapy. Symptoms typically lessen with continuous use. Reducing the frequency of application may be required. • Avoid unnecessary sun exposure. • Stop using products with benzoyl peroxide or salicylic acid if hives, itching, or difficulty breathing occurs; hypersensitivity reactions may occur (rare). • Wash hands thoroughly after application. • Due to potential systemic absorption of salicylic acid with topical use, do not use in combination with other salicylic acid products.

(*continued*)

TABLE 64–2 Ingredients of known efficacy for selected over-the-counter (OTC) classes. (Continued)

OTC Category	Generic Name (Brand Example)	Labeled Use	Warnings	Considerations
Allergy preparations	Chlorpheniramine (Chlor-Trimeton) Clemastine (Dayhist Allergy) Cetirizine (Zyrtec) Diphenhydramine (Benadryl Allergy) Fexofenadine (Allegra 12 hour, Allegra 24 hour) Levocetirizine (Xyzal Allergy 24HR) Loratadine (Alavert, Claritin)	Temporary relief of the following symptoms due to hay fever or upper respiratory allergies: sneezing, runny nose, itchy, watery eyes, itching of nose or throat.	Avoid use: in children <2 years of age; in combination with other sedatives and alcohol as sedative effects may be potentiated. Use caution when driving or operating machinery. Adverse effects include: drowsiness, dizziness, fatigue, nausea, headache, and urinary retention. Antihistamines are contained in many OTC preparations in combination with analgesics, decongestants, and expectorants.	• Diphenhydramine is the most sedating antihistamine. • Consult product labeling before use in children ages 2–11 years. • First-generation antihistamines (chlorpheniramine, clemastine, diphenhydramine) may cause excitability in children. • Second-generation antihistamines (cetirizine, fexofenadine, levocetirizine, loratadine) have minimal anticholinergic effects and are associated with lower chances of sedation.
Analgesics and antipyretics	Systemic: Acetaminophen (Tylenol) *Nonsteroidal anti-inflammatory drugs (NSAIDs)* Aspirin (Ecotrin) Ibuprofen (Advil, Motrin IB) Naproxen (Aleve) Topical: Diclofenac (Voltaren gel)	Temporary reduction of fever and temporary relief of minor aches, pains, and headaches.	*Acetaminophen* Avoid use: in combination with other drugs containing acetaminophen; in patients drinking 3 or more alcoholic beverages daily due to an increased risk of severe liver damage. Adverse effects include: drowsiness, hepatotoxicity (dose related), nephrotoxicity (with chronic overdose), and hypersensitivity reactions (rare). *Aspirin and other NSAIDs* Avoid use in patients with: underlying gastrointestinal bleeding disorders; heart failure; renal insufficiency; hepatic insufficiency; asthma; high blood pressure; cardiac disease; in children or teenagers with chickenpox or flu-like symptoms due to an increased risk of Reye syndrome (aspirin only). Adverse effects include: dyspepsia, nausea, gastric ulceration, duodenal ulceration, renal insufficiency, hypersensitivity reactions (rare), edema, and tinnitus (dose-related with aspirin). *Diclofenac Topical* Avoid use in patients with known hypersensitivity; history of asthma, urticaria, heart failure, renal insufficiency, or other allergic reaction to aspirin or NSAIDs; in the setting of coronary artery bypass graft surgery. Adverse effects include: dyspepsia, nausea, gastric ulceration or perforation, skin reactions, and edema.	*Acetaminophen* • Maximum recommended adult dose for OTC use is 3000–3250 mg/24 h (4000 mg/24 h under medical supervision). • Many products may include acetaminophen, which can lead to unintentional overdose. *Aspirin and other NSAIDs* • Use can increase risk of severe gastrointestinal hemorrhage in individuals: age 60 or older; with peptic ulcer disease or coagulation abnormalities; taking anticoagulants, corticosteroids, or other NSAIDs; who consume ≥3 alcoholic beverages daily; who take the products for a longer time than directed. • Liver damage may occur if NSAIDs, including topical diclofenac, are used for longer than directed. • Maximum recommended adult daily dose for OTC use: aspirin (3900 mg); ibuprofen (1200 mg); naproxen (660 mg). • May reduce the effectiveness of medications used to treat high blood pressure. • Long-term continuous use of ibuprofen or naproxen may increase the risk of myocardial infarction and stroke. This risk is likely lower with naproxen. • Frequent or regular use of ibuprofen may interfere with the cardioprotective effect of aspirin. • Patients should minimize exposure to natural or artificial sunlight on areas treated with topical diclofenac. • Concomitant use of topical and oral NSAIDs should be avoided. A higher rate of hemorrhage, more frequent creatinine, urea, and hemoglobin abnormalities has been documented.

(*continued*)

TABLE 64–2 Ingredients of known efficacy for selected over-the-counter (OTC) classes. (Continued)

OTC Category	Generic Name (Brand Example)	Labeled Use	Warnings	Considerations
Antacids	Aluminum hydroxide (generic only) Calcium carbonate (Tums) Magnesium hydroxide (Milk of Magnesia) Sodium bicarbonate/ citric acid (Alka-Seltzer Heartburn) Aluminum hydroxide/magnesium hydroxide/ simethicone (Mylanta Maximum Strength)	Temporary relief of upset stomach with heartburn, acid indigestion, and sour stomach. Products containing simethicone are used for relief of bloating, pressure, or gas symptoms.	Avoid use in patients with: severe renal impairment (aluminum- and sodium-containing products); heart failure or high blood pressure (sodium-containing products). Adverse effects include: diarrhea (magnesium preparations) and constipation (aluminum preparations).	• Combinations of magnesium and aluminum hydroxide are less likely to cause constipation or diarrhea and offer high neutralizing capacity. • With prolonged use, antacids may cause "acid rebound" (paradoxical acid hypersecretory state associated with increased gastrin levels). • Antacids can significantly reduce the absorption of many prescription drugs.
Antidiarrheal agents	Bismuth subsalicylate (Kaopectate, Pepto-Bismol) Loperamide (Imodium A–D)	To control symptoms of diarrhea (including traveler's diarrhea). Bismuth-containing products are also used to relieve upset stomach symptoms (indigestion, heartburn, nausea, gas, belching).	*Bismuth-containing products* Avoid use in patients: taking salicylate products; with allergies to aspirin; with bleeding disorders; with peptic ulcer disease; with bloody or black stool; in children or teenagers with chickenpox or flu-like symptoms due to an increased risk of Reye syndrome. Adverse effects include: fecal discoloration (black, tarry), tongue discoloration (darkening), and tinnitus (dose-related and more likely when coadministered with aspirin). *Loperamide* Avoid use in: children <12 years of age; patients with bloody or black stools. Adverse effects include: abdominal pain, nausea, constipation, drowsiness, dizziness, dry mouth, Torsades de pointes and cardiac arrest (with higher than recommended doses).	• Antidiarrheal agents should not be used if diarrhea occurs with fever >100°F or if blood or mucus present in stool. • Bismuth-containing products may be used as part of combination therapy for *Helicobacter pylori* eradication therapy. • Loperamide, a synthetic opioid, is not considered a controlled substance but is sometimes abused in high doses for euphoric opioid-like effects. Taking more loperamide than directed may cause serious heart problems or death.
Antifungal preparations (topical)	Butenafine (Lotrimin Ultra) Clotrimazole (Lotrimin AF) Miconazole (Desenex, Lotrimin AF) Terbinafine (Lamisil AT) Tolnaftate (Tinactin)	Relieves itching, burning, scaling, chafing, and discomfort associated with tinea pedis (athlete's foot), tinea cruris (jock itch), and tinea corporis (ringworm).	For external use only. Avoid contact with eyes, nose, mouth, or other mucous membranes. Avoid use: in children <2 years of age (clotrimazole, miconazole, tolnaftate) or children <12 years of age (butenafine, terbinafine). Adverse effects include: erythema, irritation, itching, and burning.	• For treatment of athlete's foot, apply product to spaces between toes and change shoes and socks daily. • Avoid occlusive dressings. • Do not use on nails or scalp. • Stop use and contact doctor if no improvement after 4 weeks (athlete's foot or ringworm) or 2 weeks (jock itch).

(*continued*)

TABLE 64–2 Ingredients of known efficacy for selected over-the-counter (OTC) classes. (Continued)

OTC Category	Generic Name (Brand Example)	Labeled Use	Warnings	Considerations
Antifungal preparations (vaginal)	Clotrimazole (Gyne-Lotrimin) Miconazole (Monistat-1, Monistat-3, Monistat-7, Vagistat-3) Tioconazole Monistat 1-Day Treatment	Treatment of vaginal yeast (candidiasis) infections and for the relief of external vulvar itching and irritation associated with vaginal yeast infections.	For vaginal use only. Avoid use: in children <12 years of age; if patient has lower abdominal, back, or shoulder pain, or fever, chills, nausea, vomiting, or foul-smelling vaginal discharge; in combination with tampons, douches, spermicides, or other vaginal products. Adverse effects include: vaginal itching, burning, vaginal soreness, and swelling.	• Topical vaginal antifungals should only be used for treatment of recurrent vulvovaginal candidiasis in healthy, nonpregnant women who were previously diagnosed by a clinician. • Therapy should be discontinued if symptoms do not improve within 3 days or if symptoms persist after 7 days of treatment. • Vaginal products (7-day therapy preferred) can be used for treatment in pregnant women. • Products with similar brand names may contain different antifungal products; read labels and instructions for use carefully. • Condoms and diaphragms may be damaged by the products and fail to prevent pregnancy or sexually transmitted disease.
Antitussives	Dextromethorphan (Delsym, Robitussin 12-Hour Cough Relief, Vicks Formula 44)	Temporary relief of cough due to minor throat and bronchial irritation with the common cold or inhaled irritants.	Avoid use: in children <4 years of age; in patients taking a monoamine oxidase inhibitor (MAOI), or for 2 weeks after discontinuation of an MAOI. Use with caution in patients with a chronic cough that occurs with smoking, asthma, and emphysema and in patients with cough with production of excessive mucus. Adverse effects include: confusion, excitement, irritability, nervousness, and serotonin syndrome (uncommon).	• Dextromethorphan is a nonopioid congener of levorphanol without analgesic or addictive properties. Health care providers should be alert for problems of abuse or misuse. • Often used with antihistamines, decongestants, and expectorants in combination products. • Notify provider if symptoms do not improve in 7 days or are accompanied by fever, rash, or persistent headache.
Decongestants, topical (intranasal)	Oxymetazoline (Afrin, Vicks Sinex Severe) Phenylephrine (Neo-Synephrine)	Temporary relief of nasal congestion due to common cold, hay fever, upper respiratory allergies, or sinus congestion and pressure.	Avoid use: in children <6 years of age; for durations >3 days. Use with caution in patients with: heart disease; high blood pressure; thyroid disease; diabetes; trouble urinating due to an enlarged prostate. Adverse effects include: sneezing, burning, stinging, dryness, and rhinorrhea.	• Long-acting agents (oxymetazoline-containing products) are generally preferred. • Topical decongestants should not exceed 3 days to prevent rebound nasal congestion (eg, worsening or recurrence of congestion symptoms).
Decongestants, systemic	Phenylephrine (Sudafed PE) Pseudoephedrine (Sudafed)	Temporary relief of sinus congestion and pressure. Temporarily relieves nasal congestion due to the common cold, hay fever, or other upper respiratory allergies.	Avoid use: in patients taking an MAOI or for 2 weeks after stopping the MAOI. Use with caution in patients with heart disease; high blood pressure; diabetes; thyroid disease; trouble urinating due to an enlarged prostate gland. Adverse effects include: arrhythmias, tachycardia, high blood pressure, anxiety, headache, dizziness, tremor, and insomnia.	• May be found in combination with antihistamine, antitussives, expectorants, and analgesic products. • Extended-release pseudoephedrine products should not be used in children <12 years of age. • Federal regulations established to discourage the illicit manufacture of methamphetamine specify that all drug products containing pseudoephedrine must be stored in locked cabinets or behind the pharmacy counter and can only be sold in limited quantities to consumers after they provide photo identification and are entered into a registry. • Notify providers if symptoms do not improve in 7 days or are accompanied by fever, rash, or persistent headache.

(*continued*)

TABLE 64–2 Ingredients of known efficacy for selected over-the-counter (OTC) classes. (Continued)

OTC Category	Generic Name (Brand Example)	Labeled Use	Warnings	Considerations
Emergency contraceptive	Levonorgestrel (Plan B One-Step)	To prevent pregnancy following unprotected intercourse or possible contraceptive failure.	Avoid use in the case of known or suspected pregnancy. Do not use for regular birth control. Adverse effects include: heavier menstrual bleeding, nausea, lower abdominal pain, fatigue, headache, dizziness, and breast tenderness.	• Available only by prescription for women <17 years of age. • Should be taken as soon as possible within 72 hours after unprotected intercourse. • If vomiting occurs within 2 hours of taking the tablet, the dose may need to be repeated. • Use backup contraceptive after administration. Any form of previous contraceptive method can be immediately resumed; however, a barrier method should be used for 7 days.
Expectorants	Guaifenesin (Mucinex)	Used to help loosen phlegm (mucus) and thin bronchial secretions to make cough more productive.	Avoid use in children <2 years of age. Adverse effects include: nausea, vomiting, stomach pain, and dizziness.	• The only OTC expectorant recognized as safe and effective by the FDA. • Often used with antihistamines, decongestants, and antitussives in combination products. • Administer with a large quantity of fluids for best results. • When used for self-care, do not use extended-release tablets in children <12 years of age; discontinue use if symptoms do not improve in 7 days.
Laxatives	*Bulk formers* Polycarbophil, psyllium, and methylcellulose preparations (Citrucel, Fibercon, Metamucil) *Hyperosmotics* Glycerin (Fleet Glycerin suppositories) Polyethylene glycol 3350 (Miralax) *Stool softeners* Docusate sodium (Colace, Dulcolax Stool Softener) Docusate calcium (Surfak) *Stimulant laxatives* Bisacodyl (Dulcolax, Ex-Lax) Senna (Senokot, Ex-Lax) *Saline laxatives* Sodium phosphate (Fleet enema)	Temporary relief of occasional constipation and irregularity.	*Bulk formers* Avoid use in patients with difficulty swallowing. *Polyethylene glycol 3350* Avoid use in patients with kidney disease. *Stool softeners* Avoid use in patients taking mineral oil. *Stimulants* Adverse effects include: stomach discomfort, rectal burning, and mild cramps. *Saline laxatives* Do not use more than one enema in a 24-hour period. Use with caution in patients on a sodium-restricted diet; in patients with kidney disease. *All laxatives* Use with caution in patients with a sudden change in bowel habits that persist for 2 weeks; in patients with abdominal pain, nausea, or vomiting. Adverse effects include: nausea, abdominal bloating, cramping, and flatulence.	• The safest laxatives for chronic use include bulk formers and stool softeners. • While all laxatives should be taken with adequate amounts of fluid for optimal effect, the bulk formers in powder formulations must be taken with adequate fluid to avoid choking.

(*continued*)

TABLE 64–2 Ingredients of known efficacy for selected over-the-counter (OTC) classes. (Continued)

OTC Category	Generic Name (Brand Example)	Labeled Use	Warnings	Considerations
Overactive bladder treatment	Oxybutynin transdermal system (Oxytrol for women)	Treatment of overactive bladder for women with symptoms of urge incontinence and urinary urgency and frequency for at least 3 months.	Avoid use in: men; women <18 years of age; patients with symptoms of a urinary tract infection (pain or burning when urinating, blood in urine, unexplained lower back pain, urine that is cloudy or foul smelling). Adverse effects include: sleepiness, dizziness, confusion, dry mouth, constipation, application site irritation, and blurred vision.	• Women should consult with their physician about symptoms before using this product. • Women who only experience accidental urine loss when coughing, sneezing, or laughing may have stress incontinence; this product is not effective for this condition. • The OTC patch formulation contains the same dosage as the prescription product. • One patch should be applied to abdomen, hips, or buttocks every 4 days; alternating sites. • When combined with lifestyle modifications, it takes approximately 2 weeks for symptom relief to occur.
Pediculicides (lice treatment)	Permethrin (Nix) Pyrethrins combined with piperonyl butoxide (RID) Ivermectin lotion (SKLICE)	Treatment of head lice (permethrin-containing products and ivermectin); and pubic and body lice (piperonyl butoxide-containing products).	For external use only. Avoid use: if allergic to ragweed; in children <2 months (permethrin), <6 months (ivermectin) and <2 years of age (pyrethrins combined with piperonyl butoxide); near the eyes; inside the nose, mouth, or vagina; on lice in eyebrows or eyelashes. Adverse effects include: itching and redness at the application sites.	• Proper use requires careful inspection and thorough application of the products (10 minutes) to the affected areas. • Following application, lice and nits (eggs) should be removed with a fine-tooth comb. Nit combing is not necessary with ivermectin. • Kills live lice (neurotoxic), but is not effective for eggs (nits). Therefore, repeat process in 7–10 days to kill newly hatched nits. • Clothing, bed linens, and other items that the infested person wore or used during the 2 days before treatment should be washed using the hot water (130°F) cycle and dried using the high heat cycle.
Sleep aids	Diphenhydramine (Nytol, Sominex) Doxylamine (Unisom)	Reduces difficulty in falling asleep.	Avoid use in: children <12 years of age; combination with alcohol, other antihistamines, or sedatives; individuals with angle-closure glaucoma; men with trouble urinating due to an enlarged prostate gland. Use caution when driving or operating machinery. Adverse effects include: dizziness, constipation, and dry mouth.	• Insomnia persisting for >2 weeks may be a sign of a serious underlying medical condition.
Smoking cessation aids	Nicotine polacrilex gum (Nicorette) Nicotine polacrilex lozenge (Nicorette) Nicotine transdermal patch (Habitrol; Nicoderm CQ)	Reduces withdrawal symptoms (including nicotine craving) associated with quitting smoking.	Avoid use in: children <18 years of age; women who are pregnant or breastfeeding; individuals with temporomandibular joint disease (gum only); individuals with allergies to adhesive tape (patch only). Use patch with caution in patients with a history of dermatologic conditions (eczema, psoriasis, ectopic dermatitis). *Gum & Lozenge* Adverse effects include: mouth and throat irritation, hiccups, dyspepsia, nausea, jaw soreness (gum only). *Transdermal patch* Adverse effects include: local skin reactions (erythema, pruritis, burning), headache, and sleep disturbances (abnormal/vivid dreams, insomnia).	• Nicotine replacement products in addition to behavioral support approximately double the long-term cessation rates compared with placebo. • Nicotine replacement products can be used in combination to improve long-term abstinence rates. • The patch may aid in improved adherence (once-daily dosing). • Do not use lozenge if allergic to soya (soy beans).

the ingredients and on the principles set forth in the following paragraphs.

1. Select the product that is simplest in formulation; in general, single-ingredient products are preferred. Combination products may contain effective doses of some ingredients and subtherapeutic doses of others. Furthermore, there may be differing durations of action among the ingredients, and the clinician or patient might not be aware of the presence of certain active ingredients in the product.
2. Select a product that contains a therapeutically effective dose.
3. Consumers and providers should carefully read the "Drug Facts" label (an example is given in Figure 64–1) to determine which ingredients are appropriate based on the patient's symptoms, underlying health conditions, and whatever is known about the medications the patient is already taking. Many products with the same brand name contain different ingredients that are labeled for different uses. For example, multiple products (with different active ingredients) carry the Fleet name, including Fleet laxative enema (sodium phosphate), Fleet lubricant laxative (mineral oil), Fleet stimulant laxative (Bisacodyl), and Fleet suppository (glycerin).
4. Recommend a generic product if one is available.
5. Be wary of claims of specific superiority over similar products.
6. For children, the dose, dosage form, and palatability of the product are important considerations.

Certain ingredients in OTC products should be avoided or used with caution in selected patients because they may exacerbate existing medical problems or interact with other medications

Drug Facts

Active ingredient (in each tablet) — **Purpose**
Chlorpheniramine maleate 2 mg .... Antihistamine

Uses temporarily relieves these symptoms due to hay fever or other upper respiratory allergies:
■ Sneezing ■ Runny nose ■ Itchy, watery eyes ■ Itchy throat

Warnings
Ask a doctor before use if you have
■ Glaucoma ■ A breathing problem such as emphysema or chronic bronchitis
■ Trouble urinating due to an enlarged prostate gland

Ask a doctor or pharmacist before use if you are taking tranquilizers or sedatives

When using this product
■ You may get drowsy ■ Avoid alcoholic drinks
■ Alcohol, sedatives, and tranquilizers may increase drowsiness
■ Be careful when driving a motor vehicle or operating machinery
■ Excitability may occur, especially in children

If pregnant or breast-feeding, ask a health professional before use.
Keep out of reach of children. In case of overdose, get medical help or contact a Poison Control Center right away.

Directions

Adults and children 12 years and over	Take 2 tablets every 4 to 6 hours; not more than 12 tablets in 24 hours
Children 6 years to under 12 years	Take 1 tablet every 4 to 6 hours; not more than 6 tablets in 24 hours
Children under 6 years	Ask a doctor

Other information store at 20–25°C (68–77°F) ■ Protect from excessive moisture

Inactive ingredients D&C yellow no. 10, lactose, magnesium stearate, microcrystalline cellulose, pregelatinized starch

FIGURE 64–1 Typical FDA-required labeling for an over-the-counter antihistamine. The label must contain, in the following order: active ingredient(s), including the amount in each dosage unit; purpose of product (pharmacologic action); use(s) for product (indication); specific warnings, including when the product should not be used and pregnancy information; when the patient should seek care of a health care provider; side effects and substances or activities to avoid; dosage instructions (when, how, and how often to take medication); and inactive ingredients. Additional requirements include, but are not limited to, the following: type size must be large enough to be easily read, >6-point font type for information in drug facts section; bullets must be solid square or circle 5-point type; and directions in table format for dosage instructions when presented for three or more age groups or populations. (Reproduced from U.S. Food & Drug Administration. www.fda.gov/Drugs/ResourcesForYou/Consumers/ucm143551.htm.).

the patient is taking. The presence of many of potentially harmful OTC ingredients may be unexpectedly hidden in products (Table 64–3). Although OTC medications have standardized label formatting and content requirements (see Figure 64–1), many consumers do not carefully read or comprehend this information. Lack of awareness of the ingredients in OTC products and the belief by many patients and providers that OTC products are ineffective and harmless may cause diagnostic confusion and compromise therapeutic management. For example, innumerable OTC products, including analgesics and allergy, cough, and cold preparations, contain sympathomimetics. These agents should be avoided or used cautiously by patients with type 1 diabetes and patients with hypertension, angina, or hyperthyroidism. Aspirin should not be used in children and adolescents for viral infections (with or without fever) because of an increased risk of Reye syndrome. Aspirin and other NSAIDs should be avoided by individuals with active peptic ulcer disease, those with certain platelet disorders, and patients taking oral anticoagulants. Cimetidine is a well-known inhibitor of hepatic drug metabolism and can increase the blood levels and toxicity of agents such as phenytoin, theophylline, and warfarin.

Overuse or misuse of OTC products may cause significant medical problems. A prime example is rhinitis medicamentosa or "rebound rhinitis," a condition that manifests as nasal congestion without rhinorrhea, associated with the regular use of topical decongestant nasal sprays for more than 3 days. The improper and long-term use of some antacids (eg, aluminum hydroxide) may cause constipation and even impaction in the elderly, as well as

TABLE 64–3 Hidden ingredients in over-the-counter (OTC) products.

Hidden Drug or Drug Class	OTC Class Containing Drug	Selected Product Examples
Alcohol (percent ethanol)	Cough syrups, cold preparations	Theraflu ExpressMax (10%); Vicks NyQuil Cold & Flu Liquid (10%); Vicks NyQuil Cough (10%)
	Mouthwashes	Listerine (27%); Cepacol (14%)
Antihistamines	Analgesics	Advil PM; Excedrin PM; Goody's PM Night time Powder; Tylenol PM
	Menstrual products	Midol Complete; Pamprin Multisymptom
	Sleep aids	Nytol; Simply Sleep; Sominex; Unisom
Aspirin and other salicylates	Antacids	Alka-Seltzer Original; Alka-Seltzer Heartburn Relief Extra Strength
	Antidiarrheals	Pepto-Bismol (bismuth subsalicylate); Kaopectate (bismuth subsalicylate)
	Menstrual products	Pamprin Maximum Strength
	Cold/allergy preparations	Alka-Seltzer Plus Severe Cold
Caffeine (mg/tablets or as stated)	Analgesics	Alka-Seltzer Hangover Relief (65) Anacin (32); BC Original (65/powder); BC Arthritis (65/powder); Excedrin Extra Strength (65); Excedrin Migraine (65); Excedrin Tension Headache (65/tablet); Goody's Headache Powder (33 mg/powder); Goody's Hangover (150); Stanback Headache (65/powder)
	Menstrual products	Midol Complete (60); Pamprin Maximum Strength (65)
	Stimulants	NoDoz Maximum Strength (200); Vivarin (200)
Local anesthetics (usually benzocaine or lidocaine)	Antitussives/lozenges	Cepacol Sore Throat Lozenges; Chloraseptic Sore Throat
	Dermatologic preparations	Bactine (many); Dermoplast; Solarcaine
	Hemorrhoidal products	Americaine; Preparation H Rapid Relief; Tronolane
	Toothache, cold sore, and denture pain products	Anbesol (gel, liquid); Kank-A; Orajel Formulations (many); Zilactin-B
Sodium (mg/tablet or as stated)	Analgesics/antacids	Alka-Seltzer Effervescent Tablet Formulations: Original (568); Alka-Seltzer Heartburn Relief Extra Strength (586); Alka-Seltzer Hangover Relief (371); Alka-Seltzer Gold (309)
	Cold/cough preparations	Alka-Seltzer Plus Effervescent Tablet Formulations: Severe Cold (356); Severe Cold & Cough (356); Sinus Congestion & Pain (356); Cold Original (356); Severe Cold & Flu (355)
	Laxatives	Fleet Enema (4439 mg/197mL)
Sympathomimetics (ephedrine, epinephrine; phenylephrine)	Analgesics	Sine-Off; Tylenol Sinus
	Asthma products	Bronkaid Max; Primatene Mist; Primatene Tablets
	Cold/cough/allergy preparations	Alka-Seltzer Plus (many); Dimetapp (many); PediaCare Multisymptom Cold; Robitussin (many); Sudafed (many); Theraflu (many); Tylenol Cold & Flu (many); Tylenol Sinus (many)
	Hemorrhoidal products	Preparation H (cream, gel, ointment, suppository, wipes)

hypophosphatemia. Long-term laxative use can result in abdominal cramping and fluid and electrolyte disturbances. A condition known as laxative abuse syndrome is often observed in women with anorexia nervosa. Insomnia, nervousness, and restlessness can result from the use of sympathomimetics or caffeine present in many OTC products (see Table 64–3). The long-term use of analgesics containing caffeine may trigger rebound headaches upon discontinuation. OTC products containing aspirin, other salicylates, acetaminophen, ibuprofen, or naproxen may increase the risk of hepatotoxicity and gastrointestinal hemorrhage in individuals who consume three or more alcoholic drinks daily, and long-term use of these products has been associated with interstitial nephritis. Acute ingestion of large amounts of acetaminophen by adults or children can cause serious, and often fatal, hepatotoxicity (see Chapter 4). Antihistamines may cause sedation or drowsiness, especially when taken concurrently with sedative-hypnotics, tranquilizers, alcohol, or other central nervous system depressants.

Finally, use of OTC cough and cold preparations in the pediatric population has been under scrutiny by the FDA based on a lack of efficacy data in children less than 12 years of age and reports of serious toxicity in children. Following a thorough review, the FDA recommends that OTC cough and cold agents (eg, products containing antitussives, expectorants, decongestants, and antihistamines) not be used in infants and children younger than 2 years old because of serious and potentially life-threatening adverse events associated with accidental overdose including arrhythmias, hallucinations, and encephalopathy. Drug information sources for OTC products include the *Handbook of Nonprescription Drugs,* the most comprehensive resource for OTC medications. It evaluates ingredients contained in major OTC drug classes and lists the ingredients included in many OTC products. *Facts and Comparisons eAnswers* is an online, subscription reference that is updated monthly; it provides detailed OTC product information and patient counseling instructions. Any health care provider who seeks more specific information regarding OTC products may find useful the references listed below.

REFERENCES

Consumer Healthcare Products Association: www.chpa.org.

Krinsky DL et al: *Handbook of Nonprescription Drugs: An Interactive Approach to Self-Care,* 20th ed. American Pharmacists Association, 2020.

US Food and Drug Administration: Over-the-Counter OTC Nonprescription Drugs. www.fda.gov/drugs/how-drugs-are-developed-and-approved/over-counter-otc-nonprescription-drugs.

US National Library of Medicine: DailyMed. dailymed.nlm.nih.gov/dailymed.

Wolters Kluwer Health: Facts and Comparisons eAnswers (requires subscription). www.wolterskluwer.com/en/solutions/lexicomp/facts-and-comparisons.

CASE STUDY ANSWER

Combination OTC "cold and flu" medications typically contain analgesics (eg, acetaminophen, aspirin), antihistamines (eg, chlorpheniramine, diphenhydramine), antitussives (eg, dextromethorphan), expectorants (eg, guaifenesin), and nasal decongestants (eg, phenylephrine, pseudoephedrine). AH's chronic medications include an analgesic that provides 3900 mg of acetaminophen. Over the past few days, he has initiated two additinonal OTC acetaminophen-containing products including Alka-Seltzer Plus Day Cold & Flu (650 mg acetaminophen/2 gel caps) every 4 hours and Alka-Seltzer Night Cold & Flu (650 mg acetaminophen/2 gel caps) at bedtime. The clinician should obtain a detailed medication history to determine the actual total dose of acetaminophen consumed, but it is likely that AH has ingested 6–7 g of acetaminophen daily over the past 72 hours. This cumulative dosage, coupled with AH's chronic ethanol consumption (three shots of bourbon daily), significantly potentiates the risk for acetaminophen hepatotoxicity. In the USA, unintentional acetaminophen overdose is a leading cause of acute liver failure. The warnings section on all OTC acetaminophen-containing products clearly state that severe liver damage may occur when consumers: (1) take dosages >4000 mg in 24 hours; (2) use acetaminophen in combination with other drugs containing acetaminophen; or (3) take acetaminophen and drink three or more alcoholic beverages daily. Unfortunately, many consumers do not carefully read OTC medication labels, and many do not appreciate the amount of acetaminophen "hidden" in OTC products.

CHAPTER

65

Dietary Supplements & Herbal Medications*

Cathi E. Dennehy, PharmD, &
Candy Tsourounis, PharmD

CASE STUDY

A 53-year-old woman with a history of knee osteoarthritis, high cholesterol, type 2 diabetes, and hypertension presents with new onset of hot flashes and a question about a dietary supplement. She is obese (body mass index [BMI] 33), does not exercise, and spends a good portion of her workday in a seated position. She eats a low-sugar diet and regularly eats packaged frozen meals for dinner because she doesn't have time to cook regularly. Her most recent laboratory values include a low-density lipoprotein (LDL) cholesterol that is above goal at 160 mg/dL (goal <100 mg/dL), her kidney function is normal, and her hemoglobin A_{1c} is well controlled at 6%. Her blood pressure is high at 160/100 mm Hg. Her prescription medications include simvastatin, metformin, and benazepril. She also takes over-the-counter ibuprofen for occasional knee pain and a multivitamin supplement once daily. She has heard good things about natural products and asks you if taking a garlic supplement daily could help to bring her blood pressure and cholesterol under control. She's also very interested in St. John's wort after a friend told her that it helped alleviate her hot flashes and could also help improve mood. How should you advise her? Are there any supplements that could increase bleeding risk if taken with ibuprofen?

The medical use of plants in their natural and unprocessed form undoubtedly began when the first intelligent animals noticed that certain food plants altered body functions. The World Health Organization estimates that 80% of the world's population in developing countries currently use plants as medicines. These practices, however, are very different from the plant- and non-plant-derived dietary supplements (DS) that are available to consumers living in the USA. In 2021, sales of DS in the USA generated more than $32 billion in revenue, making the production and sale of DS extremely profitable. DS manufacturers market new formulations regularly with little regulatory oversight by the US Food and Drug Administration (FDA). This has led to much unreliable information because of unknown or poor-quality natural product formulations, poorly designed clinical studies that do not account for randomization errors or confounders, and—most importantly—a placebo effect that can contribute 30–50% of the observed response. Since the literature surrounding dietary supplements is evolving, reputable evidence-based resources should be used to evaluate claims and guide treatment decisions. An unbiased and regularly updated compendium of basic and clinical information regarding botanicals is *Natural Medicines* by Therapeutic Research Center (see *Natural medicines* in the references), which includes content review by an international, multidisciplinary, collaborative review committee of experts. The recommendations in this database are limited by the quality of the existing research and the quality of the DS used at the time of the research. As a result, all statements regarding positive benefits should be regarded as preliminary, and conclusions regarding safety should be considered tentative.

For legal purposes, DS are distinguished from prescription drugs derived from plants (eg, morphine, digitalis, atropine) by virtue of

*The US Food and Drug Administration (FDA) recognizes "herbal medication" and "botanical medication" as "dietary supplements." For the purposes of this chapter, they are identical.

being available without a prescription and, unlike over-the-counter medications, are legally considered dietary supplements or food products rather than drugs. This distinction frees the manufacturer from the need for proof of clinical efficacy and safety prior to marketing, and products are assumed to be safe when used as directed, based on the manufacturers' instructions for use and a historic precedent of safety of any ingredient unless the DS contains a "new dietary ingredient" never before marketed. For a new ingredient, the FDA requires some safety data from the manufacturer before marketing. Under current law, the FDA must prove that a DS is harmful before it can be removed from the market, or its use can be restricted. Furthermore, marketed DS are not commonly tested for dose-response relationships or toxicity, and there is a lack of adequate testing for mutagenicity, carcinogenicity, and teratogenicity. Although manufacturers are prohibited from marketing unsafe or ineffective products, the FDA has met significant challenges from the DS industry largely due to the strong lobbying effort by manufacturers and the variability in interpretation of the **Dietary Supplement Health and Education Act (DSHEA, 1994).** The DSHEA defines dietary supplements as vitamins, minerals, herbs or other botanicals, amino acids, or DS used to supplement the diet by increasing dietary intake, or concentrates, metabolites, constituents, extracts, or any combination of these ingredients. For the purposes of this chapter, plant-based substances and certain synthetic purified chemicals will be referred to as DS. Among the purified chemicals, glucosamine, coenzyme Q10, and melatonin are of significant pharmacologic interest. Ephedrine, the active principle in ma-huang, is discussed in Chapter 9.

This chapter provides some historic perspective and describes the evidence provided by randomized, double-blind, placebo-controlled trials, meta-analyses, and systematic reviews involving several of the most used agents in this class. Health care providers should adhere to the principles of "do no harm" but also, because patients are strongly influenced by popular opinion and media reports, be open to therapies that support "integrative health" safely and responsibly. Maintaining an open attitude toward patients who use DS increases the likelihood that they will feel comfortable disclosing DS use. Unproven therapies that are marketed as "alternatives" to conventional medicine should be viewed with caution, but therapies that are supported by evidence-based medicine and have been assessed for benefits and risks when used in combination with conventional medicine can be viewed favorably, especially if a patient expresses an interest in, and a determination to utilize, dual treatment approaches.

HISTORIC & REGULATORY FACTORS

Under the DSHEA, DS are regulated as foods intended to supplement the diet and maintain health. DS frequently use "Structure-Function" claims on the product label, which describes an intent to "maintain the normal structure or function" of the body. Consumers, however, may use DS in the same fashion as drugs and even use them in place of drugs or in combination with drugs.

In 1994, the US Congress, influenced by growing "consumerism" as well as strong manufacturer lobbying efforts, passed the DSHEA. The DSHEA required the establishment of Good Manufacturing Practice (GMP) standards for the supplement industry; however, it was not until 2007 that the FDA issued a final rule on the proposed GMP standards. This 13-year delay allowed supplement manufacturers to self-regulate the manufacturing process and resulted in many instances of adulteration, misbranding, and contamination. For example, a study using DNA barcoding to confirm botanical content evaluated 44 botanicals containing 30 plant species and found product substitutions in 32% of samples (Newmaster et al, 2013). Therefore, much of the criticism regarding the DS industry involves problems with botanical misidentification, a lack of product purity, and variations in potency and purification, which continue to be problematic even with GMP standards in place. When the new GMP standards are met, DS manufacturers should be in compliance with this legislation. However, the FDA has limited resources to investigate and oversee compliance with manufacturing standards, particularly since many ingredient suppliers are based overseas. Furthermore, the DS ingredient supply chain is complex, and federal regulators are not able to inspect all manufacturing facilities in a timely and efficient manner. Finally, the financial incentive to maximize sales is very great, regardless of lack of evidence of product safety or efficacy.

Because of the problems that resulted from self-regulation, another law, the Dietary Supplement and Nonprescription Drug Consumer Protection Act, was approved in 2006. This law requires manufacturers, packers, or distributors of supplements to submit reports of serious adverse events to the FDA. Serious adverse events are defined as death, a life-threatening event, hospitalization, a persistent or significant disability or incapacity, congenital anomaly or birth defect, or an adverse event that requires medical or surgical intervention to prevent such outcomes based on reasonable medical judgment. These reports identify trends in adverse effects and help to alert the public to safety issues.

CLINICAL ASPECTS OF THE USE OF BOTANICALS

Many US consumers have embraced the use of DS as a "natural" approach to their health care. Unfortunately, misconceptions regarding safety and efficacy of the agents are common, and the fact that a substance can be called "natural" does not of course guarantee its safety. In fact, botanicals may be inherently inert or toxic. If a manufacturer does not follow GMP, this can also result in intentional or unintentional plant species substitutions (eg, misidentification), adulteration with pharmaceuticals, or contamination. Therefore, GMP standards must be followed by ingredient suppliers, manufacturers, and distributors, and continuous compliance is critical to ensuring the continued safety of marketed DS.

Adverse effects have been documented for a variety of DS; however, underreporting of adverse effects is likely since consumers do not routinely report, and do not know how to report, an adverse effect if they suspect that the event was caused by consumption of a DS. Furthermore, chemical analysis is rarely performed on the products involved. This leads to confusion about whether the primary ingredient or an adulterant caused the adverse effect. In some cases, the chemical constituents of the herb can clearly lead to toxicity. Some of the herbs that should be used cautiously or not at all are listed in Table 65–1.

TABLE 65–1 Various supplements and some associated risks.

Commercial Name, Scientific Name, Plant Parts	Intended Use	Toxic Agents, Effects	Comments
Aconite *Aconitum* species	Analgesic	Alkaloid, cardiac and central nervous system effects	Avoid
Aristolochic acid *Aristolochia* species	Traditional Chinese medicine; various uses	Carcinogen, nephrotoxicity	Avoid
Black cohosh *Cimicifuga racemosa*	Menopausal symptoms	Hepatotoxicity	Avoid[1]
Borage *Borago officinalis* Tops, leaves	Anti-inflammatory; diuretic	Pyrrolizidine alkaloids, hepatotoxicity	Avoid
Chaparral *Larrea tridentata* Twigs, leaves	Anti-infective; antioxidant; anticancer	Hepatotoxicity	Avoid
Coltsfoot *Tussilago farfara* Leaves, flower	Upper respiratory tract infections	Pyrrolizidine alkaloids, hepatotoxicity	Avoid ingestion of any parts of plant; leaves may be used topically for anti-inflammatory effects for up to 4-6 weeks
Comfrey *Symphytum* species Leaves and roots	Internal digestive aid; topical for wound healing	Pyrrolizidine alkaloids, hepatotoxicity	Avoid ingestion; topical use should be limited to 4–6 weeks
Ephedra, Ma-huang *Ephedra* species	Diet aid; stimulant; bronchodilator	Central nervous system toxicity, cardiac toxicity	Avoid in patients at risk for stroke, myocardial infarction, arrhythmia, hypertension, seizures, general anxiety disorder
Germander *Teucrium chamaedrys* Leaves, tops	Diet aid	Hepatotoxicity	Avoid
Gland-derived extracts (thymus, adrenal, thyroid)	Hormone replacement	Risk of bacterial, viral, or prion transmission; variable hormone content	Avoid
Human placenta derivatives	Antirheumatic; anti-inflammatory	Risk of bacterial, viral, or prion transmission	Avoid
Jin Bu Huan	Analgesic; sedative	Hepatotoxicity	Avoid
Kava-kava	Anxiety	Hepatotoxicity	Avoid
Kratom *Mitragyna speciosa*	Energy, chronic pain, opiate withdrawal, psychoactive properties	Risk of dependence and withdrawal, respiratory depression, hallucinations, seizures, hepatotoxicity, death	Avoid
Pennyroyal Extract of *Mentha pulegium* or *Hedeoma pulegioides*	Digestive aid; induction of menstrual flow; abortifacient	Pulegone and pulegone metabolite, liver failure, renal failure	Avoid
Poke root *Phytolacca americana*	Antirheumatic	Hemorrhagic gastritis	Avoid
Royal jelly of *Apis mellifera* (honeybee)	Tonic	Bronchospasm, anaphylaxis	Avoid in patients with chronic allergies or respiratory diseases; asthma, chronic obstructive pulmonary disease, emphysema, atopy
Sassafras *Sassafras albidum* root, bark	Blood thinner	Safrole oil, hepatocarcinogen in animals	Avoid

[1]Cases of hepatotoxicity have occurred; these cases are rare given the widespread use of black cohosh.

An important risk factor in the use of DS is the lack of adequate testing for drug interactions. Since botanicals may contain hundreds of active and inactive ingredients, it is very difficult and costly to study potential drug interactions when they are combined with other medications. This may present significant risks to patients.

■ BOTANICAL SUBSTANCES

ECHINACEA (*ECHINACEA PURPUREA*)

Chemistry

The three most widely used species of *Echinacea* are *Echinacea purpurea*, *E pallida*, and *E angustifolia*. The chemical constituents include flavonoids, lipophilic constituents (eg, alkamides, polyacetylenes), water-soluble polysaccharides, and water-soluble caffeoyl conjugates (eg, echinacoside, cichoric acid, caffeic acid). Within any marketed echinacea formulation, the relative amounts of these components are dependent upon the species used, the method of manufacture, and the plant parts used. *E purpurea*, the purple coneflower, has been the most widely studied in clinical trials. Although the active constituents of echinacea are not completely known, cichoric acid from *E purpurea* and echinacoside from *E pallida* and *E angustifolia,* as well as alkamides and polysaccharides, are most often noted as having immune-modulating properties. Most commercial formulations, however, are not standardized for any particular constituent.

Pharmacologic Effects

1. *Immune modulation*—The effect of echinacea on the immune system is controversial. In vivo human studies using commercially marketed formulations of *E purpurea* have claimed increased macrophage activation, phagocytosis, total circulating monocytes, neutrophils, and natural killer cells, effects indicative of general immune modulation. In vitro, Echinaforce, a standardized ethanol extract of the aerial (above-ground) parts of *E purpurea,* inhibited the rise in pro-inflammatory cytokines and interleukins 6 and 8 (IL-6 and IL-8), and also inhibited mucin secretion caused by exposure to rhinovirus type 1A in a 3D tissue model of human airway epithelium. This type of model is intended to mimic what would be seen in vivo. The extract had no effect on cytokine actions.

2. *Anti-inflammatory effects*—Certain echinacea constituents have demonstrated anti-inflammatory properties in vitro. Inhibition of cyclooxygenase, 5-lipoxygenase, and hyaluronidase may be involved. In vitro, the alkamide dodeca-2E,4E-dienoic acid isobutylamide decreased calcium influx and mast cell degranulation, resulting in a 47% reduction in mast cell histamine release. *E purpurea* root extract with a high alkamide content showed similar activity, while the same extract with little to no alkamide content showed no effect. Alkamides from *E purpurea* significantly reduce the production of pro-inflammatory cytokines (IL-6 and IL-8) in keratinocytes in vitro. In animals, application of *E purpurea* prior to application of a topical irritant reduced both paw and ear edema. A preliminary trial of topical *E purpurea* extract cream (WO3260) compared to an emollient, Imlan Creme Pur, in 60 persons with eczema, showed favorable results over 3 months with greater absolute reduction in symptoms at 85 days. Both treatments showed benefits at 4 and 8 weeks.

3. *Antibacterial, antifungal, antiviral, and antioxidant effects*—In vitro studies have reported some antibacterial, antifungal, antiviral, and antioxidant activity with echinacea constituents. For example, Echinaforce demonstrated virucidal activity against influenza A and B, parainfluenza virus, and herpes simplex virus in vitro and bactericidal activity against *Streptococcus pyogenes*, *Haemophilus influenzae*, and *Legionella pneumophila* in human bronchial cells. In vitro, Echinaforce inactivated both avian influenza virus (H5N1, H7N7) and swine-origin influenza virus (H1N1) at doses consistent with recommended oral consumption. The extract blocked key steps (ie, viral hemagglutination activity and neuraminidase activity in vitro) involved in early virus replication and cellular entry. It was less effective against intracellular virus. Newer in vitro research demonstrates that Echinaforce has dose-dependent virucidal activity against common cold human coronavirus (HCoV) 229E. Using a re-constituted three-dimensional nasal epithelium model, 50 mcg/mL of Echinaforce protected five of eight respiratory epithelial cultures from infection by HCoV 229E. Virucidal activity against severe acute respiratory syndrome (SARS)-CoV-1 and (SARS)-CoV-2 was similarly observed with 50 mcg/mL of Echinaforce. The mechanism involved the extracellular phase, prior to viral entry into the cell, not the intracellular phase. In vitro, bactericidal activity and inhibition of secretion of inflammatory cytokines produced by *Propionibacterium acnes* in human skin fibroblasts has also been observed with Echinaforce.

Clinical Trials

Echinacea is most often used to enhance immune function in individuals who have colds and other respiratory tract infections and is available in fresh, freeze-dried, and alcoholic extracts. Recent reviews have assessed the efficacy of echinacea for this primary indication. A review by the Cochrane Collaboration involved 24 randomized, double-blind trials with 33 comparisons of echinacea mono-preparations (single-ingredient echinacea preparations) and placebo. Trials were included if they involved echinacea for cold treatment or prevention, where the primary efficacy outcome was cold incidence in prevention trials and duration of symptoms in treatment trials. Overall, the review did not find significant evidence of benefit for echinacea (among all species) in treating colds. Preparations made from the aerial parts of *E purpurea* plants and prepared as alcoholic extracts or pressed juices were discussed as possibly being preferred to other formulations for cold treatment in adults, but still having a weak overall treatment effect. In prevention trials, pooling results suggested a small relative risk reduction of 10–20%, but no statistically significant benefit within individual trials.

A meta-analysis involving 14 randomized, placebo-controlled trials of echinacea for cold treatment or prevention found that echinacea decreased the risk of developing clear signs and symptoms of a cold by 58% and decreased symptom duration by 1.25 days. This review, however, was confounded by the inclusion of four clinical trials involving multi-ingredient echinacea preparations, as well as three studies using rhinovirus inoculation versus natural cold development.

The most recently published systematic review and meta-analysis used methodology similar to that of the Cochrane review and included randomized, double-blind, placebo-controlled trials using an echinacea preparation assessing prevention (9 trials), duration (7 trials), and safety (16 trials) in upper respiratory tract infection. An overall benefit for cold prevention was observed, with a relative risk ratio of 0.78 (95% confidence interval [CI], 0.68–0.88). Short-term safety also was observed, but there was no reduction of cold duration.

A supportive role in cold prevention was also recently observed in a randomized, blinded, controlled clinical trial in 200 healthy pediatric children ages 4–12 years. Echinaforce junior tablets 1200 mg/day was superior to 150 mg/day of vitamin C over 4 months and showed a significant reduction in cold development (odds ratio [OR], 0.52; 95% CI, 0.30–0.91; $p = 0.021$), cold complications (otitis media, sinusitis, or pneumonia), and need for and duration of antibiotic use.

Echinacea has been studied for enhancement of hematologic recovery following chemotherapy. It has also been used as an adjunct in the treatment of urinary tract and vaginal fungal infections and post-treatment relapse of genital condylomatosis from HPV infection. These indications require further research before they can be accepted in clinical practice. *E purpurea* is ineffective in treating recurrent genital herpes.

Adverse Effects

Adverse effects reported with oral commercial formulations are minimal and most often include unpleasant taste, gastrointestinal upset, or allergic reactions (eg, rash). Short-term use (eg, 10–14 days) is likely safe. In one large clinical trial, pediatric patients using an oral echinacea product were significantly more likely to develop a rash than those taking placebo. In a small Norwegian mother and child cohort study, 0.5% of women reported taking any formulation of echinacea during early-stage (conception up to pregnancy week 17) or late-stage pregnancy and had no adverse pregnancy outcomes compared to pregnant women who did not use echinacea. Herbal supplements, and particularly those made from alcoholic extracts, should only be used in pregnancy and lactation after consultation with the health care provider.

Drug Interactions & Precautions

Until the role of echinacea in immune modulation is better defined, this agent should be avoided in patients with immune deficiency disorders (eg, AIDS, cancer) or autoimmune disorders (eg, multiple sclerosis, rheumatoid arthritis). Although there are no well-documented herb-drug interactions for echinacea, in theory, it should also be avoided in persons taking immunosuppressant medications (eg, organ transplant recipients). In one study, coadministration of an echinacea product containing *E purpurea* and *E angustifolia* root had no effect on warfarin pharmacodynamics, platelet aggregation, or baseline clotting in healthy subjects. Human studies have shown no effect of varied *E purpurea* preparations on the pharmacokinetics of lopinavir, ritonavir, etravirine, and darunavir.

Dosage

It is recommended that patients follow the dosing on the package label, as there may be variations in dose based on the procedure used in product manufacture. Standardized preparations made from the aerial parts of *E purpurea* (Echinaforce, Echinagard) as an alcoholic extract or fresh-pressed juice may be preferred in adults for common cold treatment if taken within the first 24 hours of cold symptoms. It should not be used on a continuous basis for cold treatment longer than 10–14 days. Preventative use for 4 months has also been studied.

GARLIC (*ALLIUM SATIVUM*)

Chemistry

The pharmacologic activity of garlic involves a variety of organosulfur compounds. Dried and powdered formulations contain many of the compounds found in raw garlic and will usually be standardized to **allicin** or **alliin** content. Allicin is responsible for the characteristic odor of garlic, and alliin is its chemical precursor. Dried powdered formulations are often enteric-coated to protect the enzyme alliinase (the enzyme that converts alliin to allicin) from degradation by stomach acid. Aged garlic extract (AGE) has been studied in clinical trials but to a lesser degree than dried, powdered garlic (GP). AGE contains no alliin or allicin and is odor-free. Its primary constituents are water-soluble organosulfur compounds, and packages may carry standardization to the compound *S*-allylcysteine.

Pharmacologic Effects

1. *Cardiovascular and metabolic effects*—In vitro, allicin and related compounds inhibit HMG-CoA reductase, which is involved in cholesterol biosynthesis (see Chapter 35), and exhibit antioxidant properties. Several clinical trials have investigated the lipid-lowering potential of garlic. A general review of health outcomes assessed 6 meta-analyses for metabolic outcomes with garlic consumption (Wan et al, 2019). The median dose and duration of garlic or garlic-related supplements were 900 mg/d and 12 weeks, respectively. Patients with dyslipidemia and healthy participants showed a weighted mean difference (WMD) in total cholesterol of −15.25 mg/dL, LDL WMD −6.41 mg/dL, and HDL WMD +1.49 mg/dL. Triglycerides were not significantly affected. Persons with baseline dyslipidemia showed greater benefits in all lipid parameters compared to the WMD, while those with total cholesterol ≤200 mg/dL had no significant change in serum total cholesterol. Therapy duration beyond 8 weeks was important for effect in dyslipidemia. Diabetic but not healthy patients showed a lowering of fasting blood glucose (WMD −10.90 mg/dL) and HbA_{1c} (WMD −0.60 mg/dL). While the benefit of garlic in lowering total cholesterol and LDL cholesterol appears to be clinically relevant, optimal prescription drug therapy is far more efficacious (see Chapter 35).

Clinical trials report antiplatelet effects (possibly through inhibition of thromboxane synthesis or stimulation of nitric oxide synthesis) following garlic ingestion. A majority of human studies also suggest enhancement of fibrinolytic activity. These effects in combination with antioxidant effects (eg, increased resistance to LDL oxidation) and reductions in total cholesterol might be beneficial in patients with atherosclerosis. A randomized, controlled trial among persons with advanced coronary artery disease who consumed GP for 4 years showed significant reductions in secondary markers (plaque accumulation in the carotid and femoral arteries) as compared with patients on placebo, but primary endpoints (death, stroke, myocardial infarction) were not assessed. AGE preparations have similarly shown favorable effects in small (≤104 patients) randomized, double-blind, placebo-controlled trials in reducing coronary artery calcification (CAC) progression over 1 year, inclusive of patients on co-medication with a statin therapy. IL-6 was also significantly reduced in the largest trial at 1 year. All trials involved patients with known coronary artery disease (CAD) or who were considered medium to high risk for CAD at baseline. A reduction in low-attenuated plaque has also been reported with aged garlic extract 2400 mg/day compared to placebo in a prospective, randomized, double-blind study in patients with metabolic syndrome.

Garlic constituents may affect blood vessel elasticity and blood pressure. Several mechanisms have been proposed (eg, stimulation of nitric oxide synthase, inhibition of angiotensin 1 converting enzyme, increased production of hydrogen sulfide). Twenty placebo-controlled studies using single-ingredient preparations of GP (13 studies), AGE (5 studies), or other preparations (2 studies) were included in the most recent meta-analysis (Ried, 2016). Significant reductions in systolic blood pressure (SBP) and diastolic blood pressure (DBP) were present when all trials were considered. Benefits were most pronounced in subjects with baseline hypertension (mean SBP reduction of 8.6 ± 2.2 mm Hg and DBP reduction of 6.1 ± 1.3 mm Hg), and no significant effect was observed in subjects who had normal or prehypertensive blood pressures (<140/90 mm Hg) at baseline. A Cochrane review on the effect of garlic monotherapy for prevention of cardiovascular morbidity and mortality in hypertensive patients also identified a significant reduction in systolic and diastolic pressure compared with placebo. A separate Cochrane review of the effect of garlic on peripheral artery occlusive disease found insufficient support for this indication.

2. *Antimicrobial effects*—The antimicrobial effect of garlic has not been extensively studied in vivo. Allicin has been reported to have in vitro activity against some gram-positive and gram-negative bacteria as well as fungi (*Candida albicans*), protozoa (*Entamoeba histolytica*), and certain viruses. The primary mechanism involves the inhibition of thiol-containing enzymes needed by these microbes. A Cochrane review studying the effect of garlic on cold prevention and treatment found a significant reduction in total number of colds using a garlic supplement (with 180 mg allicin content) once daily for 12 weeks. Limited conclusions can be drawn regarding the effects observed, because only one trial met inclusion criteria. Given the availability of safe and effective prescription antimicrobials, the usefulness of garlic in this area appears limited.

3. *Antineoplastic effects*—In rodent studies, garlic inhibits procarcinogens for colon, esophageal, lung, breast, and stomach cancer, possibly by detoxification of carcinogens and reduced carcinogen activation. An umbrella review of meta-analyses for multiple health outcomes (Wan et al, 2019) assessed cancer and tumor outcomes in populations with specific allium vegetable intake. These studies were primarily epidemiologic cohort and case-control studies. Narrowing the analysis from varied allium vegetables to only those for garlic or garlic powder consumption showed a reduced odds ratio of gastric cancer of 0.51 (95% CI, 0.44–0.57) and of prostate cancer of 0.77 (95% CI, 0.64–0.91). Current anticancer studies are focused on specific organosulfur garlic compounds in in vivo animal models of cancer and in vitro effects on human cancer cell lines.

Adverse Effects

Following oral ingestion, adverse effects of garlic products may include gastrointestinal complaints such as stomach upset, nausea, bloating, flatulence (6%), hypotension (1.3%), allergy (1.1%), and bleeding (rare). Breath and body odor have been reported with an incidence of 20–40% at recommended doses using enteric-coated powdered garlic formulations. Contact dermatitis may occur with the handling of raw garlic.

Drug Interactions & Precautions

Because of reported antiplatelet effects, patients using anticlotting medications (eg, warfarin, newer oral anticoagulants, aspirin, ibuprofen) should use garlic cautiously. Additional monitoring of blood pressure and signs and symptoms of bleeding is warranted. Garlic may reduce the bioavailability of saquinavir, an antiviral protease inhibitor, but it does not appear to affect the bioavailability of ritonavir.

Dosage

Dried, powdered garlic products should be standardized to contain 1.3% alliin (the allicin precursor) or have an allicin-generating potential of 0.6%. Enteric-coated formulations are recommended to minimize degradation of the active substances. A daily dose of 600–900 mg/d of powdered garlic is most common. This is equivalent to one clove of raw garlic (2–4 g) per day. A garlic bulb can contain up to 1.8% alliin. Doses of AGE most often range from 600 to 1800 mg/d, but doses up to 7200 mg daily have been safely used in clinical trials for up to 6 months.

GINKGO (*GINKGO BILOBA*)

Chemistry

Ginkgo biloba extract is prepared from the leaves of the ginkgo tree. The most common formulation is prepared by concentrating 50 parts of the crude leaf to prepare one part of extract. The active constituents in ginkgo are flavone glycosides, terpenoids (including ginkgolides A, B, C, J, K, L, M, N, P, and Q), and bilobalide.

Pharmacologic Effects

1. *Cardiovascular effects*—In animal models and some human studies, ginkgo has been shown to increase blood flow, reduce blood viscosity, and promote vasodilation, thus enhancing tissue perfusion. Enhancement of endogenous nitric oxide effects (see Chapter 19) and antagonism of platelet-activating factor have been observed in animal models. In vitro, four biflavones (ginkgetin, isoginkgetin, bilobetin, and amentoflavone) and five flavonoids (luteolin, apigenin, quercetin, kaempferol, and isorhamnetin) were found to inhibit human thrombin at IC_{50} values of 8.05–82.08 μM.

Ginkgo biloba has been studied for its effects on mild to moderate occlusive peripheral arterial disease. Among 11 randomized, placebo-controlled studies involving 477 participants using standardized ginkgo leaf extract (EGb761) for up to 6 months, a nonsignificant trend toward improvements in pain-free walking distance (increase of 64.5 meters) was observed ($P = .06$). The authors concluded that the standardized extract lacked benefit for this indication.

The Ginkgo Evaluation of Memory (GEM) study and the GuidAge study evaluated cardiovascular outcomes as well as incidence and mean time to Alzheimer dementia associated with the long-term use of ginkgo for 5–6 years in approximately 3000 elderly (age ≥70) adults with normal cognition or mild cognitive impairment. Daily use of 240 mg/d EGb761 did not affect the incidence of hypertension or reduce blood pressure among persons with hypertension or prehypertension. No significant effects in cardiovascular disease mortality, ischemic stroke or events, or hemorrhagic stroke were observed.

2. *Metabolic effects*—Antioxidant and radical-scavenging properties have been observed for the flavonoid fraction of ginkgo as well as some of the terpene constituents. In vitro, ginkgo has been reported to have superoxide dismutase-like activity and superoxide anion- and hydroxyl radical-scavenging properties. The flavonoid fraction has also been observed to have antiapoptotic properties. In some studies, it has also demonstrated a protective effect in limiting free radical formation in animal models of ischemic injury and in reducing markers of oxidative stress in patients undergoing coronary artery bypass surgery.

3. *Central nervous system effects*—In animal models of aging, chronic administration of ginkgo for 3–4 weeks led to modifications in several central nervous system receptors and neurotransmitters. Receptor densities increased for muscarinic, α_2, and 5-HT_{1a} receptors, and decreased for β adrenoceptors. Increased serum levels of acetylcholine and norepinephrine and enhanced synaptosomal reuptake of serotonin and dopamine also have been reported. Additional possible effects include inhibition of amyloid-beta fibril formation and protective effects of Egb761 on hippocampal neurons against cell death induced by beta-amyloid.

Ginkgo has been used to treat cerebral insufficiency and dementia of the Alzheimer type. The term *cerebral insufficiency*, however, includes a variety of manifestations ranging from poor concentration and confusion to anxiety and depression as well as physical complaints such as hearing loss and headache. For this reason, studies evaluating cerebral insufficiency tend to be more inclusive and difficult to assess than trials evaluating dementia. A meta-analysis of ginkgo for cognitive impairment or dementia was performed by the Cochrane Collaboration. They reviewed 36 randomized, double-blind, placebo-controlled trials ranging in length from 3 to 52 weeks. Significant improvements in cognition and activities of daily living were observed at 12 but not 24 weeks. In contrast, improvements in clinical global assessment, were observed at 24 but not 12 weeks. The authors concluded that the effects of ginkgo in the treatment of mild cognitive impairment and dementia were unpredictable and unlikely to be clinically relevant. However, recent meta-analyses of randomized controlled trials using EGb761, 22–26 weeks in duration, that limited inclusion criteria to patients with Alzheimer dementia (eight studies), vascular or mixed dementia type (six studies), or dementia with neuropsychiatric features (four studies) showed favorable results. Significant improvements in cognition and activities of daily living were observed for ginkgo compared to placebo. Clinical global assessment of improvement also was significantly improved when EGb761 doses of 240 mg/d were used, but not doses of 120 mg/d. Because of the stricter inclusion criteria used when determining a benefit in patients with dementia, the overall methodologic quality of these studies was higher than those in the Cochrane review. This suggests that benefit is more likely to be detected in patients with a diagnosis of dementia than in patients with more mild cognitive impairment. A consensus statement (Kandiah et al, 2019) also concluded that EGb761 can be used as a single agent, where deemed appropriate, in certain patients with AD or vascular dementia and can be used as an add-on to conventional dementia therapies (acetylcholinesterase inhibitors, memantine) but should not be used for prevention of dementia. In the GEM and GuidAge studies that included persons with normal or mild cognitive impairment, the effects of ginkgo as a prophylactic agent to prevent progression to dementia were assessed. No benefit was observed with 5–6 years of ginkgo treatment.

4. *Miscellaneous effects*—Ginkgo has been studied for its effects in schizophrenia, generalized anxiety disorder, tardive dyskinesia, allergic and asthmatic bronchoconstriction, short-term memory in healthy adults, acute ischemic stroke, type 2 diabetes mellitus, erectile dysfunction, tinnitus and hearing loss, and macular degeneration. Preliminary data from eight randomized, double-blind, placebo-controlled trials involving 1033 patients suggest that EGb761 can significantly reduce total and negative symptoms of chronic schizophrenia when used in combination with standard treatment (eg, clozapine, haloperidol, olanzapine). These trials were conducted in China, so firm conclusions about benefit in a broader population are lacking. There is insufficient evidence to warrant clinical use for the other conditions listed.

Adverse Effects

Adverse effects of ginkgo have been reported with a frequency comparable to that of placebo. These include nausea, headache, stomach upset, diarrhea, allergy, anxiety, and insomnia. A few case reports noted bleeding complications in patients using ginkgo. Some of these patients were also using either aspirin or warfarin, so monitoring for bleeding in persons taking ginkgo is advisable.

Drug Interactions & Precautions

Ginkgo may have antiplatelet properties and should not be used in combination with antiplatelet or anticoagulant medications. Other single case reports have noted mood dysregulation after ginkgo use in a patient with schizophrenia, virologic failure when ginkgo was combined with efavirenz, sedation when combined with trazodone, priapism when combined with risperidone, and seizures when combined with valproic acid and phenytoin; all warrant further pharmacokinetic studies before firm conclusions can be drawn. Seizures have been reported as a toxic effect of ginkgo, most likely related to seed contamination in the leaf formulations. Uncooked ginkgo seeds are epileptogenic due to the presence of ginkgotoxin. Ginkgo formulations should be avoided in individuals with preexisting seizure disorders.

Dosage

Ginkgo biloba dried leaf extract is usually standardized to contain 24% flavone glycosides and 6% terpene lactones. The daily dose most commonly studied and associated with a benefit in clinical trials of dementia is 240 mg daily of the dried extract in two divided doses.

GINSENG

Chemistry

Ginseng may be derived from any of several species of the genus *Panax.* Of these, crude preparations or extracts of *Panax ginseng,* the Chinese or Korean variety, and *P quinquefolium*, the American variety, are most often available to consumers in the United States. The active principles appear to be the triterpenoid saponin glycosides called ginsenosides or panaxosides, of which there are approximately 30 different types. It is recommended that commercial *P ginseng* formulations be standardized to contain 4–10% ginsenosides. *P ginseng* is metabolized by intestinal flora through phase I reactions, and the deglycosylation of several ginsenosides results in the formation of 20-O-β-D-glu-copyranosyl-20(S)-PPD (compound K), which is considered a primary metabolite with pharmacologic effects. In human pharmacokinetic studies, compound K is observed in blood 4 hours after administering *P ginseng* powder and reaches peak concentrations 9–14 hours later. Plasma concentrations of compound K do show human subject variability due to different gut microbiomes.

Other plant materials are commonly sold under the name ginseng but are not from *Panax* species. These include Siberian ginseng (*Eleutherococcus senticosus*) and Brazilian ginseng (*Pfaffia paniculata*). Of these, Siberian ginseng may be more widely available in the USA. Siberian ginseng contains eleutherosides but no ginsenosides. Currently, there is no recommended standardization for eleutheroside content in Siberian ginseng products.

Pharmacologic Effects

An extensive literature exists on the potential pharmacologic effects of ginsenosides. Unfortunately, the studies differ widely in the species of *Panax* used, the ginsenosides studied, the degree of purification applied to the extracts, the animal species studied, the doses or concentrations involved, and the measurements used to evaluate the responses. Reported beneficial pharmacologic effects include modulation of immune function (induced mRNA expression for IL-2 and IL-10, interferon γ, and granulocyte-macrophage colony-stimulating factor; activated B and T cells, natural killer cells, and macrophages). Central nervous system effects included reduced activity of acetylcholinesterase, reduced levels of amyloid B protein, increased proliferating ability of neural progenitors, and increased central levels of acetylcholine, serotonin, norepinephrine, and dopamine in the cerebral cortex. Miscellaneous effects included antioxidant activity; anti-inflammatory effects (inhibited tumor necrosis factor α, IL-1β, and vascular and intracellular cell adhesion molecules); antistress activity (ie, stimulated pituitary-adrenocortical system, agonist at glucocorticoid receptor); analgesia (inhibited substance P); vasoregulatory effects (increased endothelial nitric oxide production, inhibited prostacyclin production); cardioprotective activity (reduced ventricular remodeling and cardiomyocyte apoptosis in animal models of myocardial ischemia); antiplatelet activity; improved glucose homeostasis (reduced cell death in pancreatic beta cells; increased insulin release, number of insulin receptors, and insulin sensitivity); and anticancer properties (inhibition of angiogenesis, stimulation of apoptotic cell death). Such extensive claims naturally require careful replication.

Clinical Trials

Ginseng is most often claimed to help improve physical and mental performance or to function as an "adaptogen," an agent that helps the body to return to normal when exposed to stressful or noxious stimuli. Some randomized controlled trials evaluating "quality of life" and "cognition" have claimed significant benefits in some subscale measures of behavior, cognitive function, or quality of life but rarely in overall composite scores using *P ginseng*. Better results have been observed with *P quinquefolium* and *P ginseng* in lowering glucose indices. This was the subject of a meta-analysis in which 20 randomized controlled studies involving 1295 participants (675 cases and 620 controls) in individuals with pre-diabetes and type 2 diabetes mellitus were evaluated. Fasting plasma glucose (FPG) was significantly reduced with ginseng use compared to placebo (WMD, –7.03 mg/dL; 95% CI, –10.89 to –3.17; p <0.0001). No significant benefit was seen for HgA1c and oral glucose tolerance test between groups. Subgroup analysis showed that benefits were only reduced in subjects with an FPG ≥126 mg/dL. Some randomized, placebo-controlled trials have reported immunomodulating benefits of *P quinquefolium* and *P ginseng* in preventing upper respiratory tract infections. Use of ginseng for 2–4 months in healthy seniors may reduce the risk of acquiring the common cold as well as the duration of symptoms. Because of heterogeneity in these trials, however, the findings are insufficient to warrant a recommendation of ginseng for cold prevention. To assess effects on cardiovascular health, a systematic review and meta-analysis of 17 randomized controlled trials involving predominantly *P ginseng* (12 studies) and *P quinquefolium* (5 studies) species in persons with and without hypertension was performed. Over a mean period of 9 weeks, no significant effect of ginseng was observed on SBP, DBP, and mean arterial pressure compared with controls. A separate systematic review and meta-analysis was conducted to assess the effect of *P ginseng* supplementation on blood lipid profile. Patient populations primarily had metabolic syndrome (10 of 18 randomized, controlled studies), and subgroup analysis of this population noted improved blood total cholesterol (mean difference –2.30 mg/dL [95% CI, –3.79 to –0.80] and LDL cholesterol profile –1.47 mg/dL [95% CI, –1.90 to –1.05]) compared to placebo with no effect on HDL cholesterol or triglycerides at a median dose of 3 g/daily for 8 weeks duration. This is unlikely to offer a clinically meaningful benefit compared to prescription drug antihyperlipidemics. Finally, two case-control studies and a cohort study suggest a non-organ-specific cancer-preventive effect with long-term administration of *P ginseng*. Significant benefits in some cancer-related fatigue (CRF) symptoms have been observed in both a dose-finding study and a multisite, double-blind, randomized trial using *P quinquefolium*, 2 g daily, versus placebo over a 2-month period. *P ginseng* 2 g daily also significantly improved CRF over 4 months in a phase 3 randomized trial in colorectal cancer patients. Trials involving both *P ginseng* and *P quinquefolium* at doses of 1 g daily or less have shown minimal to no benefit in reducing CRF. Studies in China have reported on a highly concentrated ginsenoside Rg3 capsule formulation (95% Rg3) that is not available in the USA. When Rg3 capsules (20 mg; Shenyi, China) were administered twice daily for 30 days and in combination with gemcitabine and cisplatin in 60 patients with advanced esophageal cancer, significant improvements were observed in 1-year survival and quality of life compared to controls receiving chemotherapy alone. Similar benefits were observed in randomized controlled studies for patients with either stage III or IV non-small cell lung cancer using Rg3 capsules, 20 mg twice daily, for 6–24 weeks with chemotherapy, compared to chemotherapy alone. A meta-analysis of 20 of these trials showed that Rg3 significantly improved response rates, overall survival, and quality of life when combined with chemotherapy (671 subjects) compared to chemotherapy alone (644 subjects).

In summary, the strongest support for use of *P ginseng* or *P quinquefolium* currently relates to its effects in cold prevention, lowering postprandial glucose, nonspecific cancer prevention, and alleviating CRF. Studies using 95% Rg3 capsules (available in China) also show benefits when used in combination with chemotherapy in certain types of cancers.

Adverse Effects

Vaginal bleeding, mastalgia, and gynecomastia in an adolescent male have been described in a case report, suggesting possible estrogenic effects. Central nervous system stimulation (eg, insomnia, nervousness, mania) and hypertension have been noted in case reports involving *P ginseng*. Methylxanthines found in the ginseng plant may contribute to this effect.

Drug Interactions & Precautions

Irritability, sleeplessness, and manic behavior have been reported in psychiatric patients using ginseng in combination with other medications (phenelzine, lithium, neuroleptics). Ginseng should be used cautiously in patients taking any psychiatric, estrogenic, or hypoglycemic medications. Ginseng has antiplatelet properties and should not be used in combination with antiplatelet or anticoagulant medications or used in large amounts peri- or post-operatively. *P quinquefolium* was reported to reduce the anticoagulant effect of warfarin but a similar herb-drug interaction was not reported for *P ginseng*, Cytokine stimulation has been claimed for both *P ginseng* and *P quinquefolium* in vitro and in animal models. In a randomized, double-blind, placebo-controlled study, *P ginseng* significantly increased natural killer cell activity versus placebo with 8 and 12 weeks of use. Immunocompromised individuals, those taking immune stimulants, and those with autoimmune disorders should use ginseng products with caution. In a pharmacokinetic study in healthy men, single- and multiple-dose *P ginseng* administered for 15 days with single doses of caffeine, losartan, omeprazole, dextromethorphan, midazolam, or pitavastatin revealed no clinically relevant drug interactions and good tolerability.

Dosage

A dose of 1–2 g/d of the crude *P ginseng* root or its equivalent is considered standard dosage. Two hundred milligrams of standardized *P ginseng* extract are equivalent to 1 g of the crude root. The trademarked preparation Ginsana has been used as a standardized extract in some clinical trials and is available in the USA. Raw *P ginseng* root may also be cultivated and sold as fresh ginseng, peeled and air-dried "white ginseng," steam-treated and air-dried "red ginseng," or steam-treated nine times "black ginseng."

MILK THISTLE (*SILYBUM MARIANUM*)

Chemistry

The fruit and seeds of the milk thistle plant contain a lipophilic mixture of flavonolignans known as silymarin. Silymarin constitutes 2–3% of the dried herb and is composed of three primary isomers: silybin (also known as silybinin or silibinin), silychristin (silichristin), and silydianin (silidianin). Silybin is the most prevalent and potent of the three isomers and accounts for 50–70%

of the silymarin complex. Oral bioavailability of silybin is poor, and this has resulted in development of newer formulations such as highly bioavailable oral silybin nanoparticles (SB-NP), which have not yet been well studied in humans. In rodents, SB-NP show higher serum levels than unmodified silybin. In vitro, SB-NP reduced HCV infection rates in human hepatocytes. Silybin-phosphatidylcholine formulations have also been shown to improve bioavailability compared to non-complexed silybin in humans. Silybin undergoes enterohepatic circulation and biliary excretion. Milk thistle products should be standardized to contain 70–80% silymarin. When evaluating clinical trials it is important to distinguish formulations that have used oral milk thistle and those that have used intravenous silybin, considering silybin's poor oral bioavailability.

Pharmacologic Effects

1. *Liver disease*—In animal models, milk thistle purportedly limits hepatic injury associated with a variety of toxins and drugs, including *Amanita* mushrooms, galactosamine, carbon tetrachloride, acetaminophen, antituberculosis drugs, radiation, cold ischemia, and ethanol. In vitro studies and some in vivo studies indicate that silymarin reduces lipid peroxidation, scavenges free radicals, and enhances glutathione and superoxide dismutase levels. This may contribute to membrane stabilization and reduce toxin entry.

Milk thistle appears to have anti-inflammatory properties. In vitro, silybin strongly and noncompetitively inhibits lipoxygenase activity and reduces leukotriene formation. Inhibition of leukocyte migration has been observed in vivo and may be a factor when acute inflammation is present. Silymarin inhibits nuclear factor kappa B (NF-κB), an inflammatory response mediator. NF-κB is known to be activated in liver conditions such as alcoholic and non-alcoholic fatty liver disease, viral hepatitis, and biliary liver disease. One of the most unusual mechanisms claimed for milk thistle involves an increase in RNA polymerase I activity in nonmalignant hepatocytes but not in hepatoma or other malignant cell lines. By increasing this enzyme's activity, enhanced protein synthesis and cellular regeneration might occur in healthy but not malignant cells. In an animal model of cirrhosis, oral silymarin reduced collagen accumulation, and in an in vitro model using human hepatic stellate cells, it reduced expression of the fibrogenic cytokine transforming growth factor β. If confirmed, milk thistle may have a role in the treatment of hepatic fibrosis.

In animal models, silymarin has a dose-dependent stimulatory effect on bile flow that could be beneficial in cases of cholestasis. To date, however, there is insufficient evidence to warrant the use of milk thistle for these indications.

2. *Chemotherapeutic effects*—Preliminary in vitro and animal studies of the effects of silymarin and silybinin have been carried out with several cancer cell lines. In murine models of skin cancer, silybinin and silymarin were said to reduce tumor initiation and promotion. Induction of apoptosis has also been reported using silymarin in a variety of malignant human cell lines (eg, melanoma, prostate, colon, leukemia cells, bladder transitional-cell papilloma cells, cervical and hepatoma cells). Inhibition of cell growth and proliferation by inducing a G_1 cell cycle arrest has also been claimed in cultured human breast and prostate cancer cell lines. The use of milk thistle in the clinical treatment of cancer has not yet been adequately studied, but preliminary trials in patients undergoing chemotherapy show that it may improve liver function (ie, reduced liver transaminase concentrations in blood). There are insufficient data to support use in patients with cancer. The antioxidant potential of milk thistle should be taken into consideration prior to administration with chemotherapeutic agents that may be affected by antioxidant compounds.

3. *Lactation*—Historically, milk thistle has been used by herbalists and midwives to induce lactation in pregnant or postpartum women. In female rats, milk thistle increases prolactin production. As such, it is possible that it could have an effect on human breast milk production. Clinical trial data are lacking, however, for this indication, as are safety data on nursing mothers and infants. Until further data become available, milk thistle should not be used for this indication.

Clinical Trials

Oral milk thistle has been used to treat acute and chronic viral hepatitis, alcoholic liver disease, and toxin- and drug-induced liver injury in human patients. A systematic review of 13 randomized trials involving 915 patients with alcoholic liver disease or hepatitis B or C found no significant reductions in all-cause mortality, liver histopathology, or complications of liver disease with 6 months of use. A significant reduction in liver-related mortality was claimed using the data from all the surveyed trials, but not when the data were limited to trials of better design and controls. It was concluded that the effects of oral milk thistle in improving liver function or mortality from liver disease are currently poorly substantiated. A multicenter, double-blind, placebo-controlled clinical trial in patients with hepatitis C refractory to interferon treatment failed to show a benefit with 24 weeks of milk thistle, 420 mg/d and 700 mg/d, on reduction of serum alanine aminotransferase levels. Milk thistle also had no effect on mean serum hepatitis C virus (HCV) RNA levels at 24 weeks. In contrast, the intravenous use of silybinin succinate has shown some benefit in reducing HCV RNA levels and alanine aminotransferase levels in patients with treatment-resistant hepatitis C infection. Prospective pilot studies have also shown benefits with intravenous silybinin before and after liver transplantation treatment in patients with HCV cirrhosis. Potent antiviral activity was demonstrated with significant reductions in HCV-RNA levels during treatment compared to placebo or nontreated controls when given for at least 14 days before transplantation and 7 days after liver transplantation. HCV-RNA relapsed, however, after silybinin withdrawal. This suggests that formulation and poor oral bioavailability may influence treatment outcomes. Lastly, milk thistle was studied in non-alcoholic steatohepatitis (NASH) without cirrhosis in doses of 480 mg and 700 mg over 48 weeks in 5 medical centers in the USA. This exploratory, randomized, double-blind, placebo-controlled study evaluated the effect of oral standardized silymarin. The study proved inconclusive, however, due to low completion rates in all groups and a substantial number of participants not meeting histologic entry criteria. Another randomized, double-blind, controlled trial using higher doses of oral standardized silymarin, 2100 mg/d for 1 year, in adults with biopsy-proven NASH, did not reduce histologic scores by 30% or more, but did reduce markers of liver fibrosis and stiffness. This may suggest that higher dosing is needed due to low bioavailability of silybinin.

Although milk thistle has not been confirmed as an antidote following acute exposure to liver toxins in humans, intravenous silybinin is marketed and used in Europe as an antidote (Legalon SIL) in *Amanita phalloides* mushroom poisoning. This use is based on favorable outcomes reported in case-control studies.

Adverse Effects

Milk thistle has rarely been reported to cause adverse effects when used at recommended doses. In clinical trials, the incidence of adverse effects (eg, gastrointestinal upset, dermatologic, headaches) was comparable to that of placebo. At high doses (>1500 mg), it can have a laxative effect caused by stimulation of bile flow and secretion.

Drug Interactions, Precautions, & Dosage

Milk thistle does not significantly alter the pharmacokinetics of other drugs transported by the P-glycoprotein transporter or metabolized by cytochrome enzymes. In a recent review, the impact of the herb was listed as "posing no risk for drug interactions in humans." Recommended oral dosage is 280–420 mg/d, calculated as silybinin, in three divided doses.

ST. JOHN'S WORT (*HYPERICUM PERFORATUM*)

Chemistry

St. John's wort, also known as hypericum, contains a variety of constituents that might contribute to its claimed pharmacologic activity in the treatment of depression. Hypericin, a marker of standardization for currently marketed products, was thought to be the primary antidepressant constituent. Recent attention has focused on hyperforin, but a combination of several compounds is probably involved. Commercial formulations are usually prepared by soaking the dried chopped flowers in methanol to create a hydroalcoholic extract that is then dried.

Pharmacologic Effects

1. *Antidepressant action*—The hypericin fraction was initially reported to have MAO-A and -B inhibitor properties. Later studies found that the concentration required for this inhibition was higher than that achieved with recommended dosages. In vitro studies using the commercially formulated hydroalcoholic extract have shown inhibition of nerve terminal reuptake of serotonin, norepinephrine, and dopamine. While the hypericin constituent did not show reuptake inhibition for any of these systems, the hyperforin constituent did. Chronic administration of the commercial extract has also been reported to significantly down-regulate the expression of cortical β adrenoceptors and up-regulate the expression of serotonin receptors (5-HT_2) in a rodent model.

Other effects observed in vitro include sigma receptor binding using the hypericin fraction and GABA receptor binding using the commercial extract. Prevention of the release of glutamate and protection of hippocampal cells from glutamate induced cell death may also play a role in the anti-depressant effect of St John's wort based on in vitro studies.

***a. Clinical trials for depression*—**A large systematic review and meta-analysis involved 29 randomized, double-blind, controlled trials, including: 18 comparing St. John's wort with placebo, 5 with tricyclic antidepressants, and 12 with selective serotonin reuptake inhibitors (SSRIs). Only studies meeting defined classification criteria for major depression were included. St. John's wort was reported to be more efficacious than placebo and equivalent to prescription reference treatments including the SSRIs for mild to moderate major depressive disorder but with fewer side effects. Most trials used 900 mg/d of St. John's wort for 4–12 weeks. Depression severity was mild to moderate in 19 trials, moderate to severe in 9 trials, and not stated in 1 trial. In another systematic review of 35 studies examining 6993 patients with major depressive disorder of mild to moderate severity, administration with St John's wort for 4 weeks or more showed moderate quality evidence of a significant improvement in depression severity compared to placebo and comparable efficacy to prescription antidepressant medications. These data and the mechanism of action data reported above suggest a potential role for St. John's wort in relieving symptoms of mild to moderate major depression. Due to the short study duration of these clinical trials, efficacy beyond 12 weeks still requires further study. Adverse effects were comparable to placebo and less than those of prescription antidepressants.

***b. Other mood-related conditions*—**St. John's wort has been studied for several other indications related to mood, including premenstrual dysphoric disorder, climacteric complaints, somatoform disorders, and anxiety. For most of these indications, studies are too few in number to draw any firm conclusions regarding efficacy. Evidence for climacteric complaints was the subject of a meta-analysis. Six trials were included: two used mono-preparations of St. John's wort and four used combinations of St. John's wort and black cohosh, *Cimicifuga racemose* (note black cohosh warning in Table 64-1). St. John's wort significantly reduced hot flashes (severity, duration, and frequency) compared to placebo when used for up to 16 weeks. Heterogeneity in these trials limits drawing firm conclusions on efficacy for this indication.

2. *Antiviral and anticarcinogenic effects*—The hypericin constituent of St. John's wort is photolabile and can be activated by exposure to certain wavelengths of visible or ultraviolet A light. Parenteral formulations of hypericin (photoactivated just before administration) have been used investigationally to treat HIV infection (given intravenously) and basal and squamous cell carcinoma (given by intralesional injection). In vitro, photoactivated hypericin inhibits a variety of enveloped and nonenveloped viruses as well as the growth of some neoplastic cells. Inhibition of protein kinase C and inhibition of singlet oxygen radical generation have been proposed as possible mechanisms. The latter could inhibit cell growth or cause cell apoptosis. These studies were carried out using the isolated hypericin constituent of St. John's wort; the usual hydroalcoholic extract of St. John's wort has not been studied for these indications and should not be recommended for patients with viral illness or cancer.

Adverse Effects

Photosensitization is related to the hypericin and pseudohypericin constituents in St. John's wort. Consumers should be instructed to wear sunscreen and eye protection while using this product when exposed to the sun. Rarely, mild gastrointestinal symptoms, fatigue, sedation, restlessness, dizziness, headache, and dry mouth have been observed. Hypomania, mania, and autonomic arousal also have been reported in patients using St. John's wort. When compared to SSRIs, St. John's wort appears to be better tolerated when used to support medical treatment of major depression.

Drug Interactions & Precautions

Inhibition of reuptake of various amine transmitters has been highlighted as a potential mechanism of action for St. John's wort. Drugs with similar mechanisms (ie, antidepressants, stimulants) should be used cautiously or avoided in patients using St. John's wort due to the risk of serotonin syndrome (see Chapters 16 and 30). The hyperforin constituent of St. John's wort has been shown to activate the pregnane X receptor (PXR), which ultimately leads to many drug interactions by inducing hepatic CYP enzymes (3A4, 2C9, 1A2) and the P-glycoprotein drug transporter. Another constituent, hypericin, which may not be present in all commercial formulations, does not have any effect on PXR, CYP, or P-glycoprotein. Case reports involving the use of St. John's wort have suggested that the herb resulted in subtherapeutic levels of numerous drugs, including digoxin, birth control drugs (and subsequent pregnancy), cyclosporine, HIV protease and nonnucleoside reverse transcriptase inhibitors, warfarin, rivaroxaban, irinotecan, tacrolimus, theophylline, and anticonvulsants. Without knowing which constituent is present in a St. John's wort formulation, indiscriminate combined use with other medicines should be avoided.

Dosage

The most common commercial formulation of St. John's wort is the dried hydroalcoholic extract. Products should be standardized to 2–5% hyperforin, although most still bear the older standardized marker of 0.3% hypericin. The recommended dosing for mild to moderate depression is 900 mg of the dried extract per day in three divided doses. Onset of effect may take 2–4 weeks. Long-term benefits beyond 12 weeks have not been well studied.

SAW PALMETTO (*SERENOA REPENS* OR *SABAL SERRULATA*)

Chemistry

The active constituents in saw palmetto berries are not well defined. Phytosterols (eg, β-sitosterol), aliphatic alcohols, polyprenic compounds, and flavonoids are all present. Marketed preparations are dried lipophilic extracts that are generally standardized to contain 85–95% fatty acids and sterols.

Pharmacologic Effects

Saw palmetto is most often promoted for the treatment of benign prostatic hyperplasia (BPH). Enzymatic conversion of testosterone to dihydrotestosterone (DHT) by 5α-reductase is inhibited by saw palmetto in vitro. Specifically, saw palmetto shows a noncompetitive inhibition of isoforms I and II of this enzyme, thereby reducing DHT production. In vitro, saw palmetto also inhibits the binding of DHT to androgen receptors. Additional effects observed in vitro include inhibition of prostatic growth factors, blockade of α_1 adrenoceptors, and inhibition of inflammatory mediators produced by the 5-lipoxygenase pathway.

The clinical pharmacology of saw palmetto in humans is not well defined. One week of treatment in healthy volunteers failed to influence 5α-reductase activity, DHT concentration, or testosterone concentration. Six months of treatment in patients with BPH also failed to affect prostate-specific antigen (PSA) levels, a marker that is typically reduced by enzymatic inhibition of 5α-reductase. In contrast, other researchers have reported a reduction in epidermal growth factor, DHT levels, and antagonist activity at the nuclear estrogen receptor in the prostate after 3 months of treatment with saw palmetto in patients with BPH. Recent reports suggest that daily saw palmetto, as compared to daily tamsulosin (see Chapter 10), has greater anti-inflammatory activity on infiltrating prostatic cells in men with BPH-related lower urinary tract symptoms at 3 months. The anti-inflammatory effects on infiltrating prostatic cells may serve as a link between hormonal changes and the remodeling process promoted by growth factors. The anti-inflammatory effects of saw palmetto also raise questions as to the value of early initiation of BPH therapy as well as the value of early combination therapy with 5α-reductase inhibitors (see Chapter 40).

Clinical Trials

A large review involved 32 randomized controlled trials in 5666 men with symptoms consistent with BPH. Seventeen trials compared saw palmetto monotherapy with placebo and found no significant improvement in most urologic symptoms (eg, international prostate symptom scores, peak flow, prostate size). This review included varied formulations of saw palmetto extracts, and the authors concluded that their results may not be generalizable to proprietary products. A more recent review that included all available published data for a proprietary hexane extract (Permixon) involved 15 randomized controlled trials and 12 observational studies and studied a dose of 320 mg once daily for patients with lower urinary tract symptoms associated with BPH. The extract significantly improved nocturia and maximal urinary flow compared to placebo. The extract showed significant improvements in the International Prostate Symptom Score (IPSS) (mean of 5.73 points) from baseline and exceeds the threshold of 3.1 points, at which a patient would be likely to see a clinically meaningful improvement. The study authors noted that the improvements in IPSS are comparable to that of an alpha blocker and the improvements in maximal urinary flow are comparable to that of tamsulosin. Overall, these findings shed new light on the hexane extract of saw palmetto as a preferred formulation. The 2020 Guidelines of the American Urological Association do not mention saw palmetto, whereas the European Association of Urology lists the hexane extract as a consideration for men with lower urinary tract symptoms (LUTS) who wish to avoid possible adverse effects such as sexual dysfunction.

Adverse Effects

Adverse effects are reported with an incidence of 1–3%. The most common include abdominal pain, nausea, diarrhea, fatigue, headache, decreased libido, and rhinitis. Saw palmetto has been associated with a few rare case reports of pancreatitis, liver damage, and increased bleeding risk, but due to confounding factors, causality remains uncertain. In comparison to tamsulosin and finasteride, saw palmetto was claimed to be less likely to affect sexual function (eg, ejaculation).

Drug Interactions, Precautions, & Dosage

No drug-drug interactions have been reported for saw palmetto. Because saw palmetto has no effect on the PSA marker, it will not interfere with prostate cancer screening using this test. Recommended dosage of a standardized dried extract (containing 85–95% fatty acids and sterols) is 160 mg orally twice daily. A preferred formulation is the proprietary hexane liposterolic extract known as Permixon or a similarly prepared formulation, whereas data for the ethanolic and supercritical CO_2 extracts are insufficient to recommend at this time.

■ PURIFIED NUTRITIONAL SUPPLEMENTS

COENZYME Q10

Coenzyme Q10, also known as CoQ, CoQ10, and ubiquinone, is found in the mitochondria of many organs, including the heart, kidney, liver, and skeletal muscle. After ingestion, the reduced form of coenzyme Q10, ubiquinol, predominates in the systemic circulation. Coenzyme Q10 is a potent antioxidant and has been heavily promoted for this reason. It may have a role in maintaining healthy muscle function, although the clinical significance of this effect is unknown. Reduced serum levels have been reported in Parkinson disease.

Clinical Uses

1. *Hypertension*—In clinical trials, small but significant reductions in systolic and diastolic blood pressure were reported after 8–10 weeks of coenzyme Q10 supplementation. The exact mechanism of coenzyme Q10 is unknown but might be related to the antioxidant and vasodilating properties on nitric oxide–mediated smooth muscle relaxation and effects on vascular endothelium. Within previous randomized, placebo-controlled trials, coenzyme Q10 was reported to significantly lower systolic and diastolic blood pressure by 11 mm Hg and 7 mm Hg, respectively, compared with no change in the placebo groups. However, an exaggerated treatment effect may have occurred as adequate randomization, blinding, and concealment of allocation have been questioned for these studies. In addition, unreported concomitant antihypertensive medications may have played a role. A meta-analysis found that coenzyme Q10 was effective in reducing blood pressure in patients with metabolic disorders, and these effects are more pronounced in people with diabetes or dyslipidemia. The current evidence suggests that coenzyme Q10 may result in small reductions in systolic and diastolic blood pressure compared to placebo. Whether coenzyme Q10 can be used to lower blood pressure in all patients either alone or in combination with other antihypertensive medications therefore remains unclear.

2. *Heart failure*—Energy depletion within mitochondria is a contributing factor to loss of heart muscle contractile function. Therefore, low plasma and mitochondrial coenzyme Q10 levels have been associated with worse heart failure outcomes, but this association is likely because low levels are a marker for more advanced heart failure, rather than a predictor of disease. Despite these findings, coenzyme Q10 is often promoted to improve heart muscle function in patients with heart failure. According to the most recent meta-analysis, coenzyme Q10 was shown to improve ejection fraction by 3.7% when used short term (2–28 weeks). It is unclear whether this small improvement in ejection fraction is applicable to all patients with heart failure, including those receiving the current standard of care. There is moderate-quality evidence to suggest that coenzyme Q10, when used as an adjunctive treatment for heart failure, has resulted in a reduction in hospitalization due to heart failure exacerbations, a reduction of cardiovascular mortality and all-cause mortality compared to the placebo group (relative reduction, 42%), and a reduction in NYHA functional class at 2 years. More research is required to better characterize the role of coenzyme Q10 in heart failure and its impact on disease severity across a more diverse patient population particularly in patients with concomitant prescription medications.

3. *Ischemic heart disease*—The effects of coenzyme Q10 on coronary artery disease and chronic stable angina are modest but appear promising. A theoretical basis for such benefit could be metabolic protection of the ischemic myocardium by reducing proinflammatory markers (including IL-6 and C-reactive protein) that contribute to oxidative stress. Double-blind, placebo-controlled trials have suggested that coenzyme Q10 supplementation improved a number of clinical measures in patients with a history of acute myocardial infarction (AMI). Improvements have been observed in lipoprotein (a), high-density lipoprotein cholesterol, exercise tolerance, and time to development of ischemic changes on the electrocardiogram during stress tests. In addition, very small reductions in cardiac deaths and ra te of reinfarction in patients with previous AMI have been reported (absolute risk reduction 1.5%). Many of these studies suffer from bias and imprecision, providing low-quality evidence as to whether coenzyme Q10 influences the risk of myocardial infarction or stroke.

4. *Prevention of statin-induced myopathy*—Statins reduce cholesterol by inhibiting the HMG-CoA reductase enzyme (see Chapter 35). This enzyme is also required for synthesis of coenzyme Q10. Initiating statin therapy has been shown to reduce endogenous coenzyme Q10 levels, which may block steps in muscle cell energy generation, possibly leading to statin-related myopathy. It is unknown whether a reduction in intramuscular coenzyme Q10 levels leads to statin myopathy or if the myopathy causes cellular damage that reduces intramuscular coenzyme Q10 levels. A meta-analysis evaluating the effect of coenzyme Q10 on statin-induced myopathy as measured by muscle pain and plasma creatine kinase activity found that coenzyme Q10 supplementation (30 days to 3 months) did not demonstrate any benefit in reducing statin-induced myopathy. More information is needed to determine which patients, if any, with statin-related myopathy might benefit from coenzyme Q10 supplementation, especially as it relates to the specific statin, the dose, and the duration of therapy.

Adverse Effects

Coenzyme Q10 is well tolerated, rarely leading to any adverse effects at doses as high as 3000 mg/d. In clinical trials, gastrointestinal upset, including diarrhea, nausea, heartburn, and anorexia, has been reported with an incidence of less than 1%. Cases of maculopapular rash and thrombocytopenia have very rarely been observed. Other rare adverse effects include irritability, dizziness, and headache.

Drug Interactions

Coenzyme Q10 shares a structural similarity with vitamin K, and an interaction has been observed between coenzyme Q10 and warfarin. Coenzyme Q10 supplements may decrease the effects of warfarin therapy. This combination should be avoided or very carefully monitored.

Dosage

As a dietary supplement, 30 mg/d of coenzyme Q10 is adequate to replace low endogenous levels. For cardiac effects, typical dosages are 100–600 mg/d given in two or three divided doses. These doses increase endogenous levels to 2–3 mcg/mL (normal for healthy adults, 0.7–1 mcg/mL).

GLUCOSAMINE

Glucosamine is found in human tissue, is a substrate for the production of articular cartilage, and serves as a cartilage nutrient. Glucosamine is commercially derived from crabs and other crustaceans. As a dietary supplement, glucosamine is primarily used for managing the pain and discomfort associated with knee osteoarthritis. Sulfate and hydrochloride forms are available, but recent research has shown the hydrochloride form to be ineffective.

Pharmacologic Effects & Clinical Uses

Endogenous glucosamine is used to produce glycosaminoglycans and other proteoglycans in articular cartilage. In osteoarthritis, the rate of production of new cartilage is exceeded by the rate of degradation of existing cartilage. Supplementation with glucosamine is postulated to increase the supply of the necessary glycosaminoglycan building blocks, leading to better maintenance and strengthening of existing cartilage.

Many clinical trials have been conducted on the effects of both oral and intra-articular administration of glucosamine. Early studies reported significant improvements in overall mobility, range of motion, and strength in patients with osteoarthritis. More recent studies have reported mixed results, with both positive and negative outcomes. One of the largest and best-designed clinical trials, which compared glucosamine, chondroitin sulfate, the combination, celecoxib, and placebo, found no benefit for glucosamine therapy in mild to moderate disease. Unfortunately, the investigators studied the glucosamine hydrochloride formulation, which has been shown to be inferior to the sulfate formulation. The formulation of glucosamine appears to play a critical role with regard to efficacy, and this may be a factor contributing to the variability observed across published studies. Some research suggests that use of a crystalline formulation of glucosamine sulfate leads to less pain, functional improvements in knee osteoarthritis, and an improvement in joint space narrowing at 3 years. Currently, national orthopedic and rheumatic societies recommend against using glucosamine for knee osteoarthritis primarily because of formulation variability and study heterogeneity. More research is needed to better define the ideal glucosamine formulation and patient populations that stand to benefit from glucosamine sulfate.

Adverse Effects

Oral glucosamine sulfate is very well tolerated. In clinical trials, mild diarrhea, heartburn, abdominal cramping, and nausea were occasionally reported. Tolerability may vary by manufacturer, and recommending a different formulation may be one way to alleviate adverse effects and improve tolerability. Cross-allergenicity in people with shellfish allergies is a potential concern; however, this is unlikely if the formulation has been properly manufactured and purified. Glucosamine sulfate does not have analgesic properties, and it is unclear if glucosamine sulfate is helpful for symptoms in other cartilage-containing joints.

Drug Interactions & Precautions

Glucosamine sulfate may increase the international normalized ratio (INR) in patients taking warfarin, increasing the risk for bruising and bleeding. The mechanism is not well understood and may be dose-related as increases in INR have occurred when the glucosamine dose was increased. Until more is known, the combination should be avoided or very carefully monitored.

Dosage

The oral dosage used most often in clinical trials is 500 mg three times daily or 1500 mg once daily. Glucosamine does not have direct analgesic effects, and improvements in function, if any, may not be observed for 1–2 months.

MELATONIN

Melatonin, a serotonin derivative synthesized by tryptophan by the pineal gland and some other tissues (see also Chapter 16), is believed to be responsible for regulating sleep-wake cycles. Release coincides with darkness; it typically begins around 9:00 PM and lasts until about 4:00 AM. Melatonin release is suppressed by daylight. Melatonin has also been studied for a number of other functions, including contraception, infertility, protection against endogenous oxidants, prevention of aging, treatment of depression, HIV infection, and a variety of cancers. Currently, melatonin is most often used as a dietary supplement to prevent jet lag and to induce sleep.

Pharmacologic Effects & Clinical Uses

1. *Jet lag*—Jet lag, a disturbance of the sleep-wake cycle, occurs when there is a disparity between the external time, ie, hours of daylight or darkness, and the traveler's endogenous circadian clock (internal time). The internal time regulates not only daily sleep rhythms but also body temperature and many metabolic systems. The synchronization of the circadian clock relies on light as the most potent "zeitgeber" (time giver).

Jet lag is especially common among frequent travelers and airplane crew members. Typical symptoms of jet lag may include daytime drowsiness, insomnia, frequent awakenings, and gastrointestinal upset. Symptoms are most prevalent during first 1–2 days following arrival at the new destination. Clinical studies of melatonin given at night have reported subjective reduction in daytime fatigue, improved mood, and a quicker recovery time (return to normal sleep patterns, energy, and alertness). These outcomes are also supported by a systematic review that showed melatonin was better than placebo in helping patients fall asleep faster and to sleep better at their destination. When traveling across five or more time zones, jet lag symptoms are reduced when taking melatonin close to the target bedtime (10:00 PM to midnight) at the new destination. The benefit of melatonin is thought to be greater as more time zones are crossed. In addition, melatonin appears more effective for eastbound travel than for westward travel. Finally, maximizing exposure to daylight on arrival at the new destination can also aid in resetting the internal clock and reducing jet lag symptoms.

2. *Insomnia*—Melatonin has been studied in the treatment of various sleep disorders, including insomnia and delayed sleep-phase syndrome. It has been reported to improve sleep onset, duration, and quality when administered to healthy volunteers, suggesting a pharmacologic hypnotic effect. Melatonin has also been shown to increase rapid eye movement (REM) sleep. These observations have been applied to the development of ramelteon, a prescription hypnotic that is an agonist at melatonin receptors (see Chapter 22).

Clinical studies in patients with primary insomnia have shown that oral melatonin supplementation may alter sleep architecture. Melatonin appears effective in some patients who develop insomnia from β blockers. Subjective and objective improvements in sleep quality and improvements in sleep onset and sleep duration have been reported. Specifically, melatonin taken at the desired bedtime, in a dark environment with bedroom and other sources of light turned off, has been shown to improve morning alertness and quality of sleep compared with placebo. These effects have been observed in both young and older adults (18–80 years of age). Interestingly, baseline endogenous melatonin levels were not predictive of exogenous melatonin efficacy.

3. *Pre- and postoperative anxiety in adults*—Melatonin given as a premedication has been shown to reduce preoperative anxiety in adults. Melatonin may be as effective as midazolam in reducing anxiety before a surgical procedure (measured 50–100 minutes after administration). The effect of melatonin on postoperative anxiety in adults is mixed, but studies support an overall reduction in anxiety compared to preoperative anxiety levels.

4. *Female reproductive function*—The presence of melatonin within the female reproductive system appears widespread in mammals, and research suggests it plays a role in reducing oxidative stress. Melatonin receptors have been identified in ovarian granulosa cell membranes, and significant amounts of melatonin have been detected in follicular fluid. Some studies suggest it can be used as an adjunctive therapy in the treatment of infertility during in vitro fertilization by reducing oxidative stress and thereby improving the quality of oocytes and embryos during ovulation induction and egg retrieval. Melatonin requirements increase during pregnancy, and researchers are evaluating the role of melatonin in preeclampsia and neonatal neurologic morbidity. Importantly, melatonin has been shown to lack teratogenic effects when taken during pregnancy. Melatonin supplementation may decrease prolactin release in women and therefore should be used cautiously or not at all while nursing.

5. *Male reproductive function*—Melatonin receptors have been identified on spermatozoa, suggesting melatonin may play a role in sperm function. When melatonin was added to semen samples, sperm motility was increased and early apoptosis was inhibited. These findings suggest that melatonin may be important in male fertility; however, more research is needed.

Adverse Effects

Melatonin appears to be well tolerated and is often used in preference to over-the-counter "sleep-aid" drugs. Although melatonin is associated with few adverse effects, some next-day drowsiness has been reported as well as fatigue, dizziness, headache, and irritability. Transient depressive symptoms and dysphoria have been reported rarely. Melatonin may affect blood pressure, as both increases and decreases in blood pressure have been observed. Careful monitoring is recommended, particularly in patients initiating melatonin therapy while taking antihypertensive medications. Melatonin manufacturing has been problematic when formulated as an oral tablet, leading to dissolution delays and a resulting lack of effect.

Selecting a chewable or sublingual formulation may be an alternative approach in this case.

Drug Interactions

Melatonin drug interactions have not been formally studied. Various studies, however, suggest that melatonin concentrations are altered by a variety of drugs, including nonsteroidal anti-inflammatory drugs, antidepressants, β-adrenoceptor agonists and antagonists, scopolamine, and sodium valproate. The relevance of these effects is unknown. Melatonin is metabolized by CYP450 1A2 and may interact with other drugs that either inhibit or induce the 1A2 isoenzyme, including fluvoxamine. Melatonin may decrease prothrombin time and may theoretically decrease the effects of warfarin therapy. A dose-response relationship between the plasma concentration of melatonin and coagulation activity has been suggested according to one in vitro analysis. If combination therapy is desired, careful monitoring is recommended especially if melatonin is being used on a short-term basis. Melatonin may interact with nifedipine, possibly leading to increased blood pressure and heart rate. The exact mechanism is unknown.

Dosage

1. *Jet lag*—Daily doses of 0.5–5 mg appear to be equally effective for jet lag; however, the 5-mg dose resulted in a faster onset of sleep and better sleep quality than lower doses. The immediate-release formulation is preferred and should be given at the desired sleep time (10:00 PM to midnight) upon arrival at the new destination and for 1–3 nights after arrival. A dark room environment is important when taking melatonin and when possible, room lights should be turned off. The value of extended-release formulations remains unknown, as evidence suggests the short-acting, high-peak effect of the immediate-release formulation to be more effective. Exposure to daylight at the new time zone is also important to regulate the sleep-wake cycle.

2. *Insomnia*—Doses of 0.3–10 mg of the immediate-release formulation given orally once nightly have been used. The lowest effective dose should be used first and may be repeated in 30 minutes up to a maximum of 10–20 mg. Sustained-release formulations are effective and may be used but, as noted above, may be inferior to immediate-release formulations. Sustained-release formulations are also more costly.

REFERENCES

Abenavoli L et al: Milk thistle (*Silybum marianum*): A concise overview on its chemistry, pharmacological and nutraceutical uses in liver diseases. Phytother Res 2018;32:2202.

Al Saadi T et al: Coenzyme Q10 for heart failure. Cochrane Database Syst Rev 2021;2:CD008684.

Apaydin EA et al: A systematic review of St John's wort for major depressive disorder. Syst Rev 2016;5:148.

Ardjomand-Woelkart K, Bauer R: Review and assessment of safety data of orally used echinacea preparations. Planta Med 2016;82:17.

Birks J, Evans JG: *Ginkgo biloba* for cognitive impairment and dementia. Cochrane Database Syst Rev 2009;1:CD003120.

Buck AC: Is there a scientific basis for the therapeutic effects of *Serenoa repens* in benign prostatic hyperplasia? Mechanisms of action. J Urol 2004;172:1792.

Burlou-Nagy C: *Echinacea purpurea* (L.) Moench: Biological and Pharmacological Properties. A Review. Plants (Basel) 2022;11:1244.

Chen TR et al: Biflavones from *Ginkgo biloba* as inhibitors of human thrombin. Bioorg Chem 2019;92:103199.

Chen X et al: Efficacy and safety of gingko biloba as an adjunct therapy in chronic schizophrenia: A systematic review of randomized, double-blind, placebo-controlled studies with meta-analysis. Psychiatry Res 2015;228:121.

Choi M-K, Song I-S: Interactions of ginseng with therapeutic drugs. Arch Pharm Res 2019;42:862.

David S, Cunningham R: Echinacea for the prevention and treatment of upper respiratory tract infections: A systematic review and meta-analysis. Complement Ther Med 2019;44:18.

Fatemeh G et al: Effect of melatonin supplementation on sleep quality: a systematic review and meta-analysis of randomized controlled trials. J Neurol 2022;269:205.

Foley HM, Steel AE: Adverse events associated with oral administration of melatonin. A critical systematic review of clinical evidence. Complement Ther Med 2019;42:65.

Fried MW et al: Effect of silymarin (milk thistle) on liver disease in patients with chronic hepatitis C unsuccessfully treated with interferon therapy. JAMA 2012;308:274.

Geller AI et al: Emergency department visits for adverse events related to dietary supplements. N Engl J Med 2015;373:1531.

Gillessen A, Schmidt H: Silymarin as supportive treatment in liver disease: A narrative review. Adv Ther 2020;27:1279.

Gravas S et al: Management of non-neurogenic male LUTS. uroweb.org/guidelines/management-of-non-neurogenic-male-luts. Accessed September 28, 2022.

Hansen MV et al: Melatonin for pre- and postoperative anxiety in adults. Cochrane Database Syst Rev 2015;4:CD009861.

Hernandez-Garcia D et al: Efficacy of *Panax ginseng* supplementation on blood lipid profile. A meta-analysis and systematic review of clinical randomized trials. J Ethnopharmacol 2019;243:112090.

Herxheimer A, Petrie KJ: Melatonin for the prevention and treatment of jet lag. Cochrane Database Syst Rev 2002;2:CD001520.

Ho MJ et al: Blood pressure lowering efficacy of coenzyme Q10 for primary hypertension. Cochrane Database Syst Rev 2009;4:CD007435.

Imaizumi VM et al: Garlic: A systematic review of the effects on cardiovascular diseases. Crit Rev Food Sci Nutr 2022;23:1.

Kandiah N et al: Treatment of dementia and mild cognitive impairment with or without cerebrovascular disease: Expert consensus on the use of *Ginkgo biloba* extract, EGb 761. CNS Neurosci Ther 2019;25:288.

Kantor ED et al: Trends in dietary supplement use among US adults from 1999–2012. JAMA 2016;316:1464.

Karsch-Völk M et al: Echinacea for preventing and treating the common cold. Cochrane Database Syst Rev 2014;2:CD000530.

Kholghi G et al: St John's wort (*Hypericum perforatum*) and depression: what happens to the neurotransmitter systems? Naunyn-Schmiedebergs Arch Pharmacol 2022;395:629.

Kim JW et al: Korean red ginseng for cancer-related fatigue in colorectal cancer patients with chemotherapy: A randomized phase III trial. Eur J Cancer 2020;130:51.

Komishono AM et al: The effect of ginseng (genus *Panax*) on blood pressure: A systematic review and meta-analysis of randomized controlled clinical trials. J Hum Hypertension 2016;30:619.

Linde K et al: St. John's wort for major depression. Cochrane Database Syst Rev 2008;4:CD000448.

Liu YR et al: *Hypericum perforatum L.* preparations for menopause: A meta-analysis of efficacy and safety. Climacteric 2014;17:325.

Mancuso C, Santangelo R: Panax ginseng and Panax quinquefolius: From pharmacology to toxicology. Food Chem Toxicol 2017;107:362.

Mastron JK et al: Silymarin and hepatocellular carcinoma: A systematic, comprehensive, and critical review. Anticancer Drugs 2015;26:475.

Mortensen SA et al: Q-SYMBIO study investigators the effect of coenzyme Q10 on morbidity and mortality in chronic heart failure: Results from Q-SYMBIO: A randomized double-blind trial. JACC Heart Fail. 2014;2:641.

Naseri K et al: The efficacy of ginseng (Panax) on human pre-diabetes and type 2 diabetes mellitus: a systematic review and meta-analysis. Nutrients 2022; 14:2401.

Navarro VJ et al: Silymarin in non-cirrhotics with non-alcoholic steatohepatitis: A randomized, double-blind, placebo controlled trial. PLoS One 2019;14:e0221683.

Newmaster SG et al: DNA barcoding detects contamination and substitution in North American herbal products. BMC Med 2013;11:222.

Nicolussi S et al: Clinical relevance of St John's wort drug interactions revisited. Br J Pharmacol 2020;177:1212.

Nicolai SP et al: Ginkgo biloba for intermittent claudication. Cochrane Database Syst Rev 2013;6:CD006888.

Ogal M et al: Echinacea reduces antibiotic usage in children through respiratory tract infection prevention: a randomized, blinded, controlled clinical trial. Eur J Med Res 2021;26:33.

Qaseem A et al: Nonpharmacologic versus pharmacologic treatment of adult patients with major depressive disorder: A clinical practice guideline from the American College of Physicians. Ann Intern Med 2016;164:350.

Rabanal-Ruiz Y et al: The use of coenzyme Q10 in cardiovascular diseases. Antioxidants (Basel) 2021;10:755.

Rambaldi A et al: Milk thistle for alcoholic and/or hepatitis B or C virus liver diseases. Cochrane Database Syst Rev 2007;4:CD003620.

Ried K: Garlic lowers blood pressure in hypertensive individuals, regulates serum cholesterol, and stimulates immunity: An updated meta-analysis and review. J Nutr 2016;146(suppl):389S.

Schergis JL et al: Panax ginseng in randomized controlled trials: A systematic review. Phytother Res 2013;27:949.

Seida JK et al: North American (*Panax quinquefolius*) and Asian ginseng (*Panax ginseng*) preparations for prevention of the common cold in healthy adults: A systematic review. Evid Based Complement Alternat Med 2011;2011:282151.

Sharma M et al: The efficacy of echinacea in a 3-D tissue model of human airway epithelium. Phytother Res 2010;24:900.

Shi C et al: Ginkgo biloba extract in Alzheimer's disease: From action mechanisms to medical practice. Int J Mol Sci 2010;11:107.

Signer J et al: In vitro virucidal activity of Echinaforce®, an *Echinacea purpurea* preparation, against coronaviruses, including common cold coronavirus 229E and SARS-CoV-2. Virol J 2020;17:136.

Soleimani V et al: Safety and toxicity of silymarin, the major constituent in milk thistle extract: An updated review. Phytother Res 2019;33:1627.

Tacklind J et al: *Serenoa repens* for benign prostatic hyperplasia. Cochrane Database Syst Rev 2012;12:CD001423.

Tan MS et al: Efficacy and adverse effects of ginkgo biloba for cognitive impairment and dementia: A systematic review and meta-analysis. J Alzheimers Dis 2015;43:589.

Therapeutic Research Center: Natural Medicines. Therapeutic Research Center, Somerville, MA. Available from: naturalmedicines.therapeuticresearch.com. Subscription required.

Vaclav T et al: Systematic review of pharmacokinetics and potential pharmacokinetic interactions of flavonolignans from silymarin. Med Res Rev 2020;17:2195.

Van Vijven JP et al: Symptomatic and chondroprotective treatment with collagen derivatives in osteoarthritis: A systematic review. Osteoarthritis Cartilage 2012;20:809.

Vela-Navartete R et al: Efficacy and safety of a hexanic extract of *Serenoa repens* (Permixon®) for the treatment of lower urinary tract symptoms associated with benign prostatic hyperplasia (LUTS/BPH): Systematic review and meta-analysis of randomized controlled trials and observational studies. BJU Int 2018;122:1049.

Vellas B et al: Long term use of standardized ginkgo biloba extract for the prevention of Alzheimer's disease (GuidAge): A randomized placebo-controlled trial. Lancet Neurol 2012;11:836.

Wan Q et al: Allium vegetable consumption and health: An umbrella review of meta-analysis of multiple health outcomes. Food Sci Nutr 2019;7:2451.

Wei H et al: Effects of coenzyme Q10 supplementation on statin-induced myopathy: a meta-analysis of randomized controlled trials. Ir J Med Sci 2022;191:719.

Wlosinska M et al: The effect of aged garlic extract on the atherosclerotic process—a randomized, double-blind, placebo controlled trial. BMC Complement Med Ther 2020;20:132.

Wu D et al: Efficacies of different preparations of glucosamine for the treatment of osteoarthritis: A meta-analysis of randomized, double-blind, placebo-controlled trials. Int J Clin Pract 2013;67:585.

Yang Z et al: Effects and tolerance of silymarin (milk thistle) in chronic hepatitis C virus infection patients: A meta-analysis of randomized controlled trials. Biomed Res Int 2014:2014:941085.

Yennurajalingam S et al: A double-blind, randomized, placebo-controlled trial of *Panax ginseng* for cancer-related fatigue in patients with advanced cancer. J Natl Compr Canc Netw 2017;15:1111.

Zhao D et al: Dose-response effect of coenzyme Q10 supplementation on blood pressure among patients with cardiometabolic disorders: A GRADE-assessed systematic review and meta-analysis of randomized controlled trials. Adv Nutr 2022;13:2180.

CASE STUDY ANSWER

Garlic has shown significant benefits in lowering total cholesterol, LDL, and systolic and diastolic blood pressure, but the effects are moderate and unlikely to be large enough to lower this patient's values into the normal range. While this patient's diabetes is under control, her hypertension places her at risk for microvascular complications of diabetes, thus making it necessary to reevaluate her current medication adherence, doses of benazepril for hypertension and simvastatin for hyperlipidemia, and duration of therapy. She would benefit from meeting with a nutritionist because packaged frozen dinners can be high in sodium, and this may be elevating her blood pressure. Increasing physical activity could also help with weight control, blood glucose management, and overall cardiovascular health. The data supporting benefits of St. John's wort in patients with hot flashes are preliminary but show promise. Good data support use of the herb to alleviate symptoms of mild to moderate depression when used for up to 1 year. However, this patient is not a good candidate for St. John's wort (a cytochrome P450 1A2, 2C9, 3A4 inducer) because of her prescription drug use and the potential for herb-drug interactions. Several dietary supplements reviewed in this chapter (garlic, ginkgo, and ginseng) may have antiplatelet effects that could be additive with ibuprofen. If this patient were also taking warfarin, additional interactions could occur with coenzyme Q10 (vitamin K–like structure), St. John's wort, and melatonin (in vitro decreased prothrombin time), leading to a decreased warfarin effect, or with glucosamine (increased international normalized ratio), leading to an increased warfarin effect.

CHAPTER

66 Rational Prescribing & Prescription Writing

Paul W. Lofholm, PharmD, &
Bertram G. Katzung, MD, PhD

Once a patient with a clinical problem has been evaluated and a diagnosis has been reached, the practitioner can often select from a variety of therapeutic approaches. Medication, surgery, psychiatric treatment, radiation, physical therapy, health education, counseling, further consultation (second opinions), and no therapy are some of the options available. Of these options, drug therapy is by far the one most frequently chosen. In most cases, this requires the writing of a prescription. A written prescription is the prescriber's order to prepare or dispense a specific treatment—usually medication—for a specific patient. When a patient comes for an office visit, the physician or other authorized health professional prescribes medications 67% of the time, and an average of one prescription is written per office visit because more than one prescription may be written at a single visit. On average, patients receive 12.3 prescriptions per year.

In this chapter, a plan for prescribing is presented. The physical form of the prescription, common prescribing errors, and legal requirements that govern various features of the prescribing process are then discussed. Finally, some of the social and economic factors involved in prescribing and drug use are described.

RATIONAL PRESCRIBING

Like any other process in health care, writing a prescription should be based on a series of rational steps as follows:

1. **Make a specific diagnosis:** Prescriptions based merely on a desire to satisfy the patient's psychological need for some type of therapy are often unsatisfactory and may result in adverse effects. A specific diagnosis, even if it is tentative, is required to move to the next step. For example, in a patient with a probable diagnosis of rheumatoid arthritis, the diagnosis and the reasoning underlying it should be clear and should be shared with the patient.
2. **Consider the pathophysiologic implications of the diagnosis:** If the disorder is well understood, the prescriber is in a much better position to offer effective therapy. For example, increasing knowledge about the mediators of inflammation makes possible more effective use of nonsteroidal anti-inflammatory drugs (NSAIDs) and other agents used in rheumatoid arthritis. The patient should be provided with the appropriate level and amount of information about the pathophysiology. Many pharmacies, websites, and disease-oriented public and private agencies (eg, Arthritis Foundation, American Heart Association, American Cancer Society) provide information sheets suitable for patients.
3. **Select a specific therapeutic objective:** A therapeutic objective should be chosen for each of the pathophysiologic processes defined in the preceding step. In a patient with rheumatoid arthritis, relief of pain by reduction of the inflammatory process is one of the major therapeutic goals that identify the drug groups that should be considered. Arresting the course of the disease process in rheumatoid arthritis is a different therapeutic goal, which might lead to consideration of additional drug groups and prescriptions.
4. **Select a drug of choice:** One or more drug groups will be suggested by each of the therapeutic goals specified in the preceding step. Selection of a drug of choice from among these groups follows from a consideration of the specific characteristics of the patient and the clinical presentation, a selection process that has been emphasized as part of "**precision medicine.**" For certain drugs, patient characteristics such as age, other diseases, and other drugs being taken (because of the risk of duplicative therapy or drug-drug interactions) are extremely important in determining the most suitable drug for management of the present complaint. As the tools of precision medicine provide more detailed information (eg, mutations of drug metabolizing enzymes—pharmacogenomics), the selection process will become more focused. In the example of the patient with probable rheumatoid arthritis, it would be important to know whether the patient has a history of aspirin intolerance or ulcer

disease, whether the cost of medication is an especially important factor and the nature of the patient's insurance coverage, and whether there is a need for once-daily dosing. Based on this information, a drug would probably be selected from the NSAID group. If the patient does not have ulcer disease but does have a need for low-cost treatment, generic ibuprofen or naproxen would be a rational choice.

5. **Determine the appropriate dosing regimen:** The dosing regimen is determined primarily by the pharmacokinetics of the drug in that patient. If the patient is known to have disease of the organs required for elimination of the drug selected, adjustment of the average regimen is needed. For a drug such as ibuprofen, which is eliminated mainly by the kidneys, renal function should be assessed. If renal function is normal, the half-life of ibuprofen (about 2 hours) requires administration three or four times daily. The dose suggested in this book, drug handbooks, and the manufacturer's literature is 400–800 mg four times daily.
6. **Devise a plan for monitoring the drug's action and determine an endpoint for therapy:** The prescriber should be able to describe to the patient the kinds of drug effects that will be monitored and in what way, including laboratory tests (if necessary) and signs and symptoms that the patient should report. For conditions that call for a limited course of therapy (eg, most infections), the duration of therapy should be made clear so that the patient does not stop taking the drug prematurely and understands why the prescription probably need not be renewed. For the patient with rheumatoid arthritis, the need for prolonged—perhaps indefinite—therapy should be explained, including how to obtain refills. The prescriber should also specify any changes in the patient's condition that would call for changes in therapy. For example, in the patient with rheumatoid arthritis, development of gastrointestinal bleeding would require an immediate change in drug therapy and a prompt workup of the bleeding. Major toxicities that require immediate attention should be explained clearly and calmly to the patient.
7. **Plan a program of patient education:** The prescriber and other members of the health team should be prepared to repeat, extend, and reinforce the information transmitted to the patient as often as necessary. The more toxic the drug prescribed, the greater the importance of this educational program. The importance of informing and involving the patient in each of the above steps must be recognized, as shown by experience with teratogenic drugs (see Chapter 59). Many pharmacies routinely provide this type of information with each prescription filled, but the prescriber must not assume that this will occur.

THE PRESCRIPTION

Although a prescription can be written on any piece of paper or in electronic format (as long as all of the legal elements are present), it usually takes a specific form. A typical printed prescription form for outpatients is shown in Figure 66–1.

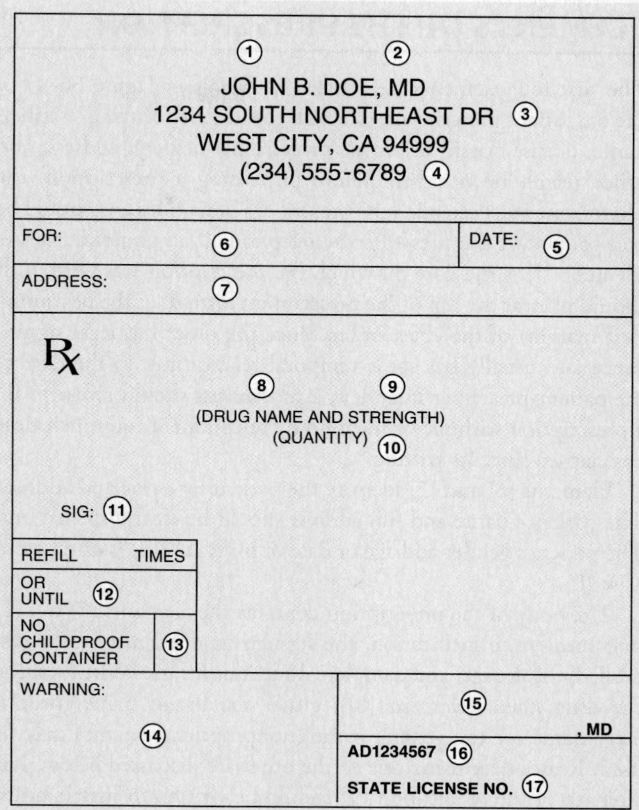

FIGURE 66–1 Common form of outpatient prescription. Circled numbers are explained in the text.

In the traditional hospital setting, drugs have been prescribed on a particular page of the patient's hospital chart called the **physician's order sheet (POS)** or **chart order.** In the electronic medical records environment, prescriptions are executed via **electronic order entry**. The contents of that prescription are specified in the medical staff rules by the hospital's Pharmacy and Therapeutics Committee or similar authority. The patient's name is typed or written on the form; the orders consist of the name and strength of the medication, the dose, the route and frequency of administration, the date, other pertinent information, and the signature of the prescriber. If the duration of therapy or the number of doses is not specified (which is often the case), the medication is continued until the prescriber discontinues the order or until it is terminated as a matter of policy routine, eg, a stop-order policy.

A typical chart order might be as follows:

3/12/2022
10:30 A.M.

(1) Ampicillin 500 mg IV q6h 5 days
(2) Aspirin 0.6 g per rectum q6h prn temp over 38.3 C (101F)
[Signed] Janet B. Doe, MD

Thus, the elements of the hospital chart order are equivalent to the central elements (5, 8–11, 15) of the outpatient prescription.

ELEMENTS OF THE PRESCRIPTION

The first four elements (see circled numerals in Figure 66–1) of the outpatient prescription establish the identity of the prescriber: name, license classification (ie, professional degree), address, and office telephone number. Before dispensing a prescription, the pharmacist must establish the prescriber's bona fides and should be able to contact the prescriber by telephone if any questions arise. Element [5] is the date on which the prescription was written. It should be near the top of the prescription form or at the beginning (left margin) of the chart order. Since the order has legal significance and usually has some temporal relationship to the date of the patient-prescriber interview, a pharmacist should refuse to fill a prescription without verification by telephone if too much time has elapsed since its writing.

Elements [6] and [7] identify the patient by name and address. The patient's name and full address should be clearly spelled out. The patient's gender and age or date of birth (DOB) is often listed as well.

The body of the prescription contains the elements [8] to [11] that specify the medication, the strength and quantity to be dispensed, the dosage, and complete directions for use. When writing the drug name (element [8]), either the brand name (proprietary name) or the generic name (nonproprietary name) may be used. Reasons for using one or the other are discussed below. The strength of the medication [9] should be written in metric units. However, the prescriber should be familiar with both systems now in use: metric and apothecary. For practical purposes, the following approximate conversions are useful:

1 grain (gr) = 0.065 grams (g), often rounded to 60 milligrams (mg)
15 gr = 1 g
1 ounce (oz) by volume = 30 milliliters (mL)
1 teaspoonful (tsp) = 5 mL
1 tablespoonful (tbsp) = 15 mL
1 quart (qt) = 1000 mL
1 minim = 1 drop (gtt)
20 drops = 1 mL
2.2 pounds (lb) = 1 kilogram (kg)

The strength of a solution is usually expressed as the quantity of solute in sufficient solvent to make 100 mL; for instance, 20% potassium chloride solution is 20 grams of KCl per deciliter (g/dL) of final solution. Both the concentration and the volume should be explicitly written out.

The quantity of medication prescribed should reflect the anticipated duration of therapy, the cost, the need for continued contact with the clinic or physician, the potential for abuse, and the potential for toxicity or overdose. Consideration should be given also to the standard sizes in which the product is available and whether this is the initial prescription of the drug or a repeat prescription or refill. If 10 days of therapy are required to effectively cure a streptococcal infection, an appropriate quantity for the full course should be prescribed. Birth control pills are often prescribed for 1 year or until the next examination is due; however, some patients may not be able to afford a year's supply at one time; therefore, a 3-month supply might be ordered, with refill instructions to renew three times or for 1 year (element [12]). Some third-party (insurance) plans limit the amount of medicine that can be dispensed—often to only 1 month's supply. Finally, when first prescribing medications that are to be used for the treatment of a chronic disease, the initial quantity should be small, with refills for larger quantities. The purpose of beginning treatment with a small quantity of drug is to reduce the cost if the patient cannot tolerate it. Once it is determined that intolerance is not a problem, a larger quantity purchased less frequently is sometimes less expensive. It should be noted that some insurance companies and states now limit the quantity of opiates per prescription.

The directions for use (element [11]) must be both drug-specific and patient-specific. The simpler the directions, the better; and the fewer the number of doses (and drugs) per day, the better. Patient noncompliance (also known as nonadherence, failure to adhere to the drug regimen) is a major cause of treatment failure. To help patients remember to take their medications, prescribers often give an instruction that medications be taken at or around mealtimes and at bedtime. However, it is important to inquire about the patient's eating habits and other lifestyle patterns, because many patients do not eat three regularly spaced meals a day.

The instructions on how and when to take medications, the duration of therapy, and the purpose of the medication must be explained to each patient both by the prescriber and by the pharmacist. (Neither should assume that the other will do it.) Furthermore, the drug name, the purpose for which it is given, and the duration of therapy should be written on each label so that the drug may be identified easily in case of overdose. An instruction to "take as directed" may save the time it takes to write the orders out but often leads to noncompliance, patient confusion, and medication error. The directions for use must be clear and concise to prevent toxicity and to obtain the greatest benefits from therapy.

Although directions for use are no longer written in Latin, many Latin apothecary abbreviations (and some others included below) are still in use. Knowledge of these abbreviations is essential for the dispensing pharmacist and often useful for the prescriber. Some of the abbreviations still used are listed in Table 66–1.

Note: It is always safer to write out the direction without abbreviating.

Elements [12] to [14] of the prescription include refill information, waiver of the requirement for childproof containers, and additional labeling instructions (eg, warnings such as "may cause drowsiness," "do not drink alcohol"). Pharmacists put the name of the medication on the label unless directed otherwise by the prescriber, and some medications have the name of the drug stamped or imprinted on the tablet or capsule. Pharmacists must place the expiration date for the drug on the label. If the patient or prescriber does not request waiver of childproof containers, the pharmacist or dispenser must place the medication in such a container. Pharmacists may not refill a prescription medication without authorization from the prescriber. Prescribers may grant authorization to renew prescriptions at the time of writing the prescription or over the telephone or electronically. Elements [15] to [17] are the prescriber's signature and

TABLE 66–1 Abbreviations used in prescriptions and chart orders.

Abbreviation	Explanation	Abbreviation	Explanation
ā	before	PO	by mouth
ac	before meals	PR	per rectum
agit	shake, stir	prn	when needed
Aq	water	q	every
Aq dest	distilled water	qam, om	every morning
bid	twice a day	qd (do not use)	every day (write "daily")
c̄	with	qh, q1h	every hour
cap	capsule	q2h, q3h, etc	every 2 hours, every 3 hours, etc
D5W, D_5W	dextrose 5% in water	qhs	every night at bedtime
dil	dissolve dilute	qid	four times a day
disp, dis	dispense	qod (do not use)	every other day
elix	elixir	qs	sufficient quantity
ext	extract	rept, repet	may be repeated
g	gram	Rx	take
gr	grain	s̄	without
gtt	drops	SC, SQ	subcutaneous
h	hour	sid (veterinary)	once a day
hs	at bedtime	Sig, S	label
IA	intra-arterial	sos	if needed
IM	intramuscular	s̄s̄, ss	one-half
IV	intravenous	stat	at once
IVPB	IV piggyback	sup, supp	suppository
kg	kilogram	susp	suspension
mcg, μg (do not use)	microgram (always write out "microgram")	tab	tablet
mEq, meq	milliequivalent	tbsp, T (do not use)	tablespoon (always write out "15 mL")
mg	milligram	tid	three times a day
no	number	Tr, tinct	tincture
non rep	do not repeat	tsp (do not use)	teaspoon (always write out "5 mL")
OD	right eye	U (do not use)	units (always write out "units")
OS, OL	left eye	vag	vaginal
OTC	over-the-counter	i, ii, iii, iv, etc	one, two, three, four, etc
OU	both eyes	ʒ (do not use)	dram (in fluid measure 3.7 mL)
p̄	after	℥ (do not use)	ounce (in fluid measure 29.6 mL)
pc	after meals		

other identification data such as National Provider Identification (NPI), Drug Enforcement Administration (DEA) number, or State License number.

PRESCRIBING ERRORS

Unfortunately, prescribing errors are common. Several groups provide online information regarding practices designed to reduce or document such errors, eg, Institute for Safe Medication Practices (ISMP; www.ismp.org) and National Coordinating Council for Medication Error Reporting and Prevention Program (MERP; www.nccmerp.org/about-medication-errors).

All prescription orders should be legible, unambiguous, dated (and timed in the case of a chart order), and signed clearly for optimal communication between prescriber, pharmacist, and nurse. Furthermore, a good prescription or chart order should contain sufficient information to permit the pharmacist or nurse to discover possible errors before the drug is dispensed or administered.

Certain types of prescribing errors are particularly common. These include errors involving omission of needed information;

poor writing perhaps leading to errors of drug dose or timing; and prescription of drugs that are inappropriate for the specific situation.

OMISSION OF INFORMATION

Errors of omission are common in hospital orders and may include instructions to "resume pre-op meds," which assumes that a full and accurate record of the "pre-op meds" is available; "continue present IV fluids," which fails to state exactly what fluids are to be given, in what volume, and over what time period; or "continue eye drops," which omits mention of which eye is to be treated as well as the drug, concentration, and frequency of administration. Chart orders may also fail to discontinue a prior medication when a new one is begun; may fail to state whether a regular or long-acting form is to be used; may fail to specify a strength or notation for long-acting forms; or may authorize "as needed" (prn) use that fails to state what conditions will justify the need.

POOR PRESCRIPTION WRITING

Poor prescription writing is traditionally exemplified by illegible handwriting. However, other types of poor writing are common and often more dangerous. One of the most important is the misplaced or ambiguous decimal point. Thus ".1" is easily misread as "1," a 10-fold overdose if the decimal point is not unmistakably clear. This danger is easily avoided by always preceding the decimal point with a zero. On the other hand, appending an unnecessary zero after a decimal point increases the risk of a 10-fold overdose, because "1.0 mg" is easily misread as "10 mg," whereas "1 mg" is not. The slash or virgule ("/") was traditionally used as a substitute for a decimal point. This should be abandoned because it is too easily misread as the numeral "1." Similarly, the abbreviation "U" for units should never be used because "10 U" is easily misread as "100"; the word "units" should *always* be written out. Doses in micrograms should always have this unit written out because the abbreviated form ("μg") is very easily misread as "mg," a 1000-fold overdose! Orders for drugs specifying only the number of dosage units and not the total dose required should not be filled if more than one size dosage unit exists for that drug. For example, ordering "one ampule of furosemide" is unacceptable because furosemide is available in ampules that contain 20, 40, or 100 mg of the drug. The abbreviation "OD" should be used (if at all) only to mean "the right eye"; it has been used for "every day" and has caused inappropriate administration of drugs into the eye. Similarly, "Q.D." or "QD" should not be used because it is often read as "QID," resulting in four doses per day instead of one. Acronyms and abbreviations such as "ASA" (aspirin), "5-ASA" (5-aminosalicylic acid), "6MP" (6-mercaptopurine), etc, should not be used; drug names should be written out. Unclear handwriting can be lethal when drugs with similar names but very different effects are available, eg, apixaban and aripiprazole, methotrexate and metolazone. In this situation, errors are best avoided by noting the indication for the drug in the body of the prescription, eg, "acetazolamide, for glaucoma." Pharmacy and Therapeutics committees have developed some additional principles to lessen errors, such as a High-Alert Medication list (www.ismp.org) and using a comma (in the USA) when the dose exceeds 999.

INAPPROPRIATE DRUG PRESCRIPTIONS

Prescribing an inappropriate drug for a particular patient often results from failure to recognize contraindications imposed by other diseases the patient may have, failure to obtain information about other drugs the patient is taking (including over-the-counter drugs), or failure to recognize possible physicochemical incompatibilities between drugs that may react with each other. Contraindications to drugs in the presence of other diseases or pharmacokinetic characteristics are listed in the discussions of the drugs described in this book. The manufacturer's package insert usually contains similar information. Many of the important drug interactions are listed in Chapter 67 of this book as well as in package inserts and drug interaction databases.

Physicochemical incompatibilities are of particular concern when parenteral administration is planned. For example, certain insulin preparations should not be mixed. Similarly, the simultaneous administration of antacids or products high in metal content may compromise the absorption of many drugs in the intestine, eg, tetracyclines. The package insert and the *Handbook on Injectable Drugs* (see References) are good sources for this information.

ELECTRONIC PRESCRIBING (E-PRESCRIBING)

Seventy percent of prescriptions in the USA are now e-prescribed. Congress has passed legislation related to e-prescribing, including Medicare Improvement for Patients and Providers Act (MIPPA) and the Medicare and Medicaid Electronic Health Record Incentive Program or the "meaningful use program." Electronic medical record systems (EMRs) have been mandated by the market and have been both praised and vehemently criticized. It is not necessarily a bad policy but, importantly, it has changed the way prescribers practice. Prescribers have become data collectors at the cost of reduced time for clinical history taking and, ultimately, taking care of patients.

E-prescribing provides an electronic flow of information between the prescriber, intermediary, pharmacy, and insurance health plan. The health plan can provide information on patient eligibility, formulary, benefits, costs, and sometimes, a medication history. The prescriber selects the medication, strength, dosage form, quantity, and directions for use and the prescription is transmitted to the pharmacy where the appropriate data fields are populated. The pharmacist reviews the order and, if appropriate, dispenses the prescription. The electronic system must be Health Insurance Portability and Accountability Act (HIPAA)-compliant, and there is often a business association agreement between the parties involved.

Prescribers can obtain decision support information such as disease-drug and drug-drug interaction information or cost information prior to prescribing as part of the health plan information. Prescriptions can be clear in their writing, but pull-down drug lists can create new errors. Prescription renewals can be processed electronically, and drug misuse or abuse may be identifiable. Theoretically, time to process prescription orders should be reduced and patients would have their medication ready when they arrive at the pharmacy.

The DEA has issued rules for e-prescribing of controlled substances. Currently, only registered prescribers can e-prescribe, and there will be several independent identification proofing sources required: a unique pin number, or retinal scan, or a fingerprint. The objective is to prevent drug diversion. DEA registrants, including pharmacies and physicians, can order a controlled drugs inventory via computer using a specific form once they are certified (Controlled Substances Ordering System, CSOS).

COMPLIANCE

Compliance (also called adherence) is the extent to which patients follow treatment instructions. There are four types of noncompliance leading to medication errors and increased health care costs as given below:

1. The patient fails to obtain the medication. Some studies suggest that one third of patients never have their prescriptions filled. Patients usually leave the hospital without obtaining their discharge medications because the hospital is not reimbursed for them by the insurer; others leave the hospital without having their prehospitalization medications resumed. In many cases, patients cannot afford the medications prescribed if the drug is not covered by the patient's insurance plan.
2. The patient fails to take the medication as prescribed. Examples include wrong dosage, wrong frequency of administration, improper timing or sequencing of administration, wrong route or technique of administration, duplication, or taking medication for the wrong purpose. This usually results from inadequate communication between the patient, the prescriber, and the pharmacist. In the USA, medication reconciliation should occur whenever a patient changes levels of care (hospital discharge) and at each office visit. At that time the medication list is reviewed in order to identify duplication of therapy, and to clearly communicate what to take, a current drug history is reviewed.
3. The patient prematurely discontinues the medication. This can occur, for instance, if the patient incorrectly assumes that the medication is no longer needed because the bottle is empty or symptomatic improvement has occurred.
4. The patient (or another person) takes medication inappropriately. For example, the patient may share a medication with others for any of several reasons.

Several factors encourage noncompliance. Some diseases cause no symptoms (eg, hypertension); patients with these diseases therefore have no symptoms to remind them to take their medications. Patients with painful conditions such as arthritis may continually change medications in the hope of finding a better one. Characteristics of the therapy itself can limit the degree of compliance; patients taking a drug once a day are much more likely to be compliant than those taking a drug four times a day. Various patient factors also play a role in compliance. Patients living alone are much less likely to be compliant than married patients of the same age. Packaging also may be a deterrent to compliance—elderly arthritic patients often have difficulty opening their medication containers. On the other hand, pharmacists can supply compliance packaging to aid in patient compliance, eg, "bingo cards" or strip packaging organized by date and time. Lack of transportation as well as various cultural or personal beliefs about medications are likewise barriers to compliance. For example, some parents refuse to allow their children to be vaccinated because of a misguided fear of autism or other toxic effects. Politically motivated misinformation about the safety of vaccines has led to the reemergence of previously abolished diseases such as poliomyelitis.

Strategies for improving compliance include enhanced communication between the patient and health care team members; assessment of personal, social, and economic conditions (often reflected in the patient's lifestyle); development of a routine for taking medications (eg, at mealtimes if the patient has regular meals); provision of systems to assist taking medications (ie, containers that separate drug doses by day of the week, or medication alarm clocks that remind patients to take their medications); and mailing of refill reminders by the pharmacist to patients taking drugs chronically. The patient who is likely to discontinue a medication because of a perceived drug-related problem should receive instruction about how to monitor and understand the effects of the medication. Compliance can often be improved by enlisting the patient's active participation in the treatment.

LEGAL FACTORS (USA)

The US government recognizes two classes of drugs: (1) over-the-counter (OTC) drugs and (2) those that require a prescription from a licensed prescriber (Rx Only). OTC drugs are those that can be safely self-administered by the layman for self-limiting conditions and for which appropriate labels can be written for lay comprehension (see Chapter 64). Half of all drug doses consumed by the American public are OTC drugs. In 2021 $603 billion was spent in the USA on prescription drugs and $151 billion was spent on OTC drugs, more than any other country. The average "specialty" drug cost was $270 per prescription, and these drugs (eg, antibodies) are driving up overall costs. However, drug makers continue to push the cost of generic drugs higher.

Physicians, osteopaths, dentists, podiatrists, and veterinarians—and, in many states and for certain indications, specialized pharmacists, nurses, physician's assistants, and optometrists—are granted authority to prescribe certain drugs (those bearing the federal legend statement, "Rx Only") on the basis of their training in diagnosis and treatment (see Box: Who May Prescribe?). Depending on the state, mid-level practitioners may prescribe/furnish prescriptions. Pharmacists are authorized to dispense prescriptions pursuant to a prescriber's order provided that the medication order is appropriate and rational for the patient.

Nurses are authorized to administer medications to patients subject to a prescriber's order.

Because of the multiplicity of third-party payers (health insurers) in the USA and Medicare and Medicaid claimants, the concept of electronic processing of prescriptions ("e-prescribing") is common. (Further information about e-prescribing may be found at www.cms.gov/Medicare/E-Health/Eprescribing/.) To further standardize electronic prescription transmission and billing, the Centers for Medicare and Medicaid Services (CMS) issued regulations effective in 2008 requiring all US health care providers to obtain a National Provider Identification (NPI) number. This 10-digit identifier is issued by the National Plan and Provider Enumeration System (NPPES) at NPPES.cms.hhs.gov. The purpose of the NPI is to identify all health care transactions (and associated costs) incurred by a particular practitioner with a single number.

In addition to a health care provider's unique identification number, some states require that prescriptions for controlled substances be written on tamper-resistant security prescription forms or e-prescriptions. The purpose of this legislation is to prevent forgeries and to tighten the control of prescription order forms.

Who May Prescribe?

The right to prescribe drugs has traditionally been the responsibility of the physician, osteopath, dentist, podiatrist, or veterinarian. Prescribing now includes—in a number of states and in varying degrees—pharmacists, nurse practitioners, nurse midwives, physician's assistants, and optometrists (see below; Table 66–2). Further changes have occurred in the wake of the COVID-19 pandemic (see below). Physical therapists may be licensed to prescribe drugs relevant to their practice in some states. The development of large health maintenance organizations has greatly strengthened this expansion of prescribing rights because it offers these extremely powerful economic bodies a way to reduce their expenses.

The primary organizations controlling the privilege of prescribing in the USA are the state boards, under the powers delegated to them by the state legislatures. Many state boards have attempted to reserve some measure of the primary responsibility for prescribing to physicians by requiring that the ancillary professional work with or under a physician according to a specific protocol. In the state of California, this protocol must include a statement of the training, supervision, and documentation requirements of the arrangement and must specify referral requirements, limitations to the list of drugs that may be prescribed (ie, a formulary), and a method of evaluation by the supervising physician. The protocol must be in writing and must be periodically updated.

The following rules govern prescribing by non-physicians in the various states.

In almost all states, nurse practitioners (NPs) and physician assistants (PAs) may prescribe—with or without physician supervision depending on the state. Likewise, optometrists may prescribe selected formulary drugs for ophthalmologic indications.

Pharmacists can initiate prescriptions in 15 states: California, Colorado, Florida, Hawaii, Maryland, Montana, New Hampshire, New Mexico, North Dakota, North Carolina, Oregon, Tennessee, Utah Washington, and West Virginia. New Mexico grants prescribing authority to medical psychologists with advanced training.

The COVID pandemic brought changes to the health care delivery system. Resources were stretched, access to care was reduced, and a new model for primary care emerged. Testing was inadequate, and vaccines were in short supply and controlled by local public health departments. Many hospitals were overwhelmed by sick patients. Some 70% of the COVID tests and vaccinations were administered by pharmacists. The shortage of personnel led to pharmacists being granted authority to test and treat symptomatic COVID-positive patients using Paxlovid under tight protocol.

Other examples of expanded authority for pharmacists include all CDC-approved vaccines, nicotine-replacement therapy, hormonal contraception, naloxone furnishing, and travel medicine furnishing. In addition, pharmacists can furnish HIV pre-exposure prophylaxis (PrEP) and post-exposure prophylaxis based on CDC guidelines and clinical training. In July 2022 the FDA authorized pharmacists with state licenses to prescribe Paxlovid (nirmatrelvir and ritonavir) to eligible patients with certain limitations to ensure appropriate assessment (renal, hepatic, and drug interaction possibilities) with prescribing of Paxlovid. Testing and prescribing within 5 days of the onset of COVID symptoms was considered essential.

The concept of a "secure" prescription form was expanded by the federal government in 2008 to all prescriptions written for Medicaid patients. Any prescription for a Medicaid patient must be written on a security form if the pharmacist is to be compensated for the prescription service. For controlled drugs, an online electronic transmission system was established: the Prescription Monitoring Program (PMP). The dispensing party submits orders for Schedule II, Schedule III, Schedule IV, and V prescriptions electronically, whereby they are stored and analyzed. In California, it is called the CURES program (Controlled Substances Utilization Review and Evaluation System). Prescribers are provided with a record of who prescribed when and which controlled drug to which patient. Additional information about CURES may be found at oag.ca.gov/cures.

In the USA, prescription drugs are controlled by the US Food and Drug Administration (FDA) as described in Chapter 1. The federal legend statement as well as the **package insert** are part of the packaging requirements for all prescription drugs. The package

TABLE 66–2 Prescribing authority of certain allied health professionals in selected states.

State[1]	Pharmacists	Nurse Practitioners	Physician's Assistants	Optometrists
California	Yes, under protocol[2]; must be trained in clinical practice; Advanced Practice Pharmacist	Yes[3]	Yes, under protocol[2]	Yes; limited to certain drug classes
Florida	Yes, according to state formulary; protocol not required; collaborative practice agreement	Yes[3]	Yes[3]	Yes; limited to certain drug classes
Iowa	Collaborative drug therapy management; yes with written protocol	Yes	Yes	Yes, limited
Idaho	Yes, notify MD in 5 days For 8 categories of medications; state formulary	Yes	Yes	Yes, limited
Michigan	Yes, under protocol; must be specially qualified by education, training, or experience	Yes[3]	Yes[3]	Yes; limited to certain drug classes
Mississippi	Yes, under protocol in an institutional setting	Yes,[3] under narrowly specified conditions	No	Yes; limited to certain drug classes
Nevada	Yes, under protocol, within a licensed medical facility	Yes	Yes[3]	Yes; limited to certain drug classes
Montana	Clinical Pharmacist Practitioner; collaborative practice agreement with physician	Yes	Yes	Yes, limited
Massachusetts	Collaborative drug therapy management agreement in place	Yes[3]	Yes	Yes, limited
New Mexico	Yes, under protocol, must be "pharmacist clinician"	Yes; do not need physician supervision	Yes[3]	Yes; limited to certain drug classes
New York	Collaborative drug therapy management; facility-based only	Yes[3]	Yes	Yes, limited to topically applied drugs
North Carolina	Yes, under physician supervision; Clinical Pharmacist Practitioner			Yes; limited to certain drug classes
North Dakota	Yes, consult agreement within a facility	Yes	Yes	Yes, limited
Ohio	Yes, consult agreement	Yes[3]	Yes	Yes, limited
Oregon	Yes, under guidelines set by the state board, formulary	Yes; do not need physician supervision	Yes[3]	Yes; limited to certain drug classes
Texas	Yes, under protocol set for a particular patient in an institutional setting	Yes; do not need physician supervision	Yes	Yes; limited to certain drug classes
Washington	Yes, under guidelines set by the state board	Yes; do not need physician supervision	Yes[3]	Yes; limited to certain drug classes

[1]Since the United States Supreme Court overturned Roe vs. Wade in 2022, each state will now have jurisdiction on where abortions are permitted or not permitted, under what circumstances, and by what method. At the time of writing, it is not clear how this will apply to the prescription of drugs for medical abortion (mifepristone and misoprostol).

[2]Under protocol; see Box: Who May Prescribe?

[3]In collaboration with or under the supervision of a physician.

insert is the official brochure setting forth the indications, contraindications, warnings, and dosing for the drug. Warnings of special importance (**black box warnings**) are displayed in a box for emphasis in the package insert. These warnings list particularly dangerous adverse effects and necessary safety information. In addition to patient safety, these warnings are of medicolegal significance.

The prescriber, by writing and signing a prescription order, controls who may obtain prescription drugs. The pharmacist may purchase these drugs, but they may be dispensed only on the order of a legally qualified prescriber. Thus, a **prescription** is actually three things: the **prescriber's order in the patient's chart,** the **written order to which the pharmacist refers** when dispensing, and the patient's **medication container with a label affixed.**

Whereas the US FDA controls the drugs and their labeling and distribution, the state legislatures control who may prescribe drugs through their licensing boards, eg, the Board of Medical Examiners. Prescribers must pass examinations, pay fees, and—in the case of some states and some professions—meet other requirements for relicensure such as continuing education. If these requirements are met, the prescriber is licensed to order dispensing of drugs.

The FDA Amendments Act of 2007 gave the FDA authority to require a **Risk Evaluation and Mitigation Strategy (REMS)** from manufacturers to ensure that the benefits of a drug or biological product outweigh its risks. The goal of this strategy is to inform physicians of the emphasized risks and benefits. Furthermore, some drugs have "boxed warnings" to elucidate their risks as part of FDA-mandated labeling.

TABLE 66–3 Classification of controlled substances. (See Inside Front Cover for examples.)

Schedule	Potential for Abuse	Other Comments
I	High	No accepted medical use; lack of accepted safety as drug.
II	High	Current accepted medical use. Abuse may lead to psychological or physical dependence.
III	Less than I or II	Current accepted medical use. Moderate or low potential for physical dependence and high potential for psychological dependence.
IV	Less than III	Current accepted medical use. Limited potential for dependence.
V	Less than IV	Current accepted medical use. Limited dependence possible.

The federal government and the states further impose special restrictions on drugs according to their perceived potential for abuse (Table 66–3). Such drugs include opioids, hallucinogens, stimulants, depressants, and anabolic steroids. Special requirements must be met when these drugs are to be prescribed. The Controlled Drug Act requires prescribers and dispensers to register with the Drug Enforcement Agency (DEA), pay a fee, receive a personal registration number, and keep records of all controlled drugs prescribed or dispensed. Every time a controlled drug is prescribed, a valid DEA number must appear on the prescription. In the USA, there is an opioid epidemic with an increase in overdoses. To combat this public health trend, prescriber education, tracking of prescribing patterns, limitations on amounts prescribed, and targeted education are being instituted.

Prescriptions for substances with a high potential for abuse (Schedule II drugs) cannot be refilled without a new prescription. However, multiple prescriptions for the same drug may be written with instructions not to dispense before a certain date and up to a total of 90 days. Prescriptions for Schedules III, IV, and V can be refilled if ordered, but there is a five-refill maximum, and in no case may the prescription be refilled after 6 months from the date of writing. Schedule II drug orders may not be transmitted over the telephone, and some states require a tamper-resistant security prescription blank to reduce the chances for drug diversion (see inside front cover).

These restrictive prescribing laws are intended to limit the amount of drugs of abuse that are made available to the public. Unfortunately, the inconvenience occasioned by these laws—and an unwarranted fear by medical professionals themselves regarding the risk of patient tolerance and addiction—continues to hamper adequate treatment of patients with terminal conditions. This has been shown to be particularly true in children and elderly patients with cancer. *There is no excuse for inadequate treatment of pain in a terminal patient; not only is addiction irrelevant in such a patient, it is actually uncommon in patients who are being treated for pain* (see Chapter 31). Unfortunately, the initiative begun several years ago to manage pain more actively has led to the overuse of opioids in non-terminal patients with chronic pain, a condition that does not respond well to these drugs. Chronic use of oxycodone, hydrocodone, and methadone has resulted in a marked increase in habituation, overdoses, and deaths. As a result, most professional authorities now advise limiting the use of any opioid in non-terminal patients to acute pain only and suggest the use of NSAIDs and other nonaddicting therapies in chronic conditions.

Some states have recognized the underutilization of pain medications in the treatment of pain associated with chronic and terminal conditions. In California, upon receipt of a copy of the order from the prescriber, eg, by fax, a pharmacist may write a prescription for a Schedule II substance for a patient under hospice care or living in a skilled nursing facility or in cases in which the patient is expected to live less than 6 months, provided that the prescriber countersigns the order (by fax); the word "exemption" with regulatory code number is written on a typical prescription, thus providing easier access for the terminally ill.

Labeled & Off-Label Uses of Drugs

In the USA, the FDA approves a drug only for the specific uses proposed and documented by the manufacturer in its New Drug Application (NDA) (see Chapter 1). These approved (*labeled*) uses or indications are set forth in the package insert that accompanies the drug. For a variety of reasons, these labeled indications may not include all the conditions in which the drug might be useful. Therefore, a clinician may wish to prescribe the agent for some other, unapproved (*off-label*) clinical condition, often on the basis of adequate or even compelling scientific evidence. Federal laws governing FDA regulations and drug use place no restrictions on such unapproved use.*

Even if the patient suffers injury from the drug, its use for an unlabeled purpose does not in itself constitute "malpractice." However, the courts may consider the package insert labeling as a complete listing of the indications for which the drug is considered safe unless the clinician can show that other use is considered safe by competent expert testimony.

Drug Safety Surveillance

Governmental drug-regulating agencies have responsibility for monitoring drug safety. In the USA, the FDA-sponsored **Med Watch** program collects data on safety and adverse drug effects (ADEs) through mandatory reporting by drug manufacturers and voluntary reporting by health care practitioners. Practitioners may submit reports on any suspected adverse drug (or medical device) effect using a simple form obtainable from www.fda.gov/safety/medwatch-fda-safety-information-and-adverse-event-reporting-program (Form FDA 3500). The FDA is expected to use these

*"Once a product has been approved for marketing, a physician may prescribe it for uses or in treatment regimens or patient populations that are not included in the approved labeling. Such 'unapproved' or, more precisely, 'unlabeled' uses may be appropriate and rational in certain circumstances, and may, in fact, reflect approaches to drug therapy that have been extensively reported in medical literature." …FDA Drug Bull 1982;12:4.

data to establish an adverse effect rate. It is not clear that the FDA has sufficient resources at present to carry out this mandate, but they are empowered to take further regulatory actions if deemed necessary. A similar vaccine-reporting program is in place to monitor vaccine safety (the vaccine adverse event reporting system, VAERS). The homepage on vaccine adverse reaction reporting may be found at vaers.hhs.gov.

The FDA has also increased requirements for labeling on drugs that carry special risks. Dispensers of medications are required to distribute "Med Guides" to patients when these medications are dispensed. These guides are generated by the manufacturers of the medications. In addition, pharmacists often provide patient educational materials that describe the drug, its use, adverse effects, storage requirements, methods of administration, what to do when a dose is missed, and the potential need for ongoing therapy.

SOCIOECONOMIC FACTORS

The Cost of Prescriptions

Lacking universal health care in the USA, many persons have private health insurance and drug insurance. The drug insurance plans are administered by organizations called **pharmacy benefit managers (PBMs)**. PBMs were originally designed to bring insurance companies and pharmacies together in a network for the purpose of providing pharmacy services. PBMs have expanded their activities to control what is prescribed, to control how much is prescribed, and to require prior authorization (from the PBM) for drugs that are not covered. The vehicle for controlling drugs is the drug formulary. Because drug utilization has value to manufacturers, they offer rebates to incentivize the PBM to select their product and increase market share. The prescriber is left with dealing with PBM-determined prescribing rules. In some cases, the prescriber writes an order and the PBM dictates what the patient will receive, the quantity or number of days' supply, and for specialty drugs, where the prescription can be filled.

Multiple factors are involved in the pricing of pharmaceuticals. Research costs, marketing costs (such as PBM rebates), production costs, shipping costs, regulatory costs, direct-to-consumer advertising costs, and profit all contribute to a drug's price. Generally, insurance companies pay for most drugs because an extensive formulary is mandated by regulations. For older patients, federal law and regulations require Medicare Part D pharmacy and therapeutics committees to make prescription drug coverage decisions based on scientific evidence and standards of practice, and also to prevent discrimination in a patient's drug therapy. Because these companies are publicly owned, the shareholders exert a strong influence to maximize profits. While the cost to make the drug may be 20% (or less) of the wholesale price, the aforementioned costs contribute to the cost of the drug to the pharmacist or physician. Greed and the excessive influence of shareholder funds (as opposed to the interests of consumers) add another component of cost and have sometimes resulted in startling increases in the price of long-established drugs (which have no current development costs) as well as newer ones. In the case of pyrimethamine, a simple and long-established small molecule drug used for toxoplasmosis, the US price increased from approximately $13/tablet to $750/tablet in 2015 when a new company acquired the rights to this drug. In 2016, the price of the formulation of epinephrine most commonly used for anaphylaxis (Epi-Pen) increased from $50 to $300 per single dose, even though no changes were made in the drug, the vehicle, or the injection unit. Acthar gel (corticotropin) increased in price from $40 in 2001 to $40,000 recently. Even digoxin's price has increased dramatically, as there is a lack of competition amongst manufacturers.

Specialty Drugs

A more complex situation applies to the pricing of new, complex molecules (so-called specialty drugs) that, unlike the above examples, required massive research, development, and manufacturing investment, eg, the new agents used for hepatitis B and C. These agents for hepatitis are extremely expensive in the USA ($24,000–75,000 for one course of treatment), but the manufacturers justify the cost as being less than the alternative (which is often a liver transplant) and the drug may be curative. In fact, specialty drugs represent over one-half of the drug spending in the USA. Furthermore, specialty drugs with no competition and restricted pharmacy access and very high costs are driving spending up even further. Drugs make up 10% of the total health care expense in the USA.

Because the US federal government limits price negotiations by the largest purchasers of drugs, the public has no protection from excessive pricing by manufacturers. Thus drug expenses constitute a large and growing burden to patients, Medicare, and private health insurers. Federal legislation signed into law in 2022 (Inflation Reduction Act-IRA) will allow the Federal Government to negotiate prices for a select number of drugs.

Generic Prescribing

Generic drug dispensing represents 10% of the total US drug expense but 90% of the drugs dispensed. Prescribing by generic name offers the pharmacist flexibility in selecting the particular drug product to fill the order and offers the patient a potential savings when there is price competition. For example, the brand name of a popular sedative is *Valium*. The generic (public nonproprietary) name of the same chemical substance adopted by United States Adopted Names (USAN) and approved by the FDA is *diazepam*. All diazepam drug products in the USA meet the pharmaceutical standards expressed in the *United States Pharmacopeia (USP)*. However, there are several manufacturers, and prices vary. For drugs in common use, the difference in cost between the trade-named product and generic products varies from less than twofold to more than 100-fold. For drugs with a limited market (eg, pyrimethamine, Epi-Pen), the incentive for generic manufacturing and marketing is very low, so only one or two generics (or none) may be available, and price competition is low or absent.

In most states and in most hospitals, pharmacists have the option of supplying a generically equivalent drug product even if a proprietary name has been specified in the order. If the prescriber wants a particular brand of drug product dispensed, handwritten instructions to "dispense as written" or words of similar meaning are required. Some government-subsidized health care programs and many third-party insurance payers *require* that pharmacists dispense the cheapest generically equivalent product in the inventory (generic substitution). However, the principles of drug product selection by private pharmacists do not permit substituting one therapeutic agent for another (therapeutic substitution); that is, dispensing trichlormethiazide for hydrochlorothiazide would not be permitted without the prescriber's permission even though these two diuretics may be considered pharmacodynamically equivalent. Pharmacists within managed care organizations may follow different policies; see below.

It cannot be assumed that every generic drug product is as satisfactory as the trade-named product, although examples of unsatisfactory generics are rare. Bioavailability—the effective absorption of the drug product—varies between manufacturers and sometimes between different lots of a drug produced by the same manufacturer. Despite the evidence, many practitioners avoid generic prescribing, thereby increasing medical costs. In the case of a very small number of drugs, which usually have a low therapeutic index, poor solubility, or a high ratio of inert ingredients to active drug content, a specific manufacturer's product may give more consistent results. In the case of life-threatening diseases, the advantages of generic substitution may be outweighed by the clinical urgency so that the prescription should be filled as written.

In an effort to codify bioequivalence information, the FDA publishes *Approved Drug Products with Therapeutic Equivalence Evaluations*, with monthly supplements, commonly called "the **Orange Book**." The book contains listings of multisource products in one of two categories: Products given a code beginning with the letter "A" are considered ***bioequivalent*** to a reference standard formulation of the same drug and to all other versions of that product with a similar "A" coding. Products not considered bioequivalent are coded "B." Of the approximately 8000 products currently listed, 90% are coded "A." Additional code letters and numerals are appended to the initial "A" or "B" and indicate the approved route of administration and other variables. The FDA also publishes the **Purple Book**, which is a list of biological products, including biosimilars and interchangeable biological products, approved or licensed by the FDA under the Public Health Services Act. It is equivalent to the Orange Book.

Mandatory drug product selection on the basis of price is common practice in the USA because third-party payers (insurance companies, health maintenance organizations, etc) enforce money-saving practices, if available. If outside a managed care organization, the prescriber can sometimes override these controls by writing "dispense as written" on a prescription that calls for a brand-named product. However, in such cases, the patient may have to pay the difference between the dispensed product and the cheaper one.

Within most managed care organizations, formulary controls have been put in place that force the selection of less expensive medications or preferred generic drugs driven by PBM rebate incentives whenever they are available. In a managed care environment, the prescriber often selects the drug group rather than a specific agent, and the pharmacist dispenses the formulary drug from that group. For example, if a prescriber in such an organization decides that a patient needs a thiazide diuretic, the pharmacist automatically dispenses the single thiazide diuretic carried on the organization's formulary. As noted below, the choice of drugs for the organization's formulary may change from time to time, depending on negotiation of prices and rebates with different manufacturers.

Other Cost Factors

Private pharmacies base their charges on the cost of the drug plus a fee for providing a professional service. There is a fee each time a prescription is dispensed. The prescriber controls the frequency of filling prescriptions by authorizing refills and specifying the quantity to be dispensed. However, for medications used for chronic illnesses, the quantity covered by insurance may be limited to the amount used in 1 month or 30 days. Thus, the prescriber can save the patient money by prescribing standard sizes (so that drugs do not have to be repackaged) and, when chronic treatment is involved, by ordering the largest quantity consistent with safety, expense, and third-party plan. Optimal prescribing for cost savings often involves consultation between the prescriber and the pharmacist. Because of continuing increases in the wholesale prices of drugs in the USA, prescription costs have risen dramatically over the past three decades, and with the passage of the Affordable Care Act (ACA), prescription volume increased while hospital services decreased. However recently the volume of prescriptions has leveled off despite the pandemic but the costs of prescriptions has risen with the burden of cost (50%) coming from specialty drugs. Is it sustainable?

REFERENCES

Adejari Adeboye: *Remington's The Science and Practice of Pharmacy*, 23rd ed. Pharmaceutical Press, 2020.

American Pharmacists Association and The National Association of Chain Drug Stores: MTM in Pharmacy Practice, Core Elements v. 2, 2008.

Bell D: A toolset for e-prescribing implementation. Rand Health, US AHRQ, 2011.

California Business and Professions Code, Chapter 9, Division 2, Pharmacy Law. Department of Consumer Affairs, Sacramento, California, 2023.

Cobaugh Danirel J, Koboutek Lisa M: ASHP Injectable Drug Information, ASHP, 2023.

Congressional Budget Office: Prices for and Spending on Specialty Drugs in Medicare Part D and Medicaid, Publication 54964, 2015.

Congressional Budget Office, Prescription Drugs: Spending, Use, and Prices, Publication 57772, January, 2022.

Cubanski J et al: Explaining the Prescription Drug Provisions in the Inflation Reduction Act. www.kff.org/medicare/issue-brief/explaining-the-prescription-drug-provisions-in-the-inflation-reduction-act/.

de Oliveira DJ et al: Medication therapy management: 10 years of experience in a large integrated health system. J Manage Care Pharm 2010;3:185.

Department of Health and Human Services: About the [opioid] epidemic. www.hhs.gov/opioids/about-the-epidemic/.

Drug Enforcement Administration: Mid-Level Practitioners Authorized by State, Title 21, Code of Federal Regulations, Section 1300.01 (b28), 5-24-16.

Dusetzina SB et al: Specialty drug pricing and out-of-pocket spending on orally administered anticancer drugs in Medicare Part D, 2010 to 2019. JAMA 2019;321:2025.

Gabriel MH: E-Prescribing Trends in the US. ONC Data Brief, 18, July, 2014.

Graber MA, Easton-Carr R: Poverty and pain: Ethics and the lack of opioid pain medications in fixed-price, low-cost prescription plans. Ann Pharmacotherapy 2008;42:1913.

Institute for Safe Medication Practices. www.ismp.org.

Iqvia Institute Report: Medicine Use and Spending in the U.S. A Review of 2018 and Outlook to 2023. May 9, 2019. www.iqvia.com/institute/reports/medicine-use-and-spending-in-the-us-a-review-of-2018-and-outlook-to-2023.

Jerome JB, Sagan P: The USAN nomenclature system. JAMA 1975;232:294.

Journal of the American Medical Association: Drug pricing. JAMA 2020;323:809 [Special Issue].

Kaiser Family Foundation: Abortion Policy Tracker. www.kff.org/other/state-indicator/abortion-policy-tracker.

Kesselheim AS et al: Clinical equivalence of generic and brand-name drugs used in cardiovascular disease: A systematic review and meta-analysis. JAMA 2008;300:2514.

Kesselheim AS et al: The high cost of prescription drugs in the United States. Origins and prospects for reform. JAMA 2016;316:858.

Levinson DR: Gaps in Oversight of Conflicts of Interest in Medicare Prescription Drug Decisions, DHHS, Office of Inspector General, March, 2013. oig.hhs.gov/oei/reports/oei-05-10-00450.pdf.

Parasrampuria S, Murphy S: Trends in Prescription Spending, 2016-2021, Washington, D.C. Office of the Assistant Secretary for Planning and Evaluation, U.S. Department of Health and Human Services, September, 2022.

Royce TJ et al: Pharmacy benefit manager reform. Lessons from Ohio. JAMA 2019;322:299.

Ruiz Jorge G, Hagenlocker Brian: E-Prescribing, AMA Journal of Ethics, June, 2006.

Schnipper JL et al: Role of pharmacist counseling in preventing adverse drug events after hospitalization. Arch Intern Med 2006;166:565.

Trissel LA: *Handbook on Injectable Drugs*, 20th ed. American Society of Hospital Pharmacists, 2018.

CHAPTER

67 Important Drug Interactions & Their Mechanisms

John R. Horn, PharmD, FCCP

One of the factors that can alter the response to drugs is the concurrent administration of other drugs. There are several mechanisms by which drugs may interact, but most can be categorized as pharmacokinetic (absorption, distribution, metabolism, excretion), pharmacodynamic (additive, synergistic, or antagonistic effects), or combined interactions. The general principles of pharmacokinetics are discussed in Chapters 3 and 4; the general principles of pharmacodynamics are discussed in Chapter 2.

Botanical medications ("herbals") may interact with each other or with conventional drugs. Unfortunately, botanicals are much less well studied than other drugs, so information about their interactions is scanty. Some pharmacodynamic herbal interactions are described in Chapter 65. Table 67–1 includes selected pharmacokinetic and pharmacodynamic interactions that may result in clinically significant adverse events in patients.

Knowledge of the mechanism by which a given drug interaction occurs is often clinically useful, since the mechanism may influence both the time course and the methods of circumventing the interaction. Some important drug interactions occur as a result of two or more mechanisms.

PREDICTABILITY OF DRUG INTERACTIONS

The designations listed in Table 67–1 are used here to *estimate* the predictability of the drug interactions. These estimates are intended to indicate simply whether the interaction will occur, and they do not always mean that the interaction is likely to produce an adverse effect. Whether the interaction occurs (precipitant drug produces a measurable change in the object drug's pharmacokinetics or pharmacodynamics) and produces an adverse effect depends on both patient- and drug-specific factors. Patient factors can include intrinsic drug clearance, genetics, gender, concurrent diseases, and diet. Drug-specific factors include dose, route of administration, drug formulation, and the sequence of drug administration. The most important factor that can mitigate the risk of patient harm is recognition by the prescriber of a potential interaction followed by appropriate action.

PHARMACOKINETIC MECHANISMS

The gastrointestinal **absorption** of drugs may be affected by concurrent use of other agents that (1) have a large surface area upon which the drug can be adsorbed, (2) bind or chelate, (3) alter gastric pH, (4) alter gastrointestinal motility, or (5) affect transport proteins such as P-glycoprotein and organic anion transporters. One must distinguish between effects on absorption *rate* and effects on *extent* of absorption. A reduction in only the absorption *rate* of a drug is seldom clinically important, whereas a reduction in the *extent* of absorption is clinically important if it results in subtherapeutic serum concentrations. Similarly, an *increase* in the extent of absorption can lead to adverse patient outcomes.

The mechanisms by which drug interactions alter drug **distribution** include (1) competition for plasma protein binding, (2) displacement from tissue binding sites, and (3) alterations in local tissue barriers, eg, P-glycoprotein inhibition in the blood-brain barrier. Although competition for plasma protein binding can increase the free concentration (and thus the effect) of the displaced drug in plasma, the increase will be transient owing to a compensatory increase in drug disposition. The clinical importance of protein binding displacement has been overemphasized; current evidence suggests that such interactions are unlikely to result in adverse effects. Displacement from tissue binding sites would tend to transiently increase the blood concentration of the displaced drug.

The **metabolism** of drugs can be induced or inhibited by concurrent therapy, and the importance of the effect varies from negligible to dramatic. Drug metabolism occurs primarily in the liver and the wall of the small intestine, but other sites include plasma,

TABLE 67–1 Important drug interactions.

Drug or Drug Group	Properties Promoting Drug Interaction	Clinically Documented Interactions
Acid-reducing agents	Antacids may adsorb drugs in gastrointestinal tract, thus reducing absorption. Some antacids (eg, magnesium hydroxide with aluminum hydroxide) alkalinize the urine somewhat, thus altering excretion of drugs sensitive to urinary pH. H_2-antagonists and proton-pump inhibitors can alter the absorption of drugs requiring gastric acidity for dissolution.	**Antivirals:** [P] Decreased absorption of antivirals that require acid for dissolution including atazanavir, fosamprenavir, indinavir, nelfinavir, and rilpivirine. **Azole antifungals:** [P] Reduced gastrointestinal absorption of itraconazole, ketoconazole, and posaconazole due to increased gastric pH. **Digoxin:** [NP] Decreased gastrointestinal absorption of digoxin. **Iron:** [P] Decreased gastrointestinal absorption of iron with calcium-containing antacids. **Kinase inhibitors:** [P] Reduced gastrointestinal absorption of acalabrutinib, belumosudil, bosutinib, ceritinib, dasatinib, erlotinib, gefitinib, neratinib, nilotinib, pazopanib, pexidartinib, and sotorasib due to increased gastric pH. **Quinolones:** [P] Decreased gastrointestinal absorption of ciprofloxacin, norfloxacin, (and probably other quinolones). **Rosuvastatin:** [P] Decreased absorption of rosuvastatin. **Salicylates:** [P] Increased renal clearance of salicylates due to increased urine pH; occurs only with large doses of salicylates. **Tetracyclines:** [P] Decreased gastrointestinal absorption of tetracyclines. **Thyroxine:** [NP] Reduced gastrointestinal absorption of thyroxine.
Alcohol	Chronic alcoholism results in enzyme induction. Acute alcoholic intoxication tends to inhibit drug metabolism (whether person is alcoholic or not). Severe alcohol-induced hepatic dysfunction may inhibit ability to metabolize drugs. Disulfiram-like reaction in the presence of certain drugs. Additive central nervous system depression with other central nervous system depressants.	**Acetaminophen:** [NE] Increased formation of hepatotoxic acetaminophen metabolites (in chronic alcoholics). **Acitretin:** [P] Increased conversion of acitretin to etretinate (teratogenic). **Anticoagulants, oral:** [NE] Increased hypoprothrombinemic effect with acute alcohol intoxication. **Central nervous system depressants:** [P] Additive or synergistic central nervous system depression. **Insulin:** [NE] Acute alcohol intake may increase hypoglycemic effect of insulin (especially in fasting patients). ***Drugs that may produce a disulfiram-like reaction:*** **Cephalosporins:** [NP] Disulfiram-like reactions are noted with cefamandole, cefoperazone, cefotetan, and moxalactam. **Chloral hydrate:** [NP] Mechanism not established. **Disulfiram:** [P] Inhibited aldehyde dehydrogenase. **Metronidazole:** [NP] Mechanism not established. **Sulfonylureas:** [NE] Chlorpropamide is most likely to produce a disulfiram-like reaction; acute alcohol intake may increase hypoglycemic effect (especially in fasting patients).
Allopurinol	Inhibits hepatic drug-metabolizing enzymes. Febuxostat will also inhibit the metabolism of azathioprine and mercaptopurine.	**Anticoagulants, oral:** [NP] Increased hypoprothrombinemic effect. **Azathioprine:** [P] Decreased azathioprine detoxification resulting in increased azathioprine toxicity. **Mercaptopurine:** [P] Decreased mercaptopurine metabolism resulting in increased mercaptopurine toxicity. **Didanosine:** [P] Decreased didanosine metabolism resulting in increased didanosine toxicity.

P, Predictable. Interaction occurs in most patients receiving the combination; NP, Not predictable. Interaction occurs only in some patients receiving the combination; NE, Not established. Insufficient data available on which to base estimate of predictability.

(*continued*)

TABLE 67–1 Important drug interactions. (Continued)

Drug or Drug Group	Properties Promoting Drug Interaction	Clinically Documented Interactions
Anticoagulants, oral	Susceptible to induction and inhibition of CYP2C9 (warfarin), CYP3A4 (apixaban, rivaroxaban), and P-glycoprotein (apixaban, betrixaban, dabigatran, edoxaban, rivaroxaban). Warfarin highly bound to plasma proteins. Anticoagulation response altered by drugs that affect clotting factor synthesis or catabolism.	***Drugs that may increase anticoagulant effect:***
		Acetaminophen: [NP] Impaired synthesis of clotting factors at higher doses.
		Amiodarone: [P] Inhibited anticoagulant elimination. Expect similar interactions with dronedarone.
		Anabolic steroids: [P] Altered clotting factor disposition?
		Antivirals: [P] Amprenavir, atazanavir, boceprevir, darunavir, delavirdine, indinavir, ledipasvir, nelfinavir, paritaprevir, ritonavir, saquinavir, simeprevir, and telaprevir can decrease apixaban, betrixaban, dabigatran, edoxaban, rivaroxaban, and perhaps warfarin elimination.
		Azole antifungals: [P] Ketoconazole, itraconazole, voriconazole, and posaconazole can decrease apixaban, betrixaban, dabigatran, edoxaban, rivaroxaban, and perhaps warfarin elimination.
		Cimetidine: [P] Decreased warfarin metabolism.
		Clopidogrel: [NP] Decreased warfarin metabolism and inhibited platelet function.
		Cyclosporine: [P] Decreased apixaban, betrixaban, dabigatran, edoxaban, and rivaroxaban elimination.
		Disulfiram: [P] Decreased warfarin metabolism.
		Efavirenz: [NP] Decreased warfarin metabolism.
		Fluconazole: [P] Decreased warfarin metabolism.
		Fluoxetine: [P] Decreased warfarin metabolism.
		Gemfibrozil: [NP] Mechanism not established.
		Lovastatin: [NP] Decreased warfarin metabolism.
		Macrolide antibiotics: [NP] Clarithromycin, erythromycin, and telithromycin may inhibit the elimination of oral anticoagulants.
		Metronidazole: [P] Decreased warfarin metabolism.
		Miconazole: [NP] Decreased warfarin metabolism.
		Nonsteroidal anti-inflammatory drugs (NSAIDs): [P] Inhibition of platelet function, gastric erosions; some agents increase hypoprothrombinemic response (unlikely with diclofenac, ibuprofen, or naproxen).
		Oxandrolone: [NP] Decreased warfarin metabolism.
		Propafenone: [NP] Probably decreases anticoagulant elimination.
		Quinidine: [NP] Additive hypoprothrombinemia, decreased apixaban, betrixaban, dabigatran, edoxaban, rivaroxaban elimination.
		Salicylates: [P] Platelet inhibition with aspirin but not with other salicylates; [P] large doses have hypoprothrombinemic effect.
		Simvastatin: [NP] Decreased warfarin metabolism.
		Sulfinpyrazone: [NP] Inhibited warfarin metabolism.
		Sulfonamides: [NP] Inhibited warfarin metabolism.
		Trimethoprim-sulfamethoxazole: [P] Decreased warfarin metabolism.
		Verapamil: [P] Decreased apixaban, betrixaban, dabigatran, edoxaban, rivaroxaban elimination.
		Voriconazole: [P] Decreased warfarin metabolism.
		See also Alcohol; Allopurinol.

P, Predictable. Interaction occurs in most patients receiving the combination; NP, Not predictable. Interaction occurs only in some patients receiving the combination; NE, Not established. Insufficient data available on which to base estimate of predictability.

(*continued*)

TABLE 67–1 Important drug interactions. (Continued)

Drug or Drug Group	Properties Promoting Drug Interaction	Clinically Documented Interactions
Anticoagulants, oral (*cont.*)		***Drugs that may decrease anticoagulant effect:***
		Apalutamide: [P] Increased metabolism of anticoagulant.
		Barbiturates: [P] Increased metabolism of anticoagulant.
		Bosentan: [P] Increased metabolism of anticoagulant.
		Carbamazepine: [P] Increased metabolism of anticoagulant.
		Cholestyramine: [P] Reduced absorption of anticoagulant.
		Dabrafenib: [NP] Increased metabolism of anticoagulant.
		Enzalutamide: [NP] Increased metabolism of anticoagulant.
		Ivosidenib: [NP} Increased metabolism of anticoagulant.
		Nafcillin: [NP] Increased metabolism of anticoagulant.
		Phenytoin: [NP] Increased metabolism of anticoagulant. Anticoagulant effect may increase transiently at start of phenytoin therapy due to protein-binding displacement of warfarin.
		Phenobarbital: [P] Increased metabolism of anticoagulant.
		Primidone: [P] Increased metabolism of anticoagulant.
		Rifabutin: [P] Increased elimination of anticoagulant.
		Rifampin: [P] Increased elimination of anticoagulant.
		St. John's wort: [NP] Increased elimination of anticoagulant.
		Tipranavir: [NP] Increased elimination of apixaban, betrixaban, dabigatran, edoxaban, rivaroxaban.
Antidepressants, tricyclic and heterocyclic	Inhibition of transmitter uptake into 5-HT and NE neurons. Antimuscarinic effects may be additive with other antimuscarinic drugs. Susceptible to induction and inhibition of metabolism via CYP2D6, CYP3A4, and other CYP450 enzymes.	**Amiodarone:** [P] Decreased antidepressant metabolism. Expect similar interactions with dronedarone.
		Barbiturates: [P] Increased antidepressant metabolism.
		Bupropion: [NP] Decreased antidepressant metabolism.
		Carbamazepine: [P] Enhanced metabolism of antidepressants.
		Cimetidine: [P] Decreased antidepressant metabolism.
		Clonidine: [P] Decreased clonidine antihypertensive effect.
		Diphenhydramine: [P] Decreased metabolism of antidepressants metabolized by CYP2D6.
		Guanadrel: [P] Decreased uptake of guanadrel into sites of action.
		Haloperidol: [P] Decreased metabolism of antidepressants metabolized by CYP2D6.
		Monoamine oxidase inhibitors (MAOIs): [NP] Some cases of excitation, hyperpyrexia, mania, and convulsions, especially with serotonergic antidepressants such as clomipramine and imipramine, but many patients have received combination without ill effects.
		Quinidine: [P] Decreased metabolism of antidepressants metabolized by CYP2D6.
		Rifampin: [P] Increased antidepressant metabolism of antidepressants metabolized by CYP3A4.
		Selective serotonin reuptake inhibitors (SSRIs): [P] Fluoxetine and paroxetine inhibit CYP2D6 and decrease metabolism of antidepressants metabolized by this enzyme (eg, desipramine). Citalopram, sertraline, and fluvoxamine are only weak inhibitors of CYP2D6, but fluvoxamine inhibits CYP1A2 and CYP3A4 and thus can inhibit the metabolism of antidepressants metabolized by these enzymes.
		Sympathomimetics: [P] Increased pressor response to norepinephrine, epinephrine, and phenylephrine.
		Terbinafine: [P] Decreased antidepressant metabolism.

P, Predictable. Interaction occurs in most patients receiving the combination; NP, Not predictable. Interaction occurs only in some patients receiving the combination; NE, Not established. Insufficient data available on which to base estimate of predictability.

(*continued*)

TABLE 67–1 Important drug interactions. (Continued)

Drug or Drug Group	Properties Promoting Drug Interaction	Clinically Documented Interactions
Antineoplastic agents. See also kinase inhibitors.	Substrates of CYP3A4 susceptible to induction and inhibition of metabolism. Abiraterone, anastrozole, aprepitant, bexarotene, bortezomib, brentuximab, cabazitaxel, cyclophosphamide, docetaxel, doxorubicin, enzalutamide, etoposide, exemestane, glasdegib, ifosfamide, irinotecan, ivosidenib, ixabepilone, ixazomib, letrozole, midostaurin, mitoxantrone, paclitaxel, panobinostat, romidepsin, sonidegib, tamoxifen, teniposide, thiotepa, toremifene, trabectedin, venetoclax, vinblastine, vincristine, vinorelbine.	**Amiodarone:** [P] Decreased antineoplastic agent metabolism. Expect similar interactions with dronedarone. **Antivirals:** [P] Amprenavir, atazanavir, boceprevir, darunavir, delavirdine, fosamprenavir, indinavir, nelfinavir, ritonavir, saquinavir, simeprevir, and telaprevir inhibit the metabolism of antineoplastic agents. Efavirenz and etravirine increase the metabolism of antineoplastic agents. **Azole Antifungals:** [P] Ketoconazole, fluconazole, itraconazole, posaconazole, and voriconazole inhibit the metabolism of antineoplastic agents. **Barbiturates:** [P] Increased antineoplastic agent metabolism. **Bosentan:** [P] Increased antineoplastic agent metabolism. **Carbamazepine:** [P] Increased antineoplastic agent metabolism. Expect similar interactions with oxcarbazepine. **Cobicistat:** [P] Decreased metabolism of antineoplastic agents. **Conivaptan:** [P] Decreased metabolism of antineoplastic agents. **Cyclosporine:** [P] Decreased antineoplastic agent elimination. **Dabrafenib:** [NP] Increased antineoplastic agent metabolism. **Dexamethasone:** [P] Increased antineoplastic agent metabolism. **Enzalutamide:** [P] Increased antineoplastic agent metabolism. **Ivosidenib:** [NP] Increased antineoplastic agent metabolism. **Kinase inhibitors:** [P] Decreased metabolism of antineoplastic agents by ceritinib, cobimetinib, crizotinib, dasatinib, duvelisib, erlotinib, idelalisib, imatinib, lapatinib, larotrectinib, nilotinib, pacritinib, palbociclib, regorafenib, ribociclib, tucatinib, and ruxolitinib. **Lumacaftor:** [P] Increased antineoplastic agent metabolism. **Macrolide antibiotics:** [P] Clarithromycin, erythromycin, and telithromycin inhibit the elimination of antineoplastic agents. **Mitotane:** [NP] Increased antineoplastic agent metabolism. **Nefazodone:** [NP] Decreased antineoplastic agent metabolism. **Phenytoin:** [P] Increased antineoplastic agent metabolism. **Rifabutin:** [P] Increased antineoplastic agent metabolism. **Rifampin:** [P] Increased antineoplastic agent metabolism. **St. John's wort:** [NP] Increased antineoplastic agent metabolism.
Azole antifungals	Inhibition of CYP3A4 (itraconazole = ketoconazole > posaconazole > voriconazole > fluconazole). Inhibition of CYP2C9 (fluconazole, voriconazole). Inhibition of P-glycoprotein (itraconazole, ketoconazole, posaconazole). Susceptible to enzyme inducers (itraconazole, ketoconazole, voriconazole).	**Antivirals:** [P] Decreased metabolism of amprenavir, atazanavir, boceprevir, daclatasvir, darunavir, delavirdine, etravirine, fosamprenavir, indinavir, lopinavir, maraviroc, nelfinavir, rilpivirine, ritonavir, saquinavir, and tipranavir. **Barbiturates:** [P] Increased metabolism of itraconazole, ketoconazole, voriconazole. **Benzodiazepines:** [P] Decreased metabolism of alprazolam, midazolam, triazolam. **Calcium channel blockers:** [P] Decreased calcium channel blocker metabolism. **Carbamazepine:** [P] Decreased carbamazepine metabolism. Potential increased metabolism of itraconazole, ketoconazole, and voriconazole. **Colchicine:** [P] Decreased metabolism and transport of colchicine. **Cyclosporine:** [P] Decreased elimination of cyclosporine.

P, Predictable. Interaction occurs in most patients receiving the combination; NP, Not predictable. Interaction occurs only in some patients receiving the combination; NE, Not established. Insufficient data available on which to base estimate of predictability.

(continued)

TABLE 67–1 Important drug interactions. (Continued)

Drug or Drug Group	Properties Promoting Drug Interaction	Clinically Documented Interactions
Azole antifungals (*cont.*)		**Digoxin:** [NP] Increased plasma concentrations of digoxin with itraconazole, posaconazole, and ketoconazole.
		Eplerenone: [P] Decreased metabolism of eplerenone.
		Ergot alkaloids: [P] Decreased metabolism of ergot alkaloids.
		Everolimus: [P] Decreased metabolism of everolimus.
		HMG-CoA reductase inhibitors: [P] Decreased metabolism of lovastatin, simvastatin, and, to a lesser extent, atorvastatin.
		Kinase inhibitors: [P] Decreased metabolism of abemaciclib, acalabrutinib, alectinib, alpelisib, asciminib, axitinib, belumosudil, bosutinib brigatinib, cabozantinib, capmatinib, ceritinib cobimetinib, copanlisib, crizotinib, dabrafenib, dasatinib, duvelisib, encorafenib, entrectinib, erdafitinib, erlotinib, fedratinib, fostamatinib, gefitinib, gilteritinib, ibrutinib, idelalisib, imatinib, infigratinib, lapatinib, larotrectinib, lorlatinib, midostaurin, mobocertinib, neratinib, nilotinib, osimertinib, pacritinib, palbociclib, pazopanib, pemigatinib, pexidartinib, ponatinib, regorafenib, ribociclib, ripretinib, ruxolitinib, selpercatinib, sorafenib, sunitinib, tepotinib, tivozanib, tucatinib, upadacitinib, vandetanib, vemurafenib, and zanubrutinib.
		Opioid analgesics: [P] Decreased elimination of alfentanil, fentanyl, methadone, oxycodone, and sufentanil.
		Quinidine: [P] Decreased metabolism of quinidine.
		Phenytoin: [P] Decreased metabolism of phenytoin with fluconazole and probably voriconazole.
		Phosphodiesterase inhibitors: [P] Decreased metabolism of phosphodiesterase inhibitor.
		Pimozide: [NP] Decreased pimozide metabolism.
		Rifabutin: [P] Decreased rifabutin metabolism. Increased metabolism of itraconazole, ketoconazole, and voriconazole.
		Rifampin: [P] Increased metabolism of itraconazole, ketoconazole, and voriconazole.
		Sirolimus: [P] Decreased elimination of sirolimus.
		Tacrolimus: [P] Decreased elimination of tacrolimus.
		See also Acid-Reducing Agents; Anticoagulants, oral; Antineoplastic agents.
Barbiturates	Induction of hepatic microsomal drug metabolizing enzymes and P-glycoprotein. Additive central nervous system depression with other central nervous system depressants.	**Antivirals:** [P] Increased metabolism of antivirals amprenavir, atazanavir, boceprevir, darunavir, delavirdine, fosamprenavir, indinavir, nelfinavir, rilpivirine, ritonavir, saquinavir, simeprevir, and telaprevir with barbiturates.
		Beta-adrenoceptor blockers: [P] Increased β-blocker metabolism.
		Calcium channel blockers: [P] Increased calcium channel blocker metabolism.
		Central nervous system depressants: [P] Additive central nervous system depression.
		Colchicine: [P] Increased metabolism and transport of colchicine.
		Corticosteroids: [P] Increased corticosteroid metabolism.
		Cyclosporine: [P] Increased cyclosporine metabolism.
		Doxycycline: [P] Increased doxycycline metabolism.
		Eplerenone: [P] Increased metabolism of eplerenone.
		Ergot alkaloids: [P] Increased metabolism of ergot alkaloids.
		Estrogens: [P] Increased estrogen metabolism.
		Everolimus: [P] Increased metabolism of everolimus.
		HMG-CoA reductase inhibitors: [P] Increased metabolism of lovastatin, simvastatin, and, to a lesser extent, atorvastatin.
		Kinase inhibitors: [P] Increased metabolism of abemaciclib, acalabrutinib, alectinib, alpelisib, asciminib, axitinib, belumosudil, bosutinib brigatinib, cabozantinib, capmatinib, ceritinib cobimetinib, copanlisib, crizotinib, dabrafenib, dasatinib, duvelisib, encorafenib, entrectinib, erdafitinib, erlotinib, fedratinib, fostamatinib, gefitinib, gilteritinib, ibrutinib, idelalisib, imatinib, infigratinib, lapatinib, larotrectinib, lorlatinib, midostaurin, mobocertinib, neratinib, nilotinib, osimertinib, pacritinib, palbociclib, pazopanib, pemigatinib, pexidartinib, ponatinib, regorafenib, ribociclib, ripretinib, ruxolitinib, selpercatinib, sorafenib, sunitinib, tepotinib, tivozanib, tucatinib, upadacitinib, vandetanib, vemurafenib, and zanubrutinib.

P, Predictable. Interaction occurs in most patients receiving the combination; NP, Not predictable. Interaction occurs only in some patients receiving the combination; NE, Not established. Insufficient data available on which to base estimate of predictability.

(*continued*)

TABLE 67–1 Important drug interactions. (Continued)

Drug or Drug Group	Properties Promoting Drug Interaction	Clinically Documented Interactions
Barbiturates (*cont.*)		**Opioid analgesics:** [P] Increased elimination of alfentanil, fentanyl, methadone, oxycodone, and sufentanil. **Phenothiazine:** [P] Increased phenothiazine metabolism. **Phenytoin:** [P] Increased phenytoin metabolism. **Phosphodiesterase inhibitors:** [P] Increased metabolism of phosphodiesterase inhibitor. **Quinidine:** [P] Increased quinidine metabolism. **Sirolimus:** [NP] Increased sirolimus metabolism. **Tacrolimus:** [NP] Increased tacrolimus metabolism. **Theophylline:** [NP] Increased theophylline metabolism. **Valproic acid:** [P] Decreased phenobarbital metabolism. *See also* Anticoagulants, oral; Antidepressants, tricyclic; Antineoplastic agents; Azole antifungals.
Beta-adrenoceptor blockers	Beta blockade (especially with noncardioselective agents such as propranolol) alters response to sympathomimetics with β-agonist activity (eg, epinephrine, albuterol). Beta blockers that undergo extensive first-pass metabolism may be affected by drugs capable of altering this process.	***Drugs that may increase β-blocker effect:*** **Abiraterone:** [P] Decreased metabolism of β blockers metabolized by CYP2D6 (timolol, propranolol, nebivolol, metoprolol, carvedilol). **Amiodarone:** [P] Decreased metabolism of β blockers metabolized by CYP2D6 (timolol, propranolol, nebivolol, metoprolol, carvedilol). Enhanced effects on myocardial conduction. Expect similar interactions with dronedarone. **Bupropion:** [P] Decreased metabolism of β blockers metabolized by CYP2D6 (timolol, propranolol, nebivolol, metoprolol, carvedilol). **Cimetidine:** [P] Decreased metabolism of β blockers that are cleared primarily by the liver, eg, propranolol. Less effect (if any) on those cleared by the kidneys, eg, atenolol, nadolol. **Cinacalcet:** [P] Decreased metabolism of β blockers metabolized by CYP2D6 (timolol, propranolol, nebivolol, metoprolol, carvedilol). **Dacomitinib:** [P] Decreased metabolism of β blockers metabolized by CYP2D6 (timolol, propranolol, nebivolol, metoprolol, carvedilol). **Diphenhydramine:** [NP] Decreased metabolism of β blockers metabolized by CYP2D6 (timolol, propranolol, nebivolol, metoprolol, carvedilol). **Duloxetine:** [NP] Decreased metabolism of β blockers metabolized by CYP2D6 (timolol, propranolol, nebivolol, metoprolol, carvedilol). **Eliglustat:** [P] Decreased metabolism of β blockers metabolized by CYP2D6 (timolol, propranolol, nebivolol, metoprolol, carvedilol). **Haloperidol:** [P] Decreased metabolism of β blockers metabolized by CYP2D6 (timolol, propranolol, nebivolol, metoprolol, carvedilol). **Mirabegron:** [P] Decreased metabolism of β blockers metabolized by CYP2D6 (timolol, propranolol, nebivolol, metoprolol, carvedilol). **Quinidine:** [P] Decreased metabolism of β blockers metabolized by CYP2D6 (timolol, propranolol, nebivolol, metoprolol, carvedilol). **Selective serotonin reuptake inhibitors (SSRIs):** [P] Fluoxetine and paroxetine inhibit CYP2D6 and increase concentrations of timolol, propranolol, metoprolol, carvedilol, and nebivolol. **Terbinafine:** [P] Decreased metabolism of β blockers metabolized by CYP2D6 (timolol, propranolol, nebivolol, metoprolol, carvedilol). ***Drugs that may decrease β-blocker effect:*** **Nonsteroidal anti-inflammatory drugs (NSAIDs):** [NP] Indomethacin reduces antihypertensive response; other prostaglandin inhibitors probably also interact. ***Effects of β blockers on other drugs:*** **Clonidine:** [NP] Hypertensive reaction if clonidine is withdrawn; this is more likely to occur with noncardioselective beta blockers. **Insulin:** [P] Inhibition of glucose recovery from hypoglycemia; inhibition of symptoms of hypoglycemia (except sweating); increased blood pressure during hypoglycemia. **Prazosin:** [P] Increased hypotensive response to first dose of prazosin. **Sympathomimetics:** [P] Increased pressor response to epinephrine (and possibly other sympathomimetics); this is more likely to occur with noncardioselective β blockers. **Theophylline:** [NP] Decreased theophylline bronchodilation especially with noncardioselective β blockers. *See also* Barbiturates.

P, Predictable. Interaction occurs in most patients receiving the combination; NP, Not predictable. Interaction occurs only in some patients receiving the combination; NE, Not established. Insufficient data available on which to base estimate of predictability.

(*continued*)

TABLE 67–1 Important drug interactions. (Continued)

Drug or Drug Group	Properties Promoting Drug Interaction	Clinically Documented Interactions
Bile acid-binding resins	Resins (cholestyramine, colestipol, colesevelam) may bind with orally administered drugs in gastrointestinal tract. Resins may bind in gastrointestinal tract with drugs that undergo enterohepatic circulation, even if the latter are given parenterally.	**Acetaminophen:** [NE] Decreased gastrointestinal absorption of acetaminophen. **Deferasirox:** [NP] Decreased gastrointestinal absorption of deferasirox. **Digitalis glycosides:** [NP] Decreased gastrointestinal absorption of digitoxin (possibly also digoxin). **Furosemide:** [P] Decreased gastrointestinal absorption of furosemide. **Leflunomide:** [NP] Decreased gastrointestinal absorption of leflunomide. **Methotrexate:** [NP] Reduced gastrointestinal absorption of methotrexate. **Mycophenolate:** [P] Reduced gastrointestinal absorption of mycophenolate. **Raloxifene:** [NP] Decreased gastrointestinal absorption of raloxifene. **Thiazide diuretics:** [P] Reduced gastrointestinal absorption of thiazides. **Thyroid hormones:** [P] Reduced thyroid absorption. **Troglitazone:** [NP] Decreased gastrointestinal absorption of troglitazone. *See also* Anticoagulants, oral.
Calcium channel blockers	Verapamil, diltiazem, and perhaps nicardipine inhibit hepatic drug-metabolizing enzymes (CYP3A4) and P-glycoprotein. Metabolism (via CYP3A4) of amlodipine, diltiazem, felodipine, nicardipine, nifedipine, verapamil, and other calcium channel blockers subject to induction and inhibition.	**Amiodarone:** [P] Decreased metabolism of calcium channel blockers. Enhanced effects on myocardial conduction with bepridil, diltiazem, and verapamil. Expect similar interactions with dronedarone. **Antivirals:** [P] Amprenavir, atazanavir, boceprevir, darunavir, delavirdine, fosamprenavir, indinavir, nelfinavir, ritonavir, saquinavir, simeprevir, and telaprevir inhibit the metabolism of calcium channel blockers. Efavirenz and etravirine increase the metabolism of calcium channel blockers. **Bosentan:** [P] Increased metabolism of calcium channel blockers. **Carbamazepine:** [P] Decreased carbamazepine metabolism with diltiazem and verapamil; possible increase in calcium channel blocker metabolism. **Cimetidine:** [NP] Decreased metabolism of calcium channel blockers. **Cobicistat:** [P] Decreased metabolism of calcium channel blockers. **Colchicine:** [P] Decreased colchicine elimination with diltiazem, nicardipine, and verapamil. **Conivaptan:** [P] Decreased metabolism of calcium channel blockers. **Cyclosporine:** [P] Decreased cyclosporine elimination with diltiazem, nicardipine, verapamil. **Digitalis glycosides:** [P] Decreased elimination of digitalis glycoside with bepridil, diltiazem and verapamil. **Eplerenone:** [NP] Decreased metabolism of eplerenone with diltiazem, nicardipine, verapamil. **Ergot alkaloids:** [NP] Decreased metabolism of ergot alkaloids with diltiazem, nicardipine, verapamil. **Kinase inhibitors:** [NP] Decreased metabolism of abemaciclib, acalabrutinib, alectinib, alpelisib, asciminib, axitinib, belumosudil, bosutinib brigatinib, cabozantinib, capmatinib, ceritinib cobimetinib, copanlisib, crizotinib, dabrafenib, dasatinib, duvelisib, encorafenib, entrectinib, erdafitinib, erlotinib, fedratinib, fostamatinib, gefitinib, gilteritinib, ibrutinib, idelalisib, imatinib, infigratinib, lapatinib, larotrectinib, lorlatinib, midostaurin, mobocertinib, neratinib, nilotinib, osimertinib, pacritinib, palbociclib, pazopanib, pemigatinib, pexidartinib, ponatinib, regorafenib, ribociclib, ripretinib, ruxolitinib, selpercatinib, sorafenib, sunitinib, tepotinib, tivozanib, tucatinib, upadacitinib, vandetanib, vemurafenib, and zanubrutinib with diltiazem, nicardipine, verapamil. Decreased metabolism of calcium channel blockers by ceritinib, cobimetinib, crizotinib, dasatinib, duvelisib, erlotinib, idelalisib, imatinib, lapatinib, larotrectinib, nilotinib, pacritinib, palbociclib, regorafenib, ribociclib, tucatinib, and ruxolitinib. **Macrolide antibiotics:** [P] Clarithromycin, erythromycin, and telithromycin inhibit the elimination of calcium channel blockers. **Nefazodone:** [NP] Decreased calcium channel blocker metabolism. **Opioid analgesics:** [NP] Decreased elimination of alfentanil, fentanyl, methadone, oxycodone, and sufentanil by diltiazem, nicardipine, and verapamil. **Phenytoin:** [P] Increased metabolism of calcium channel blockers. **Rifabutin:** [P] Increased calcium channel blocker metabolism. **Rifampin:** [P] Increased metabolism of calcium channel blockers. **Sirolimus:** [P] Decreased sirolimus elimination with diltiazem, nicardipine, and verapamil. **Statins:** [P] Decreased atorvastatin, lovastatin, and simvastatin elimination with diltiazem, nicardipine, and verapamil. **St. John's wort:** [NP] Increased calcium channel blocker metabolism. **Tacrolimus:** [P] Decreased tacrolimus elimination with diltiazem, nicardipine, and verapamil. **Theophylline:** [P] Decreased theophylline metabolism with diltiazem, nicardipine, and verapamil. *See also* Azole antifungals; Barbiturates.

P, Predictable. Interaction occurs in most patients receiving the combination; NP, Not predictable. Interaction occurs only in some patients receiving the combination; NE, Not established. Insufficient data available on which to base estimate of predictability.

(*continued*)

TABLE 67–1 Important drug interactions. (Continued)

Drug or Drug Group	Properties Promoting Drug Interaction	Clinically Documented Interactions
Carbamazepine	Induction of hepatic microsomal drug-metabolizing enzymes and P-glycoprotein. Susceptible to induction and inhibition of metabolism, primarily by CYP3A4.	**Amiodarone:** [P] Decreased metabolism of carbamazepine; increased metabolism of amiodarone. Expect similar interactions with dronedarone. **Antivirals:** [P] Amprenavir, atazanavir, boceprevir, darunavir, delavirdine, fosamprenavir, indinavir, nelfinavir, ritonavir, saquinavir, simeprevir, and telaprevir inhibit the metabolism of carbamazepine. Efavirenz and etravirine increase the metabolism of carbamazepine. Increased metabolism of antivirals by carbamazepine. **Bosentan:** [P] Increased carbamazepine metabolism. **Cimetidine:** [P] Decreased carbamazepine metabolism. **Cobicistat:** [P] Decreased metabolism of carbamazepine. **Conivaptan:** [P] Decreased metabolism of carbamazepine. **Corticosteroids:** [P] Increased corticosteroid metabolism. **Cyclosporine:** [P] Increased cyclosporine metabolism and possible decreased carbamazepine metabolism. **Dabrafenib:** [NP] Increased carbamazepine metabolism. **Danazol:** [P] Decreased carbamazepine metabolism. **Digitalis glycosides:** [P] Increased digoxin elimination. **Enzalutamide:** [P] Increased carbamazepine metabolism. **Eplerenone:** [P] Increased metabolism of eplerenone. **Ergot alkaloids:** [P] Increased metabolism of ergot alkaloids. **Fluvoxamine:** [NP] Decreased carbamazepine metabolism. **Estrogens:** [P] Increased estrogen metabolism. **Everolimus:** [P] Increased metabolism of everolimus. **Haloperidol:** [P] Increased haloperidol metabolism. **HMG-CoA reductase inhibitors:** [P] Increased metabolism of lovastatin, simvastatin, and, to a lesser extent, atorvastatin. **Isoniazid:** [P] Decreased carbamazepine metabolism. **Ivosidenib:** [NP] Increased carbamazepine metabolism. **Kinase inhibitors:** [P] Increased metabolism of abemaciclib, acalabrutinib, alectinib, alpelisib, asciminib, axitinib, belumosudil, bosutinib brigatinib, cabozantinib, capmatinib, ceritinib cobimetinib, copanlisib, crizotinib, dabrafenib, dasatinib, duvelisib, encorafenib, entrectinib, erdafitinib, erlotinib, fedratinib, fostamatinib, gefitinib, gilteritinib, ibrutinib, idelalisib, imatinib, infigratinib, lapatinib, larotrectinib, lorlatinib, midostaurin, mobocertinib, neratinib, nilotinib, osimertinib, pacritinib, palbociclib, pazopanib, pemigatinib, pexidartinib, ponatinib, regorafenib, ribociclib, ripretinib, ruxolitinib, selpercatinib, sorafenib, sunitinib, tepotinib, tivozanib, tucatinib, upadacitinib, vandetanib, vemurafenib, and zanubrutinib. Decreased metabolism of carbamazepine by ceritinib, cobimetinib, crizotinib, dasatinib, duvelisib, erlotinib, idelalisib, imatinib, lapatinib, larotrectinib, nilotinib, pacritinib, palbociclib, regorafenib, ribociclib, tucatinib, and ruxolitinib. **Lumacaftor:** [P] Increased carbamazepine metabolism. **Macrolide antibiotics:** [P] Clarithromycin, erythromycin, and telithromycin inhibit the elimination of carbamazepine. **Mitotane:** [NP] Increased carbamazepine metabolism. **Nefazodone:** [NP] Decreased carbamazepine metabolism. **Opioid analgesics:** [P] Increased elimination of alfentanil, fentanyl, methadone, oxycodone, and sufentanil. **Phenytoin:** [P] Increased carbamazepine and phenytoin metabolism. **Rifabutin:** [P] Increased carbamazepine metabolism. **Rifampin:** [P] Increased carbamazepine metabolism. **Selective serotonin reuptake inhibitors (SSRIs):** [NE] Fluoxetine and fluvoxamine decrease carbamazepine metabolism. **Sirolimus:** [P] Increased sirolimus metabolism. **St. John's wort:** [P] Increased carbamazepine metabolism. **Tacrolimus:** [P] Increased tacrolimus metabolism. **Theophylline:** [NP] Increased theophylline metabolism. *See also* Anticoagulants, oral; Antidepressants, tricyclic; Antineoplastic agents; Azole antifungals; Calcium channel blockers.

P, Predictable. Interaction occurs in most patients receiving the combination; NP, Not predictable. Interaction occurs only in some patients receiving the combination; NE, Not established. Insufficient data available on which to base estimate of predictability.

(*continued*)

TABLE 67–1 Important drug interactions. (Continued)

Drug or Drug Group	Properties Promoting Drug Interaction	Clinically Documented Interactions
Cimetidine	Inhibits hepatic microsomal drug-metabolizing enzymes. (Ranitidine, famotidine, and nizatidine do not.) May inhibit the renal tubular secretion of weak bases. See also Acid-reducing agents.	**Antivirals:** [P] Decreased metabolism of amprenavir, atazanavir, boceprevir, daclatasvir, darunavir, delavirdine, etravirine, fosamprenavir, indinavir, lopinavir, maraviroc, nelfinavir, rilpivirine, ritonavir, saquinavir, and tipranavir. **Benzodiazepines:** [P] Decreased metabolism of alprazolam, chlordiazepoxide, diazepam, halazepam, prazepam, and clorazepate but not oxazepam, lorazepam, or temazepam. **Carmustine:** [NE] Increased bone marrow suppression. **Dofetilide:** [NP] Decreased renal excretion of dofetilide. **Eplerenone:** [P] Decreased metabolism of eplerenone. **Ergot alkaloids:** [P] Decreased metabolism of ergot alkaloids. **HMG-CoA reductase inhibitors:** [P] Decreased metabolism of lovastatin, simvastatin, and, to a lesser extent, atorvastatin. **Kinase inhibitors:** [NP] Decreased metabolism of abemaciclib, acalabrutinib, alectinib, alpelisib, asciminib, axitinib, belumosudil, bosutinib brigatinib, cabozantinib, capmatinib, ceritinib cobimetinib, copanlisib, crizotinib, dabrafenib, dasatinib, duvelisib, encorafenib, entrectinib, erdafitinib, erlotinib, fedratinib, fostamatinib, gefitinib, gilteritinib, ibrutinib, idelalisib, imatinib, infigratinib, lapatinib, larotrectinib, lorlatinib, midostaurin, mobocertinib, neratinib, nilotinib, osimertinib, pacritinib, palbociclib, pazopanib, pemigatinib, pexidartinib, ponatinib, regorafenib, ribociclib, ripretinib, ruxolitinib, selpercatinib, sorafenib, sunitinib, tepotinib, tivozanib, tucatinib, upadacitinib, vandetanib, vemurafenib, and zanubrutinib. **Lidocaine:** [P] Decreased metabolism of lidocaine. **Opioid analgesics:** [NP] Decreased elimination of alfentanil, fentanyl, methadone, oxycodone, and sufentanil. **Phenytoin:** [NP] Decreased phenytoin metabolism. **Phosphodiesterase inhibitors:** [NP] Decreased metabolism of phosphodiesterase inhibitor. **Procainamide:** [P] Decreased renal excretion of procainamide. **Quinidine:** [P] Decreased metabolism of quinidine. **Theophylline:** [P] Decreased theophylline metabolism. **Tizanidine:** [NP] Decreased tizanidine metabolism. *See also* Anticoagulants, oral; Antidepressants, tricyclic; Azole antifungals; β-Adrenoceptor blockers; Calcium channel blockers; Carbamazepine.
Colchicine	Susceptible to changes in CYP3A4 metabolism and P-glycoprotein transport.	**Amiodarone:** [P] Decreased colchicine metabolism and transport. Expect similar interactions with dronedarone. **Antivirals:** [P] Amprenavir, atazanavir, boceprevir, darunavir, delavirdine, fosamprenavir, indinavir, nelfinavir, ritonavir, saquinavir, simeprevir, and telaprevir inhibit the metabolism of colchicine. Efavirenz and etravirine increase the metabolism of colchicine. **Carbamazepine:** [P] Increased metabolism of colchicine. **Cobicistat:** [P] Decreased metabolism of colchicine. **Conivaptan:** [P] Decreased metabolism of colchicine. **Cyclosporine:** [P] Decreased colchicine elimination. **Dabrafenib:** [NP] Increased colchicine elimination. **Ivosidenib:** [NP] Increased colchicine elimination. **Kinase inhibitors:** [P] Decreased metabolism of colchicine with ceritinib, cobimetinib, crizotinib, dasatinib, duvelisib, erlotinib, idelalisib, imatinib, lapatinib, larotrectinib, nilotinib, pacritinib, palbociclib, regorafenib, ribociclib, tucatinib, and ruxolitinib. **Macrolide antibiotics:** [P] Clarithromycin, erythromycin, and telithromycin inhibit the elimination of colchicine. **Mifepristone:** [NP] Decreased colchicine metabolism. **Mitotane:** [NP] Increased colchicine metabolism. **Nefazodone:** [NP] Decreased colchicine metabolism. **Ranolazine:** [NP] Decreased colchicine metabolism. **Rifabutin:** [P] Increased colchicine metabolism. **Rifampin:** [P] Increased colchicine metabolism. **St. John's wort:** [NP] Increased colchicine metabolism. *See also* Azole antifungals; Calcium channel blockers.

P, Predictable. Interaction occurs in most patients receiving the combination; NP, Not predictable. Interaction occurs only in some patients receiving the combination; NE, Not established. Insufficient data available on which to base estimate of predictability.

(*continued*)

TABLE 67–1 Important drug interactions. (Continued)

Drug or Drug Group	Properties Promoting Drug Interaction	Clinically Documented Interactions
Cyclosporine	Susceptible to induction and inhibition of elimination by CYP3A4 and P-glycoprotein. (Tacrolimus and sirolimus appear to have similar interactions.)	**Aminoglycosides:** [NP] Possible additive nephrotoxicity. **Amphotericin B:** [NP] Possible additive nephrotoxicity. **Cidofovir:** [NP] Possible additive nephrotoxicity. ***Drugs that may increase cyclosporine effect:*** **Amiodarone:** [P] Decreased cyclosporine elimination. Expect similar interaction with dronedarone. **Androgens:** [NE] Increased serum cyclosporine concentration. **Antivirals:** [P] Amprenavir, atazanavir, boceprevir, darunavir, delavirdine, fosamprenavir, indinavir, nelfinavir, ritonavir, saquinavir, simeprevir, and telaprevir inhibit the elimination of cyclosporine. **Cobicistat:** [P] Decreased cyclosporine elimination. **Conivaptan:** [P] Decreased cyclosporine elimination. **HMG-CoA reductase inhibitors:** [NP] Decreased metabolism of atorvastatin, lovastatin, and simvastatin. Myopathy and rhabdomyolysis noted in patients taking statins and cyclosporine. **Kinase inhibitors:** [P] Decreased metabolism of cyclosporine by ceritinib, cobimetinib, crizotinib, dasatinib, duvelisib, erlotinib, idelalisib, imatinib, lapatinib, larotrectinib, nilotinib, pacritinib, palbociclib, regorafenib, ribociclib, tucatinib, and ruxolitinib. Cyclosporine reduces metabolism of kinase inhibitors. **Macrolide antibiotics:** [P] Clarithromycin, erythromycin, and telithromycin inhibit the elimination of cyclosporine. **Nefazodone:** [P] Decreased cyclosporine metabolism. **Quinupristin:** [P] Decreased cyclosporine metabolism. ***Drugs that may decrease cyclosporine effect:*** **Antivirals:** [P] Efavirenz, etravirine, and nevirapine may increase the metabolism of cyclosporine. **Bosentan:** [P] Increased cyclosporine elimination. **Dabrafenib:** [NP] Increased cyclosporine elimination. **Dexamethasone:** [NP] Increased cyclosporine metabolism. **Enzalutamide:** [P] Increased cyclosporine metabolism. **Ivosidenib:** [NP] Increased cyclosporine elimination. **Lumacaftor:** [P] Increased cyclosporine metabolism. **Mitotane:** [NP] Increased cyclosporine metabolism. **Phenytoin:** [P] Increased cyclosporine metabolism. **Rifabutin:** [NP] Increased cyclosporine elimination. **Rifampin:** [P] Increased cyclosporine elimination. **St. John's wort:** [NP] Increased cyclosporine elimination. *See also* Azole antifungals; Barbiturates; Calcium channel blockers; Carbamazepine.

P, Predictable. Interaction occurs in most patients receiving the combination; NP, Not predictable. Interaction occurs only in some patients receiving the combination; NE, Not established. Insufficient data available on which to base estimate of predictability.

(*continued*)

TABLE 67–1 Important drug interactions. (Continued)

Drug or Drug Group	Properties Promoting Drug Interaction	Clinically Documented Interactions
Digitalis glycosides	Digoxin susceptible to alteration of gastrointestinal absorption. Renal and non-renal excretion of digoxin susceptible to inhibition. Digitalis toxicity may be increased by drug-induced electrolyte imbalance (eg, hypokalemia).	***Drugs that may increase digitalis effect:***
		Amiodarone: [P] Increased digoxin plasma concentrations. Expect similar interaction with dronedarone.
		Antivirals: [P] Daclatasvir, indinavir, nelfinavir, paritaprevir, ritonavir, saquinavir, and telaprevir reduce the elimination of digoxin.
		Cobicistat: [P] Increased digoxin plasma concentrations.
		Conivaptan: [P] Increased digoxin plasma concentrations.
		Cyclosporine: [P] Increased digoxin plasma concentrations.
		Lapatinib: [NP] Increased digoxin plasma concentrations.
		Macrolide antibiotics: [P] Azithromycin, clarithromycin, and erythromycin inhibit the elimination of digoxin.
		Potassium-depleting drugs: [P] Increased likelihood of digitalis toxicity.
		Propafenone: [P] Increased digoxin plasma concentrations.
		Quinidine: [P] Increased digoxin plasma concentrations; displaces digoxin from tissue binding sites.
		Spironolactone: [NP] Increased digoxin plasma concentrations.
		Tacrolimus: [P] Increased digoxin plasma concentrations.
		Ticagrelor: [P] Increased digoxin plasma concentrations.
		Valspodar: [NE] Increased digoxin plasma concentrations.
		Vemurafenib: [NP] Increased digoxin plasma concentrations
		See also Azole antifungals; Calcium channel blockers.
		Drugs that may decrease digitalis effect:
		Kaolin-pectin: [P] Decreased gastrointestinal digoxin absorption.
		Rifampin: [NP] Increased metabolism of digitoxin and elimination of digoxin.
		St. John's wort: [NP] Increased digoxin elimination.
		Sulfasalazine: [NE] Decreased gastrointestinal digoxin absorption.
		See also Acid reducing agents; Azole antifungals; Bile acid-binding resins; Calcium channel blockers; Carbamazepine.
Disulfiram	Inhibits CYP2C9. Inhibits aldehyde dehydrogenase.	**Benzodiazepines:** [P] Decreased metabolism of chlordiazepoxide and diazepam but not lorazepam and oxazepam.
		Metronidazole: [NE] Confusion and psychoses reported in patients receiving this combination; mechanisms unknown.
		Phenytoin: [P] Decreased phenytoin metabolism.
		See also Alcohol; Anticoagulants, oral.

P, Predictable. Interaction occurs in most patients receiving the combination; NP, Not predictable. Interaction occurs only in some patients receiving the combination; NE, Not established. Insufficient data available on which to base estimate of predictability.

(*continued*)

TABLE 67–1 Important drug interactions. (Continued)

Drug or Drug Group	Properties Promoting Drug Interaction	Clinically Documented Interactions
Estrogens	Estrogen metabolism (CYP3A4) susceptible to induction and inhibition. Enterohepatic circulation of estrogen may be interrupted by alteration in bowel flora (eg, due to antibiotics).	**Ampicillin:** [NP] Interruption of enterohepatic circulation of estrogen; possible reduction in oral contraceptive efficacy. Some other oral antibiotics may have a similar effect. **Antivirals:** [P] Efavirenz, etravirine, and nevirapine may reduce oral contraceptive efficacy. **Bexarotene:** [P] Increased estrogen metabolism, possible reduction in oral contraceptive efficacy. **Bosentan:** [NP] Enzyme induction leading to reduced estrogen effect. **Corticosteroids:** [NP] Decreased metabolism of corticosteroids leading to increased corticosteroid effect. Dexamethasone may increase estrogen metabolism. **Dabrafenib:** [NP] Increased estrogen metabolism, possible reduction in oral contraceptive efficacy. **Enzalutamide:** [P] Increased estrogen metabolism, possible reduction in oral contraceptive efficacy. **Griseofulvin:** [NP] Increased estrogen metabolism, possible reduction in oral contraceptive efficacy. **Ivosidenib:** [NP] Increased estrogen metabolism, possible reduction in oral contraceptive efficacy. **Lumacaftor:** [P] Increased estrogen metabolism, possible reduction in oral contraceptive efficacy. **Mitotane:** [NP] Increased estrogen metabolism, possible reduction in oral contraceptive efficacy. **Nafcillin:** [NP] Increased estrogen metabolism, possible reduction in oral contraceptive efficacy. **Phenytoin:** [P] Increased estrogen metabolism; possible reduction in oral contraceptive efficacy. **Primidone:** [P] Increased estrogen metabolism; possible reduction in oral contraceptive efficacy. **Rifabutin:** [P] Increased estrogen metabolism; possible reduction in oral contraceptive efficacy. **Rifampin:** [P] Increased estrogen metabolism; possible reduction in oral contraceptive efficacy. **St. John's wort:** [P] Increased estrogen metabolism; possible reduction in oral contraceptive efficacy. *See also* Barbiturates; Carbamazepine.
HMG-CoA reductase inhibitors (statins)	Lovastatin, simvastatin, and, to a lesser extent, atorvastatin are susceptible to CYP3A4 inhibitors and inducers; additive risk with other drugs that can cause myopathy.	**Amiodarone:** [NP] Decreased atorvastatin, lovastatin, and simvastatin metabolism. Expect similar interactions with dronedarone. **Antivirals:** [P] Amprenavir, atazanavir, boceprevir, darunavir, delavirdine, fosamprenavir, indinavir, nelfinavir, ritonavir, saquinavir, simeprevir, and telaprevir inhibit the metabolism of atorvastatin, lovastatin, and simvastatin. Efavirenz and etravirine increase the metabolism of atorvastatin, lovastatin, and simvastatin. **Bosentan:** [P] Increased atorvastatin, lovastatin, and simvastatin metabolism. **Carbamazepine:** [P] Increased atorvastatin, lovastatin, and simvastatin metabolism. **Clofibrate:** [NP] Increased risk of myopathy. **Cobicistat:** [P] Decreased metabolism of atorvastatin, lovastatin, and simvastatin. **Conivaptan:** [P] Decreased metabolism of atorvastatin, lovastatin, and simvastatin. **Cyclosporine:** [P] Decreased atorvastatin, lovastatin, rosuvastatin, pitavastatin, and simvastatin elimination.

P, Predictable. Interaction occurs in most patients receiving the combination; NP, Not predictable. Interaction occurs only in some patients receiving the combination; NE, Not established. Insufficient data available on which to base estimate of predictability.

(*continued*)

TABLE 67–1 Important drug interactions. (Continued)

Drug or Drug Group	Properties Promoting Drug Interaction	Clinically Documented Interactions
HMG-CoA reductase inhibitors (statins) (*cont.*)		**Dabrafenib:** [NP] Increased atorvastatin, lovastatin, and simvastatin metabolism. **Gemfibrozil:** [NP] Increased plasma lovastatin and simvastatin and increased risk of myopathy. **Ivosidenib:** [NP] Increased atorvastatin, lovastatin, and simvastatin metabolism. **Kinase inhibitors:** [P] Decreased metabolism of atorvastatin, lovastatin, and simvastatin by ceritinib, cobimetinib, crizotinib, dasatinib, duvelisib, erlotinib, idelalisib, imatinib, lapatinib, larotrectinib, nilotinib, pacritinib, palbociclib, regorafenib, ribociclib, tucatinib, and ruxolitinib. **Macrolide antibiotics:** [P] Clarithromycin and erythromycin inhibit the elimination of statins. **Mitotane:** [NP] Increased atorvastatin, lovastatin, and simvastatin metabolism. **Nefazodone:** [NP] Decreased atorvastatin, lovastatin, and simvastatin metabolism. **Phenytoin:** [P] Increased atorvastatin, lovastatin, and simvastatin metabolism. **Rifampin:** [P] Increased atorvastatin, lovastatin, and simvastatin metabolism. **St. John's wort:** [NP] Increased atorvastatin, lovastatin, and simvastatin metabolism. *See also* Azole antifungals; Barbiturates; Calcium channel blockers; Cyclosporine.
Iron	Binds with drugs in gastrointestinal tract, reducing absorption.	**Methyldopa:** [NE] Decreased methyldopa absorption. **Mycophenolate:** [P] Decreased mycophenolate absorption. **Quinolones:** [P] Decreased absorption of ciprofloxacin and other quinolones. **Tetracyclines:** [P] Decreased absorption of tetracyclines; decreased efficacy of iron. **Thyroid hormones:** [P] Decreased thyroxine absorption. *See also* Antacids.
Kinase Inhibitors	Substrates of CYP3A4 susceptible to induction and inhibition of metabolism: abemaciclib, acalabrutinib, alectinib, alpelisib, asciminib, axitinib, belumosudil, bosutinib brigatinib, cabozantinib, capmatinib, ceritinib cobimetinib, copanlisib, crizotinib, dabrafenib, dasatinib, duvelisib, encorafenib, entrectinib, erdafitinib, erlotinib, fedratinib, fostamatinib, gefitinib, gilteritinib, ibrutinib, idelalisib, imatinib, infigratinib, lapatinib, larotrectinib, lorlatinib, midostaurin, mobocertinib, neratinib, nilotinib, osimertinib, pacritinib, palbociclib, pazopanib, pemigatinib, pexidartinib, ponatinib, regorafenib, ribociclib, ripretinib, ruxolitinib, selpercatinib, sorafenib, sunitinib, tepotinib, tivozanib, tucatinib, upadacitinib, vandetanib, vemurafenib, and zanubrutinib.	**Amiodarone:** [NP] Decreased kinase inhibitor metabolism. Expect similar interactions with dronedarone. **Antivirals:** [P] Amprenavir, atazanavir, boceprevir, darunavir, delavirdine, fosamprenavir, indinavir, nelfinavir, ritonavir, saquinavir, simeprevir, and telaprevir inhibit the metabolism of kinase inhibitor. Efavirenz and etravirine increase the metabolism of kinase inhibitors. **Bosentan:** [P] Increased kinase inhibitor metabolism. **Cobicistat:** [P] Decreased metabolism of kinase inhibitors. **Conivaptan:** [P] Decreased metabolism of kinase inhibitors. **Cyclosporine:** [P] Decreased kinase inhibitor elimination. **Dabrafenib:** [NP] Increased kinase inhibitor elimination. **Dexamethasone:** [P] Increased kinase inhibitor metabolism. **Enzalutamide:** [P] Increased kinase inhibitor metabolism. **Ivosidenib:** [NP] Increased kinase inhibitor metabolism. **Lumacaftor:** [P] Increased kinase inhibitor metabolism. **Macrolide antibiotics:** [P] Clarithromycin, erythromycin, and telithromycin inhibit the elimination of kinase inhibitors. **Mitotane:** [NP] Increased kinase inhibitor metabolism. **Nefazodone:** [NP] Decreased kinase inhibitor metabolism. **Phenytoin:** [P] Increased kinase inhibitor metabolism. **Rifabutin:** [P] Increased kinase inhibitor metabolism. **Rifampin:** [P] Increased kinase inhibitor metabolism. **St. John's wort:** [NP] Increased kinase inhibitor metabolism. *See also* Azole antifungals; Barbiturates; Calcium channel blockers; Carbamazepine; Colchicine.

P, Predictable. Interaction occurs in most patients receiving the combination; NP, Not predictable. Interaction occurs only in some patients receiving the combination; NE, Not established. Insufficient data available on which to base estimate of predictability.

(*continued*)

TABLE 67–1 Important drug interactions. (Continued)

Drug or Drug Group	Properties Promoting Drug Interaction	Clinically Documented Interactions
Levodopa	Levodopa degraded in gut prior to reaching sites of absorption. Agents that alter gastrointestinal motility may alter degree of intraluminal degradation. Antiparkinsonism effect of levodopa susceptible to inhibition by other drugs.	**Clonidine:** [NE] Inhibited antiparkinsonism effect. **Haloperidol:** [NP] Inhibited antiparkinsonism effect. **Metoclopramide:** [NP] Inhibited antiparkinsonism effect. **Monoamine oxidase inhibitors (MAOIs):** [P] Hypertensive reaction (carbidopa prevents the interaction). **Papaverine:** [NE] Inhibited antiparkinsonism effect. **Phenothiazines:** [P] Inhibited antiparkinsonism effect. **Phenytoin:** [NE] Inhibited antiparkinsonism effect. **Pyridoxine:** [P] Inhibited antiparkinsonism effect (carbidopa prevents the interaction).
Lithium	Renal lithium excretion sensitive to changes in sodium balance. (Sodium depletion tends to cause lithium retention.) Susceptible to drugs enhancing central nervous system lithium toxicity.	**ACE inhibitors (ACEIs):** [NP] Reduce renal clearance of lithium; increase lithium effect. **Angiotensin II receptor blockers (ARBs):** [NP] Reduce renal clearance of lithium; increase lithium effect. **Diuretics (especially thiazides):** [P] Decreased renal clearance of lithium; furosemide may be less likely to produce this effect than thiazide diuretics. **Haloperidol:** [NP] Occasional cases of neurotoxicity in manic patients, especially with large doses of one or both drugs. **Methyldopa:** [NE] Increased likelihood of central nervous system lithium toxicity. **Nonsteroidal anti-inflammatory drugs (NSAIDs):** [NP] Reduced renal lithium excretion (except sulindac and salicylates). **Theophylline:** [P] Increased renal excretion of lithium; reduced lithium effect.
Macrolides	The macrolides clarithromycin and erythromycin are known to inhibit CYP3A4 and P-glycoprotein. Azithromycin does not appear to inhibit CYP3A4 but is a modest inhibitor of P-glycoprotein.	**Benzodiazepines:** [P] Decreased metabolism of alprazolam, midazolam, and triazolam. **Eplerenone:** [P] Decreased metabolism of eplerenone. **Ergot alkaloids:** [P] Decreased elimination of ergot alkaloids. **Opioid analgesics:** [P] Decreased elimination of alfentanil, fentanyl, methadone, oxycodone, and sufentanil. **Phosphodiesterase inhibitors:** [P] Decreased metabolism of phosphodiesterase inhibitor. **Pimozide:** [P] Increased pimozide concentrations. **Quinidine:** [P] Increased serum quinidine concentrations. **Theophylline:** [P] Decreased metabolism of theophylline. *See also* Anticoagulants, oral; Calcium channel blockers; Carbamazepine; Colchicine; Cyclosporine; Digitalis glycosides; HMG-CoA reductase inhibitors; Kinase inhibitors.
Monoamine oxidase inhibitors (MAOIs)	Increased norepinephrine stored in adrenergic neuron. Displacement of these stores by other drugs may produce acute hypertensive response. MAOIs have intrinsic hypoglycemic activity.	**Amphetamine:** [P] Severe reactions (hyperpyrexia, coma, death) have been reported. **Anorexiants:** [P] Hypertensive episodes due to release of stored norepinephrine (benzphetamine, diethylpropion, mazindol, phendimetrazine, phentermine). **Antidiabetic agents:** [P] Additive hypoglycemic effect. **Buspirone:** [NP] Possible serotonin syndrome; *avoid* concurrent use. **Cocaine:** [P] Severe reactions (hyperpyrexia, coma, death) have been reported. **Dextromethorphan:** [NP] Severe reactions (hyperpyrexia, coma, death) have been reported. **Guanethidine:** [P] Reversal of the hypotensive action of guanethidine. **Opioid analgesics:** [NP] Some patients develop hypertension, rigidity, excitation; meperidine, tramadol, and pentazocine more likely to interact than morphine, codeine, oxycodone, or fentanyl; *avoid* concurrent use. **Phenylephrine:** [P] Hypertensive episode, since phenylephrine is metabolized by monoamine oxidase.

P, Predictable. Interaction occurs in most patients receiving the combination; NP, Not predictable. Interaction occurs only in some patients receiving the combination; NE, Not established. Insufficient data available on which to base estimate of predictability.

(*continued*)

TABLE 67–1 Important drug interactions. (Continued)

Drug or Drug Group	Properties Promoting Drug Interaction	Clinically Documented Interactions
Monoamine oxidase inhibitors (MAOIs) (*cont.*)		**Selective serotonin reuptake inhibitors (SSRIs):** [P] Fatalities have occurred due to serotonin syndrome; contraindicated in patients taking MAOIs; *avoid* concurrent use. **Serotonin norepinephrine inhibitors:** [P] Fatalities have occurred due to serotonin syndrome; contraindicated in patients taking MAOIs; *avoid* concurrent use. **Sibutramine:** [NE] Possible serotonin syndrome; *avoid* concurrent use. **Sympathomimetics (indirect-acting):** [P] Hypertensive episode due to release of stored norepinephrine (amphetamines, ephedrine, isometheptene, phenylpropanolamine, pseudoephedrine). *See also* Antidepressants, tricyclic and heterocyclic; Levodopa.
Nonsteroidal anti-inflammatory drugs (NSAIDs)	Prostaglandin inhibition may result in reduced renal sodium excretion, impaired resistance to hypertensive stimuli, and reduced renal lithium excretion. Most NSAIDs inhibit platelet function; may increase likelihood of bleeding due to other drugs that impair hemostasis.	**ACE inhibitors (ACEIs):** [P] Decreased antihypertensive response. **Angiotensin II receptor blockers (ARBs):** [P] Decreased antihypertensive response. **Furosemide:** [P] Decreased diuretic, natriuretic, and antihypertensive response to furosemide. **Hydralazine:** [NE] Decreased antihypertensive response to hydralazine. **Methotrexate:** [NP] Possibly increased methotrexate toxicity (especially with anticancer doses of methotrexate). **Selective serotonin reuptake inhibitors (SSRIs):** [P] Increased risk of bleeding due to platelet inhibition. **Thiazide diuretics:** [P] Decreased diuretic, natriuretic, and antihypertensive response. **Triamterene:** [NE] Decreased renal function noted with triamterene plus indomethacin in both healthy subjects and patients. *See also* Anticoagulants, oral; β-Adrenoceptor blockers; Lithium.
Opioid analgesics	Opioid analgesics that are substrates of CYP3A4 (alfentanil, fentanyl, hydrocodone, oxycodone, sufentanil, and to a lesser extent methadone) are susceptible to inhibitors and inducers. Methadone is primarily metabolized by CYP2B6. Additive central nervous system depression with other central nervous system depressants.	**Amiodarone:** [NP] Decreased CYP3A4-dependent opioid metabolism. Expect similar interactions with dronedarone. **Antivirals:** [P] Amprenavir, atazanavir, boceprevir, darunavir, delavirdine, fosamprenavir, indinavir, nelfinavir, ritonavir, saquinavir, simeprevir, and telaprevir inhibit the metabolism of CYP3A4-dependent opioids. Efavirenz and etravirine increase the metabolism of CYP3A4-dependent opioids. Efavirenz increases the CYP2B6 metabolism of methadone. **Bosentan:** [P] Increased CYP3A4-dependent opioid metabolism. **Cobicistat:** [P] Decreased metabolism of CYP3A4-dependent opioids. **Conivaptan:** [P] Decreased metabolism of CYP3A4-dependent opioids. **Cyclosporine:** [P] Decreased CYP3A4-dependent opioid elimination. **Dabrafenib:** [NP] Increased CYP3A4-dependent opioid elimination. **Dexamethasone:** [P] Increased CYP3A4-dependent opioid metabolism. **Enzalutamide:** [P] Increased CYP3A4-dependent opioid metabolism. **Ivosidenib:** [NP] Increased CYP3A4-dependent opioid metabolism. **Kinase inhibitors:** [P] Decreased metabolism of CYP3A4-dependent opioids by ceritinib, cobimetinib, crizotinib, dasatinib, duvelisib, erlotinib, idelalisib, imatinib, lapatinib, larotrectinib, nilotinib, pacritinib, palbociclib, regorafenib, ribociclib, tucatinib, and ruxolitinib. **Lumacaftor:** [P] Increased CYP3A4-dependent opioid metabolism. **Mitotane:** [NP] Increased CYP3A4-dependent opioid metabolism. **Nefazodone:** [NP] Decreased CYP3A4-dependent opioid metabolism. **Phenytoin:** [P] Increased CYP3A4-dependent opioid metabolism. **Rifabutin:** [P] Increased CYP3A4-dependent opioid metabolism. **Rifampin:** [P] Increased CYP3A4-dependent opioid metabolism. **St. John's wort:** [NP] Increased CYP3A4-dependent opioid metabolism. **Ticlopidine:** [NP] Decreased CYP2B6 metabolism of methadone. *See also* Azole antifungal agents; Barbiturates; Carbamazepine; Cimetidine; Macrolides; Monoamine oxidase inhibitors.

P, Predictable. Interaction occurs in most patients receiving the combination; NP, Not predictable. Interaction occurs only in some patients receiving the combination; NE, Not established. Insufficient data available on which to base estimate of predictability.

(*continued*)

TABLE 67–1 Important drug interactions. (Continued)

Drug or Drug Group	Properties Promoting Drug Interaction	Clinically Documented Interactions
Phenytoin	Induces hepatic microsomal drug metabolism. Susceptible to inhibition of metabolism by CYP2C9 and, to a lesser extent, CYP2C19.	***Drugs whose metabolism is stimulated by phenytoin:***
		Corticosteroids: [P] Decreased serum corticosteroid levels.
		Doxycycline: [P] Decreased serum doxycycline levels.
		Mexiletine: [NP] Decreased serum mexiletine levels.
		Quinidine: [P] Decreased serum quinidine levels.
		Theophylline: [P] Decreased serum theophylline levels.
		See also Calcium channel blockers; Cyclosporine; Estrogens; Kinase inhibitors, Opioid analgesics.
		Drugs that inhibit phenytoin metabolism:
		Amiodarone: [P] Increased serum phenytoin concentration; possible reduction in serum amiodarone concentration.
		Capecitabine: [NP] Increased phenytoin plasma concentrations.
		Ceritinib: [P] Increased phenytoin plasma concentrations.
		Chloramphenicol: [P] Increased phenytoin plasma concentrations.
		Cimetidine: [NP] Increased phenytoin plasma concentrations.
		Delavirdine: [P] Increased phenytoin plasma concentrations.
		Disulfiram: [NP] Increased phenytoin plasma concentrations.
		Felbamate: [P] Increased phenytoin plasma concentrations.
		Fluconazole: [P] Increased phenytoin plasma concentrations.
		Fluorouracil: [NP] Increased phenytoin plasma concentrations.
		Fluoxetine: [NP] Increased phenytoin plasma concentrations.
		Fluvoxamine: [NP] Increased phenytoin plasma concentrations.
		Isoniazid: [NP] Increased serum phenytoin; problem primarily with slow acetylators of isoniazid.
		Metronidazole: [NP] Increased phenytoin plasma concentrations.
		Miconazole: [NP] Increased phenytoin plasma concentrations.
		Sulfamethoxazole: [P] Increased phenytoin plasma concentrations.
		Ticlopidine: [NP] Increased phenytoin plasma concentrations.
		Voriconazole: [P] Increased phenytoin plasma concentrations.
		See also Azole antifungals; Cimetidine; Disulfiram.
		Drugs that enhance phenytoin metabolism:
		Bosentan: [P] Decreased phenytoin plasma concentrations.
		Carbamazepine: [P] Decreased phenytoin plasma concentrations.
		Dabrafenib: [NP] Decreased phenytoin plasma concentrations.
		Dexamethasone: [NP] Decreased phenytoin plasma concentrations.
		Enzalutamide: NP] Decreased phenytoin plasma concentrations.
		Ivosidenib: [NP] Decreased phenytoin plasma concentrations.
		Nelfinavir: [NP] Decreased phenytoin plasma concentrations.
		Rifampin: [P] Decreased phenytoin plasma concentrations.
		Rifapentine: [P] Decreased phenytoin plasma concentrations.
		St. John's wort: [NP] Decreased phenytoin plasma concentrations.
		See also Barbiturates.

P, Predictable. Interaction occurs in most patients receiving the combination; NP, Not predictable. Interaction occurs only in some patients receiving the combination; NE, Not established. Insufficient data available on which to base estimate of predictability.

(*continued*)

TABLE 67–1 Important drug interactions. (Continued)

Drug or Drug Group	Properties Promoting Drug Interaction	Clinically Documented Interactions
Pimozide	Susceptible to CYP3A4 inhibitors; may exhibit additive effects with other agents that prolong QT_c interval.	**Antivirals:** [P] Amprenavir, atazanavir, boceprevir, darunavir, delavirdine, fosamprenavir, indinavir, nelfinavir, ritonavir, saquinavir, simeprevir, and telaprevir inhibit the metabolism of pimozide. Efavirenz and etravirine increase the metabolism of pimozide. **Bosentan:** [P] Increased pimozide metabolism. **Carbamazepine:** [P] Increased pimozide metabolism. Expect similar interactions with oxcarbazepine. **Cobicistat:** [P] Decreased metabolism of pimozide. **Conivaptan:** [P] Decreased metabolism of pimozide. **Dabrafenib:** [NP] Increased pimozide metabolism. **Dexamethasone:** [P] Increased pimozide metabolism. **Enzalutamide:** [P] Increased pimozide metabolism. **Ivosidenib:** [NP] Increased pimozide metabolism. **Kinase inhibitors:** [P] Decreased metabolism of pimozide by ceritinib, cobimetinib, crizotinib, dasatinib, duvelisib, erlotinib, idelalisib, imatinib, lapatinib, larotrectinib, nilotinib, pacritinib, palbociclib, regorafenib, ribociclib, tucatinib, and ruxolitinib. **Lumacaftor:** [P] Increased pimozide metabolism. **Mitotane:** [NP] Increased pimozide metabolism. **Nefazodone:** [NP] Decreased pimozide metabolism. **Phenytoin:** [P] Increased pimozide metabolism. **Rifabutin:** [P] Increased pimozide metabolism. **Rifampin:** [P] Increased pimozide metabolism. **St. John's wort:** [NP] Increased pimozide metabolism. *See also* Azole antifungals; Cyclosporine; Macrolides.
Potassium-sparing diuretics (amiloride, eplerenone, spironolactone, triamterene)	Additive effects with other agents increasing serum potassium concentration. Eplerenone is a substrate for CYP3A4 and is susceptible to inhibition and induction. May alter renal excretion of substances other than potassium (eg, digoxin, hydrogen ions).	**ACE inhibitors (ACEIs):** [NP] Additive hyperkalemic effect. **Amiodarone:** [P] Decreased eplerenone metabolism. Expect similar interactions with dronedarone. **Angiotensin II receptor blockers (ARBs):** [NP] Additive hyperkalemic effect. **Antivirals:** [P] Amprenavir, atazanavir, boceprevir, darunavir, delavirdine, fosamprenavir, indinavir, nelfinavir, ritonavir, saquinavir, simeprevir, and telaprevir inhibit the metabolism of eplerenone. **Barbiturates:** [P] Increased metabolism of eplerenone. **Bosentan:** [P] Increased metabolism of eplerenone. **Carbamazepine:** [P] Increased metabolism of eplerenone. Expect similar interactions with oxcarbazepine. **Cobicistat:** [P] Decreased metabolism of eplerenone. **Conivaptan:** [P] Decreased metabolism of eplerenone. **Cyclosporine:** [P] Decreased eplerenone elimination. **Enzalutamide:** [P] Increased eplerenone elimination. **Kinase inhibitors:** [P] Decreased metabolism of eplerenone with ceritinib, cobimetinib, crizotinib, dasatinib, duvelisib, erlotinib, idelalisib, imatinib, lapatinib, larotrectinib, nilotinib, pacritinib, palbociclib, regorafenib, ribociclib, tucatinib, and ruxolitinib. **Lumacaftor:** [P] Increased metabolism of eplerenone.

P, Predictable. Interaction occurs in most patients receiving the combination; NP, Not predictable. Interaction occurs only in some patients receiving the combination; NE, Not established. Insufficient data available on which to base estimate of predictability.

(*continued*)

TABLE 67–1 Important drug interactions. (Continued)

Drug or Drug Group	Properties Promoting Drug Interaction	Clinically Documented Interactions
Potassium-sparing diuretics (amiloride, eplerenone, spironolactone, triamterene) (*cont.*)		**Macrolide antibiotics:** [P] Clarithromycin, erythromycin, and telithromycin inhibit the elimination of eplerenone. **Nefazodone:** [NP] Decreased eplerenone metabolism. **Phenytoin:** [P] Increased eplerenone metabolism. **Potassium-sparing diuretics:** [NP] Additive hyperkalemic effect. **Potassium supplements:** [NP] Additive hyperkalemic effect; especially a problem in presence of renal impairment. **Rifabutin:** [P] Increased eplerenone metabolism. **Rifampin:** [P] Increased eplerenone metabolism. **St. John's wort:** [NP] Increased eplerenone metabolism. *See also* Azole antifungals; Digitalis glycosides; Macrolides; Nonsteroidal anti-inflammatory drugs.
Probenecid	Interference with renal excretion of drugs that undergo active tubular secretion, especially weak acids. Inhibition of glucuronide conjugation of other drugs.	**Clofibrate:** [P] Reduced glucuronide conjugation of clofibric acid. **Methotrexate:** [P] Decreased renal methotrexate excretion; possible methotrexate toxicity. **Pralatrexate:** [P] Decreased renal pralatrexate excretion; possible pralatrexate toxicity. **Penicillin:** [P] Decreased renal penicillin excretion. **Salicylates:** [P] Decreased uricosuric effect of probenecid (interaction unlikely with less than 1.5 g of salicylate daily).
Quinidine	Substrate of CYP3A4. Inhibits CYP2D6. Renal excretion susceptible to changes in urine pH. Additive effects with other agents that prolong the QT_c interval.	**Acetazolamide:** [P] Decreased renal quinidine excretion due to increased urinary pH; elevated serum quinidine. **Amiodarone:** [NP] Increased serum quinidine levels; additive prolongation of QT_c interval. **Antivirals:** [P] Amprenavir, atazanavir, boceprevir, darunavir, delavirdine, fosamprenavir, indinavir, nelfinavir, ritonavir, saquinavir, simeprevir, and telaprevir inhibit the metabolism of quinidine. Efavirenz and etravirine increase the metabolism of quinidine. **Bosentan:** [P] Increased quinidine metabolism. **Cobicistat:** [P] Decreased metabolism of quinidine. **Conivaptan:** [P] Decreased metabolism of quinidine. **Cyclosporine:** [P] Decreased quinidine elimination. **Dabrafenib:** [NP] Increased quinidine metabolism. **Dexamethasone:** [P] Increased quinidine metabolism. **Enzalutamide:** [P] Increased quinidine metabolism. **Ivosidenib:** [NP] Increased quinidine metabolism. **Kaolin-pectin:** [NP] Decreased gastrointestinal absorption of quinidine. **Kinase inhibitors:** [P] Decreased metabolism of quinidine with ceritinib, cobimetinib, crizotinib, dasatinib, duvelisib, erlotinib, idelalisib, imatinib, lapatinib, larotrectinib, nilotinib, pacritinib, palbociclib, regorafenib, ribociclib, tucatinib, and ruxolitinib. **Lumacaftor:** [P] Increased quinidine metabolism. **Mitotane:** [NP] Increased quinidine metabolism. **Phenytoin:** [P] Increased quinidine metabolism. **Rifabutin:** [P] Increased quinidine metabolism. **Rifampin:** [P] Increased quinidine metabolism. **St. John's wort:** [NP] Increased quinidine metabolism. **Thioridazine:** [NP] Decreased thioridazine metabolism; additive prolongation of QT_c interval. *See also* Anticoagulants, oral; Antidepressants, tricyclic; Azole antifungals; Barbiturates; Cimetidine; Digitalis glycosides; Macrolides; Phenytoin.

P, Predictable. Interaction occurs in most patients receiving the combination; NP, Not predictable. Interaction occurs only in some patients receiving the combination; NE, Not established. Insufficient data available on which to base estimate of predictability.

(*continued*)

TABLE 67–1 Important drug interactions. (Continued)

Drug or Drug Group	Properties Promoting Drug Interaction	Clinically Documented Interactions
Quinolone antibiotics	Susceptible to inhibition of gastrointestinal absorption. Ciprofloxacin inhibits CYP1A2 and, to a lesser extent, CYP3A4.	**Abametapir:** [P] Ciprofloxacin inhibits abametapir metabolism. **Albendazole:** [P] Ciprofloxacin inhibits albendazole metabolism. **Alosetron:** [P] Ciprofloxacin inhibits alosetron metabolism. **Asenapine:** [P] Ciprofloxacin inhibits asenapine metabolism. **Bendamustine:** [P] Ciprofloxacin inhibits bendamustine metabolism. **Bupropion:** [P] Ciprofloxacin inhibits bupropion metabolism. **Caffeine:** [P] Ciprofloxacin inhibits caffeine metabolism. **Clozapine:** [P] Ciprofloxacin inhibits clozapine metabolism. **Cyclobenzaprine:** [P] Ciprofloxacin inhibits cyclobenzaprine metabolism. **Duloxetine:** [P] Ciprofloxacin inhibits duloxetine metabolism. **Frovatriptan:** [P] Ciprofloxacin inhibits frovatriptan metabolism. **Lidocaine:** [P] Ciprofloxacin inhibits lidocaine metabolism. **Ramelteon:** [P] Ciprofloxacin inhibits ramelteon metabolism. **Rasagiline:** [P] Ciprofloxacin inhibits rasagiline metabolism. **Riluzole:** [P] Ciprofloxacin inhibits riluzole metabolism. **Ropinirole:** [P] Ciprofloxacin inhibits ropinirole metabolism. **Ropivacaine:** [P] Ciprofloxacin inhibits ropivacaine metabolism. **Sucralfate:** [P] Reduced gastrointestinal absorption of ciprofloxacin, norfloxacin, and probably other quinolones. **Tacrine:** [P] Ciprofloxacin inhibits tacrine metabolism. **Theophylline:** [P] Ciprofloxacin inhibits theophylline metabolism. **Tizanidine:** [P] Ciprofloxacin inhibits tizanidine metabolism. **Zileuton:** [P] Ciprofloxacin inhibits zileuton metabolism. **Zolmitriptan:** [P] Ciprofloxacin inhibits zolmitriptan metabolism. *See also* Acid-reducing agents; Anticoagulants, oral; Iron.
Rifampin	Inducer (strong) of hepatic microsomal drug-metabolizing enzymes and P-glycoprotein. Similar interactions seen with rifabutin.	**Corticosteroids:** [P] Increased corticosteroid hepatic metabolism; reduced corticosteroid effect. **Mexiletine:** [NE] Increased mexiletine metabolism; reduced mexiletine effect. **Sulfonylurea hypoglycemics:** [P] Increased hepatic metabolism of tolbutamide and probably other sulfonylureas metabolized by the liver (including chlorpropamide). **Theophylline:** [P] Increased theophylline metabolism. *See also* Anticoagulants, oral; Antidepressants, tricyclic and heterocyclic; Antineoplastic agents; Azole antifungals; β-adrenoceptor blockers; Calcium channel blockers; Carbamazepine; Colchicine; Cyclosporine; Digitalis glycosides; Estrogens; HMG-CoA reductase inhibitors; Kinase inhibitors; Opioid analgesics; Phenytoin; Pimozide; Quinidine.

P, Predictable. Interaction occurs in most patients receiving the combination; NP, Not predictable. Interaction occurs only in some patients receiving the combination; NE, Not established. Insufficient data available on which to base estimate of predictability.

(continued)

TABLE 67–1 Important drug interactions. (Continued)

Drug or Drug Group	Properties Promoting Drug Interaction	Clinically Documented Interactions
Salicylates	Interference with renal excretion of drugs that undergo active tubular secretion. Salicylate renal excretion dependent on urinary pH when large doses of salicylate used. Aspirin (but not other salicylates) interferes with platelet function. Large doses of salicylates have intrinsic hypoglycemic activity.	**Carbonic anhydrase inhibitors:** [NP] Increased acetazolamide serum concentrations; increase salicylate toxicity due to decreased blood pH. **Corticosteroids:** [P] Increased salicylate elimination; possible additive toxic effect on gastric mucosa. **Heparin:** [NP] Increased bleeding tendency with aspirin, but probably not with other salicylates. **Methotrexate:** [P] Decreased renal methotrexate clearance; Increased methotrexate toxicity (primarily at anticancer doses). **Selective serotonin reuptake inhibitors (SSRIs):** [P] Increased risk of bleeding due to platelet inhibition. **Sulfinpyrazone:** [P] Decreased uricosuric effect of sulfinpyrazone (interaction unlikely with less than 1.5 g of salicylate daily). *See also* Acid-reducing agents; Anticoagulants, oral; Probenecid.
Selective serotonin reuptake inhibitors (SSRIs)	SSRIs can lead to excessive serotonin response when administered with other serotonergic drugs (eg, MAOIs). Some SSRIs inhibit various cytochrome P450s including CYP2D6, CYP1A2, CYP3A4, and CYP2C19.	**Codeine:** [P] Reduced analgesic effect due to inhibition of codeine metabolism to morphine by fluoxetine and paroxetine. **Theophylline:** [P] Decreased metabolism of theophylline by fluvoxamine-induced inhibition of CYP1A2. *See also* Anticoagulants, oral; Antidepressants, tricyclic and heterocyclic; β-Adrenoceptor blockers; Carbamazepine; Cisapride; Colchicine; Cyclosporine; HMG-CoA reductase inhibitors; Monoamine oxidase inhibitors; Nonsteroidal anti-inflammatory drugs; Phenytoin; Pimozide; Salicylates.
Theophylline	Susceptible to induction and inhibition of hepatic metabolism by CYP1A2 and CYP3A4.	**Smoking:** [P] Increased theophylline metabolism. **Tacrine:** [NP] Decreased theophylline metabolism. **Ticlopidine:** [NP] Decreased theophylline metabolism. **Zileuton:** [NP] Decreased theophylline metabolism. *See also* Barbiturates; Beta-adrenoceptor blockers; Calcium channel blockers; Carbamazepine; Cimetidine; Lithium; Macrolides; Phenytoin; Quinolones; Rifampin; Selective serotonin reuptake inhibitors.

P, Predictable. Interaction occurs in most patients receiving the combination; NP, Not predictable. Interaction occurs only in some patients receiving the combination; NE, Not established. Insufficient data available on which to base estimate of predictability.

lung, and kidney. Induction of cytochrome P450 isozymes in the liver and small intestine can be caused by drugs such as barbiturates, bosentan, carbamazepine, efavirenz, nevirapine, phenytoin, primidone, rifampin, rifabutin, and St. John's wort. Enzyme inducers can also increase the activity of phase II metabolism such as glucuronidation. Enzyme induction does not take place quickly; maximal effects usually occur after 7–14 days and require an equal or longer time to dissipate after the enzyme inducer is stopped. Inhibition of metabolism generally takes place more quickly than enzyme induction and may begin as soon as the tissue concentration of the inhibitor is sufficient to cause reduced enzyme activity. However, if the half-life of the affected (object) drug is long, it may take a week or more (3–4 half-lives) to reach a new steady-state serum concentration. Drugs that may inhibit the cytochrome P450 metabolism of other drugs include amiodarone, androgens, atazanavir, chloramphenicol, cimetidine, ciprofloxacin, clarithromycin, cyclosporine, delavirdine, diltiazem, diphenhydramine, disulfiram, erythromycin, fluconazole, fluoxetine, fluvoxamine, furanocoumarins (substances in grapefruit juice), indinavir, isoniazid, itraconazole, ketoconazole, metronidazole, mexiletine, miconazole, omeprazole, paroxetine, quinidine, ritonavir, sulfamethizole, sulfamethoxazole, verapamil, voriconazole, zafirlukast, and zileuton.

The **renal excretion** of active drug also can be affected by concurrent drug therapy. The renal excretion of drugs that are weak acids or weak bases may be influenced by other drugs that affect urinary pH. This is due to changes in ionization of the object drug, as described in Chapter 1 under Ionization of Weak Acids and Weak Bases; the Henderson-Hasselbalch Equation. For some drugs, active secretion into the renal tubules is an important elimination pathway. P-glycoprotein, organic anion transporters, and organic cation transporters are involved in active tubular secretion of some drugs, and inhibition of these transporters can inhibit renal elimination with attendant increase in serum drug concentrations. Many drugs are partially eliminated by P-glycoprotein, including digoxin, cyclosporine, dabigatran, colchicine, daunorubicin, and tacrolimus. The plasma concentration of these drugs can be increased by inhibitors of P-glycoprotein including amiodarone, clarithromycin, erythromycin, ketoconazole, ritonavir, and quinidine. To access more than 200 brief reviews of specific drug interactions, visit www.hanstenandhorn.com/news.htm.

PHARMACODYNAMIC MECHANISMS

When drugs with similar pharmacologic effects are administered concurrently, an additive or synergistic response is usually seen. The two drugs may or may not act on the same receptor to produce such effects. In theory, drugs acting on the same receptor or process are usually additive, eg, benzodiazepines plus barbiturates, until the receptor is saturated, or the effect is maximal. However, two drugs competing for the same binding site may result in less than an additive effect. The drug with the lower potency will act as a partial agonist, which appears to act as a competitive antagonist of the drug with the greater potency. Drugs acting on different receptors or sequential processes may be synergistic, eg, nitrates plus sildenafil or sulfonamides plus trimethoprim. Conversely, drugs with opposing pharmacologic effects may reduce the response to one or both drugs. Pharmacodynamic drug interactions are relatively common in clinical practice, but adverse effects can usually be minimized if one understands the pharmacology of the drugs involved. In this way, the interactions can be anticipated and appropriate counter-measures taken.

COMBINED TOXICITY

The combined use of two or more drugs, each of which has toxic effects on the same organ, can greatly increase the likelihood of organ damage. For example, concurrent administration of two nephrotoxic drugs can produce kidney damage, even though the dose of either drug alone may be insufficient to produce toxicity. Furthermore, some drugs can enhance the organ toxicity of another drug, even though the enhancing drug has no intrinsic toxic effect on that organ.

REFERENCES

Boobis A et al: Drug interactions. Drug Metab Rev 2009;41:486.

DeGorter MK et al: Drug transporters in drug efficacy and toxicity. Annu Rev Pharmacol Toxicol 2012;52:249.

Hansten PD, Horn JR: *The Top 100 Drug Interactions. A Guide to Patient Management.* H&H Publications, 2021. www.hanstenandhorn.com.

Hillgren KM et al: Emerging transporters of clinical importance: An update from the international transporter consortium. Clin Pharmacol Ther 2013;94:52.

Horn JR et al: Proposal for a new tool to evaluate drug interaction cases. Ann Pharmacother 2007;41:674.

Hukkanen J: Induction of cytochrome P450 enzymes: A view on human in vivo findings. Expert Rev Clin Pharmacol 2012;5:569.

Konig J et al: Transporters and drug-drug interactions: Important determinants of drug disposition and effects. Pharmacol Rev 2013;65:944.

Meng Q, Lin K: Pharmacokinetic interactions between herbal medicines and prescribed drugs: Focus on drug metabolic enzymes and transporters. Curr Drug Metab 2014;15:791.

Pelkonen O et al: Inhibition and induction of human cytochrome P450 enzymes: Current status. Arch Toxicol 2008;82:667.

Roberts JA et al: The clinical relevance of plasma protein binding changes. Clin Pharmacokinet 2013;52:1.

Shah SN et al: Comparison of medication alerts from two commercial applications in the USA. Drug Safety 2021;44:661.

Thelen K, Dressman JB: Cytochrome P540-mediated metabolism in the human gut wall. J Pharm Pharmacol 2009;61:541.

Tissot M et al: Epidemiology and economic burden of "serious" adverse drug reactions: Real-world evidence research based on pharmacovigilance data. Therapie 2022;77:291.

Zakeri-Milani P, Valzadeh H: Intestinal transporters: Enhanced absorption through P-glycoprotein-related drug interactions. Expert Opin Drug Metab Toxicol 2014;10:859.

Appendix 1: Vaccines, Immune Globulins, & Other Complex Biologic Products

Harry W. Lampiris, MD, & Daniel S. Maddix, PharmD*

Vaccines and related biologic products constitute an important group of agents that bridge the disciplines of microbiology, infectious diseases, immunology, and immunopharmacology. A list of the most important preparations used in the USA is provided here. The reader who requires more complete information is referred to the sources listed at the end of this appendix. At the time of writing, many vaccines for the SARS-CoV-2 virus were in development, and several were in phase 2 or phase 3 trials. See Funk et al and Lurie et al in the references section for additional information.

ACTIVE IMMUNIZATION

Active immunization consists of the administration of antigen to the host to induce formation of antibodies and cell-mediated immunity. Immunization is practiced to induce protection against many infectious agents and may utilize either inactivated (killed) materials or live attenuated agents (Table A–1). Desirable features of the ideal immunogen include complete prevention of disease, prevention of the carrier state, production of prolonged immunity with a minimum of immunizations, absence of toxicity, and suitability for mass immunization (eg, inexpensive and easy to administer). Active immunization is generally preferable to passive immunization—in most cases because higher antibody levels are sustained for longer periods of time, requiring less frequent immunization, and in some cases because of the development of concurrent cell-mediated immunity. However, active immunization requires time to develop and is therefore generally inactive at the time of a specific exposure (eg, for parenteral exposure to hepatitis B, concurrent hepatitis B IgG [passive antibodies] and active immunization are given to prevent illness).

Duration of immunity tends to be longer with live vaccines than with inactivated vaccines. The duration of immunity may be life-long with some live vaccines, but in many infections natural immunity decreases over time. The need for booster doses of vaccines is an indication of the limited duration of immunity.

The development and availability of effective vaccines is a major success story in the battle against infectious diseases and in impact on public health is rivaled only by the availability of clean drinking water. Successful immunization programs are now being challenged by the anti-vaccination movement. Through the first 5 months of 2019, there were more cases of measles reported in the United States than in any year since 2000, when the disease was declared eradicated. Many clusters of infection have involved undervaccinated populations in association with international travel to countries with endemic measles. The majority of cases occurred in patients who were not vaccinated. Measles causes death in 1–2 of 1000 patients who contract the disease, and more than 100,000 people throughout the world continue to die annually from this highly communicable disease. Patient education and mandatory vaccination legislation are tools to combat the anti-vaccination movement.

Current recommendations for routine active immunization of children are given in Table A–2.

PASSIVE IMMUNIZATION

Passive immunization consists of transfer of immunity to a host using preformed immunologic products. From a practical standpoint, only immunoglobulins have been used for passive immunization, because passive administration of cellular components of the immune system has been technically difficult and associated with graft-versus-host reactions. Products of the cellular immune system (eg, interferons) have also been used in the therapy of a wide variety of hematologic and infectious diseases (see Chapter 55).

Passive immunization with antibodies may be accomplished with either animal or human immunoglobulins in varying degrees of purity. These may contain relatively high titers of antibodies

*Deceased.

TABLE A–1 Materials commonly used for active immunization in the United States.[1]

Vaccine	Type of Agent	Route of Administration	Primary Immunization	Booster[2]	Indications
Diphtheria tetanus acellular pertussis (DTaP)	Toxoids and inactivated bacterial components	Intramuscular	See Table A–2	None	For all children
Haemophilus influenzae type b conjugate (Hib)[3]	Bacterial polysaccharide conjugated to protein	Intramuscular	One dose (see Table A–2 for childhood schedule)	Not recommended	1. For all children 2. Asplenia and other at-risk conditions 3. Hematopoietic stem cell transplant (HSCT): three-dose series 4 weeks apart 6–12 months after successful transplant
Hepatitis A	Inactivated virus	Intramuscular	One dose (see Table A–2 for childhood schedule) (administer at least 2–4 weeks before travel to endemic areas)	At 6–12 months for long-term immunity	1. Travelers to hepatitis A endemic areas 2. Men who have sex with men (MSM) 3. Injection or noninjection illicit drug use 4. Chronic liver disease or clotting factor disorders 5. Persons with occupational risk for infection 6. Persons living in, or relocating to, endemic areas 7. Household and sexual contacts of individuals with acute hepatitis A (with additional gamma globulin in select patients) 8. For all children 9. Unvaccinated persons who anticipate close personal contact with an international adoptee during the first 60 days after arrival in the USA from a country with high or intermediate endemicity 10. Homelessness
Hepatitis B	Inactive viral antigen, recombinant	Intramuscular (subcutaneous injection is acceptable in individuals with bleeding disorders)	Three doses at 0, 1, and 6 months (two-dose series for adjuvanted vaccine at 4 weeks apart) (see Table A–2 for childhood schedule)	Not routinely recommended	1. For all infants 2. Hepatitis C virus infection 3. Persons with occupational, lifestyle, or environmental risk 4. Diabetic adults <60 years of age 5. Persons with end-stage renal disease, HIV, or chronic liver disease 6. Postexposure prophylaxis 7. Household and sexual contacts of individuals with acute and chronic hepatitis B
Human papillomavirus (HPV)	Virus-like particles of the major capsid protein	Intramuscular	See Table A–2	None	1. For unvaccinated females between 9 and 26 years of age; and for unvaccinated males aged 9–21 years. three-dose series if started after age 14 2. MSM through age 26 years 3. Immunocompromised persons through age 26 years
Influenza, inactivated	Inactivated virus or viral components	Intramuscular; an intradermal vaccine is available for adults aged 18–64 years; a high-dose formulation or adjuvanted vaccine are options for adults ≥65 years	One dose (babies and children age 6 months to 9 years who are receiving influenza vaccine for the first time should receive two doses administered at least 4 weeks apart.)	Yearly with current vaccine	1. All adults >18 years 2. All children aged 6 months to 18 years

Influenza, live attenuated	Live virus	Intranasal	Split dose in each nostril. (Babies and children age 2–9 years who are receiving influenza vaccine for the first time should receive two doses administered at least 4 weeks apart.)	Yearly with current vaccine	Healthy persons aged 19–49 years who desire protection against influenza. May be substituted for inactivated vaccine in healthy children 2–18 years except (1) asthmatics, and (2) those aged 2–4 years with wheezing in the past year
Measles-mumps-rubella (MMR)	Live virus	Subcutaneous	See Table A–2	None	1. For all children 2. Lack of evidence of immunity in adults born after 1956 and in special situations
Meningococcal conjugate vaccine ACWY	Bacterial polysaccharides conjugated to diphtheria toxoid	Intramuscular	One or two doses (see Table A–2 for childhood schedule)	Every 5 years if there is continuing high risk of exposure	1. All adolescents 2. Travel in countries with hyperendemic or epidemic meningococcal disease 3. College freshmen aged <22 years who live in dormitories 4. Military recruits 5. Individuals with HIV infection, anatomic or functional asplenia, complement deficiency, or eculizumab use (two-dose series) 6. Microbiologists who are routinely exposed to *Neisseria meningitidis*
Meningococcal serogroup B vaccine[4]	Recombinant protein	Intramuscular	2–3 doses[4]	None	1. Anatomic or functional asplenia, complement deficiency, or eculizumab use 2. Microbiologists who are routinely exposed to *Neisseria meningitidis*
Pneumococcal conjugate vaccine	Bacterial polysaccharides conjugated to protein	Intramuscular	See Table A–2	None	1. For all children 2. Adults with immunocompromising conditions, anatomic or functional asplenia, chronic renal failure, nephrotic syndrome, malignancy, iatrogenic immunosuppression, cerebrospinal fluid leaks, or cochlear implants 3. Adults ≥65 years who have not been vaccinated previously
Pneumococcal polysaccharide vaccine	Bacterial polysaccharides of 23 serotypes	Intramuscular or subcutaneous	One dose	Repeat after 5 years in patients at high risk	1. Adults ≥65 years 2. Persons at increased risk for pneumococcal disease or its complications
Poliovirus vaccine, inactivated (IPV)	Inactivated viruses of all three serotypes	Subcutaneous	See Table A–2 for childhood schedule. Adults: Two doses 4–8 weeks apart, and a third dose 6–12 months after the second	One-time booster dose for adults at increased risk of exposure	1. For all children 2. Previously unvaccinated adults at increased risk for occupational or travel exposure to polioviruses
Rabies	Inactivated virus	Intramuscular	**Preexposure:** Three doses at days 0, 7, and 21 or 28 **Postexposure:** Four doses at days 0, 3, 7, and 14; immunosuppressed patients should receive a 5th dose at day 28	Serologic testing every 6 months to 2 years in persons at high risk	1. **Preexposure** prophylaxis in persons at risk for contact with rabies virus 2. **Postexposure** prophylaxis (administer with rabies immune globulin in previously unvaccinated individuals)

(continued)

TABLE A–1 Materials commonly used for active immunization in the United States.[1] (Continued)

Vaccine	Type of Agent	Route of Administration	Primary Immunization	Booster[2]	Indications
Rotavirus	Live virus	Oral	See Table A–2	None	For all infants
Tetanus-diphtheria (Td or DT)[5]	Toxoids	Intramuscular	Two doses 4–8 weeks apart, and a third dose 6–12 months after the second	Every 10 years	1. All adults 2. Postexposure prophylaxis if >5 years has passed since last dose
Tetanus, diphtheria, pertussis (Tdap)	Toxoids and inactivated bacterial components	Intramuscular	Substitute one dose of Tdap for Td in all adults	None	All adults; pregnant women should receive a dose with each pregnancy (preferred during 27–36 weeks of gestation)
Typhoid, Ty21a oral	Live bacteria	Oral	Four doses administered every other day	Four doses every 5 years	Risk of exposure to typhoid fever
Typhoid, Vi capsular polysaccharide	Bacterial polysaccharide	Intramuscular	One dose	Every 2 years	Risk of exposure to typhoid fever
Varicella	Live virus	Subcutaneous	Two doses 4–8 weeks apart in persons past their 13th birthday (see Table A–2 for childhood schedule)	Unknown	1. For all children 2. Persons past their 13th birthday without a history of varicella infection or immunization 3. Postexposure prophylaxis in susceptible persons
Yellow fever	Live virus	Subcutaneous	One dose 10 years to 10 days before travel	Every 10 years	1. Laboratory personnel who may be exposed to yellow fever virus 2. Travelers to areas where yellow fever occurs
Zoster	Recombinant	Intramuscular	Two doses 2–6 months apart	None	All adults ≥50 years of age

[1]Dosages for the specific product, including variations for age, are best obtained from the manufacturer's package insert.

[2]One dose unless otherwise indicated.

[3]Three Hib conjugate vaccines are available for use: (1) oligosaccharide conjugate Hib vaccine (HbOC), (2) polyribosylribitol phosphate-tetanus toxoid conjugate (PRP-T), and (3) *Haemophilus influenzae* type b conjugate vaccine (meningococcal protein conjugate) (PRP-OMP).

[4]Two meningococcal serogroup B vaccines are available for use: (1) MenB-4C (Bexsero) administered as a two-dose series at least 1 month apart and (2) MenB-FHbp (Trumenba) administered as a three-dose series at 0, 1–2, and 6 months.

[5]Td is tetanus and diphtheria toxoids for use in persons ≥7 years of age (contains less diphtheria toxoid than DPT and DT). DT is tetanus and diphtheria toxoids for use in persons <7 years of age (contains the same amount of diphtheria toxoid as DPT).

TABLE A–2 Recommended routine childhood immunization schedule.

Age	Immunization	Comments
Birth to 2 months	Hepatitis B vaccine (HBV)	**Infants born to seronegative mothers:** Medically stable infants weighing at least 2000 grams should receive one dose within 24 hours of birth with the second dose administered 1–2 months after the first dose. Infants weighing <2000 grams should receive one dose at age 1 month or hospital discharge. **Infants born to seropositive mothers:** Should receive the first dose within 12 hours of birth (with hepatitis B immune globulin), with 3 additional doses of vaccine beginning at age 1 month.
2 months	Diphtheria and tetanus toxoids and acellular pertussis vaccine (DTaP), inactivated poliovirus vaccine (IPV), *Haemophilus influenzae* type b conjugate vaccine (Hib),[1] pneumococcal conjugate vaccine (PCV), rotavirus vaccine (RV)[2]	
1–2 months	HBV	The second dose should be given at least 4 weeks after the first dose.
4 months	DTaP, Hib,[1] IPV, PCV, RV[2]	
6 months	DTaP, Hib,[1] PCV, RV[2]	The third dose of RV is only necessary if RV-5 is used for one or two of the first two doses.
6–18 months	HBV, IPV, influenza	The third dose of HBV should be given at least 16 weeks after the first dose and at least 8 weeks after the second dose, but not before age 24 weeks. Influenza vaccine should be administered annually to children aged 6 months to 18 years. Two doses separated by at least 4 weeks should be administered to previously unvaccinated children 6 months to 8 years of age. Live attenuated influenza vaccine cannot be administered until age 2 years.
12–15 months	Measles-mumps-rubella vaccine (MMR), Hib,[1] PCV, varicella vaccine	The first dose of MMR may be administered at 6–11 months before departure from the USA for international travel. These infants should receive two additional doses at the usual interval. Children ≥12 months of age should receive a second dose at least 4 weeks after the first dose before departure from the USA for international travel.
15–18 months	DTaP	DTaP may be given as early as age 12 months if there has been at least 6 months since the third dose.
12–23 months	Hepatitis A vaccine	Two doses ≥6 months apart.
4–6 years	DTaP IPV, MMR, varicella vaccine	The second dose of MMR should be routinely administered at age 4–6 years but may be given during any visit if at least 4 weeks have elapsed since administration of the first dose.
11–12 years	Tetanus, diphtheria, pertussis (Tdap) vaccine, human papillomavirus vaccine (HPV),[3] meningococcal conjugate vaccine (MCV) ACWY	Three doses of HPV should be administered to all adolescents at 0, 1–2, and 6 months if started at age 15 years or older or a two-dose series (0 and 6–12 months) if started prior to age 15 years (may be started as early as age 9 years). Administer one dose of Tdap to pregnant adolescents during each pregnancy at 27–36 weeks of gestation. A booster dose of MCV should be given at age 16 years.

[1]Three Hib conjugate vaccines are available for use: (1) oligosaccharide conjugate Hib vaccine (HbOC), (2) polyribosylribitol phosphate-tetanus toxoid conjugate (PRP-T), and (3) *Haemophilus influenzae* type b conjugate vaccine (meningococcal protein conjugate) (PRP-OMP). Children immunized with PRP-OMP at 2 and 4 months of age do not require a dose at 6 months of age. PRP-T should only be used for the booster dose in children aged 12–15 months.

[2]Two RV vaccines are available for use: (1) RV-1 (Rotarix) monovalent live, oral, human attenuated rotavirus vaccine is approved for a two-dose series, and (2) RV-5 (RotaTeq) pentavalent live, oral, human-bovine reassortant rotavirus vaccine is approved for a three-dose series.

[3]Three HPV vaccines are available for use: (1) quadrivalent vaccine (HPV4), (2) 9-valent vaccine (HPV9) for the prevention of cervical, vaginal, and vulvar cancers (in females) and genital warts (in males and females), and (3) bivalent vaccine (HPV2) for the prevention of cervical cancers in females.

Data from Kim DK, Hunter P. Advisory Committee on Immunization Practices Recommended Immunization Schedule for Adults Aged 19 Years or Older—United States, 2019, MMWR Morb Mortal Wkly Rep 2019 Feb 8;68(5):115–118.

directed against a specific antigen or, as is true for pooled immune globulin, may simply contain antibodies found in most of the population. Passive immunization is useful for (1) individuals unable to form antibodies (eg, congenital agammaglobulinemia); (2) prevention of disease when time does not permit active immunization (eg, postexposure); (3) for treatment of certain diseases normally prevented by immunization (eg, tetanus); and (4) for treatment of conditions for which active immunization is unavailable or impractical (eg, snake bite).

Complications from administration of *human* immunoglobulins are rare. The injections may be moderately painful, and rarely a sterile abscess may occur at the injection site. Transient hypotension and pruritus occasionally occur with the administration of intravenous immune globulin (IVIG) products, but generally are mild. Individuals with certain immunoglobulin deficiency states (IgA deficiency, etc) may occasionally develop hypersensitivity reactions to immune globulin that may limit therapy. Conventional immune globulin contains aggregates of

TABLE A–3 Materials available for passive immunization.[1]

Indication	Product	Dosage	Comments
Anthrax	Anthrax immune globulin	Consult the manufacturer's dosing recommendations	Treatment of inhalational anthrax in combination with appropriate antimicrobials
Black widow spider bite	Antivenin (*Latrodectus mactans*), equine	One vial (6000 units) IV or IM. Some patients may require a repeat dose.	Only symptomatic patients require treatment.
Bone marrow transplantation	Immune globulin (intravenous [IV])[2]	500 mg/kg IV on days 7 and 2 prior to transplantation and then once weekly through day 90 after transplantation.	Prophylaxis to decrease the risk of infection, interstitial pneumonia, and acute graft-versus-host disease in adults undergoing bone marrow transplantation.
Botulism	Botulism antitoxin heptavalent equine, types A–G	Consult the CDC.[3]	Treatment of symptomatic botulism. Available from the CDC.[3] Incidence of serum reactions is <1%.
	Botulism immune globulin (IV)	100 mg/kg IV.	For the treatment of patients <1 year of age with infant botulism caused by toxin type A or B.
Chronic lymphocytic leukemia (CLL)	Immune globulin (IV)[2]	400 mg/kg IV every 3–4 weeks. Dosage should be adjusted upward if bacterial infections occur.	CLL patients with hypogammaglobulinemia and a history of at least one serious bacterial infection.
Cytomegalovirus (CMV)	Cytomegalovirus immune globulin (IV)	Consult the manufacturer's dosing recommendations.	Prophylaxis of CMV infection in bone marrow, kidney, liver, lung, pancreas, and heart transplant recipients.
Diphtheria	Diphtheria antitoxin, equine	20,000–120,000 units IV or IM depending on the severity and duration of illness.	Early treatment of respiratory diphtheria. Available from the CDC.[3] Anaphylactic reactions in ≥7% of adults and serum reactions in ≥5–10% of adults.
Hepatitis A	Immune globulin (intramuscular [IM])	**Preexposure prophylaxis:** 0.01 mL/kg IM for anticipated travel of up to 1 month, 0.02 mL/kg for anticipated travel up to 2 months, 0.2 mL/kg for travel >2 months (repeat every 2 months). **Postexposure:** 0.1 mL/kg IM as soon as possible after exposure up to 2 weeks. Not needed if hepatitis A vaccine was administered at least a month before exposure.	Preexposure and postexposure hepatitis A prophylaxis. The availability of hepatitis A vaccine has greatly reduced the need for preexposure prophylaxis.
Hepatitis B	Hepatitis B immune globulin (HBIG)	0.06 mL/kg IM as soon as possible after exposure up to 1 week for percutaneous exposure or 2 weeks for sexual exposure. 0.5 mL IM within 12 hours after birth for perinatal exposure.	Postexposure prophylaxis in nonimmune persons following percutaneous, mucosal, sexual, or perinatal exposure. Hepatitis B vaccine should also be administered.
HIV-infected children	Immune globulin (IV)[2]	400 mg/kg IV every 28 days.	HIV-infected children with recurrent serious bacterial infections or hypogammaglobulinemia.
Idiopathic thrombocytopenic purpura (ITP)	Immune globulin (IV)[2]	Consult the manufacturer's dosing recommendations for the specific product being used.	Response in children with ITP is greater than in adults. Corticosteroids are the treatment of choice in adults, except for severe pregnancy-associated ITP.
Kawasaki disease	Immune globulin (IV)[2]	400 mg/kg IV daily for 4 consecutive days within 4 days after the onset of illness. A single dose of 2 g/kg IV over 10 hours is also effective.	Effective in the prevention of coronary aneurysms. For use in patients who meet strict criteria for Kawasaki disease.
Measles	Immune globulin (IM)	**Normal hosts:** 0.25 mL/kg IM. **Immunocompromised hosts:** 0.5 mL/kg IM (maximum 15 mL for all patients).	Postexposure prophylaxis (within 6 days after exposure) in nonimmune contacts of acute cases.
Primary immunodeficiency disorders	Immune globulin (IV)[2]	Consult the manufacturer's dosing recommendations for the specific product being used.	Primary immunodeficiency disorders include specific antibody deficiencies (eg, X-linked agammaglobulinemia) and combined deficiencies (eg, severe combined immunodeficiencies).

(continued)

TABLE A–3 Materials available for passive immunization.[1] (Continued)

Indication	Product	Dosage	Comments
Rabies	Rabies immune globulin	20 IU/kg. The full dose should be infiltrated around the wound and any remaining volume should be given IM at an anatomic site distant from vaccine administration.	Postexposure rabies prophylaxis in persons not previously immunized with rabies vaccine. Must be combined with rabies vaccine.
Respiratory syncytial virus (RSV)	Palivizumab	15 mg/kg IM once prior to the beginning of the RSV season and once monthly until the end of the season.	For use in infants and children <24 months with chronic lung disease, hemodynamically significant congenital heart disease, or a history of premature birth (≥35 weeks of gestation).
Rubella	Immune globulin (IM)	0.55 mL/kg IM.	Nonimmune pregnant women exposed to rubella who will not consider therapeutic abortion. Administration does not prevent rubella in the fetus of an exposed mother.
Scorpion sting (*Centruroides*)	Scorpion Immune F(ab)2	3 vials IV over 10 minutes. Additional 1-vial doses may be given every 30–60 minutes as needed.	Use as soon as possible after scorpion sting in symptomatic patients.
Snake bite (coral snake)	Antivenin (*Micrurus fulvius*), equine	At least 3–5 vials (30–50 mL) IV initially within 4 hours after the bite. Additional doses may be required.	Neutralizes venom of eastern coral snake and Texas coral snake. Serum sickness occurs in almost all patients who receive >7 vials.
Snake bite (pit vipers)	Antivenin (Crotalidae) polyvalent immune Fab, ovine	An initial dose of 4–6 vials should be infused intravenously over 1 hour. The dose should be repeated if initial control is not achieved. After initial control, 2 vials should be given every 6 hours for up to three doses.	For the management of minimal to moderate North American crotalid envenomation.
Tetanus	Tetanus immune globulin	**Postexposure prophylaxis:** 250 units IM. For severe wounds or when there has been a delay in administration, 500 units is recommended. **Treatment:** 3000–6000 units IM.	Treatment of tetanus and postexposure prophylaxis of nonclean, nonminor wounds in inadequately immunized persons (less than two doses of tetanus toxoid or less than three doses if wound is >24 hours old).
Vaccinia	Vaccinia immune globulin	Consult the CDC.[3]	Treatment of severe reactions to vaccinia vaccination, including eczema vaccinatum, vaccinia necrosum, and ocular vaccinia. Available from the CDC.[3]
Varicella	Varicella-zoster immune globulin	**Weight (kg) — Dose (units)** ≥2 — 62.5 IM 2.1–10 — 125 IM 10.1–20 — 250 IM 20.1–30 — 375 IM 30.1–40 — 500 IM ≥40 — 625 IM	**Postexposure prophylaxis** (preferably within 48 hours but no later than within 96 hours after exposure) in susceptible immunocompromised hosts, selected pregnant women, and perinatally exposed newborns.

[1]Passive immunotherapy or immunoprophylaxis should always be administered as soon as possible after exposure. Prior to the administration of animal sera, patients should be questioned and tested for hypersensitivity.

[2]See the following references for an analysis of additional uses of intravenously administered immune globulin: Ratko TA et al: Recommendations for off-label use of intravenously administered immunoglobulin preparations. JAMA 1995;273:1865; and Feasby T et al: Guidelines on the use of intravenous immune globulin for neurologic conditions. Transfus Med Rev 2007;21(2 Suppl 1)S57.

[3]Centers for Disease Control and Prevention, 404-639-3670 during weekday business hours; 770-488-7100 during nights, weekends, and holidays (emergency requests only); www.cdc.gov/laboratory/drugservice/formulary.html. Clinicians who suspect a diagnosis of botulism should immediately call their state health department's 24-hour emergency number.

IgG; it will cause severe reactions if given intravenously. However, if the passively administered antibodies are derived from *animal* sera, hypersensitivity reactions ranging from anaphylaxis to serum sickness may occur. Highly purified immunoglobulins, especially from rodents or lagomorphs, are the least likely to cause reactions. To avoid anaphylactic reactions, tests for hypersensitivity to the animal serum must be performed. If an alternative preparation is not available and administration of the specific antibody is deemed essential, desensitization can be carried out.

Antibodies derived from human serum not only avoid the risk of hypersensitivity reactions but also have a much longer half-life in humans (about 23 days for IgG antibodies) than those from animal sources (5–7 days or less). Consequently, much smaller doses of human antibody can be administered to provide therapeutic concentrations for several weeks. These advantages point to the desirability of using human antibodies for passive protection whenever possible. Materials available for passive immunization are summarized in Table A–3.

LEGAL LIABILITY FOR UNTOWARD REACTIONS

It is the physician's responsibility to inform the patient of the risk of immunization and to use vaccines and antisera in an appropriate manner. This may require skin testing to assess the risk of an untoward reaction. Some of the risks previously described are, however, currently unavoidable; on balance, the patient and society are clearly better off accepting the risks for routinely administered immunogens (eg, influenza and tetanus vaccines).

Manufacturers should be held legally accountable for failure to adhere to existing standards for production of biologicals. However, in the present litigious atmosphere of the USA, the filing of large liability claims by the statistically inevitable victims of good public health practice has caused many manufacturers to abandon efforts to develop and produce low-profit but medically valuable therapeutic agents such as vaccines. Since the use and sale of these products are subject to careful review and approval by government bodies such as the Surgeon General's Advisory Committee on Immunization Practices and the US Food and Drug Administration, "strict product liability" (liability without fault) may be an inappropriate legal standard to apply when rare reactions to biologicals, produced and administered according to government guidelines, are involved.

RECOMMENDED IMMUNIZATION OF ADULTS FOR TRAVEL

Every adult, whether traveling or not, should be immunized with tetanus toxoid and should also be fully immunized against poliomyelitis, measles (for those born after 1956), and diphtheria. In addition, every traveler must fulfill the immunization requirements of the health authorities of the countries to be visited. These are listed in *Health Information for International Travel*, available from the Superintendent of Documents, US Government Printing Office, Washington, DC 20402. A useful website is wwwnc.cdc.gov/travel/. *The Medical Letter on Drugs and Therapeutics* also offers periodically updated recommendations for international travelers (see *The Medical Letter*, 2019;61:153). Immunizations received in preparation for travel should be recorded on the International Certificate of Immunization. *Note:* Smallpox vaccination is not recommended or required for travel in any country.

REFERENCES

Ada G: Vaccines and vaccination. N Engl J Med 2001;345:1042.

Advice for travelers. Med Lett Drugs Ther 2019;61:153.

Cantor JD et al: Mandatory measles vaccination in New York City—reflections on a bold experiment. N Engl J Med 2019;381:101.

Centers for Disease Control and Prevention websites: www.cdc.gov/vaccines/ and wwwnc.cdc.gov/travel/.

Funk CD, Laferriere C, Ardakani A: A snapshot of the global race for vaccines targetting SARS-CoV-2 and the COVID-19 pandemic. Front Pharmacol 2020;11:937.

Gardner P et al: Guidelines for quality standards for immunization. Clin Infect Dis 2002;35:503.

General recommendations on immunization. Recommendations of the Advisory Committee on Immunization Practices (ACIP). MMWR Morb Mortal Wkly Rep 2011;60(2):1.

Hill DR et al: The practice of travel medicine: Guidelines by the Infectious Diseases Society of America. Clin Infect Dis 2006;43:1499.

Keller MA, Stiehm ER: Passive immunity in prevention and treatment of infectious diseases. Clin Microbiol Rev 2000;13:602.

Kim DK, Hunter P: Advisory Committee on Immunization Practices recommended immunization schedule for adults aged 19 years or older—United States, 2019. MMWR Morb Mortal Wkly Rep 2019;68:115.

Lurie N et al: Developing Covid-19 vaccines at pandemic speed. N Engl J Med 2020;382:1969.

Pickering LK et al: Immunization programs for infants, children, adolescents, and adults: Clinical practice guidelines by the Infectious Diseases Society of America. Clin Infect Dis 2009;49:817.

Robinson CL et al: Advisory Committee on Immunization Practices recommended immunization schedules for children and adolescents aged 18 years or younger—United States, 2019. MMWR Morb Mortal Wkly Rep 2019; 68:112.

Rubin LG et al: 2013 IDSA clinical practice guideline for vaccination of the immunocompromised host. Clin Infect Dis 2014;58:309.

Zumula A et al: Travel medicine. Infect Dis Clin North Am 2012;26:575.

Index

Note: In this index, the letters "*b*," "*f*," and "*t*" denote text box, figures, and tables, respectively.

G

H

M

O

Q

T